Chapter 35
Assessment Guide Child With Cardiovascular Problems
Nursing Care Guide Child After Cardiac Catheterization
Nursing Care Plan Child With a Ventricular Septal Defect

Chapter 36
Assessment Guide Child With a Problem of Hematologic Composition
Nursing Care Guide Child With Sickle Cell Crisis
Nursing Care Plan Child With Classic Hemophilia A

Chapter 37
Assessment Guide Child With an Immune System Dysfunction
Nursing Care Guide Child in Protective Isolation
Nursing Care Plan Child With Juvenile Rheumatoid Arthritis

Chapter 38
Assessment Guide Child With a Gastrointestinal Problem
Nursing Care Guide Child Undergoing Colostomy or Ileostomy
Nursing Care Guide Child Undergoing Abdominal Surgery
Nursing Care Plan Child With Cleft Lip and Cleft Palate

Chapter 39
Assessment Guide Child With a Genitourinary Problem
Nursing Care Guide Child Following Genitourinary Surgery
Nursing Care Guide Child With Acute Renal Failure
Nursing Care Plan Child With a Neurogenic Bladder

Chapter 40
Assessment Guide Child With Altered Hormonal Regulation
Nursing Care Guide Child With Diabetes Insipidus
Nursing Care Plan Child With Diabetes Mellitus

Chapter 41
Assessment Guide Child With a Skeletal Condition
Nursing Care Guide Child With a Cast
Nursing Care Guide Child in Traction
Nursing Care Plan Child Recovering from Spinal Fusion

Chapter 42
Assessment Guide Child With a Neurologic Impairment
Nursing Care Guide Rehabilitation for the Child With Neurologic Impairment
Nursing Care Guide Postoperative Care of the Child Following Neurosurgery
Nursing Care Guide Child With a Seizure Disorder
Nursing Care Plan The Comatose Child

Chapter 43
Assessment Guide Child With Impaired Sensory Function
Nursing Care Guide Child Undergoing Eye Surgery
Nursing Care Guide Postoperative Management of the Child With Myringotomy
Nursing Care Plan Child With Hyphema

Chapter 44
Assessment Guide Child With a Problem of the Integumentary System
Nursing Care Guide The Burned Child During the Emergent Phase
Nursing Care Plan Child With a Burn

Chapter 45
Assessment Guide Child With Cancer
Nursing Care Guide Child With Bone Marrow Suppression
Nursing Care Plan Child With Leukemia

Nursing Care of Children and Families

A Holistic Approach

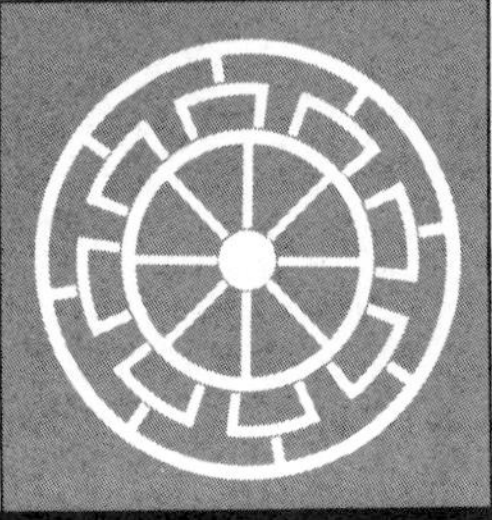

Nursing Care of Children and Families

A Holistic Approach

Sandra R. Mott, RN, MSN

Nancy Fiero Fazekas, RN, MN

Susan Rowen James, RN, MSN

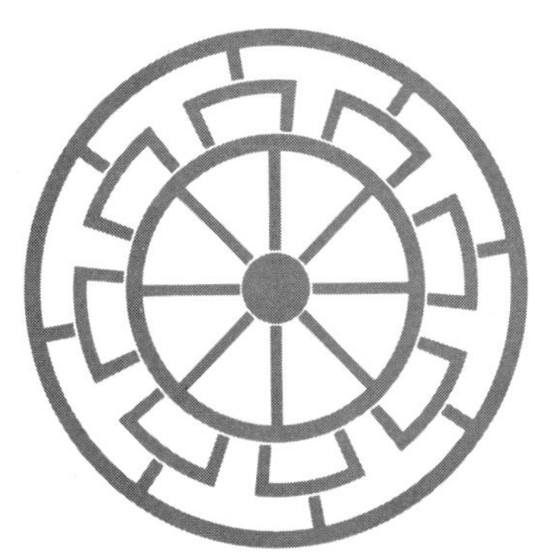

Addison-Wesley Publishing Company
Nursing Division, Menlo Park, California

Reading, Massachusetts ▪ Don Mills, Ontario ▪ Wokingham, UK
Amsterdam ▪ Sydney ▪ Singapore ▪ Tokyo ▪ Mexico City
Bogota ▪ Santiago ▪ San Juan

Sponsoring Editor: Thomas Eoyang
Production Supervisor: Glenda Epting
Developmental Editors: Debra J. Osnowitz, Katherine Sterling, Jonas Weisel
Book designer: Janet Bollow
Cover designer: Michael A. Rogondino
Manuscript editors: Dorilee Bingham, Thomas Szalkiewicz
Illustrations: Susan Strawn, Nori Tolson
Photographers: William Thompson, George Fry III, and Joseph Greco

Library of Congress Cataloging in Publication Data

Mott, Sandra R., 1942–
Nursing care of children and families.

Includes index.
1. Pediatric nursing. 2. Holistic medicine.
I. Fazekas, Nancy Fiero, 1943– . II. James, Susan Rowen, 1946– . III. Title. [DNLM: 1. Child Health Services—nurses' instruction. 2. Holistic Health—nurses' instruction. 3. Pediatric Nursing. WY 159 M921n]
RJ245.M68 1985 610.73'62 85–1289
ISBN 0-201-14054-3

Photo Credits: Chapter opening photo for Chapter 23 is courtesy of Community Association for Retarded, Inc., Palo Alto, California
Part Two chapter opening photo by Suzanne Arms

The authors and publisher thank the following institutions and agencies for their kind permission to photograph many of the children and families who appear in this book:
Children's Hospital at Stanford, Stanford, California
Community Association for Retarded, Inc., Palo Alto, California
Peninsula Center for the Blind, Palo Alto, California
Peninsula School, Menlo Park, California
Valley Medical Center, San Jose, California

The authors and publishers have exerted every effort to ensure that drug selections and dosages set forth in this text are in accord with current recommendations and practice at the time of publication. However, in view of ongoing research, changes in government regulations, and the constant flow of information relating to drug therapy and drug reactions, the reader is urged to check the package insert for each drug for any change in indications of dosage and for added warnings and precautions. This is particularly important where the recommended agent is a new and/or infrequently employed drug.

BCDEFGHIJK-MU-898765

Addison-Wesley Publishing Company, Inc.
Nursing Division
2725 Sand Hill Road ■ Menlo Park, California 94025

To those whose faith, love, support, and belief in us endured throughout the years of making our dream a reality, and whose understanding and encouragement sustained us as we edged closer toward our goal, we give our heartfelt appreciation and thanks.

We dedicate this book to those whom we love and with whom we share our lives, our memories, and our future.

Contents in Brief

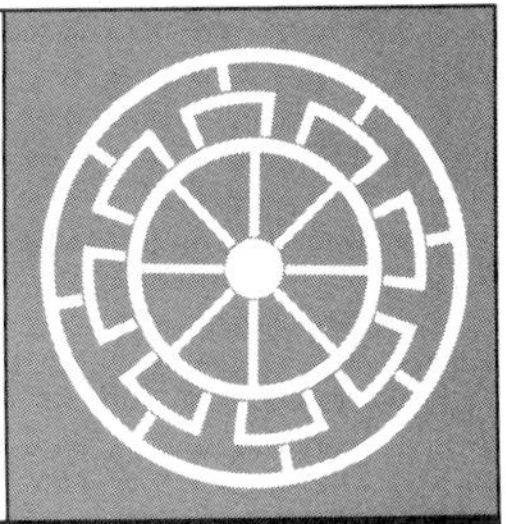

Contents in Detail

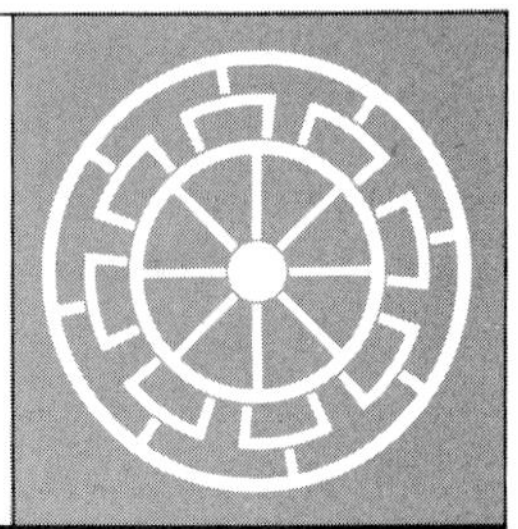

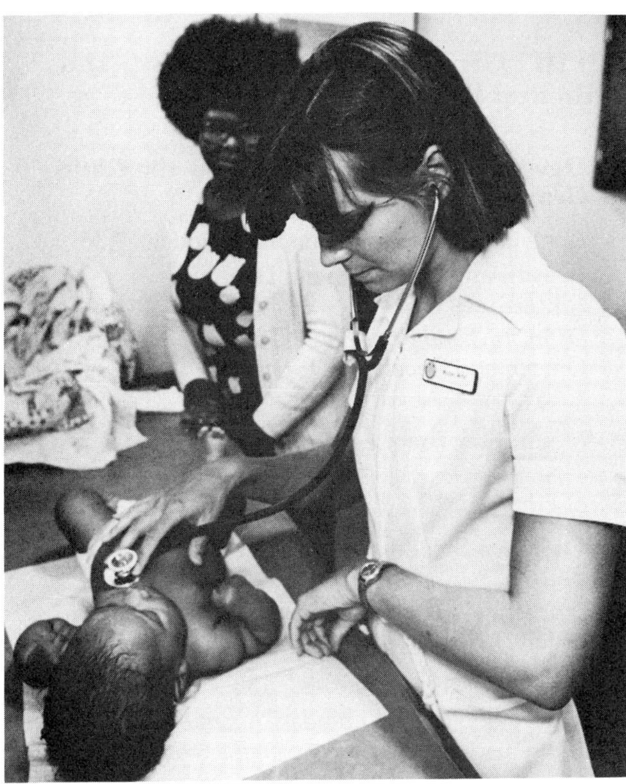

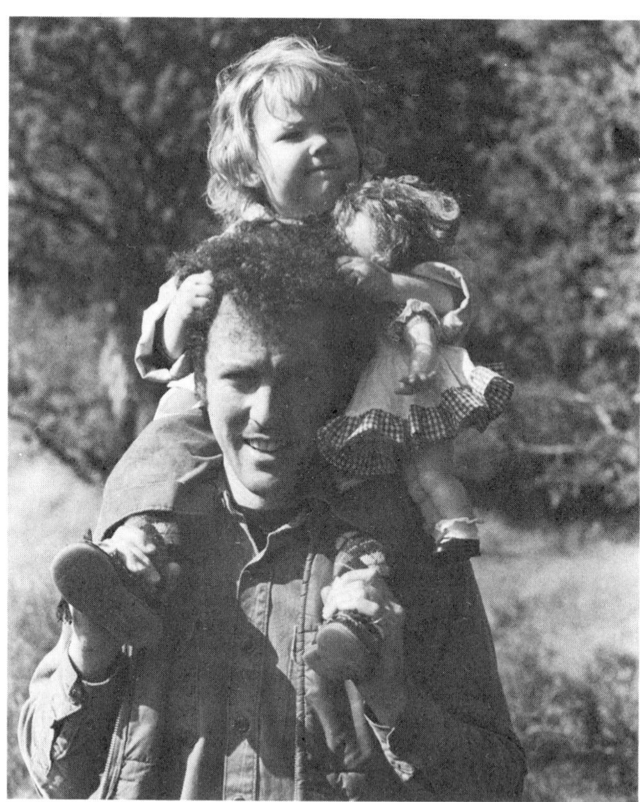

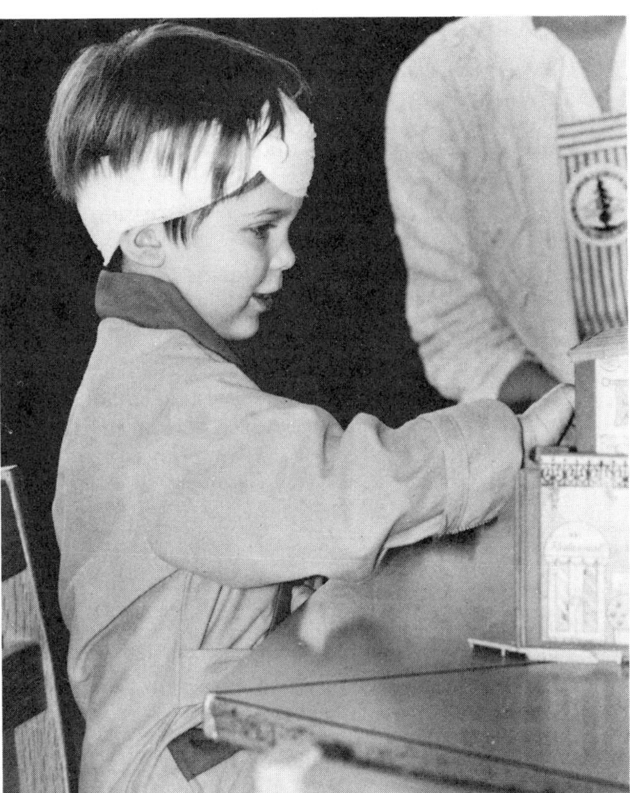

Preface

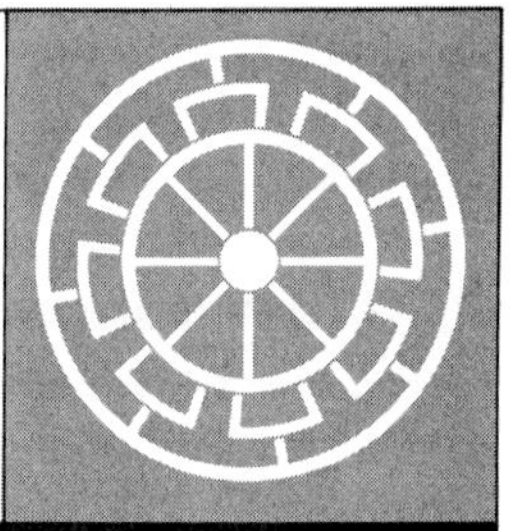

Nursing Care of Children and Families emphasizes the well child, health maintenance, and anticipatory guidance for parents. The text also consistently draws attention to the importance of the emotional needs of the child and family, discharge preparation, and anticipating home problems and adjustments. With so many themes to thread together, the text presents the information within the context of a conceptual framework that can be applied to each nursing care situation. The text's goals are (1) to provide the student with a basic ability to assess the factors affecting the child's and family's responses to health maintenance measures, illness, injury, and/or hospitalization; and (2) to use this knowledge in formulating and implementing nursing care to meet the unique physical, cognitive, and psychosocial needs for both the immediate situation and the related future.

Conceptual Framework

This text is built on four major components to the conceptual framework:

1. Nursing process
2. Systems theory
3. Orem's self-care model
4. Integration of growth and development

1. **Nursing process** The five-step nursing process (assessment, nursing diagnosis, planning, implementation, and evaluation) is applied in a consistent manner throughout the text. The application of the nursing process to child health nursing is discussed in Chapter 2. A fully developed care plan addressing the nursing care appropriate for the well child follows this chapter and exemplifies the integration of all the elements of the text's conceptual framework into the nursing process.

The chapters in Unit IV offer specific tools and guidelines for in-depth physical, nutritional, developmental, and family assessment. Serial **Case Studies* of three children are presented in all four chapters. After the last chapter, one of these children is the subject of the second well-child care plan, which demonstrates how a comprehensive assessment leads to individualized nursing diagnoses and interventions for a child and family with routine health concerns.

2. **Systems theory** We present systems theory as a framework for holistic nursing care. Children are affected by the environment of which they are a part, especially by the family's perceived needs, strengths, and limitations. Every individual interacts with the resources of his or her environment as part of the process of living. Children, because of their relative immaturity, may be more reliant on, or vulnerable to, the impact of these resources, especially in the areas of health and illness. It becomes all the more important that the nurse understand the interplay between the individual and the various resources significant for that individual.

Specific resources that we address in this text include the immediate and extended family, culture, socioeconomic status, values, religion, environment, previous experiences, coping patterns, heredity, health status, and growth and developmental level.

3. **Orem's self-care model** We have adopted the concept of self-care as one of the primary goals of nursing intervention. Rather than administer care to passive "patients," nurses, we feel, should seek to involve all clients—even children—as much as possible in the decisions and activities connected with their own health maintenance and restoration. A corollary emphasis is placed on the importance of the child's and family's own perceptions of health, illness, and injury in planning nursing care. Through this model we will also stress the importance of the nurse's teaching role, which is a major thread of the entire text.

4. **Integration of growth and development** Rather than discuss health deviations under specific age groups where they are deemed likely to occur, we have elected to discuss a given health problem in a single place, as much as possible, and to incorporate the variations of and reactions to this health problem as it affects children and adolescents. This approach allows us to highlight in a consistent manner such general themes as assessment, prevention, acute and chronic care needs, and principles of nursing care, while clearly identifying the different expressions a health problem can have in children of different ages and developmental levels. This approach also permits easier access to information about a specific problem than does the sometimes arbitrary and misleading assignment of a disease to a specific age category.

Organization and Content

The organization of this text moves from wellness to illness, and from the general to the specific (or, in systems theory terms, from suprasystems to subsystems). The book is thus divided into three parts:

- Framework for Child Health Nursing
- Health Promotion and Maintenance of the Child and Family
- Health Restoration of the Child and Family

Framework for Child Health Nursing

Part One consists of three units that present the concepts at the core of child health nursing.

Unit I, "Overview of Child Health Nursing," sets contemporary child health nursing in its historical context, explains the child health nurse's legal and ethical responsibilities, delineates the nurse's various roles, and presents the conceptual framework for the text as described earlier.

Unit II, "Influences on Human Growth and Development," forms a prelude to child development by discussing the social, cultural, genetic, and familial influences on the child.

Unit III, "Growth and Development: The Child and Family," presents a comprehensive and theoretically current exposition of growth and development for the child and family. A look at the coping strategies of children and at parenting rounds out the development perspective in this unit.

Health Promotion and Maintenance of the Child and Family

Part Two deals with assessment, prevention of illness and injury, and psychosocial threats to health.

Unit IV, "Child and Family Assessment," covers physical, nutritional, developmental, and family assessments and concentrates on normal findings for the healthy child. The unit ends with the well-child care plan described earlier.

Unit V, "Preventive Child Health Nursing: Strategies for Health Promotion," presents preventive measures in illness, injury, and poisoning. Each chapter is organized according to an epidemiological framework, identifying characteristics of the host, agent, and environment that predispose the child to health risks. The nurse's role in both primary and secondary prevention is identified. Capping this unit is a summary chapter on "Anticipatory Guidance" that explains how to synthesize the information on growth and development, assessment, and prevention that the text has presented to that point, with the goal of providing health teaching and parent counseling that will promote wellness for both the child and family.

Unit VI, "The Child and Family at Psychosocial Risk," deals with conditions that pose real or potential threats to health. Among these are dysfunctional parenting situations such as child neglect and abuse and adolescent parenting. Other health threats are mental retardation and dysfunctional behavior patterns such as eating disorders, substance abuse, and runaway behavior. This unit also includes an authoritative treatment of psychiatric and social disorders in childhood.

The psychosocial factors discussed in this unit are presented from the perspectives of both the community and the acute care setting, with an emphasis on prevention through detection of early cues to potential problems, and on the expanding role of the nurse in dealing with these problems.

Health Restoration of the Child and Family

Part Three deals with the impact of illness and the nursing implications of specific physiologic alterations.

Unit VII, "The Impact of Illness on the Child and Family," applies general principles of nursing care to the ill child in home and hospital settings, to the chronically ill child, to the sick newborn, and to the dying child. Special consideration is given to adaptations of play as part of nursing care. We stress that the nurse needs to be attentive to the viewpoints of the child, parents, and siblings in assessing the effects of hospitalization on the ill child and family unit. We also discuss the principles of teaching and preparation of the child and family for the return home.

Unit VIII, "Nursing Care of the Ill Child," concerns the nursing care of children with specific health problems, grouped by physiologic alteration. The unit begins with a chapter on fluid and electrolyte balance, because the theories and applications of this important concept are relevant to pathology in almost all body systems. The remaining chapters build on the student's previous learning in courses, such as anatomy and physiology, pathophysiology, and health assessment, where the content is also presented through a similar organization.

Emphasizing nursing assessment and principles of care, each chapter in this final unit reflects the holistic perspective of the book's conceptual framework. Building on the nursing process, systems theory, and self-care, the chapters consistently reinforce the nurse's synthesis of the interacting and complementary dynamics of each system. As conditions within one system cause changes in another, explanations and cross-references will be given.

Each chapter begins with a brief review of the normal anatomy and physiology of the body system. Nursing assessment, including relevant laboratory data, follows, emphasizing signs and symptoms of pathophysiology (in contrast to the normal findings discussed in the chapter on physical assessment) and illustrating how physical examination skills are used. This information is pulled together and highlighted in the **Assessment Guide*.

Nursing management for specific treatments and procedures are then discussed, followed by principles of nursing care, which are divided into acute care, nutritional, developmental, emotional, and health maintenance needs. The commonalities of nursing care for each type of physiologic alteration are thus learned before the specific details of each disease entity are presented. The remainder of each chapter considers the most common and significant physiologic deviations, explaining specific treatment and nursing interventions for each condition. The narrative also supports, through examples and cross-references, our emphasis on the need for seeing the child and family as a unit dependent on its resources, and for adapting nursing care accordingly.

Nursing Care Features

For bringing the principles of nursing care down to specifics and for presenting a role model of creative and individualized use of the nursing process in child health, four nursing care elements are consistently presented throughout this text:

1. *Case Study
2. *Assessment Guide
3. *Nursing Care Guide
4. *Nursing Care Plan

All these nursing care elements have been specially accented by the symbol found on the cover so they can be easily located.

The **Case Studies* and **Nursing Care Plans* present children with specific health problems or concerns and demonstrate the progression from gathering assessment data to identifying nursing diagnoses, goals, and interventions. The **Case Studies* show how assessment data are systematically organized to identify problems and priorities, while the more fully developed **Nursing Care Plans* provide rationales for interventions and evaluation criteria.

The **Assessment Guides,* as discussed earlier, pull together the significant assessment findings for physiologic alterations in each body system and present the related nursing management.

**Nursing Care Guides* offer guidelines for more generic nursing management of particular conditions that can result from disease or other threats to health. The care guides address situations such as the child with bone marrow suppression, the child following genitourinary surgery, or the child in a cast.

Learning Aids

In addition to a wide variety of tables and boxes that pull together essential information or topics of related interest, the standard pedagogical features of each chapter include a chapter outline, a list of objectives, a summary list of key concepts, references, and additional readings. To aid access to the content, a special "Cross-Reference Box" is placed in certain chapters to indicate where discussion of a related topic can be found. We have used this device for topics that the reader might reasonably expect to find in one chapter but which in fact are found in another.

Supplements

The supplemental package for this text includes an Instructor's Manual, a student study guide, and a slide package. A computerized test bank will be made available to adopters of the text.

The *Instructor's Manual* includes teaching objectives keyed to the text and to exercises in the student workbook; discussion and review questions; in-class and out-of-class activities; suggested clinical objectives; and a list of audiovisual resources. The *Manual* also includes transparency masters of important line art and pedagogical material from the text. A bank of test questions is available in booklet form and as part of a computerized test authoring program that allows instructors to create examinations based on a number of categories keyed to the text.

Nursing Care of Children and Families: A Workbook will provide students with a tested and proven tool to reinforce learning of essential content. Questions require both factual recall and applied problem solving.

A slide package provides the opportunity to show significant line art *and* photographs from the text for lecture and discussion purposes and will be available to adopters of the text.

Acknowledgements

Nursing Care of Children and Families has come to fruition after many delays and as a result of much patience and enthusiastic comment from all involved with this project. We would especially like to acknowledge the extraordinary efforts of the following people who have helped us immensely throughout:

- Thomas Eoyang, who served as our sponsoring editor and who worked many long hours not only managing the many tasks involved but also contributing his creative writing and editorial talents in an effort to produce an exceptionally polished manuscript.

- Debi Osnowitz, our talented and committed developmental editor, whose total dedication and encouragement were inspiring, particularly during times of discouragement.
- Kathy Sterling and Jonas Weisel, developmental editors who assisted with a truly overwhelming job in order that we might complete this project.
- Dori Bingham, who served as the principal copy editor and whose conscientious attention to detail facilitated our efforts.
- Tom Szalkiewicz, who served as copy editor and whose efforts are greatly appreciated.
- William Thompson, RN, principal photographer for the project, whose pictures provide a visual expression of the theoretical concepts we wished to present.
- Helene Harrington, who managed the line art, and Susan Strawn and Nori Tolson, the artists who have effectively conveyed our ideas through their artistic talents.
- Glenda Epting and the entire production staff at Addison-Wesley who undertook such a massive manuscript and applied creative production strategies to make this book a reality.
- Barry Moore, Pat Waldo, and Deborah Gale, who initiated this book and without whom we would not have undertaken this effort.
- Nick Keefe, Nancy Evans, and the other supportive people at Addison-Wesley whose patience and enthusiastic response to this book have allowed us to express our vision and commitment to high quality nursing care for children and families.
- The many helping hands who typed portions of this manuscript.
- The many reviewers whose expertise and comments were so valuable in our efforts to present a comprehensive approach to the nursing care of children and families: Joan Hagan Arnold, Adelphi University, Garden City, New York; Ruth Best, Sacramento City College, Sacramento, California; Barbara Bordeaux, University of North Carolina, Chapel Hill, North Carolina; Sue Boyer, University of Illinois, Chicago, Illinois; Marion Broome, Medical College of Georgia, Augusta, Georgia; Alice Burton, St. Olaf College, Northfield, Minnesota; Janet Chorpenning, Indiana University, Indianapolis, Indiana; Stephanie Clatworthy, Wayne State University, Detroit, Michigan; Martin Cogan, University of California, San Francisco, California; Monica Collins, Eastern Maine Medical Center, Bangor, Maine; Cherrill Colson, Columbia University, New York, New York; Diane Courney, University of Texas, San Antonio, Texas; Mary Coward, Borough Manhattan Community College of CUNY, New York, New York; Athleen Coyner, University of Utah, Salt Lake City, Utah; Kathryn Crisler, University of Colorado, Denver, Colorado; Barbara Dean, Miami Valley Hospital, Dayton, Ohio; Judy Donlen, Children's Hospital of Philadelphia, Philadelphia, Pennsylvania; Susan Erickson, Presbyterian Hospital, San Francisco, California; Gloria Essoka, Hunter College-Bellevue School of Nursing, New York, New York; Sharon Fulling, Mississippi County Community College, Blytheville, Arkansas; Diane Goldman, University of California, San Francisco, California; Beatrice Harris, Southwestern Michigan Health Care Association; Peggy Harris, Southeastern Louisiana University, Hammond, Louisiana; Duane Jeffrey, Brigham Young University, Provo, Utah; Barbara Joyce, Adelphi University, Garden City, New York; Betsy Joyce, Indiana University, Indianapolis, Indiana, Susanna Juarez, University of Texas, Austin, Texas; Carolyn Kaiser, Lake Michigan College, Benton Harbor, Michigan; Nanette Kanoff, Essex Community College, Baltimore County, Maryland; Joan Klemballa, University of District of Columbia, Washington, D.C.; Kathleen Krauser, Indiana University, Indianapolis, Indiana; Annette Lipschitz, Nassau Community College, Garden City, New York; Marcia London, Beth-El School of Nursing, Colorado Springs, Colorado; Diane Martin, Children's Hospital of Los Angeles, Los Angeles, California; Mary Ellen Meade, Indiana University-Northwest Division of Nursing, Gary, Indiana; Diana Melancon, San Antonio College, San Antonio, Texas; Barbara Michaels, El Centro College, Dallas, Texas; Donna Middaugh, Children's Hospital-Santa Rosa Medical Center, Santa Rosa, California; Gayle Pearson, Rutgers College of Nursing, Newark, New Jersey; Elizabeth Poster, University of California, Los Angeles, California; Betty Pugh, Rush-Presbyterian St. Luke's Medical Center, Chicago, Illinois; Janice Selekman, Thomas Jefferson University-College of Allied Health Sciences, Philadelphia, Pennsylvania; Phyllis Semas, California State University, Sacramento, California; Mary Lou Steffen, Westminster College-St. Mark's, Salt Lake City, Utah; Ruth Stephenson, University of North Carolina-College of Nursing, Charlotte, North Carolina; Kathleen Stolzenberger, Felician College, Lodi, New Jersey; John Stubbs, San Francisco State University, San Francisco, California; Susan Theobald, Jefferson Community College, Louisville, Kentucky; Frances Thurber, University of Pennsylvania, Philadelphia, Pennsylvania; Sharon Valente, University of Southern California, Los Angeles, California; Kathleen Vandenberg, Children's Hospital, Oakland, California; Judith Vessey, University of Pennsylvania, Philadelphia, Pennsylvania; Patty Villarreal, University of Texas-Health Science Center, San Antonio, Texas; Judith Wakim, Austin Peay State University, Clarksville, Tennessee; Jennie Walls, Kingsport Family Practice, Kingsport, Tennessee; Virginia Whalen, Pasadena City College, Pasadena, California; Susan Wilkins, Anne Arundel Community College, Arnold, Maryland; Doris Wilson, St. Elizabeth Hospital, Wash-

ington, DC; Eileen Wright, University of Michigan, Ann Arbor, Michigan; and Sheila Zerr, University of Ottawa, Ontario, Canada.

Finally, we would like to thank our many colleagues in nursing from whom we have received suggestions, information, and advice; our students and patients who have taught us much over the years; and our families and friends for their love, support, and encouragement especially during the times when our preoccupation with this project took from them attention which they so rightly deserve.

Editors

Sandra R. Mott, R.N., M.S.N.
Assistant Professor
School of Nursing
Boston College
Chestnut Hill, Massachusetts

Nancy Fiero Fazekas, R.N., M.N.
formerly Assistant Professor, School of Nursing
Doctoral Student
Boston College
Chestnut Hill, Massachusetts

Susan Rowen James, R.N., M.S.N.
formerly Instructor, School of Nursing
Boston College
Chestnut Hill, Massachusetts

Contributors

Carole C. Arenge, R.N.
Head Nurse
The Children's Hospital
Boston, Massachusetts

Michelle Burns, R.N., M.S., C.P.N.P.
Hillsdale, New Jersey

Carolyn Clayton Cahn, R.N., M.S.N.
Lecturer, Pediatrics
Department of Nursing
California State University
Fresno, California

Annette Calvi, R.N., M.S.N.
Clinical Specialist, Pediatric Pulmonary
University of Colorado Health Science Center
Denver, Colorado

John Conley, R.N., B.S.N.
Senior Staff Nurse, Child & Adolescent Psychiatry
Medical College of Georgia
Augusta, Georgia

Diane Holditch Davis, R.N., M.S.
Doctoral Candidate
University of Connecticut
Storrs, Connecticut

Cynthia E. Degazon, R.N., M.A.
Doctoral Candidate
New York University
New York, New York

Maureen De Maio, M.S.
Assistant Professor
Doctoral Candidate
Rutgers College of Nursing
Newark, New Jersey

Margaret Marusek Dozois, R.N., M.S.N.
Clinical Specialist, Pediatric Pulmonary
National Jewish Center for Respiratory and Immunology Research
Denver, Colorado

David J. Driscoll, M.D.
Associate Professor, Pediatrics
Consultant, Pediatric Cardiology
Mayo Medical School, Mayo Clinic
Rochester, Minnesota

Deanna Edwards
Lecturer, author, composer, and singer
Provo, Utah

Mary Jo Eoff, R.N., M.S.N.
Associate Professor
School of Nursing
Indiana University
Indianapolis, Indiana

Wendy J. Fibison, B.S.N., M.H.Sc., C.P.N.P.
Doctoral Candidate, Human Genetics
University of Pennsylvania
Philadelphia, Pennsylvania

Juanita W. Fleming, R.N., Ph.D., F.A.A.N.
Professor and Associate Dean
Director of Graduate Education
College of Nursing
University of Kentucky
Lexington, Kentucky

Beverly Piper Giordano, R.N., M.S.
Endocrine/Diabetes Clinical Specialist
The Children's Hospital
Denver, Colorado

Cathryn L. Glanville, R.N., M.A., M.Ed.
Associate Professor, Chairperson
Parent/Child Nursing Department
Medical College of Georgia
Augusta, Georgia

Janet A. Grossman, M.S.N., C.S.
Program Coordinator, Child Psychiatry
Rush-Presbyterian-St. Luke's Medical Center
Chicago, Illinois

Christine Herrmann, R.N., M.S.
Clinical Nurse Specialist, Child Mental Health
Milwaukee Children's Hospital
Milwaukee, Wisconsin

June Andrews Horowitz, R.N., M.S., Ph.D.
Associate Professor
School of Nursing
Boston College
Chestnut Hill, Massachusetts

Nancy Houlder, R.N., B.S.N.
Staff Nurse
Rocky Mountain Poison Control Center
Denver General Hospital
Denver, Colorado

Cynthia B. Hughes, Ed.D., C.P.N.P.
Assistant Professor
Rutgers College of Nursing
Newark, New Jersey

Mary Virginia Jacobs, R.N., M.S.N., C.F.N.P.
Family Nurse Practitioner
Yoakum Medical Clinic
Yoakum, Texas

Lorna N. Kaufman, M.Ed.
Doctoral Candidate
Boston College
Boston, Massachusetts

Gretchen L. Kelly, R.N., M.A.
Assistant Professor, Psychiatry and Nursing
Clinical Nurse Specialist, Child Psychiatry
University of Virginia Medical Center
Charlottesville, Virginia

Elizabeth B. Laliberte, R.N., M.S.N.
Assistant Professor of Nursing
University of Connecticut
Storrs, Connecticut

Barbara J. Leonard, R.N., Ph.D.
Assistant Professor, Maternal and Child Health
School of Public Health
University of Minnesota
Minneapolis, Minnesota

Betty M. Lovelace, B.S.N., M.S.
Director of Pediatric Play Therapy
Stanford University Medical Center
Stanford, California

Noreen Mahon, M.S., Ph.D.
Chairperson, Chronicity Department
Rutgers College of Nursing
Newark, New Jersey

Lyn Marshall, R.N., M.S.N.
Clinical Leader, Eating Disorders Program
Northwestern Memorial Hospital, Institute of Psychiatry
Chicago, Illinois

Bonnie A. McMillin, R.N., M.N.
Head Nurse, Emergency Room
Rochester Methodist Hospital
Rochester, Minnesota

Karen Mitchell, M.S.N., Ph.D.
Editor, *Pediatric Nursing*
Anthony J. Janetti, Inc.
Pitman, New Jersey

Kathleen Hardin Mooney, R.N., M.N., Ph.D.
Associate Professor
College of Nursing
University of Utah
Salt Lake City, Utah

Gayle Doerner Olsen, R.N., M.S., P.N.P.
Associate Professor
Department of Nursing
Winona State University
Rochester, Minnesota

Jean A. O'Neil, R.N., M.S.
Associate Professor, School of Nursing
Doctoral Candidate, Education
Boston College
Chestnut Hill, Massachusetts

J. Craig Peery, Ph.D.
Department of Family Sciences
Brigham Young University
Provo, Utah

Joy Hinson Penticuff, R.N., M.S.N., Ph.D.
Associate Professor, School of Nursing
Coordinator, High-Risk Perinatal Clinical Specialist Program
University of Texas
Austin, Texas

Bobbie Jean Perdue, M.S.N.
Assistant Professor, Doctoral Candidate
Director, Educational Opportunity Fund and Nursing Development in Urban Settings
Rutgers College of Nursing
Newark, New Jersey

Joan Pernice, R.N., M.S., C.P.N.P.
Assistant Professor
School of Nursing
Boston College
Chestnut Hill, Massachusetts

Margo Pinney, R.N., M.S.N.
Clinical Specialist, Pediatric Pulmonary
University of Colorado Health Science Center
Denver, Colorado

Marva Mizell Price, R.N., M.PH., C.F.N.P.
Nursing Consultant
North Carolina Department of Human Resources
Raleigh, North Carolina

Virginia Prout, R.N., M.S.
Doctoral Candidate
Boston College
Chestnut Hill, Massachusetts

Frances Ward Quinless, R.N., Ph.D.
Assistant Professor
Rutgers College of Nursing
Newark, New Jersey

Robert G. Riedel, Ph.D.
Licensed Consulting Psychologist
Professor, Clinical Psychology
Southwest State University
Marshall, Minnesota

Gwendolyn C. Robinson, R.N., M.A., C.P.N.P.
Director, Child Development Associates
Tolland, Connecticut

Jean Marie Rockenhaus, R.N., M.S.N.
Assistant Professor of Nursing
Montana State University
Billings, Montana

Mary Ann Scoloveno, Ed.D., P.N.P.
Chairperson, Primary Health Care Department
Rutgers College of Nursing
Newark, New Jersey

Ellen Shuzman, M.S.
Assistant Professor
Doctoral Candidate
Rutgers College of Nursing
Newark, New Jersey

Rosemary A. Simkins, R.N., M.N.
Associate Director of Nursing, Pediatrics
National Jewish Center for Respiratory and Immunology Research
Denver, Colorado

Margaret P. Smith, R.N., M.S.
Health Care Coordinator
Kennedy Memorial Hospital for Children
Brighton, Massachusetts

Charlotte M. Spicher, R.N., Ph.D.
Associate Professor, Parent–Child Nursing
College of Nursing and Health
University of Cincinnati
Cincinnati, Ohio

Sandra K. Spiller, R.N., B.S.N.
Program and Projects Coordinator
Rocky Mountain Poison Control Center
Denver General Hospital
Denver, Colorado

Judith A. Surveyer, R.N., M.S.
Coordinator, Surgical Liaison Program
The Children's Hospital
Boston, Massachusetts

Mary Walker, R.N., Ph.D., F.A.A.N.
Lecturer, School of Nursing
Director, Texas Rural Health Field Services Program
University of Texas
Austin, Texas

Patricia A. Woodbury, R.N.C., M.S.N., C.P.N.A.
Assistant Professor, Program in Public Health Nursing
School of Public Health
University of Minnesota
Minneapolis, Minnesota

Kathleen M. Wruk, R.N., B.S.N.
Associate Director
Rocky Mountain Poison Control Center
Denver General Hospital
Denver, Colorado

FRAMEWORK FOR CHILD HEALTH NURSING

PART ONE

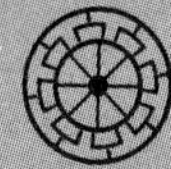

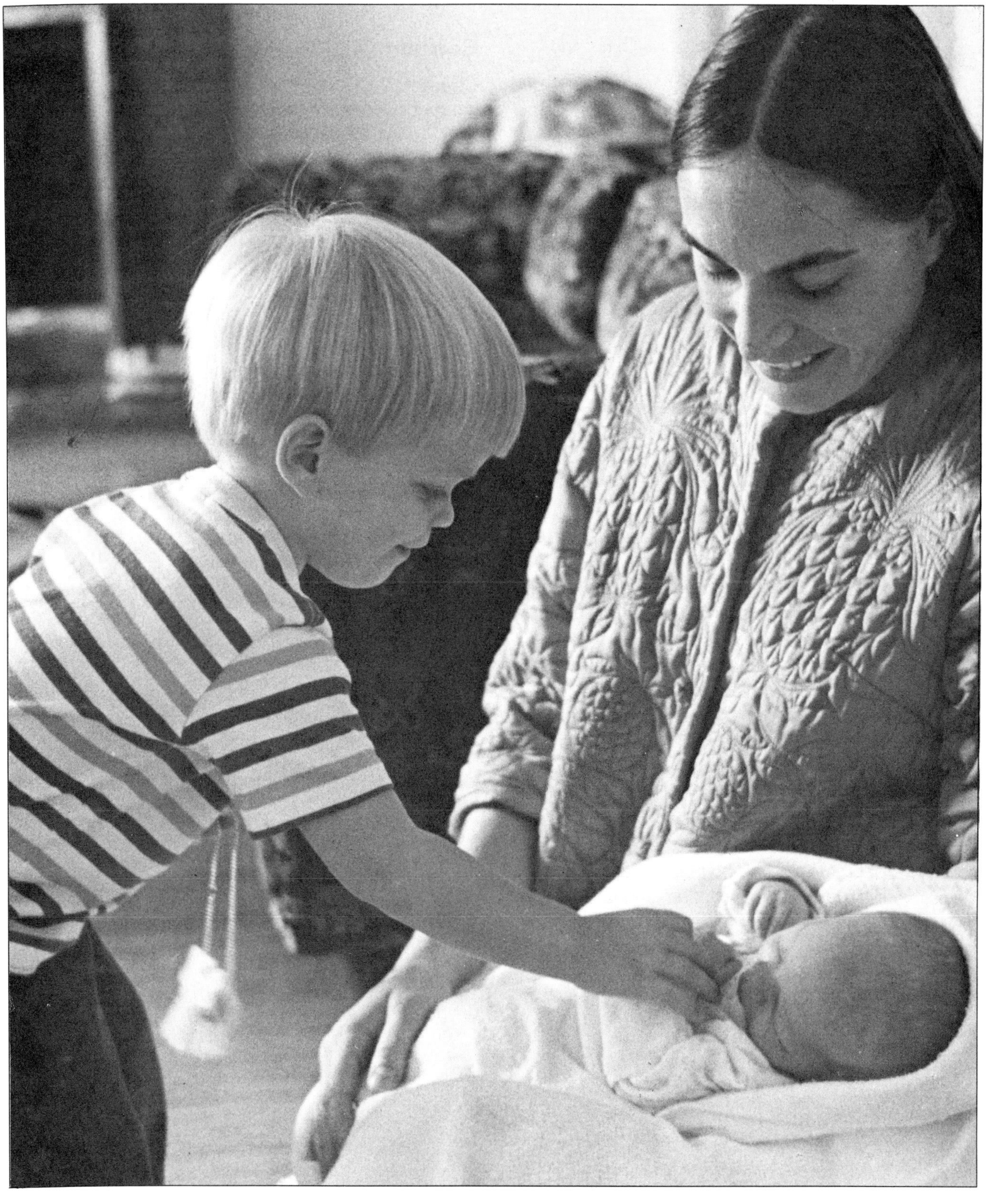

UNIT I OVERVIEW OF CHILD HEALTH NURSING

A multifaceted profession of child health nursing evolved along with improvements in the health care of children and families. Unlike pediatric nursing of the past, so named because of its association with the pediatric medical specialty, child health nursing of the present meets the needs of children and families in a variety of situations, at all levels of prevention, and in a holistic manner. Emotional, social, cultural, and developmental needs are considered as important as physical needs.

Our past is rich with examples of nurses striving to improve the health of children. Since we better understand the present by evaluating past events, in Chapter one we describe the evolution of child health nursing. We examine the past and the present varied roles of child health nurses and the settings in which they practice. In addition, we explore current influences on practice and future trends in child health nursing.

The growth of the nursing profession has generated both research and the development of nursing theory as a basis for practice. Although we recognize that no one theory as yet is accepted in its entirety by all members of our profession, we strongly feel that our professional practice must be based on a theoretical framework that can be applied to the care of children. Therefore, in Chapter two we delineate the operational basis for our book, an eclectic mixture of systems theory and Dorothy Orem's self-care model. The systems approach allows us to view children and their families as dynamic units with individual needs and varying potentials for meeting these needs. It permits holistic nursing care derived from observations and assessments of the needs of children and families as they interact with each other and their environment. Orem's theory allows us to focus on the child health nurse's role in teaching, promoting individual responsibility for self-care, and preventing disease and its consequences.

Contents

Perspectives in Child Health Nursing

1

Susan Rowen James

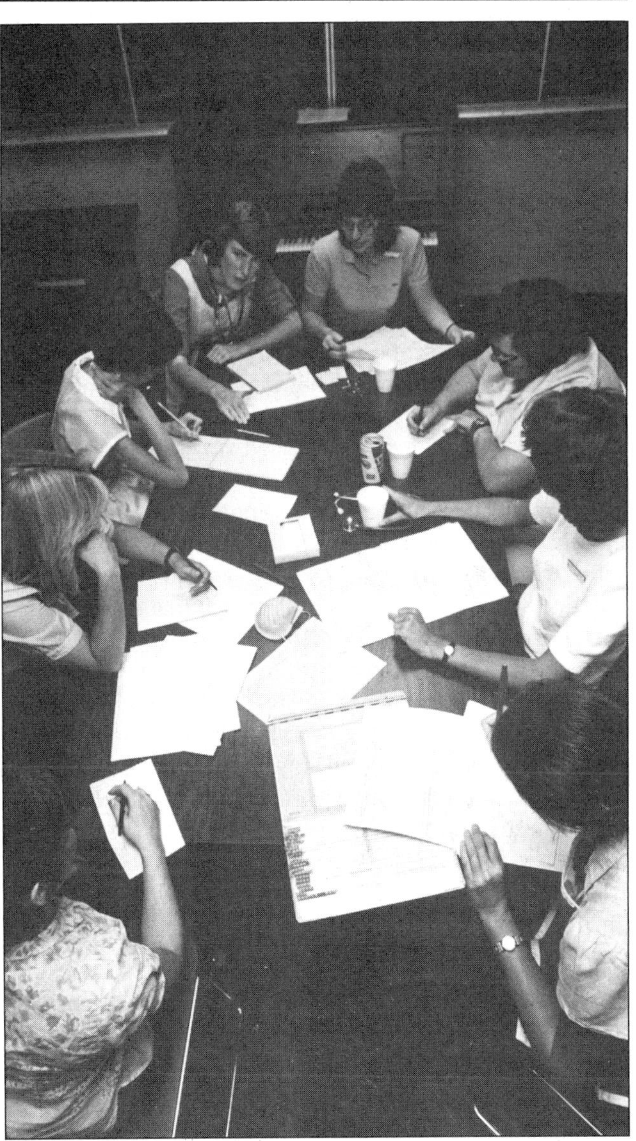

Chapter Outline

Objectives

- Describe the origins of child health nursing and its subsequent evolution.
- Explain how social and economic changes and advances in medical science helped determine the role of child health nurse.
- Describe the roles and expanded roles of the child health nurse.
- Discuss the legal and ethical ramifications affecting the nursing of children and families.
- Identify future trends in child health care.

In the past 150 years a remarkable shift of emphasis has occurred in health care, particularly in the care of the child. Historically, although it was recognized that both children and adults needed medical assistance, children were considered to be the property of their parents, and their value was essentially economic. That view contrasts significantly with the current feeling that children are the future of the world and therefore are entitled to health care that acknowledges their special needs.

The evolution of this attitude is apparent when we examine the changes in child health care over the last two centuries. Child health care has altered its focus from a strictly curative approach to a holistic approach that encompasses every aspect of health—physical, emotional, social, and environmental—and not just the absence of disease. Nowhere is this approach more noticeable than in the emerging role of the nurse, who has become a child advocate rather than simply a child caretaker.

In this chapter, we chart the development of nursing care for children. Pediatric nurses, so named for the medical specialty to which they are related, have become child health nurses in acknowledgment of the total care provided to the child and family. Child health nurses have moved from total dependence on medical supervision to become interdependent members of the health care team, having a separate area of expertise and professional accountability.

Development of Pediatrics and Pediatric Nursing

Child Health: Some Background Statistics

To appreciate where child health nursing care has been and where it is going, it is helpful first to examine the statistical data related to child health care from the turn of the twentieth century to the present. Throughout this time, birth rates have ranged from a high in 1910 to an unprecedented low in 1980. Figure 1-1 illustrates this change, showing the commonly accepted trends of wartime lows, postwar boom, and recent decline. Although the birth rates have been inconsistent, the ratio of male to female births has remained steady (Table 1-1).

Mortality rates have declined consistently. The circumstances that made life precarious for children in 1900 (62 deaths per 1000 children versus 4.1 deaths per 1000 children in 1982) (Figure 1-2) have changed, concurrent with improvements in medical and nursing care.

In 1900 the leading cause of death in children was gastroenteritis, followed closely by pneumonia (Table 1-2). Subsequent to the mandatory pasteurization of milk and the discovery and use of antibiotics, the significance of both problems decreased. The most common cause of childhood deaths today (aside from neonatal deaths due to congenital or mechanical problems) is accidents. As children

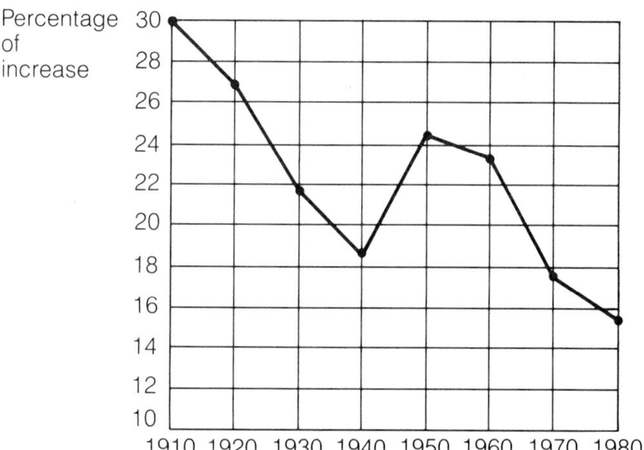

Figure 1-1 Birth rates, 1910–1980. The birth rate is the number of live births per total population, or the rate at which the population increases.

TABLE 1-1 Differences by Sex—Male to Female Ratio of Birth

Year	Male	Female
1940	1055	1000
1950	1054	1000
1960	1049	1000
1970	1066	1000
1980	1053	1000

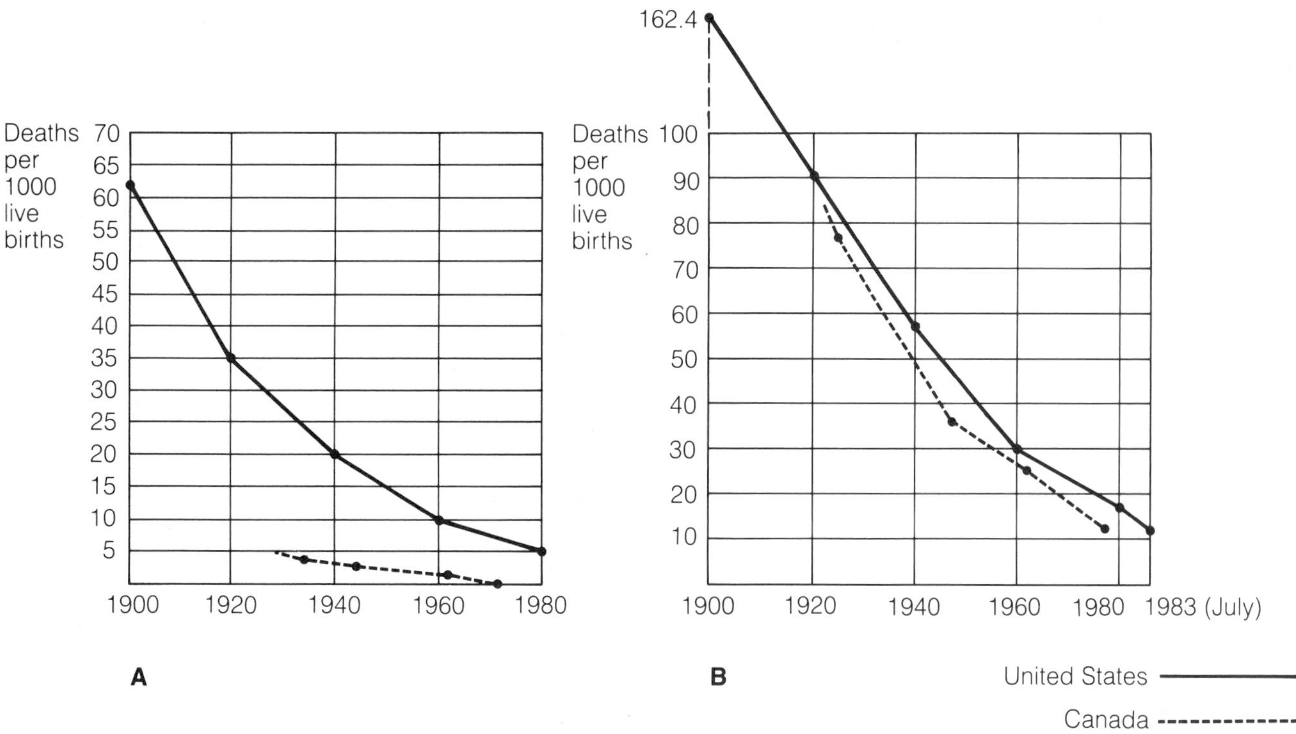

Figure 1-2 Infant and child mortality rates in the United States and Canada, 1910–1980. *A.* Childhood mortality (for children under 14). *B.* Infant mortality.

are raised in a more complex world, the potential increases for household and environmental hazards to be the instruments of death. Prevention is the only cure for this type of epidemic (Table 1-3).

Infant mortality rates also have declined dramatically, although both the United States and Canada have lagged behind many of the European countries. In 1978, at 13.8 deaths per 1000 infants in the United States and 12.4 deaths per 1000 infants in Canada, these two nations followed Sweden, Norway, Switzerland, and Denmark, among others (WHO, 1982). More current statistics show that the United States has an infant mortality rate of 11.0 deaths per 1000 infants (US Department of Health and Human Service, 1983). Better prenatal care and parent education programs have contributed to these improved rates, as have improved neonatal intensive care facilities. Medical care for mothers and children has become more available. Nursing care, particularly health supervision, has improved as the roles and functions of nurses have expanded. These factors will continue to affect mortality rates positively.

Because the decreasing mortality rates have been affected by the dramatic improvement in child health care, it is helpful to examine the evolution of child health nursing to see how it has affected children's health.

TABLE 1-2 Leading Causes of Childhood Deaths—United States*

1900	1920	1940	1960
Gastroenteritis	Pneumonia	Pneumonia	Congenital malformations
Pneumonia†	Gastroenteritis	Congenital malformations	Pneumonia
Tuberculosis	Tuberculosis	Gastroenteritis	Accidents‡
Cardiovascular disorders	Syphilis	Accidents	Gastroenteritis
Cancer	Cancer	Syphilis	Cancer

*Includes causes of infant death.

†Pneumonia includes influenza and other respiratory problems.

‡Accidents includes motor vehicle accidents.

SOURCE: Information from US Department of Health and Human Services. *1900–1980 Vital Statistics Rates in the United States*, 1983.

TABLE 1-3 Leading Causes of Childhood Death—1982

Age	Cause of death
0–1	Birth associated
	Congenital anomalies
	Other causes
	Immaturity associated
	Sudden infant death syndrome
1–14	Accidents—other than motor vehicles
	Motor vehicle accidents
	Cancer
	Birth defects
	Homicide
	Influenza and pneumonia
15–24	Motor vehicle accidents
	All other accidents
	Homicide
	Suicide
	Cancer
	Heart disease

SOURCE: US Department of Health and Human Services. *Monthly Vital Statistics Reports, 1983.* August, 1983.

Child Health Care Before the Twentieth Century

Child health care in the western hemisphere took root in the mid-seventeenth century when Augustine and Ursuline nuns and the Sisters of St. Joseph de la Fleche emigrated from France to Quebec, Canada to establish an orphanage and school for the children of the settlers. Upon arriving in Quebec, the nuns confronted rampant disease. The settlers had not totally adjusted to their new environment, and living conditions were poor. The orphanage project was abandoned in favor of the more urgent need to establish a hospital to care for the ill settlers. Through the end of the seventeenth century and the beginning of the eighteenth century, hospitals were established in other parts of North America, although during this period, medical care did not distinguish between children and adults (Jamieson, 1966).

New York Hospital, founded in 1771, was one of the first teaching hospitals in the United States. The nurses were ill-trained, and their responsibilities emphasized maintaining hygiene in the face of poor conditions. Death from communicable disease was widespread, and measures to prevent the spread of disease were unknown. Dr. Valentine Seaman, a physician at the hospital, recognized the nurses' lack of formal training and organized the first classroom presentations designed specifically for nurses. Lectures included the nursing care of children.

Specialty hospitals did not emerge until approximately 1800. The Hospital for Sick Children in London, established in 1851, was one of the first hospitals dedicated to the care of children and catering to the poor. With the hospital's publication in 1854 of one of the earliest known pediatric nursing textbooks, *How to Nurse Sick Children,* formal pediatric nursing education advanced another step (The Children's Hospital of Philadelphia, 1974).

The Hospital for Sick Children also inspired the founding in 1855 of the first children's hospital in the United States, the Children's Hospital of Philadelphia. Philadelphia, like other cities, had a high incidence of communicable disease from poor and overcrowded living conditions. Many children lived in homes that were so unsanitary that the children either died from or were left debilitated by disease. Physicians, accepting the premise that strong children become healthy adults, recognized the need for medical care aimed specifically at children. Children's Hospital was established in response to that need. It provided free medical care to children who were victims of illness or accidents (The Children's Hospital of Philadelphia, 1974).

The founding of other pediatric institutions soon followed. Children's hospitals opened in Boston, Denver, San Francisco, and other towns and cities. The care of ill children and research into childhood diseases became a rapidly expanding medical specialty.

For example, the Boston Floating Hospital (1894) was one of the more unusual institutions for the care of children. Boston had a high mortality rate in children from summer diarrhea. Physicians felt that relief from the heat would reduce disease incidence and subsequently converted a boat to accommodate sick children. The boat left the docks of Boston daily for Boston harbor carrying ill children, their

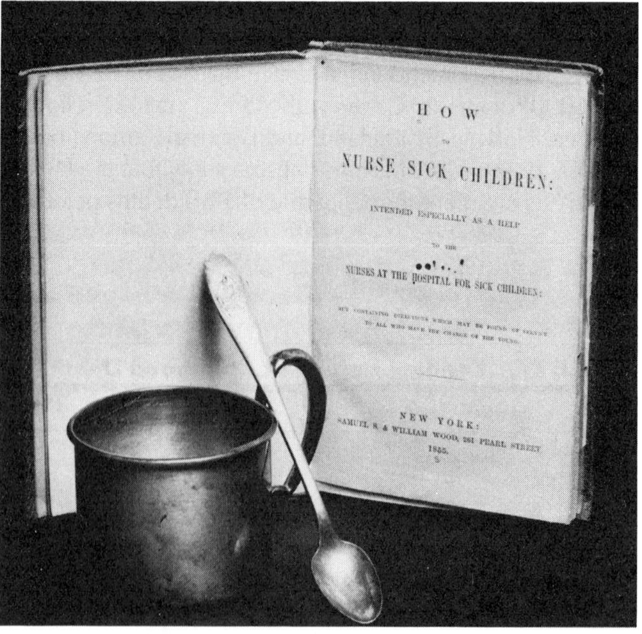

Nursing textbook, 1855.

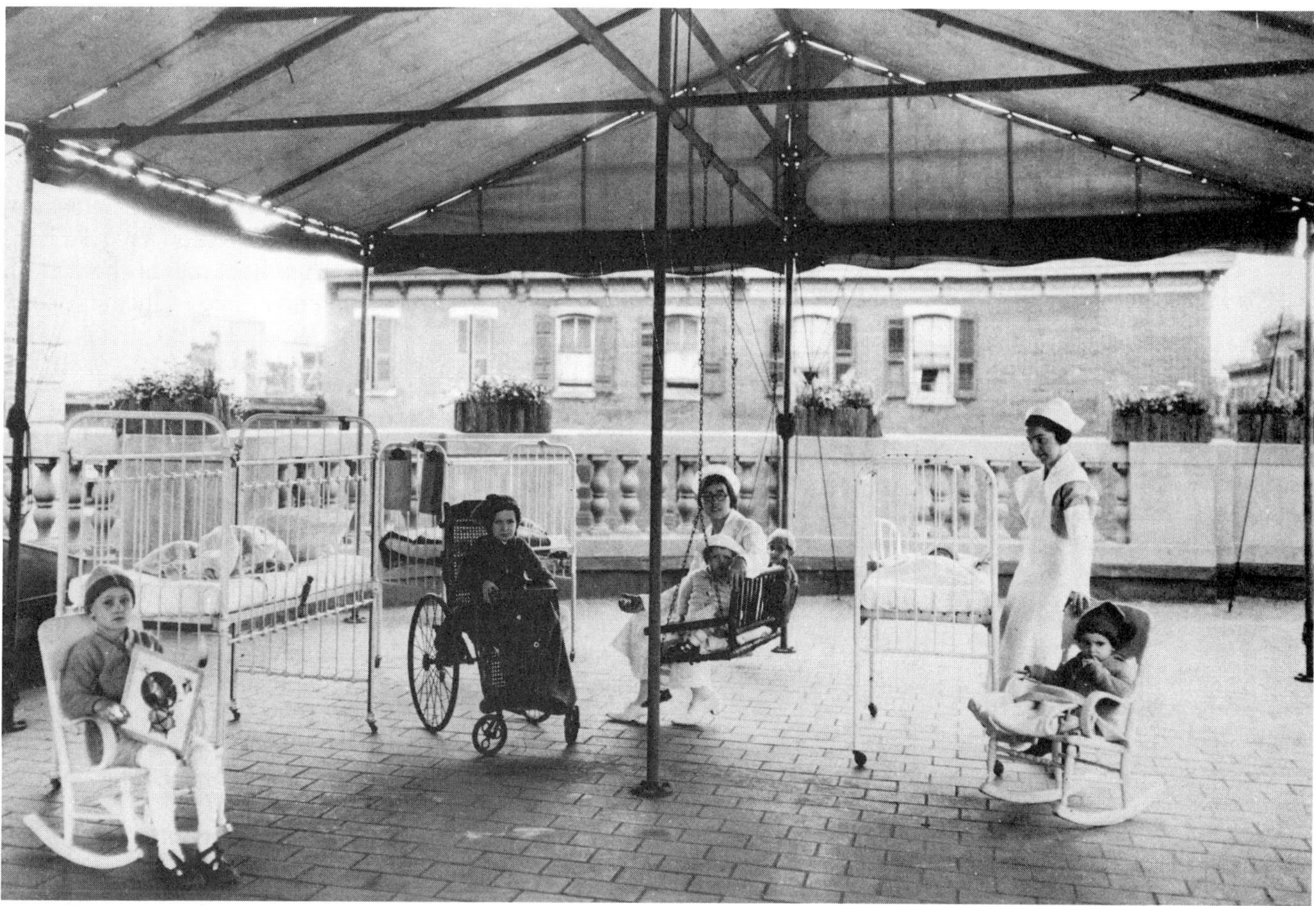

Roof Garden, 1921, The Children's Hospital of Philadelphia.

mothers, and a medical and nursing staff. Early research into the causes of and cures for gastroenteritis was conducted on the boat (Beaver, 1957). At a later date, this hospital moved to a permanent location in Boston.

The Development of Pediatric Nursing as a Specialty

The growth of pediatric nursing as a specialty paralleled the rapid expansion of medical pediatrics. In 1860 Florence Nightingale opened her first school of nursing, which was connected with St. Thomas' Hospital in London.

The Nightingale approach was radical for its day. It rejected the prevalent reliance on ignorant and uneducated nurse-servants and stressed the importance of acquiring a substantial body of knowledge and appropriate technical ability, the latter to be acquired at hospitals situated close to the training schools (Stewart and Austin, 1962).

In 1873 three schools of nursing were begun in the United States that adopted the Nightingale plan—Bellevue Training School for Nurses, Boston Training School, and the Connecticut Training School. St. Catherine's Training School in Ontario, established in 1874, was Canada's first nurses' training program to follow the Nightingale method.

Because the training schools were located in hospitals, children's hospitals developed schools to educate nurses in the care of ill children. Children's Hospital Training School in San Francisco offered formal classes in 1880 (Jamieson, 1966).

Although a pediatric nursing specialty existed during this period, the nursing role was still essentially that of child caretaker. Pediatric nurses were responsible for feeding the child and maintaining the child's nutritional status, hydration, and hygiene. They also played a significant role in preventing the spread of communicable disease, primarily through sanitation measures. These nurses worked in an era in which two of the leading causes of death were pneumonia and influenza. Pasteurization of milk was not mandatory, and antibiotics had not been discovered. Pediatric nurses followed physicians' orders and attempted to provide for the basic physical needs of the children to whom they were assigned. Nursing emphasis at this time, like the medical practice it supported, was curative rather than preventive.

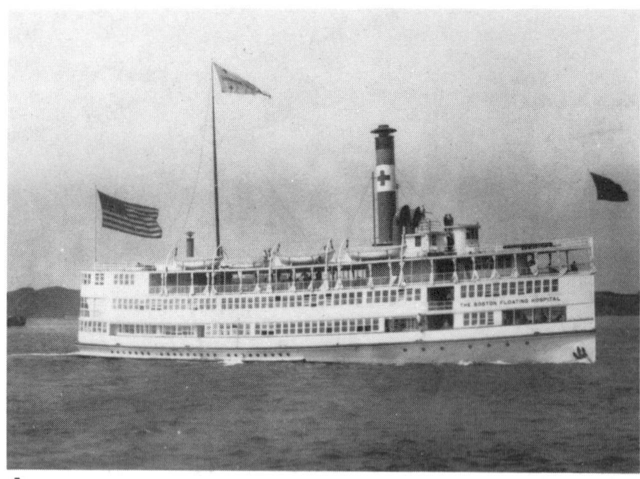

A

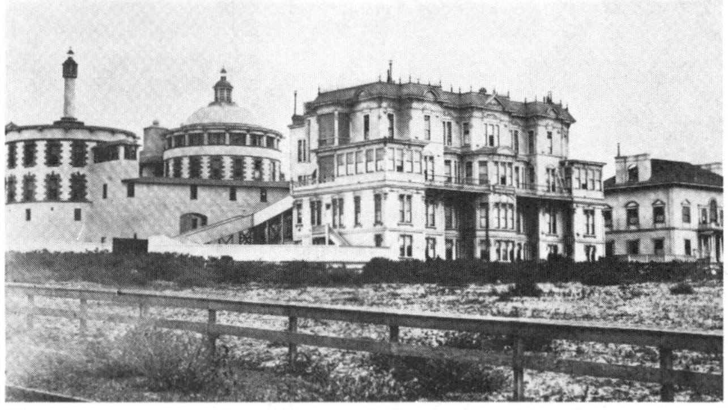

B

Teaching hospitals for early nursing education. *A.* Floating Hospital in Boston harbor. *B.* Children's Hospital in San Francisco.

Social Influences on Nursing at the End of the Nineteenth Century

By the mid-1800s, many women were attempting to improve their educational opportunities, particularly with an eye toward increasing the occupational avenues for those who were self-supporting. This factor, along with a general societal movement toward humanitarianism, fanned the development of nursing education. Better-educated nurses were needed not only to provide care for hospitalized individuals but also to do private nursing in the community (Dolan, 1978).

Visiting nursing was a new field open to educated nurses by 1886. Its development was prompted by a recognized need to provide better health care to the poor. Visiting nurses were prepared for their specialty by being educated in the hospital training programs. They provided health teaching in areas of hygiene, sanitation, child care, and the prevention of disease. Visiting nurses were somewhat autonomous, working in their clients' homes without direct physician supervison.

The settlement house concept was an outgrowth of the visiting nurse field. In 1893 Lillian Wald opened the Henry Street Settlement House. Originally designed to provide better-quality health care to the poor, it expanded its services to include not only medical care but also other social, cultural, and educational programs. It prompted a new perspective in health care—that of personal responsibility and individual accountability for health.

At Lillian Wald's instigation, nurses from the Settlement House visited the New York City schools on a regular basis begining in 1902. These early school nurses checked on the health of schoolchildren and inspected them for communicable disease.

Nursing at the Turn of the Twentieth Century

There were three legitimate nursing opportunities in the early 1900s—hospital nursing, visiting nursing, and private nursing. The growth of humanitarianism and the effects of the women's movement provided the impetus for an increase in the numbers of nurses. Positions in hospitals were limited, so many nurses chose private nursing. It was routine at that time for ill people to be cared for in their own homes. Because private nurses had very little supervision, quality control was minimal. This factor, combined with the proliferation of largely untrained "practical nurses," prompted the development of a system of nurse registration (Stewart and Austin, 1962).

The registration of nurses began in 1903 and resulted in the establishment of the State Boards of Nurse Examiners. Standards were developed that were directed toward protecting the public from undereducated, inept nurses (Dolan, 1978).

Another movement toward improving the quality of nursing and nursing education was the development of professional organizations. In response to the inconsistent standards of the nurse training schools, the American Society of Superintendents of Training Schools was formed in 1893. This organization, later the National League for Nursing, helped set standards of nursing education by establishing an accreditation system for nursing schools. Its members directed training school programs (Dolan, 1978).

A second professional organization originated in 1896—the Nurses' Associated Alumnae of the United States and Canada. In 1911 this became the American Nurses' Association, whose purpose was "To foster high standards of nursing practice and promote the welfare of nurses so all people may have better nursing care" (Dolan, 1978, p. 269).

During the early 1900s, nursing education took a step forward. Agitation from within and without the nursing community prompted a new look at nursing education, resulting in recommendations that the education of nurses be removed from the hospital and become a separate process. Nurses were to be educated not trained. Teachers' College at Columbia University instituted some classes for nurses in 1907. In 1909 the University of Minnesota at

Minneapolis established a basic nursing program. These programs were followed by others. In 1923, following a 3-year survey of nursing education, the report *Nursing and Nursing Education in the United States* was released. This report, known as the Goldmark Report, advocated the upgrading of nurse educators, as well as the educational system itself. This would prepare nurses who were qualified to teach methods of preventive health care and improve the curative focus of health care.

Functional Nursing Versus Preventive Health Care

Hospital nursing in the early years of the twentieth century became less patient centered and more task oriented. Tasks, or functions, were delegated to various nurses, resulting in fragmented nursing care. Hospital nursing did establish, however, the foundations for nursing research as nurses sought to improve the efficiency of their tasks. Research conducted at that time included studies directed toward improved care for both mothers and children. Studies that focused on the prevention of ophthalmia neonatorum, for example, resulted in better training and higher health standards for nurse midwives (Dolan, 1978).

Functional nursing continued until the beginning of World War II, as did the somewhat autonomous practice of nursing in the neighborhood centers. Also, during those years, school nursing developed further as a specialty, continuing the shift in emphasis in child health care toward health promotion and disease prevention. The activities of the school nurse in the 1930s included such duties as health screening and health education. The nurse was not, however, allowed to give treatments in the school or to perform any follow-up care (Igoe, 1980).

Changes in Child Health Care Following World War II

World War II drastically changed health care and nursing practices. Educated nurses were recruited by the armed services and were replaced by unskilled auxiliary personnel. In the United States this nursing shortage caused the closure of the neighborhood health centers and a fundamental change in the performance of nursing care. Team nursing was the response to the shortage of professional nurses. The educated nurse supervised teams of auxiliary caregivers and managed nursing units, thus becoming somewhat removed from direct patient care. Because tasks were delegated to various auxiliary personnel, the fragmentation of care continued. With the discovery and use of antibiotics, pediatric medical care again emphasized a strictly curative approach, ignoring the preventive aspects of health care for a time (McCarty, 1977).

In spite of this trend during the postwar period, several events in the1950s set the stage for the emergence of modern child health nursing. First, the discovery of the polio vaccine in the 1950s eradicated a major childhood disease. Although vaccines against other illnesses already were available, this discovery seemed to prompt more active research into disease prevention. A resurgence of the neighborhood health center concept, along with federal assistance, stimulated the development of well-child clinics where nurses not only administered vaccines but also performed other health screening and educational functions. The use of child health nurses in well-child conferences facilitated their independence. The increased contact of nurses with parents required the active use of the principles of health education.

In the early 1950s researchers also added new dimensions to child health care. They developed theories about the growth and development of children and correlated these theories with children's reactions to hospitalization. John Bowlby conducted longitudinal studies to determine children's reactions to maternal separation, a common occurrence in children's hospitals. He reported to the World Health Organization in 1951 that children need continuous contact with their mothers for healthy development (Bowlby, 1955). His studies were repeated and expanded by such researchers as James Robertson and Dane Prugh, both of whom examined the effects of hospitalization on children. The results of these studies eventually changed nursing's approach to the care of the hospitalized child. The reasons for rigid visiting hours and the exclusion of parents from participating in their child's care no longer seemed valid. As these theories became understood and accepted, nurses began to see hospitalized children as parts of family units and to alter hospital facilities to accommodate these changing concepts. In actively seeking better-quality care for their clients, they initiated what was to become the nurse-advocate role.

The 1960s: A Decade of Advances in Child–Family Nursing

The social upheaval of the 1960s did not neglect the health care field. During this decade, child health nursing began to diverge from its traditional attachment to the physician. Nurses not only demanded changes in the approach to the hospitalized child but also developed a separate body of knowledge and unique practice.

As a result of the studies by Bowlby and others, nurses became more aware of the child's response to maternal separation. Also, parents were more vocal and knowledgeable about their right to be with their children. Many hospitals subsequently relaxed visiting restrictions, some even allowing parents to remain with their children during the night.

Boston Floating Hospital opened its Family Participation Unit, an experimental unit that was federally funded to explore new approaches to pediatric hospital care (Katz, 1964). When a child was admitted to this unit, it was understood that the parents would be assisted by the nurse to assume as much responsibility for the child's care as they felt capable of. The parent performed certain treatments and assisted the nurse in preparing the child for medical procedures. With this project, family-centered child health care became a reality. Child health nurses increased the scope of their activities. They included in their care anticipatory guidance, discharge teaching, and referral to other resources within the community. The ill child became the child who happened to be ill.

During the 1960s, awareness grew that quality health care must become more available to children in rural areas. In response to this, Henry K. Silver, MD and Loretta C. Ford, RN, PhD established a program at the University of Colorado that was designed to educate a new category of health worker, the pediatric nurse practitioner. The nurse practitioner role filled a gap caused by the physician's increasing attention to the complex curative aspects of pediatric care. Nurse practitioners collaborated with physicians to provide better health care for children and families and became primary contact persons for children in the health care system. They conducted health screenings, gave well-child care, managed simple medical problems, and provided support during medical emergencies. Nurse practitioners learned how to perform a physical assessment using some of the tools that formerly were used only by physicians (Ford, 1976).

As originally envisioned, the pediatric nurse practitioner would provide care in rural areas of the country where physician accessibility was limited. The program at the University of Colorado was followed closely by programs in other areas of the country. These programs prepared practitioners to function not only in rural areas but also in urban health centers and physicians' offices. The pediatric nurse practitioner was the prototype for other expanded nursing roles in a variety of specialities. Equally important, it continued the movement to change the focus of nursing from curative to preventive.

Finally, recognition of the unique needs of children prompted greater concentration on easing their adjustment to illness. The child's routine use of play became a useful nursing tool, not only for preparing a child for hospitalization but also as a method of preventing the adverse effects of hospital procedures. Some hospitals initiated diversional programs for children, whereas others supported nurses in their efforts to include play as a routine part of care to facilitate normal growth and development. Nurses used theories of therapeutic play in a structured situation to teach children or to encourage the expression of negative feelings. Community health nurses also used theories of play both in developmental assessments and in teaching situations. They taught parents to use play to stimulate normal growth and development.

In no other decade in the history of nursing did so much change occur so rapidly. The 1960s were years of social movements that affected nursing to a degree not seen since Florence Nightingale. The child was recognized as an individual with unique needs and problems; the family was included in the decision-making process; and child–family nurses assumed their responsibility as vital contacts in the health care system. These movements in nursing facilitated the development of a separate body of knowledge and resulted in the holistic approach to the health care of children.

In 1966 the American Nurses' Association, keeping pace with the changes in nursing practice, established specialty divisions within its membership. Each division constructed standards for optimal nursing practice in its specialty. The current standards for maternal–child health nursing practice are summarized in the box following.

The 1970s: The Growth of Holistic Health Care and Nursing Autonomy

Although the groundwork for a body of knowledge in child–family nursing was developed in the 1960s, the specialty underwent significant changes during subsequent years. A major influence on the process at the time was the emerging concept of holistic health. As the term suggests, health is a more comprehensive concept than suggested by the traditional definition, which indicates merely the absence of disease. When viewed holistically, the client consists of several subsystems (biophysical, cognitive, affective, and social). Together, these interacting components form a unit that in turn interacts with a larger external system—society. (For an in-depth discussion of this general systems theory, see Chapter 2.)

This notion of a holistic approach had great significance for health care. It suggested that focusing on a specific malfunction or organ system in isolation neglected the broader health needs of the client. To understand the effect the holistic approach to health care had on child health care, it is helpful to examine the emergence of the nursing process.

The effectiveness of the holistic approach relied on an efficient communication network among members of the health care team. The vehicle for communication was the nursing care plan, which was based on a formal, cognitive assessment of client needs. As nurse scholars became more sophisticated in their interpretation of the holistic approach, they began to identify and describe diagnoses that were accepted for use in the development of nursing care plans (see Chapter 2).

The identification of these diagnoses is made possible by assessing clients' needs using a holistic framework. Appropriate interventions are developed, which are evaluated for effectiveness and revised when needed. The assessment,

Standards of Maternal–Child Health Nursing Practice

Standard I—The nurse helps children and parents attain and maintain optimum health.

Standard II—The nurse assists families to achieve and maintain a balance between the personal growth needs of individual family members and optimum family functioning.

Standard III—The nurse intervenes with vulnerable clients and families at risk to prevent potential developmental and health problems.

Standard IV—The nurse promotes an environment free of hazards to reproduction, growth and development, wellness, and recovery from illness.

Standard V—The nurse detects changes in health status and deviations from optimum development.

Standard VI—The nurse carries out appropriate interventions and treatment to facilitate survival and recovery from illness.

Standard VII—The nurse assists clients and families to understand and cope with developmental and traumatic situations during illness, childbearing, childrearing, and childhood.

Standard VIII—The nurse actively pursues strategies to enhance access to and utilization of adequate health care services.

Standard IX—The nurse improves maternal and child health nursing practice through evaluation of practice, education, and research.

American Nurses' Association, Division on Maternal & Child Health Nursing Practice. Copyright © 1983 by American Nurses' Association. Reprinted by permission.

development, and evaluation of the care plan comprises the nursing process.

The nursing process has been used by child health nurses in a variety of settings. This promoted autonomy in their practice because the greater reliability of nursing data increased nurses' capabilities for intelligent decision making. Children were assessed holistically, with a particular focus on their family and peer relationships, adjustment to hospitalization, and use of play.

The final aspect of the complex role of the child–family nurse has been the development of child advocacy. As nurses have become more autonomous and secure in their positions as contributing members of the health care team, they have been able to direct more energy toward securing better-quality health care for children and families. In their roles as advocates, nurses strive for improvements, not only in their work settings but also in health care legislation, community affairs, and worldwide assistance programs.

Current Aspects of Child Health Care

Child Health Care: The 1980s and Beyond

Essential to an understanding of how a child health nurse functions in the 1980s is an understanding of primary health care. In an age of increasing medical specialization, the role played by the general practitioner came to be sadly neglected. As a result, clients no longer had a primary contact person in the health care system, and their health concerns became scattered among specialists, none of whom viewed clients as whole persons. Primary health care, which provided the client with a practitioner who took a more comprehensive and humanistic overview, as well as a point of entry to more specialized components of the health care system, became a rarity.

As consumers became more vocal about the lack of a primary contact person in the system, medical schools developed family practice specialties that prepared physicians for the family doctor role. Meanwhile, child health nurses expanded their roles, adding health promotion activities to their acute care practice. It was obvious that nurses in the community were the ideal persons to administer primary health care to clients. As part of the nursing process, they obtained health histories, assessed client needs, performed health screening procedures, and developed comprehensive plans of care. They were able to handle common health concerns and make referrals. Community nurses met the health needs of the well client in addition to the sick. They coordinated care. At present, child health nurses fulfill the need for primary care in a number of ways.

Settings and Roles of Primary Nurses in Child Health Care

The primary nurse is essentially a contact person for the child and family in various health care settings. All nurses perform similar functions. In addition to obtaining nursing histories, they assess child growth and development, family interactions, patterns of parenting, and general life-style, including the family and child's response to stress. They recognize problems and intervene to correct them before further complications occur. Nurses perform health education activities and refer children and families to appropriate community resources. They are autonomous in their nursing practice, within the states' Nurse Practice Acts, and are accountable for their actions. In their role as child advocate, nurses initiate changes for better-quality health care. Many role definitions probably are somewhat idealistic, but many nurses function well within the framework and strive for excellence in care.

Primary Care Nursing in the Community

The Community Health Nurse Community health nurses follow children from infancy throughout the life cycle and have a unique opportunity to observe them in their natural environment. They assess children within their family structure and intervene to assist children and families to develop positive health habits. At well-baby clinics, they perform simple screening tests, administer immunizations, observe and record developmental progress, and provide anticipatory guidance for normal developmental problems. Community health nurses receive referrals from hospitals and other sources to care for acutely ill children in the home. They are particularly knowledgeable about specialized community resources. They communicate information about medical progress to the other members of the health team and are accountable for nursing actions.

The School Nurse The school nurse is gaining increasing recognition as a primary provider of health care. In the past the school nurse's role was more or less restricted to the administration of minor first-aid and emergency care. Because it is recognized that children need more comprehensive health care during the school years and because greater numbers of children with special needs are being placed in the mainstream of the school environment, the role of the school nurse has gained new dimensions.

The responsibilities of school nurses include the following:

1. Maintaining a health record for all schoolchildren, including an assessment and identification of special health problems
2. Communicable disease follow-up, including the maintenance of immunization records
3. Counseling children and families with physical, emotional, or social difficulties
4. Managing accidents and illnesses occurring in school
5. Recognizing and counseling pregnant adolescents, substance abusers, and victims of domestic violence
6. Collaborating with the school physician in conducting routine physical examinations of schoolchildren, including screening for visual or hearing impairments, scoliosis, and other health problems
7. Identifying potential health and safety hazards in the school environment

School nurses also play an active role in health promotion. They became involved with the school health education program by teaching about stress reduction, diet and exercise, and other principles for healthful living. They provide information related to problems of substance abuse, pregnancy, sexuality, and domestic violence. School nurses confer with teachers about health problems occurring in the classroom and assist teachers in the management of children with special needs (Igoe, 1980).

The Camp Nurse Nurses in camp settings function autonomously within a medical framework devised by the attending physician. The camp nurse is responsible for maintaining the health of campers and staff, administering ordered prescriptions, and managing acute illness and emergencies under the medical director's standing orders. While assessing campers upon their arrival, camp nurses identify health problems and needs for anticipatory guidance. Because children in new settings often exhibit maladaptive behaviors unknown to the parents, communication between the parents, staff, and nurse is essential for a unified approach to problem resolution. Camp nurses communicate directly with the camp administration about unsafe conditions, especially regarding high-risk areas such as the waterfront and archery and riflery ranges.

The Office Nurse Office nurses, although capable of using all the skills previously mentioned, traditionally have been assigned routine tasks such as obtaining measurements, immunization administration, routine specimen collection, and office paperwork. In the past pediatricians have been reluctant to allow nurses to assume more responsibility for health promotion. As nurses have become better educated and more prepared to be autonomous, they have assumed greater responsibility for child health care. Office nurses perform preliminary assessments, counsel parents by phone, and assist parents to cope with normal developmental difficulties. Nurse practitioners functioning in an office setting or health maintenance organization conduct well-child examinations and manage less acute illnesses. The nurse practitioner often will handle "call-in time" (scheduled time when parents may call to discuss problems their child may be experiencing) and answer the health concerns of parents.

Primary Care Nursing in the Hospital

Because a child's contact with the health care system is often through hospitalization, the child health nurse working in an acute-care setting becomes the primary contact person. Because of the development and refinement of the nursing process, these nurses are much more qualified to plan for the comprehensive health needs of clients. The increased emphasis on baccalaureate and master's degree level education for nurses helped result in better-quality primary health care.

The role of the child health nurse in an acute-care setting encompasses the holistic assessment of the child's needs, as well as use of the nursing process to facilitate recovery. Nurses assist the child and family in adjusting to a threatening situation. In addition to following a medical regimen designed to correct an existing medical problem, they view each child as an individual and attempt to incorporate as much of the child's normal routine as possible in the care plan. Child health nurses include parents in the care of their children, providing information about the disease, hospital procedures, and general health. They also coordinate the efforts of other members of the health care team to promote an optimal environment for recovery. Discharge preparation is an important function of the child health nurse, easing the transition from the hospital to the home environment.

The nurse's role in a chronic or rehabilitative hospital is similar to that in an acute setting. Greater emphasis is placed on the maintenance or improvement of the child's ability to function at maximum potential. Here, too, nurses use anticipatory guidance (see Chapter 21) for health promotion. Child health nurses are concerned with the needs of the handicapped child, and they collaborate with members of the community to ease the child's adjustments to daily living. Most important is the skill with which the nurse can assist the child and family to adjust emotionally to a chronic illness.

Primary nursing is a staffing pattern that facilitates the execution of primary health care in the hospital setting. In essence primary nursing is a system whereby the health needs of clients are met on a 24-hour basis. Children and parents seem to respond more rapidly if they can identify with one nurse. Primary nurses obtain nursing histories and construct care plans for their clients. They are accountable for the care they give and for seeing that the plans are followed and evaluated.

Expanded Roles in Child Health Nursing

Two additional roles of pediatric nurses need to be emphasized here because their influence prompted the development of autonomous nursing practice. The pediatric nurse practitioner already has been mentioned. Other expanded roles are those of the pediatric clinical specialist and the school nurse practitioner.

Clinical Nurse Specialist Clinical specialties originated at a time when nursing was functional and fragmented. Nursing leaders envisioned a nurse who would function as a coordinator of care but also one who would demonstrate expertise in a specialized area of nursing (Kinsella, 1973). This clinical nurse specialist would act as a role model and a change agent, improving the quality of care. Initially, the role was ill-defined. At present, a clinical specialist is defined as a nurse educated at the master's-degree level in a specialty and prepared to function with an increased depth of knowledge and capacity to make high-level nursing judgments. In child health care, specialists concentrate on the general care of children or on the nursing care problems generated by alterations in specific body systems. Both concentrations include the responsibility for consultation, application of change theory, research design, role modeling, and expertise in the specialty field.

Those specializing in general child health care usually practice in community hospitals, where patients are few and the disease entities less acute. Specialists act as liaisons between the hospital and community, planning care for clients as they move through the health care system. Their major focus is the quality and continuity of care. Specialists are mobile, following clients from the community to the hospital and vice versa. Their referrals come from other nurses, physician colleagues, or are self-initiated. Specialists maintain continuous, updated records on their clients and communicate essential information to other members of the health care team. Participation in staff educational development and in research to improve nursing care is implicit in the role. As Nurse Practice Acts change and third-party insurers recognize the value and cost-effectiveness of the clinical specialists, more of these nurses will establish independent nursing practices as primary caregivers.

Specialists who focus on a narrower aspect of child health care usually practice in the larger teaching hospitals. They are experts in a single aspect of care such as oncologic nursing. They, too, are physician colleagues, often working closely with the physician in research and publication. In addition to providing expert nursing care, these specialists assist the nursing staff by conducting care conferences and by coordinating care for individual clients.

School Nurse Practitioner As previously mentioned, the pediatric nurse practitioner program at the University of Colorado was the prototype for other nurse practitioner programs, most notably programs to train school nurse practitioners. Programs for school nurse practitioners emphasized the problems of well-child care and health and developmental screening. They originally varied in length from several months to 2 years, depending on the educational result. A certificate was awarded on completion of the program. In recent years the education of nurse practitioners generally has been incorporated into nursing programs at the graduate level to prepare better primary care nurses. In addition to screening and health supervision activities, the nurse practitioner can order laboratory tests, prescribe selected medications, and diagnose and treat minor illnesses and emergencies using established protocol. School nurse practitioners also assist teachers in identifying and treating children with learning or perceptual disorders. They are actively involved with community planning for handicapped children and for those with other special needs. Nurse practitioners are found in both urban and rural areas (Silver, 1971).

Initially, the role of the nurse practitioner appeared to combine traditional roles of medicine and nursing because the activities of health screening and health promotion were superseded by an emphasis on assessment tools to nursing—the otoscope, ophthalmoscope, palpation, and auscultation. As pediatric nurse practitioners continue to define their roles, however, a wide range of nursing services will be offered to children and families that are unique and separate from medicine.

Legal and Ethical Considerations

Rights of the Child and Family

In any discussions of child health care, some of the important legislative landmarks facilitating improvements in the health and welfare of children should be considered. Some of the basic rights of the child and family need to be examined as well.

In 1912, at the instigation of Lillian Wald, President Grover Cleveland created the Children's Bureau, the functions of which were as follows:

1. To recognize the rights of children for a safe birth and optimal health development to adulthood
2. To remove obstacles impeding the achievement of this goal
3. To prevent harmful conditions (Dolan, 1978, pp. 255–256)

Future White House Conferences on children and youth (held approximately every 10 years) created state divisions on maternal–child health, modified child labor laws, accepted federal responsibility to assist in the development of healthy children, made it mandatory to report certain health problems, such as phenylketonuria (PKU) and child abuse, and directed attention to minorities and the handicapped (Dolan, 1978).

The United Nations declared the year 1979 as the International Year of the Child, stating, "The main objective of the year—to encourage raising significantly the level of services benefiting children on a permanent basis–ultimately implies an increase in financial resources dedicated to this end" (International Year of the Child 1978, p. 244).

In preparation for the International Year of the Child, the United Nations reaffirmed the *Declaration of the Rights of the Child,* which calls for freedom, equality of opportunities, the social and emotional benefits of love and security, and the enhancement of maximum potential for all children. Nurses have been working toward these goals as long as pediatrics has been recognized as a specialty. Nurses care for children in developing countries. As child advocates, they have vastly improved health services to the poor and underprivileged. When applying the principles set forth in the *Declarations of the Rights of the Child,* it is evident that there are specific health rights that can be applied to both children and families. These rights include provisions for adequate medical and dental care, including preventive and prophylactic treatment, regardless of the family's ability to pay. The access to adequate nutrition, whether at school or at home, also is of primary importance for good health (Parks, 1982).

The United States has enacted legislation to attain the goals listed in the *Declaration of the Rights of the Child.* The improvement in maternal and child health service (MCH) was guaranteed when written into the Social Security Act of 1935. Since then, the federal government has supported improved accessibility of services for women and children through additional legislation: Crippled Children's Services, Maternal Infant Care Project (1963), Children and Youth Project (1965), and Medicaid, among others (Table 1-4). At present, many of these programs have been taken over by state and local governments under the Block Grant Services. Block Grants are awarded by the Office of Human Development Services, Administration for Children, Youth and Families, US Department of Health and Human Services.

In addition to basic human rights, children and families also possess legal rights that are particularly relevant for health personnel. An extensive coverage of legal rights would be impossible within the limits of this chapter because over the years the courts have defined and redefined rights as society has become increasingly complex. While children contend with societal problems such as venereal disease, drug addiction, birth control, and abortion, the courts have been interpreting the laws to ensure the child's access to adequate health care. Although children previously were regarded as possessions of their parents and therefore under total parental control as to decisions regarding health care, the courts recently have reinterpreted this assumption to give some children more freedom to seek treatment or counseling.

Generally, children hold certain legal rights in the medical system: the right to expect confidentiality, the right of access to medical records, and the right to participate in their care (Burgdorf, 1979). Included in the last right is the right to a certain amount of self-determination in decisions affecting health (Parks, 1982). It is important for nurses who work with children to recognize this right and incorporate it into their care of children and families.

Problems often occur in ill-defined areas, particularly those subject to interpretation of the laws. Two of these areas are particularly important to nurses: (1) minors' consent for treatment and (2) children's participation in research (Burgdorf, 1979).

The definition of the following two terms is essential in understanding the first issue:

Emancipated minor—a child not living at home, self-supporting, or whose parents have voluntarily or involuntarily surrendered their rights (Holder, 1977, p. 139)

Mature minor—a child over 15 years of age and able to understand medical interventions and risks (Holder, 1977)

United Nations Declaration of the Rights of the Child

Preamble

Whereas the peoples of the United Nations have, in the Charter, reaffirmed their faith in fundamental human rights, and in the dignity and worth of the human person, and have determined to promote social progress and better standards of life in larger freedom,

Whereas the United Nations has, in the Universal Declaration of Human Rights, proclaimed that everyone is entitled to all the rights and freedoms set forth therein, without distinction of any kind, such as race, color, sex, language, religion, political or other opinion, national or social origin, property, birth or other status,

Whereas the child, by reason of his physical and mental immaturity, needs special safeguards and care, including appropriate legal protection, before as well as after birth,

Whereas the need for such special safeguards has been stated in the Geneva Declaration of the Rights of the Child of 1924, and recognized in the Universal Declaration of Human Rights and in the statutes of specialized agencies and international organizations concerned with the welfare of children,

Whereas mankind owes to the child the best it has to give

Now therefore the general assembly proclaims

This Declaration of the Rights of the Child to the end that he may have a happy childhood and enjoy for his own good and for the good of society the rights and freedoms herein set forth, and calls upon parents, upon men and women as individuals and upon voluntary organizations, local authorities and national governments to recognize these rights and strive for their observance by legislative and other measures progressively taken in accordance with the following principles:

Principle 1

The child shall enjoy all the rights set forth in this Declaration. All children, without any exception whatsoever, shall be entitled to these rights, without distinction or discrimination on account of race, color, sex, language, religion, political or other opinion, national or social origin, property, birth or other status, whether of himself or of his family.

Principle 2

The child shall enjoy special protection, and shall be given opportunities and facilities, by law and by other means, to enable him to develop physically, mentally, morally, spiritually and socially in a healthy and normal manner and in conditions of freedom and dignity. In the enactment of laws for this purpose the best interests of the child shall be the paramount consideration.

Principle 3

The child shall be entitled from his birth to a name and a nationality.

Principle 4

The child shall enjoy the benefits of social security. He shall be entitled to grow and develop in health; to this end special care and protection shall be provided both to him and to his mother, including adequate pre-natal and post-natal care. The child shall have the right to adequate nutrition, housing, recreation and medical services.

Principle 5

The child who is physically, mentally or socially handicapped shall be given the special treatment, education and care required by his particular condition.

Principle 6

The child, for the full and harmonious development of his personality, needs love and understanding. He shall, wherever possible, grow up in the care and under the responsibility of his parents, and in any case in an atmosphere of affection and of moral and maternal security; a child of tender years shall not, save in exceptional circumstances, be separated from his mother. Society and the public authorities shall have the duty to extend particular care to children without a family and to those without adequate means of support. Payment of state and other assistance toward the maintenance of children of large families is desirable.

continued on next page

Principle 7

The child is entitled to receive education, which shall be free and compulsory, at least in the elementary stages. He shall be given an education which will promote his general culture, and enable him on a basis of equal opportunity to develop his abilities, his individual judgment, and his sense of moral and social responsibility, and to become a useful member of society.

The best interests of the child shall be the guiding principle of those responsible for his education and guidance; that responsibility lies in the first place with his parents.

The child shall have full opportunity for play and recreation, which shall be directed to the same purposes as education; society and the public authorities shall endeavor to promote the enjoyment of this right.

Principle 8

The child shall in all circumstances be among the first to receive protection and relief.

Principle 9

The child shall be protected against all forms of neglect, cruelty and exploitation. He shall not be the subject of traffic, in any form.

The child shall not be admitted to employment before an appropriate minimum age; he shall in no case be caused or permitted to engage in any occupation or employment which would prejudice his health or education, or interfere with his physical, mental or moral development.

Principle 10

The child shall be protected from practices which may foster racial, religious and any other form of discrimination. He shall be brought up in a spirit of understanding, tolerance, friendship among peoples, peace and universal brotherhood and in full consciousness that his energy and talents should be devoted to the service of his fellow men.

Emancipated minors may give consent for treatment. College students may or may not be emancipated minors, depending on their financial status. Mature minors may give consent for treatment under some circumstances, particularly in emergency situations when parents are unavailable. If minors give their own consent for treatment, they become financially responsible for the treatment given (Eldridge, 1979). Certain issues are sensitive, and children often are unwilling to discuss them with parents. States differ as to when treatment can be given without parental consent. Most states allow minors to obtain treatment for venereal disease and drug abuse and access to birth control without parental consent. Abortion is a more difficult issue, and laws concerning abortion vary by state (Eldridge, 1979). Generally, strict adherence to confidentiality is the rule when children seek treatment for any of the preceding reasons. Recently at issue, however, is whether parents should be informed after the treatment has taken place. Sources differ as to the appropriateness of breaches of confidentiality; however, it is generally accepted that if the physician feels duty-bound to inform parents about treatment, the child should be told before treatment begins (Holder, 1977).

Young children in the care of their parents cannot legally seek medical treatment on their own. Also, if the child is in the care of parents, other adults—such as relatives or school personnel—cannot initiate treatment without parental consent except in emergency situations. A physician who treats a child in a nonemergency situation without consent is liable and can be sued (Holder, 1977).

If a child can be treated without parental consent, that child also has the right to refuse treatment. Young children therefore are subject to the wishes of parents and cannot legally refuse treatment if the parents have requested it (Holder, 1977). It then becomes a nursing challenge to recognize the self-determination rights of children and reconcile them with parental wishes. Creativity in incorporating the wishes of the child and family in all aspects of care will optimize the treatment process.

Children also have rights when decisions are made to include them in research projects. Even very young children can understand explanations about treatments, and it is common practice to enlist their cooperation in their care. When considering whether to include a child in research, decisions need to be made about whether the research will directly benefit the child and whether the research procedure is painful. Generally speaking, parents can give consent for the child to be a research subject in a project that will benefit the child directly, even if that research is invasive. In almost all cases, however, it is preferable to enlist the cooperation of the child. If the research is to benefit society or another individual, the child's right to refuse participation assumes greater importance. This becomes a difficult issue, particularly in organ transplants where the child's refusal to donate could result in later expressions of guilt.

TABLE 1-4 Health Care Legislation Affecting Children

Title	Year	Purpose
Social Security Act	1935	Provide matching state and federal funds to encourage quality care for mothers and children as well as crippled children. Support health promotion (screening, immunizations, and so on)
Maternal Child Health Maternal Infant Care Project	1963	Reduce infant handicaps and complications due to inadequate care of childbearing women. Decrease infant and maternal mortality. Provide diagnostic services and treatment for women for whom care is inaccessible
Children and Youth Project	1965	Meet health needs of children from targeted low-income areas or those for whom care is inaccessible
Medicaid	1965	State aid to low-income families to provide reimbursement for medical care
Crippled Children's Services	1965	Locate, diagnose, and treat handicapped children under 21 years of age
National School Lunch Act and Child Nutrition Act	1966	Provide meals to children from low-income families for free or a reduced price according to income guidelines

NOTE: Most of these programs formerly under the US Department of Health, Education, and Welfare are now administered by Block Grants to the states under the supervision of the US Department of Health and Human Services.

SOURCE: Adapted from Lopata H (editor): *Family Factbook*. Marquis Who's Who, Appendix C, 1978.

Options must be presented carefully, so that the best decision for all can be made (Van Eys, 1978).

In cases where the research is nontherapeutic, such as screening procedures, young children have the right to refuse participation after receiving adequate information (Van Eys, 1978). It should be mentioned that if the children or parents refuse to participate or choose to withdraw from a research study, it cannot affect the quality of care they receive.

Legal Accountability of the Child Health Nurse

All nurses are responsible for maintaining high-quality standards of care regardless of the age of the client. Child health nurses are in a special position because of children's integral relationships with their families. The child health nurse is accountable for care given to the child within the family unit because rarely is a child seen as separate from family. Nurses giving less than high-quality care to the child–family unit are accountable for their actions to all members of the unit.

In addition to practicing high standards of health care, child health nurses must consider the previously mentioned rights of clients in the health care system, most specifically those of confidentiality, privacy, and self-determination. Nurses are responsible for maintaining accurate and descriptive records and for respecting the confidentiality of communications with their clients. In a child health-care setting, respecting privacy and maintaining confidentiality can be difficult. Health professionals differ in their attitudes toward children, some not really accepting the premise that children have the right to privacy. Behaviors such as talking freely about the child's problem with others or examining the child in front of others can become commonplace. Nurses need to be advocates for children's rights under these circumstances and can be held accountable if they are not. Another problem with maintaining confidentiality often occurs in crowded settings. Well-meaning parents will ask questions about other children they see, placing nurses in the position of finding an acceptable method for tactfully avoiding answers that would compromise other patients' privacy.

As discussed previously, children have certain rights of self-determination. Because some children will refuse treatments or medications, nurses need to use acceptable choices creatively in their care to allow the child to maintain control while still accepting necessary care. To force a child to accept a treatment can be construed as assault or battery, and the nurse can be liable for consequences (Cazalas, 1978). The overuse of restraints also is included in this category (Cazalas, 1978). The child health nurse must be certain that restraints are necessary for the protection of the child and others and that the minimum amount of restraint is used.

Nurses also are accountable for reporting certain problems peculiar to children. For example, some communicable diseases (such as venereal disease and salmonella, among others) must be reported to state public health departments. A positive test for phenylketonuria (PKU) also should be reported (Cazalas, 1978).

Most states make it mandatory to report suspected child abuse or neglect (see Chapter 22). The emphasis is on the word suspicion. Nursing personnel must report any case of suspected child abuse to the appropriate agency. In their child abuse laws most states also protect the informant from prosecution if the report is made with a sincere interest in protecting the child from harm (Holter, 1979).

The final legal issue unique to child health nurses concerns the accountability of nurses who assume expanded roles. The increasing numbers of certified nurse practitioners have forced states to reexamine their Nurse Practice Acts to accommodate these expanded roles. There is still an ill-defined overlap in some states between the medical and nursing duties of the nurse practitioner. This has caused different interpretations of legal accountability. It should be emphasized, however, that all nurses are accountable for their actions and are autonomous regarding nursing decisions. As nurse practitioners establish their practice as nurses in an expanded role and not physician extenders, Nurse Practice Acts will adjust accordingly. Meanwhile, it is the mandate of all nurses, regardless of their role, to be familiar with the provisions of the Nurse Practice Acts in their states (Murchison, Nichols, and Hanson, 1978; Nichols, 1980).

Future Directions in Child Health Nursing Care

The future directions of child–family nursing are rooted in its past. Child health nursing as a specialty has affected the entire health care system. Large children's hospitals provide care for critically ill children, whereas the community hospitals manage children with less life-threatening medical conditions. Nursing, regardless of the setting, is becoming increasingly challenging and complex. When caring for children, nurses must view themselves as primary client contacts and demand greater continuity of care. Many facilities still linger in the past, refusing to relax visiting hours and ignoring the fact that primary nursing facilitates the recovery and improved health care of the child–family unit. In their role as child advocates, nurses need to initiate changes and to accept the responsibility and accountability for the future directions of child health care.

Children growing and developing in a fast-paced world must be able to cope with the stresses of everyday living. Child health nurses will assume a more active teaching role in the hospital and community in their contacts with children of all ages. They will teach a variety of concepts designed to assist children and families in developing and using effective coping mechanisms. These concepts will include the following:

1. The importance of self-care activities in becoming responsible for one's own health
2. The interrelationship between mind and body—emotional and physical health
3. The effects of proper diet and exercise
4. The avoidance of health hazards and harmful substances
5. Stress reduction techniques

The emphasis will be on disease prevention. Nurses will be more creative, structuring health teaching to the child's age. They will more actively secure clients, both in a structured setting and as independent practitioners. Nurses will effect changes in health care through consumer education in the same way they have demonstrated the value and cost-effectiveness of health promotion.

In addition to health promotional activities, nurses will expand their role in the early identification of and intervention with high-risk families, particularly those with the potential for child abuse. Early prenatal and postpartum management of teenage mothers and their children will be essential because the incidence of teenage pregnancies is rising dramatically. The greater number of single parents is a consequence of the increasing divorce rate and incidence of unwed mothers. Additional concern is needed for the special needs of single-parent households, both within the community and when a child from this type of family is hospitalized (Barnsteiner, 1976).

Greater attention to the additional needs of children and youth is an important nursing goal. These "unmet needs" were described by an American Nurses' Association special committee in 1979 and include exploration into the problems of child abuse, substance abuse, adolescent sexual behavior, including the incidence of adolescent pregnancy and venereal disease, mental health and suicide, and other more common health problems (Durand, 1979).

Computer Applications in Health Care

Hospitals are entering the computer age, heralding great changes in the delivery of health care. Nurses in large children's medical centers will need to be experienced in handling computers. Computerized medical information will facilitate communication among members of the health care team and may lead to greater mobility and effectiveness of nurses. Children's health records retained in computer data banks will facilitate a continuous monitoring of children's health status. Much more information will be available to the child–family nurse, enabling better care planning. Researchers will have access to lifelong health information, which they will use to identify the positive and negative influences contributing to health and disease. This stored information can vastly improve the continuity of care. Consequently, however, more ethical questions will need to be addressed. Nurses must be aware that the dangers of the computer age are similar to those of the mechanized age: that the uniqueness and humanness of clients will be lost without careful attention to their personal needs.

Advances in Nursing Research

To ensure a future of improved health care for children, advances must take place in the area of nursing research. Nursing research has been conducted for years, but its focus has changed as its quality has improved. Historically, researchers investigated specific nursing procedures, curriculum theory, nurse–client relationships, and hospital management effectiveness (Gortner, 1980). Future research needs to encompass more. It needs to be more comprehensive, examining the holistic approach to health care and consumer involvement in the health care system. Research will contribute to nursing theory.

Studies need to be conducted that evaluate the effectiveness of therapeutic intervention. Nursing's theory base should be defined further by the scientific replication of research (Gortner, 1980). Nurse researchers need to examine children's reactions to stress and the appropriate interventions to set patterns for good health practices and disease prevention. New techniques of nursing practice in nurses' relationships with children and families should be evaluated and their practicality and cost-effectiveness tested.

Faced with an imminent nursing shortage, researchers can discover innovative approaches to increasing job satisfaction and generating new interest in nursing. Perhaps one of the major goals of nursing research should be "nurse advocacy." A definite, methodologic approach is needed to create and retain interest in nursing. If the profession is to survive, concerted efforts must be directed toward this end.

Key Concepts

- In the past 150 years child health care has altered its focus from a strictly curative approach to a holistic approach that encompasses every aspect of health.
- Child health nursing has evolved as a specialty keeping pace with the changes in child health care.
- Over the years statistical data relative to child care have demonstrated a variable birth rate along with a steadily declining infant and child mortality rate.
- The most common cause of childhood death in the United States today is accidents.
- Hospital care in the western hemisphere began in Canada in the mid-seventeenth century.
- Hospitals for children emerged in the mid 1800s.
- Care in early children's hospitals was directed toward controlling communicable disease and alleviating social problems contributing to disease.
- Pediatric nurses were originally child caretakers responsible for feeding the child and maintaining the child's nutritional status, hydration, and hygiene.
- The end of the nineteenth and beginning of the twentieth centuries saw increased opportunities for women and therefore for nurses.
- Nurse registration was initiated in 1903, and it, along with the founding of professional organizations for nurses, helped to provide quality control and development of nursing standards.
- Hospital nursing in the early years of the twentieth century became less patient-oriented and more task-oriented, although the foundations for nursing research were laid at this time.
- Nursing in neighborhood health centers in the early 1900s was autonomous and contributed to the shift in emphasis toward health promotion and disease prevention.
- After World War II, health care advances, such as the discovery of the polio vaccine and studies examining effects of hospitalization on children, assisted with the change in focus from curative to preventive child health care.
- New approaches to the delivery of health care to children in the 1960s included less restrictive hospital visiting hours, establishment of the pediatric nurse practitioner role, and the increased emphasis on play as a tool of child health nursing.
- Child health nurses gained greater autonomy in their practice in the 1970s as a result of improved communication techniques, increasing concern with holistic health care, and the emergence of their role as child advocates.
- The child health nurse of the present may function autonomously in a variety of roles in both the community and the hospital, including the expanded roles of clinical specialist and nurse practitioner.
- Children in this society hold certain basic and legal rights, which child health nurses are responsible to protect.
- Child health nurses are accountable for their actions and have a responsibility to maintain high-quality standards of care regardless of the age of the child.

continued on next page

- Future directions in child health nursing include expanding such activities as promoting self-care within a holistic framework, advocating a clean and healthy environment for children, reducing child and family stress, effecting changes in health care delivery through consumer education, and intervening with high-risk families.

References

Barnsteiner J: Bicentennial forecast—pediatric nursing. *RN* 1976; 39(11):21–32.

Beaver P (editor): A history of Boston Floating Hospital. *Pediatrics* 1957; 19:629–638.

Bowlby J: *Child Care and the Growth of Love*. Penguin Books, 1955.

Burgdorf M: Legal rights of children. *Nurs Clin North Am* 1979; 14:405–416.

Cazalas MW: *Nursing and the Law*. Aspen Systems Corporation, 1978.

Children's Hospital of Philadelphia *The Children's Hospital of Philadelphia in Perspective—1855-1974*. Children's Hospital of Philadelphia, 1974.

Dolan J: *Nursing in Society*. Saunders, 1978.

Durand B: The ANA hearings on the unmet needs of children and youth. *Am J Matern-Child Nursing* (November/December) 1979; 6–8.

Eldridge T: Adolescent health care—the legal and ethical implications. *Pediatr Nurs* 1979; 51–52.

Ford LC: U.S. circa 1976: Change and challenges in nursing education and practice. *Aust Nurses' J* 1976; 5:26–30.

Gortner S: Nursing research: Out of the past and into the present. *Nurs Res* 1980; 29:204–207.

Holder A: *Legal Issues in Pediatrics and Adolescent Medicine*. Wiley, 1977.

Holter J: Child abuse. *Nurs Clin North Am* 1979; 14:417–427.

Igoe J: Changing patterns in school health and school nursing. *Nurs Outlook* 1980; 28:487–488.

International Year of the Child 1979. *Nurs J India* 1978; LXIX:244.

Jamieson E: *Trends in Nursing History*. Saunders, 1966.

Katz G: Mothers help care for sick children in an experimental unit. *Hospitals* 1964; 38:37–42.

Kinsella C: Who is the clinical nurse specialist? *Hospitals* 1973; 47:72.

McCarty E: Description of primary health care needs. In: *Primary Care by Nurses: Sphere of Responsibility and Accountability*. American Nurses' Association, 1977.

Murchison I, Nichols T, and Hanson R: *Legal Accountability in the Nursing Process*. Mosby, 1982.

Nichols A: Physician extenders, the law, and the future. *J Fam Pract* 1980; 11:101–108.

Parks P: Student nurses' attitudes toward children's health rights: Implications for advocacy. *Child Health Care* (Summer) 1982; 11:25–29.

Silver HD: The school nurse practitioner program. JAMA 1971; 216:1332–1334.

Stewart I, Austin A: *A History of Nursing*. Putnam, 1962.

U.S. Department of Health and Human Services: *Monthly Vital Statistics Reports*, August 11 and October 18, 1983.

Van Eys J (editor): *Research on Children*. University Park Press, 1978.

World Health Statistics Annual—1982. World Health Organization, 1982.

Additional Readings

Andrews P, Yankauer A: The pediatric nurse practitioner. *Am J Nurs* 1971; 71:304–308.

Austin P: The primary system for pediatric nursing care. In: *Current Practice in Pediatric Nursing*. Brandt P, Chinn P, Smith ME (editors). Mosby, 1978.

Barton P: Play as a tool of nursing. *Nurs Outlook* 1962; 10:163–164.

Brown MS: Pediatric nurse practitioner: A primary manager of well-child care. *Nurs '76* 1976; 6:70–72.

Chinn P: Activities of daily living for the hospitalized child. In: *Current Practice in Pediatric Nursing*. Brandt P, Chinn P, Smith ME (editors). Mosby, 1978.

Cushing M: Legal lessons on patient teaching. *Am J Nurs* 1984; 84(6):721–722.

Davis A, et al: Ethical dilemmas in nursing research. In: *Communicating Nursing Research*. Vol II: *New Approaches to Communicating Nursing Research*. 1978.

Dietz LD: *History and Modern Nursing*. Davis, 1962.

Erikson F: The need for a specialist in pediatric nursing. *Nurs Forum* 1965; 4:24–31.

Facteau L: Self-care concepts and the care of the hospitalized child. *Nurs Clin North Am* 1980; 15:145–155.

Fagin C: Pediatric rooming-in: Its meaning for the nurse. *Nurs Clin North Am* 1966; 1:83–93.

Ford L: The changing role of the nurse in child health care. *Am J Dis Child* 1974; 127:543–545.

Freeman B, et al: How do nurses expand their roles in well child care? *Am J Nurs* 1972; 72:1866–1871.

Griffin C, Handler F: Bridging services from hospital to home. *Child Today* 1972; 1:30–32.

Hemelt MD, Mackert ME: *Dynamics of Law in Nursing and Health Care*. 2nd ed. Reston, 1982.

Hoskins C: Nursing research: Its direction and future. *Nurs Forum* 1979; 2:175–186.

Hymovich D: The effects of primary nursing care on children's, parents' and nurses' perceptions of the pediatric nursing role. *Nurs Res Rep* 1977; 12:6–7.

Jameton A: *Nursing Practice: The Ethical Issues*. Prentice-Hall, 1984.

Lopata H (editor): *Family Factbook*. Who's Who, 1979.

Moran P: Parents in pediatrics. *Nurs Forum* 1979; 3:24–37.

Mundinger MO: *Autonomy in Nursing*. Aspen Systems Corporation, 1980.

National League for Nursing. *The Realities of Primary Nursing Care: Risks, Roles, Research*. National League for Nursing Publication No. 52-1716, 1978.

Nelms BC, Mullins R: Evolution of holistic practice in nurse practitioners. *Pediat Nurs* 1980; 6:27–31.

Siegel E, Bayson S: A redefinition of the role of the public health nurse in child health supervision. *Am J Public Health* 1963:1015–1023.

Vaughan B: Role fusion, diffusion, and confusion. *Nurs Clin North Am* 1973; 8(4):703–713.

Yankauer A, et al: The practice of nursing in pediatric offices—challenge and opportunity. *N Eng J Med* 1970; 15:843–847.

Nursing Process for Child Health

2

Sandra R. Mott

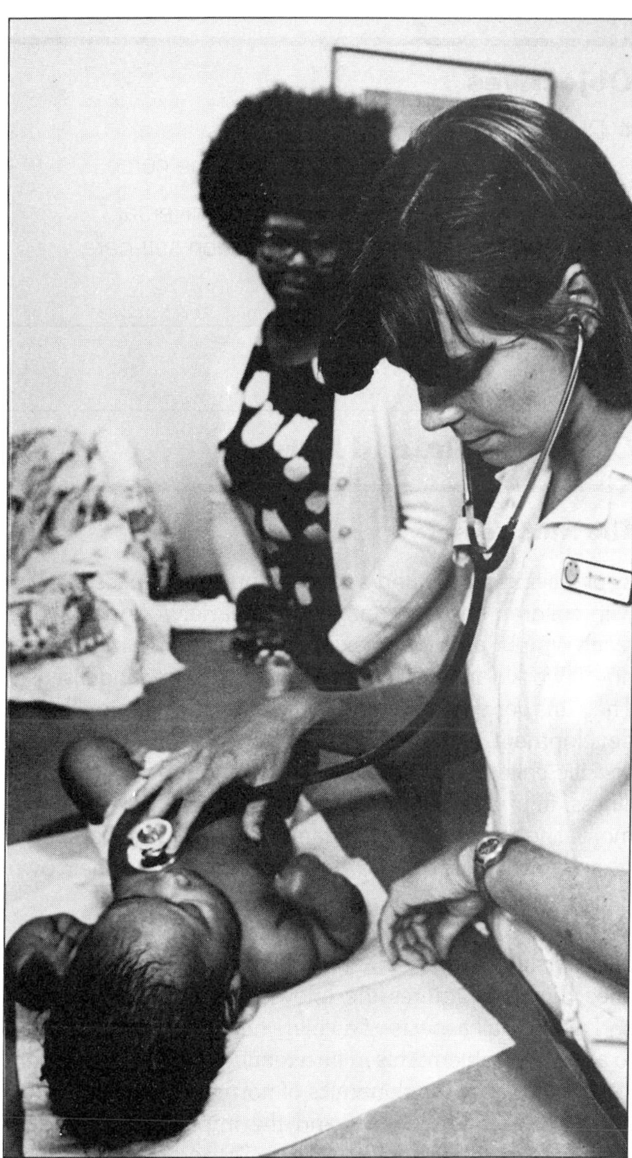

Chapter Outline

continued on next page

Objectives

- Discuss the relationship between system, suprasystem, and subsystem and the nurse.
- Discuss the relationship between universal, developmental, and health-deviation self-care requisites and the nurse.
- Define the phases of the nursing process—assessment, diagnosis, planning, intervention, and evaluation.
- Describe how nursing theory relates to the nursing process.

Child, Family, and Nurse

The Nurse's Role

In practicing the art and science of nursing, nurses interact with children and their families in a variety of ways. They teach simple and complex facts about the human body, how it works, and how to protect it from injury and disease. They answer questions about the principles of growth and development and how they apply to the problems of a specific child. They provide care during times of a child's illness, injury, or recovery. Nurses also are instrumental in motivating children and their families to take personal charge of and make responsible decisions concerning their own health.

Art and science often are seen as opposites, but in the best nursing care, they are combined creatively. As a science, nursing requires the knowledge and skill to assess and analyze all aspects of a child's health and the response to a health problem; this in turn requires a thorough understanding of both the dynamics of normal physiologic function as the child matures and the impact of pathologic processes on that function in specific body systems. The nurse also must know how normal developmental crises, illness, and injury affect children of different ages and how to identify the resources—both within the child and in the surrounding environment—that can help the child respond in the most effective way to a given health problem.

The art of nursing lies in the skill with which each nurse applies the necessary knowledge anew to each individual child. Just as no two children are alike, so no two children will respond in the same way to a health problem. As much as adults, children respond to events and people in ways that reflect their own personalities, past experiences, growth and developmental levels, cultural heritages, coping patterns, and current states of health. The nurse needs to take these factors into account when adapting the principles and details of nursing care to the unique requirements of each child. The more the nurse knows about each of these factors, the more sensitive, appropriate, and complete the nursing care will be. The essence of the nursing process is to use skillfully all aspects of the art and science of nursing to identify the child's and family's response to a health-related concern and to adapt nursing actions accordingly.

Understanding the Individual Child

Being attentive to the values, beliefs, customs, and rituals of patients is important regardless of age, but in the case of children this attention can present special challenges to the nurse. In addition to bridging the gaps that normally exist between any two adults—language, life-style, education, traditions, and the like—the nurse also must be sensitive to the fact that a child is not a "little adult" but is living through a period of rapid development in all respects: physical, emotional, cognitive, and social. Although nurses often can rely on certain shared assumptions and understanding with other adults simply as a result of having been socialized into the "grown-up" world, a child is in the process of discovering those shared assumptions and achieving an adult understanding.

This process takes place through the child's interaction with the surrounding environment—sending messages or presenting behavior to significant others and obtaining feedback about the appropriateness, expectedness, or adequacy of the behavior or message. The child then interprets this information and either maintains the behavior or communication pattern or adjusts it accordingly. This constant, dynamic, feedback process begins in childhood and continues throughout life, although the environment and the people in it change over time. In an adult, however, such learning generally becomes more consciously selected and disciplined, whereas a child seems to develop simultaneously in many directions with a rapid and undiscriminating abandon that can be wondrous to the observer.

Nurses should therefore be particularly alert to a child's unique characteristics when assessing needs and establishing a therapeutic relationship. For instance, the level of cognitive understanding is a critical factor in the child's response to care. One nurse described the case of a 4-year-old girl who seemed to be unreasonably terrified of vomiting and became upset when it happened. Later it was discovered that she equated this experience with the stuffing falling out of her torn rag doll. Reassurance and a simple explanation to the girl that her body was not made the same way as her rag doll's and about the true cause of vomiting dispelled her fears (Pontious, 1982).

A child's inner abilities and developmental status are part of the resources available to that child. The nurse also will identify additional resources, such as education, prior health care, religion, relatives, friends, socioeconomic status, and community services, that might contribute to the child's response to illness and nursing care. The child might interact with resources from any or all of these areas, which comprise both the immediate environment and society as a whole and which influence the child's interpretation of and response to the events of daily life. Perhaps none of these external factors, however, will be as significant as the support, love, and caring found with the child's own parents and siblings.

Including the Family

Nursing a child always involves that child's family. From birth, a child is continually influenced by the beliefs, values, rituals, traditions, attitudes, and practices of the family. The nurse can thus look to the family for much of the information needed to understand the child accurately. "The family is the transmitter of biological and genetic endowment, and a contributor to the psychological strength or vulnerability of its members. Furthermore, the family shapes social and moral values, whether these values are a function of ethnicity, socioeconomic class, or personal preference" (Miller and Janosik, 1980).

The family is a primary resource for the child. The nurturing and support a family provides can be crucial factors in determining how well a child responds to a health problem and to the nursing care provided. Each member of the family may contribute something to the child's abilities to cope with the health problem, and the strong, supportive interactions of the family as a whole can provide the child with a foundation of security and love, which is an extremely important resource.

On the other hand, the child's health problem and inability to function in the usual or expected manner have definite effects on the other family members, both individually and collectively. Latent problems with family members or family functioning might be brought to the fore by a crisis in the child's health. Such problems, if neglected, might not only impair the family's ability to provide the needed support for the child but could have long-term implications for the family's continued and healthy development.

It is therefore important for the nurse to include the family in the various aspects of nursing management, both by involving the family directly in the decisions and activities of the child's care and by considering the family itself as a client in potential need of nursing care. The charge to nurses in a pediatric setting is thus to focus on all family members while providing direct nursing care for a specific member; to assess the impact of the child's illness on individual family members; to assess also the relationship among and between individual family members; to appreciate and utilize the cultural heritage and values of the family; and to promote the health and growth of the family, both during and after the child's illness and recovery.

Systems Theory: A Pattern for Assessment

Rationale

To achieve the kind of multifaceted nursing care described in the previous section, a conceptual framework is necessary to provide guidance in collecting data about the child and family, categorizing and analyzing that data to arrive at specific nursing actions, and identifying priorities that will result in the most effective nursing care. Then, as information about the child, family, home, and environment is gathered, it is not just a collection of so many interesting facts but can be organized into an effective plan for translating theory into action. Such a framework is an important tool for achieving holistic nursing care.

The framework developed in this text to understand the variety of influences in a child's life is adapted from general *systems theory*. The rationale for choosing this theory is its logic, inclusiveness, and adaptability to the nursing process. General systems theory was first described by Ludwig von Bertalanffy as a theoretical, conceptual approach to facilitate the understanding of interactions between observed entities (von Bertalanffy, 1968). The key to systems theory is the focus on the interrelatedness of the various parts in the working of the whole rather than on the analysis of each part individually.

Systems theory can seem abstract and complex; therefore, it is important to note that the concepts and terminology of general systems theory are not important in and of themselves but only insofar as they assist the understanding of nursing care of children. Systems theory, or any conceptual framework, can be seen as a kind of filing system, which, like alphabetic, numeric, or other filing systems, is merely a way of organizing information in the most useful way to achieve a certain goal. A real estate agent, for example, might file information on the houses for sale alphabetically by the street address; customers might be better served, however, if such information were filed by the house's selling price, size, or location if these are the more useful qualifying features for them.

Nursing care is a much more complex undertaking than selling houses, and the factors involved are very likely more numerous and unpredictable. Nurses do not just need to retrieve information according to what a client wants but also need to synthesize widely diverse kinds of information into the basis for a plan of care. Although a single circumstance, such as infection, denial, or cultural bias, may be similar in one child to what the nurse has encountered in other children, its combination with other circumstances may create a situation that the nurse has never encountered before, every child being unique.

If a particular circumstance or fact is not placed in a framework along with other facts, its implications for nursing care may not become clear. Moreover, it may not become truly useful unless it is placed appropriately within the framework. For instance, the problem of the girl who was terrified of vomiting might easily have been classified as an affective disorder because the visible evidence was obviously a strong emotion. A plan of care prematurely based on the assumption of an emotional problem might have led in useless and even harmful directions for the child, whereas locating the root of the girl's distress in a problem of cognitive functioning led to a more appropriate resolution.

Overview

Systems theory describes the interaction of an entity with other entities and of an entity with its component parts. The entity in question is called a *system,* which is defined as a developing, responsive, nonstatic unit made up of interdependent components. A system is distinguishable from what is external to it and from its own component parts.

That which is external to the system, its surrounding environment, is organized into *suprasystems,* or larger, enveloping systems that interact with the system in question and provide a context for it. If the system in question is a child, the suprasystems can be either immediate and intimate, such as family, extended family, school, or friends, or they may be more distant, impersonal entities such as the community, ethnic group, governmental agencies, or the nation (see Figure 2-1A).

The component parts of a system are called *subsystems,* which are simply smaller internal systems that, through their interaction and interrelation, make up and define the system. If a school is the system being studied, two examples of its subsystems would be the faculty and the students. If the system under discussion is the human body, the circulatory system is an important subsystem. Subsystems and suprasystems are systems in their own right, and attention also can be focused on them, their component parts, and their surrounding environment. Between each system and another is a *boundary,* which keeps each system separate from the others and helps to establish its unique identity. Across that boundary an exchange of matter, information, or energy takes place that constitutes all interaction between systems. Between the family system and the economic suprasystem money and goods are exchanged; between the school system and the student subsystem information is exchanged; and between the human body system and the digestive system food and energy are exchanged. The boundary is thus permeable, and the system regulates its various exchanges by controlling that permeability. All living systems permit such exchanges across their boundaries and are thus considered *open systems.*

The different aspects of the exchange between one system and another are categorized as input, output, and feedback. *Input* is simply the matter, information, or energy that goes into a system, and *output* is that which comes out. In a factory system what goes in are raw materials and what comes out are finished goods. In a human being inputs such as food, information, and supportive nursing care can result, respectively, in outputs such as energy, skill, and adaptive coping strategies.

Feedback is a process that allows the system to regulate itself by receiving and responding to reactions to its own output. The system can then modify its output (for instance, its behavior), or it can change the way it selects its input. For example, a company that discovered it was producing too much of an item could cut back on its production; a child who learned that hitting a friend usually results in being hit back might alter the hitting behavior or might wish to change friends.

The structure of a system is the arrangement or organization of its components, whereas its function consists of the purposes, actions, and results of actions that the system undertakes to promote its own continued existence and growth. In the human body anatomy would be the structure and physiology would be the function. In the family system the structure would be the members of the family and their interrelationships, whereas the function would include the activities that promote the family's well-being and growth such as employment of the parents, education of the children, and recreational activities.

Equilibrium, or steady state, is a balance of the components of a system. There is no one ideal state of balance for any individual, or system; rather, the balance changes as the goals and needs of the system change. This factor distinguishes open systems from closed systems. *Closed systems* do not allow for change and development within the systems model (Stevens, 1984). An open system model is the only position possible when dealing with living people—

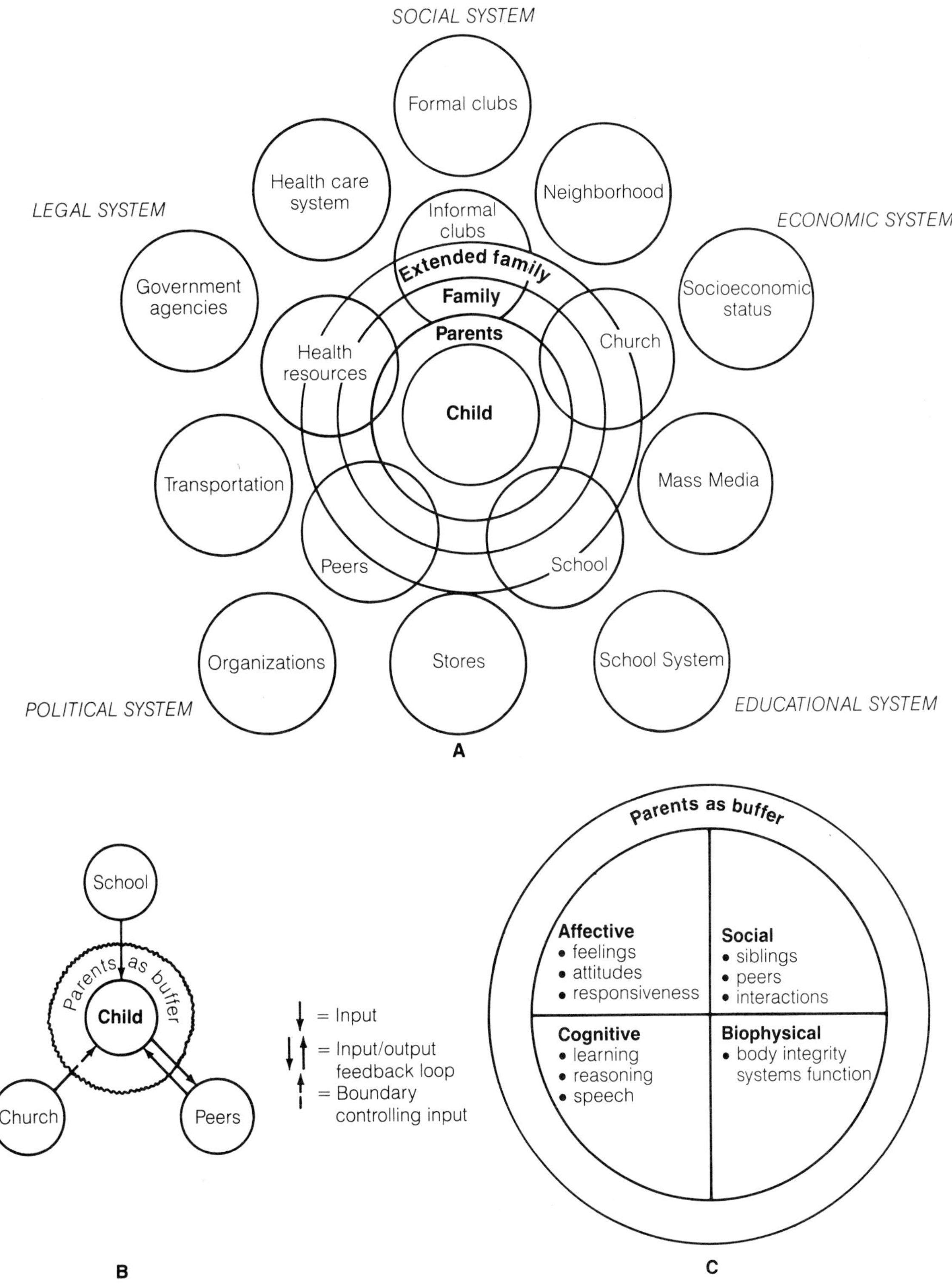

Figure 2-1 Using general systems theory to view the child and family. *A.* The child, viewed as a system, interacts with the surrounding suprasystems. Because of different degrees of distance from the child, interaction between the child and the suprasystems may be direct or indirect. *B.* Parents serve as a buffer during the developmental years. The parent–child unit form a boundary that regulates input from the environment. Input from environment may come from sources of information, such as school, or from feedback in response to output from the system, as in the peer–child feedback loop. *C.* The child's four basic subsystems (internal structure of the system) that combine to define the child's unique characteristics.

Definitions of Systems Theory Terminology

System An interacting unit made up of interdependent parts that endure over time, such as the legal system, the human being, and the respiratory system

Suprasystem Suprasystems are the larger, external environments of which the system is a part. These environments interact with the system in a process of give and take

Subsystem Subsystems are the smaller, internal, interacting components of the system that define the system

Structure The arrangement of component parts, that is, the system, suprasystems, and subsystems

Function Function of the system includes the purposes and goals manifested by the activities necessary to assure the survival, continuity, and growth of the system

Degree of openness The degree of openness of a system refers to the extent of interaction or energy exchange with the surrounding environment (suprasystems). An open system is characterized as one in which there is an exchange of information between the environment and the system. All living systems are open

Boundary Each system is surrounded by a discrete boundary that separates it from other systems within the environment. The boundary, however, is porous, thus permitting a constant exchange of information or energy between the system and its environment. The system regulates this exchange and maintains stability by selecting input from the environment and output to the environment

Input Information or energy that the environment gives to the system for processing

Output Information or energy that the system gives to the environment as a result of processing. The behavior of the system

Feedback The process that allows the system to be self-directing. Feedback involves receiving and responding to input resulting from the system's own output

Equilibrium The balance among component parts—a balanced relationship of parts that is not dependent on any fixed point or level

Stressors Any stimulus that produces stress

Stress Any response to a stressor that thwarts, frustrates, or creates obstacles to maintaining equilibrium. Any demand on the system, whether social, developmental, cultural, or physiologic, that requires response.

or, indeed, with any truly open system. The state of emotional balance that exists between child and parents, for instance, clearly will be redefined if those parents divorce. The divorce would put *stress* on the emotional relationship of the child and the parents (and would therefore be identified as the *stressor*), stress in this example being defined as the state of disturbance within the system caused by an external change. Illness, such as gastroenteritis, places stress directly on the internal systems of digestion and metabolism and thus alters the equilibrium among all of the body's systems as they respond to this change in function. In this example the disturbance within the system results from an internal change.

Application

Child as System Because any system can be the focus of attention or study, other systems can be identified as subsystems or suprasystems in relation to it. For the purposes of this text, however, it obviously makes sense to center on the child as the system around which the framework is constructed, as shown in Figure 2-1. In this scheme the parents and family are not shown as simply another suprasystem, along with peers, school, and church, but as a much more intimate and important "buffering" system around the child (Fig. 2-1B). As such, the family can constitute part of the boundary between the child and the other suprasystems and may permit direct, unmediated interactions, as with friends and peers, or may select, edit, and interpret input according to its own traditions and values, as might happen with the child's interaction with the church.

As an infant, the child is dependent on the parents to supply basic needs and to make decisions. With growth and maturity, the child becomes increasingly independent and able to make personal decisions. Because parents generally select, interpret, reinforce, and explain the social and environmental influences on the child until the child is able to do so personally, the older child's decisions usually will reflect those previously made by the parents. This is why the nurse needs to understand the parents and the parent–child interaction to understand each individual child.

Spheres of Influence—Suprasystems Beyond the child and family, the suprasystems of the surrounding environment act as spheres of influence. Suprasystems themselves can be seen as part of still larger systems and so on in an ever-expanding hierarchy that ends with the view of the whole world as a single system.

The kinds of interaction between the system and suprasystems vary according to the situation. As mentioned previously, some interactions are mediated by the parents, whereas in other forms of interaction the child is a direct participant. Some suprasystem interactions, such as those with peers, may be more conducive to output from the child than others because the opportunities for interaction are removed from direct parental supervision.

A system is not uniformly receptive to all input from the suprasystems. The system decides the type and amount of input that it is willing to incorporate. A simple example would be the child who is full and stops eating. One can view the boundary that admits some input and not others as the means by which the system selects what is acceptable. The parents may be an important part of this boundary in infancy and early childhood, but as children grow older, their own beliefs and values—whether derived directly from parents or not—tend to play an increasingly significant role in deciding what input is beneficial to their own growth, development, and functioning; that is, they tend to take charge of their own boundary. Thus, the system—whether child or child within the family—attributes relative significance to the various suprasystems in the environment. For example, religion and the values of an ethnic culture may be of paramount significance to one family, whereas another family may place more value on material comfort and social status.

The nurse who hopes to deliver appropriate and comprehensive care to the child and family will therefore need to identify their suprasystems, observing and analyzing the interactions that take place between them and the suprasystems, and evaluating which suprasystems are significant to them and might be used to support the goals of nursing care.

Internal Characteristics—Subsystems Another key concept of systems theory is that different components constitute the system. For the purposes of this text, these components are identified as areas of growth and development, the biophysical, cognitive, affective, and social subsystems (Fig. 2-1C). A more detailed analysis might also define personality and moral subsystems as areas of growth and development (see Chapters 7-11). The attributes of the child are the result of the combined functioning of these four subsystems. These areas, or subsystems, are useful in categorizing, defining, and describing the main aspects of growth and development that characterize each child. Growth and development is a continual process, with each subsystem interacting with the others to give each child a unique personality. When the child is healthy and development is progressing smoothly, steady growth occurs in all areas. If, however, illness creates dysfunction within the biophysical subsystem, the other three subsystems and the system or child as a whole are affected. Each subsystem in its own way attempts to offset the dysfunction of another subsystem by employing coping or compensating behaviors.

For example, bacteria invade a child's oral pharyngeal area, causing a sore, inflamed throat and other signs and symptoms of illness (stress on the biophysical subsystem). The white blood cells increase in number to wall off and ingest the bacteria, and fever develops in response to the inflammation (response of the biophysical subsystem). The pain being specific, the child limits swallowing to protect the sore throat but also restricts talking and alters eating habits and other activities (effects on the social subsystem).

Other subsystems also are affected as they attempt to compensate for the biophysical system dysfunction. The cognitive subsystem tries to interpret or rationalize the reason for these changes and resulting discomfort; it may try to find ways to reduce the discomfort by using past experiences or employing new ideas or suggestions. The affective subsystem may use such behaviors as sadness, irritability, patience, or courage as coping strategies to deal with the miserable feelings caused by the illness. The social subsystem may withdraw from play and peer interaction and reach out to others, perhaps the parents, for help and comfort. The behavior of the individual system when ill is thus the result of the combined responses of these subsystems. The biophysical subsystem dysfunction causes a "system disturbance rather than the loss of a single function" (Abbey, 1970).

The amount of compensatory energy from within the subsystems available to the child is an important determinant in the recovery process. If the child has one or more concurrent chronic or acute dysfunctions in any of the other subsystems, there may not be sufficient energy within the system as a whole to deal with the new threat. Subsystem composition is discussed in depth in Chapters 6–11.

Systems Theory in Nursing Care

The framework of systems theory provides a guide for assessing and analyzing the individual system. Using the framework helps the nurse to avoid making generalizations and incorrect assumptions and to arrive at correct interpretations of the behavior and communication of the child and parents. The framework also can serve as a reminder of the categories of data that need to be gathered and analyzed before the appropriate nursing goals can be formulated. The following example shows how failure to gather adequate data and to analyze it systematically resulted in thwarted nursing care goals.

A child recovering from a bacterial infection was being treated with an antibiotic, which was to be administered in specific doses over a period of time. The nurse gave careful instructions to the mother concerning the importance of the antibiotic, how and when to give it to the child, and where to store it. Five days later the child returned to the hospital with the same presenting symptoms. The nurse who had discharged them initially found out that the antibiotic had not been administered after the first day. Although it turned out that the bottle had fallen and broken, the nurse still felt frustrated that the careful explanations and instructions had been ignored and that the family had waited so long to try to obtain more medicine. Further probing revealed knowledge deficits on both sides.

The child was from a working-class family whose finances were adequate for basic necessities but little else. It was January, and the family had spent too much during Christmas and had no extra money. The father, who played the dominant role and made all the decisions in this family, believed that health was simply being well enough to do one's job, that modern medicine was ineffective, that doctors prescribed medicine simply for profit, and that his own mother's folk remedies were more beneficial. The child's mother, although she provided all of the child care, was submissive and always followed her husband's instructions. The family was very religious and believed in prayer and faith-healing.

When the bottle broke and all the medicine was lost, the parents could not afford to buy more, and, because the symptoms had abated as a result of the initial doses, the father did not think it important to continue with the medicine. When the symptoms returned, the family prayed and administered some of the grandmother's home remedies. The father refused to seek professional help, however, because he felt the medicine had failed to cure the child, which seemed to reinforce his lack of faith in health professionals. Only when the child's temperature remained high, her symptoms and irritability increased, and all food was refused did he consent to take her back to the health care provider.

The nurse realized that the father's role as decision maker and his personal biases had not been properly identified. Had the father's role and the parents' belief and values been incorporated into the initial nursing care plan, the following concerns would have been addressed: the father's authority and need for teaching, the scientific rationale as to why the medicine was necessary even after the fever subsided, incorporation of the family's religious beliefs, the use of the antibiotic in conjunction with the home remedies, and the financial needs resulting from the child's illness.

Using a systems framework, the nurse could have assessed and analyzed these factors and created an individualized care plan that promoted not only recovery for the child but also understanding for the parents and growth for the family as a whole.

Self-Care: A Goal for Intervention

Overview

The concept of function is included in systems theory. Because function refers to the purpose and activities of the system, a thorough explanation of function is important to understanding the system (child). A theory relevant for this purpose is Dorothea Orem's theory of self-care (1980). Her description of universal self-care requisites, developmental requisites, and health-deviation requisites also can be referred to as the functions of the system.

Her theory also is uniquely nursing in focus and easily expands to include the child and the family and health maintenance as well as health deviation. In Orem's theory, the person, whether it be the individual as self-care agent (person taking action) or the parent as child-care agent, assumes the role of decision maker about the activities to pursue to maintain health and promote growth and development. "Self-care is a practical response to an experienced demand to attend to oneself. . . . The demand as experienced is a stimulus to which the person responds in some manner" (Orem, 1980). Thus, the parents' awareness of their own or their children's universal, developmental, or health-related needs prompts action. The nurse's role is to "assist individuals in the exercise of their rights and responsibilities regarding health care for themselves and dependent others" (McIntyre, 1980). Putting this in a holistic context, the nurse responds to each situation according to the expressed needs for assistance, information, or support to promote health as perceived by the individual.

Universal Self-Care Requisites

An individual's means of satisfying the universal *self-care requisites* identified by Orem also could be termed activities of daily living, for they are behaviors basic to human existence, functioning, and development. This is also an area where nursing has a special interest because it emphasizes the themes of health maintenance, health promotion, and disease prevention. In performing routine activities of daily living, the child initiates self-care activity. "Ways of determining and meeting one's self-care needs are not inborn . . . the activities of self-care are learned according to the beliefs, habits, and practices that characterize the cultural way of life of the group to which the individual belongs" (Orem, 1980). It is in the area of self-care that nurses have

Key Terms in Orem's Theory of Self-Care

Self-care Activities performed on one's own behalf to maintain life, health, and well-being and to promote growth

Universal self-care requisites Actions required by the individual to sustain and maintain the personal structure and function of the human body

Developmental self-care requisites Actions required to support the normal process of growth and development or specialized processes associated with conditions resulting from inadequate environment, health, or support

Health-deviation self-care requisites Actions that exist for those who are ill, injured, or being treated for acute or chronic health-related conditions

Therapeutic self-care demands Performance of self-care behaviors that result in effective fulfillment of self-care requisites as defined and prescribed by the individual

the opportunity to teach the principles of health and to assist children and families to identify and utilize their resources for obtaining health. The nurse, however, needs to understand the interplay between the inputs from the environment (suprasystems) and the individual system before commencing any plan of management. Before introducing new ideas or suggesting changes in self-care activities, the nurse must assess whether this change would upset the balance of the system.

According to Hollen, "health is choice" (Hollen, 1981). Individuals have their own definitions of health and make their own decisions about seeking health information or assistance. Health is a subjective state of wellness. If health is a choice, nursing plays an important role in preparing children and families to make that choice. Their sharing of information and example should emphasize the decision-making process, including the analysis of the components involved, the results of possible options, and the influence of culturally transmitted values and beliefs. "Health implies the fullest possible utilization of life experiences. It is total functioning in the physical-mental-social-spiritual dimensions (i.e., the holistic inference). All of these dimensions are directly related to the capacity of the individual in a dynamic process of interaction. This interaction involves both the external environment and the internal, genetically based one" (Hollen, 1981).

"Self-care action is practical in orientation. Performing a self-care measure involves a decision, a choice" (Orem, 1980). The eight subcategories of universal self-care requisites defined by Orem and discussed in the following sections represent those areas required by all individuals throughout the life span. Choices made within each of these subcategories are based on the assumption that individuals have an inherent desire to promote their own health and make choices accordingly, choices that are based on the ideas and ideals of their cultural traditions, beliefs, and socioeconomic resources (Fig. 2-2).

Intake of Air Air refers to the essential exchange of gases in the lungs and within the cells. The need for air includes the adequacy of respirations, the mechanical process of inspiration and expiration, as well as the capacity of the alveoli to exchange carbon dioxide and oxygen. It includes the quality of the air being breathed, its oxygen content, the partial pressure under which it is being breathed, and the presence of pollutants. It also includes the body's ability to use the oxygen to metabolize hemoglobin. This demand for air alerts the body that more oxygen is needed as a result of increased metabolism due to exercise, digestion, or stress or the result of an inadequate supply of oxygen in the air being breathed. Self-care is the therapeutic response to this demand. It would include behaviors such as avoiding an area contaminated by a high concentration of pollutants in the air, minimizing activity in high altitudes, or resting after running until one's usual respiratory rate is restored.

Intake of Water Water is essential for life. The sensation of thirst is the means by which the body is alerted to its need for additional fluid intake. The body responds to both internal and external conditions and attempts to maintain fluid balance by stimulating or depressing the thirst sensation. Demands for fluid vary considerably from day to day depending on activity and the amount of insensible fluid lost via increased respirations and perspiration; thermal conditions and fluid lost by perspiration when internal and external temperatures rise; and dietary intake and increased demands from salty foods or those foods that encourage diuresis. The positive response to thirst, the appropriate intake of fluid, is therapeutic self-care.

Intake of Food The consumption of food is also essential to life and health. Food is necessary for growth and the repair of body tissue. The body is alerted to its need for food through the sensation of hunger. The appropriate response to hunger, eating, is therapeutic self-care. This means the intake of nutritious food in a well-balanced diet. Understanding food values; the daily requirements of protein, carbohydrates, fats, vitamins, and minerals; and food metabolism is an essential part of self-care.

Self-care activities in providing for each of the above three essential ingredients begins at birth. The neonate cries

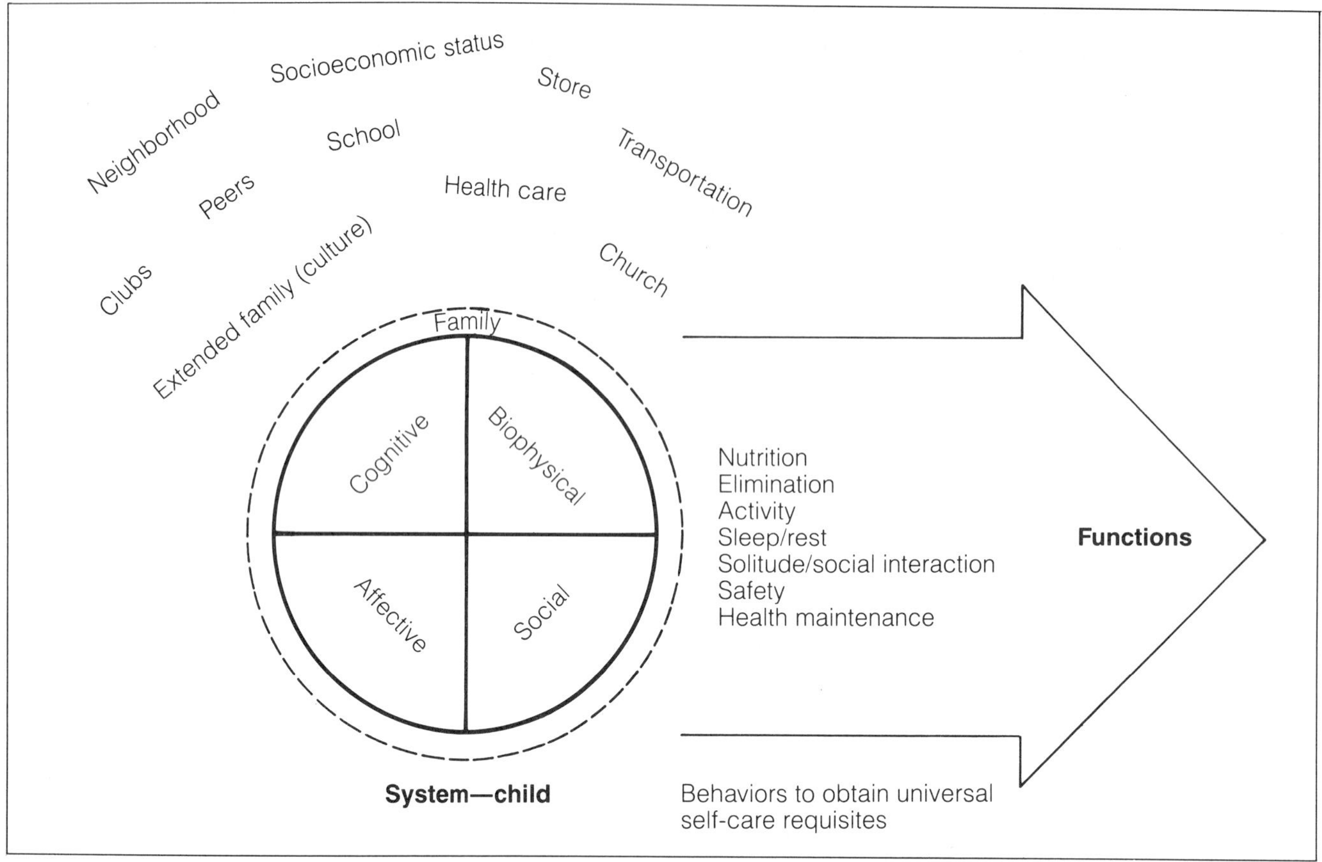

Figure 2-2 Structure and function of the system that describes a child. Structure refers to the subsystems and suprasystems and their contributions. Function refers to the child's behaviors, or activities of daily living, which characterize the child's interactions.

to let the caregiver know that sensations of thirst or hunger are present. Reflexes alert the neonate to a lack of oxygen, and appropriate responses such as yawning, crying, or rapid breathing follow. As the infant grows and develops, self-care activities change. With maturation comes an increased physical ability to provide for some of these needs. The transmission of culturally approved methods, rituals, and behaviors also influences how one responds to these needs. How well one is able to meet these requisites depends on the knowledge and understanding one has concerning the importance of the quality and quantity of air, fluids, and foods; the means by which each of these is metabolized in the body, resulting in its normal integrated functioning; and the approved methods of consumption. During the time that the child is gaining this knowledge, the parents assist and either provide the necessary relief or teach and guide the child in obtaining personal relief. The parents are vital to the child's learning because through them the ideas and ideals of the cultural, religious, and ethnic groups are interpreted. The parents also initially provide for these requisites and begin teaching the child by example and by making certain types of foods and fluids available. These guidelines are then internalized and used by the child when making choices. Children need the opportunity gradually to assume increased responsibility for their choices and eventually become their own self-care provider.

Elimination Products that are the end result of metabolism and those for which the body has no further need are eliminated. These include urine, feces, perspiration, menstrual flow, and seminal fluid. For the infant, voiding and defecation are involuntary behaviors that are done to relieve discomfort. As growth and development progress, the child learns that voluntary control is socially preferred, that there are appropriate places and conditions for elimination, and that subsequent hygiene is an essential component of elimination.

Self-care behaviors are both personal and social. With additional knowledge and understanding of the physiologic process of elimination and of the broader aspects of health and health maintenance, the individual learns to take responsibility for the care of the environment as well as the rights and responsibilities of others in the practice of personal self-care. Community health concerns also need to be included. The proper disposal of excrements, maintenance of sewage and sanitation facilities, and removal of related health hazards, such as vermin, are necessary to prevent the spread of disease.

Activity and Rest Activity may be defined as the expenditure of physical, psychologic, or intellectual energy. It includes such activities as walking, skating, running, playing games, studying, calculating, and expressing emotions. Rest is a change from one type of activity to another that results in refreshment or restoration of energy. The individual needs a balance of rest and activity for optimal health.

The activity-rest pattern of the infant is achieved partially by the infant's ability to habituate. (*Habituation* is an infant's ability to reduce or eliminate a response to stimulus following repeated or continuous exposure to it). The overstimulated infant also becomes irritable, thus indicating a need for rest and change. Sensitive parents respond to this signal and provide their infant with a restful atmosphere.

Children are not always as well tuned in to their bodies' needs. They would rather respond to the urgings of their peers to continue an activity even when they are fatigued. Long hours of intense studying tax one's intellectual energies. Rest in this situation may be a good swim. Intense emotional states of fear or anger are also energy depleting and need to be followed by a change that will restore balance and allow rest.

Responding to the body's need for rest or activity is not automatic. At times, external demands conflict with internal needs such as the child who, although exhausted, remains in the game at the request of friends. Parents initially supervise the activity and rest needs of the child. The parents interpret their child's behaviors that signal a need for an activity change. They prescribe the child's activity change, be it reading a story, taking a nap, or playing alone quietly. As the child grows, parents continue to supervise such things as bedtime, the number and type of extracurricular activities allowed, and the time for homework. Gradually, the child learns to assume responsibility for balancing activity and rest. The examples and rationale provided by parents set the tone for this decision-making process. Therapeutic self-care for this requisite is the process of making choices and decisions concerning when and how energy is expended and restored.

Self-care in this area includes "(a) Selecting activities that stimulate, engage, and keep in balance physical movement, affective responses, intellectual effort, and social interactions; (b) Recognizing and attending to manifestations of needs for rest and for activity; (c) Using personal capacities, interests, and values as well as culturally prescribed norms as bases for development of a rest-activity pattern" (Orem, 1980).

Solitude and Social Interaction This requisite, like that of activity and rest, involves complementary activities. The dynamics of being alone or being with others contribute to healthy development. The child needs contacts with a variety of other people, both adults and children. An important aspect of socialization is this exchange and interchange with others. Through contact with a variety of adults, children learn about their environment, about people, and the types of jobs significant to the daily maintenance of order and the provision of goods and services. Children also learn how to share, express themselves, and cooperate by interacting with both adults and peers. Peer activities also help children cope with the demands of life as they act out and participate in real or imagined situations through play.

Children also need time alone: time to regroup their emotions and thoughts, daydream, and think. Wise parents provide children with quiet times, encourage them to think about their feelings and attitudes, and reflect with them about the beliefs, values, traditions, and rituals that are part of their heritage.

Self-care for this need is a process of making choices, of learning how to balance the necessities for solitude and social contact. Achieving this balance is important for one's mental health and includes attaining a realistic self-concept, respecting the individuality of others, establishing meaningful friendships, and developing personal talents. Therapeutic self-care for this demand is a lifelong process with its roots in the initial parental care of the infant and thereafter in the fostering of the child's sense of autonomy and identity.

Safety Safety includes all aspects of preventing hazards such as acute disease and accidents. Self-care in this area involves the ability to protect oneself, maintain human integrity, and promote normal function and development. It means making the necessary decisions and taking the appropriate actions that will either prevent encountering hazardous events or protect oneself from uncontrolled hazards.

The infant is cared for, sheltered, and protected by the parents. As growth and development progress, the child gradually becomes more responsible for personal health habits and the observance of safety rules. The parents' role evolves from protector to educator as they teach their children the various dimensions of staying healthy. Such behaviors as personal hygiene; the avoidance of known infectious agents; car, bike, pedestrian, and water safety; and self-control are included in therapeutic self-care. The child who learns to think before acting, to take the time to assess the situation and consequences rather than "show off" to peers, is practicing self-care. The more knowledgeable the child, the fewer the chances that a careless behavior will be performed. For the well-informed child, some health habits become second-nature such as washing the hands before eating or not using someone else's glass or toothbrush. Healthy living requires practice and the opportunity to make responsible choices.

Being Normal Being normal includes being physically and mentally healthy. What is considered normal or preferred is culturally relative and interpreted differently based on each group's beliefs and values. In many ways this requisite influences the behaviors of some of the other areas. If being normal is being slender, physically active, intelligent, productive, and socially popular, this will determine the quantity and quality of food consumed, the type and amount of activity in which the child or adolescent engages, and the ratio of time spent in groups to that spent in solitude. The norms to which one is compared or to which individuals compare themselves are those that are accepted and interpreted to them by family, peers, and other authorities.

The maintenance of health would include such activities as following a recommended schedule of physical and dental examinations, keeping immunizations up to date, and practicing good personal hygiene.

Developmental Self-Care Requisites

Developmental requisites are specific self-care behaviors associated with the different developmental stages. These behaviors are particularly important for children, whose growth, development, and maturation are continually progressing to higher levels of achievement with resultant changes in perspective and abilities. These changes relate to the type of self-care actions parents and children take for health maintenance and the prevention of illness. "Because self-care is a developmental process, the nurse explores data that provides a basis from which predictions about capabilities and limitations can be made. Nurses need to know what children are doing, thinking, feeling, and understanding to evaluate and teach self-care skills" (Eichelberger, et al., 1980). Thus, evaluating the child's or parents' skills in self-care activities related to developmental requisites includes assessing the growth and developmental status of the child in the areas of physical, cognitive, affective, and social being and the integrated functioning of the whole system.

Biophysical Development Biophysical growth not only means the increase in height and weight but also the attainment of gross and fine motor skills. This increase in strength and coordination is necessary for participation in games, hobbies, and schoolwork. An example would be the progression of fine motor control the child gains in the use of crayons, pencils, and paints and how these are used for school assignments, art projects, and various games. Walking and running are examples of gross motor control, which, combined with the increased length and muscular developmental of the legs, allow for endurance and speed. Developmental theorists have established standards, or norms, that identify approximate ages at which children should accomplish specific skills. Parents and others compare the child's abilities against these standards to determine if the child is normal or developing at the expected rate. This kind of assessment enables those working with the child to plan activities and skills that are within the child's functional capacity.

Cognitive Development Cognitive development involves the process of learning. The child accumulates information about the environment and uses it to gather additional knowledge. The child's ability to learn is related to genetic endowment, as well as to opportunities to explore, manipulate objects, experiment, and create. The acquisition of concepts and their use in systematic thinking and problem solving is a means of assessing the child's cognitive abilities. The learning process of the young child initially is very basic (for example, throwing objects repetitively to identify which ones bounce and which do not). As the child's repertoire of knowledge expands, so does the ability to manipulate this information in the process of problem solving. The child's thinking advances along a continuum beginning with reflexive and sensory experiences and advancing to magical explanations for events, which then are replaced by actual experiments to explain cause-and-effect relationships and finally by thinking and problem solving in hypothetic terms.

Cognitive development begins at birth and continues throughout life. Learning experiences may be planned and carefully organized, such as school, music lessons, or teaching/learning situations, or they may be informal and self-initiated such as exploring the environment, either alone or in a group. The use of language to communicate is another cognitive skill. The child initially uses language to proclaim a need or make a request. As cognitive growth proceeds, language becomes the medium for expressing ideas, opinions, and rationales for the solutions to problems.

Developmental theorists have devised norms by which cognitive development may be assessed. These norms include measurements of the child's understanding and use of language, concepts, and operations. These standards are helpful in identifying the child's level of development and adapting interactions and expectations accordingly.

Affective Development A third area of development is the affective, which may be defined as development of the ego and *self-concept.* Self-concept is the way in which a person perceives others' views of that person's looks and actions (see Chapter 6 for a discussion of theories that address affective development.) Children who feel good about themselves, who eagerly participate in activities to the best of their ability, and who know their strengths and limitations have achieved a realistic sense of their personal identity. Achieving this state means that the previous developmental tasks and psychosocial crises have been resolved positively. It means that the child, supported adequately by parents and significant others, has established a sense of trust, which became the foundation for further growth. Trust is essential as the child begins to interact with people and the environment. As the young child experiments with newly learned skills of locomotion and verbalization, a beginning sense of identity is achieved.

The support the child receives and the manner in which this new sense of identity is used in areas of power and control are related to affective development. The nature of the child's experiences with disappointment, fear, frustration, or aggression (and the guidance the child is given regarding the appropriate expression of emotions) provides some of the means by which the child gains a positive self-concept. The presence of an empathetic listener who encourages self-expression, admits to having had similar experiences and emotions, or suggests alternative responses also helps to foster a positive self-concept. When children are helped to think positively about themselves and what they do and when they are praised for being good, for obeying, or following directions, healthy growth is fostered in this area. Children for whom obedience is expected and no recognition given have insufficient feedback to develop a positive self-concept, especially if strong negative recognition is given for all disobedient acts. The ability of children to achieve their goals (and eventually their ability to achieve their goals as adults) is related to their self-concept. The person who was thwarted as a child and made to feel incapable of success finds it difficult to take the necessary risks to achieve a goal. The fear of failure and the inability to rise above the fear become inhibiting factors that prevent goal realization.

The child's affective development is related to opportunities to interact with the environment. From these interactions and the whole process of maturation, the child gradually acquires a sense of personal identity. This identity influences future interactions by selecting what the child will respond to and what form that response will take. Some guidelines have been developed for assessing ego development, notably the application of the theories of Erik Erikson (see Chapter 6).

Social Development Social development is the child's ability to interact with others in ways that are considered appropriate by the society or culture; it is the ability to get along with others. This includes behavior with peers, as well as interactions with adults. Whether the child is in a formal situation, such as school, or an informal situation, such as neighborhood play, there is a prescribed code of conduct that is to be followed. This code of conduct reflects the ethical principles of the particular society.

Social development is learned through experience, imitation, parental guidance, and instruction as the child's actions and reactions become tempered and adapted to the expectations of others and the individual's self-identity. It evolves from the very simple, instinctive responses of the infant to the highly complex responses of adults, who consider the possible consequences of several behaviors before deciding how to respond. Learning to express one's feelings responsibly is part of social development, as are learning to respect the rights and feelings of others, to respect the work and belongings of others, and to respect and care for the environment and natural resources that are everyone's collective property.

Standards for social development are difficult to define precisely because they are interpreted arbitrarily. Even within a given culture, a wide range of different expectations are placed on the growing child. One aspect of behavior that demonstrates growth, however, is the child's ability to adapt to the expectations of a particular situation. This adaptation includes internalizing appropriate manners and actions and an attitude of respect for and sensitivity to others, which combine to guide social interactions. This adaptive capacity can be used by others to measure the child's growth and by the child to increase the ability to get along with agemates and adults in various settings.

Health-Deviation Self-Care Requisites

There are times when the self-care activities of the child or parental caretaking activities have to be altered because of disease or injury. The extent of this alteration is related to the severity or complexity of the health deviation or its management. Some situations are relatively minor, such as a head cold, and the child and/or parent have the knowledge and experience to cope. When this is the case, adjustments are made to meet the requisites of self-care activities until the disease or injury is healed and health is restored. At other times, the health deviation might exceed the parent and/or child's knowledge, experience, or ability to handle, and the child might need to become a receiver of health care.

According to Orem (1980), self-care is limited to the activities the individual initiates and performs to maintain and promote health and well-being. It does not encompass the more liberal definition of self-care, which includes self-diagnosis or self-treatment. Self-care requisites for health deviation then implies "a personal awareness of the factors involved in one's [or one's children's] health, which are many, and a personal 'ownership' of the right and responsibility to manipulate those factors in a manner congruent with personal values and beliefs" (McIntyre, 1980). The child and parents are assisted to assume a decision-making role in matters of health and activities of daily living, and they likewise have the right and, with assistance, the ability to assume the same role in decisions concerning the actions to be taken in events of injury or illness.

Health deviation results in subtle or obvious changes in the child's appearance, functioning ability, and/or feelings of well-being. The nature of the deviation may be corrected quickly, with few if any aftereffects, or a prolonged healing time may be required with many episodes of pain and disability. "The characteristics of health deviations as processes extending over time determine the kinds of care demands that individuals experience as they live with the effects of pathological or abnormal processes and live through the duration of the process" (Orem, 1980).

When an illness or injury is beyond their ability to manage, parents seek assistance from health care professionals. They exercise self-care in assuming responsibility and deciding whose advice to seek. Medical diagnostic tests and treatments may necessitate changes in behavior and limit freedom of choice such as having to take medication or change dietary habits. Surgical procedures usually result in pain, limitation of mobility, an intentional wound, and a temporary or permanent change in appearance with resultant modifications in self-concept. Some medical treatments require either permanent or temporary changes in activity to bring about the desired results.

The nature of the treatment determines in part the role of the child or parents. Some treatments exceed their abilities and require the skill and knowledge of professionals such as surgical interventions and intensive medical and nursing management. Many other treatments or procedures can benefit from the child's and/or parents' participation, either as active participants or as informants about preferences and dislikes.

Certain changes in routine self-care or child-care activities can result from illness, injury, or its treatment. These changes may require minimal adjustments and be easily worked into the daily routine, or they may require major alterations and revisions of the child's and family's routines. The nature and extent of change are related to the ability and support the child and parents have (1) to adapt to new ways of meeting universal and developmental self-care requisites; (2) to establish new techniques of self-care; (3) to modify expectations and self-image; (4) to revise the routines of daily living; (5) to develop a new life-style compatible with the health deviation; and (6) to cope with the effects of the health deviation or its medical management.

Decision and Control in Self-Care

Deliberate Action Self-care infers that the child or parent takes an active role in the decision-making process and then follows through with behaviors that are directed toward achieving the desired goal or end result. According to social learning theory, individuals use several criteria to make decisions. The first criterion is the value placed on the outcome and the importance attached to a positive outcome. Second, the present situation is appraised for its potential successful resolution by comparing it with similar past events and situations. This generalization of past events, experiences, and expectations influences how individuals perceive present and future situations. Third, the results of previous experiences and reinforcements of behaviors provide guidance and help to define the potential result of the current decision. "Deliberate action is essentially action to achieve a foreseen result that is preceded by investigation, reflection, and judgment to appraise the situation and by a thoughtful, deliberate choice of what should be done" (Orem, 1980).

Making Decisions Decision making is a learning experience that begins during childhood and continues throughout adulthood. This experience helps to advance the child from depending on parents as child-care agents to independence as a self-care agent. The child becomes aware of the meaning, significance, and/or insignificance of events from experiences, from observing role models, and from education. "Children learn responsible self-care when they are allowed to choose from alternatives, take action, and evaluate consequences" (Eichelberger, et al., 1980). This doesn't mean that the child's decision will always be the best one. It does, however, afford the child the opportunity to interact with guidelines, limits, information, and observed behaviors; to make a choice; and then experience and evaluate the results.

Parents initially select situations for the child's learning that correspond to the child's growth and developmental level, awareness level, and ability to comprehend the alternatives. For example, the child may be given the opportunity to choose whether to finish lunch before returning to play, with the condition that there are no snacks, only water, for those who don't finish lunch. If this child recently decided not to finish lunch and experienced intense hunger at midafternoon that wasn't relieved until supper, the past event probably would influence this current decision. During this learning phase, it is important for parents to help children evaluate and learn from their experiences. These experiences give them a valuable resource on which to draw for future decisions.

Coupled with experience is the need for awareness. Parents and nurses have a responsibility to provide children with information about their bodies, how they grow and function, and the roles food, rest, exercise, sleep, and social interaction play in being healthy. Approached developmentally, the parents assess the child's readiness, interests, goals, and abilities and direct teaching accordingly. It is ineffective to teach a 4-year-old the importance of eating a well-balanced diet and how to select foods from the basic four food groups. The information is too complex, and the child developmentally is operating on an egocentric level; therefore, when given a choice, the child will select favorite foods regardless of what food groups they represent.

Often parents and other role models wish that the proverbial statement, "Do as I say and not as I do" had greater effectiveness than it does. Children imitate actions more than words. They look to parents and other family members, friends, and significant people as role models—as demonstrators of self-care behaviors. The actions and responses children observe tend to be the ones they choose when the decision-making responsibility is theirs.

Decisions are made as a result of assessing and evaluating the many factors relevant to the situation and the individual's self-image. The choices made reflect the individual's awareness, experience, and role models at the time. Self-care judgments are not static but change along with the growth, maturity, and resources of the individual. Illness, fatigue, stress, anxiety, or inexperience affect the individual's ability to make a decision because they interfere with the ability to concentrate or evaluate. At these times, help or guidance may be necessary for the person's safety.

Taking Action Action refers to the behaviors that result from the decision; essentially, action is the follow-through, or enactment, of the decision. The actions continue until the demands of the decision are met. "Deliberate action is always self-initiated, self-directed, and controlled in regard to presenting conditions and circumstances" (Orem, 1980).

The ability to act on a decision, however, requires the knowledge and skills necessary to perform the action; the motivation and commitment to continue acting until the desired results are accomplished; and the available energy, health, and mental well-being required to initiate action, assign it appropriate priority, and evaluate its success.

Just as making decisions is a learning experience, so too is taking action. An increase or advancement in knowledge and skill comes from education, experience, and developmental maturity. The ability to initiate and sustain action to achieve a desired result requires insight and perseverance, both of which are gained from growth and development in all four areas—cognitive, affective, social, and physical development.

Learning and performing the behaviors necessary for self-care and maintaining one's health require both knowledge and experience. As the child learns self-care behaviors, the parents' ability to provide opportunities to perform these skills and their ability to give guidance and support during these experiences are vital to the child's sense of accomplishment and acquisition of knowledge necessary to guide future self-care actions. The combination of knowledge and experience applied to the performance of specific self-care behaviors usually results in positive reinforcement and continuation of the behaviors.

Any deficit in experience, knowledge, or ability will affect performance adversely. It might result in the parent or child identifying the need for education, practice, or experience in a certain area followed by the active seeking of appropriate resources to meet the need. Assistance might be needed to overcome the deficit and accomplish the desired behavior. When the deficit is related to the individual's health status, nursing might be of assistance.

Self-care therefore is the result of making decisions to meet universal, developmental, and health-deviation self-care needs and of taking appropriate action based on the decisions made. The human system, be it the child or child–parent unit, and the nurse interact around self-care issues in several ways. The interaction may be primarily one of education, support, various degrees of assistance, or a combination of these factors.

Modes of Promoting Self-Care

Each individual within a family thinks, acts, feels, and responds to health-related events in a particular manner because of previous experiences and relationships and the continuous feedback process between environment (suprasystems) and self (system). The goal of nursing then is to assist each family member to attain the highest level of health possible according to personal definition, perspective, or ability. Systems theory focuses on the environment and its contributions to the child's and parents' characteristics, whereas Orem's self-care theory focuses on the unique internal attributes of the child–parent unit. The environment and child–parent unit form a functional whole that determines the manner and method in which self-care requisites are met.

The nurse interacts with the child and family in three major ways: "(a) helping people to make decisions about health; (b) substituting [providing] for health-seeking behaviors when necessary; and (c) helping people to promote, maintain, and restore health behaviors" (Lunney, 1982). In most situations the nursing action is some combination of the three methods. The nurse's intention in giving assistance is to interact with empathy to foster trust and encourage growth. One positive outcome of nursing intervention is an increase in the knowledge, skill, and coping mechanisms in health-related matters, so that parents and children can continue to provide for their self-care, including self-care behaviors related to health deviation.

The concept of preventive health care is a useful means of combining the ideas of health, disease (alterations to health), and health care. There are three levels of preventive health care.

Primary Level of Prevention Nursing activities at the *primary level of prevention* are directed toward the prevention or elimination of stressors that cause illness or injury to the system. Giving information that enhances the self-care abilities of the child, adolescent, or child–parent unit is an important activity of nursing. At this level, the nursing care plan focuses on increasing the child's responsibility for self-care and decision making. The parents and nurse help the child to identify which activities are beneficial and which are not. "Guidelines and limits must be provided by either parents or nurses to protect children from irresponsible actions, yet allow them the opportunity to practice and experience increasing independence in self-care" (Eichelberger, et al., 1980). Before an individual can become independent and achieve total self-care, education and practice concerning the ways and means of providing such care is needed.

Sharing information about health and health-related activities should be a vital part of the child's annual physical examination. In this way children can be encouraged to help themselves stay healthy and to begin habits of good nutrition, rest, and exercise early. Details of self-care related to illness and injury prevention are discussed in Chapters 18, 19, and 20.

At the primary prevention level, the nurse uses the data from the physical, nutritional, growth and developmental, and activities of daily living assessments to identify areas where additional information is needed, where additional resources are required to strengthen the child's resistance to stressors, or where coping behaviors need to be expanded. The nurse evaluates the methods being practiced to meet universal and developmental self-care requisites for their therapeutic qualities within the cultural context.

Some self-care measures related to infant and child care, such as swaddling, feeding, group care, or isolation, are effective and therapeutic for that culture. Outsiders' attempts to change these practices usually result in harm rather than help. Orem (1980) cautioned nurses functioning at this level to distinguish between behaviors that are different and those that are ineffective or do not promote general well-being. Potential problems or misunderstandings can be avoided if together the child and/or parent discuss with the nurse the meaning of identified stressors and previous experiences and mutually decide on goals to increase self-care abilities.

Secondary Level of Prevention The majority of nurses function within the *secondary level of prevention.* This is the area of acute care—the consequences of a stressor invading the system and creating disequilibrium, thus necessitating health-deviation self-care measures. At this level, the nurse temporarily takes over or assists the child or the parent to perform certain functions.

If the dysfunction is minor, the nurse may be able to teach the necessary adaptations in the activities of daily living that will support recovery. Many other times, however, the dysfunction or perception of the dysfunction prevents or limits self-care ability. The child and parent require assistance from someone else. The nurse provides treatment and care until the child once again regains the previous state of health.

"Nursing, then, is a helping or assisting service to persons who are wholly or partly dependent . . . nursing is the complex ability to accomplish or to contribute to the accomplishment of the person's usual or therapeutic self-care by compensating for or aiding in overcoming the conditions or disabilities . . ." (Orem, 1980). Although the activity is one of doing for, the nursing care plan is oriented toward the return of the system's ability to perform the usual activities of daily living. The nurse also aims to make the experience as beneficial as possible and to motivate the system to an even higher state of health as a result of the compensatory, supportive, and educative interactions. Principles of nursing interactions at the secondary level are described in Chapter 29.

Tertiary Level of Prevention The *tertiary level of prevention* is frequently described as rehabilitation. At this level, the nurse assists the child and/or family to modify the usual methods of functioning to compensate for a chronic dysfunction. The nursing emphasis is to promote the adaptation of self-care activities to enable the child to be as independent as possible. The interaction between the nurse and individual focuses on ways to use internal and external resources in new combinations to offset those areas that are not fully functional. The goal at this level is to achieve a "dynamic state of adaptation to [chronic] stressors in the internal and external environment, integrating all factors for optimum use of total resources" (Neuman, 1974). When this is accomplished, the child is able to be as actively involved as possible in performing self-care and maintaining a reasonable, adaptive level of functioning. Nursing interactions for children with chronic conditions are further explained in Chapter 30.

The ultimate goal of nursing is the same regardless of the level at which the interactions occur: the health and well-being of the child. To this end, nursing provides the assistance needed for the child or child–parent unit to function to their fullest capacity. Because the child has various developmental limitations, depending on age and experience, it is necessary for the parents to be an integral part of the nursing care plan and, at times, the focus of the care plan. A plan of care at the primary, secondary, or tertiary level that involves the child, the parents, and the nurse as active participants and is adapted to the significant environmental and societal influencing factors, as well as focusing on the child's ability to perform activities of daily living, supports the child's acquisition of insight and understanding about health, its maintenance, and its restoration. Before this goal can be achieved, the nurse must first understand the individual, the organization or structure of subsystems and suprasystems, and the characteristics of the system's functions, including self-care abilities and deficits and the availability and flow of energy to maintain or restore equilibrium.

The Nursing Process: Systems and Self-Care

When the concepts of self-care and systems theory are synthesized with the nursing process, the end result is a conceptual tool that will promote a systematic, holistic, and comprehensive approach to nursing care. The nursing process has been defined as "a problem-identification and problem-solving approach to client care. It is the basis for a helping relationship characterized by knowledge, reason, and caring. Structurally, the nursing process is adapted from the scientific approach to solving problems" (Gordon, 1982). The five phases of the nursing process are assessment, nursing diagnosis, planning, intervention, and evaluation.

Although the words "process" and "phase" may imply a linear progression, it should be emphasized that each step activity is itself an ongoing process and very often will be carried out concurrently with the others (Fig. 2-3). For instance, when performing a specific intervention, such as teaching the parent the skills to treat a child's illness at home, the nurse also might be evaluating the parent's understanding of the disease process itself (the goal of a prior intervention) and gathering data (assessing) on potential problems that might affect compliance with the therapy at home. The use of a systems perspective, with its focus on interrelatedness and feedback, can promote a dynamic understanding of the nursing process itself—where input is the assessment information; output is the use of this information in formulating the nursing diagnosis, planning, and intervention; and feedback provides evaluation of the output, which results in reassessment, revision, or continuation of the nursing plan.

Assessment

The *assessment,* or data collection and analysis phase of the nursing process, is the most obvious application of systems theory. The nurse continually gathers factual information about the child, both formally and informally. The following is an approach to gathering data for making a holistic assessment of the child–parent unit:

- Introduction
  - Brief health history
  - Current health needs
- Subsystems (growth and development)
  - Biophysical (physical examination)
  - Cognitive
  - Affective
  - Social
- Suprasystems (environment)
  - Family (immediate and extended)
  - Culture (language, traditions)
  - Religion
  - Peers
  - Clubs, hobbies, organizations
  - Socioeconomic status
  - Community
  - Housing
  - Play space
  - School
- System Functions (activities of daily living—self-care)
  - Nutrition (food and fluids)
  - Elimination
  - Activity
  - Solitude and social interaction
  - Rest and sleep
  - Safety
  - Health maintenance
    - Hygiene
    - Physical check-ups
    - Immunizations
    - Dental care
  - Health deviation
    - Response to alteration in function
    - Response to treatment

For this activity to be meaningful and result in a coherent approach to the child and parent, a systematic method of obtaining and organizing the data is needed. Because assessment should be holistic, the dynamic framework supplied by systems theory offers a better alternative than would a narrower, more static framework.

Data Collection Using a systems theory framework, then, a nurse would assess the child with reference to the relevant subsystems and suprasystems. For example, the nurse would assess the biophysical subsystem for the child's ability to perform appropriate gross and fine motor skills. Other parameters, such as height, weight, anatomic proportions and functions, and physiologic functioning and intactness, as well as general health status, also would be assessed. (Physical assessment methods and parameters are discussed in Chapter 14.)

The cognitive subsystem would be assessed for the child's acquisition of knowledge, logical thinking, and ability to learn related to the developmental level. Information also would be obtained concerning the child's adaptability to change, ability to cope with stress and challenge, or any dysfunction such as delays, regressions, or disabilities in using and processing information. (Chapter 6 describes developmental theories, and specific developmental characteristics are discussed in Chapters 7–11.)

Data from the affective subsystem will convey to the nurse either the steady growth and development of the child's personality coupled with positive feelings of identity and selfhood or a dislike of self that may include feelings of anger and dissatisfaction with the self's abilities and identity (see Chapters 6–11).

Finally, from assessing the social subsystem, the nurse will learn about such characteristics as the child's ability to interact with others, preference for peers or adults as companions, and the contribution of social interaction on the child's growth in the affective and cognitive subsystems.

Whichever subsystem is being assessed, both assets and deficits are identified, as well as the actual or potential contribution each subsystem can make to offset deficits in another subsystem, thereby maintaining equilibrium in the system as a whole.

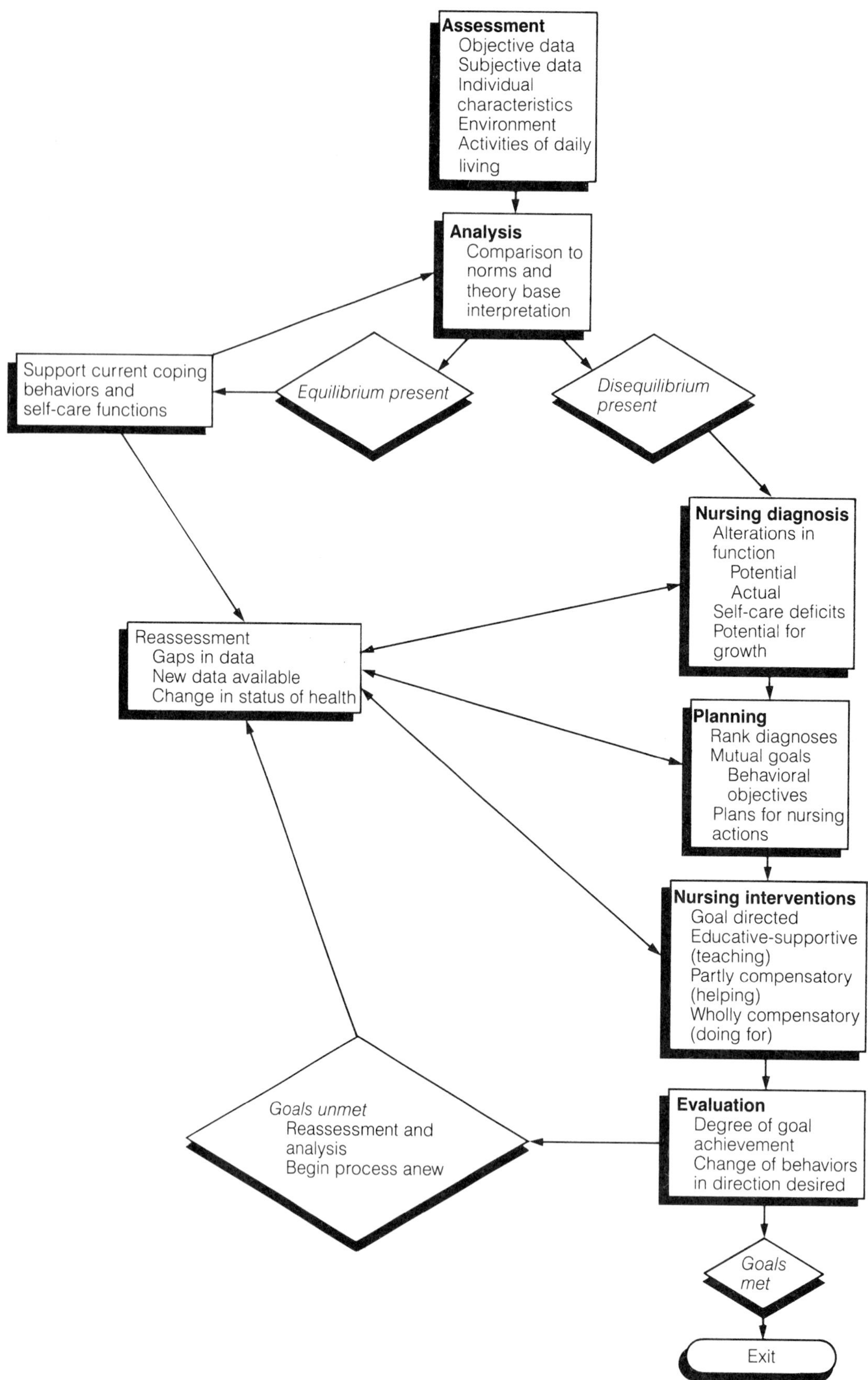

Figure 2-3 The interrelated phases of the nursing process.

Equally important is information gathered about the suprasystems, especially the parents, their roles, parenting style, and process of interacting with the child and with each other. The core of assessment data is further amplified by data from the other suprasystems. Additional information such as religion—type, use, and importance to the individual and family; culture, including nationality, language spoken at home, traditions, rituals, beliefs, folklores, and definition of health; extended family members—their presence, influence, support, and relation to the child and family; socioeconomic status, living conditions, and financial concerns and priorities; and the hierarchy of values for both the child and the family, especially the place of health in that hierarchy, can be valuable. It is essential, then, that the nurse have a working knowledge of, or an available resource that describes, the important beliefs and traditions of the various religions, cultures, and socioeconomic groups. The nurse also must have a theoretic knowledge of family roles and dynamics that can be applied to specific families.

One way of observing the child's use of internal and external resources is to assess behavior related to the activities of daily living. It is in the individual's performance of these basic functions—Orem's universal and developmental self-care demands—that characteristic choices and behaviors are demonstrated (see Fig. 2-2).

The nurse uses all available methods in collecting data, including observation, communication, inspection, palpation, auscultation, percussion, and laboratory results. The sources of these data include the child, family, friends, environment, health records, and other members of the health care team. Whatever the source or method, the cooperation and trust of the child or family is important because to be valuable, the information must be accurate.

The nurse also is careful to gather both subjective and objective data and, in particular, to take into account the client's own perception of the data as determined by personal values, cognitive abilities, or cultural background. "It is vitally important for each health care professional to recognize not only what areas need to be included in the data base but also to recognize that the approach to gathering data must be one that is congruent with the culture of the patient" (Paxton, Ramirez, and Walloch, 1976). The nurse learns from the child or significant others how facts are perceived and what they mean to those involved and tries to answer the following questions:

1. What are the child's or family's attitudes, perceptions, values, or beliefs about health?

2. What are the significant influences from culture, socioeconomic status, education, or past experience?

3. Does this particular encounter with the health care professional represent a crisis for the child or family?

4. What are the child's and family's typical coping behaviors and available resources?

Analysis Analysis is the cognitive ability, combining inductive and deductive reasoning, that leads from assessment to the nursing diagnosis. It is the act of taking the assessment data, sorting them according to a conceptual framework, comparing them with accepted norms, identifying areas of potential or actual deficit and areas of strength, and, finally, identifying the diagnostic description that best fits the data.

A nurse's analytic and diagnostic skills should develop as experience accumulates and they are based on the theoretic and factual knowledge acquired in the biologic, behavioral, and social sciences. This knowledge base provides the norms against which the nurse can assess variations and their significance. Thus, a broad knowledge base that allows for a holistic view of the individual as an open system within the larger system of the environment, with the capacity to adapt to life's stressors, constitutes the basis for the nurse's analytic interaction with the child (Brodish, 1982).

In performing the task of analysis, the nurse necessarily will be influenced to some extent by personal perceptions, values, attitudes, and expectations. Value, which is an explicit or implicit conception of what is desirable, can subtly influence a nurse's choice of one action from various alternatives, just as it influences a child's and family's choices (Kluckholn, 1951). For this reason, the nurse should be as conscious as possible about personal values and biases to ensure that they are not substituted for those of the child and family (see Chapter 3). If the nurse obtains insufficient data from the various resources during assessment, there is a greater likelihood that gaps will exist and some of the information will be interpreted from a personal perspective rather than from the child's or parent's viewpoint. The perspectives may or may not coincide, but the nurse must be alert to the possibility that there may be a difference.

Nursing Diagnosis

The product of assessment and analysis is the *nursing diagnosis,* the second phase of the nursing process. The nursing diagnosis is a comprehensive summary statement of the actual or potential altered health status or self-care deficits. This statement is the result of the nurse's analysis of the data, identification of patterns of behavior by grouping assessment information, and comparison with relevant theories and expected norms. The summary statement is chosen by referring to the list of accepted nursing diagnoses.

The diagnostic categories are not complete and generally are oriented to adult situations. Sometimes the diagnostic category is too general and needs a modifying statement to make it appropriate for the child. Occasionally, the nurse needs to construct a new diagnosis because of the unique characteristics of the child's health situation. Child–family nurses can contribute to the development and formulation of nursing diagnoses by defining those that are specific for the health status of the developing child and family. One

Accepted Nursing Diagnoses from the Fifth National Conference on the Classification of Nursing Diagnoses

Activity intolerance
Airway clearance, ineffective
Anxiety
Bowel elimination, alteration in, constipation
Bowel elimination, alteration in, diarrhea
Bowel elimination, alteration in, incontinence
Breathing patterns, ineffective
Cardiac output, alteration in, decreased
Comfort, alteration in, pain
Communication, impaired verbal
Coping, ineffective individual
Coping, ineffective family, compromised
Coping, ineffective family, disabling
Coping, family, potential for growth
Diversional activity deficit
Family processes, alteration in
Fear (specify)
Fluid volume deficit, actual
Fluid volume deficit, potential
Fluid volume excess
Gas exchange, impaired
Grieving, anticipatory
Grieving, dysfunctional
Health maintenance, alteration in
Home maintenance management, impaired
Injury, potential for (specify): poisoning, suffocation, trauma
Knowledge deficit (specify)
Mobility, impaired physical
Noncompliance (specify)
Nutrition, alteration in, less than body requirements
Nutrition, alteration in, more than body requirements
Nutrition, alteration in, potential for more than body requirements
Oral mucous membrane, alteration in
Parenting, alteration in, actual
Parenting, alteration in, potential
Powerlessness
Rape-trauma syndrome
Self-care deficit: total, feeding, bathing/hygiene, dressing/grooming, toileting
Self-concept, disturbance in
Sensory perceptual alteration: visual, auditory, kinesthetic, gustatory, tactile, olfactory
Sexual dysfunction
Skin integrity, impairment in, actual
Skin integrity, impairment in, potential
Sleep pattern disturbance
Social isolation
Spiritual distress
Thought processes, alteration in
Tissue perfusion, alteration in: cerebral, cardiopulmonary, renal, gastrointestinal, peripheral
Urinary elimination, alteration in patterns of
Violence, potential for

SOURCE: Kim MJ, McFarland GK, McLane AM: *Classification of Nursing Diagnoses: Proceedings of the Fifth National Conference, St. Louis.* Mosby, 1984.

diagnosis that is encountered frequently, for instance, is developmental delay (see Chapter 16). This general category, then, needs to be individualized by stating the nature of the delay, such as cognitive, biophysical, or a combination of several areas, and by providing relevant assessment criteria. Another example would be parental anxiety or parental fatigue caused by the child's health deviation or its treatment and the resulting change or increased demands placed on the parent.

"The ability to derive nursing diagnoses depends upon identifying the discriminating cues for each diagnosis. Consequently . . . once identified [they] can be utilized . . . in formulating a nursing diagnostic taxonomy" (Matthews and Gaul, 1979). Although, as noted previously, the current taxonomy is incomplete, it still provides a valuable source of categories that have a common meaning and implication for subsequent nursing actions. In addition, "no diagnostic classification scheme is ever complete, owing to increasing knowledge and precision in differentiating various syndromes" (Mallick, 1983).

"Nursing diagnoses are a result of nurses' ability to make an appropriate application of theoretical knowledge to the clinical setting, to interpret, to evaluate, to categorize and to make inferences based upon the utilization of cues" (Matthews and Gaul, 1979). They are an integral part of the nursing process and the means by which nurses communicate with each other concerning the identified health alterations or self-care deficits for which nurses assume responsibility and therapeutic decision making. "Nursing diagnoses provide a method for synthesizing and communicating nurses' observations" (Gordon, 1982).

Price (1980) suggested the following five questions the nurse could ask to validate the nursing diagnosis formulated:

1. Is the data base sufficient, factual, accurate, and conceptually based?
2. Is there a pattern to the data as analyzed?
3. Is the child's or parent's data base consistent with that of the nursing diagnosis?
4. Does the nursing diagnosis correspond to scientific nursing knowledge and clinical experience?
5. Would the majority of other nurses concur with the diagnosis?

Nursing diagnosis is a high-level skill that involves arriving at conclusions based on judgments related to a broad base of empiric and theoretic knowledge from the physical, behavioral, and social sciences. The responsibility to bring about changes through goal-directed nursing interactions is inherent in making a diagnosis. The assembled cluster of cues that enables the nurse to diagnose actual or potential health-related alterations or self-care deficits also gives direction as to the type of assistance required by the individual, so that nursing activities can focus on stated goals.

Nursing diagnoses are distinct from medical diagnoses. Medical diagnoses focus on pathologic processes and the means of cure, whereas nursing diagnoses focus on the child's and/or parent's response to the physical, psychosocial, or cognitive effects of the health deviation or its treatment. (See Table 2-1 for a comparison of other characteristics of the two models.)

The nursing diagnostic statement is comprised of two parts. The first part is the response—the category label corresponding to the pattern of cues as identified from the assessment data. The second part defines the contributing factor as it relates to the response. The following examples are illustrative:

Impaired mobility (response) related to bilateral corrective leg casts (contributing factor)

Potential for poisoning (response) related to developmental stages and presence of lead paint (contributing factors)

Parental anxiety (response) related to anticipation of child's surgery (contributing factor)

Knowledge deficit (response) related to nutritional needs of infant (contributing factor)

Nursing diagnoses are holistic and include responses resulting from the child's interaction with various aspects of the environment (suprasystem) that contribute to disequilibrium. Air pollution created by industrial wastes, for example, may result in an ineffective breathing pattern for the child with asthma. Disequilibrium is related to the interaction between the industrial/economic suprasystem and the child.

TABLE 2-1 Characteristics of Medical and Nursing Diagnoses

Medical diagnosis	Nursing diagnosis
Describes a specific disease process	Describes an individual's response to a disease process, condition, or situation
Is oriented to pathology	Is oriented to the individual
Remains constant throughout the duration of illness	Changes as the patient's responses change
Guides medical management, some of which may be carried out by the nurse	Guides independent nursing care, ie, nursing orders (therapies) and evaluation
Is complementary to the nursing diagnosis	Is complementary to the medical diagnosis
Has a well-developed classification system accepted by the medical profession	Has no universally accepted classification system; such systems are in the process of development

SOURCE: Kozier B, Erb G: *Fundamentals of Nursing*. 2nd ed. Addison-Wesley, 1983.

Deficits related to inability or a lack of knowledge are the contributing factors to diagnostic categories that reflect a disequilibrium between the self-care requisites and the ability to meet them. This area has particular importance for the child–family nurse, whose role often includes teaching, role modeling, and supporting learning behaviors.

Once nursing diagnoses are formulated, the nurse can develop a plan of care that is appropriate, individualized, and promotes health.

Planning

The next phase of the nursing process, planning, is to develop a nursing care plan that will assist the individual to maintain or regain equilibrium. This is a dynamic, goal-oriented process that involves the individual and the nurse. The plan should be specific; should relate to the stated diagnosis; and should reflect the child's and/or parent's participation.

Having the individuals contribute to the plan for their health care management encourages cooperation and the coordination of activities. When the plans are not arbitrarily made but consider the individual's values, ideas, beliefs, and resources, communication is improved and the nursing perspective will be more holistic. The nurse and child and/or parent discuss and agree about the assessment data, its analysis, and the nursing diagnosis. Together they define and set mutual short-term and long-term goals. Goal setting gives direction to the actions of both the nurse and child–parent unit. Decisions are made as to desired outcomes and the means by which to achieve them.

Short-Term and Long-Term Goals Short-term and long-term goals are constructed for each nursing diagnosis. These should be realistic and attainable, as well as mutually agreeable and compatible with the desired result. "Goals are stated in broad terms in order to identify effective criteria for evaluating nursing action. These goals can pertain to rehabilitation, prevention of complications associated with stressors, and/or ability of the client to adapt to these stressors" (Stanton, Paul, and Reeves, 1980).

Short-term goals are specific behaviors or changes in behavior that will enable the child or parent to reach the goal. Short-term goals should be stated as observable and measurable actions or responses that are clearly defined and understood by all. Short-term goals change as some are attained and others identified or as the individual's health status, altered function, or self-care deficit changes. It is necessary therefore that short-term goals be ranked according to priority. The nurse and child or parent determine priorities by considering input from scientific principles, nursing knowledge, past experiences, basic needs, individual perspectives, and the parent's value system. (See the nursing care plan at the end of this chapter for specific examples.)

The active participation by the child and parent in helping to define goals and objectives, determine priorities, request additional information, or be involved in decisions about treatment is an important component of planning. Nurses are learning that power and control cannot be equated with cures and care and that individuals usually are less resistant to therapy and demonstrate less stress and anxiety when they have contributed to the decision. Nurses play a vital role in this area as they establish rapport and learn the child's and/or parent's perceptions and interpretations of health and illness. This is especially true when children are involved, as will be explained in greater detail in Units VII and VIII.

Nursing Care Plan The second aspect of planning is the identification of appropriate nursing actions that will assist the child or parent to reach the objectives and goals and thus resolve the problems necessitating the nursing diagnoses. The planning phase enables the nurse to organize the interventions, so that they are purposeful, thorough, and based on scientific principles. The plan provides direction, so that nurses can utilize their time and energy efficiently and effectively. Together the nurse and child or parent discuss each nursing diagnosis and decide whether (1) no intervention is required at this time; (2) another resource or health team member is more appropriate (for example, social worker for financial concern, minister for spiritual problem); or (3) nursing intervention (assistance, support, teaching) is indicated.

Usually, several nursing interventions are required for each diagnosis. Based on knowledge, previous experience, and scientific principles, the nurse formulates and writes the care plan (nursing orders). "They should describe specific nursing actions that include time and frequency of interventions as well as the date the nursing orders were [written] updated or cancelled (Price, 1980). The written plan serves as a means of communication, so that nursing interventions are consistent, individualized, and goal directed.

The nursing care plan illustrates these phases. It is more thorough and precise than what is practical for actual situations. Its purpose, however, is to demonstrate the thought processes involved in progressing from general information intake to identifying what is pertinent and how it leads to planning for nursing interventions.

Interventions (Implementing the Plan)

Interventions may be thought of as the doing, or action, part of nursing. This action is not routine but is "intellectual, interpersonal, and technical in nature" (Stanton, Paul, and Reeves, 1980). Orem (1980) divided the extent of nursing interventions into three general categories: wholly compensatory, partly compensatory, and supportive-educative.

While performing interventions, the nurse continually evaluates their appropriateness in relation to the individual's abilities and health status. This ongoing assessment guides the nurse in the selection and extent of interventions required by the individual (Table 2-2).

Wholly Compensatory The individual who is totally dependent because of age or health status requires someone else to meet universal, developmental, and health-deviation requisites. The infant requires total care, as does someone who is unconscious or severely ill. In most cases the situation is temporary because as the infant grows and the ill recover, the nurse uses other interventions that begin to involve the individual in self-care. At other times, the ill person does not regain the ability for self-care and requires total care until death.

Partly Compensatory In these situations the nurse and child–parent unit work together to meet universal, developmental, and health-deviation requisites. For example, the child and/or parent provides self-care except for the technical maneuvers necessitated to treat the illness or injury.

The nurse's role varies and is related to "(1) the patient's actual or medically prescribed limitations for ambulation and manipulative activities, (2) the scientific and technical knowledge and skills required, of (3) the patient's psychological readiness to perform or learn to perform specific activities" (Orem, 1980). In the event of illness or injury, the parent and child usually continue as much as possible to maintain the same caregiving and receiving relationship

TABLE 2-2 Extent of Nursing Assistance Required*

	Wholly compensatory	Partly compensatory	Supportive-developmental
Individual	Passive—unable to provide self-care or health related care; may or may not be able to verbalize preferences	Able to meet all or most self-care needs but not health-related or technical care needs; learning new or better ways to meet basic needs	Meets self-care and health-related needs
Nurse	Active—does for or takes care of individual so universal, developmental, and health-related needs are met—supports individual in independent role	Supports and guides individual learning; provides technical care; assists in decision making about health-related concerns; performs care for unmet self-care needs	Teaches, supports, guides individual in decision making related to health
Examples	Infant or young child when parent is absent—unconscious individual; total paralysis; severe, acute, or degenerative illness; major trauma	Mild to moderate acute or chronic illness or injury; growing, developing child learning self-care activities; adaptive behaviors being learned	Primary level care consultation

*The respective assistance in terms of nursing actions according to individual limitations, alterations, or deficits in providing self-care.

SOURCE: Adapted from Orem DE: *Nursing: Concepts of Practice*. McGraw-Hill, 1980.

while the nurse performs and/or teaches the parents about the technical aspects of care necessitated by the child's changed health status. Included in this concept would be the nurse's assessing breath sounds, monitoring or adjusting equipment providing increased humidity, and evaluating the hydration status and adequacy of gas exchange for an infant with a respiratory infection while the parent feeds, changes, comforts, and plays with the infant.

At other times, nursing action is required to assist the parents as they learn to provide for their children's care. Examples of this would be children who have chronic health-deviation conditions occurring from congenital or inherited conditions or acquired as the result of illnesses or injuries. In these situations the nurse initially performs and demonstrates the prescribed care and procedures as they are adapted and individualized to the particular situation. Support and assistance are then provided until the parents are psychologically and technically ready to perform the care.

Supportive-Developmental (Educative) This category of nursing action consists primarily of teaching-learning activities. The participants are capable of providing for their self-care needs but require additional information, guidance, or direction to do so. As nurses interact with parents and children, they continually assess self-care activities, provide direction when change is required, and offer support and anticipatory guidance regarding developmental and safety issues. "Self-care with its goal of promoting health and preventing disease, and its emphasis on patients as active participants and decision makers, requires that nurses assist patients in arriving at informed decisions and in developing behaviors to improve health" (Chang, 1980). It is in this role that nurses assist individuals in decision making. The focus frequently centers on health promotion, with all areas of human functioning being considered. When a health-related question arises, parents seek the advice and counsel of the nurse, whose knowledge, experience, and judgment they respect.

The nurse continues to teach and support to a greater or lesser extent as the child's condition or ability changes but adapts the extent of intervention to meet changing needs. The ideal is for the children and parents to be self-sufficient, well informed, and able to provide their own care or care of their dependent child. Nursing in some respects is like wise parents, who take care of their infants and provide basic necessities during the dependent years but also teach the children how to provide for their own needs and become independent. Knowledgeable and capable, the parents step aside, yet remain available for consultation and additional help if and when needed and requested by the children. So too, nursing adjusts its involvement according to individual need, as illustrated in Figure 2-4.

The nurse assists the individual to utilize internal and external assets to realize maximum health. If there are more deficits than assets, the nurse provides interventions at the needed level until the self-care limitations are overcome or coping behaviors and resources effectively compensate. "Nursing has social, interpersonal, and technological dimensions. Nursing's primary work involves designing, managing, and maintaining . . . therapeutic self-care for individuals unable to manage their own self-care" (Chance, 1982).

Evaluation

Evaluation is a continual part of the nursing process. In evaluating, the nurse determines whether the goals are being met or whether a new approach is indicated. If the results are those desired and change is in the planned direction, the interventions continue as planned. If the results are not

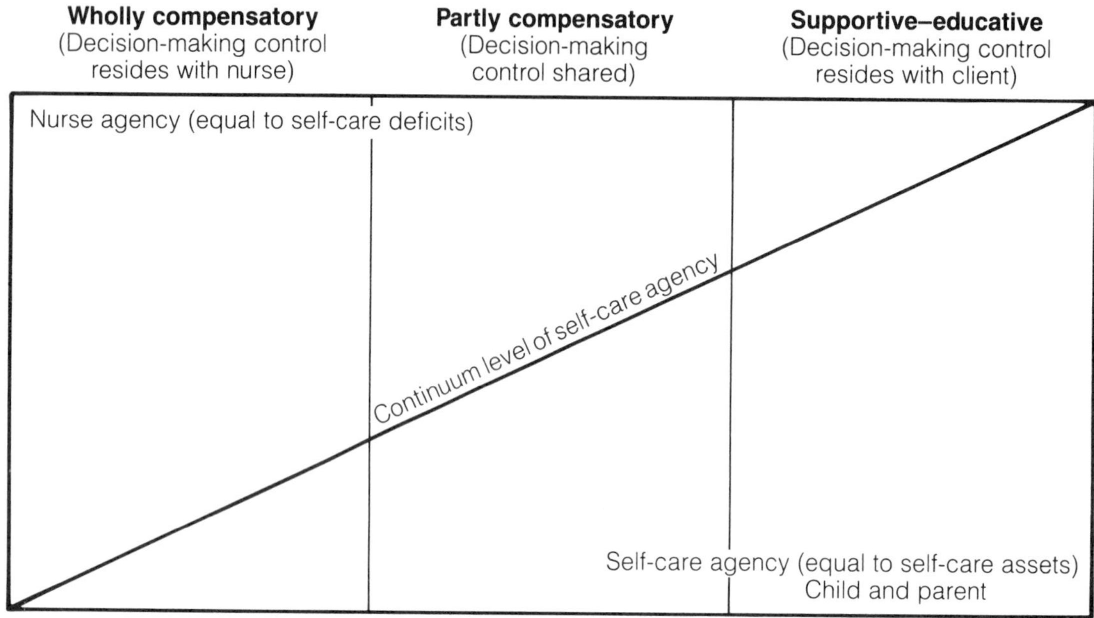

Figure 2-4 Extent of nursing interventions according to the needs presented by child–parent unit for meeting universal, developmental, and health-deviation self-care requisites. (Adapted from Bilitski, JS: Nursing science and the laws of health. *Adv Nurs Sci* 1981; 4(1):23 Reprinted with permission of Aspen Systems Corporation, © 1981.)

those desired, the process is restarted, beginning with a reassessment and concluding with new interventions and further evaluation. Evaluation includes both objective and subjective measurements. The child and parent provide an important means of evaluation as the nurse scrutinizes the care plan and determines whether the child and parent were assisted most effectively in gaining equilibrium or resuming self-care activities.

The overall goal that directs all nursing action is "the individual's need for self-care action and the provision and management of it on a continuous basis in order to sustain life and health, recover from disease or injury, and cope with their effects" (Orem, 1980). Interacting with the child and parent to provide care, the nurse continuously assesses their responses. These responses are compared with the stated objectives to ascertain whether the nursing actions selected are assisting the child and parent to meet the objectives and goals and eventually resolve the nursing diagnoses. The feedback gathered from their responses directs further nursing action.

Evaluation is central to the nursing process because it informs the nurse whether behavioral changes are occurring and whether they are occurring in the desired direction. Table 2-3 summarizes the phases and activities of the nursing process.

Implications of the Framework

The use of this framework requires gathering and integrating a considerable amount of assessment data because the environmental resources, the functioning of the child (human system), and the characteristics of the parent–child interactions are all considered significant. One example of suprasystem input to guide nursing actions would be the school-age child, Tommy, with a chronic disease who tells the nurse that hospitals are sometimes preferable to home because "it's easier." In the hospital everyone is accepting because they know that certain appearances and activity limits are part of the disease. There might even be other children with similar conditions who know what it's really like. At school, on the playground, and in the neighborhood, the other children tease or avoid him because he is different. His family is ambivalent, at times resentful and at other times remorseful because of the time demands of his care. Often, family roles, activities, and finances change as a result of his health status and their interpretation of his disease and resulting limitations. He interacts with all of these environmental inputs plus the internal changes of the subsystems affected by the disease. The influence of these suprasystems are important and contribute to the individual's ability to overcome limits to self-care.

What seemed so simple—instructions or adaptations so easily managed in a supportive atmosphere—became insurmountable obstacles when the environment changed. Tommy found it less stressful in the hospital than at home. He could cope with the disease but not the related changes in peer and family interactions. Had this information been included as a nursing diagnosis at the time of the first hospitalization, much grief could have been avoided. Through puppet or doll play the nurse could have given him ideas about what to say to other children who asked questions or teased him. By consulting with the schoolteachers and

TABLE 2-3 Definitions and Activities Associated with the Nursing Process

Term	Definition	Activities
Nursing process	A series of planned steps or phases directed toward assisting patients and their support persons; the underlying scheme or methodology of nursing practice	
Assessment	Obtaining and organizing essential information about a client	Data collecting History Nursing examination Reviewing records Interviewing Data Analysis Comparing with standard Relating data collected Identifying gaps in information
Nursing diagnosis	A statement about the patient's response to actual or potential health problems and the etiologic and contributing factors	Sorting data Grouping data into patterns Identifying alterations in function or deficits in meeting self-care requisites Comparing patterns to taxonomy of diagnostic categories Identifying response
Plan	A written guide for nursing intervention assisting the client to meet health needs and coordinating the care of nursing staff	Priority setting Goal setting Developing nursing orders Forming a nursing care plan Determining evaluation criteria
Intervention	Putting the nursing care plan into action (wholly compensatory, partly compensatory, or supportive-educative care)	Updating the data base Reviewing the plan with the patient Adjusting the plan as necessary Identifying and providing for safety precautions Determining needs for assistance Intervening as per the plan Analyzing feedback Communicating findings
Evaluation	Assessing the patient's response against predetermined standards	Identifying the appropriate standard Collecting and organizing the data Comparing the data with the criteria Establishing conclusions

SOURCE: Adapted from Kozier B, Erb G: *Fundamentals of Nursing*. 2nd ed. Addison-Wesley, 1983.

discussing the impact of the disease from Tommy's perspective, the nurse could have helped them prepare the other children and talk about some of the "what if" situations and what to do or not to do. A more thorough exploration of community resources as well as the economic situation of the family might have discovered an acceptable form of assistance to lessen the effects of the time and financial stressors on the family.

Nursing diagnoses that are the result of a thorough assessment of the interaction between the child–parent unit and the environment and that include the assets and deficits of each will delineate which of the self-care behaviors in each group (universal, developmental, and health-deviation) require nursing intervention. The interventions of the nurse will then complement the internal and external resources to restore equilibrium by adapting activities of daily living to self-care limitations. This process constitutes a holistic approach that begins with the child and/or parent, progresses to the environment as perceived and utilized by them, and demonstrates the interrelatedness of the two in their interpretation and support of health maintenance and restoration.

The nursing care plan at the end of this chapter is a systematic guide to the collection, analysis, and use of assessment data. This guide enables the nurse to delineate the components and thus analyze their contribution to the whole. Potential or actual problems of disequilibrium and self-care deficits can be identified. Clusters of similar concerns are noted and nursing diagnoses identified. Long-term and short-term goals are stated as child and/or parent behaviors and interventions planned and implemented that are in harmony with their resources, abilities, and needs for nursing assistance. These interventions are evaluated continuously and changed as needed. The criteria for evaluation are the goals and objectives and whether the interventions are assisting the child and parent to meet the long-term and short-term goals.

By using the combined systems and self-care approach within the nursing process, the nurse, child, and parent together think through what is right in each situation. There is no single set of rules or standard care plan. The nurse draws on knowledge, skills, experiences, resources, sense of self-respect, concern, commitment, and flexibility to adapt nursing interventions to the unique requirements of each situation. The common goal is health, which correlates with optimum functioning as defined by the child and/or parent.

What initially seemed like an insurmountable task becomes manageable when the nurse has an organizing framework as a guide. The challenge of adapting nursing intervention to the unique situation of each individual can be likened to setting out on a journey through a forest no one has traveled before. The trees in this particular forest have leaves and branches as do trees in other forests; water flows through the streams as it does elsewhere; and the rocks are as cold and hard as other rocks. Taken all together, however, the shapes, configurations, sounds, smells, and natural pathways of this forest are subtly different from those of any other, and to find the way successfully, the traveler must build on what is known of forests in general, while remaining alert to the peculiar twists and turns of this particular forest.

Likewise, the nurse maps the terrain of the child and family, gathering data about the subsystems, suprasystems, and system functions, and in so doing defines the nursing role. The nurse identifies the best ways to give assistance. This is then communicated to others—the map is passed on—so that continuity can be maintained. Once the paths are defined, that is, once the nursing diagnoses and goals are stated, the journey becomes manageable and familiar as the nurse, child, and parent travel together toward the goal of health.

In the chapters that follow, and especially those in Unit VIII, detailed consideration will be given to the nursing diagnoses, interventions, and evaluations appropriate to specific alterations in human functioning and the performance of activities of daily living.

Key Concepts

- The best nursing care creatively combines science and art: science as the knowledge of human biology, pathophysiology, and psychology, and art as the creative and specific application of this knowledge to the health care needs of each individual child and family.
- The nurse involves the family in the decisions and activities of the child's care, and considers the family itself as a client in potential need of care.
- General systems theory can be considered a framework for the collection and analysis of assessment data because it focuses on the interrelatedness of the various parts in the working of the whole.
- A *system* is a non-static unit, composed of component *subsystems*, and enveloped by the *suprasystems* of its environment.
- Across the boundaries between systems exchanges of matter, information, or energy take place. These exchanges are categorized as *input, output,* and *feedback*.
- Looking at the child as a system, the nurse sees the family as a suprasystem of crucial significance, acting as an important "buffering" system around the child and therefore as part of the boundary between the child and other systems.
- The attributes of the child are the result of the combined functioning of the four component subsystems: the biophysical, cognitive, affective, and social domains of growth and development.
- Orem's theory of self-care can be used to describe the functions of the child as system, and therefore to identify appropriate goals for health maintenance and restoration.

- Nursing has an important role in preparing children and families to make choices with regard to health. These choices can be categorized into the eight universal self-care requisites defined by Orem.
- For the child, whose rapid rate of maturation is one of the most important characteristics, the nurse's assessment of the growth and development status with respect to physical, cognitive, affective, and social development is crucial.
- Health deviations affect the child and family's capacity for self-care and may require new adaptations and techniques to meet universal and developmental self-care requisites.
- Self-care is the result of making decisions to meet universal, developmental, and health-deviation self-care needs, and of taking appropriate actions based on the decisions.
- The concepts of primary, secondary, and tertiary prevention describe the modes in which the nurse can promote self-care for the child and family.
- Combining systems theory and self-care concepts into a framework for the nursing process can promote a systematic, holistic, individualized, and comprehensive approach to nursing care.
- Assessment, or data collection, addresses the child's relevant subsystems and suprasystems, identifying both assets and deficits, and uses a variety of methods such as observing the child's own activities of daily living, physical assessment techniques, and assessment of family functioning.
- Nursing diagnoses are comprehensive summary statements of actual or potential alterations of health status, and are the means by which nurses communicate with each other about the identified health deviations or self-care deficits for which they assume responsibility and make decisions.
- Planning for the child's health care involves cooperation and agreement by the child and/or parent in setting mutual goals, identifying appropriate nursing actions to help the child or parent to reach these goals, and synthesizing these into a systematic and prioritized nursing care plan.
- Intervention, or implementing the plan, can fall into one of three categories, as described by Orem: wholly compensatory, as for an infant who requires total care, partly compensatory, as for the child or parent who can participate in some aspects of self-care, and supportive-developmental (educative), which consists of teaching and learning activities.
- Evaluation, a continual part of the nursing process, is the means by which the nurse determines whether the interventions were adequate or appropriate to meet the stated goals.

References

Abbey JC: A general systems approach to nursing. Pages 19–29 in: *General Systems Theory Applied to Nursing*. Putt M (editor). Little, Brown, 1978.

Brodish MS: Nursing practice conceptualized: An interaction model. *Image* (Feb/March) 1982; 14:5–7.

Chance S: Nursing models: A requisite for professional accountability. *Ad Nurs Sci* (Jan) 1982; 5:57–65.

Chang BL: Evaluation of health care professionals in facilitating self-care: Review of the literature and a conceptual model. *Adv Nurs Sci* (Oct) 1981; 3:43–58.

Eichelberger KM et al: Self-care nursing plan: Helping children to help themselves. *Pediatr Nurs* (May/June) 1980; 6:9–13.

Gordon M: *Nursing Diagnosis Process and Application*. McGraw-Hill, 1982.

Hollen P: a holistic model of individual and family health based on a continuum of choice. *Adv Nurs Sci* (July) 1981; 4:27–42.

Kluckhohn CKM: Values and value orientations in the theory of action. Pages 921–976 in: *Toward a General Theory of Action*. Parsons T, Shils EA (editors). Harvard University Press, 1957.

Lunney M: Nursing diagnosis: Refining the system. *Am J Nurs* (March) 1982; 82:456–459.

McIntyre K: The Perry model as a framework for self-care. *Nurse Pract* (Nov/Dec) 1980; 5:34–38.

Mallick MJ: Patient assessment—Based on data, not intuition. *Nurs Outlook* (Oct) 1981; 29:600–605.

Matthews CA, Gaul AL: Nursing diagnosis from the perspective of concept attainment and critical thinking. *Adv Nurs Sci* (Oct) 1979; 2:17–26.

Miller JR, Janosik EH: *Family-Focused Care*. McGraw-Hill, 1980.

Neuman B: The Betty Neuman health-care systems model: A total person approach to patient problems. Pages 99–110 in: *Conceptual Models for Nursing Practice*. Riehl JP, Roy C (editors). Appleton-Century-Crofts, 1974.

Orem DE: *Nursing: Concepts of Practice*. McGraw-Hill, 1980.

Paxton P, Ramirez MC, Walloch EC: Nursing assessment and intervention. Pages 148–191 In: *Providing Safe Nursing Care for Ethnic People of Color*. Branch MF, Paxton PP (editors). Appleton-Century-Crofts, 1976.

Pontious SL: Practical Piaget: Helping children understand. *Am J Nurs* (Jan) 1982; 82(1):114–117.

Price MR: Nursing diagnosis: Making a concept come alive. *Am J Nurs* 1980; 80(4):668–671.

Stanton M, Paul C, Reeves JF: An overview of the nursing process. In: *Nursing Theory: The Base for Professional Nursing Practice*. Nursing Theory Conference Group. Prentice-Hall, 1980.

Stevens, BJ: *Nursing Theory: Analysis, Application, Evaluation.* Little, Brown, 1984.
von Bertalanffy L: *General Systems Theory: Foundations, Development, Applications.* Braziller, 1968.

Additional Readings

Allison SE: Framework for nursing in a nurse-conducted diabetic management clinic. *J Nurs Admin* 1973; 3:53–60.
Arakelian M: An assessment and nursing application of the concept of locus of control. *Adv Nurs Sci* (Oct) 1980; 3:25–42.
Aspinall MJ, Jambruno N, Phoenix BS: The why and how of nursing diagnosis. *Matern Child Nurs J (Nov/Dec)* 1977; 2:354–358.
Auger JR: Behavioral Systems and Nursing. Prentice-Hall, 1976.
Avant KC, Walker LO: The Practicing Nurse and Conceptual Frameworks. *Matern Child Nurs J* 1984; 9(2):87–90.
Bilitski JS: Nursing science and the laws of health: The test of substance as a step in the process of theory development. *Adv Nurs Sci* (Oct) 1981; 4:15–29.
Bloch D: Some crucial terms in nursing: What do they really mean? *Nurs Outlook 1974;* 22(11):689–694.
Bower F: *The Process of Planning Nursing Care.* Mosby, 1972.
Buckley W: *Sociology and Modern Systems Theory.* Prentice-Hall, 1967.
Calley JM et al: The Orem's self-care nursing model. Pages 302–314 in: *Conceptual Models for Nursing Practice.* 2nd ed. Riehl JP, Roy C (editors). Appleton-Century-Crofts, 1980.
Chapman JE, Chapman HH: *Behavior and Health Care.* Mosby, 1975.
Chinn PL (editor): Application of theory. *Adv Nurs Sci* 1982; 5(1):1–88.
Chinn PL (editor): Nursing theories and models. *Adv Nurs Sci* 1980; 3(1):1–92.
Chinn PL (editor): Practice-oriented theory. Part II. *Adv Nurs Sci* 1979; 2(1):1–90.
Chinn PL (editor): Nursing diagnosis. *Adv Nurs Sci* 1979; 2(1):1–93.
Chinn PL (editor): Practice-oriented theory. Part I. *Adv Nurs Sci* 1978: 1(1):1–95.
Coleman LR: Orem's self-care concept of nursing. Pages 315–328 in: *Conceptual Models for Nursing Practice.* 2nd ed. Riehl JP, Roy C (editors). Appleton-Century-Crofts, 1980.
Crawford G, Dufault K, Rudy E: Evolving issues in theory development. *Nurs Outlook* 1979; 27(5):346–351.
Donley R: Why has nursing been slow in developing a theoretical base? *Image* 1980; 12(1):2.
Eichelberger KM et al: Self-care nursing plan: Helping children to help themselves. *Pediatr Nurs* 1980; 6(3):9–13.
Fawcett J: A framework for analysis and evaluation of conceptual models of nursing. *Nurse Educator* 1980; 5(6):10–14.
Flaskerud JH, Halloran EJ: Areas of agreement in nursing theory development. *Adv Nurs Sci* (Oct) 1980; 3(1):1–8.
Forti TJ, Hyg MS: Advice: A well-intentioned ineffectual notion. *Nurse Pract* 1981; 6(1):25–27.
Friedman MM: *Family Nursing Theory and Assessment.* Appleton-Century-Crofts, 1981.
Fueler SS: Holistic man and the science and practice of nursing. *Nurs Outlook* 1978; 26(11):700–704.
Goodwin JO: A cross-cultural approach to integrating nursing theory and practice. *Nurse Educator* 1980; 5(6):15–20.
Grier MR: Decision-making about patient care. *Nurs Res* 1976; 25(2):105–110.
Hall BA: The change paradigm in nursing: Growth versus persistence. *Adv Nurs Sci* 1981; 3(4):1–6.
Hall JE, Weaver BR: *Distributive Nursing Practice: A Systems Approach to Community Health.* Lippincott, 1977.
Hamdi M, Hutelmyer C: A study of the effectiveness of an assessment tool in identification of nursing care problems. *Nurs Res* 1970; 19(4):354.
Hardy M: Perspectives on nursing theory. *Adv Nurs Sci* 1978; 1(1):37.
Hauck MR, Roth D: Application of nursing diagnosis in a pediatric clinic. *Pediatr Nurs* 1984; 10(1):49–52.
Henderson V: Nature of nursing. *Am J Nurs* 1961; 61(8):62–68.
Hurley PM: Family assessment: Systems theory and the genogram. *Children's Health Care* 1982; 10(3):76–82.
Jacoby MK, Adams DJ: Teaching assessment of client functioning. *Nurs Outlook* 1981; 29(4):248–250.
Johnson DE: Behavioral System Model for Nursing. Pages 207–216 in: *Conceptual Models for Nursing Practice.* 2nd ed. Riehl JP, Roy C (editors). Appleton-Century-Crofts, 1980.
Jones PE: A terminology for nursing diagnoses. *Adv Nurs Sci* 1979; 2(1):65–72.
Joseph LS: Self-care and the nursing process. *Nurs Clin North Am* 1980; 15:131.
Keller JJ: Toward a definition of health. *Adv Nurs Sci* 1981; 4(1):43–64.
Kilchenstein L, Yakulis IM: The birth of a curriculum: Utilization of the Betty Neuman health care systems model in an integrated baccalaureate program. *J Nurs Educ* 1984; 23(3):126–127.
Kim MJ, McFarland GK, McLane AM: *Classification of Nursing Diagnoses: Proceedings of the Fifth National Conference.* Mosby, 1984.
King C: The self-help/self-care concept. *Nurs Pract* (June) 1984; 5(6):34.
King IM: *A Theory for Nursing Systems, Concepts, Process.* Wiley, 1981.
Kinlein ML: Self-Care Concept. *Am J Nurs* 1977; 77(4):598–601.
Klir GJ (editor): *Trends in General Systems Theory.* John Wiley, 1972.
Kritek PB: Commentary: The development of nursing diagnosis and theory. *Adv Nurs Sci* 1979; 2(1):73–80.
Kritek PB: Generation and classification of nursing diagnoses: Toward a theory of nursing. *Image* 1978; 10(3):33–40.
Lamonica EL: *The Nursing Process: A Humanistic Approach.* Addison-Wesley, 1979.
Lewis L: This I believe . . . about the nursing process—Key to care. *Nurs Outlook* 1968; 16:26–29.
Little DE, Carnevali DL: *Nursing Care Planning.* Lippincott, 1979.
McCain RF: Nursing by assessment—Not intuition. *Am J Nurs* 1965; 65(4):82–84.
McCloskey JC: Problem-oriented record vs. the nursing care plan. *Nurs Outlook* 1975; 23(8):492–495.
McMurrey PH: Toward a unique knowledge in nursing. *Image* 1982; 14(1):12–15.
Marriner A: *The Nursing Process, A Scientific Approach to Nursing Care.* Mosby, 1978.
Matthews CA, Gaul AL: Nursing diagnosis from the perspective of concept attainment and critical thinking. *Adv Nurs Sci* 1979; 2(1):17–26.
Miller JR, Janosik EH: *Family-Focused Care.* McGraw-Hill, 1980.
Mikhail B: The health belief model: A review and critical evaluation of the model, research, and practice. *Adv Nurs Sci* 1981; 4(1):65–82.
Mooney MM: The ethical component of nursing theory. *Image* (Feb) 1980; 12(1):7–9.
Newman M: *Theory Development in Nursing.* Davis, 1979.
Norbeck JS: Social support: A model for clinical research and application. *Adv Nurs Sci* 1981; 3(4):43–59.
Norris CM: Self-Care. *Am J Nurs* 1979; 79(3):486–489.
Nursing Development Conference Group: *Concept Formalization in Nursing.* 2nd ed. Little, Brown, 1979.
Nursing Theories Conference Group: *Nursing Theories.* Prentice-Hall, 1980.
Orem D: *Nursing: Concepts of Practice.* 2nd ed. McGraw-Hill, 1980.
Patterson JG, Zerad LT: *Humanistic Nursing.* Wiley, 1976.
Putt AM: *General Systems Theory Applied to Nursing.* Little, Brown, 1978.
Rawls AC: Evaluation of the Johnson behavioral model in clinical practice. *Image* 1980; 12(1):13–16.
Riel JP, Roy C: *Conceptual Models for Nursing Practice.* 2nd ed. Appleton-Century-Crofts, 1980.

Rodgers, JA: Health is not a right. *Nurs Outlook* (Oct) 1981; 10:590–591.

Romano C, McCormick KA, McNeely LD: Nursing documentation: A model for a computerized data base. *Adv Nurs Sci* 1982; 4(2):43–56.

Rotter, JB: Generalized expectancies for internal versus external control of reinforcement. *Psychological Monographs* 1966; 80(1):1–28.

Ruben BD, Kim JY: (editors). *General Systems Theory and Human Communication.* Hayden, 1975.

Ryan BJ: Nursing care plans: A systems approach to developing criteria for planning and evaluation. *J Nurs Admin* 1973; 3(3):50–57.

Sarbin TR, et al: *Clinical Inference and Cognitive Theory.* Holt, Rinehart and Winston, 1960.

Sciarillo WG: Using Hymovich's framework in the family-oriented approach to nursing care. *Am J Matern Child Nurs* 1980; 5(4):242–248.

Sloboda S: Understanding patient behavior. *Nursing '77* 1977; 7(9):74–77.

Smith DM: Writing objectives as a nursing practice skill. *Am J Nurs* 1971; 71(2):319–320.

Smith MC: Proposed melaparadigm for nursing research and theory development: An analysis of Orem's self-care theory. *Image* 1979; 11(5):75–79.

Taylor JW: Outcome criteria as a measurement of nurse performance. *Nursing Digest* 1975; 3(5):41–45.

Thomas MD, Coombs RP: Nursing diagnosis: Process and decision. Reprinted from *Nursing Forum* 5(4):50–64 in *The Nursing Process: A Humanistic Approach.* Lamonica EL (editor). Addison-Wesley, 1979.

Ujhely G: *Determinants of the Nurse-Patient Relationship.* Springer, 1968.

Vincent P: Some crucial terms in nursing: A second opinion. *Nurs Outlook* 1975; 23(1):46–48.

Walker LO, Avant KC: *Strategies for Theory Construction in Nursing.* Appleton-Century-Crofts, 1983.

Ware A: Using nursing prognosis to set priorities. *Am J Nurs* 1979; 79(5):921.

Yura H, Walsh MB: *The Nursing Process: Assessing, Planning, Implementation, Evaluating.* 3rd ed. Appleton-Century-Crofts, 1978.

Zimmer JJ: Quality assurance for outcomes of patient care. *Nurs Clin North Am* (June) 1974; 9:305–325.

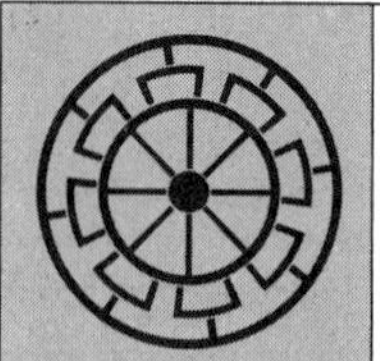

Nursing Care Plan   Applying the Nursing Process

Assessment Data

Name: Daniel
Age: 12 months
Family Composition: Mother, father, sister Linda, 3 years old
Previous Health History: Unremarkable; Healthy except for an upper respiratory tract infection three times
Current Concern: Routine examination

Assessment	Child's Abilities, Characteristics, Interpretation	Parental Assistance, Characteristics, Interpretation	Nursing Analysis, Comparison to Theory
SUBSYSTEMS (Growth and development)			
Biophysical			
Gross motor	Daniel stands by himself; pulls himself to standing position; sits from standing position. Walks holding onto furniture, walls, or parents' hands. Creeps forward or backward at will, creeps upstairs but not down.	Parents walk Daniel and encourage independent walking. Pleased with his progress; anticipate walking and have childproofed house from sister.	Normal development (creeps 9–12 mo; walks 10–15 mo). Parents knowledgeable and provide appropriate stimulation. Parents anticipate next accomplishment. Equilibrium present.
Fine motor	Good pincer grasp; scribbles with crayon—also "puts everything in mouth." Transfers toy from hand to hand; drops and picks up toys at will. Coordination improving when playing peek-a-boo and pat-a-cake, claps hands, covers eyes. Drinks from cup with minimal spilling.	Provides appropriate toys that stimulate eye-hand coordination; spends time playing games. Monitors small objects, especially sister's toys—expresses frustration about Linda's carelessness and her need to be constantly present. Expressed fear that one of the children, especially Daniel, would choke.	Normal development (pincer grasp 9–10 mo; mouthing of objects typical at 10–14 months). Parents knowledgeable and provide toys, sense of responsibility. Potential safety problem—small objects around and child puts everything in mouth.
Physical examination (head to toe; see Chapter 14)	Weight—10.2 kg: 50th percentile; length—76 cm: 50th percentile; temperature—37°C.		Normal growth curve.
Head	Cephalic, no lumps or lesions; anterior fontanel open, posterior fontanel closed. Full range of motion in neck. Hair clean, silky, evenly distributed.		Normal appearance and function.
Face	Symmetric features; alert and responsive; dimple on right cheek.		

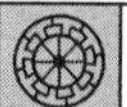

NURSING CARE PLAN Applying the Nursing Process (continued)

Assessment	Child's Abilities, Characteristics, Interpretation	Parental Assistance, Characteristics, Interpretation	Nursing Analysis, Comparison to Theory
Nose	Symmetric—centered; no discharge or inflammation.	Parent states Daniel had a cold three times during past year. Concerned about frequency of and how to prevent colds, length of contagious time, loss of mother's time from employment.	Illness (even minor) results in family disequilibrium. Health maintenance concerns.
Mouth/throat	Mucous membranes moist, smooth, and pink—occasional dry lips from drooling. Six white teeth (four upper, two lower). Lower lateral incisors hard, white areas. Tongue without coating and freely movable. Tonsils large, noninflamed.	Parent relates that Daniel is irritable when teething. Questions how to relieve pain and irritability and sleep disturbance.	Teething discomfort creates minor disequilibrium. Requesting assistance and information. Teething discomfort and behavior within normal limits—is painful.
Eyes	Symmetric, no strabismus. Fixate on object and follow full range horizontally and vertically. Conjunctiva free of irritation. Pupils equal and reacting to light. Sclera are white. Red reflex visualized, uniform.	Parent questions about possibility of strabismus—family history.	Parent knowledgeable about familial relation. Requesting information for reassurance. Normal appearance and function.
Ears	Normal appearance and position; responds to sounds and name. Small amount of soft cerumen; tympanic membrane is pearly pink, translucent; landmarks visualized bilaterally.	Parent questions purpose of "wax" in the ear canal and how to cleanse because it looks dirty.	Normal appearance and function. Requesting health maintenance information.
Skin	Normal color; turgor good; texture smooth and warm; no rashes or irritated areas; nails pink and smooth.	Parent states that Daniel is prone to diaper rash, which sometimes responds to ointment and sometimes to air—requests best method of treating and why rashes are so frequent.	Requesting health maintenance information; diaper rash is fairly common, especially with plastic pants or diapers; skin is otherwise healthy.
Lymph nodes	No cervical, axillary, or inguinal nodes palpable.		Normal finding.
Chest	Sternum has midline appearance; symmetric.		Normal finding.
Lungs	Respiratory rate—30 breaths/min; regular, quiet; no use of accessory muscles; breath sounds clear; no adventitious sounds.	No severe respiratory distress reported, only nasal congestion.	Normal appearance and function (normal respiratory rate is 20–40 breaths/min); equilibrium.

continued on next page

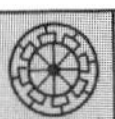

NURSING CARE PLAN Applying the Nursing Process (continued)

Assessment	Child's Abilities, Characteristics, Interpretation	Parental Assistance, Characteristics, Interpretation	Nursing Analysis, Comparison to Theory
Heart	Apical pulse—120 beats/min; blood pressures is 96/50; S_1 S_2 clear and distinct; rhythm regular; no murmurs or thrills; normal size by percussion.	No concerns; no shortness of breath with activity; no color changes.	Normal function (normal pulse is 80–150 beats/min; blood pressure: systolic 96 ± 30, diastolic 66 ± 25); equilibrium.
Abdomen	No obvious distention; no illnesses; good appetite; normal elimination.	No history of regurgitation or vomiting.	Normal function; equilibrium.
Genitalia	Normal male; no masses or irritation.	No history of urinary tract infection.	Normal function and appearance; equilibrium.
Spine—extremities	Upper back straight; range of motion complete in all extremities; arms even—uses both in play, beginning to show preference for left hand; digits of normal length and placement; legs even—slight outward curve, no extra fat fold; toes of normal length and placement; broad base of support and tottering gait when walking.	No concerns or history of injury/illness.	Normal appearance and function (legs initially curved slightly, straighten with maturation and bone growth); wide-based gait provides support and balance when learning to walk; equilibrium.
Neurologic	Normal reflexes; cranial nerves intact.	No history of seizures.	Normal function; equilibrium.
Cognitive			
Piaget	Daniel beginning to use words—Mama, Dada, bye, up; babbles and uses jargon; searches for hidden object where last found—follows visible sequential displacement; removes barrier to get to another toy; uses toys to achieve desired result; purposefully explores surroundings—curious.	Parents talk to Daniel all the time—use normal speech; spend time playing "thinking-type" games with him; allow him to explore surroundings and manipulate toys and objects.	Evidence of behavior reflects Piaget's sensorimotor stage, substages 4 and 5—coordination of secondary circular and early tertiary circular behaviors; normal expectation.
Learning style	Imitates sister and parents; learns by watching and doing.	Parents reinforce desired behaviors and offer praise for new achievements.	Appropriate use of reinforcement and child's use of imitation.
Coping	Cries when tired or frustrated; uses favorite blanket when sad or tired; clings to parents when in strange surroundings; uses cute attention-getting tricks to get own way/coy.	Parents aware of Daniel's need for parental support and use of blanket to cope; assess his crying as a need to be picked up or to "cry it out."	Normal use of coping for 1-year-old; equilibrium.

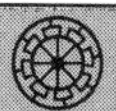

NURSING CARE PLAN Applying the Nursing Process (continued)

Assessment	Child's Abilities, Characteristics, Interpretation	Parental Assistance, Characteristics, Interpretation	Nursing Analysis, Comparison to Theory
Affective			
Erikson	Attached to parents, cries when they leave; very affectionate toward family; trusts family—especially parents, and prefers them to all others; shows emotions of pleasure, anger, and fear; comfortable when in a routine.	Parents respond to Daniel's needs for attention and affection; verbalize feelings of anxiety when he cries for babysitters; parents strive to maintain routine, dependable environment.	Erikson's first stage of trust vs. mistrust; trust well established with parents; secure in their presence.
Ego development	Egocentric.	Parents foster independence.	Gaining sense of self/separate identity; equilibrium.
Social			
Peers (interaction)	Loves other children, especially sister and "friends" at day care; spends time watching their activities and imitating but little interaction.	Many opportunities to be with other children.	Peer interactions normal for age; solitary or parallel interaction.
Strangers (reaction)	Strangers visually inspected; will respond positively if parent is holding, otherwise cries and is difficult to calm.	Parents knowledgeable about normality of stranger anxiety and limit experiences when they are not also present; babysitters only problem; questions how long to expect the behavior and what to do to decrease Daniel's anxiety.	Normal anxiety—requesting information for health maintenance.
Play activities	Manipulative and exploratory play; favorite toys make music or other noise—likes to get results from actions; interactive play with adults—ball rolling, peek-a-boo, pat-a-cake; turn play, putting block in basket, shape finders.	Provide appropriate articles to explore, foster curiosity; play interaction-type games.	Normal play-type activity well supported for growth and future interactions; equilibrium.
SUPRASYSTEMS (Environment)			
Family			
Immediate and extended; roles	Comfortable with grandparents and relatives; no preference for one parent over the other.	Father works full-time as salesman; travels within local district; no overnight trips; mother works part-time as music teacher in school system; parents share household and child-care tasks; satisfied with	Nuclear family, supportive relations; current equilibrium.

continued on next page

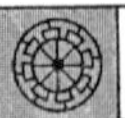

NURSING CARE PLAN Applying the Nursing Process (continued)

Assessment	Child's Abilities, Characteristics, Interpretation	Parental Assistance, Characteristics, Interpretation	Nursing Analysis, Comparison to Theory
		this arrangement; maternal parents live nearby and babysit occasionally—both involved in own activities; visit every Sunday afternoon; relationship viewed positively and described as noninterfering; paternal parents live out of state; visit yearly for several weeks—good relationship; siblings involved in college and personal careers—infrequent visits—contact mostly via telephone and short visits; close-knit family in event of crisis (none at present); generally accepting of each other's independence.	
Religion	Attends church nursery; quickly settles with familiar routine and people providing care.	Protestant—attend church regularly; value religion highly—friends at the church—active in related groups and organizations; source of moral and ethical decisions.	Value and source of support for family; equilibrium.
Culture Rituals, traditions lifestyle, values, language	Becoming socialized within family—participates in family activities and rituals; learning language.	English language spoken; value system reflects dominant American (WASP) orientation—busy, structured life; hard work and career advancement valued highly; children valued and time spent playing with them daily (mother in morning, and father before supper); Possessions important; mother works so extras can be obtained; health a value—desire for adults and children to function optimally; spend money for prevention—regular exercise; no health problems currently; both parents college graduates; college	Health a value and reflected in efforts to stay healthy; achievement oriented—material objects important; "American" culture (middle class) espoused; equilibrium present; many assets—health, education, finances, attitudes about health, children; potential stress—excessive work to get ahead.

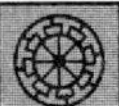

NURSING CARE PLAN Applying the Nursing Process (continued)

Assessment	Child's Abilities, Characteristics, Interpretation	Parental Assistance, Characteristics, Interpretation	Nursing Analysis, Comparison to Theory
		bank accounts started for each child—want them to go to the best school possible; family traditions center on holidays, family gatherings, weekend visit from grandparents; food is strictly "American"—meat and potatoes; occasional fast food or frozen dinners—try to eat well; cleanliness and appearance important—well dressed; money important to purchase desires, saving is done for specifics; little time spent in leisure—"too much to do."	
Peers/friends	Neighborhood contacts beginning; day-care children and personnel.	Large circle of friends associated with work, neighborhood, church, organizations; mostly social; small group of close friends; find each other and family their best friends and are satisfied.	Adequate—no tension; equilibrium.
Clubs, organizations, hobbies	No real clubs yet—swimming lessons at the local YMCA.	Members of local country club and civic organizations; attend symphony concerts; no time for hobbies.	Busy family—limited leisure time a potential stressor to health.
Socioeconomic status	Adequate—dependent on parents.	Finances adequate—concern is with purchasing wants not needs (own own home); insurances cover all potential needs; work and activities done for advancement and recognition.	Middle-class, upwardly mobile family; current equilibrium.
Community	Supportive for desired development.	Suburban area of single-family homes, reported to have good schools, expected to attain certain living style; area of professionals and upwardly mobile, business-related families; many clubs; nearby shopping centers; no public transportation other than train to city.	Middle-class community with many supportive facilities; current equilibrium.

continued on next page

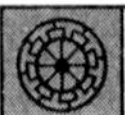

NURSING CARE PLAN Applying the Nursing Process (continued)

Assessment	Child's Abilities, Characteristics, Interpretation	Parental Assistance, Characteristics, Interpretation	Nursing Analysis, Comparison to Theory
School	Day care when mother is teaching—five afternoons; no problem going, seldom cries.	Satisfied with arrangement; child is happy, toys and space clean and safe; children are well supervised, staff show love and patience; positive response to school system in town but no personal experience.	Satisfactory day care and potential school programs; current equilibrium.
Housing	Has own room and lives in new (5-year-old) house.	Own (mortgaged) own home, purchased when new; four bedrooms; adequate furnishings; space adequate for needs.	Current equilibrium; home meets needs.
Play space	Large yard—safe play area with sandbox and swing set; each child has own room; large playroom; each child has own toys as well as shared ones; quiet street—yard is fenced; playground two blocks away.	Parents monitor play when outdoors; because Daniel "puts everything in his mouth," he is not outside alone; house safe and prized possessions out of reach; only problem is stairs, so mother tries to keep Daniel with her when doing housework.	Play space adequate; child's limited ability presents potential safety factor with stairs; current equilibrium (safety covered later).
FUNCTIONS OF SYSTEM (Activities of daily living—self-care)			
Nutrition			
Food and fluid	Sits in high chair for meals; prefers to feed self—does well with finger foods; learning to use a spoon—frequent spills, turns spoon over; drinks from cup at snack and mealtime—some spills; bottle of juice or milk taken at bedtime (240 ml each time); favorite foods—eggs, cheese, yogurt, beans, carrots, fruit, potatoes, and crackers; has six teeth, bites, chews, and gums table food—has trouble with meat unless ground; refuses prepared infant foods; appetite generally good.	Parents knowledgeable about nutrition and child's needs from basic four food groups; restrict sweets and empty-calorie snacks; parents assist Daniel with eating to ensure adequate intake; allow him to feed himself and learn from experience; accept value of self-feeding; mother comments, "It's just another mess to clean up" and "Hard to keep things neat and clean with two children."	Adequate food and fluid intake; one- to three-year-old needs 125 ml/kg/; Daniel needs 1250 ml/day; one-year-old needs 75–152 calories/kg/day; Daniel needs 750–1520 calories/day; potential health maintenance problem with dental caries and bedtime bottles; mother ambivalent about mess from self-feeding—potential stressor.
Elimination	Wears diapers; daily bowel movement; normal bladder functioning—wet every 2–3 hours.	Parents cleanse and change Daniel as necessary; use front-to-back technique when cleaning him.	Normal function; knowledgeable care; equilibrium.

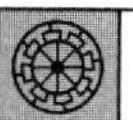

NURSING CARE PLAN Applying the Nursing Process (continued)

Assessment	Child's Abilities, Characteristics, Interpretation	Parental Assistance, Characteristics, Interpretation	Nursing Analysis, Comparison to Theory
Activity	Has become increasingly active and curious—into sister's play and toys; sits and plays short periods of time (5–10 minutes) with toys requiring shape-matching or manipulations to make 'sounds work'; crawls everywhere, concentrates on walking; short attention span—goes quickly from one toy or activity to another; does not watch television routinely.	Parents provide Daniel with toys and encourage learning new skills; understand that interference with sister is part of sibling relation—able to distract fairly well; parents monitor television closely, prefer to read books.	Normal activity level and attention span; parents knowledgeable; equilibrium.
Solitude and social interaction	Has quiet play times by himself or alongside parent; much social interaction with day-care children; free to do as desires at home.	Parents satisfied with Daniel's time spent alone in play—see creative potential; time with others is more than adequate; pleased with time available to spend with adults—parents, relatives, and day-care personnel.	Good balance; current equilibrium.
Safety	Dependent on others.	Parents maintain safe home environment; safety plugs on outlets; gate at stairway, which sister leaves open: "I have to check that gate constantly, I'm so afraid Daniel will fall"; medicines, poisons, and household cleansers kept in high cupboards; appliances and cords kept out of reach and behind things; no extension cords used; very small and fragile objects kept high except for some of sister's toys—mother is very afraid of child's choking on something; tablecloths removed; use seat belts and car seat whenever in the car; secure Daniel in high chair; keep crib side up.	Parents knowledgeable; children's immaturity a deficit—potential safety problem.
Rest and sleep	Naps for 2 hours during early afternoon—usually at day care; sleeps through the night (7 P.M.–7 A.M.).	Parents help Daniel maintain nap and sleep routine; they are alert to sign of fatigue and promote rest or quiet activity.	Sleep needs met; normal sleep for 1-year-old is 14–15 hr/day.

continued on next page

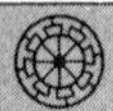

NURSING CARE PLAN Applying the Nursing Process (continued)

Assessment	Child's Abilities, Characteristics, Interpretation	Parental Assistance, Characteristics, Interpretation	Nursing Analysis, Comparison to Theory
Health maintenance			
Hygiene	Dependent on others.	parents keep him clean—daily bath and shampoo; allow water play in tub; finger and toenails cut and clean; clean clothes/frequent changes.	Parents knowledgeable; current equilibrium.
Physical check-ups	Dependent on others.	Parents value health highly; take Daniel for all assessments and examinations as scheduled; follow suggestions for care during illness episodes; seek help for maintenance.	Parents knowledgeable; seek help as needed; current equilibrium.
Immunizations	Up to date—3 DPT; 3 TOPV.	Parents knowledgeable.	Equilibrium.
Dental	Dependent on others.	Parents do not brush his teeth; questioned when to begin and how to do them; water is fluoridated.	Health maintenance concern about dental care; inadequate at present.
Health-deviation demands (limitations on self-care)		These currently do not apply because Daniel is healthy. They would be developed in the event of illness, injury, or need for other health care interventions. Examples are given in later chapters when such conditions are discussed.	
Impact of disease/injury/disability/disfigurement			
Impact of medications			
Impact of treatments			
Impact of hospitalization			
Impact of surgery			

Nursing Diagnoses and Goals

1. **Nursing diagnosis:** Potential alteration in health maintenance related to a knowledge deficit about aspects of child care specified by the child's parents.

   Long-term goal: Parents will provide for Daniel's universal and developmental requisites.

   Short-term goals: (a) Parents will list five ways of preventing colds. (b) Parents will discuss relation between increased peer contact and illness. (c) Parents will list one other child-care resource when incidence of illness is high at Daniel's day-care center. (d) Parents will list five appropriate toys that can be used as teething aids. (e) Parents will discuss possible harm from fluid-filled teething aids. (f) Parents will discuss how to use medicine that is rubbed on the gums to relieve teething pain. (g) Parents will state difference between normal eyes and strabismus. (h) Parents will state relation between fatigue and signs of strabismus. (i) Parents will state the purpose of earwax, will describe how to clean the external ear without touching the ear canal, and will demonstrate how to put liquid glycerin into the ear to soften wax. (j) Parents will discuss the relationship of diaper rash to Daniel's diet, type of diaper, and other changes in care. (k) Parents will use protective covering between diaper changes. (l) Parents will check Daniel at least every 2 hours and change diapers when needed. (m) Parents will discuss nature of their anxiety about Daniel's crying. (n) Parents will discuss four ways to decrease Daniel's anxiety and crying when they leave him.

2. **Nursing diagnosis:** Potential alteration in safety related to the immaturity of children and Daniel's growth and developmental stage.

Long-term goal: Daniel will not have any serious falls,

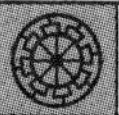

NURSING CARE PLAN Applying the Nursing Process (continued)

ingest household substances, or experience other household-related accidents.

Short-term goals: (a) Parents will discuss ways to teach Daniel to crawl down the stairs. (b) Parents will discuss the value of teaching Daniel some simple safety habits rather than blaming Linda for safety problems. (c) Parents will list names of poisonous plants. (d) Parents will demonstrate how to care for a choking child.

3. **Nursing diagnosis:** Potential alteration in dental health maintenance related to bedtime bottles and inadequate brushing of teeth.

   Long-term goal: Daniel will not have excessive dental caries.

   Short-term goals: (a) Parents will discuss the relation of dental caries and putting Daniel to bed with a bottle of milk or juice. (b) Parents will describe the process of tooth decay. (c) Parents will demonstrate how to care for Daniel's teeth. (d) Parents will start to have Daniel brush his own teeth.

4. **Nursing diagnosis:** Potential alteration in health maintenance of parents related to ambitions and limited leisure time.

   Long-term goal: Parents will not have stress-related illnesses.

   Short-term goal: (a) Parents will discuss potential health factors related to increased stress. (b) Parents will spend time each week in leisure activities that they enjoy. (c) Mother will identify two ways to lessen her concern about having a "mess-free" house.

Interventions	Rationale	Evaluation
1. Give parents information about ways to prevent illness (eg, adequate rest, good nutrition, exercise, avoiding becoming overheated, rapid changes in temperatures, exposure, careless disposal of tissue, not covering nose and mouth when coughing, sneezing, or blowing nose).	Infants have limited immunity and need extra external protection until 5 years of age, when the child's level of immunity equals that of the adult.	Parents remember and practice cold prevention measures.
Advise parents to avoid crowds when incidence of illness is high; not to share glasses, utensils, food, or toothbrushes; and to teach child to cover mouth and nose when coughing or sneezing. Discuss possibility of other child-care arrangements during times of high incidence of illness at the day-care center. Discuss relation of illness and close contact between the two children at play. Encourage parents in their presently good health practices for Daniel, especially those that will help him resist infection.	The only ways at present to limit the number of colds are good hygiene, rest, diet, exercise, and avoiding others with colds.	Child's exposure to others with colds is limited.
Discuss ways to relieve discomfort from teething (eg, use of cold, wet washcloths, hard toys for chewing, silver teething toys).	Teething causes some pain and consequent irritability. Cold, pressure, or rubbing seems to relieve pain most satisfactorily.	Parents remember to use articles from list.
Warn parents not to use fluid-filled teething aids because fluid is often contaminated.	Teething does not cause illness, but colds or other viral illnesses may be present at the same time.	Parents will not use fluid-filled toys. Parents will separate symptoms of cold or illness from teething process.
Discuss cautious use of over-the-counter rub-on medication to relieve pain. Note that effectiveness of such medication is variable.	Use of rub-on medication may help a parent who feels the need to relieve pain more than it helps the child, but it may be effective.	Parents will state whether medicine rubbed on gums helped to relieve teething pain.

continued on next page

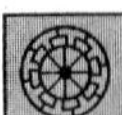

NURSING CARE PLAN Applying the Nursing Process (continued)

Interventions	Rationale	Evaluation
Praise parents for their concern and realization of familial tendency.	Strabismus is familial. Children with broad bridges of the nose or widely set eyes often appear to have strabismus but do not.	Parent will explain differences.
Demonstrate test for strabismus (light reflection in pupils).	If light is reflected in centers of both pupils when shone at a distance from the center of the nose, no strabismus is present.	Parents will monitor Daniel's eye position and movement at home.
Offer reassurance. Test Daniel carefully during succeeding visits. Explain ways to monitor use of eyes at home.	Monitoring child at home includes watching the ability to judge depth perception when picking up small objects with one eye covered, a test that can be carried out by parents.	
Discuss the purpose of earwax, explaining that it is normal and part of the ear's protection.	Parents should know that the waxy material in ears is to protect and lubricate the ear canal and that it serves to remove dust, dirt, and debris when the flow is not impaired.	Parents are less concerned about appearance and able to explain the purpose of earwax.
Discuss the proper cleaning of the external ear and danger of cotton-tipped applicators or anything small in the ear. Discuss the use of liquid glycerin to loosen hard wax (if there are no other signs of infection or earache). Explain the need to allow oil to drain out with softened was.	Parents should know that cleaning with small objects pushes wax back and often results in wax buildup, pain, and dimenished hearing ("never use anything 'smaller than an elbow' in the ear"). Wax may be softened if it is hard. Liquid glycerin softens wax and then allows oil and wax to drain out by themselves. (This technique should never be used if any indication of other drainage, infection, or pain is present.)	Parents will be able to clean the child's ears properly.
Discuss Daniel's tendency to have diaper rash and any relation to citrus foods such as orange juice and tomatoes. Discuss relation of rash to detergent or other washing aids and discuss possible need to change brand of disposable diapers.	There are many types of rashes—allergic, ammonia, bacteria, yeast, or contact. Rashes vary in type and location. Those that are not in the creases or buttocks usually are some type of contact rash. A change in detergent, extra rinsing, or change in the type of diaper used may be necessary.	Child will have fewer problems with diaper rash; parents will identify specific causes of rash and will be able to make necessary adjustments.
Discuss use of plastic pants and advise parents to avoid them. Advise parents to increase Daniel's intake of water. Discuss relation of new foods, especially some that are hard to digest, and changes in stool patterns. Avoid foods that are suspected of being related to rash. Discuss changing diapers more frequently, use of medicated powder or ointment with diaper changes, avoiding the use of powder with talc, and use of baking soda in bath water. Always apply pro-	Plastic pants keep the skin wet and more susceptible to rash. Increased intake of water helps to avoid concentrated urine. Allergic rash related to foods eaten will be seen shortly and consistently after such food is consumed; parents should therefore be able to identify foods that cause rash. Stool changes such as diarrhea can result from sensitivity to particular foods. Yeast rashes are seen in creases and buttocks and are more common when skin is moist. Skin	Parents will make necessary changes to prevent diaper rash.

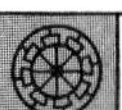

NURSING CARE PLAN Applying the Nursing Process (continued)

Interventions	Rationale	Evaluation
tective covering in thin film and always clean thoroughly between diaper changes.	needs frequent cleaning and drying. Ointment to protect the skin from moisture may be needed if rash worsens from initial appearance. Cornstarch is a medium for yeast growth and should not be used.	
Discuss when rash or diapers can be exposed to air for drying. Advise parents to pin or fasten diapers loosely.	Ammonia rashes are most common after the first few months and may resolve faster with exposure to air; the best way to rid diapers of ammonia is to hang them outside on a sunny day so that the sun kills the spores. Loose diapers allow air to circulate.	
Discuss how often parents leave children with a sitter.	Exposure of children to babysitters and a chance for parents to have time together are important. Discussion ascertains whether parents' anxiety is due to the infrequency of the experience or the reverse.	Child will be less fussy when parents leave, and parents will be less concerned about crying episodes that are brief.
Discuss the parents' concern about leaving while Daniel is crying. For example, are guilt feelings associated with this? Does it spoil their evening, cause concern for the sitter, create a bad reputation as parents, or affect the child's reputation? Discuss their trust and confidence in the sitter.	The child gains a sense of object permanence and knows that he has only one mother and one father and will protest when a familiar person is not present. This is a normal part of development, as the child lets the parents know how important and needed they are. If the child senses that the parent trusts the sitter, this often reduces some of the child's anxiety.	Parents will have a consistent, reliable babysitter.
Advise parents to have something special for children, such as ice cream cones or cookies, and be sure the child's needs are met before leaving (for example, that the child is clean, dry, and fed, if possible). If parents are leaving later in the evening, advise them to have Daniel in pajamas with a story read and to have the sitter read an extra story (as a "treat"). Suggest telling Daniel earlier in the day that the sitter will be coming and leaving at the stated time without going back to check. Advise calling to relieve parental anxiety.	The more familiar and routine the process, the less the fuss. Children at this age do best with familiarity.	Parents will incorporate familiar routine into daily routine with babysitter.
2. Praise parents for their awareness and concern. Advise parents to teach Daniel to crawl downstairs backward and to put pillows or cushions at the bottom of the stairs while Daniel is learning.	One-year-olds are curious and have no sense of what is dangerous and what is not. It is better to childproof an area than to follow the child around and constantly say "no." It is safer to teach the child to manage steps by demon-	Parents will teach Daniel to crawl down the stairs.

continued on next page

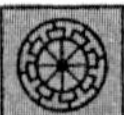

NURSING CARE PLAN Applying the Nursing Process (continued)

Interventions	Rationale	Evaluation
	strating how to crawl down them and then helping the child to do the same than it is to rely on someone else to close the gate. The process can be repeated until it is learned, as crawling is best learned by imitation.	
Assess size of Linda's toys for possibility of choking. Suggest that Linda play with them in her room with the door closed and that otherwise they be put away, out of reach.	Limiting access to a sibling's toys removes the possibility of a child's swallowing and choking on small objects.	Toys that may be dangerous will be out of Daniel's reach.
Review with parents what to do in event of a child's choking. Demonstrate the Heimlich maneuver.	Knowing the Heimlich maneuver may save a life.	Parents will be comfortable and confident of their knowledge and skills about what to do if their child chokes.
Advise parents to use nontoxic crayons that are also washable. Advise parents to check the outdoors for poisonous plants or sharp objects that could be dangerous. Give parents a list of poisonous plants. Advise parents to have syrup of ipecac on hand and to have phone numbers for the doctor and poison control center next to the phone.	Poisonous plants should be hung out of reach or removed. A list should be available for reference. Syrup of ipecac and phone numbers for the doctor and poison control center should be accessible for emergencies.	Parents will be comfortable and confident of their knowledge and skills in handling an emergency if their child swallows something poisonous. Plants that are poisonous will be moved to safe, high places.
3. Discuss what happens when food or sugar is held in the mouth during sleep, which occurs when Daniel goes to sleep while sucking on a bottle of milk or juice. Explain that saliva flow decreases during sleep so that milk carbohydrates or sugar from the juice remains on the teeth, initiating the formation of acid, which breaks down tooth enamel. Suggest switching Daniel to a bottle of water at night. Begin by diluting juice with water and increase the amount of water by 1 oz each night so that by the end of the week, the bottle contains only water.	Food, especially carbohydrates and sugar, are damaging to dental enamel if allowed to remain on teeth. Children who fall asleep with milk or juice bottles have sugar or carbohydrates on their teeth. The enzyme that breaks these substances down also destroys tooth enamel and causes dental caries. During sleep, this process happens faster because of lesser amounts of saliva.	Daniel will go to bed with a bedtime bottle containing water.
Have Daniel drink water after each meal to rinse the food from his mouth. Advise parents that care for Daniel's teeth includes cleaning the teeth with gauze wrapped around a parent's finger. Note that parents should delay actual brushing until 18 months of age.	Rinsing his mouth after eating removes any leftover pieces of food. Cleaning the teeth with a piece of gauze is the best way to clean tender teeth. Gingival teeth are tender, so brushing should be delayed until 18 months of age.	Parents will clean Daniel's teeth after each meal.

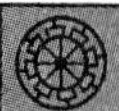

NURSING CARE PLAN Applying the Nursing Process (continued)

Interventions	Rationale	Evaluation
Introduce the toothbrush and allow Daniel to "brush" his teeth so that he can begin to learn with time to play and practice.	Dental care should begin when teeth first appear. Brushing that is introduced as fun should be a positive experience. Time to play and experiment allows the child to learn by imitating. Parents will need to brush child's teeth until around 5 years of age because the child's fine motor coordination is still immature.	Daniel will start to use a toothbrush.
4. Discuss with parents the importance of leisure activities to reduce stress, making the connection between stress and illness and noting that some illnesses can be avoided by reducing stress. Discuss the importance of time to enjoy and not just care for the children. Discuss doing an enjoyable family activity together once a week or every other week. Suggest activities or help parents identify enjoyable activities; suggest having children participate with suggestions when they are old enough.	Children are sensitive to the stresses and pressures of parents and respond accordingly, so it is important to be relaxed when interacting with a child. Research has demonstrated a relation between stress and excessive self-imposed demands and increased incidence of illness, especially cardiovascular disease. Leisure activity for enjoyment and relaxation is important and different from exercise for the sake of exercise.	Parents will spend time each week in leisure activities, either as a couple or as an entire family.
Suggest that mother designate one room for children to use for play and not clean that room until the end of the day. Suggest one or two rooms in which quiet play only is allowed.	A source of tension between parents and children can be parental concern for neatness and the child's lack of concern. Compromise is better than frustration. It is important to find ways to accommodate a child's needs to manipulate, explore, and play while accommodating a parent's needs for a sense of satisfaction in homemaking. Using specific rooms or times for certain activities is often a successful solution.	Daniel's mother will find a compromise between needs for play and neatness.
Put newspapers under high chair. Use plastic tablecloths.	These measures should lessen the cleanup after meals.	Parents will find mealtime less stressful.

UNIT II

INFLUENCES ON HUMAN GROWTH AND DEVELOPMENT

Each child is a unique combination of characteristics resulting from the interplay of nature (heredity) and nurture (environment). Both nature and nurture are important to the child's growth and development, as the child's inherited potential can be realized only in a supportive environment. In Unit II our purpose is to acknowledge the important contributions and supporting role that each one plays in the total developmental picture of the child.

In Chapter 3 we explore the many ways in which culture—as expressed in belief systems, values, rituals, and traditions—influences the family's child-rearing practices, orientation toward health, as well as the prevention and treatment of disease. We also examine the ways in which the socioeconomic factors of environment contribute to the availability of community resources for the child and family. The nurse who understands the role played by social and cultural factors can plan interventions that complement rather than conflict with a family's beliefs, traditions, and resources.

In Chapter 4 we focus on the family and describe variations in type, structure, function, and style of interaction. The discussion of the importance of family roles, communication patterns, and development in relation to family dynamics is followed by illustrations of how the nurse uses this information when teaching and working with children and their families.

In Chapter 5 the fundamentals of heredity are reviewed, and specific facts about transmission of inherited characteristics or conditions are illustrated. We discuss the steps of cell division, formation of DNA, and protein synthesis. We also include the consequences of alterations in the genetic code whether at the gene or chromosome level. The role of the nurse in genetic counseling concludes this chapter.

Contents

Social and Cultural Influences on the Child

3

Virginia Prout

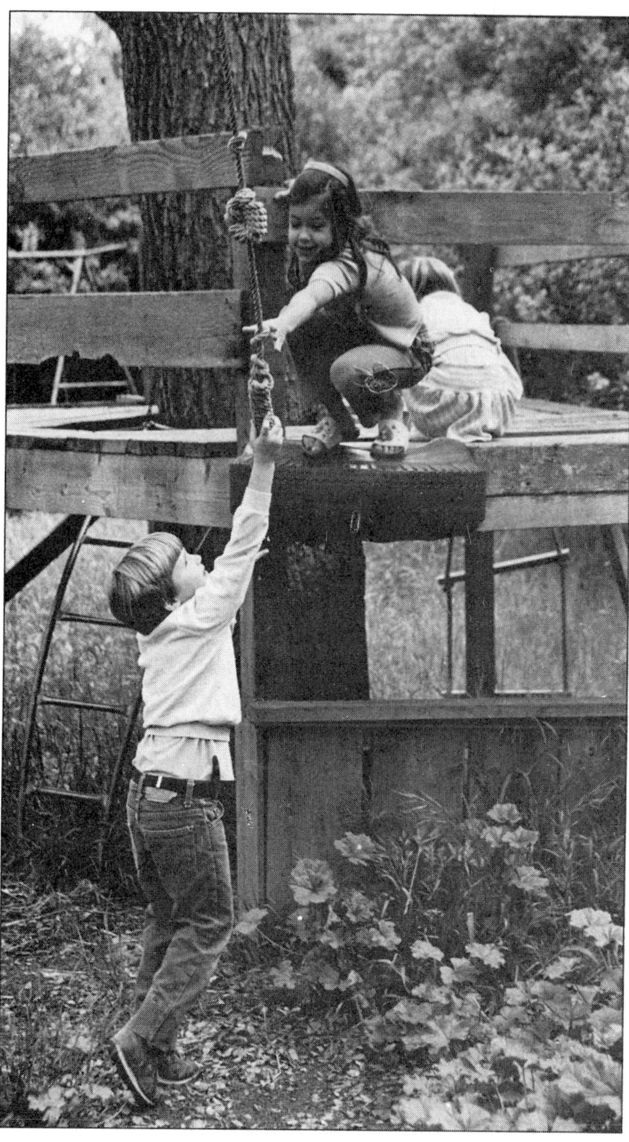

Chapter Outline

Objectives

- Define culture, ethnicity, and socioeconomic class.
- Discuss how the suprasystems of family, peers, and school; local structures; and society at large influence the socialization of the child.
- List the components of a cultural assessment.
- Explain the relation of ethnic folk traditions and health response behaviors.
- Define the responsibility of the nurse in relation to communication, research, and providing health care and teaching.

In Chapter 2 we discussed general systems theory as a useful framework for guiding the collection and organizing of data to establish a nursing diagnosis and manage care. The value of this approach is that it increases the nurse's understanding of the significance of the child's behaviors and interactions with the family and others. The acts and events that occur in the lives of children and their families take place in a broad social and cultural context. The more complete the understanding of that context, the more realistic and accurate will be the view of the developing child and the more humanistic and holistic will be the nursing management of that child's health problems.

In this chapter, we explore the social and cultural aspects of the child's world. The social sphere includes people, such as the child's family, peers, and members of the larger community, and institutions that make up such systems as school, media, health care, government, and the economy. The cultural atmosphere encompasses more intangible entities such as norms, values, beliefs, morals, customs, knowledge, and attitudes. American society is extremely diverse ethnically, and it would be difficult to specify a single, uniform culture; rather, the immigration of various groups, from colonial settlers to the more recent political refugees, has created a complex fabric in which some elements of culture may be shared among most or all of the various ethnic or racial groups, whereas other elements remain unique for a specific group. Effective nursing care of children and their families includes an understanding of and sensitivity to the complexity of cultural variation in American society.

Systems Model for Studying the Environment

Several models for systems analysis have been developed and used in diverse disciplines, including the study of the child and family. Bronfenbrenner (1977) and Brim (1975) have developed a particularly useful model for describing the various influences on child development, placing the child in the total context of culture and society and not just in relation to the immediate surroundings of family, school, and community. In this model the environment can be visualized as a series of concentric circles, with the inner circle representing the child's immediate systems of contact and the outer circles consisting of the larger systems that influence and guide the inner circles to a greater or lesser degree (Fig. 3-1).

Family, Peers, and School

The first circle in the scheme presented in Figure 3-1 includes individuals who directly impinge on and influence children and their development. Of these, the family is the most important contact.

Family as Boundary As discussed in Chapter 2, the family can be seen not only as the most intimate suprasystem surrounding the child but also as part of the boundary that controls the dynamic exchange between the child and other parts of the environment. The boundaries of the family system will determine how exchanges with other systems will influence and modify the family's life, which, of course, includes the child. If the family's being assimilated into the wider culture is acceptable to the family, the boundaries of the family system will become more permeable to unfamiliar values and behaviors. If, on the other hand, the family resists what it perceives as threatening influences from the environment, its boundaries becomes less permeable and its integration into the surrounding culture more gradual. The family's perception of its place within the wider culture, which might be heavily influenced by its ethnic heritage, must be understood by the nurse to define client needs more effectively and to adjust intervention strategies more sensitively. The family, its structure and function and its influence on the child, is discussed in more depth in Chapter 4.

The Role of Peers The child's social horizons broaden as the young child's experiences with a larger group of individuals outside of the family increases and new relationships with peers and other adults are formed. The child's level of language development, cognition, and motor skills provide the vehicles for this social exchange and entry into a world outside the family. This expanded environment provides the young child with a wide range of experiences in which to learn to adapt to a real and varied world.

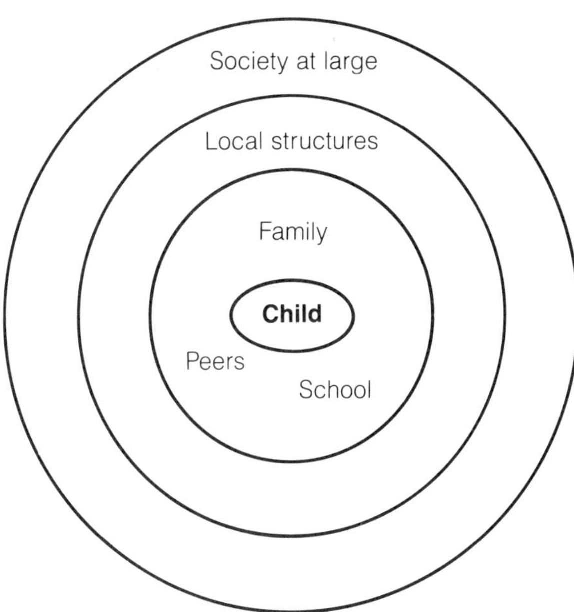

Figure 3-1 Social and cultural systems that influence the child. Inner circles represent systems with direct influence. Outer circles represent larger systems of influence.

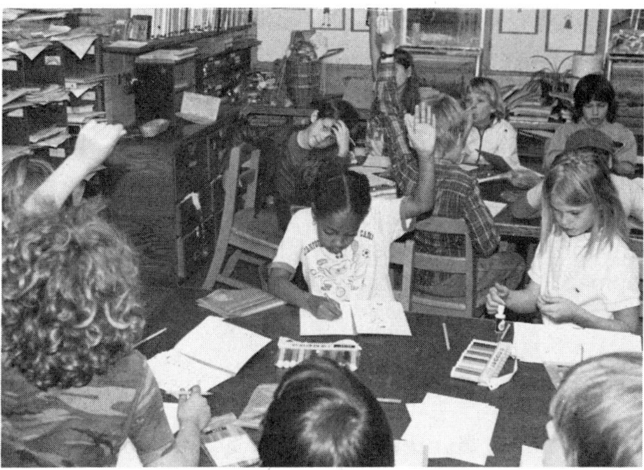

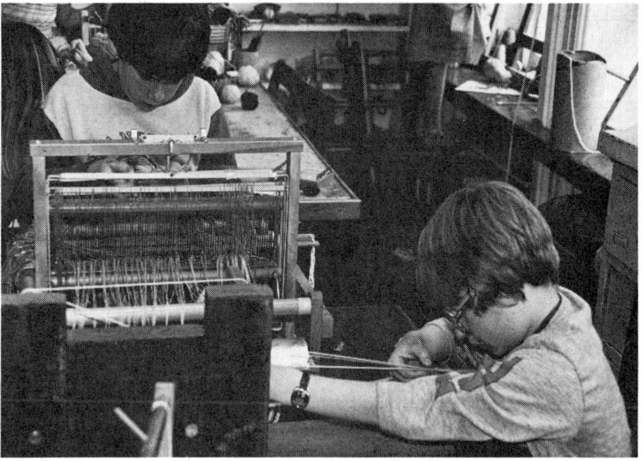

Schools are a major force for socialization, although teaching methods differ. Compare traditional classroom to nontraditional classroom settings.

For most children, their peer group is a significant socializing force in which roles are practiced and perfected. The reinforcement (input) that children receive from one another that either supports or negates their actions and behaviors is mediated and processed (throughput) to influence subsequent perceptions and expectations of behavior approval and acceptance by the child (feedback). New skills are shared and the role modeling of behavior abounds as children imitate each other's actions and responses.

Children's play activities are not only fun and enjoyable but also serve as an arena for testing and exploring the environment, developing a sensitivity to the feelings of others, and refining skills and interactive abilities.

The Role of School Schools are one of the major forces of socialization in Western countries. Most children spend 12 or more years in formal schooling. School affects the lives of children in many ways, including role transition (from son or daughter to pupil), change in setting (from home to classroom), and adaptation to a different authority figure (from parent to teacher). Each child perceives school differently and builds on both positive and negative experiences as they contribute to the totality of personal development.

Yussen and Santrock (1982) noted that many schools have middle-class standards and expectations and are thus a powerful socializing force because only one view is presented. "It often seems as though one of the major functions of schools in this country is to train children to function in and contribute to middle-class society, since politicians who vote on school funding are usually middle class, school-board members are predominantly middle class, and principals and teachers are often middle class" (p. 500).

Curriculum decisions concerning textbooks and teaching methodology often reflect the beliefs and perceived ideology of the dominant culture. The textbooks selected frequently portray happy, intact, two-parent, white families working or playing together. The actual diversity of family life and its numerous forms is often overlooked. The existence of frustration, loneliness, fear, sadness, or anger, which is a reality for many children, may be ignored.

Some studies indicate that teachers have different expectations and goals for the students vis-à-vis the school setting. This may be reflected in their attitude, the time and energy they are willing to spend on the students' learning, and their efforts to communicate with the parents. Children usually attempt to meet adult expectations. Children who have high aspirations most likely have parents and teachers reaffirming them.

School promotes the child's cognitive development (learning), but it also contributes in a significant way to the child's social and affective development. The feedback that occurs between teacher and student and between peers and student communicates approval or disapproval for the student's output as expressed in attention, behavior, and class participation. When approval is present, the child is motivated to excel; when disapproval is present, the child may become discouraged or disruptive. The classroom environment and atmosphere influence the child's development, attitude toward learning, and self-concept.

Local Structures

Community Systems Systems at the local level (Fig. 3-1), although they may not impinge directly on the individual child, have a strong influence on the immediate settings that the child inhabits. Examples of these community systems are local governments, local health-care agencies, local school systems, and locally based religious organizations. The interaction among the various systems at this level results in relationships and qualities that have a direct effect on the life-style of the family and on its support system. These include the nature and requirements of the parents' work, the characteristics of the local neighborhood, the relations between the school and community, social networks, modes of transportation and communication, and patterns of recreation and social life. Nurses are in a key position to observe the issues, deficits, and strengths of the components of this second level as they affect the health of the child and family. Taking advantage of this position by learning and understanding the child's relationships to the suprasystems at this level will support the nurse's goal of individualized care.

One example of the response of systems at this level to the needs of children and their families is the establishment of work-site day-care programs provided by major employers. Placing a day-care facility within the work setting allows the parent to return to work while remaining available to the infant, decreases the length of daily separation of parent and child by allowing visits during coffee breaks and lunch hour and involves the parent more actively in the design and management of the agency caring for the child. The interaction of parent and day-care staff yields less obvious but equally significant benefits. The staff gains increased understanding of the child's background and idiosyncracies, whereas the parent has more frequent opportunities to be close to the child, maintain the child's confidence, and share the child's experiences. Day-care staff and parents also can collaborate to locate other community resources that can diminish the potential isolation felt by working families. By supplementing the nurturing of the child, such an arrangement can supplement the nurturing of the family itself. (Guidelines for selecting a day-care facility are included in Chapter 21.)

Local Support Systems Environmental conditions, such as substandard housing, inadequate child care, and the lack of available support systems, are significant influences on child health and development (Provence, Naylor, and Patterson, 1977; Glickman and Springer, 1978; Kagan, Kearsley and Zelazo, 1978). To support the goals of self-care for the child and family, nurses need to be informed about such environmental conditions at the local level. Helping local health-care programs and agencies identify and meet children's health-care needs—whether the need is for preventive well-child visits or for special programs—is a contribution nurses are well equipped to make. An appropriate nursing activity at the local level is involving the community, school, church, government, and health-care agency in the assessment, planning, implementation, and evaluation of comprehensive programs. Likewise, the nurse can be alert to other issues such as gaps in service, overlap of programs, and the dangers of bureaucratic complexity.

The media, too, can play an increasingly effective role in alerting the public to local environmental issues and available services and is thus an invaluable resource to the nurse. Some local broadcasting networks and newspapers have now established hotlines for consumers that help with a variety of issues, from dealing with a negligent landlord to locating a special educational program for a handicapped child. Whereas a family with a learning-disabled child may not have specific information on or direct access to appropriate services, the nurse, by keeping informed and involved in local systems, can promote the freer exchange of information and energy between that family and the systems that supply needed services and care.

Society at Large

The outermost of the circles in Figure 3-1 represents the composite system that embraces all of the others such as the social system, economic system, political system, legal system, and health care system. Embedded in this composite system are the common cultural patterns that underlie our daily lives such as the value placed on education, the work ethic, monogamy, democratic government, the rights of the individual, and the rights of groups.

The most significant forces that influence child development at this level stem from large-scale governmental policies and priorities. Major statistical surveys and field reports regarding child health needs are primarily sponsored and conducted by federal and state agencies. This information provides the basis for large subsidies, legislative policy changes, and other major actions that can affect the milieu in which children develop. In 1980 a US Congressional Select Panel (of child health and development experts) prepared a report on the promotion of better child health as a national strategy. The results of this three-volume report were published by the US Department of Health and Human Services (Report of the Select Panel for the Promotion of Child Health). This report and others like it help to establish priorities in child research, health care, and education and to initiate immunization and nutritional programs.

The allocation of government resources for programs and services that promote child health is subject to national and international fluctuations in politics and the economy. The real issue remains, however, the ability of private, local, and governmental agencies to provide quality service and maintain continuity of care for the children and families they serve.

Nursing is discovering the important role to be played in the process of deciding how resources are to be allocated. As nursing has gained recognition as a profession, it has become more organized and effective in advocating and developing innovative and efficient programs essential both to today's children and to the well-being of future generations. Nurses, because of their numbers and because of their role as front-line health workers, can offer an important and needed perspective on policies that govern health care. Individual or collective participation in the political and other systems at this level can be an effective way for nurses to promote the health of all children and their families. Membership in professional nursing organizations, such as the American Nurses' Association, and participation in its local specialty units, such as maternal–child health, can be an important step in keeping abreast of and having a say in the major legislative and lobbying efforts of that organization. Wider participation by nurses in such professional groups can strengthen nursing's voice in determining national priorities and budget allocations. Keeping current on the major issues and events at the national, state, and local levels can enhance the nurse's understanding of the influences on child and family health that emanate from the suprasystems at these levels.

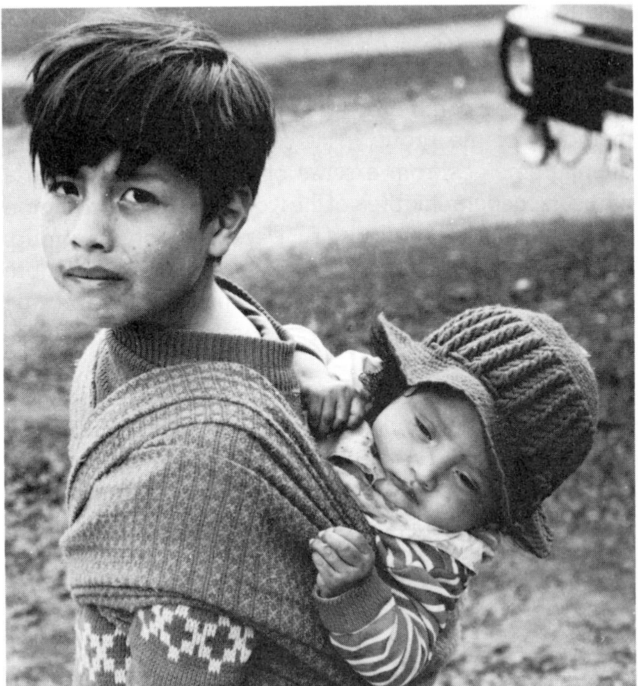

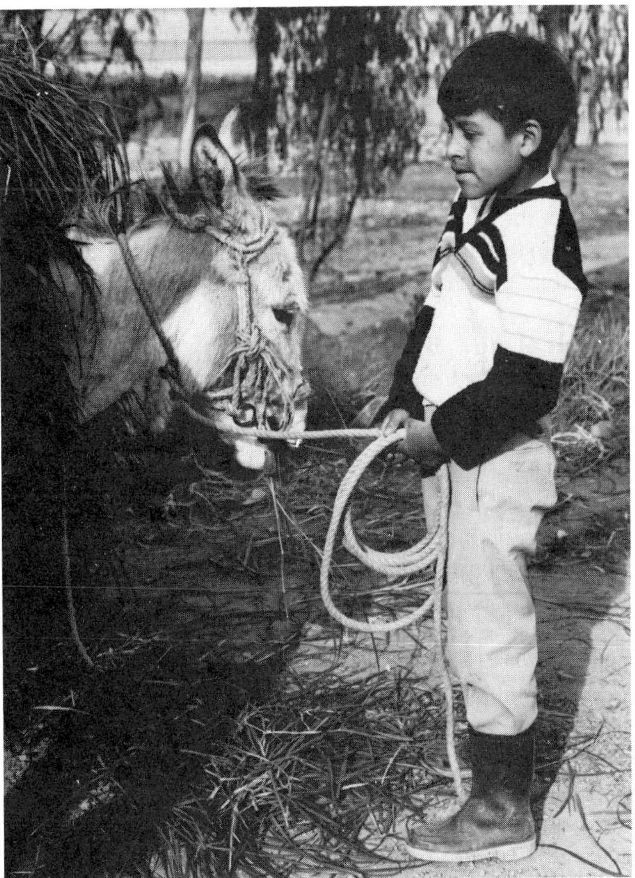

In some cultures, older children are responsible for assuming some adult responsibilities. Caring for younger siblings may be the responsibility of the older child, and children may help to support the family economically.

Ethnicity and Culture

Race, ethnicity, and culture are terms that are often confused with each other, but important distinctions must be made among their actual meanings. *Race* refers to the classification of human beings into groups based on particular physical characteristics such as skin pigmentation, head form, and stature. Caucasoid, Mongoloid, and Negroid are the three racial types generally recognized. *Culture,* on the other hand, is the learned patterns of behavior and thinking shared by a particular group and transmitted over time by group members to other group members. These patterns provide tested and acceptable solutions to the problems of living (Orque, Bloch, and Monrroy, 1983, p. 10). *Ethnicity* is the condition of belonging to a group whose members share a unique cultural, social, and linguistic heritage (Henderson and Primeaux, 1981).

Each child, as a member of an ethnic group, shares to some degree a common background and culture with other members of the group. This common background frequently emerges from a sense of shared beginnings in a particular geographic area of the world and from a common language, religion, and history. Depending on the group, one or another of the common elements will have more significance; for example, religious characteristics are the main features that distinguish the Amish and Mennonites from the larger culture.

The ways in which significant behavioral and personality characteristics evolve depend to a large measure on these ethnic traditions. The sex-role development of the child, attitudes toward competition, and willingness to accept or reject the attitudes, practices, and values of the dominant culture are just a few examples of how the subsystems are influenced by the child's ethnic background.

Impact of Ethnicity on Health Care

There are many good reasons why nurses who care for children should increase their understanding of ethnic variation among people. Included in these reasons are the variations in physical and behavioral norms that define health for a particular group, the differences in how children are viewed from one culture to another, the impact of healing beliefs and practices on a client's health behaviors, and the effect of the nurse's understanding (or lack of it) on participation in therapy. Table 3-1 summarizes a variety of health-related factors that may affect nursing care.

Physical and Behavioral Norms The assessment phase of the nursing process involves not only collecting data but also comparing these data to the established healthy norms. If the norms chosen are not appropriate for the individual—if, for example, an Asian child's growth is assessed on the basis of norms for white children—the assessment will not result in an accurate nursing diagnosis.

"A nurse who cares for people of another culture needs to know certain basic biological concepts in order to give not only adequate care, but also nonharmful care" (Overfield, 1977). There is a range of physical variation among people of different races with regard to growth rate, dentition, body structure, blood group, and susceptibility to certain diseases, to mention just a few variables. Although a thorough and detailed knowledge of every physical variation among racial groups is beyond the abilities of any one nurse, the important concept to emphasize is simply that biologic variations exist (Overfield, 1977).

Similarly, standards of behavior can differ from one ethnic group to another. For instance, individuals brought up in a more traditional Asian culture may be much more formal than is usual in American society. A nurse caring for the child of Asian heritage may never succeed in getting to a first-name basis with the family and will need to understand that the more formal address is a sign of mutual respect and appropriate personal distance (Orque, Bloch, and Monrroy, 1983, p. 28).

Psychologic characteristics, such as self-concept, also can differ along ethnic lines. These characteristics can be the result of centuries of cultural development, or they may be the products of specific, more recent historical events such as the adjustments forced on Vietnamese immigrants by years of violent upheaval (Orque, Bloch, and Monrroy, 1983, p. 262).

How Children Are Viewed Ethnicity also will affect the value placed on children, the child's role within the family structure, and which adult members of the family are most likely to assume child-care responsibilities. Economic necessity also has a major influence on these matters. It would benefit the nurse caring for children of varying ethnic backgrounds to know something, for example, about the childrearing attitudes that stem from the Confucian value system of some Asian families (Orque, Bloch, and Monrroy, 1983, p. 203) or about the more active role played by extended family members (grandmothers, aunts, cousins, and older siblings) in the socialization of black children (Friedman, 1981, p. 286).

Impact of Health Beliefs One of the cultural beliefs to which many nurses subscribe is that the western, scientific conception of health and disease, with its technologically advanced medical system, is the most effective model for health restoration. This view is not necessarily shared, however, by people from other cultures, who may have developed comprehensive models of their own that have little in common with the western model. Herbs, folk remedies, the evil eye, spiritualism, and the Yin/Yang dualism are all examples of particular beliefs or practices rooted in the culture of a particular ethnic group. Although these beliefs and practices may not have been scientifically validated, they can nevertheless have a powerful influence on what a client believes to be an accurate description of an illness or an effective method of cure. "Although folk medicine may be defined as primitive by outsiders, it is functional for the persons within a culture" (Henderson and Primeaux, 1981, p. 175).

The more nurses learn about the ethnically derived health beliefs and practices of the children and families in their care, the better able they will be to create a relationship of mutual respect and trust, which is necessary for effective health care.

Effect on Participation "Allegiance to an ethnic group results in certain structural and functional variations in family organization which are durable because they are valued"

TABLE 3-1 Comparison of Health-related Factors and Subcultures

	Definition of health	Cause of illness—is prevention possible; if so, how?	Name of healer, healing practices	Problems of entry to health care system	Communication patterns	Sexuality and family life	Beliefs about death
Navajo Indian	Harmony between individual, earth, and supernatural, as well as the ability to survive difficult circumstances[1,2]	Disease is disharmony and can be caused by violating taboo or attack by witch; illness prevented through elaborate religious rituals; do not believe in germ theory[1,2]	Medicine man, who is more than average human being, is therefore influential figure; medicine man diagnoses and treats problem; treatments include yucca root, massage, herbs, and chanting; his chant states person will get well, and person believes him[1,2]	Language; will first visit medicine man; general beliefs are not compatible with health care system and structure; problems also include money and past experiences of disrespect; fear of spirits of dead may influence decision to leave hospital early[1,2]	Time of silence after each speaker to show respect and reflection on what they said; little eye contact; time orientation not very strict; recording of conversation invasion of privacy[1,2]	Family, extended family, and tribal ties strong; cooperation emphasized; consider children as individuals as soon as they can talk, therefore can make own decisions[1,2]	Fear of spirits of dead; children and family should be with dying person[1]
Hispanic-American	Gift from God also good luck; can tell healthy person by robust appearance and report of feeling well[1,3,4]	Illness is punishment from God for wrongdoing, to be suffered; it can be prevented by eating well, praying, being good, and working; wearing medals may help; physically, illness is an imbalance between "hot" and "cold" properties of body[1,3,4]	Healer called curandero; cures hot illness with cold medicine and reverse; classification of hot and cold diseases varies; penicillin is hot medicine; massages and cleanings are common[4]	Language; will first go to woman for advice, then if needed, to "señora," then to curandero, then to physician; many migrant workers are Hispanic, and frequent moves may make access to medical care difficult; belief that hospital is place to go to die causes underuse of system; modesty may result in woman bringing friend to physician with her[1,3,4]	Confidentiality and modesty important; too many questions are insulting; it is more acceptable to make tentative statement to which they can respond; time orientation not strict; politeness essential[1,3-5]	High degree of modesty, may prefer home births for this reason; men are breadwinners, women homemakers; women are healers, men make all decisions[1,3-5]	Afterlife of heaven and hell exists

continued on next page

TABLE 3-1 continued

	Definition of health	Cause of illness—is prevention possible; if so, how?	Name of healer, healing practices	Problems of entry to health care system	Communication patterns	Sexuality and family life	Beliefs about death
Traditional black	Harmony with nature, no separation of mind and body[4]	Disease is disharmony caused by spirits and demons; it can be prevented through good diet, rest, cleanliness, and laxatives to clean out system; some use of copper and silver bracelets for prevention	Some belief in voodoo still prevalent; religious healing practiced; geophagia (eating of clay) and pica (eating of starch) practiced[4,6]	May seek folk or religious healer first; money and type of service affect decision; emergency room frequent entry point; black women have high "non-compliance" rate[4,6]	Racism toward blacks still prevalent; common names for symptoms should be known by health worker; time orientation not strict	Matriarchy prevalent; almost 30% of black families have woman head of household; therefore women make decisions[4,6]	Death is passage from evils of this world to another state; blacks have shorter life expectancy than national average[6]
Chinese-American	Balance of yin and yang (negative and positive energy forces); healthy body is gift from parents and ancestors[4,7,8]	Illness caused by imbalance of yin and yang, which may be due to overexertion or prolonged sitting; disease is prevented through better adaptation to nature[4,7]	Acupuncture and moxibustion (which is a therapeutic application of heat to skin) restore balance of yin and yang; herbal remedies such as ginseng used for many illnesses; healer is called physician[4,7]	Language; traditional Chinese physicians were paid to keep their patients well and cared for sick without fees because illness indicated they had failed in their job; Chinese physicians are available in community and may encourage patients to use Western physician; family spokesman may accompany patient to Western physician[4,7]	Open expression of emotions not acceptable; therefore might not complain about pain or symptoms; may smile when does not understand[4,7]	Women subservient to men; patriarchal family; ancestor worship and respect for obedience for parents observed; divorce considered disgrace[1,4,5]	Reincarnation[7]
Low income	Functional definition; if you can work, you are healthy[5,9]	Belief that illness is not preventable; fatalism common; future orientation minimal because present problems are too great[1,5,9]	Will often rely on folk healers and remedies because of belief and problems gaining access to health care system[5]	Use of public funding may limit access and type of care; present time orientation and beliefs about prevention may cause delay in obtaining care; inability to afford health insurance; may lose day's pay to go to physician[5,9]	May use slang and language of subculture; may view providers as authoritarian; time orientation not strict[5]	Many single-parent families with woman head of household[9]	Depends on culture and religion

TABLE 3-1 continued

	Definition of health	Cause of illness—is prevention possible; if so, how?	Name of healer, healing practices	Problems of entry to health care system	Communication patterns	Sexuality and family life	Beliefs about death
High income	No data available	General belief in prevention of illness through diet, exercise, and good health habits; motivators such as previous experience or family tradition are influential in actual practice of prevention[5]	Combination of traditional practices of religion and culture, frequent use of health care system and self-help information[5]	Access not too difficult, usually through private physician; most have health insurance through employer[5]	Most like health care culture; cannot be expected to understand jargon	Women more likely to have career by choice than financial necessity	Depends on culture and religion
Health care culture	Optimal level of functioning; more than absence of disease; physical, emotional, social, and mental health included[5]	Scientific approach to cause of illness; prevention involves periodic physical examinations, laboratory studies, innoculations, as well as avoiding smoking and overeating, etc.[4]	Healing done by physician, usually takes place in office or hospital; treatments based on scientific knowledge and are frequently embarrassing or uncomfortable; often emotional component of disease is ignored[4]	Physician is main access to system; focus is basically curing illness rather than prevention; encouragement given to population to seek care as soon as symptoms appear; consider health care system as only provider	Widespread use of jargon and specialized language; large percentage of workers from middle class; often expect gratitude for care given; time orientation strict; written records kept[4]	Hierarchy, with physicians making decisions	Death usually means workers have failed to do their job; elaborate means are used to keep people alive; ethical and legal questions are being discussed and tested

[1]Data from Brownlee, A. T.: 1978. Community, culture, and care: a cross-cultural guide for health workers. The C. V. Mosby Co., St. Louis.

[2]Data from Wood, R.: 1976. The American Indian and health. In Ethnicity and health care. NLN publ. no. 14–1625, pp. 29–35.

[3]Data from Gonzales, H.: 1976. Health care needs of the Mexican American family. In Ethnicity and health care, NLN publ. no. 14–1625, pp. 21–28.

[4]Data from Spector, R.: 1979. Cultural diversity in health and illness. Appleton-Century-Crofts, New York.

[5]Data from Murray, R., and Zentner, J.: 1975. Nursing assessment and health promotion through the life span. Prentice-Hall, Englewood Cliffs, N.J.

[6]Data from Martin, B.: 1976. Ethnicity and health care: Afro-Americans. In Ethnicity and health care. NLN publ. no. 14–1625, pp. 47–55.

[7]Data from Wang, R.: 1976. Chinese Americans and health care. In Ethnicity and health care. NLN publ. no. 14–1625, pp. 9–18.

[8]Data from Channing, G.: 1955. What is a Christian Scientist? In Rosten, L., editor: A guide to religions of America. Simon & Schuster, New York.

[9]Data from Fromer, M.: 1979. Community health care and the nursing process. The C. V. Mosby Co., St. Louis.

SOURCE: Gingrich-Crass J: Structural variables: Factors affecting adaptation. In: *School nursing: A framework for practice.* Wold SJ. Mosby, 1981, pp. 136–141. Copyright 1981. Reprinted with permission of the C. V. Mosby Co.

(Miller and Janosik, 1980, p. 59). Behaviors and attitudes that relate to family customs, rituals, priorities, and ideals are values that endure over time because they provide a sense of identity, belonging, and continuity. No one is born with these values; rather, they are learned through verbal and nonverbal exchanges with society as its members represent the cultural and ethnic traditions. Value acquisition is a dynamic process that begins at birth and continues throughout life.

As the family interacts with others in the external environment, its boundary regulates the amount and type of input from other systems. In this way the family decides what coincides or is acceptable and what is not (what is ignored and what is rejected). How rigid or porous the family boundary is varies greatly within ethnic groups, as well as from one type of ethnic group to another. The more porous the family boundary, the greater the assimilation of attitudes, beliefs, and values from the new culture, with a corresponding decrease in the commitment to the ethnic heritage of the family.

In the United States today there is a growing recognition and pride in ethnic diversity and less support for its total assimilation as previously promoted by supporters of the "melting pot" perspective. This increased ethnic awareness is of significance for nurses. Unless nurses adapt their teaching and implementation of nursing actions to the family's ethnic characteristics, they risk inappropriate and ineffective care. "When family values differ markedly from those of the larger system, there is a likelihood of conflict between the two systems" (Miller and Janosik, 1980, p. 59). An individual's customs seem perfectly natural to that individual; likewise, the customs and beliefs of children and families from different cultural and ethnic traditions are valued as a natural and important part of their lives. Sometimes, for example, the dietary preferences of a family can influence childrearing values and compliance with specified protocol.

As a case in point, a young mother continued to feed her 15-month-old child strained, prepared baby food rather than table food, as she had been advised. The nurse was concerned about the child's nutritional status and opportunity for independent feeding experiences. It occurred to the nurse that the ethnicity of this family might offer some clues. This was validated when the nurse learned that the family was of West Indian heritage and that their dietary preference was for food that was highly spiced with curry and pepper. The mother had remembered an earlier admonition by the nurse to restrict salt and spices for the child and therefore felt she was complying with the advice that had been given to her. The nurse then worked with the mother to identify ways to serve the child table foods prepared prior to the addition of strong spices. The mother was encouraged to participate in finding methods to meet the child's dietary needs and was happy to comply with the eventual plan.

The particular characteristics of several major cultural and ethnic groups in the United States will be described in the following sections: the black family, the Hispanic family, the Asian family, the Arab family, and the Native American family. These categories are obviously broad, and the subgroups within each description certainly deserve further discussion: the various Native American tribes; the Chinese, Japanese, Vietnamese, and other Asian groups; and the various black populations of Caribbean and African origin. Every ethnic group and subgroup has its own historical and contemporary details that are fascinating and that influence health care beliefs. When the nurse is knowledgeable about these specific values and beliefs, health-related information can be adapted to achieve congruence between it and the family system. When congruence occurs, cooperation and understanding usually follow.

The following discussion is restricted to general categories. The references cited in the section entitled "Additional Readings" at the end of this chapter are intended to provide supplementary information. The best resource for learning about the ethnic characteristics of a family, however, is from the family members themselves. The careful collection of data, as described in Chapter 2, is a valuable guide for making nursing decisions.

The Black American Family

The black American family is one of the most conspicuous ethnic groups in the United States and as such has undergone considerable analysis and study. The results of these efforts have received mixed reviews. Some of the criticisms leveled at these reports include oversight of the "institutional effects" of racism and the "adaptive mechanism" of the black American family (Greathouse and Miller, 1981), which perhaps have contributed to the long-standing position of many black families apart from the mainstream of society. Particular disparity appears to exist between the analytic results of black and white social scientists. Many white social scientists see the black family as disorganized and unstable, whereas black social analysts point out the diversity of black family structure, the tenacity of its folklore and religion, and the inappropriateness of comparing a subcultural family life with a set of white, middle-class family norms (Turner, 1973).

A brief, historical review shows the damaging effects the system of slavery had on the heritage and family forms of Afro-Americans. Tribal groups were dispersed, which forced slaves to learn English and adapt to new foods and customs to survive. The owners viewed the slaves as property to be bought and sold as they desired. Marriage and family life often were forbidden; however, they were valued highly by the slaves, who devised novel ceremonies to legitimize a relationship. Regardless of the meaning of marriage to the blacks, the white owner felt no obligation to honor it and would separate couples or family members by selling or using one of them sexually.

Following emancipation in 1865, family life, especially in the agrarian South, gained some stability. Although legally free, life was a struggle because many blacks did not have the skills, finances, farmland, or support to provide for their basic needs. Some blacks saw migration to the northern urban centers as their salvation. Unfortunately, this move had as many negative components as remaining in the south because racism, limited job opportunities, and degrading living conditions awaited them.

The black family has a long history of survival through adaptation to a hostile environment. They are perhaps the least understood and most frequently stereotyped ethnic group. The dominant culture has found it easier to forget or deny the harsh psychologic, sociocultural, and economic conditions, both past and present, that have necessitated family adaptation behaviors that differ from those of the prevailing culture.

The impression that black families are matriarchal, disorganized and loosely bonded is a stereotype much disputed by social scientists (Hill, 1972; Gutman, 1976). The following are some of the factors contributing to this perception:

1. Slave owners tended to keep mothers and children together but bought and sold males regardless of their status as spouse or father
2. A high proportion of women were employed prior to and during the industrial era because of the availability of domestic work. Although they were underpaid and exploited, they learned managerial skills as cooks, nursemaids, and household organizers that they transferred to their own families
3. Many black males in urban areas experienced low-status and irregular employment

Hill's (1972) research noted that although they were at times unable to operationalize their values, the black families adhered to such sacrosanct American values as the family unit, honest work, achievement, and religion. Unique survival traits, which included strong kinship systems and role flexibility, however, placed them outside of the mainstream of acceptable role performance. Women were often required to perform several roles well, including parent, worker, and household manager.

Ostracized for years from craft unions, equal education, and opportunities for advancement, black males often suffered as second-class citizens. The limited employment opportunities for men contrasted with the somewhat more available ones for women and resulted in role redefinition. In many black families the woman is the sole, primary, or collateral breadwinner. "Problems attending blackness in a racially biased society undoubtedly have contributed to inadequate role performance among black men, decreased the importance of matrimony, and increased the divorce rates" (Miller and Janosik, 1980, p. 89).

The number of black households headed by women is high—over 30%. This is more of a socioeconomic phenomenon than an ethnic preference. Epstein (1974) observed that the family structure as altered by the effects of racism has affected the socialization of black children, especially boys. The girls are given preferential treatment because there are more opportunities for them to be upwardly mobile. Consequently, boys lose their incentive to excel academically and to take responsibility and plan for their future. Development of a positive self-image by all their children is a crucial goal of black parents.

This is far from the only structure for black family life, however. Variations exist according to geographic, economic, social, and educational experiences of the family (Greathouse and Miller, 1981). According to the US Department of Commerce, as many as 61% of black families live in a nuclear family structure with two parents. There also remains a historical emphasis on strong bonds of kinship, the importance of the extended family, and the role of religion and friends for mutual, social, emotional, and economic support.

Major issues still confronting many black children and their families center on economic disadvantages, a high rate of unemployment, particularly among adolescents, and the problems that result: more limited access to health promotion resources, substandard housing, and infant mortality.

A variety of folk medicine beliefs and practices have evolved for the black community and should be understood by the nurse. According to Greathouse and Miller (1981), some of the common preventive measures employed by black mothers include tying a black string around the child's wrist to prevent straining and minimize discomfort from constipation and applying a belly band around the infant's abdomen to prevent umbilical hernias. Spector (1979, pp. 236–238) lists the following home remedies relatively common in the black community:

1. Sugar and turpentine are mixed together and taken by mouth to get rid of worms. This combination can be also used to cure a backache when rubbed on the skin from the navel to the back.
2. Numerous types of poultices are employed to fight infection and inflammation. The poultices are placed on the part of the body that is painful and/or infected, in order to draw out the cause of the affliction.

   One type of poultice is made of potatoes. The potatoes are sliced or grated and placed in a bag, which is placed on the affected area of the body. The potatoes turn black and, as this occurs, the disease goes away. It is now believed that, as these potatoes spoil, they produce a penicillin mold that is able to destroy the infectious organism. Another type of poultice is prepared from cornmeal and peach leaves that are cooked together and placed either in a bag or in a piece of flannel cloth. The cornmeal ferments and combines with an enzyme in the peach leaves. The antiseptic from the fermented cornmeal and the enzyme destroy the bacteria and hasten the healing process. A third poultice, made with onions, is used to heal infections, and a flaxseed poultice is used to treat earaches.
3. Herbs from the woods are used in a multitude of ways. Herb teas are prepared—for example, from goldenrod root—to treat pain and reduce fevers. Sassafras tea is frequently used to treat colds. Other herbs that are boiled to make a tea include the root or weed of rabbit tobacco.
4. Bluestone, a mineral found in the ground, is used as medicine for open wounds. The stone is crushed into a powder and sprinkled on the affected area. It prevents inflammation and is also used to treat poison ivy.
5. To treat a "crick" in the neck, two pieces of silverware are crossed over the painful area in the form of an X.
6. Nine drops of turpentine nine days after intercourse act as a contraceptive.
7. Cuts and wounds can be treated with sour or spoiled

milk that is placed on stale bread, wrapped in a cloth, and placed on the wound.

8. Salt and pork (salt pork) placed on a rag can also be used to treat cuts and wounds.
9. A sprained ankle can be treated by placing clay in a dark leaf and wrapping it around the ankle.
10. A method for treating colds is with hot lemon water with honey.
11. When congestion is present in the chest and the person is coughing, he can be wrapped with warm flannel after his chest is rubbed with hot camphorated oil.
12. An expectorant for colds consists of chopped raw garlic, chopped onion, fresh parsley, and a little water, all mixed in a blender.
13. Hot toddies are used to treat colds and congestion. These drinks consist of hot tea with honey, lemon, peppermint, and a dash of brandy or whatever alcoholic beverage the person likes and is available. Vicks Vaporub is also swallowed.
14. A fever can be broken by placing raw onions on the feet and wrapping them in warm blankets.
15. Boils are treated by cracking a raw egg, and peeling the white skin off the inside of the shell, and placing it on the boil. This brings the boil to a head.
16. Garlic can be placed on the ill person or in the room to remove the "evil spirits" that have caused the illness.

Some folk beliefs are magical such as the wearing of amulets or charms to ward off disease. In some locations voodoo is practiced to remove spells and hexes believed to cause illness. Most folk medicine is associated with procedures such as warm applications, massages, the use of herbal teas to treat colds, pain, or fever, and numerous types of poultices to treat inflammation and infection (Bullough and Bullough, 1982).

As with many groups in which economic hardship and the scarcity of food have been long-standing problems, great emphasis is placed on feeding the young child. Solid foods are often introduced early because the parent equates being full with being happy. The family may be more concerned that the child eat and not be hungry than that the child receive adequate nutrition.

Patterns of discipline vary widely and are related more to the social, educational, and economic level of the parents than their ethnicity. In one study the tendency of black middle-class parents to be less restrictive and directive, to interact more verbally, and to stress feelings and motives was similar to those of white middle-class parents. Black lower-class parents were less verbal, more restrictive, and more directive, as were their white counterparts (Zegiob and Forehand, 1975). It must be noted, however, that these definitions of class can be arbitrary, and that several others exist (working class, capitalist class, etc.).

Rearing a child in a subculture that differs from the dominant culture is a special challenge to the black family because feelings of ambivalence, hostility, and pride exist. Although material possessions may be less available, the child is encouraged to participate in the adults' activities. Children are welcome, and the sharing of child-care tasks by siblings and other family members is assumed. This exposure to adult roles and responsibilities encourages the child's role modeling behavior. The adult role is learned early, and peer groups are cherished as the arena for testing and discussing these new roles (Comer and Poussaint, 1975).

Peer group learning is significant for black children. In this context they learn communication patterns and ebonics (black English), codes of conduct, skills, and sex-role behaviors. Black parents try to control the peer group influence by supervising contacts, forbidding interactions with individuals judged to be trouble-makers, or even moving to a different neighborhood.

Despite racism and economic hardships, black parents strive to provide their children with love, security, a sense of belonging, independence, and the incentive to succeed. The male in particular is socialized to be independent, aggressive, and strong. Sports and athletic abilities are valued highly and considered by many blacks to be their "ticket to success."

Childrearing, socialization, and attitudes about health are culturally related. The nurse must be sensitive to this relationship between the ethnic and religious values of the black child and family and their unique strengths and limitations as they relate to health-seeking and response behaviors.

The Hispanic Family

The term "Hispanic" is used to refer to several unique subcultural groups that share a common language and Spanish heritage. The predominant Hispanic groups in the United States include the Mexican- Americans (Chicanos) and the Puerto Rican-Americans. Individuals who can trace their families to Cuba and South and Central America are also referred to as Hispanics (Queen and Habenstein, 1974).

Many of the Mexican-American families in this country populate areas in the west and southwest, particularly New Mexico, Texas, and California. Puerto Rican families have tended to settle in Northern urban areas such as New York City and Boston. The proximity of Florida to Cuba has attracted Cuban families to this area.

The historical backdrops to the settlement of these groups in the United States vary according to the economic and political conditions of the areas they left. For the Chicano and Puerto Rican groups, economic hardship and the need for labor in this country were the chief attractions leading to immigration. Many Cuban-American families came here for political reasons, whereas others came for economic reasons.

The settlement and assimilation of Mexican-American families in this country is closely tied to the availability of work and the economic hardships of life in Mexico (Ehling, 1981). A common misconception, however, is that most of these people are employed as migrant farm workers (Spector, 1979). That the initial influx of Mexican workers into the southwest was farm laborers is well documented, as well as the hardships, economic abuses, and prejudices that many experienced. More recently, a gradual shift in the geographic and labor movements of the Mexican-American family has occurred, and today the majority live in large cities. Unfortunately, they must grapple with the same realities of crowded urban living that face many other subcultural groups, including the blacks and Puerto Ricans (Queen and Habenstein, 1974).

Generalizations regarding the characteristics, attitudes, and beliefs of the Hispanic family and their childrearing practices cannot do justice to the variety and richness of these groups. Certain characteristics, however, are predominant and can be cited.

The family of Hispanic ancestry, in fact, shares a common bond with several other subcultural groups in terms of its strong sense of family (nuclear and extended). Many groups whose origins can be traced to the Mediterranean area of the world (Hispanic, Italian, Greek, and Portugese) exhibit similar characteristics in their sexual role definitions, emphasis on respect and discipline, and open displays of affection toward their children. Hispanic and Italian families also share a belief in the evil eye (mal ojo), special social and religious ties to a child's godparents, and the value of the firstborn male child (Gambino, 1974; Ehling, 1981; Lacay, 1981).

The Hispanic father is viewed as the ultimate authority, but his involvement in the day-to-day activities of childrearing is minimal; child care is the mother's responsibility (Queen and Habenstein, 1974). Children are highly valued, and their health and well-being are attended to with a variety of rituals, customs, and folk practices. The gradual assimilation of the Hispanic-American family into American society, however, has changed some of these practices and the value attached to them. According to Ehling (1981), the Mexican practice of "la dieta," for example, where mother and infant are restricted indoors for 40 days, has diminished in popularity. Nevertheless, a wealth of folk practices and health beliefs have been retained. Special care of the child's head, particularly the fontanel, is stressed, and the use of medicinal herbs and potions is common. Olive oil is particularly valued for its preventive and healing properties, and drafts and chills are to be avoided (Ehling, 1981).

As with the black American family, some Hispanic mothers may use a belly band to prevent umbilical hernias. The feeding of the infant is important, and adding cereal to the bottle is a common practice because a fat infant is thought to be a healthy one.

The structure of the Hispanic family and the involvement of a large number of relatives in the child's care have important implications for the nurse in understanding the patterns of interactions, socialization, and discipline experienced by the child. Respect, politeness, and modesty are highly valued as the child interacts daily with several adult relatives and family friends. In the Mexican-American family less emphasis is placed on rigid rules, harsh punishments, and rigorous toilet training, whereas Puerto Rican families place more value on the discipline of the child. With adolescence, differences in these patterns become more obvious. Boys more often are encouraged to develop relationships outside the home and allowed a wider range of experience, whereas the girls are carefully protected, being allowed to date only when chaperoned. These patterns are gradually changing as social and peer pressure conflict with traditional roles and young girls resist the restrictive authority of their parents (Queen and Habenstein, 1974).

It is important for the nurse working with Hispanic family groups to be familiar with their culture. Only then is it possible to give assistance that is both well-intentioned and culturally appropriate. Brownlee (1978) noted that every group has its visible parts—dress, housing, language, and food—and its invisible parts—traditions, attitudes, beliefs, and customs. The invisible parts are the most valued and the most likely to be misinterpreted by outsiders. Many Hispanic families use a combination of folk and western health resources. Whenever possible, the nurse should incorporate the folk health care practices into the teaching and care provided.

Characteristics of the family structure and function must be considered when interacting with Hispanic families. The authority for decision making often resides with the father or an older female member and not the mother. It is important for the decision maker to be present when communications and instructions are given. It is not unusual for a Hispanic person to seem to comprehend information when in reality such understanding does not exist. During early childhood, Hispanics are taught to respect authority; therefore, they will feign understanding so as not to offend the nurse. For most Hispanics, family privacy is valued highly. They resent questions that they interpret as intrusive. They believe that personal family problems should remain within the family and that it is shameful to disclose them to an outsider. The nurse must be tactful and considerate of this fact when collecting data during the assessment phase of the nursing process. Their religious beliefs also contribute to their motivation to seek health care. Good health is perceived as a gift from God and illness as punishment for wrongdoing. Some Hispanics delay seeking medical care because they assume that they must endure the illness as restitution for some evil deed. Religious commitment varies in intensity, but there is always a sense that disease and recovery are God's will.

The Asian Family

Asian populations in this country include several diverse subcultural groups who can trace their origins to China, Japan, Vietnam, Hawaii, the Philippines, and other areas in the Far East. Chinese-Americans have a long history of settlement in the United States, whereas the Vietnamese are more recent immigrants to this country.

The cultural and social attitudes, beliefs, and values of the Asian-American family are grounded in a long history and strong religious traditions. For several of these groups, Confucianism has played a major role in shaping these values and beliefs. "Confucianism was based on two themes: (1) common people or the lower class should be in an entirely subordinate position, and (2) patriarchy and the family are a unit for social action" (Sodetani- Shibata, 1981, pp. 103–104).

The length of time that a family has been in the United States and the number of generations that have been reared here play a significant part in shaping the apparent role distributions, patterns of interaction, and childrearing practices of the Asian-American family. The Japanese, in fact, have given specific names to each succeeding generation in this country (Sodetani-Shibata, 1981). Traditionally, parents held authoritative positions within the family unit, and the children were required to make many filial expressions of duty and respect toward the parents. Verbal communication among family members was less frequent in Asian-American families than in some other subcultural groups, although more emphasis, perhaps, was placed on nonverbal behaviors and indirect expressions of affection (Suzuki, 1980).

The gradual assimilation over time of these groups into American society has resulted in some changes (Arkoff, Meredith, and Iwahara, 1967). The remnants of their beliefs and values persist to greater or lesser degrees in Asian-American families, however. For each group, the family unit is the primary social unit, and filial duty toward one's parents and older relatives is expected. In the Chinese family ancestor worship may be practiced. Stoicism, humility, modesty, and loyalty are important virtues that color much of the overt behavior of the Asian-American.

These virtues also underlie the childrearing practices of the family. Although the infant and young child is generally indulged and readily appeased, the parent adopts sterner forms of discipline as the child matures, thus instilling values and desired behaviors. Clear, gender-related childrearing practices are noticeable even in those families who have been influenced by the dominant western culture in this country. Traditional cultural customs, language, and maternal attitudes tend to foster determination and ambition in male children and modesty and passivity in female children (Suzuki, 1980). The nature of the extended family, the role of the elders in the family, and the importance of the child respecting the parent has resulted, to a large extent, in this phenomenon.

Early toilet training is valued in the traditional Chinese family and perhaps can be related to the emphasis that this culture places on self-control (Char, 1981). Many Vietnamese mothers believe that a fat infant is a healthy infant and may need to be guided in their feeding practices. Generally, however, the food practices of the Asian-American family are well balanced and admired by western nutritionists for their low cholesterol content and high fiber and bulk.

Each subcultural Asian group has its own set of folkways, health beliefs, curatives, and preventive health practices. For the Chinese, the balance between the "Yin and Yang," or darkness and light, is considered vital to good health. The Japanese and Vietnamese also view illness as a result of disharmony with the universe or nature. Special foods, herbs, and acupuncture are utilized, although often in conjunction with traditional western health practices.

The Arab Family

The number of Arab families in the United States has increased, particularly in the last 20 years (Meleis and Sorrell, 1981). The countries of origin for these people are primarily Lebanon, Syria, Iraq, Egypt, and other countries near the Persian Gulf. Each of these areas lends its own flavor to the life of the particular Arab family, as does the family's religion (Christian or Islamic). Several cultural values and characteristics, however, transcend the geographic and religious differences that may exist. Other variables, such as socioeconomic level, education, experience, and the length of time the family has been in the United States, all affect the family's "Arabism" (Meleis and Sorrell, 1981).

The Arab family, like that of several other immigrant and minority groups, is the central point around which much in the child's life revolves. Strong relationships exist beyond the nuclear family and include extended family members and close friends. These significant others provide support and caring to the family and serve as adjuncts to the family in times of need. Although the social nature of Arab family life is adult-centered, children are not excluded from participating in a wide range of adult activities and celebrations. According to Meleis and Sorrell (1981), the Arab family focuses on the here and now and places less emphasis on planning for the future. This may be a result of a long history of adversity in the Arab world. Punctuality is also less important to most Arabs than some other ethnic groups. These characteristics may have implications for the health care professional in assessing a child's development, health, and family milieu.

The gender-related differences in the adult role responsibilities and prohibitions are conveyed early on to the children in an Arab family. Boys are encouraged to be self-confident, strong, and able to function in the world outside the family. Girls are required to be circumspect in their demeanor and dress and are more closely held within the family unit and the home. Male children, particularly first-born males, are particularly valued in the traditional Arab family.

The Arab family, like many Mediterranean groups, also believes strongly in the power of the evil eye. Arabs might suspect someone who praises or compliments the baby as being capable of casting the evil eye on the child. Therefore, the nurse should be careful to focus her praise on the mother's skills rather than the child's attributes (Meleis and Sorrell, 1981).

As with other cultures, the Arab family brings with it a host of myths, folkways, rituals, and practices to either prevent or ward off illness. Stoicism with pain is not valued. The use of touch and human contact, however, is more highly valued for the reduction of stress and discomfort than some of the more traditional western approaches.

The differentiation of parental roles, the importance of the extended family, and the experience of the child and family in its unique social situation must be considered by the nurse in providing care to the Arab child and family. Religious taboos and culturally based values, beliefs, and attitudes must be understood and incorporated into the care plan.

The Native American Family

To do justice to the richness and variety of Native American family life would require an in-depth discussion of each of the nearly 300 different Indian tribes (Farris and Farris, 1981). Regional and specific tribal differences are numerous and influence everything from the methods of defining lineage within an extended family to food preferences and dietary habits.

Generally, the Native American family is the primary social unit for the young child. The family, however, can consist of aunts, uncles, and grandparents. The availability and close proximity of these relatives to the nuclear family makes the sharing of child-care responsibilities more likely and increases the opportunities for the child to observe a variety of role relationships and interactions. The requirements and restrictions imposed by the federal government on Indian life throughout American history have, in some instances, weakened and rocked the traditional stability of Indian family life.

The values and beliefs that transcend specific tribal custom and provide a direct influence on the Native American child include the following:

1. A belief in and respect for the harmony and interrelatedness of man and nature
2. Food as a social vehicle
3. The use of ceremonies and rituals for purification and religious purposes
4. The transmission of the history and ways of the tribe and its role responsibilities by the elders to the youths
5. Egalitarian relationships among various age groups within the tribe
6. The right to privacy and self-determination (Spector, 1979)

Life for many modern Native American families can be difficult because of poverty, substandard living conditions, and the erosion of traditional family and tribal ways (Farris and Farris, 1981). These factors have increased family stress, created ambivalent value systems within the family, and increased feelings of alienation and isolation. These factors have obvious implications for the nurse working with these families and the systems that address their needs (Sevcovic, 1973).

The health care needs of any group are best met when the provider has a comprehensive understanding of that group's culture. For example, there is a Native American medicine man who works in conjunction with his wife (a white physician) to provide comprehensive and appropriate health care to an Indian population. The blending of these traditions has resulted in higher compliance, improved health, and increased interaction between the ways of the "white man" and the Indian. This kind of creativity exemplifies how understanding, respect, and cooperation can make a significant difference in the role that the health care professional can play with culturally diverse clients.

Socioeconomic Culture

A cultural system can be identified not just along ethnic lines but also according to social and economic factors that may make the client's assumptions and values significantly different from those of the nurse. Most nurses are personally familiar with the socioeconomic realities of the working and middle classes. Although ethnic, racial, and cultural backgrounds are as diverse in the nursing profession as in any other, the advanced education and training that nurses receive results in a relatively secure socioeconomic position. Moreover, despite the various backgrounds of individual health care workers, it can be argued that the health care system as a whole reflects dominant middle-class values (Orque, Bloch, and Monrroy, 1983, p. 40). Nurses need to learn and understand the conditions and needs of those children and families who may occupy social strata different from their own in order to overcome cultural biases in the delivery of nursing care. Children become aware of social class differences at an early age, particularly as they enter school (Elkin and Handel, 1978, p. 76). The realities of lifestyle and the subsequent forces that affect the child of an affluent family are often as unfamiliar to the nurse as the pressures and stressors affecting the child who lives in poverty. Robert Coles, in his series on *Children of Crisis,* addressed the issues that influence both privileged and poor children in separate volumes of his work (Coles, 1977). Stereotyped beliefs and prejudices affect both of these seemingly diverse groups. This is an irony that transcends social class.

Poverty

One definition of social class is the unequal distribution of material goods, power, and prestige that cuts across society. A sense of powerlessness may accompany poverty and can be a major obstacle to the nurse–client relationship and the self-care abilities of the poor family. "The feeling of powerlessness which characterizes the culture of poverty stems from poor peoples' dependency on organizations to meet their socio-economic and health care needs" (Robertson, 1969, p. 44).

For the child growing up in poverty, there may be a consistent lack of material advantage, a continuing sense of powerlessness, a narrowly confined world of experience, and a constant sense of frustration. Conditions of substandard and insufficient housing and sanitation, poor nutrition, and inadequate or inappropriate stimuli can all seriously impair a child's health and general well-being.

In addition to these direct consequences of these conditions for health maintenance, poverty can have further implications for those seeking to maintain or restore health. For various reasons, the poor may not use the health care system to the same extent or in the same ways as do people from other economic strata. A poor family may feel that the quality of care available to them is not as good as that available to those able to pay more. They may not seek treatment for a health problem for several reasons: lack of funds, fear of lost time from work, unawareness of services, or the need to maintain pride of self-sufficiency. Educational disadvantage may impair their recognizing the severity of a particular health problem or the ineffectiveness and dangers of some health practices (Orque, Bloch, and Monrroy, 1983, pp. 39–41). A poor family may simply be excluded from the health care delivery system by being priced out of the medical care market. Finally, access to quality health care may be problematic. "Many rural and urban poor lack qualified professionals to attend to them. Even in the cities, health care facilities are not always located where the poor can reach them. At present there has been significant improvement in health care services for the poor, but we still have a significant way to go, both in delivering effective health care and in getting the poor to effectively utilize what is available" (Bullough and Bullough, 1982, p. 154).

Even when a poor family is able to obtain health care, the contrast between the health care facility and the family's home environment may induce culture shock or lower self-esteem. A sterile, quiet, and orderly hospital may bewilder a family from a dirty, noisy, chaotic slum neighborhood (Henderson and Primeaux, 1981). A less effective nurse–client relationship may result from such a reaction. However, the nurse can help to mitigate their reaction through alert, sensitive, and individualized care. The key lies in acknowledging the strengths of the family and using this knowledge to help empower them. The goal is to promote optimal health.

Affluence

Although a wealthy family would not seem to lack the resources to take effective advantage of and have access to the health care system, there are other potential risks of which the nurse should be aware. For one thing, less is known about the very rich than about other groups. "Anthropologists have put in a lot of time with Indians and Eskimos but they have not studied upper-middle-class or wealthy American families. . . . Where are the long scholarly bibliographies that tell us about the values and ideals, the customs and habits, the beliefs and practices of the well-off, the quite well-off, the almost rich, and the rich indeed?" (Coles, 1977, p. 559).

The child from a wealthy home may be subject to inconsistent or apathetic care given by a succession of nannies or governesses. Large, isolating homes may limit the social contacts and attachments available to the child and result in poor communication and dispersed attachments (Prout, 1980). A strong sense of family heritage and explicit codes of behavior are often strengths for these families; but they may also impair the development of close, continuous child–parent relationships. For example, the work and social demands of affluent parents may encroach on their time and availability to nurture their children.

It would, however, be incorrect to assume that wealth and poverty in and of themselves necessarily impair the development of children or create problematic family relationships. Obviously, many people from both economic strata have developed, achieved, and prospered. How the family perceives and copes with their economic situation is as important as the structural facts of that situation. Completely different economic facts may result in the same risk factor affecting the child's health. A child's isolation, for example, may result from the parent's need to earn a subsistence income, in the case of the poor family, or, in the case of the wealthy family, to maintain a certain level of social or financial success. The relative stability of family life has been found to be an important factor in predicting the chances of a child growing up to have problems that might be classified as dysfunctional (Bullough and Bullough, 1982, p. 163). Such stability can be undermined in an affluent family as well as in a poor one.

Cultural Assessment

The assessment of social and cultural factors can greatly influence the eventual outcomes of the nurse's relationship with the child and family. Many aspects of an individual's life are the direct result of social and cultural factors. For example, religious customs, the use of language, food preferences, manner of dress, styles of parenting, and response to pain are all directly related to the customs, norms, and values of an individual's social and cultural milieu. Rules regarding discipline, methods of communication, plans for the future, goals and aspirations, and the degree of trust or mistrust of outsiders (including health care workers and agencies) also will be influenced by social and cultural forces.

An awareness of ethnicity is important in the nursing assessment because part of that assessment is comparing collected data with norms, and physical and behavioral norms may vary from one ethnic group to another, as discussed earlier. "If the nurse is not aware of the patient's culture, [the nurse] is likely to misjudge the impact of the patient's culture on health care" (Orque, Bloch, and Monrroy, 1983, p. 9).

Two conceptual frameworks have been developed to assess the social and cultural subsystem of the child, one by Madeleine Leininger (1970) and another by Modesta Orque and colleagues (1983).

Leininger's Framework

Leininger cited three dimensions of the social and cultural subsystem: the normative subsystem, the practice subsystem, and the interpersonal relationship subsystem. The *normative subsystem* is the explicit and implicit norms that govern behavior. Norms rely on explicit rules that describe what individuals within the group should do *(prescribed norms)* and should not do *(proscribed norms)*. The second dimension, or *practice subsystem,* refers to the actual behavior of the group member as an expression of what the group thinks and believes. These behaviors are directly observable. Health-related behaviors such as eating practices, hygiene, and exercise patterns are observable examples of behaviors included in this dimension.

The third dimension is the most important. The *interpersonal relationship subsystem* is the foundation on which most of the group's behaviors and actions are based. The form that interpersonal relationships take and the methods of communication that arise between members of a group, such as the family, are the major determinants of group solidarity, stability, and functioning. Among the major facets of this dimension are the use and distribution of power within the system, social status and prestige characteristics motivating group members, the roles that group members assume or assign to one another, and the methods of communication and system of shared meanings that the members have evolved for their interactions.

Orque's Framework and Bloch's Assessment Guide

Orque's ethnic/cultural system framework contains eight categories of solutions to the problems of meeting basic human needs. Each component can affect other components and the cultural system as a whole. The relative importance of each component also will vary from person to person and from family to family. The eight components are as follows:

1. Family life processes
2. Diet
3. Religion
4. Art and history
5. Value orientations
6. Social group's interactive patterns
7. Language and communication process
8. Healing beliefs and practices

Building on Orque's framework, Bloch (1983) developed an assessment guide for ethnic/cultural variation. Both Orque's framework and Bloch's assessment guide are built on a concept of basic human needs that applies to both the nurse and the client. The four major data categories of Bloch's assessment guide are the cultural, sociologic, psychologic, and biologic/physiologic. These categories parallel the four subsystems of the individual child discussed in Chapter 2: the biophysical, cognitive, affective, and social.

The cultural data category includes ethnic origin and racial background, the value orientation of time, and alternative healing beliefs and practices. The importance that cultural factors have for the client also must be assessed. A family that has immigrated to the United States within the last 10 years, for instance, may hold more strictly to the values and beliefs of its native culture than one that has lived in this country for several generations.

In looking at the sociologic data, the nurse examines such factors as the family's economic situation, level of education, social network, and valued social institutions. In this data category the effects of wealth and poverty are appropriately placed.

The effect of a family's ethnic and cultural background on the self-concept of its members is a major factor assessed under the psychologic data category. Although it might be easy to assume that self-esteem would be generally lower for groups who feel alienated from the mainstream of society, some families feel their own ethnic heritage to be superior to the relatively brief tradition of "American" culture.

Biophysical variations among ethnic minority groups will have an important influence on the results of the nurse's physical assessment of a child. Skin assessment is a clear example, since variations in skin color are similar to those seen in certain pathologic conditions. In addition, certain ethnic groups may be more susceptible to certain diseases or may be more exposed to disease-causing agents in the environment than other groups. Other variations, such as lactose deficiency among Asians, will have implications for nutritional and other nursing interventions.

Key Assessment Questions

The foregoing discussion of Leininger, Orque, and Bloch's conceptualizations of ethnic and cultural variation make clear the importance of assessing these subsystems for effective nursing care of the child. A complete assessment of the social and cultural subsystems of the child and the child's family therefore should include answers to the following questions:

1. What is the ethnic/racial/religious background of this child and family?
2. How are children incorporated into this family?
3. How do ethnicity, religion, and race shape the parents' role(s) and those of the children in this family?
   a. How comfortable are the child and family in interacting outside the cultural subsystem?
   b. Do language barriers exist?
   c. How is this family's ethnic/racial heritage viewed by the larger culture?
   d. How does this child/family view its place in the larger culture?
   e. Is assimilation a goal?
   f. Is isolation a goal?
4. How does this family define member roles and child roles in terms of gender? How does the sex of this child influence the interactions and inputs that the child receives from the family and community in which it resides?

These questions should supply the nurse with a sufficient basis to begin the necessary exploration of the ethnic and cultural variables that will affect a child's and family's response to illness.

Other Implications for the Nurse

The social and cultural influences on children and their families also have a major impact on the role nurses play in their health care. Unlike some workers, whose functions are based on a more limited set of skills—typists, for example, or plumbers—nurses assume and fulfill their "roles" much as actors do: nursing care requires not just manual skill or applied knowledge but the participation of the nurse's entire person. It follows that understanding and preparing that person is essential to effectively performing in the role. It also would seem to be important to examine the nature of the role itself, that is, how the nurse's role relates to the child and family and to the society at large, with respect to the social and cultural influences that have been the subject of this chapter.

Personal Preparation

Every person is the product of a long process of socialization that lasts a lifetime—a process by which individuals learn how those around them expect them to behave and what behaviors they expect and value in others (Goode, 1964). It is important therefore not only to define and enact the many roles of the nurse but also to acknowledge, modify, and use as best as possible the strengths and attributes, weaknesses, and human frailties that each individual brings to an encounter. In their personal and professional lives, nurses' beliefs, values, and attitudes are enmeshed in their behavior and actions, views of health and illness, and decisions about themselves and others. How well nurses understand themselves has a direct effect on how well they will understand and care for others.

Acknowledging Biases The practice of nursing is directed toward meeting the needs of the individual, family, and community in an ever-changing society. Essential to this practice is an understanding of how individuals and groups of individuals interact and adapt over time and in a series of social contexts. As society changes, the needs of individuals also change. The role of the nurse in child health therefore includes the identification and individualization of those interventions that address the changing nature of society and the experiences that these changes create for the individual child, family, and community.

Significant to this practice is the ability and willingness of the nurse to acknowledge and understand personal cultural beliefs, values, and attitudes. This acknowledgment can free the nurse to provide truly holistic and humanistic care to all children and their families from a variety of cultural and ethnic backgrounds.

Unfortunately, it is all too easy to view and interpret the behaviors and life-styles of others from one's own cultural biases. Labeling, stereotyping, and imposing one's own values can significantly alter the ultimate effectiveness of the nurse–client interaction and may result in the alienation and possible withdrawal of the child and family from the health care system. The likelihood of this occurring might be minimized if greater attention is paid to the cultural differences that may exist between the nurse and the client.

Clarifying Values The provision of optimal and humanistic health care requires that nurses first understand the value system that they bring to a situation. Clearly, a multicultural society, such as the one present in the United States, consists of several dominant cultures and subcultures that specify the desirable behaviors and attitudes of their members. Each person belongs and ascribes to a unique set of norms and values on which assessments, decisions, and actions are based. The key is to recognize and accept the uniqueness, freedom, and autonomy of one's self and others in a situation.

Values clarification has been described as a process by which the individual explores the multiple attitudes and beliefs that govern personal behavior. The goal of this process is to discover those conceptions and misconceptions that color actions and attitudes, thereby freeing the professional to enter a nurse–client relationship with greater objectivity and sensitivity.

Several frameworks have been developed to clarify one's values for greater self-awareness and objectivity. The philosopher Martin Buber (1958) defined one approach as the "I-Thou" relationship. The focus of the nurse–client relationship, based on the "I-Thou" framework, requires a sensitivity to and acceptance of the differences between the cultural contexts that each person brings to an encounter.

Another framework that has been applied to values clarification is symbolic interactionism. This framework comes from social psychology. In essence symbolic interactionism focuses on the uniqueness of each individual and the dynamic nature of the interactions and activities in which people engage (Charon, 1979). Proponents of using this framework for values clarification believe it can improve the appreciation that one has for another's perspective by exploring the meaning attached to the symbols and cues inherent in interactions.

Numerous other frameworks for values clarification also have been developed. Although each may identify a different series of steps or strategies, the ultimate goal of each method is a clearer understanding and appreciation of the values and attitudes of one's self and others. This kind of awareness can free the nurse to empathize and relate to the human condition of the client and, in so doing, act as a true advocate and effective health provider. This process can assist in distinguishing assessments that are perhaps value-laden and based on cultural biases from assessments that are based on objective, scientifically supported rationales.

Client Interactions

If nurses continue to work toward improving their cultural and ethnic sensitivity, three beneficial effects will enhance the interaction with children and their families: an informed awareness on the part of the nurse, more effective nurse–client communication, and greater flexibility in making appropriate accommodations.

Awareness Many of the assessments and interventions that nurses employ in caring for clients are imbued with the values of the health care system, which may differ sharply from those of the clients. How often have nurses provided nutritional guidelines to clients based on their own dietary practices or those of the dominant culture? How much more effective nutritional guidance would be if it were provided in the context of the family's customs and food preferences—one in which meals and methods of preparation were discussed in more appropriate terms and with familiar ingredients.

Childrearing practices also are heavily laden with cultural values and norms. Those practices that may conflict with the values of the health care provider and the dominant culture may be diagnosed as alterations in parenting and subject to planned nursing strategies for modification. The intent of the provider may well be to facilitate parenting behavior and enhance the child's growth and development through well-planned interventions. The actual outcome, however, may be the withdrawal of the family from the health care system and the alienation of this group to further health care interventions. Discussions regarding such common issues as toilet training, discipline, and sleeping arrangements should reflect an awareness of the cultural beliefs and values of the child and family. Assessments and interventions should then be planned and enacted with these factors in mind. Whenever possible, alternatives and modifications should be designed and presented in the context of cultural awareness and empathy for the conditions that the child and family share. The direct involvement of the parents in developing the plan can help to ensure its relevance and appropriateness.

Communication In some ethnic and cultural groups, members are free to vocalize their pain and clearly convey their feelings of physical discomfort. People from Oriental cultures, however, respond to pain much more subtly—stoicism in response to physical discomfort is a cultural expectation. This is just one example of how culture and ethnicity can affect nurse–client communication.

Perhaps the most significant barrier to effective nurse–client interactions is the confusion and misunderstanding that can result from the process of communication. Communication is affected by culture in a variety of ways. The appropriateness of terms, the nuances of meaning, and the contextual aspects of the interaction are vital aspects to any relationship. For most people, the concept of space and the distance between individuals as they speak is an important cultural factor. The dominant culture of North America deemphasizes the personal and physical contact that is integral to the communication process of several other groups. In addition, the use of voice tones, hand and arm movements, and other nonverbal cues illustrates carefully prescribed differences from one culture to another.

For each family, methods of communicating, loving, disagreeing, and sharing develop. The ways in which they convey to each other information, support, a sense of urgency, or calm understanding messages are vital to each family's integrity. These very basic behaviors, which are essential to daily living, frequently, however, may be at odds with the expectations of individuals outside the family unit. Once again, it is imperative that the various patterns of communication that groups use be assessed in the total context of their situation. Systems analysis can be most useful for assessing this aspect of daily living. It is helpful, for example, for the nurse to ascertain who has the authority for decision making, how disagreement with this authority is expressed, and what the acceptable methods are of expressing feelings of respect and love between members in the family. In Italian families, for example, the father is viewed as the central authority, whereas true power regarding major household and childrearing decisions lies with the mother. This has clear implications for the parental roles that each parent adopts. When admiring Mexican-American infants, it is essential to include touch. Otherwise, the mother is convinced that the infant will develop symptoms of mal ojo, which consists of fitful crying, fever, diarrhea, and vomiting. They believe that nurses who do not touch an infant cannot be trusted.

Accommodation For the nurse to work with the child–family system, accommodations must be made to the unique expressions of the sociocultural dimensions that exist within the group. Direct and indirect observation of group interaction, knowledge of cultural values, and familiarity with a variety of subcultural practices will enhance the interventions implemented. The child–family unit therefore must be included when formulating the plan of care. Specific health care beliefs, taboos, and rituals can be accommodated by this approach.

Nurses who are sensitive and evaluate all forms of communication objectively are an important link between the family and the health care establishment. They are in the unique position of being informed about both the health care system and the family system and able to interpret the one to the other. Many of the folk traditions are an integral part of the cultural response to a health need, some are basic childrearing practices, and some have religious significance. Whenever possible, and this is most of the time, these traditions should be included in the nursing care plan.

For example, a Laotian infant was hospitalized because of diarrhea and dehydration. The nursing staff initially viewed the mother as uncooperative because every night she would take the infant out of the crib and into her cot to sleep with her. The staff feared for the infant's safety, and it created a slight inconvenience when monitoring the infant's treatment during the night. Some of the staff even questioned whether this mother might be resistant in other aspects of her infant's health care regimen because she had several herbal combinations at the bedside and performed various rituals "to appease the errant spirit." Fortunately, a part-time nurse who knew the cultural traditions was available. She explained the Laotian customs and beliefs to the staff, who then were able to understand and incorporate them into the plan of care. The herbs were for the mother's back pain from a fall and were not being used to treat the infant's condition; the rituals were related to the belief that illness is disharmony with the universe. Furthermore, parents in this culture always sleep with their young children. The nurse also interpreted the medical regimens and goals to the mother. With improved communication, the mother and nursing staff respected and trusted each other and cooperated in the infant's care.

Most accommodations, such as this one, may create a minor change in nursing routine, which, in reality, is inconsequential when one's goal is to provide holistic health care. "At one time or another in history each model—magic, religion, and science—has been perceived as the panacea, the ultimate. However, no system with its unique methods has solved all problems for all people for all times. All systems function for most people some of the time" (Deck and Folta, 1979, p. 422).

Participating in Research

Part of the nurse's role is to support the scientific basis of nursing care through research. This includes both applying research findings to nursing practice and engaging in research activity to increase the body of knowledge that forms nursing's scientific basis.

Application to Practice It is essential that the nurse keep up with the literature in other disciplines, as well as in nursing, that addresses the social components of the various cultures and structures in which children live. One study, published by Lambert, Hamers, and Frasure-Smith in 1979, focused on childrearing values and practices among several ethnic groups cross-nationally (Lambert, Hamers, and Frasure-Smith, 1979). This study pointed up the differences and similarities in several ethnic groups both within the countries of origin and within Canada. The stresses of assimilation and gradual adoption of the ways of the dominant culture were noted. This has important implications for the kinds of guidance that nurses provide as a family enters and proceeds through the health care system. Clearly, a respect for the cultural values and beliefs of that family should be incorporated into the plan of care. Respecting food preferences and taboos, religious rituals, and patterns of social etiquette can advance significantly the development of a trusting relationship and reduce noncompliant health-related behaviors.

Engaging in Nursing Research The Select Panel Report commissioned by the US Congress recently defined and prioritized national strategies for improving child health (Report of the Select Panel for the Promotion of Child Health, 1979). Some of the major concerns cited in this report include (1) the unequal distribution of health services to certain socioeconomic, ethnic, and regional groups; (2) the need to focus greater attention to the psychologic, social, and behavioral factors that influence child health; (3) the need to identify family stressors and changes that impact on child health; and (4) the need for more research into the possible correlation between background (demographic), family, and social factors and the incidence of behavioral and psychosocial problems in children.

This report clearly shows the continued need for clarifying the social indicators that exist and impinge on the child and family systems, both directly and indirectly, through well-planned and conducted research investigations. To be most useful, this research should reflect an ecologic view of the child's environment as a series of continually interacting systems and subsystems. Both deductive research, which starts with a theoretic question and moves from the particular to the general, and inductive research, such as field research and participant-observational studies, in which theory is derived from data, are necessary and relevant to this process.

Data gathered from individual children and families can supply the nurse with a wealth of information on which to design researchable questions and identify tentative assumptions. Pursuing these questions, testing these assumptions, and sharing the results of analysis can improve the understanding of child development and the methods for enhancing it.

Key Concepts

- The process of socialization for children includes interactions with the primary suprasystems of family, peers, and school plus the more general suprasystems of local structures and generalized environment, including culture, race, and ethnicity.
- Childrearing practices are intimately related to the cultural beliefs and traditions of the family; consequently, there are many equally good but different ways to perform the same task or approach the same problem.
- Cultures are composed of numerous subcultures, all of which have various interpretations of rituals and practices. Therefore, it is important for nurses not to generalize but to be sensitive to the unique characteristics of each subculture.
- The response to health needs often involves a combination of traditional folkway treatments plus those of modern health care.
- Socioeconomic class differences envelop all cultures and influence childrearing and health-related behaviors in specific ways, including attitudes and practices regarding preventive measures.
- Cultural assessments are an essential aspect of assessment data and should include family life processes, diet, religion, art and history, value orientations, language, interactive patterns, and healing beliefs and practices, as emphasized by Modesta Orque's framework.
- Nurses play a pivotal role in interpreting the family's traditional folkway system and the western medical scientific health care system to each other to enhance mutual understanding and decrease mutual fear and mistrust because of a knowledge deficit.
- Accommodating nursing interventions to include the family's belief systems benefits the client and enhances participation.
- Nurses need to discover their own values and explore the relationships among their values, perceptions, actions, and method of processing information as the first step in the process.
- An assessment guide developed by Bloch and based on the eight categories of Orque is a valuable guide that corresponds to the four subsystems of the human being described in Chapter 2, thus noting the interrelatedness of culture and human development.
- To practice holistic nursing, the nurse must keep current and be personally involved in research that contributes to the understanding of the intricate network of cultural and ethnic and environmental influences that are played out in childrearing and health-related roles.

References

Arkoff A, Meredith G, Irvohara S: Generation differences in values: Americans, Japanese-Americans, and Japanese. *J Soc Psychol* 1967; 71: 169–175.

Bloch B: Bloch's assessment guide for ethnic/cultural variations. In: *Ethnic Nursing Care: A Multicultural Approach*. Orque MS, Bloch B, Monrroy LSA (editors). Mosby, 1983.

Brim O: Macrostructural influences in child development and the need for childhood social indicators. *Am J Orthopsychiatry* 1975; 45: 516–524.

Bronfenbrenner U: Toward an experimental ecology of human development. *Am Psychol* 1977; 32:513–529.

Brownlee AT: *Community, Culture and Care: A Cross-Cultural Guide for Health Workers*. Mosby, 1978.

Buber M: *I and Thou*. Smith RG (translator). Scribner, 1958.

Bullough VL, Bullough B: *Health Care for the Other Americans*. Appleton-Century-Crofts, 1982.

Char E: The Chinese American. In: *Culture and Childrearing*. Clark A (editor). Davis, 1981.

Charon J: *Symbolic Interactionism*. Prentice-Hall, 1979.

Coles R: *Privileged Ones*. Vol V: *Children in Crisis*. Little, Brown, 1977.

Comer JP, Poussaint A: *Black Child Care: How to Bring up a Healthy Black Child in America*. Simon & Schuster, 1975.

Deck ES, Folta JR: Problem solving: Magic, religion, and science. In: *A Sociological Framework for Patient Care*. Folta JR, Deck ES (editors). Wiley, 1979.

Ehling MB: The Mexican American (El Chicano). In: *Culture and Childrearing*. Clark A (editor). Davis, 1981.

Elkin F, Handel G: *The Child and Society: The Process of Socialization*. (3rd ed.) Random House, 1978.

Epstein CF: Successful black women. In: *Changing Women in a Changing Society*. Juber J (Editor). University of Chicago Press, 1974.

Farris LS, Farris CE: The Native American. In: *Culture and Childrearing*. Clark A (editor). Davis, 1981.

Friedman MM: *Family Nursing: Theory and Assessment*. Appleton-Century-Crofts, 1981.

Gambino R: *Blood of my Blood*. Doubleday, 1974.

Glickman B, Springer N: *Who Cares for the Baby?* Schocken, 1978.

Goode W: *The Family*. Prentice-Hall, 1964.

Greathouse B, Miller V: The black American. In: *Culture and Childrearing*. Clark A (editor). Davis, 1981.

Gutman R: *The Black Family in Slavery and Freedom 1700–1925*. Pantheon Books, 1976.

Henderson G, Primeaux M: *Transcultural Health Care*. Addison-Wesley, 1981.

Hill R: *The Strengths of Black Families*. Emerson Hall, 1972.

Kagan J, Kearsley R, Zelazo P: *Infancy*. Harvard University Press, 1978.

Lacay G: The Puerto Rican in mainland America. In: *Culture and Childrearing*. Clark A (editor). Davis, 1981.

Lambert W, Hamers J, Frasure-Smith N: *Childrearing Values: A Cross-National Study*. Praeger, 1979.

Leininger M: *Nursing and Anthropology: Two Worlds to Blend*. Wiley, 1970.

Meleis AJ, Sorrel L: *Arab American women and their birth experiences. Am J Matern Child Nurs* (May/June) 1981; 6:171–176.

Miller JR, Janosik EH: *Family Focused Care*. McGraw-Hill, 1980.

Orque MS, Bloch B, Monrroy LSA: *Ethnic Nursing Care: A Multicultural Approach*. Mosby, 1983.

Overfield T: Biological variation: Concepts from physical anthropology. *Nurs Clin North Am* 1977; 12:19–26. Reprinted In: *Transcultural Health Care*. Henderson G, Primeaux M (editors). Addison-Wesley, 1981.

Prout V: Emotional deprivation and the privileged child. In: *A Call for Action on Behalf of Children*. American Nurses' Association, Publication No. MCN 11:11–12, March, 1980.

Provence S, Naylor A, Patterson J: *The Challenge of Day Care*. Yale University Press, 1977.

Queen S, Habenstein RW: *The Family in Various Cultures*. Lippincott, 1974.

Report of the Select Panel for the Promotion of Child Health: *Better Health for our Children: A National Strategy. Vol. 1*. Public Health Service Publication No. 79-55071. US Department of Health and Human Services, 1980.

Robertson HR: Removing barriers to health care. *Nurs Outlook* 1969; 17:43–46.

Sevcovic L: Health care for mothers and children in an Indian culture: *Family Centered Community Nursing: A Sociocultural Framework*. Reinhardt AM, Quinn MD (editors). Mosby, 1973.

Sodetani-Shibata AE: The Japanese-American. In: *Culture and Childrearing*. Clark A (editor). Davis, 1981.

Spector R: *Cultural Diversity in Health and Illness*. Appleton-Century-Crofts, 1979.

Strengfellow-Liem N, Liem L: The Vietnamese in America. In: *Culture and Childrearing*. Clark A (editor). Davis, 1981.

Suzuki R: The Asian-American Family. In: *Parenting in a Multicultured Society*. Fantini MD, Cardenas R (editors). Longman, 1980.

Turner, W: A position on the question of ethnical neutrality in social science. J Afro-American Issues 1973; 3:323–330.

Yussen SR, Santrock JW: *Child Development: An Introduction*. Brown, 1982.

Zegiob LE, Forehand R: Maternal interactive behavior as a function of race, socioeconomic status and sex of the child. *Child Dev* 1975; 46(2):564–568.

Additional Readings

Anderson W: Cultural strategies. In: *High-Risk Parenting*. Johnson SH (editor). Lippincott, 1979.

Auger JR: *Behavioral Systems and Nursing*. Prentice-Hall, 1976.

Bee H: *Social Issues in Developmental Psychology*. Harper & Row, 1978.

Bowlby J: Attachment and Loss. Vol. 1. *Attachment*. Basic Books, 1969.

Brosman J: A proposed diabetic educational program for Puerto Ricans in New York City. In: *Transcultural Nursing: A Book of Readings*. Brink P (editor). Prentice-Hall, 1976.

Burr W, et al.: *Contemporary Theories About the Family: Research-Based Theories*. Free Press, 1979.

Carpio B: The adolescent immigrant. *Can Nurse* (March) 1981; 77(3): 27–29.

Clark A (editor): *Culture and Childrearing*. Davis, 1981.

Cohen A, Hodges H: Characteristics of the lower blue collar class. *Soc Prob* (Spring) 1963; 10:303–334.

Davies M, Yashida M: A model for cultural assessment. *Can Nurse* (March) 1981; 77(3).

Drakulic L, Tanaka W: The East Indian family in Canada. *Can Nurse* (March) 1981; 77(3).

Fantini MD, Russo A: Parenting in a pluralistic society: Toward a policy of options and choices. In: *Parenting in a Multicultural Society*. Fantini MD, Cardenas R (editors). Longman, 1980.

Garbarino J: *Children and Families in the Social Environment*. Aldine, 1982.

Grosso C: The Vietnamese American family . . . and Grandma makes three. *Am J Matern Child Health Nurs* (May/June) 1981; 6:177–180.

Hall E, Whyte WF: Intercultural communication: A guide to men of action. In: *Transcultural Nursing: A Book of Readings*. Brink P (editor). Prentice-Hall 1976.

Joe V: A new lifestyle in a new land. *Can Nurse* (March) 1981; 77(3).

Kodama K: Nursing in Japan. *Can Nurse* (March) 1981; 77(3).

Lamb M: What can research experts tell parents about effective socialization? In: *Parenting in a Multicultural Society*. Fantini MD, Cardenas R (editors). Longman, 1980.

Leyn RB: The challenge of caring for child refugees from Southeast Asia. *MCN* (May/June) 1978; 3:178–182.

Mercer E: A "professional" approach to helping immigrants and refugees. *Can Nurse* (March) 1981; 77(3).

Moore LE, et al: *The Biocultural Bases of Health*. Mosby, 1980.

Staples R, Mirandi, A: Racial and cultural variations among American families: A decennial review of the literature on minority families. In: *Family in Transition*. Skolnick AS, Skolnick JH (editors). Little, Brown, 1983.

Swanson AR, Hurley PM: Family systems: Values and value conflicts. *J Psychosoc Nurs Men Health Serv* 1983; 21(7):24–30.

Tizard JB: The institution as an environment for development. In: *The Integration of the Child in a Social World*. Richard MP (editor). Cambridge University Press, 1972.

Tripp-Reimer T, Brink PJ, Saunders JM: Cultural assessment: Content and process. *Nurs Outlook* (March/April) 1984; 32(2):78–82.

Family Influences on the Child

4

Virginia Prout

Chapter Outline

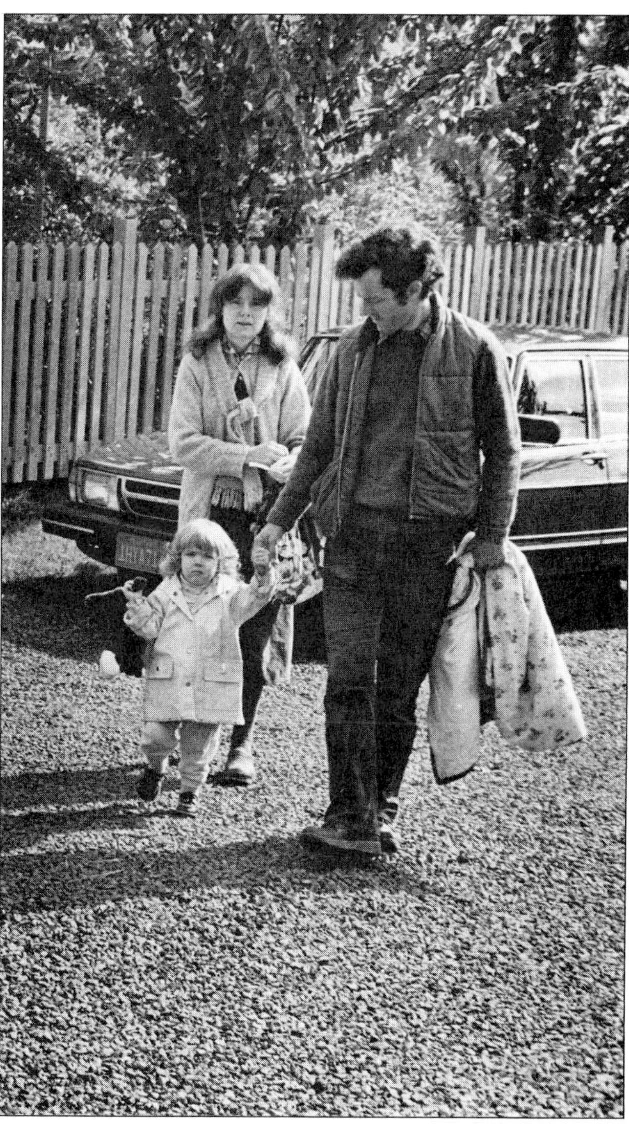

Objectives

- Describe the evolution of the family.
- List the influences affecting families today.
- Explain how the concepts of family structure and function can be used to describe families.
- Explain the process by which family roles serve to socialize children for adult roles.
- Describe the ways in which families develop and maintain a family system.
- Explain the components of family communication.
- Define current types of families and the needs they commonly present to the nurse.

Socialization of the child is a dynamic process in which each child's unique characteristics and endowments interact with and influence others. The family is the earliest and primary environment in which socialization takes place because it is here that the child first experiences human interaction (Elkin and Handel, 1978).

Beginning at birth and through an intricate interweaving and meshing of events and interactions, socialization of the child transmits what it means to be male or female, what constitutes acceptable social behavior, and what society values in terms of roles and achievements—in other words, an entire frame of reference that will allow the child to share a common conception of reality with the world at large. The microcosm of the family translates this frame of reference as it is received from the macrocosm of society into the daily behaviors and communications that make up the socialization process.

Although other determinants of a child's social development include the child's age, gender, ethnic or racial background, religious upbringing, socioeconomic status, and parents' level of education, no discussion of this process would be complete without a look at where socialization begins. The burgeoning literature on the concepts of attachment and bonding clearly indicate that socialization begins with the first relationships that the neonate experiences (see Chapter 7).

In receiving care and experiencing the reciprocal stimulus of infant cues and caregiver responses, the infant first develops a sense of self and other persons. For most children, these first relationships occur within the family, thereby making the family the child's primary socializing agent. The family, to a large degree, mediates the forces and conditions that affect the child and acts as a screening device for cultural influences and experiences.

In this chapter, we address the question of family definition by looking at both past and present definitions of the family. We analyze the subsystems that are part of family life, and we examine current types and family configurations and future trends.

Defining Families

Each child comes from and belongs to a family. Identifying the family, in personal terms, is relatively easy for most people. The state of families and family life in today's world, however, is much researched and debated. Although statistics and studies indicate that families are changing, theorists struggle with the seemingly simple task of defining a family in broader contexts.

Is a family a unit composed of parents and children, or is it a more extended unit that includes grandparents, aunts, uncles, and cousins? Is a family always defined biologically, or can it encompass biologically unrelated people who share a residence? Can the family include "surrogate parents" and "significant others," and, if so, who are they and where do they belong in relation to the family? What, finally, are the commonalities that define each of these groups that are called a family?

A biologic view of the family, in its simplest form, includes the relationship of a couple and their offspring. This definition, however, loses sight of the multitude of emotional and social characteristics and relationships that hold people together, either in conjunction with their biologic ties or despite their lack of them. Definitions should therefore also include those who are not biologically related but view themselves and are viewed as a unique social unit. This perspective allows the inclusion of such phenomena as divorce and adoption, which are widely accepted in many cultures, into an analysis of the family because, although a family may exist as a social unit and vice versa, effective parenting and the socialization of children does not depend on biologic ties or relationships. They depend instead on three broader considerations: (1) the goals and values of the parents; (2) the characteristics of the child; and (3) the practices and mores of the family culture and subculture. The terms "parenting" and "socialization" may be used as synonymous concepts describing all that occurs within the family unit which influences the child's growth and development (Lamb, 1980).

Families, no matter what external form they take, are therefore the basic social units that hold people together in ways that no other social grouping can accomplish. They are important socializing vehicles that transmit the family's values, knowledge, skills, and culture from one generation to the next. The form that a family takes, the way it is organized, and the priorities it sets mediate much of these experiences for the child. A useful method for beginning to explore the effects of these factors is to look at the historical evolution of the family from some of its earlier beginnings to the many varieties of families that exist today.

Historical Evolution of the Family

Although the origin of the family is speculative because of limited records, the chances are that language and family were invented about the same time and developed together over a long period (Gough, 1971, reprinted in Skolnick and Skolnick, 1983). Families, according to Bronowski (1973), have undergone four major transitions during the span of human existence. This history of humankind is divided unequally. First is biologic evolution, which distinguishes humans from their ape ancestors and which took place over the span of several million years. Fossil records indicate that apes, gorillas, and chimpanzees lived in Europe, Asia, and Africa 12–28 million years ago. Evolution then progressed through various phases until the appearance of modern Homo sapiens about 70,000–50,000 years ago.

Gough (1971, reprinted in Skolnick and Skolnick, 1983) noted that the majority of anthropologists believe that family life, as well as domestic dwellings, tool use, cookery, and language, were developed prior to the time of Neanderthal man—200,000–100,000 years ago. In fact, the first use of fire is thought to have occurred among the cave-dwelling hominids at Choukoutien near Peking 500,000 years ago.

Second is our cultural history—a progressive advance in civilization that separates people from their more primitive human ancestors. The early hunting and gathering societies were widespread before the cultivation and domestication of animals occurred—about 15,000–10,000 years ago. In many ways these primitive societies are similar to the modern hunting and gathering societies that have been studied in Oceania, Asia, Africa, and America.

These societies lived in groups of 20–200 people that were divided into families, most of which were nuclear, some extended, and occasionally some polygynous. Division of labor existed within the household because of necessity, and each member contributed to the well-being of the others. The men did the hunting and fishing with spears or bows and arrows while the women and children (especially girls) gathered wild berries, fruits, plants, and nuts. They also processed and prepared the food. Dwellings were simple and movement frequent as food supplies became diminished and new ones had to be sought (Gough, 1971, reprinted in Skolnick and Skolnick, 1983). The lives of women in nomadic tribes were narrowly defined—first to produce children (particularly males) and second to tend to the repetitive everyday activities necessary to the survival of the tribe. The life of the nomadic family was therefore stark and simple and allowed little room for either innovation or emotional attachments to places or people. These early nomads based family ties on a belief in a single founding father (Bronowski, 1973).

Aspects of the cultural transition occurred within the last 10,000 years, during which time the nomadic life of these humans was changed by agriculture (Bronowski, 1973). As land and animals became domesticated, the tribes became larger, more complex, and more organized. The primary method for organizing people to ensure greater productivity was kinship. These large households were common in the agrarian states of ancient Greece, Rome, India, China, and the Islamic empires.

A major change in the lives of some families thus occurred with the cultivation of wheat and herds of animals. Families then settled in an area together, worked the land, and shared a sense of loyalty and a commitment to the past and the present, with each family member working toward the future.

According to Bronowski, the family underwent the third transformation 5000 years ago when cities developed in western Europe and along the fertile crescent. Craft specialization and trade emerged, which led to the gradual exploration of the world. These larger societies created central political leadership with various ranked allegiances along kinship lines, which then formed the basis for the distribution of goods, services, and power. With the rise of the state, the woman's role became less central to the family's economic welfare.

This state of affairs was followed by a fourth transition, the industrial revolution and its extension in ongoing technologic production. With the influx of industry and capitalism, the primary work place for the man was away from the home. The woman meanwhile stayed at home to care for the children and tend to domestic responsibilities.

With the rising technologic level of the society, whether in Europe, the United States, Canada, Japan, or Russia, both urbanization and bureaucratization occurred. As the family roles and functions became redefined, kinship ties were an even more important resource, providing mutual assistance and reciprocal services.

Throughout each of these general transitions, social and economic factors played a role in the resultant changes in the structure and function of the family. A look at the recent history of the family in the western world during the sixteenth and seventeenth centuries shows that strong generational ties to common property still existed and that marriage often was seen as a practical solution for economic stability or growth. During this time, necessity and material advantage frequently took priority over marriages based on love and self-fulfillment. Nevertheless, the family provided a strong sense of purpose coupled with strong ties to the past. New generations were expected to carry on cultural traditions.

The disadvantages of this cohesiveness included little mobility and little privacy. The boundaries between families and the community were permeable, as family and community life were closely woven together. Relationships outside the family were strong, and socialization frequently occurred within the extended family and local community. Other basic differences existed as well. The rates of infant and child mortality, for example, were high, and the parent–child relationship was strongly influenced by the basic struggle for survival. Strong bonds of affection were withheld until the parents were certain that the child would live. Parents had many children to protect themselves from possible loss.

Major shifts in philosophies, religions, and political systems occurred in the seventeenth and eighteenth centuries. The age of enlightenment heralded an emphasis on the rationalization of institutions and a focus on the rights of individuals—both concepts that have influenced today's institutions. The more traditional European hierarchies—church, monarchies, and the generational family inheritance—were changed by these shifts. In America waves of immigration were facilitated by the promise of economic prosperity. Family ties and the rigid boundaries of communal village life were thus loosened as some members left to seek freedom, fame, or fortune in a new land. Initially, many early immigrants reestablished familiar patterns of family life, but these patterns were modified to accommodate various changes within the economic, political, and social structures as they were constructed in the new world.

The advent of the industrial revolution in the early nineteenth century brought with it major economic shifts that in turn influenced other social systems and institutions. These changes dramatically affected family life. Changes in family roles; patterns of authority, mobility, and stability; and values, beliefs, and attitudes that shaped family interactions paralleled changes in the wider environment.

The change from an agricultural to an industrial economy, for example, meant that the family was no longer a self-sufficient economic unit. Previously, the family household was a busy work place, where family life and work were integrated and labor was shared among all its members. The family also functioned as the school, church, workshop, hospital, and social center. As family members were employed in mass production, they were increasingly separated from each other, and the interdependence of the family economy gave way to a wage economy. The decline in family based enterprise thus altered the boundaries of the family system and led to changes in the family structure. In addition, the expansion of industry and improved methods of transportation resulted in a period of rapid urbanization.

These changes were gradual and, according to Hareven (1982), varied among social classes and ethnic groups. The rural and working-class urban families maintained the preindustrial patterns longer. These families continued to function as collective units, and even if everyone worked outside the home, they all contributed their earnings for the well-being of the family.

Industrialization had a greater impact on the middle class and, to a certain extent, was responsible for the growth of the middle class. Home and work were separate, leading to the concept of the male as the wage-earner and good provider for his family. The woman, freed from economic-related functions, could devote herself to domestic responsibilities and the children. The unique stage of life now known as childhood is a direct result of this emergence of the middle-class family. The children were no longer needed as laborers on the farm or in the factory and were perceived as dependent beings requiring nurture and protection.

The cult of domesticity originated in the middle class but invaded other classes and by the late nineteenth century was the ideology of the larger society. Nevertheless, "a majority of working-class and ethnic families continued to adhere to the earlier way of life; most importantly, they maintained a collective view of the family and its economy" (Hareven, 1982, p. 455).

Today, many families still strive to maintain ties to the past and to the extended family. Immigrants often work hard to preserve old and familiar ways, yet their children, the second generation, want to be like their peers whose cultural and social background may be very different from that of their parents (Gambino, 1974). Peer groups are an important socializing influence, but the result of their influence is sometimes tension between their suprasystems, representing new and different sets of values, traditions, beliefs, and behaviors, and those of the child's family. Parents encourage their children to go to school, to get ahead, and grow but at the same time are faced with the dilemma of not wanting their pasts and values dismissed. "The major historical change in family values has been a change from a collective view of the family to one of individualism and sentiment" (Hareven, 1982, p. 456).

Questions of definition still remain. Is family evolution a cyclic phenomenon? Are today's transitions a natural evolutionary pattern of family adaptation, or do modern changes in family life indicate a breakdown of the family as a system? Are parents losing control over children, especially adolescents, or is adolescent rebellion just an aberration of American culture? Did the bonds of property and religion hold men and women together better in the past than the bonds of sex and sentiment do today? Are families today really so different from the traditional families in the past?

Influences on Today's Families

Current concerns focus on mechanisms to support family continuity and cohesiveness. As economic realities are propelling women into the work force, new roles are being explored and tried. The mass media frequently refers to the problems of alienation and isolation that result from family relocation and mobility. Some would question the consequences of increasing governmental involvement in daily life, suggesting that more decision making might best be retained by the family. Laws regarding compulsory education and immunization are just two examples of programs that, although well intended and necessary, do illustrate a loss of family control over the lives of family members.

Significant legal decisions regarding the sexual behavior of family members are now being made by powers external to the family unit. The controversies regarding abortion and contraception, parental rights, and adolescent rights indicate a shift from control of the family over individual behavior to control by the individual to make choices. The ethical ramifications of these debates are complex, not only because of traditional religious prohibitions but also because of questions over the rights and obligations of family members. These issues indicate that the forces outside the family are influencing some of the most intimate relationships within the family.

Even so, the family remains a primary environment for socialization. The bonds that hold its members persist, and the strength of family life may be its ability to endure and change without being destroyed. The resilience of families has allowed them to be restructured, adapt, and survive from the earliest forms to the variety of forms that exist today. The assets and strengths of families do not rest on the particular structure or form that they take, the culture in which they exist, or the values that they hold. Rather, their strength is their ability to nurture their members, meet their physical, emotional, and social needs, develop group norms, and adapt to stress and change.

The form that a family takes and the style that it adopts are unique characteristics for each family. The nurse needs to understand the variations of family styles and organization to help families function effectively.

Assessing the family includes looking at its "psychosocial interior" (Elkin and Handel, 1978). This psychosocial interior includes (1) the family's characteristic coping mechanisms in response to stress (whether maturational or situational) and (2) internal family functioning such as decision-making processes, role expectations and assignments, patterns of communicating and responding to individual needs, family cohesiveness, the willingness to share in family group tasks, and shared family values and goals.

In assessing the family, the nurse views the family within its own social, economic, and cultural contexts. The ethnic and religious influences are significant (see Chapter 3), and the educational and economic position of the family plays a key role in the family's identity. The family's interaction with the community and its use of community resources are important considerations. Just as the relationship between child and family is interdependent and reciprocal, the relationship between the family and the community is dynamic, as it changes and shifts over time. The psychosocial pattern of a given family is therefore determined by the dynamic interplay between suprasystems and subsystems. Conflict and tension within the family affect the adaption of the family to its community as well as its functioning. (Family assessment is further discussed in Chapter 17.)

Framework for Studying Families

A set of specific properties and characteristics is difficult to assign to the notion of "family" because this term has been used to describe different configurations of human relationships. Nurses do, however, need tools with which to identify useful and appropriate strategies for defining, assessing, and working with families. Several theories and frameworks have been developed, and nursing therefore has approached the study of families in a variety of ways.

The medical model primarily categorizes families as normal or abnormal. Medical terminology labels families as adaptive or maladaptive and bases interventions on those definitions. This dysfunctional, or problem-focused, view of families has several limitations. The most obvious limitation is its potential for subjective bias and diagnosis based on the nurse's own values. The subsequent placement of families in labeled categories creates the danger that the nurse will lose sight of the family's strengths.

More holistic approaches in child and family nursing have been derived in part from the earlier emphasis of family study in each of the traditional nursing specializations (Knafl and Grace, 1978). Maternity nursing was a forerunner in looking at the total family and its strengths. Family–child nursing tended to focus on the mother–child dyad. Community health nursing addressed family centered care but frequently focused on what were defined as problematic families or families from disadvantaged or minority backgrounds. Psychiatric nursing often focused on the dysfunctional emotional development of one or more family members, whereas medical-surgical nurses dealt with the effects of health and illness on the family's adult members. In each specialty area early nursing approaches tended to view families in situational or developmental crises and, to a lesser degree, viewed the concept of family life in its totality and on a continuum.

Current nursing practice in child health nursing and in other nursing specialties has been enhanced by the incorporation of several theoretic frameworks from other disciplines and by the development of more comprehensive and appropriate models for nursing practice. The systems model of this text and the development and use of a taxonomy of nursing diagnosis (see Chapter 2) illustrate this point. Other considerations in describing families include an analysis of family structure and function, analysis of family roles, theories of family development, and analysis of family communications.

Family Structures and Functions

The theory of structural functionalism views the family as one of the component parts of the greater social system. The family interacts with and contributes to the continued operation of the social system. At the same time, the social system consisting of its institutions, collectivities, norms, and values, influences the socialization of the family. Of even greater significance is the cultural system, which encompasses the available knowledge, symbols, and ideas that guide institutionalized patterns of interaction and internalized aspects of personality. Thus, the suprasystems provide the ideas and objects of orientation that result in the family's moral standards (norms and values), organization, and patterning of relationships (Parsons, 1951; Knafl and Grace, 1978). The *structure* of the family refers to the number of family members and the relation of each of the family members to the others. For example, parent–child and sister–brother relationships are part of a family's structure.

Family interaction is complex because of the various interpersonal relationships within a family. Dyadic relationships increase in the order of triangular numbers with each additional member (Fig. 4-1). The following formula is helpful in determining the number of interpersonal communications possible in a family:

$$x = \frac{y^2 - y}{2}$$

where x is the number of dyads or interpersonal relations and y is the number of persons. Thus, for a family of four, six dyads are possible, whereas the number of dyads increases to ten for a family of five.

The *functions* of a family are not, as the term might indicate, simply the tasks performed by family members. Rather, function refers to the *consequences* that a family's interrelated motives and subsequent behaviors have for the family as a unit (Ritzer, 1983). Manifest functions are those consequences that are intended by the family and serve a purpose (Merton, 1968). Latent functions are those consequences that are unintended but nonetheless beneficial. For example, the manifest function of the intended consequence, of both parents working outside the home may be financial stability. The latent function, the unintended consequence, may be a more flexible and equitable delineation of household and childrearing responsibilities between parents. Possible dysfunction may be caused by increased stress for the working mother if she continues to shoulder complete responsibility for household and childrearing tasks.

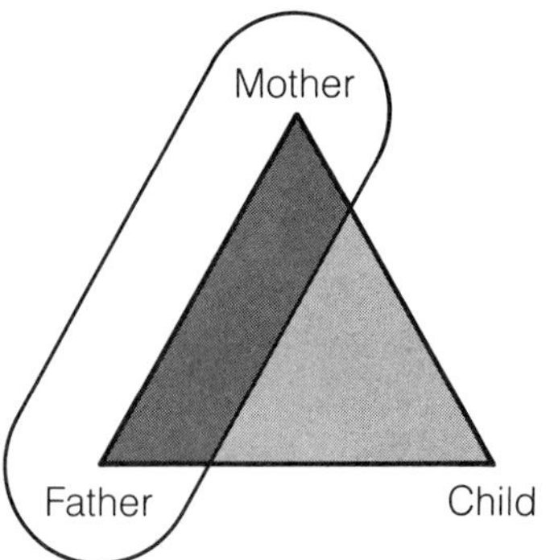

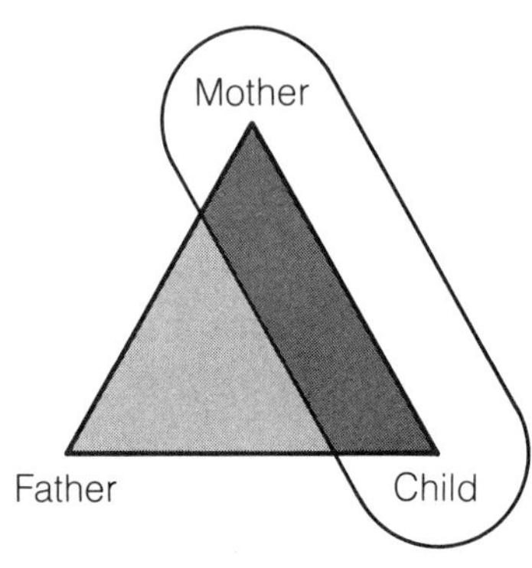

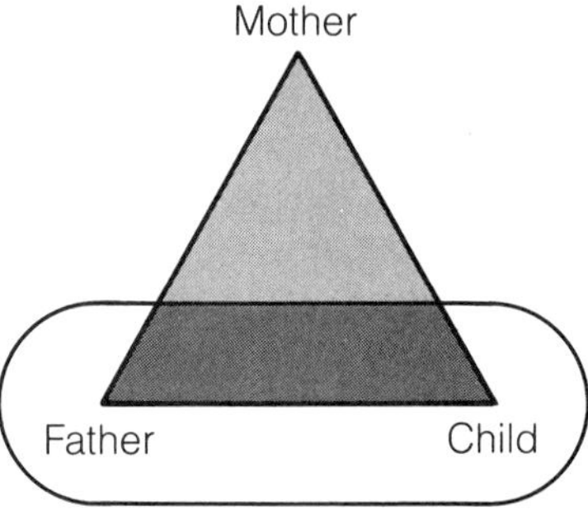

Figure 4-1 Dyadic relationships within a triangular family structure. (From Wilson, H., and Kneisl, C. 1983. *Psychiatric Nursing.* 2nd ed. Menlo Park, CA: Addison-Wesley, p. 614.)

The assumption in any such analysis is that families have certain functional requirements and that these functions serve purposes for individual family members, the family as a unit, and the family's society. Functions can be broadly grouped into six categories: (1) affective functions; (2) socialization and social placement functions; (3) functions of providing physical care and necessities; (4) reproductive functions; (5) economic functions; and (6) family coping functions (Friedman, 1981).

Family Roles

The concept of a *role* includes a set of behaviors, attitudes, beliefs, principles, and values that characterize the occupant of a given social position or status. Roles prescribe a set of cultural expectations for persons in standard situations. Roles may be acquired in several ways. They may be ascribed on the basis of a quality such as sex, age, or birth order. They may be achieved as a result of performance, choice, or effort such as spouse, parent, lawyer, or nurse. A role sometimes is adopted temporarily for a specific purpose or in designated situations such as that of a victim or party clown. Finally, a role may be assumed. Children assume various roles in their games as they pretend to be different family, community, or media-related people (Robischon and Scott, 1969).

A number of roles, each composed of a set of behaviors normatively prescribed and proscribed, are involved in each social position (or status). Learning the behaviors associated with these positions is integral to the process of socialization for the child. Role theory focuses on what people do, why they do what they do, and what strains and conflicts arise.

Nye (1976) identified eight areas in which roles were important: marriage/parenthood/family provider; household maintenance; child care; child socialization; sexuality; recreation; therapy (care of ill family members); and kinship. Although some of these roles historically have been associated with either father or mother, the current trend is for both parents to assume these roles. Thus, these roles are parts of a position but not limited to a single position. Roles are dynamic in that some decline while others emerge over time. The traditional role expectation that the father is the good provider for his family's economic needs has declined in importance, and often this role is shared with the wife. In some families the role assignments are reversed and new responsibilities emerge, such as when the father assumes the housekeeper and child caretaker roles and the wife takes on the role of sole provider.

Among family members roles overlap. For example, the roles of parent and child and husband and wife intersect. The woman in her role as a mother functions differently than she does in her role as a wife. These two roles overlap, however, in that any change in her role relationship with her spouse or child will result in changes in the other relationship. It also will result in changes within the family system because the family system is the interdependent whole composed of multiple subsystems and role relationships.

Role relationships involve unique responsibilities and activities both within and across the boundaries of the family. The expected behavior of each family member in these reciprocal arrangements permits social interaction to proceed in an orderly manner. Equilibrium for both the conjugal and kinship network depends on the complementarity of roles.

The role arrangements of a family refer not only to the relationship of the family members to one another (mother–child or aunt–niece) but also to the relationships between and among these individuals. For example, Mary Smith may be a mother, but she must have a child to assume that role. Role perceptions and role expectations are conceptual tools that help define how family members perceive their roles and how their actions (as a result of these perceptions) fit the expectations that other family members have of them. Discrepancies between role perceptions and role expectations can result in family conflict or disharmony. Mary Smith may perceive her position as a mother to include sole responsibility for the roles of child caretaker, child socializer, and housekeeper. Her husband, in his position as father, may expect to share these roles and participate in domestic and child-care activities. These opposing expectations may create disharmony. Because roles are defined culturally, the wife and husband may not hold the same set of normative definitions, and each spouse may have different expectations about role norms, sanctions, and enactment.

Many fathers feel a sense of ambiguity about their role. The role modeled for them by their fathers or the role they observe enacted by their peers may conflict with what their wives want or what they desire to do with respect to child care and domestic activities. The media does not help in this regard. The majority of television programs portray the more traditional family of the father as the primary provider and the mother as the homemaker who may or may not have an ancillary career. Until recently, the behavioral science literature neglected the father's contribution in any of the so-called nurturing responsibilities of the family. It was almost as if the father had become an appendage to the main body of mother and children. His job took him away from the family in more than the obvious physical ways. The traditional father's image of himself and of his career as a father was based on his work performance, ability to provide for the family's economic future, and present level of material comfort.

Since the 1970s there has been a shift in emphasis, and the father's role has become the focus of many studies and reports, particularly looking at the nurturing role of fatherhood (LeMasters and DeFain, 1983, p. 154). An early example of this changing emphasis can be seen in the response of Benjamin Spock to severe criticism from feminist groups concerning his classic text *Baby and Child Care.* He now argues that "the father—any father—should be sharing with the mother the day-to-day care of the children from birth onward . . . including housework to teach the children that it is as vital, worthy and challenging as his job" (1974, pp. 242–243).

For the child, adequate parental role models are essential for the transmission of adult role behaviors. Early on, children begin to associate certain activities with particular people. As children play, they identify some of these roles and explore the acts of doing and being. The relative cohesiveness of relationships among family members, the ease with which adults in the family enact and share role responsibilities, and the degree to which family members find satisfaction in their intimate and broader personal and work relationships will, in large measure, shape the child's view of adult functioning and interpersonal relationships. Conflict and tension over role responsibilities, lack of clarity as to who does what, and confused patterns of communication and hidden messages may serve to distort the child's eventual role perceptions and potential enactment of those roles in later life. Sex role development and achievement motivation in particular are influenced by observing and imitating adult behavior (Giele, 1974).

Family Development

Like the variety of developmental theories that describe the child (see Chapter 6), theories of family development provide a way of analyzing components of family life. Each theory sheds some light on the developmental process as applied to the family.

Theory of Duvall The concept of a developmental task is central to a synthesis of theories of child and family development. Evelyn Duvall described eight tasks that are common to all families. These are (1) physical maintenance; (2) allocation of resources; (3) division of labor; (4) socialization of family members; (5) maintenance of order; (6) placement of members in the larger society; and (7) maintenance of motivation and morale (Duvall, 1977).

Duvall also specified certain stage-critical events that occur during the family life cycle:

> Critical events such as being married, bearing children, releasing them as teenagers and young adults and continuing as a couple through the empty nest and aging years propel a family into and through each new stage in its history. Each new developmental crisis necessitates new adaptations and imposes new responsibilities at the same time that it opens up new opportunities and poses new challenges (Duvall, 1977, p. 178).

The successful completion of these tasks results in continued growth and satisfaction. Failure to accomplish a developmental task may result in dissatisfaction, disruption, and societal disapproval. Each period in the life of a family thus presents different challenges and requirements.

The family life cycle as proposed by Duvall consists of eight successive stages, beginning with the married couple followed by the childbearing family and thereafter based on the age and school placement of the oldest child (Table 4-1). Although stages overlap when there is more than one child in the family, the family is pushed into new unknowns with its oldest child and repeats the stage with subsequent children.

TABLE 4-1 Duvall's Eight-Stage Family Life Cycle

Stage	Description
I	Married couples (without children)
II	Childbearing families (oldest child between birth and 30 months)
III	Families with preschool children (oldest child 2½–6 years old)
IV	Families with school children (oldest child 6–13 years old)
V	Families with teenagers (oldest child 13–20 years old)
VI	Families launching young adults (first child gone to last child's leaving home)
VII	Middle-aged parents (empty nest to retirement)
VIII	Aging family members (retirement to death of both spouses)

SOURCE: Duvall EM: *Marriage and Family Development,* 5th edition. (JB Lippincott). © 1977 by Harper & Row, Publishers, Inc. Reprinted by permission of the publishers.

Developmental Tasks For child health nurses, an analysis of the family as a system may be readily integrated with theories of family development. Four tasks are common to each stage in the life of a family. The nurse therefore assesses the family's current ability to accomplish each of the following developmental tasks:

1. Assisting each family member to meet individual developmental tasks (see Chapter 6)
2. Integrating the family system and individual family members into their wider environments (for example, work, school, community)
3. Meeting the physical needs of the family
4. Establishing and maintaining the internal family system

In assessing a family's ability to assist individual members with their developmental tasks, the nurse explores how the family provides consistent nurturing and how the family initiates and adapts to change. For instance, a child's growth to adolescence can be particularly problematic for a family striving to balance nurturance of teenage children and adaptation to the many changes that adolescence brings.

In assessing a family's ability to integrate itself and its individual members into its wider environments, the nurse explores the amount and type of involvement that the family has with schools, religious organizations, and health care facilities. The family's patterns of leisure activities are also important.

In assessing the family's ability to meet physical needs, the nurse looks at the family's ability to supply the basic necessities for family maintenance (food, shelter, clothing, and health care). Here, the nurse's awareness of resources that can assist families to meet these basic needs is important.

Assessment of the internal components of the family system includes determining whether communication and interaction among family members serve to maintain or adjust values, goals, and behaviors as needed. Methods of decision making, the distribution of power, boundary maintenance, and adaptations to crises and change are vital factors to the family's internal system. The degree to which each member perceives the individual and collective needs of other family members, respects other members as important, and attempts to gratify other members' needs determines family harmony. In addition, each member's interaction with the rest of the family is modified by temporary variables, such as illness, fatigue, stress, or being busy, and more stable variables such as personality, resources, education, and experience.

Family Communication

Clear communication occurs within the family when the feelings and actual messages that individuals convey are similar (Satir, 1967). Communication is often simultaneously verbal and nonverbal. Clear communication results when verbal and nonverbal messages are similar or when family members are able to question and clarify perceived discrepancies.

Communication theories are useful tools for analyzing patterns of interaction within a family. For the nurse, this means assessing how messages are conveyed, perceived, and interpreted by family members. Components of family communication can be assessed according to patterns of (1) sending and receiving messages; (2) expressing feelings; (3) expressing power; and (4) resolving conflicts (Satir, 1972; Friedman, 1981).

Patterns of Communication Clearly sent messages reflect a congruence between what is actually said and how it is said (facial expressions, voice tone, posture). The content of the message is explicit, and feedback from the recipient of the message is sought for verification (Friedman, 1981). For example, "I'm worried that the amount of time Susie is spending on the telephone is interfering with her school work. What do you think?" Concluding the statement with a specific question is a clear indication that a response is expected. The response may be either a statement or another question that seeks to ascertain more information such as, "Are you concerned because her grades have gone down?" or "How much time a day does she talk on the telephone and to whom?"

A clearly received message requires that the receiver listen actively to what is being said and allow the sender to complete the statement. It also requires a flow of information from the recipient as feedback to the sender signifying that the message was either received as intended (validation) or asking for clarification (Friedman, 1981). Expressive patterns of communication (feelings, power, conflict) are vital to healthy family communication (Friedman, 1981). Such expressions may be verbal and nonverbal messages of affection, responsibility and obligation, and differences.

The nurse needs to understand that family communication is a relative phenomenon and as such is always subject to dysfunction. Healthy communication in a family is, by definition, more functional than dysfunctional. According to Friedman (1981), clear communication in a "well-functioning family" only occurs one third of the time. Dysfunctional communication can be caused by the sender or receiver. A dysfunctional sender may send unclear messages, for example, by using sarcasm or silent anger instead of making a clear statement of feeling. A dysfunctional receiver may not listen carefully to what is said or may cut the sender off before the message is completed.

Boundaries Affecting Communication Family communication outside its immediate environment depends on how open or closed the family's boundaries are. The relative permeability of the boundaries regulates the amount of information the family receives. At times, a family needs to reduce the number or intensity of inputs so that it can attend to more immediate needs. For example, new parents may have to screen out the multitude of well-intentioned yet conflicting suggestions they receive about handling their infant. Families that are bombarded with information may have difficulty making choices and setting priorities. Difficulties also can arise when the family system receives insufficient input. These families may not receive the information and support that they need to function.

If the family is overloaded with information from the surrounding environment, it sends out messages that it will not accept further input. For example, a family that is served by several health and social service providers may find itself receiving contradictory or inconsistent information. Confused and unable to comply with all the advice, the family may decide to miss an appointment.

A family receives and interprets information through the lens of such factors as language, culture, emotional stability, and intellectual capacity. These factors influence how information is received, interpreted, used, or discarded. Situational stressors also can play a role in this process. For example, the Jones family moved from Chicago to Boston. Several of their new neighbors stopped by to greet them the day that they arrived. Initially, the Joneses were thrilled to find themselves in such a congenial neighborhood. Their two school-age children were quickly distracted and enticed to join newfound friends in a variety of play activities. Meanwhile, Mr. and Mrs. Jones found themselves conducting several tours of the house as their neighbors stopped by to say hello. Although several of the neighbors offered to lend a hand, Mr. and Mrs. Jones refused, thinking that their neighbors were just being polite. As the day progressed, little unpacking occurred. By dinner time, Mr. and

Mrs. Jones found themselves with no cookware in the kitchen, their children scattered throughout the neighborhood, and their new neighbors long since gone to enjoy a leisurely dinner at their own homes. Confused, frustrated, and hungry, Mrs. Jones stopped at a neighbor's house to ask whether her children were there. Because she looked harassed, the neighbor invited her in for tea. Mrs. Jones declined. The neighbor, sensing Mrs. Jones's tension, asked if anything was wrong. Mrs. Jones described the day's events, the family's current state of confusion, and the need to prepare a meal. The neighbor helped Mrs. Jones to track down her children and escorted them home. She insisted on staying to help them unpack and arranged for her husband to bring over a platter of cold cuts for dinner.

In this instance feedback, the process by which the family assesses how it has actually functioned and how it could function more effectively, would affect the family's boundaries in the future. Mr. and Mrs. Jones learned through their experiences that their initial behavior contributed to their dilemma. Fortunately, Mrs. Jones' ability to state her needs, seek and accept help appropriately, and use help when it was offered served to reinforce a sense of acceptance within the new neighborhood. In addition, the next time someone offers to lend a hand, Mr. and Mrs. Jones will be less quick to decline the offer.

"A study of the family as an institution must relate it to the context of the particular society in which it functions, because relationships within the family and its pattern of life must be to some extent congruent with the demands that the community makes upon its members" (Coser, 1974, p. xiii). Thus, when nurses gather data about a family and assess its ability to provide care for dependent children, a variety of theories and frameworks must be considered. No single theory completely explains the complexity of interactions and dynamics that characterize a family.

Types of Family Configurations

There are probably as many forms of the family as there are of society. For the purposes of this chapter, the discussion will be limited to the American family (Table 4-2). The American family has undergone significant changes in the role structure of its members and in its patterns of childrearing. Historically, mothers shared childrearing responsibilities with nearby members of the extended family, including grandparents, aunts, cousins, and older children. Today, the nuclear family and its variations have emerged as the predominant form of family life. An increasingly mobile and urban society has also in many instances resulted in the decline in the number of extended family structures (Cohen, 1974).

Industrialized society assigned the childrearing role to women and the economic-provider role to men. Gronseth (1972) contended that "this social arrangement meshes well with the demands of industry. Moreover, this pattern is the basis for most of the sex-role divisions and of their consequences in modern society. Without a major restructuring of this division of labor it will be impossible to achieve an end to other destructive sex-role divisions" (p. 175). Any change within the social structure is difficult and occurs slowly, especially when power is at stake and the direction of change results in a loss of power for the changing group. The innate resistance to change then is even greater. William Goode's (1982) study noted the ways in which men's lives are affected by the changes that have been initiated by the women's movement and their stubborn resistance to these changes. The point of greatest resistance is in participating in domestic tasks. Women's work has become so effectively devalued that to share in it is contrary to most men's self-concept. The man's identity often is equated with his profession or occupation, and his family and children follow his work in his priority system. The resistance to change also hinges on the apparent inevitable results of an ideology of patriarchalism that supports the sex-role power bias. This ideology assumes that men are superior in all areas except child care and domestic responsibilities and therefore should be entitled to greater power and prestige.

The values and realistic choices available to the American family have changed. Educational and career opportunities for women have become increasingly realistic options. This shift in educational and career advantages has prompted many women to seek modes of expression and fulfillment outside the home. The number of single-parent families also has risen, creating new patterns in family life and new needs for resources.

The requirements of the capitalist economy have necessitated other changes. The family has become even more isolated and private, having one or more cars for personal transportation. Television and other electronic media provide a ready escape into a world of entertainment. At the same time, the family has become increasingly consumer oriented. The increase in leisure time and money and the thrust of advertising encourage the family to participate in impulse buying for the instant gratification of needs or wants.

Nuclear Families

The *nuclear family* commonly is defined as a small, functional group composed of a mother, a father, and their children. The primary socialization process of the child in a nuclear family is the shared responsibility of two parents. Although the nuclear family generally is considered traditional, some researchers view this style of family life as restrictive and deficient in the range of possible role models (Elkin and Handel, 1978). In the nuclear family parent–child relationships are more intense. Parents are concerned and feel responsible for their child's future and recognition

TABLE 4-2 Types and Percentages of Different Family Forms in the United States

Traditional variant family forms	Nontraditional, experimental variant family forms
The most prominent traditional types of variant family forms now existing are 1. Nuclear family—dual career, husband, wife, and children living in same household (16%) 2. Nuclear dyad—husband and wife alone: childless or no children living at home (10%) a. Single career b. Dual career 1. Wife's career continuous 2. Wife's career interrupted 3. Single-parent family—one head as a consequence of divorce, abandonment, or separation (with financial aid rarely coming from the second parent) and usually including preschool and/or school-age children (16%) a. Career b. Noncareer 4. Single adult living alone (20%) 5. Three-generation family—may characterize any variant of family forms 1, 2, or 3 living in a common household (5%) 6. Middle-aged or elderly couple—husband as provider, wife at home (children have been launched into college, career, or marriage) (13%) 7. Kin network—nuclear households or unmarried members living in close geographic proximity and operating within a reciprocal system of exchange of goods and services 8. "Second career" family—the wife enters the work force when the children are in school or have left home	Emerging (experimental) variant family forms (4%) include 1. Commune family a. Household of more than one monogamous couple with children, sharing common facilities, resources, and experiences; socialization of the child is a group activity b. Household of adults and offspring—a "group marriage," where all individuals are "married" to each other and all are parents to the children. Usually there is a charismatic leader 2. Unmarried parent and child family—usually mother and child, where marriage is not desired or possible 3. Unmarried couple and child family—usually a common-law type of marriage with the child their biologic issue or informally adopted 4. Cohabiting couple—unmarried couple living together 5. Homosexual unions—persons of same sex living together as "marital partners"

SOURCE: Reprinted from "Types and Percentages of Different Family Forms in the United States." Family Systems in the 1970s: Analysis, Policies and Programs by Marvin B. Sussman in volume no. 396 of THE ANNALS of The American Academy of Political and Social Science. © 1971 by The American Academy of Political and Social Science.

of special needs. This peculiar combination of being both the authority figure and provider of emotional comfort creates tension in the parental role. The absence of community assistance and support or even sociability, however, is considered to be the norm. Thus, parents and children become dependent on each other for need fulfillment.

Dual-Career Families Although the nuclear family persists as a family form, it has undergone significant alterations. The most notable change is the increasing number of mothers who, either by choice or economic need, are entering the work force. This has created a need for child-care alternatives, which have in turn exposed the children to a wide range of people and experiences.

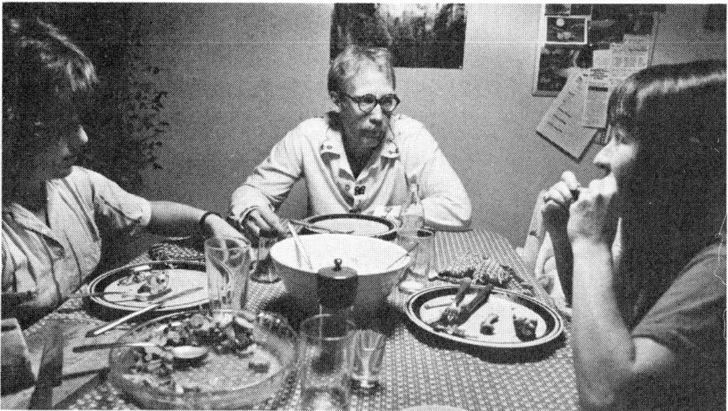

In nuclear families, a mother and father are traditionally responsible for the socialization of their children.

Since the 1950s society's macrocosmic structures have changed, with resultant economic implications. Many more families need a second income to exist. The declining infant mortality rate and increased longevity of both sexes has changed the population distribution and concomitantly its needs (Skolnick and Skolnick, 1983).

In the 1960s men who were also fathers were making choices that exemplified a change in ideas. These choices were counter to the norm but were tempered in degree, extent, and visibility of deviance. These men had wives who also had a permanent career, as opposed to working temporarily to help out during times of financial need. Consequently, these fathers shared in the domestic and child-care responsibilities and activities. For years, the father has been socialized away from child-care responsibilities. This is changing, and fathers are learning to nurture their children in ways similar to those traditionally associated with mothers. To do this, fathers are spending more time with their children.

An early study of dual-career couples done by Rapoport and Rapoport described this process of creating a balance between the strains and benefits of change as representative of "creative variants." "These couples worked at creating a new form of family and career structure which they felt to be in some sense better" (1982, p. 27). In essence they carved out a new niche for themselves that differed from the niche defined by the prevailing social milieu but that better fit their personalities and visions.

The roles of fatherhood and motherhood have institutionalized definitions that convey general meanings for the society as a whole. These general role definitions are taught to succeeding generations (for example, that the father is the provider of goods and the head of the household and the mother is the homemaker and the one who provides for the basic needs of the children). At the microscopic level, however, the meanings of father and mother may be quite different in the context of the individual family or even of the community group because the institutionalized definition no longer fits the reality. This new definition of shared roles and responsibilities gradually becomes objectified and externalized within the group, internalized by the children of the group, and eventually finds its way into society as a whole. As society adapts to this change, the abstract becomes concrete and new realities are constructed. The roles of fatherhood and motherhood are being redefined. The new definition and image of the father as one who is capable of nurturing, expressing love and concern, and who is responsible for family service activities is emerging, together with the new role of the mother as an economic provider and a decision maker with equal power and privileges. Policy changes are on the horizon as they follow the impact these role changes have at the macroscopic level of society.

Reconstituted Families In recent years the relative stability of the nuclear family has been rocked by an increasing number of marital separations and divorces, often resulting in a variation on the nuclear family known as the *reconstituted family* (Fantini and Rossi, 1980). Reconstituted, or blended, families are established through remarriage and in many instances result in larger kinship systems for the child. Research on the effects of these arrangements has not yet determined what impact, if any, these changes have on the developing child and what factors can be brought into play to mediate possible untoward effects.

Recent research indicates that there is a greater risk for separation or divorce in remarriages that follow a divorce (Cherlin, 1978). The 1976 US Bureau of the Census reported a 7% greater divorce rate in remarriages than in first marriages. The higher divorce rate suggests that for some families, the maintenance of the family unit is more precarious in remarriage after divorce.

Research also has found that when the second marriage included children from either one or both of the first marriages, the probability of a second divorce increased. If there were children from the second marriage, the probability decreased (Cherlin, 1978). One of the problems experienced by blended families is the limitations imposed by language (Cherlin, 1978). By what term do children address their mother's new husband or father's new wife? Symbols are used to define coordinate roles. The term stepparent originally was reserved for the parent who replaced a deceased parent; however, in situations of divorce the child has an additional parent or even two additional parents.

Many times, mothers and fathers have commented that their children refused to allow the new spouse's children to call them "mom" or "dad." The enforced distinction made it difficult for them to enact the parent role equally toward both sets of children. Family relationships are complex, and few guidelines are available to help with the problems that arise. Clearly, there are more questions than answers, and each family has to work out its own destiny with limited supports or guidance.

Extended Families

The extended family consists of two or more nuclear families arranged either across generations to include grandparents or among siblings to include aunts, uncles, and cousins. Today, few children grow up in extended families in which related adults other than two parents comprise the household and provide additional support on a regular basis. Even more typical in the past was the individual nuclear household with extended family members living nearby or within the same town. The current emphasis on mobility necessitated by school or occupation often separates kinship families by hundreds of miles or more. Although physical separation exists, emotional attachment and loyalty remain high in most situations. There is a special relationship between grandparents and grandchildren and among cousins, aunts, and uncles. For example, 4-year-old Mark was hesitant to talk with adults or play with children that he did not know. When some relatives visited whom he had seen only once before when he was an infant, however, he immediately interacted with them as if they were best friends. His mother commented that Mark placed relatives in a different category and that if someone were family, they were special. This attitude was true for the parents as well.

Today, kinship ties are important more for friendship and emotional support than for economic cooperation. Of all types of visiting and socializing activities, the most common are visiting with relatives. The intensity and extent of kinship ties vary with each nuclear family and the absence of such ties is often explained on the basis of personality differences. For some families, the trend for mothers to return to work has revived the practice of depending on relatives, albeit those living in separate households, to care for children while the parents are working. In fact, over 30% of child care in the United States is provided by relatives (Fantini and Rossi, 1980).

Therefore, although the number of extended families has decreased, several cultural groups continue to rely heavily on their relatives, and many other families are rediscovering the advantages of well-maintained kinship systems. The extended family form has more often persisted relatively unchanged among certain lower-income or less culturally assimilated families.

Communal Families

For some families, the attributes of an extended family lifestyle have been sought by establishing communal living arrangements. The result is a *communal family* and shared childrearing, which is neither a new nor an exclusively American phenomenon. Communal childrearing arrangements have been documented in many societies and in the United States from its early beginnings. The number of communal families and children reared in them, however, rose significantly during the 1960s and 1970s. Many of these arrangements have since dissolved; however, some continue to exist and new ones to emerge.

Communal families exist in a variety of settings and forms but generally are defined as a group of unrelated adults who come together to form a committed unit. The structure of and functions in these families vary considerably from formal and defined patterns of roles and relationships to informal groupings with diffuse relationships and roles. The Israeli kibbutzim exemplify the structured and functionally defined approach to communal childrearing (Rabin, 1965; Bettelheim, 1969; Spiro, 1975). A less-structured and less-defined pattern of role relationships is the "hippie" commune, as described by Sara Davidson (Davidson, 1971).

In general, communal families are established as alternatives to the family forms that these family members reject. Particular ideologies and a search for belonging and kindred relationships often have been the impetus for establishing communal arrangements. The belief in children's potential and the need for freedom to become and create is a value of many communal groups (Lynn, 1977). Most communal family members regard themselves as an extended family that contains nuclear family units (Berger, 1971). Usually, the tie between infant and mother is fostered, but as the child grows, the importance of the child's relationships with other adults in the group assumes greater significance. Ambiguity may exist regarding child–parent relationships, and conflicts among adults concerning the consistency of child discipline and guidance are evident (Berger, 1971). Because of the wide variation that can exist in these arrangements, however, it is impossible to define any specific general characteristics and influences on child development. Rather, the nurse needs to assess each child and family individually to determine the structural, functional, social, and affective variables influencing that child.

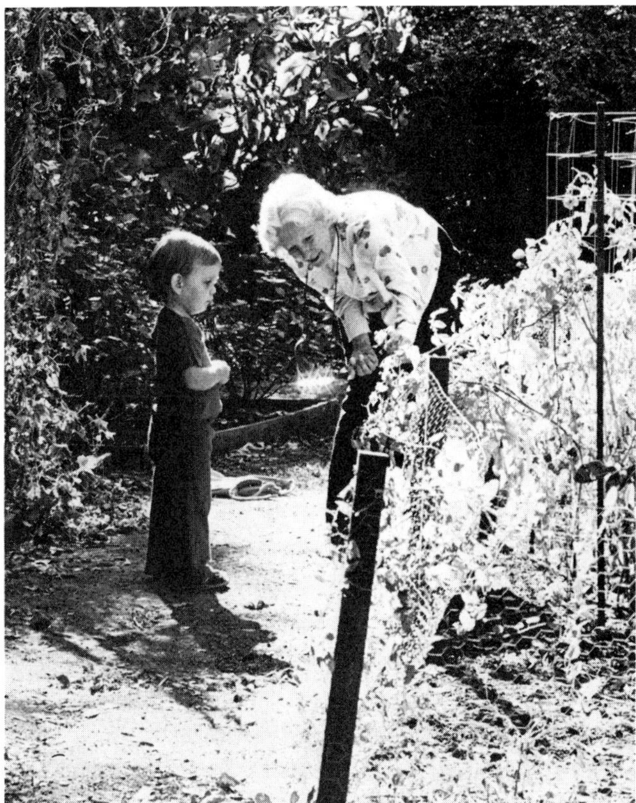

In extended families, grandparents and children develop special relationships.

Single-Parent Families

Single-parent families, in which children have day-to-day contact with only one parent, usually result from the death of one parent, marital separation, divorce, or birth of a child to an unmarried woman. A recent trend has been for unmarried individuals to adopt a child. In most instances single-parent families are headed by a female parent. For many of these families, issues of companionship and support for the available parent, financial solvency, and role modeling of adult interactions in a family setting are sources of concern for future child development.

Lamb (1980) found that nuclear families were more effective and reliable as socializing agents than single-parent families but only when the marital relationship and overall emotional milieu of the nuclear family were harmonious. Additional issues or sociocultural factors for the single-parent family either facilitate or impede effective parenting, but these factors need further study. For some cultural groups, single-parent households have been traditionally and effectively structured as the dominant family form and have resulted in relatively satisfactory child development. What seems to be significant for the health professional therefore is that this family structure is not deviant from the traditional nuclear family form but rather should be viewed in the

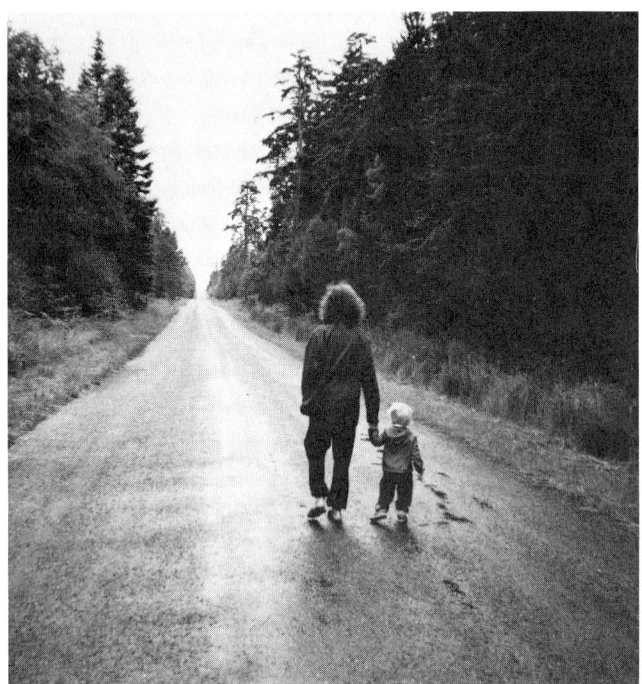

When single parents have the necessary supports, single-parent families can be effective and reliable in socializing young children.

context in which it occurs and the coping ability that it manifests. Concerns center on available supports during times of parental stress, parental coping strategies, sharing of responsibilities within the family unit, childrearing attitudes, beliefs, and values, and the overall functional stability of the family.

Because of the number of marriages that end in divorce, many young children must cope with the disruptive and separating effects that divorce brings. The actual crisis of the divorce is often preceded by a long period of conflict and discord within the family, and, at times, the child may be torn between conflicting allegiances. For some children, the divorce actually brings a sense of relief as tempers calm and battles end.

The actual divorce process may be a complex and lengthy legal procedure. The divorcing partners and their children need to begin to cope with the difficulties inherent to loss, separation, and a sense of failure throughout the period of separation and divorce. New patterns of relationships must be defined as the system's boundaries and channels of communication change. For some families, the stigma that they perceive to be associated with the divorce may intensify the closing of the family's boundaries. For others, the boundaries become more permeable as the individuals recognize the need for support and help in dealing with their stress.

In all instances the children of the divorcing parents find themselves in a situation that significantly affects them but over which they feel they have no control. This sense of powerlessness for many children is translated into self-doubt and guilt because they cannot comprehend that they did not somehow contribute to the problem. Confusion and anger result as the child finds it necessary to assign blame and form allegiances and take sides. Coping strategies that children use to deal with separation are discussed in Chapter 12.

The risks involved in the single-parent family headed by the unwed adolescent parent are of particular concern to the health care professional, even though attitudes toward unwed pregnancy in society are changing. Several problems that still confront this family include

1. Fostering the adaptive development of the adolescent parent by making referrals to special school programs and supportive social services
2. Helping the adolescent to cope with the conflicting demands of normal adolescent development and parental role development
3. Monitoring and facilitating the healthy development of the child
4. Providing appropriate ongoing anticipatory guidance, health care, and health and/or parenting education

Continuity of care, careful follow-up, and inclusion of the father when appropriate and possible should be part of the nurse's goals when working with the adolescent parent. The special needs of both adolescent parents and single-parent families without adequate supports are discussed in Chapter 22.

Gay Families

An area of recent study and professional attention is the developmental, social, and cultural implications of childrearing within a *gay family* in which the adults are the same sex. The dilemma of the gay family is similar to that of several other minority groups in the United States (Martin and Lyon, 1972). The prejudice and discrimination inherent in minority group status is, however, only one of the complex issues to consider in relation to this family form. Children and parents living in gay families also must cope with such issues as social or family disapproval, the trauma of divorce or separation, and conflicts in sexual role adoption and enactment.

Homosexuality and lesbianism are still condemned by many people. For the health care professional, sensitivity and acceptance are necessary prerequisites to helping these families cope with the day-to-day issues of childrearing and health maintenance. Patterns of relationship, real or perceived stressors, and resources within the family unit must all be assessed to facilitate healthy child and family development. In some communities several organizations and support groups can assist the gay family in achieving its goals and carrying on its everyday activities with dignity, self-acceptance, and self-awareness. The nurse should be aware of these resources for potential referral and as repositories of current literature that can be used when working with these families.

Foster-Care Families

As many as 266,000 children currently are living in foster homes in the United States. Foster care placement has almost entirely replaced the institutional placement of children whose natural parents are unable or unwilling to care for them (Keniston, 1977). (The legal system that affects foster care is discussed in Chapter 22.) Some of the important issues and dilemmas relative to the foster-care family include

1. The lack of formal parental rights for foster parents
2. The ambiguity of the foster parents' role
3. The potential incongruity between paid foster-care services and the provision of a warm, loving home
4. The constant possibility of removal of the child from the foster-care home, which often prevents the foster parents from "becoming too attached" (LeMasters and deFrain, 1983)

Because a child's family is the base from which the child ventures to explore the world and initially develops an awareness of affectional bonds to others, a foster-care experience can have considerable impact on a child. Understanding this impact also invites a closer examination of foster-care programs that can facilitate a child's development during a temporary breakdown within the child's natural family.

Various documented effects and consequences result from separation of the young child from the primary caregiver, and analysis of these effects has contributed to an understanding of the nature of human bonds (Bowlby, 1969). These bonds or ties eventually influence the child's perception of self as a social entity, the child's trust of the world, and the autonomy and independence needed to venture out confidently and effectively into the world beyond the family. The shock of sudden separation, for which there has been no preparation or transitional process, gives rise to several behavioral responses by the young child. In her writings about her observations of young children, particularly those under 4 years of age, suffering various separation experiences during World War II, Anna Freud described the shock of sudden separation as creating feelings of loneliness and abandonment, which were manifested by gestures, facial expressions, tearfulness, and anger (Freud, 1968). She also documented the need for specific interventions to ease the child's transitional adjustment to these separations and for alternative child-care arrangements.

The level of development that a child can attain in a foster-care setting therefore depends in part on complex factors that, if properly known and knowledgeably implemented, can create an enriching environment for the child. The relationships that the child develops with substitute caregivers (foster parents) is a major factor. Particularly important are the aspects of predictability and continuity. The importance of these factors is very evident from the research that has been done in residential childrearing settings. Frequent changes in staff in institutional childrearing settings often resulted in children who had diffuse attachments with no specific preference for a single individual (Tizard, 1972); however, in extended families of multiple caregivers, healthy attachments occurred. The significant difference was that in the extended families care was provided by warm, loving people on a regular basis and in a personal way. These multiple caregivers were stable in their personal care as well as their composition. Studies of Israeli kibbutzim also point out that the essential variables for minimizing the effects of separation of the child from the parent lie in the consistency and quality of care the child receives and the attention given to sustaining the child's relationship with the natural parents (Rabin, 1967).

What can be learned from these studies and applied to the foster-care setting involves the incorporation of factors most likely to reduce the stress of separation and provide an opportunity for child development and enrichment of the child–family relationship. The following factors emerge as significant:

1. Placement of the child in a warm, accepting environment
2. Incorporation of familiar routines, foods, and so on
3. Encouraging feelings of belonging
4. Reassurance of eventual parental reunion, if realistic
5. Helping the child to separate reality and fantasy
6. Appropriate and consistent discipline
7. Opportunities to discuss parents and home
8. Preventing further separations by avoiding frequent changes in foster-care placement
9. Contact with the natural parent(s) when possible

Trends in the Evolution of Families

The rate of change within the structure and function of the family system has been attributed to an ever-increasing rate of change in the systems that surround and intersect the family. Large numbers of families from diverse backgrounds have been assimilated into single societies, yet these societies continue to retain the rich cultural heritages and influences that the people brought with them. Current concerns regarding families are the rising divorce rate, economic hardships, and an increase in the number of mothers working outside their homes. The family has changed, but despite these changes, the family continues to exist as a vital force in the social and emotional fabric of life. Many reasons may account for this vitality, not the least of which are the unique role that the family plays and the social and intimate needs of people.

Other factors also have contributed to the durability and continuity of family structures. Several disciplines have studied families, and from each of these disciplines has grown a large body of knowledge that has been incorporated by professionals working with children and their families. Health care agencies and their personnel have increasingly encouraged and supported network systems between parents whose children share similar problems. Families also have taken a more active role in identifying their needs and availing themselves of the services that best meet them. Day-care services have increased in number and improved in quality. Cooperative centers with active parental involvement have been designed. Community agencies have set up referral centers for parents in need of help and consultation. Parents with special needs have joined together to provide mutual support, education, and political leverage for the issues that concern them.

Key Concepts

- The family is the earliest and primary environment in which socialization of the child takes place.
- Definitions of the family in today's society vary widely and are sometimes controversial.
- The evolution of the family is a result of social, political, economic, and philosophic changes.
- The nurse views the family as an open system and considers both the dynamics within a family and the influences on it.
- Family structure describes the number of family members and the relation of each family member to the others; family function describes the effects of family behaviors on the family system.
- Family roles determine relationships among family members and are a primary socializing influence on the child.
- Family development may be defined by a set of developmental tasks that the family undertakes at various times.
- Communication within the family is a significant indication of family functioning; communication outside the family is affected by the permeability of its boundaries.
- Types of families common today include nuclear and reconstituted families, extended families, communal families, single-parent families, gay families, and foster-care families.

References

Berger H, et al: Childrearing practices of the communal family. In: *Family in Transition.* Skolnick AS, Skolnick JH (editors). Little, Brown, 1971.

Bettelheim B: *Children of the Dream.* MacMillan, 1969.

Bowlby J: *Attachment and Loss.* Vols 1 and 2. Basic Books, 1969.

Bronowski J: *The Ascent of Man.* Little, Brown, 1973.

Cherlin A: Remarriage as an incomplete institution. *Am J Sociol* 1978; 84(3):634–649.

Cohen D: *Serving Preschool Children.* DHEW Publication No. OHD. US Department of Health, Education, and Welfare, 1974.

Coser RL (editor): *The Family: Its Structure and Functions.* 2nd ed. St. Martin's Press, 1974.

Davidson S: The hippie alternative: Getting back to the communal garden. In: *Family in Transition.* Skolnick AS, Skolnick JH (editors). Little, Brown, 1971.

Duvall E: *Marriage and Family Development.* Lippincott, 1977.

Elkin D, Handel G: *The Child and Society: The Process of Socialization.* Random House, 1978.

Fantini MD, Rossi A: Parenting in a pluralistic society: Toward a policy of options and choices. In: *Parenting in a Multicultural Society.* Fantini MD, Cardenas R (editors). Longman, 1980.

Freud A: *The Writings of Anna Freud.* Vol. IV. International Universities Press, 1968.

Friedman M: *Family Nursing: Theory and Assessment.* Appleton-Century-Crofts, 1981.

Gambino R: *Blood of My Blood.* Doubleday, 1974.

Giele J: Changes in the modern American family: Their impact on sex roles. In: *The Family: Its Structures and Functions.* 2nd ed. Coser RL (editor). St. Martin's Press, 1974.

Goode WJ: Why men resist. In: *Rethinking the Family: Some Feminist Questions.* Thorne B, Yalom M (editors). Longman, 1982.

Gough K: The origin of the family. Reprinted in: *Family in Transition.* Skolnick AS, Skolnick JH (editors). Little, Brown, 1983.

Gronseth E: The breadwinner trap. In: *The Future of the Family.* Howes LK (editor). Simon & Schuster, 1972.

Hareven TK: *American Families in Transition: Historical Perspectives on Change in Normal Family Processes.* Walsh F (editor). Guilford Press, 1982.

Keniston K, and the Carnegie Council on Children. *All Our Children: The American Family Under Pressure.* Harcourt Brace Jovanovich, 1977.

Knafl RA, Grace HK: *Families Across the Life Cycle.* Little, Brown, 1978.

Lamb M: What can research experts tell parents about effective socialization? In: *Parenting in a Multicultural Society.* Fantini MD, Cardenas A (editors). Longman, 1980.

LeMasters EE, DeFrain J: *Parents in Contemporary America.* Dorsey Press, 1983.

Lynn D: Cultural experiments in restructuring the family. In: *Contemporary Readings in Child Psychology.* Heatherington EM, Parke R (editors). McGraw-Hill, 1977.

Martin D, Lyon P: *Lesbian Women.* Bantam Books, 1972.

Merton R: Latent and manifest functions. In: *Social Theory and Social Structure.* Free Press, 1968.
Miller JR, Janosik E: *Family Focused Care.* McGraw-Hill, 1980.
Nye FI: *Role Structure and Analysis of the Family.* Sage Publications, 1976.
Parsons T: *The Social System.* Free Press, 1951.
Rabin AJ: *Growing Up in the Kibbutz.* Springer, 1967.
Rapoport R, Rapoport RN: Three generations of dual-career family research. In: *Dual-Career Couples.* Pepitone-Rockwell F (editor). Sage Publications, 1982.
Ritzer G: *Contemporary Sociological Theory.* Knopf, 1983.
Robischon P, Scott D: Role theory and its application in family nursing. *Nurs Outlook* 1969; 17:52–57.
Satir V: *Conjoint Family Therapy.* Science and Behavior Books, 1967.
Satir, V: *Peoplemaking.* Science and Behavior Books, 1972.
Skolnick AS, Skolnick JH (editors). *Family in Transition.* Little, Brown, 1983.
Spiro M: *Children of the Kibbutz.* Harvard University Press, 1975.
Spock B: *Raising Your Child in a Different Time.* Norton Press, 1974.
Tizard JB: The institution as an environment for development. In: *The Integration of the Child in a Social World.* Richard MP (editor). Cambridge University Press, 1972.

Additional Readings

Aguelera D, Messick J: *Crises Intervention.* Mosby, 1974.
Ainsworth M, Bell S: Attachment, exploration and separation. In: *Readings in Child Development and Relationships.* Smart R, Smart M (editors). MacMillan, 1972.
Averbach A: *Parents Learn Through Discussion.* Wiley, 1968.
Bandura A: *Social Learning Theory.* Prentice-Hall, 1977.
Bebbington AC: The function of stress in the establishment of the dual-career family. *J Marriage and Family* (August) 1973; 35:530–537.
Brim O: *Education for Childrearing.* Russell Sage Foundation, 1959.
Cain A: Assessment of family structure. In: *Family Focused Care.* Miller J, Janosik E (editors). McGraw-Hill, 1980.
D'Antonio WV, Aldous J: *Families and Religions: Conflict and Change in Modern Society.* Sage, 1983.
de Mause L: *The History of Childhood.* Psychohistory Press, 1974.
Fein G, Clark-Steward A: *Day Care in Context.* Wiley, 1973.
Foley V: *An Introduction to Family Therapy.* Grune & Stratton, 1974.
Fox MF, Hesse-Biber S: *Women at Work.* Mayfield, 1984.
Garbino J: *Children and Families in the Social Environment.* Aldine, 1982.
Gathorne-Hardy J: *The Unnatural History of the Nanny.* Dial Press, 1973.
Green E: Losses in the family system. In: *Family Focused Care.* Janosik E, Miller J (editors). McGraw-Hill, 1980.
Grollman C (editor): *Explaining Death to Children.* Beacon Press, 1967.
Hardy M, Conway M: *Role Theory: Perspectives for Health Professionals.* Appleton-Century-Crofts, 1978.
Harley B: Socialization for roles. In: *Role Theory: Perspectives for Health Professionals.* Hardy M, Conway M (editors). Appleton-Century-Crofts, 1978.
Hilliard A: Respecting the child's culture. *Child Today* (Jan/Feb) 1979; 8:21.
Horowitz JA, Perdue BJ: Single-parent families. *Nurs Clin North Am* (Sept) 1977; 12:503–511.
Hymovich DP, Chamberlin RW: *Child and Family Development.* McGraw-Hill, 1980.
Kimball G: *The 50-50 Marriage.* Beacon Press, 1983.
Kelly J, Wallestein JJ: Brief interventions with children in divorcing families. *Am J Orthopsychiatry* 1977; 47:23–39.
Kubler-Ross E: *On Death and Dying.* Tavistock, 1970.
Lein L, Blchar MC: Working couples as parents. In: *Family in Transition.* Skolnick AS, Skolnick JH (editors). Little, Brown, 1983.
Lewis M: The social network systems model. In: *Review of Human Development.* Field TM, et al (editors). Wiley, 1982.
Mead DE: *Six Approaches to Childrearing.* Brigham Young University Press, 1977.
Minuchi S: *Families and Family Therapy.* Harvard University Press, 1974.
Montagu A: *Culture and Human Development.* Prentice-Hall, 1974.
Olson DH, McCubbin HI: *Families: What Makes Them Work.* Sage, 1983.
Profence S, Naylor A, Patterson J: *The Challenge of Day Care.* Yale University Press, 1977.
Prout V: Emotional deprivation and the privileged child. In: *A Call for Action on Behalf of Children.* American Nurses Association, Publication No. MCN 11:11–12, March, 1980.
Queen S, Habenstein RW: *The Family in Various Cultures.* Lippincott, 1974.
Robertson HR: Removing barriers to health care. *Nurs Outlook* 1969; 17:44.
Sahler O (editor): *The Child and Death.* Mosby, 1978.
Satir V, Stachowick J, Taschman H: *Helping Families to Change.* Jason Aronson, 1977.
Thorne B, Yalom M (editors). *Rethinking the Family: Some Feminist Questions.* Longman, 1981.
Werner E: How children influence children: The role of peers in the socialization process. *Child Today* (March/April) 1979; 8:10–11.
Williams J: The terminally ill parent. In: *High-Risk Parenting.* Hall S (editor). Lippincott, 1979.
Wiltse K: Foster care in the 1970s: A decade for change. *Child Today* (May/June) 1979; 8:10–14.

Developmental Implications of Heredity

5

Wendy J. Fibison Susan Rowen James

Chapter Outline

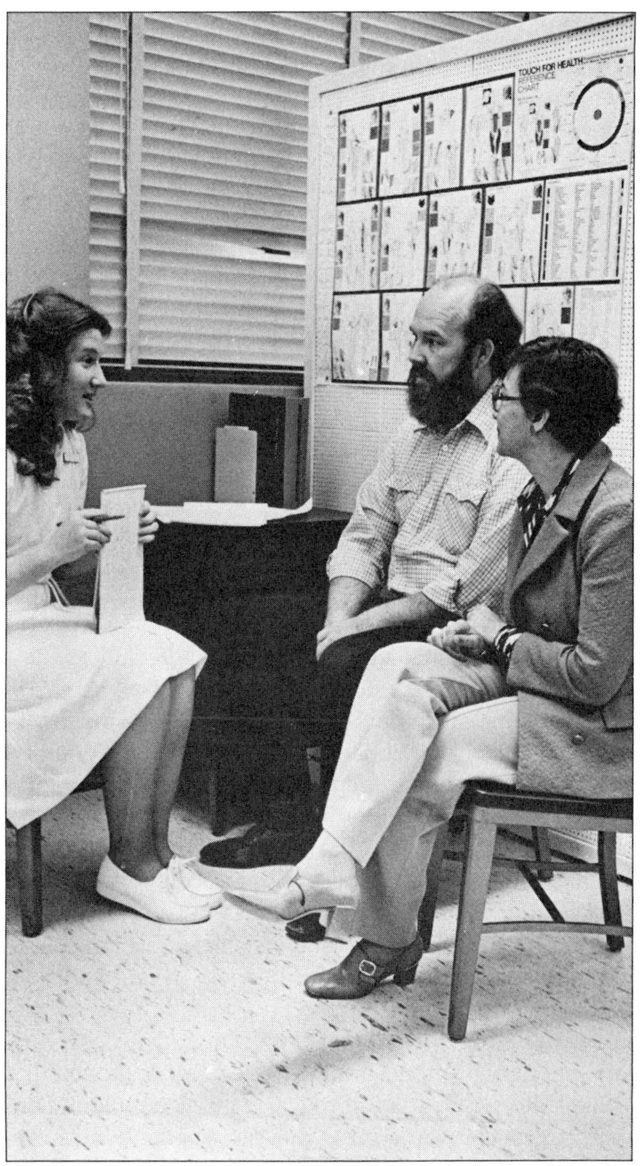

Objectives

- Describe the components of an individual cell that are directly related to heredity.
- List the steps involved with DNA and RNA replication and protein synthesis.
- State the major modes of the inheritance of traits.
- Relate the use of twin studies to investigations of multifactorial inheritance.
- Explain some of the underlying genetic mechanisms related to metabolism and the development of immune components.
- Identify the child health nurse's role in intervention with families at risk for genetic disorders.

The pattern and progress of human childhood development beginning before conception has long fascinated scientists, health professionals, and parents. Investigations have ranged from rigorous scientific research in laboratories to parental observations and informal exchanges. For example, geneticists examine the influence of chromosome number and arrangement on development; psychologists address such issues as birth order and environment; and parents look often to their own behavior and treatment of the child. In seeking to understand developmental influences, they all share a common goal—to identify factors that would support and enhance the developmental potential of any given child.

Both environment (suprasystems) and heredity (subsystems) contribute to the normal development of the child. Environmental factors are physical as well as emotional. The health and nutritional status of the mother prior to conception and during pregnancy influence the development of the fetus. Once born, infants require not only food but love and affection for their progress to be normal. As the child becomes more mobile and social, opportunities to practice new skills are necessary. Without practice, reinforcement, and encouragement, the child's developmental potential may not be reached. In more severe cases of deprivation, development may be arrested. Much of the knowledge of these needs has been acquired by observing what happens when environmental factors go wrong.

Similarly, what scientists have learned about human heredity stems in large part from examining how genetic mechanisms can err, resulting in congenital disorders and health problems.

The techniques for examining the role of heredity in development are continually being refined as the complex mechanisms of genetic regulation are revealed piece by piece. Genetic engineering, recombinant DNA techniques, sequencing, and gene mapping are some of the tools available to the geneticist in the search for the keys to heredity influences on development. Scientists are just beginning to probe the depths of the genetic contribution to normal development. Sorting out what is the result of heredity, what is the effect of environment, and what the interactions are between the two is a complex challenge.

This chapter concerns the genetic component of the child's normal development. Relevant research findings are reviewed. Although the discussion assumes previous exposure to the principles of human genetics, including cell structure and division, a brief review of protein synthesis and the modes of inheritance seems appropriate. More information on the genetic factors in specific health problems, such as phenylketonuria, diabetes mellitus, and mental retardation, can be found in the primary discussion of those problems in the appropriate chapters.

The Genetic Code

Proteins

Body growth and many body functions are dependent on the synthesis of proteins. Proteins are large organic molecules that vary in size, shape, and function. One or more chains of amino acids—polypeptides—fold and coil into the three-dimensional structure of the protein molecule. Twenty different amino acids are found in protein structures, and their proper sequence is necessary to provide a biologically functioning protein.

The specific sequencing of amino acids allows the chains to fold, and the folded configuration gives the molecule strength, as well as the ability to interact with its environment. There are several types of proteins, each with specific functions:

1. *Enzymes*—affect biochemical and metabolic reactions in the cell and in the organism as a whole
2. *Hormones*—aid in metabolism and sexual development and function
3. *Antibodies*—part of the body's defense against illness
4. *Structural*—building blocks of the body—include proteins that function singly (collagen) and those that are bound with other elements such as
   a. nucleoproteins (nucleic acid)
   b. glycoproteins (polysaccharides)
   c. lipoproteins (fats)
   d. transport proteins (metal), for example, hemoglobin

Proteins are synthesized in most cells. The timing of a protein's production and the amount of protein produced play a crucial role in development. Certain proteins may be synthesized only during embryonic development, and other proteins are produced only in the adult. The factors responsible for this activating mechanism currently are under intensive study.

Protein Synthesis

Nomenclature Protein synthesis in the cell is directed by a genetic code that translates a message from a particular gene into a sequence of amino acids comprising a polypeptide chain. To understand this mechanism a definition of appropriate terms is indicated.

The *gene* is considered the biologic unit of heredity. Its function is to code for the synthesis of a protein, an RNA molecule, or other genes. Genes are composed of chemical building blocks called *nucleotides.* Each nucleotide unit contains a pentose sugar, a phosphate, and a nitrogenous base, all of which are joined by chemical bonds. Two strands of nucleotides in specific sequences form the double-helix configuration of the *DNA* molecule, deoxyribonucleic acid (Fig.5-1).

Four nitrogenous bases have been identified as part of the DNA molecule: adenine (A), guanine (G), cytosine (C), and thymine (T). The molecule looks like a twisted ladder, with the rungs being the nitrogenous bases—two bases linked by hydrogen bonds form each rung. In the DNA molecule the bases pair in a specific pattern—A always matches with T and G with C. The two strands of DNA, then, are always complementary. The sequence of nucleotides on the DNA strand determines the protein it will synthesize. Because there are four different bases that can array themselves in an almost limitless sequence, the potential number of proteins is enormous. There can be millions of nucleotides in a human DNA strand (Ayala and Kiger, 1984).

Genes situate themselves on *chromosomes.* Chromosomes are located in the cell nucleus and are formed by DNA molecules winding themselves around protein molecules like thread around a spool (Jenkins, p. 73) (Fig. 5-2). The gene is located at a specific position, or *locus*, on a chromosome. There may be 50–100,000 gene loci in human chromosomes, although only 1200 gene loci have been accurately identified (Jenkins, 1983). The human cell has 46 chromosomes in its nucleus, half donated by the mother and half contributed by the father during fertilization. Twenty-two pairs are *autosomes*, chromosomes other than the *sex chromosomes.* The remaining two chromosomes are sex chromosomes, XX producing a female and XY creating a male. During cell division, individual chromosomes can be identified by size, shape, and banding patterns produced by biologic stains. A *karyotype* (Fig. 5-3) is a pictorial array of chromosomes used for analysis.

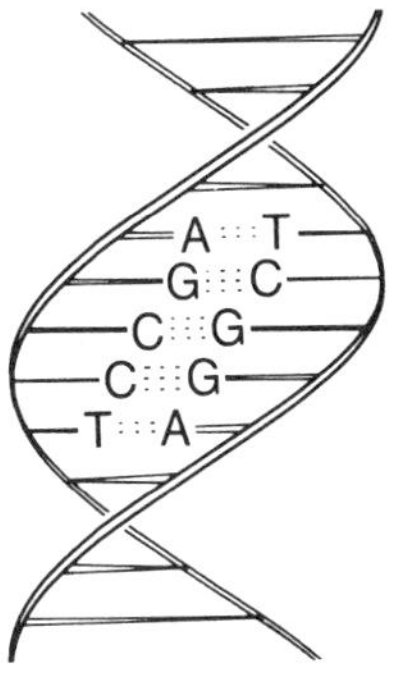

Figure 5-1 Structure of DNA strand. (From Jenkins JB: *Human Genetics.* Benjamin/Cummings, 1983.)

Before a cell undergoes mitotic division, chromosomes reproduce themselves, thus ensuring that identical genetic information is carried to each of the two newly created cells.

RNA and ribosomes are essential to an understanding of protein synthesis. *RNA*, or ribonucleic acid, is a single-stranded structure, in contrast to the double-helix structure of DNA. The constituents of RNA are phosphoric acid, a sugar (D-ribose), and bases (adenine, guanine, cytosine, and uracil). Several types of RNA have been observed in the nucleus and cytoplasm of the cell, three of which are involved in protein synthesis. *Messenger RNA* (mRNA) is transcribed from DNA in the nucleus and transmits the genetic information to the cytoplasm. Only mRNA actually is translated into the polypeptide chains that form the proteins. When the shorthand DNA–RNA–protein is used, mRNA is assumed. Once in the cytoplasm, mRNA complexes with ribosomal RNA (rRNA), which in part forms the *ribosomes*, the "factory" in which protein synthesis occurs. Transfer RNA (tRNA) acts as a retriever, obtaining the necessary amino acids from the cytoplasm and aligning them in the proper sequence for the protein to be synthesized.

Genetic Information Transfers Genetic information is transferred in three ways:

1. DNA to DNA by replication
2. DNA to RNA by transcription
3. RNA to protein by translation

The DNA molecule of the gene replicates itself with the assistance of enzymes, using an RNA molecule as a primer. The chemical bonds between the nitrogenous bases are weakened at nucleotide initiation points, and the molecule comes apart to form two separate but complementary strands (Fig. 5-4). Each strand serves as a template for the synthesis of a new strand. Each new strand is the complement of the template; that is, new A links to template T and new G to template C, forming two complete molecules that are identical to the original. Only precise replication ensures accurate function of the gene.

For the message on the gene to be translated into an amino acid sequence, it first must be transcribed onto an

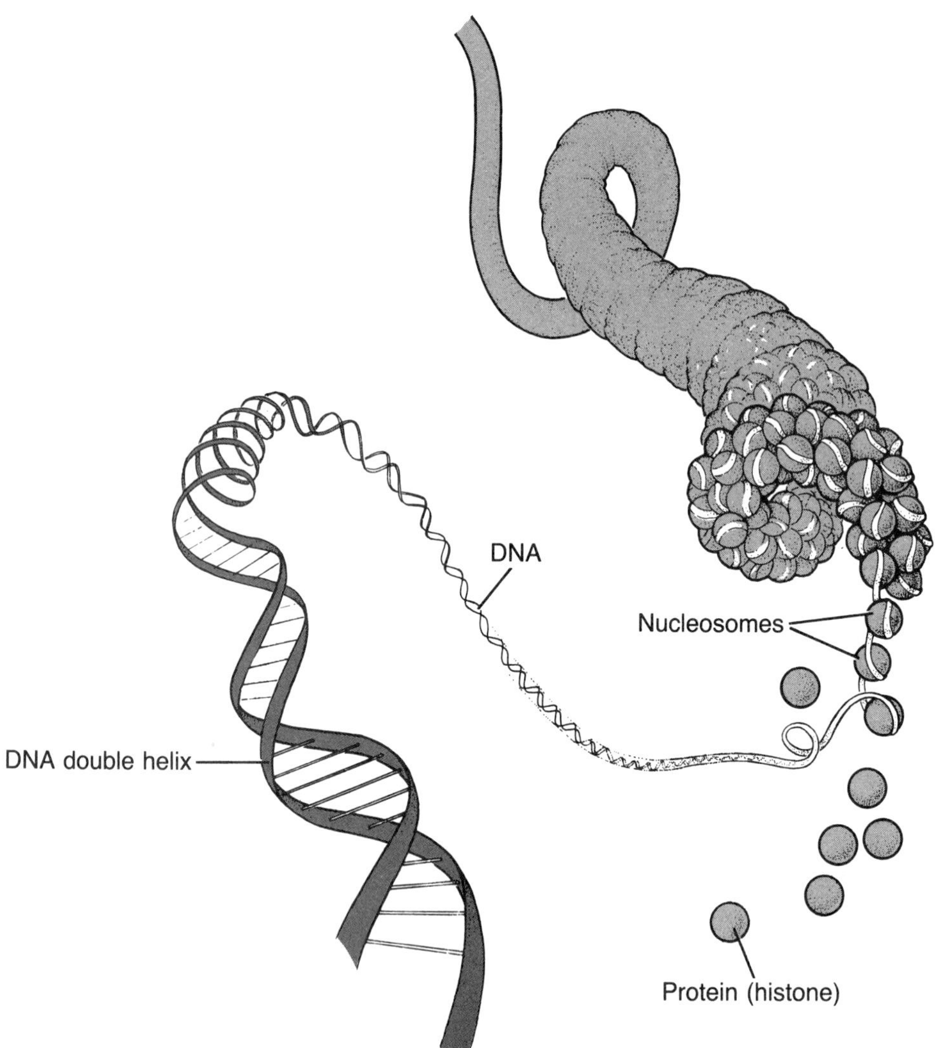

Figure 5-2 Chromosomes are formed by DNA molecules winding themselves around protein molecules like thread around a spool. (From Jenkins JB: *Human Genetics*. Benjamin/Cummings, 1983.)

RNA molecule. The mechanism of transcription occurs in the following sequence:

1. An enzyme, RNA polymerase, binds to a nucleotide region on the DNA molecule (promoter), which is located at the beginning of a gene

2. The DNA strands unwind and separate at the bases, and one DNA strand serves as a template for the RNA that is being synthesized. The new RNA is the complement of the DNA template, but with the U linking to A since RNA contains uracil instead of thymine

3. The synthesis terminates at a signal nucleotide at the end of the gene, the RNA and polymerase separate from the DNA, and the DNA strands reconnect (Jenkins, 1983) (Fig. 5-5).

Interspersed among the nucleotide sequences that are transcribed onto mRNA are segments of DNA that are not translated. These segments, or *introns*, are usually excised enzymatically from mRNA before translation. Their function is not yet understood (Gilbert, 1981).

All types of RNA are synthesized in the nucleus but then pass through pores in the nuclear membrane to the cytoplasm, where protein synthesis occurs.

The sequence of the nucleotides determines the sequence of the 20 different amino acids in the synthesis of a protein molecule. The mRNA picks up the sequence during transcription. The *genetic code* refers to the correspondence between a sequence (or *codon*) of three nucleotides in DNA or RNA and the amino acid that that codon is specifying in the process of protein synthesis. This is a linear relationship, meaning that the sequence of nucleotides in DNA and RNA is translated into a corresponding sequence of amino acids. Given that there are 64 possible combinations of condons, and that there are only 20 amino acids, different codons can result in the same amino acid.

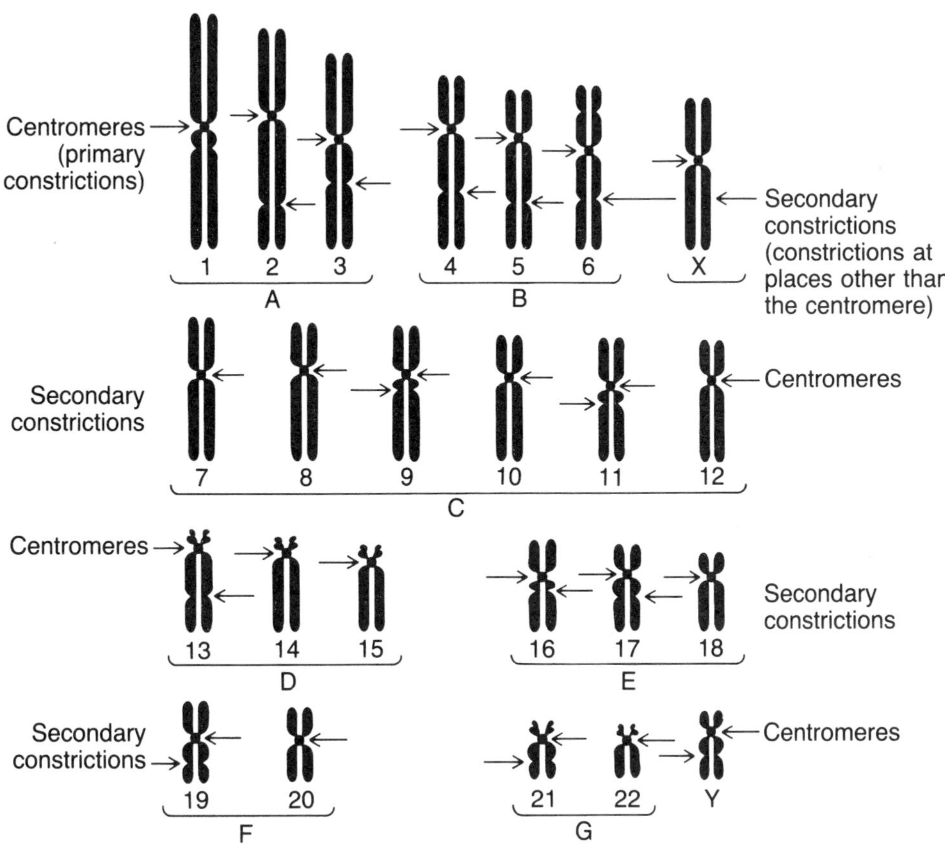

Figure 5-3 Normal male karyotype (chromosome makeup). Only one member of each pair of autosomes (nonsex chromosomes) is shown. The X and Y chromosomes are grouped with the autosomes according to size and centromere position. (From Jenkins JB: *Human Genetics.* Benjamin/Cummings, 1983.)

The mRNA cannot translate directly into an amino acid sequence. The translation is mediated by tRNA and occurs on the ribosome. The ribosome attaches to the mRNA and begins to "read" the code at a start codon. The tRNA has a unique cloverleaf structure with two attachment areas—one area at the "stem" binds to an amimo acid in the cytoplasm, whereas the opposite "leaf" has a region, called an *anticodon* (three nucleotides), which binds to the complementary codon in the mRNA (Fig. 5-6). Protein synthesis occurs as the ribosome moves down the mRNA molecule one codon at a time. A tRNA molecule binds an appropriate amino acid to its stem and binds to the mRNA at its anticodon site. Another tRNA brings a second coded amino acid, which is joined to the first amino acid by a peptide bond. After bonding, the first tRNA is released to obtain another amino acid, and so on. Amino acids are joined by peptide bonds to make a peptide chain until a termination codon is reached, and the peptide chain and RNA are released from the ribosome (Fig. 5-7) (Jenkins, 1983).

These mechanisms for protein synthesis are still being studied intensively. Scientists formerly thought that one gene

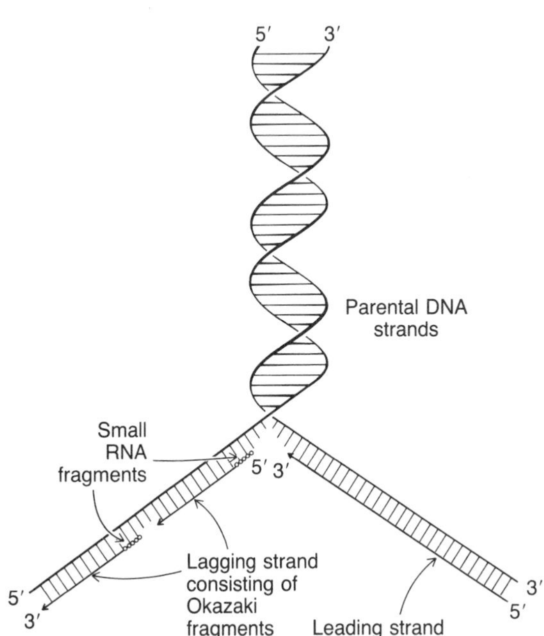

Figure 5-4 DNA replication. (From Jenkins JB: *Human Genetics.* Benjamin/Cummings, 1983.)

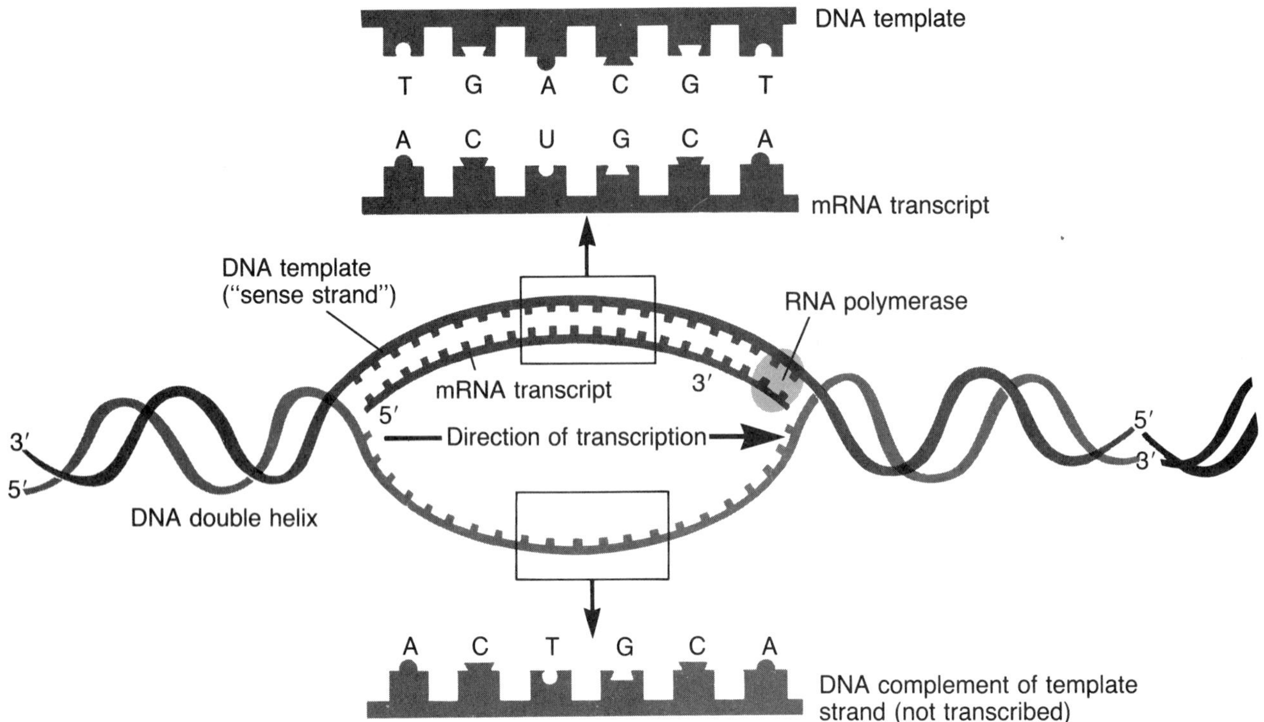

Figure 5-5 RNA transcription. (From Jenkins JB: *Human Genetics.* Benjamin/Cummings, 1983.)

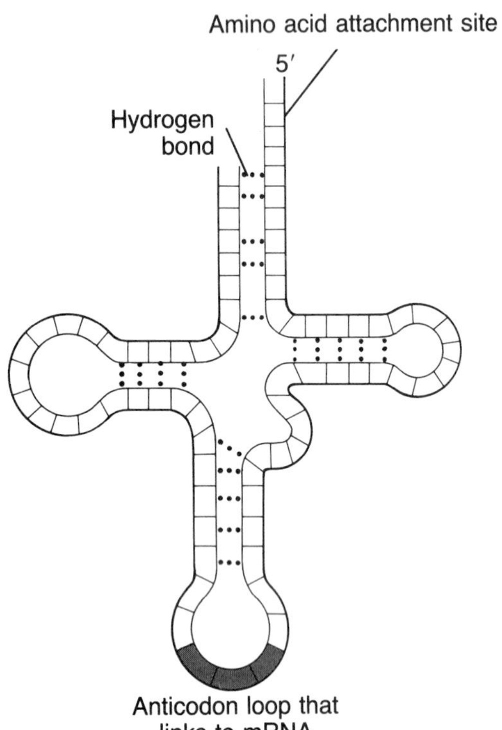

Figure 5-6 Cloverleaf structure of transfer RNA. (From Jenkins JB: *Human Genetics.* Benjamin/Cummings, 1983.)

coded for one polypeptide chain. In some proteins (specifically immunoglobulins) it has been theorized that more than one gene is involved or that segments of genes are spliced together to form mRNA, thus providing many combinations through gene rearrangement (Marx, 1981).

Protein synthesis in the cell occurs during the interphase portion of the cell's life cycle, as does DNA replication. These activities eventually increase the size of the cell to the point where cell division is initiated. Chromosomes, with their surrounding DNA, coil and become thicker and shorter in preparation for division (Fig. 5-8). As a consequence of DNA replication and chromosome division, genes are reproduced exactly in daughter cells. These cells then begin protein synthesis anew. If for some reason a nucleotide in the DNA or RNA molecule is changed, that change (mutation) will be passed to the daughter cells, and the structure and function of the resulting protein will be altered irrevocably.

Development From Conception to Birth

The human organism begins as a *zygote,* a cell resulting from the union of the sperm and egg that normally contains

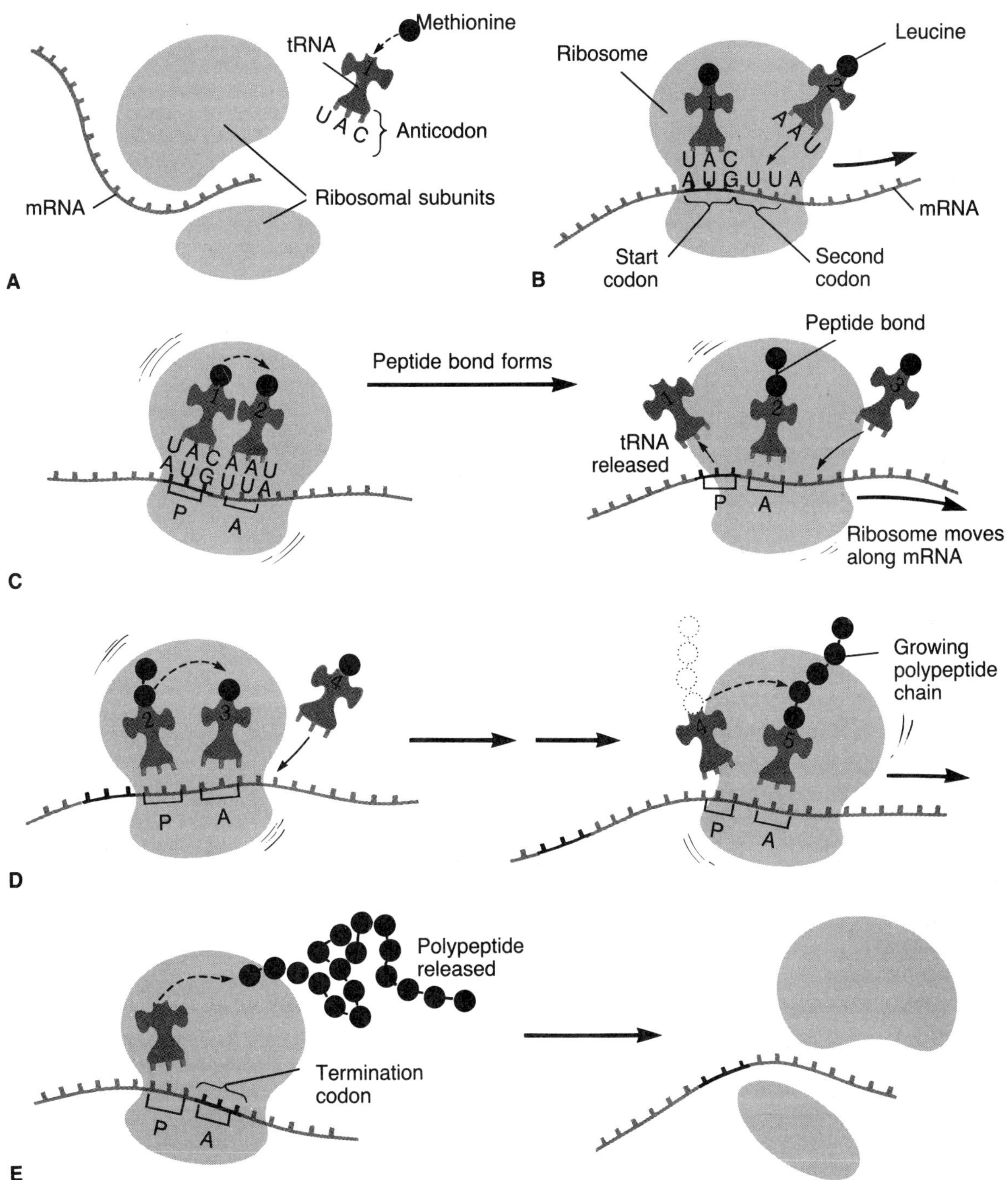

Figure 5-7 Information transfer. (From Jenkins JB: *Human Genetics*. Benjamin/Cummings, 1983.)

all the necessary genetic material. The development of a human being from a zygote involves complicated, interrelated processes through which the structural and functional organization of the system is realized progressively. It is an ordered process, each step depending on the successful completion of the previous step. Embryologic development of the organism from the zygote has several basic aspects: multiplication of cells, cell movement, differentiation of cells (cytodifferentiation), the formation of tissues and organs, and increase in mass.

Shortly after fertilization, the zygote beings to undergo cell division, or *mitosis*. Each daughter cell receives the same complement of genes as the zygote from which it has descended, except that the gametes (sperm and ova), which

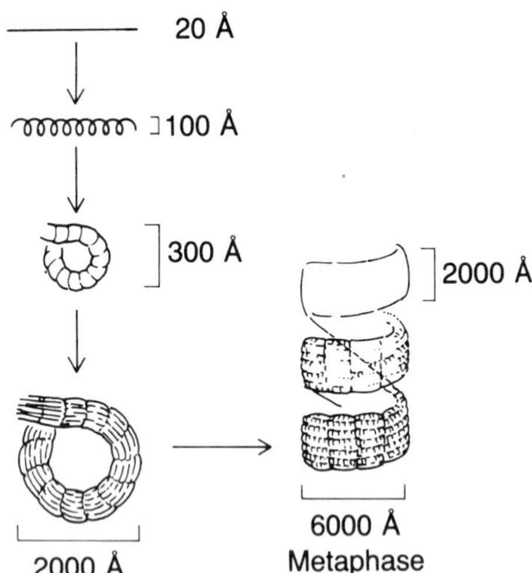

Figure 5-8 Chromosomes coiling in preparation for mitosis. (From Ayala FS, Kiger JA: *Modern Genetics*. 2nd ed. Benjamin/Cummings, 1984.)

will develop later, will have half the number of chromosomes as a result of meiosis. During embryogenesis, many genes become active or inactive at specific stages in development. The result of this is that cells become differentiated into a variety of cell types, for example, skin, nerve, bone, and gland cells. With additional division, cell function becomes progressively restrictive until complete differentiation occurs (Fig. 5-9). Although their genetic makeup (or *genotype*) is identical, the cells differ in their form and function (or *phenotype*) because only a specific number of genes are expressed in each cell. For example, all somatic cells (that is, cells other than the germ cells) contain the genes for synthesizing the protein hemoglobin. These genes, however, are only expressed in erythrocytes.

Development is a complex process about which scientists are learning more all the time. They are attempting to identify what regulatory mechanisms are responsible for turning genes on and off at the proper time. They also are trying to unravel the mystery of why many genes are expressed in only one tissue or, at most, in a limited number of tissues.

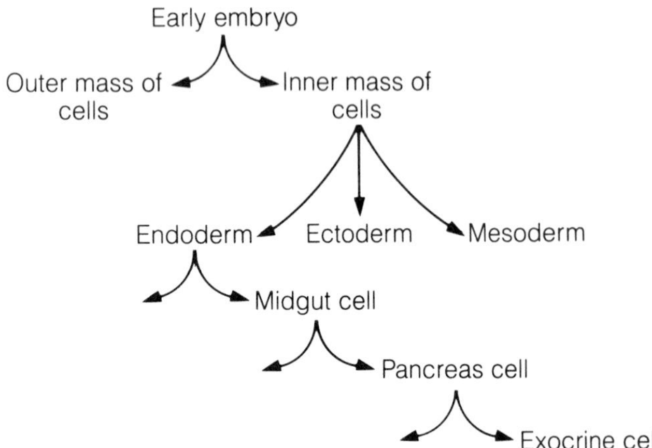

Figure 5-9 Cell differentiation. (From Jenkins JB: *Human Genetics*. Benjamin/Cummings, 1983.)

Morphogenesis, the formation of tissues and organs, occurs at a more complex stage of development. The initiation and regulation of these developmental stages and the role of genes in these processes presently are under study. Many researchers in this area are hoping to find answers that will give clues to the role of heredity in congenital malformations.

Another aspect of embryogenesis is cell movement. It has been demonstrated, for example, that cells of the neural crest migrate extensively from their origin on the dorsal surface of the neural tube to various distant parts of the embryo. Once localized, the cells differentiate into a variety of cell types, including some sensory cranial nerves, the adrenal medulla, and sympathetic ganglia. The initiation and control of cell migration is another aspect of development that is being scrutinized. Congenital anomalies such as spina bifida and cleft palate are believed to result from abnormal cell movements during this critical stage of development.

Cellular death and its timing are also critical in embryogenesis. This phenomenon is necessary to the formation of lumens, such as the intestine, and in processes such as the separation of fingers and toes. It is postulated that cellular degeneration is gene-controlled and can therefore be altered by defective gene action during critical stages of development, producing, for example, the webbed fingers or toes seen in many families. Because many organs develop concurrently in the embryo, a defect in one organ can result in an associated defect in another. This is why when one congenital defect is present, additional defects should be suspected.

Changes in the levels of cellular proteins (enzymes) during embryogenesis reflect changes in the activity of specific genes. Specific enzymes appear at characteristic times during development; this occurrence must reflect the activation of previously inactive genes. Measuring these gene products gives one a relatively useful indicator of the gene control of differentiation. Knowledge of differential gene action also has clinical applications. Many enzymes are known to increase near the time of birth, such as enzymes that indicate surfactant production in the lungs, and these can be used to measure fetal maturity.

Modes of Inheritance

Definition of Terms

The nature of gene activity and its effect on protein synthesis has been examined in this chapter. It is evident that the gene must be expressed in some observable manner in the developing organism. *Genotype* refers to the genetic makeup of an organism (the collection of genes in the organism's chromosomes) or it may refer to an individual locus that is, the genotype for blood group A might be $I^A i$. The genotype remains relatively stable throughout the organism's lifetime. Alternate forms of a gene are called *alleles*. They are generated by mutation and may result in normal or abnormal expression. A *trait* is an observable manifestation of a gene or combination of genes such as eye and hair color. The sum of the traits characterizes a person and contributes to the *phenotype*. Whereas genotype refers to the precise genetic composition of a cell, phenotype is what is actually manifested. Phenotype is the expression of genes—the entire physical, biochemical, and physiologic makeup of an organism—and it implies an interaction with the surrounding environment.

The more varied the environmental conditions, the more diverse might be the phenotype developed from any one genotype. A gene requires a biologic environment that allows the information to be expressed, and much is yet to be learned about the nature of that environment, the interactions between gene products and the environment, and the initiation and regulation of gene activity. Scarr and Kidd (1982) reiterated the following three points when summarizing the relationship of genotype to phenotype in human development:

1. Different genotypes can, and often do, produce different phenotypes
2. Different genotypes can, and often do, produce phenotypes that are indistinguishable
3. The same genotype often is capable of producing more than one phenotype, depending on environmental conditions

A trait that is an expression of a genotype is inherited as genes are passed on during fertilization. For a given pair of genes, one allele is contributed by the mother and one is passed on by the father. If the two alleles for a given gene are identical, the person is said to be homozygous for that gene or the trait associated with that gene. For instance, cystic fibrosis is an inherited trait. The gene for this trait has two alleles: *C*, the normal allele, and *c*, the allele that can result in the disease. If a person has identical alleles, either *CC* or *cc*, the person is *homozygous* for that gene. If the alleles are different, that is, *Cc*, the person is *heterozygous* for that gene.

An allele is *dominant* if its trait is expressed when only one copy is present in the genotype—$I^A i$ is a genotype for blood group A, I^A being the dominant allele. A trait is *recessive* when two alleles are required for its expression in the phenotype—ii results in blood group O. Codominance occurs with the genotype combination of two different dominant alleles, neither of which can subdue the other—$I^A I^B$ results in blood group AB.

Two additional concepts are applicable here. *Penetrance* is defined as "the proportion of individuals (with the same allele) showing the expected phenotype" (Ayala and Kiger, 1984). *Expressivity* is the degree to which the trait is manifested in the individual. For example, complete penetrance and full expressivity would result in all individuals with identical alleles expressing the trait in the identical manner—all individuals with $I^A i$ will have blood group A.

Incomplete penetrance and variable expressivity would lead to only some individuals expressing the trait, and those that did would express it at a different time or in a different manner. Although many traits are inherited according to classic Mendelian rules, penetrance and expressivity can affect the way the traits are expressed in the phenotype. There are other ways that genes modify the phenotypic expression of traits that are not necessarily applicable to this discussion but are explained more fully in genetics texts.

Many traits for disease conditions are inherited. One mechanism for the nurse to identify an inherited disease pattern in a particular family is to use a *genogram*. A genogram is a diagramatic form of recording a family history using standard symbols (Fig. 5-10). The extent of the pedigree depends on the disorder being considered. Minimally, the nurse includes the affected child through whom a family comes to the attention of the investigator, siblings, and preceding and succeeding generations. Consanguineous or multiple marriages should be carefully documented. Information on each member should include age, health, live births, stillbirths, and miscarriages. If a member is dead, the age of death and the cause are documented. The place of birth or origin of a family can be important. For example, the incidence of Tay-Sachs disease is higher in Ashkenazic Jews than in Puerto Ricans. A well-constructed genogram can give clues to genetic etiologies and modes of inheritance. Knowledge of inheritance patterns permits health professionals to predict the risk that a particular trait or disorder will occur in an offspring or other relatives.

Autosomal Inheritance

The inheritance of traits that are controlled by genes located on autosomes is called autosomal inheritance. Most of the well-understood cases of autosomal inheritance in humans involve traits controlled by single gene loci. Autosomal inheritance can follow either dominant or recessive patterns. In the dominant pattern the allele responsible for the trait is the dominant one, and the trait will be expressed regardless of what the other allele is. In the *recessive* pattern the allele responsible for the trait will not result in the expression of the trait if the other allele in the pair is dominant. An autosomal recessive trait will be expressed only when the alleles specifying it are homozygous.

Genetic disorders caused by *autosomal dominant inheritance* are relatively rare. Examples are achondroplasia (dwarfism), Huntington's disease, neurofibromatosis, and osteogenesis imperfecta. According to Mendelian rules, if an individual is heterozygous for the allele of any of these disorders, the disease will be expressed and there is a 50%

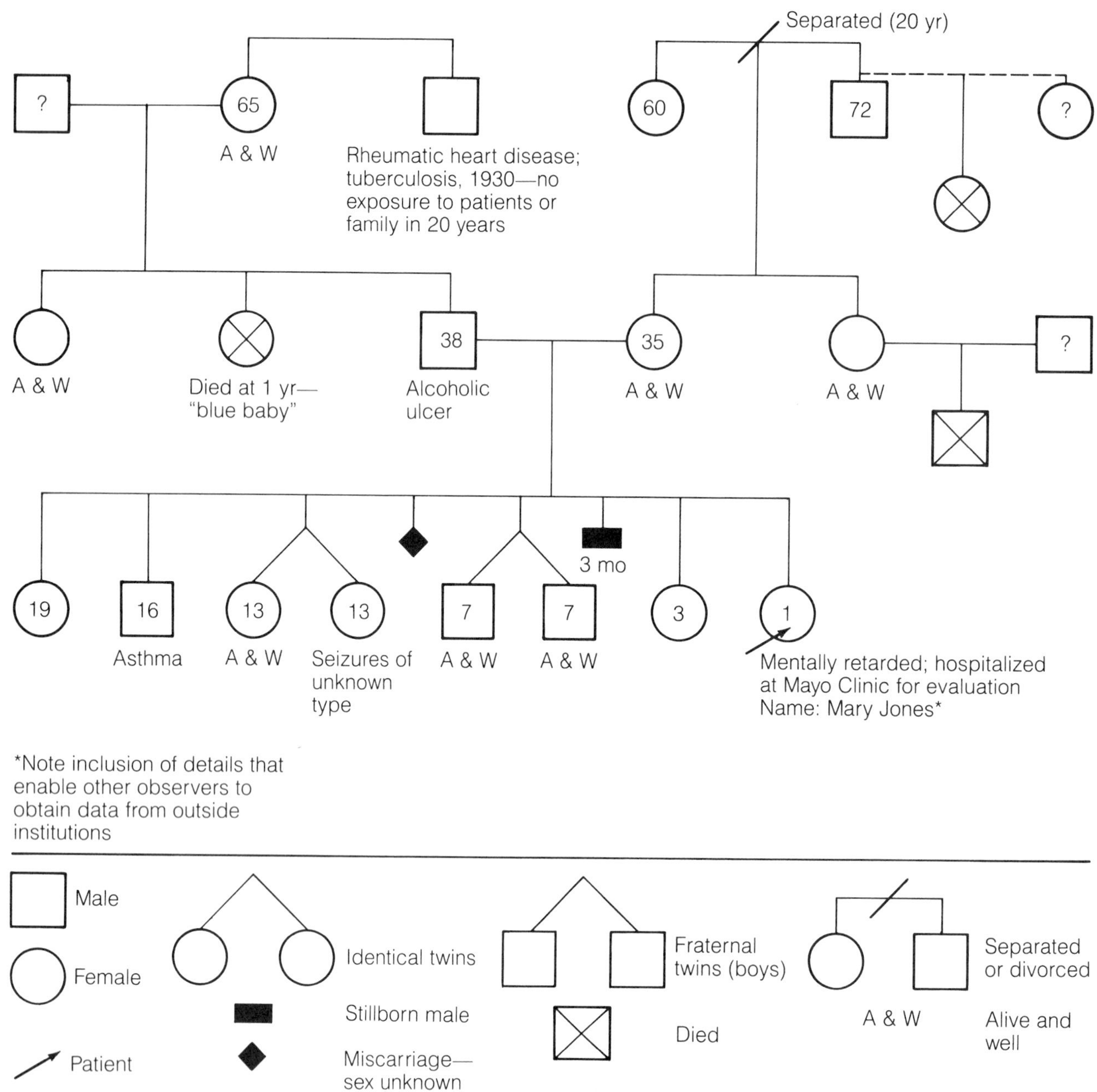

Figure 5-10 Genogram used to diagram a family history.

chance that the individual will pass it on to an offspring (Fig. 5-11 and Table 5-1). Some autosomal dominant defects occur as new mutations.

Examples of *autosomal recessive* disorders are Tay-Sachs disease, cystic fibrosis, and phenylketonuria. When children have one of these disorders, they have inherited two copies of the deleterious allele, one from each parent. Each parent is a *carrier* of the trait and phenotypically is essentially normal. When both parents are carriers of cystic fibrosis, for example, each child they have has a 25% risk of manifesting the disease, a 25% chance of not inheriting the gene from either parent, and a 50% chance of becoming a carrier (Table 5-2 and Fig. 5-12).

TABLE 5-1 Autosomal Dominant Disorders

Disorder	Affected System	Description	Nursing Implications
Achondroplasia	Musculoskeletal	Failure of cartilage cell proliferation, premature closure of growth plates, dwarflike appearance with arms and legs too short for body. Many affected fetuses die in utero or shortly after birth; others live in good health to old age but have short stature, usually shorter than 5½ ft	No known medical intervention. Assist parent with grief work if child dies as a neonate (see Chapters 31 and 32). Give counseling as the child grows older to assist with development of a positive body image.
Huntington's disease	Neuromuscular	Onset between 20 and 50 years of age. Delusions, paranoia, abnormal eye movements, mental deterioration. Death after 10 to 15 years from onset. Progressive deterioration of the nervous system causing uncontrolled movements of the limbs	The genetic marker recently has been identified and will eventually enable the affected child to know of the condition in advance. This will assist in appropriate decision making for marriage and family planning
Sickle cell disease	Hematologic	Crescent-shaped erythrocytes	(see Chapter 36)
Hemolytic anemias	Hematologic	Abnormality of erythrocytes results in red cell destruction and consequent anemia	(see Chapter 36)
Thalassemia	Hematologic	Mild anemia with heterozygous form. Cooley's anemia (homozygous, recessive inheritance) appears in late infancy when fetal hemoglobin is depleted. Pallor, facial irregularities including protruding maxilla, enlarged spleen with severe anemia. Death by age 20 in most cases	Seen primarily in children of Mediterranean heritage (see Chapter 36)
von Willebrand's disease	Hematologic	Type of Factor VII hemophilia with dominant inheritance pattern, severe epistaxis the most common symptom	(see Chapter 36)
Spherocytosis	Hematologic	Spherical shape of red blood cell due to increased permeability to Na+. Shift of fluid into cells causes rupture. Severe anemia from cell destruction. Aplastic crisis—extreme anemia from bone marrow shut-down and consequent decrease in red blood cell production. Enlarged spleen	Splenectomy during early childhood relieves the disorder
Marfan's syndrome	Skeletal	Elongated extremities associated with occular defects, especially of the lens. Spinal deformities occur during growth. Death may occur from cardiovascular defects	Ongoing assessment for cardiovascular difficulties

Sex-Linked Inheritance

Sex-linked inheritance includes X-linked and Y-linked inheritance. At present, there is no known example of a genetic locus on the Y chromosome other than those thought to be associated with male sex determination. The X chromosome carries many genes related to traits other than sex. If an X chromosome with a defective gene is passed on to a male, even if the gene is recessive, it can manifest itself because there is no normal gene on the Y chromosome to mask its effects. In contrast, in a female a recessive deleterious gene on one X chromosome might be masked by a dominant normal gene on the other X chromosome. If a

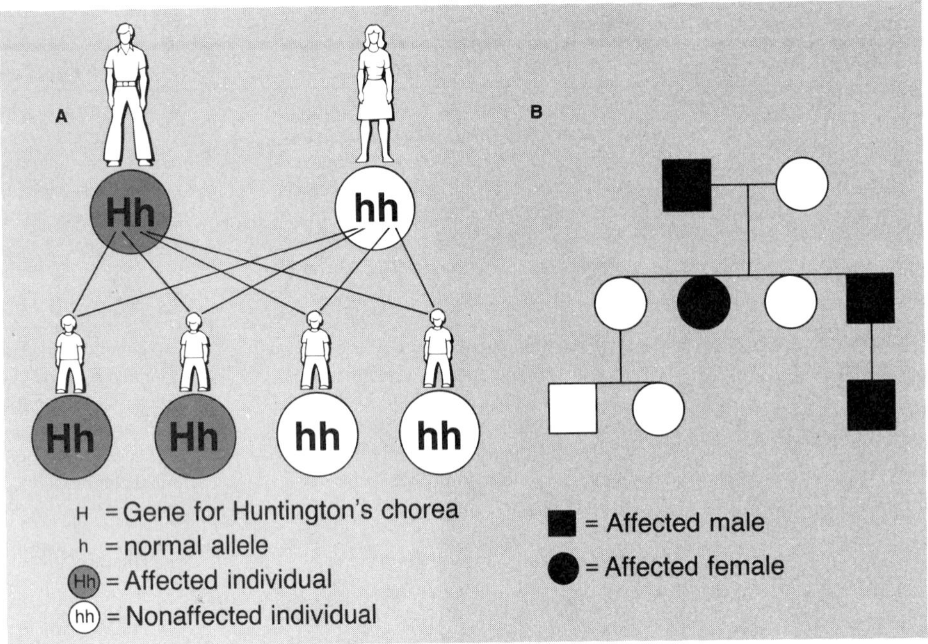

Figure 5-11 Autosomal dominant pattern. (From Olds S: *Maternal-Newborn Nursing*. 2nd ed. Addison-Wesley, 1984.)

woman is a carrier for an X-linked condition, each son she produces has a 50% chance of inheriting the abnormal gene and manifesting the disease and a 50% chance of being normal (Fig. 5-13). Each daughter she produces has a 50% chance of becoming a carrier herself, capable of transmitting the disease to her sons. Factor VIII hemophilia, red-green color blindness, and Duchenne's-type muscular dystrophy are examples of disorders transmitted by X-linked inheritance (Table 5-3).

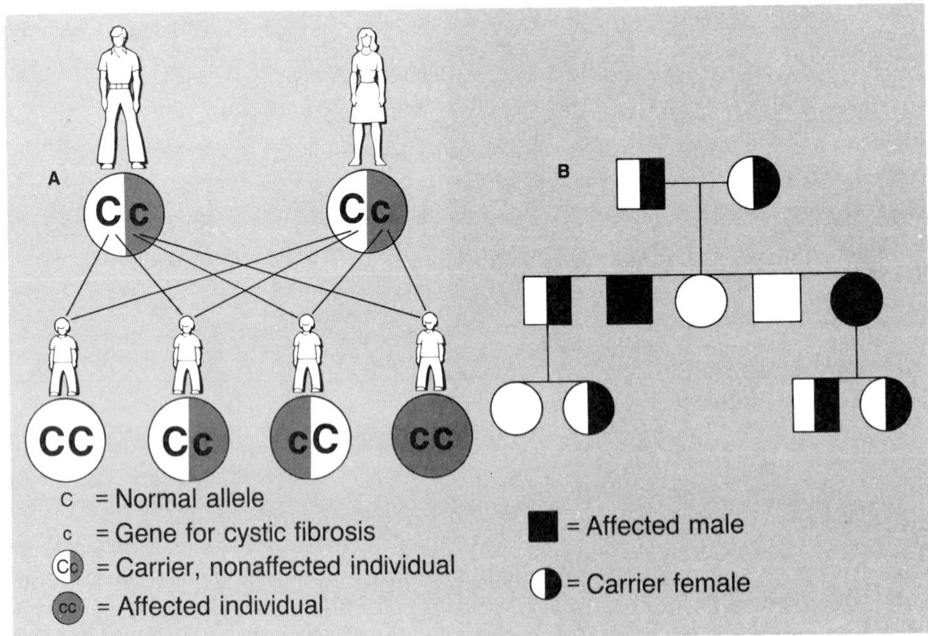

Figure 5-12 Autosomal recessive pattern. (From Olds S: *Maternal-Newborn Nursing*. 2nd ed. Addison-Wesley, 1984.)

TABLE 5-2 Autosomal Recessive Disorders

Disorder	Affected System	Description	Nursing Implications
Adrenogenital syndrome	Metabolism	Overproduction of androgen results in premature virilization in boys (usually before age 5) and pseudohermaphroditism in girls, loss of sodium in some cases	Early treatment will lead to normal sexual maturation in girls (see Chapter 40)
Cystic fibrosis	Respiratory Metabolism Digestive	Abnormal function of the exocrine glands resulting in thickened secretions and abnormal Na+ and Cl− levels in sweat. Chronic pulmonary disease, pancreatic enzyme deficiency, and fibrosis	(see Chapter 38)
Galactosemia	Metabolism	Increased levels of galactose from inability to metabolize lactose products. Manifested by feeding problems, vomiting, diarrhea, and failure to thrive. Associated liver enlargement and cataracts. Death or mental retardation	Diet free of milk products can improve the condition
Phenylketonuria	Metabolism	Mental retardation from build-up of phenylalanine in blood. Children are usually blond, blue eyed due to interference in production of melanin. Urine has musty odor. Possible seizures	Milk-free diet; low dietary intake of protein. Children can be detected shortly after birth through blood and urine testing that is mandated in most areas. Emotional problems may result from dietary restrictions (see Chapters 23 and 38)
Tay-Sachs disease	Neurologic	Caused by an enzyme defect; at approximately 6 months, deterioration of nerves and muscles causes muscle spasticity, seizures, vision loss, mental retardation. Death occurs in early childhood	Most common occurrence is among Jewish people of European origin (see Chapter 23)
Albinism	Integumentary	Defect in melanin formation results in fair skin, white hair, and pigmentless eyes; associated with visual difficulties and photophobia	Children are usually of normal intelligence; may need support for visual problems
Sickle cell disease	Hematologic	Crescent-shaped erythrocytes with decreased hemoglobin; cells cannot pass freely through small blood vessels and therefore buildup in various organs including the liver and the spleen. Child with trait may have abnormal cells but not enough for symptoms. Child with the disease experiences pain, swelling of hands and feet, pain in abdomen from splenic involvement, severe anemia	(see Chapter 36)

Chromosome Alterations

Deviations from the normal chromosome complement can be categorized into those involving a numeric change and those involving a structural change. Numeric changes can affect the autosomes or sex chromosomes and result in more than or less than 46 chromosomes. Trisomy 21 syndrome (Down's syndrome) results from an extra number 21 chromosome. Turner's syndrome (XO) is an example of a numeric change affecting a sex chromosome, with the resultant number of chromosomes being 45.

Several factors are associated with an increase in the occurrence of numerical aberrations. Late maternal age is a major factor associated with Trisomy 21, for example, and to a lesser extent with other trisomies. It has been suggested that paternal age over 55 years is also a contributing factor (Stene et al., 1977). A correlation between high-thyroid autoantibody levels and chromosomal anomalies has been observed in families of children with Trisomy 21. The conclusion is that autoimmune disease seems to have some role in nondisjunction (Thompson and Thompson,

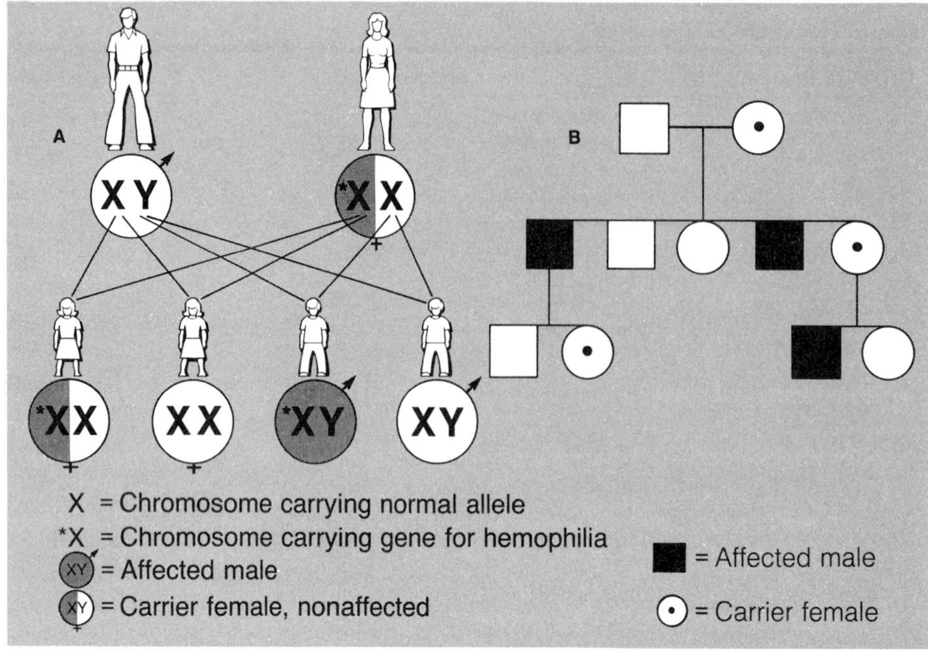

Figure 5-13 Sex-linked recessive pattern. (From Olds S: *Maternal-Newborn Nursing*. 2nd ed. Addison-Wesley, 1984.)

1980). Radiation exposure, neoplastic drugs, viruses, and chromosome abnormalities themselves are associated with nondisjunction events.

Alterations of chromosome structure involve a loss, gain, or rearrangement of genetic material. The change may involve only a small segment of DNA (that is, a few base pairs) or entire chromosome arms. Phenotypes of individuals with chromosome alterations vary greatly. All clinically significant chromosome abnormalities can be identified by routine cytogenetic techniques (Stephenson and Weaver, 1981). Amniocentesis during the first trimester of pregnancy can provide couples with information about the chromosome complement of the fetus (Table 5-4).

TABLE 5-3 X-Linked Inherited Disorders

Disorder	Affected System	Description	Nursing Implications
Color blindness	Senses	X-linked disorder in which females are carriers and male children are affected. Three types include red, blue, green; green, purple; and yellow, blue	Children unable to discriminate certain colors. May need support in school setting
Hemophilia A	Factor VIII deficiency	Bleeding tendency and abnormal bruising become evident as gross motor skills develop in the child. Prolonged bleeding even with mild trauma; Hemorrhages into joints can cause pain and degeneration	(see Chapter 36)
Hemophilia B	Factor IX deficiency (Christmas disease)	Wide range of severity according to factor blood level	
Duchenne's muscular dystrophy	Neuromuscular	Early signs of difficulty in motor activity leads to weakness and muscle wasting. May be associated with mental retardation. Death usually occurs before adolescence	

TABLE 5-4 Disorders Related to Chromosome Alterations

Disorder	Genetic Alteration	Description	Nursing Implications
Down's syndrome	Trisomy 21	Most common chromosome disorder occurring in 1:600 to 1:1000 births. Phenotypic features include epicanthal folds, simian creases on palms, hypotonia, flat nasal bridge, protrusion of the tongue. Various degrees of mental retardation	Associated with other conditions such as cardiac disease and hematologic disorders, among disorders of other systems. (see Chapter 23) Retardation
Edward's syndrome	Trisomy 18	Mental retardation. Almost all organ systems affected. Appearance of small head, low-set ears, small features. Abnormal flexion of fingers. Only 13% infants live beyond one year; most die within 10 weeks	Assessment for organ involvement (see Chapter 23)
Pateu's syndrome	Trisomy 13	Most severe malformations of all chromosomal abnormalities. Mental retardation. Small head, small malformed eyes, spasmodic seizures, deafness, extra digits, split tongue. Only a few infants live longer than one year; most die soon after birth	(see Chapter 23)
Cri-du-chat syndrome	Deletion of short arm of chromosome 5 (5p-)	Infants up to 1 year of age have a characteristic cry of a cat due to abnormal laryngeal development. Severe mental retardation, microcephaly, widely spaced eyes, broad nose, low-set ears. Congenital heart anomalies present in about 25% of cases. Children survive better than with trisomies, and some survive into adulthood	IQ is so low (less than 35) that institutionalization may be required (see Chapter 23)
Klinefelter syndrome	Additional X chromosome (47,XXY) Variants include XXYY, XXXY, XXXXY	Small testes, sterility, abnormally long legs; 50% of individuals develop breasts, female distribution of body hair. Slight mental retardation, though some individuals have IQ in the normal range	(see Chapter 23)
Turner's syndrome	Monosomy X (XO)	Failure to develop normal secondary female sexual characteristics at puberty. Low hairline. Wide chest with broadly spaced nipples. Narrowing of aorta. Puffy feet in newborns. High palate. No apparent mental retardation.	(see Chapter 40)
XYY syndrome	Additional Y chromosome	Nearly all males with this karyotype are phenotypically normal. They tend to be taller than XY males but with lower muscular strength and poorer coordination and may be susceptible to severe acne. Sexual development is normal. IQ may be somewhat lower, but within normal range	Occurs in 1 of 700 live male births (Jenkins, 1983). Suspicion that these children exhibit greater impulsivity and delinquent behavior is controversial

continued on next page

TABLE 5-4 continued

Disorder	Genetic Alteration	Description	Nursing Implications
Wilms' tumor	Deletion of short arm of chromosome 11 (11p−)	A type of renal cancer in young children. Strong association with absence of irises in the eyes. Other physical defects affect the gastrointestinal and genitourinary systems. Some mental retardation	(see Chapter 45)

Multifactorial Inheritance

Multifactorial inheritance (polygenic inheritance) is more difficult to analyze than the classic Mendelian modes of inheritance. Multifactorial inheritance refers to a trait that is determined by the interaction of a number of genetic loci and environmental factors. It accounts for much of the normal variation in families such as in stature and intelligence. Intelligence, for example, is a trait that shows continuous variation in the general population. It is not a matter of having intelligence or not having intelligence but rather where one falls along a continuum. In the general population intelligence extends from retardation (IQ less than 70) to exceptional (IQ greater than 130). The majority of people have IQs within the 90–110 range, the mean being 100. Intelligence is affected by environment and genes. Most of the differences among normal human beings demonstrate continuous variation.

Multifactorial inheritance also accounts for many common disorders and congenital malformations. A multifactorial disorder (Thompson and Thompson, 1980) is one that is "determined by a combination of genetic and environmental factors" without reference to the nature of the genetic component(s). Congenital hip dysplasia, pyloric stenosis, congenital heart disease, spina bifida, and cleft lip and palate are included in this category. Multifactorial traits and diseases tend to cluster in families, but there is no clear-cut, predictable genetic pattern in individual families. In general, once a couple has had one affected child, the chance of having another child with the same defect is between 2% and 5%. After having two affected children, the risk increases again because the second birth indicates that the parents may have more predisposing factors than originally suspected. These risk figures may vary in different geographic areas and should be checked prior to counseling a couple regarding the risk of recurrence.

Because the developing person is never separate from an environment it is nearly impossible to determine accurately those portions of a behavior that are genetic and those that are environmental. The concept of *heritability* is a tool for defining this distinction.

Heritability is a mathematical proportion correlated with the amount of variation for a specific trait in a given group. It may be due to either genetic or environmental factors. For instance, if members of a group, genetically identical for a trait, were placed in widely different environments, any variation in the expression of the trait would be solely due to environment. The heritability factor would be zero (0). If members of a group with different genotypes for a trait were placed in an identical environment, any variation in the expression of the trait would be genetic, and the heritability would be one (1). A group with members having different genotypes placed in different environments would demonstrate heritability somewhere between 0 and 1 (Jenkins, 1983; Ayala and Kiger, 1980).

Heritability does not measure the amount of genetic influence on a particular trait, but instead measures only the portion of the variation in the trait's expression which is a result of genetic variation. There are two corollaries to this:

1. Heritability is a measure of a specific population in a specific environment.
2. If heritability is high, the variation is not necessarily genetic. Given two different environments the trait will vary in its expression between environments, but the heritability will be high (Jenkins, 1983)

For example, given a nurturing environment, all members of a group generally will flourish although variations among group members will have a high heritability because the environment is constant. In a poor environment the members generally will be poorly developed, but again the variations within the group will demonstrate a high heritability (Jenkins, 1983).

Although heritability can be and is used in the study of polygenic or multifactorial inheritance, it is evident that its use is limited and will not prove genetic causation for the expression of a trait.

Twin Studies in Multifactorial Inheritance

Both genetic and environmental factors affect development. The only reliable way to determine whether either set of factors has an important role in development or the expression of traits is to find a way to hold one variable constant while changing the other. If the observed trait then varies, it can be concluded that the altered factor plays an important role. The study of twins is one way to approach the problem. In 1875 Galton introduced the twin method as a way to study the effects of "nature and nurture." Since then, twin studies have been used to study the influence of genetic and environmental factors on intelligence, behavioral and psychologic characteristics, and disease conditions.

The twin method is based on the fact that monozygous (MZ), or identical, twins originate from a single fertilized ovum (zygote). Within the first 14 days after fertilization, the zygote divides into two embryos, which are identical with respect to genotype. Because they have identical genotypes, MZ twins can be used to assess whether some feature, which shows variation in humans, has a basis in heredity.

Dizygotic (DZ), or fraternal, twins occur when two ova are shed in the same menstrual cycle and are fertilized by two separate sperm. On the average, fraternal twins have half their genes in common, making them just as similar genetically as ordinary siblings. Their phenotypic differences are the result of dissimilar genotypes and environmental influences. Frequently, DZ twins of the same sex are used as a control group in twin studies.

Concordance

When twins manifest the same specific trait, for instance, hair color, they are said to be concordant. When they differ in a specific trait, they are said to be discordant. If there is a genetic component in producing a certain trait, concordance in MZ pairs should exceed that in DZ pairs. The stronger the genetic influence, the greater the difference between MZ and DZ pairs is likely to be. Therefore, the difference in concordance between MZ and DZ twins can be used to determine whether genetic variability plays a role in a given disease or a specific trait.

Certain traits in twins have been examined and established for concordance. For example, eye color has a concordance of 99% in MZ twins and 38% in DZ twins. The large discrepancy between concordance in the MZ and DZ pairs indicates a strong genetic influence. A communicable disease such as measles had a concordance of 95% in MZ twins and 87% in DZ. The concordance difference between groups was so slight that evidence points to environmental factors (Jenkins, 1983).

Other research approaches have been used in addition to twin studies. For example, unrelated children reared in the same home are being studied to see to what extent a common environment increases similarities. Different families are being compared, and members of the same family are compared for a number of specific traits.

Limitations of Twin Studies

Twin studies have several obvious limitations, the most prominent being the size of samples, which historically have been small. It is recommended that at least 100 pairs each (MZ and DZ) of same-sex twins be studied to have validity in the area of concordance.

Researchers need to establish that twin sets are definitely MZ by a check of genetic markers (for instance, blood antigens). Even then, there is no guarantee that a genetic mutation may not have occurred in the trait being studied (Jenkins, 1983).

Although MZ twins result from the division of a single ovum, their prenatal environments usually differ. Because prenatal environment is uncontrollable, innate environmental differences will exist. For example, the phenotype of MZ twins may differ by as much as 1000 g in birthweight due to varied nutrient access in utero.

Assumptions of consistency in the postnatal environment are not necessarily valid. For instance, when the examination of personality traits shows MZ twins to be significantly more alike than DZ twins, it may be concluded that the greater concordance of the MZ twins may be due to the identical genotype. Environmental pressures, however, often affect the personality of MZ twins. Because they look alike, there may be many subtle environmental pressures to dress and act alike, thus skewing results that seem to point to the genetic causation of a trait. In examining the environments of twins reared apart, it has been suggested that because of similar genotype, MZ twins seem to seek out similar environments. If this is true, the importance of environmental influences will be somewhat minimized.

These criticisms of the twin studies draw attention to the complexity of the problem. Although it is extremely difficult to delineate genetic versus environmental influences on aspects of development, twin studies still are valuable in drawing attention to the possibilities of genetic contribution.

A major controversial issue in the study of multifactorial inheritance is the genetic influences on intelligence. Awareness of the controversial aspects of this issue is important for nurses. Although there has been no definitive proof of genetic determination of intelligence, genes do control the physiological processes that control certain aspects of behavior and personality. Because genes code for protein synthesis, they are implicated in the production of neurotransmitters (acetylcholine, norepinephrine, dopamine, etc.) and the production of hormones that control behavior. A simplification of this concept would be that genes control the potential for intelligence while environment modifies its expression.

Mange and Mange (1980) suggested criteria that can be used as guidelines when considering the issue of multifactorial inheritance. At least two important criteria, taken together, are necessary to establish a genetic probability:

1. The trait must occur more often among relatives of the identified person than the general population

2. The trait must not spread to unrelated persons exposed to similar environmental situations. (This helps to exclude infections and nutritional deficiencies that may run in families or be prevalent in local populations)

Mange and Mange noted that these two criteria are necessary but not always sufficient. The following additional observations will further support a genetic basis:

3. The trait appears at a characteristic age without any obvious precipitating event
4. The trait varies in frequency between populations
5. Identical (MZ) twins share the trait more often than do fraternal (DZ) twins
6. A human trait resembles a trait known to be inherited in experimental or farm animals

Genetic Effects on Aspects of Physical Development

Metabolism

Body homeostasis is maintained by regulatory mechanisms, some of which affect the biochemical pathways. Just as genes code for the production of neurotransmitters that control behavior, they also direct the synthesis of enzymes that regulate metabolism.

A biochemical pathway is a series of steps in which a final product depends on a specific sequence of events. Each step in the process depends on the successful completion of the previous step (Fig. 5-14). It follows, then, that a defect in the sequence will result in an abnormality. For example, in phenylketonuria (PKU) the gene that codes for the enzyme that converts phenylalanine to tyrosine is defective, and the enzyme is not produced. Phenylalanine accumulates in the blood and eventually causes brain damage, with a resulting decrease in IQ and small head size (Ayala and Kiger, 1984, p. 634). Children with PKU tend to have light hair because tyrosine is later converted to melanin. It can be seen then that a single defective gene can cause multiple problems in the phenotype by interfering in a biochemical pathway. It should be mentioned here, however, that the determination of the final phenotype in children with PKU is environmental. Early detection by screening can prevent brain damage if it is followed by nutritional therapy (see Chapter 38).

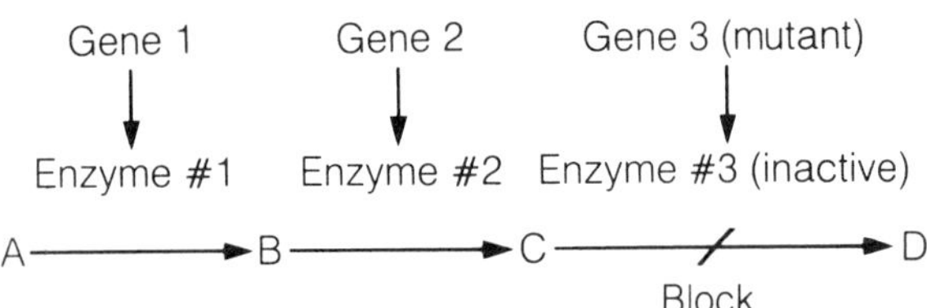

Figure 5-14 Biochemical pathway. (From Jenkins JB: *Human Genetics*. Benjamin/Cummings, 1983.)

Galactosemia is another disease where the absence of a necessary enzyme blocks the normal process of metabolism and results in the buildup of a substance, in this case galactose, that can have fatal effects on the child. In galactosemia, as with PKU, restricting the intake of the substance in question can prevent the negative effects, but early recognition of the disorder is required.

Other enzyme defects do not become apparent except as a reaction to certain drugs. Serum cholinesterase is an enzyme that does not appear to play a crucial part in normal development, but it is necessary in the breakdown of succinylcholine, a drug used as a muscle relaxant. If the normal form of the enzyme is not present, the person usually does not suffer any ill effects unless succinylcholine is administered. In the absence of the normal enzyme, the drug does not break down quickly, and the effects, instead of being temporary muscle relaxation, involve total paralysis.

In these examples of inborn errors of metabolism, it can be seen how a genotype can result in a life-threatening phenotype but only if a certain interaction with the environment takes place. The intake of phenylalanine, galactose, and succinylcholine are examples of such interactions; if the person with the aberrant genotype can be identified early enough and these interactions eliminated, the negative effects of the genetic alteration can be avoided.

The following major regulatory mechanisms affect biochemical pathways:

1. *Positive control system*—regulatory enzyme initiates the biochemical pathway
2. *Negative control system*—halts an activity that would normally proceed
3. *Feedback*—the final product of the pathway regulates the initiating step

There is both positive and negative feedback. In positive feedback the final product reinitiates the sequence and increases the rate of reaction. Negative feedback occurs when the final product ceases the activity. There are other control mechanisms affecting biochemical pathways, and there are thousands of pathways in every cell (Jenkins, 1983). These regulatory mechanisms promote homeostasis in both individual cells and the body as a whole.

Immune System—Development of Antibodies

Genes play an important role in the proper functioning of the body's immune system. Before the genetic mechanism can be understood, a brief review of terms is helpful. (See Chapter 37 for further information on the immune system.) An *antigen* is a substance foreign to the body that elicits an immune response. Examples of antigens are microbial organisms or toxic substances such as poisons. *Antibodies* are proteins synthesized by cells to bind with and destroy antigens. Also known as *immunoglobulins*, each antibody is specific to the antigen that triggered its synthesis (Jenkins, 1983).

Two types of lymphocytes function in the immune response:

T-lymphocytes—recognize viruses, fungi, parasites, cancer cells, and toxins and bind with them for elimination

B-lymphocytes (plasma cells)—synthesize antibodies to attack the antigens and clump them together to be destroyed by macrophages

On the cell surfaces of both types of lymphocytes are sites, which act as antigen receptors. The cells recognize corresponding antigens and bind them to the receptor site.

According to the clonal selection theory, both B- and T-lyphocytes are committed to recognizing and destroying one particular antigen even before exposure to any. This means that in the human millions of antigen-specific cells exist to correspond with the enormous variety of antigens. Exposure to its specific antigen causes each type of cell to divide and mature into an effective antigen-destroying lymphocyte (Jenkins, 1983).

The study of the genetics of antibody formation and of the immune system in general recently has offered exciting insights not only into the basis of the immune system but also into gene behavior. Although the various theories proposed are too involved for the present discussion (for further details, see Jenkins, 1983, pp. 300-305), they all attempt to shed light on the question of how antibody genes can produce the rich diversity of antibodies of which the human body is capable. What is unquestionable is that genetic activity underlies the formation of antibodies and thus controls the function of the immune system itself. Consequently, it is important to understand the principles of genetics as they underlie defects in the immune system.

Current research is uncovering many connections between disease, or susceptibility to disease, and the genetics of the immune system. Three areas in particular are the HLA gene complex, autoimmune diseases, and diseases of immunologic deficiency.

The tissues of every individual can be distinguished from the tissues of every other individual by proteins on the cell surface called *histocompatibility antigens*. These antigens are responsible for the acceptance or rejection by the body of tissue grafts and organ transplants. Many of the genes that code for histocompatibility antigens are found in a single region on chromosome 6 called the *human lymphocyte A* complex, or *HLA*. Antigens coded by HLA are being associated with an increasingly large number of diseases, although the direct causal relationship has not been clarified. The more common of these diseases in children include herpes infections, malignancies such as Hodgkin's disease and acute lymphatic leukemia, juvenile rheumatoid arthritis, insulin-dependent diabetes mellitus, and celiac disease.

Some of the HLA-associated diseases are considered autoimmune diseases. Autoimmune diseases occur when the immune system responds inappropriately to a person's own body tissue. Normally, an individual's lymphocytes should have built up a tolerance to that individual's "self-antigens," but circumstances may result in an unfamiliar self-antigen that will stimulate an autoimmune reaction. Autoimmune diseases associated with HLA include juvenile rheumatoid arthritis and juvenile diabetes mellitus (see Chapter 37).

There are several rare genetic disorders, called immunologic deficiency diseases, in which the immune system is unable to respond to antigens. Many but not all of the genetically determined immunologic deficiency diseases are X-linked and usually occur in infancy, between 6 months and 2 years of age. These infants are highly susceptible to recurrent infections. One example of an immunologic deficiency disease, Swiss type agammaglobulinemia, is the result of an autosomal gene mutation and is commonly fatal for the child, who usually succumbs to infections within the first 4 years of life. Another disease, acquired immune deficiency syndrome, or AIDS, has been the object of much publicity and research recently, and cases have been identified among children as well as the more highly publicized populations at risk. It is theorized that AIDS may have a genetic component but the genetic link has not been established. (See Chapter 37.)

Nurse's Role

It can be seen from this discussion of genetics that genes influence the normal growth and development of the person either directly or indirectly. The final expression of the genetic message is influenced in many areas by the environment. Traits, as individual expressions of genes, can be simple (for instance, enzyme production) or complex (for instance, intelligence), each having its own hereditary pattern and modification by the environment. Defects in the genetic message can produce ineffective function in one or more body systems. Because many of these defects are predictable, genetic counseling can be of great benefit to parents.

Prenatal Screening

Prenatal screening is now available that can diagnose a number of genetic problems in utero, thus enabling the woman to make decisions regarding the best options for her particular situation. Amniocentesis, ultrasound, alpha fetoprotein determinations, and fetoscopy are a few of these available tests.

Women over age 35 are at greater risk for bearing children with chromosome alterations, and amniocentesis early in pregnancy is a useful diagnostic tool. Estimates indicate, however, that one- to two-thirds of women over 35 years of age postpone their first prenatal visits until it is too late for amniocentesis to be performed (Fibison, 1983). Reasons for choosing not to undergo the procedure are many. Some may fear what will be discovered or the decisions involved in bearing a defective child. There may be a lack of knowledge about age-related genetic defects or a conscious decision to live with the consequences of defect, regardless of whether the problem is diagnosed in utero. Some women unconsciously avoid making any decision, and consequently make a decision by default. Regardless of the reasons, nurses need to be accepting of personal attitudes regarding prenatal diagnosis, while encouraging prospective parents to be aware of what is available.

In many settings nurses are able to identify and refer for counseling families at risk for genetic defects. In acute-care settings, chronic-care settings, well-child clinics, or schools, child health nurses can identify families who would benefit from counseling.

The indications for referral for genetic counseling may include the following:

1. Congenital anomalies, including mental retardation in child or family
2. Familial disorders such as diabetes
3. Known inherited disease
4. Metabolic disorders
5. Chromosomal abnormalities

The need for information or for prenatal diagnosis, especially in women over the age of 35, is an additional indication for referral (Olds, 1984). Unfortunately, many couples give birth to a child with a genetic defect before they are aware of a need for counseling. Referral for these couples will give them access to predictive information that can be used to plan future pregnancies.

Genetic Counseling

Inevitably, parents ask, "Will this happen to us again?" If they do not wish to have more children, they may be asking the question for healthy siblings or other relatives. It is important that the health professional responding to this question be well versed in genetics. This means understanding the modes of inheritance, communicating scientific information to clients, and recognizing the impact that this information may have on the families. The counselor should have updated information on the disorder in question with regard to mode of inheritance, therapies and prenatal diagnostic capabilities. Modes of inheritance for some disorders, like diabetes mellitus are not clear cut. The counselor also should be knowledgable about procreative alternatives if the couple does not wish to risk another pregnancy themselves. Good interpersonal skills are therefore a necessity.

The nursing role in genetic counseling will depend on the practice setting the nurse's level of preparation. If the mode of inheritance is fairly straightforward (for example, PKU), the counseling may be done in the primary-care setting. For more complicated situations, referral to a genetic clinic is in order.

General guidelines for a nursing role are as follows:

Assessing the couple's level of understanding of the genetic information (can parents explain the mode of inheritance? What recurrence risks were explained to them?)

Identifying how each parent interprets the information (the parent's view the recurrence risk as low or high? How will this information affect their decision regarding more children?)

Clarifying information and correcting misconceptions

Identifying how the genetic component of the information has affected the feelings of each parent (what is the meaning of "carrier"; does a parent feel stigmatized or guilty?)

Reassuring the parents that it is not their "fault," that each individual carries six to eight deleterious genes

Assisting the parents with decision-making as necessary (Decisions related to genetic information may include changing to a more reliable birth control method, becoming pregnant again, adoption, informing relatives who also may be at risk)

Finding resources that the couple may need (for example, prenatal diagnosis, artificial insemination by donor, additional counseling or therapy)

Educating the public for the early recognition and prevention of genetic defects

A major nursing role in genetic counseling is to provide support to families who either have a defective child or who have predictable chances for having one in a future pregnancy. Many issues are involved with providing compassionate nursing care, and nurses need to be aware of problems that can result from the spector of having a defective child.

Underlying most parents' aspirations for a successful pregnancy is the ability to have a healthy child. Any threat to this normal expectation can result in a threat to the parents' self-esteem. Fear can result in the use of such coping mechanisms as denial, projection, and displacement (Tishler, 1981). Occasionally, feelings of fear or guilt in one parent are displaced onto the spouse, resulting in marital stress and depression.

Fear of future pregnancies after the birth of a defective child brings out ethical issues of birth control, abortion, sterility, and right to life (Tishler, 1981). Anxiety regarding these issues must be expressed before any effective, genetically focused information is understood. Otherwise, important information may be lost because anxiety interferes with its processing. Parents who have given birth to defective children need to go through the grieving process before they can adequately prepare to plan for the future. (The process of grieving for children with chronic conditions is discussed in Chapter 30.) Children who are at risk for developing genetic disorders, such as Huntington's disease later in life should be given the opportunity to express their feelings and obtain supportive nursing care.

To provide support to parents nurses need to have clarified their own feelings about the ethical issues involved. Nurses too have difficulty with some of these issues but need to understand their feelings before they can provide unbiased, professional nursing care. Learning that something in one's genes is responsible for a disorder in a child is very difficult, even when it is something that is clearly beyond the control of the individual. A knowledgable, compassionate nurse can help these people accept genetic information and make realistic and appropriate decisions for future childbearing.

Key Concepts

- The influence of heredity on the developing person is complex and in many instances cannot be removed from environmental factors (suprasystems). Optimal body growth and the proper functioning of body subsystems depends on the synthesis of proteins.
- The mechanism of protein synthesis is regulated by genes via DNA and RNA replication, transcription, and translation.
- Development of the embryo is accomplished by the processes of cell multiplication, cell movement, cell differentiation, organ formation, and increase in mass. Developing processes in the embryo are controlled genetically, although the mechanisms are not totally understood.
- Any genetic defect occurring in the embryo will affect proper growth and function of the system involved.
- The genetic makeup of an organism—genotype—is expressed in the phenotype—the sum of observable traits.
- Traits are inherited through various modes, including autosomal, sex-linked, and multifactorial.
- Twin studies have been used by researchers to examine the proportional effect of multifactorial inheritance on certain behavioral characteristics. Because genes control protein synthesis, they directly affect body function such as in metabolic pathways and the development of antibodies.
- Nurses need to be aware of the genetic role in development to intervene appropriately with families at risk for genetic defects.
- The child health nurse can intervene by identifying and referring high-risk families for appropriate counseling, as well as by educating the public regarding the importance of prevention.

References

Ayala FJ, Kiger JA: *Modern Genetics.* 2nd ed. Benjamin/Cummings, 1984.

Fibison WJ: The nursing role in the delivery of genetic services. *Issues in Health Care of Women* 1983; 4:1–13.

Gilbert W: Gene sequencing and gene structure. *Science* (Dec 18) 1981; 212:1305–1312.

Jenkins JB: *Human Genetics.* Benjamin/Cummings, 1983.

Mange A, Mange E: *Genetics: Human Aspects.* Saunders College, 1980.

Olds S: *Maternal-Newborn Nursing,* 2nd ed. Addison-Wesley, 1984.

Scarr S, and Kidd K: Developmental behavior genetics. In: *Mussen Handbook of Child Psychology.* Haith M, Campos J (editors). Wiley; 1982.

Stene J et al: Paternal age effects in Down's syndrome. *Ann Hum Genet* 1977; 40:299–306.

Stephenson SR, Weaver DD: Prenatal diagnosis—a compilation of diagnosed conditions. *Am J Obstet Gynecol* 1981; 141:319.

Thompson J, Thompson M: *Genetics in Medicine.* Saunders, 1980.

Tishler CL: The psychological aspects of genetic counseling. *Am J Nurs* 1981; 81:733–734.

Additional Readings

Applewhite S, Busbee D, Burgaonkar D (editors): *Genetic screening and counseling in Multidisciplinary Perspective.* Thomas, 1981.

Bakwin H: Lateral dominance. *J Pediatr* 1950; 36:385.

Brown MS, Murphy MA: *Ambulatory Pediatrics for Nurses.* McGraw-Hill, 1975.

Cudworth AG, Woodrow JC: Genetic susceptibility of diabetes mellitus: analysis of the HLA association. *Br Med J* 1976; 2:846.

Erlenmeyer-Kimling L, Jarvik L: Genetics and intelligence: A review. *Science* 1963; 142:1477–1479.

Ganda OP, Soeldner SS: Genetic, acquired and related factors in the etiology of diabetes mellitus. *Arch Intern Med* 1977; 137:461.

Holden C: Identical twins reared apart. *Science* (March 20) 1980; 207:1323–1328.

Illingworth R: *The Development of the Infant and Young Child: Normal and Abnormal.* Churchill Livingston, 1975.

Kelly P: *Dealing with Dilemma.* Springer-Verlag, 1977.

Kelly T: *Clinical Genetics and Genetic Counseling.* Year Book, 1980.

Lowrey GH: *Growth and Development of Children.* Year Book, 1978.

McKusick V: *Mendelian Inheritance in Man.* 6th ed. Johns Hopkins University Press, 1982.

Marx J: Antibodies: Getting their genes together. *Science* (May 29) 1981; 212:1015–1017.

Merrit H: A Textbook of Neurology. 6th ed. Lea & Febiger, 1979.

Nance WE (editor): *Progress in Clinical and Biological Research: Twin Research.* Part A: *Psychology and Methodolgy.* Part B: *Biology and Epidemiology.* Part C: *Clinical Studies.* Alan R. Liss, 1978.

Neel JV: The genetics of juvenile-onset-type diabetes mellitus. *N Engl J Med* 1977; 297:1062.

Nelson WE: *Nelson Textbook of Pediatrics,* 12th ed. Vaughn V, McKay J, Behrman R (editors). Saunders, 1983.

Newman H, Freeman F, Holzinger K: *Twins: A Study of Heredity and Environment.* University of Chicago Press, 1937.

Osborne R, DeGeorge F: *Genetic Basis of Morphological Variation.* Harvard University Press, 1959.

Rimland B, Munsinger H: Burt's IQ data. *Science* 1977; 195:248.

Rowe D, Plomin R: The Burt controversy: A comparison of Burt's data on I.Q. with data from other studies. *Behav Genet* 1978; 8:81–84.

Rubenstein P, et al: Genetics and juvenile diabetes mellitus. A recessive gene closely linked to HLAD and with 50 percent penetrance. *N Engl J Med* 1977; 297:1036.

Scarr S, Weinberg R: I.Q. test performance of black children adopted by white families. *Am Psychol* 1976; 31:726–739.

Scarr S, Weinberg R: The influence of "family background" on intellectual attainment. *Am Sociol Rev* 1978; 43:674–692.

Shields J: *Monozygotic Twins Brought Up Apart and Brought Up Together.* Oxford University Press, 1962.

Sutton H: *An Introduction to Human Genetics.* 3rd ed. Saunders College, 1980.

Wilson R: Twins and siblings: Concordance for school-age mental development. *Child Dev* 1977; 48:211–216.

UNIT III GROWTH AND DEVELOPMENT: THE CHILD AND FAMILY

The intricacies of a child's growth and development are the subject of this unit. Understanding the physical, cognitive, affective, and social characteristics of the child is essential to a complete understanding of the child as an individual.

By discussing normal growth and development in a single unit we are able to identify fundamental principles as well as describe sequential stages and phases. We also emphasize such themes as the progression and fine tuning of skills; the obvious and subtle changes in qualitative and quantitative thought; the acquisition of self-esteem, autonomy, and personal identity; and the change in orientation from family to peers as the child enters school and engages in an increasing variety of social contacts.

Chapter 6 reviews the work of the major developmental theorists such as Piaget, Freud, Erikson, Gesell, Skinner, and Bandura. The more particular contributions of theorists such as Fowler on faith development and Kohlberg on moral development are also discussed.

Chapters 7 through 11 incorporate these theories to present a composite sketch of the child within designated age spans. Chapter 7 describes the rapid development of the infant from birth through 18 months. Chapter 8 discusses the child from 18 months to $4\frac{1}{2}$ years and looks at both the accomplishments and limitations experienced in this phase. In Chapter 9 we examine how school attendance and increased peer interaction open up a new world for the child. The exposure to different authority figures and value orientations and a new sense of responsibility for one's behavior characterize middle childhood, the years from $4\frac{1}{2}$ to 8. Occurring around age 8, the cognitive and other changes described in Chapter 10 translate into a greater interest in learning and motivation to complete projects in both school and play. This increased independence and the associated adult expectations characterize late childhood, the years between 8 and 12. The stress and storm of adolescence begins with puberty and continues through the high school years, approximately ages 12 to 18. Chapter 11 presents these years as a struggle for definition, as the adolescent experiments with roles, begins to use hypothetical thought, and deals with the conflicts between dependence and independence.

Two topics of growth and development are discussed separately because of their importance and the difficulty of restricting specific behaviors to certain ages. In Chapter 12 we explore the great variety of coping strategies children use to deal with developmental, environmental, and situational stressors. Because a major focus of this text is the family and the pivotal role played by parents in fostering the child's growth and development, Chapter 13 presents parenting styles and such concerns as discipline, temper tantrums, and responsibilities.

Contents

Developmental Theories:
How the Child Grows

Sandra R. Mott

6

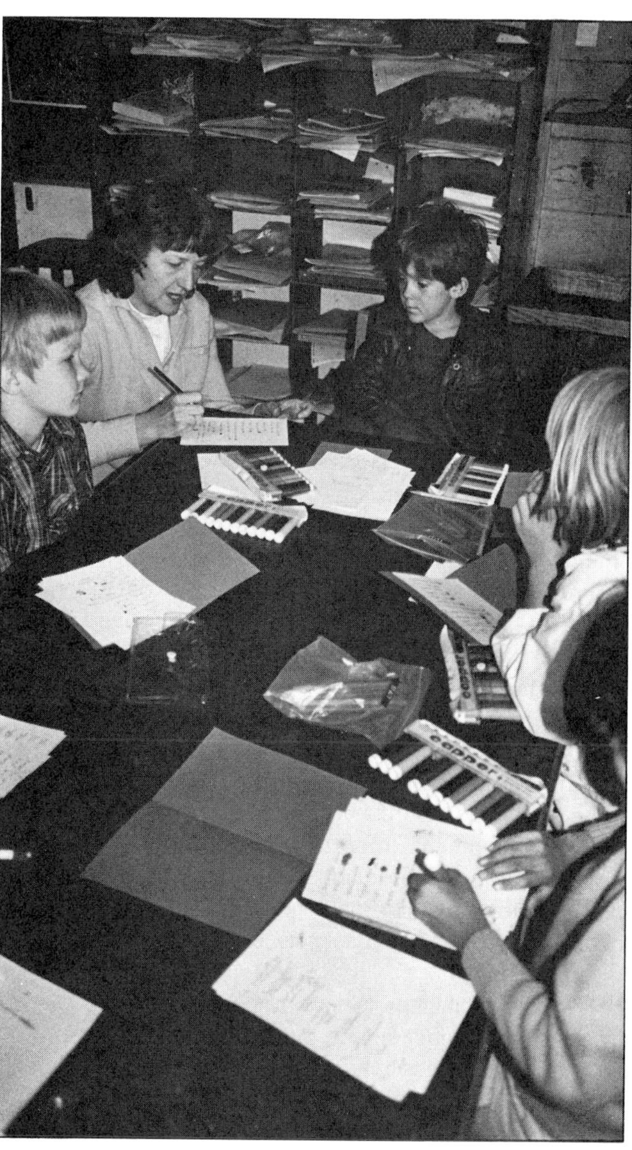

Chapter Outline

Objectives

- Define the concepts that underlie growth and development theories.
- Relate the principles of growth and development theory to the child's personality, behavior, and skill levels.
- Explain the importance of growth and development theories to child health nursing.
- Identify the principal growth and development theorists.
- For each of the principal theorists, explain the assumptions, terms, areas of interest, research methods, and findings that support the theory.
- Compare the major theoretic approaches to human growth and development by comparing assumptions, terminology, areas of interest, research methods, and explanations.
- Define the stages of growth and development that serve as a framework for understanding the developmental process.
- Identify general patterns and expectations of physical, cognitive, affective, and social development of the child from birth through adolescence.

Human growth and development, the unfolding of the child's personality, characteristics, and potential, are processes that are unique to each child yet follow an orderly process that is guided and influenced by both genetic endowment and the environment and includes contributions from the child's family, culture, and community. To understand these processes, researchers always study more than the child because the child does not and cannot develop in a vacuum. Various sociologic factors are discussed in Chapters 3 and 4, in which it is noted that society and some of its structures and interactions affect the child directly and that others add a more subtle yet significant contribution to the child's development. Important as these factors are, they are not sufficient. In addition to these nurturers of socialization, a number of internal regulators also moderate how the child perceives and interprets, organizes, and responds to stimuli.

Developmental theorists have proposed many hypotheses to explain these phenomena. Some researchers have contributed new theories, whereas others have discussed new interpretations or applications of a theory or combinations of theories. Most theorists have studied one aspect of development, such as ego development, cognitive development, moral development, biophysical development, or psychosocial development in great detail. Each of these aspects is important in understanding related behaviors and characteristics of the child; one must keep in mind that the child does not develop in isolated parts. Rather, development occurs as a whole that is always greater than the sum of its individual parts.

In this chapter, we will not present all of the many developmental theories, but we will describe and compare the major theories that are applicable to nursing practice. These major theories are also applied in subsequent chapters as we describe specific profiles of children at each developmental stage.

Applying Theories to Nursing Practice

Theories provide guidelines or possible explanations for behavior, responses to events, or adult–child interactions. They are the ways in which data are organized and presented by the researcher for use by others.

Developmental theorists basically seek to answer the questions of how the human organism grows and develops and why certain characteristics tend to appear at certain ages or in similar situations. In an attempt to answer these questions, theorists select certain facts and discard others, and in so doing they identify the facts they consider as important to the phenomenon of development. The facts they select relate in part to the theorist's educational and experiential background as well as the methodology used to collect data. This is one reason why there are so many theories and why it is necessary to know both the limitations and contributions of each theory.

Theories can be useful to nurses in providing insight into the child's thinking, capabilities, and probable responses. As such, a theory can direct interaction, provide a rationale for behavior, or assist the nurse in understanding a child's thought processes, verbal expressions, and actions.

At the same time, theories can be limiting, usually not so much for what is said but for what is left unsaid or assumed. Theorists describe according to their method of analysis or as a result of their data sample. They identify the usual or expected milestone accomplishments in a child, changes in a child's quality of thinking, and a child's development of a sense of self or acquisition of acceptable responses to others in various situations. The nurse may expect, however, to find exceptions or other ways of defining the usual. Growth and development are complex processes, and seldom can a situation be explained by a single theory. Rather, human communication, whether expressed by acts or words, must be understood as a synthesis of biologic, cognitive, affective, and social processes. At any time, one or another process might be more dominant, but all have an influence on the growing child. These influences, although similar in some respects, are different for each child. Thus, as nurses apply the theories that explain growth and development, they always take into account individual differences.

Nurses use the understanding of growth and developmental sequences to assess the child's health status; "growth and development has been termed, appropriately, the basic science of child health" (Haggerty, in Valadian and Porter, 1977). Variations in the child's growth pattern or plateaus in development may be cues to underlying problems of biologic, cognitive, or psychosocial significance. For example, the nurse may attribute the child's failure to gain weight as anticipated to a nutritional deficit, hormonal deficiency, or parental neglect. Additional information and diagnostic tests would be needed to identify the cause of the variation, but an altered growth pattern often is a clue that something is amiss and that further investigation is needed.

Knowledge of usual growth and development patterns and sequences also provides the basis for the nurse's anticipatory guidance to parents. When parents are informed about what to expect next from their children, they are better prepared to take measures to support their children's progress. Parenting is a learned role; nurses can aid parents in this endeavor by providing them with appropriate information and guidance (see Chapter 21). The nurse thus assists and directs the parents so as to facilitate the child's optimal growth and development. For example, children who are able to pull themselves to a standing position will soon be walking, first by holding onto objects and eventually on their own. A parent who is aware of this sequence and the child's needs will prepare for the child's safety, provide encouragement and practice for the child to master this skill, and remain sensitive to the child's readiness and learning pace. A knowledgeable parent is better able to participate in and enjoy a child's accomplishments and learning.

Nurses need to help parents interpret the various theories and apply the information accessible to them. The collection of "how to" literature is vast, and parents, especially first-time parents, often seek answers and guidance from a variety of resources. This variety might result in confusion and even more uncertainty as the advice of one source contradicts that of another. The guidelines given also might be so superficial that they cannot be implemented or so exact that they fail to account for child and parent differences. Parents might establish unrealistic standards, and children might feel defeated or imperfect if they cannot meet such standards. Nurses who understand the intent of developmental theories can convey their purpose to the parent, thereby helping parents to understand themselves and their children better. In this way the nurse can be instrumental in helping both parent and child develop together in a way that accommodates and enhances the self-concept of each.

Growth and Development: Dynamic Processes

Growth and development are lifelong processes. In some periods, such as infancy and adolescence, the processes are more rapid and obvious than in others, but they are just as significant or important during other periods. Growth and development are dynamic processes in that their hallmarks are interaction and change, during which the child is influenced constantly by both internal and external factors. The ongoing assessment and manipulation of these factors by the child and others enhances growth and development and thus promotes health. Each child is affected by the environment and in turn interacts with and affects the environment in a reciprocal process (Fig. 6-1).

Definitions and Principles

Growth and development are terms that are often used together because they are not synonymous and interchangeable. The terms identify independent processes; however, they are interrelated and refer to complex phenomena occurring in the human body.

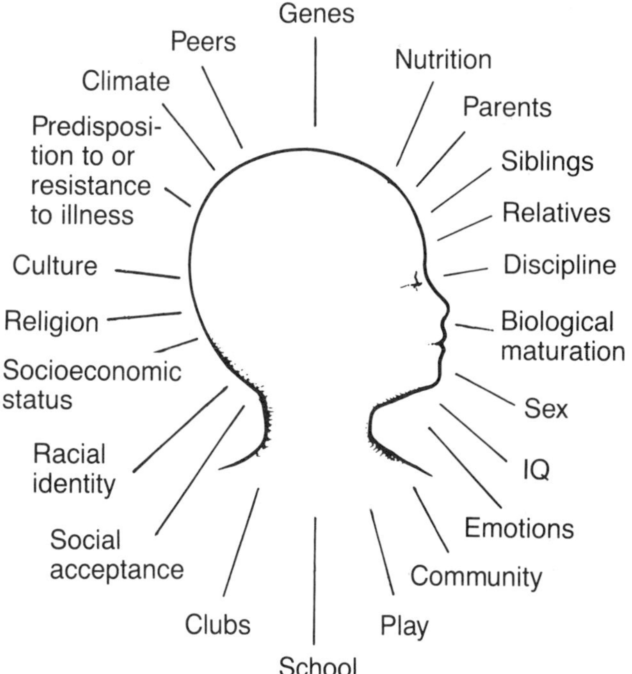

Figure 6-1 Interplay of heredity and environment in the development process. A multitude of influences shapes personality.

Although noticeable physical growth may ease or cease with adulthood, development continues. Because human life is an ever-changing experience and challenge, new skills and necessary adaptations to different situations are learned as the child adjusts to internal and external changes and events.

Nine specific principles are also helpful in providing a framework for interpreting the changes that occur in the child from birth through adolescence. They are intended only as guidelines, however, because each child's profile is the result of the interaction between genetic potential and environment.

Principle 1: Growth and development are orderly and sequential. A child's maturation is predictable and follows a generally universal timetable. Certain universal characteristics are common to the human species. These include such changes as rapid growth during the first year, slow growth during middle and late childhood, the loosening of primary teeth during middle childhood, and the appearance of secondary sex characteristics during early adolescence. The onset, length, and effects of each phase vary with each child, but the basic developmental sequence is the same for all children.

Principle 2: Growth and development are related to environment. Family, peers, and community are among the important factors creating the social and emotional climate for the child. Family and community settings vary considerably and, as a result, so do their rules and regulations, institutions, economics, values, mores, definitions of play and work, sex-role expectations, and resources. As the children grow and interact with others, they are socialized as parts of environmental groups in which appropriate values and behaviors are learned. Because cultures and environments differ, these values and behaviors also differ. What is true and correct behavior for one cultural group and setting may not be so for another. For example, in most western cultures competitiveness is recognized as a positive virtue, but the same competitive behavior is viewed negatively in some eastern societies.

Principle 3: The pace of growth and development is specific for each child. Although growth and development are essentially continuous, they are not synchronous. Each body system has a timetable for increments in size, weight, and complexity of function. For instance, the nervous and cardiovascular systems have early accelerations both because they are essential and because other systems depend on them. Likewise, changes in appearance, behavior, and skill acquisition vary with each individual child. Frequently, a child seems to develop in one area while other areas show a developmental plateau. A child who is learning to walk, for example, devotes much energy and time to this task, while fine motor skills and talking seem to progress slowly or even not at all. Each child's timetable for all aspects of growth and development is unique; therefore, the great variation among children requires nurses to consider their overall behavior and not only their specific skills. The same rationale explains the wide age span for developmental norms on most assessment guides. It is the combination of development in the various areas—biophysical, cognitive, affective, and social—that results in a child's uniqueness.

Principle 4: Growth and development occur in a cephalocaudal direction. This means that the areas closest to the brain or head develop first and are followed by the trunk and then the legs and feet. The direction of growth is evident at birth as the head is disproportionally large, comprising one quarter of the infant's length. During the embryonic state, the brain and central nervous system also develop

Key Terms for Growth and Development

Growth an increase in size of either the whole organism, as evidenced by an increase in height and weight, or any of its parts, such as bones or organs. Growth can be measured quantitatively (Lowrey, 1978).

Development an increase in the complexity of function and skill progression (Lowrey, 1978). These are qualitative changes such as the older infant's ability to digest and metabolize meats and vegetables, the acquisition of eye-hand coordination to master self-feeding, the building of block towers during early childhood, or the perfection of fine motor control during middle childhood. In essence, development is the fine tuning and perfecting of functions.

Maturation the sequence of physical changes that are related to genetic factors. These changes occur in healthy children. They are independent of environment, but their timing may be influenced by environmental factors. For example, children are able to walk once myelinization is complete, but the stimulated child will accomplish this task earlier than the deprived or malnourished child.

Adaptation the body's adjustment and accommodation to environmental factors. These may be momentary, such as the eye's iris widening upon entering a dark room, or they may be permanent such as the enlargement of the remaining kidney following a nephrectomy.

first and most rapidly, thus accounting for the infant's appearance. Further developmental progress follows myelinization and muscle maturation, thus explaining the advances in motor ability that progress from head control to sitting to crawling to standing and finally to walking (Fig. 6-2).

Principle 5: Growth and development occur in a proximal-distal direction. Controlled movements closest to the center of the body occur before controlled movements that are distant to the body axis. The infant rolls over before skillfully using a pincer grasp to pick up a raisin. Proximal-distal development is also evident in the child's interpretation of the world, which changes from egocentricity to a view that is broader and more socially related and ultimately to an outlook that is other-centered (Fig. 6-2).

Principle 6: Growth and development become increasingly differentiated. In all aspects of development mass, or generalized, responses progress to skilled, or specific, responses. The infant's early responses to stimuli involve total body activity. The newborn cries with the whole body: legs kick, arms thrash, shoulders twist, and the face becomes red and contorted. The older child cries only with the eyes and face. The young child responds in general when unhappy, in pain, delighted, excited, or afraid. With maturation and experience, these emotions and feelings become better defined, and the child's responses become more refined and specific.

Principle 7: Growth and development become increasingly integrated. Behavior and function progress from simple to complex as the child gains new skills and combines previously learned skills to accomplish more difficult tasks. For instance, the young child learning to drink from a cup first combines eye-hand, grasping, and hand-mouth coordination; then, once the cup reaches the mouth, the child adds controlled tipping and mouth, lip, and tongue movements to drink and swallow the liquid. What seems so natural to the adult is, for the child, the result of considerable prior effort in connecting previously learned single behaviors to the attainment of new skills. Childhood is a foundation, a period during which basic learning and skills are acquired, combined, and perfected in preparation for the increasingly complex functions and skills required by the growing organism.

Principle 8: Certain periods are critical during growth and development. This principle is often not well understood but has a variety of applications. For instance during times of rapid cell division and growth, the organism is most vulnerable to insults from abnormal conditions. The increased incidence of congenital anomalies in children of mothers exposed to certain viruses, chemicals, or drugs during the first 10–12 weeks after conception is evidence of this. Early malnutrition also results in cognitive deficits, whereas later nutritional deprivation does not have the same deleterious effects.

Whether critical periods exist for other learning and skill

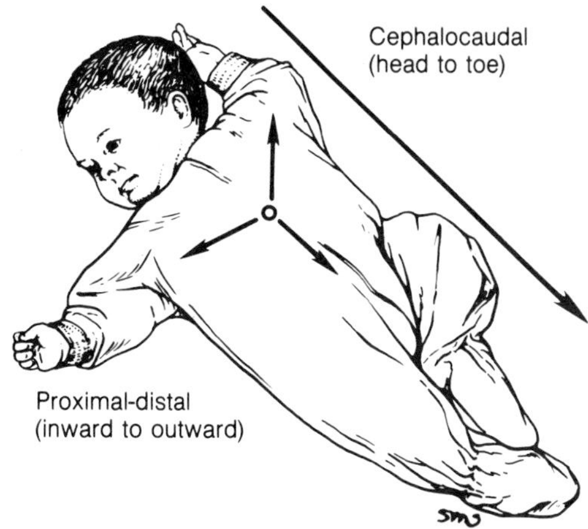

Figure 6-2 Principles of development: Cephalocaudal (head to toe) and proximal-distal (inward to outward).

development is a question requiring additional research. The work of Konrad Lorenz, in which he demonstrated a period of imprinting with young birds (Lorenz, 1970), is one study that suggests similar developmental periods in humans. Researchers interested in maternal–infant bonding have proposed that there is a sensitive period immediately after birth during which the close relationship that develops between an infant and the primary caregiver begins. Researchers have questioned both the nature and timing of this phenomenon and whether the critical period is related to the infant or the parent. Human resiliency that compensates for less-than-ideal conditions and children's common patterns of development also need further investigation (Gewirtz, 1961; Tulman, 1981). In the areas of affective and social development, the increased adaptability and flexibility of the human organism might increase the so-called critical period significantly. There does seem to be some validity to the concept of sensitive periods for learning new skills and tasks. Although learning is not precluded beyond this time, it occurs with greater difficulty (Nelms and Mullins, 1982).

Principle 9: Growth and development are continuous and are influenced by many factors. Although both environment and the many genetic and maturational factors influence growth and development, this last principle emphasizes the total picture of a complex, multidimensional, ongoing process. To understand the growth and development of the human organism, it is necessary to identify the way in which a multitude of factors combine and contribute to the whole. The growth and development process is integrated, the result of the interaction of biophysical, psychologic, and environmental factors. Heredity and environment work together in important ways, and genetic factors provide the potential and set in motion the process that is stimulated and nurtured by the environment and the many experiences that affect the degree to which the individual's potential is fulfilled.

Concepts Integral to Growth and Development Theories

Many theories offer explanations of the various facets of growth and development but none answers all the questions about the nature of being human, the how and why individuals are both similar and dissimilar, and the relative roles of biology and environment. Each theory, however, describes a segment of the growth and development process and is helpful in understanding the process as a whole. One might think of the individual as a house with the window shades pulled and the doors closed. As information and insight are gained from each theory, a door opens or a shade is raised, thus shedding light on the human condition and the human capability of interacting uniquely with others.

Studying and then synthesizing the many growth and development theories provides the nurse with a framework within which to comprehend the dynamic organization of internal and external stimuli. Individuals relate both phylogenetically and genotypically to their environments. Such a synthesis, therefore, requires an examination of each theory and a clarification of what it does and does not reveal about human growth and development.

The Theorist's Assumptions A theorist's assumptions provide some basic information about that particular theorist's beliefs concerning the human condition. Before understanding or putting a theorist's ideas in perspective, the nurse needs to know the aspect of development on which the theorist focused, the methodology for data collection and analysis, the theorist's philosophic and a priori convictions, and the ways in which these beliefs contributed to the results. A theorist's assumptions might be a response to another theory that might have been adopted, modified, or even rejected. Theoretic assumptions also might be the result of experience or deeply held beliefs. Whatever the case, assumptions about the nature and progression of development are important and influential components of the framework upon which the theory is built.

Identifying the significance of these underlying assumptions provides an understanding of the theorist's view of being human and the nature of interaction between the individual and the environment. The essential question is not which view is right or wrong but rather what the consequences are of these basic premises and how they influence decision making for growing and developing children.

Malleability Beliefs concerning the relative roles of heredity and environment in the developmental process are evident in the degree to which the theorist assumes that behavior and personality are formed at birth. The degree to which behavior and personality are considered changeable determines the degree of human *malleability* assumed by the theorist. This is sometimes referred to as the controversy between nature and nurture, between heredity and social control, or between maturation and learning. Theorists tend to fall into one of three general groups: (1) those who claim that genetics determines most, if not all, of development; (2) those who claim that the child's experiences and thus the child's environment is the predominant determiner; and (3) those who credit both heredity and environment as significant and interacting contributors, each one operating to a greater or lesser extent during various aspects of development (Fig. 6-3A).

A theorist's beliefs about the child's malleability correspond to the value that theorist attaches to culture, community, and family as socializing agents. Environmental factors make little difference if a predetermined genetic capability and timetable are responsible for the manner and quality of development, but they are crucial factors if individual development is the result of experiences with a variety of people and situations.

A theorist's assumptions on malleability are important for understanding not only the theory but also the theory's application in supporting different philosophic and political stances. In general, proponents of the more conservative stances prefer and use the findings of those theorists who favor heredity as the determining factor. Among these findings are the work of Jensen (1969), who attempted to equate intellectual capacity to racial differences, and the more recent research done by ethologists in their quest to find a link between genetic principles and behavior development. For example, Hess (1970) concluded from a series of experiments examining visual responses that women are more attracted to and therefore have a biologic predisposition to infants that is not present in men. Can it then be inferred that women, and not men, should be the primary caregivers of infants? Such a finding can be used and abused to promote one's ideology.

More liberal stances, on the other hand, point to those theorists who stress environment as a determining factor in behavior. Proponents of this belief are more likely to suggest the need for social programs to enhance and support the learning climate for special populations. Longitudinal studies of early Head Start classes, for example, indicate the effectiveness of these programs in aiding the intellectual and psychosocial development of children from low-income families (Lazar, 1979). This assumption is the impetus for other social programs, such as the Supplemental Food Program for Women, Infants, and Children (WIC) (Berkenfield and Schwartz, 1980) and the Early Intervention programs directed toward parents and high-risk infants, which are intended to create an environment that enhances learning and responsiveness (Ramey, Campbell, and Finkelstein, 1983). Such political recommendations are based on theoretic assumptions about the possibilities for human change.

Between these two opposing views are numerous other stances that use findings from both sides of the controversy. Interactional theorists, for example, claim that, to varying degrees, environmental and maturational factors interact to

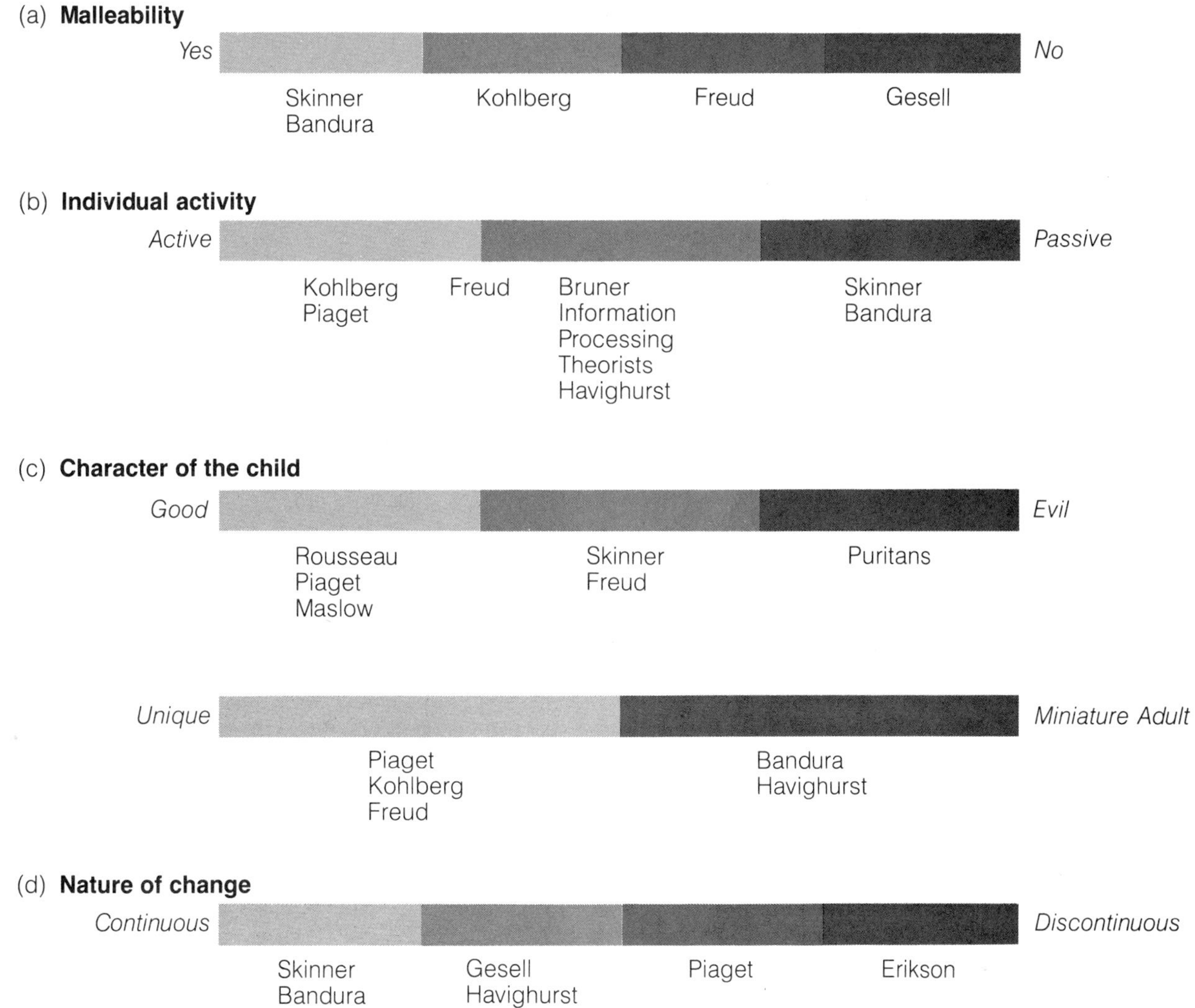

Figure 6-3 Comparison of assumptions underlying the findings of developmental theorists.

influence the quality of development. For instance, the nutritional health of a woman prior to and during pregnancy is related to her developing fetus. A healthy mother in turn is more likely to have healthy genes that will be expressed to their potential in a supportive, well-nourished environment (Zeskind and Ramey, 1978). Other theorists have studied reciprocal behaviors between the infant and parents and have concluded that "The infant, then, appears to be genetically programmed to respond to and learn about and become attached to that aspect of his environment that is most likely to ensure his survival—namely, another person" (Lewis, 1982).

These debates about the correct view of development and the relative contributions of genetics and environment are not as important as identifying the underlying theoretic assumptions. Nurses, in applying theories of growth and development while caring for children, need to determine how these assumptions influence various theories and how the resulting theories are used by others.

Individual Activity A second assumption to identify is the theorist's beliefs concerning the child's contribution to personal development and the learning process. Is the child an active participant or a passive recipient? Does motivation for learning come from within, from an innate curiosity and desire to know the meaning and symbols of the environment, or does motivation come from without, supplied by others? Theorists such as Freud and Piaget credit inner needs with the thrust that directs the child's interaction with animate and inanimate objects in the environment. These theorists believe that the child develops and learns by actively constructing reality from these multiple encounters and interactions with the environment. Maturation then advances the child's ability to reason and handle complex pieces of information. According to these theorists, a supportive environment is an asset, but it is the child who formulates reality; the environment does not tell the child what to learn.

Behaviorists such as Skinner and Bandura, however, claim that the motivating force that directs the child's learning comes from the environment. They postulate that the child reacts to stimuli provided by others and is a product of a society that supplies and directs children's learning about their culture and their world.

Once again, between these two polar stances is a third group of theorists, represented by learning theorists such as Bruner and Montessori, who emphasize that both the child's motivation and the environmental teachers are needed for learning (Fig. 6-3B). For them, the ability to learn and the process of relating information so that it becomes meaningful comes from the child, but parents and teachers are responsible for providing ideas and instruction about the culture and world. The child's potential cannot be realized without direction and influence from others skilled in the transmission of knowledge.

How one views the role of environment in the process of development and learning is significant in the determining of public policy. A community that believes in the value of early education and well-qualified teachers will quote from theories that support the role of environment. Their opponents will cite theories that emphasize the child's inherent maturation and autonomous learning and thus reduce the importance of environmental issues and perhaps the school budget as well.

Character of the Child Two questions are important to this assumption. The first is the moral condition of the child. Although this issue was once of greater importance, it still influences the way in which motives and wrongdoings are attributed to children today. In the seventeenth century the Puritans believed that children were born evil and needed definitive guidance from adults to acquire goodness. In contrast Rousseau and, later, Piaget attributed innate goodness to the child and suggested that significant adults are charged with the responsibility of protecting the child from the evils of society, which has the potential to corrupt the child. Freud considered the child to be amoral, neither good nor evil, but with the capacity to internalize society's values and thus a sense of right and wrong. For Freud, moral sense is culturally acquired rather than innate (Fig. 6-3C). A parent's interpretation of an infant's cry may demonstrate one of these views. Is the infant crying because of selfishness, self-centeredness, and desire for pleasure, or is the cry a means of communication and interaction? The way in which parents and others answer this question influences how they respond to the infant.

The second aspect of the child's character is whether a child is developmentally different from an adult or is instead a kind of miniature adult. Is childhood a particular, unique time of life, or is it simply time spent learning to become an adult? Theorists who assume the child's uniqueness focus on the ways in which change occurs, the ways that children integrate new and old information, and the quality of change in their thinking and relationships with their environment. Theorists who view childhood as a proving ground for adult behavior are more interested in quantitative changes and the rapidity with which children learn to respond in socially approved ways.

Adults' goals for children are, in essence, related to the value they place on childhood as a unique time of life. Some adults think it is important that the child read by 3 years of age, whereas others are content that the child is developing gross and fine motor coordination while playing with peers. The essential question is whether the child's learning is special and whether it should be respected as such or be considered inefficient if not structured to accomplish the acquisition of more facts in less time. How parents and educators answer this question is important for determining educational goals and such decisions as the age at which subject matter is introduced in a school curriculum.

Nature of Change The final assumption to consider is the manner in which a theorist believes that developmental changes occur. Again, there are two essentially distinct views, one that development occurs in definite, sequential stages and the other that development is continuous (Fig. 6-3D). Behaviorists promote the idea of small, continuous increments of change and deny any identifiable difference in thinking or behavior as the child progresses to adulthood.

Other theorists believe in defined stages that mark simultaneous changes in the child's thinking about the world and relating to others. These stages progress in an orderly fashion, and each successive stage is the result of a greater integration of past and present experiences into more complex behaviors and responses. Some theorists, such as Piaget and Erikson, consider these stages to be universal and unvarying. They assume that children of all cultures develop in similar ways and pass through the same sequence of cognitive and psychosocial growth patterns, although individuals may display characteristics of more than one stage during transitional phases. At these times, some behavior and thinking is typical of the stage into which the child is moving, whereas other thought patterns and actions are reminiscent of the stage the child is leaving.

Many theorists have identified stages, or levels of growth and development, that occur as the child develops. Some, such as Gesell, correlate stage with chronologic age, whereas other theorists do not. Some, such as Piaget and Erikson, consider only one aspect of development, whereas other theorists, such as Havighurst, look at multiple aspects and attempt to present a total picture of the child at a particular stage. Other questions that theorists might or might not discuss are the rate of progression through each stage, regression to a previous stage, or fixation at any one stage. These questions relate to concerns of normal or abnormal development and how the theories can provide insight into approaching such problems.

Research Design In applying the many theories of growth and development, the nurse also finds it helpful to ascertain the theory's breadth of application, extent of prediction, and degree of control. These variables define the limits, potential insights, and methodology of the theory. Figure 6-4 organizes the different theorists' research according to their research design.

The breadth of application for any theory essentially determines the extent to which the theorist seeks or is able to answer specific questions. For example, Piaget devised his theory because he wanted to discover why students gave incorrect answers on the intelligence test developed by Binet.

The extent to which a theory measures cause and effect describes the limits of the theory in predicting the child's future behavior. Most theories therefore describe trends and usual reactions but not absolutes. The theorist's degree of control is measured by how the data were gathered, which may have been through field studies, controlled laboratory experiments, or a combination of the two.

Maturation Theories

Maturation theorists emphasize the role of genetics as the determiner of how and in what order developmental changes occur. Dating back to Jean Jacques Rousseau, the French philosopher of the late seventeenth century, this theoretic view was proposed as one that coincided with the natural growth of children. By providing guidelines to parents and tutors, Rousseau popularized the idea that each aspect of development—physical, cognitive, and psychosocial—had its own internal, predetermined, maturation timetable. Teaching done before the predetermined time was therefore wasted and could even be detrimental because the child was not ready to learn. The questions pondered by Rousseau still engage developmental researchers today (Thomas, 1979). Is there a critical period for learning, when the maturation factors are primed for the intake of new information? Are there upper and lower limits to this time? What really happens if instruction is given too early or late?

Although other theorists have since modified and amplified Rousseau's ideas and his explanations of children's growth and development, he laid the foundation for changes in the way adults, especially educators, have viewed both the child and their own role as teachers. Rousseau insisted that the child is good (moral), unique, and a being whose genetic potential requires firsthand experiences with seeing, doing, touching, experimenting, and problem solving in order to learn.

Later, the maturationists further explained development as autogenetic, suggesting that the child plays the active role and the environment the supportive role. In such theoretic constructs the environment provides the stage for the expression of genetically endowed physical, cognitive, and psychosocial skills as they become evident in the mannerisms, interactions, abilities, orientation to life, and construction of experiences by the child. In essence the child is seen

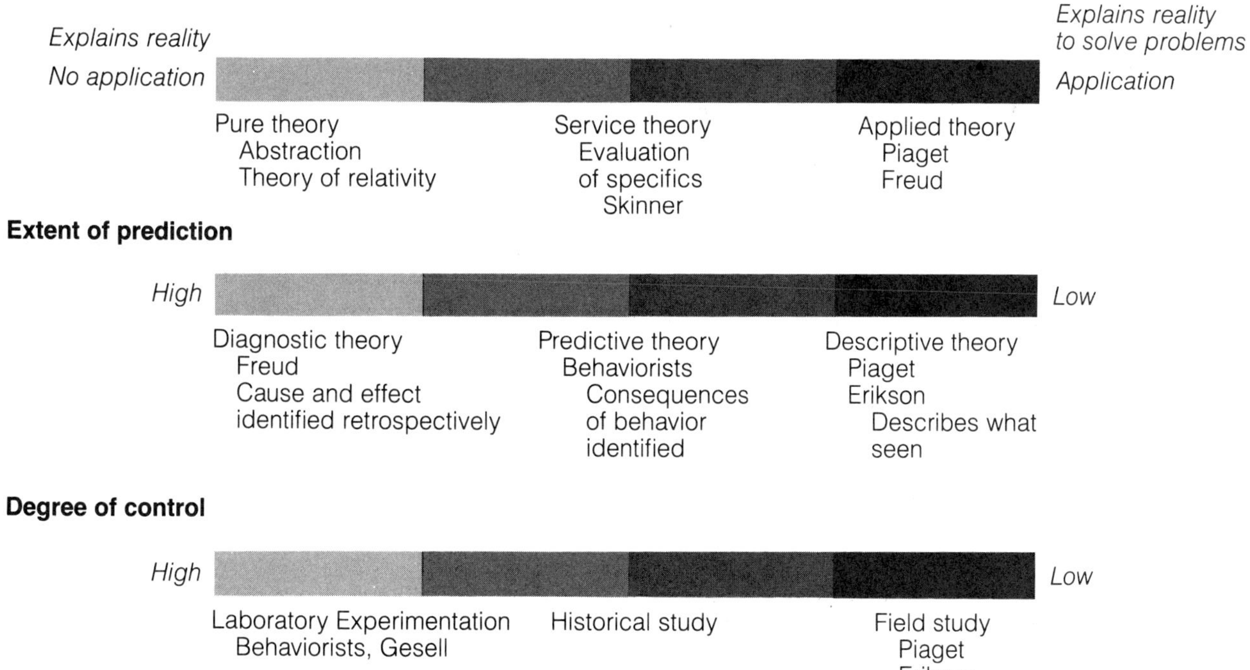

Figure 6-4 Comparison among the parameters of research design for developmental theorists.

as actively attempting to actualize his or her genetic potential fully. Mastery of one skill provides the impetus toward learning another, more complicated skill; the process then repeats itself and thus becomes self-generative.

Theory of Gesell

Arnold Gessell (1880–1961) is the theorist credited with adopting the term *maturation* to refer to the developmental changes that result from the genes. His initial fascination with the orderly, sequential patterns of embryonic development motivated him to study human development over time in an effort to verify that the same processes continued after birth. Gesell dedicated his life to observing and gathering detailed, descriptive, longitudinal data of characteristic behavior and skills of infants, children, and adolescents through 16 years of age. He noted that behavior becomes progressively organized as the child grows, and he attributed this organization to the unfolding of the child's genetic inheritance. He was impressed that similar skills and behaviors seem to appear at about the same time in all children. This finding provided him with evidence of the progressive maturation of the neuromuscular system, a process that enables the child to perform and organize motor skills and other behaviors.

Gesell studied twins and ultimately concluded that phylogenetic skills are preprogrammed and that prior practice or teaching makes little, if any, difference in the time of their appearance. His studies involved dividing identical twins so that one twin would be permitted to develop naturally while the other twin would be given special practice and experience with a skill such as walking. Gesell found no significant differences in the timing with which each pair of twins walked without assistance. Special practice could not be proven to be beneficial, thereby reinforcing Gesell's belief that readiness for change is genetically controlled and follows a predetermined program.

Gesell and his assistants did not limit their observations to one method or one aspect of development. They used observations, films, and interviews with parents to collect data that presented a composite picture of each child studied. This multitude of data was then categorized into ten major areas for which gradations of maturity were correlated with specific traits. These areas and their subheadings are outlined in Table 6-1; taken together, they form a data base for a personality profile.

Gesell described cycles of behavioral trends that tended to coincide with chronologic ages. With each cycle, a characteristic pattern alternating between equilibrium and disequilibrium occurs. Times of equilibrium are defined as years in which the child is in good balance, "having relatively little difficulty within himself or with the world about him" (Ilg and Ames, 1960, p. 20). These are followed by periods when behavior becomes disorganized, and the child appears to be "at odds with his environment and with himself" (Ilg and Ames, 1960, p. 21). As a result of their analysis, Gesell and his group outlined ages and stages, each lasting from 6 months to 1 year, in a sequence in which better and worse times follow each other repetitively. Each stage and corresponding age were described as though it brought its own personality, clearly definable and resulting from maturational changes. Because the theory predicted that better years would follow worse years, the phrase, "It's just a stage," became popular, and parents were admonished to be patient and tolerant of difficult times because these times were only temporary (Table 6-2).

TABLE 6-1 Areas of Behavior Observed for Personality Profiles

Type of behavior	Observable traits
Motor characteristics	Body activity; eye and hand movements
Personal hygiene	Eating, sleeping, elimination; bathing and dressing; health and somatic complaints; outlets for tension
Emotional expression	Affective attitudes; crying and related behaviors; assertion and anger
Fears and dreams	—
Self and sex	—
Interpersonal relations	Maternal–child interactions; child–child interactions; groups in play
Play and pastimes	General interests; reading; music; radio; cinema
School life	Adjustment to school; classroom demeanor; reading; writing; arithmetic
Ethical sense	Blaming and telling alibis; responses to directions, punishment, praise, or reason; sensing good from bad; understanding truth and property
Philosophic outlook	Attitudes toward time, space, language, thought, war, death, deity

SOURCE: Gesell A, Ilg FL: *Child Development: An Introduction to the Study of Human Growth*. Harper & Row, 1949, p. 69.

Gesell and colleagues acknowledged individual differences but linked them with genetic inheritance as expressed in the child's body build. The theory of somatotypes developed by William Sheldon (1940, 1942) was used to account for the observed variations in personality types. (Sheldon equated personality types with physical characteristics.) The skills and behaviors that typified each were those observed in the most children and reflected the normative pattern of development. Children who did not fit this description were assumed to belong to one of the groups that bordered the norm.

At one end of the scale were children who were thin, fragile, and petite, similar to Sheldon's ectomorphic type.

TABLE 6-2 Gesell's Cycles of Behavior

Age in years			Description
Cycle 1	*Cycle 2*	*Cycle 3*	
2	5	10	Smooth, consolidated
$2\frac{1}{2}$	$5\frac{1}{2}$–6	11	Breaking up
3	$6\frac{1}{2}$	12	Rounded, balanced
$3\frac{1}{2}$	7	13	Inwardness
4	8	14	Vigorous, expansive
$4\frac{1}{2}$	9	15	Inwardness-outwardness troubled, "neurotic"
5	10	16	Smooth, consolidated

SOURCE: Adapted from Ilg FL, Ames L B: *The Gesell Institute's Child Behavior.* Dell, 1960, p. 22.

Their personalities tended to be restrained, oversensitive, inhibited in social situations, intense, and quick to react. At the other end of the scale were children with opposite appearances and personalities. These children were similar to Sheldon's endomorphic type in that they were soft, round, overweight, had poor musculature, and loved comfort, sleep, relaxation, food, and the approval of others. Thus, Gesell and colleagues presumed that the inherited distribution and proportion of muscle, fat, and bone density rather than the environment accounted for temperament and personality differences.

Although still assuming the predominant importance of heredity, some of Gesell's followers later accepted the idea that the environment has some influence on development. "All of this does not mean that human behavior is *entirely* determined by hereditary factors. What it does mean is that the body structure provides the raw material out of which personality is formed: that is the instrument upon which the life forces, both internal and external, play" (Ilg and Ames, 1960).

Their painstakingly constructed atlas of chronologic growth and development according to motor, affect, language, and social domains (Table 6-3) serves as a guide for parents to assess the current status of their children and to anticipate a child's next stage. Although Gesell's behavioral profiles are subject to criticism because of his small sample size and the similar socioeconomic backgrounds of his subjects, the idea of cataloguing the expected appearance of skills and their order laid the foundation for the various developmental assessment guides currently in use (see Chapter 16).

Theory of Sociobiology

Sociobiology is a recently emerged, genetically oriented field in which theorists are interested in determining the causes of human behavior and believe that biologic forces are more important than was formerly thought. Sociobiologists postulate that survival of the species is the underlying motivator of behavior. Edward O. Wilson defined sociobiology as the "systematic study of the biological basis of all social behavior" (Wilson, as quoted in Thomas, 1979). The sociobiologists' premise suggests that if responses to environmental factors are biologically based, they are similar over time and across cultures.

This theory relates differences that appear among ethnic and racial groups to genetic factors rather than environment or culture, thus explaining Bayley's (1965) finding of racial differences in data from motor and mental tests for 1- to 15-month-old infants. When other factors were controlled, black children consistently scored higher on motor tests but scored equally with white children on mental tests. A sociobiologist would conclude that blacks genetically are programmed differently from whites; differences in maturation of motor development is then both logical and consistent with their sociobiologic theory.

Tanner (1961, 1973) has noted that some basic traits of development are not altered, even though modifications in the environment may be responsible for changing other traits. For example, when the diets of Asian children were improved, their height and weight dimensions correlated more closely with American children, but there was no change in their characteristic facial and trunk-limb proportions. These traits were seen as genetically based and resistant to environment. Skeletal growth and the maturation of motor skills appears to be more closely linked to genetic factors than to environment.

In the quest to understand more about the complex phenomena of how and why children grow and develop as they do, the sociobiologic theory provides some new ways of assessing heredity and the role it may play in social behavior. The theory serves as a reminder of the possible importance of genetic factors, but nurses and other health professionals need to exercise caution when attempting to apply it in the context of today's complex society.

Theory of Ethology

Ethology is defined as the study of animal behavior and its correlation to and revelations about human behavior. Like sociobiology, ethology affirms the contributions made by heredity in determining the nature of the human being. Ethologists insist that certain environmental events invoke innate responses and that these responses are not learned and seem to be universal. For example, the infant's smile may be an unlearned response as part of an exchange of favors between persons. Aggression is another innate response, with similarities in fighting and aggression rituals in the animal kingdom that are analagous to schoolyard altercations (Yussen and Santrock, 1982).

Ethologists study their subject matter in a natural environment and remain nonparticipating observers. Data collected on any subject, such as schoolyard aggression, come

TABLE 6-3 An Example of Gesell's Developmental Schedules

54 months	Key age 60 months	72 months
	Motor Development	
Hops on one foot	Skips using feet alternately	Jumps from height of 12 in; lands on toes
Articulation not infantile	Stands on one foot for more than 8 seconds	Ball: advanced throwing
Drawing: traces cross	Walking backwards: 6 cm board, no step off	Stands on each foot alternately with eyes closed
	Pellets: 10 into bottle in 20 seconds	Walking backwards: length 4 cm board
		Drawing: copies diamond
	Adaptive Development	
Manipulates cubes: makes gate from model	Manipulates cubes: builds two steps	Manipulates cubes: builds three steps
Drawing: copies square	Drawing: Unmistakable man with body and so forth	Drawing: man with neck, hands, clothes
Drawing: three bubbles correct	Drawing: copies triangle	Drawing: man's legs are two-dimensional
Geometric forms: points to nine	Drawing: copies rectangle with diagonal at 66 mo	Drawing: copies diamond
Counts four objects and answers "how many?"	Drawing: adds seven parts to incomplete man	Drawing: adds nine parts to incomplete man
Aesthetic comparison: correct	Drawing: four bubbles correct	Weights: five weights, no error, best trial
Missing parts: two correct	Counts: 10 objects correctly	Missing parts: all correct
Digits: repeats four (one of three trials)	Counts: 12 objects correctly at 66 mo	Digits: four correct (two of three trials)
	Weights: only one error in five block test (at 72 mo)	Fingers: correct no. 1 hand; on both hands
	Fingers: correct no. on each hand	Adds and subtracts within 5
	Personal–Social	
Communication: calls attention to own performance (at 60 mo)	Dressing: dresses and undresses with no assistance	Dressing: ties shoelaces
Communication: relates fanciful tales (at 60 mo)	Communication: asks meaning of words	Communication: differentiates A.M. and P.M.
Communication: bosses and criticizes (at 60 mo)	Play: dresses up in adult clothes	Communication: knows right and left (three of three) or complete reversal (six of six)
Play: shows off dramatically (at 60 mo)	Play: prints a few letters at 60–66 mo	Communication: recites numbers to 30s

NOTE: Four different areas of development are examined: motor, adaptive (fine motor), language, and personal-social.

SOURCE: Bigner J J: *Human Development*. Macmillan, 1983, p. 16. Reproduced from various copyrighted books by Arnold Gesell and associates, all rights reserved. The Psychological Corporation, 304 East 45th St., New York, N.Y. 10017.

from a variety of settings and cultures and are analyzed for evidence of innate responses. The genetic inheritance of the human species is regarded as both the controller and inventor of social behavior.

One well-known ethologist is Konrad Lorenz, whose work with young goslings demonstrated a phenomenon he termed *imprinting*. Lorenz found that shortly after hatching, young goslings will follow the first moving object that comes into view. They then "imprint" the object and are willing to follow its lead. Normally, the first moving object a newly hatched gosling sees is the mother goose, but Lorenz found that if he substituted himself for the mother, the goslings would then follow him. Similar experiments with other animals suggested that there is a sensitive period in the life of a young animal in which imprinting takes place (Thomas, 1979). Ethologists may surmise, therefore, that imprinting is related to the phenomenon of attachment that is evident in the human species.

Both the ethologist and the sociobiologist credit environment with a formative role in the child's development. They assume that individuals adapt to their environment because of their genetic endowment and this ability ensures survival of the species. Their emphasis on survival indicates that these theories are a refined form of Darwin's theory of evolution. Their goal is to discover the biologic foundation for the origins of child behavior from comparative studies conducted on animal behavior. Although ethologic theory sometimes is criticized as being simplistic, there is now a growing interest in acquiring advanced knowledge concerning the limits and contributions of the genes for individual development at all levels.

Cognitive-Structural Theories

The focus of cognitive-structural theories is the manner in which children learn to think, reason, and use language. Cognitive-structural theorists are interested primarily in defining the developmental patterns of intelligence, that is, the orderly progression of mental thought and problem solving as it advances from simple to complex.

Cognitive theorists study qualitative changes in children's thinking from illogical to logical thought and finally to their ability to handle abstract concepts. They describe and analyze how children learn rather than what they learn, which includes the child's experiences and processing of information. Unfortunately, the study of these processes is limited to inferences made from observable behaviors; there is no other way for the theorist to "see" what is transpiring in the child's mind.

Cognitive theorists propose that development in cognition is the result of the child's active interaction with the environment together with maturation, especially maturation of the central nervous system. The rate of and potential for growth is assumed to be determined genetically, an assumption that partly accounts for individual differences. The continuous, repetitive interaction between one's genetic endowments and environment results in growth. "One cannot progress beyond the biologically determined levels, but the individual can function maximally within these levels if the environment is optimally supportive" (Schuster and Ashburn, 1980).

Theory of Jean Piaget

The most widely read and well known of the cognitive theorists is Jean Piaget (1896–1980). His cognitive development theory has provided the basis for other theories such as Kohlberg's theory of moral development and Fowler's theory of faith development. Although Piaget primarily is considered a child psychologist and educator, his work is not concerned with predicting behavior or promoting pedagogic principles. He might more appropriately be described as a genetic epistemologist, that is, a scientist who studies how knowledge is acquired and how learning takes place. Piaget was interested in defining and explaining systematically the growth and development of intellectual structures and knowledge. His theory reflects his scientific concern for the careful collection and classification of observations and his philosophic interest in seeking logical, internally consistent systems.

Piaget's theory initially resulted from field studies of children, first his own and neighborhood children and later those of other cultures and countries. He viewed "development as an inherent, unalterable, evolutionary process; yet within this developmental process he locate[d] a series of distinct developmental phases and subphases" (Maier, 1965). For Piaget, the gnawing question on which his hypotheses were based was how the child adjusted to the world. He sought to gain insight into the steps and process of discovery, reinvention, understanding, and the acquisition of knowledge. In successive studies Piaget explored the growth of intelligence, attainment of moral perspective, and concept of physical reality as they develop during childhood. He concluded that a child's knowledge is neither inborn nor passively constructed by society; rather, children construct their own intelligence through actions performed on objects, thus creating or recreating logical principles.

Piaget then proposed that learning follows development and is the result of the active manipulation of objects and internal structuring of the event that resulted in the child's manipulating operations. According to Piaget, operations are actions characterized by their great generality; they are reversible, and never isolated but rather are always capable of coordination into overall systems (Piaget and Inhelder, 1969). This possession of operations, of special mental processing, is the heart of intellectual growth.

Intellectual growth is therefore not only an accumulation of facts. The child is not an empty vessel into which information is funneled about how the world functions. Rather, learning is an internal action that enables the child to know, modify, and transform objects and to understand the process of the transformation and thus the construction of the object (Piaget and Inhelder, 1969). Intellectual growth occurs when the newly learned operations are lasting, generalized, and the result of progressively higher levels of problem-solving ability.

Intellectual development, the process of restructuring knowledge, occurs in a series of five steps, as follows:

1. Initial level, or the child's way of thinking or structural unit for comprehension
2. External disturbance or situation that does not fit into the old structure or way of thinking and creates a conflict or disequilibrium
3. Compensation, which occurs when the problem is solved by intellectual activity
4. New way of thinking, or different organizational pattern now that previous patterns are sensed as inferior and absorbed in a new, superior pattern
5. Equilibrium

As the child interacts with the environment, new objects are discovered and new problems uncovered. This creates disequilibrium, to which the child adjusts or adapts by constructing solutions that result in a permanent system of compensations and a higher level of cognitive behavior (Piaget and Inhelder, 1969). A child's developing intelligence is therefore born of action and grows within the child as the result of two continual processes, assimilation and accommodation (Fig. 6-5.) *Assimilation* is the continuous

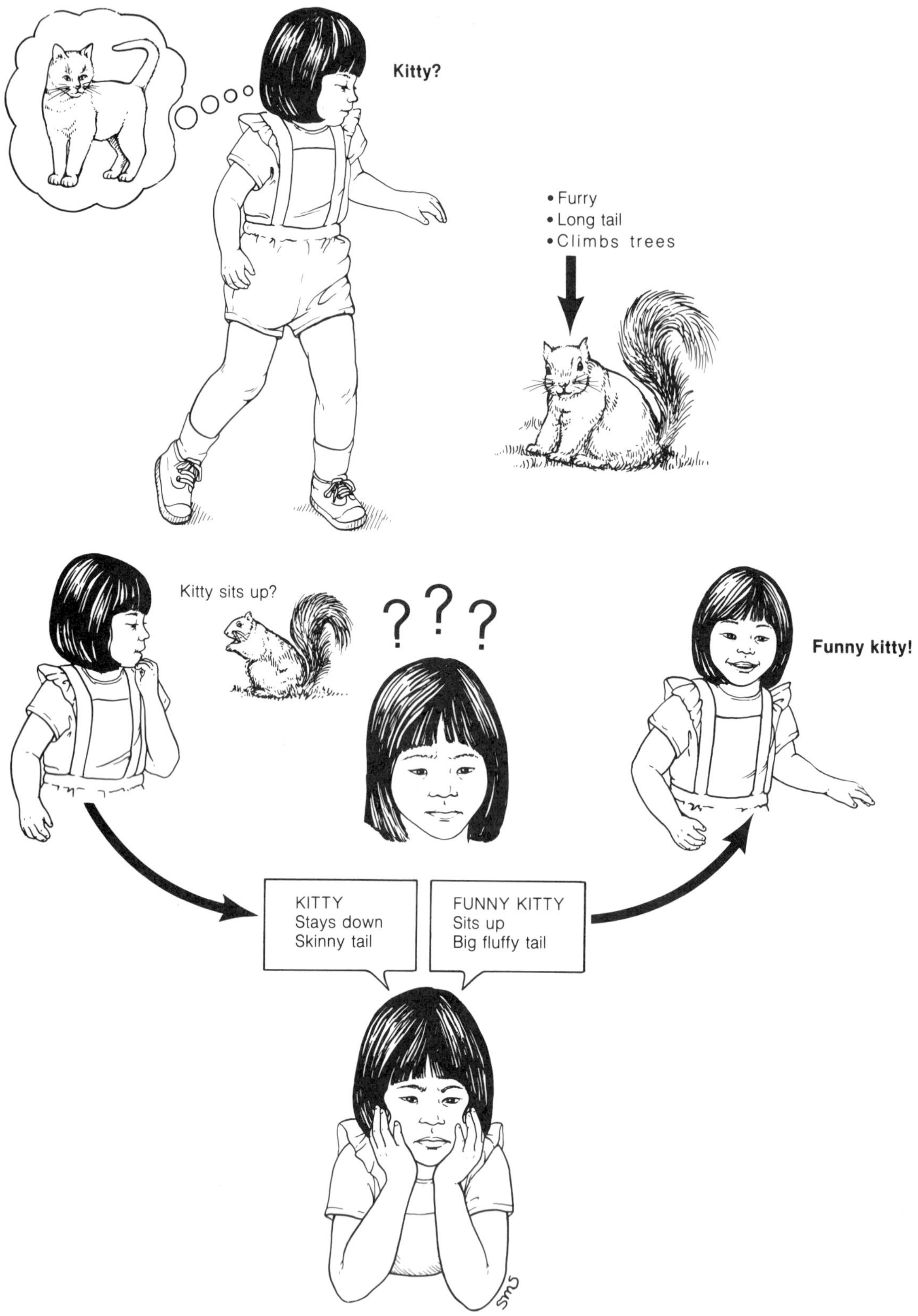

Figure 6-5 Process of accommodation, by which the child alters cognitive structures to comprehend new data from the environment.

process by which the child integrates new experiences into already-existing schemes; one might compare a scheme to a balloon and assimilation to putting more air into the balloon (Wadsworth, 1979). The process of *accommodation* is used when a child is confronted with a new stimulus and is unable to assimilate it into an existing scheme, necessitating modification of the scheme or creation of a new scheme.

Piaget identified a combination of four areas that allow cognition to develop. They are (1) maturation of motor and perceptual abilities; (2) experience with physical objects in the environment; (3) experience in social interactions with peers, parents, other adults; and (4) equilibration. *Equilibration* is defined as self-regulation and, as such, is the coordinator of the three other areas; it is a balance between assimilation and accommodation, the condition toward which the organism constantly strives (Fig. 6-6). Piagetian terms are defined in Table 6-4.

Piaget believed that cognitive growth and development proceed in this way at all levels of development, from birth through adulthood, so that the developmental schemes of the adult are built on those of the child. According to Piaget, the quality of a child's thinking changes with progressive development. This is not an abrupt change but is gradual and signifies the process of adaptation to the environment and new organization of structures of thought. Children of similar ages respond to intellectual tasks in a similar manner, and their responses are reflections of their levels of reasoning. Piaget therefore postulated the following principles of development:

1. All development proceeds through the same sequence of phases
2. All development progresses from simple to complex
3. Development begins from experience with concrete objects and situations and proceeds to abstraction only after mastery of the concrete
4. Personality development includes experience with the physical world, then the social world, and finally the world of ideas
5. Personality development begins with an egocentric orientation and progresses to objective assessment and finally to an internal sense of reality

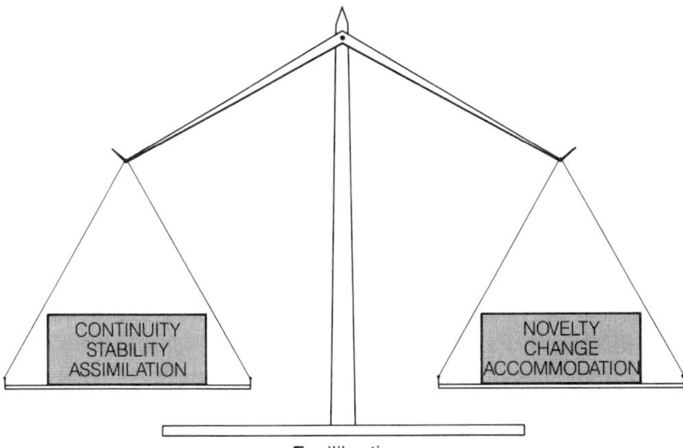

Figure 6-6 Equilibration consists of complementary processes operating simultaneously.

TABLE 6-4 Definition of Piagetian Terms

Term	Definition
Adaptation	Active process of achieving equilibrium between self and environment
Cognitive functions	Invariants that guide cognitive behavior; namely, organization and adaptation
Cognitive structures	Shape and pattern of intelligent acts that are characteristic of a given level of mental growth. They are neither innate nor static
Assimilation	Process by which the organism interprets/adjusts information to fit the present level of cognitive structure. Child subjectively interprets environmental events
Accommodation	Converse of assimilation. Process by which cognitive structures are changed to handle increasingly complex information from the environment. Incorporation of experiences as reality and change in subjective interpretation to coincide
Scheme	Cognitive structure by which child assimilates information. Active organizational principle underlying frequently repeated behavior. Sequence characterized by minimum change. Increase in number and diversity with age and integration of reality
Equilibration	Self-regulation—process by which narrow, immature definitions and ways of thinking about the world evolve into broader, more inclusive and mature thought patterns
Operations	Mental activity developed from overt behavior practiced, internalized, and carried out representationally. The process of active transformation and interpretation of reality, which is the goal of cognitive development. They are characterized by being organized, reversible, and following logical rules and regulations.
Systems	Related operations, including actual and potential ones that characterize a certain level of development

SOURCE: Adapted from Brainerd CH: *Piaget's Theory of Intelligence*. Prentice-Hall, 1978, and Labinowicz, ed: *The Piaget Primer*. Addison-Wesley, 1980.

6. Intellectual behavior begins with activity and progresses to activity and thought and then to thought with minimal activity

Four phases and related subphases mark this sequence of development and maturation of intellectual thought. Between each phase is a period of transition in which a combination of behaviors exists. At the end of each phase is a brief time of equilibrium characterized by distinct, sequential changes in the way that thinking is organized. Imbalance quickly resumes as the child finds new ways of problem solving and is dissatisfied with the old answers to questions or old methods of stucturing thought.

The four phases are (1) the *sensorimotor phase*, a time of relating and organizing sensations and motor movements; (2) the *preoperational phase*, a time of increased use of symbolism but limitation in logical thinking to the here and now; (3) the *concrete operational phase*, a time of rapid gains in logical thinking about concrete things; and (4) *the formal operational phase*, a time of unlimited thought, including abstractions, hypotheses, and propositions. As thought becomes increasingly complex, the child will try to solve new and more challenging problems (Fig. 6-7).

The phases represent the increased integration of structures from the first to the last. Prior thought patterns become increasingly organized into a comprehensive system. The phases are sequential, but each child passes through them at that child's own pace; therefore, the ages commonly associated with each phase are only approximations.

According to Piaget, the sensorimotor phase, which comprises the first 2 years of life, is the time during which the foundation for future cognitive functioning is laid down. Piaget defined this phase as a series of discrete and qualitatively different subphases in which the child responds to the environment in increasingly complex ways, leading to early problem-solving ability. Piaget's phases of sensorimotor development are as follows:

1. The reflexive stage, the first month of life, during which the infant's innate reflexive responses, such as sucking and grasping, become more efficient and more generalized
2. The primary circular reaction stage, from about 1 to 4 months of age, during which the infant performs more and more complex behaviors, which appear as repetitive (circular) responses to initial chance events; these behaviors center on the infant's own body
3. The secondary circular reaction stage, from about the fourth to the eighth month of life, during which the infant's behaviors begin to show some understanding of objects, and the infant's interactions with the environment seem almost intentional, that is, done for the results that follow such as shaking a rattle for the sound it makes
4. The coordination of secondary schemes, from about 8 to 12 months of age, during which the child learns to direct actions toward an intended goal and better understands concepts of space and object permanence
5. The tertiary circular reaction stage, from about 12 to 18 months of age, during which the infant comes to under-

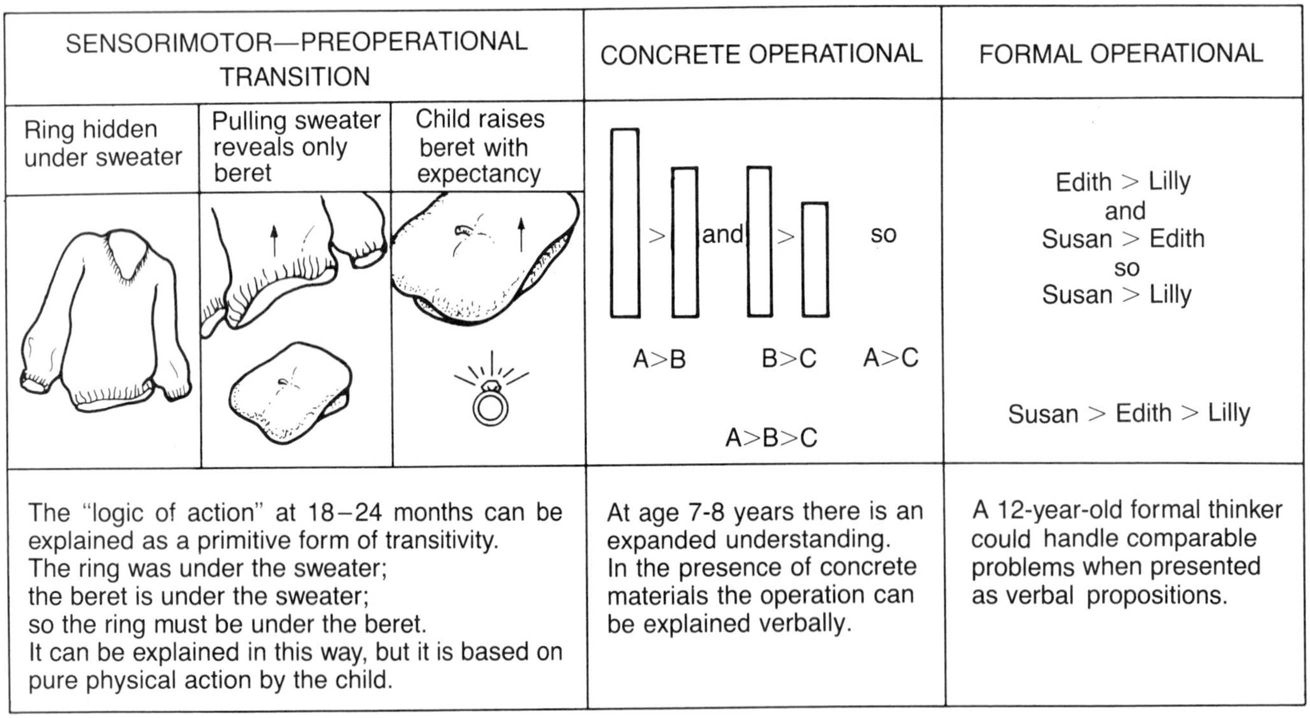

SENSORIMOTOR—PREOPERATIONAL TRANSITION			CONCRETE OPERATIONAL	FORMAL OPERATIONAL
Ring hidden under sweater	Pulling sweater reveals only beret	Child raises beret with expectancy	> and > so A>B B>C A>C A>B>C	Edith > Lilly and Susan > Edith so Susan > Lilly Susan > Edith > Lilly
The "logic of action" at 18–24 months can be explained as a primitive form of transitivity. The ring was under the sweater; the beret is under the sweater; so the ring must be under the beret. It can be explained in this way, but it is based on pure physical action by the child.			At age 7-8 years there is an expanded understanding. In the presence of concrete materials the operation can be explained verbally.	A 12-year-old formal thinker could handle comparable problems when presented as verbal propositions.

Figure 6-7 Comparative complexity of problems solved at each of Piaget's operational stages.

stand causality and object permanence, recognizing that objects placed out of sight continue to exist

6. The mental combinations stage, from about 18 to 24 months of age, in which children are able to think before they act and are able to use memory for early problem solving

Table 6-5 describes the changes that occur in several aspects of development during the sensorimotor phase. Taken together, these aspects create a multidimensional description of the infant's cognitive development.

Piaget suggested that in early childhood children learn to think and understand by characterizing new experiences according to past experiences. A child might, for example, try to bounce a new ball because an old ball bounced when it was dropped. This preoperational phase is a time of trial-and-error learning, which Piaget divided into two phases:

1. The preconceptual phase, from about 2 to 4 years of age, which is characterized by the increased use of symbols, especially language, and by representational thought, egocentrism, assimilation, and symbolic play

2. The intuitive phase, from about 4 to 7 years of age, during which the child demonstrates increased symbolic functioning, with a more sophisticated use of language, decreasing egocentrism, more exact imitation of reality through symbolic play, better balance between assimilation and accommodation, and incessant questioning. Piaget further defined and illustrated a number of characteristics that are specific to this phase of cognitive development (Table 6-6).

Children in Piaget's concrete operational phase learn by manipulating concrete objects but are still unable to perform mental operations requiring abstraction. They may, for example, understand the principles of addition but will recognize that $8 + 7 = 15$ only after previous manipulation of the numbers represented by tangible objects. Logical thinking is therefore limited to tangible, known, or directly perceived information.

Children learning at the concrete operational stage do understand the concept of relation. They are able to classify objects according to two or more characteristics (at first, color and size are used, then shape and other properties become included); they are able to comprehend hierarchic arrangements, and they come to understand the concept of seriation, or the ordering of a series of objects according to a given principle. A child at this stage may, for the first time, be able to arrange a group of pencils according to size. Children in this phase understand the principle of conservation—that is, that certain properties of objects, like volume or mass, remain constant (are conserved), even though the shape or appearance of an object may change. Examples of this developing logical thinking are shown in Figure 6-8.

The following are further characteristics of concrete operational thought:

1. Understanding the rules of reversibility

2. Understanding the concept of number through improved spatial operations and object identity

3. Ability to focus on several dimensions of a situation simultaneously, a principle that Piaget called decentration

4. Decreased egocentrism and ability to see another's perspective

5. Imitation of details, often manifested through intricate rules for collective games

6. Improved sense of equality and justice in which wrongdoing is punished and the wrongdoer must compensate for damage done

Piaget's formal operational phase, which begins at about 11 years of age, corresponds with the beginnings of adolescence. This is the phase in which children learn to evaluate the environment without relying on concrete phenomena. Adolescents develop logical thinking, the ability to work with abstract ideas, and the ability to speculate. Their mental capacities now allow them to follow a train of thought to a logical conclusion and to test hypotheses with deductive reasoning. Adolescents' reasoning abilities are increasingly multidimensional, and they are able to synthesize and integrate concepts into larger systems and can manipulate facts, ideas, and consequences.

Other characteristics of the formal operation phase are as follows:

1. Understanding of mathematics and scientific principles such as concepts of variables and proportion

2. Evidence of reflective, futuristic thinking

3. Establishing personal rules and values based on a more developed sense of equality

Theory of Information Processing

Although Piaget has contributed a wealth of ideas and insights into the process of cognitive development during childhood, contemporary theorists have, in their research and replication studies, identified inconsistencies and difficulties with Piagetian theory. Theorists such as John Flavell and Robert Siegler have built on Piaget's theory but have also extended his work, focusing more on describing the step-by-step development of specific intellectual capabilities (Yussen and Santrock, 1982).

The *information-processing theory*, as represented by Flavell (1963), Siegler and colleagues (1973), Yussen and Santrock (1982), and others, is another way of viewing mental activity. This theory concentrates on how children select stimuli and on the processes involved in interpreting and using the information for problem solving. The child first encodes the problem into key parts by identifying the

TABLE 6-5 Sensorimotor Phase: Multidimensional Development at Each of Six Stages

Stage	Object permanence	Means-ends relations	Schemes
1. Reflective, ready-made schemes Characterized by predictable, innate, survival reflexes (0–1 mo)	No expectations; out of sight, out of mind, egocentric	No intentionality; unable to distinguish between need and action; adapts to world through reflexes that change as a function of experience	Looking; hearing; sucking; rooting; grasping
2. Primary circular reactions Characterized by stereotyped repetition; own body center of interest (1–4 mo)	Visual pursuit; no motor pursuit but visual following of object to point of disappearance, expecting it to reappear	Different responses to objects; visually directed grasping; acquisition of elementary habits without distinguishing means from ends; rudimentary distinction of need and action	Mouthing; attentive; looking; grasping-letting go; hand-mouth coordination; beginning distinction of assimilation and accommodation
3. Secondary circular reactions Characterized by environment and objects as center of attention; acquired adaptations (4–8 mo)	Recognizes partially visible object and will search briefly for partly hidden ones at location of disappearance	No intentional goal-directed behavior; functional differentiation between need and act; repeats behaviors found novel or interesting	Hand-eye coordination; multiple schemes capable of producing interesting results: hitting; kicking; shaking; pulling; patting; grabbing
4. Coordination of secondary schemes Characterized by intentionality—goal in mind prior to any action; consolidation and coordination of schemes (8–12 mo)	Beginning to internalize conceptions of objects; systematic search for object hidden under single barrier in same place; unable to sustain search through multiple barriers or displacements	Differentiation of means and ends; behaviors repeated with intended goal in mind at onset; disinguishes objects from related activity; active problem solving; beginning of intelligence	Addition of breadth to previously acquired schemes to increase adaptation and intentionality: dropping; throwing; examining
5. Tertiary circular reactions Characterized by interest in novelty, creativity; discovery of new means by active experimentation (12–18 mo)	Follows series of visible displacements in search for hidden object; retains image of visible moving object	Trial-and-error learning; discovery of new means through experimentation; use of objects in systematic ways to discover new possibilities; modifies means (discovers new ways) of reaching same end (goal); accommodation	Social schemes showing systematic creation of new schemes for specific situations; coordinates schemes; generalizes existing schemes to fit variety of situations
6. Inventions of new means through mental combinations Beginning of thought; mental problem solving ends dependence on overt trial and error (18–24 mo)	Awareness of permanency of objects; follows series of invisible displacements; retains mental image of absent object	Discovery of new means by internalized combinations resulting in insight; uses objects for their innate qualities; foresight in problem solving—mentally manipulate event prior to acting	Invent new schemes through mental representations of symbols and their combinations; increased capacity for and use of mental symbols; naming

question and the information available. Next, the child devises a plan for using the information to solve the problem or answer the question. Finally, the child assesses or evaluates the results. It is the ability to understand each of these steps that determines the results of the child's attempts to solve problems. Young children often do not encode the question properly and thus give a "wrong" answer. Age and experience enable children to increase the amount of stored information that is then available for creating solutions to the problems they confront.

TABLE 6-5 continued

Causality	Objects in space	Imitation	Play
No real signs of understanding causal relationships	Alternate glancing; no appreciation of relationships; objects do not have definite boundaries	Immediate reflexive imitations; no true imitation	Practice or exercise of basic reflexes
Magical-phenomenalist, believes that self is cause of all action; exact repetition of accidental or random self-initiated event that brought pleasure—diffuse connection between action and result	Localization of sound begins; heterogeneous, unrelated centered spaces on infant's body (perceptual systems); no distinction between internal and external stimuli	Pseudoimitation; reproductive assimilation—self-imitation of behaviors already possessed (ie, sounds and gestures)	Repetitive practice of new results of behavior for pleasure; apparent voluntary repetition of actions
Observes actions and consequences and repeats those that bring pleasure; separates actions from internal feelings; formation of action patterns with external world	Increasing awareness of own behavior acting on different objects—separates objects spatially according to actions; separates self from environment; differentiates internal and external stimuli; follows trajectories of objects dropped anticipating landing spot	Imitation (true) of familiar sounds and gestures already a part of infant's repertoire	Repetition of interesting actions applied to familiar objects
Conceives of end results, then acts to achieve result; aware that objects other than self cause results; anticipates events and actions of others	Improved space concept; able to assign objects spatial locations independent of own actions; object constancy—object exists outside of perception	Use of generalized schemes to express unfamiliar sounds and gestures	Beginning of ritualization in actions; means becomes enjoyable and prolonged as end in themselves
Recognizes independent causality—outside of infant's wishes; able to view cause-and-effect relations more objectively; solicits adult help to cause desired action; other people seen as autonomous actors	Understands relationships between objects and their use; spatial relations further refined and objectified; combines and relates objects in different spatial configurations, reversals, and rotations	Quicker, more precise, true imitation based on ability to discern differences between objects; confined to action phase of model; unable to internalize familiar words, invisible gestures	Expressive function; repetition of learned behavior for self-satisfaction; repetition of action phase—activity to amuse; predominance of assimilation
Searches for independent causality; infer cause when observes effect—predict effect when observes causes	Symbolic representation of spatial features of objects; able to locate objects in familiar space—solve detour problems; relates objects to each other through internal system of representation	Capable of delaying the imitation for several days; imitation of complex, inanimate, and/or absent models, unfamiliar words, invisible gestures	Increased possibilities of play activities through mental representation; symbolically reenact event with objects at hand to represent reality; ritualized symbolic play begins

Information processing might be simplified and diagrammed as in Figure 6-9. Each major step also may be composed of several substeps. Major steps may overlap, and the flow of information does not need to follow any specific route. Problem solving might be defined as the last step, or the outcome of the process, or it might be defined as the whole process (Fig. 6-10).

Attention is, as the term suggests, the child's noticing or spending time observing an object or participating in an event. With maturation, the time spent on a single activity

Conservation Tasks	Establish Equivalence	Transform or Rearrange	Conservation Question and Justification
Conservation of number Number is not changed despite rearrangement of objects.	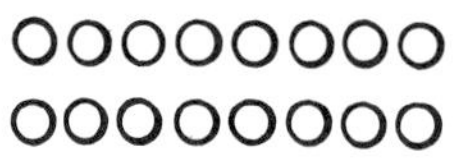 OOOOOOOO OOOOOOOO	Rearrange one set.	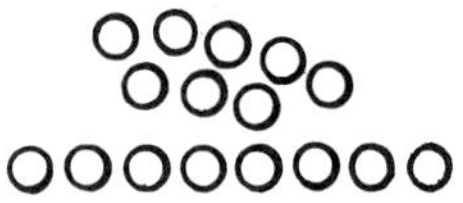 Are there the same number of red and green chips or. . . ?
Conservation of length The length of a string is unaffected by its shape or its displacement.		Change shape of one string.	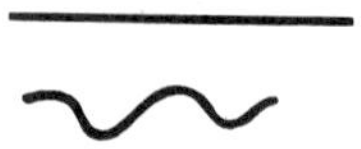 Will an ant have just as far to walk, or. . . ?
Conservation of liquid amount The amount of liquid is not changed by the shape of the container.	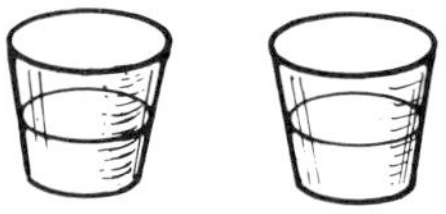	Transfer liquid.	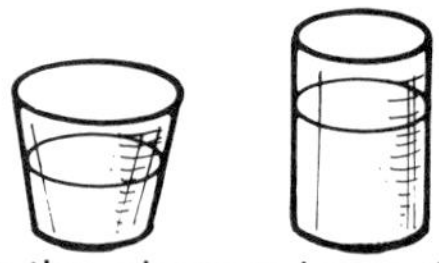 Do the glasses have the same amount of water, or. . . ?
Conservation of substance (solid amount) The amount of substance does not change by changing its shape or by subdividing it.	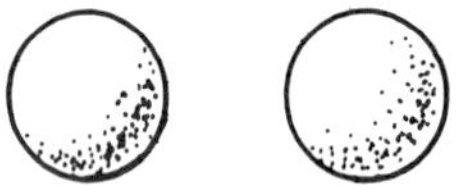	Roll out one clay ball.	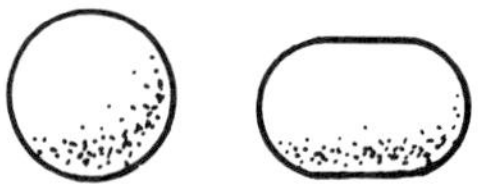 Do you still have the same amount of clay?
Conservation of area The area covered by a given number of two-dimensional objects is unaffected by their arrangement.	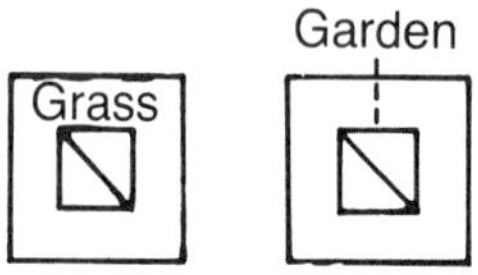 Grass Garden	Rearrange one set of triangles.	Is there still the same amount of "room" for planting, or. 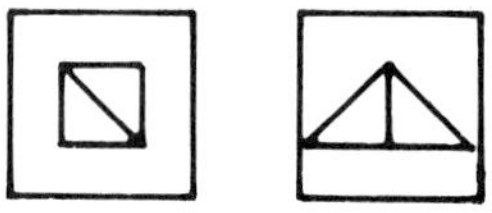 . . ? Is there still the same amount of grass to eat, or. . . ?
Conservation of weight A clay ball weighs the same even when its shape is elongated or flattened.	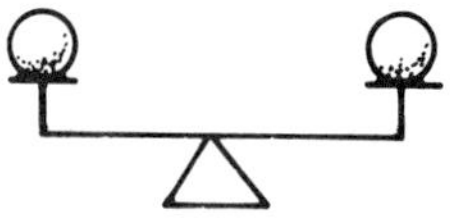	Change shape of one ball.	Do the balls of clay still weigh the same, or. . . ?
Conservation of displacement volume The volume of water that is displaced by an object is dependent on the volume of the object and independent of weight, shape, or position of the immersed object.	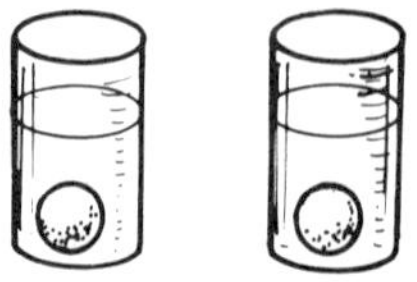	Change shape of one ball.	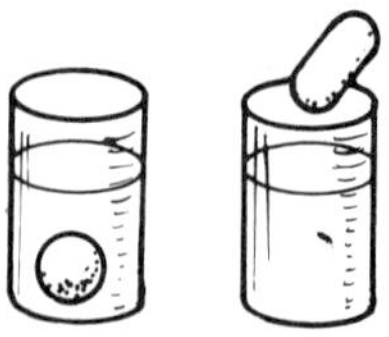 Will the water go up as high, or not?

Figure 6-8 Piaget's concrete operational phase (7–11 years), in which logical thinking is demonstrated in the ability to conserve and justify response. (From Labinowicz E: *The Piaget Primer.* Addison-Wesley, 1980, p. 94.)

TABLE 6-6 Characteristics of the Piagetian Phase of Preoperational Thought

Term	Definition
Egocentrism	Inability to take role or perspective of another; viewing the self as the center of reality
Centration	Focus on one aspect of situation; inability to manipulate two dimensions at the same time; child easily deluded by appearance
Animism	Belief that inanimate objects have human feelings and are capable of human actions
Artificialism	Belief that everything that exists in the world has been created either by human beings or by a supernatural force specifically for humans and in the same manner as humans build things
Finalism	Belief that every question has a simple and direct answer, every event a direct cause, and that nothing happens spontaneously or by chance
Imminent justice	Sense that world is equipped with built-in system of law and order so that things can punish as well as humans
Transductive thinking	Specific to specific thinking. Difficulty understanding comparisons or relational terms; the child concentrates on either the parts or the whole but is unable to relate the two
Monologue	Talking to oneself out loud for a prolonged period of time without regard for the presence of a listener
Collective monologue	Talking "at" instead of "with" another person; two or more conversations occurring simultaneously, each at an egocentric level, neither child taking account of the other's words
Irreversibility	Inability to reverse an action, situation, or physical properties of an object. Associating a change in appearance with a qualitative or quantitative change in the identity of the object or event. Focusing on the end result
Nonconservation	Inability to retain identity of two dimensions at the same time. Influenced by perceptual changes; difficulty understanding compensation (eg, when one dimension changes, a corresponding offsetting change occurs in another dimension)
Symbolic play	Pretend or imaginary play; use of one object or self to represent that of another (eg, block can be a boat, car, or building). Play-acting events experienced in everyday living; often with role change or extension. Blending of fantasy with reality

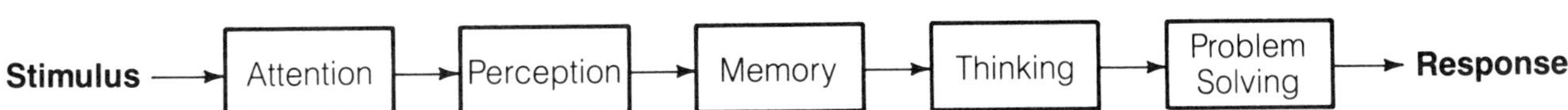

Figure 6-9 Hypothetical series of steps of information processing in which problem solving is the outcome of a linear progression. (From Yussen SR, Santrock, JW: *Child Development: An Introduction.* Wm. C. Brown, 1982.)

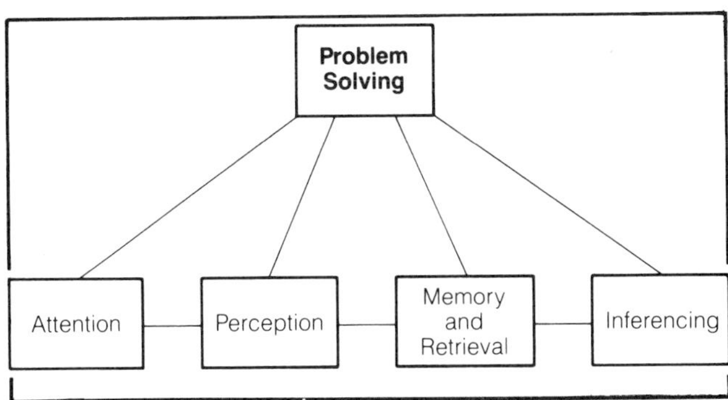

Figure 6-10 Hypothetical model of information processing in which problem solving regulates the process. (From Yussen SR, and Santrock JW: *Child Development: An Introduction.* Wm. C. Brown, 1982.)

lengthens, and the child becomes less distractable, more selective, and more organized in searching for helpful cues. Figure 6-11 exemplifies a problem that requires attention to a number of details before a child can answer the question.

Perception is the meaning attached to the information received from the senses about the environment; it is inter-

For example, an infant may be observed trying to pick up the strawberries printed on the kitchen tablecloth. Limited experience in visually judging depth and knowledge of cues

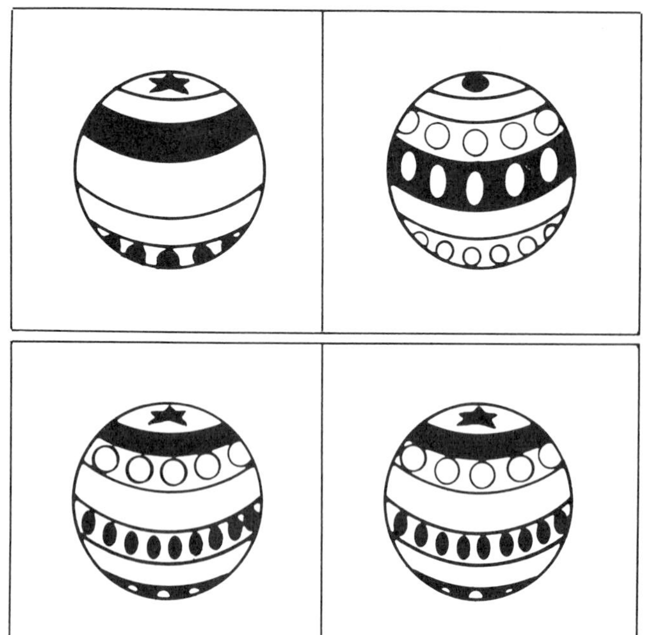

Figure 6-11 Which two are alike? Attention to detail, spacing, and design is needed to answer the question. The child needs to study the balls, not just guess, and the studying takes time.

has, for this infant, caused confusion between two-dimensional drawings and three-dimensional objects.

Memory is the means by which the child stores information for later use. Memory is a complex phenomena that has been classified according to different kinds—recognition, recall, and paired associates—or different levels—sensory register, short-term, and long-term (Table 6-7).

Inference is a relation drawn between two events that is not directly stated but can be assumed. It might have a logical basis, so that the child might reason that (1) heavy objects fall faster than light ones, (2) the blue block is heavier than the green one, (3) therefore, the blue block will be the first to land when both are dropped from an equal height. It also might have an empiric basis, so that the child will relate experience or special knowledge to specific events. An empirically related inference is either literal, which then involves closely related and easily made associations, or nonliteral, which then demands considerable prior knowledge about similar events that can be recalled and transposed to facilitate understanding the subject at hand. For example, Sam liked to swim. He followed Joe to the middle of the lake. Joe sent Sam home because he barked. Inference here is more difficult because of limited cues. Sam barks and swims and so is probably a dog. Joe went to the middle of the lake and did not want Sam there because of the noise he made. This may mean that Joe is fishing. From previous experience, the child may know that fish do not like noise or splashing and that larger fish live in deeper water, which is usually in the middle of the lake. Therefore, the child may infer that Joe wants Sam to leave so that the fish will bite.

The process of making inferences simply might be termed thinking. It is the selective use and combination of current and retained information to formulate new relations between events. *Problem solving*, a particular form of thinking, can then be defined either as the end result or the monitoring of the flow of information. Solving the problem or providing the answer is the goal toward which the flow of information is regulated. In addition to identifying the goal, problem solving also necessitates step-by-step planning and ongoing evaluation of the process. Older children are more efficient problem solvers because they have greater knowledge and insight about themselves, objects, events, and interactions.

Information processing explains learning as a continuous mental activity involving progressively more sophisticated ways of handling information. The steps involved define the specific ways information is organized for this process. In this way the theory attempts to resolve some of the inconsistencies of Piaget's theory without negating his valuable insights concerning cognitive development.

TABLE 6-7 Memory—How Information is Retained

Kinds of memory	**Method of retention**
Recognition	Identifying from another source the situations or events that previously were experienced or known
Recall	Remembering without other aids certain events, lists, dates, numbers, names from past (recent or distant) experiences
Paired associates	Remembering items in pairs and recalling the second item when the first is given
Levels of memory	**Method of retention**
Sensory register	Immediate recall only lasting seconds
Short-term	Brief retention of information—also called working memory
Long-term	Prolonged retention of information lasting from several minutes to years. Various methods of grouping, reviewing, and organizing data are employed to achieve this type of retention

Theory of Lawrence Kohlberg

Lawrence Kohlberg (1927–) studied one aspect of development, the changes that occur in the child's thinking about moral judgments or the process by which the child acquires reasoning about what is right or wrong, approved or unapproved ways of interacting with others, or behaving in social or personal situations. Unlike Piaget, who based his study of moral development on the concept of rules and respect for rules, Kohlberg identified morality with justice. He stressed that the orientation to justice is defined as "relations of liberty, equality, reciprocity, and contract between persons" (Kohlberg, in Lickona, 1976, p. 40) and that this relation distinctively defines morality.

Moral behavior is culturally related and as such reflects the extent of internalization of societal rules and expected behaviors. Although moral judgments are but one subset of values, Kohlberg felt that they differed from the others by tending "to be universal, inclusive, consistent, and based on objective, impersonal or ideal grounds" (Kohlberg, 1968, p. 490).

On the basis of responses given by research volunteers; ages 10 through 28, to a series of stories containing different moral dilemmas, Kohlberg isolated three levels of thinking according to the criteria that respondents used for making judgments. Within each level, two stages were further defined (Table 6-8). This study allowed Kohlberg to establish four characteristics of stage development that remain unchanged. These are (1) that the six stages must occur in successive sequence; (2) that individuals cannot comprehend a stage that is further than one stage beyond their own; (3) that individuals are attracted to the next higher stage; and (4) that disequilibrium and conflict result in evaluation and usually aspiration to the next stage (Duska and Whelan, 1975).

Stages 1 and 2 comprise the preconventional level of moral development and include preadolescent children and some adults. At stage 1, punishment and obedience orientation, the motivation is fear of punishment. Actions are the consequence of fear of authority's disapproval. At stage 2, instrumental relativist orientation, the motivating force changes to accommodate pleasure seeking. The hope of receiving a reward often will overcome fear. Duska and Whelan summarized the characteristics of the preconventional level as "egoism or self-interest which arises from a cognitive disposition to judge things completely according to their consequences" (1975, p. 58).

The second level of moral development is the conventional level. This level involves recognition of the values of a group and respect and allegiance to these ideals regardless of the consequences. At stage 3, interpersonal concordance of "good boy-nice girl" orientation, the child gains the ability to see another person's point of view and acts without a promise of reward. The opinions and approval of a group become very important, and the peer group often determines right from wrong.

TABLE 6-8 Stages of Moral Development According to Kohlberg

Stage	Definition
Preconventional level	Behavior abides by cultural rules because of punishment or reward consequences
Stage 1—punishment and obedience orientation	Good and bad and right and wrong are thought of in terms of consequences of an action; avoidance of punishment
Stage 2—instrumental realistic orientation	Right action is whatever satisfies one's own needs and occasionally the needs of others; exchange of favors; "do for me and I do for you"
Conventional level	Behavior is self-controlled due to expectations of others and desire to conform to and accept social expectations
Stage 3—interpersonal acceptance of "good boy," "nice girl" social concept	Good behavior is what pleases and is approved by others; response to stereotype; social units are loose and flexible
Stage 4—The "law and order" orientation	Right behavior accepts and shows respect for authority; doing one's duty for the good of the social order; laws are permanent and not likely to change
Postconventional, autonomous, or principles level	Effort to define moral values and principles that are valid beyond the authority of the group and even beyond the self
Stage 5—social contract, utilitarian orientation	Adherence to legal rights commonly agreed on by society but with laws subject to interpretation and change in terms of rational consideration for the rights of the individual while maintaining respect of self and others
Stage 6—universal ethical principle orientation	Right behavior is defined in terms of ethical principles based on logical comprehensiveness, universality, and consistency and respects the inherent dignity of human beings as individuals

SOURCE: Data from Kohlberg L: Stage and sequence: The cognitive-development approach to socialization. In: *Handbook of Socialization: Theory and Research*. Gaslin D (editor). Houghton Mifflin Company, 1969.

Stage 4, law and order orientation, involves the development of an abstract concept of a moral law that is overall and all-encompassing. This is seen as a resolution to the many conflicting rules of different groups. Kohlberg maintained that most adults are at this stage because they think abstractly and see themselves as members of society. They "can sympathize with a person who breaks a law, but their sympathy will be overridden by a concern to uphold the social order which requires a strict adherence to rules and proper authority" (Duska and Whelan, 1975, p. 65).

Kohlberg's third level of moral development is the principled thinking, or postconventional level. Kohlberg originally thought that this level was attained when one finished high school. Later, however, he realized that although adults can comprehend stage 5, most do not actually live in this autonomous fashion. He proposed three conditions that must be met for a person to achieve such autonomy: (1) skepticism, or the tendency to be intellectually disillusioned by the supposed benefits of society's laws; (2) egoism, or a sense of deciding in one's own mind what is right and wrong; and (3) relativism, or the ability to see how certain rules are relative to the beliefs and needs of a particular society (Duska and Whelan, 1975, p. 70). Stage 5, social-contract legalistic orientation, involves the ability to examine society's laws and then rationally reason whether that law is acceptable for one's standards or whether it is self-defeating by interfering with the needs of the person it is meant to aid.

In stage 6, universal ethical principle orientation, the person's concern is with the dignity and equality of all human beings. The reasoning as to why something is right or wrong is again the province of the individual thinker, and the person's standards for justice are set even higher and more equitably than those set by society. At times it may mean overriding societal views.

The consequences of an action for Kohlberg are not as important as the reasoning or motivations behind the action. Does one give to charities because it is a tax incentive or because it is not right for any human to be deprived of basic needs for food, shelter, clothes, or medical care? The results are the same, but Kohlberg's scheme indicates that the moral reasoning providing the rationale for the action is really very different.

Lewis (1982) identified factors involved in making moral decisions as intelligence, ability to anticipate the future, empathy, controlled attention, containment of fantasies, self-esteem, and self- confidence. The child's capacity to make moral decisions is related to the whole complex process of socialization. This includes learning rules, observing models, and taking different roles, first vicariously in play and later during life events. Although environment and interaction are important, Kohlberg viewed the maturation process of cognition as the primary determiner of moral development.

Within Kohlberg's sequential stages, each successive stage builds on the previous stage and adds one or two new dimensions. The stages do not correspond to any chronologic age. Rather, they describe an orientation to morality that is based on "normative order, utility consequences, justice or fairness and ideal-self" (Kohlberg, in Lickona, 1976, p. 40). These terms are defined as follows:

1. *Normative order*—orientation to prescribed rules and roles of the social or moral order. The basic considerations in decision making center on the element of rules
2. *Utility consequences*—orientation to the good or bad welfare consequences of action in the situation for others and/or the self
3. *Justice or fairness*—orientation to relations of liberty, equality, reciprocity, and contract between persons
4. *Ideal-self*—orientation to an image of the actor as a good self, or as someone with a conscience, and to his or her motives or virtue (relatively independent of approval consequences from others) (Lickona, 1976, p. 40)

As cognitive development advances, so does the individual's ability to make moral judgments. In a study of children Kohlberg (1969) found that industrial societies demonstrated a positive correlation among age, social participation, intelligence, and responses to moral judgment questions, correlations that did not appear in nonindustrial societies. Perhaps, therefore, the stages of moral thinking he described have a more integral relation to culture than was previously assumed.

Kohlberg's theory is interesting but not problem-free. Because it is difficult to assess and/or eliminate the role of culture, his analysis of moral development seems to be more characteristic of western civilizations than of other civilizations, which presents problems for the claim of universality in moral behaviors. Furthermore, the theoretic emphasis on reasoning as the sole determiner for developmental stage excludes the importance of human behavior and feelings. Other theorists have noted a considerable variance between what one thinks is the right decision and what one actually does.

The dilemmas Kohlberg suggested also are not relevant for children, who are concerned with friendships, peer relations, or parent and family relations that involve them. Posing more realistic dilemmas could help in assessing the decision-making processes in children's moral judgments. Finally, Kohlberg's theory was formulated according to the responses of a group of 50 males aged 10–28 years. Carol Gilligan (1982) has noted that females' thoughts and actions involve significantly different dimensions with different objectives and goals. For example, relationships may be more highly valued by women, which may be reflected in the rationales they use in confronting moral dilemmas.

Theory of James Fowler

One of the many dimensions that contribute to the whole person is that of faith. James Fowler has developed a theory that describes the development of faith, or the spiritual dimension of human life irrespective of religious affiliation. "The word faith points to a reality, however vague or ambivalent in conception it might be" (Fowler and Keen, 1980). Fowler uses faith as a verb, thus making it an active force that gives meaning to the individual's life. He also describes faith as a relational phenomenon. "Faith is an active 'made-of-being-in-relation' to another or others in which we invest commitment, belief, love, risk and hope" (Fowler and Keen, 1980).

Fowler posits not only a commitment (allegiance) to persons but also to their values, ideals, or causes, thus creating a triadic relationship (Fig. 6-12). This relationship provides a sense of order and direction to life, which is lived in response to one's constructed "ultimate environment," (Fowler's metaphor for the Judeo-Christian "Kingdom of God" or Teilhard's "The Divine Milieu") (Fowler and Keen, 1980, p. 24). Faith is seen as a key element in the individual's self-system and identity; as such, it plays a significant role in personality development.

In many ways Fowler was influenced by the work of Piaget and Kohlberg. He assumed that development is an interactional process, that the child actively constructs knowledge through interchanges with a dynamic environment. His is a structural-developmental theory. In each stage new patterns of thought and value formation are added to those previously held; hence, the stages must come in a definitive sequence without any skips. Faith stages, however, are distinct from cognitive stages in that they develop from an integration of knowledge and values, an integration that demonstrates the additional influence of Erik Erikson.

The influence of Piaget and Kohlberg is further demonstrated by Fowler's assertion that the individual constructs new ways of knowing and behaving to meet new environmental challenges. Faith development is a process of relinquishing and rebuilding, which is in many ways aided by life crises, challenges, and the kinds of disruptions that theologians call revelations. These challenges, or crises, make

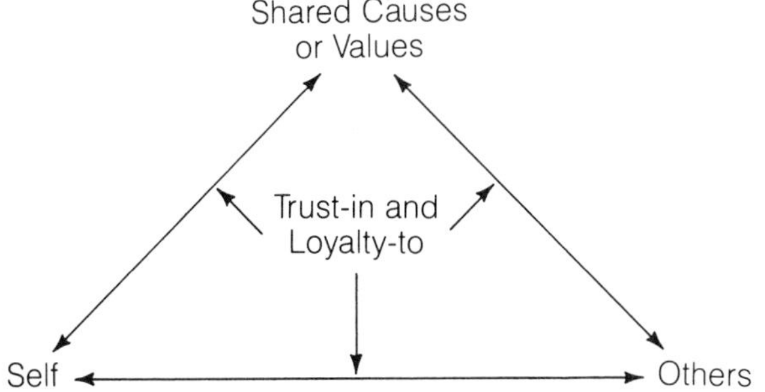

Figure 6-12 Triadic relation of faith-in-being as described by James Fowler. (From Fowler J, Keen S: *Life Maps: Conversations on the Journey of Faith.* Edited by Jerome Berryman, copyright © 1978. Reprinted with permission of Word Books Publishers, Waco, Texas 76796. Word Book, 1978, p. 20.)

the old methods inadequate for coping with the current reality; thus, the progression to new methods begins.

Through the process of conducting semiclinical interviews with a representative cross section of Americans from ages 4 through 84 years of age, Fowler proposed a theory of six separate stages (and a prestage) in the process of faith development (Table 6-9). These stages explain the patterns of value formation and interpretation that underlie faith development. Fowler theorized that the age at which a stage occurs varies considerably among individuals but that the sequence does not. He also noted that a lifetime equilibrium may occur at any point, beginning with stage 2.

According to Fowler, these stages are a way of interpreting this dynamic and complex process. He suggested that the individual passes from stages of simple and undifferentiated structures to stages characterized by complex and differentiated structures. Each stage is a structural whole containing identifiable variables about the way in which a world view is constructed. Stages are not marks of intelligence or achievement but rather references to which certain aspects of valuing, thinking, relating to events, and interacting with others can be better understood. Table 6-9 presents the structural characteristics of each stage as both a synthesis and elaboration of contributing theories and patterns of faith development.

Fowler's theory has directed the attention of health professionals to an often overlooked area of development, one that is essential for holistic health care. Faith development encompasses both cognitive and affective dimensions of shaping responses; it responds to life events and orients goals and motives with respect to a transcendent force or ultimate environment, the self and others.

Psychodynamic Theories

Psychodynamic theorists are interested in the emotional forces reflected in the individual's personality. Early psychodynamic theorists sought to define and describe the motivations and inner workings of the mind as they were manifested and developed during the individual's lifetime. The question they sought to answer was related to the origins and development of the personality.

Personality is an extremely complex term to define, and there are probably as many definitions as persons attempting to formulate the same. A very basic and admittedly too simple definition is that personality is the outward expression of the inner self. "Personality encompasses temperament, mood, character traits (like honesty, dependability, independence, and physical appearance and behavior) . . . Personality also involves the ability to interact with others as well as modes of adjustment to life changes" (Fong and Resnick, 1980, p. 351). Personality development as

TABLE 6-9 Faith: The Structural-Developmental Approach

Stages	Form of logic*	Form of world coherence	Role-taking†
Undifferentiated			
Intuitive-projective	Preoperational	Episodic	Rudimentary, empathy
Mythic-literal	Concrete; operational	Narrative-dramatic	Simple perspective-taking
Synthetic-conventional	Early formal operations	Tacit system; symbolic mediation	Mutual role-taking (interpersonal), "third person" perspective
Individuative-reflective	Formal operations (dichotomizing)	Explicit system; conceptual mediation	Mutual role with self-selected group or class
Paradoxic-consolidative	Formal operations (dialectic)	Multisystemic; symbolic and conceptual mediation	Mutual, with groups, classes and traditions other than one's own
Universalizing	Formal operations (synthetic)	Unitive actuality, "one beyond the many"	Mutual, with the commonwealth of being

described by psychodynamic theories also includes self-esteem and self-concept. As explained in Chapter 2, the way in which a person feels, personally looks, and acts is *self-esteem*. The way a person thinks others perceive his or her looks and actions is *self-concept*.

Psychoanalytic theorists argue that personality development begins during infancy and that during this formative time adults, especially the caregivers, are instrumental in shaping the future adult personality. Personality development then seems to be related to the degree of need fulfillment, satisfaction, and pleasure that the infant and young child are able to obtain.

Theory of Sigmund Freud

One of the earliest developmental theories and the one that has influenced thinking and theory formation since its inception is that of the Viennese neurologist-psychoanalyst Sigmund Freud (1856–1939). In an effort to identify the etiology of the puzzling physical symptoms that were without known medical cause in some of his patients, Freud became interested in the seemingly powerful but consciously unknown influences that early experiences had on a person's behavior or physical complaints. His study and research focused on describing and verifying the existence

TABLE 6-9 continued

Locus of authority	Bounds of social awareness	Form of moral judgment‡	Role of symbols
Located in and derivative of child's attachment/dependent relationships to parents or parent-like adults. Criteria of size, power, and visible signs of authority	Family, primal others	Punishment-reward	Magical-numinous
Located in incumbents of authority roles and made (more or less) salient by personal proximity and trust-inspiring qualities	"Those like us" (in familial, ethnic, racial, class, and religious terms)	Instrumental; hedonism	One-dimensional, literal
Located in tradition or consensual perspective of valued group and in persons authorized or recognized as personally worthy representatives	Conformity to class norms and interests	Interpersonal concord (law and order)	Multidimensional, conventional
Located in personally appropriated pragmatic or ideologically established perspectives and in spokespersons or group procedures or outlooks consistent with such perspectives	Self-aware adherence to chosen class norms and interests	Reflective relativism or class-biased universalism	Critical translation into ideas
Located in the dialectic between critically self-chosen beliefs, norms, and values and those maintained in the reflective claims of other persons and groups and in various expressions of cumulative human wisdom	Critical awareness of and transcendence of class norms and interests	Principled higher law (universal-critical)	Postcritical rejoining of symbolic nuance and ideational content
Building on all that went before, authority now located in the judgment purifed of egoic striving and attentive to the requirements of being	Transclass awareness and identification	Loyalty to being	Transparency of symbols

*Modified from Piaget.

†Modified from Solmon.

‡Modified from Kohlberg.

SOURCE: Fowler J, Keen S. *Life Maps: Conversations on the Journey of Faith* (Berryman J, editor). Word Books, 1978, pp 96–99. Copyright © 1978; used by permission of Word Books, Publishers, Waco, Texas 76796.

of a connection between the mind and the body. Freud hypothesized that this connection was related to the idea of the unconscious, which he defined as a deep depository for ideas, emotions, problems, fears, and pains within the mind. According to Freud, the individual was not cognizant of these feelings, yet they influenced and often determined behavior and personality characteristics (Freud, 1923).

The *unconscious*, which is present at birth, was to Freud the source of instinctual drives. The two dominating drives motivating behavior and competing for supremacy are the life and death instincts (Freud, 1923). The life instinct, with its psychic energy, libido, is responsible for behavior that expresses love, self-presentation, and constructive conduct. On the other hand, the death instinct is manifested in self-centered, cruel behavior, aggression, hate, and destructive conduct. Freud referred to this basic self-serv-

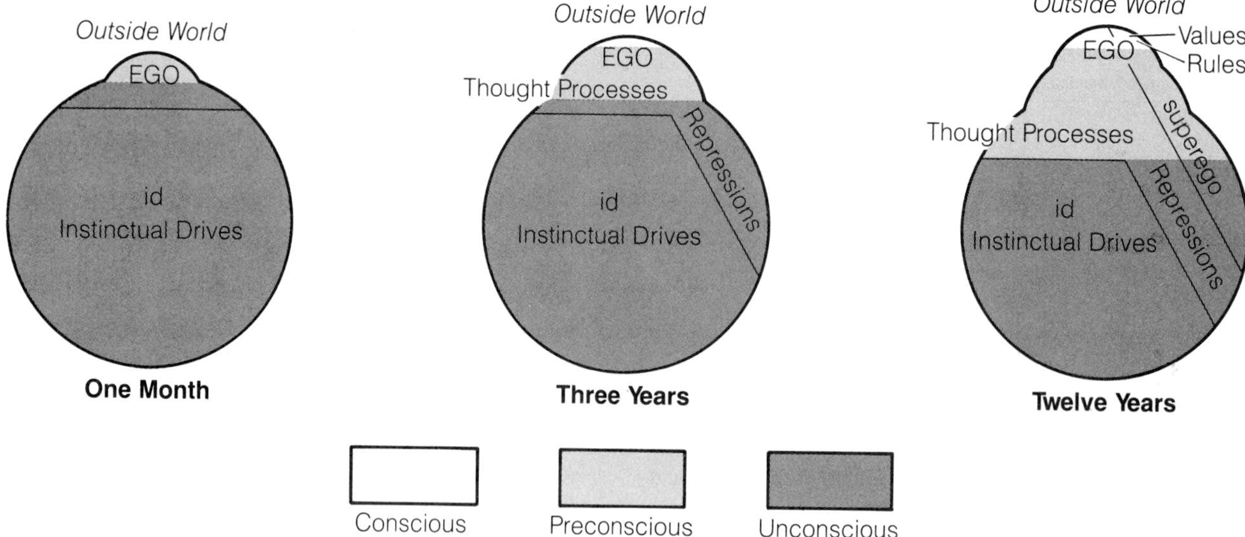

Figure 6-13 Developmental forces in the structure of the mind. (From Murray TR: *Comparing Theories of Child Development.* © 1979 by Wadsworth Publishing Company, Inc. Reprinted by permission of Wadsworth Publishing Company, Belmont, California 94002.)

ing level of mental functioning as the *id* and postulated that the id drives the individual to seek self-pleasure as quickly as possible and at any expense. Pain and discomfort result when an instinctual need is unfulfilled.

The newborn's behavior is one example of the response to instinctual needs. Whenever hungry, wet, or uncomfortable, the newborn cries until the need is met. Freud noted, however, that with time, repetition of familiar patterns, and interaction, the demand for immediate gratification is modified. This is related to the development of the ego and to reasonable ways to achieve need fulfillment.

Freud described the *ego* as a mediator, or reality principle. The ego takes the demands of the id, rechannels them, and makes them compatible with other people and events. Functioning on the conscious level, the "ego consists of rational thoughts, perceptions, and plans to help the child cope with reality" (Yussen and Santrock, 1982, p. 20). In Freudian terms then the development of problem-solving skills is the result of continual negotiation between the id's internal needs and the ego's growing awareness of the necessity for practical solutions within a complex external world, together with the physical maturation of organs and body systems.

The ego exists on the conscious level; it is the force aware of the here and now, or the mainstream of thought and action. Because this level is limited in the amount of information it can contain, Freud added a third level, the *preconscious*, which exists between the conscious and unconscious. Information and images stored at the preconscious level are easily recalled and are controlled by the ego. The preconscious also might be thought of as the processing center, where the mind mentally manipulates vague id requests and translates them into meaningful messages for the conscious ego, so that it can search its memory bank for the most suitable match before allowing its overt expression.

The *superego* develops from the ego and is related to the child's experiences of praise for obeying and punishment for disobeying. Freud conceived of the superego as those rules and values that become internalized and function as the conscience (what not to do) and ego ideal (what to do). Once the superego is functional, it serves as disciplinarian by creating feelings of guilt and remorse for transgressing rules and pride and self-praise for adhering to rules. Freud did not cast these developmental forces as a sequence of stages, although he did occasionally diagram his conception of their development within the mind (Fig. 6-13).

Freud described the process of socialization and personality development as a lifelong struggle among the instinctual pleasure drives of the id, the reality of environmental expectations and demands for acceptable behavior as sensed by the ego, and the moral standards, beliefs, values, and rules incorporated from significant people by the superego. In the event that the id's impulses could not be satisfied, Freud created escape valves in the form of defense mechanisms. Some of these defense mechanisms are compensation, regression, projection, sublimation, and displacement. Their purpose, according to Freud, is to repress threatening thoughts or painful experiences from these unmet needs.

Freud elaborated on the steps of personality development by identifying five stages of pleasure seeking or psychosexual growth. Each stage related to the body part, called an erogenous zone, which brought primary pleasure

TABLE 6-10 Freud's Stages of Psychosexual Development

Stage	Age range	Erogenous zone	Sexual activity
Oral	0–18 months	Mouth, lips, tongue, teeth	Sucking, swallowing, chewing, biting
Anal	8 months–4 years	Anus, buttocks	Expulsion and retention of waste products
Phallic (Oedipus complex)	3–7 years	Genitals	Masturbation
Latent	5–12 years	—	—
Genital (Oedipus complex)	12–20 years	Genitals	Masturbation, sexual intercourse, feelings for others

SOURCE: Fong C, Resnick R: *The Child*. Benjamin/Cummings, 1980, p. 352.

during that phase of growth and development. Table 6-10 summarizes these five stages.

Freud viewed the reduction of tension during the *oral stage* as both pleasurable and critical for infant survival. Sucking and mouthing of objects was also important for early learning about the environment. The *anal stage* was seen as a major hurdle in the child's life because this was the first time that delay of gratification became required and expected through toilet training. Knowledge of gender differences, identification with one's own gender, and conflict and then identification with the parent of the same sex constituted the *phallic stage*. During this stage, Freud posited the famous *Oedipus complex* (derived from the Greek tragedy, *Oedipus Rex*), which appears when sons have an incestuous desire to have intercourse with their mothers. The *Electra complex* is the corresponding phenomenon in girls, in which they have incestuous feelings toward their fathers (Fong and Resnick, 1980). A period of transition, the resolution of sexual conflict and investment in other interests and peers, occurred during *latency*, and a rekindling of earlier sexual (Oedipal) conflicts marked the *genital stage*. During this time, Freud theorized that the individual vacillated between dependence and independence, eventually establishing personal autonomy and adult relationships.

Freud built this theory on the retrospective memories of his maladjusted patients, and this has created difficulties for others trying to reproduce his results. Many other theories have therefore been based on psychoanalytic assumptions (Thomas, 1979), but because so much of Freud's theory depends on the unconscious, instincts, and defense mechanisms, it fails to meet scientific criteria for validity. It did and still does, however, remind nurses and others of the importance of childhood and its role in developing adult personality characteristics.

Theory of Erik Erikson

The developmental theory of Erik Erikson was based on and expanded from Freudian analysis. Erikson acknowledged the contribution of biologic factors to the developmental process, but he emphasized the equally significant role of the cultural and social aspects of environment. He proposed a theory of psychosocial development of the healthy individual from birth to death that stressed the complex interrelationships between physical and emotional variables throughout the individual's lifetime.

Erikson maintained that each individual has the unique capacity to create a personal life-style beginning in childhood. He saw the individual as active and having the potential to be either good or bad. For him, development was a lifelong process or a series of beginnings. "An individual has neither a personality nor a character structure; a person is always a personality in the making, developing and redeveloping" (Maier, 1978).

The psychosocial development of the ego was for Erikson an interactive process whereby the individual reconciles current internal polar struggles and establishes a new orientation to self and society. This process is continuous, for each mastery of opposing "pulls" provides only temporary relief from tension as new incentives for development and a different set of polarities soon become evident, signifying the equation between development and dynamic continuous change. Erikson suggested that all new development is rooted in prior accomplishments, experiences, and behaviors while also providing the impetus for the additional acquisition of skills and the opportunity to correct or improve earlier skills.

Erikson believed that although development is a continuous process, it also has distinct phases characterized by the achievement of developmental goals. Each phase or

Stage	1	2	3	4	5	6	7	8
Maturity								Ego Integrity vs. despair
Adulthood							Generativity vs. stagnation	
Young adulthood						Intimacy vs. isolation		
Puberty and adolescence					Identity vs. diffusion			
Latency				Industry vs. inferiority				
Locomotor Genital			Initiative vs. guilt					
Muscular Anal		Autonomy vs. shame						
Oral Sensory	Trust vs. mistrust							

Figure 6-14 Erikson's phases of psychosocial crisis in ego development.

stage presents a developmental crisis to be mastered. These crises are represented in the eight stages of life that describe the development of the self in relation to the demands and expectations of society. The stages form the life span, beginning with birth and concluding with old age and death. Erikson was one of the first theorists to acknowledge that development continues during adulthood and is not completed with adolescence.

Childhood for Erikson was the beginning of a growing process that culminated in the achievement of ego identity. He saw the process as a series of steps with gradually increased differentiation. Ego identity consists of two aspects, an inner-focused aspect that involves personal knowledge and acceptance of oneself and an outer-focused aspect that includes the sharing of group values and ideals or "some kind of essential character with others" (Erikson, 1968).

Erickson's theory was based on Freud's psychosexual concepts but expanded to include adult development and the role of the environment, especially the interplay between the self and significant others. Erikson created a grid to illustrate the process of ego development. Each step represented the psychosocial crisis or conflicting personality traits that characterized that stage (Fig. 6-14).

Erikson also extended to psychosocial development the epigenetic principle accepted for physical development. This principle simply states that the child is preprogrammed to accomplish certain skills and tasks in a definite order and within a certain time period. "In short, Erikson proposed that it is the nature of the human species to pass through an identifiable series of psychosocial stages as the individual grows up, stages determined genetically, regardless of the culture in which the growth occurs. The social environment, however, does have a significant effect on the nature of the crises arising at each stage and on the success with which the child and adolescent will master the stage" (Thomas, 1979).

The resolution of each crisis could result in either positive growth and preparation for future crises or frustration and difficulty in coping with the crisis in subsequent stages. Failure to succeed at any one of the developmental tasks does not doom the child to failure for life. There is always the hope that mastery will be attained, even though at a delayed rate. Difficulty at any one stage may slow progress through the other stages, but Erikson's theory is essentially optimistic, and he believed that the child eventually would develop the necessary competencies for healthy functioning in society.

The approximate ages of the first five stages of Erikson's theory correspond to those of Freud's. They integrate the psychosexual focus of the developing child with biologic instincts, and this concept then is expanded to emphasize

TABLE 6-11 Erikson's Timetable of Developmental Stages

Stage	Psychosocial crisis	Radius of significant others	Theme
I.	Trust vs. mistrust	"Maternal" person	To get; to give in return
II.	Autonomy vs. shame/doubt	"Paternal" person	To hold on; to let go
III.	Initiative vs. guilt	Family	To make; to make like—play
IV.	Industry vs. inferiority	"Neighborhood," school, instructive adult	To make things; to make together—complete
V.	Identity vs. role confusion	Peer groups (In and out groups)	To be oneself; to share being oneself or not being oneself
VI.	Intimacy vs. isolation	Partners in friendship, sex, competition	To lose and find oneself in another
VII.	Generativity vs. self-absorption	Partner	To make be; to take care of
VIII.	Integrity vs. despair	Humanity	To be, through having been; to face not being

SOURCE: Adapted from Erikson, EH: Identity and the life cycle: A Review. By permission of W.W. Norton & Company, Inc. Copyright © 1980 by W.W. Norton & Company, Inc. Copyright © 1959 by International Universities Press, Inc.

the process of self-development in relation to others and to general societal expectations. Erickson's last three stages deal with adult development and are therefore not applicable to child health nursing, although an important aspect of Erikson's theory is not concluded with adolescence (Table 6-11).

Trust Versus Mistrust This first stage involves the period of infancy. During this time, the infant's important task is to establish mutual giving and getting between the self and the caregivers. The infant learns to trust both self and environment because of the consistency with which the basic needs of food, comfort, and warmth are met. "The general state of trust, furthermore, implies not only that one has learned to rely on the sameness and continuity of the outer providers, but also that one may trust oneself and the capacity of one's own organs to cope with urges . . ." (Erikson, 1963).

Mistrust may result if needs are met unpredictably or inadequately. When caregivers are inconsistent or convey a sense of confusion and chaos, the infant is unable to feel that the world is a safe and reliable place but rather feels that the environment must be regarded with wariness and mistrust.

Autonomy Versus Shame and Doubt This stage spans the initial years of early childhood and involves the child's newly developing physical and mental skills. The child begins to discover the many things that can be accomplished with motor skills and language. Self-assertiveness and an intense desire to practice and perfect these new skills characterize this stage. As parents support the child and allow for gradually increasing independence in such tasks as eating, dressing, toileting, and bathing, they enhance the child's sense that muscles, impulses, self, and the environment can be controlled for mutual cooperation and benefit.

Shame and doubt are the result of the parent's always doing for the child the things that are being learned. The child treated in this way is thus made to feel inadequate or incapable. A parent who overly criticizes a child and expects perfection rather than making allowance for learning and mistakes also conveys a sense of shame and doubt about the child's ability to control self and the world.

Initiative Versus Guilt The later years of early childhood involve the crisis of initiative, the instigating of activity rather than imitating or responding to the actions of others. The skills perfected previously and the sense of self-confidence gained now motivate the child to initiate activities and ask questions. The child spends time inventing new ways to use known skills, trying out new combinations, and imagining how it would feel to be someone or something else. This is also a time of learning to take responsibility for one's behavior.

Guilt is the negative side of this stage and is the result of frequent reprimands for using initiative. Children who are severely restricted in their activities and whose questions are belittled and unanswered will develop a sense of guilt about their thoughts and actions. Guilt developed during this stage may be manifested as passivity and reluctance or even a refusal to initiate any action requiring motor or language skills.

Industry Versus Inferiority During the middle and later childhood years, the challenge is sufficient mastery of skills to create and complete projects. Whereas the doing was of utmost importance in the previous stage, the satisfactory completion of the project is now all important. The social world of the child involves peers, which is often the group that plans and produces the result. Children become increasingly competitive both in school and play because the sense of industry is benefited by being first, best, smartest, or fastest.

Children who can never measure up to adult expectations or are ridiculed by their peers are likely to develop a sense of inferiority. Their status within their group and their self-evaluation becomes endangered once they believe that whatever they do or however much they try is not good enough.

Erikson noted that at this time the child spends as much time outside the home as in it. This allows for negative feedback given by those at one place to be countered with support and sensitivity at the other place. By this time, parents, teachers, and peers all contribute to the development of industry or inferiority.

Identity Versus Identity Diffusion The task of the adolescent is to achieve a stable sense of who the self really is. This is accomplished by integrating the past knowledge of using tools and social interaction with the present development of physical and sexual maturity. "The growing and developing youths, faced with this physiological revolution within them, are now primarily concerned with what they appear to be in the eyes of others as compared with what they feel they are, and with the question of how to connect the roles and skills cultivated earlier with the occupational prototypes of the day" (Erikson, 1963).

Adolescence is a time of trying on different roles to evaluate how they "fit"—how one feels playing the role and how others, especially peers, respond to the role. Identity formation is a crucial point in an adolescent's life because it affects the quality of decisions and commitments that one will make as an adult.

Although identity occurs eventually in most cases, identity diffusion may be the result if the adolescent is unable to acquire a sense of self, direction, or place in the world. Erikson stated that in the contemporary world, "We are witnessing a situation where youths sport identity confusion very openly and almost mockingly, for they prefer to find their own way to new ethical commitments" (Maier, 1978, p. 86). This attitude is related to the rapid social and technologic changes that make it more difficult for one to find continuity from the past to the present to the future. Such times involve a longer adolescence because of the increased difficulty experienced in integrating ideals and reality, past events, and future possibilities.

Although Erikson's stages are distinct, he made allowances for development to move in either direction at any time during the individual's lifetime. His theory is a tribute to his perceptive observations and descriptions of human development. It lacks scientific measures and statistics; however, the sensitivity with which he conveys the individual's relation to self, others, and society as a whole and his commonsense approach are to be applauded. Recognition of the complexity and diversity of the human personality is the reason why he emphasized that life is constant change. That is why crises confronted at one stage of life may reappear at another, why crises not completely resolved may return for new and better resolutions, and why failure to achieve a positive balance between the two traits the first time does not mean that the individual will not have a second chance to do so.

Theory of Margaret S. Mahler

Margaret Mahler studied the maternal–infant dyad and the development of independence. Her clinical studies included infants from birth through 36 months of age, and her assumptions reflected those of the psychoanalytic tradition, which views the infant as narcissistic and driven by instincts that demand satisfaction. The mother is viewed as the primary source of satisfying these instincts and so becomes the love object.

To gain independence, the infant progresses through a series of steps in a process Mahler termed *separation-individuation*. The infant first separates from the symbiotic relation experienced with the mother when physical maturation enables independent movement. The attainment of individual characteristics or individuation is a gradual process that involves practice together with maternal support and encouragement. As a result, the child becomes an autonomous, independent self, which is then consolidated as personal identity (Table 6-12).

The first 4 months of life are the precursors of the process. During this time, the infant is totally self-centered and convinced that the world revolves around the search for this "niche" in the environment, which takes place as the result of instinct gratification. After this "niche" is secured, the infant becomes aware of the person providing this gratification and vaguely senses a difference between stimuli arising from internal and external sources. This is the optimal time for the infant to become more responsive to the caregiver (the mother according to Mahler), who provides a large percentage of these external stimuli in the form of caressing and en face activities.

The process of separation follows. It begins with differentiation, during which the infant explores, through all the senses, the physical features of the parent. The infant thus becomes aware of the difference and separateness between self and parent. Differentiation, or "hatching," which appears with the infant's ability to sit and turn away at will, infers that a degree of self-entity is present.

The second phase is practicing, which corresponds to the infant's increased mobility and interest in learning about the world and its objects. Movement in and out of the care-

TABLE 6-12 Mahler's Intrapsychic Separation-Individuation Process

Phase	Age	Characteristics of child
Precursors of process		
Normal autism	Birth–1 month	"Absolute primary narcissism." Lack of awareness of mothering agent. Unaware of self-other differentiation. "Primitive hallucinatory disorienation." Physiological rather than psychological processes dominate behaviors. Energies focused toward physiological need satisfaction and maintenance of homeostasis. Minimal response to external events.
Normal symbiosis	1–5 months	"Sociobiological interdependence." Primary narcissism now includes mothering agent. Sees mother as a part of self—a dual unity with a common boundary. Dimly aware that he cannot meet his own needs. Beginning to be aware of and attend to external events, but unable to distinguish between internal and external experiences.
Subphases of process		
Differentiation ("hatching")	5–9 months	"Lap baby." Specific bond between the infant and his primary caretaker emerges. Explores her face and body. Begins to distinguish and differentiate between own and mother's body, self-nonself, and mother–not mother. Molds to body of caretaker. Begins to alter behavior in response to mother's cues. Curiosity and wonderment with novel experiences. Much visual inspection of both people and the environment.
Practicing Early (Crawling) Late (walking)	9–14 months	Elated investment in his own burgeoning physical autonomy. Begins to move away from mother physically. Becomes absorbed in own activities, but mother needs to be present as an anchor for safe exploration of the environment. Many "emotional refueling" behaviors. May have a transitional toy or object.
Rapprochment	14–24 months	Uses mother as an extension of self. Recognizes own physiological separateness from mother. Wants to share each new accomplishment with her. Shadowing and darting away behaviors. Stranger shyness and adverse reactions to separations may be due to a growing sense of vulnerabilty. Increased "emotional refueling" behaviors.
Consolidation	24–36 months	Establishment of affective object constancy—ability to separate from mother without extreme anxiety. Emergence of core gender-identity. Play becomes more purposeful and constructive. Symbolic play emerges. Able to wait for need gratification.

SOURCE: Schuster CS, Ashburn SS: *The Process of Human Development: A Holistic Approach.* Little, Brown, 1980, p. 188. Adapted from Mahler MS, Pine F, Bergman A: *The Psychological Birth of the Human Infant.* © 1975 Mahler MS. Basic Books, Inc., Publishers.

giver's presence is possible now, but the infant tends to keep checking, thereby maintaining at least visual contact. With continued development and secure relations, the tolerance for separation increases and the need for rechecking, or "refueling," is less intense.

Rapprochement is a time in which the young child's need for the parent and the parent's love is heightened because the increased physical and cognitive abilities of the child are a source of both pleasure and anxiety. Thus, the child needs to share and show all these new discoveries and obtain the necessary emotional "refueling" before returning to the world of play and discovery.

The final phase is the consolidation of individuality. During this phase, the young child gains the cognitive ability to retain a mental image, which facilitates "refueling" without the actual presence of the parent. The child attains emotional constancy, which enables the child to experience a new sense of self-awareness. Adaptation and conflict are dealt with in an individual manner, which in turn becomes characteristic of the child (Mahler, Pine, and Bergman, 1975). The child gains self-assurance and confidence in the ability to act and relate with others.

Theory of Harry Stack Sullivan

As a neo-Freudian, Harry Stack Sullivan (1892–1949) emphasized the reduction of tension, both biologic and social, as a pivotal aspect of personality development. His focus was on interpersonal relations, and he identified these as the motivator for behavior and the source of psychosocial health. His theory is an outgrowth of Freud's, but rather than further developing concepts of the id, ego, and superego, Sullivan postulated that self-concept was the key to personality development. His theory not only acknowledged the presence of environment but actually emphasized the role of social approval and disapproval in the child's formation of a self-concept. He concluded that obtaining a positive self-concept is as important as fulfilling physical needs.

He used an analytic method in studying the basis for human personality. He reasoned that "bad" interactions with the environment can cause tension and anxiety, of which individuals are constantly trying to rid themselves, and that a good social relationship can give rise to security, which is a major goal in life. Accordingly, Sullivan suggested

TABLE 6-13 Sullivan's Stages of Healthy Interpersonal Development From Birth to Maturity

Phase	Level of interacting, communicating, and comprehending
Infancy	Experiences maternal tenderness and intuits maternal anxieties. Struggles to achieve feelings of security and to avoid anxiety
Childhood	Modifies actions to suit social demands in sex-role training, peer play, family events. Uses movement and language to avoid anxiety
Juvenile	Learns to accept subordination to authority figures outside the family. More concept of self-status, and role
Preadolescence	Capable of participating in genuine love relationships with others. Develops consideration and concerns outside the self
Early adolescence	Heterosexual contacts enter into personal relationships. Attempts to integrate sex with other personal relationships
Late adolescence	Masters expression of sexual impulses. Forms satisfying and responsible associations. Uses communication skills to protect self from conflicts with others

SOURCE: Freiberg K L: *Human Development: A Life-Span Approach*, 2nd ed. Copyright © 1983 Wadsworth, Inc. Reprinted by permission of Wadsworth, Health Sciences Division, Monterey, California.

that human personality develops as an individual develops actions or tools to gain security and to avoid anxiety. If anxiety arises from a situation in an environment, "dissociation from personality awareness of those tendencies of the personality which are not included or incorporated in the approved structure of the self arises" (Sullivan, 1953, p. 46). The principle of the self-system develops as the self becomes dynamic in preserving security.

Sullivan's model defines the first cultural environment, the one most crucial in forming the individual, as the home, of which the main component is the parent. This also constitutes the first phase of Sullivan's theory of interpersonal development, which occurs from birth through adolescence in six successive phases (Table 6-13). The progression toward mature relations hinges on communication skills and the integration of experiences. As a result of positive, growth-producing experiences, the adolescent has a stable self-concept and can adapt through the adroit use of communication to protect the self from conflict, whatever the situation.

To a great extent, self-concept is developed in the child as the parent reflects approval or disapproval for behaviors and relates positive or negative feelings about life. Sullivan described the infant as initially experiencing the world at a "prototaxic" level. Life is a series of unconnected events, and each event occurs in isolation from the others. As the infant begins to organize these various events and to discriminate among them, the level of experience advances to "parataxic." Meaning is now attached to objects and persons, and their use or action is anticipated. Parental emotion or mood are communicated and incorporated as "good me" or "bad me" personification. A bottle is no longer an isolated object; it means food and usually a parent's holding or giving of the bottle to the infant. Meanings become attached to objects through the experience associated with them. The infant also attaches meaning to the person who helps reduce tension. To some extent, this level of experience continues throughout life. The final level is "syntaxic" and occurs when the child has acquired language. At this level, meaning is attached to such symbols as words and gestures. Communication is now possible, and the world is defined as either good or bad.

Sullivan claimed that the parent plays an influential role in portraying to the child a positive or negative evaluation of the developing self. As early events and their meanings are portrayed and result in either a "good me" or "bad me" personification, this fuses into the self-concept around the onset of the juvenile phase. From this point, however, the self is still capable of influence and change by situations and interactions with others in the environment. Development of self-concept for Sullivan is continuous.

In many respects Sullivan's theory deviates from traditional psychoanalytic theory and encompasses aspects of sociology and social psychology because of the emphasis on social interactions. Sullivan also was convinced that personality can and does change during childhood. In other words the interchange between parent and infant does not necessarily determine adult personality. Peers and other adults also play influential roles, and the cultural environment contributes to the shaping of self-concept.

Behaviorism

Behaviorism explains human actions and interactions as the result of learned responses to environmental stimuli. The behaviorist does not research individual personality development as much as general laws of human behavior that can be applied to everyone. Behavorial research largely is conducted in a laboratory, where variables can be controlled. Behaviorists eschew the vague concepts of mind and mental functions because these cannot be seen or measured. In addition, the confusion and variety of ideas presented by the many theorists make behaviorists skeptical of such speculations. The task of psychology as defined by the behaviorists is to "identify the observable conditions that influence human behavior" (Thomas, 1979, p. 383).

Behaviorists concentrate on the present and on ways to alter or control the environment to change, modify, or teach

TABLE 6-14 Behaviorist Terminology

Term	Definition	Example
Stimulus (S)	An event that immediately precedes a response and evokes or elicits it	Picture, person, spoken word
Response (R)	Reaction to stimulus, an activity displayed by an individual	Smiling, talking, "yes," "eh"
Contingency	The relationship between a response and its consequence	A correct response will be followed by "good"; an incorrect response will be followed by "bad"
Reinforcement	The process of increasing the frequency of a response by controlling consequent events	The presentation of "good," or candy or money given after desired response
Reinforcement schedule	A predetermined rate of delivery of a consequent event	One star for one response; one check for three responses; one point for 2 minutes of sitting at the table
Continuous reinforcement schedule	The delivery of a reinforcer for each response or specified time unit of responding	One chip for each response; one star for each response; one point for each 3 minutes of sitting at the table
Variable reinforcement schedule	The delivery of a reinforcer for an average number of responses or time units intermittently	One chip for an average of five responses given five times during 25 correct responses
Primary reinforcers	Things used as reinforcers that supply survival needs	Food, warmth, water
Secondary reinforcers	Things used as reinforcers that are pleasurable but not related to survival	Money, stickers, trinkets, praise
Extinction	One process of *de*creasing the frequency of a response by withdrawing all consequences	Stop doing anything after response
Positive reinforcer	A consequent event that increases the frequency of a behavior if presented	"Good," "right," money, candy
Negative reinforcer	A consequent event that decreases the frequency of a behavior if presented	"No," "wrong," "say it again"
Chaining	The process whereby several responses are joined in a single response	"I," "I want," "I want a," "I want a ring"
Shaping	The process of teaching new behaviors by rewarding approximations of the desired response	Lifting the spoon, "good," lifting the spoon and opening mouth, "good," lifting the spoon and opening mouth, spoon in mouth, "good"

SOURCE: Adapted by permission of CRM Books, a division of Random House, Inc. from Schell RE, Hall E: *Developmental Psychology Today*, 3rd ed.

desired behaviors. The past is not considered the root of all behavior, as it is for the psychodynamic theorist. Maturation is not as central to learning as the cognitive-structuralists would have one believe. The environment and its relation to the person's influence on it is what is definable and measurable, and only these relations allow psychiatrists to predict human behavior.

Theory of B. F. Skinner

The vocabulary (Table 6-14) of behaviorism was popularized by B. F. Skinner (1904–). Assuming that the child is a passive recipient of environmental influences and therefore malleable, Skinner believed that learning could be controlled by proper structuring and response to the child's action. For Skinner, learning is defined as the result of responses received from the environment. Because the child is considered to be a miniature adult and all learning is cumulative, adults are responsible for creating optimal conditions so that the desired learning can be achieved.

Skinner postulated that there are two types of *conditioning*, or behavioral responses to a *stimulus*. The first response is the classic relationship documented by Pavlov and his well-known experiments with dogs in which a stimulus that causes an unconditioned response is linked with a second stimulus. After several times with both stimuli, the original stimulus is eliminated, and only the second one is used. *Classic conditioning* is thus a procedure in which conditioned reflexes are established by the association of one stimulus with another stimulus that is known to cause an unconditioned reflex. The resulting response is the conditioned response to the unrelated conditioned stimulus (Fig. 6-15).

The second type of response is what Skinner referred to

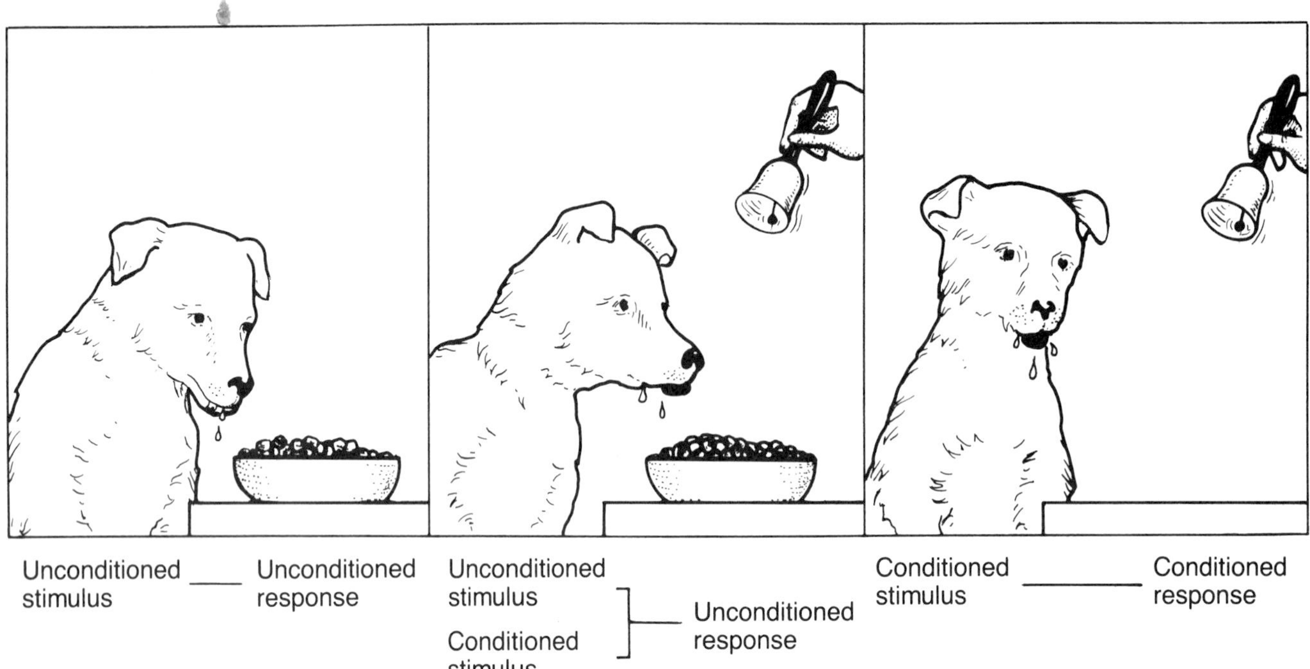

Figure 6-15 Pavlov's classical conditioning paradigm. Pairing of unconditioned stimulus (food) and unconditioned response (salivation) with conditioned stimulus (bell) results in a conditioned response when food is eliminated and the only stimulus is the bell ringing.

as *operant conditioning*, a procedure by which the frequency of a response can be increased or decreased, depending on when, how, and to what extent it is reinforced. Convinced that humans, like animals, will always repeat an action that brings pleasure, Skinner noted that the consequences of action, what he termed *reinforcement*, are all important. If the stimulus is difficult to decipher, it is not significant; what is critical is the result of the behavior. Positive consequences will foster repetition of the action (Fig. 6-16).

To demonstrate his theory, Skinner designed cages with electronic levers that delivered food when they were pressed. The animal learned that the two events were related through the repeated consequence of a primary reinforcer that rewarded its pushing the lever. Thus, whenever desirous of food, attention, or relief from boredom, the animal would push the lever, fully expecting some food to appear (Fig. 6-17).

Skinner and his associates later discovered that learning was more permanent if reinforcers were provided intermittently rather than continuously. They also concluded that time, patience, and steps that were carefully graded from simple to complex were needed when teaching complicated behaviors.

Skinner did not exclude factors of genetic inheritance from his theory. In his novel, *Walden Two* (1948), the children were very different and represented all levels of intelligence, even though their environment for their first decade of life had been identical. What he emphasized, however, was the role of environment in transforming the potential

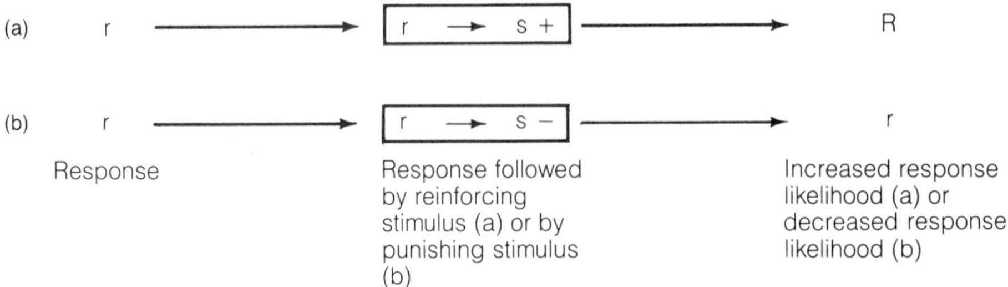

Figure 6-16 Operant conditioning, in which the stimulus follows the response. Skinner's concept of learning postulates that the consequence of a behavior is all-important in determining the repetition of the behavior. (From Yussen SR, Santrock, JW: *Child Development: An Introduction.* Wm. C. Brown, 1982, p. 133.)

for learning into actual learning. Because behavior, its consequences, and its repetition or lack of repetition are observable, he considered his theory to be more scientific than other developmental theories. Skinner also emphasized that his theory explains why a behavior occurs and does not simply describe what occurs.

Nurses can use the principles of behaviorism to change certain actions of some children. For example, if a group of participants repeatedly arrives late for appointments or a health education class, the nurse first speaks to them about this and then commends them for attempts to arrive on time. The first few times this praise may be for being 7 minutes late instead of 10. The reinforcer is then given only for being even more punctual until punctuality finally becomes the norm. The principle is that positive cooperative behavior is praised and rewarded rather than disobedience punished.

A negative behavior may, however, become inadvertently rewarded and thus conditioned. The small child who cries for candy at the store may be given some candy to stop the crying and to decrease parental embarrassment. The next time the parent and child go to the store the child will cry for candy again because last time that behavior (crying) was successful in obtaining the desired object. The parent may once again comply with the child's wishes or anticipate the wish and provide the candy even before the behavior begins. Denying the request and ignoring any outbursts begins the process of *extinction*, in which the behavior is "unlearned" because the reinforcement has been removed. Extinction does, however, take longer; it requires greater effort to extinguish the behavior than to condition it.

Skinner is credited with introducing concepts of programmed instruction (Fig. 6-18) and computer learning. With programmed instruction methods, the immediate feedback provides the reinforcer, either positive or negative, for the child's efforts and thus encouragement to go on or to try again.

Critics claim that Skinner's theory is too simplistic and reductionist and that the learning that occurs is memorization and cannot be applied to other situations. Table 6-15 compares behaviorism with cognitive theory. Sociologists, on the other hand, are quick to point out the very powerful influence that environment has on the acquisition of behavior, attitudes, and background experiences, which comprise the rules for each member of the society and by which each member lives and makes decisions.

Theory of Albert Bandura

Although he agreed with the concepts of conditioned learning as amplified by Skinner, Albert Bandura (1925–) was not convinced that all learning had to occur in such a trial-and-error fashion. He therefore proposed that many behaviors were the result of imitation. His *social learning theory* is a set of behavioristic concepts and principles that

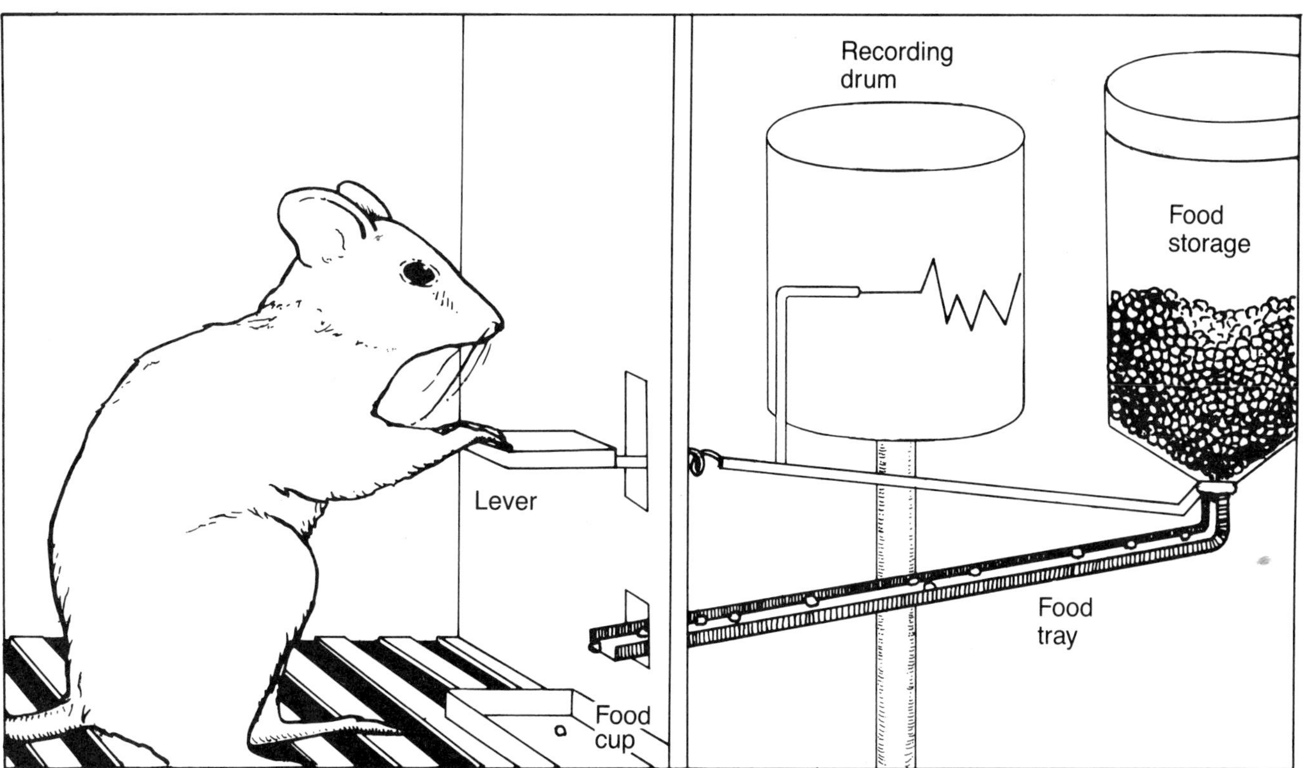

Figure 6-17 Schematic representation of a "Skinner box" used for conditioning animals.

The sequence is usually based solely on the logical thinking of the adult developers.

One-exposure learning: a single strategy is artificially isolated and practiced. Children's creative capacities are suppressed.

The instructional sequence moves from the least difficult to the most difficult examples. The steps are often so small that it is not possible to get an overall view.

The direction is linear. New information is simply added to the existing information.

Intellectual conflict is discouraged. The steps are so small that success is guaranteed and the responses are almost automatic.

Immediate feedback is given to the children's responses. The evaluation is external.

Figure 6-18 Principles of programmed instruction. (From Labinowicz E: *The Piaget Primer*. Addison-Wesley, 1980.)

frequently are used in describing and explaining personality characteristics and social behavior. It emphasizes the social variables and the ways in which they are responsible for the child's behavior. An important variable is whether observed actions are rewarded or punished; two other variables are the similarity of the imitated model to the self and the degree of prestige accorded the model. Thus, two concepts that are central to Bandura's research are (1) *imitation*, the principle and the process by which an individual copies or reproduces what has been observed, and (2) *modeling*, a principle and a process by which an individual learns by observing the behavior of others.

In a study designed to assess delayed imitation of deviant models in the absence of the models, Bandura assigned nursery school children to one of the following groups: aggressive adult models, nonaggressive adult models, human aggression on film, aggression on filmed cartoons, or a control group. For the groups assigned to aggressive model and filmed human aggression, the model demonstrated various acts of physical and verbal aggression toward a large, inflated plastic doll. The model in the cartoon film was a cartoon character participating in pranks and fights aimed at overpowering another character. The nonaggressive model sat quietly in the room and ignored both the doll and the instruments of agression that were present. After viewing the model's behavior according to their assigned groups, the children were mildly frustrated. The researchers then counted the number of imitative and nonimitative aggressive behaviors each child performed in a setting identical to the one previously viewed but without the model present.

The children who observed the aggressive models had many aggressive behaviors in their repertoires, many of which imitated precisely those they viewed. The children in the nonaggressive and control groups demonstrated few aggressive acts. Furthermore, those in the nonaggressive group displayed inhibited behavior characteristic of their model to a greater extent than did the control children. The children not only demonstrated that modeling occurs in the later absence of the model but also showed that film-mediated models are as effective as real-life models in transmitting social attitudes, values, actions, beliefs, and behaviors that may be appropriate or deviant (Bandura and Walters, 1963).

Bandura also examined the influence of the sex of the model and the sex the child on the concept of imitation. He found that "boys showed significantly more imitative aggression than girls, but the sexes did not differ in the extent to which they reproduced the model's verbal aggression. In addition, the male model was a more potent influence on male subjects than was the female model" (Bandura and Walters, 1963, p. 105). Another interesting note was that the children performed considerably fewer aggressive behaviors when the nonaggressive model was a male rather than a female.

In another study Bandura assigned nursery school children randomly to one of four groups: (1) a group in which the aggressive model was rewarded; (2) a group in which the aggressive model was punished; (3) a control group without models; or (4) a control group with expressive nonaggressive models.

Children who observed the aggressive model rewarded imitated many more verbal and physical aggressive acts than did those who saw the model punished. The latter group did not differ significantly from the control groups, thus demonstrating the inhibitory effect of exposure to punishment. On the basis of the response-consequences interpretation of modeling effects, Bandura predicted that if the behavior of an aggressive model is rewarded, the child will be more likely to imitate it than if the behavior is punished.

To a greater or lesser extent, imitative behaviors occur

TABLE 6-15 Comparison of Piagetian and Behaviorist Positions

	Behaviorist position	Constructivist-interactionist
Goals	Pass on knowledge	Develop knowledge
	Emphasis on past/present	Emphasis on present/future
	Training for short-term objectives	Education for long-term goals
Learning	Knowledge is structured externally	Knowledge is structured internally
	Knowledge is a copy of reality	Knowledge is interpretation of reality
	Linear/cumulative	Nonlinear; restructuring necessary
	Passive learner	Active learner
	Lack of understanding due only to lack of relevant experiences	Lack of understanding is due to lack of relevant experiences within developmental constraints
	Small steps—smooth ride on paved road	Varied steps—roller coaster ride
	Predictable behavior	Less predictable behavior
Intelligence	Fixed	Developing
	Collection of skills	Organized, coherent, whole structure
Teaching	Can teach any subject effectively in some intellectually honest form to any child at any age of development by arranging for prerequisite experiences	Basic notions are accessible to children 7–10 years of age, provided that they are divorced from their mathematical expression and studied through materials that a child can handle
	Teaching by telling is an accepted method	Teaching by telling is deemphasized; emphasis is placed on experiences to give meaning to the words prior to their use
	Correct answers are reinforced; wrong answers are not accepted	All responses are accepted and are related to the materials under study to extend understanding or to develop thinking process
	Locus of evaluation is external—correct answer is only in teacher's head or in the textbook	Locus of evaluation is internal—feedback is available from materials and logical consistency
	Promotes extrinsic motivation	Promotes intrinsic motivation
	Stress memorization	Stresses development of understanding
Curriculum	Rigid—structured by adults in a tight sequence that is logical to them, requires knowledge of subject matter, usually structured in small steps to encourage immediate success	Flexible—structured by adults and/or children; when structured by adults it involves the juxtapositioning of children's incomplete thinking patterns; requires much knowledge of child development and knowledge of subject matter; steps are of varied size to encourage involvement in the equilibration process
Outcomes	Fosters child dependence	Fosters child independence
	Ill-adapted to changing world	Well-adapted to changing world

SOURCE: Reza R, Post T: *The Mathematics Laboratory: Theory to Practice*, Prindle, Weber, Schmidt, 1973 and Labinowicz E: *The Piaget Primer: Thinking, Learning, Teaching*. Addison-Wesley, 1980, p. 267.

throughout the life span, but not all learning or acquisition of new behaviors can be accounted for by imitation. Social learning theorists have difficulty explaining creativity and changes in thinking about moral dilemmas. Nevertheless, Bandura distinguished between the acquisition of a response set and the actual performance of the behavior. The child may acquire a new way of thinking or responding to a situation but may save it for a more appropriate time (Fig. 6-19). Just because the child does not demonstrate and imitate performance does not mean that imitation has not occurred. Imitation is therefore more than mere mimicking; it is learning a whole behavior pattern from observing and evaluating another's behavior. Thus, the child's personality and character are learned through a process of gradually acquiring values and beliefs, response sets, and patterns of experience.

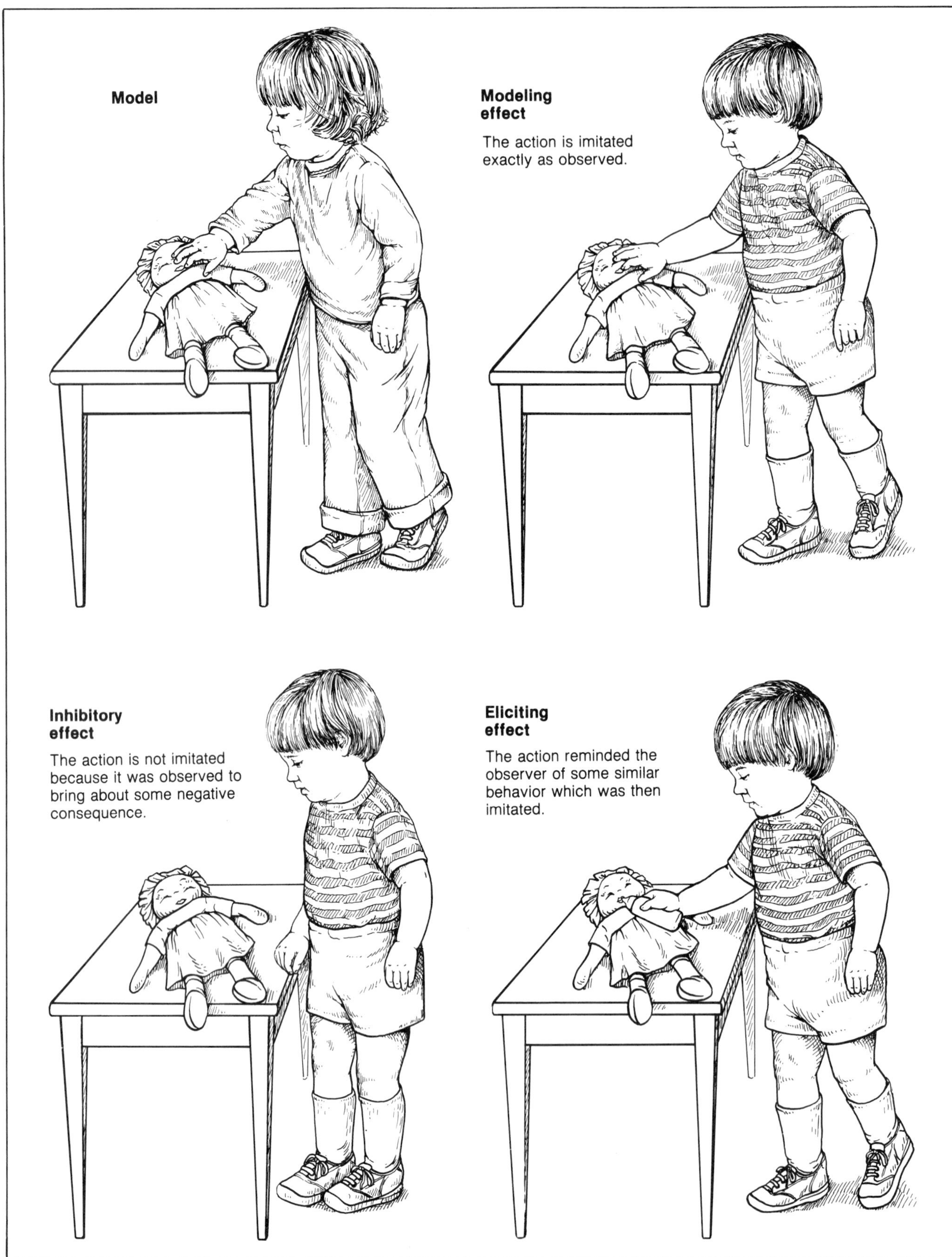

Figure 6-19 Bandura's modeling effects on social learning.

Theory of Robert Sears

Robert Sears (1908–) was one of a group of theorists who restructured one theory into another. Sears analyzed the various concepts of Freudian theory from a behaviorist perspective; one such concept was *identification*, the process by which the child obtains a sense of self by behaving, reacting, and feeling like somebody else, usually the parent.

Parents provide children with the early consequences of behavior, consequences that a behaviorist defines as positive or negative reinforcement. These consequences, often produced unconsciously, influence the child's development. The parent is thus the earliest and most frequent model for the child and the one with whom the child identifies. The parental model is viewed as powerful and rewarding because most, if not all, of the child's initial need gratification results from parental care. As the child grows and becomes more independent and less in need of parental care, the child achieves need satisfaction by observing and imitating the parent. The mental image sustained by the child then becomes self-reinforcing and rewarding.

Sears attempted to link childrearing practices with types of behavior exhibited by children. This attempt promoted the idea of *determinism*, the notion that parental behaviors determined the child's personality and behavior. These studies created more questions than they answered, but they did demonstrate an interesting combination of two theories to explain a concept. When viewed as one of the ways in which children learn about societal expectations, the concept of parents as primary role models is significant.

Parents and nurses both know that the old familiar admonition, "Do as I say and not as I do," often seems to fall on deaf ears. Is this the case because of the powerful influence of behavior observation on behavior performance? Observation allows the child to learn without formal teaching. The child first learns from the home environment, which provides initial reinforcement of approved behaviors that are, to some extent, imitative of parental behaviors; these begin with smiles, cooing, and babbling sounds and progress to more sophisticated social responses.

Sears described the cumulative result of learning identification as taking place in three phases. The first two phases are closely associated with the parents, and the final phase extends to peer and other extrafamilial relations. Phase one is rudimentary behavior. It relates to reflexes and the survival needs for food and warmth. Early on, the infant relates the comfort experienced from having these needs met with parental actions. Phase two is secondary motivational systems—family centered learning. During this phase, children use their parents as role models. They learn how to think, act, and feel by observing, imitating, and then adopting parental responses. The children identify with their parents because the result is generally positive. The parents provide rewards when their children respond to situations in appropriate ways. Children view parents as powerful and desire to be like them. They figure that one way to accomplish this is to behave as much like their parents as possible. As parents fulfill their children's dependency needs and provide affection and security, they foster this process of identification.

Phase three is secondary motivational systems—extrafamilial learning. This phase includes all of the nonfamily persons who influence the child such as friends, teachers, classmates, club leaders, and others. As time and experience away from home increase during middle childhood and thereafter, decisions and behavior become increasingly influenced by these important people. As in the case of parents, it is from these people that the child desires recognition and approval. One way to receive such attention is to behave, think, and feel similarly.

Other Developmental Theories

Developmental Tasks: Theory of Robert J. Havighurst

The concept of developmental tasks as a way of organizing the process of living is the work of many theorists and developmental psychologists. Robert Havighurst is recognized for organizing and promoting the concept during the 1950s. Stated very simply, a *developmental task* is whatever a person is learning, doing, and perfecting at a given stage during the life span. A more precise definition, according to Havighurst, is "a task which arises at or about a certain period in the life of the individual, successful achievement of which leads to his happiness and to success with later tasks, while failure leads to unhappiness in the individual, disapproval by society, and difficulty with later tasks" (Havighurst, 1953).

Developmental tasks include all aspects of development— cognitive, physical, affective, and social. They reflect the culture and therefore vary from culture to culture to portray the values and beliefs that are important and appropriate. They provide a general method of assessing the child's progress at each stage and define a standard progression through defined stages. They provide a general guideline for teachers and other adults in identifying what can be expected of children at various stages and how to mesh expectations and abilities.

A developmental task originates from one of three sources. It may have a biologic basis and reflect physical maturation and the acquisition of growth and developmental skills. It may be the result of cultural expectation and mirror the particular belief system of which the child is part. It may be based in individual values and aspirations for personal achievement.

The popularity of the theory can be attributed to its reasonableness and logic. The wide age range included in each

TABLE 6-16 The First Three Developmental Tasks According to Havighurst

Stage	Developmental tasks
Infancy and early childhood	Learn to walk
	Learn to take solid food
	Learn to talk
	Control elimination of body wastes
	Learn sex differences and sexual modesty
	Form concepts and learn language to describe social and physical reality
	Get ready to read
	Learn to distinguish right and wrong and begin to develop a conscience
Middle childhood	Learn physical skills necessary for ordinary games
	Build wholesome attitudes toward oneself as a growing organism
	Learn to get along with age-mates
	Learn an appropriate masculine or feminine social role
	Develop fundamental skills in reading, writing, and calculating
	Develop concepts necessary for everyday living
	Develop conscience, morality, and a scale of values
	Achieve personal independence
	Develop attitudes toward social groups and institutions
Adolescence	Achieve new and more mature relations with age-mates of both sexes
	Achieve a masculine or feminine social role
	Accept one's physique and use body effectively
	Achieve emotional independence from parents and other adults
	Prepare for marriage and family life
	Prepare for economic career
	Develop an ideology—a set of values and an ethical system as a guide to behavior
	Achieve socially responsible behavior

SOURCE: Havighurst R J: *Developmental Tasks and Education* 3rd ed. Copyright © 1972 by Longman Inc. Reprinted by permission of Longman Inc., New York.

stage fosters a general impression of normative behavior. Table 6-16 illustrates the tasks for the first three stages only because the final three stages relate to adult development. Havighurst's theory is continuous, and he assumed that learning is cumulative. The child is viewed as immature and involved in the process of becoming a mature adult.

The idea of the so-called "teachable moment" evolved from this theory. Because each stage encompasses a wide age range, the period of time correlated with the "teachable moment" is fairly well accepted. "If the task is not achieved at the proper time, it will not be achieved well and failure in this task will cause partial or complete failure in the achievement of other tasks yet to come" (Havighurst, 1953).

The advantage of the concept of developmental tasks is the neat, composite picture it paints of the development of the child. The disadvantage is that the elements of the picture are so large that individual steps are lost. To be truly useful, therefore, it must be used in conjunction with the other more detailed and specific theories.

Hierarchy of Needs: Theory of Abraham Maslow

Humanistic psychology is concerned with the human response to life. Rather than focusing on one specific aspect of development and attempting to be objective and scientific, humanists view behavior as the total individual response to life and living. They are concerned with subjective feelings and responses and define development from a personal perspective. Humanists recognize contributions from

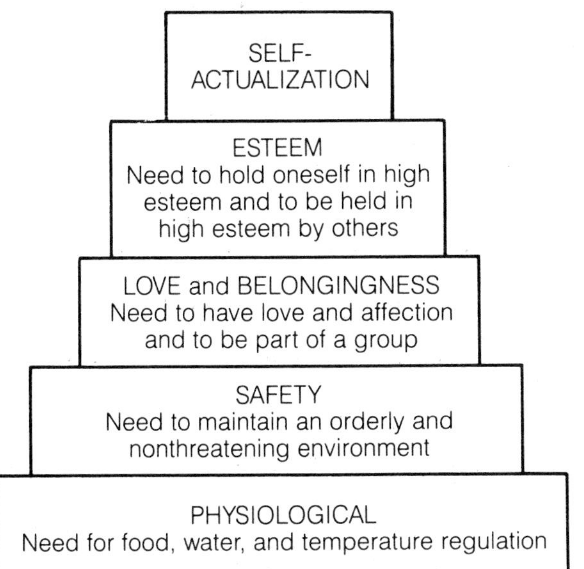

Figure 6-20 Maslow's needs hierarchy, from lower-order requirements to higher-order desires. (From *Human Development: A Life Span Approach,* 2nd ed. by KL Freiberg, p. 66, Monterey, California. Wadsworth Health Sciences Division, 1983.)

both heredity and environment and suggest that the challenge is to interact with the child so as to foster the optimal development of human potential.

As the result of observing and interacting with his own children, Abraham Maslow (1908–1970) became convinced that the inner nature of children is good or at least neutral but is definitely not evil. He then postulated that the role of adults, and especially parents, is to assist the child to express and live in harmony with the self.

Rather than a theory of ages and stages and specific accomplishments, Maslow's theory is one of becoming, or of the interplay between fulfilling basic foundational needs and having resources available so that the individual may realize the full potential of personal abilities. To this end, much attention is given to the child's perceptions, feelings, and values. It is not so much a theory that specifies the steps of growth and development of the child as it is a goal toward which all theories should be directed. Maslow assumed that a child's personality is not determined by the past or early infant experiences but that all experience has an important part in fulfilling initial physiologic needs so that self-growth can continue. The young child has more than biologic and cognitive needs; there are also the needs to be loved and respected for who one is at that moment.

Maslow (1968) identified two types of needs that the child, and later the adult, seeks to fulfill. The first he called deficiency needs. These included basic physiologic needs for food, drink, rest, and warmth; needs for safety and security, defined as the need to be free from fear and protected from harm and danger; the need for a sense of belonging, of love and affection from family and friends; and needs for self-esteem, self-concept, and positive respect from others. The lower needs in Maslow's list had to be satisfied before the higher needs, culminating in self-actualization, could be approached.

The second type of needs are growth or self-actualization needs. Although more ambigious and difficult to describe, Maslow (1968) defined the need for self-actualization as a striving to realize one's potentials, capacities, and talents and "an unceasing trend toward unity integration or synergy within the person."

Maslow thus conceived of need fulfillment as a hierarchy, as illustrated in Figure 6-20. The lower-level needs appear at the base of the pyramid, and these must be satisfied before there can be any movement to the upper-level needs. One need tends to be predominant at a time, thus demanding fulfillment before further growth can occur.

Maslow envisioned the self as a composite of values and beliefs incorporated from others in the environment, together with an intrinsic sense of right and wrong. The individual therefore is self-motivated toward positive, healthy, self-fulfilling growth. Although not generally thought of as a child development theorist, Maslow does challenge nurses working with children and seeking to understand them in a holistic framework. His needs theory suggests that nurses should be cognizant of children's immediate deficiency needs and their fulfillment as the first step toward fostering children's potential development.

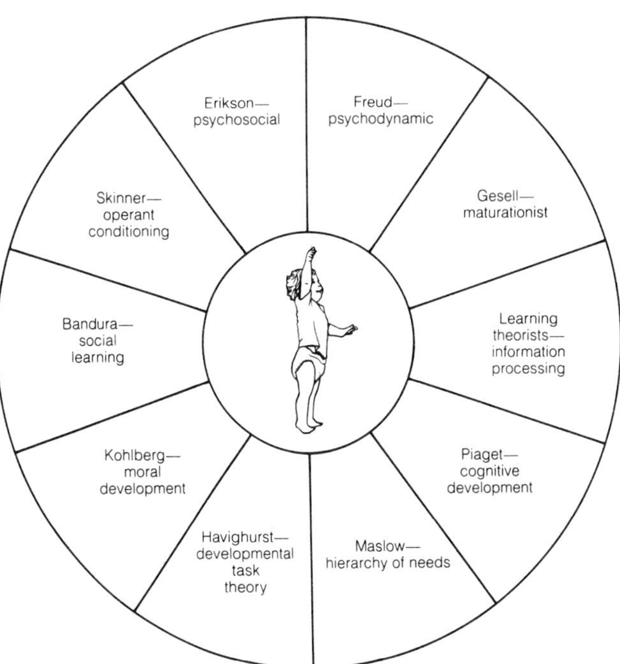

Figure 6-21 Human development as a composite of various theories. Each sheds light on the process and helps explain human behavior and personality.

TABLE 6-17 Comparison of Major Developmental Theories

Developmental stage	Erikson (psychosocial development)	Piaget (logical and cognitive development)
Infancy	Trust vs. mistrust	Sensorimotor period Substage 1—pure reflex adaptations Substage 2—primary circular reactions Substage 3—secondary circular reactions Substage 4—coordination of secondary schemes Substage 5—tertiary circular reactions
Early childhood toddler	Autonomy vs. shame and doubt	Substage 6—invention of new solutions through mental combinations Transition—early preconceptual
Preschool	Initiative vs. guilt	Preoperational stage Preconceptual—uses representational thought to recall past, represent present and anticipate future Intuitive—Increased symbolic functioning; able to see simple relationships
Middle childhood	Industry vs. inferiority	Concrete operations—categoric classification; reversible concrete thought
Later childhood	Industry vs. inferiority (continued)	Formal operations Substage 1—relations involving the inverse of the reciprocal (ability to form negative classes and to see relations as simultaneously reciprocal)
Adolescence	Identity vs. role diffusion	Substage 2—capacity to order triads of propositions or relations
Mid	Identity vs. role diffusion (continued)	Substage 3—true formal thought; construction of all possible combinations of relations; deductive hypothesis testing
Late	Identity vs. role diffusion (continued)	(Note: all relations between Piaget and Kohlberg are that attainment of the logical stages is necessary, but not sufficient, for attainment of the moral stage)

Framework for Developmental Stages

The various child development theories discussed in detail in this chapter provide an analysis of the child from nearly every possible angle (Table 6-17). Each theory contributes to a better understanding of the child and the process of development (Fig. 6-21). Chapters 7 through 11 focus on the application of these theories to children in the various stages of development.

Infancy, the first phase, is the period of birth and early

TABLE 6-17 continued

Kohlberg (development of moral reasoning)	Freud (psychosexual development)	Sears (social learning and identification)	Integration of theories
	Oral stage	Rudimentary behavior	Phase 1—establishing primary independence from parent; focus on motor and sensory experiences
Stage 0—the good is what I want and like	Anal stage	Secondary motivational—family centered learning	Phase 2—establishing self as independent decision maker concerning use of acquired skills; focus on increased mobility and use of language for communication; doing for the sake of doing; increased learning about the environment and relation of self to it
Stage 1—punishment—obedience orientation; obey rules to avoid punishment	Phallic stage (Oedipus complex; Electra complex)		
Stage 2—instrumental; hedonism and concrete reciprocity; conform to obtain rewards, favors	Latent stage	Secondary motivational—extrafamilial learning	Phase 3—establishing self in new relations with peers and goals for project construction; focus on the satisfactory completion of the project; use of fine motor skills
Stage 3—seeking good relations and approval of family group; oriented to interpersonal relations of mutality	Latent stage (continued)	Continuation of extrafamilial learning (little research beyond this point by Sears)	Phase 4—establishing self as a logical thinker and problem solver with the ability to expand one's perspective to others, focus on concrete problems and their solutions; sophisticated motor and social skills involving group cooperation and organization.
Stage 4—obedience to law and order in society; maintenance of social order—show respect for authority	Genital stage		Phase 5—establishing new ways of relating to parents and peers; increased attraction to opposite sex; new ways of thinking and ability to solve hypothetic problems and think about the future; focus on resolution of dependence vs independence in all modes of behavior
Stage 5A—concern with individual rights and legal contract; social contract; utilitarian lawmaking perspective	Genital stage (continued)		
Stage 5B—higher law and conscience orientation; orientation to internal decisions of conscience but without clear rationale or universal principles	Genital stage (continued)		

beginnings in the life of the child. An infant is essentially a preverbal child, generally from 0 to 18 months of age. During this time, the child experiences rapid growth in all parameters, the most noticeable of which is physical growth. The infant's initial social interactions are formed, and the sense of trust in self and others is developed; learning about the environment is closely related to motor and sensory experiences.

Early childhood is the time from 18 months through $4\frac{1}{2}$ years old. Physical skills and gross motor activities become well learned, and fine motor activities are being learned. For the child in this phase, language has opened new horizons in thought and interaction, but understanding is still limited, and the world is perceived from an egocentric perspective. Social interactions continue to develop, and the child becomes increasingly independent. No longer dependent on others, the child increasingly wants to do things without help and to decide when and how to do them.

Early childhood encompasses the phase of toddlerhood, with its beginning assertion for self-recognition and independent mobility and the continuation and refinement of these during the preschool phase. Children in western cultures increasingly have early social and peer group experiences away from home and are exposed to early learning of language and mathematical concepts. This progressive learning effectively compresses this early period into one more homogenous period rather than two separate phases.

Middle childhood is the time of the early school-age child. The first 4 years of school, from kindergarten through third grade, are times of new discoveries. New learning and ways of thinking occur as the child becomes less tied to fantasy and more realistic. New fine motor skills are learned and others perfected. Social relations expand as the child becomes increasingly peer-oriented. The child's sense of self is gained from satisfaction in tasks performed and recognition from others.

Late childhood is the time in which the child becomes increasingly sophisticated in thinking, behavior, and interactions. The ability to think logically and solve problems is, for this later school-age child, both fun and challenging. Competition with the self and others is a motivating force, but instead of thinking only about the self, the child can now take the perspective of others and respond accordingly. This phase includes children from about 8 years, or fourth grade, until the beginning of preadolescence (about 12 years of age).

Adolescence is the time from prepubescence through high school. The key characteristics of this phase are the physical changes associated with hormonal changes and development of secondary sexual features. Changes in thinking and reasoning become evident, and the child is now able to solve abstract and hypothetic problems.

The growth and development of the child from a helpless newborn to an independent, self-functioning adolescent are marvelous, yet complex, phenomena that are only partially understood. The more nurses understand these ongoing processes, however, the more effectively they can be involved in planning interventions, whether in the areas of teaching, prevention, or providing care.

Key Concepts

- Developmental theorists seek to answer how human beings grow and develop and why identifiable characteristics appear at certain ages or in similar environments.
- Developmental theories can direct nursing actions and explain a child's behavior or thought processes as long as the nurse considers children's individual differences.
- Each theory describes a segment of the development process and provides part of the nurse's understanding of the process as a whole.
- Theories are limited by the theorist's underlying assumptions, research design, and method of analysis.
- Theoretic assumptions include notions about the child's degree of malleability, contribution to self-development, and character and beliefs about the nature of change.
- Growth and development occur as orderly, sequential processes, although their pace varies from child to child.
- Growth and development are continuous processes influenced by a variety of factors involving both suprasystems and subsystems.
- Maturation theorists, such as Arnold Gesell, emphasize the role of genetics as the determiner of how and in what order developmental stages occur; Gesell, for example, concluded that development of some skills is preprogrammed to occur at certain ages.
- Sociobiologists and ethologists are concerned with the biologic basis of social behavior but also acknowledge the role of environment; ethologists such as Konrad Lorenz study the correlation between animal and human behavior.
- Cognitive-structural theorists study the qualitative changes in children's thinking, reasoning, and language skills by observing behaviors and making inferences; information-processing theory, for example, defines learning as continuous mental activity leading to problem-solving ability.

- Jean Piaget, a cognitive-structural theorist, defined learning as an active process in which the child develops intelligence and logic skills by manipulating the environment.
- Lawrence Kohlberg, a cognitive-structural theorist, studied moral development and identified a series of stages, or levels, of moral judgment through determining the motivation and decision-making process.
- James Fowler developed a cognitive-structural theory of faith development that examines commitment to persons, values, ideals, or causes, which in turn influence individual coping strategies.
- Psychodynamic theorists examine the emotional forces reflected in personality; for example, both Margaret Mahler and Harry Stack Sullivan studied parent–child interaction and its role in the development of independence and self-concept.
- Sigmund Freud, an early psychodynamic theorist, studied unconscious motivation and defined the stages of personality development that were related to psychosexual growth.
- Erik Erikson expanded on Freud's work by analyzing the role of the environment and past experience in influencing personality development.
- Behaviorists such as B. F. Skinner, Albert Bandura, and Robert Sears explained development as the result of learned responses to environmental stimuli.
- B. F. Skinner defined learning as a process of conditioning, or response to a stimulus, and thereby suggested principles that nurses can use in influencing behaviors of some children in some situations.
- Albert Bandura explained behavior as a result of social learning, which functions through imitation and the evaluation of others in the environment.
- Robert Sears examined the process of identification, through which children learn from experiencing the consequences of behavior and come to identify the self with the parent.
- Robert J. Havighurst defined the concept of developmental tasks, which suggests that each stage of development involves a series of tasks that reflect the essential aspects of development at that stage.
- Abraham Maslow, in examining the human response to development, identified a series of needs, which he arranged in a hierarchy to suggest that lower-level needs must be met before higher-level needs can be addressed.
- The variety of developmental theories, taken together, suggest a series of developmental stages; at each stage, the child makes critical progress in one or more areas of development.

References

Bandura A, Walters R: *Social Learning and Personal Development.* Holt, Rinehart & Winston, 1963.

Bayley N: Comparisons of mental and motor test scores for ages 1–15 months by sex, birth order, race, geographical location and education of parents. *Child Dev* 1965; 36:379–411.

Berkenfield J, Schwartz JB: Nutrition intervention in the community—the "WIC" program. *N Engl J Medi* 1980; 302(10):579–580.

Bigner JJ: *Human Development—A Life-Span Approach.* Macmillan, 1983.

Brainerd CJ: *Piaget's Theory of Intelligence.* Prentice-Hall, 1978.

Duska R, Whelan M: *Moral Development, A Guide to Piaget and Kohlberg.* Paulist Press, 1975.

Erikson E: *Childhood and Society.* Norton, 1963.

Erikson E: *Identity: Youth and Crisis.* Norton, 1968.

Flavell J: *The Developmental Psychology of Jean Piaget.* Van Nostrand, 1963.

Fong BC, Resnick MR: *The Child: Development Through Adolescence.* Benjamin/Cummings, 1980.

Fowler J, Keen S: *Life Maps: Conversations in the Journey of Faith.* Word Books, 1978.

Freiberg KL: *Human Development: A Life-Span Approach.* Brooks/Cole, 1983.

Freud S: Beyond the Pleasure Principles. In: *The Standard Edition of the Complete Psychological Works of Sigmund Freud.* Vol 18. Strachey J (editor). Hogarth, 1957.

Freud S: *The Ego and the Id.* Hogarth, 1974. (Translation of 1923 work.)

Gesell A, Ilg FL: *Child Development: An Introduction to the Study of Human Growth.* Harper & Row, 1949.

Gewirtz JL: A learning analysis of the effects of normal stimulation, privation, and deprivation on the acquisition of social motivation and attachment. In: *Determinants of Infant Behavior.* Floss BM (editor). Wiley, 1961.

Gilligan C: *In a Different Voice: Psychological Theory and Women's Development.* Harvard University Press, 1982.

Haggerty R: Foreword. In: *Physical Growth and Development.* Valadian I, Porter D (editors). Little, Brown, 1977.

Havighurst RJ: *Human Development and Education.* Longmans Green, 1953.

Havighurst RJ: *Developmental Tasks and Education.* McKay, 1972.

Hess EH: Ethology and developmental psychology. In: *Carmichael's Manual of Child Psychology. vol 1 Mussen H (editor), Wiley, 1970.*
Ilg FL, Ames LB: *The Gesell Institute's Child Behavior.* Dell, 1960.
Jensen AR: How much can we boost IQ and scholastic achievement? *Harvard Educational Review* 1969; 39:1–123.
Jensen AR: *Educability and Group Differences.* Harper & Row, 1973.
Kohlberg L: Moral development. In: *International Encyclopedia of the Social Sciences.* Macmillan, 1968.
Kohlberg L: Stage and sequence: The cognitive-development approach to socialization. In: *Handbook of Socialization: Theory and Research.* Goslin D (editor). Rand McNally, 1969.
Kohlberg L: Moral stages and moralization: The cognitive-developmental approach. In: *Moral Development and Behavior.* Likona T (editor). Holt, Rinehart & Winston, 1976.
Labinowicz E: The Piaget Primer. Addison-Wesley, 1980.
Lazar I, Darlington R: *Lasting Effects After Preschool.* Final Report, HEW Grant 90C-1311. US Department of Health, Education, and Welfare (DHEW Publication No. (OHDS) 79-30179), 1979.
Lazar I: *The Persistence of Preschool Effects, Education Commission of the States.* US Department of Health, Education, and Welfare (DHEW Publication No. (OHDS) 78-30130), September, 1977.
Lewis M: *Clinical Aspects of Child Development.* Lea & Febiger, 1982.
Lickona T (editor): *Moral Development and Behavior: Theory, Research, and Social Issues.* Holt, Rinehart & Winston, 1976.
Lorenz K: Companions as factors in the bird's environment. In: *Studies in Animal and Human Behavior.* Harvard University Press, 1970.
Lowrey GH: *Growth and Development of Children.* Year Book, 1978.
Mahler MS, Pine F, Bergman A: *The Psychological Birth of the Human Infant: Symbiosis and Individuation.* Basic Books, 1975.
Maier HW: *Three Theories of Child Development.* Harper & Row 1965.
Maier HW: *Three Theories of Child Development: The Contributions of Erik H. Erikson, Jean Piaget, and Robert R. Sears and their Applications.* Revised ed. Harper & Row, 1978.
Maslow AH: *Motivation and Personality.* Harper & Row, 1970.
Maslow AH: *The Farther Reaches of Human Nature.* Viking, 1971.
Nelms BC, Mullins RG: *Growth and Development—A Primary Health Care Approach.* Prentice-Hall, 1982.
Piaget J, Inhelder B: *The Psychology of the Child.* Basic Books, 1969.
Ramey CT, Campbell FA, Finkelstein NW: Course and structure of intellectual development in children at high risk for developmental retardation. In: *Learning and Cognition in Mental Retardation.* Brooks P, Baumeister A (editors). University Park Press, 1983.
Schell RE, Hall E: *Developmental Psychology Today.* 3rd ed. Random House, 1979.
Schuster CS, Ashburn SS: *The Process of Human Development: A Holistic Approach.* Little, Brown, 1980.
Sheldon WH: *Varieties of Physique.* Harper & Row, 1940.
Sheldon WH: *Varieties of Temperament.* Harper & Row, 1942.
Siegler RS, Liebert DE, Liebert RM: Inhelder and Piaget's pendulum problem. *Developmental Psychology* 1973; 9:97–101.
Skinner BF: *Beyond Freedom and Dignity.* Knopf, 1971.
Skinner BF: *Walden Two.* Macmillan, 1948.
Sullivan HS: *Conceptions of Modern Psychiatry.* Norton, 1953.
Tanner JM: *Education and Physical Growth.* University of London Press, 1966.
Tanner JM: Growing up. *Sci Am* 1973; 229(3):34–43.
Thomas RM: *Comparing Theories of Child Development.* Wadsworth, 1979.
Tulman LJ: Theories of maternal attachment. *ANS* 1981; 4(3):7–14.
Wadsworth B: *Piaget's Theory of Cognitive Development.* Longman, 1979.
Yussen SR, Santrock JW: *Child Development: An Introduction.* Brown, 1982.
Zeskind PS, Ramey CT: Fetal malnutrition: An experimental study of its consequences on infant development in two caregiving environments. *Child Dev* 1978; 49:1155–1162.

Additional Readings

Baldwin AL: *Theories of Child Development.* Wiley, 1968.
Campbell SF: *Piaget Sampler.* Wiley, 1976.
Field TM et al: *Review of Human Development.* Wiley, 1982.
Flavell JH: Wohlwill J: Formal and functional aspects of cognitive development. In: *Studies in Cognitive Development.* Eldird D, Flavell J (editors). Oxford University Press, 1969.
Fowler JW: *Stages of Faith: The Psychology of Human Development and the Quest for Meaning.* Harper & Row, 1981.
LaBarba RC: *Foundations of Developmental Psychology.* Academic Press, 1981.
Omery A: Moral development: A differential evaluation of dominant models. *ANS* 1983; 6(1):1–17.
Piaget J: *The Development of Thought.* Viking Press, 1977.
Schell RE, Hall E: *Developmental Psychology Today.* Random House, 1983.
Selman RL: *First Things: Social Reasoning.* Guidance Associates, 1974.
Sullivan HS: *The Interpersonal Theory of Psychiatry.* Norton, 1953.
Sullivan HS: *The Fusion of Psychiatry and Social Science.* Norton, 1964.
Vurpillot E: The development of scanning strategies and their relation to visual differentiation. *J Exp Child Psychol* 1968; 6:632–650.
Watson R, Lindgren HC: *Psychology of the Child and the Adolescent.* Macmillan, 1979.
Zeskind PS, Ramey CT: Preventing intellectual and interactional sequelae of fetal malnutrition: A longitudinal, transactional, and synergistic approach to development. *Child Dev* 1981; 52:213–218.

Infancy

J. Craig Peery Sandra R. Mott

7

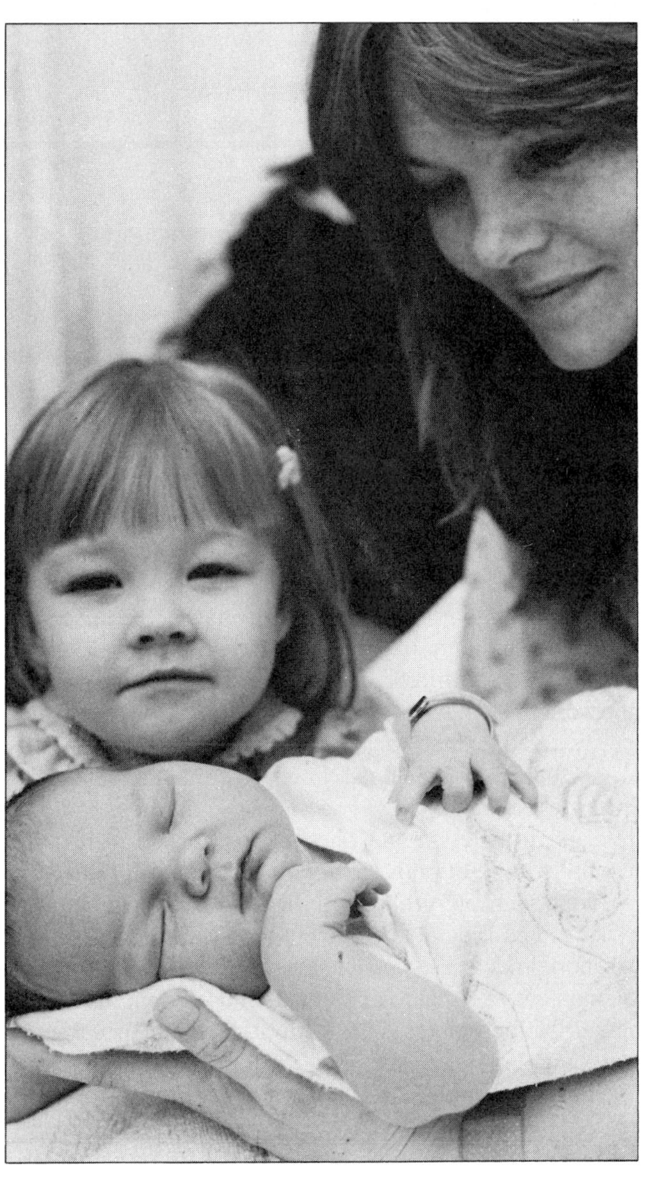

Chapter Outline

continued on next page

Objectives

- Explain the influences of suprasystems and subsystems on infant development.
- Define the major criteria for neonatal assessment.
- Define the major parameters of development in infants.
- Explain the essential biophysical changes that occur in infancy.
- Describe the principal theoretic explanations for sensory-perceptual, cognitive, personality, communicative, and social development in infancy.
- Identify the basic health care needs for infants.

The word "infant" is derived from Greek and Latin and means literally "one who does not speak." Infancy usually is defined as the time from birth to about 18 months of age, when children begin to speak in sentences consisting of two words. At fertilization, the tiny zygote weighs less than one millionth of an ounce. During gestation, the fetus grows into an infant weighing approximately 6 billion times more than the original cell from which it started. During infancy, the rate of growth decelerates from the gestational rate; nevertheless, rapid physical growth and maturation continue to be of primary importance.

Along with physical growth, the infant develops motor skills and considerable coordination of sensorimotor organization. Infants also begin to learn to communicate and to take an active social role. The rate of developmental progress in all these areas is more rapid during infancy than at any other time of life.

Shortly after birth, the infant appears to be relatively helpless. A number of reflexes are initially part of the infant's behavior repertoire, and infants have some rudimentary control over eye and head movements, but few other physical skills are present. During the first few months, the infant progresses from this relatively helpless state to a level of substantial skill and ability in both motor coordination and mobility. By the end of infancy, the child can sit up, crawl, walk, and even run. Infants can reach out and grasp objects to examine them, pass them from hand to hand, and manipulate them with increasing skill. The combination of neuromuscular maturation and practice leads to psychomotor coordination, which the infant quickly puts to practical use, and by the end of infancy, children can feed themselves with utensils and manipulate and play with toys in ways that were entirely impossible a few short months before.

Language development and communication progress from the ability to cry to the ability to babble in a broad range of sounds and then to the ability to imitate sounds common to the language spoken in the environment. When the child begins to put words together into two- and three-word sentences, the preverbal phase concludes, and the infant progresses to early childhood.

In this chapter, we capsulize the many changes that infancy involves. We review the various suprasystem influences, which for the infant are principally the family and its culture, expectations, and members' roles. We examine the various aspects of subsystem development—biophysical, sensory-perceptual, cognitive, personality, communication, and social—and we note the expected changes that are part of the infant's development in the first 18 months of life.

Developmental Changes in Infancy

During the first 18 months of life, the infant develops a number of social skills and abilities. A warm and deep relationship with the parent is soon translated and expanded into relationships with relatives, caregivers, or siblings. Infants show a beginning ability to enjoy peer socializing at a very simple level. In the beginning the infant's personality predominantly is evident in the satisfying of immediate needs: eating when hungry, being changed when wet, sleeping when tired. This natural egocentrism begins to broaden during the first few months, and the infant comes to recognize and respond to the emotional communication received from others. This is preparation for an emerging sense of self and for the struggle for autonomy and independence during early childhood, when children express their individual views of the world by saying "no" to virtually every proposition.

The transitions from the intrauterine environment to the outside world and then from a neonate to a walking, talking person at 18 months of age encompasses a wide variation of developmental rates and personality styles. On one hand, the development of motor skills and personality characteristics proceeds in a relatively ordered and sequential fashion. First infants roll over, then they crawl, and then they walk. A neonate will respond to all caregivers but prefers the parent after a few days, and by 9 months of age may have a substantial aversion to strangers. Within this normal sequence, each child finds a niche and forges a unique path across the developmental landscape. A precocious infant may start walking at 8 months, whereas next door, the infant born fifth into a busy family may not begin to walk until 13 months of age. However, these two individuals eventually may play side by side on their high school basketball team. The infant born as the fifth child in a family of active older siblings may never exhibit stranger anxiety because a wide range of family, friends, neighbors, and extended family is always available in the environment. Next door, the baby born first in the family might exhibit substantial stranger anxiety at 9 months. Once again, however, both may be perfectly well-adjusted children when they enter preschool together.

For all the changes and developments that take place in infancy, the development of most infants proceeds remarkably well. The nurse's role is often first to understand the sequences of development and discuss them with the parent and then to help the parent appreciate and facilitate these stages. This is an important aspect of primary prevention. Likewise, analysis of developmental delays is critical because such delays can indicate biophysical or psychosocial difficulties. Astute observations compared with the developmental history provide important cues as to the infant's overall development as well as the accomplishment of specific tasks (see Chapter 16).

Influences of the Suprasystems

Family Infants are sensitive to the social and cultural environmental influences of the suprasystems (see Chapters 3 and 4). They are innately attractive to adults, and parents tend to lavish them with attention and care without any encouragement. A firstborn infant can be a source of delight and wonder for parents, but firstborn children also are subjected to first-time parental errors, occasional overconcern, and sometimes unrealistic expectations. With subsequent infants, the parents' skills are more readily developed, but the time spent with the parents frequently is decreased. Older siblings often come to play a significant role in the social interaction and socialization process of subsequent infants. Extended family, grandparents, aunts and uncles, and close family friends also can provide an enriching and expanded network of caregiving and socialization. These individuals constitute a fabric of social influence into which the infant can be integrated.

Parents perceive their infants in substantially different ways because the effects infants have on parental values and life situations vary. Most parents eagerly await the arrival of their infants and anticipate this event as a positive, life-enhancing experience. A relatively high proportion of infants, however, are "unplanned" in that their parents were not trying actively to conceive when the pregnancy occurred. Sometimes, these infants interrupt career plans, come in the middle of schooling, or add an undesired burden on family finances and resources. Parents' reactions to their infants can also vary with the infant's temperament. A "good baby," one who is placid and makes few demands, might be easy to manage but potentially easy to ignore in the midst of pressing demands from family and other outside sources. An active, vocal, and intrusive infant can be more difficult to manage and may try parents' patience when demanding 2 A.M. feedings shortly after birth, but this infant may also move quickly into the family and be a source of enjoyment to all while insisting on taking a place within the family structure.

For example, one happy, easygoing infant seldom cried to be fed. Abby was content to watch the constant stream of activity provided by her older siblings. They adored her and spent time playing, holding, and interacting with her. Unfortunately, she was too content, and her mother found that if she did not set the alarm, Abby might miss a feeding. The older children had been very demanding as infants. Like clockwork, they cried to be fed every 3 hours, and their mother would stop whatever she was doing and take care of them. With Abby's complacency and her mother's busy schedule managing a large family, 5 or 6 hours would slip by between feedings. Abby's mother commented that it was a major transition to adapt to this infant's placid temperament.

Social and economic differences also affect parents' motivations for having an infant. For some parents, having a baby fulfills the primary purpose of marriage; for others, especially unmarried teens, the value of an infant is the increase in status and attention from society that the mother enjoys for a time. For some families, the increased demands on parental resources (both time and money) are easily accommodated; for others, these demands are sources of stress. Auxiliary and support services sometimes are available for infant care and for other household tasks, making the adjustment easier. Increased demands on time and financial stresses may, however, put a substantial strain on a marriage and try the coping skills of all the family members.

For example, the unplanned pregnancy for a couple who thought that they had completed their family and were starting to prepare for college tuitions and long-delayed travel plans resulted in a crisis. Instead of the mother obtaining a part-time job as planned, she stayed home to care for this new infant. The father took a second job to supplement their income, which necessitated weekend and evening work. The family was seldom together, the older children resented the infant, whom they blamed for changing all their plans, the mother was tired and felt "tied down" all over again, and the father did not have the energy to play games or the time to attend the numerous events in which the older children participated. The parents finally realized that changes had to be made if the family was to survive. Family life had deteriorated to the point where each member was living and acting as if no one else mattered. Fortunately, this family was able to identify that they had a problem and were willing to work together to solve it and restore the happy times of the past.

When the mother has a career or needs to be employed for financial reasons, infant care must be provided by someone else during her absence. In two-parent families, the parents may be able to accommodate each other's needs and arrange for one of them to be home to provide care. This necessitates careful planning and good communication between the parents. Sometimes, relatives live nearby and can be of assistance. Many parents, however, do not enjoy the convenience of having a family member who is capable and willing to be a caregiver and must find other resources. Such sources may be a friend, acquaintance, or someone recommended by one of them who provides infant and child care either in her own home or is willing to come to the infant's home. Nannies are gaining in popularity in the career-oriented families of the upper middle class. In fact, a few schools recently have opened to teach these skills to individuals interested in becoming a nanny. Day care is another resource that is available; however, some day-care centers do not accept infants, some limit the number of consecutive hours or total weekly hours that the infant can be there, and some are very expensive. (Criteria for selecting a day-care center and a baby-sitter are listed in Chapter 21.)

The student who has not completed high school or is in college and who decides to keep her infant may be forced to stay home rather than return to school if family members cannot assist with the infant's care. The other options are often too expensive. Some urban high schools have provided an alternative to encourage the mother to complete her education and also to serve as a resource for an elective course. The school provides facilities for day care for the infants and young children of the students and staff during school hours. The day-care site in turn provides the field work experience for a course in marriage and the family. A few colleges and universities have similar arrangements. Such on-site day care also benefits the staff and faculty who have infants or young children. Some factories and businesses have responded to their employees' requests and have made similar arrangements for on-site day care. When day care is located at the same site as the parent, there is the additional benefit of parent–child interaction during breaks and lunch. It helps the nursing mother, who can continue her classes or job and still provide for her infant's nutrition.

Another creative alternative some parents have developed is a child-care co-op in which a group of families trade equal child-care time. This is a cost-saving method but penalizes families in which the adults work full-time. Parents find it difficult to find another 40 hours in a week when child care is needed unless some adults are employed during the second or third shift and need assistance during those hours. A child-care co-op is, however, a convenient and economical method for families with part-time work commitments.

The economic position of the family determines to a large extent how infant care needs are met. Whether the infant is the firstborn or the fourth, the impact on the family is considerable. Plans and roles must consider the needs of this dependent member. It has been estimated that a child costs at least $2000 a year without any extras such as day care or private school. One mother figured that she spent as much on day care per year as she would sending the child to a mid-priced private college.

Some families adapt easily and consider the infant as a planned extension of their life and an experience to share. Other families find the infant's arrival to be a stressor that creates anxiety and turmoil and severely taxes their ability to cope. Nurses need to recognize the behaviors, questions, and comments that indicate stress. Assessment, planning, and intervention to assist and support the family then can follow (see Chapters 17 and 21).

Culture and Ethnicity The birth of an infant represents different norms and expectations for various cultural and ethnic groups. For some groups, it is a time of religious celebration, and the entire family gathers around while the infant is baptized or given a blessing by the father in a formal religious service. In some cultures taking care of the infant is strictly "women's work," and fathers keep their distance. In some American subcultures taking care of an infant becomes largely an extended family proposition. This is especially likely when a single teenage mother decides to keep her baby and live at home. Young teenagers, who are only partially grown themselves and still have substantial schooling ahead of them, frequently rely on their own parents and other extended family members to assist in childrearing. Whereas in some families this arrangement is an expected part of normal family development, in other families an unwed mother is a source of substantial family embarrassment and even shame.

Each of these variations in the suprasystem provides the infant with a different socialization experience, and family dynamics can influence personality and social development; however, infants are remarkably robust and flexible and each adapts to variations in care and social environment brought about by differences in family values and resources or differences in cultural and religious practices. Infants thrive in the snowbound wilderness environment of the Eskimo family and on the tropical islands of Fiji. There is more than one way to raise a child successfully and a wide variation in the social and emotional environments that are healthy and wholesome for an infant. Even in less-than-ideal circumstances, infants adjust remarkably well. Nurses assessing infants and their families therefore need to distinguish between unusual or less-than-optimal family environments and families that are genuinely at risk such as those extreme cases of abuse or neglect so severe that the infant will fail to thrive and severe damage may result (see Chapter 22).

Subsystem Assessment

Transition at Birth During the first few days of life, the neonate makes the transition from the warm, secure, fluid-filled intrauterine environment to the outside world, which is filled with sounds, sights, and a variety of new experiences. This transition is not without substantial adjustments; it is both abrupt and traumatic. During labor and delivery, the neonate is literally forced through the pubic opening in the pelvis and through the birth canal by the muscular contractions of the uterus. The pressure on the head is frequently so great that it is elongated and stretched at the leathery fontanels.

In addition to the abrupt environmental change at birth, the neonate must experience abrupt physiologic changes. For the first time, the heart takes on the full responsibility for pumping blood through the circulatory system; for the first time, the bronchoioles and air sacs in the lungs fill with air, and the lungs begin to supply oxygen to the blood; with the first few breaths, comes the possibility of making a sound with the vocal cords and of hearing the sound of one's own voice.

An hour or so after birth, the neonate frequently drifts off into a deep sleep that can last for many hours. Like the mother, the neonate seems to welcome the opportunity to rest after the stressful and difficult experience of labor and birth. Far from looking like the "Gerber baby," the neonate's skin is frequently red, wrinkled, covered with fine, light hair and a white, cheesy coating, and looks one or two sizes too large. Some neonates have heads full of hair (which sometimes falls out during the first few months), whereas others are completely bald. During the first few days, when the neonate is making the transition from a completely dependent to an independent person, certain specific characteristics and abilities aid in supporting the infant's psychologic status and developmental maturity. Figure 7-1 indicates the variety of developmental changes that occur from birth to about 56 weeks of age.

Neonatal Assessment A number of measurements and test procedures frequently are employed to evaluate the neonate—the Apgar evaluation (Apgar, 1953); birthweight and length; physical assessment, including a neurologic examination (for example, Prechtl and Beintema, 1964); and the Brazelton Neonatal Behavioral Assessment Scale (Brazelton, 1973).

Assessment Guides The *Apgar evaluation* was developed by Virginia Apgar (1953) and is particularly sensitive to oxygen deprivation, which may have occurred during labor and delivery or is evident in infants with neurologic or respiratory disorders. The Apgar evaluation is administered at 1 minute and again at 5 minutes after birth to evaluate the neonate's ability to support vital functions. Five variables—heart rate, respiratory effort, muscle tone, reflex irritability, and body color—are given a score of 0, 1, or 2 (Table 7-1). A high score of from 8 to 10 at 5 minutes indicates that the neonate is in good condition in that the blood is oxygenated. A score of 3 or lower indicates that immediate emergency steps may be necessary to help the infant survive.

The standard physical assessment parallels the physical examination (Chapter 14), whereas the neurologic examination evaluates the gestational age and neuromuscular response of the neonate. The *Brazelton Neonatal Behavioral Assessment Scale* (BNBAS) (1973) includes some elements of the neurologic examination and some fundamental social interaction behaviors. It has been found to predict developmental vulnerability and developmental delays reasonably well, and it is used increasingly in a number of professional settings (see Chapter 16).

Birthweight and Length The birthweight for neonates is between 2500 and 4300 g (5.5 and 9.5 lb). Birth length is between 46 and 56 cm (18 and 22 in), with the average being 50 cm (20 in) (Schuster and Ashburn, 1980, p.118). Birthweights above 4550 g (10 lb) may be an indication of problems with developmental physiology or problems associated with the mother's physiology during the last weeks of pregnancy. A low birthweight is considered to be less than 2500 grams (5.5 lb). A low birthweight frequently indicates some kind of developmental problem during gestation and is associated with multiple risk conditions (see Chapter 31). The frequency of low birthweight is higher for minority women, those with lower socioeconomic status, and those who have experienced complications during pregnancy.

Reflexes Although neonates appear to be fragile and perhaps slightly alien, their behaviors are very well directed. Behaviors that initially seem to have little to do with mature human functioning are closely related and even predictive of later-developing perceptual and motor skills. Among the best evidences of the sophistication of the neonatal nervous

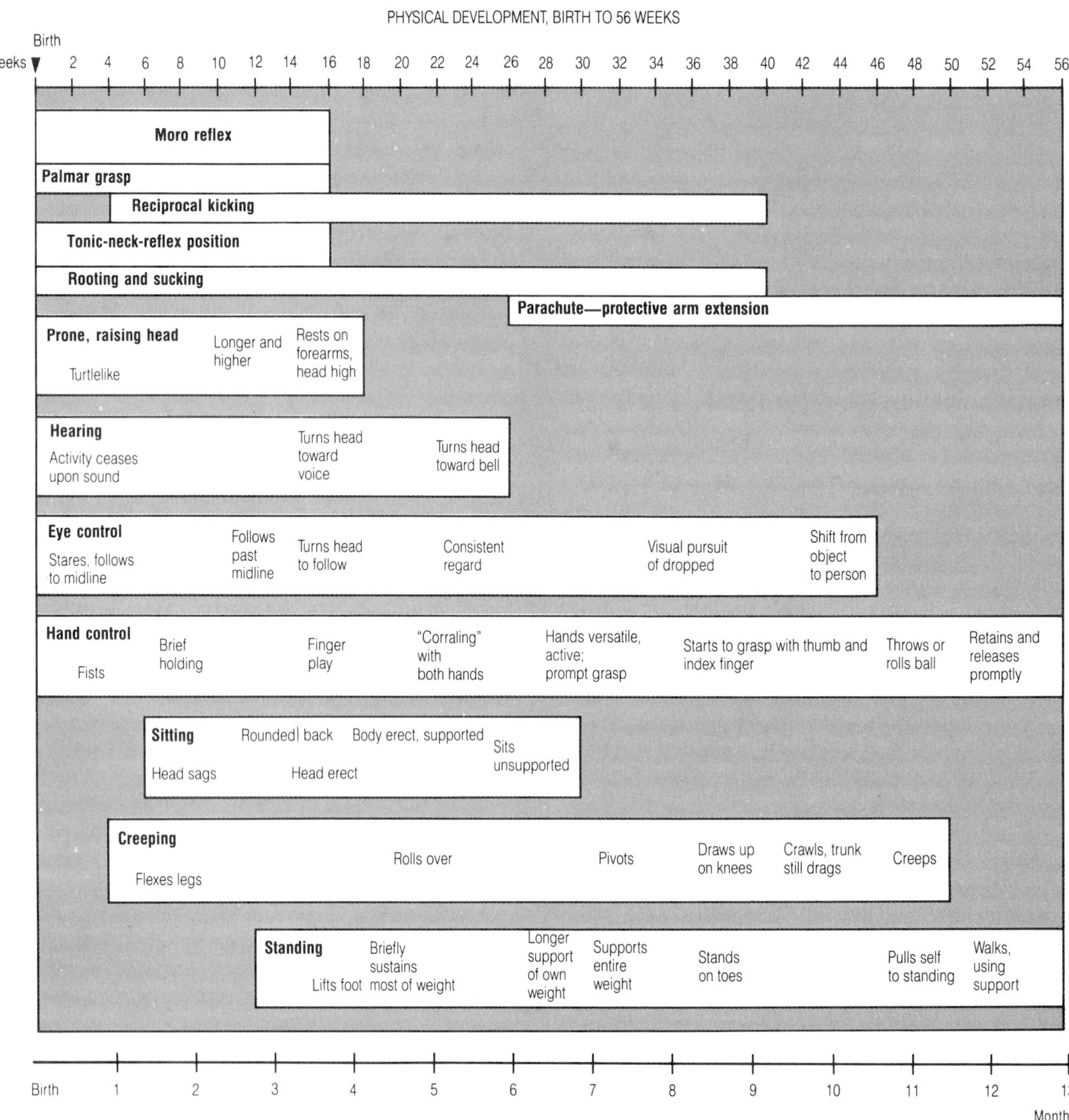

Figure 7-1 Developmental changes from birth to 56 weeks of age.

system are the neonate's reflexes. Reflexes are specific patterns of behavioral response to directly focused stimulation. Table 7-2 indicates some of the most common reflexes.

Alterations in these reflexes resulting in consistent weakness, absence, or asymmetry may indicate defects or neurologic damage in the areas tested. Reflex testing is, consequently, included in the standard neurologic and behavioral examinations. Some reflexes have obvious adaptive purposes, and some are directly related to later-developing competencies. The pupillary and blinking reflexes, for example, are lifelong and serve an obvious protective function for the visual system. Grasping and walking reflexes, although initially strong, fade after the first couple of months, and these tasks have to be relearned later. Rooting and sucking reflexes also have great survival value. Some reflexes, such as the Babinski, abdominal, and tonic neck reflexes, are not obviously tied to later-developing behaviors. They are, nevertheless, helpful in assessing the functioning and

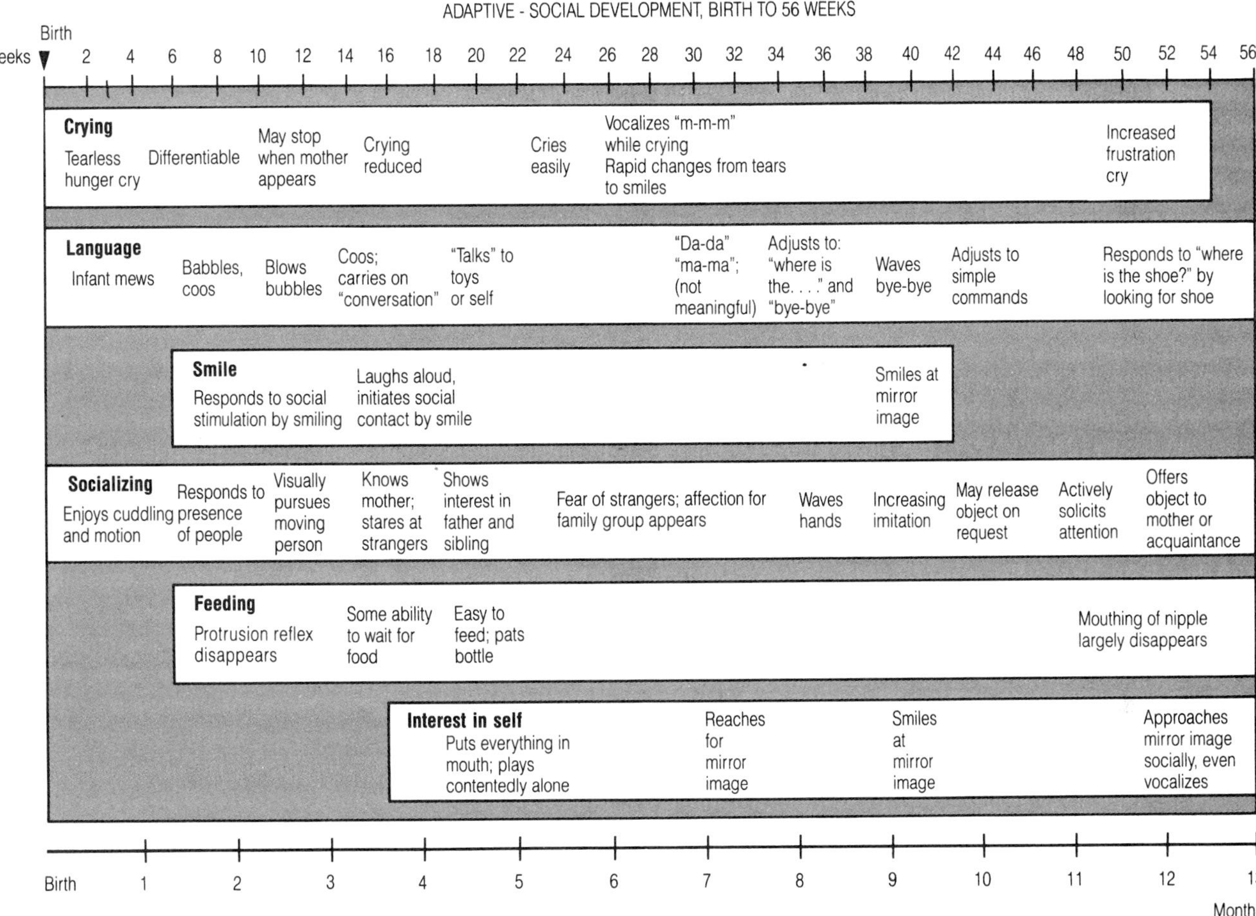

maturation of the neonate's central nervous system (Florentino, 1973).

As the infant makes the transition from the prenatal environment through birth, these reflexes facilitate emerging from one kind of world into another. At birth, the cerebral cortex is not fully capable of controlling the infant's body and giving meaningful direction to behavior. Reflexes provide some necessary involuntary responses and give the brain and central nervous system time to mature and begin to take over the controlled coordinated behaviors. During the neonatal transition phase, many of these reflexes are prominent enough to have predictive value for later levels

TABLE 7-1 Apgar Scoring Chart for Evaluating the Status of the Newborn

Sign	0 points	1 point	2 points
Heart rate	Absent	Slow (less than 100)	Greater than 100
Respiratory effort	Absent	Slow, irregular	Good strong cry
Muscle tone	Limp	Some flexion of extremities	Extremities well flexed, active motion
Reflex—irritability (response to catheter in nostril)	No response	Grimace	Cough, sneeze, or cry
Color	Blue, pale	Body pink, extremities blue	Completely pink

SOURCE: Apgar VA: The newborn (Apgar) scoring system. *Pediatr Clin North Am* 1966; 13:645. W.B. Saunders Company. Reprinted by permission.

TABLE 7-2 Common Reflexes of the Neonate

Reflex name	Evoking stimulus	Response
Blinking reflex	Light flash	Closing eyelids
Pupillary reflex	Light flash	Constriction of the pupil to brighter light
Rooting reflex	Light touch of finger on cheek close to mouth	Head rotation toward the stimulation; mouth opening and attempt to suck finger. Disappears by about 4 months of age
Sucking reflex	Finger (or nipple) inserted into mouth	Rhythmic sucking
Moro reflex	Infant lying on back with head slightly raised; head is suddenly released. Or infant is held horizontally, then lowered quickly about 6 in and stopped abruptly	Arms extended out, head thrown back, fingers spread wide; arms then brought back to center convulsively with hands clenched; extension of spine and lower extremities. Disappears by about 6 months of age
Startle reflex	Loud noise	Similar to Moro reflex flexion in arms; fists clenched
Grasping reflex	Finger placed in palm of hand	Infant's fingers closed around and grasped
Babkin reflex	Infant lying on back, pressure applied on both palms	Head turned to midline, mouth open, eyes closed. Disappears by about 4 months of age
Tonic neck reflex	Head turned to one side while infant lies on back	Arm and leg extended on the side the infant faces. Opposite arm and leg are flexed
Abdominal reflex	Tactile stimulation or tickling	Contraction of the abdominal muscles
Withdrawal reflex	Slight pinprick to the sole of the infant's foot	Leg flexes
Walking reflex	Infant supported in an upright position with feet lightly touching a flat surface	Rhythmic stepping movement. Disappears at about 4 months of age
Babinski reflex	Gentle stroking on the sole of the foot	Fanning and extension of the toes (adults respond with flexion of toes to this stimulation)
Plantar, or toe-grasping, reflex	Pressure applied with the finger against the balls of the infant's feet	A plantar flexion of all toes. Disappears by the end of the first year of life
Swimming reflex	Infant placed prone in 2 in of water (avoid water in nose and mouth)	Arm and leg swimming-like movement

of functioning and are more predictive than similar behavioral examinations conducted later in infancy. Some abnormal functioning that can be detected using reflexive evaluations may not appear for several months or even years. Although these abnormalities can be detected in the neonate, they may disappear during a "silent" period until they emerge as problems in later development (Prechtl and Beintema, 1964) (see Chapter 16).

The Moro reflex may serve as a barometer of central nervous system functioning. Its presence, absence, and hyper- or hyporesponsiveness at various ages is often a clue that some other problem may exist. Because the Moro reflex is strongest for a full-term normal infant during the first 8 weeks of life, the nurse should be suspicious if there is an obvious diminished response during these weeks. Diminishment of the reflex might indicate a birth injury, postbirth injury, or a congenital anomaly that has caused cerebral pressure. Sometimes, the cerebral pressure is related to cerebral edema or other factors present at birth. In these situations the Moro reflex may be absent initially and gradually appear as the edema decreases or other factors, such as hemorrhage, are treated.

There is a normal transition in the characteristics of the Moro reflex. Around $2-2\frac{1}{2}$ months of age, the vigorous, total-body, easily elicited response becomes more controlled, deliberate, and refined. Then, with the increased

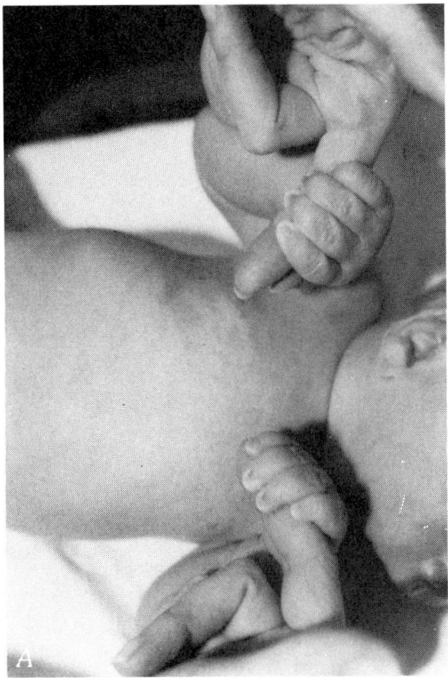

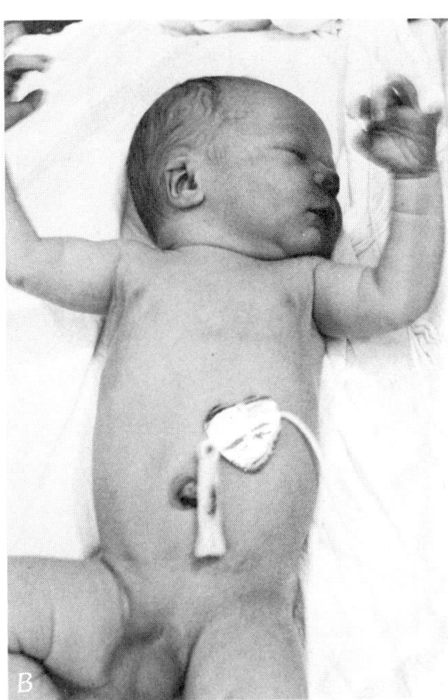

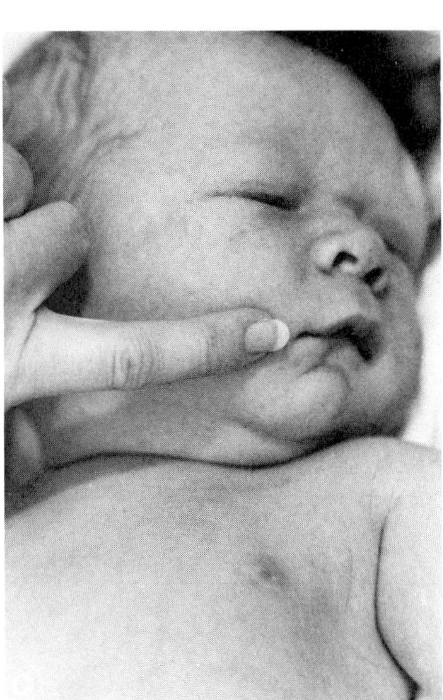

Neonatal reflexes. *A*. Grasping reflex. *B*. Moro reflex. *C*. Rooting reflex. (From Swearingen PL: *The Addison-Wesley Photo-Atlas of Nursing Procedures*. Addison-Wesley, 1984.)

maturation of the central nervous system and better integrative capacity of the 3-to $3\frac{1}{2}$-month-old, the response becomes a simple body-jerk denoting the appropriate waning of the reflex. By 6 months of age, the Moro reflex should no longer be present (Haynes, 1977). When the reflex persists after 6 months, it could have developmental or neurologic significance. Paine (1964) noted the abnormal, extended presence of the Moro reflex in some children with spastic tetraparesis and in some children who later developed athetosis.

More important than any one indicator or single abnormal reflex pattern is the presence of a cluster of warning signs. Primitive reflexes present at birth should give way to righting reflexes (neck, head, and body righting), which are followed by protective reactions (parachute reflex) and finally by equilibrium or balance reactions (sitting, standing). There is a standard age when the reflexes should disappear or appear (Fig. 7-2). The infant's pattern can be compared with the standard to assess neuromotor development.

Subsystem Interaction Progressive development is complex and involves more than neuromotor behaviors, as demonstrated by reflex responses to various stimuli. Development evolves from the interplay of the subsystems as they interact and mutually support task accomplishment. Growth and development of all subsystems occurs simultaneously with the maturation of the neurophysical system. The infant actively learns about the environment and its properties while assimilating experiences into innate schemes or modifying the schemes to accommodate the events and objects that are different. In addition, the infant's subjective experience and perception of events further contributes to behavior organization. Korner (1979) wondered if this repeated self-interpretation and self-experience might be responsible for continuity in the development of a sense of self. The social subsystem also is influential as the infant develops in response to interactions with the environment and especially the parents. These early parent–child interactions may be synchronous, leading to positive results, and thus confirm the child's sense of being able to influence the environment. If, however, interactional asynchrony occurs, the child has limited feedback and is then unable to identify a consistent response to expressed needs. The presence of synchrony or asynchrony affects the infant's future attempts to achieve need satisfaction, attention, and mutual regulation.

Development is never one-dimensional; rather, it is the amalgamation of the infant's characteristics, original tendencies, and responses to intricate environmental influences. A lag in physical development, for example, may be the result of an unresponsive or chaotic social environment. Gesell (1954) commented that an infant cannot learn to smile in response to a smiling person if a smiling person seldom is present.

As the subsystems work together to maintain homeostasis, a consistency of expression, style, tempo, and intensity develops that tends to recur with each new developmental acquisition. For example, infants respond differently but consistently to changes in blood glucose level and hunger sensations. Each infant has a unique pattern, including

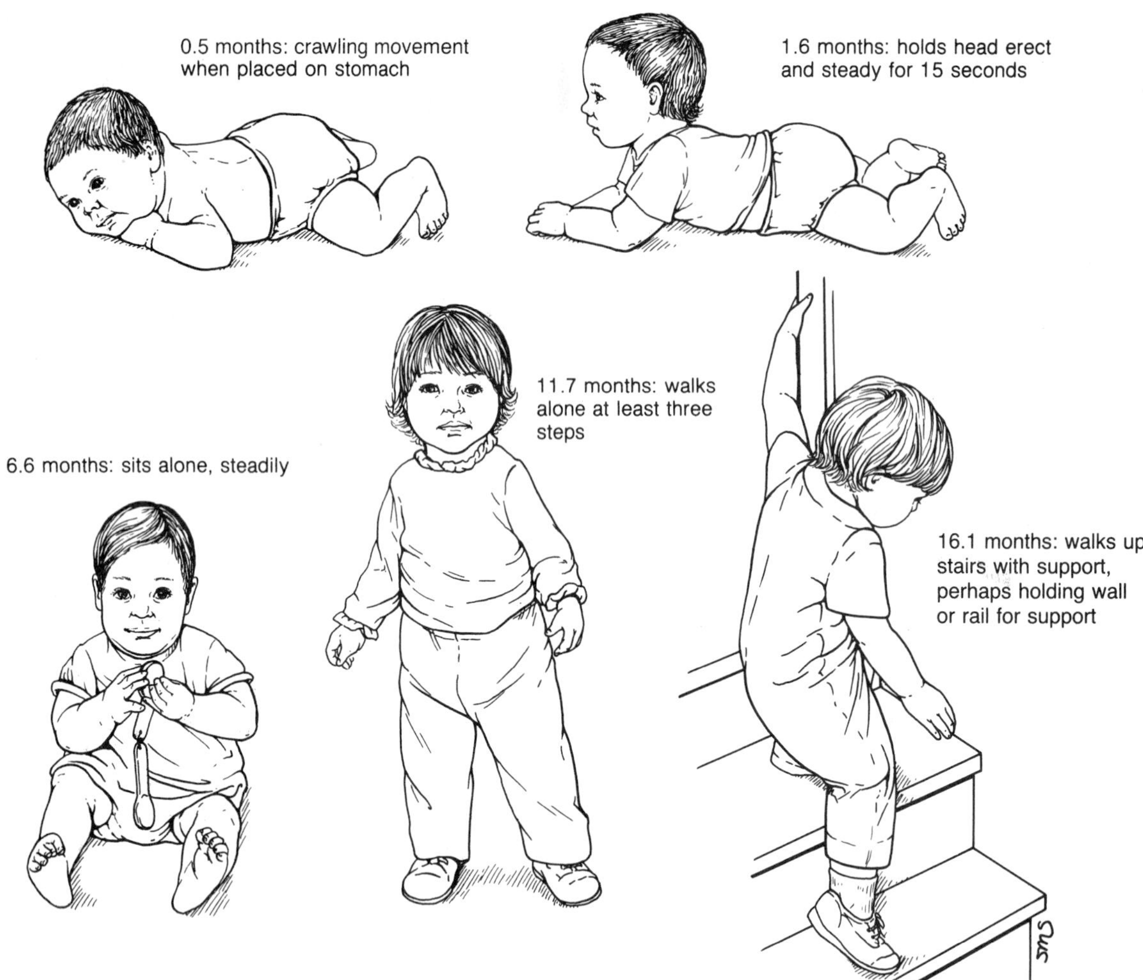

Figure 7-2 Sequence of motor development with average ages at which infant achieves coordination.

intensity of reaction, ability to delay gratification, self-comforting behaviors, ability to elicit assistance from others, and skills or resources for diversion. This combined interplay becomes evident in what has been described and generalized as the quiet, average, and active infant (Brazelton 1970). Some infants move rapidly from one new skill to another. Each challenge is attacked vigorously with instant success sought so the next challenge can be confronted. These infants may walk at 9 or 10 months of age. Other infants tend to practice and delight in each skill attained and have no desire to hurry on to the next one. They may not walk until they are 15 or 16 months old. The third group, or average infants, progress from skill to skill at a rate somewhere between the two extremes. Although enjoying each new skill, they are eager for a new challenge and are usually walking around 12–13 months of age. All three groups are developmentally normal expressions of generalized response patterns, thus demonstrating mutual subsystem influence and support.

Parameters of Infant Development

Biophysical Development

Length and Weight Following birth, infants lose 5%–10% of their birthweight until they stabilize within a few days, establish fluid balance, and start to gain weight. The median birthweight is 3.23 kg (7 lb) for girls and 3.27 kg ($7\frac{1}{4}$ lb) for boys. Within a week or two after birth, the birthweight is achieved, and increments continue at about 2 lb (0.9 kg) per month for the first 3 months. By approximately 5 months of age, the birthweight has doubled and weight gain slows slightly to 1 lb (0.45 kg) per month until 1 year of age. Most infants triple their birthweight in the first year. The amount of weight gained is important, but even more critical is whether the increments are steady and continue along their percentile curve on the growth chart (see Appendix A). Infants who are below the tenth percentile or above the ninetieth percentile or who deviate two percentile groups from their previously established curve require further assessment and evaluation (Lowrey, 1978).

At birth, the median length is 49.9 cm ($19\frac{3}{4}$ in) for girls and 50.5 cm (20 in) for boys. Length increments average 1 in (2.54 cm) per month for the first 6 months and then slow. By 1 year of age, the increase in length is 50% of birth length, although, again, the actual numbers are influenced by a host of genetic and environmental factors. The important consideration is the steady gain along the infant's designated percentile as established soon after birth (Lowrey, 1978).

On the average, girls are slightly shorter and weigh slightly less than boys, although the differences between the sexes in both weight and stature become more pronounced with age. The average weight for girls is about 1 lb (0.45 kg) less than that for boys at 1 year of age. At 1 year, girls are also approximately $1\frac{1}{2}$–2 in (3.80–5.80 cm) shorter than boys, but by 2 years of age, girls have caught up and are about the same average height (National Center for Health Statistics, 1979).

Birthweight is influenced by the mother's size and by the internal capacity of the uterus, one of the reasons that birthweight does not differ much between the sexes. Some infants are genetically "programmed" to be physically large; it is as if they have "big genes." Because birthweight is influenced by maternal factors, however, infants who have a genetic predisposition to be large but are born to small mothers make rapid weight and length gains during the first few months of life. This phenomenon is known as "birth catch-up." Because the first few months allow the infant to manifest genetic tendencies for size and stature, correlations of birth stature and ultimate adult height are not as reliable as correlations made during early childhood.

Never at any time during life, not even during the adolescent growth spurt, do physical stature and weight increase at such an accelerated rate. This is most obvious to parents, who witness the rapid rate at which infants grow out of clothes. Stretchy jump suits and sleepwear can be more practical than clothing made of nonelastic material, which will likely be worn for only a month or two at most.

An infant's proportions are substantially different from those of an adult. Two months after conception, the fetus' head is approximately half of the length of the body. At birth, the head still takes up one quarter of the infant's body length, as compared with only about one eighth of the adult's body length. Infants are large-headed because the neurons in the brain develop before birth. The eyes, for example, are approximately adult size.

Median head circumference at birth is 34.3 cm ($13\frac{1}{2}$ in) for girls and 34.8 cm ($13\frac{3}{4}$ in) for boys. This circumference of the head is larger than the circumference of the chest, but at approximately 1 year of age, the chest and head are equal in circumference, and thereafter the chest is always larger. About half of adult height is the length of the legs. An infant's legs are approximately one third of the body length, and they tend to be slightly curved or bowed during the first few months of life. Both legs and trunk grow about equally during the first year, but then the legs begin to accelerate and grow more rapidly. Neonates who seem skinny and wiry rapidly add fatty tissue and, later on, muscle tissue, so that all infants appear cherubic.

Neurologic Maturation The first period of histologic development of the brain involves neuroblastic multiplication. During this period, which is completed about midway through prenatal development, the fetus attains the actual number of adult nerve cells. Normal brain development, however, involves much more than the potential number of neurons.

The second period of development consists of the rapid growth of neurons. *Neurons* are the nerve cells of the brain and comprise about 10% (or 12 billion cells) of brain tissue. Neurons, whose number is complete at birth, are responsible for consciousness, memory, voluntary and involuntary sensory and motor responses to stimuli, and thought control. During infancy, the size of the neurons increase but not their number. The third period begins during the latter half of prenatal development and continues through the fourth year of life. This phase includes an increase in the number and size of the *glial* cells (otherwise known as the supporting cells, which account for 90% of brain tissue), myelinization, and increase in length of the *axons* and elaboration of the branchings and number of dendrites (Lowrey, 1978: Freiberg, 1983).

Young infants have few *dendrites*, that is, the branched extensions surrounding the nucleus and cytoplasm of the neuron that receive nerve impulses from other nearby neurons. The proliferation of dendrites during infancy allows for better transmission of sensory and motor nerve impulses from one axon across a *synapse* to the dendrite of another neuron. Concurrently, the process of myelinization, begun around the fourth prenatal month, progresses to the afferent nerve fibers that transmit motor impulses to produce voluntary movement or speech. By birth, most of the afferent nerves (transmitters of sensory impulses) and the nerves of the brain stem are fairly well myelinated. This accounts for the early domination of reflex activity in the infant.

Myelinization is the encasement of the axon (the single long impulse transmitter of each neuron) by a white, fatty substance. Myelin increases the speed of nerve impulses and improves the accuracy with which they reach their destination. Both factors are important for efficient, sophisticated brain activity. The order in which the neurons are myelinated corresponds to the sequence of development; for example, myelinization of the spinal cord follows the cephalocaudal direction. From birth to 2 years of age, the

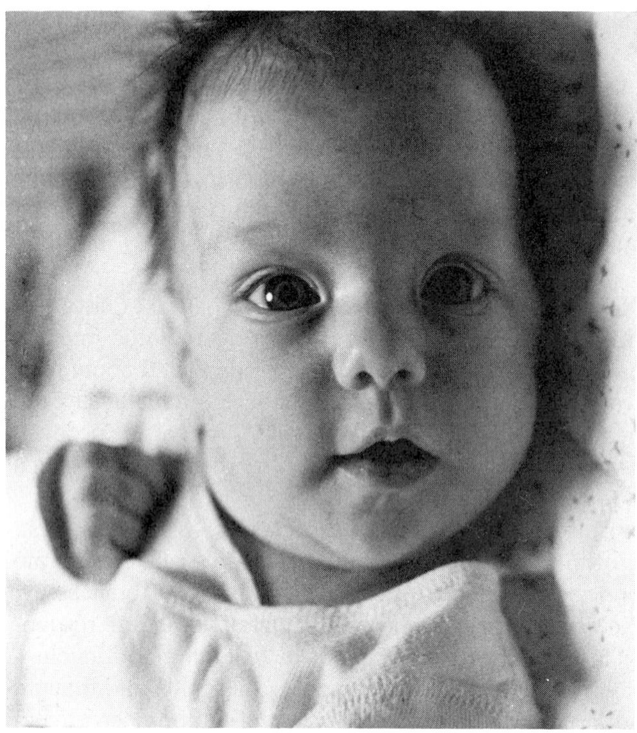

The neonate's random motion develops so that movements are increasingly directed.

cerebral cortex is rapidly myelinated, thus facilitating sensorimotor coordination, as evidenced in walking, running, manipulating small objects, or tossing a beach ball. As myelinization continues to the cortical association areas, early perceptual symbolic functioning appears in speech and the symbolic use of toys in play. Development in this area continues during early childhood (Yussen and Santrock, 1982).

These factors—the number of neurons, number of glial cells, amount of myelinization, dendritic proliferation, and synaptic connections—singly and jointly create the conditions necessary for the development of higher mental functions. Each factor performs a role. Its exact nature is unknown, but the result is significant and evident in the developing person's capacity for thought and behavior.

An indicator of this maturation process is the increase in size and weight of the brain. At birth, the average brain weight is 325 g (0.7 lb), increasing to 1000 g (2.2 lb) at 1 year of age. Thereafter, growth slows, and the average adult brain weight is 1400 g (3.1 lb). Actual brain cell development depends mostly on diet, first during pregnancy and lactation and then increasingly for the infant as other foods are introduced as weaning takes place. Adequate nutrition is therefore essential throughout the entire period of infancy to ensure proper brain growth.

Gross Motor Skills Related to actual growth in brain weight is a remarkable increase in the infant's ability to perform increasingly complex behavioral tasks. Abilities both with gross motor behaviors involving major combinations of muscle systems and fine motor behavior involving more precise and purposeful movements of selective muscle groupings occur simultaneously and rapidly during infancy (Fig. 7-2).

Two major principles—the cephalocaudal and the proximal-distal principles (see Fig. 6-2)—describe the development of gross and fine motor behavior during infancy. The neonate has substantial control over eye, head, and mouth movements. Control over the upper body, torso, and legs develops in that order during infancy, thus demonstrating the cephalocaudal principle. The neonate randomly flails both arms or moves them in synchrony to sound. The infant develops sequentially the ability to swing one or both arms in a desired direction, then the ability to strike an object, usually a toy dangling within reach, with one hand, and finally the ability to reach out and grasp.

Fine Motor Skills The cephalocaudal principle therefore defines much of gross motor behavior. The proximal-distal principle, on the other hand, defines the development and coordination of fine motor skills. These begin with uncoordinated thrashing of the arms and legs and progress to purposeful arm, wrist, hand, and finger movements.

The ability to reach out and handle objects—*visually directed reaching*—is an important skill that enables the infant personally to explore the surroundings. Visually directed reaching coupled with an infant's innate tendency to put everything into the mouth requires that the infant be monitored closely at all times. Small or dangerous objects that might be aspirated (for example, marbles or grapes) or that could do damage if swallowed (for example, safety pins or coins) should be kept out of reach. On the positive side, visually directed reaching and increasing fine motor

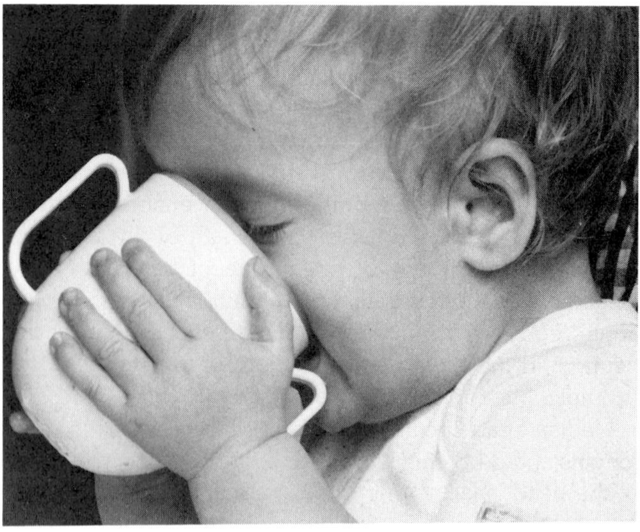

The ability to reach, grasp, and control an object is indicative of developing fine motor skills.

coordination enable the infant to feed himself or herself, initially using hands and fingers and then advancing to the use of a spoon. It also encourages practicing the newly acquired skills of grasping toys of different shapes and weights, using the pincer grasp to manipulate small objects as picking up a raisin or holding a block in each hand while alternately inspecting and banging them together.

A child who is especially slow in developing motor skills may be at risk. Assessment guides were, in fact, developed to identify infants with serious lags in normal development so that further testing could determine the cause of the developmental delay.

For the overwhelming majority of children and parents, however, monitoring physical skills as they develop is a source of delight and satisfaction and sometimes even of surprise as the persistent infant makes a tremendous effort to develop skills that older children and adults take for granted.

Assessing Motor Skills Chapter 16 covers the principal developmental criteria nd guidelines for assessing gross motor development. In measuring any infant against normative milestones for motor development, the nurse should recognize that individual variation is likely for any infant and that the normal range of variation for the development of most of these behaviors lasts several months. For example, just because infants usually don't roll over until the end of the second month doesn't mean that any particular infant won't roll over before that. One startled mother left her infant on the changing table for a moment to get a clean diaper and was surprised to hear a thump followed by screams from the infant, who had just rolled over for the first time and rolled off the changing table in the process.

Another major advance is the infant's self-initiated and actively pursued exploration of the world that occurs with crawling and walking. For the first time, mobility provides independent access to portions of the world that the infant has only examined from afar. Although the first steps are frequently a source of family excitement, they also herald potential stress and risk. Nothing is safe as the curious infant moves quickly from room to room discovering the previously hidden treasures inside of cupboards, on top of coffee tables, in bookcases, and under beds. Sometimes the infant examines costly and fragile treasures with disastrous results long before the parent anticipated they would be discovered. Accidents also are all too common in infancy and include falling down steps, getting into the road, or climbing into a bathtub full of water. Infants who are developing these self-locomotion skills need increased and constant supervision when they are in circumstances that could be dangerous.

Cardiovascular System Birth initiates several changes in the cardiovascular system. Once born, the infant has to be self-sufficient in transporting oxygen and nutrients to the cells and waste products from the cells to the appropriate system for excretion. Once the umbilical cord is clamped, the umbilical vessels have no purpose and become fibrotic within 2–5 days. This shift in blood flow away from the placenta and to the general circulation causes the diameter of the inferior vena cava to increase (Fig. 7-3).

Similarly, the size of the aortic arch increases with the closure of the ductus arteriosus. With closure, the blood flow through the ascending aorta increases because it is the only outflow source of the left ventricle, whose volume and pressure increase in response to physiologic changes at birth. The ductus arteriosus takes as long as several weeks to close completely, resulting in transient shunting of blood during the first week or so of life. Closure is related to the increased degree of oxygen saturation of the blood. The volume of blood flow is also greater because of the increased size of the pulmonary vascular bed.

The foramen ovale also ceases to have a function after birth. With independent respiration for resultant oxygen transport, the pulmonary vasculature requirements increase considerably. No longer is blood shunted away from this site. From the moment of the first breath, the pressure changes in the atria. It rises in the left and falls in the right secondary to decreased pulmonary resistance and diminished placental venous return. Although functionally closed shortly after birth, anatomic closure takes several weeks.

These particular transformations result in the overall change from an essentially singular or mixed pattern of circulation to a well-defined, two-sided circulation—the right side consisting of unoxygenated blood and waste products and the left side consisting of oxygenated blood and nutrients.

The neonate's heart lies horizontally in the thoracic cavity. With growth and increased capacity, the heart gradually shifts to a more vertical position. The right ventricle initially is more muscular and weighs 13% more than the left ventricle; this reflects the direction of the fetal cardiac work load. After birth, however, the muscle mass of the left ventricle increases at a greater rate, which reflects a switch in the direction of the work load. By 4–5 months of age, the

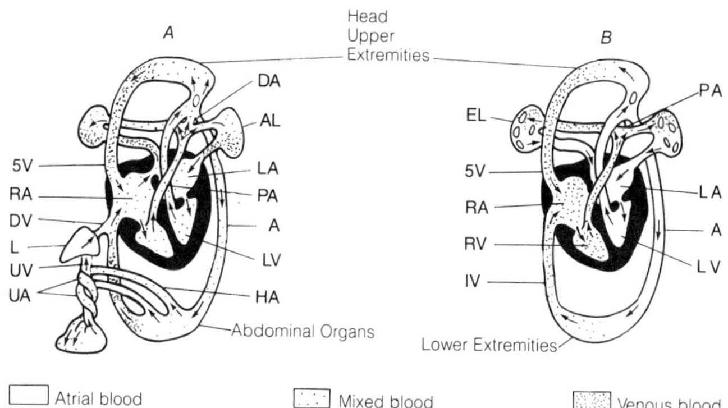

Figure 7-3 Circulatory changes at birth. *A*. Fetal circulation. *B*. Normal postpartum circulation.

weight of the ventricles is equal, and thereafter the left ventricle is thicker, eventually reaching the adult ratio of two to three times as thick as the right ventricle (Lowrey, 1978).

The total size and weight of the heart increases rapidly and, in fact, doubles during the first year of life. This phenomenon results in greater efficiency of each contraction, as chambers can accommodate and pump a greater volume and therefore do not have to contract as frequently. The neonate's heart rate averages 120–140 beats/min, whereas the heart rate of a 1-year-old is 115 beats/min. As the heart rate slows, there is a corresponding rise in blood pressure from a systolic pressure of 78 at birth to 96 at 1 year of age. Obtaining accurate readings is extremely difficult, because the heart rate is controlled by the involuntary nervous system, and the wide variation in readings depends on whether the infant is awake, crying, or asleep. Activity results in a more active heart rate and sleep or rest in a slower heart rate.

At birth, the neonate's ability to stabilize body temperature is immature. It takes several weeks for the small capillaries to expand and contract appropriately in response to the external temperature. Thus, the parent must dress the neonate to provide the necessary warmth or cooling. With maturation, the hormones and involuntary nervous system take control, and the capillaries work efficiently. Another indication of immature capillary function is the phenomenon of *acrocyanosis,* the cyanotic appearance of the feet, hands, and sometimes the lips. These peripheral parts are also cool to touch. Acrocyanosis disappears during the first month as the capillary response to temperature change improves.

The neonate's circulating blood volume is directly related to the length of time between birth and clamping of the umbilical cord. Late clamping results in an increase of blood volume by as much as 60% over early clamping. The average volume is 80–110 ml/kg in the neonate and declines slowly to 75–90 ml/kg in the older infant. Blood values reflect blood volume and the maturity of the hematopoietic process. The red blood cells and hemoglobin levels are highest after birth, fluctuate during the first 6 months of life, and attain fairly steady levels by 1 year of age.

Respiratory System Birth inaugurates respiration. The stimulus for the onset of respiration is believed to be anoxia resulting from a lack of placental oxygenation when the umbilical cord is clamped. The anoxia in turn causes chemical changes at various sites such as the medulla and aortic and carotid chemoreceptors.

The first breaths expand the collapsed alveoli. The vigorous cries of the neonate are important as these first breaths are perhaps the most difficult because of the resistance of the smaller bronchi and alveoli. The number of alveoli rapidly increases during the first 6 months of life, and their weight doubles during that time. By 1 year of age, the weight of the lungs is triple that of birth (Lowrey, 1978).

Infants use accessory muscles, especially the diaphragm, for breathing, and their pattern of respiration is therefore termed *diaphragmatic.* The rate, depth, and rhythm of an infant's respiration are variable and related to immaturity.

The other anatomic features of the respiratory system are significant because of their relative size. The trachea is only 4 cm long at birth and its diameter is one-fourth that of the adult's. The supporting cartilage is softer, and the epiglottis is located higher (at the first cervical vertebra), as is the bifurcation of the trachea (at the third to fourth thoracic vertebra), all of which make the infant more vulnerable to respiratory distress (Valadian and Porter, 1977; Lowrey, 1978).

The neonate's respiratory rate is rapid. This is due in part to the presence of anatomic dead space where air moves but without gas exchange. In addition, the high metabolic rate increases the demand for gas exchange, further supporting the rapid rate. With maturation, the rate decreases gradually from 40 to 60 to 30 to 40 breaths/min.

Infants are obligatory nose breathers from birth until 3–4 months of age. Mouth breathing must be learned, an important concern when an infant experiences any nasal congestion or obstruction. Before they learn to mouth-breathe, infants take single gasps or respond to anoxia by crying but then close their mouths and breathe through their noses until anoxia once again results.

Gastrointestinal System Aided by the rooting, sucking, and swallowing reflexes, the neonate is capable of ingesting and digesting breast milk or its equivalent. Some infants have strong sucking reflexes immediately after birth, whereas others will take up to 4 days to develop an effective suck. The neonate's sucking reflex is different from the older infant's. The mouth is specially shaped, with a longer soft palate and shorter distance from the mouth to pharynx to facilitate sucking and swallowing without aspiration, anatomic differences that help the young infant learn to coordinate sucking, swallowing, and breathing. By 6 months of age, the mouth is proportioned like that of an adult.

The suck of the young infant also is aided by the tongue thrust reflex, by which the infant's tongue is thrust against and underneath the nipple to express the milk. This reflex gets in the way and is often misinterpreted by a parent feeding an infant solid foods for the first time. When cereal is added to the diet, the young infant has to learn a new way of handling food, that is, pushing it to the back of the mouth. The tongue thrust reflex disappears around 6 months of age, at the same time that lateral jaw movements become coordinated. Many infants are then able to respond favorably to solid foods.

Saliva is present at birth, but many of the salivary glands do not start producing saliva until the third month. Increased saliva production is evidenced by an increase in drooling. Few neonates have diets high in starch, so they do not need large amounts of the enzyme ptyalin that is present in saliva.

So little of the neonate's food stays in the mouth for any length of time that the enzyme is essentially ineffective at this stage, although it is present in adequate supply by the time most infants start to eat solid foods.

The capacity of the neonate's stomach is approximately 90 mL (3 oz). The stomach grows rapidly during the first 3 months of life and then grows more slowly, so that by 1 year of age, the capacity is 210–360 mL (7–9 oz) (Lowrey, 1978). Young infants require feeding every $2\frac{1}{2}$–4 hours because their stomachs are smaller and empty more rapidly. Other factors that promote stomach emptying are food that is too cold or high in carbohydrates, large quantities of food at one time, and positioning the infant on the abdomen or right side after feeding. Many infants have poor muscle tone in the lower esophageal sphincter, which results in their spitting up. Maturation and more time spent in an upright position are usually all that is required to cure this problem.

Some breakdown of protein in the stomach is caused by hydrochloric acid and rennin, but most digestion takes place in the small intestine. The length of the gut grows by 50% during the first year, and most of the digestive enzymes, such as the pancreatic amylase, lipase, and trypsin, together with bile, reach adult proportions by 1 year of age.

The young infant has many stools, often following each feeding. This is due in part to the composition of the feeding but also to the immature large intestine. Water is not well absorbed, so that the stools are soft, liquid, and frequent. With maturation, the addition of solid foods, and increased bacterial flora, stools become less frequent and firmer. The nature and frequency of stools are related to the infant's diet. The neonate's first stool is *meconium*. This greenish-black, sticky substance is a combination of bile, cast-off epithelial cells, other digestive juices, and amniotic fluid. Meconium is present for a couple of days and gradually changes to the soft, yellow stools, which are lighter for breast-fed infants and darker yellow or brownish for formula-fed infants. The addition of new food is often evident in changes in the stool. Various vegetables, for example, may offset the stool's color and sometimes its consistency.

The musculature of the anal sphincter develops as the infant becomes more upright. By the end of this developmental phase, some regularity in the timing and number of stools usually is evident. Release is still involuntary, however, and most infants are not yet ready for or capable of responding to toilet training.

Genitourinary System The neonate's excretory system is anatomically complete but functionally immature. The musculature of the bladder is not well developed, and the involuntary release of urine occurs throughout infancy.

Bladder capacity is only 15 mL, and the bladder is emptied involuntarily whenever this amount is attained. Involuntary voiding results in 20 or more voidings per day, which explains why parents complain that the infant is always wet. The immature infant is still unable to concentrate urine so it appears like water—colorless, odorless, and with a specific gravity around 1.008.

Although the infant can produce urine, urination occurs at the expense of a large turnover of water. Reabsorption and filtration functions in the renal tubules are limited, but these functions are essentially attained by 6 months of age. Some of the epithelium of the kidney is very thick and is thus an inefficient filter. As the epithelial layer thins, it becomes capable of reabsorbing the urinary filtrates for bodily use, thereby concentrating the urine.

The infant's kidneys are primarily responsible for maintaining fluid and electrolyte balance and filtering wastes from the blood. Initially, the infant's fluid requirement is greater than the adult's because a greater proportion of liquid is excreted. By the same token, the infant cannot tolerate excessive fluid intake, and there is a precarious between adequate hydration and dehydration (60–75 mL/kg/24 hr) on one hand and overhydration on the other hand (over 160 mL/kg/24 hr). With maturation, increased tubular size, and a functional epithelium, the kidneys become more efficient and are able to make internal adjustments in response to external factors and fluid load.

Integumentary System The neonate's skin is thinner and more sensitive than that of the older infant and certainly that of the adult. The infant is susceptible to blistering, chafing, and rashes caused by rough surfaces, friction, or irritation. Evaporation of water through the skin is greater because the epidermal barrier is less effective, an important factor because of the infant's relatively high fluid needs and propensity to dehydration when fluid requirements are not maintained.

Of the three types of sweat glands, only the sebaceous glands are active during the fetal period and early infancy. These glands are located all over the body, except in the palms of the hands and soles of the feet. They produce the vernix caseosa, which covers the skin prior to birth and continues to lubricate the infant's skin, accounting for the soft, smooth skin that typifies this period. Sebaceous retention cysts are *milia*, the tiny, whitish, opalescent spots present around the nose and chin during the first weeks of life. They disappear spontaneously, and, although unflattering to the neonate, they are benign. The activity of the sebaceous glands decreases after infancy and resumes again with puberty.

The apocrine glands (sweat glands responsible for body odor) are present but remain small and dormant until prepuberty. The eccrine glands, sweat glands that respond to changes in temperature and emotional stimuli, are functional but immature during infancy. The skin and sweat glands work together to protect the body from bacterial invasion, a protective function that increases with maturation.

Hair follicles become active at birth, so that hair grows, especially on the scalp. Hair present at birth often falls out and is replaced by hair of a different color or texture. The presence and amount of hair varies greatly, not only during infancy but also throughout life.

Infants have long, thin fingernails and toenails. These grow fast, and infants frequently scratch themselves or others accidentally. Nails are best trimmed while the infant is sleeping because there is always the risk of cutting the nail too short or even cutting an infant who is resisting or crying.

Immune System The infant's protection from infectious sources takes a variety of forms. Whereas the skin and sebaceous glands provide a physical barrier of resistance, the mucosa of the respiratory, intestinal, and genitourinary tracts serve as barriers by both their physical structure and enzyme production. Various blood cells serve as phagocytes, which engulf and devour bacteria and viruses.

Near the end of gestation, the fetus also receives passive immunity from the mother. The neonate therefore is born with the mother's immunities, either obtained by immunization or clinical exposure to various illnesses. This passive immunity lasts from 3 to 6 months and protects the infant from major childhood diseases such as diphtheria, pertussis, measles, rubella, and poliomyelitis. Although passive immunity provides initial protection, it is not permanent, and the infant needs to receive active immunization against these conditions according to an established immunization schedule (see Chapter 18).

Breast-fed infants receive some additional antibodies to influenza, mumps, and chickenpox. Breast milk has large quantities of immunoglobin A, which provides additional protection against infection that is unavailable to formula-fed infants.

Gradually, as the infant is exposed to various bacteria and viruses, antibodies are formed, and the infant becomes more resistant to infections. Like everything else, this system is initially immature but develops rapidly during the first year of life (Fig. 7-4).

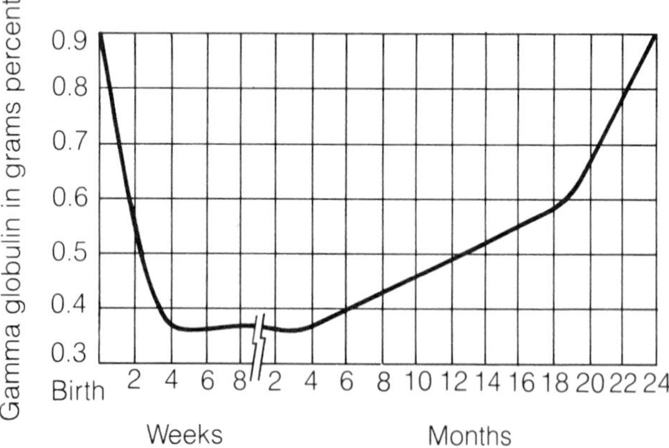

Figure 7-4 The rapid fall in gamma globulin levels increases the infant's susceptibility to illness. The levels rise slowly and reach adult levels by 2 years of age.

Sensory-Perceptual Development

Infants' perceptual abilities are remarkably well organized, even from birth. The neonate is sensitive to light, sound, touch, and other kinds of tactile stimulation, all sensory abilities that are used to assess the infant's neurologic status. During the first few months of life, these rudimentary sensory and perceptual abilities mature rapidly. Infants quickly become highly sophisticated in perceiving conditions and changes within their environments and use input from their sensory organs. For example, the neonate scans the outline of faces, but the 7-month-old infant recognizes specific features and identifies the face as either familiar or unfamiliar. The neonate discriminates between loud and soft sounds, whereas the 10-to 12-month-old infant quickly and precisely locates sounds and relates hearing and sound production by imitating common sounds.

Vision Physiologically, the eye of the neonate is prepared for discriminating both brightness and color, and the neural activity in the retina of a newborn is similar to that of an adult (Chow, et al., 1979). The neonate's eyes respond to increases in the brightness of lights by pupil constriction.

Even moderately bright lights may evoke this pupillary response (Mann, 1964). Sensitivity to brightness develops rapidly in the first 2 months of life, and infants can discriminate between differences in brightness as small as 5% (Peeples and Teller, 1975). By 3 months of age, infants probably are able to discriminate between different colors (Bornstein, 1976). By 4 months of age, infants show a difference in attention to successive presentations of different colors and seem to perceive the color spectrum in a way that is similar to the ability of adults to discriminate blue, green, yellow, and red (Bornstein, Kessen, and Weiskopf, 1976). Infants at this age seem to prefer reds and blues to yellows and greens (Bornstein, 1975).

Sensitivity to differences in brightness is much greater when a figure and a background are presented simultaneously. Kessen and Bornstein (1978) found that 4-month-old infants did not discriminate between visual presentations that were either twice as bright or half as bright as an original field when they were presented in sequence.

Visual Accommodation At birth, the ciliary muscles, which change the shape of the lens in the eye for focusing, are immature (Mann, 1964). *Visual accommodation,* or the ability to focus on distant objects as well as close ones, is therefore limited in the neonate.

Determining an infant's ability to perceive distance and depth is a difficult proposition because infants have only a limited behavioral repertoire with which to respond. In a carefully controlled experiment in which objects were perceived to be falling toward an infant's face, White (1963) demonstrated that 8-week-old infants blinked as the falling object approached. Infants younger than 8 weeks did not blink.

Bower and colleagues (1970) demonstrated that 10-day-old infants respond to objects approaching their faces by rotating their heads and raising their arms defensively. Ball and Tronick (1971) also demonstrated that 1-week-old infants avoid what appear to be impending collisions by turning their heads and raising their arms, but if the object appeared to be bypassing the infant's head and thus preventing collision, the avoidance behavior was not elicited.

Avoiding an impending collision, technically called *looming* with an approaching object is a behavior common to many lower animals as well. Peery (1980) found that 1-day-old infants can participate with adults in a mutual approach-withdrawal pattern of facial behavior that also has been observed in older infants (Stern, 1971) and during early childhood (Peery and Crane, 1980). Such reactions are thought to be important for developing and regulating reciprocal interaction and a sense of personal space.

Brazelton (1979) observed the cyclic attention-withdrawal behavior in 2-to 24-week-old infants during interactions with their parents. During periods of attention, the infant approached the parent with smooth, motoric body movements and an intent gaze. This attention was followed immediately by withdrawal such as gaze aversion or closing of the eyes. The parents who were in tune with their infants would then initiate behaviors such as gentle touching, smiling, or vocalizing to contain their infant and restore attention. This reciprocal interaction supported the infant's cycle of energy-expending approach initiatives, such as eye-brightening, smiling, or cooing, followed by a brief recovery of quiet inattention or rest and return to active, attentive involvement. Parental interaction that responded to the infant's cycle resulted in a smooth, homeostatic curve of reciprocal involvement and recovery. When parent and infant respond in harmony, the feedback loops are positive, thus establishing a pattern of behavior that enhances both physiologic and affective development. This reciprocal intent attention lays the foundation for learning and the formation of interpersonal relationships of mutual respect.

Not only do young infants have fundamental capacities of depth perception, but depth perception also is translated rapidly into behavioral regulation, as has been demonstrated in experiments using a "visual cliff." Gibson and Walk (1970) devised a visual cliff apparatus consisting of a table with a strong plexiglass top and a checkerboard material affixed to the bottom of the plexiglass. Halfway across the table, the checkerboard material dropped several feet from the surface of the table to the floor, giving the visual impression of a drop-off. In experiments, infants between 6 and 14 months of age showed substantial reluctance to cross the "cliff" part of the table, even though they could feel the plexiglass beneath them. Campos and colleagues (1978) demonstrated that infants between 2 and 4 months of age displayed heart rate deceleration and increased attention when placed on top of a visual cliff; their reactions suggested they could perceive the "drop-off," although they did not appear to be frightened by it. Nine-month-old infants, however, displayed heart rate acceleration when placed on the deep side, which indicated that they were afraid (Campos, 1976).

Richards and Rader (1981) observed that infants who learned to crawl before they were $6\frac{1}{2}$ months old crossed the cliff without fear. They hypothesized that these infants were guided in their crawling by tactile sensations, whereas infants who learn to crawl after $6\frac{1}{2}$ months of age depend on visual information for their guidance.

Once infants are capable of visually directed reaching, at about 4 months of age, they make more reaching movements toward rattles and toys that are within their grasp than toward ones that are more than an arm's length away. Once again, research indicates that infants who are quite young perceive space and depth (Bower, 1972; Field, 1976; Gordon and Yonas, 1976).

Visual Acuity A neonate's *visual acuity*, or ability to perceive objects clearly, ranges between 20/600 and 20/800 (Fantz, 1961b) and combines with limited visual accommodation, or ability to focus on objects of varying distances. The neonate has a fixed focal length of about 8–12 in, with 9 in as optimum, and can see objects at that distance with reasonable clarity. By 4 months of age, visual accommodation equals that of the adult's, thus increasing the amount of visual stimulation (Haynes, White, and Held, 1965). Visual acuity at 16 weeks of age improves to 20/200–20/300.

Neonates are able to follow moving objects with their eyes, and eye movement is coordinated so that both eyes move together. Young infants seem to prefer moving objects to stationary ones (Kessen, Haith, and Salapatek, 1970). Visual pursuit and tracking in the neonate initially is jerky and not well controlled, but smooth control usually is achieved by about 6 weeks of age (Dayton et al., 1964). In studies of visual pursuit using patterns of blinking lights moving in a sequence, infants from 1 to 4 months of age are not only able to track movement but, after observing the cycle several times, also can anticipate the direction of the movement. They seem to learn the "rules of the game" in that their eyes return to the first light, and they wait for it to go on after reaching the end of the row (Nelson, 1968; Bower, Broughton, and Moore, 1971). It is as though they assume a single object causes the lights to blink, and they follow the invisible, circular trajectory that such an object would take. Their eyes therefore are focused on the first light when it blinks again.

In addition to substantial visual perception, infants seem to have built-in visual preferences. They generally seem to prefer more complex to simpler stimuli and will look at a patterned surface longer than a plain one (for example, a checkerboard longer than a single color) (Fantz, 1965) (Fig. 7-5). This preference for visual complexity seems to develop as infants grow older (Greenberg, 1971). Fantz (1963) demonstrated that infants prefer a bull's eye to newsprint

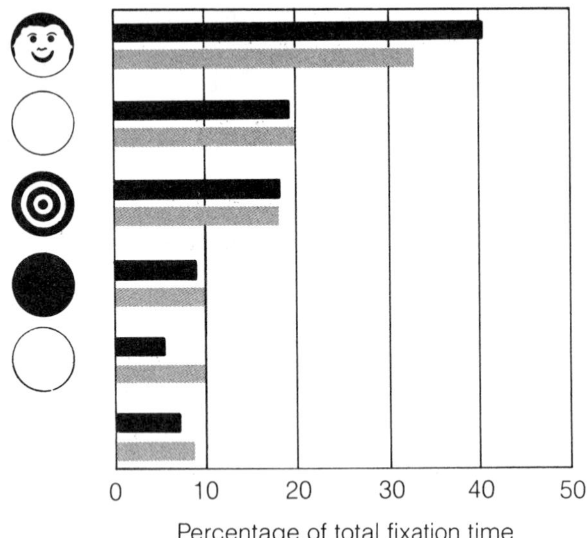

Figure 7-5 Infant's perceptions of patterns. The importance of pattern rather than color or brightness is demonstrated by the infant's responses to a face, a piece of printed matter, a bull's eye, and a plain, multicolored disk. (From Fantz R L: The Origin of Form Perception. *Sci Am* May 1961. Copyright 1961 by Scientific American, Inc. All rights reserved.)

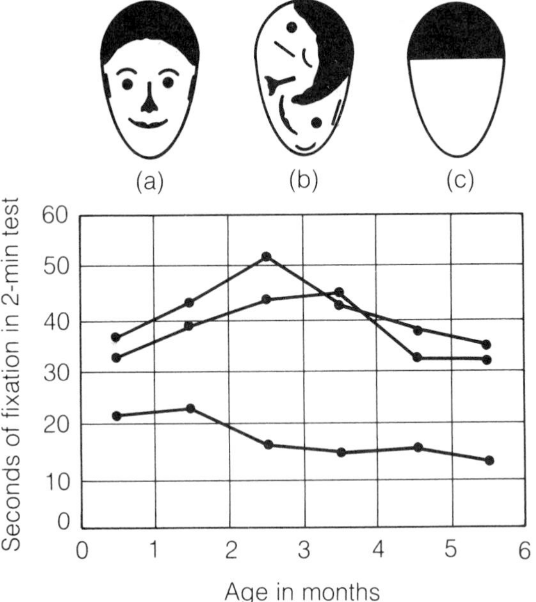

Figure 7-6 Infant's viewing preferences for faces. The adaptive significance of form perception is indicated by the infant's preference for a real face (a) over a scrambled face (b) and for both over a control figure (c). The charted results show average fixation times for infants of various ages. (From Fantz R L: The Origin of Form Perception. *Sci Am* May 1961, p. 72. Copyright 1961 by Scientific American, Inc. All rights reserved.)

and seem most attracted by a cartoon of a human face. By 5–7 months of age, infants not only recognize facial representations accurately but also can make very fine discriminations in slight changes in facial presentations, indicating that they are sensitive to facial forms of nonverbal communication (Fagan, 1979) (Fig. 7-6).

Scanning patterns also seem to change during the first few months of life. One-month-old infants primarily scan the perimeters of objects and focus on contrasts such as the squares of a checkerboard or the contrast between the iris and the white of an eye (Salapatek and Kessen, 1976). Two-month-old infants pay more attention to the interior of an object (Salapatek, 1975) and concentrate on facial features such as the eyes and the mouth (Maurer and Salapatek, 1976) (Fig. 7-7).

Hearing The infant's ear is well developed at birth. The anatomic structures are intact, only smaller than those of the adult's ear. The major difference is the shorter, wider, more horizontal eustachian tube, which provides a direct passageway for organisms to travel from the nasopharyngeal area to the middle ear. This structural difference combined with the reclining position assumed for drinking during infancy predisposes the infant to middle ear infections (see Chapter 26).

The fetus is sensitive to sound as much as 2 months before birth. Neonates can discriminate between differences in pitch (Weir, 1976), and they can detect the direction of the source of sound (Leventhal and Lipsitt, 1964). Soft, high-pitched noises have a calming effect; shrill noises are likely to alarm the infant. They are especially responsive to the human voice, that is, a frequency of 200–500 cycles/sec and a sound length of 5–15 seconds. They tune out many of the other environmental sounds (Eisenberg, 1970). This ability to discriminate allows infants as young as 3 days old, for example, to tell the difference between their mother's voice and the voice of another woman (DeCasper and Fifer, 1980).

Infants respond differently to sounds of contrasting pitch. Multifrequency tones in the higher range of the female voice tend to quiet and focus their attention, whereas very high or very low frequencies create distress and alarm-like responses. By 3–5 months of age, infants can imitate various musical notes produced by their mothers in response to their vocalizations (Kessen, Levine, and Wendich, 1979).

Many parents have noticed that as they speak, their infant tends to move in synchrony to their voice. Slow-motion cinematography has been able to capture visually the smooth, rhythmic movements of the infant's body and extremities as they respond to inflection, articulation, and rapidity of parental speech. This illustrates the infant's ability to separate human sounds from other environmental sounds.

Hearing is important for language acquisition. In addition to differentiating among sounds of various frequency, duration, and intensity, infants learn to identify familiar word combinations. By 1 year of age, the infant distinguishes between nonsense sound combinations and frequently heard words. Kagan and colleagues (1971) demonstrated that 1-year-olds became alert and babbled more in response to

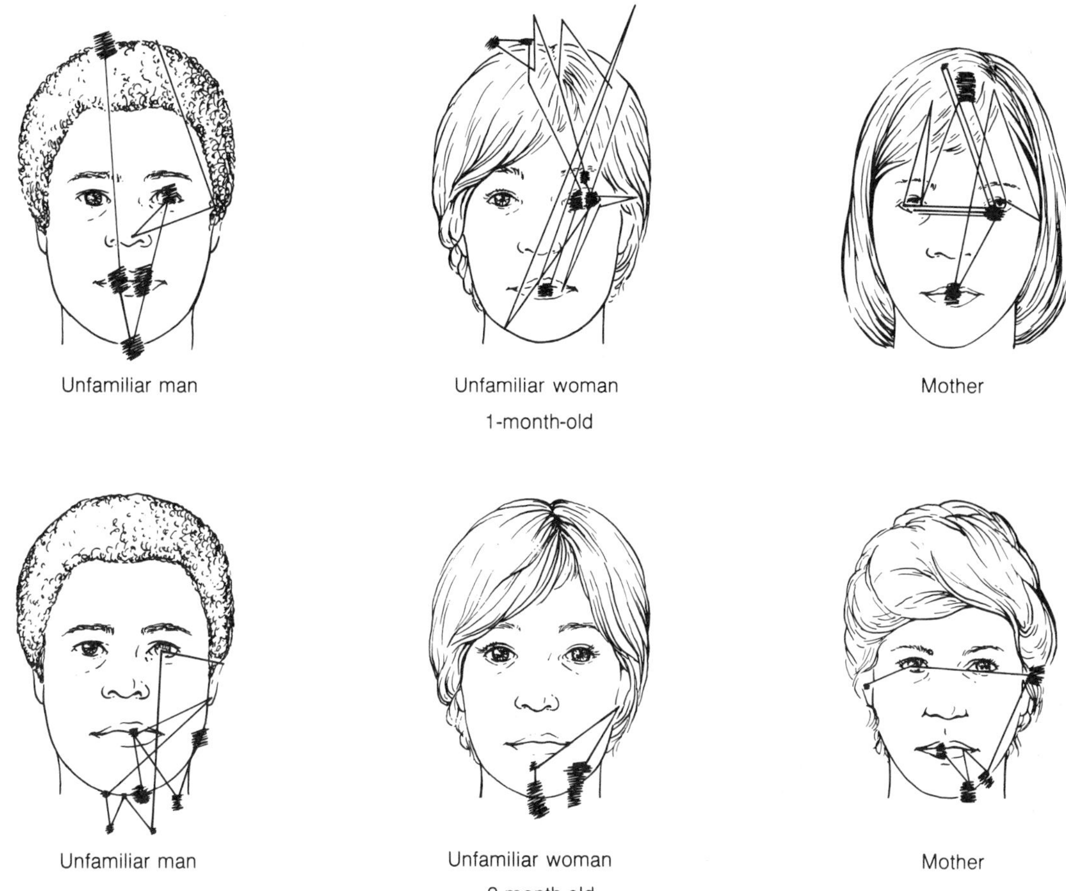

Figure 7-7 Differences in scanning patterns in 1- and 2-month-old infants. At 1 month of age, infants tend to fixate on general features but show more attention to the eyes and mouths of their mothers. At 2 months of age, infants show more interest in facial features, such as the eyes, nose, mouth, ears, and hair of unfamiliar males and females, but they still pay more attention to the eyes and mouths of their mothers.

sentences that included commonly heard words, such as "mommy," "daddy," and "smile," than to sentences that were nonsensical.

Taste and Smell Measuring an infant's reaction to taste and smell is much more difficult than the other senses, although these senses also are functional shortly after birth. A neonate can detect sweetness and will turn away from strong noxious odors (Lipsitt, Engen, and Kaye, 1963). Infants also learn to distinguish the smell of their mother's milk, and the infant will turn toward the mother (Macfarlane, 1975). Infants alter their sucking in response to different tastes, sucking less when the liquid is unsweetened, more when the liquid is sweet, and minimally when the liquid is salty. The mother's breast milk, which is unsweetened, loses its appeal if the infant has just tasted glucose water.

Tactile Sensitivity A neonate's sensitivity to a pinprick is one of the variables used in the Brazelton Neonatal Behavioral Assessment Scale, but the neonate also is sensitive to much less noxious stimuli and can even feel a puff of air (Young and Douthitt, 1974) or a thread pressed against the infant's skin (Rose, Schmidt, and Bridger, 1976). An infant's responsiveness to tactile stimulation can be a function of the infant's state of arousal (Lewis, Bartels, and Goldberg, 1967) and can change according to the level of hunger (Pomerleau-Malcuit and Clifton, 1973) (see Chapter 16).

Salient responses to touch include the rooting and sucking reflexes and the defensive maneuvers that infants demonstrate when restrained or when objects interfere with respiration. All of these reactions are critical for survival. Infants also respond to gentle, soothing patting or stroking by relaxing and cuddling. Coldness, wetness, abrupt pats, or jostling, on the other hand, increase tension and distress.

Cognitive Development

Cognition, one of the most frequently studied aspects of infant development, is defined by two distinguishable, although not necessarily opposing, theoretic approaches.

The primary difference between these approaches is their theoretic view of how cognition and learning occur.

The first approach, put forward by Jean Piaget, is based on his observations and subsequent construction of a theory denoting stages of cognitive development. The second approach has its roots in behaviorism and learning theories associated with more traditional psychology. Both approaches are important and help in understanding the nature of infant behavior. (Growth and development theories are discussed in Chapter 6.)

Learning and Behavior According to Piaget (1952, 1969), an infant's thinking does not go much beyond rudimentary reflexive behaviors during early infancy. Gradually, the infant develops a repertoire of behaviors and learns to accommodate existing schemes to new situations, thereby developing internal cognitive memory and representations. During infancy, the tie between the infant's ongoing behavior and cognitive experience of the world is very direct. This tie between behavior and thought distinguishes Piaget's approach to infant thinking and is the source of many of his insights about learning in the first months of life.

Behavioristic principles suggest that young infants learn through operant conditioning (see Chapter 6). Infants respond to a number of reinforcers, including colored lights and novel sounds, an opportunity to be tickled or talked to by a smiling parent, or an opportunity to taste a sweet liquid. One of the primary concerns of those interested in operant conditioning with infants has been the age at which an infant is capable of learning in this way. Piaget concluded that it was not until Stage 4 of the sensorimotor period, between 8 and 12 months of age, that an infant became clearly aware that self-initiated behavior could cause changes in the environment and began to understand the difference between means and ends.

Regardless of whether an infant fully understands the difference between means and ends, a number of researchers have demonstrated that infants much younger than 8 months of age can learn by operant conditioning. Three-day-old neonates will control the rate of their sucking, for example, to have an opportunity to hear their parents' voices (DeCasper and Fifer, 1980). In a series of systematic and carefully controlled studies, Papousek (1967) found that infants as young as 3 weeks of age can produce stable, conditioned responses to the sound of a bell by turning their heads (Papousek, 1967). Very young infants are difficult subjects for conditioning experiments because neonates have a limited behavioral repertoire and because the amount of energy required for a given response may be more than the infant is willing to expend given the insignificant and trivial nature of some of the reinforcers.

Certain situations are, however, conducive to infant learning. Infants who receive attention, are talked to, tickled, played with, and generally stimulated by a normal home environment learn faster and learn a wider variety of things than infants in institutional settings (Clarke-Stewart and Apfel, 1979).

Stages of Cognition Piaget divided cognitive development into several stages (see Chapter 6). The first of these stages, the sensorimotor stage, is in turn divided into six substages of developing cognitive ability.

During the first month of life, the infant learns little but does exercise innate reflexes in bringing about basic adaptations like feeding, which are necessary for survival. By exercising these reflexive behaviors (called *schemes*), the infant begins to develop some fundamental control over body activity but has no understanding of the world, no understanding of cause-and-effect relationships, and no concept of object permanence or stability.

The primary circular reactions stage (1–4 months of age) is the time during which behaviors occur at random but give rise to pleasant sensations and so are repeated. Wiggling the legs or sucking the thumb, for example, may occur initially in a random way but then are repeated because they bring intrinsic enjoyment. They are centered on the body, therefore are "primary," and they are circular because they repeat patterns of behavior that initially had no specific meaning.

Secondary circular reactions (occurring at approximately 4–8 months of age) change the focus of the infant's attention from centering on the body to centering on items of interest in the environment. For the first time, the infant understands that behavior can have an effect on the environment. For example, the infant may be wiggling one foot and accidentally tap the side of the crib, producing an interesting sound, or the infant may accidentally wiggle a mobile. The behavior of this crib knocking is repeated to produce a sound or a visual experience and is secondary because the response affects the environment.

During the next stage, the purposeful coordination of means and ends (at approximately 8–12 months of age), the infant begins to coordinate more than one scheme to reach a goal. For example, looking, reaching, and grasping become coordinated to facilitate reaching out and grasping a desired object. Although this coordination is not combined with an understanding of time or permanence, infants recognize familiar objects and people. When a toy is hidden under a blanket, the infant makes no attempt to remove the blanket to obtain the toy. Piaget believed that this means that, for the infant, the toy ceases to exist once it is out of sight.

Also, during this stage, infants demonstrate what is called the A-not-B phenomenon. This is manifested experimentally by placing a ball in a cup to the infant's right side and letting the infant reach in and take the ball out. After several trials, the ball is placed in a cup on the left side. Even though the infant can see the ball being placed in the cup on the left and can see the ball, the infant still will attempt to find the ball in the cup on the right-hand side (Fig. 7-8). This kind of behavior lends credence to Piaget's hypothesis that thinking and cognition have their roots in motor behavior. According to Piaget, an infant at this stage does not differentiate between the concept of the ball and the concept of reaching for the ball in the cup on the right side. The ball and reaching for the ball are one, so that the infant is not able to displace the ball mentally into the cup on the left.

During the first four stages, the infant's primary means of adapting to the environment is assimilation. With the development of tertiary circular reactions (at approximately 12–18 months of age), the infant begins to develop accommodation. No longer are behaviors repeated identically for their own sake; rather, the repetition includes modification of the behavior to produce new results or sounds. For example, the infant may say "dadda" and then practice the new sounds "daddy," "dad," and so on. These modifications are called tertiary because they are modifications in the behaviors themselves to produce novel ends. The infant is coming to understand that an important factor in bringing about change in the environment is personal action and interaction. Insights arising from experimenting with new behaviors become incorporated into the ability to deal more effectively with the world. Infants are now capable of responding to simple requests such as obtaining a toy from another room.

Mental representation (at approximately 18–24 months of age) is the sixth and final stage of the sensorimotor period. It is really a transition from sensorimotor intelligence to a cognitive intelligence that relies less directly on repeated behaviors and is more of an internal cognition that begins to resemble what adults consider thought. Rather than going through the process of trial and error in solving the A-not-B problem, for example, the older infant can anticipate that the ball will be found in the left cup after seeing it put there. The emerging abilities of mental representation are crucial in developing to the next stage, or preoperational thought (see Chapter 8).

One of the major difficulties in studying cognitive development in infants is understanding what it is that an infant is "thinking" and then designing experiments that allow the researcher to draw inferences about thought from the infant's behavior. Another difficulty with studying cognitive development in infancy is the need to divide "perception" from "conception." A great deal of attention has been given to the skills and abilities that enable the infant to perceive the environment using sensory modalities. "Conception" in

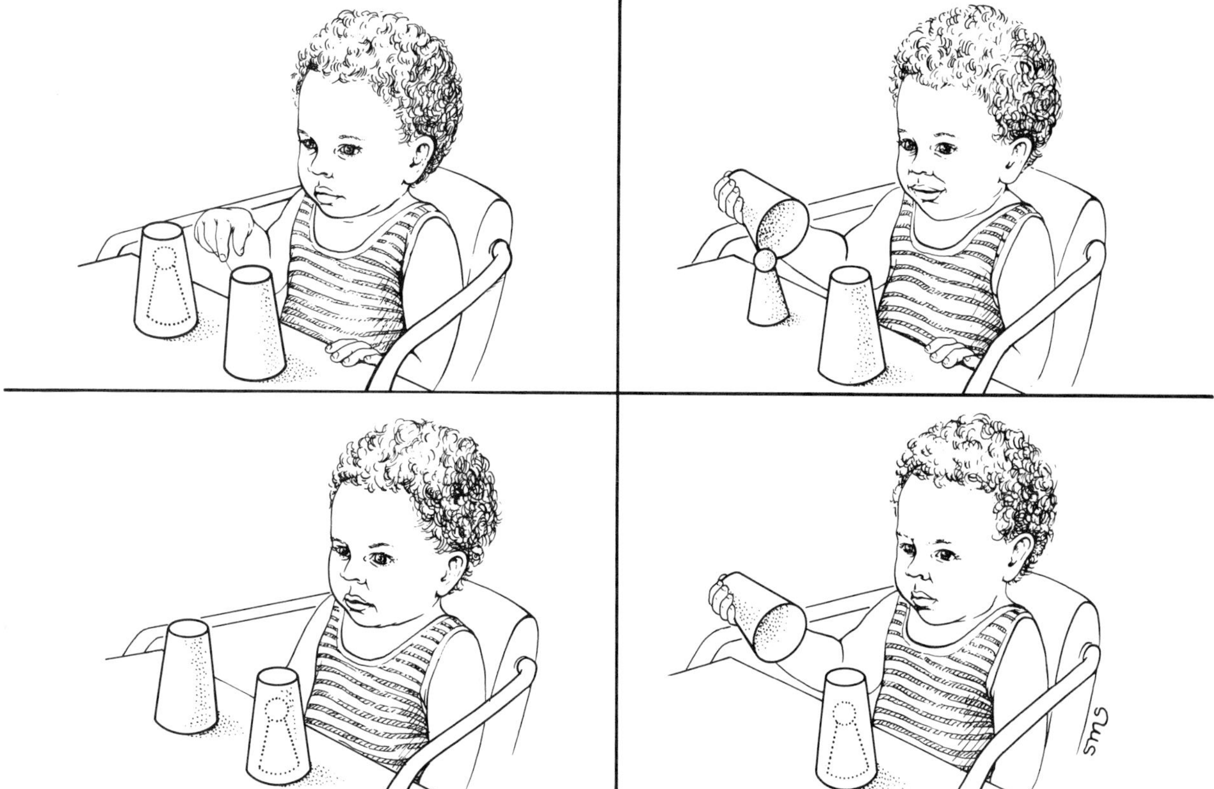

Figure 7-8 The search for a hidden object. The infant looks for an object where it is first hidden and does not look further. Piaget suggested that the infant is not yet able to differentiate between the object and the act of reaching for it. This is an example of A-not-B phenomenon.

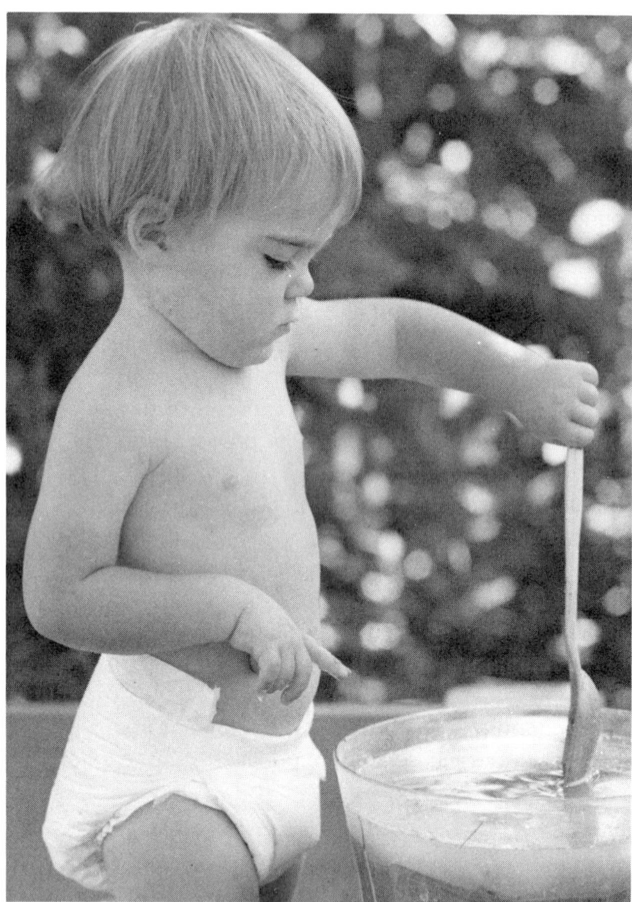

From 12 to 18 months, the infant develops accommodation and learns to repeat behaviors to produce desired results.

adults is the process of using these rudimentary perceptions as a basis for developing higher-order constructs about the world. These constructs are concepts that are the hallmark of "thinking." Piaget went beyond the reconstruction of percepts into concepts and said that thinking is rooted in motor behavior. Piaget believed that the infant actively integrates perceptual experiences with developing motor behaviors to develop concepts about how the world operates.

The rudimentary concept studied most intensively is object permanence. According to Piaget, an infant in the secondary circular reaction substage does not understand that an object exists when it is not seen. Piaget explained the infant's thinking as follows: when the mother leaves the bedroom where the infant is playing and the infant then crawls out into the kitchen and sees the mother there, it is as if there were two mothers—one for the bedroom and one for the kitchen. As mentioned earlier, a toy hidden under a blanket may "cease to exist" for an infant under 8 months of age, and if a young infant is shown an object that suddenly seems to change shape (for example, a sphere changing into a cube), the infant will not be particularly surprised (Bower, 1977).

The development of object permanence seems to occur at some point between the third and ninth month of life. Evidence actually shows that it occurs somewhat before Piaget originally thought. For example, a 3-month-old infant who is simultaneously presented with three mothers (with the use of mirrors) is quite delighted, but a 5-month-old infant presented with three mothers simultaneously shows signs of distress. Bower (1974) concluded that this kind of distress indicates that a child is beginning to understand that there is only one mother for any given place and time.

Infants also do not understand spatial relationships like "on and in" and "in front of and behind" until 10 or 11 months of age. For example, if a small toy is held in front of a 5-month-old, the infant reaches to try to obtain it. If the toy is placed on top of a small platform in front of the infant, there is a puzzled expression and little attempt to retrieve it. Infants show the same kind of difficulty with the concepts of "in front of" and "behind," particularly when the distance between the two objects is small. If a toy is placed in front of a screen by several inches and within reach, the infant has no difficulty in reaching out to grasp it. But if the toy is placed right next to the screen, the infant has more difficulty, almost as though there is no understanding that the toy is separated from the screen and still available to be picked up (Bower, 1977).

Although some psychologists have questioned Piaget's contention that there is no intercoordination between sensorimotor schemes until 8–12 months of age (Lamb and Campos, 1982), Piaget's original observations about infants and the concepts he derived from those observations have been remarkably resilient to empiric demonstration.

Memory All kinds of learning require the capacity for memory (see Chapter 6, Table 6-7). Even a rudimentary kind of memory is required for habituation to take place.

Piaget argued that recall memory is not possible during the first year, yet infants as young as a few days old show a preference for their mother's voices, indicating that they have a memory that lasts over a relatively long term (when compared with their life span of just a few days). Other studies have shown that infants younger than 1 year of age show preferences for and illustrate recognition of objects that are familiar in their lives. For example, they recognize familiar individuals and toys. Because of the difficulty in having infants respond in ways that are unambiguous and easy to interpret, no one is sure exactly what their memory limits are. It does seem clear, however, that in addition to the memory required in learning and social development tasks, the capacity for longer-term memory increases throughout infancy and that memory serves social development when the infant memorizes faces and voices. This was evidenced by one infant who responded with a special chuckle whenever she heard or saw her brother, resulting in a special relationship between them. Memory also is manifested in intellectual development by a capacity to understand and use language, play, and be effective in gaining control over the environment.

Personality Development

Just as Piaget provided the basic theoretic framework for understanding cognitive development in infancy, Sigmund Freud provided the first theoretic model for understanding personality development in infancy (see Chapter 6).

According to Freud (1969), birth is a traumatic experience. Emerging from the womb, the neonate is overwhelmed and frightened by sights and sounds. This first trauma provides a basis for regression to infantile behavior when faced with overwhelming instinctual or environmental stimulation in later life. According to Freud, an easier birth would diminish the traumatic shock and create less fear in the young child. Leboyer (1975) and other proponents of "gentle birth" also are concerned with reducing birth trauma to the infant.

Egocentricity According to Freud's psychodynamic model, the neonate is driven primarily by the id. The ego functions emerge only gradually during the first year (Freud's oral stage of development), and the infant has no superego at this time. The neonate's primary concern is having instinctual needs for food and comfort met. The younger infant is egocentric and does not understand the relationship between self and environment. The infant's primary mode of interacting with the environment is *incorporation,* the process by which needs are met through the mouth (hence the oral stage). If the infant's needs for care, food, cuddling, warmth, and comfort are met, movement through the oral stage is relatively smooth. If needs are not met, serious conflict develops. After the first few months of life, an emerging ego begins to develop that distinguishes between "self" and "not self." The infant begins to understand that the performance of certain behaviors leads to the gratification of desires. A parent becomes a primary source of "goods and services," and thus infants develop a primary dependency on their parents, although at the same time parents are seen as separate individuals.

There are some similarities in the ways Freud and Piaget viewed the young infant. Both saw the infant's mental capacity as extremely limited. Both saw infants as predominantly egocentric and unaware of how the world operates. Both felt that infants became capable of developing concepts and learning behaviors during the first year of life, and both saw the first year as a very primitive, rudimentary stage of development.

Erik Erikson (1963) also saw early life predominantly as a conflict between inborn motivations and social control (see Chapter 6). Erikson (1977) believed that the child is preprogrammed to develop certain psychologic capacities at different ages (the *epigenetic principle*), but whether the outcome of these stages is successful or frustrated depends on the kind of social environment the infant experiences.

The first stage is the stage of basic trust versus basic mistrust and lasts through the first year or so. Like Freud, Erikson saw the infant as fundamentally dependent and egocentric, demanding the satisfaction of basic biologic needs without understanding how those needs are met. According to Erikson, if an infant is fed, caressed, and cared for when uncomfortable, hungry, cold, or wet, the world is seen as a fundamentally friendly place that can be trusted and relied on to satisfy one's needs. A basic sense of trust then develops. If, by contrast, the infant experiences frustration, punishment, confusion, and deprivation when attempting to have needs met, the world is seen as a harsh, capricious, and unreliable place, and a basic sense of mistrust is developed.

Erikson also believed that experiences in each stage have a major, long-lasting influence on personality. If an infant develops a basic sense of mistrust, that sense can be diminished by later positive experiences but never thoroughly eliminated, and vestiges of that mistrust will be seen in the individual's adult personality.

The psychodynamic models of both Freud and Erikson agree that it is important for an infant during the first year to live in an environment that is warm, supportive, and capable of meeting the infant's egocentric demands and biologic needs. Both theorists also agree that it is unrealistic to make demands requiring cognitive skills of infants when the necessary personality characteristics are not yet available. In this they agree with Piaget.

Temperament *Temperament* is the child's basic behavioral style, which affects that child's interactions. The psychodynamic view of personality development emphasized the importance of internal drives and parental responses; therefore, if parents make mistakes in raising their children, their mistakes could damage the child's personality permanently.

Partly in reaction to this parent-centered view and partly in response to parents who sought counseling and advice because they attributed all of their children's negative characteristics to their mistakes, Stella Chess, Alexander Thomas, and Herbert Birch, and other researchers began studying the infant's innate characteristics in the early 1950s. They wanted to determine whether characteristics evident in an infant were relatively stable throughout development and relatively resistant to environmental influences. The New York Longitudinal Study (NYLS) was designed to examine this question about the persistence of personality characteristics even at a young age. Thomas and colleagues (1963) determined that infants do have individual characteristics even as neonates and that these characteristics differentiate infants one from another. After studying a large number of young children, these researchers identified nine characteristics of child temperament (Table 7-3).

TABLE 7-3 Characteristics of Child Temperament

Temperamental Factor	Description
Activity level	Some infants are wiggly—they splash in their bath, thrash around in their beds, and don't sit still for a minute. Some infants are placid—they lie still, sit quietly and observe for long periods, and manifest a low activity level
Rhythmicity	Some infants quickly and readily adopt a schedule for life: feeding at regular intervals, sleeping at regular intervals, and resisting changes in these schedules. By contrast, other infants sleep and eat at irregular hours and do not develop a rhythmic pattern for life processes
Approach or withdrawal as a reaction to novelty	Some infants are drawn toward new toys; they never show stranger anxiety and readily move into new situations. Some infants hold back from playing with a new toy or seem hesitant when faced with new people or situations; they withdraw from novelty
Adaptability	Some infants adjust easily to new situations, changes in schedule, taking a bath. Infants with low adaptability may persistently have difficulty in adjusting to changes and may never like being left with baby-sitters
Sensory threshold	Some infants seem remarkably sensitive to changes in temperature; they respond to a cold or a stomachache with intense crying; they awaken easily from a nap at the slightest noise. Other infants seem to have a much lower sensory threshold; they can sleep through a rocket blast, cry little when they fall down and hurt themselves, and don't overreact to an earache
Intensity of reaction	Some infants give everything when they respond; they laugh hysterically when their father makes faces at them; they cry and scream if they can't have a cookie. Infants with low-intensity reactions whimper when they are hungry or never object strongly when they are requested to do things they don't want to do
Positive or negative mood	Some infants seem to be happy and easygoing, responding to most of life with a cheerful disposition. Some babies seem to be innately disgruntled and pessimistic about much of what goes on
Distractibility	When found playing with a forbidden item, some infants can be distracted easily to playing with a plastic bowl or a rattle. Other infants demand to be fed immediately when they are hungry and will not be put off by an alternative activity
Attention span persistence	Some babies will play with a favorite toy for long periods of time or lie on their backs and watch mobiles. Other infants flip from one activity to another at the slightest frustration; toys or blocks are cast aside in favor of a rubber ball or an opportunity to look out the window

SOURCE: Adapted from Chess S, Thomas A: Temperament and the parent-child interaction. *Pediatr Ann* 1977; 6:26–45.

Thomas, Chess, and Birch determined that combinations of these different temperamental characteristics frequently would appear in clusters that defined the characteristics of a child. They grouped these characteristics into three classes: (1) the easy child; (2) the difficult child; and (3) the slow-to-warm-up child (Table 7-4). The easy child has a positive mood, is high on rhythmicity and adaptability, and often reacts positively to new toys. This child makes little fuss when a family schedule is changed and is as adaptable to traveling on vacation as to staying at home with the baby-sitter. The difficult child is irregular, does not adapt to new routines, has a high intensity of reaction and negative moods, and frequently responds negatively to new stimuli. The difficult child spits out new food, cries when left with the baby-sitter, and fusses during a first car trip and during subsequent trips as well. The slow-to-warm-up child also reacts negatively to novel stimuli but has a low intensity of reaction and tends to have irregular habits. This child may respond in an initially negative way to changes in life patterns or circumstances but will eventually adjust and adapt positively.

Temperament theory has generated considerable interest, and another researcher, William Carey (1982), devised screening instruments for infant and child temperament (see Chapter 16). Every parent with more than one child knows that the differences between children are not strictly caused by differences in parenting. "They are as different as night and day" is an expression commonly used by parents when

TABLE 7-4 Personality Types and Temperament

Type of child	Activity level (proportion of active periods to inactive ones)	Rhythmicity (regularity of hunger, excretion, sleep, and wakefulness)	Distractibility (degree to which extraneous stimuli alter behavior)	Approach-withdrawl (response to a new object or person)	Adaptability (ease with which a child adapts to changes in environment)	Attention span and persistence (amount of time devoted to an activity, and the effect of distraction on the activity)	Intensity of reaction (energy of response, regardless of its quality or direction)	Threshold of responsiveness (intensity of stimulation required to evoke a discernible response)	Quality of mood (amount of friendly, pleasant, joyful behavior as contrasted with unpleasant, unfriendly behavior)
"Easy"	Low to moderate	Very regular	Varies	Positive approach	Very adaptable	High or low	Low or mild	High or low	Positive
"Slow to Warm Up"	Varies	Varies	Varies	Initial withdrawal	Slowly adaptable	High or low	Mild	High or low	Slightly negative
"Difficult"	Varies	Irregular	Varies	Withdrawal	Slowly adaptable	High or low	Intense	High or low	Negative

Note: temperament of a child allows classification as "easy," "slow to warm up," or "difficult" according to the rating in certain key categories in the nine-point personality index. The categories are only a general guide to temperament. Of the 141 subjects, 65% could be categorized, but 35% displayed a mixture of traits. Such a child might, for example, be rated "easy" in some ways and "difficult" in others.

SOURCE: Thomas A, Chess S, Birch HG: The origin of personality. *Sci Am* 1970; 223(2):106–107.

describing their children. In fact, subtle differences related to the vigor of the infant's suck, ease of consolability, and preferred position are noted at birth and provide clues to this infant's temperament as compared with those of the infant's siblings. Children do seem to have their own personalities and their own approaches to dealing with the world, and these characteristics do seem to persist over time. Unfortunately, both the nine temperamental constructs postulated by Thomas, Chess, and Birch and other temperamental constructs postulated by other researchers have not proven to be consistent or externally verifiable when examined in other research studies.

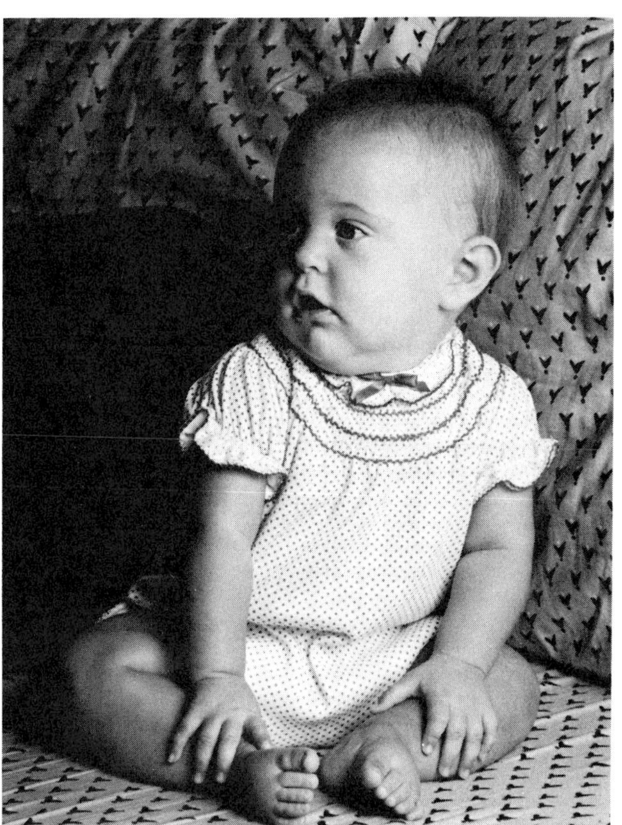

Infants show temperamental characteristics that indicate developing personality differences.

A review of the research literature relating to temperament raises questions about the instruments used to measure temperament and their ability to satisfy the scientific requirements of validity and reliability. Therefore, although temperament remains an intriguing approach to understanding individual differences and certainly has considerable validity for those working with individual infants, the research on understanding exactly how temperamental factors can be identified and how they influence a child's behavior over time is still in its "infancy," and much remains to be learned.

Communication and Language Development

Nonverbal Communication Among the most important milestones in infancy is the development of the ability to communicate with others. During most of infancy, communication is nonverbal, and young infants develop considerable skill in communicating without the use of language. During the second year of life, these nonverbal communication skills become matched with verbal communication skills, so that by the end of infancy, even though their actual vocabulary is limited, the infant's capacity for communication is well developed for many of the practical social encounters that occur daily. Nonverbal communication takes place using five different modalities: moving, gazing, managing interpersonal space, facial expression, and physical attractiveness.

Condon and Ogston (1967) established that when two adults converse, the listener's body moves in synchrony with the speaker's speech. Condon and Ogston called this simultaneous coordination of movement between speaker and listener *interactional synchrony*. In analyzing the effect of adult speech on neonatal movement, Condon and Sander (1974) discovered that the body of a neonate also moves in synchrony with adult's speech, regardless of the language that the neonate is hearing. This fundamental ability to respond to language by coordinating neonatal movement with spoken stresses is one of the earliest forms of social interaction, an important step in social communication.

The fetus can hear before birth and has a considerable opportunity to experience the rhythms of human speech by listening to the mother before birth. In infancy, therefore, what appears to be thrashing and wiggling is instead coordinated with adult speech when adults are close enough to be heard.

The infant's actual amount of movement increases with age, particularly between 9 and 15 months of age (Kagan, Kearsley, and Zelazco, 1978). Because adults tend to infer that movement is related to the infant's happiness, they may unconsciously reinforce this behavior by further stimulation and interaction. Infants therefore might soon learn that moving and wiggling are likely to bring adult attention.

Because vision is controlled voluntarily from birth, gazing is an important part of an infant's nonverbal communication. Eye contact is important social communication (Goffman, 1963), and early eye contact makes a significant difference in a parent's feelings toward a child. Eye contact is thought to be one of the cardinal factors in developing parent–infant attachments. By 3 months of age, the coordination of adult–infant gazing shows some remarkable similarities to the interactional synchrony of adult dialogue. Neurologic mechanisms that control gazing and dialogue might therefore be similar, and the gaze and vocal communication might share some fundamental properties of human communication that are evident in the infant's gaze long before language develops (Jaffe, Stern, and Peery, 1971).

Parents and infants engage in long mutual gazes during play and feeding activities. Gazing then becomes integrated with touching and vocalizing behaviors, and both parent and infant participate in the mutual regulation of social play behavior during the early months (Stern, 1974). Head turning and gazing can be important parts of regulating the intensity of social contact (Peery, 1980), and gaze aversion and head turning become integrated in increasingly complex ways into social interaction as the child matures (Stern, 1971). As the infant becomes able to turn toward adults and engage them visually and then turn away and avert the gaze, the infant develops fundamental control over the intensity of social involvement. Head turning therefore might be the child's first expression of "no" or "yes."

Touching, also a form of communication, has not been researched. When adults communicate warmth and affection to their children by using touching, stroking, patting, and kissing, infants respond positively (Stern, 1974; Newman and Newman, 1978). An infant's touch or a pat on the parent's leg can, however, be a way of seeking adult attention. Just as 4-month-old infants first reach to touch inanimate objects with developing fine motor control, so they will reach out and touch an adult's face or put their fingers in an adult's mouth when they are being held. This expression of interest may be an early form of communication.

Adults usually are interested in an infant's facial expressions, especially smiling (Bower, 1977). Infants begin smiling about 3–5 weeks after birth (Dittrizhova, 1969), but these smiles might not be a form of social interaction. Infants do smile, for example, during their sleep. This early smiling is not, as commonly supposed, an expression of "gas pains" but rather the relaxation of facial muscles. The 6-week-old infant's smile clearly results from human stimulation. Infants first smile when presented with parts of human faces, and they particularly enjoy smiling human faces. Infants might smile for many reasons and with great variation in the degree of emotional involvement. Behaviors associated with smiling range from bright-eyed attention to laughing and giggling at 9 or 10 months of age. They also learn that smiling and laughing prolong adult attention and play.

Infants also might present very sad and distressed faces when crying. An infant's crying face combined with the compelling sound of an infant cry is a very powerful mechanism for communicating displeasure and is virtually impossible for adults to ignore. Adult responses to crying also are clear reinforcers for the crying behavior, so that infants learn early that crying brings the gratification of needs. Crying is therefore the infant's first form of communication. (Parental responses to crying and colic in infancy are discussed in Chapter 13.)

Physical attractiveness is an innate characteristic that infants use to communicate with adults. The ethologist Konrad Lorenz (1943) first theorized that the young of many species share facial characteristics that identify them as babies and make them particularly attractive. This "babyness" phenomenon consists of large eyes, a large forehead, a small pug nose, a relatively small mouth, and small ears, as compared with adult features. Baby birds and many baby mammals, including dogs and cats, share these facial characteristics in common with human babies.

Lorenz believed that this configuration of facial characteristics evoked both attention and a positive emotional response from adults. The person who says "isn't that cute" and then picks up a puppy is responding to the attractiveness of this facial configuration. Fullard and Reiling (1976) conducted research on children between second and twelfth grade and confirmed that Lorenz's hypothesis seems to be correct. Before adolescence, boys and girls show little preference for babies' faces in comparison with other kinds of human faces, but during and after adolescence (when children become capable of having their own children), they come to express a clear preference for baby faces. This preference emerges between sixth and eighth grade for girls and between tenth and twelfth grade for boys.

Verbal Communication During the first 8 or 9 months of life, infants develop substantial ability at nonverbal communication. They can express happiness, laughter, sadness, or frustration; they can obtain attention from adults and participate with adults in closely regulated social interaction without ever saying a word. Before infants are able to speak, they are apparently able to understand communication and language. An infant's first words usually are spoken around 10–12 months of age, and a few months later, the infant begins to develop rudimentary phrases (Lenneberg, 1966).

Before actually using language, however, infants progress through universal stages of prespeech development. Babbling, cooing, and gurgling accompany the infant's smiling at 1 month of age. Infants soon begin to produce the sounds of their native language in a sequence that Jacobson (1968) believed to be invariant from culture to culture. By 6 months of age, infants engage in verbal dialogue that is somewhat similar to adult speech; adults and infants also play together using vocalizations and this familiarizes children with patterns of adult speech (Stern, et al., 1975; Schaffer, 1971). These fundamental speech sounds, which occur in the earliest months, are transformed into *morphemes,* or sounds that carry meaning, and into words at about 8–10 months of age.

A number of theories explain the transitions from basic speech sounds to words and then to more complex use of language. Skinner (1957) proposed that infants learn adult forms of speech through reinforcement for speech-like production. Others (Chomsky, 1957; Bloom, 1970; Brown, 1970) have proposed that the ability to understand and generate a language is part of the child's neurologic development and that children begin to form language that is typical of children in other cultures rather than typical of adults in their environment.

Early language is *holophrastic speech,* in which the infant uses a single noun to convey the entire meaning of the sentence. For example, a child will use "car" to mean "I want to go in the car," "There is our car," "Where is my toy car?" The infant then progresses to *telegraphic speech,* which is produced by eliminating the connective words and focusing on the content words. A child of 18 months will say "more cookie" or "mommy sock" to communicate meanings that require much more refined language structures in adult speech (Brown and Belugi, 1964). This is the stage of language development that marks the end of infancy and the beginning of early childhood.

Social Development

Attachment The theoretic understanding of attachment, an affectional tie between the infant and a primary caregiver, has several historical roots. Freud and Erikson theorized that neonates are dominated by survival instincts but can do little to provide the means necessary to assure survival. Infants therefore manifest wants by crying and demonstrate satisfaction by sleeping and rudimentary playing. Because parents are the primary sources of the infant's needs, the infant comes to associate parents with need fulfillment. Thus, the infant becomes dependent, both physically and emotionally, on the parents for meeting needs, and need fulfillment becomes the foundation for building a basic sense of trust.

Early studies by Renee Spitz (1945, 1946) demonstrated that infants placed in foundling homes and deprived of warm, consistent, loving relationships did extremely poorly as compared with infants who were raised by their parents. They were more susceptible to infection and disease and showed retarded physical development, as well as delays in toilet training, speech development, and various other measures of social development.

Using monkeys to test the Freudian hypothesis that infants depend on their parents, Harry Harlow and colleagues (1959, 1966) discovered that it is more than supplying food that makes an infant attached. Harlow's classic studies involved using two kinds of "surrogate mothers" in raising infant monkeys. The surrogate mothers had wire bodies, one covered with terry cloth and one with a wire mesh.

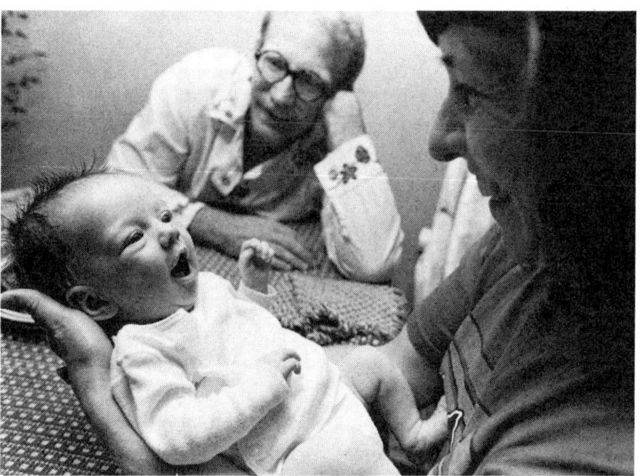

Eye contact between infants and parents is important in the process of attachment.

Harlow discovered that infants preferred clinging to and associating with the "terry cloth mother" even though they might be fed exclusively by a bottle in the "wire mother." The infant monkeys would cling to the terry cloth mother when frightened and use the terry cloth mother as a secure base of operations (Fig. 7-9). This finding emphasized the importance of tactile stimulation and bodily contact. It also contradicted behaviorist learning theory and the Freudian hypothesis that attachments developed exclusively because of the provision of primary reinforcers such as food.

Research in Scotland by Schaffer and Emerson (1964) found that 7-month-old infants began to develop specific attachments to parents and that by 10 months of age, most seem to be attached to their parents and become distressed when left alone, particularly in a strange situation. John Bowlby (1969) reviewed the findings relating to parent–infant relationships and developed the most elegant theory of attachments up to that time. Combining the Freudian idea of dependence with the ethologist's information about imprinting and sensitive periods for developing parent–child relationships in lower animals, Bowlby hypothesized that the child's primary attachment was essential for developing emotional well-being. He then identified basic behaviors that the infant used to enhance and encourage attachment (Table 7-5). Primary caregivers provide nurturance, warmth, social stimulation, and a secure base from which infants can reach out and begin to explore their world.

Other researchers, most notably Mary Ainsworth (1973), have expanded the theories of attachment and explored parent–infant interaction in a variety of experimental settings. Probably the most well-researched experimental paradigm for demonstrating attachment is the parent–infant separation model first used by Schaffer and Emerson (Ainsworth, et al., 1979) (Table 7-6). Research on the parent–infant dyad shows that between 9 and 24 months of age, the strength of attachment can be measured by the infant's attempt to seek proximity when left alone in a room by the parents. Contact-seeking and proximity-maintaining behavior seems to peek at around 18 months of age and then decrease (Fig. 7-10). Kotelchuck (1976) used the separation paradigm to demonstrate that infants are more attached to both fathers and mothers than they are to strangers and that this attachment behavior seems to be a cross-cultural phenomenon.

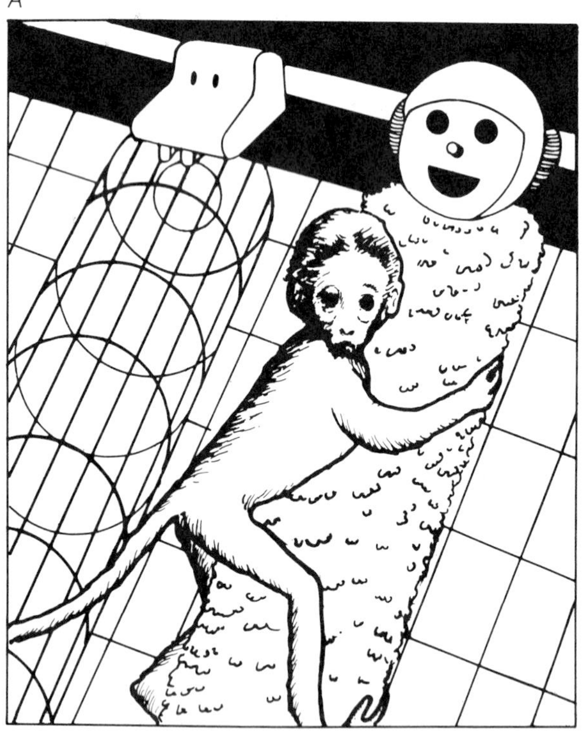

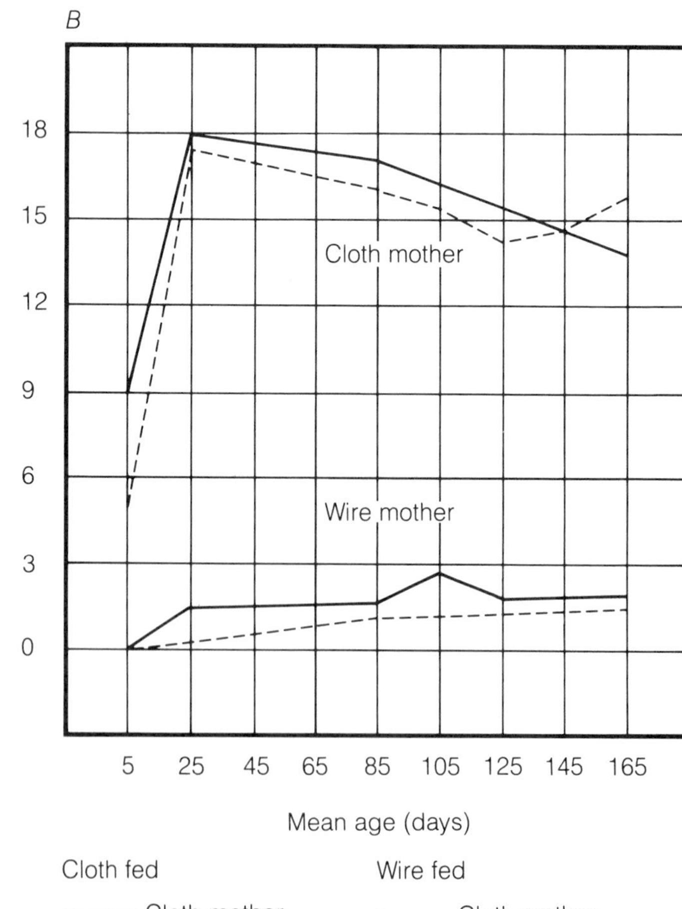

Figure 7-9 The infant monkey clings to the terry cloth "mother" rather than the wire surrogate. *B.* Comparison of the time spent with terry cloth and wire "surrogate mothers." Infants show a clear preference for the terry cloth surrogate, no matter which surrogate feeds them, indicating the relation between care and comfort in the needs of infant monkeys. (From Harlow H F: *American Psychologist* 1958; 13:273–685. Copyright 1958 by the American Psychological Association. Reprinted by permission of publisher.)

TABLE 7-5 Bowlby's Attachment Process and Behaviors

Behavior system	Descriptions
Fixed-action behaviors Crying Smiling	These infant behaviors activate parental responses that bring the adult into close proximity with the infant. Infant crying and smiling behaviors during early infancy (usually after the first year) are called "fixed-action" systems. Fixed-action behaviors are those that promote proximity but that are not altered or changed by the infant in relation to adult responses. For example, crying may continue at the same level of intensity even though the adult may be about to pick up the infant
Goal-corrected behaviors Sucking Following Clinging	Sucking, following, and clinging also generate parental responses that bring both infant and parent closer together. These three behaviors are called goal-corrected behaviors because the infant takes an *active* role in maintaining proximity by adjusting its responses to the parent's behavior (eg, the infant may "cling" more tightly to the parent when the parent attempts to put the child down than simply while being held by the parent)

SOURCE: Schiamberg LB, Smith KU: *Human Development.* Macmillan Publishing Company, New York, 1982, p. 252.

TABLE 7-6 Ainsworth's Stages of Infant Attachment

Stage	Age	Characteristics
Stage 1	0–3 months	Infant uses sucking, rooting, grasping, smiling, gazing, cuddling, and visual tracking to maintain closeness with caregiver
Stage 2	3–6 months	Infant is more responsive to familiar figures than to strangers
Stage 3	7 months to 2 years	Infant begins actively to seek proximity with the object of attachment
Stage 4	Toddlerhood and beyond	Infant uses a variety of behaviors that influence the behavior of the object of attachment to satisfy the need for closeness

SOURCE: Ainsworth MDS: The development of infant–mother attachment. In: *Review of Child Development Research.* Vol 3. Caldwell B, Ricciuti H (editors). University of Chicago Press, 1973.

At around 8–9 months of age, many infants develop stranger anxiety and negative reactions to strangers, usually at the same time that parental attachment first develops. Infants recognize familiar faces as different from strange ones, and they become centered on primary caregivers; they feel distress when these primary attachment figures are not present or are replaced with unfamiliar figures. This also is related to the fact that they have become increasingly aware of their dependence on their parents and, likewise, their vulnerability when their parents are not present. Although stranger anxiety is not manifested by all infants, it is thought to be related to the infant's emerging understanding that parents have a permanent relationship with them. Infants who have been surrounded by many people such as extended family members or friends of older siblings, tend to manifest less distress when parents leave. Although they prefer their parents, these infants have learned that other familiar, and even not so familiar, persons can meet their needs. For example, one young mother was concerned that her 10-month-old infant seldom complained when she left. She also was both pleased and puzzled that he readily interacted with strangers. This infant had several health problems that were being treated and monitored by physical therapists, nutritionists, and visiting nurses. He had become accustomed to positive experiences from a variety of people and thus did not have that sense of vulnerability experienced by infants who have received all their care from their parents.

Research in attachment presents a number of difficulties, one of which is measuring the attachment itself. During infancy, contact-seeking and proximity-maintaining behaviors seem to be a sensitive measurement, but, by 2 years of age, the child's separation protest has begun to decline (Lewis, Weinraub, and Ban, 1972). The 2-year-old also has developed a greater repertoire of coping behaviors, sense of self-confidence, and cognitive understanding. When parents leave, telling the child they will return after lunch, it is accepted because that is exactly what happened on previous occasions. The ability to remember past experiences helps the child to cope confidently with current, similar experiences. By 4 years of age, separation anxiety disappears altogether, except for children who seem to be particularly insecure (Peery and Aoki, 1982). Consequently, measuring attachment or love for one's parents across a life span is still awaiting an elegant methodologic solution.

Recent research suggests that attachment should not be the central focus of parent–infant emotional and social development. Some researchers feel that attachment should be included in broader considerations of many aspects of parent–child interaction and the complexities of the infant's

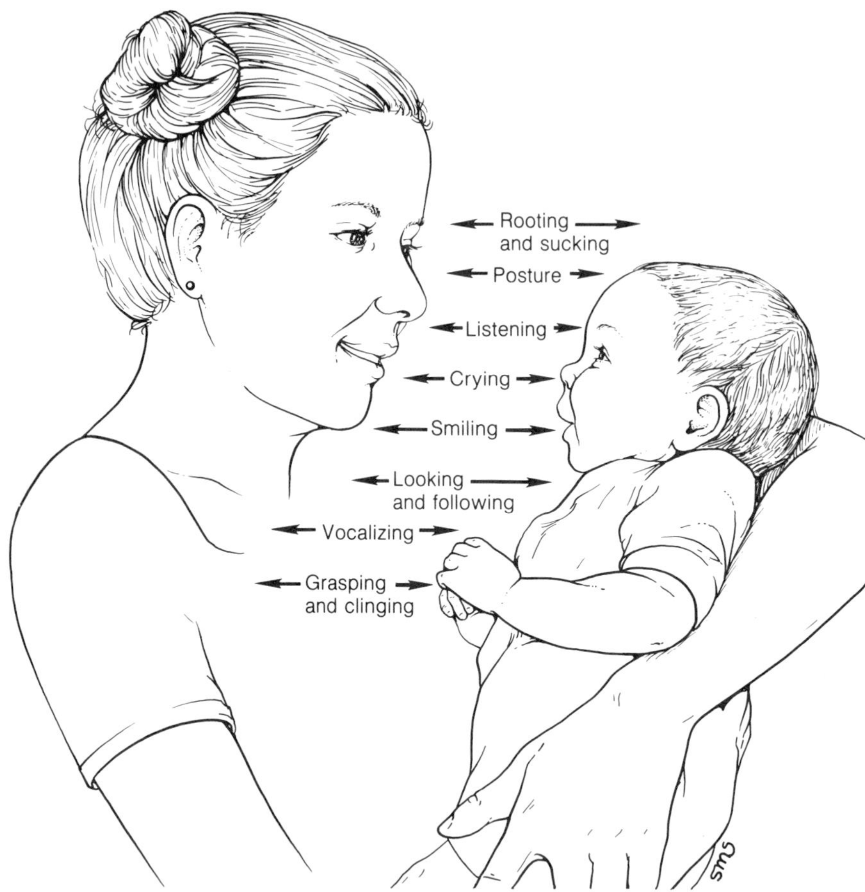

Figure 7-10 Ainsworth's components of attachment and their interaction in specific areas.

social network (Weinraub, et al., 1977). If infants are understood to engage in a variety of complex interactions, not only with their parents but also with other family members, strangers, and friends, the emotional bond between the parent and child becomes only one of the important variables that should be considered in trying to understand infant social development (Table 7-7).

Siblings and Peers Birth order is an influencing factor in family dynamics because parents often spend more time and give more attention to the firstborn infant than they do to subsequent infants (Boronson, 1973), and parents have higher expectations for the accomplishments of the firstborn child (Rothbart, 1971). Parents also tend to "practice" with their firstborn child and frequently make many parenting mistakes with this infant.

Siblings sometimes are assigned to infant caregiving, especially in large families where the older siblings are considerably older than the new infants. Little is known about sibling interaction during infancy, but research on social interaction between peers during infancy has yielded interesting results. Early in the first year, infants will begin to respond to social advances made by other infants. Infants who have older brothers and sisters seem to have more social skill and to be more responsive to these social advances by their peers. Initially, infant play seems to be object-centered, and infants pay more attention to toys than to each other. During the second year, this gradually decreases, and actual social interaction begins to increase (Eckerman, Whatley, and Kutz, 1975). Social interactions during the latter half of the second year, however, frequently involve acts of aggression—taking toys, pulling hair, and hitting (Mueller and Vandell, 1979). Cooperative social play is a development that occurs considerably later (see Chapter 8).

Parents, older siblings, and peers may all serve as models for the infant's behavior and may have a powerful influence in helping the infant to learn (Bandura, 1977). Aggression and positive social interactions demonstrated to children can be adopted quickly into their behavioral systems. Models for behavior can come from television and motion pictures as well as the live models a child sees at home and with peers. Considerable research has documented the importance of modeling as a way of fostering social behavior with

TABLE 7-7 Behaviors and Interactions With Others That Influence the Process of Socialization

Behavioral system	Social behaviors
Attachment	Staying near, asking to be held, crying. The presence of a caring adult to whom the infant is strongly attached provides a sense of protection
Fear, wariness	Avoidance of objects, persons, and situations that might be harmful. Most infants older than 7 or 8 months are cautious of or distressed by strangers. Wariness declines as the infant grows older (over 2 years) and begins to interact with strangers
Affiliative	Smiling, vocalizing, and showing toys to persons other than those to whom infants are strongly attached
Exploratory	Presence of attachment figures lends security to infants' first "voyages" of exploration. Based on initial strong attachment to a caregiver, as infants grow older they gain more confidence in "going it alone"

SOURCE: Lawton JT: *Introduction to Child Development.* Wm C. Brown, 1982.

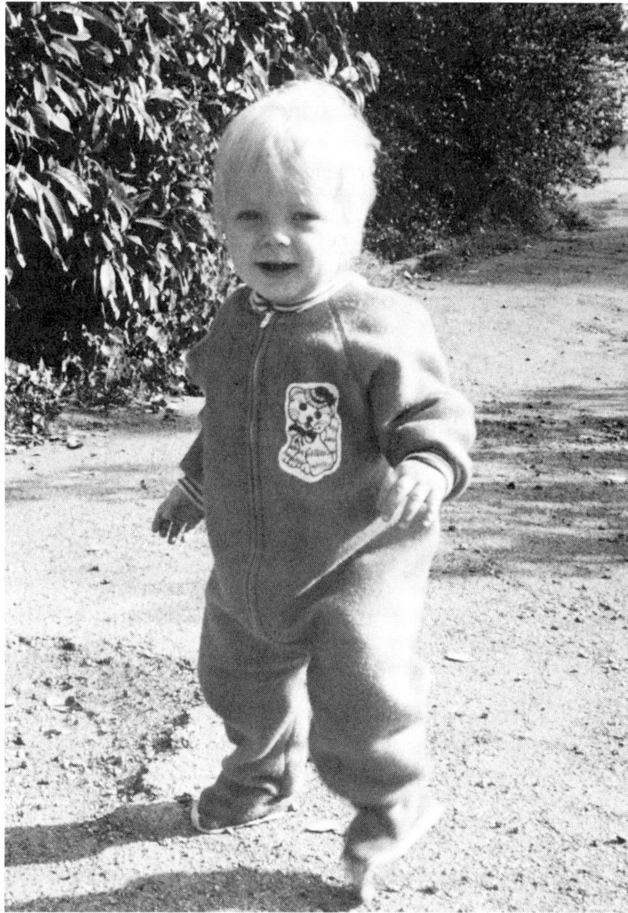

Developing motor skills allows the infant to explore the environment and practice new skills.

children in early childhood. Although less formal research has been done with infants, infants do learn substantially from watching the social interactions in their families. Although they do not understand language, infants are clearly sensitive and responsive to nonverbal communication and learn from the behavior exhibited in their social environment.

Integrating Development Through Play

Play during infancy is an important way of becoming acquainted with the environment. Playing first with the parents and family and then with toys and peers, the infant learns about cause and effect, interactions and expectations, and personal skills and abilities. Play, moreover, is fun. It is repetitious activity that is done for the sole enjoyment of practicing a known or comfortable pattern of behaviors.

Piaget (1962) noted that play during infancy involved the pure assimilation of sensorimotor actions because they are enjoyed. The infant will pick up the rattle, shake it, and watch the movement and listen to the sound and then drop the toy, look around, and repeat the action. Why? Because it brings pleasure and is fun. The schemes of reaching, grasping, lifting, and shaking are so well mastered that they are done without effort. The activity is no longer work but pleasure. It is the means to the end or just the activity itself that is satisfying.

Play begins as soon as the sensations are enjoyed. Play is the link that enables the infant to become a social being. From the early smile in response to parental coaxing to total involvement in a world of toys and their manipulations, the infant learns and practices becoming like others in the environment.

Themes of Play

There are many different theories about the process of play and its value. Psychodynamic theorists tend to describe play around its theme. Early play focuses on the infant's own body. The fascination of moving, touching, and intertwining one's own fingers or hands or of bringing them into sight singly or together and then watching them will occupy an infant for long periods of time. This activity might be accompanied by babbling or cooing sounds that express additional pleasure. These positive experiences are repeated over and over again for their kinesthetic sensation satisfaction. This type of play allows infants to increase their awareness and control of desired actions involving their own bodies. Theorists have termed this play *autoerotic* (Anna Freud, 1965) or *autocosmic* (Erikson, 1963). It also corresponds to Mahler's description of the autistic infant, which simply refers to the centering of interests, actions, and pleasure on the self.

As the infant becomes aware that the parent is not an extension of the self, there is a shift in the theme of play. Now the infant extends play to the parent, with face patting or poking and, unfortunately, hair pulling. Mahler referred to this phase as symbiotic (Mahler, Pine, and Bergman, 1975). Play is enhanced by the parent's participation and willingness to be the "object." Vocalizations are involved in play as well as the infant masters the production of various sounds and their combinations. Sounds are created and utterances and squeals of various pitch and intensity are practiced solely because of their intrinsic enjoyment.

Toward the end of the first year, the infant extends the play world to objects, which serve as an extension or substitute for the parent when the parent is not present. In addition, little games such as pat-a-cake and peek-a-boo are added. The infant would play these games endlessly and often begs for them to be continued long after the adult has tired of the activity.

Toys as objects to manipulate and work out themes gain importance at the beginning of the second year. Erikson defined this play as the microsphere stage. The infant uses small objects and toys to work out or manage larger events experienced in the real world. The world is put in order and better understood as the older infant controls these small toys and thus achieves a sense of mastery. While playing with a dollhouse, a toy gas station, cars, trucks, dolls, stuffed animals, or puppets, the older infant becomes engrossed in creating and controlling events. This type of play becomes more elaborate during early childhood. Erikson viewed this fantasy type of play as preparatory for interaction with peers.

Toys increasingly become a medium for play and skill perfection. The push-pull and dump-fill activities popular with infants at this age provide for the practice of fine and gross motor behaviors, manipulation of objects at will, and trial-and-error experiences with objects of different sizes and shapes. Thus, doing things with and to objects becomes the theme of the play. Peller (1954) noted that play also was used to overcome the fear of parental loss when object permanence was acquired. The peek-a-boo game, retrieval of rolled or tossed objects, and doll play were seen as means of playing out this fear.

Older infants increasingly enjoyed play with the parent using toys as a medium. Rolling a ball back and forth, mutual stacking of shapes or blocks, shape-sorter toys involving searching and finding the right hole for the shape, top spinning, and looking at picture books are but a few activities that encourage parent–infant play.

Content of Play

Theorists who prefer to focus on the content of play note the exploratory nature of infant's first play (Hurlock, 1978). Initial exploration is visual, and the 1-to 3-month-old infant spends long periods of time staring at objects and people, especially faces. It is not uncommon for parent and infant to spend several minutes locked into each other's gaze as if trying to absorb all the details of each other's appearance.

As neuromuscular maturation progresses, infants gain control over arms, hands, and upper body and use them to explore both their own body and other objects. The manipulation of objects is influenced by maturation and coordination. First, things are patted or swiped at as the young infant finds hours of enjoyment hitting the mobile or cradle gym and watching the result, which usually includes both sound and movement. Improved coordination permits better eye-hand-mouth control, and objects soon are grasped, maneuvered, and brought to the mouth for further exploration. The infant delights in the increased voluntary control over self and objects. Time is passed happily surrounded by toys, which are picked up, mouthed, banged, shaken, and dropped, and the same or similar actions are repeated on another toy. As mobility improves, the object world and its combinations become even greater.

Early play, as defined by Smilansky (1968) is primarily functional and includes aspects of sensorimotor experience. The infant, according to the level of maturation and skill in coordination, interacts spontaneously with the environment. As these infants move quickly and freely from one activity to another, their thorough enjoyment of whatever they are doing is play. There are no extrinsic goals—blocks are stacked, not to see how high they can make the tower, but just for the fun of picking up one block and putting it where the infant wants it to go.

Gross motor play encourages the exploration of the physical self in relation to the environment. The older infant walks back and forth because the skill that had once been work is now mastered, and pure delight is taken in this accomplishment. Once a skill has been mastered, there is a magnetic attraction to practice it again and again. Many parents have expressed frustration over the fact that once climbing is perfected, nothing is safe. The infant climbs up stairs but cannot get down, up onto a chair or couch and from there to the windowsill or lamp table, but once there is both proud and helpless.

Fine motor activities are another aspect of functional play that generates coordination and the control of more precise movements. Toys and other external objects are manipulated. The repetitive building and knocking down of the block tower facilitates the use of a mastered skill involving the precision of motor-perceptual movement.

Near the end of infancy, play becomes constructive. The skill acquired in the manipulation of objects and understanding their function is now put to use in creating structures. This encourages the expression of feelings and the use of self as the creator of the event. Play construction helps children to create a world through their own eyes and according to their own style.

The content of play has been discussed by Sutton-Smith (1971) in his analysis of play activities. Early play activity involves imitating what has been previously mastered by exploratory or self-testing activities or what has been observed from others. Imitated play involves those actions and behaviors perceived as fun and within the infant's repertoire.

Exploratory play is an extension of exploration activities. Exploration activities are directed toward learning and therefore require effort and concentration. Exploratory play is doing or practicing what has already been learned purely for the pleasure the activity brings. Initially matching shapes is a learning process, and finding the right spot for a circle, square, or triangle is difficult. A few weeks later, this same infant quickly matches all objects and shapes and is ready to repeat the performance. The early exploration activity has now become exploratory play. When parental attention is being given, this infant may tease and purposefully place a circle over the square hole, mischievously look up at the parent for a response, laugh, find the correct hole, and repeat the game just created.

Research done by Clarke-Stewart (1973) illustrated that infants were interested in objects for what could be done to and with them. They used their senses to explore the object as a whole and in its individual parts. If a toy had a cord that, when pulled, caused other parts to move, the action of pulling and watching the movement would be repeated several times followed by separate inspection of the cord and each movable part.

Interest in specific toys peaks and wanes in relation to the infant's own interest, sense of achievement, and desire to practice new skills. A toy that has multiple uses will return to a favored spot as the infant discovers each new use to which it can be put.

Structure of Play

The final approach to the categorization of play is that of structure. Piaget (1962) acknowledged play themes and content, but because of his interest in how infants learn, he focused on the cognitive complexity of games. The complexity of infant's play is related to the complexity of the available materials and the infant's cognitive development. Piaget noted that some principles form distinct systems of cognitive functioning and can be attributed to rules about the structures of things. An infant must first learn the properties of objects such as roundness. Then, putting a round form into a circular hole can be repeated endlessly for the sheer joy of it.

Practice games appear during Stage 2, or primary circular actions (see Chapter 6). The initial play consists of the repetition of self-initiated vocal or visual schemes, which is a continuation of assimilation. Practice games occupy all of infancy because, as Piaget noted, learning about the environment and its properties occurs by actively interacting with it.

Uzgiris (1967) noted the pattern of schemes used by infants in relation to exploration and the use of objects. Table 7-8 shows the progressive sequence the infant employs in learning about an object and its properties. Practice games are demonstrated by infants shaking, grasping, throwing, clapping, winding up the jack-in-the-box or the music box, running, or climbing for the pleasure of the activity itself. Play in this sense is the process of reexperiencinig, reexploring, and reinvestigating the familiar because it is there to be done.

TABLE 7-8 Progression in Schemes Used by Infants to Explore Objects in Their Environment

Behavior observed in the majority of infants	Age in months
Mouthing	2
Holding	2
Visual inspection	3
Hitting	4
Shaking	5
Examining	6
Pulling, tearing, rubbing	6
Squeezing, sliding	6
Pushing	7
Dropping	8
Throwing	9
Socially instigated behaviors	10
Showing	14
Naming	18

SOURCE: Uzgiris IC: Ordinality in the development of schemas for relating to objects. In: *Exceptional Infant. The Normal Infant.* Vol 1. Helmuth J (editor). Bruner/Mazel, 1967.

Symbolic play appears near the end of infancy. It contains the element of make-believe and pretend while providing the opportunity for imaginary games and fantasy reenactment. It has no limits; anything can become what is desired. A block is a car, a plane, a house, or a bed because of the power of magical assignment. One knows what the object is because of the sounds or functions associated with it rather than its appearance.

Parental Actions to Facilitate Play

Parents provide a supportive role with respect to the infant's play. Some of the dimensions of play are determined by the physical nature of the materials. If there is never anything to see or to reach, why bother? If the object grasped is not interesting in terms of color, noise, or movement, there is little incentive to keep reaching out for it. Objects or toys do not have to be expensive; some of the best toys are those created by the parent. Universally favorite toys seem to be boxes, pots and pans with lids, wooden spoons, and other kitchen-related containers. For several months, a 1-year-old will spend hours playing with a large plastic dishpan, a bag of potatoes, a wooden spoon, and a dishtowel. Some actions are ritualistically performed and others are newly created, but the playing process of pretending, exploring, manipulating, and fantasizing is engaged in freely and obviously enjoyed.

Another important supportive role of the parent during this stage is playing with the infant. The first games involve visual gazing and responding to facial interactions. The parent who enjoys an activity with the infant encourages the infant to be perceptive and responsive. The complex interactional process that is established between the parent and child around play is usually positive. Parent and child enjoy each other mutually. They orient each other to the environment, specific stimuli, causal relations, and social conventions.

Health Care Needs of Infancy

Hygiene

The infant depends on the parent for skin care and cleanliness. During early infancy, sponge baths are appropriate because the infant does not need to be immersed daily in a tub. For both infants and parents, bath time is usually a time for playful interaction. The frequency of baths depends on the condition of the infant's skin, whether dry, moist, or oily, temperature of the environment, and the infant's schedule. Few infants require a daily bath, and applying lotion or petroleum is preferred for infants with dry skin. For all infants, the diaper area should be cleansed carefully with each diaper change. After feeding, hands and faces may need to be cleaned, depending on the infant's age and neatness in eating.

Miliaria—Prickly Heat During hot, humid summer days, infants are prone to a rash that is technically termed *miliaria* and commonly called prickly heat. It appears suddenly and can disappear just as quickly once the skin is cooled. The rash is caused by inflamed or blocked sweat glands and consists of tiny, pinhead-sized erythematous, papular lesions with vesicles in the center. Because infants do not perspire until after the first month of life, neonates are particularly susceptible. Miliaria also occurs throughout the life span and is harmless. It develops whenever body warmth is excessive because of the weather, indoor overheating, or overdressing. Removing excess clothing, leaving an overheated room, finding a cool, shady spot outdoors, or giving the infant a tepid sponge bath will decrease body warmth and reverse the appearance of prickly heat. Powder, if used, should be applied in a thin layer, and cornstarch, creams, and ointments should not be used. Gently patting the infant's skin to keep it dry and changing damp clothing and bed linen also helps.

Seborrheic Dermatitis—Cradle Cap Although the infant is clean and the head and hair are washed frequently, seborrheic dermatitis, or cradle cap, may occur. Its cause is unknown but appears to be related to activity of the sebaceous glands. The scalp is the most frequent site, but it also might be found on the eyebrows and eyelids, behind the eyelids, behind and in the ears, on the sides of the nose, and in the inguinal region. Cervical lymph node enlargement may also be associated with the condition.

Cradle cap appears as thick, yellowish, oily, scaly, nonpruritic patches. Often, the area of greatest involvement is the anterior fontanel. Parents need to be reassured that the "soft spot" is not fragile but similar to skin and will not be harmed by routine washing. A simple method of removing the scaly patches is to use a cotton ball to apply baby oil on each site, allow the oil to penetrate the crusts, and then thoroughly wash the scalp with a dandruff-control shampoo. Fine-tooth combing or brushing with an old toothbrush then removes the flakes from the hair. Daily shampooing should follow. This same procedure can be used for other sites except the eyes. Parents need to be cautioned not to pick at the crusts to remove them but to first soak them and wash the site thoroughly.

In most instances the condition is temporary. It appears sometime between 2 and 12 weeks of age and usually disappears by 8–12 months of age. If the sites become infected, the physician should be consulted because additional treatment is necessary.

Diaper Dermatitis—Diaper Rash Experienced parents say that it is easier to prevent *diaper dermatitis,* or diaper rash, than to treat it. It is the nurse's responsibility to emphasize to all parents the importance of thoroughly cleansing the perineal area with each diaper change as the best way to prevent diaper rash. Sponging the area with warm water or mild soap and water followed by gentle drying is recommended. Other measures that help to promote dryness and adequate aeration of the area include the frequent changing of wet or soiled diapers; the limited use of plastic or rubber pants because they retain moisture (making the perineal area wet and warm—a perfect medium for bacteria growth); and exposing the perineal area to the air for 5–10 minutes, three or four times a day. This often can be accomplished around diaper changing times. In addition, applying a thin film of medicated powder helps to promote dryness. Powder must be used carefully. It should not be shaken vigorously because inhaling the powder dust can cause respiratory problems (Chow, et al., 1979). Excess powder is a hazard because it will cake in the body creases, particularly the groin, and result in skin excoriation. Rather, a small amount of powder should be put in the parent's hand and then lightly rubbed onto the infant's skin so that a thin film covers the entire diaper area. Medicated powder is preferred over powder containing talc because talc does not absorb water and has no antifungal or antibacterial properties.

Cornstarch, creams, and petroleum jelly generally are contraindicated. Any ointment or powder containing boric acid must never be used because of the associated risk of systemic poisoning. Petroleum jelly, once a favorite, is no longer used because it is too occlusive and does not allow adequate aeration. Its use results in excessive softening and thinning of the protective layers of the skin, predisposing that area to yeast infections. Cornstarch tends to cake once wet, which irritates the skin and promotes skin breakdown. With any loss of skin integrity in a wet, warm, dark environment, bacteria and fungi thrive. Preventing this combination is the goal of providing for the infant's hygiene needs.

Diaper rash has numerous causes, including contact with external irritants, bacterial or fungal infections, ammonia irritation, and reaction to certain foods ingested. To a large extent, the management of a diaper rash resembles the measures recommended for its prevention. Identifying the causative agent is especially helpful in preventing a recurrence of the rash. Parents are usually good detectives and can identify what has been changed or is new and different in the infant's routine and care. Known irritants are soaps, fabric softeners, disposable diapers, acid from urine and feces, certain breakdown products from foods, such as orange juice and tomatoes, and the use of plastic pants, cornstarch, excess powder, or ointments. One mother concluded that although disposable diapers were more convenient when traveling, they were not worth the diaper rash her infant experienced after they were used. Another parent discovered that orange juice, even when diluted with water, was the guilty irritant.

There are some distinguishing characteristics among the diaper rashes. Contact rash has patches of erythema, skin softening and thinning, and eventual breakdown along the groin, inguinal region, buttocks, and, sometimes, abdomen. Management of this type of rash includes the preventive measures previously discussed, elimination of the irritant, and careful application of a healing ointment, which can be purchased without prescription. The nurse should advise the parent to reapply a thin film of ointment with each diaper change. The previously applied ointment must be carefully washed off first. The use of mineral oil can facilitate the removal of some ointments. These ointments must be used cautiously because they are potential sensitizers. It is necessary to warn parents that each infant's rash responds differently, and sometimes more than one ointment must be tried before satisfactory results are obtained.

Fungal infections present as smooth, bright red, shiny, raised lesions, which are circumscribed and the size of a pinhead. The lesions are found in the inguinal region and may spread to the buttocks and abdomen. If the infection is mild, it can be controlled by following the preventive measures and using a medicated powder. If the rash is severe, the addition of an antifungal cream is required.

An ammoniacal diaper rash is seen more frequently in infants over 7 months of age. The rash is located on the buttocks, abdomen, and inner thighs. It is an erythematous, papulovasicular rash, and the urine smells strongly of ammonia. Management includes preventive measures, the careful use of healing ointments, increasing the infant's water intake to dilute the urine, and adding 1–2 oz of cranberry juice to the infant's daily fluid intake to acidify the urine. If cloth diapers are used, the addition of bleach or vinegar to the final rinse cycle also helps to acidify the diapers.

Some infants are more prone to diaper rash than others. Infants with fair complexions tend to have more sensitive skin and be less tolerant of wet diapers and irritants in general. Many times, an infant who has a diaper rash is uncomfortable. The addition of a wet diaper can be painful, resulting in increasing restlessness and irritability.

The nurse can advise the parents that by instituting preventive measures from the beginning, they quickly become routine. The advantage is a happy infant with few, if any, diaper rashes.

Sleep and Rest

Sleep patterns during infancy vary greatly. The neonate averages 16 hours of sleep a day, with some neonates requiring as little as 10 hours and others as much as 22 hours. Sleep patterns vary from infant to infant, and sleep-wake routines vary from month to month for individual infants. The neonate sleeps in a series of naps. Some naps last 30 minutes, whereas other naps last 3–4 hours. Approximately half of the neonate's sleep time is spent in REM sleep. Rapid-eye-movements (REM) sleep is characteristic of Stage 1, or light, sleep. During this stage of sleep, involuntary muscle movements and dreaming occur, which accounts for the many coughs, gurgles, sighs, squirms, and squiggles the young infant makes while sleeping. When the nurse shares this information with parents, it helps them to understand that the sounds their infant makes are not necessarily waking-up sounds. Therefore, it is best to wait until the infant is obviously awake before picking him or her up to be changed or fed. Adults who are awakened frequently during REM sleep become increasingly fatigued and irritable. There is some indication from limited studies that the same phenomenon may be true for infants (Levine, et al., 1983).

During infancy, the organization of sleep and wakefulness changes significantly, whereas the total amount of sleep decreases only by 2–3 hours. The average sustained sleep of the neonate seldom exceeds 4 hours; it increases to 7 hours for the 5-month-old and 11–12 hours for the 18-month-old. With longer sleep periods come longer times of wakefulness. Instead of the six naps a day needed by the neonate, the older infant does well with only one or two naps. The sleep-wake patterns tend to be a stable characteristic for the individual infant. The 18-month-old who required less-than-average sleep as a neonate continues to thrive on less sleep, whereas the infant who required more than an average amount of sleep as a neonate still does (Jacklin, et al., 1980).

One indicator of maturation appreciated by parents is sleeping through the night. Moore and Ucko (1957) found in their study of 104 infants that 70% slept through the night (midnight–5 A.M.) at 3 months of age, 83% at 6 months of age, and 90% at 1 year of age. Having an infant begin to sleep through the night, however, does not mean an end to night wakings. It is common for infants to awaken during the night between 5 and 9 months of age and again during their second year of life, even after months of having slept through the night. Various factors that have been identified as contributing to night wakings include low sensory threshold, temperament (Carey, 1975), history of perinatal stress such as prolonged labor (Bernal, 1973), sleeping in the same room as the parents (Traisman, Traisman, and Garri, 1966), teething, and continued breast-feeding after 6 months of age (Osterholm, Lindeke, and Amidon, 1983).

Factors that do not influence night waking are the early introduction of solid foods (Beal, 1969), age, sex, sleeping in the same room as a sibling, parental expectations, and motor development (Osterholm, Lindeke, and Amidon, 1983). The developmental component involved is the diurnal organization of REM sleep and the transitions from REM to non-REM sleep. The maturation process of these aspects of sleep appears to be associated with night wakings (Levine, et al., 1983).

Whether night wakings are considered to be problematic depends on the parent's perception. Some parents find themselves so tired from being awakened at night that they are irritable during the day, whereas other parents are able to tolerate the sleep interruptions better. For example, one mother commented that her daughter showed considerable intelligence at 5 months of age because she had already figured out the family routine. The infant would sleep from 6–9 P.M. every evening while her parents were busy helping the older children to do their homework and get ready for bed. When the others were settled, she would awaken for her special time, often staying up until midnight. She and her parents enjoyed this time of individualized attention. She would awaken next at 5 A.M., and one of her parents would bring her to their bed so she could breast-feed before the others got up for the day. This mother admitted that, although this routine worked well for them, it would not be ideal for everyone.

Parents vary in their sleep-wake needs just as infants do. Some parents become very discouraged when an infant who has been sleeping through the night starts to awaken again during the night. When assessing an infant's total sleep time, it is important to relate these sleep-wake patterns to those of the family and the ways in which each member is affected when they do not coincide.

It is often helpful to reassure parents that night wakings are common and that they appear to be related to maturational, temperamental, and environmental factors. Each situation needs to be assessed and changes planned to fit with the needs and life-style of the family. Like so many aspects of parent–child interactions, there is no one "right way" but rather as many variations as there are actors. The goal is to establish a good fit between the parent and infant so that the relationship can thrive.

Nutrition

Infant nutrition is a subject that combines current research and a plethora of information with cultural attitudes and traditions about food and feeding routines, together with the socioeconomic factors that influence food choices. The child health nurse not only needs to be well informed about traditional or middle-class ways of meeting nutritional requirements but also must be knowledgeable about cultural and ethnic preferences as well as individual variations. Good nutritional habits begin in infancy and are one of the best preventive health care practices available. Nutrition education therefore must be directed to parents during the prenatal period. Often, a first step is examining the belief that fat babies are healthy babies or the stereotype that good parents have fat babies. Infantile obesity has become a major concern, especially because it may jeopardize optimal development. Chapter 15 discusses nutritional requirements and nutritional concerns, such as weaning, in infancy.

The food of choice for infants under 6 months of age is milk, either human milk or prepared formula. Adequate intake of either one provides all known nutritional requirements, with the possible exception of vitamin D and fluoride for breast-fed infants, and an optimal balance of carbohydrate, protein, and fat in readily digested forms (American Academy of Pediatrics, 1980). The addition of solid foods prior to 6 months of age only adds excess calories and imposes a heavy renal solute load while increasing water demands (American Academy of Pediatrics, 1976a and b). A variety of prepared formulas are available, including some formulas to accommodate infants who are allergic to milk or who have specific nutritional needs (Table 7-9). Human milk has the additional advantages of providing protection against disease in the form of immune factors and resistance to antigen absorption from the small intestine (Gulick, 1983). Infants, furthermore, are rarely allergic or unable to digest and metabolize their mothers' milk.

The American Academy of Pediatrics (1976) has recommended that infants receive either human milk or prepared formula during their first year of life. The use of homogenized cow's milk during the first year places the infant at risk for iron-deficiency anemia. The iron in cow's milk is poorly absorbed, and intake in excess of a quart per day may cause intestinal bleeding and occult blood loss.

Around 6 months of age the infant is physiologically and developmentally ready to have solid foods added to the diet. An indicator on which to base an infant's nutritional care is the development of motor functions (Table 7-10). For example, the normal neonate initially is capable of rooting, sucking, and swallowing fluids; at first, the sucking is an up-and-down tongue movement that matures to a back-and-forward tongue movement. Nutritional care plans depend on an understanding of these developmental changes, so that the nurse can help the parent to recognize specific behaviors. For instance, the strong tongue extrusion reflex during the first 6 months of life inhibits an infant from accepting spoon feeding but assists in the intake of breast-milk or formula. Infants can better learn solid food feeding once they can sit up, reach, grasp, and exercise lateral tongue movements and good hand-to-mouth coordination. Waiting until 6 months of age to introduce solids not only allows neuromuscular maturity but also development of the digestive system's ability to handle foreign proteins with the enzymes necessary for the absorption and use of specific nutrients. By 6 months of age, most infants need an external source of iron because prenatal stores have been depleted. Iron-fortified cereals are recommended at this time and are continued daily at least until the child is 18 months old. Three level tablespoons of dry cereal diluted with milk or formula make a serving of about 60 g, providing 7 mg of iron (Fomon, et al., 1979). The RDA for iron for infants 6–12 months of age is 15 mg; therefore, if the infant takes two feedings of cereal per day, this would adequately meet the daily requirement. The infant who has been on an iron-fortified formula need not start with cereal but may choose to take fruits or vegetables.

Traditionally, the sequence in which foods are introduced is (1) cereals, particularly rice for its nonallergenic properties; (2) fruits such as peaches, pears, or applesauce; (3) vegetables, with yellow vegetables such as squash, sweet potatoes, or carrots (being careful to avoid a buildup of carotene) being given before green vegetables like peas or beans; and (4) strained meats such as nonallergenic lamb or veal. High-protein foods such as meats are never given before 6 months of age because of the increased chance of an allergic reaction. In families with histories of allergies the nurse advises parents to read all baby food jar labels carefully. Many strained fruits are preserved with orange juice, and many of the meat and vegetable dinners contain tomato, both of which are allergenic. The potentially allergic infant should not be given orange juice until after the first birthday (see Chapter 37 for discussion of allergies). By 7–9 months of age, teething allows the infant to chew, and the infant has a mature swallowing ability that makes it possible to experience foods with different textures. By 9–12 months, the infant indicates a readiness to self-feed appropriate finger food. Finger foods might include sliced and peeled apple, sliced peach, a piece of cheese, or a few pieces of dry cereal. These foods are readily softened by saliva, thereby preventing choking. Peanuts, popcorn, or hard candy, which can be inhaled or choked on, should be avoided at this age.

It is most important that the parent be advised to introduce one new food at a time and no faster then once every 5 days so that any symptoms of intolerance can be traced. The more simple the choice of foods, the less is the chance of providing excess calories. The infant can tolerate the simplicity and limited choices better than the parent. Parents should know that prepared dinners provide more starch fillers than meat and vegetables and that desserts, although attractive, offer no more than empty calories. Strained fruits offer mostly carbohydrate and some vitamin C. Vegetables are a good source of vitamin A. Strained meats contain protein and minerals. Orange juice and other juices are good sources of vitamin C. Juices are best offered from the cup and initially diluted with water to assist in eventual weaning. Eggs yolks are a poor source of iron and need not be offered until the infant reaches 1 year of age.

Manufacturers of commercially prepared infant foods recently have reduced or eliminated the sugar and salt from their products because of concern about the development of hypertension and obesity in later life. Home-prepared infant foods, which some parents prefer, usually have a higher caloric density because of lower water content and may have significant amounts of added salt if parents are not guided in the preparation of these foods.

TABLE 7-9 Pediatric Formulas

Formula (Company)	Carbohydrate	Protein	Fat	Stool characteristics	Explanation
Enfamil (Mead Johnson)	Lactose	Nonfat milk	Soy, coconut oils	Formed, greenish-brown with very little free water around stool	Can be used with infants with fat intolerance. Appropriate formula for normal infants who have no special nutritional requirements
Similac (mRoss)	Lactose	Nonfat milk	Soy, coconut, corn oils	Formed, greenish-brown with very little free water around stool	Iron may be added to any of these formulas to supply a dependable daily intake; for premature infants; for offspring of anemic mothers; for infants of multiple births; for infants with low birthweights and those who grew rapidly; for infants who have lost blood
SMA (Wyeth)	Lactose	Electrolyzed whey, nonfat milk	Coconut, safflower, soybean oils	Similar to breast-milk stools: small volume, pasty yellow, some free water	
Isomil (Ross)	Sucrose, cornstarch, corn syrup solids	Soy protein isolates	Soy, coconut corn oils	Mushy, yellow-green with more free water than cow's milk stools	Used for children with milk allergies
Neomulsoy (Syntex)	Sucrose	Soy protein isolates	Soy oil		
Nursoy (Wyeth)	Sucrose, corn syrup	Soy protein isolates	Coconut, oleic, safflower, soybean oils, and soy oil		
Prosobee (Mead Johnson)	Sucrose, corn syrup	Soy protein isolates	Soy oil		Metabolic defects, eg, galactosemia
Lofenalac (Mead Johnson)	Corn syrup solids, tapioca starch	Hydrolyzed casein (most of phenylalanine removed)	Corn oil	Similar to cow's milk formula: formed, greenish-brown with very little free water around stool	Used in children with phenylketonuria in whom a low phenylalanine diet is needed
Lanala (Mead Johnson)	Lactose	Casein	Coconut oil	Similar to cow's milk formula stool	Sodium-free. Used in infants with severe renal/cardiac disease. Not recommended for long-term use without a sodium supplement
Similac PM 60/40 (Ross)	Lactose	Demineralized whey and nonfat milk	Coconut and corn oil	Similar to cow's milk formula stool	Cow's milk base. Low renal solute base. Low-sodium but supplies daily sodium requirements. Used in long-term renal/heart disease patients
Portagen (Mead Johnson)	Sucrose, corn syrup solids	Sodium caseinate	Fractionated coconut oil, corn oil	Similar to cow's milk formula	Indicated in a child with liver or pancreatic disease because the medium-chain triglycerides are absorbed into the portal system and do not require bile and

TABLE 7-9 continued

Formula (Company)	Carbohydrate	Protein	Fat	Stool characteristics	Explanation
					pancreatic enzymes for digestion, eg, cystic fibrosis
Nutramigen (Mead Johnson)	Sucrose, tapioca starch	Enzymically hydrolyzed 8 casein	Corn oil	Low-volume, green stools with some mucus	Used in protein hyper-sensitive disorders where intact proteins are not tolerated; this formula's proteins are broken into amino acids and poly-peptides, eg, congenital galactosemia. Also used in cases of multiple food allergies
Pregestimil (Mead Johnson)	Dextrose, tapioca starch	Enzymically hydrolyzed 8 casein	Fractionated coconut oil, corn oil	Low-volume, green stools with mucus	Used in some cases of fat or carbohydrate mal-absorption because for-mula is composed of simple structures that are easily absorbed, eg, cystic fibrosis. High intestinal osmolarity; therefore may result in diarrhea. Must be started at half-strength and gradually increased to full-strength. Can be used for protein supple-mentation
Cho-Free (Syntex)	None	Soy protein isolate	Soy oil	Similar to soy formula stools	Carbohydrate-free for-mula. Provides 12 calo-ries/oz. Used in short-term carbohydrate intol-erance
Lytren (Mead Johnson) Pedialyte (Ross)	—	—	—	—	Used for dehydration, loss of electrolytes, and the replacement and prevention of electro-lytes. Indicated in diar-rhea and vomiting. Post-operative fluid for oral electrolyte replacement. Contraindicated in infants with impaired renal function

Infants respond differently to the introduction of solid food. Some infants adapt quickly to the new tastes and textures, whereas others initially resist and only gradually make the adjustment to eating solids. When the infant refuses a food, it is best to stop and try again in a few days. Force-feeding at this stage paves the way for mutual frustration and future power plays involving food. When solids are introduced at 6 months of age, most infants progress rapidly to table foods. Soft foods, such as mashed potatoes, cooked carrots, squash, beans, canned fruits, yogurt, toast, cereals, soups, and cottage cheese, are managed well. Foods that splinter, such as raw carrots and celery sticks, should

TABLE 7-10 Infant Feeding Behaviors

Age	Hunger behavior	Feeding behavior	Satiety behavior
Birth to 13 weeks (0–3 months)	Cries; hands fisted; body tense	Rooting reflex; medial lip closure; strong suck reflex; suck-swallow pattern; tongue thrust and retraction; palmomental reflex; gags easily; needs burping	Withdraws head from nipple; falls asleep; hands relaxed; relief of body tension
14–24 weeks (4–6 months)	Eagerly anticipates; grasps and draws bottle to mouth; reaches with open mouth	Aware of hands; generalized reaching; intentional hand-to-mouth; tongue elevation; lips purse at corners—pucker; shifts food in mouth—prechewing; tongue protrudes in anticipation of nipple; tongue holds nipple firm; tongue projection strong; suck strength increases; coughs and chokes easily; preference for tastes	Tosses head back; fusses or cries; covers mouth with hands; ejects food; distracted by surroundings
28–36 weeks (7–9 months)	Reacts to food preparation sounds; vocalizes hunger; reaches out	Biting (first teeth); turns palm toward face; draws lower lip with food; thumb-finger grasp and palmar grasp; increased dexterity of hands; lateral tongue movement; mature swallow; chewing begins—vertical jaw protrusion; sucking decreases; holds bottle; handles cup awkwardly	Changes posture; closes mouth; shakes head "no"; plays with and throws utensils
40–52 weeks (10–12 months)	Vocalizes; grasps utensils	Tongue licks food from lower lip; holds and transfers to mouth; drinks from cup with spillage; lateral chewing movements; sticks out tongue; demands to feed self	Shakes head "no"; sputters

be avoided because of the danger of aspiration. Commercially prepared strained or junior meats or home-pureed meats need to be continued until the infant has an adequate chewing ability because meat is such an important source of iron.

By 9 months of age, the infant should be eating three meals a day and drinking about 24 oz of formula. If breast-feeding, the number of feedings should decrease to around four per day. At 1 year of age, the infant can be completely fed on table food and the daily milk intake decreased to 18–24 oz.

Feeding Difficulties The hallmark of good parenting is the contented, thriving infant. When the infant appears to be hungry all the time or refuses to eat, parents, particularly the breast-feeding mother, are under stress. Parental anxiety transmitted to the infant sets up a cycle that creates a real dilemma for the family. In assessing this situation the nurse should first ascertain whether the infant gained 4–7 oz/week for the first 6 months of life. Next, the adequacy of fluid intake and output should be determined. The infant should have at least six wet diapers per day, and, if adequately nourished, the infant should fall quietly asleep for several hours after a feeding.

Breast-feeding mothers who are having difficulty feeding their infants are concerned immediately about the adequacy of their milk production. Supporting the nursing mother requires that the nurse transmit knowledge and confidence. The signs of successful lactation include milk dripping from the breast before feeding at the sight or sound of the baby, milk dripping from the opposite breast during the feeding, uterine cramps during the feeding, cessation of any nipple discomfort during the feeding, milk dripping during sexual arousal, and a tingling sensation of the nipple seconds after the feeding starts. These signs all indicate the presence of a good "let-down reflex," which is essential for successful lactation. The initiation of the let-down reflex requires a strong suck from the infant.

Regurgitation Regurgitation, or spitting up, of predigested milk frequently occurs in the early months but can continue for most of the first year. One advantage of breast-feeding is that the regurgitation is odorless, whereas regurgitated formula smells sour. Although regurgitation can be most disconcerting to parents, it is not necessarily indicative of a nutritional problem. Evidence of a satisfactory growth pattern often reassures the family.

The amount, force, and character of the contents of regurgitation should be investigated, however, to rule out any significant gastric problem. Observing a feeding is helpful in determining any changes to suggest. The nurse might, for example, encourage adequate burping during the feeding to eliminate air bubbles. The neonate should be burped after every ounce of formula or every 5 minutes of breast-feeding. The infant should be held in a relaxed, comfortable position and the bottle tipped so that milk fills the nipple to prevent swallowing air. If regurgitation is caused by an immature gastric sphincter, placing the infant in a semi-upright position, as in an infant seat, following the feeding allows the milk or food to settle.

Gastrointestinal Changes Constipation can be a concern for parents, particularly if they do not understand the normal bowel patterns of infants. Breast-fed and formula-fed infants are rarely constipated. Parents first need to know that it is the consistency and not the frequency of the stool that characterizes constipation. A hard, formed, marble-sized, dry, hard-to-pass stool is descriptive of a constipated condition. Most infants have stools at least once a day. Some infants may have stools as infrequently as once every 2–3 days and still have a normal stool pattern if the stool is a normal, soft consistency. If the infant does have an occasional hard stool, the nurse might recommend an increase in fluid intake, or, if the infant is on solid foods, an increase in fruits and fruit juices.

A very watery stool occurring more than five times in a day is diarrhea. Parents sometimes confuse diarrhea with the frequent, loose, yellowish, seedy stool of the breast-fed infant or the use of certain types of formula (Table 7-9). Because diarrhea is unusual in the breast-fed infant, it suggests an infection, and the parent should be referred for medical diagnosis. For the bottle-fed infant, the nurse first might want to investigate the formula preparation, source of water supply, and possibility of contamination. If the infant is on solids, it may reflect the introduction of a new food, fruit juice, or excess fruit intake. For mild diarrhea, which lasts only a day or two, the cessation of solid food may be indicated along with diluting the formula with water, either half-and-half water or one quarter of formula to three quarters of water. Diarrhea in infants, particularly under 6 months of age, is considered serious because it may lead to dehydration. The nurse therefore should seek medical supervision for the parent and child.

Dentition

The first tooth appears at about 6 months of age. The timing of tooth eruption is hereditary. Some infants get their first tooth for their first birthday. Additional studies should be done if the infant is born with a tooth. It may be either a normal or supernumerary lower deciduous tooth. Supernumerary teeth are loose, have no roots, and need to be removed because of their defective structure and chance of being aspirated.

The teething experience is different for each infant. Some parents are surprised to discover that the first tooth has erupted because there was no noticeable change in their infant's behavior. Other parents have anxiously awaited the tooth's eruption because their infant has been irritable, uncomfortable, awake at night, and eating fussily for several weeks. After the first tooth erupts, a new one follows at intervals of approximately 1–2 months (Table 7-11). Dental development coincides with the general pattern of skeletal development (see Chapter 14).

When teething occurs, the infant's gums are red, swollen, and sensitive. Having the gums rubbed with a clean, wet cloth or gauze or chewing on hard objects seems to relieve the tension and discomfort felt in the gums. Hard rubber teething rings, beads, ridged toys, or teething pretzels seem to be favorites for chewing. One infant kept a hard rubber bead necklace in his mouth for hours at a time while cutting his lateral incisors. He would secure the toy behind his present teeth and then massage his sore gums by constantly biting down on the beads.

TABLE 7-11 Sequence of Tooth Eruption

Location of tooth	Approximate age	Range
Lower central incisors	6 mo	5–11 mo
Lower lateral incisors	7 mo	6–15 mo
Upper central incisors	8 mo	6–12 mo
Upper lateral incisors	9 mo	7–18 mo
Lower first molar	12 mo	10–30 mo
Upper first molar	14 mo	10–20 mo
Lower cuspid	16 mo	11–24 mo
Upper cuspid	18 mo	11–24 mo
Lower second molar	24 mo	13–31 mo
Upper second molar	26 mo	13–31 mo

Sometimes infants find comfort in toys that have been cooled in the refrigerator. One parent provided relief by freezing water in popsicle containers and then rubbing the infant's gums with it. The plastic, liquid-filled teething toys are not recommended. The infant may puncture the plastic with a sharp tooth and ingest the liquid, which is often contaminated.

Primary teeth are important for speech development, maintaining space for permanent teeth, and the proper development of the facial muscles and ligaments that support upper and lower jaw development. It is essential to provide good care of the primary teeth. Loss of primary teeth may cause overcrowding when the permanent teeth erupt. Early dental care consists of following meals and the intake of sweetened liquids with a drink of water. In addition, several times a day the parent should gently rub the teeth with gauze wrapped around a finger. (See Chapter 15 for a discussion of "bottle-mouth syndrome.") Good nutrition is also important for healthy teeth and gums. Teeth require calcium, phosphorus, vitamins C and D, and fluoride for the growth and formation of enamel. Chewing helps to develop strong teeth. The inclusion of crackers, cereals, raw fruits, and hard rolls provides the infant with opportunities for strenuous chewing.

Coincidental to teething is the lowered resistance to infections that results from the depletion of maternal antibody reserves. Teething does not cause illness. Fevers, diarrhea, or other signs of illness need to be assessed separately and medical care sought.

Exercise

The kicking, stretching, crying infant is an exercising infant. Crying is a normal discharge of tension and way of maintaining homeostasis; therefore, it has both physiologic and psychosocial benefits. Infants enjoy movement and exercising the large body muscles. Some infants are very active and seem to be in perpetual motion. One concerned young mother needed to be reassured by the visiting nurse that she was a good mother because she thought her daughter, although healthy, was too thin. The nurse spent a few hours observing them at their home and assessing the infant's growth history and food intake. It was noted that the infant was thin only in relation to a neighbor's infant but was gaining weight and following her own growth curve. This girl was very active, always kicking, reaching, rolling over, waving her arms, and squealing, in contrast to the more passive activity engaged in by the neighbor's infant. The nurse demonstrated the infant's firm extremity muscles and strong neck and abdomen muscles by pulling her up to a sitting position, having her resist to a toy being pulled away, and other similar games. Together, the nurse and mother concluded that this infant was never going to be "fat" but was healthier for all of her spontaneous exercising.

Young infants who do most of their exploring visually benefit from parent-guided exercises. These can be done at bath time, and some communities have special postnatal exercise programs for the infant and mother. For the infant, the program begins with a passive range of motion exercises, frequently done to music or nursery rhymes. Other activities then are added to enhance muscle development and flexibility such as pull-ups, roll-ups, playing airplane, and, later, wheelbarrow walking.

Infant movement, activity, and play have the added advantage of fostering social interaction and learning about the environment. Young infants can exercise better when placed on a firm surface. Older infants who have started to crawl need safe spaces in which to practice and further develop the associated muscles. Playpens are actually more appropriate for the young infant because they provide a safe, firm surface and nearby toys for stretching and reaching exercises than for the older infant, who needs a larger area for optimal development.

Safety

The infant is unaware of safety factors and totally dependent on adult caretakers to provide a safe environment. As motor control progresses, the infant becomes increasingly vulnerable. The nurse's role is to prepare parents for the infant's next sequence of development and to alert them to potential injuries. Safety-related behaviors that are practiced from the beginning soon become habits that can protect the developing infant. For example, always securing the safety belt around the infant when on the changing table means that an initial rolling over will not result in a fall from the changing table to the floor.

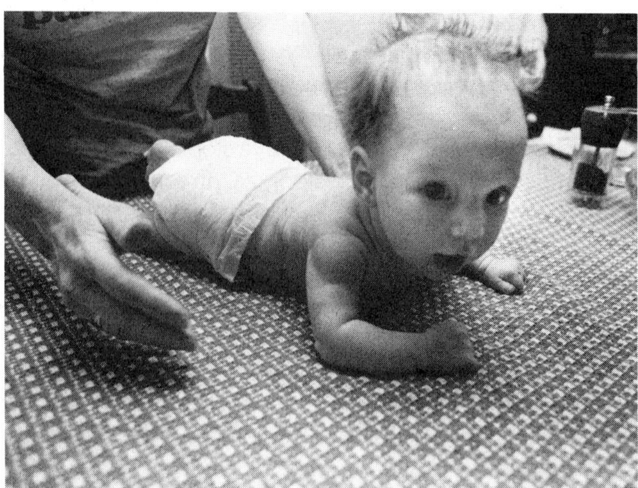

As infants develop motor skills, parents need to develop safety-related behaviors to protect the child.

"Expect the unexpected" is a good rule of advice to give to parents. There are only a few short months of relative inactivity before the curious, mobile infant is into everything. One mother commented that she was so glad she had taken the time to safety-proof the house before her twins were born because since their birth she had not had the time. It also was easier to cope with the initial inconvenience of looking up instead of down for cleaning supplies and dish detergent before the infants were there to compete for her time and attention. Toy safety, automobile safety, environmental safety, and other specific safety factors are discussed in Chapters 19 and 20.

Transition to Early Childhood

The first 18 months of a child's life are marked by rapid development in all areas. The horizontal neonate is now an active, vertical child. Secure with the gross motor skills of walking, climbing, and running, it is now time to practice coordination and fine motor skills. The once-dependent neonate has become secure in the immediate environment and is ready to exert some control over it. Through exploration and play, objects have acquired meaning and relationships to other objects or events. The infant has become increasingly aware of self—self as an individual, as an actor, and as a creator of action. In addition, the infant is beginning to acquire language and the ability to use symbols.

Language opens up a whole new world to the child. It brings "an all-pervasive transformation of perceiving, feeling, thinking and general intelligence" (Stone and Church, 1975). The ability to communicate through language marks the end of infancy and the beginning of early childhood.

Key Concepts

- Developmental progress during infancy involves major changes in the infant's biophysical, affective, cognitive, and social subsystems.
- Infancy encompasses the developmental phase from birth until the beginnings of language (around 18 months of age).
- The family is the major supersystem directly impacting on the infant's life; however, the family acts according to the beliefs, values, and traditions of its culture.
- As a result of growth, development, and maturation, the infant progresses from reflexive behaviors to independent mobility.
- The infant initially communicates by crying but rapidly adds cooing, babbling, monophasic sounds, and then words.
- The infant develops a sense of self; the neonate views the self and environment as one, then gradually differentiates between the two through a process of individuation.
- The infant learns to trust the self, the environment, and the caregivers through the consistent response to and satisfaction of needs.
- Attachment to caregivers is a process that consists of interaction and the chain of events related to the reduction of tension and discomfort.
- Exploration and active experimentation with objects in the environment enable the infant to begin to learn the properties of objects.
- The concept of object permanence is learned during Stage 5 of Piaget's sensorimotor phase of development. The infant now searches for the hidden object in more than one place.
- The neonate's body's systems all function but are immature. Most systems (except the reproductive system) achieve near mature levels of functioning by the end of infancy.
- The sensory capacities of the neonate are more highly developed than was once thought. Vision is adequate at a distance of 8–12 in, and by 3 weeks of age, an infant distinguishes the mother's face from that of a stranger.
- Until 4 months of age the infant prefers soft, high-pitched voices; after 4 months of age any human voice is preferred. Infants are alarmed by shrill sounds.
- Research has demonstrated that infants have definite senses of smell, taste, and touch.
- Play is an important part of infancy; the infant develops gross and fine motor skills through practice play.
- Play also helps the infant to learn spatial relationships because it involves motion and interaction with objects.
- The content of play includes the infant's own body, others' bodies, toys, exploratory play, repetitive play, and early symbolic play.
- Developmental theorists characterize infancy as a time of the rapid acquisition of developmental skills and growth. Piaget emphasized the infant's use of reflexes, emerging motor capacities, and sensory abilities to learn actively about the environment. Erickson noted the foundation of trust established between parent and infant and its relation to the gratification of oral needs.
- Dependence also characterizes the infant. For example, the parent needs to provide for hygiene and skin care needs, especially preventing diaper rash.
- Sleep patterns mature and consolidate so that longer sleep periods occur at night. This coincides with longer wakeful periods during the day.
- Good nutrition is essential for optimal development. Human milk or formula are sufficient for the first 6 months of life, after which solids are added to the infant's diet.

- The first tooth erupts around 6 months of age, and teething continues until 20 deciduous teeth are present.
- The prevention of injuries is the parents' responsibility because the infant is unaware of dangers. Parents benefit from anticipatory guidance about safety practices.

References

Ainsworth MDS: The development of infant-mother attachment. In: *Review of Child Development Research.* Vol 3. Caldwell BM, Riccuiuti HN (editors). University of Chicago Press, 1973.

Ainsworth MDS, et al: *The Strange Situation: Observing Patterns of Attachment.* Erlbaum, 1979.

American Academy of Pediatrics, Committee on Nutrition: Commentary on breast-feeding and infant formulas, including proposed standards for formulas. *Pediatrics* 1976a; 57:278–285.

American Academy of Pediatrics, Committee on Nutrition: Iron supplementation for infants. *Pediatrics* 1976b; 58(5):765.

American Academy of Pediatrics, Committee on Nutrition: On the feeding of supplemental foods to infants. *Pediatrics* 1980; 65:1178–1180.

Apgar VA: A proposal for a new method of evaluation of the newborn infant. *Curr Res Anesthes Analg* 1953; 32:260, 267.

Apgar VA: The newborn (Apgar) scoring system. *Pediatr Clin North Am* 1966; 13:645.

Ball W, Tronick E: Infants' response to impeding collision: Optical and real. *Science* 1971; 171:818–820.

Bandura A: *Social Learning Theory.* Prentice-Hall, 1977.

Beal V: Termination of night feeding in infancy. *J Pediatr* 1969; 75:690–692.

Bernal J: Night waking in infants during the first 14 months. *Develop Med Child Neurol* 1973; 15:760–769.

Bloom L: *Language Development: Form and Function in Emerging Grammars.* MIT Press, 1970.

Bornstein MH: Infants are trichromats. *J Exp Child Psychol* 1976; 21:425–445.

Bornstein MH: Qualities of color vision in infancy. *J Exp Child Psychol* 1975; 19:401–419.

Bornstein MH, Kessen W, Weiskopf S: Color vision and hue categorization in young infants. *J Exp Psychol [Hum Percept]* 1976; 2:115–129.

Boronson W: First born—fortune's favorite? Pages 192–196 in: *Readings in Human Development 73–74.* Dushkin, 1973.

Bower TGR: *Development in Infancy.* Freeman, 1974.

Bower TGR: Object perception in infants. *Perception* 1972; 1:15–30.

Bower TGR: *A Primer of Infant Development.* Freeman, 1977.

Bower TGR, Broughton JM, Moore MK: Infant responses to approaching objects: An indicator of response to distal variables. *Percept Psychophysics* 1970; 9:193–196.

Bower TGR, Broughton JM, Moore MK: The development of object concept as manifested by changes in the tracking behavior of infants between 7 and 20 weeks of age. *J Exp Child Psychol* 1971; 11:182–183.

Bowlby J: *Attachment and Loss.* Vol I. Hogarth Press and Institute for Psychoanalysis, 1969.

Brazelton TB: *Infants and Mothers.* Delacorte Press, 1970.

Brazelton TB: *Neonatal Behavioral Assessment Scale.* Clinics in Developmental Medicine. No 50. Spastics International Medical Publications and Lippincott, 1973.

Brazelton TB: Behavioral competence of the newborn infant. *Sem Perinatol* 1979; 3(1):35–44.

Brown R: *Psycholinguistics.* Free Press, 1970.

Brown R, Belugi V: Three processes in the child's acquisition of language. In: *New Directions in the Study of Child Language.* Lennenberg EL (editor). MIT Press, 1964.

Campos J: Heart rate: A sensitive tool for the study of emotional development. In: *Developmental Psychobiology: The Significance of Infancy.* Lipsitt L (editor). Erlbaum, 1976.

Campos J, et al: The emergence of fear on the visual cliff. In: *The Origins of Affect.* Lewis M, Rosenblum L (editors). Plenum, 1978.

Carey WB: A simplified method for measuring infant temperament. *J Pediatr* 1970; 77:2, 188–194.

Carey WB: Breast-feeding and night waking. *J Pediatr* 1975; 87:327–329.

Carey WB: Clinical appraisal of temperament. In: *Developmental Disabilities: Theory Assessment and Intervention.* Lewis M, Taft L (editors). S. P. Medical and Scientific Books, 1982.

Chess S, Thomas A: Temperament and the parent-child interaction. *Pediatr Ann* 1977; 6:26–45.

Chomsky N: *Syntactic Structures.* Mouton, 1957.

Chow MP, et al: *1979 Handbook of Pediatric Primary Care.* Wiley, 1979.

Clarke-Stewart KA: Interactions between mothers and their young children: Characteristics and consequences. *Monographs of the Society for Research in Child Development* 1973; 38:153, 6–7.

Clarke-Stewart KA, Apfel N: Evaluating parental effects on child development. In: *Review of Research in Education.* Vol 6. Shulman LS (editor). Peacock, 1979.

Condon WS, Sauder LW: Neonate movement is synchronized with adult speech. *Science* 1979, 183:99–101.

Condon WS, Ogston NWD: A segmentation of behavior. *J Psychiatr Res* 1967; 5:221–235.

Dayton G, et al: Developmental study of coordinated eye movements in the human infant. *Arch Ophthalmol* 1964; 71:865–875.

DeCasper A, Fifer W: Of human bonding: Newborns prefer their mothers' voices. *Science* 1980; 208:1174–1176.

Dittrizhova J: In: *Brain and Early Behavior.* Robinson RJ (editor). Academic Press, 1969.

Eckerman CO, Whatley JL, Kutz SL: Growth of social play with peers during the second year of life. *Dev Psychol* 1975; 11:42–49.

Eisenberg RB: The development of hearing in man: An assessment of current status. *J Am Speech Hearing Assoc* 1970; 12:119–123.

Erikson EH: *Childhood and Society.* Norton, 1963.

Erikson E: *Toys and Reason.* Norton, 1977.

Fagan JF: Origins of facial pattern recognition. In: *Psychological Development from Infancy.* Bornstein MH, Kessen W (editors). Erlbaum, 1979.

Fantz RL: A method for studying depth perception in infants under 6 months of age. *Psychol Record* 1961a; 11:27–32.

Fantz RL: The origins of form perception. *Sci Am* 1961b; 204:66–75.

Fantz RL: Visual perception from birth as shown by pattern sensitivity. *Ann NY Acad Sci* 1963; 118:793–814.

Fantz RL: Visual perception from birth as shown by pattern selectivity. *Ann NY Acad Sci* 1965; 118:739–814.

Field T: The adjustment of reaching behavior to object distance in early infancy. *Child Dev* 1976; 47:304–308.

Florentino MR: *Reflex Testing Methods for Evaluating C.N.S. Development.* Thomas, 1973.

Fomon SJ, et al: Recommendations for feeding normal infants. *Pediatrics* 1979; 63:52–59.

Freiberg KL: *Human Development: A Life-Span Approach*. Brooks/Cole, 1983.

Freud A: The concept of developmental lines. In: *Normality and Pathology in Childhood: Assessment of Development*. Freud A (editor). International Universities Press, 1965.

Freud S: *The Complete Psychoanalytic Works of Sigmund Freud*. Norton, 1969.

Fullard W, Reiling AM: An investigation of Lorenz's "babyness." *Child Dev* 1976; 47:1191–1193.

Gesell A: *The First Five Years of Life*. Harper, 1940.

Gesell A: The ontogenesis of infant behavior. In: *Manual of Child Psychology*. Carmichael L (editor). Wiley, 1954.

Gibson EJ, Walk RD: The "visual cliff." *Sci Am* 1960; 202:64–71.

Goffman E: *Behavior in Public Places*. Free Press, 1963.

Gordon FR, Yonas A: Sensitivity to binocular depth information in infants. *J Exp Child Psychol* 1976; 22:413–422.

Greenberg DJ: Accelerating visual complexity levels in the human infant. *Child Dev* 1971; 42:905–918.

Gulick EE: Infant health and breast-feeding. *Pediatr Nurs* 1983; 9(5):359–362.

Harlow HF, Zimmerman RR: Affectional responses in the infant monkey. *Science* 1959; 130:420–431.

Harlow HF, Harlow MH: Learning to love. *Am Sci* 1966; 54:244–272.

Haynes H, White BL, Held R: Visual accommodation in human infants. *Science* 1965; 148:528–530.

Haynes U: *A Developmental Approach to Casefinding*. DHEW Publication No. (HSA) 77-5210. US Government Printing Office, 1977.

Hurlock EB: *Child Development*. McGraw-Hill, 1978.

Jacklin C, et al: Sleep pattern development from 6 through 33 months. *Pediatr Psychol* 1980; 5:295–303.

Jacobson R: *Child Language, Aphasia, and General Sound Laws*. Keiler AR (translator). Mouton, 1968.

Jaffe J, Stern DN, Perry JC: "Conversational" coupling of gaze behavior in pre-linguistic human development. *J Psycholinguist Res* 1971; 2:321–329.

Kagan J, Kearsley RB, Zelazco PR: *Infancy, its Place in Human Development*. Harvard University Press, 1978.

Kagan J, et al: *Change and Continuity in Infancy*. Wiley, 1971.

Kessen W, Bornstein MH: Discriminability of brightness change for infants. *J Exp Child Psychol* 1978; 25:526–530.

Kessen W, Haith MM, Salapatek PH: Human infancy: A bibliography and guide. In: *Carmichael's Manual of Child Psychology*. Mussen PH (editor). Wiley, 1970.

Kessen W, Levine J, Wendich KA: The imitation of pitch in infants. *Infant Behavior and Development* 1979; 2:93–100.

Korner AF: Conceptual issues in infancy research. In: *Handbook of Infant Development*. Osofsky JD (editor). Wiley, 1979.

Kotelchuck M: The infant's relationship to the father: Experimental evidence. In: *The Role of the Father in Child Development*. Lamb ME (editor). Wiley, 1976.

Lamb ME, Campos JJ: *Development in Infancy*. Random House, 1982.

Lawton JT: *Introduction to Child Development*. Brown, 1982.

Leboyer F: *Birth Without Violence*. Knopf, 1975.

Lenneberg EH: Speech development. In: *Brain Functions III*. Carteretle EC (editor). University of California Press, 1966.

Leventhal AS, Lipsitt LP: Adaptation, pitch discrimination and sound localization in the neonate. *Child Dev* 1964; 35:759–767.

Levine MD, et al: *Developmental-Behavioral Pediatrics*. Saunders, 1983.

Lewis M, Weinraub M, Ban P: Mothers and fathers, girls and boys: Attachment behavior in the first two years of life. In: *Research Bulletin* (RB 72-60). Educational Testing Services, December 1972.

Lewis M, Bartels B, Goldberg S: State as a determinant of infants heart rate response to stimulation. *Science* 1967; 155:486–488.

Lipsitt LP, Engen T, Kaye H: Developmental changes in the olfactory threshold of the neonate. *Child Dev* 1963; 34:371–376.

Lorenz KZ: Die angebarenen formen moglichev Er faliruny. *Z Tierpsychol* 1943; 5:235–409.

Lowrey GH: *Growth and Development of Children*. Year Book, 1978.

MacFarlane A: Olfaction in the development of social preferences in the human neonate. In: *Parent-Infant Interaction*. CIBA Foundation Symposium, 33, 1975.

Mahler MS, Pine F, Bergman A: *The Psychological Birth of the Human Infant: Symbiosis and Individuation*. Basic Books, 1975.

Mann I: *The Development of the Human Eye*. British Medical Association, 1964.

Maurer D, Salapatek P: Developmental changes in the scanning of faces by young infants. *Child Dev* 1976; 47:523–537.

Moore T, Ucko LE: Night waking in early infancy: Part I. Arch Dis Child 1957; 32:333–342.

Mueller EC, Vandell D: Infant-infant interaction. In: *Handbook of Infant Development*. Osofsky J (editor). Wiley, 1979.

National Center for Health Statistics. *Vital and Health Statistics*. Health Services and Mental Health Administration, US Government Printing Office, Series 11, 1979.

Nelson KE: Organization of visual-tracking responses in human infants. *J Exp Child Psychol* 1968; 6:194–201.

Newman BM, Newman PR: *Infancy and Childhood—Development and its Contexts*. Wiley, 1978.

Osterholm P, Lindeke LL, Amidon D: Sleep disturbance in infants aged 6 to 12 months. *Pediatr Nurs* 1983; 9(4):269–271.

Paine RS: The evolution of infantile postural reflexes in the presence of chronic brain syndromes. *Dev Med Child Neurol* 1964; 6:345.

Papousek H: Experimental studies of appetitional behavior in human newborns and infants. In: *Early Behavior: Comparative and Developmental Approaches*. Stevenson NW, Hess EH, Rheingold NC (editors). Wiley, 1967.

Peeples DR, Teller DY: Color vision and brightness discrimination in two-month-old human infants. *Science* 1975; 189:1102–1103.

Peery JC: Neonate-adult head movement: No and yes revisited. *Dev Psychol* 1980; 6:245–250.

Peery JC, Aoki E: Leave-taking behavior between preschool children and their parents. *J Genet Psychol* 1982; 140:71–81.

Peery JC, Crane PM: Personal space regulation: Approach-withdrawal-approach proxemic behavior during adult-preschooler interaction at close range. *J Psychol* 1980; 106:63–75.

Peller LE: Libidinal phases, ego development and play. In: *Psychoanalytic Study of the Child*. Vol 9. International Universities Press, 1954.

Piaget J: *The Origins of Intelligence in Children*. International Universities Press, 1952.

Piaget J: *Play, Dreams and Imitation in Childhood*. Gattengo C, Hodgson FM (translators). Norton, 1962.

Piaget J, Inhelder B: *The Psychology of the Child*. Basic Books, 1969.

Pomerleau-Malcuit A, Clifton RK: Neonatal heart-rate response to tactile, auditory and vestibular stimulation in different states. *Child Dev* 1973; 44:485–496.

Prechtl H, Beintema D: *The Neurological Examination of the Full-Term Newborn Infant. Clinics in Developmental Medicine*. No 12. Spastics Society and Heinemann, 1964.

Richards JE, Rader N: Crawling-onset age predicts visual cliff avoidance in infants. *J Exp Psychol [Hum Percept]* 1981; 7:382–387.

Rose SA, Schmidt K, Bridger WH: Cardiac and behavioral responsivity to tactile stimulation in premature and full-term infants. *Dev Psychol* 1976; 12:311–320.

Rothbart MK: Birth order and mother-child interaction in an achievement situation. *J Pers Soc Psychol* 1971; 17:113–120.

Salapatek PH: Pattern perception in early infancy. In: *Infant Perception from Sensation to Cognition*. Vol 1. Cohen LB, Salapetek P (editors). Academic Press, 1975.

Salapatek P, Kessen W: Visual scanning of triangles by the human newborn. *J Exp Child Psychol* 1966; 3:155–167.

Schaffer HR: *The Growth of Sociability*. Penguin Books, 1971.

Schaffer HR, Emerson PE: The development of social attachments in infancy. *Monographs of the Society for Research in Child Development* 1964; 29(3): series 94.

Schiamberg LB, Smith KU: *Human Development*. Macmillan, 1982.

Schuster CS, Ashburn SS: *The Process of Human Development*. Little, Brown, 1980.

Skinner BF: *Verbal Behavior*. Appleton-Century-Crofts, 1957.

Smilansky S: *The Effects of Sociodramatic Play on Disadvantaged Pre-School Children*. Wiley, 1968.

Spitz RA: Hospitalism: An inquiry into the genesis of psychiatric conditions in early childhood. In: *The Psychoanalytic Study of the Child*. Vol 1. Eissler RS, et al (editors). International Universities Press, 1945.

Spitz RA: Hospitalism: A follow-up report. In: *The Psychoanalytic Study of the Child*. Vol 2. Eissler RS, et al (editors). International Universities Press, 1946.

Stern DN: A micro-analysis of mother-infant interaction. *J Am Acad Child Psychiatry* 1971; 10:501–517.

Stern DN: The goal and structure of mother-infant play. *J Am Acad Child Psychiatry* 1974; 13:402–421.

Stern DN, et al: Vocalizing in unison and in alternation: Two modes of communication within the mother-infant dyad. *Annal of the New York Academy of Science: Developmental Psycholinguistics and Communication Disorders* 1975; 263:89–100.

Stone T, Church J: *Childhood and Adolescence*. Random House, 1975.

Sutton-Smith B: Children at play. *Natural History* 1971; 80(10):54–60.

Thoman EB, Liederman PH, Olsen JP: Neonate-mother interaction during breast-feeding. *Dev Psychol* 1972; 6:110–118.

Thomas A, et al: *Behavioral Individuality in Early Childhood*. New York University Press, 1963.

Traisman A, Traisman H, Garri A: The well baby care of 530 infants. *J Pediatr* 1966; 68:608–614.

Uzgiris IC: Ordinality in the development of schemas for relating to objects. In: *Exceptional Infant*. Vol I: *The Normal Infant*. Bruner/Mazel, 1967.

Valadian I, Porter D: *Physical Growth and Development From Conception to Maturity*. Little, Brown, 1977.

Weinraub M, Lewis M: The determinants of children's response to separation. *Monographs for the Society for Research in Child Development* 1977; 42(2).

Weinraub M, Brooks J, Lewis M: The social network: A reconsideration of the concept of attachment. *Hum Dev* 1977; 20:31–47.

Weir L: Auditory frequency sensitivity in the neonate: A signal detection analysis. *J Exp Child Psychol* 1976; 21:219–225.

White BL: Development of perception during the first six months. Paper presented at the American Association for the Advancement of Science. December, 1963.

Young RK, Douthitt TC: Newborn responses to threshold tactile stimulation. *Child Dev* 1974; 45:237–242.

Yussen SR, Santrock JW: *Child Development: An Introduction*. Brown, 1982.

Additional Readings

Bell RQ: Contributions of human infants to caregiving and social interaction. In: *The Effect of the Infant on its Caregiver*. Lewis ML, Rosenblum LA (editors). Wiley, 1974.

Barnet AB, Lodge A, Armington JC: Electroretinogram in newborn infants. *Science* 1965; 148:651–654.

Beard R: *Piaget's Developmental Psychology*. Mentor-New American Library, 1969.

Bernard S, Sontag LW: Fetal reactivity to tonal stimulation: A preliminary report. *J Genet Psychol* 1947; 70:205–210.

Brown R: *A First Language: The Early Stages*. Harvard University Press, 1973.

Campos JJ, Langer A, Krowitz A: Cardiac responses on the visual cliff in prelocomotor human infants. *Science* 1970; 170:196–197.

Caputo DV, Mandell W: Consequences of low birthweight. *Dev Psychol* 1970; 3:363–383.

Conel JL: *The Postnatal Development of the Human Cerebral Cortex*. Vols 1, 5, and 6. Harvard University Press, 1939, 1955, 1959.

Diekman WJ, et al: Observations on protein intake and the health of the mother and baby. *J Am Diet Assoc* 1951; 27:1046–1052.

Dobbing J: *Biologic and Clinical Aspects of Brain Development*. Mead Johnson Symposium on Perinatal and Developmental Medicine, No 6. Mead Johnson, 1975.

Dobbing J, Sands J: The quantitative growth and development of the human brain. *Arch Dis Child* 1973; 48:757–767.

Doris J, Casper M, Porsky R: Differential brightness thresholds in infancy. *J Exp Child Psychol* 1967; 5:522–535.

Frankenberg WK, Dodds JB: The Denver Developmental Screening Test. *J Pediatr* 1967; 71:181–191.

Hutlenlocher J: The origins of language comprehension. In: *Theories in Cognitive Psychology*. Solso RL (editor). Erlbaum, 1974.

Hutt C, Onstead C: The biological significance of gaze aversion with particular reference to the syndrome of infantile autism. *Behav Sci* 1966; 11:346–356.

Ludington-Hoe SM: What can newborns really see? *Am J Nurs* 1980; 83(9):1286–1289.

Maddi S: *Personality Theories: A Comparative Analysis*. 4th ed. Dorsey Press, 1980.

Mills M, Melhuish E: Recognition of mother's voice in early infancy. *Nature* 1974; 252:123–124.

Osofsky J (editor): *Handbook of Infant Development*. Wiley, 1979.

Peery JC: Effect of different situations on mother-infant gazing. *Child Study J* 1978; 8:111–121.

Peery JC, Ingoldsby B: Body activity, psychological state and psychiatric diagnosis. *Hillside J Clin Psychiatry* 1980; 2:87–94.

Peery JC, Stern DN: Gaze duration frequency distributions during mother-infant interaction. *J Genet Psychol* 1976; 129:45–55.

Peery JC, Stern DN: Mother-infant gazing during play, bottle-feeding, and spoon-feeding. *J Psychol* 1975; 91:207–213.

Piaget J: *The Construction of Reality in the Child*. Basic Books, 1954.

Robson KS: The role of eye-to-eye contact in maternal-infant attachment. *J Child Psychol Psychiatry* 1967; 8:13–25.

Russell MJ: Human olfactory communication. *Nature* 1976; 260:520–522.

Salapatek PH, Kessen W: Visual scanning of triangles in the human newborn. *J Exp Child Psychol* 1966; 3:155–167.

Wagner TJ, Hindi-Alexander M: Hazards of baby powder? *Pediatr Nurs* 1984; 10(2): 124–125.

Zelazo PR, Zelazo NA, Kolb S: "Walking" in the newborn. *Science* 1972; 176:314–315.

Early Childhood

Cynthia B. Hughes June Andrews Horowitz

8

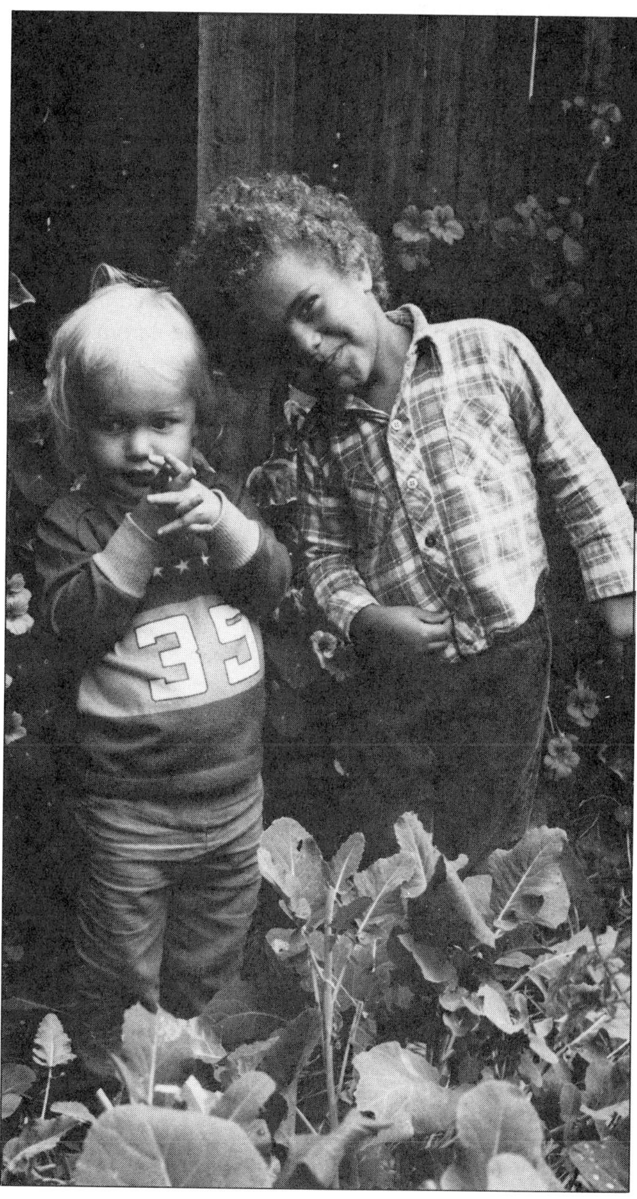

Chapter Outline

Objectives

- Explain the influences of both suprasystems and subsystems on development during the early childhood phase.
- Define the major parameters of development in early childhood.
- Explain the essential biophysical changes that occur in early childhood.
- Describe the principal theoretic explanations for personality, cognitive, language, moral, and social development in early childhood.
- Explain the purpose of play in early childhood.
- Identify the basic health care needs of preschool children.

Locomotion and language distinguish early childhood (the time from about 18 months to 4½ years of age) from infancy. These skills enable the young child to move beyond complete dependence on the significant parenting figures. The ability to walk and talk are important self-enhancing skills that positively affect children's abilities to interact with their environment. They become distinct individuals, no longer totally dependent on parents. Around 18 months of age, language and locomotion are accompanied by an increased intellectual awareness of self in relation to others, particularly significant others.

This awareness of self, of "me," is, however, accompanied by emotional turmoil and tension. The child's behaviors demonstrate a need for separation from the parent, be it physical or emotional. This need is characterized by running from the parent, by saying "no" to all requests, and by temper tantrums. Paradoxically, the drive for independence frequently is accompanied by increased dependence, demands for parental attention, and/or hesitancy with strangers.

In this chapter we examine the influences of both suprasystems and subsystems on the child's development. We look specifically at the suprasystems of family and community as they interpret the culture, values, ethnic background, sex role expectations, and socioeconomic resources that they bring to the child's experience. As children interact with these suprasystems, they begin to develop unique characteristics that contribute to the shaping of their personalities.

We further examine those parameters of subsystem development that are most prominent in early childhood. The child at this stage acquires the ability to symbolize, or use words, to describe the outer and inner worlds. The acquisition of language thus frees the child from having to communicate only through experience. The ability to use words to describe external or internal events gives the child a powerful tool in exploring and manipulating the environment. This newly found ability to communicate is a catalyst for the child's cognitive, moral, and psychosocial development. Integration of these developmental changes is achieved primarily through play.

Because early childhood is also a time of significant growth and physiologic change, we discuss the major changes in the child's biophysical subsystems and the essential health care needs that concern both parents and nurses.

Developmental Changes in Early Childhood

The transition into early childhood is marked by disequilibrium. Parents often remember the period from 18 to 36 months as one of the most challenging times for parenting. Negativism, tantrums characterized by cries of "me do it," and rebellion against food and bedtime alternate with clinginess, shyness, separation anxiety, and scrupulous adherence to rituals. The first phase of early childhood is marked by incredible growth and developmental changes. During this stage, the child first tries to control the environment while not being controlled by it. Such efforts reflect the child's dilemma—the need to hold on and yet to let go—although the desire for independence still is not matched by an ability to be independent. Fortunately for parents, a calmer, more delightful period follows. Although the 3- to 4½-year-old does have periods of disequilibrium (particularly at 3½ and 4½ years of age), these are tempered by the acquisition of important self-care skills, greater problem-solving skills, and more emotional and social maturity. The responses of the 3 to 4½-year-old are more than just a negative version of the parent's wishes. The child at this age bursts into a time of creativity, imagination, and fantasy, all of which result in an amusing, delightful companion. Eventually, the parent can relinquish full-time duty as the child's superego, or disciplinarian, as the child begins to recognize and set personal limits.

The increased mobility and feeling of independence characteristic of this period culminate in such behaviors as the child's ability to walk to school. A child about to enter school has achieved a relative degree of independence in communication, locomotion, and self-care.

Influences of the Suprasystems

Family The child, as an open system, interacts with the environment, which in turn contributes to the child's uniqueness. During early childhood, the child's environment is primarily the immediate family, and therefore children experience and interpret events, activities, and decisions as their families perceive these aspects of living. As observed by Erikson and other theorists, the child's world of significant others extends first to the immediate family, then to the extended family, and next to early peer relations.

Therefore, during early childhood the intense infant–parent bonds are transformed into broader relationships, but the safety, trust, and stability provided by the family remain critical. Not until middle childhood, however, does the child step beyond the family and develop truly independent relationships.

Through the family, the child is introduced to society and to the rituals and traditions that become associated with holidays, annual events, or celebrations. Although today's children are introduced to society outside their families at earlier ages, families are still primary socializers, and they play predominant teaching roles and provide necessary continuity. As the child learns and adapts to the social milieu, the availability of parental support is pivotal. Children who have learned about trust from the nurturing, consistent responses of parents are able to trust others. They have acquired basic knowledge and information from parental teaching, are able to learn from teachers, and have experimented with adapting their behavior to family members' and others' expectations. These children are then able to adapt to different standards or demands of others because they have achieved some self-control and sense of self and can now begin to learn goal-directed and appropriate self-initiated activity.

The family structure sets the stage for reciprocal family interactions and includes both membership and role relations. A firstborn child may, at this time, need to adapt to a younger brother or sister, or a second or third child may be part of a family that is expanding and adjusting to incorporate a new member. Children with brothers and/or sisters learn about social power, the significance of age and sex, and the ways these items are used to achieve status or to discriminate. The firstborn who enters this phase as an only child has learned to interact with adults and seeks to gain their approval. For this child, interacting with peers may be difficult initially (Bigner, 1979).

The first experiences of having to share toys, adults' attention, or play ideas can be rather traumatic. For example, 4-year-old David was an only child in a nuclear family and experienced a rude initiation when he attempted to join his neighborhood peer group. At first, these children were curious about David, his toys, yard, house, and family. They asked many questions while exploring the area. They then took over and told David what he could do, what toys he could use, and that he had to be the baby when they played "house." David made some initial attempts to comply, but soon he could be heard to say, "But my daddy always lets me be the boss," and "Mommy bought that truck for me, it's mine, and I want it now. I'll tell my mommy." Frustrated, he ran into the house and informed his mother that he did not like these children and wanted to play with only her or daddy because they were nicer.

In extended families more family members may be psychologically, socially, and/or physically present for the developing child. A network of close relationships expands the complexity of interactions, diffuses intense parent–child ties, and broadens social support systems. In extended families the child has more role models and a greater diversity of occupations and personalities to imitate through play.

A child growing up in an extended family has grandparents, aunts, uncles, and cousins available either within the same house or nearby such as next door, around the corner, or on the next farm. If a parent is busy, another adult can be found to help or to listen as needed. For example, 4-year-old Susie likes her big family because she never has to be alone. If her parents are busy, she goes downstairs to her grandparents, and one of them usually has time to play a game or talk. Although she is the youngest in her family, she thinks she knows all about caring for and playing with infants because she spends a lot of time with her 6-month-old cousin, who lives next door. She talks to another aunt about being a schoolteacher and visits her uncle while he is working at the bank. She knows all about tools and carpentry because her grandfather is a carpenter, and together they built her dollhouse. When her siblings and cousins play ball, she is right there, learning what to do and how to do it. The extended family provides a great variety of resources, role models, and teachers for the child.

Patterned family behaviors are passed on from previous generations and encompass the developing child. A "family script" that expresses expectations for this child is influenced by cultural, social, or ethical values. The young child growing up in an extended family that is both psychologically and physically close will have experiences that are different from those of the child in a more isolated family.

Comparing the experiences of Susie and David as described above helps to illustrate the difference in orientation experienced by children from extended families and those from small nuclear families. David's play activities and approval-seeking were oriented toward his parents. Susie's sphere of orientation involved a variety of adults and children of different ages. David was exposed to one set of standards and expectations from his parents, who also were responsible for fulfilling all of the other numerous roles related to family maintenance. Susie related intimately with several families and observed different interpretations of the same standards and different ways of performing similar roles. She had a larger radius of people from whom to receive recognition or approval. In Susie's situation the extended family was supportive and a positive experience; unfortunately, this is not always the case. Sometimes extended families have more negative, competitive experiences than positive ones.

Culture, Ethnicity, and Values A society or culture's views of life and a child's role in it are all influenced by suprasystems, or patterns, larger than the family. The framework for these patterns is laid down in these early identity-building years. The cultural, ethnic, or value suprasystems influence how the child is seen in family life. In preindustrial times, for example, children were like family employees, being part of a family work force and therefore valued (Kephart, 1961).

In many cultures the child is a symbol of familial vitality, or what Erikson called generativity (see Chapter 6). Children are valued for providing continuity through the generations, and childrearing values and styles are part of the culture transmitted from generation to generation. For the child, important factors are fitting in, identifying with the family culture, and belonging to the reference group (Brink, 1982). Nurses do not therefore consider one parenting style as being superior or inferior to another.

During the early childhood phase, children incorporate the mores and beliefs of these suprasystems—family culture, ethnicity, and values—principally through their parents. Parental teaching and expectations that convey social norms thus enable the child to become an accepted member of a social group. These are the years during which the child observes and imitates the behavior of others. Symbols, whether gestures or words, develop specific meanings and become vehicles for transmitting ideas. The significance of learning developmental tasks also reflects society's values. Tasks related to toilet training, feeding habits, and disciplinary patterns are culturally induced. Also related to culture and socioeconomic suprasystems are values ascribed to success, money, competition, and cooperation (Kagan, 1974).

Children acquire a taste and preference for certain foods and styles of cooking because they become familiar with them as they learn to become a member of a given social group. Likewise, a child learns to use chopsticks, a wooden spoon, a fork, or a bowl for eating by imitating elders. The concepts of rules and manners are introduced during this phase, and parents generally expect children to know and follow such rules by the time they enter school. The parent's pattern of childrearing is important because it communicates to the child the expectations of the greater society. Parental choices determine whether the child can or cannot participate in adult conversation, whether there are different or similar expectations of behavior for boys and girls, and the extent to which the child is expected to contribute to the household chores, attend school, or play with peers.

In some families, for example, the adage "children should be seen and not heard" is strictly adhered to, whereas in other families adult conversation is secondary to that of the children's. In most German families correct table manners and respect for parents are expected behaviors, and children are considered to be rude if they do not observe them. In some Italian families, on the other hand, table manners are not as important as finishing the food served and praising the one who prepared it. In Oriental cultures male children are preferred to female children and given a higher status and more privileges. In many cultures there are different expectations for firstborn children than for subsequent children. Although claiming to be egalitarian, many North American parents tend to restrict their daughters more than their sons in such things as the distance allowed from home when playing with friends and the use of tools such as hammers and saws.

The child learns about behaviors, feelings, and different perspectives by imitating adult models though play. In turn, the adults' responses reflect approval or disapproval of these actions back to the child, and this feedback serves to reinforce behaviors. Through imitation and adults' responses, the child develops a self-concept. Role playing for children is both anticipatory socialization, in which roles that might become reality are acted out, and also fantasy, during which the child takes on behaviors of hypothetic or imaginary characters for pleasure and for new experiences (Stone, 1962).

Gender-Related Roles The child's social experience within the family is influenced by birth order, sex, and family member roles in relation to other suprasystems. Attitudes toward the sex of the child are derived partly from the values of the ethnic group and partly from the socialization practices and sex stereotyping that prevail in society. Stereotyping often is evident in the chores assigned to children during this stage. Boys begin to take out the trash and help their fathers rake leaves or shovel snow, whereas girls begin to set the table and help their mothers bake a cake or dust the furniture.

Whereas rigid expectations concerning appropriate gender-related roles were once endorsed, these prescriptions gradually have relaxed, especially for the middle class. Social change, notably the advent of the women's movement in the 1960s and the dramatic increase in the number of women working outside their homes from the 1970s to the present, has changed the once-assumed definitions and role responsibilities of each sex. To some degree, it is now acceptable for boys to adopt some traditionally feminine traits, such as being sensitive to others' feelings, and for girls to adopt some traditionally masculine traits such as being assertive and work oriented. One study showed that girls tended to adopt masculine traits in conjunction with feminine traits, so that the endorsement of traditional masculine traits did not mean that girls considered themselves less feminine (Horowitz, 1981). This trend is not likely to result in identical sex role identities for girls and boys. Rather, it appears that greater diversity will be allowed and, perhaps, encouraged.

Although it is true that the differences in childhood experiences and opportunities to explore the socioemotional area of their personalities is no longer as great between boys and girls, Rubin (1976) noted that there are still considerable class differences. Middle-class children of both sexes are provided more freedom and receive more acceptance for their exploration of the expressive aspects of personality. In working class families the young boys are made to understand that they are to be men, which means that they do not cry, nurture, or reflect. Rubin observed that the 4½-year-old son of a working- class family would shake his father's hand as he bid him goodnight, whereas the middle-class 4½-year-old would crawl up into his father's lap and exchange a goodnight hug and kiss (Rubin, 1976).

Because women and men today are extending and expanding the roles they are willing and able to assume, internal family life is affected. Tasks once delegated solely to homemakers (once only wives and mothers) are more often now shared among family members. These role changes affect the family and consequently affect the child. For example, increased demands are placed on communities to provide alternatives for child care when both parents are employed.

Socioeconomic Resources Family members take on roles such as the breadwinner, caregiver, teacher, parent, and sibling, and these roles are further related to larger systems. Family breadwinners are in turn assigned status or position in society based on income, education, and occupation. Both the child's and the family's role in a community are influenced by these factors.

This is evident by the section of town in which the family lives; the child's opportunities to participate in various activities such as music lessons, swimming, or art; the presence of a second or third vacation home; and the type, amount, and quality of toys available. There are also more subtle indicators such as the manner in which the town bankers, merchants, or officials respond to the family (especially the father). The amount of attention, level of expectation, and degree of responsiveness from nursery school teachers, as well as the school attended, provide other cues to the child's status in the community (Coles, 1977).

The family's employment status and thus the larger economic suprasystem facilitates or inhibits their access to resources. The degree to which the family is economically secure is related to the educational success and achievement of children (Keniston, 1977), as well as their access to material and nonmaterial resources (see Chapters 3 and 4).

Neighborhood schools, the living and play environment, the ecologic quality of the community, the educational resources of parents in the community, and the provision and quality of health care are related directly to the economic resources and the ideology of the family and community. The community's resources for young children have the potential to provide quality early childhood experiences. These resources might include nursery schools, a Head Start program, child care for working parents, or YWCA-YMCA programs, all of which positively affect the child. A community that chooses to provide such resources enriches the lives of its young children by providing positive interaction with the surrounding environment.

Other suprasystems, such as the health care system and the criminal justice system, also influence parenting and act as parenting agents. The quality and diversity of screening, counseling, and intervention programs available for children and their families enhance or inhibit healthy development.

Many communities provide tax-supported health services through federal, state, or local monies. Communities differ in their ability to provide and philosophy about providing screening programs as one of the health services. Early childhood is the ideal time to detect the precursors of some diseases and identify certain correctable disorders. For screening programs to be of value, they must be convenient, free or of minimal cost, well advertised, and include a follow-up program when problems are detected. Providing screening programs subsumes the commitment to health education, prevention, and early intervention rather than the traditional practice of crisis intervention. This progressive philosophy conveys the community's concern for the quality of life of its residents and a willingness to spend the resources of time, money, and energy to achieve a better-quality life.

In the past immunization programs were the most widely known and accepted means of preventing illnesses. These are still important today but other, equally important, programs have been added. Newer approaches to improve and maintain health during the early childhood years include blood tests to screen for anemia, lead levels that are too high, sickle cell trait or disease; vision screening to detect strabismus, amblyopia, and color blindness; auditory and speech screening to identify hearing loss or articulation problems; and developmental screening to assess gross and fine motor skills, including coordination and balance.

The extent to which these programs are accessible before the child enters school is significant. Vision, hearing, speech, or other physical disorders can adversely affect the child's ability to learn. In addition, the child's achievement of a positive self-concept is thwarted if others tease, mock, or make fun of an existing deficiency. The availability of these health services is related to social values and whether community leaders consider such services in terms of free enterprise or in terms of health as the right of all. Those with the latter view are more likely to provide free clinics for immunizations and screening than are those who favor the traditional "fee-for-service" system (Read, 1973).

Similarly, a community's protective systems (legal and legislative) offer parenting alternatives for children in health- or life-threatening situations. Such services are evident in the child protection agencies and the relationship between these agencies and the courts. The efforts and resources utilized for providing adequate care for poor, abused, or neglected children reveal whether their situation is thought to be the result of the parent's psychologic limitations or because of broader underlying social structural factors. When social conditions, such as poverty, unemployment, or inadequate housing, are seen as contributing agents, there is a greater degree of community support for programs to combat these conditions and help those victimized by them. The goal of such programs on a local, state, or even national level is to integrate these families into the community and to provide the essential services that are important during the formative years of early childhood. Support for such concrete programs tends to decrease when the community believes in the psychodynamic theory and considers parental problems and limitations to be the main reason for poor and abused young children (Pelton, 1981).

Interactions Among Subsystems

A child's internal environment also can be described as being composed of interacting subsystems. Each subsystem develops and matures according to key genetic and phylogenetic phases. The interaction among subsystems and with the external environment results in a unique product—a human being. For example, the temperament of the child results from the interaction of the child's cognitive, perceptual, affective, neurophysiologic, and psychologic subsystems. This internal interaction, however, may be affected by significant external or environmental relationships.

Genetic endowment and the child's interaction with the external and internal environments contribute to each child's unique growth pattern. The direction and phases of growth, however, are predictable. Normal children reach developmental milestones, such as walking, language acquisition, and bladder and bowel control, within a certain time frame. The patterns of the separate behaviors that lead to these milestones may differ, but the results are stable and consistent for all children. (Developmental norms and commonly used tools for nursing assessment are discussed in Chapter 16.)

Because of the interaction among subsystems, growth in one subsystem influences growth in another. Social growth in the toddler is facilitated by language acquisition, cognitive growth, and fine and gross motor skills. Similarly, motor skills such as bicycling and ballplaying may be facilitated by social interactions. Emotional growth, evidenced by learning to tolerate separation anxiety, is made easier by the mental achievement of what Piaget termed object permanence, or the ability to hold an image in one's mind of the "lost object" (see Table 6-5). The child who cried at 9 months when a parent or caregiver was out of sight can now understand that objects that have disappeared from view are not gone forever.

The age at which children normally reach their milestones varies widely. Children progress at paces that are optimum for them.

Parameters of Early Childhood Development

The parameters of early childhood development describe the basic aspects of the developmental subsystems. Included in this chapter are the areas most commonly analyzed and discussed by developmental theorists. As these areas interact with each other, they contribute to the uniqueness of each child's appearance, personality, skill level, creativity, and coping style.

Biophysical Development

Biophysical development encompasses the growth and development of the body and its organ systems. This development includes genetic inheritance, anatomic structures, chemical balances, and physiologic processes. The smooth functioning of the combined systems that comprise this general area is important for health maintenance and the maximization of the child's potentials.

Musculoskeletal System The short, squat, bowlegged, potbellied, swaybacked toddler is replaced at 5 years of age with a slimmer, straighter, more flat-tummied, leggy preschooler. Ossification of the skeletal system, an indication of skeletal maturity, advances during this period, as does growth of the long bones. From 2 to 5 years of age, approximately 45 foci of ossification appear, and growth of the legs occurs faster than growth of the trunk, so that after the first year, 66% of the child's increase in height is leg growth. The change in height ranges from 30 to 46 in (75–117 cm) during this period. During early childhood, growth averages 2–3 in/yr, and few differences in growth between the sexes are evident (Schuster and Ashburn, 1980).

Muscle growth occurs more slowly during early childhood than during infancy, but this is balanced by a decline in the proportion of weight that consists of adipose tissue. As adipose tissue accumulation declines, the child becomes thinner and muscle tone also improves. Differences in muscle development at this age may be attributed to environmental and genetic influences because hormonal influences will not affect muscle size until puberty. The child's weight increases, on the average, from about 22.5 to 45 lb, or 10–20 kg (Schuster and Ashburn, 1980). After about

2 years of age, variations among children's weights may be greater. (See Appendix A for representative standards of height and weight curves for this age group.)

Respiratory System Growth of the respiratory system in early childhood parallels growth in the rest of the body. The barrel-shaped infant's chest changes to approximate the adult-shaped chest, which has a greater transverse than anterioposterior diameter. Breathing continues to be abdominal until about 7 years of age, but as lung size increases, the vital capacity and maximum breathing capacity increases.

The rapid and irregular rate of respirations found in infancy has stabilized and gradually slowed. (See Appendix B for normal respiratory rates in this age group.) The average respiratory rate at 2–3 years of age is 20–30 breaths/min. Respiratory and pulse rates are more labile in children than in adults and thus are more likely to change in response to crying, illness, and exercise. Nurses assessing young children therefore need to consider these factors. Because of immune and structural immaturity, respiratory illness is more common during childhood (see Chapter 34).

Cardiovascular System The cardiovascular system also grows and matures in early childhood, although the heart grows more slowly than the rest of the body. With increasing size and increased blood volume, the heart becomes a more efficient pump and the pulse rate decreases, so that at 2 years of age the average heart rate is 90–110 beats/min. Palpation of the carotid artery or auscultation of the apical pulse provides the most reliable measurement of heart rate in this age group.

Blood pressure also increases with age, along with increasing stroke volume and cardiac output. Systolic blood pressure increases from 90 to 95 mm Hg at 3 years of age to about 100 mm Hg at 5 years of age (Chow, et al., 1979). Diastolic blood pressure changes from about 60 to 65 mm Hg between 3 and 5 years of age. (See Appendix B for a summary of pulse and blood pressure values.)

Sensory System The senses mature with age. Fused, binocular vision begins at 9 months and continues to develop until 6 years of age. The gradual changes occurring in the size of the eyeball and the refractive power of the lens and cornea do little to refine the child's vision. Hyperopia, or farsightedness, remains predominant throughout early childhood, and the child finds it hard to focus on fine, small letters or pictures.

By 18 months of age, convergence of the eyes is well established and accommodation to near and far objects is well developed, although localization of distant objects is still crude. Vision is about 20/70 at 2 years of age, 20/50 at 3 years of age, 20/40 at 4 years of age, and 20/30 at 5 years of age (Nelms and Mullins, 1982).

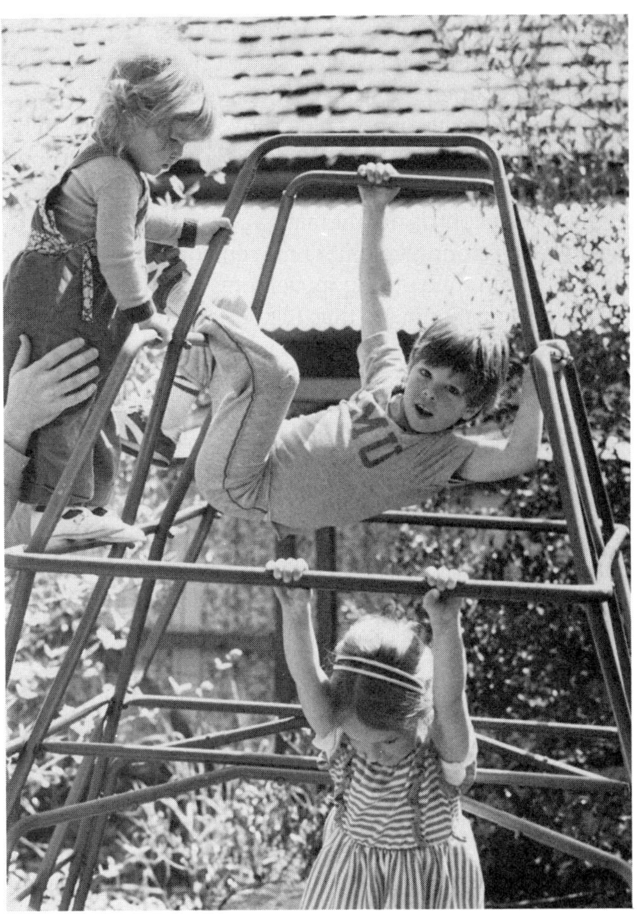

Gross motor development in early childhood. The 2-year-old needs adult support. The 4-year-old has gained the coordination and dexterity to use the playground equipment alone.

Lack of coordination between the muscles of the eyes (a condition known as strabismus) results in the child focusing with only one eye. This enables the child to avoid the diplopia resulting from the failure of binocular vision. Central vision of the other eye may be suppressed, resulting in amblyopia, a dimness of vision caused by disuse, and, if uncorrected, total, permanent loss of central vision in one eye. Treatment should begin by 2 years of age (see Chapter 43 for a more complete discussion of disorders of the eye).

Hearing in the preschool child is at adult levels, but because of the immaturity of the structure of the ear, the child is more prone to infection and fluid accumulation in the middle ear, which can alter hearing acuity. Hearing can be evaluated in the toddler through the assessment of language development and behavioral response to speech or environmental noise. Depending on maturity level, the child will be able to participate in audiometric testing at 3 or 4 years of age. Responses to an audiogram will, however, be affected by the child's attention span, perseverance, and level of environmental distraction.

Neuromuscular System Neuromuscular growth in the young child is a complex process that results from neural maturation, genetic factors, and environmental interactions. Certain milestones, such as locomotion, seem to be attained through neural maturation but still respond to environmental influences.

One indication of neural maturation is the cessation of the child's mirroring voluntary movements on one side of the body with involuntary movements on the other side. One-sided functioning is thus fully established by 4 years of age. Neural tissues grow as rapidly during early childhood as they did in infancy. Ninety percent of the adult size of the brain is achieved by 2 years of age. Myelinization of the cortex, brain stem, and spinal cord follows the cephalocaudal, proximaldistal principle (see Fig. 6-2).

Increasing complexity and refinement of both gross motor and fine motor skills characterize early childhood development. Neuromuscular behaviors have therefore been incorporated into various screening tools for nursing assessment during early childhood (see Chapter 16).

From the age of about 18 months, a child can build a tower of two to four blocks and scribble spontaneously. By the age of 4½ years, many children can draw a five-part human figure and build a tower of eight or more blocks. Similarly, developing from pulling off a sock or hat at 18 months of age, many 4½-year-olds can tie a shoe and dress themselves. A 2-year-old can jump with both feet off the ground. A 4½-year-old can hop, skip, and walk a straight line with heel-to-toe placement.

Personality Development

Characteristics of the child's personality take form during the early childhood period. During infancy, temperamental differences coupled with environmental and genetic influences account for individuality, but around 18 months of age, the child exhibits more complex and unique personality traits.

Self-Control and Limit Setting A variety of personality theories explain the course of early childhood development (see Chapter 6). Psychoanalytic theory, with its roots in Sigmund Freud's work, describes the motivational forces behind behavioral phenomena. The toddler phase of early childhood corresponds to Freud's second stage of sexual development, the anal phase. Freud thought that this maturation was responsible for this shift in focus, although he suggested that parental views and demands regarding toilet training and cleanliness were also contributing factors (Chess and Hassibi, 1978).

Parents of toddlers often recognize the way the child attempts to control powerful others, usually parents, by withholding and expelling during toilet training. One 2-year-old girl, for example, learned that she could refuse to "go potty" before a family outing and then subsequently cause great upset by demanding to stop for a bathroom trip once the journey had begun. Related to this withholding characteristic is the toddler's tendency to say "No." Little children constantly hear prohibitions against their actions during this time of increased locomotion and exploration, and they begin to mimic parents with automatic recitals of "No" in response to every request or demand. Once they have learned the power of the word, they use it to test limits. Parents of toddlers need tremendous patience and an understanding of the interplay of developmental tasks as their children attempt to discover and define their place. The young child needs to be given a small measure of control, and the consequences of the child's actions must be clearly and consistently presented and demonstrated. It is during this phase that the child becomes increasingly capable of exploring the environment, discovering new motor and adaptive behaviors, and learning how to communicate with others. Erik Erikson's theory suggests that the environment may support the child's autonomy through these experiences or may engender feelings of shame and doubt (see Chapter 6). Parental attitudes and behaviors, which are a significant part of this environment, therefore influence the child's sense of self. If socializing experiences, such as toilet training, eating correctly, and self-dressing, are fraught with anxiety and become a battle of wills, the child is likely to feel shame and doubt. If, however, the child is encouraged and supported in these developmental tasks, a realistic and positive sense of autonomy results.

One of the more frequently heard demands is "Me do it." One 2½-year-old astonished her proud grandmother in front of a group of friends at church. This young girl loudly insisted that she was going to put on and button her new coat, and offers of help were refused defiantly. The wise grandmother stepped aside and covertly watched as the child struggled for 20 minutes until she got the coat on and partly buttoned. Proudly she showed her grandmother, who praised her accomplishment.

Parents often find that they need to allow extra time before an outing so that young children can express their autonomy in dressing; otherwise, a battle of wills is likely to ensue and the children chastised for making everyone late.

A major issue for the young child is the development of self-control. Toilet training, limits on behavior, and peer interactions all require the child to curb impulses and shape actions. Some youngsters engage in a battle of wills and resist parental guidance, so that temper tantrums are fairly common during this period. Children become enraged that their wishes are not gratified. These outbursts of screaming, thrashing, and kicking are triggered even more quickly if children are tired or hungry. When parental limits are consistent and reasonable, most children will learn to cope with frustrations and modify expectations and temper tantrums will cease.

Children who find grocery shopping to be uninteresting and restrictive attempt to compensate by pestering for some treat or special purchase. When this verbal plea does not produce the desired results, they resort to temper tantrums, which often are successful because of the parental embarrassment they create. Parents then placate the child to save face. Once success is attained, the behavior is more likely to be repeated. One mother recalled her humiliation when her 3-year-old son screamed the entire time during one shopping trip when she refused to buy him some candy because it was too close to lunch. The next week, she shopped after lunch, her son again requested candy, and she refused; after one or two more tries, he accepted her answer. She attributed his not resorting to a temper tantrum to the combination of not being hungry and not having success with that tactic the previous week.

To achieve the upcoming tasks of the school years, the child begins to learn how to interact appropriately with others in various situations. This necessitates self-control over the undisciplined expression of self- centered feelings.

Personality theorists consider the early childhood period to be crucial in the development of a healthy self-concept. "Self-concepts are thought to be complex integrations of feelings and attitudes that are formed as reactions to social learning situations which take place" (Nelms and Mullins, 1982, p. 389). Self-esteem is considered to be the evaluative component of self- concept and is a measure of how competent, pleased, worthy, and loved the child feels. Children require support to gain a realistic sense of their abilities and limitations. The development of self-esteem, which continues during this phase, forms the basis for trying out new things and relationships in this and later developmental stages. Children with a high degree of self-esteem are more active and demonstrate more leadership and self-confidence than those with low self-esteem.

Children assume that what adults tell them about themselves is true. A child who fears water is not helped to develop a positive self-concept if significant others make comments such as, "See, Amy is your age and she is not afraid of the water, so why are you?" or "Last year you went in up to your chin and now you are afraid to get your feet wet, what is wrong with you."

Seymour Epstein (1973) proposed that the self-concept theory is really a theory about the self, which has its initial construction during childhood by the child in response to the information received from others. In this process the child attempts both to enhance self-esteem and to select social interaction situations that provide positive feedback. As Sullivan (1953) noted (see Chapter 6) the child validates feelings of "good me" or "bad me" through relationships with other people. Thus, parents, siblings, teachers, peers, community leaders, and society all play a role in the way a child organizes temperament, personal attributes, and feelings to achieve positive feedback. If the child is unable to please the significant others or if the effort to do so is judged too costly, a sense of failure and feelings of "bad me" result. Adults who are insensitive to the young child's perspective and belittle childhood fears may contribute to the development of a negative self-concept. If, on the other hand, the child receives approval, love, and support from significant others, a positive self-concept is engendered.

Freud's theory postulates that successful mastery of the tasks of toilet training gradually shifts the child's attention to the genital zone. The ensuing Oedipal phase is the period in which children discover anatomic differences between the sexes. Libidinal investment is then focused on the boy's penis or girl's clitoris, and, according to Freud, this discovery and interest are related to concerns over threats or fears of harm and castration among boys and envy and sadness over the absence of visible male genitalia among girls. Freud's theory of the Oedipus complex further claimed that the healthy outcome of this conflict is that the young boy represses his unacceptable wishes for his mother and identifies with his father. Although Freud failed to develop a completely satisfactory description of this process for the young girl, he theorized that girls follow a similar course as the girl's desire for her father leads her to view her mother as a rival. Realistic limitations and fear of retaliation by the parent of the same sex help the child to reject these desires and to identify with the same-sex parent (Freud, 1969).

When parents are comfortable with their own sexuality and recognize that behavior associated with the Oedipal period is normal, problems need not result. For example, one 4-year-old boy told his mother that he hoped Daddy would never come home and he would be the "new Daddy." The mother understood the child's message and let him know that she was glad to have him care for her but that it would be wonderful for the entire family to see Daddy again. When the father returned, the mother was careful to include the son in tales of the business trip so that he would not feel threatened by his father's renewed presence.

The development of the superego, which Freud equated with conscience and punishment, coincides with the Oedipal phase. Freud (1969) described the superego as the "heir" to the Oedipus complex, meaning that the superego can only be formulated after that complex has been resolved. As he grows older, the 4-year-old who wanted to replace Daddy will therefore be more likely to identify with his father and less likely to express similar desires.

Independence Common to the theoretic perspectives of early childhood are several central concepts that facilitate understanding the young child's developing personality. During early childhood, the child begins a gradual shift from complete dependence to a beginning independence. From a small infant completely reliant on caregivers, the child develops by exploring the surroundings and communicating wishes. Locomotion and language thereby allow the child a small measure of self-reliance.

The toddler's sense of independence is, however, a fragile thing. Protection, nurturance, and the provision of basic needs are still parental responsibilities. The typical toddler may excitedly examine a new object or corner of the house only to break into tears when suddenly noticing that a parent is no longer nearby.

From 3 to 4½ years of age, the child is faced with increasing challenges that help to develop independence. During this time, the child's social world begins to expand beyond the family boundaries to the playground, neighborhood, and nursery school. The environment then requires that the child tolerate separation from parents and learn to play with other children. In addition to the developing superego, the limit-setting function of the parents assists the child in controlling unacceptable impulses and behavior. Erikson's theory defines the psychosocial issue of this stage as initiative versus guilt. As in the previous stage, protective and supportive limits encourage the child to initiate interactions and foster self-esteem. Overly restrictive controls and global prohibitions tend to create a sense of guilt, dampen the child's initiative, and lower self-esteem. A child who has internalized appropriate limits is consequently developing a healthy self-concept.

The child's ability to take pride in new accomplishments and to have that pride validated by parental approval provides the basis for a sense of initiative. The mother who praises her daughter's early attempts at selecting her clothes and dressing herself encourages autonomy and supports initiative, whereas the mother who criticizes the daughter's combination of colors or uneven buttoning of her blouse paves the way for a sense of guilt and fear of failure in meeting expectations. "From a sense of self-control without loss of self-esteem comes a lasting sense of good will and pride; from a sense of loss of self-control and of foreign overcontrol comes a lasting propensity for doubt and shame" (Erikson, 1973).

As more mothers work outside the home, independence may be learned at an even earlier age. The young child's learning to function without the constant support of an adult is crucial in making a successful transition to school and middle childhood.

Related to independence is the development of a sense of separation or personal boundaries. The young child moves from the normal mother–child symbiosis of infancy to a separate identity. Although emotional connections remain, the child begins to feel like an individual with feelings, reactions, and abilities attributed to no other person. For example, the child no longer bursts into tears when a peer is distressed but can differentiate between personal distress and that of someone else.

As the young child begins to explore the environment and make tentative moves toward independence, the stage is set for what Margaret Mahler (Mahler, Pino, Bergman, 1975) termed the *separation-individuation* phase of development.

The healthy process of separation-individuation involves the toddler's ability to move away from the total protection of the parent and the parent's ability to provide a safe and caring atmosphere for exploration, thus fostering the child's sense of self as a separate and unique being. Successful completion of this process allows the young child to enter the world of peer interactions in early childhood. The child learns that initiative and exploration are rewarding and, at the same time, learns that the secure parent–child relationship need not be sacrificed when the network of relationships is expanded.

Cognitive Development

Reasoning and Logic The child's ability to learn about the consequences of actions and to manipulate the environment is fundamental to development. Cognitive development is not an isolated phenomenon. It springs from the child's genetically inherited characteristics, life experiences, and social interaction, related factors that support and contribute to each other. For example, the 3-year-old child who manipulates pebbles is learning by experience. By feeling, dropping, and tossing the pebbles, the child learns about some of their properties; by counting and ordering the pebbles in a row, the child learns about ordering objects, not about the pebbles themselves, and thus develops skills involving logic and mathematics.

During early childhood, a major change in cognition takes place: the child begins to use symbols to represent the outside world, a phase that Piaget (Piaget and Inhelder, 1969) labeled the *preoperational phase* of thought (see Chapter 6). For the first time, the child can view the course of an event without actually experiencing it.

Early in this stage, the child experiences severe limitations in internalizing events, and because the child cannot yet form abstractions or generalizations, cognition is mostly restricted to concrete actions. In addition, children learn sequences and routines, so that once the sequences of steps begins, the child's mental review proceeds systematically, step-by-step, with little variation. For example, the child cannot state what number follows eight without counting from one to eight first and then responding with the answer nine.

The child's ability to classify objects is another important aspect of preoperational thought. Early in this phase, the child is not aware of the characteristics that unite all members of a class. For example, when 2- or 3-year-olds place all blue blocks in a pile, they are not necessarily demonstrating their ability to categorize; rather, they are responding to the dominant characteristic—the blue color. This ability to classify objects is limited because the child's inductive reasoning tends to deal with a limited range of available information. Lindsay and Norman (1977) provided an apt description of the preoperational child's system of categorization: "A child is likey to group a bat with a ball (because you play with them), then a tomato with a ball (because they are round), and then put a rose with the tomato (because they are red). An adult does not do this. Rather, adults insist on finding one single rule that applies to all objects.

During this stage, children are described as *egocentric*, that is, viewing everything in relation to themselves. They are intolerant when told, "I don't understand you" because they have not learned that another's views or perceptions may be different. Nor can the young child imagine how an object would look from another position or even conceive that other experiences or feelings are possible. For example, when told not to take the truck from his friend, Johnny replied, "But it's mine." When told, "But Lee is sad and crying," Johnny responded, "But it's mine, and I need it." At this age, Johnny is unable to be objective. The egocentric behavior of early childhood means that he is unable to consider that Lee also might want the truck.

Another important aspect of preoperational cognition is *irreversibility*, the ability to anticipate the consequences of an action, but the inability to reverse the process and return the object to its original state. The thought process itself is perceived as a real action that, once completed, cannot be mentally reversed.

Piaget's familiar water glass problem illustrates the concept of irreversibility. Three glasses are set side by side. One glass is tall and narrow, and the other two glasses are low and wide. The two wide glasses are filled with equal amounts of water. Next, the water is poured from one wide glass to the narrow glass; the level of the water rises to a higher point. When the child is asked whether the narrow glass has the same amount of water as the other wide glass or whether the water level would be the same if the water were poured back to the empty wide glass, the answer is likely to be "no." Some children will explain that the level is higher so there is more water; others will say that there is less water because the width is thinner. In preoperational thought the concept of conservation of volume does not yet have meaning (Piaget, 1952).

Play and Fantasy Preoperational thought also is characterized by *symbolic play*, in which the child pretends and reenacts events. Part of the delight of children at this stage is their ability to pretend and fantasize. A broomstick becomes a motorcycle, a stack of pillows a fort, a doll a crying baby to comfort. Although thought is symbolic, the symbols are not necessarily organized into a cohesive set of concepts and rules. That stage of development occurs during the subsequent period of concrete operations. For these children, reality and fantasy are partly interchangeable, but a gradual shift begins to mark the difference between pretending and reality. Children then seek more realistic props for play; for example, they come to prefer toys that are realistic replicas of real objects.

The young child's understanding of dreams also blends the real world and fantasy. In dreams real events seem to be happening in a real place. After a frightening dream, the child may be reluctant to return to his or her room because "the bad dream is still in there."

For example, for weeks after being scared by a birthday party clown and subsequently having a bad dream about it, one 3-year-old girl made her mother chase all of the clowns out of her room every night before turning off the light. A 4-year-old boy had a recurring dream about a vicious dog. He would escape to his parents' room and refuse to return to his room until both of them joined him in inspecting his room to make certain that the dog was not there. Then he would have them double check the window to be sure that it was locked, leave the light on, and close the door.

Imaginary playmates also are created from the young child's active imagination and serve as examples of the child's cognitive processes. Estimates indicate that 20%–50% of children 4 and 5 years of age have imaginary companions (Stone and Church, 1975). The invisible playmate may serve a specific need by expressing feelings that the child is unable to verbalize safely such as resentment or hostility.

Frequently, children who have imaginary playmates are characterized as imaginative and bright, although this phenomenon occurs at all intellectual and socioeconomic levels. Imaginary playmates often serve as the scapegoat for a child's lapses in behavior, as in "Susie spilled the milk," or paradoxically, as the developing conscience or superego that guides the child's behavior. The playmate embodies the child's conscience by reminding what should or should not be done and by gently scolding when infractions are committed. One researcher suggested that these playmates are introduced during times of stress or developmental tension and represent a healthy way of coping with this stress (Nagera, 1969).

For example, to cope with the realities of learning right from wrong, one boy created an imaginary adult friend. "Mrs. Legger" told his mother when she could go downstairs or outside and where she could walk in his room. He also used her when he wanted something, such as, "Mrs. Legger wants Robert to have a drink of juice and a cracker now."

Imaginary playmates serve to reduce loneliness and provide the child with an opportunity to try out interaction styles and to control the outcome of play. Many parents relate how they had to dress, set the table, or hold the hand of some imaginary friend. The child often becomes very upset if the parent does not cooperate. For example, 3-year-old Sarah would not get in the car because her mother had left Amy (her imaginary friend) in the shopping cart in the store. They had to go back and get Amy, who (according to Sarah) was crying because she had been left and thought no one loved her. Once Amy was retrieved, all was fine and Sarah was her happy self once again.

Self-Awareness

Inherent in the child's ability for preoperational thought is the developing capacity for self-awareness. Children can now study their own actions and separate them from events in the environment. They also might sense their own vulnerability because danger or harm can be imagined. Ages 4 and 5 usually are characterized by a sudden explosion of fears (Stone and Church, 1975). For instance, the child may imagine scary figures in the shadows on the wall at night and demand that a light be left on. A minor illness or medical procedure sometimes leads to the expression of panic and fear of mutilation or dying. Support by parents, caregivers, and health professionals can assist the young child during times of stress or illness (see Chapter 29). The child's active imagination may be used effectively in mastering the frightening situation; for example, doll play with a syringe can ease the child's fear of receiving an injection (see Chapter 28).

The capacity for self-awareness and rudimentary classification skills are fundamental to developing gender identity. Early in this period, the child labels himself or herself as a boy or girl, a vital task in psychosexual development. Concurrently, the young child begins to learn stereotypic and gender-related traits.

Equilibration, the Piagetian process of self-regulation, is significant at the end of early childhood. At this time, the child becomes uncomfortable with some previously accepted reasons or answers to questions about the nature of things. The notion of *compensation* illustrates how a child actively regulates this thinking to restore equilibrium to disequilibrium. If clay is shaped into a sausage, the child focuses on one dimension, either width or length. When the clay is reshaped to make it shorter, the child is likely to refocus on the opposite dimension. Eventually, the child will come to recognize the relation between width and length. Compensation thus occurs when the child is able to focus on more than one dimension at a time. This self-regulation process was described by Piaget as "the fundamental factor in the acquisition of logical-mathematical knowledge" (Piaget, 1972).

Memory New knowledge is stored in memory schemes. For most young children, recognition memory surpasses recall memory, and both abilities improve with age. An 8-year-old usually will be able to recall about eight of a set of 12 objects shown but will identify all 12 if they are included in a larger group of objects. In contrast, the 4-year-old child shown the same objects would recall three or four objects and would recognize 10 or 11 of them (Mussen, Conger, and Kagan, 1979).

The reason for this improvement in memory, especially in recallability, is not known. One important factor, however, is that as the child's store of knowledge grows, new information can be related to previously acquired information. The young child begins to code the information in a form that makes retrieval possible and tries to remember by rehearsing the information. This process clearly is related to language development and the ability to use symbols and codes. Adults have few, if any, conscious memories of events in their lives prior to 2 or 3 years of age. Limited knowledge, lack of language and symbolic thought, and only a developing sense of self are factors that help to explain why memory storage and/or retrieval is hampered in early life. Infants and very young children also might store information in ways that are different from methods used after language and classification skills are learned. If this is so, then the older child or adult is unable to retrieve knowledge stored in infancy because the key to the storage system is lost.

Creativity Cognitive gains are evident in the creativity of young children. A rich imagination and the ability to make new things out of seemingly unrelated parts characterize the highly creative child.

Creativity and cognitive changes can be demonstrated in young children's drawings. Table 8-1 illustrates how children progress from random markings (common to 2-year-olds) to the creation of symbolic representations of imagined and real objects. Drawings not only delight adults but also provide a window to the child's thoughts.

Language Development

Changes in Children's Speech One of the most dramatic developments in childhood—the beginning of language—occurs during the second year of life. Names of objects and a few simple verbs are learned first, and by the end of the second year, the child has a vocabulary of about 50 words. From this basic language, the young child begins to construct two-word sentences.

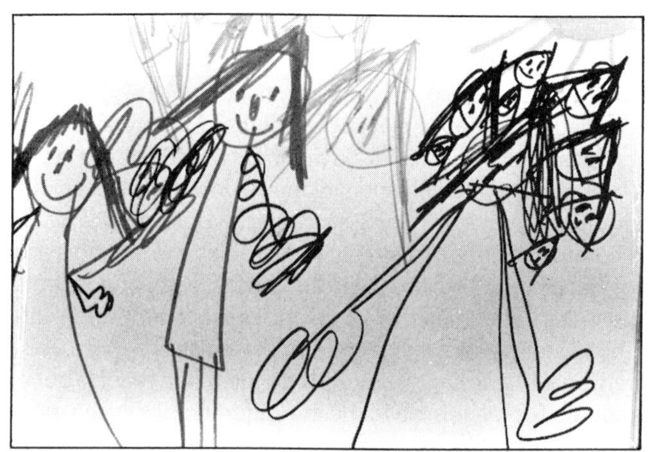

In early childhood, drawings are symbolic representations of the child's thoughts.

TABLE 8-1 Sequence of Skills in Children's Drawings

Age	Skill
2 years	Scribbling various positions on paper
	Single- and multiple-line drawings
	Varieties of scribbling patterns
3 years	Space on paper often enclosed
	Simple crossed lines
	"Suns" with lines emanating from them
	Beginning of crudely drawn human figures
4 years	Circles and squares
	Crude houses and cars
	Trees and animals
5 years	More complex drawings of people, buildings, trees, and animals

SOURCE: Gibson J: *Living: Human Development Through the Lifespan*. Addison-Wesley, 1983. Adapted from Kellog R, O'Dell S, *Analyzing Children's Art*. National Press Books, 1969.

A 2-year-old puts two to three words together using primarily nouns and verbs. A 4½-year-old speaks in complex sentences, using and understanding all forms of grammar. These early sentences are telegraphic, or shortened versions of adult sentences, composed of nouns and verbs with an occasional adjective. These short sentences can express a range of meanings and have been found in the speech of young children from various cultures speaking different languages. The following meanings have been identified in telegraphic speech (Slobin, 1972; Lindsay and Norman, 1977; Mussen, Conger, and Kagan, 1979).

Identification: see car
Location: Mommy there
Repetition: more candy
Nonexistence: milk all gone
Negation: not doggie
Possession: my ball
Attribution: small baby
Agent-action: Daddy sit
Action-object: take teddy
Agent-object: Mommy bag
Action-location: lay bed
Action-recipient: give kitty
Action-instrument: go car
Question: where Daddy?

After the child gradually learns to use sentences, vocabulary appears to increase suddenly. By about 30 months of age, the child no longer uses "baby talk" or babbling; all verbal output has communicative intent, and the young child begins to show frustration if adult listeners cannot interpret his or her meaning. Sentences become longer and may include from three to five words.

New elements begin to enter the young child's speech. Sentences become more complex and are characterized by some prepositions, particularly "in" and "on"; occasional articles, such as "an"; forms of the verb "to be," including "is" and "are"; nouns with plural and possessive endings; and some verb tense inflections such as the past (ed) and the progressive (ing). These linguistic additions (called grammatical morphemes) are developed gradually over a period of 2–3 years (Mussen, Conger, and Kagan, 1979). A 20-month old asks, "Mommy, change Carolyn?" Six months later the same question is asked as, "Mommy, did you just change Carolyn?"

By about 3 years of age, the young child has a vocabulary of some 1000 words and approximately 80% of communication is understandable, even to strangers. Although grammatical mistakes occur, the child's speech takes on the quality of colloquial adult speech. Nurses assessing children's language development therefore need to know that young children will learn basic grammar from the colloquial language they hear and not according to textbook guidelines. Thus, their language competence should be assessed in light of the language forms and communication styles to which they have been exposed.

Although many formal grammatical rules are not learned until the school-age years, the child's language is well established by about 4½ years of age. Deviations from the spoken adult language appear more in word selection and variety than in grammar. At the end of the preschool period, the child's speech includes complex sentences that are constructed by joining two simple sentences with the conjunction "and" or by placing one simple sentence or thought within another (for example, "I see you go"). Some errors still occur in questions that involve inserting the question word (why, who, what, where) and inverting the subject and part of the verb, but the child has nearly mastered the proper use of negation, so that even double negatives and the omission of the auxiliary form of "to be" do not interfere with the child's meaning. Some grammatical forms usually do not appear until the child reaches school age; these forms include the conjunctions "if" and "so," the verb "have," passive constructions, personal pronouns, and nominalization (using verbs as nouns, as in "running is fun") (Mussen, Conger, and Kagan, 1979).

Theories of Language Acquisition Various theories have been proposed to explain the fascinating mystery of language acquisition among children. Some theorists, particularly B. F. Skinner and other behaviorists, view language as a behavior that is learned through operant conditioning. Behaviorist learning theory suggests that the child's attempts at speech are selectively reinforced by adults who encourage sounds that mimic adult speech. For example, a mother who hears her child first say "mama" is likely to be pleased and will encourage and reinforce the child's behavior in making the sound.

Other theorists reject the assumption that language acquisition is a learned behavior. Noam Chomsky, a noted linguist, has developed a biologic, or natavistic, theory of language development. He has suggested that humans possess an innate language structure, which he dubbed a *language acquisition device (LAD)*. The LAD is thought to enable the young child to process what is heard (linguistic input), to make rules, and to understand and produce grammatical speech. Chomsky's theory therefore contends that the human ability to communicate through speech is innate and not learned and that all children eventually will learn to express thoughts with more complex speech. Although such a theory is very difficult to prove or refute, the universal nature of language development suggests that it depends both on maturation and on changes in the brain (Chomsky, 1957; Lavatelli and Stendler, 1972).

Active problem solving has been shown to be part of language acquisition. In one study 2-year-old children given a statement were able to repeat it by using their own grammatical repertoire (Slobin and Welsh, 1971). In another investigation children speaking black English were able to translate sentences from standard English into their own colloquial speech (Labov, et al., 1971). The children's ability to solve problems and adapt language illustrates Piaget's concept of self-regulation.

Research has not clearly shown that adult intervention can influence the process of language acquisition. After reviewing the available data concerning the influences of teaching, modeling, and reinforcement on children's language development, Mussen, Congers and Kagan (1979) concluded that none of these learning methods had a significant impact on the acquisition of grammatical competence. Children apparently learn a system of rules for a particular language, not a universal language, indicating that the environment must have some effect.

Adults may be able to assist children in learning language by simplifying their own speech when engaging young children in verbal exchanges. As the speech of adults gradually becomes richer and more complex, young children then shape or modify their language accordingly. This can happen in the classification of categories; for example, a young child will understand "car" but not "automobile," and a proper name is easier to identify than a pronoun, that is, "Mommy" instead of "I" or "me." Adults can help the child's conversation to progress by using both words and as the child gets older, using only the more complex word. Active encouragement and placing value on verbal communication are additional parental factors that may enhance the child's language development.

Moral Development

During early childhood, children begin to learn rudimentary standards of behavior and a sense of right and wrong. Psychoanalytic theory proposes a psychodynamic explanation of moral development as the emergence of the conscience or superego. Cognitive theory, as specified by Kohlberg (1969), offers insight into another aspect of moral development (see Chapter 6).

The 2-year-old is just starting to learn that some actions are forbidden and others rewarded. Sometimes characterized as the "no" stage, this period is the time in which the child gains a simple understanding that actions have consequences and that some limits must be learned. Three- and 4-year-olds are also in Kohlberg's premoral, or preconventional, stage of moral development, but they have developed a larger repertoire of moral judgments. They can judge behavior as good or bad according to the rewarding or punitive response it will elicit. They learn not to repeat a behavior, such as throwing sand in the sandbox, because it results in parental disapproval, which is expressed in their being punished such as having to spend time in the house or losing a privilege.

At 4½ years of age, children are just starting to evaluate actions according to inherent labels of good and bad, and they are beginning to understand moral concepts beyond reward and punishment. Transition to Kohlberg's conventional moral stage is gradual, and the consistent conformity to rules that characterizes this stage does not appear until middle childhood.

Fowler (1978) noted that the simple religious beliefs that are often taught to children during the early childhood years foster the development of faith (see Chapter 6). Part of moral development in many families also includes learning about God and the moral teachings of a religion. For some children, moral development is fostered by the parents' faith and by participating in major religious practices or holidays.

Social Development

Social development involves learning the customs and mores of society and adopting culturally defined behaviors or roles. The tasks of social development are interwoven with those of personality and cognitive development. Havighurst's (1972) view of the developmental tasks of early childhood demonstrates the links among these aspects of development: to form simple concepts of social and physical reality; to learn to relate oneself emotionally to parents, siblings, and other people; to learn to distinguish right and wrong; and to develop a conscience.

Imitation, the observing and copying of a model's actions, is a major component of social development in early child-

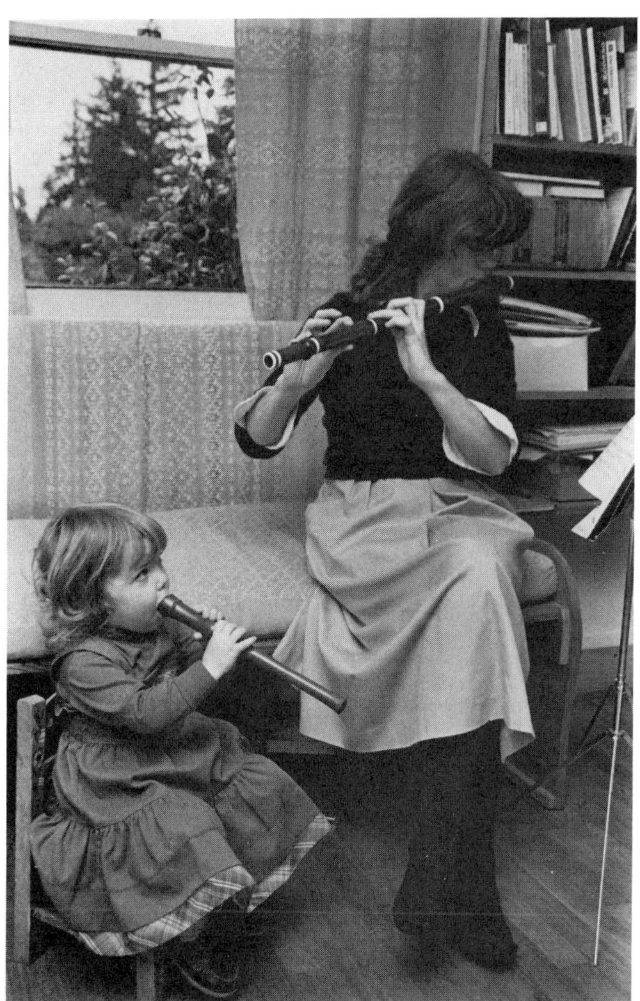

Imitation is an essential part of social development in early childhood.

hood. Gewirtz and Stingle (1972) built on modeling theory and proposed a process called "generalized imitation." They suggested that the first imitative behaviors occur by chance, through assistance, or direct training. When the child reproduces these responses, they are strengthened by positive reinforcement from socializing agents, particularly the parents. Gradually, the child adopts a set of varied but "functionally equivalent" behaviors that are maintained by intermittent reinforcement. Over time, the behaviors take on intrinsic value and will be reproduced without direct reinforcement from the model. Occasional reinforcement from the social milieu will support continued demonstration of the behavior.

The child first learns to say "Thank you" by responding to parental direction to do so. After being rewarded verbally or with a show of affection for saying "Thank you," the behavior is extended to a variety of situations. Soon the child is heard to say "thank you" when given something or when thanking someone for holding open a door. Imitation encourages a child to identify with adults, usually a parent.

One outcome of identification during the early childhood years is the child's adoption of gender-related traits, attitudes, and behavior. By the onset of this developmental phase, around 2 years of age, the young child should have a clear sense of gender identity; that is, "I am a girl" or "I am a boy." From 3 to 4½ years of age, the next task is to adopt characteristics, views, and behaviors that are consistent with culturally prescribed roles of males and females. Through identification with the parent of the same sex and reinforcement by parents and others, children gradually develop male or female identities.

Integrating Development Through Play

The various components of a child's development—biophysical, emotional, cognitive, and social—are all subsystems that interact to produce a unique child. Growth in one sphere influences growth in another. Social growth in the toddler is facilitated by the acquisition of language, cognitive growth, and fine and gross motor skills. Similarly, motor skills, such as bicycling and ballplaying, may be facilitated by social interactions. Emotional growth, such as learning to tolerate separation anxiety, is made easier by the mental achievement of object permanence.

Play is an important mechanism through which such integration occurs, but play was not always considered the meaningful part of childhood that it is now. Throughout history, some cultures and religions have considered play devilish, frivolous, or worthless. Today, however, play is understood to be a valuable tool that enhances growth and aids in the development of fine motor skills as well as sensory and perceptual capabilities. Play enhances emotional coping and releases tension. Play allows the child to reenact and reconstruct events and interactions that occur in daily life. The child masters the physical and psychosocial domain through play and develops social skills in interaction, cooperation, sharing, and assertiveness. The child learns and assimilates cultural norms and adult occupational, family, and sex roles. Moral and ethical questions of right and wrong are evaluated and safely experimented with through play.

Types of Play

Play ideas vary. Samples are "Let's play house. I'll be the mommy, you be the big sister," "Let's pretend our mother is dead and we're lost in the woods," "Let's play school and do homework" (this after a day at nursery school or kindergarten), "Let's play war," "Let's pretend we're turkeys," "Let's be birds or airplanes" (this when jumping off the living room couch), and "I'm making presents for Holly and Andrea." From this potpourri of play ideas, work and

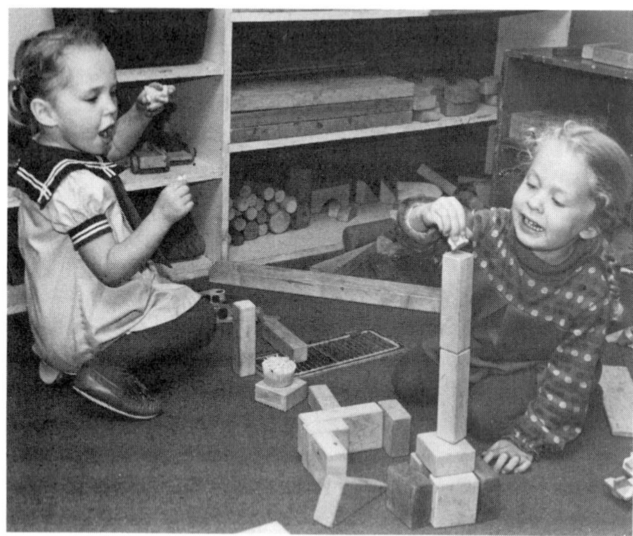

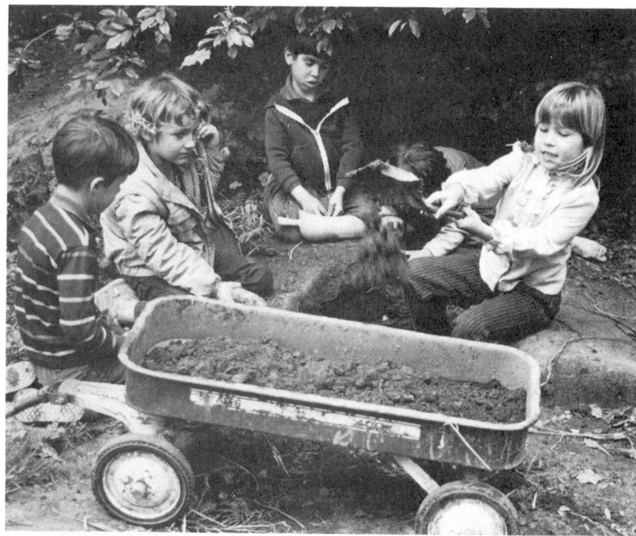

Play in early childhood takes various forms. Parallel play does not involve cooperation between children, while cooperative play involves more interactive activity, with clearly delineated roles.

family roles are assumed; separation and aggression issues are played out; and fine and gross motor skills are practiced. Fun, high spirits, and silliness are a part of some, but not all, play scenes.

A traditionally accepted categorization of play is the one developed by Parten and Newhall (1943), who described play according to the relationship between the players. *Unoccupied behavior* is at one end of a continuum. Here, the child is not involved in any activity that teaches or furthers development and attention drifts. Two-year-olds normally spend 10%–12% of their time this way, and normally developing 3-year-olds spend 7%–8% of their time doing this. In *onlooker play,* the child observes others' activities. Included in this category is time spent watching television as well as watching other children play. Television watching often increases during early childhood because of reinforcement from peers or parents, and its effect on children has interested researchers. Although the findings are inconclusive, some of the evidence certainly points to an alarming proportion of time spent in this form of play, which diminishes the time spent in more active types of play.

Solitary play, in which children are engrossed in their own independent play with toys or projects, is apparent at all levels of development. The younger child, who is limited in the social, psychologic, and cognitive skills necessary for more advanced and prolonged interaction, spends a greater proportion of time in this type of play. Nevertheless, it is equally important for the 4½-year-old to spend some time in this form of play because having privacy and personal space has been linked to creativity in children (White, 1975).

Parallel play is characteristic of the 2-year-old, who plays alongside others without interacting or cooperating. Although 2-year-olds frequently engage in this type of play, they are not limited to it. Similarly, 4-year-olds, who are better able to engage in cooperative play, also enjoy activities like coloring, which is a form of parallel play.

Associative play involves interaction and a common activity within a loosely structured environment. Several 2- and 3-year-olds may enjoy and weave in and out of a simple ball game or play together with a truck. The time and tolerance for this kind of play increases with age. *Cooperative play,* often considered the most complex form of play because it involves a common interactive activity, is characterized by a variety of roles assigned through interaction among children. In cooperative play tasks are all allocated, and the plot is delineated; children clearly belong or do not belong to the play. The 4-year-old will begin to get involved in the casting and directing of this type of play. A younger child is frequently assigned the part of the baby and plays it very well.

Play also might be described according to the type of activity (Piers, 1972). *Functional play,* or physical play, is action play and may be social, boisterous, and competitive or it may be manipulative and include doing jigsaw puzzles, practicing word or sound combinations, or exerting social control over others. Physical or sensorimotor play occurs in infancy and continues at a more advanced level throughout early childhood. *Symbolic play*—pretending, make-believe, or fantasy—is a type of play in which reality is transformed through language, action, or physical objects. Symbolic play can occur as early as 18 months of age but certainly is evident by 3 years of age and increases steadily thereafter.

Games that mutually involve the participants and include taking turns and repeating behavior are a final way of characterizing play. Although recent evidence and opinion suggest that gamelike interaction occurs during infancy, rudimentary game-playing is certainly established in the 3- to

4-year-old. Hide-and-seek, tag, and some simple board games (such as Candyland® and Winnie the Pooh®) exemplify this kind of play. Play for children can be characterized further as fun and as an end in itself. Play is more than what it appears to be; it should therefore provide a reasonable challenge for the child and take place in a relaxed setting.

Parental Actions to Facilitate Play

How can parents facilitate or enhance their children's play? Experts agree that the freedom allowed in a child's environment is a chief ingredient in successful play. This freedom implies reasonable physical freedom (that is, some reasonable space without excessive rules regarding the use of the space). If the child's only play space is in the living room, the many "no's" and comments like "don't touch" and "don't climb" restrict the child's freedom. The child in play also should have the freedom to make mistakes, be imperfect, be silly, regress—in short, to be socially and emotionally free of parental evaluation.

How adults play with children is also important. Both increased imagination and complexity of play result from parents who play with their children. Children also learn from parents who elaborate the play of their children. In other words, parents who add buildings to a town or help expand a farm started by a 3 or 4-year-old are elaborating on the play of their children.

What types of toys are appropriate for children during early childhood? To facilitate all aspects of development, play should involve large muscle groups, fine motor skills, imagination, and creativity, and it should be at different times active, quiet, associative, and solitary. Many different kinds of toys are appropriate for early childhood. Toys or household articles that accomplish more than one kind of play can serve the child well. Building blocks can enhance fine motor skills and creativity while the child engages in solitary or associative play. Swings, slides, or balls encourage gross motor activity and associative kinds of play. Crayons, scissors, and paper encourage fine motor skills and creative activities. Props that allow for creative and dramatic play include dress-up clothes, toy stoves, dishes, refrigerator, store, puppets, and doctor and nurse kits.

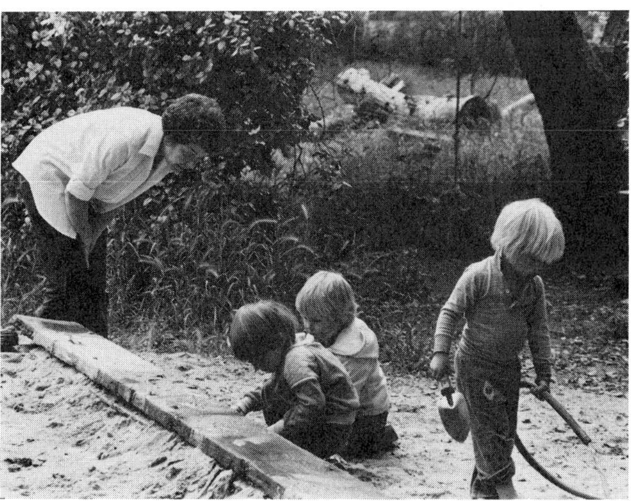

In early childhood, children learn from adults facilitating play.

Imaginary companions are also certainly a normal part of early childhood. Although a parent should not rearrange the family for this new member, parents can certainly play along and accommodate these temporary visitors. (Chapter 13 discusses additional parenting concerns and parent–child interactions.)

Health Care Needs of Early Childhood

Hygiene

The change from dependence to independence occurs dramatically in a relatively short time. The 18-month-old who can pull off socks and diapers learns in the next few years to dress, button, zipper, select clothes, and even tie shoelaces. The young child who splashes instead of washes hands in the sink (with some supervision) becomes one who can brush teeth, take care of toileting, basic hygiene, and even help wash hair. The spoon- and finger-feeder is replaced by a knife and fork user and even part-time assistant kitchen helper in setting the table, buttering bread, or baking. The 2-year-old who absolutely refuses to go to bed or take a nap is replaced by a fairly logical, reasonable participant in limit-setting decisions, although this child is still occasionally illogical and unreasonable.

One of the important and stressful milestones of self-care in early childhood is control of the bowel and bladder. Readiness for toilet training is a composite of neurophysiologic, personal-social, adaptive and cultural characteristics of the child. Because of the enormous amount of folk wisdom passed down from generation to generation about when and how to toilet train, nurses need to anticipate this milestone much earlier than readiness criteria might otherwise indicate.

Brazelton (1962) reported in his survey of toilet training among 672 boys and 491 girls that the average age of completion of both bladder and bowel training was 33.3 months. Daytime training was achieved somewhat earlier, at 28.5 months. Girls were trained on an average of 2.46 months earlier than boys.

Some parents begin toilet training at a much earlier date than these figures would indicate. The nurse can introduce the concept of readiness and encourage the parents to look for the following adaptive and psychomotor readiness signs: the ability to walk well, the balance and ability to climb and sit on a potty chair, and the ability to undress oneself. Standing and walking indicate myelinization of the spinal tract to the level needed for bowel and bladder sphincter control. Behavioral readiness is reflected in the child's awareness of the need to urinate or defecate. These signs include a word, increased fussiness, clinginess, silence, or actual movement toward the bathroom. The child's ability to imitate people and maintain an attention span of at least 5 minutes as well as letting go of a toy when requested are also readiness signs.

Parents must be "ready" too. Toilet training requires time, consistency, patience, and understanding. Optimally, there is congruence between the child's readiness and that of the parent's. Before discussing methods for toilet training, the nurse must assess the readiness of the entire family suprasystem. Overly high expectations about toilet training from family members may result in overly rigid or harsh toilet-training methods. A new sibling in the family may significantly alter a child's readiness. A family with two working parents may well have to involve the child's other caregiver(s) in toilet-training methods (Schuster and Ashburn, 1980).

Brazelton (1962) advocated individual child-oriented toilet training based on readiness criteria and beginning with the introduction of a potty chair. Powell (1981) encouraged the parent to reinforce immediately, consistently, and positively the child's appropriate elimination acts. Ignoring accidents or inappropriate toileting acts is more satisfactory than slapping, spanking, threatening, or bribing the child.

Sleep and Rest

Sleep needs during the early childhood period slowly decrease. The 2-year-old needs 12–14 hours of sleep per day (including naps), but unlike the infant, most of this sleep is at night, although one afternoon nap of 1–2 hours is still common. The percentage of rapid-eye-movement, or REM, sleep has decreased to 25% (Powell, 1981). Behavioral problems related to rest and sleep needs frequently occur, and resistance to going to bed may reach an all-time high. Equilibrium is assisted by adhering to repetitive or patterned behavior in the form of rituals. Consistent rituals around bedtime help make the transition from awake to sleep easier, although attempts to prolong these indefinitely warrant parental limit-setting.

The sleep needs of the 3- to 4-year-old decreases to 10–12 hours per day. This is the time when a nap frequently is eliminated, and all of the sleep takes place at night. Although REM sleep decreases to 20%, vivid dreams and nightmares may result in night terrors or awakening during this period (Powell, 1981).

In contrast to the infant's normal awakening during the night and parents' social and cultural willingness to tend to infants at night, the young child who awakens at night is considered a problem. Developmentally, sleep is a form of separation from parents, and separation at this stage is sanctioned culturally by most families in the United States. Because one of the developmental themes of this stage is separation-individuation, nurses can assist parents in looking at their child's sleep habits from this perspective.

Children generally love to sleep with their parents if they are allowed to do so, and such habits as having a parent present while falling asleep frequently become problematic for this age group. The young child who is acquiring a more sophisticated repertoire of coping and cognitive abilities can participate in a routine nighttime plan. Generally, parents can plan and explain a bedtime ritual with the children (for example, brush teeth, hear a story, hug goodnight, then lights out). The parent also can reassure the child that someone will comfort him or her if need be in the middle of the night. "Daddy will come to pat you on the back and see if you're ok, but you must stay in your bed and sleep in your own bed all night, then Daddy will go back to bed." Crucial to any communication with the child is consistent, appropriate, and congruent behaviors that reinforce the spoken message.

Illingsworth (1966) suggested that sleep problems are related to parent behaviors, particularly those of overanxiety and overpermissiveness. Parents can promote good sleep habits by creating a consistent and nurturing environment in which firm expectations about good sleep habits for the whole family are upheld.

Nutrition

The National Research Council lists the Recommended Dietary Allowances for toddlers and preschoolers (Table 8-2). Table 8-3 translates these nutrient requirements into the number of required servings in the basic four food groups for this age. During this period, activity increases, but the overall growth rate slows. Calorie requirements decrease to an average of about 100 kcal/kg (45 kcal/lb) (Hussey and Kanoff, 1979). Behaviorally, this decrease in growth in the 10–24-month-old period is manifested as a physiologic anorexia. Appetite decreases, and meals may be skipped. Food, when taken, may be patterned to reflect strong food preference. *Food jags*, as they are commonly called, may result in requesting some chosen food three times a day.

Some of the tensions of this developmental era are often manifested during meals. The child's need for rituals may result in food jags. The child's ability to say no is frequently practiced at mealtime by refusing food. One child had a peanut butter and jelly sandwich and a glass of milk or juice three times a day for 6 months. Whenever any other food was offered, the answer was "no," but the sandwich was always happily eaten.

Usually, these strong food likes or dislikes will disappear if they are ignored. The intrusiveness and talkativeness of the 3-year-old may manifest itself by not allowing anyone else to control dinner conversation. The physically active

TABLE 8-2 Meeting Daily Nutrition Requirements

RDAs	Age 1 to 3	Age 4 to 6	Foods to meet RDAs
Energy (kcal)	1300	1700	All foods
Protein (g)	23	30	Meat, eggs, fish, peanut butter
Vitamin A (μgRE)*	400	500	Liver, yellow vegetables, dark green vegetables
Vitamin D (IU)	400	400	Fortified milk
Vitamin E (IU)	5	6	Corn oils, leafy vegetables, red meat
Ascorbic acid (mg)	45	45	Citrus fruits, tomatoes, fortified beverages
Folacin (μg)	100	200	Organic meats, green leafy vegetables, yeast
Niacin (mg)	9	11	Meat, poultry, legumes, peanut butter
Riboflavin (mg)	0.8	1.0	Milk, dairy products, organic meats, enriched cereals
Thiamine (mg)	0.7	0.9	Cereals, grains, liver
Vitamin B_6 (mg)	0.9	1.3	Bananas, liver
Vitamin B_{12} (μg)	2.0	2.5	Lean meat, liver, eggs, fish
Calcium (mg)	800	800	Milk and milk products
Phosphorous (mg)	800	800	Milk, eggs, nuts, legumes
Iodine (μg)	70	90	Iodized salt, milk
Iron (mg)	15	10	Organic meats, dried legumes, shellfish, muscle meats, nuts, green leafy vegetables, fortified cereals
Magnesium (mg)	150	200	Nuts, soybeans, whole grains, legumes
Zinc (mg)	10	10	Seafood, milk, meats

SOURCE: Reproduced from *Recommended Dietary Allowances*, 9th edition, 1980, with permission from the National Academy Press, Washington, DC 20418.

*1 retinol equivalent = 1 μg retinol or 6 μg carotene.

and intense 4-year-old may have to leave the table for bathroom expeditions and may fidget frequently. Table manners at this age are only minimally acceptable.

Despite these immaturities, the nutritional habits of the young child reflect the independence and skill observed in other areas. Hussy and Kanoff (1979) summarized the developmental skills of feeding as follows:

Fifteen to eighteen months—child holds own spoon, although spilling occurs because of lack of wrist and hand coordination; child holds a cup and drinks well from it

Twenty-four months—wrist-hand coordination is established; child eats well with spoon and drinks from glass

Two and one-half years—rotary chewing skills are established; corn and meats are therefore acceptable

Three to four years—child can begin to use a fork

Four years—child uses a fork well; may begin to cut soft foods

Five to six years—child uses a knife to cut soft foods

Because of food jags, physiologic anorexia, and negativism during early childhood, parents frequently worry about their children's nutritional intake. Some health professionals recommend assessing the child's diet for a week to determine the number of servings eaten in the basic four food groups. This can reassure parents and encourage them not to focus unduly on individual mealtimes. Parents can be reassured that the refusal to eat all food at all meals is normal. As long as frequent high-carbohydrate snacks are not responsible for a diminished appetite, parents can avoid power struggles by not insisting that the child eat everything.

Pipes (1981) suggested that most well-developing children seem to get all their required nutrients at mealtimes and do not need many snacks. Others recommend smaller, more frequent feedings for young children, emphasizing that meals and snacks should contain high-quality protein, fiber, and vitamin-rich foods. For snacks, protein and fiber might be provided by cheese squares, peanut butter on celery, apples, or milk; vitamins might be obtained from fresh fruits, fruit juices, or raw vegetables such as carrot sticks, celery, or green pepper.

Children in early childhood enjoy simple, attractively colored and served food. Giving the child small portions sets reasonable expectations that the child will be able to finish the meal. Children often refuse casseroles and mixed foods but enjoy raw vegetables and finger foods. Meats are often not a favorite food, and parents must substitute other high-protein foods.

Feeding habits and attitudes toward food patterns of mealtime socialization are formed in these early years. Food can easily take on secondary meanings that can interfere with the concept of healthful nutrition. Food can become a bribe or a pacifier for tired, irritable, or bored children. Parents are heard to coax compliance by saying, "If you are good, I will buy you an ice cream cone" or "Finish your vegetables and you can have an extra cookie." Food can become a weapon against well-meaning parents. Even food given as love can lead to obesity and overall poor nutrition because of the over-representation of certain food groups. Mealtime can become a time of family exchange and communication or a time when anger and hostilities are vented.

Parents can achieve sound nutritional habits by following some simple rules (Hussey and Kanoff, 1979):

1. Avoid confrontations over disliked foods and table manners

TABLE 8-3 Recommended Daily Food Groups

Food group	Daily servings: 2 to 4 years	Daily servings: 4 to 6 years	Portion size
I. Milk and cheese group (1.5 oz cheese = 1 cup of milk)	3 to 6	3 to 4	4 oz of milk or milk substitute
II. Meat, eggs, poultry, fish, peanut-butter group (protein high here)	3	3	Meat, fish and poultry = 1 to 2 oz Eggs = 1 Peanut butter = 1 to 2 tbsp Legumes = $\frac{1}{4}$ to $\frac{1}{3}$ cup cooked
III. Fruit and vegetable group	4 to 5 Include one green leafy vegetable or yellow vegetable One citrus fruit or other vegetable or fruit rich in ascorbic acid	4 to 5	Cooked vegetables = 2 to 4 tbsp Raw vegetables = few pieces Canned fruit = 4 to 8 tbsp Fruit juice = 3 to 4 oz Raw fruit = $\frac{1}{2}$ to 1 small
IV. Cereal and bread group	3	3	Bread = $\frac{1}{2}$ to 1 slice Cooked cereal = $\frac{1}{4}$ to $\frac{1}{2}$ cup Dry cereal = $\frac{1}{2}$ to 1 cup Pasta = $\frac{1}{4}$ to $\frac{1}{2}$ cup Crackers = 2 to 3
Fats—bacon, butter, or vitamin A fortified margarine	3	3 to 4	Bacon = 1 slice (not to be substituted for meat) Butter or margarine = 1 tsp
Desserts	As needed to meet calorie demands		$\frac{1}{4}$ to $\frac{1}{2}$ cup

SOURCE: Adapted from The Institute of Home Economics, U.S.D.A.: *Four Food Groups of the Daily Food Guide*. Publication No. 30. Children's Bureau of the U.S. Department of Health, Education, and Welfare.

2. Give nutritious, appropriate-sized, well-timed, between-meal snacks
3. Avoid tensions at the table
4. Avoid the inappropriate use of food
5. Include the child in dinnertime conversations
6. Offer a well-balanced variety of nutritious food types that are colorful and attractively served
7. Avoid introducing sugared desserts as a necessary part of the meal
8. Develop reasonable expectations about eating (for example, the child cannot have a dessert if other foods are not touched)

The most frequent dietary insufficiencies in this age group are iron, ascorbic acid, calcium, and vitamin A; iron is the most frequent deficiency (Hussey and Kanoff, 1979). Parents and nurses can therefore examine children's diets particularly for these deficiencies and can make subsequent adjustments. (Nutritional assessment is covered in Chapter 15.)

Dentition

All 20 deciduous or primary teeth normally have erupted by 30 months of age. The cuspids and the bicuspids (first and second molars) are usually the teeth erupting during the second year. The care of primary teeth is important because of their role in the development of good speech habits, their need for proper eating habits, their importance for cosmetic purposes related to body image, and their relation to the health of the permanent teeth (diseased primary teeth can seriously affect the structure of permanent teeth). Brushing of teeth should begin in infancy, and children should increasingly assume partial responsibility for brushing their teeth. Children need supervision by parents because they lack the fine motor skills and persistence to brush their teeth well. Nevertheless, young children should be allowed to initiate and participate in toothbrushing.

One of the crucial variables contributing to dental health is the child's diet. Poor nutritional habits, such as the nursing bottle syndrome, have been linked to dental diseases. Some studies have shown that (1) carbohydrate consumption (mostly sugar) increases tooth decay; (2) the risk of caries is greater if the sugar is in a form that will be retained (for example, caramel or candy); and (3) the risk of caries is related to the frequency of between-meal snacks containing sugar. The total amount of sugar consumed per day is therefore not as important as the form of carbohydrate or the frequency with which it is ingested (Wei, 1981).

Optimal fluoride intake improves dental health. The consumption of fluoridated water is a preventive dentistry regimen; a fluoridated dentifrice is another source of fluoride in the growing child (Wei, 1981). If the water in a community does not meet the minimum standards for fluoridation, a system of fluoride supplementation may be needed.

Suggestions to parents vary about the optimal age for a routine check-up by the dentist. Three-year-olds or certainly 4-year-olds should have the maturity to cooperate with the dental examination and teeth cleaning. Good preparation for the visit can come from role-playing, doll-playing, stories, or a visit to the dentist with an older sibling.

Parents can promote fine dental health by (1) carefully monitoring the diets of their children, particularly with regard to the frequency and quality of carbohydrates; (2) getting information about the fluoridation levels of water in the community; (3) taking their preschoolers for a dental examination; and (4) introducing a self-care regimen of early and frequent toothbrushing.

Exercise

The image of busy children with parents running after them may make structured or organized exercise seem superfluous or humorous. Nevertheless, physical activity is important for muscular development, gross motor skills, and social skills, as well as an outlet for tension. Exercise also benefits the circulatory system.

During early childhood, there is no difference in muscle size between the sexes; however, children show wide differences in muscle tone and the amount of adipose tissue, both directly related to exercise. Obesity may begin to develop in these early years, as lifelong patterns and attitudes toward exercise are being formed.

Children of this age, if given the opportunity and encouragement, love the vigorous exercises of running, jumping, going down slides, or swinging. Older children refine their exercise skills by adding skipping, hopping, tumbling, bicycling, and swimming. Engaging in these exercises helps develop muscle strength, balance, coordination, and social skills (to the extent that the exercise is done with other children). Exercise helps consume the child's seemingly endless energy and is particularly important for very active children. Exercise also serves as a tension outlet for bored, irritable, pent-up children. After vigorous exercise, chldren are emotionally and mentally better able to deal with challenging cognitive tasks, practice fine motor skills, or to engage in solitary play.

Parents need to provide this kind of outlet for their children on a daily basis. For children who seem clumsier or more tentative in the outdoors, parents need to encourage and reinforce this kind of activity. Just bringing children to play areas with other children encourages exercising. Peer pressure is an excellent aid for those children who need to overcome their shyness or reluctance. Wise parents also alternate these vigorous exercise periods with quiet periods. For the 2-year-old, this quiet time may be a nap or solitary play; for the 4-year-old, quiet time may be time spent coloring or looking at a book. Parents need to be alert to the clues in their children's behavior that signal overfatigue. Parents particularly need to help children over transitional periods. Children of this age frequently have difficulty making transitions from one type of activity to the next, from active, boisterous play to quiet play.

Safety

Accidents are the leading cause of death in the early childhood period (Monthly Vital Statistics Reports, August 11, 1983). Early childhood is the time when parents move from total supervision and responsibility for their children's safety to relinquishing some of these controls and allowing their children to assume some responsibility for their own safety. This is an important and necessary milestone.

Motor vehicle deaths account for the greatest number of accidental deaths of children. For children under 3 years of age, these occur primarily when children are passengers. After age 3, they also occur when children are pedestrians. The second largest category of death occurs from fires or burns. Burns may occur from an uncovered heating apparatus, matches, spilled hot liquids, or electrical currents. The third cause of accidental deaths is drownings. Falls and poisoning are both fourth because they occur about equally. Falls, particularly down stairs or from open windows, account for most of this group of accidental deaths, whereas poisonings result from cleaning fluids, medicines, insecticides, and cosmetics that children ingest. Prevention and treatment of accidental poisoning is discussed in Chapter 20.

Most accidents are preventable, unlike malignancies, blood dyscrasias, and other forms of serious diseases, and parents can protect their children's health by creating a safe environment. Parents can promote an awareness of safety in their children through education and the reinforcement of safe behavior. (Nursing inverventions to prevent injuries to children are discussed in Chapter 19.)

Transition to Middle Childhood

The theme of early childhood is the child's progress toward independence, self-care, responsibility, and accountability. Although the 4½-year-old emerging from this stage is by no means an adult, important social, cognitive, cultural, and psychomotor skills have been acquired. At the end of the early childhood period, a distinct personality has been formed, and the 4½-year-old is ready to venture out into the world of school feeling good about it.

Genetic, environmental, and interpersonal factors contribute to the development of each child as a unique person. The early childhood years are a wonderful time of discovery and learning. Nurturance, encouragement, and support by caring adults are necessary ingredients for making this a "magic" period of development.

Key Concepts

- The developmental progress during early childhood involves major changes in the child's biophysical, affective, cognitive, and social subsystems.
- The process of maturation and experiences with objects and obstacles in the environment result in the learning and mastery of many gross motor skills and fine motor skills.
- Early childhood encompasses the developmental phase between early language and locomotion and formal school in kindergarten.
- The suprasystems—especially those of family, culture, and ethnicity—play a major role in the socialization process and relate to the child the expected behaviors, use of language, and relation with adults and peers.
- Gender identity is intimately related with cultural definitions and the imitation of significant role models.
- The child becomes increasingly independent in physical abilities and responsibility for self as expressed in self-care behaviors.
- Early childhood is filled with crises related to development such as toilet training, learning to share, and learning to control impulses in response to parental admonitions.
- The acquisition of self-concept and self-esteem is an important aspect of development; adults who are supportive of children's questions, needs for increased reassurance, and expression of initiative communicate to the child a positive self-concept.
- Early childhood is characterized by incessant questioning as the child learns about the organization and functioning of the environment.
- The ability to use information is limited by the lack of concrete experiences, and the child accepts any answer whether it is logical or not.
- The child fuses fantasy and reality in searching to understand the world, but increasingly distinguishes between them.
- The learning of language and its use to express needs, requests, ideas, or plans develops rapidly and includes all speech parts and the ability to construct complex sentences by the end of early childhood.
- Moral development begins as children learn right from wrong in response to punishment and reward.
- Rituals help children gain some control over events and put their lives in order.
- Developmental theorists characterize early childhood as a time of egocentricity, limited logical thinking, and active and creative imagination (Piaget); a time of developing autonomy and initiative leading to either a positive sense of self or a negative sense of self (Erikson); and a time of gender and role identification with the parent of the same sex following resolution of love for the parent of the opposite sex (Freud).

- Play enhances all types of learning and enhances all aspects of development through the use and practice of motor, mental, and social skills.
- The child engages in various types of play such as solitary, onlooker, parallel, and by the end of early childhood including associative and cooperative.
- These are important years for learning about basic self-care activities and participating in screening programs to detect any potential problems, especially those that are correctable with early intervention.
- The parent's role in protecting and educating the child changes as the child gains independence and spends time away from home.
- Parents must provide a safe environment for dependent, impulsive 2-year-olds, gradually allow 3- and 4-year-olds to participate in self-care decisions and be independent in play, and prepare 5-year-olds to be responsible for following safety guidelines and hygiene practices as taught.

References

Bigner JJ: *Parent-Child Relations.* Macmillan, 1979.

Brazelton TB: A child-oriented approach to toilet training. *Pediatrics* 1962; 29:121–128.

Brink P: An anthropological perspective on parenting. In: *Parenting Reassessed: A Nursing Perspective.* Horowitz J, Hughes C, Perdue B (editors). Prentice-Hall, 1982.

Chess S, Hassibi, M: *Principles and Practice of Child Psychiatry.* Plenum, 1978.

Chomsky N: *Syntactic Structures.* Mouton, 1957.

Chow M, et al: *Handbook of Pediatric Primary Care.* Wiley, 1979.

Coles R: *The Privileged Ones.* Little, Brown, 1977.

Epstein S: The self-concept revisited: Or a theory of a theory. *Am Psychol* 1973; 28:407.

Erikson EH: *Childhood and Society.* Norton, 1973.

Fowler J, Keen S: *Life Maps: Conversations in the Journey of Faith.* Word Books, 1978.

Freud S: An outline of psychoanalysis. In: *The Complete Psychoanalytic Works of Sigmund Freud.* Norton, 1969.

Gewirtz JL, Stingle KG: Learning of generalized imitation as the basis for identification. In: *Readings in Child Behavior and Development.* Lavatelli CS, Stendler F (editors). Harcourt Brace Jovanovich, 1972.

Havighurst RJ: *Developmental Tasks and Education.* McKay, 1972.

Horowitz JA: *The Relationship of Father Absence/Presence and Daughter's Perception of Mother's Gender-Related Traits to the Daughter's Views of her own Gender Related Traits and Women's Roles.* (Doctoral Dissertation.) New York University, 1981.

Hussey C, Kanoff N: Toddler and preschool nutrition. In: *Maternal and Child Nutrition Assessment and Counseling.* Slatterly J, Pearson G, Torre C (editors). Appleton-Century-Crofts, 1979.

Illingsworth RS: Sleep problems of children. *Clin Pediatr* 1966; 5:45–58.

Kagan J: The psychological requirements for human development. In: *Raising Children in Modern America.* Talbot N (editor). Little, Brown, 1974.

Keniston K and the Carnegie Council on Children: *All Our Children: The American Family Under Pressure.* Harcourt Brace Jovanovich and the Carnegie Corporation, 1977.

Kephart WM: *The Family, Society and the Individual.* Houghton-Mifflin, 1961.

Kohlberg L: Stage and Sequence: The cognitive-development approach to socialization. In: *Handbook of Socialization: Theory and Research.* Goslin D (editor). Rand McNally, 1969.

Labov W, et al: A study of non-standard English of Negro and Puerto Rican speakers. In: *Cooperative Research Reports.* Vol 1. US Regional Survey, 1971.

Lavatelli CS, Stendler F (editors): *Readings in Child Behavior and Development.* Harcourt Brace Jovanovich, 1972.

Lindsay PH, Norman DA: *Human Information Processing: An Introduction to Psychology.* Academic Press, 1977.

Mahler MS, Pine F, Bergman A: *The Psychological Birth of the Human Infant: Symbiosis and Individuation.* Basic Books, 1975.

Mussen PH, Conger JJ, Kagan J: *Child Development and Personality.* Harper & Row, 1979.

Nagera H: The imaginary companion. *The Psychoanalytic Study of the Child* 1969; 24:165–196.

Nelms BC, Mullins RG: *Growth and Development—A Primary Health Care Approach.* Prentice-Hall, 1982

Parten MB, Newhall S: Social behavior of preschool children. In: *Child Behavior and Development.* Baker BG (editor). McGraw-Hill, 1943.

Pelton LH (editor): *The Social Context of Child Abuse and Neglect.* Human Sciences Press, 1981.

Piaget J: *The Origins of Intelligence.* International Universities Press, 1952.

Piaget J, Inhelder B: *The Psychology of the Child.* Basic Books, 1969.

Piaget J: Development and learning. In: *Readings in Child Behavior and Development.* Lavatelli CS, Stendler F (editors). Harcourt Brace Jovanovich, 1972.

Piers MW (editor): *Play and Development.* Norton, 1972

Pipes PL: *Nutrition in Infancy and Childhood.* Mosby, 1981.

Powell ML: *Assessment and Management of Developmental Changes in Children.* Mosby, 1981.

Read DA: *The Concept of Health.* Holbrook Press, 1973.

Rubin LB: *Worlds of Pain.* Basic Books, 1976.

Schuster CS, Ashburn SS: *The Process of Human Development.* Little, Brown, 1980.

Slobin DL: Seven questions about language development. In: *New Horizons in Psychology.* No 2. Dodwell PC (editor). Penguin Books, 1972.

Slobin DL, Welsh CA: Elicited imitation as a research tool in developmental psycholinguistics. In: *Language Training in Early Childhood Education.* Lavatelli CS (editor). University of Illinois Press, 1971.

Stone GP: Appearance and the early emergence of the self. In: *Readings in Social Psychology.* Lindesmith AR, Strauss AL, Denzin NK (editors). Dryden Press, 1962.

Stone LJ, Church J: *Childhood and Adolescence: A Psychology of the Growing Person.* Random House, 1975.

Sullivan HS: *Conceptions of Modern Psychiatry.* Norton, 1953

US Department of Health and Human Services: *Monthly Vital Statustics Reports,* August 11, 1983.

Wei S: Nutrition, diet, fluoride and dental health. *Pediatr Basics* 1981; 30:5

White B: *The First Three Years of Life.* Prentice-Hall, 1975.

Additional Readings

Bandura A: The role of modeling processes in personality development. In: *Readings in Child Behavior and Development.* Lavatelli CS, Stendler F (editors). Harcourt Brace Jovanovich, 1972.

Brill E, Kilts D: *Foundations for Nursing.* Appleton-Century-Crofts, 1980.

Caplan F (editor): *The First Twelve Months of Life.* Grosset & Dunlap, 1973.

Chance P: *Learning Through Play.* Gardner Press, 1979.

Chomsky C: Language development before age six. In: *Readings in Child Behavior and Development.* Lavatelli CS, Stendler F (editors). Harcourt Brace Jovanovich, 1972.

Duvall EM: *Marriage and Family Development.* Lippincott, 1980.

Heilbrun AB: Sex-role identity in adolescent females: A theoretical paradox. *Adolescence* 1968; 3:80.

Horner M, McClellan M: Toilet training: Ready or not? *Pediatr Nurs* 1981; 7:12–18.

Hughes CB: *Stressors, Roles, Strain, and Coping Mechanisms in the Continuously Employed Nurse-Mother.* (Doctoral Dissertation.) Columbia University, 1980.

Lenneberg EH: *Biological Foundations of Language.* Wiley, 1967

Kohlberg L: The development of children's orientations toward a moral order: Sequence in development of moral thought. *Vita Humana* 1963; 6:311–333.

Kohlberg L: Development of moral character and moral ideology. In: *Review of Child Development Research.* Vol 1. Hoffman ML, Hoffman LW (editors). Russell Sage Foundation, 1964.

Lichtenberg P, Norton DG: *Cognitive and Mental Development in the First Five Years of Life.* National Institute of Mental Health, 1970.

Lidz T: *The Person: His Development Throughout the Life Cycle.* Basic Books, 1968.

Liss M: *Sex Roles and Children's Play.* Academic Press, 1983.

Mahler MS, Gosliner J: On symbiotic child psychosis: Genetic, dynamic and restrictive aspects. In: *The Psychoanayltic Study of the Child.* Vol X. International Universities Press, 1955.

Mitchell S: Imaginary companions—friend or foe? *Pediatr Nurs* 1980; 6:30.

Piaget J: *The Grasp of Consciousness: Action and Concept in the Young Child.* Harvard University Press, 1976.

Middle Childhood

Bobbie Jean Perdue   Cynthia E. Degazon   Sandra R. Mott

9

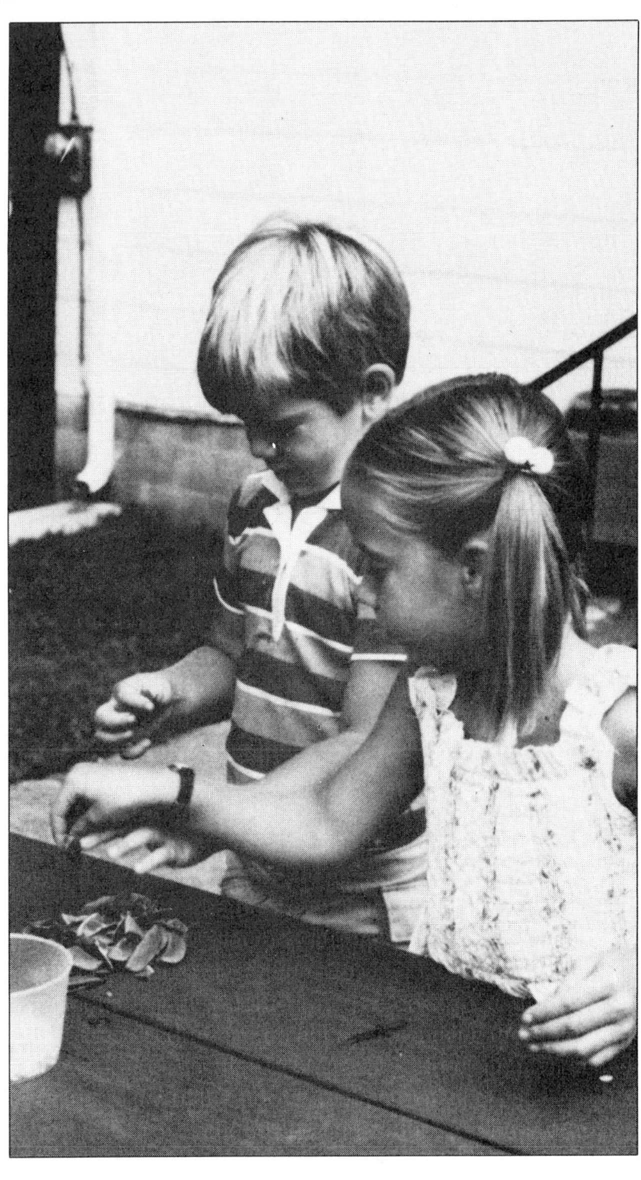

Chapter Outline

Objectives

- Explain the influences of both suprasystems and subsystems on middle childhood development.
- Define the major parameters of middle childhood development.
- Explain the essential biophysical changes that occur in middle childhood.
- Describe the principal theoretic explanations for personality, cognitive, language, moral, and social developments in middle childhood.
- Explain the purpose of play in middle childhood.
- Identify the basic health care needs of children in middle childhood.

The literature and statistics on middle childhood do not agree on a uniform age span for the period. Most child developmental specialists define middle childhood as the early school-age stage, before the child enters the later school grades or adolescence. Given the major changes in cognitive skills and the effects of these changes on school and peer group activities for most American children, we have elected to use 4½–8 years as the age range for middle childhood. The physical and cognitive changes that occur between these ages seems to account for the corresponding new social roles adopted during middle childhood (Kenny, 1983).

Middle childhood is a time of transition during which the child is away from the protection of the home or nursery school for a greater portion of each day. The child entering school is challenged to learn new skills and adapt to new environments. Relationships with authority figures change as the child is expected to conform to the expectations of teachers and school rules. In the school environment the child is exposed to new peer groups and learns increasingly to identify with representatives of suprasystems outside the family.

In this chapter we analyze the changing and expanding nature of the suprasystems influencing the child's socialization and the many biophysical, cognitive, affective, and social subsystem changes that affect development in this stage. We define the conflicts, tasks, and norms associated with the developmental parameters of middle childhood, and we identify the basic health care needs common to children in this age range.

Developmental Changes in Middle Childhood

The transition from early to middle childhood is a more drastic change than many people realize. Children enter middle childhood with many skills and therefore feel that when they command, the world will obey. During this period, they will continue to acquire significant abilities in language, thought, feeling, symbolism, moral consciousness, independence, and self-awareness.

Growing self-awareness, however, allows children at this age to see more clearly the challenges confronting them, challenges that test the child's sense of omnipotence. At least one theorist (Havighurst, 1953) considered these changes equal in significance to those encountered in puberty. Among these challenges are (1) the search for independence; (2) the need to become part of a group; and (3) the need to succeed in school. Children may be particularly uncertain about the problems of socialization, while they more easily realize that physical and cognitive skills are acquired through maturation and practice and are therefore more subject to their will. The structures that children enter at this time force them to include peers and teachers in their social system and therefore to confront their limitations in social skills.

To meet these challenges, children become resourceful in using their energies and their developing assets to complete the tasks they set for themselves. Many other factors influence the successful completion of these tasks, in addition to the child's intrinsic strengths. Family characteristics, socioeconomic conditions, ethnic and cultural heritage, and the values shared by family, school, and community all play a vital role in the child's ability to master the immediate environment.

Influences of the Suprasystems

In contrast to early childhood, middle childhood socialization is characterized by greater contact with adults and children who reside outside the home (Fig. 9-1). During middle childhood, children become part of new suprasystems, expanding their networks to include new social relationships. A child's interaction with adults and children in each of the new environments forms the basis for the development of an emerging self-concept and internalizing of standards in areas of competence.

Family The socializing functions of the family continue to be important during middle childhood but also might change in relation to the child's total socialization experience. The child spends increasingly larger blocks of time away from home where additional attitudes, knowledge, and skills necessary for societal participation are gained.

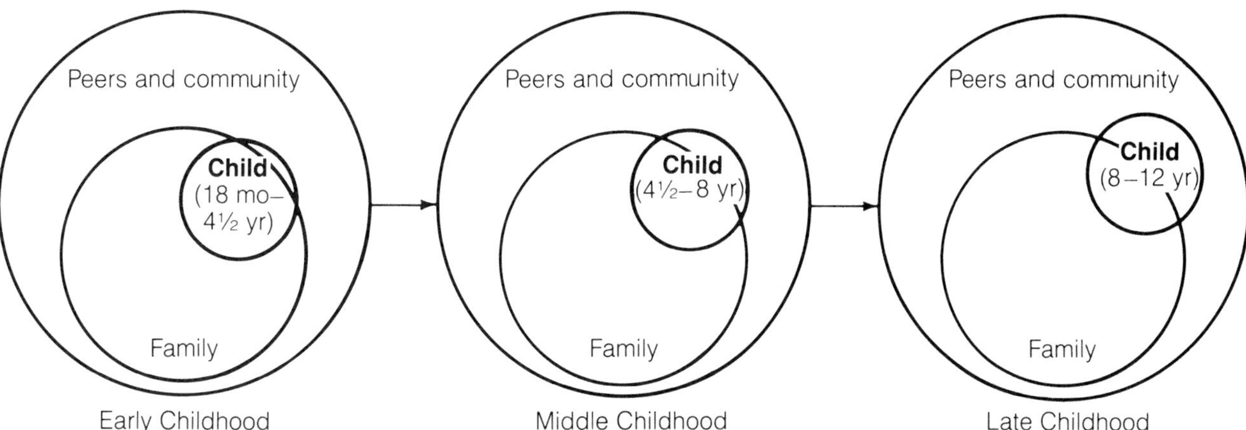

Figure 9-1 With age and maturity the child gradually progresses through the boundary of the family to immediate interaction with the environment.

Although the socializing responsibility now is shared, the family's contribution still is critical in such areas as the development of the child's self-concept, self-esteem, sex-role identification, interpersonal skills, social role as a family member, and social norms—particularly as they are interpreted by the family.

During middle childhood, the family's support is invaluable as the child embarks on new experiences. The family provides stability and security in a world where everything else seems to be changing. Within the family context, the child feels free to express the tensions, fears, and anger that would be unacceptable in front of peers or teachers. One 5-year-old, for example, eagerly left for kindergarten every morning accompanied by her sibling and friends. When she returned home at noon, however, she needed some special "love time," when she would sit on her parent's lap and recount the morning's experiences.

Children who feel secure with their family know that someone who understands them will be there to help them in times of difficulty. Knowing this enables them to cope with new experiences, problems, or demands when away from home. Once they return to the secure confines of their home and family, however, they become free to express their feelings of anger, disappointment, or self-doubt. They no longer have to work at meeting someone else's expectations but rather know that they can reveal their true emotions and still be loved and accepted. Parents sometimes need to be reassured that this "Dr. Jekyll and Mr. Hyde" phase of personality development is a characteristic expression of the struggle during middle childhood to integrate new ideas, facts, behaviors, and attitudes with those previously known and accepted. Thus, the child begins a process of self-evaluation and self-acceptance in a world now comprised of a multiplicity of rules and values.

Children in this age group tend to hold the family in high regard. When children are exposed to alternative ways of doing things or different attitudes, they reduce their tension by reaffirming to others that "My mom or dad said to do it this way." Parents are idealized, and their manner of performing their roles is accepted as the best way. This loyalty may range from basic skills, such as how to throw or catch a ball, to life-style decisions. For example, one young girl commented that when she grew up she was going to go to the office just like her mommy. When asked why, she quickly replied that otherwise she would have to stay home and she wants to be like her mommy because only a smart mommy can take care of both an office and children. She added that she had "the best mommy in the world." In this way children begin to internalize the social values presented by their parents.

Parents who have given their children freedom within consistent guidelines and explained the rules and limits imposed on behavior and the rationales for their expectations and values have prepared their children for new experiences and the judgments of others. Siblings who may have difficulty getting along with each other at home help and defend one another in unfamiliar or troublesome situations because of family love and loyalty. These children know how their parents expect them to behave when they are at school, a friend's house, or a community activity. Commonly, however, these children misbehave and become demanding or whiny when they return home to relieve the tension generated by consciously performing within parental guidelines. Explaining this tendency to parents helps them to understand why their children behave the way they do and the importance of the family. The angel at school who becomes a hellion at home does so because of the trust and security already established within the family. The child also anticipates that the family will limit "out-of-bounds" behavior and help sort out and put into perspective confusing ideas and feelings. In this way the family contributes to the child's growing sense of reality and the internalization of values.

In his research on self-esteem, Coopersmith (1967) noted a correlation between certain family experiences and the development of high self-esteem during middle childhood.

He concluded that the consistent enforcement of a rather expansive set of rules contributed to the child's sense of reality and self-confidence in decision making. Parents who were comfortable in their parental role, confident of their abilities, and self-reliant conveyed to their children the importance and benefits of showing respect to others. These parents also were sensitive to their children's needs and abilities and had close, loving relationships with them. The children realized that they were important as individuals because their parents took the time to share in joint activities such as a card game, school project, or family outing.

Children who received positive feedback from significant adults also developed high self-esteem. Parents who had definite values and standards of behavior and who took the time to communicate them to their offspring tended to have children capable of making good judgments and feeling good about themselves. The parental role in this area should not be underestimated. It demands considerable time and effort because parents must have confidence in presenting and enforcing their beliefs, as well as set examples or act as role models. Although children in this age group are increasingly influenced by others, they still look to their parents for guidance.

Parenting styles do make a difference, as was shown in the Fels study done by Kagan and Moss (1962). Parents who were restrictive and authoritarian required strict adherence to rules but took little time to explain each rule and its importance or to discover their child's unique needs and abilities. Their children tended to be passive, shy, socially inept, immature, and dependent. Parents who were more permissive or authoritative, that is, democratic, provided opportunities for children to make choices. These parents generally discussed rules and agreed with their children about rules before enforcing them. Their children tended to be more creative, autonomous, socially adept, and self-directed. (See Chapter 13 for a more complete discussion of parenting styles.)

Although parents have a very significant influence on the developing child because of their power and authority, the relationship is reciprocal. The child's personality contributes equally to parent–child relations. The feedback loops of behavior output and individual responses are complex and different for each family. Although some general statements can be made, it is impossible to predict how parental characteristics and practices will affect the individual child (see Chapter 13).

Siblings Siblings also exert some influence on the child's behavior. During middle childhood, the number of siblings present and the number of years between their ages are important components of the home setting in which the child is socialized. The social learning environment is different for the firstborn child, the middle child, and the last child born. The most obvious difference is the number of members and the variety of personalities and ages comprising the family unit.

Researchers have made some generalizations concerning parental interactions with children of different birth order. Parents tend to be more involved, participate in more play activities, and have higher expectations for their firstborn child (Sutton-Smith and Rosenberg, 1970; Dunn and Kendrick, 1982). Parents appear to be more casual and less demanding of their successive children. Later-born children also have the advantage of older siblings with whom to identify. This identification sometimes takes the form of competition, as when each strives to excel in the same activity and to receive parental recognition for being the best.

In the process of trying to perform better than each other, they earn one another's respect. Older siblings are motivated to set high standards especially in their areas of strength, thereby hoping not to be surpassed. Intending to be as good or even better, younger siblings accept the challenge, respect the older ones' accomplishments, and follow their examples for success. Older siblings in turn respect the efforts of the younger ones. For example, one boy, who was the oldest in his family, commented that he sometimes thought his younger brother was special because he could do so many things better than other children his age. This younger brother meanwhile expressed pride in the recognition his older brother received and determined to be his equal.

For other children, this process of identification often results in the purposeful development of different characteristics and behaviors. The younger child strives to develop a unique identity. In one family of three children, for example, the youngest child was described as different from and yet in some respects an interesting combination of the two older children. By meshing personal characteristics with a few highly rewarded traits from each sibling, the youngest child benefited from the experiences of the older siblings while claiming a special spot within the family unit. During this developmental phase, children become more aware and selective of how they present themselves to others. Much learning occurs informally by observing and imitating those behaviors of others that are rewarded and repeating other behaviors discovered by chance to have positive results. For example, 6-year-old Carolyn quickly realized that it was to her advantage not to retaliate when her older brother teased her. When she ignored him, he stopped because it was not as much fun as when she reacted by screaming at him. This response helped her to cope at school when children teased her. When she remained calm, it became more obvious to the teacher which child had initiated the interaction. The child doing the teasing was then reprimanded, and Carolyn was praised. In addition, she became popular by befriending children who did not know how to respond to teasing.

Culture, Ethnicity, and Values As children branch out from the home, they become more aware of the significance of their heritage. The process of learning social norms and roles continues, but now other individuals share in their transmission. The goal of socialization is to maintain a patterned response by learning to live within a group, perpetuate a group's history, and promote its mastery over the environment.

By middle childhood, cultural rituals, values, beliefs, language, and customs begin to have a greater impact than biologic maturation on the child's growth and development. The input from these suprasystems accounts for the attitudes, behaviors, skills, and relationships that are unique to each culture.

One of the cultural characteristics of western civilizations in general and the United States in particular is competition. The overarching, unspoken motivating factor is to learn a skill as quickly and completely as possible because those who are best are rewarded. This achievement orientation contrasts with the more cooperative orientation of nonindustrialized countries. In an extensive study of 104 societies, Barry and colleagues (1959) observed that obedience and responsibility were more highly valued in nonindustrialized societies, whereas achievement was more highly valued in industrialized societies. Other cross-cultural comparisons (Kagan and Madsen, 1972; Holtzman, et al., 1975) have resulted in similar conclusions. These findings have led some anthropologists and developmental theorists to question whether the strong, early emphasis placed on competition and achievement supports optimal mental health during middle childhood.

In school this phenomenon is manifested by the awarding of stickers, spending time at special-interest tables, or having extra quiet-reading time. The child quickly concludes and the teacher confirms that those who are most skilled and the first to finish assigned work are rewarded. The child works for the reward rather than for the joy of learning. Such a child, for example, might read books at home only when the school holds a reading contest because reading is perceived as a worthwhile activity only if rewarded by teacher and peers rather than as a stimulating activity in itself.

Athletic contests are another area in which competitiveness is emphasized. The child learns that there are personal goals and group goals; however, if personal goals are overemphasized, the value of cooperation to attain group goals quickly becomes muted. For example, one elementary school physical education teacher decided to have a track meet consisting only of relay races. In this way groups of four to six children cooperated, and winning became a group rather than an individual effort.

In many cultures middle childhood is the time when children are given increased responsibilities. In rural areas these tasks might include feeding the chickens and doing farm-related chores, either alone or with a parent. Rural children also might be expected to care for younger siblings, pick food from the garden, gather firewood, or tend to the care and security of the animals. Thus, they begin to practice their future roles by learning skills and participating in various aspects of the adult world. In the Niger Republic, for example, 7-year-old boys join the camel herdsmen and learn the geography of the country, the traits of the animals, and the tasks of being a herdsman. In urban cultures the child's chores might consist of taking out the trash, sweeping the stairs and sidewalk, filling the birdfeeders, walking the dog, or setting and clearing the table for supper. Participation in family tasks increases the child's sense of responsibility for each family member's well-being. As one 8-year-old girl explained to her younger sister, "If we help clean up after supper, Mommy and Daddy will have time to play a game with us. If we run off and play, they won't have as much time to spend with us." Experience had taught this child that when family members helped each other, everyone benefited.

Religion Several faiths include children in middle childhood in certain of their rituals, reflecting the increased ability of the child at this age to deal with concepts such as religious faith and morality. In many Protestant denominations this is the time when children receive their own Bible and participate in communion. The Catholic church believes that 7-year-olds can tell right from wrong and therefore should begin to participate in confession and take their first communion. Children thereafter are expected to attend church and participate in religious activities with the adults.

Television Television has become an integral part of the American culture and, as such, influences the child's growth and development. When used appropriately, television can enrich the child's world, introducing new ideas and concepts. However, television also can have a negative impact on the child's development. Children in this age group have difficulty distinguishing reality from fiction, and thus the violence seen on television has its greatest negative effect on them. Children tend to internalize and act out what they see on television. Although research findings are inconclusive as to the long-term effects on children of viewing aggressive behavior (Watson and Lindgren, 1979), parents should monitor the television shows their children select to ensure that development will be enriched and not inhibited.

Another detrimental aspect of television is the behavior it prevents. Bronfenbrenner (1972) noted that television is one of a host of factors that conspire to isolate children from parents, peers, and society in general. When the television is turned on, family discussions, questions and answers about the day's events, games, festivities, and even arguments lose their significance. The opportunity and incentive for meaningful human contact is replaced by this technologic invention that casts its spell on whomever is willing to be enchanted. Children need to have contact and interaction with others to participate in the process of character building, to learn firsthand from others about values and the give and take of relationships, and to use the power of imagination in creative play experiences. Even when television is watched with another person, it too often is a passive, lonely experience. There is a very real danger that during the impressionable phase of middle childhood, children receive more input from the mass media than from interpersonal communication (Kittrell, 1978).

Unfortunately, too many television programs still portray stereotypic roles related to race, sex, age, and religion. Young, white men more often are cast as dominant, competent, and powerful, whereas women, the elderly, and minority-group members are given subsidiary roles. Television also paints an unrealistic picture of life in that problems are easily and quickly solved, what is good and right prevails, violence is permissible when used by police, and pain or suffering is short-lived.

To help offset these obvious disadvantages, television has some positive aspects. Through television, children can be exposed to a variety of places, events, and viewpoints not available otherwise. At its best, television provides facts and scenes about wildlife, people, customs, and the landscape of other countries, information about how the human body functions, how food is grown and processed, or how clothing is manufactured. Some programs socialize as well as entertain. They focus on prosocial behaviors and deal with attitudes, including fairness, equality, unselfishness, and honesty. Sensitive but relevant topics, such as divorce or death, sometimes are highlighted.

Television is a powerful socializing force on children, and the child's social attitudes and behavior are affected by it. Whether the influence is more positive than negative or vice versa remains a question for social scientists (Comstock, 1978). Television, however, does provide models that children emulate and material that influences their values, beliefs, expectations, and actions.

Social Class Middle childhood, with the beginning of formal education, organized clubs, such as Brownies or Cub Scouts, and greater exposure to world and regional events, often is the first time that children become aware of the various life-styles and living conditions of individuals with different backgrounds. Social class is a process "by which different social relations to the means of production are inherited and reproduced under capitalism" (Rapp, 1982: p. 171). As such, there are numerous inequities relating to educational and occupational opportunities, access to power, levels of community influence, and economic resources. Children become aware of these differences as they compare their clothes, toys, houses, or vacations with those of their more or less affluent peers.

Social class distinctions influence the child's behavior and self-concept. During middle childhood, children are introduced to the meaning of social class in general and their own social class in particular. Through personal contact, television, books, or school, they learn that other children may have a very different standard of living from their own.

Children of different social classes generally are raised differently. For wealthy children, the emphasis is on learning the skills needed for their future roles as wealthy adults. This training commonly is stereotyped by sex, probably because the parents' roles typically are defined on the basis of sex. A boy generally follows his father's lead in learning about finances and business, whereas a girl emulates her mother, learning to manage household matters, fulfill social obligations, and engaging in charitable activities.

During middle childhood, wealthy children begin to appreciate the connection between their parents' life-style; frequent absences from the home for business, charitable, or social reasons; and the meaning of activities that connote power and prestige in the community and in the nation. Wealthy parents might be too busy to spend much time with their children or to invest a great deal emotionally in their children. They can, however, offer some compensation in the form of material advantages, including the best education, opportunities for travel, and the lessons or equipment for any interest.

Affluent children learn that to be wealthy is an ambiguous collection of responsibilities, power, comfort, fulfilled dreams, and fears. The children sense that in some vague way they also are accountable for their family's status. For some this means accepting the care and discipline given by a strict nanny so that the family will continue to have a good reputation. For others it may mean tolerating loneliness while being surrounded by things but not by friends with whom to share them. For some affluent children much time is spent with adults in organized activities selected by their parents. Parental fears may also be transferred to the children. Parents may fear losing valuable collections to thieves or large sums of money because of an incorrectly calculated business transaction. Children then learn that fears of loss are a normal part of life.

At the opposite extreme are the millions of children growing up in poverty. Their lives contrast starkly with those of the very rich. Poor children have few choices, become keenly aware that they are powerless, are often labeled as different or intellectually limited, and have to learn early how to survive in a hostile world. Poor children generally are taught to be obedient, respectful, and conform to authority. Their parents tend to be fatalistic, feeling that others control their lives and that only luck or good fortune can change their situation. As a result, the children may have a poor self-image and feel that achieving success or recognition in the same areas as do their contemporaries from the other income groups is impossible. For example, a child may have a low self-esteem in English class compared with the more verbal and expressive middle-class peers but compensate for this with feelings of high self-esteem during music class because of an excellent singing voice.

Many poor children enter school at a distinct disadvantage as they have had limited exposure to books, magazines, or art supplies. They soon realize that other children easily accomplish tasks that they must struggle to learn. Their enthusiasm for learning wanes as they become easily discouraged with hard work and sparse rewards. Instead they invest energy in other tasks for which they receive more immediate recognition and consequently view as more valuable.

Children internalize their parents' and peers' values. Lower-class parents are more likely to feel pressured and discouraged from trying to provide for the family with insufficient income, crowded housing, inadequate laundry facilities, total child-care responsibility, and the constant worry about having enough food and clothing for everyone. Their limited resources with which to cope with these concerns compounds the problem and reduces their tolerance for anything that might mean more work. In her extensive, comparative study, Feshbach (1973) noted that lower-class parents talked less to their children, were less tolerant of misbehavior, more critical of mistakes, and used negative reinforcement more frequently than did middle-class parents. The lower-class children, consequently, were not encouraged to explore, ask questions, or experiment—activities that foster learning; rather, they were encouraged to conform to parental directives.

Believing the future to be too unpredictable, lower-class parents tend to focus more on the present. The immediate gratification of needs or wants, although difficult to achieve, is strongly desired. Poverty has more than its share of anxieties, illnesses, and frustrations, and there is little incentive to save money. The child learns that any money saved might have to be spent on basic necessities of food or clothing and never get to be used for the desired treat. The child usually spends the dime found on the sidewalk for some "penny" candy rather than save the dime until there is enough money to buy the preferred ice cream sundae.

Most children belong to the middle class. This diverse class includes children whose parents are professionals and those whose parents are clerks at a local store. It is this group that is depicted on television and to which industry addresses its production and advertising its sales pitches. Although the spectrum of financial resources is broad in this class, the goals middle-class parents have for their children are similar. Education generally is valued highly as a means of getting ahead in life. Middle-class children usually are prepared for school, having had stories read to them at home, educational games played with them, and toys that fostered learning as well as enjoyment.

These children are generally in good health, as it too is a value. Parents provide plenty of nutritious food for meals and snacks. Appropriate amounts of rest and activity are emphasized, and parents monitor bedtime and ensure a quiet environment for sleep. Homes often are spacious, and many children have their own rooms. They also are taught to value and respect their own belongings, space, and the rights of others to their own property and privacy. Parents model behaviors that include achievement-oriented goals and planning for the future. Middle-class children are also encouraged to start saving their money at an early age.

Middle-class children move from home and family into school and neighborhood groups that have similar values, standards, and expectations. They are encouraged and rewarded for competition, the ability to delay gratification, curiosity, eagerness to learn, hard work, and respect for authority. The subtle message conveyed to most middle-class children is that achievement and success are the result of honest work, consistent effort, and cooperation. It is important to spend money wisely, which includes saving for the future as well as purchasing the goods and services that serve to identify the so-called "good life." Children eventually are granted many of their requests for toys and entertainment because material possessions and being entertained are means of communicating success.

The differences among social classes exist more in economics than in personalities. It is important not to stereotype children and families according to their socioeconomic class because as many similarities exist across classes as differences exist within a class. The nurse therefore assesses each child and family according to their own strengths and weaknesses.

Socioeconomic class is only one of many suprasystems that influences the development of a child. Value orientation, self-esteem, and self-concept are acquired in a variety of ways and from many resources. The nurse therefore determines how each resource operates in the child's and family's life. Nurses frequently discover that different values and life-styles are not automatically better or worse than those of the majority; rather, it is how these values and life-styles contribute to personal and family growth that is important. (Family assessment is discussed in greater detail in Chapter 17.)

The suprasystem that comprises culture is a broad, indirect source of information. Prior to middle childhood, the family is the primary interpreter and representative of cultural traditions. As children begin to interact with other social organizations and institutions, such as school, clubs, and community groups, they are exposed to the greater collection of beliefs, values, norms, rituals, rules, and expectations that influence behaviors, attitudes, and opportunities. Middle childhood opens the door to new learning experiences.

School Despite the continuing importance of the family environment, many socialization functions are transferred from home to the playground and classroom. For the first time since the child's birth, parents may find that they are competing with teachers and other children for their children's attention. In these suprasystems of education and community, the child finds new models to imitate, thus increasing the opportunities to acquire new cognitive, social, physical, and affective skills.

The function of education is twofold: to perpetuate the culture and to stimulate thinking, learning, and creativity. The beginning of formal schooling is a rite of passage for children in modern industrialized countries. It also coincides with the phase in cognitive development in which children begin to think more logically. Formal schooling provides the child with a landmark in the growing-up process. Interests and energy become shared among family, school, and peers. The educational community now actively participates in the transfer of information and skills such as reading, writing, problem solving, and interpersonal relations. To the extent that the family and school agree on the role and value of education, there is congruence in the purposes and goals formulated for the child, which in turn fosters the child's adaptation to the new environment.

Schools vary in intent, size, and character. A 5-year-old might first learn socialization skills in a neighborhood school center, a federally funded or private day-care or preschool program, an elaborate child development laboratory, or a church school. Kindergarten and preschool programs facilitate the transition from family life and relatively unstructured activities to the more organized, cooperative, and structured needs of group learning. Introducing children to learning, following directions, and working alone or in a group are all functions of early school experiences. Social skill acquisition is as important a goal as the development of cognitive skills. Educators have found that children need to develop independence, social competence, and a sense of self before they can begin to accumulate and use basic facts and communication skills (Edwards, 1968). One kindergarten teacher encouraged the children's development of self by creatively using the music of *Marlo Thomas and Friends* from the album "Free to Be You and Me" (Arista Records). These children learned to value their rights and abilities as unique individuals who were free not to conform to sex-role stereotypic behaviors but to pursue their own interests and develop their own talents.

Teachers, like parents, are powerful people, and the kind of teachers that children have greatly influences whether the school experience will be a source of reward, happiness, and encouragement or a source of failure, frustration, and shame. Success in school fosters feelings of self-pride and contributes to a sense of industry. Positive feelings about school are enhanced by warm, encouraging teachers who instill confidence in children, involve them in classroom activities, and are constructive in criticizing behavior.

Children often view their first teachers as a substitute parent. Baumrind (1972) noted that the three different parenting styles regarding discipline that were identified in parents (see Chapter 13) were found also in teacher–student relations. She argued that the authoritative teaching style best fostered learning because it encouraged individual initiative, social responsibility, and self-esteem. This teaching style directs the children's learning while encouraging verbal give and take, curiosity, and cognitive exploration. Studies have found that children seem to benefit from teachers who are sensitive, supportive, and encouraging. Children from such classes tend to be more resourceful when confronted by possible failure and more involved in classroom activities (Schiamberg and Smith, 1982).

Speculation about the relationship between teacher's expectations and children's performance in school suggests that teachers are highly influential in children's achievements. Although the "Pygmalion hypothesis" has not always been supported when tested under rigorous conditions, teachers clearly do, as in the myth of Pygmalion, play a creative role in shaping children's expectations and self-concepts. For example, teachers have been found to spend more time with children they feel to be high achievers than they do with low achievers (Brophy and Good, 1970). They encourage high achievers to interact more and to accept greater responsibility for their actions, and they tend to give extra work and extra rewards to high achievers (Rosenthal, 1973).

The transition from home to school is a significant milestone in the young child's life. It involves learning new skills considered basic to life, namely, reading and writing. It also entails becoming familiar with a new environment, schedule of activities, peers, and authority figures. How successful the child is in making these initial adjustments influences future school-related experiences. Children's attitudes toward school and toward adult authority figures in general are correlated with their level of school achievement and their teachers' expectations.

Peer Groups It is in the peer group that children learn to interact with age-mates and participate in both competitive activities and cooperative projects. In a peer group the 4½- to 8-year-old child's friends are playmates. This group tends to be informal and transient, consisting of small groups of children who usually are of the same sex. The peer group provides a supportive environment for the child's move from family to school and community. Initially, the peer group consists of those children who are in close physical proximity to each other. Children play together because they live near each other, attend the same school, participate in the same religious education class, or are in the same swimming, ballet, or gymnastics class. Later, these children become more selective and seek friends with common interests and abilities.

The peer relationship is dynamic and necessitates mutual give and take. Friendships are earned; they are not acquired automatically. Children quickly learn that peers have more options and different opinions about how a game is played, a skill performed, or a task completed than do siblings. Children who insist on doing everything their way soon find themselves left out of games and activities. They learn that they must adapt, share ideas, and then follow mutually agreed on rules if they want to be included. Sometimes these games are traditional, such as tag, hide-and-seek, or hopscotch, whereas at other times, they imitate television programs or aspects of family life. At still other times, they are pure fantasy, with roles and action created by active imaginations. Whatever the game, cooperation and adherence to the ground rules are essential. Otherwise, the game disintegrates and arguments and hurt feelings result.

For example, while investigating the rising crescendo of an argument, one parent discovered that five girls who wanted to play "neighbors" could not agree on the location of their houses. It seemed that one girl was threatening the harmony of the group by insisting on locating her house in someone else's "pretend" driveway. This violated their rule that the houses had to be far apart so that no one could spy on another's "dress up" plans. Sometimes such disagreements can be resolved if the other children allow an exception or reach a compromise. Often, the children go their separate ways, complaining that a friend does not play fairly, always has to be the boss, or is selfish and spoiled. During middle childhood, children tend to be very expressive and fairly uninhibited when justifying their behavior with their friends.

During this developmental phase, the child adapts to the contrast between adult–child relations and peer relations. The warm, nourishing, and intimate relationship experienced with adults is not present with peers. With adults the child assumes a more dependent role, whereas with peers it is important for the child to be independent. Peer relations are characterized as being sociable, aggressive, experimental, and somewhat calculated. The child has to concentrate on enacting prosocial behaviors with peers; adults encourage and support these actions (Santrock, 1983). Children meet each other as equals, their physical, cognitive, and psychosocial development at a similar level. Hence, they understand each other from a different perspective than does the adult. During middle childhood, it is more important to maintain face or status with peers than with adults. For example, at home, Leah, 5 years old, cried whenever there was a thunderstorm, was afraid of animals, and refused to go to sleep without a night-light. These fears temporarily disappeared when she slept overnight during a rainstorm with her best friend, Karen, who had a dog and no night-light. She later told her mother that she was not afraid because Karen was not afraid but that she still did not like storms. She continued to express these fears at home, where it was safe to do so.

In group play children learn how to accommodate their plans and desires with those of others. Peers also help organize and refine the child's self-concept. Negative feedback from an adult who views the child's rock and bottle cap collections as "silly" might be offset by positive recognition from peers, as certain behaviors or skills are evaluated differently by peers than by adults. For example, a child's sense of humor or antics might not be appreciated by serious-minded adults, but peers might applaud such behavior and view the child as a leader. By providing positive feedback in this way, peers help a child to bolster a faltering self-concept and to categorize certain behaviors as appropriate for adults and other behaviors as appropriate for peers.

Peers also help each other to become less egocentric and to think about situations from another person's perspective. Social interaction with age-mates is necessary for the development of this skill. Isolated children who have minimal peer contact are limited in their ability to understand other viewpoints (Fischer and Lazerson, 1984). Another social skill that the middle childhood peer group begins to foster is conformity to social norms and expectations. In this respect the peer group is a powerful agent for cultural continuity. It is within the context of the peer group that children learn what to expect from each other and subsequently how to maintain harmony in a variety of situations.

Sex-Role Identification During middle childhood, the child's awareness and understanding of culturally defined roles for males and females increases. Through peer group associations and play, children learn what behaviors and responses are expected of them by others because of prevailing sex-role stereotypes. Although many of these stereotypes are ambiguous and currently inappropriate, they are difficult to change. They were created originally to provide a semblance of order and predictability in an extremely complex world and have become accepted as social norms. Attitudes and behaviors must change before the stereotypes are modified.

The behavior of boys and girls during middle childhood in industrialized countries is more alike than different. This is partly explained by growth and development processes, such as improved coordination, opportunities to participate in sports, more homogeneous expectations by teachers, and the development of problem-solving skills. It also reflects the gradual shift in societal norms and the child's increased exposure to successful women who are achievement and career oriented. Furthermore, there is a growing recognition that many sex-role stereotypes are culturally learned and reinforced. As parents and teachers communicate this concept to children, their understanding that these stereotypes are not absolutes increases.

Male aggressiveness and female dependency seem to be learned rather than innate behaviors. When children quarrel, parents frequently reprimand their sons for being too rough or aggressive with their weaker, defenseless sisters, even though the sisters might be older. Parents also tend to be more comfortable with rough-and-tumble play from boys than from girls. Thus, girls and boys are given cues that influence their interests and foster socialization into roles that conform, at least in part, to the cultural stereotypes.

Interactions Among Subsystems

The suprasystems provide the context in which the child interacts in the developmental process. Each child develops in a unique way that reflects the interaction of the various suprasystems and the child's individual assets. These assets are the child's identifying characteristics and include physical skills, personality features, social behaviors, and cognitive abilities. The development that has occurred and is occurring in each of these areas helps the child to interact with and learn from the various suprasystems.

The developmental tasks of middle childhood push the child outward into more concentrated interactions with the environment. Physically, the child begins engaging in games and other activities requiring practice and coordination. Socially, the child moves from home and family to the world of school, peers, and playground, learning social skills and how to get along with age-mates. Cognitively, the child learns how to communicate symbolically and question the "how's" and "why's" of life.

Parameters of Middle Childhood Development

Biophysical Development

Unlike the rapid growth that occurs between birth and early childhood and the growth that characterizes the prepubertal years, the biophysical changes that occur during middle childhood basically are unremarkable. The muscular changes that primarily do occur involve the refinement of muscular development rather than cellular growth. Children learn to combine motor activities into games and to be goal directed. For example, they incorporate throwing and hitting a ball and running in games like kickball and soccer. If children in middle childhood are well nourished, they appear to be at their healthiest, full of energy and play.

Children at this stage grow at their own rates, within the limits of typical growth patterns (see Appendix A). Hereditary and environmental factors are responsible for the individual differences (see Chapter 5).

Musculoskeletal System Height and weight are two measures of the child's health status. Taken together, they tell whether the child is developing according to established guidelines. During middle childhood, these standards are unaffected by sex. The average annual increase in weight is 2.3 kg (5 lb), and the average annual increase in height is approximately 5 cm (2 in). The acceleration in both weight and height during this time is minimal, and the growth curves appear to reach a plateau. During this time, the child's weight and height might remain stationary for weeks at a time and is not a cause for concern. Growth retardation is pronounced only when it occurs at times when growth normally is accelerated such as during infancy and adolescence. Racial and socioeconomic conditions do, however, account for differences in growth patterns among children. The child from an advantaged family tends to be taller and heavier than a child from a disadvantaged family.

Growth in the musculoskeletal system accounts for most of the weight increase during middle childhood. "Baby fat" is replaced by muscle, bone tissue replaces cartilage, and length is added to the long bones of the extremities and the facial bones. The child acquires a thin and lean appearance. The weight of the 5-year-old is about twice that of the 1-year-old; at 7 years of age, the child weighs seven times the birthweight. Two additional mnemonics for growth from 4½ to 8 years are weight in pounds equals approximately six times the age plus 12 and height in inches equals two and one-half times the age plus 30 (Lowrey, 1978).

Healthy children should maintain their position on the percentile curves from age to age during middle childhood. Failure to maintain a pattern of growth for the age range may indicate health problems in the child because growth deviations usually accompany or follow disease.

Posture improves as the pelvis leans backward and the abdominal muscles become stronger. The cervical spine begins to take on a curvature in the thoracic area, and the vertebral curves continue to develop. Not until late childhood, however, does the child develop voluntary control of these curves and the ability to improve posture. Exercise and physical activity are necessary to help maintain flexibility and strength and to foster muscular development. The child's posture during middle childhood is a reflection of nutritional status, fatigue, and body growth.

The mandible and maxilla increase in overall length, height, and width. The chin also becomes more developed. The facial dimensions of a 6-year-old are approximately 80%–83% those of the adult. This elongation in the structure of the jaw accommodates the corresponding dental changes. During middle childhood, usually around 6 years of age, permanent molars erupt. About this time, the child begins to lose primary teeth, which are replaced by larger secondary (permanent) teeth. The central incisors are the first teeth to be lost and account for the "toothless gap" appearance of many first-graders and the introduction of the myth about the tooth fairy. One first-grader felt very left out because he had not yet lost a tooth, an event regarded as a status symbol by his classmates. His greater concern, however, was that the tooth fairy might run out of money before he had a chance to collect.

The age at which children lose teeth is variable and related to genetic factors. Girls tend to lose teeth earlier than do boys. Prolonged undernutrition might delay eruption of secondary teeth.

Respiratory System Changes in the respiratory system are related to maturation and overall body growth. The lungs' slow descent into the thoracic cavity continues. It is thought that alveolar multiplication is complete around 8 years of age; thereafter, dilation and widening account for the increase in lung growth. Lung weight increases from 211 g at 5 years of age to 290 g at 8 years of age (Johnson, Moore, and Jeffries, 1978). This increase in lung tissue results in more adultlike (vesicular) breath sounds.

With maturation the respiratory system becomes more efficient. Tidal volume (the amount of air exchanged with each breath) increases during middle childhood, which enables the child to participate in more vigorous and prolonged activity without becoming breathless or oxygen deprived. In addition, the child's vital capacity (total of inspiratory reserve volume, tidal volume, and expiratory reserve volume) increases significantly: from 1140 mL at 5 years of age to 1890 mL at 8 years of age for males and from 1010 mL at 5 years of age to 1615 mL at 8 years of age for females (Johnson, Moore, and Jeffries, 1978).

Two other characteristics of respirations during middle childhood are a slower respiratory rate (20–24 breaths/min) and increased use of the costal muscles for respiration. Prior to this time, the diaphragmatic muscles are more prominent.

Cardiovascular System The changes occurring in the cardiovascular system during middle childhood complement those in the respiratory system in facilitating the child's increased tolerance and resilience for activity. The mean weight of the heart increases slightly from 90 g to 110 g during middle childhood (Johnson, Moore, and Jeffries, 1978) and takes a more vertical position within the thoracic cavity. The 5-year-old's heart is four times the size it was at birth. This growth is essential to accommodate the increased oxygen and circulatory needs associated with growth and development. By 7 years of age, the left ventricle is as thick as an adult's, and the muscle mass is two to three times greater than that of the right ventricle. The heart rate declines steadily and averages 95 ± 30 beats/min during this age span (see Appendix B).

The heart sounds continue to have a high pitch during this period. About 50% of children in this age group will have an innocent heart murmur at some time, with a peak incidence around 6–9 years of age. These soft, systolic murmurs have no other cardiac symptomatology and are the result of normal turbulence and the vibration of blood passing over valves or through vessels close to the surface. Innocent murmurs frequently disappear with a change in position. A functional murmur, on the other hand, indicates a pathologic process, although not necessarily within the heart. Certain disorders, such as anemia, will result in a functional murmur (Silver, 1978).

Unlike the declining heart rate, blood pressure increases in the middle childhood years, averaging 105–95/65–60 mm Hg. Boys and girls have essentially the same blood pressure readings until the onset of puberty. Blacks have been found to have a lower blood pressure, although the incidence of hypertension is higher for blacks (Londe, et al., 1977). Hemoglobin and hematocrit levels increase slightly, and the white blood cell count is reduced somewhat.

Sensory System Sensory organs enable the child to recognize what is happening in the environment and to respond through reflex action. In middle childhood, however, the sensory system is not developed in all of these areas. The child's senses of smell and taste develop early in infancy and are fully mature by middle childhood. The sense of touch continues to develop as the child interacts with and interprets the environment, and both vision and hearing undergo significant changes at this stage.

During middle childhood, the child's vision begins to change from hyperopic to normal. Normal, or 20/20, vision means that a child is able to see an object 20 feet away with normal acuity. Changes in visual acuity during middle childhood reflect the focusing of images on the retina. By developing the ocular muscles and controlling eye movements, the child attains normal vision. Children with poor vision do not normally complain of vision problems because they have never had normal vision and do not know the difference. Screening tests for possible vision impairment and further examination are therefore important in this age range.

Hearing and language development are clearly correlated in middle childhood. As children learn to discriminate fine differences between articulated sounds and voice pitch, they also learn to duplicate phonetic utterances and understand translations. Middle childhood is therefore the prime time to introduce a child to a foreign language because the child is able to learn a foreign language quickly and speak as fluently as a native speaker and usually without an accent. For example, the 5- and 7-year-old girls of a family who moved to the United States from France learned English with a minimum of difficulty. Within a couple of years, their speech was fluent and lacked any trace of an accent. Their parents, on the other hand, were still having difficulty hearing and subsequently producing certain sounds.

Although the eustachian tube has grown longer, narrower, and slanted, a small percentage (3%–4%) of children develop hearing defects associated with chronic middle ear infections. This percentage increases significantly (18%–20%) for children of lower socioeconomic backgrounds, suggesting that screening tests for schoolchildren are a valuable tool in detecting hearing impairments before any unrecognized conditions cause learning problems. (Hearing and vision impairments are discussed in Chapter 43.)

Gastrointestinal System As the stomach enlarges, the child becomes able to ingest increased amounts, thus reducing the frequency of eating. The child also tolerates different kinds of foods better and develops preferences. The child's nutritional intake must, however, meet the demands of growth and metabolic needs, and hence parents must supervise food selection. By the time children begin school, they have learned to control elimination. Stools are well formed, and they have one to two bowel movements per day.

Genitourinary System The increase in renal tubular mass during middle childhood increases the weight of the kidneys. The size of the bladder differs among children, but girls tend to have larger bladders. The frequency of urination varies depending on the amount of fluids ingested, temperature, humidity, time of day, and the child's emotional state. The average 6-year-old has an output of about 1000 mL/day, and the constituency of the urine and its specific gravity are similar to those of an adult. In boys the genitourinary system is mainly for urination; hormonal activity has not begun to influence the reproductive glands.

Immunologic System The development of the immunologic system is accelerated during middle childhood. The child resynthesizes antibodies with each exposure to the same antigen. In spite of this protective mechanism, 71% of school absenteeism is related to infections developed during these years (Holm, 1978). Immunity levels increase through this process, however, and the incidence of symptomatic illnesses decreases. The high incidence of infections during the first year or two of school is related to the increased number of exposures to ill children, careless hygiene practices, and the still-developing immunologic system. Teaching about health and the prevention of illness is an important function of the school nurse when interacting with children in the early grades (see Chapter 18).

The lymphatic system, especially tonsillar tissue, enlarges during middle childhood. This enlargement is considered a normal physiologic function and part of the body's defense mechanism. Enlarged tonsils and adenoids are not surgically removed unless they compromise physiologic functions or become abscessed. This lymphatic hyperplasia ceases around 7 years of age; consequently, the tonsils and adenoids appear to be small in the adult in comparison.

Neuromuscular Function By the time the child reaches middle childhood, the development of the nervous system has slowed from its rapid growth of infancy and early childhood. The brain is about 90% of the adult size and weighs about 1200 g. The maturation of the central nervous system permits children to perform increasingly more complex gross and fine motor skills, to process all incoming stimuli, and to have greater control over their bodies. Children gradually progress from clumsy and uncoordinated movements to graceful and agile ones.

Cerebral dominance is established, and a definite hand preference is evident by 4½ years of age. The neurologic center for speech usually is localized in the left hemisphere. Speech patterns provide a guide to the intactness of the neurologic system.

Gross Motor Skills Beginning with middle childhood, children have greater control over their movements. They are more dextrous in stopping, turning, running, climbing, and jumping. By rearranging their foot patterns and using an overhead motion instead of a horizontal arm and body movement, they add momentum to the objects they throw. The right-handed child, for example, now transfers body weight to the right rear foot in preparation to throw and then takes a step forward onto the leading left foot before releasing the object. Most children are proficient overhand throwers by 6 years of age. Boys tend to be better at long-distance throwing than girls (Corbin, 1980). Skills developed at an earlier age continue to be refined throughout this development phase. Children become more coordinated, have better balance, and exert greater strength in performing activities such as throwing a ball. They bask in the wonderful discovery of their ability to perform so many physical skills such as bicycle riding, tree climbing, and roller skating. Any activity that entails the use of balance is desired. At this time, they focus more on gross motor activities than on fine motor activities. These newfound abilities are so enthralling that children often play until they are exhausted.

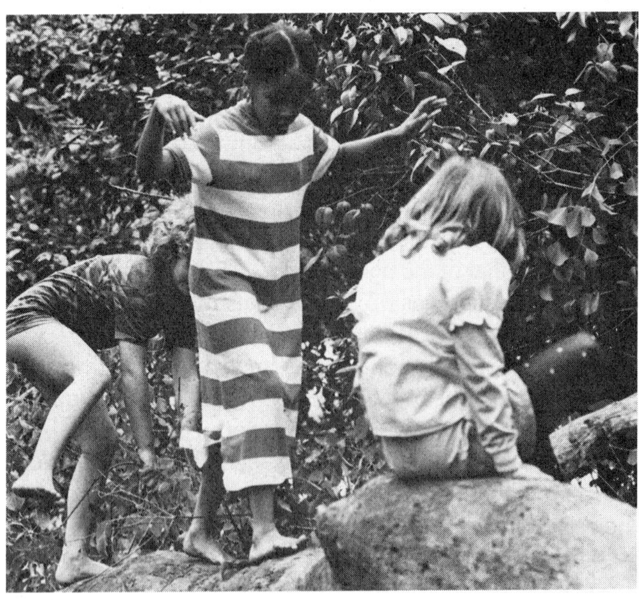

In middle childhood, children gain greater control of gross motor skills.

Five- and six-year-olds are full of energy. They find sitting still and prolonged quiet activities difficult to tolerate because they yearn to practice their skills and exercise their developing muscles. They have learned to hop, skip, tandem walk, and catch and throw a ball smoothly. Some even know how to swim, roller skate, or ride a bicycle. Their improved balance also permits them to walk along narrow objects such as curbs, stone walls, logs, the wooden sides of sandboxes, and balance beams. They combine their physical skills with the social skills involved in playing with others and play games such as dodge ball and follow the leader and spend many hours in fantasy games.

Seven- and eight-year-old children begin to show conscious awareness of their activities. They are more goal oriented; for example, they run to reduce the time it takes to get somewhere and use bicycles adroitly to run errands. They show more caution in performing gross motor skills than they did the year before. They continue to have high energy levels, but they also select activities that include sitting still and resting. Their attention span is also increased.

Fine Motor Skills The fine motor skills of middle childhood reflect a maturing central nervous system. With increased mastery of more complex skills and the child's finer dexterity, better control over writing instruments such as crayons and pencils is achieved.

Five-year-old children can tie knots, manipulate buttons in buttonholes, paint, and color. They can write letters and numbers and use crayons and pencils with more confidence. In addition, they can draw recognizable human figures showing details of eyes, ears, and other major parts of the body. Because they now handle tools with greater precision, they enjoy using scissors to cut out objects, and they also can comb their hair and brush their teeth.

Six-year-olds perform various tasks using tools. These tools might be associated with writing, carpentry, or eating. Although they use tools awkwardly, they are keenly interested in manipulation for its own sake and less interested in what they create. The boat or car they create by nailing several pieces of wood together actually does resemble the desired object; however, they take more pride in the acts of sawing, nailing, and perhaps painting than in the finished product. They perform activities rapidly, coordinating the use of hands and eyes. For example, a 6-year-old spends much time and concentration on the task of fitting together small building blocks but is not always successful. The rapidity with which the blocks are stacked might cause the alignment to be off, and the blocks often fall. In the same way the child can print capital letters, but sometimes in reverse.

At 7 years of age, some letters and numbers might first be written in reverse, but the child recognizes the error and makes the correction. Seven- and eight-year-olds love to write and enjoy writing and receiving letters. They practice their new skill by using their imagination to create stories or plays for which they compose the script. As fine motor skills develop, they hold pencils with a tighter grasp near the point and with their forefingers curved in. As they write across the page, they tend to reduce the size of the letters. By 7 years of age, they can readily draw triangles, and by 8 years of age, they can draw diamonds. (Developmental assessment is discussed in more detail in Chapter 16.)

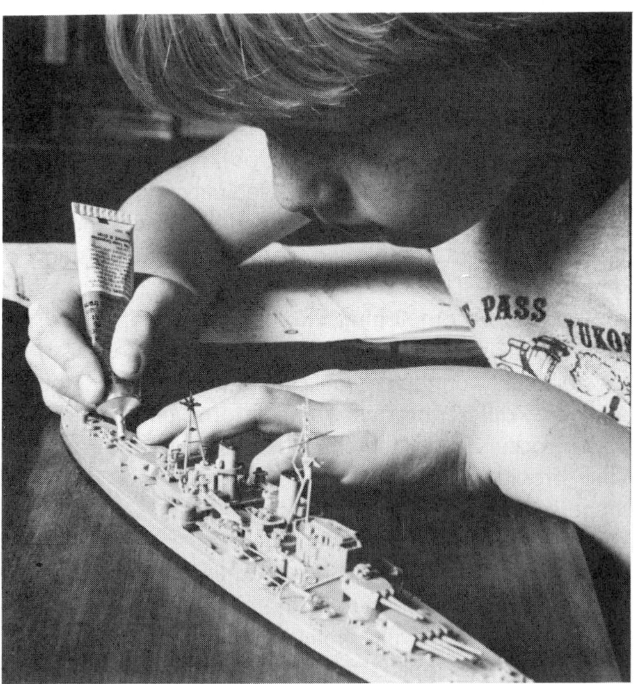

In middle childhood, children's activities reflect developing dexterity and increasing refinement in fine motor skills.

Personality Development

Personality development in childhood correlates highly with development in other areas. As in infancy and early childhood, the personality attributes of 4½- to 8-year-old children influence their thought processes. As the child's development progresses, personality traits remain a factor in decision making, even though cognition and social awareness take on additional meaning.

The affective qualities demonstrated by a child in middle childhood stem from an emerging self-identity based on the internalization of values learned at home. Love, friendship, and satisfaction, for example, are positive emotional expressions that contribute to feelings of psychologic well-being among children of this age. Fear, anger, and anxiety are expressions of negative emotion.

Gender Identification Middle childhood is a time when gender and social identity become solidified. Lamb (1978) explained that gender identity is not secure until the child is satisfied and feels comfortable being male or female. Once this occurs, the child identifies first with the same-sex parent and then with other role models, imitating their behaviors and thus taking on stereotypic sex-role attitudes and actions.

This explanation of the process of identification is a refinement of Freud's concept (1969). He presented identification as the resolution of the Oedipal complex (or Electra complex in females) and claimed that it was the major task the child accomplished during the phallic stage of development. The recognition of sex differences is a prerequisite to accomplishing the task (see Chapter 6). For Freud, identification, broadly defined as the process whereby the child takes on the desirable attributes of beloved people, takes two different forms. The first form, *anaclitic identification,* occurs when the child identifies with the caregiver who provides sustenance. The second form, *defensive identification,* occurs when the child identifies with a powerful figure to escape punishment.

Freud assumed that this powerful figure was the child's father and that the young boy therefore passed from identifying with a caregiving mother to imitating a more powerful father. As applied to young girls, however, Freud's analysis of gender identification in childhood was far less specific.

Defensive identification is, for Freud, the basis for the development of the superego in the 4- to 5-year-old child. Once children learn to identify with their parents, they judge actions as right or wrong on the basis of how their parents evaluate these actions. This developing conscience in turn influences how children act in situations involving moral judgment.

Freud assumed that by the time the child reached 6 years of age, the Oedipus complex is usually resolved and the child enters the latency period. During latency, the development of intellectual skills becomes paramount. Kohlberg (1966), on the other hand, noted that gender identity is a two-step process. The child first acquires a basic sense of identity. This usually occurs in early childhood, when, for example, Mark will identify himself as a boy and his sister, Lisa, as a girl. The second step occurs during middle childhood and entails the concept of gender constancy. Now, Mark affirms that boys will always become men and girls will always become women and that this fact can never change. Even if a boy grew his hair long and wore dresses and makeup, he would still be a boy. Thus, the child has an intellectual grasp of the concept and meaning of gender.

Although they have more freedom to choose friends, games, and activities, children during middle childhood tend to prefer to be with others of the same sex. They play games, establish rules, and assign roles that often are exclusive and reflect their future roles. Boys will participate in such play activities as football, police, or space rangers and temporarily take the names of their heroes. Girls will play house, school, or television studio, assigning names and roles accordingly. The two groups often stake out their own territory and post "No Girls Allowed" or "Entrance Limited to Boys Only" signs. Each group regards their sex as superior, more intelligent, and more talented. In their peer group, characterized by its separation of interests and activities, boys and girls develop their skills, values, and roles with others most like themselves. This division according to gender facilitates the socialization process, aids in the attainment of competence, and reduces the risk of failure. Children gain a better sense of who they are by establishing who they are and are not like. Likeness is rooted in gender identity and the internalization of behaviors, roles, attributes, and mannerisms of the same-sex role models.

Sense of Self The contribution to the child's development that others in the environment make is a consistent theme in the theory of Erik Erikson (see Chapter 6). During middle childhood, developmental tasks focus on interacting appropriately and creatively with the environment. According to Erikson (1973), the 3- to 6-year-old child must resolve the dilemma of initiative versus guilt by learning to explore beyond the self (see Chapter 6). Children's initiative can be seen in the increasing number of questions they ask and in the make-believe world they create. Through fantasy, the children's newfound confidence in their abilities and the support they receive at home and at school are conveyed by the enthusiasm with which they approach new experiences.

How the parents and other adults react to the child's inquisitive posture is important because they influence the child's leaning toward initiation or guilt. Cohen (1974) summarized the salient points that Erikson made about how the family assists the child who is striving to master initiative. The family should (1) teach the child where play ends and responsibility and purpose begin; (2) clearly define the do's and don'ts with reference to words and actions; and (3) develop a mutually loving relationship between father and son or mother and daughter based on worth and acceptance, thereby fostering behaviors that are similar to those of the same-sex parent.

Feelings of satisfaction stimulate the child first in the development of initiative and second in the production of work, or industry. Constructing new behaviors is satisfying. Children derive pleasure from building, discovering new knowledge, and learning. Discovering new twists to old behavior patterns also creates excitement. Initially, the child is rewarded by approval received for beginning a task. For example, as the sense of initiative is acquired, the child's energy turns toward narrowing the difference between the mental image and the actual appearance of a block city or drawing of a house. The final product now becomes important, and the child works to replicate reality or transcribe a creative idea accurately.

Erikson saw the child's conflict after 6 years of age as one of industry versus inferiority. As children apply their newly learned skills to the playground and school, they attain a sense of industry, but if they fail to meet the tasks at hand, children acquire a sense of inferiority. At this stage, children develop skills in deductive reasoning and playing games according to established rules. Parent, teacher, and peer evaluation of a child's "work" are influential in establishing self-worth. Armed with newly acquired, although sometimes transient, concrete operational skills, the 7-year-old begins the task of mastering school tasks.

As children interact with others and accomplish the tasks of middle childhood, they refine their sense of self. They are able increasingly to understand how they are seen by others. Their self-concept reflects how others respond to them, what others appear to think of them, and how others evaluate their skills. Susan Harter (1982) described a developmental approach to the study of self-concept. During middle childhood, the child's self-concept is a composite of views received from many people—parents, teachers, peers, neighbors, and relatives. The child progresses within the structure of simple descriptions from first thinking about self as being good or bad in everything to being able to differentiate aspects of self that are more skillful or appreciated than others. The content of behaviors from which the child gathers a sense of self begins with physical attributes (for example, beautiful hair, tallest in the class), progresses to behaviors or skills (for example, best runner, neatest penmanship), and from there to the psychologic dimensions of emotions or feelings (for example, happy, fearful), motives or intentions (for example, reward, honor), and cognitions or thought processes (for example, altruism, competition).

The acquisition of self-concept is a complex process that is influenced by the expectations of many others and therefore does not follow a smooth continuum. The child often is found to be at a different structural level of thinking depending on the content dimension being assessed. The structural changes, each with two levels of thinking, roughly correspond to cognitive levels, with simple descriptions coinciding with preoperational thought, trait labels with concrete operational thought, single abstractions with formal operational thought, and higher-order abstractions with adult thought.

The child with a positive self-concept feels capable, worthy, important, and likeable, which translates into self-respect and self-confidence. Children with a negative self-concept feel unacceptable, doubt their ability to do well or to have friends, and develop a sense of inferiority.

Another aspect of children's developing sense of self is self-control, that is, learning to cope with frustrations and control feelings of aggression. Along with self-control and self-concept is a sense of self-worth. The child's sense of acceptance and competence is related to the ease and success with which school-related skills are accomplished. When children are praised for their reading, writing, and mathematic skills, they feel proud and positive about their abilities. They will inform others that they are in the top reading group or have the most stickers for excellent papers. The child who has problems learning the assigned skills, experiences failure, or is constantly being told to try harder has difficulty liking or promoting the self. This child is also likely to be timid, easily discouraged, and hesitant to participate with peers in class discussions or projects.

In several interesting studies discussed by Santrock (1983), it was noted that improvement of a negative self-concept is best achieved by the child's learning basic skills and thus changing behavior. This is an important fact for nurses to remember, especially when caring for children with chronic illnesses or handicapping conditions. It is more beneficial to teach such children the skills that will help them to function optimally than to give them a falsely inflated view of themselves.

Fears Middle childhood is the time when early childhood fears wane, to be replaced by new fears. As the child matures, imagination and fantasy are replaced by more realistic thinking. Between the ages of 4½ and 6 years, fears related to physical injury increase, whether from animals, especially dogs, activities such as swimming that relate to drowning, or active imaginations that recreate or invent threatening creatures and harmful situations. The child naturally is fearful of things that are different, unexpected, or not understood. Children from advantaged environments tend to have a higher proportion of fears related to personal safety and health, whereas children from disadvantaged environments generally are more fearful of supernatural happenings.

Nurses especially need to be cognizant of the child's fears, respect them as real, be patient and understanding of their influence on the child's behavior, and must never belittle the child or ignore the fear. It is common for children to be very fearful of the strangeness of the personnel and environment in health care facilities.

Around 7 or 8 years of age these fears for personal well-being become replaced by anxieties and fears about school and social relationships. Jersild (1975) found that 7-year-old children were anxious about (1) school performance; (2) peer acceptance; (3) teacher acceptance; and (4) school conduct.

Interpersonal Relationships Temperament influences the ease with which a child in middle childhood successfully completes the tasks of this stage. Temperament, as conceived by Chess and Thomas (1977), is the characteristic pattern of responding and reacting. Temperament is present at birth and probably is genetically determined (Watson and Lindgren, 1979). Although temperamental patterns affect all aspects of behavior, in middle childhood they are most evident as the child develops interpersonal relationships.

Children who are 4½ years old enter middle childhood eager to engage in cooperative play and express themselves more freely. Before children can enjoy their newfound playmates, however, they must first learn to become emotionally competent by developing inner controls. They must be able to reflect on events before responding. Their outbursts of aggression therefore become more verbal and less physical. In addition, they discover that altruism reinforces friendships and that aggression destroys them.

They learn from the give and take of peer interactions that there are times when being competitive gains approval such as running one's fastest to win the race. At other times, however, cooperation is preferred such as being a teammate and working together to win a soccer game. One 6-year-old boy learned that he reaped more praise for passing the soccer ball to a teammate, even though she was a girl, who was open and scored easily. Previously, when he had ignored her and attempted to score the goal himself and failed, his teammates rebuked him and called him selfish.

At 4 or 5 years of age, children act in response to their feelings. The concept of social etiquette is not part of their repertoire (Harter, 1981). Younger children also emphasize simpler and more superficial aspects of personality development as a basis for friendship (Selman and Selman, 1979). At 4 years of age, children thought that admiration should be the basis for friendship. At 5 years of age, loyalty and commitment were valued. Six-year-olds wanted their friends to be genuine and recipients of their aid. At 7 and 8 years of age, children were more concerned with more complex friendship qualities such as the potential for intimacy, sharing similar interests, and sharing the same attitudes and values.

The friendships that children develop with peers in the neighborhood, at the playground, or in school physically draw them away from their families. The benefits of peer relations are many: (1) the opportunity to test out newly acquired skills; (2) the opportunity for practicing these skills among equals at the child's own pace; and (3) the opportunity for transitional experiences from the stable world of people, from the familiar and dependable world of the family to the unfamiliar world outside the home, and from dependence on the "giants" who are adults to independence among equals, that is, one's peers.

Humor, a way of reacting to the satisfaction of peer interactions, is noticeable during the middle childhood years. Jokes, rhyming of words, and spontaneous laughter in a group are forms of humor among 5- to 8-year-olds. Most of their jokes are judged to be boring or ridiculous by their older siblings and adults. Many children enjoy jokes that involve puns or taboo subjects such as jokes about elimination. Some of their favorite humor includes "knock-knock" jokes or elephant jokes, which they repeat ad nauseum. They gradually learn that a joke is funniest the first time told and does not get the same positive response thereafter. One 5-year-old repeated an elephant joke she had heard her brother tell. She derived much egocentric pleasure in telling it, noting the positive response its punch line received; however, she did not understand it. Finally, she asked her mother why people laughed about the elephant crying. The joke was "what does a grape say when an elephant sits on it? Nothing, it just lets out a little wine." The fact that she did not understand the joke did not interfere with the pleasure she derived from telling it.

Seven- and eight-year-olds entertain each other by reading riddles and jokes. Their improved memory enables them to increase their repertoire by remembering what they read as well as what they hear. One boy who thoroughly enjoyed humor made weekly trips to the library until he had read all of the joke and riddle books in the children's section.

Cognitive Development

Piaget's concepts of assimilation and accommodation are useful for explaining learning and thinking during middle childhood (see Chapter 6). According to Piaget, children 4–7 years of age are in the intuitive stage, in which the child seems to understand intuitively the rules that govern the social environment. In reality the child is more able to cope with the physical world than to understand how it is governed. The child's thinking processes are still governed by the perceptual appearance of things, egocentricity, and illogical reasoning. Even so, children at this stage are less egocentric than in the preconceptual stage and can distinguish between their own perception of the real world and the reality of the physical and social environment (Piaget, 1973).

The child constantly questions why events occur, such as why the sun shines in the daytime and the moon at night. Because they are unable to comprehend the concept of planetary rotation, they explain the event in terms familiar to them, such as saying that the sun gets tired and goes to bed at night and the moon takes its place.

Intuitive thought processes are characteristic of *transductive thinking.* A precursor of inductive reasoning, transductive thinking involves drawing conclusions from one specific, current event to another equally specific and immediate event. For example, the child who sees the wind blowing leaves away might conclude that it is possible for children to be blown away by a strong wind. Until the child is able to classify or discern similar from dissimilar objects, conclusions about their operations might be illogical.

Much learning in middle childhood occurs by imitation but without tangible rewards or punishments. Bandura and Walters (1963) viewed this type of modeling as more complex than operant conditioning because it occurs in social situations. Therefore, any analysis of learning must include social interactions, the social situation, and the personalities of the persons involved to determine whether learning has occurred. Practice opportunities also must be available. Piaget noted that imitation without practice can be insufficient.

Imitation and Behavior Social learning theories have integrated some aspects of both behaviorism and psychosocial stage theories. Whereas Freud and Erikson focused on dependence and identification as the antecedents for learning, social learning theorists stress imitation and reinforcement. To social learning theorists, a child 4–7 years old learns when behavior is reinforced. Other social learning theorists go further and suggest that observing another person might be sufficient to lead to a learned response.

Bandura (1963) argued that when placed in social situations, children often learn much more rapidly by observing the behavior of others. Observational learning is a cognitive process that teaches the child the outcomes of the behavior without the child's having experienced the outcomes firsthand. The child's experience with the model reflects an experience that may be direct or indirect, real or symbolic, but the child interprets the model's behavior and selects the knowledge to retain. Learning in middle childhood might therefore be a vicarious process in which the child need not directly experience the reinforcer to learn.

Children particularly observe models who are rewarded, have personal characteristics that are favorable, and who are somewhat similar to them. The 6-year-old taking gymnastic lessons might watch Olympic or national competition on television and then try to perform similar tricks. A young boy who met a professional basketball star decided to pursue a career in basketball. He spent hours practicing, trying to imitate everything this player did. As a result, he was the best player on his midget basketball team. In essence, Bandura postulated that cognition is influenced by the child's own motivation. Hence, learning through modeling varies from child to child.

Sears suggested that the child's behavior is primarily the product of experiences and that motivation in middle childhood incorporates learning from sources outside the family (Sears, Maccoby, and Levin, 1957). During this stage, the child's dependence on the family shifts to a wider social environment, and the child transfers dependence from the family to teachers, peers, and community organizations.

Egocentricity Egocentric children believe that everyone perceives and interprets the world in exactly the same way that they do. In middle childhood egocentricity is not an intentional act of disregarding but rather the inability to see another person's point of view. During the intuitive phase, egocentric thinking is less intense than in the preconceptual phase. Four-year-old children have difficulty comprehending such concepts as "share," "fair," "right," or "wrong." Not until they reach 6 years of age and begin to recognize that other people have personal reasons for their behavior can they fully understand socially prescribed rules.

Before 4 years of age, there is no evidence that children can understand another's point of view. Four-year-olds, however, can show empathy toward others who are placed in unfortunate situations (Smart and Smart, 1977). Significant changes occur in the child's ability to take another's perspective as the child advances toward concrete operational thinking. By 6 years of age, the child is less egocentric and realizes that another person might have a different view of the same event. The 6-year-old child also can begin to understand whether another person's actions are accidental or intended and recognizes that other people might act on the basis of their own personal feelings. Role taking necessitates development of the cognitive skills that enable the child to understand other people, their emotional states, their perspectives, and the differences between these perspectives and the child's point of view.

Egocentricity is a source of both joy and sadness. As a source of joy, it contributes to the child's refreshing and uncensored evaluation of the situation at hand, but sadly, the egocentric child cannot assess the consequences of actions on others. As the child gradually learns about others through interaction with peers, teachers, and neighbors, egocentric thinking decreases. For example, while playing with blocks in school, 4-year-old Jack decided he needed another large yellow block. He looked around for one, but none were in sight. Then he saw a long row of them where Carolyn was playing. Quickly he went over to that area and took two of the blocks. As she attempted to reclaim them, an argument ensued. Jack shouted that he needed them to complete his building, and Carolyn protested that he had taken her yellow brick road. Neither child could understand the other's point of view, and both children were outraged that someone was interfering with their project.

Self-knowledge, or the development of conscious awareness of self, progresses during the early phase of middle childhood, when the child's emphasis is on images of physical events, to the latter phase of middle childhood, which is the beginning of Piaget's concrete operational stage (see Chapter 6). Children learn to organize and interpret stories, dreams, and images. Initially, when children tell a story or relate a dream, they omit large portions because they assume that the listener shares their perspective. In fact, they have little tolerance if the listener requests additional information. By 6 or 7 years of age, they realize that the listener only knows what they relate and thus provide detailed accounts of the events.

Animism, Realism, Causality, and Fantasy *Animism* is the belief that the world of objects is alive and has personality and purpose; it is the illogical process of equating movement with life. During middle childhood, children often attribute human features to any object that moves. Leaves, for example, are assumed to be alive. Animism possibly facilitates the projection of children's feelings and attitudes onto external objects, provides an explanation of events and happenings in understandable, familiar terms, and assists in the child's development from egocentricity to an awareness of others.

Pulaski (1971) identified four stages in the decline of animism, two of which are seen in middle childhood, or Piaget's intuitive phase. The first stage is a shift from the child's attributing animism to all objects to attributing animism just to moving objects. The second stage is the child's attributing human qualities to invisible propelling forces such as wind or thunder.

For example, by attributing human qualities to thunder, the child might project fear and anger about the noise by defining the thunder as angry clouds growling and fighting or as "cloud people" throwing rocks against a mountain. These explanations provide reasons for the noise in ways the child understands. The child also begins to realize that events occur independently and are not necessarily caused by the child's will or actions.

Another aspect of the child's thinking is realism. *Realism* in middle childhood is the belief that all things are tangible and concrete, including objects, pictures, dreams, and words. (It is also an expression of egocentricity.) When children begin to separate mental thoughts from the physical world, their use of realism lessens. The child eventually comes to understand that names are arbitrary and are not the object itself. For example, a dog is called a dog but could also be called a pet, hound, or pooch. Most children in middle childhood have grasped this much but do not yet realize that names bear no relationship to the items they describe.

Causality in middle childhood is the belief that a causal relationship exists between two things or events because they appear or occur close together. Things do not happen by chance in the child's world. Every event must have a cause, whether logical or not. Many of the child's explanations use the self as a model, such as the candle is awake and happy when lit but sad and sleeping when not lit. If two things happen in succession, they are often related as cause and effect in the child's mind, regardless of whether such explanations are logical. For example, a 4½-year-old might provide the following rationale for why an ice cube melted: "The ice cube melted because it got tired of standing up." A 7-year-old, however, might state that it melted because the sun was too hot but would be unable to explain how the changes in its state occurred. As the child questions, observes, and attempts to relate cause and effect to events, reality gradually gains precedence over fantasy as the more plausible explanation.

Fantasy in middle childhood is undirected, free, and symbolic thinking that is difficult to put into words. Research in children's thinking shows that fantasy plays an essential role in the development of adaptive ways to cope with life's problems (Fraiberg, 1959; Mitchell, 1980). Fantasy is a way of dealing with reality. Through fantasy, children direct their thoughts to a limited extent, but this free-roving, personal, inner method of symbolic play is their tool for learning. It is through fantasy that the child develops the capacity to move from a personal, subjective, and egocentric point of view to a more other-centered perspective.

Fantasy is evident in the stories that children tell and the games they play. As the child grows, so does the amount and richness of the fantasy. Even at this age, however, gender differences are evident. Boys' tales tend to be more active, have more themes of aggression, use a greater variety of characters, and have more objects from transportation, electronics, and nature. Girls' stories tend to be more intensive, detailed, and involved with feelings, people, home, and the here and now.

Conservation, Centration, and Irreversibility The notion that objects can be transformed from one state to another and still preserve their integrity is foreign to the 4- and 5-year-old. At this stage, children simply cannot comprehend that two equal quantities remain equal as long as nothing is added or subtracted. The child has not grasped the principle of *conservation,* that certain properties of objects remain the same despite transformations.

Lack of conservation is best demonstrated with 4- and 5-year-olds when two equal-size balls of clay are put before them. Children of this age correctly respond that the balls have the same amount of clay. When the perceptual properties are changed by rolling one into a sausage shape in front of the children, they will change their minds, select the longer of the two pieces, and state that it has more clay. Piaget (1969) said that children in the intuitive phase think that if things look different, they must be different.

At approximately 6 or 7 years of age, children begin to comprehend conservation of substance. To gain an understanding of this concept, children first focus on only one aspect or dimension of the object without recognizing relationships among such dimensions as height, weight, length, and width. This lack of multidimensional perception is termed *centration.* Because they cannot recognize reversibility, they also are easily deceived by appearance. They do not mentally reverse the process, that is, change the sausage shape back into the ball shape. Eventually, children vacillate in comprehending this concept and might be able to focus on more than one dimension simultaneously but without understanding the relationships among the dimensions observed. At this point, the child will be able to recognize that the mound of clay is the same but can do so only by concrete experimentation. Logical explanations for such phenomena usually are not given until the child is 10–12 years old and can reason abstractly.

Until abstraction is possible, the child can understand events in the present but is limited by irreversibility and is unable to retrace the process (see Chapter 6). Another example of irreversibility is a 5-year-old child who is able to tell his teacher that he has a brother but when asked whether his brother has a brother, he replies "No." Most 6- and 7-year-olds are in transition. They can reverse familiar, concrete events that they have experienced or when they have the objects to manipulate back and forth. One child moved childlike characters back and forth between a toy vehicle and doll house while verbally problem solving: "In the car you are crowded, in the house you have lots of room, but there are the seven in the car and seven in the house so there must be more room in the house and less room in the car."

The child's ability to conserve begins with the conservation of number. The 4-year-old preconserver focuses on a single dimension. If 20 coins are arranged in two rows of ten so that the rows are of equal length, the child will identify them as equivalent. If one row is then pushed together, the child will center only on the length of the rows and claim that the longer (original) row has more coins than does the pushed-together row. The 5-year-old generally is at the transitional phase, which is characterized by inconsistency of response. By 7 years of age, most children have the mental ability to count and a basic understanding of addition and subtraction. Instead of focusing on the length of the rows, they count the number of coins. If the number is the same, they know the rows are equivalent even though the rows are of different lengths. In addition to number, conservation tasks that are mastered during middle childhood include length, liquid amount, solid amount, and sometimes area. The final conservation task involves displaced volume and is not gained until the end of late childhood.

Time, Space, Seriation, and Classification Like all learning during middle childhood, children's experiences with time are perceptual. By 4 years of age, children are able to remember time sequences and the repetition of events in particular places. They have also mastered such concepts as next summer, last summer, daily events, and months. Concepts such as the time of day and clock time are developed around 5 or 6 years of age (Santrock, 1983).

Piaget (1973) maintained that spatial knowledge develops so that the child eventually can locate an object in reference to other objects and without self-reference. Before this is possible, however, the child must first represent space by formulating a cognitive map and placing objects in relation to self. When 4-year-olds are shown a community scene and then asked to place the doll figures in their model scene in the positions that they had observed them, they will place the figures in the same general proximity. However, they will not be concerned with replicating left–right or before–behind distances. Five- and six-year-olds demonstrate a heightened awareness of spatial relations and will place the dolls more exactly. If the model is turned 180°, they will place the dolls in relation to themselves as if the rotation had not occurred. Egocentric children are unable to conceive of another point of view. Until egocentricity diminishes, objects are assumed to be positioned in relation to the child. Seven-year-olds have a better understanding of relationships in space and are able to account for the rotation and replicate the model when positioning their dolls (Labinowicz, 1980).

During middle childhood, children master such quantitative terms as more, less, all, some, none, and another. According to Gelman (1978), children in this age group follow five principles when counting and quantifying objects:

1. One-to-one correspondence, in which each item is given a tag
2. Stable order, in which the tag given must be from an ordered list
3. Cardinal principle, in which the last tag given designates the number of items in the array counted
4. Abstraction, in which any set of items can be counted
5. Order irrelevance, in which the item to be counted can be tagged in any order as long as each is tagged once and only once

The ability to arrange objects according to increasing or decreasing size is *seriation*. The 4½-year-old can identify which of two sticks, labeled A and B, is longer. If A, the longer stick, is replaced by a very short stick, C, the child then will identify B as longer than C. If asked whether A or C is longer, this child would have to guess at the answer because the ability to order events mentally that occur sequentially has not been attained. The child also has not mastered the concept of greater than or lesser than and thus lacks a principle to which to refer to solve the problem. The 7-year-old has no difficulty answering the question. This child can reason that if A is longer than B and B is longer than C, then A is longer than C.

During middle childhood, children learn to classify objects according to their properties. Among 4- and 5-year-olds, objects are grouped perceptually rather than according to a category. Many studies demonstrate that these children are more likely to group objects on the basis of color rather than form. If given blocks in various shapes, sizes, and colors, the child is likely to put a yellow cube next to a yellow block and a green triangle next to a green block. This kind of classification, in which each object is related to the one beside it but without an overall relationship tying them together is called *chaining*. The shift from color preference to form preference occurs at about 5 years of age. Most 6-year-olds, after having grouped objects on the basis of color, will further subgroup them on the basis of shape and then size.

The 5-year-old has difficulty understanding that something might be included in more than one class. The child focuses on one property of the object and is unable to mentally abstract and compare two of its properties. For example, if there are five oranges and two apples in the bowl, the child will state that apples are a fruit and oranges are a fruit. When asked whether there is more fruit or more oranges, the child confidently answers more oranges. By 8 years of age, the child usually is able to mentally retain and compare several properties of an object and will answer that apples and oranges are both fruits so there is more fruit.

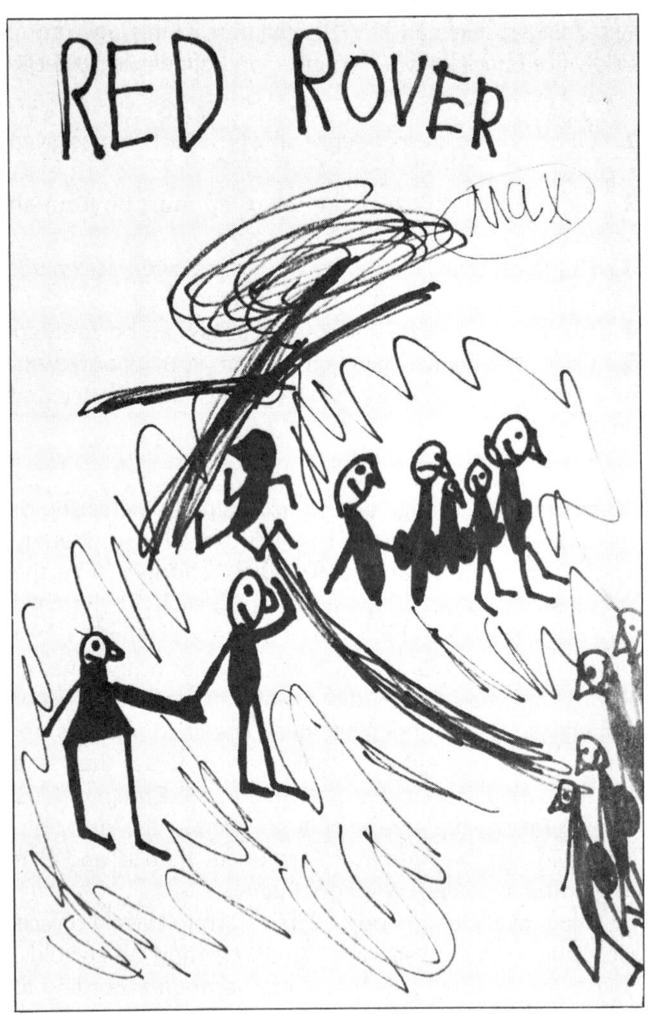

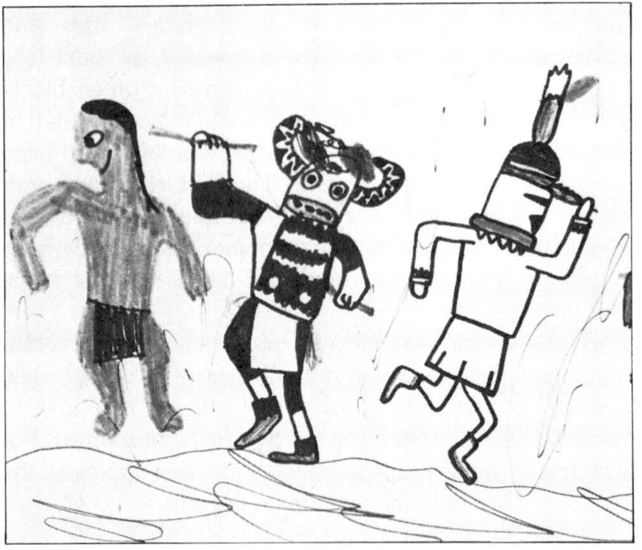

Creativity in middle childhood shows a developing perception of detail and form. Drawing done by a 6-year-old shows elementary sense of human form, while drawing done by the same child two years later reflects awareness of detail in dress and position.

Another way to explain the process by which children learn the concept of class inclusion is provided by the information processing theorists (see Chapter 6). This theory analyzes the steps the child must perform before obtaining an answer. An error in any one of these steps results in an incorrect response. First, the child must decipher the key parts of the question, that is, sort out critical from extraneous information. In the example just cited, the oranges, the definition of fruit, and the concept of group with more must be remembered, and the exact number of apples does not alter the response. Second, a plan to answer the question must be formulated. The child decides what to count and whether to count some things more than once. Third, the child counts the number of oranges and the amount of fruit and compares these numbers (Trabasso, 1977). The answer depends on the child's ability to remember the problem, perform the steps, and compare the results.

Memory and Attention By the time children are 5 years old, they have excellent recognition memory and can readily identify objects they have seen before. Both quantitative and qualitative memory have improved. Children at this age can recall and repeat back an increasing amount of information, and the repeated information is increasingly accurate. With their developing cognitive abilities, they begin to create strategies for remembering, such as repeating the list, grouping objects, and relating an event to the situation.

Major advances in memory occur during middle childhood. The child learns to use relations to recall the sequence of observations and some social interactions. Fantasy and imitative play might help them to remember how to behave or perform certain skills. This freedom to practice remembering during play fosters better retention and practice in monitoring their memories. For example, when Sam is sent to the store for milk, butter, and bread, he memorizes the list by repeating the items several times, holding up three fingers, each one representing a different item, or mentally visualizing the items. When he gets to the store, he repeats the list as he obtains the items. If he were to forget an item, he would attempt to remember it by repeating his original method for memorizing the list.

Although children's attention spans are short, they are able to concentrate on activities for longer periods of time. They are not as easily distracted by other children, toys, and noise. Improved attention enables them to organize the input of information better, that is, more systematically. This in turn facilitates memory retention.

Creativity The creativity evident throughout early childhood prepares children for concrete operations. As children creatively fashion their own world, they constantly modify and change the external environment to correspond to their internal world. Young children are always seeking new experiences to exercise old skills and develop new ones; they use creativity to achieve this task. Children who experience success and have high self-esteem are more adventuresome and creative. They do not relate conformity to approval to the same extent as do children with low self-esteem (Coopersmith, 1967).

The creative child will derive pleasure from inventing a tune on the piano, such as expressing joy by lightly playing a series of high notes or expressing sadness by playing the low notes slowly and methodically. A less creative child will attempt to play a known tune rather than experiment with something new. Art is another area where the creative child expresses mood, feeling, and ideas or experiments with color and design. The more self-confidence and self-esteem children have, the freer they feel to invent, experiment, and create.

A valuable medium for assessing creativity in children is art. According to Durio (1975), children's creativity follows three stages of development. The first stage is manipulation. The child explores the media and learns its capabilities. The second stage is intuitive design. The child who is exploring the art medium will pay attention to a shape or form in the material. For example, a roll of clay might suggest a snake. In the third phase, representational design, the child decides in advance what to make and then acquires the material needed to perform the task. A child can vacillate back and forth among the three stages or remain at any one stage for a given period of time.

Creativity and intelligence are not to be equated. Both are concepts composed of multiple parts and difficult to define, but their focus is different. Guilford (1967) described creativity as *divergent thinking,* that is, a type of thinking that formulates many ways to answer one question. *Convergent thinking,* on the other hand, seeks to identify the one best answer for each question. The key to fostering creativity in children is for adults to encourage flexibility, the exploration of ideas, and imagination.

A commonly held stereotype is that creativity declines with age because of social pressures to conform. As middle childhood moves toward late childhood, the manner of expressing creativity changes. Feeling and imagery do not disappear from the child's work but are complemented by realistic perceptions of the world. Spontaneity takes on more complexity in its revelation but is not decreased as the child's thinking becomes more concrete (Dudek, 1974).

Language and Development

At 5 years of age, the child's language is well developed and bears a striking resemblance to what is spoken in the immediate environment. Grammatic structure and voice control of the 4½-year-old match the meaning of what is said. These children have the ability to put sentences together indicating future and past tense. They can also blend sounds together, a prerequisite for learning to read. All children's speech, however, assumes the characteristics of what is spoken by their parents and other familiar adults and reflects such variables as socioeconomic class and geographic region. This includes regional accents such as the broad "a's" of people living in Boston or the slow drawl of someone living in southern Georgia.

Within a language are variations called dialects. Some dialects are blends of English and a second language such as Spanish or Native American. The most common blend is known as black English. Although linguistically similar to formal English, black English has some differences that are thought to hinder the child's learning to read. Some of the skills needed for phonetic analysis are not used in black English (Baratz, 1973). The casualness of communication is marked by a general acceptance of nonagreement in person and number between a subject and verb, the dropping of some sounds ("clof" for "cloth"), and the merging of words ("dondodat" for "do not do that").

By 5 years of age, the child's vocabulary increases to 2500 words and is understandable to all adults. Dale (1976) suggested that 5-year-old children should have the following uses of language:

1. *Instrumental*—children understand that language is a tool for getting things done. Messages such as "I need," which convey children's wishes and desires, should be a common part of their vocabulary.
2. *Regulatory*—children realize that language can be used to control their behavior. In turn, children can use language to influence the behavior of other children and adults. The regulatory function takes the form of rules stated in words.
3. *Interactional*—children use language to organize and define relationships with other people (for example, defining a make-believe playmate's role).
4. *Personal*—children who practice the use of language gain an awareness of individuality.
5. *Heuristic*—children discover a dimension of reality (for example, asking a question in a certain way will get desired results).
6. *Imaginative*—children can use language in pretend play, games, and with combinations of real and made-up words.
7. *Representational*—children can use language to represent certain aspects of reality. Through the use of representative language, children develop a system of mutually understood symbols that facilitates communication with others.

By 6 years of age, when the child enters first grade, the child's vocabulary approaches 3000 words. Children in kindergarten and first grade use words as tools to explore the social environment of school. Additional improvements in the child's speech patterns develop as a result of the linguistic stimuli produced by television and other informal teaching media.

The increase in vocabulary is significant because words aid the child in moving away from egocentricity. Three- and four-year-old children in particular use the names of objects to make inferences about the world. Their inferences can

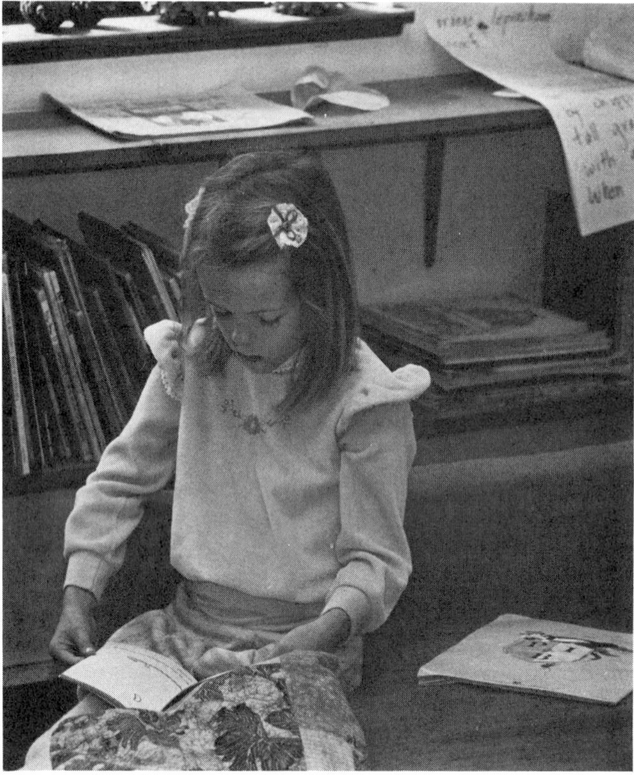

In middle childhood, the environment affects the child's developing use of language.

result in their making connections between objects and actions. Thus, a dog becomes a "bow wow" and a cow a "moo moo." Naming itself, however, is a stimulus for learning. A study conducted by Weir and Stevenson (1959) on 3-, 5-, 7-, and 9-year-old children suggested that children are more successful in learning to distinguish among various kinds of objects if they are taught to name the objects. The children in this study were trained to perform a task that required them to discriminate between correct and incorrect members of paired pictures of animals. Children in the experimental group also were instructed to say the name of the animal before they selected a picture. The children in the control group received the same training but were not requested to say the animal's name. After the children had attained the same level of success at the task, they were given similar but more complicated sets of problems to perform. Results indicated that the children who had been asked to verbalize performed more successfully.

Parents in particular, but also other significant adults and peers, influence the type of words their children use. Researchers have observed that in families where parent–child interactions were characterized by the parent's verbalizations about objects rather than feelings or relationships, the child's language also reflected the parent's emphasis. Moreover, parents adjust their speech to their children's in their choice of topics and length of utterances (Moerk, 1976), and they adapt their use of language to their children's performance and achievement levels.

The educational level and socioeconomic status of the parents is reflected in their speech. Children from better educated and advantaged families are more likely to have a larger vocabulary and be more fluent in expressing themselves. Children adapt the speech patterns of their environment, not only their geographic surroundings but also their social surroundings. The speech patterns and words chosen when speaking to adults often are less casual and quite different from those used when conversing with peers.

Children who live in a bilingual environment usually speak one language at home and English at school. In some European countries two or more languages are learned by everyone. Some educators debate whether the child is confused by having to learn two words and grammatic forms for everything, or if the child benefits from the intellectual stimulation such learning provides. Research with bilingual children in Geneva, Switzerland indicated that language confusion is minimal when children only speak the second language with specific people and at specific places (Dale, 1976). For example, if French is spoken at home with the family and at play with peers and English is spoken only at school, there does not appear to be any delay in acquiring cognitive skills such as reading and writing. Additional research, however, is needed to determine whether there are other cognitive or psychosocial aspects of bilingualism that might influence the child's development (Schuster and Ashburn, 1980).

Moral Development

As children progress through middle childhood, they learn, organize, and internalize the values of significant adults as a basis for decision making. Moral development is a process that involves stimulation from the social environment and transformation of cognitive thought patterns. It is more than the imprinting of rules and virtues from adults to child.

Piaget and Inhelder (1969) observed a heteronomous obedience to rules in children from 4 to 7 years old, as if the rules were sacred and therefore unalterable. Although these children would verbalize an obligation to the rules of a game, they were unable to practice these rules consistently while playing the game. Their egocentricity and limited ability to think abstractly prevented them from applying the rules except by imitation.

For example, while playing a board game, Chris recited the rules exactly. When she noticed that she was behind, however, she changed some of the rules to her advantage. When confronted by her father, she claimed that she and her brother always played the game as she had redefined it. She did not perceive that she was altering the rules.

During middle childhood, the child is primarily self-centered and can consider other people's welfare only if it is personally beneficial. Such children behave in morally acceptable ways in the presence of enforcement agents, but they lack the internal controls necessary to act responsibly when left on their own.

Gradually, as the result of cooperative play and the maturation of cognitive thought processes, children view rules as a code for social behavior rather than laws handed down by some authority. Robert Selman (1976) noted that there is a definite relationship between a child's moral development and the development of perspective-taking abilities. During middle childhood, children usually function at level 1, subjective perspective taking. The child becomes aware that self-perspective is different from another's perspective and thus acquires a new awareness of the thoughts, ideas, feelings, and intentions of others.

With maturation, the child transfers authority from the caregiver to peer group. At this stage, the child conforms to all the rules of the group and assumes an absolute stance when interpreting the rules of the game. The child has a less egocentric understanding of morality and experiences guilt and shame when violating the group norm.

The 7- to 10-year-old, according to Piaget and Inhelder (1969), recognizes that rules are necessary to regulate the game and facilitate fair competition. Rules are no longer viewed as absolute but as flexible according to the situation. Once the rules are agreed on, however, everyone must adhere to them. Children of this age have a very strong sense of justice.

As children become able to take another's perspective, they judge wrong according to intention rather than degree of material damage. They begin to understand that the important difference is whether someone intended to do wrong (cheat, steal, lie) rather than the extent of damage resulting from the act. Prior to 8 years of age, guilt is assigned regardless of motive. As children become able to identify with others, they start to compare intentions. Gradually, their attitudes change, and guilt is defined in terms of intention.

According to Kohlberg (1969), the majority of children during middle childhood operate at the second stage of the preconventional level (see Chapter 6). "Taking care of number one" is the objective of the child at this stage. A wrong act is defined as one that elicits punishment, whereas a correct act is rewarded. The criteria used to determine right or wrong are related to cultural rules, adult responses, and the desire to satisfy the child's own needs. Children do what is expected or requested of them if it is in their own interests. For example, Tommy told his friend on the way to school that the only reason he was going to school that day was because he wanted to play outside after school. Earlier that morning his mother had warned him, when he started complaining about vague aches and pains, that if he did not go to school, he could not play outside after school. Once he heard that ultimatum, Tommy decided it was more advantageous to go to school even though he did not feel like going that particular day.

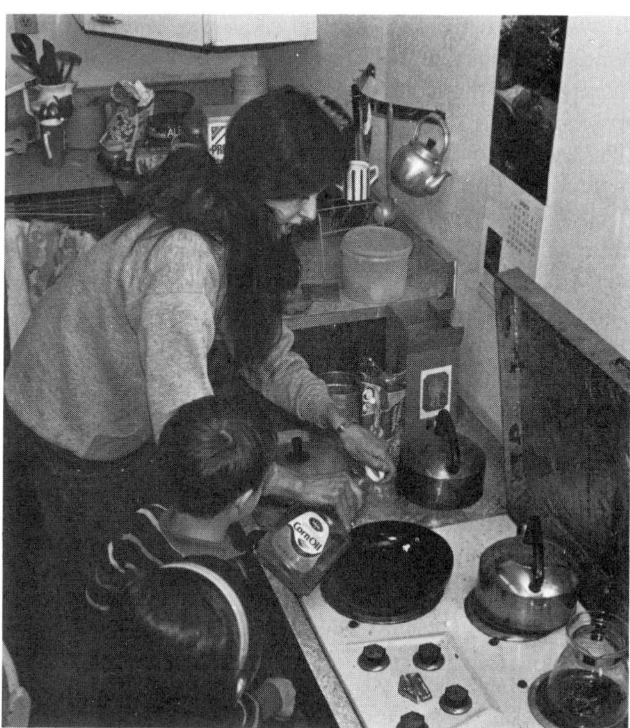

Parents continue to be important agents of socialization as children in middle childhood learn new skills and participate in family functioning.

Preconventional stage 2 is also characterized by the exchange of favors, that is, "Do for me and I will do for you." For example, children bargain and trade with others to obtain a desired object. During recess, one boy who forgot his snack was overheard making a deal to satisfy his hunger. In exchange for a cookie, he offered his friend two baseball cards. Children's motivations for doing right, sharing, and being kind are based on the positive response they receive from others.

Social Development

Havighurst's theory of developmental tasks (see Chapter 6) suggests that the developmental tasks of middle childhood are the result of (1) the thrust of the child out of the home and into the peer group; (2) the thrust of the child into the world of games and work, which requires the acquisition of new muscular skills; and (3) the thrust of the child into the world of adult concepts, logic, symbolism, and communication. Havighurst's theory further suggests that by the end of middle childhood the child has incorporated a unique style and achieved a personal level in all three areas (Havighurst, 1979).

Nine developmental tasks have been identified for the middle childhood period. The first task is mastering the physical skills necessary for ordinary games. To accomplish these tasks, the child must learn physical skills such as throwing and catching, kicking, climbing, swimming, and handling simple tools. Success at these tasks, however, requires that the neuromuscular system reach the corresponding level of maturation. Children learning physical skills are praised by peers when they succeed and ridiculed by them when they fail.

Havighurst's second task is the building of wholesome attitudes toward oneself. Completion of this task leads to a well-balanced personality, good health habits, physical neatness and orderliness, and positive attitudes about one's gender. The child's biophysical development is part of this task because physical growth means that muscles are developing rapidly, permanent teeth are replacing deciduous teeth, and posture is improving. Both peers and adults show approval for the child's developing physique and physical skills.

Havighurst's third task is learning to get along with age-mates. The child with a wholesome self-attitude feels secure enough to establish good relations with peers. Acceptance by peers is crucial to the child's development because it is at this time that the child's dependence begins to shift from parents to peers and community. Moreover, social habits developed during middle childhood provide the basis for future interactions.

The fourth of Havighurst's tasks is learning an appropriate masculine or feminine social role. Even though anatomic differences between boys and girls are not evident until after middle childhood, expectations for sex roles and gender identity form the basis for social behavior. Children imitate sex roles that are expected for their social class.

Developing fundamental skills in reading, writing, and calculating is Havighurst's fifth task. As children in middle childhood refine their fine motor skills, they gradually obtain these skills, although skills development continues through late childhood. Emphasis on skills is influenced by the child's social environment. Middle-class parents are more likely to encourage and support the achievement of a higher level of these skills in their children than are parents of lower-class backgrounds. Parents who have the time and resources might begin teaching their children at home, so that, although schools are responsible for teaching children these skills, many children start school having acquired the basic reading skills.

Developing the abstract concepts necessary for everyday living, such as time space, number, temperature, height, and speed, is Havighurst's sixth task and is related to skills development. Not until the child's brain has reached a particular level of maturation can the child begin to formulate concepts that involve perceptions with some level of abstraction. Concept formulation during middle childhood evolves from the child's real or fantasized experiences, enhanced by cognitive skills. From concepts developed in middle childhood, the child develops a view of the world.

Developing conscience, morality, and a scale of values is Havighurst's seventh task and is clearly connected to moral development. The process of developing a conscience continues from the earlier periods of infancy and early childhood. The child begins to learn right from wrong, good from evil, and happiness from pain. These concepts, generally taught by parents and reinforced by other authority figures, provide the basis for the child's developing moral conduct and a system of values that will guide future ethical decisions.

In achieving personal independence, Havighurst's eighth task, the child begins to learn that adults (parents and teachers) are not infallible and can be wrong at times. Although this process continues throughout all stages of development, children in middle childhood begin to think of themselves as future adults, making decisions about activities to perform around the home, books to read, games to play, and those with whom to play. They gradually spend longer periods away from home and might, for example, spend a night with a friend. At a relatively early stage, American children are encouraged to develop personal independence. Parents with high expectations for achievement tend to expect their children to grow up fast, get ahead, be alert, and take the initiative.

In middle childhood the child also develops attitudes toward social groups and institutions, Havighurst's ninth developmental task. Children learn attitudes by imitating people whom they believe to have prestige and associating simple, deeply emotional, pleasant or unpleasant experiences with given objects or situations.

Attitudes toward religious, social, political, and economic groups are formed after the child starts interacting with the world outside the family. Such attitudes are an outgrowth of experiences with the family, teachers, and peers and knowledge gained from movies, radio, television, books, and the larger community.

Younger children (4–6 years of age) have a global, undifferentiated concept of their religious identity. They group people as either religious or not religious, based on whether or not they go to church. It is as if God makes people of different denominations as well as of different skin colors (Elkind, 1978). The child's knowledge of religion is a combination of what significant others have said and personally formulated and imagined ideas and descriptions. These descriptions often relate to a concrete object. For example, when asked to describe or draw a picture of God, children frequently will equate Him with their grandfather or an elderly friend.

The 7- and 8-year-old is able to distinguish religious fact from fantasy. Ideas about religion in this age group are based on concrete, objective experiences. They take on characteristic beliefs and observances that symbolize their religion such as baptism, communion, attendance at church or synagogue, and observance of feast or holy days.

Fowler and Keen (1978) noted, however, that although children expressed a more orderly, concrete view of the world, they had a private, speculative fantasy view also.

They drew on this fantasy world to explain abstract concepts such as evil and events such as death. Events beyond their understanding were rationalized by assigning them to "God's power," creating a mythic, powerful character, or expanding on an idea about space or UFOs seen on television or at the movie theater. The child is able increasingly to make sense out of the world but must rely on concrete experiences to do so.

Integrating Development Through Play

Middle childhood is a transitional time in which the child has gained basic gross and fine motor skills and is now in the process of perfecting these skills; language is now used as a tool; and although language is initially limited to speech, the child at the end of this phase has learned the significance of written words.

During this time, children participate in cooperative play as they explore their environments and learn about their cultures. Their play becomes more realistic and complex. They enact roles with greater detail and accuracy through sociodramatic play, which in turn allows the child to resolve conflicts, fill in gaps of understanding, change roles or power structures, change outcomes, or invent new problems to solve. This is a time of increased peer interaction and the challenge of learning to get along with others both in pairs and in groups. Cognitive skills are developing, and the child is entering a transitional phase of thinking. Gradually, the limitations of preoperational thought are giving way to an increased awareness of objects, their transformations, and their reversibility. Numbers and letters become meaningful as they also become useful. Games with rules are increasingly important because they lend order and structure to play and provide a neutral means of settling arguments.

Play in middle childhood is both associative and cooperative. Children learn to share, borrow, and lend toys, and they eventually learn to cooperate with three or four people in a highly organized way. Play also contributes to the refinement of gross and fine motor skills and sensory and spatial perception, the release of emotional tension, the positive imitation of powerful others, and the development of leader and follower skills. Favorite games include tag, hide-and-seek, jump rope, rhythmic games such as ring-around-the-rosy and farmer-in-the-dell, follow-the-leader, red-rover, and fruit-basket upset. Their improved fine motor coordination enables them to manipulate objects such as clay, models, paints, small construction blocks, and needle and thread. From initially exploring the possibilities with these objects, they advance to the satisfactory completion of their project. At first, the clay might be pounded and rolled into a simple ball or snake, but eventually the child learns to make a bowl, basket, seal, or dog with the clay. Likewise, the threaded needle is first pulled in and out of the cloth haphazardly. Then a design is made on the cloth and the child carefully follows the outline, creating a picture with the stitching.

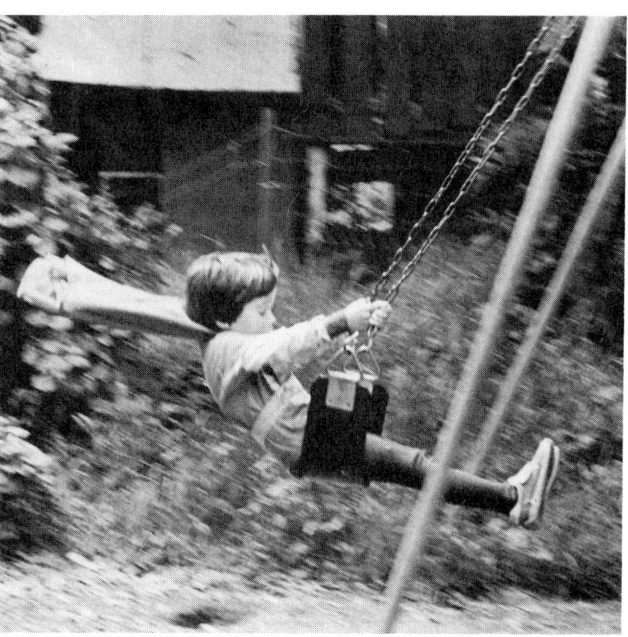

Play in middle childhood contributes to the development of motor skills while providing the child with an outlet for fantasy.

Symbolic play, in which symbolic thought is used to simulate reality, is a significant part of middle childhood. Ideas, rather than features of objects, govern the child's thinking about a particular toy. Aided by fantasy and imaginary playmates, 4- and 5-year-old children are capable of creating realms of play from a single object just by pretending. The discarded appliance box becomes a fort, clubhouse, or spaceship according to the group's desire. Once the game is decided, roles are assigned, and children imitate and create actions to correspond to their role's expected performance.

Although a few games with rules are mastered by 4½ years of age, the ability to master games with complex rules rarely occurs before 7 years of age. Parents who foster inner controls in their children provide a supportive environment for their children's play activities. Children want to win and experience intense emotions in game situations. Parents who help their children put into perspective the short-term consequences of a game versus long-term friendships and lessons learned from being a good loser help prepare them for life experiences. Play facilitates the important developmental tasks of learning to cope with defeat, controlling one's emotions, and praising another's skills.

With adequate reinforcement for independent mastery during middle childhood, the child learns to internalize two crucial systems: a self-reward system and a system of standards. The self-reward system allows children to praise and reinforce themselves for successes, and children also internalize the standards of the socializing agents who have rewarded or punished them. As the internalization process occurs, the need for and dependence on external social reinforcement decreases (Harter, 1981).

Health Care Needs of Middle Childhood

Hygiene

The 4½-year-old child shows beginning competence in self-care, which is continually refined during middle childhood. By time children reach 6 years of age, they are toilet trained and perform the activities associated with toileting, that is, manipulating their clothing, wiping themselves, flushing the toilet, and washing their hands. The female child should be taught to wipe from front to back (toward the rectum) after urination and defecation to decrease the possibility of introducing bacteria into the vagina or urethra.

At this age, children may be too busy with play to perform self-care activities, and parental monitoring is therefore essential. Parents must ensure that children caring for themselves properly wash their hands, face, ears, and body when taking baths; however, children should not be expected to give themselves complete baths until they are 7 years old. Children can dress and undress themselves when their clothing is simple and at 7 years of age can graduate to combing their hair.

Parental guidance aids children in self-care activities. Left alone, the child will wear the same clothing repeatedly. Therefore, the selection of clothing appropriate for activity and weather requires parental assistance. A child of this age can change clothes at will, but if unsupervised, the child will leave clothes wherever they were removed. This requires frequent reminders from the parent to return clothes to their correct location.

Sleep and Rest

Children in middle childhood require about 12 hours of sleep per night, particularly during the school year. Failure to obtain adequate sleep can lead the child to daytime irritability, fatigue, poor attention span, and poor learning. The 4½- to 6-year-old might still require a daytime nap or quiet period to restore their energy levels.

Most children in this age range dislike bedtime. They might be immersed in play or television, or they might use stalling tactics to keep from going to bed. The parent can help the child prepare for bed by setting a time limit for the child and assisting the child to meet it by issuing reminders as the time approaches for bed, enabling the child to conclude activities gradually; incorporating relaxing activities such as stories, religious readings, prayers, and loving, affectionate confidences; selecting appropriate television shows that do not introduce excessive stressors; and restricting games that may be too stimulating.

Just as children need time to prepare for bed, they also need time to prepare for the start of the day's activities. Upon wakening, children usually are still very sleepy and stumble around before they are fully awake. Therefore, children should be awakened early and given adequate time to get ready for the day without being rushed.

Nutrition

As children grow, their nutritional requirements change. Requirements per unit of body weight decrease while total intake increases. The 5-year-old requires about 90 calories/kg of body weight, whereas the 8-year-old needs about 80 calories/kg of body weight.

Growth in this age group is slow and steady. Children need a nutritional intake that will facilitate growth and development to meet the basal metabolic needs and keep the body functioning at an optimal level, meet the body's growth needs, allow for cellular growth, meet cellular replacement needs, and meet cellular repair needs (Schuster and Ashburn, 1980).

By the time the child reaches middle childhood, nutritional patterns and habits have been formed and are strongly associated with cultural and socioeconomic identification. For example, in Puerto Rican families red beans are a common source of protein, whereas rice and fish provide protein for Vietnamese children. Several studies have shown positive correlations between the child's socioeconomic status and height and weight. Children from families with fewer economic resources or less education tend to be shorter and leaner.

Because the focus for children in middle childhood is play, they are little interested in spending time at the table eating. They frequently use their fingers to pick food up off their plates, stuffing it in their mouths, and swallowing without thoroughly chewing. They talk with their mouths full of food and at times cause accidents. At breakfast, they eat in a hurry and sometimes rush off without completing the meal. Lunch may be served in school or brought from home, but the child frequently is free to select what to eat. The 6- and 7-year-old can select food from vending machines.

Recognizing that the child in this age group is extremely active, parents should refrain from imposing too rigid an environment at mealtime. It is important to balance teaching the child table manners with promoting a healthy atmosphere conducive to eating. The child also should be taught to select nutritious snacks, including fresh and dried fruits, vegetables, cheese, peanut butter, nuts, and granola. Snacks high in refined sugar should be avoided. Between 4¼ and 8 years of age close parental monitoring of nutrition is crucial. Children need continuous nutritional supervision to obtain the right nutrients and in the proper amounts so that excess weight does not become a problem.

Dentition

Oral hygiene is part of the child's daily needs. Toothbrushing helps to remove bacteria, carbohydrates, and other leftover food materials from the teeth. If these residues are not removed, plaque forms in the child's mouth. The two methods of oral hygiene for this age period are brushing and flossing the teeth.

Using a medium-bristle toothbrush, the child should brush the teeth immediately after eating both meals and snacks. When this is not practical, the child should be taught to "swish and swallow" as an alternative to brushing after eating. The technique consists of taking mouthfuls of water and swishing it around and through the teeth to remove excess food particles from the mouth. Not until they reach approximately 9 years of age can children fully master the technique of flossing, so flossing during middle childhood should be performed by parents. Dental floss should be placed between the teeth in areas where the toothbrush cannot reach. Flossing should be done at least once per day (at bedtime).

Self-care activities must be promoted if children are to develop proper dental health, but until they are able to manipulate a toothbrush adequately, parents must brush their teeth for them. The selection of a toothbrush and dentifrices are important aspects of oral hygiene and should not be underplayed. When teaching oral hygiene, the parent should emphasize the frequency of brushing and the role carbohydrates play in the development of dental caries. Appointments with the dentist should be made every 6 months to ensure that dentition is following a normal course and to assess any need for corrective work.

Children are somewhat anxious and fearful about dentists. Parents can promote a positive attitude about a trip to the dentist, so that children will be more relaxed. Parents also can monitor their children's diets to ensure adequate intakes of calcium and vitamin D, which are necessary for the calcification of teeth.

One of the most striking biophysical changes occurring during middle childhood is the process of replacing deciduous (baby) teeth with permanent teeth. This process begins at about 5 years of age, and unless children are prepared, the experience can be very frightening. Once prepared, children view the experience very positively because they associate it with receiving gifts from the "tooth fairy" and because it indicates that they are finally beginning to enter the adult world.

The first permanent teeth erupt when the child is between 5 and 7 years of age. The new central incisors usually appear much too large for the child's mouth and face, but as nasomaxillary and mandibular growth continue, the child assumes a more adult face to accommodate the permanent teeth. Teeth tend to erupt a few months earlier in girls than in boys. Cultural factors also play a crucial role in determining when children cut their first permanent teeth. For example, American children get their first incisors at about 6.5 years of age, children from Ghana at 5.3 years of age, and children in Hong Kong at 6.2 years of age.

Malocclusion in middle childhood occurs when the upper and lower teeth do not meet properly in the horizontal or vertical position. As a result, the child's normal chewing and biting are impaired. A National Health Examination Survey of children between 6 and 11 years of age reported that about two-thirds of children have normal occlusion. Fourteen percent of the remaining one-third of children had problems related to appearance, chewing, or speech (Kilman and Helpin, 1983). For the child in this age group, malocclusion develops from three major sources: oral habits, tooth crowding, and trauma. Oral habits are mainly thumb and finger sucking that continue after the eruption of permanent teeth. Crowding, which starts when the child is between 5 and 6 years of age, occurs when the new permanent teeth crowd out the remaining primary teeth. This situation should be monitored closely by a dentist. It might be temporary and disappear with growth and elongation of the maxilla and mandible. If crowding persists, braces might be necessary. Another dental concern during middle childhood is crossbite, that is, the lower teeth crossing over the upper teeth when the mouth is closed. This condition usually necessitates braces early, before the bones of the maxilla are fused. The braces stretch the upper jaw until the bite is corrected. Good oral hygiene is essential with braces, and gum, toffee, and caramels are forbidden.

Exercise

Children in middle childhood are constantly on the move. Exercising influences normal growth and increases the size of bones and the degree of mineralization. The child's cardiovascular, skeletal, and neuromuscular systems benefit from maximum physical activity. The child needs space to run, jump, and skip and needs freedom from parental restriction to exercise.

Even so, the play activities of children in middle childhood must be monitored. Because these children are so energetic and always willing to play, they do not always recognize their own capacities and will play continually unless asked to take breaks. The child who fails to take breaks and allow the body to reenergize can become overtired and exhausted. The 6-year-old is goal oriented and will use energy to complete specific tasks. The 7-year-old is conservative and will plan games that permit periods of sitting and resting. Unless children are assigned rest periods, they will not normally rest on their own. Parents should learn to recognize cues of fatigue or irritability before overexertion occurs.

Safety

Safety is important for children of all age groups (see Chapter 19). During middle childhood, children begin to spend more time away from home, thereby diminishing available parental supervision. Children are also more active than in earlier years; they are more daring and adventurous and hence are exposed to more hazards.

Parents have support systems to help in providing safety for children, including crossing guards, police, firefighters, and older children. In school, children are instructed on safety in preparation for interaction with the external environment, but parents do need to reinforce these instructions routinely with their children.

Six- and seven-year-olds love to ride bicycles. They use bicycles both for play and for errands. Parents must instruct them on the rules to be followed when riding in the streets with other vehicles. Children must be confined to safe areas. Safety instructions for bicycle riders should include the dangers of carrying another passenger on the bicycle and the importance of stopping at street signs, looking in both directions before crossing the street or coming out from behind a parked car, crossing at street signs, and not riding the bicycle on busy streets.

Children in this age range also should be cautioned about using drugs from unmarked bottles or without reading labels. They should not be permitted to use drugs without parental guidance. Parents should not transfer medications out of original bottles and should keep all medications out of children's reach. In case of an emergency, parents should have in a handy location a list of antidotes and the telephone numbers of the pediatrician and/or emergency room of the nearest hospital and the regional poison control center (see Chapter 20).

Children in middle childhood should not be left unsupervised when swimming. Children should be given the do's and don'ts about playing in the water and should be instructed about water safety measures. Children enjoy climbing trees, but when climbing a tree, the child should inspect each branch before proceeding on it. Young branches and dead branches break easily and are dangerous. Electrical poles, water towers, wire fences, and other structures are dangerous, and the child should be taught to avoid them.

Guns are also dangerous and should be kept in a locked place and out of a child's reach. Ammunition should never be kept in the firearm. Parents cannot be with children to protect them at all times and must therefore teach safety practices so that children can avoid the pitfalls themselves. If faced with a dangerous situation, children should have the knowledge to make wise decisions.

Transition to Late Childhood

The theme of middle childhood is the child's movement from the family to peers and community, along with growth toward independence and responsibility for self-care and decision making. New skills, maturing cognitive structures, and orientation toward others mark the child's emergence from egocentricity toward taking another's perspective. The child now is less imaginative and able to separate reality from fantasy. Answers to questions that were illogical but satisfactory no longer make sense. Advances in cognitive thought motivate the child to find more logical, rational answers to questions about everyday reality.

The child's venture into the world of school results in meeting new friends, learning new concepts, and exploring new surroundings. The child learns to communicate through the written word as well as the spoken one. Stories are created and written and adventures and fantasies are read and then shared with others.

Physical skills and coordination improve during this stage and prepare the child for more serious competition. The social and emotional skills that are learned also prepare the child for smooth interaction with others.

For each child a unique set of genetic and environmental factors combine to foster development. During middle childhood, children learn more about their culture, religion, values, and socioeconomic status, as well as those of other groups. Supportive adults who take the time to answer children's many questions will encourage open, honest curiosity and an eagerness and pleasure in learning throughout life.

Key Concepts

- Middle childhood is characterized by the child's movement from the home and family as a primary resource to that of school, peers, and community.
- The family remains critical, although its role has changed to one of behind-the-scenes support.
- Children gain new insights and understanding about their culture, ethnicity, and values as well as those of others with whom they play and attend school.
- Children learn that society has certain expectations for behavior and role performance, many of which are gender stereotyped.

- The peer group becomes an increasingly important influence, and friends are chosen on the basis of similar interests rather than physical proximity.
- Physical growth slows during middle childhood. The long bones continue to grow, which gives the child a more adultlike appearance.
- Primary teeth are lost and replaced by permanent teeth.
- Gross motor skills are perfected and used in combination for games, advanced skills, and competition.
- Fine motor skills are refined, and the child uses these skills in writing, model building, crafts, and projects.
- Personality characteristics are fairly well established during this developmental phase. Self-concept continues to be developed as a result of social interaction with a wider spectrum of people.
- Fears relate more to performance at school and play than to personal safety.
- At the beginning of middle childhood, the child is egocentric and possesses limited cognitive thought structures. By the end of this stage, the child is able to take another's perspective.
- The advance in cognitive skills is related to increased attention and improved memory.
- The child internalizes roles, values, expectations of behavior, and an understanding of right and wrong and good and evil from the words and actions of significant adults.
- Initially, the child does right (follows rules) for fear of punishment or desire of reward; with increased understanding and experience, the child views rules as social organizers to ensure justice.
- Moral and faith development continue to be linked to concrete experience and the imitation of others.
- Play takes on more organization, and games involve groups. Competition between teams is introduced. Gross and fine motor skills and social interaction behaviors of sharing, coping with disappointment, and controlling emotions are developed through play.
- Games that mix fantasy and reality remain popular, but now the children know where one leaves off and the other begins.
- Self-care activities related to hygiene, dress, nutrition, rest, and exercise increase as the child becomes more independent and spends more time away from home.
- Children need to be taught how to select nutritious foods and to practice safety rules when walking, bicycling, and swimming.

References

Bandura A, Walters R: *Social Learning and Personality Development.* Holt, Rinehart & Winston, 1963.

Baratz J: Teaching reading in an urban Negro school system. In: *Language and Poverty.* Williams F (editor). Markam, 1973.

Barry H, Child IL, Bacon MK: Relation of child training to subsistence economy. *Am Anthropol* 1959; 61:51–63.

Baumrind D: Socialization and instrumental competence in young children. In: *The Young Child.* Vol. 2. Hartup WW (editor). Washington, DC: National Association for the Education of Young Children, 1972.

Bronfenbrenner U: *Influences on Human Development.* Dryden Press, 1972.

Brophy JE, Good TL: Teacher's communication of differential expectations for children's classroom performance: Some behavioral data. *J Educat Psychol* 1970; 61:365–374.

Chess S, Thomas A: Temperament and the parent–child interaction. *Pediatr Ann* 1977; 6:26–45.

Cohen S: Early childhood. In: *Human Development.* Lugo JO, Hershey GL (editors). Macmillan, 1974.

Comstock GA: The impact of television on American institutions. *J Communication* (Spring) 1978; 28:12–18.

Coopersmith S: *The Antecedents of Self-Esteem.* Freeman, 1967.

Corbin CB: *A Textbook of Motor Development.* 2nd ed. Brown, 1980.

Dale P: *Language Development: Structure and Function.* Holt, Rinehart & Winston, 1976.

Dudek S: Creating in young children—attitude or ability. *J Creative Behav* 1974; 8(4):282–292.

Dunn J, Kendrick C: *Siblings: Love, Envy and Understanding.* Harvard University Press, 1982.

Durio HF: Mental imagery and creativity. *J Creative Behav* 1975; 9(4):233–244.

Edwards E: Kindergarten is too late. *Sat Rev* (June 15) 1968; 68–80.

Elkind D: *The Child's Reality: Three Developmental Themes.* Erlbaum, 1978.

Erikson E: *Childhood and Society.* Norton, 1963.

Feshbach ND: Reinforcement patterns in children. In: *Minnesota Symposium on Child Psychology* Vol 7. Pick A (editor). University of Minnesota Press, 1973.

Fischer KW, Lazerson A: *Human Development.* Freeman, 1984.

Fowler J, Keen S: *Life Maps.* Word Books, 1978.

Fraiberg S: *The Magic Years.* Scribner, 1959.

Freud S: *The Complete Psychoanalytic Works of Sigmund Freud.* Norton, 1969.

Gelman R: Cognitive development. *Annu Rev Psychol* 1978; 29:297–332.

Guilford JP: *The Nature of Human Intelligence.* McGraw-Hill, 1967.

Harter S: Developmental perspectives on the self-system. In: *Carmichael's Manual of Child Psychology*. Vol IV. Hetherington EM (editor). Wiley, 1982.

Harter S: A model of mastery motivation in children: Individual differences and developmental change. In: *Minnesota Symposium on Child Psychology*. Vol 14. Collins, WA (editor). Erlbaum, 1981.

Havighurst RJ: *Developmental Tasks and Education*. McKay, 1979.

Holm VA: *"Childhood" in The Biologic Ages of Man*. Smith DW, Bierman EL, Robinson NM (editors). Saunders, 1978.

Holtzman WH, Diaz-Guerrero R, Schwarz, JD: *Personality Development in Two Cultures: Cross-Cultural and Longitudinal Study of School Children in Mexico and the United States*. University of Texas Press, 1975.

Jersild AT: *Child Psychology*. Prentice-Hall, 1975.

Johnson TR, Moore WM, Jeffries JE (editors). *Children Are Different: Developmental Physiology*. Ross Laboratories, 1978.

Kagan J, Moss HA: *Birth to Maturity*. Wiley, 1962.

Kagan S, Madsen MC: Experimental analysis of cooperation and competition of Anglo-American and Mexican children. *Develop Psychol* 1972; 6:49–59.

Kay P: The imaginary companion. Review of the Literature. *Matern Child Nurs J* (Spring) 1980; 9:8–11.

Kenny SL: Developmental discontinuities in childhood and adolescence. In: *Levels and Transitions in Children's Development* (New Directions for Child Development, No 21). Jossey-Bass, 1983.

Kilman C, Helpin ML: Recognizing dental malocclusion in children. *Pediatr Nurs* 1983; May/June:204–208.

Kittrell E: Children and television: The electronic fix. *Child Today* (May–June) 1978; 7:20–37.

Kohlberg L: A cognitive-developmental analysis of children's sex-role concepts and attitudes. In: *The Development of Sex Differences*. Maccoby EE (editor). Stanford University Press, 1966.

Kohlberg L: Stage and sequence: The cognitive-developmental approach to socialization. In: *Handbook of Socialization: Theory and Research*. Goslin D (editor). Rand McNally, 1969.

Labinowicz E: *The Piaget Primer*. Addison-Wesley, 1980.

Lamb ME: *Social and Personality Development*. Holt, Rinehart & Winston, 1978.

Londe S, et al: Blood pressure and hypertension in children: Studies, problems, and perspectives. In: *Juvenile Hypertension*. Neal MI, Levine LS (editors). Raven, 1977.

Lowrey GH: *Growth and Development of Children*. Year Book, 1978.

Mitchell S: Imaginary companions: Friend or foe. *Pediatr Nurs* 1980; 6(6):29–30.

Moerck EL: Process of language teaching and training in the interactions of mother–child dyads. *Child Develop* 1976; 47:1064–1078.

Piaget J: *Child and Reality*. Grossman, 1973.

Piaget J, Inhelder B: *The Psychology of the Child*. Basic Books, 1969.

Pulaski M: *Understanding Piaget*. Harper & Row, 1971.

Rapp R: Family and class in contemporary America. In: *Rethinking the Family*. Thorne B, Yalom M (editors). Longman, 1982.

Rosenthal R: The Pygmalion effect lives. *Psychol Today* (September) 1973; 7:56–58.

Santrock JW: *Life-Span Development*. Brown, 1983.

Schiamberg LB, Smith KU: *Human Development*. Macmillan, 1982.

Schuster CS, Ashburn SS: *The Process of Human Development*. Little, Brown, 1980.

Sears R, Maccoby E, Levin H: *Patterns of Childrearing*. Harper & Row, 1957.

Selman R: A developmental approach to interpersonal and moral awareness in young children: Some education implications of levels of social perspective-taking. In: *Values and Moral Development*. Thomas C, Hennessy SJ (editors). Paulist Press, 1976.

Selman RL, Selman AP: Children's ideas about friendship: A new theory. *Psychol Today* (October) 1979; 9:71–80.

Silver GA: *Child Health, America's Future*. Aspen, 1978.

Smart MS, Smart RC: *Children: Development and Relationships*. Macmillan, 1977.

Sutton-Smith B, Rosenberg BG: *The Sibling*. Holt, Rinehart & Winston, 1970.

Trabasso T: The role of memory as a system in making transitive inferences. In: *Perspectives on the Development of Memory and Cognition*. Kall RV Jr, Hagen JW (editors). Erlbaum, 1977.

Watson RI, Lindgren HC: *Psychology of the Child and the Adolescent*. Macmillan, 1979.

Weir MW, Stevenson HW: The effects of verbalization in children's learning as a function of chronological age. *Child Develop* 1959; 36:173–178.

Additional Readings

Albinson JG, Andrew GM: *Child in Sport and Physical Activity*. University Park Press, 1976.

Bandura A: *Social Learning Theory*. Prentice-Hall, 1977.

Bigelow B, LaGaipa J: Children's written descriptions of friendship: A multidimensional analysis. *Devel Psychol* 1975; 2(6):857–858.

Birren JE, et al: *Developmental Psychology*. Houghton Mifflin, 1981.

Bordzinsky D: Sex differences in children's expression and control of fantasy and overt aggression. Child Develop 1979; 50(2):372–379.

Bullock M, Gelmen R: Preschool children's assumptions about cause and effect: Temporal ordering. *Child Develop* 1979; 50(1):89–96.

Chomsky N: *Language and Mind*. Harcourt Brace Jovanovich, 1968.

Coles R: *Children of Crisis*. Dell, 1967.

Coles R: *Privileged Ones*. Little, Brown, 1977.

Crain W: *Theories of Development*. Prentice-Hall, 1980.

Fishbach H, Lewis S, Keiffer R: Children's understanding of perspectives. *Develop Psychol* 1972; 1(1):21–33.

Flavell J: *The Developmental Psychology of Jean Piaget*. Van Nostrand, 1965.

Garvey C: *Play*. Harvard University Press, 1977.

Gibbs JC: Kohlberg's stages of moral judgment: A constructive critique. *Harvard Educat Rev* 1977; 47(1):43–61.

Goodnow J: *Children's Drawing*. Harvard University Press, 1977.

Mitchell C, Ault R: Reflection, impulsivity and the evaluation process. *Child Develop* 1979; 50(4):1043–1049.

Moore K: Childhood enuresis. *Can Nurse* (March) 1984; 80:38–42.

Murphy LB, Moriarity AE: *Vulnerability, Coping and Growth*. Yale University Press, 1976.

Mussen PH, Conger J, Kogen J: *Child Development and Personality*. Harper & Row, 1974.

Nelson K: Concept, word and sentence: Interrelations in acquisition and development. *Psychol Rev* 1974; 81:267–285.

Piaget J: *The Child's Conception of Physical Causality*. Harcourt Brace Jovanovich, 1930.

Piaget J: *Play, Dreams, and Imitation in Childhood*. Norton, 1962.

Rubin Z: *Children's Friendships*. Harvard University Press, 1980.

Schell RE, Hall E: *Developmental Psychology Today*. Random House, 1983.

Shatz M, Gelman R: The development of communication skills: Modification in the speech of young children as a function of the listener. *Monogr Soc Res Child Dev* 1973; 38:152.

Tauber M: Parental socialization techniques and sex differences in children's play. *Child Dev* 1979; 50(1):225–234.

Tulkin SR, Kagan J: Mother–child interaction in the first year of life. *Child Develop* 1972; 43:31–41.

Late Childhood

10

Maureen de Maio Ellen Shuzman Sandra R. Mott

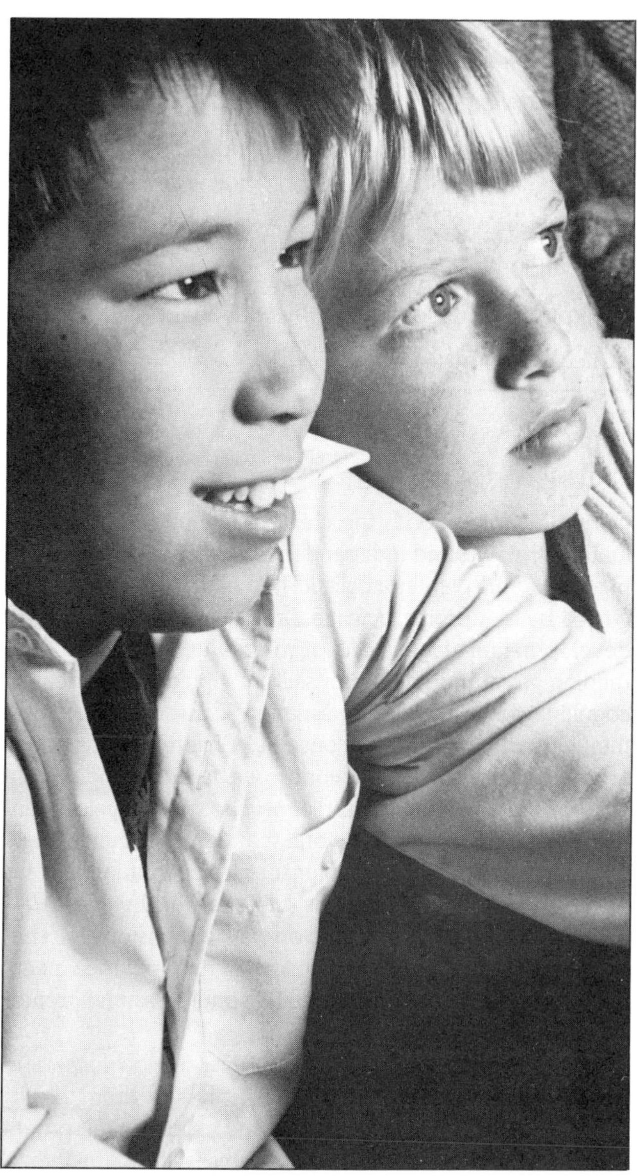

Chapter Outline

continued on next page

Objectives

- Explain the influences of both suprasystems and subsystems on late childhood development.
- Define the major parameters of late childhood development.
- Explain the essential biophysical changes that occur in late childhood.
- Describe the principal components of personality, cognitive, language, moral, and social development in late childhood.
- Explain the purpose of play in late childhood.
- Identify the basic health care needs of children in late childhood.

During late childhood, the child's experiences are accentuated by newfound independence and the ability to solve problems and plan strategies. The child's world is characterized by friendships, activities, and new experiences. This developmental stage is one of mastering, integrating, and refining gross and fine motor skills, coupled with increased cognitive powers involving seriation, conservation, logical thinking, and space–time concepts. Children in this phase are more oriented to the world outside the home. These children consolidate their earlier psychosocial development with their present world, a world that becomes increasingly diverse and complex as they encounter new situations and people with differing opinions, attitudes, and values. Parents, teachers, and peers take on new dimensions for children during this time. Parents lose their omnipotence, peers become more important, and other adults assume greater influence.

In late childhood the child lives in a world of ups and downs, and transitions occur frequently and dramatically. From about 8 to 12 years of age, the child's development is a continuous, complex process. This is a dynamic, exuberant period in which the child moves away from being mostly dependent on the home and family and toward entering the world of adolescence.

Most significant in this process is the growing influence of school and peer groups in shaping the child's development. In this chapter, we examine the pervasive effect of these suprasystems on the child's personality, cognitive, moral, and social development. We consider the biophysical changes and health care needs that characterize late childhood, and we discuss the function of play in integrating and enhancing the many aspects of development at this stage.

Developmental Changes in Late Childhood

Influences of the Suprasystems

Family The family continues to be an important source of influence, comfort, and support for the child in late childhood. Parenting and the reciprocal relationship developed between the parent and child remains fairly stable (Kagan and Moss, 1962). Although the basic relationships continue, the child's need for attention decreases, and parents find themselves moved to the background and mainly giving guidance and support, monitoring activities, and providing assistance when requested. Parents are accepted as participants in family activities but not in peer group activities.

By 8 years of age, children no longer think of their parents as omnipotent. These children have been exposed to other perspectives, are more equipped cognitively to make decisions, are more independent, and view their parents more realistically. They will ask their parents for advice or help with homework problems or a project, but they do not appreciate it if parents try to do the work for them. Relations between parent and child become delicate and complicated. Parents often comment that they never know when to help or how much assistance to give. The 8-year-old is torn between wanting parental advice but being unable to tolerate criticism or suggestions. It takes patience and tact to gain the child's confidence during this struggle to develop a sense of industry and accomplishment. The 10-year-old is able to tolerate constructive criticism and may be self-critical. At this age, children are more independent and responsible for themselves and for completing their projects. They are also more respectful of their parents' knowledge and abilities.

As children demonstrate increased maturity and independence, their parents' expectations usually increase. Assigned chores might become more numerous, complicated, or time consuming. Family responsibilities and peer activities may conflict, necessitating difficult decisions. For example, a 12-year-old boy was given the job of splitting and stacking some wood for the wood-burning stove used to heat the house. His friends were going sledding and urged him to join them. Although the snow was perfect for sledding and he had the fastest sled in the neighborhood, this boy knew that if the wood was not split, his house would not be warm. Difficult decisions such as this become more frequent during late childhood.

Family composition can change during this period. A new sibling might be born, an elderly grandparent move in, the parents separate or divorce, or one parent dies. Family roles sometimes change if the mother begins working outside the home or if a parent goes to school or changes jobs. How well children adapt to these changes depends on how well they are prepared, whether they are included in family discussions, and their ability to understand the reasons for the change. Once children are able to consider alternative points of view, they can perceive and respond to the needs and attitudes of others. For example, in one family the father decided to change careers, which meant that he had to return to school. Family discussions were held during the decision-making period, and the children were encouraged to voice their opinions, questions, and concerns. Although initially angry about the plan because it necessitated moving and a change in life-style, the 9-year-old and 11-year-old children were able to understand their father's reasoning and future goals, to place the decision within a realistic time perspective, and look for the positive aspects of the plan.

Children whose parents separate or divorce during this developmental period seem to cope better with the experience than do younger children. Conflict, hurt, and confusion exist, especially during the first painful year or two following the separation; however, children at this age do not experience the strong sense of guilt and responsibility that younger children feel. The increase in cognitive and perspective-taking abilities enable the 8- to 12-year-old child to view the process more realistically, resolve feelings of loyalty, and assign responsibility more objectively (Wallerstein and Kelly, 1980). The end of conflict between the parents and the provision of adequate support systems, both financial and emotional, appear to be key factors in how well children cope with divorce. One study found that children living in a harmonious single-parent family functioned better than children living in a conflict-laden nuclear family. The presence or absence of conflict appears to be

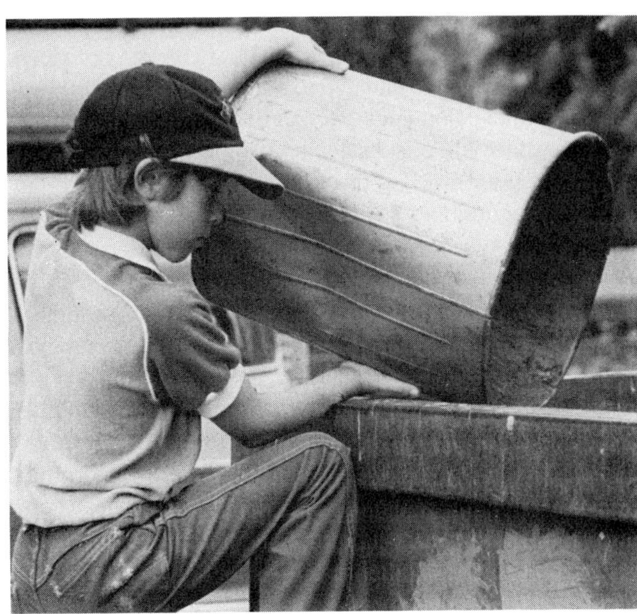

In late childhood, children are able to assume some responsibility for family chores.

a more critical variable than family composition in the child's ability to interact with others, accept responsibility, and cope with stress (Hetherington, Cox, and Cox, 1978).

Many studies have examined the relationship between the patterns of parenting and the child's self-concept (Baumrind, 1965; Coopersmith, 1967). Self-confident and independent children usually have parents who are warm, supportive, directive, trusting, minimally punitive, and who provide opportunities for autonomy and responsibility. Dependent children with low self-confidence frequently have parents who are restrictive, punitive, fearful, aloof, and who provide few opportunities for autonomy or experimentation (Yanni, 1982). The foundation parents provide for their children's experiences in greater society and continuing parental support are key factors in the child's ongoing socialization.

Culture, Ethnicity, Socioeconomic Resources

To a large extent, the child's social environment is determined by the community in which the family lives, whether urban, suburban, rural, affluent, or disadvantaged. The child's schooling and leisure-time activities are likewise influenced by the environment. The values, beliefs, rituals, and goals transmitted to children from their parents reflect the family's life-style and experiences. Affluent children might be sent to boarding or private schools to attain the best education available and to prepare them for entry into prestigious prep schools and colleges. Children from disadvantaged communities may be struggling to mesh conflicting values between home and school. Schools with discipline and motivational problems are more prevalent in disadvantaged areas. Children whose mothers work are likely to have more responsibilities because their help is needed for the household to function smoothly. Most children are given chores, which might be limited to being responsible for their bedroom and belongings or might include being responsible for other aspects of the household. Some children earn money by mowing grass, shoveling snow, delivering papers, or babysitting. Whether they are expected to share that money, save it, or spend it as they desire depends on family needs and values.

The child's peer groups and leisure activities also reflect environmental resources. Whereas certain sports, such as basketball and baseball, are more egalitarian and include children from all social strata, other sports, such as tennis and golf, necessitate expensive lessons and generally exclude those from lower socioeconomic families. Some communities have recreational organizations that are partially supported by public funds and provide group activities and lessons. Parents from suburban communities tend to encourage their children to join clubs, take music or dance lessons, and participate in sports programs. Some children have little free time for spontaneous neighborhood play.

Watching television is a popular leisure-time activity. Much concern has been verbalized by developmentalists about the influences of television on the child's attitudes and behaviors (see Chapter 9). Children at this age often imitate the values and behaviors, both positive and negative, they see played out before them on television. Ryan (1976) noted that children who lived in lower socioeconomic areas spent more time watching television than children in more affluent suburban areas. For many of these disadvantaged children, living in housing projects or high-rise rent-to-income apartments, watching television is a more attractive alternative than standing around hallways or street corners.

School By late childhood, children have developed fundamental skills in spelling, reading, handwriting, phonics, arithmetic, and arts and crafts. They have some familiarity with the natural sciences and geography (for example, students plan nutritional meals, talk about the earth and solar system, and make maps of their rooms). By 8 and 9 years of age, children's education broadens as history, social studies, and current events become part of the school curriculum. Children at this age learn to use maps, discuss distant countries and their cultures, and debate current issues.

Initially, these subjects are difficult for most students to learn. Children's personal experiences provide few examples that are similar to those of the ancient Greeks or Romans or to those of the people and governments that characterized medieval times. In addition children who have done little traveling might know their own towns or cities but only vaguely understand the size of their states, the locations of state capitals, the names of neighboring states, and the names and locations of other countries. In late childhood, it is still difficult for children to relate events that

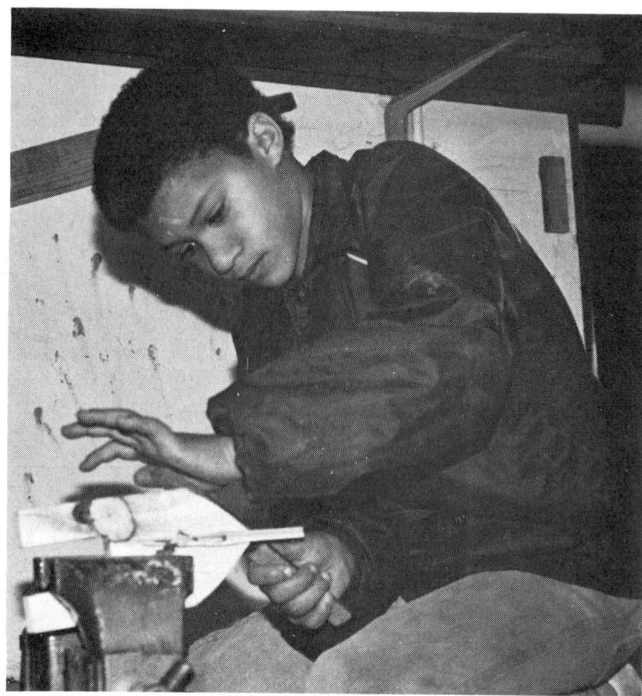

During late childhood, the child continues to develop and refine skills.

happened in the past or in other locations to their present or future lives. The child therefore still needs concrete examples, often supplied by visual aids and other creative means.

For example, when studying about the Far East, one third grade class rearranged their classroom to resemble an Oriental home. They then invited their families to join them for a program to demonstrate what they had learned, including a typical meal prepared in advance by the children.

By 11 years of age, the child can deal with abstract concepts beyond actual experiences and can work with new problems. Older children are therefore able to learn about other parts of the world without the aid of models and simulated experiences.

Early in this developmental period, language is a major focus. Children learn to describe events and work with numbers in both oral and written form. The acquisition of language is a vital component of more complex learning such as problem solving and interpreting the natural and social sciences. Language is needed for creative writing, following directions, play, and socialization.

Mathematics and geometry deal with patterns and relationships. Children learn to recognize the patterns and relationships between addition and subtraction and multiplication and division. Later, they can deal with spatial arrangements and find the areas of triangles, squares, and rectangles. Learning mathematic concepts is evident as the child begins to note these patterns and relationships outside the classroom. A child at this stage can manage an allowance, monitor game scores and players' averages, and know which glass really does contain more lemonade.

Children need little extrinsic prompting to learn about the natural sciences. They are inquisitive and readily ask questions about causes and effects. Among others, children ask questions about trees, insects, rain, water, rocks, life, birth, death, and sexuality. The child learns about the natural sciences through experimentation and by rediscovering what others before have discovered. Children collect insects, play with rocks, and build model cars; they explain phenomena and point out items of interest to peers and siblings.

Although children can have difficulty in learning about geography, history, and current events, they demonstrate an awareness of societal problems, politics, and values. Children might not fully understand poverty or a congenital disease, but they will collect money for charities or donate a part of their allowance, demonstrating that they have learned social rules and values. They observe game rules, classroom rules, and parental rules. They detest cheating among peers. By the end of late childhood, they have developed more sophisticated notions of morality.

In some school systems sixth grade is part of middle school, whereas in other systems sixth graders remain in elementary school and enter junior high school in seventh grade. The transition from elementary school to either middle school or junior high school usually includes being exposed to new teaching styles, meeting new classmates and teachers, becoming familiar with a new setting, and adapting to new expectations. These schools often are considerably larger than the smaller, more familiar elementary schools, and this is a major adjustment for many children. The experiences of a sixth grader in elementary school are quite different compared with those of a sixth grader in middle school. One study noted that middle school sixth-grade girls were more interested in boys and had a higher level of self-esteem than elementary school sixth-grade girls (Yussen and Santrock, 1982). Conversely, elementary school boys had a higher level of self-esteem, and there was little or no difference in their interest in girls. This finding corresponds to the difference in the onset of puberty between the sexes. The more adolescent-like atmosphere of middle school promotes the girls' earlier developmental changes. In fact, sixth-grade girls might begin telephoning boys and arranging for mixed-group activities. Boys, especially those who are late developers, shy, or immature, may find this transition difficult. Status among boys frequently is measured by physical strength or athletic ability. As they compare themselves to the older boys in middle school, feelings of inferiority might increase in sixth-grade boys, whereas in elementary school they are the oldest and usually the strongest and most competent in sports.

Peer Groups Peer groups are an important aspect of development during late childhood. More and more time is spent with peers. The 8- to 10-year-olds spend most of their time with peers of the same sex. The 11- and 12-year-olds begin to venture into activities and organizations in which both sexes participate. Most children find that doing things with another person, especially a best friend, is far more fun than doing things alone. Two boys found that mowing grass changed from being a weekly chore to fun when they did it together. Some children prefer to have one or two close friends, whereas other children are happiest in a crowd.

Children acquire much information about themselves from peer interactions. They also learn that to have friends, they have to be a friend, that is, be trustworthy, empathetic, happy, and modest. For example, one 9-year-old girl was feeling lonely and sorry for herself because her best friend was away at camp for the summer. One day while riding her bike around the neighborhood, she stopped to help a girl who had fallen. Although she initially did not know this girl, she soon discovered that they were the same age and both lonely because the injured girl was new in town. The summer brightened for both as they discovered mutual interests and learned from each other. When the other girl returned from camp, they became a happy trio.

The peer group is also a strongly influential group that controls its members by promoting conformity to group norms, style of dress, and activities. As 8- to 12-year-olds assume responsibility for hygiene practices, they become interested in their appearance. Interest in current fads and fashions becomes a favorite pastime and is fostered by the mass media, which beckons children in this age group to buy and wear designer jeans, shoes, and other status symbols. The urge to conform, which is so much a part of socialization in late childhood, makes the children a ready target for such marketing efforts.

Cultural differences are evident in the ways children during late childhood view the roles played by peers and adults. Bronfenbrenner (1967) found that children from Russia were more loyal to adult standards of behavior than were American children. American children were more likely to follow peer standards than adult rules, reflecting the importance of peer acceptance and approval. Bronfenbrenner asked both groups of children whether they would participate in a minor act of mischief in school. The response of the two groups was similar when they thought their parents and teachers would be informed. If no one or only peers were informed, the two groups responded differently, illustrating the powerful role played by peers in the American child's socialization. An earlier study by Boehm (1957) found that American children were more likely to ask a peer for help than were Swiss children. When help was needed to decorate a classroom for a surprise party, 92% of the American children said that they would ask a peer who was well known for artistic talent to provide assistance. In the same situation 70% of the Swiss children said they would ask the teacher for help.

Although cultural differences are real, within the culture, adult and peer norms coincide more frequently than they conflict. Most adults in the United States view childhood as a time to have fun before being required to take on many responsibilities. It is a time to learn how to interact with others within the greater society.

Sex Roles Sex-role stereotypes are still rampant in American culture, although flexibility is increasing as more men and women become involved in careers held almost exclusively by one or the other sex in the 1960s. Many 10-year-olds understand that stereotypes are not absolute and that alternatives are possible. As they begin to think about their future, the more women they see in executive or business roles and repair or mechanic roles and the more men they observe assuming nursing or allied health, elementary education, or secretarial roles, the more feasible these options become.

Prior to the onset of puberty, most girls are not interested in traditionally feminine activities. The inclusion of girls on school and community sports teams not only transcends a stereotype but enhances their gross and fine motor development as well as socialization. Their inclusion in competitive games and activities provides motivation and opportunities for achievement. Adults who expect children to do well and provide honest encouragement and support help both boys and girls to relate achievement to their own efforts. Socialization experiences during late childhood are of critical significance to the adolescent's and adult's achievement orientation. The traditional patterns of socialization followed sex-role stereotypes and assigned a boy's failure to external causes and a girl's failure to lack of ability. This pattern is changing as now both boys and girls are given opportunities to assign success to ability and failure to external causes (Santrock, 1983).

Subsystem Interactions

Growth and development during late childhood emphasizes the refinement of coordination. The motor skills the child struggled to learn earlier are now performed smoothly and masterfully. To these skills are added new cognitive structures that enable these children to be more efficient at problem solving. The newfound ability to manipulate information, conserve facts, and reverse a process helps to answer questions that earlier were puzzling. Much attention is given to the social aspect of development, in which all other facets of growth play a role. During late childhood, the amount of time spent with peers and adults other than family increases. The results of these experiences and interactions are related to the integration of physical, cognitive, and psychosocial skills.

Parameters of Late Childhood Development

Biophysical Development

During late childhood, children begin to lose their willowy appearances and exhibit the adult proportions they will possess when they are older. Each child grows at an individual pace, which explains the diversity in height and weight seen throughout late childhood. In addition, the variations in height and weight are sex related and reflect genetic and environmental factors. Boys initially tend to be slightly heavier and the same height or somewhat taller. Girls, however, begin their growth spurt around 10 years of age and quickly surpass the boys in both height and weight until the boys catch up around 13–14 years of age during their growth spurt. Growth during late childhood is highly individualized, and generalizations are difficult to make. Prior to their respective growth spurts, there is little difference in body contour between girls and boys. The average weight gain is 3–3.5 kg (5–7 lb) and the average height increase is 5–6.4 cm (2–2.5 in) per year. As was the case during middle childhood, the weight gain is related to increased muscle mass and strength. Continued long bone growth accounts for the increase in height.

Musculoskeletal System Bone growth is relatively slow during late childhood, although the long bones and facial bones become more prominent. Ossification continues to occur, with the bones becoming longer and denser. Skeletal system development becomes synchronized with the maturation of the reproductive system. Approximately 1–2 years before the onset of puberty, children (particularly girls 10–12 years old) experience a growth spurt.

The child's head attains 95% of its adult size by the age of 8 or 9 years (Cooke, 1968). Rapid growth in the sinal cavities occurs until 12 yeras of age, when the sinuses are nearly adult size. Sinuses strengthen the structural formation of the face, reduce the weight of the head, and add resonance to the voice (Schuster and Ashburn, 1980). There is little change in the size of the skull, but the face appears larger because of changes in the facial bones. The roundness of the face is gradually lost as the mandible and chin become more prominent and the alignment of the mouth changes to accommodate the permanent teeth. The central and lateral incisor deciduous teeth have been replaced by larger permanent teeth by the time most children are 9 years old. The first permanent teeth to appear are the 6-year molars. They erupt when the child is approximately 7 years of age (see Chapter 14).

Children often appear gangly, awkward, and clumsy during this period of development. Several factors contribute to this typical awkward appearance. The loss of deciduous teeth gives the child an occasional "toothless" look; the long bones grow faster than the adjacent muscles; and the shoulders remain unchanged, sloping and rounded, despite broadening of the chest.

Although the muscular system remains relatively immature, muscle tone does increase. The abdominal muscles become taut, and the curvature of the spine lessens. There is more flexibility in the lower extremities, allowing the child to become more adept at activities such as gymnastics, dancing, or sports.

Muscular injuries are common during late childhood. As they grow stronger and more coordinated, children become involved in various activities that demand more strength and endurance, and their bodies are not always able to meet the demands placed on them.

Cardiovascular System Cardiovascular maturation continues during late childhood, and by 9 years of age, the heart is six times its birthweight. Cardiac output increases to meet the increased oxygen and circulatory requirements. The pulse rate approaches adult norms as the cardiac rate decreases. Pulse rates vary with each child and are related to age, gender, size, and activity (see Appendix B). Systolic blood pressure increases as the heart grows.

Respiratory System Maturation of the respiratory system occurs, and the respiratory rate decreases to approach adult norms (see Appendix B). Lung capacity is proportional to the size of the child. Respiratory tissues mature and tidal volume doubles between 5 and 10 years of age. These factors facilitate increased endurance for active games and sports. Upper respiratory problems are somewhat less common in late childhood; however, there may be an increase in sinus infections. The rapid growth of the sinuses provides warm, moist, dark areas for bacterial growth. (Respiratory disorders are discussed in Chapter 34.)

Sensory System Growth and development of the eye is essentially complete by 6 years of age. However, some children's eyes may have a growth spurt just prior to puberty, resulting in myopia (nearsightedness). Visual acuity and ocular muscle movements plus peripheral vision and color discrimination are fully developed by 7 years of age. Depth perception improves as the brain learns to fuse the images of each eye (Chinn, 1979). Large print is no longer necessary for these children to either see or read.

Other perceptual skills, such as those related to hearing, touch, smelling, and tasting, are fully developed prior to late childhood.

Skin Until the child reaches prepubescence, the appearance of the skin changes little. As children reach prepubescence, the sebaceous glands become more active. Vasomotor instability is also common, and children frequently experience uncontrollable blushing.

Gastrointestinal System The gastrointestinal system achieves adult functional maturity during the late childhood years. Stomach capacity increases, and children are increasingly able to tolerate different foods. The shape of the stomach also changes, but not until 10–12 years of age does the stomach take on the "bagpipe" adult proportional shape (Holm, 1978).

Genitourinary System During late childhood, the kidneys develop to twice their neonatal length to accommodate the increased metabolic functions of the body. Fluid and electrolyte balance is stabilized because the more mature renal system can adequately conserve water. Bladder capacity is increased, especially in girls. Nocturnal enuresis can become a chronic problem for the child or only an occasional mishap (see Chapter 24). The results of a urinalysis done on a child during this time would closely resemble adult norms.

Sexual development begins at approximately 10–12 years of age for the prepubescent female, although some girls show no signs of secondary sexual characteristics during late childhood. Pubertal changes such as breast enlargement, pubic hair, and menstruation begin to appear in some girls. Only a small percentage of males who experience accelerated growth will exhibit outward signs of secondary sexual characteristics such as increased genital size or short, downy, pubic hair. Most of these changes occur during adolescence (see Chapter 11).

Neuromuscular Function Myelinization continues during this time, further improving the conduction of nerve impulses. This improved transmission of nerve impulses together with increased experience transforms the awkwardness of middle childhood into the dexterity that is evident by the end of late childhood. The central nervous system also matures, and the older child consistently demonstrates refined gross and fine motor skills. Coordination improves so that children perform skills with more balance and smoothness. The prepubescent child enters the world of adolescence with highly developed gross and fine motor skills.

Gross Motor Skills The world for children in late childhood is very exciting as they become involved with activities that are both enjoyable and rewarding. Gesell and colleagues (1956, 1977) described the characteristics of motor improvement for children at this stage. Eight- to twelve-year-old children exhibit less of the diffuse high energy associated with middle childhood as gross motor skills become controlled by cognitive processes and purposeful actions. Basic skills learned previously are practiced until

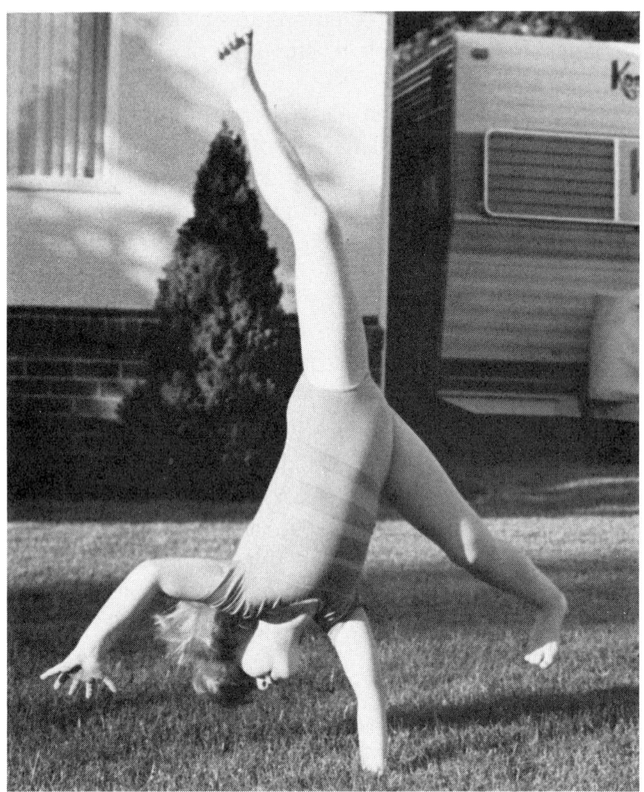

As gross motor skills become more controlled, the child practices until a skill is mastered.

perfected. The child spends hours, either alone or with peers, working to master a particular gymnastic exercise, hit the baseball farther, shoot free throws consistently, or perform various ballet movements. Strength, endurance, rhythm, and gracefulness are added to their performance. These children are no longer content merely to accomplish the skill; they set high standards and demand self-mastery.

For example, one 11-year-old Little League baseball player measured his enjoyment of the game by how well he performed in both fielding and batting. If he did well, it was a good game even if his team lost. If he did not get a hit or made fielding errors, it was a bad game regardless of whether his team won or lost.

A sense of competition is high as children attempt to outdo each other in activities requiring strength, speed, and endurance. They will challenge each other to feats of tree climbing, weight lifting, or jumping rope. They invent tricks with skateboards, bicycles, or swings to prove their superiority and ability to master a complex skill. Whatever their forte, they seek opportunities to demonstrate this acquired skill to others, hoping (expecting) to be much admired.

Fine Motor Skills During late childhood, children do have spurts of high energy, but the perfection of fine motor skills accompanied by increased cognitive ability allows children at this age to enjoy activities that require concentration and coordination such as video games, sewing, crafts, or more quiet, intricate board games. Eye–hand coordination improves to include speed and smoothness, and children generally prefer writing to printing. They now possess some of the flexibility and coordination needed to learn the more intricate skills required to play musical instruments.

Children of 9 and 10 show improved eye–hand coordination to the extent that each hand can be used independently. Children can now engage in activities that require concentration and differentiation. Art, sports, scouting activities, and gymnastics become favorite pastimes. Writing becomes smaller, and the child can write for longer periods of time. Quieter activities, such as model building, reading, and drawing, become more enjoyable. Children of 11 and 12 have almost attained the skillful movements of the adult. Skills are now perfected through practice and increased self-confidence. Energy levels remain intense. Children of this age become more involved with complex tasks; hence, the child who enjoyed doing simple artwork now enjoys working on intricate patterns when making handicrafts.

Immunologic System The maturity of the immunologic system is reflected in the body's ability to localize infections better. The amount of lymphoid tissue (which produces antibodies) peaks at approximately 7 years of age. Thereafter, it decreases as the child gets older. Allergic conditions are also common and may be severe (Bridgewater, Voignier, and Smith, 1978).

Personality Development

Self-Concept Self-concept, the mental picture of oneself formed in the process of growing and developing, is composed of psychologic, sociologic, and physiologic experiences. Children learn about themselves through self-exploration, comparison to others, and response from others.

Blaesing and Bruckhaus (1972) pointed out that as the child's environment broadens to include both home and school, the child might be subjected to feelings of inadequacy and inferiority. For instance, a child might note that other children speak better, run faster, and perform more effectively. Children might ostracize peers who are exceptionally slow or exceptionally bright. Children who have actual or imagined limitations can develop negative self-concepts because they do not meet the expectations of themselves or others. Even wearing corrective glasses can lead to a disturbance in the body image.

Blaesing and Bruckhaus (1972) also noted that children who fail to develop positive self-concepts require a greater degree of physical stimulation. These children often meet this need independently through rocking, clapping hands, and initiating other stimulating actions. A positive self-concept emerges for those children who develop friendships and are able to perform physical and cognitive tasks at levels relatively equal to their peers. Self-concept in late childhood is closely related to gender, and gender-role identification develops from an increasing awareness of self-concept. Sexual self-exploration and comparison of one's genitals with another's helps to sharpen self-concept as well as sexual identity. As multiple body changes begin to occur at the end of late childhood, the emerging adolescent focuses much attention on the body (see Chapter 11).

Sexuality Human sexuality does not denote only physical actions but includes the concept of self-identity. Freud (1962) believed that late childhood is characterized by a period of sexual latency, that is, a period in which sexual impulses are suppressed and diverted into other outlets.

Freudian theory holds that latency occurs as a result of the child's attempt to alleviate the fear of castration and dissolve the Oedipal and Electra complexes (see Chapter 6). Freud also believed that biologic factors and, at times, education promote latency. Other psychoanalysts (Fredland, 1975) claimed that children are fearful of being humiliated and in attempting to deal with this fear, they relinquish the Oedipal and Electra goals and concentrate on gaining mastery and skill in other areas. Latency is characterized by the suppression of sexual impulses and channeling of energies into the acquisition of new skills, learning new roles, mastering educational tasks, and developing moral and ethical standards.

Freud (1962) did not equate latency with complete cessation or lack of sexual activity but noted that sexual impulses are present throughout late childhood. Although the child learns to deny the direct sexual or instinctual gratification, masturbation, thumb sucking, and other sensual activities can persist. Tension and frustration might induce sexual impulses. Tackling a difficult task or studying for an examination might stimulate the child sexually, but the child may react with disgust, shame, and guilt when these impulses are overt.

At 8 or 9 years of age, children are no longer satisfied with simple answers about sexuality and reproduction. They want to know about respective male and female roles and often will wait for an appropriate time and then ask a barrage of questions about birth and procreation (Boettcher and Boettcher, 1978). Because late childhood is characterized by a concern for body image and integrity, it is also a time when children become concerned about how birth occurs. They might have been told that the baby leaves the woman through an orifice, but even at 9 years of age, some children believe that babies are born through the mother's abdomen. The older child wants explicit information and will ask peers if unable to obtain this information from parents.

Sexual awareness and curiosity increase for both sexes. Children are more exposed to nudity, sexual innuendos, and behavior from television, music, radio, and movies than their parents were. The implications of increased exposure and decreased restraint concerning topics related to sex are open to speculation. In some families the children feel more free to ask questions and discuss what they have heard or seen with their parents. Parents can then clarify or correct any misconceptions. In other families the children feel embarrassed to mention sexual issues, especially if they think their parents might disapprove.

Among peers, children share information, giggle, whisper, or create codes for words dealing with elimination and sex. There is considerable variation in the age at which pubertal changes begin. Eleven-year-old girls may or may not evidence signs of breast development. The early maturing girl might attempt to hide her breasts by wearing large sweatshirts or loose blouses while the late maturing girl observes her with envy, dreaming of the day when she will be able to wear a brassiere. Boys experience few pubertal changes during late childhood, although some boys experience initial growth in their genital organs.

As they begin to experience changes in their bodily appearance, personality traits, feelings, and moods, children become more interested in the relationship of these changes to puberty. Sometime before puberty and usually around 10 years of age, children need to be given the basic information about menstruation, intercourse, and reproduction. Although it is best that they get this information from their parents or responsible adults, studies continue to indicate that the majority of youth acquire their knowledge about sex from peers (Kaluger and Kaluger, 1984). Sometimes the child's curiosity is not satisfied by factual information. Children might ask if they can watch their parents have intercourse, or might attempt to peek through the keyhole into the parents' bedroom. One ingenious child put a tape recorder under the parents' bed.

Self-Esteem Self-esteem becomes increasingly important to children as their growing cognitive powers permit them to gain and master new skills. Sieman (1978) pointed out that a child's feelings of self-worth can be encouraged by (1) a high degree of acceptance by family and others; (2) clearly defined and consistent limits; and (3) flexibility within those limits to permit individual activity.

Depending on their self-esteem, children will differ in their reactions to new situations, praise, or criticism. Children with high self-esteem can accept criticism, feel more confident, and usually think they will be successful. Children with low self-esteem will demonstrate opposite behaviors.

During late childhood, the child's feelings of self-esteem are influenced by many factors. Parents, teachers, and peers are most crucial; success and achievements, no matter how small, are increasingly vital. Lavishing sincere praise for a chore or task well done increases the child's perception of self-worth. Children depend on encouragement and praise from significant persons to facilitate mastering skills and personal development. Next to the parents, teachers are influential persons during this time, and their sensible use of their authority, education, and knowledge aid in developing the child's feelings of self-worth. Teachers also help children to learn acceptable behavior by teaching them to control aggressive impulses and by directing children's energies into constructive activities. Erik Erikson (1963) called this phase of development the stage of "industry vs. inferiority" and viewed it as the "entrance into life" (see Chapter 6). This developmental stage is marked by the child's determination to master particular tasks and experiences that enable more competent, more accomplished, and less dependent behavior. Children acquire distinctive patterns of characteristic behaviors and skills that foster their sense of industry. The concept of industry is delineated by self-control, cooperation, and compromise, which go beyond playful expressions.

Children want to be recognized for their accomplishments. Erikson suggested that the child forms basic attitudes toward work during this period in response to systematic instruction provided by society. Such instruction often includes the skills, such as reading and writing, needed to become a useful, productive member of the society. Children are eager to learn at this stage, and successful learning increases their self-esteem.

Children are motivated by peer approval and such extrinsic stimuli as grades, material rewards, and privileges. It is not only important to be able to manipulate the environment but also to do so successfully. If children do not succeed in accomplishing these tasks, they develop a sense of inadequacy or inferiority, often losing status among their peers. This may discourage them from identifying with peers and other aspects of their society.

Erikson proposed that unsuccessful or delayed resolution of this psychosocial crisis results in the child acquiring a sense of inferiority. Children also may feel inferior if they have not achieved adequate separation from their families and spend their energy on maintaining family bonds, leaving them no energy to interact with the outside environment of peers, school, and society. This behavior may reflect incomplete resolution of previous psychosocial crises or limited parental support and encouragement for independent behaviors.

For example, the only recognition that satisfied one 10-year-old girl was the occasional praise she received from her mother. To her, it seemed that everything her mother did was perfect and everything she herself did, whether it was making her bed, baking a cake, running a race, or writing a story, made her susceptible to criticism. She labored over simple projects for hours to earn a rare positive comment from her mother. She therefore had little time, energy, or interest in exerting similar efforts to obtain recognition from others. She also discounted praise received from others if her effort had not been affirmed by her mother.

A sense of inferiority also may occur if children feel defeated, if they have difficulty, or if they are unable to learn certain tasks, often because of physical disabilities or unrealistic goals set up by the child's family or school. Children with a sense of inferiority might never finish a task for fear of failing or will sometimes be afraid to try mastering a new task for fear of being shamed. All children will feel some degree of inferiority with some particular skills, despite a positive attitude toward themselves and their work; however, success or mastery of one task can compensate for others they perform less well. How children perceive their success or failure at mastering certain tasks depends on the reinforcements provided by significant persons. As children begin to master any task, they need both constructive criticism and positive reinforcement. Both parents and teachers should instill a sense of accomplishment and self-esteem during this period.

Lack of self-esteem, Erikson pointed out, also may be caused by the child's constricting the world and focusing entirely on mastering one particular skill, such as playing a musical instrument, and thereby neglecting relationships with other people. Personality development by late childhood is closely related to social development and the child's interaction with the various suprasystems. Ideally, the environment provides a balance between mastering developmental tasks or skills and strengthening interpersonal skills. Without this balance, the child might develop a poor self-concept and a sense of inferiority, which will lead to difficulty in mastering the tasks of adolescence.

Independence Although the development of independence begins during infancy, late childhood is a period during which the child makes great strides toward becoming independent. Increased cognitive power coupled with refined gross and fine motor skills provide the necessary tools for becoming self-reliant. During their struggle for independence, however, children are extremely dependent on their families for encouragement and support.

During late childhood, a child can assume more responsibilities that are relatively complex such as helping with household chores, caring for younger siblings, and doing simple errands. A gradual increase of responsibilities helps children learn new skills and gain confidence—both vital to the development of self-reliance. In addition, learning to be responsible for completing chores and assignments creates a sense of being a contributing member of the family system. It provides a prelude for becoming a cooperative, reliable, and productive member of adult society.

At times, attempts to be independent and self-reliant meet with frustration and failure. These episodes should be viewed as potential growth experiences rather than lost opportunities. For example, one 11-year-old boy worked hard one summer mowing grass. By the end of the summer, he had earned over $100. His parents told him that he could decide what he wanted to do with his money. Initially indecisive, this boy spent a considerable portion of his savings on a spur-of-the-moment trip to an amusement park with some of his friends. He had a wonderful time and considered the money well spent until a month later when he wanted to buy a new bike. He wished that he had not spent his money so freely at the amusement park when he discovered that he did not have enough money left to purchase the bike he wanted. He realized the consequences of spending his money without first considering carefully the options. The experience provided a good lesson in making decisions as he learned to take responsibility for his actions. Because the decision had been his, he could not blame someone else, and although frustrated, he accepted the outcome.

The child will aspire to success with every new situation, task, or opportunity. Some of these goals will be met, whereas others will not, resulting in feelings of frustration. With the encouragement of family, friends, and schoolteachers and counselors, children can learn to be self-reliant and to deal with the frustration that may result from unmet aspirations.

Cognitive Development

Concrete Operations Until late childhood, action and egocentric thought are the child's primary methods for coping with the world. During late childhood, a transition occurs, and the child begins to develop what Piaget called "concrete operations." This transition appears after the child has demonstrated the ability to represent mentally what has been perceived and to view the self and actions objectively (Piaget and Inhelder, 1969) (see Chapter 6). The attainment of concrete operations, along with the decrease in egocentricity and increase in language skills, allow the child to think, act, and interact at a more sophisticated level.

Concrete operations, which relate directly to objects and not to expressed propositions or statements, concern the child's grouping actions, objects, and events according to general coordinating structures and relationships (Piaget and Inhelder, 1969). The child's ability to group falls into the following categories:

1. *Closure or composition grouping*—two or more classes may be combined to produce a general inclusive class (Piaget and Inhelder, 1969; Inhelder, 1979). For example, children may combine cats and dogs into the class of animals and apples and oranges into the class of fruit.
2. *Tautology grouping*—a class may be added to itself to yield the same class (Schilder, 1970; Blaesing and Bruckhaus, 1972) (for example, apples plus apples equals apples), although this type of action does not hold true for numbers (for example, 2 plus 2 equals 4, not 2).
3. *Inverse relationships or reversibility groupings*—all classes formed are reversible (that is, may be transformed back into their original, less-inclusive classes) (Beard, 1969; Piaget and Inhelder, 1969). The child who has mastered this concept is able to subtract when addition was previously performed or divide when multiplication was carried out (for example, fruit minus apples equals oranges). Reversibility, a factor in effective problem solving, enables the child to anticipate the results of actions.
4. *Identity grouping*—a class united with its opposite is obliterated (Piaget and Inhelder, 1969; Piaget, 1974). This type of grouping is apparent in subtraction (for example, ten apples minus ten apples equals zero apples). Grouping by identity operates in the concept of conservation. The child learns that 10 oz of water is 10 oz of water whether the water is in a short, wide glass or a long, thin glass.
5. *Association grouping*—three or more elements may be combined in any manner to produce the same result (Beard, 1969; Piaget and Inhelder, 1969). For example, $(2 + 1) + 3 = 2 + (1 + 3)$. The child thus understands the properties of addition but at 8 years of age might not yet know that this grouping does not hold true for all actions, for example, $3\,(3) - 2 = 7$, but $3\,(3 - 2) = 3$.

Classification Children in late childhood learn to group items according to shared characteristics. The child can easily divide classes into subclasses and thus form a hierarchy (Beard, 1969). For example, when presented with groups of animals, children can construct the following hierarchy:

- Animals
  - Dogs
    - Beagles
    - German Shepherds
  - Cats
  - Rabbits

They also can respond correctly to questions such as, "Are there more beagles or more dogs?" "If all the dogs ran away, would there be any animals left?" "Are rabbits and cats both animals?" and "If all the animals died, would there be any rabbits?" Eight- and nine-year-olds are able to construct hierarchies only when they can visualize the actual objects, whereas 10- to 12-year-olds can construct hierarchies when given verbal representations of the objects.

The ability to classify and sort items indicates that the child can identify a concept and mentally represent the concept prior to taking action. When children under 7 or 8 years of age are asked to sort items according to shape or size, they approach the task by comparing one item with another and rarely look at the whole. Children who have mastered concrete operations, however, examine the whole and consider more than one concept at a time to arrive at a decision. As the child's operational skills increase, double classifications become common (that is, classifications that are based on more than one shared characteristic such as size and shape or function and color).

Classification is manifested in many of the activities of children. Most common is the proliferation of collections in late childhood: stamps, baseball cards, stickers, posters,

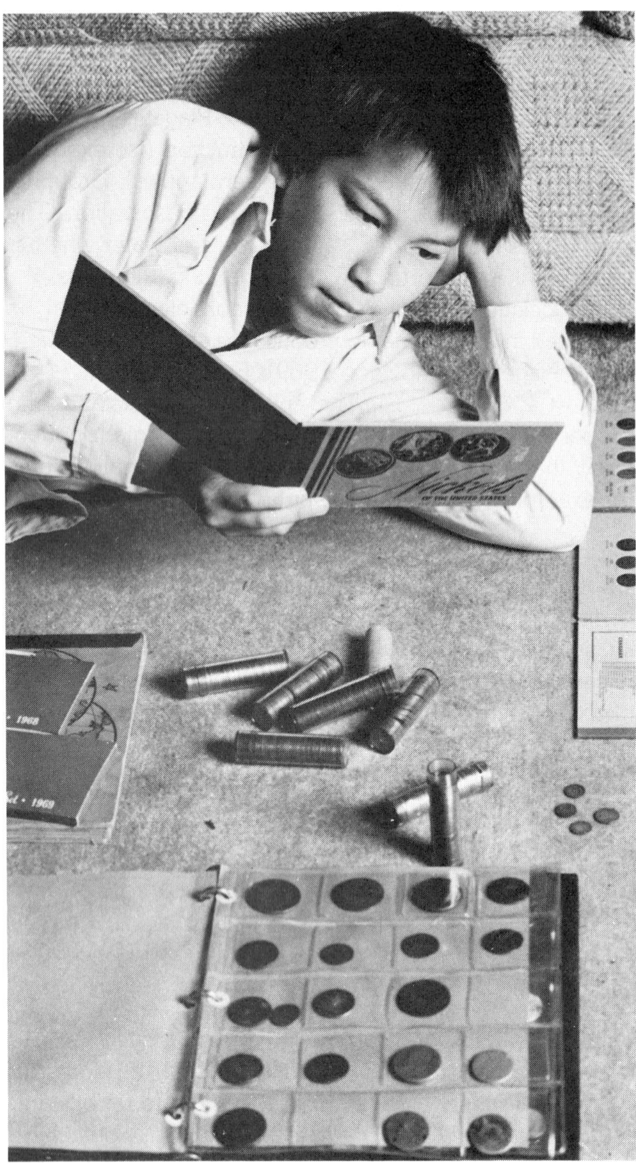

Coins are just one of the many collections in late childhood.

seashells, records, T-shirts, postcards, coins, and magazines. In school, children learn to classify countries according to geographic location, population, type of government, economics, and natural resources.

Seriation Prior to 7 or 8 years of age, children learn to build a limited sequence of objects in successive, related pairs. In late childhood this process develops into *seriation,* in which objects and events are arranged and related according to distinguishing characteristics (Piaget and Inhelder, 1969). For instance, children often rank members of their peer group according to toughness or degree of success in a given sport. They select members of a baseball team on the basis of seriation and often line up in school in an order based on height. In school children learn to read maps, interpret graphs, and compare gradations in color intensity, all of which require viewing the whole, comparing the concepts, and arriving at a conclusion. With increasing skill, the child begins to seriate in more than one dimension or with more than one set of characteristics.

Conservation The concept of conservation is one of the complex operations that is mastered during late childhood. Piaget demonstrated that the child's ability to grasp the concept of conservation progresses in late childhood. By 8 years of age, children use their logical capacities of compensation, identity, and reversibility to perform the operation necessary to understand the concept of conservation of liquid. Experiments using the conservation of weight instead of liquid demonstrated that the former operation was not learned until 9 or 10 years of age (Labinowicz, 1980). At 11 or 12 years of age, children recognize that volume is conserved regardless of the size or shape of the container, and the 12-year-old does not merely know that volume has been conserved but also can explain the concept of conservation (Piaget and Inhelder, 1969).

Understanding the concept of conservation is essential if the child is to perform mathematic skills, solve problems, and comprehend other operations involving space, time, movement, and speed. For example, substitution is a form of conservation and may be expressed mathematically by the equation $3 + 1 = 4 = 2 + 2$. In problem solving, however, children need to recognize how different combinations or equivalents may be used. One child who collected coins, for example, learned the concept of conservation by determining how many and which types of coins were equal amounts of money.

Numbers At 7 or 8 years of age, the child learns to use numbers to measure quantity, weight, time, and space through classification and seriation. After the child perceives that each number has a meaning, regardless of the various characteristics of the elements, the child is prepared to examine relationships that are expressed numerically. The child can tell time, manipulate numbers for solving mathematic problems, and understand monetary figures, making it possible to go to the store and purchase an item independently or manage an allowance.

Space, Time, Movement, and Speed With the ability to classify, seriate, conserve, and comprehend the meaning of numbers, the child begins to examine the concept of space, an understanding that remains limited during most of late childhood. Not until 12 or so years of age does the child usually come to appreciate space as an abstraction.

Children first learn to make spatial measurements by dividing a line into segments and measuring the distances between them. Children in late childhood comprehend geometric space (that is, the measurements of length and angles) but cannot incorporate space successfully into their activities. A child might, for example, understand that a given triangle consists of two smaller triangles, but when attempting to replicate the triangles precisely, the child fails because of difficulty in applying concepts without a concrete object for reference. Children learn to appreciate proximities, distances, openness, closedness, and the coordination of positions. They learn to read and draw maps. They deal with geography and astronomy in school and, by 9 years of age, can appreciate projections (Piaget, 1962). The child can imagine or draw shadows, the projections for simple objects, sticks, disks, and rectangles and by 11 and 12 years of age can draw more complex objects.

In late childhood time is initially sequential and purposeful. The child at 7 years of age is time conscious and likes to wear a watch and within a year is acutely aware of time. Up until 9 years of age, the child uses time to plan the day, but with maturation, time becomes a conceptual measurement for planning not only activities of daily living but also future events.

As soon as time becomes a functioning operation, the child can comprehend the concept of speed (Piaget, 1970). First, the child merely assumes that a moving object is in motion longer than another if it has traveled a longer distance, but using the concept of time, motion can be viewed temporally. The child then understands speed as a function of time and distance.

Intelligence and Creativity The child exposed to a large and varied environment masters concrete operations, acquires a command of numbers and words, and exercises new cognitive structures. By 8 years of age, the child relinquishes animistic and egocentric thought and inquires about the causes and effects of natural phenomena (see Chapter 9). The child is open to the opinions of others and is capable of dealing with events and facts with minimal distortion.

Their increased capacities for logical thinking enable children at this age to respond to a situation as a whole rather than being limited to the part affecting them. In describing a science experiment such as the pendulum problem, they accurately describe the results of each trial regardless of who did it. They vary the length of string, the weight, and occasionally the point of release to determine which variables make the pendulum swing the fastest. Although they are precise observers and no longer view the impetus of the swinging action as the contributing factor, they have difficulty systematically eliminating variables to arrive at a conclusion.

The child's conclusions are the result of multiple trial-and-error attempts to find by chance which variable makes the difference. Gradually, the child learns to deal with multiple stimuli of varying complexity. Initially, the child can deal only with abstractions that resemble actual experiences, but eventually, the child understands representative concepts removed from actual experiences.

The 8-year-old develops an appreciation for logical reasoning and the implications of events and actions. At 9 years of age, the child is intrigued with details and at 11 years of age is inquisitive. Eight- and nine-year-olds can understand the physical sciences, but children do not grasp more complex concepts such as morality, social relationships, and death until 10 or 11 years of age. As children grow older, they manifest the intellectual ability to deal with abstractions, an intellectual ability that is developed further in adolescence and adulthood.

Intelligence has numerous different facets. Piaget defined intelligence as the qualitative changes that occur in the child's thinking as a result of maturation and experience. Psychometricians measure intelligence quantitatively by means of various tests. Definitions of intelligence therefore vary depending on what aspect is being studied. Wechsler (1958) defined intelligence as "the global capacity of the individual to act purposefully, to think rationally, and to deal effectively with the environment."

Intelligence seems easier to define than to measure because it is strongly influenced by the environment, home, culture, and school. During late childhood, various group tests are given in school to assess the child's ability to perform at grade level and the appropriateness of advanced placement. A major problem in intelligence testing is cultural bias. In general, the tests reflect the vocabulary and culture of the educated, middle-class, white society. Children from minority and low-income groups score lower even with nonverbal tests because subtle cultural biases influence the child's performance (Vernon, 1965). Although widespread testing continues, psychologists and educators are quick to point out the limitations of standard intelligence tests. The narrow range of cognitive functioning that is tapped by such tests relates primarily to the content taught at school. Many of the other facets of intelligence, such as social adaptability, everyday problem solving, and general work performance, are not tested. If administered and interpreted carefully, intelligence tests are useful measurements of one aspect of the child's mental capacity; however, they are abused when they are used to label children.

Some children who demonstrate intellectual superiority and academic achievement in school participate in special programs. These programs usually take one of three forms: enrichment, grouping, or acceleration. Enrichment programs seek to broaden the child's academic experience to include advanced courses, independent study, and exposure to the fine arts. Grouping is the same concept as tracking, a plan that groups children of similar abilities together. Although this might benefit the better students, it deprives the others, especially minority and disadvantaged children, from the classroom stimulation provided by the questions and discussions of these more academically adept students. Acceleration occurs when the student skips a grade or compresses a grade into a semester.

Another component of intelligence and one not measured by the standard tests is creativity. In fact, historically, some of the world's most creative individuals were thought to be unable to learn. Perhaps this was because their inquisitive minds took them beyond the basic, more simple answer requested by their teacher. "Creativity is the process of first identifying a problem and then carrying through until the results of the problem solving are communicated" (Santrock, 1983). This entails developing ideas and hypotheses, following each to a logical conclusion, and then modifying, retesting, or formulating new plans by which to solve the problem. Exercises in creative thinking are part of many classroom activities. Brainstorming and playing with improbabilities are two techniques frequently used to foster creative thinking. Both of these techniques encourage the free flow of ideas, release from conventional answers, and freedom to fantasize.

Creativity tends to wax and wane as the child progresses through each developmental phase. This coincides with Piaget's observation that egocentrism increases at the beginning of each new phase of cognitive skills (Piaget and Inhelder, 1969). Pressures to conform are heightened when learning a new skill or manner of thinking. Once the skill or thought process is mastered, the child is free to experiment with it, thus thinking more creatively. Creativity can be stifled if not allowed expression. Children need to be permitted and even encouraged to follow through with their ideas even though they might seem silly to an adult. Teachers and parents who provide opportunities for creative expression sustain an atmosphere that supports curiosity and investigative problem solving, skills beneficial for learning during adolescence. Putting words and sentences together to form poems, rhymes and stories is a manifestation of creativity. The following was written by a nine-year-old.

> Snowfights
> fun, exciting
> turning faces red
> ducking, dodging, and throwing
> Exciting.

Memory During late childhood, the child uses short-term memory frequently in school. For example, the child looks at a word and repeats the spelling. If only short-term memory existed, however, the child would lose the ability to spell the specific word. Long-term memory therefore allows the child to learn and store information, but it requires organizing information into a purposeful form, a process called *encoding* (Gagne, 1977). Encoded information is and may be retrieved when external or internal stimuli are matched appropriately. A new problem might, for example, stimulate information retrieval.

By late childhood, information may be organized as concepts, visual representations, and verbal complexes. Seven-year-olds accurately remember familiar words but cannot spell well. At 9 years of age, the child has vacillating immediate recall ability (Gesell, Ilg, and Ames, 1956), but the 10- to 12-year-old is able to retrieve information to apply to new situations.

Long-term memory is crucial for the child to succeed in school and at play. Words, numbers, concepts, and rules must therefore be encoded and retrieved. To facilitate learning, teachers write on the blackboard, use audiovisual materials, assign homework, provide books, and administer tests.

Motivation Motivation for learning is a component of all learning theories. Sources of motivation can be intrinsic or extrinsic to the child. The need to achieve a sense of industry, gain independence, bolster self-esteem, and attain aspirations motivates children to learn. The child learns to read and no longer needs to have an adult or older sibling read a bedtime story. The child swings a bat and strikes the ball into the field, thus gaining peer approval and a sense of pride. Mastery of a task often leads to such positive reinforcement as being praised or receiving an excellent grade. Motivation can take the form of an intrinsic desire to achieve. Children often attempt complicated and difficult tasks to prove that they are capable (for example, constructing a model that contains numerous parts). Needs also motivate children. The desire to be accepted by peers stimulates the child to work on scholastic or athletic tasks. No one likes to be ostracized as the "dumb kid" or the "clumsy kid."

Cognitive Conceit Cognitive conceit is a manifestation of the child's new cognitive powers (Elkind, 1974). In early and middle childhood, prior to concrete operational thought, children perceive adults as powerful, omnipotent beings. During late childhood, that aura of power begins to dissipate. Children are delighted when they discover that their parents or teachers can make mistakes, and they take this discovery a step further with the notion that all adults are stupid or foolish. For example, a teacher who makes a little mistake in the class might cause the children to roar with laughter almost uncontrollably.

Cognitive conceit is also evident in children's stories that are made up, read in comics or books, or seen on television and in movies. Adults play inconsequential roles in stories in which superheroes are featured. Children perceive themselves as having all the answers and skills necessary in life, whereas adults, those bungling fools, lack those talents.

Language Development

A child's language at the beginning of late childhood differs from an adult's because of dissimilar patterns of thought, a less sophisticated vocabulary, and fewer experiences to draw on. Prior to 7 years of age, thought is egocentric and symbolic (see Chapters 8 and 9). Language in early and middle childhood is a vehicle for reinforcing the child's activity and is less integrated with socialization than it is in late childhood.

By 8 years of age, children begin to depend more on speech and use fewer gestures to communicate. The telephone becomes a social activity. Children may play with language and they sometimes make up words or speak pig latin. Piagetian theory questions whether the 8-year-old can communicate solely through language because children at this age are first connecting cognitive images with words. Piaget (1974) found that when children up to 8 years of age are asked to tell a story, they disregard the order of events and interchange pronouns inappropriately. These children expect that others will understand them unconditionally. Two children can communicate verbally only after they have developed similar sets of behaviors and vocabularies. Beginning at 8 years of age, children begin to put order into their storytelling, and at later ages they narrate events in order and use appropriate pronouns.

During late childhood, children encounter and learn new words and concepts. Mastery over complex sentence structure occurs, and they make fewer grammatical errors. Vocabulary increases rapidly, partly because of the more advanced reading level and exposure to new words within the context of familiar ones. Children 9–12 years old are more adept at spoken language than younger children because older children are more prone to ask questions about what is unfamiliar. Older children also have developed the ability to use concrete operations and can analyze and interpret language. At the end of late childhood, spoken language resembles that of adults.

Schooling facilitates the child's use of language, especially as a means of exchanging and processing information. The child learns general techniques for organizing and solving problems because language gives meaning to the properties of objects, thereby enabling the child to explain the rationale for a decision, the rules of a game, or the steps for conducting a science experiment.

During late childhood, the child's ability to understand the meaning of sentence forms in which the deep structure is not the same as the surface structure improves significantly. Carol Chomsky (1969) found that although 7- and 8-year-old children had less difficulty comprehending sentences in which there was a mismatch between surface and deep structural order, understanding this altered relation of subject–action–object was not complete until they were 9 or 10 years old. A surface-structure sentence is one that follows the common English form of noun phrase followed by verb phrase (for example, "The dog ran after the cat"). A deep-structure sentence does not follow the common interpretational rule (for example, " The dog is hard to see at night"). In this sentence the subject is not clearly stated but implied. The first noun (dog) is not constructed to be the subject, which poses problems for children who initially want to apply the same interpretational rule consistently to all sentences. With experience and increased cognitive skills, the child learns to interpret variations in sentence structure.

Mastering the ambiguities of language and sentence structure sets the stage for jokes and riddles. Table 10-1 shows how these ambiguities are used to create humor. This improved comprehension of word usage enables children to manipulate meaning and structure to their advantage. They delight in creating riddles and repeating traditional ones.

Moral and Faith Development

During late childhood, the child's cognitive and moral development evolve simultaneously. Prior to late childhood, children tend to adopt parental standards as they abandon their relative hedonism. They are confined by external sanctions, where rewards or punishments govern their behavior. Adults are assumed to be right, and there is little understanding of the reasoning behind certain judgments. The older child now is able to judge an act with some reasoning. For the first time, a child can see beyond the result of an action.

Piaget (1965, 1969), well known for his work on both cognitive and moral reasoning, defined his first stage of

TABLE 10-1 Jokes and Riddles of Late Childhood, Classified by Type of Language Ambiguity

Type of Ambiguity	Joke	Riddle
Lexical (word formation)	"Order! Order in the court!" "Ham and cheese on rye, please, Your Honor."	"Why did the farmer name his hog 'Ink'?" "Because he kept running out of the pen."
Phonologic (speech sound)	"Waiter, what's this?" "That's bean soup, ma'am." "I'm not interested in what it's been, I'm asking what it is now."	"Why did the cookie cry?" "Because its mother had been a wafer so long."
Surface structure (regrouping of words to give two meanings)	"I saw a man-eating shark in the aquarium." "That's nothing. I saw a man eating herring in the restaurant."	"Tell me how long cows should be milked." "They should be milked the same as short ones, of course."
Deep structure (two different relations between noun and verb possible)	"Call me a cab." "You're a cab."	"What animal can jump as high as a tree?" "All animals; trees cannot jump."

SOURCE: Adapted from Gibson J: *Living: Human Development Through the Lifespan.* Addison-Wesley, 1983.

moral development as "morality of restraint." (According to Piaget, this stage lasts from about 3 to 12 years of age, or until adolescence.) The concept of justice and the child's respect for rules are part of the stage of morality of restraint. During this stage, the child's concept of justice progresses from a rather rigid idea of right and wrong to the notion of equity in moral judgments. Thus, from 8 to 11 years of age, a progressive idea of egalitarianism evolves. The older child making a judgment now takes into account others' interpretations and viewpoints. Still governed by rules, these children now have more insight into the rationale for those rules.

Children begin to demonstrate their understanding of right and wrong in all aspects of their lives. Lying is one way to exhibit the ability to conceptualize right and wrong. For the 8-year-old, lying is natural to protect one's self-interest. The 8-year-old definitely knows that certain acts result in punishment. The child therefore avoids punishment by lying, but the lie is not an intentional, planned deception. For example, two sisters were describing their afternoon of neighborhood play experiences. The older sister described in detail how her younger sister had not shared her ball and teased one of their friends. The younger sister, aware that punishment follows when rules of conduct are broken, explained the incident quite differently and blamed the afternoon quarrel on their young friend. At 10 years of age, the older sister had a better understanding of the importance of mutual cooperation and the need to tell the truth, whereas the 6-year-old viewed lying as a way of avoiding punishment and something for which one was punished only if one were caught.

The older child also relinquishes egocentric thought processes and develops the ability to relate to others. Through experience and cooperative activity, the child develops an understanding of the rationale for rules. Prior to playing a game, these children will spend considerable time reviewing the rules to ensure mutual consent. Rules tend to have minor changes depending on the group and situation; however, the aim of these children is for mutual consent and cooperation so that play can proceed. They no longer consider themselves submissive to rules but create and use rules to organize the game and ensure fair play. During this period, therefore, children tend to be more forgiving as rules of conduct focus on cooperation or mutuality, but not until children reach the second stage of "morality of reciprocity" are they able to view morality and such concepts as justice abstractly.

Continuing with Piaget's work, Lawrence Kohlberg (1973) studied cross-cultural moral development and noted that children from 8 to 12 years of age tended to demonstrate characteristics of his stage three, "interpersonal acceptance of 'good boy, nice girl' social concept," and stage four, "the 'law and order' orientation" (see Chapter 6). These two stages, which are in turn part of Kohlberg's defined "conventional level of morality," suggest that up to about 10 or 11 years of age, children seem to interpret right and wrong according to physical consequences or the physical power of authorities (Kohlberg, 1969). From 8 to 10 years of age, moral development consists of seeking and gaining approval. Children during this time also need to establish and maintain good relationships with their peers, teachers, and families. From 10 to 12 years of age, children's moral reasoning is characterized by concern for showing respect for authority and maintaining rules and social order. Children are now concerned with demonstrating the ability to be responsible and accountable for their actions. They view rules more objectively and genuinely understand their implications. Adults and the authority they hold at home, school, or within religious groups take on special importance for children during this period. Children try to emulate these authority figures and the power they yield.

When questioned why they have to go to school, the response of children who reason at Kohlberg's stage three will demonstrate their concern for doing what is expected of them by others. For example, one boy stated simply that he went to school because everyone expected him to—his friends, parents, and teachers. Being good is important and that means being kind, showing respect, helping others, obeying, and being trustworthy. A stage-four child will add that school attendance is part of obeying the law. As one boy commented, "whether you like it or not, you have to attend school until 16, that is the law." Doing right is related to observing laws. Upholding the law is viewed as a social duty and one way of contributing to the good of society.

Because laws are made by adult authorities, these people are highly respected. During late childhood, children often claim that they want to be like a teacher, minister, coach, or club leader. They daydream of what they would do with such power if they were in a similar leadership position or if they were a parent.

The child's world during this period encompasses family, peers, school, and the larger society, and children in late childhood struggle to understand the differences in relationships and values. They begin to look beyond behavior and try to understand what motivates it and the potential consequences of their actions. In the process a deeper sense of social responsibility begins to emerge and blossom.

In describing faith development, Fowler (1974) observed that 8-year-olds may still subordinate the religious attitudes of peers to those of their family. They conceptualize God or the Supreme Being in human terms, sometimes as a kindly, benevolent being who grants their requests when they are good and at other times as a judge who doles out punishment for wrongdoing. The 11- and 12-year-olds are exposed more to different religious beliefs and tend to question the rightness or wrongness of beliefs that differ from theirs. They usually seek advice from some authority figure, whether their minister, Sunday school teacher, or youth group leader. These children often find it difficult to resolve conflict in belief systems because they are striving for acceptance and conformity in other parts of their lives. They resolve this conflict either by dismissing all other beliefs as wrong and being convinced that theirs is the only true religion or by excluding religion as a basis for their friendships.

Social Development

During late childhood, children want to be accepted by their peers and feel that friendships are important. By 8 years of age, children have best friends, most often of the same sex. As the child approaches adolescence, friendships with the opposite sex reappear, and gangs of friends begin to form.

Competition and Compromise Harry Stack Sullivan (1953) studied the concept of competition in the socialization process and concluded that competition appears among all children, regardless of culture, at approximately 6 years of age. He viewed competition as a natural phenomenon that is highly valued and vigorously encouraged in western technologic society, so much so that a child who cannot compete because of physical or mental limitations is labeled nonfunctional. During late childhood, children must learn to deal with the forms of competition that are accepted within their society. These range from such competitive situations as the spelling bee in school to team sports. Children like to set up situations where they either win or at least meet their self-prescribed goals. When children play together, the child who expects to win usually sets up the challenge. In the game of "hide and seek," for example, the child who volunteers to be "it" usually expects to find everyone.

The alternative to competition is compromise, which, according to Sullivan, means learning to give and take. Through compromise, children learn the rules of the game and understand that they will sometimes win and sometimes lose. Children often make their own rules and require strict adherence to those rules within either the game or the relationship. Reciprocity is typical in late childhood, and "If you do this for me, I'll do this for you" is a common comment. In this way both parties define themselves as winners and therefore maintain self-esteem. Children's rules involve strict adherence; those who break the rules are "cheaters," and fights between cheaters and noncheaters are common.

With compromise also comes cooperation, which is essential for a child's developing sense of industry. Sullivan pointed out that compromise and competition should be balanced so that neither becomes a troublesome trait. The person who is only competitive and feels a vital need to be ahead of everyone else will have problems with social functioning, as would the person who is always willing to defer to almost anyone.

The very competitive child frequently is intense and self-demanding in all that is undertaken, whether it is a game, schoolwork, or home project. Recent studies (Allen, 1983) have assessed children for the presence of Type A and B behavior patterns. A Type A behavior pattern is defined as "a characteristic action–emotion complex which is exhibited by those individuals who are engaged in a relatively chronic struggle to obtain an unlimited number of poorly defined things from their environment in the shortest period of time, and, if necessary, against the opposing efforts of other things or persons in the same environment" (Friedman, 1969). A Type B behavior pattern is the relative absence of Type A behaviors. Although many questions surround the emergence, development, and stability of Type A behavior patterns in children, there is growing evidence that altering certain behavioral characteristics of the pattern will promote a more healthy life-style for these children.

Siegal and Matthews (1983) hypothesized that there are four general ways that parents, teachers, and health care personnel can help children alter some of these behaviors, especially excessive anger and overachievement. First, children should be advised to exercise, eat a balanced, low-cholesterol diet, and not to smoke. During late childhood, children begin to eat more meals away from home and experience peer pressure. Knowing what foods and activities are good for them and having adult support and role models as guides will help them in the decision-making process (see Chapter 18). Second, these children need guidance to identify appropriate times and settings to be competitive. They might need to learn how to have fun. For example, one boy who was an excellent swimmer and on a youth swim team had to learn to have fun swimming. Whenever he went swimming, he wanted either to race or to challenge someone in distance swimming. With guidance, he realized that it was healthier to limit competition to the practices and swim meets and to enjoy water games and relaxing swimming with his friends. Third, these children need assistance in formulating well-defined goals.

Characteristically, they tend to push themselves beyond their abilities, strength, and endurance because there is no defined goal or identifiable end. For example, a sixth grader who stayed up later and later each evening to complete her homework was tired and grouchy during the day. Upon investigation, her parent discovered that she not only was doing her homework but extra credit work as well. She and her parent discussed family expectations and academic achievement in concrete terms and together set well-defined, reachable goals. Fourth, these children need help in identifying and dealing with anger in constructive ways. When challenged, they respond aggressively and impatiently in an attempt to control the situation. They benefit from learning relaxation techniques (see Chapter 18).

Sullivan (1963) identified two other factors contributing to social development during this period: social subordination and social accommodation. *Social subordination* is a redefinition of the authorities to whom the child must answer. At this stage, the family is no longer the only authority, and other authorities such as teachers, counselors, or crossing guards have become a part of the child's environment. These people have limitations on their authority, however, and children must understand their power and how this differs from family authority at home. *Social accommodation* is the process by which children learn that the environment consists of people different from each other and from themselves. Children first label such differences as right or wrong but begin to learn to approach a person or situation with some degree of flexibility.

During this time, however, children's social accommodation is incompletely developed, and they are often cruel to other children who are considered different. Children with eyeglasses or dental braces, those who are poor students or clumsy athletes, or those whose skin color, name, religion, or style of dress varies from that of the majority are common targets for ridicule.

Children who are bused to different neighborhoods for school find the experience a mixture of positives and negatives. Their obvious minority status subjects them to isolation, teasing, and curiosity. Teachers and counselors can create a mutually beneficial situation in which both groups learn from each other so that each group becomes more flexible and accepting of others.

Through social accommodation, children form peer subgroups such as clubs or gangs. These may facilitate socialization, or they may generate rebellion against parental figures or other authorities. Children at this time often discover what other children can or cannot do, what they can get away with, and what they get punished for. They see differences in their peers' parents' expectations that they never imagined could exist. Children now integrate competition, compromise, social accommodation, and social subordination into their personal development, and they gain a more accurate and realistic self-image.

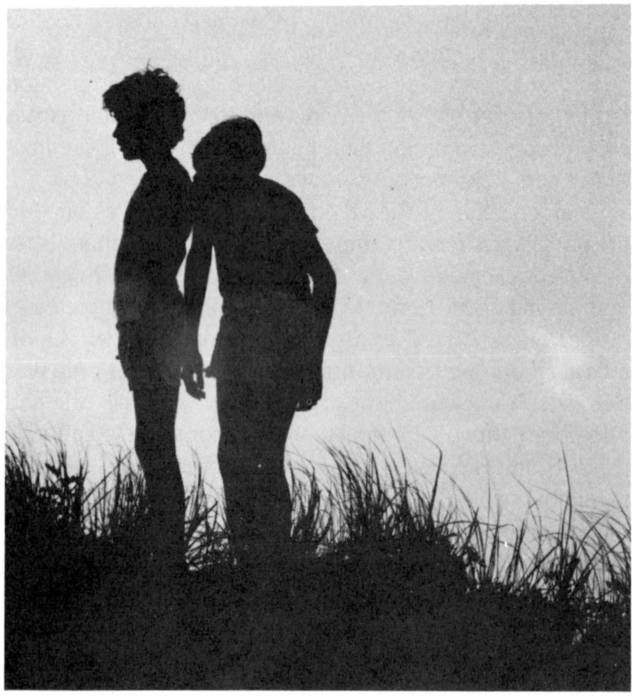

Late childhood is a time of close same-sex friendships, or "chumships," which are part of the process of social accommodation.

Solitude and Social Interactions At times during late childhood, the child needs solitude and respite from a complex and changing world; at other times, social interactions are crucial to development and survival within the growing complex of suprasystems that involve the child. Most children seek moments of solitude through such activities as reading, playing in their own rooms, or fantasizing in private. Social interactions vary depending on the child's environment and companions; interactions take place at home, on the playground, or in school. Social interactions are a testing ground for their newly acquired skills, and each child handles interactions in a characteristic way. Whether timid or aggressive, each child incorporates both solitude and interaction into social development.

Developmental Tasks Robert S. Havighurst (1972) defined the principal developmental tasks of late childhood as gaining mastery over one's own body and developing intrapersonal and interpersonal skills (see Chapter 6). Specifically, developmental tasks at this stage are as follows:

1. Learning the physical skills necessary for ordinary games
2. Building wholesome attitudes toward oneself as a growing person
3. Learning to get along with age-mates
4. Learning an appropriate masculine or feminine role
5. Developing fundamental skills in reading, writing, and calculating
6. Developing the concepts necessary for everyday living
7. Developing conscience, morality, and a scale of values
8. Achieving personal independence
9. Developing attitudes toward social groups and institutions

Mastering one's body is important to the child's self-image. Children concentrate on developing the dexterity and control needed to master new tasks or skills. Late childhood is a time when children ally themselves with those most like themselves. Same-sex peers become increasingly important as children develop their feminine and masculine roles. Now that the once-rigid differentiation in gender-related roles has changed, both boys and girls cross the boundaries traditionally set up by families, cultures, or societies. For example, many Little League and soccer teams are comprised of both boys and girls. In school and organized clubs everyone is required to learn sewing, cooking, and carpentry.

Integrating Development Through Play

During late childhood, play strengthens the child's self-concept, self-esteem, and emerging sexuality. Play, alone or with peers, provides an environment in which a sense of industry can develop. The child takes pride in new tasks mastered in play; for example, riding a bicycle as well as or better than peers promotes self-concept, self-esteem, and a sense of industry.

Organized play can promote or diminish a child's self-esteem. Little is more humiliating than being the last one selected to play a team sport. Such a child usually is seen to have little talent or few friends, and for this child, organized play is dreaded and contributes to a sense of inferiority. On the contrary, being the first child selected or the team captain who does the selecting provides the child with a sense of accomplishment or a new role to try.

Creating gender-specific roles in play and creating fantasies concerning male–female relationships promote the child's developing sexuality. Fantasy is also a vehicle for the child to consider new roles. Daydreams and make-believe play allow the children to be heroes or heroines and superstars. Goals and wishes are attained through fantasy.

Play also maintains and promotes body functions and physical skills. Riding, jumping, team sports, and other vigorous activities promote circulation, metabolism, muscle tone and strength, and elimination. Drawing, coloring, cutting paper dolls, and sewing promote fine motor skills. Coloring between the lines, playing baseball, and other ball games develop hand–eye coordination.

Play both reflects and promotes cognitive development. Creativity is manifested through building sand castles and snow sculptures, erecting towers, or sewing a simple doll's dress. The child who has mastered concrete operations often collects various objects. Mastery in arithmetic and reading allows children to play board games (for example, Monopoly® or Careers®). Moral and social development are fostered through adhering to the rules of the game because dishonesty among friends is not tolerated. As the child's vocabulary increases and spelling improves, word games such as Scrabble® or Boggle® become popular. Children comprehend space, time, movement, and speed through relay races and swimming meets; they play with time in make believe, such as playing combat and synchronizing imaginary 24-hour watches.

During late childhood, the social component of play takes on a new dimension. Solitary play is often a conscious choice, and interest also develops in group play, as children join baseball and soccer teams, Boy or Girl Scouts, Boys Club, Girls Club, 4-H clubs, as well as nonstructured group play. Team sports help to develop the sense of competition and compromise as children learn to work together to

Appropriate Activities, Games, Crafts, and Hobbies for Late Childhood

Ages 7–8

- Tops, drawing, coloring, painting
- Listening to or reading reality and fantasy stories
- Joining organized clubs
- Beginning team sports
- Games of "it," "tag," and "hide-and-seek"
- Swimming, skating, biking, free-flow dance
- Making simple collages and doll's clothing
- Clay work, sawing wood, and nailing wood together
- Easy board games
- Collecting

Ages 9–10

- Individual play
- Drawing geometric figures, making jewelry
- Dressing up in discarded adult clothing
- Collecting
- Team sports, hopscotch
- Putting on shows and plays, such as a circus or puppet show
- Running a lemonade stand
- Designing a tower or airplanes and other objects out of household items (eg, houses out of ice cream sticks)
- Ballet lessons, piano lessons
- Hiking, skating, biking
- Complicated board games
- Reading folk tales, stories of everyday life, comic books

Ages 10–12

- Sewing, weaving baskets, wood work, metal work, plastic work
- Carving, kite making, knitting
- Designing, drawing
- Collecting
- Singing, attending concerts and museums
- Reading adventure stories, scientific discovery, fantasy, biography, history, mysteries, and westerns
- Gymnastics
- Fishing
- Games that include board games, vocabulary games (eg, crossword puzzles, number games, cards, and knowledge games)

accomplish a goal. If the team wins, each child feels responsible, and self-esteem is increased; if the team loses, self-esteem need not be hampered because team members can commiserate over the loss together.

Health Care Needs of Late Childhood

Hygiene

Children past 6 or 7 years of age are capable of carrying out personal hygiene practices daily. They can be held responsible, in varying degrees, for bathing, grooming, dressing, and properly discarding soiled clothing. Depending on the child's dexterity and ability to manipulate the environment, an adult might be needed to assist the child in activities of daily living. For example, in the early part of late childhood, children may be able to bathe part of their bodies but need help with their back; however, most children can bathe themselves and either fill the bathtub with water or take a shower by 8 or 9 years of age. Because brushing teeth, cutting nails, and cleaning under nails require manual dexterity, children up to 9 years of age might need assistance.

Young children need to be reminded frequently to carry out hygienic practices, but as they grow older, children need fewer reminders and may resent reminders that are too frequent and forceful. By 9 and 10 years of age, many children can assume full responsibility for personal hygiene. They can select their own clothes and place soiled clothing in the proper receptacle. Many children by 11 and 12 years of age, and especially girls, become conscious of fashionable clothes and hair grooming.

Throughout late childhood, children strive for independence and are busy with play and other activities; therefore, parents might meet varying resistance concerning hygienic practices. At 8 years of age, a child may need to be reminded to bathe; at 9 years of age, the child bathes willingly; at 10 years of age, the child bathes infrequently; and at 11 and 12 years of age, the child begins to set a routine for bathing. As the child matures and becomes aware of the body changes brought about by adolescence, grooming and cleanliness become important.

Sleep and Rest

Despite their abundance of energy, children in late childhood do tire and need to restore and repair their bodies. The 8-year-old needs about 10–11 hours of sleep each night (Gesell, Ilg, and Ames, 1977). Bedtime is usually at 8 or 9 P.M., although children seldom fall asleep immediately. Some children read, daydream or talk privately before drifting off to sleep. Others might want a parent to read a story or tuck them into bed. In the morning they awaken spontaneously.

As they grow, children deny or are unaware of the need for sleep. The child might resist bedtime to finish an activity or go to bed later than a younger sibling. Bedtime is progressively delayed, so that although the 8-year-old might go to bed at 8 P.M., the 9- or 10-year-old might not go to bed until 10 P.M. By 10 years of age, less sleep is required, and in some households 10-, 11-, and 12-year-olds have the same bedtimes as an adult. By 12 years of age, the child also resists going to bed less and enjoys quiet, private moments. From 8 or 9 years of age on, listening to the radio or reading a book becomes a common presleep activity. Although sleep time is delayed, children might waken purposefully early so that they can play alone, watch television, or read before going to school. By late childhood, the child's awakening time depends on bedtime and personal preference.

In general, sleep is peaceful during late childhood. Occasional nightmares are often the result of a scary television program or event. Children often independently choose not to watch a scary television program to avoid nightmares.

Nutrition

Nutrition during late childhood is no longer closely monitored by the parents. The child, whose world has expanded and who spends more time outside the home, is influenced by others' eating habits and dietary intake. Children in this age group begin to determine their own nutrition. Mealtime is a social event. The child still enjoys eating with the family and by 10 or 11 years of age, might help prepare part of the meal. Children particularly enjoy preparing recipes learned at school or taken from cookbooks written especially for children. The child gradually learns table manners and might criticize the manners of others, especially those of younger siblings.

At school, friends are also meal partners, and children frequently share or swap parts of their lunches with their friends. Because conformity is the social norm, a child usually wants to buy lunch at school if friends do.

Children have definite food likes and dislikes, but by 7 or 8 years of age, they will try new foods or foods previously not liked. In general, children prefer plain foods to gourmet foods, but as they mature, their food likes resemble those of adults.

The 7-year-old's appetite might still be minimal, but by 8 years of age, children have greater appetites, and by 10 years of age, their appetite is similar to that of an adult. Despite their increasing appetites, children seldom voluntarily interrupt play and other activities for meals. If unsupervised, they might either neglect to eat a meal or simply grab high-carbohydrate snacks until the next meal, which diminishes their appetite for it. Sometimes they are so eager to return to their game or to meet a friend that they hurry through their meal, not taking time to eat a well-balanced meal or satisfy their bodily needs. When hunger and fatigue return, they might become irritable and disagreeable or resort to snacks, usually of the high-carbohydrate variety. Poor eating habits might result in obesity, a fairly common problem during late childhood that is often related to replacing balanced meals with frequent empty-calorie snacks. To promote growth and development, children need at least four servings of milk and cheese, three servings of meat and eggs, four servings of fruits and vegetables, and four servings of breads and cereal. Boys and girls between 7 and 10 years of age require approximately 2400 calories per day. Boys over 11 years of age require an additional 400 calories per day (Pearson, 1979). (See Chapter 15 for a discussion of nutritional assessment in late childhood.)

Dentition

During late childhood, the permanent teeth erupt, and therefore, dietary and hygienic habits in this period will have a lasting effect on the teeth in later years.

Dental caries are extremely common in late childhood. Plaque, a film composed of bacteria and waste products, forms and hardens on tooth enamel (Slattery, 1976). The accumulation of plaque attracts fermentative carbohydrates and provides bacteria with a nutritive environment in which to grow. The interaction of plaque, carbohydrates, and bacteria promotes tooth decay. Plaque is removable. If the plaque has been allowed to harden, a dentist or dental hygienist needs to remove it, but because plaque does not harden immediately, frequent toothbrushing may remove a large portion of it. Children should be taught to brush their teeth after meals and snacks and to use dental floss between their teeth once a day. Frequent brushing is rarely practiced either by children or their adult role models, so that children up to 9 or 10 years of age need to be reminded to brush and floss their teeth and taught how to do both properly. Slattery (1976) noted that children under 10 years of age often lack the manual dexterity to brush the posterior teeth correctly; therefore, parents should assist.

Fluoride in toothpaste and fluoridated water impede tooth decay. Children should be taught to use an appropriate toothpaste and encouraged to drink fluoridated water. Children's diets and eating patterns also should be carefully monitored. Snacks should not be overloaded with soda pop, dark chocolate, cakes, and cookies. Snacks composed of carbohydrates and sugars should be followed by toothbrushing. Frequent dental screening and early treatment of problems will help keep the child's teeth healthy.

Exercise

Most children engage in sufficient physical activity to support normal structure growth. Many children walk to and from school, participate in various sports or play games that involve running, climbing, jumping or bike riding. In addition, some schools have a daily exercise program in which all students perform progressive sets of exercises. Physical activity increases mineralization and bone width, which are important for both muscle and skeletal strength.

Attitude, interests, and habits regarding exercise are developed during childhood. Active children often are active adults, whereas inactive children become sedentary adults. Many adult health problems, especially those related to obesity and cardiovascular diseases, have been related to inactivity in childhood. The adult's functional capacity, motivation, and performance expectations are formulated during childhood (Albinson and Andrew, 1976).

The types of activities children choose are related to the social systems in which they participate. Peer pressure, adult expectations, and role models influence values and behavior. A child with a talent for a particular motor skill will not develop it if the peer groups spend their free time playing video games at the neighborhood arcade. Parents still need to supervise their children's activity to ensure a balance between active exercise, whether in sports or games, and quiet activity. Children benefit when parents support them in their activities. They usually want to have family members watch them participate in races or ball games. If parents are unable to attend, the child is eager to tell them about the race or game afterward.

Parents must have realistic expectations of their children's abilities, otherwise the children can become discouraged and feel inferior. The child experiences physical, cognitive, and social maturation between 8 and 12 years of age, which contribute to improved coordination, speed, understanding of events, and ability to plan strategies. Activities and expectations must coincide with development. Adults might need to help the child comprehend this concept as well. Children frequently place unrealistic demands on themselves to either win or perform beyond their abilities. This self-demand might be as true for video and computer games as for active games and organized sports.

Safety

Much of the child's recreation time is spent in physical activity and sports, which contribute to growth and development, but are potentially harmful. Injuries sustained from physical activity and sports range from minor to fatal (see Chapter 19). A child runs down the street, trips, and scrapes a knee. A boy climbs a high fence, his pants get caught on the wire, and as he tries to free himself, he falls, fracturing the bones in his legs. A girl riding a bicycle tries to catch up to her friends across the street, neglects to look for traffic, collides with a car, and is killed. A child's eye is injured by a thrown baseball. A child unable to swim walks out into the water too far and drowns. The list of injuries, accidents, and casualties is endless.

Despite the potential dangers, children should not be discouraged from partaking in physical activity or sports, but education, guidance, and frequent safety reminders are warranted. During late childhood, the cognitive ability to grasp and use the concepts of safety is present. Children can be taught the rules of safety and prevention just as they can be taught the rules of a game. Simple reminders such as "look both ways before you cross the street" and "no pushing on the ice" help to reinforce safety rules. Prevention is best carried out through proper instruction. Coaches, knowledgeable in team sports, can educate children about the body mechanics involved in a given sport. Swimming or skating lessons might prevent casualties. Making certain that children are wearing the appropriate attire for a given sport or activity might prevent injury (for example, wearing sneakers on a gym floor, wearing jogging shoes to run). Health screening might identify those children whose health dictates that they should be excused from certain activities.

Transition to Adolescence

The theme of late childhood is the child's growing independence and responsibilities for self-care, decision making, and perfecting motor skills. It is also a time for learning new combinations of physical skills and mental powers and of understanding the successes and failures of human life. It is a time when adults outside the home exert an increasing influence on children and peers take on increased value. During late childhood, children attempt to master the roles and responsibilities needed for socialization in their culture, with the comfort of knowing they can still enjoy being a child at the same time. Through school, play, and interpersonal relationships within the home environment and the outside world, children perfect the first steps they took as younger children to walk into adolescence with a sense of accomplishment, self-esteem, independence, industry, and affiliation.

Key Concepts

- Late childhood is a time of coordinating, perfecting, and using the skills gained through earlier experiences and learning and increased independence as the child spends more time away from home at school, clubs, lessons, and play.
- Peers become constant companions, selected on the basis of similar interests, compatible personalities, and traits such as honesty and trustworthiness.
- The child interacts increasingly with the suprasystems that characterize the community, learning in the process that the beliefs, rituals, and values others subscribe to might differ from the child's.
- The family remains a significant influence in the child's life, but it moves to the background as peers and other adults assume greater importance.
- During late childhood, the child's biophysical, affective, cognitive, and social development continue to be refined.
- Biophysical growth continues at a steady, although slower, pace. Organs have reached maturity in structure and function. Motor skills are expanded and refined, enabling the child to perform more complex tasks.
- Major changes occur in the child's cognitive thought processes. Piaget refers to this stage as the concrete operational phase.
- The cognitive problem-solving that occurs is related to concrete objects and is the transition from action necessary in earlier phases to the verbal hypothetical ability yet to develop.
- Late childhood is characterized by a general decentering of cognitive thought processes. The child can take the perspective of another, can reverse or reconstruct the events or problem to reach a solution.
- Children use language to express thought, explain the logic they used to solve the problem, and communicate new knowledge.
- During late childhood, operations of seriation, class inclusion, reversibility, and conservation of length, weight, and volume are mastered.
- Formal schooling provides the setting and motivation for children to develop and use their skills in reading, writing, mathematics, and information processing.
- Short-term and long-term memory improves during late childhood, allowing children to use and apply previously learned material more efficiently.

- Moral and faith development advance to include the social implications of behavior.
- The child in this phase spends much energy completing projects and accomplishing goals. Success is judged by the recognition received from others.
- Self-esteem grows when the child is successful in some endeavor; feelings of inferiority grow if success and recognition are not attained.
- Children with high self-esteem are more autonomous and creative and less likely to conform.
- Sexual awareness increases, as does the need for accurate information about pubescent changes and reproduction.
- Friendships become extremely important. Friends provide feedback and comfort.
- Responsibilities increase as children participate in household chores such as mowing grass and taking care of younger siblings.
- Health care maintenance becomes the child's responsibility. Children at this age need to be reminded less to perform hygiene and dental care practices because their appearance becomes more important to them.
- Children in late childhood make more decisions about nutrition, and they eat more and more meals away from home.
- Late childhood is an active and generally healthy phase. Basic exercise habits and endurance as well as attitudes toward exercise are formulated.
- During late childhood, children learn more about themselves, their interests, and abilities and begin to prepare for adolescence.

References

Albinson JG, Andrews GM: *The Child in Sport and Physical Activity.* University Park Press, 1976.

Allen MT: An overview of the Type A behavior pattern in children and adolescents. *Pediatr Nurs* (Nov/Dec) 1983; 9(6):407–412.

Baumrind D: Parental control and parental love. *Children* 1965; 12:230–234.

Beard R: *An Outline of Piaget's Developmental Psychology for Students and Teachers.* Mentor Books, 1969.

Blaesing S, Bruckhaus J: The development of body image in the child. *Nurs Clin North Am* (Dec) 1972; 7:560–592.

Boehm L: The development of independence: A comparative study. *Child Dev* 1957; 28:85–92.

Boettcher J, Boettcher K: Sex education for fifth and sixth graders and their parents. *Am J Matern Child Nurs* (July/Aug) 1978; 3(4):218–220.

Bridgewater SC, Voignier RR, Smith, CS: Allergies in children: Recognization. *Am J Nurs* (April) 1978; 78(4):613–621.

Bronfenbrenner U: Response to pressure from peers versus adults among Soviet and American school children. *Int J Psychol* 1967; 2:199–207.

Carpenter F: *The Skinner Primer.* Free Press, 1974.

Chinn PL: *Child Health Maintenance: Concepts in Family Centered Care.* 2d ed. Mosby, 1979.

Chomsky CS: *The Acquisition of Syntax in Children from 5 to 10.* MIT Press, 1969.

Cooke RE (editor): *The Biological Basis of Pediatric Practice.* McGraw-Hill, 1968.

Coopersmith S: *The Antecedents of Self-Esteem.* Freeman, 1967.

Elkind D: *Children and Adolescents: Interpretative Essays on Jean Piaget.* 2nd ed. Oxford University Press, 1974.

Erikson EH: *Childhood and Society.* 2d ed. Norton, 1963.

Fowler JW: Toward a developmental perspective on faith. *Relig Educ* 1974; 69:207–219.

Fredland M: Latency: Its tasks and its settings: An overview. In: *Sexuality and Psychoanalysis.* Adelsons E (editor). Brunner/Mazel, 1975.

Freud S: *Three Essays on the Theory of Sexuality.* Basic Books, 1962.

Gagne R: *The Conditions of Learning.* 3rd ed. Holt, Rinehart & Winston, 1977.

Gesell AL, Ilg FL, Ames, LB: *The Child from Five to Ten.* Harper & Row, 1977.

Gesell AL, Ilg, FL, Ames LB: *Youth: The Years from Ten to Sixteen.* Harper & Row, 1956.

Havighurst RJ: *Developmental Tasks and Education.* 3rd ed. McKay, 1972.

Hetherington EM, Cox M, Cox R: The aftermath of divorce. In: *Mother–Child/Father–Child Relations.* Stevens JH, Matthews M (editors). National Association for the Education of Young Children, 1978.

Holm VA: Childhood. In: *The Biologic Ages of Man.* Smith DW, Bierman EL, Robinson NM (editors). Saunders, 1978.

Inhelder B: Memory and intelligence in the child. In: *Studies in Cognitive Development: Essays in Honor of Jean Piaget.* Elkind D, Flavell J (editors). Oxford, 1979.

Kaluger G, Kaluger MF: *Human Development.* Mosby, 1984.

Kohlberg L: Continuities in childhood and adult moral development revisited. In: *Life-Span Developmental Psychology: Personality and Socialization.* Bates PB, Schaie KW (editors). Academic Press, 1973.

Kohlberg L: Stage and sequence: The cognitive–development approach to socialization. In: *Handbook of Socialization: Theory and Research.* Goslin D (editor). Rand-McNally, 1969.

Labinowicz E: *The Piaget Primer.* Addison-Wesley, 1980.

Pearson G: Nutrition during the middle years of childhood. In: *Maternal and Child Nutrition: Assessment and Counseling.* Slattery J, Pearson G, Torre C (editors). Appleton-Century-Crofts, 1979.

Piaget J: *The Child's Conception of Movement and Speed.* Ballentine Books, 1970.

Piaget J: *The Child's Conception of Space.* Basic Books, 1962.

Piaget J: *The Child's Conception of Time.* Norton, 1967.

Piaget J: *The Language and Thought of the Child.* Meridian Books, 1974.

Piaget J: *The Moral Judgment of the Child.* The Free Press, 1965.

Piaget J, Inhelder B: *The Psychology of the Child.* Basic Books, 1969.

Ryan TJ: Psychosocial development and activity in middle childhood. In: *Child in Sport and Physical Activity.* Albinson JG, Andrew GM (editors). University Park Press, 1976.

Santrock JW: *Life-Span Development.* Brown, 1983.

Schilder P: *The Image and Appearance of the Human Body.* International Press, 1970.
Schuster CS, Ashburn SS: *The Process of Human Development.* Little, Brown, 1980.
Siegal JM, Matthews KA: Type A behavior, achievement striving and their childhood origins. In: *Advances in School Psychology.* Vol 3. Kratochwill TR (editor). Erlbaum, 1983.
Sieman M: Mental health in school age children. *Am Matern Child Nurs* (July/Aug) 1978; 3(4):215.
Slattery J: Dental health in children. *Am J Nurs* (Feb) 1976; 76(2):1159–1161.
Sullivan HS: *The Interpersonal Theory of Psychiatry.* Norton, 1953.
Vernon PE: Ability factors and environmental influences. *Am Psychol* 1965; 20:723–733.
Wallerstein JS, Kelly JB: *Surviving the Breakup: How Children Actually Cope with Divorce.* Basic Books, 1980.
Wechsler D: *The Measurement and Appraisal of Adult Intelligence.* Williams & Wilkins, 1958.
Yanni MIY: Perception of parent's behavior and children's general fearfulness. *Nurs Res* (March/April) 1982; 31(2):79–82.
Yussen SR, Santrock JW: *Child Development.* Brown, 1982.

Additional Readings

Betz CL: Faith development in children. *Pediatr Nurs* (March/April) 1981; 7:22–25.
Cohen DH: *The Learning Child.* Vintage Books, 1972.
Fischer KW, Lazerson A: *Human Development.* Freeman, 1984.
Friedman M: *Pathogenesis of Coronary Artery Disease.* McGraw-Hill, 1969.
Gelfand DM: *Social Learning in Childhood.* 2nd ed. Brooks/Cole, 1976.
Kagan J, Moss H: *Birth to Maturity.* Wiley, 1962.
Magnusson D, Allen VL: *Human Development.* Academic Press, 1983.
McCown DE: Moral development in children. *Pediatr Nurs* (Jan/Feb) 1984; 10:42–45.
Oda DS: Community nursing in schools: Developing a specialized role. In: *Community Health Nursing.* Archer S, Fleshman R (editors). Duxbury Press, 1979.
Omery A: Moral development: A differential evaluation of dominant models. *Adv Nurs Sci* (Oct) 6(1):1–17.
Salzinger K: *Psychology: The Science of Behavior.* Springer, 1969.
Sarnoff C: Normal and pathological psychological development during the latency age period. In: *Development in Normality and Psychopathology.* Bemporad J (editor). Brunner/Mazel, 1980.
Singer JL: *The Inner World of Daydreaming.* Harper & Row, 1975.
Strickland D: Friendship patterns and altruistic behavior in preadolescent males and females. *Nurs Res* (July/Aug) 1980; 30(4):222, 228, 235.
Tuan Y: *Landscapes of Fear.* Pantheon Books, 1979.
Yelen SL, Weinstein A: Theories of learning. In: *A Teacher's World.* Weinstein A, Yelen SL (editors). McGraw-Hill, 1977.

Adolescence

Jean A. O'Neil

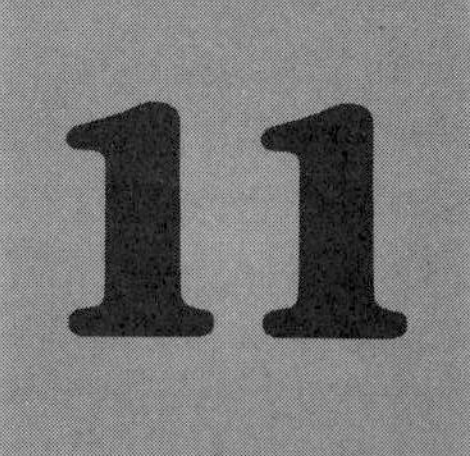

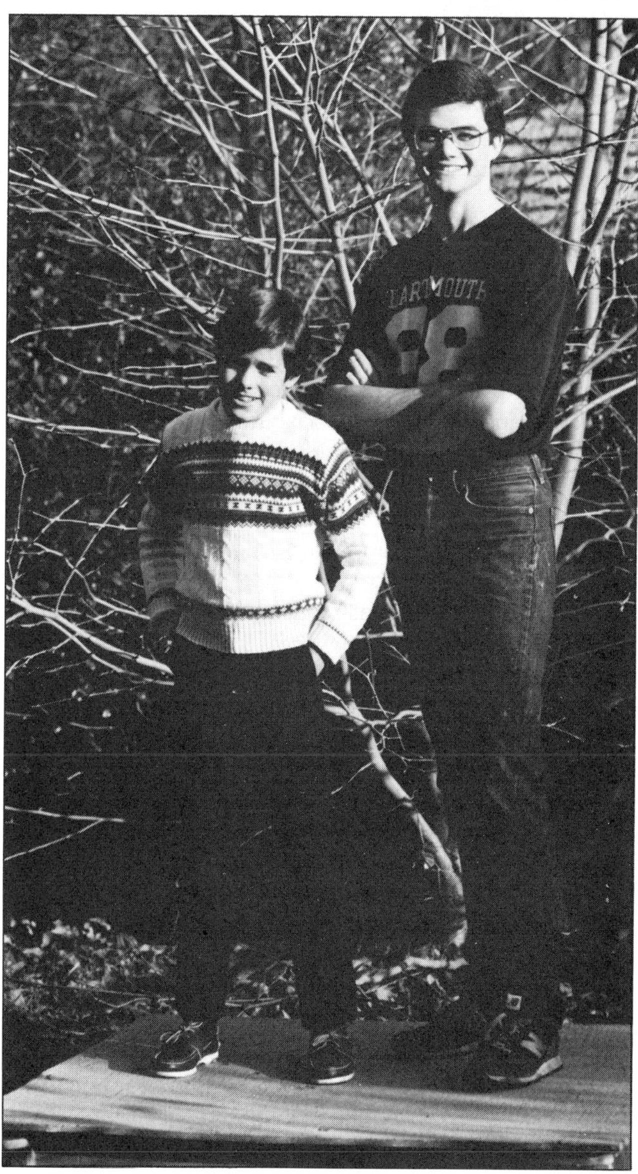

Chapter Outline

Objectives

- Explain the influences of both suprasystems and subsystems on the adolescent's development.
- Define the major parameters of development in adolescents.
- Explain the essential biophysical changes that occur in adolescence.
- Describe the principal theoretic explanations for personality, cognitive, language, moral, and social development in adolescence.
- Define the criteria that distinguish adolescence from adulthood.
- Identify the basic health care needs of adolescents.

Adolescence is the longest developmental stage and the most difficult to define. Some authorities define it chronologically as the teenage years or the years when the reproductive system matures, a process that might begin as early as age $8\frac{1}{2}$ and extend into the 20s. Others define adolescence as a time of emerging legal and economic independence and place it in a social framework. If that social framework is the school system, adolescence in the United States may begin in the sixth or seventh grade, or middle school or junior high school, and may end after graduation or withdrawal from senior high school or college, depending on the person's legal age, maturity, or occupational attainment. Psychologically, adolescence is an optimistic time of rapid growth in physical, intellectual, and social achievement, but it is also a period of moodiness, rebellion, or even a sad loss of childhood innocence and ease.

The universally recognized biologic changes that mark the transition from childhood to adulthood are more extensive than popular literature, which tends to focus on size, strength, and reproductive system changes, would lead one to believe. In adolescence metabolic and hormonal changes affect almost every subsystem, and psychosocial development is further affected by the interaction of physical, cognitive, and emotional capacities. Physical growth and development do merit detailed discussion, but physical development does not occur in isolation from psychosocial development.

In this chapter, we cover both the physical, cognitive, and psychosocial parameters of adolescent development. We analyze the impact of the suprasystems on shaping the adolescent's emerging sense of identity, and we review the health care needs of adolescents along with the nurse's role in promoting self-care.

Developmental Changes in Adolescence

Many words used to describe this phase of life are biologically based. The most general term, *maturation,* applies to the physical changes that occur as a result of internal body processes or internal regulation (Valadian and Porter, 1977). For example, rapid height increments are evidence of a growth spurt and signify maturation. Such physical growth is related more closely to age than to environment, but suprasystems and subsystems do interact. For example, an adolescent's decision to use weights to build muscles does not spur maturation, but muscle size and strength-building efforts will not succeed unless they coincide with maturation of the muscular system. Social environment and age consequently are both factors in the physical changes that occur at this stage.

The terms *pubescence* and *puberty* are less well defined. Both derive from the Latin "pubescere," which means to be covered with hair (Katchadourian, 1977), but are applied to various aspects of sexual maturation. *Pubescence* is similar to maturation but is more specific in that it covers the process of internal physiologic changes involved in reproductive system maturation. *Puberty* may describe a process involving numerous changes and a considerable amount of time or it may be defined by a specific event (Sommer, 1978). For example, puberty as an event is definitely signaled in the female by menarche, or the first menstrual period. In the male puberty is signaled to some by the presence of pigmented pubic hair and to others by the first ejaculation.

The difference between puberty and pubescence is therefore related to process. Puberty involves the relationship between physiologic and psychologic changes occurring as early as age $8\frac{1}{2}$ in the preadolescent period and reaching a peak in the mid or late teens. *Nubility,* a term applied to the late phase of puberty, or the outcome of pubescence, refers to the attainment of reproductive maturity and fertility. This word is derived from the Latin "nubilis," meaning of marriageable age (Katchadourian, 1977) and marks what is currently recognized as the last phase of the process of adolescence.

Although the sequence of maturation is universal, the rate is highly variable between sexes and among individuals of the same sex. The average age of onset of puberty is 2 years earlier in females than in males, but factors other than sex differences affect pace. Some authorities feel that body type differences often are correlated with the tempo of maturation. Terminology describing distinctive or predominant characteristics of body types in both sexes is based on the germinal layers of embryonic development used in medical and psychologic literature (Sheldon, Stevens, and Tucker, 1940; Tanner, 1962).

The first body type to complete maturation is the *mesomorph,* a body type characterized by rectangular shape, hardness, apparent bone and muscle development, and strength (Lindzey and Hall, 1978). Individuals with this body type tend to be taller and fatter before puberty but may be the same height or even shorter than age and sex peers at nubility (Tanner, 1962). At the opposite extreme is the linear, fragile, flat-chested, thin, lightly muscled, large-brained *ectomorph* (Lindzey and Hall, 1978). When late-maturing, the ectomorphic individual may reach the greatest height. In the middle is the *endomorph,* who is soft, spheric, low in muscle and bone development, but high in digestive system development. The endomorphic individual may begin puberty before the mesomorphic person and end it after the ectomorphic individual, taking the longest time for pubescence (Tanner, 1962).

Even with standard differences between the sexes, a female ectomorph, or late-maturing girl, may begin maturation later than a male mesomorph, or early-maturing boy.

Influence of the Suprasystems

Culture and Ethnicity The community's recognition of the change from child to adult status is specific in the *rites of passage,* or initiation ceremonies marking the start of adulthood, that are common to many societies worldwide. Vestiges of transitional rituals remain in certain religious practices and in the significance attached to certain social events, school progressions, and laws. For example, Christian confirmation and Jewish Bar and Bat Mitzvah reflect the need and ability of an adolescent to affirm through personal decision a belief in the religious doctrines he or she has been taught. The laws governing the assumption of adult rights and responsibilities, such as the legal age for marriage, consent for health care, compulsory education, employment, driving, military service, criminal procedures, and drinking alcoholic beverages, vary but are also forms of recognition of adult status.

The needs and aspirations of some cultural and ethnic groups may conflict with these laws. For example, migrant workers frequently violate compulsory education and child labor laws; the Amish religious sect also obtains exemptions from compulsory education laws to preserve its traditions (Stone and Church, 1973).

Socioeconomic Resources Social class, particularly income level and the interaction patterns associated with it, seems to be more influential than race or ethnicity in determining the social involvement and achievement of adolescents. Lower levels of employment, lower salaries, shorter school enrollment, increasing numbers of families where fathers are absent, increasing frequency of premarital pregnancies, and early marriages are documented characteristics that affect adolescent development in lower-class and working-class families (Gordon, 1972).

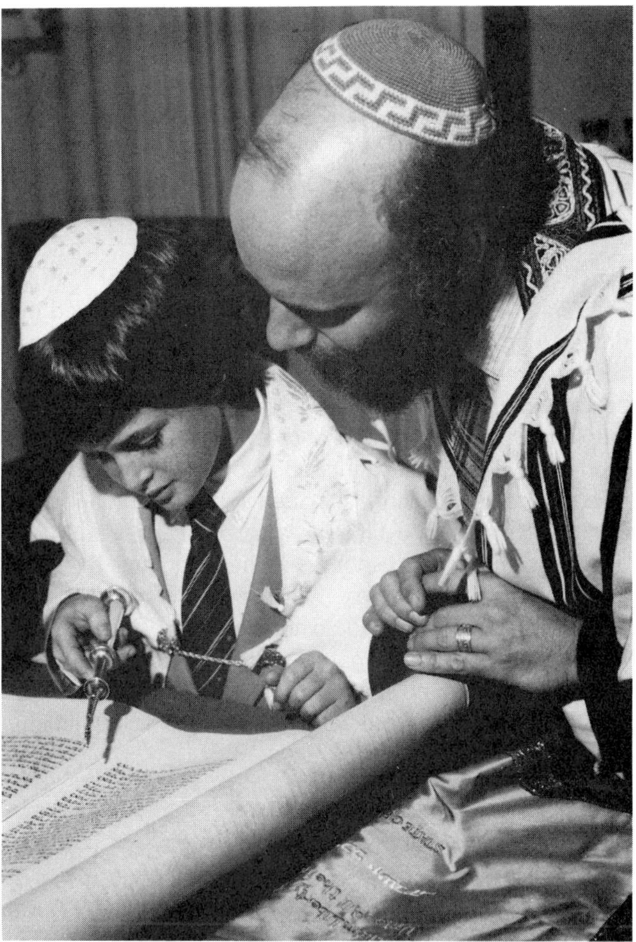

Rites of passage, such as the Jewish bar mitzvah, traditionally mark the transition to adulthood and are common to many cultures.

Because basic necessities are of paramount importance, these factors intrinsically affect the quality of the adolescent's life. Adolescents in the lower socioeconomic classes are often needed to help support the family financially. This necessitates after-school employment or even increased school absenteeism. School work suffers, leading to failure and/or dropping out. The adolescent may be unable to participate in enriching extracurricular activities. Opportunities for peer activities and involvement in school clubs or projects are limited.

The lower-class adolescent is influenced by family expectations that encourage early adulthood. As a result of this, the adolescent might perceive school as drudgery and leave at the first available opportunity. Expectations of adolescents at the upper-income level emphasize that the child not embarrass the family. It is not essential for the child to be brilliant, and school may be seen as a place to have a good time. For those adolescents who are intellectually motivated, however, belonging to an upper socioeconomic level gives them educational advantages and parental support helpful to goal achievement. Demographic forecasts predict that greater proportions of the adolescent population will be found in lower socioeconomic groups and in urban centers in the near future (Gordon, 1972).

More directly, the prolonged schooling of postindustrial societies, which marks the social framework of adolescence, is a pattern of deferred gratification that conflicts with the needs, goals, and actions of people involved in a daily struggle for economic survival. Schools are not successful in meeting all the adolescents' needs for acceptance and achievement. Social class lines, often influenced by the amount of money available for dress and membership dues, tend to be rigidly drawn in school social groups and activities. The early tracking of students into vocational paths also might accentuate differences in potential development, as well as emotional responses to the judgments that decisions about education imply (Kagan, 1972). Because courses in vocational schools often do not parallel those in standard high schools, the vocational student's opportunities to redirect goals are limited. Later tracking would facilitate more accurate decisions about career directions without limiting opportunities.

Family Family structure, interaction, and aspirations are consistently believed to be more influential than schooling factors in achievement motivation (Gordon, 1972). Socioeconomic class-related family styles also might present problems. Communication patterns, educational attainments of parents and siblings, and parental aspirations are repeatedly noted to correlate with adolescent achievement in education (Rosen, 1969).

In a family it is often apparent that one or more of the children will follow in the career footsteps of the parents, provided that the parents are satisfied with their own career choices. Years ago, when there were limited opportunities for women, this was more evident. If the mother were a housewife, nurse, or teacher, the daughter often would choose the same occupation. With expanding opportunities for women, adolescent girls, while using the mother as a role model, also might consider the father's occupation as a valid career choice.

Size of the family is reported to be significantly related to achievement, with more success demonstrated by children from small families or older children from large families. Adolescents from families where parents and/or siblings have demonstrated high achievement levels tend to follow the same course. Small families often can more easily promote intellectual growth and achievement because more individual attention generally is given to each child. This is more difficult in larger families. The oldest child initially receives a great deal of attention and stimulation. As the others arrive, time constraints usually make it impossible to do the same for successive children. Oldest children therefore may be more motivated than their siblings to pursue advanced education.

Another important factor is the *role modeling* of adult behavior, a form of imitation common to adolescents. Role models for behaviors are diverse and important at this stage (Bandura, 1969). Other relatives or esteemed adults, such as teachers, Scout leaders, coaches, religious leaders or political leaders, serve as role models for occupational choices that the adolescent may choose to pursue. If the adult is positive about the career and the rewards are obvious, the likelihood of the adolescent's following an early interest in a similar career is increased.

The adolescent's searching for explanations of cultural, ethnic, socioeconomic, and family structure differences leads to a recognition of the values held and expressed by the parents. Happiness, honesty, consideration, and dependability are values reported by both middle-class and working-class parents, but the differences in childrearing illustrate different emphases between future-oriented goals and standards.

Middle-class childrearing patterns, aimed at aiding the young to achieve self-control, autonomy, and concern for others, focus on the intent of a person's actions. The give and take of communication necessary to evaluate intent is a kind of analysis that helps to foster verbal ability. Verbal ability alone ranks above parental aspirations, social class, and self-esteem as factors correlated with the educational aspirations of adolescents.

Working-class families, on the other hand, are reported to use stricter, more authoritarian childrearing patterns that focus on achieving respectability, as demonstrated by obedience to situational rules (Duvall, 1977). For example, in making judgments about whether to use alcohol the adolescent from the middle-class family is more apt to examine the options and discuss the advantages and disadvantages of the situation with family members. Thus, the final decision ultimately is made by the adolescent, with the understanding that consequences of the decision are accepted. Conversely, the adolescent from the more authoritarian environment faces preset guidelines or rules, thus diminishing the capacity for decision making. This adolescent may demonstrate behavior extremes of conformity or rebellion.

School Socially, the school years expand the child's peer interactions. A progression occurs from same-sex, informal play groups to more structured competitive and cooperative group activities and then to exclusive, same-sex partnerships or "chumships" (Sullivan, 1953). All of these interactions precede apparent interest in the opposite sex. Expressed interest in the opposite sex and in marriage as a goal frequently is concurrent with the onset of puberty (Mussen, Conger, and Kagan, 1974).

From the learning tasks of late childhood, the child gains confidence in personal achievement and the ability to initiate and achieve projects and to complete or cooperate with peers (Gruen, 1964). These outcomes foster a sense of industry, as described by Erikson (1963) (see Chapter 6). This or the opposite outcome, which Erikson termed a sense of inferiority, affects the ability or willingness to plan for adult roles, further education, or occupation.

School as a suprasystem has a multifaceted effect on the adolescent because it provides an environment suitable for promoting task completion. In addition to encouraging cognitive development, schools establish a climate of social interaction. Adolescents, in contacts with their peers and teachers in the school setting, validate thoughts and test new ideas in the process of developing unique identities. During the high school years, adolescents assume responsibility for learning (one hopes). These years are a time for finding and developing the self and being accountable for personal behavior.

The learning climate in the schools allows adolescents to explore avenues of future goals and directions while being guided by significant others outside the family structure. During the high school years, many adolescents make preliminary decisions about vocations or careers and take definite steps toward achieving their goals such as applying for college admission, obtaining job experience, or receiving vocational training.

Extracurricular activities offered by most school systems allow the adolescent opportunities to engage in team participation or the in-depth pursuit of a hobby or other constructive activity. Some schools offer a variety of sports as well as theater groups, bands, newspapers, television and radio studios, ski clubs, and more. These activities not only promote special interests but also provide structured opportunities for contacts with members of the opposite sex in nonthreatening situations. These opportunities promote the development of a sense of confidence in future heterosexual relationships.

Peers Perhaps at no other stage in development do one's peers have as major an influence as during adolescence. As children mature and begin to separate from the family, the peer group becomes important as a judge of ideas, morality, mode of dress, and activity participation. It becomes extremely important for the adolescent to become "one of the group." Popularity seems to be an important goal. In any setting, however, the groups vary according to informal standards established by the members. For instance, the most popular adolescents in one group may be those who wear designer clothing and are judged to be the most physically attractive. Other groups may have an activity, such as sports, auto mechanics, or computer programming, in common, or they all may be particularly talented in music, art, dance, or science. Even those who are considered unpopular by their peers might be members of a group whose basis is their unpopularity. The sense of belonging is a basic need.

Peer groups provide a dilemma for many adolescents, however, because in an attempt to live up to the standards of the group or to become more popular, they may feel forced to depart from the family standards. Decisions about whether to engage in substance abuse or to participate in sexual relations, for example, are major decisions with far-reaching consequences (see Chapters 24 and 39). The ability to resist peer pressure at the risk of losing popularity requires a consistently supportive attitude from parents and teachers. Adolescents eventually learn to internalize standards but often as a result of trial and error. Unfortunately, in some cases experimentation as a result of peer pressure has undesirable and even tragic consequences such as teenage pregnancy and deaths from drunk driving. A successful beginning in developing standards eases the transition into adulthood, where peers more often are judged by their unique qualities than by a common appearance or actions.

Interactions Among Subsystems

A *secular trend* is a phenomenon manifested through many years or generations; it has no connotations of or opposition to religion (Katchadourian, 1977). Secular trends related to adolescence are (1) increasingly earlier ages of onset of puberty and (2) attainment of greater height and weight during puberty. For example, since 1900, research in western countries has demonstrated that average menarche occurs 4 months earlier, height has increased 1.0–2.5 cm, and weight has increased 0.5 kg (Tanner, 1972). The trend toward the earlier onset of puberty does, however, seem to be leveling off.

Some researchers are concerned that the earlier onset of puberty may interfere with the attainment of physical, social, and cognitive skills needed for adult roles. Although Freud designated the preadolescent school-age years as a latency period free from the conflict of sexual drives, more recent research has renewed interest in childhood accomplishments (Hall, 1954). The nurse's knowledge of earlier developmental progress is therefore useful in assessing the impact of puberty. Children may experience relatively short or long periods of slow growth, during which they may direct energy into motor skill coordination, competence, and satisfaction in peer relationships and both formal and informal pursuit of knowledge. All of these areas of human development are challenged in adolescence. Specific, definite expectations of self and others are more uncertain in adolescence. Even social opportunities are influenced by variations in the pace of puberty, a phenomenon over which the adolescent has no control.

During late childhood, the child becomes more graceful and coordinated as body proportions slim, legs lengthen, and posture straightens. Longer legs and arms and a lower center of gravity aid gross motor skills of running, reaching, climbing, and bike riding. Continued myelinization of the nervous system enhances achievement in writing and other fine motor skills. Then, certain features of the adolescent growth spurt disrupt steady progress in the attainment of these gross and fine motor skills. First, a disproportionate phase occurs during the growth spurt, and, second, the outward manifestations of change increase self-awareness.

Physiologically, developmental age is calculated by skeletal age and not chronologic age. Although trunk growth eventually accounts for 60% of the adolescent's increase in height, the sequence of growth begins in the extremities, with closure of the epiphyseal growth plates in the long bones under the influence of sex-specific hormones. During this sequence, members of either sex may appear and feel awkward and uncoordinated; both sexes may worry about sex-inappropriate changes. For example, girls may worry about their temporary appearance of having disproportionately large hands and feet. Young people need reassuring information about expected growth patterns during this period of *asynchrony* (maturation of different body parts at different rates) (Valadian and Porter, 1977).

Restlessness, moodiness, and fluctuations between independence and dependence are signals of transition that reflect a *lability*, or lack of stability in emotions and behavior. Lability is often made evident by spoken desires unmatched by preparation (Elkind and Weiner, 1978). Lability of impulse control may relate to loss of body control. In puberty, both sexes must deal with body functions over which they initially have no control: menstruation in the female and penile erection in the male. Again, young people need information to explain and validate what is "normal."

Parameters of Adolescent Development

Biophysical Development

Musculoskeletal System Growth is a major characteristic of adolescence; in fact, more growth occurs during this period than at any time since infancy. Height and weight changes are particularly noticeable because they follow the plateau of slow childhood growth from the ages of 5 to 10 years. This peak in the incremental growth curve corresponds with breast development and precedes menarche in girls; it usually occurs between 10 and 18 years of age. In boys the growth spurt follows testicular enlargement and corresponds with penile elongation; it usually occurs between 12 and 20 years of age. The trunk is the fastest-growing portion of the body and accounts for 60% of the height increase (Valadian and Porter, 1977).

The influence of sex hormones on epiphyseal (growth plate) closure in the long bones of the extremities causes a close relation between the pace of maturation and eventual height. A very early or very late onset of puberty corresponds to extremes of short or tall stature unless this factor is counteracted by a genetic base for shortness or tallness. Adolescents who reach puberty at the mean (average) age are usually at the mean for height and weight of corresponding sex and age (Katchadourian, 1977). Both height and weight increase during the sudden or drawn-out growth spurt of adolescence, but height increases are more pronounced (Valadian and Porter, 1977). The predominant female sex hormone, estrogen, stimulates the accumulation of more subcutaneous fat in girls, creating a softer, curved appearance. Testosterone, the important male sex hormone, stimulates greater growth in denser bone and muscle tissue and therefore causes a greater weight gain in males.

The sequence of bone growth also is based on the effects of sex hormones on the epiphyseal plates of the long bones. An outcome of pubescence is the fusion of these primary and secondary ossification centers, a process called *epiphyseal-diaphyseal fusion.* This fusion occurs first in the distal end of the long bones and then in the proximal end, a sequence opposite to the proximal-distal development in infancy. Each shafted bone follows a similar pattern but on a different timetable. The universality of the sequence makes assessing developmental age a matter of determining skeletal rather than chronologic age (see Chapter 16).

Attainment of full bone length begins in the feet and proceeds to the calves, then the thighs, then to the hands, and then forearms to upper arms. Trunk growth follows a similar pattern: first the length and breadth of hips, then the chest and shoulders, and finally the length of the trunk increase (Katchadourian, 1977). Females gain weight from the accumulation of subcutaneous fat, but males show a greater weight gain because of their denser bone and muscle tissue.

During the disproportionate phase of this process, the young person may need to be assured about the normality and sex-appropriateness of these changes. For example, the 2-year lag in the onset of the growth spurt between females and males is counterbalanced later by the greater height attained by males, which is attributed to a longer preadolescent growth period and greater growth velocity.

Sex differences are apparent in body proportions as well as in height and weight gains. The straightening of the facial profile, with greater projection of the nose and more prominence of the jaw, is more marked in males. Male growth also results in broader shoulders, with relatively narrower hips and larger legs in proportion to trunk length. The shoulders of females are narrower, the hips are wider, and the legs are shorter in relation to the trunk length.

Lymphatic System Although the adult continues to produce immunoglobulins at a steady daily rate and at an increased rate in response to different forms and quantities of antigens, lymphoid tissue is the first to mature and regress. The tonsils, adenoids, spleen, and scattered lymph nodes reach maximum volume a few years before puberty. The thymus, the major lymph node, which serves as the primary producer of lymphocytes in the neonate, begins involution at puberty as the lymphocytes of other nodes become self-sustaining (Valadian and Porter, 1977).

Cardiovascular System As the heart grows, the pulse rate decreases. The heart rate, which dropped rapidly in early childhood, decreases more slowly until nubility. From pubescence on, the heart rate in females is slightly faster than that of males, although many factors of health and activity affect the actual rate.

The blood pressure similarly is affected by many variables. The general trend is for both systolic and diastolic blood pressure to rise between $2\frac{1}{2}$ and 18 years of age. The systolic blood pressure might increase from 85 to 112 mm Hg during this time, whereas the diastolic blood pressure might increase from 55 to 70 mm Hg. Males demonstrate a slightly higher systolic blood pressure; there is no sex difference in the diastolic blood pressure (Valadian and Porter, 1977).

Red blood cell mass and hemoglobin rise as both sexes approach nubility, but the increase is greater in males because of the action of testosterone. Between menarche and menopause, the female has a lower red blood cell mass and hemoglobin level. The effect of cyclic menstrual flow on the female may contribute to this phenomenon (Katchadourian, 1977).

Respiratory System Increases in lung capacity and the efficiency of oxygen–carbon dioxide exchange are due to an increase in both the number and size of alveoli from birth to maturity. As all respiratory structures grow during this time, the respiratory rate decreases, ranging from 40 to 60 breaths/min in normal neonates and from 15 to 20 breaths/min in adults. Respiratory efficiency is greater in males when it is measured as respiratory exchange, maximum breathing capacity, or vital capacity (Valadian and Porter, 1977).

Sensory Organs According to the studies of Arnold Gesell (Gesell, Ilg, and Ames, 1956) and the Oakland and Berkeley growth studies (Jones, 1965), the major motor accomplishment of adolescence is visual. The Gesell group (1956) described a series of changes: (1) fixation, or seeking and holding an image; (2) focus, or discriminating and defining an image; and (3) fusion, or identifying, synthesizing, unifying, and interpreting the image. Gesell related age to the steps in this sequence. For example, fixation seems to be dominant at 10 years of age, but focus becomes dominant at 11 years of age. The child then alternates between fixation and focus before finally fusing the two functions.

During periods of growth, the eyeball lengthens. Many instances of myopia (nearsightedness) are discovered during adolescence because eyeball lengthening may result in the visual images coming into focus in front of the retina (see Chapter 43). Most adolescents, however, simply outgrow childhood hyperopia (Valadian and Porter, 1977). Fourteen years of age is a good time to appraise vision because the adolescent is cooperative and the visual skills are well organized and efficient for near-distance tasks. The appraisal may include eye following, mobility of accommodation, ocular pickup, convergence, associated postural and prehensive responses, and visual adjustments to varying distances in space. At midadolescence (15 years of age), visual fatigue is common, but it is followed by decreased effort and greater smoothness in reading performance by 16 years of age (Gesell, Ilg, and Ames, 1956).

Positive changes in hearing result from a greater ability to pay attention and to discriminate among sounds (Gesell, Ilg, and Ames, 1956). There is no physiologic reason for a loss of hearing, but pathologic processes, such as chronic serous otitis media or cholesteatoma, and the use of certain ototoxic drugs, such as streptomycin sulfate, can cause permanent hearing loss.

Endocrine System The signal to start the sequence of puberty originates in the brain and not in the pituitary gland; nevertheless, endocrine system activity increases significantly. For maturation to begin, certain internal changes must occur. The pituitary output of gonadotropins begins to increase under the influence of the hypothalamus. The gonads grow and produce increasing quantities of sex-specific hormones. Several theories attempt to explain the timing of these changes.

The former prevailing theory was based on the physiology of the feedback mechanism in endocrine system function and on empiric data about the influence of genetics and nutrition on the timing of maturation (Tanner, 1972). Similar timing in the onset of puberty is observed between mother and daughter and identical twins unless stress or nutritional differences occur. According to this theory, the hypothalamus, which has been sensitive to minute quantities of hormones produced by the immature boy's testes and girl's ovaries, becomes less sensitive to such feedback. Rather than shut down releasing factor production, the hypothalamus keeps stimulating the pituitary gland until a new equilibrium is reached in late adolescence, when neural growth, testicular and ovarian maturation, and hormone production are all in balance (Vick, 1984).

Although feedback operates as a control, the control exerted through the central nervous system is now known to be more important. This explains why external factors such as stress or fear of pregnancy result in irregular menstrual cycles or amenorrhea. Researchers have also learned that ovulation, which depends on a "burst" release of luteinizing hormone (LH), does not occur if the neural pathways from the genitals are severed (Vick, 1984).

Another theory is derived from research noting the metabolic rate and mean weight at menarche; this is a "critical weight" hypothesis applied to females. It describes a critical weight of 47.8 kg (105 lb) that is accompanied by an alteration in the metabolic rate. The altered metabolic rate disturbs the equilibrium between the hypothalamus and gonads or reflects another set of factors that stimulate the increased production of releasing factor. The feedback mechanism is assumed, but the theory is based on observations of the mean weight at menarche noted in longitudinal growth studies, where weight was constant despite variations in age at menarche, the secular trend of increasing body size and earlier menarche, and the effects of malnutrition in delaying menarche (Peterson, 1979).

The hypothalamus, a small area of the brain located inside the cerebrum (under the thalamus, and partly in front of the midbrain), provides the neuroendocrine linkage that signals the onset of puberty. It has both nerve and blood vessel pathways to other parts of the body. Its relation to the pituitary gland lies in the blood vessel connections. Hypothalamic releasing factors, or pituitary-regulating factors, are tiny amounts of chemicals carried to the anterior pituitary gland. Three of these factors are directly related to sexual maturation. Two are releasing factors that stimulate the pituitary gland to release follicle-stimulating hormone (FSH) and LH; the third is an inhibitory factor that prevents the pituitary gland from releasing prolactin, the hormone that stimulates milk production (Katchadourian and Lunde, 1975).

Five hormones produced by the anterior pituitary gland are known to influence growth and development. Four are called "trophic" hormones because they regulate hormone production by other endocrine glands. These are titled by their target glands: (1) thyrotropin; (2) adrenocorticotropin; (3) two gonadotropins; and (4) mammotropin or lactotropin. The fifth, pituitary growth hormone, acts directly on body tissue, both by directly influencing the processes of protein anabolism and by interacting with other hormones, especially thyroid hormone, to promote growth from postfetal life through adolescence. Although controversy exists as to whether its secretion increases at puberty, pituitary growth hormone is known to facilitate the actions of testosterone and estrogen (Katchadourian, 1977).

The two gonadotropins are essentially the same chemical substances in both males and females but are named for their functions in female sexual maturation. The first of the gonadotropins, FSH, is secreted cyclically in the postpubescent female in coordination with the second gonadotropin, LH. FSH stimulates the maturation of an ovarian follicle. Through a feedback mechanism, increased estrogen levels increase LH levels, and LH supports the follicular response to FSH, ovulation, and formation of the progesterone-producing corpus luteum. In the male FSH promotes the maturation of sperm in conjunction with adequate levels of thyroid hormone and testosterone and an optimal thermal environment. LH may be called interstitial cell-stimulating hormone (ICSH) in the male because it influences the Leydig cells, or interstitial cells of the testes, to produce testosterone (the primary androgen, or male sex hormone). High levels of circulating testosterone will inhibit LH/ICSH secretion in the male through a feedback mechanism to the pituitary gland, but the mechanism of male FSH regulation is unknown.

At puberty, the cortex of the adrenal gland, stimulated by pituitary adrenocorticotropic hormone, will secrete increased amounts of steroid hormones—androgens and small amounts of estrogen—in both sexes. This increase is more important in the female because the adrenal androgens influence the growth of pubic and axillary hair, the development of the clitoris, and the general growth spurt.

Reproductive System The sequence of reproductive system maturation is more predictable than the age or rate at which it occurs.

Hormonal Influence Between menarche and menopause, the cells of the ovarian follicles secrete two hormones, estrogen and progesterone, to support the female role in reproduction. The primary female sex hormone, estrogen, is present in small amounts in both sexes; the amount rises at puberty but at a greater rate in the female. Female estrogen is secreted by the maturing ovarian follicle. Estrogen has both direct and indirect effects on sexual organ maturation and on general growth. It directly influences the growth and development of the ovaries, uterus, and vagina and the enlargement of the breasts. Estrogen is involved in several associated changes that are called *secondary sex characteristics*, including the nature and distribution of axillary and pubic hair, the darkening of the skin of the nipples and genital region, and the shaping of female body contours through fat distribution. In addition, estrogen both aids growth of the skeleton and promotes epiphyseal maturation, or the cessation of bone growth.

The remains of a mature follicle that has extruded its egg (the corpus luteum) secrete progesterone and a smaller amount of estrogen; the combined hormones prepare the lining of the uterus to sustain an embryo. If fertilization and implantation occur, the placenta takes over the function of progesterone secretion. If fertilization does not occur, both estrogen and progesterone production decrease rapidly and menstruation (the shedding of the uterine lining, or endometrium) occurs (Fig. 11-1). Ovarian hormones have both behavioral and physiologic effects. Estrogen increases sexual responsiveness, whereas increased levels of progesterone tend to reduce sexual desire (Katchadourian and Lunde, 1975). Increased sexual desire in women also is correlated with high androgen levels.

The interstitial, or Leydig, cells interspersed between the seminiferous tubules in the testes are the major producers of the primary androgen, or male sex hormone, testoster-

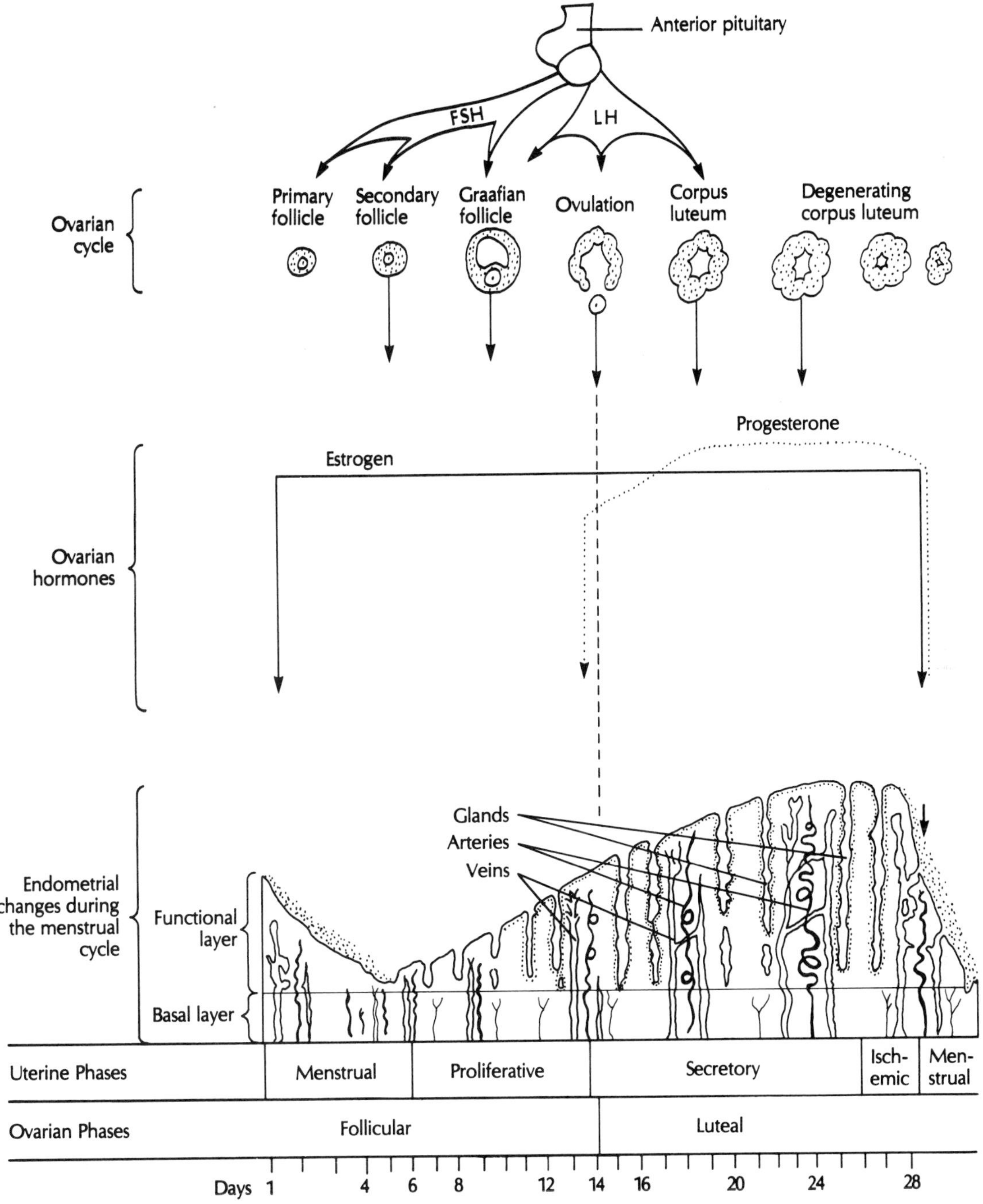

Figure 11-1 Female reproductive cycle: Interrelationships of hormones and the four phases of the uterine cycle and the two phases of the ovarian cycle.

one. The small amounts of testosterone present in both sexes before puberty originate in the adrenal glands. Testosterone, like estrogen, has both direct and indirect effects on male reproductive maturation and on general growth.

Testosterone also produces behavioral effects, including sexual drive and potency. Its direct influences on male reproductive organs include sex and growth effects, which are apparent in enlargement of the scrotum and elongation of the penis. Within the scrotum, the nonfunctioning solid seminiferous tubules of the testes become active sperm-producing structures for fertility. Testosterone influences secondary sexual characteristics of the male in voice changes, the character and distribution of pubic, axillary, facial, and body hair, and a predisposition to acne. Testosterone has an anabolic, or growth-promoting, effect on height, the number and size of muscle cells, and, eventually, the clo-

TABLE 11-1 Hormonal Control of Growth and Maturation

Hormone	Location	Function
Releasing factors (luteinizing releasing hormone, LRH)	Hypothalamus	Stimulates the pituitary release of FSH and LH
Inhibiting factor	Hypothalamus	Prevents the release of prolactin
Thyrotropin	Hypothalamus	Causes the thyroid to secrete T_3 and T_4, which affect metabolism
Adrenocorticotropin	Anterior pituitary gland	Stimulates the adrenal glands to produce steroid hormones, androgens, and estrogen
Follicle-stimulating hormone (FSH)	Anterior pituitary gland	Female: stimulates maturation of the ovarian follicle with LH; male: promotes maturation of sperm
Luteinizing hormone (LH)	Anterior pituitary gland	Female: supports ovulation and the formation of the corpus luteum; male: influences testicular production of testosterone
Pituitary growth hormone	Anterior pituitary gland	Influences anabolism, promotes growth; facilitates the action of testosterone and estrogen
Testosterone	Testes	Affects male reproduction and growth, including the appearance of secondary sex characteristics
Estrogen	Ovaries	Affects sexual organs of both male and female; promotes the growth and maturation of female reproductive organs and secondary sex characteristics
Progesterone	Ovaries	Readies the uterine lining for growth of the embryo

sure of the epiphyseal plates in the long bones (Katchadourian and Lunde, 1975) (Table 11-1).

Female Growth Sequence Breast growth is the first visible sign of female sexual maturation and usually coincides with the beginning of the growth spurt (Fig. 11-2). A mild asymmetry in this growth is normal. There are five stages of breast growth: (1) elevation of the nipple; (2) enlargement of the areola, the darkened area around the nipple; (3) enlargement of the breast; (4) projection of the areola and nipple; and (5) recession of the areola, leaving only the nipple projecting. (The 2-year transient breast growth that occurs in males reaches only the second stage.) (Valadian and Porter, 1977.)

The second sign, pubic hair growth, sometimes precedes breast development (Fig. 11-3). Again, five stages have been distinguished: (1) no true pubic hair during puberty; (2) pale, fine hair, mainly at the sides of the labia in the female; (3) darker, coarser, curled hair; (4) hair of adult character; and (5) hair of adult quantity with an inverted triangle at the mons pubis. In the final stage hair covers the sides of the labia and the perianal area. Stages 2 to 4 take 2 years; stages 4 to 5 may take 4 to 5 years. The rate of axillary hair growth corresponds to the growth of pubic hair (Valadian and Porter, 1977). The external female organs are called the vulva, or pudendum. They include the mons pubis, the labia majora and labia minora, clitoris, and the vaginal opening, which is usually partly covered by the hymen in virgins. During puberty, these organs, especially the clitoris, become enlarged and increase in erotic sensitivity. The internal organs, the paired ovaries and fallopian tubes, the uterus, and vagina, increase in weight and musculature at this time. The cellular changes of the vagina, which cause its lining to thicken and the organ to enlarge, are the first internal changes of puberty. The vaginal contents also become acidic.

Finally, the onset of menstruation and the establishment of menstrual cycles provide a definite observable sign of reproductive maturation, although the first cycles may be anovulatory. For menstruation to occur, both the uterus and the ovaries undergo changes. The inner lining of the endometrium expands, with longer, thicker muscles, to become functional (Valadian and Porter, 1977).

Male Growth Sequence The male's first visible sign of sexual maturation is testicular enlargement, which begins between 10 and 13 years of age and is completed between 14 and 18 years of age (Fig. 11-4). Two associated events follow testicular growth, but their timing is highly variable. The first is postpubertal orgasm, a neuromuscular event that is usually accompanied by the second event, ejaculation, the discharge of semen. Ejaculation is necessary for fertilization. Adolescent ejaculation most often is elicited by masturbation and less frequently occurs as nocturnal emission (Katchadourian and Lunde, 1975).

The growth of male pubic hair follows stages similar to

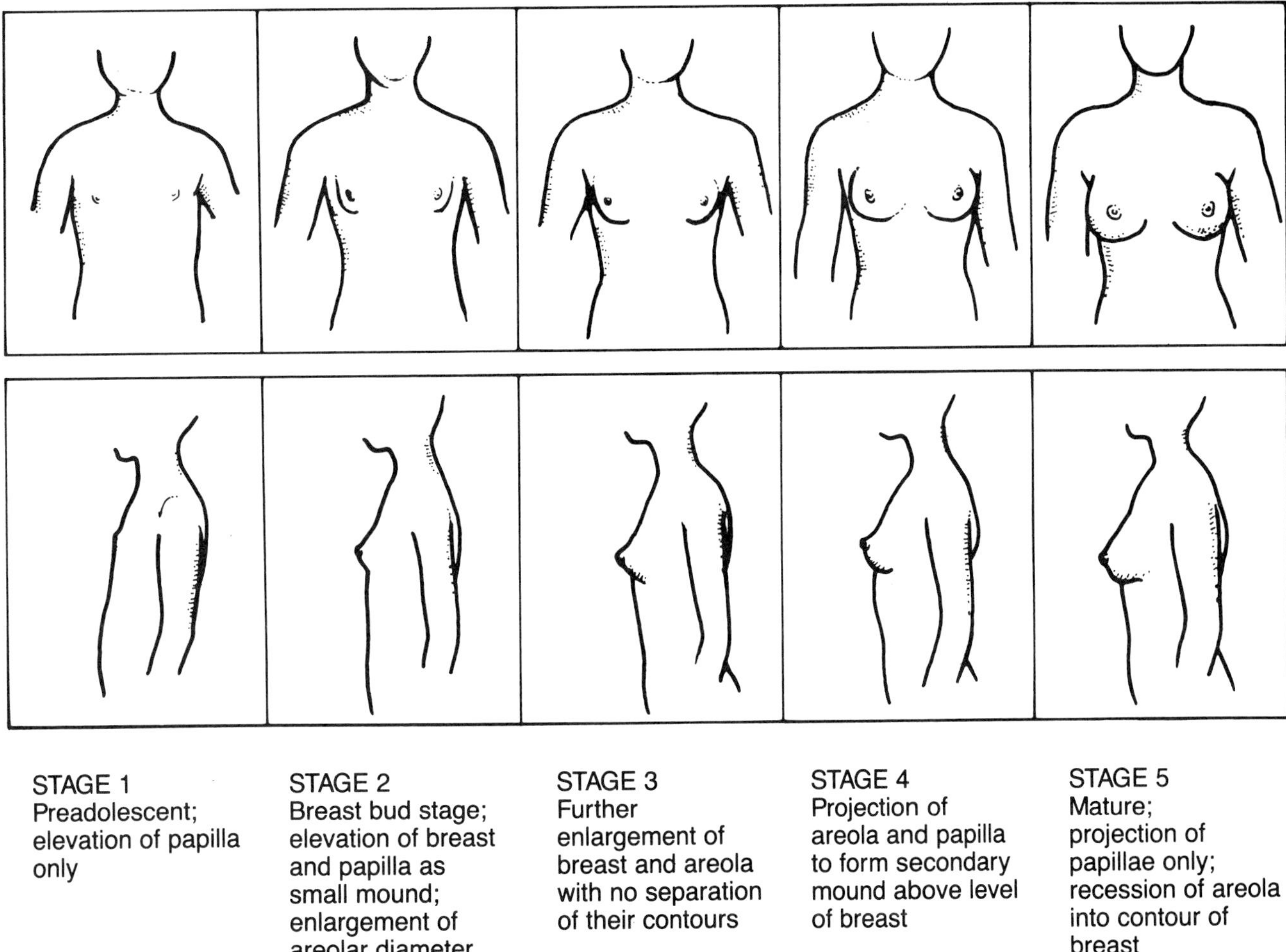

Figure 11-2 Maturational stages of female breast development.

those of the female, but the hair initially is distributed at the base of the scrotum, then the base of the penis, and eventually spreads over the pubic area.

The male external genitalia are the penis and scrotum. A four-stage sequence of growth progresses from (1) prepubertal consistency in the size of both organs; (2) scrotal sac enlargement and a coarsening, wrinkling, and a reddening (darkening) of the scrotal skin, which indicates enlargement of the enclosed testes; (3) penis lengthening; and (4) further enlargement of the penis and darkening of the scrotal sac. It is common for one side of the scrotum to grow faster than the other side. Penile growth occurs later than testicular and scrotal growth (Valadian and Porter, 1977). Approximately 40% of males also experience enlargement of the nipple area of the breast as a transient, 2- to 3-year phenomenon (Valadian and Porter, 1977).

Neuromuscular Function Gesell, Ilg, and Ames (1956) described an age-related sequence of gross motor development during adolescence. By 12 years of age, less spontaneous gross motor activity occurs, but the legs are still active. Each following year activity becomes more balanced and the need for relaxation increases. For example, extreme efforts to perfect an athletic skill give way to a more natural pattern of activity, although explosive bursts of action persist into midadolescence.

The sequence of muscle maturation roughly parallels the growth spurt, with some differences occurring between the sexes. Muscle growth in males coincides with the peak of the growth spurt; in females muscle growth rate peaks 6 months after the peak of height growth. In addition, the influence of testosterone in males accounts for their greater muscle growth and strength, especially in the upper extremities. Both sequential and sex differences are demonstrated in gross motor skill accomplishments such as running and lifting, but in both sexes muscle growth and strength basically are stimulated by muscle use.

There is no physiologic basis for sex differences in fine motor skills. For both sexes, visual maturation is probably the greatest contributor to the improved eye-hand coordi-

STAGE 1
Preadolescent
No pubic hair
STAGE 2
Sparse growth of long, downy, straight, slightly dark hair, chiefly along labia
STAGE 3
Darker, coarse, curly hair, spreading slightly
STAGE 4
Hair adult in type, but area covered smaller than in adult
STAGE 5
Hair adult in quantity and area

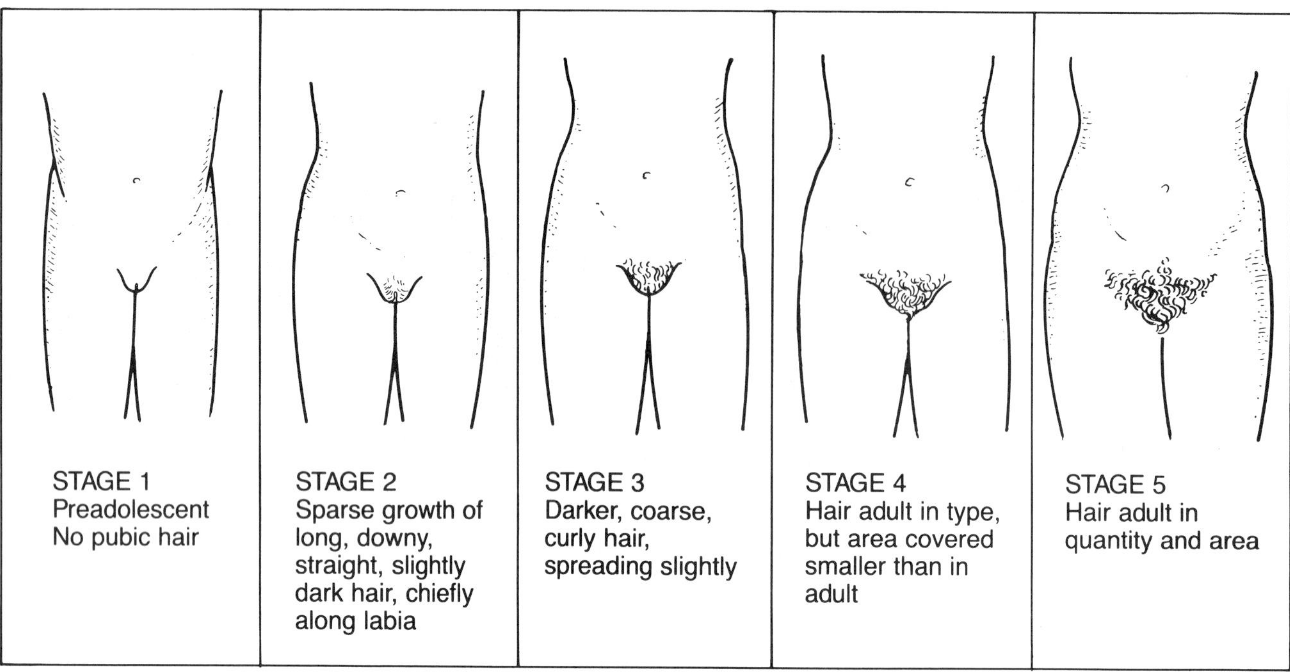

Figure 11-3 Maturational stages of female pubic hair development.

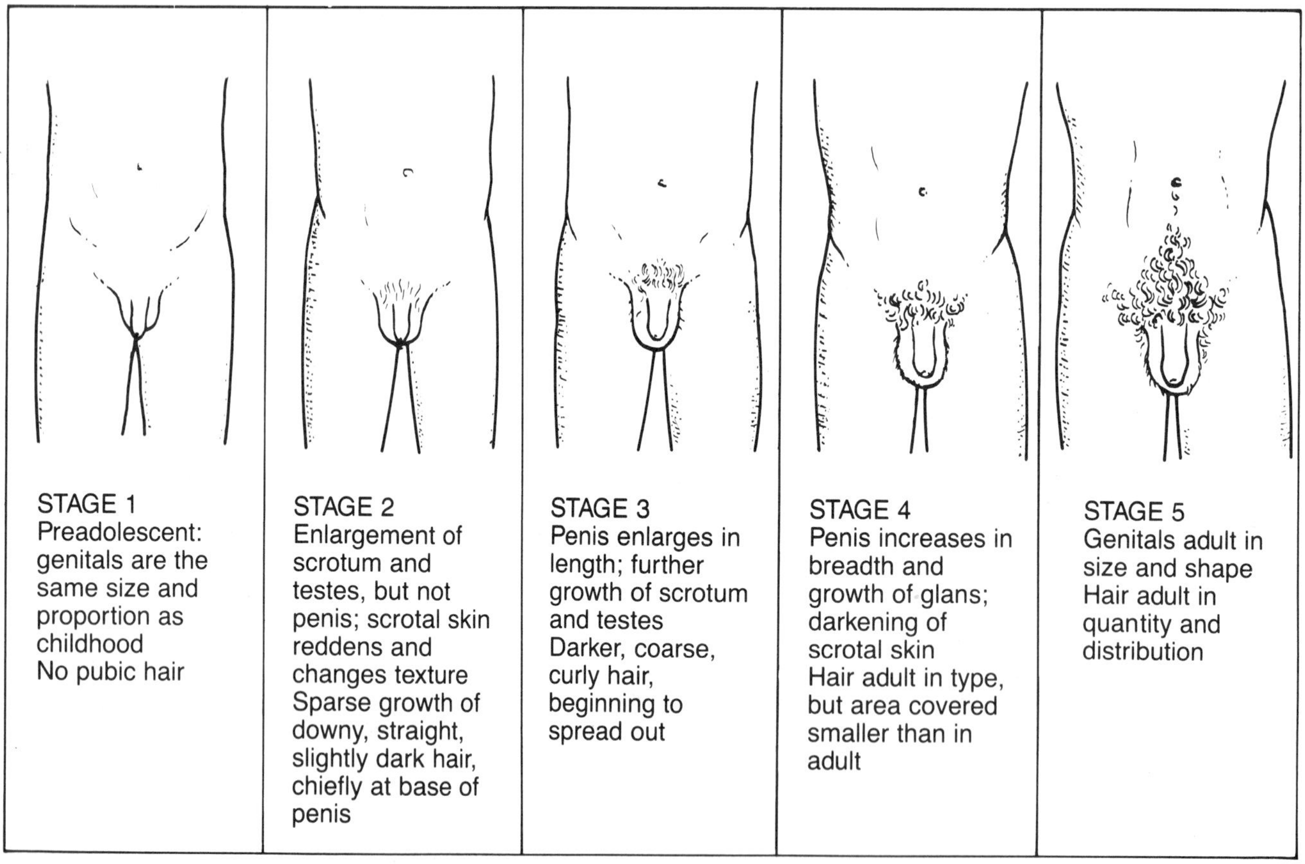

STAGE 1
Preadolescent: genitals are the same size and proportion as childhood
No pubic hair
STAGE 2
Enlargement of scrotum and testes, but not penis; scrotal skin reddens and changes texture
Sparse growth of downy, straight, slightly dark hair, chiefly at base of penis
STAGE 3
Penis enlarges in length; further growth of scrotum and testes
Darker, coarse, curly hair, beginning to spread out
STAGE 4
Penis increases in breadth and growth of glans; darkening of scrotal skin
Hair adult in type, but area covered smaller than in adult
STAGE 5
Genitals adult in size and shape
Hair adult in quantity and distribution

Figure 11-4 Maturational stages of male genital development.

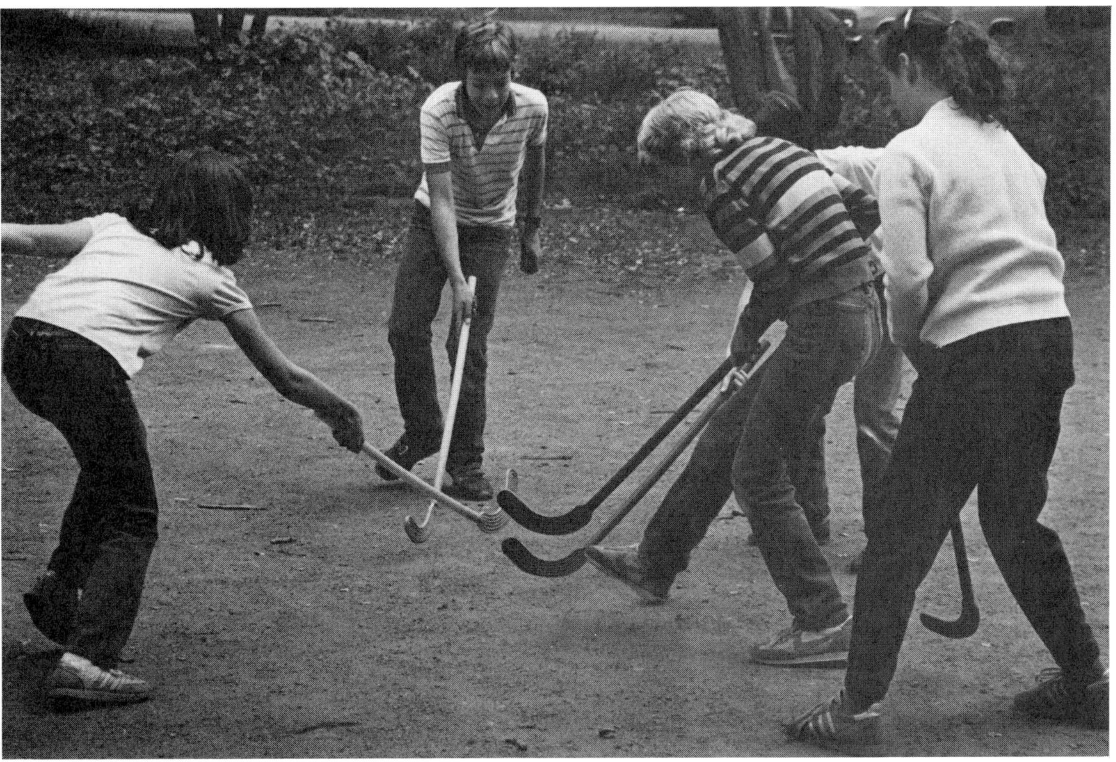

Gross motor development in adolescence leads to developing athletic skill, as evidenced by participation in team sports.

nation evidenced by adolescents' interest and skill in arts and crafts. The sense of accomplishment resulting from the refinement of such skills may release tension and contribute to self-esteem.

Personality Development

Several leaders in psychodynamic thinking have made important contributions to understanding adolescent personality development. Personality theorists recognize unconscious and conscious elements from both past and present experiences in the following functions:

1. *Sexuality*—to integrate gender, affection, and genital function, the adolescent reviews earlier identifications and attractions to parents, expands and intensifies friendships with same-sex peers, and experiments with opposite-sex relationships.
2. *Leader/follower role*—adolescents use peer group activities to test their interpersonal influence and their needs for others to achieve goals.
3. *Response to authority*—an appearance of rebellion against authority might mask an unconscious desire for control (Miller, 1974). The adolescent might challenge limits and appreciate them at the same time. The adolescent seeks guidelines but must experience decision making and its consequences.
4. *Values*—experiments in role playing from the superficial level of appearance to more essential human behaviors are used to test both self-image and the response of others to self. Such role playing represents an effort to resolve confusion about values in practice. Adolescents carefully observe adults for the consistency of stated values and action behavior.
5. *Emotional control*—appropriate outlets for the release of tension, as well as physical maturation, resolve the problems of emotional lability that are most pronounced in early adolescence.
6. *Self-esteem*—self-definition and self-evaluation, the essential components of self-esteem, require involvement in interpersonal relations in which the self can be seen through the reactions of others.
7. *Belonging*—the adolescent turns from family acceptance, which may be taken for granted, to choice and a new level of mutual closeness in relationships outside the family. This may involve a search for belonging, for being accepted by chosen others.
8. *Self-assertion*—the adolescent learns to share thoughts and feelings, first to validate them and later to contribute to human interactions.
9. *Daydreams*—the reverie of daydreams for anticipation, review, and tension release can facilitate development but needs to be controlled. An excessive daydreamer may with-

draw from human relations. Fantasy life may interfere with the use and evaluation of real interpersonal relations or create ideals that human interactions cannot achieve.

Physical and emotional changes in adolescence have a profound impact on personality development in the adolescent. In addition, familial and societal attitudes impinge on the teenager and might exacerbate the inner turmoil the young person is experiencing.

The psychodynamic theory of Sigmund Freud presents a biologically based model of psychosexual development in which the maturation of certain body zones contributes to conflicts among the unconscious drives of the id, the conscious ego, and the unconscious superego sanctions. Freud's final stage of psychosexual development, the genital stage, occurs at puberty. He believed that to successfully complete this stage, the genital stage, the sexual drive that is an initial focus of libido (energy) on one's own genital activity must be turned to a person of the opposite sex outside one's family. The second major drive, the aggressive drive, must be channeled into productive work to benefit society and into hobbies to sublimate energies (Hall, 1954).

Freud concentrated mainly on early adolescence. Another psychotherapist, Derek Miller (1974), offered a three-stage description of adolescence. This description is roughly age-related and encompasses five factors: (1) physiologic base; (2) emotional control; (3) self-esteem; (4) activities; and (5) relationships. Miller's conception of early adolescence, corresponding to ages 11–15, is characterized by turmoil. This turmoil has a physiologic basis in the body changes, loss of body control, and hormonal influence on the emotions. According to Miller, adolescents are consciously aware of restlessness and tension and unconsciously look for control. Therefore, overt defiance of parents and other authorities may be manifested. Miller described boys as experiencing physical discomfort that they release in jokes, physical play, and masturbation. At this stage, the boy denies his father as a model. Miller cautioned the mother to avoid sexually stimulating action on her part. Girls demonstrate shy embarrassment and defensive behavior such as hostile giggling. The girl may seek solitude but can use both diaries and friends to draw herself out. Miller stressed the importance of the father's reaction to the girl's development, encouraging him to express verbally his appreciation of her attractiveness. Similarly, Peter Blos (1962) discussed aggression and possessiveness as Oedipal regressive characteristics in the relations of early adolescent girls to members of the opposite sex. He also noted the implication of pregenital bisexuality in the "tomboy" behavior of girls. In boys the regression he described is more extreme, more action-oriented, and more concrete: a derisive turning away from the opposite sex. Middle and late adolescence are discussed below.

In his more recent work on early adolescence, Blos (1972) emphasized the importance of the latency, or preadolescent, period for extending and strengthening ego functions such as cognition, memory, anticipation, tension tolerance, self-awareness, and the ability to distinguish between reality and fantasy (action and thought). These ego functions must be reliable to resynthesize the ego and achieve ego autonomy during adolescence. Anna Freud (1966), Muss (1975), and Blos (1962, 1972) all stressed the need for parents to understand rather than oppose the behaviors of the young adolescent to support progression in the mastery of conflicts.

Extremes in hairstyles or modes of dress are obvious examples of the adolescent's urge to achieve autonomy. Punk haircuts may be irritating or embarrassing to parents. Adolescents themselves may not even like the look but feel compelled to try it. If parents understand the directive force that prompts the adolescent behavior, they can be supportive rather than authoritative until the phase passes, which it eventually does.

Interpersonal Relationships Harry Stack Sullivan, a psychiatrist who explained human development according to interpersonal relationships (see Chapter 6), described first an interaction called "chumship" and second the psychodynamics of the integration of lust, both of which he considered essential to early adolescent development. Chumship is a special relationship with one same-sex friend, which marks the transition from juvenile indifference to peers except as competitors or task helpers to adolescent interpersonal intimacy (nongenital closeness) (Sullivan, 1953). Two major benefits are gained from chumship: (1) one gets a look at oneself through the chum's eyes, and (2) one learns about another because it is of great interest to observe and analyze one's experiences with the other. Sullivan (1953) deemed chumship a prerequisite for eventual heterosexual intimacy and mature sexuality.

Accordingly, only later in adolescence should the need for intimacy be directed to a person of the opposite sex. Fondness for a special friend can manifest itself in common interests and activities, as well as modes of dress, hairstyles, and makeup. Close friends often are inseparable. Adolescents have an opportunity to see themselves reflected honestly and can practice communication techniques that can be used later in a heterosexual relationship. Girls in early adolescence might support one another and exchange confidences. They often can be seen dancing together at junior high school dances while prompting one another to be the first to ask a boy to dance. Very often, close friends will have parents with similar expectations of behavior, and the friends can insulate each other from social ostracism if their social mores do not match those of their peers.

To Sullivan (1953), orientation to living included lust and a need for intimacy, interwoven but not identical drives. His concept of the integration of lust into personal identity involved (1) acknowledgment of genital-based urges for heterosexual unity; (2) organization of the individual system of motives that get a person involved with others or lead to avoidance of others; and (3) organization of an appropriate heterosexual interpersonal situation of choice.

Middle adolescence, at approximately 14–18 years of age, features, according to Miller (1974), identification of "what I am" and self-realization. Although physical changes are stabilizing, two problems reach their peak: (1) acne affects appearance, and (2) adolescents face the possibility of pregnancy. The middle adolescent's sense of sexual power might be overwhelming and the young person made anxious by overpermissive parents. "Adolescence finds sexually mature young persons trying to cope with new situations and sensations while they are still psychologically immature" (Olds, London, and Ladewig, 1984). Sexual activity at this time is more apt to be a testing of oneself and responding to peer pressures than a loving relationship. Miller designated this period the peak of the need for adult models other than parents because middle adolescents tend and need to test the quality of people in their environment. Middle adolescents need to bounce ideas, values, and feelings about morality and sexual desires against significant adults other than family members. In this way adolescents determine ways to be similar as well as different, thus further developing autonomy and clarifying identity.

In late adolescence, the years from 17–20 (or later for those in college), the characteristic described by Miller (1974) is coping. The late adolescent needs the opportunity to try out the personality structure confirmed in middle adolescence. Here, the adolescent might forgive parents for parental failures and omissions or rebel, depending on how the young person's first steps into adulthood were confirmed by the parents.

A first child may have more difficulty in this respect than subsequent children. Coping with separation and confronting parents with its inevitability is difficult for the late adolescent. For example, an adolescent who has chosen to pursue a career in a different part of the country may encounter opposition tactics from parents such as, "You don't have a job," "Whatever do you want to go there for? The weather's terrible," "Wouldn't you be happier . . . (anywhere else)?" The root of the problem is not the "where" but the fact that the adolescent is going and leaving the family behind. After a confrontation on the adolescent's part, the situation might either result in a traumatic rupture of the family structure or the parents' support.

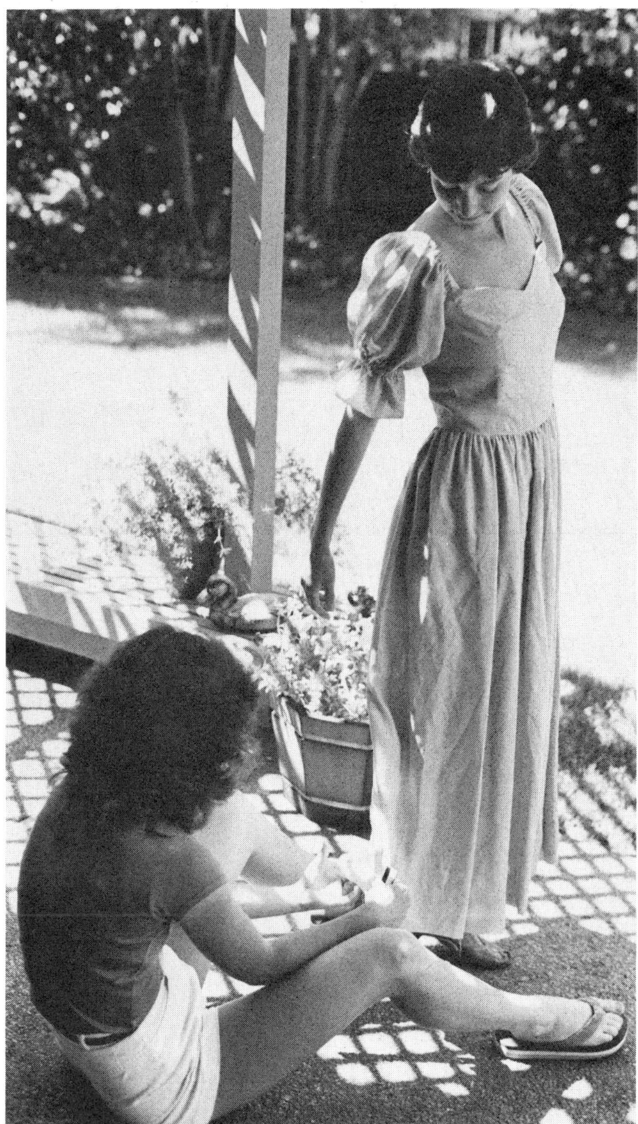

"Chumship" in adolescence is a special relationship with a same-sex friend and marks the transition to interpersonal intimacy.

Identity Crisis The identification that Miller suggested characterizes midadolescence is similar to the "identity versus role diffusion" psychosocial crisis of adolescence described by Erikson (1968) (see Chapter 6). According to Erikson's view of human development, adolescent identity achievement depends on a favorable resolution in each prior psychosocial crisis. The consequent ego strengths achieved during infancy and early and middle childhood can be used in resolving the new crisis.

Erikson's concept of identity has several components of self-definition and self-evaluation: (1) a temporal perspective that enables a person to realize continuity of identity, that is, being the same person in the past, present, and future; (2) a value orientation based on personal decision and commitment; (3) vocational orientation with active preparation for a work goal; and (4) specific gender sexuality of being male or female (Gallatin, 1975). To resolve the identity crisis, the adolescent may experiment with several roles. Erikson cautioned parents and other authorities not to react too strongly to such experimentation because some adolescents are so fragile that they will accept a label and fixate in a role that gains attention. Successful progress in resolving the adolescent identity crisis fosters the ego strength of fidelity (Erikson, 1968). The person then finds someone and something to be true to.

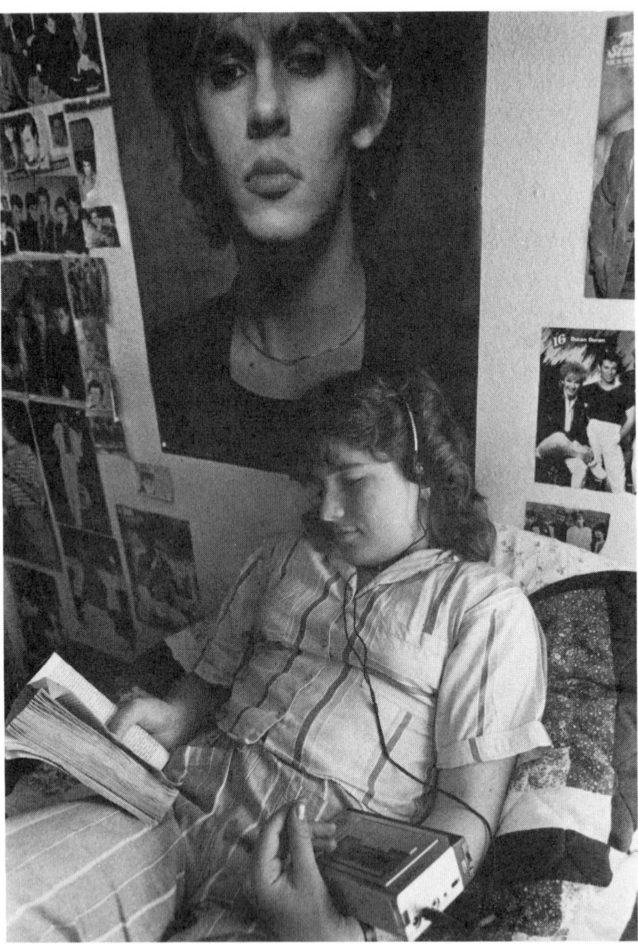

Adolescence is a time of questioned identity. Adolescents need time to consider and reflect in the process of self-definition.

Whether evidence of resolution of the adolescent identity crisis can be found in young adults is the question posed by James Marcia (1966, 1980). He used two criteria: (1) crisis, in the sense of dealing with questions and doubt, and (2) commitment, meaning a personal decision. Marcia applied two of Erikson's components of identity, the vocational and the value orientation, in his studies. His initial work with male college students included questioning each subject about how certain he was about the appropriateness of his chosen major and whether he had ever doubted his religious beliefs. Marcia (1966, 1980) found the following four types of identity crisis outcomes:

1. *Identity achievement*—subject experienced crisis (questions) and reached commitment (personal decision)
2. *Moratorium*—subject is experiencing crisis and has not yet reached but expects to reach a commitment
3. *Foreclosure*—subject has never experienced crisis but is strongly committed to a goal or value fostered by family or other external influence
4. *Diffusion*—subject might have experienced a crisis but is not interested in commitment

For example, the high school student considers many different roles when attempting to decide on a career. Some entering college may choose a liberal arts program to postpone making any commitment to a specific academic area. Even those who make a commitment because the program requires it, such as nursing, often experience a period of disequilibrium as specialty courses begin. The final outcomes of this crisis are either a commitment to the chosen profession, change in the subject area, or a continuing search.

Regression and Conflict Resolution Anna Freud (1967) and Peter Blos (1972) focused principally on early adolescence and described regression in development as a form of conflict resolution. They explained that the surge of sexual urgency experienced by the adolescent may overwhelm the sublimations (socially approved channels of drive direction) developed during the pregenital phases. Peter Blos (1962) perceived adolescence as a time of turmoil and echoed Sigmund Freud in recognizing that puberty intensifies both the aggressive and libidinal drives.

Anna Freud (1967) discussed "phase adequate regression to early levels," where regressive behavior occurs but is not beyond the norm for the individual's stage of development. These regressive behaviors demonstrate the urgency of the adolescent's body needs. Adolescents have a need to idealize personal desires and thus demonstrate ambivalence in relationships. They may cling to and control love objects, especially parents, in the service of the final resolution to the Oedipal conflict. This resolution enables the young person to transfer ties from the family to same-sex peers and eventually to a person of the opposite sex. In this way a child's integration into groups and the community as a whole is fostered.

Cognitive Development

Formal Operations Cognitive theorists relate important advances in thinking to the physical and social maturation of the adolescent. Piaget's theory of cognition describes operations of cognition as activities through which the individual attempts to transform reality by applying procedures to various data (see Chapter 6) (Piaget, 1952; Flavell, 1963). According to Piaget, maturation of the nervous system, combined with material and social experience and personal activity, enables the adolescent to achieve formal operations. Piaget's formal operations stage is defined by the ability to reason from the possible to the actual.

Formal operational thought possesses several characteristics. First, the individual learns to hypothesize, or to use propositional thinking, which is free from the evidence of experience essential to earlier concrete operations. At this stage, the adolescent is able to imagine several alternatives to the same phenomenon. An adolescent need not believe an alternative thesis to consider it. Formal operations enable a person to decenter thinking, to adopt alternative frames of reference. A person with formal operational thinking can imagine a view from various spatial positions and eventually can think about an abstract concept from another person's point of view.

Formal operations and the ability to hypothesize facilitate scientific problem solving. The adolescent can envision multiple relations of cause and effect, can control variables mentally, and can plan a systematic combination of possibilities prior to actual experimentation. This abstract thinking requires some caution because of the danger of losing touch with reality. This problem, known as *cognitive slippage,* may occur in adolescents who push thinking to its limits in mentally constructing an ideal world (Ginsburg and Opper, 1979). This ideal world expresses a utopian existence that is free from day-to-day problems and stresses, a world of equal social classes without poverty and greed. The problem with this fantasy is that adolescents may then experience major difficulties adjusting to the futility of attaining this utopia.

Second, formal operations, exemplified by what Piaget called the INRC group of transformations (identity, negation, reciprocity, correlation), enable the person to call on many available operations and therefore to be flexible (Piaget, 1954; Ginsburg and Opper, 1979; Neimark, 1975). For example, the Piagetian concept of conservation (see Table 6-4) is no longer restricted to the immediate, testable environment. Also, through formal operational, or abstract, thinking, the individual can order relations, such as big, bigger, biggest, without tangible evidence.

Piaget's transition from concrete to formal operations usually is assumed to occur in early adolescence but is not age specific. In fact, some people never achieve formal operations, and most people achieve formal operations on limited types of data.

> An example of the shift from concrete to formal operations may be taken from the work of E. A. Peel. Peel asked children what they thought about the following event: "Only brave pilots are allowed to fly over high mountains. A fighter pilot flying over the Alps collided with an aerial cableway, and cut a main cable causing some cars to fall to the glacier below. Several people were killed." A child at the concrete-operational level answered: "I think that the pilot was not very good at flying." A formal-operational child responded: "He was either not informed of the mountain railway on his route or he was flying too low. Also his flying compass may have been affected by something before or after take-off, thus setting him off course causing collision with the cable."
>
> The concrete-operational child assumes that if there was a collision the pilot was a bad pilot; the formal-operational child considers all the possibilities that might have caused the collision. The concrete-operational child adopts the hypothesis that seems most probable or likely to him. The formal-operational child constructs all possibilities and checks them out one by one (Kohlberg and Gilligan, 1971, reprinted with permission).

Motivation and Learning In North America organizing and understanding information are emphasized more than the acquisition and memorization of facts, especially in the higher school grades. Basic academic subjects, however, also include formulas and rules for processing information. Piagetian theory deals more with the first type of learning. Learning theories that apply to the acquisition of information originally focused on behavior shaping, or external control of an individual's learning. Current theories suggest that the learner is active both in the decision to undertake a learning task and in the evaluation of his or her success (Smart and Smart, 1977).

Personal responsibility for learning requires motivation, which is linked with enjoyment of school and/or with perceived immediate or long-term rewards for the effort expended. For most adolescents, family-derived motivating factors predominantly influence the duration of school enrollment and degree of achievement. In the school setting the relevance of school studies to occupational goals is more effective for motivation, especially when studies are combined with actual work experience. For example, research on the process of vocational choice demonstrates a gradual transition during adolescence from fantasy about potential occupational goals to a realistic appraisal of one's own abilities and interests in comparison with the demands of different occupations (Borow, 1976; O'Hara and Tiedeman, 1969). Planning for the future is part of the experience of most high school students.

Social learning theorist Albert Bandura (1977), whose experiments concentrated on the response to the role modeling of behavior, believed that motivation could be affected by external factors such as observing other peoples' behavior and its consequences. According to Bandura, creating an environment that is conducive to learning is the responsibility of adults. Adolescent learners then observe, remember, judge, decide, and create a response according to their own values.

For example, an adolescent often will use a teacher as both a role model and a motivational influence. As motivating factors, teachers' methods of presentation (discussion, didactic, audiovisual) are as important as an enthusiastic approach to students. Adolescents are more highly motivated to learn in an atmosphere that fosters excitement about the subject area. Students motivated in this way become self-motivated in other areas and expand their interests.

Memory Some personal capabilities important to school learning peak in adolescence. For example, research on human memory, which is certainly important to knowledge acquisition, demonstrates that memorization is a more active process than originally thought. The adolescent's efficient use of mnemonic schemes or memory aids is an indication of the active nature of memory (Smart and Smart, 1977).

For example, one 14-year-old girl used mnemonic devices to aid her memory in various schoool subjects. She remembered the sons of Leah for her theology class with the phrase, "Reuben saw lice (or lines) just in zebras." This gave her the first letters of the names Reuben, Simeon, Levi, Judea,

Issachar, and Zebulun. She remembered the formula for the slope of a line, y = mx + b, by saying to herself, "y is over there, mx stands for missiles, and b = Brian" (her brother). So, y = missiles Brian means y = mx + b. She remembered that "per" in Latin means "through" with reasoning that, as she said, "doesn't make any sense, but that's how I remember it." "Everything was handed down through the sun, so 'person' means 'through the sun,' and therefore 'per' means 'through.' "

Creativity The adolescent who achieves abstract thinking differs from the child intent on fact collection and convergent thinking, or finding the one right answer. Formal operations are therefore conducive to the definition of creativity as divergent thinking or producing many possible answers to a problem. The adolescent who achieves formal operations demonstrates thought and can switch readily from purposeful thinking to fantasy (Smart and Smart, 1977). Fantasy, in turn, is part of the adolescent's process of setting long-term goals. The literature that is popular with adolescents also indicates their enjoyment of fantasy as a leisure-time pursuit. To nourish their creativity, adolescents need time for reflection and planning. Reflection leads to better self-awareness and personal insight in many adolescents.

Large, long-term studies of people considered to be creative in adolescence show good health and social adjustment as well as academic and career productivity, findings that contradict the stereotype of someone becoming creative to compensate for a physical or social handicap. Research has identified both inhibitors and facilitators of creativity (Terman, 1954; Torrance, 1969). Some of the inhibitors are an extremely peer-oriented culture, sanctions against questioning and exploring, and overemphasis on stereotypic sex roles. Facilitators of creativity include a social setting in which a variety of talents and achievements are rewarded, assistance with social skills so that creative individuals interact with peers and are less isolated, attention to the development of values, and aid in coping with fears. Overall, an environment that respects unusual questions and unusual ideas and provides opportunities for self-initiated and unevaluated learning is rewarding to creative thinking.

Recently, high school students are being encouraged more and more to demonstrate creative thinking. Creative problem-solving courses are available through some school systems, which result in such competitions as "Olympics of the Mind." These competitions confer status on the creative child and increase the subsequent acceptance by peers. Nurses can assist parents to encourage artistically, athletically, or intellectually creative adolescents. Nurses need to be aware of the adolescent's creative interests. For instance, fantasy games involving unstructured play and the use of imagination as well as strategy are popular with adolescents. In an acute-care setting nurses can encourage group contacts to promote creative interaction among adolescents. Incorporating specific interests into the therapeutic regimen encourages participation in self-care.

Language Development

As cognitive abilities develop in adolescence, so does the learning of new words, structures, and purposes of language. For example, reading, writing, and speaking depend on the coordination of visual skills, maturation, and experience. Adolescents develop skills in written language, involving both the style of writing and the expression of personality characteristics. Greenfield and Bruner (1966) correlated formal thought in societies with schools to education in written language. In writing a person separates the abstract from the concrete, might let symbolic processes outdistance concrete facts, and thus enhances the capacity to think about possibilities. Writing used in this way becomes an extension of thought and therefore reflects cognitive development.

Writing in adolescence may be used to put thoughts about self on paper for evaluation in a diary or journal. For many adolescents, the evaluation process is a private one. In the hospital setting the nurse must respect the limits that adolescents set (see Chapter 29).

Health problems require communication, and language barriers must be surmounted. Professionals often acquire a protective language in the same way succeeding generations of adolescents have been noted to adapt words and phrases to meanings that adults cannot decipher. Special vocabulary and other variations of language may be used in peer dialogue (Elkind and Weiner, 1978). Most important to nursing is a vocabulary that permits the comfortable discussion of body changes between the adolescent and nurse. To achieve this, adolescents can learn anatomic terms, and the nurse can learn lay terms to refer to body parts and functions (Bell, 1981). Inquiring about a student's school progress may indicate the level of language skills to the nurse who is selecting health teaching methods and materials for the adolescent.

Moral Development

Piaget's (1932) theory of cognition involves a component of moral development. Piaget described a progression from a heteronomous morality, in which the young child believes rules are made by authority and cannot be broken, to an autonomous morality based on social experiences with peers. This progression brings the child to realize that people make and change rules, and a centered moral scheme is a sign of preadolescent maturity.

In Kohlberg's theory (Kohlberg, 1963, 1976), the common achievement of moral reasoning in adolescence is the second, or conventional, level (see Chapter 6, Table 6-8). The two stages at this level are Stage 3, an orientation to interpersonal relations of mutuality, sometimes called a "good boy, good girl" conception, and Stage 4, in which the theme is the maintenance of social order, fixed rules, and authority. This is often called the "law and order" stage. Both stages of moral reasoning at this level require a formal operational level of cognition to adopt alternative frames of reference or understand the viewpoints of others.

Kohlberg's Stage 3 is the stage in which the adolescent focuses on the approval of others and often looks to the peer group to determine norms for approval. This is the time of confirming, in which moral dilemmas are solved by appealing to a group standard. The adolescent who cheats on a test may justify cheating in this way: "Everybody does it; besides, I wouldn't have been allowed to stay on the team if I hadn't passed and that would have let the team and the coach down." Adolescents at Kohlberg's Stage 4 are inclined to do what the law or their own sense of duty requires. Some might, for example, register for the draft "because that's the law," regardless of their personal views or group expectations.

Kohlberg's educational experiments also were intended to stimulate the development of moral reasoning. His experiments with high school students included discussions of moral issues in groups where members could be exposed to the next higher level of reasoning from their own. Findings suggest that education can foster moral reasoning in adolescents. Kohlberg and Turiel's (1971) studies have demonstrated that individuals understand reasoning at or below their own dominant levels and are interested in and attracted to the next higher level. For instance, the student who would register for the draft "because that's the law" can discuss the consequences of being drafted with a veteran. A veteran of a war such as Vietnam, which evoked many conflicting moral issues, can provide an alternate viewpoint for the adolescent's consideration.

Faith Development

James Fowler (1976) extended the psychosocial developmental theories of Erikson, Piaget, and Kohlberg in describing faith development (see Chapter 6). Fowler linked his description of Stage 3, synthetic-conventional faith, with early adolescence, and he linked Stage 4, individuating-reflexive faith, with late adolescence. In synthetic-conventional faith (Stage 3), "Coherence and meaning are created by people as authorities or the authority of consensus among respected people. The person does not yet have to take on the burden of world synthesis for himself/herself" (Fowler, 1976).

In the transition from this stage to Stage 4, the individual begins to assume responsibility for his or her own commitments, life-style, beliefs, and attitudes. The person at Stage 4 faces the tensions between individuality and belonging to community, between subjectivity and objectivity, between self-fulfillment and service to others, and between the relative and the absolute (Fowler, 1976). An example of this would be the crisis of faith common in the adolescent period. Being exposed to values and beliefs that may differ from those held by the family often precipitates questioning and exploring in an attempt to apply these beliefs to one's own life. This exploration causes tension, as conflicts with family and long-held traditions arise. The outcome is the ability to extrapolate and use what most closely fits the life-style the individual has chosen.

Social Development

Developmental Tasks In his theory of developmental tasks, R. J. Havighurst (1972) placed adolescence third in six life phases for which he identified particular developmental tasks (see Chapter 6). Havighurst's developmental tasks are derived from a constellation of pressures arising from physical maturation and the development of individual values and goals in the context of cultural expectations.

Havighurst (1972) described eight tasks of adolescence, as follows:

1. Achieving new and more mature relations with age-mates of both sexes
2. Achieving a masculine or feminine social role
3. Accepting one's physique and using one's body effectively
4. Achieving emotional independence from parents and other adults
5. Preparing for marriage and family life
6. Preparing for an economic career
7. Developing an ideology—a set of values and an ethical system as a guide to behavior
8. Achieving socially responsible behavior

Albert Bandura (1977) emphasized the continuity of adolescence rather than its disruptions. His views are based on studies that demonstrated harmonious, if not completely communicative, parent–child relations. He criticized the mass media for sensational depictions of troubled individuals as role models for adolescents. Bandura, like Erikson, cautioned against overinterpretation of superficial signs of nonconformity such as fashion fads. He deplored the tendency to focus attention on negative role models of adolescent behavior because of the hazard of self-fulfilling prophecies, a phenomenon in which people behave in the way they believe others expect them to behave.

Maturation and Social Interaction Differences in psychologic and social adjustments between early and late maturers are either more pronounced or more frequently studied in males (Jones and Bayley, 1950; Jones and Mussen, 1958; Weatherly, 1964). The results of short- and long-term studies yield more questions than conclusions. For example, personality characteristics, such as the tendency for late-maturing girls to be withdrawn and to attempt to be inconspicuous in group activities, may be evaluated by some researchers as negative behaviors and by others as compensating behaviors. Only a few studies consider the social suprasystem surrounding, supporting, or making demands on the individual.

Studies do show that early maturers of both sexes demonstrate more positive self-concepts and that late maturers demonstrate more anxiety. The expanded social opportunities available to girls seem to be limited to early adolescence but continue for early-maturing boys. Parents and peers accept maturity and readily provide opportunities to assume responsibility and leadership to early-maturing males. Although dating opportunities are available earlier to early-maturing girls, parents may be anxious about premature sexual activity and its possible consequences. Whereas late maturers appear more childlike and are treated as children, the early maturers are rated by peers to be more attractive and desirable as dates. Thus, development-stimulating opportunities are rewarded on the basis of physical characteristics. By late adolescence, physical differences are less apparent, but late maturers report more negative feelings about themselves and seek more attention and affection.

The interaction of social and psychologic factors is more pronounced in the findings from the longitudinal studies (Jones, 1965). Early developers continue to be socially successful in adulthood but tend to be conforming and somewhat overcontrolled. Some positive findings appear among late maturers, who appear to benefit from adaptive compensation by being insightful, exploring, independent, and spontaneous. An additional hypothesis is that late maturers have happier marriages because of their greater psychologic insight.

Integrating Development Through Play

Adolescence is the period when the child's conceptions of play develop into those of the adult. Erikson (1963) aptly described this difference by defining play as the work for a child in contrast to the adult's use of play as an escape from work pressures. Many forms of play do contribute to growth in the child and perhaps to preservation of function in all ages. Speed of reaction, strength, endurance, and coordination are all aspects of physical fitness that are enhanced by physical play in the form of gross motor skills. Bone growth, muscle size and strength, and the blood's oxygen-carrying capabilities are a few body functions that need to be stimulated by regular exercise. Fine motor precision and dexterity may be enhanced by arts and crafts. On both the physical and the psychic level, excess anxiety or tension may be relieved by a balance between work and play that supports the interaction of the complementary branches of the autonomic nervous system, the stress-stimulated sympathetic responses, and the restorative-maintenance parasympathetic functions.

Three types of play predominate in adolescence. Cooperative play is exemplified in games, clubs, and dating; team play in organized sports; and construction and creativity in hobbies. The content of play includes fantasy through daydreaming, art, reading, and dramatics; role playing in dramatics and some games, club activities, and dating; and both cognitive and motor skills in hobbies, sports, and arts and crafts (Farina, Furth, and Smith, 1959). Research on gender differences in team sports reveals that girls are less apt to participate in games requiring motor skills of organized teamwork after the onset of puberty. Many girls thus miss opportunities for learning to respond to criticism and to settle disputes, to organize activities, and to compete in a structured environment. They also miss the chance for improved physical fitness that exercise provides. Male concentration on organization and competition in team sports may, however, deny boys the opportunities to develop a sense of intimacy or commitment. These findings would seem to indicate that the expectations, interest, and assistance of parents in the play activities (as well as in the education of both boys and girls) need to be evaluated critically in light of the life challenges to be faced by both sexes (Rivers, Barnett, and Baruch, 1979).

As adolescents begin dating, sex-role experimentation and appraisal of self in male–female interaction become more important. Developing relationships is usually the stated purpose of dating among older adolescents. Younger adolescents tend to describe dating simply as participation in socially desirable activities (Douvan and Adelson, 1969).

Because parents of adolescents, at least middle-class parents, tend to stress the importance of preparing for future goals, such as getting good grades in high school to get into college, nurses may need to remind them of the adolescent's need for real play and relaxation. Any tendency for parents to overidentify or compete with their children also might impinge on certain activities, such as sports or dating, and interfere with the adolescent's emerging sense of identity.

Health Care Needs in Adolescence

Basic physical and health care activities during adolescence require some modifications because of maturational changes and because parents need to foster independent decision making by the adolescent.

Hygiene

Complete self-direction in the area of hygiene is achieved by midadolescence. Skin care concerns are intensified first because of the increased activity of the sebaceous glands. This factor, over which the adolescent has no control, contributes to acne. These glands produce sebum, a mixture of fatty acids, lipids, and sterols, which helps to keep the skin moist by inhibiting the evaporation of water. The environment influences the amount of secretion; more sebum is produced in hot, humid climates. Androgens also stimulate glandular activity, so that more secretion occurs in males (Valadian and Porter, 1977).

Acne can produce skin lesions, including varying numbers and combinations of comedones (blackheads), papules (inflamed tissue), pustules (pus-containing lesions), and cysts (fluid-filled sacs). These lesions are caused by a plug of sebum blocking the hair follicles and by the inflammatory response of surrounding tissue. The areas affected are the face, upper chest, back, shoulders, and forehead. The earlier the onset, the more severe will be the manifestations; the average ages of the onset of acne are 14–17 years in girls and 16–19 years in boys. Nurses might find that adolescents must be told to avoid handling or squeezing the lesions to prevent further infection and scarring. Cleanliness and attention to dietary elements that aggravate the condition might help, but medical care often is needed. Parents sometimes blame adolescents' diets or hygienic practices for the occurrence or severity of acne; nurses might need to explain that acne cannot be blamed solely on diet or hygiene (see Chapter 44).

Increased sweat gland activity requires careful cleansing of the body and airing and cleaning of clothes. Deodorants and body powders become necessary because of the interaction of bacteria with the secretion of the newly active apocrine sweat glands, resulting in a pungent odor. The choice of appropriate deodorants or antiperspirants is based on effectiveness, cost, and any existing allergies. A deodorant or antiperspirant that causes a skin irritation should be discontinued, and a girl who shaves axillary hair should not apply a deodorizing agent immediately after shaving.

The third concern, menstrual hygiene, requires special attention because the irregularity of girls' early menstrual cycles often leads to embarrassment caused by soiled clothes. Second, exposure of this body secretion to air and/or stasis of the secretion on unchanged absorbent materials results in odor. Finally, menstrual flow conveys a sense of the unknown and lack of control, because it is secreted from the vagina, which is located in a less visible body area and surrounded by the hair-covered labia. Girls can achieve some control by learning the signs that forecast the menstrual period such as skin eruptions, tender breasts, weight gain, and unusual hunger. A variety of comfortable, unobtrusive, absorbent materials are available for use during menstrual periods, for anticipated periods, or for midcycle discharges. External absorbent materials, usually called sanitary pads but also referred to as napkins, towels, or cloths, are constructed with a waterproof backing and hydrostatic packing to draw fluid away from the vulva. Some are biodegradable, easing disposal problems. They are available in various sizes, thicknesses, and shapes to accommodate varying ages, amounts of flow, and body configurations. They may be secured by belts or, more recently, by adhesive attachment to close-fitting panties.

Internal absorption may be achieved by inserting a plug of absorbent material, called a tampon, into the vagina, but the recently demonstrated incidence of a serious, sometimes fatal, systemic illness called toxic shock syndrome (TSS) has drawn attention to factors affecting tampon use in women of all ages. Estimates indicate that 95% of documented cases of TSS occur during menses, and a significant relationship has been found between tampon use and the development of TSS. Tampon users of all ages are advised to be cautious in tampon use. Women may alternate tampon use with external sanitary pads; current advice is to use an external pad at night or during sleep. Pad use during the lighter first and last days of menses decreases the trauma potential of these days, when tampon insertion is more difficult because of less lubrication. Thorough handwashing before insertion, perineal cleansing, frequent changing of tampons, and careful and complete removal of tampons can decrease local infection with *Staphylococcus aureus,* a possible antecedent to TSS (see Chapter 39). Baths, showers, and soap and water cleansing of the genital area, with separate wiping from front to back, offer sufficient cleaning of the vulva so that douching is not needed.

Parents need to understand the involuntary and often confusing nature of these hygienic concerns. Ridicule and blame are destructive to the self-esteem of the young person, who is trying to gain control over a changing body and, at the same time, trying to be accepted in peer social interactions. Parents may seek resources or refer young people to health professionals for current, accurate information. The best assistance is offered by alertness to signs of the onset of puberty and anticipatory guidance.

Sleep and Rest

During adolescence, the range of bedtimes becomes more variable. As adolescents become more aware of body needs, they go to bed because they think they need sleep, and they dawdle less. Some adolescents spend the entire evening in their bedrooms. Adolescents find more pleasure in sleeping and will sleep late when possible. They often have problems getting up (Gesell, Ilg, and Ames, 1956).

Parents can encourage the greater awareness of body needs occasioned by fatigue. Parents also can use bedtime and awakening time as opportunities for adolescents to exercise control and recognize the consequences of their decisions. Alarm clocks usually decrease family tension and increase individual responsibility if arousal is a problem. The major complaint of parents of teenagers probably is that teens sleep too much.

Nutrition

The energy allowances for males between 11 and 18 years of age range from 2000 to 3900 kcal, depending on height, weight, and activity; for females in the same age range, the energy allowance is 1500–3000 kcal, using the same criteria. These ranges are based on median energy intakes of these age groups followed in longitudinal growth studies. Median male height in these studies ranged from 157 cm (62 in) in the 11–14 age range to 176 cm (69 in) from ages 15–18. Males ranged in weight from 45 to 66 kg (99 to 145 lb) over the same age range. Females ranged in height from 157 to 163 cm (62 to 64 in), and female weight ranged in the 12 to 15 age range from 46 to 55 kg (101 to 120 lb) (see Appendix A). These are averages; variations depend on both body build and activity patterns.

Especially during the growth spurt, adolescents show a markedly increased need for calories. The observation that teens, especially males, seem to be hungry and eating all the time may relate to an imbalance between the size of the stomach and the amount of calories needed. Nutrient intake is important for growth, energy, emotional control, appearance, and the health of the next generation. Problems in this area may be mild and easily solved or complex and controlled only with professional help. (Nutritional assessment is discussed in Chapter 15.)

Three problems of insufficient nutritional quality may occur. The first is the problem of empty calories, evidenced by the popularity of snacks, soft drinks, chips, and candy in North American culture. Such an intake often leads to a sufficient calorie intake but a deficiency of nutrients. The problem is intensified if it is derived from a lifelong pattern of poor eating habits and lessened if it is a temporary adaptation to peer culture. Second, some adolescents select vegetarian diets, which can be adequate with careful planning but are more frequently inadequate in protein. The third dietary concern is weight control, where excessive or inadequate intake may be caused from or may itself cause both psychologic and physical problems.

Nurses can help parents to focus on the adolescent's need to make individual decisions in many areas of life and to prevent food intake from becoming the center of an independence–dependence struggle. For example, parents may refer to nutritionists for information in planning a nutrient-adequate diet and to consumer groups to influence the quality of snacks available in schools. Severe problems such as anorexia nervosa or bulimia require both psychiatric and medical treatment (see Chapter 24). Milder problems, such as obesity, may be resolved within community support groups.

Dentition

If malocclusion exists, it is usually advisable to correct it during adolescence. Later correction is possible but physical, psychologic, and social factors make it more difficult. The eruption of third molars ("wisdom teeth") during this period may intensify the degree of malocclusion.

Self-direction in the care of teeth usually has been established by midadolescence, but the adolescent might need to be reminded to obtain regular professional care. An increased incidence of dental caries between the ages 14 and 17 years is thought to be due to maturational changes (Valadian and Porter, 1977). Parents are urged to provide regular dental checkups and treatment of problems but to avoid blaming dietary or self-care practices of teens for the seemingly involuntary increase in caries in this age group.

Exercise

Research demonstrates that physical activity is necessary to support normal growth, especially of bones and muscles; to prevent adult health problems, especially arteriosclerotic vascular disease; to motivate lifelong activity involvement; and to enhance learning in the classroom. Therefore, regular habits of exercise through individual or group activities yield short- and long-term physical and psychologic benefits. Parents can set examples that benefit themselves as well as their offspring. Current reports of participation indicate that parents may need to encourage girls and academically oriented adolescents to increase the balance between sedentary and active pursuits in favor of more exercise. Parents also might need to urge a greater range of activity for girls.

Safety

Major potential dangers in adolescence are unplanned pregnancy (see Chapter 22) and sexually transmitted disease (see Chapter 39). The incidence of both is increasing as 55% of adolescents 13–19 years of age are sexually active (Zelnik and Kantner, 1980). Improved methods of contraception and the increased provision of sex education in public schools reach only a small percentage of the adolescents. Cognitive and emotional development for the adolescent involves integration of sexuality into a continuous personal and social identity and the need for social support and responsible decision making.

Parents and professionals need to recognize cognitive, emotional, social, and physical development in planning sex education. Many of the typical adolescent's perceptions of sexual intercourse are myths and stereotypes about how to be popular with peers, to achieve adult status, and to prove one's identity. During routine examinations the nurse therefore assesses the young adolescent's knowledge about sex, intercourse, contraception, and reproduction. Being well-informed and understanding the personal and physiologic dynamics of a heterosexual relationship are the first steps in prevention. The knowledgeable adolescent is less likely to take risks thinking that "it (pregnancy) can't happen to me" or that "my partner would use some protection." Adolescents must know the facts but also must be aware of the personal responsibility each has regarding sexual activity. Education in the use of contraceptives is secondary, for example, to efforts to enhance the adolescent's self-concept and the ability to refuse unwanted sexual intercourse. Similarly, a responsible decision to be sexually active when one is socioeconomically unable to care for a child requires that contraception be considered. The nurse needs to explain the advantages, disadvantages, and effectiveness of each contraceptive method and then needs to support the adolescent in the proper use of the method chosen. Table 11-2 provides a perspective of the various contraceptive methods available.

Adolescent participation in sports also presents safety concerns. To participate safely in sports, the teenagers must make choices concerning the level of activity and their maturity and physical condition. Health professionals increasingly direct attention to protecting vulnerable body areas in violent, contact, and combative sports and to preventing the complications of injuries (see Chapter 19).

Adolescents often seem to be in constant motion, with boys and girls ranging over extensive spaces in their activities. Bikes enable teenagers to cover greater distances, but in American culture, the prized achievement in adolescence is obtaining a license to drive. The hazards associated with mobility are reflected in mortality statistics for adolescents, with motor vehicle accidents far outdistancing any other cause of death in this age group (Smith, Bierman, and Robinson, 1978). In the early years the victims are pedestrians or, more frequently, bike riders; later, they are car drivers or passengers.

Teenagers' ability to drive increases the need for personal responsibility for their own safety and for that of others. Nurses may contribute to accident prevention by participating in safety education programs in schools. More frequently, nurses will care for accident survivors, who may require long-term hospitalization and who may be suffering grief as well as physical injuries. Basic driver education is minimal preparation for an activity that requires foresight and self-discipline as well as skill. Trial and error in the assumption of lesser responsibilities is helpful preparation for the independence achieved in the role of car driver or operator of any motor vehicle.

Alcohol, tobacco, and drug use also represent important health hazards to adolescents. Although more information is available to young people today about the dangers of these practices, greater numbers of adolescents are involved in them and at younger ages. Role modeling by adults, peer pressure, and the motivation to achieve adult status or independence from adults in some areas are factors associated with the use of all three agents. Peer support groups seem to be more successful than authoritarian practice in prevention and recovery programs, illustrating the complexity of individual and social interaction.

TABLE 11-2 Advantages, Disadvantages, and Effectiveness of Different Forms of Contraception

	Theoretical effectiveness*	Use effectiveness*	Inexpensive	No major side effects	No medical exam or follow-up	Protects against sexually transmitted diseases	Disposable	Partner cooperation needed	Increased body awareness	Avoidance of "artificial substances"	Can predispose to major health problems	Can cause major infections	Can cause minor irritations	Can be expelled or dislodged	Can initiate menstrual problems	Can cause discomfort to wearer	Coital related	Must manipulate genitals
Tubal ligation	0	0.04								X								
Vasectomy	0	0.15								X								
Oral contraceptives	0.1	0.3									X		X		X			
Intrauterine device (IUD)	2	5									X	X	X	X	X	X		X
Diaphragm with spermicide	3	15		X		X							X	X			X	X
Condoms	1	5	X	X	X	X	X	X		X			X	X		X	X	X
Foams or jellies	5	20	X	X	X	X	X						X	X		X	X	X
Rhythm (calendar)	14	35–40	X	X	X			X	X	X								
Withdrawal	3	15–23	X	X	X			X	X	X							X	X
Mucous (ovulation method)			X	X	X			X	X	X								X
Cervical cap	3	15		X						X			X	X		X		X
Douche		35–40	X	X	X		X			X			X				X	X

SOURCE: Olds SB, London ML, Ladewig PA: *Maternal-Newborn Nursing*. Addison-Wesley, 1984, p. 121. Adapted from Romney SL, et al: *Gynecology and Obstetrics: The Health Care of Women*. McGraw-Hill, Blakiston, 1975, p. 552 and from Tatum HJ, Connell-Tatum EP: Barrier contraception. *Fertil Steril* (July) 1981; p. 5.

*Number of pregnancies per 100 woman-years of use.

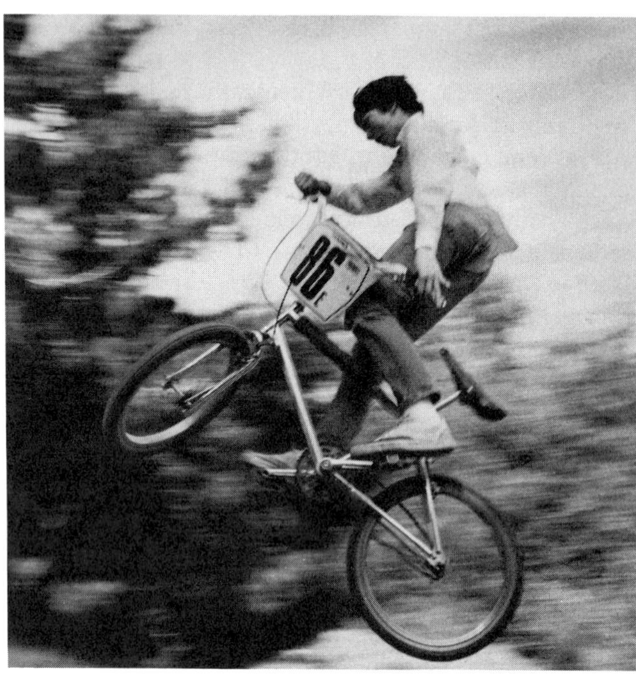

Adolescents need to learn to take responsibility for their own safety.

The nurse becomes actively involved with the prevention of substance abuse, particularly in the school setting. Nurses' contacts with adolescents on a day-to-day basis facilitate their active involvement. (See Chapter 21 for anticipatory guidance and Chapter 24 for specific information concerning substance abuse.)

Transition to Adulthood

The prime objective of adolescence, recognized by all theorists, is achieving a sense of self or personal identity. The definite and obvious changes of puberty, the cognitive development of an increasing ability to think about one's own thinking, and the highly variable rate of development among individuals of the same age challenge the teenager's sense of self. The adolescent's physical, and especially reproductive, maturation occurs in a context of economic dependence, creating an individual who is neither wholly child nor adult and causing both grief and anticipation at some level of consciousness.

The adolescent might achieve a sense of continuity of self and a positive self-concept with ease or turmoil. The social setting, and especially the responses of significant people in this setting, influence the adolescent's progress. Nurses might interact with adolescents or the significant people, such as parents and teachers, to provide information and clarify misconceptions about many issues of human growth and development. Nurses also have to consider how health problems affect the adolescent's ongoing efforts to confirm personal identity.

Key Concepts

- Adolescence involves definite changes that affect every subsystem and the person's interactions with the suprasystems, especially those of family, peers, and school.
- Health problems may arise from the expansion of the parameters of human existence during adolescence or, arising from other sources, may interfere with parameter expansion. For example, the increasing range, skill, and independence of mobility may lead to accidents.
- The preadolescent transitional phase is noted for its importance as a time for building physical coordination and cognitive information processing skills, as well as comfort in peer interactions.
- Some physical and psychologic signs of the onset of puberty are evident and some are less obvious. Physical signs include maturation of the sweat glands and sexual organs, as well as changes in body configurations. Psychologic changes are evident in behavior.
- The onset of puberty is a major transition and is often associated with disequilibrium.
- Male and female reproductive systems follow specific patterns of maturation that are related to the interaction of neurologic and hormonal controls.
- The early adolescent regression theories of Anna Freud and Peter Blos are related to the basic concepts of psychoanalytic theory. An interpersonal focus has been added by Harry Stack Sullivan, who described an interaction called chumship.
- A review of the central concepts of affective-personality development helps to define and understand sexuality, leader–follower roles, response to authority, values, emotional control, self-esteem, belonging, self-assertion, and daydreaming.
- Social development includes a consideration of the developmental tasks derived from the interaction of maturation with the goals of the individual and the

cultural expectations of the social environment, as described by Havighurst.

- The varied purposes and forms of play, including dating, in adolescence are exemplified by cooperative play, team play, and constructional play.
- The temporal, value, vocational, and specific gender sexuality components of self-image and self-concept are challenged in the psychosocial crisis of adolescence described by Erik Erikson as a conflict resolution between identity and identity diffusion or confusion.
- Adolescents need to experiment with several roles to achieve identity. James Marcia developed a method for evaluating identity achievements by applying the components of vocation choice and value orientation.
- Characteristics of formal operations have been described by Jean Piaget. Learning theories are related to school tasks of adolescents, with special attention to motivation and memory.
- Language development is linked to cognitive development, school tasks, and self-concept development. Likewise, the moral development theories of Jean Piaget and Lawrence Kohlberg and the faith development theory of James Fowler are related to cognition and affective-personality development.
- Hygienic concerns in adolescents include special attention to skin care, sweat gland activity, and menstrual hygiene. Development concerns relate to sleep and rest, nutrition, dental care, and exercise. Safety concerns include sexual activity, sports participation, motor vehicle operation, and use of alcohol, tobacco, and drugs.

References

Bandura A: The stormy decade: Fact or fiction? In: *Issues in Adolescent Psychology.* Rogers D (editor). Appleton-Century-Crofts, 1969.

Bandura A: Social Learning Theory. Prentice-Hall, 1977.

Bell R: *Changing Bodies, Changing Lives: A Book for Teens on Sex and Relationships.* Random House, 1981.

Blos P: *On Adolescence: A Psychoanalytic Interpretation.* Free Press, 1962.

Blos P: The child analyst looks at the young adolescent. In: *Twelve to Sixteen: Early Adolescence.* Kagan J, Coles R (editors). Norton, 1972.

Borow H: Career development. In: *Understanding Adolescence.* 3rd ed. Adams JF (editor). Allyn and Bacon, 1976.

Brown LK: Toxic shock syndrome. *Matern Child Nurs J* 1981; 4:57–59.

Douvan E, Adelson J: American dating patterns. In: *Issues in Adolescent Psychology.* Rogers D (editor). Appleton-Century-Crofts, 1969.

Duvall EM: *Marriage and Family Development.* Lippincott, 1977.

Elkind D, Weiner IB: *Development of the Child.* Wiley, 1978.

Erikson EH: *Childhood and Society.* Wiley, 1963.

Erikson EH: *Identity: Youth and Crisis.* Wiley, 1968.

Farina AM, Furth SH, Smith JM: *Growth and Play.* Prentice-Hall, 1959.

Flavell J: *The Developmental Psychology of Jean Piaget.* Van Nostrand, 1963.

Fowler J: Stages in faith: The structural-developmental approach. In: *Values and Moral Development.* Hennessy T (editor). Paulist Press, 1976.

Freud A: *The Ego and the Mechanisms of Defense.* International Universities Press, 1967.

Gallatin JE: *Adolescence and Individuality: A Conceptual Approach to Adolescent Psychology.* Harper & Row, 1975.

Gesell A, Ilg F, Ames LD: *The Years From Ten to Sixteen.* Harper & Row, 1956.

Ginsburg HJ, Opper S: *Piaget's Theory of Intellectual Development.* Prentice-Hall, 1979.

Gordon C: Social characteristics of early adolescence. In: *Twelve to Sixteen: Early Adolescence.* Kagan J, Coles R (editors). Norton, 1972.

Greenfield PM, Bruner J: Culture and cognitive growth. *Int J Psychol* 1966; 1:89–107.

Gruen W: Adult personality: An empirical study of Erikson's theory of ego development. In: *Personality in Middle and Late Life.* Neugarten B (editor). Atherton Press, 1964.

Hall CS: *A Primer of Freudian Psychology.* New American Library, 1954.

Havighurst RJ: *Developmental Tasks and Education.* 3rd ed. McKay, 1972.

Jones IH: The history of sanitary protection. *Nurs Times* (March 6) 1980; 76:407–408.

Jones MC: The later causes of boys who were early or late maturing. *Child Dev* 1957; 28(1):113–128.

Jones MC: A study of socialization patterns at the high school level. *J Genet Psychol* 1958; 93:87–111.

Jones MC: Psychological correlates of somatic development. *Child Dev* 1965; 36:899–911.

Jones MC, Bayley N: Physical maturing among boys as related to behavior. J Educ Psychol 1950; 41:129–148.

Jones MC, Mussen PH: Self conceptions, motivations, and interpersonal attitudes of early and late maturing girls. *Child Dev* 1958; 29:491–501.

Kagan J: A conception of early adolescence. In: *Twelve to Sixteen: Early Adolescence.* Kagan J, Coles R (editors). Norton, 1972.

Katchadourian H: *The Biology of Adolescence.* Freeman, 1977.

Katchadourian H, Lunde D: *Fundamentals of Human Sexuality.* Holt, Rinehart & Winston, 1975.

Kohlberg L: Moral development and identification. In: *Child Psychology.* Stevenson H (editor). University of Chicago Press, 1963.

Kohlberg L: Moral stages and moralization: The cognitive-developmental approach. In: *Moral Development and Behavior: Theory, Research and Social Issues.* Lickona T (editor). Holt, Rinehart & Winston, 1976.

Kohlberg L., Gilligan C: The adolescent as a philosopher: The discovery of self in a post-conventional world. *Daedalus* (Fall) 1971; 100:1051–1086.

Kohlberg L, Turiel E: Moral development and moral education. In: *Psy-*

chology and Educational Practice. Lesser GS (editor). Scott Foresman, 1971.

Lindzey C, Hall C: *Theories of Personality.* Wiley, 1978.

Marcia J: Development and validation of ego-identity status. *J Pers Soc Psychol* 1966; 3:551–558.

Marcia JE: Identity in adolescence. In: *Handbook of Adolescent Psychology.* Adelson J (editor). Wiley, 1980.

Miller D: *Adolescence: Psychology, Psychopathology and Psychotherapy.* Jason Aronson, 1974.

Muss RE (editor): *Adolescent Behavior and Society: A Book of Readings.* Random House, 1975.

Mussen PH, Conger JJ, Kagan J: *Child Development and Personality.* Harper & Row, 1974.

Neimark ED: Intellectual development during adolescence. In: *Review of Developmental Research.* Vol 4. Horowitz FD (editor). University of Chicago Press, 1975.

O'Hara R, Tiedeman D: Vocational self-concept in adolescence. In: *Issues in Adolescent Psychology.* Rogers D (editor). Appleton-Century-Crofts, 1969.

Olds SB, London ML, Ladewig PA: *Maternal-Newborn Nursing.* Addison-Wesley, 1984.

Peterson AC: Can puberty come any faster? *Psychol Today* (Feb) 1979; 12:45–46.

Piaget J: *The Construction of Reality in the Child.* Cook M (translator). Ballantine Books, 1954.

Piaget J: *The Moral Judgment of the Child.* Gabain M (translator). Free Press, 1965.

Piaget J: *The Origins of Intelligence in Children.* Cook M (translator). International Universities Press, 1952.

Rivers C, Barnett R, Baruch G: *Beyond Sugar and Spice: How Women Grow, Learn and Thrive.* Putnam, 1979.

Rosen B: Family structure and achievement motivation. In: *Issues in Adolescent Psychology.* Rogers D (editor). Appleton-Century-Crofts, 1969.

Sheldon WH, Stevens SS, Tucker WB: *The Varieties of Human Physique.* Harper & Row, 1940.

Smart MS, Smart RC: *Children: Development and Relationships.* Macmillan, 1977.

Smith DW, Bierman EL, Robinson N: *The Biologic Age of Man From Conception Through Old Age.* Saunders, 1978.

Sommer BB: *Puberty and Adolescence.* Oxford University Press, 1978.

Stone LJ, Church J: *Childhood and Adolescence: A Psychology of the Growing Person.* Random House, 1973.

Sullivan HS: *The Interpersonal Theory of Psychiatry.* Perry HS, Gavel ML (editors). Norton, 1953.

Tanner JM: *Growth of Adolescence, With a General Consideration of the Effects of Hereditary and Environmental Factors Upon Growth and Maturation from Birth to Maturity.* 2nd ed. Blackwell, 1962.

Tanner JM: Sequence, tempo, and individual variation in growth and development of boys and girls aged twelve to sixteen. In: *Twelve to Sixteen: Early Adolescence.* Kagan J, Coles R (editors). Norton, 1972.

Terman LM: The discovery and encouragement of exceptional talent. *Am Psychol* (June) 1954; 9:221–230.

Torrance EP: Fostering creative thinking during the high school years. In: *Issues in Adolescent Psychology.* Rogers D (editor). Appleton-Century-Crofts, 1969.

Valadian I, Porter D: *Physical Growth and Development from Conception to Maturity.* Little, Brown, 1977.

Vick RL: *Contemporary Medical Physiology.* Addison-Wesley, 1984.

Weatherly D: Self-perceived rate of physical maturation and personality in late adolescence. *Child Dev* 1964; 35:1197–1210.

Zelnick M, Kantner JK: Sexual and contraceptive experience of young unmarried women in the United States, 1976 and 1971. In: *Adolescent Pregnancy and Childbearing.* Chilman CS (editor). US Department of Health and Human Services Publication No. (NIH) 81-2077, Dec. 1980.

Additional Readings

Bailey DA: The growing child and the need for physical activity. In: *School-Age Children: Development and Relationships.* Smart MI, Smart RC (editors). Macmillan, 1978.

The Boston Women's Health Book Collective: *Our Bodies Ourselves: A Book By and For Women.* Simon & Schuster, 1976.

The Boston Women's Health Book Collective: *Ourselves and Our Children: A Book By and For Parents.* Random House, 1978.

Coles R: *Privileged Ones: The Well-Off and the Rich in America.* Little, Brown, 1977.

Comer JP, Poussaint AF: *Black Child Care: How to Bring Up a Healthy Black Child in America: A Guide to Emotional and Psychological Development.* Simon & Schuster, 1975.

Comfort A, Comfort J: *The Facts of Love: Living, Loving and Growing Up.* Crown, 1979.

Douvan E, Adelson J: *The Adolescent Experience.* Wiley, 1966.

Dwyer JT, et al: Adolescents' attitudes towards weight and appearance. *J Nutr Educ* 1969; 1:14.

Elkind D, Weiner IB: *Development of the Child.* Wiley, 1978.

Erikson EH: *Childhood and Society.* Norton, 1963.

Erikson EH: *Identity: Youth and Crisis.* Norton, 1968.

Erikson EH: *Youth: Change and Challenge.* Basic Books, 1963.

Frisch RE: Weight at menarche: Similarity for well-nourished and under-nourished girls at differing ages and evidence for historical constancy. *Pediatrics* 1972; 50:445–501.

Frisch RE, Revelle R: Height and weight at menarche and a hypothesis of menarche. *Arch Dis Child* 1971; 46:695–701.

Guttmacher A: *Teen Pregnancy: The Problem that Hasn't Gone Away.* The Alan Guttmacher Institute, 1980.

Haimowitz MQ, Haimowitz NR (editors): *Human Development: Selected Readings.* 3rd ed. Harper & Row, 1973.

Kagan J, Coles R (editors): *Twelve to Sixteen: Early Adolescence.* Norton, 1972.

Katchadourian H: *The Biology of Adolescence.* Freeman, 1977.

Katchadourian H, Lunde D: *Fundamentals of Human Sexuality.* Holt, Rinehart & Winston, 1975.

Maire HW: *Three Theories of Child Development.* Harper & Row, 1969.

Mussen PH, Jones MC: The behavior-inferred motivations of late and early maturing boys. *Child Dev* 1958; 29:61–67.

Mussen PH, Jones MC: Self-conceptions, motivations and interpersonal attitudes of late and early maturing boys. *Child Dev* 1957; 28:243–256.

Neimark ED: Adolescent thought: Transition to formal operations. In: *Handbook of Developmental Psychology.* Prentice-Hall, 1982.

Nelms BC: What is a normal adolescent? *Am J Matern Child Nurs* (Nov./Dec.) 1981; 6(6):402–406.

Rivers C, Barnett R, Baruch G: *Beyond Sugar and Spice: How Children Grow, Learn and Thrive.* Putnam, 1979.

Robertiello RC: *Hold Them Very Close, Then Let Them Go: How to Be an Authentic Parent.* Dial Press, 1975.

Rogers D (editor): *Issues in Adolescent Psychology.* Appleton-Century-Crofts, 1969.

Rubin LB: *Worlds of Pain: Life in the Working-Class Family.* Basic Books, 1976.

Scheff RE, Hall E: *Developmental Psychology Today.* Random House, 1978.

Schestowsky B: Helping your adolescent client become more physically fit. *Can Nurse* (April) 1983; 79:24–25.

Schowalter JE, Anyan R: *The Family Handbook of Adolescence.* Knopf, 1979.

Schuster CS, Ashburn SS: *The Process of Human Development: A Holistic Approach*. Little, Brown, 1980.
Sheldon WH, Stevens SS, Tucker WB: *The Varieties of Human Physique*. Harper & Row, 1940.
Shipman WG: Age of menarche and adult personality. *Arch Gen Psychiatry* 1964; 10:155–159.
Smart MS, Smart RC: *Children: Development and Relationships*. Macmillan, 1977.
Smart MS, Smart RC: *Readings in Child Development and Relationships*. Macmillan, 1972
Smith EA: The date. In: *Issues in Adolescent Psychology*. Rogers D (editor). Appleton-Century-Crofts, 1969.
Valadian I, Porter D: *Physical Growth and Development From Conception to Maturity*. Little, Brown, 1977.
White JE: Initiating contraceptive use: How do young women decide? *Pediatr nurs* 1984; 10: 347–352.
Yeaworth RC, et al: The development of an adolescent life change event scale. *Adolescence* 1980; 15(57):91–97.

Coping Strategies of Children

Noreen Mahon Mary Ann Scoloveno

12

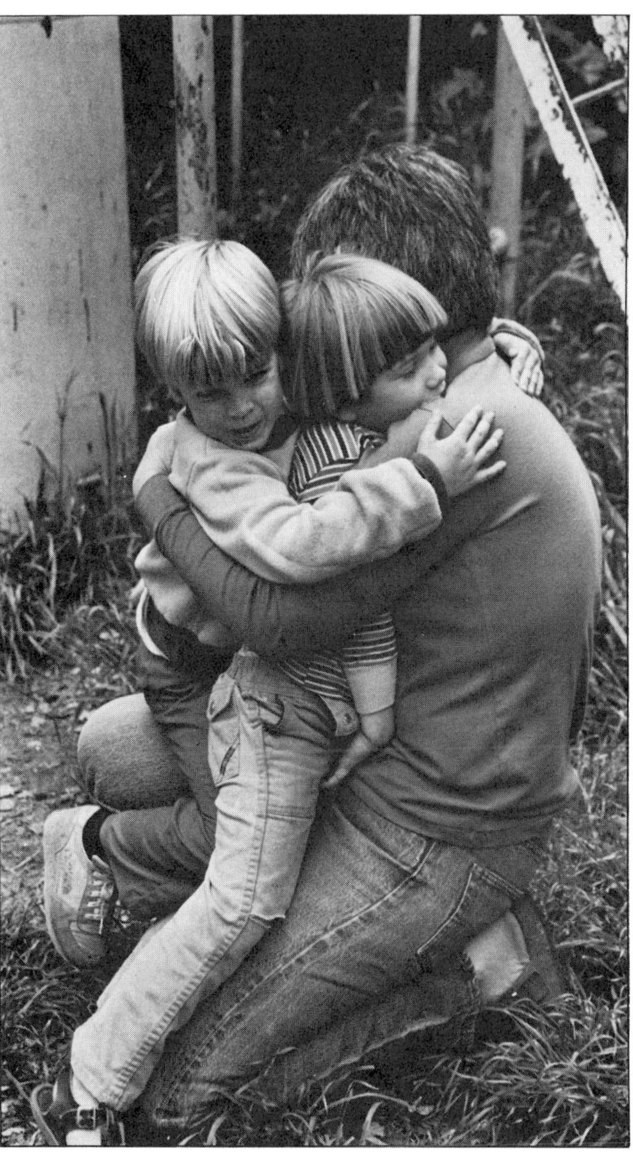

Chapter Outline

Objectives

- Define the types of coping behaviors that children use to adapt to stress.
- Identify the factors that influence coping strategies.
- Define the principal coping strategies used by children.
- Explain the common stressors that create the necessity for adaptation at various developmental stages.
- Identify coping behaviors common to each developmental stage.
- Explain how the styles of coping change as the child matures.
- Explain how coping strategies are acquired.
- Define basic techniques that can assist children in learning to cope.

Bobby, 4 years old, sits and talks to Stewie, his friend. Bobby is the only one who communicates with his playmate because Stewie is imaginary, a product of Bobby's fantasy. Beth, 2 years old, has a temper tantrum when she is in the store shopping with her parents. She falls to the floor, kicking and crying. If these behaviors were displayed by adults, they would be considered inappropriate, but in children they are effective coping strategies.

Our purpose in this chapter is to focus on children's coping strategies. We discuss methods of coping as behavior used to adapt to stress; we consider how children acquire these behaviors; and we look at the factors that influence coping styles. We also examine children's ways of adapting to common stressors and the variety of coping behaviors at different developmental stages.

Coping as Adaptation

Children use coping strategies throughout childhood to achieve growth and gain equilibrium. In the course of developing children learn to cope with maturational and situational stressors and to manage their world better. *Coping strategies* are learned behaviors that are influenced by the child's prior experiences, stage of development, environmental demands, areas of vulnerability, and significant role models. Some authorities view coping behavior on a continuum from adaptive to maladaptive (Zeitlin, 1980). Adaptive coping behaviors generate learning that can be added to the child's repertoire and used later to cope with new situations. Maladaptive coping strategies, on the other hand, increase stress and interfere with new learning. Maladaptive coping strategies also lead to dysfunctional behavior (see Chapter 24).

Coping strategies are specific behavioral sequences that are used to deal with challenges or problems. Normal children use several adaptive, age-appropriate strategies to make their dependence more tolerable. Murphy and Moriarty (1976) analyzed children's coping behaviors over an 18-year period and classified these behaviors on the basis of factor analysis as either environmental coping or self-coping. *Environmental coping* is essentially the ability to cope with environmental opportunities, challenges, frustrations and threats. *Self-coping* is the ability to adapt personal relations to the environment so as to maintain integrated functioning (Murphy and Moriarty, 1976). Children's perceptions are important to both environmental coping and self-coping. Children usually base their perceptions on their own observations, on what is presented to them by significant people in the environment (usually their parents), and on fantasy.

Coping behaviors are thus learned behaviors that are influenced by the interaction of children of all ages with the environment. Lazarus and Launier (1978) added that coping requires intrapsychical and action-oriented efforts to deal with internal and environmental demands.

Equilibrium and Disequilibrium

Gesell, Ilg, and Ames (1956, 1977) identified major cycles of growth that occur at certain intervals throughout the life span (see Table 6-2). These alternating patterns are defined as periodic equilibrium and disequilibrium. Although each child has a unique pattern of growth, basic profiles often characterize a child's behavior. Therefore, periods of disequilibrium are predictable times of stress that require the child to learn coping behaviors as a form of adaptation.

Gesell identified times of equilibrium as times when the child seems balanced and consolidated such as at ages 2, 5, and 10 years. Periods of disequilibrium reflect anxiety and an inward focusing such as can be seen in the $2\frac{1}{2}$-year-old, at 6 years of age, and at 11 years of age. As children grow older, they seem to be in equilibrium at certain developmental stages. Children in equilibrium are easygoing and secure. At other stages, disequilibrium results in wanting too much, trying new things, and dissatisfaction.

For example, $2\frac{1}{2}$-year-olds are assertive and emotionally labile in their attempts to achieve physical control and deal with the frustrations of limited verbal skills. Natural curiosity leads them into inappropriate situations, and their protests against parental limits are frequent and clamorous. As 3-year-olds, they are more secure, the inner frustrations of the earlier period no longer as evident. Children will move from the apparently equitable world of the 5-year-old to the tumultuous world of the 6-year-old. Six-year-olds in a state of disequilibrium want to control the environment but have not yet developed a secure sense of themselves. They are characteristically brash and aggressive and can be very rigid and demanding. Adjustment to school is often followed by a state of equilibrium and emotional calm. During this time, the child's role becomes more clearly defined, and emotional outlets take on more socially acceptable forms.

From 7 to 10 years of age, children alternate periods of equilibrium with periods of disequilibrium. The 7-year-old lives in a calmer world and may cope with stress by withdrawing. The 8-year-old tends to confront challenges and faces a world that is expansive and fast-moving. Eight-year-olds are more sensitive and interested in relationships, leading to increased self-esteem and independence as friends take on greater importance. Ten-year-olds find themselves in a predictable, secure equilibrium, with an increased attachment to family, whereas 11- and 12-year-olds enter adolescence in a period of disequilibrium.

Types of Coping Behaviors

Pearlin and Schooler (1978) identified three general types of coping behaviors that are common to developmental stages. The first category includes behaviors that are used in attempts to modify a stressful situation, a type of coping strategy that allows the child to seek help from others. Because adults usually consider themselves self-reliant, children probably use this coping strategy more often than adults. The child who is frightened, for example, may run to the parent for assistance.

The second type of coping strategy identified by Pearlin and Schooler consists of those behaviors that allow the child selectively to ignore a threatening situation or to make the threat an unvalued aspect of life. Adults use this strategy often, but children have difficulty with it because they often have trouble determining the significance of problems and arranging them in order of priority. For example, children who are having difficulty with fractions may have trouble relegating the difficulty to a low priority, especially if parents and teachers emphasize its importance.

Pearlin and Schooler's third type of coping strategy includes those behaviors that assist children in managing the threat of stress rather than the stressor itself. For example, children use coping strategies to deal with impending doctor's visits so that they can cope when such visits actually occur.

Children use a variety of coping strategies throughout their development. Broadly defined, coping strategies include defense mechanisms, which aid the child with both environmental coping and self-coping. *Defense mechanisms* are psychologic processes that temporarily assist the child to reduce stress levels. Children use defense mechanisms in situations that involve excessive stress and conflict with which the child cannot deal directly. The use of defense mechanisms is evident across developmental levels. The temporary use of defense mechanisms gives the child the opportunity to organize resources for successful coping with stress and conflict. When a child is unable or unwilling to master new demands or stresses, the defense mechanisms help the child to maintain a state of equilibrium (Hurry and Sandler, 1971).

Although coping strategies can be viewed across age levels, patterns of coping behavior also change with developmental stage (Chess and Thomas, 1976). Coping strategies in early and middle childhood generally are expressed on an overt behavioral level—temper tantrums, for example. With increasing cognitive development, which brings a capacity for understanding symbols and the beginning of a sophisticated self-image, coping strategies reflect the normal transition from action to ideation. Behaviors are thus less overt, and defenses are increasingly internalized. Adolescents, for example, are more likely to use sublimation than regression.

Factors Influencing Coping

A variety of influential, interacting variables influence the coping behaviors of children and adolescents. Among these variables are age, personality, and previous experiences with stress and role models. These factors influence the methods of coping as the child grows and develops.

Age Age is an important variable in influencing coping behavior because age carries with it a level of cognitive and psychosocial development that enables the child to deal with stress. The concept of separation-individuation (see Chapter 6) illustrates the importance of age and corresponding developmental stage as variables in coping because researchers attribute significance to this component of the child's development and its relationship to dealing with stress at a later time.

Mahler and colleagues (1971) divided separation-individuation into four subphases. The first subphase, differentiation, occurs at approximately 5–10 months of age, when infants recognize themselves as separate and different from others. The infant at this time can tolerate increasing separation from the parent but becomes anxious if the parent is not available. The second subphase, according to Mahler, is practicing, which occurs at 10–15 months of age. The infant in this phase is curious and exploratory, practicing motor skills and accepting strangers more readily. Rapprochement, the third subphase, occurs from 15–22 months of age, with the child actively resisting separation from the parent. The fourth subphase, consolidation, occurs at 18–36 months of age, when the child develops the ability to retain a mental image of the parents, as well as a beginning sense of time in activities of daily living.

The concept of separation-individuation demonstrates that children between approximately 6 months and 3 years of age will be vulnerable to separation from the parent for prolonged periods of time. Infants younger than about 6 months of age do not view themselves as separate from parents and are relatively immune to the stressor of separation. In early childhood, as children approach 4 years of age, the vulnerability to separation decreases because they are at a cognitive stage in which they are able to perceive object permanence.

Temperament Temperament reflects the style of behavior used to cope with anxiety or stressful demands. The child's temperament usually reflects the kind of interactions that exist within that individual's environment. Children who routinely are exposed to screaming or fighting, for example, are most likely to react with the same behavior to any perceived or real threat, anxiety, or stressor. The intensity of the reaction, however, may differ in relation to those around them. Some children are always loud and boisterous, whereas others can be quiet or shy. Some children are open and take immediate risks with new people and situations, whereas other children are cautious.

Depending on their temperaments, children have their own characteristic ways of releasing tension. Gesell's studies suggest that a child's temperament determines, in part, the child's choice of emotional outlets (see Chapter 6). Six-year-olds, for example, tend to kick furniture and swing legs, bite their nails, stutter, and make faces. Temper tantrums occasionally characterize the 6-year-old. The 7-year-old, with fewer emotional outlets, tends to internalize much of the stress and anxiety associated with new people or situations. Eye blinking and complaints of headaches are common with this age group.

Eight-year-olds tend to become dramatic in releasing tensions, and earlier patterns of behavior may reappear. Crying, especially when tired, is very common in this age group. The 9-year-old's temperament often is characterized by stamping feet, growling, and muttering. These children also use fine motor activities such as fiddling with clothes or hair. They tend to be short-tempered and impatient. Tension outlets for the 10-year-old are less obvious, but finger-to-mouth activity increases. Eleven-year-olds demonstrate increased motor activity when anxious or under stress, and they tend to stumble a lot. Making faces and eye blinking are also common. The 12-year-old's temperament shows a decreasing intensity. Less-intense coping behaviors are common by this time. Thomas, Chess, and Birch (1969) studied the temperament of children from birth to 10 years of age and found differences among children in the following nine areas:

1. Activity level
2. Adaptability to changes in routine
3. Intensity of responses
4. Tendency to approach or withdraw
5. Persistence
6. Distractibility
7. Regularity of sleeping patterns
8. Regularity of eating patterns
9. Sensitivity

A child's style of behavior in these nine categories provides a basic definition of that individual's temperament. Although children's temperamental features change as they become older, these features play an important role in determining interactions with the environment (Rutter, 1981).

These findings demonstrate that most children accept new experiences easily and adjust well to changes in routine. Other children, however, are slower to adjust to new situations, and still others react negatively to new experiences and changes in routine (Chess, Birch, and Thomas, 1969). Rutter (1981) suggested that these temperamental features could either protect children or place them at risk because of their effects on parent–child interaction. Temperament then is an important factor in influencing coping style, and parents need to be aware of children's different behavioral styles and focus on positive interactions as both parents and children learn to cope with differences in behavior.

Previous Experiences As children grow and develop, they experience many stressful situations. Rutter (1981) suggested that stress early in childhood may sensitize the child to the effects of later stressors and help in learning to overcome stress later in life. The long-term effects of stressful events also are related to the ways in which the child has dealt with stress previously and whether the child adapted successfully at those times.

Stress adaptation is related in theory to Erikson's epigenetic principle, which further indicates that previous experiences determine coping behavior (see Chapter 6). If, as Erikson asserted, psychologic capacities develop at appropriate ages and development is a result of interactions with the environment, the child's experience with influential suprasystems affects the child's behavior patterns. Successful resolution of stress at one developmental stage should therefore lead to successful resolution of similar situations during a subsequent developmental stage.

Role Models Social networks and role models, as essential components in the child's environment, are also important to the achievement of children's coping repertoires. Parents are the most significant people in young children's environments. Parents may act protectively, thereby modifying the stressful situation, and young children learn to imitate parental behavior in response to stress. Nurses therefore intervene with the entire family when helping children to cope with stressors.

As children develop and enter school, peer groups become both role models and social support networks. Rutter (1981) documented the effect of the social peer group in altering children's perception of and reaction to stress. Peer group support, as well as personal relationships with family members, peers, and teachers, protect children as they develop coping repertoires. Personal success at home, in school, and with the peer group helps children to develop the self-esteem needed to cope with stressful life events at particular developmental levels.

Specific Coping Behaviors

Regression

Regression is the return to a behavior used in an earlier stage of development in order to cope with a threatening situation. Three-year-olds who are toilet trained, for example, may begin soiling their pants in an effort to cope with the introduction of a new baby into the home. Regression also can affect adolescents. For example, Mike, a 15-year-old boy, is small for his age. His fear of being unable to cope with adolescent social situations has resulted in regression. His friends are boys younger than himself and his activities with them allow him to avoid the stress of initiating friendships with girls. The purpose of regressive behavior is to return the child to a less stressful level of functioning.

Displacement

Displacement is used to shift emotional energies from a stressful object or situation to one that is less threatening. If the child's needs cannot be met adequately because of physical and social limitations, the child may direct feelings and energies into new channels that provide gratification in a different form (Lazarus, 1976). This permits the child to cope with frustrations. For example, the adolescent who is angry with a parent for setting limits may punch a door rather than the parent in an effort to substitute a nonthreatening object for a threatening person. For example, 5-year-old David was always well behaved in school until his parents adopted a baby. Suddenly, he became aggressive, pushing and hitting other children to be first in line or closest to the teacher. He appeared to feel that the baby had taken over first place in his parents' affections. Aggression toward his peers was less frightening than aggression toward the new baby would be, and releasing his anger at school allowed him to cope at home.

Denial

Denial involves suppressing an awareness of people or events that could be threatening. The child copes with the threat by denying its existence (Lazarus, 1969). When using denial, the child often rejects reality. Children sometimes use denial when they are doing poorly in school, thus refusing to face the threat of possible failure.

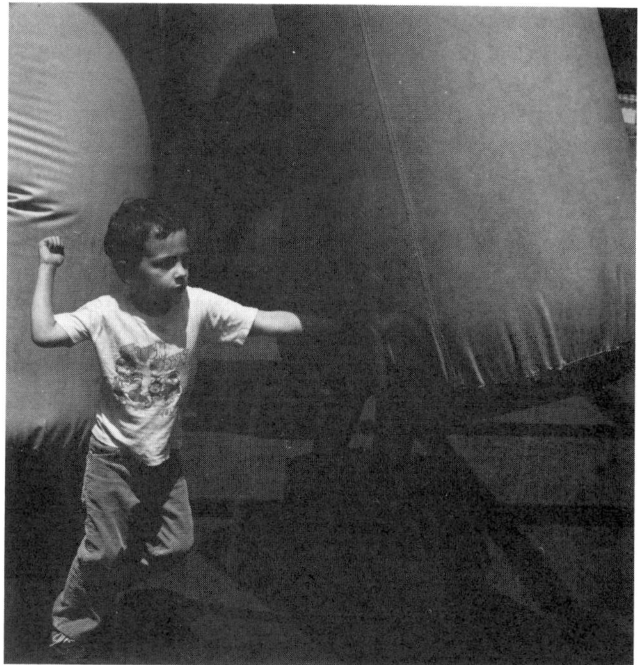

The releasing of a child's feelings of aggression can be channeled into less harmful and more acceptable directions.

Denial often is seen in the newly toilet-trained child who has a toilet accident and does not acknowledge it or in the adolescent who brags about social conquests to avoid dealing with social insecurity. By denying the perceived failure, the child avoids having to deal with the resulting stress.

Projection

Projection is the attribution of negative feelings and qualities to others while denying that they originate in oneself. The child using projection thus denies the responsibility for conflict and may attribute an impulse or feeling to another person instead of accepting it (Lazarus, 1976). In early childhood projection is evident in play, through which the child projects blame and anger on an inanimate object such as a doll or an imaginary friend.

Projection often is evident when children use puppets to express stressful feelings. For example, 6-year-old Richard's puppets were deathly afraid of loud noises, particularly smoke alarms. Richard had accidentally triggered a fire alarm when he was 4 years old. His fear of loud noises was reflected in his puppets' responses, allowing him to appear to be in control.

Rationalization

Rationalization is the development of a false justification for behavior to hide an anxiety-provoking situation. Children who do not participate in team sports because they fear that they will do poorly may claim that they are too busy with schoolwork to join the team. This rationalization might help them to continue functioning until they can enlist someone's help in developing sufficient skill to make them feel comfortable with team participation (Chess and Thomas, 1976).

One of the most common phrases associated with rationalization in children is, "The other kids told me to do it." This is the classic attempt to justify behavior that is contrary to a parental directive. For instance, 3-year-old Mary came in the house with marigolds in her mouth, necessitating a call to the poison control center. She said her friend David had told her to eat the flowers and she did, despite having been warned repeatedly not to eat anything she found outdoors. Her own actions thus were given an excuse that she thought her parents might find acceptable.

Sublimation

Sublimation is behavior that focuses attention on a substitute for an unacceptable feeling. When sublimating, children divert energies toward socially acceptable rather than destructive activities. Feelings of anger, for example, may be diverted into such activities as running and participation in sports. Artistic expression also can be a form of sublimation. Certainly, musical masterpieces express the feelings of their composers. Feelings of anger can be diverted into creative energy, whether it be pounding piano keys or nails or punching clay. Children of all ages should have outlets available to them for directing emotions into acceptable channels.

Attack

Verbal or physical *attack* is often a child's response to fear. The aggressive behavior is analagous to a "fight or flight" mechanism in which the child perceives that someone or something is a threat to personal well-being. For example, during a physical examination, young children often try to take the equipment away from the examiner or hit, bite, and scream in an effort to gain control over a threatening situation.

Identification

Identification is the socialization process by which a child takes on or internalizes characteristics of another, particularly a parent. This mechanism is important in the healthy development of the child's personality and is a part of the child's developing gender identity (Lazarus, 1976). Freud postulated that identification is a form of defense against powerful authority figures. By taking on the characteristics of the authority figure, the child avoids punishment.

In early or middle childhood, for example, a boy may state that he will be a lawyer like his father; later on he may identify with teachers and want to become an educator. Often, the identification is so complete that, to their dismay, parents can see their more embarrassing qualities in the actions of their children. For example, 2-year-old Amy was seen with her hands on her hips talking to her doll: "If you don't stop that right now, I'm going to spank your bottom." Her mother was chagrined to see the imitation, which was identical, even to voice inflection.

Temper Tantrums

Temper tantrums are a natural developmental phenomenon. Infancy and early childhood involve the frustration of newfound independence and concomitant limitations imposed by the inability to express oneself in adult ways through language. When children are having difficulty with self-control, coordination, decisions, or fears, they use temper tantrums as a coping strategy. In these early years children cannot communicate in more acceptable ways because they do not have the past experiences or language development to do so. Tantrums vary in intensity from mild screaming to full-scale kicking, pounding, and breath-holding.

The number and extent of tantrums depends on the child's temperament and parental reactions. Some children, although capable of excellent language skills, use tantrums frequently to protest imposed limits. Others may use this strategy only once or twice in an attempt to release frustration and exert control over the environment. Tantrums, particularly when associated with breath-holding, can be frightening for parents to watch. Whereas temper tantrums may be an effective coping strategy for the 2-year-old, the same behavior will not work for the 12-year-old who, for example, is having difficulty with a math problem. Developmental level is an important variable in determining whether the selected strategy will be successful. (The parental management of temper tantrums is discussed in Chapter 13.)

Play

Although children do not have the same experiences with coping as adults, they do have a mode of expression that enables them to master the environment. This mode of expression is play, which serves to integrate development at each stage (see Chapters 7–11).

Fantasy *Fantasy*, a form of play, involves some type of role change and appears to help children tolerate their dependent and relatively helpless status more easily and to prepare them for their adult role (Volmut, 1979). Children can tolerate frustrations if they can achieve imaginary gratification through fantasy. Witte (Volmut, 1979) found that by 2 years of age, children are capable of engaging in fantasy because they can partially distinguish real events from those that are imaginary. Fantasy is one of the most useful mechanisms of children's coping. It is a form of expression that can provide insight into a child's actual concerns.

According to Freudian psychodynamic theory, fantasizing permits primarily sexual or aggressive drives to be satisfied. Fantasizing does allow children to try new roles, solve problems, obtain independence, and seek refuge from unpleasant situations or environments. During late childhood, for example, fantasy serves as a kind of imitation. Children mimic the behavior and speech of their adult role models and take on a variety of imaginary roles. They may be mothers, fathers, cowboys, spacemen, spacewomen, superhuman beings, and combat soldiers. They simulate parental arguments, fight wars, battle space creatures, and love a doll as one loves a child. A girl may fantasize that she is a princess in love with a prince, a type of fantasy that reflects her maturing sexuality. The younger child may converse out loud with her prince, and the conversations provoke the child to continue the fantasy. As the child matures, these conversations are internalized because of authoritative disapproval and the ever-increasing attention demands of school. Diaries allow for the written expression of fantasies and are often used by early adolescents in place of conversations. (Play and fantasy as coping mechanisms for hospitalized children are discussed in Chapter 28.)

Daydreaming *Daydreaming,* a form of fantasy, is used as a coping mechanism throughout development. Like the adult who dreams about winning a lottery, children daydream about becoming important people. This form of fantasy is a method of obtaining omnipotence so that one can cope with feelings of vulnerability (Schuster and Ashburn, 1980). During most of late childhood, daydreams are internal. Only when alone or during certain forms of play does the child act out the daydream.

Daydreaming in school from the second grade on, however, is serious. Frequent daydreaming in school might reflect an inability to cope with schoolwork, boredom, or perhaps a learning disability. Daydreaming or imaginary play might reflect emotional disturbances. Indeed, child therapists have used make-believe play to determine what troubles a child, but daydreaming is still a vital part of normal development. A teacher once complained to a father about his son's daydreaming. The father replied, "Miss Smith, where would we be if no one ever daydreamed of faraway lands, of planets, of electricity. . .?"

Stressors and Common Coping Behaviors

Childhood is a time for adapting to new situations that present maturational challenges such as the mastery of a developmental task, addition of a sibling into the home, or going to school. Children also commonly confront such situational stressors as separation from principal attachment figures, illness, and injury. Children respond to stressful situations in a variety of verbal and nonverbal ways, often combining specific coping strategies into complex behavior patterns. Responses to stress also have certain age-typical characteristics that can guide the nurse in caring for children and their families. Stressors and coping behaviors common to specific developmental stages are summarized in Table 12-1.

Separation

The child's concept of separation follows that of object permanence and temporary separation but precedes the understanding of death. During infancy, the child learns that if an object is removed from sight, the object might reappear, yet the infant also learns that some objects do not reappear (for example, "milk all gone"). The infant's reaction to being separated from an object depends on the degree and the nature of the attachment to the object. As children mature, they are confronted with more frequent experiences of separation, most of which are temporary or involve separation from objects that are readily replaceable. A child loses a ball, a glove, or a boot, all of which can be replaced. Unless the child had developed an attachment to the object or the object is irreplaceable, little importance is given to the loss or separation.

Some life situations, however, are manifested by painful separation. Parents divorce; a friend moves; a pet dies; and a child graduates from school. Children may react to these separations with bereavement, fear, guilt, and curiosity. For the infant, the parent is of primary importance, and separation from the parent is a major source of stress. Coping with separation is therefore directly related to the infant's attachment experiences (see Chapter 7). To cope with separation, infants initiate interactions and begin demonstrating more control over their environment. In an effort to cope with displeasure the infant displays anger by crying and turning away. As they grow older, infants use temper tantrums as a coping strategy.

Robertson and Bowlby (1951) described three phases of response to separation: (1) protest; (2) despair; and (3) detachment. In the initial phase of protest the child cries, calls, and searches for the attachment figure, while rejecting the comfort measures of others. In the second phase, despair, the child becomes more withdrawn, and if separation continues, detachment, the third phase, may occur. Robertson and Bowlby's findings indicate that when the attachment figure returns after prolonged separation, the child's attachment behaviors may be minimal. The duration of the child's detachment is therefore directly related to the length of the separation, as well as to the child's developmental level. Ability to cope with the stress of illness also is related to the proximity of the attachment figure (see Chapter 27).

TABLE 12-1 Stressors and Coping Strategies Common to Specific Developmental Stages

Developmental stage	Common stressors	Possible coping behaviors
Infancy	Separation	Crying, temper tantrums, withdrawal
Early childhood	Separation	Temper tantrums, crying, regression
	Inability to communicate with adults	Fantasy (eg, imaginary playmate), transitional objects, ritualism, identification
	Inability to distinguish reality from fantasy	Protest, attack
	Fears—bodily harm	Protest, attack, projection, ritualism, fantasy
	Introduction of sibling	Regression, attack
Middle childhood	Fears—loss of control, unknown phenomena	Role play, denial, projection, identification
	School phobias (see Chapter 24)	Meticulousness, lying, cheating, rationalization
	Separation	Attack, regression, displacement
Late childhood	School phobias (see Chapter 24)	Lying, cheating
	Separation	Displacement, withdrawal
Adolescence	Need for independence—fear of failure	Rebellion, sublimation, denial, rationalization
	Developing adult roles	Fantasy, withdrawal, daydreaming, identification

Divorce The divorce rate in the United States has risen so sharply that divorce is a common source of stress for children of all ages. Divorce usually provokes a crisis for all family members, and children cope with their emotions in ways that are specific to their developmental levels and ages.

For example, 8-year-old Linda's parents became divorced after months of trial separations and reconciliations. The custody battle was bitter in that both parents sued for full custody. Eventually, a joint custody arrangement was established, with Linda spending portions of the week with each parent. The two houses were in the same neighborhood to allow Linda to maintain friends and have uninterrupted schooling. At first, Linda fantasized about a permanent reconciliation between her parents. When it became evident that this would not occur, she became angry and verbally aggressive toward both parents. She exhibited frequent tantrums during the settling-in process as she struggled to cope with a back and forth existence. She saw the custody differences as a rejection of her by both parents. Several years later, although she seems to have coped successfully with her new life, her behavior with her parents is chameleon-like. She appears to assume the characteristics of the parent she is with and is still struggling with her own identity. Linda's behavior is an example of the array of coping mechanisms employed by a child in a divorce. She used many strategies to decrease the situational stress, and these would differ if she were at a different developmental level.

In early childhood the child has difficulty understanding what is happening and may have varied reactions to the divorce. Fear and anxiety are evidenced in these children by their worrying about who will care for them. Anger and aggression are exhibited by increased irritability and temper tantrums. Children may project aggressive impulses onto others and become fearful that others will harm them. Early childhood is a time of vulnerability to guilt feelings. The child may believe that something he or she did or failed to do caused the divorce, and feelings of pervasive sadness, evidenced by crying or sobbing and bewilderment are common. Regression often is used to cope with the divorce. Some regressive behaviors include thumb-sucking, an increased need for a security blanket, lapses in toilet training, and reverting to infantile play (Haber, et al., 1982).

In middle childhood the child is able to understand the meaning of divorce and its impact on the family. Children at this stage tend to worry about the many changes in their lives and often fantasize about the deprivations that may accompany these changes. A common reaction to the divorce is anger—both boys and girls tend to become angry and blame their mothers for the divorce. Children in middle childhood may cope with the stress of the divorce in maladaptive ways such as by eating compulsively or by hoarding and demanding new possessions (see Chapter 24). In this age period the child tends to idealize the noncustodial parent (Haber, et al., 1982).

In later childhood intense anger is a common reaction to divorce. The anger often is focused on the parents' irresponsibility in dissolving the family structure. Children experience feelings of rejection and loneliness and may feel ashamed about the divorce. Some children defend themselves against divorce by aligning with one parent against the other. A common coping strategy is increased school and recreational activities. Children at this stage may expend considerable energy in working for parental reconciliation (Haber, et al., 1982).

The adolescent also experiences a high degree of anger toward parents, anger that may be used as a defense against sadness and feelings of vulnerability. The adolescent is resentful about the divorce and its impact on family life. Coping strategies vary but are likely to include increased participation in sports, hobbies, and schoolwork. Antisocial behavior and deliberate violation of family rules also occur. Adolescents do, however, have the advantage of being able to express their feelings verbally and channel their feelings into organized activities (Kelly and Allenstein, 1977).

The emotional impact of divorce is clearly a major consideration for the health professional working with these families. Parents not only may need to be supported themselves but also need guidance in how to support their children through their loss and its attending grieving period. The parent who has custody, usually the mother, also needs reassurance that she is competent and able to function as a single parent. Economic and social changes must be considered and negotiated. The following therapeutic guidelines are useful in helping children cope with divorce:

1. Assess the strengths and limitations of the family system
2. Assess the relationships of the significant parties within and without the family system
3. Identify what changes the divorce has caused in the social, emotional, interactional, and economic aspects of the family's life
4. Be available as a listener without taking sides or being judgmental
5. Help the family to assess realistically the situation and the options that are available
6. Talk with the children; identify how they perceive what is happening; be open to cues regarding changes in their social and school activities
7. Help parents and children to communicate openly and honestly
8. Refer to or seek collaboration/consultation from other professionals when warranted

(Family assessment is discussed in Chapter 17. Nursing care for families at risk is discussed in Chapter 22.)

The nurse's role can be vital to the child's coping with the divorce experience because the parents' energies may be caught up in their own feelings and concerns during the crisis. Many studies and much literature have been written on the effects of divorce on the child and family, and the nurse should use these data to understand more fully the crisis of divorce and its impact on the family system and the children in it. The nurse also might recommend books about divorce that are written for the age and understanding of the child. Most local libraries can be of assistance in compiling a useful list.

Kelly and Allerstein (1977) offered particularly useful information for nurses working with children experiencing divorce, suggesting the data that the nurse should assess and offering concrete interventions according to age groups.

Death Death and loss are inevitable experiences for all families. The alterations and disruptions that occur in the family system require redirection of the energies within the system as structures and functions change. New role responsibilities and relationships must be defined and methods of communication repatterned. The healthy resolution of a loss experience is important for the future development of the child. The events that surround the crisis are poignant memories for many children. No one, at any age, can experience a serious loss without having to make major adjustments. A period of bereavement and its accompanying feelings of denial, anger, and depression are inevitable in working through the stress of such a crisis. Some people, whether children or adults, require assistance to progress through the grief process and to reestablish equilibrium. If the child is not allowed to express these feelings adequately and share them in an accepting and understanding environment, the child may adopt dysfunctional methods for coping with grief, such as eating disorders, antisocial behavior, or depression.

Adequate coping strategies and supports are essential in resolving grief. Withdrawal, aggression, fears, and physical changes are just some of the coping strategies that children may exhibit. The nurse's understanding of these behaviors according to the child's level of development and family context is essential to facilitating the child's progress through the bereavement period. (The process of grieving is discussed in Chapter 32.)

The concept of death, like the reaction to any phenomenon, depends on the child's level of cognitive and personality development. The infant has no conception of time or perception of the meaning of death. Before the development of attachment relationships and demonstration of separation anxiety, death or loss has little or no significance, yet separation from a significant caregiver may be analogous to a death experience for the infant once parent–child attachment is established. Infants thus respond to separation by crying and clinging to their caregivers.

By early childhood, the child's egocentric thinking and ritualistic behavior may cause the child to speak about the dead person as if nothing has changed because the person lives on in the child's fantasy world. At $1-2\frac{1}{2}$ years of age, vague distinctions between fantasy and reality make it impossible to understand death. Coping patterns used to deal with the death of a significant person center on the need for ritualistic behavior. Behaviors such as visits to the grave site and either anger or intense sadness in response to any changes in the dead person's former living environment typify reactions at this stage. Parental understanding of the need for ritual and simply pointing out reality without contradicting the child's fantasies surrounding death help the child to cope with death and loss.

In the later phase of early childhood and into middle childhood, children acknowledge death but believe that the power of magical thought can cause events. They therefore associate death with guilt, shame, and punishment. Because they have fewer coping strategies for dealing with loss, they may react to a less significant loss with more outward grief than they show in response to a more significant loss. In so doing the child may be using denial to deal with the overwhelming reactions to death. In early childhood guilt and self-blame are common whenever a parent dies after the child has misbehaved. The child may believe that the parent's death is a punishment and interpret literally statements the parent made in the past when reprimanding the child (for example, "You'll be the death of me yet"). The child's inability to understand the cause of death coupled with magical thought evoke guilt and blame. The child believes that wishing someone were dead is enough to cause death. Coping behaviors at this age also include regression, giggling, and attention seeking. Understanding and support during this period help the child to resolve the loss over time. In middle childhood death is associated with a form of punishment that can be avoided by "being good." Anger also might be apparent in the child's coping repertoire. By late childhood, most children have an adult concept of death, and their attitudes are influenced by those who support them. As the child reaches 10 and 11 years of age, death is viewed as a permanent and irreversible phenomenon. In late childhood and adolescence, however, adult awareness and understanding of death mean that the child is less likely to accept death than the younger child. The adolescent yearns for the one who is lost and occasionally hopes that the significant person will return. Some adolescents have been observed searching for their lost loved ones or have described a sense of the dead person's presence. The adolescent who recognizes that this cannot happen experiences sadness. Frequently, the adolescent experiences anger about the death, as well as feelings of guilt and fear, and may be anxious and clinging, engaging in behaviors that are difficult to understand (Bowlby, 1980). The care and support of a parent or significant person is essential in assisting the adolescent to resolve these feelings about death.

Moving The feelings of loss and separation in children are sometimes the result of moving away from friends. Although some reactions to moving are evident at early ages, children in middle and late childhood and in adolescence have the most difficulty coping with this type of loss. The peer group is important to these children, so that grieving about the loss of friends because of moving is significant. They often cope by displaying signs of loneliness, boredom, withdrawal, hostility, and displaced anger.

For example, Jean, a 16-year-old girl, recently moved into a small town and enrolled in the local high school. At her former school, which had twice as many students, she was a popular and accepted member of several groups. Her first weeks at the new school were lonely ones. Any overtures on her part seemed to be ignored by her classmates, who already were in established peer groups. Two months into the school year found her sitting alone in the cafeteria, no longer interested in attempting to make friends, and displaying an attitude of aloofness to protect herself from the hurt of rejection. Although her protective shell helped her cope with her feelings of separation, it made her much less approachable to concerned classmates, thus prolonging her adjustment to her new environment.

Fears

Fears, like separation, are common stressors that are evident throughout the life span and generally develop from actual or perceived threatening stimuli and events. They may be manifested either overtly or symbolically but become increasingly sophisticated as the individual matures. With experience, fears are discarded or transformed and reorganized.

Fear of Unknown Phenomena Early childhood is a time of fears, principally fears of bodily harm. Using what Piaget calls preoperational thought, these children are influenced by outside phenomena such as the media and thereby perceive that certain situations are real and can threaten them. The child is caught between the egocentricity of infancy, which was itself protective, and logical thought that provides explanations for phenomena (Piaget, 1928). Because their thinking processes are thus "magical," these children fear harm from imagined phenomena that seem real to them. They will cope with these fears by protests and cries similar to those of infants, but because they have begun to acquire a more mature use of language, they are also able to explain their fears.

Young children who become preoccupied with the fear may reach for help and plan a method of attack or escape. Their aggressive behavior becomes more goal directed than the behavior of the infant. In early childhood temper tantrums are a common coping strategy, and children may attack and physically resist a situation they view as threatening. Fear of bodily injury and deviation from familiar rituals mean that a visit to the doctor's office, for example, may be stressful for both the child and the parent because the child may physically attack the examiner and kick and scream. Play helps young children to cope with the environment; nurses should therefore use play when attempting to assist these children cope with threatening situations. Knowing the child's rituals also allows the hospital nurse to incorporate them in the plan of care (see Chapter 28).

In early childhood children have limited resources for dealing with stress and therefore often resort to fantasy in efforts to cope with their fears. It is through fantasy that children are able to deal with the stresses of daily living and come to understand themselves in relation to the people and the environment around them. Some children will create imaginary playmates in response to their needs and may use these companions as friends, scapegoats, or models. An older child described his imaginary companion and his coping strategy in this way:

> I once had a friend named Stewie. No one could see or hear him but me. Stewie did everything with me. When I felt sick, Stewie was sick. When I moved, Stewie moved too. When I went to the hospital, Stewie came with me. When I was happy, Stewie was happy. Sometimes Stewie was bad, and I had to explain to him what being good was like. Stewie was my friend. He does not live with me anymore because I grew up, and I don't need him anymore.
>
> Bobby, age 11

Like imaginary playmates, inanimate objects, such as blankets or toys, may be the focus of a child's fantasy. Fantasy used in this way enables children to cope with an ever-changing world and plays an essential role in the child's coping repertoire. Griffith's (1935) research identified fantasy and symbolic thinking of 5-year-olds as a useful method of coping with life's problems. Imagination and fantasy are thus useful coping strategies in helping the child manage the environment.

Children in middle and late childhood have a variety of fears such as fear of animals, fear that a significant person will die, and fear of physical harm. Many of these fears have been learned through actual experience or repeated parental warnings. For instance, children are told at an early age to be careful while on or near the stairs because they might fall and be injured. Fear of bees may be due to an actual experience in which the child was stung or it may be the result of watching the reactions of others when bees are nearby.

The 7-year-old experiences visual and spatial fears—shadows are misinterpreted as monsters, ghosts, and other creatures. The mass media and social forces may stimulate the formation of fears. The child may insist that the closet door be closed because spies and burglars lurk there but deals with these fears by putting a light on before entering a dark room. The 8-year-old has less fear of natural elements, such as rain and thunder, and less fear of the dark but may exhibit a marked fear of death, with an awareness that death is an irreversible and final outcome for everyone. Many children fear being buried alive, which is often a fear of suffocation. To deal with the fear of death, many children undertake role play by pretending to be dead and burying themselves under garments.

With increasing maturity, fears become personal and private. The child can mock old fears. Nine-year-olds will try to scare each other and take pride that they don't scare easily. The 10- to 12-year-old has still fewer fears, although fears specific to a particular child may persist.

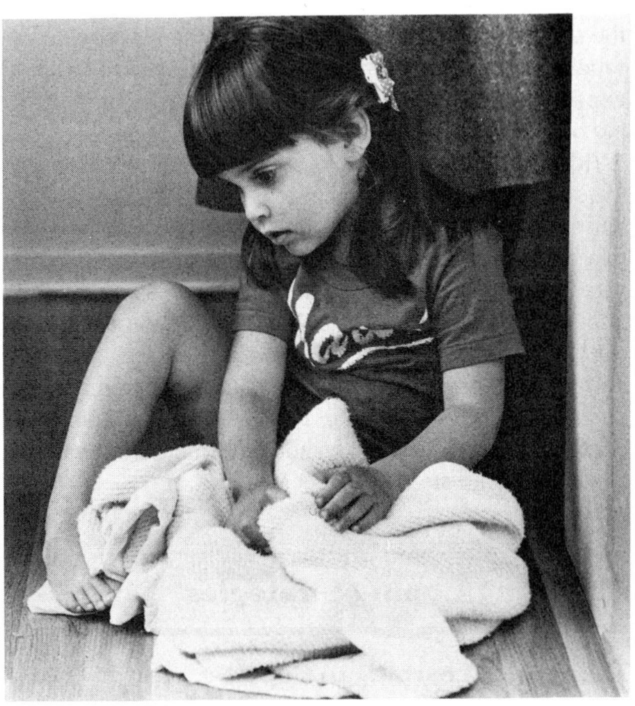

Inanimate objects such as blankets can be a focus or agent of a child's fantasy life, thus providing a source of security against fears and stressors.

Fears of Failure In middle and late childhood a common fear is loss of self-control. As the child's environment expands to include peer groups and teachers, attachment to people outside the child's immediate family causes separation from earlier attachment figures, and grieving and a sense of loss may follow. Because success in school and in competitive activities are now important, children of this age group learn to cope with situations by cooperating in group standards and rules. The child may use such coping strategies as meticulousness and care about details in schoolwork to become successful and thus control the stress.

In middle and late childhood coping strategies to control fear of failure include lying and cheating. If children feel that they are not measuring up to the expectations of parents, teachers, and peer groups, they may lie or cheat in an attempt to obtain perceived success in a difficult situation. At times, lying may be part of the child's fantasy formation.

In the earlier years of late childhood, lying is the practical alternative the child employs to avoid parental or authoritative anger and disapproval. The child is usually fully aware of reality but chooses to ignore or conceal the truth. Lying to avoid anger, punishment, and unpleasantness often continues throughout adulthood.

To cope with the loss of self-control in school or during illness or injury, these children also may also display loneliness, hostility, or displaced anger. Adolescence brings with it the task of self-identity and the associated fear of failing at this essential developmental task. Adolescents cope with the stress of attempting to establish independence through rebellion and fantasy formation, in which adolescents experiment with different roles, clothing styles, and seeming omnipotence.

Adolescents use a variety of coping strategies to deal with this stress. Coping is directly related to societal expectations and sex-role identity. For example, the adolescent boy may join a football team instead of a debating team if his perception is that playing football is more "masculine" than debating. Other coping behaviors include eating and other oral behavior, "goofing off," physical exercise, retreating into fantasy and daydreaming, boasting, asking questions, and talking it out (Menninger, 1963). Adolescents also might display signs of loneliness, withdrawal, and boredom when confronted with stress.

Acquiring Coping Strategies

Theories of Learning to Cope

Coping strategies are learned behaviors. As with any other learned response, the learning of coping strategies depends on the child's cognitive development. What the child learns is what works in situations that are stressful.

Cumulative learning theory, as proposed by Gagne (1970), postulates that more complex learning depends on more primitive learning, a theory applicable to the learning of coping behaviors. The infant learns signals that provide a response to a stimulus such as hunger. Children eventually progress to the problem-solving abilities found in the adolescent by building on the learning of earlier stages.

The infant then progresses from responding primarily through reflex activity to beginning to organize activity in response to the environment (Piaget and Inhelder, 1969). Trial-and-error learning is too sophisticated for the infant, yet infants find that certain interactions occur through such behaviors as crying, clinging, sucking, and smiling. In early childhood the egocentric child also learns that certain coping responses will elicit interaction with people in the environment, yet language skills are not fully developed, so that young children often resort to coping behaviors that include temper tantrums to elicit responses from significant people in relation to stressful situations.

According to Piaget (1928), early childhood is a time of preoperational thought, during which children are able to verbalize their mental processes but also are influenced by outside phenomena (see Chapter 8). These children learn that fantasy assists them in managing their world and coping with stress. They learn by imitating significant people in their environment. This type of learning continues throughout adolescence, and the imitation of models such as parents, teachers, and peers contributes to the coping repertoire. Identifying a person's *locus of control* is a way of explaining how that person exhibits control over the environment (Phares, 1976). A child with an internal locus of control learns to cope with stress positively by responding actively to the stressor. A child with an external locus of control learns to see outside forces as responsible for events and therefore tends to use avoidance behaviors as coping strategies. Significant persons in the child's environment reward logical problem solving in stressful situations. A child who is taught that any attempt to cope with environmental threats is useless because the stressor cannot be controlled will learn to submit blindly to the wishes of others.

Techniques for Learning Coping Strategies

Children can learn to reduce stress by responding actively to it. Bensen described stress reduction as a *relaxation response,* which he defined as an integrated, psychologic response to stressors that engender a "fight or flight" reaction. A person copes with stress by relaxing rather than fighting or fleeing. According to Bensen, all relaxation techniques include a comfortable position, a quiet environment, repetition of a word or phrase, and adoption of a passive attitude (White, 1975). With help, children can learn to elicit this response. For example, when a child is displaying aggressive behavior, prescribing a quiet "time out," in which the child goes to a designated place, encourages and teaches relaxation as a coping strategy. Such interventions must, however, be appropriate to the child's developmental stage. (Parenting techniques for managing behavior and teaching children appropriate responses are discussed in Chapter 13.)

Meichenbaum and Goodman (1969) used the principles of the relaxation response when dealing with impulsive children and found that children who are taught to talk to themselves using positive statements become more self-controlled. Some of the stress-coping thoughts that can help the child quiet negative arousal include the following (Davis, et al., 1980):

Preparation for stress

- There's nothing to worry about
- I'm going to be all right
- I've succeeded with this before
- What exactly do I have to do?
- I know I can do each one of these tasks
- It's easier once you get started

Confronting stress

- Stay organized
- Take it step by step; don't rush
- I can do this; I'm doing it now
- I can only do my best
- I can get help if I need it
- It's O.K. to make mistakes

Meichenbaum proposed a theory of cognitive self-control, which involves three stages: (1) self-observation; (2) incompatible thoughts; and (3) behaviors and cognitions concerning change. Through practice, children learn effective coping strategies when aroused by stress (Schwartz and Shapiro, 1976).

During infancy and early childhood, children will not have the problem-solving abilities or language development to practice cognitive self-control, but they do have support systems, such as parents and family members, who can promote positive coping behaviors. If these significant persons, who make up the child's support network, learn to cope with stress in a positive manner, they will be able to assist children to do so as well. Parents also might need assistance with coping, and the nurse often is called on to assist parents in coping with the tasks of parenting (see Chapter 13). Parenting groups may be formed to help parents learn effective methods of assisting children to cope with stress and for making parenthood more pleasurable.

Parents also must learn those age-appropriate responses that are directly related to a child's developmental level. Children imitate effective listening and coping behaviors, so parents may first need to cope with their own stress. Parents and other significant persons in the child's environment must be able to call on nurses for assistance in coping with the maturational and situational stressors that occur in their lives. They also must know the resources that are available to assist them in coping with the stresses of parenting and daily living.

Key Concepts

- Coping strategies are learned behaviors that the child uses to adapt to stress.
- Coping behaviors that are age-appropriate and that help the child adapt to the environment are a normal part of development.
- Coping is a way in which the child responds to the disequilibrium that is part of normal growth and development.
- Although specific coping strategies are evident across developmental stages, patterns of coping do change with the child's development.
- A child's coping behaviors are influenced by age, temperament, and the role models and experiences to which the child has been exposed.
- Specific coping behaviors include regression, displacement, denial, projection, rationalization, sublimation, attack, identification, temper tantrums, and play.
- Stressors that give rise to coping behaviors may be part of a normal developmental stage, or they may be situations, such as parental divorce or a death in the family, that can occur at any time in the child's development.
- The nurse's role in recognizing coping behavior can be important in helping both the child and the family to adapt to stress.
- The way in which a child copes with fear usually typifies the child's response to a real or perceived threat.
- Children learn coping strategies by trial and error, with consequent reinforcement, and by developing the communication skills that are a part of normal development.
- Children can learn adaptive coping strategies through such techniques as relaxation.

References

Bowlby J: *Attachment and Loss.* Vol 3. Basic Books, 1980.

Chess S, Birch HG, Thomas A: *Temperament and Behavior Disorders in Children.* New York University Press, 1969.

Chess S, Thomas A: Defense mechanisms in middle childhood. *Canadian Psychiatric Association Journal.* 1976; 21:521.

Davis M, Eshelman E, McKay M: *The Relaxation and Stress Reduction Workbook.* New Harbinger Publications, 1980.

Gagne RM: *The Conditions of Learning.* 2nd ed. Holt, Rinehart and Winston 1970.

Griffiths R: *A Study of Imagination in Early Childhood.* Routledge and Kegan Paul, 1935.

Haber J, et al: *Comprehensive Psychiatric Nursing.* 2nd ed. McGraw-Hill, 1982.

Hurry A, Sandler J: Coping with reality: The child's defenses against the external world. *Brit J Med Psychol* 1971; 44:380.

Kelly J, Allerstein J: Brief interventions with children in divorcing families. *Am J Orthopsy* 1977; 47:23.

Lazarus RS: *Psychological Stress and The Coping Process.* McGraw-Hill, 1969.

Lazarus RS: *Patterns of Adjustment.* McGraw-Hill, 1976.

Lazarus RS, Launier R: Stress-related transactions between person and environment. *Perspectives in International Psychology.* Pervin LA, Lewis M (editors). Plenum, 1978.

Mahler M: A study of the separation-individuation process and its possible application to the borderline phenomena in the psychoanalytic situa-

tion. In: *The Psychoanalytic Study of the Child.* Vol 26, Eissler RS et al (editors). Quadrangle, 1971.
Meichenbaum D, Goodman J: Reflection-impulsivity and verbal control of motor behavior. *Child Devel* 1969; 40:785–797.
Menninger K: *The Vital Balance.* The Viking Press, 1963.
Murphy L, Moriarty A: *Vulnerability, Coping and Growth.* Yale University Press, 1976.
Pearlin LI, Schooler G: The structure of coping. *J Soc Behav* (Mar) 1978; 19:2–18.
Phares EJ: *Locus of Control in Personality.* General Learning Press, 1976.
Piaget J: *Judgment and Reasoning in the Child.* Harcourt Brace Jovanovich, 1928.
Piaget J, Inhelder B: *The Psychology of the Child.* Basic Books, 1969.
Robertson J, Bowlby J: Responses of young children to separation from their mothers. *Courrier du Centre International de L'Enfance* 1951; 2:131–142.
Rutter M: Stress, coping and development: Some issues and some questions. *J Child Psychol Psychiatry* 1981; 22:337.
Schuster CS, Ashburn SS: *The Process of Human Development: A Holistic Approach.* Little, Brown 1980.
Schwartz GE, Shapiro D: *Consciousness and Self-Regulation.* Vol 1. Plenum Press, 1976.
Volmut J: Fantasy in the nursing of children. *Perspectives in Psychiatric Care.* 1979; 17:211.
White KL: Prevention as a national health goal. *Prev Med* (Sept) 1975; 4(3):247–251.
Zeitlin S: Assessing coping behavior. *Am J Orthopsychiatry* (Jan) 1980; 50(1):139.

Additional Readings

Ainsworth MDS, Whittig BA: Attachment and exploratory behaviors of one-year olds in a strange situation. In: *Determinants of Infant Behavior.* 4th ed. Methuen, 1969.
Ainsworth MDS, Whittig BA: The development of infant-mother attachment. In *Review of Child Development Research.* Vol 3. Caldwell BM, Ricciuti HN (editors). University of Chicago Press, 1973.
Bowlby J, Robertson J: The nature of the child's tie to his mother. *Int J Psychoanalysis.* 1958; 39.
Erickson E: *Identity, Youth and Crisis.* W. W. Norton, 1968.
Erickson E: *Childhood and Society.* 2nd ed. W. W. Norton, 1980.
Felice M, Friedman S: The adolescent as a patient. *J Contin Educ Ped* (Oct) 1978.
Fine LL: What's a normal adolescent? *Clin Ped* (Jan) 1973; 12.
Ginsberg H, Opper S: *Piaget's Theory of Intellectual Development.* Prentice-Hall, 1969.
Klaus MH, Kennel JH: *Maternal-Infant Bonding.* Mosby, 1976.
Kohlberg L: The development of children's orientation toward a moral order: Sequence in the development of moral thought. *Vita Humana* 1963; 6.
LaMontagne L: Three coping strategies used by school-age children. *Ped Nurs* (Jan/Feb) 1984.
Piaget J: *The Psychology of Intelligence.* Routledge and Kegan Paul, 1950.
Piaget J: *The Moral Judgment of the Child.* The Free Press of Glencoe, 1960.
Sander LW: Issues in early mother-child interaction. *J Am Acad Child Psychiatry* 1962; 1.

Parenting

Karen Mitchell

13

Chapter Outline

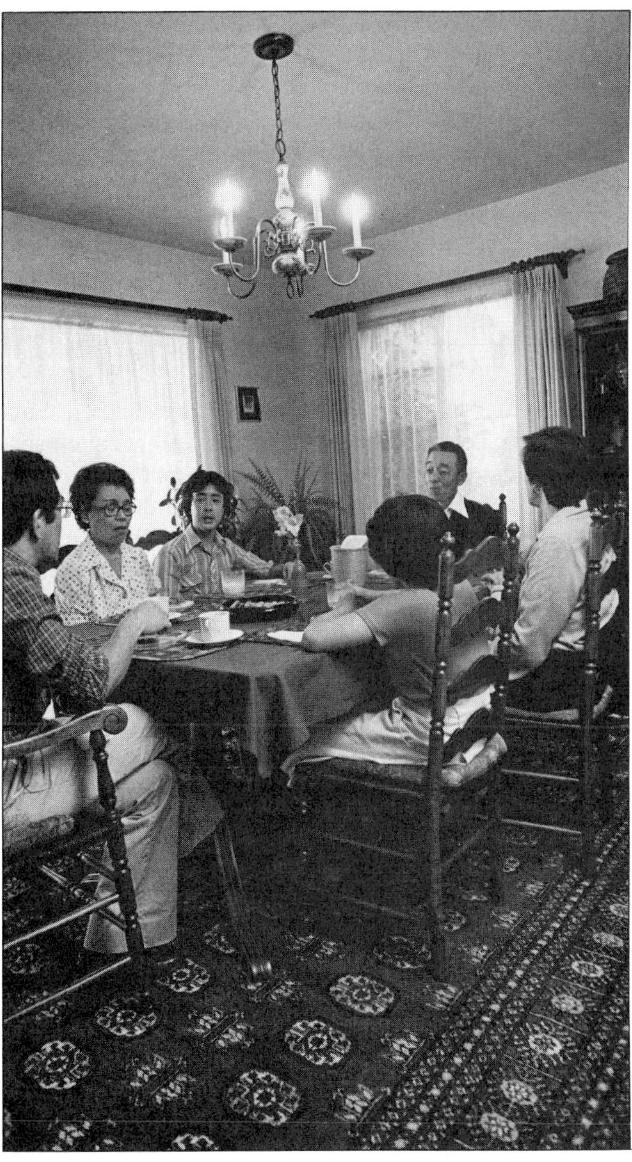

Objectives

- List the tasks associated with parental development at each developmental stage.
- Define the process by which the child is helped to move from the pleasure principle to the reality principle.
- Identify the types of support available to parents.
- Explain the guidelines for effective communication between parents and children.
- Describe the methods by which parents can minimize unacceptable behavior.
- Define authoritative, authoritarian, and permissive parenting.
- Define the approaches to the parental management of a behavioral problem.
- Describe the specific methods and applications for behavior modification.
- Describe the assessment and management process for specific behavioral concerns.

The attachment between parents and their children may be the strongest of human relationships. Parents often see children as extensions of themselves, personifying parental hopes and dreams. Through this unique and caring relationship, parents and children develop the ability to love each other deeply, and parents in turn provide the nurturance and warmth essential for the development of the child's self-concept.

This unique partnership between parents and children involves the crucial development of mutuality, the coordination of giving and receiving. Parents influence and are influenced by their children. This interrelationship among family members reflects the concept of the family as a system in which each part affects the others. The dynamic interplay among family members involves continuing changes in both the parents and their children so that whenever one individual develops or changes in any respect, other family members accommodate and develop in response.

In this chapter, we see that what Erikson (1964) called the "cogwheeling" of life cycles, which involves the mutual development of strengths in parents and children. As children enter particular developmental stages and struggle with each stage's developmental tasks, parents also grapple with their own anxieties and tensions. Each developmental task the child faces presents the parents with an opportunity to reexamine and rework previous experiences and behavior patterns. For example, the parent attempting to assist the 2-year-old to establish a sense of autonomy in the face of frequent doubts also reanalyzes and reworks a personal sense of autonomy, despite past doubts or shames. The parent's vitality and self-concept ideally are also strengthened through interactions with the child, so that as parents assist their children along the continuum toward self-actualization, they too may be activated to higher levels of development.

Parenting, although not an exact science, does encompass skills that can be learned. Parents who wish to develop their parenting skills can practice effective communication and can learn to promote acceptable behavior in their children. In this chapter, we analyze the components of effective parenting, and we examine the variety of parenting styles and methods of discipline that the nurse needs to understand in caring for children and their families.

Parental Development

According to Friedman and Friedman (1977), parents progress through identifiable developmental stages and undertake developmental tasks as they attempt to accommodate themselves to their child's development. During infancy, a key parental task is learning cues and interpreting an infant's needs. Blood (1972) suggested that the difficulty at this stage is defined by the infant's inability to use language and the initial parental frustration with "translation" problems.

Parents frequently become extremely anxious when their infant cries and they feel unable to determine what the infant wants or needs. The parent feels tremendous responsibility for the well-being of this small newcomer. Parents need to be reassured that they really are reacting appropriately and meeting the infant's needs. When the parent begins to feel secure in reading the infant's cues and interpreting needs, that parent may state confidently, "He is sleepy" or "She is hungry now" rather than, "I think he is sleepy or hungry." Parents then become spokespersons for their infants and interpret their infants' needs and wants to others.

The ability to meet another's needs successfully is extremely rewarding and motivates parents to invest even more time and energy in their children. This early interaction in turn tends to foster the infant's sense of trust and hope for future pleasant experiences. Parents need empathy and support as they attempt to meet their infants' tremendous needs for nurturance. If parents receive support during this period and become confident of their abilities to read their infants' cues, they may find infancy extremely rewarding and pleasurable. If parents are unable to meet their infants' needs for affection and nurturance, however, and if they feel overwhelmed by their infants' dependence, they may experience feelings of helplessness, anger, guilt, or exhaustion.

During early childhood, a primary parental task is learning to accept the child's growth and development by accepting some loss of control while at the same time maintaining necessary limits. As young children struggle to become more autonomous by exerting their wills, they often struggle against the wishes of others, particularly their parents. The child's "no" characterizes speech at this stage. The child vacillates between dependence and independence, "wanting to be a baby" one moment and wanting to do everything alone the next moment. Parents may simultaneously welcome their children's independence while missing the cuddly, dependent infant of a few months before. Parents who are insecure about their own authority and autonomy might perceive their children's refusals and negativism as disrespectful and threatening.

Parents of young children need reassurance that their children do still love them and need them very much despite the negative outbursts or refusals to accept parental help. Parents need to understand that children develop their individual identities by asserting themselves only with those people they trust and on whom they rely. Therefore, the child's ability to express needs and wishes honestly reflects a sense of trust that the parent will understand and not leave, regardless of the child's behaviors. At the same time, children need reassurance from their parents that there is order in such a disorderly world. They need their parents to maintain limits that protect them from danger or from unnecessary failures. In the process the child develops a realistic sense of autonomy while learning the family's definition of socially acceptable behavior.

During middle childhood, one parental task is learning to become separate from the child and allowing independent development while demonstrating appropriate standards through role-modeling. Because of children's imagination and creativity in words and movement, parents are now able to converse at length with their children and face an endless barrage of questions. Children incorporate adult values and standards into their lives and are most aware of any discrepancies between values preached and practiced; therefore, parents need to provide both role models of appropriate behavior and standards and opportunities for the child to initiate activities with a sense of purpose. Parents who resist their children's efforts to become self-sufficient instead foster closer dependence on the family.

During late childhood, a parental task is learning to accept rejection without abandoning the child. As children become more competent and autonomous, seek more freedom, and spend more time outside their families, parents who have been completely absorbed in their role as physical caregivers may experience difficulty in adjusting to the children's increasing self-sufficiency and to the addition of other adults and institutions in their children's lives. Parents are needed now more as psychologic support than as actual caregivers. As children develop a sense of industry, parents become acutely aware of expectations for their children and may focus on achievement and ethical standards of conduct. Parents need to provide a secure base of support, love, and guidance while fostering their children's involvement in activities outside the family. Indicators of parental difficulties in this stage are two extremes: (1) abandonment of any rules or involvement or (2) restriction of the child to the family to the exclusion of outside involvements.

During adolescence, a parental task is learning to build a new life by adjusting to altered family roles and relationships established during the adolescent's identity crisis. While attempting to communicate and deal successfully with adolescents, parents must concurrently prepare for their children's eventual departure from the home. Both adolescent upheavals and thoughts of children leaving home may create distress for parents. Adolescents, undergoing stringent self-appraisals of who they are and what they want to be, also might examine parents critically. Both parent and child might thus be questioning values and contesting rules. Adolescence is in some ways similar to early childhood, when the young child sought autonomy, as parents must again deal with issues of independence and self-direction by providing security and reliability through clear limits and expectations for acceptable behavior. Parents now are faced with children who are maturing sexually; they are confronted with social and sexual issues with which the parents might not feel comfortable. Parents must attempt to provide the nurturance and guidance needed to launch an adolescent into young adulthood while simultaneously rethinking family roles and marital relationships.

Fostering Healthy Development in Parents and Children

As children become increasingly involved with the environment, parents play an essential role in assisting their movement from the pleasure principle to the reality principle. Psychodynamically, infants and young children are described as operating under the *pleasure principle,* or desiring immediate satisfaction of their needs with little ability to consider extenuating circumstances or to delay gratifications. The child must learn to account for others' needs and maintain self-control until needs are met before becoming an accepted and maturely functioning member of society. With parental assistance, the child learns to face reality and establish self-control during times of stress. The child becomes aware of the *reality principle* and learns to delay gratification until appropriate circumstances arise.

Parents generally hope to establish pleasant, mutually rewarding relationships with their children. They want to help their children become healthy, well-adjusted adults. At the same time, a parent wants to maintain a sense of personal and social well-being. The difficulty arises in determining effective methods for accomplishing these goals.

Although parenting can be a tremendously rewarding and pleasurable experience, it can become a terribly trying and demanding job if suddenly thrust on unprepared individuals. Parenting is a 24-hour-per-day, 365-day-per-year career that is assumed by many persons who are totally unaware of the job accountabilities. Thus, parents may need assistance in understanding their children's behavior and in learning skills to facilitate communication and effective family functioning.

Parental influence in role modeling can never be underestimated. True to the ancient adage, actions always speak louder than words. If parents hope to foster healthy self-concepts in their children, they too must develop and display positive aspects of themselves. Parents who continually deny their own needs for the satisfaction of others are not particularly healthy models to follow nor are parents who never compromise with others and instead meet only their own needs. Therefore, parents might first need to value self-assertion, volition, and independence in themselves before they can value these qualities in their children. Nurses might need to encourage parents to relax and enjoy their children. They might need to reassure parents that over the years everyone makes a variety of mistakes or less-than-ideal responses but that individual actions are not traumatic in themselves. Rather, a loving, caring attitude, willingness to admit mistakes, and overall honesty are most important.

Defining the Parenting Role

Parenting is the process by which a child within a family is supported in learning about the norms, rituals, and requirements of becoming a contributing member of a social group. Whether or not they are acting consciously, parents adopt various models of behavior for raising their children. The model selected often reflects the parent's experience as a child, perceived societal expectations, and awareness of the parent and child's personalities.

Brink (1982) found, in her research with parents and children, that the most important ingredient for good parenting was giving the child a sense of belonging to a particular family group. Children need love, but even more they need to know that they are securely attached to someone. Good parenting can be accomplished in different ways, depending on the model of parenting behavior adopted, but good parenting is healthy and growth-producing. Specific parenting behaviors are therefore not as important as the degree of fit between parental actions and parental beliefs and abilities.

Since the 1970s the emphasis has shifted from childrearing, in which study focused on the child, to parenting, in which the parent is the focus of study. As a result, communication patterns, leadership styles, behavior requirements, and personal awareness are criteria used to define parenting.

In her study analyzing parental preconceptions of the parenting role, Newberger (1977) identified four conceptions of parenting, which she defined as developmental levels. These levels relate to the parent's views of the child, the parent–child relationship, and personal functioning as a parent. The four levels demonstrate a progression in comprehensiveness, flexibility, and reciprocal awareness of parenting. They are

1. *Egoistic parental conceptions*—At this level parents view children according to the child's response to the parent's need. Parenting is defined as concrete childrearing tasks. Success is measured by the child's behavior that brings satisfaction or recognition to the parent. The parent–child relationship is described according to what each does for the other.
2. *Conventional parental conceptions*—Parents at this level do not see their children as unique individuals but as part of the general category of children. The parent–child relationship is one of defined roles that each is obliged to fulfill. Guidelines for responding to their children come from tradition and cultural standards that prescribe correct methods. Success is having the child internalize the culture and behave according to traditional norms.
3. *Subjective-individualistic parental conceptions*—Parents at this level view each child as unique and attempt to understand the child's perspective and experience. The parent–child relationship shows obvious emotional exchange, and this provides the basis for actions and role enactment. The parenting role is modified to fit the child.
4. *Analytic parental conceptions*—At this level the parent views the child as a complex self-system of interactions. The parent–child relationship is one of stability and shared feelings, experiences, and appreciation of each other's views and needs. The parental role is viewed as a process to facilitate personal growth for both child and parent.

By understanding how parents view their role as parents in general and their relationship to their children in particular, nurses can adapt their interventions to the parent's needs. For example, the nurse might respond to a parent's questions about discipline or sibling rivalry by first noting the parent's expectations for the child's behavior. The nurse needs to recognize, however, that parental awareness at that lower levels does not mean lack of love or attention but rather limitations in flexibility. Parents functioning at these levels are often less willing to use a variety of approaches to solve parenting-related problems. (See Chapter 17 for a discussion of the nurse's role in family assessment.)

Of primary importance to parenting is the understanding that both parents and children are human and should not be expected to perform superhuman feats. Sometimes, people enter parenthood with an unhealthy attitude, thinking that they must relinquish their rights and responsibilities as persons and attempt to assume the single role of parent. This parental role is evidenced by overprotection and may progress to that of a martyr who relishes self-sacrifice and always exhibits a kind, benevolent attitude of fairness, regardless of personal feelings or needs. This facade of saintliness is transparent to children and impossible to maintain for long periods without frequent outbursts of tension and resentment.

Likewise, parents who strive to be seen as godlike and all-knowing are destined for conflict with their children. Parents fall swiftly from self-appointed pedestals as children accurately identify flaws in the performance. The parent who adopts this stance also presents the child with an unrealistic view of people and unconsciously encourages the child to mock this omnipotence and to suppress feelings rather than attempt to deal honestly with them.

Styles of Parenting

Childrearing is a complex socialization process that is expressed uniquely by every family. Many factors determine how a specific family will carry out its childrearing responsibilities. The social expectations of the society in which the family lives define the acceptable limits of behavior, whereas the cultural, religious, and emotional characteristics of the family shape its approach to this goal. Cross-cultural analyses of childrearing practices reveal a wide variation in the types of parental behaviors that successfully achieve the behavioral expectations of the cultures and subcultures in which they occur. Some societies have extensive, complex, kinship systems and family patterns where designated relatives provide child care so that the parents can pursue other tasks. The history of societies that practice polyandry or polygyny reveal that definite role behaviors and divisions of labor are assigned to the various partners. The essential factor is not the style of parenting but that someone is institutionally sanctioned and supported to provide child care. Even so, the experiences and outcomes vary for each child, even for children within the same family.

Each child brings to a family a particular set of characteristics that affect both that child's behavior and the behaviors evoked in others. The personality traits, birth order, and gender of the child are a few of the child's characteristics. The parent's response to these attributes, the way in which the parent interacts with the child, and the parent's methods of discipline are the characteristics of that individual's style of parenting. The parental behaviors and childrearing practices that make up a parenting style generally can be broadly categorized as authoritative, authoritarian, or permissive (sometimes termed laissez-faire).

In practice most parents mix parenting styles. Some parents actually vary their responses so often that children receive both authoritarian and permissive messages at the same time. Nurses therefore need to know the working definitions of parenting styles to recognize them in both their pure and mixed forms. Parents sometimes need nurses to explain that any style of parenting can be effective as long as the expectations for children's behavior are consistent and age-appropriate.

Authoritative Parenting According to Baumrind (1979), the most effective parenting style is authoritative. *Authoritative parenting* involves guiding the child's behavior in a rational, issue-oriented manner. Parents who interact with their children in this way set standards and establish limits that are clearly conveyed. In addition to valuing disciplined behavior, parents encourage self-assertion and independence by respecting the children's actual abilities and capacities. Authoritative parents try to be open and receptive to children's thoughts and feelings and respect children's opinions and rights to disagree, but they retain ultimate control when a particular behavior is deemed unacceptable. Rules are tempered with reasonable flexibility and an understanding of the child's developmental stage and abilities. Explanations appropriate to the child's age and level of understanding are offered when disagreements arise so that parental empathy, sensitivity, and responsibility are balanced.

For example, if a 16-year-old girl asked her parents for permission to attend a weekend party, the parents might respond authoritatively by asking whether there would be adult supervision or by determining whether their daughter had met her responsibilities at home and at school during the week. An authoritative response to an adolescent would therefore involve consistent behavioral norms and clear explanations for parental limits.

Authoritarian Parenting In contrast, parents with an *authoritarian parenting* style value obedience over independent development and rely on many inflexible rules and regulations to govern behavior. Authoritarian parents seek to shape the child according to a series of rigid, clearly defined rules and limits. The parent retains strict control over definitions of acceptable behavior. Discipline often is achieved by punishing the child rather than by explanation or positive example. Deference and respect for parental authority are expected, and little room is left for questioning or choice.

An authoritarian response to the same 16-year-old girl's request might therefore be based on a predetermined rule. For instance, the parents might arbitrarily choose to limit their daughter's social activities to two parties a month and would base their decision on the number of parties she had attended so far that month.

Permissive Parenting *Permissive parenting* takes many forms, but in the extreme it refers to the absence of restraints and maximum freedom for the child, with little or no parental input. Permissive parents provide little direction to their children's behavior. Limits usually are not clearly defined, if they are defined at all. Punishments also are rare because the child is encouraged to develop personal standards of behavior. A permissive response to this same adolescent girl's request, on the other hand, is likely to be a question asking the child whether she wants to attend the party.

Some permissive parents emphasize happy homes and assume that their children will develop according to behavioral norms. Permissive parenting may allow older children to learn to make their own decisions, but some children do not always welcome such freedom or are not yet mature enough to accept complete responsibility for their actions. Conflicts also might arise for young children who are suddenly confronted by teachers, peers, and others who have clear expectations for their behavior. Children who are unused to acting within prescribed limits, for instance, often find socialization at school particularly difficult.

Advising Parents

Sources of Advice Parents, like children, often seek all-encompassing rules to follow in their attempts to make their lives predictable and secure. Mandates from "experts" or professionals assume tremendous power as parents, like small children, search for order within a disorderly world. Life, however, is not clearly defined by rights and wrongs, and an uncomfortable area of ambiguity exists between these extremes. Parental honesty about actions and feelings may be more significant than the specific parenting behavior or technique exhibited.

Hollen (1982) found that parents use a variety of support systems for advice and information about parenting. Her study suggested that a parent's spouse was likely to be the most often used parental support. Relatives were next, followed by books and consultants (Table 13-1). Her study also pointed to the mother's greater need for support in parenting, thereby suggesting that single mothers have a greater need than other parents for support.

All categories of parental support have limitations. Relatives, for example, can undermine discipline by tolerating behaviors that the parent prefers to minimize. One grandmother repeatedly allowed her adolescent grandson to borrow her car and use the entire tank of fuel without refilling it. Books and consultants also might cause parents problems if parents are advised merely to follow a trend, to make abrupt transitions in parenting style or acceptable norms, or to limit their perspective on parenting to address a narrow range of preconceived concerns.

The Nurse's Role When parents enter the health care system through the hospital, community health clinic, or physician's office, they arrive with some preconceived notions about those problems or issues that nurses are equipped to handle. They often assume that nurses are interested solely in illness or physical complaints because traditionally these have been considered the concerns of health care providers. Therefore, the parent who may have an array of psychosocial concerns frequently presents only those physical problems perceived as appropriate to the situation.

Nurses therefore need to convey to parents that they are interested in learning about and assisting with all concerns parents may have about their children, whether these are physical or psychologic, major or minor. The nurse assists the parent to clarify those key concerns regarding the child, so that, from a parent's diffused, nonspecific feeling of concern, specific target behaviors for intervention can be delineated. Therefore, the first step in analyzing a parenting concern is identifying the major issues or concerns.

When focusing on the family as the client, the nurse must be aware that the child's behavior problems may be symptomatic of larger difficulties within the family. If the parent is under stress, normal childhood behaviors may be perceived as abnormal and disruptive. Children may be reacting to unrealistic parental expectations or stressful events within the home or community. Therefore, the nurse needs to understand the complete context of the child's family, school, and community environment to assess the possible reasons for the child's behavior. Recognizing that within the family each family member's behavior influences the other members, nurses focus on those behaviors that need to be altered to achieve smooth family functioning. (Nursing care of the family at risk is discussed in Chapter 22.)

Parenting Skills

Communication

Human beings cannot survive without some sort of attachment to each other. Families can provide this needed foundation of warmth and support. Parents and children alike need to learn to be more responsive to each other. Responsiveness, however, requires a certain degree of self-esteem, self-confidence, comfort, and support from others.

Listening to Children Empathy and effective communication enhance parent–child interactions. Empathy involves accepting another's communication and identifying with that person's feelings, thoughts, and perceptions

TABLE 13-1 Books and Multimedia Resources for Parents

Title	Topic
Lendon Smith, *The Encyclopedia of Baby and Child Care,* Prentice-Hall	Basic information about growth and development and childhood diseases
Benjamin Spock, *Baby and Child Care,* Simon & Schuster	Classic book with information about both childrearing and childhood illness
Burton White, *The First Three Years of Life,* Prentice- Hall	Effects of parenting practices on young children
Bill R. Wagonseller, Mary Burnett, Bernard Salzberg, and Joe Burnett, *The Art of Parenting,* Research Press	Five-session multimedia workshop program on communication, assertiveness, and behavior management
Bill R. Wagonseller and Richard L. McDowell, *You and Your Child,* Research Press	Building a trusting relationship between parents and children
Thomas Gordon, *Parent Effectiveness Training,* Peter H. Wyden	Ways of using communication rather than punishment with children
A. S. Neil, *Freedom—Not License,* Hart Publishing	Appropriate use of permissive parenting
Richard C. Robertiello, *Hold Them Very Close, Let Them Go,* Dial Press	Psychodynamic methods of childrearing
James Dobson, *Dare to Discipline,* Tyndale House	Conservative methods of discipline involving parental firmness and commitment
James Dobson, *Hide or Seek,* Fleming H. Revell	Ways to raise confident and psychologically healthy children
Melvin L. Silberman and Susan A. Wheelan, *How To Discipline Without Feeling Guilty,* Research Press	Methods of discipline that are both effective and humane
Wesley C. Becker, *Parents Are Teachers,* Research Press	Types of reinforcement to teach discipline for both home and school
Gerald R. Patterson, *Living With Children,* Research Press	Minimizing unacceptable behavior in young children
Bruce L. Baker, et al., *Behavior Problems,* Research Press	Steps to minimize behavior problems, especially for children with special needs
Bruce L. Baker, et al., *Toilet Training,* Research Press	Step-by-step guide to toilet training
Bruce L. Baker, et al., *Play Skills,* Research Press	Play programs to develop skills in young children

(Guerney, 1979). It does not require agreeing with the other person's view but simply attending to and listening respectfully. A receptive rather than punitive or judgmental attitude is essential for empathetic listening by the parent.

Actual behaviors also might convey an empathetic attitude. Guerney (1979) offered five guidelines for what not to do in parent–child communication:

1. Parents should try not to ask questions while children are speaking. Questions may divert children's attention from their main thoughts or may bring up areas that children are not yet comfortable or ready to discuss.
2. Parents should avoid presenting an opinion about what children are saying; this tends to close the discussion immediately. Parents instead can share their feelings when children are finished.
3. Parents should not interpret children's speech or try to explain what the children really mean, because children may feel their opinions or ideas are inferior or that parents misconstrue their meanings.
4. Parents should not recommend solutions or changes in views.
5. Parents should not make judgments or evaluations while children are speaking.

Active listening by parents has may advantages (Gordon, 1975). It allows the free catharsis of feelings in children, so that children become more aware of their feelings and are able to release pent-up emotions with their parents. Empathetic listening also enhances feelings of warmth between parents and children. The feelings of being heard and truly understood are deeply satisfying and create a desire for more intimate discussions between the parent and child. Parents also feel great reward as they appreciate their children's thoughts, fears, and dreams and feel that they are sharing important moments in their children's lives. Active listening by parents fosters problem solving in children by allowing alternatives to be explored.

Skillful listening may assist children to become more empathetic with their parents and others. Children may be more able and willing to listen to another's viewpoints when they first experience receptive listening from their parents. Empathetic listening conveys a sense of parental trust in children's ability to be self-directive and accountable for their actions. Thus, skillful empathetic listening facilitates openness and honesty in parent–child communications and promotes healthy development in children.

Speaking With Children In addition to empathetic listening, the skillful expression of ideas and feelings fosters positive parent–child relations. A goal of parental communication is to express thoughts and feelings clearly and honestly without eliciting unnecessary defensiveness in the child. Before sharing views, parents must recognize that children have their own perceptions of parental conversations. Both children and parents desire to protect and defend their own self-concepts. A parent should therefore avoid attacking a child's self-concept; this prevents unnecessary defensiveness and hostility.

Parents can learn specific techniques for effective parent-child communication (Gordon, 1975; Guerney, 1979). For instance, statements that are less hostile may be phrased subjectively to reflect the parent's own needs and feelings. One way to do this is to express "I messages" rather than "you messages." For example, "You had better stop running in and out of the back door; you are making too much noise" is a "you message." A parallel "I message" might be, "I can't read my magazine with so much commotion; I need peace and quiet so either play outside or play a quiet game inside." The "I message" clearly identifies the parent's needs and expectations of the child and avoids terms such as "good," "right," "best," or "true." The child–parent interaction is thus limited to what the parent thinks or feels, regardless of global values or standards.

"I messages" are less likely to elicit power struggles and hostility from children because they do not threaten or attack the child's self-concept. Instead, they communicate that it is the child's responsibility to modify behavior. The honesty of an "I message" provides the child with a model for honest communication about ideas and feelings and requires the parent to express human needs, thus fostering intimacy between the parent and child (Gordon, 1975).

Effective expression also avoids overgeneralizations of character criticisms of the child. Instead, the parent can describe the specific incidents or behaviors that trigger a reaction. Overgeneralizations and accusations such as "you always" or "you never" are likely to anger the child and also to diminish the parent's credibility. Statements recounting the exact behavior or incident allow the child to respond appropriately.

Another aspect of effective expression is for the parent to describe his or her feelings if these feelings should be taken into account in dealing with the situation. Children, like adults, often are unaware of the impact of their behavior. When parents acknowledge feelings, children might then modify their behavior to be more thoughtful and more responsive to others. For example, a parent might appropriately share feelings by saying, "I feel angry because I have so little quiet time to read or listen to music. I feel I have the right to some moments of privacy just as you do. I need to find a time when I can be totally uninterrupted." Such a statement can open the door for the child to participate in relieving the situation.

Expressing basic positive feelings about the child also helps to blunt any implied criticisms in the parent's statement. For instance, "I feel you have really tried harder this week to allow me some quiet time. I realize you are trying to be considerate, but I still am frustrated that I can't read the newspaper without arguments or questions when I arrive home. I want to read the paper from 5:30 to 6:00, and then I will feel like talking."

Such a clear statement of the parent's expectations indicates the behaviors that the parent desires from the child. In describing the desired behavior change specifically, the parent also describes the positive feelings that will be evoked by this behavior change. For example, the parent might explain, "I feel frustrated when I am interrupted while talking on the phone. I would like you to be quiet while I'm on the phone and hold your questions or requests until I finish. If I can finish a conversation without interruption, I won't be so irritable and will be happy to talk with you when I hang up." This is essentially an "I message" that honestly expresses the parent's needs by describing a behavior change without implying character criticisms. By sharing expectations, the parent allows the child to correct undesirable behavior or offer alternative solutions.

Empathizing with the child while expressing parental feelings or expectations further assists the child in maintaining self-esteem. The parent should therefore try to appreciate the possible reasons for the child's behavior. For example, saying, "You must want to say something right now, but you'll have to wait for a few minutes until I'm off the phone" indicates that the parent understands the child's needs.

Minimizing Unacceptable Behavior

Modifying the Environment Many parent–child difficulties can be prevented by designing a home environment that encourages children's independence and provides opportunities for learning and recreation. Parents can provide interesting and stimulating environments that are appropriate to the developmental level and interest of the child. Enriching the environment might mean providing fingerpaints or modeling clay during early childhood and providing interesting books, building sets, or play houses during middle childhood. Children need specific areas at home that serve as their private places to pursue activities they enjoy.

When young children need to wind down and relax before mealtimes or bedtime, the environmental stimuli might need to be restricted. These periods should be limited to quiet, sedate activities such as being read to or reading books or listening to records. Rough, boisterous activities, such as wrestling or playing chase, should be avoided to prevent overstimulating the child.

To provide opportunities for children to exercise independence and responsibility, parents can provide self-care activities that children can easily perform. For young children, parents can buy clothes that slip on rather than button or zip, thus assisting children to dress themselves. In-between meal snacks can be placed on the lowest level of the refrigerator or kitchen cabinet so that children can feed themselves when they are hungry between meals. During late childhood, children can learn to prepare simple foods for themselves or to handle the stereo correctly when listening to music. Adolescents might use their own alarm clocks to schedule themselves and learn to wash and dry their own clothes. Thus, each family member is able to perform at the highest level of self-care and shares the responsibility for smooth family functioning.

Parents also can design the home environment to prevent injuries and decrease their "security-watch" role. "Childproofing" the home thus serves not only to prevent accidents but also to allow parents and children to relax at home (see Chapter 19). For instance, parents of infants and young children can remove any fragile or dangerous objects from the child's reach by clearing the coffee tables of favorite vases and placing kitchen cleaners and medicines in high, locked cabinets. During early and middle childhood, parents need to continue to remove dangerous articles from reach but can also begin to stress the child's role in avoiding danger. Parental warnings at this stage include cautioning children about playing near the street or getting into water without an adult present. During late childhood, parents emphasize the child's role in self-protection by teaching safety rules about activities like swimming and bicycling. By adolescence, parents hope to see evidence that the child has learned safety, but this may be a difficult time for parents if adolescents value adventurousness or daring without regard to risks. Parents of adolescents can express their concern and emphasize the role of responsible behavior in determining the limits of freedom.

Setting Limits Children, like adults, need to feel a sense of order, continuity, and security within their families. From a secure home, children feel free to explore and develop their potentials. Firm, consistent limit setting or discipline fosters competence in children (Baumrind, 1979; Gordon, 1979; White, 1979), which is reflected in such characteristics as social responsibility, independence or self-direction, curiosity, language ability, and intelligence.

To provide clear, consistent limit setting, parents and other family members must first discuss their expectations for the child. When family members disagree about what is expected of the child and what should happen when these expectations are not met or if family members are unable to agree about expectations for the child's behavior, the child senses this confusion and may play one family member against another. Too often in such situations, one family member is forced to assume the "tough guy" or "heavy" role. More important than the parenting style or specific limits set is the need for agreement and support among family members regarding the major expectations of the child.

As agreement is reached, each family member should consistently enforce the limits, but because parents are human and imperfect and children are growing and changing, complete agreement and consistency is not always possible. As children grow, issues and limits evolve and change. Family members may not even anticipate a new issue until it is upon them and their judgment is required instantly. They often do not have time to mull over an issue and decide on an approach that can be applied with a "united front" when a particular situation arises. Working out and adhering to basic principles and applying, adjusting, and reapplying specific approaches helps children reap the benefits, security, and freedom of relative consistency.

A key factor in determining the effectiveness of limit setting, or discipline, appears to be whether the parent provides issue-oriented reasons for the limits and explains the consequences of violating these limits. If the child shares the parent's problem-solving processes and is allowed to verbalize feelings and thoughts, the child may be increasingly able to solve problems and assume responsibility for behaviors. Young children using preoperational thought tend to judge the rightness or wrongness of an act by its consequences and not by the actor's intention, a perception that Piaget (1965) demonstrated by presenting the child with a story that involves a dilemma. Piaget's classic story is of two children; one breaks 12 dishes while helping his mother and the other breaks only one dish while being disobedient. When asked which child in the story was naughtier, the child typically chooses the one who broke 12 dishes even though his intentions were clearly admirable.

The parent also should try to separate disapproval of certain behaviors from acceptance of the child as a person by conveying love but explaining that particular behaviors are unacceptable. Whether children, especially young children, can differentiate between parental feelings about their actions and feelings about themselves is open to question. Children are helped to separate actions and feelings if parents do not discipline when angry but wait until they are in control of their feelings about the misbehavior.

Protestations of love and affection can also appear to be insincere at the time when a parent is expressing any form of disapproval. Parents therefore need to observe carefully their children's responses to disciplining and explanations, remembering that having to listen to an explanation can in itself be a punishment. The young child often does not understand a parent's words and meaning, and the older child clearly is faced with parental criticism and is therefore unable to avoid, sidestep, or forget that a wrong was committed. For differing reasons, both young and older children often become very uncomfortable, fidgety, and distracted as a parent carefully expresses disapproval of the child's behavior. Despite drawbacks, however, dissapproval of behavior is far preferable to disapproval of the whole child. A parent must simply try to handle a child's reactions but cannot assume that feelings of self-worth will remain intact.

As adolescents attempt to become more independent, parents sometimes have difficulty letting go. Adolescents often want complete freedom from responsibilities and limit setting but also want unlimited use of a car and a generous allowance, creating conflicts that may be interpreted by the parents as defiance and insubordination on the part of the adolescent. Conflicts and communication problems are common during this stage of development.

Avoiding Win or Lose Conflicts Conflict is inevitable in any human relationship. The key is not whether conflict occurs but how the conflict is resolved. Conflicts between parents and children are not only inevitable but are likely to be frequent. Conflicts may even be healthy because they allow parents and children to accept disagreements and to recognize the need for mediation and compromise.

Despite the positive opportunities conflict can provide, parents are often well advised to reduce the potential for conflict whenever possible. Parents can allow children as much responsibility for self-care as is appropriate for their developmental abilities so that responsibility for such functions as feeding and hygiene rests with the children, thus helping to remove parents from possible power struggles. Parent and child may carefully select those areas for which the parent will assume responsibility and those areas that can be under the child's care. The child's choices can be selected to minimize unnecessary parental involvement and to provide the child with opportunities to be independent and exercise some rights. For example, adolescents might be allowed to set their own sleeping and waking routines, although they may need guidance in setting their own bedtimes. Adolescents usually have their own alarm clocks and can be responsible for getting to school and to other activities on time. If the adolescent's late-night behavior begins to result in difficulty in getting to school on time, poorer grades, or difficulties in sports, the adolescent, with parental guidance, would then be responsible for correcting the problem by modifying the behavior.

When conflict does occur, problems may arise if parents and children think only of "win or lose" resolutions. The win or lose frame of mind pits one individual against another, with each wanting to force needs and wants on the other. The "winner" feels satisfaction after achieving the goal or coming out ahead, whereas the "loser" often feels defeated and angry. When conflict is expressed this way, the resolution does not have the mutual support of parent and child (Gordon, 1975).

More advantageous is a "no-lose" resolution. The "no-lose" method of conflict resolution involves mutual discussion and compromise. Both parents and children identify the problem areas and conflicts and discuss possible solutions. Problem solving occurs with input from parents and children, so that resolutions are mutually acceptable compromises that depend on family support. The "no-lose" method has many advantages. Parents and children must take time to share thoughts and feelings and thus may become more empathetic with each other. Children are more motivated to carry out their parts of the solutions because they participated in the decision-making process. Allowing input from both parents and children also encourages problem solving, so that decisions may be made more appropriately. Hostility can be reduced if children feel that they understand a situation better and also are responsible for resolving the conflict. Group decision making eliminates a power struggle by requiring the cooperation of each family member (Gordon, 1975).

Finding Time Together Like any other human relationship, the parent–child relationship requires energy, effort, and time. Without uninterrupted periods of sharing between children and parents, building a relationship is difficult. Regardless of the hectic nature of family schedules, some time each day should be allotted exclusively to children. The time does not have to be scheduled, nor does it have to be lengthy, but it must be appropriate to the situation. For example, it would be inappropriate to state that every night from 7:00 to 7:30 is play time regardless of the circumstances. Instead, all might agree that the time after supper is family time when the family plays games, works on puzzles, or talks together. Situations such as a late supper, the presence of company, or time demands on individual family members, however, necessitate exceptions that may or may not be anticipated. These exceptions are taken in stride when a pattern of mutual give and take has been established as a result of previous family life experiences.

Parents need to communicate that they are available as "consultants" for talking or sharing whenever the child feels the need and the parent is able. Sometimes, the parent may need to explain that a job started has to be completed before the child may talk. At the same time the parent conveys interest in learning what the child has to say so as not to discourage the child.

Time for enjoyable contact is essential. Whether parents are dropping their activities to play with small children or listen to older children or setting weekly dates for fun activities, such as sports or movies, ongoing, pleasurable moments together are important.

Discipline

When a parent brings concerns about a child's behavior to the nurse's attention, that parent frequently feels embarrassed or guilty. A parent may feel responsible for the problem or frustrated at being unable to handle the concern without assistance. Nurses need to reassure all parents that they have done their best and that all parents need support and assistance. Parents also can be reminded that only truly concerned and committed parents make the efforts to provide guidance and discipline for their children. The nurse and parent can then evaluate management approaches for

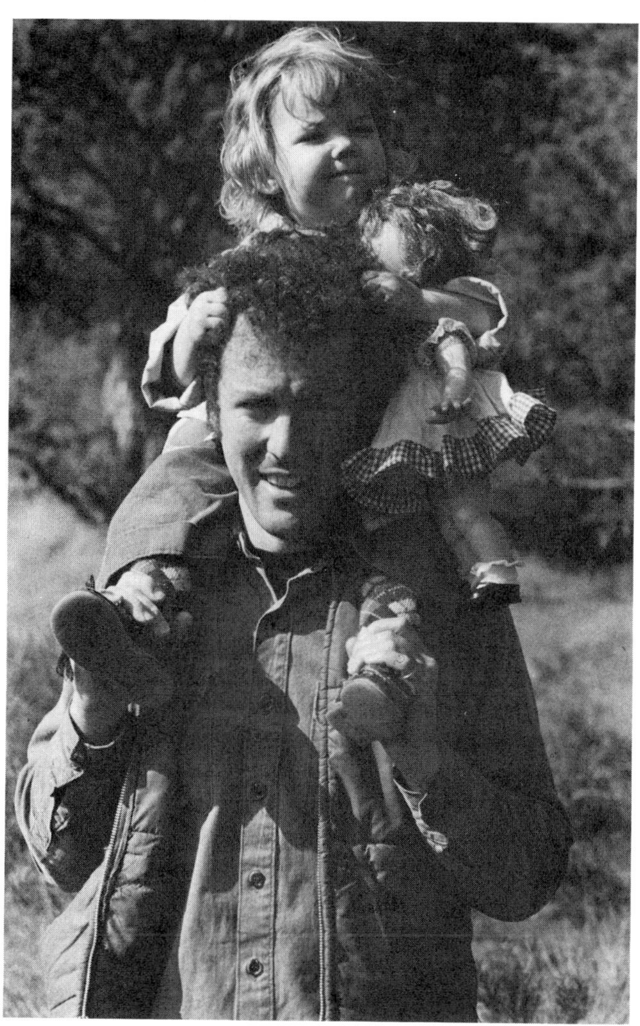

Building time into family schedules for pleasurable moments together is important for developing the relationship between parent and child.

their appropriateness for an individual family's values and parenting styles.

Corporal Punishment One traditional management approach used by many American families has been corporal, or physical, punishment, primarily spanking. Various sources contend that as many as 90% of parents use physical punishment at some time with their children, and some authorities state that general American values support punitive practices. Many parents feel that they have a moral obligation to control their children and require obedience and that physical punishment is the most effective means of control (Steinmetz and Straus, 1974; Pratt, 1976). The greater use of corporal punishment in lower socioeconomic groups has been documented; however, recent studies have revealed smaller differences among social classes than researchers previously thought (Erlander, 1974).

Corporal punishment refers to nonbrutal physical punishment in response to a child's unacceptable behavior. This is in marked contrast to arbitrary brutal punishment, which has been shown to be associated with antisocial characteristics such as aggression or withdrawal in children. Baumrind (1979) postulated that occasional spankings or other nonbrutal physical actions are not harmful in themselves but that the harmful effects of punishment are related to parental attitudes that are hostile, aggressive, and restrictive. Corporal punishment, judiciously administered, according to Baumrind, can allow the parent to release pent-up emotions without harming the child. The child also might feel less guilty about an unacceptable behavior after being punished for it. The punishment is most effective when given as soon as possible after the unacceptable behavior and when accompanied by the parent's reasons for punishment and reminders about acceptable behaviors that must be substituted.

Many experts disapprove of physical punishment as a behavior management approach. They argue that no positive learning results from corporal punishment. Children might respond simply out of fear and do not learn to solve problems or work out conflicts without resorting to physical aggression. Children might tend to avoid the person who administers corporal punishment, and the parent–child relationship might be damaged. If punishment is delayed until one parent arrives home, the punishment probably will be less effective and also will create more psychologic disturbances than an immediately administered spanking.

Corporal punishment also tends to require increasing severity to produce the same results. The child does not gain any insight or self-control with this method alone and may learn detrimental lessons from this role-modeling of aggressive behavior (Ginott, 1961; Azrin and Holz, 1966; Piuck, 1975; Murphy, 1976; Hammer and Drabman, 1981). Most parents at some time have used physical punishment in the form of a light spank on the bottom. It may occasionally be recommended, as when an 18-month-old runs into a street. Nurses, however, need to understand the pros and cons of this method and discuss them with parents. Nurses also can assist parents to consider alternative measures of tension relief, such as taking a brisk walk around the house, when the urge to spank or hit occurs.

Psychodynamic Intervention A second method of discipline is a strictly psychodynamic approach (Fraiberg, 1959; Ginott, 1961). This approach focuses on insight into the reasons for the child's behavior and is based on the notion that all behavior originates in past development, although also influenced by current circumstances. The assumptions are that the many unconscious motivations within people frequently make them unaware of the causes for their behavior and that problematic behavior results when the child is unable to express emotions or conflicts directly. Negative emotions then become repressed or are expressed inappropriately or symbolically. Psychodynamic management involves seeking to understand the meaning underlying the child's behavior and to facilitate the child's expression of feelings, so that, through insight and catharsis, the child's behavior can be altered.

The professional therapist's role in the psychodynamic treatment of troubled families is far different from the parents' use of psychodynamic principles in relation to their children. In applying psychoanalytic principles to the parent–child relationship, parents emphasize the importance of open communication and the expression of feelings but do not begin to "analyze" the child or attempt to treat major family difficulties.

Psychodynamic skills that are helpful to parents include active empathetic listening and the skillful expression of thoughts and feelings. Parents encourage children to share feelings and provide opportunities for the relaxed sharing of thoughts and feelings among family members. Parents try to be responsive to their children's needs and to act as a realistic "sounding board" when appropriate.

Active listening is sometimes inappropriate, and parents need to be aware of these occasions. Children might not be ready to share feelings and might require more time for introspection. Parents should be able to recognize the child's need for privacy and simply offer to listen whenever the child is ready to talk. Forcing a conversation does not demonstrate respect for the child's feelings and may only add to the child's frustration.

Active listening is also inappropriate when there is no time to listen to a complete expression of the child's feelings. Parents are not helpful if they only allow the child to begin sharing before they close the conversation. Hit-and-run or "quickie" emotional encounters are frustrating and ineffective. Therefore, parents should let the child know if there is no time for exploring the problem at a particular time and should determine a future time when it will be appropriate to talk. For example, if a child is complaining about going to school as the family is walking out the door, the parent may say, "I understand that you are unhappy with school, but it is now time to leave for school. We can talk about your feelings at another time." The parent thus acknowledges the child's feelings but also reinforces the limit of getting to school on time.

Other psychodynamic approaches that are helpful to parents are play activities that facilitate the child's expression of feelings and parallel stories that are relevant to the child's feelings or experiences. Expressive play activities might be modeling clay or messy fingerpaints for the young child or punching bags for an aggressive child. Fantasy play activities with doll houses or puppets also can provide young children with acceptable means of releasing their emotions (see Chapter 28).

Parallel stories are stories created by the parents about feelings or experiences that are relevant to the child. For example, a young child who was upset with the arrival of a new baby sister was told this story: "Once there was a little boy named Bobby. He was the only little boy in his family. He lived in a house with his Mom and Dad. He liked being the only child because he got all of his parents' and grandparents' attention. Then one day, his mother had to go to the hospital to have a baby and when she came home, she brought a baby sister named Ann. Ann was very tiny and needed lots of attention. Ann cried and made lots of noise so Bobby's parents held her a lot. Bobby felt sad and mad that Ann took so much of his Mom and Dad's time. Bobby didn't know for sure he was still special to his Mom and Dad, but they loved him more than ever. They were so glad to have a son." Following the story, the parent could ask, "How do you think Bobby felt?" "What could his Mom and Dad do to help Bobby feel better?" "What things can Bobby do that his little baby sister might wish she could do?"

The purpose of the parallel story is to allow the child to identify safely with a character in a story and to express feelings that might be frightening or too intense to be acknowledged openly. Children can learn that thoughts are not actions and that unacceptable feelings and thoughts are normal but that they do not have to result in unacceptable actions. The story allows the child to judge actions or feelings from a third-person perspective. When the feelings of the story become too intense, the child can stop the storytelling (Weisberger, 1975).

Logical Consequences Another method of discipline with which a number of parents are familiar is based on the work of Alfred Adler (1978a, 1978b), a psychiatrist who was concerned with problems in parenting and educating children. Adler primarily viewed childhood behavior problems as evolving from the conflicts of equality and freedom in a democracy without concurrent responsibility and accountability.

Adler's method is based on the assumption that the parent's primary goal is viewed as facilitating the child's social development. Parents facilitate this social development in three basic ways: (1) children are taught to respect order and accept social rules; (2) power struggles with children are avoided; and (3) parents provide constant encouragement for their children (Dreikurs, 1958).

A key technique in the Adlerian approach for instilling respect for order or social rules is termed *logical consequences,* although the concept of logical consequences is certainly not unique to Adler. The theory of logical consequences involves allowing children to experience the natural results of their misbehavior. Thus, children learn that it is more satisfying and pleasurable to respect the rules or guidelines than to violate them (Dreikurs and Grey, 1970). For example, the parent warns 5-year-old Bobby that if he plays in the mud puddle after getting dressed, he will be wearing soggy clothes and shoes to kindergarten. Bobby promptly jumps in the puddle. Without criticizing or nagging, the parent simply locks the house and takes Bobby to kindergarten in his wet outfit and shoes.

To use logical consequences, the parent allows the child to choose between acceptable and unacceptable behavior. This may require great restraint and does demand that the parent respect the child. The parent provides guidance and encouragement in the child's decision making, but the child becomes accountable for actions. Logical consequences are most effective in dealing with attention-getting behaviors such as dawdling. It is inappropriate for use in dangerous situations that require immediate prohibition and the removal of the child. When a 3-year-old runs into the street, the parent first removes the child and states the danger of the situation. Parents might say, "You will have to remain in the backyard until you are ready to stay away from the street." The child is thus protected from injury but also reminded of the consequences of action.

Whereas punishment stresses the power of personal authority (that is, "because I said so"), logical consequences conveys the reality of the social order and not the power of the authority figure. The child becomes aware of the rules of social living that enable people to function effectively in society. When an older child is demanding and bossy with neighborhood children, the parent may discuss with the child how other people perceive being told what to do. Parents may explain that this behavior is not fun for the other children and that they will probably want to avoid and not play with a child who continues to act this way. If the child persists and is no longer invited to play with the others, that child may decide to become more cooperative to rejoin the group.

Logical consequences, unlike arbitrary punishment, is related to the misbehavior. If the schoolchild dawdles and misses the bus, receiving a tardy slip and school authority disapproval are to be expected. Children can become acutely aware of their responsibility for the results of their actions. Logical consequences should not involve a moral judgment, whereas punishment usually evokes guilt. The results of certain actions are neither "good" nor "bad," they simply are either pleasant or unpleasant to the child. Children's actions are not interpreted as indicators of their basic human worth but simply as effective or ineffective in assisting them to achieve satisfaction or fulfillment.

Rather than deal with past actions, the parent using logical consequences as a technique is concerned only with what happens now and allows the child to predict what will result if such behavior occurs again in the future. Children begin to see the cause-and-effect processes of daily life and accept responsibility for the consequences of their behavior.

Parents can be more objective and less emotionally distressed when they use logical consequences than when they use punishment. They are not the harsh judges determining appropriate punishments but rather allow the natural results of behavior to occur. Using logical consequences, parents focus on facilitating children's development as responsible, socially acceptable members of society. Parents and children learn to appreciate being responsible for their individual actions and for general family functioning. Power conflicts are avoided between authoritarian, godlike parents and dependent children who have little control over their actions or the consequences of those actions. The realities of the social order therefore assist children to develop as accountable, autonomous individuals.

Behavior Modification A fourth method of discipline is social learning, or behavior modification (Patterson, 1976; O'Neil, McLaughlin, and Knapp, 1977; Hammer and Drabman, 1981). This method is based on the principles of behaviorism, with its emphasis on changing behavior by manipulating the response, or reinforcement, evoked by the behavior. Rewards and punishment are two kinds of reinforcement. (Principles of behaviorism are discussed in Chapter 6.)

Reinforcement Positive reinforcement may be nonsocial (food, money, toys) and social (smiles, hugs, kisses). As it becomes associated with the positive reinforcer, a behavior may in itself become satisfying and motivating and its frequency will increase. If a behavior is never reinforced, its frequency will decrease. Immediate rewards or positive reinforcement are the most effective, and these rewards should occur often when the child is first learning a new behavior. A child also should be rewarded with each step in the learning process of a new behavior. Once a behavior is learned, it is likely to be sustained even if it is not reinforced every time it occurs but is instead managed on an intermittent schedule of positive reinforcement.

Negative reinforcement, or the association of an unpleasant or painful experience with the behavior, causes the child to avoid the experience or to decrease or stop the unwanted behavior. For example, if failing to do his homework is the son's undesirable behavior, the parent may take away his television privileges on those evenings when the homework is not finished. A negative reinforcer may simply be the withdrawal of any reinforcer (for example, ignoring the behavior) or the application of an aversive stimulus (such as saying "No, that is wrong" or using criticism). Theoretically, a behavior decreases when a negative reinforcer follows.

With behavior modification, the parent focuses only on the observable, currently occuring behaviors and pays little or no attention to their motivations. The assessment of each behavioral concern—by analyzing its timing, duration, frequency, and associated circumstances—is essential to successful behavior modification. In particular, identifying those aspects of the situation that serve unintentionally to reinforce inappropriate behavior is the key to planning environmental changes that would eliminate such reinforcement.

General treatment plans for behavioral concerns include the following guidelines:

1. The parent should ignore the unwanted behavior if possible and respond positively to the child's desirable behaviors
2. The parent needs to be aware that the child's behavior initially worsens when the parent ignores the unacceptable behavior

As in all parenting approaches, consistency is essential for behavior modification to be effective.

To use behavior modification effectively, it is important to be accurate in identifying what will be a positive reinforcer and what will be a negative reinforcer from the child's perspective. It is also important to be attentive to what behavior is being reinforced, whether positively or negatively. For example, a child stands under her mother in the kitchen and whines until the mother surrenders and gives her a cookie before supper. The child then stops whining. Although the mother may feel that she stopped the whining behavior effectively, she is in fact positively reinforcing the behavior of whining to obtain a desired end. The child learns that whining does obtain the cookie after all and will use this strategy again. In another case the child may not perceive a punishment such as spanking as a negative reinforcer if, in fact, the child's desired goal was to obtain the parent's attention.

Ignoring unacceptable behaviors may be very difficult for parents. If the parent can interpret a behavior as attention getting, however, and can realize that the increase in frequency of the behavior is proportionate to the amount of frustration demonstrated by the parent, the parent may be able to ignore the behavior by temporarily leaving the child's presence. For example, a child may have a temper tantrum as the parent tries to read the evening paper. The parent can simply leave the room without comment and find a quiet place, such as a bedroom, to escape.

A worsening of behavior, or "response burst," is a brief initial increase in the inappropriate behavior as the child suddenly discovers that the current amount of misbehaving no longer obtains the desired attention. The child therefore escalates the intensity or frequency of behavior in an attempt to retrieve the lost attention. If no attention results during this burst, the frequency of the behavior will decrease and eventually disappear. Parents must understand what causes the response burst, so that they do not simply assume that ignoring the behavior is ineffective and resume previous strategies. Children need to realize what will result when unacceptable behavior occurs.

Responding positively to the child's desirable behaviors is also important in any treatment plan. Too often, parents only give their children attention when they are misbehaving and neglect to "catch them being good" (Christophersen, 1979) and compliment them on pleasant behaviors. For example, when a child is playing quietly, the parent need not avoid the child but can simply take a few seconds to say, "Thanks for playing so nicely while I read the paper. I really appreciate it."

The "Time-Out" Plan A treatment plan called "time out" is recommended for those behaviors that cannot be allowed simply to decrease over time (such as fighting or hurting others) or those behaviors that appear to be motivated by attention from others or are self-rewarding to the child. The term *time out* is abbreviated from "time out from reinforcement." It is an intervention that is designed to place the child in a bland environment that is unpleasurable and unstimulating to the child. Because time out does not involve physical pain and the parent is removed from the unpleasant experience itself, this technique does not have the problems and side effects associated with physical punishment (Hammer and Drabman, 1981). Time out is primarily effective with young children, but it is not without adverse effects. Parents must try to be aware of the devastating effects some unstimulating environments might have on the child. A child might, for example, be very afraid of a dimly lit, lonely environment. Placing the child in such an area then becomes a more severe punishment than the parent anticipated.

In using the time-out technique, parents must understand and consistently observe the following steps. First, the parent selects one problem behavior, although time out may later be applied to other inappropriate behaviors. Second, the child must be aware of the expectations for behavior (the "house rules"), as well as the consequences of any misbehavior. The child must understand these expectations and consequences prior to beginning the time-out procedure. Third, the parent must work out in advance each detail of time out. A small cooking timer should be available and a special area designated for time out. The time-out area should be as bland as possible (for example, the bathroom or laundry room) to serve the purpose of providing time out from pleasurable activities. For the purpose of time out, sending children to their rooms is usually ineffective because they may find pleasure in toys or books. If children simply need to calm down and regain control, however, being sent to their rooms may be very helpful, although the bedroom ideally should not be associated with punishment or unpleasant events. Fourth, the parent should allow no loopholes in time out. When the inappropriate behavior occurs, time out immediately follows, regardless of any excuses or interruptions in dinner or playtime.

The time-out procedure itself occurs as follows:

1. The child is made aware of the expectations for behavior and the consequences of misbehavior
2. The parent tells the child what to do or stop doing (for example, "Tommy, stop jumping on the couch now")
3. If the child does not immediately comply, the parent warns the child of the consequence of continued misbehavior (for example, "Tommy, if you don't stop jumping on the couch now, you go to time out"). This statement should be made firmly but nonemotionally, without begging, yelling, or threatening
4. If the child still does not comply, the parent places the child in time out. The child under 5 years of age is generally

placed in time out for five minutes and the child over 5 years old for 10 minutes.

5. The child is told, "You stay here until the timer rings"

The difficulties that parents frequently encounter when using time out may include refusal, resistance to the time-out procedure, or aggressive behavior. If the child refuses to go to time out, the parent warns the child that the timer will be reset for an additional 5 minutes unless the child immediately goes to time out. If the child continues to refuse to go, the parent should give the young child two firm spanks on the behind or legs and physically place the child in time out. If the child leaves the time-out area, the same procedure should be followed. The child also might scream and cry loudly when placed in time out. Behavior such as singing or talking is allowable, but screaming and kicking are unacceptable. If such unacceptable behavior occurs, the child is told that the timer cannot be set until the unacceptable behavior stops. The child who starts to make a mess during time out should be warned that the timer will have to be reset after the mess is cleaned up and that any time already spent in time out will not be counted.

The key to time out, as in other discipline techniques, is consistency. Certain difficult situations might require modification of the procedure. The child's misbehavior might, for example, occur in a public place such as church or the supermarket. In these situations the parent "marks time out" by marking with a pen on the child's hand the number of time-out periods earned upon arriving home (Drabman and Creedon, 1979, pp. 99–100). Another difficult situation occurs when children dawdle and cause themselves to get to bed late. In this situation Drabman and Creedon recommended that parents employ "beat-the-buzzer" by setting the timer for a realistic period in which the child must get ready (Drabman and Creedon, 1979). If the child beats the buzzer by being ready before it rings, the parent will read a book or play a game with the child until bedtime. For each minute or part thereafter that the child is late, the child must go to bed one half-hour earlier than usual the following evening.

If used consistently, time out can be an extremely helpful device in controlling inappropriate behavior in young children. The parent avoids unpleasant screaming matches and power struggles with the child. Discipline is achieved with the parent portraying a calm, self-controlled role model. With older children, or after approximately 8 or 9 years of age, attempting to utilize time out can precipitate a power struggle. The older child usually is better taught by the methods of logical consequences or reinforcement.

Managing Specific Behavioral Concerns

Crying and Fussiness During Infancy One of the most frequent and frustrating of parental concerns involves the inevitable crying periods that occur during infancy. The infant's crying often is misinterpreted as a rejection of the parent or a signal that the parent is failing to meet the child's needs. Parents must be reassured of their positive efforts while being offered possible explanations for their infants' behavior.

To assist parents, the nurse can first assure the parent that crying is extremely common in infancy and then assess the nature and pattern of the crying. Specific information also should include the following:

1. The time of day that the crying occurs
2. The duration of each crying episode
3. The onset of the crying: "When did the parents begin to consider the crying a problem?"
4. Situational factors: "What is going on when the crying occurs?" "How is feeding related to these crying episodes?"
5. Feeding techniques: "Are you bottle-feeding or breast-feeding?" "Are any solid foods or cereals being given?" "How is the baby being fed?" "How is formula prepared?" "Is the bottle propped or held?" "What is the size of the nipple holes?" "How often do you burp the baby?"
6. Pattern of elimination: "Does the infant experience diarrhea, constipation, passage of gas, or flatus?"
7. Parent's reaction to the crying (level of anxiety, fatigue, depression): "How do you feel when the child cries?"
8. Handling of the crying by parents and others: "What has been tried?" "What has worked?" "What has not worked?"
9. The infant's behavior pattern when not crying: "Is the child's behavior easy and predictable, extremely alert, or unpredictable?"

In addition to questioning the parent, the nurse also might observe the parents' interaction with the infant (see Chapter 16). The nurse should observe a feeding and perhaps suggest ways of decreasing the infant's air ingestion (see Chapter 7). It also is helpful to compliment the parents about positive responses to the infant in feeding and holding.

Brazelton (1976) noted that a crying period occurring in infants from 3 to 10 weeks of age is extremely common at the end of each day and is a possible precursor to the social period of infancy. Brazelton further stated that a 2-hour period of crying daily during these early weeks can be expected and will only resolve with time. He felt that infants seem to need this crying period to release energies and will stop this behavior when they are able to participate in interesting activities.

If feeding or other physical problems can be ruled out as reasons for the crying, parents can be reassured that the crying is a normal, although frustrating, part of the infant's development. The nurse first encourages the parent to try comforting techniques to quiet the child (such as rocking, cuddling, changing diapers). If none of these techniques works, the parent should try not to become agitated because this simply increases the crying. When the parent feels anxiety mounting, the parent should place the child in a safe place, such as the crib, while "tuning out" by undertaking some pleasurable activity. The infant might, for instance, be placed in the crib while the parent takes a 5- to 10-minute break in a more relaxed part of the home. Parents should identify activities they will use to comfort themselves during their infants' crying jags (such as listening to a favorite record, working in a flower bed, or walking briskly around the yard). Frantic attempts to quiet an infant only worsen the situation.

The nurse also can assist the parent in assessing the general temperament of the child (see Chapter 16) and developing appropriate parenting strategies. Some infants usually are more receptive to external stimulation than others and respond with increased crying and activity. If an infant is overreactive, the parent should develop a calm, orderly routine and avoid unnecessary bombardments of sensory stimulation.

Colic *Colic* is unexplained periods of crying within the first 3 months of infancy associated with abdominal distention, spasms, and/or the passage of flatus or gas (Chow, et al., 1979). The symptoms usually occur late in the day. The infant cries loudly, clenching fists, extending legs, and acting as if searching for food; however, feeding does not quiet the infant. From a usual 2–3 hours of daily crying, colicky infants can cry 8–12 hours per day. With crying, the infant's entire body becomes tense and hyperactive. Crying then causes the further ingestion of air, and the vicious cycle of abdominal distention and pain results (Brazelton, 1976). Research has yielded little agreement on the specific causes of colic. Possible explanations include feeding problems, parental tension and anxiety, milk allergy, physiologic immaturity of the gastrointestinal system, and hyperactivity and overresponsiveness of the infants themselves. Colic usually disappears when the infant is 3 or 4 months old (Brazelton, 1976; Rudolph, 1977; Chow, et al., 1979).

Colic, like its primary symptom, crying, is nerve-wracking, frustrating, and terribly stressful to parents. The nurse again observes parent–child interactions and feeding procedures. As organic causes are ruled out, management may include adaptive feeding methods that eliminate as much air ingestion as possible. These might include feeding the formula-fed infant upright with the bottle held and not propped; adequate-size nipple openings; frequent burping during and after the feeding, and propping the infant up for 5–10 minutes after the feeding. Some formula-fed infants may be changed to soy milk or another special formula. If the infant is breast-fed, the mother should avoid all foods that she notes cause gas. Breast-feeding mothers also might transmit cow's milk protein through their milk; therefore, mothers who are breast-feeding colicky infants may need to eliminate all milk products from their diets (Jakobsson and Lindberg, 1978). (Nutritional concerns in infancy are discussed in Chapter 15).

Comfort measures, such as wrapping the infant warmly and providing rhythmic activities, might be tried. Activities might include walking, rocking, or riding in a car. Restructuring the environment in a calm, quiet manner is recommended. Brazelton (1976) noted success with the following treatment regimen:

1. Allow 20 minutes of crying
2. Spend 10 minutes offering sugar water and comforting the infant
3. Allow 20 more minutes of crying

Brazelton's method decreased the amount of crying and limited it to two predictable periods, one in the early morning and one in the evening, for a daily total of only 2 hours of crying.

Parents of colicky infants need great reassurance and support. They should understand that their infants are not ill and will stop this behavior when they are approximately 3 months of age. Guilt feelings should be acknowledged and the possible explanations for colic explored. Parents should be encouraged to designate free time for their enjoyment to decrease their anxiety and frustration.

Toilet Training Although frequently a source of great parental anxiety, toilet training may be viewed as an educational process that assists children to attain increased control over bodily functions and to progress toward becoming socially acceptable members of society. If perceived as a developmental process that should be inherently rewarding to children as they progress toward maturity, conflict can be avoided, and toilet training can be achieved relatively easily.

The first premise of toilet training is that the process occurs according to the child's own speed and level of readiness. Readiness for toilet training includes the following:

1. The child has passed the excitement of walking and running for their own sake and is now able to sit quietly for short periods
2. The child understands words associated with the toilet and uses them before needing to go to the bathroom
3. The child is able to remove pants and underwear
4. The child imitates behaviors such as brushing teeth or wiping up spills
5. The child enjoys placing toys or clothes where they belong
6. The child is able to stay dry for a few hours at a time
7. The child urinates a large amount at one time rather than dribbling continually (Azrin and Fox, 1981; Brazelton, 1976)

The management of toilet training is based on the child's readiness and the family's cultural practices (see Chapter 4). The nurse might need to discourage attempts to toilet train before 18 months of age because the child is not physiologically able to control sphincter muscles until 18–

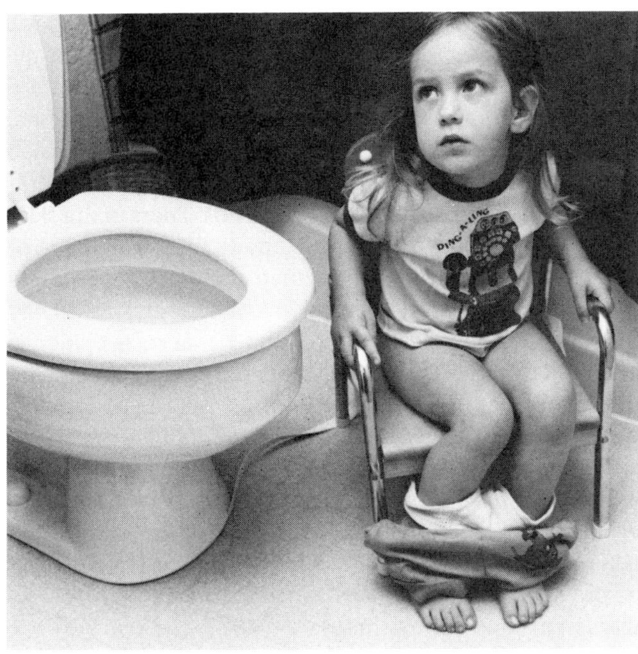

Emphasis on the child's independence and self-care, and attentiveness to the child's physiologic and psychologic readiness can make toilet training a nonstressful experience.

24 months of age. Between 18 and 30 months of age, the child can be observed for readiness signals.

Reasonable expectations for toilet training are indicated by Brazelton's (1962) 10-year study of 1170 children, which revealed that

1. Twelve percent of the children achieved bowel training first
2. Eight percent achieved bladder training first
3. Eighty percent achieved bowel and bladder control simultaneously
4. Most were trained by 27–29 months of age
5. Forty percent were still bedwetting at 4 years of age and 30% were bedwetting at 5 years of age
6. Two-year-olds voided about 12 times per day, with about 2 oz per voiding
7. Three- to 6-year-olds voided about eight times per day, with about 3 oz per voiding

Parents must have realistic expectations for their children regarding toilet training and should adapt their practices accordingly. Because the expectations of the parents are crucial to the process, the nurse should assess these as well. Preferably, the nurse should explore attitudes about toilet training with the parent when the child is 9–12 months old. Questions should involve the parent's plan to toilet train (when and how), the parent's experiences with toilet training, cultural or family pressures about toilet training, the parent's understanding of bowel and bladder maturity, and the parent's attitudes toward modesty and cleanliness. The nurse should respect the parent's ideas but may suggest other ideas for consideration.

Once readiness is determined, the parent may begin toilet training in a manner that the family finds comfortable. One method uses the following steps. First, a potty chair is placed in the bathroom, and the child is informed that this chair is the child's. The deflector provided for male potty chairs should be removed because it can hurt the child getting up and down. Once daily, with all clothes on, the child is taken to sit on the chair for a few minutes and allowed to get up whenever desired. The parent tells the child what is supposed to happen in the chair (for example, "This is where you dudu"). Second, once accustomed to the chair, the child can be taken to sit on it without clothes or diapers. This should be done at a time when a bowel movement might be expected. When the child does have a bowel movement in the diaper, the parent undoes the diaper and places it in the chair, saying something like, "One day you will be able to dudu in the chair."

Third, if the child begins to become interested, the parent takes the child to the chair several times a day to see whether the child can urinate or have a bowel movement. The parent can praise the child for positive results. Fourth, once the child seems ready to monitor his or her own actions, the parent can allow the child to remain undressed from the waist down as much as possible with the potty chair handy in the room or yard. The child is reminded that this is the child's business but that the parent will help remind the child to go. Eventually, training pants, which are easy for the child to pull up and down, can be worn.

This method is only one of many options available to families. An important concept in evaluating methods of toilet training is its appropriateness for the individual child and family. Regardless of the particular method chosen, parents need to remember that children should be rewarded for successful efforts but not punished for unsuccessful attempts.

Toilet training should be a nonstressful experience in which the parent emphasizes independence and self-care for the child. If parents can relax and delay toilet training until the children are physiologically and psychologically ready, they might toilet train themselves by observing and imitating family members or playmates. As with any other function, children might regress by having accidents in times of stress or change. Parents can become perplexed and frustrated when accidents occur, and the nurse needs to reassure them that regression is a normal part of the child's development and that such "slip-ups" or "accidents" do not indicate failure or a lack of effort on the child's part. Children need encouragement and patience during these periods until they are able to resume the desired control.

Noncompliance Noncompliance is a child's refusal to cooperate, seemingly constantly, through words or actions. Commonly known as "not minding," this behavior is often extremely frustrating and aggravating for parents. The parent frequently makes requests repeatedly before the child even responds. If the behavior continues, a grand power struggle results.

By refusing to comply immediately, the child actually controls the parents attention for significant periods of time. This holding of the parent's attention reinforces the child for exhibiting negativistic behavior. Regardless of the specific noncompliant behaviors exhibited (for example, refusing to eat or not picking up toys or clothes until reminded five or six times), similar management techniques can be applied in all situations.

Key guidelines for parents who are concerned about noncompliant behavior are consistent limit setting and avoiding power struggles whenever posssible. Parents need to agree about expectations for their children's behavior and to respond consistently. Limits are provided while children are encouraged to exercise as much self-care and responsibility as appropriate. By encouraging children's responsibility for their own behavior, parents may eliminate the potential for many power struggles. When conflict does occur, parents may employ the "no-lose" method of conflict resolution, which involves mutual discussion and compromise (Gordon, 1975).

The simple allowance of choices, encouragement of autonomy, and clear expression of limits does not, however, always prevent or eliminate inappropriate behavior. When noncompliant behavior occurs, parents may allow children to experience the consequences of their actions, or parents may remove the attention awarded the behavior through time out. Parents must be very careful to assess the child's situation fully to decrease undue stress for the child and to meet the child's larger needs.

A common noncompliant behavior is a refusal to eat. If the child refuses to eat food prepared for the rest of the family, the parent can simply state that this is the only food available. The child most likely will refuse several meals, but the parent should be firm and continue to offer food at mealtimes. The child is engaged in a power struggle and will continue to refuse food as long as attention results. The nurse needs to assure the parent that the child will not starve and that, if hungry enough, the child will eat. The key to managing noncompliant behavior with this approach is removing all the attention the child gains by this undesirable behavior. This can be a true challenge for parents because many find the temptation to scold and lecture very great.

Another common noncompliant behavior involves personal hygiene (for example, toothbrushing). The parent might then state, "Fine with me, but because candy and cookies destroy unbrushed teeth, you get no sweets as long as you don't brush." When the child desires a cookie, toothbrushing should resume without a comment needed from the parent. Another management technique might be to state that it is the child's decision to stop brushing, but that if there are any cavities at the next dental visit, the child will have to resume brushing or perhaps pay a portion of the dental bill.

Another common hygiene concern involves personal cleanliness habits of late childhood. Children at this stage are experiencing early sexual development and maturational changes involving body odor and oiliness of the skin. If parents become concerned about the cleanliness or attractiveness of their children, they might need to reassess their expectations and discuss them with the children. They may find solace in learning that this behavior is epidemic in this age group. For example, many children, upon being questioned about why only one or no pairs of underpants were in a week's laundry pile, have contributed a stack of clean underwear to the wash. These children are becoming increasingly assertive and independent, and gradually they will assume responsibility for self-care and experience the consequences of their behavior. Again, clear limits should be provided while involving the children in problem-solving discussions and compromises.

Noncompliant behavior also might involve a refusal to pick up clothes or toys. One technique is to place these items in a special Saturday box in the parent's bedroom and allow the child to retrieve them only at the end of each week. Therefore, the child might be forced to go without favorite toys or to wear less-than-favorite clothes until the week is over. Many parents survive this stage by ignoring a child's room except during periodic clean-ups.

Another common example of noncompliant behavior is dawdling in the morning and refusal to get dressed promptly, which, like any noncompliant behavior, requires an assessment of the entire situation. If the child dawdles, the cause could be that the child is tired or the home is extremely hectic or chaotic. If the child is tired and dawdling while getting ready in the morning, an earlier bedtime might be needed. If the family is in chaos, more time might be needed to allow everyone to get ready in a more relaxed manner. Many families find that they need to awaken earlier as their children become older and more independent. The children need more time than the parents to ready themselves for the day. Simple organizational techniques to save time might include setting out clothes at night or providing cereal or oatmeal that each family member can prepare. An alarm clock could be provided for the child, and the child reminded of the responsibility for being on time. When late, the child would receive the consequences of being tardy. The "beat-the-buzzer" technique of behavior modification also might be a helpful incentive to be on time.

Aggressive Behavior Many children commonly engage in aggressive behavior such as fighting. Such behavior as hitting, biting, and scratching is definitely antisocial and not productive in building healthy relationships.

Parents should agree on limits and make these clear to children. Parents need to explore the motives for their children's behavior and attempt to deal with the underlying stresses and anxieties. During an aggressive episode, the parent may remove the child to another place for cooling off, and after calm is restored, the parent may listen to the child's feelings. The child may be reminded that angry thoughts and feelings are normal and acceptable but that acting out this anger is unacceptable. The child and parent might explore alternative coping methods when anger occurs; these might include walking away to cool off or hitting a punching bag or pillow.

Parents might be well advised to stay out of a situation unless it is obviously dangerous. Thus, parental attention would be removed as a motivation for this behavior, and children would be required to resolve their conflicts alone. When tempers are hot and persons become irrational, however, external measures such as behavior modification might be appropriate. The time-out procedure is also useful with younger children to avoid parental nagging or scolding.

Bedtime Difficulties Sleep problems that sometimes occur in early childhood are related to autonomy. Young children often protest being placed in bed, even when exhausted, and may awaken during the night and continue to protest. If the parent gives in to the child's demands, the resulting pattern of behavior might be difficult to break. Sleep problems also might be related to separation because some children find separation from the parent at night to be long and painful and attempt to reestablish contact during the night. If the parent also finds the separation difficult, the parent might subtly foster this behavior by getting up with the child or taking the child into the parent's bed, patterns that indicate overdependence and make the struggle for autonomy particularly difficult. Nightmares also might occur during this stage, and children who become very frightened by their dreams may need parental reassurance.

Many parents express frustration over the seemingly endless bedtime theatrics involved in getting a child to bed, as well as keeping the child there once tucked in. Several general principles may facilitate the process. First, a bedtime hour must be determined and consistently enforced. Before-bedtime activities for young children should be limited to calming, peaceful activities that are not too disturbing or stimulating. Desirable activities might be quiet and imaginative play, artwork, or children's games and stories. Rough-housing, active physical sports, and watching violent or exciting television shows might tend to keep the child awake. Thirty minutes before bedtime, a young child should be reminded that there are 30 minutes more to play and be with the family. Older children might choose activities that are pleasurable or relaxing to them such as listening to the stereo or reading. Evening also might be an appropriate time for parents and children to unwind by discussing the day's events.

If children have difficulty going to sleep, parents might need to explore and attempt to alleviate any possible causes of stress or anxiety. A child can be placed in bed but allowed to play quietly there or read until asleep. Parents need to leave both young and older children alone after tucking them in for the night to avoid reinforcing "staying-awake" behavior.

Children should know what is expected of them and be allowed some control in the bedtime transition. If the child protests at bedtime or awakens during the night and demands attention, the parents' response should be assessed. By 2 years of age, most children can fall asleep and stay asleep with only occasional attention from a parent (see Chapter 8).

Using behavior modification, a parent might try the following steps. After tucking the child in and completing all bedtime rituals (such as stories, a drink of water, going to the toilet, and being told where the parent will be), the parent instructs the child to stay in bed and warns the child that getting up will result in going to time out for 2–5 minutes. The child also is told that by staying in bed all night, there will be an extra bedtime story the next night and that if the child gets up, there will be no story the next night. The child's crying and calling for the parent should be totally ignored. A child who gets out of bed is quickly placed in time out with no comment. If these steps are followed consistently, desired bedtime behaviors should result within 2–3 weeks.

Another bedtime difficulty has been referred to as the "midnight intruder" (Patterson, 1976), which is when the child crawls into bed with the parent. If this behavior is undesirable, the parent should simply return the child to bed with such statements as, "Mom and Dad sleep in their bed, and you sleep in yours." Before tucking the child in, the parent can say, "If you stay in bed all night, I will come to your bed in the morning and read you two stories." Another method would be to remind children that if they stay in bed all night, they can play with a favorite toy the next day but that if they get up, they cannot have the toy.

Another bedtime difficulty is the problem of nightmares and fears. Many preschoolers are afraid of the dark. Parents should respect these fears and attempt to assist the child by providing a nightlight or flashlight for the child to hold. When awakened by a nightmare, children should simply be told by parents that they were only dreaming and that they are fine. Parents may remind the children that a parent is always nearby. Discussions of the dream can be saved for the next day when the child is totally awake. If chronic nightmares occur, the parent should explore possible causes of stress, anxiety, or overstimulation and alleviate these factors whenever possible.

Temper Tantrums Temper tantrums elicit extreme parental responses due to the ear-splitting noise and usual elaborate performances in such public places as supermarkets or stores. Tantrums are most common in children 18 months to 3 years of age and signal the child's negativism and struggle for autonomy (see Chapter 8). Regardless of the motives, this behavior is socially unacceptable and intolerable to the nerves of most parents.

Temper tantrums in early childhood are most common when the child must cope with frustration (See Chapter 12). The frequency, intensity, and duration of tantrums are influenced by the precipitative events, temperamental characteristics, and parental response. The nurse therefore should explore these variables to understand the child's behavior and parental perceptions.

Most parents with a shouting child feel the urge to punish the child physically. A light tap on the bottom might relieve the parents' frustration but might also be ineffective in preventing recurrent outbursts. The parents might need reassurance that the child's behavior is attention seeking and is reinforced by any attention given.

If possible, an effective technique involves ignoring the behavior and remaining calm. If using behavior modification, parents warn children that temper tantrums are unacceptable and that each tantrum therefore results in, for example, time out. If young children have tantrums in public, they can receive "time-out" marks on their hands and are placed in time out upon returning home.

Many children calm down if sent or taken to their rooms until they have settled down. A more difficult technique for the parents is ignoring the behavior. If the child falls to the floor in a tantrum, the parent simply leaves the room without comment. Parents are probably well advised to find some means of relaxing or discharging tension at these times. Ignoring tantrums in public places is almost impossible for most parents because they feel great embarrassment and guilt about the child's performance. If parents can ignore the public display, however, they simply leave the children at the scene and relocate nearby until the tantrum is over.

Because tantrums tend to occur when children are hungry or tired, parents should try to plan family activities and outings for times when the children are rested and recently fed. Parents need to be sensitive to their children's developmental and tempermental abilities and minimize situations that are overtaxing or overstimulating.

Masturbation Masturbation is a normal exploration of the body, particularly the genital area. Almost all children engage in touching or exploring themselves. Masturbation usually begins in infancy, and parents might express concern about the behavior during early or middle childhood. Masturbation is pleasurable and might be used for the sensation itself or to release anxiety or tension.

Parents' values concerning modesty and sexuality are crucial to handling this behavior. Parents might need to understand that children's touching of themselves in private might best be ignored to prevent unnecessary attention or anxiety. Nurses can reassure parents that this is a normal process that often increases around 4 years of age and disappears if ignored. The parent should, however, differentiate between masturbation in private and in public. Without causing fear or guilt in the child, the parent can simply let a child know that touching oneself is not appropriate in front of other people. The child, already incorporating the concepts of pride and modesty, usually will accept this advice without difficulty.

Sibling Rivalry Competition among siblings and an intense need to validate equal, just, and fair treatment and recognition from the parent are the most pervasive characteristics of sibling relationships. Sibling rivalry occurs in almost every family with more than one child. It is most common in families where the age range between children is small, with brothers close in age having the least harmonious relationship of sibling pairs (Yussen and Santrock, 1982). Firstborn siblings appear more dominant in all situations, especially when the firstborn is also female. Sibling rivalry tends to be more severe in families with few children

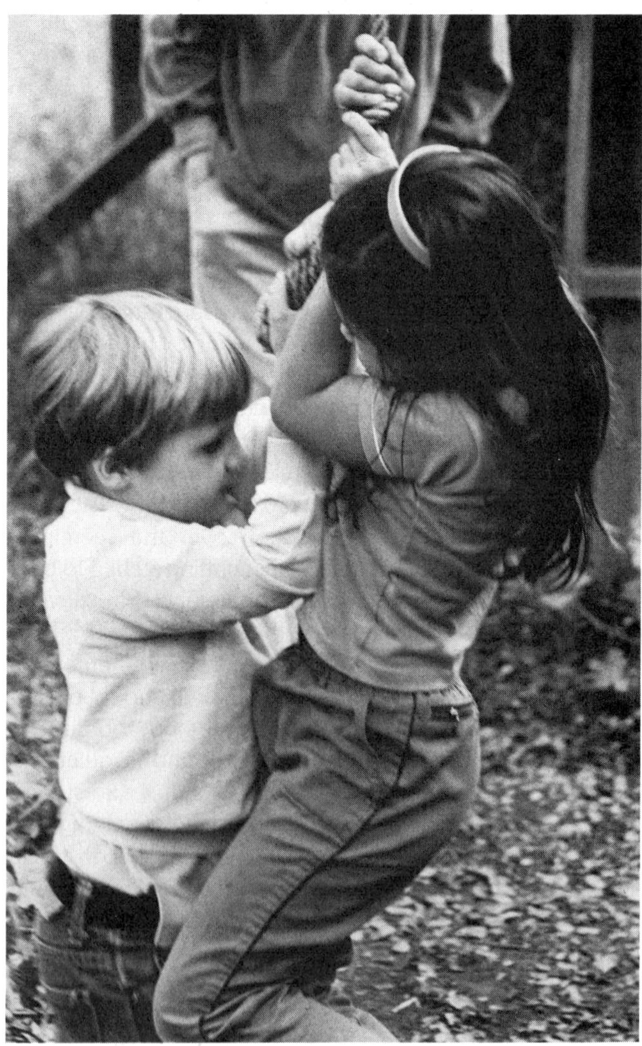

In sibling rivalry, firstborn siblings appear more dominant in all situations, especially when they are female.

vying for parental attention and in single-parent families with few adults as role models. It is somewhat less prevalent in large families with many children because the rivalry between individual children is diluted by the influence of many family members.

In families with children whose ages are widely spaced, older children are likely to assume roles as "surrogate parents" and often assume many parenting tasks as well. Some older children resent these additional responsibilities, whereas others may resent either the relaxed attitude with which some parents raise their later-born children or the privileges that younger children might enjoy. The potential for resentment and jealousy is most acute in reconstituted families in which a younger child is the product of the remarriage. Younger children with much older siblings express rivalry or jealousy. A young child may feel pressured to live up to an older sibling's reputation and to match or exceed the older child's accomplishments. One 4-year-old boy, for example, was delighted to learn that he could expect one day to be taller than his 18-year-old sister.

For most families, however, sibling rivalry is typified by behavior problems among children who are close in age. Parents who want to count on their older children to stop or limit inappropriate behavior are then faced with a dilemma in which they might wonder whether to expect the same standards of behavior in both the older and the younger child. In most situations the solution is to reinforce age-appropriate behavior in both children without blaming either child for the behavior problem. For many parents, this is not always easy because children are often quick to point out what they perceive as another child's preferential treatment. For instance, one 13-year-old boy balked when told that he must eat a large breakfast before going to school and complained that his 16-year-old sister was allowed to sleep a little later and eat only orange juice and toast.

Parents faced with similar situations often need to explain to their children that fairness does not necessarily mean that each child is treated in exactly the same way. Differences in children's temperaments, needs, and family environment may dictate different standards. A parent may, for example, need to explain to the 13-year-old that a fast-growing adolescent boy needs a large breakfast to stay alert and concentrate on schoolwork.

Younger children are more likely to fight with each other over toys than to challenge differences in parental standards. In minimizing the unacceptable behavior, parents need first to define what is acceptable and age appropriate. If, for instance, the older of two young children has been taught to share, this behavior might be reinforced by rewarding that child for sharing the toy. It also might be necessary to modify the environment by separating the children and taking the toy away.

Parents who find time for each of their children also minimize sibling rivalry. Children often fight to compete for parental attention but are less likely to do so if they feel individually loved and appreciated. Finding time to give each child singular attention is especially difficult in single-parent families, in which one parent must divide what time is available among the children. For all parents, however, time spent actively listening to the child and communicating about expectations minimizes the occurrence and the severity of behavior problems.

Key Concepts

- Parents progress through developmental stages and undertake developmental tasks as they accommodate themselves to their children's development.
- An essential developmental task for parents is helping children move from the pleasure principle to the reality principle.
- Parents need to define their roles to their children so that the children understand that they are both parents and people.
- The variety of support systems available to parents includes spouses, relatives, friends, books, and nurses, but parents ultimately must take responsibility for their decisions.
- Skillful communication with children requires active and empathetic listening, "I messages" that express parents' needs without criticizing a child's character, and clear expressions of both parents' expectations and positive feelings about their children.
- Unacceptable behavior can be minimized by modifying the environment, setting clear limits, avoiding win or lose conflicts, and finding time for parents and children to spend together.
- Clear, consistent limit setting reflects an authoritative style of parenting.
- Approaches to behavior management include corporal punishment, psychodynamic management, logical consequences, and behavior modification.
- A frequently effective method of behavior modification is the "time-out" plan, in which the young child is placed in a nonstimulating environment to neutralize positive reinforcement for unacceptable behavior.

- Crying, fussiness, and colic during infancy may require a variety of parental interventions but are usually resolved over time.
- Toilet training is best undertaken when the child is physiologically and psychologically ready; the nurse's guidance is based on an assessment of the family's expectations and attitudes.
- Noncompliance, aggressive behavior, bedtime difficulties, and temper tantrums are best handled with parental consistency, clear limit setting, and avoidance of power struggles with the child.
- Parents need to allow themselves chances to "cool off" when children's misbehavior cause stress and anxiety.
- Masturbation is a normal behavior that nurses should urge parents to ignore when done in private.
- Sibling rivalry can be minimized by reinforcing positive behaviors in all children and by providing each child with individual attention.

References

Adler A: *Education of Children.* Regnery-Gateway, 1978a.

Adler A: *Understanding Human Nature.* Fawcett, 1978b.

Azrin NH, Holz WC: Punishment. In: *Aberrant Behavior: Areas of Research and Application.* Honig WK (editor). Appleton-Century-Crofts, 1966.

Azrin NH, Fox RM: *Toilet-Training in Less Than a Day.* Pocket Books, 1977.

Baumrind D: Parents as leaders: The role of control and discipline. In: *Families Today.* DHEW Publication No. 79-815. US Department of Health, Education, and Welfare, 1979.

Blood RO: *The Family.* Free Press, 1972.

Brazelton TB: *Doctor and Child.* Delacourte Press/Seymour Lawrence, 1976.

Brazelton TB: A child-oriented approach to toilet training. *Pediatrics* 1962; 29:121–128.

Brink PJ: An anthropological perspective on parenting. In: *Parenting Reassessed: A Nursing Perspective.* Horowitz JA, Hughes CB, Perdue BJ (editors). Prentice-Hall, 1982, pp. 66–84.

Chow MP, et al: *Handbook of Pediatric Primary Care.* Wiley, 1979.

Christophersen ER: Behavioral pediatrics. In: *Family Health Care.* Hymovich DP, Barnard MU (editors). McGraw-Hill, 1979.

Drabman RS, Creedon DL: Marking time-out. *Child Behav Ther* Spring, 1979; 1:99–101.

Drabman RS, Creedon DL: Beat-the-buzzer. *Child Behav Ther* Fall, 1979; 1:295–296.

Dreikurs R: *The Challenge of Parenthood.* Hawthorn Books, 1958.

Dreikurs R, Soltz V: *Children: The Challenge.* Hawthorn Books, 1964.

Dreikurs R, Grey L: *A Parents' Guide to Child Discipline.* Hawthorn Books, 1970.

Erlander HS: Social class and corporal punishment in childrearing: A reassessment. *Am Sociol Rev* 1974; 39:68–85.

Fraiberg SH: *The Magic Years.* Scribner, 1959.

Friedman AS, Friedman DB: Parenting: A developmental process. *Pediatr Ann* 1977; 6(9):564–572.

Ginott HG: *Between Parent and Child.* Macmillan, 1961.

Gordon T: *Parent-Effectiveness Training.* New American Library, 1975.

Gordon I: Improving parent skills. In: *Families Today.* DHEW Publication No. 79-815. US Department of Health, Education, and Welfare, 1979.

Guerney BG: Fortifying family ties. In: *Families Today.* DHEW Publication No. 79-815. US Department of Health, Education, and Welfare, 1979.

Hammer D, Drabman RS: Child discipline: What we know and what we can recommend. *Pediatr Nurs* (May/June) 1981; 7:31–35.

Jakobsson I, Lindberg T: Cow's milk as a cause of infantile colic in breastfed infants. *Lancet* 1978; 2:437–439.

Murphy MA: When parents ask about discipline. *Pediatr Nurs* (Nov/Dec) 1976; 2(6):28–32.

Newberger CM: *Parental Conceptions of Children and Child-Rearing: A Structural-Developmental Analysis.* (Dissertation.) Harvard University, Cambridge, Mass, 1977.

O'Neil SM, McLaughlin BN, Knapp MB: *Behavioral Approaches to Children With Developmental Delays.* Mosby, 1977.

Patterson G: *Living With Children.* Research Press, 1976.

Piaget J: *The Moral Judgment of the Child.* Free Press, 1965.

Piuck CL: Child-rearing patterns of poverty. *Am J Psychother* 1975; 29(4):485–502.

Pratt L: *Family Structure and Effective Health Behavior.* Houghton Mifflin, 1976.

Rudolph AM (editor): *Pediatrics.* Appleton-Century-Crofts, 1977.

Steinmetz SK, Straus MA (editors): *Violence in the Family.* Dodd, Mead, 1974.

Weisberger E: *Your Young Child and You.* Dutton, 1975.

White BL: Developing a sense of competence in young children. In: *Families Today.* DHEW Publication No. 79-815. US Department of Health, Education, and Welfare, 1979.

Yussen SR, Santrock JW: *Child Development: An Introduction.* Wm. C. Brown, 1982.

Additional Readings

Brink RE: How serious is the child's behavior problem? *Matern Child Nurs J* (Jan/Feb) 1982; 7:33–36.

Chamberlin RW: Parenting styles, child behavior and the pediatrician. *Pediatr Ann* 1977; 6(9):584–591.

Graubard PS: *Positive Parenthood.* New American Library, 1977.

Keniston K and The Carnegie Council on Children. *All Our Children: The American Family Under Pressure.* Harcourt Brace Jovanovich, 1977.

Miller JR, Janosik EH: *Family Focused Care.* McGraw-Hill, 1980.

Vaughan VC, Brazelton TB (editors). *The Family—Can It be Saved?* Year Book, 1976.

Webster-Stratton CW, Kogan K: Helping parents parent. *Am J Nurs* (February) 1980; 80:240–244.

Wilson AL: Parenting in perspective. *Fam Community Health* 1978; 1(3):65–77.

HEALTH PROMOTION AND MAINTENANCE OF THE CHILD AND FAMILY

PART TWO

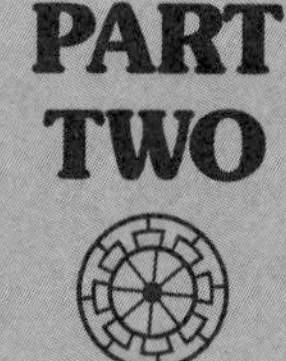

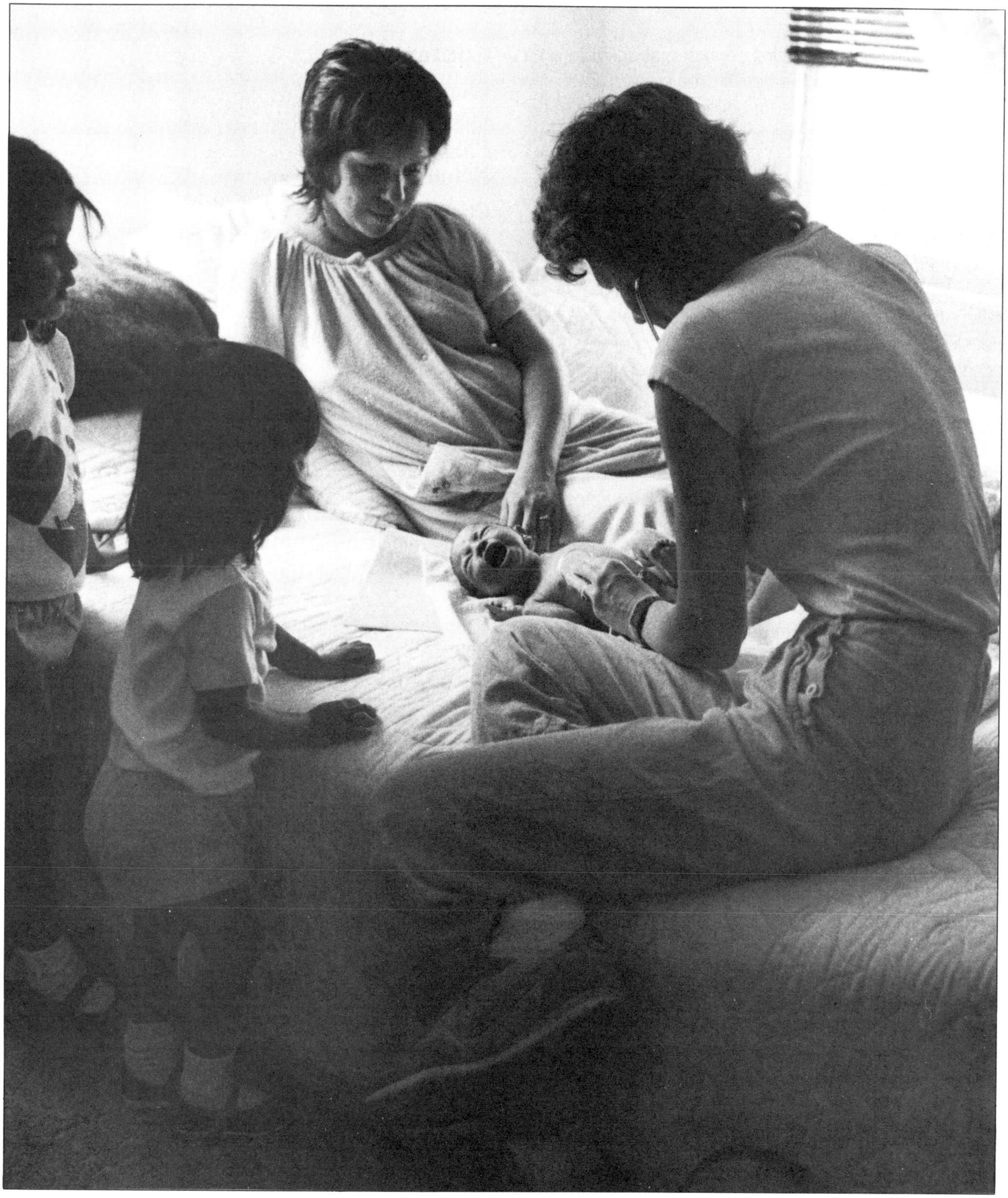

UNIT IV CHILD AND FAMILY ASSESSMENT

The nurse is often the first contact that children and families have with the health care system. The nurse is often responsible for collecting health data, interpreting the data for early identification, intervention, and prevention of health problems, and for making necessary referrals to other members of the health care team. Assessment is therefore a vital part of the child health nursing process.

As discussed in this unit, a comprehensive health assessment of a child not only provides data that reflect the child's current physical, nutritional, developmental, and family status, but also places that child on a continuum that includes past health, effects on current functioning, and clues about future level of functioning. In the absence of specific medical problems, nursing responsibilities during regular visits for well-child care include anticipatory guidance, assessment of developmental progress, and help for the family in dealing with childrearing problems and minor emotional difficulties. The nurse thus implements preventive care for the child and family before major problems arise and lead to long-term disabilities. In this unit we reflect the nurse's role in preventive care as it has expanded over the past decades.

The assessment skills necessary for comprehensive preventive nursing care involve data collection about physical (Chapter 14), nutritional (Chapter 15), developmental (Chapter 16), and family (Chapter 17) health parameters. This unit also presents the nurse with interviewing skills for taking a family health history, physical examination skills, and communication skills that allow both child and family to participate fully in the planning and evaluation of their health care.

In each of the chapters three representative children and their families are presented as case studies. Each case study illustrates the use of an assessment tool for data collection, analysis of the data, and appropriate nursing diagnoses and interventions. At the end of the unit, one of these serial case studies is the basis for a care plan that integrates all the data and nursing diagnoses and demonstrates how the nurse uses assessment data to provide comprehensive nursing care.

Contents

Physical Assessment

Joan Pernice

14

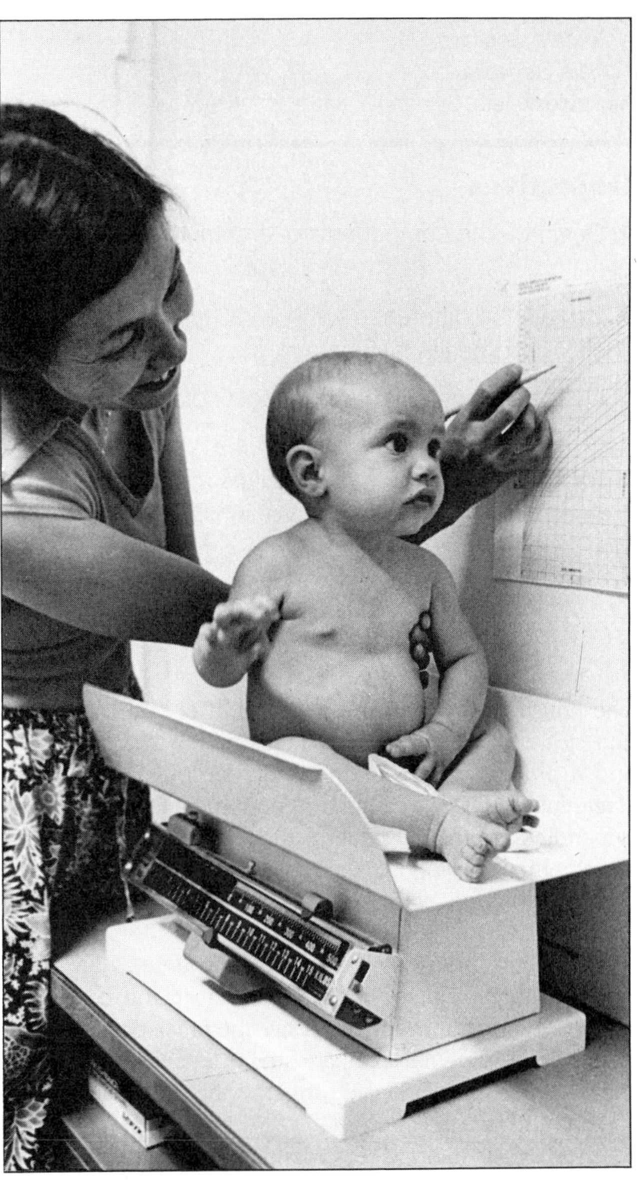

Chapter Outline

continued on next page

Objectives

- Describe the components of a complete health history.
- Explain the difference between a well-child and a sick-child health history.
- Define the health screening tools commonly used in physical assessment.
- Identify the factors that determine the nurse's approach to the physical examination.
- Explain the methods used to reduce the child's anxiety in the physical assessment setting.
- Identify the body systems assessed by the physical examination.
- Identify the assessment criteria associated with each body system.
- Describe the four basic physical examination techniques.
- Name the signs and symptoms associated with alterations from normal expectations for each body system.

The physical assessment, a component of both well-child and sick-child health care, includes both a health history and a physical examination in conjunction with physical screening tests. The emphasis and methods used vary depending on the purpose of the visit and the age and developmental level of the child. The nurse therefore plans the assessment according to the needs of both the child and family.

The physical assessment process is continuous and actually begins with the nurse's initial contact with the child and parent. During the health interview, the nurse observes the child's developmental level, the quality and effectiveness of the parent–child relationship, and the child's overall growth pattern and health status.

A systematic method for organizing the physical assessment ensures thoroughness and consistency in performing and recording physical findings. Whereas the actual written document is the format used by physicians, the nursing assessment is specifically intended to lead to a nursing diagnosis, which is followed by planning and intervention for nursing problems.

In this chapter we discuss the components and methods of a physical assessment. We describe the process of interviewing parent and child, observing, and then documenting data. We define the procedures and purposes for essential health-screening tools, both measurements and laboratory data, and we describe the assessment criteria and likely findings for each phase of the physical examination.

Health History

Interviewing

The health history is an important part of the health assessment. Studies have shown that 60% of medical conditions in children can be diagnosed by history alone (Bernstein and Bernstein, 1980). The information obtained in a health history often determines the part of the examination that requires special emphasis and the laboratory tests that are indicated. Historical data provide the background for the interpretation of physical examination and laboratory findings.

The ability to obtain a good health history is an important skill that a nurse develops with practice. All learned styles and patterns of communication are brought to the clinical interview. Research substantiates that the nurse who has a good relationship with the client is likely to obtain the complete and accurate data necessary for a correct diagnosis (Korsch, 1973). The verbal and nonverbal exchange of information between the client and nurse is necessary and basic to the nursing process, and the quality of that communication directly affects nursing outcomes. Attentive and sensitive listening occurs best in private. Furthermore, clients who are provided privacy are likely to trust that what they share will be kept confidential.

Depending on the type of information needed, the nurse may use either open-ended questions or closed, direct questions. Open-ended questions are broad questions that leave the client (child and/or parent, as appropriate) free to describe the situation or problem. For example, "What can I do for you today?" or "Tell me about your problem" are broad questions that allow a range of responses. The nurse notes the way in which the client describes problems, why the client is concerned, and whether problems are related to specific life events. The nurse strengthens rapport by expressing interest, offering encouragement, or asking for clarification. This takes time because the client might give unnecessary or irrelevant information and also might avoid talking about the issue at hand. A person with limited verbal skills might fear this type of question and require another approach.

The closed, direct question does not encourage the client to talk freely but asks instead for specific responses to specific questions. "How old is the baby?" and "What medication did you take?" are closed, direct questions. This format is necessary during a sick-child visit but generally is used in combination with the open-ended approach. The wording of questions is thus a component of nursing care and involves the nurse in initial planning and evaluation of the client's response.

From birth until adolescence, children are accompanied to the health center by a parent, guardian, or other relative, and the nurse therefore needs to interview the adult and child in a variety of creative ways. With the nonverbal infant and the young child, the interview is between the adult and nurse, with the nurse observing the child in play and in interaction with the adult (see Chapter 16 for assessment guidelines). As the child matures, the nurse includes the child in the history taking to the extent that is developmentally appropriate. Children like to be asked what their favorite foods are or what game they like the best and who their best friends are. This integration of the child into the interview gives the child a feeling of having some control over the situation, acclimates the child to the environment, and helps the child to begin to trust the nurse. Conversing with the child also gives the nurse important information about the child's speech patterns, cognitive and developmental levels, and relationship with the adult.

Adolescents, especially older adolescents, may come to the health center by themselves. The nurse then focuses the interview and history taking on the adolescent's concerns, asking questions about information that the adolescent is likely to know. When an adolescent is accompanied by a parent or other adult, the nurse needs to assess whether the two should be seen together or separately. If seen separately, each should know that confidentiality is assured. If an issue arises that the nurse feels ought to be shared, the nurse suggests that the adolescent and adult meet together but does not revoke confidentiality.

Content and Format of the Health History

Child health nursing involves several health history formats: the complete health history, the interim health history, and the acute health history. Although the categories of information obtained in each format are similar, the specific information that is sought differs (Table 14-1).

Identifying Data This phase of the health history involves a limited amount of information recorded concisely. Much of the data already might be included on the child's chart and need only verification. The informant (mother, father, child, grandparent, neighbor, and so on) is noted, along with an assessment of the informant's reliability in providing accurate data.

This section of the health history always includes the child's age, date of birth, and sex. Frequently, the child's race is included, but this information is useful only when the child may be at risk for diseases that occur more frequently in a particular racial group. For example, certain anemias, such as thalassemia and sickle cell trait or disease, occur most often in dark-skinned people of African, Arab, or Mediterranean descent.

If the child's and family's primary language is not English, the nurse notes the extent to which the family does understand and speak English to assess the need for an interpreter. Some clients, although not fluent in English, can use the language to some extent, but this might be problematic if the client understands only a small portion of the whole interaction. If an interpreter is involved in the interview, this should be noted with the data about the informant.

Chief Complaint The chief complaint is a brief description of the specific reason for, or the client's perception of, the primary reason for the visit. It should be recorded as a concise statement or statements in the client's own words. For example, if the opening question is "What may I do for you today?" or "Tell me why you came here to the clinic" and the client responds with "We are here for a checkup," the nurse records "well-child care" or "health maintenance." If the client is seen for assessment and care of an illness, the chief complaint then includes the symptoms and their duration as described by the client. The nurse might need to guide the client to describe the most relevant and pertinent symptoms; asking which one problem or symptom brought the client to the clinic or office often helps.

The duration of the chief complaint indicates whether the problem is acute or chronic and also is useful in assessing its severity. For instance, if a client describes having "headaches for 3 years" and the symptoms are not congruent with the urgency of the visit, there might be underlying reasons for the visit. The nurse then asks further exploratory questions to uncover the real problem.

TABLE 14-1 Child Health History Adaptations for Purpose of Visit

Acute Illness Visit	Well-Child Interim Visit
Identifying information	Identifying information
Source of information	Source of information
Chief concern	Chief concern (if any)
Definition of chief concern	Definition of chief concern
Onset—sudden or gradual, previous episodes Location of complaint—anatomically precise Quality—dull, sharp, aching, burning, itching, etc. Quantity—intensity and degree of discomfort Chronology—previous health, onset of problem, duration, frequency, change over time Setting—home or school	Current health history Any health related problems since last visit Nutrition Elimination Sleep Development—gross motor, fine motor, language, cognitive, social-emotional, concepts of sex and death Environmental factors—safety, pollution, etc. Immunization status and reaction to previous immunizations
Alleviating or aggravating factors Associated symptoms Associated changes in child's or family's life Actions taken to relieve problem Epidemiologic information—exposure, contacts, travel	Update or add to family, psychosocial, past medical history only as necessary
Family, psychosocial, past medical and current health status sections of history not included unless relevant to defined problem	Review of body systems
Review of body systems	

History of Present Illness The history of a present illness (HPI) is the detailed narrative of the client's chief complaint. This portion of the health history is not usually included in a health maintenance visit unless the client presents a specific physical or psychosocial problem. In analyzing symptoms the nurse proceeds in an orderly manner, including the major components: total duration, date of onset, characteristics at onset or at any other time, aggravating or relieving factors, treatments tried and the results, and course since onset.

Total duration refers to the client's recall of the day the problems began and is recorded as the date of onset or the last time the client felt well. The nurse ascertains the manner of onset by asking, "How did the problem start?" and "Was it gradual or sudden?" Asking about the child's state of health immediately before the illness provides data about family health patterns and general well-being. Depending on the nature of the chief complaint, the nurse also might assess any precipitating and/or predisposing factors related to onset. These might include emotional disturbances, infections (for example, exposure and incubation period), allergies, physical exertion, fatigue, and environmental factors.

Characteristics at onset or any other time usually refers to a description of pain or discomfort because these usually denote a physical problem. The nurse might, for example, ask, "Is the pain sharp, dull, or aching?" Having the child point to, or the parent describe, the location and radiation of the pain also is useful. Children should attempt to describe the intensity of the pain and its temporal character in their own words. To facilitate the child's description, the nurse asks whether the pain is continuous, intermittent, sharp, throbbing, aching, or stabbing. Finding out how the pain has affected the child's normal eating, playing, and sleeping behaviors is a good method of assessing the severity of the problem.

Aggravating factors or relieving factors cause a change in the type, location, severity, or duration of the pain (aggravating factors worsen and relieving factors lessen the client's perception of pain). They need to be documented in the client's words, usually by asking what made the client feel worse or better. The course since onset includes the circumstances related to the problem: whether it is a single, acute attack; recurrent acute attacks; or daily, periodic, or continuous occurrences. The nurse notes whether the child or parent reports that at the time of the visit the problem is better, worse, or unchanged and records data about the medical attention provided, if any, and its effects.

Past Health History and Birth History The section for past health history and birth history includes the client's neonatal history and the mother's obstetric history. Because events during pregnancy and in the perinatal period can have long-range organic and psychologic effects, the details of the birth history are important in planning health maintenance and problem management.

An older child or adolescent who has had no serious medical or psychologic problems need not be asked detailed questions, but these clients may be asked whether they have ever been told anything about their births. A negative response generally indicates no problems.

Pregnancy, labor, and delivery histories begin with open-ended questions such as, "How was your pregnancy?" Often, beginning the history taking in this way, with the mother's own health, enlists her cooperation and assistance with the remainder of the history and examination. Direct questions then can be used to obtain the relevant information regarding the onset and frequency of prenatal care, status of prenatal health, and events of labor and delivery (including the client's APGAR, if known, and the time spent in the hospital). An assessment of the parent–child relationship, an important component in child development, is best begun by assessing parental feelings toward the pregnancy. (Developmental history and assessment are discussed in Chapter 16.)

Any illnesses, hospitalizations, surgery, and accidents should be included specifically, with details of the events. Equally important is the child's reaction to these events. Most parents recall only serious medical problems and need to be asked directly about common childhood diseases such as chickenpox, strep throat, and tonsillitis. Also important is historical information about childhood injuries such as falls, cuts, or burns, which parents might not consider serious accidents. Such incidents might suggest a need for parental guidance and education regarding childhood safety. (Chapters 18 and 19 discuss the prevention of illness and injury.)

Allergies are recorded with details about symptoms, etiology (if known), treatment, and results. The nurse also asks about any unusual reactions to food, drugs, or environmental agents, even if the reaction was an isolated incident. A single reaction may indicate an early allergic predisposition, or a seasonal cycle may suggest an allergy (for example, "Every spring she gets sick"). Current medications are documented by listing all prescribed or nonprescribed drugs taken and the reason for their use. Immunizations are documented on the child's immunization schedule. Most parents have a separate record that can be copied into the chart. If the parent is a reliable informant and states that the child's schedule is complete, this is noted as such in the chart.

Family Health History This section of the health history is best introduced to the parent by stating its purpose for inclusion. Most parents understand that the child's health might be affected by family health, especially congenital or familial health problems. A simple statement such as, "I would like to ask you some questions about the health of family members" is appropriate. Significant features of the medical histories of all immediate family members are then documented; for any serious problems, details about the diagnosis, cause, treatment, and management are included. A family history of medical problems also might have psychologic ramifications due to the stress, financial burdens, or turmoil for the family. A genogram concisely shows the health, ages, and relationships of family members (see Fig. 5-10). A narrative format is used commonly to describe the family and its environment. The purpose of this section is to begin assessment of the family in which the child is a member. Depending on the data collected, a further, in-depth family assessment might be needed, especially if preliminary data reveal problematic family relationships or social, psychologic, or financial concerns (see Ch. 17).

Review of Body Systems The review of body systems is a thorough checklist of any and all possible medical problems the child has experienced. If the review contains a previous problem, the nurse documents the duration, frequency, intensity, course, associated factors, and results of treatment. It is extremely important to review body systems thoroughly for any past or current health deviation or concern. Any significant positive response needs to be recorded.

Because most parents and children are not familiar with medical terminology, the nurse phrases questions in appropriate ways. For example, "Has Johnny had any ear infections?" might be understood but "Has Johnny had any otitis media?" might not.

The review of body systems is also a good time to integrate health teaching with the assessment. For example, if the parent reports that the child has had frequent bladder infections, the nurse discusses preventive management and assesses the parent's understanding of the causes and treatment of the problem.

Current Health The section about current health includes the child's habits of eating, eliminating, and sleeping, as well as a current developmental profile. With an older child or adolescent, this includes any use of or experimentation with alcohol, drugs, and cigarettes. Given a supportive, trusting relationship, the nurse can discuss openly with the child the reasons for this behavior and its potential consequence (see Chapter 18).

Health Screening

In the physical assessment process, screening and laboratory tests are useful in augmenting the health history and physical examination findings. They provide quick, inexpensive measures for detecting those children most likely to have a specific problem. Screening and laboratory tests often provide valuable information about the accuracy of the entire health assessment and have become common and accepted practice.

Caution is needed in the use of screening tests because false-positive and false-negative results can cause overreferrals or underreferrals for a more complete diagnostic workup. For example, some children show positive test results, even though they do not have the condition for which they are being tested; this in turn causes overreferrals to diagnostic specialists. False-negative test results cause

(text continued on p. 374)

Child Health History

Date and Initial Data

Identifying Information

1. Name (nickname or preferred name)
2. Age, birthdate
3. Sex
4. Primary care and other health resources

Source of Information (Referral Source)

1. Parent, child, or other (medical records)
2. Reliability of source

Chief Concern (CC)

1. Any concern of child, family, or other person working with family
2. Usually described in a brief statement, using the patient's words

Definition of CC or History of Present Illness (HPI)

1. Onset—sudden or gradual, previous episodes
2. Location of complaint—anatomically precise
3. Quality—dull, sharp, aching, burning, itching, etc.
4. Quantity—intensity and degree of discomfort
5. Chronology—previous health, onset of problem, duration, frequency, change over time
6. Setting (home, school)
7. Alleviating or aggravating factors
8. Associated symptoms
9. Associated changes in child or family's life
10. Actions taken to relieve problem
11. Epidemiologic information—exposure, contacts, travel

History

Birth History

Pregnancy—gravida, para, abortions, miscarriages, onset and place of prenatal care

1. Duration—EDC, number of weeks
2. Complications and time of occurrence
 a. Drugs—self-prescribed, prescribed by doctor, street drugs, alcohol, tobacco
 b. Exposure to infectious disease—STD (sexually transmitted disease), rubella, other
 c. X-ray exposure
 d. Kidney infection
 e. Vaginal bleeding
 f. Hypertension
 g. Swelling of extremities
 h. Excessive or inadequate weight
 i. Diet during pregnancy
 j. Trauma, surgery
 k. Ultrasound
 l. Amniocentesis
3. Was pregnancy planned?
4. Emotional adjustment to pregnancy.
5. Problems with previous or subsequent pregnancies

Labor and Delivery—Hospital

1. Length of labor
2. Rupture of membranes
3. Medications
4. Presentation of infant
5. Type of delivery
6. Forceps
7. Complications—bleeding, fever, etc.
8. Did infant breathe spontaneously?
9. Apgars, if available

Neonatal History

1. Birthweight, height, and OFC (occipital frontal circumference)
2. Complications: jaundice, cyanosis, apnea, incubation, seizures, skin eruptions, vomiting, refusal to eat, weight loss or gains during hospital stay, other
3. Temperament of infant
4. Any abnormalities

Infancy

1. Temperament of infant
2. Feeding pattern—type, frequency, addition of new foods and reaction
3. Problems in infancy—illnesses, excessive crying, vomiting, etc.
4. Parental response

Development

1. Motor: sat alone, crawled, walked, tricycled, prehension, weaned, self-feeding, toilet training
2. Language: babbled, single words, sentences (one word, two words, or more), easy or difficult to understand
3. Psychosocial behavior: smiles, fears, tantrums, detachment, transitional object, toleration of separations

Illnesses—Age when each occurred and treatment received; pneumonia, croup, asthma, high fevers; childhood diseases; meningitis, nephritis, etc.; any complications or sequelae

Hospitalization—Date, cause, child's reaction

Surgery—Date, hospital, doctor, reason for surgery, any complications

Accidents or Injuries

Allergies—Drugs, foods, other items; type of reaction; skin, respiratory, behavioral, neurologic, other

Medications—Over the counter, prescribed, or home remedies; taken in past; taking presently

Immunization—Dates, reactions

Family History

Family Members—Age and state of health (parents, siblings, grandparents, maternal and paternal aunts and uncles)

1. EENT—deafness, blindness, glaucoma, cataracts, myopia, strabismus, nosebleeds, sinus problems
2. Cardiovascular and respiratory—TB, asthma, hay fever, emphysema, hypertension, heart disease, strokes, rheumatic fever, anemia, leukemia
3. GI—ulcers, colitis, other problems
4. GU—kidney infections, kidney stones, bladder problems
5. Musculoskeletal—arthritis, multiple sclerosis, muscular dystrophy, congenital hip or foot problems, other problems
6. Neurologic—seizures, epilepsy, nervous disorder, mental retardation, learning disorders or problems
7. Chronic—diabetes, cancer, tumors, serious allergies, thyroid problems, birth defects, substance abuse
8. Miscellaneous—any other medical problem not mentioned

Psychosocial Family History

1. Education of parents
2. Occupation of parents
3. Living arrangements—type of housing, number of rooms, persons in household, sleeping arrangements, water supply tested?, proximity to playground, schools, transportation
4. Religious affiliation and/or philosophical outlook
5. Racial or ethnic background
6. Financial status, particularly method of payment for medical expense
7. Family crises or stress—recent death, divorce, separation, hospitalization, accidents, natural disasters
8. Family profile—how family members relate to each other, family activities, social outlet for members, support system, philosophy of parenting
9. Family's use of health care resources, attitudes and participation in preventive health
10. School and community involvement

Review of Body Systems

Pertinent Negatives Related to CC

1. General—overall state of health, ability to perform normal daily functions
2. Head—trauma, headaches, size, fontanelles
3. Eyes—redness, drainage, unusual movements, visual acuity, strabismus, cataracts, tearing, infections, photophobia
4. Ears—infections, drainage, hearing, care habits, ringing
5. Nose—drainage, congestion, bleeding, smelling ability, sinus pain
6. Mouth—condition of teeth, lesions on mouth or tongue, palate, condition of gums, pattern of dental care, odor
7. Speech and voice—hoarse, stridor, voice changes, articulation problems, fluency problems
8. Throat—frequent sore throats, tonsillitis
9. Neck—stiffness, masses, tenderness, goiter
10. Lymph—swollen nodes, tenderness, inflammation, pain
11. Breasts—discharge, masses, pain, self-examination pattern
12. Respiratory—cough, sputum, wheezing, dyspnea, pain, smoking, hemoptysis, stridor, pain, shortness of breath, pneumonia, other infections, cyanosis
13. Cardiac—exercise intolerance, pain, murmurs, cyanosis, syncopal episodes, hypertension
14. GI—appetite, swallowing difficulty, constipation, diarrhea, abdominal hernia, thirst, pain, jaundice, changes in bowel habits, food intolerances, nausea, vomiting, hemorrhoids
15. GU—urgency, frequency, dysuria, polyuria, nocturia, dribbling, enuresis, hematuria, STD, vaginal or penile drainage, menarche, menstrual history, pruritis, OB history
16. Musculoskeletal—pain, redness, swelling of joints, limitation of movement, fractures, edema
17. Skin—texture, lesions, bruising, petechiae, hair loss, dryness, itching, care habits

continued on next page

18. Neuro—seizures, ataxia, unconsciousness, loss of sensation, unusual movements as twitches or tremors, slow learning, clumsiness, memory loss

Current Health

Habits

1. Nutrition
   a. Diet—frequency of meals, amount and types of food
   b. Eating habits—likes and dislikes
   c. Vitamins—kind, how often, how much, iron, fluoride

2. Elimination
   a. Urine—frequency, color, odor, character of stream
   b. Bowel—frequency, character, and color of stools
   c. Toilet training—age, accidents, day or night

3. Sleep
   a. Difficulty putting to bed
   b. Hours
   c. Disturbances—nightmares, night terrors (if so, what does the parent do?)
   d. Day-time naps

Development

1. Client's view of development—how does child compare to siblings and peers? What can child do now?
2. Gross motor—timing of achieved major milestones (rolling over, walking, biking)
3. Fine motor—feeding self, writing, copying, coloring, using scissors, tying shoes
4. Language—words, vocabulary, articulation, fluency
5. Cognitive—general understanding level, curiosity, major interest in learning (not necessarily in school), academic performance, grades in school, concepts of sex and death
6. Social
   a. Emotions
   b. Temperament
   c. Trust and attachment to parents
   d. Independence in activities—feeding, toileting, hygiene; ability to entertain self; ability to go around neighborhood; ability to separate from parents; self-concept; self-control (management of impulses and feelings such as love, anger, aggression, fear, jealousy); social relationships with parents, siblings, peers; reaction to new situations; response to discipline, type of discipline; responsibilities; general interests and activities (indoors, outdoors); annoying or deviant behaviors (tantrums, lying, stealing, meanness, thumbsucking)

Sexual Understanding of Adolescents Birth control methods if appropriate

Environmental Factors

1. Pollutants—noise, air, chemical
2. Safety risks

underreferrals because children sometimes pass screening tests, even though they have the condition for which they are being tested. Therefore, it is most important when doing an assessment to perform screening tests accurately, repeat the tests at prescribed intervals, and record the results accurately to decrease the risk of false-positive and false-negative results.

Measurements

Because children grow rapidly, measurements of height, weight, and head circumference are significant. Failure or delay in any one of these parameters might be an early indicator of a serious problem, especially because failure in one area eventually affects the others.

Measurements of height, weight, and head circumference document the child's rate of growth and changes from previous examinations; therefore, they need to be taken periodically and plotted on a graph.

Height Height usually is measured at every well-child visit; the method used varies with the age of the child. Measuring the length of a young infant usually requires two people; one person secures the child's head as the child lies flat, and the other person extends the child's legs and marks the length between the head and heel. The distance is then measured using a metal or paper tape and recorded. Cloth

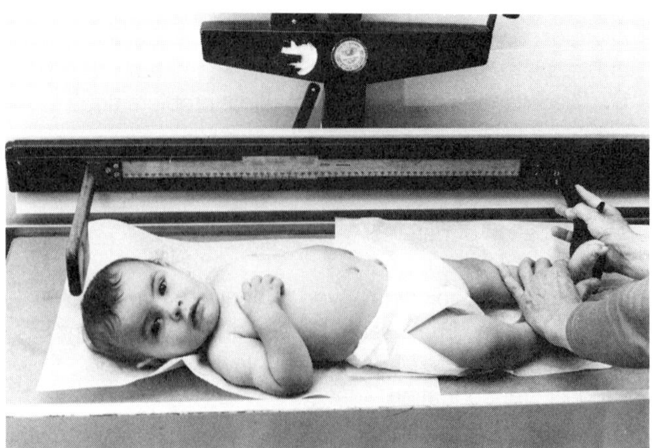

An infant's length is measured from crown of head to heels of feet, with legs fully extended. (From Kozier B, Erb G: *Techniques in Clinical Nursing*. Addison-Wesley, 1982.)

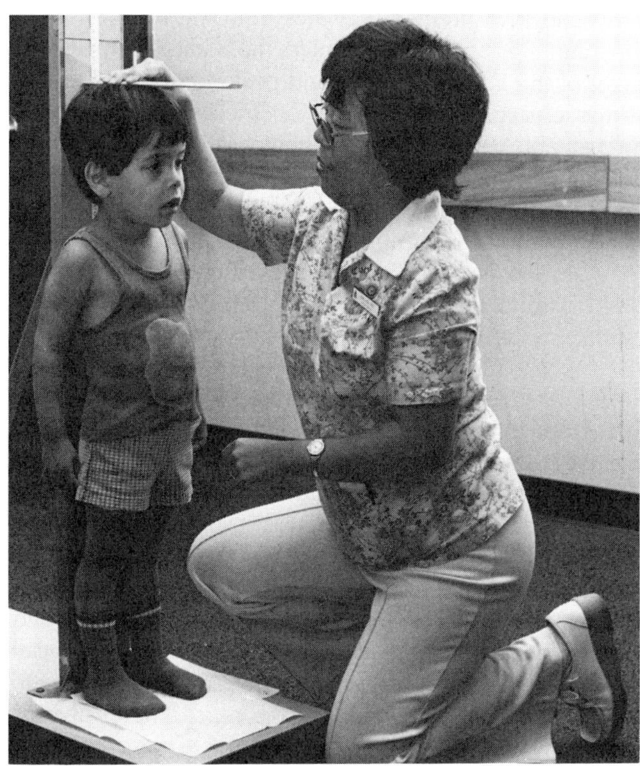

A child's height is measured by having the child stand straight, without shoes, and by placing the measuring marker on top of the child's head. (From Kozier B, Erb G: *Techniques in Clinical Nursing*. Addison-Wesley, 1982.)

tapes should not be used because they stretch. For older children who can stand, height measurement is easier and more accurate because they can be positioned on a standard scale. The child is instructed to stand straight and quietly in stocking or bare feet as the attached tape measure is placed on the top of the head. As a safety measure, the base of the scale should be against the wall, and the nurse should steady the scale as the child stands on it.

Height is generally a familial trait; therefore, a child who has tall parents and grandparents and is healthy and well nourished is likely to be tall. The height percentile at birth often remains the same throughout development. Short stature also is genetically determined, but abnormally short stature can be due to chronic illness such as heart or kidney disease, allergies, malnutrition, or growth hormone deficiencies.

Weight Weight is another important index of the child's general growth and nutritional status and is therefore measured at every well-child visit. Because sudden and often drastic fluctuations can occur, weight also should be checked at every sick-child visit.

Infants are weighed without any clothing, including diapers, on a balanced infant scale. The infant should be protected from direct contact with the scale by cloth or paper. Infants should be protected from falls and should not extend beyond the length of the scale. Young children who are walking usually can be weighed on the adult standing scale and should be weighed with all clothing removed except underpants. Older children can remain clothed but without shoes and be weighed on the standing scale.

As with height, the weight measurement is plotted on a growth chart (Appendix A). Weight generally follows the same percentile from one visit to the next, and any sudden decrease or increase should therefore be evaluated. The most common cause of a significant weight increase is obesity; endocrine disorders are rare, as are renal or cardiovascular dysfunction. Weight decrease usually is caused by chronic disease, acute infections, emotional problems, malnutrition, diabetes, and dehydration.

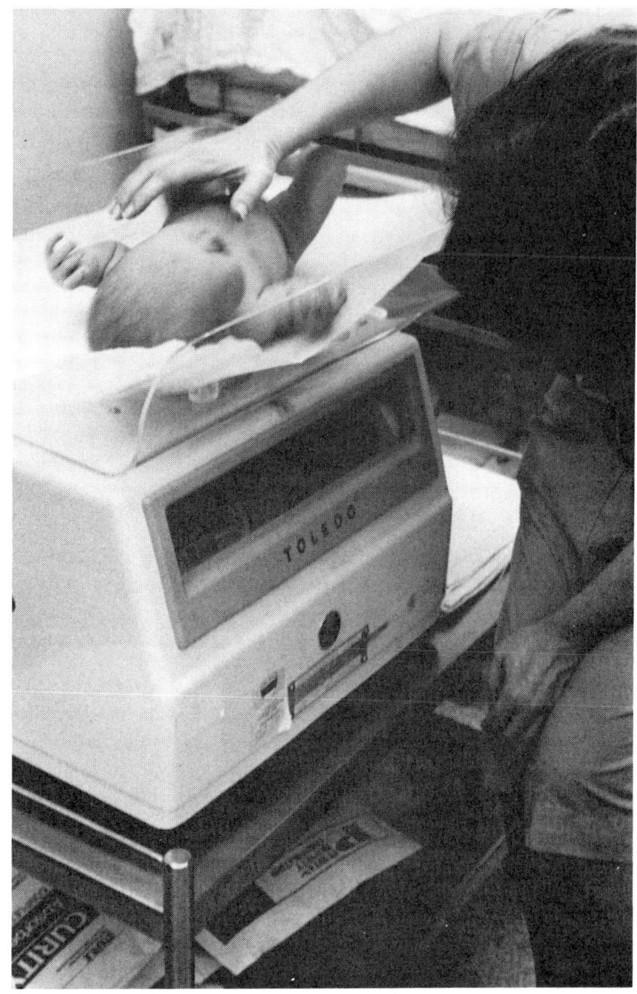

Infants are weighed on a draped balanced scale and are protected from falls at all times. (From Swearingen PL: *The Addison-Wesley Photo-Atlas of Nursing Procedures*. Addison-Wesley, 1983.)

Head Circumference Most health practitioners include head circumference measurements in every well-child visit from birth to 2 years of age, whereas some practitioners continue noting this measurement up to 3 years of age. Head circumference is documented in centimeters and often is recorded as "OFC" in children's health records to indicate occipital frontal circumference. Special conditions, such as failure to thrive, craniostenosis, and hydrocephalus, warrant more frequent head circumference measurements.

The most reliable method for obtaining the head circumference is to measure with a metal or paper tape three times and record the largest measurement on a head circumference graph (Appendix A). The tape should be held securely on the child's head over the forehead and the occipital protuberance. It should not cover the ears. Although it is often not possible, having the same practitioner measure the head circumference at every well-child visit further ensures accuracy.

In general, the neonate's head circumference is slightly larger than chest circumference, and this ratio is fairly constant until the child is 2 years old, when the chest circumference becomes greater than head circumference.

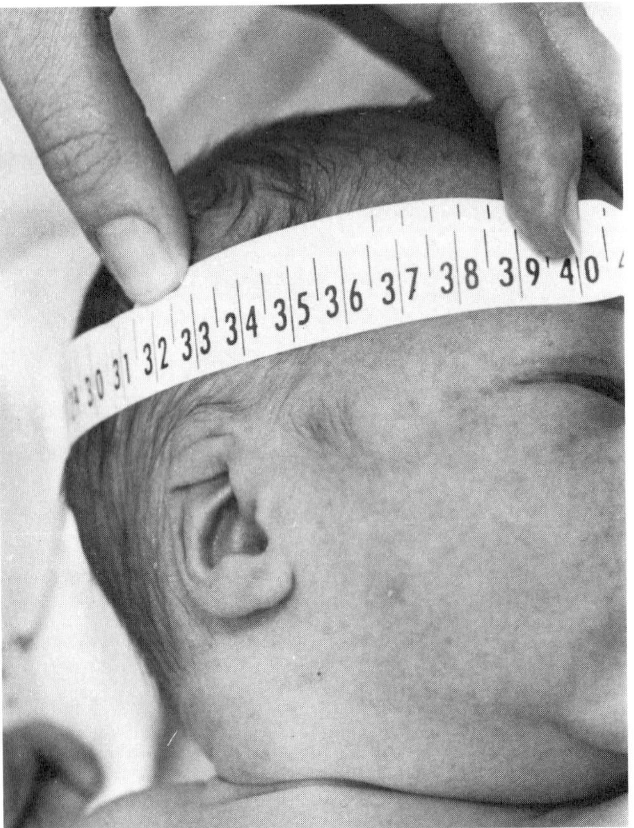

Head circumference is measured with a paper or metal tape held securely over the child's forehead and occipital protuberance. (From Swearingen PL: *The Addison-Wesley Photo-Atlas of Nursing Procedures*, Addison-Wesley, 1983.)

If head measurement deviates from the norm or from the infant's established percentile, the additional measurement of the infant's anterior and posterior fontanelles becomes crucial. At birth, both fontanelles and all sutures are palpable, and the anterior fontanelle is easily measured in centimeters on vertical and horizontal planes. The anterior fontanelle is 1–2 in across and closes at some time between 9 and 18 months of age. The posterior fontanelle may be closed at birth or closes by 3 months of age; it is one-fourth to one-half inch across. Premature or delayed closing can cause or indicate serious neurologic problems.

Vital Signs The frequency with which vital signs are assessed on well children varies from clinic to clinic, but most nurses follow general guidelines. Temperature might not necessarily be taken at every well-child visit during infancy but should be taken during the older child's annual physical examination. The choice of taking an oral, axillary, or rectal temperature depends on the child's age, cooperation, and general health. For example, infants usually have rectal temperatures taken while lying on their backs or sides with their legs gently restrained and the nurse's hand holding the thermometer. Older children also might have their temperatures taken rectally if there is any question of safety or if a health problem warrants this method. Generally, a 6-year-old can understand the procedure for oral temperature taking and can be trusted not to bite off the end of the thermometer. Axillary temperatures also are used when rectal and oral temperatures are contraindicated, as with diarrhea or rectal irritation. Recent research indicates that axillary temperature measurement might be as accurate as rectal measurement and might be preferable, both physically and psychologically (Barrus, 1983).

Pulse and respiration should be measured at every well-child visit because they directly indicate functioning of the cardiac and respiratory systems. The pulse should be auscultated in the apical area of the heart, palpated in the radial and femoral areas, and assessed for rate and rhythm. It often is necessary to assess the pulse in the femoral and dorsal pedal areas when there is a question of a cardiac vascular problem as, for example, in coarctation of the aorta. Femoral pulse is important for the young infant as a detection measure; the dorsal pedal pulse might not be easily felt. Pulses should be taken for a full minute.

The rate, rhythm, and depth of a child's respiratory pattern should be observed at every well-child visit and especially at sick-child visits. Infants and children should be observed and their respirations counted for a full minute with their upper clothing removed. Older, more cooperative children can be observed as they sit quietly on the examining table during examination of the chest and lungs.

Blood pressure also should be measured at every well-child visit because of the increased prevalence of hyper-

TABLE 14-2 Guidelines for Blood Pressure Cuff Selection

Age	Size
Neonate	2.5–3 cm
Infant	4–5 cm
1- to 4-year-old	6–7 cm
5- to 10-year-old	8–10 cm
10-year-old and older	10–12 cm

tension in children. The blood pressure cuff must be the correct size for the child. It should be 1.5 times the diameter of the part of the extremity to be measured or no less than one-half and no more than two-thirds of the part of the extremity to be measured (Table 14-2). If there is a family history of hypertension, cardiovascular disease, or atherosclerosis, some health practitioners routinely monitor the child's blood pressure from infancy with a Doppler.

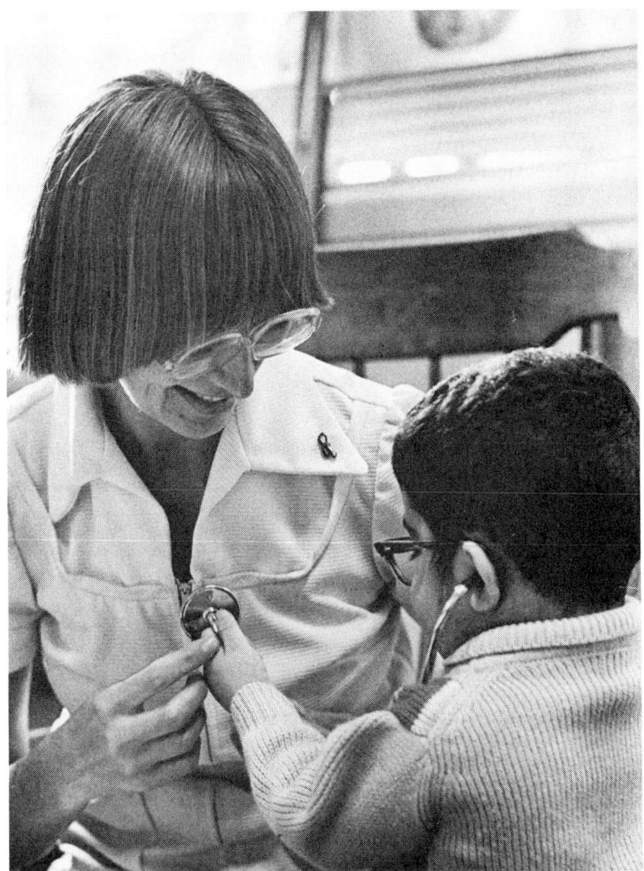

Children are less fearful if they are allowed to manipulate equipment before the nurse takes vital signs.

Laboratory Tests

Although the nurse's role in screening blood and urine tests varies from one setting to another, all nurses should be familiar with how these tests are performed, how specimens are obtained and tested, and how results are interpreted.

In ambulatory settings protocols for well-child visits usually involve hematocrit, hemoglobin, lead screen, urinalysis, and urine tests for culture and sensitivity as routine laboratory tests. Children who are at risk for sickle cell trait or disease, thalassemia, glucose-6-phosphate-dehydrogenase deficiency (G_6PD), or galactosemia are screened at the appropriate time, as determined by the characteristics of the potential disease and the reliability and validity of the screening test.

For screening, the blood and urine tests determine whether a child is within a normal range or whether intervention is required. For example, anemia in childhood may first only be detected through a routine hematocrit and hemoglobin check or a complete blood count. An asymptomatic urinary tract infection in a 4-year-old-girl would be detected through a routinely scheduled urine test for culture and sensitivity and treated before more serious upper urinary tract disease could occur. When obtained in conjunction with subjective and objective findings, laboratory tests used as screening aids or diagnostic tools provide comprehensive data.

Physical Examination

Adaptations for Children

The "systems approach," the head-to-toe physical assessment technique recommended for adults, is often not feasible with children, although its format is generally the outline used to document assessment findings. For children, the nurse's approach to assessment depends on the developmental and chronologic age of the child, the amount of stress and anxiety the child associates with the examination, the amount of trust developed in the nurse–child–parent relationship, and the child's state of health or illness.

The nurse must first consider these factors and then adjust the approach to fit the needs of the child and parent. Performing a physical assessment in a supportive, nonthreatening, and educative environment is an art that should be a nursing goal in providing comprehensive health care. A guide for approaching the pediatric client during physical assessment is provided in Table 14-3. Such a guide, however, is only a starting point for assessing the child's and parent's physical needs, cognitive understanding, and emotional functioning.

Those parts of the examination that require a quiet child, such as auscultation of the heart and lungs, should be done

TABLE 14-3 Approaches to Health Assessment During Childhood

Age	Preparation and Position	Sequence of Examination
Infancy (0–18 months)	In a warm examination room completely undress infant leaving only diaper on. Gain parent's cooperation in holding infant and keeping infant quiet and comfortable. For a young infant, examination can be done on parent's lap with infant supine or prone. As infant sits alone, examination can be done with child sitting on parent's lap or sitting on table with parent standing nearby. For uncooperative child, use appropriate restraints with the child lying on examination table.	With a quiet infant, begin with auscultation of heart, lungs, and abdomen. Palpate and percuss if infant remains relaxed. Proceed with a toe-to-head approach, examining each body system using gentle and then more invasive techniques. Terminate examination with the most traumatic procedures; such as examination of eyes, ears, and mouth (EENT). Neurologic assessment can be integrated into examination, left until the end, or done just before the EENT examination.
Early Childhood (18 months–$4\frac{1}{2}$ years)	During history interview with parent, have child become familiar with environment by having appropriate play toys available. Before examination begins, allow child to see, feel, and play with stethoscope and otoscope. If this increases anxiety, proceed as quickly as possible. Some children may not become unduly upset by getting completely undressed; others may do better by having articles of clothing removed as that body part is examined. It is usually best to have child's underpants on throughout the examination.	Begin to observe child playing in the room during the history interview. Much of the musculoskeletal and neurologic examination can be done by astute observation of the child in play. Inspect and palpate as much as possible by playing with the child. Auscultate heart, lungs, and abdomen. Then proceed in a toe-to-head approach, palpating and percussing all remaining body parts. All traumatic procedures (such as the EENT examination) should be left until the end.
Middle Childhood ($4\frac{1}{2}$–8 years)	These children often like to become involved and can be very cooperative when given responsibility for answering a few questions during history interview. It is usually best to let children undress themselves; leaving underpants on and putting on gown. *Briefly* explain each procedure while examining child, allowing child first to manipulate equipment if that seems to decrease anxiety. Younger children may still prefer to sit on parent's lap; older children may like to be examined sitting on table or standing next to parent.	This age group can be cooperative and allow examination to proceed in head-to-toe sequence, but it is often wise to leave ear and throat until the end.
Late Childhood (8–12 years)	Older children usually do not mind getting undressed but often prefer to be left alone in the room to do so. Gowns should be provided; and child usually prefers to keep underwear on. If females have begun to wear bras, these can be removed as the breast examination is to be done. Children of this age like to have everything explained to them and should be encouraged to be involved in the history interview and examination as much as possible. Some children prefer that their parents remain in the room; others (especially preadolescents) may prefer having their parents wait outside. It is best to discuss this with both parent and child.	Examination usually can proceed in head-to-toe sequence, with examination of the genitalia done at the end. If a neurodevelopmental exam is to be done, then that is best done at the beginning of the process. Health education should be incorporated into appropriate sections by discussing knowledge of health behaviors (for example, skin care, diet, sports injuries, sexual development).
Adolescents (12–19 years)	Adolescents require privacy in undressing and in being examined. Often parents wait outside during the examination and sometimes during the history interview but both the adolescent and parent should meet with the clinician together to discuss appropriate health issues. Usually, adolescents are familiar with the equipment and procedures. Most important to them is the immediate feedback of the exam results. They like to know that everything is "normal."	Examination proceeds in head-to-toe sequence with genitalia usually left until the end, although some female adolescents often like to have the pelvic examination (if one is to be done) first. They should always be asked for their preference. Health education should be included. Adolescents are often receptive to anticipatory guidance on such issues as sexual maturity, drugs, and school behaviors.

first with infants and young children who are initially cooperative. The nurse then proceeds from the least traumatic procedures, engaging the child in the examination as much as possible. Adequate preparation increases the child's sense of security; for example, providing time for the child to manipulate stethoscopes and switch the "flashlight" of the otoscope on and off can ensure a quick and efficient examination later on.

Combining knowledge, skill, and sensivity to the child's and parent's physical and emotional needs, the nurse can execute a complete physical appraisal. Enlisting the help of the parent is of utmost importance, but respecting the parent's needs is also crucial. Therefore, although it might be best to have the parent help to gently restrain the child's head for an ear examination, the child's behavior might make the parent anxious, and it might be best to enlist the help of a colleague. For the 1- to 2-year-old, the entire examination often is best performed while the child sits on the parent's lap.

When a child is ill or in pain, the nurse assesses the healthy body systems first and then proceeds to the areas associated with the health problem. For example, a child whose history documents a potential ear infection should have chest and lungs evaluated first to rule out respiratory involvement before the more traumatic and possibly painful otoscopic exam.

Whenever the nurse's assessment findings deviate from the normal or expected findings, referral is made to the physician for further evaluation.

Physical examination uses four assessment skills: (1) inspection; (2) palpation; (3) percussion; and (4) auscultation. Details of these techniques are presented in Table 14-4.

General Appearance

The physical examination should begin with an overall impression of the child. This is a cumulative, subjective impression of the child's physical appearance, nutritional status, and such behavioral and developmental parameters as the degree of activity, gait, posture, coordination, and emotional state.

Physical appearance usually includes a description of the child's facial expression because it may give clues about a child who is in pain, extremely frightened, or happy. Symmetry and coordination of body movement also are noted, with attention to posture and types of body movement. A child might favor a painful body part, and movements might be stiff and awkward. A child who is fearful might not physically interact with the environment, whereas a secure, happy child might play freely with the available toys or sit in a straight, upright, well-balanced posture.

Also important is the child's state of cleanliness or hygiene. The condition of the child's hair, nails, skin, teeth, and feet can give clues to the home environment. Appropriateness of dress can indicate the parent's knowledge of children's needs, as well as the family's financial resources.

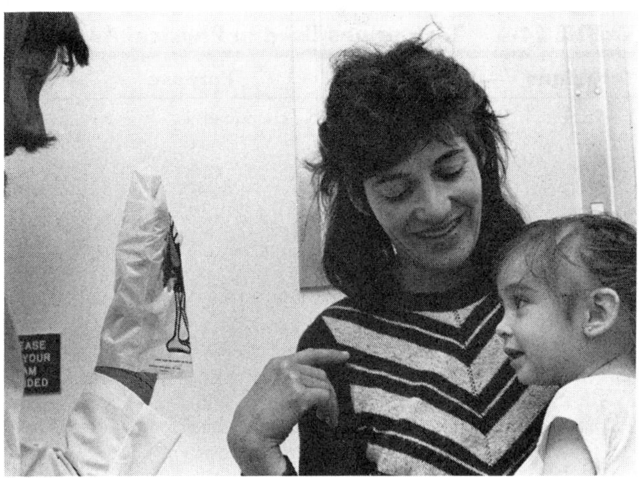

With adequate preparation and the help of the parent, the nurse can gain the child's cooperation during the examination.

General appearance also should include an impression of the child's nutritional status. The nurse observes body size and shape, noting the relationship between the child's height and weight. The nurse's impression of the child's nutritional state should be compared with the parent's history of feeding practices; any discrepancy may be an indication for nutritional counseling. (Nutritional assessment is discussed in Chapter 15.)

An assessment of the child's behavior and elements of the child's personality encompasses the child's activity level, interactions with others, and response to new situations. These data are documented as part of general appearance but are part of a larger developmental assessment (see Chapter 16).

A complete developmental assessment should be included as part of every health assessment for well-child care, but general developmental impressions guide the nurse in sequencing the physical examination and provide clues to specific systems that might need further testing. For example, a statement recorded about general appearance might be, "cooperative, smiling 3-year-old, well developed, well nourished, playing with toys, in no acute distress."

Skin

Skin is an important part of the physical assessment because a change in this system can be a response to changes in the external bodily environment. The skin protects the deeper tissues from injury and the invasion of antigens, regulates body temperature, provides an avenue for excretion, and is involved in sensations of touch, heat, or cold. Physical assessment of the skin involves evaluating the skin's ability to perform these functions. Skin is assessed systematically

TABLE 14-4 Techniques Used in Physical Assessment

Technique	Purpose	Comments
Inspection	Evaluation of visible characteristics	First step in assessment Adequate exposure of area inspected and good direct lighting necessary Nurse uses eyes to examine thoroughly and unhurriedly the area inspected, may also use senses of smell and hearing Most valuable but most difficult to learn; requires sensitivity and keen observations Each body part inspected for color, tone, texture, firmness, masses, hair distribution, movement, and symmetry
Palpation	Hands used to touch or feel area being assessed for temperature, texture, vibration, size, or position Light palpation is gentle pressure applied with the fingertips or palms Deep palpation is firm pressure applied with the fingertips to evaluate organs within the abdomen; deeper palpation is achieved by placing the fingers of one hand over the fingers of the hand that is palpating Ballottement is application of pressure by tapping or bouncing of several fingers to note pressure within an organ (for example, ocular pressure) or rebound tenderness (for example, of the abdomen or specific organ)	Temperature (for example, of the skin) assessed best with the dorsum of the fingers Texture, size, or position (for example, texture of the hair, size or position of an organ or mass) best assessed with palmar surface of the fingertips; also assessed are moisture, consistency, pressure (for example, pulses) form, and movement Vibration or pulsation (for example, air or sound moving through the lungs or cardiac thrills) assessed best with the palms Validates visual impression used to assess organs, glands, bones, muscles, hair, skin, and mucosa The child must be relaxed to assess adequately internal organs. Tight, tense muscles act as a barrier
Percussion	Rapping motion used to determine the density of an area assessed or the borders of a specific organ Blunt or direct percussion done by striking the surface assessed with a partially flexed finger (usually the middle finger) Bimanual or indirect percussion accomplished by placing the middle finger of one hand on the surface to be percussed (other fingers should not rest on the surface to be percussed as this will diminish the sound created by percussion); the middle finger or index and middle fingers of the other hand strike the middle finger resting on the body surface on the upper phalange; only the very tip(s) of the striking finger(s) used	Direct percussion used most often to percuss the nasal sinuses or tendons or inflamed organs; indirect percussion used to percuss any area of the body Percussion sounds include resonance, hyperresonance, tympany, dullness, flatness (see Table 14-9)
Auscultation	Listening to or studying sounds arising from organs through the direct contact of the ear on the body surface over the organ or, more commonly, with the aid of a stethoscope The diaphragm (flat side) of the stethoscope picks up high-frequency sounds and is used for auscultation of most organs Bell (curved or cupped side) of the stethoscope when applied lightly picks up low-frequency sounds such as heart murmurs	Done over the lungs, heart, and abdomen to determine the functional status of these organs; the skull, thyroid gland, and carotid arteries are auscultated for bruits (swishing sounds) Requires concentration, listening to only one sound at a time, disregarding all others; then systematically proceeding from one area to another

through inspection and palpation for color and pigmentation, turgor, moisture, texture, temperature, sensitivity, and the presence of any lesions. Hair, nails, and mucous membranes also are included in this assessment.

The skin is examined generally as a whole to assess the client's overall condition, then specifically as each body part is examined. For example, as the head and face are examined, the skin also is assessed, first by general inspection of the area, then more specifically as the scalp and areas of the face are assessed. Although the skin is assessed throughout the complete examination, the findings are recorded under one heading for skin.

Color and Pigmentation Skin color varies from whitish-pink to shades of brown depending on race; within a specific race, color variations are found. Dark-skinned children, such as those of American black, native American, Mexican, Mediterranean, Latin, or Asian descent, have various pigmentations from brown to red, bluish, and olive-green skin tones. For example, Oriental children may appear

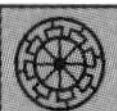

CASE STUDY Multiple Ecchymoses

Assessment

Mark, 3 years old, was brought to the clinic by his mother for evaluation of his growth and development. His mother reports that although small for his age, Mark is a very strong-willed, active child, more so than his older siblings were at this age. He seems to "get into everything" and "doesn't pay attention to where he is walking."

Family

Mark, his parents, and his older siblings recently moved into the area. Father is a salesman; mother is a homemaker. All family members are healthy and generally get along well with each other. Maternal and paternal grandparents were all short, ranging from 4 ft 10 in to 5 ft 7 in.

Child

Mark sits quietly on his mother's lap and plays with some toys. His mother comments that in the past several months he has been learning to ride a tricycle and most recently has been learning to climb the ladder apparatus on the side of his swing set.

Environment

The family owns its own home, and Mark has his own room. The yard is fenced, and, according to his mother, Mark has an abundance of toys but prefers to play imaginative games with a parent.

Clinical Data

Physical Assessment Data Mark's physical examination is within normal limits in all areas including a detailed neurologic assessment. He is small for his age, but his growth is steady along the tenth percentile. His general health is good. Mark has, however, many small ecchymotic (less than 1 cm) areas on both legs, and there are two larger (2 cm) ecchymotic areas on his right forearm. There are no other skin lesions, petechiae, lacerations, or abrasions. According to his mother, Mark seldom complains about his bumps when he collides with furniture or falls. His mother has not noted any injuries that seem to bleed for a long time.

Laboratory Data Routine complete blood count is within low normal range (hemoglobin 12 mg/ml and hematocrit 34%). Serum lead level is 20 (normal < 40).

Comparison to Standard

Mark appears to be a busy, curious, imaginative young boy with multiple bruises from his physical activities. It is important, however, to rule out blood dyscrasias and hemolytic problems and to validate the relation of activity to bruising.

Nursing Diagnoses

1. Potential alteration in health related to multiple ecchymotic areas
2. Potential alteration in family process related to the mother's concern about Mark's "being different"

Plan for Interventions

Goals

1. Mark's growth and development will progress without incident and be supported by family
2. Mother will adapt her expectations of Mark's behavior to that of his personality

Interventions

1. Refer to physician for further evaluation and possible laboratory studies related to bruising
2. Discuss with Mark's mother that his bruises are normal for an active, imaginative boy
3. Reassure parent that height is inherited and that this probably accounts for Mark's short stature
4. Discuss aspects of normal growth and development and differences in temperament among children
5. Allow mother to express her concerns about Mark's being "different" from his older siblings
6. Encourage mother to set some limits on Mark's physical activities by planning quiet-time activities, such as reading to him

jaundiced, as compared with white children, because of the yellow pigmentation of their skin. Black children may have a normal bluish pigmentation to their gums, buccal mucosa, and nail beds. In making an accurate assessment, the nurse therefore considers the amount of melanin genetically inherited among children of different races. If the child looks different from the parent, the nurse asks about the other parent.

Skin color also changes in response to the body's adjustment to heat and cold. Children may seem to have a reddish pigmentation when they are flushed from *hyperthermia* (raised body temperature). *Hypothermia* (lowered body temperature), which may be caused by excessive exposure to cold, can cause a child to look abnormally pale. In this situation it can be difficult to determine whether this pallor is temporary and due to cold or caused by a more serious nutritional anemia. Edema also decreases the skin tone and sometimes produces a false pallor. Skin color therefore is most reliably assessed in a well-illuminated, temperature-regulated room. The color of the examining room is impor-

ke a white child appear slightly jaun- ake the child appear slightly cyanotic. pects a change in skin color, the best is to assess those areas of the body where the ast melanin is produced: the sclera, conjunctiva, lips, palate, nail beds, and mucous membranes. Pallor and cyanosis are most readily evident in these areas. *Pallor,* or paleness due to a decrease in hemoglobin content, might be a sign of anemia, chronic disease, or shock. In white-skinned persons, pallor is a loss of pink coloring; in black-skinned persons the skin becomes ash-gray. *Cyanosis,* or bluish discoloration, caused by reduced hemoglobin in the capillaries, can result from cardiac disease, respiratory decompensation, or excessive exposure to cold. *Erythema,* or redness of the skin, might be caused by local infection, systemic infection, sunburn, skin irritation, or allergy. The degree of erythema reflects the amount of increased blood flow to the area. Erythema should be described by its location, size, presence or absence of warmth, type of distribution (diffuse or circumscribed), and the presence or absence of lesions.

Jaundice, or yellowish color, which is caused by an increase in bilirubin, is seen in the skin of children with hemolytic blood disease or liver disease. Jaundice must be differentiated from skin that is yellowish due to *carotenemia,* an excessive intake of vitamin A. The skin should be inspected for *hyperpigmentation* (abnormally increased pigmentation) or *hypopigmentation* (abnormally decreased pigmentation). If either condition is present, the abnormality should be described according to its location, size, and the involvement of surrounding areas. Hyperpigmentation is associated with Addison's disease, during pregnancy, or in hyperthyroidism. Hypopigmentation is seen in children with *vitiligo,* the absence of melanin.

Turgor Tissue turgor refers to the amount of elasticity and recoil in the skin. It is one of the best indications of nutrition and hydration in children. Normal skin turgor is elastic and taut. It is assessed by grasping the skin on the abdomen, pulling it up and taut, and quickly releasing it. Skin with good turgor resumes its normal shape without residual marks. Depending on the amount of dehydration or malnutrition, the skin will maintain its pinched shape or fall back slowly onto the abdomen. Other causes of poor or decreased skin turgor are muscle disorders, excessive exposure to ultraviolet rays, and chronic disease.

Both pitting and nonpitting edema are caused by excessive retention of water in the body tissues and should be evaluated with turgor. Edema is identified by pressing a thumb over the body surface that appears edematous. After releasing the finger, any sign of indentation that lasts several seconds indicates *pitting edema*; puffiness that does not remain indented is *nonpitting edema.* Edema often is seen in the periorbital area of the face when it is due to crying, sleeping, allergies, or kidney disease. *Dependent edema,* seen in the buttocks and lower extremities, often indicates kidney or cardiac anomalies. The nurse therefore assesses the symmetry of the edema in the corresponding body part and the color of the edematous area.

Moisture Normal skin is subtly moist. Any increase in moisture is seen as clamminess or perspiration; any decrease in moisture, evidenced by dry, parchment-like skin, should be evaluated. The nurse palpates all areas of the skin, assessing any variations in moisture from one body area to another. Dry skin only on the hands, lips, or genitalia may indicate a contact dermatitis, whereas generalized dry skin may indicate poor nutrition, overexposure to the sun, or overbathing.

Texture Inspection and palpation of the skin for texture assesses the quality and character of the skin surface. Normally, children's skin is smooth, not oily or clammy, and of even temperature. Skin that is rough and dry might indicate an endocrine problem or might be the result of overbathing, overexposure to the weather, or poor hygiene.

Flaky skin or scaling between the fingers or toes might be a sign of a fungal infection, dermatitis, eczema, or inflammation of the skin that may cause scaling on the extensor and flexor surfaces of the arms (elbows) and legs (knees), cheeks, and behind the ears. Seborrheic dermatitis ("cradle cap") is seen as oily, scaly patches on the scalp or along the hairline. Skin texture should be assessed for the crackling sensation seen in children with subcutaneous emphysema. Any marks or scars are palpated and the surface characteristics recorded. Some children may form excessive scar tissue, called *keloid,* which is palpated as a raised, hypertrophied scar.

Temperature Palpation of the skin to evaluate temperature is best done by symmetrically feeling each body part and comparing each side with the other and upper with lower body parts. Localized hyperthermia might be the result of a burn or infection and indicates an increased blood flow to the area. Generalized hyperthermia might be the result of fever, sunburn, or a brain disorder. Localized hypothermia might be caused by peripheral arterial sclerosis or from inadequate clothing for climatic conditions. Children in shock often have generalized hypothermia.

Sensitivity In assessing the sensitivity of a child's skin, the nurse needs to rely on both nonverbal and verbal clues to the child's discomfort. Any body area that has abnormal findings for color, turgor, texture, and temperature is assessed for pain or abnormal sensations such as burning, itching, tingling, or throbbing. If possible, the child should describe the feeling. Otherwise, the nurse documents the child's nonverbal responses while palpating sensitive areas. Children typically protect a painful area or pull away from the nurse, cry, or fuss.

TABLE 14.5 Common Childhood Skin Lesions

Primary Lesion	Description
Macule	Flat, circumscribed, usually smaller than 1 cm; color differs from surrounding skin, seen in rubella, scarlet fever rubeola
Papule	Raised, solid, sharply circumscribed small (0.5 cm to 1 cm in diameter) and colored in various shades of pink to red, seen in rosea and psoriasis
Nodule	Small (1–2 cm), solid, in dermal layer of skin or subcutaneous tissue; one example is dermatofibroma
Tumor	Solid, larger than 1–2 cm, soft or hard consistency, may lie deep in tissues
Wheal	Circumscribed, flat-topped, relatively transient with irregularly shaped borders, seen in allergic reactions, hives, insect bites
Cyst	Nontender, fluid-filled mass, may be ganglion or tumor
Vesicle	Small, less than 0.5–1 cm in diameter, circumscribed, elevated, fluid-filled, seen in herpes simplex, herpes zoster, poison ivy, varicella
Bullae	Larger than a 1-cm vesicle, seen in second-degree burns or on soles and palms in scarlet fever
Pustule	Vesicle that contains purulent exudate seen in acne, impetigo, and staphylococcal infections

Secondary Lesion	Description
Scales	Thin flakes of exfoliated epidermia seen in psoriasis, seborrhea, and tinea capitis
Crusts	Dried serum, blood, or purulent exudate seen in eczema, impetigo
Excoriation	Mechanical removal of the epidermis; one example is a scratch mark or scrape
Erosion	Moist, often-depressed lesion from loss of the superficial epidermis, seen as a result of chickenpox
Ulcer	Deeper loss of skin surface often to dermis and subcutaneous layers; examples include decubitus ulcer and syphilitic chancre
Fissure	Deep, linear cleavage extending into the dermis, seen in fungal infection such as athlete's foot
Lichenification	Thickened and roughened skin with increased visibility of skin furrows, seen in atopic dermatitis or as a sequela to eczema
Atrophy	Thinning of skin
Scar	Dense connective tissue resulting from destruction and healing of skin
Keloid	Hypertrophied scar
Striae	Pale, white, thin stripes, although purple during initial stretching, seen in rapid gain and/or loss of weight and in pregnancy

Lesions Any lesion noted on the skin is described in detail for size, shape, color, location, surface characteristics, anatomic distribution, and morphologic features. Lesions are classified as primary, secondary, and vascular. *Primary lesions* arise from previously healthy normal skin and are the initial lesions in a disease process. They may begin as a color change to the skin, as a macule or nonraised lesion. Other primary lesions involve the skin, such as solid masses of various sizes and shapes, papules (raised lesions), nodules, or fluid-filled masses such as vesicles, bullae, and pustules.

Secondary lesions result from changes in primary lesions. They may be caused by loss of skin from erosions, ulcers, or fissures or deposits on the skin, such as crusts and scales, or they may fall into a separate category of secondary lesions caused by lichenification, atrophy, excoriation, scars, and keloids.

Vascular lesions are intravascular, as in cherry angiomas, spider angiomas, or venus stars, or extravascular, as in petechiae and ecchymoses. Vascular lesions also are seen in the neonate at birth or shortly thereafter; these include the port-wine stain (nevus flammeus), hemangioma simplex (strawberry mark), infantile hemangioma (stork-bite mark), and cavernous hemangioma. Cafe-au-lait spots and nevi also should be assessed, and referral for further evaluation is warranted if lesions are numerous or extensively involve the body surfaces. Table 14-5 lists the skin lesions and describes them according to size, shape, color, surface characteristics, and morphologic features.

Hair A child's hair covers the entire body except the palms and soles, inner surfaces of the labia in girls, and inner surfaces of the prepuce and glans penis in boys. Hair is assessed for distribution, color, texture, amount, and quality. Children's scalp hair is usually soft, pliable, shiny, and strong. The scalp hair should be inspected for cleanliness and for lice. Genetic factors affect a child's hair and are

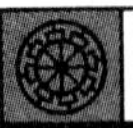

CASE STUDY Diaper Dermatitis

Assessment

Family

Katy, four months old, is brought to the clinic by her mother for a routine well-child visit. Mother appears competent but insecure regarding infant care and anxiously comments about noticing a "rash" on Katy's buttocks that has become progressively worse. She changes Katy's diapers frequently and thoroughly cleanses the diaper area with warm water and a mild soap.

Child

Mother reports Katy urinates six or seven times a day and has soft stools two to three times a day. No history of loose stools. Urine does not have a particularly strong or offensive odor. Katy is breast fed and does not receive any supplements. Mother has been using disposable diapers.

Clinical Data

Physical Assessment Data Katy's perineum and buttocks are fiery red; redness extends into her inguinal area and along her umbilicus. There is a diffuse scattering of macules and papules over the area with clusters of papules in the skin folds of the inguinal area and along the demarcating borders of the rash. There is no evidence of pustules. Katy's physical examination otherwise is normal. She is growing along the fiftieth percentile and appears to be developmentally on time.

Laboratory Data None

Nursing Diagnosis

1. Alteration in skin integrity
2. Potential for secondary skin infection in afflicted areas related to unresolved, chronic diaper rashes causing changes in epidermal layers of the skin

Plan for Intervention

Goals

1. Katy's diaper rash will resolve
2. Katy will have no evidence of superimposed skin infection

Interventions

1. Encourage mother to continue appropriate skin cleansing
2. Encourage use of cloth diapers that have been presoaked and washed in mild soap or detergent
3. Discuss reasons for not using rubber or plastic pants over diapers
4. Suggest using absorbent lap pad when holding Katy
5. Discuss keeping Katy's buttocks exposed to air and sunlight as often as possible
6. Discuss increasing Katy's fluid intake by adding a 4 oz ½-strength apple juice bottle during acute phase of diaper rash
7. Discuss findings with pediatrician so antifungal ointment prescription can be written
8. Discuss how to apply ointment in a thin layer over all afflicted skin surfaces three times a day after the skin has been cleansed and well dried
9. Have mother telephone in three to four days to report if there are or are not noticeable effects from prescribed regimen
10. Inform Katy's mother that the diaper rash should begin to respond to skin cleansing and medication in that time with complete resolution within ten days
11. Advocate that mother continue modified regimen to protect Katy from repeat of the diaper rash

---

responsible for curliness or coarseness, as well as color and distribution. Some dark-skinned children have hairlines that normally extend down the neck and below the midforehead; this familial trait should be noted because children with cretinism might exhibit a similar hair pattern. Hair that is dry, brittle, fragile, or depigmented might indicate a nutritional deficiency. Loss of hair, or *alopecia,* might be caused by tinea capitis, hair pulling, or the child's lying in the same position for an extended period of time.

Other types of hair that should be evaluated in addition to head hair include body hair, beard hair, axillary hair, and pubic hair. Eyebrows, eyelashes, and any hair on the face should be evaluated. Chest, axillary, and pubic hair should be evaluated as part of the assessment of the development of secondary sexual characteristics. The spine and buttocks should be inspected for hair tufts, which might be seen in children with spina bifida.

Nails Nails are examined for color, shape, and condition. Such characteristics as clubbing of digits, curving, and spooning of nails are noted. Clubbing often is seen in children with congenital heart disease or chronic respiratory disease. Convex or concave curving might be hereditary or due to injury, poor nutrition, or infection. Cuticles should be assessed for intactness and smoothness, noting any signs of infection. The nurse also notes any evidence of nail biting, skin picking, or thumb sucking.

Lymph Nodes

The lymphatic system—with its intricate network of capillaries that collect lymph from organs and tissues, collecting vessels that carry lymph to the bloodstream, and lymph nodes that act as filters for the collecting vessels—is a major contributor to the immunologic and metabolic processes of the body (Fig. 14-1). The lymphatic system is involved in the formation of macrophages and lymphocytes and in the process of phagocytosis. As such, it indicates (1) local or systemic infection or inflammation; (2) disorders in metabolism; (3) metastatic cancer; (4) hypersensitivity reactions; and (5) homeostatic dysfunctions related to the cleaning of debris and red blood cell hemolysis.

In the physical examination of lymph nodes, the nurse assesses the presence or absence of *lymphadenopathy* (disease process involving the lymph nodes) because a large lymph node or generalized lymphadenopathy may be the first sign of disease. Lymph nodes are found in clusters or chains; they seldom occur singly. They are either in the subcutaneous connective tissue (*superficial lymph nodes*) or are beneath muscular fascia and in body cavities (*deep lymph nodes*). Table 14-6 summarizes important information concerning each lymphatic system chain. Lymph nodes are evaluated as the part of the body in which they are located is assessed.

Lymph nodes are palpated with the distal portion of the fingers (fingerpads) by gently but firmly pressing in a circular, rotary motion along the regions in which lymph nodes are normally present. In the examination of the cervical area, it is often easier to have the child tilt the head 10–20° toward the side being examined. Children are often ticklish and might need to be distracted to prevent them from hindering the examination by becoming rigid. Nodes in the axillas are best palpated with the child's arms relaxed and slightly adducted. Epitrochlear nodes are best examined with the child's arms slightly flexed; the popliteal nodes are best palpated with the child's knees bent at a 40° angle to relax the tendons and muscles.

Lymph nodes palpated during the examination are described and assessed by noting the following characteristics:

1. *Location*—specify the exact chain palpated
2. *Skin*—palpable nodes in children are often normal, and nodes 3 mm to 1 cm in size, especially in cervical and

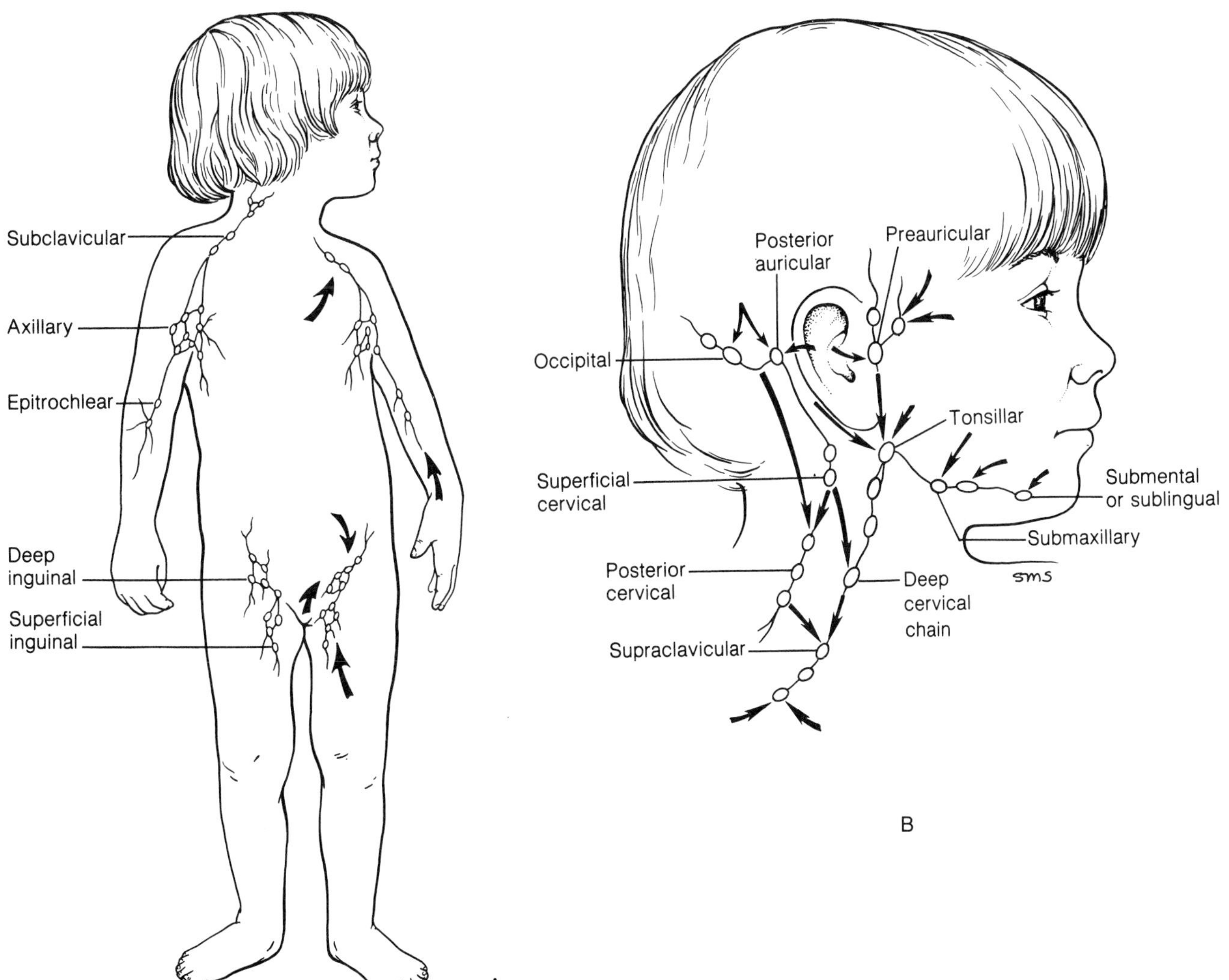

Figure 14-1 *A.* Location of lymph nodes. *B.* Direction of flow of lymph.

TABLE 14-6 Lymphatic System

Chain	Location	Areas Drained	Clinical Significance of Enlargement
Occipital	At nape of neck (lower occipital bone)	Occipital region of scalp	Pediculosis, seborrhea, tick bites, chickenpox, rubella, external otitis, scalp lesions
Posterior auricular	Mastoid, behind ear	Posterior part of temporoparietal region, pinna, posterior part of external acoustic meatus, scalp, facial skin	Rubella, skin lesions in area drained, external otitis, chickenpox, pediculosis
Preauricular	Directly in front of ear (anterior to tragus), temporal	Face, eye, lateral surface	Lesions of the eyelids (chalazions), conjunctivitis, infectious skin disorders of the face
Superficial cervical	Chain over sternocleidomastoid muscle at upper section of neck superficially	Tongue, tonsils, pinna, parotid scalp, neck, thorax	Scalp infections, pediculosis, lesions in areas drained, scarlet fever
Deep cervical (jugular)	Begins with tonsillar node at the angle of jaw and continues under sternocleidomastoid muscle, ending posterior to this muscle in supraclavicular chain	Most of tongue, tonsils, pinna, parotid, oropharynx, nose, paranasal sinuses, palate, larynx, trachea, esophagus, middle ear	Tonsillitis, pharyngitis, thyroid disease, inflammatory process of areas drained, scarlet fever
Submaxillary (submandibular)	Beneath body of mandible midway between chin and ear	Medial conjunctiva, cheek, side of nose, upper lip, lateral part of lower lip, gums, submaxillary gland, anterior margin of tongue	Stomatitis, conjunctivitis
Submental	Beneath chin	Central portions of lower lip, floor of mouth, apex of tongue	Dental infections
Tonsillar	The first of the deep cervical chain at angle between ear and jaw	Mouth, pharynx, principal node for tonsil	Tonsillitis, pharyngitis
Parotid	Parotid gland; lateral wall of pharynx at junction of mandible and maxilla; occasionally in subcutaneous tissue over parotid gland	Parotid gland, tissues of face, root of nose, tympanic cavity, eyelids, frontotemporal region, external auditory canal	Parotitis, mumps, tumors
Supraclavicular	Directly over medial area of clavicle	Head, abdomen, breast, thorax, arm, lung	May be first node enlarged with Hodgkin's disease
Posterior cervical	Along anterior border of trapezium muscle	Scalp and neck	Pediculosis, scalp infections
Infraclavicular	Below clavicle	Breast, anterior thoracic wall	Breast cancer, infection
Lateral axillary	Along head of humerus	Entire arm except that which drains into epitrochlear	Infection or disease of hand, arm
Central axillary	Adipose tissue of central axilla at base	Arm, breast, anterior and posterior thoracic wall, lateral, posterior and anterior axillary nodal groups	Infection or disease of arm, chest, breast
Subscapular (posterior axillary)	Posterior wall of axilla fossa and lateral edge of scapulae	Skin and muscles of neck and thoracic wall	Infections or disease of skin of neck and thorax
Pectoral (anterior axillary)	Lateral border of pectoralis minor	Anterior and lateral thoracic wall and breast	Infection or disease of thorax or breast
Subclavicular (medial)	Superior to and posterior to pectoralis minor	Upper portion of breast, other axillary nodes	Disease or infection of breast or other areas drained by axillary nodes
Epitrochlear	Medial aspect of inner elbow just above medial epicondyle of the humerus	Ulnar surface of forearm; little, middle, and ring finger; medial portions of the hand	Arm, hand, finger infection, congenital syphilis, cat scratch disease

TABLE 14.6 continued

Chain	Location	Areas Drained	Clinical Significance of Enlargement
Horizontal inguinal	Parallels inguinal ligament, runs diagonally towards perineum	External genitalia (excluding testes), perineum, glutei, abdominal wall below umbilicus, anus	Infections of perineum or genitalia, STD, lice, diaper rash
Vertical inguinal	Runs vertically at upper, inner aspect of the thigh	Drains most of the leg and buttocks and aspects drained from horizontal inguinal	Infections of legs, feet, genitalia, anus, STD, lice, diaper rash
Popliteal	Popliteal fossa	Drains areas of muscles, joints and tendons of knee and leg, feet	Infections of knee joint and heel and lateral aspect of posterior half of foot

SOURCE: Adapted from Alexander M, Brown M: *Pediatric History Taking and Physical Diagnosis for Nurses.* McGraw-Hill, 1979.

inguinal areas, commonly are seen in healthy children. These small nodes are called "shotty nodes" and usually indicate past infections. Past respiratory infections will cause shotty nodes in the cervical area; a resolved diaper rash may be the cause of palpable nodes in the inguinal area

3. *Surface characteristics*—palpable nodes are evaluated for smoothness, nodularity, or irregularity

4. *Consistency and symmetry*—nodes are described as firm, soft, spongy, cystic, round, or oval

5. *Mobility or fixation*—nodes are noted as feeling attached or unattached to underlying fascia

6. *Heat, tenderness, erythema*—nodes are rated as warm to the touch, painful, and red

Whereas shotty, nontender, firm, mobile nodes are a sign of a resolved past infection, a warm, reddened, frequently tender, enlarged node signals a current infection. This inflammation of the lymph nodes, or *lymphadenitis,* is due to an infectious process, either viral, bacterial, or fungal. It needs to be differentiated from acute *lymphangitis,* which is an infection of the lymph vessels themselves and involves pain and redness in the affected area.

Common childhood diseases that cause lymphadenopathy are rubella, which causes enlarged occipital, posterior cervical, and posterior auricular node chains, and tonsillitis and pharyngitis, which usually cause cervical lymphadenitis. Tinea pedis, or ringworm, on the legs would cause inguinal lymphadenopathy. Generalized lymphadenopathy is typical of mononucleosis, measles, and leukemia; the nodes are discrete and firm to the touch.

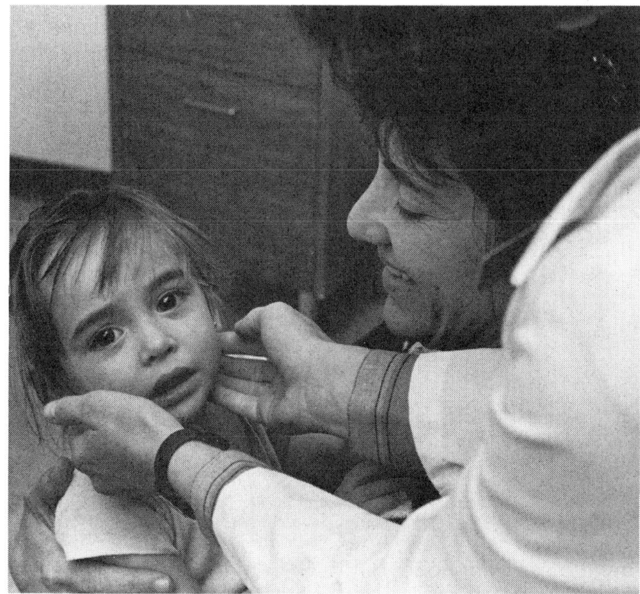

Lymph nodes are palpated gently, with a firm, circular motion.

Head, Face, and Neck

Head The head is inspected and palpated for size, shape, symmetry, deformities, control, movements, position, and, in infants for fontanelles and sutures. Normal head circumference is between 32 and 38 cm at birth and is generally 1–2 cm larger than the chest until after the first year of life. Head size then approximates chest size, but chest growth begins to exceed head size during early childhood until the head is 5–7 cm smaller than the chest. Any significant discrepancy in head circumference as measured and plotted on the head circumference graph warrants further evaluation to rule out health problems such as craniosynostosis, microcephaly, or hydrocephaly.

The shape of a neonate's head may be asymmetric because of the birth process, but any prominent bulges or swellings should be noted. *Cephalohematoma* (bleeding below the periosteum of the skull bones, normally restricted to one bone), and *caput succedaneum* (edema that generally crosses suture lines) may be seen immediately after birth. Generally, however, heads are described as normocephalic. The range of norms is hereditary; thus, the child's normal head circumference and shape will be similar to the parents'.

A thorough examination for any asymmetry or deformities of the head involves inspecting the head from all angles. The nurse might be able to do this as the child sits on the parent's lap, or the child might need to stand up for clearer visualization. At the same time, the nurse can inspect head control and movements. Because infants attain head control from a lying to sitting position by 4 months of age, significant head lag after 6 months of age signifies the need for referral to evaluate possible cerebral injury.

Range of motion is evaluated by asking the older child to look in each direction (up, down, and to either side) or by manually putting the child through each position. Infants can be shown a bright toy to follow horizontally from side to side. Any lateral limitations in head movement may indicate *torticollis,* or twisting of the neck, which is caused by shortening or injury to the sternocleidomastoid muscle. Hyperextension of the head and neck, termed *opisthotonos,* with pain on flexion is an indication of meningeal irritation or brain damage, as in Tay-Sachs disease.

In the infant the scalp is inspected and palpated for fontanelles and sutures, scaliness, infections, and hair. Infants are born with six fontanelles, but generally only the anterior and posterior fontanelles are palpated (Fig. 14-2). The fontanelles are assessed for size, pulsations, and tenseness, that is, bulging, flattened, or sunken appearance. The nurse notes whether the fontanelles are clean because some parents are afraid to touch them, having heard myths that doing so could cause brain damage. The anterior fontanelle is palpated in two dimensions and recorded as "anterior fontanelle 1.5 cm by 2 cm." This fontanelle generally closes between 9 and 18 months of age. Any premature or delayed closing warrants further evaluation and referral. The posterior fontanelle, which may not be readily palpable at birth or shortly after, closes by 3 months of age. Fontanelles are normally flat with slight pulsations. Any significant bulging, sunken appearance, or great pulsations when the infant is quiet require further evaluation and referral. Sutures, which may appear as prominent ridges at birth because of the birth process, usually flatten by 6 months of age and should not be palpable or overriding.

In older children, the scalp is assessed for lesions, scaliness, cleanliness, evidence of infections such as those caused by ticks or lice, and signs of trauma such as ecchymosis or scars.

Face The face is inspected and palpated for symmetry, movement, spacing of features, color and texture, temperature, and tenderness. Looking at the child from several angles or observing the child laughing, frowning, and smiling allows the nurse to observe symmetry, movement, and the placement of features. The eyes should not be widely set, a condition termed *ocular hypertelorism,* or unusually close together, a condition called *ocular hypotelorism.* The nose should be midline with symmetric nares; the mouth and lips should be symmetric. The child's ears should be located at the same level, and the top of the pinna should

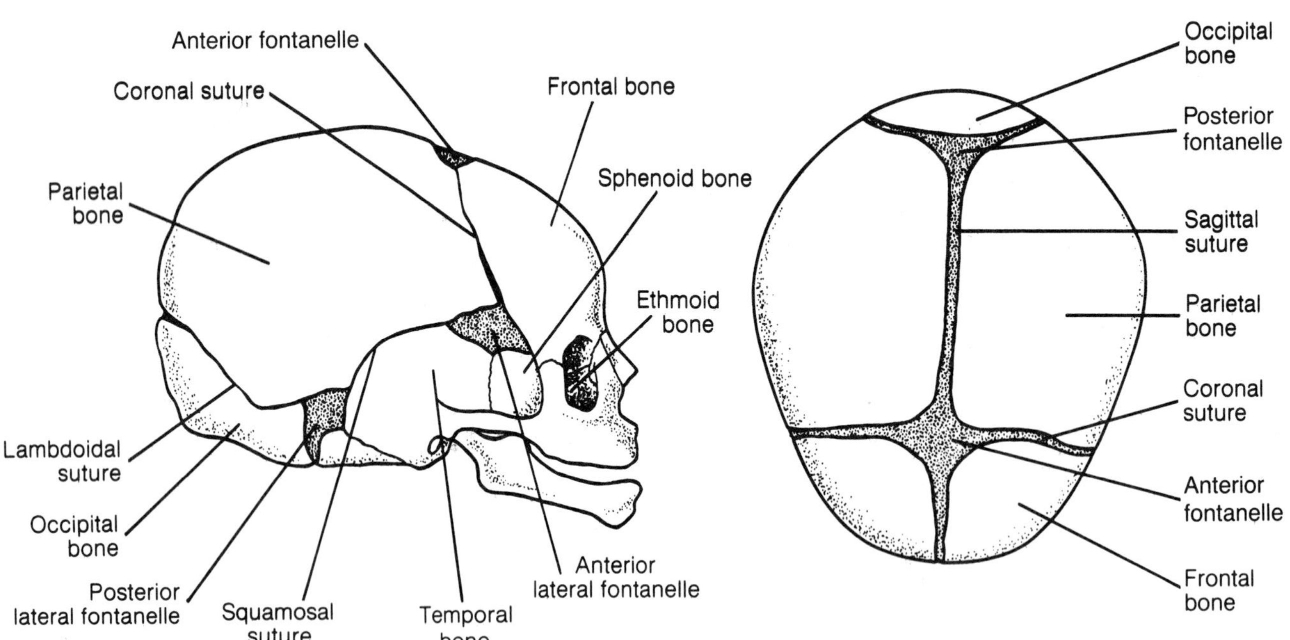

Figure 14-2 The bones of the skull showing the fontanelles and suture lines (From Kozier B, Erb G: *Fundamentals of Nursing.* 2nd ed. Addison-Wesley, 1983.)

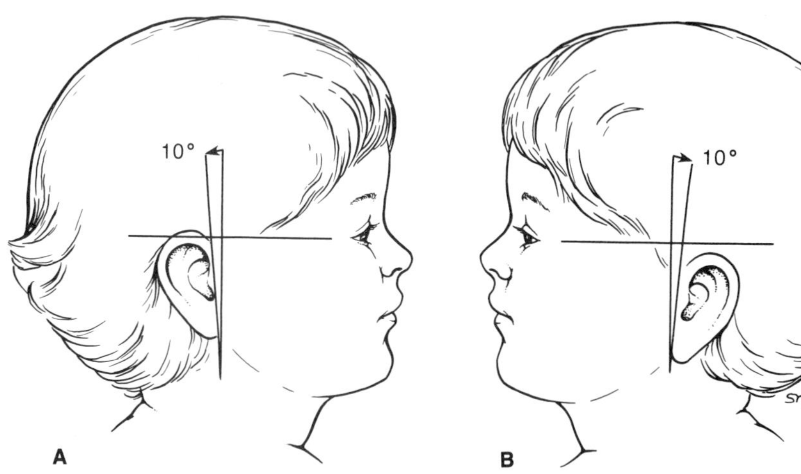

Figure 14-3 Alignment of ears. *A.* Normal ears. *B.* Low-set ears.

cross an imaginary line drawn from the occiput to the lateral corner of the eye (this is termed the *eye-occiput line*). Low-set ears may indicate renal anomalies or Down's syndrome (Fig. 14-3).

While observing the child's facial movements, the nurse assesses the symmetry of the nasolabial folds. Any asymmetry may indicate Bell's palsy or paralysis of cranial nerve VII. Any edema, twitching, and tics also are observed and palpated and may be caused by a nervous disorder or a disease process.

Neck The neck is inspected and palpated for position, movement, size and shape, and the position of the trachea and thyroid gland and auscultated for bruits or pulsations (Fig. 14-4). The neck should be symmetric from all angles. Observation of any extra folds of posterior skin, or webbing, warrants further evaluation to rule out certain syndromes (for example, Turner's syndrome).

Movement and control are assessed by turning the child's head from side to side and up and down. Strength, tone, and integrity of the sternocleidomastoid muscle is tested by

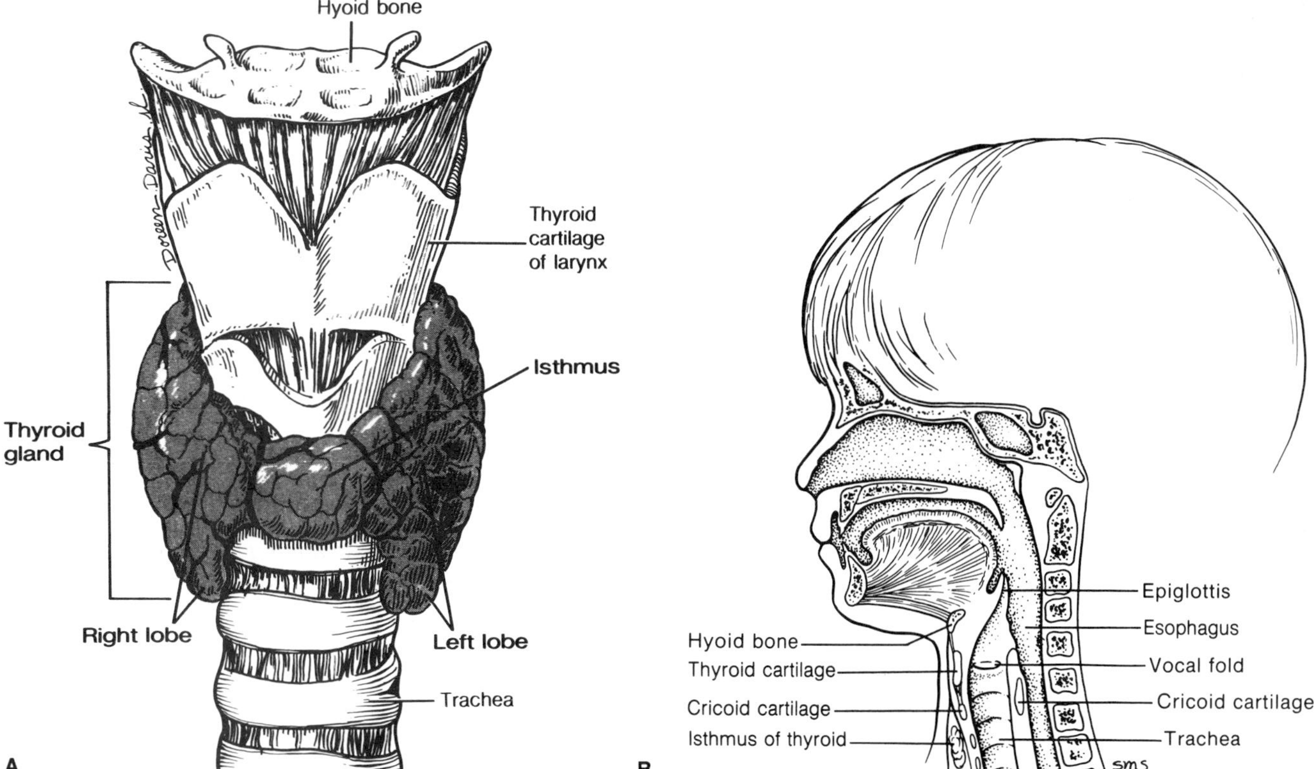

Figure 14-4 *A.* Ventral view of the thyroid gland. (From Spence AP, Mason EB: *Human Anatomy and Physiology*, 2nd ed. Benjamin/Cummings, 1983.) *B.* Lateral view of the thyroid gland.

having the child turn the head against the nurse's resisting hand. The trapezius muscle is likewise tested against resistance by having the child shrug the shoulders up while the nurse's hand pushes down.

The trachea is inspected and palpated to determine its normal midline position. With the child's neck hyperextended, the nurse palpates the tracheal rings, with the thumb on one side and index finger on the other. Beginning at the suprasternal notch and moving upward, the nurse can assess the position of the trachea.

The larynx and trachea are then palpated with the nurse either in front of or behind the child. From either position, the nurse first locates the hyoid bone and the thyroid and cricoid cartilages of the larynx. The hyoid bone lies just below the mandible; the thyroid cartilage, shaped like a shield, lies in the neck at the level of the bifurcation of the common carotid artery. The cricoid cartilage is palpable just below the thyroid cartilage and is the lowermost cartilage of the larynx. The thyroid gland and isthmus are then palpated on either side just below the cricoid cartilage.

The thyroid examination requires that the child swallow, causing the gland to move upward. The nurse's one hand palpates behind the sternocleidomastoid muscle and pushes inward and toward the trachea while the other hand pushes in against the first hand, feeling the size, shape, and surface characteristics of the thyroid. In normal, healthy children a thyroid gland is often not palpable.

The neck is auscultated to identify any bruits (soft rushing sounds), pulsations, or murmurs. The bell of the stethoscope is placed over the carotid arteries. Any bruits, excessive pulsations, or murmurs may be signs of cardiovascular problems.

Eyes

The primary methods for examining the eyes are inspection and sometimes palpation of the external structures for size, symmetry, and color and inspecting the interior structures to assess the retinal structures. A complete eye examination also includes a series of tests of visual acuity.

Vision screening often is done at the beginning of either the physical examination after measurements are taken or as the first part of the eye examination. It is the least intrusive procedure in the eye assessment, and children are most familiar with it. Vision screening should begin in infancy and continue throughout life at regular intervals. In infancy vision is tested by observing the child's ability to follow a light or a brightly colored toy. Most parents are sensitive to an infant's sense of sight and should be asked whether they believe their child can see.

Light perception in neonates is tested by noting a blinking response as a light is shined into the child's eyes. In early childhood visual acuity can be tested with a picture test such as Allen cards, which are black pictures of familiar objects (horse, birthday cake, house, and so on) on white cards. After ascertaining that the child can correctly name the objects, the nurse shows the cards while slowly moving away from the child. A 3-year-old should achieve a score of 20/50; a 4-year-old should obtain a score of 20/40. That is, the 3-year-old should identify the pictures correctly at 20 ft that someone with normal visual acuity could identify at 50 ft. The fraction denotes the resolving power of the eye. A child who cannot identify the pictures or has a 5-ft difference between eyes should be referred.

Children who are unable to read letters, including those for whom English is not the first language, may have their vision tested with the Snellen E test. The child indicates which direction the E is pointing (up, down, right, or left) either by pointing a hand in the same direction or by identifying the direction by referring to concrete items placed in the environment (for example, table, door, ceiling, floor).

The Snellen Alphabet Chart is used for children and adults who can identify letters. Whatever test is used, the nurse must follow the directions correctly to ensure an accurate assessment. Adequate lighting is essential. There should be no glare, and the chart should be placed at the child's eye level. The child should be provided with a large paper cup, index card, or eye patch to help occlude the eye not being tested. The occluding object is placed against the midline of the child's nose, not directly against the eye or eyeglasses, if worn. Children often need to be reminded several times to keep both eyes open, even the eye that is covered. After the child clearly understands the procedure, the nurse tests the child's vision as far down the chart as the child is capable of reading. Reading more than half the letters is a passing score. The child should be started on line 20/40 or 20/50 and moved up or down depending on the results. The results are then recorded immediately in the child's chart.

Expected visual acuity for various ages is listed in Table 14-7. Any child who does not have age-appropriate visual acuity or a two-line difference between eyes should be referred for further evaluation.

Color vision also should be assessed in every child, usually in early childhood, once colors have been learned. Color blindness is hereditary; therefore, a positive family history warrants a careful examination of the child. Most 3- and 4-year-old children know their colors and can simply be asked to name the color of their clothing or of colored blocks or toys (see Chapter 16). The Ishibara Plates are a standardized color vision test that can be used with children who are able to discriminate among letters, numbers, geometric figures, and a figure background. A color-blind child and the child's parent will need counseling for such safety purposes as interpreting traffic signals.

External Eye The external eye examination begins with the eyelashes. They should be assessed for distribution, direction of growth, and pigmentation. Lashes that turn inward can cause conjunctival irritation. The examination continues with the eyelids (Fig. 14-5). The lids are observed

TABLE 14-7 Visual Acuity at Various Ages

Age	Visual Acuity
Birth	Fixates on objects 8–12 inches away, may follow object briefly if in alert, quiet state (20/600—20/800)
2–3 months	Fixates and follows objects in horizontal and vertical directions (20/300)
1 year	20/100
2 years	20/70
3 years	20/50
4 years	20/40
5 years	20/30–20/20

for edema, color, position, the presence of any exudate or infection, and the ability to open and close completely. Edema of the lids can be the result of systemic disease (for example, nephrosis) or a local response such as from an insect bite. Any ecchymosis should be noted.

The lids are inspected for proper placement on the eye. When the eye is open, the upper lid should fall somewhere between the upper iris and the pupil. Any lag of the lid that causes dropping over more of the pupil is called *ptosis* and might be a familial trait or might be acquired through paralysis of the oculomotor cranial nerve by disease or trauma. Other malpositions of the eyelids are *entropion* (inversion of the lid, causing the eyelashes to rub onto the eye) and *ectropion* (outward turning of the lid, exposing the conjunctiva). Either condition needs careful assessment to rule out damage to the eye structures and potential infection and loss of vision.

Epicanthal folds are vertical folds of skin on the lid and often cover the inner canthus (Fig. 14-6). They give the child the appearance of "slant eyes." Epicanthal folds might be present in Asian children and some Caucasian neonates. They also might be a sign of Down's syndrome, glycogen storage disease, or renal agenesis and are then seen with other physical characteristics of these conditions.

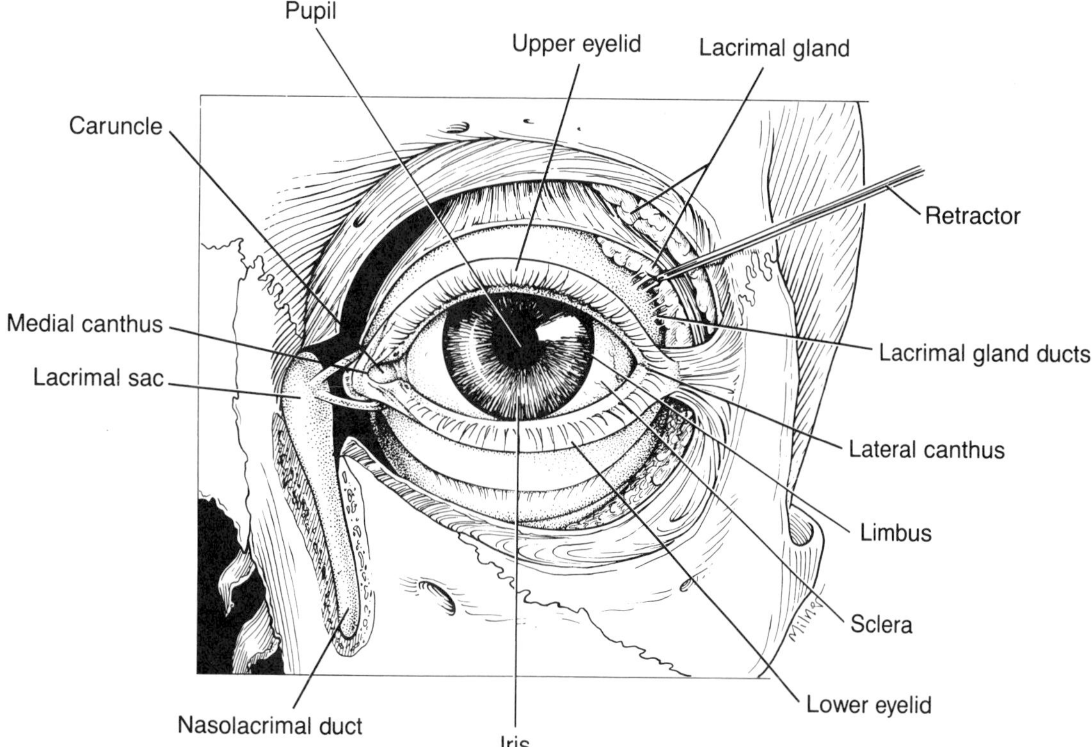

Figure 14-5 Structure of the eye with lacrimal gland retracted to show ducts. (From Spence AP, Mason EB: *Human Anatomy and Physiology*, 2nd ed. Benjamin/Cummings, 1983.)

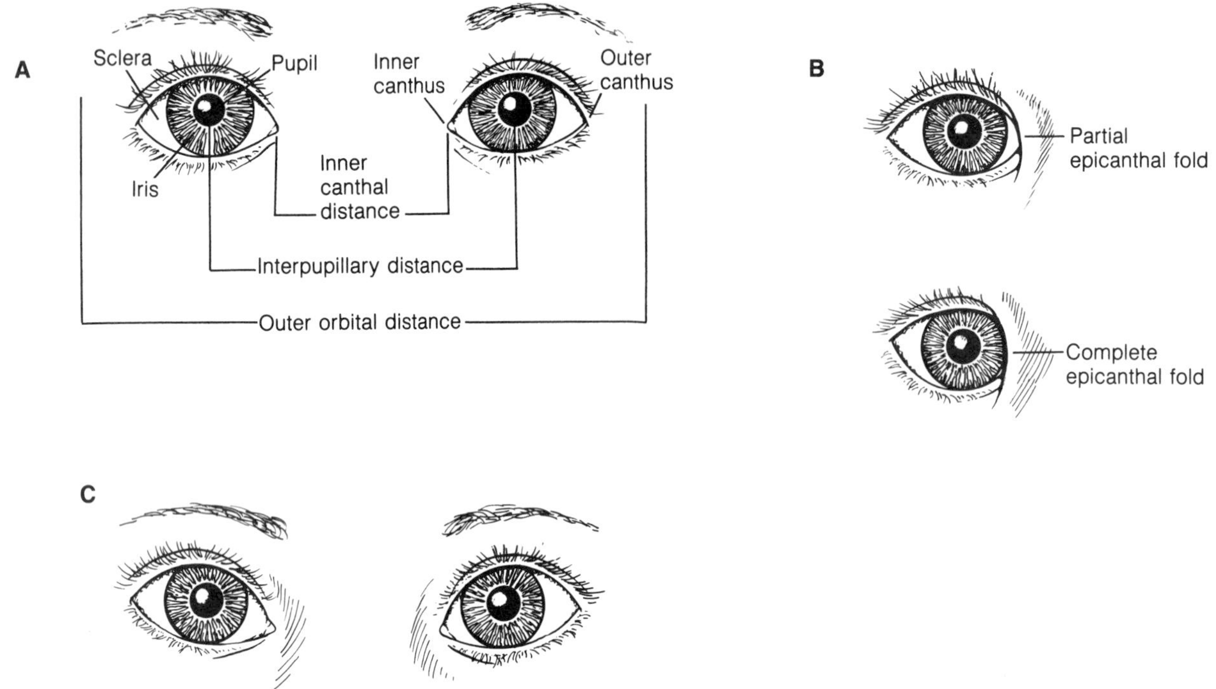

Figure 14-6 *A*. Anatomic landmarks of the eye. *B*. Epicanthal folds. *C*. Upward palpebral slant ("almond-shaped eyes").

Dacryocystitis, or inflammation of the lacrimal sac or duct, with swelling, redness, and a purulent discharge, is a common infection of young infants and children. It often is caused by a blocked duct, or *dacryostenosis,* which is present from birth. Neonates cry without tears. Infants usually begin to tear by 3 months of age, and the persistent absence of tears may indicate a blocked duct. Marginal blepharitis is seen as inflammation of the lid, with scaly, crusted lid edges. It may occur as a result of severe seborrheic dermatitis and resolves with treatment of the scalp condition. A hordeolum, or stye, is an inflammation of the sebaceous glands near the lashes. It usually is seen as a painful, red, swollen area. A chalazion, or a granuloma of the meibomian glands (sebaceous glands), is a nonpainful, discrete swelling that moves freely under the skin.

The nurse inspects the conjunctiva for color, hemorrhages, and inflammation. The palpebral conjunctiva is the lining of the lids. The upper conjunctiva is best examined by gently everting the lid as the child looks down. A cotton-tipped applicator can be placed over the upper lid and the lashes gently grasped and rolled over to expose the conjunctiva clearly. The lower conjunctive is more easily inspected by gently pulling the lid down as the child looks up. Normal conjunctiva is pink and glassy. Inflammation of the conjunctiva, causing redness and often discharge, can be due to bacterial or viral infections, allergy, or chemical or mechanical irritations. A "cobblestone" appearance of the conjunctiva often is seen in children with severe or chronic allergies.

The bulbar conjunctiva covers the eye up to the junction of the cornea and sclera. It should be transparent, and the white color of the underlying sclera should be visible. Redness is due to dilation of blood vessels and may indicate eye strain, irritation, or bleeding disorders. An overgrowth, or hypertrophy, of conjunctival tissue, often extending over the cornea is called a *pterygium.* A yellowish, triangular growth on either side of the cornea that does not interfere with vision is called a *pinguecula.* Both conditions are seen occasionally in children.

The sclera, or white covering of the eyeball, should be clear. Jaundice causes a yellowish sclera; a bluish tone might indicate glaucoma or might be a late sign of increased bilirubin. Dark-skinned children might have tiny black marks, which are normal. The cornea, or covering of the iris and pupil, should be crystal clear, without any inflammation, ulceration, or opacity. Corneal abrasions are often a result of eye trauma and should be properly treated to prevent more serious corneal ulcerations. The best way to test for abrasions is with staining, but they also can be seen by shining a light obliquely toward the cornea.

The iris is observed for color and inflammation. The permanent color of the iris is seen by 6 months of age in 50% of children and in all children by 1 year of age. *Heterochromia,* or irises of different colors, can be normal or associated with congenital syndromes or chronic low-grade infections of the iris. Brushfield's spots (a light or white speckling of the iris) might occur in normal children but is seen most often in children with Down's syndrome or other syndromes associated with mental retardation. *Iritis,* or inflammation of the iris, is seen as dulling of the color of the iris, ciliary flush, and pain. It often is seen in individuals with juvenile rheumatoid arthritis.

The pupils are examined for pupillary response and size. Pupil size should be equal, and pupils should be responsive to light both directly and consensually. A pupil reacts to light directly if the pupil into which the light is shone constricts; it reacts consensually if it constricts when the light is shone in the opposite eye. Accommodation, or constriction when focusing on a nearby object, and dilation when looking into the distance also are tested. Difference in pupil size (*anisocoria*) can be normal, but any sudden differences noted require a complete neurologic evaluation.

The lens should be evaluated with examination of the iris and pupil. The nurse assesses the lens for cataracts and dislocations. Cataracts or opacities of the lenses can be seen by flashing a light into the eye, preferably at an oblique angle. A red reflex should be visible. Any patient with a possible cataract or dislocated lens should be referred to an ophthalmologist.

The final part of the external eye examination is observation of extraocular movements (Fig. 14-7). The nurse assesses the child for nystagmus, strabismus, and peripheral fields. *Nystagmus* involves involuntary, rapid, jerky movements of the eye as the child is observed through the six cardinal fields of gaze. The direction of the nystagmus should be recorded. *Strabismus* involves deviation of one or both eyes. A paralyzed extraocular muscle or nerve causes paralytic (noncomitant) strabismus. It is present only in the field of action of the involved muscle or nerve. Nonparalytic (concomitant) strabismus occurs when the eyes do not move simultaneously in any quadrant. Strabismus that occurs only intermittently, for example, when the child is fatigued, is a *phoria*; an overt strabismus is a *tropia*. The movement of the eyeball is observed for deviation outward, *exo,* or deviation inward, *eso.* Therefore, a child with overt strabismus in which the eye deviates inward during examination of extraocular movements through the fields of gaze is described as having esotropia. Strabismus that remains undetected can cause amblyopia, reduction or dimness of vision, or even blindness.

Two screening tests are used to detect phoria types of strabismus. The corneal light reflex test is performed by shining a light at the bridge of the child's nose as the child looks straight ahead, fixating on an object. The light reflex normally should fall at the same point on the pupils; any deviation indicates strabismus. This test requires the cooperation of an older child who can follow directions. The cover test may be performed on younger children who can be kept in a quiet, alert state. It is done by first getting the child to fixate on an object about 12 in away, then quickly covering one eye, making sure both eyes remain open, and observing any inward or outward movement of the uncovered eye. The occluded eye is then uncovered and inspected for any movement. The test is repeated with the opposite eye. Normally, no deviation occurs in either eye; any deviation is recorded according to the direction of the eye movement. The child with this condition should be referred for further testing to prevent the development of amblyopia.

Children who have wide nasal bridges or epicanthal folds may appear to have strabismus, a condition referred to as *pseudostrabismus.* Negative cover and light reflex tests rule out this condition.

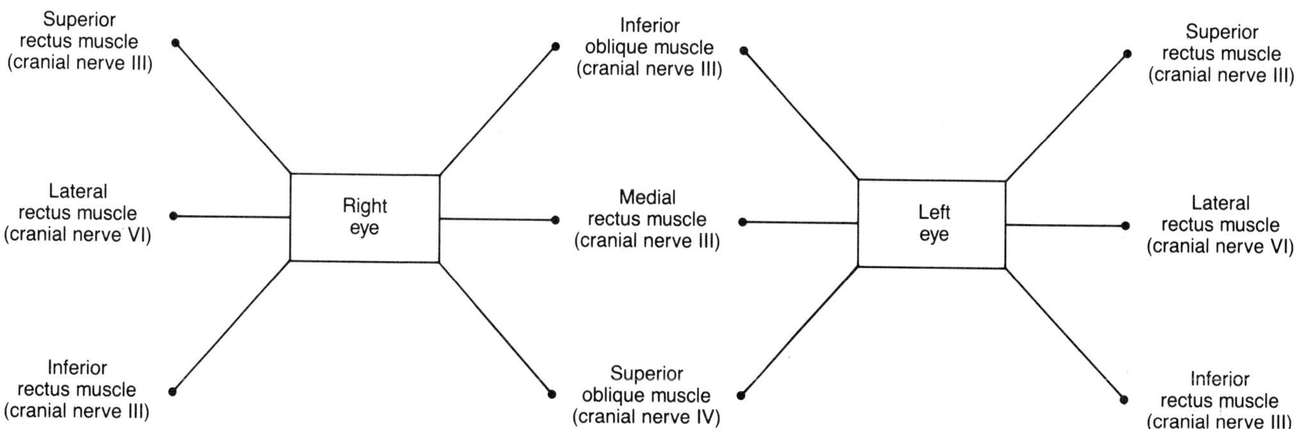

Figure 14-7 Visual fields of extraocular movement. If the child's eyes cannot move to a given position, dysfunction of a muscle or cranial nerve is indicated.

Internal Eye The internal eye examination involves assessment of the optic disk, retinal vessels, macula, and general background with an ophthalmoscope. This part of the eye examination requires patience to learn and a cooperative child who can sit quietly in a semidarkened room. An ophthalmoscope has from 15 to 20 diopters in the black (positive lens) and in the red (negative lens). (A diopter is the refractive power of the lens with a focal distance of 1 m.) The refractive ability of the child's and the nurse's eyes determines the diopters to be used during the examination. The red numbers, or negative lens, compensate for nearsightedness, and the black numbers, or positive lens, compensate for farsightedness.

The ophthalmoscope generally is dialed to 0. At a distance of 12 in, the nurse centers the light on the child's eye and assesses the red reflex. Gradually moving closer to the child and turning the dial to the red negative numbers, the examiner assesses the cornea, aqueous chamber, lens, and vitreous chamber. With the nurse and child's foreheads almost touching, the nurse examines the fundus, arteries, and veins. The optic disc is then located and observed for size, shape, color, margins, and physiologic cup. Normally, the optic

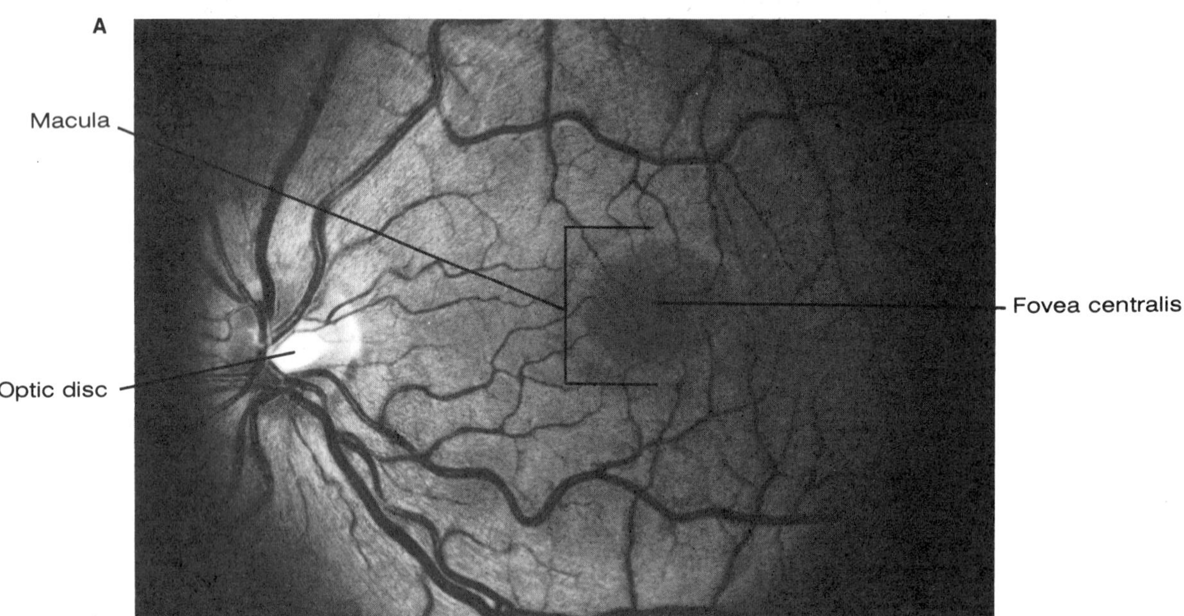

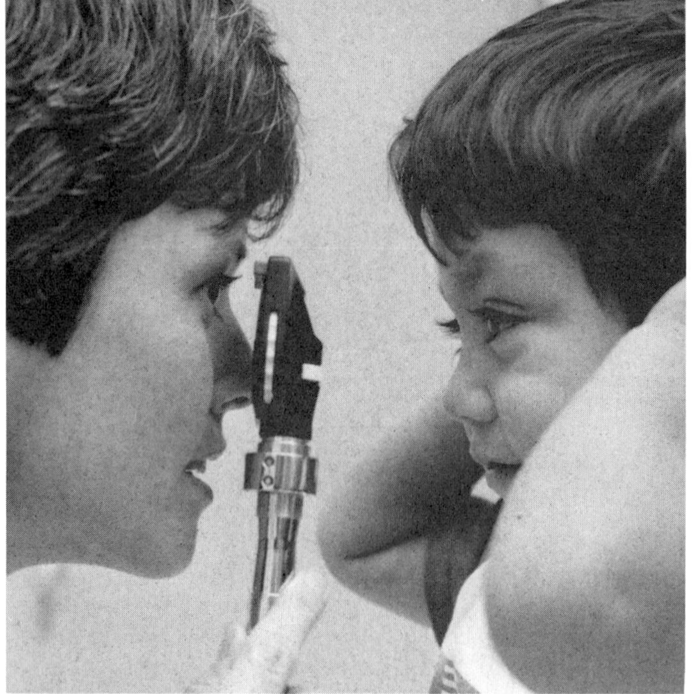

A. Retinal vessels of the internal eye. (From Spence AP, Mason EB: *Human Anatomy and Physiology*. 2nd ed. Benjamin/Cummings, 1983.) *B*. Inspection of the external eye. Keeping both eyes wide open, holding the ophthalmoscope 12 in. from the child and steadying it against the nose, the nurse uses the right eye to examine the child's right eye and vice versa.

disc is creamy white to pinkish, 1.5 mm in diameter, and round to oval, with sharp, clear margins. A depression slightly temporal of the center is the physiologic cup.

The retinal vessels are observed for color, size, and regularity. Normal arteries are one-fourth the size of veins and brighter in color, exhibiting a light reflex from the center. Veins are darker and may pulsate near the optic disc. They should both be observed for any narrowing, dilatation, tortuosity, or nicking. Any abnormality warrants referral for further evaluation.

The fundus, or general background, is assessed for pigmentation and integrity. The color varies depending on skin and hair pigmentation but is normally an orange-red color and uniform throughout, with no signs of hemorrhagic areas, scars, or punctate spots, which would indicate diabetic retinopathy. The macula lies near the temporal side of the fundus, two disc diameters away, and is one disc diameter in size. It is brighter than the optic disc, and the gleaming light in the center is the fovea centralis. This is the most light-sensitive part of the eye, and the nurse often can locate it by asking the child to look briefly into the light on the ophthalmoscope. This, however, may cause the child some discomfort, which is why it is the last part of the eye examination.

Ears

External Ear The ear examination begins with an assessment of the position, size, shape, color, and symmetry of the ears (Fig. 14-8). Any lesions or deformities are noted. The pinna should cross the eye-occiput line. It is inspected for the normal skin tone, color, and such structural anomalies as ear tags; it is palpated for nodules, lesions, or masses and for turgor. The mastoid, the bony prominence posterior to the earlobe, is observed for color, temperature, tenderness, and lesions.

The external auditory canal (Fig. 14-9) is observed for color, edema, discharges, amount and texture of cerumen (earwax), lesions, masses, or foreign bodies. (The nurse also notes whether cerumen is fresh or old.) Any serosanguineous discharge may be from a perforated tympanic membrane, a foreign body irritation, or scratching. A purulent discharge usually means serious otitis caused by either a fungal or bacterial infection.

Middle Ear The middle ear is examined with an otoscope. The largest speculum that can comfortably fit in the child's ear should be used. The otoscopic examination generally is not painful unless there is an external otitis or furuncle in the ear canal. Children, however, become easily frightened and anxious during this part of the examination, although adequate preparation and a secure environment might alleviate these problems. Any child who cannot cooperate needs to be securely restrained to prevent traumatic damage to the ear during the examination.

Children who cannot be trusted to remain still should be restrained gently in one of two general positions. The first position is to have the child seated on the parent's lap, with the child's head resting securely against the parent and the child's arms held along the sides. The other position is to have the child lie on the abdomen, arms along each side

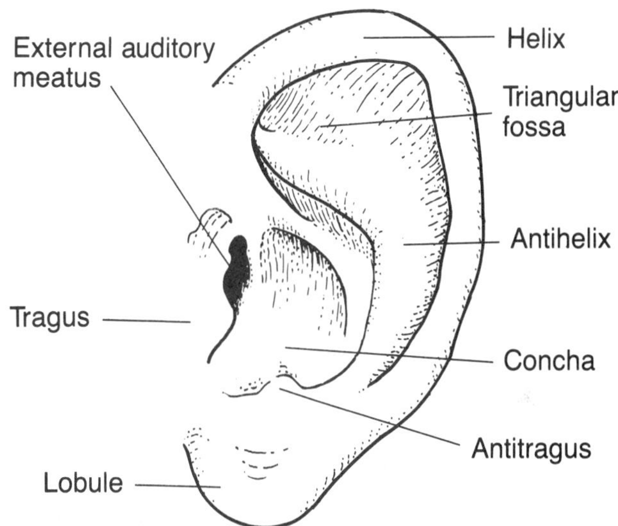

Figure 14-8 Structures of the external ear.

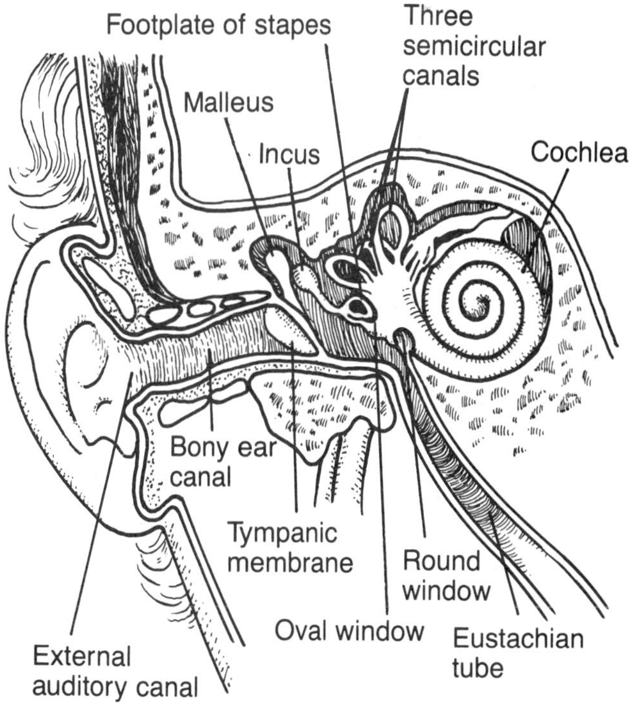

Figure 14-9 External auditory canal, middle ear, and inner ear.

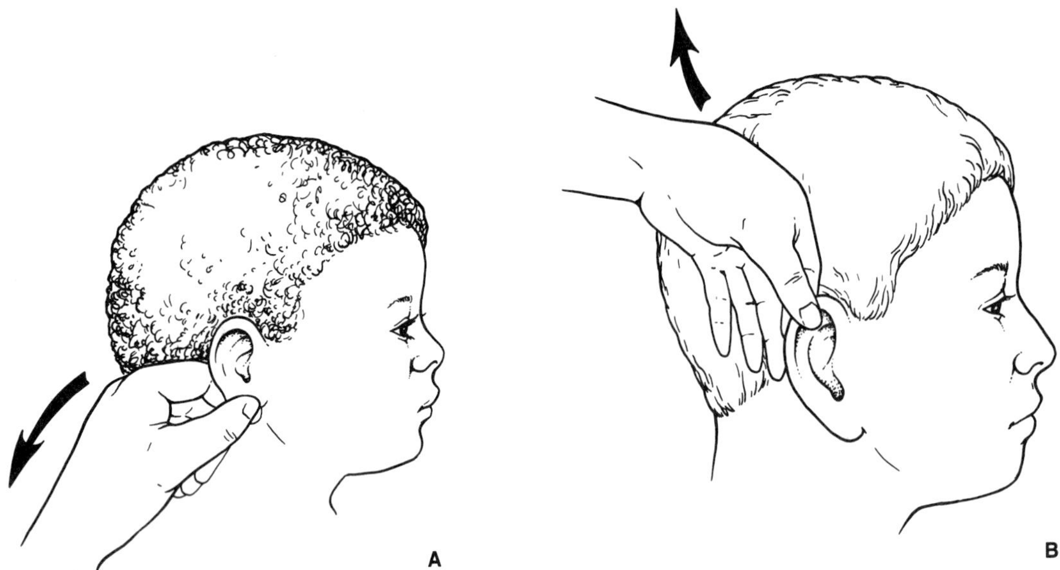

Figure 14-10 Straightening the external auditory canal for insertion of otoscope. *A.* Infant. *B.* Adolescent.

or held above the head, with the head turned and securely held by the examining nurse and the lower body held by the parent. The older child who can sit still on the examination table needs only to tilt the head to one side for better visibility.

Once the child is adequately restrained, the otoscope can be placed inside the ear canal. Ear canals of infants and young children curve upward, so the ear lobe is pulled gently down and out for visibility. Ear canals of older children and adults are longer and curve downward; therefore, the top of the pinna is grasped up and back (Fig. 14-10).

The external canal is then examined internally for any erythema ("swimmer's ear"), furuncles, foreign bodies, lesions, or discharges. The amount, color, and texture of the cerumen is noted and described.

Examination of the middle ear consists of observation of the tympanic membrane and landmarks (Fig. 14-11). The tympanic membrane is assessed for color, light reflex, and mobility. Normally, it is pearly gray. Any erythematous membrane indicates a middle ear infection but also might be seen in a child who is crying. A dull gray-to-yellowish color often is seen with serous otitis. The light reflex is a triangular cone of light located at the inferior anterior quadrant, to the right of the umbo. A diffuse, spotty, or absent light reflex indicates a middle ear disease. Mobility is then tested with a pneumatic bulb attached to the otoscopic head. Slight instillation of air will cause a normal tympanic membrane to move smoothly. Jerky, sluggish, or absent mobility is another sign of middle ear disease.

Landmarks assessed during the examination are the umbo, short and long processes, and cannulas. The pars flaccida and the anterior and posterior malleolar folds also are assessed, although these structures are not always clearly visible. In an acute suppurative ear infection, the landmarks might not be visible because of bulging of the eardrum. Serous otitis that causes negative pressure in the middle ear and retraction of the eardrum may cause the long process to appear more forward than normal or the malleus itself to be more accentuated.

The tympanic membrane is then observed for any perforations or scars. Perforations commonly are seen along the cannula; scars might be seen anywhere on the eardrum.

Hearing Screening Hearing is an essential part of examining the senses and should be included in every well-

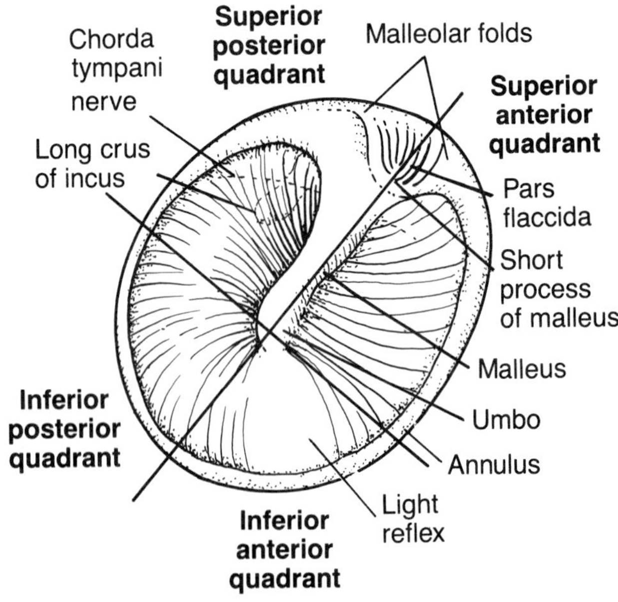

Figure 14-11 Anatomic landmarks of the middle ear.

child physical examination. The development of speech and language depends on adequate hearing. The two major causes of hearing loss are (1) sensorineural loss, which is a disorder in the inner ear (caused by ototoxic drugs or meningitis), the auditory cranial nerve, or the brain, and (2) conductive loss, which is an external or middle ear disorder (caused by chronic bilateral otitis media or trauma).

Children who are at risk for hearing problems are those who have had multiple middle ear infections, have a familial history of congenital hearing impairment, had a cleft palate, were exposed prenatally to infections such as rubella, were premature, had birth anoxia, or who took ototoxic drugs during infancy (for example, neomycin, streptomycin). These children require early and periodic hearing evaluations.

Hearing is best assessed in infants by eliciting the startle reflex with a bell. The nurse also notes the infant's ability to localize sound. The parent is usually reliable in assessing an infant's ability to hear. Young children who can sit quietly and respond to directions such as "Give me the truck" most likely have no significant hearing problem. The child who seems to ignore parental requests or listens to the television or radio turned up loudly may need audiometric testing.

An audiometer measures the threshold of hearing for pure-tone frequencies and loudness. It determines both the severity of the hearing loss and the sound cycles involved. Tuning forks also are used to identify hearing loss. The Weber test is performed by placing a vibrating tuning fork on top of the child's head and asking whether the child can hear the vibrations in both ears, a normal response, or in only one ear (for example, "Where do you hear the tuning fork?"). If the sound is lateral to only one ear, the child has a conductive hearing loss in that ear or a sensorineural hearing loss in the opposite ear. Lateral sound in the affected ear occurs because extraneous noise, which is blocked out by a middle ear problem, does not interfere with bone vibration, and the child hears the sounds more loudly in the affected ear. If the inner ear or auditory nerve is affected, bone vibrations are not detected, and the sounds are heard better in the unaffected ear.

The Rinne test is performed by placing a vibrating tuning fork first on the mastoid process. When the child can no longer hear the vibration, the fork is brought forward to the external auditory canal, and the child is asked whether it can be heard again. A normal response is that the child can now hear it. Air conduction is greater than bone conduction; therefore, if no ear problem exists, the Rinne test is positive. Any child who cannot hear the sound through air conduction with the tuning fork at the external auditory canal should be referred. An external auditory canal blocked by hardened or crusted cerumen may be the cause of a decrease in hearing.

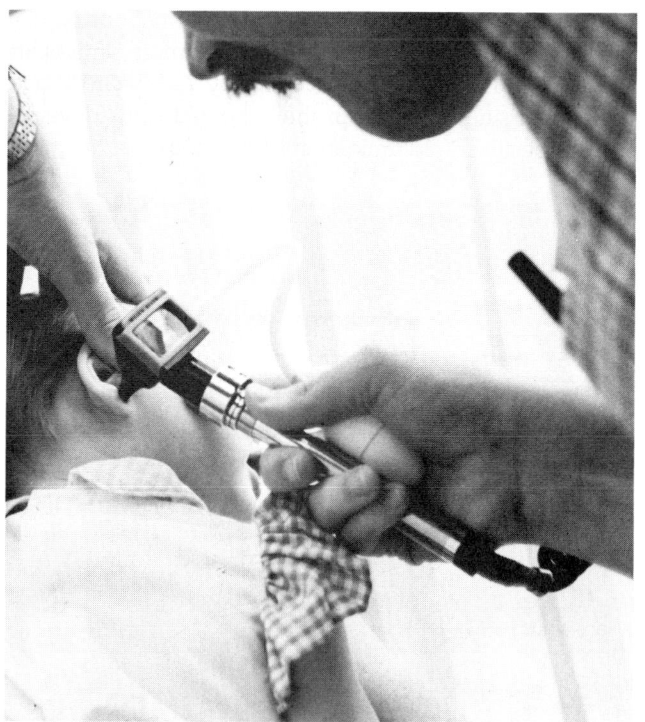

A

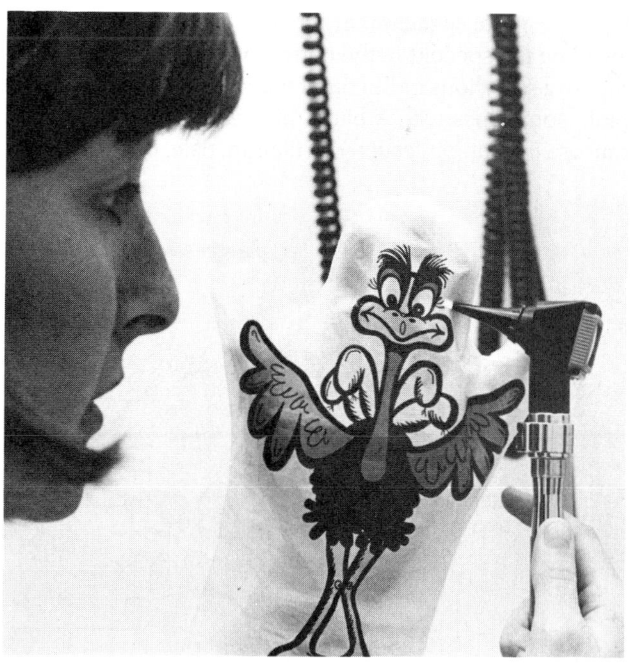

B

A. The infant's head is held against the mother while the ear is examined. (From Kozier B, Erb G: *Techniques in Clinical Nursing.* Addison-Wesley, 1982.) *B.* During early and middle childhood, preparation for ear examination helps in gaining the child's cooperation.

Nose

The nose is responsible for temperature control of the air, humidification, and filtration of the first passageway to the respiratory tract. It is also the sensory organ of smell. Each of these functions depends on the patency of the mucosal lining of the nasal cavity. The nurse assesses the health and integrity of the nose and its structures principally by inspection.

The nose is examined for size and shape, patency of nares, color of mucous membranes, and the absence or presence of discharge, masses, or polyps. Although the size and shape of a child's nose may be determined by heredity, several unusual shapes need to be noted. A flat nose may indicate congenital anomalies (for example, cleft palate) or other conditions. Children with chronic allergies develop a crease across their noses as a result of pushing up against the tip of the nose in response to itching or rhinitis.

Patency of the nares is assessed by placing the diaphragm of the stethoscope under one nare while blocking the other nare. As the child breathes, a film appears on the diaphragm. An infant who does not have patent nares will demonstrate respiratory distress with flaring of the nares and respiratory retractions. Infants are obligatory nose breathers. A child who breathes through the mouth may have enlarged adenoids, nasal polyps, allergies, or a deviated septum.

Internal examination of the nose requires either a penlight or a nasal speculum attached to the otoscope. Gently inserting the speculum, the nurse observes the color, integrity, and secretions of the nasal mucosa. Normal mucosa is pink, sometimes with a bluish hue, and moist. Reddened mucosa indicates infection or irritation; pale, boggy mucosa indicates allergies; and gray, swollen mucosa indicates chronic rhinitis. Watery discharge may be caused by allergies or upper respiratory infections. Purulent discharges are common with sinus infections or foreign bodies. Blood-stained discharge may indicate nasal bleeding occurring at the anterior tip of the septum. Allergy, trauma, a dry climate, nose picking, or blood dyscrasias will cause epistaxis.

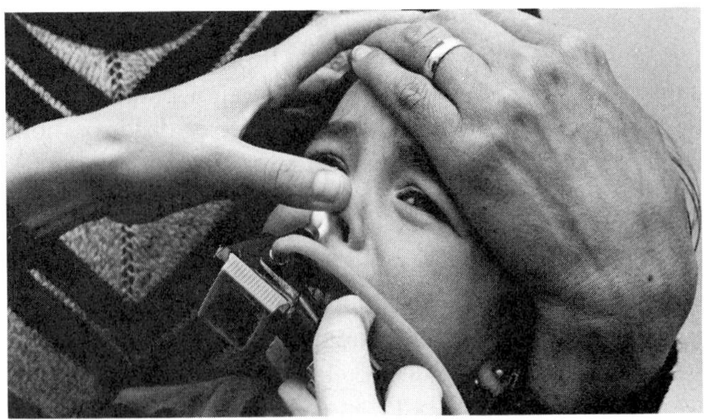

Inspection of the internal structures of the nose.

The vestibule of the nose is assessed for such lesions as furuncles. The inferior and middle turbinates are assessed for patency and discharges. The anterior portion of the septum is assessed for any septal deviation.

Palpation and percussion of the sinuses are also performed (Fig. 14-12). Normally, the sinuses cannot be felt, but a child with sinusitis may complain of pain or tenderness on palpation. The maxillary and ethmoid sinuses are the only sinuses developed at birth. By 7–8 years of age, the frontal sinuses develop; the sphenoid sinus develops after puberty. Transillumination of the sinus also might be

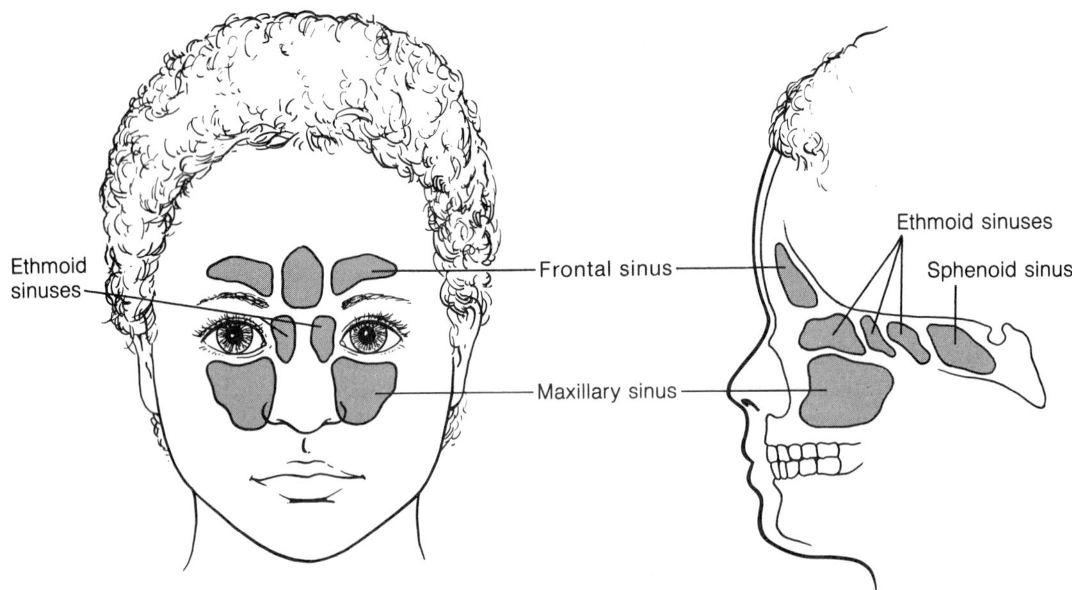

Figure 14-12 Front and lateral views of the facial sinuses.

done, but this procedure is limited in that only the maxillary and frontal sinuses can be transilluminated. It also is not very successful in children because of the small size of the sinuses.

Mouth and Throat

Evaluation of the mouth and throat is best left until the end of the examination because it is often difficult for the child (Fig. 14-13). With a cooperative child, almost the entire examination can be done without a tongue blade. Playing games with the child, asking the child to open wide, and shining a penlight to examine the structures often suffices for a complete assessment. Infants and younger or uncooperative children, however, need adequate restraints. A tongue depressor and penlight are usually essential for visualization.

The examination should proceed in an orderly manner from the external structures, from the lips to the gums, teeth, tongue, buccal mucosa, palate, and oropharynx. The lips are inspected for symmetry, color, moisture, the presence of any fissures or lesions, and edema. The surrounding area also is inspected for pallor or cyanosis. Asymmetry of the lips, with drooping of one side, indicates involvement of the facial (VII) cranial nerve. Pale lips may indicate uremia, and cherry-red lips are seen in children with acidosis or carbon monoxide poisoning. Any chancre, herpes simplex, or other lesion is noted and described. Mouth odor also should be assessed at this time. Unusual odors may be present in children with poor oral hygiene, nasal obstruction due to allergies, foreign bodies, or polyps, diabetic acidosis, diphtheria, and malnutrition.

Teeth are inspected for number, location, type (deciduous or permanent), malocclusions, color, caries, and

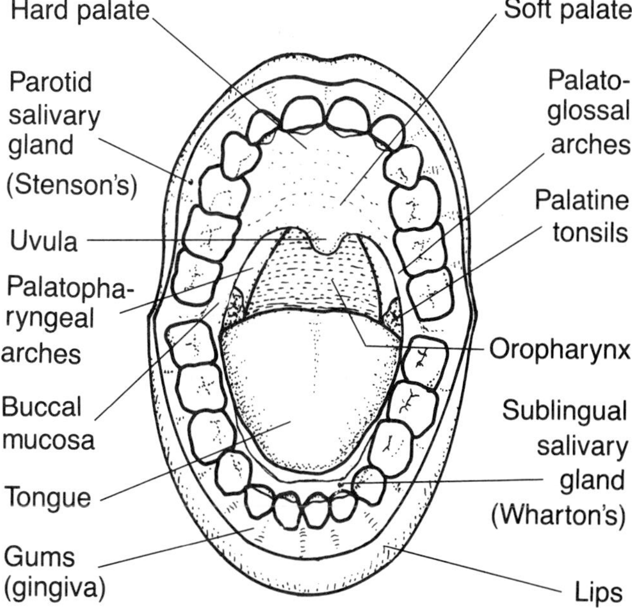

Figure 14-13 Internal structures of the mouth.

hygiene. The first teeth erupt at about 6 months of age; all 20 deciduous teeth have erupted by 30 months of age. Permanent dentition begins at about 6 years of age and continues until all 32 teeth have erupted (Fig. 14-14).

Teeth with flattened surfaces may be due to bruxism (teeth grinding); notches may be due to trauma. Malocclusion can be caused by persistent thumb sucking or overcrowding of teeth in the mouth. Normal occlusion occurs when the upper central incisors just overlap the lower incisors. Teeth that are mottled or pitted are seen in children who have ingested an excessive amount of fluoride; green or black discoloration of the teeth is caused by antibiotic ingestion (for example, tetracycline) or iron ingestion. The teeth also should be inspected for evidence of caries, and any dental work should be inspected for intactness. The nurse might want to incorporate dental hygiene counseling at this point in the examination. Children should begin to be exposed to dental hygiene by 2 years of age by being taught to hold a toothbrush to clean their teeth (see Chapter 8). Dental radiographs are contraindicated until 5 years of age.

The gums (gingiva) are inspected for color, inflammation, recession, swelling, bleeding, tenderness, and ulcerations. Gums may be affected by the ingestion of medications such as iron, anticonvulsants, and tetracycline, much as the teeth are affected. A black line may indicate lead poisoning, although this line may be normal in dark-skinned children. Inflammation, swelling, and bleeding may be secondary to infection, poor oral hygiene, or poor nutrition. Hypertrophied or receding gums should be noted.

The buccal mucosa is inspected for color, moisture, condition of the salivary ducts, and the presence of lesions and masses. Normal buccal mucosa is pink and moist, but brown or black areas may be seen in dark-skinned children. Koplik's spots are bright red spots with bluish white specks in their centers and may be seen in the prodromal stage of measles. Candidiasis (thrush) is evidenced as white patches that cannot be scraped off. These usually occur on the tongue and hard palate and are caused by fungal infections.

The salivary glands, Stensen's duct (parotid gland), opposite the upper second molar, and Wharton's duct (submaxillary gland), at the base of the tongue on opposite sides of the frenulum, are assessed for patency. Any blockage or swelling could indicate an infection.

The tongue is assessed for color, texture, size, movement, position, and the presence of masses or lesions. The normal tongue is pink and has a normal configuration of papillae. A gray tongue with exaggerated grooves is called a "geographic tongue" and might be normal, or it might indicate allergies, fever, or drug ingestion. A red, inflamed tongue ("strawberry tongue") is seen in scarlet fever. Vitamin deficiencies also can cause a tender, red tongue. Tremors of the tongue are seen in children with cerebral palsy, chorea, and hypothyroidism. Excessive protrusion of the tongue, or *glossoptosis,* is seen in mental retardation or in children

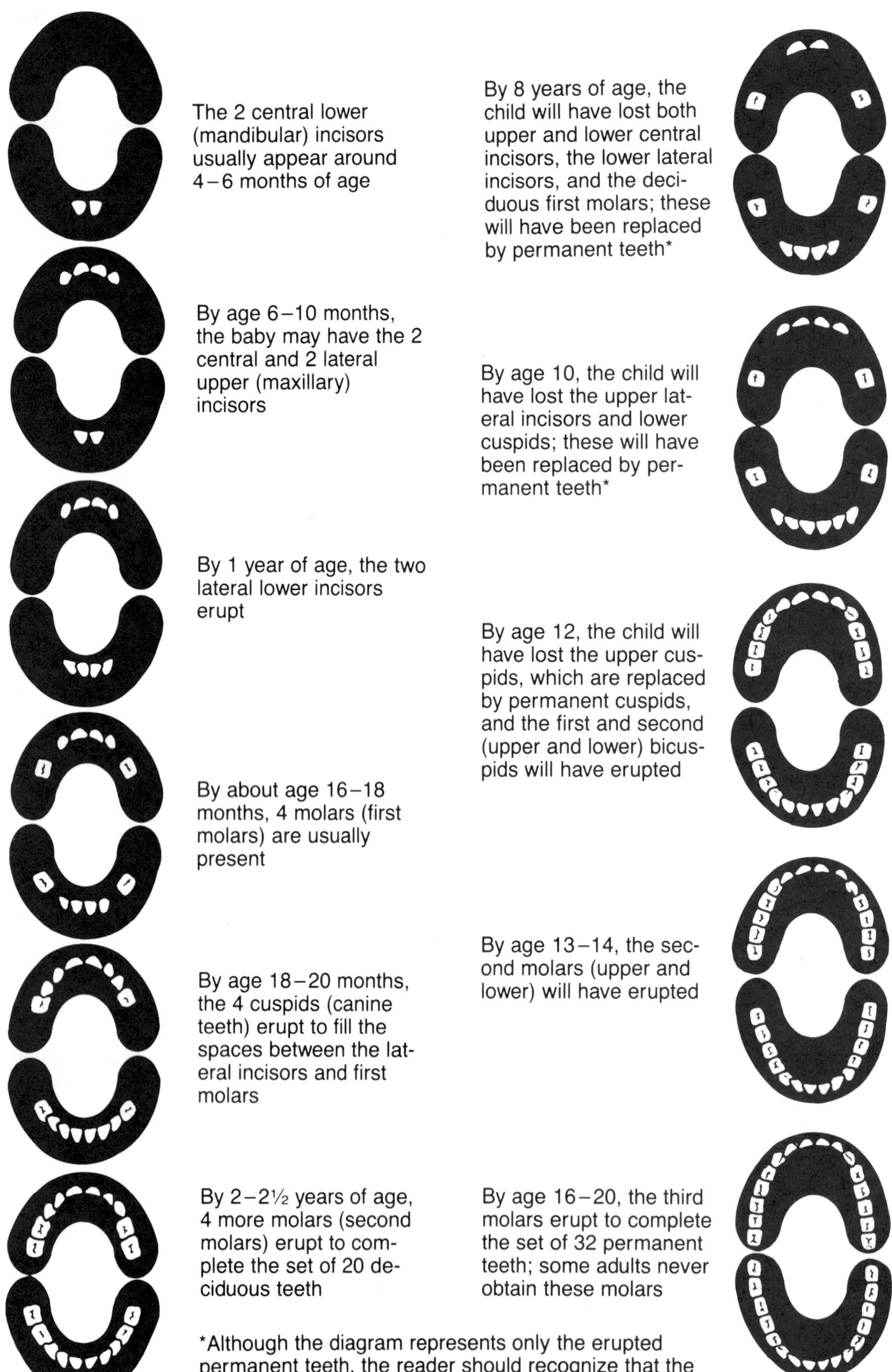

Figure 14-14 Progression of dental development.

for whom the mouth cavity is too small for the normal-size tongue. The attachment of the tongue to the frenulum linguae is assessed to determine whether the child is "tongue-tied."

The hard and soft palates and the pharynx are inspected and palpated for color, shape, position, condition of the tonsils, and the presence of exudate, lesions, and masses. Any cleft in the soft or hard palate is noted, and the height of the palatal area is assessed. An abnormally high arch may cause speech problems and is often associated with congenital disorders. Epstein's pearls, found in neonates, are white nodules in the midline of the palate and are insignificant.

The uvula is inspected for movement and symmetry as the child says "ahhh" or gags. The uvula should remain midline, and the soft and hard palates should rise upward symmetrically. Abnormal movement or absence of movement may indicate paralysis of glossopharyngeal or vagus nerves or diphtheria.

Tonsils, if present, are inspected for color, edema, size (noted as 1+ to 4+), symmetry, and the presence of exudate or crypts. (Tonsillar crypts are scars from past infections.) Tonsils are normally large during childhood but begin to shrink by the time a child reaches puberty. Reddened, enlarged tonsils covered with exudate indicate infection.

The posterior pharynx is assessed for color, edema, and the presence of exudate, lesions, and petechiae. Enlarged adenoids may be seen as lymphoid hyperplasia; viral infections often cause petechiae, ulcers, or vesicles. Postnasal discharge may indicate an allergy or sinus infection. At the end of the examination, the child's gag reflex is tested by stroking the posterior pharynx with the tongue depressor. If the nurse suspects one of the croup syndromes, especially epiglottiditis, this test is contraindicated. Epiglottiditis is evidenced by an acute, sudden onset, drooling, and resistance to lying down (see Chapter 34).

Chest

The chest is examined by inspection, palpation, percussion, and auscultation. Knowing the landmarks of the thorax is important in identifying the underlying structures and describing the exact location of abnormalities. The lines of reference are the midsternal line; the midclavicular lines; the anterior, mid-, and posterior axillary lines; the scapular lines; and the vertebral lines. The landmarks used as points of reference are the manubrium and body of the sternum, the xiphoid process, and the scapula. The angle of Louis, just below the sternal notch, is an important landmark because the second rib articulates there and the trachea bifurcates into the right and left bronchi (Fig. 14-15). The 12 pairs of ribs (the first seven pairs articulate with the sternum; the next three pairs articulate with the ribs above them; and the last two pairs are floating with no direct attachment) can then be palpated laterally to the sternum, taking care to avoid the costochondral junctions. The nurse needs to be familiar with locating and palpating each rib

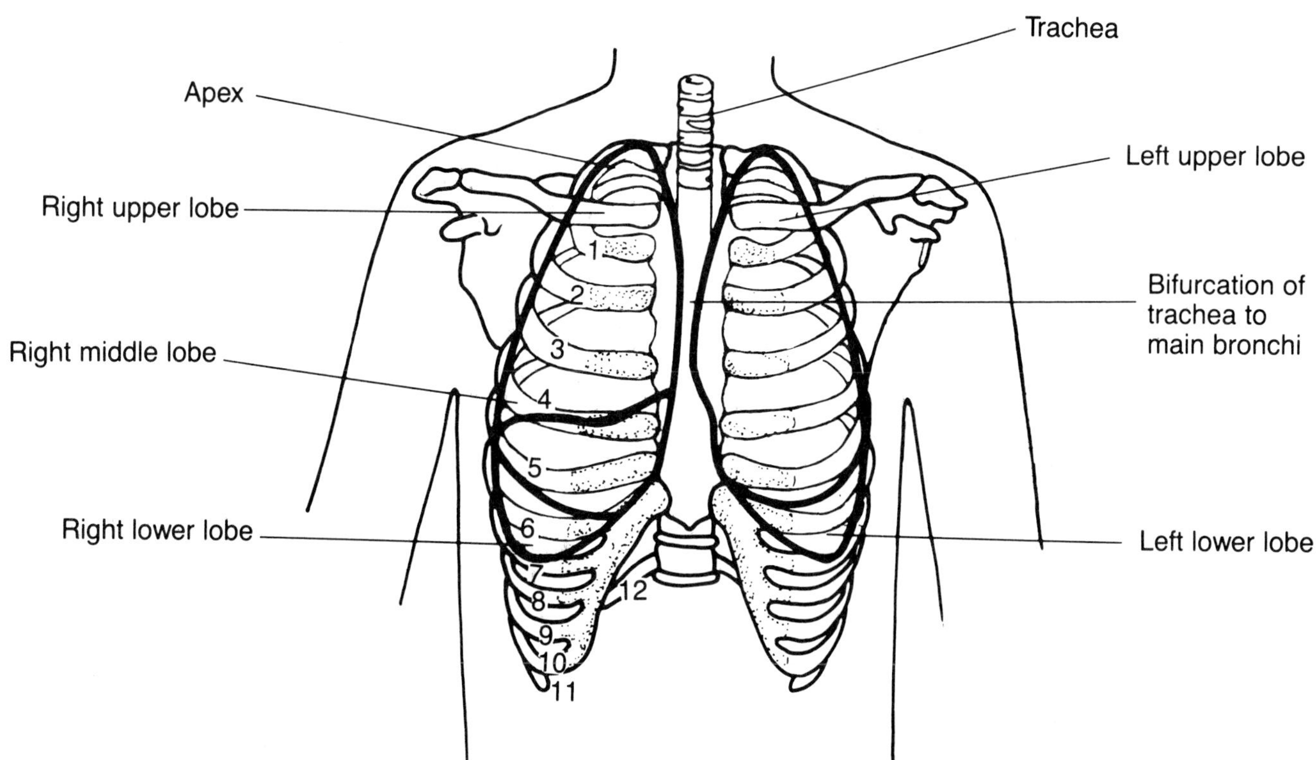

Figure 14-15 Anatomic areas of the chest.

because ribs are anatomic landmarks for palpating, percussing, and auscultating the underlying organs. The space beneath the second rib is the second interspace. Posteriorly, the tip of the scapula is at the sixth to eighth rib, depending on scapular deviation.

The chest is inspected and palpated for skin color, texture, and the presence of lesions and masses. Supernumerary nipples 5–6 cm below the nipples or on the milk line might be noted. Any scar should be described according to size, shape, and location. The chest is inspected for shape. The neonate's chest is round with the anteroposterior diameter equaling the transverse diameter. With growth, the chest assumes a more oval shape, with the transverse diameter greater than the anteroposterior diameter. Marked disproportions in the chest are checked by measuring chest size and comparing it with head size. The relationship between the two will be altered by abnormal chest shapes such as a barrel chest.

Any kyphosis or scoliosis, which affect the shape of the chest, is noted. Atrophy or hypertrophy of chest muscles should be further evaluated to ascertain the cause. Asymmetry of the chest might be caused by tumors, the congenital absence of some chest muscles, precordial bulging or enlargement of the heart, or pneumothorax. Abnormal chest structures are noted and described as "pigeon chest" (sternum protruding from the chest wall and with a series of vertical depressions along the costochondral junction), "barrel chest" (ribs forming circles), and "funnel breast," or pectus excavatum (depression of the sternum). The posterior chest wall also is inspected for symmetry of the scapulas; any deformities are noted.

Lungs The chest should be inspected and palpated during inspiration and expiration (Fig. 14-16). Respiratory motion is observed during quiet and deep respiration. It is important to note the type, rate, rhythm, and depth of respiration. Any use of accessory neck muscles or the presence of retractions is described. With normal inspiration, the chest expands, the sternal angle increases, and the diaphragm descends. With normal expiration, the chest diminishes, the sternal angle decreases, and the diaphragm rises.

The nurse assesses respiratory excursion by placing the hands with fingers slightly spread out at the lower costal borders anteriorly or at the tenth rib posteriorly. During respiration, the nurse's hands will move with the chest wall. The nurse therefore notes any divergence of the thumbs on expiration. In children under 6 or 7 years of age, respiratory movements are abdominal (diaphragmatic); in older children costal (thoracic) movements are observed during respiration. Abdominal breathing in an older child indicates respiratory problems or fracture of one or several of the ribs. Decreased movement on one side of the chest may indicate a pneumothorax, pneumonia, atelectasis, or an obstructive foreign body. Marked retractions are noted, and locations are described as intercostal (between the ribs), suprasternal (above the sternum), substernal (below the sternum), or supraclavicular (above the clavicles).

The character of the respirations is noted and described as normal, unlabored breathing or as dyspnea (labored breathing). The nurse assesses respiration for a full minute because episodes of irregular respirations are normal during infancy. Abnormal respirations should be described as listed in Table 14-8.

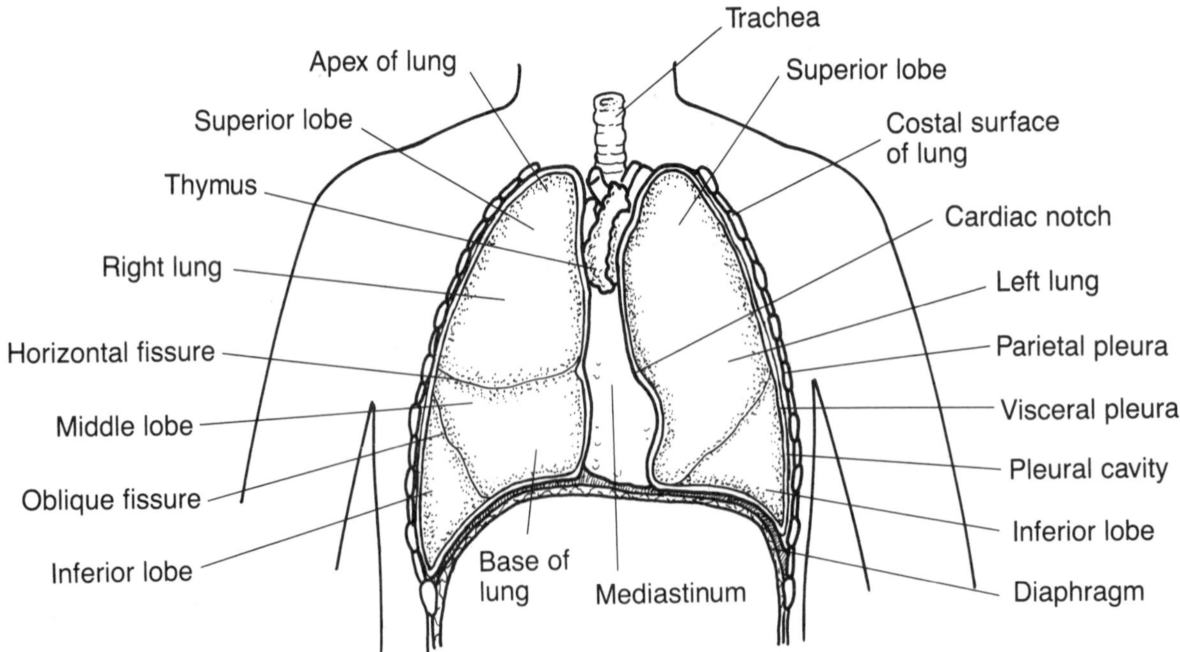

Figure 14-16 Internal structures of the chest cavity.

TABLE 14-8 Various Respiratory Patterns

Pattern	Definition
Biat's breathing	Rapid, irregular breathing; shallow then deep
Cheyne-Stokes respiration	Predictable pattern followed by a pause and then several breaths; hyperpnea, shallow breathing, apnea (may be normal in children)
Kussmaul breathing (hyperpnea)	Deep gasping, hyperventilation
Alkalotic breathing	Slow, shallow breathing
Amphoric breathing	Hollow, low-pitched breathing
Cogwheel breathing	Jerky inspiration
Bradypnea	Abnormally slow respirations, respirations less than normal
Tachypnea	Rapid respirations, faster than normal
Apnea	Cessation of breathing 15–20 seconds or more

Tactile fremitus, the palpation of voice conduction through the thorax, is felt as a vibration on the chest as the child speaks. With the palmar surfaces of the hand, the nurse palpates the child's chest wall, moving symmetrically on either side of the sternum anteriorly and the vertebral column posteriorly. As the child speaks the words "ninety-nine" or "blue moon," the vibrations are felt under the nurse's hands. Tactile fremitus normally is more palpable in infants, thin children, and at the regions of the thorax where the trachea and bronchi are closest to the surface; as the nurse's hands progress downward, the sound decreases and is least palpable at the base of the lungs. Absent or decreased tactile fremitus occurs in disease processes or conditions that cause bronchial blockage such as asthma, pneumothorax, pleural effusion, or aspiration of a foreign body. Increased tactile fremitus occurs when a solid mass is present as a result of pneumonia or atelectasis. When present, as in a lung abscess or occasionally in pneumonia, pleural friction rubs also can be palpated and feel like fine vibrations that cause a tingling sensation on the nurse's fingers. Crepitation, which is actually a sound, is felt where the subcutaneous tissue contains air, as in subcutaneous emphysema. It gives a coarse, crackly sensation.

The chest is percussed to determine the relative amounts of air, liquid, and solid material in the underlying lung and to determine the position and landmarks of organs. Percussion penetrates to a depth of about 5–7 cm, and the sound that emanates depends in part on the amount of muscle and fascia present. The indirect method of percussion is best used to percuss the chest and should proceed in an organized, symmetric manner from side to side in sequence to compare the sounds, then slowly progressing downward, interspace by interspace. Percussion should be performed over the intercostal spaces, just lateral to the sternum anteriorly and the spine posteriorly, avoiding bony prominences. Anteriorly, percussion should begin at the apices of the lungs between the neck and shoulder muscles.

Resonance, a low, loud, long sound, normally is heard over all lung surfaces. Dullness is normal at the fourth to fifth right intercostal space at the midclavicular line (because of the liver) and at the fifth left intercostal space medially to the midclavicular line to the cardiac borders. Tympany, a high, loud, long, musical sound, is normal at the sixth left intercostal space because of the air-filled stomach. Any deviations from these expected sounds is noted and warrants referral. Posteriorly, percussion begins at the shoulders and proceeds in the same symmetric manner. The posterior lung fields should be heard as resonance, with dullness of the diaphragm heard at the level of the eighth to tenth ribs. Hyperresonance, or a deep, dull sound in unexpected areas, warrants referral. Hyperresonance might indicate excess air in the lung tissue or an increase in density (for example, pneumothorax, asthma, emphysema, or pneumonia). See Table 14-9 for a description of percussion notes.

The chest and lungs are auscultated using the diaphragm of the stethoscope because most of the sounds are of high frequency. Auscultation is performed to assess breath sounds, adventitious sounds, bronchopathy, and whispered pectoriloquy. Breath sounds are evaluated for pitch, intensity, quality, duration, and location. The types of breath sounds are listed in Table 14-10. Breath sounds are caused by the motion of air through the upper respiratory tract, trachea, and main bronchi. These sounds are then filtered and altered as they pass through small airways and lung tissue. Therefore, breath sounds vary in healthy and disease states as the underlying lung is altered by the disease process.

Adventitious respiratory sounds (additional sounds not normally heard) are superimposed on normal breath sounds and are not alterations of normal breath sounds. They are classified as either rales or rhonchi and, if noted, are described. Rales result from the passage of air through secretions present in the alveoli. Rhonchi are continuous sounds produced by the passage of air through edematous or spasmodic airways or through bronchi laden with secretions. Wheezes result from partial obstruction caused by

TABLE 14-9 Percussion Notes

Note	Description	Examples
Tympany	High pitch, loud intensity, long duration, musical quality	Gas-filled organs such as stomach or intestines
Hyperresonance	Deep pitch, loud intensity, prolonged duration	Overinflated parts of the lung
Resonance	Low pitch, loud intensity, long duration	Normal parts of the lung
Dullness	Medium pitch, intensity, and duration	Liver, spleen, mass density of an organ
Flatness	High pitch, soft intensity, very short duration	Bone

the narrowing of the lumen of a respiratory passageway (Table 14-11).

Children having adventitious sounds are referred for further evaluation. Absent or diminished breath sounds are always abnormal and also need further investigation. An obstructed airflow can be caused by a foreign body, fluid, air, or mucus.

Voice sounds also are part of the normal auscultation of the lungs. They are elicited in the same manner as tactile fremitus except that the nurse uses the stethoscope. Normal voice sounds or resonances are heard as muffled, indistinguishable sounds. Hearing clear, distinct words on auscultation is abnormal. Whispered pectoriloquy occurs when the child whispers and the nurse listens to the chest through the stethoscope. The nurse should not understand the child's whispered syllables. Bronchophony occurs when the nurse listens as before but the child speaks in a normal volume and tone. Any condition that causes increased fremitus, such as consolidation (for example, from pneumonia or a solid tumor), also results in the verbalized syllables being clearly distinguishable.

Breasts The breasts should be examined in girls and boys as part of the routine well-child examination. The examination can best be incorporated into the inspection and palpation of the skin surface of the chest. If the nurse provides a relaxed and comfortable environment, most children, even pubertal-age children, will cooperate with the examination.

The nipples should be assessed for color, symmetry, spacing, and the presence of any lumps. The darker pigmented areola also should be assessed. Pubertal breast development usually begins in girls between 10 and 14 years of age. One breast may develop before the other, and the child might need to be reassured that this is normal. Precocious breast development in both boys and girls might be normal but requires further evaluation. In males gynecomastia often causes anxiety and conflicts of body image, and the nurse needs to explore the child's feelings. Delayed breast development should be evaluated along with the development of any other secondary sexual characteristics.

The breasts are assessed for size and symmetry, contour, skin color, temperature, tenderness, and the presence of

TABLE 14-10 Characteristics of Breath Sounds

Type	Description	Location
Vesicular Loud Soft	Medium-to-low pitch, low intensity; breezy, swishing, or rushing quality; inspiration three times longer than expiration, seen as 3:1 or 5:2 ratio	Periphery of lung fields except over sternum and scapulae
Bronchovesicular Loud Soft	Medium-to-high pitch; moderate intensity; blowing, muffled sound; inspiration equal to expiration	Normally over upper one-third of sternum and intrascapular area, abnormal in areas where normal vesicular heard, usually indicates a mixture of aerated and consolidated lung
Bronchial Soft Loud	High pitch, loud intensity, harsh and tubular quality expiration twice as long as inspiration and separated by a brief pause, seen as 2:1 ratio	Normally over trachea and manubrium, abnormal over lung periphery and heard in disease states

NOTE: Breath sounds in children seem louder than in adults because of the thinness of the chest wall.

TABLE 14-11 Adventitious Breath Sounds

Type	Description	Etiology
Rales		
Fine (crepitant)	High pitch, soft, crackling or popping noises, noncontinuous, heard at end of inspiration located at periphery of lung fields	Pneumonia, early pulmonary edema, congestive heart failure
Medium (subcrepitant)	Medium pitch, loud, wet, moist, noncrackling, heard on early or midinspiration, clear with coughing located in the bronchioles	Pulmonary edema, increased accumulated secretions
Coarse (bubbling)	Low pitch, loud, bubbling, heard on expiration, clear with coughing located in the trachea or bronchi	Bronchitis, resolving pneumonia
Rhonchi		
Sibilant	High pitch, loud wheezing or musical, mid or late expiration, located in the trachea, bronchi, or bronchioles	Anatomical narrowing of respiratory tract, asthma
Sonorous	Low pitch, loud, snorelike, throughout respiratory cycle, cleared with coughing, located in the larger bronchi or trachea	Upper respiratory tract infections, bronchitis
Pleural friction rub	High pitch, moderately loud, jerky and leathery, most frequently at end of inspiration	Irritated or inflamed pleural surfaces
Wheezes		
Inspiratory	Either more sonorous or musical, heard during inspiration	High obstruction (for example, laryngeal edema or foreign body aspiration)
Expiratory	Whistle or sighing sound heard during expiration resulting from turbulence of airflow	Low obstruction (for example, asthma, bronchiolitis)

masses or lesions. The breasts are palpated with the child in a supine position with the arm on the side to be examined under the head and a pillow under the shoulder. Proceeding from the nipple and progressing in a counterclockwise manner in concentric circles, the nurse palpates lightly with the fingertips in a rolling, circular motion. The entire breast and surrounding area up to the axillas should be palpated. The procedure is then repeated with the opposite breast.

Breasts should be examined in various positions: (a) with the child sitting with arms at the sides; (b) with the child sitting with arms raised above the head; (c) with the child sitting with arms on hips pushing down; and (d) with the child leaning forward with arms extended. With all of these positions inspection for asymmetry, dimpling, masses, and discharge is possible.

Any palpable nodules are described according to location (by quadrant or clock method in centimeters from the nipple), size, shape (round or discoid, regular or irregular), consistency (soft, firm, hard), circumscribed or merging with surrounding tissues, mobility or fixedness, and tenderness.

During the breast examination, the nurse can use the opportunity to discuss sexual maturation and the importance of routine self-examination, especially in adolescent females who have reached sexual maturity. This includes

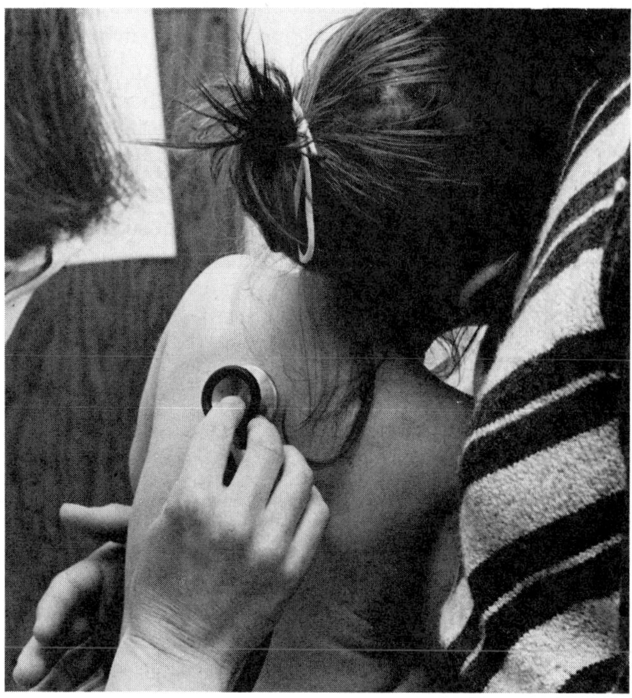

The chest and lungs are auscultated with the diaphragm of the stethoscope.

demonstrating the palpation technique and the most appropriate time of the month to perform breast self-examinations (a few days following menstruation). Estrogen and progesterone hormones might cause benign palpable cysts during preovulatory and ovulatory periods, but these hormones are at their lowest level just after menstruation.

Heart The heart is examined using inspection, palpation, percussion, and auscultation. Percussion to outline the size and shape of the heart may be done using the direct or indirect method. Much practice is required to master either technique. Auscultation provides the most significant data on cardiovascular status and is a useful technique for nurses.

Overall cardiac assessment involves a comprehensive evaluation of the pulses, blood pressure, respiratory function, and general physical growth and development. The nurse therefore palpates the following pulses: superficial temporal, carotid, radial, bronchial, femoral, popliteal, and dorsal pedalis. The normal ranges for these pulses are listed in Appendix B. The various types of pulses that usually are abnormal and require further evaluation are listed in Table 14-12.

The precordium is inspected and palpated to assess precordial bulging, thrills, lifts or heaves, precordial friction rubs, and the point of maximal impulse (PMI). The normal chest is symmetric and quiet, but in thin children the PMI, or apical pulse, may be seen or felt as a slight pulsation. With children 8 years of age and above, this pulse usually is located at the fifth left intercostal space at the midclavicular line (Fig. 14-17). In younger children the PMI may be located higher and more medially because the heart lies slightly more horizontally with the apex to the left of the nipple line. The PMI should be sustained throughout systole and should not be diffuse. As the nurse feels for the PMI, any vibratory thrills and precordial friction rubs are noted. Thrills feel similar to the belly of a purring cat and are caused by forced blood flow from one chamber of the heart to another through narrowed or abnormal openings. Precordial friction rubs are high-pitched grating sounds that are not affected by changes in respiration. In children holding their breath, a precordial friction rub will not cease, whereas a pleural friction rub will stop. Observations of cardiac functioning also include assessing for any clubbing of fingers, peripheral cyanosis, distended neck veins, edema, and bounding pulse pressures.

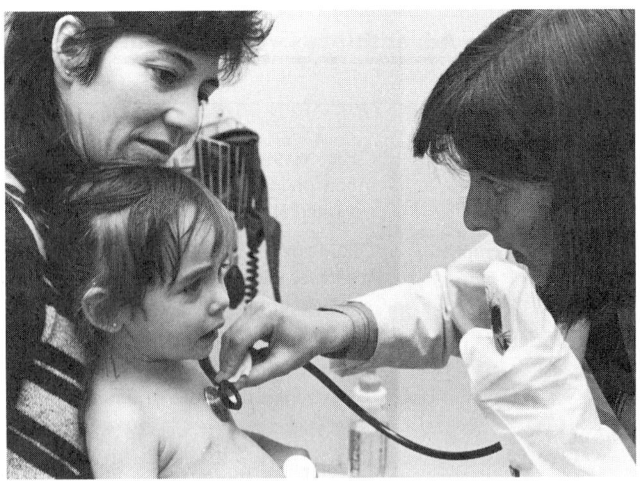

Ausculation of the heart includes the intensity, quality, duration, and location of heart sounds.

The clinical appraisal of a child's cardiovascular status is based to a large extent on the findings made during auscultation of the heart. The heart sounds heard are produced by the opening and closing of heart valves and the vibration of blood against the walls of the heart and vessels (Fig. 14-18). In an organized manner, using both the bell (low frequency) and the diaphragm (high frequency), the nurse assesses the auscultatory areas of the heart as follows:

Sternoclavicular area at the right and left sides of the sternum

Aortic area at the second right interspace adjacent to the sternum

TABLE 14-12 Patterns of Abnormal Pulse

Term	Description
Pulsus alternans	One strong beat followed by one weak beat
Carrigan's pulse (Water hammer pulse)	Forceful, bounding pulse at radial and femoral areas with an increase in pulse pressure
Pulsus bisferiens (Dicrotic pulse)	Double radial pulse for every apical beat
Pulsus bigeminus	Coupled rhythm with the beat felt in pairs
Pulsus paradoxes	Waxing and waning, intensity of pulse decreasing with inspiration
Sinus arrhythmia	Rate increasing with inspiration, decreasing with expiration (a normal arrythmia)
Bradycardia	Decreased rate
Tachycardia	Increased rate

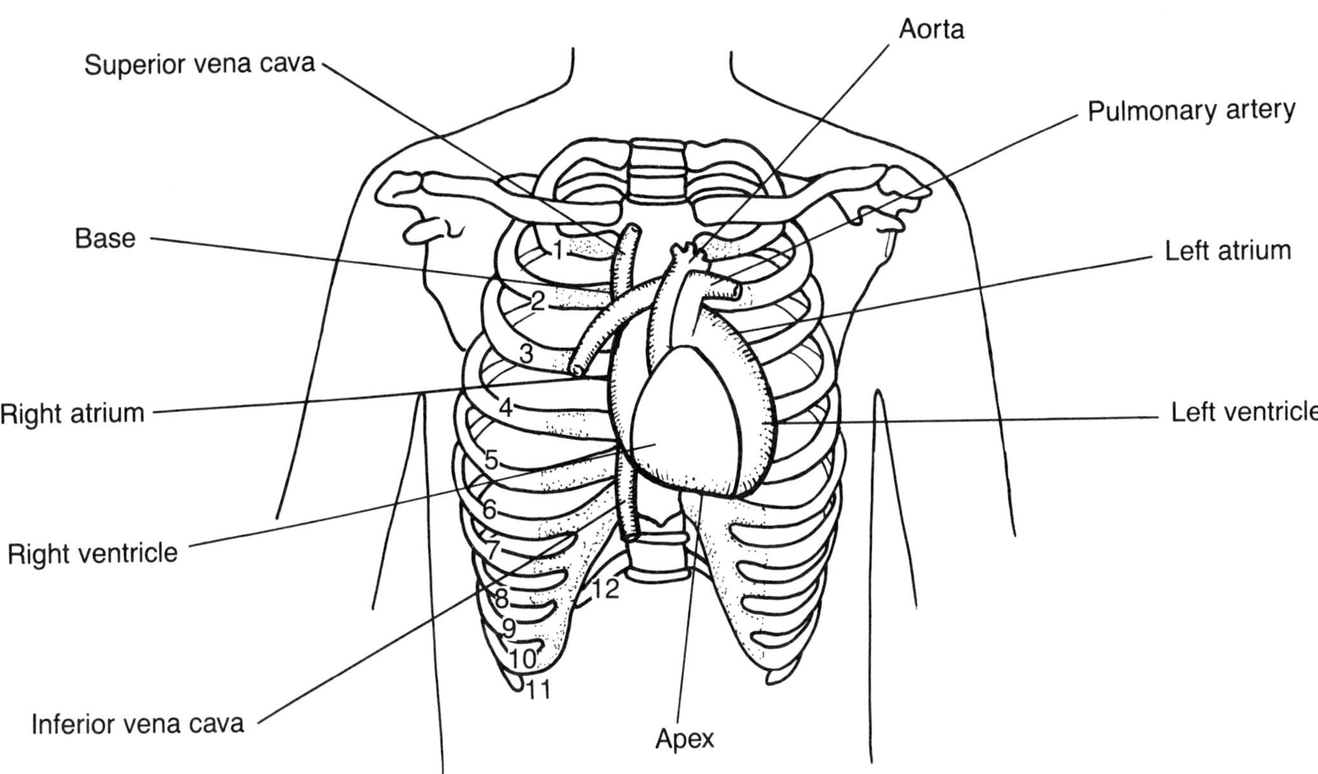

Figure 14-17 Structures of the heart.

Pulmonic area at the second and third interspaces next to the sternum

Anterior precordium

Erbs's point, or ectopic area, at the third, fourth, and fifth right interspace and sometimes to the left and directly over the sternum

Mitral or apical area at the fifth interspace at the mid-clavicular line

The nurse also should auscultate the area around the left lower sternal border because this is often where functional murmurs are heard best.

Auscultation should include assessment of the intensity, quality, duration, and location of the heart sounds. The point at which they are loudest and whether any splitting is present also should be noted. Under normal circumstances, only two sounds are produced during each cardiac contraction. The first heart sound (S_1), the "lub," is the result of vibrations transmitted from the area of the mitral and tricuspid valves as they close at the onset of ventricular systole. This first heart sound is synchronous with the carotid pulse. The nurse can time the heart sounds by simultaneously palpating the carotid pulse and auscultating the apical pulse. The first heart sound is normally louder at the apex and is long and low pitched. The mitral valve closes slightly ahead of the tricuspid valve but is not normally audible. The second heart sound (S_2), the "dub," results from closure of the aortic and pulmonic valves (semilunar valves). Aortic valve closing occurs slightly ahead of pulmonic valve closing and may be audible. S_2 is shorter and higher pitched than S_1. With closure of the semilunar valves, blood flows into the aorta and the pulmonary artery.

The aortic valve closure is heard best in the second intercostal space to the right of the sternal border. The pulmonic valve closure is heard best in the second intercostal space to the left of the sternal border. The tricuspid valve is heard best in the fourth and fifth intercostal space to the left of the sternal border and also to the right of the sternum. The mitral valve is heard best in the fourth and fifth intercostal space just to the left of the mid-clavicular line. The examiner should also listen over the carotid area in the neck, over and under the clavicle, along both the right and left sternal borders, and over the left anterior chest, the left lateral thorax, and the left and mid back. Auscultation should be done with the child in the upright position, the recumbent position, and the left lateral decubitus position.

The interval between S_2 and S_1 is the diastole, or heart relaxation. A split of these sounds in S_2 often is distinguishable as a widening of the sounds during inspiration because inspiration prolongs ventricular filling and delays pulmonary valve closure. It is considered normal in children and should disappear when children are asked to hold their breath. "Fixed splitting," in which the split in S_2 does not change during inspiration, is abnormal and warrants referral.

Two other heart sounds, S_3 and S_4, may be auscultated. S_3 is heard early in the diastole at the apical area and is the result of vibrations produced during ventricular filling. It is

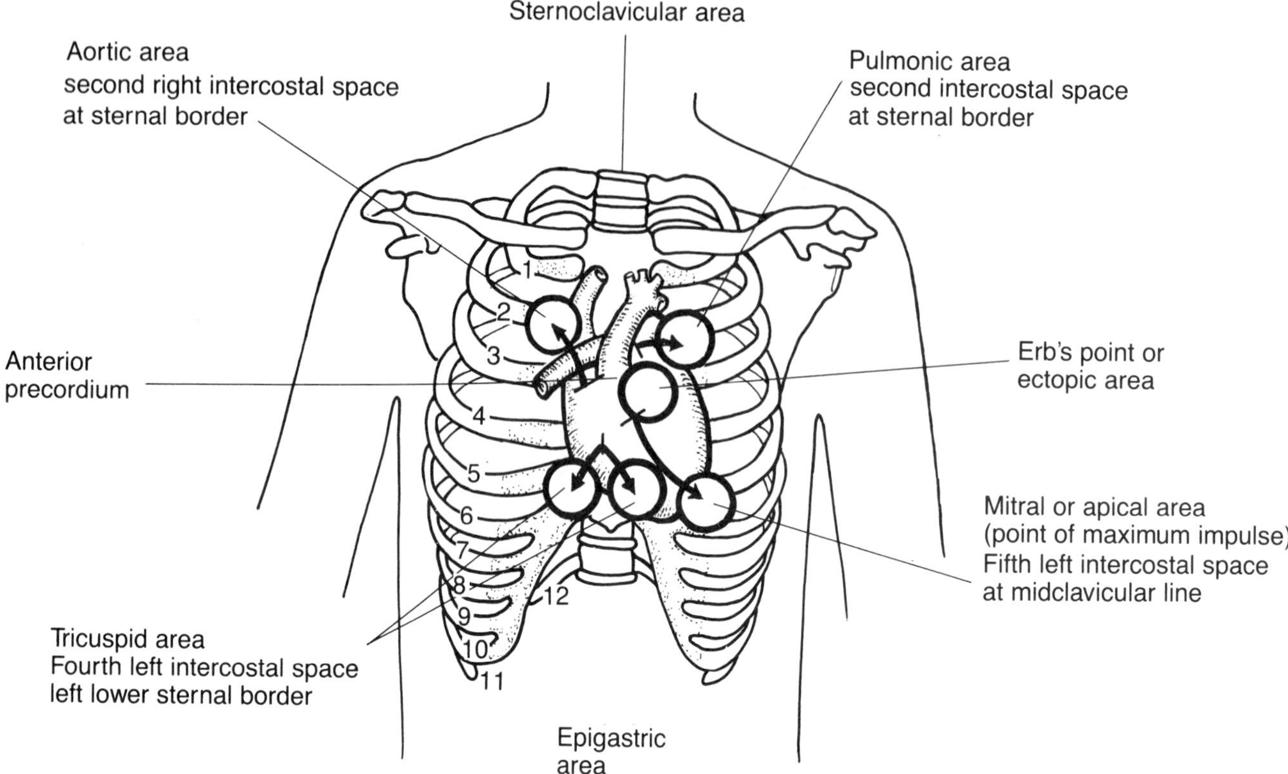

Figure 14-18 Sites for auscultation of the heart.

normal in children and young adults, especially in conjunction with a slow heart rate, but is abnormal in older adults unless they are active athletes. S_4 is a presystolic heart sound caused by an audible atrial contracton as a result of ventricular overload. It is considered abnormal and requires further evaluation. Table 14-13 summarizes the characteristic of heart sounds.

Heart sounds should be auscultated with the child in a supine position, in a left lateral lying position, and in a sitting position. If abnormal heart sounds are heard, the child should then also be evaluated when standing and when leaning forward. Specific abnormal heart sounds are louder in certain positions. Ejection clicks, which are most often caused by aortic or pulmonic stenosis, are high-pitched sounds

TABLE 14-13 Heart Sounds

Heart Sound	Cause	Location	Characteristics
S_1	Closure of the mitral and tricuspid valves, which occurs at the beginning of systole	Apex of the heart	Slight split may be heard as mitral valve closes slightly before the tricuspid and occurs simultaneously with carotid pulse
S_2	Closure of the aortic and pulmonic valves, which occurs at the beginning of diastole	Base of the heart	Split sound may be heard as aortic valve closes slightly before pulmonic valve. Normal "physiologic split" is wider on inspiration and narrower on expiration. A wide split or a "fixed split" (no variance with respiration) is not normal and is associated with atrial septal defect
S_3	Thought to be caused by rapid blood flow from atria to ventricle. Heard early in diastole	Near the apex of the heart with the bell in the left lateral decubitus	Referred to as "gallop rhythm." May be normal in children but also is a symptom of congestive heart failure
S_4	Heard late in diastole, just before S_1		May be normal in children but usually requires further evaluation

TABLE 14-14 Grading of Intensity of Heart Murmurs

Grade	Description
I	Very faint, frequently not heard if child sits up or has just exercised
II	Usually audible in all positions, louder than Grade I
III	Loud but not accompanied by a thrill
IV	Loud, accompanied by a thrill
V	Loud enough to be heard with stethoscope barely on chest wall and accompanied by a thrill
VI	Often heard with ear, loud enough to be heard with stethoscope not touching chest wall, accompanied by a thrill

occurring early in the systole and are abnormal. An opening snap, another abnormal heart sound, is a brief, high-pitched sound that occurs early in the diastole and is caused by mitral or tricuspid valve stenosis.

Murmurs are another category of heart sounds. Murmurs are caused by turbulent blood flow, which results from (1) blood trying to flow past a partial obstruction; (2) an irregularity within a blood vessel; (3) increased blood flow due to fever, anemia, or hyperthyroidism; (4) the flow of blood into a dilated chamber; (5) regurgitant blood flow due to incompetent valves; or (6) blood going from high pressure to low pressure, as in a septal defect. Murmurs should be described according to their timing or the point at which they occur in the S_1-S_2 cycle. Timing then is noted as early, middle, or late systolic or diastolic. Murmurs are described further by their location, or the point at which the sound is heard best on the chest (for example, pulmonic, aortic); by their radiation, or the point to which the sound radiates when auscultated from loudest to faintest areas; and by their grade, or intensity (Table 14-14).

There are two types of murmurs: innocent (functional) and organic. Although definitive diagnosis requires referral to a physician, the nurse might be able to differentiate the two types. Innocent murmurs are generally systolic, of short duration, not transmitted to other areas of the heart, low pitched, and musical. They are usually Grade III or lower, do not increase over time, and vary according to position. They do not affect normal growth and development. (Organic murmurs are pathologic and discussed in Chapter 35.)

Abdomen

The abdomen usually is examined beginning with inspection and then proceeding to auscultation, percussion, and palpation. Depending on the age and cooperativeness of the child, the sequence may be altered. Auscultation frequently follows the evaluation of heart and lung sounds if the child remains quiet. Inspection can occur whenever the child is undressed, and palpation might be left for the end of the examination, when the child is more comfortable with the nurse. A thorough abdominal evaluation requires that the nurse be familiar with the location of the abdominal organs and their normal size, shape, and consistency (Fig. 14-19).

In inspecting the abdomen the nurse assesses abdominal movement, size, symmetry, contour, skin color and integrity, the umbilicus, and the presence of any masses. Because the respiratory pattern of the young child is abdominal, the nurse can observe movement of the abdomen with inspiration and expiration. A child in this age group who is not following the abdominal breathing pattern needs to be assessed for peritoneal irritation. Older children (6–8 years of age or older) who are using abdominal muscles to breathe need to be assessed for respiratory problems. Peristalsis is not normally visible and, if observed, might indicate such intestinal obstruction as pyloric stenosis, malrotation of the bowel, or duodenal stenosis. Pulsations in the epigastric

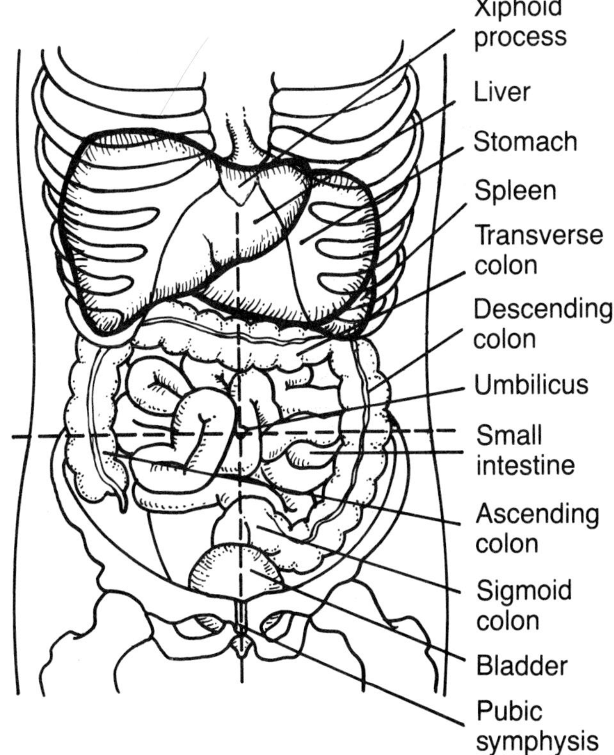

Figure 14-19 Abdominal structures.

area might be normal aortic pulsations. These are especially evident in thin children but should be assessed to rule out an aortic aneurysm.

A child's abdomen should be symmetric, but the contour varies depending on the child's age, muscular development, and general nutritional status. The normal abdomens of infants and young children have a prominent "potbelly" appearance. By 4–5 years of age, this potbelly shape begins to disappear, and the child's abdomen has a flatter contour. A scaphoid (concave) abdomen is seen in children who are thin or undernourished. A large, prominent, flabby abdomen often is seen in obese children. Any protuberant abdomen needs to be evaluated for tumor, *organomegaly* (enlargement of an organ), ascites, feces, flatulence, or pregnancy, all of which can cause abdominal distention. The abdomen should be inspected from all sides to determine the extent and location of the distention; it is then percussed and palpated.

The umbilicus is inspected for position, herniation, inflammation, discharge, and odor. A bluish umbilicus might occur with intra-abdominal hemorrhage; a nodular umbilicus might signify abdominal cancer. An everted umbilicus without a hernia might be caused by increased intra-abdominal pressure, whereas an inverted umbilicus might be normal or caused by obesity. An umbilical calculus is a hard mass of debris that is the result of poor hygiene; a granuloma is a small, red, solid button deep in the umbilicus and is seen in neonates.

Protrusion of the umbilicus might indicate a herniation. The nurse should palpate the size of the opening. Most hernias close by the time the child is 1 year of age, but can be seen in children up to 2 or 3 years old. Treatment is variable, but at no time are such "home remedies" as belly binders or belly tapes helpful. The muscles strengthen with maturation and increased activity, especially walking.

Diastosis recti abdominis (splitting) of the rectus muscles of the abdomen, which leaves the central portion of the abdomen uncovered, is not uncommon. As long as the muscle is not herniated and only 1–2 in of width are bulging, this condition can be considered normal.

Drainage from the umbilicus should be assessed for odor, color, amount, and consistency, and periumbilical redness should be examined. Any drainage should be cultured. The drainage might be caused by infection, a patent urachus, or a urachal cyst.

Auscultation follows inspection so that bowel sounds are not disturbed by percussion and palpation. Bowel sounds, the result of peristalsis, are the short clicks and gurgles heard through the stethoscope. They occur every 10–30 seconds, and their frequency is recorded as the number per minute (for example, five bowel sounds per minute). *Borborygmus,* or "stomach growls," the loud grumbling noises often heard without a stethoscope, can occur as frequently as 15–34/min. High-pitched, hyperactive sounds are heard in children with gastroenteritis, diarrhea, and intestinal obstruction. The absence of peristalsis might indicate paralytic ileus or peritonitis, but bowel sounds might be irregular; therefore, the nurse must listen for at least 5–10 minutes before judging that they are absent. The frequency and character of bowel sounds should be auscultated in each quadrant. Various other sounds, usually vascular sounds, might be auscultated and are described for pitch, intensity, and location. Bruits, rubs, and hums warrant referral for further evaluation.

The abdomen is percussed to delineate the location, size, and contour of specific organs. With the child in a supine position, either on the examining table or on the parent's lap, the abdomen is percussed using indirect percussion. The nurse follows a pattern beginning on one side and proceeding around to all four quadrants. Liver dullness is percussed at the sixth interspace anteriorly, the midaxillary line, and the ninth interspace posteriorly. The lower border of the liver often is percussed 2–3 cm below the costal

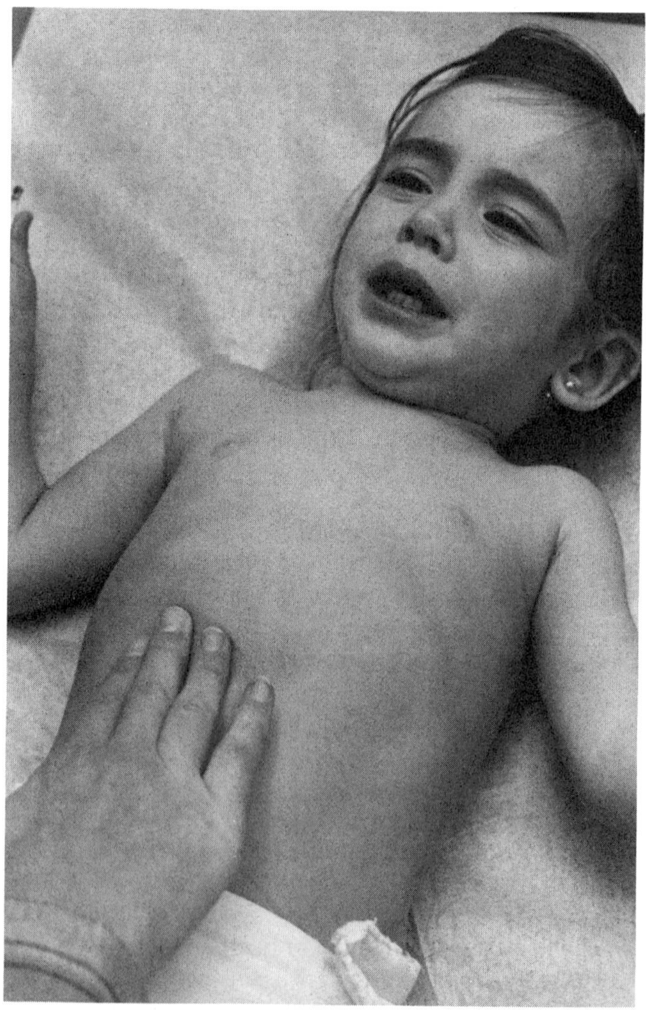

Superficial palpation involves lightly palpating the abdomen using the fingertips as points of pressure to identify areas of tenderness, muscle tone, or presence of lesions.

margin. The best technique for assessing the size of the liver is to percuss downward from lung resonance to dullness at the midclavicular and midaxillary lines and up from tympany in the lower quadrant to dullness of the lower borders. The spleen generally is percussed between the ninth and eleventh interspaces in the left midaxillary line. An occasional tympanic note is percussed where the lung overlies the splenic flexure. Tympany generally is heard over the stomach and the rest of the abdomen. Any other percussed areas of dullness might indicate masses or excessive obstruction with feces and requires careful evaluation.

The final method of assessment is palpation. There are two types of palpation: superficial and deep. Superficial palpation of the abdomen involves lightly palpating each quadrant, noting any areas of tenderness, assessing muscle tone, and noting the presence of any superficial lesions. It is best done by placing the examining hand flat onto the skin and using the fingertips as points of slight pressure. Tenderness elicited during superficial palpation might be caused by visceral pain, somatic pain, or rebound tenderness. *Visceral pain* is pain from an organic lesion or organ dysfunction. It is dull, poorly localized, and difficult to characterize. *Somatic pain* arises from involvement of somatic structures such as the peritoneum of the abdominal wall. It is a sharp, bright pain and is well localized. *Rebound tenderness* is the phenomenon of pain occurring when the fingers are removed during palpation. It may suggest peritoneal inflammation or appendicitis.

Deep palpation is performed to detect any organomegaly (of the spleen, liver, kidneys, or part of the colon) and any masses. Masses are described by their size, location, consistency, contour, mobility, and tenderness. Deep palpation requires warm hands and a relaxed child. The nurse might find it helpful to have the child flex the knees to relax the abdominal musculature or to divert the child's attention by playing games or asking interesting questions.

Deep palpation is best done during deep inspiration and deep expiration. The nurse might use one hand to support the posterior structures while placing the examining hand on the abdomen. Another method is to place one hand on top of the other to provide guidance and firmer pressure. If a child has complained of pain during superficial palpation, that area of the abdomen is deeply palpated last. Deep palpation usually begins in the lower left quadrant and then proceeds to the lower right quadrant and upward so that an enlarged spleen or liver is not missed.

The spleen normally can be palpated 1–2 cm below the left costal margin in infants and young children. It often is not palpable in older children. Normally, only the tip of the older child's spleen is felt during inspiration as it descends into the abdominal cavity. Ballottement, or palpating for the spleen between two hands, one placed against the back and the other pushing frontward, is often useful in locating the spleen. Special care must be taken when inflammation of the spleen is likely (for example, in infectious mononucleosis or erythroblastosis) because it is possible to rupture an inflamed spleen.

The liver edge normally can be palpated 1–3 cm below the right costal margin in infants and young children. In older children the liver might not be palpable. It is best felt by palpation beginning below and easing toward the costal margin, pressing in and up as the child inspires or holds the breath in. Normally, the liver descends during inspiration as the diaphragm moves downward, and its sharp edge can be felt on the flat palpating fingers. Liver tenderness occurs in children with infectious hepatitis, liver abscesses, or infectious mononucleosis.

The kidneys are only significantly palpable in neonates. The kidneys are rarely felt at any other time because they lie too deep in the abdominal cavity. If they are palpable, only a normal lower pole of the right kidney is often felt, but it is important to rule out hydronephrosis, polycystic disease, and Wilms' tumor.

The bladder, if distended, is palpable above the symphysis pubis. Occasionally, the cecum, a soft, gas-filled mass, is palpable in the right lower quadrant. The sigmoid colon also might be palpated as a sausage-shaped mass that is freely movable and often tender in the left, lower quadrant. The sigmoid colon must not, however, be mistaken for intussusception, which involves pain.

The inguinal canal should be inspected and palpated for hernias during the routine examination. Inguinal hernias are protrusions of peritoneum through the abdominal wall in the region of the inguinal canal. An indirect inguinal

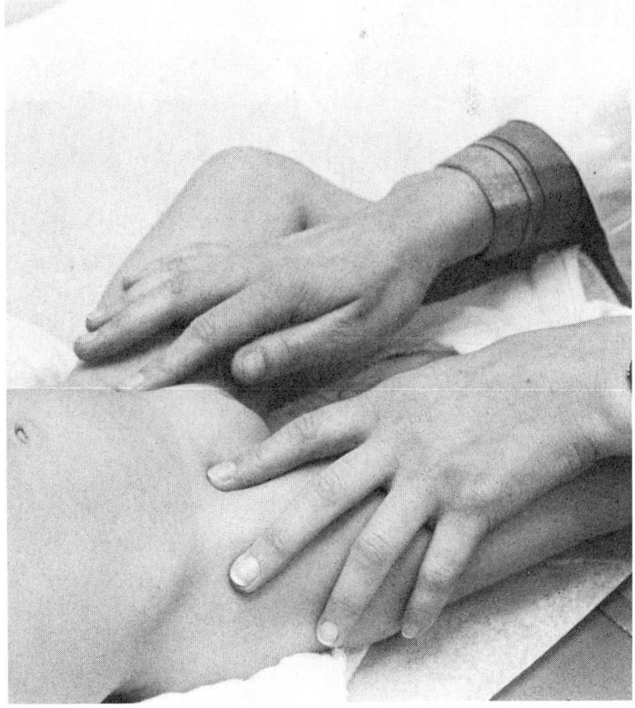

Palpation for a femoral hernia, which may be found about two fingerbreadths inside the femoral artery.

hernia passes through both the internal and external inguinal rings and transverses the inguinal canal. It is nine times more frequent in boys and often becomes quite large and descends into the scrotum. It is seen at birth or by 2–3 months of age. Palpation for inguinal hernias involves sliding the little finger into the external ring at the base of the scrotum following the spermatic cord. A direct inguinal hernia bulges through the posterior wall of the inguinal canal of Hesselbach's triangle, directly behind the external ring. It is palpated as a bulge at the area of the inguinal canal and is frequently an acquired hernia in males. A femoral hernia is found about two fingerbreadths inside the femoral artery and is common in females. It is palpable as a small, soft mass in the femoral canal, on the anterior surface of the thigh.

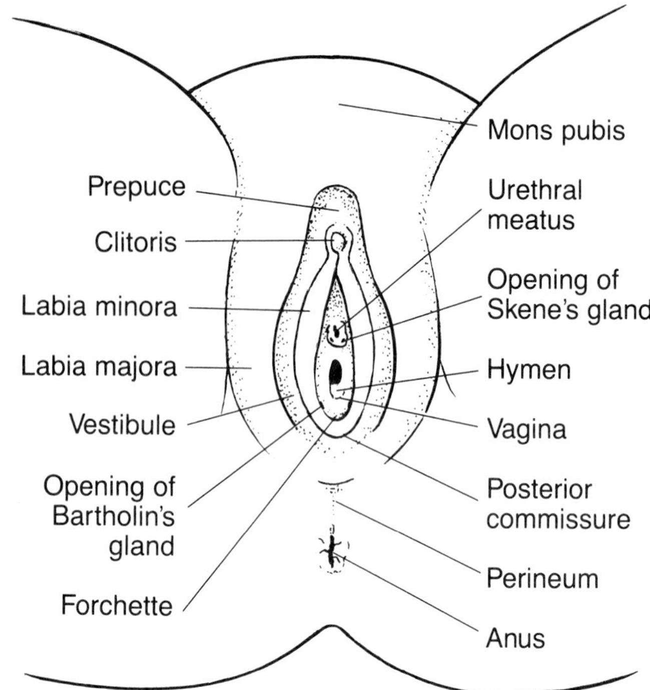

Figure 14-20 External female genitalia.

Genitalia

Female Genitalia Assessment of the female genitalia should be part of every routine well-child examination. It often follows the abdominal assessment while the child is still in the supine position. Adolescents, because of their concern and modesty, might request that the examination be done either at the beginning or at the end of the physical assessment. It is best to proceed quickly with the examination and to reassure both child and parent if everything appears normal. The nurse may wear examining gloves during inspection and palpation of the genitalia.

The external female genitalia are examined for any masses or lesions on the mons pubis (Fig. 14-20). The presence or absence of pubic hair is noted, and hair is described according to its distribution, color, quantity, and quality. The labia majora and labia minora are inspected for skin integrity, color, size, and the presence of any masses. In infants the labia minora usually is larger than the labia majora. Any swelling and redness in an older child might signify an infection, masturbation, or foreign-body or sexual molestation. Any skin lesions, such as chancres or warts (condyloma acuminatum), are noted. The clitoris, normally about 2 × 1 cm, is assessed for size. It might normally be large in the neonate, however, because of maternal hormones. Any enlarged clitoris should be further evaluated to rule out pseudohermaphroditism or labioscrotal fusion.

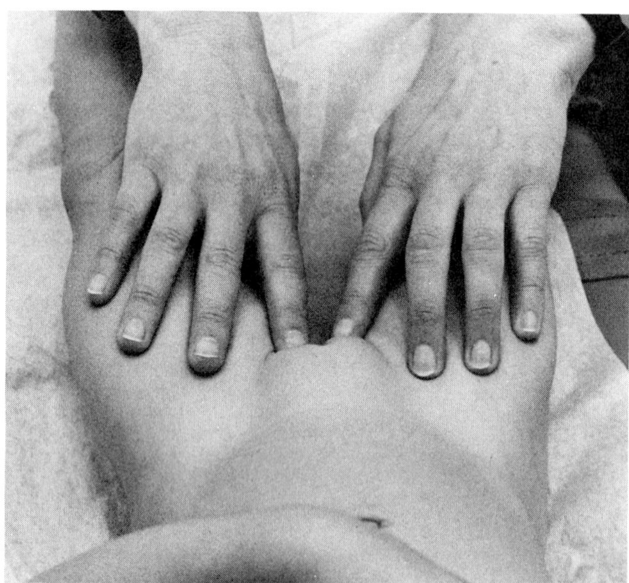

Assessment of the genitalia generally follows the abdominal assessment and includes inspection and palpation for any abnormalities.

The urethral meatus should be assessed for erythema (indicative of urethritis), edema, and discharge. If Bartholin's and Skene's glands are palpable, an infection (usually a sexually transmitted disease) is present and requires further evaluation. The vestibule should be inspected and palpated for lesions and masses. In sexually active adolescents the urethral meatus frequently is the site of venereal lesions.

The vaginal opening is assessed for size, adhesions, erythema, edema, and discharge. Congenital absence of the vagina or an imperforate hymen are noted if either condition is present. Redness and foul-smelling discharge indicates an infection, a foreign body, or pinworms. A cheesy, white, thick discharge is characteristic of a candidal infection.

A pelvic examination also is performed on sexually active adolescents, girls requesting oral contraceptives, older adolescents whose mothers received diethylstilbestrol (DES), and adolescents with primary amenorrhea. Younger children with histories of sexual abuse and trauma might require speculum examinations of the walls of the vagina.

Male Genitalia As with girls, the genitalia examination of boys should proceed in an efficient, nonchalant, and relaxed manner (Fig. 14-21). Reassuring the child and parent that the findings are normal reduces anxiety and fearfulness.

The penis is assessed for skin color, texture, and integrity. An enlarged penis may be due to precocious puberty or testicular cancer. In uncircumcised neonates the foreskin remains tight and is not freely retractable until 1–2 years of age. After 2 years of age, the prepuce, or foreskin, of uncircumcised boys should be assessed for retractability. It normally retracts easily from the glans. Phimosis is present when the foreskin is not freely retractable and prevents observation of the glans and interior surface of the prepuce.

Adhesions sometimes are seen in males as the result of the circumcision or the traumatic retracting of a tight foreskin. Lesions, such as chancres, warts, such as condyloma acuminatum, and nodules palpated on the dorsomedial surface of the penis require further evaluation.

The urethral meatus is assessed for position, shape, ulceration, and discharge. Normally, it is positioned centrally on the tip of the glans. *Hypospadias* is a condition in which the meatal opening is on the ventral side of the penis; *epispadias* is a meatal opening on the dorsal side. If possible, the child's urinary stream should be observed, or information from the child or parent should be obtained on the strength and steadiness of the urinary stream. In neonates it is important to observe the urinary stream to assess the possibility of bladder neck obstruction or a malformed urethra. A short urethra could lead to future kidney or bladder infections.

The shaft of the penis is inspected for size, varicosities, and masses. The infant's penis is approximately 2–3 cm long; a smaller penis may indicate pseudohermaphroditism. During puberty, the penile shaft enlarges to adult size and pubic hair develops. Pubic hair should be described for its distribution, color, quantity, and quality.

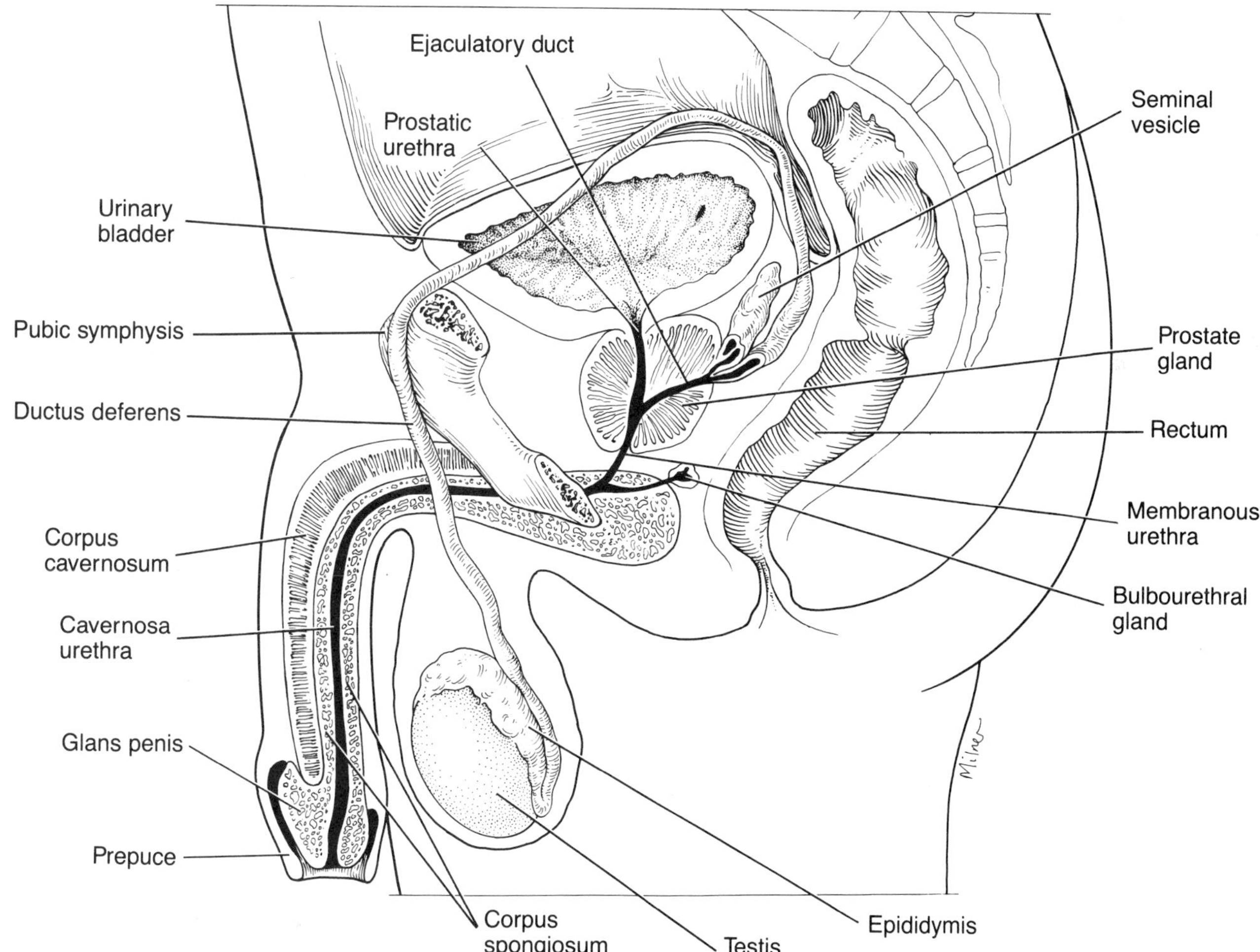

Figure 14-21 Sagittal section of the male pelvis. (From Spence AP, Mason EB: *Human Anatomy and Physiology*, 2nd ed. Benjamin/Cummings, 1983.)

The scrotum is inspected and palpated for size, symmetry, edema, masses, and lesions. The scrotum enlarges with the development of secondary sexual characteristics, and the number of rugae increases. The scrotum may appear asymmetric because the left testis is generally lower than the right testis in the scrotal sac. Any lesions should be noted; firm, yellow-to-white, nontender sebaceous cysts frequently are seen. The scrotum should be palpated bilaterally for the testes. The testes are evaluated for size, shape, and consistency; they should be equal in size, regularly smooth, freely movable, and slightly sensitive to compression. To palpate the testes, the nurse holds one finger over the inguinal canal, occluding it while palpating the scrotum with the other hand. The procedure is then repeated on the opposite side. The normal cremasteric reflex causes the testes to ascend into the inguinal canal, making them inaccessible to palpation. The absence of testes in the scrotum is called *cryptorchidism* and warrants referral if the child is over 3 years of age. Most undescended testes descend by that time; if not, surgical intervention might be required.

The epididymis is palpated as a vertical ridge of soft, nodular tissue behind the testes. It is evaluated for size, shape, consistency, and tenderness. The spermatic cord is palpated by grasping it between the thumb and forefinger; it should be traced from its origin in the testes up to the pelvic cavity. Normally, these last two structures are difficult to assess and often are not readily palpable to the beginning practitioner.

Hernias also might be assessed as part of the genital examination. Assessment of femoral pulses and regional lymph nodes also should be included at this time.

Musculoskeletal System

The musculoskeletal system is responsible for the support of the body and movement as muscles attached to the bones shorten in contraction and lengthen in extension. The examination of the musculoskeletal system begins as the child is observed walking, sitting, rising from sitting, playing, and performing such tasks as dressing and undressing. The examination should proceed from general to specific inspection.

General inspection should include observations for general body alignment and symmetry of movements; the nurse notes any clumsy, awkward, or involuntary movements. Any deformities are often immediately obvious, and any shortenings or lengthenings of the extremities should be described. Unusual postures might be evident and should be assessed completely during the regional examination of the spine. Every inch of the spine and extremities should be palpated to gather complete data. Bones are palpated for general shape and outline. Any thickening, abnormal prominences, or indentations are noted. The skin over the joints is palpated for temperature, tenderness, pain, and swelling. Both sides of the body should be compared. Active and passive motion of the joints should be assessed and findings described by normal range of motion, restricted motion, severe weakness, or paralysis. Muscles are inspected and palpated for symmetry, mass, tone, strength,and paralysis. Muscle tone normally is felt as slight resistance when a relaxed limb is moved passively. Muscle tone is described as normal, rigid, spastic, or weak; strength and power are assessed with gravity, against gravity, and against resistance. A simple test is to place both the nurse's hands in the child's and ask the child to squeeze hard. Another test is to have the child attempt to pull away as the examiner firmly grasps both hands.

Inspection and palpation of the upper extremities begins with assessment of the head and neck. The clavicles and scapulas are palpated for size and symmetry, and any fractures or abnormalities are noted, especially in the neonate. The neck is placed through a range of motions, and any trapezius muscle spasm or neck swelling is noted. The hands and wrists are tested for range of motion, and the joints are palpated for warmth and tenderness, which may indicate rheumatoid arthritis or redness and bony enlargement. The length of the fingers is assessed as long, narrow, short, stubby, or clubbed. The number of fingers is counted and any *polydactylism* (extra digits) or *syndactylism* (webbed digits) noted.

Widening of the wrist bones may indicate rickets and is therefore noted. Creases of the hands are inspected for the normal crease pattern (*dermatoglyphics*). The simian crease seen in individuals with Down's syndrome also is seen in 5% of the normal population; it may be normal but is noted. The elbows are assessed for swelling, inflammation, tenderness, nodules, and the carrying angle. The arms normally form a smooth, continuous line of approximately 180°. If the lower arm is bent forward, decreasing the angle, the child is said to have an increased carrying angle. The child's shoulders also should be assessed for pain and motion; the nurse attempts to push the child's arms down as the child resists by extending the arms in front.

The lower extremities are inspected and palpated, beginning at the hips. The range of motion of the hips is very important in childhood and must be assessed from the neonatal period throughout development. Undiagnosed hip contractures, which may be preventable, can cause lifelong disability. The neonate's hips are therefore assessed for adduction and abduction to rule out congenital dislocation or subluxation of the hip. Ortolani's maneuver is used to assess a neonate's hips. It is done by placing the infant in the supine position. While flexing the infant's hips and knees to a 90° angle, the nurse's middle finger is placed opposite the lesser trochanter and the thumb is placed in the inguinal area. The infant's thighs then are moved into abduction while thumb pressure is applied forward and inward over the lesser trochanter. This maneuver will demonstrate dislocation of the hips if a palpable "click" is felt as the femoral head relocates in the acetabulum. The hips of older children can be tested for contracture (flexion deformity) by having the child lie supine and alternately flex each hip by bending the knee and pulling it up towards the chest. If a hip flexion contracture is present, the hip opposite the bent knee will flex up also, which indicates a positive Thomas test.

The knees are inspected and palpated for normal hollows above the patella. Any loss of normal contours might indicate fluid in the knee. Several maneuvers test for fluid in the knee; the bulge sign is a bulge of fluid medial to the patella after milking the patella on either side in an upward direction and tapping lateral to the patella. This test is particularly useful with small amounts of fluid. For larger amounts of fluid, ballottement of the knee is more useful. This is done by pushing downward above the patella, then tapping the patella briskly against the femur. If an audible or palpable tap results, the sign is positive, indicating fluid under the kneecap. The knees also should be assessed for injuries such as torn medial or collateral ligaments and torn miniscus.

The legs are assessed for symmetry, shape, strength, and equality of length. *Genu varum,* or "bowlegs," is a lateral bowing of the tibia. It may be normal in toddlers and should disappear as the child begins to walk but may persist up to $3\frac{1}{2}$ years of age. Genu varum is present when, as a child stands, the medial malleoli are in opposition, and the knees are greater than 1 in apart. *Genu valgum,* or "knock knees," is seen if knees touch and when the medial malleoli are more than 1 in apart from each other. It appears between 3 and 4 years of age. If it persists, however, it should be further evaluated.

Tibial torsion, or abnormal rotation or bowing of the tibia, also might be seen in young children (Fig. 14-22). One test is to have the child sit with the legs hanging over the side of the examining table. Normally, as a plumb line is drawn from the great iliac crest through the middle of the knee, it intersects between the second and third toes, and only the anterior edge of the lateral malleoli is seen. If one-half to three-fourths of the malleolar circle are seen, tibial torsion is present, and the child should be referred. The child's feet are assessed for *pes cavus* (high arch) and *pes planus* (flatfeet). Both conditions might be normal, depending on the child's age, but referral is warranted if they are causing pain or problems with proper shoe fit. Normally, the nurse is able to place one finger under the child's medial arch as the child stands. An arch that does not allow the one finger is considered flat, and an arch that allows more than one finger is considered high. The feet also are inspected for size and position. *Pes valgus,* or toeing out, may cause tibial torsion; *pes varus,* or toeing in, can cause or be caused by an anteverted femur or by tibial torsion. *Metatarsus adductus, or metatarsus varus,* is turning in of the forefoot only; the knee is straight and midline. This condition often is seen in neonates and young infants.

The child's feet should be observed for shape and position. Clubfoot, or *talipes,* is described according to the position of the foot. *Talipes equinovarus* is seen as forefoot

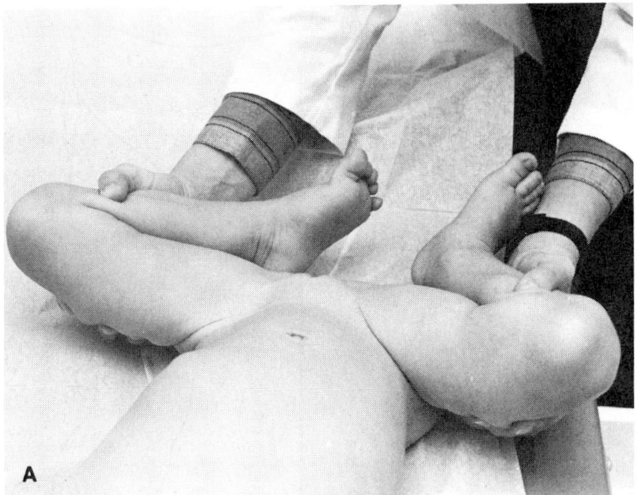

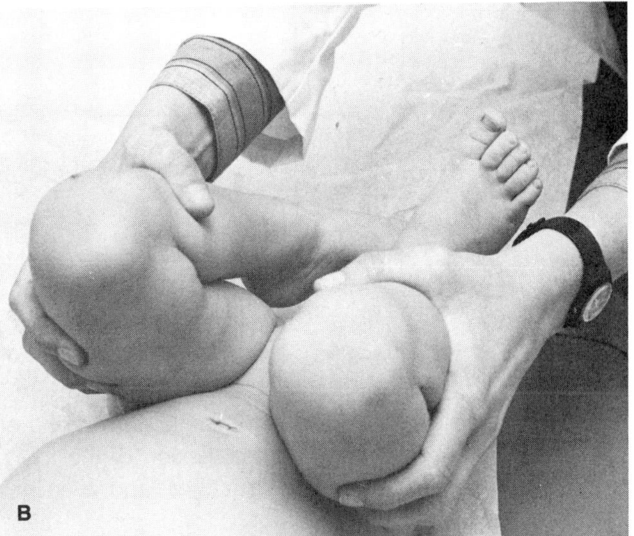

Testing for hip contractures and range of motions. *A.* Abduction. *B.* Adduction.

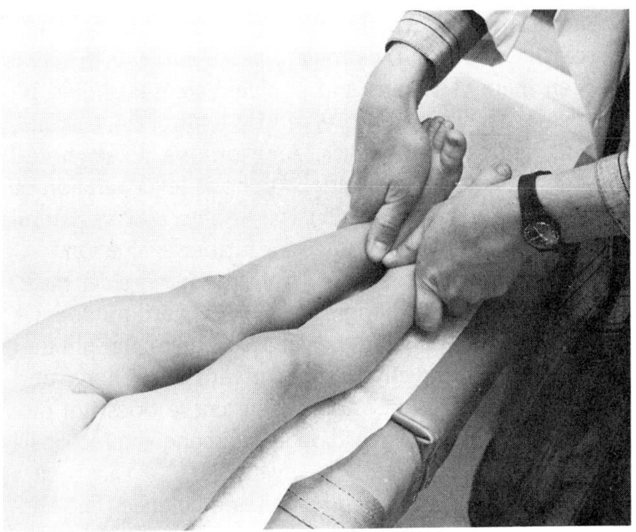

Measuring for equality of leg length.

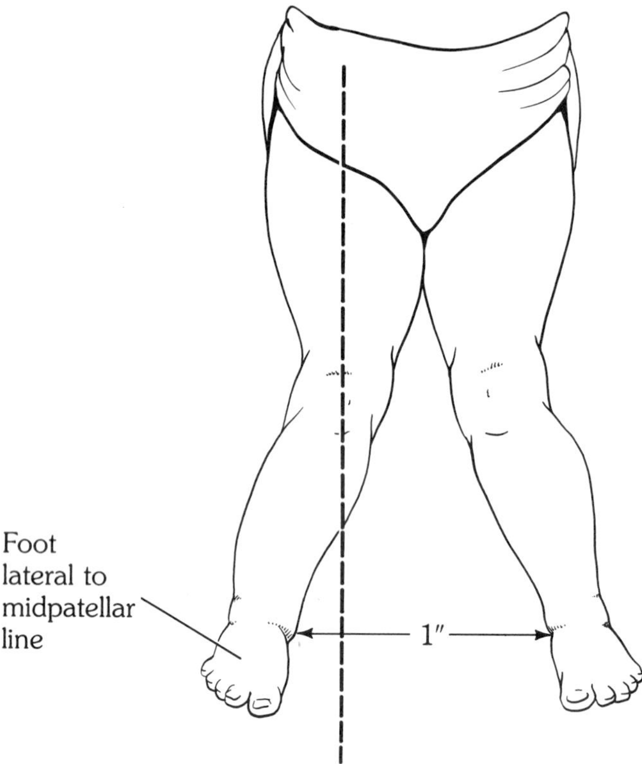

Figure 14-22 Tibial torsion. Plumb line from iliac crest should intersect toes and only anterior edge of lateral malleoli is seen.

adduction, inversion of the heel, and plantar flexion of the foot. *Talipes calcaneovalgus* is dorsal flexion of the foot, contracted and elongated ankle structures, and eversion and lateral deviation of the forefoot.

The spine is inspected and palpated for position, curvature, and lesions. As the child stands erect, the head normally is centered on the spine, so that if a plumb line is dropped from the occiput, it falls directly to the midline of the sacrum. The level of the shoulders should be equal and the scapulas should be symmetric, with a 3- to 5-in distance between them. The hips and popliteal creases should be symmetric. The spine is observed for the normal cervical, thoracic, and lumbar curves. Any *lordosis* (exaggerated anterior convexity of the spine), *kyphosis* (exaggeration or angulation of the posterior spinal curve), or *scoliosis* (lateral curvature of the spine) is noted for further evaluation.

Posture should be observed from the front, side, back, and when the child is bending forward toward the toes. A spinal curve evident when the child is standing upright that disappears when the child bends forward is functional and usually indicates poor posture. If the curve does not disappear, the child may have idiopathic or congenital scoliosis and needs to be referred.

The child also is observed for gait and balance. The toddler typically has a broad-based gait with poor balance. By 4–5 years of age, the gait is narrow based, well balanced, and can be assessed for components. The stance phase begins with heel strike, followed by midstance and push-off stages. The swing phase begins with acceleration, followed by "swing through" and deceleration. Smoothness of movement and the position of the child's arms and legs should be noted as the child walks, runs, skips, and follows a straight path.

Neuromuscular Function

Neurologic assessment usually is integrated into the total health assessment as the nurse proceeds in a systematic and organized approach. For example, as the child's face is being examined, the nurse may assess the cranial nerves.

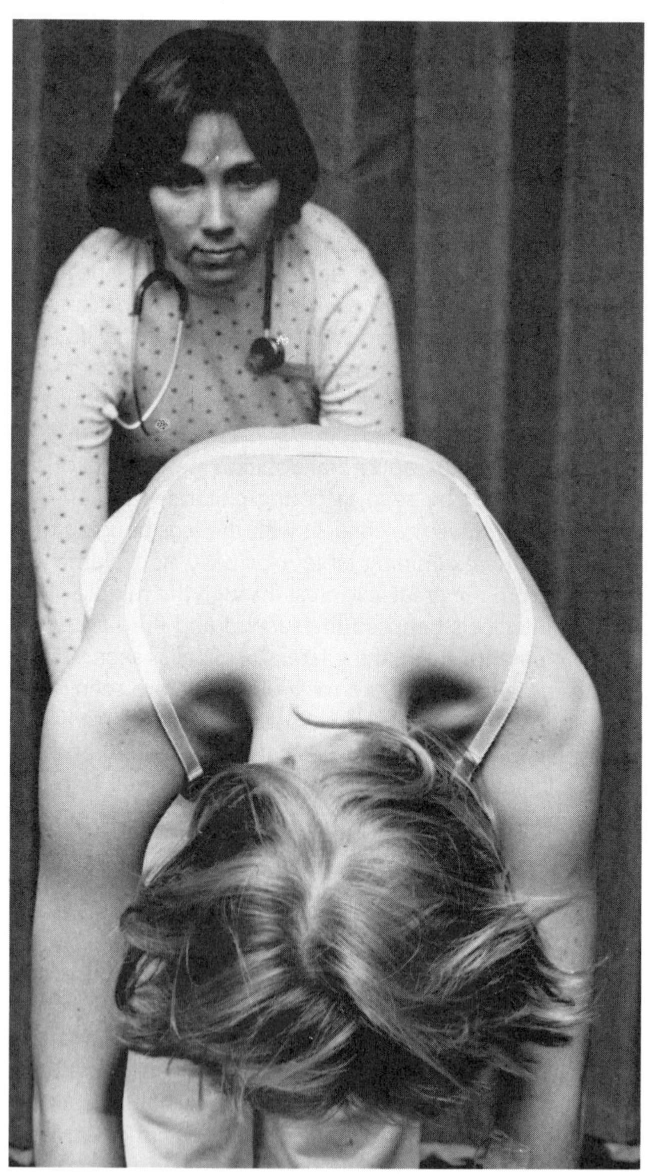

Inspection of the spine should indicate any curvature, which may suggest poor posture or a skeletal disorder, such as scoliosis.

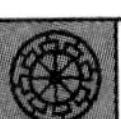

CASE STUDY Functional Spinal Curve

Assessment

Pam, age 12, and her mother are requesting an annual physical examination to complete school forms for junior high school. Pam's mother states that her only concerns about Pam's health are her weight and "bad posture"; Pam walks "hunched over" to hide her height and early development. There is a negative family history for musculoskeletal problems.

Family
Pam and her mother live together in a small apartment. Pam's parents are divorced, and her older sister is married. Her father has hypertension and is obese, and her mother has a thyroid condition and also is obese.

Child
Pam does not verbalize any concerns other than being overweight. She sits slouched down in her chair. Her poor posture detracts from her attractive facial features. Pam volunteers that she participates in bike riding and swimming activities.

Clinical Data
Physical Assessment Data Negative physical examination in all systems except musculoskeletal. Pam has complete range of motion and good strength in upper and lower extremities. No evidence of muscle atrophy or weakness. Deep tendon reflexes are intact. Observations of Pam's spine indicate a slight lateral curve when standing straight that disappears when Pam bends over forward. Spine also appears straight on side bending with no exaggerated kyphosis or lordosis; no asymmetry of scapula heights, hip levels, or popliteal skin folds; and no evidence of skeletal deformities.

Comparison to Standard
Preliminary assessment indicates a functional or nonstructural spinal curve due to poor posture. Nonstructural scoliosis that is postural needs to be ruled out from idiopathic or structural scoliosis that is associated with a rotary deformity of the spine.

Nursing Diagnoses

1. Potential for back and leg pain with continued poor posture and subsequent likelihood of muscle weakness in affected areas
2. Alteration in nutrition related to imbalance of caloric intake and expenditure evidenced in obesity

Plan for Interventions

Goals

1. Pam will discontinue her habits of poor posture and increase physical activity to improve muscle strength and coordination
2. Pam will increase physical activity to increase caloric expenditure

Interventions

1. Conduct thorough nutritional assessment
2. Consult with physician to rule out structural scoliosis
3. Encourage Pam to correct posture consciously when walking and sitting
4. Encourage Pam to increase biking and swimming activities
5. Discuss physical fitness exercises or aerobic dancing to increase activity and coordination
6. Ask Pam to return in 6 months for reevaluation of posture and position of spine

---

The nurse observes the child at play and assesses gross and fine motor functioning, balance and coordination, strength, and muscle tone. It is often necessary and appropriate, however, to perform a neurologic examination as a separate and complete element in a total health assessment. This consists of assessing the child's intellect and language ability, cerebellar function, motor function, sensory function, reflexes, and "soft" neurologic signs (minor neurologic signs that may or may not be indicative of a serious problem).

Data from the health history help the nurse to determine whether a complete and separate neurologic exam is warranted. For example, any historical information that includes reports of seizures, headaches, vertigo, changes in visual acuity, changes or loss of hearing, loss of sensation, muscular weakness, or involuntary movements may be neurologically significant and indicate the need for a specific neurologic evaluation. In addition, any child with a history of behavioral, developmental, or learning problems should have a complete neurological examination and specific developmental and educational tests (see Chapter 16).

Because of the variability in maturation of the nervous system, assessment of neurologic integrity of the infant or young child requires modification of most testing approaches as well as in the interpretation of findings. Variabilities in physical endurance of young infants and children and in their abilities to cooperate requires a modified method for valid testing. A standard neurologic examination generally is not appropriate (or likely to be successful) before middle childhood.

The neurologic examination involves assessment of function in six major areas: the cerebrum, the cranial nerves, the cerebellum, the motor system, the sensory system, and reflex action.

General Cerebral Function The assessment begins with general observations of the child's appearance, posture, facial movements, speech, behavior, and movements. These observations are made by the nurse during history taking or examination of the other body systems. Marked variations are noted and guide the remainder of the examination and the choice of specific additional tests.

Assessment of general cerebral functions includes evaluation of the child's state of consciousness, intellectual performance, and mood. The older child can be examined for orientation to time, place, and person. While asking the child questions to assess these areas of cerebral function, the nurse keeps in mind the child's cognitive, speech and language, and general developmental levels. (Developmental assessment is discussed in Chapter 16.)

Memory is another part of general cerebral function, and recall, short-term, and long-term memory are therefore evaluated (see Table 6-7). Immediate recall, the retention of an idea or thought for a brief time, is tested by having the child repeat numbers. A 4-year-old child usually can repeat three numbers (for example, 3, 2, 1), whereas a 5-year-old can repeat four numbers, and a 6-year-old usually can repeat five numbers. Recent memory is memory that lasts slightly longer than immediate recall and is tested by showing the child a familiar object. Later during the examination, the child is asked what object was shown earlier. Remote memory is memory for longer periods of time. To assess this, the child can be asked about projects that were done in school.

Specific Cerebral Function Three specific cerebral functions should be evaluated: (1) cortical sensory interpretation; (2) cortical motor integration; and (3) language. Many of the tests for cortical sensory and cortical motor evaluation can be presented as games to the child and are useful in establishing rapport with the child by eliciting cooperation and trust.

Cortical sensory interpretation is the ability to recognize objects through the senses. The inability to do this is called *agnosia.* Tactile sensory interpretation, or *stereognosis,* is evaluated by placing a familiar object in the child's hand and asking the child to identify the object with eyes closed. Familiar objects used are often coins, keys, or paper clips. *Graphesthesia,* the ability to identify familiar shapes traced in the palm or on the back of the hand, is also tested. By middle childhood, children usually can identify numbers, especially 0, 1, 3, or 8. Younger children usually can identify geometric shapes such as circles or parallel lines.

Visual sensory interpretation is tested by asking the child to hand the nurse a familiar object. The child is instructed to retrieve the object from an assortment of three or four objects. Auditory sensory evaluation is tested by having the child listen, with eyes closed, and identify familiar sounds such as a bell or a whistle. Cortical motor integration, the ability to perform responsive acts, is tested in several ways. One way of testing this specific cerebral function is to have the child copy various designs. A 3-year-old child usually can draw a circle, a 4-year-old can draw a square, and a 5-year-old can draw a triangle. Older children usually can draw diamonds or more complicated forms. Another way of testing motor integration is to have a child 6 or more years old fold a piece of paper to fit and be placed inside an envelope. The inability to perform such tasks is termed *apraxia.*

The child's ability to use language, both receptively and expressively, also is tested. Screening tests for articulation and speech might be used, but the nurse also tests the child's ability to follow directions, discriminate between two similar words, and repeat nonsense syllables. (Language assessment is discussed further in Chapters 7, 8, and 9.)

Cranial Nerves Evaluation of the 12 pairs of cranial nerves is the next component of the neurologic assessment, although if a complete neurologic examination is not done, this evaluation can be integrated into the physical examination of the face, neck, eyes, and ears.

Complete assessment of the cranial nerves depends on the cognitive and developmental level of the child; the nurse can only test functions for which the child is able to understand and therefore cooperate in the testing. The cranial nerves, functions, and procedures for testing are listed in Table 14-15.

Proprioception and Cerebellar Function Tests for proprioception and cerebellar function involve assessing posture, balance, and coordination. The nurse can assess these functions through standardized developmental tests that evaluate gross and fine motor abilities and balance and coordination. Knowing the expected developmental level of a child at any given age is necessary to interpret the child's abilities appropriately (see Chapter 16). For example, in early childhood the child usually can stand well balanced on one foot for 5 seconds; by middle childhood, the child can do so for 15 seconds and usually can hop on one foot staying in place and maintaining balance. Younger children have more difficulty with hopping, usually until $4\frac{1}{2}$ years of age.

General cerebellar function begins with an examination of the child's gait. Gait is evaluated by having the child first walk normally and then walk a straight line by walking heel-to-toe. Balance is tested by having the child stand unsupported, feet together, eyes open and then with the eyes closed. This test of cerebellar integrity, the Romberg test, is positive if the child sways significantly, although a slight-to-minimal sway is normal. Safety measures, usually standing close to the child, should be taken to prevent injury if the child falls.

Coordination generally can be assessed by observing the child's ability to stack blocks, dress and undress, and throw and kick a ball. Specific tests for coordination are finger-to-nose, fingers-to-thumb, heel-to-shin, and rapid alternating motions such as supination and pronation of the child's

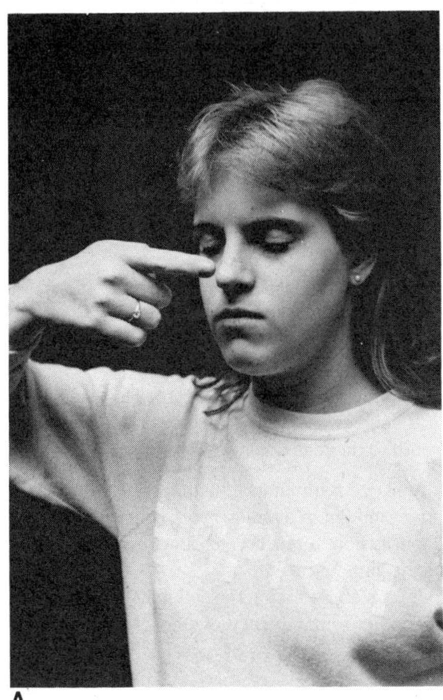
A

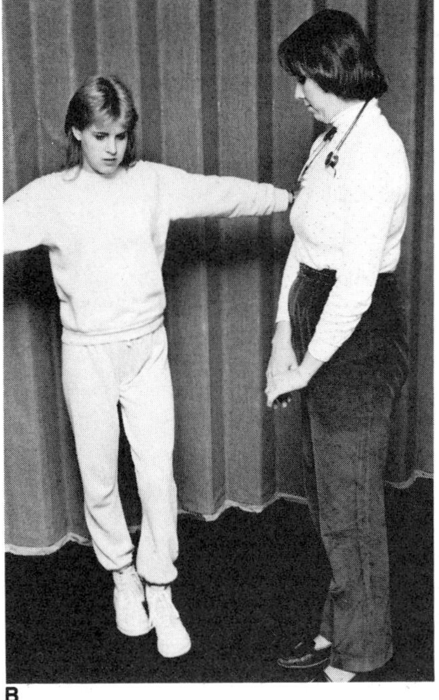
B

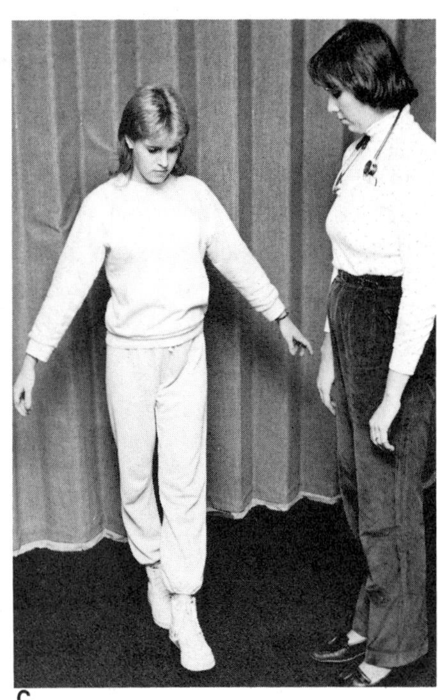
C

Neurologic function may be assessed by testing for coordination. *A.* The child touches the nose with a finger. *B.* The child stands on one foot. *C.* The child demonstrates a heel-to-toe walk.

hands. In the finger-to-nose test, the child is asked to touch the nose with the index finger first on one hand and then the other, first with the eyes open and then with the eyes closed. The child should be "on target," and any miss should be documented. The fingers-to-thumb test is done by asking the child to touch each finger of one hand to the thumb of the same hand as rapidly as possible; the nurse observes the smoothness and accuracy of the responses, noting any missing movements in the opposite hand or any additional movements elsewhere in the body, especially the face as lip smacking, eye twitching, or facial grimaces.

In the heel-to-shin test, the child lies supine and is asked to place one heel rapidly down the shin of the opposite leg from knee to ankle. Any uncoordination or inaccurate movements are documented. Rapid alternating movements are tested by asking the child to pat the knees with the palms of the hands and then the backs of the hands as rapidly as possible. Any clumsiness of movement or irregular timing is noted.

Motor Function Evaluation of the motor system includes a gross examination of muscle size, tone, strength, and any abnormal muscle movements. Most of the motor system is evaluated during the musculoskeletal examination, but any abnormality is assessed in relation to both the neurologic and musculoskeletal systems.

Muscle size and tone are assessed for any hypertrophy, atrophy, and asymmetry. Muscle strength is assessed in upper and lower extremities and evaluated for any asymmetry or involuntary movement when put through such stressful maneuvers as hand grasping or leg raising. Any twitching, choreic movements, tremors, or tics are abnormal.

Senses Assessment of the senses includes evaluation of superficial sensation (pain, temperature, and light touch) and deep sensation (vibration sense, position sense, deep pain, and discrimination). Assessment must be done on symmetric body parts for comparison, and any suspected sensory loss is mapped out from most affected to least affected area.

Superficial sensation is assessed by stroking body parts (for example, the face, trunk, arms, or legs) with a wisp of cotton and, with the child's eyes closed, having the child point to or verbally identify the area touched. Superficial pain is evaluated by using blunt and sharp tips of a safety pin on body parts and asking the child to identify the pin as either dull or sharp. (This is often traumatic for a child and may be omitted if the sensation of light touch is intact.) Temperature sensation often is not evaluated, but if it is, the child is asked to indicate hot or cold sensations as they are felt in test tubes filled with cool and warm water.

Deep sensation is evaluated by testing vibration sense over long prominences such as the sternum, elbows, knees, and iliac crests. The child is asked to note when the vibrating tuning fork stops, and the nurse tests the validity of the child's response by placing the tuning fork on the nurse's own corresponding body part. Position sense is tested by grasping the child's distal phalanx of the finger or toe digit

TABLE 14-15 Cranial Nerves

Nerve	Function	Normal Response
Cranial I: olfactory (sensory)	Smell	With eyes closed, the child correctly differentiates familiar odors with each nostril
Cranial II: optic (sensory)	Visual acuity	Child accurately calls out letters of 20/20 test line of eye chart
	Color vision	Child differentiates between red and green lines on Snellen chart
	Near vision	Child is able to read newsprint at distance of 1 ft. or 30 cm
	Peripheral vision	Child identifies object 60 degrees toward nose, 50 degrees upward, 90 degrees temporally, and 70 degrees downward
Cranial III: oculomotor (motor and proprioception)	Pupillary reactivity	Pupil size symmetrical, neither widely dilated nor pinpoint in average room light. Prompt constriction in reaction to direct and consensual light stimulus
	Eyelid elevation	Child is able to retract eyelid fully on command
	Movement of eye upward and outward, upward and inward, and medially	Smooth, symmetrical movements through all six cardinal positions of gaze
Cranial IV: trochlear	Movement of eye downward and inward	
Cranial V: trigeminal	Sensation of face	Child shows brisk blink response to touch of cornea
	Ophthalmic branch: cornea, ciliary body, conjunctiva, nasal cavity, sinuses; skin of eyebrows, forehead, and nose Maxillary branch: skin on side of nose, lower eyelid, cheek, upper lip Mandibular branch: skin of temporal region, external ear, lower face, lower lip, mucosa of anterior two-thirds of tongue, mandibular gums, and the teeth	With eyes closed, child indicates facial and oral tactile perception. Child correctly identifies facial pain stimulus and distinguishes hot and cold applications over three regions
	Movement of muscles of mastication (masseter, temporalis, pterygoideus)	Symmetrical tension in muscles of clenched jaw. Child is able to move jaw laterally against resistance
Cranial VI: abducens (motor and proprioception)	Movement of eye laterally	Normal eye movement
Cranial VII: facial (mixed)	Taste to anterior two-thirds of tongue Secretion of sublingual and submaxillary salivary glands	Child perceives sweet, sour, bitter, and salty tastes with each side of anterior tongue
	Movement of facial muscles, scalp, ears, forehead, around eyes, lips	Child is able to elevate eyebrows, frown, close eyes tightly, show teeth. With jaw closed, child can whistle, puff cheeks and smile symmetrically
Cranial VIII: acoustic (sensory)	Cochlear branch: hearing	With opposite ear masked, child hears whispered voice from 2 ft (60 cm) and correctly repeats words whispered With opposite ear masked, child hears watch tick from same distance at which examiner just able to hear it Weber test: no lateralization (see Chapter 43) Rinne test: air conduction longer than bone conduction (see Chapter 43) Schwabach test: duration of client's bone conduction equal to that of examiner

SOURCE: Adapted from Berger KJ, Fields WL: *Pocket Guide to Health Assessment*, 1980. Reprinted by permission of Reston Publishing Company, a Prentice-Hall Company, 11480 Sunset Hills Rd., Reston, VA 22090.

TABLE 14-15 continued

Nerve	Function	Normal Response
	Vestibular branch: balance	Child is able to tandem-walk, stand with feet together without postural deviation. Child is able to appose finger to nose or finger to finger without past pointing
Cranial IX: glossopharyngeal (mixed)	Position of palate and uvula	Uvula elevates midline*
	Sensation of mucosa of pharynx and palatine tonsils. Taste in posterior one-third of tongue Secretion of parotid salivary gland Movement of pharynx	Perceives touch stimulus on pharyngeal mucosa* Salivation in response to spicy food Gag reflex intact*
Cranial X: vagus (mixed)	Movement of palate, pharynx, and larynx	Able to phonate without hoarseness or articulation difficulty Child is able to swallow without regurgitating and breathe with ease
Cranial XI: accessory (motor and proprioception)	Movement of trapezius and sternocleidomastoid muscles	Child is able to raise shoulders against resistance. Child is able to turn head side to side Child is able to strongly oppose resistance to attempt to return chin to midline
Cranial XII: hypoglossal (motor and proprioception)	Movement of the tongue	Tongue protrudes to midline No tremors, fasciculations, atrophy Child is able to oppose resistance Pronunciation of "R" words intact (rugged, ragged, third, riding)

*Nerves IX and X both participate in this response.

on its lateral surfaces and moving it up or down. The child, with eyes closed, is asked to identify whether the finger or toe is in an up or down position.

Deep pain can be evaluated by strong pressure on the calf or forearm muscles, but this usually is not warranted unless clinically indicated, as in decreased levels of consciousness. Sensory discrimination is tested through stereognosis and graphesthesia. In addition, another test for discriminatory sensation is one-point discrimination. One part of the body is touched, and the child is asked to point to that area. This can be done with a wisp of cotton and is easily integrated into the primary sensation testing.

Deep Tendon Reflexes Assessment of the deep tendon reflexes (DTRs) provides the nurse with information about the function of the reflex arcs and spinal cord segments of those muscles stretched without complicating other cord segments or higher neural structures. The DTRs evaluated are the biceps reflex, the triceps reflex, the brachioradialis reflex, the patellar reflex, and the Achilles tendon reflex. Superficial reflexes, such as the abdominal reflexes, the cremasteric reflex, the gluteal reflex, and the plantar reflex, also are evaluated, as is the Babinski reflex.

Reflexes usually are graded as follows:

4+ = brisk, hyperactive clonus
3+ = brisker than normal
2+ = normal, active
1+ = low normal, slightly diminished response
0 = no response, absent

Reflexes are evaluated for strength and symmetry from side to side and from upper to lower extremities. In eliciting deep tendon reflexes, the tendon should be slightly stretched and briskly tapped with a reflex hammer. Methods for eliciting the deep tendon reflexes and expected normal responses are listed in Table 14-16.

The superficial reflexes are also listed in Table 14-16. The abdominal reflex is elicited by stroking the four quadrants of the abdomen toward the umbilicus. A normal response is that the umbilicus moves toward the stimulus. The cremasteric reflex, present in males, is elicited by stroking the inner aspect of the thigh; the nurse then observes whether the testes move into the inguinal canal (a normal response). The gluteal reflex is elicited by stimulating the perianal area and observing for contraction of the anal sphincter. The plantar reflex is elicited by stimulating the

TABLE 14-16 Assessment of Reflexes

Reflex	Test	Normal Response
Deep tendon reflexes		
Biceps reflex	Hold child's arm by placing partially flexed elbow in hand with thumb over antecubital space. Strike own thumbnail with hammer	Partial flexion of forearm at the elbow
Triceps reflex	Abduct arm, supporting upper arm and let the forearm hang freely. Strike triceps tendon above the elbow	Partial extension of forearm
Brachioradialis reflex	With arm and hand in relaxed position, strike above the styloid process of the wrist	Flexion of arm at elbow and at forearm
Patellar reflex	With child sitting on edge of table or on parent's lap and with lower leg flexed at the knee and dangling freely, tap the patellar tendon just below the kneecap	Partial extension of lower leg
Achilles reflex	With child sitting on edge of table or on parent's lap and with lower leg flexed at the knee, support the foot lightly in one hand and strike the Achilles tendon with the hammer	Plantar flexion of the foot (foot pointing downward)
Superficial reflexes		
Abdominal reflex	In the upper abdomen, stroke the skin over the lower thoracic cage, from the midaxillary line toward the midline. In the midabdomen, stroke toward the midline at the umbilical level. In the lower abdomen, stroke from the iliac crest toward the midline of the hypogastrium	Ipsilateral contraction of the muscles in the epigastric abdominal wall, or umbilical deviation toward the stimulated side
Cremasteric reflex	In males, stroke the inner aspect of the thigh	Elevation of the cremaster with prompt elevation of the testis on the ipsilateral side
Plantar reflex	Scratch the sole of the foot near the lateral aspect, from heel to toe	Plantar flexion of the toes or entire foot (toes or foot pointing downward)
Superficial anal reflex	Stroke the skin or mucosa of the perianal region	Contraction of the external and anal sphincters

A

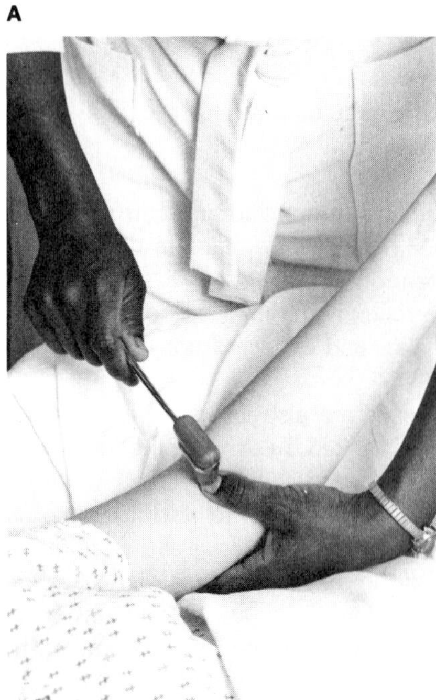

B

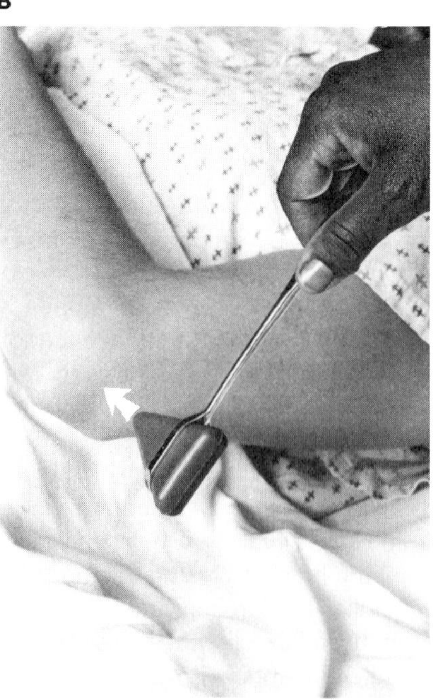

C

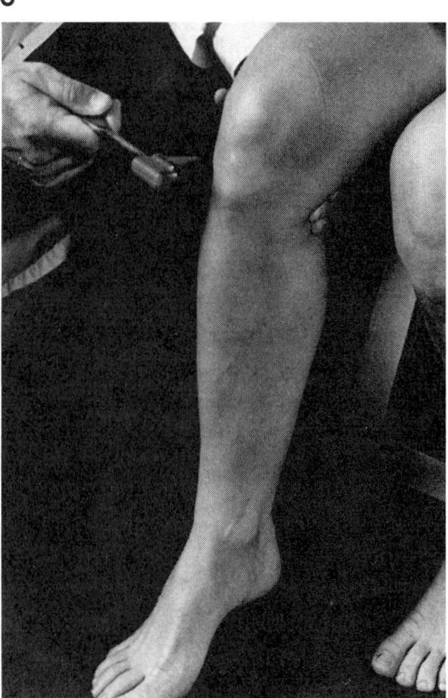

lateral border of the sole of the foot, starting at the heel and continuing to the ball of the foot and then proceeding over toward the great toe. The normally observed response is flexion of all of the toes. The Babinski reflex can be tested by observing for dorsiflexion of the great toe and fanning of the other toes when the sole of the foot is stroked.

Neurologic "soft" signs refer to signs whose significance is not understood fully but which tend to alert the nurse to possible difficulties in school, attention-requiring tasks, and coordination. These include such signs as clumsiness, hyperactivity, inconsistencies in perceptual development, language disturbances, balance disturbances, and mixed or confused laterality. Much research is being done in this area to ascertain whether these signs are predictive of future learning difficulties. If they are, early intervention when first noted is desirable.

Facing page: Assessment of deep tendon reflexes. *A.* Biceps reflex. *B.* Triceps reflex. (From Swearingen PL: *The Addison-Wesley Photo-Atlas of Nursing Procedures.* Addison-Wesley, 1983.) *C.* Patellar reflex.

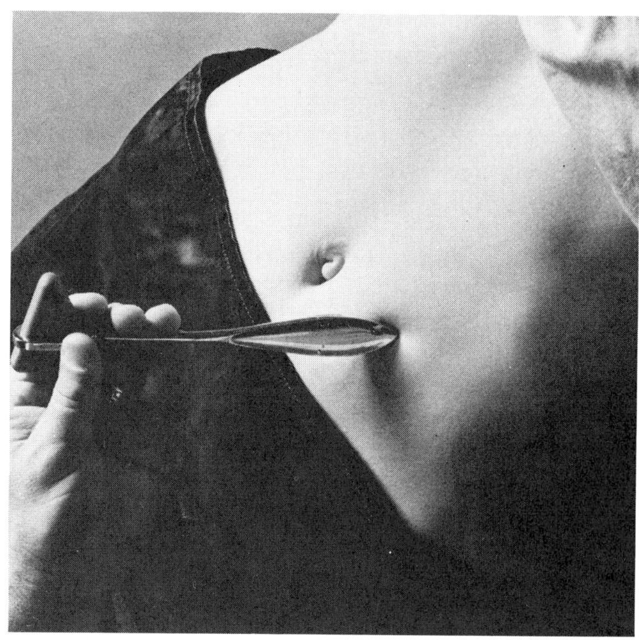

The abdominal reflex is elicited by stroking the abdomen toward the umbilicus so that the umbilicus moves toward the stimulus.

Key Concepts

- A health history requires effective interviewing skills and a systematic method for documentation.
- A health history includes identifying the purpose of the visit; the history of the present illness (if any); the past, birth, and family health history; and the child's current state of health.
- Health-screening tools, principally physical measurements and laboratory tests, are useful in augmenting and validating the assessment findings and in identifying children likely to have specific problems.
- The nurse plans the sequence of and health teaching associated with the physical examination according to the needs of both the parent and child.
- Essential skills for performing a physical examination include inspection, palpation, percussion, and auscultation.
- Physical examination begins with an assessment of the child's general appearance, which includes the nurse's impression of the child's nutritional status and developmental progress.
- Assessment of the skin, which includes hair and nails, may reveal evidence of injury, underlying pathologic processes, nutritional deficiency, or need for health teaching.
- Assessment of the lymph nodes proceeds throughout the physical examination and might reveal signs of infection or inflammation, metabolic disorders, metastatic cancer, hypersensitivity reactions, or homeostatic dysfunction.
- The head, face, and neck are assessed for symmetry, control, and movement and associated signs of congenital defects or underlying pathologic processes.
- Eyes and ears are assessed for the level of function and any evidence of defects or infection; vision and hearing screening are important parts of the physical examination.
- The nose, mouth, and throat are examined for the degree of function and any evidence of abnormalities or infection.
- Examination of the chest—lungs, breasts, and heart—includes assessing function, developmental progress, and signs of underlying pathologic processes.

- Examination of the abdomen involves assessing the abdominal organs and identifying any symptoms of dysfunction.
- Genitalia are examined for developmental progress and any evidence of dysfunction.
- The musculoskeletal system is assessed for the level of function and for any developmental anomalies.
- Assessment of neuromuscular function involves a neurologic examination that includes the reflexes and sensory, cerebral, cerebellar, and motor functions.

References

Barrus, D. H. "A comparison of rectal and axillary temperatures by electronic thermometer measurement in preschool children." *Pediatr Nurs* 1983; 7:424–425.

Bernstein, L., and Bernstein, R. *Interviewing: A Guide for Health Professionals.* Appleton-Century-Crofts, 1980.

Korsch, A. "Pediatric interviewing techniques." *Curr Prob Pediatr* 1973 (May); 3(7):00.

Additional Readings

Alexander, M. M., and Brown, M. S. "Physical examination. Parts 1–17." *Nursing '73* 1973; (July, Aug., Sept., Oct., Dec.): *Nursing '74* 1974; (Jan., Feb., April, July, Aug.): *Nursing '75* 1975; (Jan.): *Nursing '76* 1976; (Jan., Feb., March, April, June, July).

Anyan, W. *Adolescent Medicine in Primary Care.* Wiley, 1978.

Barnard, M., et al. *The Handbook for Comprehensive Pediatric Nursing.* McGraw-Hill, 1980.

Barness, L. *Manual of Pediatric Physical Diagnosis.* 4th ed. Year Book, 1973.

Bates, B. *A Guide to Physical Examination.* Lippincott, 1974.

Brown, M., and Murphy, M. *Ambulatory Pediatrics for Nurses.* 2nd ed. McGraw-Hill, 1981.

Chinn, P. *Child Health Maintenance.* Mosby, 1974.

Chow, M., et al. *Handbook of Pediatric Primary Care.* Wiley, 1979.

Committee on Children with Handicaps. "Vision screening of preschool children." *Pediatrics* 1972; 50(6):966–967.

DeAngelis, C. *Pediatric Primary Care.* 2nd ed. Little, Brown, 1979.

Downs, M., and Silver, H. "The A, B, C, D's to H.E.A.R.—early identification in nursery, office and clinic of the infant who is deaf." *Clin Pediatr* 1972; 11(10):563–565.

Emans, S. J., and Goldstein, D. *Pediatric and Adolescent Gynecology.* Little, Brown, 1977.

Eoff, J. J., and Joyce, B. "Temperature measurements in children." *Am Nurs* 1981; 81:1010–1011.

Ferholt, J. D. L. *Clinical Assessment of Children: A Comprehensive Approach to Primary Pediatric Care.* Lippincott, 1980.

Green, M., and Haggarty, R. J. *Ambulatory Pediatrics.* Saunders, 1978.

Jarvis, C. M. "Vital signs—how to take them more accurately and understand them more fully." *Nursing '76* 1976; 6(4):31–37.

Jarvis, C. M. "Perfecting physical assessment. Parts 1–3." *Nursing '77* 1977; (May, June, July).

Lehmann, J. "Auscultation of heart sounds—where to listen, how to listen and what to listen for in the identification of heart sounds." *Am Nurs* 1972; 72(7):1242–1246.

Malasanos, L., et al. *Health Assessment.* Mosby, 1977.

Moss, J. R. "Helping young children cope with the physical examination." *Pediatr Nurs* 1981; 7(2):17–20.

Murphy-Alexander, M., and Brown, M. *Pediatric History Taking and Physical Diagnosis for Nurses.* McGraw-Hill, 1979.

Osborn, L. M. "Group well-child care: An option for today's children." *Pediatr Nurs* 1982; 8(5):306–308.

Park, M., Kawabori, I., and Guntherath, W. "Need for an improved standard for blood pressure cuff size." *Clin Pediatr* 1976; 15(9):784–787.

Patient Assessment Program Instruction. *Am J Nurs* 1974; (Sept., Nov.): 1975; (Jan., March, May, Sept., Nov., April): 1976; (Sept., Nov.): 1977; (Feb.): 1978; (Oct., Nov.).

"Recommendations of the task force on blood pressure control in children." *Pediatr* (Suppl):799–820.

Redman, J., and Bissada, N. "How to make a good examination of the genitalia of young girls." *Clin Pediatr* 1976; 15(10):907–908.

Silver, H., Kempe, C., and Bruyn, H. *Handbook of Pediatrics.* Lange, 1973.

Thompson, J., and Bower, A. *Clinical Manual of Health Assessment.* Mosby, 1980.

Yoos, L. "A developmental approach to physical assessment." *Am J Matern–Child Nurs* 1981; 6(3):168–170.

Nutritional Assessment

15

Patricia A. Woodbury

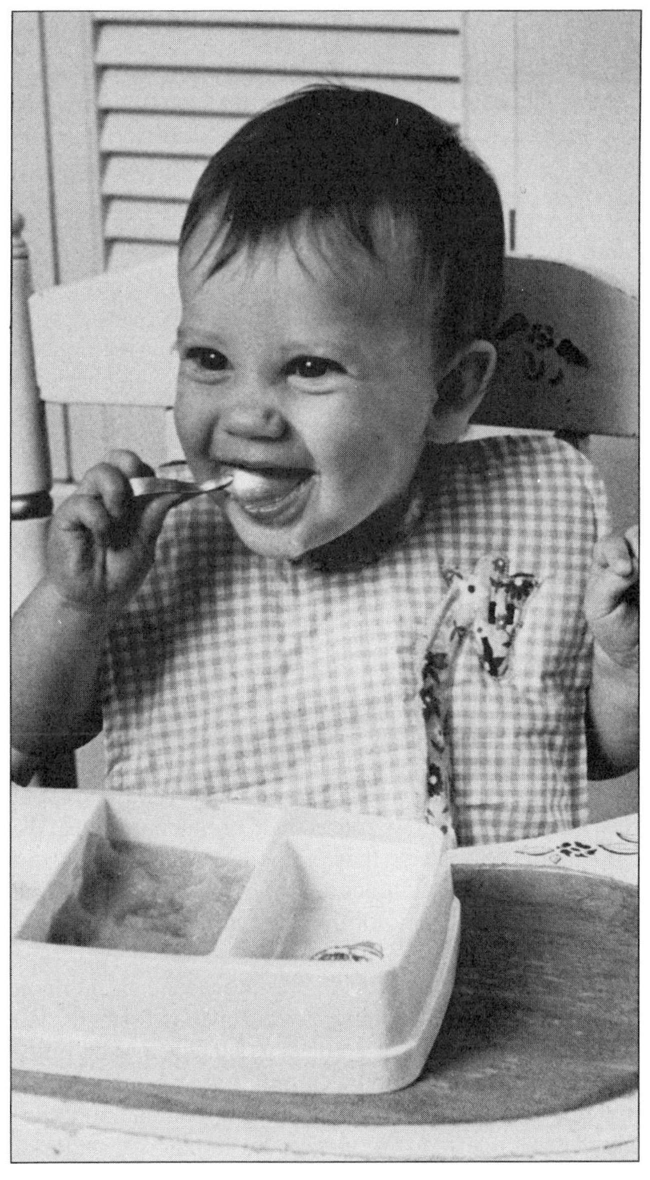

Chapter Outline

Objectives

- Define the nutritional assessment.
- Identify the factors that affect nutritional status.
- List the components of the nutritional assessment.
- Describe the methods of data collection and analysis used in the nutritional assessment.
- Describe the nutritional concerns that are common in childhood.
- List the interventions that address the common concerns of childhood nutrition.

Assessment of nutritional status is becoming increasingly more prominent in primary health care. The relationship of nutrition to health and disease has become the subject of much research and consumer interest. Nurses' experience with nutrition varies widely, but the current emphasis on the early recognition and prevention of health problems has made nutritional assessment an integral part of nursing care. As primary health care providers, nurses play an important role in the identification and management of food habits. Nutritionists, who work actively with nurses, are important resources for nurses in the nutritional care of clients.

While we do not know whether the adults of today would be in better health if their dietary habits as children had been better, we do know that certain diseases are related to food habits. Prevention and the early detection of health problems are therefore major goals among health care providers. Children are susceptible to nutritional deficiencies because they are growing and developing. The more rapid their growth, the more critical their nutritional status. We may therefore assume that promoting optimum nutrient intake and positive attitudes toward eating in childhood will improve the well-being of the adult in later years (Knittle and Hirsch, 1967).

In this chapter we provide the knowledge of nutrition necessary to nurses making a nutritional assessment. We define basic concepts of and factors influencing the nutritional assessment, including current nutritional trends. We describe the assessment process both generally and specifically as it relates to the various developmental stages of children. We apply assessment to the nursing process, explain the role of nutrition in planning nursing interventions, and discuss the concerns of children and families in providing adequate nutrition.

Purpose of the Nutritional Assessment

The nutritional assessment, as part of preventive health care, leads to the early identification of nutritional problems and concerns. Assessment is the first step in determining the goals of or needs for nutritional adaptations and in identifying behaviors, symptoms, or misconceptions about food habits or intake that could lead to nutritional health problems later in life. A nutritional assessment profiles the child's and family's eating habits, attitudes, and life-style, all of which are important in the development of a specific health care plan.

In assessing the child's nutritional status, the nurse therefore (1) determines the amount and variety of food intake and the feeding practices of both the child and family; (2) obtains baseline data about the intake of essential nutrients according to the child's metabolic needs; (3) determines the child's and family's concerns about nutritional well-being, whether these are related to food intake, feeding behaviors, attitudes, energy level, or development; and (4) determines whether nutritional intake is sufficient to promote physical growth.

As an integral part of the total health assessment, the nutritional assessment complements physical, developmental, and family assessments. In the process the nutritional assessment involves a comprehensive review of the subsystems and suprasystems that influence the child and often determine what is consumed.

The early identification of health care needs occurs at the primary health care level. In recent years the nursing profession has begun to encompass primary health care in community health settings such as schools, private offices, and hospital outpatient departments. The nurse is often the primary health care provider—the health professional who first sees the child, often when the child enters the health care system. The nurse also might have continuing and ongoing contact with the child and family during the child's growth and development. The nurse is in a key position to influence basic health care practices, including how and what children and their families eat. Child health nurses and nurse practitioners can and do handle such well-child care in child health practice. Communicating basic nutritional needs of children is therefore a major role for the nurse.

Nurses can be influential in establishing dietary and feeding practices early in life. Because consumers tend to turn to the health care system for information about nutrition, nurses are often able to exert influence through nutritional counseling. For example, one study of 270 families in a prepaid medical insurance program in New York indicated that mothers look to pediatricians for advice on how to feed their infants (Andrew, Clancy, and Katz, 1980) but suggested that pediatricians were not using their position fully to influence feeding practices.

According to Morse and colleagues (1979), many previous studies have indicated that physicians exert a strong influence on infant-feeding practices, particularly in advising about prepared formulas and vitamin supplements, the cessation of breast-feeding, and the early introduction of solids. In their study of 131 mothers in private practices in Pennsylvania, these researchers found that knowledge of nutrition was clearly correlated with the mother's cooperation with specific feeding recommendations. Mothers who breast-fed their infants also tended to be more informed about nutrition and more independent in deciding when to add solids or modify their infant's intake. Recognizing that consumers are becoming more knowledgeable about nutrition, nurses have an essential role to play in nutritional counseling.

Factors Affecting the Nutritional Assessment

Callaway (1981) suggested that confusion regarding the language used to describe nutrition might be clarified by identifying commonly agreed-on definitions and basic concepts. Callaway's 12 principles suggest the following basic concepts pertaining to the nutritional assessment:

- Dietary requirements are based on scanty research.
- The data collected are limited by problems of reliability and recall.
- Dietary patterns are a result of cultural and emotional influences.
- Nutritional status is a multifaceted condition.
- Interventions related to dietary habits should be directed toward adaptation rather than direct change.
- The human body is remarkably adaptable to variations in nutrient intake.

Nutrition Research

Since the 1970s, the surge of interest in nutrition has spurred nutritional research but has sparked controversy among nutritional researchers. Because much research is done on laboratory animals and experiments with human subjects are limited for ethical and economic reasons, the results of many studies are questionable. The rodent, for example, is not an appropriate animal for all aspects of nutrition research (Winick, 1971; Williams, Tanner and Hughes, 1974). Indeed, the results obtained with any animal model used in nutritional research should not be applied directly to human nutrition. Dietary concerns and requirements for children more accurately can be extrapolated from adult requirements; however, this method might not account adequately for social and cultural differences. Until all the data have been compiled, health educators must deal with incomplete scientific evidence and the uncertainty of some findings.

Related to the applicability of research are questions of reliability. Most methods of determining food intake involve lengthy, time-consuming interviews, which require cooperation on the part of the interviewee. Recording eating patterns over several days also might encourage the subject to change the normal eating habits, and a brief, 1-day recall might not be typical of other days and might reflect an over- or underestimate of intake. Therefore, the nurse who is collecting data should recognize the limitations in these methods and refrain from making judgments solely on the basis of recall.

National Surveys Before the late 1960s, few regional or national nutritional status studies were conducted. In 1967 the US Department of Health, Education, and Welfare responded to a legislative mandate and undertook a study of the incidence of serious hunger and malnutrition in the United States. Although this was the first, largest, and most comprehensive attempt to survey the nutritional status of Americans, the study was limited to ten states and the lowest economic groups of the urban and rural populations. This study, the "Ten-State Nutritional Survey of 1968–1970," did not identify acute malnutrition but, in focusing on protein intake, found inadequate and faulty nutrition. The major dietary problem was not the improper selection of foods, as expected, but an inadequate total energy intake. Thus, the quantity of food, not the quality, was deficient (Lowe, et al., 1975).

In addition, family income was found to be directly related to the amount of food available, and this ultimately was reflected in children's growth. Significant dental caries were associated with an increased consumption of refined carbohydrates. Iron intake was uniformly below dietary standards for all age groups, particularly for adolescent boys. This study also found "overnutrition" and noted a need for the weight standard to include the percentage of allowable fat. "Race standards" that differentiated racial variations in growth were another significant need that was identified.

In the same time period another survey, the "Preschool Nutrition Survey," examined the nutritional status of a cross section of children under 6 years of age. This survey had findings similar to the Ten-State Nutritional Survey in that it identified a lack of sufficient quantity of food rather than of nutritional quality (Owens, et al., 1974). Iron-deficiency anemia again was unrelated to income. An impressive number of children received vitamin supplements, a factor correlated with increased socioeconomic status and decreased age.

This study looked not only at the clinical manifestations of nutrition, of which there were few, but also at feeding behaviors and practices. Supermarkets were mainly used except by low-income families, who were more likely to shop at small grocery stores where prices were higher and selections limited. Mothers had the greatest influence on food purchasing and attitudes, and most mothers purchased high-energy foods. When income was limited, the family tended to buy fewer fruits and vegetables, which are expensive but are good sources of vitamins. Food patterns varied according to socioeconomic level, with higher-income families tending to have more routine daily habits and lower-income families allowing unlimited snacking.

In 1970 the US Department of Health, Education, and Welfare announced plans to establish a national surveillance system of the nation's health and nutrition under the direction of the National Center for Health Statistics. The Health and Nutrition Examination Survey (HANES) therefore was created to measure, report, and record the nutritional status of American citizens (Green and Harry, 1981). To determine nutritional status, this organization designed a study that involved examining 30,000 persons aged 1–74 years every 2 years to analyze two requirements of good health—adequate intake and use of nutrients—and determine whether they are being met in the representative sample. Although all the data from the first sample obtained between 1971 and 1974 have not been analyzed and interpreted, the findings do indicate that iron is the nutrient most often at or below the standard in all population groups. The mean protein intake for both blacks and whites of all age groups approached or exceeded the standard in all income groups (Green and Harry, 1981).

Thus far, none of the surveys has discovered significant clinical manifestations of malnutrition other than perhaps the indications of growth failure and obesity. The Ten-State Nutritional Survey noted specific populations at risk—the very poor, migrant workers, and Native Americans. Those individuals at greater nutritional risk also are likely to be pregnant, very young, adolescent, or elderly. More recently, hospitalized patients have been determined to be at increased nutritional risk.

Since 1936, the US Department of Agriculture has conducted, approximately every 10 years, a survey of food consumption patterns in the United States. The most recent survey, conducted in 1977–1978, sampled 1500 households. In comparison to the previous survey conducted in 1965, the results of this study demonstrated the following:

1. A 10% decrease in caloric intakes in all age groups without an accompanying loss of weight.
2. Protein intakes were unchanged except that the consumption of such foods as pork, luncheon meats, eggs, and dried beans decreased. Beef, poultry, fish, and nut consumption increased.
3. The consumption of such carbohydrates as breads, cereals, milk products, and concentrated sweets such as sugar, syrup, jelly, and candy decreased. The intake of soft drinks, sugared desserts, and fruit punches increased.
4. Fat intake declined for all ages because of the decreased use of fats, oils, milk products, bacon, and luncheon meats.
5. The average intake of vitamins and minerals met or exceeded the 1974 recommended daily allowance (RDA), with the exception of calcium and iron. Females over 12 years of age consumed fewer milk products and therefore had a lower calcium intake. Although the iron intake increased in infants because of iron-fortified formulas, the iron intake in 1- to 2-year-olds and females 12–15 years old continued to be low (Pao and Cronin, 1980).

National Guidelines As a result of the national surveys of malnutrition, the US Department of Agriculture update on food consumption patterns in the past decade, and the scientific advances in research on diet and disease, government concern and participation have increased in the area of food, nutrition, and health. In 1974 the Senate Select Committee on Nutrition and Human Needs requested the National Nutrition Consortium to issue guidelines for a national nutrition policy. In 1977 the National Nutrition Consortium presented the Dietary Goals of the United States (Green and Harry, 1981). These goals are to reduce the caloric intake related to caloric expenditure, increase the consumption of complex carbohydrates, reduce fat consumption, particularly saturated fat, and reduce the intake of cholesterol, refined sugars, and salt. These goals were the subject of some controversy among professionals and confusion among consumers.

In an effort to reduce the public's confusion, the US Departments of Agriculture and Health and Human Services distributed *Dietary Guidelines for Americans* in 1980. These guidelines were developed to advise people about how to stay healthy by maintaining a proper diet, to dispel some of the misinformation, and to help Americans make informed decisions about the foods they eat (General Mills, 1980). These guidelines are as follows:

1. Eat a variety of foods—There is general agreement on this recommendation.
2. Maintain ideal weight (see Appendix A)—This has unanimous support.
3. Avoid too much fat, saturated fat, and cholesterol—Both the National Academy of Sciences (NAS) and the American Medical Association (AMA) feel that the evidence is not strong enough to recommend that all healthy adults reduce their intakes of cholesterol, total fat, and saturated fat.
4. Eat foods with adequate starch and fiber—There is some support for the increase of complex carbohydrates and plant fibers at the expense of simple sugars, but the Federal Trade Commission (FTC) does not support fiber labeling because, at present, dietary fiber has not been defined.

5. Avoid too much sugar—The NAS does not believe that most people need to reduce their sugar intake. The only known harmful effect of sugar is dental caries, which is correlated with the frequency of sugar intake and the amount of sugar in contact with the teeth rather than the amount of sugar consumed.
6. Avoid too much sodium—No one disputes that reducing the intake of sodium might be helpful in the prevention of hypertension. The recommended intake is 3–8 g/day of iodized salt or a maximum of 8 g/day.
7. Alcohol, if used, should be consumed in moderation—This recommendation had general agreement.

Dietary Trends

Many of the dietary goals and guidelines described in the previous sections reflect an overall change in the American population's life-style. Although Americans tend to be sedentary, particularly since the industrial revolution, interest in regular exercise and activity programs has increased.

The individual's activity level depends on age, personality, and life-style. Most studies have shown that obese people expend less energy than thin people when carrying out the same activity (MacLean and Graham, 1982). Likewise, an active child is more likely to expend more energy and require a higher caloric intake than less active peers.

The increased expenditure of energy often makes body-conscious, health-conscious persons also want to change their eating habits. Another current trend is the quest for natural foods, which has generated public interest in obtaining scientific information about food and some misleading information as well.

Related to these trends is the variety of vegetarian diets, which are becoming increasingly common. Food consumption patterns are partly the result of changed parenting styles and group living arrangements. Who prepares the meals and how and when food is consumed in any one household are now assessment criteria.

Males and females of different ages also vary in their food preferences. In one study of school children (Lamme and Lamme, 1980), boys listed hamburgers as a favorite supper, whereas girls preferred spaghetti or chicken. Macaroni and cheese was preferred more by children 6–8 years old than by younger or older children. At different ages or developmental stages, the quantity of children's intake varies depending on the demands of their physical growth.

Adaptability Most people cannot accept a complete change in aspects of their life-styles, particularly in their food habits. People who are motivated might be able to adapt or add to their current practices if they perceive the value of the change. Nondietary factors can be equally important. For example, a family without a full-time homemaker is likely to eat more prepared and convenience foods. Advertisers appeal to this need for convenience and promote prepared foods. To overlook this factor in nutrition intervention would most likely frustrate the client and promote resistance to suggestions.

People can and do remain healthy and function effectively with a variety of diets that are far different from the scientific ideal (Dubos, 1979). Most people have adaptive mechanisms such as metabolic and enzymatic changes that respond to dietary variations, although ranges of tolerance for these variations depend on such factors as genetics and pathologic and physiologic alterations (Callaway, 1971). This is fortunate for humanity, but it makes nutrition education even more difficult for the nurse because clients often are inclined to feel that there is no reason to change or improve their dietary habits.

A person's current pattern of food use is based on past experiences and is essentially a set of learned behaviors. Many of these behaviors are established early in life and are influenced by the family, cultural, and social groups to which a person belongs. The nurse is therefore careful not to express approval or disapproval for what or how a client eats because judgments might trigger emotional reactions and inhibit the nurse–client relationship.

Availability of Food Why people eat what they eat is a complex question, but the availability of food in a region or neighborhood is certainly a strong determinant of the food consumed. Food is usually more available to the people who live in the area in which it is grown. Today, however, foods that were once seasonal are available throughout the year. Where food is purchased and by whom also determines availability. The small corner grocery store tends to be more expensive and have less variety, although it is more convenient. Shopping there can limit the amount and variety of potential nutrients that a family receives. The method of food preparation also might increase or decrease the availability of food nutrients. The regularity of meals and types of snack foods consumed also influence nutrients available to children.

The ability to pay for food determines usage patterns (Green and Harry, 1981). Because the modern world is linked by transportation systems and technology, food can be sent quickly to locations far from its origin. Consumption patterns in turn affect food choices, making some foods less expensive and more readily available. Even so, inadequate income does dictate the variety and quantity of food available, and poor people tend to buy high-energy foods that are less expensive than such foods as fruits, vegetables, and meats.

Social and Cultural Patterns Because a woman's nutritional status is as important as her nutrient intake during pregnancy, nutrition and consumption patterns influence fetal development and the eventual status of the infant. Feeding behaviors and practices begin to develop from the time a child is first fed, and they continue to develop as long as the child depends on others to provide food and to make decisions about how and what foods should be eaten (Gifft, Washbon, and Harrison, 1972).

The infant first responds to internal stimuli that dictate hunger. As feeding becomes associated with human interaction, food takes on a significance beyond the satisfaction of physiologic needs and becomes a means of finding love, comfort, and security. By kindergarten, children have developed definite food habits and have learned much about the role food plays in their family's cultural and socioeconomic environment.

Older children might find that mealtime is a happy occasion when family members communicate and share with each other or might learn that food is a reward for good behavior and that the loss of it is a consequence of bad behavior. The older child might find eating a source of satisfaction when lonely, sad, or frustrated or may use food as a means of buying friends or getting back at parents. Clearly, some of these reasons for eating can cause significant problems such as anorexia nervosa or obesity.

Cultural influences on food habits are related to ethnic, economic, religious, and educational differences (see Chapter 3). A family's attitudes toward food, its significance, and the definition of good nutrition and health arise from these cultural sources. Because of the variety in ethnic groups in the United States, the nurse should assess the consumption pattern of each child and family without assuming that a particular ethnic background determines food preferences. For example, Chinese, Mexican, and "soul" foods are popular with a cross section of Americans. Perhaps only the fast-food hamburger can accurately be called an indigenous "American food" (Green and Harry, 1981).

State of Health Nutritional status is a health condition that is influenced by the intake and use of nutrients. Nutritional status is determined by correlating data from physical, biochemical, clinical, and dietary studies (Christakis, 1973), as well as accounting for social, economic, and cultural influences. These factors are the assessment criteria that determine an individual's nutritional status.

A self-limiting acute illness temporarily increases nutritional requirements, but decreased intake caused by decreased appetite, weakness, nausea, or the pain that might be associated with the illness can prevent the body from meeting these requirements. If an illness is short-lived, regaining proper nutrition after recovery rehabilitates the nutrient needs and body stores. Chronic diseases and disabilities produce changes that might influence nutritional status differently. Chronic conditions can affect digestion, use, storage requirements, and destruction and excretion of nutrients. Special therapeutic diets frequently are part of medical interventions to prevent further deterioration of nutritional status and provide the energy for health restoration. (Specific conditions are discussed in Chapter 34–45.)

The Process of the Nutritional Assessment

Data Collection

To be efficient and pertinent to nursing diagnoses and interventions, the process of nutritional assessment must be systematic. The step-by-step approach incorporates history taking, dietary recall, physical measurements, and laboratory tests. The nutritional concern directs the process and the amount and depth of the data collected.

Nutritional Concern The sooner the nutritional concern is known, the more efficient and direct the assessment process can be. Unfortunately, in many well-child visits, nutritional concerns might not be elicited until late in the assessment process, and the nurse and client might then need to review portions of the health history. A client's nutritional concern can be expressed directly, for instance, about a particular food source or intake. Nutritional concerns, however, often are expressed more indirectly as concerns about growth, behavior, activity, illness, or even food processing and preparation.

Questions related to family composition and resources, such as child care, group living arrangements, or single-parent families, often reveal a nutritional concern. Vague responses to questions about family routines and specific religious and health preferences should alert the nurse to potential nutritional concerns and suggest the relevant historical information that is needed.

History A nutritional history focuses on three pertinent areas: (1) demographic and environmental characteristics; (2) family food and eating practices; and (3) the child's specific nutritional patterns. Although these areas sometimes are subsumed by other aspects of a health assessment, specifically worded questions might be needed to elicit responses that describe the environmental influences on nutrition and the child's and family's consumption patterns.

Assessment questions might include the following:

- Is the child or family currently adhering to any special diet?
- Who in the family is employed and what do they do?
- What industries are part of the community?
- How is the family's water supplied and is the water fluoridated?
- Where does the family purchase food and are family members receiving any food subsidies or assistance?

The specific amount of family income usually is not as significant as employment status and income assistance (for example, food stamps) because these factors also might indicate the level of education in the family, which in turn is helpful in planning interventions. Community health problems might be related to the industry or water supply in the community. For example, one young child in a rural community experienced a dramatic slowing in weight gain and periodic diarrhea after being weaned from the breast. Extensive testing revealed that the bacteria count of the water supply was borderline and sometimes exceeded allowable limits. The child's sensitivity to this particular bacteria caused the growth failure, and when bottled water was used, growth resumed and the diarrhea ceased. Determining whether the water supply is fluoridated is important information with respect to dental health. Whether the family obtains food from supermarkets, small grocery stores, or home growing is important in understanding the variety of nutrients available.

Other important family information includes the size of the family, a history of diseases affecting the family, who prepares the meals, how meals are scheduled, and the cooking and food preparation facilities. (Family assessment is discussed further in Chapter 17.)

The parent's impression of the child's development is a clue to the family's awareness and value of growth measurements, especially height and weight, which indicate nutritional status. Establishing the parent's perception of the child's past nutritional intake and eating habits provides background for any needed adaptation of food intake. The following are some specific questions that can be asked:

1. Has the child recently gained or lost weight?
2. How much time does a typical meal take?
3. Was (or is) the infant breast-fed or bottle-fed?
4. How is formula prepared?
5. At what age were solid foods introduced?
6. How much does the child eat, and how much time elapses between feedings?
7. Has the child had any food intolerances characterized by vomiting, diarrhea, colic, weight loss, or skin rash?
8. Does the family eat together, separately, or in shifts?

Parental statements regarding the child's appetite and ability to self-feed are important, although the value of this past feeding information is best determined by the age of the child and the presenting concern. The child's past illnesses support the current nutritional assessment and overall health status, and the nurse therefore should inquire about any illnesses, treatment, or hospitalization. Information about the mother's health and nutritional status during pregnancy should be included in the assessment of a younger child.

To obtain information about the child's current eating habits, the nurse might consider asking for a description of a typical day's activities, including when meals occur, from the time the child arises until the child goes to bed. Part of this description involves data about feeding utensils, where food is eaten, and the people with whom the child eats. These data indicate the degree of nutritional support for a growing and maturing child and the type and quality of the social experiences surrounding food. The nurse assesses the child's attitude toward food by asking both parent and child about food preferences. The parent's attitudes toward food also help in understanding the child's developing food preferences and attitudes.

In addition, the nurse should be familiar with specific cultural dietary habits, likes, dislikes, and beliefs. Traditional western food is regarded as bland and unacceptable by other cultures. Besides obtaining information about the child's food intake, it is helpful to determine the role of food and meal patterns in the context of the family's religious or ethnic tradition.

For example, Jewish dietary laws are based on interpretations of the Bible. In current practice the food habits of Jews are influenced to a great extent by how orthodox they are. Orthodox Jews might observe all dietary and ceremonial laws regarding food. Conservative or reform Jews might observe some laws, none at all, or only on religious holidays. Consequently, when working with Jewish families, it is imperative that the nurse know how strictly a family adheres to these dietary laws. The country from which the Jewish client comes also might influence the food habits.

The Jewish dietary laws are as follows:

1. Meat and dairy products may not be eaten at the same meal. Eggs and fish may be eaten with meat or dairy products.
2. Butter, a dairy product, cannot be served or combined with meat or meat products. Conversely, suet or poultry fat cannot be combined with dairy products. Margarine prepared without milk solids may be used with milk or meat products (package marked with "U").
3. Separate utensils must be used in preparing meat meals and dairy meals.
4. All meat and poultry must be specially killed and treated according to religious laws (kosher). Only the forequarters of the animals may be used. The animals must be those that have a cleft hoof and chew their cud. Thus, pork and its products are prohibited.
5. Milk or milk products cannot be eaten until 6 hours after the ingestion of meat.
6. Only fish with scales and fins may be eaten. Shellfish are prohibited.
7. Poultry traditionally is served on the Sabbath or holidays.
8. There are no religious laws pertaining to vegetables or fruits.
9. Blood is forbidden on food because blood is synonymous with life.
10. Food can be "koshered" at home. This is the process of soaking the meat in water, salting it thoroughly, allowing it to drain, and washing it three times to remove the salt.
11. Milk and milk products may be eaten immediately before a meat meal.

Among ethnic groups, regional differences in eating habits also exist. In a large country, such as China, it is important to know the regional origin of the family. Styles of Chinese cooking vary and are known as Mandarin (northern), Shanghai (central), and Cantonese (southern). In general, Chinese cooking involves much preparation, whereas the actual cooking time is brief. Methods of cooking are steaming, boiling, or stir-frying in a small amount of hot fat. Ovens are not used.

The eating habits of the Chinese are influenced by a belief in the importance of balancing the intake of "hot" and "cold" foods—hot and cold relating to the reaction a food has within the body and not to temperature or seasoning.

Puerto Ricans also have characteristic dietary practices related to balancing "hot" and "cold" food. Certain foods are given during times of illness to balance the body's reaction to disease. When native foods are unavailable or too expensive, these families hesitate to use substitutes that are more common to western nutrition. Table 15-1 describes the food habits of Chinese and Puerto Ricans and suggests ways in which nutrition can be improved in these two groups.

TABLE 15-1 Relationship of Culture to Diet and Food Choices

	Puerto Rican diet pattern		**Chinese diet pattern**	
	Characteristics of food habits	*For better nutrition and economy*	*Characteristics of food habits*	*For better nutrition and economy*
Milk group	Milk might be used in insufficient quantities because of economic conditions or intolerance. Although milk might not be consumed as such, a cup of "cafe con leche" can contain 2–5 oz of milk	The use of milk as a beverage and in cooking might need to be encouraged, including evaporated milk. Nonfat dry milk can be used in cooking, puddings, and on cereals. Low-lactose milk is available, which is better tolerated	Restricted use of milk or milk products beyond infancy is caused by traditional scarcity and expense. Milk is considered a luxury item. For some, milk is unacceptable and disliked	Milk can be mixed into cereals such as oatmeal. "Steamed eggs" using milk are well liked. (This product is like a pudding or custard, prepared the Chinese way in a covered dish on a rack over water)
	Domestic American cheese is used in limited quantities. Native white cheese (resembling farmer cheese but firmer and saltier) is used but is expensive	Greater emphasis can be placed on the use of cheese	Cheese is rarely used, but a cheese-type product made from goat's or cow's milk is eaten in northern China	Encourage milk cheese, which is usually acceptable, and ice cream, which is popular. Bean curd is high in calcium and protein and usually is both well liked and economical
Meat group	Chicken is eaten frequently; often in combination with other foods Expensive cuts of pork and beef are selected more often than other meats and usually are fried	Emphasize lean, less tender, and less expensive cuts of meat and long, slow cooking methods for the less tender cuts.	The amount of meat used is very limited. In China only the upper middle class is likely to eat meat daily. In the United States it is more common for all Chinese to have some meat daily, usually in mixed dishes. Pork, fish, and eggs are popular. Chicken and shellfish are used less frequently but are generally well liked	Encourage the increased use of meat, fish, poultry, and eggs. For babies, "baby food meat" may be introduced. Encourage the use of minced and chopped meats for appropriate age groups to become accustomed to taste and usage
	Ham butts and sausage are used to flavor different dishes. The intestine of the pig is eaten, either fried (cuchifritos) or stewed with native vegetables (salcocho) and chick peas	Suggest that the use of expensive cuchifritos be limited to special holidays. If salcocho is used, encourage larger quantities of vegetables and chick peas		
	Fish is used in limited amounts; salt codfish is a common choice	Suggest the more frequent consumption of fish—fresh, frozen, and canned		

TABLE 15-1 (continued)

	Puerto Rican diet pattern		Chinese diet pattern	
	Characteristics of food habits	*For better nutrition and economy*	*Characteristics of food habits*	*For better nutrition and economy*
	Eggs are used more often in cooking than as a main dish. The highest priced eggs are often purchased. Fried and scrambled eggs are popular	Greater use can be made of eggs as a main dish and as a meat substitute. Medium rather than large eggs often are a better value		
	Beans are eaten almost every day, either cooked or served with rice. A sauce called "refrito" (green pepper, tomato, garlic, lard) is served with the beans and rice. Pigeon and chick peas are very popular	The use of larger amounts of beans than rice may be desirable. Some milk, meat, chicken, cheese, or fish should be eaten with the bean meal to provide complete protein. Pigeon peas are more expensive than chick peas. The use of chick peas should be encouraged because their protein is almost as good as that of the soybean		
Vegetable and fruit group	Expensive imported vegetables, such as yautia, apio, malanga, name, and plantain are frequently used. In addition to being high in starch, these vegetables have fair amounts of B vitamins, iron, and vitamin C. Pumpkin, carrots, green pepper, tomatoes, and sweet potatoes are well liked. Pumpkin is used to thicken and flavor foods	Encourage the use of less expensive vegetables such as carrots, beets, yellow squash, or yellow or white turnips. Root vegetables may be prepared and served the same way as the Puerto Rican tubers (plantain, yautia, yucca, name)	A wide variety of vegetables are used. Many farms produce familiar and favorite Chinese vegetables. Widely used vegetables include spinach, broccoli, leeks, various greens (only recently grown in this country), bok toy (cabbage), carrot, pumpkin, sweet potato, mushrooms (as seasoning), soybeans, brussel sprouts, turnip, radish, watercress	Continued use of a variety of vegetables and fruits for all members of the family and at all times is desirable. Discussion of the cost comparison of fresh, frozen, and canned fruits and vegetables and seasonal fluctuations in price may be helpful
	Head lettuce, cabbage, fresh tomatoes, and onions are often basic salad ingredients. Lettuce is believed to be very nourishing	Stress the greater use of canned tomatoes, except when fresh tomatoes are plentiful and less expensive. Urge the use of more cooked and raw, dark green, leafy vegetables. Stress a greater intake of other salad greens and green cabbage rather than iceberg lettuce for salads	Regional additions in China are: corn (northern); kohlrabi, white eggplant (central); yautia, eggplant, bamboo shoots, and snowpeas (a delicacy) (southern)	
	Long cooking of vegetables, as in stews, is common	Emphasize the correct method of cooking vegetables: a small amount of boiling water, a covered pot, and a short cooking time	Fruits considered to be a delicacy may be used as a snack food and not a dessert. (Some fruits are reserved for men)	Encourage the use of some fruits or vegetables high in vitamin C daily as a "snack" or a dessert

continued on next page

TABLE 15-1 (continued)

	Puerto Rican diet pattern		Chinese diet pattern	
	Characteristics of food habits	*For better nutrition and economy*	*Characteristics of food habits*	*For better nutrition and economy*
	Potatoes are eaten in small amounts and most often in stews or soups or fried	Greater use of potatoes cooked in the skin can be suggested	Northern fruits are persimmon, peaches, plums, pears, and large dates. Central fruits are apples, figs, and winter melon. Southern fruits are abundant and include bananas, mango, red tangerines, papaya, pineapple, orange, litchi nuts, figs, and small dates	
	Imported fruits are used often. Oranges are being used more than formerly. Bananas and fresh pineapple are quite popular and are frequently eaten. Fruit cocktail, canned pears, and peaches are liked very much	Oranges, grapefruit, and citrus juices, fresh, frozen, and canned, can be used in greater amounts. Encourage the use of bananas and fresh pineapple in season, as well as apples and pears and other fruits in season. Recommend the use of fruits, canned in light rather than heavy syrup, because these are often better buys		
	Peach, apricot, and pear nectars are commonly used	Point out that nectars are expensive and offer minimal food value		
Bread and cereal group	Bread may be used in only small amounts. Plantain is often eaten in place of bread. French bread, rolls, and crackers are the most frequent choices.	Encourage the use of whole grain and enriched breads and the use of enriched or brown rice to replace white polished rice.	In China regional differences in consumption exist. In the north mostly wheat products are eaten, including noodles and steamed bread. Millet and rice are also used. In the central region rice is the predominant food. In the south rice, rice flour, and "sticky rice" are used extensively.	Encourage the use of enriched or brown rice
	The use of breakfast cereals, especially for children, is increasing. Oatmeal, farina, cornmeal, and cornflakes are the ones most commonly eaten. Cereals often are cooked in milk instead of water	The use of breakfast cereals, especially whole grain and enriched ones, should be encouraged, as well as the practice of cooking cereal in milk. The use of sugar-coated cereals should be discouraged		
Miscellaneous	Butter is used in small amounts and only on bread Lard and salt pork are used to flavor many dishes, often in large amounts	Suggest margarine in place of butter and corn, cottonseed, or soybean oils to season vegetables and other dishes, rather than lard and salt pork	Soybean oil, peanut oil, and lard are used	Affirm the practice of the limited use of fats and encourage liquid types

TABLE 15-1 (continued)

Puerto Rican diet pattern		Chinese diet pattern	
Characteristics of food habits	*For better nutrition and economy*	*Characteristics of food habits*	*For better nutrition and economy*
Expensive oils are used on vegetables and salads. Olive oil is a favorite			
Sugar is used very liberally in sweetening beverages and prepared desserts. Cakes, pies, guava, orange, and mango pastes, and boiled papaya preserves are favored often between meals	Encourage the less frequent use of sugar and sugar-rich desserts. Guava and mango pastes retain some of the vitamin C even after boiling but are expensive	Sweets used are sugar, molasses, brown sugar, and occasionally preserves. The seasonings used most often are salt, ginger, garlic, scallion, parsley, red and green pepper, sugar, and vinegar. More highly seasoned foods are eaten by northern Chinese families.	
Black malt beer is a favorite beverage. It is believed to be very nourishing and is combined with beaten egg for convalescents and pregnant women. In addition to being quite high in calories, it contains a fair amount of iron and some of the B vitamins	Recommend the use of other nourishing beverages, such as milk and fruit juices, rather than the expensive black beer		
Canned soups, such as chicken and vegetable, are often served as the main dish	Stress meal planning around a main dish made of a protein food rather than soups of low protein value		

Food Intake Records The assessment of food intake is the distinguishing part of the nutritional assessment process and is often the nurse's starting point. Several methods of collecting food intake data are available to the nurse. The 24-hour recall is one of the most common, least time consuming, and easiest methods to perform. This method is viewed as a screening tool because it does not provide a reliable estimate of the child's usual intake. The parent or child is asked to recall all the food and drink consumed in the last 24 hours. The parent or child must indicate the time of food intake, the type or brand of food, the method of preparation, and the amount consumed in standard measures (Table 15-2). Vitamin supplements are also included. The nurse usually follows this report by asking the parent or child whether this last 24-hour period was typical. If it was not, the nurse asks what was unusual about that day (for example, eating at a restaurant, being ill, or having another food preparer). Because people rarely eat the same quantity or quality of foods each day, the validity of the 24-hour recall can be strengthened by obtaining recall reports for several days, including both weekdays and weekends.

A 3- to 7-day dietary record kept by the parent or child requires a certain degree of cooperation and is frequently biased by an attempt to improve the diet for the record. Parents are instructed to measure or weigh portions of foods and record the amounts consumed, a difficult burden for most people, who also often unintentionally omit such foods as condiments and snacks. Even if the data are not precise, however, recording intake for several days might be more revealing and valuable to the consumer than to the nurse.

A third method is recording food frequency. With it, the parent or child fills out a form indicating how frequently specific foods are eaten in a day or week. This checklist method does not reveal how much food is eaten and therefore does not allow the nurse to quantify nutrient intake, but the data can be analyzed by a computer for an average daily or weekly nutritional intake related to the various food categories. If it were incorporated into the health interview, this method would be more time consuming.

Clinical Data The clinical assessment consists of the physical examination, related measurements, and labora-

TABLE 15-2 Sample Food Intake Record

Time	Food	Type or preparation	Amount
9:00 A.M.	Egg	Soft boiled	1
	Bread	whole wheat (homemade)	2 slices
	Margarine		2 tsp
	Orange juice		8 oz
12:30 P.M.	Soup, chicken with vegetables	Homemade	4 oz
	Cheese	Cheddar	1 oz
	Bread	Whole wheat (homemade)	1 slice
	Peanut butter	Commercial	1 tbsp
	Jelly	Commercial	2 tsp
	Milk	2%	6 oz
4:30 P.M.	Soda crackers	Commercial	2
	Apple juice	Commercial	4 oz
6:00 P.M.	Ground beef	Broiled	2 oz
	Peas	Frozen	1 tbsp
	Milk	2%	8 oz
	Applesauce	Commercial	4 oz

tory tests (see Chapter 14). The clinical findings might be indicative of nutrient deficiency (Table 15-3), but this is rare unless severe, or third-level, malnutrition is present.

Malnutrition can be defined more broadly to include overnutrition as well as undernutrition. Malnutrition has a characteristic course of development with a series of well-defined levels. The first level is low dietary intake of one or more nutrients, as determined by an intake review. If the low intake continues, the body stores of nutrients become depleted, and second-level malnutrition is evident in laboratory values. The third and final stage of malnutrition is the appearance of physical signs or symptoms.

Important in the physical assessment is inspection of posture, mental alertness, and emotional state, which for some children might indicate low energy, illness, or possible undernutrition. Any positive clinical signs are recorded along with pertinent subjective data.

Measurements The several methods of assessing growth in relation to age and sex include height, weight, head circumference, skinfold thickness, bone age, dental age, and sexual age. The most common, most efficient, and least expensive measurements assess height, weight, head circumference, and skinfold thickness. Measurement of height, weight, and head circumference are discussed in Chapter 14. The accuracy with which growth measurements are obtained is essential to the reliable interpretation of the data.

The skinfold thickness measurement assesses subcutaneous fat. When the weight for length or height ratio is increased, the cause of the weight increase cannot be determined conclusively with a regular body weight measure. The cause might, for example, be excess fat, heavy bone structure, or increased muscle mass. A skinfold thickness measurement determines whether the amount of subcutaneous fat is excessive for the child's age by comparing the measurement against a standard.

Skinfold thickness is assessed by measuring the subcutaneous tissue over the triceps or posterior aspect of the upper nondominant arm. Other areas, such as the scapular and thoracic muscles, can be used, but they are not as convenient as the triceps area. The standards for triceps skinfold thickness are given in Table 15-4.

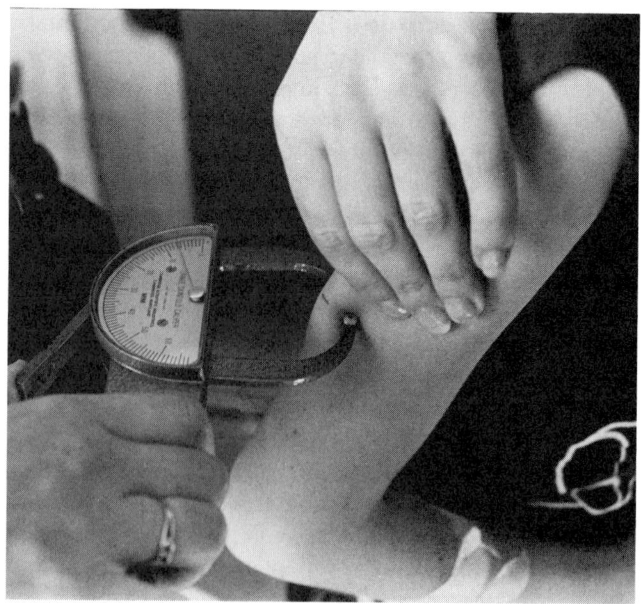

Measurement of skinfold thickness.

TABLE 15-3 Clinical Signs of Nutritional Disorders and Possible Causes

Affected body area	General population standard	Signs of nutritional disorders	Possible nutrition-related causes
Hair	Shiny, firm, not easily plucked	Lack of natural shine; dryness, dullness; ease of plucking; thinness, sparseness; changed color (flag sign)	Protein-calorie deficiency
Face	Skin smooth, with color uniform, according to cultural heritage. No edema	Loss of skin color; dark skin over cheeks and under eyes; scaling of skin around nostrils; edematous face (moon face)	Iron deficiency; inadequate caloric intake; lack of B-complex vitamins; protein deficiency
Eyes	Bright, clear, shiny, with pink, moist membranes. No lesions or tissue mounds.	Pale conjunctiva	Iron deficiency
		Dull cornea; soft cornea; Bitot's spots	Vitamin A deficiency
		Redness and fissuring of eyelid corners	Riboflavin, niacin, pyridoxine deficiency
Lips	Smooth; no edema; no lesions	Redness and edema of mouth and lips, angular fissures	Niacin, riboflavin deficiency
Tongue	Deep pink; no edema; papillae visible	Edema; redness, rawness; fissures	Folic acid, niacin, vitamin B_{12}, pyridoxine deficiency
		Magenta color	Riboflavin deficiency
		Pale color	Iron deficiency
		Atrophy of papillae	Niacin, folic acid, vitamin B_{12}, iron deficiency
Teeth	White; free of pain and caries	Mottled enamel, occasionally with brown spots	Excess fluoride during development
		Caries	Poor dental hygiene; excess sugar
Gums	Deep pink; do not bleed easily; no edema	Sponginess; prone to bleeding easily; receding	Ascorbic acid deficiency
Glands	No edema or tenderness	Thyroid edema	Iodine deficiency
		Parotid enlargement	General malnutrition; protein deficiency
Skin	No lesions, dark or light spots; no rashes	Dryness, sandpaper feel of skin (follicular hyperkeratosis)	Vitamin A deficiency; deficiency in unsaturated and essential fatty acids
		Red, swollen pigmentation of exposed areas (pellagrous dermatosis)	Niacin or tryptophan deficiency
		Petechiae	Ascorbic acid deficiency
		Hyperpigmentation	Vitamin B_{12}, folic acid, niacin deficiency
		Lack of subcutaneous tissue	Prolonged calorie deficiency
Nails	Firm, with pink nail beds; not brittle	Spoon-shaped nails that are brittle and ridged	Iron deficiency
Musculoskeletal system	Pain-free during the usual activities of daily living	Muscle atrophy; dependent edema	Protein-calorie deficiency

continued on next page

TABLE 15-3 (continued)

Affected body area	General population standard	Signs of nutritional disorders	Possible nutrition-related causes
		Thin, soft, frontal and parietal bones; soft, thin, infant skull bones; epiphyseal swelling; knock-knees; bowlegs	Vitamin D deficiency
		Small bumps on both sides of chest wall (beading on ribs)	Vitamin D and calcium deficiency
Neurologic system	Intact muscle innervation and tactile senses	Burning-foot syndrome	Pantothenic acid deficiency
		Tetany; neuromuscular irritability	Magnesium deficiency
		Mental confusion, irritability	Thiamine, niacin deficiency
		Sensory loss; loss of vibratory sensation, particularly in feet and ankles; calf tenderness	Thiamine deficiency

SOURCE: Green ML, Harry J: *Nutrition in Contemporary Nursing Practice.* John Wiley & Sons, 1981.

TABLE 15-4 Triceps Skinfold Percentiles (millimeters)

	Male					Female				
Age	**5th**	**15th**	**50th**	**85th**	**95th**	**5th**	**15th**	**50th**	**85th**	**95th**
0–5 mo.	4	5	8	12	15	4	5	8	12	13
6–17 mo.	5	7	9	13	15	6	7	9	12	15
$1\frac{1}{2}$–$2\frac{1}{2}$ yr.	5	7	10	13	14	6	7	10	13	15
$2\frac{1}{2}$–$3\frac{1}{2}$	6	7	9	12	14	6	7	10	12	14
$3\frac{1}{2}$–$4\frac{1}{2}$	5	6	9	12	14	5	7	10	12	14
$4\frac{1}{2}$–$5\frac{1}{2}$	5	6	8	12	16	6	7	10	13	16
$5\frac{1}{2}$–$6\frac{1}{2}$	5	6	8	11	15	6	7	10	12	15
$6\frac{1}{2}$–$7\frac{1}{2}$	4	6	8	11	14	6	7	10	13	17
$7\frac{1}{2}$–$8\frac{1}{2}$	5	6	8	12	17	6	7	10	15	19
$8\frac{1}{2}$–$9\frac{1}{2}$	5	6	9	14	19	6	7	11	17	24
$9\frac{1}{2}$–$10\frac{1}{2}$	5	6	10	16	22	6	8	12	19	24
$10\frac{1}{2}$–$11\frac{1}{2}$	6	7	10	17	25	7	8	12	20	29
$11\frac{1}{2}$–$12\frac{1}{2}$	5	7	11	19	26	6	9	13	20	25
$12\frac{1}{2}$–$13\frac{1}{2}$	5	6	10	18	25	7	9	14	23	30
$13\frac{1}{2}$–$14\frac{1}{2}$	5	6	10	17	22	8	10	15	22	28
$14\frac{1}{2}$–$15\frac{1}{2}$	4	6	9	19	26	8	11	16	24	30
$15\frac{1}{2}$–$16\frac{1}{2}$	4	5	9	20	27	8	10	15	23	27
$16\frac{1}{2}$–$17\frac{1}{2}$	4	5	8	14	20	9	12	16	26	31
$17\frac{1}{2}$–$24\frac{1}{2}$	4	5	10	18	25	9	12	17	25	31

SOURCE: Adapted from Frisancho, A: Triceps skin fold and upper arm muscle size norms for assessment of nutritional status. *J Clin Nutr* 27:1052, 1974.
NOTE: These percentiles were derived from data obtained on white subjects in the United States Ten-State Nutritional Survey of 1968–1970. In this survey obesity in adults was defined as a fatfold greater than the 85th percentile.

Midarm circumference is a measurement of the arm halfway between the shoulder and elbow; it reflects the quantity of body fat and muscle mass. Midarm muscle circumference has been shown to correlate with other measures of total muscle mass (Gray and Gray, 1980). Because muscle serves as the major protein reserve of the body, this measurement can be considered an index of the body's protein reserves. The upper arm muscle circumference is calculated by using the following formula:

$$\text{Arm muscle circumference} = \text{arm circumference} + (3.14) \times \text{triceps skinfold (in centimeters)}$$

The recommended standards in percentiles are from the Ten-State Nutritional Survey and are presented in Table 15-5.

Laboratory Tests Laboratory results comprise the third component of the clinical data included in the nutritional assessment. Biochemical studies are a means of determining the subclinical nutrient deficiencies, or second-level malnutrition, before the physical or clinical manifestations become apparent. The number and types of laboratory tests depend on the history and physical findings. Hemoglobin evaluation is routine to identify any iron-deficiency anemia. In most well-child populations, however, unless the knowledge of the community or the family's religion, lifestyle, or economics indicate a possible nutritional deficiency, a battery of laboratory tests has a low yield of useful data and is not cost effective. The most critical time for this concern in young children is between 4 and 6 months of age and again during adolescence.

Depending on the results of these screening tests, additional tests might be ordered to confirm anemia. These tests might include the serum iron level, iron-binding capacity, level of free erythrocyte blood porphyrins, transferrin saturation, or serum ferritin level. Hemoglobin, protein, cholesterol, and vitamin A levels in the blood are fairly stable and reflect long-term dietary influences. If community, family, or child data indicate the likelihood of any deficiencies, additional biochemical studies certainly are indicated. In contrast, levels of water soluble vitamins in blood or urine might fluctuate with dietary intake and may not be as reliable as biochemical indices. This is particularly true of vitamin C, carotenes in plasma, and thiamine, riboflavin, and other B vitamins, which are all excreted in urine.

Analysis

A nutritional assessment includes not only data about food intake but also data about environment, family, and lifestyle. A complete assessment of nutritional status includes physical assessment data as well as biochemical screening tests.

TABLE 15-5 Arm Muscle Circumference Percentiles (centimeters)

	Male					Female				
Age	**5th**	**15th**	**50th**	**85th**	**95th**	**5th**	**15th**	**50th**	**85th**	**95th**
0–5 mo.	8.1	9.4	10.6	12.5	13.3	8.6	9.2	10.4	11.5	12.6
6–17 mo.	10.0	10.8	12.3	13.7	14.6	9.7	10.2	11.7	12.8	13.5
1½–2½ yr.	11.1	11.7	12.7	13.8	14.6	10.5	11.2	12.5	14.0	14.6
2½–3½	11.4	12.1	13.2	14.5	15.2	10.8	11.6	12.8	13.8	14.3
3½–4½	11.8	12.4	13.5	15.1	15.7	11.4	12.0	13.2	14.6	15.2
4½–5½	12.1	13.0	14.1	15.6	16.6	11.9	12.4	13.8	15.1	16.0
5½–6½	12.7	13.4	14.6	15.9	16.7	12.1	12.9	14.0	15.5	16.5
6½–7½	13.0	13.7	15.1	16.4	17.3	12.3	13.2	14.6	16.2	17.5
7½–8½	13.8	14.4	15.8	17.4	18.5	12.9	13.8	15.1	16.8	18.6
8½–9½	13.8	14.3	16.1	18.2	20.0	13.6	14.3	15.7	17.6	19.3
9½–10½	14.2	15.2	16.8	18.6	20.2	13.9	14.7	16.3	18.2	19.6
10½–11½	15.0	15.8	17.4	19.4	21.1	14.0	15.2	17.1	19.5	20.9
11½–12½	15.3	16.3	18.1	20.7	22.1	15.0	16.1	17.9	20.0	21.2
12½–13½	15.9	16.9	19.5	22.4	24.2	15.5	16.5	18.5	20.6	22.5
13½–14½	16.7	18.2	21.1	23.4	26.5	16.6	17.5	19.3	22.1	23.4
14½–15½	17.3	18.5	22.0	25.2	27.1	16.3	17.3	19.5	22.0	23.2
15½–16½	18.6	20.5	22.9	26.0	28.1	17.1	17.8	20.0	22.7	26.0
16½–17½	20.6	21.7	24.5	27.1	29.0	17.1	17.7	19.6	22.3	24.1
17½–24½	21.7	23.2	25.8	28.6	30.5	17.0	18.3	20.5	22.9	25.3

SOURCE: Adapted from Frisancho, A: Triceps skin fold and upper arm muscle size norms for assessment of nutritional status. *Am J Clin Nutr* 27:1052, 1974.

NOTE: These percentiles were derived from data obtained on white subjects in the United States Ten-State Nutritional Survey of 1968–1970.

The analysis in the nutritional assessment should reflect the reasons for doing the assessment. When the assessment reveals concerns that the child or family might have about growth and nutrition, these concerns must be included in the analysis along with the child's nutritional status.

Following data collection, the nurse first determines the significance of the data base. The data must be compared with some standard or guideline that has been deemed valid through research with an appropriate reference population. Although experience frequently might be the basis of a judgment, for purposes of consistency and clarity, guidelines such as the Recommended Daily Allowances (RDAs) and the National Center for Health Statistics (NCHS) growth grids (see Appendix A) are more acceptable professionally. Knowledge of the development, standardization, strengths, and limitations of such guidelines makes the nurse's analysis of the data more reliable.

The simplest guide is the basic four food groups, published many years ago by the US Department of Agriculture and since published by the National Dairy Council under the title *Guide to Good Eating*. This guide (Table 15-6) suggests a means by which a nutritious diet can be obtained every day if adequate amounts of food are selected from the four main groups—namely, milk, meats, fruits–vegetables, and grains. This pattern provides variety and ten leading nutrients necessary for a healthful diet. This guide also describes the number of servings from each food group and serving size needed for each population (for example, child, teenager, adult pregnant woman, and lactating woman) (Table 15-7).

Using this guide, the nurse can quickly assess the quality and variety of the diet in relation to the food groups and nutrients. Although it does not indicate total calories consumed and the percentage of major nutrients in the diet, this is a good screening device to determine the need for a more detailed assessment.

When the data suggest that a more detailed assessment is indicated, food intake can be calculated by using one of the many food composition tables published by the US Department of Agriculture (for example, *Handbook Number 8*). The calculations require looking up each food on the composition table and comparing the nutrient values per amount of intake. Today, with the large variety of prepared foods that are available and the many ways of preparing foods, calculating nutrients might be difficult, and the nurse should judge and compare the food consumed

TABLE 15-6 Nutrients for Health

Nutrient	Important sources of nutrient	Some major physiologic functions		
		Provide energy	*Build and maintain body cells*	*Regulate body processes*
Protein	Meat, poultry, fish Dried beans and peas Egg Cheese Milk	Supplies 4 calories/g	Constitutes part of the structure of every cell, such as muscle, blood, and bone; supports growth and maintains healthy body cells	Constitutes part of enzymes, some hormones and body fluids, and antibodies that increase resistance to infection
Carbohydrate	Cereal Potatoes Dried beans Corn Bread Sugar	Supplies 4 calories/g Major source of energy for central nervous system	Supplies energy so protein can be used for growth and maintenance of body cells	Unrefined products supply fiber—complex carbohydrates in fruits, vegetables, and whole grains—for regular elimination; assists in fat utilization
Fat	Shortening, oil Butter, margarine Salad dressing Sausages	Supplies 9 calories/g	Constitutes part of the structure of every cell; supplies essential fatty acids	Provides and carries fat-soluble vitamins (A, D, E, and K)
Vitamin A (retinol)	Liver Carrots Sweet potatoes Greens Butter, margarine		Assists formation and maintenance of skin and mucous membranes that line body cavities and tracts, such as nasal passages and intestinal tract, thus increasing resistance to infection	Functions in visual processes and forms visual purple, thus promoting healthy eye tissues and eye adaptation in dim light

TABLE 15-6 (continued)

		Some major physiologic functions		
Nutrient	**Important sources of nutrient**	*Provide energy*	*Build and maintain body cells*	*Regulate body processes*
Vitamin C (ascorbic acid)	Broccoli Orange Grapefruit Papaya Mango Strawberries		Forms cementing substances, such as collagen, that hold body cells together, thus strengthening blood vessels, hastening healing of wounds and bones, and increasing resistance to infection	Aids in utilization of iron
Thiamine (B_1)	Lean pork Nuts Fortified cereal products	Aids in utilization of energy		Functions as part of a coenzyme to promote the utilization of carbohydrate; promotes normal appetite; contributes to normal functioning of nervous system.
Riboflavin (B_2)	Liver Milk Yogurt Cottage cheese	Aids in utilization of energy		Functions as part of a coenzyme in the production of energy within body cells; promotes healthy skin, eyes, and clear vision
Niacin	Liver Meat, poultry, fish Peanuts Fortified cereal products	Aids in utilization of energy		Functions as part of a coenzyme in fat synthesis, tissue respiration, and utilization of carbohydrate; promotes healthy skin, nerves, and digestive tract; aids digestion and fosters normal appetite
Calcium	Milk, yogurt Cheese Sardines and salmon with bones Collard, kale, mustard, and turnip greens		Combines with other minerals within a protein framework to give structure and strength to bones and teeth	Assists in blood clotting; functions in normal muscle contraction and relaxation and normal nerve transmission
Iron	Enriched farina Prune juice Liver Dried beans and peas Hamburger	Aids in utilization of energy	Combines with protein to form hemoglobin, the red substance in blood that carries oxygen to and carbon dioxide from the cells; prevents nutritional anemia and growth retardation	Functions as part of enzymes involved in tissue respiration

SOURCE: Courtesy National Dairy Council.

TABLE 15-7 Basic Four Food Groups Recommendations

Stage	Food	Number of servings	Serving size
Infant (10–18 months)	Milk	2	1 cup
	Meat	2	1–1½ oz
	Vegetables–fruits	4	½ cup vitamin C fruit or vegetable, 2–3 tbsp others
	Bread–cereal	4	½ slice bread, ½ oz cold cereal, ¼ cup cooked cereal
Early childhood (1½–4½ years)	Milk	2–3	1 cup
	Meat	2	2 oz
	Vegetables–fruits	4	½ cup vitamin C fruit or vegetable, ¼ cup others
	Bread–cereal	4	1 slice bread, 1 oz cold cereal, ½–¾ cup cooked cereal
Middle childhood (4½–8 years)	Milk	2–3	1 cup
	Meat	2	2–2½ oz
	Vegetables–fruits	4	½ cup vitamin C fruit or vegetable, ⅓ cup others
	Cereal–bread	4	1 slice bread, 1 oz cold cereal, ½–¾ cup cooked cereal
Late childhood (8–12 years)	Milk	3 or more	1 cup
	Meat	2	2–3 oz.
	Vegetables–fruits	5	½ cup vitamin C fruit or vegetable, ⅓ cup others
	Bread–cereal	4	1 slice bread, 1 oz cold cereal, ½–¾ cup cooked cereal
Adolescence	Milk	4	1 cup
	Meat	2½	2–3 oz, 7-oz total
	Vegetables–fruits	5	½ cup
	Bread–cereal	5	1 slice bread, 1 oz cold cereal, ½–¾ cup cooked cereal
Adulthood	Milk	2	1 cup
	Meat	2	2–3 oz
	Vegetables–fruits	4	½ cup
	Bread–cereal	4	1 slice bread, 1 oz cold cereal, ½–¾ oz cooked cereal
Pregnancy	Milk	3	1 cup
	Meat	2½	2–3 oz, 5- to 7-oz total
	Vegetables–fruits	5	½ cup (two servings vitamin C fruit or vegetable)
	Bread–cereal	4	1 slice bread, 1 oz cold cereal, ½–¾ cup cooked cereal
Lactation	Milk	4	1 cup
	Meat	3	2–3 oz (6- to 9-oz total)
	Vegetables–fruits	6	½ cup (two servings vitamin C fruit or vegetable)
	Bread–cereal	5	1 slice bread, 1 oz cold cereal, ½–¾ cup cooked cereal

SOURCE: Courtesy National Dairy Council.

to the food that is most similar on the composition table. After all the nutrients have been calculated, the total amount of each is tallied.

The nutritional standards most frequently referred to in the United States are the RDAs prepared by the Food and Nutrition Board of the National Research Council (Tables 15-8 to 15-10). The RDAs are defined as the levels of intake of essential nutrients considered to be adequate for meeting the known nutritional needs of practically all healthy persons (Committee on Dietary Allowances, 1980). The RDAs do not represent minimal requirements; the estimates generally exceed the needs of most people. In evaluating individual diets the RDAs are therefore a relative index of adequacy, and diets that equal or exceed the RDAs are probably adequate; however, a diet less than the RDAs cannot be assumed to be inadequate. The RDAs provide guidelines for modifying or improving the nutritional value of a diet and are an important source of comparison when analyzing assessment data. The result of analysis is the definition of the problem, or the nursing diagnosis based on an interpretation of the data (see Chapter 2). The nursing diagnosis usually is a statement categorizing nutritional adequacy based

TABLE 15-8 Recommended Dietary Allowance for Protein, Fat-Soluble and Water-Soluble Vitamins, and Minerals*

		Weight		Height				Fat-soluble vitamins		Water-soluble vitamins							Minerals					
	Age (years)	kg	lb	cm	in.	Protein (g)	Vitamin A (μg R.E.)†	Vitamin D (μg)‡	Vitamin E (mg α T.E.)§	Vitamin C (mg)	Thiamine (mg)	Riboflavin (mg)	Niacin (mg N.E.)‖	Vitamin B_6 (mg)	Folacin¶ (μg)	Vitamin B_{12} (μg)	Calcium (mg)	Phosphorus (mg)	Magnesium (mg)	Iron (mg)	Zinc (mg)	Iodine (μg)
Infants	0.0–0.5	6	13	60	24	kg × 2.2	420	10	3	35	0.3	0.4	6	0.3	30	0.5#	360	240	50	10	3	40
	0.5–1.0	9	20	71	28	kg × 2.0	400	10	4	35	0.5	0.6	8	0.6	45	1.5	540	360	70	15	5	50
Children	1–3	13	29	90	35	23	400	10	5	45	0.7	0.8	9	0.9	100	2.0	800	800	150	15	10	70
	4–6	20	44	112	44	30	500	10	6	45	0.9	1.0	11	1.3	200	2.5	800	800	200	10	10	90
	7–10	28	62	132	52	34	700	10	7	45	1.2	1.4	16	1.6	300	3.0	800	800	250	10	10	120
Males	11–14	45	99	157	62	45	1000	10	8	50	1.4	1.6	18	1.8	400	3.0	1200	1200	350	18	15	150
	15–18	66	145	176	69	56	1000	10	10	60	1.4	1.7	18	2.0	400	3.0	1200	1200	400	18	15	150
	19–22	70	154	177	70	56	1000	7.5	10	60	1.5	1.7	19	2.2	400	3.0	800	800	350	10	15	150
Females	11–14	46	101	157	62	46	800	10	8	50	1.1	1.3	15	1.8	400	3.0	1200	1200	300	18	15	150
	15–18	55	120	163	64	46	800	10	8	60	1.1	1.3	14	2.0	400	3.0	1200	1200	300	18	15	150
	19–22	55	120	163	64	44	800	7.5	8	60	1.1	1.3	14	2.0	400	3.0	800	800	300	18	15	150
Pregnant						+ 30	+ 200	+ 5	+ 2	+ 20	+ 0.4	+ 0.3	+ 2	+ 0.6	+ 400	+ 1.0	+ 400	+ 400	+ 150	**	+5	+25
Lactating						+ 20	+ 400	+ 5	+ 3	+ 40	+ 0.5	+0.5	+ 5	+ 0.5	+ 100	+ 1.0	+ 400	+ 400	+ 150	**	+10	+50

SOURCE: *Recommended Dietary Allowances,* 9th edition, 1980, with permission from the National Academy Press, Washington, DC 20418. See Table 8-2 for suggested foods to meet RDAs for each nutrient.

*The allowances are intended to provide for individual variations among most normal persons as they live in the United States under usual environmental stresses. Diets should be based on a variety of common foods to provide other nutrients for which human requirements have been less well defined.

†Retinol equivalents. 1 retinol equivalent = 1 μg retinol or 6 μg β-carotene.

‡As cholecalciferol. 10 μg cholecalciferol = 400 IU vitamin D.

§α tocopherol equivalents. 1 mg d-α-tocopherol = 1 α T.E.

‖N.E. (niacin equivalent) is equal to 1 mg of niacin or 60 mg of dietary tryptophan.

¶The folacin allowances refer to dietary sources as determined by *Lactobacillus casei* assay after treatment with enzymes ("conjugases") to make polyglutamyl forms of the vitamin available to the test organism.

#The RDA for vitamin B_{12} in infants is based on average concentration of the vitamin in human milk. The allowances after weaning are based on energy intake (as recommended by the American Academy of Pediatrics) and consideration of other factors such as intestinal absorption.

**The increased requirement during pregnancy cannot be met by the iron content of habitual American diets nor by the existing iron stores of many women; therefore the use of 30–60 mg of supplemental iron is recommended. Iron needs during lactation are not substantially different from those of nonpregnant women, but continued supplementation of the mother for 2–3 months after parturition is advisable to replenish stores depleted by pregnancy.

TABLE 15-9 Estimated Safe and Adequate Daily Dietary Intakes of Additional Selected Vitamins and Minerals*

		Vitamins			Trace Elements†						Electrolytes		
	Age (years)	*Vitamin K (μg)*	*Biotin (μg)*	*Pantothenic acid (mg)*	*Copper (mg)*	*Manganese (mg)*	*Fluoride (mg)*	*Chromium (mg)*	*Selenium (mg)*	*Molybdenum (mg)*	*Sodium (mg)*	*Potassium (mg)*	*Chloride (mg)*
Infants	0–0.5	12	35	2	0.5–0.7	0.5–0.7	0.1–0.5	0.01–0.04	0.01–0.04	0.03–0.06	115–350	350–925	275–700
	0.5–1	10–20	50	3	0.7–1.0	0.7–1.0	0.2–1.0	0.02–0.06	0.02–0.06	0.04–0.08	250–750	425–1275	400–1200
Children	1–3	15–30	65	3	1.0–1.5	1.0–1.5	0.5–1.5	0.02–0.08	0.02–0.08	0.05–0.1	325–975	550–1650	500–1500
and	4–6	20–40	85	3–4	1.5–2.0	1.5–2.0	1.0–2.5	0.03–0.12	0.03–0.12	0.06–0.15	450–1350	775–2325	700–2100
Adolescents	7–10	30–60	120	4–5	2.0–2.5	2.0–3.0	1.5–2.5	0.05–0.2	0.05–0.2	0.1 –0.3	600–1800	1000–3000	925–2775
		50–100	100–200	4–7	2.0–3.0	2.5–5.0	1.5–2.5	0.05–0.2	0.05–0.2	0.15–0.5	900–2700	1525–4575	1400–4200

SOURCE: *Recommended Dietary Allowances*, 9th edition, 1980, with permission from the National Academy Press, Washington, DC 20418.

*Because there is less information on which to base allowances, these figures are not given in the main table of the RDA and are provided here in the form of ranges of recommended intakes.

†Because the toxic levels for many trace elements may be only several times the usual intake, the upper levels for the trace elements given in this table should not be habitually exceeded.

TABLE 15-10 Mean Heights and Weights and Recommended Energy Intake

Category	Age (years)	Weight kg	Weight lb	Height cm	Height in	Energy needs (with range) kcal	MJ*
Infants	0.0–0.5	6	13	60	24	kg × 115 (95–145)	kg × .48
	0.5–1.0	9	20	71	28	kg × 105 (80–135)	kg × .44
Children	1–3	13	29	90	35	1300 (900–1800)	5.5
	4–6	20	44	112	44	1700 (1300–2300)	7.1
	7–10	28	62	132	52	2400 (1650–3300)	10.1
Males	11–14	45	99	157	62	2700 (2000–3700)	11.3
	15–18	66	145	176	69	2800 (2100–3900)	11.8
	19–22	70	154	177	70	2900 (2500–3300)	12.2
Females	11–14	46	101	157	62	2200 (1500–3000)	9.2
	15–18	55	120	163	64	2100 (1200–3000)	8.8
	19–22	55	120	163	64	2100 (1700–2500)	8.8
Pregnancy						+ 300	
Lactation						+ 500	

SOURCE: *Recommended Dietary Allowances*, 9th edition, 1980, with permission from the National Academy Press, Washington, DC 20418.

NOTE: Energy allowances for children through age 18 are based on median energy intakes of children of these ages followed in longitudinal growth studies. The values in parentheses are 10th and 90th percentiles of energy intake.

*One thousand kilocalories equals 4.184 megajoules (MJ).

on documented nutrient intake. A statement of growth and developmental status that specifically corresponds to the child's nutritional status and any environmental problems, family or community, that affect the child's nutritional status also should be stated. Possible nursing diagnoses include existing or potential alterations in nutrition, which often are related to how the child's nutritional needs for physical growth are being met and the contributing influences of the family or social environment.

Nutritional Requirements

Infancy

The first few months of life are a critical time for growth and development, and nutrition plays a major role in the outcome of that growth period. Nurses can provide nutritional education to parents by evaluating the infant's growth and using it as a guide to individual nutritional needs. Nutritional interventions always depend on the physical and developmental characteristics of each child.

The first year is a critical period for brain growth, evidenced by the increased head circumference, which accounts for approximately 80% of the total anticipated adult brain growth. This is a significant measure because postnatal undernutrition interferes with brain cell division during the first year of life (Winick, 1978).

In addition, the major organs of the body, such as the heart, lungs, liver, and kidneys, follow the same pattern; the period of fastest overall growth is during infancy. Because the digestive and renal systems are immature at birth and for nearly a year thereafter, however, certain nutrients, especially the concentrated proteins in meats and eggs, are not handled easily by the infant. Obesity in infancy, although its relation to adult obesity is controversial, is related to hyperplasia (increased number of cells) of adipose cells, which occurs normally in the first 9 months of life and peaks at 6 months of age (Salans, Cushman, and Weisman, 1973). (See Chapter 7 for other specific increments in growth.)

The infant's energy needs are mainly based on caloric expenditure resulting from basal metabolism, growth, and activity. The caloric expenditure requirement for basal metabolism is 50% of the total caloric intake in the first 4 months of life (Pipes, 1981). This energy need is highest during infancy because of the greater proportion of body surface area to weight. The energy required to maintain the functions of rapidly growing and developing body organs is greatest during infancy. The action, or increased heat production, needed to digest and absorb the major nutrients is also part of the infant's basal energy needs.

Twenty-five percent of caloric expenditure goes into growth needs during infancy (Pipes, 1981). This percentage decreases as the rate of growth slows and does not normally increase again until puberty. The other 25% of caloric expenditure is attributed to physical activity. The activity patterns of infants show great variation among individuals over time. Table 15-11 shows how caloric requirements change according to age and specific bodily function. By 1 year of age, activity needs increase, growth needs decrease, and basal metabolism or maintenance requirements begin to slow because the growth of organs slows; growth of muscle, bone mass, and fat require less energy.

The required number of calories is expressed per body weight in kilograms. The calories required for normal full-term infants in the first year range from 90 to 120 calories/kg of body weight. The lower the birthweight, the higher the caloric need in the early months. By 12 months of age, the caloric need is closer to 90 calories/kg.

The three major nutrient sources of energy are protein, carbohydrate, and fat; the recommended distribution of these nutrients in the young infant's diet is based on human milk as a standard. The distribution of these nutrients in human milk is protein, 7%; carbohydrate, 38 to 44%; and fat, 49 to 55%.

Fat is roughly one-half the total calories, reflecting its importance in carrying fat-soluble vitamins, providing essential fatty acids, and affecting development of the nervous system, especially myelinization. Increased fat intake in infants spares protein as an energy source and provides satiety. Less than 30% fat makes the diet unpalatable and places the infant at risk for delayed myelinization (Winick, 1978); the upper limit for fat should be 50%. Excessive carbohydrate in an infant's diet causes diarrhea; decreased carbohydrate causes protein (amino acids) and fats to be metabolized for energy. Protein in excess of 20% increases the renal solute load and the total body water requirement.

Water is also an essential component because it transports nutrients to and waste products from the cells; it also helps to regulate body temperature. Water is lost from the body by evaporation through the skin and lungs, as well as through feces and urine. Under normal conditions, infants do not need additional water. The infant's average water requirement is between 120 and 160 mL/kg/day. Most infant foods, such as breast milk, formula, and strained, commercially prepared food, contain 80%–90% water. When more calorically dense foods, such as strained meat and egg yolks, are introduced, additional water is needed. In unusual circumstances, such as during hot weather, fever, illness with diarrhea and vomiting, or improperly diluted formulas, additional water is needed to offset the reduced fluid intake and increased extrarenal losses.

TABLE 15-11 Total Caloric Requirement Per Day (calories/kg)

	8 weeks	10 months	4 years	14 years	Adult
Basal	55	55	40	35	25
Standard daily activity	7	7	6	6	6
Excreta	11	10	8	6	6
Additional activity	17	20	25 ±	20 ±	10 ±
Growth	20	12	8–10	14	0
Total	110	104	87–89 ±	81 ±	47 ±

SOURCE: Reproduced with permission from Lowrey, G. H.: *Growth and Development of Children*, 7th ed. Copyright © 1978 by Year Book Medical Publishers, Inc., Chicago.

Foods Sources Infants are fed a variety of foods in a variety of ways, and whether these differences in infant feeding practices have any effect on eventual health is still unknown. The consequences might be too subtle to be detected by casual observation or may be of long-term rather than short-term significance (Fomon, et al., 1979).

Milk Several forms of milk are available: (1) human milk, which, from a well-nourished woman, offers nutritional, immunologic, and psychologic benefits to the infant; (2) commercially prepared formulas; and (3) evaporated milk formula. Unmodified cow's or goat's milk is not recommended for infants in the first year of life because it contains more protein and increases the renal solute load.

In recent years the trend has been to encourage breast-feeding. One study showed that 90% of pediatricians recommended breast-feeding (Gerber Products Company, 1978); a 1979 survey indicated that the percentage of infants receiving breast milk either alone or in combination with infant formula has been increasing since 1971 (Martinez and Nalezienski, 1979). The benefits of breast-feeding actually begin immediately after birth with the production of a yellowish fluid called *colostrum*. Colostrum has a significant nutritional content and supports growth. It contains more protein (3%–5%) and less fat, carbohydrate, and calories (60 calories/dL). The mineral content of sodium, potassium, chloride, and zinc is high, as is the vitamin A and E content. Colostrum provides a rich source of antibodies to protect the neonate against enteric infections, and it has a laxative effect, which helps to clear the gut of meconium. It also makes the intestines less permeable to foreign proteins.

About the tenth day following delivery and depending on the onset of breast-feeding and the strength of the sucking stimulus, the breast-fed infant receives mature milk. The composition of breast milk varies considerably from woman to woman and depends on such factors as period of lactation, hour of expression, amount secreted, maternal age, and parity. Generally, the maternal diet does not affect the nutrient composition of the breast milk, except for vitamins A, C, and E and riboflavin, thiamin, and saturated fatty acids. Lactating mothers are encouraged to drink orange juice and to eat yellow vegetables, liver, and grains. An increase in fat in the maternal diet is also reflected in the breast milk. Inadequate maternal nutrition with prolonged lactation affects the quantity more than the quality of the milk.

As shown in Table 15-12, human milk and cow's milk provide essentially the same amount of calories (approximately 20 calories/oz) and the same amount of water; their major sources of energy, however, are somewhat different. The protein content of human milk is lower, but the content of whey protein (lactoglobulin and lactoferrin) is higher, as compared with the greater amount of casein (large-curd protein molecule) found in cow's milk. A calf needs the higher protein content because it grows faster than the human infant. Human tolerance of cow's milk, particularly for infants, is facilitated by the homogenization of cow's milk, which modifies the large protein curd and makes it more digestible. The protein in human milk (and therefore the whey) is of higher nutritional quality and is absorbed more efficiently because of its digestible curd. The major albumin, actoglobulin, provides a host resistance factor in the intestines of the infant.

As compared with cow's milk, human milk has more of the amino acids cystine and taurine, which are essential for growth. Lactose is the prominent carbohydrate in human milk, and its higher concentration, as compared with cow's milk, has two major benefits: lactose increases the absorption of calcium and stimulates the growth of beneficial microorganisms in the infant's gut by producing organic acids, creating an acid environment, and checking the growth of pathologic bacteria, such as *Escherichia coli* and *Shigella* (Pipes, 1981).

Although the total fat content of human milk and cow's milk is similar, the lipids of human milk are better absorbed because of the fatty acid composition (Nutrition Committees of the Canadian Pediatric Society and American Academy of Pediatrics, 1978). Unsaturated fatty acids predominate in human milk, whereas the saturated fatty acid concentration is higher in cow's milk. Linoleic acid, which is important for the maintenance of skin integrity in the infant, is higher in human milk (4%) than in cow's milk (1%). The higher amount of cholesterol in human milk is

TABLE 15-12 Comparison of Mature Human Milk to Unmodified Cow's Milk

Human milk	Cow's milk
Similar caloric content (71 calories/dL)	Similar caloric content (60 calories/dL)
Similar water content (85.2%)	Similar water content (87.4%)
Less protein (7% of total calories); casein/whey ratio = 40:60	More protein (20% of total calories); casein/whey ratio = 82:18
More lactose (CHO) (42% of total calories)	Less lactose (30% of total calories)
More cholesterol and linoleic acid (4%)	Less linoleic acid (1%)
More vitamin C	Less vitamin C
More vitamin E	Less vitamin E
Fewer minerals	More minerals (calcium, phosphorous)

considered necessary for the development of the enzyme system, which is needed to maintain cholesterol homeostasis later in life.

Both human milk and cow's milk provide adequate quantities of vitamin A and B complex vitamins (Pipes, 1981). Human milk from well-nourished mothers contains more vitamin C and E. Breast-fed infants of strict vegetarian mothers should receive multivitamin supplements because there is no known vegetable source for vitamin B_{12} (MacLean and Graham, 1982). The availability of vitamin D in human milk is somewhat controversial, but rickets is uncommon in the breast-fed, full-term infant, even though human milk contains a small amount of this vitamin. One possible explanation is that the vitamin D in human milk is in the form of an easily absorbed sulfate analogue. Therefore, the Committee on Nutrition of the American Academy of Pediatrics recommends that if the mother's vitamin D nutrition has been inadequate and if the infant does not benefit from sunlight because of dark skin color or limited exposure, supplements of 400 IU/day of vitamin D are indicated (Committee on Nutrition, 1980).

The mineral content of cow's milk is several times greater than that of human milk. Cow's milk contains more than three times as much calcium and six times as much phosphorus as human milk. This higher calcium to phosphate ratio has been implicated in hypocalcemic tetany in the neonate (Pipes, 1981). Although the calcium content is lower in human milk, two-thirds of it is absorbed because of the presence of lactose. The iron content of human milk has been reported to be as little as 0.3 mg/L, but about half of this iron is absorbed, as compared with an absorption rate of 10% for iron from other foods. Cow's milk may cause gastrointestinal bleeding with occult blood loss. This contributes to iron deficiency during infancy (Nelms and Mullins, 1982). The better availability of iron in human milk may be due to the lower content of protein and phosphorous and the higher levels of lactose, vitamins C and E, and copper. Iron deficiency rarely develops before 4–6 months of age because the infant's stores can supply the major portion of iron needs during this period. The addition of iron-fortified cereals to the diet after 6 months of age supplies adequate amounts of iron (Committee on Nutrition, 1980).

Another controversial issue is the availability of fluoride in human milk. Evidence shows that fluoride supplementation early in life alters the prevalence of dental caries in the permanent dentition and fosters mineralization of the teeth early in infancy. Some authorities feel that the low level of fluoride present in human milk is sufficient in early infancy. The Committee on Nutrition of the American Academy of Pediatrics recently favored initiating fluoride supplements shortly after birth in breast-fed infants but also recognized that fluoride supplementation could be initiated at 6 months of age (Committee on Nutrition, 1980). In deciding whether to recommend fluoride supplementation for the breast-fed infant, the nurse also should consider the family's access to fluoridated water and whether the infant is given water between feedings.

Commercially prepared formulas (see Chapter 7 for a list) often utilize nonfat cow's milk and closely simulate human milk. Normal full-term infants who consume adequate amounts of formula do not need any additional nutrient supplementation in the first 6 months of life. The caloric content of formulas is 67 calories/dL or 20 calories/oz. The protein and mineral content of the cow's milk is reduced to avoid the increased solute load and intestinal blood loss that can occur in young infants who are fed untreated cow's milk. The fat in the formula is provided in the form of vegetable oils (polyunsaturated fat), which are more easily absorbed. Vitamins and minerals have been added in the recommended amounts, except for iron. Some brands of formula are marketed both with and without iron. Iron-fortified formulas contain 12 mg of iron per 32 oz, as compared with a trace of iron in nonfortified formulas. Some authorities feel that there are few indications for feeding commercially prepared formulas that are not fortified with iron (Fomon, et al., 1979) because untoward reactions associated with iron, such as fussiness, colic, constipation, or diarrhea, have not been firmly established.

Soy-based formulas made from vegetable protein are available for infants who are thought to be sensitive to cow's milk. This formula is similar to the other formulas except for the protein and carbohydrate. Sucrose from corn syrup replaces lactose if lactose intolerance is suspected.

In recent years the popularity of evaporated milk formulas has decreased, but evaporated milk formulas are acceptable for feeding the young infant. The milk is heat treated to reduce the protein molecule, contains cholesterol, and can be fortified with vitamins A and D. To prepare the formula, 2–3 oz of milk are added to 3–4 oz of water, with 2 tsp of corn syrup, or 13 oz of milk (one can) and 18 oz of water with 2 tbsp of corn syrup. Evaporated milk formula is less expensive than commercially prepared formulas. An infant fed with this formula should receive supplements of vitamin C and iron.

Solid Foods The trend today is to introduce solid foods to the infant no sooner than 5–6 months of age to establish better participatory eating habits in the infant and to avoid overfeeding, obesity, and the development of allergies. When solid foods are introduced, the infant usually reduces caloric intake from milk and substitutes calories from the carbohydrates in solid food. Before 5–6 months of age, the infant's neuromuscular abilities prevent voluntary participation in the feeding process. (Feeding a 2-month-old infant solid food virtually requires forced feeding, with the infant a compliant victim.) By 6 months of age, the infant is more aware of the environment, shows an interest in other foods, and can physically participate in feeding. (The guidelines for introducing solid foods are discussed in Chapter 7.)

Assessment Criteria A detailed history of the mother's health both before and during pregnancy provides important data about fetal growth and development. Birth data, including the height and weight of the mother and/or infant, might suggest the specific maternal influence of prenatal health.

The dietary history focuses on specific food intake and the parent–child interaction. Infant feeding generally is an emotional investment for the parent, and the nurse's questions reflect this understanding. If the infant is being breastfed, the nurse asks the following questions:

1. How often is the child fed and for how long?
2. Do you alternate breasts?
3. How are you and the infant enjoying this experience?
4. How do you recognize satiety in the infant?
5. How do you recognize hunger?
6. How often is the infant burped?
7. How many breaks does the infant take?
8. What does your diet consist of?
9. How would you describe the infant's sleeping and elimination patterns?
10. Do you have any concerns?

If the infant is being bottle-fed, the nurse enquires about the kind of milk being used and notes whether it is prepared formula (ready-to-feed, concentrated, or powder, iron fortified or plain), evaporated milk, or cow's milk (whole, 2%, or skim). Other questions include the following:

1. How many cans of formula do you use each week?
2. Do you prop the bottle while feeding?
3. What brand of milk (formula) is being used?
4. How is the milk (formula) prepared?
5. How often is the infant fed?
6. How much is taken at each feeding and during a 24-hour period?
7. How do you feed the bottle to the infant?
8. Is the formula fortified with iron?
9. Do you have any concerns?

Also significant are supplemental vitamins, iron, or fluoride. If these are given, the parent should be asked how much and why. The nurse also should ask whether any other foods or fluids are given to the infant and, if so, how much, when, and why.

The infant's specific abilities during the first year are determined by asking how the parent perceives growth, describes appetite, and describes the infant's activity, personality, and temperament (see Chapter 16). A placid, less active infant probably does not need the same amount of calories as an active, highly volatile infant.

Identifying the infant's skills and potential needs for developmental stimulation can help the parent incorporate these needs into feeding activities. For example, if the infant has developed a forefinger grasp or is poking fingers at small objects, the parent might try introducing some safe finger foods to encourage both eating skills and fine motor coordination.

Early Childhood

Because caloric needs are reduced in early childhood (for example, 1300 calories, 45 calories/lb, or 100 calories/kg), these must be quality calories. The recommended intake of protein is 1.8 g/kg of body mass. A 13-kg (29-lb) child therefore needs 23 g of protein, less than the protein in three glasses (24 oz) of milk (8 oz provide 8 g of protein) and 2 oz of meat (1 oz provides 7 g of protein) (Enders and Rockwell, 1980).

By 4 years of age, the child requires about 39 calories/lb, or a total allowance of approximately 1300–2300 calories/day. Protein requirements based on the RDA are 1.5 g/kg for the 4- to 6-year-old. Two cups of milk (16 g of protein) and 2 oz of meat (14 g of protein) supply this protein requirement and also help to meet the child's calcium and riboflavin needs (Enders and Rockwell, 1980).

With the development of bones and teeth, calcium intake becomes important. Two or three glasses of milk (560–840 mg of calcium) per day will meet the daily requirement of 800 mg of calcium. Whole milk or milk with 2% fat content should be consumed and skim milk avoided until after 2 years of age because of its deficiency in essential fatty acids needed for myelin development. Other sources of calcium, such as cheese, yogurt, and ice cream, can be used as substitutes for milk.

To maintain 15 mg of iron per day during this frequently iron-deficient period, children should be encouraged to eat iron-fortified infant cereals and other high-iron food sources like liver (2 mg of iron per ounce), legumes, green vegetables, and enriched and whole-grain products. Although the RDA for iron is reduced to 10 mg for 4- to 5-year-olds, the discontinuation of iron-fortified infant cereals makes it difficult for the child to obtain an adequate amount of dietary iron. The next best substitute is cooked cereals (for example, Cream of Wheat, oatmeal), although children frequently prefer sugar-coated dry cereals that are not iron fortified. Once the child can chew, meats are a good source of iron.

A daily source of vitamin C is also important becase it facilitates iron absorption and might be helpful in preventing and fighting infections. The RDA of 40 mg can be met easily through $\frac{1}{2}$ cup of orange juice or other citrus juice. Vitamin A (2000 IU/day) is usually met through a variety of foods, particularly yellow and green vegetables. Although parents might express interest, supplementary vitamins and minerals are not particularly beneficial if the child is receiving a varied and nourishing diet; the exception is the child who is on a strict vegetarian diet. Many children's vitamins also contain high levels of sugar.

Food Sources During early childhood, there are few nutritional problems. In general, the child's diet resembles that of the parent's, except that the quantity is less. Early childhood appetites are erratic, and a parent might worry that the child is not eating enough food. The child's metabolic needs, however, have decreased and growth has slowed so that the child's bodily needs are not as great. The child's lower nutrient needs, increased ability to self-feed, and greater range of food likes facilitate meal planning and the inclusion of the young child during meals.

MacLean and Graham (1982) noted that children from advantaged socioeconomic backgrounds tended to be taller and heavier. Because the percentage of protein intake (% protein/kcal) for most socioeconomic groups is generally above the 8% of energy recommended, the growth difference appears related to the quantity of food consumed. Significant undernutrition in this age group tends to be rare in the United States.

In a study assessing the nutritional status of young children among poor migrant farmworkers in the midwest, it was observed that the majority of these children consumed less than the RDAs in all four food groups (Paredes-Rojas and Solomons, 1982). The weights of these children were misleading because they were average or above average. This, however, was related to the large amount of empty calories consumed in the form of candy and soda. Although not malnourished, these children were undernourished because of their parents' lack of knowledge and misconceptions about foods. Nurses play a critical role in assessing intake and teaching about healthful eating.

Food preferences in this age group tend to be for easy-to-eat foods such as cheese, yogurt, fruits, cereals, breads, cookies, and fruit drinks (Pipes, 1981). Meats other than hamburger, frankfurters, and chicken are avoided because of the time required and difficulty to chew. Children also tend not to like casseroles, cooked vegetables, and liver.

Assessment Criteria During early childhood, children are more selective about their food and the way it is served. The child's erratic appetite, definite likes and dislikes, and insistence on certain rituals often cause the parent to wonder about the child's nutritional health. Many parents express concern about their children's apparently limited choices of food.

The nurse often finds it helpful to review with the parent the child's eating habits throughout the day. Children often consume several snacks during the day, sometimes at planned intervals, such as midmorning and midafternoon, which coincide with nursery school or day care activities. If the child is at home, snack times may coincide with an older sibling's return from school. Many children also have snacks whenever they become hungry or thirsty, see a peer eating, or watch a food commercial. Some children appear to nibble their way through the day, never eating a substantial meal but constantly eating something.

It is important to identify the child's total intake to determine whether the child is eating the proper amounts of basic nutrients. Questions to ask the parent might include the following:

1. What are the child's preferred foods? What foods does the child refuse to eat?
2. Approximately how many times a day does the child drink milk? How much milk is consumed each time?
3. What fruits and vegetables does the child like? How frequently are these foods eaten? Will the child eat raw and cooked vegetables? Is fresh or canned fruit preferred?
4. What types of meat does the child eat? How often does the child eat cheese or peanut butter on bread or crackers?
5. Does the child have a pattern of snacking before meals? If so, what does the child request? What is the child given?
6. What rituals, if any, has the child developed with food? (For example, does the child expect a sandwich to be cut, certain foods to be placed on prescribed places on the plate, or certain foods eaten first?)
7. How often during the day does the child eat a snack? What is the usual snack?
8. Does the child have to request food, or is food available for the child to select and eat at will?

Answers to these questions enable the nurse and parent to understand the child's total intake. Frank and colleagues (1977) noted that snacks might provide one-fourth of the child's total calories and one-fifth of the calcium and ascorbic acid requirements.

The nurse also assesses the child's energy and activity levels. The very active child probably meets energy and nutrient requirements prior to the evening meal. By supper time, fatigue has a greater influence on behavior than hunger. A small, simple meal therefore is tolerated better than a gourmet meal or one prolonged by family conversation.

Middle and Late Childhood

The middle–late childhood periods are characterized by slow, continual growth, both in size and proportion. The average American child at 6 years of age is 46 in tall and weighs 48 lb; by 12 years of age, height has increased to about 60 in and weight to 85 lb (Slattery, Pearson, and Torre, 1979). A skinfold-thickness measurement becomes important because weight problems can begin in middle childhood. The child expends significant energy, both in the required mental activities of schoolwork and in the many recreational and sports activities in which the child engages. Infection, increased because of the high degree of exposure, periodically affects nutrient intake.

The child generally has a good appetite, likes variety, and is usually not fussy but may maintain previous food preferences and aversions. A progressive picture of a child's eating habits shows the changes associated with increasing maturity.

> The first grader tends to talk a lot at the table, spill food, grasp for food across the table, speak with a mouth full of food, and shovel a lot of food into the mouth at one time. Napkins are not generally used at this age. By 7 years of age, the child usually is willing to try new foods and might even begin to eat foods that were previously rejected. The 8-year-old has a ravenous appetite and strong preferences for certain foods. Manners tend to be improved but are displayed more often in public than in the home. By this age, the child is neater while eating and begins to use a napkin. By 9 or 10 years of age, the child has a keen interest in food and likes to help prepare it. The fifth grader is positive in food preferences and will eat most items, but plain foods are still preferred. Food that is attractively served and that smells and looks good makes a positive impression and will often stimulate the appetite. The 10-year-old child will eat an adult meal and have adult table manners (Slattery, Pearson, and Torre, 1979, p. 104).

Perhaps every parent needs to pin this description to the refrigerator door as a reminder that the behaviors they try to correct are normal and that change is inevitable. This might alleviate many of the eating problems of this age group, which are related more to how the child eats than to what the child eats.

The RDA (1980) for calories for children ages 7–10 years of age is 2400, or approximately 80 calories/kg of body mass. The RDAs for most of the nutrients are increased during this period, except for vitamins D and C, calcium, iron, zinc, and phosphorus. More appropriate allowances for individual children might be evident from observations of appetite, activity, growth, and weight gain in relation to deposits of subcutaneous fat (Committee on Dietary Allowances, 1980). Although this may be a period of relatively slow growth, adequate calories are needed for maintenance and activity. If the caloric intake is low, proteins are used for energy rather than for tissue building. The physical indications of nutritional status are listed in Table 15-13.

Food Sources By middle and late childhood, the frequency of meals is reduced to four to five per day; portion sizes gradually increase (Table 15-14). Breakfast is an important meal for this age group because the child needs a high-protein, nutritious meal in the morning to provide the energy needed to perform academically. Many children prefer fortified, ready-to-eat cereals but also should have orange juice and a protein such as a hard-boiled egg or peanut butter or cheese on toast because these prevent low blood sugar, which lowers efficiency. Active children need snacks, particularly after school, and usually accept cheese, fruit, yogurt, raw vegetables with cream cheese dip, or peanut butter. Instead of soda pop, children should be encouraged to drink fruit juices, flavored milks, or ice cream drinks, which provide quality calories and a better source of nutrients.

Once the child enters school, both peers and teachers influence the child's food consumption and provide new ideas about nutrition. Peers encourage the child to taste new foods and to assume new food preferences. As the child becomes increasingly independent, the purchasing and selecting of food, especially at school, become a matter of personal choice.

The School Lunch Act of 1945 provided hot meals at a nominal cost for schoolchildren. School lunches were to provide one-third of the RDA, including 8 oz of milk (whole, flavored, or low fat), two or more servings of vegetables or fruit, 2 oz of protein, and a bread or bread substitute. More recently, the program has encouraged students and parents to reduce food waste and more flexibility has allowed portions more appropriate for each age group. Yperman and Vermeersch's study (1979) found that in middle childhood participation in the school lunch program was likely to be due to influences from home such as the mother's full-time employment, whereas in late childhood participation was due to the child's desire to choose a lunch menu comparable to a friend's.

Because of children's many activities, they sometimes have trouble finding time to eat. They often stop for a quick meal and run back to their games or activities, only to return later for another snack. Many children prefer to watch television while eating. The challenge for parents is to provide quick but nutritious meals and snacks to offset the effects of this pattern of food intake, which is a contemporary problem.

Because snack patterns are not only a way of life but play a significant nutritional role, snacks which should be encouraged are those that supply nutrients and not merely calories, such as dried or fresh fruits, raw vegetables, crackers and cheese, peanut butter, nuts, whole-grain breads, milk and milk products, such as yogurt and puddings, and unsweetened fruit juices.

Assessment Criteria Because the maturing child is increasingly influenced by the community, the nurse should assess the child's nutritional status in conjunction with the community environment. A walk through a neighborhood supermarket determines the availability of fortified foods such as commercially prepared breads and cereals, whole milk fortified with vitamin D, margarine fortified with vitamin A, and low-fat milk fortified with vitamins A and D. Enquiring about the use of iodized salt and the fluoride content of the water is important to the assessment. If foods and water are obtained from atypical sources, such as health food stores, local farms, or a private well, the nurse needs to understand the differences in available nutrients.

Questions about intake usually are addressed to the parent, but the nurse might want to ask 10- to 12-year-olds to report this information. The nurse's discussion with the child might provide a learning experience for both child and parent. Steady growth and seemingly unproblematic health sometimes mask potentially significant nutritional problems such as overnutrition and undernutrition. Because the child

TABLE 15-13 Physical Indications of Nutritional Status in Middle and Late Childhood

Physical aspect	Well-nourished child	Malnourished child	Deficiency
Height and weight	Within growth norms—steady gain and increase from year to year	Above or below growth norms—failure to gain or excessive weight gain each year	Protein, calorie, other essential nutrients
Skin	Clear, smooth, elastic and firm	Rough, dry, scaly, xerosis	Vitamin A
	Reddish-pink mucous membranes	Petechiae, ecchymoses, poor wound healing	Vitamin C
		Depigmentation of skin	Protein, calorie
		Lesions	Riboflavin
		Dermatitis, sensitivity of skin to sunlight	Niacin
		Pallor	Vitamin B_{12}, iron, folacin
Musculoskeletal	Well-developed, erect posture Shoulder blades flat Arms and legs straight Skull and jaw well developed Firm muscles with good tonus Moderate amount of fat	Head sags, winged scapula, bowed legs, costochondral beading, cranial bossing	Calcium, vitamin D
		Epiphyseal enlargement of wrists	Vitamins D, C
		Small flabby muscles, muscle weakness	Phosphorus, protein
		Faulty epiphyseal bone formation	Vitamin A
		Pretibial edema bilateral	Protein, calorie, thiamine
Head	*Hair*—Smooth, good amount, lustrous	Dull, dry, depigmented, abnormal texture, easily pluckable, thin	Protein, calorie
	Eyes—Clear and bright	Dull with dark circles and hollows. Bitot's spots, conjunctivitis, xerosis, night blindness (nyctalopia), light sensitivity (photophobia)	Vitamin A, riboflavin
	Mouth—Pink, moist lips; pink, firm gums; full set of teeth	Cracking and scaling lips, cheilosis, fissuring of mouth corners	Riboflavin
		Spongy, swollen gums, bleed easily (gingiva)	Vitamin C
		Irregular or missing teeth with cavities; defective tooth enamel	Vitamin D, A
		Glossitis	Folacin, B_{12}, niacin, iron
		Tongue fissuring	Niacin
Neck	Normal size	Enlarged thyroid	Iodine
		Enlarged parotids	Protein, calorie
Neurologic		Listless	Protein, calorie
		Loss of ankle- and knee-jerk reflexes, motor weakness, sensory loss	Thiamine
		Headache	Niacin, thiamine
		Polyneuritis, motor weakness	Thiamine
Abdomen	Flat	Distended, protrudes, hepatomegaly	Protein, calorie
Cardiac	Normal heart size and sounds	Cardiac enlargement and tachycardia	Thiamine, potassium

SOURCE: Pearson GA: Nutrition in the middle years of childhood. from *Matern Child Nurs* (Nov/Dec), Vol. 2:6.

TABLE 15-14 Daily Food Guide for Middle and Late Childhood

Types of food	Recommended amounts	Average Servings (6–9 years)	Average Servings (10–12 years)	Foods included	Contribution to diet
Milk and cheese (1.5 oz cheese = 1 cup of milk) 1 cup = 8 oz or 240 g)	4 servings per day	$\frac{3}{4}$–1 cup	1 cup	Milk—fluid, whole, skim, evaporated; cheeses (natural or processed); ice cream	Calcium, magnesium, riboflavin, protein, phosphorus, vitamins A and B_{12}, and vitamin D, if milk is fortified
Meat group (protein foods) Egg Lean meat, fish, poultry (liver once a week) Peanut butter Dried beans	3 or more servings per day	1	1	Beef; veal; lamb; pork; variety meats such as liver and sausages; poultry; fish; shellfish; eggs. Alternates include dry beans, dry peas, lentils, nuts, peanut butter	Protein, iron, thiamine, riboflavin, vitamins B_6 and B_{12}, phosphorus, and niacin
Fruits and vegetables	At least 4 servings, including:				Vitamins C, A, riboflavin, folic acid, iron, and magnesium
Vitamin C source	1 or more (twice as much tomato as citrus)	1 medium orange	1 medium orange	Citrus fruits, berries, tomato, cantaloupe, mango	
Vitamin A source	1 or more	$\frac{1}{4}$ cup	$\frac{1}{3}$ cup	Green or yellow fruits and vegetables	
Other vegetables or	2	$\frac{1}{3}$ cup	$\frac{1}{2}$ cup	Potatoes, legumes	
Other fruits		1 medium	1 medium	Apple, banana	
Bread and cereals (whole grain or enriched)	At least 4				Protein, iron, thiamine, riboflavin, niacin,
Bread		1–2 slices	2 slices		vitamin E, and food energy
Ready-to-eat cereals		1 oz	1 oz		
Cooked cereal		$\frac{1}{2}$ cup	$\frac{3}{4}$ cup	Includes macaroni, spaghetti, rice, grits, noodles	
Fats and carbohydrates	To meet caloric needs				
Butter or margarine (1 tbsp = 100 calories)		2 tbsp	2 tbsp	Mayonnaise, oils	Vitamins A and E
Desserts and Sweets		3 portions	3 portions	100 calorie portion = $\frac{1}{3}$ cup of pudding or ice cream, 2 cookies, 1 oz of cake, $1\frac{1}{3}$ oz of pie, 2 tbsp of jelly, jam, honey, or sugar	

SOURCE: Adapted from US Department of Health, Education and Welfare. Four food groups of the daily food guide. USDA Institute of Home Economics and Publication No. 30, Children's Bureau, 1977.

is rarely seen for health care except when ill, the growth pattern and nutrient intake can be overlooked. Subtle symptoms of poor appetite, weight loss, irritability, or poor posture can indicate a significant underlying pathologic condition. The nurse therefore should approach each health care encounter holistically to avoid overlooking a preventable nutritional problem.

Adolescence

Adolescence is a nutritionally vulnerable time because of the increase in physical growth and the changes in life-style and food habits. Because of the adolescent's process of development, nutrition education seldom affects eating practices. Eating and food choices are reactions to a variety of physical, emotional, and psychosocial motivations or impulses.

Nutritional requirements are closely related to the rate and timing of the adolescent growth spurt, which begins in males at about 12 years of age and peaks at around 14 years of age and begins in females at approximately 10 years of age and peaks at around 12 years of age. During the growth spurt, males increase their lean body tissue and skeletal mass while concurrently decreasing total body fat; females gain proportionately more fat, so that by 20 years of age, they have about twice as much body fat as males. Males have a later, larger, and more prolonged growth period (National Dairy Council, 1981).

Because of their larger and longer growth period, the nutrient requirements of adolescent males are greater than those for adolescent females. These requirements vary not only with sex but also with age, body build, activity, and physiologic state. Males generally increase their caloric intake with greater physical maturity, whereas females decrease their caloric intake because their growth precedes sexual maturity. The 1980 RDAs for average caloric intakes based on chronologic age are as follows:

Females 11–14 years—2200 calories
Males 11–14 years—2700 calories
Females 15–18 years—2100 calories
Males 15–18 years—2800 calories

After 10 years of age, energy allowances decline to 45 calories/kg for adolescent males and 38 calories/kg for adolescent females (Committee on Dietary Allowances, 1980). After 11 years of age, the allowances for most of the nutrients are increased, as follows:

Protein—56 g for males and 46 g for females
Vitamin A—1000 μg for males and 800 μg for females
Vitamin C—60 mg
Calcium—1200 mg
Iron—18 mg
Zinc—15 mg

These significant increases come at a period in life in which the eating habits may be poorest. Calcium and iron are most important because of the increase in skeletal mass, the expansion of blood volume and muscle mass in the male, and iron loss in the female menstrual flow. Adolescents should be advised to increase their milk intake to four servings a day and to select high iron-containing foods, such as animal proteins, to meet these increased nutrient needs. Males usually are better able to meet their nutrient requirements because of larger food intake; most females are calorie conscious and are not willing to consume a larger amount of food.

Food Sources Despite claims that adolescents have the poorest dietary intake of the general population, the findings of past national surveys show no evidence of extensive nutrient deprivation for adolescents (National Dairy Council, 1981). Nutrients most often consumed in inadequate amounts are iron, calcium, riboflavin, and vitamin A. Calcium and riboflavin are generally associated with a decrease of dairy food in the diet and the drinking of soft drinks rather than milk. Most people also find it difficult to consume 18 mg of iron each day when their caloric intake is low, as is particularly common with adolescent females.

Food habits most common among adolescents involve skipping meals, particularly breakfast, snacking between meals, and eating away from home, especially at fast-foods restaurants. Skipping meals seems to be related to busy schedules and social activities, getting up late, having no time to fix anything, and not being hungry generally. Snacking does not have to create nutrient deficiencies if the foods chosen contribute to the RDAs. For the rapidly growing and active teenager, frequent eating is physiologically important.

Youth are caught up in the well-documented societal trend of fast-food consumption. A 1976 survey of 1400 United States households indicated that fast-food restaurants were patronized by members of 73% of American households, and nearly one-third of the respondents ate in a fast-food restaurant at least once a week (Young, Brennan, and Irving, 1981). Fast foods are reported to be high in calories, protein, fat, and sodium and low in vitamins A and C and crude fiber. In an attempt to overcome these deficiencies and still eat the fast food, the adolescent can be encouraged to include two glasses of milk (low-fat milk fortified with vitamins A and D for the calorie-conscious adolescent), one serving of a dark green leafy vegetable, and one glass of orange juice ($\frac{1}{2}$ cup, or approximately 50 mg, or one orange, which has 70–75 mg of vitamin C) or another citrus fruit to enhance the absorption of any iron consumed (Slatter, Pearson, and Torre, 1979).

Assessment Criteria If the adolescent is reliable and cooperative, historical information about nutritional intake reveals concerns regarding nutritional risk. The nurse needs to ask about food habits, likes and dislikes, frequency of food intake, attitudes about food, settings in which foods are eaten, and a typical day's schedule and activities. Because of sporadic eating patterns, a 24-hour recall does not usually provide a typical day's diet but is still practical and less time consuming. Routine physical assessment data such as hemoglobin and hematocrit and a skinfold thickness measurement are also part of the assessment.

In addition, the nurse needs to know about the adolescent's life style, employment, use of oral contraceptives and possible pregnancy, sports participation, and/or drug use. Any history of nutritional problems contributes to the nurse's understanding of the adolescent's current nutritional needs. These problems can be related to such health conditions as weight deficit or excess, anemia, chronic disease, infections, or psychologic stressors. The nurse can develop a more complete and specific nutritional care plan by determining the adolescent's perception of nutritional status, level of satisfaction with current body image, previous attempts to change food intake, and motivation to accept additional suggestions for change.

The pace and the dynamism of adolescence poses a challenge for the nurse. Special interest, understanding, and a willingness to listen is required for the nurse to participate in nutritional education and planning with the adolescent. Nutrition knowledge and food habits during adolescence have long-range effects in adult life.

Concerns in Childhood Nutrition

Assessment of nutritional concerns might lead to the identification of disorders that require both medical and nursing intervention.

Weaning

Weaning historically refers to the infant's loss of the mother's milk, although it can refer to a change from breast milk to cow's milk formula, a change from bottle to cup, or the introduction of solid food in the diet. Weaning should be a mutually satisfying experience for both parent and child. Infants feel strong emotional attachments related to the security surrounding the original source of nourishment, be it breast or bottle. The transition to other sources and means of food intake must therefore be easy and comfortable. The nurse guides and encourages the parent to recognize the infant's cues of readiness for weaning.

Weaning usually occurs sometime during the last half of the first year, but it is also determined by parental preference. Prepared formula is best continued throughout the first year. If the parent wants to feed the infant cow's milk during the first year, whole (3% fat) cow's milk is advised only for infants older than 9 months of age. Once cow's milk is the infant's main source of milk, it should be limited to 1 qt/day, although if the infant is already receiving a significant amount of calories from solid food, milk intake will have decreased. Cup feeding can be introduced at about 5 months of age, when the infant can place the lips at the rim of a cup. Many infants who are breast-fed until at least 7 or 8 months of age are weaned directly to a cup with no intervening bottle feeding.

Another option during weaning is to use the cup at mealtimes and allow a bottle before naps and bedtime, taking care to prevent "bottle–mouth syndrome." Many parents find that diluting the formula or milk with gradually increasing amounts of water is a convenient method of weaning. They begin with a dilution of three parts formula to one part water, after a few days advance to half formula and half water, follow that with one part formula and three parts water, and then plain water. Some children initially want the security of going to bed with their bottle; however, few enjoy drinking water and willingly substitute a stuffed toy or blanket for the bottle.

Dental Caries

Development of caries, or "bottle–mouth syndrome," in infancy is associated with feeding sweetened liquids (formulas, fruit juices, human milk, cow's milk) or a sugared pacifier when the infant is falling asleep. The liquids pool around the maxillary incisors and mandibular molars, which are not protected by the extruded tongue. Because the infant has ceased sucking, the saliva is inactive, and the carbohydrate continues to contact the teeth and bacterial plaque, thus creating an environment for the development of caries. Preventing this condition includes feeding while holding the infant and not allowing an infant to take a bottle with sweetened liquids to bed. After the teeth have begun to erupt, offering water after feeding and before bedtime is a good method of early dental care.

By early childhood, the child should be seen by a dentist to assess and maintain good oral and dental development. Determining whether the parent has started some form of oral hygiene with the child is important in assessing the maintenance of a healthy dentition and fostering good nutrition. Fluoride becomes very important with the erupting of deciduous and permanent teeth. Supplements are not indicated unless the water supply is not fluoridated.

Dental caries interferes with good nutrition if chewing creates oral discomfort. Children will avoid foods such as meats, raw vegetables, and fruits, preferring soft breads and dairy products. This practice deprives them of essential nutrients, vitamins, and minerals. Caries occur frequently during middle and late childhood in children with poor nutrition or poor dental hygiene. This is a critical problem because permanent teeth are erupting at this time. Frequent intake of sugary snacks should be avoided, and brushing the teeth after snacks or meals should be encouraged. The availability of fluoridated water in the community is the most cost-effective prevention method. By this time, children should be seeing dentists on a regular basis and receiving appropriate dental education. Dental health also is frequently incorporated in the health education curriculum in elementary school.

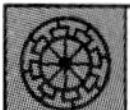

CASE STUDY Weaning

Assessment

Katy is a 4-month-old infant who was brought to the clinic for a routine well-child visit. She has been breast-fed since birth, and her mother wants to know about introducing solid foods and weaning Katy to formula bottle-feeding.

Family

Katy is the firstborn of two young parents. There are no significant medical problems in either parent's family. Her father is regularly employed and participates in Katy's care, and her mother plans to go back to work soon. A neighbor will take care of Katy. The family has no unusual dietary preferences. Katy's mother says she maintains a balanced diet for herself, is not on any reduction diet, and does daily exercises.

Child

Katy was a full-term, $6\frac{1}{2}$-lb infant who had an uncomplicated gestational period. She has had no illnesses and is currently beginning to reach and grasp. She has strong sucking movements and holds her head steady. She urinates six or seven times a day and has soft stools two or three times a day. She has been sleeping through the night for the past 3 weeks.

Environment

The family has access to the city water supply, which is fluoridated. The family purchases food from a nearby supermarket and lives in a three-bedroom house in a suburban housing development.

Food Intake

Katy is breast-fed every 3–4 hours for approximately 10–15 minutes at each breast. Her mother has not fed Katy any foods or other milk but does express her breast milk for an occasional bottle. Katy is described as having a good appetite. She receives supplemental vitamins A, C, and D, and the mineral fluoride once a day.

Clinical Data

Physical Assessment Data Katy is an alert, smiling, cooing infant. Her physical examination revealed no abnormal clinical findings.

Growth Katy's height is 62 cm ($24\frac{1}{2}$ in); her weight is 6 kg (13 lb, 2 oz); her head circumference is 41 cm ($16\frac{1}{2}$ in). She has doubled her birthweight and has gained approximately 2 lb/mo for the past 3 months.

Comparison to a Standard

In a breast-fed infant the principal standard is growth. According to the National Center for Health Statistics growth charts, Katy is at the fiftieth percentile for height, weight, and head circumference. The maternal diet is adequate for lactation, and there is no reported concern about reduced intake or nutrient deficiencies as a result of a special diet or health condition. Katy is therefore a breast-fed 4-month-old with adequate nutrition and growth and developmental behaviors appropriate for her age.

Nursing Diagnosis

1. Potential for alterations in nutrition: less than body requirements related to proposed weaning.

Plan for Interventions

Goal

1. Katy will be weaned to formula and introduced to solid foods to maintain the nutrient intake needed for her ongoing growth and development.

Interventions

1. Recommend changing to an iron-fortified formula. For her age and weight, Katy should have 34 oz of formula per 24 hours. (From 3–6 months of age, 52 calories/lb is the recommended intake according to the National Academy of Sciences.) (Markesberry and Wong, 1979.)
2. Discuss formula preparation and storage. Formula may be prepared as needed. (Liquid concentrate is diluted 1:1 with water, or several bottles may be prepared in advance and then refrigerated.) Suggest offering Katy 5–6 oz of formula six times a day.
3. Provide the mother with information about the care of her breasts and the possible discomfort from sensations of fullness. Advise her to substitute bottle feedings for breast feedings gradually, offering the bottle at one feeding for several days before substituting a second bottle feeding.
4. Teach the mother developmental behavioral cues indicating a readiness for solid food (eg, tongue protrusion reflex diminishing, improved head control and ability to lean forward and backward to accept or reject food, and independent movements of tongue and lips).
5. Advise feeding Katy dry infant cereal (rice) mixed with formula twice a day when she is ready for solid food.
6. Telephone Katy's mother in 1 week to see how weaning is progressing.
7. Provide support for the mother.
8. Measure Katy's growth, development, and food intake again to see whether the goals have been met.

Malnutrition

Malnutrition is defined as either overnutrition or undernutrition. In poor communities and developing countries, the problem is undernutrition, whereas in middle-class communities the problem is overnutrition, as evidenced by obesity. Undernutrition has a variety of causes, all of which result in inadequate intake or usage of essential nutrients (Fig. 15-1). Any possibility of malabsorption problems, as indicated by changes in the gastrointestinal tract, warrant an investigation. Alterations in absorption frequently involve the major nutrients—protein, carbohydrate, and fat. (Chapter 38 discusses the management of the gastrointestinal problems involving nutrition.)

Marasmus When the intake of all nutrients and calories is insufficient to meet the body's needs for maintenance, growth ceases and a state of balanced starvation, or *marasmus,* exists. The onset of marasmus is gradual, resulting from inadequate energy intake rather than a single nutrient deficiency.

Marasmus occurs in infants and children and may be the result of physiologic diseases, psychosocial problems, or a combination of the two (Table 15-15). When calories are inadequate, growth first slows, resulting in stunting (low height for age), and then ceases; eventually, weight is lost, resulting in wasting (low weight for age). As the condition becomes more acute, irritability, listlessness, and passivity increase. The chronicity of marasmus allows the body to adapt. Most laboratory findings are nonspecific. Usually, mild anemia is present, the metabolic rate is low, and oxygen consumption is low.

Once the cause of the undernutrition is identified, interventions can be coordinated to provide an adequate and usable dietary intake. The cause and severity of marasmus dictates how cautiously to proceed and in what form to add calories. Too many calories too quickly cause diarrhea. The

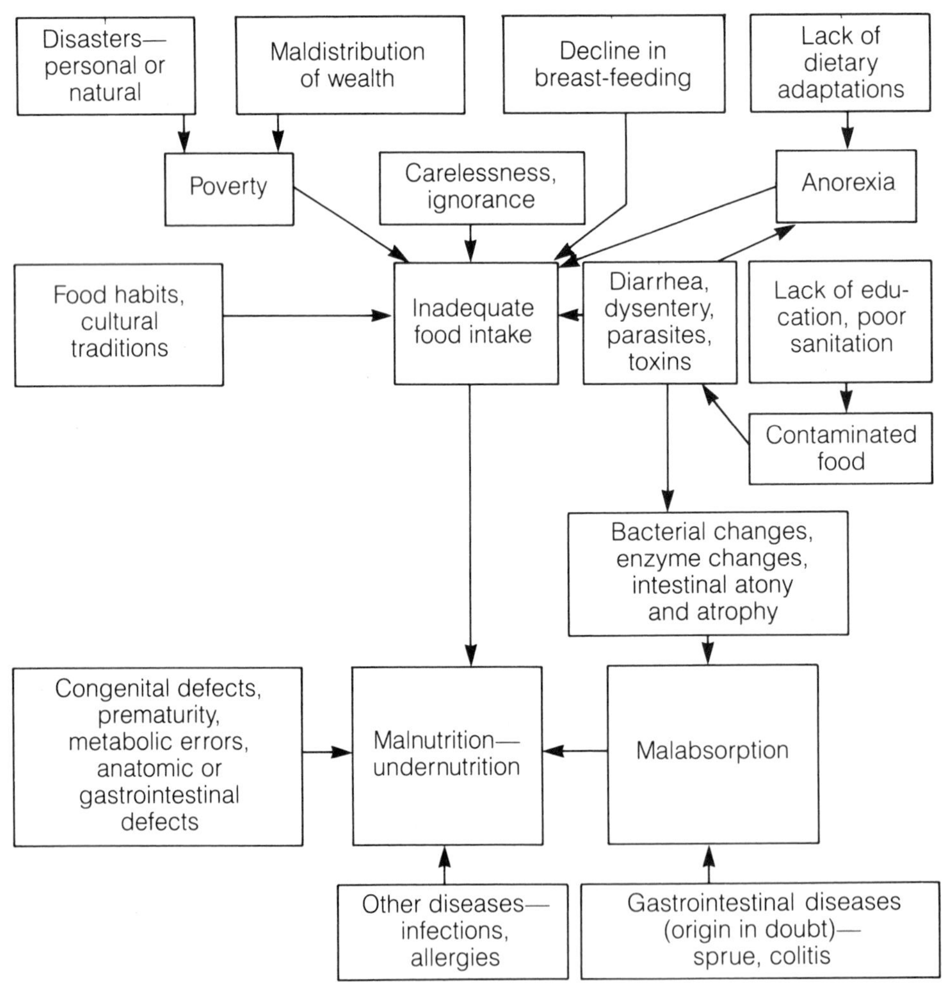

Figure 15-1 Factors resulting in inadequate intake or use of nutrients, leading to malnutrition in children. (Adapted from Williams CD: Malnutrition. *The Lancet* 1962; 2:342–44, and Moore JA, Glittenberg A: *Biocultural Basis of Health*. Copyright © 1980 by Lorna G. Moore, Denver, CO.

TABLE 15-15 Common Causes of Marasmus

Cause	Example
Inadequate intake	Abuse or neglect Errors in formula preparation—overdilution Psychosocial dwarfism Congestive heart failure Anorexia of chronic renal disease, chronic infection Elimination diets—suspected food allergy, chronic nonspecific diarrhea Vegetarian or natural foods—bulkiness, low energy density Chronic vomiting—chalasia, achalasia, rumination, pyloric stenosis Anorexia nervosa
Inadequate absorption	Postintestinal resection Decreased surface area—chronic diarrhea, celiac disease, Crohn's disease Pancreatic disease—cystic fibrosis, Schwachman-Diamond syndrome Chronic liver disease Poor digestibility of foods—pure vegetarian, some natural foods
Increased requirements	Hypermetabolic states—for example, hyperthyroidism Increased "work," as with chronic lung disease, cardiac failure, and spasticity, or with competitive athletics

SOURCE: Adapted from MacLean WC, Graham GG: *Pediatric Nutrition in Clinical Practice.* © 1982, Williams & Wilkins Co., Baltimore, 1982.

nurse plays a vital role in teaching and supporting the child and family during this transition to different dietary patterns.

Kwashiorkor When the intake of protein is inadequate with respect to calories and other nutrients, the protein–energy deficiency is known as *kwashiorkor.* Few children in developed countries have this deficiency because they receive more than 8% of their calories from protein. When the protein–energy percentage is reduced, such as occurs in children from developing countries and in situations in which intravenous glucose and high-calorie formulas must be used for a prolonged period of time, the body responds by catabolizing stored proteins.

Kwashiorkor can occur from inadequate intake, absorption, or utilization. It may be related to chronic conditions, such as cystic fibrosis, or acute conditions such as bacterial sepsis. Whatever the cause, the characteristic signs and symptoms appear. The child is irritable, listless, and edematous. Edema ranges from mild swelling of hands and feet to marked peritoneal fluid accumulation. There is loss of pigmentation in the skin and hair (for example, black hair turns red). Hair becomes silky and sparse and is easily pulled from the scalp. A nondescript skin rash appears, and the skin flakes off, leaving raw areas. The liver enlarges as a result of fatty infiltrates.

As with marasmus, treatment is determined by the cause and severity of the condition. Because the onset of kwashiorkor is more sudden, the body has had less time to adapt and is in a more precarious state. The nurse plays a pivotal role in assessing the child's tolerance to treatment and the reintroduction of oral intake.

Food Sensitivity

Food Allergy Twenty-five percent of the population suffers from some type of allergic disease, and 50% of these diseases are due to food allergy, which occurs more often among children than among adults (Brenneman, 1979). (Specific allergies and their associated management are discussed in Chapter 37.) Food allergy is manifested by respiratory, gastrointestinal, and skin symptoms. True allergies are a result of antibodies responding to specific antigens or foreign proteins that are consumed. The most common of the offending proteins are milk, egg whites, and wheat.

With infants, cow's milk is a common food allergy, most often manifested by vomiting, diarrhea, skin rash, or irritability and abdominal cramping. Special formulas are available for allergic infants such as soybean preparations and meat-based and hydrolyzed casein-based formulas. Infants with a strong family history of allergy or those who have already reacted to cow's milk should be monitored carefully when solid foods are introduced. Wheat and eggs should be delayed, and hypoallergenic rice cereal frequently is the first food for all infants.

When a food sensitivity is suspected, a thorough history of food intake, food preparation, and suspected reactions is reviewed. A simple elimination diet may be used to identify positively the suspected food. To do this, the child eats a regular diet, except that the suspected offending food is eliminated. The child is then observed to see whether symptoms subside or appear. If the food is not known, the child is put on a regular diet, except that all known allergenic foods are eliminated. With a major elimination diet, the child eats only the hypoallergic foods for 2 weeks. Other foods are then added, one at a time, and the child is observed for symptomatic reactions. Some common highly allergenic foods are wheat, eggs, chocolate, seafood, and nuts; slightly allergenic foods include fresh fruit (peaches, pears, apples, apricots), chicken, and beef. Common hypoallergic foods are rice and rice products, pears or peaches (frozen, canned, or cooked), lamb, carrots, gelatin desserts, and lettuce (Slattery, Pearson, and Torre, 1979).

Food Additives A *food additive* is any substance that, when added directly or indirectly, becomes a component of food or affects the functional characteristics of the food (Green and Harry, 1981). Food additives have become a recent concern, particularly in regard to processed foods. Additives are used in food not only as a preservative but also to improve various functional properties such as flavor, odor, texture, and nutritional quality, and because the demand for out-of-season foods and easy-to-fix processed foods has become a way of life. It is difficult to eat without ingesting food additives.

Natural foods are not necessarily better. If foods do not have added preservatives, they develop mold or turn rancid more quickly, making them potential agents of disease. Some natural foods, like certain mushrooms, are poisonous. Lima beans and apricot pits contain cyanide and spinach and beets have nitrates, which convert to nitrites and can be harmful in high doses. Spinach and beets also are not recommended for children under 3 months of age. Most foods containing certain chemicals or toxins, however, are eaten in small quantities and as part of a balanced diet and thus they are safe. Although some authorities argue that natural foods are better, neither the human body nor a chemist can distinguish a synthesized vitamin from those that occur naturally (Stare and Whelan, 1976).

The controversial and noted Dr. Benjamen Feingold (1975) has claimed that chemicals added to food can affect children's behavioral patterns, particularly by increasing their activity level. He recommends eliminating foods containing natural salicylates, artificial colors and flavors, and certain preservatives. For most families, however, this intensive food monitoring creates a major change in family life-style. Scientific evidence is inconclusive, including some positive, some negative, and some mixed findings in the completed research (Fine, 1980). At present, the strongest evidence supporting a direct relationship between food consumption and hyperactivity in children comes from parents.

Some adherents of the dietary management of childhood hyperactivity propose that certain foods and food additives act as drugs, increasing the neurologic responses to stimuli (Brenner, 1977). Children who adhere to the strict elimination of offending foods evidence improved behavior and ability to concentrate. Although some children respond favorably to dietary management, others do not, underscoring the fact that more research is needed to better understand the relationship between diet and behavior.

Recent interest in the relationship between food and disease has led to concern about certain food additives, such as saccharin and nitrates, which might produce cancer. Food additives are tested by the Food and Drug Administration for toxicologic effects on laboratory animals before the additives are approved for use, but such tests are expensive and take 3–4 years to complete (Green and Harry, 1981). The nurse involved in nutritional assessment and nutrition education therefore needs to be aware of current findings and recommendations.

Iron Deficiency

Iron deficiency is the reduction of iron in the body stores, as documented by a decreased serum iron, or ferritin, level, decrease in transferrin saturation to less than 16%, an increase in free erythrocyte protoporphyrin (FEP) to greater than 50 μg/dL of red blood cells, and a decrease in mean corpuscular volume (MCV) (Fomon, 1976). If the deficiency continues, a hyprochromic microcytic anemia results, which is indicated by a decrease in hemoglobin to less than 11.0 g/dL and a hematocrit of less than 33%. (The nursing management of iron deficiency is discussed in Chapter 36.)

Iron deficiency is quite common in the United States and is unrelated to socioeconomic factors, as indicated by national nutritional surveys. Infants between the ages of 6 and 24 months are prone to iron deficiency because their stores of maternal iron are depleted, and they are dependent on external sources. Low-birthweight infants, infants fed unmodified cow's milk in the first 6 months of life, adolescent males in their growth spurt, and menstruating females are also subject to iron deficiency. Normal full-term infants have sufficient iron stores to last until they are 4–6 months of age, at which time external iron intake is needed. Preterm or low-birthweight infants deplete their iron stores by 2 months of age and usually require an iron supplement (Committee on Nutrition, 1976).

Iron deficiency is a preventable condition, and regular monitoring of food intake and routine hematologic values in children promotes the early identification and possible prevention of anemia. Any family history of anemia and special dietary practices, such as vegetarianism, should be determined. The child's growth parameters should be measured. Any change in growth or eating habits and unusual behavior (for example, pica) could be symptomatic of iron deficiency. Pallor of the mucous membranes and skin is an early sign of iron-deficiency anemia. When the hemoglobin drops below 6 g/dL of blood, such symptoms as irritability, inability to concentrate, anorexia, and decreased activity are present; these are followed by cardiac symptoms and systolic murmurs (Vaughn, McKay, and Behrman, 1979).

The infant requires 8 mg/day of iron; this is best obtained from breast milk, which is 50% absorbable, from iron-fortified formula, which has 12 mg of ferrous sulfate per quart and which is 4% absorbable, from iron-fortified dry infant

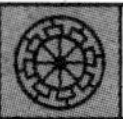

CASE STUDY Iron Deficiency

Assessment

Mark is a 3-year-old male who was brought to the clinic by his mother because of concern about his weight and poor food intake.

Family

Mark is the youngest of three children. His father is a salesman with a large company. The family recently transferred to the area. The mother has few friends and feels that the neighbors are very cautious about new residents. There are no significant family health problems. The parents are of average height, but both have short relatives in their families.

Child

Mark was $7\frac{1}{2}$ lb, 19 in at birth. He was bottle-fed formula with no difficulty and has no food intolerances. His appetite is usually fair, but he was never a big eater. He feeds himself using a combination of fingers and utensils. He has had few colds, no serious illnesses, no injuries, and no hospitalizations. His immunizations are up to date. He is described as active and doing the things that most children his age do. He sleeps well, has no history of gastrointestinal problems, and has a daily defecation of a soft, brown, formed stool. He has seen a dentist twice, and his teeth are in good condition and developing well.

Environment

The family has a community water supply, which is believed to be fluoridated. Family members shop at the local supermarket. The family eats supper together, which is described as a pleasant social experience. Breakfast and lunch are eaten together on the weekends but not during the week because of school and work time constraints. They have no special food preferences, dietary habits, or special diets.

Food Intake—24-hour recall

Breakfast	4 oz orange juice (concentrate diluted 3:1) $\frac{1}{2}$ cup Cheerios with 4 oz of 2% milk 1 slice of raisin toast with pat of margarine
Snack	4 oz of 2% milk or 4 oz of fruit-flavored yogurt
Lunch	2 slices of white bread with 1 oz of Velveeta cheese 1 apple 6 oz of 2% milk
Snack	Peanut butter cookie (1) 4 oz of 2% milk
Supper	1 piece of baked chicken thigh $\frac{1}{2}$ cup of applesauce Few potatoes 4 oz of 2% milk $\frac{1}{2}$ cup of vanilla ice cream

The mother described this day's intake as typical, except that Mark sometimes has an egg for breakfast instead of cereal. She said he likes breads, dairy products, and canned fruits but does not eat vegetables and other meats such as steak and pork. The parents have tried unsuccessfully to make him sit at the table until he eats his vegetables, or to punish him by putting him to bed, or to coax him by reading stories at the table. The mother states that she is discouraged and wonders what to try next. Her other children were not problem eaters.

Clinical

Physical Assessment Data Mark is a cooperative, alert, thin boy with good color. His temperature was 36.8 C axillary. He had no abnormal physical findings.

Growth Mark's height is 90 cm (26 in); his weight is 13 kg ($28\frac{1}{2}$ lb); his head circumference is 49 cm ($19\frac{1}{2}$ in).

Laboratory Tests Hemoglobin is 12 g/dL, hematocrit is 34%; urinalysis is normal.

Comparison to a Standard

According to the National Center for Health Statistics growth charts, Mark is at the 10th percentile for height, weight, and head circumference. Mark's food intake, compared with the basic four food groups, revealed that he had adequate servings of milk, bread, and meat but that his intake was low in the fruit and vegetable group. By comparing food intake with the food composition tables and calculating the nutrient values, it was determined that, for this day, Mark took in approximately 1210 calories, 1259 mg of calcium, 636 μg of vitamin A, 3.5 mg of iron, and 60 mg of vitamin C. According to the Recommended Daily Allowances, this caloric intake is adequate because the range for 1- to 3-year-old children is 900–1800 calories/day. Mark has an adequate or excessive intake of most of the selected nutrients except iron.

Nursing Diagnoses

1. Potential risk for decreased iron stores related to an inadequate intake of iron.
2. Potential for alterations in parenting related to a new environment and lack of support.

Nursing Interventions

Goals

1. Iron deficiency will be prevented through dietary counseling.
2. The mother will become comfortable about parenting skills through support and education about normal child development.

Interventions

1. Recommended high-iron foods: liver, legumes, raisins, leafy green vegetables, vegetable soups, vegetables mashed up and mixed in with mashed potatoes, and iron-fortified cereals.
2. Recalculate diet, with several dietary recalls, to document deficiency.
3. Praise the mother for the quality of the food choices and lack of empty-calorie foods.

continued on next page

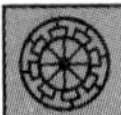

CASE STUDY Iron Deficiency (continued)

4. Suggest giving raw vegetables as snacks and serving larger portions of meat.
5. Allow the mother to express concerns about the new environmental situation and suggest community groups she might be interested in attending.
6. Discuss Mark's behaviors and compare them with expected 3-year-old behavior.
7. Suggest other developmental areas the mother can focus on regarding Mark's developing skills.
8. Arrange another clinic visit, at which time the mother will bring in a 3-day diet record to evaluate further Mark's nutrient intake.
9. Begin developmental counseling with the mother at that time and include a further assessment of family concerns and needs.

cereals, which are 4% absorbable, and from strained meats. The young child can receive 4–6 mg of iron per 1000 calories.

Unfortunately, a continued increase in milk intake and the introduction of poor-quality snack foods often prevents the intake of high-iron and iron-fortified foods. Most Americans can obtain 6 mg of iron per 1000 calories in their diets. The adolescent male is most likely to obtain 15 mg of iron because he consumes an average of 2500 calories/day. This is still less than the recommended 18 mg of iron; therefore, the nurse needs to educate children and parents about high-iron foods. Adolescent females average about 1750–2000 calories/day and therefore rarely obtain their required iron intake. Most often, this population should take iron supplements until they reach 17 years of age (Fomon, 1976).

Although iron deficiency is preventable, it is rarely diagnosed until anemia is noted by the routine blood tests of hemoglobin or hematocrit. Because the body can adapt to iron deficiency, the incidence of anemia is not as great as the incidence of iron deficiency would suggest. Dallman (1979) has said that the percentage of iron absorbed varies among individuals and depends on the amount of iron in the diet and the body's iron stores. The more iron ingested, the lower the percentage absorbed; the lower the body's iron stores, the greater the percentage of iron absorbed (Dallman, 1979).

Iron absorption from food depends on the presence of heme iron found in meats; nonheme iron found in cereals, eggs, legumes, and vegetables; ascorbic acid; and the combination of food consumed. Dairy products, tea, and phosphorus salts decrease absorption. For example, the iron in dry infant cereals is absorbed better if the cereal is mixed with juice rather than with milk (Stewart, 1978). Foods that are good sources of iron include meats, poultry, fish, nuts, eggs, green vegetables, whole wheat flour, legumes, and enriched cereals.

Vegetarian Diets

Vegetarians are persons who live principally on vegetable or plant food and abstain from eating meat, poultry, fish, or other animal products. The three primary forms are lacto-ovovegetarians, who include dairy products and eggs in their nonflesh diet; lactovegetarians, who consume milk or milk products but exclude meat, poultry, fish, seafood, and eggs; and total vegetarians, or vegans, who consume no animal products, eggs, or dairy products (American Dietetic Association, 1980). The lactovegetarian and lacto-ovovegetarian diets are nutritionally similar to the usual American diet, and therefore the nurse can expect the growth and development of children with these diets to be normal. The stricter vegetarian, or vegan, however, is more susceptible to a variety of nutritional deficiencies. These diets might be high in bulk, but energy needs may not be met. Their lower caloric intake might result in protein being used to provide energy, and plant foods are not a good source of vitamins B_{12} and D. Fortified foods such as soybean milk or meat analogues are a good source of these vitamins. Vitamin D also can be obtained by exposing the skin to sunlight or with supplements such as cod liver oil. For the total vegetarian, the nurse should encourage the regular and ample intake of dark green vegetables, legumes, fortified soybean milk, nuts, and seeds to provide calcium and riboflavin. Infants of vegans should be given fortified soybean formula to get adequate protein, vitamins, and minerals. Although iron is available from some plant foods, it is not as absorbable as heme or animal sources of iron.

In counseling vegetarians, the nurse needs to recommend good food sources of iron and emphasize the inclusion in each meal of a food high in ascorbic acid to enhance the availability of nonheme (plant food) iron (American Dietetic Association, 1980). Table 15-16 lists the four food groups and suggested daily intakes for lactovegetarians and lacto-ovovegetarians. With the vegan diet, care must be taken to obtain complete proteins. For example, some complementary proteins include cereal grains and legumes, beans and corn tortillas, rice and lentils, or rice and soy products. This diet is not recommended for infants and young children because of potential deficits in iron, calories, vitamin B_{12}, calcium, riboflavin, and zinc (Johnston, 1984).

The diet and nutritional status of infants and children in vegetarian families will be variable. Dietary styles for each child must be assessed individually before judging nutri-

TABLE 15-16 Four Food Groups and Suggested Daily Intakes for Vegetarian Diets

Food group	Food sources and recommended intake
Grains, legumes, nuts, and seeds	Six servings or more. Include several slices of yeast-raised, whole-grain bread, a serving of beans, and a few nuts or seeds
Fruit	One to four pieces. Include a raw source of vitamin C such as citrus fruits, strawberries, or cantaloupe
Vegetables	Three servings or more. Include one or more servings of dark, leafy greens such as romaine lettuce, spinach, or chard
Milk and dairy products	Two or more glasses of fresh milk for adults, three or more for children. (Children under 9 years of age use smaller glasses.) Other dairy products can be used to meet part of the milk requirement.
(Eggs)	(Eggs are optional—up to four per week—and may be included for lacto-ovovegetarians)

tional adequacy or deficiencies. Many people who become vegetarians do so gradually and often evolve toward stricter forms. The nurse therefore should enquire not only about the preference for vegetarianism but also about the family's changing patterns in dietary habits (MacLean and Graham, 1980). A thorough report of the specific foods consumed, their brands, and their methods of preparation is particularly important in assessing a vegetarian diet. In addition, other factors about the family life-style should be determined, as listed in Table 15-17.

Obesity

Because Americans generally are overfed, obesity is prevalent in 10–30% of the population (Forbes, 1979), and some reports suggest that 40% of the population is overweight (Green and Harry, 1981). Obesity exists when there is an energy imbalance and when energy intake exceeds the energy needs for growth, maintenance, and activity for a period of time. Obesity is distinguished from being overweight by an excessive (greater than 20% of ideal weight) deposition of adipose tissue, or body fat. Weight in excess of the standard for a given height can be a result of increased lean body mass, adipose tissue, or both.

The assessment process includes specific questions to provide the nurse with information indicating the extent of an overweight problem or whether a child is at risk for obesity. During the history taking, questions are asked about family health history in regard to specific diseases because obesity can predispose to such major health hazards as hypertension, cardiovascular disease, diabetes mellitus, gallbladder disease, and degenerative joint disorders. The incidence of obesity in the child is higher when both parents are obese.

TABLE 15-17 Factors Influencing Vegetarians' Nutritional and Health Status

Characteristic	Useful indicators
Diet	Extensiveness of animal food avoidances
	Extensiveness of other food avoidances (attention should be paid to the frequency and amount of foods eaten rather than simply whether they are or are not consumed)
	Willingness to use special foods (either enriched, fortified, or naturally occurring sources rich in nutrients, which may be problematic) or specific vitamin-mineral supplements
	Time on the regimen
	Nutritional knowledge (for dietary planning)
	Groups with high needs that make them especially vulnerable (eg, infants, young children, adolescents, women during pregnancy and lactation, the ill, or those recovering from illness)
Related health practices	Use or disuse of tobacco, alcohol, licit and illicit drugs
	Use of orthodox medical advice (is it on an ongoing basis or only as a last resort in acute crises?)
Coexisting disease states	Is a special therapeutic diet or supportive therapy necessary for coexisting health problems?
Other social characteristics	Living arrangements—communal or single–family unit (may be relevant for spread of infectious disease)
	Income and educational level
	Affiliation with groups having special teachings about diet or other aspects of life-style

SOURCE: Factors influencing vegetarians' nutritional and health status. Copyright The American Dietetic Association. Reprinted by permission from *Journal of the American Dietetic Association*, Vol. 77:61, 1980.

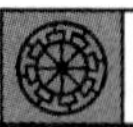

CASE STUDY Obesity

Assessment

Pam is a 12-year-old junior high school student who has come to the nurse's office for advice about weight reduction. The nurse notes that she is significantly overweight. Pam admits she has tried to lose weight but without success.

Family

Pam is the youngest of two girls. Her older sister, who is also overweight, is married and no longer lives at home. Pam's parents are divorced. Her father is also overweight and has hypertension. Pam's mother works to support herself and Pam, is overweight, and has a thyroid condition.

Child

Pam is in the seventh grade; her grades are average. She has few friends. She rides her bike to and from school and takes swimming lessons once a week. She watches a lot of television. Menarche occurred when Pam was 11 years of age.

Environment

The family lives in a small house in the city, near a major shopping center.

Food Intake—24-Hour Recall

Breakfast	2 waffle squares with 2 tbsp of syrup and 2 pats of margarine
Lunch (at school)	2 cups of chicken chow mein with rice and noodles 1 roll with 1 pat of margarine 1 cup of canned peaches 8 oz of skim milk
Snack	2 chocolate chip cookies and 20 oz of soda pop
Supper	$\frac{1}{2}$ large pizza with cheese and tomato 20 oz cola
Snack	1 apple

Clinical Data

Physical Assessment Data Pam is an alert but sad-appearing, overweight, pubescent female; her blood pressure is 120/80.

Growth Pam's height is 163 cm ($64\frac{1}{2}$ in); her weight is 92.8 kg ($206\frac{1}{4}$ lb); her triceps skinfold is 25 mm.

Comparison to a Standard

According to the National Center for Health Statistics growth charts, Pam's height is at the 95th percentile, her weight is greater than the 95th percentile, and her triceps skinfold is at the 95th percentile. Pam's intake is low in milk and meat, high in fruits, vegetables, and bread, with no citrus fruit this day. For this day, Pam took in approximately 3092 calories. The Recommended Daily Allowance range for 11- to 14-year-old females is 1500–3000 calories. Most of these calories are from carbohydrates and protein. Her vitamin A intake was 1105 μg (RDA is 800 μg); vitamin C was 16 mg (RDA is 50 mg); calcium was 1568 μg (RDA is 1200 μg); and iron was 21.8 mg (RDA is 18 mg).

Nursing Diagnosis

1. Alteration in nutrition: more than body requirements related to excess intake.
2. Potential for adult hypertension and hypothyroidism related to adolescent obesity and family history.

Nursing Interventions

Goals

1. Pam will increase her caloric expenditure and decrease her caloric intake.
2. Pam will lose 0.5 lb/wk until her optimal weight is attained.
3. Pam will not develop any disorders related to obesity.

Interventions

1. Encourage Pam to increase her bicycling and swimming activities by 30 minutes/day. Suggest she attend "free swim" every afternoon in addition to her weekly lesson.
2. Encourage the addition of one citrus fruit in the daily intake of fruits and vegetables.
3. Increase skim milk intake for vitamin D content. Replace soda consumed as a snack and at supper with 8 oz of skim milk.
4. Decrease sugared drinks and soda with the goal of complete elimination.
5. Select the salad bar at school instead of the entree.
6. Refer Pam to her family physician for a complete medical assessment.
7. Refer Pam for laboratory tests for hemoglobin, hematocrit, urinalysis, serum cholesterol and triglyceride levels, and complete thyroid studies.
8. Suggest that Pam attend weekly meeting at the junior high formed by other girls on weight-reduction plans.
9. Establish a routine and have Pam come in weekly for weight checks and to report on food intake and physical activities.
10. Discuss with Pam how to keep a diary of food intake to determine food choices and resources to learn about the nutrient content of these choices.
11. Devise a reward system to use for successes in weight loss or changes in eating and physical activity habits such as not eating while watching television.
12. Coordinate goals and interventions with the family physician.

Family eating habits also are assessed. Those habits that contribute to weight problems include eating while watching television, eating high-calorie snacks, particularly at bedtime, eating fast foods, fried foods, and desserts frequently, food deprivation as a form of punishment, and eating when depressed or angry. Family activity patterns also are assessed. Parents who do not encourage physical activity but do encourage more sedentary interests help to establish a child's lifetime activity patterns. Any indication of current stress or emotional difficulty in the family should alert the nurse to ask about the effects on food habits because eating is a means of handling stress for some people.

The nurse also assesses the child's past growth pattern. Data include birthweight, rate of growth, past eating habits, bottle- or breast-feeding, timing of the introduction of solid foods, and any feeding problems. Although not firmly determined, rapid weight gain, encouraging the infant to finish the bottle at every feeding, and the early introduction of solid foods might contribute to later weight problems. The importance of food in family life and how it is used (for example, as a reward for good behavior) might be significant in overeating.

The child is inspected visually for signs of overweight (fat rolls and soft, doughy skin texture) in the abdomen, buttocks, and upper thighs. Monitoring the rate of growth is most important in all children. Comparison of weight to height does not specify the amount of adipose tissue, but if this is greater than the 95th percentile on the NCHS growth charts, further evaluation for obesity is indicated (see Appendix A). A helpful guide for assessing nutritional status with regard to growth and the relation of weight to length during the first year is found in Table 15-18. This guide is particularly useful when assessing breast-fed infants, in whom the amount of intake cannot be measured. Skinfold thickness measurements of the triceps are helpful in distinguishing adipose tissue from muscle mass. Measures greater than the 95th percentile on the skinfold thickness standards indicate a greater-than-normal increase in adipose tissue (see Table 15-4).

The early identification of children at risk for obesity is mainly subjective. Knowing the factors associated with obesity and interviewing the child and/or parent with sensitivity to eating patterns help to make an appropriate nursing diagnosis and effective care plan. An important aspect of the assessment is whether the child or parent is concerned with the obesity. If not, any plan will fail, but if they are concerned, involving them in the planning is the first nursing intervention.

TABLE 15-18 Tentative Definition of Obesity

	Males		Females	
Age (months)	**Length (in) Less than**	**Weight (lb) More than**	**Length (in) Less than**	**Weight (lb) More than**
1	20.4	9.3	20.3	8.8
	20.9	9.9	20.6	9.5
	21.3	10.4	21.1	10.1
	21.7	11.3	21.5	10.6
3	22.8	13.2	22.4	12.4
	23.3	14.1	22.8	13.0
	23.7	15.2	23.3	13.7
	24.2	16.1	23.7	14.5
6	25.8	17.0	24.9	16.5
	26.2	18.0	25.7	17.6
	26.7	19.9	26.1	18.5
	27.2	21.2	26.7	19.6
9	27.6	20.1	26.9	19.6
	27.9	21.4	27.4	20.7
	28.5	23.6	28.0	21.8
	29.0	24.7	28.8	22.9
12	29.0	22.5	28.5	21.8
	29.4	24.0	28.8	23.1
	30.1	25.6	29.6	24.5
	30.7	27.6	30.3	25.6

SOURCE: Adapted with permission from Markesbery BA, Wong WM: Watching baby's diet: A professional and parental guide. *Matern Child Nurs* (May/June) 4:3. Copyright © 1979 American Journal of Nursing Company, and Foman SJ: *Infant Nutrition.* W.B. Saunders, 1974.

NOTE: A rule of thumb about weight gain is that 7–8 oz/wk is usual but that 5–12 oz/wk also might be normal.

Key Concepts

- The goal of the nutritional assessment is to identify existing or potential nutritional problems by reviewing the child's health status, attitudes toward food, activity patterns, and eating habits.
- The process of the nutritional assessment includes identifying the quantity and quality of food intake and the eating patterns of both the child and family.
- Nutritional assessment criteria depend on nutritional research, which relies heavily on surveys, and dietary trends, which are related to the choice of food, adaptability to change, availability of food, social and cultural patterns, and health status.
- Data collection for the nutritional assessment encompasses history taking, dietary recall, physical measurements, and laboratory tests.
- The nurse encourages the parent or child to express any nutritional concerns early in the assessment process, so that specific data about growth, eating behavior, activity patterns, food preparation, and family preferences can be collected to address the concern.
- Types of food intake records include a 24-hour recall of dietary intake, for which the parent or child relies on memory, and a dietary record kept by the parent or child over several days.
- Clinical data relevant to nutritional status include physical assessment findings (especially growth measurements), skinfold thickness and midarm circumference measurements, and laboratory data.
- Malnutrition includes both overnutrition and undernutrition and occurs in three levels: (1) low dietary intake; (2) depleted body stores; and (3) appearance of physical signs and symptoms.
- Following data collection, the nurse analyzes the data to determine whether nutritional intake is adequate to promote growth. Recommended daily allowances and standard growth charts, together with any nutritional concerns and information about the family and community, are the criteria for analysis and nursing diagnosis.
- In infancy more calories are needed for metabolism, growth, and activity than at any other developmental stage.
- Infants receive their nutrients—principally protein, carbohydrates, fat, and water—from milk, which can be human milk, commercially prepared formula, or evaporated milk formula.
- Unmodified cow's milk is not recommended for infants under 6 months of age.
- Solid foods are best introduced to an infant no earlier than 5–6 months of age.
- In early childhood nutrient deficiencies often include iron, calcium, and vitamin C; nutritional problems resulting from insufficient quantities of food are also prevalent in some populations.
- Middle and late childhood are characterized by slow, continuous growth and an increased need for calories to maintain high levels of activity.
- Because schoolchildren are influenced by the school environment as well as their families, parents might need to provide nutritious snacks to meet nutritional requirements, and nurses may need to advise parents about nutritional needs.
- Nutritional needs in adolescence are related to the rate and timing of the adolescent growth spurt.
- Dietary patterns in adolescence, especially fast-food consumption, suggest that food habits are an essential part of the nutritional assessment, and specific interventions might be needed to prevent deficiencies.
- Obesity can occur at any age, including infancy, and might require interventions planned for both the child and the family to modify eating and activity patterns.
- Iron deficiency, or the reduction of iron in body stores, is a preventable condition that can be treated with the adequate dietary intake of iron.
- Food sensitivities include food allergies, which are treated by avoiding the offending food.
- Weaning, or the change in infancy from breast- or bottle-feeding to a cup, usually occurs in the last half of the first year but is determined by parental preference and infant readiness.
- Dental caries can be avoided by limiting the intake of sweetened foods, not allowing the infant to fall asleep with a bottle, and providing dental care beginning in early childhood.

References

Abraham S et al: *Preliminary Finding of the First Health and Nutrition Examination Survey, United States 1971–1972: Dietary Intake and Biochemical Findings.* US Department of Health, Education, and Welfare, January, 1974.

American Dietetic Association: Position paper on the vegetarian approach to eating. *J Am Diet Assoc* (July) 1980; 77:61–68.

Andrew M, Clancy KL, Katz MG: Infant feeding practices of families belonging to a prepaid group practice health care plan. *Pediatrics* (May) 1980; 65:978–988.

Brenneman JC: Food allergy. *Contemporary Nutrition.* (March) 1979; 4(3).

Brenner A: A study of the efficacy of the Feingold diet on hyperkinetic children. Some favorable personal observations. *Clin Pediatr* 1977; 16:652–656.

Callaway CW: Bridging the gaps in human nutrition. *Nutr News* (April) 1981; 44:5–6.

Christakis G: Nutritional assessment in health programs. *Am J Public Health* (Nov) 1973; 63(Suppl): 80.

Committee on Dietary Allowances, Food and Nutrition Board, National Research Council: Page 28 in: *Recommended Dietary Allowances.* 9th ed. National Academy of Sciences, 1980.

Committee on Nutrition: Iron supplementation for infants. *Pediatrics* (Nov) 1976; 58:763–765.

Committee on Nutrition: On the feeding of supplemental foods to infants. *Pediatrics* (June) 1980; 65:1178–1180.

Committee on Nutrition: Practical significance of lactose intolerance in children. *Pediatrics* (Aug) 1978; 62:240–244.

Committee on Nutrition: Vitamin and mineral supplement needs in normal children in the United States. *Pediatrics* (Dec) 1980; 66:1015–1021.

Dallman PR: Nutritional anemias. In: *Pediatric Nutrition Handbook.* Committee on Nutrition. American Academy of Pediatrics, 1979.

Dubos R: Keynote address: Nutritional adaptations. *Am J Clin Nutr* (Dec.) 1979; 32:2623–2626.

Enders, JB, Rockwell, RE: *Food, Nutrition, and the Young.* Mosby, 1980.

Feingold BF: Hyperkinesis and learning disabilities linked to artificial food flavors and colors. *Am J Nurs* May 1975; 75(5): 797–803.

Fine MJ (editor): *Intervention With Hyperactive Children.* Spectrum, 1980.

Forbes GB: Obesity. In: *Pediatric Nutrition Handbook.* Committee on Nutrition. American Academy of Pediatrics, 1979.

Fomon SJ: *Nutritional Disorders of Children: Prevention, Screening, and Followup.* HEW Publication No. 77–5104. US Department of Health, Education, and Welfare, 1976.

Fomon SJ, et al: Recommendations for feeding normal infants. *Pediatrics* (Jan) 1979; 63:52–58.

Frank GC, et al: Dietary studies of rural-school children in a cardiovascular study. *J Am Diet Assoc* 1977; 7:31.

General Mills: Toward a national nutrition policy. *Nutrition Policy Issues,* No. 9, Dec 1980.

Gerber Products Company: *Market Research Study.* Gerber Products Company, 1978.

Gifft HH, Washbon MB, Harrison GG: *Nutrition, Behavior and Change.* Prentice-Hall, 1972.

Gray GE, Gray LK: Anthropometric measurements and their interpretations: Principles, practices, and problems. *J Am Diet Assoc* (Nov) 1980; 77:534–538.

Green M, Harry J: *Nutrition in Contemporary Nursing Practice.* Wiley, 1981.

Johnston PK: Getting enough to grow on. *Am J Nurs* (March) 1984; 84(3):336–339.

Knittle JM, Hirsch J: Infantile nutrition as a determinant of adult adipose tissue, metabolism and cellularity. *Clin Res* 1967; 15:323.

Lamme AJ III, Lamme, LL: Children's food preferences. *J School Health* (Sept) 1980; 50:397–402.

Lowe CU, et al: Reflections of dietary studies with children in the Ten-State Nutritional Survey of 1968–1970. *Pediatrics* (Aug) 1975; 56: 320–326.

MacLean WC, Graham GG: *Pediatric Nutrition in Clinical Practice.* Addison-Wesley, 1982.

MacLean WC, Graham, GG: Vegetarianism in children. *Am J Dis Child* (May) 1980; 134:513–519.

Martinez GA, Nalezienski JP: The recent trend in breast-feeding. *Pediatrics* (Nov) 1979; 64:686–692.

Morse W, Sims LS, Guthrie HA: Mother's compliance with physician's recommendation on infant feeding. *J Am Diet Assoc* (Aug) 1979; 75:140–148.

National Dairy Council: Nutritional concerns during adolescence. *Dairy Council Dig* (March/April) 1981; 52:7–11.

Nelms BC, Mullins R: *Growth and Development—a Primary Health Care Approach.* Prentice-Hall, 1982.

Nutrition Committee of the Canadian Pediatric Society and the Committee on Nutrition of the American Academy of Pediatrics: Breastfeeding. *Pediatrics* (Oct) 1978; 62:591–601.

Owens GM, et al: A study of nutritional status of preschool children in the United States, 1968–1970. *Pediatrics* (April) 1974; 53(Suppl): 53:597–646.

Pao EM, Cronin FJ: USDA's food consumption survey: Nutritional implications. *Nutr News* (April/May) 1980; 43:5–6.

Paredes-Rojas RR, Solomons HC: Food for thought: impact of a supplemental nutritional program on low-income preschool children. *Pediatr Nurs* (July/Aug) 1982; 8(4): 315–317.

Pipes PL: Page 141 in: *Nutrition in Infancy and Childhood.* 2nd ed. Mosby, 1981.

Salans LB, Cushman S, Weisman RE: Studies of human adipose tissue. Adipose cell size and number in nonobese and obese patients. *J Clin Invest* 1973; 52:929–941.

Slattery JS, Pearson GA, Torre, CT: Page 104 in: *Maternal and Child Nutrition: Assessment and Counseling.* Appleton-Century-Crofts, 1979.

Stare FJ, Whelan EM: Panic over food additives. *Pediatr Basics* (Jan) 1976; 14:12–14.

Stewart RA: Improving the bioavailability of iron. *Pediatr Basics* 1978; 20:3.

Vaughn VC III, McKay RJ, Behrman RE: Page 1376 in: *Nelson's Textbook of Pediatrics.* 11th ed. Saunders, 1979.

Williams JPG, Tanner JM, Hughes PCR: Catch-up growth in male rats after growth retardation during suckling period. *Pediatr Res* 1974; 8:149-154.

Winick M: Cellular growth during early malnutrition. *Pediatrics* (June) 1971; 47:969–978.

Winick M: Nutrition and nerve cell growth. *Fed Proc* (Oct) 1978; 62:591–601.

Young EA, Brennan EH, Irving GL: Update: Nutritional analysis of fast food. *Public Health Curr* (May/June) 1981; 21.

Yperman AM, Vermeersch JA: Factors associated with children's food habits. *J Nutr Educat* (April-June) 1979; 11:72–76.

Additional Readings

Caghan SB: The adolescent process and the problem of nutrition. *Am J Nurs* (Oct) 1975; 75:1728–1731.

Charney E, et al: Childhood antecedents of adult obesity. Do chubby infants become obese adults? *N Engl J Med* 1976; 295:6–9.

Dansky KH: Assessing children's nutrition. *Am J Nurs* (Oct) 1977; 77(10):1610–1611.

DuRant RH, Linder CW: An evaluation of five indices of relative body weight for use with children. *J Am Diet Assoc* (Jan) 1981; 78:35–40.

Grant A: *Nutritional Assessment Guidelines.* Cutter Medical Laboratories, 1979.

Gulick EE: Infant health and breast-feeding. *Pediatr Nurs* (Sept/Oct) 1983; 9(5):359–362, 389.

Halpern SL: *Quick Reference to Clinical Nutrition.* Lippincott, 1979.

Jonides L: Childhood obesity: A treatment approach for private practice. *Pediatr Nurs* (Sept/Oct) 1982; 8(5):320–322.

Kreutler P: *Nutrition in Perspective.* Prentice-Hall, 1980.

Mandelbaum JK: The Food square: Helping people of different cultures understand balanced diets. *Pediatr Nurs* (Jan/Feb) 1983; 9(1):20–21.

Markesbery BA, Wong WM: Watching baby's diet: A professional and parental guide. *Matern Child Nurs J* (May/June) 1979; 4:177–180.

Mattes J, Gittelman-Klein R: A crossover study of artificial food colorings in a hyperkinetic child. *Am J Psychiatry* 1978; 135:987–988.

McMillan JA: Iron absorption from human milk, simulated human milk, and proprietary formulas. *Pediatrics* (Dec) 1977; 60:896–897.

McNutt KW: How contemporary is our nutrition education? *Contemp Nutr* (June) 1981; 6(6).

Moore LG, et al: *The Biocultural Basis of Health.* Mosby, 1980.

Pearson GA: Nutrition in the middle years of childhood. *Matern Child Nurs J* (Nov/Dec) 1977; 2(6):378–384.

Rudy CA: Vegetarian diets for children. *Pediatr Nurs* (Sept/Oct) 1984; 10(5):329–333.

Stahl MD, Guida DA: Slow weight gain in the breast-fed infant: Management options. *Pediatr Nurs* (March/April) 1984; 10(2):117–120.

Stephenson M: The confusing world of health foods. *FDA Consumer* (July/Aug) 1978; 12:18–23.

Sundberg MC: Framework for nursing invervention in the treatment of obesity. *Issues Ment Health Nurs* (Fall) 1978; 1:25–44.

Wenck DA, Baren M, Dewan SP: *Nutrition: The Challenge of Being Well Nourished.* Reston, 1980.

White JE, Owsley VB: Helping families cope with milk, wheat, and soy allergies. *Maternal Child Nursing* (Nov/Dec) 1983; 8(6):423–428.

Williams CD: Malnutrition. *Lancet* 1962; 2:342–344.

Winkelstein ML: Overfeeding in infancy: The early introduction of solid foods. *Pediatr Nurs* (May/June) 1984; 10(3): 205–208, 236.

Developmental Assessment

16

Gayle P. Olsen Bonnie McMillin

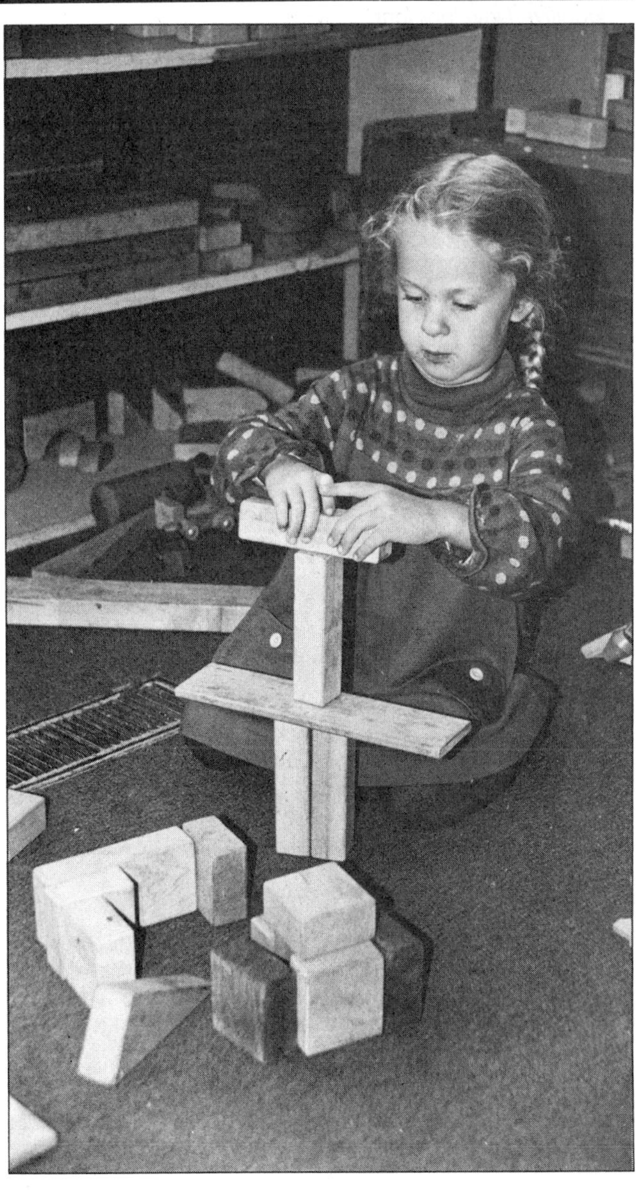

Chapter Outline

continued on next page

Objectives

- Explain the purpose of a development assessment and its role in the nursing process.
- Identify developmental milestones for specific ages.
- Define the components of a developmental history.
- Identify the developmental areas for both structured and unstructured observations.
- Identify the standard assessment tools associated with specific ages.
- Explain the distinction between assessment and screening.
- Define the developmental norms and assessment techniques for specific ages.

Human development is a multidimensional process influenced by both the subsystems and the suprasystems that affect each child. Each infant is born with an internal drive or motivation to develop, but the child's environment influences progress, either enhancing and promoting or inhibiting and undermining development. Research has demonstrated many factors that affect development; some of these factors are characteristics of the child and parent, relationships within the family, the home environment, nutritional status, socioeconomic status, and family cultural practices.

The developmental assessment is complex because not only are the child's innate characteristics considered but also the external factors that may affect the child's developmental progress. Nurses investigate how children think, act, relate, and view themselves and the world in which they live. They examine not only these subsystems of the child's development but also the suprasystems—the relationships and environment that influence development.

In Chapters 7 through 11 we discuss the developmental norms that correspond to each developmental stage. In this chapter we discuss the assessment criteria that the nurse uses to verify normal development and correct possible problems. To facilitate comparisons across age stages, we focus on standard developmental areas and the changes that are evident as the child matures.

Purpose of the Developmental Assessment

The developmental assessment is one part of the nursing assessment that provides the basis for nursing management. The nurse uses the information gained during a developmental assessment to plan comprehensive care for the child and family. Essentially, a developmental assessment should accomplish the following:

1. Validate that the child is developing normally or detect problems early.
2. Provide anticipatory guidance and counseling for both the child and parent.
3. Help the parent understand the child's behavior.
4. Identify the child's fears and concerns.
5. Help the child and parent prepare for new experiences.
6. Foster optimal development.

Both the nurse and the parent need to understand that what is "normal" represents a wide range of behaviors at any given age. The behavior of two children the same age might be quite different, yet both children may be well within the normal range. The active, determined 1-year-old might be adept at walking and is attempting to master running. The quiet, contented 1-year-old, on the other hand, is happy to sit and watch the action. The latter child is satisfied with creeping and is in no hurry to walk. Both children are healthy, and both are functioning within the normal range of expected skills for their age.

The parent who has an opportunity to discuss concerns with the nurse and participate in the child's developmental assessment is better able to recognize normal development. This recognition reassures the parent not only that the child is doing well but also that the parent is doing a good job as a parent. Such reassurance, however, is not validated until the parent has had an opportunity to discuss fully all concerns. Without such an opportunity, reassurance will be less effective because the parent is likely to feel that the nurse does not understand the parent's situation.

A developmental assessment also should detect developmental problems as early as possible. In many cases, although not all, identifying developmental problems early can lead to interventions that significantly improve outcomes and minimize deleterious sequelae. For example, a delay in language development is often the first sign of a hearing impairment. Over time, poor speech might result in teasing by other children, thus affecting the child's social relationships and self-esteem. By identifying and treating the problem early, the nurse gives the child time to improve language skills and learn to communicate normally. If the problem is not identified and allowed to persist, the child will fall further behind in language skills, and the damage to the social relationships and self-esteem is likely to be more severe.

A *developmental delay* is a parameter of development that lags behind the normal range for a given age. Developmental delay, with or without mental retardation, is another condition that can be influenced positively by early identification and treatment. Although mental retardation usually cannot be reversed or "cured," special help can maximize the retarded child's potential. (Nursing care of the mentally retarded child is discussed in Chapter 23.)

Parental Concerns

By assessing the child's developmental changes and the parent's responses to these changes, the nurse can determine the type of guidance that would be most helpful to the parent and child. Just as each child's temperament, personality, responses, and priorities are different from other children of the same age, parents also respond in different ways. Some parents are more sensitive than others to a child's changing needs; some parents are more supportive of normal developmental changes and are ready to adapt their own behavior in response to the changes in their children, whereas other parents resist changes in both their children and themselves. Variations in the behavioral patterns of children and parents are therefore taken into account when planning effective anticipatory guidance or counseling.

Some parents, for example, thoroughly enjoy the dependency of the neonate and young infant. The child's development, especially the acquisition of skills associated with independence such as mobility and language, is accepted but not eagerly anticipated. These parents might not respond positively, for example, to their 11-month-old child's early attempts to walk, refuse food, or demand a certain toy. Other parents might find the dependent stage difficult and push their children to accomplish tasks before they are ready or have the necessary skills. Most 1-year-olds participate in their feeding during mealtimes; however, their limited ability to manipulate utensils indicates that they are not ready to perform this task independently. Encouraging and expecting the child to perform beyond the child's capabilities in any respect creates tension within the parent–child dyad, and this is an area in which the parent is out of tune with the child's development. Nurses thus help parents recognize developmental changes in their children, understand the child's changing behavior, and evaluate their own responses. In providing such anticipatory guidance, the nurse can do much to foster optimal development in the child.

Parents often express concern about "behavior problems," which are frequently developmental and might represent the child's attempt to negotiate a particularly difficult developmental phase. Determining the child's developmental status allows the nurse to judge whether a particular behavior is related to a developmental issue.

For example, the parents of one 18-month-old boy complained of "terrible tantrums that last 5–10 minutes." They reported that their 4-year-old had never acted like this. A developmental assessment revealed that the boy's temperament had been somewhat labile and intense since birth. His moods changed quickly, so that when he was happy, he was very happy, but when he was unhappy, he was very unhappy. The assessment further revealed that the boy was attempting to master many new tasks such as building block towers and climbing, and that his tantrums frequently occurred after he failed in these attempts. He also displayed a lot of "go away, come closer" behavior with his parents, seeming to desire close contact but pushing the parents away when the closeness was offered. He was very motivated to do things for himself and frequently became furious when someone tried to do things for him.

The developmental history therefore clarified a behavior pattern, showing that the child's tantrums were related to his attempts to establish autonomy and the frustration caused by a perception that his attempts were being threatened. The pattern of intense responses explained why his temper tantrums were longer and more vigorous than another child's. With this understanding, the nurse could guide his parents to appropriate interventions such as giving the boy opportunities for self-determination, allowing him to do as much as possible for himself, and providing experience with skills he could master.

Children's Concerns

When confronted by a stressful situation such as illness, hospitalization, divorce, or death, the child's perceptions and responses will, to a great extent, be determined by developmental level. A developmental assessment thus helps the nurse to understand the child's perceptions and coping behaviors (see Chapter 12).

When children are hospitalized, for example, the differences in their reactions are due in part to differences in development (reactions to hospitalization are discussed in Chapter 27). For example, one normal 2-year-old was particularly energetic, involved in mastering motor skills, and not very responsive to verbal explanations and stories. The nurse responsible for this child's care provided periods for vigorous physical activity. Another 2-year-old, also normal, was more interested in language and responded well to verbal explanations and to stories about hospitalization, which in turn determined the nursing interventions for this child. Some children cope with stress by regressing, and the nurse uses this information to plan interventions. Treating such children as if they were functioning at their normal developmental level is inappropriate; the nurse recognizes the need temporarily to regress to an earlier stage but also encourages and motivates the child to resume functioning at a more appropriate level.

To prepare a child effectively for new experiences, the nurse must have a good understanding of the child's developmental status to gear explanations to the appropriate level. If the developmental assessment shows, for example, that a child consistently has had difficulty in adjusting to new situations, the nurse uses this information and helps the child adjust to hospitalization by allowing the child more time to become familiar with the environment and by not introducing the child to too many persons or places at first. Such a child initially might be overwhelmed by a busy place like the playroom but may do well playing with one or two children in another room and then gradually progressing to the playroom (see Chapter 28).

A developmental assessment can provide information for the nurse to help the parent plan activities that maintain and promote the child's developmental progress. By determining the child's capabilities and identifying developmental interests, the nurse can help the parent provide activities, toys, and experiences that will stimulate further development.

The Developmental Assessment Process

Both nurses and physicians sometimes are lulled into assuming that a child who looks normal or acts normal really is normal. Research by Bierman and colleagues (1964), for instance, concluded that pediatricians who relied on clinical impressions without systematic assessments identified only 3 out of 11 retarded children. Such serious oversights make clear that each child deserves a thorough assessment. Korsch and colleagues (1961) found that physicians consistently failed to identify children with significant developmental problems. For example, one child under 3 years of age was autistic but appeared normal. Performance in cognitive skills, especially classification and memory tasks, and motor skills indicated that this child was even precocious. If the nurse had not explored the child's social, affective, and language development carefully, the diagnosis of this severe developmental disability would have been delayed even further.

The developmental assessment should include all the subsystems—biophysical (especially gross and fine motor skills) cognitive, language, social, and affective—and must be systematic and comprehensive. Without an organized approach, important data might be missed, and the detection of potential problems may be delayed.

All areas of development are interrelated and interdependent, although nurses commonly organize data about development into different categories (motor, cognitive, social, affective, and so forth). This categorization is useful, but it should never obscure the recognition that the child is a single organism and that development in one area directly affects development in other areas. An 18-month-old child, for example, is working on achieving autonomy. In early childhood, developing motor ability aids the quest for autonomy by providing the child with the means to ambulate independently and separate physically from the parents. Increasing competence with language allows this child to express dissenting opinions on matters of concern ("No no," "Me do," or "Go away"). A secure parental relationship provides a support base from which the child can venture away independently and return with confidence. Motor, language, and social aspects of development all contribute to the child's quest for autonomy, and the need for autonomy itself motivates efforts in motor, language, and social development. Because development in these subsystems is mutually reinforcing, problems in one area are likely to affect other areas.

Developmental Milestones

Some nurses assess development by surveying the child's achievement of major milestones. *Milestones* are standards of reference based on the assumption that a child should undertake certain tasks or display certain behaviors by a given age. If the child does this, all is assumed to be well. Comparing the child's behavior with well-known developmental milestones is a useful technique that is employed by nearly all child health professionals; however, when used alone, this technique is not sufficient.

This approach must be combined with a careful history and sensitive attention to the child's temperament, home and school environment, self-esteem, approach to people, approach to tasks, and parent–child relationship. Developmental milestones are therefore a useful reference but should only be a starting point for identifying developmental concerns.

Factors Conducive to Optimal Development

Love, security, and the avoidance of criticism

Acceptance and praise for the child

Firm, loving emphasis on teaching acceptable behavior

Encouraging exploring and trying new things; structuring experiences to provide success

Encouraging independence and avoiding overprotection

Tolerating normal negativism and aggressiveness

Providing good behavior examples (reading, television programs, efforts to find the cause of things)

Expecting success for the child but avoiding overambition

Instilling a tolerant attitude toward others

Providing suitable play materials

Encouraging accuracy, thoroughness, and self-confidence

Allowing the child to learn from mistakes

Encouraging persistence

Encouraging curiosity and questioning

Providing linguistic stimulation

Emphasizing discovery rather than role learning

Emphasizing self-control and responsibility

SOURCE: Adapted from Illingsworth RS: *The Development of the Infant and Young Child—Normal and Abnormal*. Churchill-Livingstone, 1972.

Timing the Assessment

The extent of a developmental assessment varies depending on the circumstances, but serial assessments generally are more reliable than one-time assessments. The American Academy of Pediatrics recommends that the developmental assessment be included in each well-child visit. Although recommendations vary, many clinics conduct well-child developmental assessments at the following ages: 2 weeks, 2, 4, 6, 9, 12, 18, and 24 months, and every year thereafter.

A good developmental assessment need not be time consuming. At some time, preferably the first well-child visit, a thorough developmental history should be obtained. After that, the history need only be updated by making pertinent observations related to development during a routine visit. If any problems or concerns arise, time must be provided for an additional assessment.

Any concerns expressed by the parent or child about developmental issues should be explored fully as they arise and should not be postponed. One clinic visit might not provide time for this, however, so the nurse may need to plan subsequent visits. When a child is at risk for a developmental problem or has a suspected problem, the assessment must be detailed and complete. A thorough assessment involves a team approach, as the nurse, physician, developmental scientist, speech pathologist, psychologist, and educator participate in the evaluation. The team members share their findings and contribute jointly to a plan of management. The risk factors for developmental problems are listed in Table 16-1. (Family-related risk factors are discussed in Chapter 22).

The nurse also completes a developmental assessment for any child who is hospitalized. The data obtained are essential in developing an individual plan of care. If the

TABLE 16-1 Risk Factors for Developmental Disabilities

Type of risk	Specific concerns
Prenatal factors	Maternal disease (diabetes mellitus, hypertension, infections, toxemia, anemia)
	Maternal malnutrition
	Maternal age
	Exposure to chemicals (environmental, drugs, alcohol, tobacco)
Intrapartum factors	Prolonged or precipitous labor
	Fetal distress
	Interruption of oxygen
	Significant blood loss
Neonatal factors	Low birthweight (premature or small for gestational age)
	Neonatal asphyxia
	Low Apgar evaluation
	Birth defects
	Sensory malfunction (eg, blindness or deafness)
	Disease (hypoglycemia, sepsis, respiratory distress syndrome, meningitis, hypothyroidism)
	Kernicterus
Social factors	Poverty
	Poor attachment between parent and child
	Over- or understimulating environment
Genetic factors	History of mental retardation, learning problems
	Genetic disorders, birth defects in blood relatives
Factors in older child	Serious illness (such as meningitis)
	Head trauma
	Chronic illness
	Psychologic trauma (eg, abuse, separation, multiple losses)
	Malnutrition (decreased protein intake, skim milk intake during first 6 months of life, inadequate caloric intake for bodily needs)

child is too ill to participate in the assessment process, the nurse depends largely on historical data provided by the parent.

Developmental Assessment and the Nursing Process

The first question to be answered following an assessment is whether the child's overall development is within the normal range. Although this question may appear very simple and straightforward, it does imply that each and every concern about the normality of the child's developmental progress has been categorically ruled out. To make a nursing diagnosis of normal development, the nurse must document answers for the following specific questions about each area of development:

1. *Quality of information.* Do I have enough information? Does any of the information conflict? Are my observations compatible with the history given? Did the parent and/or child express any concerns about this area of development?
2. *Indication of risk.* What are the child's strengths and weaknesses in each area of development? Does any part of the history, observations, or testing suggest that this child is at risk for developmental delays? Has the child experienced difficulties in the past in this area of development?
3. *Suprasystems and subsystems.* What effect does the child's temperament, environment, health, nutritional status, family relationships, or stress have on this area of development?

Any area in which the child does not perform within the standard normal range should be examined closely, often by retesting at another time to validate findings or by collecting additional data. Consistent evidence that the child's performance is below expectations for age suggests developmental delay and warrants further investigation. The nurse may then need to determine whether this is a primary problem or symptomatic of a more encompassing situation or problem. Delayed development of a gross motor skill such as sitting unassisted might, for example, be secondary to the cultural tradition of being swaddled for the first 6 months of life or a compensation for the limited availability of oxygen for growth, as experienced by some infants with cardiac anomalies. On the other hand, the delay might be primary, such as in children with neuromuscular disease. In an older child stuttering might be secondary to a poor self-image or a primary condition, the aftermath of a head injury.

Related to these assessment criteria are questions about the child's environment. Is the parent aware of a possible problem? Has the parent expressed concern or seemed to deny the existence of a problem? How are the environment, family, and child's temperament affecting this developmental problem? How is this developmental problem affecting the family, child's temperament, or environment? How is the child compensating for the problem?

Developmental delays often are the result of a complex etiology that the nurse can identify only through detailed data collection and analysis. For example, the child with poorly developed fine motor skills because of a neurologic problem is vastly different from the child whose equally poor fine motor skills result from an impoverished or hostile environment. This illustrates the necessity of including assessment data from all sources that might either foster or hinder a child's development.

Nursing Diagnosis Three general kinds of nursing diagnoses are likely to follow a developmental assessment. These are (1) that the child's development is within normal limits; (2) that the child is at risk for developmental problems and thus exhibits developmental vulnerability; and (3) that the child's development in one or more areas is not within normal limits and the child therefore might exhibit developmental delays. These are not, however, mutually exclusive categories. For example, the 3-year-old child with normal motor capabilities, delayed language skills caused by a hearing loss, and the risk of psychosocial problems caused by a difficult family situation does not necessarily fit neatly into one of these three categories, and the nurse needs to formulate multiple diagnoses and a multifaceted plan of care.

After exploring each area of development, the nurse should be able to make a nursing diagnosis that reflects the child's present developmental status. This statement or statements describe the child's present functioning in each area of development, emphasizing the observed strengths. If the child is felt to be developmentally at risk, this is stated and the reasons listed. Any deviation from the norm is thus described fully and the cause identified, if possible. Suggested nursing diagnoses for the 3-year-old described briefly in the preceding paragraph are as follows:

1. Developmental delay in language and the formation of speech sounds related to a hearing loss
2. Potential for developmental delay in cognitive, affective, and social areas related to the hearing loss and limited ability to interact with others
3. Developmental vulnerabililty related to the difficult family situation, which is now complicated by child's need for special support teaching and experiences with others to compensate for the hearing loss

Developmental Vulnerability Vulnerability of any kind is caused by lowered resistance. A child's developmental progress is vulnerable when the effects of the child's interacting subsystems and suprasystems cause enough stress to place the child's normal development at risk. A child might, for example, be developmentally at risk because of rapid growth, immature coping strategies, or changes in the family system. Children are often developmentally vulnerable when increased stress overtaxes their abilities to cope and thus lowers their resistance. Developmental vulnerability might therefore lead to maladaptive coping and dysfunctional behavior (see Chapter 24).

For instance, an adolescent female experiencing a normal growth spurt much earlier than her peers might be at risk for delays in social development and may be further at risk for dysfunctional behaviors caused by the stress of not "fitting in." The 5-year-old who enters school after 2 years of repeated hospital stays might exhibit vulnerability in social and cognitive development. In phrasing the nursing diagnoses, the nurse might therefore note the regression common to hospitalized children and the stress of repeated separation from parents.

Developmental Delays The diagnosis of developmental delay is usually a complex process that involves a multidisciplinary team approach and extensive assessment of both the child and family. The nurse's suspicion, however, might be the first step in this process. A nursing diagnosis indicating a potential for developmental delay is often the basis of the initial referral to a developmental specialist or diagnostic center.

Developmental delays might be caused by a complex etiology and require long-term multidisciplinary management. A child might, for example, exhibit learning problems during the first year of school, which may in turn indicate mild or borderline mental retardation (see Chapter 23). Some children exhibit developmental delays that are caused by problems in family dynamics or by dysfunctional parenting (see Chapter 22). In all such instances the nurse's role is first to refer the child for further testing and second to participate in planning the child's care.

Some developmental delays are caused by a parental lack of knowledge or misinformation. A child's motor skills might be delayed if a parent, thinking the infant too young to play, does not provide any toys. For example, one child showed delayed social development in the area of peer interaction. Assessment revealed that the parents, recent immigrants from India, had isolated their daughter from other children to prevent her from losing her cultural identity as a member of the Brahman caste. In both of these examples, the developmental delays were secondary to other factors. The parents of these children stated that they knew very little about normal development and wanted to be good parents for their children. The children were healthy and capable of developing normally, but needed the opportunity for experience. The nurse spent time with the parents, providing them with information, guidelines, support, and encouragement as they modified their parenting styles. In these two situations the child's delayed development was easily rectified by correcting parental misconceptions. It is important to assess parenting practices for information about the child's performance. A child should never be labeled as developmentally delayed too quickly. What appears to be delayed development might only be a delay in experience.

Planning After formulating a diagnosis of actual or potential developmental vulnerability or delay, a plan for intervention must be outlined. If intervention is to be helpful to the child and family, the plan must address the individual child's history, temperament, culture, and family environment. It must include an assessment of the family's and child's acceptance of the proposed intervention. Acceptance usually is obtained by enlisting the help of the family in planning. Including parents and children in the planning process also lets them know that they are participating members in a team effort and should improve cooperation and promote positive results. Interventions and suggestions need to be carefully planned around the family's life-style. Involving the family in this phase will help the nurse to determine what might or might not work for this family.

Once a definitive diagnosis has been established and the etiology determined, the professionals are identified who will be part of the health care team. If the developmental concern is related to environmental influences, such as a poor parent–child relationship, an unstimulating environment, or a death or divorce, the nurse might well be the primary organizer of care. If the concern is physical or medical, such as a neurologic deficit, cerebral palsy, or autism, referrals to appropriate professionals are also necessary. Multidisciplinary management is common and often advantageous in that it provides several viewpoints and ideas for management. In many settings a consistent, primary caregiver who has good rapport with the family and child is required. This person is often the nurse, who then coordinates, interprets, and communicates the team's suggestions.

Planning interventions means setting realistic goals. For example, if the child is capable only of maintaining the present level of functioning in an area, this should be the goal. Accepting a child's limitations might be very difficult for some parents. The family might need time to accept a problem. (Family coping with chronic conditions is discussed in Chapter 30).

Encouraging family members to express their feelings might help them to move toward acceptance. Along with an explanation of the problem, the nurse might help by emphasizing the child's normal development and strengths. Labeling the child as learning disabled or retarded should be avoided if possible. Anticipatory guidance should cover not only the problem but also normal developmental concerns and issues (see Chapter 21).

Intervention If the child's present development is within normal limits, these findings need to be communicated to the parent and child, emphasizing the child's identified strengths. Parents need to be praised for positive parenting. Environmental factors that foster or hinder parenting and the child's development should be discussed. Anticipatory guidance should include future developmental issues, suggestions for stimulating various areas of development, and a discussion of the effects of such suprasystems as peer relationships, school, and family on the child's development. Any parental concerns need to be discussed and either resolved or included in ongoing interventions.

The child who is developmentally vulnerable, for whatever reason, will need to be reassessed at frequent, regular intervals. When explaining the necessity for frequent follow-up to the parent and child, the nurse details the reasons for concern and the potential implications these factors have on the child's development. That the child's present development is normal should be emphasized, however, and the child's strengths noted. In addition, the nurse provides anticipatory guidance and emphasizes beneficial environmental factors and positive parenting actions, thus providing reinforcement.

When a child's development is abnormal in one or more areas of development, the first step in the plan is to confirm the diagnosis as definitively as possible. Screening tests are repeated to ensure their accuracy. More definitive diagnostic testing might be needed, and referral to an appropriate professional may be warranted. Referrals for developmental concerns often are made to developmental specialists, a developmental diagnostic center, psychologists, speech therapists, audiologists, pediatricians, and neurologists.

After referral, the nurse might serve a number of functions in the multidisciplinary management of a child with delayed development. In general the nurse coordinates services, professionals, and appointments, translates complicated medical diagnoses and treatments into understandable lay terms, acts as a resource for child development and parenting concerns, is a teacher and a child and family advocate in the health care setting, and is a trusted health care professional with whom family members can share their feelings.

Each team member plays a significant and cooperative role in the intervention plan. General goals are defined, as well as specific goals related to the skills of the specialists involved. Teamwork is essential so that the goals and intervention plan for one problem are not counterproductive to those planned for another problem. Someone, frequently the nurse, then coordinates the plans to ensure their smooth and orderly enactment.

First Steps in a Developmental Assessment

The assessment process begins with the collection of data, both careful history (subjective data) and pertinent observations (objective data). Standardized developmental tests are a useful adjunct but are no substitute for careful history and observation.

In some settings developmental screening or testing is delegated to a paraprofessional who reports the results to the nurse. Paraprofessionals are often trained to administer standard tests and might be able to identify children who need further developmental assessment. Although this is an option, the nurse does not get the opportunity to observe the parent and child during testing and might miss some data. For instance, some children approach a task with confidence, whereas some are anxious; some children have long attention spans, whereas others are easily distracted. The child's reactions to success or failure at a task can be significant. Some children approach tasks rigidly, some are

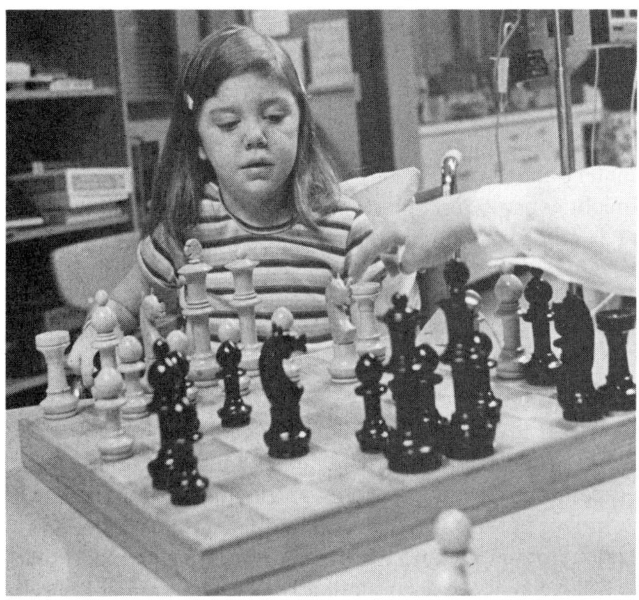

Games using abstract thinking are ways of assessing formal operations.

flexible, some are impulsive, and others are reflective. Parents might be encouraging and helpful; other parents might criticize or inhibit the child. Some parents allow the child to proceed independently; other parents attempt to take over and tell the child how to proceed. Parental reactions to the child's success or failure might be significant. Much of this more subjective data would be unavailable to the nurse who delegates this part of the assessment.

Ensuring Cooperation The quality of the relationship between the nurse and family affects the accuracy and the completeness of the data obtained. Both parent and child need to feel that the nurse is a caring, capable, and trustworthy person before they will share their thoughts, feelings, and experiences. The nurse must be able to communicate warmth, concern, competence, and acceptance. Nonverbal communication is as important as verbal communication. A nurse who cares always addresses and talks about the child by name, remembers little idiosyncrasies such as a preferred position, food, or toy, and takes the time to provide comfort when the child is distressed or stimulation when the child is bored.

For example, one father commented that he felt comfortable talking about his fears, concerns, and dreams with one particular nurse because this nurse sat and listened as if he and his child were the most important people in the world. By discussing these topics with a trusted nurse, this father was helped to put them into perspective, and the nursing care for this family reflected the staff's efforts to be sensitive to the father's needs as well as those of the child's.

Interviewing Parent and Child As much as possible, the child should be included in the assessment process. Children as young as 2 years of age can participate by answering simple questions. Parents and children of all ages should be seen together for at least part of the interview so that the nurse can observe their interaction. The nurse also might want to see the parent and child separately; separate interviews are almost essential for adolescents.

If the nurse feels uncomfortable explaining the need for separate interviews and asking one family member to leave the room, this can best be accomplished by explaining matter-of-factly that separate interviews are standard procedure. Parents are often reluctant to discuss concerns or talk about children who are present, and likewise, children might not share their concerns or thoughts in the presence of a parent. The nurse assures each party of confidentiality but might suggest to the family members that they discuss issues of importance within the family. Observing how the child handles separation from the parent and behaves without the parent can also be enlightening.

The concerns that either parent or child chooses to discuss when the other is absent can be revealing. Some families communicate openly and discuss problems directly, and family members do not discuss new concerns during separate interviews. Other families do not discuss concerns openly with each other, and during separate interviews, these family members might bring up topics they were hesitant to discuss in front of each other.

For example, an adolescent girl who had a chronic illness but was comparatively healthy and doing well in school mentioned to the nurse that she wished her parents would give her more freedom. She knew they loved her and wanted her to be happy, but at the same time she thought their fears and restrictions were extreme. She cooperated because she did not want to hurt them but admitted to feeling increasingly resentful. After further discussion of her concerns, the nurse suggested that she talk to her parents about this matter, and together they identified some areas where it would be appropriate for this girl to have additional responsibility for making decisions. When interviewing the parents, the nurse discussed normal adolescent growth and development and asked the parents to give their impressions of their daughter's developmental status. This provided an opportunity for the nurse to suggest ways in which they could comfortably foster their daughter's independence and sense of identity. The nurse also encouraged the parents to discuss this idea with their daughter. In this way the nurse was able to help the family members gain new insights into their own and each other's viewpoints and, more important, to suggest ways to enhance individual and family development.

To assess development, the nurse needs the child's cooperation. This is usually not difficult with older children but may be a problem with a younger child. As young children observe their parents interacting with the nurse, they usually are reassured that the nurse is a "safe" person. If the nurse approaches interaction gradually, respecting the child's right to control the level of involvement, the child is further reassured. Allowing the child to play with assessment equipment helps to prepare the child for subsequent testing. Another way to gain cooperation is first to present tasks that the child can do, presenting more difficult tasks after the child has succeeded at the first tasks. This prevents the child from becoming discouraged by an inability to succeed at a certain task and refusing to do any other tasks.

If the nurse is unable to establish rapport and gain cooperation, the complete assessment might need to be delayed. The nurse might have to interact with the child a few times so that the child will become familiar and comfortable in the nurse's presence before attempting to complete the assessment.

It is useful to begin the assessment process by asking for the parent's perception of the child's developmental progress. This might indicate which areas need to be explored in greater depth. Questions that can be asked to elicit this information include the following:

1. What concerns do you have about your child's development?
2. How would you describe your child's development?
3. How does this child's development compare with that of any brothers and sisters?

If a parent has a particular concern about a child's development, it is helpful to discover this early in the assessment process by obtaining an exact description of the concern or problem and exploring what the parent thinks the problem means. The nurse determines when the parent first became concerned and whether the problem has seemed to improve or worsen. Any factors that appear to make the problem better or worse should be noted. It is important to determine whether this is the only problem or whether the child has developed other related symptoms. The nurse explores any recent changes in the child's or family's life (such as moving, separation, death, divorce, illness), the impact of the problem on the family and child, what measures the family has taken to deal with the problem, and whether any of these measures have been effective. Useful questions to ask include the following:

1. How do family members see the problem? Do all family members agree it is a problem?
2. How does the child see this problem?
3. How has this problem affected the functioning of the family (for example, disrupted sleep patterns, caused marital arguments, prevented parents from going out)?

The Developmental History

The developmental history provides a detailed profile of the child in a familial and social context and includes a survey of the child's personality and skills and the nature of the child's interpersonal relationships. Because medical, social, or family problems might affect the child's development, the developmental history is part of the overall health history. Problems in the prenatal, natal, and postnatal periods often have long-term effects on the child and might cause or contribute to developmental disabilities.

In some settings written questionnaires are used to obtain a developmental history. The parent is asked to answer specific written questions about the child prior to seeing the nurse. These questionnaires can be helpful in ensuring that all areas of assessment are covered and can indicate problem areas, but they are not a substitute for the interaction between the parent and nurse. These questionnaires also have significant disadvantages. Questionnaires seem impersonal to many parents and might hinder the establishment of rapport between the nurse and parent. Parents might not understand the meaning of a question and unintentionally give inaccurate information. They might find it difficult to reduce complex behaviors to a simple "yes" or "no" answer, as questionnaires often demand. Because parents do not have a chance to explain their answers, the nurse may not understand what the parent wishes to communicate. Questionnaires also are clearly inappropriate for parents who are limited in their ability to read and/or write.

Several factors influence the accuracy of the historical data obtained from parents (Hokelman, Kelly, and Zimmer, 1976). Parents recall recent events more accurately than past events and recall concrete facts such as birthweight most accurately. Some parents tend to exaggerate the developmental abilities of their children, particularly the firstborn child, whereas parents with several children are less likely to recall specific information correctly. Parents also tend to recall major developmental milestones, such as smiling, sitting up, and walking, better than less significant milestones such as rolling over and pulling up to a standing position. The components of the developmental history are summarized in Table 16-2.

The nurse also explores the child's behavior and the parent–infant relationship during infancy. The infant's temperament and early behavior can affect a parent's attitude and behavior in many ways. Questions that might elicit this information include the following:

1. How would you describe the child as a baby?
2. What was it like for you taking care of the baby in the early weeks?
3. What happened when the baby cried? How often did the baby cry?

The nurse then explores any problems elicited by asking more detailed questions such as the following:

1. How did you handle the problem?
2. How did you feel about this?
3. When (if ever) was the problem resolved?

TABLE 16-2 Components of the Developmental History

Developmental factor	Specific criteria
Parental view of the child's development	
Concern of some aspect of the child's development	Definition of the concern Chronology (when the parent first became concerned, whether the problem has improved or worsened) Aggravating or alleviating factors Associated symptoms Associated changes in the child's life Impact of the problem on the child and family Actions taken to deal with the problem
Prenatal factors*	Duration of pregnancy Exposure to chemicals Exposure to infectious agents or radiation Complications (bleeding, hypertension, toxemia, excessive or inadequate weight gain, diabetes, malnutrition) Emotional adjustment to pregnancy
Intrapartum factors*	Length of labor Rupture of membrane Presentation and type of delivery Complications (precipitous or prolonged labor, bleeding, fever, fetal distress) Condition of infant (Apgar evaluations, need for resuscitation) Parental reactions and perceptions regarding labor and delivery
Neonatal factors*	Birthweight, height, and occipitofrontal circumference Birth defects or injuries Complications (respiratory problems, jaundice, cyanosis, apnea, sepsis, poor suck, meningitis, lethargy) Behavioral characteristics of the infant (alertness, state changes, consolability) Parental responses and perceptions of the infant
Family history*	Mental retardation, genetic disorders, learning disabilities, "slow" development, birth defects in blood relatives (including grandparents, aunts, uncles, and cousins)
Past development	Parental perceptions of past development Problems in infancy (excessive crying, colic, poor feeding, poor weight gain) Parental reaction to infant and feelings about parenthood Ages of major milestones (smiling, rolling over, sitting alone, crawling, walking, first word, first sentences, prehension, toilet training)

Developmental factor	Specific criteria
Temperament	Activity level Regularity of body functions Ease of adaptability Approach and withdrawal reactions to new situations Responsiveness to stimuli Quality of mood (usually positive or usually negative) Intensity of mood Distractability Persistence Parental response to child's temperament
Gross motor skills	Survey of child's gross motor abilities (sitting, walking, climbing, sports)
Fine motor skills	Survey of child's fine motor skills (reaching for objects, grasping, copying, coloring, writing)
Opportunities for child to develop fine motor skills	
Language development	Receptive language (ability to comprehend the spoken word) Expressive language (ability to communicate through symbols, vocabulary, grammar) Speech (articulation, fluency) Opportunities to develop language skills
Cognitive development	Characteristics of the thought process Problem-solving ability Interest in learning Academic performance Type of school experience Parental awareness of child's interests Opportunities for development of cognitive skills
Social development	Relationships (parent–child, sibling, peer, teacher, grandparent) Self-concept (child's view of self, perceptions of strengths and weaknesses) Level of responsibility Independence (eating, sleeping, decision making, time management, reaction to separation) Self-control (management of emotions and impulses) Discipline (method used, child's responses)

NOTE: The specific data for each component depend on the age of the child.
*Often obtained elsewhere in the health history.

The nurse then surveys developmental milestones and explores any delays in their achievement. Because the accuracy of this information is often limited, records in baby books are often useful in helping parents to remember. If significant developmental delays were present earlier, however, manifestations might still be evident. If there are no current manifestations, the earlier delay most likely was not significant.

The child's behavioral characteristics (temperament) plays a significant role in determining how the child approaches and interacts with the environment. Thomas and Chess (1977) provided nine categories for describing temperamental differences. They are as follows:

1. Activity level
2. Regularity of biologic function
3. Adaptability (ability to adapt to changes)
4. Approach or withdrawal reactions to new experiences
5. Responsiveness to stimuli (how sensitive the child is to stimuli)
6. Predominant mood (usually positive or usually negative)
7. Intensity of mood (how positive or negative responses are)
8. Distractibility
9. Persistence

Thomas and Chess further described three different combinations of temperamental characteristics:

1. The easy child is characterized by regular biologic function (sleep, defecation, and so forth), a generally positive mood with mild to moderate intensity, easy adaptability to change, and a positive approach to new situations.
2. The difficult child is characterized by irregular body functions, withdrawal responses in new situations, negative mood with high intensity, and slow adaptability to change.
3. The slow-to-warm-up child is characterized by withdrawal responses in new situations, slow adaptability to change, negative mood with mild to moderate intensity, and regularity in body functions.

Few children fit exactly into one category, but most children tend to resemble one or another. No quality judgment about the child's "goodness" or "badness" is implied because each temperamental characteristic has positive and negative aspects. Temperament itself is not good or bad, but specific situations might make it seem so. For example, persistence might be a positive attribute when a child is learning to walk and persists in the effort in spite of repeated falls, but persistence might seem negative when the child continues negative behavior such as crying or throwing food. The parents' perception of the child's temperament might be more significant than the child's temperament itself. For example, a mother who had difficulty conceiving might be delighted with her "difficult" infant and may overlook the trouble the child causes her. On the other hand, a woman whose career was interrupted by an unplanned pregnancy might find caring for her "easy" infant to be difficult and unrewarding (Carey, 1972).

Temperamental characteristics do play a large role in the developmental process, but cognitive abilities, personal motivation, and the supportiveness of the environment all combine with temperament to create a reciprocal process that shapes each child's development (Chess and Thomas, 1977).

Another area to explore is family stress. The nurse attempts to discover any factors that might disrupt the family unit, and if such stressors exist, the nurse assesses the family members' perceptions, coping strategies, and support systems. The impact of stress on the child should be assessed in depth. (Families at risk are discussed in Chapter 22.)

Observations of Development

Direct observations of both the child and family are an extremely important part of the developmental assessment. Virtually all behavior of both children and families provides data; therefore, nurses need to note even seemingly minor incidents. Not all behavior is significant, but the nurse will not be able to make judgments if the behavior was not first observed.

There are two types of observation: structured and unstructured. *Unstructured observations* result when the nurse observes the behavior of the child throughout the entire visit. *Structured observations* result when the child is asked to perform certain tests or tasks. Both types of observation are important (Fernholdt, 1980). Because the child's behavior in an unfamiliar setting might not be representative of usual behavior, the nurse should validate observations with the parent.

Structured observations can be a source of anxiety for both the parent and child, so the nurse needs to establish rapport prior to presenting specific tasks. The parent and child should be told that the child will be given some easy tasks first and then be given some more difficult tasks, not all of which children of this age are expected to do. To prevent the parent from coaching, the nurse explains to the parent that if the child needs help with a certain task, the nurse will provide it.

Unstructured observations supplement and validate the information obtained during the history. Clinicians sometimes note discrepancies between what was told to them in the history and what they observe themselves during the visit. A parent might tell the nurse that the child is doing fine and has no problems, but the nurse may observe behavior such as clumsiness, squinting, or inarticulate speech that indicates potentially significant problems. Occasionally, a parent deliberately attempts to mislead the nurse, but more often, the parent is unaware that certain behavior indicates a problem or has become so used to the behavior that it is not noticed anymore. An occasional parent might even feel so guilty or ashamed that the problem is denied (Fernholdt, 1980).

Observations made during a clinic visit or a hospital stay usually are made in conjunction with a history, and the combined data are sufficient to evaluate a child's development. In some instances, however, a visit to the child's home, day-care center, or school might be necessary to gain a clearer picture of events in these settings and how they affect the child.

During the course of contact with the child and family, the nurse often develops an overall impression, which should be neither accepted nor rejected but should be validated or invalidated by the careful collection and assessment of data. Impressions, although not scientific and objective, are often significant. The nurse might develop a "certain feeling" about a child, which although not accepted as fact, might indicate certain areas to explore in depth. Table 16-3 summarizes the observations and assessment questions that correspond to the areas of development.

Temperament The nurse notes both the child's activity level and factors such as anxiety or fear that might affect the activity level. The nurse usually can identify the child's mood and its intensity during the visit, but a one-time observation, especially when the child is in an unfamiliar situation, might not be representative of the child's usual mood. For instance, an infant who cries during the visit and is very difficult to comfort displays an intense mood that the nurse can validate by asking the parent whether this is typical.

The assessment setting itself provides an excellent opportunity to observe how the child reacts in new situations (for example, whether the child uses predominantly approach or withdrawal behaviors). The way in which the child handles transition, such as leaving the waiting room and entering the examination room or stopping one activity and starting another, often demonstrates the child's adaptability. The nurse also notes the child's sensitivity to stimuli in the assessment setting. For instance, does the child notice every little sound, movement, and touch, or do only stronger stimuli capture the child's attention? The child's persistence can be evaluated by noting how much time the child spends in one activity. For example, one young boy told his mother he wanted to leave. When the mother explained that it was not yet time to leave, he accepted this and began another activity. A more persistent child might have continued to pester the mother with repeated requests to leave. The nurse also can assess distractibility by observing whether the child is able to attend to certain tasks or whether the child's performance is frequently disrupted when distracted by other things.

Motor Skills Many observations about gross and fine motor development can be made simply by observing the child's movements in the assessment setting. As the child walks, runs, and climbs, the nurse observes strength and coordination. The way the child handles toys, crayons, and small objects is important in assessing fine motor abilities. Specific structured tasks are often administered at certain ages. The standard neurologic exam (Chapter 14) also provides a wealth of information about motor development.

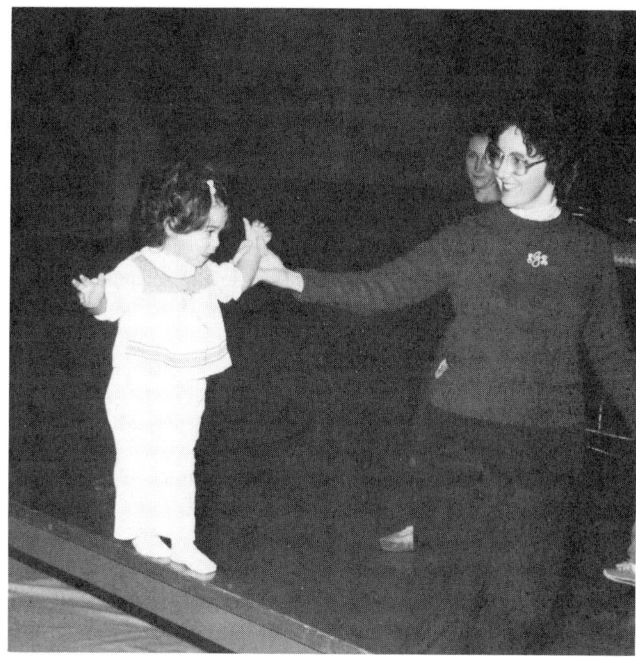

Precocious development of motor skills.

Language Development The nurse observes the child's ability to listen to comments and instructions by engaging the child in conversation and noting the child's use of words and grammar, articulation and fluency of speech, and quality of voice. Standardized tests also are available to assess these abilities. The nurse should pay particular attention to the verbal interchange between the parent and child to note whether the parent responds positively to the child's efforts with language. Also significant is whether the parent explains things to the child and whether the parent gives commands and restrictive messages most of the time.

Cognitive Development The nurse assesses cognitive development by observing the child's general interest in the surroundings. Also helpful are observations about the child's use of objects and toys. Structured tests are used for specific ages. The nurse notes how the parent responds to the child's exploratory efforts and whether the parent fosters cognitive growth by providing encouragement and explanations.

Social and Affective Development Observing the parent–child interaction provides a wealth of data about how the parent and child relate and how this affects the

TABLE 16-3 Observations of Development

Developmental area	Specific observations	Assessment questions*
General observations	Posture Appearance Correlation between history and appearance	
Temperament	Activity level during assessment Mood and intensity Reactions to assessment setting Reaction to transition from one activity to another Responsiveness to stimuli (sound, touch, lights, odors) Desire to persist at task Distractability	Does your child usually get tired about the same time each day? (Get hungry?; Wake up?; Defecate?) How active is your child? If interested in an activity, how long is the child able to hold still? Does the child usually walk or run? How long does it take your child to adjust to a new situation? (Deal with changes in routine?; React to surprise?) Does your child usually notice colorful things, bright lights, mild odors, soft noises, wet diapers? Does your child seem generally happy or sad? (Have a good time playing?; Look forward to new events?) How does your child react to frustration? Does your child show strong preferences for people, places, or situations? How does your child behave when frustrated or excited? Does the child usually finish tasks? Does the child practice a skill repeatedly or give up after several tries? If upset, how long before the child gets over it? When busy with one activity, can the child be directed to another easily? When busy playing, does the child become distracted by people nearby?
Gross motor skills	Refer to age-specific guidelines Large muscle actions Mastery level of action	When did the child accomplish specific skills? Was each skill easily achieved or was considerable time and effort required? How does the child compare with any siblings in the timing with which skills were developed?
Fine motor skills	Refer to age-specific guidelines Small muscle actions Coordination and dexterity of movements	
Language development	Ability to listen and understand Ability to communicate Vocabulary and grammar Articulation and fluency Quality of voice Quality of verbal interchanges between parent and child	What sounds or words does your baby say? How does your child let you know what's wanted? Does your child seem to listen to what you say? Does your child seem to understand what you mean? When your child speaks, are you able to understand? Are strangers able to understand your child?
Cognitive development	Ability to answer questions Use of toys and/or equipment Performance of age-specific tasks Curiosity and exploratory behavior Parental response to exploratory behavior Parental behavior to foster cognitive development	How curious would you say your child is? What is the child most interested in learning about recently? How well does your child remember? Short term? Long term? What ways have you found to help your child learn these things? How well does your child read and comprehend reading? How does your child go about solving problems? How does your child do in school? How does your child like school?

TABLE 16-3 continued

Developmental area	Specific observations	Assessment questions*
		What type of school is it? Open or traditional classroom? Graded or ungraded? What standardized tests have been done in school?
Social and affective development	Parent–child relationship Characteristics of interactions Sensitivity to needs of each other Reactions to separations, if any Responsiveness Management of conflict, if any Whether child or parent answers child's self-description	How would you describe your relationship with your child? How much time do you spend together? What do you do when you are together? Tell me about your child's relationship with your husband (wife)? Does the child seem to be closer to one or the other parent? How does the child react when left by you for a period of time? How does your child feel about teachers? How does your child get along with a babysitter? How often is the child left with a babysitter? What do you like the most about your child? What is the most difficult thing about raising your child at this age? What things make you angry with your child?
	Sibling relationship (if siblings are present) Child's ability to relate to other children	How do brothers and sisters get along? Which sibling is the child closest to? Where there is conflict between siblings, how is it handled? How does the child get along with other children? How does the child act when meeting a new child for the first time? Does the child have a special friend? Why is this friend special? What opportunities does the child have for peer contact? Are the child's friends the same age, younger, or older?
	Child's self-concept, self-esteem Approach to tasks Reaction to success or failure Description of self	How does the child seem to feel about himself or herself? What words would the child use to describe this? What would you say the child is especially good at? What is the child not too good at? What does the child seem to worry about? Does the child ever get mad at or ashamed of himself or herself? Why? How do you handle this? Is the child a leader or follower? Is the child happy with himself or herself or want to be someone else?
	Management of emotions Range of emotions displayed Ability to manage feelings and fears appropriately Parental responses to child's emotions Parental disciplinary measures, if any Child's response to discipline	What things seem to make the child happy? (Sad? Angry? Embarrassed?) How does the child usually act if sad or? How does the child express emotions? How do family members react? How do adult family members deal with sad or angry feelings? What things is the child most afraid of? How is the child usually disciplined? What things does the child do that usually require discipline?

continued on next page

TABLE 16-3 continued

Developmental area	Specific observations	Assessment questions*
Social and affective development (cont.)	Management of Emotions (cont.)	How often does the child get punished? How consistent are disciplinary measures? How does the child react to disciplinary measures? Do family members agree on when and how to discipline?
Independence	Ability to proceed independently with tasks Parental ability to foster independence	Does your child help with household chores? What chores does your child do? How reliable is the child about doing chores? Is your child able to handle feeding? (Dressing?) How is bedtime managed? Is the child able to fall asleep alone, or does the child need attention? Does the child sleep all night? If the child awakens at night, what happens? How does the child react when separated from parents? What decisions does the child make unaided? How does your child manage time? Is the child able to plan to get jobs or homework done?

*Questions can also be rephrased and directed to the child directly if the child is old enough to respond.

child's development. In particular, the nurse should observe both the parent's and child's sensitivity to each other's cues. The parent's ability to understand the meaning behind the child's behavior and respond appropriately is important in providing an atmosphere conducive to development, and the nurse should be alert for positive or negative exchanges between the parent and child. If negative feelings or conflicts develop, the nurse should then note how the parent and child handle them.

A child's self-concept and self-esteem are difficult to measure directly, but observing how the child approaches tasks (that is, with confidence, hesitancy, or apprehension) provides valuable insight. The child's response to success or failure at tasks also provides useful data.

When a range of emotions is displayed during the assessment, the nurse observes carefully how the child manages feelings. Some children lose control under stress, other children are able to articulate their feelings, whereas other children cling to their parents for support. How the parent responds to the child's expression of emotion is also important. If the parent must discipline the child, the nurse uses this opportunity to observe the parent's ability to recognize inappropriate behavior, set reasonable limits, and enforce appropriate consequences.

The nurse also notes the child's level of independence in the assessment setting. The parent's ability or inability to allow the child some independence is significant in the development of autonomy and confidence. Separating parent and child gives the nurse an excellent opportunity to observe how each handles the situation.

Developmental Assessment Tools

Once a developmental history has been completed, the nurse may choose to use an established developmental tool to assess either a particular area or various aspects of the child's development. *Screening* might be part of the assessment, but the two processes are not the same. Developmental screening tests are generally inexpensive, easy to administer, standardized tests that can be used to detect possible developmental delays or deficits in large populations. A developmental assessment encompasses standard screening tests but includes the judicious use of the more detailed tests for psychologic and intellectual functioning (Table 16-4) in conjunction with a thorough history and observations of development, health, environment, and family relationships. Differences between screening and assessment are outlined in Table 16-5.

Generally, developmental screening tests are designed to assess one or more areas of development, in which the child's performance on certain tasks is then compared to a standardized norm. Standardized screening tests are helpful in focusing on an area in which the nurse can observe the child's functioning, but they have limitations. Standardized tests are not entirely reliable; some children with developmental problems pass a test, whereas some normal children fail it. Screening tests do not provide the background with which to interpret the results, they do not involve a developmental history, and the cause of any developmental delay cannot be determined from the screening test alone. Some developmental delays are temporary, the result

TABLE 16-4 Some Commonly Used Psychologic and Intelligence Tests

Age group*	Test	What it measures
Infancy (birth–2 years)	Bayley Scales of Infant Development (Psychological Corporation, 1969)	General intelligence
	Cattell Infant Intelligence Scale (Psychological Corporation, 1950)	General intelligence
	Vineland Social Maturity Scale (American Guidance, 1965)	Social development
Preschool (2–5 years)	Columbia Mental Maturity Scale (Psychological Corporation, 1972)	General intelligence (requires no verbalization)
	Frostig Developmental Tests of Visual Perception (Consulting Psychologists' Press, 1961)	Visual Perception
	Illinois Test of Psycholinguistic Abilities (ITPA) (University of Illinois Press)	Language development
	Merrill Palmer Scale (Merrill Palmer, 1963)	General intelligence
	Peabody Picture Vocabulary Test, Revised (PPVT-R) (American Guidance, 1981)	Language development
	Stanford-Binet Intelligence Scale, Form L-M (Houghton Mifflin Co., 1960)	General intelligence
	Vineland Social Maturity Scale (American Guidance, 1965)	Social development
	Wechsler Preschool and Primary Scale of Intelligence (Psychological Corporation, 1967)	General intelligence
School age (6 + years)	Children's Apperception Test, Revised (CAT) (Psychological Corporation, 1980)	Projective personality
	Columbia Mental Maturity Scale (Psychological Corporation, 1972)	General intelligence (requires no verbalization)
	Bender Visual-Motor Gestalt Test for Children (Western Psychological Services, 1962)	Visual-motor development; used as psychologic measure
	Frostig Developmental Tests of Visual Perception (Consulting Psychologists' Press, 1961)	Visual-motor development
	Peabody Picture Vocabulary Test (American Guidance, 1981)	Language development
	Stanford-Binet Intelligence Scale (Houghton Mifflin Co., 1960)	General intelligence
	Vineland Social Maturity Scale (American Guidance, 1965)	Social development
	Wechsler Intelligence Scale for Children—Revised (WISC-R) (Psychological Corporation, 1974)	General intelligence
	Wepman Auditory Discrimination Test (Language Research Associates, 1958)	Language discrimination
	Wide Range Achievement Test (WRAT) (Psychological Corporation, 1965)	Reading, spelling, and arithmetic

SOURCE: Darling RB, Darling J: *Children Who Are Different*. Mosby, 1982.
*Children functioning above or below their chronologic age level might be given tests listed for other age ranges.

of prematurity, cultural traditions of child care, or correctable congenital anomalies. For example, a 4-year-old boy had developmental delays in gross motor skills before his cardiac defect was corrected surgically. Within a year after surgery, he was performing all age-appropriate skills well. Screening tests are not diagnostic but rather suggest delays or strengths. Children who appear to have delays generally are retested at a later date to confirm the accuracy of the results and to verify that the results were not caused by extraneous factors such as the child's mood, interest level, or fear. If a second test indicates the same delay, more extensive diagnostic tests and appropriate referrals might be warranted.

Screening tests are administered according to an instruction manual to ensure valid results, and parents and children therefore need to be instructed carefully about the test's purpose, procedures, and results. Screening tests generally are not predictive of future development or performance but are indicative of the child's present performance level. Serial measurements of some tests, such as the Denver Developmental Screening Test, are more useful than a one-time screening because serial measurement allows development to be observed over time. Screening tests used serially provide objective data about a child that can substantiate or weaken the developmental assessment.

Temperament Questionnaires Four questionnaires are available to assess the child's temperament. These are as follows:

1. The Infant Temperament Questionnaire—for infants 4–12 months of age (Carey and McDevitt, 1978)
2. The Toddler Temperament Scale—for children 1–3 years of age (Hegvick, McDevitt, and Carey, 1982)
3. The Behavioral Style Questionnaire—for children 3–7 years of age (McDevitt and Carey, 1978)

4. The Middle Childhood Questionnaire—for children 8–12 years of age (Hegvick, McDevitt, and Carey, 1982)

Each questionnaire consists of series of descriptions to which the parent responds by indicating the behavior that best describes the child. Sleep, feeding, elimination, and play behaviors are but a few of the behaviors described in the questionnaires (Fig. 16-1). Each item is categorized into one of nine aspects of temperament: activity, rhythmicity, adaptability, approach, sensory threshold, intensity, mood, distractability, and persistence. Responses to each item are put in the appropriate category; according to the scores, the child is identified as having certain temperamental characteristics.

Each test is easy to administer and generally takes no longer than 10 minutes for parents to complete. Information obtained is based on the parent's perception of the child's temperament, how this perception compares with the perception of other children of the same age, and whether the child's temperament is a problem. These tools can be useful as a basis for discussions of differences in temperament and individual needs and suggestions for dealing with children with difficult temperaments. Helping parents to understand a child's temperament can enhance positive parent–child relationships and facilitate meeting the child's developmental needs (see Chapter 13).

TABLE 16-5 Developmental Screening Versus Nursing Assessment

Developmental screening	Nursing assessment
Often used when large numbers of children are to be evaluated in a limited amount of time	Done on an individual basis with each child and family
Assesses only selected representative factors and behaviors	Comprehensive and systematic assessment of all relevant factors, includes both history and observations
Indicates a possible problem and need for further assessment	Defines the nature of a problem and contributes to an understanding of the cause
May be done by a paraprofessional	Done only by a qualified professional
Usually uses a standard form or checklist and thereby runs the risk of being situationly or culturally biased	May include standard tests as appropriate, including psychologic and detailed intellectual tests. Is based on sound knowledge of child development and an in-depth analysis of the individual child and family
Generally inexpensive and easy to administer	In-depth, time-consuming, expensive procedure

Denver Developmental Screening Test The Denver Developmental Screening Test-Revised, or DDST-R (Frankenberg, Goldstein, and Camp, 1971), is a widely used standard developmental screening test for children from birth to 6 years of age (see Appendix C). It is used to screen children for possible developmental delays, identify developmental delays objectively, and monitor children who are at risk of developmental delays. The DDST-R is not an IQ test, nor does it predict present or future intellectual performance. A child with a questionable or failing score should be referred for further testing.

The four broad areas of development assessed in the DDST-R are (1) personal–social; (2) fine motor–adaptive; (3) gross motor; and (4) language. For each behavior an age range is given that indicates when 25%, 50%, 75%, and 90% of the children perform the task. The test usually is administered by asking the child to perform tasks of increasing difficulty according to standard instructions. A few items are scored according to the parent's report. Because scoring and instructions are connected, nurses who use this tool must study the instruction manual carefully and review the material periodically for their results to be valid. The DDST-R is a valuable test to use whenever some aspect of a child's development seems inappropriate or parents express concern about their child's progress. The form quickly identifies how the child's abilities and behavior compares with the norm for that age, either offering reassurance or suggesting the need for referral.

Denver Prescreening Developmental Questionnaire Another tool that is helpful in assessing a child for developmental vulnerability is the Denver Prescreening Developmental Questionnaire (PDQ) (Fig. 16-2). Designed for use in situations that do not allow for even the 15- to 20-minute application of DDST-R, the PDQ is valuable to the nurse because of its brevity and the information it provides about the parent's awareness of the child's behavior.

The PDQ consists of 97 questions, which are grouped according to age, and only the ten questions that correspond to the child's age are answered by the parent. When compared with other screening tools and methods, the PDQ reliably identified 80% of children at risk for developmental delays, regardless of the setting (Frankenburg, 1975).

Brazelton Neonatal Behavioral Assessment Scale The Brazelton Neonatal Behavioral Assessment Scale (BNBAS), developed by T. Berry Brazelton (1973), focuses on the behavior of neonates. The scale assesses the neonate's responses to the environment and to changes in the environment. The BNBAS measures 27 behavioral responses and 20 elicited responses, including neurologic capabilities and responses to certain stimuli (Fig. 16-3). The items on the scale are organized into six categories of

INSTRUCTIONS TO PARENT

1. There are *no right or wrong* or good or bad answers, only descriptions of your child.
2. Please base your ratings on the child's *recent* and *current* behavior (the last *four* to *six weeks*).
3. Rate each question *separately*. Do not purposely try to present a consistent picture of your child.
4. Use *extreme ratings* where appropriate. Try to avoid rating only near the middle of each scale.
5. Rate each item *quickly*. If you cannot decide, skip the item and come back to do it later.
6. *Rate every item*. Please circle any item you are unable to answer due to lack of information or any item that does not apply to your child.
7. Consider only *your own* impressions and observations of the child.

The infant, 4–12 months (95 total questions)

☐	The infant plays continuously for more than 10 minutes at a time with a favorite toy.	almost never	1	2	3	4	5	6	almost always
☐	The infant accepts his/her bath any time of the day without resisting it.	almost never	1	2	3	4	5	6	almost always
☐	The infant takes feedings quietly with mild expression of likes and dislikes.	almost never	1	2	3	4	5	6	almost always
☐	The infant wants and takes milk feedings at about the same times (within one hour) from day to day.	almost never	1	2	3	4	5	6	almost always
☐	The infant is shy (turns away or clings to mother) on meeting another child for the first time.	almost never	1	2	3	4	5	6	almost always
☐	The infant eats about the same amount of solid food (within 1 oz) from day to day.	almost never	1	2	3	4	5	6	almost always
☐	The infant is fussy on waking up and going to sleep (frowns, cries).	almost never	1	2	3	4	5	6	almost always
☐	The infant plays with a toy for under a minute and then looks for another toy or activity.	almost never	1	2	3	4	5	6	almost always

The 1–3 year old (97 total questions)

☐	The child continues an activity in spite of noises in the same room.	almost never	1	2	3	4	5	6	almost always
☐	The child shows strong reactions (cries, stamps feet) to failure.	almost never	1	2	3	4	5	6	almost always
☐	The amount of milk or juice the child takes at mealtime is unpredictable from meal to meal (over 2 oz difference).	almost never	1	2	3	4	5	6	almost always
☐	The child practices physical activities (climbing, jumping, pushing objects) for under 5 minutes.	almost never	1	2	3	4	5	6	almost always
☐	The child vigorously resists additional food or milk when full (spits out, clamps mouth closed, bats at spoon, etc.).	almost never	1	2	3	4	5	6	almost always
☐	The child stops to examine new objects thoroughly (5 minutes or more).	almost never	1	2	3	4	5	6	almost always
☐	The child spends over an hour reading a book or looking at the pictures.	almost never	1	2	3	4	5	6	almost always
☐	The child watches TV for under 10 minutes, then turns to another activity.	almost never	1	2	3	4	5	6	almost always

continued on next page

Figure 16-1 Samples of questions asked on the temperament questionnaires. Parents are given the appropriate age-range tool and the directions stated in this figure. Following each questionnaire, the parent is asked to summarize the child's temperament relative to general categories and to compare the rating with other children of the same age. Reprinted by permission of the authors.

The 3–7 year old (100 total questions)

☐ The child leaves or wants to leave the table during meals.	almost never	1	2	3	4	5	6	almost always
☐ Changes in plans bother the child.	almost never	1	2	3	4	5	6	almost always
☐ The child notices minor changes in mother's dress or appearance (clothing, hairstyle, etc.).	almost never	1	2	3	4	5	6	almost always
☐ The child reacts strongly (cries or complains) to a disappointment or failure.	almost never	1	2	3	4	5	6	almost always
☐ The child approaches children his/her age that he/she doesn't know.	almost never	1	2	3	4	5	6	almost always
☐ The child plays quietly with his/her toys and games.	almost never	1	2	3	4	5	6	almost always
☐ The child moves about actively when he/she explores new places.	almost never	1	2	3	4	5	6	almost always
☐ The child likes to go to new places rather than familiar ones.	almost never	1	2	3	4	5	6	almost always

The 8–12 year old (99 total questions)

☐ Responses to parent's instructions are predictable.	almost never	1	2	3	4	5	6	almost always
☐ Remains pleasant (smiles, etc.) even when tired.	almost never	1	2	3	4	5	6	almost always
☐ Looks up right away from play when telephone or doorbell rings.	almost never	1	2	3	4	5	6	almost always
☐ Moves right into a new place (store, theater, playground).	almost never	1	2	3	4	5	6	almost always
☐ Adjusts within a day or two to changes in routine (different bed time, new chores, etc.).	almost never	1	2	3	4	5	6	almost always
☐ Follows a consistent routine after school (snack-play-dinner; play-dinner-homework; etc.).	almost never	1	2	3	4	5	6	almost always
☐ Happy and pleasant on short trips in the car or on the bus.	almost never	1	2	3	4	5	6	almost always
☐ Approaches new visitors in the home.	almost never	1	2	3	4	5	6	almost always

Figure 16-1 continued

behavior, including habituation, orientation, motor maturity, variability, self-quieting abilities, and social behaviors.

The infant's score for each item is based on the best performance and not on the average. Several attempts at each item are encouraged, and the best performance is recorded. The infant's state is an integral part of the assessment and a consideration in most items. The term *state* or *sleep-wake state,* refers to the infant's state of arousal as determined by the infant's initial behavior and ability to modify behavior response to stimuli. The Neonatal Behavioral Assessment Scale divides the neonate's sleeping and waking patterns into six different and distinct states as follows:

1. Quiet sleep—regular respirations, no rapid eye movements, little spontaneous muscle movement
2. Active sleep—irregular respirations, rapid eye movements, occasional movements of body
3. Drowsiness—semidozing, variable activity level with possible vocalization
4. Quiet alertness—bright eyes, alertness, attention to selected stimuli, suppression of motor activity
5. Active waking—increased motor activity, fussing, less attention to stimuli
6. Crying—loud crying, jerky muscle movements, limited response to stimuli

The neonate's states of arousal, abilities to deal with environmental stimuli, and movement from one state to another are very important concepts for nurses to integrate in the

DENVER PRESCREENING DEVELOPMENTAL QUESTIONNAIRE

4 year

Please read each question carefully before you answer. Circle the best answer for each question. YOUR CHILD IS NOT EXPECTED TO BE ABLE TO DO EVERYTHING THE QUESTIONS ASK.

YES—CHILD CAN DO NOW or HAS DONE IN THE PAST
NO —CHILD CANNOT DO NOW, HAS NOT DONE IN THE PAST or YOU ARE NOT SURE THAT YOUR CHILD CAN DO IT

Child's Name
Date
Birthdate

R —CHILD REFUSES TO TRY
NO-OPP—CHILD HAS NOT HAD THE CHANCE TO TRY

4 year check — Answer 71 through 80

71. Can your child pedal a tricycle at least ten feet? If your child has never had a chance to ride a tricycle his size, circle NO-OPP. YES NO R NO-OPP

72. After eating, does your child wash and dry his hands well enough so you don't have to do them over? Circle NO-OPP if you do not allow him to wash and dry his hands by himself. YES NO R NO-OPP

4 year, 3 month check — Answer 73 through 82

73. Does your child put an "s" at the end of his words when he is talking about more than one thing such as blocks, shoes, or toys? YES NO R NO-OPP

74. Without letting your child hold onto anything, have him balance on one foot for as long as he can. Encourage him by showing him how, if necessary. GIVE HIM THREE CHANCES. Estimate seconds by counting slowly. Did your child balance 2 seconds or more? YES NO R NO-OPP

75. Without letting your child take a running jump, ask him to jump lengthwise over this paper. Did he do this without landing on the paper? YES NO R NO-OPP

76. Have your child draw this figure in the space below. DO NOT SAY "CIRCLE." *Do not help or correct your child.* Say to your child, "Draw a picture just like this one," and point to the picture on the right.

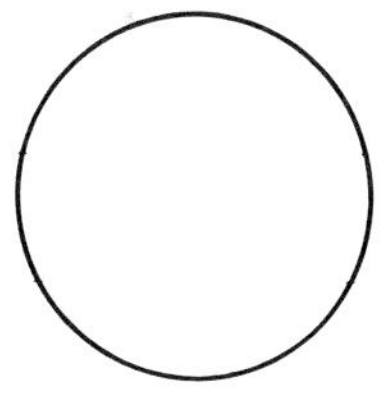

Look at these examples when scoring your child's drawing.

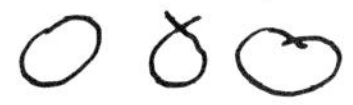

Answer YES

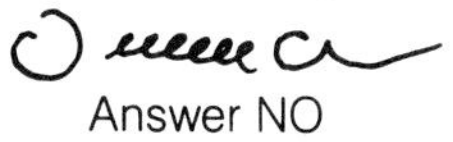

Answer NO

Did your child draw a circle? YES NO R NO-OPP

4 year, 6 month check — Answer 77 through 86

77. Can your child put *eight* blocks on top of one another without the blocks falling? This applies to *small* blocks about 1 inch in size and not blocks more than 2 inches in size. YES NO R NO-OPP

4 year, 9 month check — Answer 78 through 87

78. Does your child play hide-and-seek, cops-and-robbers or other games where he takes turns and follows rules? YES NO R NO-OPP

79. Can your child put jeans, shirt, dress or socks on without help except snapping, buttoning and belts? YES NO R NO-OPP

80. *Without your coaching or saying his name so he can repeat it,* does your child say both his first and last name? Nicknames may be used in place of first name. Circle NO if he only gives his first name or is not easily understood. YES NO R NO-OPP

Figure 16-2 Prescreening Developmental Questionnaire. Reprinted with permission of William K. Frankenburg, MD, University of Colorado Medical Center.

Behavioral and Neurological Assessment Scale

Date Hour

Infant's name .... Sex .... Age .... Born ....
Mother's Age .... Father's Age .... Father's S.E.S. ....
Apparent Race ....
Examiner(s) .... Place of examination ....
Conditions of examination: Date of examination ....
Birth weight .... Current weight .... Length .... Head circ. ....
Time examined .... Time last fed .... Type of feeding ....
Type of delivery .... Apgar ....
Length of labor .... Birth order ....
Type, amount and timing of medication given mother ....
....
Anesthesia? ....
Abnormalities of labour ....

Initial State: observe 2 minutes

1	2	3	4	5	6
deep	light	drowsy	alert	active	crying

Predominant states (mark two)

1	2	3	4	5	6

Elicited Responses

	O*	L	M	H	A†
Plantar grasp		1	2	3	
Hand grasp		1	2	3	
Ankle clonus		1	2	3	
Babinski		1	2	3	
Standing		1	2	3	
Automatic walking		1	2	3	
Placing		1	2	3	
Incurvation		1	2	3	
Crawling		1	2	3	
Glabella		1	2	3	
Tonic deviation of head and eyes		1	2	3	
Nystagmus		1	2	3	
Tonic Neck reflex		1	2	3	
Moro		1	2	3	
Rooting (intensity)		1	2	3	
Sucking (intensity)		1	2	3	
Passive movement					
Arms R		1	2	3	
Arms L		1	2	3	
Legs R		1	2	3	
Legs L		1	2	3	

*O = response not elicited (omitted)
†A = asymmetry

Descriptive Paragraph (optional)

Attractive	0	1	2	3
Interfering variables	0	1	2	3
Need for stimulation	0	1	2	3

What activity does he use to quiet self?
hand to mouth
sucking with nothing in mouth
locking onto visual or auditory stimuli
postural changes
state change for no observable reason

COMMENTS:

Behavior Scoring Sheet

Initial State ....
Predominant State ....

Scale (Note State)	1	2	3	4	5	6	7	8	9
1. Response decrement to light (2,3)									
2. Response decrement to rattle (2, 3)									
3. Response decrement to bell (2, 3)									
4. Response decrement to pinprick (1, 2, 3)									
5. Orientation inanimate visual (4 only)									
6. Orientation inanimate auditory (4, 5)									
7. Orientation animate visual (4 only)									
8. Orientation animate auditory (4, 5)									
9. Orientation animate visual & auditory (4 only)									
10. Alertness (4 only)									
11. General tonus (4, 5)									
12. Motor Maturity (4, 5)									
13. Pull-to-sit (3, 5)									
14. Cuddliness (4, 5)									
15. Defensive movements (4)									
16. Consolability (6 to 5, 4, 3, 2)									
17. Peak of excitement (6)									
18. Rapidity of buildup (from 1, 2 to 6)									
19. Irritability (3, 4, 5)									
20. Activity (alert states)									
21. Tremulousness (all states)									
22. Startle (3, 4, 5, 6)									
23. Lability of skin color (from 1 to 6)									
24. Lability of states (all states)									
25. Self-quieting activity (6, 5 to 4, 3, 2, 1)									
26. Hand-mouth facility (all states)									
27. Smiles (all states)									

Figure 16-3 Scoring sheet for the Brazelton Neonatal Behavioral Assessment Scale (BNBAS). From Brazelton TB (1984): *Neonatal Behavioral Assessment Scale*, 2nd ed. London: S.I.M.P. with Blackwell/Philadelphia: Lippincott.

administration and interpretation of assessment data. The BNBAS is not a simple screening test but rather a fairly in-depth assessment tool requiring considerable time to achieve reliability in administration.

The assessment should be done in a quiet and somewhat darkened room and should be begun midway between feedings with the infant sleeping, dressed, and covered. The examination takes 20–30 minutes to administer and another 10–15 minutes to score. Demonstrating portions of the examination to parents usually helps them to understand their infant's capacities, how the infant reacts to stimuli, and the states in which the infant is most receptive to stimuli. Parents are then able to recognize and modify their responses and expectations, making this an excellent teaching aid by which parents can gain insight into their infant's behavior patterns, temperament, and state changes.

Washington Guide to Promoting Development in Young Children An easily administered and evaluated assessment tool is the Washington Guide to Promoting Development in the Young Child. Designed in 1966 by A. Paulus and Kathryn Barnard (Powell, 1981), the Washington Guide provides a general assessment framework covering eight areas of developmental functioning: (1) motor skills; (2) feeding skills; (3) sleeping behaviors; (4) play skills; (5) language skills (receptive and expressive); (6) discipline skills; (7) toilet training; and (8) dressing skills. These skills and behaviors are assessed according to age, within 3-month range groups up to 52 months, and evaluated against established norms. Age-appropriate tasks and suggested activities to promote the acquisition and maintenance of these skills are listed in opposite columns to facilitate easy administration.

As a teaching tool, the Washington Guide is helpful in providing specific suggestions to augment development and parenting skills. It does not include administration or scoring criteria but instead helps to identify a functional age and note general areas of delays through direct observation of the child performing specific tasks.

Goodenough–Harris Drawing Test The Goodenough–Harris Drawing Test (originally the Goodenough-Draw-A-Man Test, 1926) is a standard nonverbal developmental test that is used with children from 3 to 15 years to assess intellectual maturity. It is, however, entirely dependent on fine motor control, which might influence the results. The test is administered by instructing the child to draw three pictures: a man, a woman, and a self-portrait. The child is asked to do his or her best and draw the whole person. Younger children might need a break between pictures, but in general, the test takes about 15 minutes to administer and can be given to groups of children simultaneously or to individual children. The drawings are scored individually using the manual for specific item standards. A raw score is then obtained and used to calculate a percentile for age (Harris, 1963).

The test provides a means to assess how the child visualizes a person, how this visualization is organized and interpreted, and how it is then reproduced. In addition to conveying information about a child's mental capacities, it might inadvertently provide cues about biophysical, especially neuromuscular, and affective aspects of development (Coleman, Iscoe, and Brodsky, 1959).

Bakwin and associates (1948) developed a modified Draw-a-Man Tool, with 28 criteria for scoring, eliminating scores for aspects of the drawing that seemed more related to fine motor and artistic abilities (Fig. 16-4).

Denver Articulation Screening Examination The Denver Articulation Screening Examination (DASE) (Fig. 16-5) is an easily and quickly administered screening examination to assess the speech of $2\frac{1}{2}$- to 6-year-olds. No special training is needed, and the directions are printed on the form. The nurse asks the child to repeat each of 22 words that represent vowel sounds, consonant sounds, and blends, as well as various locations of the sound within the word. The nurse assesses for the articulation of the sounds and the intelligibility of the child's speech. Retesting is done in 2 weeks if the results are abnormal. A child who has a second abnormal test should be referred for a thorough developmental assessment and speech evaluation.

Peabody Picture Vocabulary Test The Peabody Picture Vocabulary Test assesses verbal intelligence for children $2\frac{1}{2}$ years of age to adulthood. It is not a timed test but generally requires about 15 minutes to administer. The test is administered individually; the child is shown a page with four pictures on it. The examiner then reads the stimulus word (for example, carrying), and the child is instructed to point to the picture that best portrays that word. The child begins with a plate specified according to age; 150 plates are arranged in order of difficulty. Plates of increasing difficulty are presented until the child scores six incorrect responses in eight consecutive plates. A raw score is then calculated, and standard tables are used to obtain an intelligence quotient, percentile score, and developmental age (Dunn, 1965).

Developmental Indications for the Assessment of Learning A standard screening tool for the assessment of prekindergarten children is the Developmental Indication for the Assessment of Learning (DIAL) (Mardell and Goldenberg, 1975). The purpose of the DIAL is to identify children in need of a more thorough assessment. It is designed to screen large numbers of children in a relatively short period of time (25–30 minutes). The DIAL is administered by a team of operators with special, limited

Hypothetical Drawings

Credits, 1, 2, 4, 5, 11, 12.
Total score 6
Mental age = $4\frac{1}{2}$

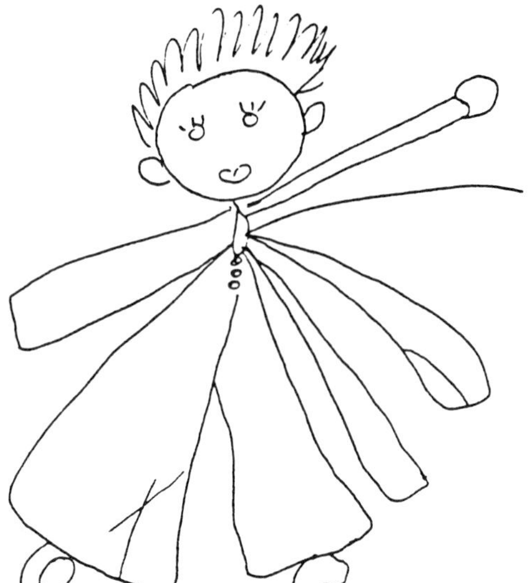

Credits 1, 2, 3, 4, 7, 11, 13, 16, 18, 19, 23, 25, 27
Total score 13
Mental age = $6\frac{1}{2}$

Criteria

1. Head present
2. Legs present
3. Arms present
4. Trunk present
5. Length of trunk greater than breadth
6. Shoulder indicated
7. Both arms and legs attached to trunk
8. Legs attached to trunk and arms to trunk at correct point
9. Neck present
10. Outline of neck continuous with that of head or trunk or both
11. Eyes present
12. Nose present
13. Mouth present
14. Both nose and mouth in two dimensions, two lips shown
15. Nostrils indicated
16. Hair shown
17. Hair on more than circumference of head, nontransparent, better than scribble
18. Clothing present
19. Two articles of clothing, nontransparent
20. Entire drawing with sleeves and trousers shown, free from transparency
21. Four or more articles of clothing definitely indicated
22. Costume complete without incongruities
23. Fingers shown
24. Correct number of fingers shown
25. Fingers in two dimensions, length greater than breadth, angle subtended not greater than 180 degrees
26. Opposition of thumbs shown
27. Hand shown as distinct from fingers or arms
28. Arm joint shown with elbow, shoulder, or both

Scoring

To score the approximate mental age of a child, the basal age is three. For each four criteria met by the drawing, the child is credited with one additional year. The total number of years credited is added to the basal age, and the sum represents the mental age of the child.

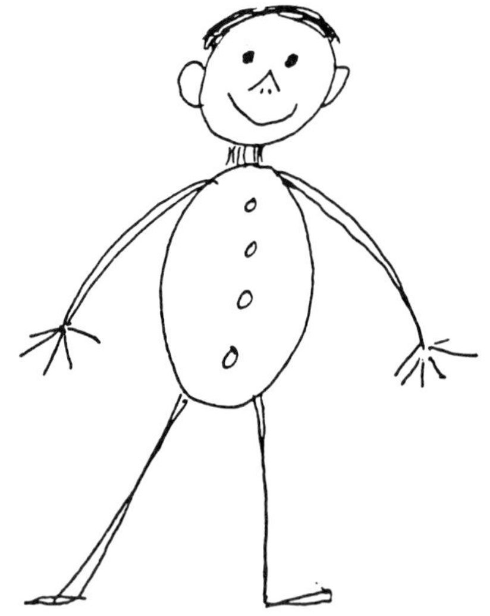

Credits, 1, 2, 3, 4, 5, 7, 8, 9, 11, 12, 13, 15, 16, 18, 23, 24
Total score 16
Mental age = 7

Figure 16-4 Modification of the Goodenough Drawing Test. (From Bakwin RN, Weider A, Bakwin H: Mental testing in children. *J Pediatr* 1948; 33:384. The C.V. Mosby Co.)

training. Stations are set up to screen gross motor skills, fine motor skills, concepts, and communication skills; the child rotates through each station.

Pediatric Examination for Educational Readiness The Pediatric Examination of Educational Readiness (PEER) is a standardized observation system developed for use by health care professionals and requires special training (Levine, et al., 1980). It is designed for prekindergarten children (4–6 years of age) and combines a physical assessment (10–15 minutes) with a neurodevelopmental and behavioral assessment (20–30 minutes). Areas assessed in the PEER include physical status, dressing and undressing, attention–activity level, behavioral adaptation, space–body awareness, gross and fine motor skills, visual processing, auditory processing, and language. The PEER is intended to generate a profile of a child's strengths, weaknesses, and behavioral style. An absolute is not obtained, and the PEER is organized to avoid specific labels. The intent is to estimate the child's educational readiness and identify any needs for special support or services.

Vineland Adaptive Behavior Scales The acquisition of social skills at appropriate intervals in childhood is a major developmental task. An application of Orem's self-care model, the Vineland Adaptive Behavior Scales are useful in measuring individual differences in development and in measuring a child's rate of growth and change in acquiring social skills (Fig. 16-6). Developed in 1936 and revised repeatedly since then, the Vineland Adaptive Behavior Scales provide an easy-to-use and reliable tool in assessing self-care. With a retest reliability reported at 0.92 (Anastasi, 1982), the Vineland Adaptive Behavior Scales are used with individuals from birth to 18 years of age or older.

The assessment involves interviewing the parent or primary caregiver about both the frequency of selected social behaviors and the opportunities the child has to use them. Average ages for the acquisition of certain behaviors are placed in a successive order on the scoring sheet and marked using designated symbols that indicate the child's performance of behaviors and how frequently they occur. The specific items sample such aspects of social development as self-direction, social participation, and self-sufficiency. Although not rating scales, the Vineland Adaptive Behavior Scales do assess the child's ability to look after practical needs. The five domains of social adaptation measured are as follows:

1. Communication
2. Daily living skills
3. Socialization
4. Motor skills
5. Maladaptive behavior

Deficits in each of these areas are identified and might be assessed further to identify specific patterns of disability. The Vineland Adaptive Behavior Scales are useful with clients who are too young to communicate effectively, too unreliable to describe themselves accurately, or unable to provide data because of illness or developmental delay.

Intelligence Tests The intelligence quotient (IQ) test has been equated erroneously with general intelligence, although it is no more than the score on a test. Intelligence tests often measure already acquired skills, facts, or knowledge. The Stanford–Binet test and the Wechsler Intelligence Scale for Children are two such tests. The Stanford–Binet test operationally defines IQ according to mental age versus chronologic age. The Wechsler Intelligence Test for Children compares the performance of one child with that of peers the same age.

Educators and parents have used the IQ scores as indicators of success in school. Although the IQ score does reflect specific cognitive abilities, it does not reflect school performance or potential. Motivation, role models, and self-evaluation influence success in school as well as the IQ score, and those children who desire to do well scholastically often succeed if they do not have a significant cognitive handicap. Parents and educators also influence IQ scores; therefore, children who are expected to do well make an honest effort to succeed while taking examinations and intelligence tests, whereas children who are expected to fail do poorly on tests.

Self-Esteem Inventory The Self-Esteem Inventory (Fig. 16-7), developed by Coopersmith (1967), is a series of statements about family, school, peers, self, and general social activities. The inventory is designed to assess the self-esteem of children from grades four through twelve. Self-esteem is the evaluation the child makes and maintains of the self; it relates to the attitudes of approval and disapproval internalized from others and the degree to which the child views the self as capable, significant, successful, and worthy. Essentially, the tool conveys a self-judgment of worthiness (Coopersmith, 1967).

There are two forms of the Self-Esteem Inventory: the long form (58 questions) and the short form (25 questions). The short form consists of the 25 questions which demonstrated the highest item score relationships and correlates favorably with the long form.

The child is instructed to check the column labeled "Like me" if the statement describes common or frequent feelings. The child is reminded that there are no right or wrong answers. After the child completes the inventory, the number of responses indicative of high self-esteem are counted and multiplied by 4 ($25 \times 4 = 100$). Instead of exact criteria, Coopersmith (1967) employed an index of relative

(text continued on p. 496)

DENVER ARTICULATION SCREENING EXAM
for children 2 1/2 to 6 years of age

Instructions: Have child repeat each word after you. Circle the underlined sounds that he pronounces correctly. Total correct sounds is the Raw Score. Use charts on reverse side to score results.

NAME

HOSP. NO.

ADDRESS ____________

Date: ________ Child's Age: ________ Examiner: ____________ Raw Score: ________
Percentile: ________ Intelligibility: ____________ Result: ____________

1. table	6. zipper	11. sock	16. wagon	21. leaf
2. shirt	7. grapes	12. vacuum	17. gum	22. carrot
3. door	8. flag	13. yarn	18. house	
4. trunk	9. thumb	14. mother	19. pencil	
5. jumping	10. toothbrush	15. twinkle	20. fish	

Intelligibility: (circle one) 1. Easy to understand 2. Understandable 1/2 the time. 3. Not understandable 4. Can't evaluate

Comments:

Date: ________ Child's Age: ________ Examiner: ____________ Raw Score ________
Percentile: ________ Intelligibility: ____________ Result: ____________

1. table	6. zipper	11. sock	16. wagon	21. leaf
2. shirt	7. grapes	12. vacuum	17. gum	22. carrot
3. door	8. flag	13. yarn	18. house	
4. trunk	9. thumb	14. mother	19. pencil	
5. jumping	10. toothbrush	15. twinkle	20. fish	

Intelligibility: (circle one) 1. Easy to understand 2. Understandable 1/2 the time. 3. Not understandable 4. Can't evaluate

Comments:

Date: ________ Child's Age: ________ Examiner: ____________ Raw Score ________
Percentile: ________ Intelligibility: ____________ Result: ____________

1. table	6. zipper	11. sock	16. wagon	21. leaf
2. shirt	7. grapes	12. vacuum	17. gum	22. carrot
3. door	8. flag	13. yarn	18. house	
4. trunk	9. thumb	14. mother	19. pencil	
5. jumping	10. toothbrush	15. twinkle	20. fish	

Intelligibility: (circle one) 1. Easy to understand 2. Understandable 1/2 the time. 3. Not understandable 4. Can't evaluate

Comments:

Figure 16-5 Denver Articulation Screening Examination. Reprinted with permission of William K. Frankenburg, MD, University of Colorado Medical Center.

To score DASE words: Note Raw Score for child's performance. Match raw score line (extreme left of chart) with column representing child's age (to the closest previous age group). Where raw score line and age column meet number in that square denotes percentile rank of child's performance when compared to other children that age. Percentiles above heavy line are ABNORMAL percentiles, below heavy line are NORMAL.

PERCENTILE RANK

Raw Score	2.5 yr.	3.0	3.5	4.0	4.5	5.0	5.5	6 years
2	1							
3	2							
4	5							
5	9							
6	16							
7	23							
8	31	2						
9	37	4	1					
10	42	6	2					
11	48	7	4					
12	54	9	6	1	1			
13	58	12	9	2	3	1	1	
14	62	17	11	5	4	2	2	
15	68	23	15	9	5	3	2	
16	75	31	19	12	5	4	3	
17	79	38	25	15	6	6	4	
18	83	46	31	19	8	7	4	
19	86	51	38	24	10	9	5	1
20	89	58	45	30	12	11	7	3
21	92	65	52	36	15	15	9	4
22	94	72	58	43	18	19	12	5
23	96	77	63	50	22	24	15	7
24	97	82	70	58	29	29	20	15
25	99	87	78	66	36	34	26	17
26	99	91	84	75	46	43	34	24
27		94	89	82	57	54	44	34
28		96	94	88	70	68	59	47
29		98	98	94	84	84	77	68
30		100	100	100	100	100	100	100

To Score intelligibility:

	NORMAL	ABNORMAL
2 1/2 years	Understandable 1/2 the time, or, "easy"	Not Understandable
3 years and older	Easy to understand	Understandable 1/2 time Not understandable

Test Result: 1. NORMAL on Dase and Intelligibility = NORMAL

2. ABNORMAL on Dase and/or Intelligibility = ABNORMAL

* If abnormal on initial screening rescreen within 2 weeks. If abnormal again child should be referred for complete speech evaluation.

Figure 16-5 continued

ITEM SCORES
2 Yes, usually
1 Sometimes or partially
0 No, never
N No opportunity
DK Don't know

Age	Item	INTERPERSONAL RELATIONSHIPS	PLAY & LEISURE TIME	COPING SKILLS	COMMENTS
<1	1. Looks at face of caregiver.	☐			
	2. Responds to voice of caregiver or another person.	☐			
	3. Distinguishes caregiver from others.	☐			
	4. Shows interest in novel objects or new people.		☐		
	5. Expresses two or more recognizable emotions such as pleasure, sadness, fear, or distress.	☐			
	6. Shows anticipation of being picked up by caregiver.	☐			
	7. Shows affection toward familiar people.	☐			
	8. Shows interest in children or peers other than siblings.		☐		
	9. Reaches for familiar person.	☐			
	10. Plays with toy or other object alone or with others.		☐		
	11. Plays very simple interaction games with others.		☐		
	12. Uses common household objects for play.		☐		
	13. Shows interest in activities of others.		☐		
	14. Imitates simple adult movements, such as clapping hands or waving good-bye, in response to a model.	☐			
1, 2	15. Laughs or smiles appropriately in response to positive statements.	☐			
	16. Addresses at least two familiar people by name.	☐			
	17. Shows desire to please caregiver.	☐			
	18. Participates in at least one game or activity with others.		☐		
	19. Imitates a relatively complex task several hours after it was performed by another.	☐			
	20. Imitates adult phrases heard on previous occasions.	☐			
	21. Engages in elaborate make-believe activities, alone or with others.		☐		
3	22. Shows a preference for some friends over others.	☐			
	23. Says "please" when asking for something.			☐	
	24. Labels happiness, sadness, fear, and anger in self.	☐			
	25. Identifies people by characteristics other than name, when asked.	☐			
4	26. Shares toys or possessions without being told to do so.		☐		
	27. Names one or more favorite television programs when asked, and tells on what days and channels the programs are shown. N MAY BE SCORED.		☐		
	28. Follows rules in simple games without being reminded.		☐		
	29. Has a preferred friend of either sex.	☐			
	30. Follows school or facility rules.			☐	
5	31. Responds verbally and positively to good fortune of others.	☐			
	32. Apologizes for unintentional mistakes.			☐	
	33. Has a group of friends.	☐			
	34. Follows community rules.			☐	
6	35. Plays more than one board or card game requiring skill and decision making.		☐		
	36. Does not talk with food in mouth.			☐	
	37. Has a best friend of the same sex.	☐			
	Count items before basal as 2, items after ceiling as 0.	☐	☐	☐	Sum of 2s, 1s, 0s page 7

INTERPERSONAL RELATIONSHIPS

PLAY & LEISURE TIME

COPING SKILLS

COMMENTS ____________________

SOCIALIZATION DOMAIN

Figure 16-6 Vineland Adaptive Behavior Scales. Reprinted with permission of the American Guidance Service, Inc., Circle Pines, Minnesota.

SOCIALIZATION DOMAIN

ITEM SCORES
- 2 Yes, usually
- 1 Sometimes or partially
- 0 No, never
- N No opportunity
- DK Don't know

	Item	INTERPERSONAL RELATIONSHIPS	PLAY & LEISURE TIME	COPING SKILLS	COMMENTS
	38. Responds appropriately when introduced to strangers.			☐	
7, 8	39. Makes or buys small gifts for caregiver or family member on major holidays, on own initiative.	☐			
	40. Keeps secrets or confidences for more than one day.			☐	
	41. Returns borrowed toys, possessions, or money to peers, or returns borrowed books to library.			☐	
	42. Ends conversations appropriately.			☐	
	43. Follows time limits set by caregiver.			☐	
	44. Refrains from asking questions or making statements that might embarrass or hurt others.			☐	
	45. Controls anger or hurt feelings when denied own way.			☐	
	46. Keeps secrets or confidences for as long as appropriate.			☐	
10, 11	47. Uses appropriate table manners without being told. DO NOT SCORE 1.			☐	
	48. Watches television or listens to radio for information about a particular area of interest. N MAY BE SCORED.		☐		
	49. Goes to evening school or facility events with friends, when accompanied by an adult. N MAY BE SCORED.		☐		
	50. Independently weighs consequences of actions before making decisions.			☐	
	51. Apologizes for mistakes or errors in judgment.			☐	
12, 13, 14	52. Remembers birthdays or anniversaries of immediate family members and special friends.	☐			
	53. Initiates conversations on topics of particular interest to others.	☐			
	54. Has a hobby.		☐		
	55. Repays money borrowed from caregiver.			☐	
15 to 18+	56. Responds to hints or indirect cues in conversation.	☐			
	57. Participates in nonschool sports. N MAY BE SCORED.		☐		
	58. Watches television or listens to radio for practical, day-to-day information. N MAY BE SCORED.		☐		
	59. Makes and keeps appointments.			☐	
	60. Watches television or listens to radio for news independently. N MAY BE SCORED.		☐		
	61. Goes to evening school or facility events with friends, without adult supervision. N MAY BE SCORED.		☐		
	62. Goes to evening nonschool or nonfacility events with friends, without adult supervision.		☐		
	63. Belongs to older adolescent organized club, interest group, or social or service organization.	☐			
	64. Goes with one person of opposite sex to party or public event where many people are present.	☐			
	65. Goes on double or triple dates.	☐			
	66. Goes on single dates.	☐			

Count items before basal as 2, items after ceiling as 0.

	INTERPERSONAL RELATIONSHIPS	PLAY & LEISURE TIME	COPING SKILLS	
1.				Sum of 2s, 1s, 0s page **8**
2.				Sum of 2s, 1s, 0s page **7**
3.				Number of Ns pages **7** and **8**
4.				Number of DKs pages **7** and **8**
				SUBDOMAIN RAW SCORE (Add rows 1—4 above)

COMMENTS ____________________

Figure 16-6 continued

Short Form SEI
Total score = # correct
(xy if 100 desired)
Total score correlates 0.86 with total scores of long form
No subscales

NAME ______________________ School ______________________

Class ______________________ Date ______________________

Please mark each statement in the following way:

If the statement describes how you usually feel, put a check (√) in the column "Like Me."

If the statement does not describe how you usually feel, put a check (√) in the column "Unlike Me."

There are no right or wrong answers.

	LIKE ME	UNLIKE ME
Example: I'm a hard worker.		
1. I often wish I were someone else.		
2. I find it very hard to talk in front of the class.		
3. There are lots of things about myself I'd change if I could.		
4. I can make up my mind without too much trouble.		
5. I'm a lot of fun to be with.		

Figure 16-7 Self-Esteem Inventory (first 5 questions—sample only). Reproduced by special permission of the publisher, Consulting Psychologists Press, Inc., from the Self-Esteem Inventory, by Stanley Coopersmith, PhD, copyright 1968.

self-esteem, with a score in the upper quartile (75–100) indicating high self-esteem, a score in the middle two quartiles (25–75) indicating medium self-esteem, and a score in the lower quartile (0–25) indicating low self-esteem.

By assessing general self-esteem and noting how the child responded to specific questions, the nurse can pinpoint areas of uncertainty or attitudes of self-dislike and include this information when planning nursing care.

Developmental Assessment for Specific Ages

The Neonate

The neonatal period, from birth to 30 days of age, is one of transition and adaptation as the infant begins to interact with the extrauterine environment. The birth process is marked by intense physical stress, after which the infant faces new stimuli and major physiologic changes. For parents, the neonatal period is also a time of transition.

Genetic endowment, prenatal events, duration of labor and delivery, type of delivery, maternal medication in labor, and perinatal events all influence infant behavior. The traditional view that the neonate is passive, helpless, and vulnerable has been supplanted by the recognition that neonates have tremendous capabilities and play an active role in adapting and responding to their environment. Newborn infants are able to see—although focal length is limited and nystagmus (wandering eye movements) is present—hear, attend selectively to stimuli, suppress motor activity and reflexes that inhibit the ability to attend to stimuli, shut out offending stimuli, and elicit responses from the environment that promote development.

In a developmental assessment, the nurse therefore seeks to identify the infant's capabilities and vulnerabilities, as evidenced by the child's interaction with the environment. Although infant behavior was once thought to be shaped by the parent, researchers now recognize that infants also shape the behavior of their parents or other caregivers (Lewis and Rosenblum, 1974). The nurse therefore closely observes parent–infant interactions, assessing both the infant's and the parent's behavior. The nurse assesses the parent's ability to adapt to a new person and a new role (parenting) by closely noting parent–infant behavior and provides an opportunity for the parent to discuss thoughts and feelings.

The guidelines for developmental assessment of the neonate are presented in Table 16-6. Many of the items listed are adapted from the Neonatal Behavioral Assessment Scale

(Brazelton, 1973). Although the proper administration of this scale requires special training, a nurse who has not received formal training might find items from the scale useful, although the results are not as valid or reliable as when the assessment tool is used.

A neonatal assessment is best done in a quiet, dimly lit environment because the noise and light of a normal nursery might be overwhelming and cause the infant to retreat defensively into sleep or lose control and scream. Performing the assessment at the mother's bedside with the father present is generally the ideal. This minimizes offending stimuli for the infant and gives the parents an opportunity to observe the assessment procedure and learn about the infant.

State The infant's responses to stimuli depend on the infant's state. The nurse therefore considers the infant's state in determining the significance of the infant's responses.

Neonates actively use different states by shutting out disturbing stimuli or attending to positive stimuli. For example, immediately after painful procedures such as injection or circumcision or following an exhaustive episode of crying, many infants go into a deep sleep, an adaptation to a painful experience. Pain, hunger, immaturity, and physiologic problems might, however, affect the infant's ability to use state to respond to stimuli. Premature infants cannot afford to compromise their limited energy by maintaining a quiet alert state, and if such a state is achieved briefly, sleep quickly follows.

In assessing a neonate the nurse pays particular attention to two aspects of the infant's state control. The first aspect is the infant's ability to attain and maintain the quiet alert state and the rapidity and frequency with which the infant changes state. The infant's ability to remain quiet and alert is important because this is the state in which the infant is best able to interact with the environment. The parent usually finds interaction most gratifying when the infant is quiet and alert. If the infant does not attain this state spontaneously, the nurse might help by providing gentle vestibular stimulation such as holding the infant at a 30° angle and gently rocking to and fro or placing the infant over the shoulder. If the infant still does not readily attain a quiet alert state, the nurse might need to assess the infant more than once to determine whether this is due to the infant's inability or the technique or timing of the assessment. The second aspect is that some infants rapidly progress from a sleeping to a crying state, whereas other infants progress more gradually. Some infants are able to maintain themselves in certain states for a long time, whereas others seem to change unpredictably from one state to another. The pattern and frequency with which the infant changes state are therefore important criteria.

Habituation Habituation is the infant's ability to shut out disturbing stimuli and is related to the infant's control of state (see Chapter 7). Habituation can be assessed by presenting stimuli (for example, a flashlight to the eyes, rattle, or bell) to the infant during light sleep or drowsiness and observing the response is repeated several times. The infant typically reacts markedly to the first presentation but reacts less and less to each subsequent presentation until a minimal or no response is noted. The phenomenon of diminishing response is referred to as *response decrement.*

An infant who has a limited ability to habituate continues to display a marked response each time the stimulus is

TABLE 16-6 Guidelines for the Assessment of the Neonate

Developmental area	Expected behaviors
Perinatal history	
Assessment of gestational age	
State control	Attain and maintain the quiet alert state Changes state gradually rather than abruptly
Habituation to offending stimuli	Response decrement to shining of light in eyes during light sleep, noise of rattle and bell during light sleep
Consolability	Consoles self or accepts consolation from adult
Visual orientation	Fixates on object and/or face Follows object or face with eyes Attains eye contact with adult
Auditory orientation	Attends to rattle and/or voice Turns toward source of sound
Motor skills	Predominantly positioned with arms and legs flexed Moves symmetrically Moves smoothly Moves purposefully Reflexes present, normal response to elicitation
Social development	
Infant	Gives clear cues Responds with eye contact, attending to adult face and/or voice, accepting feeding readily, displaying satisfaction, cuddling close to adult when held
Parent	Perceives infant positively May feel some ambivalence toward infant Displays sensitivity to needs and cues of infant by recognizing and responding to infant's signals, recognizing infant's alert periods and attempting interaction; using en face position and attempting eye contact; holding infant close to trunk, speaking positively about or to infant Showing awareness of infant's capabilities

presented. This lack of response decrement represents a decreased ability on the infant's part to control state; such infants tend to be overreactive and show a limited ability to modulate their responses (Als and Brazelton, 1981).

Consolability *Consolability,* the infant's willingness to be comforted when crying, is another measure of the infant's control of state. When the infant is upset and crying, the nurse observes the infant's behavior and notes any attempts at self-consolation (for example, flexion of the arms and legs to body, attending to stimuli, putting hand to mouth).

For infants who are unable to console themselves, the nurse uses a progressive series of maneuvers to console the infant. For example, the nurse might (1) face the infant directly in the infant's line of vision; (2) present both face and voice; (3) proceed to place a hand on the infant; (4) enfold the infant's arms onto the chest; (5) pick the infant up; and (6) rock, talk, and walk with the infant. The nurse then notes how much external intervention, if any, the infant requires to be comforted.

Visual Orientation Visual ability is best assessed when the infant is in the quiet alert state. The nurse is interested in the infant's ability not only to fixate on an object visually but also to suppress motor activity so that random movements do not interfere with attending to visual stimuli. The nurse might begin by presenting a colorful object in the infant's line of vision, 8–9 in from the face, and observing the infant's response. If the infant fixates on the object, the nurse might move the object slowly to each side to see whether the infant's eyes follow it. The nurse then presents his or her face to the infant, attempts to have the infant fixate on the face, and moves from side to side to assess the infant's following ability. If the infant does not fixate on the face alone, the nurse might present face and voice together in an attempt to engage the infant.

The nurse notes the infant's willingness to make eye contact because some infants readily make eye contact, whereas other infants avert their gaze and avoid eye contact. Parents usually find eye contact positive and gaze aversion disconcerting, and some parents interpret gaze aversion as rejection. Actually, the stimulation of direct eye contact might be too much for some infants to handle, and averting their gaze is a protective measure (Greenspan and Lieberman, 1980).

Auditory Orientation As with visual orientation, the nurse is interested not only in the infant's ability to respond to auditory stimuli but also in the infant's ability to suppress motor activity that would interfere with the ability to attend to stimuli.

Auditory orientation is best assessed with the infant in the quiet alert state. The nurse first presents an interesting noise, such as a rattle, at the infant's side. The infant generally becomes alert and listens to the noise, and some infants turn their heads toward the source of the noise. The nurse also presents verbal stimuli. Infants seem to prefer a higher-pitched, female voice and more readily look toward the source of a higher voice than a lower voice if given a choice. Offensive verbal stimuli (too loud or too high-pitched) elicit a defensive response of crying or habituation.

Motor Skills The standard neurologic exam for neonates provides much information about the infant's motor system, including muscle tone, strength, and primitive reflexes (see Chapter 7). In addition to this information, the following aspects of the neonate's motor system should be evaluated during a developmental assessment:

1. *Posture.* Neonates typically maintain a posture with their arms and legs flexed close to the trunk most of the time. When the arms and legs are often extended and/or limp and in an asymmetric position, this is a cause for concern, and appropriate referral is needed to a developmental specialist or pediatrician.
2. *Symmetry of movement.* The amount and range of movement of the infant's arms and legs should be about equal on each side. Moving only one extremity or moving one extremity less than the other suggests a disorder.
3. *Smoothness of movement.* A neonate whose central nervous system is intact generally has smooth and free motor movements most of the time. All infants occasionally show some jerky movements (as in the Moro reflex), but these movements should not predominate. Tremulousness, jitteriness, or jerkiness might be caused by an immature or disorganized central nervous system or another organic cause (such as hypoxia or hypocalcemia). As the infant recovers from physical insults, motor movement often becomes more smooth and fluid.
4. *Purposeful movements.* The normal neonate is capable of purposeful motor activity such as bringing the fist to the mouth to suck on it. The infant also has purposeful defensive movements. The nurse can assess this ability by placing a small cloth over the infant's face. After a few initial movements, the infant should attempt to swipe at the cloth and remove it.

Social and Affective Development In assessing the social dimension of neonatal development, the nurse focuses on the parent–infant interaction, determining what each individual brings to and takes from the interaction. Normal infant development requires affectionate, reciprocal responses between the parent and child, a process of attachment that takes time to develop (see Chapter 7).

Bonding, the first step in the attachment process, refers to the powerful attraction and entrainment with the infant that a parent experiences. Ideally, bonding between the parent and infant occurs in the first few hours and days of the neonatal period and is initiated prenatally as the parent plans for the arrival of the developing fetus. After birth,

A. Neonate shows intense interest in the human face. *B*. Infant follows a red ball. *C*. Infant turns head to follow a human face. (From Avery, ME, Talusch, HW: *Diseases of the Newborn*. 5th ed. Saunders, 1984.) Reprinted by permission.

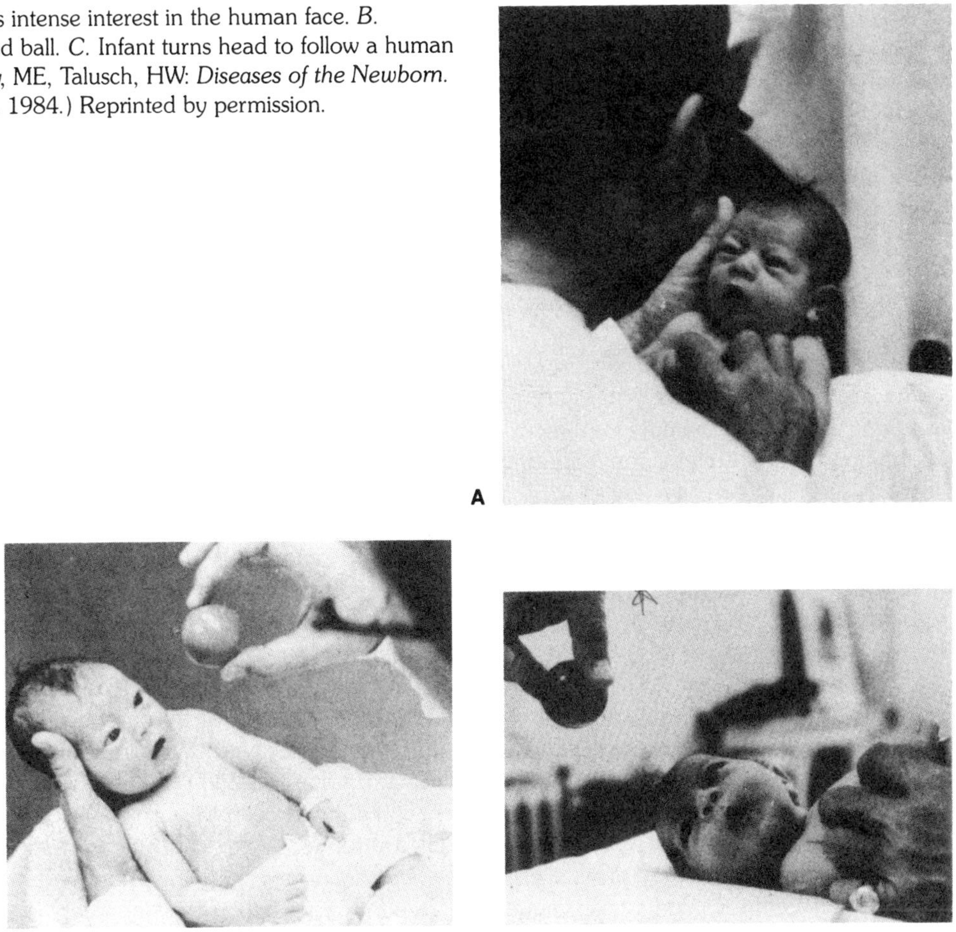

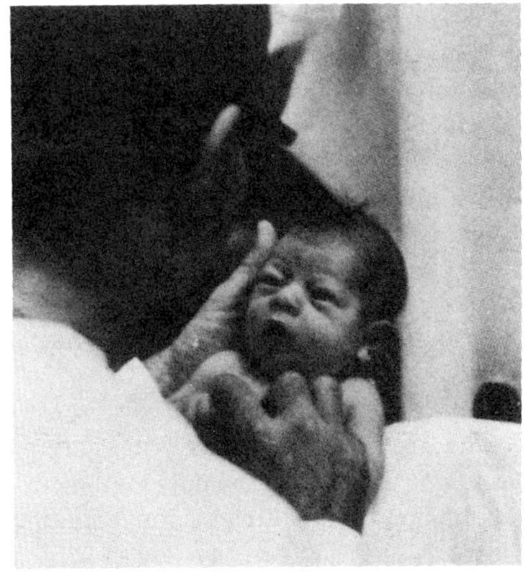

A

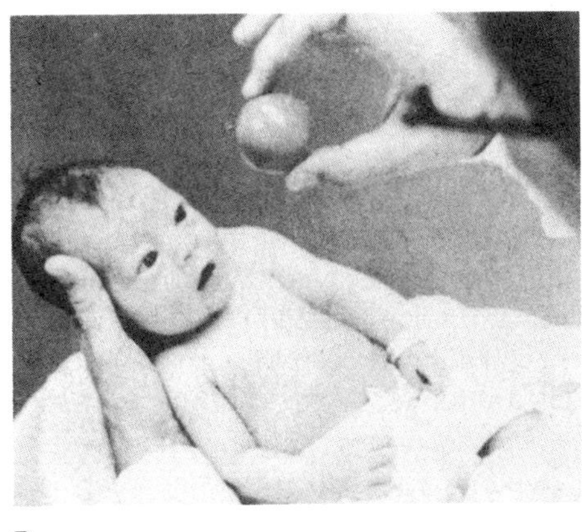

B

C

parent–infant contact elicits a variety of mutually pleasurable and rewarding responses. If bonding does not occur in the first few days, for example, if parent and child are separated because of illness, a positive and strong attachment can still occur.

Bonding is facilitated by a supportive environment; therefore, the nurse assessing the neonate notes any factors that might affect the bonding process negatively. These negative factors include neonatal prematurity or illness, separation of the mother and infant after birth, a birth defect in the infant, a nonsupportive environment, and family stress (Klaus and Kennel, 1976).

Robson and Moss (1970) studied the process of attachment from birth to 4 months of age and described several stages that mothers typically experienced in relation to their infants. These stages are as follows:

Labor. The mother is concerned mainly with herself, having a peripheral interest in the infant.

1–4 days. The mother describes vague and strange feelings of a strong protectiveness toward the infant, makes positive comments, but has difficulty describing the infant.

1–4 weeks. The mother feels tired and expresses difficulty in communicating with the infant.

4–6 weeks. The mother expresses an increasingly positive feeling; the infant "begins to be a person" (this corresponds with the infant's increasing social behavior, especially smiling).

6–9 weeks. The mother feels that the infant recognizes her.

16 weeks. The mother expresses an intense love for the infant.

Parents' feelings and perceptions about their infants are the first major focus in the assessment process because as parents begin to learn about their infants, they experience a variety of emotions. Ambivalence and anxiety are common and expected reactions. Parents who have difficulty describing their infant usually are still becoming acquainted with the infant. Although ambivalence is expected, a predominantly negative attitude is a cause for concern and close follow-up. Specific areas to assess include the following:

1. Attitudes toward pregnancy

2. Expectations of labor and delivery as compared with perceptions of the actual experience
3. Expectation of the infant prenatally as compared with perceptions of the actual infant
4. Perceptions of positive and negative characteristics of the infant (for example, the infant's sex)
5. Concern regarding self or spouse
6. Concern regarding the infant
7. Feelings of adequacy or inadequacy as a parent
8. Supportiveness of spouse and/or other significant persons

A second major area to assess is the parent's sensitivity to the infant's cues because a parent's ability to interpret the infant's behavior and respond appropriately is the cornerstone of optimal parent–infant interaction. Specific behaviors that reflect this sensitivity are as follows:

1. Recognition of hunger, satiety, fatigue, and distress signals from infant
2. Recognition of alert periods and attempts to interact with the infant
3. En face positioning and attempts to engage the infant in eye contact
4. Holding the infant close to the trunk
5. Speaking positively to the infant

In assessing this aspect of the parent–infant interaction, the nurse also evaluates the clarity of the infant's cues. Some infants give clear cues that they are hungry, tired, alert, satisfied, or distressed, whereas other infants give vague and unclear cues, so that parents have difficulty in interpreting the meaning of their behavior. A new parent generally finds great satisfaction in understanding an infant's behavior and meeting an infant's needs; therefore, parents who feel unable to read their infant's cues often feel frustrated and lose confidence. To assess the infant's ability to interact, the nurse also pays close attention to the infant's responsiveness to the parent. The infant's ability to eat well and display satisfaction are socially significant behaviors that affect parent–infant interaction.

A third focus of assessment is the parent's awareness of the infant's capabilities and adeptness and competence in caring for the infant, which influence how the parent relates to the infant. The parent who is unaware of the infant's perceptual and behavioral abilities might not provide an environment that is most conducive to optimal development. For example, a parent who believes a newborn infant cannot see well probably will not attempt to achieve eye contact with the infant.

The nurse uses the data collected to help the parent recognize the capabilities and strengths of the infant. Demonstrating these capabilities is a very captivating and powerful intervention. One study involving high-risk teenage mothers, for example, showed that a demonstration of their infant's capabilities and capacities for interaction resulted in a greater awareness of infant cues and a more sensitive mother–infant interaction (Olsen, et al., 1981). The nurse also might alert parents to infant behavioral patterns they anticipate, thereby helping them to develop strategies to deal with infant behavior. Nurses can thus support parents as they endeavor to reach out to care for and enjoy their new infants. Many new parents lack smoothness and confidence in handling an infant, yet their sincere efforts to meet their infants' needs are a significant strength.

Although neonates do not fit neatly into specific categories, some patterns of neonatal behavior require special attention. The first special concern is the overresponsive infant who demonstrates much activity, hypersensitivity to stimuli, and poor control of state. "This type of infant is easily roused to intense motor activity and responds to almost all stimuli by marked crying. Thus aroused, such an infant tends to perpetuate, in a cyclical manner, the overresponse to stimuli and the uncontrolled motor behavior for prolonged crying periods" (McCarthy and Brazelton, 1980). Overresponsive infants show little ability to be consoled either by themselves or by others. They are likely to cause considerable stress for new parents, who generally feel inadequate and blame themselves for the infant's behavior.

The nurse can help the parent to understand that the sensitivity and activity of the infant is part of a behavioral style and not a reflection of parental inadequacy. The parent can then proceed to learn ways to help the infant learn self-control.

The second special concern is the unresponsive infant. Brazelton described these neonates as "difficult to rouse from sleep states and when they do finally come to an awake state, they remain difficult to alert and are relatively inactive. They reacted dully to visual and auditory cues to which an average baby would have responded in an excited way. After they were awakened, they maintained a dull awake state for long periods, which seemed to prevent them from getting back down to a normal sleep. These rather poorly organized states inevitably affected their environments. Mothers reported that they found the babies 'unpredictable' and 'difficult to understand.' They complained they were never sure they were reaching them and their inclination was to leave them alone." Such infants thus might set the tone for failed interactions (Brazelton, Parker, and Zuckman, 1976). Infants who are small for gestational age often fit this category, although as they grow older they might develop a more hyperresponsive style.

The nurse again can help the parent see that the infant's behavior reflects individual makeup and not parental failure. Unresponsive infants often need more stimulation and structure. Parents can then learn to help their infants attain and maintain alertness.

The third special concern is the premature infant. Premature infants have certain characteristics that depend on their gestational age and physiologic stability. Premature infants who are younger and sicker have poorly defined states and limited control of state. They have a limited ability to habituate to stimuli and tend to respond in a cyclical fashion, having difficulty in terminating a response. Premature infants are thus at the mercy of their environments, more so than normal neonates. As the premature infant develops, a predictable pattern of progress emerges. The infant displays increasing control of physiologic functions as pulse and respirations become more stable and vasomotor instability diminishes, and the infant then gains control of motor functions. With increasing central nervous system maturity, the infant develops better control of state and an increased capacity for interaction (Brazelton, Tronik, and Adamson, 1975). (Care of the high-risk infant is discussed in Chapter 31.)

It is also impossible to predict the long-term developmental outcomes based on perinatal events and neonatal behavior. The central nervous system of the young infant is both plastic and resilient. Infants with a major physiologic insult, although at increased risk, might develop normally if raised in a supportive environment with appropriate stimulation, whereas infants with only minor insults and at relatively low risks might have poor developmental outcomes if raised in a disorganized and unsupportive environment such as a family with multiple stressors and limited resources.

Most important in assessing infants with special behavior patterns is the match between the infant's behavior and the parent's expectations. A hyperactive, hyperresponsive infant might be perceived as difficult by some parents and exciting by others. Likewise, a quiet, unresponsive infant might be disconcerting for some parents but ideal for others. (Chapter 22 discusses the assessment and detection of the family at risk.)

The 1- to 3-Month-Old Infant

During the first year of life, the infant's biologic growth and developmental maturation is rapid and exciting; progress can be recognized almost daily. Guidelines for the assessment of the 1- to 3-month-old infant are summarized in Table 16-7.

Temperament Between 1 and 3 months of age, as the infant becomes more predictable and the parent becomes more familiar with the infant, certain patterns of behavior begin to emerge. Most parents begin to identify the unique personality and behavioral traits of their infant, but it is still too early to make definitive statements about an infant's temperament or to consider the infant's behavior stable and predictive of later behavior. The nurse therefore can only begin to assess obvious temperamental characteristics for these infants.

Initial assessment data can be obtained by asking parents to describe the infant's activity level. Some infants are markedly active, wiggling and kicking vigorously much of the time, whereas others are more quiet and less active. Parents generally can describe whether an infant seems happy or unhappy most of the time, but their perceptions might change as the infant matures. For example, infants between 1 and 3 months of age often display an increase in crying. As they begin to cry less after about 3 months of age, parents might view the infants' mood somewhat more positively.

By 3 months of age, the biologic functions of most infants are somewhat predictable. Regular feeding and sleeping schedules generally are established, although infants who have not yet developed fairly regular schedules eventually might do so. The nurse does, however, need to assess the environment of infants whose schedule is still erratic at this age to identify any difficulties. Some infants are unable to establish a regular schedule in spite of the best parental efforts, whereas other infants might not have had an opportunity to develop a reasonable schedule because of a disorganized and unpredictable environment.

The nurse elicits the parents' perceptions of and reactions to a range of temperamental characteristics. If the infant's behavior is different from the parent's expectations and desires, the nurse must explore this carefully. When an infant does not fit parental expectations, considerable frustration, guilt, and resentment might develop. Parents often blame themselves, assuming that difficult infant behavior is a result of parental incompetence and inadequacy. The nurse then might need to help the parent to understand that the infant's temperament is innate and to develop appropriate strategies for dealing with the infant.

Comments that might be helpful in initiating a discussion of parent–infant interaction include the following:

1. Tell me what a day with the baby is like.
2. How have your feelings about the baby changed over the last few weeks?
3. Show me how the baby 'talks' to you.
4. What happens when the baby cries?
5. How does the baby act with the father (mother)?
6. How does the baby act with the sitter?

Not all parents develop appropriate behavior. Functional and dysfunctional parenting behaviors are summarized in Table 16-8. (See Chapter 22 for a discussion of dysfunctional parenting.)

Gross Motor Skills The infant's degree of head lag when pulled to a sitting position is an important measure of gross motor development. As the infant matures, the amount of head lag decreases, so that by 3 months of age, most infants display minimal head lag. When prone, the neonate can lift the head and turn it from side to side. The 2-month-old infant is able to raise the head 45°; the 3-month-old infant raises the head 90°. When supported in a sitting position, the 3-month-old infant can hold the head erect, occasionally bobbing forward.

TABLE 16-7 Guidelines for the Assessment of the 1-to 3-Month-Old Infant

Developmental area	Expected behaviors	Assessment techniques
Temperament	Parent perceives the infant's temperamental characteristics	Ask the parent about the infant's temperament
Gross motor skills	Minimal head lag when pulled to a sitting position Head bobs when supported in sitting position	Observe and provide performance opportunity
1 month	Lifts head and turns from side to side when prone	Ask the parent about the infant's daily opportunity for development of motor skills
2 months	Lifts head 45 ° when prone	
3 months	Lifts head 90° when prone	
Fine motor skills	Palmar grasp present but fading Hand-to-mouth tendency Hands open (not clenched) most of time Follows object 180° with eyes by 3 months Swipes at objects suspended above eyes Becomes excited by object but is unable to grasp unless put in hand	Observe the infant's visual response to objects and whether followed by reaching, touching, and grasping attempts Ask parent about infant's opportunity for development of fine motor skills (eg, presence of cradle gym, mobile, or reachable hanging toys
Language development	Attends to noises and voices Responds differentially to voice of primary caregiver Pattern, pitch, and intensity of cry varies Begins prelanguage vocalization (small throaty noises and early cooing) Vocalizes more to primary caregiver	Listen to the infant's vocalizations in response to the parent or toy Ask whether the parent can differentiate pain and hunger Assess the quality and quantity of language stimulation
Cognitive development	Begins to replace reflex activity with more deliberate behavior Begins to repeat pleasurable chance movement (eg, thumb sucking, swiping at musical toy)	Observe difference in response between pacifier and thumb Observe ability to locate sound Ask the parent about quality and quantity of environmental stimulation
Social and affective development		
Infant	Watches faces intently and engages in eye contact Shows preferential behavior toward primary caregiver Occasionally smiles (birth to 6 weeks) Shows consistent social smile (6 to 8 weeks) Follows caregiver around room with eyes Shows increasingly predictable behavior and routines Cues increasingly clear Cries for increased periods Begin reciprocity in interaction with parents	Observe infant–parent interaction, the infant's attempts to initiate attention Ask the parent if infant is awake and alert for increasing periods
Parent	Holds the infant closely and securely Shows sensitivity to the infant's cues and responds appropriately Interacts reciprocally with the infant Maintains eye contact with the infant Takes pleasure from interacting with the infant Continues to feel fatigued because of night feedings Reports frustration caused by increased crying	Observe the parent's response to the infant's movements and vocalizations Ask the parent about adjustments to infant care

TABLE 16-8 Functional and Dysfunctional Parenting Behaviors

	Functional behaviors	Dysfunctional behaviors
Feeding	Offering appropriate amounts and/or types of food to the infant	Providing inadequate types, amounts, or temperatures of food for the infant
	Holding the infant in a comfortable position during feeding	Not holding the infant or holding the infant in an uncomfortable position during feeding
	Burping the infant during and after feeding	Not burping the infant
	Preparing food appropriately	Preparing food inappropriately
	Offering food at a comfortable pace for infant	Offering food at a pace that is too rapid or slow for the infant's comfort
		Propping the bottle
		Not responding to cues of satiety
Infant stimulation	Providing appropriate verbal stimulation for the infant during visit	Providing no stimulation or only aggressive verbal stimulation for the infant during visit
	Providing tactile stimulation for the infant at times other than during a feeding or moving the infant away from danger	Not providing tactile stimulation or providing only aggressive handling of the infant
	Providing age-appropriate toys	No evidence of age-appropriate toys
	Interacting with the infant in a way that satisfies the infant	Frustrating the infant during interactions
Infant rest	Providing a quiet or relaxed environment for the infant's rest, including scheduled rest periods	Not providing a quiet environment or a consistent schedule for rest periods
	Ensuring that the infant's needs for food, warmth, and/or dryness are met before sleep	Not attending to the infant's needs for food, warmth, and/or dryness before sleep
Perception	Demonstrating realistic perceptions of the infant's capacities, health, and safety needs	Showing unrealistic perceptions of the infant's capacities, health, and safety needs
	Realistic expectations of the infant	Unrealistic expectations of the infant
	Recognizing the infant's developing skills or behavior	No awareness of the infant's development
	Showing realistic perceptions of own parenting behavior	Showing unrealistic perceptions of own parenting behavior
Initiative	Initiative in attempts to manage the infant's problems, including actively seeking information about infants	No initiative in attempts to meet the infant's needs or to manage problems, not following through with plans
Recreation	Providing positive outlets for own recreation or relaxation	Not providing outlets for own recreation or relaxation
Interaction with other children	Demonstrating positive interaction with other children in the home	Demonstrating hostile or aggressive interaction with other children in the home
Nurturing role	Expressing satisfaction with parenting	Expressing dissatisfaction with parenting
	Speaks positively about the infant	Resents the time required for the infant's care

SOURCE: Adapted from Harrison L: Nursing intervention with a failure-to-thrive family. Copyright © 1974 American Journal of Nursing Co. Reproduced with permission from *Maternal/Child Nursing*, Vol. 1, No. 2.

The nurse assesses the infant's opportunities for practicing gross motor skills. Most parents automatically provide such opportunities in the following ways:

1. Placing the infant in the prone position at various times during the day
2. Supporting the infant in an erect or semierect position periodically (such as lap or an infant seat)
3. Pulling the infant to the sitting position occasionally

Other gross motor activity is still under reflex control

Fine Motor Skills As the infant approaches 3 months of age, the hands are open most of the time; prior to this the fists often are clenched. The palmar grasp reflex usually is gone or greatly diminished. The infant is likely to become excited when an object is presented, swiping at it and behaving as if wanting to grasp it; most infants, however, are unable to do this unless the object is placed in the hand. The infant is able to hold an object for a short time before dropping it. By 3 months of age, most infants can follow an attractive moving object for 180°.

The nurse assesses the activities that parents provide to support the development of fine motor skills and might encourage some parents to provide support for fine motor development. Opportunities routinely available in most homes to support fine motor development include the following:

1. Moving colorful objects slowly from side to side in the infant's line of vision (for example, mobiles)
2. Dangling toys within the infant's reach so that the infant can practice reaching
3. Allowing the infant to be with the family to observe people and activities

Language Development By 3 months of age, the infant attends carefully to noises and voices and responds differently to the familiar voice of the caregiver. The infant is able to coo and is likely to coo more for a familiar person. Parents often report that they can tell the difference between cries related to hunger and those caused by pain.

The nurse observes parental behavior that fosters language development. Such behaviors include the following:

1. Responding positively to the infant's attempts at vocalization
2. Encouraging the infant to vocalize by making simple sounds and waiting for the infant to "talk" back
3. Answering the infant's cues promptly

The speech that parents use when speaking to their infant is usually different from the speech used with other people. This special type of speech has been called "motherese" (Horowitz, 1982) and often involves a high-pitched voice, repetitive syllables, and special words. This special speech seems to be particularly attractive to infants and, when combined with gestures, serves to acquaint the infant with language.

Cognitive Development By 3 months of age, the infant has entered what Piaget termed the primary circular reactions stage (Piaget and Inhelder, 1969) and begins to replace reflexive behavior with deliberate activity (see Chapter 6). For example, the neonate generally turns to and attempts to suck any object that touches the lips or cheeks (such as a blanket), but by 3 months of age, infants are more discriminating and do not suck on objects that do not provide satisfaction, although they continue to put everything in their mouths. At this age, the infant also displays a beginning sense of causality and predictable sequence. For instance, a 2-month-old infant who is crying because of hunger often stops crying and begins sucking when the parent is heard approaching; the infant appears to anticipate eating. Infants generally find new sights and sounds exciting, and their hand–mouth movements generally have become smooth.

The nurse assesses the parent's awareness of the infant's emerging abilities and developing curiosity. Questions to open discussion might include the following:

1. What activity does your infant seem to enjoy the most?
2. What new things is the baby learning?

Social and Affective Development The progress of social development in the first 3 months of life is evident as the infant becomes more alert and responsive; these changes are very gratifying to the parent. Many infants occasionally smile during the early weeks of life, but a consistent social smile, which most parents find irresistible, generally appears around 8 weeks of age. The infant's cooing behavior is also exciting to parents, and many parents feel that the infant's preferential smiling and cooing is a reward for the hard work of the first weeks.

By 2–3 months of age, the infant sleeps longer at night, is awake more during the day, and is more alert when awake. The infant's patterns of eating, sleeping, and reacting to people, objects, and events are also more predictable. Infants are able to express their needs with better-differentiated cues that are read more easily by parents. Parents begin to recognize a wide variety of expressions—a happy face, a frown, a look of surprise, and expressions of soberness or wariness (Mendell and Yogman, 1982).

The increased clarity of the infant's cues and the parent's increasing ability to read the cues promote the development of a reciprocal relationship in which the parent and infant take turns attending and responding to each other. The sensitivity, intensity, and timing of these responses increases as parents learn to modify their behavior in response to their infant's cues. When a parent is sensitive to the infant and responds appropriately, the infant begins to act deliberately to influence the environment.

The nurse assesses the parents' sensitivity to the infant by noting their awareness of the infant's behavior and ability to recognize cues of hunger, fatigue, distress, or joy. As parent and child engage in a face-to-face interaction, the infant periodically becomes excited and might need to look away from the parent to control this excitement. After a short time, the infant will be ready to begin interacting again. A sensitive parent recognizes the infant's need to recover from the peak excitement and does not attempt to interact again until the infant shows readiness.

When infants are learning new skills, they sometimes persist in a behavior and are unable to stop themselves from repeating the activity until they begin to cry. Parents might need to learn to recognize such obligatory behavior and intervene before the infant becomes frustrated (Horowitz, 1982). For instance, a 2-month-old infant lying prone might repeatedly raise both head and chest to look around and may continue to do this even after becoming fatigued. The parent who recognizes the infant's inability to redirect activity intervenes and does this for the infant.

The nurse also assesses the impact of the infant on the parents' relationship and their relationships with any older children. The period of adjustment to new roles and expectations can be very stressful, and parents often give up doing activities together as they focus on the infant. Parents might need assistance in remaining sensitive to each other's needs and in nurturing their relationship. Older siblings might feel more threatened as the infant becomes more responsive and attracts more attention. Parents might feel guilty because they have less time to spend with older children, or they may begin to expect more of an older child.

If the infant is left with a caregiver other than a parent for a significant period of time, the nurse explores the quality of care the child receives.

The 3- to 6-Month-Old Infant

Normal behaviors associated with developmental areas are summarized in Table 16-9.

Temperament From 3 to 6 months of age, definite individual differences appear in the infant. The nurse therefore explores the infant's daily schedule, sleep habits, reactions to new foods (if these have been started), reactions to new people, situations, and objects, general activity level, and usual mood. The nurse directly observes the infant's response to being undressed and to procedures. At this stage, the Infant Temperament Questionnaire (Carey and McDevitt, 1978) might be useful in assessing temperament. This assessment tool asks parents to focus on specific infant behaviors and therefore provides some objectivity in a description of the infant, which can then be compared with the parent's more subjective report. If the parent's verbal description differs significantly from the objective description, the nurse needs to explore this discrepancy.

Because parents see that many of their infant's characteristics are not necessarily a result of their parenting, the nurse can use this analysis of the infant's temperamental qualities to help the parent better understand the infant's behavior.

Gross Motor Skills Between 3 and 6 months of age, the infant makes significant progress in gross motor development. Increased muscle strength allows the infant to hold the head steady, to sit, first with support and then briefly unassisted, to bear partial weight on the legs when held in a standing position, and to roll over, which allows the infant greater variety in position and activity.

The nurse might want to assess the parent's view of the significance of motor development. Because gross motor activity is so readily observable, it is often a standard by which parents compare children. Parents might become concerned if their infant's progress, although normal, is slower than another infant's. They might need reassurance that differences in the rates of development, within certain limits, are expected and that an infant who is less accomplished in one area of development generally is more accomplished in another area. Racial factors also might affect developmental rates, for example, gross motor development often is accelerated in black infants (Bayley, 1965).

Fine Motor Skills During this 3-month period, the infant makes significant gains in fine motor skills, progressing from clumsy and inaccurate batting maneuvers to reaching and grasping movements that are often successful. The increased ability to handle and explore many objects allows the infant to learn about the world. During assessment, the nurse can dangle interesting objects near the infant and observe the infant's ability to reach and grasp. Objects also can be placed near the infant and the infant's effort to obtain them observed.

The nurse also assesses the parent's awareness of the infant's fine motor skills and explores the kinds of objects available to the infant for exploration; these might include toys attached to the sides of the crib or objects stretched across the crib.

Language Development The infant continues to be interested and responsive to noises in the environment, and by 5 months of age is able to localize sounds made below the level of the ear. Infants use an increasing variety of tones, sounds, and intensities in their efforts to vocalize, but control over these variables might not be well established, and the young infant might become startled by making a noise that is louder than intended. The younger infant might try hard to make noise but be unable to produce audible sounds in the first attempts.

The nurse continues to assess the quality of verbal interchange between the parent and infant, noting whether the parent pays attention to the infant's vocalizations and evaluating the parent and infant's reciprocal responsiveness.

Cognitive Development Specific behaviors are often subtle and variable in infants 3–6 months of age, but the infant's ability to recognize familiar persons or objects is usually observable. The infant who sees a familiar object or person becomes excited and acts as if a particular event is anticipated. For example, if the infant sees and hears a parent approach, the infant is likely to become excited in anticipation of a pleasurable interchange. The infant also commonly demonstrates an awareness of his or her own body by gazing at the hands and touching the hands together, exploring one hand with the other. Infants in this stage are said to engage in activity more for the pleasure of the act than for the result. For example, young infants often vigorously and repeatedly kick their legs, even though the action does not produce any observable external response, which indicates that the act of kicking itself is pleasurable for the infant.

At about 4 months of age, the infant is likely to engage in an activity because it produces an interesting result. Piaget

TABLE 16-9 Guidelines for the Assessment of the 3- to 6-Month-Old Infant

Developmental area	Expected behaviors	Assessment techniques
Temperament	Parental perceptions of infant's temperamental characteristics	Ask the parent about the infant's temperament
Gross motor skills		
3 months	Minimal head lag Back rounded when supported in sitting position	Observe the infant's movements when prone, supine, and pulled to a sitting or standing position Ask the parent about the infant's opportunities to develop gross motor skills
4 months	Decrease in reflexes, increase in controlled movements Head steady when supported in sitting position Back less rounded when sitting Raises head and chest when prone, supporting weight on arms	
5 months	Rolls over intentionally Back straight when in a sitting position Bears most of weight when held in a standing position No head lag when pulled to a sitting position	
Fine motor skills		
3 months	Regards hand Grasp reflex disappears Begins to hit at objects, missing often Begins to reach for objects but does not usually obtain them	Ask the parent about the infant's opportunities to develop fine motor skills—types of toys preferred and available Observe the infant's ability to manipulate rattle, blocks, toys of different sizes
4 months	Brings hands together to midline Holds objects intentionally but is unable to let go Plays with object in hands Puts objects in mouth Begins to pick up objects, often misses Uses both hands when attempting to pick up object	
5 months	Picks up objects voluntarily, misses less frequently Alters hand position to accommodate size of object If holding one block, drops it to pick up another Plays with toes Regards hand less Begins thumb opposition in picking up object, but skill is not refined	
Language development		
3 months	Squeals, coos "Talks" when spoken to Searches for sound in room Localizes sound by turning head to side	Listen to the infant's verbalizations while playing with a toy or interacting with parent Ask the parent if the infant imitates sounds and differentiates human sounds
4 months	Laughs aloud Begins to use consonant sounds (h, n, k, g, p, b) Varies tone and intensity of vocalizations Varies quality of vocalizations with mood	
5 months	Localizes sound made below level of ear Uses simple vowel sounds such as "ah-goo"	Ask the parent about the quality and quantity of verbal interaction with the infant

TABLE 16-9 continued

Developmental area	Expected behaviors	Assessment techniques
Cognitive development		
3 months	Repeats behaviors found to be interesting Engages in activity more for the pleasure of the activity than the result Recognizes familiar faces and objects (such as a bottle or toy) Discovers parts of own body Does not search for objects dropped from sight	Observe the infant's use of objects, imitation of gesture Observe the infant's response to a hidden object Ask the parent to describe the infant's environmental stimulation, for example, how and where the infant spends day, toys, and individuals available for interaction
4–5 months	Directs interest toward result of action Attempts to maintain interesting events discovered by chance Becomes more skilled at grasping, mouthing Shows interest in novelty	
Social and affective development	Reciprocal interaction in parent–infant relationship (turn taking, infant's expecting response from parent, parental sensitivity to infant's cues) Preferential response to family members and especially primary caregiver Discriminates familiar persons from strangers Might show early stranger wariness	Observe parental response to infant distress and the infant's response to parental comforting

called this behavior secondary circular reaction (see Chapter 7). For example, if the infant accidentally kicks a mobile and causes a bell to ring, the infant attempts to kick the mobile again to reproduce this interesting result. Infants are aware of novelty in their environment and often regard new persons or objects with interest.

The nurse therefore assesses the parent's awareness of the infant's learning and attempts to support learning. Because cognitive changes are subtle, the parent might not recognize the infant's progress or understand the significance of new behavior. When the nurse demonstrates and interprets developing behaviors, the parent might find these new behaviors a source of pleasure and excitement.

Questions useful in assessing the parent's awareness of the infant's learning needs include the following:

1. What new things is the baby learning?
2. What type of activities does the infant seem to enjoy most?

In assessing the parent's responses, the nurse is also alert for signs of overstimulation or understimulation. Understimulation can occur when the infant is left to play alone for extended periods of time and has limited opportunities for interaction; overstimulation can occur when the infant is overwhelmed by a steady barrage of stimuli. Overstimulation makes it difficult for the infant to sort out significant from irrelevant occurrences. To some extent, overstimulation and understimulation are relative terms, and infants vary in their needs for amounts and types of stimulation. For example, the stimulation appropriate for an average infant might be too much for the hyperresponsive infant who has a low sensory threshold.

Social and Affective Development Reciprocity should be clearly evident in the parent–child interaction during this period because the infant and parent exhibit characteristic behaviors as they interact with each other. The infant's behavior with the parent is significantly different from the infant's behavior with a stranger, as the 6-month-old infant might begin to exhibit stranger wariness.

Brazelton and colleagues (1975) have studied the behavior of mothers and infants engaged in face-to-face encounters. These interactions are characterized by a marked sensitivity of each to the behavior of the other. The infant anticipates a specific type of interaction with the mother; therefore, the interaction has a certain rhythm of give and take. Three distinct phases mark this interaction as follows:

1. Engaging in the interaction with initial vocalization and smiles as faces brighten
2. Conducting a play dialogue that might include smiling, baby talk, and touching, which leads to great excitement on the infant's part
3. Disengaging briefly as the infant looks away and attempts to recover from the excitement

This characteristic cycle of engagement and disengagement might occur several times a minute and is a sign of positive attachment. Brazelton and colleagues (1975) also have studied what happens when the mother does not respond as the infant expects. When the mother presents

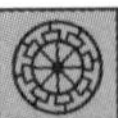

CASE STUDY Temperamentally Easygoing Four-Month-Old Infant

Assessment

Katy is a 4-month-old infant who was brought to the clinic for a routine well-child visit.

Family

Katy is the firstborn child of a nuclear family. The pregnancy was planned, and the parents read many books in preparation for her birth. The mother expresses concern about conflicting ideas presented in different books. She has no family members nearby to give advice or answer her questions. She asks whether Katy is progressing normally, because her neighbor's child, who is 5-months-old, seems to be doing many more things than Katy. The mother had no experience with infants prior to Katy.

Child

Katy was a full-term, healthy infant. She has grown steadily in weight and length, has remained healthy, has a good appetite, and has started sleeping through the night. The mother describes her as a "good, easy baby."

Environment

The family has recently purchased a 10-year-old house in a suburban neighborhood. Katy sleeps in a crib in her own bedroom. The mother describes Katy's room as colorful; there is a musical mobile on the crib and another above the changing table. Katy accompanies her mother to the store and on errands. She always is secured in an infant car seat when in the car or secured in her stroller when taken for a walk. Katy has a large variety of rattles, music boxes, stuffed animals, and other infant toys.

Clinical Data

Temperament: Katy is described as a happy infant who has a fairly predictable schedule for feeding, sleeping, and play periods. She has adapted well to new places and people and is easy to take visiting. The mother thinks that Katy prefers quiet, verbal games to active ones such as being bounced or swung in someone's arms.

Growth: Katy's length is 62 cm (24½ in); her weight is 6 kg (13 lb, 2 oz); her head circumference is 41 cm (16½ in).

Gross Motor Skills: Katy displays a very slight head lag when pulled to a sitting position. Generally wobbly, back rounded, but head steady when held by hands, Katy can be maintained in a sitting position briefly. She raises her chest up, supports self on arms, and looks around when placed prone. She turns from her back to side.

Fine Motor Skills: Katy looks at her hands, brings them together in front of her face, and puts them in her mouth. She reaches for and attempts to grasp a rattle but drops it; however, she grasps the rattle tightly when it is placed in her hand. She intently follows a toy for 180°. Katy manipulates a soft squeeze toy by bringing it to her mouth and turning it around in her hands.

Language Development: Katy squeals, coos, laughs, and plays with her voice. She varies the pitch and intensity of sounds in verbal play with her mother.

Cognitive Development: Katy demonstrates a preference for a new toy. She repeatedly shakes a small rattle that makes a musical sound. She obviously recognizes her mother. She searches briefly (looking around) for a dropped toy, then redirects her interest to another toy.

Social and Affective Development: The mother holds Katy securely and is sensitive to her needs and mood. There is reciprocal interaction between Katy and her mother, and they obviously enjoy playing together.

Comparison to a Standard

Katy's development at 4 months of age, when compared with the assessment guide and the standardized Denver Developmental Screening Test, is well within normal expectations. In addition, her general growth and health have been excellent, which further indicates that she is thriving.

Nursing Diagnoses

1. Potential for growth related to Katy's normal development, easy temperament, and positive reciprocal parent–child relationship.
2. Parental knowledge deficit related to lack of previous experience with infants, absence of nearby family members for consultation, and conflicting ideas obtained from books.

Plan for Interventions

Goals

1. Katy will continue to develop within normal expectations.
2. The mother will express confidence that Katy is developing normally.
3. The mother will express satisfaction with her parenting skills and understanding of normal growth and development.

Interventions

1. Discuss with Katy's mother her concerns about Katy's progress.
2. Discuss the individual differences in temperament, developmental progress, and the significant changes that occur within 1 month during the first year of life.
3. Demonstrate how Katy compares with the Denver Developmental Screening Test.
4. Praise the mother for positive parenting behaviors such as verbal play and sensitivity to Katy's cues.
5. Suggest pulling Katy up to a sitting position after diaper changes and supporting her in that position for a time while playing with her to strengthen her back muscles for sitting.
6. Provide anticipatory guidance about Katy's development during the next few months.
7. Encourage the mother to call if she has any questions or concerns about Katy or what she reads.
8. Invite the mother to attend a community group meeting of parents with young children.

a still and unresponsive face, the infant becomes concerned, tries to draw her into an interaction, and finally shows distress and confusion at her unresponsiveness and withdraws. This study suggests that infants clearly expect certain types of interaction with their parents.

Interactions between fathers and infants has not been studied as extensively as mother–infant interaction, but research indicates that reciprocity is also evident in the father–infant relationship, although mothers and fathers might interact differently with the infant. For example, mothers tend to use soft, repetitive talking more than fathers. Fathers tend to use more rhythmic tapping, poking, and physical games than mothers (Parke, 1979).

By this age, infants generally are on a predictable schedule and sleep through the night. Their cues usually are clearer, and parents have little trouble interpreting their infant's meaning. In assessing social development, the nurse therefore carefully observes the interaction between the infant and parent, eliciting information by comments such as the following:

1. Tell me what a day with the baby is like?
2. Show me how the baby talks to you.

The nurse also observes the parent's response to the infant's distress. Most parents display protectiveness and concern, and they attempt to comfort an infant quickly. The nurse then notes the infant's response to comforting. The nurse can further observe the infant's reaction to the nurse, who is a stranger; the infant usually prefers to interact with the parent, although some infants tolerate or even enjoy interacting with the nurse.

The 6- to 9-Month-Old Infant

The guidelines for assessing development in infants 6–9 months of age are summarized in Table 16-10.

Temperament By 6 months of age, definite temperamental characteristics usually are evident, and the parent is aware of the infant's individuality. The nurse assesses the infant's activity level; predictability of daily routine; sleep–wake patterns; responses to new situations, food, toys, and persons; general mood; responses to changes in surroundings; and ability to be distracted when engaged in interesting activities. The Infant Temperament Questionnaire (Carey and McDevitt, 1978) is a useful adjunct to the development history and the nurse's observations.

When describing their infant to the nurse, parents often appreciate having their perceptions validated. Nurses therefore might want to assure parents that they see the same temperamental traits the parents have described. The nurse also helps the parent to understand both positive and negative aspects of the infant's temperament. For example, persistence might seem negative when a child persists in screaming or refusing food, but the same quality is an asset as the child learns new skills. The persistent infant does not, for instance, give up trying to learn how to crawl after a few frustrating attempts to move to a desired destination such as following a favorite toy rolling across the floor.

As infants' emotions become more clearly expressed, they are able to communicate their likes and dislikes more effectively. Joy is evident as the infant interacts with a familiar person. Anger is often evident when play is interrupted.

Gross Motor Skills The ability to sit alone without support for long periods of time is an important milestone that allows the infant to use both hands to explore objects. The infant, who is also becoming increasingly mobile, is able to roll, shimmy, hitch, or crawl, so that, although the exact method of locomotion might vary, most infants manage to move purposefully. At 6 months of age, the infant crawls by pushing with the hands, moving backward; by 9 months of age, forward movement is accomplished.

Fine Motor Skills By 6–9 months of age, reaching and grasping are well developed, and the infant is learning new skills such as using the hands independently, unilateral reaching, and transferring objects from one hand to the other. These skills are assessed by a series of structured observations. The nurse first places two small blocks in front of the infant to see whether the infant will pick up both blocks. If the infant can do this, the nurse provides a more complex task by offering one small block to the infant. When the infant has grasped the block, the nurse then offers a second block within reach of the hand already holding the block. To take the second block, the infant must transfer the first block to the empty hand.

The nurse also observes the infant's ability to pick up a small object by placing a raisin on a table and observing whether the infant is able to grasp the raisin. At 6 months of age, infants use a raking movement that involves all the fingers, but by 9 months of age, they have mastered the pincer grasp.

Language Development Infants between 6 and 9 months of age are able to locate sounds accurately and begin to recognize familiar words, including their own name. Infants often seem to enjoy listening to their own voice.

The infant begins to combine vowels and consonants and to combine some syllables such as "mama" and "dada," although these sounds are not used in a meaningful way. Many infants begin to imitate such sounds as coughing or such easy syllables as "dada." The nurse might observe this ability by asking the parent to try to get the infant to repeat a sound because the infant more likely will imitate a familiar person.

The nurse should observe how the parent responds to the infant's vocalizations. Positive parental behaviors include

TABLE 16-10 Guidelines for the Assessment of the 6- to 9-Month-Old Infant

Developmental area	Expected behaviors	Assessment techniques
Temperament	Parental perceptions of the infant's temperamental characteristics	Ask the parent about the infant's temperament
Gross motor skills	Bears weight on legs when held No head lag when pulled to a sitting position Sits alone without suppport Stands holding on (75% of infants are able to do this by 9 months) Moves around by hitching, rolling, crawling, and creeping	Observe the infant sitting; ask the parent to estimate the length of time the child is able to sit before falling over Observe the infant's activity when prone; ask the parent about the infant's skill performance
Fine motor skills	Reaches and grasps well Picks up two blocks Transfers object from hand to hand Obtains small object using raking motion of fingers Improved finger–thumb opposition Turns wrists to better examine objects	Observe the infant's hand positions when reaching, grasping objects of different sizes Ask parent about the environment and opportunities to learn and practice new behaviors
Language development	Laughs and squeals Enjoys listening to own voice Combines vowels and consonants ("ga," "ba") "Talks" to toys Imitates sounds Combines syllables ("mama," "dada") Recognizes familiar words—own name Vocalizes emotions	Listen to the infant's vocalizations; assess the infant's ability to imitate sounds Observe the parent–infant verbal interaction Ask the parent how much time is spent "talking" to the infant
Cognitive development	Uses well-developed behaviors for mouthing, shaking, banging, and dropping when examining objects Looks for object that is dropped from sight Wary of strangers Imitates simple sounds and gestures Develops awareness of means-ends relationships Obtains object by pulling on string	Observe the infant's response to a hidden object Observe the infant's ability to repeat actions purposefully Ask the parent about the infant's play opportunities and the introduction of new toys or objects
Social and affective development	Reciprocity evident in parent–child relationship Displays more initiative in interactions and explorations Increasingly interested in objects Begins finger feeding of simple foods such as crackers Plays peek-a-boo Enjoys looking at self in mirror Demonstrates clear emotional states Communicates likes and dislikes Displays joy and anger Shows displeasure if activity is interrupted Aware of strangers	Observe parental response to the infant's initiative and infant's interest in objects Ask the parent how time is spent with infant, nature of activities, interaction

acknowledging the emotional tone of the baby's vocalization, naming objects of interest, and engaging in imitative verbal play with the infant.

Cognitive Development While continuing to learn specific behaviors for individual objects, the infant's repertoire for exploring these objects becomes more complex. The infant commonly mouths, pats, shakes, bangs, and drops objects while learning about their properties. In this stage the infant, who is beginning to grasp the concept of object permanence, recognizes an object when only part of it is visible, although this ability is still limited. For example, if a favorite toy is partially covered by a cloth, the infant recognizes certain visible parts and retrieves the object.

If part of a bottle is hidden but the nipple is showing, the infant is likely to recognize the bottle, but if only the middle of the bottle is exposed, recognition is less likely. The infant's focus is obtaining the object (result) independent of the means employed; any combination of means is used until the result is achieved.

Stranger awareness, which is primarily a social behavior, depends on cognitive development. A young infant views a stranger with interest but without wariness; however, between 6 and 9 months of age, the infant begins to react to a stranger with sober study, attempting to fit this new face into the scheme of faces that are already familiar. The infant who is unable to do this becomes anxious. Some infants become distressed and cry when a stranger appears.

The infant also demonstrates the ability to imitate simple behaviors and sounds. These behaviors might be difficult to elicit during an assessment, but parents frequently are able to report imitative behavior such as hand clapping, rattle shaking, or patting a pet.

Social and Affective Development After 6 months of age, the infant begins to display more initiative in eliciting and maintaining an interaction (Sanders, 1976). Reciprocity is still evident in the parent–infant relationship, but the nurse is likely to observe the infant taking the lead in games, such as toy toss or drop and fetch, stretching out arms to be picked up, and reaching up to play with the mother's face during feedings.

Infants also display more initiative in exploring the environment. As infants become more interested in their surroundings, their parents might feel that they are less interested in them. For example, an infant who previously was quiet and contented during a feeding is likely to interrupt the feeding to attend to some distraction in the environment. Infants who begin to use their fingers to feed themselves also generate ambivalence in their parents, who are excited by the infant's new development but also feel some sadness as the infant begins to show independence.

The nurse therefore assesses not only the infant's initiative in interactions and interest in objects but also the parent's response to these behaviors. Discussions of the infant's mobility or feeding behavior might provide relevant information. The nurse also observes the infant's initiative in exploring the assessment setting and observes the parent's response to the infant's efforts. If this exploration does not occur spontaneously, the nurse might place an interesting object near the infant and watch the infant's response, which also might provide a means of discussing the parent's feelings about the infant's interests and explorations.

If the infant is regularly cared for by a babysitter or at a day-care center, the nurse assesses the infant's response to being left, the parent's response to leaving the infant, and the infant's interactions with the babysitter or day-care center staff.

The 9- to 12-Month-Old Infant

Guidelines for assessing the 9- to 12-month-old infant are summarized in Table 16-11.

Temperament Although the infant's temperamental characteristics are fairly stable by 9 months of age, the manifestations of these characteristics change as the infant matures, and at each age, the infant's temperamental characteristics present new issues and challenges for the parent. For example, high activity levels might cause parental concern. A young infant who is temperamentally active typically does a lot of arm waving, leg kicking, rolling, and wiggling, but the parent usually manages these activities satisfactorily. As this infant approaches 1 year of age and begins to crawl or walk, however, the parent faces new challenges. An active infant, whose judgment obviously is limited, is likely to encounter hazardous situations and can cause stress for the parent.

The nurse assesses both how the infant's temperament affects the infant's approach to developmental tasks and how the parent perceives and responds to the infant's behavior. Some infants typically withdraw in new situations and have difficulty adapting to change. When such an infant enters this stage of development, in which stranger wariness is common, the infant's responses might seem more extreme, and the infant may take longer to adjust to new people. The Infant Temperament Questionnaire (Carey and McDevitt, 1978) is a useful assessment tool for this age.

Gross Motor Skills Most infants at this stage creep with their stomachs off the ground, but some infants continue to crawl on their stomachs, and some progress directly to walking without ever really creeping. Whatever the method, however, the infant's mobility opens new areas for exploration and provides new learning experiences.

Infants at this age are very skilled at sitting and can lean and twist without losing their balance. Pulling up to a standing position and walking along holding onto furniture then become exciting activities. Some parents report that their infants even practice these skills at night in the crib, waking the parents up when they pull themselves up to stand and are unable to sit down again.

The nurse can readily assess these behaviors by giving the child time to become accustomed to the surroundings and the freedom to move around. Most infants usually spontaneously demonstrate motor accomplishments as they move from one area to another exploring the environment and investigating new objects. Also important is the parent's responses to the infant's motor skills. Most parents find these skills exciting, but some parents are disturbed by their infant's explorations and might try to limit their activity by using a playpen or by discipline. The nurse then might have to explain that exploring is a necessary part of the infant's developmental progress.

TABLE 16-11 Guidelines for the Assessment of the 9- to 12-Month-Old Infant

Developmental area	Expected behaviors	Assessment techniques
Temperament		Assess the infant's temperamental characteristics; discuss parental perceptions
Gross motor skills	Sits steadily; twists around without falling, rights self if falls	Place the infant in a sitting position, place an interesting object on side and toward back of the infant; observe whether the infant obtains the object
	Gets to a sitting position from a lying position	Observe; ask the parent whether the infant does each behavior
	Pulls to a standing position; sits down with a bump	
	Stands alone either momentarily or longer	
	Creeps with abdomen off the floor	
	"Walks" holding onto furniture	
	Walks with help	Hold the infant's hands and observe walking, assess parental responses to increased motor activity
	Might take first step	
Fine motor skills	Bangs two objects together	Give the infant two blocks and observe activity; may demonstrate activity first
	Thumb–finger grasp	Place a small object such as a raisin on the table and observe how the infant picks up the object
	Puts objects into a container	Provide small objects and a container and see whether the infant puts objects into the container
Language development	Might say "mama" and "dada" specifically	Observe; ask the parent about the infant's vocabulary
	Uses expressive sounds	
	Continues to imitate speech sounds	Have the parent present simple speech sounds and see whether the child repeats the sounds
	Understands simple words (5 words by 12 months of age)	Ask the parent whether the infant consistently responds to specific words
		Assess the quality of communication between the parent and infant
Cognitive development	Continues to be interested in environment	Observe exploratory behavior and assess parental response to the infant's exploratory efforts
	Displays intentional behavior	See whether the infant purposefully seeks an interesting experience
	Imitates novel behavior	Ask the parent to perform simple activity (something the infant does not ordinarily do) and to get the infant to imitate
	Associates symbols with events	Ask the parent whether the infant understands simple expressions like "pat-a-cake" and "bye-bye"
	Differentiates means and ends	Place a toy out of reach of the infant with a string attached to the toy and near the infant, see whether the infant obtains the toy
	Searches for a hidden object	Show an interesting toy to the infant, then cover it with a cloth, see whether the infant uncovers the object
		Assess opportunities for cognitive growth
		Assess parental awareness of the infant's developmental interests
Social and affective development	Many infants show a heightened attachment to mother	Assess parent–child interaction, assess the infant's use of the parent (especially the mother) as a resource, assess parental response to the infant's focus on primary caregiver
	Shows separation anxiety	Discuss the infant's behavior at separation with the mother; discuss parental responses to separations

TABLE 16-11 continued

Developmental area	Expected behaviors	Assessment techniques
	Protests at bedtime or awakens during night	Assess sleep patterns, discuss how the parent manages protest at bedtime or night waking (if these are concerns)
	Begins self-feeding	Discuss with parent whether the infant feeds self
	Shows sensitivity to approval or disapproval	Assess the infant's response when the parent says "no"; assess parental perceptions of and response to infant "misbehavior"
	Affection	Observe interaction
	Enjoys simple games	

Fine Motor Skills The infant at this age should be able to bang two blocks together. The nurse tests this ability by putting a block in each of the infant's hands, demonstrating the banging maneuver, and observing the infant's actions.

To test the infant's grasping ability, a small edible object such as a raisin or piece of prepared cereal (for example, Cheerios®) can be placed on the table in front of the infant. The nurse then notes the precision with which the infant picks up the object. By 12 months of age, the infant should use a neat pincer motion of the thumb and index finger.

The nurse further tests fine motor function by having the child put small objects into a container with a 2- to 3-in opening, a skill that can be demonstrated first so that the child gets the idea.

Language Development Much of language assessment depends on reports from the parent because most infants do not freely verbalize in a strange situation. Most infants use "mama" and "dada" appropriately by 12 months of age, and some infants also use other single words. At 12 months of age, a five-word vocabulary consists mostly of nouns. Infants continue to imitate speech, and imitation often becomes a favorite game. In observing this behavior the nurse has the parent present the sound to be imitated because the infant is more likely to imitate sounds for a familiar person.

Infants at this age use expressive jargon, which often sounds conversational except that the words are unintelligible. Variations in tone, inflection, volume, and rhythm are all present. Because understanding (receptive) language precedes using (expressive) language, infants often comprehend several simple words such as "bye-bye" and "no, no." The parent can report to which words the infant consistently responds.

An infant who does not respond to verbalizations and does not babble actively should be assessed for hearing loss. The nurse also assesses the quality of communication between the parent and child, noting both the parent's and infant's awareness and responsiveness. The content of the parent's speech to the child also should be noted. Some parents provide rich explanations that enhance language development, whereas other parents use more restrictive communication, with few explanations and many commands.

Cognitive Development Curiosity is a predominant characteristic and is usually evident if the child is given the freedom to explore. During the assessment, the nurse might have a couple of safe and attractive objects available to the infant. The nurse observes how the infant approaches the objects and how the parent responds (whether the parent encourages the infant to attain and explore the objects or curtails the infant's activity). The infant's approach to examining objects is fairly systematic and commonly includes mouthing, banging, and shaking.

Infants at this stage are clearly purposeful in seeking an interesting object. Earlier, the infant discovered interesting actions by chance and then repeated or maintained those actions; now the infant aggressively pursues and manipulates the object with the intent of eliciting an interesting response. If something is in the way, the infant will work to get around it. Intentionality is also evident in the parent–infant relationship. For example, the infant who feels that the parent might be leaving acts intentionally to make the parent stay. The parent can be asked, "How does your infant behave when you are preparing to go out alone?" In addition to providing information about the infant's cognitive strategies, this also elicits information about the parent–infant relationship and how each manages separation.

At this age, the infant can imitate novel behavior, which is best elicited by a familiar person. The nurse therefore asks the parent to perform a specific behavior for the infant to imitate. Any number of behaviors are appropriate to elicit imitation as long as the infant does not routinely do them and they are not too complex. Patting a doll, patting the stomach, and making simple sounds are all appropriate.

Simple differentiation of means and ends is evident when the infant pulls on a string to obtain a toy. For a younger infant, the string is only a string. For the infant at this stage, the string is a means to get the toy. The nurse can test this by placing a toy out of reach, leaving the string near the child's hand, and observing the infant's behavior.

The nurse also might observe how the infant associates symbols with certain events. For example, the words "pat-a-cake" might elicit the typical clapping behavior; "bye-bye" might be associated with someone leaving.

Finally, the nurse assesses the child's learning environment. This would include the parent's response to exploratory behavior, the types of objects available for exploration, the infant's freedom to explore, parental awareness of the infant's development and learning needs, and how parents promote infant learning.

Assessment questions might include the following:

1. What new things is the child learning?
2. What is the child most interested in?

Social and Affective Development From 9 to 12 months of age, the infant demonstrates increasing interest in the environment. Many infants also display a heightened attachment to the parent or, as Sanders (1976) termed it, "refocalization on the mother." The infant displays a desire for frequent and close contact and is often very demanding of parental attention, particularly during periods of stress. Some infants clearly prefer their mothers over other family members, and, although they might previously have accepted care and comfort from other family members, they are now satisfied only with their mothers.

If this behavior occurs, the nurse explores the parent's reactions. Some mothers find this intense type of relationship with the infant satisfying and respond with flexibility to the infant's demands. Other mothers might find the infant's expectations overwhelming and resent the infant's demands on their attention and time. Some mothers might fear that the infant's clinginess or dependency at this stage will become a permanent personality trait. Such mothers might resist meeting the infant's demands and may actually back off from their infant emotionally. Although some limit setting is appropriate at this stage, a mother who does not make herself somewhat available to the infant may not be providing the secure base an infant needs to be able to explore freely in the future.

In addition, the nurse assesses other family members' feelings about the infant's intense focus on the mother. Fathers might feel left out or rejected. Other siblings may resent the amount of time and attention the mother devotes to the infant and might become jealous. In the assessment setting the nurse can use the infant's stranger wariness and dependence on the parent as a focus for discussing these issues.

Separation becomes a key issue in this stage (see Chapter 7). Infants often protest vigorously when parents prepare to leave. After the parents have left, some infants continue to cry during the entire separation. Some infants act sad and despondent, whereas others resume their normal functioning. The more familiar the babysitter, the less severe the reaction, but parents generally are distressed about leaving an infant who is so obviously upset. Some parents feel guilty about going away and choose not to leave at all. The nurse therefore explores how the infant reacts to separations, how the parents feel about separations, and what measures the parents use to minimize the infant's distress.

The nurse also assesses the infant's sleep behavior at this age. Bedtime is a form of separation, and many infants react to it as such. Infants might protest at bedtime. Some infants awaken during the night and cry for attention, seeking to reestablish contact with the parent. Ideally, parents should not reinforce this behavior, encouraging the infant instead to return to sleep alone.

Autonomy begins to become important at this stage. Infants usually are interested in self-feeding, and parents should allow the infant independence in this area. Many parents and infants work out a compromise in which the infant self-feeds certain types of food while the parent interjects spoonfuls of other foods.

The nurse assesses how the parent perceives and handles the infant's "misbehavior." Infants at this age usually are quite sensitive to approval or disapproval of others. They commonly understand the meaning of "no" and might feel very distressed if scolded. They do not, however, recall which actions are forbidden or have the self-control to regulate their actions.

The 12- to 24-Month-Old Child

The guidelines for assessing the 1- to 2-year-old are summarized in Tables 16-12 and 16-13.

Temperament As the child begins to struggle with the issue of autonomy, common behavioral expressions include negativism and emotional lability. A temperamentally negative child might seem particularly difficult. Likewise, a child who has difficulty adjusting to change might seem rigid and inflexible. Children between 1 and 2 years of age are often considered hyperactive by their parents, who sometimes need to understand that activity and ritualistic behavior are normal and that these particular characteristics are neither good nor bad.

The nurse begins to assess the parent's perceptions of the child's temperamental qualities with questions such as, "What are the qualities you like the most in your child?" or "What things about your child do you find to be most troublesome?"

Gross Motor Skills Between 12 and 15 months of age, most infants begin to walk. By 18 months of age, children generally walk well, although they may have difficulty walking around corners, stopping suddenly, or navigating around obstacles. By 15 months of age, nearly all children can stoop and recover objects from the floor without holding onto a support.

Between 18 and 24 months of age, most children learn to run, walk backward, and kick a ball without falling. They

TABLE 16-12 Guidelines for the Assessment of the 12- to 18-Month-Old Infant

Developmental area	Expected behaviors	Assessment techniques
Temperament		Assess temperamental characteristics of the infant; discuss parental perceptions of temperament
Gross motor skills	Stands alone	Observe the infant in a standing position
	Walks well	Observe the infant's gait
	Creeps up stairs	Ask the parent whether the infant creeps up stairs or climbs on furniture
	Stoops to recover an object on the floor	While the infant is standing, drop a toy on the floor near the feet and observe how the child obtains toy
	Throws objects but might fall in the process	
	Has difficulty walking around corners or stopping suddenly	Discuss with the parents the infant's opportunities to develop gross motor skills
Fine motor skills	Builds tower of two blocks	Present two blocks and demonstrate how to stack, observe the infant's ability
	Drinks from cup	Observe or ask the parent how well the infant drinks unaided
	Uses spoon without rotating the wrist, spills when bringing utensils to mouth	Observe or ask the parent whether the infant uses a spoon and the amount of spillage
	Scribbles spontaneously	Offer paper and crayon or pencil
	Removes shoes and socks	
	Turns pages in heavy cardboard book	Offer child heavy cardboard book and observe
Language development	Uses expressive sounds	Listen to the quality of verbalization
	Uses gestures to ask for objects	Ask the parent how the infant indicates wishes and observe the infant's gestures
	Shakes head "no"	Observe or ask the parent
	Says several intelligible words	Observe for the use of words, ask the parent whether the infant uses words
		Observe parental response to verbalization and the quality of parent–infant verbal interactions
Cognitive development	Continues curiosity and exploration	Ask the parent about the infant's exploratory efforts; assess how parent feels about the infant's explorations and the amount of freedom the infant is given to explore
		Assess parental awareness of child's development
	Interest in books	Offer child simple, colorful book and observe response
	Finds hidden object with successive visible displacements	Place an interesting, visible toy under cover; then move under another cover and drop while infant watches and with toy visible; see whether the infant locates the toy; allow several tries if necessary
	Inserts circle into formboard or puzzle	Present formboard without circle and see whether the infant can insert the circle into the formboard
	Imitates behavior of parent (such as housework)	Ask the parent for examples of imitations
		Assess opportunity for cognitive growth
		Assess parental response to exploratory behavior
Social and affective development	Increasing autonomy	Assess parental feelings regarding the infant's increasing autonomy
	Ventures away from parent to explore but returns frequently for reassurance	Observe the infant's exploratory behavior in the assessment setting
	Tolerates separations better than before	Discuss with the parent how the infant reacts to separations, how parents feel about separations, and how frequently separations occur; observe separation directly, noting the behavior of both the parent and child during leave taking, behavior of both during separation, and child's ability to play, interact,

continued on next page

TABLE 16-12 continued

Developmental area	Expected behaviors	Assessment techniques
Social and affective development (cont.)		and be comforted in the absence of the parent; note their behavior when reunited
	Temper tantrums might occur	Assess frequency and intensity of tantrums, assess parental response
	Feeds self, usually refuses attempts of others to feed	Discuss mealtime behavior; assess parental attitudes regarding infant's self-feeding
	Protests at bedtime	Assess sleep behavior, noting especially protest or night waking and parental reactions
	Notices strangers but is less wary than before	Observe child's reaction to nurse
	Affectionate and loving; might kiss and hug parent	Observe interaction, noting affectionate interchanges, who initiates them, and how the infant and parent respond
	Changes moods quickly and frequently (emotional lability)	Assess parental reaction to the infant's mood changes
	Begins to be provocative; purposely does things that are forbidden and watches for parental response	Assess parental reactions to "misbehavior"; discuss parental discipline and the infant's response, observe parental limit setting and reactions to the infant's breaking the limit

are generally able to walk up stairs with one hand held but often crawl down stairs. During this time, children also learn to sit on small chairs or objects, a difficult task because the child cannot look at the chair and sit down on it at the same time. Children spend considerable time and energy mastering this skill.

The parent can describe the child's ability to climb, but the nurse often can observe this skill in the assessment setting. Because children generally learn to climb up before they can climb down, they periodically find themselves stranded. The nurse might find teaching about safety especially important at this stage (see Chapter 19). Most children at this age are so motivated to master motor skills that they use any and all opportunities to do so.

The nurse assesses the parent's attitude toward the child's motor development. Some parents find it difficult to tolerate the child's constant activity and might attempt to limit it with a playpen or other device. Although these might be convenient for parents, they may not provide the assumed measure of safety because many children learn to climb out of them. In addition, excessive use of these devices might affect the child's development adversely by limiting the opportunities to practice motor skills. Some parents are concerned about their children's many falls and might attempt to limit motor activity to protect the child, a type of overprotection that also may affect the child's development adversely. If they are to master basic motor skills, children need opportunities to practice.

Fine Motor Skills Between 9 and 12 months of age, the infant masters prehension; between 12 and 18 months of age, the infant masters the ability to control the release of an object, a skill most easily demonstrated by stacking blocks. The infant must pick the block up correctly, place it appropriately, and release it carefully. The 18-month-old infant should be able to stack one block on another.

Infants 12 to 18 months old who have been exposed to paper and pencil usually can scribble spontaneously. They also can turn the pages of a heavy cardboard or thick plastic book. By 16 months of age, most infants drink well from a cup. They also can use a spoon but often spill as the spoon approaches the mouth. They also are able to remove their shoes and socks.

By 24 months of age, prehension and release are well controlled. The 2-year-old can stack three to four blocks and pick up very small objects using precise prehension. Some children can draw straight lines as well as scribble and can use spoons with little spillage. They also are able to turn the thin pages in a book or magazine, perhaps two to three at a time.

Language Development Language development marks the transition from infancy to early childhood (see Chapter 8). The average 12-month-old uses expressive jibberish much of the time and speaks perhaps one or two words. By 24 months of age, the average child uses about 300 words, and most children of this age are able to combine two to three words in a phrase. Between 12 and 15 months of age, most infants gesture for what they want and usually are able to shake their heads "no." By 24 months of age, most ask for what they want by name. The 2-year-old should be able to point to a part of the body when asked. Many children between 18 and 24 months of age can name common objects when shown pictures (ball, dog, etc), and some children are able to follow simple directions such as "give the ball to mommy." Because the child must

TABLE 16-13 Guidelines for the Assessment of the 18- to 24-Month-Old Child

Developmental area	Expected behaviors	Assessment techniques
Temperament		Discuss temperamental characteristics of the child and parental perceptions
Gross motor skills	Runs clumsily	Observe the child's running or ask parent to describe
	Pushes and pulls toys	Provide push toy for the child
	Seats self on small chair	Provide small object for the child to sit on or ask parent whether child does this
	Walks backward	Observe the child walking backward
	Kicks ball forward	Demonstrate kicking a ball and tell the child to do this
	Walks up steps with one hand held	Ask the parent how the child manages stairs
		Discuss with the parent the child's opportunities to develop gross motor skills
Fine motor skills	Builds tower of three to four blocks	Provide blocks and demonstrate stacking
	Grasp and release are well controlled	Observe the child picking up a small object and the release of blocks when stacking
	Attempts to imitate drawing straight line	Provide paper and crayon, demonstrate a line, and ask the child to draw
	Uses spoon with little spilling	Ask the parent to describe the child's skill at eating
	Turns pages in book, may turn two to three at a time	Provide book and observe how the child handles it
Language development	Uses several single words	Listen to the child's verbalizations and ask the parent what words the child uses
	Combines two words in a phrase	Ask the parent whether the child combines two or more words
	Points to body part	Ask the child (or have the parent ask the child) to point to eyes or nose
	Names an object	Show the child a picture of a common, interesting object and ask the child to name it
	Follows simple directions	Tell the child to "take the ball (or other object) to mother"; "give it to me," or "put the ball on the table"
		Observe the quantity and character of the verbal interchanges between the parent and child
Cognitive development	Dumps a raisin from a bottle spontaneously or with demonstration	Place a raisin in a bottle and tell the child to get it out, may demonstrate
	Locates hidden object with invisible displacements	Place a small screen in front of the child, put a toy in a small cup, put the cup behind a screen and dump the toy, show the child the empty cup and observe the child's reaction; the child should locate the toy behind the screen; ask the parent whether the child goes through cupboards to get objects
	Obtains an object by using a tool	Place an interesting toy on a table just out of reach, place a toy rake or stick near the child and observe whether the child uses a rake to obtain the toy; may demonstrate; ask the parent whether the child drags a chair across the room to climb and obtain an object that is out of reach
	Deferred imitation	Ask the parent whether the child imitates nonpresent behaviors
	Begins to "pretend"	Ask the parent whether the child does any simple "pretending" behaviors
	Infers a cause while only seeing an effect	Watch for behavior during assessment

continued on next page

TABLE 16-13 continued

Developmental area	Expected behaviors	Assessment techniques
		Assess the child's learning environment (parental encouragement, appropriate toys, books)
		Assess parental response to exploratory behavior
Social and affective development	Increasing autonomy but continues marked dependence on parent	Assess parental feelings about child's increasing independence
	Insists on self-feeding	Assess feeding situation, noting particularly whether the child feeds self independently and how the parent handles food refusal
	Beginning negativism, temper tantrums	Ask the parent whether the child is becoming more negative, assess the frequency and intensity of temper tantrums, assess parental response
	Separation anxiety but the child is learning to cope better	Discuss the child's behavior during separation, ask the parent to compare the child's current behavior with behavior at an earlier age to identify evidence of more adaptive coping, assess the parental reaction to separation
	Uses "transitional objects" for comfort	Ask whether child has a "security" object and the situations in which it is used, assess the parents' perception of a transitional object
	May begin to be ritualistic	Ask the parent about family routines and how the child responds if routines are altered
	Changes moods rapidly and frequently (emotional lability)	Discuss the child's mood changes with the parent, assess parental perceptions and reactions
	Understands most limits but does not have self-control	Discuss with the parent the limit set, how the child responds, and what happens if the child disobeys and assess the parent's perception of the child's "misbehavior"
	Begins to be possessive	Ask the parent whether the child demonstrates possessiveness, ask the child to give the nurse an object (shoe or toy) and see how the child responds
	May indicate readiness for toilet training	Discuss parental views concerning toilet training techniques and how to handle accidents; assess the child for signs of readiness

hear clearly to develop language skills, the nurse is alert for any signs of hearing impairment.

The quality of language to which the child is exposed is a significant determinant of the child's language skills. Children whose parents use language well, talk frequently to the child, name objects, explain events, and read stories develop better language abilities than children whose parents do not support language development in these ways.

Cognitive Development During this stage, which Piaget termed tertiary circular reactions (see Chapter 6), the infant is interested in exploring the environment and discovering new means of solving problems. The infant uses trial and error in learning about relationships between things. By 18 months of age, most children are able to locate a hidden object, although between 12 and 18 months of age, the infant must watch the object being hidden in one location and then in another to locate the object correctly in the second location because a mental image of the object can be retained only when the object is visible. During this stage, infants also are increasingly aware of geometric shapes. By 15–18 months of age, the infant should be able to insert a circle in a formboard and imitate more complex behavior such as housework.

Between 18 and 24 months of age, the child learns to solve problems through what Piaget called mental combinations. The child is thus able to begin to find solutions mentally. For example, when given a small-necked bottle with a raisin inside, a younger child typically tries to remove the raisin by poking a finger into the bottle or shaking the bottle, but the 2-year-old more often examines the bottle and then dumps the raisln out.

Between 18 and 24 months of age, children can readily differentiate means from ends and can use tools to obtain an object. The nurse assesses this skill by placing a toy on a table within sight but out of reach of the child. A toy rake or stick is then placed near the child, and the nurse observes whether the child uses the tool to reach the object. Parents also might report that their child use tools at home. A child might, for example, drag a chair over to a counter and climb on it to obtain something out of reach.

The child between 18 and 24 months of age also is able to locate a hidden object without having seen it hidden. To assess this ability, a small screen is placed in front of the child, and an interesting toy is placed in a cup. The cup is then placed behind the screen, and the toy is dumped out. The child is unable to see what has happened behind the screen, but the empty cup is shown to the child, who should be able to locate the toy. To do this successfully, the child must be able to follow the progress of the toy and infer its location. Parents often report evidence of object permanence, noting that children know where certain household items are stored and where to go to find them.

The child's ability to imitate also becomes more refined in this stage; therefore, children imitate not only new behaviors but also previously witnessed behaviors, a skill termed *deferred imitation*. For example, the child might observe another child sitting on a potty chair and imitate this behavior a few days later. Deferred imitation requires that the child be able to remember the behavior and imitate it from memory. The ability to use mental representations (that is, to symbolize) is further evident in children's simple pretend games. For example, the child might put a doll to bed and cover the doll with a small cloth, indicating the ability to recall and imitate a behavior pattern.

Two-year-olds can discern simple cause-and-effect relationships, a skill that can be tested by using a toy activated by a squeeze bulb. The child watches the toy move when the bulb is squeezed and should relate the squeezing and movement well enough to make the toy move it in the same way. The child might need several tries to accomplish this.

Social and Affective Development Because autonomy is the major issue in the second year of life, the child's struggle for self-determination is reflected in much day-to-day behavior. Autonomy is an emotionally charged issue for both the parent and child; therefore, the nurse needs to assess their handling of the issue. Children attempt to define themselves as separate and independent from their parents, but they continue to be dependent on their parents and to need parental attention, approval, and acceptance (see Chapter 8).

Many parents feel somewhat ambivalent about their children's increasing independence. Some parents express sadness that the child is "growing up so fast" and is no longer a baby but also might be excited and pleased by the child's increasing competence and new skills. Parents who find it hard to relinquish the closeness of infancy might attempt to prolong that closeness and in the process undermine the child's attempts at autonomy. Questions that may open this area for discussion include the following:

1. As you watch your child becoming more independent, how does it make you feel?

2. Have you noticed changes in your relationship with your child?

The child ventures farther from the parent but continues to seek frequent contact and reassurance. Research by Ainsworth (1973) suggested that a stable relationship between the parent and child provides a secure base from which the child may explore but to which the child can return with confidence. The nurse observes the extent of the child's exploratory behavior, how far the child ventures from the parent, and how the child maintains contact with the parent. This information should be interpreted carefully, however, because unfamiliar surroundings and the presence of a stranger might inhibit the child's normal behavior.

Negativism, one manifestation of autonomy, appears around 15 months of age as most infants begin to shake their heads "no." By 18–20 months of age, most children are likely to say "no" even when their actions indicate "yes" (see Chapter 8). Parents might become confused, uncertain, or upset as they watch agreeable, pleasant infants become negative and resistant. The nurse therefore assesses the parent's interpretation and response to the child's negativism and resistance. Parents who understand that negative behavior is a manifestation of the child's attempts to be more independent are likely to allow the child to do things unaided and prevent unnecessary frustrations by maintaining appropriate limits. Parents who view negativism as a challenge to their authority might react by "cracking down" and insisting on compliance, resulting in more intense resistance or in the child's suppressing the quest for autonomy. Parents who feel threatened by this behavior might give in to unreasonable demands to avoid a confrontation; the child, however, is unable to make reasonable decisions and needs adults to set limits, without which autonomy can be frightening. (Parental management of temper tantrums is discussed in Chapter 13.)

Questions that address these concerns include the following:

1. What is the most difficult thing about having a child this age?
2. Does the child say 'no' yet? How often? In what situations?
3. Why do you think the child does this?
4. How do you handle it when your child refuses to do something you feel is important?

Feedings are times in which the child usually strives for independence. The 12- to 14-month-old infant might be fed willingly; however, by 18 months of age, most children insist on feeding themselves. In discussing feeding the nurse often learns how the parent feels about and responds to the child's developing autonomy and increased demands. The nurse assesses mealtime practices such as who feeds the child and what happens if the child refuses to eat either a particular food or a whole meal. Parents are encouraged to allow children to feed themselves in spite of the messiness and to refrain from coercing children to eat what they do not like or want. On the other hand, children should not dominate mealtime and can adhere to reasonable limits such as not eating sweets until the end of the meal and not throwing food.

Most infants between 12 and 15 months of age are ready to give up the bottle and take pride in using a cup. When a child over 18 months of age is using a bottle, the nurse needs to assess the reasons. (Weaning is discussed in Chapter 15.) The child should no longer need a bottle for the gratification of sucking and should be able to use a cup, but children occasionally use the bottle as a comfort measure. The parent might find it easier to use a bottle to deal with the child's demands than to give more appropriate forms of attention or may use the bottle to keep the child a "baby."

The nurse explores bedtime routines, how the family responds to the child's protests, and how the family responds if the child awakens during the night. (Parental management of bedtime problems is discussed in Chapter 13.) Frequent nightmares or night terrors should be investigated more thoroughly.

If separation continues to be difficult, the nurse assesses how the child reacts before, during, and after separation. Equally important are parental feelings and reactions about separation, the frequency with which separations occur, and the quality of care provided during the parent's absence. Children who are left consistently with a warm and nurturing caregiver might show little distress when separated from the parent, but a child who is rarely separated from the parent may react much more strongly. A young child's protest at separation is usually an appropriate, adaptive coping strategy, which the parent should recognize as such (see Chapter 12). Most children are better able to tolerate separations as they approach 2 years of age. They realize that their parents continue to exist after leaving and learn that their parents always return. Developing language skills (for example, "Mama bye bye") also helps the child to control the experience and anticipate the parent's return.

The nurse might ask the parent to leave the room to observe the response to separation directly. This should be done only at the end of the assessment because reestablishing rapport with the child might be difficult. Such direct observation might clarify separation issues. For example, one mother described her child's negative reactions to separation at length and stated that the child made such a scene that it was not worth trying to leave him. The nurse asked the mother to leave the room for a few minutes so the nurse could assess the child's behavior. The mother spent a lot of time telling the child she would leave but would be back soon, hugged the child several times, and then returned for one more hug just before leaving. After the mother left, the child cried for a short time but accepted comfort from the nurse. He looked frequently toward the door where his mother had left but continued to play. The mother opened the door twice during the 5 minutes to see whether the child was all right, and each time his play was disrupted, he cried and reached for her. The assessment clarified to the nurse that the mother was so uncomfortable about separation that it seemed to be more of a problem for her than for her son. These observations led to a discussion between the nurse and mother that revealed the mother's ambivalence and guilt about leaving the child while she worked and her fear that her absence eventually would harm the child emotionally. Direct observation thus provided data essential to understanding the problem and developing an effective intervention strategy.

Transitional objects are another way in which a child copes with stress at this stage. The use of "security" objects (blankets, toys) or comfort measures (sucking thumbs, curling hair) provide a source of comfort to the child when the parent is unavailable for support and are useful as an adaptive strategy (see Chapter 8). The nurse might need to assess how the parent views such an object; an occasional parent discourages this strategy because it seems "babyish."

The assessment setting provides an ideal opportunity to observe the parent's attempts to control the child's behavior and how inappropriate behavior is handled. For example, if the child attempts to open an equipment drawer, the nurse can observe how the parent intervenes. Does the parent allow the child to explore until there is an actual risk of damage or danger, or does the parent attempt to inhibit the behavior immediately? Does the parent verbally reprimand the child and expect instant obedience or reinforce the verbal message by removing the child from the situation? Is the parent gentle, firm, forceful, or harsh? Does the parent use distraction to direct the child to a new activity, and if so, how does the child respond? Is the child angered or dejected, persistent in the misbehavior, or accepting of a new direction?

Because toilet training is one of the major tasks of early childhood, the nurse discusses the parent's plan for helping the child develop bowel and bladder control and assesses the child's readiness for toilet training. (Methods of toilet training are discussed in Chapter 13.)

The 2- to 4-Year-Old Child

Developmental norms and assessment techniques for 2- and 3-year-olds are summarized in Table 16-14.

Temperament The reactions of the parents and others modify the child's behavior just as the child's temperament influences others in the child's environment. The assessment of both temperamental characteristics and parental perceptions of temperament provides a basis for more effective guidance for the family. The characteristics of the child's temperament (as defined earlier in this chapter) continue to be evident as the child seeks to gain autonomy and control of motor skills.

(text continued on p. 525)

TABLE 16-14 Guidelines for the Assessment of the 2- and 3-Year-Old Child

Developmental area	Expected behaviors		Assessment techniques	
	2-Year-old	*3-Year-old*	*2-Year-old*	*3-Year-old*
Temperament			Assess temperamental characteristics of the child and discuss parental perceptions of the child's temperament	Assess temperamental characteristics and parental perceptions
Gross motor skills	Jumps in place	Alternates feet going up stairs	Tell the child to jump, demonstrate if necessary	Observe or ask the parent to describe
	Broad jumps 8 in	Rides a tricycle	Place sheet of paper on the floor and tell the child to jump over it	Ask the parent whether the child pedals a tricycle
	Tip-toes		Tell the child to walk on tiptoes, demonstrate if necessary	
	Goes up and down stairs alone; places both feet on each step		Ask the parent to describe how the child manages stairs, observe if possible	
	Balances on one foot for 1 second	Balances on one foot for 2 seconds	Tell the child to stand on one foot for as long as possible; demonstrate if necessary	Tell the child to stand on one foot as long as possible; may demonstrate if necessary
Fine motor skills	May copy a circle	Copies circle Copies cross	Show the child a circle but do not let the child observe the circle being drawn and do not name the circle; ask the child to "draw one just like this" and see whether the child draws an enclosed shape that is not necessarily perfectly round	Show the child a circle but do not let the child observe the circle being drawn and do not name the circle, ask the child to "draw one just like this." Use the same technique as with the circle but with a cross
	Imitates a circle		Allow the child to watch the circle being drawn and tell the child to "draw one just like this"	
	Imitates a vertical line		Allow child to watch a line being drawn and tell the child to "draw one just like this"	
	Builds tower of seven to eight blocks	Builds "bridge" from blocks	Provide 1-in cubes and tell the child to build a tower, may demonstrate	Assemble a bridge and tell the child to build one
	Holds pencil with fingers rather than fist	Puts pellets into a narrow-necked bottle	Observe how the child uses pencil or crayon	Provide a narrow-necked bottle and pellets and tell the child to put the pellets into the bottle, may demonstrate

continued on next page

TABLE 16-14 continued

Developmental area	Expected behaviors		Assessment techniques	
	2-Year-old	*3-Year-old*	*2-Year-old*	*3-Year-old*
Fine motor skills (cont.)	Turns doorknobs		Observe the child opening a door or ask the parent whether the child does this	
			Assess the opportunities for the development of fine motor skills	
Language development	Combines two and three words	Speaks in sentences using adverbs and adjectives	Listen to the child's spontaneous speech, ask the parent for examples of the child's word combinations	Listen to the child's speech and sentence structure
	Names pictures of common objects		Present realistic pictures of common objects such as a dog, cat and ball and ask the child to name them	
	Follows simple directions Uses plurals Uses "I," "Me," and "You" Knows one color	Understands "up" and "down" Understands "loud" and "soft" Gives first and last name Understands "tired," "cold," and "hungry" Asks many questions, very talkative Knows two colors Improved articulation	Tell the child to "Give the ball to mommy," "Put the ball on the table," and "Put the ball on the floor" and see whether the child can do two of three tasks Listen to the child's spontaneous speech for the use of plurals; place several blocks on the table, ask the child, "What are these," and listen for "s" at the end of blocks; ask the parent whether the child uses plurals Listen to the child's speech, ask the parent whether the child uses these words at home Place blocks of different colors on the table and ask child to give the nurse the red block (or another color) Assess the quality of verbal interaction between the parent and child	Tell the child to put hands "up" and then "down" Tap an object softly or loudly on the desk and ask the child to describe Ask the child to say his or her whole name Ask the child, "What do you do when you are tired?" "Cold?" "Hungry?" and expect two of three appropriate answers Assess the quality of the interaction between the parent and child, assess parental responses to the child's questions Place blocks of different colors on the table, ask the child for the red (blue, yellow, or green) block Should be able to understand half of the child's speech
Cognitive development	Dumps a raisin from a bottle spontaneously	Imaginative play	Place a raisin in a bottle and tell the child to get it out; the child should be able to do so readily	Discuss with the parent the child's evidence of imagination

TABLE 16-14 continued

Developmental area	Expected behaviors		Assessment techniques	
	2-Year-old	*3-Year-old*	*2-Year-old*	*3-Year-old*
	Places circle, square, and triangle in formboard Unscrews lid Infers cause from observing effect Characteristics of thought: egocentricity, animism, transductive thinking, perception-bound thinking, and magical thinking	Repeats three digits States own sex Classifies according to one characteristic Characteristics of thought include egocentricity, transductive thinking, animism, perception-bound thinking	Present formboard with three forms and tell the child to place the forms in the right places Provide a small jar with a screw top, place a toy inside and tell the child to obtain the toy Allow the child to see a wind-up toy in action but do not allow the child to observe the toy being wound up, give the toy to the child and see whether the child can wind the toy up Listen to the child's spontaneous speech and observe spontaneous activities, engage the child in conversation and attempt to elicit the child's perceptions	Ask the child to repeat three single numbers (should do so in two of three trials) Ask whether the child is a boy or a girl Present 12 forms: four triangles (two red, two blue), four squares (two red, two blue), and four circles (two red, two blue; ask the child to put, like forms together Observe the child's speech and activity; engage the child in conversation and attempt to elicit perceptions
Social and affective development	Increased independence from parents but still needs "refueling"	Depends less on parents but needs reassurance and support	Observe parent–child interaction, noting the child's ability to function alone and to use the parent as a resource, discuss parental reactions to the child's increasing independence	Assess parent–child interactions, noting how independently the child functions, how the child approaches tasks, and whether the parent allows the child to perform a task without interference
	Undresses self and attempts to dress self Independent, refuses certain foods Protests at bedtime, awakens during night Separation anxiety, but child is better able to tolerate separations May continue use of transitional objects Achieves bowel and bladder control during day Remains dry at night	Activity initiates many projects and explorations but does not necessarily complete them Performs simple tasks around the house Tolerates separations from parent for short periods Demonstrates an awareness of sex role behavior and family roles	Observe the child's dressing and undressing directly, ask the parent to describe who dresses and undresses the child, who selects the clothes, and how willing the child is to accept help Assess feeding behaviors and parental response to food refusal Assess sleep behaviors and parental response Discuss the child's behavior before, during, and after separation; discuss parental feelings about separation; may ask parent to leave room and observe separation behavior directly	Assess the child's behavior in exploration and interaction, note how the child approaches tasks, assess parental feedback to the child Discuss with the parent what tasks the child does; assess parental satisfaction with the child's performance Discuss the child's behavior before, during, and after separation; assess parental reactions; discuss the extent of these with the parent Ask the child such questions as, "What do mommies do?" and "What do daddies do?"

continued on next page

TABLE 16-14 continued

Developmental area	Expected behaviors		Assessment techniques	
	2-Year-old	*3-Year-old*	*2-Year-old*	*3-Year-old*
Social and affective development (cont.)			Discuss with the parent whether and how toilet training has been established	
			Assess the frequency of "accidents" and how these are managed; assess the child's reactions to training procedures and accidents	
	Negativism continues but begins to decrease as child becomes more secure about autonomy	Negativism and ritualism are significantly decreased	Observe the child for instances of negativism, discuss parental perceptions of the child's negative behavior and note whether the parent sees change; assess parental response to negative behavior	
	Temper tantrums begin to diminish as the child develops more mature strategies to cope with conflict and frustration		Discuss the occurrence of tantrums with the parent and note precipitating factors, the child's behavior, and parental responses	
	Ritualism (begins to diminish)		Discuss the child's special routines and reaction to disruption of routine	
	Dawdling		Observe for dawdling in assessment setting and observe parental response	
	Indicates an understanding of unacceptable behavior but has limited self-control	Shows a willingness to conform to parental expectations Exerts more self-control but is not reliable, continues to need supervision	Observe limit setting by the parent and the child's response to the limit; discuss parental responses to "misbehavior"; ask the parent to describe the limits set at home, how these are enforced, and the responses when the child breaks a limit	Observe limit setting by the parent and observe the child's response to limits Discuss with the parent any concerns about misbehavior; type of discipline usually used, and child's response
	Demonstrates specific fears	Evidences specific fears	Discuss with the parent whether the child has special fears and how the parents respond	Ask whether the child is especially fearful of anything and how the parent responds
	Parallel play with other children	Associative play, begins to share, plays interactive games with other children but with little regard for rules	Observe the child's play; discuss with the parent how the child interacts with other children, assess opportunities for peer relationships	Ask the parent to describe the child's interaction with peers and siblings

Gross Motor Skills The 2- to 3-year-old child shows significant progress in coordination and balance. By 3 years of age, the clumsy running style of the 2-year-old is controlled. The 3-year-old is able to start and stop quickly and negotiate corners safely and is also developing greater skills in jumping, climbing, and balancing. Children at $2\frac{1}{2}$ years of age generally are able to go up and down stairs while holding onto a rail or person for support. Two-year-olds place both feet on each step; by 3 years of age, the child alternates feet when going up stairs and may also do so when going down stairs.

Although 2- and 3-year-olds enjoy gross motor activity for its own sake, gross motor skills are important to other areas of development. As the child's gross motor skills improve, the child is able to be increasingly independent and explore more widely. Gross motor abilities therefore also affect psychosocial and cognitive development.

Fine Motor Skills Tasks used to assess fine motor development actually involve much more than just fine motor coordination. They require accurate visual perceptions, good eye–hand coordination, and such cognitive abilities as comprehending imitation and cause-and-effect relationships.

As the child builds a tower of blocks, the nurse notes the ease with which the child grasps the blocks, the accuracy of the placement of the blocks, and the ability to control the release of the blocks. This task also provides information about the child's cognitive abilities. To build a tower, the child must understand the principle of properly placing one block precisely on top of another. By 36 months of age, the child should be able to stack seven to eight blocks and by 48 months of age should stack nine to ten blocks.

By $3\frac{1}{2}$ years of age, the child should be able to build a "bridge" of three blocks. In assessing this skill the nurse first assembles a bridge, being sure to leave a space between the two bottom blocks, and then gives three blocks to the child, asking the child to build a bridge that looks the same. When completed, the child's bridge should also have a space between the bottom blocks. If it does not, the nurse asks the child whether the two structures look exactly the same.

The nurse can present paper and pencil tasks to the child at this stage, making sure that the child is comfortably seated near an appropriate writing surface. The nurse first notes how the child grasps the pencil; a 3-year-old should hold the pencil with the fingers and not with the fist. There are two different kinds of tasks: those that require copying and those that require imitation. A copying task requires the child to reproduce a preformed shape; the child does not watch the nurse draw the shape. With an imitation task, the nurse demonstrates how to draw the shape and then asks the child to perform the same action. Most children find it more difficult to copy than to imitate. When copying a preformed shape, the child must be able to conceptualize the steps that result in the correct shape; when imitating, the child can first watch the actions necessary to achieve the result. By 3 years of age, most children can imitate a vertical line and a circle. By $3\frac{1}{2}$ years of age, most children can copy a circle. Some 3-year-olds also are able to copy a cross.

A motor task that children commonly master by this age is turning doorknobs. This task requires both coordination for simultaneous grasp and wrist rotation and a cognitive understanding of the relationship between turning the knob and releasing the door. Three-year-old children also should be able to place small pellets into a narrow-necked bottle. The nurse notes the precision with which the child picks up the pellets and the accuracy with which they are released into the bottle. By questioning the parent about the availability of crayons, paper, clay, and the like at home, the nurse can further assess the child's opportunities for developing fine motor tasks.

Language Development The child makes tremendous progress in language ability between 2 and 4 years of age. The average 2-year-old has a vocabulary of 200–300 words. By 3 years of age, the child's vocabulary is likely to include 900–1000 words, and the child might seem to talk all the time. The 2-year-old combines two and three words into meaningful phrases; the 3-year-old speaks in short sentences using both adverbs and adjectives.

By $2\frac{1}{2}$ years of age, the child should be able to name a picture of a common object if the picture is realistic and the child is familiar with the object. The 3-year-old should be able to name several common objects such as a dog, cat, house, man, chair, ball, horse, bird, woman, and doll.

By $2\frac{1}{2}$ years of age, children generally use the pronouns "I," "me," and "you" correctly and refer to themselves by "I" or "me" rather than by name. All 3-year-olds and many 2-year-olds use plural forms correctly. The child of this age should be able to follow two of the following commands:

1. Give the ball to mommy.
2. Put the ball on the table.
3. Put the ball on the floor.

The nurse needs to give each command separately because the average 2-year-old is not able to follow two commands at once.

By 3 years of age, the child can identify one color; by 4 years of age, the child can identify two colors. The nurse tests this ability by placing four blocks of different colors on the table and asking the child to give the red one (or blue, yellow, or green) to the nurse. The child should be able to select the correctly colored block. A more difficult task is to name the color of an object, although many 3-year-olds also are able to do this.

The 3-year-old child usually is able to understand "up" and "down." The nurse tests this by asking the child to put both hands "up" and then to put both hands "down." Nurses should be careful not to give cues by raising their own

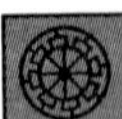

CASE STUDY Active, Busy Three-Year-Old

Assessment

Three-year-old Mark was brought to the clinic because his mother was concerned about his small size, small appetite, and food rituals.

Family

Mark's family, consisting of a mother, father, and two older sisters, moved to the area 6 months previously. Both parents and the sisters are of average height and in good health. The mother comments that the girls always did what they were requested but that Mark has been a difficult child because of his strong will. Mealtime is a battle to get Mark to eat unless his mother feeds him. For a while the girls could coax him to eat, but that no longer works; Mark screams and refuses their attention.

Child

Mark always has been small for his age but is active and a quick learner. The mother's record of his developmental milestones mirrors those of his sisters. Mark has had a few colds but no serious illnesses or hospitalizations. The mother is worried that Mark's picky eating habits have gotten worse since the move. She thinks that the move has been particularly difficult for him and that he misses his friends. He spends most of his day with her, wants her to play games with him, and no longer allows his sisters to watch him when she goes to the store but insists on joining her. She also has to sit in his room at night until he goes to sleep; otherwise he has a tantrum.

Environment

The family lives in a four-bedroom home that has a large, fenced-in yard. Mark has a wading pool, swing set, sandbox, and tricycle, plus a room full of toys, stuffed animals, and books.

Clinical Data

Once reassured that his mother would remain, Mark agreed to participate in the assessment. He skillfully performed all of the gross and fine motor skills requested. His speech usually was understandable; but he spoke very quietly, so it was difficult to hear him. When asked to repeat an answer, he refused. His mother responded that he was shy, became embarrassed easily, and never repeated anything. He identified shapes, colors, and grouped like shapes together. He counted to ten and demonstrated comprehension of the concept of numbers one through five. He gave satisfactory definitions of six adjectives and stated his full name when asked. He remained close to his mother while performing skills and looked to her for approval after each task.

Mark's mother had no concerns about his overall development. She thought that he was a bright child, only small. While his mother was being interviewed, Mark initiated many attention-getting behaviors. She responded each time by interrupting the interview to meet his request, which included asking the nurse if he could play with a stethoscope and reflex hammer. Mark seldom has been asked to do any household chores, including picking up his toys. His mother commented that the children usually got their own way when they were young, but that this was probably more true for Mark than it had been for his sisters. Mark has not responded positively to any of the discipline measures that the parents have used, and his mother hopes that he will "grow out of it" and be more cooperative (eg, dress and undress himself, brush his teeth, and be obedient) and less demanding in another year.

Comparison to a Standard

When Mark's development is compared with the expected behaviors, he is at or above his age level in all areas except social and affective development. He remains very dependent on his mother and does not tolerate separation well. He demands to have his own way and does not accept behavioral limits, nor is he willing to conform to parental expectations. He has had minimal help in learning appropriate ways of expressing autonomy and initiative.

Nursing Diagnoses

1. Developmental delay in the area of social and affective development related to parental inexperience and insufficient guidance.
2. Potential for continued ineffective coping related to positive feedback for regressive behaviors and lack of consistent limits and appropriate responsibilities.

Plan for Interventions

Goals

1. Mark will separate from his parents without incident (tantrum, crying).
2. Mark will join a community or church peer group activity.
3. Mark will do one household task (eg, picking up his toys) before bedtime every evening.
4. Mark will demonstrate independent self-care behaviors (eg, feed himself).
5. The parents will have clear, consistent, and age-appropriate expectations for Mark's behavior.
6. The parents will explain to Mark the rationale for limiting a socially unacceptable or unsafe behavior as soon as it is done.

Interventions

1. Discuss with the parents the process of growth and development and the child's needs to learn how to compromise, take turns, and channel energy appropriately.
2. Use the Prescreening Developmental Questionnaire to validate general assessment data.
3. Encourage the parents to leave Mark with his sisters or a babysitter to go shopping or to a movie.
4. Encourage the mother to formulate a bedtime ritual with Mark that does not include her sitting in his room until he goes to sleep.

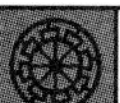

CASE STUDY Active, Busy Three-Year-Old (continued)

5. Discuss with the parents and Mark what "jobs" he can do at home and the expectation that it be done daily.
6. Suggest laying out Mark's clothes so that he can dress himself. Set a time to be dressed such as before or after a certain television program in the morning.
7. Explore with the parents the availability of playgroups or community activities for children Mark's age.
8. Encourage the parents to take Mark to the neighborhood playground so that he can meet and play with other children.
9. Have Mark help around the house alongside his parents. Specify "work" and "play" times.
10. Praise Mark for age-appropriate behaviors, being careful not to bribe him to perform.
11. Discuss the principles of discipline—consistency, immediacy, realistic expectations, and clear explanations.
12. Recognize the parents' frustration and encourage them to try different approaches such as limited choices, diversion, and incentives (eg, when you finish your meat, we'll play a game).
13. Suggest that the parents keep a diary of how long and how consistently an approach was tried and how Mark responded.
14. Discuss the decrease in appetite and reliance on food fads that typify Mark's age. Review the principles of nutrition, timing of snacks, and ways of making food attractive to children.
15. Refer the parents and Mark to a nutritionist for nutrition counseling.
16. Refer the parents and Mark to a pediatrician to evaluate the appropriateness of further studies, including growth hormone studies.

hands or raising their eyes. The child also should understand the distinction between "loud" and "soft." In assessing this an object is tapped loudly and then softly, and the child is asked, "Did that sound loud or soft?" The nurse repeats the test several times to see whether the child consistently responds correctly.

By the time they reach 4 years of age, children understand the concepts "cold," "hungry," and "tired." The nurse therefore tests the 3-year-old's understanding by asking, "What do you do if you are cold?" "Hungry?" "Tired?" The child should answer appropriately two of the three concepts.

The nurse also assesses the quality of verbal interchange between the parent and child. The ideal is open and elaborative communication in which the parent attends to what the child says and responds with explanations for events and rationales for limits. More closed and restricted communicators are likely to inhibit the child's speech by instructing the child to be quiet, offer fewer explanations, and present fewer concepts. Because the child's language skills depend on the amount and quality of language used at home, the opportunities to communicate and the responses the child receives when using language are important assessment criteria.

The nurse also assesses the child's articulation of speech sounds. By 3 years of age, 50%–75% of the child's speech should be intelligible to nonfamily members. A child whose speech is difficult to understand might have a hearing loss or other problems. Mild dysfluency, such as stuttering, however, is common in young children.

Cognitive Development Two- and three-year-olds demonstrate an increased use of symbols, which is reflected in language development and imaginative play. Imaginative play might involve substituting an object or person for another object or person. For example, the child might find a stick and say, "Let's pretend this is a hammer." In proceeding to use the stick as a hammer, the child is mentally attributing the qualities of a hammer to the stick, even though those qualities are not really present.

Imitation becomes increasingly complex and sophisticated as the child learns to imitate the behaviors of others. For example, children pretending to be fathers or mothers are able to imitate many behaviors displayed by their own parents. Problem-solving abilities also improve as the child is able to conceptualize the correct solution to a simple problem without having to try several possible solutions first.

In assessing problem-solving skills, the process the child uses to reach the solution is as significant as the solution itself. By 3 years of age, most children can correctly place simple forms into a formboard on the first try, without resorting to trial and error. Another task for assessing problem-solving skills is to place a small toy into a clear screw-top jar and ask the child to get the toy. The nurse then observes the strategies the child uses to open the jar. Most 3-year-olds readily unscrew the lid.

Children at this age are able to infer a cause from observing its effect. To test the child's understanding of this concept, the nurse shows the child a wind-up toy in action without allowing the child to see the actual winding procedures. After the toy has wound down and stopped, the child is asked to make the toy go again. The child usually assumes that some mechanism initiates the action and tries various strategies until discovering the correct one. The nurse then continues to observe whether the child discovers the association between repeated winding and prolonged action.

Memory improves during this stage. To test immediate recall, the nurse might say three single numbers and ask the child to repeat them. The average 3-year-old is able to do this on two out of three trials. Three-year-olds often can recite simple nursery rhymes or songs, a further demonstration of memory.

Three-year-old children can classify objects according to a single characteristic. One way to test this is to present 12 simple forms (circles, squares, and triangles colored red and blue) and ask the child to put the like objects together. Young children usually classify only by color, putting all the blue shapes in one pile and all the red shapes in another pile. Older children are able to classify according to more than one characteristic, by placing the red triangles in one pile, the blue triangles in another pile, and so on.

The skilled observer usually finds spontaneous demonstrations of the child's egocentricity but also might question the child. For example, the nurse might use a question that requires the child to consider the nurse's need for information such as, "If I were walking on your street, how would I know which house was yours?" The young child might answer, "Because I live there," unable to see that the nurse does not have the same perspective as the child. As the child matures and becomes less egocentric, the child becomes able to consider another's need for information, and the response might be, "It's a blue house, and my red tricycle is in the front yard." Transductive thinking is evident in responses to such questions as, "Why does it rain?" or "Why do people get sick?" The child is likely to have very personal and often unrealistic ideas of causality.

The child's perception-bound thinking can be assessed by placing six buttons widely spaced in a row and six buttons closely spaced in another row. When asked which row has more buttons, the child responds that the row with widely spaced buttons has more, a characteristic of preoperational thought (see Chapter 6). Even if the nurse carefully demonstrates that there are really the same number of buttons, the child is unable to alter the perception and insists that the longer row has more buttons.

Social and Affective Development For the 2-year-old child, the establishment of autonomy remains a central issue, and negativism, tantrums, and ritualistic behavior often continue until $2\frac{1}{2}$ to 3 years of age. As the child's autonomy becomes more secure, these behaviors begin to diminish. Three-year-olds continue to assert their independence and might exhibit these behaviors occasionally but not to the extent of the younger child. If the child does not display autonomous behaviors, the nurse should be concerned.

Occasionally, a parent might fear that as the child becomes more independent, the closeness of the parent–child relationship will diminish. Conflict between the parent and child, which is normal at this age, might be seen as a threat to the relationship, and negative behaviors may be very difficult for the parent to manage. For example, one young, single mother of a 2-year-old was very closely involved with her son and had few other significant relationships in her life. The relationship with her son provided a major source of closeness and gratification for her. As the child began to assert himself and demonstrate some negativism, the mother feared that this closeness would be lost. The child's negative behavior became so threatening to her that when the child protested at bedtime or staged a tantrum, the mother immediately gave in to his demands. When he cried at bedtime, she took him to her bed; if he became upset, she offered him a bottle. At 3 years of age, this child continued to sleep with his mother, to use his bottle frequently during the day, and protest vehemently if separated from his mother. Although the mother's behavior met her needs to maintain a close, dependent relationship, her responses were clearly detrimental to the child.

In assessing the parent–child interaction, the nurse therefore observes the following:

1. Opportunities for the child to make choices and to proceed independently
2. Parental response for independent activity
3. The way the child approaches a task (independently or with parental assistance)
4. Whether the parent allows the child to proceed with the task or interferes
5. The child's use of the parent for support
6. The parent's availability to the child for support and encouragement
7. Parental response to negative behaviors

Another aspect of developing autonomy is the child's self-care abilities. Two-year-old children generally feed themselves, although they continue to need help in such tasks as cutting food or buttering bread. Food refusal is common in this age group, so the nurse assesses what happens when the child refuses to eat certain foods. Does the parent perceive this as a problem? Does the parent attempt to force the child to eat, bribe the child, or ignore the behavior?

Two-year-old children are able to undress themselves and button some of their own clothes; three-year-olds generally are able to dress themselves with supervision, except for buttons or tying shoes. The 3-year-old knows the front from the back of clothes. The nurse assesses the child's self-dressing ability, how much assistance the child needs, and the child's willingness to accept help. How the parent and child negotiate these issues is as significant as who actually dresses the child. Negotiating takes time, and a parent whose time is limited because of other responsibilities might find it easier to dress the child, avoiding conflict but also thwarting the child's learning a self-care skill. Several nursery school teachers whose program includes gym and swim lessons commented that one of their major tasks each year is teaching children how to dress themselves. One parent solved the dressing problem by laying the child's clothes out the prior evening, choosing easy pull-on pants and tops and tube socks. Together, parent and child decided that in the morning the parent would tie the shoes and that at other times the child could practice tying knots and bows.

Between the ages of 2 and 3 years, most children achieve bowel and bladder control during the day, and some children remain dry at night as well. (Toilet training is discussed in Chapter 13.) Once the child is toilet trained, the nurse asks the parent to describe the child's toileting habits and inquires about the frequency of accidents and how the child reacts to accidents. The parent's perceptions of the causes of the accidents and response to accidents might be significant. Also helpful is asking parents how toilet training was accomplished and how the child reacted to training procedures.

The nurse also assesses any problems related to bedtime and sleep. Most families with 2- and 3-year-old children have special routines that ease the transition at bedtime and alert the child that bedtime is near. (Parental management of bedtime problems is discussed in Chapter 13.)

Although parents remain central figures in children's lives and separation continues to be painful, children who mature socially and cognitively are increasingly able to tolerate short separations (see Chapter 8). Two-year-olds might continue to protest separations vigorously, but by 3 years of age, many children are able to accept parental absences calmly. The nurse assesses how the child behaves before, during, and after a separation; what the parent does to minimize the stress of separation; and whether the child has developed more mature strategies to deal with separation. If problems continue to be associated with separations (such as vehement protest when the parent leaves, inconsolable or withdrawn behavior while separated, rejection of or lack of interest in the returning parent), the nurse assesses the parent's feelings about separation. If the parent is feeling ambivalent, anxious, or guilty about leaving the child, these feelings might be picked up by the child, and the child may react more to the parent's unspoken negative cues than to the actual separation itself.

Children at this stage might develop real or imagined fears, sometimes triggered by an actual or perceived event. For example, the child may become frightened when a big dog comes too near, even though the dog is clearly friendly. The child might even begin to fear all animals because of this one event. The child usually can imagine scary events but does not possess the logic to deal with fears realistically. The nurse therefore asks whether the child has any specific fears, how troublesome these fears are, and how the parents handle them. (Coping strategies that children use to manage fears are discussed in Chapter 12.) The 3-year-old typically devotes considerable energy to broader explorations and the mastery of new skills and uses imaginative play to learn about various social roles. Three-year-olds initiate many projects but may have little interest in completing them. This may be a matter of concern to some parents, but it is a normal pattern in 3-year-old children. In assessing the child's initiative, the nurse observes whether the child feels free to explore, imagine, and communicate and whether the child receives mostly positive or negative reinforcement for these behaviors.

The nurse notes a need for further evaluation if the child feels overly guilty for thoughts and wishes, is afraid to play spontaneously for fear of negative outcomes, or is made to feel bad about normal exploration and exuberance.

Two-year-old children are developing notions of body image and usually can state whether someone is a boy or a girl, although they might not always be accurate and the criteria they use in making the distinction may be questionable (such as long hair versus short hair, dresses versus pants). Three-year-olds show an increased awareness of sex role behavior, and the nurse might ask such questions as the following:

1. How can you tell if someone is a girl or a boy?
2. What do mommies do?
3. What do daddies do?

Young preschoolers often imitate behaviors of both sexes, although behaviors of their own sex usually predominate. The nurse can ask parents whether the child tends to imitate one or both parents. Parents occasionally express concern if their children imitate behaviors that the parents feel are appropriate only for the opposite sex; some parents are especially concerned if little boys imitate their mothers, although this is generally normal behavior. If the child consistently imitates only opposite-sex behavior, however, an in-depth family assessment might be indicated (see Chapter 17).

Two-year-old children have an increased understanding of what is acceptable and unacceptable behavior, but self-control remains limited. Two-year-olds cannot be trusted to "obey" and usually challenge parental limits in spite of the consequences. Once the autonomy issue is more or less resolved, the child becomes more willing to conform to parental expectations. Three-year-olds have better self-control but are still not reliable and need continued supervision. In assessing disciplinary patterns the nurse needs direct observation of misbehavior, limit setting by the parent, and subsequent responses by the child. (Methods of discipline are discussed in Chapter 13.)

Dawdling is a common behavior in young children and seems to be related to children's ambivalence about complying with parental wishes. When faced with a parental demand, 2- and 3-year-olds might not disobey but may not exactly obey either. When the child resists by doing nothing, the parent is likely to be frustrated. The nurse therefore assesses whether a child uses dawdling as a strategy for dealing with parental pressure and how the parents manage this behavior.

By this stage, the child's interactions with other children, both siblings and friends, are important. The nurse therefore explores with the parent the child's opportunities to interact with other children and ability to get along with other children. If a child is overly aggressive or unusually withdrawn with peers, a more thorough assessment is indicated.

The nurse also discusses how siblings get along and how conflicts between siblings are managed. Questions that may be helpful include the following:

1. How do your children get along?
2. How often do they argue?
3. What usually starts the conflict?
4. How do the conflicts usually end?

Even young children are able to perform helpful tasks around the house. Two-year-olds are able to put toys away and pick up clothes, although they need frequent reminders and close supervision. Three-year-olds can be responsible for some simple tasks on a regular basis, although they too need reminders. The nurse asks whether the child is responsible for certain tasks, how the child handles the responsibility, and how the parent perceives the child's performance. Being praised for tasks that they do fosters self-esteem in children.

The 4- to 5-Year-Old Child

Developmental norms and assessment techniques for 4- and 5-year-olds are summarized in Table 16-15.

Temperament As the child prepares to enter elementary school, certain temperamental characteristics might help or hinder the transition to formal education such as activity level, adaptability to change, reaction to new situations, persistence, and distractability. Children who might need special help in making the transition to school are particularly active or passive, have typically been slow to adjust to change, have tended to withdraw in new situations, and are distractable. Such temperamental characteristics are not necessarily "problems," but information about the child's responses might be used to plan interventions to ease the transition.

For example, if a child has tended to withdraw in new situations or to have difficulty adjusting to changes, arranging for several short visits to the new classroom before the start of school might be helpful. Two or three short visits with the teacher on a one-to-one basis might reduce some of the child's anxiety. Simply alerting the teacher to the child's response pattern also allows the teacher to plan special strategies for the child.

Gross Motor Skills As the child matures, motor skills become more refined. Four-year-old children generally are able to balance on one foot for at least 5 seconds; five-year-olds generally can balance for 10 seconds. In the assessment setting the child should have three trials and should succeed in two, and with all gross motor tasks, the nurse's demonstration helps elicit the child's best performance. Four-year-old children should be able to perform a forward heel-to-toe walk for at least four steps, and five-year-olds should be able to do a backward heel-to-toe walk. A line on the floor for the child to follow is helpful; a piece of tape about 4 ft long serves this purpose.

By 4 years of age, most children alternate feet when going up and down stairs and can climb up and down jungle gyms, slides, and other playground equipment. Four-year-olds should be able to hop twice; five-year-olds usually are able to skip and jump rope and might ride a bicycle with training wheels. A 5-year-old also can catch a bounced and tossed ball with two hands on two of three trials. A basic neurologic examination also provides information about the child's gross motor abilities (see Chapter 14).

Fine Motor Skills The ability to perform the fine motor tasks reflects more than coordination of the small muscles. The child must have adequate eye–hand coordination and the cognitive ability to imitate and reconstruct. To draw a person, the child must be able to translate the mental image of a person to a representative drawing without the benefit of copying or imitating.

As the child proceeds with the tasks, the nurse notes (1) how the child holds the pencils or scissors; (2) the precision with which the child picks up and releases the objects; (3) the accuracy with which items are copied; and (4) the presence of tremors, excessive clumsiness, or poorly formed shapes. Children of this age who are able to print letters often reverse similar letters (such as "b" instead of "d" or "p" for "g"). Parents who have read about dyslexia (a perceptual problem that causes reading and writing disorders) might need reassurance that in the 4-, 5-, or 6-year-old child, letter reversals are common and acceptable.

Fine motor skills are essential in the early elementary grades, and skills like tying shoes are important. Maturation plays a role in the child's ability in this area, and not all children develop those skills at the same age. The nurse therefore assesses the opportunities for practice at home. These opportunities might include the use of tools such as crayons, pencils, and scissors that aid in developing fine motor skills. A child who is clumsy or has difficulty with eye–hand coordination or copying might need special help, but the child's development should not be labeled as a "problem," and special help should not become a stigma for the parent or child.

Language Development Whereas 4-year-olds can speak in sentences of five to six words, 5-year-olds use longer sentences and should use nouns, pronouns, verbs, articles, prepositions, adjectives, and adverbs correctly. Children 4 and 5 years of age normally have difficulty with

(text continued on p. 537)

TABLE 16-15 Guidelines for Assessment of the 4- and 5-Year-Old Child

Developmental area	Expected behaviors		Assessment techniques	
	4-Year-old	*5-Year-old*	*4-Year-old*	*5-Year-old*
Temperament			Assess temperamental characteristics and parental perceptions	Assess temperamental characteristics of child and parental perceptions
Gross motor skills	Balances on one foot for 5 seconds May balance on one foot for 10 seconds	Balances on one foot for 10 seconds	Tell child, "Do this as long as you can," while demonstrating; time the number of seconds the child can balance and expect the child to balance for 5 seconds on two of three trials	Tell child, "Do this as long as you can," while demonstrating; time the number of seconds the child can balance and expect the child to balance for 10 seconds on two of three trials
	Hops twice on one foot	Jumps rope	Tell the child to hop on one foot, demonstrate if necessary	Ask the child to jump rope; may demonstrate if necessary
	Forward heel-to-toe walk, heel within 1 in of toe, for at least four steps Runs with good leg–arm coordination	Performs heel-to-toe walk, toe within 1 in of heel, for at least four steps backwards	Tell the child to do heel-to-toe walk, demonstrate if necessary, helpful to have line on floor for the child to follow	Tell the child to do backward heel-to-toe walk, may demonstrate if necessary; helpful to have line on floor for the child to follow
	Goes up and down stairs using alternating feet; begins climbing jungle gyms and other playground equipment	Runs on toes Skips by alternating feet Becomes proficient at climbing playground equipment	Observe the child or ask the parent to describe how the child manages stairs and playground equipment	Observe the child or ask the parent about the child's running, skipping, and playing on playground equipment
	Catches bounced and tossed ball with arms; may trap ball against body	Catches bounced ball; catches small tossed ball with hands	From a distance of 3 ft, have the child catch a bounced ball and a tossed ball; note if catching or trapping ball with arms and body; expect the child to either catch with arms or trap ball on two out of three attempts	Tell the child to stand 3 feet away and catch a bounced ball with hands (not with arms or by trapping against body); expect the child to catch two of three throws but do not count poor throws that the child misses; do again except tossing instead of bouncing ball.
		Rides bicycle with training wheels		Ask the child and parent about bicycle riding abilities
Fine motor skills	May imitate square after demonstration	Copies square and triangle	First see whether the child can copy a square from a picture without being shown; if not, demonstrate how to draw a square by drawing two opposite sides first and then the other two sides; corners should be about 90°	Show the child a square and a triangle but do not let the child see the shapes being drawn and do not name the forms; tell the child to draw one like each of the pictures
	Copies cross		Show child a cross but do not let the child see it being drawn and do not name it, tell the child to	

continued on next page

TABLE 16-15 continued

Developmental area	Expected behaviors		Assessment techniques	
	4-Year-old	*5-Year-old*	*4-Year-old*	*5-Year-old*
Fine motor skills (cont.)			draw one like the picture; lines need not be straight to pass	
	Draws a person with three identifiable parts; draws house crudely	Draws a person with at least six parts; improved drawing of house	Tell the child to draw a person but do not tell the child which parts to draw; the child's picture should include three identifiable body parts, but if one part of a pair (eyes, arms) is not drawn, that part does not count	Tell the child to draw a person but do not tell the child which parts to draw; the child's picture should contain six identifiable parts; if one part of a pair (eyes, arms) is not drawn, that part does not count
	Uses scissors	Cuts along a straight line for 6 in	Provide the child with scissors and paper with the outline of a simple shape and tell the child to cut out the shape; ability to use the scissors effectively is more important than precision in cutting	Give the child a piece of paper 6 in wide with a line drawn straight across and tell the child to cut along the line
		May print a few letters or even simple words (such as own name)	Assess the child's opportunities to practice fine motor skills	Ask the child whether he or she can print letters or name, expect letter forms to be clumsy and reversals to be common
		Begins to tie shoelaces		Tell the child to tie shoelaces—either own or on doll
Language development—expression and comprehension	Uses sentences of four to five words	Uses complete sentences with nouns, pronouns, verbs, adverbs, adjectives, prepositions, and articles	Listen to the child's spontaneous speech	Listen to the child's spontaneous speech; noting the child's ability to listen and to comprehend verbal messages throughout the assessment
	Understands prepositions such as "under," "on top of," "behind," "in front of"	Defines words according to shape, composition, or general category	Ask the child to place an object in various positions (eg, "Place the block on top of the table"); the child should perform three of four trials correctly	Ask the child to define words, one at a time, with such questions as "What is a ________?" and words such as ball, lake, house, shoe, desk, banana, ceiling; expect the child to define most words (six of nine) appropriately
	Understands analogies	Decodes verbal messages	Ask the child the following: "If fire is hot, ice is ________?" "Mother is a woman, Daddy is a ________" "A house is big, a mouse is ________?"; the child should perform two of three trials correctly	Say to the child, "Guess what I have. It is long and hard and you write with it." "It is made of paper, it has pictures and stories and pages in it" or use other examples

TABLE 16-15 continued

Developmental area	Expected behaviors: 4-Year-old	Expected behaviors: 5-Year-old	Assessment techniques: 4-Year-old	Assessment techniques: 5-Year-old
		Identifies the composition of objects		Ask the child what a spoon (shoe, door, etc) is made of
		Follows three commands		Tell the child to do three simple actions and give the commands at one time (eg, "Put the pencil on the table; bring me the book; pick up the block")
	Recognizes three colors	Identifies four colors	Place four colored blocks on a table, ask the child to give the nurse the red (blue, green, or yellow) one, replace the block on the table and repeat using another color; ask for four colors; the child should perform three correctly	Place colored blocks on the table, point to the blocks, and tell the child to identify the color or to give the red (blue, yellow, etc) block to the nurse
		Identifies basic geometric shapes		Show the child a circle, triangle, and square and ask the child to name each shape
				Assess the verbal interaction of the parent and child
Cognitive development	Understands concepts of "long" and "short"	Repeats ten-word sentence	Present two lines, one of which is longer; ask the child to point to the longer line; change the position of the lines; the child should consistently choose the longer line	Tell the child to "listen carefully to what I say and then say what I say. We are going to the store to buy some bread" or use another simple sentence
	Understands "heavy" and "light"	Reproduces a pattern of four objects in the correct order	Present two objects, one of which is noticeably heavier; ask the child to hold the objects and say which is heavier	Place a block, pencil, ball, and book on the table, ask the child to name each object, then scramble the objects and tell the child to put them back the way they were
	Repeats four digits		Tell the child to listen carefully, then say four single digits and ask the child to repeat; the child should succeed in one of three trials	
	Counts three objects		Present ten blocks and tell the child to "take two blocks and put them here" indicating a place on the table; put the blocks back into the group and tell the child to "take three blocks" and so on	

continued on next page

TABLE 16-15 continued

Developmental area	Expected behaviors		Assessment techniques	
	4-Year-old	*5-Year-old*	*4-Year-old*	*5-Year-old*
Cognitive development (cont.)		Classifies objects according to similarities in relationship		Ask the child, "How are bread and milk alike?" "How are a jacket and hat alike?" and expect the child to identify similarities between the objects
	Continues to classify objects according to one characteristic	May be able to classify objects according to more than one characteristic	Present 12 forms: four triangles (two red, two blue), four squares (two red, two blue), and four circles (two red, two blue); ask the child to put like forms together	Present 12 forms: (four triangles (two red, two blue), four squares (two red, two blue) and four circles (two red, two blue); ask the child to put like forms together, first according to color and then according to shape
	Does not perceive conservation of matter		Present two identical glasses with the same amount of water in each; as the child watches, pour the water from one glass into a tall, narrow glass; ask the child which glass has more water; present two balls of clay the same size; roll one ball into a long, narrow shape; ask the child which shape has more clay	
	Continues to be imaginative, tells stories mixing fantasy and reality but with little regard for accuracy	Shows imagination but accurately describes events	Discuss the child's imaginative play with the parent; ask whether the child exaggerates or "tells tales"	Discuss the child's imaginative play with the parent; ask how often the child exaggerates or "tells tales"
		Shows more realistic sense of causality		Ask the child such questions as, "Why do people get sick?" "Why does it rain?" and expect ideas to be inaccurate but less fanciful than the younger child's
	Considers others' perspectives (less egocentric)		Observe for spontaneous examples of the ability to consider another's point of view during the assessment	
Social and affective development	Demonstrates independence in daily activities, dresses and undresses without supervision, buttons clothes (except in back); knows front from back	Independently dresses, washes, and performs toileting	Observe how child dresses and undresses self in assessment, discuss with the parent and child who selects clothes and dresses child and how much help the child needs	Discuss the child's daily habits with both the parent and child, assess how the child performs these tasks during the assessment exam and whether the parent interferes

TABLE 16-15 continued

Developmental area	Expected behaviors: 4-Year-old	Expected behaviors: 5-Year-old	Assessment techniques: 4-Year-old	Assessment techniques: 5-Year-old
	Washes own face and hands		Discuss with the parent how the child handles hygiene	
	Manages toileting without help, remains dry at night with an occasional "accident"		Inquire about toileting habits and assess frequency and responses to accidents	
	Generally separates easily from parents	Separates easily from parents	Discuss with the parent how the child reacts to separation and how the parent feels about separation; ask the parent to leave the room and observe how the child and parent react to separation	Discuss with the parent how the child handles separation and how parents react to separation (school entry may temporarily cause renewed separation anxiety)
	Verbalizes feelings	Verbalizes feelings	Observe how the child handles feelings during the assessment, observe parental responses, ask the child such questions as, "What is the happiest (saddest, scariest) thing you can think of?" and discuss with the parent how the child acts when sad, angry, or frightened	Observe how the child handles feelings during assessment; observe parental responses; ask the child such questions as "What is the happiest (saddest, scariest) thing you can think of?" and discuss with the parent how the child acts when sad, angry, or frightened
	Fears about body integrity emerge; other fears may remain or diminish		Discuss with the parent any concerns about the child's fears and how the parent responds	
	Judges acts according to consequences but does not take intention into account	Judges acts according to consequences but does not take intention into account	Present a moral dilemma to child and observe the child's behavior in the assessment setting, note parental limit setting and the child's response	Present a moral dilemma to the child, observe the child's behavior, noting parental limit setting and the child's response
	Defines acceptable and unacceptable behavior but might not always accept limits; controls behavior in assessment setting	Controls behavior in assessment setting, defines acceptable and unacceptable behavior	Discuss with the parent how the child responds to limits, what happens if the child breaks a limit, what type of discipline the parent uses, and how the child responds; explore the child's perceptions of discipline	Discuss with the parent how the child responds to limits, what happens if the child breaks a limit, what type of discipline the parent uses, and how the child responds; explore the child's perceptions of discipline
	Regularly performs household tasks but might need reminders	Habitually performs certain household tasks	Discuss with the parent and child what jobs the child does around the house	Discuss with the parent and child what jobs the child does around the house
		Displays sex stereotypic behavior		Explore the parent–child relationship according to how the child interacts with each parent, the time spent with each parent, and typical activities with each parent; ask

continued on next page

TABLE 16-15 continued

Developmental area	Expected behaviors		Assessment techniques	
	4-Year-old	5-Year-old	4-Year-old	5-Year-old
Cognitive development (cont.)				the parent whether the child seems to imitate one parent more than the other
	Displays sexual curiosity and interest in bodily differences between girls and boys; may have own private theories to explain sexual differences and reproduction	Displays sexual curiosity; may have own private theories to explain sexual differences and reproduction	Ask child such questions as, "How can you tell if someone is a girl or a boy?" "Why are girls and boys different?" "Where do babies come from?" and ask the parent whether the child has engaged in sexual exploration of self or others; discuss parental response	Ask the child questions such as, "How can you tell if someone is a boy or a girl?" "Why are boys and girls different?" "Where do babies come from?" and ask the parent whether the child has engaged in sexual exploration of self or others; discuss parental response
	Shows strong attachment to parent of opposite sex	Looks for parental support and encouragement	Discuss the parent–child relationships, including how the child gets along with each parent, whether the child prefers one parent or the other in certain situations, how much time each parent spends with the child, and the types of activities parents and child do together	Note parental response to child's performance, whether the parent allows the child to proceed independently or intervenes; note whether parent makes encouraging or discouraging comments
	May exhibit jealousy of siblings	May exhibit jealousy of siblings	Discuss the relationship between the child and siblings, noting how the child gets along with each sibling, the incidence of conflicts, and how conflicts are resolved; may ask the child directly, "What do you like best about your brother (sister)?" "Is there anything you don't like about ________?" "Do you ever fight with ________?" "What happens then?"	Discuss the relationship between the child and siblings, noting how the child gets along with each sibling, the incidence of conflicts, and how conflicts are resolved; may ask the child directly, "What do you like best about your brother/sister?" "Is there anything you don't like about ________?" "Do you ever fight with ________?" "What happens then?"
	Engages in cooperative play with peers; shares but frequently reminds others of ownership of objects	Engages in cooperative play Relates appropriately to adults outside family	Discuss with the parent how the child interacts with other children, what types of play the child engages in, and the child's ability to share; assess opportunities for the child to interact with peers	Discuss with the parent how the child interacts with other children, what types of play the child engages in, and the child's ability to share; assess opportunities for the child to interact with peers Note the child's response to the examiner

TABLE 16-15 continued

Developmental area	Expected behaviors		Assessment techniques	
	4-Year-old	*5-Year-old*	*4-Year-old*	*5-Year-old*
	Looks for parental support and encouragement		Note parental response to the child's performance, whether the parent allows child to proceed independently or intervenes; note whether the parent makes encouraging or discouraging comments	
	Displays confidence in approaching tasks	Displays confidence in approaching tasks	Observe how the child approaches tasks during the assessment; note any hesitancy, carelessness, expectation of success or failure, use of parent as a resource, and reaction to successful or unsuccessful performance	Observe how the child approaches tasks during the assessment; note any hesitancy, expectation of success or failure, use of parent as a resource, and reaction to successful or unsuccessful performance

past and future tenses of irregular verbs. For example, the child might say, "I eated the apple" instead of "I ate the apple." Four-year-olds should be able to understand such prepositions as "over," "under," "behind," and "in front of."

The 4-year-old should be able to identify at least three colors, and the 5-year-old should identify at least four colors. The nurse can expect the 4-year-old to recognize colors by pointing to them and can ask the 5-year-old to name colors. The 5-year-old should be able to name basic shapes (circle, square, and triangle). The child approaching 6 years of age also should know the composition of common objects such as a spoon, shoe, or door and might give several correct answers to each of those items. For example, a spoon might be made of silver, metal, plastic, or wood; a shoe might be made of leather, plastic, rubber, cloth, or wood; and a door can be made of wood, metal, or glass.

The 4-year-old should be able to use simple analogies, which depend on the child's understanding of the relationships between concepts. The nurse assesses this skill by asking the child to complete a sentence that requires an analogy; such a sentence might be, "If fire is hot, ice is (   )?" The nurse presents the sentences exactly, without giving the child clues (for example, "What do you keep in the freezer at home?").

The 5-year-old should be able to decode verbal messages and name an object that is described. To respond correctly, the child must understand the words, use the words to construct a mental image, and translate the image into a verbal response. Similar abilities are needed to listen and follow directions, an important skill for the young child entering school because much information is given in the form of spoken directions. To assess this skill, the nurse can give three simple commands at the same time and observe the child's ability to remember the commands and carry them out correctly. All three commands might be repeated together a second time if the child is unable to remember.

The speech of 4- and 5-year-olds should be understandable to those outside the family. The child should be able to articulate clearly all speech sounds. A helpful tool for screening is the Denver Articulation Screening Examination. Occasional, mild stuttering in preschool children is not abnormal, but consistent or excessive stuttering warrants a more thorough evaluation.

The quality of the verbal interaction between the parent and child is an important part of language assessment. The nurse notes the following:

1. The amount of verbal interaction between the parent and child
2. Whether the parent listens to the child's comments
3. Parental response to the child's verbal messages (positive or negative feedback)
4. The content of the parent's verbal statements (vocabulary, grammar, ability to present and elaborate on concepts)
5. The child's ability to listen and respond to the parent

Cognitive Development The 4-year-old should be able to remember and repeat four single digits. Given three trials, the child should succeed in at least one. The 5-year-old generally can repeat a ten-word sentence, but if the child is unable to repeat the sentence on the first try, the nurse may present another sentence. The nurse can assess visual memory by arranging four common objects in a row and instructing the child to look at the objects carefully. Then the objects are scrambled, and the child is asked to put them back in the original order.

Four-year-old children are able to understand the difference between long and short. To assess this, two lines, one of which is considerably longer, are shown to the child, and the child is instructed to point to the longer line. The lines should be turned upside down and sideways as well, and the child should be able to select the longer line regardless of its position. The 4-year-old also is generally able to use the concepts of heavy and light. The child can be given two objects of similar size and asked which is heavier. The differences in weight must be readily apparent because the young child will be unable to identify subtle differences. Objects used might include a marshmallow and a rock or a ping-pong ball and a solid rubber ball.

Four-year-olds continue to classify according to one characteristic (see Chapter 9). When presented with circles, triangles, and squares of different colors and asked to put like objects together, most 4-year-olds will sort the objects by color. If shown how to classify the objects by shape, many will do this as well. Some 5-year-olds are able to sort by both color and shape when asked to do so. The nurse initially might ask the child to put like objects together and then ask the child to focus on one group of sorted objects and to group like objects together again to form subgroups (such as to divide the group of red objects into groups of red circles, red squares, and red triangles).

Five-year-old children can classify objects according to their relationship. The nurse might, for example, ask the child, "How are a jacket and a hat alike?" and expect the child to identify similarities such as, "They both keep you warm" or "You wear them when it's cold." The child's ability to conceptualize classes and subclasses is, however, still limited. For example, when the nurse shows the child a picture of five jackets and two hats and asks whether there are more items of clothing or more jackets, the child is likely to answer that the picture contains more jackets because jackets are not yet classified as a subgroup of clothes.

Children at this stage make considerable progress in understanding numeric concepts. Four-year-olds often can count to ten by rote, but most children at this age understand the concepts of numbers up to three and can correctly identify three objects. Five-year-olds often can correctly count and identify eight to ten objects. By this time, children know how old they are.

Because the thought processes of these children are influenced more by perception than by logic, 4- and 5-year-olds usually are unable to understand the concept of conservation (see Chapter 9). To test this, the nurse can use two balls of clay that are the same size. One ball of clay is then rolled into a long, thin shape, and the child is asked which shape has more clay. The child, using what Piaget termed preoperational thought (see Chapter 6), chooses one or the other because it looks "longer" or "fatter." The child is unable to reason that the amount of clay was not altered and that only the shape was changed. The same concept also can be tested by pouring the same amount of water from a short, fat glass into a tall, thin glass. Again, the child usually is unable to reason that the amount of water has not changed. In both tasks the child is more likely to answer correctly if allowed to pour the water or manipulate the clay. Some investigators feel that asking the child initially, "Which has more?" and then changing the form of the matter and asking, "Now which has more?" implies that the answer should be different and unfairly pushes the child toward an incorrect answer. A better assessment technique is to allow the child to watch as the nurse pours the water and manipulates the clay and then ask the child, "Was there more water (clay) before I poured (changed) it, after I poured (changed) it, or the same?"

Both 4- and 5-year-olds continue to use imaginative speech and play. Whereas the 4-year-old mixes fantasy and reality with little regard for accuracy, the 5-year-old is able to describe situations accurately. The 5-year-old might continue to tell fanciful tales but is able to realize which part of the tale is accurate and which is not.

Five-year-olds are also less egocentric and better able to consider another point of view. The nurse can observe spontaneous evidence of this throughout the assessment but also might ask a question requiring the child to consider the nurse's perspective such as, "What would be a good present to buy for your 1-year-old brother?" The 5-year-old should be able to consider the 1-year-old's perspective in answering, "A bike wouldn't be good because he couldn't ride it yet."

The child's understanding of causality becomes more realistic with maturation. The ideas might not be accurate, but they are likely to be less fanciful than a younger child's. Questions such as, "Why do people get sick?"; "How do kites fly?"; and "Why does it rain?" will produce interesting answers such as "People get sick because they go out in the rain"; "Kites fly because the wind blows them"; and "It rains to make things grow."

Social and Affective Development Children 4 and 5 years of age are proud of their abilities and eager to do things on their own. They are generally independent in self-care (see Chapter 9). The nurse observes how the child manages dressing and undressing in the assessment setting and should note whether the child performs these tasks independently or relies on the parent for help. The nurse also can discuss with the parent how hygiene and dressing tasks are managed at home.

Most 4- and 5-year-olds also are quite independent in toileting but might need occasional help wiping themselves. Most children at this age remain dry both day and night with only occasional accidents. About 10%–15% of 5- and 6-year-olds have nocturnal enuresis, although the frequency varies from once or twice a month to almost nightly. Although most children with nocturnal enuresis do not have underlying organic or psychologic problems, a careful assessment is indicated (see Chapter 24). Daytime wetting is not common in 4- and 5-year-olds and requires a thorough evaluation. Daytime wetting should be resolved before the child enters school to avoid teasing and social repercussions. The nurse explores whether accidents occur, how frequently, how the child responds, and how the parent manages the situation.

Four- and five-year-olds generally are able to separate quite easily from their parents and can play independently. In times of stress, however, the presence of a parent is very important. School entry, hospitalization, divorce, death, and other stressful situations might cause the child to regress to earlier forms of separation anxiety (see Chapter 27). The nurse might ask the parent to leave the room for a few minutes to see how both the child and parent handle the separation. If separation is a concern, the nurse explores how both the parent and child react. Assessment questions might include the following:

1. How long has the problem with separation been occurring?
2. How do you feel when you see the child crying?
3. What things have you tried to make the separations easier?
4. How does the child act when knowing that you must leave?
5. How does the child act after you leave?
6. How long does it take the child to adjust after the separation?

By 4 years of age, most children are able to express their feelings, and the nurse therefore notes throughout the assessment how the child handles emotions and how the parent responds. The nurse also might discuss with the parent how the child's emotions are handled at home. Questions might include the following:

1. How can you tell if the child is sad?
2. What does the child usually do if angry?
3. What type of things make the child angry (sad, frightened, etc)?

In assessing the child's awareness of emotions, the nurse might ask the following:

1. What is the scariest (happiest, saddest) thing you can think of?
2. What is something that makes you really mad?

Four-year-olds might continue to have unrealistic fears. Five-year-olds also might have specific fears, but because of their ability to distinguish reality from fantasy, they are more likely to evaluate their fears more logically (see Chapter 9).

Both 4- and 5-year-olds are able to recognize acceptable and unacceptable behavior, at least in familiar settings, although they do not always behave in acceptable ways. Most children control their behavior in an assessment setting, so the nurse observes the child's behavior throughout the assessment and notes overactivity, withdrawal, aggressiveness (verbal or physical), destructiveness or other acting-out behaviors.

The nurse also observes how the parent sets limits on the child's behavior, noting whether the parent is consistent, states the limit clearly and firmly, and enforces the limit.

Equally important are how the parent enforces limits and how the child responds. (Discipline and limit setting are discussed in Chapter 13.) The nurse also might discuss whether the behavior in the assessment setting is typical of the child's behavior at home.

In exploring the child's perceptions of discipline, the nurse might ask the following:

1. What is the very naughtiest thing a 4- (or 5-) year-old girl (or boy) could ever do?
2. Why would that be so naughty?
3. If you were a mommy (or daddy) and your little girl (or boy) did something very naughty, what would you do?
4. If you were naughty, what would your mommy and/or daddy do?

Because children of this age need opportunities to develop a sense of responsibility and pride in accomplishment, the nurse discusses the tasks the child is responsible for and how the child handles the responsibility. Children of this age often need reminders.

The nurse might determine the child's level of self-confidence by observing how the child approaches the tasks presented during the assessment. The nurse notes whether the child proceeds independently and seems to expect success, uses the parent as a resource if difficulty is encountered, hesitates, withdraws, refuses to perform, or otherwise seems to expect failure. The nurse notes how the child responds to success or failure at a specific task and how the parent reacts to the child's performance.

Four- and five-year-olds commonly display curiosity about sexual matters and typically are aware of the bodily differences between girls and boys. They might, however, have their own theories to explain sexual differences and reproduction. Questions to elicit the child's sexual perceptions include the following:

1. How can you tell if someone is a boy or a girl?
2. Why are girls and boys different?
3. Are you a girl or boy?
4. Where do babies come from?

The nurse might ask the parent whether the child has engaged in sexual exploration of self or others and may need to discuss further the parent's response to questions related to the child's sexual curiosity. In communicating with children both the nurse and parent need to use proper names for body parts and avoid characterizing any bodily function as dirty or bad.

The nurse also explores the parent–child relationship, noting such variables as the amount of time the child spends with each parent and with others in the family and the type of activities they do together. Children often imitate parents of both sexes, and parents might express concern if the child imitates behavior that the parents feel is appropriate only for the opposite sex (see Chapter 9). Although such imitation is normal, consistent imitation only of opposite-sex behavior requires further assessment.

Because sibling rivalry is common in families, the nurse discusses the child's relationship with siblings, inquiring about the frequency of conflicts, the precipitating factors, and how conflicts are resolved. Questions to address directly to the child include the following:

1. What do you like best about your brother (or sister)?
2. Is there anything you don't like about ?
3. What things does your brother (or sister) do that makes you mad (or sad)?
4. Do you ever fight?
5. What happens then?

Most 4- and 5-year-olds enjoy playing with peers and are able to play cooperatively. Because the ability to relate to peers is crucial for the child entering school, the nurse always explores this question with 4- and 5-year-olds. The nurse can discuss with both the parent and child how the child gets along with peers, what types of activities the child engages in, and the child's ability to share.

Questions to assess the child's social sense might include, "What would you do if you were playing with a toy and another child came and grabbed it?" If the child answers, "I'd tell him to give it back" or "I'd get my mom," the child is likely to have developed a mature social sense. Answers such as, "I'd cry," "I'd kick him," or "I'd let him play with it" might indicate less maturity and suggest a need for further observation.

School attendance requires the child to be able to relate to adults outside the family (see Chapter 9), a skill that can be assessed by noting how the child relates to the nurse. The nurse also might discuss with the parent how the child typically responds to new adults.

The 6- to 12-Year-Old-Child

Table 16-16 summarizes the developmental norms for children 6–12 years of age.

Motor Skills Motor development during middle and late childhood includes steady improvements in coordination speed, accuracy, and balance, which are refined as a result of maturation and the practice of activities requiring these skills. Running, climbing, jumping, and throwing are common components of children's games that require some skill for participation and acceptance in many group activities.

Eye–hand coordination also improves and aids in the development of fine motor skills. Handwriting, for example, requires some refinement of fine motor skills and hand–eye coordination, as do drawing, cutting, painting, working complex puzzles, playing a musical instrument, doing woodwork, needlework, or other crafts, and playing video games or using a computer terminal.

Many motor skills are demonstrated objectively in a neurologic examination (see Chapter 14) (such as walking, running, hopping, tandem walking, heel-and-toe walking, Romberg's maneuver, finger pursuit, putting finger to nose, using rapid alternating hand movements, and rapid finger tapping). Fine motor skills can be assessed by having the child write sentences, letters, numbers, draw progressively complex shapes, draw pictures, or work puzzles. These tasks provide a general assessment of the child's coordination and motor ability. In general, children of this age group are cooperative and enjoy doing such tasks. Successful completion is very important to them, so the nurse reinforces each attempt the child makes to perform each task.

The developmental history often provides much information about the child's aptitudes, interests, and progress. Additional assessment questions serve to update this history and detect any changes in developmental patterns. Questions addressed to the parent might include the following:

1. What kind of physical activities does the child enjoy? Any organized sports? What? How often?
2. Is the child involved in any of the following activities: gymnastics, cycling, swimming, baseball, soccer, or track?
3. How would you describe the child's performance in physical activities? Does the child keep up with the other children? If not, please elaborate. How would you describe the child's coordination?
4. Is the child's performance in physical activities and coordination different now from a year ago? In what ways?
5. Does the child take music and dance lessons? How are these progressing?
6. What kinds of quiet activities does the child enjoy?
7. How would you describe the child's handwriting and drawing? Have you noticed any changes in the child's performance in these areas over the last year? In what ways?
8. Has the child experienced any difficulties learning skills that require small movements such as tying shoelaces, cutting, or buttoning? If so, please elaborate.
9. Do you have any concerns about the child's development of physical skills and/or fine motor skills? If so, what are they?

The nurse might want to rephrase and direct many of these questions to the child. If the child does not participate in any sports activities or does not practice gross motor skills, the nurse can explore the cause with both the parent and child. The child might, for example, have no interests in these areas or may not have been allowed to do physical activity.

(text continued on p. 544)

TABLE 16-16 Guidelines for the Developmental Assessment of the 6- to 12-Year-Old Child

	Expected behaviors		
Developmental area	*6- to 8-Year-olds*	*8- to 12-Year-olds*	**Assessment techniques**
Temperament			Assess the child's temperamental characteristics and parental perceptions Ask how easily the child becomes upset and how the child responds to disappointments, being teased, and new experiences
Gross motor skills	Rides bike without training wheels	Does tricks on bikes; has races; begins to use bike for transportation	Ask questions to elicit child's interest and participation in sports, dance lessons, and physical activity
	Runs, skips, hops, jumps, climbs with increased speed and improved accuracy (can walk a 2-in wide balance beam, jump and hop into small squares); learns to climb trees and an interval-knotted rope and roller skate	Increased skill fluidity, and control of skipping, running, hopping and jumping actions; running speed increases to 5 m/sec, broad jump distance reaches 4–5 ft, and vertical jump height measures 8–10 in; adept at tree climbing; learns to shinny up a rope	Observe or inquire about the child's coordination in running, skipping, jumping, climbing, or hopping Question the child's perception of ability and performance in physical activities Ask the parents about their expectations in relationship to the child's performance and participation in activities
	Learns to swim	Improves swimming and adds new strokes	
	Improved coordination allows activities to be more purposeful such as dance lessons, gymnastics, relay races, and kickball	Continued improvement in coordination and ability to participate in organized competition, either individually or as a team member Increased stamina, identification, and practice of individual skills	
Fine motor skills	Prints numbers, letters, and words; printing becomes smaller and more accurate; learns cursive writing	Fluent printing of numbers and letters in correct alignment; cursive writing improves	Ask child about writing skills; may have child print or write name
	More precise in artwork, including drawing, coloring, painting, and cutting; chosen designs and projects are reproduced more accurately	Uses tools increasingly well; more advanced art, carpentry, and crafts projects	Ask the child and parent about crafts, artwork, and other projects that might be hobbies or special interests
	Improved hand–eye coordination for board games, puzzles, and playing musical instruments	Increased precision and speed in manipulating small objects into place such as stamps in an album; improved skill and finger dexterity in playing musical instruments	Assess hand–eye coordination by the child's performance on the neurologic examination
	Can throw small ball about 40 ft fairly accurately	Can catch and/or intercept pathways of small balls when thrown from a distance; throws ball overhand and underhand	Ask what the child can do best when playing ball and what aspect (throwing or catching) needs work

continued on next page

TABLE 16-16 continued

Developmental area	Expected behaviors: 6- to 8-Year-olds	Expected behaviors: 8- to 12-Year-olds	Assessment techniques
	Most children can tie a bowknot by the time they are 8 years old	Proficient at tying bowknots	Ask the child to tie a bowknot
Language development—expression and comprehension	Oral vocabulary of 2500 words by 6 years of age; sentence length approximately five words in length	Increased expansion of oral vocabulary to 7200 words; greater use of language for socialization; reading vocabulary of 50,000 words; speech is entirely understandable	Listen to the child's speech and use of grammar and syntax
	Makes use of all the various parts of speech	Improved grammar and correct use of parts of speech	
	Asks questions that indicate a quest for information about the purpose of objects	Uses language to solve problems; talks through options before making a decision	Note the child's ability to listen and follow directions
	Able to arrange stories of events objectively and begins to write "pretend" stories	Oral and written stories become more logical; characters and events are described in detail; able to create suspense; uses metaphors and personifications	Ask the child to relate some event in school or at an after-school activity; note sentence structure, objectivity, and whether the story is told logically
	Defines words according to their related action (eg, apple = something to eat)	Gives precise, dictionary-type definition to words	Ask the child to define several words such as orange and snow
Cognitive development	Increased attention span allows for improved visual discrimination and processing of information from the environment	Major advancement in ability to do more complex intellectual tasks; improved attention fosters focusing on details	Ask the child about school and ability to listen and follow directions; may use drawing of four objects, each slightly different, and ask the child to identify the differences
	Takes an interest in learning facts and solving problems	Wants to acquire large store of facts because they're useful and interesting; enjoys reading the Guinness World Record books; may focus on a special interest	Ask the child to solve problems; include both written and oral problems
	Knows number combinations up to ten; can count by 1, 2, 5, or 10; has basic idea of addition and subtraction; can tell time	Multiplication and division concepts fairly well mastered; uses numbers beyond 100 with understanding; uses and understands simple fractions	
	Is learning to read	Gathers factual information for reports from a variety of sources; is interested in learning about foreign places	Ask the child and parent about the types of books the child enjoys reading
	Knows comparative value of coins	Makes change for small amounts of money	Have the child identify various coins and then ask child to provide change for word problem about buying milk or something else that costs less than the money given to the salesperson
	Memory improves; remember best the material that is meaningful to them; beginning to use imagery as a memory aid	Develops strategies and uses a greater variety of memory aids, including rehearsal and organization	Ask the child to recite the Pledge of Allegiance; show a box with ten objects, then cover the box and ask the child to name as many objects as possible; ask the child to explain the method used for remembering
	Able to differentiate fantasy and reality but still thinks that radio and television characters are real	Skeptical of "realness" of television and radio programs	Ask the child if events that happen on a favorite program are real and why

TABLE 16-16 continued

Developmental area	Expected behaviors: 6- to 8-Year-olds	Expected behaviors: 8- to 12-Year-olds	Assessment techniques
	Developing a sense of humor; tells a joke repeatedly	More sophisticated sense of humor; uses double meanings and metaphors; enjoys riddles; begins to read comics in newspaper	Ask the child to repeat a riddle or joke and assess the type of humor
	Preoperational to concrete operational thinking; able to perform mental operations of conservation of liquid amount and solid amount	Concrete operational to beginning of formal operational thinking; able to perform additional mental operations of conservation of area, weight, and solid volume	Use the Piagetian task for conservation; may use two clay balls—roll one into a sausage shape and ask the child if the amount of clay has changed; ask the older child if the weight of the clay balls has changed
	Has acquired operations of reversibility, basic class inclusion, class hierarchy of visible objects, seriation of visible objects	Has acquired additional operations of class inclusion, hierarchy of representation; seriation tasks presented verbally are accomplished by 12 years of age	Have the younger child place a series of blocks in order according to descending size; observe for frequency of size comparison; ask the older child a representation question, "If Karl's red shirt is darker than Matthew's, and Karl's shirt is lighter than Adam's, who has the darkest shirt?"
	Does not understand relationships among time, speed, and distance; solves problems by trial and error; has difficulty verbalizing rationale for solution; considers two factors simultaneously but not more	Understands relationships among time, speed, and distance; still uses trial-and-error approach to problem solving but is more logical in approach; has difficulty verbalizing answer; considers two and maybe three factors by 12 years of age but may omit the fourth factor	Provide the child with a small balance and series of weights; request the child to position the weights so that the sides balance, then ask the child why it balanced and how things are related
	Less egocentric, able to take another's viewpoint; can consider someone else's feelings or needs; internalizes sense of conscience; follows rules to avoid punishment	Better able to take another's perspective; focuses on the intention of a behavior rather than on the act itself; follows conscience in decision making; obeys rules because they are instrumental; expects favor in return, views rules as instruments for own or other's satisfaction of needs	Tell the child about someone who cheated by going out of turn while playing a game because of wanting to win so badly and someone else who won by forgetting a penalty and ask what should be done; assess how the child solves the problem and the use of rules
Affective and social development	Expands social environment because of school and peer-group activities; peer group gains importance; usually same age and boys and girls play together	Social environment expands with activity; involvements, friends outside of immediate neighborhood; peer group influences become stronger; usually same-age, same-sex peers	Ask the child to name and describe friends and their favorite activities
	Learns to relate to new authority figure; notices differences in cultural, ethnic, and religious traditions; friends often reside in neighborhood; beginning to be more selective in choosing friends	Increase in new authority figures with organized club and team membership; increased interest in sociocultural differences; tends to categorize peers according to skills; more selective in friends—choose friends who have similar interests and skills; friendships usually loosely knit with boys and more tightly knit for girls	Ask the child and parent about the child's adjustment to school, new expectations from teacher, ability to relate to children of different backgrounds

continued on next page

TABLE 16-16 continued

Developmental area	Expected behaviors		Assessment techniques
	6- to 8-Year-olds	*8- to 12-Year-olds*	
Affective & social development (cont.)	Becoming self-critical—wants to do things well, complete projects; becomes upset if performance not up to personal expectations	Self-critical, proud of accomplishments, refuses to accept recognition perceived as undeserved	Have the child draw a picture and explain what is good, what needs improvement, and why; assess the child's demand on self to do well
	Begins collections and hobbies	More invested in hobby or collection	Ask the child to describe any hobbies or collecting; assess interest and use for self-concept
	Learns and begins to use social manners of greeting	Gradual improvement of social manners but might use selectively	Ask the parent to evaluate the child's manners
	Able to complete chores with reminding at times; may bargain to get paid for work around the house	Able to assume more responsibilities but tends to argue about what parents expect done; constant comparison with peers	Ask the parent about the child's cooperation in completing tasks, need for reminders, and response when reminded
	Awareness of individual attributes; further development of sense of self-esteem	Self-concept redefined in relation to peer's and new authority figures' perspectives; self-esteem related to self-perception of skill mastery	Have the child describe self; note the statements that indicate positive or negative attitudes about self
	Delay of gratification possible; can control emotions and assume responsibility for own behavior but has difficulty if tired or hungry	Able to delay gratification; controls and expresses emotions more appropriately and takes responsibility for own behavior	Ask the child about own behavior if someone teases, picks an argument or fights, or does not complete their work and the child has to do it; have the child compare what ideal and actual responses are and note the child's ability to accept responsibility
	Fears decreasing but may be stimulated by reading, television, or movies; might fear shadows or strange noises; worries about being late for school, not being liked, and not having someone to play with at recess	Fears more appropriate and reasonable such as exams, school or sport performance, or personal failure; fears body injury or pain	Ask whether the child is afraid of certain objects, animals, the dark, injury, or pain and note the child's response
	Understanding of sexuality more realistic	Understands human reproduction	Ask the child about reproduction and differences between the sexes, and note the child's understanding of facts
	Precausal ideas about reasons for illness	Understands health concepts	Ask the child why someone gets sick and note the child's response and understanding of realistic, logical, or scientific cause-and-effect relationships

Language Development The developmental history provides useful information concerning language development. The child's first words and any previous speech difficulties, chronic otitis media, hearing loss, or family history of speech and/or hearing difficulties are all factors that affect the child's present language level. Asking the parent about any concerns in the child's speech or language development is always helpful. The nurse listens objectively to the child's speech and conversation. Observations include whether the child is articulate, whether all words and sounds are clear and understandable, and whether the syntax and grammar are appropriate. The nurse determines whether the child communicates clearly without stuttering or stammering and whether the child's conversation is understandable, appropriate, and stated clearly and logically. If the child is quiet during much of the visit, the nurse might try

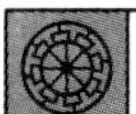

CASE STUDY Obese Adolescent

Assessment

Pam, 12-years-old, and her mother came to her primary health care nurse for a routine health assessment and advice concerning how to lose weight. Pam has gained 10 lb in the last 3 months, and her clothes no longer fit.

Family

Pam lives with her mother, who works full time. Her parents separated a year ago and are now divorced. She has an older sister, who is married and lives out of state. Pam's immediate family members are all obese, her father also has hypertension, and her mother has a hypothyroid condition.

Child

Pam always has had a weight problem and remembers being teased and called names such as "fatty" and "two-ton." She likes to eat and has developed many bad habits related to food intake (eg, eating while watching television, upon returning home from school, when doing homework, when lonely, and when bored). Her activities have decreased because she does not enjoy doing things alone. She and her sister used to take long bike rides, but now Pam only rides her bike to and from school. She swims once a week and enjoys that. Most of Pam's free time is spent watching television. She is an honor-roll student at school. She began menstruating when she was 11 years old.

Environment

Pam and her mother live in a second-floor apartment in a small house in the city.

Clinical Data

Temperament: Pam appears sad, tired, and self-conscious about her weight. She holds a magazine in front of her chest to hide the buttons pulling apart on her blouse. She sits slouched over to minimize her height.

Growth: Pam's height is 163 cm (5 ft, 7 in), which places her at the 95th percentile. Her weight is 92.8 kg (204 lb, 3 oz), which also places her above the 95th percentile.

Gross and Fine Motor Skills: Pam's motor skills are acceptable. Her fine motor skills are well coordinated, as evidenced by her small, neat handwriting. She exhibits some awkwardness with gross motor tasks because her weight makes movement and balance difficult to combine.

Cognitive Development: Pam's academic performance has been her strength. She hides in her books and likes learning. Her favorite subjects are English and social studies. She daydreams about living in another country.

Social and Affective Development: Pam has few friends, only many acquaintances. She helps her peers with their homework, but it seldom results in her gaining a friend. Her sister was her best friend until she moved away. Pam does not like being fat and is ready to try anything to lose weight. She says that she feels even more left out of things at the junior high school than at the grammar school and adds, "How can anyone like me when I am so ugly?"

Comparison to a Standard

According to National Center for Health Statistics growth charts, Pam is considerably overweight. Her score on the Self-Esteem Inventory was 20, which placed her in the low self-esteem quartile. Social development is limited, with school defined for mental education only. Pam participates in only a few activities with peers, and then her relationship is one of "alongside of" rather than "chumship." Pam's gross and fine motor skills are appropriate for her age level, and her cognitive skills are excellent.

Nursing Diagnoses

1. Alteration in self-concept related to negative feedback from peers and lack of friends.
2. Alteration in self-esteem related to disturbed body image secondary to obesity and height.
3. Developmental vulnerability related to social isolation by peers and self-defeating behaviors with regard to weight control.

Plan for Interventions

Goals

1. Pam will join the weight reduction club at school.
2. Pam will lose 0.5–1.0 lb/wk.
3. Pam will modify her eating habits and eliminate high-calorie snacks and junk foods.
4. Pam will offer academic help to peers, thus increasing her contacts and emphasizing her strengths.
5. Pam will take an interest in her appearance by dressing neatly, wearing clothes that fit, and keeping hair clean and combed.
6. Pam will walk, stand, and sit with good posture.

Interventions

1. Provide Pam with information about available resources at the junior high school to assist her in losing weight such as the weight reduction club, school nurse, and school nutritionist.
2. Encourage Pam to join the weight reduction club to obtain peer support for her efforts.
3. Discuss with Pam ways to increase her caloric expenditures such as swimming every day and adding a half hour to the time she spends riding her bike.
4. Discuss with Pam and her mother other possible after-school activities or clubs (eg, the Girl's Club, YMCA activities, Girl Scouts) that Pam might be interested in joining.
5. Review growth and development, informing Pam that the majority of her height already should be attained because menarche has occurred.

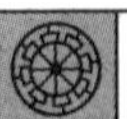

CASE STUDY Obese Adolescent (continued)

6. Discuss the different rates at which girls mature and Pam's perceptions about being an early maturer.
7. Explain to Pam the importance of good posture with respect to appearance and the prevention of muscular weakness.
8. Discuss the relationship of caloric intake and caloric expenditure with respect to weight loss.
9. Discuss with Pam ways to change her pattern of eating between meals (eg, keeping busy with after-school activities, putting signs on the cupboards and refrigerator reminding her not to snack, decreasing the amount of time she spends watching television).
10. Give Pam and her mother a list of foods and their calories to help them to plan Pam's diet better.
11. Review nutrition principles and the need for foods from the basic four food groups.
12. Advise Pam to eat smaller quantities at meals, to eat salads with no or low-calorie dressing instead of casseroles and creamed dishes for lunch at school, to eat fruit instead of cookies, ice cream, or pastry for dessert, and to drink skim milk.
13. Discuss with Pam's mother ways to prepare food to reduce the caloric content such as broiling or boiling instead of frying.
14. Refer Pam to a pediatrician to rule out any disease process contradicting weight loss.
15. Discuss the benefits of losing weight slowly and by changing eating habits, the types of food eaten, and the exercise routine.
16. Discuss clothing styles and general appearance with an emphasis on how to detract from weight and focus on Pam's attractive facial features and hair.
17. Discuss with Pam and even role-play ways to make friends. Suggest that she initiate helping some students with homework or in-class assignments.
18. Have Pam and her mother keep a record of their food intake and activities and bring it with them for weekly weight checks and conferences.
19. Suggest that Pam and her mother devise a reward system for every 10 lb Pam loses.

asking the child to describe his or her home, room, school, hobbies, vacation, or friends. A discussion can reveal much about the child's skills at expression and speech patterns.

Cognitive Development Assessment of cognitive development in middle and late childhood involves subjective and objective data that might include school interests, performance, difficult subjects, interest and ability in word and/or mathematic problems, and ability to reason and understand concepts. The nurse generally asks both the parent and child for any concerns about cognitive ability and/or school performance.

Objective data about cognitive development are available throughout the assessment. The nurse notes whether questions are answered appropriately and whether the child answers questions directly or initiates conversation, perhaps by asking questions about the equipment or the assessment.

Cognitive development can be measured concretely. The child's understanding of reversibility, for example, can be tested by having the child count forward and backward or do some addition and subtraction problems. Classification tasks might require various skill levels. For instance, a set of blocks of different colors and shapes are useful for the younger child, whereas a group of pictures of various birds, reptiles, mammals, or plants are appropriate for the older child.

Children normally find these tasks enjoyable and are eager to participate. Concrete tests provide much more information about cognitive processes, however, if the nurse encourages the child to explain the actions or thinking used to reach answers. Because cognitive development is gradual, children often operate in more than one stage of development.

Children's experiences in school and more structured learning situations help them to organize and develop strategies for remembering information (see Chapters 9 and 10). Activities and problem-solving experiences in which the child participates are remembered best. Various types of memory are used by the child in the learning process. For example, in learning to read the child uses visual memory for recognizing sight words, auditory memory for sound–symbol relationships in phonetic analysis, and recall memory for word definition.

Six-year-olds begin to use imagery (association of a visual image with the word) as a memory strategy and by 9 years of age demonstrate considerable skill in memorizing information using this technique. Categorizing information is seldom done by 6-year-olds but is a frequently used method of 10-year-olds. Older children also make greater use of rehearsal memory because learning by rote or drill enables them to remember lists of facts such as historical dates, chemical elements, poems, or the locations of countries and cities.

Social and Affective Development Objective data collection concerning psychosocial development usually is limited without observing peer interaction and/or school contact. Observation of the child's posture, eye contact, degree of comfort with the interview, and the interactions between the parent and child can, however, offer valuable clues concerning the child's self-concept and self-esteem.

Historical data provide a framework for a psychosocial assessment in middle and late childhood. The child's past and present exposure, experiences, and reactions to other children indicate the nature and extent of peer relationships. Children can describe their friends, whether they have a best friend, and whether they would rather play with friends or be alone. Children usually are eager to describe their participation in organized groups (scouts, sports, youth clubs, bands, etc), what these groups are like, or what they do after school and on weekends.

Of special interest are questions about school. These questions might include the following:

1. What's school like?
2. What's the best (or worst) part of school?
3. What kinds of things are you learning at school now?
4. Is school difficult? If so, in what ways?

Questions specifically addressed to the parent might include the following:

1. Does the child enjoy going to school?
2. Does the child have any problem getting up in the morning or not wanting to go to school?
3. How much school has the child missed and for what reasons?
4. Do you have any concerns about the child's school adjustment and performance?

Having the parent describe the child's relationships with other children and the family provides an added dimension. The parent might point to changes in peer and/or family relationships, which may in turn require further assessment.

In assessing the parent–child relationship, the nurse interviews both the family and child for information concerning the home environment and relationships. Questions for discussion might involve how much time the family is at home, what the family does at home, and what family members do together. In separate interviews the nurse might ask both the parent and child whether they talk about problems, what kinds of conflicts they have, how these conflicts are resolved, what the parent and child like and dislike about each other, and what the child's strengths and weaknesses are. Asking both the parent and child to describe the relationship also provides useful data for comparison.

The Adolescent

Table 16-17 summarizes the developmental norms for adolescents. The adolescent might be seen in a health care setting for any number of reasons, routine physical examinations, sports examinations or injuries, accidents, birth control information, screening for sexually transmitted diseases, or illness. Nurses who interact with adolescents need a basic understanding of the developmental issues that are important in the adolescent years. Because adolescents are involved with school and peer relationships outside the home and family, the adolescent is more likely to be seen in the assessment setting without the parent. Those who feel that their concerns are confidential might first need assurances that the nurse can be trusted not to reveal what they disclose.

Motor Skills Physical growth is so rapid during these years that adolescents commonly experience periods of clumsiness. Accelerated growth of the extremities, hands, and feet might precede trunk growth, which results in awkward motor coordination. This problem is short-lived, however, because trunk growth quickly catches up.

The adolescent's motor function should be comparable to an adult's. The adolescent actually is able to withstand stress and strain equal to or exceeding that of an adult, primarily because of increased muscle size and strength, which is more pronounced in males than in females. Fine motor coordination, evidenced by handwriting and the manipulation of small objects, also should be as refined as in adults.

Assessment of adolescent motor development is similar to assessment of motor development in late childhood. Subjective data include interest and participation in physical activities and sports, along with self-assessment of physical strength, endurance, abilities, injuries, limitations, or restrictions. Interest and ability in such activities as drawing, model building, needlework, carpentry, or typing are helpful in assessing fine motor control.

Historical data about developmental milestones assess motor development, whereas the medical history might provide clues to any previous, present, or future motor limitations. A thorough neurologic examination provides appropriate and objective data concerning gross and fine motor maturation and control (see Chapter 14).

Because adolescents are self-conscious about their bodies and abilities, the nurse needs to be careful to explain procedures and their significance fully. Explaining the assessment findings is also important to reassure adolescents that they are functioning normally.

Cognitive Development Subjective assessment of cognitive development includes questions concerning school interests, hobbies, and school performance. Also helpful are questions directed toward what the adolescent perceives as personal strengths and weaknesses. Much of this information can be obtained by engaging the adolescent in a conversation about daily routine, feelings about school, and special interests. Related to cognitive development at this stage are data such as first words, sentences, language difficulties, school adjustment, previous school performance, and school attendance.

TABLE 16-17 Guidelines for the Developmental Assessment of the Adolescent

Developmental area	Expected behaviors	Assessment techniques
Temperament		Ask adolescent and parent, if present, to describe adolescent's temperamental characteristics discipline and response
Gross motor skills	Progressing from awkward, clumsy stage to adult-like motor skills; activity level varies—may become involved in organized and/or competitive sports; choice of activities is influenced by personal preferences	Ask the adolescent about participation in physical activities; have adolescent state activity preferences and why they are favored; have the adolescent assess own perception of performance; ask about parental perceptions of child's skills, use of talents, choice of activities
Fine motor skills	Refined fine motor skills; Hand–eye coordination adultlike	Assess the adolescent's performance during a neurologic examination
	Precise movements when building models and doing fine sewing or other crafts; speed and individuality in handwriting; capable of small printing or writing; art skills perfected if interested; improved dexterity in fingers for playing musical instruments	Ask about any hobbies, interests, crafts; have the adolescent describe and evaluate abilities
Language development	Speech and writing totally understandable; expansion of oral and reading vocabulary; reading and writing complex sentences; follows abstract ideas; enjoys fantasy and scientific literature; peer dialect commonly used	Ask about favorite or current book being read
Cognitive development	Concrete to formal thinking; works with decimals; increased ability to reason abstractly; understands abstract ideas—"justice", "honesty"; aware of moral codes	Ask the adolescent about school, academic performance, and favorite subject; ask the adolescent to define justice and relate the concept to a recent event
	Able to generate hypothesis—to consider "possible" and follow idea through to a logical conclusion	
	Systematically solves verbal and mental problems using the scientific method	Present the pendulum problem and observe the process used to solve it; note the adolescent's ability to consider and systematically eliminate variables
	Plans ahead—oriented toward personal future such as college, career; tends to be idealistic	Discuss future goals—assess adolescent's perception of options
	Capable of imaginative, creative, inventive thinking; of mentally testing the hypothesis and critically evaluating it	Ask the adolescent, "If you could change the world in only one way, what would that change be and why?"
Social and affective development	Establishing sense of self-identity; may try out different roles in the process	Ask such questions as, "Do you like yourself?" "Do you fear being rejected?"
	Introspective; demands privacy and spends time daydreaming	Discuss importance of time alone to daydream
	Emotionally labile	May ask if moody, tense, easily angered, or anxious
	Establishes sexual identity; knowledgeable of bodily changes and implications for relationships	Ask the adolescent to provide a word picture of personal characteristics; favorite and disliked traits and behaviors; goals and aspirations
	Adopting life-style that fits with sense of self and goals for future; concentrates on special interests	
	Predominant orientation is the peer group; becomes increasingly involved with peers and "excuses" self from family activities; chooses own friends of both sexes; contacts widen with increased mobility	Ask the adolescent about friends, favorite activities, and frequency of group activities; might ask if it is easy or difficult to make friends
	Vacillates between independent and dependent behavior; family stress might be present	Discuss the adolescent's relationship with the family, especially the parents; ask, "What is the best thing about your parents, what 'bugs' you the most?"; note the adolescent's responses
	Might opt to follow rules and values of peers over those of society; generally decides right and wrong according to the rules of the majority	

TABLE 16-17 continued

Developmental area	Expected behaviors	Assessment techniques
	Formulates personal beliefs and values; may or may not explain them to others, especially parents	Present moral dilemma such as, "Your brother tells you a secret. He was going to a rock concert but was telling the parents he was going to a friend's house. Later, there is a need to contact your brother. Should you tell your parents where he is? Why?"
	Establishing own identity within family; moving to more adult relationship of love and respect but independence; process of establishing identity one of storm and stress	Discuss with the parent the adolescent's behavior and attitude at home, relationships with siblings and adults in family

Objective data collection might involve experiments to demonstrate the adolescent's ability to think abstractly or form hypotheses. For example, the adolescent might be presented with a pail of water and a number of objects small enough to fit within the pail. The adolescent is then asked to classify the objects according to whether they float and to explain the basis of this classification. The adolescent is encouraged further to manipulate the objects and explain why some objects assigned to one or the other classification did not fit the prediction made about floating or sinking. Finally, the adolescent is asked to propose a theory that links all the floating objects together. The adolescent, who is at Piaget's stage of formal operations (see Chapter 6), is capable of integrating several properties and can successfully complete the experiment. (At the earliest stage of concrete operations, the child has difficulty classifying when one property, such as size or weight, does not hold true for all the objects.)

Because cognitive and social development are closely related by adolescence, the nurse also might present several different social situations and ask the adolescent to define the possibilities. For example, an adolescent might be asked about a social or political event, which provides another opportunity to observe the adolescent's thinking patterns and reasoning abilities.

Social and Affective Development Assessment of adolescent social development results from the nurse's interaction with the adolescent. Some questions that might provide needed information include the following:

1. Tell me about yourself. Any hobbies or special interests?
2. How do you spend your free time? Tell me about your friends. What are they like? What do you do together? How much time do you spend with your friends? What do you like to do for fun?
3. What do you like (or dislike) about yourself? What are your strengths (or weaknesses)?
4. What do you like about your friends? Parents? School? What are things like at home? Tell me about your relationship with your parents. What are they like? Can you talk to them about problems, school, friends, sex?
5. If you were a parent, what would you do that is different from what your parents are doing?
6. Who can you talk to about your problems?
7. Have you thought about what you'll do when you leave home? Any plans for college or vocational school? Any fears you will not be accepted or able to do the work? Any career or work plans?
8. Do you date? What's that like for you? Are your friends dating? Are you sexually active? (A sexual history here might be appropriate.)
9. Do you use drugs? Tobacco? Alcohol? If so, what? How often? How much? Do you drink or use drugs with your friends or when you're alone? How do you feel when you use drugs or alcohol? Do your friends and/or parents use alcohol and/or drugs?
10. Are you afraid of being different? Being teased? Being lonely?
11. Do you fantasize about the future?

Because many of these questions can be very threatening to an adolescent, they must be approached carefully and only after trust and rapport have been established. Listening, accepting, spending time with the adolescent, and refraining from judgmental comments help to build rapport. Issues concerning drugs and sex, for instance, might be better left until later in the interview, after trust has been established.

Objective data come principally from the adolescent's presentation in the assessment setting. Observations of posture, eye contact, nervous habits, and ease in speaking, language, and social skills give the nurse an idea of the adolescent's self-concept and social skills. Observable interactions with family or peers also provide valuable data.

Family relationships can encourage or restrict development; therefore, the nurse needs to explore this area with the parent as well as the adolescent. Many characteristics common to adolescents, such as constant questioning of values, peer group conformity, dating, or daydreaming, might be stressful to the family.

Questions directed to the parent frequently supply a wealth of information concerning present family relationships (see Chapter 17). Further questions might center on discipline, responsibilities, limits, family activities, the adolescent's strengths and weaknesses, school performance, perception of the parents, dating, or peer relationships. What the parents like and dislike about the adolescent also provides more information concerning the parent–adolescent relationships. Asking whether the parent has any concerns about the family's relationship with the adolescent reveals additional psychosocial information.

Key Concepts

- A developmental assessment should foster optimal development by validating that the child is developing normally or detecting problems early so that necessary interventions can be planned.
- A systematic developmental assessment, which includes all subsystems of development, prevents the nurse from overlooking developmental problems that are not immediately evident.
- Developmental milestones are a useful standard of reference in determining whether a child's behaviors are normal for a given age, but the achievement of milestones does not always indicate normal development.
- Serial developmental assessments require at least one thorough developmental history and pertinent observations of development at each well-child visit.
- In formulating a nursing diagnosis following a developmental assessment, the nurse considers the quality of information, any indications of risk, and the effect of specific suprasystems and subsystems on the child's development.
- Interventions planned to address a child's developmental needs may vary from anticipatory guidance for normal development and health promotion to extensive multidisciplinary management for serious developmental problems.
- The nurse includes both the child and parent in the assessment process and might need to interview the child and the parent separately to ensure open communication.
- To assist the child in cooperating and performing well with assessment tasks, the nurse proceeds slowly, allows the young child to play with equipment, and structures tasks to progress from simple to complex.
- Open-ended questions addressed to both the parent and child assist the nurse in identifying developmental concerns early in the assessment interview.
- Observations of development might be structured or unstructured and include data about temperament, motor skills, language development, cognitive development, and social and affective development.
- Developmental screening might be part of the assessment but is distinctly different in that it depends on standard, easy-to-administer tools that compare a child's development in one or more areas with a standard of reference.
- Common tests for developmental screening include the Carey Temperament Questionnaires, the Denver Developmental Screening Test, the Goodenough–Harris Drawing Test, the Brazelton Neonatal Behavioral Assessment Scale, the Peabody Picture Vocabulary Test, the Developmental Indications for the Assessment of Learning, the Pediatric Examination for Educational Readiness, and a variety of intelligence tests.
- In assessing the neonate the nurse seeks to identify the infant's capabilities and vulnerabilities evident in the infant's interactions with the environment.
- The infant's state of arousal is a means by which the infant responds to stimuli; other assessment criteria include the infant's habituation, consolability, visual and auditory orientation, motor skills, and social and affective responses.
- The nurse assesses the parent–infant attachment by observing parental responses to infant behaviors and awareness of the infant's cues.
- Between 1 and 3 months of age, the infant's behavior becomes more predictable, and the infant develops a palmar grasp, attends to noises and voices, and develops early social responses to caregivers.
- Between 3 and 6 months of age, infants develop temperamental differences, learn to sit with support, can direct reaching and grasping toward objects, begin vocalizing, can recognize people and objects, and develop reciprocal social interactions.

- Between 6 and 9 months of age, the infant's temperament becomes increasingly evident, and the infant learns to sit alone, use reaching and grasping to achieve goals, make sounds and recognize words, and explore the environment.
- Between 9 and 12 months of age, infants become more active, are aware of strangers, reach and grasp precisely, speak single words, demonstrate intentional and directed behaviors, and show intense attachment to parents.
- Between 12 and 24 months of age, children show marked temperamental differences, learn to walk, control grasping and release of objects, communicate through language, and struggle with their needs for both independence and security during separation from parents.
- Between 2 and 3 years of age, children develop coordination and balance, improve sensory perception, learn to use paper and pencil, develop their vocabulary and improve their ability to respond to speech, and learn to interact with peers.
- Between 4 and 5 years of age, children refine their motor skills, learn to speak in sentences, develop abilities to memorize and classify objects, and can control their behavior within prescribed limits.
- Children from 6 to 12 years of age continue to develop coordination and their abilities to reason and understand concepts, learn to write and communicate ideas, and develop interpersonal skills by interacting with teachers and peers.
- Because adolescents experience rapid physical growth together with cognitive, social, and affective development, nursing assistance might be needed to help them understand developmental norms.

References

Ainsworth M: The development of infant–mother attachment. In: *Review of Child Development.* Vol 3. Caldwell B, Ricruiti H (editors): University of Chicago Press, 1973.

Als H, Brazelton TB: A new model of assessing the behavioral organization of preterm and full-term infants. *Am Acad Child Psychiatry* 1981; 20: 239–263.

Anastasi A: *Psychological Testing.* 5th ed. MacMillan, 1982.

Bakwin RN, Weider A, Bakwin H: Mental testing in children. *J Pediatr* 1948; 33:384.

Bayley N: Comparisons of mental and motor test scores for ages 1–15 months by sex, birth order, race, geographical location and education of parents. *Child Dev* 1965; 36:379–411.

Bierman JM, Vaage M, Hoznik MD: Pediatrician's assessment of the intelligence of two-year-olds and their mental test scores. *Pediatrics* 1964; 34: 680–690.

Brazelton TB: *Neonatal Behavioral Assessment Scale.* Lippincott, 1973.

Brazelton TB, Tronik E, Adamson L, et al: Early mother–infant reciprocity. In: *Parent–Infant Interaction.* CIBA Foundation Symposium 33, 1975.

Brazelton TB, Koslowski B, Main M: The origin of reciprocity: The early mother–infant interaction. Pages 49–76 in: *The Effect of the Infant on Its Caregiver.* Lewis M, Rosebloom LA (editors). Wiley, 1974.

Carey W: Clinical applications of infant temperament measurements. *J Pediatr* 1972; 81.

Carey W, McDevitt S: Revision of the Infant Temperament Questionnaire. *Pediatrics* 1978; 61: 735–739.

Coleman JM, Iscoe I, Brodsky M: The "draw-a-man" test as a predictor of school readiness and as an index of emotional and physical maturity. *Pediatrics* (Aug) 1959; 24:275.

Coopersmith S: *The Antecedents of Self-Esteem.* Freeman, 1967.

Dunn LM: *Expanded Manual for the Peabody Picture Vocabulary Test.* American Guidance Service, Inc.,1965.

Ferholdt JD: *Clinical Assessment of Children: A Comprehensive Approach to Primary Pediatric Care.* Lippincott, 1980.

Frankenburg WK: The Denver Prescreening Development Questionnaire. LADOCA Project and Publishing Foundation, Inc., 1975.

Frankenburg WK, Sciarillo W, Burgess D: The newly abbreviated and revised Denver Developmental Screening Test. *J Pediatr* 1981; 99(6):995–999.

Frankenberg WK, Goldstein AD, *Camp B:* The revised Denver Developmental Screening Test: Its accuracy as a screening instrument. *J Pediatr* 1971; 79:988–995.

Goodenough FL: *Measurement of Intelligence by Drawings.* World Book, 1926.

Greenspan SI, Lieberman AF: Infants, mothers and their interaction: A quantitative clinical approach to developmental assessment. In: *The Course of Life: Psychoanalytic Contributions Toward Understanding Personality Development.* Vol 1. *Infancy and Early Childhood.* Greenspan SI, Pollock GH (editors). National Institute of Mental Health. US Department of Health and Human Services, 1980.

Harris DB: *Children's Drawing as Measures of Intellectual Maturity.* Harcourt Brace Jovanovich, 1963.

Hegvik R, McDevitt S, Carey W: The Middle Childhood Temperament Questionnaire. *J Dev Behav Pediatr* 1982; 3: 197–200.

Hokelman RA, Kelly J, Zimmer AW: The reliability of maternal recall. *Clin Pediatr* 1976; 15: 261–265.

Horowitz FD: Child development for the pediatrician. *Pediatr Clin North Am* 1982; 29: 359–376.

Klaus M, Kennel J: *Maternal–Infant Bonding.* Mosby, 1976.

Korsch B, Cobb K, Ashe B: Pediatricians' appraisals of patients' intelligence. *Pediatrics* 1961; 27: 990–1003.

Levine M, et al: The pediatric examination of educational readiness: Validation of an extended observation procedure. *Pediatrics* 1980; 66: 341–349.

Lewis M, Rosenblum LA: *The Effect of the Infant on its Caregiver.* Wiley, 1974.

Mardell C, Goldenberg D: *Manual for Developmental Indicators for the Assessment of Learning.* Childcraft Educational Corporation, 1975.

McCarthy J, Brazelton TB: Neonatal behavioral assessment. *Drug Ther* (Feb) 1980; 103–115.

McDevitt S, Carey WB: The measurement of temperament in 3- to 7-year-old children. *J Child Psychol Psychiatry* 1978; 19: 245–251.

Mendell F, Yogman M: Developmental aspects of well child visits. *J Dev Behav Pediatr* 1982; 3: 118–121.
Olsen, et al: Use of the Brazelton Neonatal Behavioral Assessment as an intervention. Unpublished manuscript, 1981.
Parke R: Perspectives on father–infant interaction. In: *Handbook of Infant Development.* Osofsky J (editor). Wiley, 1979.
Piaget J, Inhelder B: *The Psychology of the Child.* Basic Books, 1969.
Powell M: Page 184 in: *Assessment and Management of Developmental Changes and Problems in Children.* 2nd ed. Mosby, 1981.
Robson, KS, Moss HA: Patterns and determinants of maternal attachment. *J Pediatr* 1970; 77: 976–985.
Sanders L: Issues in early mother–child interaction. In: *Infant Psychiatry: A New Synthesis.* Rexford EN, Sander LW, Shapiro T (editors). Yale University Press, 1976.
Thomas A, Chess S: *Temperament and Development.* Brunner/Mazel, 1977.

Additional Readings

Brazelton TB: Crying in infancy. *Pediatrics* 1962; 29: 579–588.
Caldwell B: *Instruction Manual—Inventory for Infants (Home Observation for Measurement of the Environment).* University of Arkansas at Little Rock, 1970.
Carey W: Measuring infant temperament. *J Pediatr* 1972; 81: 414–418.
Carey W: A simplified method for measuring infant temperament. *J Pediatr* 1970; 77: 188–194.
Casey P, Bradley R: Developmental screening for the pre-school-age child: Practical recommendations. *J Arkansas Med Soc* 1980; 77: 175–179.
Casey P, Bradley R: The impact of the home environment on children's development. *J Dev Behav Pediatr* 1982; 3: 146–152.
Chess S, Thomas A: Temperament and the parent–child interaction. *Pediatr Ann* 1977; 6: 26–45.
Cohn DH, Stern V: *Observing and Recording the Behavior of Young Children.* Teachers College Press, 1978.
Darling RB, Darling J: *Children Who Are Different.* Mosby, 1982.
Douglas H, Spietz A: The feeding and teaching scales. In: *NCAST Learning Manual.* Barnard K (editor). University of Washington, 1978.
Erickson E: *Childhood and Society.* Norton, 1963.
Erickson M: *Assessment and Management of Developmental Changes in Children.* Mosby, 1980.
Flapan D, Neubauer P: Issues in assessing development. *J Am Acad Child Psychiatry* 1970; 9.
Funk J, Ruppert E, Jurs S: Assessing the predictive validity of developmental milestones. *J Dev Behav Pediatr* 1982; 3: 143–145.
Ginsberg H, Opper S: *Piaget's Theory of Intellectual Development.* Prentice-Hall, 1969.
Goodnow J: *Children Drawing.* Harvard University Press, 1977.
Golden GS: The developmentally disabled child: Detection, assessment, referral and treatment. *Child Care Newsletter* 1984; 3(1):8–11.
Greenspan SI: *The Clinical Interview of the Child.* McGraw-Hill, 1981.
Harrison LL: Nursing intervention with the failure-to-thrive family. *Matern Child Nurs J* (March/April) 1976; 1(2):111–116.
Hart H, Bax M, Jenkins S: The value of a developmental history. *Dev Med Child Neurol* 1978; 20: 442–452.
Illingworth RS: *The Development of the Infant and Young Child, Normal and Abnormal.* Churchill-Livingstone, 1972.
Kolberg L: Moral stages and moralization: The cognitive and developmental approach. In: *Moral Development and Behavior.* Lickona T (editor). Holt, Rinehart & Winston, 1976.
Lewis M, Taft LT: *Developmental Disabilities. Theory, Assessment and Intervention.* SP Medical and Scientific Books, 1982.
Lichtenstein R, Ireton H: *Preschool Screening.* Grune & Stratton, 1984.
Littman B, Parmalee AH: Medical correlates of infant development. *Pediatrics* 1978; 61: 470–474.
McCall R: A hard look at stimulating and predicting development: The cases of bonding and screening. *Pediatr Rev* 1982; 3: 205–212.
Nelms C, Mullins G: *Growth and Development. A Primary Health Care Approach.* Prentice-Hall, 1982.
Piaget J: *The Construction of Reality in the Child.* Ballantine Books, 1954.
Smart M, Smart R: *Children: Development and Relationships.* MacMillan, 1977.
Sroufe A: Socioemotional development. In: *Handbook of Infant Development.* Osofsky J (editor). Wiley, 1979.
Strangler S, Huber C, Routh D: *Screening Growth and Development of Preschool Children—A Guide for Test Selection.* McGraw-Hill, 1980.
Szumowski E, Chamberlin R: Typical behaviors of one-year-old children and their mothers. *J Dev Behav Pediatr* 1980; 1:122–127.
Tronick E, Brazelton TB: Clinical uses of the Brazelton Neonatal Assessment. In: *Exceptional Infant: Assessment and Intervention,* Vol III. Friedlander EZ (editor). Brunner/Mazel, 1975.
Vaughn B, Deinard A, Egeland B: Measuring temperament in pediatric practice. *J Pediatr* 1980; 96: 510–514.
Ventura JN: Parent coping behaviors, parent functioning and infant temperament characteristics. *Nurs Res* (Sept-Oct) 1982; 31(5):269–273.

Family Assessment

Joan Pernice Lorna Kaufman

17

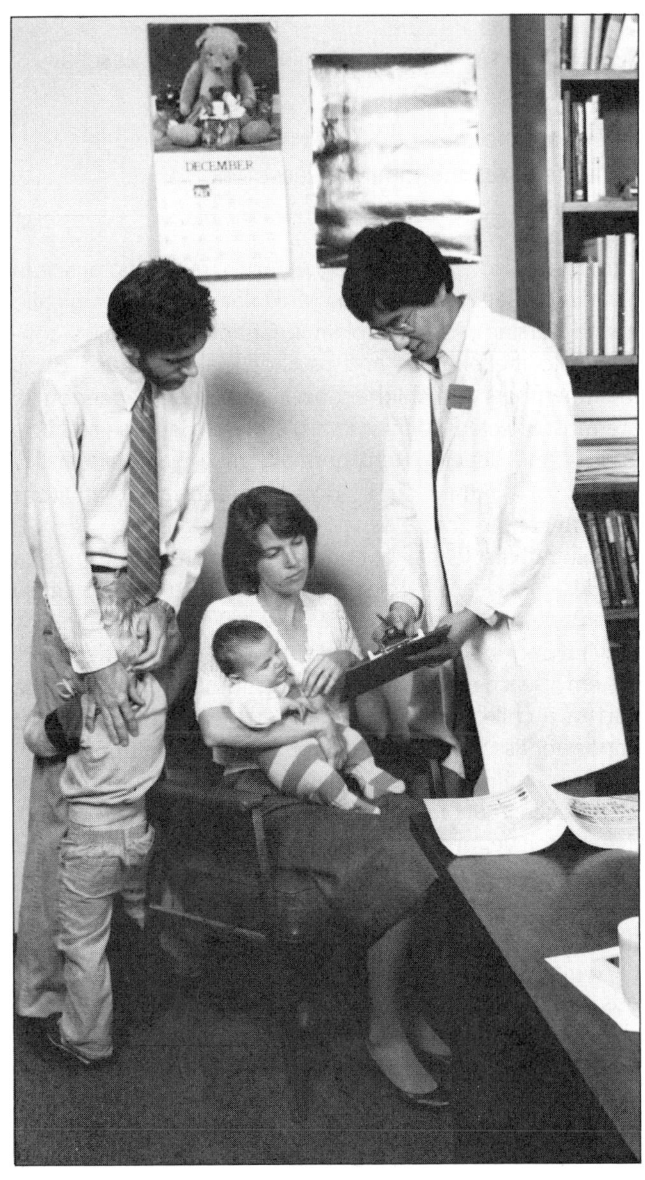

Chapter Outline

Objectives

- Explain the role of the nurse in family assessment.
- Define the criteria the nurse uses to assess the family.
- Describe the settings in which the family assessment takes place.
- Explain the methodology with which the nurse approaches the family assessment.
- List the assessment tools commonly used in family assessment.
- Relate the goals of family assessment to the nurse's role in establishing a care plan.

Family assessment is an integral part of nursing practice in a variety of settings, but it has particular significance in child health nursing. As we explain in Chapter 4, families contribute to the physical and psychosocial well-being of all their members, but children, because of their dependence, are most affected by their family system. Because a child's growth and development normally take place within the context of a family, family dynamics and family environment affect the child's developmental progress.

Children first learn about human relationships from their families. They learn behaviors and roles from watching family members, and they learn patterns of communication as they interact with parents, siblings, and others in the family system. Learned behaviors and patterns in turn become part of a child's developmental course and are therefore important assessment criteria for the child health nurse.

In promoting optimum health the nurse assesses the child by collecting data not only about the child's physical, affective, cognitive, and social development but also about the family system that affects these developmental subsystems. In Chapter 4 we define types of families and present a framework for studying family functioning. In Chapter 13 we define styles of parenting and describe common methods of discipline that parents often use in response to their children's behavior. In this chapter we consider the importance of family dynamics and parenting in the process of family assessment, and we discuss the role of family assessment in planning interventions for the child's health.

Purpose of the Family Assessment

Family assessment is the process of gathering and analyzing data about a family and its members. This process is characterized by continuous data collection accompanied by professional judgments that determine the significance of the data and direct the nurse toward areas of concern. Effective family assessment is dynamic and flexible. Its hallmark is the ongoing acquisition and interpretation of information. Although the nurse may choose to use available assessment tools to collect and organize data, unstructured observations and informal discussions may be equally useful. These techniques often provide the nurse with the information needed to plan interventions that promote family functioning and child health.

Data collection for family assessment thus comes from many sources: client interviews, structured and unstructured observations, subjective appraisals by family members and others, and information provided by referral sources, agencies working with the family, and other members of the health team. The information requested depends on the setting and context for assessment. In a well-child setting family assessment directs the nurse in anticipatory guidance and health teaching (see Chapter 21). In a hospital setting information about the family assists the nurse in discharge preparation and planning follow-up care (see Chapter 29).

In child health nursing family assessment is not to be confused with family therapy. Although family therapy also requires data collection and emphasizes the role of the family system in child development, its purpose is quite different. Family therapy focuses on the family as a whole. It usually involves more formal interviewing and treatment processes and often identifies problems that require long-term therapy. In contrast, family assessment focuses on a family's characteristics, concerns, roles, and relationships as they affect child health. Its purpose is to identify needs for teaching and referral and, in the process, to promote family growth.

The following factors should be included in a family assessment according to Robischon and Smith (1977):

Family boundary definition
Family roles
Family arrangement
Amount of available energy
Power structure
Ability to change
Communication patterns
Physical environment
Economic resources

Incidence of family illness
Parental behavior
Family self-care ability

The Family Assessment Process

Applying Family Theories

Family assessment in nursing draws on the methods and theories of many other disciplines. Sociologists and psychologists, for example, tend to view family structure and function by analyzing family members' interactions and responses to situations together with the cultural norms and institutions (education, health care) that affect the family system. Other disciplines focus on the economic, legal, or religious influences on the family (Hill and Hanson, 1960; Nye and Bernardo, 1966).

Although all of these views may help the nurse to understand a particular family, none by itself provides all of the information necessary for a comprehensive assessment. Miller and Janosik (1980) recommended an eclectic approach to family assessment that combines many available theories into a general framework with a broad application. They concluded that a general systems framework is not restrictive because it deals with the multiple aspects of family life, including family social systems.

In nursing Duvall's (1977) descriptions of family stages and family developmental tasks provide the theoretic bases for many assessment criteria. (Family development is discussed in Chapter 4.) In the same way that theories of child development provide the nurse with a frame of reference, theories of family development define norms that the nurse can use in analyzing data about a specific family. Like the many theories of child development, each family theory provides the nurse with some insight into a family's expectations, capabilities, and needs. In effect, the theory provides a standard of comparison, although no theory should be applied so rigidly that it prevents the nurse from identifying strengths, weaknesses, or needs that the theory does not address.

No two families are alike; the combination of experiences, personalities, relationships, and ambitions is unique to each family. Each family develops and maintains its own homeostasis that provides a sense of predictability, security, tradition, and purpose. "Power, mutual expectations, repetitive and reciprocal patterns of behavior, roles, rules, communication, and boundaries are the essential components which maintain homeostasis in the family" (Phipps, 1980). Therefore, every family responds to change, challenge, or crisis differently because their expectations of other family members are different, their roles and function within the family are specific to their situation, and they have adapted their method of communication to the personalities and relationships that comprise their family. Families also respond to new or stressful situations in different ways depending on their stage of development and the degree to which earlier developmental tasks were achieved.

For example, assessing the adjustment of a young couple who have recently become parents requires more than gathering data about general aspects of family development and the family's success in achieving new developmental tasks. The assessment data also should include information about the family's cultural and socioeconomic orientation and how this couple defines their individual roles within these suprasystems. In addition, it is valuable to identify the family structure before the infant's birth and note if and how it has changed with the infant's arrival. A woman who is actively pursuing her own career may or may not find her role as a mother to be disruptive. How she responds to the changes necessitated by her new role depends on available resources, planning and adjustments made prior to the infant's birth, her own personality, the infant's temperament and characteristics, expectations of spouse, family, and friends, the cultural and ethnic meaning attached to children, and her relationship and ability to communicate with her spouse and family. The key to helping individuals grow as parents is not simply to compare them with some standard or theory but rather to understand how they define and enact their role, what their perceived satisfaction is, and what their concerns are. Only then does assessment data have meaning because it then directs the plan for intervention.

The manner in which women combine the roles of parent and professional cannot be assumed. For example, one nurse was concerned because the mother's response to questions about the infant's routines and behavior were vague, although the mother and infant appeared to have a good reciprocal relationship. At the following well-child visit, the father also was present. Following customary practice, the nurse addressed questions about the infant's characteristics and abilities to the mother. The mother, however, deferred to the father, who answered each query in detail. Finally, the nurse asked why the father seemed to know more about the infant's routines than the mother did. The parents explained that their personal goals and the demands of their careers were such that the father could take time off and work at home more easily than the mother could. They also did not want their relatives, who did not approve of their decision, to care for their infant. They believed that, contrary to the traditional stereotype, either parent could nurture and provide for the infant's needs and that it was healthier for both of them to be involved in childrearing. They knew and accepted the fact that at various times one or the other of them would be more involved and more knowledgeable about the infant's routines than the other. The nurse supported their decision to share child care and made a note in the infant's records to involve both parents when obtaining data, to assess both parent's adaptation to and satisfaction with their parenting role, and to support

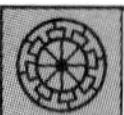

CASE STUDY Combining Parenthood and Career

Assessment

Katy is a 4-month-old infant who appears healthy. Her mother plans to return to work and have a neighbor take care of Katy. She wonders whether this will interfere with Katy's future development in any way.

Family

This nuclear family consists of a father, age 26, a mother, age 25, and Katy, 4 months. There are no extended family members living within a 100-mile radius. Both parents were only children and have had minimal experience with infants. The pregnancy was planned, and Katy's birth was eagerly anticipated. There were no prenatal complications, but a cesarean delivery was necessary because of prolonged labor. The family's insurance policy did not fully cover the longer hospitalization. The father is employed full-time now that he has completed his education. The mother taught school until 1 week prior to Katy's birth.

Child

Katy is a healthy, happy infant who is developing according to expected norms. She is breast-fed, gaining weight, and increasing in length appropriately. She responds well to the mother. The mother reports that the father participates in Katy's care and that their relationship is positive.

Environmental

The family has recently purchased a three-bedroom home in the suburbs. Being homeowners has taken more time, money, and energy than they had anticipated. Financial concerns especially have mounted during the past year.

Clinical Data

Structure and Function: There are three members in this nuclear family, a 26-year-old father, 25-year-old mother, and 4-month-old daughter. No extended family live nearby. The mother reports that relations with the extended family on both sides have been good in the past, although her plans to return to teaching instead of staying home with Katy have been a source of recent friction.

The couple share household tasks as other time constraints permit. The mother said that she has been doing the majority of household tasks since Katy was born because she was home and her husband was just beginning his career. In fact, he often brought work home to finish in the evening. He did spend the weekends working around the house.

Family roles: The mother commented with a tone of resentment that she and her husband seemed to have slipped into stereotyped sex roles since moving into their own home and Katy's birth. They had shared more tasks before, but then there had been more to do, and previous routines, such as going to the laundromat, were no longer necessary. They often had combined work and fun such as browsing at used book stores while the clothes were washing. She hoped they could do more things together as a couple as Katy got older.

Communication Patterns: The mother commented that she and her husband communicated well with each other. She missed other adult conversation during the day and was beginning to think that she never talked about anything other than Katy, which was exactly what she had vowed would not happen. Although they had less time together now, she described her marital relationship as one of "best friends," each spouse knowing the other so well they could share their thoughts and concerns. They had agreed that she should return to teaching, both for her personal and professional well-being and for financial reasons.

Economic Resources: Finances are a matter of concern, but poverty is not an issue. The family has incurred many debts related to education, home purchase, and the extended hospital stay when Katy was born.

Parental Behavior: Katy's mother appears to be developing a good reciprocal relationship with Katy. Throughout the interview, however, the mother's greatest concern seemed to be her inexperience and consequent doubts about providing appropriate child care. She wanted to return to teaching but feared that it would be too great an adjustment for Katy. It seemed as if she were searching for specific information and evaluation guidelines so she could grade her parenting behaviors. She had read many books, but these had confused her because each author had a slightly different parenting philosophy.

Comparison to a Standard

This family has many strengths and the members appear capable of providing for each other's needs. They compare favorably in all assessment areas related to the tasks of family development. They are providing for Katy's basic needs but need recognition and increased self-confidence to achieve satisfaction in their new role. The parents are concerned about continuing to meet Katy's affective needs when the mother returns to teaching.

Nursing Diagnoses

1. Knowledge deficit about parenting role related to inexperience with children, confusion from books read, and inadequate feedback from others.
2. Family coping—potential for growth related to family strengths of communication and sensitivity to each other's needs.
3. Potential alteration in parenting related to financial concerns and plans for mother to resume teaching and Katy to be cared for by a neighbor.

Plan for Interventions

Goals

1. Parents will state their philosophy about parenting.
2. Parents will identify cues from Katy that her developmental needs are being met.
3. Each parent will identify a time to spend playing with Katy every day.
4. Parents will express confidence in the babysitter's ability to care for Katy in their absence.

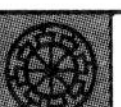

CASE STUDY **Combining Parenthood and Career (continued)**

Interventions

1. Explore with the family their ideas about parenting, experiences as parents, and confusion about advice received.
2. Encourage the parents to formulate their own philosophy of parenting and to discuss how they want to approach various parenting concerns such as discipline, bedtime routines, feeding patterns, and toys.
3. Emphasize the uniqueness of each child and parent–child relationship and the importance of "fit" rather than rigid adherence to outside advice or frequent comparison to another's way of parenting.
4. Provide parents with information about normal growth and development, thereby helping them to anticipate Katy's needs and behaviors.
5. Have parents describe the ways that Katy communicates her satisfaction with their care, her pleasure with their interactions, or when she is unhappy and their ability to soothe her and encourage them to accept these behaviors as indicators that they are good parents.
6. Support the parents by telling them to call any time they have a question or concern about Katy or their parenting role.
7. Tell them to schedule a special time for playful interaction with Katy and to emphasize quality in the time they are together because the quantity of time will decrease.
8. Encourage the parents to discuss household tasks and the need to share the work load at home when both are working outside the home.
9. Praise the parents for their open communication with each other and emphasize its value during times of change and adaptation to new roles.
10. Suggest that the mother leave Katy with the babysitter for short times before she actually goes back to work so the babysitter and Katy get to know each other.
11. Tell the mother to write down Katy's schedule, likes, dislikes, favored positions, and play activites for the babysitter so Katy's routine can be maintained.
12. Provide the babysitter with telephone numbers where Katy's mother, father, and primary health care provider can be reached.
13. Offer to initiate a referral if the family's financial concerns become burdensome.
14. Show parents their favorable comparison to family assessment tools such as Assessment of Family Strengths and Family Developmental Tasks to provide further feedback regarding their parenting skills.

their decision to continue their careers and share child-rearing responsibilities.

Collecting Data

The process of data collection provides the nurse with a mechanism for establishing rapport with family members. A trusting relationship with mutual respect and open, honest communication also sets the stage for a comprehensive assessment in which family concerns are addressed. At the same time, the nurse guides the family into an active role in health care by providing both parents and children with opportunities to ask and answer questions.

Preparing for the Interview Rapport and communication are enhanced when the nurse is prepared for the family's visit. This requires reading available records and anticipating needs, which in turn requires a knowledge of normal child and family development.

Careful preparation also helps the nurse to remain flexible in response to family members' questions and concerns. Although the nurse begins the interview with an "agenda" that includes general assessment criteria and likely concerns for the family and child, family members' questions and responses might direct the nurse to unanticipated areas. In such instances adhering rigidly to a series of questions might limit the scope and depth of the family's answers. If, however, the nurse is prepared for a variety of issues, family members are more likely to see the nurse as a responsive person, a resource, and an advocate rather than an examiner.

Parental concerns sometimes are different than those anticipated by the nurse. The parent might use the well-child visit for one child to discuss concerns about another child or to introduce an unexpected topic. If the nurse demonstrates genuine interest, appears calm and unhurried, sits down, and asks the parent some general questions about the family, it helps to set the tone of the interview.

For example, one nurse's agenda was to continue teaching a family about the care required by their daughter, who was a newly diagnosed diabetic. The nurse initiated a discussion about the relationship of diet, insulin, and activity for this girl but quickly sensed that the family's thoughts were elsewhere. Rather than continue with the planned agenda, the nurse asked a general question about the other family members. A long pause followed, and then the father admitted to being preoccupied. Their oldest son had been involved in an accident, and although no one had been seriously hurt, the accident was the result of deliberate disobedience. The parents were confused and uncertain about what to do next. They inquired about how to discipline their son effectively, how to meet the needs of each one of their children without showing favoritism, and how to communicate with children who want to listen to their peers instead of their parents. While listening to the parents, the nurse concluded that the homeostasis that once existed for this family had been disrupted. Previous patterns of communication had broken down, role expectations had been violated, and the family did not have the necessary resources to cope with the dual crises of their daughter's chronic illness and son's defiant behavior. The nurse referred the parents to a family therapist for further help and counseling, commended them for their concern, and reassured them that there was plenty of time to learn about their daughter's care when they were ready and able to concentrate on the subject.

In this situation the nurse referred the family to appropriate resources. The rapport and trust previously established between the nurse and the family, however, conveyed to the family the appropriateness of asking questions and sharing their concerns.

Facilitating Communication The nurse encourages family members to communicate by showing sensitivity to individual feelings, listening rather than judging, and acknowledging the importance of questions and concerns. Providing helpful information and assistance throughout the interview often convinces the family that the nurse is supportive. Integrating questions into the flow of conversation helps to create a relaxed, nonthreatening interaction.

Open-ended questions also help to stimulate thought and encourage family members to express their concerns. For example, the nurse might ask a child, "How have things been going with your family?" rather than, "Do you get along with your parents?" The closed question is likely to elicit a quick "yes" or "no" response but is less likely to help the nurse identify specific problems or possible solutions. Open-ended questions, on the other hand, sometimes lead to momentary silences as the child or parent considers an answer. The nurse might need to learn to wait without speaking to avoid the awkwardness that silence creates, so that family members can choose their own words and take an active part in the conversation. In the same way the nurse allows the family to help set the pace of the interview, which gives the family some control over the process and might lead to more honest, thoughtful responses.

Even when the nurse is not asking a question or providing information, well-worded responses can encourage family members to share information. For example, the nurse might respond to a parent's anxiety by saying, "I'm concerned about your problem and would like to know more." Simply expressing concern tells the parent that the problem is valid, and the request for more information allows the parent to direct the interview toward areas that require further attention.

Observing Nonverbal Cues Throughout the assessment process, the nurse watches for nonverbal cues that reinforce or contradict spoken or written information. Family members seldom come prepared to describe their concerns fully or to respond to the nurse's questions with well-constructed answers. A look or a gesture sometimes tells the nurse more about family interaction than family members are willing or able to describe.

For example, if a husband looks angry, acts impatient, or seems not to listen as his wife speaks, the nurse might infer that he disputes what she is saying or that he resents her acting as spokesperson for the family. Further questions, perhaps suggesting that he respond to what his wife has said, would then assist the nurse in interpreting his behavior. If, for instance, a talkative 5-year-old girl suddenly becomes quiet and withdrawn when her mother enters the room, the nurse needs to determine the cause of the child's silence. Perhaps it is an expression of fear or the result of having been taught to speak only when expressly told to do so.

In identifying the feelings and needs that these behaviors suggest, the nurse may determine who in a family is dominant and who is submissive, what kinds of interactions are encouraged or tolerated, and whether family members are open to intervention.

Asking the Parent to Describe the Child Encouraging parents to describe their children also might provide useful data. Parents' choice of words, what they say, and what they do not say might offer additional insight into parent–child relationships. The nurse might use the parent's description to begin an assessment interview or might help the parent to consider the child's strengths and weaknesses in new ways.

For example, the mother of a quiet 8-year-old boy described him as "sensitive, artistic, and considerate of others," whereas his father described him as a "sissy" because he did not want to play competitive sports and preferred to take piano lessons. The parents' separate descriptions of their son thus illustrated a conflict in their values and expectations. Helping them to recognize the mixed messages the child was receiving also helped to explain the child's low self-esteem and problems with social development.

A parent's description of a child also might uncover the predominant parenting style. The parent who defines a 12-year-old's behavior as consistently disobedient might be saying as much about assumptions related to parenting as about the child. The parent who expresses concern about discipline and setting age-appropriate limits might be observing the same behavior but perceiving the parenting role in a different way. (Styles of parenting are discussed in Chapter 13.)

To complete the picture, the nurse asks for examples of what the parent means by terms such as "undisciplined" or "consistently disobedient." Parental expectations sometimes are in conflict with the child's abilities, or the definition the child and parents have of obedience is different. For example, when the father tells his son to shovel the sidewalk, the son interprets the message as having to do the job sometime that day, whereas the father intends for the job to be done immediately. When the son does not obey instantly, the father concludes that it is another example of consistent disobedience. The father sometimes might feel that his role within a male-dominant structured family is being threatened as his son approaches adolescence. Occasionally, there is a great discrepancy between the chores assigned to a child and what the child's friends have to do, or sometimes a family is inflexible about family functions, which creates conflictual situations. For example, if one of the child's chores is to mow the grass on Saturday morning and the child's baseball team plays a game every Saturday morning, this sets up a conflict. Once the nurse obtains more specific data about the parent's perception of the child, the information can be placed in perspective and interpreted according to guidelines provided by theoretic norms.

Assessment Criteria

Family Structure, Function, and Roles The nurse usually can outline family structure by observing family interaction and asking family members to describe their family. These data enable the nurse to identify the composition of the family, its organization, and the relationships among family members. Each family member is identified according to age, gender, and relation (for example, father, son, brother). The family also is identified according to its composition, that is, nuclear, extended, single-parent, or reconstituted. Next, the nurse describes the ways in which family members interact with each other that characterize the family's pattern of relationships. "These include communicating, problem solving, meeting family members' needs for affection and intimacy, resolving conflict, and dealing with loss and change" (Cain, 1980).

For example, when updating a family assessment during a well-child visit, one nurse asked, "What changes have occurred in your family during the past year?" The mother responded that her husband's parents now lived with them but that everything was essentially the same. The nurse then turned to the 13-year-old daughter, Lisa, and said, "Tell me what it is like to have your grandparents live with you." Lisa gave some vague answers about always having someone home after school and someone else to watch her younger brother, but she then paused for a few minutes, looked down, clenched her fists, and said, "But they are so unfair. They never stop finding chores for me to do around the house, but the boys never have to do anything." The mother looked surprised, stating that she thought Lisa was proud of all the housework she had been doing. Lisa admitted to being pleased with the results but hating the process and feeling left out while her friends did things together. The nurse continued to ask questions and gather data from Lisa and her mother. Apparently, the grandparents believed that girls needed to help in the house because that was their future role, they were opposed to women having careers, and they criticized Lisa's mother for working. The boys, aged 10 and 5, were supposed to learn how to be men, which the grandparents believed was accomplished by peer interaction. The parents did not share these attitudes, but their respect and cultural reverence for their elders prevented them from saying anything.

Thus, by asking a few questions and taking the time to explore the situation, the nurse learned that a change in this family's composition also meant major changes in their relationships and that the potential for family dysfunction existed. The nurse encouraged Lisa and her mother to make a list of chores that would be Lisa's responsibility and a list of chores that her brothers would be responsible for doing. Lisa thus would have more free time to attend some after-school functions. The mother was encouraged further to discuss these plans tactfully with her husband and his parents. The nurse also made a follow-up appointment for Lisa to return to discuss how the plan was working.

Questions that elicit information about family structure include the following:

1. What are the names, genders, and ages of immediate family members?
2. Do other relatives (grandparents, uncle, aunt, cousin) live in the house?
3. Do other relatives participate in family life on a regular basis?
4. What is the relationship of immediate family members (stepparent, stepchild)?
5. Is one child special for any reason (health status, handicapped, youngest, oldest, only girl or boy)?
6. Does any adult seem more sensitive to or relate better with one child than the others?

The nurse assesses family function, or the effects of the family's roles, allocation and completion of tasks, and the presence of harmony or disharmony within the family system, by assessing habits and the activities of daily living. If family members help each other solve problems, meet challenges, and share feelings, the family system is supporting its members (that is, is relatively functional). Family dysfunction might appear in response to a variety of stressors from inside or outside the family and might in turn place the family at risk. (Nursing care of the family at risk is discussed in Chapter 22.)

Other aspects of family function include family members' awareness of each other's needs, their emotional closeness, their health care practices, and their ability to communicate with each other. Individual perceptions of these aspects of family function might vary among family members; therefore, the nurse who suspects that family members disagree might want to interview them separately.

The bonds or attachments between family members influence the roles and rules that organize family life, facilitate adaptation to change, and determine to a large extent

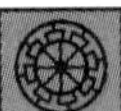

CASE STUDY Coping with a Move to a New Area

Assessment

Three-year-old Mark, who appears small for his age, has recently moved into the area with his father (age 40), his mother (age 35), and two older sisters (ages 10 and 12). Mark clings to his mother during the interview. The mother answers the nurse's questions completely but appears tired and discouraged; her voice is monotonous and her facial expression is serious. She does smile and respond affectionately to Mark.

Family

The family moved to this northern city 6 months previously. Prior to this, they lived in the same small southern town the mother had lived in as a child and near where both parents' families still live. They moved because her husband was transferred. He has a sales position with a large company, and this move meant a sizeable promotion. He has been very busy in his new job, frequently staying at the office until 7 or 8 PM. In addition, he has had to do more traveling in his new position. The two older children appear to have made the adjustment to the north and the larger city without any difficulties. They found friends in the neighborhood who were their age and had similar interests. Changing schools in the middle of the year actually was an asset because they met their friends through school activities.

Mark's mother states that her life is lonely. She used to know everyone, and now she knows no one. At first it was fun fixing up the new house, but now that that is done she finds that time drags. The neighbors seemed friendly when they first moved in, but she is convinced that it was only cautious politeness. They all seem too busy or preoccupied now to care if she even exists. She has made a few friends from church, but they work, which makes getting together problematic. She describes herself as shy and finds it difficult to make new friends. She admits to feeling homesick, is self-conscious about her southern accent, and is tired all the time.

Child

Mark is the result of an unplanned but not unwanted pregnancy. His mother states that she loves babies and would have a dozen if she could; however, complications during Mark's delivery necessitated her having a hysterectomy, so Mark is their last child. She describes Mark as a special child because he is the youngest and the only boy. His sisters claim he is spoiled, but the mother does not agree, stating that it is only the age difference that makes it seem that way. Although Mark stayed very close to his mother during the interview, his mother reports that he is very active at home. There are no children Mark's age in the neighborhood, so the two of them spend a lot of time together. She describes Mark as a somewhat difficult child unless he gets his own way, but then he is a pleasure. He states that he misses his friends and the games they played.

Environment

The family has purchased a new home. There are no financial concerns. There is a playground two blocks away, and the girls walk to their respective schools. The mother describes the neighborhood as unfriendly.

Clinical Data

Family Suprasystems: The change in environment from south to north, from small town to city, and from familiarity to unfamiliarity has influenced this family's patterns of functioning. The husband and two older children appear to be thriving with the change. They have become involved in work, school, and community. In contrast, the mother and son have viewed the new environment as threatening and have kept themselves at home. She has taken him to the playground only once, preferring instead to buy him his own swing set.

The family attends a church of the same denomination as the one they attended in the south, but the mother thinks the service is too formal. She, however, has made her only friends thus far in this group, and Mark enjoys the Sunday school.

The subtle changes between the culture of southern hospitality as defined by the mother and the northern wariness and aloofness have caused her to insulate herself and Mark from others.

Family Subsystems: The boundaries of the subsystems in which the mother is a member have become blurred. There is no clear differentiation between the spouse subsystem and the parent–child subsystem. Mark and his mother have become very close and in many ways are each other's best friend. Although Mark has always been special, the mother states that their relationship has become exceptionally close since the move.

The mother states that her husband has been too busy to spend much time with her or the children. He derives great satisfaction from his work and friendships there. She describes him as an ambitious person. His drive to succeed has made the adjustment to this move all the more difficult.

The girls have formed a special sibling subsystem. They seem to understand and enjoy each other. The mother thinks that they tend to "gang up" on Mark, so she listens to his side of the story more carefully and gives in to him. The father has found time to attend the girls' school performances and recitals. The mother has not attended these because of Mark's sleep needs. The mother describes the girls as being ambitious like their father.

Comparison to a Standard

The subsystem boundaries in this family have been altered and blurred instead of remaining well defined. The mother is seeking the friendship from her son that she should be seeking from her husband. This behavior is further separating her son from his sisters in the sibling subsystem. The sisters have formed their own subsystem within the sibling subsystem because of the distinct difference in their relationship with their mother and that of their brother and mother. The father seems to have withdrawn from his subsystem and is functioning as an individual.

Participation in the suprasystems of work, school, community, church, or recreation is limited. Three family members participate fully while two members hardly participate at all.

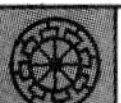

CASE STUDY Coping with a Move to a New Area (continued)

Nursing Diagnoses

1. Alterations in parenting related to blurring of subsystem behaviors and inadequate interaction with available suprasystems.
2. Ineffective family coping related to move, transition to new environment, and few supports.

Plan for Interventions

Goals

1. Parents will reestablish complementary behaviors within the spouse subsystem.
2. Mother will become involved in some activities requiring interaction with the available suprasystems.
3. Mark will become involved in some peer group activities.
4. The sibling subsystem will be unified.
5. The parent–child subsystem will be stabilized, and the children will report no favoritism.

Interventions

1. Discuss with the mother her feelings of loneliness and isolation. Validate their legitimacy because of the move and related change in life-style and activities plus the lack of familiar resources for support. It may be helpful for the mother to complete an assessment form such as the Feetham Family Functioning Survey to pinpoint any area of dysfunction.
2. Discuss with the mother ways to reestablish the activities she and her husband previously enjoyed as a couple and to redefine their values and beliefs about the family and its priority.
3. Offer to discuss the mother's needs for companionship with her and her husband together.
4. Suggest that husband and wife plan "Saturday night dates" again, some of which may include his friends from work.
5. Encourage them to spend time talking together every evening about their day, topics of interest, future plans, or whatever.
6. Discuss with the mother her interests, hobbies, and recreational preferences and provide her with information that can help her replace the previous suprasystem interactions with new options.
7. Contact and inform the minister of the church they attend about the mother's loneliness and need for friends and activities.
8. Encourage Mark and his mother to visit the playground two to three times a week.
9. Explore with the mother the idea of nursery school for Mark in September so he can benefit from a peer group.
10. Help the mother to redefine her relationship to Mark, to spend specified times interacting with him, but to encourage independent play times as well.
11. Suggest planning special family activities such as picnics, sightseeing trips, museums, and beach outings; have the children take turns selecting an activity.
12. Encourage the mother to spend specified times with each daughter, to take an interest in their activities, and to attend their programs.
13. Discuss with the mother her tendency to cater to Mark and the effect it is having on her daughters. Suggest she concentrate spending equal time listening to their complaints.

by whom and how decisions are made. A family that is functional demonstrates role consonance, that is, harmony and compatibility among family members concerning their ascribed and achieved roles (see Chapter 4). There also is communication and flexibility; for example, if the child who usually sets the table and makes the salad has band rehearsal one evening, either a parent or a sibling will complete the task. The key to whether harmony or discordance results in the family is the degree of similarity between what should be done by whom and what is being done by whom.

For example, if the family has agreed to share household tasks and the children are supposed to make their beds and clean their rooms but either do not do it or fail to meet the mother's expectations, tension results. The mother might continue to do these chores for the children, all the while resenting being overloaded with work, or interaction between the mother and children will be one of conflict. When assessing family functioning, the nurse needs to clarify the role expectations family members have for themselves and for each other.

Questions that elicit information about family function include the following:

1. How much help does your family give you when you have a problem?
2. How much time does your family spend together?
3. In what ways does your family support or resist your personal choices?
4. How do members of your family express their feelings for each other?
5. How does your family divide household tasks?
6. How are child-care responsibilities divided?

Related to the assessment of family function are the roles that family members assume. The nurse must avoid imposing personal assumptions about family members' roles on a client family. For example, the stepmother of the children in a reconstituted family might be the disciplinarian, even though she is neither the birth parent nor the "man of the house."

(Text continues on p. 565)

TABLE 17-1 Developmental Tasks and Family Assessment

Developmental subsystem	Family tasks	Family systems assessment
Infancy		
Biophysical development Normal fine and gross motor milestones	Provide safe, comfortable environment with proper nutrition and health care Maintain a nurturing relationship with infant by parent through mutual regular feeding and sleeping patterns Learn to care competently for infant	Is the environment safe, with adequate food and clothing? Does the family have a regular source of medical care and an adequate income? Does family provide muscle activity, toys, or equipment to enhance motor development? Does parent restrict infant's physical movement? Is child at an appropriate weight?
Cognitive development Sensorimotor stage	Provide environment with appropriate level of interaction and stimulation for sensorimotor development (auditory, visual, and tactile stimulation) Spend time with infant to enhance language and sensorimotor development	Does parent consciously encourage language development through labeling and verbal interchanges with the infant? Does parent invest time and interest in enhancing developmental milestones? Does parent provide appropriate toys to foster sensorimotor development (books and toys that require eye–hand coordination)?
Affective development Oral stage Trust vs. mistrust	Develop attachment between infant and caregivers Provide an environment that consistently satisfies infant's needs	Does parent have appropriate perceptions and expectations of the infant? In what ways does parent spend time on a regular basis interacting with infant? Is there a continuity and consistency in caregivers? Is the home free of conflict?
Social development	Maintain relationship with relatives and community Have sources of emotional and tangible support	Does the family see or communicate with relatives at least once a month? Is family involved in community organizations (church, leisure activities, etc)? Is the parent pleased with the role of parent?
Early childhood		
Biophysical development Development of gross and fine motor control; use of utensils to feed self; beginning self-dressing; scribbling; copying simple geometric designs; toilet training accomplished during this period; eating habits might become idiosyncratic	Provide safe environment to allow child an opportunity for motor development Encourage gross and fine motor activity through appropriate toys, permitting required space to experiment with walking and other movements Facilitate beginning skills in self-care (feeding, dressing, and toileting) Encourage gradual independence in self-care activities (dressing, bathing) Provide opportunities for successful toilet training Adjust family meal and sleep patterns to include child	Has the home been childproofed? Is parental supervision adequate for activity levels of this age? Is the child allowed to move around the home? How much time is spent in crib, playpen, or highchair? Does the family provide approriate toys or equipment to enhance both fine and gross motor development? Does child receive regular medical care? Does the family respect the child's food likes and dislikes? Is there respect and consideration for changing sleep needs? What are the family's accident prevention behaviors?
Cognitive development Ability to solve new problems through representation; object permanence with invisible displacement; prediction of cause-and-effect relationships; development of spoken language (egocentric speech) with eventual	Encourage language development through continual verbal interaction with child by labeling objects and reading Encourage sensorimotor development through appropriate toys Take the child into areas of the community that provide variety and stimulation	Do family members spend time talking to the child? Do parents have any structured play time with the child? Do parents read to the child? What do parents do to consciously encourage cognitive development? How much time is spent on this?

TABLE 17-1 continued

Developmental subsystem	Family tasks	Family systems assessment
mastery of speech; preoperational stage of development of such conceptual modes of thought as transformation, concentration, reversibility, and conservation; thought becomes representational		Is the child included in family activities and outings? Does the child get out of the house regularly? Do parents provide appropriate toys? How do the parents support/encourage the child in beginning decision making and responsibility for actions and behavior? To what extent is the famly involved with a preschool experience, nursery school, organized day care, or a play group?
Affective development Autonomy vs shame and doubt Initiative; ability to use physical and emotional energy for self-direction, self-exploration, and experience with a multitude of new adventures; development of the superego through resolution of the Oedipal or Electra conflict; continued emergence of the child's ego structures; development of gender identity	Provide ratio of control to freedom in toilet training, mobility, and satisfaction of needs Be available to help child deal with conflicts between mental images and reality Provide appropriate ratio between restrictions and permissiveness Reinforce child's appropriate sense of body image	Are parents either overly restrictive or overly permissive in toilet training, allowing mobility, and "messy" play activities? How does the family handle the child's fears? What role does the "imaginary playmate" have in the family? What are the discipline practices? How are fathering and mothering roles delineated in the family? How do these roles support and affect the child's identification process?
Social development Development of autonomy through self-control	Provide child with opportunities to interact with other children Provide opportunities to visit with relatives Help child in learning how to share and interact with others Set appropriate limits on child's behavior Plan for family oriented extracurricular activities Support interactions with larger social environment and interactions to validate the child's emerging perceptions of the larger social world	If child is in day care, is amount of time acceptable? Is it quality day care? Is the child in a play group? What is the size, frequency, and supervision? How is time spent with siblings? Does the child have regular visits with relatives? How do parents assist the child with social interactions? What is the family mode of discipline? How frequently do parents punish? What are the specific opportunities available to the child for engaging with a wider social environment? How do the family members relate to the child's larger world?
Middle and late childhood		
Biophysical development Lower growth rate but increased self-awareness of bodily changes and increased efficiency in motor skills	Continue to meet child's nutritional and physical needs Be sensitive to changes in eating and sleeping patterns of the child	Does the parent allow the child a choice in foods occasionally? Is there negotiation on bedtime when appropriate? Does the family provide an environment that supports expanding motor skills? (ie, amount of play space available, use of public playgrounds, involvement in cooperative sports)?
Cognitive development Period of concrete operations; cognitive ability to use logic; use of symbols, classification of information; social communication; Preconventional stage of moral development	Foster child's emerging cognitive style (the way the child organizes information and finds solutions to problems)	Does the family reinforce and support the learning that is taking place in school? Is attention paid to the child's homework? Is the parent involved in the child's school activities and communicating with teachers regarding the child's progress?

continued on next page

TABLE 17-1 continued

Developmental subsystem	Family tasks	Family systems assessment
Middle and late childhood (con't.)		
Affective development Industry vs. inferiority	Provide for and support the child's entrance into larger society and school, social organization (community, sports, clubs, etc.) and peer groups	Does the home/school environment provide a wide array of opportunities and materials for creative and productive work?
Social development Development of self-concept, self-esteem	Be sensitive to child's developmental abilities and limitations Foster child's developing ego through unconditional acceptance, continued love, and affective nurturance	Are family members honest with the child? Does the family guide the child into setting limits to behavior (eg, taking turns with others or caring for own room and personal belongings)? Does the family provide age-appropriate play materials? Do play materials differ for sons and daughters? In what ways does the family allow the child to test out new ideas and concepts? What are the family's attitudes toward and practice of television viewing, video games, and other media? How do the family members perceive the child's developing sense of right and wrong? What is their style of discipline toward the child? Do they allow the child limited responsibility for actions? How does the family foster the child's strivings for personal accomplishments? Do family members encourage and support involvement in extracurricular activities, membership in organizations, or self-expression through individual interests? How do family members convey acceptance to the child? Do they set clear and consistent limits to behavior? Is there flexibility with these limits to permit individual changes? Are the family members sensitive to the importance of the child's peer group? How accepting are they of the child's peer group?
Adolescence		
Biophysical development Growth spurt with development of primary and secondary sexual characteristics	Provide health education to adolescent regarding physical bodily changes Provide sex education and/or seek out health care providers to assist in this task	Is there an open, honest approach toward sexuality? How do family members feel about sexual identity? How is love and affection expressed?
Cognitive development Period of formal operations (ie, abstract mental functioning) Conventional stage of moral development		How does family encourage and/or support adolescent in vocational or professional pursuits? In what ways does the family help prepare the adolescent for adult work life? How does the family give the adolescent an opportunity to act on own problem-solving strategies?
Affective development Identity (ie, clarifying and becoming aware of one's personal self) vs. diffusion	Appropriately adjust family roles to move from parental protectiveness and sole responsibility to guided and increased adolescent individuality, independence, and autonomy	What are methods of parental control (ie, authoritative, permissive, or bureaucratic parenting styles)?

TABLE 17-1 continued

Developmental subsystem	Family tasks	Family systems assessment
Social development Self-definition, personal uniqueness, and independence	Continue stability in family acceptance and affection within atmosphere of mutual trust	How does the family exhibit an atmosphere of mutual trust? How do family members handle the issue of privileges (ie, use of family car, dating, and choice of social activities)? How has family handled issues of sexuality, drinking, and drugs? How does the parent handle the adolescent's swings in behavior from childlike to adultlike? How does the parent react to the adolescent's increasing dependence on the peer group and decreasing dependence on the family?

Other questions to ask include the following:

1. How are decisions made within the family?
2. Which family members are consulted when a decision has to be made? Who has the final say?
3. How are disagreements resolved?
4. In what ways are each of the children involved in resolving disagreements?
5. Who decides what method of discipline to use?
6. What do you see as the role of each family member?
7. Are family roles a source of agreement or conflict?'

Family Suprasystems and Subsystems Identifying a family as vulnerable to dysfunction means identifying the family as the client. The nurse thus applies the nursing process not only to the child but also to the family (Table 17-1). Assessing the suprasystems that influence the family provides the nurse with clues about existing or potential needs for support. Questions about schoolwork, employment, community interactions, and recreational activities might give family members the opportunity to express concerns. The nurse then notes any existing needs that might be met by referral to appropriate community resources.

Because a family system also is influenced by its subsystems, the nurse needs to assess the values, beliefs, expectations, and parenting style, which are all part of the family system. These aspects of family life often suggest family priorities or possible support systems that family members might have overlooked.

For example, one mother expressed her belief in the importance of caring for aging parents and described her difficulties in dividing her time between caring for her mother, who was increasingly dependent, and caring for her active 3-year-old son. For this mother, a home health aide might provide the needed support or, perhaps, a nursery school program would give her adequate time to fulfill all her responsibilities.

Minuchin (1974) defined three major subsystems within the family system. They are the spouse subsystem (husband–wife), parental subsystem (parent–child), and sibling subsystem (sister–brother; brother–brother; sister–sister). The structure and relationships within each of these subsystems are unique and strictly bounded in the healthy family. If the boundaries become blurred so that there is little differentiation between the subsystems (for example, the mother relating to daughter as a sister), a dysfunctional family pattern may be indicated.

Phipps noted that being a member "within a particular subsystem influences a family member's power, influence, and even specific skills developed" (1980:39). Each family member belongs to multiple subsystems and generally uses different skills, behaviors, and roles in each one. For example, within his nuclear family, a man, as a husband, belongs to the spouse subsystem and as a father belongs to the parental subsystem; in the extended family this man belongs to a sibling subsystem, and as a son belongs to another parental subsystem. The manner in which this man fathers his children is related to how he was fathered and the values, beliefs, rituals, and traditions he wants to pass on to his children. The pattern of interactions within a family thus is complex, which emphasizes the importance of doing a thorough assessment and resisting the temptation to arrive at quick conclusions.

Knowledge of Child Care Assessing a parent's knowledge of normal growth and development, expectations for children's needs, and available child-care resources enables the nurse to identify knowledge deficits and provide anticipatory guidance (see Chapter 21). Encouraging questions about developmental norms and health care needs often allows the parent to ask about specific developmental problems.

A parent's knowledge of child care is especially important during times of transition in the family's development. The

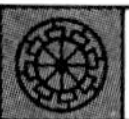

CASE STUDY Communicating Expectations

Assessment

Pam is an obese, sad-appearing 12-year-old girl. Her parents are divorced, and she lives with her mother. Her older sister is married and lives 500 miles away.

Family

The family has experienced considerable stress during the past 4 years, which ended with the separation and divorce of Pam's parents. Following the divorce, Pam's mother (age 50) had to begin working. She works full-time on an assembly line for a toy-manufacturing factory. The work is tiring and the rewards few. When she returns home each evening, she does not want to cook, go shopping, play games, or even talk. Although the mother is overweight, she claims that she cannot lose weight and especially not now that she has to work so hard. She blames her former husband, who "drank too much," for the divorce. She describes him as having a vicious temper that he could not control and being self-centered and insensitive to others. She is glad for the divorce but not for the consequences.

She describes herself as passive, somewhat a loner, and chronically tired. She complains that Pam does not do enough to help around the house. She especially would like Pam to cook supper every evening, feeling that while she sits at home watching television, she might as well be doing something constructive.

Pam's sister got married last year and moved out of the state. The mother states that Pam and her sister were opposites, with Pam more like the mother and the sister more like the father. The sister writes and visits frequently. No one has heard from the father since he moved out of the house. There are a few close friends and relatives nearby who help as needed.

Child

Pam appears apathetic, answers questions as briefly as possible, and fidgets in her chair. Pam resents her mother's having to work and not being there when she gets home from school. Pam compensates for her loneliness by eating. Although she is a good student, Pam waits to do her homework until her mother returns home so the mother can help if she is needed. Pam admits that she does very little around the house but does not think she should have to do much because her friends do not have to do many chores. She mentions that her mother is always complaining that she does not do anything but that her mother never tells her what to do. Pam quickly adds that if her mother wants her to cook, she has to teach her first.

Pam states that she misses her sister and father. She and her sister had become close friends and would spend long periods of time talking because of the parental arguments. She is glad her sister is happy and envies her. Pam doesn't miss the shouting and arguments, but she does miss the times she used to spend with her father, talking and playing games before supper. Now she has no one with whom to talk, share concerns and ideas, or ask questions about growing up. Her mother always is too tired to talk.

Pam has few friends. Sometimes peers telephone about an assignment or to request assistance with a homework problem but seldom to ask Pam to join them for an activity or party. Because of her weight problem and inability to wear the clothes other 12-year-olds are wearing, Pam does not like herself. Because her mother is working and not at home after school, she cannot invite anyone over. She looks forward to her swimming lesson, which is the only after-school activity her mother allows, because it gives her something to do after school.

Environment

The family lives in an apartment on the second floor of a small house in the city. The street in front of the house is always noisy and congested with traffic. There is a small backyard where a few flowers grow. The family rents their apartment and walks three blocks to the laundromat every week and one block to the grocery store. The mother does not have a car but uses public transportation to get to work. Pam rides her bicycle to and from school.

Clinical Data

Communication Patterns Pam and her mother live together but communicate only when absolutely necessary. There is a brief exchange in the morning as Pam is getting up and her mother is leaving for work. Pam waits for her mother to initiate conversation in the evening, stating that she has learned the hard way not to talk until her mother is ready to do so. Sometimes they even complete their tasks before supper in silence. The mother states that she has a lot on her mind and does not want to burden Pam with "adult worries." The mother mentions that she shares these worries with her sister, who lives nearby. She wishes that Pam had a close friend to confide in and is concerned about Pam's lack of friends.

Weekends are better than during the week. Pam and her mother both say that they enjoy each other's company while doing the laundry and shopping together. The conversations, however, are "light," about other people and events of the past week. Pam is not allowed to talk about her father or the divorce, but unresolved questions about the past 4 years haunt her. She has often thought about writing to her sister but does not want to bother her.

Patterns of Power: The mother is the decision maker in all areas. Pam follows direct commands, such as not having friends over when her mother is not home, cleaning her room, setting and clearing the table, and helping with the weekend chores of laundry and shopping. She passively resists following up on any of the mother's hints about making supper or doing more to help around the house.

When they go shopping for food or clothes, her mother decides what to buy. Pam has learned to request, not suggest, purchasing something she particularly likes. Pam daydreams of the time when she has more freedom and can decide what clothes to purchase for herself.

Comparison to a Standard

The outstanding characteristic of this family is their strained patterns of communication and the one-sided distribution of power. Direct communication is limited to necessary conver-

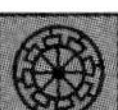

CASE STUDY Communicating Expectations (continued)

sation when the mother is "ready." Two-way communication really only occurs on the weekends, and even then both mother and daughter agree that the mother initiates the conversation. Communication is closed. Pam is not allowed to talk about the subjects that concern her the most (her father and the divorce), and the mother does not share her feelings with Pam.

The mother exerts her will concerning the use of resources and division of labor. When there is conflict, Pam gives in to her mother, realizing that she has no choice because her mother is her only parent.

Nursing Diagnoses

1. Alteration in parenting related to the change in roles due to the divorce and the mother's need to work.
2. Dysfunctional family process related to ineffective communication patterns and the inability to share personal concerns.

Plan for Interventions

Goals

1. Pam and her mother will communicate with each other in a meaningful way and discuss the pain of the divorce.
2. Pam will demonstrate initiative in helping her mother.
3. Pam's mother will give Pam more freedom to make decisions about her clothes and choice of activities.

Interventions

1. Discuss with Pam her routine day and how she would like to change it.
2. Discuss the pain of divorce with both mother and daughter, the presence of unresolved issues, and their anger about the consequences.
3. Refer each to a self-help group that meets every week at the library, which is within walking distance from their apartment. Children of Divorced Parents meet after school, and Parents Without Partners meets in the evening.
4. Encourage the mother to allow Pam to participate in more supervised after-school activities such as the Girls' Club and free swim at the YMCA.
5. Discuss with Pam ways that she could help around the house. Have her initiate the ideas and suggest she do it as a surprise for her mother.
6. Suggest that Pam's mother either borrow from the library or purchase an inexpensive children's cookbook for Pam and use it together, allowing Pam to select some recipes.
7. Suggest that Pam be allowed to choose specific food or clothing items within a given price range.
8. Encourage Pam and her mother to include some recreational activities in their weekend chores and to take turns selecting what to do.
9. Suggest that the mother might find it helpful to take a 30-minute nap when she comes home from work.
10. Suggest that Pam and her mother work out a plan about how to accomplish household chores.
11. Encourage Pam and her mother to discuss what they want and expect from each other as well as what aggravates them about each other. Have them contract to do or not to do certain behaviors, such as nag or pout, and return in 1 week to discuss how the week went.

birth of a child, for example, regardless of whether it is the first child, presents new challenges and stressors for all family members. New parents might be unaware of the changes a child will bring to the family. Parents expecting an additional child might not anticipate the needs of siblings and the difficulties of meeting the needs of both an infant and one or more older children. The nurse's knowledge of typical family stressors and family development is therefore important in identifying potential needs during times of additional stress.

Family Assessment Tools

In much the same way that the nurse might choose to use a standard tool to assess a child's development, the nurse also might use a variety of tools designed to collect data for family assessment. Assessment tools also might assist the nurse in organizing and analyzing data, but the tool itself is not a complete assessment. Data collected in this way need to be considered together with structured and unstructured observations and the results of discussions with family members. In this way the nurse can consider the data obtained with an assessment tool in conjunction with other relevant information not obtained by the tool.

The time required to use family assessment tools and the settings in which they are used vary. Some tools, like the Home Observation for Measurement of the Environment (HOME), are designed to assess parent–child interaction in the home environment and cannot be used in a clinical setting. Others, like the Family Environment Scale (FES), are useful in a variety of clinical settings and can be used to identify areas that need more complete assessment. Many tools are questionnaires that the nurse might use with all members of a family to provide a ready means of comparison.

Neonatal Perception Inventory The Neonatal Perception Inventory (NPI) is a two-part questionnaire that allows the nurse to compare a parent's expectations for an

NEONATAL PERCEPTION INVENTORY I
AVERAGE BABY

Although this is your first baby, you probably have some ideas of what most little babies are like. Please check the blank you think best describes the AVERAGE baby.

How much crying do you think the average baby does?

______	______	______	______	______
a great deal	a good bit	moderate amount	very little	none

How much trouble do you think the average baby has in feeding?

______	______	______	______	______
a great deal	a good bit	moderate amount	very little	none

How much spitting up or vomiting do you think the average baby does?

______	______	______	______	______
a great deal	a good bit	moderate amount	very little	none

How much difficulty do you think the average baby has in sleeping?

______	______	______	______	______
a great deal	a good bit	moderate amount	very little	none

How much difficulty does the average baby have with bowel movements?

______	______	______	______	______
a great deal	a good bit	moderate amount	very little	none

How much trouble do you think the average baby has in settling down to a predictable pattern of eating and sleeping?

______	______	______	______	______
a great deal	a good bit	moderate amount	very little	none

NEONATAL PERCEPTION INVENTORY II
YOUR BABY

You have had a chance to live with your baby for a month now. Please check the blank you think describes your baby.

How much crying has your baby done?

______	______	______	______	______
a great deal	a good bit	moderate amount	very little	none

How much trouble has your baby had feeding?

______	______	______	______	______
a great deal	a good bit	moderate amount	very little	none

Figure 17-1 Neonatal Perception Inventory (NPI) at 2 days and at 1 month. Each time the parent completes two forms, one representing the average baby and one representing the parent's baby.

How much spitting up or vomiting has your baby done?

a great deal	a good bit	moderate amount	very little	none

How much difficulty has your baby had in sleeping?

a great deal	a good bit	moderate amount	very little	none

How much difficulty has your baby had with bowel movements?

a great deal	a good bit	moderate amount	very little	none

How much trouble has your baby had in settling down to a predictable pattern of eating and sleeping?

a great deal	a good bit	moderate amount	very little	none

DEGREE OF BOTHER INVENTORY

Crying	a great deal	somewhat	very little	none
Spitting up or vomiting	a great deal	somewhat	very little	none
Sleeping	a great deal	somewhat	very little	none
Feeding	a great deal	somewhat	very little	none
Elimination	a great deal	somewhat	very little	none
Lack of a predictable schedule	a great deal	somewhat	very little	none
Other (specify):				
______	a great deal	somewhat	very little	none
______	a great deal	somewhat	very little	none
______	a great deal	somewhat	very little	none
______	a great deal	somewhat	very little	none

SOURCE: Brousard ER, Hartner MS: Further considerations regarding maternal perceptions of the first born. In: *Exceptional infant studies in abnormalities.* Vol 2. Hellmuth J. Brunner/Mazel, 1971.

Figure 17-1 continued

"average" infant with that parent's perceptions of his or her own infant at 2 days and at 1 month of age (Fig. 17-1). The questionnaire rates the parent's perception of the infant's crying, feeding, spitting up, sleeping, bowel habits, and general routine on a scale from 1 to 5. The scores of the two parts are compared and the difference between the parent's perceptions of the average infant and the actual infant is the score. A larger score therefore means a larger

Models for Family Assessment Criteria

Horton (1977)—Horton's model addresses (1) family structure; (2) family function; and (3) family processes (adaptation, integration, and decision making).

Helvie (1981)—Helvie's model analyzes structure and processes in families in conjunction with the type of family configuration (eg, single parent, nuclear). He applies four characteristics: (1) organization; (2) boundary; (3) differentiation and specialization; and (4) territoriality.

Clark (1978)—Clark proposes 11 areas of assessment, ranging from basic criteria such as family members present at the visit to more abstract concerns such as anxiety levels, norms, roles, functional and dysfunctional relationships, disruptions, atmosphere, and phases of interaction.

Clemen, Egsti, and McGuire (1981)—Clemen, Egsti, and McGuire use a two-pronged model that addresses (1) structural parameters (division of labor, distribution of power, boundaries, relationships outside the family, rituals, symbols); and (2) process parameters (methods that determine family structure, decision making, and maintenance).

Friedman (1981)—Friedman presents a modified structural–functional model consisting of four basic areas: (1) identifying data; (2) environmental data; (3) family structure; and (4) family function. This umbrella framework provides a useful means of organizing data for nursing-related interventions.

Grace and Camilleri (1981)—Grace and Camilleri analyze normality, disturbance, and techniques for intervention within the family system.

Edison (1979)—Edison advocates specific guidelines that include family constellation, finances, transportation, daily activities, avocations and recreational interests, health history, dental care, sexuality, health resources, strengths and coping mechanisms, weaknesses and problems, and goals.

discrepancy between the actual and the imagined infant and suggests that the parent–child relationship might in some way be at risk. The 1-month score is considered to be the better predictor of the parent–infant relationship (Broussard and Hartner, 1971).

At the 1-month interview, the parent also completes the Degree of Bother Inventory, in which the parent ranks how troublesome specific infant behaviors and activities are. Blank lines are provided for the parent to include additional behaviors that are not specified.

This tool provides valuable information concerning the developing parent–child relationship. It helps to quickly identify areas on which the nurse needs to focus in providing teaching, support, counseling, anticipatory guidance, or other interventions such as encouraging attendance at parent groups or referrals to enhance parental skills.

Maternal Attachment Assessment Strategy The Maternal Attachment Assessment Strategy, developed by Patricia Avant, provides a system of observing maternal–child behavior and establishing a profile of the mother's attachment behaviors (Avant, 1982). Developed for use with primigravidas, its reliability has been established at 0.99. Administration involves a time-sampling procedure, in which the observer watches the mother's feeding behaviors for 20 seconds and records the data on a scale for the remaining 40 seconds in a series of 15 1-minute periods. Behaviors such as the mother's distractibility and whether she looks at and talks to the infant are noted, along with the infant's behavioral state. Although not a predictive scale, the four scores the Maternal Attachment Assessment Strategy yields—(1) affectionate behavior; (2) maintaining proximity; (3) care-giving skills; and (4) overall attachment—produce a profile of maternal attachment behaviors that might indicate problem areas.

Mother–Infant Play Interaction Scale The Mother–Infant Play Interaction Scale (MIPIS) is another useful tool for assessing potential family vulnerability (Walker and Thompson, 1982). A relatively new tool developed by Thomas and colleagues at the University of Texas in 1977, the MIPIS is designed to measure response reciprocity between mother and infant during unstructured play. Observations are made for 5 minutes, scored on a 16-item scoring sheet, and then divided into three subscales—the maternal, infant, and dyadic subscales. The results are uniquely useful in improving the examiner's observation skills by increasing sensitivity to specific aspects of interaction. After observing at least five interactions, the examiner can begin to see a pattern that can be used in conjunction with the mother's perceptions as a basis for discussion and teaching.

Home Observation for Measurement of the Environment The Home Observation for Measurement of the Environment (HOME) inventory was designed to sample certain aspects of the quantity and quality of social, emotional, and cognitive support available to a young child within the home (Elardo, Bradley, and Caldwell, 1975; Bradley and Caldwell, 1976; Bradley and Caldwell, 1979).

The HOME assesses the animate and inanimate aspects of the child's environment that either foster or impede growth and development. This functional approach identifies the interactions of these various characteristics of the child's environment (see Appendix D).

Based on clinical observations and observations in the home, Caldwell and colleagues devised two inventories that measure the environmental characteristics that might be associated with favorable developmental outcomes for the child. Both inventories (birth to 3 years and 3 to 6 years) offer a framework for systematically and objectively collecting information about aspects of a child's environment that can be used for the mutual benefit of both child and parent.

The HOME (birth to 3 years) measures the following six subscales: (1) emotional and verbal responsivity of the mother; (2) avoidance of restriction and punishment; (3) organization of the physical and temporal environment; (4) provision of appropriate play materials; (5) maternal involvement with the child; and (6) opportunities for variety in daily stimulation.

The HOME (3 to 6 years) attempts to measure the changing environment of the older child. It consists of seven subscales: (1) provision of stimulation through equipment, toys, and experiences; (2) stimulation of mature behavior; (3) provision of a stimulating physical and language environment; (4) avoidance of restriction and punishment; (5) pride, affection, and thoughtfulness; (6) masculine stimulation; and (7) independence from parental control.

The HOME inventories evaluate the environment as the child lives it by profiling a typical day for that child within a specific home environment. The inventories provide data about the stimulating or inhibiting activities the child experiences from the environment and who in the family provides various aspects of care to the child.

This information is important to the nurse's understanding of the impact of the family on the child's developmental progress. It suggests that an environment either fosters growth and is supportive of the child's cognitive, physical, and psychosocial needs or is deficient in one or more areas. This helps the nurse to identify strengths and weaknesses in a family and to assess the emotional climate. Inadequate support might place the family at risk for dysfunctional parenting (see Chapter 22) or the child at risk for dysfunctional behavior (see Chapter 24).

Family APGAR The Family APGAR is a screening questionnaire that is designed to identify the ways in which a member of the family perceives the functioning of the entire family. (It is not comparable to the Apgar physical screening tests for neonates.) Areas in which family functioning are assessed involve family interaction such as marital satisfaction, feelings of happiness and closeness, communication, and problem solving. These areas of family

TABLE 17-2 Family APGAR

Component	Definition	Assessment questions
Adaptation	Use of intra- and extrafamilial resources for problem solving when family equilibrium is under stress	"How have family members aided each other in time of need?" "In what way have family members received help or assistance from friends and community agencies?"
Partnership	Sharing of decision-making and nurturing responsibilities by family members	"How do family members communicate with each other about such matters as vacations, finances, medical care, large purchases, and personal problems?"
Growth	Physical and emotional maturation and self-fulfillment achieved by family members through mutual support and guidance	"How have family members changed during the past years?" "How has this change been accepted by family members?" "In what ways have family members aided each other in growing or developing independent life-styles?" "How have family members reacted to your desires for change?"
Affection	Caring or loving relationship among family members	"How have members of your family responded to emotional expressions such as affection, love, sorrow, or anger?"
Resolve	Commitment to devote time to other members of the family for physical and emotional nurturing; also usually involves a decision to share wealth and space	"How do members of your family share time, space, and money?"

functioning are designated with the terms Adaptation, Partnership, Growth, Affection, and Resolve (Smilkstein, 1978). These components, which are considered basic to family functioning, are assessed with suggested open-ended questions (Table 17-2).

Specifically, adaptation is measured by the sharing of resources or the degree to which a family member is satisfied by the amount of assistance received from family resources. Partnership is measured by the sharing of decisions and mutuality in problem solving. Growth is measured by the flexibility with which the family changes roles and attains physical and emotional growth or maturation. Affection is viewed as a member's satisfaction with the intimacy and emotional interaction within the family. Resolve is the way time is shared or the family member's satisfaction with the time commitment that has been made to the family by its members.

Through open-ended questions, the nurse documents specific responses about each of the five basic components. Then, by using the Family APGAR Questionnaire, the nurse obtains a qualitative measure of a family member's satisfaction with each of those functional components (Fig. 17-2). The questionnaire provides baseline data about the level of family functioning and each member's interplay within the family.

Family Assessment Tool for School Nurses and Other Professionals The Family Assessment Tool (FAT) uses the nursing process to collect developmental data about children in school (Fig. 17-3) (Holt and Robinson, 1979). The focus of FAT is the child as a member of a family and in a home environment, but the tool draws on systems theory to interpret the interactions among family, school, and community. The goals of the FAT are to assist school personnel in understanding the child and the family and to involve the family in the evaluation of and decision-making process regarding the child.

The FAT organizes data about the child's home and sociocultural environment, family interaction styles, the child's growth, developmental, and health history, and the family's health and social history. The data are then interpreted and summarized as a nursing assessment with a list of priorities indicating family problems and family strengths and weaknesses.

Although this tool initially was designed to provide a methodology and organization for school nurses as they collected information on children with school problems, it is appropriate for use by nurses in community settings and is especially beneficial for data collection and assessment during home visits.

Family Environment Scale The Family Environment Scale (FES) developed by Moos and colleagues (1974) is an assessment tool that can be used by nurses in community, hospital, or outpatient clinic settings to collect data about an individual's perception of family life. It is a 90-item questionnaire that assesses the social environment of a family. It provides data with which the nurse can compare parent and child perceptions, compare actual and preferred family milieus, and assess and facilitate change in family environments.

As an assessment tool, the FES can be used by nurses to make comparisons within the family, among family members, and among families. Such a scale provides a means for assessing significant dimensions of the family system (Eichel, 1978).

The FES is structured in an easily understandable format that collects a great deal of information about the family in a relatively quick and efficient way. A family member's perceptions of the family are assessed by asking the family member to measure and describe interpersonal relationships among family members and the directions of personal growth emphasized within the family and to identify the basic organizational structure of the family.

The significance of the FES in a nursing family assessment is that it can (1) provide a systematic method for the collection of data about a child's family system; (2) increase the nurse's knowledge of the child's family system; (3) provide information on the strengths and weaknesses of the child's family support system; and (4) provide direction in family intervention (Eichel, 1978).

Family Adaptability and Cohesion Evaluation Scales The Family Adaptability and Cohesion Evaluation Scales (FACES II) is an assessment tool that specifically tests an individual's perception of the family by examining family cohesion, or the emotional bonding of family members to one another, and the family's adaptability or ability to change its power structure, role relationships, and rules in response to situational and developmental stresses (Olson, Bell, and Portner, 1978). Specific concepts used to measure cohesion are emotional bonding, boundaries, coalitions, use of time and space and their boundaries, friends, decision making, interests, and recreation. Specific concepts used to measure adaptability are family power, negotiation style, role relationships, and relationship rules.

Designed to be given twice, once for the family members' perceptions of their family and second for their perceptions of the ideal family, the nurse can assess the level of satisfaction with the current family system by comparing the perceived and ideal responses on the questionnaires.

This tool is appropriate for all adult family members and for children as young as 12 years of age or at the seventh grade reading level. It is clinically useful in that it provides nurses with an understanding of how family members see the family and how they would like it to be. This information allows the nurse to identify the specific differences between parent and child as they function within the family system. The nurse can then plan interventions focused on those specific areas of family disengagement or discrepancy.

Family APGAR Questionnaire

	Almost always	Some of the time	Hardly ever
I am satisfied with the help that I receive from my family* when something is troubling me.	______	______	______
I am satisfied with the way my family* discusses items of common interest and shares problem solving with me.	______	______	______
I find that my family* accepts my wishes to take on new activities or make changes in my lifestyle.	______	______	______
I am satisfied with the way my family* expresses affection and responds to my feelings, such as anger, sorrow, and love.	______	______	______
I am satisfied with the amount of time my family* and I spend together.	______	______	______

Scoring: The patient checks one of three choices, which are scored as follows: "Almost always" (2 points), "Some of the time" (1) point, or "Hardly ever" (0). The scores for each of the five questions are then totaled. A score of 7 to 10 suggests a highly functional family. A score of 4 to 6 suggests a moderately dysfunctional family. A score of 0 to 3 suggests a severely dysfunctional family.

*According to which member of the family is being interviewed, the interviewer may substitute for the word "family" either spouse, significant other, parents, or children.

Figure 17-2 Family APGAR Questionnaire. From Smilkstein, G. Assessment of Family Function. In G. Rosen et al., eds., *Behavioral Science in Family Practice.* Appleton-Century-Crofts, 1980.

Feetham Family Functioning Survey The Feetham Family Functioning Survey (FFFS) (Feetham and Humenick, 1982) assesses the accomplishment of normal family tasks and functioning in a family with either an impaired or a normal child. The survey is a systematic method of assessing family functioning under stress. The assessment tool consists of 23 questions evaluating six areas of functioning: (1) household tasks; (2) child care; (3) sexual and marital relations; (4) interaction with family and friends; (5) community involvement; and (6) sources of support.

A self-reporting instrument, the FFFS takes approximately 10 minutes to complete. Its primary value is in pinpointing specific areas of dysfunction in a stressed family. By identifying a specific stressor, the nurse can proceed to

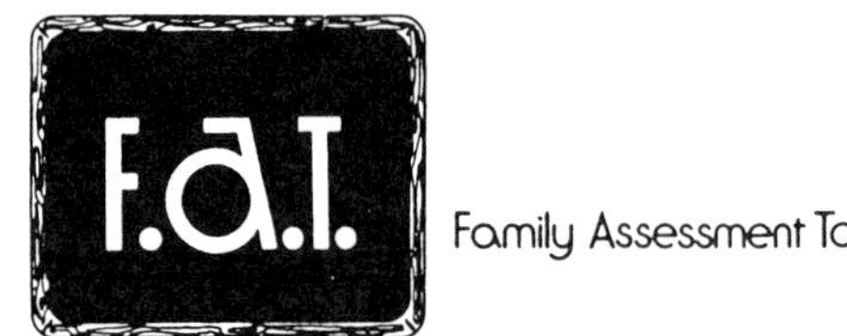

Assessment of ______________________________ Family

Child of Concern ______________________ Birthdate ____________

Address ______________________ Telephone ____________

Purpose of Assessment ______________________________

Report submitted by ______________________ Date ____________

Observations

I. Description of Home and Environment
II. Significant Socio-Cultural Influences
III. Interaction of Family Members

Area of Inquiry

I. Family's Perception
- *A. "What does the family see as a problem?"
- *B. "What has the family already tried?"
  "What does the family think might be a solution?"
- *C. "If special education is considered, how does the family feel about it?"
- *D. "Describe your child in a few sentences."
- *E. "What goals does the family have for the child?"

II. Health Interview

A. Growth and Development

Antenatal: Age and health of mother during pregnancy, other pregnancies, AP care and experiences, weight gain, drug ingestion, illnesses, blood type, length of gestation.

Natal: Length of labor, anesthesia, type of delivery, condition of baby at birth (cry, color, O_2, incubator), birth weight.

Postnatal: Problems in nursery, feeding or sleeping problems, excessive weight loss.

Development: Rolled over, sat alone, walked, talked (meaningful words, 2 word sentences), feeding history, teeth eruption, urine and bowel control, establishment of hand preference, development compared to siblings and parents, school experiences, developmental testing, developmental tasks.

Disturbances: Speech delays or irregularities, lethargy, attention disorders, hearing and vision difficulties, clumsiness of motor tasks, enuresis, encopresis, pica, thumb sucking, failure to grow or unusual growth, antisocial behavior.

Learning Patterns: Self-reliance, self-control, approach tendency, learning style.

B. Health History

Childhood diseases, illnesses, accidents, seizures, hospitalizations, ear infections, medications, allergies, immunizations. Last P.E. date? Where? By whom?

Figure 17-3 Family Assessment Tool (FAT).

C. Present Status
Eating, sleeping, elimination, interests, peer relationships, exercise/play, method of discipline, sexuality.

D. Review of Systems
Skin, Eye, Ear, Nose, Throat, Cardio-Respiratory, Gastro-Intestinal, Genito-Urinary, Musculo-Skeletal, Neurological.

III. Family History
A. Family Composition: age, sex, present status of siblings, age of parents, extended family.
B. Health Status of Family Members.
C. Educational and work experiences of parents.
*D. "How do all family members get along together?"
"What activities do they share?"

Items with asterisk [*] are subjective questions that require nurse to elicit expectations, understanding of problem, general feelings and values that family has about child of concern.

Closing Discussion with the Family

I. Review goals with family
A. Define the problems.
B. Discuss information to be shared with school staff.
C. Empahsize family sharing in decision making process.

II. Arrange for follow-up contacts.

Nursing Summary

I. Assessment
A. Interpret data and summarize impression.
B. List and prioritize problems.
C. List family's strengths and weaknesses.

II. Plan
A. Meet with staffing team and family to review information.
1. Identify problem areas.
2. Identify family, school, and community resources.
3. Discuss alternative solutions.
B. Identify a solution if possible.
1. Designate team members to be involved with the family.
2. Involve family.
C. Develop an Individualized Educational Program (IEP) with a health component.
D. Determine evaluation criteria and procedure (when, by whom, how, and where).

III. Implement Health Component of Individualized Educational Program.

IV. Evaluation — Determine success of plan based on criteria established in II. D.

Figure 17-3 continued

identify sources of support that will help to diminish the stress.

The indicators of family functioning measured by this questionnaire are as follows:

Disagreement with spouse
Discussion of concerns and problems with spouse
Emotional support from friends and relatives
Emotional support from spouse
Help from friends
Help from relatives
Help from spouse
Problems with other children
Satisfaction with marriage
Satisfaction with sexual relations
Talk with friends and relatives
Amount of time spent in household tasks
Amount of time spent in leisure recreational activities
Amount of time the respondent misses doing housework
Amount of time other children miss school
Amount of time spent with spouse
Amount of time spouse misses work
Amount of time spent with children
Amount of time spent with health professionals
Amount of time spent with neighbors
Amount of time the respondent is ill

The respondent rates statements describing each area on a scale from 1 (little) to 7 (much) according to the present situation, ideal situation, and how important the area described is to the respondent. When the importance score is compared with the discrepant score (difference between present and ideal), the direction and degree of satisfaction and dissatisfaction with family functioning can be identified and plans for intervention discussed.

Family Coping Index The Family Coping Index developed by Freeman and Lowe (1964) provides a framework for assessing the nursing needs of a family (Fig. 17-4). Designed for use by public health nurses, the index is comprised of a scoring profile sheet, a care plan note sheet, and a set of instructions, which the nurse can adapt to fit any setting. The nine areas of assessment for family functioning are as follows:

1. Physical independence
2. Therapeutic independence
3. Knowledge of condition
4. Application of principles of general hygiene
5. Attitudes toward health care
6. Emotional competence
7. Family living patterns
8. Physical environment
9. Use of community resources.

The Family Coping Index is based on nursing diagnoses determined by the family's ability to cope with family needs and adapt to health-related stress. This assessment tool defines coping as "dealing with problems associated with health care with reasonable success" (Freeman and Lowe, 1964). Families are scored on a sliding scale from 1 (no competence) to 3 (moderate competence) to 5 (complete competence) for present functioning and a second score for anticipated functioning following nursing interventions. The tool thus provides direction for intervention and guidelines for periodic evaluations.

Assessment of Family Strengths Another valuable guide for assessing family self-care was developed by Otto (1963). This framework focuses on family strengths. The twelve categories assessed are as follows:

1. The ability to provide for the physical, emotional, and spiritual needs of family members.
2. The ability to be sensitive to the needs of family members.
3. The ability to communicate thoughts and feelings effectively.
4. The ability to provide support, security, and encouragement.
5. The ability to initiate and maintain growth-producing relationships and experiences within and without the family.
6. The capacity to maintain and create constructive and responsible community relationships.
7. The ability to grow with and through children.
8. The ability to perform family roles flexibly.
9. The ability for self-help and to accept help when appropriate.
10. The capacity for mutual respect for the individuality of family members.
11. The ability to use a crisis experience as a means of growth.
12. The concern for family unity, loyalty, and interfamily cooperation.

By identifying family strengths, the focus is directed to the family resources and how they may be used to enhance family functioning.

Nursing Child Assessment Satellite Training Tools Barnard and Douglas (1976) developed several tools to assess the child's interaction with the caregiver. These tools, the Nursing Child Assessment Feeding Scales and the Nursing Child Assessment Teaching Scales, measure characteristics of both the caregiver and the child. Caregiver characteristics include sensitivity to cues, response to distress, social–emotional growth fostering, and cognitive growth

FAMILY COPING INDEX SCORING PROFILE SHEET

FAMILY NAME

COPING AREA	RATING X-STATUS O-EST. CHANGE	COPING ESTIMATE: INITIAL PERIODIC DISCHARGE
		DATE
		JUSTIFICATION
Physical independence	1 2 3 4 5 Not applicable ☐	
Therapeutic independence	1 2 3 4 5 Not applicable ☐	
Knowledge of condition	1 2 3 4 5 Not applicable ☐	
Application of principles of general hygiene	1 2 3 4 5 Not applicable ☐	
Attitudes toward health care	1 2 3 4 5 Not applicable ☐	
Emotional competence	1 2 3 4 5 Not applicable ☐	
Family living patterns	1 2 3 4 5 Not applicable ☐	
Physical environment	1 2 3 4 5 Not applicable ☐	
Use of community resources	1 2 3 4 5 Not applicable ☐	

Figure 17-4 Family Coping Index. SOURCE: Ruth B. Freeman, RN, EdD, Frederick A. Clark, MD, Marie L. Lowe, RN, PhD.

fostering. Infant characteristics include clarity of cues and responsiveness to the parent. These tools are useful in the assessment of parent–child interactions and serve as an excellent teaching guide to relationships, infant cues, feedback, or interaction styles.

Feeding is an integral and essential part of the parent–infant relationship, and observation of a feeding can provide valuable information regarding the parent–infant interaction. The feeding scale involves observing a complete feeding of an infant (birth to 1 year) and is administered most effectively in the infant's home at a regular feeding. The observer must remain silent throughout the feeding and must be able to view both parent and infant at all times.

The feeding scale has 76 items that are scored as "yes" or "no," including 50 parent behavior items such as "parent stops or starts feeding in response to child's distress" and 26 infant behavior items such as "child vocalizes to parent during feeding." Each item is categorized according to caregiver and infant characteristics. Scores are not percentiles but do give some indication of the quality of the parent–child interaction during feeding. This tool in turn provides information about parent–child attachment, the parent's role in the child's development, and the effect of the parent and child on each other.

The teaching scale is similar to the feeding scale but looks at a different aspect of the parent–child relationship. The parent is instructed to teach the child (birth to 3 years) a specific age-appropriate task. For instance, the parent of a 9-month-old infant might be instructed to teach the infant to put a small block into a cup. The parent is told to teach the task in any way that he or she chooses, and to manipulate materials and move about as needed. If the task proves to be too hard or too easy, another approved item may be selected.

The teaching scale includes 73 items, 50 parent behavior items such as "parent uses at least two different sentences or phrases to describe the task to the child" and 23 child behavior items such as "child vocalizes while looking at task materials." These items are again categorized according to the caregiver and child characteristics, and scoring is identical to the feeding scale, although the teaching usually involves a much shorter time span than the feeding observation and thus requires precise observation of the interaction. Although the teaching task might not be as natural an interaction as feeding, it does give the nurse an opportunity to observe the caregiver's style of instructing the child, the feedback given, and the frustration and adaptability of both parent and child. Again, percentiles are not calculated, but an impression about parent–child interaction and the effect of this interaction pattern is created.

With the number and variety of assessment tools available, the nurse can select the ones that will best validate general assessment data already obtained and those that will help to focus and direct nursing interventions most effectively.

Key Concepts

- Family assessment is the process of gathering and analyzing data about a family and its members; it is distinct from family therapy in that it is not a process of formal treatment.
- The overall goal of family assessment is to promote family growth by identifying needs for teaching and referral.
- Family assessment draws on a variety of disciplines and theories; these provide the nurse with a frame of reference with which to analyze the data obtained about a family.
- The process of data collection requires preparing for the interview by developing an "agenda" of likely concerns, facilitating communication through open-ended questions, observing nonverbal cues, and asking the parent to describe the child.
- In the process of assessment, the nurse collects data about family structure, function, roles, suprasystems, subsystems, and knowledge of child care.
- Assessment of family structure, function, and roles may point to problems that affect relationships within the family system.
- Assessment of family suprasystems and subsystems might reveal a family's values and priorities and suggest existing or potential needs for additional support.
- In assessing a family's knowledge of child care, the nurse considers the family's stage of development together with any transitions in the family or in the lives of any of its members.
- Family assessment tools include the Home Observation for Measurement of the Environment, the Family APGAR, the Family Assessment Tool for School Nurses and Other Professionals, the Family Environment Scale, the Family Adaptability and Cohesion Evaluation Scales, the Family Coping Index, the Feetham Family Functioning Survey, the Nursing Child Assessment Satellite Training Tools, and the Neonatal Perception Inventory.

References

Avant P: A maternal attachment assessment strategy. In: *Analysis of Current Assessment Strategies in the Health Care of Young Children and Childbearing Families.* Humenick S (editor). Appleton-Century-Crofts, 1982.

Barnard KE, Douglas HB: *Child Health Assessment. Part 1: A Literature Review.* DHEW Publication No. (HRA) 75–30 US Health Resources Administration. US Government Printing Office, 1976.

Bradley RH, Caldwell BM: Early home environment and changes in mental test performance in children from 6 to 36 months. *Dev Psychol* 1976; 1:93–97.

Bradley RH, Caldwell BM: Home environment and cognitive development in the first 2 years: A cross-logged panel analysis. *Dev Psychol* 1979; 15(3):246–260.

Broussard ER, Hartner MS: Further considerations regarding maternal perception of the first born. In: *Exceptional Infant: Studies in Abnormalities,* Vol 2. Hellmuth J (editor). Brunner/Mazel, 1971.

Cain A: Assessment of family structure. In: *Family Focused Care.* Miller JR, Janosik EH (editors). McGraw-Hill, 1980.

Clark C: *Mental Health Aspects of Community Health Nursing.* McGraw-Hill, 1978.

Clemen S, Eigsti D, McGuire S: *Comprehensive Family and Community Health Nursing.* McGraw-Hill, 1981.

Duvall EM: *Marriage and Family Development.* Lippincott, 1977.

Edison C: Family assessment guidelines. In: *Family Health Care—General Perspectives.* Vol 1. 2nd ed. Hymovich D, Barnard M (editors). McGraw-Hill, 1979.

Eichel E: Assessment with a family focus. *J Psychoc Nurs Ment Health Serv* (Jan) 1978; 11–14.

Elardo R, Bradley RH, Caldwell BM: The relation of infants' home environments to mental test performance from six to thirty-six months: A longitudinal analysis. *Child Dev* 1975; 46:71–76.

Feetham S, Humenick S: The Feetham family functioning survey. Pages 259–268 In: *Analysis of Current Assessment Strategies in the Health Care of Young Children and Childbearing Families.* Humenick S (editor). Appleton-Century-Crofts, 1982.

Freeman R, Lowe M: *The Family Coping Index.* Johns Hopkins School of Public Health and Richmond, Virginia, City Health Department, Nursing Service, Cooperative Nursing Study, 1964.

Friedman M: *Family Nursing—Theory and Assessment.* Appleton-Century-Crofts, 1981.

Grace HK, Camilleri D: *Mental Health Nursing—A Socio-psychological Approach.* 2nd ed. Brown, 1981.

Helvie C: *Community Health Nursing—Theory and Process.* Harper & Row, 1981.

Hill R, Hanson DA: The identification of conceptual frameworks utilized in family study. *Marriage Fam Living* 1960; 22:299–311.

Holt S, Robinson T: The school nurse's family assessment tool. *Am J Nurs* (May) 1979; 950–953.

Horton TE: Conceptual basis for nursing intervention with human systems: Families. In: *Distributive Nursing Practice: A Systems Approach to Community Health.* Hall JE, Weaver BR (editors). Lippincott, 1977, pp. 101–115.

Miller JR, Janosik EH: Evaluation of family progress. In: *Family-Focused Care.* Miller JR, Janosik EH (editors). McGraw-Hill, 1980

Minuchin S: *Families and Family Therapy.* Harvard University Press, 1974.

Moos R: *Family Environment Scale.* Consulting Psychologists Press, 1974.

Nye FI, Bernardo FM (editors): *Emerging Conceptual Frameworks in Family Analysis.* Macmillan, 1966.

Olson D, Bell R, Porter J: *FACES.* University of Minnesota Press, 1978.

Otto HA: A framework for assessing family strengths. In: *Family-Centered Community Nursing: A Sociocultural Framework.* Vol 1. Reinhardt AM, Quinn MD (editors). Mosby, 1973.

Phipps LB: Theoretical frameworks applicable to family care. In: *Family Focused Care.* Miller JR, Janosik EN (editors). McGraw-Hill, 1980.

Robischon P, Smith JA: Family assessment. In: *Current Practice in Family Centered Community Nursing.* Vol 1. Reinhardt AM, Quinn MD (editors). Mosby, 1977.

Smilkstein G: The family APGAR. A Proposal for a family function test and its use by physicians. *J Fam Pract* 1978; (6):1231–1239.

Walker, Thompson: Mother–infant play. In: *Analysis of Current Assessment Strategies in the Health Care of Young Children and Childbearing Families.* Humenick S (editor). Appleton-Century-Crofts, 1982.

Additional Readings

Allmond BW, Buckman W, Gofman HF: *The Family is the Patient.* Mosby, 1979.

Bradley RH, Caldwell BM, Elardo R: Home environment, social status, and mental test performance. *J Educat Psychol* 1977; 69(6):697–701.

Coser RL (editor): *The Family: Its Structures and Functions.* St. Martin's Press, 1974.

Erickson GD, Hogan TP (editors): *Family Theory: An Introduction to Theory and Technique.* Aaronson, 1976.

Folta JR, Deck ES (editors): *A Sociological Framework for Patient Care.* Wiley, 1979.

Gilliss CL: The family as unit of analysis: Strategies for the nurse researcher. *Adv Nurs Sci* 1983; 5(3):50–59.

Hansen D, Hill R: Families under stress. In: *Handbook of Marriage and the Family.* Christensen HT (editor). Rand McNally, 1964.

Knafl KA, Grace HK: *Families Across the Life Cycle.* Little, Brown, 1978.

Lewis J: *How's Your Family.* Brunner/Mazel, 1979.

Longo DC, Williams RA (editors): *Clinical Practice in Psychosocial Nursing: Assessment and Intervention.* Appleton-Century-Crofts, 1978.

Miller JR, Janosik EH (editors): *Family Focused Care.* McGraw-Hill, 1980.

Murray RB, Zentner JP (editors) *Nursing Assessment and Health Promotion Through the Life Span.* 2nd ed. Prentice-Hall, 1979.

Nye IF, Bernardo F: *The Family: Its Structure and Interaction.* MacMillan, 1973.

Nye IF (editor): *Role Structure and Analysis of the Family.* Sage Publications, 1976.

Perry SE: Parent's perceptions of their newborn following structured interactions. *Nurs Res* 1983; 32(4):208–212.

Roberts CS, Feetham SL: Assessing family functioning across three areas of relationships. *Nurs Res* 1982; 31(4):231–235.

Schless A, Mendels J: The value of interviewing family and friends in assessing life stressors. *Arch Gen Psychiatry* 1978; 35:565–567.

Sedgwick R, et al: Family health assessment. *Nurse Practitioner* 1981; 6:37.

Snyder C, Eyres SJ, Barnard K: New findings about mother's antenatal expectations and their relationship to infant development. *Am J Matern Child Nurs* 1979; 4(6):354–357.

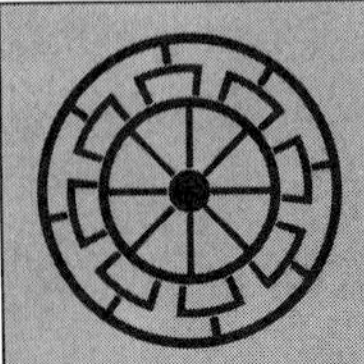

Nursing Care Plan Basing Care on Assessment

Assessment Data

Pam is a 12-year-old junior high school student who appears older than her age because of her height, early maturation with the development of secondary sexual characteristics, and obesity. Many attempts to lose weight with fad diets have been unsuccessful. Pam is unhappy with her appearance and tries to hide her size by slouching when sitting and hunching over when walking, both of which contribute to poor posture and an apparent functional spinal curve.

Pam has a history of being overweight and has developed many poor eating habits such as snacking while doing homework, when watching television, or when bored. She enjoys eating and either takes a second serving or a large first serving. Her understanding of the caloric content and nutritive value of the foods she eats is limited. Although she gets a little exercise, it does not compensate for her excess caloric intake.

Pam has several acquaintances, but since her only sister married and moved away a year ago, she is unable to name any friends. Her low self-esteem and negative self-concept prevent her from taking the initiative to make friends. Academically, Pam does very well and consistently demonstrates logical thinking and creative problem solving in her classes, skills that she thus far has been unable to transfer to her personal life.

Pam's parents divorced 6 months ago, and Pam lives with her mother in a small, second-floor apartment in the city. Since the divorce, Pam's mother has had to work full time, which she resents and finds difficult. She would like Pam to help around the house more but makes only indirect references to this desire, which Pam does not take seriously. Pam, on the other hand, feels confined to the house and wants more freedom to choose alternative activities but is afraid to ask for this privilege. Both Pam and her mother harbor considerable anger about the divorce and its consequences, but they have been unable to share their feelings with each other.

This is a routine health assessment. Pam's only concerns are her obesity and desire to lose weight.

Nursing Diagnoses and Goals

1. **Nursing diagnosis:** Alteration in nutrition—more than body requirements—related to excess intake.

   Long-term goal: Pam will increase her caloric expenditure and decrease her caloric intake.

   Short-term goals: (a) Pam will lose 0.5–1.0 lb/wk. (b) Pam will increase her activity and exercise level. (c) Pam will modify her eating habits and eliminate high-calorie snacks and junk foods.

2. **Nursing diagnosis:** Alteration in self-esteem related to disturbed body image secondary to obesity and height.

   Long-term goal: Pam will take an interest in her mature appearance, wearing clothes that fit, and accentuate her facial features and golden blonde hair.

   Short-term goals: (a) Pam will discuss growth and developmental variations between an early maturer and late maturer, recognizing herself as a normal early maturer. (b) Pam will identify styles and colors that deemphasize her weight and height, which currently compare unfavorably with peers. (c) Pam will brush her hair daily and choose a hairstyle that complements her facial features.

3. **Nursing diagnosis:** Alteration in self-concept related to negative feedback from peers and lack of friends.

   Long-term goal: Pam will investigate the weight control and fitness club at school for the dual purpose of losing weight and making friends.

   Short-term goals: (a) Pam will talk about the weight control club, its activities, and membership with someone who is an active member. (b) Pam will attend at least two club meetings before her conference next month.

4. **Nursing diagnosis:** Developmental vulnerability related to social isolation by peers and self-defeating behaviors with regard to weight control.

   Long-term goal: Pam will offer academic help to peers, thus increasing her contacts and emphasizing her assets.

   Short-term goals: (a) Pam will suggest that she and the girl who frequently calls her for assignment information study together for the next test. (b) Pam will volunteer to organize the next group project assignment in school.

5. **Nursing diagnosis:** Dysfunctional family functioning related to ineffective communication patterns secondary to an inability to share personal concerns.

   Long-term goal: Pam and her mother will communicate with each other in a meaningful way.

   Short-term goals: (a) Pam and her mother will discuss their expectations of and for each other. (b) Pam and her mother will discuss the pain of the divorce.

6. **Nursing diagnosis:** Alteration in parenting related to a change in family structure and roles because of the divorce and the mother's need to work.

   Long-term goal: Pam will demonstrate initiative in helping

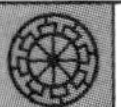

NURSING CARE PLAN Basing Care on Assessment (continued)

her mother with daily household chores and taking responsibility for decisions made.

Short-term goals: (a) Pam will make supper one evening a week. (b) Pam and her mother will list specific areas of responsibility that each of them will fulfill.

7. Nursing diagnosis: Potential for back and leg pain with continued poor posture and subsequent likelihood of muscle weakness in affected areas.

Long-term goal: Pam will discontinue her habits of poor posture and stand and sit tall with a straight back.

Short-term goal: Pam will increase her physical activity level to strengthen her muscles and improve her coordination.

8. Nursing diagnosis: Potential for adult obesity and hypothyroidism related to adolescent obesity.

Long-term goal: No underlying pathologic process will be identified.

Short-term goals: (a) Pam will not be at risk for developing complications from any existing conditions. (b) Pam will not have any untoward effects associated with losing weight.

Interventions	Rationale	Evaluation criteria
1. Discuss the relationship of caloric intake and calorie expenditure with respect to weight loss	Begin with general principles that are stated in concrete terms appropriate for a 12-year-old who is an adept concrete operational thinker	Did Pam lose 0.5–1.0 lb/wk and was it documented at her weekly weight checks?
Discuss the benefits of losing weight slowly as a result of changing eating habits, types of food eaten, and exercise routine	Successful weight loss requires a long-term commitment to a change in life-style rather than "overnight" success by a crash or fad diet plan.	
Review nutrition principles and the need to obtain food from the basic four food groups	Move from general to specific and from known to unknown information	
Advise Pam to eat smaller quantities at meals, to eat more salads using no dressing or low-calorie dressing instead of casseroles and creamed dishes for lunch at school, and to eat fresh fruit instead of cookies, ice cream, or pastry for dessert	Give specific directions about changing food habits and how to eat wisely without drastic changes. There are many hidden calories in casseroles and creamed dishes; desserts add calories but little food value	Did Pam sufficiently alter her food intake and eliminate between-meal snacking to help her lose weight?
Advise Pam to eat one citrus fruit per day or a glass of orange juice.	Best source of vitamin C	
Tell Pam to increase her skim milk intake, substitute milk for soda at mealtimes, and make milk her afternoon snack	Skim milk has the same nutritive value as whole milk minus the fat calories. By 12 years of age, brain development is complete, so there is no need for excess essential fatty acids. Milk is an excellent source of vitamin D	
Advise Pam to eliminate sugared drinks and to drink water instead	Sugared drinks and junk food offer empty calories; water is a better thirst quencher	
Give Pam and her mother a list of foods and their respective caloric content and nutritive value	Knowing food values will help in planning meals that are healthy and low in calories	

continued on next page

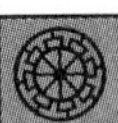

NURSING CARE PLAN Basing Care on Assessment (continued)

Interventions	Rationale	Evaluation criteria
Discuss the methods of food preparation as a means to reduce calories (broil or boil instead of fry)	One way to avoid adding unwanted calories is not to fry or cook in oil	
Discuss with Pam ways to change her pattern of eating between meals (eg, increasing after-school activities, leaving signs on the cupboards or refrigerator reminding her not to eat, decreasing the amount of time she watches television)	Breaking habits is a difficult task and is helped by changing the routines and leaving handy reminders	
Discuss with Pam ways to increase her caloric expenditures such as swimming every day and adding a half hour to the amount of time she rides her bike	To lose weight, calories must be expended, and exercise is the best way to burn up calories. Swimming and bike riding are both excellent ways to use all the muscle groups. Since she already participates in these activities, increasing the amount of time spent doing them is preferred to starting something new that she might or might not enjoy	Has Pam's exercise level increased to include at least an additional half-hour every day?
Have Pam and her mother keep a record of food intake, method of preparation, duration of activity, and description of activity	Keeping a record serves as a reminder and concrete illustration of the relationship among intake, expenditure, and balance of calories. Involving the mother gives Pam a source of encouragement and raises the mother's level of awareness concerning food choices and preparation	Has Pam's general activity involvement increased so that there is less empty time to be filled by watching television with its attendant temptation to snack?
Have Pam compare her daily intake of the four basic food groups with the standard recommended daily allowances	Comparing actual intake with the recommended intake will help Pam to plan a healthy diet	
Pam will return weekly for a weight check and conference. She will bring her records with her each time	Weekly weight checks are a good indicator of weight loss or control. Checking Pam's records facilitates the identification of positive practices and additional areas where advice might be helpful. It also reinforces the value of keeping and analyzing records as a guide in weight control	
Pam will reward herself for every 10 lb she loses or significant change in behavior (eg, not eating between meals for 2 weeks)	Rewards along the way provide the necessary motivation to continue	
2. Review growth and development and the relationship between the onset of puberty and bodily changes	Important to assess Pam's knowledge of puberty and understanding of secondary sexual changes she is experiencing and reassure that they are normal	Can Pam identify the sequence of developmental changes associated with puberty and explain the ramifications of being an early maturer?
Discuss the different rates at which girls mature and Pam's perceptions about being an early maturer	Girls who mature early often feel out of place because they are taller and more developed than their peers. They feel conspicuous and	

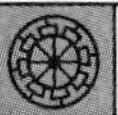

NURSING CARE PLAN Basing Care on Assessment (continued)

Interventions	Rationale	Evaluation criteria
	might try to hide breast development and height. Body image is an important aspect of self-esteem. Girls tend to cease adding height after menarche has occurred; therefore, in a year or two, Pam will no longer be obviously taller than her peers	
Discuss aspects of general appearance, emphasizing cleanliness, clothing styles, and colors that tend to hide excess weight	Self-esteem comes from how one perceives oneself, so it is beneficial to make Pam appear as attractive as possible while she is losing weight. Clothes that are dark, have vertical patterns, and fit well do not call attention to weight. Also, the use of jackets, cardigan vests, overblouses, and loose-waist dresses or jumpers helps	Is Pam wearing clothes that are clean, neat, and fit to avoid calling attention to herself when in a group?
Assess Pam's wardrobe with her for possible combinations and outfits. Emphasize that being neat and clean is more important than having a variety of clothes	It is important that Pam look nice without spending money on new clothes—the goal is weight loss, and new clothes at the beginning would be a waste of money. Cleanliness and neatness are crucial to Pam's feeling good about her appearance, and the limited variety is only temporary	
Encourage Pam to emphasize her attractive facial features and golden blonde hair. Suggest that Pam experiment with different ways of fixing her hair	It is helpful to highlight one's most positive features. New hairstyles are noticed quickly, calling attention to an aspect of Pam's appearance that is favorable	Is Pam's hair clean and neatly styled to accentuate her facial features?
3. Provide Pam with information about available resources at her junior high school to assist her in losing weight such as the weight control and fitness club, school nurse, and school nutritionist	Pam needs ready access to resources for daily information, support, and encouragement	Did Pam find out about the activities and membership of the weight control and fitness club by talking to one of its members?
Assess Pam's perceptions of the club and whether she knows any of its members (might need to provide a few names)	It is unlikely that Pam would join a club that she thought was for "fat" girls only or whose membership she disliked. Might need to clarify a wrong perception (eg, the club's membership also includes athletes and others who are interested in weight control and good nutrition)	
Encourage Pam to investigate the weight control and fitness club as a means of obtaining peer support for her efforts	Best to find out about a group before joining	Did Pam attend two club meetings before deciding whether to join?
Suggest that Pam visit the club several times and compile a list of benefits and a list of disadvantages to membership	It is better for Pam to make the decision concerning membership based on her information and sense of "fit" between the club, its goals, and membership and herself.	

continued on next page

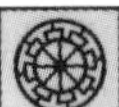

NURSING CARE PLAN Basing Care on Assessment (continued)

Interventions	Rationale	Evaluation criteria
4. Discuss with Pam her routine day and how she would like to change it	Involve Pam in planning and decision making about changes and goals	Did Pam study with another student before the test last week?
Have Pam identify what her strengths are and what she can offer to others	The first step in getting involved is to identify areas of confidence, experience, or excellence	
Discuss with Pam and even role-play ways to make friends. Suggest that Pam initiate helping some students with homework, studying together for an exam, or organizing an assigned class project	Individuals who have a negative self-concept often do not envision the possibility of making friends, especially not taking the initiative; therefore, it is helpful to have ideas or a specific plan	
5. Acknowledge the pain of divorce to both Pam and her mother, the presence of unresolved issues, and their anger about the consequences	It is helpful to have a third party put feelings into words and to give them legitimacy	Were Pam and her mother able to talk about their feelings and anger related to the divorce?
Refer Pam and her mother to a self-help group that meets locally (Children of Divorced Parents meets once a month and Parents Without Partners meets one evening a month)	Self-help groups are often therapeutic resources and are able to provide practical ideas and support from personal experience	
Encourage Pam and her mother to discuss what they want and expect from each other as well as what aggravates each of them about the other	Honest, open communication facilitates trust and understanding and often clarifies misconceptions	Did Pam and her mother discuss their expectations of each other so that misconceptions could be clarified?
Have Pam and her mother contract with each other to do or not do certain behaviors, such as nag or pout, and discuss how the week went at the weekly conference	A contract requires a conscious commitment to perform or not perform certain behaviors and usually has better results than a vague agreement	
Suggest that Pam's mother might benefit from a half-hour nap when she returns home from work	The mother's needs have to be acknowledged as well as Pam's	
6. Suggest that Pam and her mother work out a plan to see that household chores get done	By specifying certain tasks and the individual who has the responsibility to fulfill the assigned task, the household chores get done without one person feeling overburdened. Working on the plan together allows some freedom of choice as to which tasks are chosen	Did Pam and her mother identify tasks for each to fulfill and are they being responsible in fulfilling their obligation to help each other in this way?
Suggest that Pam's mother either borrow from the library or purchase an inexpensive, easy cookbook to use in teaching Pam some simple recipes of her choice	Pam might be more willing to help with meal preparation if she perceives it as fun or learning a new and useful skill. Pam is intellectually capable of following directions after initial guidance. It also provides a	Did Pam prepare a supper of her choice once a week?

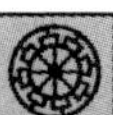

NURSING CARE PLAN Basing Care on Assessment (continued)

Interventions	Rationale	Evaluation criteria
Suggest that Pam prepare one meal a week of her choice	means to achieve success and recognition plus the chance to choose foods consistent with her diet plan	
Encourage Pam and her mother to include some recreational activities in their time together, taking turns choosing the activity	Pam and her mother need to enjoy each other as mother and daughter. A family is not all work and no play	
Discuss with Pam and her mother other possible after-school activities or clubs (eg, the Girl's Club, YMCA activities, including daily free swim, and the Girl Scouts) in which Pam might be interested and decide to join	If Pam is involved in other activities, it provides opportunities to meet new friends and gives her less time to do nothing, which not only aggravates her mother but encourages Pam to snack to relieve boredom	Did Pam investigate possible after-school activities and did she select two in which to participate?
Suggest that Pam be allowed to select her own clothes within a given price range	Having Pam select her own clothes and activities gives her freedom to make decisions and also the responsibility to choose wisely. This helps to define her role as an individual with normal developmental needs for peer interaction	
7. Explain the importance of good posture with respect to appearance and the prevention of muscular weakness	Poor posture puts undue strain on muscles, which weakens them. Good posture, while acknowledging height, helps one to appear neat and poised	Has Pam increased her physical activity and is she making a conscious effort to practice good posture?
Encourage Pam to consciously correct her posture when walking, standing, or sitting (eg, think about her posture every hour when the alarm on her digital watch rings)	Changing a habit takes effort and being reminded keeps one conscious of the habit and helps the process of change	
Discuss physical fitness exercises or aerobic dancing to increase activity and coordination	These are specific ways to strengthen muscles used to support the spine in good posture	
Consult with the family physician to rule out structural scoliosis	Although assessment indicated a functional curve resulting from poor posture, this finding must be validated	
Have Pam return in 6 months for reevaluation of posture and spinal curve	The curve will straighten with exercise and good posture; if it does not improve or worsens, further diagnostic testing will be required or a more specific program of daily exercises	
8. Refer Pam to the family physician for a complete medical assessment to rule out any conditions contraindicating weight loss by diet and exercise	Before beginning any diet plan, it is best to consult with a physician to validate the plan's safety for the individual. Obesity increases the cardiac load and risk of hypertension	Is Pam's health compatible with the weight loss plan? Is there any existing condition to contraindicate the plan?

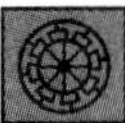

NURSING CARE PLAN Basing Care on Assessment (continued)

Interventions	Rationale	Evaluation criteria
Refer Pam to the family physician for laboratory tests for hemoglobin, hematocrit, serum cholesterol, and triglyceride levels, and complete thyroid studies	These tests indicate various aspects of body function with respect to conditions for which Pam is at risk from her family history, her age, or her obesity	
The nurse will coordinate goals and interventions with the family physician	Teamwork is essential to accomplish the goals of preventing future obesity, cardiac disease, and emotional isolation	Is Pam tolerating the plan to reduce weight by changing her habits of intake and exercise?

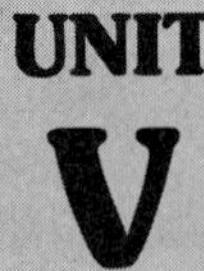

PREVENTIVE CHILD HEALTH NURSING: STRATEGIES FOR HEALTH PROMOTION

Many nurses and health professionals accept the principle that self-determination is essential to health maintenance. For maintaining optimal wellness individuals need to include practices in their daily routines that promote health and prevent illness and injury. Children are no exception to this philosophy. Child health professionals play an important role in encouraging children to become knowledgeable health consumers, willing to take individual responsibility for promotion of health and prevention of disease. The same marketing strategies used by the business community, such as the media advertising of food and toys, can be used by health professionals to develop the child's knowledge and sense of responsibility.

Consistent with our book's holistic framework and application of self-care theory, in Unit V we present four chapters dealing with prevention of illness and injury. In each chapter we illustrate prevention strategies that assist nurses and parents to prepare children to be responsible health consumers. Each chapter is constructed around an epidemiologic framework that examines the interrelationship of host, agent, and environmental factors contributing to the occurrence of disease or injury.

Chapter 18 examines the concept of optimal wellness and delineates preventive interventions directed toward parents and children. The themes of individual responsibility and the child as a health consumer are stressed. Nursing strategies at the primary and secondary levels of prevention, which include health education, screening, and health protection measures, are discussed in depth. Chapter 19 examines factors contributing to childhood injury and details accident prevention from a developmental perspective. The secondary level of prevention is addressed, with descriptions of nursing interventions for common emergencies. Chapter 20 discusses poison prevention, also from an epidemiologic perspective. The emergency management of childhood poisonings is followed by a detailed discussion of readily available poisonous substances, which the student can use as a comprehensive reference. Chapter 21 completes the prevention unit with a compact summary in table form of the previous three chapters. This chapter models a clear analysis of relevant data as a basis for a comprehensive developmental overview of health promotion and preventive nursing care.

Prevention of Illness

Gwendolyn C. Robinson

18

Chapter Outline

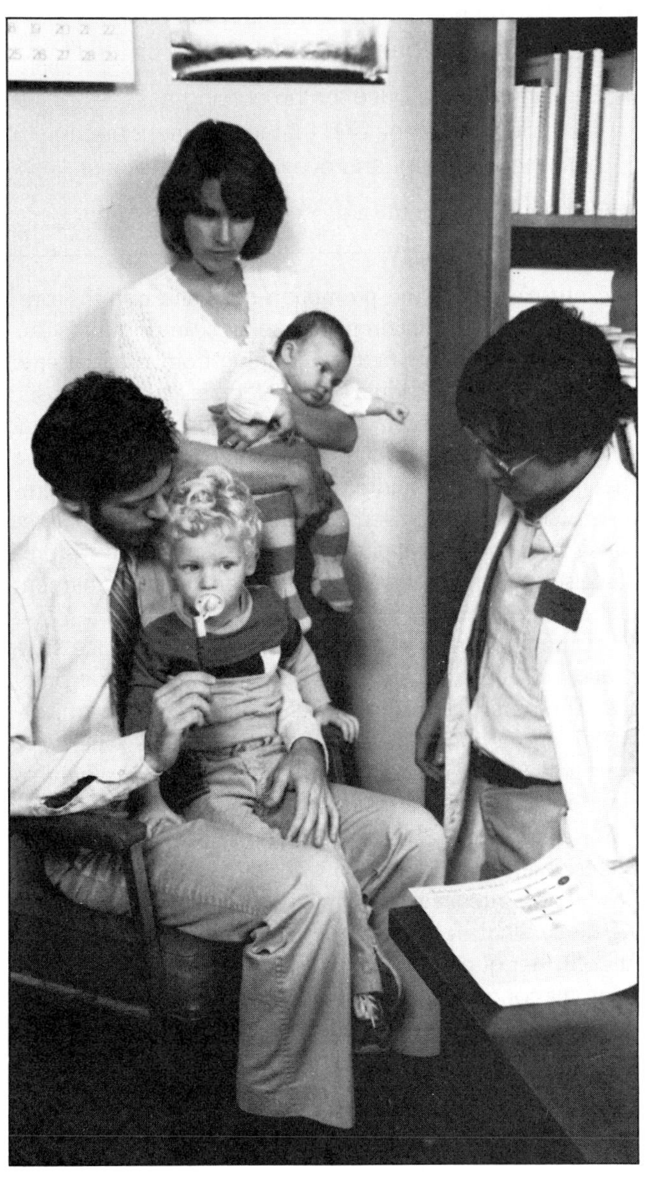

Objectives

- Discuss the concept of health within the context of an epidemiologic framework.
- Identify the nurse's role in health promotion, protection, and prevention of illness in children.
- Explain the data base for the nursing assessment of the child, the agent, and the environment during both the pre-event and event phases of illness.
- List the nursing strategies related to consumer awareness, health education, and techniques for staying healthy.
- Illustrate health protection measures affecting the child as an individual and society as a whole.
- Discuss measures to reduce the severity of an illness or to contain its communicability.
- Explain strategies to prevent infection and to reduce the complications of illness.

The nurse's role in the promotion of health and the prevention of illness in children is increasingly important today. The responsibility for health is shifting from medical care systems to the individual. Many factors, such as costs, increased worker shortages, and alterations in traditional roles of health care professionals, have necessitated the changes. The social and economic framework of contemporary culture, the limited time devoted to health maintenance, and the seemingly limitless costs of health restoration also demand that nurses strengthen their commitment to health promotion strategies in nursing practice. The assessment of individual attitudes, beliefs, and life-style relating to health must become part of professional practice. The nurse can use personal experience to encourage health promotion. Successful practice results when the practitioner can cite examples that confirm the value of a healthful life-style as a practical reality.

For example, one boy whose parents had required some extensive and painful dental work decided that bad teeth was a consequence of becoming an adult. This boy asked the nurse what he could do to keep his good baby teeth. After further questioning and discovery of the events leading to his concern, the nurse discussed with him basic facts about dental hygiene, emphasizing the importance of routine dental checkups and daily care. The boy was reassured by this information, doubly so when his parent confirmed that the present problems were the result of neglectful dental care during college and graduate school. This negative example was relevant and meaningful for the boy, who changed his routine to include brushing his teeth more often.

Children can learn to make positive health behaviors an integral part of their lives. Healthful living early in life will lower the risk of disease and the frustration of major life-style changes necessitated by a preventable health crisis. Regardless of practice setting, nurses can make a great impact on the health of children. As a role model, the nurse can positively influence parents, teachers, children, community leaders, and other health care professionals. The nurse also can provide information about how to stay healthy and can promote the effective utilization of health resources to children and their significant others.

In this chapter we discuss the concept of wellness as it relates to child health promotion. First, we review concepts such as health, wellness, illness, health promotion, and prevention of illness, then we discuss the historical perspectives on child health. Second, we describe the nursing assessment within an epidemiologic framework. We explore the influences on child health, including individual behavior, contact with adverse agents, and the role of the environment. Finally, we present nursing interventions and teaching strategies appropriate for each stage of child development, along with techniques for teaching specific health promotion and preventive behavior.

The philosophic framework for this chapter is a holistic concept of wellness. This entails a respect for individuals, their heritage, and the corresponding variety of choices available to attain maximum physical, mental, and spiritual well-being. The nurse can encourage the individual's active participation in the effective use of personal resources in the practice of health promotion. The nurse needs to identify the significance and purpose of cultural, social, familial, and economic factors and to include them in any teaching. When changes or additions are necessary, it is essential to first assess the client's level of readiness for new information and methods of incorporating related ideas and behaviors into the client's life-style. Change can be difficult, requiring a period of adjustment as the client works on developing habits, attitudes and beliefs that are positive and growth enhancing. The more positive, health-promoting habits the child establishes, the fewer negative behaviors will have to be changed when the child becomes an adult. Every nurse who comes in contact with children needs to bear this in mind.

Concepts

Health

Historically, to be healthy has meant to be free of illness or disease. Being healthy implies being able to function effectively and to respond successfully to the needs of both the internal and external environments. Currently, the World Health Organization defines health as "a state of complete physical, mental, and social well-being, and not merely the absence of disease" (Read, 1973). This implies that health is the homeostasis that occurs as a result of a person's interacting subsystems and suprasystems.

Wellness

The concept of wellness includes both health and illness. On a continuum, wellness encompasses all the possibilities of life. It views the individual as moving between the extremes of the human experience—premature death and high-level wellness (Fig. 18-1).

Wellness is a dynamic, changing phenomenon that results from the individual's successful integration of internal function with the ongoing, changing, external environment. It is influenced by genetic and environmental factors and requires constant adaptation to maintain effective and efficient regulatory activities at physical, psychological and social levels. Wellness is relative and a matter of subjectivity.

In this definition of wellness, an individual can have a disease, handicap, or any degree of physical, emotional, or spiritual deficit and still be considered well because the focus is on the individual's conscious choice to be self-directed and move toward achieving high-level wellness.

Illness

Illness is a dynamic, characteristic series of events that occur between the individual and the environment. It is influenced by genetics and environment and represents the failure of the individual to adapt successfully to internal and external stressors or to integrate biopsychosocial function with the changing environment. Illness can be either a concrete or subjective phenomenon.

Illness is a signal of imbalance. It occurs at a point on the illness–wellness continuum. Early signs of illness might be unrecognized or ignored, thus preventing the individual from realizing high-level wellness. In the illness–wellness model (Fig. 18-1), the progression is outlined as beginning with signs such as fatigue, irritability, or depression. When these warning signals are not heeded, the individual might develop symptoms of a disease, either physical or psychosocial. Lack of attention to the symptoms might eventually result in a disability such as heart disease, arthritis, cancer, or psychosis. Further debilitation might result in premature death.

Each person, or parents in the case of children, must decide on the focus for their life and choose behaviors that support their choice. A commitment to health includes a balanced life-style, with time for rest and relaxation, adequate diet, and regular exercise.

Stress

The concept of stress and its relation to illness (illness results when the individual is unable to adapt to change and maintain balance) also must be considered. Stress is defined as a general reaction pattern that occurs as a response to stimuli confronted in the activities of living. Stress is constantly present and may be either a constructive or destructive force. Three stages of reaction to stress have been identified. The first stage is *alarm:* the individual responds via biologic defense mechanisms and attempts to return to a balanced state. During the second stage, there is *resistance* to the continuing stressors and attempted adaptation via mobilization of coping resources. The third stage is *exhaustion*. The individual who cannot achieve balance becomes depleted and vulnerable. At this point, the individual is open to disease. It is important to note that the stressors can be either life supporting (eustress) or life threatening (distress) (Fig. 18-2). Positive reactions to stress depend on the individual's ability to reestablish harmony between the internal

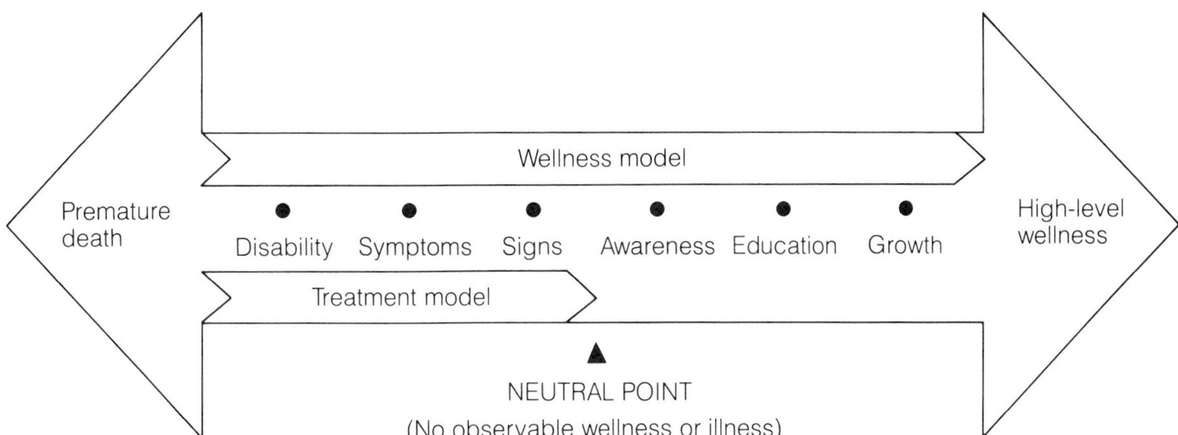

Figure 18-1 The illness-wellness continum. (From Ryan RS, Travis JW: *The Wellness Workbook*. Copyright © 1981.) Used with permission of Ten Speed Press.

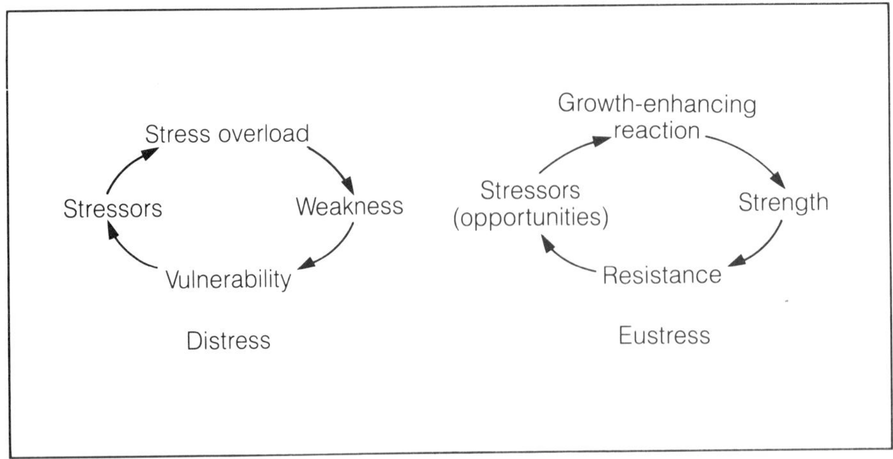

Figure 18-2 Two stress reactions: distress and eustress. (From Business Week's *Executive Health*. McGraw-Hill, Inc. © 1978. All rights reserved.)

and external environments. This process of adaptation enables the individual to retain integrity while accommodating to the realities of the environmental change. Adaptation is a matter of individual differences in perception, conditioning factors, and coping mechanisms because the same stressor, for example, entering a new school, can produce opposite effects in different people (Fig. 18-3).

People tend to view childhood as a time of pleasure without the pressures of adulthood, but children also respond physiologically to the events in their lives. Stress, and the need to adapt to stress, begins in childhood. The child can begin to develop insight about the source of stress, routine practices leading to good general health, and a repertoire of positive coping strategies. Table 18-1 outlines some of the life events that are stressors for children (Heisel et al., 1973). In addition to these events, the nurse considers a child's developmental crises and activities of daily living. Such routine activities as mealtime, toileting, bedtime, or naptime can be either a positive or a negative experience for a child. For example, Amanda is a 5-year-old, well-adjusted kindergartener. Both of her parents work at jobs each finds challenging and demanding, but they are at work from 7 A.M. to 6 P.M. daily. Amanda attends a day-care center before and after school and has direct contact with her parents between 6 P.M. and 7 A.M. each weekday and all day on weekends. Much of Amanda's experience with mealtime and rest/sleep time has been dictated by her parents' work lives.

This family situation can be either a positive, growth-producing life-style or a negative, distress-producing life-style. If the family is able to make the time together special so that it contributes to growth as a family, Amanda will interpret home and family as pleasant and joyful. If the time at home is hurried, without a plan for meals, bedtime, and other routine health-promoting daily activities, Amanda might be in a distressful environment. Routinely hurried mealtimes and daily bedtime battles are in direct conflict with a

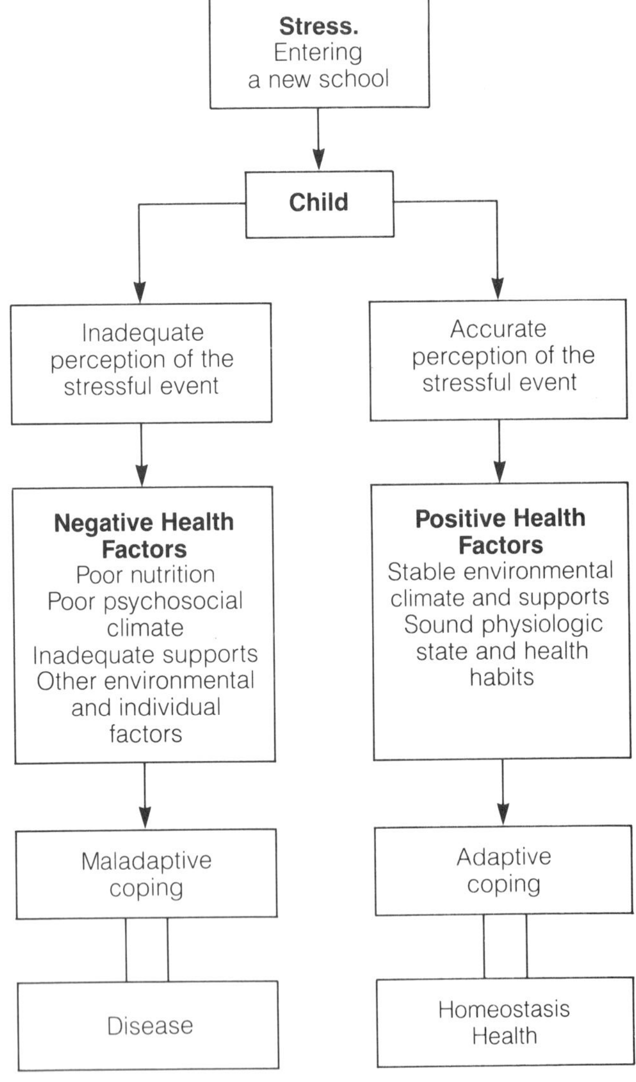

Figure 18-3. The process of adaptation and coping with stress. (Adapted from Smith M, Selye H: Reducing the negative effects of stress. Copyright © 1979, American Journal of Nursing Company. Reproduced with permission from The *Am J Nurs* (Nov); 79 (11).

TABLE 18-1 Stress Scale for Children*

Life events	Preschool age	Elementary school age	Junior high school age
Beginning nursery school, first grade, or high school	42	46	45
Change to a different school	33	46	52
Birth or adoption of a brother or sister	50	50	50
Brother or sister leaving home	39	36	33
Hospitalization of a brother or sister	37	41	44
Death of a brother or sister	59	68	71
Change of father's occupation requiring increased absence from home	36	45	42
Loss of job by parent	23	38	48
Marital separation of parents	74	78	77
Divorce of parents	78	84	84
Hospitalization of a parent (serious illness)	51	56	54
Death of a parent	89	91	94
Death of a grandparent	30	38	35
Marriage of a parent to a stepparent	62	65	63
Jail sentence of a parent of 30 days or less	34	44	50
Jail sentence of a parent of 1 year or more	67	67	76
Addition of third adult to family (ie, grandparent)	39	41	34
Change in parents' financial status	21	29	40
Mother beginning to work	47	44	36
Decrease in number of arguments between parents	21	25	29
Increase in number of arguments between parents	44	51	48
Decrease in number of arguments with parents	22	27	29
Increase in number of arguments with parents	39	47	46
Discovery of being an adopted child	33	52	70
Acquiring a visible deformity	52	69	83
Having a visible congenital deformity	39	60	70
Hospitalization of self (child)	59	62	59
Change in acceptance by peers	38	51	68
Outstanding personal achievement	23	53	65

continued on next page

TABLE 18.1 continued

Life events	Preschool age	Elementary school age	Junior high school age
Death of a close friend (child's friend)	38	53	65
Failure of a grade in school	—	57	62
Suspension from school	—	46	54
Pregnancy in unwed teen-age sister	—	36	60
Becoming involved with drugs or alcohol	—	61	70
Becoming a full-fledged member of a church or synagogue	—	25	28
Not being accepted into an extracurricular activity the child wanted to be involved in (ie, team, band)	—	—	49
Breaking up with a boyfriend or girlfriend	—	—	47
Beginning to date	—	—	55
Fathering an unwed pregnancy	—	—	76
Unwed pregnancy	—	—	95

*Different life events produce varying amounts of stress for children—the more points, the greater the stress. The chart is arranged in order of how frequently the events occur.

SOURCE: Heisel JS, et al: The significance of life events as contributing factors in the diseases of children. *J Pediatr* 1973; 83(1):119.

life-style of minimal distress and hinder the teaching of positive health behaviors to children. Specific techniques for teaching children positive ways to accomplish the necessary daily activities of life are discussed later in this chapter.

Goldberg (1978) found that when tension-producing and unpleasant life events consume more than $1\frac{1}{2}$ hours per day, the body is at risk for illness. Learning early in life to attend to the controllable behaviors is an important health promotion goal.

Daily Activity Assessment Scale

Log daily activities, including time spent on every task for 1–2 weeks. Using the following scale, assign each activity a score of 1–5:

1—pleasant, enjoyable, and relaxing
2—pleasant but taxing (perhaps hurried)
3—necessary (neither pleasant nor unpleasant) but taxing
4—unpleasant, hurried, or tension producing
5—very unpleasant, pressured, and tension producing

More than $1\frac{1}{2}$ hours spent on activities in categories 4 and 5 over several days requires an evaluation of those activities. Strive for low scores.

SOURCE: Goldberg P: *Executive Health*, McGraw-Hill, 1978.

Health Status of Children

Historically, the primary focus of child health has been on the physical and environmental factors influencing the morbidity and mortality rate in childhood (see Chapter 1). Current concerns about the health status of children have been expanded to include social and emotional perspectives as well as health promotion measures.

Historical Emphasis on Infection and Malnutrition

Children are proportionately less affected by severe chronic illness in the twentieth century than at any previous time. The advent of antibiotics and effective immunization have decreased the mortality rates for both communicable and infectious diseases. Communicable childhood diseases such as diphtheria, tetanus, whooping cough, and poliomyelitis are relatively rare. Smallpox has been eradicated. The number of cases of measles, mumps, and rubella has also dropped. Infectious diseases such as influenza and pneumonia are rarely killers of children, although they are still a problem in terms of acute illness and the need for hospitalization. Contracting communicable diseases is still a threat at present, however, and with disease comes the possibility of handicapping complications and occasionally death. The US Public Health Service has recommended as one of the goals for the 1980s specific measures to maintain the current successes in the decline in communicable diseases.

A potential major health hazard is the nutritional status of children. Nutritional status includes eating habits as well as the amount and choices of food. Child health problems related to diet and nutrition begin prenatally and continue through adolescence and throughout life. Poor nutrition or excess food intake has been reported to have at least some causal relationship to obesity, high blood pressure, dental disease, heart disease, cancer, and diabetes. Childhood problems such as failure to thrive, delayed physical and mental growth, and learning disabilities also have been linked to poor nutrition. (Nutritional assessment is discussed in Chapter 15.)

Current Emphases in Child Health Care

As children's problems from communicable diseases and poor nutrition decline, the emphasis on child health care has shifted toward the promotion of wellness and elimination of the factors contributing to illness. Health promotion and health protection are terms used to describe activities that maintain and enhance health. These terms are distinct from one another with respect to the manner of choice and control exercised by the individual.

Health Promotion Individuals make the decision and assume responsibility for activities that relate to health promotion. These activities are most beneficial when they are an active part of living, performed prior to the presence of an illness. Physical fitness programming, for example, is a health promotion measure. It advocates the adoption of specific health behaviors that may result in maintaining a state of wellness in the individual. Health promotion is internally chosen rather than externally imposed.

Health Protection Health protection refers to action that focuses on controlling environmental factors such as immunization, fluoridation of water, infectious disease control, and sanitation (Levi, 1979). In this category the responsibility is outside the individual's control and benefits the general population. The government legislates and regulates certain health protection measures. Whereas health promotion strategies benefit the individual directly, society at large benefits more from specific protection measures.

Prevention of Illness Prevention of illness encompasses both health protection and health promotion strategies that are directed toward preventing, interrupting, or minimizing the occurrence and consequence of disease. Both individuals and society benefit from strategies of illness prevention. Prevention strategies can be seen at three levels.

The primary level of prevention includes those measures taken before the presence of illness. Specific protection measures such as immunization programs are on this level, as well as many health promotional activities. The secondary level of prevention includes early recognition and treatment measures that interrupt or minimize the consequences of the disease process. Some screening procedures are included in secondary prevention measures. The tertiary prevention level includes rehabilitative measures or efforts to prevent the progression of a disability. The goal of this level is for the individual to function as well as possible (Dagg, 1981). Within the concept of wellness the individual might benefit from using all levels of prevention.

Once a family makes a commitment to a life-style that promotes wellness, its members choose behaviors in nutrition, exercise, sleep and relaxation, work and recreation, spiritual activity, and social relationships that will enhance and support their health promotion program. They will benefit from such protective primary prevention measures as obtaining proper immunization and drinking pasteurized milk and fluoridated water. Regular dental and vision screening and physical assessment will be part of their secondary prevention program. If a handicap or disability is present, attention will be given to measures designed to return the individual to an optimal level of functioning (tertiary-level behavior).

Health Promotion and Illness Prevention: An Epidemiologic Perspective

On the wellness-illness continuum there is a point at which signs of ill health appear. Strategies of health promotion and illness prevention are effective at various levels of illness manifestation. The course of a disease can be divided epidemiologically into distinct entities, or phases, that correspond to the levels of prevention: the pre-event phase, corresponding to the primary level of prevention; the event phase, corresponding to secondary prevention; and the final phase, corresponding to tertiary prevention. Factors in the pre-event phase determine whether the event will occur. Factors in the event phase affect the severity of the illness; and factors in the final phase affect the amount and extent of resulting disability (Rivara, 1982).

Factors influencing the wellness state of the child include, "lifestyle (self-created risks), environment, human biology, and the health care system" (McKay and Segall, 1983). Epidemiologically, these factors include characteristics of the host, characteristics of the agent, and characteristics of the environment. The course of each epidemiologic phase is determined by the interplay between these vital characteristics. The remainder of the chapter will focus on the nurse's role in the pre-event and event phases as it affects the promotion of health and prevention of illness.

Primary Prevention: The Nurse's Role

Nursing Contact With Children

The pre-event phase involves those factors that can be altered to prevent illness from occurring. Nurses influence children's health through their contacts with them in the community and in the schools.

Primary Health Care Nurse The nurse might be the only continuous health care professional for a child throughout childhood. This provides a unique opportunity for the child, family, and nurse to participate together in the growth process. The nurse might be an independent practitioner or part of a team. The focus of care is to help the child freely choose positive health behaviors. The child and the nurse must not only share the goal but work together to attain that goal. For example, although most parents of young children cite good health as a goal, some parents' behavior might counteract progress toward that goal. Unstructured life-styles, reliance on fast foods, irregular schedules that preclude regular rest periods, and inconsistent caregivers might be incompatible with the development of a physically and mentally healthy child. Although the stated goal might be health, the real priority in that parent's life might be economic well-being. The role of the nurse is to help the parent work out life-style patterns that will best meet the goal of economic security without compromising the goal of having a healthy child.

It is important for the nurse to consider the demands of work, family, and community and the need for personal satisfaction as they affect the parent and child. The flow of information and support must be interchangeable from client to nurse and from nurse to client. Each must view the other as a resource to be considered in meeting individual and common goals.

Regular health maintenance visits for children generally occur through 6 years of age. After this age, parents and children might not seek health counseling unless a problem exists. Other health professionals unwittingly contribute to the neglect of general health care by confining their contacts with the child to the issues central to their specialty. The tunnel vision that is sometimes part of specialized practice might hinder a view of the patient as a whole person. For example, lack of consideration for the total nutritional needs of a child might delay the healing of a surgical problem.

When contact with the child is for diagnosis or treatment purposes, the effective primary health care nurse will take the opportunity to assess the wellness level and institute appropriate strategies for health promotion. Nurses can alert other health professionals to the need to encourage parents and responsible children to seek support for wellness behavior.

School Nurse The most influential nurse from middle childhood through adolescence is the school nurse. The role of school nurses is comprehensive and includes health promotion, health teaching, health protection, and other strategies to prevent and control the spread of illness (see Chapter 1). Nurses encourage the development of positive health behaviors in children through teaching in the classroom as well as in the office. Stress-reduction techniques, the hazards of drug, alcohol, and cigarettes, and sex education are all areas where the school nurse can be an effective teacher and role model. School nurses are also role models for such self-care activities as nutrition, exercise, and preventive dental care.

School nurses promote children's awareness of health as a holistic concept. They support children in developing a personal health history. They emphasize emotional and spiritual health by helping children to clarify their values.

School nurses work with children, families, teachers, and the community to plan for the health needs of all. They are instrumental in helping both children with special needs and those who are chronically ill to enter the mainstream of school life. In addition, they can provide referrals for children needing more specialized follow-up care.

Assessment

Assessment during the pre-event phase is directed toward determining the individual characteristics of children as they relate to the environment and the agents with which they come in contact. Assessment data indicate where the child and family fall on the wellness–illness continuum. In addition, assessment enables the nurse and client to formulate diagnoses and construct a health plan that will increase the child's level of wellness.

Characteristics of the Child Some characteristics of the child include prenatal "givens" (resistance and immunity to disease, genetic predisposition to disease, and so on), emotional state (temperament), understanding of wellness concepts, health habits, and developmental skills.

A major psychosocial factor affecting child health is life-style. The effects of stress and the ability of a child to adapt to the changes in daily life are receiving more attention (Levi, 1979; Johnson, 1981). Unlike adults, children have not developed the coping strategies needed to deal with situational, societal, and personal changes (see Chapter 12 for a detailed discussion of coping strategies).

Children's understanding of wellness concepts plays an important role in developing positive health habits. Studies done to identify children's concepts of illness (Williams, 1979; Wood, 1983) found that most children have rudimentary understanding of illness. Young children usually view illness as either "germ" related or environmentally caused (weather elements such as cold, heat, rain). Children over 10 years of age can understand the concept of multiple causation. Factors seen as affecting disease occurrence most often are (1) the attitudes or actions of the children themselves, that is, "I didn't get enough sleep and got overtired," or "I was bad and I got sick" (illness as punishment); (2) physiologic agents (microorganisms); (3) outside forces such as environmental phenomena; and (4) injury.

Children's comprehension of germ theory and disease transmission varies so widely that any education must be based on the individual child's level of understanding. Assessment should identify the individual child's perception of wellness or illness. Although children comprehend their own role in disease occurrence, it does not appear that they understand their role regarding illness prevention. They need to be taught that by controlling the factors that result in disease, they can control the occurrence of disease.

Interest has been renewed in the idea of self-care as incorporated within the concept of health promotion and as a major characteristic of the child that affects the commitment to wellness (see Chapter 2). Self-care is action taken by individuals to care for or cure themselves, either acting alone or in consultation with a health care practitioner (Mattson, 1982). Critics of self-care fear that individuals might not seek professional assistance or suffer damaging effects of illness from a delay in consulting health care practitioners. Holistic health proponents claim that all experience is important as a lesson along the continuum of life, and thus the individual can learn from any experience, even an illness. The availability of a wider variety of choices allows the individual to choose the most beneficial mode of healing and the one that coincides with personal beliefs. Nursing assessment of self-care must be based on knowledge of the developmental process necessary to achieve independence in this area.

According to Dorothea Orem's theory (1980), the self-care agent for the infant is the parent (see Chapter 2). Parents respond to the universal needs of infants in general and to the specific cues given by each individual infant. The predominant responsibility of the self-care agent in infancy is to meet the universal demands, health-deviation demands, and developmental demands of infancy.

In early childhood emphasis is on the universal demands for social interaction, safety, and food. Because life-style patterns are developing in this period, special attention to habit formation is important. Establishing positive health behaviors for good nutrition, regular exercise, and adequate rest and sleep is essential.

Between the ages of 2 and 5 years, self-care increases rapidly. Children can articulate the desire for food and feed and dress themselves with assistance. Bowel and bladder control are developing, and complete self-care is possible by $4\frac{1}{2}$ years of age. Meeting self-care demands for rest and activity is individualized. Some children lie down when they are tired, whereas other children need to be directed to do so.

The child in middle childhood exhibits a large measure of autonomy in most of the universal demands, but special consideration must be given in the area of safety. Exposure to substance abuse begins at the end of this period. The role and influence of the school increases. Lewis and Lewis (1980) reported that children at this age are able to initiate their own health care visits. Children whose parents emphasize self-care will cope with many health crises by themselves.

During late childhood and throughout adolescence, the predominant universal self-care demand is safety. Because of increased participation in athletics and greater exposure to the hazards of substance abuse, the older child and adolescent are at risk for injury or illness. Although able to understand safety concepts, children at these ages need support from parents to cope with the increasing demands of peer groups, which sometimes involve unsafe or unhealthy practices.

Other characteristics of the child that the nurse assesses include the child's level of cognitive development, temperament, respect for self, spiritual and moral development, and commitment to wellness concepts, as evidenced by the presence of positive health habits.

Characteristics of the Agent Assessment data relative to the agent include the (1) length of contact with the agent; (2) transmissability of the agent; and (3) potential effect of the agent on the child's wellness level. Examples of agents are microorganisms, stress, abusable substances, and diet.

Microorganism-caused diseases are dependent on many variables, with the disease's destructive potential and mode of transmission being related to the specific agent. The characteristics of the organism include its *infectivity*—a measurement of the organism's ability to survive and multiply in any given host; *pathogenicity*—the organism's ability to produce a standard clinical manifestation after infecting a host; *toxicity*—the ability of the organism to induce toxic clinical symptoms from its chemical breakdown; *virulence*—the severity of the clinical reaction once the disease has commenced; *invasiveness*—the measure of the extent of tissue penetration and distribution; and *antigenicity*—the ability of the organism to induce an immune response (Kolff and Sanchez, 1979).

The modes of transmission include (1) *contact*—either direct (body to body—for example, sexually transmitted diseases), indirect (touching contaminated objects or substances and transferring the infection from hand to mouth), or droplet (considered to be contact because infection spread occurs within 3 ft of a contaminated individual); (2) *airborne*—transfer of extremely small organisms under certain environmental conditions (for example, influenza); (3) *vehicle*—edible substances and biologic products (blood) that convey organisms to a susceptible host (for example, botulism, hepatitis); (4) *vector*—disease-carrying arthropods that infect the host by biting or by transferring organisms onto food or the skin (for example, Rocky Mountain spotted fever) (Kolff and Sanchez, 1979).

Other disease-causing agents, however, are entirely unrelated to organism transfer. Stress, as mentioned previously, can have an adverse effect on the body in that it breaches body defenses and contributes to disease. The action of stress alters physiologic processes, specifically neuroendocrine pathways and hormonal activity. It most likely alters the immune response, although the mechanism is still being studied.

Certain chemicals produce illness. For example, asbestos, used for many years in buildings, is a known carcinogen. The saccharin controversy emphasized the uncertainty regarding agents in food. The list of suspected cancer-causing agents grows longer each year, creating problems for local and national regulatory agencies.

Not only food additives but also the foods themselves can contribute to disease—both in kind and amount (see Chapter 15). A diet high in cholesterol or low in iron can lead to a high-risk situation. Too many calories results in obesity—a known risk factor in cardiac disease. When left between teeth, food promotes bacterial growth, leading to dental caries.

Abusable substances, such as alcohol, drugs, and cigarettes, also can affect the wellness level and the occurrence of disease in the child. Alcohol, considered for years to be a socially acceptable substance, has known effects on the brain, circulatory system, and other body organs. Overuse of this substance affects the thinking processes and coordination. For this reason, alcohol is particularly dangerous in conjunction with driving. Alcohol-related deaths, particularly in adolescents, have increased dramatically. Many states in the United States have raised the drinking age to 21 and imposed mandatory jail sentences for drunk driving. Children are exposed to alcohol at a young age, particularly if it is present in the home. Inadequate role modeling and other individual and environmental factors can lead to alcoholism in the young adult. The deleterious effects of alcohol on the fetus are beginning to be discovered.

Drug availability also has increased in the last 20 years. Substances such as marijuana, cocaine, amphetamines, and tranquilizers, among others, are commonly found in high schools. Drug use among elementary school students has increased. In addition to the detrimental effects these drugs have on physical performance, addictive behavior can affect all areas of children's lives, initiating a maladaptive cycle that is difficult to break.

Perhaps the most common, although no less dangerous, substance children are exposed to throughout their lives is cigarette smoke. Heavy smoking can contribute to many cardiovascular and respiratory diseases—lung cancer being one of the more serious. The effects of smoking are felt as early as in utero, resulting in smaller birthweight babies born to mothers who are heavy smokers. Children who themselves do not smoke can still exhibit respiratory problems from the amount of smoke in their environment. Fortunately, vigorous school health programs and public campaigns and the provision of non-smoking areas in public locations have cut down the influence of smoking on nonsmokers.

Finally, environmental allergens are agents that can lead to disease occurrence in susceptible children. See Chapter 37 for a discussion of allergens.

Characteristics of the Environment Assessment characteristics in the environment include geographic factors influencing disease occurrence, facilities in the home, emotional climate, air and water quality, education of parents, and socioeconomic status. Prevention of the following health hazards are included in the US Public Health Service recommendations for national goals and objectives for child health promotion: exposure to hazardous chemicals, radiation, and lead; inadequate waste disposal; unsafe water, foods, and drugs; and accidents (US Department of Health and Human Services, 1981a).

Exposure to hazardous chemicals and radiation are especially problematic during fetal development. Such chronic disorders as growth retardation, minimal brain damage, and altered immunologic response in very young children have been linked to exposure to noxious substances. Some public health experts attribute nearly all the major chronic diseases as well as some of the acute conditions such as poisoning, gastroenteritis, and seizures in the United States to exposure to hazardous substances. A serious aspect of exposure to hazardous substances in childhood is the delayed effect. Sometimes the problems are not evident for 20 years (US Department of Health and Human Services, 1981a).

The Panel on Promotion of Child Health (US Department of Health and Human Services, 1981a) reports that 45% of radiation exposure to the general public is through medical and dental care, whereas the remaining exposure to radioactive materials is in the air, soil, and water. This panel has recommended the creation of national standards to limit medical- and dental-related exposure of pregnant women and the medical-related exposure of children under 1 year of age.

Exposure to pesticides is a problem that extends from fetal life throughout adulthood. The hazard includes exposure to dangerous chemicals in food and water as well as those in the atmosphere from aerial spraying. In children the effects are more dangerous because of the proportionately low body weight per exposure as compared with adults.

This results in problems such as birth defects, stillbirths, infant mortality, and poisoning from contaminated breast milk.

Another environmental health hazard in children is exposure to lead (see Chapter 20). Elevated lead levels are associated with brain damage, poor school performance, and slow development. Both community and family efforts are necessary to combat this problem.

The issues surrounding the disposal of hazardous waste are embroiled in political and economic controversy. Health crises due to improper waste disposal have been reported in several states. One of the first major incidents, at Love Canal, New York, was discovered after the residents reported an unusually high incidence of spontaneous abortions and birth defects. Subsequent investigations resulted in the discovery of a chemical leakage from a waste disposal site. Citizen action and long periods of working with public and private agencies resulted in a solution. Numerous other sites around the United States are being identified, however, and the problems of who is primarily responsible and what to do remain unsolved.

Although difficult to measure, the effects of social and emotional factors on health status are receiving more attention. It is generally accepted that there is a connection between these factors and physical problems. In addition, the effects of physical illness on the emotional and behavioral aspects of living are becoming better understood.

Poverty and educational status also affect attitudes about health. Parents who are unable to pay for preventive care might not consider health maintenance visits a priority. Even the availability of health care facilities does not guarantee that they will be used. Historically, the poor have been crisis oriented toward health, using the emergency room as the primary source of health care. Health promotion and illness prevention have not been part of their life-style. Economically disadvantaged parents are reported to perceive their children's health as poor (US Department of Health and Human Services, 1981b).

Even for children who are above poverty levels, access to preventive health care is limited. Most third-party payments are made for the treatment of acute illnesses. Few insurance companies compensate for well-child visits, even under major medical coverage. The growth of health maintenance organizations is a partial answer to this problem, but these are not yet widespread enough to provide for the wellness needs of most families.

Results of a recent set of studies by the National Center for Health Services Research (US Department of Health and Human Services, 1981c) indicated that of the many environmental factors contributing to children's health, the mother's educational level was particularly significant as a health determinant. Children of mothers who had received more schooling tended to be healthier, particularly in the area of dental health. The factors influencing this appeared to include not only the development of positive health attitudes through the educational process but also that these mothers tended to encourage preventive health care. In addition, smaller families enabled parents to give more individual attention to the health needs of their children.

Conditions in the home contribute to the family's state of wellness. Emotional stability, spiritual and moral values, and positive relationships between family members reduce the level of stress. Physical aspects of the home environment are important in determining comfort and family safety as well as conditions conducive to disease transmission. The characteristics of the home to be assessed are as follows:

1. Age and type of the dwelling
2. Toilet and washing facilities
3. Provision of warmth and the type of heat
4. Humidification and insulation
5. Waste disposal
6. Home safety (see Chapter 19)
7. Adequate space for the number of family members
8. Presence of allergenic or adverse chemical substances
9. Room for privacy and play

Other important variables in the home environment involve cultural approaches to health care (see Chapter 3), positive childrearing practices, and adequate role modeling.

Interventions

After assessing the characteristics of the child, agent, and environment, nurses initiate strategies that alter negative health habits and promote wellness. Optimal health can be achieved through increased participation in the health care system (by consumer awareness) and in health education. If absent, certain health protection measures will be promoted.

Consumer Awareness Manufacturers of children's toys, cereal companies, and producers of television programs have recognized for years that children comprise a major portion of the consumer block. Clever advertising policies have encouraged children to demand products from parents, and competition among peers to possess these products adds fuel to an already large fire. Unfortunately, health consumerism has not kept pace with commercialism. Recognizing that children are consumers in their own right presents the challenge of how to use consumerism and marketing techniques to promote health. Children need to be taught from an early age that greater participation in the health care system as consumers will improve the health care delivery to society as a whole.

Consumer awareness includes the right to health, the means to health, and the marketing of health. Health is a natural state. Within the context of the wellness concept, everybody possesses a measure of health, regardless of the presence of a disability or an illness. Children do not think about their health because it is natural, it is given, it is expected, and that is as it should be. Individuals who do have a particular health problem are more likely to focus on their problem rather than on health in general. However, it is important for the individual to recognize that although health is a right and is natural, it is essential to make choices to maintain health and move toward optimal potential.

There are three areas to be considered in discussing health and consumer awareness. First, there is the individual's responsibility to exercise the right to health. Second, there is society's responsibility to promote and protect the health status of everyone. Third, there is the responsibility of the health care professional, especially nurses, to make services and information available to assist consumers to make choices that are best suited to their particular situation.

Individual Responsibility It is the individual's responsibility to make choices. A heightened awareness of one's personal health status might elevate health as a priority. Individual life-style is an important variable, which to a greater or lesser degree is affected by heredity, culture, income level, age, familial attitudes, personal beliefs, and educational level (see Chapters 3 and 4). Behavior reflects belief. For example, the adolescent who lists health as a priority but eats primarily at fast-food restaurants, smokes, and doesn't exercise is in reality placing a higher value on peer acceptance than on health. The actions of this individual contradict the stated belief.

Societal Responsibility What is society's responsibility for health promotion? The efforts of society must be aimed at health protection measures that allow the best possible environment for the individual to reach personal goals. For example, the individual has very little direct control over issues such as the disposal of hazardous waste, safe roads, protection against communicable disease, and unsafe drugs and food. It is the responsibility of the private and public sectors to meet their responsibilities through safe waste disposal, healthful work conditions, and the enforcement of health regulations.

The state of the economy is related to health and the quality of life. Funds for nutritional and well-child programs might be decreased during an economic crisis. Such changes can be instrumental in increasing the risk of morbidity and mortality.

Society has a responsibility to provide the possibility of choice. Risk-taking behavior is the right of the individual, but the options must be presented. The risk involved in smoking, for example, has been widely publicized, and most children and adolescents are aware of the hazards; therefore, smokers are acting at their own risk. A societal issue of risk to nonsmokers exposed to smoke is receiving increasing attention. More nonsmokers are questioning the rights of the individual to smoke versus the rights of nonsmokers who are subjected to this hazard.

Nursing Responsibility Health education as a vehicle for information and the availability of health services as support systems are the means through which the individual can make choices. Nurses can be instrumental in health education both as consumers and professionals by modeling positive health behaviors (Mullen, 1981).

The provision of health services is a means of promoting health to the consumer. Although economics is an issue in the utilization of health services, it is not always the major barrier. More often, the greater obstacle is lack of awareness of the concepts of wellness and health promotion on the part of the consumer. Important areas for nursing are assessment of knowledge deficits and education. Parents need to be taught and supported to best fulfill their role as the primary seeker of their child's health care. Attitudes and habits learned during childhood and seen practiced by the family are the ones more likely to be retained when the individual becomes independent.

Children and adolescents also require direct information that is appropriate to their level of understanding and relates to current concerns. There are times when they have specific questions that need to be answered, and the nurse is regarded as one who is knowledgeable and approachable. Generally, these children are oblivious of the concepts of wellness and health promotion and need to be "sold" on the idea that what one eats and how one lives does make a difference.

Active participation in the health care system is a goal for children to achieve to exercise their rights and responsibilities as health care consumers. Project PACT, a program developed by nurses at the University of Colorado, is a unique program that encourages children's participation in their health care. The purpose of the program is to increase children's abilities to communicate with health care professionals. Increased communication results in children's greater participation in their own care as well as health care that is individualized to the child's own needs. It promotes the attitude that children are in control of their own health and health care. In addition, children who use these communication skills from an early age become articulate adults who are able to be critical consumers, thus improving health care delivery to society as a whole. The program encourages children to do the following:

1. Ask questions.
2. Relay information about themselves.
3. Express the need for health instruction.
4. Cooperate with health professionals in decision making and constructing a health plan.
5. Clarify their own self-care responsibilities (Igoe, 1980).

Programs such as this, together with creative marketing techniques, will create conscientious and informed health consumers.

Marketing Health Promotion The concept of marketing health promotion involves the same elements as the nursing process: assessment, planning, action, and evaluation. Levi (1979) has suggested the following criteria for preventive action:

1. Evaluate the public health significance associated with the service and education to be provided.
2. Identify the level of public awareness.
3. Identify the modifier of the behavior or situation.
4. Delineate the cost factors.
5. Describe the population.
6. Assess the availability of a change agent.

Successful marketing depends on providing the consumers with the product or service they need. Therefore, consumers must be convinced that the information or service is appropriate in a personal way. Concerning children, it becomes apparent that efforts regarding nutrition, substance abuse, or life-style education must take into account that the child or even the family might not understand or accept the need for such programs or services. For example, young children cannot understand the need to eat nutritious foods or establish regular eating habits in childhood to avoid the threat of illness in middle age. They want to know what difference it will make in running the race, learning to read, or making a snowman. It is just as difficult for children to comprehend the cause-and-effect relationship between their current lack of exercise and the development of illnesses and disease in later life. Adolescents might be aware of the negative effects of the use of alcohol, tobacco, and drugs, but the priority at that age is usually acceptance by the peer group rather than future health. The selling of health thus is a major challenge.

The media has a subtle but powerful influence on the beliefs and attitudes of children. The most obvious health-related effects are through the advertising of foods and drugs and the aggressive, sometimes violent television programming. Other influences of television on children have been noted as follows:

1. *Messages by way of benign neglect*—Programming on health issues is presented solely from a germ theory or organic cause perspective. Individual choice or responsibility for prevention is not emphasized. The relationship between attitudes and beliefs and illness is neglected. The message might say that lack of exercise contributes to obesity but omit the individual responsibility to exercise or any guidelines about resources or types of exercises.
2. *Selective reporting*—Issues that are "newsworthy" tend to focus on the sensational as it relates to a select few such as artificial heart machines, cures for catastrophic illness, organ transplants, and the like. Of major importance to the promotion of health is the effect of life-style. Recently, there have been programs or reports on the benefits of physical fitness, diet, and stress reduction on health. But the reporting is on an adult level and shows the behavior changes being practiced by adults. The idea of modeling positive health behavior during early childhood receives little attention.
3. *Traditional roles for the health care professional*—Doctors, veterinarians, and psychologists continue to be highlighted in presentations about current developments in health. It is rare for nurses to be interviewed or nursing activities described. If the role of primary health promoter belongs to the nurse, nurses must become more visible as role models, as health educators, and as resources for information about ways to reach optimum health.

Television is a primary source of information in the American culture. It is reported to be the most influential source of information other than the parents. The average child spends 27 hours a week watching television. About 20% of the time consists of advertising (Samuels and Samuels, 1982). To date, several attempts have been made by both commercial and public television to air children's health programming. The efforts have been short-lived because they are not economically rewarding. The media has a profound effect on children. Because of their great capacity for fantasy and their inability to scrutinize the information, children can be victimized by television. Some programming, such as *Sesame Street* and *Electric Company*, provide children with good self-care health promotion attitudes. Segments on cleanliness, nutrition, and resting are effective. The "Slim Goodbody" segment on *Captain Kangaroo* is an excellent health promotion model for children. The violent, aggressive behavior that is prevalent on television is not a positive influence on children, although opinions differ regarding its long-lasting effects.

Because young children are hero worshippers, health segments are more effective if current heroes are incorporated. For example, children will respond better if "Mr. T" tells them something about nutrition than they will to the words of "The Incredible Edible Egg." Encouragement of critical television viewing for children and families is a major nursing responsibility.

The printed word, primarily magazines, and radio both influence children. The message in many songs and the words and actions of some public figures idolized by the young is to get "high" by using drugs, alcohol, and sex. One avenue for communicating the message of positive health behaviors to children is the public relations requirement of the Federal Communications Commission, which dictates that all stations must allow free public information programming. This obligatory time can be used for health promotion segments directed toward children.

Although individual efforts are important, the private and public sectors also must be involved in the marketing campaign for health promotion. Environmental goals can only be met by large groups coming together and working toward a common goal.

The criteria mentioned by Levi (1979) are appropriate for working through these more encompassing health issues. One question related to cost is whether the taxpayer will be receptive to the public's being responsible for these programs. There may be less resistance to the cost of clean air, safe food and water, and immunization programs because these would clearly benefit all persons. The question still remains, though, how much responsibility each individual has for the health and safety of the whole group. The increased participation in and encouragement of creative media marketing of health by nurses will positively influence children's consumer awareness.

Health Education—Factors Influencing Teaching Health to Children Children learn about health in many ways. Although the family is the primary teacher, the influence of peers, teachers, and media is significant. Nurses and other health care providers also are important references and affect health behaviors through education, service, and role modeling. The world of children includes direct and indirect contact with people, active and passive learning about health, and how to practice health behaviors.

Parents Parents are the first model for the child. Mullen (1981) cited research on beliefs about food and disease in children and showed ways in which parents are the source of information. Behaviors such as smoking and the use of alcohol are more prevalent in children whose parents also exhibit these behaviors. In a study of child-initiated health visits to the school nurse, patterns reflected parental attitudes and beliefs about health. The behavior pattern was internalized by 12 years of age (Lewis, 1980).

The family plays an important role in the health education of children; specifically the role is as follows:

1. To set the health-related goals and objectives for the family
2. To identify the behaviors and habits that are consistent with the family's beliefs and attitudes
3. To seek information and consultation appropriate to the family's needs

Peers The influence of the peer group begins when children interact with other children outside the family unit. As early as nursery school, the ideas expressed by a young companion are considered and added to the teachings of the parents. Getting along with and being accepted by peers is a major developmental task during childhood and adolescence. There are times when peer pressure might outweigh the influence of the family. It is during adolescence that the work of early health education reaches fruition. In a study of smoking behaviors among teenagers, the habits of their peer group, especially best friends, furnished the greatest incentive to smoke; parental examples were second. More information is needed on the role of the peer group in establishing positive health behaviors as well as how to counterbalance the negative influences of peer pressure.

Teachers Although the educational community is aware that it plays a role in health education and modeling positive health behaviors, these are not considered priority matters. With the increasing emphasis on science, mathematics and technology, curricula allocate cursory time to health and creative arts instruction. Despite the national objective of physical fitness for all children, physical education time might be nothing more than a glorified recess. Only 22 states in the United States certify secondary school teachers to teach health, and no state certifies elementary teachers in health education (Mullen, 1981). Recognition that health is a lifelong process and is not limited to physical well-being is not always evident in the schools. For many educators, the response to physical or emotional distress in a student is a trip to the school nurse.

Personal health beliefs are communicated by the educator as well as the parent. Demonstrating positive health attitudes and behaviors is effective even when a health course per se is not established. Teachers often need the resources supplied by the school nurse to assist children in managing and finding answers to their health concerns.

The role of the school in health education is as follows:

1. To supplement the parents' role as the primary health educator
2. To provide instruction based on the needs of children
3. To offer supportive health services
4. To maintain a safe and healthy environment

Nurses have a professional mandate to promote health and teach positive health behaviors. Changes in attitudes and orientation have been developing in all areas of the human services. The terms holistic and wellness are evidence of these changes; however, the practice of these concepts and principles is not widespread. There is some resistance to these changes in attitude and the locus of responsibility.

The primary role of the nurse is to assist the individual to promote, maintain, or restore health. The growing interest in holistic health and self-care affords nurses the opportunity to move into the forefront as health promoters. More research must be conducted on health promotion by nurses. Nurses need to become more visible in the media, teaching health and defining their role as health providers. Nursing activities such as speaking to parent groups, participating in career awareness programs, and counseling at health fairs will provide an avenue for defining roles.

Health Education—Techniques for Maintaining Health Nurses have the opportunity to provide health education throughout the life span. Education begins during the prenatal period as the nurse assists the pregnant woman to define parameters that will not only promote the good health of the fetus but also assist the woman with optimal postpartum recovery. Education continues throughout childhood to prepare the child for an adulthood of optimal wellness. Because nursing roles overlap during some developmental periods, nurses should recognize the danger that some important information might not get to the child. This problem can be corrected through adequate communication between health professionals and families.

Life is a process, and wellness is a continuum. Child health education requires an understanding of the development of both children and adults. Learning the skills to meet the goal of high-level wellness depends on the developmental stage of the individual. Table 18-2 illustrates the teaching strategies for children at various developmental stages.

Health education is directed toward staying healthy and preventing illness. When teaching children health promotion techniques, both general and specific concepts are discussed. The health behaviors that are described in the following sections are appropriate for all children. They include the techniques for meeting all the universal needs of humans as well as health promotion measures and primary and secondary prevention measures.

Basic Concepts Nurses and clients should understand the following concepts and the rationale for their inclusion in the action plan for each health promotion technique:

1. Establish the need for the behavior to sustain life.
2. Identify the specific purpose or function of each need that, when integrated into life-style, helps to form a whole and balanced person.
3. Each of the needs should fit into a natural order or progression.
4. Commit to a regular practice of positive health behavior that will yield the desired result.

Using proper diet as an example of the first concept, the child becomes aware of the need for food on more than an automatic response level and begins to consider eating behaviors that are commensurate with meeting the goal of wellness, that is, nutritional snacks, fruits instead of candy, and so forth.

The second concept involves identifying the specific role the need plays in achieving a balanced personal life. For example, understanding that food is needed to sustain the whole person's body–mind system helps the individual to develop habits consistent with meeting that goal.

Third, all of nature works in an orderly way. The concept of order is difficult for humans to accept as a working principle. Relative to food, each nutrient is utilized in an orderly way to meet specific biologic needs and according to a natural timetable. When committed to changing dietary behaviors, the client needs encouragement to sustain the behavior until the desired result becomes evident.

Objectives for School Health Programs

1. Continuing appraisal of each child's health status.
2. Understanding of each youngster's health needs.
3. Supervision and guidance of each child's health.
4. Development of the highest possible level of health for each child.
5. Prevention of defects and disorders.
6. Detection and referral of all defects and disorders.
7. Special health provisions for the exceptional child.
8. Reduction in the incidence of communicable diseases.
9. Positive health awareness and a desire for a high level of health in each child.
10. Development of wholesome health attitudes.
11. Development of healthful personal practices.
12. Acquisition of scientific and functional knowledge of personal and community health.
13. Development of an appreciation of aesthetic factors related to health.
14. Development of a high level of self-esteem in each child.
15. Effective social adjustment.
16. Hygienic mental environment at school.

SOURCE: Anderson CL, Creswell WH: *School Health Practice*. Mosby, 1980.

It probably is most difficult for the client to practice the behavior with sufficient regularity to ensure results. However, being committed to making the health behavior a regular part of the client's life is the only way that the goal can be achieved.

Specific Concepts

Nutrition Clients should understand the role nutrition plays in their lives as well as understanding why they eat and the function of food. Next, each client should choose the types of food that will promote optimal body, mental, and spiritual function. This includes the basic nutritional requirements for each person and specific dietary practices appropriate for individuals with special needs. Understanding the relationship between food and illness helps in making positive choices if avoiding illness is a priority. Young children get their attitudes about food from adults. Food is used negatively in our culture as a pacifier, a time filler, or as an incentive. These negative uses of food must be replaced by positive ones.

Children must be taught the basic uses of food, regardless of whether they have a food-related problem. For example, children who are obese first need to learn the

TABLE 18-2 Developmental Approach to Health Education

Age	Developmental characteristics	Learning styles	Teaching strategies
Infancy (birth to 18 months)	Dependency for meeting universal health care demands; beginning cognitive development, requires stimulation; expression of needs by crying, moving, and so forth; emotional—trust vs. mistrust; beginning development of coping mechanisms	Sensorimotor (Piaget); stimulation for adequate growth; preverbal	Help parent clarify roles; encourage bonding; assist parents to meet universal self-care demands and foster a nurturing environment; teach parents health care measures—importance of regular well-child checkups, immunizations, and environment modification
Early childhood (18 months to $4\frac{1}{2}$ years)	Tendency to demand; aggressive and protest behavior; fantasy and fears; focus on control of elimination; positive or negative attitudes learned from environment; self-protection decreased due to increased curiosity	Preconceptual; trial and error; use of fantasy and drama; short attention span requires varied presentation; needs repetition to learn	Teach parents importance of continuing immunization and well-child visits; continue environmental protection; teach cleanliness and safety by role modeling; encourage beginning responsibility for self-care—bathing, dressing, dental care; teach parents appropriate criteria for choosing child or day care; encourage positive self-image; coordinate teaching with periods of optimal wakefulness and attention; encourage regular rest periods
Middle childhood (5–8 years)	High activity level; increased emphasis on physical prowess; increasing intellectual development; increasing spiritual and moral development; emphasis on following rules; awareness of socially acceptable behavior; increasing identification with peers	Beginning to be a concrete thinker and problem solver; language skills improving; learns best by manipulating objects	Continue to emphasize well-child care; encourage participatory care and control over own health; teach rules of safety; encourage self-esteem by positive reinforcement; give clear, concise answers to questions regarding death and moral issues; explore values and how they relate to peers' values; encourage independence in meeting self-care demands; encourage parents to provide a wide variety of experiences and opportunities to solve problems; beginning education in areas of sex, substance abuse, and child abuse; allow for questions; use humor as a teaching tool to gain and keep affection
Late childhood (8–12 years)	Increasing awareness of causes of disease might lead to psychosomatic complaints; peer group important; need to achieve competence in school and sports; beginning exposure to abusable substances; increased self-direction (eg, will initiate visits to school nurse)	Concrete, with beginning development of abstract conceptual thought; problem-solving capability; well-developed language skills	Focus on safety principles; use influence of peer group to alter health behaviors; encourage parental support and continued role modeling; utilize the media to encourage positive health habits; health education in the schools to continue fostering positive health habits and prevent substance abuse; use problem situations and discussion groups to teach health concepts and grapple with moral issues

TABLE 18-2 continued

Age	Developmental characteristics	Learning styles	Teaching strategies
Adolescence	Physical maturation; peer pressure most influential; accidents increase, particularly automobile; substance abuse; sexual activity—can lead to pregnancy or venereal disease; focus on social rather than healthful aspects of living	Abstract; problem solving; future oriented	Emphasize enhancing self-esteem; identify and reinforce positive behaviors; utilize peer counseling and alter group rather than individual behaviors; minimize the negative

principles of a basic diet and then the specific dietary practices that are related to obesity. A child who is a diabetic should know the basic food combinations and then learn to modify the diet to meet the specific needs for that disability. In teaching a child about nutrition, modeling is the most important technique. The use of too many facts should be minimized. The desired outcomes are as follows:

1. To understand the relationship between food and the body
2. To develop a sense of excitement and adventure in learning about food
3. To begin to develop a personal responsibility for food selection, understanding the consequences of the food choices made (Frankel, 1980)

Specific nutritional techniques include regular meals, nutritious snacks spaced between meals and at least $1\frac{1}{2}$ hours before a regular meal, and beginning the day with a wholesome breakfast. Eating slowly and complete mastication increase enjoyment and promote effective digestion.

Parents must study their own dietary habits and needs and be aware of how they are being picked up by their children. They also need to be aware of the food intake of their children, especially in the school-age period when children are not home for each meal. Attention must be given to the school lunch program and after-school snacks and, in the case of working parents, breakfast for those children responsible for getting their own meal. Some unsupervised children eat food that can alter behavior and result in poor school performance. Being aware of the role specific foods play in special problems is important. Food plays a role in the following illnesses or maladaptive situations: dental problems, obesity and its sequelae, hyperactivity, allergies, and eating disorders.

Obesity According to Samuels and Samuels (1979), the following are specific techniques for helping children deal with obesity. Children should be encouraged to:

- Be aware of their food intake by keeping a daily log.
- Develop an internal control and sense of personal responsibility. Understand the consequences of what is eaten in terms of its effects on health.
- Decrease the possibility of negative food intake by eliminating or decreasing the amount of "junk" food in the house.
- Eat low-calorie snacks.
- Develop the habit of eating when hungry and eating only until satisfied. Eat slowly to allow for the appearance of satiety. Eat only while sitting at a table.
- Limit second helpings or make decisions about the kinds of food, thereby developing the internal control discussed above.
- Limit sedentary activity, such as watching television, because it might be a subliminal prompter to eat.
- Plan physical summertime activites and incorporate exercise in daily life all year round.

(See Chapter 24 for a further discussion of the psychosocial aspects of obesity.)

Dental Problems The prevention of dental disease related to food intake focuses on sugar intake. Decreasing the intake of sugar and removing the plaque buildup by proper brushing and flossing is primary dental prevention. It is not necessarily the amount of sugar consumed but the pattern of intake. For example, eating a large amount of sweets all at one time followed by proper dental hygiene is more effective in preventing cavities than eating small amounts without brushing. Encouraging schools and other public facilities to eliminate cavity-causing foods from vending machines is another prevention method.

The avoidance of foods that commonly predispose the child to develop tooth decay is recommended. In addition to eliminating sugar-based sweets, prime offenders include sugared cereals and white bread. Milk products should not be allowed to remain in the mouth without taking the appropriate dental hygienic measures because they stimulate bacterial growth, which leads to dental caries. For this reason, parents should be encouraged not to give the infant a bottle in bed (see Chapter 7). A diet high in calcium, phosphorus, and appropriate vitamins encourages the development of strong teeth. Oral fluoride preparations reduce the later incidence of tooth decay.

In addition to diet, individual self-care behaviors include brushing the teeth with fluoride toothpaste, using fluoride rinses, and taking advantage of routine dental care. Toothbrushing in early childhood helps the child begin good dental habits early in life. Because the early morning and evening routines might be hurried, children of working parents might need extra attention and reminders to brush their teeth.

Devices such as bathroom stools, special toothbrushes, and Water Piks® enable even small children to participate fully in their dental care. Routine dental prophylaxis is recommended throughout the life span.

Sleep Recognizing the effect of sleep on daily life is important. Children have regular sleep/wake cycles that are determined by the body's natural biorhythms. A regular bedtime and a rest schedule as close to the individual's biorhythms as possible will allow the body to rejuvenate. Children can be taught to become aware of their biorhythms and to rest and relax according to the cues they receive. Young children often follow rituals such as rocking themselves to sleep or having bedtime stories read to them around sleep time. The pleasure of having a story read, a soft cuddly animal, or a blanket should be respected. The environment for rest is important. The use of low music or night-lights can calm an upset child. Decreasing activity before sleep is helpful because many children need time to wind down.

Psychosocial factors affecting sleep include the quality of the relationship with the parents or siblings and fears. In the early childhood period, fears and separation anxiety are normal. Many children are afraid to go to sleep because they are afraid to be separated from their parents or afraid of "monsters." Sleep should not be used as a punishment. When a child is threatened with bed for disruptive behavior, a negative reason is given for a positive health behavior.

Sleeping with parents has many implications, the primary one being sleep disruption for both parent and child. The underlying causes of this behavior might vary from overdependency in the child to loneliness in the parent. Some children initiate the behavior as a way to seek comfort during a nightmare or to obtain warmth. Unfortunately, sleeping with parents can become habit forming and cause stress between parent and child or between parent and spouse. Each family needs to consider the needs of both parent and child when dealing with the behavior. The nurse needs to be alert for any unstated contributing factors such as single-parent loneliness, sexual rejection by a spouse, or limited space in poor families (see Chapters 8 and 13 for a more detailed approach to the problem).

Elimination Elimination is the body's natural mechanism for ridding itself of waste through perspiration, voiding, and defecation. Generally, bowel elimination is regular and need not be assisted by laxatives. The individual differences depend on rhythm, exercise patterns, and the kind of food eaten. Attitudes toward elimination are important. To ignore such issues as readiness and the development of sphincter control or to use fear and coercion during toilet training will affect the child's attitude about defecation in the future. Certain culturally laden ideas about cleanliness and elimination must be considered. Many children will hold their urine or bowel movement because they are unable to use a toilet outside their own home or at certain times of the day. They might have inaccurate ideas about unclean toilets and disease or embarrassment over odors.

Nurses need to encourage parents to approach toilet training in a calm, nonthreatening manner to encourage positive elimination habits in their children. Parents can assess readiness for toilet training and encourage regular elimination according to the child's own natural schedule (see Chapter 13). Children can be taught how to use public toilet seats properly to avoid direct contact with the seat itself.

Children of all ages should be encouraged to take the time for proper elimination and to be in tune with their bodies' needs. Adequate water and proper nutritional intake will help promote regular elimination.

Exercise The three major forms of exercise include aerobic exercises, which increase cardiovascular function, stretching exercises, which are important to muscle and bone structure, and body-building exercises, which are not essential. To derive the most benefit from exercise the person should include exercises from both the aerobic and stretching groups in any exercise routine. Exercise should be fun so that it is incorporated more easily into one's lifestyle. For some people, exercise is a competitive activity; however, the competition is secondary to the health benefits. Proper exercise must be regular, at least three to four times a week. The safety aspects of exercise are important, and supervision is essential. Warm-up and cool-down periods need to precede and follow any strenuous exercise.

Exercise programs in the schools should be carried over to the home on weekends and during the summer. These programs should be part of the routine family activities. Family walks, hiking trips, and swimming and running together are also beneficial family activities. Many activities can be either group or solitary. Jumping rope and basketball are activities that can be done alone or with a group and can be performed from childhood through adulthood.

There has been a rebirth in the interest in exercise and its role in health. Exercise is being used for everything from curing mental problems to alleviating physical maladies. Children are happy when they are in motion, and they move naturally. Adults, from presidents to sports figures, are models for children for the positive use of exercise. Children must be taught to extend exercise into adult life.

They should know that regular exercise will affect health positively by preventing heart disease, reducing blood pressure, controlling weight, and increasing lung capacity.

For children under 6 years of age, exercise is needed for agility and to improve coordination. Cooper (1968) suggested that children over 10 years of age use adult exercise schedules in such activities as running or swimming. Exercise should be incorporated into the child's regular daily routine to establish healthful habits that will carry over into adulthood.

One danger of exercise is overuse of the body, which can result in structural or functional injury. It is essential that children be provided with proper clothing and equipment, especially footwear, to prevent this occurrence. Stretching exercises and cool-down periods should be components of all aerobic workouts to minimize adverse effects.

"Life sports," such as swimming, tennis, and biking, should be encouraged at an early age. Unlike team sports, these aerobic activities are enjoyable throughout the life span and provide optimal health benefits.

Physical Care Clothing provides protection against exposure to extreme temperatures and foreign bodies. Clothing, to promote health, must be loose and clean. Attention must be given to the role of clothing in the development of self-esteem. The need to be part of the group is related to clothing fads and fashion. In adolescence clothing gives an opportunity to develop individuality. Many children have their own style of dress. They should be allowed to experiment with the kinds of clothes and colors they enjoy.

The purpose of bathing is to prevent or protect from disease and to enhance appearance. It is also excellent for relaxation. Young children do not need to bathe every day. Twice a week and as necessary to remove visible dirt is sufficient. The face and hands need frequent washing, as well as the diaper area in infants. Too much bathing or extremely hot water can deplete body moisture. For dry skin, oils need to be replaced. For safety, the use of oil in the bath water of very young children should be monitored to prevent slipping. Parents should be reminded to check the water level and water temperature and to supervise young children during bath time.

The notion of cleanliness as a preventive measure against disease is difficult for young children to understand. Handwashing can be taught as a habit before meals and after toileting and after handling animals. As children move into school, they will learn the facts related to the spread of disease and begin to take responsibility for preventing the transfer of disease.

Children can be taught that their bodies are necessary for living, and they can develop the concepts for maximum use of the physical self. Caring for the body through cleanliness, safety, and protection against abuse are part of the proper use of the body parts. For example, maximum eye

Health Maintenance Schedule

Nursing Activities	Ages
Assessments	2 weeks; 2, 4, 6, 9, 12, and 18 months; 2, 3, 5, 8, 11, 13, 15, and 17 years
Complete history and physical examination	First visit, interval history thereafter
Immunization (DTP, OPV, MMR, Td)	According to schedule
Rubella serology	Prepuberty (unvaccinated girls)
Tuberculin (tine) test	1, 3, 5, 11, and 15 years
Hemoglobin/hematocrit	1, 4, 9, 12, 14, and 16 years
Lead screening	2 years
Urinalysis	6 months; 2, 3, 4, 5, 6, 9–10, 11–12, 13–15, and 15–18 years
Urine culture	3 and 8 years
Blood pressure	4 years and at each subsequent visit
Vision/hearing	1, 4, and 6 months; 1, 3, and 6 years and at each subsequent visit
Language	2, 3, and 5 years
Dental	6, 7–8, 13–15, and 15–18 years
Scoliosis	9–10, 11–12, and 13–15 years
Counseling (nutrition, physical care, psychosocial concerns, sex education, safety, family interaction)	Each visit

National Environmental Health Objectives

1. Control of toxic agents responsible for cancer, birth defects, respiratory disease, kidney disease, and other chronic diseases.
2. Decrease in the prevalence of lead toxicity.
3. Eradication of exposure to toxic chemicals that cause birth defects and miscarriages.
4. Reduce the risk factors caused by toxic waste.
5. Increase air quality by emission control programs.
6. Protection of community water systems.
7. Safe toxic waste disposal for industrial residential waste.
8. Elimination of dangerous pesticides, fungicides, and herbicides known to be carcinogenic or mutagenic in humans.
9. Decrease in unnecessary diagnostic radiographs in medical and dental practice.

health requires attention to diet, safety, cleanliness, proper lights, and rest. For optimal body structure, correct posture, proper nutrition, adequate rest, and exercise are essential.

Respect for one's own body and the bodies of others is an important concept to be taught to children. Parents need to provide privacy for their children and encourage them to respect the privacy of others. Healthy respect for the self increases the child's feeling of importance and allows for appropriate relationships with others.

Immunization Guidelines

1. Live viruses should be administered at least 1 month apart if not given on the same day.
2. There should be intervals of 2–3 weeks to 1 month between the administration of an inactivated virus.
3. Live viruses and inactivated viruses can be given simultaneously at different sites or together orally.
4. Live viruses may be given in licensed combinations such as MR and MMR.
5. Killed viruses may be given simultaneously at different sites.
6. If immune serum globulin has been given, a minimum of 6 weeks must elapse before a live virus can be given. It is better to wait 3 months.
7. Vaccines associated with adverse local or systemic effects should not be given simultaneously, for example, typhoid and cholera.

SOURCE: Adapted from Center for Disease Control, 1983.

Provision of Health Services Child health care includes a well-child health maintenance schedule. A comprehensive health history encompasses both the present and past history. A family profile, the child's profile, a review of body systems, and a general care history (dietary, elimination, sleep and rest, and development) form the data base. The assessment includes objective data in the form of a physical examination, necessary laboratory studies, screening procedures, such as vision and auditory screening, and the plan of action based on the data collected, client's needs, and anticipatory guidance by the nurse.

Health Protection Health protection measures are directed toward both the general population and the individual. They prevent dental and infectious diseases as well as limit exposure to toxic agents, accidents, and injuries. Protection measures include fluoridation of water, immunizations, and other strategies that will achieve national environmental health objectives.

Fluoridation Fluoridation is a dental health protection measure. Its goal is to reduce the incidence of cavities in permanent teeth and to reduce gum disease. The use of fluoride in community water, in toothpastes and rinses, and fluoride supplements are current practices. Fluoride has been used in community and school water systems and has reduced cavities up to 90% in children (US Department of Health and Human Services, 1981a).

Immunization The goal of immunization is to prevent the occurrence of an infectious disease by introducing an antigen or an antibody (see Chapter 37). Immunization programs may be started on any well child who is 2 months of age and weighs more than 10 lb. The risks of immunization include potential side effects and complications, contamination of the serum with microorganisms other than the desired antigens, and worsening of a natural disease or failure to protect against the disease. Vaccinating a person whose resistance to infection is decreased or who is allergic to the vaccine could result in death. It is also possible that vaccination might postpone the natural infection until a time when it would be worse to contract the disease (Powell, 1977).

Immunizations have greatly reduced the worldwide incidence of diseases. Smallpox, for example, has been virtually eliminated as a result of vigorous immunization policies. Cases of poliomyelitis, rubella, and rubeola have decreased markedly since the development of vaccines against these diseases. Although recent publicity regarding the safety of the pertussis vaccine has aroused public concern, the benefits of the vaccine seem to outweigh the possible adverse consequences.

The national goals for immunization include adopting standard records, reviewing procedures to identify children needing immunization, and making the services available regardless of the ability of those needing immunization to pay (US Department of Health and Human Services, 1981).

Although the incidence of communicable disease has decreased as a result of a vigorous immunization effort, the US government is still concerned with keeping the numbers of immunized people at a high level. The success of the immunization program has contributed to public apathy in this regard. The Federal Immunization Initiative of 1977 still provides access to immunization for everyone, regardless of ability to pay (Richmond, Filher, 1979).

Nurses need to take responsibility for disseminating information about immunizations through the school curriculum, during health maintenance visits, and through day-care centers and other community forums. The Centers for Disease Control's recommendations for childhood immunizations are listed in Table 18-3.

Other Health Protection Measures Additional health protection measures include water supply protection through mechanisms such as chlorination, control of animals that carry diseases, and other public health policies such as pasteurization of milk.

Education is a powerful health protection strategy in dealing with infectious diseases. The educational process changes individual health habits and environmental practices. For example, individuals and groups must be educated about venereal diseases such as gonorrhea, syphilis, and herpes. Children and their parents need information about sexually transmitted diseases to reduce the risk of contracting them. School-age children should be educated and informed before and during the time of greatest risk of contracting sexually transmitted disease. Peer counselors are effective when working with adolescents. Mass training can be effective for health professionals and laymen. Health care professionals working in clinical settings and schools need training. Improved public awareness about sexually transmitted diseases and assurance of confidentiality, along with the help of the media, has made prevention and treatment more effective. In addition to school-age children and parents, according to the Public Health Service, target populations for education and treatment related to sexually transmitted diseases are parents, homosexual groups, and women with pelvic inflammatory diseases (Hacker, Palchik-Allen, Rosey, 1980). Secondary prevention requires early detection and treatment. Community control of prostitution and the discouragement of sexual promiscuity are other protection issues in need of community support

TABLE 18-3 Recommended Schedule for Active Immunization of Normal Infants and Children

Recommended age*	Vaccine(s)[†]	Comments
2 months	DTP-1[‡], OPV-1[§]	Can be given earlier in areas of high endemicity
4 months	DTP-2, OPV-2	6-week to 2-month interval desired between OPV doses to avoid interference
6 months	DTP-3	Additional dose of OPV at this time optional for use in areas with a high risk of polio exposure
15 months[¶]	MMR**	
18 months[¶]	DTP-4, OPV-3	Completion of primary series
4–6 years[††]	DTP-5, OPV-4	Preferably at or before school entry
14–16 years	Td[§§]	Repeat every 10 years throughout life

SOURCE: New immunization guidelines issued by the CDC. *Hosp Pract* (March) 1983; 18:1000

*These recommended ages should not be construed as absolute; that is, 2 months can be 6–10 weeks, etc.

[†]For all products used, consult manufacturer's package enclosure for instructions for storage, handling, and administration. Immunobiologics prepared by different manufacturers might vary, and those of the same manufacturer might change from time to time. The package insert should be followed for a specific product.

[‡]DTP—Diphtheria and tetanus toxoids and pertussis vaccine.

[§]OPV—Oral, attenuated poliovirus vaccine contains poliovirus types 1, 2, and 3.

[¶]Simultaneous administration of MMR, DTP, and OPV is appropriate for patients whose compliance with medical care recommendations cannot be assured.

**MMR—Live measles, mumps, and rubella viruses in a combined vaccine.

[††]Up to the seventh birthday.

[§§]Td—Adult tetanus toxoid and diphtheria toxoid in combination, which contains the same dose of tetanus toxoid as DTP or DT and a reduced dose of diphtheria toxoid.

Contraindications and Precautions Related to Immunization

1. Do not immunize a child with an active infectious disease or one who has a febrile illness, with the exception of the common cold.
2. Do not administer a live-virus vaccine to a child who has a malignancy and/or is on radiation therapy, is receiving an alkylating agent or an antimetabolite, or is immune-depressed naturally or artificially.
3. Do not immunize a person who had a previous allergic reaction to the vaccine or an individual who has received a blood product within the past 8 weeks.
4. A child in a family with a known member who has an immunologic problem should not be vaccinated or immunized without consultation with a physician.
5. Although a pregnant woman should not receive rubella vaccine, susceptible children living with a pregnant woman should be vaccinated.
6. Extreme caution should be exercised in giving vaccines that are grown on fibroblast tissue cultures of chickens and ducks (such as measles, mumps, or influenza vaccines) to children with known allergies to feathers, eggs, chickens, or ducks.
7. Vaccines containing antimicrobial agents are contraindicated in people who are sensitive to antimicrobial drugs.
8. The administration of DPT vaccine to children with known neurologic problems might be contraindicated.

SOURCE: Williams L: Childhood immunization. *Pediatr Nurs* (Jan/Feb) 1982; 8:18–22.

(Bereson, 1975). (See Chapter 39 for information about detection and treatment of sexually transmitted diseases.)

Environmental protection includes dispersing information to schools and the private sector. Additional public health education facilitates disease control through safer water and food, increased technology for water sterilization, water treatment systems, improved design of health care facilities (US Department of Health and Human Services, 1981).

Health education regarding toxic substances must occur on both individual and group levels. The problems of industrial and institutional disposal of waste, air control, and clean air associated with automobile emissions have implications for the private and public sectors. The individual has less control in this area but can be effective through political action and community action. Parents must be aware of the potential threat to the family's health from exposure to hazardous substances. Children can be taught by parents and through the school health curriculum to avoid vacant lots and abandoned buildings near industrial sites and also not to eat food or drink water from unsafe areas.

Secondary Prevention: The Nurse's Role

The event phase, or secondary level of prevention, involves factors that determine the extent of illness once it has occurred. The nurse's role involves assessing the characteristics of the child, agent, and environment and intervening to prevent the disease from becoming severe or being transmitted.

Assessment data obtained from the child, agent, and environment during the event phase are similar to the data obtained in the pre-event phase. If symptoms of illness are apparent, these indicate that the pre-event health promotion and protection strategies were ineffective. Nursing strategies during the event phase are directed toward screening measures to detect and arrest health deviations, isolation and control of communicable disease, prevention of infection, and prevention of complications.

Assessment

Characteristics of the Child As in the pre-event phase, assessment of the child includes determining such factors as psychosocial and emotional health, cognitive and developmental level, understanding of disease concepts and body functions, and self-care level. Physical bodily differences in children often determine the susceptibility to and extent of illness. For example, girls are more prone to develop urinary tract infections because their anatomic structure facilitates bacterial invasion. Individual responsibility for cleanliness and positive health habits can arrest the extent of disease. Children who are reliable about handwashing after toileting are less likely to develop or spread diseases related to hand-to-mouth contact. Those children who cover their mouths when coughing or sneezing and who properly dispose of tissues can limit the extent of droplet-spread organisms.

Characteristics of the Agent The nature of microorganisms and their modes of transmission affect disease occurrence and severity. (See "Pre-event assessment: Characteristics of the Agent" for an in-depth discussion of these agents.) The extent of illness also is affected by such factors as diet, stress, environmental chemicals such as lead, abusable substances, and allergens.

Because the event phase is determined by manifestations of illness, devices used to control the severity of a problem might be considered to be agents during this phase. For example, eyeglasses and hearing aids, although used to improve the functional quality of the senses, might actually be detrimental if not maintained properly.

Conservation of energy—sleep/rest—is an important variable in preventing complications of illness and as such becomes an agent during the event phase. Other treatment measures used to alleviate disease or restore health also are considered to be agents.

Characteristics of the Environment In addition to the previously mentioned environmental factors such as air and water quality, socioeconomic status, parents' educational level, and conditions in the home, the event phase also includes access to community resources and mechanisms for referral. Groups such as the Leukemia Society, the Arthritis Foundation, and the American Lung Association, to name a few, provide assistance to children and families. This assistance might take the form of actual financial aid for medical costs or of providing group and individual support. Efforts are directed toward minimizing disease consequences and disseminating information to increase public awareness. Nurses must assess the availability of community agencies and other supports to make appropriate referrals for illness intervention.

Interventions

Screening Although health screening certainly can be considered an aspect of child health promotion, specific screening procedures are performed to detect the presence of a deficit. Abnormal screening results indicate the need for intervention to prevent a further deficit. Screening is performed on a regular basis as part of the health maintenance schedule and as needed if problems are suspected.

Vision Complete vision screening includes tests for muscle coordination, ocular disorders, color vision, and visual acuity (Krajicek and Tomlinson, 1983). The indications for referral are presented in Table 18-4. Specific vision tests are described in detail in Chapters 14 and 43. Nursing strategies for limiting vision deficits include the following:

1. Encouraging children to wear eyeglasses if they are prescribed
2. Teaching children to avoid eye strain by using proper light when reading
3. Encouraging the use of protective glasses when working with power tools or caustic chemicals
4. Teaching children not to rub their eyes, particularly when their eyes come in contact with a foreign object
5. Recommending plastic lenses for children who participate actively in sports
6. Teaching the proper care of contact lenses

Auditory Routine auditory screening is performed during infancy and childhood. Special considerations that warrant auditory screening of infants are as follows:

1. Family history of a childhood hearing deficit
2. Congenital perinatal infection such as cytomegalovirus or rubella
3. Anatomic malformations of the head and neck
4. Birthweight less than 1500 g
5. Hyperbilirubinemia at a level requiring an exchange transfusion
6. Meningitis
7. Severe asphyxia, including birth hypoxia (Krajicek and Tomlinson, 1983)

Special indications for auditory screening during childhood include the following:

1. Children with a history of frequent episodes of otitis media
2. Inattention in the classroom
3. Apparent hearing difficulties in the home environment

Table 18-5 lists the auditory screening tests and referral indications. Detailed descriptions of the tests are found in Chapters 14 and 43. Interventions directed toward limiting hearing deficits are as follows:

1. Encourage prompt treatment of an otitis episode
2. Teach proper ear care, including cleaning and the removal of cerumen
3. Discourage loud radio, stereo, or television volumes

TABLE 18-4 Vision Screening

Test	Age	Nursing implications
Direct observation for ocular pathology	All	Refer to physician if signs of Inflammation; strabismus; opacities; foreign bodies
Visual acuity tests Snellen; Allen/picture cards "E" Game	Early to middle childhood and older	Refer for further testing children 3 years if greater than 20/50; 4 years if greater than 20/40; 5 years and over, if greater than 20/30
Cover test	Older children able to fixate	Refer for evidence of strabismus
Corneal light reflex	Infants and younger children	Refer for evidence of strabismus
Hardy-Rand-Ritter; Ishihara	Late childhood	No referral for color blindness but parents and teachers need to be aware of the problem.

SOURCE: Data from Sprague (1983) and Wold (1981).

TABLE 18-5 Auditory Screening

Test	Age	Nursing implications
Reflex elicitation	Birth to 3 months	Refer if reflexes absent in response to sound
Hearing and communication questionnaire	Birth to 12 months	No referral needed if parents report child's response to their vocalizations
Crib-O-Gram	Newborn	No response to stimulus of 90 db peaking at 3000 Hz indicates failure
Tympanometry	6 months and older	Refer if there is abnormal middle ear pressure and absent acoustic reflex
Pure tone audiometry	3–5 years	Failure of child to respond to any one frequency (1000, 2000, 4000 Hz) at 25 dB indicates referral
Audiometry	Older than 5 years	Failure at any frequency indicates referral

SOURCE: Data from Downs (1983) and Wold (1981).

4. Teach children not to insert objects into their ears, especially cotton-tipped swabs

Tuberculosis Although the incidence of tuberculosis has decreased dramatically since the midtwentieth century, children, particularly those from foreign countries where the disease is still endemic, are susceptible. Tuberculosis is spread by droplets, and the incidence increases in overcrowded environments. The most common tuberculosis skin test is the tine test, which is administered at approximately 1 year of age and every several years throughout childhood. A positive tine test (2 mm of induration) warrants rescreening with purified protein derivative (PPD). Positive PPD necessitates a more comprehensive diagnostic workup, including a chest radiograph and sputum examinations. It must be remembered that children who have been immunized against tuberculosis with thė Bacille Calmette Guérin (BCG) vaccine will demonstrate a positive PPD (Kolff and Sanchez, 1979).

Lead Sources of lead in the environment vary from lead paint to the atmosphere (see Chapter 20). Lead screening is routine during early childhood because children in this age group characteristically use their mouths to explore their surroundings. The screening procedure involves a fingerstick capillary blood sample, which is tested for lead and erythrocyte protoporphyrin. The normal lead level is below 29 μg/dL (micrograms per 100 mL of whole blood). Acceptable erythrocyte protoporphyrin levels are below 49 μg/dL (Commonwealth of Massachusetts, 1983). Nurses need to encourage parents to keep children away from lead-based house paint, painted antique furniture and toys, and improperly baked earthenware—all sources of lead. Children exhibiting signs of pica (see Chapter 20) should be referred for special care.

Anemia Lowered hemoglobin and hematocrit levels indicate iron deficiency anemia (see Chapter 36). A capillary blood sample reveals the following abnormal values (American Academy of Pediatrics, 1977):

Hemoglobin	6 months to 10 years	Lower than 11 g/dL
	10 to 14 years	Lower than 12 g/dL
	Over 14 years (male)	Lower than 13 g/dL
	Over 14 years (female)	Lower than 12 g/dL
Hematocrit	6 months to 10 years	Lower than 34%
	10 to 14 years	Lower than 37%
	Over 14 years (male)	Lower than 41%
	Over 14 years (female)	Lower than 37%

Interventions are based on teaching proper dietary practices to increase iron consumption. Encouraging compliance with taking prescribed medication is an important nursing strategy.

Scoliosis Posture screening is important for all children, but particularly for preadolescent and adolescent girls. The causes of scoliosis are varied, but if unchecked, scoliosis can lead to visible structural and functional deformities (see Chapter 41). Observation of the child includes visual inspection of frontal and dorsal posture. The nurse checks for uneven hip and shoulder levels as well as for muscular disproportion. In addition to the standing posture, the child should be seen while bending loosely from the waist as if to touch the toes. Again, visible curvatures or uneven muscular development are noted. Because poor posture is a contributing factor in scoliosis, nurses should encourage proper posture and body mechanics in children. Schoolbooks or heavy objects should be carried in a backpack rather than on either hip.

Control of Communicable Disease Nursing strategies in controlling communicable diseases are directed toward containing the illness and preventing complications. Droplet-spread illnesses, such as colds, can be contained by teaching the child and family proper hygienic measures and disposal of contaminated articles. Children from an early age can be taught to cover their mouths while coughing or sneezing. Tissues that have been contaminated with nasal discharge should not be left where other family members can come in contact with them. Children should be encouraged to wash their hands frequently, and particularly after coughing. Strict isolation is not necessary, although close contact with other family members can and should be discouraged. Young children in particular need constant reminders to prevent droplet spread.

Personal and environmental cleanliness is an important deterrent to contact diseases. Examples of contact conditions are impetigo, pediculosis, fungal and parasitic infections, and sexually transmitted diseases (see Chapters 26 and 39). Children should be advised to wash their hands thoroughly after elimination and not to share articles of clothing, particularly hats and underwear. Children must be reminded continuously to develop these habits because they often feel there is too little time for such practices. In their enthusiasm they may swap baseball hats or combs, leading to the rapid spread of lice. Simple explanations of the dangers inherent in such actions will help establish positive behaviors.

Prevention of Infection and Its Complications Measures taken during the event phase will decrease the potential for disability resulting from unchecked illness. Simple prevention measures such as thorough cleaning of wounds and the application of antibacterial ointments will decrease the incidence of skin infection (see Chapter 44).

When children sustain abrasions, parents are usually informed and institute appropriate action. Nurses might need to make parents aware, however, that often the older child is too busy to stop playing to have an injury attended to. Untreated wounds might be noticed days later when the child complains of pain in the area. Nurses need to encourage parents to be observant of their children's physical state. Prompt and adequate treatment of illness and injury will prevent the appearance of more serious complications.

Key Concepts

- Children can make positive health behaviors an integral part of their lives with the help of the nurse.
- Respect for individuals and their heritage, along with choices to attain one's physical, mental, and spiritual potential, provide a holistic concept of wellness.
- The concept of health is viewed in relation to the wellness–illness continuum.
- The health status of children has improved due to a shift in emphasis from prevention, control, and the cure of infectious diseases to an internal locus of control over all aspects of health.
- Health promotion and health protection strategies are directed toward the goal of illness prevention.
- Levels of illness prevention are primary, secondary, and tertiary, corresponding to factors that prevent the occurrence of an illness, reduce its severity, and limit complications.
- Data for nursing assessment and diagnosis arise from the examination of the characteristics inherent in the child, the agent, and the environment at all levels of prevention.
- Characteristics of the child include prenatal and hereditary factors, cognitive and developmental level, emotional state, understanding of wellness concepts, and health habits.
- Characteristics of the agent encompass the nature and action of organisms and the effects of stress, toxic chemicals, abusable substances, and diet on the child.
- Important environmental factors include air and water quality, socioeconomic status, education of parents, and conditions in the home.
- Nursing strategies for health promotion in children are directed toward increasing consumer awareness and health education.
- Children as health consumers assume control over and responsibility for their own health status.
- Influential factors for successful health education of the child are the parents, peers, teachers, and health professionals.
- Health education encompasses techniques for staying healthy and for reducing the severity and spread of illness.
- Health education is geared toward the developmental characteristics and age-related learning styles of children.

- Techniques are effective in specialized areas of nutrition, obesity, dental problems, sleep, elimination, exercise, and physical care.
- Adequate health maintenance requires regular health promotion and well-child monitoring.
- Health protection measures include fluoridation of the water supply, immunization, pasteurization, and other public health policies directed toward environmental protection and the control of communicable disease.
- Health education is a powerful health protection strategy.
- Nursing interventions to reduce the severity of a child's deficit include visual, auditory, lead, anemia, tuberculosis, and scoliosis screenings.
- Nursing strategies for illness control encompass teaching an awareness of disease transmission and actions children can take to counteract communicability.
- The complications resulting from an illness can be reduced by prompt and adequate treatment and referral to appropriate community agencies.

References

American Academy of Pediatrics: *School Health: A Guide for Health Professionals*. Appendix G. American Academy of Pediatrics, 1977.

Commonwealth of Massachusetts: *Childhood Lead Poisoning Prevention Program*. Commonwealth of Massachusetts Department of Public Health, 1983.

Cooper K: *Aerobics*. M. Evans and Co., 1968.

Dagg N: Primary prevention: Health promotion and specific protection. In: *School Nursing*. Wold S (editor). Mosby, 1981.

Downs M: Early identification and intervention for auditory problems. In: *Detection of Developmental Problems in Children*. Krajicek M, Tomlinson A (editors). University Park Press, 1983.

Frankle R: It's never too early for nutrition education. *School Health* (Sept) 1980; 50(7):387–391.

Goldberg P: *Executive Health*. McGraw-Hill, 1978.

Hacker S, Palchik-Allen N, Rosey C: Factors influencing the success of a community VD program held in a university facility. *Public Health Rep* (May/June) 1980; 95:247–252.

Heisel JS, et al: The significance of life events as contributing factors in the diseases of children. *J Pediatr* 1973; 83(1):119–123.

Igoe J: Project health PACT in action. *Am J. Nurs* (Nov) 1980; 80:2016–2021.

Johnson J: More about stress and some management techniques. *J School Health* (Jan) 1981; 51:36–42.

Kolff C, Sanchez R: *Infectious Disease Management*. Addison-Wesley, 1979.

Krajicek M, Tomlinson A (editors): *Detection of Developmental Problems in Children*. University Park Press, 1983.

Levi L: Psychosocial factors in preventive medicine. In: *Healthy People: The Surgeon General's Report on Health Promotion and Disease Prevention*. US Department of Health and Human Services. PHS Publication No. 79-55071A. US Government Printing Office, 1979.

Lewis CE, Lewis M: Child-initiated health care. *J School Health* (March) 1980; 50:144–148.

Mattson PH: *Holistic Health in Perspective*. Mayfield, 1982.

McKay R, Segall M: Methods and models for the aggregate. *Nurs Outlook* (Nov/Dec) 1983; 31(6):328–334.

Mullen PD: Behavioral aspects of maternal and child health; natural influences and educational intervention. In: *Better Health For Our Children: A National Strategy*. Vol IV. *Background Papers*. US Department of Health and Human Services. US Government Printing Office, 1981.

New immunization guidelines issued by the CDC. *Hosp Pract* 1983; 18(3):100a–100h.

Orem DE: *Nursing: Concepts of Practice*. McGraw-Hill, 1980.

Powell KR: Basic principles of immunization. *Pediatr Nurs* (Sept/Oct) 1977; 3:7–11.

Read D: *The Concept of Health*. Holbrook Press, 1973.

Richmond J, Filner B: Infant and child health needs and strategies. In: *Healthy People: The Surgeon General's Report on Health Promotion and Disease Prevention*. US Department of Health and Human Services, PHS Publication No. 79-55071A. US Government Printing Office, 1979.

Rivara F: Epidemiology of childhood injuries. *Am J Dis Child* 1982; 136:399–405.

Samuels M, Samuels N: *The Well Child Book*. Summit Books, 1979.

Samuels M, Samuels N: *The Well Baby Book*. Summit Books, 1982.

Smith M, Selye H: Stress. *Am J Nurs* (Nov) 1979; 79:1953–1964.

Sprague, J: Vision screening. In: *Detection of Developmental Problems in Children*. Krajicek M, Tomlinson A (editors). University Park Press, 1983.

US Department of Health and Human Services: *Better Health for Our Children: A National Strategy* Vol 1. *Major Findings and Recommendations*. US Government Printing Office, 1981a.

US Department of Health and Human Services. *Better Health For Our Children: A National Survey*. Vol III. *A Statistical Profile*. US Government Printing Office, 1981b.

US Department of Health and Human Services. *Determinants of Children's Health*. NCHSR Research Summary Series. National Center for Health Services Research, 1981c.

Williams P: Children's concepts of illness and internal body parts. *Matern Child Nurs J* (Summer) 1979; 8(2):115–123.

Wood S: School-aged children's perceptions of the causes of illness. *Pediatr Nurs* (March/April) 1983; 9:101–104.

Wold SJ: *School Nursing: A Framework for Practice*. Mosby, 1981.

Additional Readings

Anderson CL, Creswell WH: *School Health Practice*. Mosby, 1980.

Bauman E, et al (editors): *The Holistic Health Lifebook*. And/Or Press, 1981.

Blattner B: *Holistic Nursing*. Prentice-Hall, 1981.

Chow MP, Durand BA, Feldman MN (editors): *Handbook of Pediatric Primary Care.* Wiley, 1979.

Clark CC: *Enhancing Wellness: A Guide to Self Care.* Springer, 1981.

Coates T: Adolescence: The transition years. *J School Health* (May) 1982; 52:293–294.

Cormier JF, Trammel H: Fighting tooth decay: The fluoride plan. *Pediatr Nurs* (May/June) 1979; 5:18–26.

Dwyer J: Nutrition education and information. In: *Better Health for Our Children: A National Strategy.* Vol IV. *Background Papers.* US Department of Health and Human Services. US Government Printing Office, 1981.

Eichelber KM, et al: Self-care nursing plan. Help children to help themselves. *Pediatr Nurs* (May/June) 1980; 6:9–13.

Ferguson T: *Medical Self-Care: Access to Health Tools.* Summit Books, 1980.

Foster PC, Janssens NP: Dorothea E. Orem. In: *Nursing Theories: The Base for Professional Nursing Process.* George JB (Editor). Prentice-Hall, 1980.

Grever E: A health screening project for children in preschool programs. *Pediatr Nurs* (Sept/Oct) 1976; 2:16–22.

Hollander A: *How To Help Your Child Have A Spiritual Life.* Bantam Books, 1980.

Jessor R: Problem behavior and developmental transition in adolescence. *J School Health* (May) 1982; 52:295–300.

Johnson JW: More about stress and some management techniques. *J School Health* (Jan) 1981; 51:36–42.

Joy WB: *Joy's Way, A Map for the Transformation Journey.* Houghton Mifflin, 1979.

Kilmon C, Helpin M: Update on dentistry for children. *Pediatr Nurs* (Sept/Oct) 1981; 7:41–6.

Levin LS, Katz AH, Holst E: *Self-Care: Lay Initiatives in Health.* Prodist, 1979.

Liebow P: The new-look school nurse. *Psychosocial Nurs* (March) 1984; 22(3):37–41.

Lorenz KY, et al: Toward a conceptual formulation of health and well-being. In: *Strategies for Public Health: Promoting Health and Preventing Disease.* Lorenz KY, Davis DL (editors). Van Nostrand, 1980.

Marks A: Health screening of the adolescent. *Pediatr Nurs* (July/Aug) 1978; 4:37–42.

McCrown D: TV: Its problems for children. *Pediatr Nurs* (March/April) 1979; 5:17–24.

Murray R, Zentner J: *Nursing Assessment and Health Promotion Through the Life Span.* Prentice-Hall, 1979.

Murray R, et al: *Nursing Concepts for Health Promotion.* Prentice-Hall, 1975.

Perry CL, Murray DM: Enhancing the transition years: The challenge of adolescent health promotion. *J School Health* (May) 1982; 52:307–311.

Pilch JJ: *Wellness: Your Invitation to Full Life.* Winston Press, 1970.

Pontious SL: Practical Piaget: Helping children understand. *Am J Nurs* (Jan) 1982; 82:114–117.

Redman BK: *The Process of Patient Teaching in Nursing.* Mosby, 1976.

Rhodes RL, et al: *Elementary School Health, Education and Service.* Allyn and Bacon, 1981.

Rozman D: *Meditation for Children.* University of the Trees Press, 1976.

Ryan RS, Travis JW: *The Wellness Workbook.* Ten Speed Press, 1981.

Selekman J: Immunization: What's it all about. *Am J Nurs* (Aug) 1980; 80:1440–1445.

Selye H: *The Stress of Life.* McGraw-Hill, 1976.

Selye H: Stress and the promotion of health. In: *Strategies for Public Health: Promoting Health and Preventing Disease.* Lorenz KY, Davies DL (editors). Van Nostrand, 1980.

Siemon M: Mental health in school-aged children. *Matern Child Nurs* (July/Aug) 1978; 211:217.

Taubenhaus L, Jackson A: *Vision Screening of Preschool Children.* Thomas, 1969.

Thomas RM: *Comparing Theories of Child Development.* Wadsworth, 1979.

US Department of Health and Human Services: *Promoting Health/Preventing Disease: Objectives for the Nation.* US Government Printing Office, 1980.

Vipperman JF, Rager PM: Childhood coping: How nurses can help. *Pediatr Nurs* (March/April) 1980; 6:11–18.

Watts P: The whole person concept as a part of the elementary school health education program. *J School Health* (May) 1982; 286:90

Williams L: Childhood immunizations. *Pediatr Nurs* (Jan/Feb) 1982; 8:18–22.

Prevention of Injury

Judith A. Surveyer Susan Rowen James Michelle Burns

19

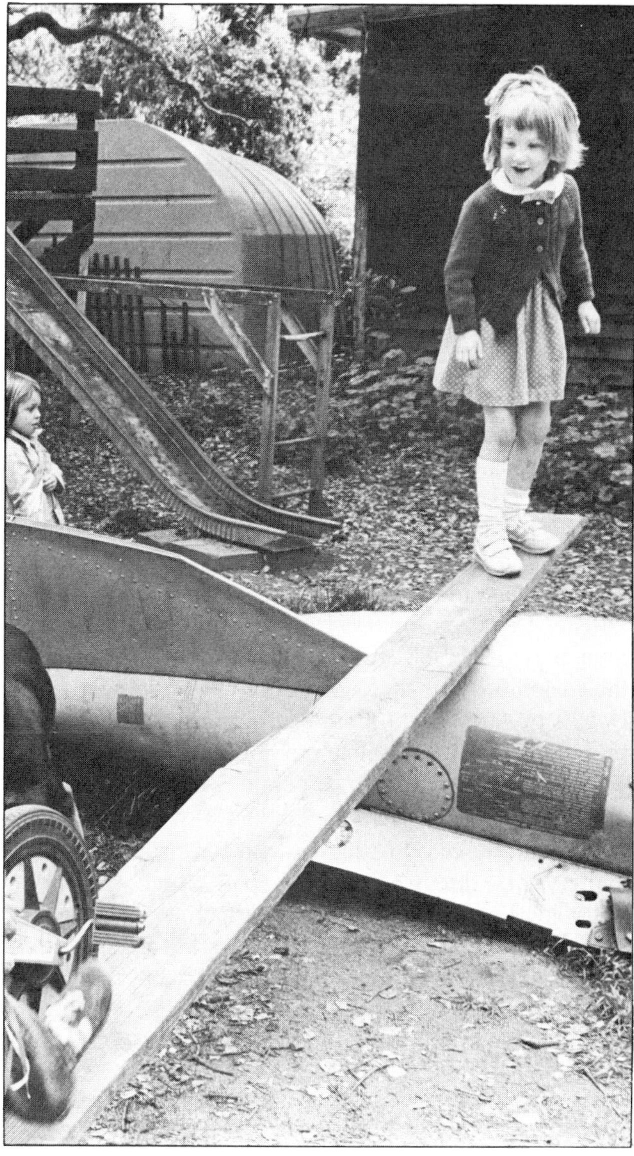

Chapter Outline

Objectives

- Describe the nursing strategies for injury prevention using an epidemiologic framework.
- List the characteristics of children that predispose them to injury.
- Delineate the various vectors of energy transfer and their relationship to childhood injury.
- Identify the environmental characteristics that contribute to childhood accidents.
- Relate the developmental characteristics of children to injury prevention strategies.
- List the components of a safe play area.
- Describe safety hazards in the home and environment and the prevention strategies to alter them.
- Describe safety education as it applies to specific injury prevention.
- List the assessment criteria and nursing interventions to reduce the severity of an injury.

Injuries are the single most important cause of childhood disease, disability, and death (Rivara, 1982). In fact, injuries are the leading cause of death among all persons between 1 and 38 years of age (Halperin, et al., 1983). Motor vehicle accidents nearly equal the total number of other fatal accidents in children 1–14 years of age. Motor vehicle accidents are the leading cause of death in the 14- to 24-year-old age group (US Department of Health and Human Services, 1983). Burns and drownings account for the majority of other deaths related to accidental injury. Deaths by any one of these causes can be prevented by proper education and safety promotion strategies. Routine well-child care should incorporate safety education at every level.

The nursing care of children who have suffered severe injury will be discussed in the chapter on the appropriate physiologic concept. For instance, treatment of burns will be presented in Chapter 44, whereas fractures and cast care will be discussed in Chapter 41. In this chapter we address the vital topic of *injury prevention*. The special concerns of poison prevention and treatment deserve special coverage and are discussed in Chapter 20.

An Epidemiologic Approach to Injury Prevention

One authority has stated, "An injury is no accident" (Doege, 1978). Everyone considers a fall from a tree, an automobile collision, or choking on a piece of food—and the injuries these cause—as "accidents," and so they are in the sense of not being intended. Injuries are not accidents, however, in the sense of being completely random occurrences. There are predisposing factors that contribute to both the actual event of an injury and to the severity of the physical consequences of the event. Manipulating these factors at the primary or secondary levels of prevention can help to prevent accidents or lessen the injuries they cause. To understand these factors, an epidemiologic framework is useful, which groups these factors into (1) characteristics of the host; (2) characteristics of the agent; and (3) characteristics of the environment.

Characteristics of the Child

As in the epidemiology of illness, the *host* is defined as the child. Many characteristics of the child can influence the incidence, type, and severity of injury. These characteristics include age or developmental stage, sex, locomotor skill, activity level, cognitive ability, and peer influence, among others. The influence of age, for example, has been suggested by research that examined the different kinds of injuries most often suffered by children in different age groups. Whereas preschool children are most likely to be injured from poisonings, burns, and home injuries, older children are at greater risk of drownings, sports injuries, and motor vehicle collisions (Rivara, 1982).

Characteristics of the Agent

The *agent* in an epidemiologic approach to injuries is not a microbe, as it would be in many illnesses, but a vector of energy transfer (Rivara, 1982). Most injuries involve some kind of energy transfer, whether mechanical energy, such as in a fall, car collision, or bullet wound; chemical energy, such as in a plant poisoning; thermal energy, such as in a burn or scalding; or electrical energy, such as in a shock or fire resulting from bad wiring. The agents in these cases would be the vectors of these energy transfers such as the tree from which the child falls, the gun, the plant, and the hot water heater. Just like microbes, these agents are ever present in the environment, and their complete elimination is not often possible. Being aware of how individuals interact with these agents and adjusting behavior appropriately are the strategies by which safety can be promoted and injury avoided.

Characteristics of the Environment

The elements of the environment that can affect the occurrence and severity of injuries can be divided into physical and sociocultural aspects. Physical aspects include such factors as how the home is arranged and whether the child is protected from potential hazards; the conditions on public streets and whether they present unusual dangers to pedestrians; and the design, maintenance, and supervision of child and youth recreation areas—playgrounds, swimming pools, schoolyards, and the like. Sociocultural factors of the environment also can affect child safety. Poverty, parenting style, family stress, the cultural emphasis placed on the values of aggression and competition, and governmental interventions, such as the 55 mph speed limit, have all been studied with regard to their effects on the frequency and severity of injuries.

The nurse's role in injury prevention requires accurate data collection at both the primary and secondary levels. The modification of factors that prevent or alter the severity of injury can only occur after thorough assessment and identification of nursing diagnoses. Nursing interventions are directed toward the individual and society, and the goal is to alter the factors that lead to an injury, either from a promotional or protective approach. For example, safety education promotes recognition of dangerous practices by the child or persons within the environment. Protection includes legislation that alters agents and the environment for the benefit of society as a whole. Both safety promotion and injury protection measures can reduce the incidence of accidental injury.

Primary Prevention: The Nurse's Role

Assessment of the Child's Characteristics

Assessment of the child involves identifying those characteristics that might lead to injury. Along with age, many other variables play an important role in determining the incidence of accidents and the type of injury that occurs. "Accident proneness" is a catch phrase formerly used to categorize those children who had repeated accidents. Studies have indicated that there is no definitive evidence that any one group is at risk for repeated accidents because of other psychogenic phenomena such as unresolved guilt (Rivara, 1982). Certain characteristics, however, might predispose a child to being an accident risk.

Curiosity Curiosity is a natural motivator for children as their senses develop. Children learn from their senses of touch, taste, sight, hearing, and smell as they explore the playground of new experiences outside their cribs. Parents must allow and encourage young children to learn while providing for their safety. Parents of an adventurous child must be even more vigilant. Children whose environment is unlimited often can find themselves in danger.

Whereas some children are adventuresome, and this spirit of adventure gets them into difficulties, other children need limits to feel secure in their environment. An environment that allows limitless freedom for exploration might result in an insecure child who takes extra risks as an attention-getting mechanism. This "stop me" behavior, although not conscious, by its very nature can lead to injury. Testing parental limits is something children do to validate parental caring. Without this validation, children will continue their attempts, sometimes finding themselves in situations beyond their control. For example, 3-year-old Bobby was allowed to roam the neighborhood at will. Eventually, he wandered out of his familiar surroundings and was seen by a family friend playing near a new house foundation. Fortunately, the friend recognized Bobby and brought him home before anything happened to him, but the injury potential was high as a result of the child's wandering out of his familiar environment.

Developmental Stage Injury risk also is determined in great part by developmental stage—physical, cognitive, affective, and social. Two-year-olds, for example, who are in a negativistic period might refuse to obey parental requests or might engage in activities their parents forbid. Rebelliousness in adolescents is similar to 2-year-old negativism in that adolescents also tend to go against parental or societal prohibitions. Adolescents also are more prone to substance abuse, and alcohol and drugs have been implicated in at least 50% of motor vehicle accidents today (Halperin, et al., 1983). Drugs and alcohol also have been implicated in other common accidents of adolescence such as drowning.

Discrepancies between the developmental skill level and ability to manipulate toys results in injuries. Children try to operate playthings that are inappropriate for their level of motor skill development (Rivara, 1982). Table 19-1 lists further developmental characteristics that predispose a child to injury.

Gender Gender is a determinant of injury incidence. Boys appear to have more accidents than girls. According to Rivara (1982), this is probably due to behavioral differences. For example, boys might take greater risks in their play activities, climbing higher, riding faster, and performing complicated moves on bicycles and skateboards. Aggressive behavior, although certainly not exclusive to boys, is a proven injury risk factor.

(text continued on p. 624)

TABLE 19-1 Developmental Approach to Accident Prevention

Age	Developmental characteristics	Potential hazards	Preventive strategies
Infancy			
0–3 months	Newborn is totally dependent on care given by parents; some head control and can move in crib; taste, sight, and hearing are developing	Can catch arms or fingers between loose-fitting mattress and frame of crib	Use crib sides and bumpers; stuff towels between mattress and crib side; cribs should have slats no more than $2\frac{3}{8}''$ apart
		Suffocation in crib	Do not use pillows or excess blankets
		Automobile accidents	Infant car seats should be used from birth
		Sudden movement leading to falls	Do not leave baby alone on high places, particularly on an adult bed or infant seat; keep a hand on baby at all times, especially during bathing when baby is slippery with soap; on stairs, hold baby with two hands
		Burns and punctures from bathing and changing; poisoning from spoiled formula	Test bath water for lukewarm temperature; be careful of sharp points of diaper pins near baby's skin; store formula in cool, dry place; protect child from sunburn
3–6 months	Good head control; can turn from stomach to back and can put hands in mouth; touch is used to learn about the properties of objects	Harmful objects within baby's immediate reach	Remove potential hazards such as hot coffee while baby is sitting on parent's lap; protect baby from hot faucet while bathing in sink; toys should have no removable parts or sharp edges that could be put in baby's mouth or eyes; do not allow access to plastic bags
		Sharp fingernails	Parents can cut baby's fingernails while baby sleeps
6–9 months	Holds own bottle; beginning to drink from cup; may sit unsupported; can pull to standing position and has pincer grasp; transfers objects; some children begin to scoot or crawl—world expands beyond nursery; like to feed themselves crackers and finger foods	Glass breakage if dropped	Use plastic bottles
		Child's range of grasp increases with mobility	Cover electrical outlets and wind cords on appliances to keep them out of reach; lock lower cabinets or remove any dangerous objects (eg, glass jars, soap powders)

TABLE 19-1 continued

Age	Developmental characteristics	Potential hazards	Preventive strategies
		Increased access to hazardous fixtures and furniture	Use gates to protect from stairways; fence off wood-burning stoves and space heaters; supervise constantly when child is in walker, swing, jumper, or high chair; wastebaskets, plants, and household cleaners contain potential poisons and should be placed out of child's reach; remove hazardous machinery such as fans and humidifiers from floor level
		As teeth develop, babies enjoy teething biscuits	Supervise for choking; do not leave baby unattended while eating
9–12 months	Can pull self to a sitting position; creeps and cruises around furniture; exhibits purposeful behavior and can reach for objects out of their grasp; some children begin to verbalize; begins to eat finger foods	Mobility and range of grasp increase further	Turn pot handles in on stove; remove stove burner dials if within reach; remove dangerous objects from counters and tables
		Hazardous fixtures become increasingly accessible	Screen windows and use gates on stairways if not already done; use playpens with sides up and corrals with net siding
		Choking from small objects	Cut food into small pieces; no peanuts or popcorn; child should eat while sitting; easy to handle eating utensils; check toys for small pieces; keep money out of reach
Early Childhood			
12–18 months	Can walk alone and navigate stairs; can stoop and retrieve; has some fine motor skills and some verbal skills	Body control not highly developed, resulting in an unsteady walk; would rather run than walk	Keep furniture with sharp edges, glass coffee tables, and the like out of child's way; keep house clutter-free; lock up poisonous substances if not previously done; pull-toy strings should not be greater than 12″ in length
		Bath—temperature of water and slippery tub	Lukewarm water at low level in tub; teach child not to stand in tub; never leave child unattended during bath time; run cold water first before mixing with hot

continued on next page

TABLE 19-1 continued

Age	Developmental characteristics	Potential hazards	Preventive strategies
18–24 months	Can run, jump, and stand on one foot; verbal skills expanding; taste, touch, and smell continue to develop	Accidents are more frequent when parents are preoccupied such as at mealtimes and in the morning	Parents can share responsibility for preparing meals and watching children; children's television programs can hold attention during meal preparation; parents should be alert to children's whereabouts
		Fire begins to be a hazard, especially charcoal fires in the summer	Parents should begin to educate children about danger of fire; place matches out of reach; teach fire safety
		Curiosity makes household and yard plants more interesting	Teach child not to put any plants, leaves, berries, etc in mouth
		Climbing accidents become more frequent, especially out of cribs	Parents can have child sleep with crib sides lowered temporarily until a bed is obtained
2–3 years	Walks on tiptoe; enjoys imitating adults; enjoys riding toys; can learn simple prohibitions; using many nouns and verbs in speech	Injury from riding toys	Parents should teach child about riding in streets or behind cars; plastic tricycles are lower to the street and slower than metal ones—but lower vehicles are harder to see by passing motorists
		Children are attracted to brightly colored objects such as pills	Child should be taught never to take pills unless given by parent; medicine should not be made to "taste good"
		Drowning—children who have been taught to swim might get careless in the water	Pools should be fenced; careful observation at beaches; even children who swim should be observed
3–5 years	Has good gross motor coordination; interested in action toys, "big wheels," and tricycles; loves to explore and experiment, especially on playgrounds	Injury from playground equipment	Safety teaching should include no walking in front of swings, no pushing and shoving off equipment
		Foreign objects in Halloween candy	Parents should check Halloween treats before allowing child to eat them; throw away any loose or open candy
		Choking	Teach children not to run with candy or other objects in their mouths
		Increasing freedom out of doors; contact with unleashed animals	Encourage cooperative play; teach street safety—looking both ways, crossing at corners, watching lights; teach children to avoid strangers and keep

TABLE 19-1 continued

Age	Developmental characteristics	Potential hazards	Preventive strategies
			parents informed of their whereabouts; teach children to walk quietly near animals and to avoid approaching them if parents are not present
Middle and late childhood			
5–12 years	Increased muscle tone; improved motor coordination enables increasingly difficult activities; sensitive to peer pressure; responds to rules; magical thinking leads to identification with superheroes	Imitates action seen on television	Parents should teach critical television viewing and talk to children about their favorite shows
		Skateboard misuse, particularly in populated areas	Caution children to remember street safety when on skates or skateboards; extra control is needed for downhill runs; discourage jumps
		Bicycle accidents are common	Teach bicycle safety
		Drowning—ice or water	Teach children water safety; do not allow skating unless ice thickness is proven safe; never swim or skate alone
		Sports injuries	Teach parents and children sports safety
		Automobiles	Require seatbelts at all times; teach child not to hide or play near cars
		Nighttime accidents increase as child is allowed more freedom	Parents should encourage children to be home before dark; wear light-colored clothing and reflective material when walking at night
		Vacant buildings, excavations, quarries, sand pits, house foundations	Teach children to avoid these areas and not to play around heavy machinery; tell child not to hide in refrigerators or piles of leaves
		Flying objects—balls, darts, arrows, stones	Any target sport should be carefully supervised; targets should be in isolated areas or against walls; teach children not to throw objects at people or moving vehicles
		Abusable substances—effect of drugs and alcohol on coordination and judgment lead to accidental injury	(See Chapters 11 and 24)

continued on next page

TABLE 19-1 continued

Age	Developmental characteristics	Potential hazards	Preventive strategies
Adolescence			
Over 12 years	Conflict between dependence and independence; increased decision-making skills; peer influence more important than parental influence; increasing goal orientation	Abusable substances	(See Chapter 24)
		Vehicle hazards—cars, motorcycles	Driver safety; parents need to set firm limits on car use, particularly regarding drinking and driving
		Outdoor activities—swimming, jogging, boating, etc no longer under direct parental supervision	Encourage adolescents to do activities in a group so others can obtain help in case of injuries
		Firearms	Teach rules for hunting and proper care of firearms; keep firearms locked up and hidden away
			Parental role modeling regarding safety and hazards leading to injury can affect their children's safety practices; open communication between parents and children is a powerful preventive measure

NOTE: These ages are arbitrary. Parents should be taught to anticipate their children's development and take preventive action according to individual developmental patterns.

Peer Pressure Peer pressure contributes greatly to accident incidence. Competitiveness is exaggerated by peers and can lead to injury in children who try to "do one better" or succumb to taking dares.

Special Needs Some children with special needs are at greater risk for injury. For example, children who are hyperactive or have high activity levels appear to be at risk. These children might be excessively stimulated by their environment. They react diffusely to stimuli, and their excessive activity can be random and without purpose. Their short attention span and inability to attend to directions leads them into accident-causing situations that they are not prepared to deal with appropriately.

Handicapped children have special problems, and normal hazards become particularly dangerous for them. For children with handicaps affecting hearing and vision, additional precautions around traffic are necessary. Children with medical problems such as seizures, diabetes mellitus, cystic fibrosis, and asthma can be at greater risk for injury, particularly when participating in competitive sports. Keeping such children in a state of maximum health can reduce the injury potential.

Assessment of the Agent: Vectors of Energy Transfer

Assessment of the agent involves identifying those agents that are hazardous and that, if altered, can prevent injury from occurring. Agents of primary importance include the automobile, bicycles, the child as a pedestrian, water, fire, toys, and infant equipment.

Automobiles Automobiles are the primary agents of injury in children and are the number one cause of death for children in some age groups (Righi and Krozy, 1983). Victims of motor vehicle accidents include not only children who are passengers but also children who are pedestrians, bicyclists, and automobile drivers.

There are two periods of impact in an accident. The first impact occurs when the automobile comes to a sudden stop in a collision. The second impact occurs when the occupant stops motion by hitting part of the car or the restraint of a seatbelt or car-restraint system. An unrestrained child in a motor vehicle is propelled forward during a collision at a speed and force comparable to a fall from a third-floor window. Head-first propulsion results from the child's body weight and distribution (Reinhard, 1980).

Assessment of automobile safety is primarily concerned with the use of seatbelts and child safety restraint systems. Seatbelts are proven to be effective in reducing injury and mortality from automobile collisions. It is said that for every 1% increase in seatbelt use, 172 lives are saved (Righi and Krozy, 1983). Effective January 1, 1978, Tennessee was the first state to legislate that children under 4 years of age or weighing less than 40 lb had to use a federally approved car restraint while riding in a car. Fifteen states followed and passed legislation within the next 3 years. Most states presently have laws governing car restraints, and many states have car safety education programs. However, compliance with the law is low (Reinhard, 1980).

As of January 1, 1981, all car restraint systems manufactured after May, 1980, must follow standards set by the Federal Motor Vehicle Safety Standards 213–80. These guidelines require the following:

1. All car restraint systems manufactured for infants and children be dynamically tested in frontal collision situations at 30 mph. The seats must protect and restrain the occupant adequately.
2. Sufficient force is required to open the harness to prevent children from accidentally releasing the clasp.
3. The directions for use must be clear and visible.
4. The restraint also must be tested under a variety of conditions of improper use.

Lists of approved car seats are available in consumer magazines or from the US Department of Transportation. Car seats are made of energy-absorbing material. They distribute pressure over the entire body and provide support for the head and neck. They are secured by the standard lap belt and often a tether (Fig. 19-1).

A safety-tested car seat is an integral part of the layette for the newborn. The infant's first experience in a car seat should be on the ride home from the hospital. The newborn will learn to associate the motion of the car with being fastened up and being secure. The seat allows the infant to be in a reclining position, secured with a regular seatbelt

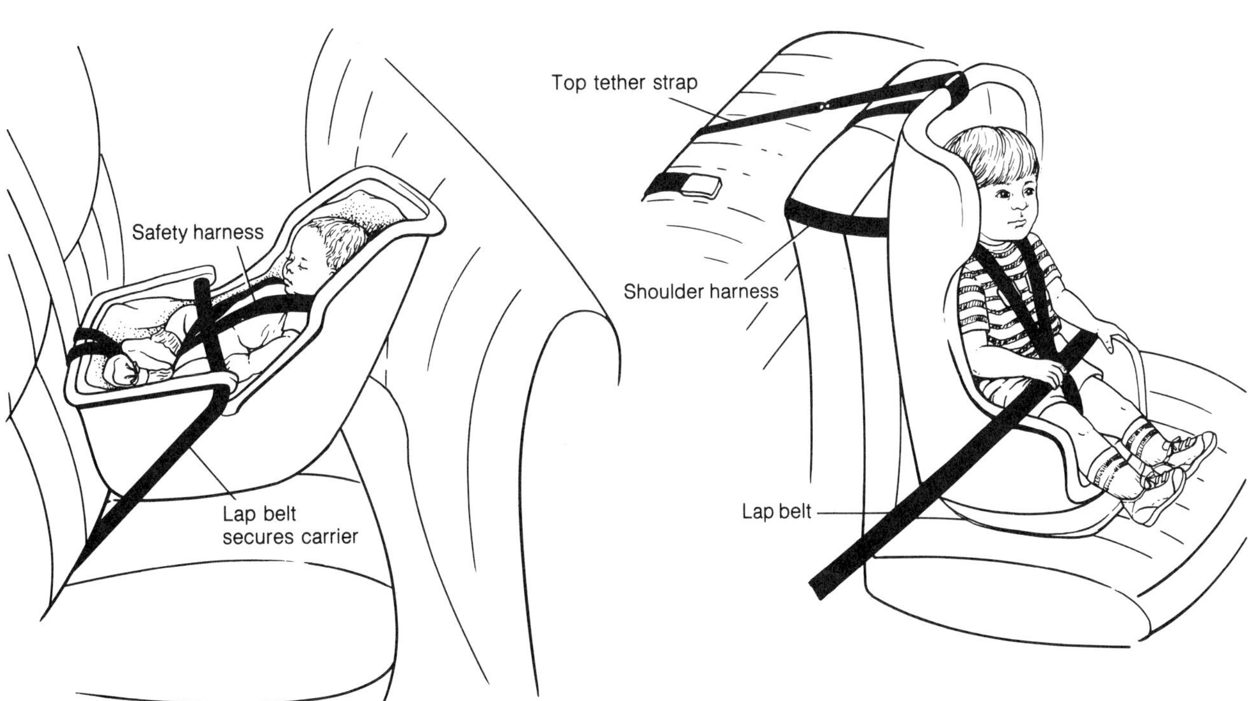

Figure 19-1 Infant restraints. *A*. Infant carrier for the infant from birth to about 12 months of age. *B*. Anchoring the top tether of an infant carrier.

and a safety harness, and facing the rear of the car. Some car seats must be anchored to the body of the car (tethering) to prevent the seat from flying forward in a crash (Fig. 19-1).

Early childhood car seats are elevated so that the child can see out the windows. Again, tethering is often necessary to prevent forward motion in a collision. The child sits in an erect position facing forward. Many car seats provide safety shields to protect vulnerable chest and abdominal organs. Parents might be frustrated by children climbing out of car seats. Children should learn that the car only moves when they are restrained in their car seats. Above 40 lb or 40 in, children may be safely restrained in regular seatbelts using cushions to keep the belts in position over their laps and to keep them from applying pressure over the abdomen.

In addition to assessing accessibility to child-restraint systems, nurses need to assess parental role modeling in relation to cars. If children do not see their parents "buckle up," they will not understand why they should be restrained. Also, parents' behavior in the automobile and while driving sets the standards for their children's later behavior.

Other problems with automobiles occur when cars are overcrowded or when children are playing near streets. Station wagons, which are often used to transport large numbers of children, are not safe when children are riding unrestrained in the back window area. Children riding in the backs of pickup trucks are at additional risk for injury. Not only are they unrestrained, but also, in the event of a collision, they will be propelled directly onto the street and might very well be run over by another vehicle. Children should not ride in a parent's lap because of the danger of being thrown forward and crushed by the parent during impact. Children also should not be allowed to play in or near parked cars.

Bicycles Since the late 1970s bicycle accidents have accounted for 1.25 million accidents, 77% of which occur to children younger than 15 years of age (Betz, 1983). The greater percentage of accidents affect children in the 5- to 14-year-old age group, although 30% of accidents occurred to children under 5 years of age (Betz, 1983).

Structural factors in the bicycles themselves, such as mechanical defects, account for only a small percentage of accidental injury (Betz, 1983). Those factors influencing accident incidence are the style of the bicycle, the type of braking device, child and size mismatch, and type of child bicycle seat. Bicycle accidents can involve collision with a motor vehicle or an environmental obstacle. Other injuries are caused by falls and by limbs caught in wheel spokes.

"High-rise" bicycles with long, thin seats and high handlebars are not suitable for beginning riders. They place the center of gravity over the rear wheel and do not give the necessary protection to the genital area. Hand brakes, which require that equal pressure be applied to both wheels, demand coordination not usually possessed by children until they are about 11 years old. Coaster brakes are the simplest and safest to operate. Assessment of a safe bicycle includes asking the parent whether the child's bike has the following: slip-resistant pedals, a strong frame, handlebars that are low and in proportion to the seat height, the center of gravity over the center of the bicycle, a bicycle flag, and reflectors on the spokes and pedals. The bicycle should not be too large for the child's size.

Bicycle seats should be used by all children over 1 year of age who are passengers on a bicycle ridden by an adult. Children under 1 year of age are not stable enough in a seat to prevent injury. A safe bicycle carrier is secured tightly to the bicycle and is constructed of durable material. The seat must protect the child's lower body and must prevent foot and hand access to the spokes. The child should be belted into the seat at all times while moving and should be encouraged to wear a protective helmet.

A minibike is a bicycle with a small motor. Although licensing laws vary, children younger than driving age may have access to minibikes. Because of this, the potential for minibike accidents in children under 15 years old is high. Minibikes are not intended for on-street operation and are misused in many instances. Because minibikes are capable of speeds up to 30 mph, helmets are necessary to prevent injuries (Consumer Reports, 1981). Minibike riders should avoid traffic situations where automobiles are traveling at speeds greater than 40 mph.

Minibikes cause injuries in several ways. The exhaust pipes can burn the legs. Many children cannot apply adequate pressure to the brake pedal, and some of the braking systems are unsafe. Because of the small design and short wheelbase, minibikes can be unstable. Some children even have experienced hearing loss from the noise of the motor.

Children as Pedestrians Children often dart into traffic from between parked cars and usually are hit within a two-block radius of their homes (American Automobile Association, 1976). Factors that contribute to the high number of pedestrian accidents in children include their natural curiosity, short attention span, and impulsiveness. These qualities often lead to poor judgment near streets. A small child's height, which averages 35–40 in above the ground, is not enough to allow clear visibility of oncoming cars (American Automobile Association, 1976). Drivers also have difficulty distinguishing very small moving objects. Children might be unaware of traffic signals or rules. A young child may not judge accurately the amount of time it will take to cross a street safely (American Automobile Association, 1976). It is natural for children to be so immersed in a game that they automatically chase a ball into the street without thinking of the dangers involved.

Assessment of children as pedestrians involves ascertaining the child's knowledge of safety as well as the child's developmental level and temperament. In pedestrian accidents the child and the car as agents combine to produce the injury.

Water Water is an agent for both drownings and burns. Drownings occur as a result of contact with a variety of water hazards, including those in common household locations such as the bathtub or toilet. According to the American Red Cross (1981), only about 40% of yearly drownings are a result of recreational activity such as swimming. Sixty percent of drownings are a consequence of accidental falls into the water, boating accidents, and accidents in the home.

Children at different ages are susceptible to different kinds of drownings. Infants less than 1 year old might drown when left unattended in a bathtub. Toddlers fall into private swimming pools and lakes. In middle and late childhood, children drown in pools and lakes while swimming. Adolescents take risks in large bodies of water. When learning to walk, children are unsteady on their feet, and extra caution is needed when they are near sources of water, particularly in the bathroom or outdoors.

Scaldings are the most common burns seen in all age groups, and children under 3 years of age are burned by hot liquids more than by any other agent. The temperature of the liquid and the duration of contact determine the degree of injury, and cooling the scald with cold water is an important immediate response. At 156° F, it takes only 2 seconds for a full-thickness burn (destruction of epidermis and dermis) to occur (Feldman, et al., 1978). Tap water is as hot as 156° F in some homes, and a pan of boiling water or freshly poured coffee is much hotter (212° F).

Very young infants are burned less frequently than those beginning to crawl or walk, but scalds do occur. An adult unwisely holding an infant while eating hot soup or drinking a hot beverage might spill some and cause a deep scald.

Typically, the older infant or toddler is burned when adults leave a cup of hot tea or coffee too close to a tabletop or counter edge. As the adult turns to replace the kettle on the stove or attend to some other task, the child reaches for the cup, upsets it, and sustains a significant scald burn. Pot handles protruding over the stovetop are another hazard, as are tablecloths and dangling electrical cords—anything a child can reach, grasp, and overturn. Common appliances such as electric coffee pots and frying pans are associated with major, disfiguring, and life-threatening burns.

Hot liquids must be kept out of reach, pan handles turned inward to the back of the stove, and electrical cords tied up and away from curious toddlers. Children should not be underfoot in the kitchen when meals are being prepared, particularly when parents are carrying pots of boiling liquids from the stove to the sink and countertops.

Bathroom tap water scalds occur when children are left unattended in or near the bathtub. The doorbell or telephone rings, and the parent leaves "for just a moment." Children might try to climb into a tub where the water is untested and too hot, or they might experiment with faucets. The rules to follow include never leaving children alone in a bathroom, always running hot water well mixed with cold, and testing the temperature of the water before placing the child in the bathtub. Children should be taught to turn cold faucets on first and then to mix in the hot water. Child abuse with scalding tap water does occur and should be considered, especially when there are no splash marks and there is an even burn. For example, a burn over the "socks area" of the feet and ankles along with a buttocks burn suggests that the child might successfully have resisted further immersion. (The nurse's role in assessing child abuse is discussed in Chapter 22.)

A less frequent but often deep and disfiguring injury is an electrical burn caused by biting through the wire or chewing on the end of a cord. Saliva, primarily water, is an excellent conductor of electricity. Because water conducts electricity, children should be taught not to bring televisions or radios into the bathroom with them and particularly not to touch an electrical appliance when they are wet.

Ice is a water hazard with a high injury potential. Children should not have small ice cubes in drinks since, if aspirated, the cube can occlude the child's airway. Also they should be discouraged from running while eating popsicles or other frozen treats on sticks. (The hazards of ice skating are discussed in the section entitled "Outdoor Environmental Hazards".)

Fire Fascination with and curiosity about fire starts at an early age, long before the child can competently handle matches, fireplaces, and stoves. As children grow, they imitate adult behavior and might attempt activities beyond their skills. For example, a 3-year-old girl watched her mother tightly wad newspaper to start a fire in the stove. She took a piece of paper herself, loosely crumpled it, and tossed it into the open flames, only to have it ignite quickly in her hands and then ignite her clothing. Flame burns are particularly serious because they almost always require skin grafting for wound closure (see Chapter 44).

Clothing does not protect the body from fire, although different fibers react differently to flame, and fabrics can be treated with flame-retardant chemicals. Synthetics melt, natural fibers (cotton, silk, wool) ignite, and combination fabrics both melt and support flames. The laws regulating the manufacture of children's sleepwear (FF3-71, FF5-740) specify that sizes 0–14 must be flame resistant, meaning that the fabric is treated with a chemical that helps it resist continued burning when brought in contact with a source of flames. Recently, TRIS (2,3 dibromopropyl phosphate), used to treat sleepwear, was banned. Bacterial studies indicated that it was mutagenic (Blum and Ames, 1977). Sleepwear in stores today does not contain TRIS but has been treated to meet flame-resistance requirements. Parents must follow laundering instructions and be advised to ask for flame-resistant materials if they make their children's pajamas or nightgowns. Studies conducted in Boston, Massachusetts, and Ann Arbor, Michigan, reported that sleepwear-related injuries have been virtually eliminated since this law was enacted (McLoughlin, et al., 1977; Feller, et al., 1980).

In assessing fire hazards in the home, the nurse includes inquiries about provisions made for the proper handling and disposal of cigarettes. Naturally, children of parents who smoke are at greater risk because of the availability of matches. Matches should be stored in metal containers and out of children's reach. Cigarette lighters are a particularly dangerous fire hazard because, depending on the type, less manual dexterity might be needed to light them than matches. Cigarettes should not be left in ashtrays within a child's reach, and they should be extinguished completely before disposal.

Gas stoves also can present a fire hazard to children. Many stoves have on and off dials within a child's reach, allowing for easy flame ignition. These dials can be removed to prevent accidental lighting. Wood stoves, radiators, heating grates, space heaters, barbeque grills, and discarded hot charcoal also can create fire hazards.

Toys Toys are a most important ingredient of a child's normal growth and development. They also can, however, be instruments of danger when inappropriately manufactured or used. At any one time, thousands of a particular toy might be recalled because of manufacturing defects. A recent example of this was a type of teddy bear for young children that lost its eyes and nose when used on a regular basis, creating the potential for choking (Pomeranz and Schultz, 1982). Most toys are directed toward a particular age group. Parents must be certain not to purchase a toy that is beyond the age level of a child. Although children might be manually capable of manipulating a toy directed at an older-age child, the toy might not be safe.

The Child Protection and Toy Safety Act of January, 1970 was instituted to identify and remove hazardous toys from the market. The US Consumer Product Safety Commission is a federal organization with the authority to ban hazardous toys from sale. Unfortunately, mechanisms for establishing safety standards for all toys before they are marketed are not yet in place. The result, then, is that dangerous toys are recalled after they have injured children (Brown, 1978). The burden of providing safe toys rests, as it always has, with the parents.

Resources concerning toy safety include pamphlets by the US Consumer Product Safety Commission and the US Government Printing Office. Information regarding toy recalls can be found in consumer magazines and newspapers.

Toys should be bought and maintained with injury prevention in mind. Nurses can assess parents' knowledge regarding toy purchasing according to the following principles:

1. Read all toy labels for age recommendations and information concerning the safety of the component materials.
2. Check all toys for sharp edges or points, small loose parts, adequate construction, loud noise, improper electrical wiring, and objects that can be propelled.
3. Avoid buying toys with flexible joints that can catch children's fingers.
4. Avoid baby teething toys that are breakable or contain liquid. Even minute cracks can precipitate bacterial growth in the liquid.
5. Electrical and chemical toys, particularly those with heating elements, are recommended for older children only (over 8 years of age) (US Consumer Product Safety Commission; Brown, 1978).

The proper maintenance and storage of toys is as important as proper purchasing. Toys should be checked on a regular basis for breakage or excessive wear. Wooden toys can be resanded and repainted with nontoxic paint. If toys are irreparable, they should be discarded. All plastic wrappers should be disposed of immediately. Balloons are particularly hazardous when broken and have been known to cause obstruction of the airway. For this reason, they should not be used by young children without supervision. Parents should use caution with toy chests because they can injure children's fingers or heads if the lid falls on the child. The nurse also needs to assess the availability of toys in families with children of various ages. It might be necessary to recommend separate play areas if the age discrepancy between the children is too wide.

Infant Furniture Prior to 1974, there were no uniform safety standards for infant cribs. As a result, many children were injured each year in crib accidents. Federal requirements for infant cribs were established, and all cribs manufactured after February 1, 1974 are required to comply with these standards (Brown, 1978). They include regulating the width of the space between crib side slats (no more than $2\frac{3}{8}$ in at any point), standardizing the interior measurements (28 in $\pm\frac{5}{8}$ in in width and $52\frac{3}{8}$ in $\pm\frac{5}{8}$ in in length), requiring special latch release features, recommending standard mattress size and thickness, and regulating the height of the crib sides in relation to the mattress support height (Consumer Reports, 1973).

Nurses need to be aware, however, that many parents purchase older cribs and playpens at yard sales and are not knowledgeable about the safety standards. If cribs are found to fail these standards, especially in the use of lead paint or the slat space width, the nurse should recommend the use of full crib bumpers until a safer alternative can be provided.

More recent attention has focused on play space. As an alternative to the traditional playpen, many parents are using expandable wooden "corrals" to confine children. The advantages of these corrals are that they allow the child greater play area and are more portable. Although generally stable, corrals have contributed to injury by providing openings for children to use as footholds for climbing. Some children have been injured by placing their heads through the openings and having the corral collapse on them. Folding play spaces with net sides or playpens with side netting decrease this type of injury occurrence. Playpens with net sides, however, are not without danger. Infants should never be left in these areas with one side left down. Doing this increases the potential for the infant to suffocate from being caught between the playpen pad and the netting.

Assessment of Environmental Characteristics

If a child is an accident repeater or if the nurse notices a discrepancy between the child's needs and parental expectations, an environmental assessment is indicated. The assessment is geared toward identifying parental factors that might be contributing to accidents as well as assessing the relative safety of the child's physical environment. The assessment should be noncritical, with the nurse emphasizing concern about the child's safety to the parents while giving support and encouragement.

If the home is particularly chaotic and the child seems to be using accident behavior as an attention-getting mechanism, further counseling and family sessions are indicated. This might need to be followed by referral for special counseling. Factors in the environment that contribute to injury include parental factors such as inattention or fatigue, general developmental expectations of children, family stability, socioeconomic status, and physical environment conditions. (Nursing care of the family at risk is discussed in Chapter 22.)

Family/Parental Factors It is generally accepted that accidents increase at times of the day when the parent is paying less attention to the child. Examples of these critical times are the morning rush, when parents are getting off to work or children off to school, and meal preparation time. After a hard working day, parents tend to "tune out" their children while trying to unwind, thus becoming relatively unaware of what their children are doing.

Parental fatigue and worry can contribute to accidents, and the nurse therefore assesses the family's support systems. Do the parents have supportive relationships that enable them to renew their own strength? Caring for children all day can be an isolating experience for a parent. Play groups, mother's groups, and babysitting co-ops represent attempts to develop supportive networks to deal with these feelings. A parent who feels personally renewed has more strength for childrearing and an increased ability to attend adequately to each child.

Other factors also contribute to parental inattention. For example, illness of a family member, which requires parental attention and concern, also may contribute to parental inattention and greater potential for injury. Children in the care of a babysitter, particularly if the sitter is an older sibling, can increase their testing behavior, which might result in an injury. Parents therefore need to caution babysitters to pay special attention to the younger children to prevent such occurrences.

Developmental Expectations Parental expectations should coincide with the child's actual developmental level. Expectations that are too low can increase injury risk. For example, a mother reported that a real estate broker showing their house cautioned her to keep the crib side up because her infant was standing up in bed. The mother's response was, "My baby cannot stand yet!" Perhaps in the chaos of moving, this child's development was temporarily ignored or perhaps the mother's expectations of the child lagged behind the child's actual development.

Expectations that are too high also can lead to injury by prompting children to attempt skills for which they are not ready. For example, a 3-year-old can learn to follow simple directions but is not able to cross a street alone or to play outside unsupervised. An infant is not ready to master steps on a steep, 14- to 20-foot stairway but can be taught on two-step plastic toy stairs. The challenge for parents is to provide a stimulating environment that promotes development but also protects from injury.

Family Stability Parental discord or family stress can predispose children to injury because any instability can distract parental attention. Family events that can cause confusion might include moving, vacations, household company, or the addition of a new family member. (See Table 18-1, which lists the stress events for young children that might contribute to both accidents and illness.)

Family relocation, either temporary, such as a vacation, or permanent, might contribute to accidental injury. Vacations often place children near unsupervised bodies of water or wooded recreational areas. The child's need to be supervised constantly might not allow parents much relaxation while on vacation. Drowning, boating accidents, fish hooks, camp fires, and sunburns, among others, pose hazards. For a child, being lost in a strange neighborhood is a terrifying experience. When on vacation, parents need to redefine boundaries and rules immediately with their children. Some parents bring their babysitters with them from home, so that their children will be watched while the parents have some free time. When moving to a new neighborhood, a tour of adjacent streets and learning the new telephone number and address can prevent a child from experiencing the trauma of being lost.

Divorce or separation creates disequilibrium within the family. Parents preoccupied by family disorganization can allow a young child to go unwatched. In some divorce situations, most notably those involving a custody dispute, children might increase acting-out behavior (see Chapter 12). In some instances this behavior leads to increased risk taking and subsequent injury.

A new child in the family causes similar family disequilibrium and decreased parental attention. Children who feel displaced often take risks to gain attention. Parents with a new infant are often exhausted and under stress and therefore not as vigilant as they might be ordinarily. Parental well-being is a significant variable in the prevention of injuries. Recognizing that parents are under stress and encouraging them to use support systems (family, friends, or babysitters) can give parents the necessary relief to cope.

Parental/Family Values The style of childrearing affects the child's risk of injury. Particularly pertinent to this issue is the promotion of autonomy. From the early childhood years, becoming independent is the child's task. Some parents, however, encourage autonomy to such a degree that safety is jeopardized. Young children are allowed to wander at will, and some children of the middle childhood stage are left at home unsupervised after school. Although children of this age might understand safety concepts, when confronted by a crisis, such as a fire, they might panic and take inappropriate actions.

The young child's decision-making skills are not highly developed. Parents should recognize that young children are not capable of seeing all sides of an issue and need to be assisted to clarify issues and understand consequences. Children who are allowed complete freedom regarding decision making will not only feel insecure but will increase their injury potential as a result of processing data incompletely.

Some families value competitiveness and aggression, and children are encouraged to develop these characteristics at an early age. The child's primary outlet for aggression and a competitive spirit is athletic participation. Unfortunately, sports and fitness-related accidents account for more than 11 million injuries each year (Southmayd and Hoffman, 1981). More than 55% of these injuries are related to biking, baseball, football, and basketball. In a study done by the Consumer Product Safety Commission (Southmayd and Hoffman, 1981), the following facts were revealed about sports injuries:

1. Seventy percent are incurred by children 10–24 years of age, and 40% are sustained by children under 15 years of age.
2. The most common type of injuries are sprains, strains, contusions, abrasions, and lacerations.
3. Injuries affect the parts of the body that are most vulnerable for a particular sport, for example, a hockey goalie's knees.

The prevention of accidents should be the focus of sports for children. An important decision for parents is to determine at what age their children can participate safely in competitive sports. Children begin to value competition at about 6 years of age. Young athletes require different rules, equipment, and coaching than adults because of the vulnerability of their growing bodies (American Medical Association, 1977). For parents, both psychologic and physical considerations are relevant. Does the enjoyment of playing as part of a team outweigh the criticisms of organized competitive sports?

Sports for young children should not be conducted like sports for older individuals. Young athletes might give up sports participation because of excessive criticism and negative reinforcement from coaches. Unfair matching, creating an unequal contest, the regimentation of training, and the psychologic pressure to win all contribute to athletic dropouts. Factors in the sports environment, such as an uneven playing field or inadequate equipment, contribute to injuries. Specific maneuvers such as high sticking in hockey or deliberate fouling in basketball are often associated with injuries. Penalties have been instituted to prevent this type of play. Young muscles and bones are also vulnerable to chronic recurring stress, often resulting in injury from excessive use. Changes in game rules, however, have prevented some of the more prominent overuse syndromes such as pitcher's elbow. Finally, physical mismatch increases sports injuries. Teams should be divided according to size and body maturation and not according to age (Pappas, 1981). Programs geared to educating coaches about new rulings and sensitivity to the young athlete are important.

Nurses can counsel parents regarding the physical and psychologic considerations of competitive sports. Some American Medical Association authorities suggest no contact sports prior to ninth grade. Contact sports include football, ice hockey, boy's lacrosse, rugby, wrestling, and diving. Authorities also advise against scoring, ranking, win or lose situations, and championships prior to 10 years of age (Schering Symposium on Sports Medicine, 1980).

Many of the traditionally all-male sports are now open to females. Prior to puberty, there is no valid reason to separate boys and girls. After the onset of puberty, bruising and collision sports for mixed competition should be eliminated. Even in individual noncontact competition, such as swimming, the size discrepancy between postpubescent boys and girls can result in unfair matching, with injury resulting from attempts to compete on an equal footing.

Injury-free sports for adolescent girls require added considerations such as equipment and clothing that adequately protect and support breast tissue and the pelvic girdle. Preseason conditioning programs help strengthen critical muscles and joints.

Sports can still be a part of life for children with chronic diseases. The Special Olympics for handicapped children allows them an opportunity to succeed in sports. Diabetic children are encouraged to participate in sports because their disease is more likely to be controlled if they are physically fit. Special considerations for children with asthma and heart disease can be checked with a physician, but participation in sports rarely is ruled out.

A preseason physical examination is necessary to detect any conditions precluding sports participation. If an injury occurs during a game, the coach must make an informed decision regarding the child's ability to continue playing. Nurses can assist coaches in the decision-making process by emphasizing the following:

1. The injury should be accurately diagnosed.
2. The person examining the child must take adequate precautions to prevent exacerbation of the injury.
3. The examiner should feel confident that the injury will not worsen with further play and that continued participation will not produce new injury.

Socioeconomic Factors Living conditions for people in lower socioeconomic groups can result in an increased incidence of accidents. The environment might be more hazardous and difficult to childproof. Trash and litter in houses or streets, dim lighting, faulty electrical wiring, steep or broken stairways, unscreened windows, or porches on second and third stories can create dangerous situations for small children. Bicycles in city traffic become very different toys than when they are used to ride on a country road.

Children often play or run into streets when yards or playgrounds are unavailable. For people in the lower socioeconomic groups, family vigilance and community activism are necessary for the child's welfare. Community groups can work toward better sanitation and improved lighting. They can put pressure on landlords to repair hazardous living conditions.

Physical Environment of the Home The home can be one of the most dangerous places for a child if it is not properly childproofed. The challenge to parents is providing a safe environment without completely suppressing the child's curiosity and sense of adventure. If parents are reluctant to confine a child in a playpen, a playroom, which can be kept separate from the rest of the house by a gate, is a viable alternative. If the child is allowed to wander freely, the entire house must be made safe. The nurse's assessment of the home environment is directed toward room-by-room safety (Fig. 19-2 and Table 19-2).

The kitchen and the bathrooms need special attention because most dangerous substances are stored in these rooms. Devastating internal and external burns can occur when corrosive household products are left within reach. The exploring child can both spill and ingest these products. Drain openers, oven cleaners, electric dishwasher powders, and low-phosphate detergents contain corrosive alkalis. There are dangerous acids in toilet bowl cleaners, metal polishes, and swimming pool cleaners. All of these chemicals must be stored high up and out of reach. Sometimes, if the child likes to climb, it is necessary to keep the chemicals under lock and key.

Food stored near the kitchen stove attracts young children. They climb close to the flame, intent only on getting to the cookies or candy. Matches or lighters left lying about might be too much of a temptation even for the child who "knows better" to resist. Other factors influencing the types of burns children receive are cultural practices such as cooking on the floor or ground, using open flames with small children about, new products like the slow-cooking electrical cookery pot, or the increase in popularity of an item like the wood-burning stove.

Bathrooms have their own particular hazards. In addition to the storage of cleaners, medications of all kinds are commonly stored in bathroom medicine cabinets. Children who can climb find these substances easily accessible. Other poisonous substances also are found in the bathroom. Many cosmetics can be poisonous if ingested, particularly astringents, which are primarily alcohol, and nail polish remover (see Chapter 20). Hairspray, if sprayed directly into the face, can cause eye injuries. Razors and razor blades are bathroom items that must be inaccessible to children.

Basements and garages contain many hazardous substances such as pesticides, fertilizers, weed killers, paints, and paint cleaning products, to name only a few items. Tools also can be a safety hazard. Poisonous and caustic substances preferably should be located in a locked cupboard. All tools must be kept out of reach. Lawn mowers should be disconnected to prevent accidental activation. Both basements and garages should be considered off limits to young children.

Young children also should be encouraged to stay away from sewing areas. Pins, needles, and thread bobbins are small enough to be ingested and cause internal damage.

Outdoor Environmental Hazards Outdoor hazards are plentiful. Parts of some common garden plants are poisonous (see Chapter 20), and children should be taught not to eat anything found outside without first checking with a parent.

Other outdoor environmental hazards that can injure children include air pollution, noise pollution, toxic substances, smoking chemicals, and carcinogens in drinking water (see Chapter 18). Testing and tracking devices used by nearby military bases can violate safe levels of radiation or noise pollution. Proximity to commercial airports can have the same effect.

Swimming pools, fresh and saltwater beaches, and farm ponds present unique problems. Young children can slip and fall into unfenced private pools. Older children can slip and fall while running on pool decks. Neck and back injuries are caused by children diving headfirst into shallow water. Extra precaution is necessary when children are visiting grandparents or families with no young children. Although the pool might be fenced, the gate may be left unlocked.

Fresh and saltwater beaches can be hazardous if children are not supervised carefully. The numbers of people frequenting beaches combined with the unfamiliar landscape

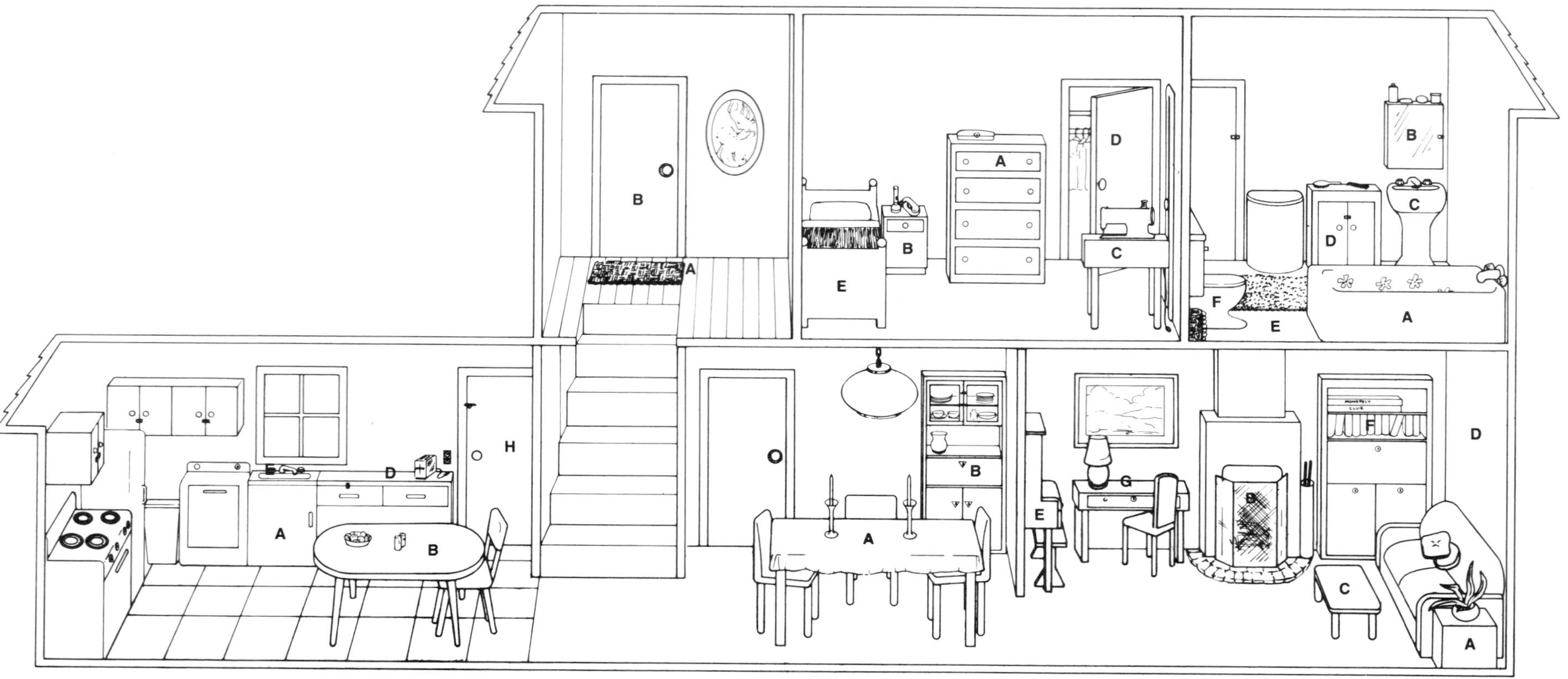

Figure 19-2 Childproofing the home: home safety check.

TABLE 19-2 Home Safety Check

Room/object	Hazard	Prevention strategies
Kitchen		
A—lower cabinets and drawers	Poisonous and corrosive substances in cabinets or on counters, including spices and extracts used in cooking	Remove and place out of reach in locked cabinet
	Alcohol or liquor in lower cabinets	Place in upper cabinets with cabinet lock
	Sharp knives, scissors, or other dangerous articles in drawers	Place in upper cabinet with cabinet lock or use drawer lock
	Breakable bowls or pie plates in lower cabinets	Remove or use cabinet lock
B—kitchen table	Pills or medicine on kitchen table or window sills	Lock up with other dangerous substances; use childproof caps

C—stove	Stove dials easily accessible	Remove until needed
	Cookies or other attractive food over the stove	Remove to another location; have fire extinguisher available
	Stove turned on when not in use	Make sure burners are off and that gas pilot is working properly; keep matches in metal container covered and out of reach
D—countertop	Food processor on counter	Remove blades to make them inaccessible; keep processor unplugged to prevent accidental activation
	Other electrical appliances on countertops—toaster, coffee pot, etc	Keep unplugged; use short cord or wind and secure cord
E—sink	Accessible disposal	Keep covered to prevent children from sticking hand in
F—floor	Wastebasket	Have a covered wastebasket to reduce curiosity; keep in closet or cabinet or in out-of-reach location
	Accessible stepstool might be used for climbing	Keep in kitchen closet; use plastic door handle covers to prevent entry
G—dishwasher	Knives within reach	Keep door closed and locked
H—door	Outside access available to children	Use simple door lock out of child's reach
Dining room		
A—table	Tablecloth hanging within reach	Remove cloth or use shorter cloth, particularly when lighted candles are on table
B—buffet with hutch	Breakables on buffet	Remove
	Glass and china items accessible in china cabinet	Use cabinet locks to prevent access
	Chafing dishes and hot trays	Keep unplugged until just before use
	Accessible wine rack	Move to higher location; keep bottles out of reach
Living room		
A—end table	Poisonous plants	Identify plants that are poisonous and remove or place out of child's reach
	Lighting fixtures	Make certain table lamps are unable and not easily displaced
B—fireplace	Fireplace or wood stove	Use fireplace screen; place gate around wood stove; dangerous fire-stoking equipment should be out of reach; do not heat water on wood stove; never cook with charcoal in fireplace; keep chimney damper open
C—coffee table and couch	Furniture edges	Sharp-edged furniture should be removed or padded
	Ashtrays	Keep ashtrays empty; dispose of cigarettes properly; keep matches and lighters out of reach
D—window	Curtains and draperies	Short draperies recommended with small children; if using long drapes, make sure drapery rod is securely fastened to wall
E—piano	Pianos and piano benches	Keep cover over keys when not in use
F—bookshelves	Stereo equipment	Stereo cabinet with locked doors recommended
	Games	Games with small pieces must be kept out of reach or in locked cabinets
	Books	Check that books cannot be pulled off shelves easily
G—desk	Desk accessories	Remove sharp objects, pencils, pens, paper clips, etc from desk top; lock drawers if possible
H—dehumidifiers and fans	Blades and motors	Check consumer magazines to purchase child-safe appliance; grates should be too narrow for little fingers

continued on next page

TABLE 19-2 continued

Room/object	Hazard	Prevention strategies
Hallways and stairs		
A—carpets	Slippery rugs	Use nonslip rug pad under rugs
B—closets	Attractive playing area	Use plastic door knob covers for all closets containing hazardous items
Bathroom		
A—tub	Slippery surface, hot water	Apply decorative nonskid strips to bottom; use flexible plastic faucet cover; keep hot water heater turned down; keep shampoo, soap, and razors out of reach
B—medicine cabinet	Dangerous substances	All medicines need childproof caps and should be in a locked cabinet. Remove any cosmetics, hair dyes, nail polish, etc and keep in a locked bathroom closet
C—Vanity and sink	Dangerous substances	Remove perfumes and powders from vanity top; electric shavers and toothbrushes should not be near water source; use outlet fillers for exposed outlets; use cabinet locks on vanity cabinets; store bathroom cleaners in locked bathroom closet; hairdryers, curling irons, and wastebaskets should be out of reach
D—linen closet	Dangerous substances	Closet should have a bolt lock or door handle cover to prevent entry; storage place for dangerous items
E—floor	Space heaters	Floor coil heaters should not be available for child's use
	Rugs	All bathroom rugs should have nonslip backing
	Clothes hamper	Hampers with covers are recommended
F—toilet	Water and dangerous chemicals	Keep toilet cover closed; avoid continuous toilet cleaners
Bedrooms		
A—bureaus	Dangerous substances and small objects	Remove cosmetics and small pieces of jewelry from bureau top; put loose change away and out of reach; keep jewelry box locked; drawers should not be easily removable
	Fans	Keep fans and air conditioners unplugged; use only when parent is around and never in children's rooms; do not place fans on floor; keep all electrical outlets filled
B—night tables	Breakable objects	Remove breakables; telephones, radios, etc should be situated in middle to prevent being pulled off; keep a flashlight here for emergencies
C—sewing table	Electrical appliance, small, sharp objects	Keep machine unplugged until needed; keep bobbins, needles, and pins in inaccessible locations
D—closets	Dangerous substances, plastic bags	Remove any mothballs or other insecticides; do not use plastic cleaner bags to store clothing in closets that are unlocked; keep clothes hangers off floors
E—beds		Do not use too much bedding or pillows for young children; keep children in sleepers if concerned about the cold; discourage children from playing on bunk beds or bunk ladders; see information about crib safety

NOTE: Be alert for dangerous items in the home. Use a commonsense approach to safety.

can result in disorientation and a lost child. Broken pieces of shells or glass lying buried in the sand can cause severe lacerations of the feet. Jellyfish and man-of-war can cause painful stings. At saltwater beaches, children need to understand safety in dealing with tides, undertows, and currents.

Boating carries the additional hazards of motors, capsizing, or being caught far from land. Although boating is thought to be a relaxing sport, children require special consideration. Constant supervision of children might inhibit a parent's pleasure.

Children always must wear life jackets while boating. Parents should check weather forecasts before leaving shore and have a radio on board. Extra life preservers, extra oars, and fire extinguishers also should be stocked for emergencies. The engine should be turned off when boarding the boat. Anyone swimming should not be near the propellers of the motor. Children should be taught how to move around in a boat and not to stand in small boats.

Farm ponds or local swimming holes frequently are used for recreational purposes. Farm ponds, which formerly were used as watering holes for animals, have been adapted for swimming by the addition of rafts, docks, and other aquatic equipment (American Red Cross, 1981). Because of uncertain depths and hazards from trash disposed of on the bottom, these areas should be used with caution. It is recommended that these ponds be fenced like private pools and that the water be tested frequently for bacterial content (American Red Cross, 1981).

Ice has accident potential, particularly when frozen ponds are accessible to children. Children should be allowed to skate only when the ice is proven to be thick enough to support the weight of a group—approximately 4 in (American Red Cross, 1981). Local police departments usually will provide information regarding ice safety on local ponds. Children should skate close to shore and never skate alone. Ice rescue equipment, such as a ladder or a flat-bottom boat, should be available where water depths are sufficient for drowning. Cold weather clothes, such as long scarfs, must be used with care because they can easily get caught and accidentally strangle a child.

Interventions: Primary-Level Strategies to Prevent Injuries

Anticipatory Guidance to Facilitate Parental Teaching Anticipatory guidance is a major nursing responsibility (see Chapter 21). During the safety assessment, the nurse listens for parents' assessment of their children's individual characteristics. The child's general activity level, responsiveness, degree of adaptability to change, and sense of independence and caution determine the need for improved safety. The nurse then can discuss the activity limits the parent is currently using and the effectiveness of these limits in light of the accident liability of the child. If the child is a risk taker and shows little sense of fear, parents might need to structure the environment more tightly.

Nurses can assist parents by providing instructional materials and helping them assess their children's capabilities and limitations according to their developmental stages. Two children of the same age may have different levels and different needs. One child might require more structure than another.

The principles of health education are described in Chapter 18. Safety education is most effective when it is directed specifically toward changing a single aspect of an agent or the environment rather then dealing with the whole problem all at once. For example, during an initial conference, the nurse might deal with the use of car restraints, or safety gates, or fire drills. Nurses need to evaluate the effectiveness of their teaching strategies during each successive conference, while remembering that the psychologic and socioeconomic aspects of the environment are as important as the physical aspects.

Community resources (library, fire and police departments) are good sources of teaching aids for parents. Poison control centers have stickers and warnings for medicines and poisonous substances. Pamphlets from the US Government Printing Office that might interest parents include *A Toy and Sports Equipment Safety Guide* #113k, *Young Children and Accidents in the Home* #121k, and *Home and Fire Safety* #201k. Discussion of the child's anticipated period of growth and development with a focus on the appropriate safety issues should be included in each well-child visit. Observing limit-setting situations and the parent–child interaction in the office can give the nurse valuable information.

During the process of maturation, safety for children changes from protection of the young child to education of the older child. A difficult issue for parents is the fine line between overprotection and allowing the child to make choices and take risks, which encourages growth. Allowing a child to ride a bicycle to the store alone or permitting an adolescent to take the family car are issues that most parents face.

Parents learn to teach children to know their own limits and responsibilities as they grow. Consistent and understandable limits enforced in a gentle, firm manner eventually teach children to make safe judgments for themselves. Children should understand parental expectations regarding rules for safety as well as comprehend the reasons for them. External limits that make sense to children gradually will be internalized by them when they are called on to make safety decisions in new situations.

Parents teach by example as well as by method. Children are keen observers, and young children tend to imitate what they see. Fastening seatbelts, looking before crossing a street, and safe driving habits are a few examples of safe practices children might imitate. All parents would like their children to learn moderation and good judgment. Consci-

Resources for Prevention of Injury

Films

Physicians for Automotive Safety: *Don't Risk Your Child's Life*. Communications Department. Rye, NY.
Visucom: *The Perfect Gift for Tamie*. Redwood City, CA.
National Safety Council: *Childsafe*. Chicago, IL.
Film Loops, Inc.: *Do You Care Enough?* Princeton, NJ.

Pamphlets

Action for Child Transportation Safety: *Car Pool Survival Kit, Kids Are Fragile, Protecting Child Passengers*, and *This is the Way Baby Rides*. Bothell, WA.
American Academy of Pediatrics Transportation Hazards Committee: *Will You Give Your Child the Perfect Gift?* Inglewood, CA.
Martens R, Seedfelt: *Guidelines for Children's Sports*. American Alliance for Health, Physical Education, Recreation and Dance, Washington, DC, 1979.
Preschool Children in Traffic. Program No 3265. American Automobile Association. Falls Church, VA, 1976.
A Toy and Sports Equipment Safety Guide. No 113k.
Young Children and Accidents in the Home. No 121k.
Home and Fire Safety. No 201k. US Government Printing Office, Pueblo, CO.
Child Safety for Injury Prevention. No G836. Ross Laboratories, Columbus, OH, January, 1982.

entious role modeling will facilitate the development of these qualities.

Nurses can instruct parents about appropriate conditions for teaching. For example, nurses need to encourage parents to discuss safety issues with children in a calm, relaxed atmosphere. Parents can then encourage children to describe how they would handle unsafe situations, that is, what to do if they smell smoke, how to get help if a friend is injured, what to do if they are lost or if a ball rolls into the street. Children are in hazardous situations before entering school and need to be taught safety at an early age. Family fire drills, learning how to reach an operator or how to dial home, knowing the home address and parents' names, and learning to ask a police officer for help are certainly useful tools for teaching children to manage crises. Indicating safe habits or safety principles to children during daily contact with them promotes safe behavior. For example, practicing crossing the street appropriately can be done every time a young child accompanies a parent on a walk. Most children will automatically incorporate these safety actions into their behavior patterns after the constant repetition and practice.

Environmental Modification: Childproofing A parent learns to adapt the environment to respond to the child's needs. These adaptations are called childproofing. Each room of the house should be made as hazard-free as possible for the specific child's developmental level and in anticipation of the upcoming levels. Devices such as safety gates for stairs, electrical outlet fillers, locks for drawers and cabinets, and plastic door handle protectors can limit the environment for an inquisitive child. Most toy stores carry child safety equipment, all of which is simple to install. The removal of the parents' favorite breakable items until the children can handle them carefully prevents parental distress and the resulting increase in pressure on the children. Room-by-room childproofing is illustrated in Figure 19-2.

Nurses may need to remind parents that the home need not be a fortress, nor should safety proofing limit the enjoyment of other family members. Young children are perfectly happy playing with household implements such as pots and pans and wooden spoons, and these should be accessible to them. Older children should have space allotted to them where they can keep their own possessions out of reach.

Nurses can assist parents to create a stimulating, attractive, and safe play area for their young children. Brightly painted shelves or cupboards for toy storage should be within the child's reach. Large, covered plastic containers can be used to hold toys with multiple pieces to prevent loss and injury to a family member who might trip on them. Play spaces made of large cartons allow children to hide and promote imaginative play. They can be painted to look like a train or a zoo cage—great for the storage of stuffed animals. Tape recorders to play children's music are simple to operate and safer than record players. Colorful wall murals come in a variety of subjects and are not only attractive but also promote learning. Equipment for activities that require parental supervision can be kept out of reach in a closet. Riding toys should be stable and low to the ground. Provision should be made for safe climbing such as toy stairs or small wooden boxes in a step structure.

By creating an attractive and interesting play area for children, parents can reduce injury because children will tend to play in the area created for them. If at all possible, this area should be close to a part of the house where a parent spends the most time so the young children will not feel isolated and be tempted to wander into an unsafe area.

Safety Education: Additional Nursing Strategies Related to Specific Hazards

Burn Prevention In the early years children's motor abilities develop at a much faster rate than their ability to protect themselves and make judgments about safety. They rely on adults to keep their surroundings safe, depending chiefly on parental knowledge, attentiveness, and love. Most burn accidents are preventable. They occur in predictable patterns for each age group. In young children burns happen when there is a temporary lapse in parental attention or a lack of knowledge regarding growth and development. In older children there can be a lack of proper parental supervision along with a lack of knowledge, on the child's part, regarding the dangers of fire and flammable liquids.

House fires cause injury and death in all age groups, and it is important to plan with children what to do in case of fire, for example, escape routes, a common meeting place, how to crawl under smoke, and how to stop, drop, and roll if clothing ignites. The very young are vulnerable in house fires because they have neither the ability nor the knowledge to escape. They also might be innocent bystanders of another child's match play or the victim in a motor vehicle accident involving fire. All too often a youngster is found crouched under a bed or in a closet, badly injured or dead, when a clear escape route was available or a window handy nearby to call for help.

Adults do not supervise children in late childhood as closely as younger children and might unwisely assign tasks such as stoking a wood stove or filling a gasoline-powered lawn mower to children who are unable to do these jobs safely. Many burns result from the careless use of or experimentation with fires and flammable liquids, most commonly gasoline. Adults, as well as children, often do not understand the dangers of gasoline. Vapors ignite, and using a flammable liquid near open flames is very hazardous. Adults must demonstrate safe behavior such as storing gasoline only when absolutely necessary, using specified containers, using gasoline only in well-ventilated areas, pouring with a funnel to avoid splashes, and storing and using gasoline away from heat sources such as clothes dryers and water heaters. They must teach their children the common dangers around the home and neighborhood.

Electricity fascinates youngsters, particularly children in late childhood. Electrical wires high above the ground are not insulated, and it is not even necessary to touch them to receive a burn because electricity arcs. Boys, especially, might climb trees and utility poles or trespass in areas where there are high-voltage wires. Electrical burns from this source result in deep damage to muscle and bone, often necessitating amputation of an arm or leg.

Clothing design sometimes is associated with types of burns. Long, flowing nightgowns worn near fireplaces, space heaters, or while cooking are dangerous. Some states allow children to have access to firecrackers. Children need to know how to handle them properly to prevent accidental explosion and injuries to the hands or face.

Parents or teachers might turn to the school nurse for help when a child is consistently playing with matches. Individual counseling with families, using visual aids such as simple posters, films, and samples of burned clothing, is often sufficient to stop this behavior. However, a session with the family might reveal deeper problems such as a troubled marriage, disturbed parent–child relationship, or a history of repeated fire setting. On-going psychologic counseling might be necessary (see Chapter 2).

Nurses in primary care agencies must include burn prevention measures in their home intervention strategies for parents. Some important points include inspecting electrical appliances for frayed or dangling cords and exposed parts, checking for accessibility of matches, lighters, flammable liquids, and caustic household products, measuring tap water with a meat or candy thermometer, and turning water heaters to a low setting. Each floor of the house needs a smoke detector, and every family member should know fire escape plans. Local fire departments can help school and community nurses with home and school-based prevention projects. Educational materials are available for school nurses to present to children and parents. PTA meetings are a good forum. Project Burn Prevention and other agencies have filmstrips for children and adults that are designed to reach each age group. The burned clothing of children who played with matches can be a dramatic visual and tactile aid. Children as young as 3 and 4 years old can comprehend that the clothing did not protect the skin from burns. Nurses can learn more about children's perceptions by asking them to draw a picture after the film and by discussing the presentation. Older children often ask questions and share their own experiences. Information about first aid fits in well with burn prevention teaching. Practicing the stop, drop, and roll sequence for clothing ignition, rehearsing what to do in case of a house fire, and practicing

Resources for Teaching Burn Prevention

Project Burn Prevention
Education Development Center
55 Chapel Street
Newton, MA 02160
617-969-7100

US Consumer Product Safety Commission
Washington, DC 20207
Toll-free Hot Line—800-638-8326

The Office of Planning and Education
US Fire Administration
Washington, DC 20472

National Fire Protection Association
470 Atlantic Avenue
Boston, MA 02210

dousing "pretend" scalds with cool water gives children concrete behaviors to rehearse that will help them in an emergency.

Prevention of Drowning Children can be taught to swim and follow the rules of water safety by about 5 years of age. If appropriately instructed, children at even younger ages can be taught to remain afloat after an accidental fall into water until help arrives. Use of the survival float (face forward taking intermittent breaths) conserves energy and is an effective method of reducing the incidence of drowning. Children who live close to natural water or pools should be taught to swim at the earliest possible age. Rules for water safety should be given with swimming instruction.

Infant swim programs have their own advantages and disadvantages. Young infants can be taught to float, but they cannot be taught safety rules. Therefore, they should never be left near the water unsupervised.

Nurses can become involved in discussing water safety with parents and children. They should be knowledgeable about local facilities that provide swimming and water safety instruction. Camp nurses should assess the safety of the camp waterfront and the adequacy and competency of the lifeguards as they assess other aspects of camp safety. Rescue equipment is necessary at all recreational swimming areas.

Water safety rules that nurses should emphasize include always swimming with a buddy, accurately assessing swimming capabilities, knowing the water depth before diving, swimming in supervised areas, not swimming during electrical storms, avoiding swimming near diving boards or diving platforms, avoiding a reliance on buoyancy devices to boost swimming ability, knowing the basic, safe, rescue techniques, and calling for help only when needed (American Red Cross, 1981).

Motor Vehicle and Bicycle Accident Prevention Nurses should reinforce the statistics that validate the need for car seats to parents. Lists of safety-tested car seats are available to help parents choose alternatives. The expense of the car restraint system ($20–60) is minimal when compared with the costs of hospitalization for injuries. Parents, clubs, and community organizations often recycle car seats. Nurses need to know what resources their communities offer. Magazines offer a multitude of ideas to distract small children on long car trips. Stops every 2 hours allow children to stretch their muscles and unwind. Parents should insist on the use of seatbelts for all car occupants. Appropriately approved car restraint systems should be used for the child under 4 years of age or weighing less than 40 lb.

Developmentally, most 6-year-olds can balance a two-wheeler bike. Many schools and neighborhoods have bicycle safety programs. School-age children enjoy participating and receiving a certificate or special recognition while learning safety.

Rules for bicycle safety to reinforce with parents include the following:

1. Ride with traffic.
2. When riding at night, wear light-colored clothes and have a light and reflectors on the bike and clothing.
3. Look to both sides when changing lanes.
4. Yield when entering a roadway.
5. Obey traffic signals.
6. Use appropriate hand signals for turns.

Street Accident Prevention Children can be taught in developmental steps how to navigate traffic and to cross the streets. A 2-year-old can learn where to play and walk, that is, only in the yard and on sidewalks or grass. A 3-year-old can learn to listen for cars and be aware if they are coming or going. A 4-year-old can begin to learn to cross the street. When learning colors, a 5-year-old can learn about traffic signals. The American Automobile Association Early Childhood Traffic Bureau offers an excellent set of booklets reinforcing traffic rules for young children.

Parents need to set clear boundaries and rules for their children about crossing streets. They need to provide safe areas for children to play (especially in cities where children often play in the street). For young children, parents might make arrangements with other parents to cross children back and forth to friend's houses. They need to teach children safety habits for dealing with traffic, that is, learning to cross with the light, looking and listening before crossing, entering and leaving a car from the curbside, and not chasing a ball or toy into a street. Caution when entering or leaving school buses is also important to emphasize to children.

Prevention of Injury for the Handicapped Some mention already has been made of hazards for handicapped children. For children with hearing and vision handicaps, increased precautions around traffic are necessary. Parents can request special signs advising motorists to watch for deaf and blind children.

Children prone to seizures have 15% higher incidence to drowning. The sudden temperature change of cold water might trigger a seizure (Livingston, 1977). Children with other chronic diseases, especially asthma, cystic fibrosis, and diabetes mellitus, are advised to keep their bodies in maximum health through physical fitness and sports.

For parents, the patience required to teach handicapped children safety can be overwhelming. The nurse needs to be aware of local organizations and support groups for handicapped persons and their families. (Nursing care for the families and child with a chronic condition is discussed in Chapter 30.)

Health Protection Related to Childhood Injury Prevention

Society is extremely concerned about the health of children. Child health protection has been alluded to throughout this chapter in reference to specific federal and state legislation enacted to increase children's safety. The child car restraint legislation, the law regulating flameproofing of children's sleepwear, and the Child Protection and Toy Safety Act are examples of health protection measures to prevent injury. It is the responsibility of the nurse to keep abreast of new legislation regarding child safety and communicating the facts to parents and the community at large.

Secondary Prevention: The Nurse's Role

When a child becomes injured, the severity of the injury often is related to the promptness and effectiveness of the initial treatment. Nurses in a variety of settings might be called on to administer first aid to an injured child. Accurate assessment of the child's condition combined with knowledgeable first-aid measures can reduce the severity of an injury or even save a child's life. The major injury crises and the corresponding nursing actions are presented in Table 19-3 (beginning next page).

In summary, the nurse plays a vital role in the prevention of accidents and injury to children. Being aware of safety hazards and knowing how to alter them are crucial to the general health and well-being of all children.

Key Concepts

- The incidence of accidental injury can be reduced by the application of appropriate prevention strategies.
- Injury prevention, like illness prevention, can be analyzed within an epidemiologic framework.
- Nurses assess the characteristics of children, agents, and the environment that contribute to accident incidence.
- The characteristics of children that contribute to injury include curiosity, developmental level, sex, peer pressure, and handicapping conditions.
- The vectors of energy transfer include automobiles, bicycles, children as pedestrians, water, fire, toys, and infant furniture.
- Agents can be altered to prevent injury (for example, the use of child car restraint systems).
- Environmental characteristics that contribute to injury are parental inattention and fatigue, improper developmental expectations, family instability, cultural values, socioeconomic status, and physical surroundings.
- Environmental aspects can be changed to reduce injury potential (for example, improved athletic facilities and equipment for children).
- Nurses can influence the childhood accident rate through anticipatory guidance and parent/child safety education.
- Childproofing in a home means creating a safe living environment for children by preventing access to hazards.
- Burns can be prevented by educating children in schools and at home and by practicing how to react in a fire.
- Drownings can be prevented by strict attention to water safety rules.
- Vehicle injuries can be reduced by the use of seatbelts in automobiles and by knowledge and practice of bicycle safety measures.
- Children can be taught pedestrian safety according to their developmental level.
- Nurses need to be aware of health protection legislation and communicate the information to families and the community in general.
- Nurses can reduce the severity of injuries by accurate assessment and effective interventions using the principles of first aid.

TABLE 19-3 First-Aid Principles for Children

Category	Assessment criteria		Nursing interventions
Airway	Child not ventilating; cyanosis of lips and nail beds	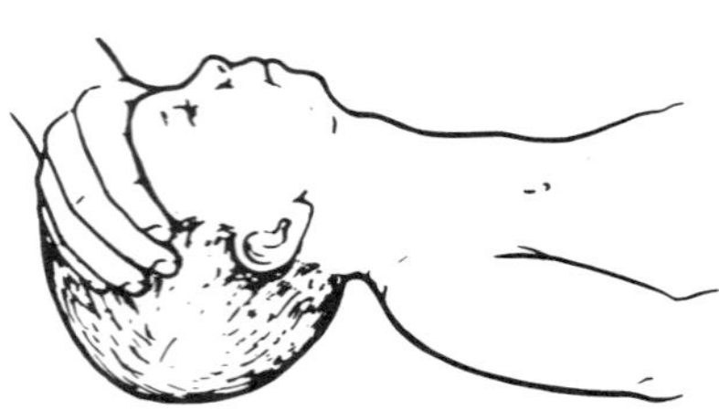 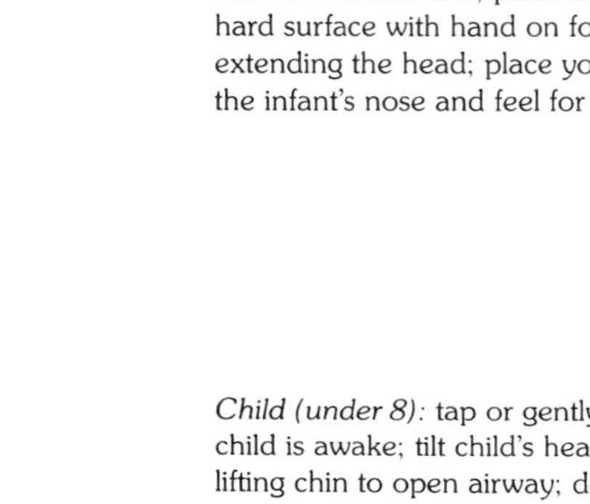	*Infants:* pinch baby's feet or gently flick the base of the sternum; place infant on a flat, hard surface with hand on forehead, gently extending the head; place your cheek near the infant's nose and feel for exhalation
		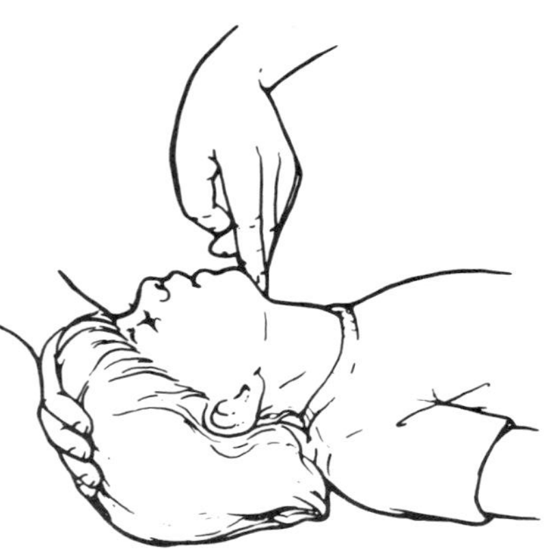	*Child (under 8):* tap or gently shake; ask if child is awake; tilt child's head back gently lifting chin to open airway; do this procedure on a flat, hard surface; observe for respiration *Child (over 8):* treat as for adult
Breathing	Child still not breathing after airway cleared	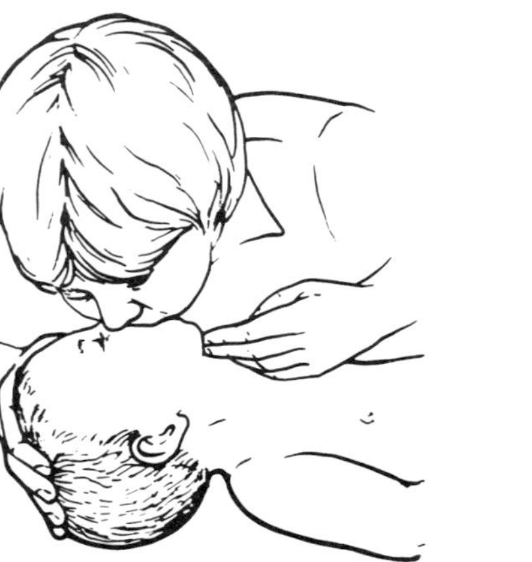	*Infant:* give four quick puffs of air using air in cheeks only; cover infant's mouth and nose with your mouth, creating a seal; check for the spontaneous resumption of breathing; if infant not breathing, check pulse at the inner aspect of elbow; if pulse is present, continue with breathing only *Rate:* one breath every 3 seconds, or 20 breaths/min

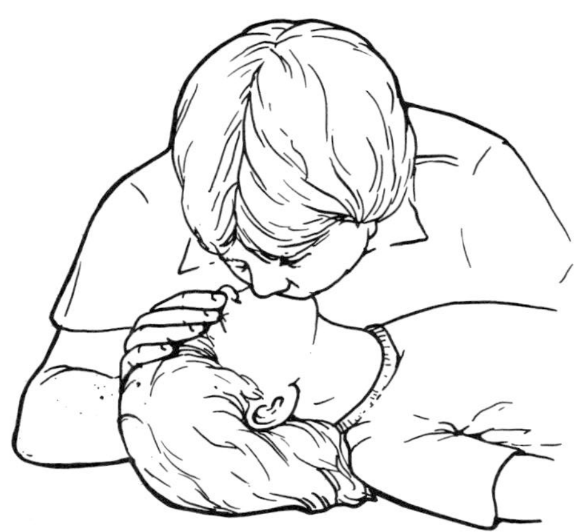

Child: give four breaths, enough to make the chest rise; pinch the nose and make a seal over the mouth only; allow for exhalation between breaths; check the carotid pulse for 5 seconds; if pulse is present but child is not breathing, continue respirations
Rate: one breath every 4 seconds, or 15 breaths/min (one breath every 5 seconds, or 12 breaths/min for child over 8 years of age)

NOTE: Check to make certain of chest rise and fall; avoid getting air into stomach

Circulation	Absent pulse; cyanosis		

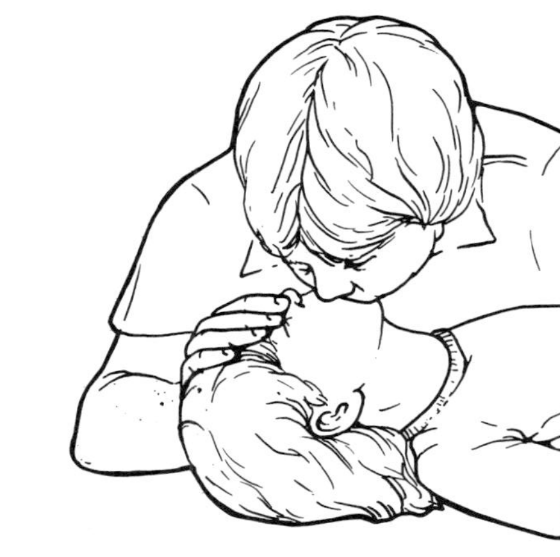

Infant: place index and middle fingers at a point halfway down the sternum; depress $\frac{1}{2}$ to $\frac{3}{4}''$ toward the backbone
Rate: 80–100 compressions/min; give one breath for every five compressions; check for the resumption of cardiac rate for 5 seconds after each minute of CPR; **do not stop CPR for more than 5 seconds**

Child: use the heel of one hand to compress sternum; depress 1 to $1\frac{1}{2}''$
Rate: 80–100 compressions/min; give one breath for every five compressions; stop periodically to check for the resumption of circulation but not for longer than 5 seconds

Older child: use two hands over lower portion of sternum for compressions; depress $1\frac{1}{2}$ to $2''$
Rate: 80 compressions/min; give two breaths after each 15 compressions; stop periodically to check for the resumption of circulation but for no longer than 5 seconds
Two-person rescue: 60 chest compressions with one breath after each five compressions

continued on next page

TABLE 19-3 continued

Category	Assessment criteria	Nursing interventions
Choking	Child appears distressed; unable to vocalize; cyanosis; older child will point to throat **NOTE:** if child is coughing and pink, WAIT and OBSERVE	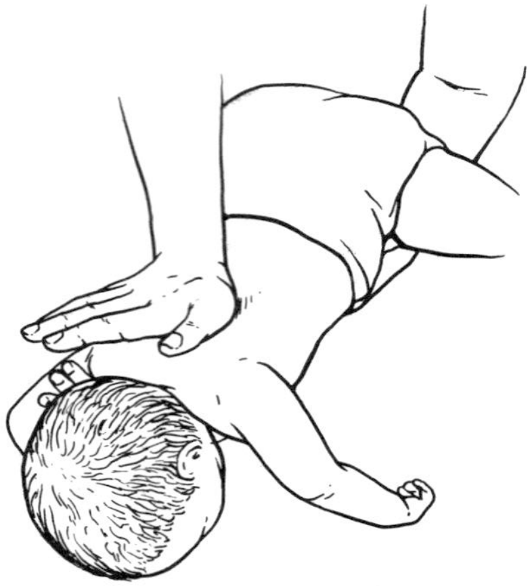 *Infant:* turn infant upside down and administer three back slaps between the scapula with the palm of the hand; if the object is not dislodged, turn the infant over and administer three chest compressions with index and middle fingers; continue alternating back blows with compressions until the object is dislodged *Child:* turn upside down or lean child forward bent from the waist to administer back blows; back blows should be adjusted to the child's size; follow back blows with chest compressions and alternate until object is dislodged
		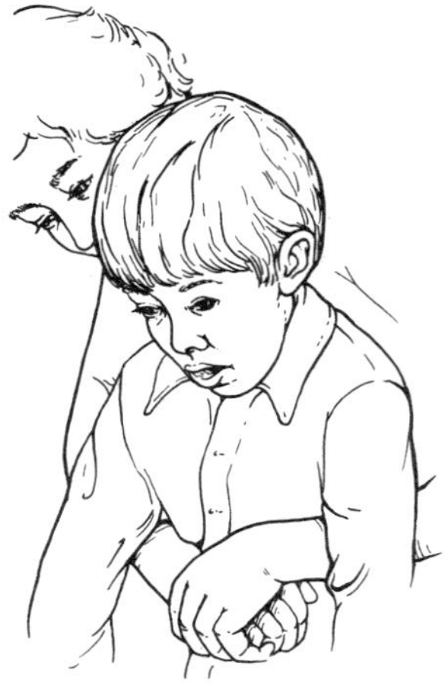 *Older child:* stand behind child, supporting chest with one hand and administering back blows with the other; if unsuccessful, reach both arms around the child halfway between the sternum and umbilicus; make a fist with one hand (thumb inside); cover with the other hand and administer four upward thrusts approximately 2 seconds apart; alternate with back blows until the object is dislodged **NOTE:** after object is dislodged, CPR might be necessary
Bleeding	Moderate bleeding from a wound	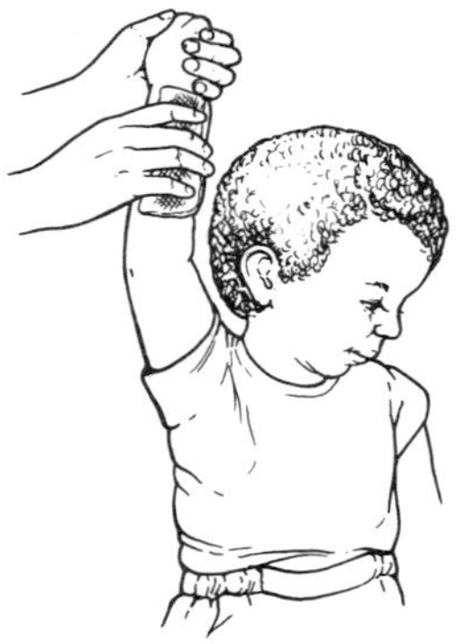 *Children of all ages:* cover the wound with a clean cloth or dressing and apply direct pressure with your hand over the dressing; if an extremity is affected, elevate it while applying the pressure; keep applying pressure for approximately 15 minutes *or* apply a pressure dressing with several layers of square pads held in place by gauze or other wrap; do not remove the dressing until medical advice has been obtained; if blood soaks through the dressing, add additional layers

	Severe bleeding from a wound that continues despite direct pressure and elevation; arterial bleeding; amputated limb	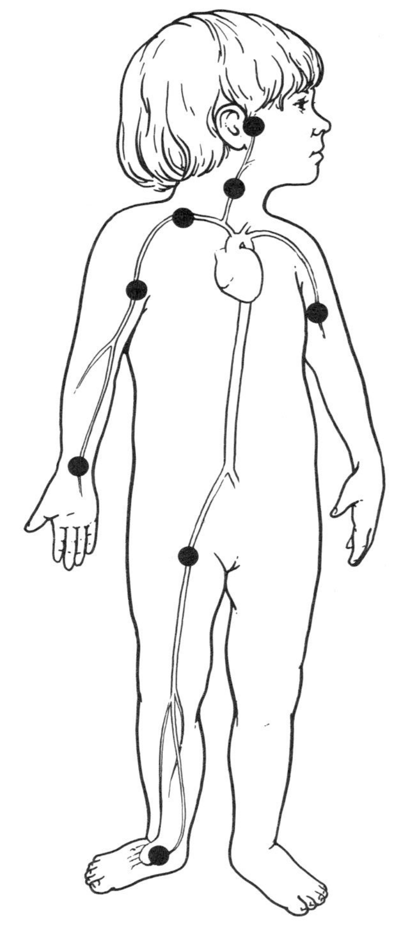	If direct pressure and elevation are unsuccessful in controlling bleeding, add pressure to pressure points with fingers and thumb; if the femoral artery is to be compressed, the heel of the hand should be used; treat for shock **NOTE:** do not use a tourniquet except as a last resort for bleeding that cannot be controlled by other methods
Head injuries	Unconsciousness; contusion on the head; projectile vomiting; headache; disorientation; alteration in pupil size and reaction; convulsions; drainage from nose or ears; tense fontanelle	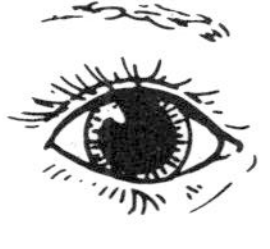 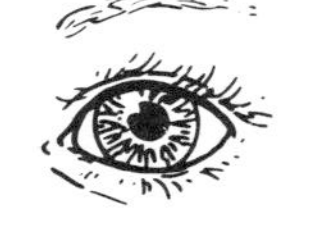	Differentiate unconsciousness from infant breath holding; apply ice to the contusion; allow the child to sleep but awaken at hourly intervals to check neurologic signs; encourage relaxation; head may be kept slightly elevated but never below level of the feet; seek medical consultation if there is a decrease in level of consciousness, convulsions, deterioration of neurologic signs, drainage from nose or ear, or bulging fontanelle

continued on next page

TABLE 19-3 continued

Category	Assessment criteria		Nursing interventions
Back and neck injury	Pain at site of injury; weakness, numbness, or paralysis below injury site; lack of movement in more than one extremity; decreased sensation in trunk or extremities	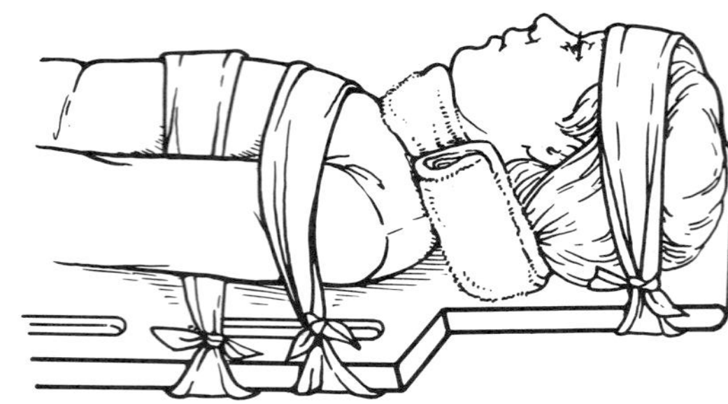 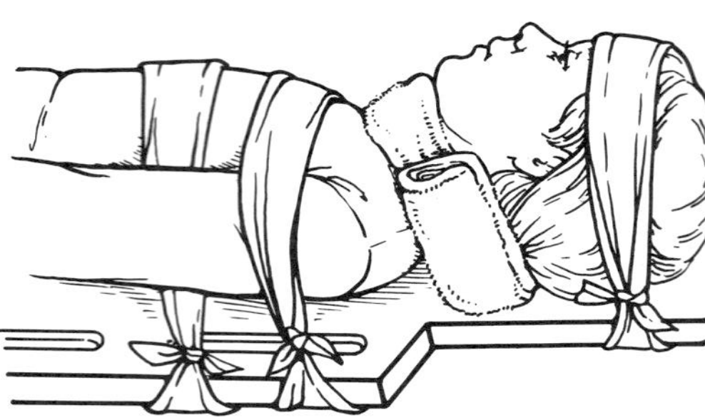	Prevent side-to-side movement of the child; preferably do not move; explain all actions to the child to ensure cooperation; if movement is necessary, the child should be secured to a firm, flat surface such as a backboard or door; pad the sides of the neck or head with rolled towels, newspapers, sneakers, etc to prevent movement; fasten the head to the board first, followed by the feet and the remainder of the body; enlist the help of several people to transfer the child to the board, so as to maintain rigid alignment; if the child is injured in the water, CPR might be necessary
Drowning	Child found floating just beneath the water or ice surface; cessation of respiration with associated cyanosis **NOTE:** time is a crucial factor; if resuscitation is initiated within the first 4 minutes of a drowning, sequelae from hypoxia will be reduced	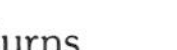	Inflate the child's lungs with four quick breaths, then remove from the water if possible; continue artificial respiration or CPR as previously described; the child might vomit; turn the head to the side to prevent aspiration; institute artificial respiration even if the length of time in water is unknown; children who have drowned are known to have been successfully resuscitated after long periods of submersion due to a reflex that traps oxygen in the body and slows down body processes; a child who has been revived needs immediate medical attention for the prevention and treatment of complications
Burns	Epidermis and part of dermis destroyed (partial thickness burns)—area is red, painful, edematous, and possibly blistered Dermal layer destroyed through subcutaneous fat (full-thickness burn)—area is pearly white, tan, brown, or black, not painful, tissue is dry Criteria for hospital admission: 1. Burns on children under 2 years of age unless minor and superficial 2. Electrical burns 3. Deep chemical burns 4. Burns complicated by fracture or soft tissue injury 5. Burns complicated by concurrent illness, eg, diabetes, renal disease, etc	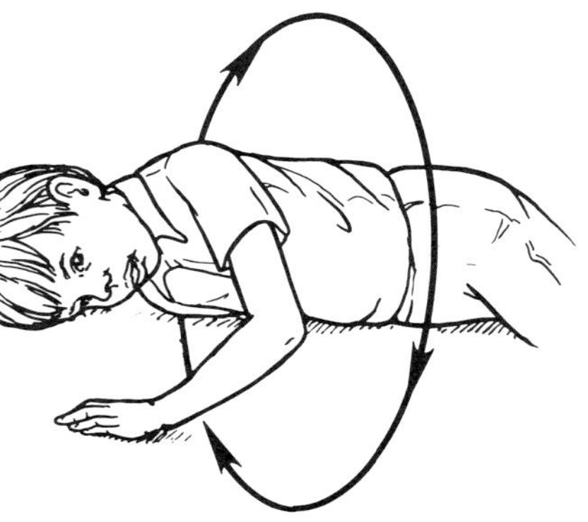	Stopping the burn process is the initial goal; smother flames by having the child do the stop, drop, and roll procedure or by wrapping the child in a blanket; douse clothing with cool water; cool down all burns from hot liquids; remove all non-adherent clothing; flush chemical burns with copious amounts of water for at least 20 minutes while en route to an emergency room; keep burned child warm because skin loss alters temperature-regulating mechanisms; if the burn is from an electrical current, switch off electricity before treating; initiate CPR as necessary and treat for shock

Frostbite	Skin will be white, hard, numb, and cold		Immerse affected area in tepid water for approximately 20 minutes or until signs of warmth return; child might experience excruciating pain in the area as it warms
Skeletal injuries	Edema, discoloration, pain, and/or alteration of movement at injury site; extreme tenderness to the touch; numbness and tingling; appearance of bone through the skin	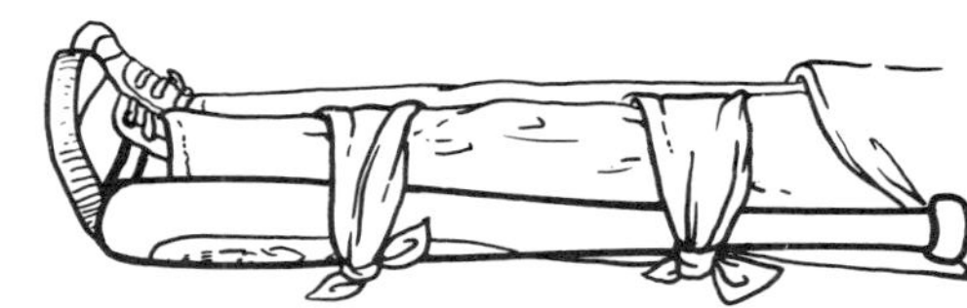	Radiography is the only method of accurately diagnosing a fracture; apply ice to the injury and elevate; if the bone protrudes, cover it with a sterile or clean dressing; immobilize joints above and below injury location by the use of splints and/or sling; folded newspapers or magazines, barrel slats, etc can be used as splints; tape an injured toe to the adjacent toes to immobilize; consult physician when fracture is suspected or in cases of severe tissue swelling
Eye injuries	Pain; watery eyes; conjunctivitis; visible object impaled in eye; blurred vision; light flashes or spots	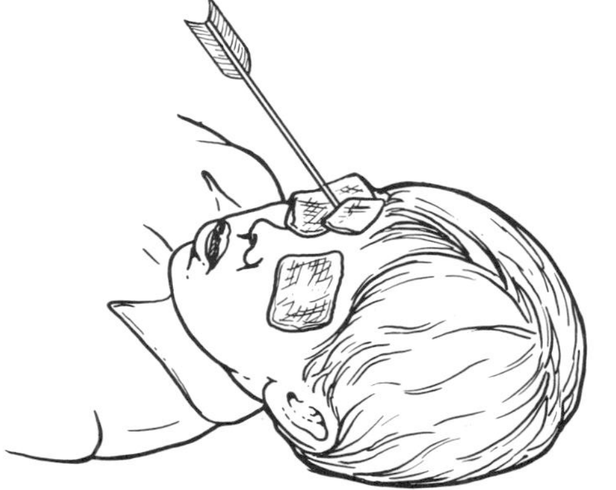	Check eye for small foreign particles by having the child look up and down; lids may be everted and the particle, if seen, removed with a saline-moistened cotton-tipped applicator; severe pain in the corneal area should be checked by an ophthalmologist; the eyes can be patched for comfort; small objects impaled in the cornea must be removed by a physician; large objects (such as an arrow, pencil, etc) should be stabilized by surrounding them with sterile gauze pads; the other eye also should be covered; explain all actions to the child to increase cooperation and decrease movement from resistance; transport child to emergency room with minimal movement; if the eye has sustained a direct blow, observe the child carefully for signs of severe pain, blurred vision, and other signs of internal injury; consult an ophthalmologist
Anaphylaxis	Generalized urticaria, bronchospasm, wheezing, laryngospasm, fainting, shock; history of recent exposure to an allergen—medication, insect sting, etc		If an insect sting, carefully remove stinger without rupturing the sac; apply a tourniquet proximal to a sting site but do not completely close off circulation; if epinephrine is available, administer 0.2 – 0.5 mL of 1:1000 strength subcutaneously or into a sting site; this may be repeated in 20 minutes; antihistamines such as diphenhydramine also can be administered; treat for shock **NOTE:** this is a life-threatening crisis requiring immediate medical attention.

References

American Automobile Association: Preschool children. In: *Traffic: Parents Guide for Action*. American Automobile Association, 1976.

American Medical Association: *Medical Evaluation of the Athlete, a Guide*. American Medical Association, 1977.

American Red Cross: *Swimming and Aquatics Safety*. The American National Red Cross, 1981.

Betz CL: Bicycle safety: Opportunities for family education. *Pediatr Nurs* (March/April) 1983; 9:101–111.

Blum A, Ames B: Flame-retardant additives are possible cancer hazards. *Science* 1977; 195:17–22.

Brown V: Providing a safe environment for children. *Matern Child Nurs J* (Jan/Feb) 1978; 3:53–55.

Consumer Reports. Welcome step toward preventing crib deaths. FDA standards for crib structure. *Consumer Reports* 1973; 38:437.

Consumer Reports. Motorized bikes and mopeds. *Consumer Reports* (May) 1981; 46:260–261.

Doege TC: An injury is no accident. *N Engl J Med* 1978; 298:509–510.

Feldman KW, et al: Tap water scalds in children. *Pediatrics* 1978; 62:1–7.

Feller I, et al: Assessing the impact of flammability standards. Presentation to the Twelfth Annual Meeting of the American Burn Association. San Antonio, Texas; 1980.

Halperin S, et al: Unintentional injuries among adolescents and young adults: A review and analysis. *J Adolesc Health Care* 1983; 4:275–281.

Livingston S: Epilepsy and drowning in childhood. *Br Med J* 1977; 2:515.

McLoughlin E, et al: One pediatric burn unit's experience with sleepwear-related injuries. *Pediatrics* (Oct) 1977; 60:405–409.

Pappas A: Children and sports. In: *Sports Health*. Southmayd W, Hoffman M (editors). Quick Fox, 1981.

Pomerantz J, Schultz D: Safe and sensible play-things. *Parents* 1982; 57:88.

Reinhard S: Nursing responsibility in infant car safety. *Matern Child Nurs J* (Jan/Feb) 1980; 5:64–65.

Righi F, Krozy R: The child in the car: What every nurse should know about safety. *Am J Nurs* (Oct) 1983; 83:1421–1434.

Rivara F: Epidemiology of childhood injuries. *Am J Dis Child* 1982; 136:399–405.

Schering Symposium on Sports Medicine. *Am J Sports Med* 1980; 5:370–384.

Southmayd W, Hoffman M (editors): *Sports Health*. Quick Fox, 1981.

US Consumer Product Safety Commission: *For Kids' Sake*. US Consumer Product Safety Commission No. CPSC-75-630-9.

US Department of Health and Human Services: *Monthly Vital Statistics Report*. Vol 32. Government Printing Office, 1983.

Welcome step toward preventing crib deaths. FDA standards for crib structure. *Consumer Rep* 1973; 38:437.

Additional Readings

National Safety Council: *Accident Facts*. National Safety Council, 1981.

Allen C: The female athlete. In: *Issues in Comprehensive Pediatric Nursing*. McGraw-Hill, 1980.

Austin G, Oliver JS, Richards JC: *The Parents' Medical Manual*. Prentice-Hall, 1978.

Baker SP: Motor vehicle occupant deaths in young children. *Pediatrics* 1979; 64:860–861.

Baker SP, Fisher RS: Childhood asphyxiation by aspiration or suffocation. *JAMA* 1980; 244:1343–1346.

Bass M: Asphyxial crib death. *N Eng J Med* 1977; 296:555–556.

Bass JL, Metha KA: Developmentally oriented safety surveys. *Clin Pediatr* 1980; 19:350–356.

Berger LR: Modern motor milestones. *Pediatrics* 1978; 62:1037–1038.

Berger LR, Rivara FP: Minibikes: A case study in under-regulation. *Business Soc Rev* (Summer) 1980; 34:41–43.

Carey RJ, et al: Sports trauma management and the high school nurse. *J School Health* 1982; 52(7):437–440.

Dershewitz RA: Home safety: Is anticipatory guidance effective? In: *Preventing Childhood Injuries. Twelfth Ross Roundtable on Critical Approaches to Pediatric Problems*. Ross Laboratories, 1982.

Dupont J: EENT emergencies. *Nursing* (Nov) 1979; 11:65–70.

Eflert H: Helping preschool children learn to be safe. *Can Nurse* 1979; 75(11):26–31.

Feck G, Baptiste MS: The epidemiology of burn injury in New York. *Public Health Rep* 1979; 94:312–318.

Feldman KW, Simms RJ: Strangulation in childhood: Epidemiology and clinical course. *Pediatrics* 1980; 65:1079–1085.

Healer C, et al: *Burn Injuries: Causes, Consequences, Knowledge, Behavior*. A Summary Report to the US Consumer Product Safety Commission. 1976.

Helfer RE, Slovis TL, Black M: Injuries resulting when small children fall out of bed. *Pediatrics* 1977; 60:533–535.

Hoffman-LaRoche: *Help for the Choking Victim*. Roche Health Care Guide No 2. Hoffman-LaRoche, 1980.

Hodgson C, Woodward CA, Feldman W: A descriptive study of school injuries in a Canadian region. *Pediatr Nurs* (May/June) 1984; 10(3): 215–220.

Hones D: *An Evaluation of the Effectiveness of Child-Resistant Packaging*. Office of Strategic Planning. US Consumer Product Safety Commission. April, 1978.

Johnson CJ, et al: Student injuries due to aggressive behavior in the Seattle public schools during the school year 1969–1970. *Am J Public Health* 1974; 164:904–906.

Miller M: Cycle trauma. *Nurs '80* (July) 1980; 10:26–31.

Nachem B, Bass RA: Children still aren't being buckled up. *Matern Child Nurs J* (Sep/Oct) 1984; 9:320–323.

Pearn JH, et al: Bathtub drownings: Report of seven cases. *Pediatrics* 1979; 64:68–70.

Pearn JH, et al: Drowning and near-drowning involving children: A five-year total population study from the city and county of Honolulu. *Am J Public Health* 1979; 69:450–454.

Peterson B: Morbidity of childhood near-drowning. *Pediatrics* 1977; 59:364.

Pless IB: Accident prevention and health education: Back to the drawing board? *Pediatrics* 1978; 62:431–435.

Rehm R: Teaching cardiopulmonary resuscitation to parents. *Matern Child Nurs J* (Nov/Dec) 1983; 8:411–414.

Reisinger KS: Smoke detectors: Reducing deaths and injuries due to fire. *Pediatrics* 1978; 62:280–287.

Robertson LS: Crash involvement of teenaged drivers when driver education is eliminated from high school. *Am J Public Health* 1980; 70:599–603.

Robertson LS, Zador PL: Driver education and fatal crash involvement of teenage drivers. *Am J Public Health* 1978; 68:959–965.

Scherz R: Fatal motor vehicle accidents of child passengers from birth through 4 years in Washington State. *Pediatrics* 1981; 68:572.

Schiller J: *Childhood Injury*. Stein & Day, 1977.

Sousa B: School emergencies—preparation not panic. *J School Health* 1982; 52(7):437–440.

Thorne B: A nurse helps prevent sports injuries. *Matern Child Nurs J* (July/Aug) 1982; 7:236–239.

Travis L, Schreiner B: Camps for children with diabetes: A philosophy and its application. *Diabetes Educator* (Spring) 1984; 10:13–20.

US Department of Transportation: *Child Restraint Systems for Your Automobile*. National Highway Traffic Safety Administration DOT HS-805-174. Jan 1980.

Prevention of Poisoning

20

Kathleen M. Wruk
Nancy Houlder
Carolyn Clayton Cahn
Sandra K. Spiller

Chapter Outline

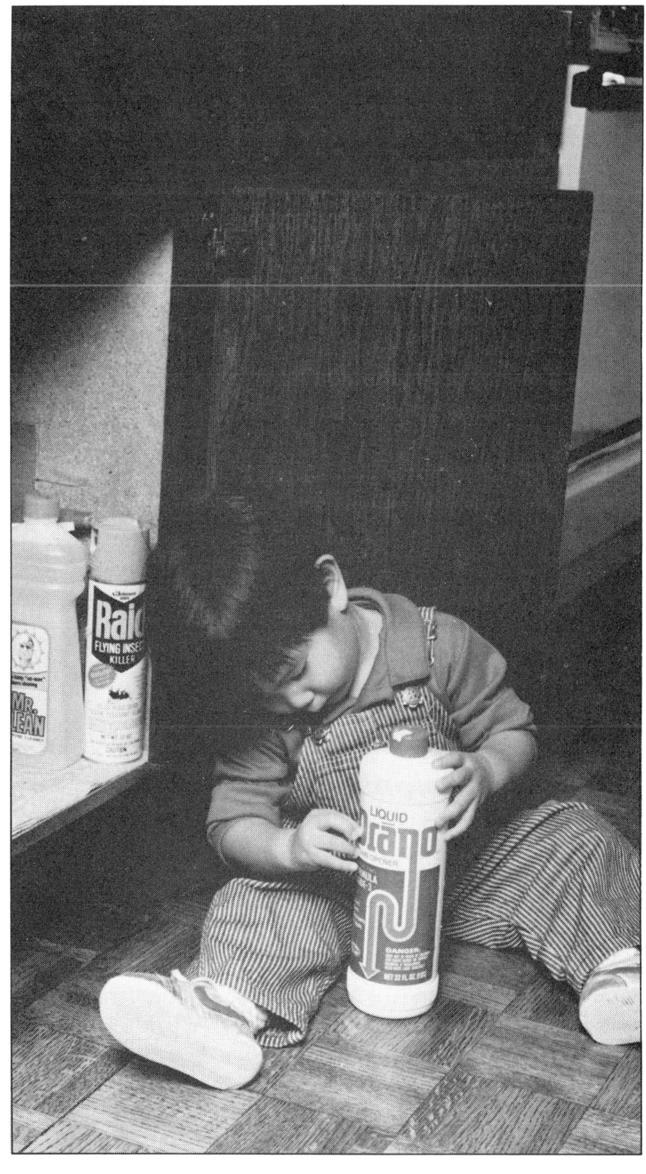

continued on next page

Caffeine
Ethanol
Ethylene Glycol
Methanol
Tetrahydrozoline
Camphor
Sedative Hypnotics
Opiates
Cyclic Antidepressants
Lomotil

Objectives

- List the factors predisposing to accidental poisoning, including the characteristics of the child, the agent, and the environment.
- Explain the characteristics of children that contribute to accidental poisoning such as their exploratory nature and knowledge deficits.
- Enumerate the characteristics of poison agents, including those most commonly found around the home.
- List the environmental factors existing in the home, the outdoors, and the schools that contribute to accidental poisoning.
- Explain the nurse's role in parent education for the prevention of childhood poisoning.
- Describe the general first-aid measures nurses should teach parents to use in the event of a poisoning.
- Explain the nurse's role in the assessment and management of the acutely poisoned child.
- Describe the facets of the nursing care of children poisoned by specific agents.

Factors Predisposing to Accidental Poisoning

Accidental poisoning occurs in an estimated 2 million children in the United States each year. Poisoning is the most common nontraumatic pediatric emergency. It accounts for 10% of all ambulance responses, 9% of all emergency room visits, and 5%–10% of all medical admissions (Micik, 1978). The most common form of poisoning is oral ingestion, but toxicity also can result from eye exposure, inhalation, topical exposure, and envenomation. The Poison Prevention Packaging Act of 1970 is a major health protection measure that has reduced the incidence of poisonings from prescription drugs by requiring the use of child resistant covers for prescription medication containers (Jacobi, 1983).

Primary Prevention: The Nurse's Role

Nursing Assessment of the Child

Exploratory Nature of Young Children Accidental poisoning occurs most frequently in children under 5 years of age (Fig. 20-1). These children are in developmental stages in which they are actively exploring and learning about their environment (see Chapters 7 and 8.) Children 2 years of age and under explore with all of their senses. They touch with their fingers, look with their eyes, and taste and feel with their mouths. Unfortunately, this characteristic can lead to accidental poisoning. Some of the first poisons encountered in the environment of a crawling child are plants. Children under 1 year of age are attracted to the patterns and shapes of the leaves and often put them into their mouths. Even mild exposure of this type to plants such as *Dieffenbachia* can cause painful blistering and swelling of the mucous membranes in the mouth.

Crawling children can find such products as drain cleaners and dishwasher detergents stored under the kitchen sink. Small amounts of these products in the mouth can cause tragic mouth and esophageal burns. Rat poisons and baits left on closet floors or behind furniture attract curious youngsters.

As the child's mobility, ingenuity, and capabilities increase so does the risk of poisoning. When children are able to stand and walk, they can find medications on the bedside table or in a purse or furniture polish on low shelves. When they start to climb, a whole new world invites their exploration. They can now reach the medicine cabinet with its rich supply of bottles and pills. They can use a chair to reach the perfumes and after-shave lotions on the dresser

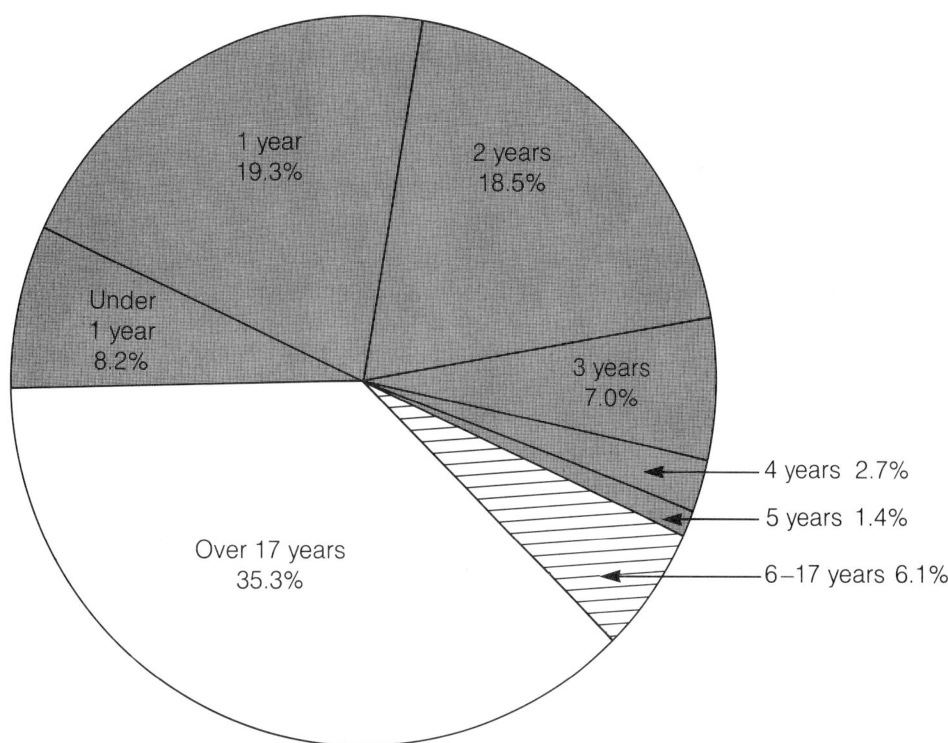

Figure 20-1 Incidence of poisoning, by age of victim.

and the aspirin by the kitchen sink. In their attempt to understand the world, children try to imitate their parents' use of these products. Lacking any concept of toxicity, they often will taste the sweet-smelling liquids and pretty-colored pills.

In rare cases young children have a condition called *pica*. Pica is manifested by a compulsion to ingest unusual substances such as dirt, matches, paint, and newspapers. Children with this condition do not merely put these substances in their mouths but actually swallow them. Pica seems to be related more to an emotional than a nutritional deficit, although many children with pica exhibit signs of nutritional deficiencies. Children with pica often manifest signs of lead poisoning.

After 3 years of age, the incidence of poisoning decreases, reflecting a higher level of cognitive understanding of potential danger. Children still can be poisoned accidentally by dangers they are unaware of such as gasoline stored in empty soda pop bottles in the garage or sweet-tasting, cartoon-character–shaped, chewable multivitamins with iron.

Knowledge Deficit in Children Regarding Poisonous Substances Children in middle and late childhood are most apt to be poisoned accidentally by materials used in play or craft activities. Pretend tea parties with unknown poisonous berries have resulted in emergency room visits. A particularly tragic form of poisoning can occur because of the tendency in this age group toward magical thinking about medicine. Children often conclude that if one pill is good, more would be better. One tragic example of this type of poisoning occurred when an $8\frac{1}{2}$-year-old boy awoke after having wet his bed and took a handful of his enuresis medication. His parents found him unconscious the next morning, and he died 12 hours after admission to the hospital (Herson, Schmitt, and Rumack, 1979).

Knowledge Deficit Regarding Drugs Adolescents are exposed to an increasingly complex and readily available supply of psychoactive drugs (see Chapter 24.) In one large study of high school seniors (Johnston, Bachman, and O'Malley, 1981), between six and seven out of every ten students (65%) reported illicit drug use some time in their lives. In addition to the magnitude of potential health problems associated with experimentation and abuse of drugs, the possibility of poisoning exists because of the total lack of quality control in their manufacture and sale. Street drugs often do not contain what they are alleged to contain. The results of a street drug pharmacologic analysis (Anonymous, 1979) revealed that only 50.6% of street samples submitted contained the same drug as alleged, 24.2% contained the alleged drug plus other drugs, and 20% contained entirely different drugs. Poisoning occurs when these drugs are taken and unexpected and dangerous effects are experienced.

Nursing Assessment of the Poison Agent

Modern society offers an almost limitless potential for toxic exposure. Over 58,000 chemical substances are manufactured, imported, or processed for commercial purposes in the United States (Environmental Protection Agency, 1982). These chemicals are combined into hundreds of thousands of products for use in industry and the home. Household cleansers, disinfectants, dishwasher detergents, pesticides, automotive supplies, art and hobby supplies, and perfumes are among the many common household products that can be toxic if used improperly.

A wide variety of pharmacologic compounds are found commonly in home medicine cabinets. Sales in the United States of over-the-counter drugs bring in $13 billion per year, and sales of prescription drugs bring in almost $8 billion per year (Wiemer, et al., 1979). Many of these medications are flavored and brightly colored, resembling candy. Adults often are unfamiliar with pediatric dosages, and chronic poisoning can occur if a child is given a slightly high dose over a period of several days. Poisoning also can occur if a child is given medication prescribed for another family member. Illegally manufactured psychoactive drugs are increasingly accessible to adolescents and in some cases younger children.

Not all poisons are manufactured by humans. Poisoning from food sources has been a concern since the beginning of recorded history (Temple and Mancini, 1980). Bites or stings from some insects, spiders, and snakes can cause serious illness. Many trees, plants, and mushrooms contain toxic compounds. The increase in the popularity of houseplants is reflected by a substantial increase in the number of accidental poisonings from plants.

TABLE 20-1 Substances Most Frequently Ingested by Children Under 5 Years of Age Reported by Poison Control Centers in 1978

Type of substance	Percentage
Plants	11.7
Soaps, detergents, and cleaners	6.2
Antihistamines and cold medications	4.3
Perfume, cologne, and toilet water	4.0
Vitamins, minerals	3.9
Aspirin	3.8
Children's	2.7
Adult	0.5

Adapted from *National Clearinghouse for Poison Control Centers Bulletin.* 1980; 24(10).

Nursing Assessment of Environmental Factors

Household The majority of accidental childhood poisonings occur in the home and involve common household products (Table 20-1). The majority of poisonings involving soaps, detergents, and related household products occur while these products are being used (Giles, 1980). Many poisonings occur when the substances are not in their original containers. The kitchen is the most frequent site for poisoning in the home, followed by the bathroom and bedroom.

Outdoors The backyard and surrounding neighborhood, with its abundance of plants, insects, pesticides, and mushrooms, is also a common site for poisoning. When children visit the home of adults without small children, they are likely to be exposed to conditions that invite accidents. Grandparents' medications frequently are left on bedside tables or by kitchen sinks. They often are taken out of their original containers for ease of administration. Relatives or adult friends without small children might not be aware of the dangers present under their sink or in their closets.

Schools Child-care centers and schools, although often careful to follow poison prevention guidelines, can be the sites of poisoning when the curiosity and inventiveness of the child override safety precautions. For example, children have been poisoned by eating berries and leaves intended for use in art collages.

Relationship to Family Parents can act as buffers preventing the curious, active, exploring child from contact with the dangers present in the environment. They can take concrete steps to limit the contact between the child and the environmental dangers. They can "poison proof" the home by storing household products and medications in areas inaccessible to the child. They can provide education through discussion and by showing the proper ways to handle dangerous materials. They can monitor a child's activities in the neighborhood and be alert to potential problems when the child visits other homes.

Poisoning occurs when the young child comes into unsupervised contact with poisonous substances. This may occur because the parents are unaware of the dangers, have not safely stored toxic products, or have not provided adequate supervision. All parents are subject to influences that can limit their effectiveness. These influences include situational, emotional, and social stresses. In some cases accidental childhood poisoning seems to be more related to parental problems and disturbed family relationships than to home safety (Sobel, 1970). When parents are under stress, they are less able to act as vigilant and effective supervisors, and the child is more likely to come into contact with the dangers in the environment.

Situational factors that demand a parent's attention can play a role in accidental poisoning. Minor events such as a ringing telephone can call a mother away as she is doing the wash and leave a toddler alone to explore the bottles of bleach and detergent. Temporary situational stresses, such as an overflowing washing machine in the laundry room or a flat tire in the garage, can expose a child to an otherwise inaccessible environment at a time when the parent's attention is focused elsewhere. More prolonged stressful situations include vacations, moving, or guests in the home.

An illness in the family can limit a parent's supervisory effectiveness. For example, it is more difficult for a parent who has been up all night with a sick baby to effectively monitor a slightly jealous 3-year-old child who is intent on tasting some of baby's pretty orange medicine.

Social and emotional stressors such as unemployment or divorce can diminish the parents' emotional energy and limit their ability to adequately supervise their child. This decreased supervision coupled with the child's increased need for attention during these crises can result in poisoning.

TABLE 20-2 Poison Prevention Education

Well-child visit	Items to be discussed with parents
1 month	Dosing—vitamins/iron
2 months	Dosing—antipyretics
4 months	Dosing—cold products
6 months	Products up/storage
9 months	Ipecac/what to do in case of a poisoning
1 year	Ipecac follow-up
$1\frac{1}{2}$ years	Child-resistant locks/storage
2 years	Child-resistant packaging
3 years	Poison symbols/poison patrols
4 years	Preschool education programs
5–12 years	School education programs

SOURCE: From Gillies, et al: Management of pediatric poisoning: Role of the nurse practitioner. *Pediatric Nursing* (Sept/Oct) 1980:6:33–35.

Principles of Nursing Management—Primary Level of Prevention

Education to Prevent Poisonings Nursing management of accidental poisoning begins with education. Nursing activities are directed toward increasing the parents' awareness and encouraging practices that decrease the chances of accidental poisoning. The discussion of poisoning should be a routine part of well-child visits (Table 20-2). Early visits can be used to familiarize parents with the therapeutic use of drugs. The correct dosages of common over-the-counter medications and the danger of overusing medications or saving and sharing medications within the family should be reviewed.

Parents need to be informed of the dangers present in the environment and the developmental characteristics of young children that make them susceptible to these toxic hazards. They should be encouraged to go through their home room by room, on their hands and knees at the child's level if necessary, and remove and safely store all potential toxins. Parents should be given a list of poisonous plants (Table 20-3) and encouraged to identify and in many cases remove all toxic plants from their home and garden. Parents must be helped to make home safety so automatic that even in times of stress their ability to protect their child will not be decreased.

The principles of poison safety should be reviewed. Most poison control centers provide educational materials on request—for example, the Mr. Yuk sticker program. In addition, various materials are available to professionals and parents at a low cost.

Poison prevention discussion should be included in a child's annual physical examination at least until the child is 5 years of age. Discussion with the child and parent can help to assess the level of understanding and degree of compliance with the suggested actions and identify areas where further teaching is required. Assessment of the family might indicate situational or stress-related factors that may increase the chances of a poisoning accident. These factors and their relationship to poisoning can then be discussed. As the child enters adolescence, a frank discussion of the problems associated with experimentation with drugs is indicated.

Education to Prepare Parents to Handle a Poisoning Accident In spite of the most conscientious program of home safety, accidental poisoning can still occur. It is vital that the nurse help prepare the parent for such an emergency. It is a terrifying experience for parents to walk into a room and discover that their child has eaten all of the children's aspirin or tasted the bleach. The nurse can help by encouraging parents to develop a plan of action before such an incident occurs.

Parents need to be alert for the signs of accidental poisoning. The most obvious indicators would be presence of poisonous items such as pills, mothballs, or plant parts in the child's hand, mouth, or in the play area. Burns, blisters, or odor around the mouth are possible signs of ingestion. Open, empty containers in the child's possession are another cause for investigation.

Less obvious signs of poisoning occur as the child begins to develop symptoms. These symptoms might include:

1. Sudden alteration in level of consciousness—sleepiness, dizziness, atonia, convulsions, coma.
2. Alterations in the rate and quality of respirations, leading to signs of respiratory distress.
3. Sudden onset of severe vomiting and diarrhea (Schiller, 1977).

TABLE 20-3 Common Poisonous Plants

Houseplants

Common name	Botanic name	Poisonous part
Boston ivy	*Parthenocissus quinquefolia*	All parts
Caladium	*Caladium*	All parts
Dumbcane	*Dieffenbachia*	All parts
Emerald duke	*Philodendron hastatum*	All parts
English ivy	*Hedera helix*	Leaves, berries
Parlor ivy	*Philodendron cordatum*	All parts
Split leaf philodendron	*Monstera deliciosa*	All parts
Umbrella plant	*Cyperus alternifolius*	All parts

Outdoor plants

Common name	Botanic name	Poisonous part
Apricot	*Prunus armeniaca*	Stem, bark, seed pits
Azalea	*Rhodendron occidentale*	All parts
Castor bean	*Ricinus communis*	Seeds, if chewed
Chokecherry	*Prunus virginiana*	Leaves, seed pits, stems, bark
Daffodil	*Narcissus*	Bulbs
Foxglove	*Digitalis purpurea*	Leaves, seeds, flowers
Hemlock (false parsley, snake root)	*Conium maculatum*	All parts, root, and root stalk
Hens-and-chicks	*Lantana*	All parts
Hydrangea	*Hydrangea macrophylla*	Leaves, buds
Jimsonweed	*Datura stramonium*	All parts
Jonquil	*Narcissus*	Bulbs
Lily of the valley	*Convallaria majalis*	All parts
Mistletoe	*Phoradendron flavescens*	Berries
Morning glory	*Ipomoea violaces*	Seeds
Nightshade	*Atropa belladonna*	All parts
Oleander	*Nerium oleander*	All parts, including dried leaves
Rhododendron	*Rhododendron*	All parts
Rhubarb	*Rheum raponticum*	Leaves
Sweet pea	*Lathyrus odoratus*	Seeds, pods
Tulip	*Tulipa*	Bulbs
Wisteria	*Wisteria*	Seeds, pods

SOURCE: Adapted from San Francisco Bay Area Regional Poison Center: *Poisonous and Non-Poisonous Plant List.* San Francisco Bay Area Regional Poison Center. 1979.

The phone number of the poison control center, the ambulance rescue squad, and the family physician should be kept in plain sight by the telephone. The parents should be encouraged to decide ahead of time which hospital they would go to and the shortest route to take. Parents should become familiar with the principles of first-aid management for poisoning, and a copy of the emergency guidelines should be posted in a medicine cabinet or on a closet door.

Every home in which small children live or regularly visit should have a 1-oz bottle of syrup of ipecac for each child under 5 years of age (see the section entitled "Gastric Emptying" in this chapter). Parents should be instructed to use syrup of ipecac only on the advice of a poison control center or physician. The nurse should remind parents to check the ipecac regularly for expiration date. Because it is used so infrequently, this might be overlooked.

There is no universal antidote. Contrary to popular belief, most poisons do not have antidotes. Alleged antidotes such as tea and burnt toast are useless. The use of home remedies to induce vomiting, such as saltwater, mustard water, or a finger down the throat, are ineffective, often harmful, and cause dangerous delays in seeking effective treatment. Antidotes and first-aid information on product labels are often incorrect and sometimes dangerous. Parents should be instructed to always call the poison control center or their physician as soon as the exposure is discovered and before administering any antidote or emetic, including syrup of ipecac. If they are unsure if the exposure is dangerous, they should not wait for symptoms to appear but call for assistance immediately.

When a poisoning has occurred, parents often feel extremely guilty. They need support and understanding from the nurse. Their correct actions, such as calling for professional help immediately, should be praised. They have now seen firsthand how easily a poisoning accident can occur and are usually eager for help in preventing its recurrence.

Safety Guidelines

1. Keep all household products out of the reach of young children when not in use. When these products are in use, they should never be out of sight of adults—even if it means taking them along when answering the telephone or the doorbell.
2. Choose cleaning supplies with childproof or hard-to-open containers. Containers should be rinsed prior to discarding.
3. Items should be kept in their original containers. They should never be stored in food containers or soft-drink bottles.
4. All products should be properly labeled, and one should read the label before using.
5. Don't save medicine. Leftover medications should be discarded by flushing them down the toilet. Current medications should be stored separately from other household products, preferably locked up. Metal boxes with locks commonly used to store checks are difficult for a child to open and can be used effectively to store medications.
6. Return medication to safe storage immediately after using. Never leave any medication (including vitamins or aspirin) by the sink or on the dining table.
7. The light always should be on when giving or taking medications.
8. Adults should avoid taking medications in front of children because youngsters tend to imitate adults.
9. Medications should be referred to as "medicine" and never as "candy."
10. Safety packaging should be used properly and closed securely after use.
11. Ask the nursery for the botanic name of any new plant purchased and record it. Avoid planting or placing poisonous plants in areas easily accessible to young children. Alert family where potentially poisonous plants are already planted and supervise children carefully when they are in those areas.

Many poison control centers send poison information to callers as a way of following up on this concern. Nurses who come into contact with parents in an acute care hospital or during a follow-up appointment should discuss the poisoning with the parents, looking for the factors that influenced the incident and working together on a plan to prevent its recurrence. There are occasions when the poisoning accident might signal the presence of more serious family problems. Nurses should be alert to this possibility and be ready to make the proper referral if their assessment indicates further action is needed.

Secondary Prevention: The Nurse's Role

Nursing Assessment of the Acutely Poisoned Child

Nurses might be dealing with poisoned children in an ambulatory setting or emergency room, or they may be giving information as members of a poison control center team. As in any other aspect of nursing care, care of the child who is the victim of an accidental poisoning begins with a thorough assessment. Time is often a crucial factor; therefore, the nurse must be skilled in obtaining the maximum amount of information in a minimum amount of time.

History When a suspected poisoning occurs, it is essential for the nurse to obtain a good history. Nurses in doctors' offices, emergency departments, and poison control centers are often called by parents of children who have been exposed to poisons. Whether it is a minor ingestion or a serious emergency, the nurse must obtain certain basic information. In cases where the poisoning is severe or potentially severe, the patient's address is important so that emergency equipment can be dispatched. In less critical situations the patient's name and telephone number must be obtained so that follow-up calls can be made if the patient is to be treated at home.

Basic Information Specific initial information should include the exact name of the product, when the exposure occurred, the approximate amount involved, route of the exposure, evidence of exposure, current symptoms, and age, weight, and gender of the patient. The caller should be asked if any treatment already has been instituted. Some treatments that used to be common can be more dangerous than the poison such as neutralization and gagging with a finger down the throat.

Age and weight are necessary to assess the potential severity of an exposure. Knowledge of age-related differences in drug effects or metabolism and the amount of the exposure on a weight basis (that is, milligrams of drug ingested per kilogram of body weight) are necessary to manage the potentially poisoned patient appropriately. Close approximation of weight is especially important in dealing with children.

An initial assessment can be made whether life is in immediate danger, potential danger, or no danger.

Secondary Information Further information might be needed before the final assessment and treatment plan are established. A secondary history should clarify the amounts involved, for example, counting pills and verifying the amount originally in the container. Other medication/

Selected Materials on Poison Prevention

We Want You to Know About Preventing Childhood Poisonings
(Three-fold leaflet, 3½" × 8¼", explaining some of the hazards of accidental poisonings and ways to prevent such accidents. Tells how to get help if a child is poisoned. Available in either English or Spanish.)

Limited quantities available from U.S. Food and Drug Administration, HFE-88, 5600 Fishers Lane, Rockville, MD 20857.

Home Safe Home
(Tips for parents on how to protect young children in the home environment. Spanish versions available.)

Up to 100 copies free. Ask for information on larger orders. The Soap and Detergent Association, 475 Park Avenue South at 32nd Street, New York, NY 10016.

Home Poisons (193.10)
(A 4-page, 3½" × 6½" leaflet containing basic information on steps to take to prevent home poisonings.)

Limited quantities. 50-499, 6.5 cents each; 500-999, 5.3 cents each; 1000-4999, 4.3 cents each. National Safety Council, 444 N. Michigan Avenue, Chicago, IL 60611.

Poison Perils in the Home (599.75)
(A 12-page, 4" × 6" booklet takes readers from room to room in their homes pointing out everyday household products that might be deadly poisons.)

50-499, 14.1 cents each; 500-999, 11.3 cents each; 1000-4999, 10 cents each. National Safety Council, 444 North Michigan Avenue, Chicago, IL 60611.

A General Approach to the Emergency Management of Poisonings
(A large wall chart displaying poisoning information as it relates to: clinical evaluation; coma; cardiac arrythmia; metabolic acidosis; seizures; gastrointestinal disturbance; elimination of poison from GI tract, skin, and eyes; elimination of absorbed substances and supportive therapy; and antidotes. Written for medical, nursing, and allied health personnel.)

$5.00 per copy. American College of Emergency Physicians, P.O. Box 61911, Dallas, TX 75261. (Payment must accompany all orders.)

First Aid for Poisoning
(An 8½" × 11" two-color flyer/poster. ARC Stock No. 320800.)

Limited quantities available through local Red Cross chapters. Larger quantities available at nominal cost.

Solid and Liquid Poisons (429.04-21)
(A 6-page data sheet containing practical information on poisons in and around the home, pointing out special dangers to children.)

10-99, 38 cents each; 100-999, 34 cents each; 1000-4999, 33 cents each. National Safety Council, 44 N. Michigan Avenue, Chicago, IL 60611.

Common Poisonous and Injurious Plants
(Information on what to do when a child has ingested parts of a plant.)

Produced by Food and Drug Administration. Up to 15 copies free. For bulk orders, Superintendent of Documents, Government Printing Office, Washington, D.C. 20402. $2.75 charge per copy.

Plants that Poison
(An illustrated chart of common poisonous plants indicating size, toxic parts, and symptoms of poisoning. Contains information on preventing plant poisoning and emergency measures.)

Single copy and quantity price list free. Send self-addressed, stamped business envelope to: The Kalamazoo Poison Prevention Council, P.O. Box 2261, Kalamazoo, MI 49003.

Emergency Action for Poisoning
(3½" × 8½" card outlining the first aid steps to take in the event of a poisoning. Produced in conjunction with the American College of Emergency Physicians.)

Up to 5 copies available free. Reproduction proof for local printing available for $5.00. American Association of Poison Control Centers. c/o Dr. A. Manoguerra, University of California Medical Center, Regional Poison Center, 225 Dickinson St., San Diego, CA 92103. Regional and local poison centers have other informational material available on request.

SOURCE: From the National Poison Prevention Week—List of Materials, March 20–26, 1983. Reprinted with permission of the Poison Prevention Week Council, Washington, D.C.

General First-Aid Principles for Parents

Immediately after the exposure has been discovered:

1. Check to be sure that the poisoned child is breathing and has a heartbeat. If not, start cardiopulmonary resuscitation. Call the fire department rescue squad or ambulance.
2. If the poison is *in the eye,* flush the eyes with lukewarm tap water poured from a cup or pitcher for at least 15 minutes. Do not use anything but water in the eye before talking to your poison control center or physician.
3. If the poison has been spilled *on the skin* or clothing, remove the clothing and flood the involved area with water. Then wash with soapy water and rinse. Call your doctor or poison control center.
4. If gas, fumes, or smoke have been *inhaled,* move the victim to fresh air as quickly as possible. Call your poison control center or physician.
5. If the poison has been *swallowed,* call your poison control center or physician immediately. Be prepared to give the exact name of the substance from the container and the details of the exposure. Estimate how much was taken and how long ago. Give the age of the victim. Look carefully for any symptoms and describe them. Save the container and any material that the child vomits.
6. Do not attempt to give anything to a victim who is unconscious or having convulsions. Call the fire department rescue squad or ambulance.
7. Do not make a person vomit unless instructed to do so by a poison control center or physician. Follow the instructions carefully and use only syrup of ipecac.

Poison Control Centers

The first poison information center was established in Chicago in 1953. During the next 20 years, the poison control center movement grew rapidly, and in 1980 there were 466 active poison control centers known to the National Clearinghouse for Poison Control Centers (Schaeffer and Lavengood, 1982).

At present, the trend is toward the consolidation of manpower and other resources from small, local centers into large, regionalized poison control centers. These regional centers are staffed with nurses and/or pharmacists who have advanced training in the recognition and management of toxicologic emergencies. They provide telephone management and follow-up for patients at home and referral and consultation services for the hospital treatment of critically poisoned patients. Most regional poison control centers are open 24 hours per day, 365 days per year and answer calls from the public and health professionals.

Most poison control centers offer poison prevention education activities for the public, including pamphlets and booklets, slide shows, special school programs, speaker's bureau, and poison warning labels. Many regional centers provide education on the recognition and management of poisoning for the region's physicians, nurses, and allied health personnel.

products included in the exposure should be ruled out. The patient's past medical history, general health, known allergies, and current medications should be determined.

In cases of childhood poisoning, the nurse always should suspect the possibility of sibling or playmate exposure. All too frequently, only the child "caught in the act" is considered to be at risk for developing toxicity. The possibility of shared adventures and of one child "feeding" another child should be considered.

Nursing Interventions in Managing the Acutely Poisoned Child

First Aid for Poisoning Once the history-taking process is complete, first aid for poisonings can be initiated. The most common routes of exposure are (1) ingestion; (2) inhalation; (3) ocular; and (4) dermal. Other less common routes are parenteral, rectal, and vaginal. Removal of substances from the gastrointestinal tract, skin, and eyes is necessary to prevent toxic effects. Ocular exposure should be treated with copious irrigation for 15–20 minutes with normal saline or water. The best way to accomplish this task in children is to "mummify" or wrap them in a bath towel with their hands at their side. The child should be held over the sink and pitchers of tepid water poured over the eyes. It is not necessary to force the child's eyes open. Given reassurances, the child will relax and blink frequently enough to let the solution irrigate the eye.

The first aid for dermal exposures is a 15- to 20-minute irrigation with water to the affected area. Assess exposed area for burns, particularly with caustic exposures.

For inhalation exposures, the victim should be removed from the exposure site. Resuscitation should not be attempted in the contaminated area. Respiratory status should be assessed by monitoring respirations. Supportive care should be given as needed.

The greatest number of poisonings involve ingestion. The initial first-aid measure for any ingestion other than medicine is the administration of milk or water, as long as the child is awake and alert. Fluids should not be given to the unconscious or convulsing child. Children should be given 6–8 oz of milk or water, whichever is readily available in the home. The American Association of Poison Control Centers has suggested that pills not be diluted by fluid intake because drug absorption might be enhanced. Neutralization, the concept of adding a strong acid to a strong base for caustic ingestions, is an outdated method of therapy. Neutralization produces an exothermic (heat-producing) reaction, which can be harmful. Milk is the first-aid remedy for ingested caustic poisons, with water as an alternative.

Evaluation and Management of the Poisoned Child Initial evaluation of the child's immediate danger and good supportive care comprise the basic management of any poisoned patient. Basic supportive care should include the following:

1. Establishment and management of the airway. The patient should be intubated if the gag reflex is lost, if seizures are present, or if the patient has lost consciousness. Oxygen should be given as needed.
2. Cardiovascular stabilization. Shock should be prevented and treated with fluids or vasopressors if necessary. Fluids should be given to hydrate the patient, using caution with the amount given to prevent pulmonary edema.
3. Establishment and management of an acid–base and electrolyte imbalance.
4. Naloxone (Narcan) can be given in any overdose situation to rule out the presence of any narcotics.
5. Glucose administration may be warranted.

Prevention of Absorption

Gastric Emptying Syrup of ipecac has been a nonprescription drug since 1966 in amounts of 30 mL or less. Because of its excellent safety record, no toxicity has ever been reported when the drug has been used in the recommended doses (Haddad and Winchester 1983: 11).

Children should be given 15 mL of ipecac followed by 6–8 oz of water. If vomiting does not occur within 20–30 minutes, the pharynx can be stimulated with a blunt instrument (for example, a spoon handle, tongue depressor, or back of a toothbrush). Gagging with a finger might cause damage to the throat as well as a bite to the finger. The dose of ipecac can be repeated once if the previous steps have been taken without results. It is not recommended to give ipecac to children under 1 year of age unless medical supervision is available.

Ipecac is contraindicated in the following situations:

1. If the child is comatose, having seizures, or has ingested a substance that has the potential to cause rapid-onset seizures or central nervous system depression.
2. In a child who has ingested a caustic substance (strong acid or base).
3. For some petroleum distillates (for example, mineral seal oil) in which the risk of aspiration outweighs the benefits of emesis.

Gastric Lavage Gastric lavage is indicated to empty the stomach if the child is unconscious, having seizures, or when a decrease in consciousness is expected. Endotracheal or nasotracheal intubation should precede the placement of an orogastric hose for airway protection. The patient should be placed in a left-lateral, head-down position.

A large-bore (28 French Ewald) tube is safe in children over 1 year of age. Smaller tubes will not adequately remove the larger fragments of material (Haddad and Winchester, 1983: 11). Repeated washings should be conducted until the returns are clear. Children should receive no more than 10 mL/kg per washing. Saline solution is recommended, and it is important to recover any lavage fluid that is instilled. When lavage is complete, the tube should be kept in the stomach for activated charcoal and cathartic instillation. When the tube is no longer needed, it should be pinched off and removed.

Whenever gastric lavage is performed, the patient should be on the left side and in the Trendelenberg position to minimize the risk of aspiration and maximize the return (Haddad and Winchester, 1983: 11). To ensure proper tube placement, air should be injected into the hose and a stethoscope used over the stomach.

The following is a list of the indications for gastric lavage:

1. When the poison is recently ingested and/or is an agent likely to slow gastric emptying.
2. When the patient is comatose, convulsing, or requires airway protection.
3. When the ingested poison is rapidly absorbed (for example, strychnine, cyanide), in which case induced emesis might be too slow to be effective or too dangerous if the patient rapidly becomes symptomatic (Burke, 1972).

Charcoal Activated charcoal is a fine black powder that is highly absorbent of most drugs and chemicals and is not itself absorbed through the gastrointestinal mucosa. Activated charcoal can be given either orally in a water slurry or via nasogastric tube. It should be given to all overdose patients after the completion of a gastric emptying procedure. Activated charcoal should not be given with ipecac because the ipecac will be inactivated by the activated charcoal.

The recommended dose of activated charcoal in children is 15–50 g. A sweetener such as 70% sorbitol can be added to the charcoal to make it more palatable for children.

Cathartics Cathartics usually are administered simultaneously with charcoal. Saline cathartics (sodium sulfate, magnesium citrate) are given in a dose of 250 mg/kg for a child and 30 g for adults.

Advanced Nursing Management The majority of poisoned patients can be managed by adhering to simple protocols such as gastric emptying, decreasing absorption, administration of charcoal and a cathartic, and basic life support. However, in certain poisonings more specific management techniques might be indicated. For a child presenting to an emergency care facility several hours after ingesting a poison and exhibiting life-threatening symptoms, gastric emptying and observation alone might not be effective. Therefore, the following discussion outlines more sophisticated techniques for managing the poisoned child and some possible indications for the clinical application of these techniques.

Forced Diuresis Forced diuresis (Poisindex, 1974) is a technique utilized to enhance elimination of drugs. There are primarily two types of forced diuresis: alkaline and acid. Both types involve maintaining or increasing a patient's urine flow to 3–6 mL/kg/hr and altering the urine pH.

An alkaline diuresis is effective in salicylate and phenobarbital poisonings. The goal of an alkaline diuresis is to achieve a urine pH of 7.5–8.5 by administering sodium bicarbonate.

Acid diuresis has been shown to enhance the excretion of amphetamines and also has been used with phencyclidine and strychnine poisonings. The goal of this type of diuresis is to acidify the urine to a pH of 4.5–5.5 using ammonium chloride. The use of acid diuresis is contraindicated in patients with suspected rhabdomyolysis.

Specific nursing care of the child undergoing forced diuresis should include careful monitoring of fluid intake and output to avoid fluid overload, hourly monitoring of electrolytes, and careful observation for symptoms of pulmonary edema.

Hemodialysis Another method of enhancing the excretion of drugs or toxins is hemodialysis, whereby toxic products are removed as the patient's blood is dialyzed against a semipermeable membrane.

Hemodialysis should be considered when the poisoned child develops any of the following life-threatening symptoms that do not respond to more conventional therapy:

1. Coma or hyperactivity caused by a dialyzable drug that cannot be treated by conservative means.
2. Acid–base and electrolyte disturbances that cannot be controlled.
3. Marked hyperosmolality that is not due to easily corrected fluid problems.
4. Marked hypothermia or hyperthermia.
5. Hypotension threatening renal or hepatic function that cannot be corrected by adjusting circulating volume.
6. Supportive care in the face of renal failure (Rumack, et al., 1981).

The effectiveness of hemodialysis in the poisoned patient depends on several pharmacokinetic parameters of the drug or toxin for which the procedure is being used. A few of the considerations for the particular drug or toxin include the volume of distribution, molecular weight, solubility, half-life, and dialysis clearance compared with total body clearance (Parker and Parker, 1983). (See Chapter 39.)

Hemoperfusion Hemoperfusion is a procedure that involves pumping a poisoned patient's blood through a column of adsorbent material (which binds specific drugs or toxins) and then recirculating the blood back to the patient. The adsorbent materials used in this procedure are activated charcoal or amberlite resin.

The popularity of this procedure has alternately waxed and waned since its introduction in 1964 (Pond, et al., 1979). Because of the variable clinical success achieved with hemoperfusion, its use is now restricted to highly selective situations. Since its introduction, this procedure has been employed for a wide variety of drugs and toxins; however, theophylline remains the most frequent poison for which this treatment technique is used.

Chelation Heavy metals such as mercury, lead, and arsenic are not readily excreted by the body; hence, the progressive accumulation of these metals leads to toxicity. Chelation is a procedure that effectively interrupts or reverses the toxicity of these substances by enhancing their excretion. This is accomplished by the administration of a specific chelating agent that binds with the heavy metal, forming a complex which can then be eliminated by the kidneys.

Some of the commonly used chelating agents include deferoxamine (Desferal), dimercaprol (BAL In Oil; BAL; British Anti Lewisite), penicillamine (Cuprimine; Depen Titratabs; D-penicillamine), and edetate calcium disodium (Calcium Disodium Versenate; EDTA).

Antidotes An antidote is a physiologic antagonist that can reverse the toxic effects of a given poison. Few antidotes actually are available for use in the poisoned patient; however, correctly administered antidotal therapy can be life saving for specific poisonings.

Care for the Child Poisoned by Specific Poisonous Agents

The following agents are those which are commonly available and may be accessible to children in their homes. Information about these poisons can be used as a reference guide for nurses and as a resource for nurses to assist parents in the removal of poisonous agents from the home.

Lead Poisoning with lead remains a concern for the young child in today's world. Lead is present in abundance everywhere in our environment. Potential sources of poisoning with lead include contaminated food and drink consumed from improperly glazed earthenware (Klaasen, 1980), exposure to the soiled clothing of lead workers (Baker, et al., 1977), and airborne lead and lead fallout in street dust and soil (Lin-Fuj, 1973). Azarcon (a folk medicine remedy), containing approximately 93.5% lead, is brought into the United States from Mexico and is another known cause of lead intoxication in children (FDA, 1983). The most frequent cause of lead poisoning in children, however, is the ingestion of paint chips from windowsills and frames painted with lead-based paint (Klaasen, 1980) and dusts containing lead.

Lead poisoning is caused by the ingestion or inhalation of lead products. However, because the body absorbs lead poorly, multiple exposures might be required to produce toxicity (Poisindex, 1974). In the early stages of lead poisoning, symptoms may be very nonspecific: listlessness, irritability, vomiting, anorexia, abdominal pain, and constipation. More advanced stages of lead poisoning might include encephalopathy, drowsiness, clumsiness, ataxia, seizures, coma, and respiratory arrest (Pincus and Saccar, 1979).

The diagnosis and treatment of lead poisoning are based on clinical and laboratory findings. In all patients with a blood level of 50–60 μg/dL or greater, treatment with chelation is recommended (Poisindex, 1974). Higher levels and/or a patient exhibiting severe symptoms might require more than one chelating agent (see the section on screening for lead in Chapter 18).

Because the early manifestations of lead poisoning are easily confused with other illnesses, an accurate diagnosis of lead poisoning might be missed. Frequently, only intensive questioning by the physician or nurse will uncover the environmental risk factors that warrant further diagnostic testing. Abdominal and skeletal radiographs and basic screening tests are useful in establishing a diagnosis.

Children are at a greater risk for lead poisoning if they have a history of pica and/or they reside in older houses with peeling paint. Lead-free paint was introduced in the 1940s (Lin-Fuj, 1973). A home nursing assessment is indicated when a child has a diagnosis of lead poisoning. Parents need to be aware of the environmental cause of lead poisoning, and appropriate environmental modifications should be undertaken.

Snake Venom The highest incidence of snake bites occurs in children (Russell, 1980). This is understandable when one examines the play of children: turning over old logs or fallen trees to see what's underneath, crawling over and around rocks and boulders, or attempting to catch a snake for a pet. Of the approximately 120 species of snakes in the United States, only 20 are considered venomous (Poisindex, 1974). These include snakes of the Crotalidae family (cottonmouths, copperheads, and rattlesnakes) and the Elapidae family (coral snakes).

When a bite occurs from a venomous snake, the degree of poisoning depends on several factors, including:

1. The nature, location, depth, and number of bites
2. The amount of venom injected
3. The species and size of the snake
4. The age and size of the victim
5. The victim's sensitivity to the venom
6. The kind of first-aid treatment and subsequent medical care the victim receives (Russell, 1980)

Snake venom poisoning can vary from minimal to very severe. Envenomation by a snake of the Crotalidae family nearly always produces immediate swelling and edema within 5 minutes of the bite (Russell, 1980). Other local symptoms include ecchymosis, vesicle formation, thrombosis of superficial vessels, necrosis, sloughing of injured tissues, and pain. Systemic effects include sweating, faintness, regional lymphadenopathy, hematologic abnormalities (hemoconcentration, decrease in red blood cells and platelets, and prolonged bleeding and clotting times), abnormal urinalysis (hematuria, glycosuria, and proteinuria), and neuromuscular findings (fasciculations, paresthesias, and weakness).

Elapids, in contrast to the Crotalids, produce only minimal toxicity locally. Systemic effects range from drowsiness, weakness, nausea, and vomiting to paralysis.

Overly aggressive first aid prior to hospitalization frequently has resulted in more serious injury to the patient than if more conservative measures had been applied. Current first-aid recommendations do not include packing an envenomated area in ice, nor are tourniquets or excising the bite advocated. Appropriate first-aid measures include reassuring the child, keeping the child quiet, cleansing the wound, and immobilizing the bite area at the heart level and in physiologic position, followed by transport to a health care facility. If the snake can be identified without further risk of envenomation, this might provide helpful information to the physician in formulating the patient care plan.

Hospital care then begins with patient assessment, providing life support if necessary, and careful observation of the patient to determine the seriousness of the envenomation. Some serious envenomations that require treatment with antivenin include patients exhibiting progressive swelling and edema involving the bite area; paresthesias of the mouth, scalp, fingers or toes; or other systemic effects (Russell, 1980) such as shock, hemorrhage, coagulopathy, or hypotension. If the child requires antivenin, it is best administered intravenously and within 4 hours of the bite. The usefulness of antivenin after 24 hours is questionable (Russell, 1980). Caution should be used in the administration of antivenin to all patients and especially those who are allergic to horse serum. Reactions to antivenin can range from a sensitivity reaction—apprehension, pruritus, dyspnea, and anaphylactic shock—to delayed serum sickness (Russell, 1980), which is manifested by reddening and swelling at the site of injection, fever, myalgia, nausea and vomiting, arthritis, lymphadenopathy, and pain (Harrison, et al., 1977). One way of determining if additional antivenin is needed is by monitoring the degree of edema produced by the bite. This is accomplished by careful measurement of the extremity 10 cm proximal to the bite and at a second proximal site every 15–30 minutes.

Initial laboratory testing following Crotalidae bites should include blood type and crossmatch, complete blood count, platelet count, protime, and urinalysis. Additional management of the venomous snake bite might also include tetanus prophylaxis, antibiotic therapy, wound debridement, and other supportive care as indicated.

Consultative services regarding the identification of snakes are provided by many zoos. Further assistance with management can be obtained by contacting the regional poison control center. Information regarding locating antivenin is maintained by the Oklahoma Poison Information Center (24-hour phone number: 405– 271–5454).

Spiders In the United States two genera of spiders, *Loxosceles* and *Lactrodectus,* are responsible for the vast majority of significant spider envenomations.

Several species of *Loxosceles* are found in the United States, and all (both male and female) are venomous. However, the species *Loxosceles reclusa* (brown recluse spider) found predominantly in the midwestern states enjoys the most notoriety. This spider is 5–20 mm in length, with very long legs, yellowish to brown in color, and is distinguished by a violin-shaped area of dark color on the dorsal side of the cephalothorax (Frazier, 1969).

Envenomation by the brown recluse spider gives rise locally to pain, bleb formation, erythema, and ecchymosis and necrosis, which leads to eschar formation and ulceration (Russell, Waldron, and Madon, 1969; Arnold, 1976). The lesion might progress to involve underlying muscle tissue. The systemic signs and symptoms that have been reported include fever, chills, malaise, weakness, nausea, vomiting, hemolytic anemia, thrombocytopenia, and other hematologic dyscrasias (Poisindex, 1974).

The treatment of *Loxosceles* envenomation might include excising the bite area (Frazier, 1969), but this procedure generally is only recommended early in the clinical course. Other treatment might involve the administration of steroids, cleansing, soaking, and debridement of the wound and any supportive care deemed necessary. Several weeks following the bite, surgical interventions and even skin grafting may be indicated.

The presence of the *Lactrodectus mactans,* or black widow spider, has been reported in every state of the continental United States. Only the female is toxic. She is described as being shiny black, with a body 1.5 cm in length, long legs, and a distinctive red hourglass-shaped marking on the ventral side of the abdomen (Frazier, 1969).

Toxic effects depend on whether envenomation has occurred. This does not always happen with all bites. Initial symptoms include a pinprick sensation at the site of the bite followed by a dull ache or numb feeling. Within 2 hours of exposure, the victim might develop muscle aches and cramping involving the large muscle groups (abdomen, back, legs, buttocks). Muscle fasciculations are also common. The toxic effects culminate in "boardlike" muscle rigidity, pain, and paralysis. Other nonspecific symptoms might include headache, weakness, prutitus, increased perspiration, nausea, and vomiting. In some cases blood pressure and cerebrospinal fluid pressure might be increased (Poisindex, 1974).

Treatment of *Lactrodectus* envenomations should be guided by the clinical presentation of the patient. Conservative measures involving muscle relaxants (diazepam and methocarbamol) and/or calcium gluconate might relieve spasms and muscle pain effectively in most patients; however, if pain is severe, narcotics (meperidine hydrochloride or APC [acetylsalicylic acid, phenacetin, and caffeine] with codeine) also might be employed. Antivenin should be considered for patients with severe signs and symptoms that do not respond to other forms of treatment. Children treated with antivenin should be observed closely for anaphylaxis and delayed serum sickness. (See the discussion of adverse effects of antivenin in the previous section on snake venom poisoning.)

Carbon Monoxide Carbon monoxide is a colorless, odorless gas that can cause poisoning in an insidious manner. It is produced by a variety of well-known sources: automobile exhaust, inadequately ventilated fireplaces, and malfunctioning gas appliances (furnaces, water heaters, stoves). Other causes include space heaters or charcoal grills that are operated improperly or with insufficient ventilation.

Carbon monoxide toxicity is due to the special affinity of the gas for oxygen. Carbon monoxide binds with the hemoglobin molecule with an affinity 250 times that of oxygen (Zimmerman and Truxal, 1981). This results in the formation of carboxyhemoglobin and ultimately prevents adequate oxygenation of all tissues of the body.

Symptoms have been categorized in terms of carboxyhemoglobin levels. Levels fall rapidly after exposure is terminated, especially when the patient is given oxygen, and symptoms are more appropriately correlated with peak carboxyhemoglobin levels. Low levels of carboxyhemoglobin (between 10% and 25%) produce minor shortness of breath on exertion, headache, nausea, and throbbing temples. Levels above 30% might cause severe headache, dizziness, weakness, and confusion. Carboxyhemoglobin levels in the 60%–70% range might produce coma, convulsions, respiratory failure, and death (Winter and Miller, 1976).

Following removal of a victim from the source of exposure, the carboxyhemoglobin level starts to diminish. When the patient breathes room air, the half-life of carbon monoxide is about 5 hours. Oxygen, the primary treatment for carbon monoxide poisoning, will reduce the half-life of carbon monoxide to 90 minutes at an FIO_2 of 100% (Zimmerman and Truxal, 1981). Oxygen competes with carbon monoxide for the hemoglobin molecule. In addition, oxygen is dissolved in the plasma for distribution to the tissues independent of the hemoglobin carriage mechanism.

Even more effective is the use of hyperbaric oxygen, which at 3 atm of pressure reduces the half-life of carbon monoxide to less than 30 minutes (Zimmerman and Truxal, 1981). Hyperbaric oxygen should be considered in comatose children or those with hypotension, acidosis, or electrocardiographic changes suggestive of ischemia. Actual improvement in morbidity and mortality with the use of hyperbaric oxygen awaits further research.

Numerous chronic sequelae have been reported following carbon monoxide poisoning, including personality changes, memory disturbances, visual perception problems, ataxia, and other abnormalities (Raskin and Mullaney, 1940; Smith, Brierly, and Brandon, 1971). Binder and Roberts (1980) discussed a case report of a child poisoned with carbon monoxide who was later evaluated for behavioral disturbances. Findings included fine and gross motor impairment, abnormal electroencephalographic results, visual–perceptual problems, and language problems. Further study by these authors suggested that more information is needed regarding the long-term effects of carbon monoxide.

Cardiac Glycosides Although cardiac glycoside poisonings in children are considered rare, they are potentially life threatening (Zucker, et al., 1982). Cardiac glycosides are found in a variety of plants such as oleander, foxglove, and lily of the valley (Poisindex, 1974). The two most commonly used pharmaceutical digitalis preparations are digoxin (Lanoxin) and digitoxin.

The therapeutic index for the cardiac glycosides is marginal; even small amounts can result in severe toxicity. The normal pharmacologic action of therapeutic doses of these drugs is to increase cardiac contractility and slow the heart rate. An overdose produces both a myocardial depressant effect and increased irritability of the heart, creating a broad spectrum of cardiac dysrhythmias, including heart block, premature ventricular contractions, bradycardia, and ventricular fibrillation. Death generally is caused by a primary myocardial dysrhythmia. Other toxic effects include nausea, vomiting, lethargy, drowsiness, and hyperkalemia (Poisindex, 1974).

Treatment not only consists of general management techniques but also involves careful monitoring of the patient's cardiac and electrolyte status. Procedures such as hemoperfusion and hemodialysis are not effective because of the high volume of distribution of these drugs. A unique aspect of treatment following cardiac glycoside poisoning focuses on the pioneering efforts of researchers to develop an antibody that enhances the elimination of these drugs. The Fab antibody fragments were utilized successfully in a human for the first time in 1976 (Smith, et al., 1976). At present, these antibodies have proven to be safe and effective in reversing the toxic manifestations of digoxin and digitoxin poisoning (Smith, et al., 1982). Their administration is governed by Federal Drug Administration approved protocol. However, because of limited production and availability, the use of Fab antibody fragments has been restricted to severely poisoned patients. Information regarding Fab antibodies can be obtained by contacting the regional poison control center.

Patient management also might include the use of atropine, lidocaine, and phenytoin and/or a cardiac pacing device. Supportive and symptomatic treatment remains the focus of therapy for digitalis poisoning.

Insecticides The potential for poisoning with insecticides is very high because of their widespread use in both the home and agriculture. The two types of insecticides probably responsible for the majority of toxic exposures in the United States today came into popular use after DDT was banned in 1973 (because of its adverse environmental effects) (National Clearinghouse for Poison Control Centers Bulletin, 1972).

The most toxic organophosphates are those prepared for agricultural use such as parathion. The least toxic are those insecticides prepared for home and garden use such as malathion (Milby, 1971; Poisindex, 1974).

The population at greatest risk for insecticide poisoning are field workers and farmers, commercial applicators, and individuals employed in the manufacture of insecticides. Also at risk are the home gardener who is careless about using proper application techniques for insecticides and children who accidentally ingest or are otherwise exposed, for example, a child playing in a recently sprayed area. Suicides with these products are also not uncommon.

Pharmacology Organophosphates and carbamates enter the body by inhalation, ingestion, or absorption by the skin and conjunctiva. Their primary physiologic mode of action is inhibition of the enzyme acetylcholinesterase at the cholinergic synapses of the nervous system. This enzyme inhibition prevents the normal metabolism of acetylcholine. The resulting accumulation of acetylcholine at the synapses initially stimulates and later inhibits synaptic transmission (Namba, et al., 1971).

The symptoms of organophosphate poisoning can be classified by three receptor groups: muscarinic, nicotinic, and central nervous system. The muscarinic effects (anorexia, nausea, vomiting, sweating, diarrhea, salivation, lacrimation, excessive bronchial secretions, dyspnea, and wheezing) generally precede the nicotinic effects, which include muscle twitching, fasciculations, increased fatigability, and generalized weakness. The central nervous system effects include tension, anxiety, headache, and drowsiness and may progress to confusion, coma, and respiratory arrest. When death occurs it is usually due to impaired respiratory function (Ganandran, 1974).

Treatment The order of treatment for poisoning of the organophosphates depends somewhat on the severity of the poisoning. Decontamination of the skin and hair with copious amounts of soap and water should be accomplished as soon as possible to prevent further dermal absorption, but this might have to be delayed until further life-support measures have been instituted and therapeutic antidotes atropine and pralidoxime (2-PAM) have been administered. Atropine rapidly reverses muscarinic and central nervous system manifestations, whereas 2-PAM reverses the muscarinic and nicotinic manifestations (Done, 1960). These two used together are very effective in organophosphate poisoning.

In addition to supportive management, antidotal therapy, and decontamination, the clinician might find that laboratory serum and red blood cell acetylcholinesterase levels are helpful in determining the severity of the poisoning.

The carbamate group of insecticides are very similar to the organophosphates in many respects. The primary difference is that the carbamates have a shorter duration of action and, in general, a lower toxicity (Levy, 1979). Treatment, if indicated, should be administered as for the organophosphates.

Many poisonings with these insecticides are preventable. In the home individuals need to be educated regarding proper application, storage, and disposal of these potentially dangerous substances. (State and local health departments can assist with disposal.) Employees who routinely work with insecticides need to understand proper decontamination procedures, not only of their own person but also of any clothing worn and equipment used. Hospital personnel also should be instructed to wear rubber gloves and use extreme precautions while decontaminating or otherwise treating the insecticide-poisoned patient (Poisindex, 1974).

As in lead poisoning, the early symptoms of organophosphate/carbamate poisonings might be easily confused with other illnesses, and the clinician must be particularly astute in identifying the patient potentially at risk for toxicity.

Aspirin The pediatric preparations contain 75–81 mg (approximately $1\frac{1}{4}$ grains) of aspirin per tablet, and the adult preparations contain 325–650 mg of aspirin. Aspirin is found in cold and allergy medicines along with antihistamines and decongestants. Sustained-release preparations are available, in which sustained high levels and prolonged absorption might be present. Methyl salicylate (oil of wintergreen) is almost 99% pure salicylate. It is absorbed quickly after oral ingestion, and the peak might appear sooner than with other aspirin products. Various sunscreen agents, tropical creams for osteoarthritis, and other rubefacients also contain salicylate. Aspirin is used for minor aches and pains, arthritic and rheumatoid conditions, analgesia, antipyresis, and anti-inflammatory conditions.

Pharmacology Hyperpnea and tachypnea are characteristic of an aspirin overdose. Direct stimulation to the medulla occurs 15–20 minutes after ingestion, producing tachypnea. An increase in the oxygen demand and increase in carbon dioxide production result from the uncoupling of mitochondrial oxidative phosphorylation. Respiration is stimulated by the increased carbon dioxide. The rate and depth of respiration result in a decreased PCO_2 as the alveolar carbon dioxide is expulsed. A respiratory alkalosis occurs, resulting in hypocapnia and an increase in the arterial pH. The kidneys compensate by excreting bicarbonate (a base) in an attempt to normalize the arterial pH.

In adult salicylate poisonings and mild to moderate overdoses in older children, respiratory alkalosis alone or in combination with an alkaluremia is seen initially. A paradoxic aciduria (an acid urine with alkaline plasma) might represent intracellular hypokalemia prior to the plasma potassium level becoming decreased.

In the severe poisonings and in chronic overdose exposures, an acidosis with accompanying aciduremia is present.

	Plasma	Urine
Phase I	Alkalosis	Alkaluremia
Phase II	Alkalosis	Aciduria
Phase III	Acidosis	Aciduria

The most profound toxic effect occurs at the cellular level with the uncoupling of mitrochondrial oxidative phospoyrylation, inhibition of the Kreb's cycle, and an increased metabolism and increased demand for glucose. The building up of organic acids with an anion gap produces a metabolic acidosis and hyperthermia. Usually, hypoglycemia is seen in children and hyperglycemia in adults (Figure 20-2).

The bleeding time is prolonged. Hemorrhage is not a common clinical sequelae in the toxic state.

Therapeutic doses of salicylates in the nursing mother are considered safe for the infant (Findlay, et al., 1981). Infants are at risk if the mother takes larger than therapeutic doses (Levy, 1978). Salicylate readily crosses the placenta, and chronic maternal ingestion may be associated with an increased incidence of stillbirths, antepartum and postpartum bleeding, prolonged pregnancy and labor, and lower birthweight infants (Corby, 1978).

Range of Toxicity The Rocky Mountain Poison Center uses the guidelines in Table 20-4 for salicylate ingestion. If the patient should become symptomatic at any point, evaluation by a health care practitioner is necessary.

Toxicity from chronic ingestion is believed to be obtained by 2 or more days of greater than 100 mg/kg/24 hours

TABLE 20-4 Aspirin Toxicity

Acute: single oral dose	Symptoms	Treatment
Mild toxicity (therapeutic)—150 mg/kg	Nausea, vomiting, tinnitus	If less than 100 mg/kg, no treatment is necessary. If 100–150 mg/kg, a cathartic should be given
Moderate toxicity—150–300 mg/kg	Mild to severe hyperpnea, lethargy, and/or excitability; neurologic involvement	Emesis should be induced at home and a cathartic given. Patient should be followed by phone for 24 hours
Severe toxicity—300–500 mg/kg	Life-threatening, metabolic acidosis, seizures, coma, and death	A physician should evaluate. Emesis or lavage should be performed and charcoal and cathartic administered. 6-hour salicylate level should be obtained.
Potentially lethal—greater than 500 mg/kg	Potentially lethal cardiovascular and respiratory shut-down—death	Emergency room evaluation of salicylate level; dialysis might be indicated

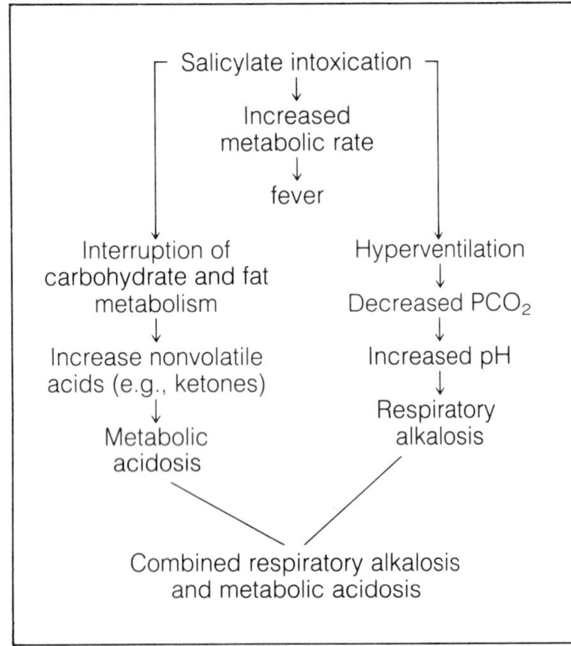

Figure 20-2 Primary physiologic outcomes occurring with salicylate intoxication.

(Temple, 1981). Frequently in pediatrics, toxicity from salicylates is the result of too frequent or too much aspirin administered for therapeutic purposes (Done, 1978). Toxicity can also develop from therapeutic administration to a child who has a decreased fluid intake and urine output, resulting in a decrease in the excretion of salicylates. The diagnosis of a chronic overdose is often missed or delayed. It should be ruled out in a patient presenting with altered mentation. The clinical findings rather than the drug levels should be used to assess toxicity.

Blood levels should be evaluated 6 hours after ingestion when the salicylate peaks (with oil of wintergreen ingestion, 2- and 6-hour blood levels should be obtained). Ingestion of a large amount of aspirin might cause a concretion to form in the stomach, and absorption may be delayed. Symptomatic patients with a low level could be the result of a chronic ingestion or of a concretion being absorbed continuously. A peak level from enteric-coated tablets might occur for up to 28 hours because of the erratic absorption. The Done nomogram (Fig. 20-3) (Done, 1960) is used to correlate salicylate levels with the time of ingestion of a single oral dose and gives the expected clinical toxicity.

Treatment Supportive care includes establishing respiration, hydration, monitoring electrolytes and arterial blood gases, and correcting acid–base imbalances.

Absorption can be prevented by emesis induced with ipecac or lavage; administration of charcoal and a cathartic are also indicated.

Enhancement of excretion is important in the patient with a salicylate overdose. The dehydration should be treated first and a good urine flow established. Bicarbonate should be administered if the patient is acidotic. The nurse should monitor hydration and the potassium level until the salicylate level is therapeutic. Alkalinization of the urine after rehydration (changing the urine pH from 5 to 8) appears to increase the excretion of salicylate twentyfold, but a pH of 8 might be difficult to maintain (Levy, 1979).

Hemodialysis should be considered if the child is unresponsive, refractory to conventional therapy, has high blood salicylate levels (greater than 130 mg/dL 6 hours after ingestion), refractory acidosis (pH less than 7.1), progressive clinical deterioration, fails after conventional therapy, or pulmonary edema or renal failure are present (Poisindex, 1974).

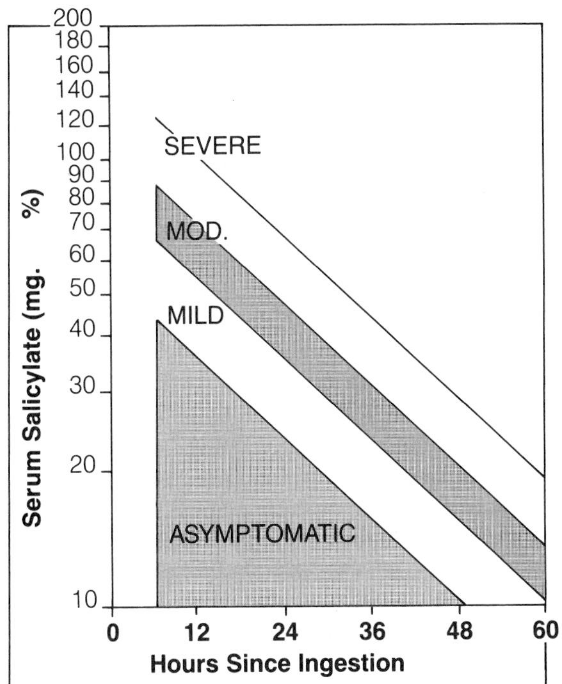

Figure 20-3 Done Nomogram for salicylate poisoning. The nomogram should be used with the following cautions: (1) The patient has taken a single acute ingestion and is not suffering from chronic toxicity. (2) The blood level to be plotted on the nomogram is drawn 6 hours after ingestion. (3) Levels in the toxic range drawn before 6 hours should be treated. (4) Levels in the nontoxic range drawn before 6 hours should be repeated to see if the level is increasing. (From *Pediatrics* [July/Dec] 1960; 26(5):805. Copyright American Academy of Pediatrics, 1960.)

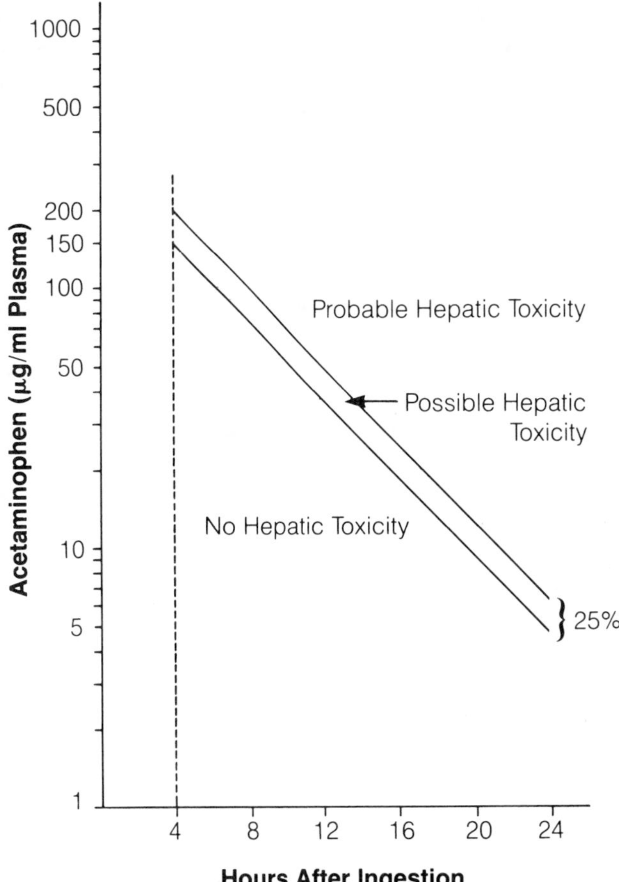

Figure 20-4 Rumack-Matthew Nomogram for acetaminophen poisoning. The nomogram should be used with the following cautions: (1) The time coordinates refer to time of ingestion. (2) Serum levels drawn before 4 hours may not represent peak levels. (3) The graph should be used only in relation to a single acute ingestion. (4) The lower solid line 25% below the standard nomograms is included to allow for possible errors in acetaminophen plasma assays and estimated time from ingestion of an overdose. Adapted from *Pediatrics* (June) 1975; 55(6). Copyright American Academy of Pediatrics 1975.

Acetaminophen There are over 200 nonprescription acetaminophen preparations in tablet, suppository, capsule, liquid, and long-acting forms. It is often found in combination with other analgesic agents.

Pharmacology Acetaminophen (APAP) is used mainly for its antipyretic and analgesic effects. Peak plasma concentrations occur within 70–160 minutes in therapeutic doses and within approximately 4 hours in the overdosed patient. The therapeutic half-life is 2–4 hours.

APAP gets into the milk of lactating mothers. Maternal use at therapeutic doses does not appear to put the nursing infant at risk (Poisindex, 1974). Therapeutic doses of acetaminophen can be used safely during pregnancy (Drugdex, 1977).

Range of Toxicity An amount of 7.5 g or more in an adult or 140 mg/kg or greater in a child is considered to be potentially toxic. The blood level is 150 µg/mL or greater 4 hours after ingestion. The level should be plotted on the Rumack–Matthew nomogram to determine toxicity in an acute overdose (Fig. 20-4) (Rumack and Matthew, 1975).

Clinical Effects Toxicity mainly affects the liver as the glutathione in the liver is depleted and the arylating metabolite covalently binds to the liver cells, resulting in cell necrosis and even death.

During phase I (up to 24 hours after ingestion), the patient might be asymptomatic or present with anorexia, nausea, vomiting, diaphoresis, and malaise.

In phase II (after 24 hours), right upper quadrant pain secondary to hepatic damage occurs. Abnormal blood chemistries and elevated liver function tests are seen. Coagulation defects, jaundice, renal failure, myocardial disorders, and hepatic encephalopathy are sequelae of hepatic necrosis and are evident in phase III (3–5 days after ingestion). Death related to hepatic failure occurs in 10% of cases of serious ingestion. Recovery occurs in the last stage.

Treatment Treatment is based on the time interval following ingestion and the history of co-ingested substances. If 100–140 mg/kg of APAP has been ingested, emesis with ipecac can be induced at home. If a toxic APAP blood level is obtained when plotted on the nomogram, the child should be treated with N-acetylcysteine (Mucomyst). At present, this treatment is considered investigational by the FDA, and the child should be placed on the Rocky Mountain Poison Center's protocol.

If there is a mixed ingestion, which is potentially toxic, charcoal and a cathartic should be given if the patient is treated before approximately 10 hours after ingestion. Clinical judgment is important as to the time of ingestion and the potential outcome of co-ingestion. The charcoal should be lavaged out after 2 hours and prior to giving the loading dose of Mucomyst because the charcoal will bind the Mucomyst, rendering it ineffective.

Hemodialysis, peritoneal dialysis, charcoal hemoprofusion, and forced diuresis are not indicated (Poisindex, 1974).

Hydrocarbons Aspiration pneumonitis is the most serious toxic effect after ingestion of a hydrocarbon. The highest risk of aspiration and toxicity is associated with the low-viscosity hydrocarbons (Kulig and Rumack, 1981). The nurse should suspect aspiration if coughing, dyspnea, tachypnea, cyanosis, rales, rhonchi, and decreased breath sounds develop. Pulmonary edema and hemoptysis might occur. Anoxia and respiratory arrest sometimes can occur with severe aspiration.

Aromatic hydrocarbons (containing a benzene ring) include toluene, xylene, and benzene. They are found in glues and nail polish removers. The toxic effects are mainly caused by the inhalation of vapors. A burning sensation in the mouth and esophagus might be seen after ingestion. Central nervous system excitation followed by depression, seizures, or coma might ensue following large ingestions. Dermal exposure produces skin irritation, whereas an eye exposure can result in corneal burns.

At one time, fluorinated hydrocarbons (freons) were commonly used in refrigerators and as propellants in aerosols. The clinical effects of toxicity are bronchial constriction, lung irritation, and decreased contractility of the heart. "Sniffing" from a bag filled with a hydrocarbon produces hypoxia. Arrhythmias caused by the fluorinated hydrocarbons are difficult to reverse.

The aliphatic hydrocarbons (straight chain) include gasoline, kerosene, and fuel oil. Aspiration pneumonitis, central nervous system depression, cyanosis, tachycardia, and hyperpyrexia might be seen post ingestion. It is unlikely for systemic effects to occur after an accidental poisoning. If aspiration occurs, it probably happened while swallowing. Nausea, vomiting, diarrhea, abdominal pain, and persistent belching are common. The gastrointestinal effects usually are self-limited, not dangerous (Kulig and Rumack, 1981), and might be relieved by administration of a cathartic.

The chlorinated hydrocarbons are perchloroethylene, trichloroethylene, different types of insecticides, methylene chloride, trichloroethane, and carbon tetrachloride. They may act as a central nervous system depressant, produce renal and hepatic damage, and defat the skin.

The following hydrocarbons are not considered harmful if ingested: asphalt and tar, lubricants (motor oil, transmission oil, cutting oil, household oil, heavy greases), mineral oil, liquid petroleum, baby oil, and liquid petrolatum (Poisindex, 1974).

Mineral seal oil, signal oil, and furniture polish oils carry the highest risk for aspiration, and therefore emesis is not recommended. There is no documentation to suggest that they are absorbed from the gastrointestinal tract (Poisindex, 1974).

Treatment Evacuation of the stomach is generally recommended for certain hydrocarbons because of their inherent central nervous system, renal, hepatic, bone, or other systemic effects. CHAMP is a mnemonic device that can be used to remember these hydrocarbons. **C**amphor can produce central nervous system depression and seizures, and therefore lavage is recommended. **H**alogenated, **A**romatic, heavy **M**etals, and **P**esticide hydrocarbons should be decontaminated by the induction of vomiting. The patient should be monitored for symptoms of aspiration. If the patient is symptomatic, a baseline chest radiograph should be obtained and a repeat radiograph obtained at 6–8 hours.

Supportive care is performed for an aspiration penumonitis. Antibiotics are reserved for specific indications and should not be used prophylactically (Steele, Conklin, and Mark, 1972).

Caustics Examples of alkaline corrosives are lye, lime, Clinitest® tablets, electric dishwasher detergents, and low-phosphate detergents. Various household bleaches contain chlorine-active compounds, which are potentially caustic. Ammonia-containing products include cleaning and bleaching agents, liniments, and aromatic spirits of ammonia. Acids are found in hydrochloric (muriatic) and sulfuric acids and Aqua Pegia (nitric and hydrochloric acids). Disinfectants, wood preservatives, and creosotes might contain phenols.

Clinical Effects Alkalis and acids produce different clinical effects after ingestion. The main effect of alkalis occurs on the lips, tongue, oral mucosa, and esophagus. Esophageal burns might be present in the absence of burns to the mouth (Cello, Fogel, and Boland, 1980). Alkalis tend to affect mainly the esophagus, with gastric involvement occurring in only about 20% of the cases (Heindle, 1926). Acids might produce mild to moderately severe oral and esophageal burns, with the more severe burns occurring in the stomach, mainly in the pyloric area. Tissue injury is caused by dehydration or the generation of excessive heat (Jelenko,

Acetaminophen Protocol

I. Brief explanation: APAP overdose can cause hepatotoxicity when the glutathione in the liver is depleted and the arylating metabolite covalently binds to the liver cells, causing cell necrosis and death.

II. Criteria for the use of the protocol:
  1. 7.5 g or more by history; 140 mg/kg for children under 12 years of age.
  2. Within 24 hours—must know time of ingestion by 2 hours.
  3. Final determinant being plasma level above 150 μg/mL 4 hours post ingestion.

III. Informed consent must be obtained because N-acetylcysteine is still an experimental drug.
  1. N-acetylcysteine is the only approved oral treatment for APAP overdose in the US. Side effects are nausea, vomiting, and diarrhea.
  2. Mixed ingestion: Lavage, charcoal, magnesium sulfate. Charcoal *must* be lavaged out.
  3. Mucomyst:
     a. Loading dose is 140 mg/kg PO of 20% × 1 dose.
     b. Maintenance dose is 70 mg/kg PO of 20% × 17 doses every 4 hours.
     c. Dilute 3:1 for 20%, 1:1 for 10%. Goal—make a 5% solution.
     d. Vomiting: If patient vomits within 1 hour, repeat the dose. If patient vomits after 1 hour, go to the next dose. For persistent vomiting use nasogastric or Miller-Abbott tube.
     e. Diluent: Use only Coke, Pepsi, Fresca, orange juice, or grapefruit juice. If PO, chill over ice, administer through straw, closed container.

IV. APAP levels:
Draw plasma levels at 4 hours post ingestion. Get two to three levels at 4-hour intervals to determine half-life.

V. Laboratory tests:
Every 24 hours: serum glutamic oxaloacetic transaminase (SGOT), serum glutamic-pyruvic transaminase (SGPT), Total bilirubin, blood ureanitrogen, prothrombin time.

VI. Miscellaneous:
  1. Pregnancy test if of childbearing age.
  2. Diet and activity as tolerated. Give N-acetylcysteine 1 hour before meals or 2 hours after meals.
  3. Avoid all medications, if possible.

VII. Follow-up:
Nontoxic—repeat liver function tests at 48 hours.
Toxic—if liver function tests are elevated, monitor daily until normal.
Toxic—if liver function tests are not elevated at the end of third day, no follow-up is required.

Financial responsibility: Patient is responsible for all expenses.

1974). Acid compounds do not tend to penetrate deeply into the tissues, as do alkalis (Knopp, 1979).

Systemically, chlorine-active compounds can produce hypotension and coma. Convulsions, coma, and liver and kidney damage can result if ammonia is absorbed. In a phenol ingestion hyperactivity, marked diaphoresis, hyperkinetic activity, convulsions, and hepatic and renal toxicity can result.

The form of the caustic material ingested (either liquid or granular) might determine the location and extent of injury. The use of liquid caustic drain cleaners in households has produced accidental injuries to the esophagus that have been more severe than those formerly seen with granular caustic drain cleaners (Leape, 1974). Solid crystals tend to adhere to the glossopharyngeal, palatal, and proximal esophageal mucosa, producing deep, irregularly arranged burns. Because they tend to adhere proximally, less damage is expected distally (Kirsh and Ritter, 1976). As a result of the easy passage of liquid caustics, diffuse damage to the esophagus may be seen (Ray, et al., 1974).

Range of Toxicity The liquid alkaline corrosives can result in 100% esophageal burns, whereas the crystalline compounds result in about 10%–30% burns (Poisindex, 1976). Ingestion of 2 oz or more of a household concentrate of a chlorine-active compound might produce burns. The concentration of ammonia is more critical than the volume. Household (5%–10%) ammonia usually does not produce burns but has irritating effects on the skin, eyes, and respiratory tract. Industrial strength (27%–30%) ammonia is likely to produce caustic symptoms. Undiluted forms of acids invariably cause damage. Two grams of pure phenol could cause death, whereas 1 or 2 mL might cause corrosive effects.

Treatment Vomiting should not be induced after the ingestion of a caustic. The single most important action is to have the victim drink milk or water immediately (Conrad, 1983). Acid or base substances should not be used in an attempt to neutralize the caustic. Emesis or lavage should be avoided. Children with symptoms should have nothing by mouth after initial dilution until after surgical consultation. Surgical consultation is indicated if the patient has dysphagia, pain, excessive drooling, or oral burns. Esophagoscopy might need to be performed within the first 24 hours. Although controversial, steroids should be started immediately if esophageal burns are present (0.1 mg/kg/day of dexamethasone [Decadron].) The steroids usually are given for 3 weeks and then tapered if burns are found or esophagoscopy is not done.

With an industrial-strength ammonia oral exposure, the patient should be assessed for shock and pulmonary edema. A tracheostomy might be necessary for glottic edema. Steroids might help prevent stricture.

If there are burns in the mouth from an acid ingestion, the esophagus must be examined. The tube should not be passed into the stomach. If a gastrointestinal obstruction is present, parenteral fluids and hyperalimentation should be given (usually for 3 weeks or longer).

Activated charcoal should be given with a phenol and related compound ingestion. The patient should be monitored for seizures and the acid–base balance. Baseline liver and renal tests should be obtained and followed if the patient is symptomatic.

The skin should be decontaminated by removing the clothing and irrigating the skin with water for 20 minutes. The burns should be treated symptomatically.

If the vapors are inhaled, first-aid management is to remove the patient to fresh air. Oxygen should be administered for severe dyspnea or hypoxemia. The patient should be assessed for oral or nasopharageal burns and monitored for chest pain, pulmonary edema, and pneumonitis. The patient's vital signs should be monitored. If pulmonary edema develops, mechanical ventilation with positive end-expiratory pressure should be considered.

An eye exposure requires immediate irrigation with tap water or preferably sterile saline for 20 minutes. An eye examination should be performed if there is persistent pain, redness, irritation, or visual disturbances to determine if the eye has been damaged.

Cold and Cough Preparations Cold and cough preparations contain a wide variety of ingredients such as anticholinergic and sympathomimetic agents, alcohol, and dextromethorphan in combination or alone.

Anticholinergic agents include antihistamines, triprolidine, chlorpheniramine maleate, brompheniramine, and diphenhydramine hydrochloride. They antagonize acetylcholine competitively at the neuroreceptor site. The anticholinergic syndrome has easily recognizable symptoms of central and peripheral effects. Central effects include anxiety, delirium, disorientation, hyperactivity, and seizures. Coma, respiratory paralysis, and death might ensue in severe intoxications. Peripheral involvement includes tachycardia, hyperpyrexia, mydriasis, vasodilatation, urinary retention, decreased gastric motility, warm, dry skin, dry mouth, and loss of secretions in pharynx, bronchi, and nasal passages. The syndrome might be cyclic and delayed. Physostigmine should be considered to treat convulsions, severe hypertension, and hallucinations.

Sympathomimetic agents include pseudoephedrine and phenylpropanolamine (PPA) (used as a nasal decongestant and a stimulant) and ephedrine (used as an oral bronchodilator). In the overdose situation the clinical effects are the result of the specific agent acting on the alpha or beta receptors. Observing the patient for 4–8 hours usually is required. Cardiac arrhythmias might be present, along with tachycardia, precordial pain, and elevated blood pressure. Anorexia, nausea, and vomiting might occur. An acute ingestion of phenylpropanolamine might result in a hypertensive crisis, resulting in cerebral hemorrhage and myocardial ischemia.

Dextromethorphan usually is found in combination with nonprescription decongestants and antihistamines. It has no analgesic or addictive activity, but the cough threshold is increased. Drowsiness, dizziness, nystagmus, ataxia, stupor, coma, hyperexcitability, vertigo, and occasionally convulsions are toxic reactions. Dextromethorphan also has anticholinergic properties. These properties might be manifested by dilated pupils, blurry vision, urinary retention, or a dry mouth.

Multivitamins Significant toxicity after the ingestion of multivitamins (without iron, vitamin A or D, or fluoride) is unlikely (Poisindex, 1974). The only expected symptoms are gastrointestinal irritation if ten or more multivitamins are consumed.

Niacin (vitamin B_3) can produce intense cutaneous flushing that lasts 2–3 hours with no other symptoms even at therapeutic doses.

The water-soluble vitamins (folic acid, thiamine [B_1], riboflavin [B_2], pyridoxine [B_6], cyanocobalamin [B_{12}], biotin, pantothenic acid) are unlikely to produce toxicity. The B vitamins can give a brilliant yellow color to the urine.

The toxicity of vitamins A and D is well established. Toxicity with vitamin A is seen following the ingestion of 100,000 units or more daily for weeks or months or an acute ingestion of 12,000 IU/kg. Symptoms include vomiting, anorexia, skin lesions, increased intracranial pressure, and hypothrombinemia (especially in infants). Chronic toxicity can result in optic atrophy and blindness. Toxic symptoms usually clear once the vitamin A is withdrawn. Vitamin A is essential for normal vision in dim light.

Vitamin D is required for the absorption of calcium and phosphorus from the gastrointestinal tract. Nausea, vomiting, diarrhea, confusion, anorexia, fatigue, headache, pruritus, weakness, renal tubular damage, and hypercalemia are toxic effects that can occur from the overingestion of vitamin D.

Iron Iron is supplied alone as ferrous sulfate or ferrous gluconate, combined with multivitamins, and included in some birth control pills (usually in the last seven, or placebo, pills). The percentage of elemental iron per tablet is important:

Ferrous sulfate, 300 mg = 60 mg of elemental iron
Ferrous gluconate, 325 mg = 39 mg of elemental iron
Ferrous fumarate, 200 mg = 66 mg of elemental iron

Iron is necessary for hemoglobin formation and the oxidative processes of the body. Two-thirds of the body's store of iron is in the form of hemoglobin, and the remainder of iron is found in the reticuloendothelial system. There are 3.5 g of iron in the body.

The major clinical symptoms of an iron overdose are stupor, obtundation, shock, acidosis, hematemesis, bloody diarrhea, and coma. The minor clinical symptoms include vomiting, diarrhea, mild lethargy, confusion, leukocytosis, and a blood glucose level greater than 150 mg/dL.

The clinical toxic state has five phases. The first phase occurs 30 minutes to 2 hours post ingestion. The patient should be assessed for lethargy, restlessness, hematemesis, abdominal pain, and diarrhea. Necrosis to the gastrointestinal tract occurs from the direct effect of iron on the mucosa. The second phase might give a false sense of security because the child appears to recover. Observation is mandatory. The third phase occurs 2–12 hours after the first phase. The patient should be monitored for the onset of shock and refractory acidosis with cyanosis and fever. The fourth phase develops 2–4 days post ingestion. Hepatic necrosis occurs, which is believed to be secondary to the direct action of iron on the mitrochondria. In the fifth phase, 2–4 weeks post ingestion, gastrointestinal obstruction caused by the gastric or pyloric scarring from the corrosive effects of iron occurs in rare cases.

Five clinical and laboratory findings have been associated with patients having serum iron levels greater than 300 mg/dL and therefore susceptible to toxicity. These findings include diarrhea, vomiting, leukocytosis (white blood cell count greater than 15, 000 cells/mm^3), hyperglycemia (blood sugar level greater than 150 mg/dL), and a positive abdominal radiograph (Lacouture, et al., 1981).

Toxicity is based on milligrams per kilograms of body weight. The toxic dose is in the range of 45–60 mg/kg. Toxicity is also based on clinical findings. Deaths have occurred from ingestion greater than 60 mg/kg. Ten ferrous sulfate tablets have proved fatal to an infant (Poisindex, 1974).

Treatment The nurse must calculate the milligrams per kilograms of body weight on the maximum amount of elemental iron possibly ingested. If ingestion is less than 20 mg/kg and the patient is asymptomatic, no treatment is necessary. Emesis with ipecac syrup is indicated for an ingestion of 20–60 mg/kg of iron with no clinical symptoms. If ingestion of more than 60 mg/kg of iron occurred or if the patient is symptomatic at any point, referral to a medical facility is warranted. The following is a list of the treatment steps for an iron overdose:

1. Absorption should be prevented by emesis or lavage.
2. Sodium bicarbonate (1%–5%) should be administered to form an insoluble complex of iron. Give 50–100 mL of the 1%–5% bicarbonate solution orally with ipecac or in the first 250–500 mL of lavage fluid. Then, 50–100 mL should be instilled and left in the stomach after emesis or lavage.
3. Abdominal radiographs should be obtained because iron is radiopaque. The radiograph might be negative if the iron has dissolved or if it is attached to the bowel wall.
4. Serum iron (SI) and total iron binding capacity (TIBC) blood tests should be obtained.
5. The indications for deferoxamine therapy are the presence of free iron (SI greater than TIBC), SI greater than 350 μg/dL with an asymptomatic child, or any symptomatic patient. The urine should be monitored for a pink to orange color, which indicates excretion of the chelated complex.

Caffeine There are numerous over-the-counter diet preparations and other drugs such as Midol, No Doz, and Excedrin that contain caffeine, and therefore abuse or accidental ingestion of these substances can lead to caffeine toxicity. Caffeine also is found in chocolate and numerous beverages. Brewed coffee has 40–180 mg/5 oz cup, brewed tea has 20–110 mg/5 oz cup, cocoa has 2–25 mg/5 oz cup, and soft drinks (Coca Cola, Pepsi Cola, and Royal Crown Cola) have 10–15 mg/dL or 35–55 mg/12 oz.

Pharmacology Caffeine causes stimulation of the central nervous system, diuresis, direct stimulation of the heart and skeletal muscle, and inhibition of the contractility of smooth muscle. Caffeine temporarily allays the sensation of drowsiness and fatigue and increases gastric acid and pepsin secretions. A vasodilation of the coronary arteries and a vasoconstriction of the cerebral arteries might occur with a slight net peripheral vasodilation.

Range of Toxicity Death is rare following a caffeine overdose. The minimum toxic dose has not been well established in the literature. The estimated adult lethal dose is 5–10 g. One gram in a single dose might produce convulsions, tremors, tachycardia, pyrexia, vomiting, and diarrhea. Toxic symptoms have been reported in several neonates who received 36–136 mg/kg of caffeine for respiratory depression (Banner and Czajka, 1980). In large doses insomnia, restlessness, tinnitus, convulsions, headache, photophobia, cardiac arrhythmias, gastrointestinal irritation, gastric bleeding, hyperglycemia, and metabolic acidosis might occur.

Treatment The following is a list of treatment guidelines for a caffeine overdose:

1. Absorption should be prevented by emesis or lavage and the administration of charcoal and a cathartic.
2. Urine output should be monitored.
3. Cardiac function and vital signs should be monitored.
4. Gastrointestinal irritation and bleeding should be assessed.

Ethanol Ethanol is present in perfumes, elixirs, beverages, mouthwashes, and other products. Denatured alcohol does not necessarily mean methanol.

Pharmacology Ethanol is rapidly absorbed from the stomach and small intestine. The peak level occurs within 30 minutes to 3 hours. The liver is primarily responsible for the metabolism of ethanol. A continuous infusion of ethanol is used to treat ethylene glycol and methanol poisonings.

An 80 proof alcoholic beverage contains about 40 g/dL of ethanol. One ounce of an 80 proof alcohol (a "shot") equals 12 g of ethanol.

Blood alcohol (mg/dL)	Symptoms in nonchronic patients
100	Intoxication
250	Coma
350	Surgical anesthesia
400	Death

The toxic clinical effects of ethanol are nausea, vomiting, mental confusion, ataxia, exaggerated mental status, muscle incoordination, hypoglycemia, and seizures. Death usually is caused by respiratory failure.

Treatment involves the prevention of absorption by ipecac or lavage, charcoal, and a cathartic. The blood glucose level must be monitored. Thiamine is used to prevent Wernicke's encephalopathy in chronic ethanol abusers and must be used concurrently with glucose. The patient should be observed for seizures. Supportive care is indicated.

Ethylene Glycol Ethylene glycol is found in permanent antifreeze, deicers, dyes and wood stains, leather goods, varnishes and enamels, lacquer and thinner preparations, and some cosmetics. It is a colorless, odorless, water-soluble liquid and is used frequently as a substitute for alcohol.

Pharmacology Ethylene glycol is metabolized by alcohol dehydrogenase to several toxic organic acids, including oxalic acid and glycolic acid. The metabolites interfere with oxidative phosphorylation, cellular respiration, and glucose metabolism, which leads to renal damage, acidosis, or death. Oxalic acid might precipitate in the urine to form calcium oxalate crystals. The peak level of ethylene glycol occurs 6–12 hours after ingestion. It is absorbed very rapidly from the gut. The percutaneous absorption of ethylene glycol is minimal. The half-life of ethylene glycol with ethanol therapy is about 3 hours. See Figure 20-5.

Range of Toxicity Any amount of ethylene glycol ingested must be regarded as potentially harmful. Levels between 20 and 50 mg/dL are associated with toxicity. Severe toxicity generally is considered to be greater than 50 mg/dL. Lethal amounts are considered to be 1.4 mL/kg in children and 100 mL in a 70-kg adult (Hunt, 1932). Although the minimal lethal dose is not well defined in the literature, death has been reported after a 60-mL ingestion (Wedman, 1946); however, survival has occurred after an ingestion of 400 mL (Seeff et al., 1970).

Clinical Effects The central nervous, cardiopulmonary, and renal systems are affected in three distinct phases (Berman, Schreiner, and Fegs, 1957). An ethylene glycol ingestion should be suspected in a child who appears intoxicated but has no smell of alcohol on the breath. Symptoms are delayed with a concurrent ethanol ingestion.

There are three main phases with an overdose. During phase 1, 30 minutes to 12 hours after ingestion, the nurse should observe for an altered mental status and a high anion-gap metabolic acidosis. Anion gap (AG) is calculated as Na − (Cl + HCO_3). The normal AG level is 12–14 mEq/L. In ethylene glycol intoxication the level frequently might be greater than 20 mEq/L. Clinical signs and symptoms include shortness of breath, tachypnea, aciduria, decreased serum bicarbonate, decreased carbon dioxide, and an elevated AG. During phase 2, 12–36 hours after ingestion, respiratory distress and pulmonary edema might ensue. If death occurs, it is usually in this phase. During phase 3, 24–72 hours after ingestion, renal failure might occur. With supportive therapy, a return to normal kidney function is expected to take up to 4 months.

The finding of a large amount of calcium oxalate crystals on urinalysis is considered indicative of ethylene glycol intoxication. However, calcium oxalate crystals are not always present, and their presence is not mandatory for the diagnosis of ethylene glycol ingestion. A diminishing urine output might be the first indication of renal involvement.

Ethanol therapy is indicated for an increased AG metabolic acidosis with a history of an ethylene glycol ingestion, a serum ethylene glycol level greater than 20 mg/dL, a symptomatic patient with a history of an ethylene glycol ingestion, and when an ethylene glycol level is not readily available but a concurrent ingestion of ethylene glycol and alcohol is suspected (Scherger, et al., 1983). The serum glucose level should be monitored because ethanol can produce hypoglycemia, especially in children.

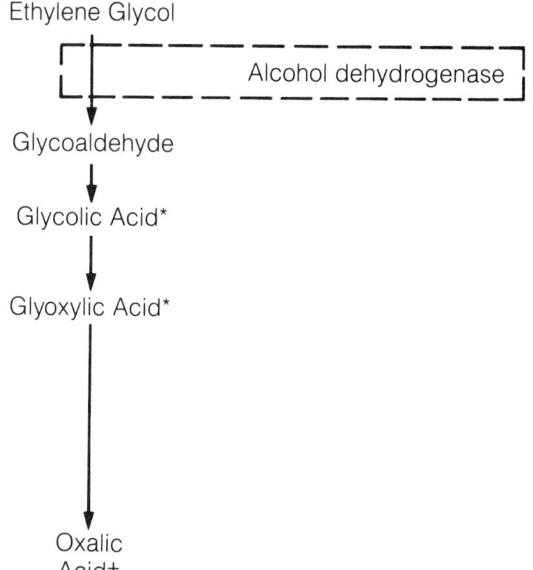

*Causes oxalemia, acidosis, renal interstitial edema
†Forms calcium oxylate crystals
Adapted from Rumack BH: Ethylene glycol management in: *Poisindex*. Micromedex, 1974–1984.

Figure 20-5 Simplified diagram of the metabolism of ethylene glycol.

Hemodialysis can be used in conjunction with the intravenous administration of ethanol. An ethylene glycol level greater than 50 mg/dL, a severe acid–base or fluid and electrolyte imbalance, and renal failure are the main indications for hemodialysis.

Treatment Absorption should be prevented, The ethylene glycol level should be obtained. Arterial blood gases should be followed to monitor pH. The patient should be observed for seizures. The nurse should monitor the patient's renal functions, watching for crystalluria. Thiamine and pyridoxine used early in the treatment can help prevent oxalate formation. Hemodialysis is indicated for peak levels of ethylene glycol greater than 50 mg/dL, severe acid–base disturbances, or renal failure. Concurrent therapy of ethanol and dialysis should not last longer than 1 day.

Ethanol effectively competes with methanol and ethylene glycol for the alcohol dehydrogenase (a hepatic enzyme), thus inhibiting the formation of toxic metabolites. The toxic metabolites of both ethanol and ethylene glycol ingestions are what produce the toxic effects.

Methanol Methanol (methyl alcohol, wood alcohol) is present in antifreeze, paint solvents, and canned fuels. Methanol is converted to formic acid. The plasma half-life of methanol is usually 8 hours.

Pharmacology Methanol is absorbed rapidly and completely. The peak serum level occurs in 1–2 hours. Small amounts can be absorbed dermally or by inhalation. Ninety-four percent of methanol is eliminated by the liver. The process of methanol conversion is as follows:

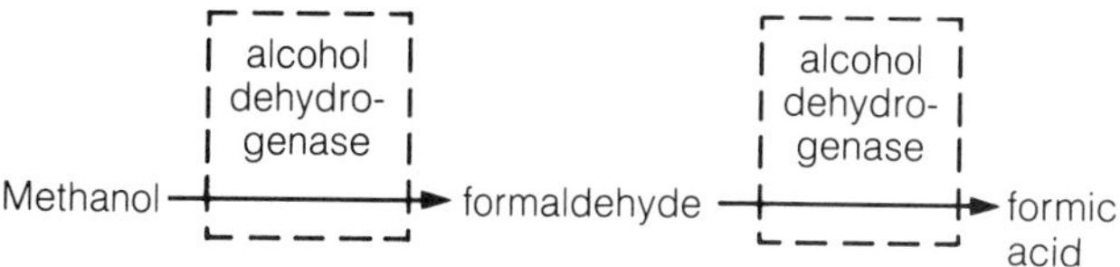

Range of Toxicity There is a wide range of toxicity. Blindness has occurred after the ingestion of 4 mL of absolute methanol (McCoy, et al., 1979). The lethal dose is thought to be between 60 and 240 mL (Gosselin, et al., 1976).

Clinical Effects The patient with an acute methanol intoxication presents with the following symptoms: central nervous system depression, severe AG metabolic acidosis, and optic changes. Generally, the symptoms are delayed about 18–24 hours after exposure. The early symptoms can resemble those of ethanol intoxication, with general malaise, headache, dizziness, gastrointestinal upset, weakness, and vertigo. In severe poisonings coma and seizures might ensue. Dyspnea might occur.

The presence of a severe AG metabolic acidosis is one of the most significant clinical findings. The plasma bicarbonate level is markedly decreased and might even be zero. Pancreatic necrosis can occur, and an elevated serum amylase may be present.

Visual disturbances might be delayed for several hours or days after an acute ingestion. Transient visual abnormalities can include blurred or double vision, constricted visual fields, changes in color perception, and seeing spots. The incidence of permanent ocular damage is related to the severity of the metabolic acidosis and amount of ethanol ingested (Dethlefs and Naraqui, 1978).

Treatment Absorption should be prevented by the administration of ipecac or lavage, charcoal, and a cathartic. If the level of methanol is 20 mg/dL or less, the patient should be observed for symptoms. Methanol and ethanol levels should be obtained. The patient should be monitored for acidosis. Ethanol therapy is indicated for peak methanol levels of 20–50 mg/dL, acidosis, and/or a strong history of ingestion, even without the corroborating methanol levels. Dialysis and ethanol therapy are indicated for levels greater than 50 mg/dL, visual impairment, acidosis not corrected by sodium bicarbonate, and renal failure. Dialysis should be used in conjunction with ethanol therapy.

Tetrahydrozoline Tetrahydrozoline is used as a decongestant for nasal and nasopharyngeal mucosa, as a topical decongestant in conjunctivitis, and for minor eye irritation.

Pharmacology Tetrahydrozoline is a potent alpha adrenergic agent. Tetrahydrozoline is rapidly absorbed from the gastrointestinal tract after oral administration. Systemic absorption might occur following administration, especially in larger than recommended doses, either intranasally or intraocularly (Martindale, 1977). Tetrahydrozoline affects the central H_2 and alpha adrenoceptors but not the H_1 or beta adrenoceptors (Sanders, Miller, and Patil, 1975).

Clinical Effects Overdose or intoxication from the oral ingestion or excessive topical administration of tetrahydrozoline can result in severe drowsiness with diaphoresis, hypertension or shock, bradycardia, respiratory depression, and coma. Younger children, especially infants, are more susceptible to toxicity (Product Information, 1981). Spontaneous recovery can be expected 24–36 hours after exposure. No permanent sequelae or deaths have been reported.

Treatment Absorption should be prevented by the administration of ipecac or lavage, charcoal, and a cathartic. The patient's vital signs and electrocardiographic status should be carefully monitored.

Camphor Camphor is found in some mothballs, topical products used for the relief of muscle aches, and some preparations used as respiratory aids and stimulants. Camphorated oils (20% camphor in cottonseed oil) were removed from the United States market in 1982 by the Food and Drug Administration because of the potential hazards.

Range of Toxicity The toxic dose of camphor ranges from 0.75 to 20 g (Aronow and Spigiel, 1976), and camphor is therefore an extremely toxic substance. It crosses the placenta and has been associated with fetal death (Weiss and Catalano, 1973).

Clinical Effects After ingestion, the patient should be observed for nausea, vomiting, and central nervous system excitation with tremors and convulsions. Central nervous system depression can follow periods of excitation, and respiratory failure might ensue (Poisindex, 1974). The onset of convulsions might be sudden and without warning (Kopelman, et al., 1979).

Treatment If the history is suspicious of ingestion of 0.5 mg of camphor in a child or 1.0 mg in an adult or if symptoms develop, the patient should be referred to an emergency department.

Lavage, with protection of the airway, should be used in the emergency department to decontaminate the gastric contents rather than ipecac administration because of the high risk of seizures. Charcoal and a cathartic should be given. If children are symptom-free for 4–6 hours, they can be discharged. If symptoms of gastrointestinal upset or neurologic signs develop, the child should be admitted to an intensive care unit where anticonvulsants are readily available. Hemoperfusion and hemodialysis might be required for severe poisonings.

Sedative Hypnotics

Barbiturates Barbiturates are of two basic types: short acting and long acting. Short-acting barbiturates include pentobarbital sodium, secobarbital sodium, and thiopental sodium. Long-acting barbiturates include phenobarbital and mephobarbital. They are used as anticonvulsants, sedatives, and hypnotics.

Pharmacology The barbiturates interfere with the transmission of nerve impulses to the cerebral cortex, causing central nervous system depression. The barbiturates have no analgesic properties and are metabolized in the liver. Short-acting barbiturates are minimally excreted by the kidney, whereas long-acting barbiturates are cleared primarily in the kidney in overdoses.

Clinical Effects The child who has ingested a toxic amount of barbiturates might develop confusion, coma, respiratory acidosis, shock, and hypothermia. Alcohol and antihistamines will enhance the toxic effects if ingested concurrently.

Treatment Prevention of absorption (by the administration of ipecac or lavage, charcoal, and a cathartic) and supportive care with careful assessment of respiratory status are indicated. Multiple-dose charcoal might significantly decrease the serum half-life and increase the clearance of phenobarbital. Alkalinization of the urine with sodium bicarbonate to a pH of 7–8 will enhance renal excretion of the long-acting barbiturates.

Benzodiazepines

Pharmacology Sedatives such as diazepam (Valium), flurazepam (Dalmane), and chlordiazepoxide (Librium) are minor tranquilizers that exhibit central nervous system depressant activity. These drugs might cause prolonged drowsiness in the overdose patient because of their prolonged half-life.

Clinical Effects Benzodiazepines cause ataxia, lethargy, slurred speech, and respiratory depression when ingested in large amounts. Following massive oral overdoses, fatalities are rare.

Treatment Absorption should be prevented by the administration of ipecac or lavage, charcoal, and a cathartic. The patient's vital signs, especially respirations, should be monitored closely.

Opiates

Pharmacology Opiates depress the central nervous system, thereby producing coma and the cessation of respiration. Addiction following chronic use of these agents is common.

Clinical Effects Opiate and opioid overdose (heroin, morphine, propoxyphene, methadone) can cause serious respiratory depression, coma, and sinus bradycardia. Pupils are usually pinpoint but might be dilated with severe acidosis, hypoxia, hypotension, bradycardia, and respiratory depression.

Treatment Good supportive care (airway, breathing, circulation) should be established simultaneous with the prevention of absorption (administration of ipecac or lavage, charcoal, and a cathartic). Naloxone (Narcan), a pure narcotic antagonist, reverses all opiates without inducing respiratory depression even in the absence of opiates. An initial pediatric intravenous dose of 0.1 mg/kg of naloxone should be given and the dose (0.1 mg/kg) repeated as needed. Higher-than-usual doses of naloxone might be required to reverse propoxyphene and pentazocine overdoses and large overdoses of other narcotics (Stahl and Kasser, 1983).

The half-life of naloxone (20–30 minutes) is significantly shorter than the half-life of most narcotics. For example, the half-life of meperidine (Demerol) is 3.2 hours. Naloxone might have to be repeated to counteract the respiratory depressant effects of these longer-acting narcotics.

Withdrawal in the Neonate The onset of symptoms of narcotic withdrawal in the neonate begin in the first 48 hours but might be delayed as long as 8 days. The clinical effects include a decreased Moro reflex, uncoordinated sucking action, tremors, a shrill, protracted cry, increased tendon reflexes, convulsion, watery diarrhea, cyanosis, dehydration, vasomotor instability, and collapse. The diagnosis of narcotic withdrawal in a neonate can be confirmed by identifying the narcotic in the urine of the mother and infant after symptoms are present.

Treatment The goal of treatment is the control of symptoms. Phenobarbital, diazepam, and chlorpromazine have all been used in the treatment of withdrawal symptoms. Camphorated opium tincture (paregoric) can be given and appeared to be more effective than phenobarbital in one controlled study (Carin, et al., 1983). (See Chapter 24 for a discussion of drug abuse.)

Cyclic Antidepressants

Pharmacology Cyclic antidepressants are prescribed to children to treat depression and to manage nocturnal enuresis. Cyclic antidepressants have both central and peripheral effects, which result from the blockage of the reuptake of norepinephrine, an atropine-like anticholinergic effect, and a direct myocardial depressant effect. The major cause of mortality is cardiotoxicity.

Cyclic antidepressants can be divided into several classifications determined by their structure, as follows:

- Tricyclics
  - Amitriptyline (Elavil)
  - Amoxapine (Asendin)
  - Doxepin (Sinequan)
  - Desipramine (Norpramin)
  - Nortriptyline (Aventyl)
- Tetracyclics
  - Maprotiline (Ludiomil)
  - Mianserin (investigational)
- Bicyclic
  - Viloxazine (investigational)
  - Zimelidine (investigational)
- Miscellaneous
  - Trazadone (Desyrel)

Clinical Effects The clinical effects of cyclic antidepressant overdoses are variable. Mild exposure can result in lethargy, tachycardia, urinary retention, and a dry mouth. Severe cyclic antidepressant ingestion can result in hypotension, convulsions, coma, and life-threatening ventricular arrythmias.

Treatment The following is a list of treatment guidelines for cyclic antidepressant overdose:

1. Absorption should be prevented by the administration of ipecac or lavage, charcoal, and a cathartic.
2. All patients should be placed on a cardiac monitor and observed for conduction defects and ventricular arrhythmias for a minimum of 6 hours. Patients with arrhythmias should be monitored until they are free of arrhythmias for at least 24 hours. Conduction defects can be managed with phenytoin administered intravenously at 15 mg/kg (up to 1 g), not to exceed a rate of 0.5 mg/kg/min. Ventricular arrhythmias might respond to concurrent alkalinization and phenytoin therapy. Arrhythmias unresponsive to this therapy might respond to lidocaine, inderal, or physostigmine.
3. Children are frequently more sensitive to antidepressants and might demonstrate symptoms at lower doses. Any history suggestive of cyclic antidepressant ingestion in

children warrants evaluation in an emergency care facility and cardiac monitoring.

4. Fatal poisonings have occurred in children following the ingestion of as little as 250 mg of imipramine, and severe toxicity with seizures and cardiac arrhythmias has occurred in a 3-year-old following the ingestion of 100 mg of desipramine (Manoguerra, 1982).

Lomotil

Pharmacology Lomotil is a combination of diphenoxylate and atropine sulfate. Diphenoxylate has a definite constipating effect.

Clinical Effects Lomotil causes serious respiratory depression, which is characterized by periods of apnea and respiratory failure. Children also might develop drowsiness progressing to coma, which might be delayed up to 6–8 hours or longer after ingestion. Anticholinergic effects include urinary retention and absence of bowel sounds (Rumack and Temple, 1974).

Treatment Suspected Lomotil ingestion should be evaluated in an emergency care facility with the prevention of absorption and assessment of vital signs. All children should be observed for 24 hours in an intensive care unit regardless of other factors. It is considered negligent to discharge a child (age 0–6 years) after Lomotil ingestion before 24 hours of observation because of the possibility of delayed symptoms. Respiratory depression and coma can be reversed with naloxone. The recommended pediatric dose is 0.1 mg/kg intravenously. If the child does not respond to this initial dose, a follow-up dose of 2 mg can be administered.

Key Concepts

- Poisoning is the most common pediatric emergency, accounting for 10% of all ambulance responses and occurring most frequently in children under 5 years of age.
- Young children normally use their mouths while exploring, which predisposes them to being poisoned.
- As children grow, the accessibility of poisonous substances increases.
- During middle and late childhood, children often have a knowledge deficit regarding poisonous substances, whereas adolescents are often ignorant about the lack of quality control in the manufacture and sale of street drugs.
- The list of poisons includes not only household products and medications but also plants and venomous snakes and spiders.
- The majority of poisonings occur in the home from common household products and poisonous substances not stored in their original containers.
- Children are exposed to greater poison hazards when visiting the homes of adults without small children such as grandparents.
- Poisonings increase when stress or family disequilibrium results in decreased supervision of the child.
- Nursing interventions at the primary level are directed toward increasing the parents' knowledge and encouraging practices that decrease the chances of accidental poisoning.
- Discussion of poisoning should be a routine part of well-child visits, informing the parents of the characteristics of the child, agent, and environment that contribute to poisoning.
- Poison-proofing the home should be a top priority for parents.
- Nurses can educate parents about the signs and symptoms of poisoning as well as the initial first aid required to minimize the resulting injury.
- Keeping syrup of ipecac in the house and having the poison control center telephone number easily accessible are important first-aid principles.
- Parents should call their nearest poison control center before treating any poison ingestion.
- Nurses should help the parents deal with their feelings of guilt following an accidental poisoning.
- Nursing care of a child following an accidental poisoning includes obtaining all possible pertinent information in the shortest possible time.
- A nursing history includes such factors as the telephone number and address of the child, circumstances and agent of the poisoning, symptoms, physical characteristics of the child, and any treatment initiated by the parent.

- The nursing assessment can be made whether life is in immediate danger, potential danger, or no danger.
- Secondary information, such as whether playmate or sibling exposure also occurred, might be obtained as well.
- First aid for ocular exposure requires flushing with copious amounts of water for 15–20 minutes; first aid for dermal exposure is the same.
- The initial measure for poison ingestion is the administration of milk or water if the child is conscious, except in instances of pill ingestion.
- Initial management of the child includes establishment and maintenance of the airway, cardiovascular stabilization, restoring any electrolyte imbalances, and the administration of naloxone (for overdose situations).
- Prevention of poison absorption is accomplished by gastric emptying, gastric lavage, charcoal, and/or cathartics.
- Advanced management of the acutely poisoned child includes forced diuresis, hemodialysis, hemoperfusion, chelation, or antidotes.
- Nurses should be familiar with or able to locate information regarding specific poison agents.

References

Arnold RE: Brown recluse spider bites: Five cases with review of the literature. *JACEP* 1976;5(4):262–264.

Aronow R, Spigiel R: Implications of camphor poisoning. *Drug Intell Clin Pharm* 1976;10:631.

Baker E, et al: Lead poisoning in children of lead workers. *N Engl J Med* 1977;296(5):260–261.

Banner W, Czajka P: Acute caffeine overdose in the neonate. *Am J Dis Child* 1980;134:495–498.

Berman LB, Schreiner GE, Fegs J: The nephrotoxic lesions of ethylene glycol. *Ann Intern Med* 1957;46:611–619.

Binder JW, Roberts RJ: Carbon monoxide intoxication in children. *Clin Toxicol* 1980;16(3):287–295.

Burke M: Gastric lavage and emesis in the treatment of ingested poisons: A review and clinical study of lavage in ten adults. *Resuscitation* 1972(I);91–105.

Carin S, et al: Neonatal methadone withdrawal. *Am J Dis Child* 1983; 137;378–382.

Cello JP, Fogel RP, Boland R: Liquid caustic ingestion. *Arch Intern Med* 1980;140:501–504.

Conrad F: Tips for treating corrosive burns. *Nursing* (Feb) 1983;13(2):55.

Corby DG: Aspirin in pregnancy: Maternal and fetal effects. *Pediatrics* 1978;62(Suppl):930–937.

Dethlefs R, Naraqui S: Ocular manifestations and complications of acute methyl alcohol intoxication. *Med J Aust* 1978;2:483–485.

Done AK: Aspirin overdose: Incidence, diagnosis and management. *Pediatrics* 1978:62(Suppl):890–897.

Done AK: Salicylate intoxication: Significance of measurements of salicylates in blood in cases of acute ingestion. *Pediatrics* 1960;26:800–807.

Drug Facts and Comparisons. Lippincott, 1985.

Drugdex. Micromedix, Inc. (Englewood, CO), 1977.

Environmental Protection Agency: *Toxic Substances Control Act Chemical Substances Inventory*. U.S. Govt. Printing Office, 1982.

FDA Drug Bull. Dept. Health and Human Services. 1983;13:1.

Findlay JWA, et al: Analgesic drugs in the breast milk and plasma. *Clin Pharmacol Ther* (May) 1981;29:625–633.

Frazier C: *Insect Allergy*. Warren H. Green, 1969.

Ganandran A: Organophosphate insecticide poisoning and its management. *Anaesth Intensive Care* 1974;2(4):361–368.

Gilles C et. al: Management of pediatric poisoning: Role of the nurse practitioner. *Pediatr Nurs* (Sept/Oct) 1980;633–635.

Gosselin RE, et al (editors): Methyl alcohol, in *Clinical Toxicology of Commercial Products*. 4th ed. Williams and Wilkins, 1976.

Haddad LM, Winchester J: *Clinical Management of Poisoning and Overdose*. Saunders, 1983.

Harrison TR, et al: *Principles of Internal Medicine*. 8th ed. McGraw-Hill, 1977.

Heindl D: Klinische beebachtungen an 137 gutartigen oespphagustenosen der I chirurgische universitatsklinik. Wein. Ztschr Exp Chir 1926;199:252.

Herson VC, Schmitt BD, Rumack BH: Magical thinking and imipramine poisoning in two school-aged children. *JAMA* 1979;241(18):1926–1927.

Hunt R: Toxicity of ethylene and propylene glycol. *Industrial Eng Chem* 1932;24:361.

Jacobi A: Preschooler's discrimination of poisonous from non-poisonous household items as identified by the Mr. Yuk poison prevention sticker. *CHC* 1983;11(3):98–101.

Jelenko C: Chemicals that "burn." *J Trauma* (Jan) 1974;14:65–72.

Johnston LD, Bachman JG, O'Malley PM: Drugs and the nation's high school students. In: *Drug Abuse in the Modern World*. Nahas GG, Frick HC (editors). Pergamon Press, 1981.

Kirsh MM, Ritter F: Caustic ingestion and subsequent damage to the oropharyngeal and digestive passages. *Ann Thorac Surg* (Jan) 1976;21:74–82.

Klaasen CD: Heavy metal and heavy-metal antagonists. In: *Pharmacologic Basis of Therapeutics*. 6th ed. Williams & Wilkins, 1980.

Kline S, Bayer M: Insecticide poisoning. TEM 1979;1(3):73–83.

Knopp R: Caustic ingestions. *JACEP* 1979;8:329–336.

Kopelman R, et al: Camphor intoxication treated by hemoperfusion. *JAMA* 1979;241:727–728.

Kulig K, Rumack B: Hydrocarbon ingestion. *Curr Top Emerg Med* 1981;3(4):1–5.

Lacouture P, et al: Emergency assessment of severity in iron overdose by clinical and laboratory methods. *J Pediatr* 1981;99(1):89–91.

Leape LL: New liquid lye drain cleaners. *Clin Toxicol* 1974;7(1):109–114.

Levy G: Clinical pharmacokinetics of aspirin. *Pediatrics* 1978; 62(Suppl):867–872.

Levy G: Pharmacokinetics of salicylate in man. *Drug Metab Rev* 1979;9: 3–19.

Levy G, et al: Evidence of placental transfer of acetaminophen. *Pediatrics* 1975;55:895.

Lin-Fuj JS: Preventing lead poisoning in children. *Child Today* 1973; 2–6.

Manoguerra AS: Tricyclic antidepressants. *Crit Care Q* 1982;43–51.

Martindale: *The Extra Pharmacopaeia.* 27th ed. Pharmaceutical Press, 1977.

McCoy HG, et al: Severe methanol poisoning. Application of pharmacokinetics model for ethanol therapy and hemodialysis. *Am J Med* 1979;67:804–807.

Micik S: Emergency medical services and poison control. *Clin Toxicol* 1978;12(3):309–317.

Milby TH: Prevention and management of organophosphate poisoning. *JAMA* 1971;216(13):2131–2133.

Namba T, et al: Poisoning due to organophosphate insecticides, acute and chronic manifestations. *JAMA* 1971;465–489.

National Clearinghouse for Poison Control Centers Bulletin. 1972;1–4.

National Clearinghouse for Poison Control Centers Bulletin. 1980;*24*(10).

Parker PR, Parker WA: Pharmacokinetic considerations in the haemodialysis of drugs. *J Clin Hosp Pharm* 1982;7:87–99.

Pincus D, Saccar C: Lead poisoning. American Family Physician (Jan) 1979;19(6):120–124.

Poisindex. Micromedix, Inc. (Englewood, CO), 1974.

Pond S, et al: Pharmacokinetics of hemoperfusion for drug overdose. *Clin Pharmacokinet* 1979;4(5):329–354.

Product Information: Tyzine. Key Laboratories, 1981.

Raskin N, Mullaney: The mental and neurological sequelae of carbon monoxide asphyxia in a case observed for fifteen years. *J Nerv Ment Dis* 1940;92:640.

Ray JF, et al: The natural history of liquid lye ingestion. *Arch Surg* 1974;109:436–439.

Rumack BH, Matthew H: Acetaminophen poisoning and toxicity. *Pediatrics* 1975;55:871–876.

Rumack BH, Temple: Lomotil poisoning. *Pediatrics* 1974;53:495–500.

Rumack BH, Sullivan J, Peterson R: *Management of Acute Poisoning and Overdose.* Rocky Mountain Poison Center, 1981.

Russell FE: Page 254 in: *Snake Venom Poisoning.* Lippincott, 1980.

Russell FE, Waldron WG, Madon MB: Bites by the *Loxosceles Unicolor* and *Loxosceles Arizonica* in California and Arizona. *Toxicon* 1969;7:109–117.

Sanders J, Miller DD, Patil PN: Alpha adrenergic and histaminergic effects of tolozoline-like imidazoles. *J Pharmacol Exp Ther* 1975;195(2):362–371.

San Francisco Bay Area Regional Poison Center: *Poisonous and Non-Poisonous Plant List.* San Francisco Bay Area Regional poison Center, 1979.

Schaffer JH, Lavengood SJ: 1980 survey of poison control centers, summary of results. *National Clearinghouse for Poison Control Centers Bulletin* 1982;26(1).

Scherger D, et al: Ethylene glycol intoxication. *J Emer Nurs* 1983;9(2):71–73.

Schiller J: *Childhood Injury.* Stein & Day, 1977.

Seeff LB, et al: Ethylene glycol poisoning: Survival after ingestion of 400 cc with 42 days of oliguria and 17 days of coma. *Med Ann DC* 1970;39:31–35.

Smith JS, Brierly H, Brandon S: A kinetic mutism with recovery after repeated carbon monoxide poisoning. *Psychol Med* 1971;1:172.

Smith TW, et al: Reversal of advanced digoxin intoxication with Fab fragments of digoxin-specific antibodies. *N Engl J Med* 1976;294:797–800.

Smith TW, et al: Treatment of life-threatening digitalis intoxication with digoxin-specific Fab antibody fragments. *N Engl J Med* 1982; 307(22):1357–1362.

Sobel R: The psychiatric implications of accidental poisoning in childhood. *Pediatr Clin North Am* 1970;*17*(3):653–685.

Stahl, Kasser IS: Pentazocine overdose. *Ann Emer Med* 1983;12:28–31.

Steele R, Conklin R, Mark H: Corticosteroids and antibodies for the treatment of fulminant hydrocarbon aspiration. *JAMA* 1972;219:1434–1437.

Temple AR: Acute and chronic effects of aspirin toxicity and their treatment. *Arch Intern Med* 1981;141:364–369.

Temple AR, Mancini RE: Management of poisoning. In: *Pediatric Pharmacology.* Yaffe SJ (editor). Grune & Stratton, 1980.

The 1977 street drug analysis results. *Clin Toxicol* 1979;14(5):619–630.

Wedman C: A few cases of ethylene glycol intoxication. *Acta Med Scand* 1946;126:295.

Weiss J, Catalano P: Camphorated oil intoxication during pregnancy. *Pediatrics* 1973;52:713.

Wiemer MB, et al: *Clinical Pharmacology and Therapeutics in Nursing.* McGraw-Hill, 1979.

Winter PM, Miller JN: Carbon monoxide poisoning. *JAMA* 1976;236:1502.

Zimmerman SS, Truxal B: Carbon monoxide poisoning. *Pediatrics* 1981;68(2):215–224.

Zucker AR, et al: Fab fragments of digoxin-specific antibodies used to reverse ventricular fibrillation induced by digoxin ingestion in a child. *Pediatrics* 1982;70(3):468–471.

Anticipatory Guidance

Joan Pernice Sandra R. Mott

21

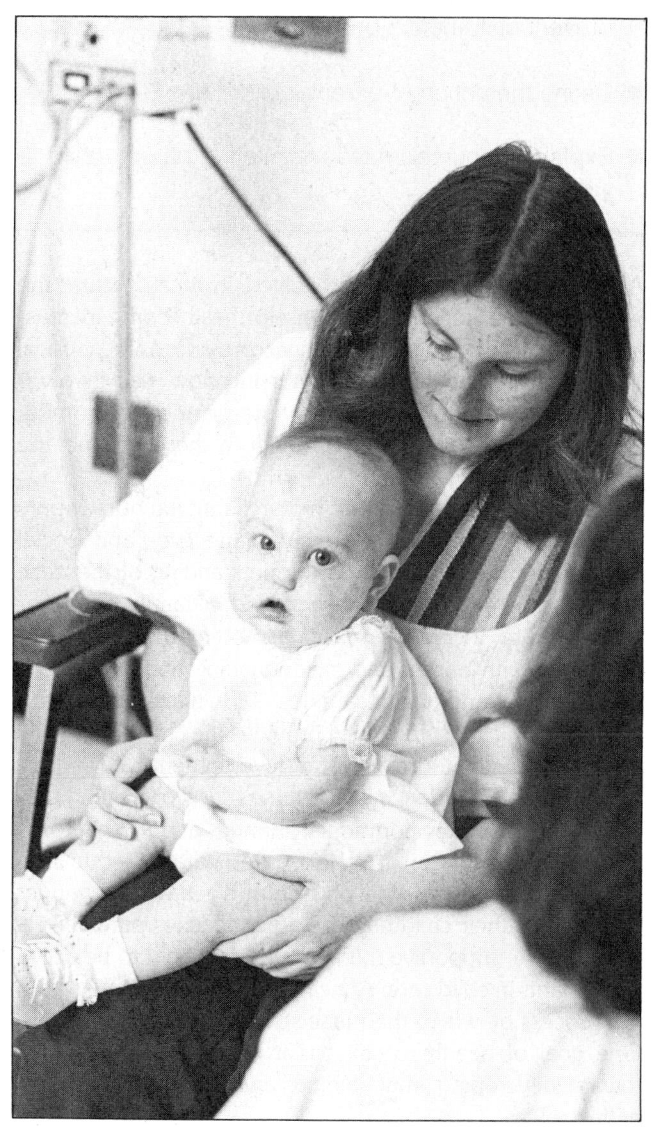

Chapter Outline

Objectives

- Define anticipatory guidance.
- Explain how anticipatory guidance can be used to prevent child health problems.
- Define the notion of parent–child "fit."
- Explain the nurse's role in facilitating parent–child interactions.
- Describe the developmental norms and common concerns about which parents often need nursing guidance.
- Relate common parenting concerns to the expected developmental stage in which each occurs.
- Describe nursing interventions that enhance parents' confidence and ability to meet their children's developmental needs.

As child health nursing has evolved in recent years, the nurse's role as teacher and counselor has become increasingly significant. Nurses no longer provide only physical care to children. Child health nursing now also involves assessment and interventions that are planned to promote the psychosocial development of both the child and the family.

Child health care therefore requires that the nurse apply knowledge of physical, cognitive, affective, and social development together with an understanding of theoretic and scientific principles to each individual family. Comprehensive care includes appropriately timed assessments combined with parent and child teaching about developmental norms and health care needs. By teaching self-care and parenting skills, the nurse provides the child and family with tools they can use to foster development.

Anticipatory guidance is the nurse's tool for helping parents prepare for developmental changes and to better understand their children. It is a form of preparatory education in which parents learn what physical and behavioral changes to expect in their children. The nurse teaches parents in a collaborative, supportive manner, allowing them to be active participants in child care. Anticipatory guidance is therefore the process by which the nurse structures health teaching. One goal of health teaching is in turn to guide parents toward developing, maintaining, and enjoying their parenting roles.

In Chapter 13 we discussed parenting styles and methods of discipline that the nurse might need to teach parents at particular stages of child development. In Chapters 7 through 11, we outlined the process of development and the basic health care needs for children at each developmental stage. Specific guidelines for assessing the family's ability to support and the child's own progress in accomplishing expected skills, tasks, and behaviors in the areas of physical growth, nutritional health, developmental milestones, and family relations are found in Chapters 14 through 17. In Chapters 18 through 20 we discussed the prevention of common childhood problems related to illness, injury, and poisoning. In this chapter we summarize the information in these preceding chapters by providing a structure for specific nursing interventions at each stage of child development, and we define the concepts that the nurse applies in providing well-child care.

Anticipatory Guidance as Prevention

Anticipatory guidance is a form of preventive child health care. Whether the nurse works with parents in an ambulatory clinic, hospital, health maintenance organization, or day-care center, the process of anticipating child health problems and intervening before they occur is a form of primary prevention.

The assessment process provides the opportunity for nurse–parent discussions about parental concerns and potential needs. Open-ended questions and active listening then help the nurse to identify areas that might require further assessment and intervention. As Chapter 16 explains, parent–child interaction is a component of the nurse's assessment of social development, and the data obtained might suggest knowledge deficits that require teaching or referral. In determining whether assessment data suggest a need for teaching, the nurse considers both parent and child behaviors. Do parental behaviors and the developmental stage of the child correspond? Is the parent realistic in perceiving the child's capabilities? Does the parent understand the need for an environment that is conducive to development of all subsystems?

Potential for Family Growth

The extent to which families maintain their functioning depends greatly on the childrearing methods practiced by the parents. Parents often express the need for affirmation or guidance in developing a flexible repertoire of skills that they can adapt to the unique qualities of their children. Nurses might therefore need to teach parents methods of discipline, managing normal developmental concerns (such as toilet training or temper tantrums), and communicating with children (see Chapter 13).

The nurse uses skills in child and family assessment to plan with the family how best to provide needed assistance to support adaptive parenting and prevent dysfunction. Knowing the normal developmental milestones and tasks for each stage allows the nurse to anticipate questions and direct discussions toward areas of potential need. The nurse then paces teaching to match the parent's readiness to learn and thus enhances parental self-esteem.

Stressors for Parents Family life has changed dramatically since the 1950s as families have been affected by technical, environmental, political, and economic forces. Children are now influenced by a variety of systems outside their families as they come in contact with television, day-care centers, government agencies, and changing schools and religious institutions. As all of these factors influence the family system, they challenge parents to monitor these factors by being informed and selective as to the influences to which their children are exposed. Parents then need to decide when to encourage or restrain their children's participation. In an increasingly complex world, some parents have difficulty teaching values, setting limits, and promoting development in ways that are consistent with the expectations of the family and the community at large.

Nurses in community-based health agencies, sometimes in collaboration with social services, might conduct parenting classes. In other settings the nurse intervenes to refer parents to educational sessions sponsored by churches, school systems, or private organizations. The nurse might, however, need to consider whether a family's financial resources make such a referral feasible or whether a social service agency can offer financial aid.

For example, if a child in a low-income family is diagnosed as having a learning disability, referring the child to an expensive private school that is equipped to handle the problem is not an appropriate solution. A better solution might be a special class within the public school system combined with a neighborhood-based after-school tutorial program where special education is offered free of charge. Advice is thus most acceptable and effective when the parent has the resources to follow it.

Another source of confusion for parents is the vast array of advice they receive. Relatives, friends, books, and other well-meaning advisors might offer conflicting solutions to problems and information about childrearing. Many parents need the nurse to help them sort through the advice and determine the solution to a specific problem or general parenting style that is most consistent with their values, cultural norms, parenting goals, and child's personality.

The nurse might find it useful to refer parents to books about parenting. An extensive body of literature is available in libraries and bookstores; therefore, the nurse will want to be familiar with the family's needs and preferences before making specific recommendations. Printed materials are also best used in conjunction with counseling sessions to provide parents with opportunities to discuss their reactions. Books that describe "how to be a parent" can be helpful, but they also can confuse parents if the information is misinterpreted, inappropriate, or followed too rigidly.

Many parents also worry about leaving their children with others, whether with a babysitter occasionally or with

Guidelines for Selecting Day Care

1. *Facilities*: Should be clean, have safe, sturdy equipment inside and sturdy playground equipment outside, and be furnished according to the size and age of the children. Rooms should be bright and cheery, with no peeling paint or wallpaper. General safety measures should be observed (eg, wall plugs, fire extinguishers, no dangling cords, kitchen area gated, smoke detector alarms, and sprinkler system).

2. *Philosophy of care*: Should have organized activities and a structured day that includes independent, free play. Assess the tools and toys available for creative expression, supervision of interactions, and willingness to discuss the child's experience with objects and tools in the act of creating. A variety of play and learning experiences should be available. Observe the nature of the discipline practiced.

3. *Organization*: Note the age divisions of the groups, how many groups, and the space allotment. Evaluate how meals are served and feeding managed. Note the type of food served and its appropriateness. Note the provision for naps and willingness to adapt to each child's need for more or less rest.

4. *Policy for illness*: Evaluate the center's plan if the child becomes ill or injured at the facility. Inquire whether the center has a firm policy about children not attending when ill with a "cold." Does the center provide transportation to a primary health care agency?

5. *Ratio between staff and children*: Assess if each infant or child is provided with sufficient individual attention. Do time and staffing allow individual or small group play and teaching experiences?

6. *Recommendations*: Be sure the center is state-approved and licensed and passes all board of health and safety regulations and fire code requirements. Obtain references from friends or relatives who have used the center.

7. *Child's response*: The best indicator is the child's reaction. Note whether the child is happy when picked up, reasonably happy to be attending, talks positively about the staff and other children, and whether the child seems to have a special or preferred staff person.

Guidelines for Picking a Sitter

1. *Recommendations*: Check with friends or relatives who have used the sitter previously. Discuss an adult sitter's qualifications with the agency or, if younger, with parents, teachers, or club leaders. Inquire about letters of reference or special classes in babysitting responsibilities.

2. *Age*: The sitter's age varies somewhat with the child's age and child-care need. Adults are preferred for extended periods of time such as weekends or for several days. Young infants require a sitter who is thoroughly familiar with infant care and demands, either an adult or an experienced high school student who has younger siblings. Elementary school children can care for young children for brief periods during the day. It is usually best if the babysitter resides in the neighborhood and his/her parents are at home. Older children might resent sitters who are close in age; best to have an adult in that situation.

3. *Experience*: It is best if the sitter has had previous experience with child care, including the care of younger siblings or relatives. If using an agency service, inquire about the sitter's employment history. If the sitter's experience is limited, begin with a short assignment.

4. *Experience with your child*: If the sitter lives in the neighborhood, evaluate interactions with the child in other situations, child's response to sitter, and sitter's ability to tend to the child's needs. If the sitter is unknown, it might be helpful to have the sitter come for an hour the day before to get acquainted with the child so that the child will view the sitter as a friend. If coming the day before is inconvenient, have the sitter arrive an hour earlier for the same purpose.

5. *Personal characteristics*: The sitter should be healthy, with no acute illnesses, have mature judgment, be responsible, and be knowledgeable about safety in general and specific safety for the child's age. The sitter should enjoy being with and playing with children and be patient. The sitter should follow the parent's directions about food, bedtime, television, clothing, and other routines and rules. The sitter should not ask to have personal friends of either sex over while sitting and should not use the telephone for social calls. The sitter should be told where the parent may be reached, if necessary, the expected return time, emergency telephone numbers, and where to put messages.

a child-care center on a regular basis. They might express concerns about safety, nutrition, cleanliness, or the overall quality of attention given by child-care providers. The nurse often can help parents choose appropriate child care by providing information. Some parents need checklists of points to consider in selecting a sitter. Others need to know about options available for child care during the day.

Some parents need to know that child-care providers, especially those who care for a child daily, also might require information about a specific child's developmental needs. For example, if an infant who is learning to crawl spends each day at a babysitter's home, the parent will need to assess that environment to determine whether the child's safety needs are being met.

Parent–Child "Fit" In the process of assessing family functioning, the nurse assesses the *parent–child "fit,"* or the extent to which both parent and child meet and adapt to each other's needs. An imperfect parent–child fit might be the result of insufficient or deficient attachment early in infancy, or it might become evident later, as the child's developing personality fails to match the parent's expectations.

The nurse assesses the parent–child fit by asking the parent about the expectations held concerning the child, whether reality and expectations are similar, and how well parent and child have adapted to each other. When the parent and child "read" each other's signals correctly, their responses are appropriate, and each feels competent.

For example, when observing the infant who is beginning to squirm and fuss, the parent changes the infant's position, provides a new toy, or spends a few minutes in play, feeling confident that those actions will satisfy the infant. The parent has learned to interpret correctly the infant's sounds and to respond in ways that are satisfying to both of them. Another mother has learned that when her young son whines and lays his head down on the table, it is better to give him a nap before the meal. He plays so hard that he is unaware of his fatigue until he sits down to eat. Her sense of competence in her ability to interpret her son's needs enables her to follow through with her decisions even when questioned or criticized by others.

At other times, a developmental history might reveal that the parent had anticipated a quiet, cuddly infant and instead had to contend with an infant who fussed a great deal and was difficult to console. The infant's temperament did not "fit" the parent's expectations. Normal development might therefore be compromised unless interventions can help the parent adapt to the behavioral pattern of the infant and experience positive reciprocal interactions with the child.

The child health nurse who meets the parent for the first time during the postpartum and neonatal period thus assesses the parent's expectations and the infant's temperamental characteristics (see Chapter 16). If expectations and temperament do not match, early detection gives the nurse the opportunity to assist the parent to adapt to the infant and learn to appreciate the positive aspects of the infant's temperament.

Potential for Meeting Developmental Needs

By understanding the child's temperament and behavioral style, the parent can approach each developmental stage in a way that is consistent and fosters growth. Parents whose expectations for their children's development are realistic come to appreciate each child's unique characteristics. Knowing developmental norms also allows the parent to promote development by providing appropriate stimulation.

For example, some 1-year-olds need special attention to verbal stimulation to help them practice language skills. Others need toys that provide opportunities to enhance gross motor development. The parent who has learned about developmental norms and who knows the child's behavior patterns, strengths, and weaknesses is more likely to be prepared for the child's developmental progress.

The nurse might need to remind some parents that children progress at different rates and that when most children concentrate on one or another area of development, they plateau or appear slower in the others. The nurse therefore explains that normal developmental milestones occur within a range and that a pace that might appear to be slow in some areas is not necessarily evidence of serious developmental delays. Some parents also might need to learn to accept their children's slower-paced development. The nurse then counsels the parents to focus on the child's strengths and to accept the child's need to learn skills at a slower pace.

In the process of developmental assessment, the nurse might therefore want to emphasize a child's strengths and achievements. For example, in assessing an infant the nurse might use the Brazelton Neonatal Behavioral Assessment Scale (BNBAS) to teach the parent about the behavioral and temperamental qualities of an infant. (The BNBAS is discussed in Chapter 16.) The nurse identifies the infant's strengths while proceeding through the assessment and describes the infant's responses as positive signs of development. The parent then learns to recognize the infant's responses as a pattern of behavior and can plan caregiving and consoling methods according to what works best for the infant's behavioral style. By facilitating this recognition, the nurse supports the parental adjustment process and enhances a positive parent–infant fit.

The assessment process also provides an opportunity for the nurse to discuss parenting and caregiving techniques that seem best suited for a particular infant. This enables parents to get a head start in learning their infant's characteristics and what methods work best, which would otherwise have to be learned through trial and error. Parents learn how best to hold their infants, what environmental stimuli engage the infants most, and how the infant expresses hunger. The assessment process might then help parents to understand and anticipate behaviors and affords them the opportunity to ask questions about problem areas.

When parents cite problems in feeding, sleeping, discipline, or dependence, the nurse's best response is usually, "What have you tried to do about it so far?" If the parent then describes a method that has failed, the nurse might ask, "Why do you think it didn't work?" As parents describe their responses, the nurse might discover that the parent did not give the method a chance or that the parent was not comfortable with the method chosen. Parenting styles and methods need to be suited to the parent as well as the child. For example, a parent who finds it difficult to allow an infant to cry unattended for a few minutes need not be encouraged to do so. The nurse might instead ask, "What would you like to do now?" and proceed to work with the parent to develop a plan for solving the problem. Likewise, the parent of a 12-year-old who is frustrated by the consistently negative reply given whenever the child is asked to help around the house can be helped to analyze why the current approach is not working and to formulate a new one. Sometimes parental expectations do not change with the child's development. The child's perception of the chores requested might be that they are for "babies" and beneath the dignity of a 12-year-old. By helping the parent and child better understand their own selves and each other, the nurse can facilitate communication between them.

Structuring Anticipatory Guidance

To teach parents about their children's upcoming developmental needs, the nurse begins each interview with a teaching plan that includes general health maintenance needs for the child's age. The teaching plan, however, is not rigid. Because many parents desire to be more informed and involved in their child's care, their needs for information are as varied as their educational and experiential backgrounds. By asking parents general open-ended questions about their child as well as questions about their specific concerns, the nurse can identify areas where additional information and discussion are needed. In addition, similar questions are asked and information obtained from the child as appropriate. The nurse then adapts teaching to match the expressed concerns and implied needs of both the child and family. Table 21-1 outlines likely health maintenance needs at each developmental stage and represents a synthesis of material covered in greater depth in the preceding chapters.

TABLE 21-1 Schedule for Child Health Maintenance Program

		Assessment area—guidelines				Anticipatory guidance		
Age	**Procedures**	**Physical**	**Nutritional**	**Developmental**	**Family**	**Safety**	**Health**	**Parenting role**
1 month	Parental concerns; lab (PKU [phenylketonuria] as indicated); prenatal, birth, and neonatal history	Growth assessment—plot length, weight, and head circumference; reflexes; complete examination, include vision and hearing	Type of feeding; total intake (ounces or length of time at breast); frequency of feedings; discuss need for fluoride, vitamins, and iron as indicated	Reflex stage—responds to object, follows to midline; hands held in fist; lifts head slightly when prone; begins cooing; sensitive to light and sounds; regards face	Bonding between parent and infant; adjustment of family to new member; parental expectations and infant's temperament as perceived by parent; participation of other family members in infant's care; parental satisfaction	Use of infant safety seat in car; secure infant on changing table and infant seat; never leave alone except in crib or playpen; crib safety (bars spaced $2\frac{1}{4}$ in or less, mattress right size, bumper pads around crib); pacifier safety	Discuss delaying solids; avoid large crowds; care not to overdress; bathing and skin care needs, especially diaper area	Appropriate stimulation (eg, talking to and holding, rocking, mobile, touching, music); interpreting infant's cry—not always hunger, may be for attention or position change; attachment versus spoiling; waking time gradually increases; guidelines for selecting a babysitter; if breast-feeding, pump or supplement feeding
2 months	Parental concerns; immunizations (DPT #1, OPV #1)	Growth assessment—plot length, weight, and head circumference; interval history; complete examination	Type and amount of feeding; frequency of feedings (schedule or feeding routine more dependable); discuss caloric needs	Better head control; head erect though bobbing when supported sitting; raises head 45° when prone; social smile; follows past midline—follows moving person; may get fist to mouth; coos, gurgles	Reciprocal interaction between parent and infant and between other family members and infant; adjustment of siblings to infant; family routines and sharing of tasks; parental perception of infant's temperament and of "fit" into family; parental satisfaction	Review car safety; emphasize securing infant, raising crib sides, and not leaving alone because infant becoming more active, will start to turn over; toy safety—large, smooth edges, nonbreakable, no small objects (pins) within reach	Possible reaction to immunizations; topical comfort measures—systemic reaction care; guidelines for indicating an infant is ill (eg, change in feeding, sleeping, disposition, fever, sneezing, vomiting, diarrhea); guidelines for contacting child health provider	Appropriate stimulation (eg, continue trust-fostering behaviors, increased interest in visual stimulation—toys, baby mirror, faces); increased alert times; move awake infant from room to room with parent; guidelines for selecting day care if appropriate; lay infant prone several times a day to strengthen neck muscles

TABLE 21-1 continued

		Assessment area—guidelines				Anticipatory guidance		
Age	**Procedures**	**Physical**	**Nutritional**	**Developmental**	**Family**	**Safety**	**Health**	**Parenting role**
4 months	Parental concerns; immunizations (DPT #2, OPV #2)	Growth assessment—plot length, weight, and head circumference; interval history; complete examination; assess disappearance of infantile reflexes (all [except sucking] should be diminishing); vision and hearing examination	Type of feeding; amount and frequency; nighttime feeding	Pulls to sit with little head lag; follows 180°; may roll over; begins reaching; hands together at midline—stares, repeats; grasps toy, brings to mouth; localizes sound; vocalizes random syllables; laughs	Responds to parent in special way; recognizes difference between family member and stranger; family function and roles with infant and each other returning to "normal"; parents have time alone	Review auto safety; increased mobility requires extra precautions—may decide to change diapers and dress infant on floor or in crib; review toy safety—puts everything in mouth, all small objects out of reach, need to caution other children; begin to lower mattress	Discuss when to start solids; begin with rice cereal, use 5–7 days before trying another; discuss response to last immunization and expected response to second one; drooling might begin—sign of salivary gland maturation; not teething	The use of jumper, high chair, swing for short intervals when able to hold head erect; stimulation needs include cradle gyms to grasp, toys to reach, grasp, shake; keep with people when awake; pull to sit after changing and support in sitting position; schedule more regular
6 months	Parental concerns; immunizations (DPT #3); lab—urinalysis	Growth assessment—plot length, weight, and head circumference; interval history; complete examination; assess disappearance of infantile reflexes (palmar grasp, tonic neck and Moro absent, parachute evolving, neck righting and reciprocal kicking diminishing, sucking present); assess vision (strabismus) and hearing; might start cutting teeth	Type of feeding; solid food started; frequency and total intake; review caloric needs; decrease in formula/breast milk when solids added	Sits—tripod positions; rolls over in both directions; transfers objects from hand to hand; imitation of familiar sounds, gestures; hand–eye coordination—purposeful reaching; separates self from environment; begins separation anxiety; vocalizes to get attention; repeats interesting behaviors	Infant more playful and responsive to family; increased interest on part of older siblings and father; plays with self-made sounds, toys, objects—imitates familiar—enjoys attention; discuss infant–parent "fit"; parenting satisfaction; family communication patterns	Review auto safety; discuss toy safety—removal of large stuffed animals from crib (use to stand on and fall); lower mattress before infant is standing; safety-proof house (location of poisons, including plants, extension cords, "breakables," tablecloths, sharp edges, stairs, wall outlets, space heaters); safe teething toys; increasingly mobile	Discuss addition of solids—emphasize importance of cereal for iron; add fruits and yellow vegetables; try each for 5–7 days before adding new to screen out allergies; only one new food at a time; no eggs or orange juice; finger foods such as crackers; introduce cup; discuss response to last immunization and expected response to third; review ill-child care	Discuss weaning if appropriate or encourage to wait until 1 year of age if breast feeding; use of formula versus cow's milk; discuss danger of bottle-mouth syndrome with bedtime bottles of formula or liquid with high sugar content; discuss separation anxiety—preference for primary caregiver; night crying might occur; teething comfort aids

continued on next page

TABLE 21-1 continued

Age	Procedures	Assessment area—guidelines				Anticipatory guidance		
		Physical	Nutritional	Developmental	Family	Safety	Health	Parenting role
9 months	Parental concerns; lab—hemoglobin/hematocrit, screening for sickle cell disease, and glucose-6-phosphate dehydrogenase (G-6-PD) deficiency as appropriate	Growth assessment—plot length, weight, and head circumference; interval history; complete examination; speech (jargon and inflected vocabulary indicates hearing intact)	Eats three to four meals a day; feeds self finger foods; starts using spoon but needs help; drinks from held cup; eats table foods that are soft, chopped, or ground; problem with meats	Sits alone; bears weight on legs when supported; crawls, scoots increasingly mobile; obeys simple commands; pincer grasp—picks up small objects; everything goes to mouth; manipulates two objects held simultaneously; claps two blocks; plays hide-and-seek and peek-a-boo; search for hidden object; jargon and consonant sounds	Parental philosophy about discipline, limit setting, rituals; incorporation of infant into family routines (eg, mealtimes); sibling jealousy might increase with child's mobility; participates in games with infant	Review auto safety; review environmental safety—home safety; removal of poisons—care when cleaning about placement of cleaning aids; have poison control center's phone number available; review toy safety and special locations for older children's small toys—use plastic bottles; discuss water safety (tub and recreational); bicycle passenger safety	Discuss eating habits—self-feeding and curiosity with food; provide ideas to cope with mess of self-feeding; review foods high in iron and vitamins B and C; discuss child's curiosity and need to explore; restriction of sugared foods at bedtime and naptime	Discuss dental care when teeth erupt; use of syrup of ipecac; prepare for change in activity, curiosity level, determination; discuss "rights" of each child to own time, space, and toys; separation anxiety continues; start bedtime and naptime rituals to give day structure for child—difficult to stop play to sleep
12 months	Parental concerns; tuberculosis (tine) test	Growth assessment—plot length, weight, and head circumference; interval history; complete examination; assess teeth and dental care; infantile reflexes have disappeared—Landau, neck righting, and parachute present; vision and hearing screening	Eats table foods; three to four meals a day; majority of milk from cup—limited to 16–20 oz per day; feeds self	Stands—pulls self to standing position; cruises around furniture; creeps; may take a few steps alone; finds hidden object with systematic search; behaviors repeated with intended goal; imitates unfamiliar sounds and gestures; may say two to three words; stacks rings on pole; builds two-block tower; wary of strangers	Review parenting philosophy—discipline, consistency, and age appropriate; areas off-limits for infant well enforced; enjoys family and family enjoys infant's games, affection; uses familiar adults to obtain wants	Review auto safety, household safety both indoors and outdoors; teach about things "hot" and causing "owies"; locks for medicine cupboard because child will start climbing and nothing is out of reach; stair safety—teach how to climb (crawl) downstairs; use low water level in bathtub—always supervise	Discuss normal decrease in appetite—need to limit milk intake to 16–20 oz per day; may use cow's milk; review dental care; review care of ill child—increase in respiratory tract illnesses likely; review judicious use of snack foods—no peanuts or popcorn because of danger of choking	Discuss the developing sense of autonomy—ways to foster independence, cope with strong will, enhance growth of ego; bedtime rituals continue; if bottle still used before sleep, it should contain water; discuss negativism; constantly getting into things; stimulation to foster speech; limit setting; fears strange people and places

TABLE 21-1 continued

Age	Procedures	Assessment area—guidelines				Anticipatory guidance		
		Physical	Nutritional	Developmental	Family	Safety	Health	Parenting role
15 months	Parental concerns; immunization (measles, mumps, rubella)	Growth assessment—plot length, weight, and head circumference; interval history; complete examination; assess teeth	Eats three to four meals a day; uses spoon as well as fingers; manages cup alone—may be completely weaned	Walks alone; stoops to recover toy; tosses and rolls ball; indicates wants by pointing; scribbles on paper; says five to six words; retains mental image of visible moving object; trial-and-error learning of object use; quicker imitation of unfamiliar, also more precise and true	Family harmony or disharmony with active, "into everything" infant; use of distraction, positive reinforcement; solicits adult help, and affection usually willingly given	Review auto, home, yard, stair, water, and toy safety; countertop safety, appliances unplugged because child is more proficient climber; aware of cords dangling because child reaches between cabinets and under furniture	Review use of syrup of ipecac; need for balance of activity and rest—exercise needs, sleep needs, and routine changes in naptimes	Discuss toys requiring matching shapes, stacking, push–pull toys, manipulative toys, and books; discuss perception of temper tantrums—how to handle; discuss readiness for toilet training; methods of training
18 months	Parental concerns; immunizations (DPT #4, OPV #3)	Growth assessment—plot length, weight, and head circumference; interval history; complete examination	Eats three to four meals a day; feeds self; uses cup well; appetite small—may refuse certain foods	Running, climbing starts; language skills increasing; comprehension better than expression; finds hidden object following several visible displacements; builds three-block tower; imitates household chores	Family routines that include infant; parental times alone—coping with active, curious, autonomous infant; consistency in expectations	Review safety needs, especially seasonal activities and play with other children; move to regular bed	Appetite varies—review basic food needs and alternatives when foods are refused; use of vitamins, continued use of fluoride	Discuss satisfaction with discipline used and effectiveness; time together in quiet and active play; interest in books, naming objects; separation anxiety present
2 years	Parental concerns; lab—hemoglobin/hematocrit, lead level screen, urinalysis; tuberculosis (tine) test	Growth assessment—plot length, weight, and head circumference; interval history; complete examination	Eats three meals a day; some may want to be fed combined with self-feeding; completely weaned	Climbs, runs, walks backward, walks stairs, kicks ball; might jump one step—both feet; builds four- to five-block tower; turns book	Child's temperament and "fit" into family; coping with child's curiosity and drive for autonomy; satisfaction with discipline; able to play	Imitates others—special precautions needed when playing with older children; may need to use gate with steep/narrow stairs; yard fenced and	Appetite fair—might be picky at times; review needs and importance of not making issue of food intake; avoid sweets and sugared foods—give	Discuss progress of toilet training; benefits of peers for play; solitary and parallel play; difficulty with sharing—sense of ownership; unable to take

continued on next page

TABLE 21-1 continued

		Assessment area—guidelines				Anticipatory guidance		
Age	**Procedures**	**Physical**	**Nutritional**	**Developmental**	**Family**	**Safety**	**Health**	**Parenting role**
2 years (*cont.*)				pages; strings large beads; puts together large-pieced puzzles; uses objects and toys symbolically; retains mental image of absent object; toilet training progressing; does simple tasks in house when requested; uses two-word sentences—vocabulary increases	"pretend" games with older siblings; consistency with family rules—imitates adults	locked gate; needs supervision or safe, enclosed area when outside; supervise with pencil, crayons (crayons should be nontoxic)	nutritious snacks; review signs of illness and ill child care; teach child to blow nose, cover mouth when coughing or sneezing	turns unless supervised; egocentric; imagination used in play; nightmares; fears increase as reality and imagination blend; importance of reading to child; preparation for new sibling if indicated
3 years	Parental concerns; lab—urine culture (girls), urinalysis; tuberculosis (tine) test	Growth assessment—plot height and weight; interval history; complete examination; vision screening, hearing screening, language screening, blood pressure	Eats three meals a day; normal diet; feeds self; use of utensils; might need help cutting meat	Rides tricycle; balances on one foot; jumps; dresses and undresses with assistance; builds bridge; copies circle; wants to please; toilet trained; uses plurals; talks constantly, tells stories; some sharing but remains egocentric; knows name and age	Fatigue level of family in keeping up with active child; peer and sibling rivalry, especially if anticipating new sibling or recent arrival of sibling; child allowed to develop at own pace	Review safety—still too small for adult seatbelts in car; safety of playground-type equipment; teach street, pedestrian safety but still supervise outdoors; not responsible; might start organized swimming lessons	Dental care—primary visit to dentist; teach to brush own teeth; adequate sleep and rest; helpful to have quiet time before meals to compensate for fatigue from play	Advisability of nursery school or organized playgroup; questioning age—wants to know why, how, when, where—give simple, concrete answers; learning logic and order of environment; fears of bodily injury; imaginary friends; television viewing

TABLE 21-1 continued

		Assessment area—guidelines				Anticipatory guidance		
Age	**Procedures**	**Physical**	**Nutritional**	**Developmental**	**Family**	**Safety**	**Health**	**Parenting role**
4 years	Parental concerns; lab—hemoglobin/hematocrit, urinalysis	Growth assessment—plot height and weight; interval history; complete examination; blood pressure	Eats three meals a day; has food jags; picky eater; normal diet	Hops on one foot, walks up stairs using alternating feet; copies cross; understands prepositions; dresses with minimal assistance; less egocentric; hand preference; uses scissors; many fears—dark, animals, water; peer play increases	Separates from family easily; family support of child's initiative; cooperates in household chores; family outings, special activities, games, trips; child's versus sibling's or parent's view of rules	Review street and pedestrian safety, auto safety, toy safety, water safety, boating safety—wear life preserver; safety around animals	Review nutritional requirements; age and appetite appropriate servings; illnesses might increase due to more peer contact; dental care—flossing of teeth	Type and amount of television viewing; own responsibilities assigned—might need reminders; plays hard to point of exhaustion; value of reading to child; early sex education
5 years	Parental concerns; lab—hemoglobin/hematocrit, urinalysis; immunizations (DPT #5, OPV #4); tuberculosis (tine) test	Growth assessment—plot height and weight; interval history; complete examination; blood pressure; vision screening; audiometric hearing check; articulation screening	Eats three meals a day; normal diet; food jags	Skips, rides bicycle with training wheels; uses pencil correctly; copies triangle; walks downstairs using alternating feet; catches ball; dresses self independently; draws figure of person (three parts); conscious of social routine	Ready for child to start school; parent's interest and participation in school activities; limit setting; opinion of peers, school adjustment; combine expectations of family and other authority figures	Review safety; add bicycle safety; emphasize pedestrian safety, especially never going with or taking food from a stranger; home fire drills	Discuss snacks and junk food; teach health habits—not to share hats, combs in school; exercise program; sleep needs; make aware of potential for sexual abuse	Time with child to talk about day at school, what child learned; having child go to school (parental readiness); questions self in world (eg, birth, death, God, religion)

continued on next page

TABLE 21-1 continued

		Assessment area—guidelines				Anticipatory guidance		
Age	**Procedures**	**Physical**	**Nutritional**	**Developmental**	**Family**	**Safety**	**Health**	**Parenting role**
6 years	Parental concerns; lab—urinalysis	Growth assessment—plot height and weight; interval history; complete examination; blood pressure; dental assessment; vision and hearing check	Eats three meals a day; less fussy about foods; better appetite; definite likes and dislikes	Increased skill and speed in running, throwing ball; rides bicycle without training wheels; draws six-part or greater person; understands number concepts 1–10; prints letters and numbers; uses all parts of speech; begins to read	Allows increased independence—use of telephone; rules for play and chores age appropriate; sibling rivalry	Review safety—school and pedestrian, bicycle, auto, roller skate; home fire drills; discuss safe play areas—define limits for riding bike	Increased responsibility for health—proper outdoor dress for recess; making healthy food choices; protect self from illnesses	Emotional—changes rapidly; easily frustrated; unable to tolerate criticism; putting world of variation of values and beliefs previously learned into perspective; sex education
7–8 years	Parental concerns; lab—urine culture (girls)	Growth assessment—plot height and weight; interval history; complete examination; blood pressure; vision screening; audiometric hearing screening; dental assessment	Normal diet—monitor milk intake	Perfects skills—tandem walk backward; dance, and gymnastics; copies diamond and square; good eye–hand coordination; tells time; counts money; concrete, logical thinking emerges; concept of reversibility and conservation; peers important—efforts to win peer acceptance; fair play very important	Relationship with parents—may have increased need for mother's attention; relationship with siblings	Review home fire drills; safety conscious around house and outdoors; more cautious in play; water safety, tool safety, and safety around animals	Food choices; use of money—junk food purchases when away from home; needs guidance in personal habits; review making aware of sexual abuse	School adjustment—more responsibilities and "work" at school and home; sex education; moral development—depends on being caught and punished; "petty theft" and lying common; school performance; summer activities; camp selection

TABLE 21-1 continued

Age	Procedures	Assessment area—guidelines: Physical	Nutritional	Developmental	Family	Anticipatory guidance: Safety	Health	Parenting role
9–10 years	Parental concerns; lab—hemoglobin/hematocrit; urinalysis	Growth assessment—plot height and weight; interval history; complete examination; blood pressure; vision and hearing check; scoliosis check	Normal diet	Perfection of skills—sports, crafts, writing; organized groups; peers very important—best friend loyalty; concrete thinker—masters concepts of class inclusion, conservation (except displaced volume); logical thinker in problem solving; moral development; beginning reciprocity for self-interest; takes pride in work	Relationship with family and multiple authority figures outside of family; begins to work alongside parent; talking about problems, asking questions within family	Review personal safety, sport or athletic safety, auto safety, bicycle and dirt bike safety, water safety, tree climbing safety, tool safety, guns and fireworks	Responsible for actions—needs guidance and reminders; light for reading and handicrafts; protect eyes when sawing or sanding wood; discuss peer influence on diet, choices, activity	Communicate with child to learn thoughts, problems, ideas; sex education; dilemmas; moral education—rights and wrongs and gray areas; school performance; television viewing patterns; mood swings
11–12 years	Parental concerns; lab—hemoglobin/hematocrit, urinalysis; tuberculosis (tine) test	Growth assessment—plot height and weight; interval history; complete examination; blood pressure; scoliosis check; early sexual development assessment; vision screening; hearing screening	Normal diet—might suddenly increase with growth	Sense of industry—works to complete (perfect) finished product; peer group and activities; fine motor skills (eg, neat handwriting); coordination in running, throwing ball long distance;	Ability to grant independent decision making; grant privacy; acceptance of peers; focus on accomplish-ments; realistic chores; family activities, rituals; examples in home on drug and alcohol use	Review safety at home, outdoors, school, sports, recreational; peer influence and doing something on a "dare" (eg, guns, fireworks, tree climbs, height jumping)	Discuss peer pressure—including smoking and drug and alcohol use; sex education, responsibility for behaviors; exercise and leisure time, sleep needs	Mood swings; dependence and independence vacillation; growth spurt; appetite increase; fatigue frequent; increased interest in opposite sex

continued on next page

TABLE 21-1 continued

Age	Procedures	Assessment area—guidelines				Anticipatory guidance		
		Physical	Nutritional	Developmental	Family	Safety	Health	Parenting role
11–12 years (*cont.*)				beginning to solve problems mentally—less trial and error and dependence on concrete objects; moral development—beginning of sense of social responsibility to conform and "be good"				
13–15 years	Parental concerns; adolescent's concerns; lab—hemoglobin/hematocrit, urinalysis, VDRL (Venereal Disease Research Laboratories) if sexually active; immunization (Td booster) tuberculosis (tine) test	Growth assessment—plot height and weight; interval history; complete examination; blood pressure; scoliosis check; vision screening; sexual development assessment; hearing screening	Normal diet—appetite varies with growth spurt; fad diets	Skill perfection—speed and accuracy; interest more focused and efforts concentrated; school achievement; peers important; mental processes to formulate ideas, test hypotheses, and draw conclusions; deductive logic; independent decisions; seeks own identity; heroes	Examples set in home regarding smoking, use of alcohol and drugs, driving habits; interest and participation in school, sport, and club activities; motivation provided to perform at highest level possible; testing of parental authority, limits; how conflicts are resolved	Review personal safety practices—being responsible; babysitting safety; teach first aid	Review personal health—nutrition, sleep, exercise, sports; skin care; discuss use and peer influence regarding alcohol and drugs; sex education and responsibility; information about venereal disease; dental care	Discuss concepts of freedom and responsibilities; ideas about future; daydreams; need for privacy, respect; moody—trying to find real self; increase in somatic complaints

TABLE 21-1 continued

		Assessment area—guidelines				Anticipatory guidance		
Age	Procedures	Physical	Nutritional	Developmental	Family	Safety	Health	Parenting role
15–18 years	Parental concerns; adolescent's concerns; lab—hemoglobin/hematocrit, urinalysis, VDRL if sexually active; tuberculosis (tine) test	Growth assessment—plot height and weight; interval history; complete examination; blood pressure; vision screening; dental assessment; sexual development assessment; hearing screening	Normal diet; fad diets to lose or gain weight	Adult skills; formal operational thinking; school progress; future plans; fears of failure; fears about future, body image, peer nonacceptance; considers viewpoints of others; flexible in thinking—increasing understanding and accumulation of facts; development of sex role—sexual identity; peers valued—regular group for social activities	Adolescent and family relations; communications; decision-making power and control shared or not; example set in daily habits and life's values; leisure activities	Auto safety as driver—responsibility for others and self versus "showing off"; review safety practices in all areas	Hygiene and skin care; personal health—body changes, responsibility for decisions; sex education—use of contraception; nutritional needs	Mood swings; independence and dependence vacillation; dating; struggle with different value orientations; use of money (present versus future orientation); television viewing

Key Concepts

- Anticipatory guidance is a form of preparatory education in which the nurse anticipates needs before they occur and teaches parents to prevent health problems.
- Because the nurse intervenes to prevent potential health problems, anticipatory guidance is a form of primary prevention.
- In preventing family dysfunction the nurse uses assessment skills to support adaptive parenting and supply needed information.
- The nurse adapts the teaching plan and the guidance offered to match parental concerns and family resources.
- Parent–child "fit" is the extent to which both parent and child "read" each other's signals and respond appropriately, resulting in a mutual sense of competence.
- The nurse prevents problems related to parent–child fit by monitoring the attachment process during infancy and by assessing parental expectations for the child together with the child's temperament.
- Identifying a child's strengths and praising adaptive parenting help the parent to appreciate the child's capabilities and meet the child's developmental needs.
- The nurse begins each assessment interview with a teaching plan based on anticipated needs and norms for growth and development at each stage.

Additional Readings

Auerback A: *Parents Learn Through Discussion.* Wiley, 1968.

Austin G, et al: *The Parent's Guide to Child Raising.* Prentice-Hall, 1978.

Blosser C: Avoiding potential behavior problems in children. *Pediatr Nurs* (May/June) 1979; 5(3):11–15.

Brim OG, Kagan J: *Constancy and Change in Human Development.* Harvard University Press, 1980.

Brim O: *Education for Childrearing.* Russell Sage Foundation, 1959.

Carey W: Clinical applications of infant temperament measures. *J Pediatr* 1972; 81(4):823–828.

Carey W, McDevitt S: Revision of the infant temperament questionnaire. *Pediatrics* (May) 1978; 61(5):735–739.

Chinn P, Leonard K: *Current Practice in Pediatric Nursing.* Vol III. Mosby, 1980.

Chow MP, et al: *Handbook of Pediatric Primary Care.* Wiley, 1979.

Clark A: Recognizing discord between mother and child and changing it to harmony. *Am J Matern Child Nurs* (March/April) 1976; 100–106.

Clark A, Alfonso D: Infant behavior and maternal attachment: Two sides to the coin. *Am J Matern Child Nurs* (March/April) 1976; 94–99.

Cochran M, Bressard J: Child development and personal and social networks. *Child Dev* (Sept) 1979; 50(3):601–616.

Farr KS: Communication pitfalls in routine counseling. *Pediatr Nurs* (Jan/Feb) 1979; 5(1):55–57.

Funke J, Irby MI: An instrument to assess the quality of maternal behavior. *J Obset Gynecol Neonatal Nurs* (Sept/Oct) 1978; 7(5):19–22.

Gazda GM, Walters RP, Childers WC: *Human Relations Development.* Allyn and Bacon, 1975.

Gordon V: Teaching concepts of good parenting. *Int Nurs Rev* (Sept/Oct) 1979; 26(5):137–138.

Gorman C, Kennedy CE: The parent–educator nurse. *Am J Matern Child Nurs* (July/Aug) 1980; 5(6):277–279.

Haggerty L, Kudzma E: Expectant parents' classes: An alternative environment for learning health maintenance. *J Nurs Educat* (Feb) 1980; 19(2):13–19.

Henrich AP, Bernheim RF: Responding to patients' concerns. *Nurs Outlook* (July) 1981; 31(7):428–434.

Hollen P: Parents' perceptions of parenting support systems. *Pediatr Nurs* (Sept/Oct) 1982; 8(4):309–313.

Horowitz J, Hughes C, Perdue BJ: *Parenting: A Nursing Perspective.* Prentice-Hall, 1982.

Jarrett GE: Childrearing patterns of young mothers: Expectations, knowledge and practices. *Am J Matern Child Nurs* (March/April) 1982; 7(2):119–127.

King M, Novik L, Citrenbaum C: *Irresistible Communication: Creative Skills for the Health Professional.* Saunders, 1983.

Korner A: Individual differences at birth—implications for child-care practices. *Birth Defects* 1974; 10(2):51–61.

Kron T: *Communication in Nursing.* Saunders, 1972.

Lamb M: Fathers: Forgotten contributors to child development. *Hum Dev* 1975; 18(4):245–266.

Linley JF: Mothers' attitudes regarding health care for their children. *Am J Matern Child Nurs* (Jan/Feb) 1984; 9(1):37–39.

Matas L, Arend R, Sroufe L: Continuity of adaptation in the second year: The relationship between quality of attachment and later competence. *Child Dev* 1978; 49(3):547–556.

McInerny T, Chamberlin R: Is it feasible to identify infants who are at risk for later behavioral problems? *Clin Pediatr* (March) 1978; 17(3):233–238.

Metzl MN: Teaching parents a strategy for enhancing infant development. *Child Dev* 1980; 51(2):583–586.

Miller DL, Baird SF: Helping parents to be parents—a special center. *Am J Matern Child Nurs* (March/April) 1978; 3(2):117–120.

Mitchell K: Helping parents enjoy parenting. *Child Care Newsletter* 1984; 3(1):5–6.

Murphy CM: *Quick Reference to Pediatric Nursing.* Lippincott, 1984.

Murray RB, Zentner JP: *Nursing Concepts for Health Promotion.* Prentice-Hall, 1979.

Myers B: Early intervention using Brazelton training with middle-class mothers and fathers of newborns. *Child Dev* 1982; 53(2):462–471.

Nelms BC, Mullins RG: *Growth and Development—A Primary Health Care Approach.* Prentice-Hall, 1982.

Norton CB: Can you hear between the lines? *RN* (Sept) 1978; 4(9):117–122.

Nugent JK: The Brazelton neonatal behavioral assessment scale: Implications for intervention. *Pediatr Nurs* (July/Aug) 1981; 7(4):18–21.

Pickarts E, Fargo J: *Parent Education: Toward Parental Competence.* Appleton-Century-Crofts, 1971.

Post CW, Robinson JG: A good beginning for families. *Pediatr Nurs* (July/Aug) 1980; 6(4):32–36.

Powell ML: *Assessment and Management of Developmental Changes and Problems in Children.* Mosby, 1981.

Pridham KF: Infant feeding and anticipatory care: Supporting the adaptation of parents to their new babies. *Matern Child Nurs J* (Summer) 1981; 10(2):111–126.

Pringle SM, Ramsey B: *Promoting the Health of Children. A Guide for Caretakers and Health Care Professionals.* Mosby, 1982.

Roberts FB: A model for parent education. *Image* (Oct) 1981; 13:86–89.

Ryberg JW, Merrifield EB: A questionnaire for assessment of parents' needs in a child health clinic. *Pediatr Nurs* (Sept/Oct) 1982; 8(5)318–319, 322.

Swendson L, Meleis A, Jones D: The family and you: Role supplementation for new parents—a role mastery plan. *Am J Matern Child Nurs* (March/April) 1978; 3(2):84–91.

Thomas A, Chess S: *Temperament and Development.* Brunner/Mazel, 1977.

Trotter S, Thoman EB (editors): *Social Responsiveness of Infants.* Johnson and Johnson Baby Products Company, Pediatric Round Table Series, 1978.

Vaughn B, Deinard A, Egeland B: Measuring temperament in pediatric practice. *J Pediatr* (March) 1980; 96(3):510–514.

Ventura JN: Parent coping behaviors, parent functioning, and infant temperament characteristics. *Nurs Res* (Sep/Oct) 1982; 31(5):269–273.

Webster-Stratton C, Kogan K: Helping parents parent. *Am J Nurs* (Feb) 1980; 80(2):240–244.

Widmayer S, Field T: Effects of Brazelton demonstration for mothers on the development of preterm infants. *Pediatrics* 1981; 67(5):711–714.

Worobey J, Belsky J: Employing the Brazelton scale to influence mothering: An experimental comparison of three strategies. *Dev Psychol* 1982; 18(5):736–743.

UNIT VI THE CHILD AND FAMILY AT PSYCHOSOCIAL RISK

In this unit we examine various factors that place children and families at psychosocial risk. The child health nurse can encounter these children and families in many situations and assume some responsibility for nursing care. The level of responsibility may be limited or primary and may range from identification and referral of those at risk to planning, implementing, and evaluating nursing care. One emphasis in the following chapters is therefore the specific role of the child health nurse in a given situation. We also focus on the interrelationship of the child, family, and larger environment.

In Chapter 22 we discuss various risk factors, assessment criteria, and nursing management for families with either a history of or a potential for emotional or physical abuse. Chapter 23 presents considerations for nursing care of the child and family when a child has an organic, mental, or developmental disorder. We detail nursing care of the child with dysfunctional behaviors in Chapter 24. Finally, in Chapter 25 we extend our discussion to the child with a psychiatric or social disorder. Using current terminology, this chapter covers nursing care appropriate for the child health nurse, rather than the psychiatric nurse specialist. Together, these chapters provide a framework for flexible and sound nursing assessment, diagnosis, intervention, and evaluation for these challenging children and families.

Contents

Nursing Care of the Family at Risk

22

Elizabeth Laliberte

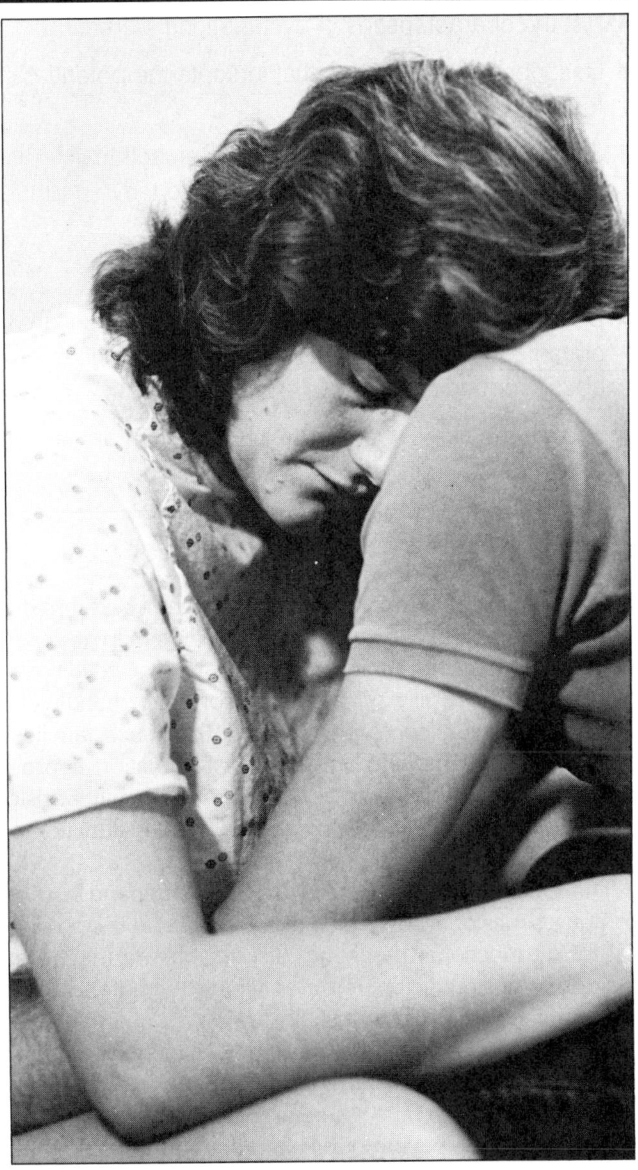

Chapter Outline

Objectives

- Relate the concept of risk to the nurse's role in preventive health care.
- List the characteristics of dysfunctional parenting.
- Describe the risk factors that indicate the potential for dysfunctional parenting.
- Explain the relationship between dysfunctional parenting and both inorganic failure to thrive and delayed development.
- Define the types of child neglect and abuse.
- Describe the process of reporting a case of child abuse and the possible legal outcomes of child abuse reports.
- Explain the nurse's role in preventing child abuse and neglect.
- List the possible community supports to which nurses might refer dysfunctional families.
- Explain the purpose of multidisciplinary management for dysfunctional families.
- Explain the nurse's role in supporting dysfunctional parents and children in dysfunctional families.
- Describe the common needs of adolescent parents.
- Explain the nurse's role in supporting adolescent parents.
- Describe the common needs and interventions for families prone to violence.
- Describe the common needs of multiproblem families.

When the development or life of a family member is threatened, the family might be described as a "family at risk." Any member of the family, whether parent or child, can place the entire family system at risk for abnormal development or dysfunction (Johnson, 1979). In such families individual members who are not able to function appropriately threaten the family as a whole. The family at risk is therefore vulnerable to being a family with dysfunctional parenting.

The extent to which a family is at risk depends on a complex series of factors that indicate stress and the potential for dysfunctional parenting. *Risk factors* are therefore indicators, not predictors, of areas where the potential for unmet needs exists. They usually are developmental and situational stressors that historically have a high correlation with dysfunction (Johnson, 1979). In assessing both the child and family, the nurse therefore identifies stressors and coping strategies, paying particular attention to those that suggest risk. Because a risk factor is not a predictor of dysfunction, however, the nurse analyzes risk factors together with other assessment data to identify areas of unmet needs for which intervention is required.

The number or severity of stressors and unmet needs places some families at high risk for dysfunction. For example, the pregnant adolescent is developme~tally vulnerable because of the combined stress of pregnancy and her own ongoing growth and development needs. Additional risk factors for this individual might include single parenthood without necessary material and personal support systems, limited experience and knowledge of child care, and social isolation. These combined developmental, sociologic, and psychologic factors create a situation of high risk for this young family.

We recommend multidisciplinary intervention for high-risk families. In this way all members of the health care team participate in providing services to improve family functioning and health promotion. Analyzing assessment data provides cues that the nurse uses to identify a troubled family and initiate multidisciplinary intervention for long-term care or supervision. The nurse applies the phases of the nursing process in planning family health care.

Nursing care for the family at risk also involves an understanding of the ways in which families and their cultural, ethnic heritage and current socioeconomic profile (see Chapter 3) influence their members. In Chapter 4 we present a framework for studying families and discuss the family's influences on the child. In Chapter 13 we describe styles of parenting and methods of discipline that nurses might need to teach parents. In Chapter 17 we discuss the role of family assessment in child health nursing, and we describe the assessment techniques that nurses use to identify family function, roles, communication, development, interaction, and potential dysfunction.

In this chapter we analyze the risk factors that contribute to family dysfunction. We discuss the patterns of dysfunctional parenting and the patterns of behavior that lead some parents to abuse or neglect their children. Holistic nursing care directs us to look at all aspects of the family system as well as the component parts. Knowing risk factors, we are able to identify potential dysfunction and through intervention prevent disruptive effects on the family. Nursing goals are then to identify the family at risk, prevent predictable dysfunctional behaviors, reduce disintegration, foster positive relationships, and provide referrals to community resources and services.

Dysfunctional Parenting

Families are supposed to be loving and nurturing and provide for the needs of their members. Many families, however, do not meet these goals. A family that is unable to provide physically and emotionally for the needs of its members is said to be a *dysfunctional family*. In the dysfunctional family the degree to which family stresses override family strengths places the family at risk. All families experience times of stress when they function well and other times when they function poorly, some even to the point of disintegration. Because children depend on their families to meet their needs, dysfunctional families are characterized by dysfunctional parenting. Determining whether the dysfunctional pattern is temporary, situational, or chronic is therefore a nursing goal for the family at risk.

Most families can cope with stress by relying on their coping mechanisms, internal resources, physical and emotional energies, and external supports. The inability to cope can lead to frustration, anger, and other inappropriate parental responses. Children witnessing such behavior might become frightened and confused. Because parents are role models, children imitate the maladaptive coping patterns they see at home, which then might result in dysfunctional behaviors that leave the child vulnerable to delays in social development.

Dysfunctional parenting thus involves a disturbance in the parent–child relationship. Dysfunctional parenting might result when the parenting style has been affected negatively by one or more stressors. Some parents, however, survive multiple stressors and remain effective parents, whereas other parents have problems with parenting when faced with only mild or temporary stress. Dysfunctional parenting also is evidenced by inconsistency or inflexibility in the parenting style. This type of parenting often takes its toll on selected children in a family. Inconsistency is evident when a parent singles out one child as a scapegoat. Inconsistency also occurs when the same behavior receives very different responses depending on the parent's mood. The child never establishes a trusting relation because care is not directed toward providing a consistent, nurturing environment to satisfy basic needs. Inflexibility might be dysfunctional if a parent is unable to adjust expectations to match the individual needs of different children.

Members of dysfunctional families experience troubled lives, and their patterns of living are usually in much chaos. They often do not plan schedules for meals, sleep, or recreation. Events might just happen, with much noise accompanying the confusion and disorganization. In dysfunctional families parents might be psychiatrically impaired (among abusive parents, 5% have evidence of psychosis [Justice and Justice, 1976]), social and economic stresses are usually high, and self-care, judgment, and future planning are deficient (Greenspan, 1982). Greenspan showed that infants in these families are at risk for increased mortality and morbidity, particularly in affective and social development, during the first years of life.

In planning care for a dysfunctional family, the nurse therefore needs to assess the family dynamics in relation to the potential for crisis: (1) the origin of the stressor(s), whether situational, transitional, or social/cultural, creating the crisis; (2) the personal reaction to the crisis as manifested by cognitive, biophysical, emotional, and behavioral responses; and (3) the support services and family resources available to facilitate coping and crisis management (Fig. 22-1).

Characteristics of Dysfunctional Parenting

Inadequate Communication Clear, functional communication patterns are one way in which families meet the emotional needs of their members. Communication, however, often is seriously limited or emotionally restrictive in the dysfunctional family. Patterns of communication might be haphazard because the individuals have difficulty stating what they think or believe. Frequently, feelings are overlooked or are not expressed either verbally or nonverbally. This in turn results in missed cues and messages so that inappropriate responses are common.

When family members fail to interact effectively, they create many problems in activities of daily living. Their use of language might be sparse or irregular and may result in members' relying on nonverbal cues to convey messages. When family members fail to listen actively to each other, they do not share achievements and goals. Mutual respect might then be lacking. For example, one boy had to wait several days until his mother read about his first-place honor in the spelling contest to discuss it. By then, his excitement over winning had passed. His mother worked at home and would scowl or ignore him if he interrupted her when she was concentrating. Her negative response occurred so frequently that he stopped sharing school events unless she initiated the topic. Although she was physically present when he returned home from school, she was emotionally distant and unable to provide consistent interaction or interest in his activities or accomplishments to support his development.

Inadequate communication usually leads to inappropriate expectations among family members. The inability to meet these expectations robs members of opportunities for self-esteem through accomplishment. The adult who lacks interpersonal skills has a minimal capacity for friendship. Coupled with the inability to trust others, these characteristics interfere with any opportunities to receive support or to support the emotional development of a child.

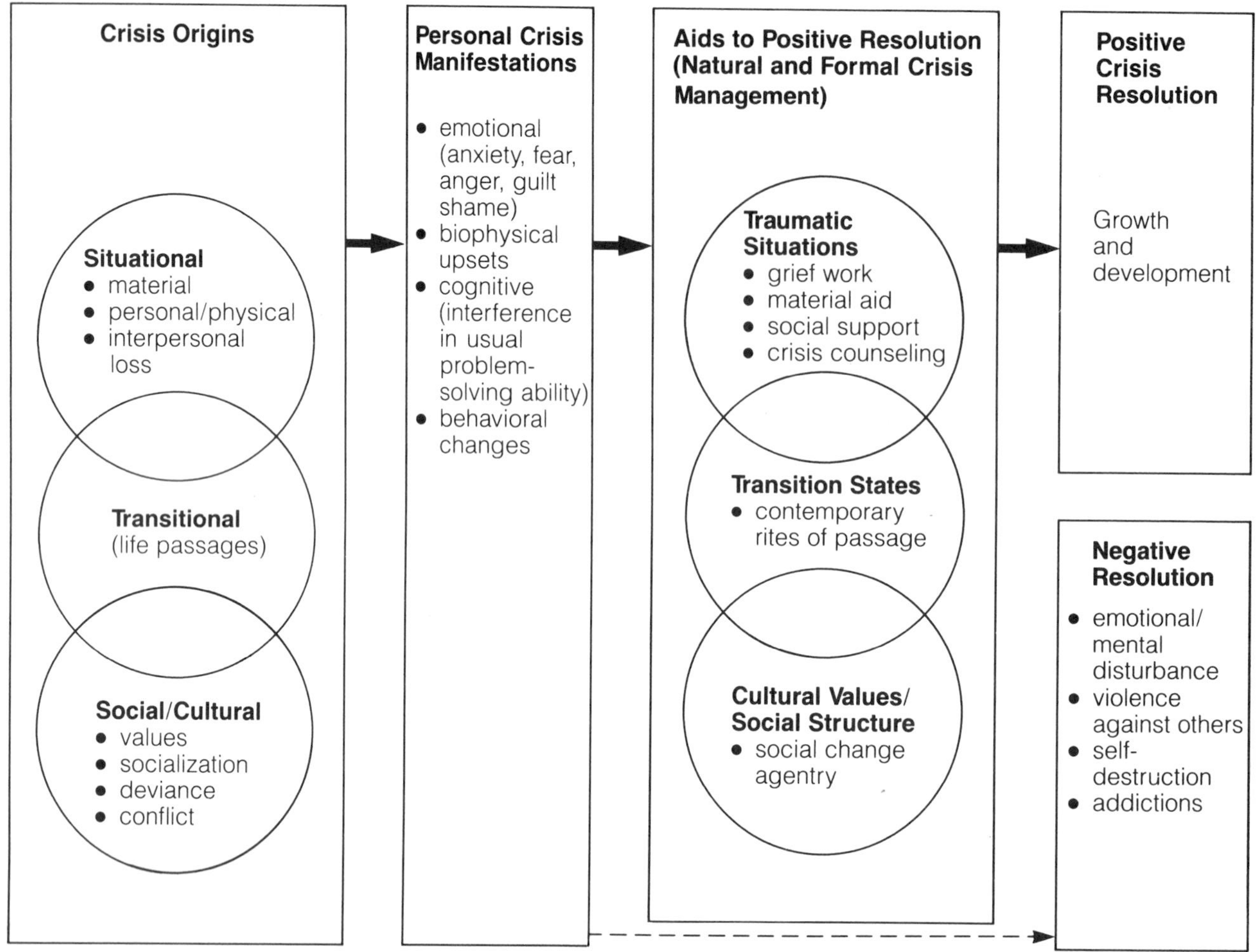

Figure 22-1 Paradigm of the interactional components of crisis and the relation of supportive resources to positive growth-producing outcomes. (From Hoff L: *People in Crisis*. 2nd ed., Addison-Wesley, 1984, p. 32.)

Parents in dysfunctional families communicate by responding only to negative behaviors in their children. Positive behaviors might be expected but are often ignored so that the pattern of response conveys a sense of unimportance to the child. Parents might verbally establish rules but not model the expected behaviors. Enforcement of rules usually is sporadic, with compliance either demanded immediately or overlooked. Disciplinary methods are not established or explained to the child. (Discipline is discussed in Chapter 13.) Extremes in behaviors, which might be either overly permissive or overly rigid, thus rob the child of problem-solving experiences.

Restrictive communication to a young, dependent child can have lasting effects. The child might learn that language is unnecessary and then may not make any efforts at verbal communication. The longest-lasting effect is that children have no insight into feelings, either their own or those of others. For example, one mother repeatedly told her daughter not to bore others with her idle chatter. If she had something important to say, she should say it as concisely as possible, but otherwise she should keep quiet. Constant reminders of this rule, which essentially allowed the communication of facts but not feelings, resulted in the girl's belief that her thoughts, questions, and ideas had little value. She gradually withdrew her attempts to verbally solve problems of relationships or put feelings into perspective, sensing that there was something inherently wrong with her for attempting to do so in the first place.

Children in dysfunctional families might behave in ways that indicate distress. Children from disorganized environments might be inattentive and tired because they lack sleep. They might be poorly nourished because of improper diet and nutrition. Family life tends to focus on parental needs. Children might be allowed to spend vast amounts of time unsupervised or watching television.

Family pressures that cause the child anxiety in turn interfere with learning, which usually is first manifested in school difficulties. Shyness, withdrawal, excessive fears, truancy, aggressiveness, school failure, psychosomatic health problems, and the inability to get along with peers all might indicate emotional problems. Sometimes, it is the child's abnormal behavior that signals problems within the family.

Multidisciplinary interventions involving counselors, parents, teachers, and nurses are often necessary. Working through unresolved feelings will promote the mental health of the child. Children who are thwarted in their attempts to express their feelings or who receive confusing and mixed messages from their family often have a mixture of unexpressed anger, aggression, resentment, self-pity, fear, and guilt. Helping the child to identify the existence of these feelings is the first step and takes time, patience, and empathy. Once identified, the reasons for the feelings should be uncovered. Sometimes, a perfectly normal emotion that was not allowed initial expression gives rise to the subsequent expression of negative feelings in socially unacceptable ways. For example, one young girl was forbidden to express anything but love and admiration for her new sibling when in reality she intensely disliked this screaming intruder who took away her parents' love and attention. She then began to compete aggressively with her peers for her teachers' attention. Her parents' insensitivity to her need to work out her jealous feelings and their desire for her to conform to their expectations had prevented her from expressing her feelings. Because negative thoughts or comments about her sibling were taboo and resulted in her being reprimanded, she sought to compensate for perceived lost attention by demanding undivided attention from other significant adults. Unable to handle feelings of jealousy, she verbally and physically contested anyone else who sought her teachers' attention.

For the nurse, dysfunctional parents are difficult to reach because the quality of parenting is a delicate issue to discuss. The nurse tries to establish trust by patiently forming a relationship of reliability and honesty and by strengthening and reinforcing positive parenting skills. Parents' unmet needs and defenses often get in the way of their ability to modify behaviors, and for parents who have been hurt before, trust comes slowly if at all. If adult members in the dysfunctional family feel a low sense of self-esteem, their ability to support one another is limited. If only one parent in a two-parent family is committed to improving family relations, the family system is at risk for disintegration.

Members of dysfunctional families usually express little thought or knowledge of feelings. Sadness or depression is generally the tone of the family, and body language might convey this message. There is little evidence of excitement and few episodes of happy laughter in the home where the mother spends the day in a daze, sitting on the couch, watching television, and smoking cigarettes, apparently oblivious to the activities and needs of her children. The children, consequently, feel no obligation or desire to share the events of their lives with her and find life dull and routine. Family members need help in voicing feelings to each other and in learning to share concerns. Because this kind of communication is often foreign, progress is usually slow and should be evaluated frequently to meet the family members' needs.

Role Confusion Among Family Members Disturbed relationships within a family can have lasting and harmful effects on all members, but the growing child is most vulnerable. For instance, if the parent is too self-centered because of insecurity and immaturity, the child becomes isolated and might feel rejected. Immature parents who, because of their own unmet needs, expect their children to become the parents they never had, create a cycle of parental dysfunction. Parents who are unable to take on adult roles fail to provide for their children both economically and emotionally.

If, in a two-parent family, either parent is competing with the children for love and attention, unhealthy relationships develop. The competing parent might feel deprived when the child is nurtured and vent anger and rage on the child rather than the spouse (Kempe and Kempe, 1978). Because children learn from their parents by imitation and identification, they need parents to maintain authority, provide guidance, and make decisions. Any deviation from these expectations is confusing to the child and results in unhealthy relationships and developmental vulnerability. The child who is cast into an adult role prematurely might begin to compete with the parent, and the parent may in turn resent the child's taking over an adult role in the family.

In dysfunctional families relationships among siblings usually mirror other troubled family relationships. Dysfunctional parenting usually causes normal sibling rivalry and competition to be far out of proportion and so intense as to be destructive rather than constructive. The siblings battle each other for recognition and the limited amount of attention they perceive as being available from their parents. Attention is more likely to be given for negative, even violent, behavior than for positive, empathetic behavior.

The role of scapegoat is also evident in some troubled families in which one child is singled out because of temperament, appearance, birth order, disability, sex, or health status as the cause of all family problems, and much activity focuses on this child. Empiric evidence has shown that if the scapegoat child is removed from the family, the parent reassigns the role to another child unless long-term family therapy helps to correct the dysfunction.

Identifying the parent who is the main decision maker and the distribution of power in a family is helpful in planning intervention. If one parent is passive and the other is dominant, certain behaviors are interdependent and might hamper one member's progress. For example, a wife who is submissive to a dominant husband might wish to initiate change but also may feel that she needs permission from her husband before taking any action. A first step in planning interventions might then be to interest the husband in making the necessary changes so that accustomed family functions are not entirely disrupted.

The nurse might find that having parents describe their own childhoods and family lives provides clues to the roles assumed within a family. Reactions to specific incidents usually correlate directly with current family functions because parents tend to follow their own parents' roles and style of childrearing (Steele, 1975).

Family members who feel negative about their roles carry invisible scars. Their unmet needs for attention, love, and recognition interfere with the identification of others' needs, leaving each member vulnerable to problems. For example, a mother craving recognition for the output of energy and accomplishment of managing a home has a difficult time giving appropriate recognition and praise to the child's initial efforts to wash the windows. In addition, a parent–child mismatch, in which the child does not seem to "fit" the parents (parent–child "fit" is discussed in Chapter 21), is sometimes the only plausible explanation for a certain child's differential treatment and might explain child abuse or neglect. People with emotional scars need much support and praise in any new venture. Because of past family problems, members of dysfunctional families are hesitant to seek new opportunities for fear of failure. If members can seek out and succeed at new opportunities, however, success will improve self-esteem.

Isolation The dysfunctional family usually is living in both physical and emotional isolation. Parents in the dysfunctional family tend to have few friends, seldom leave their homes, and have difficulty forming close personal relationships. Their apparent lack of interpersonal skills might be related to their own limited opportunities to learn them as a child. Research has noted that 2- and 3-year-olds who have been abused or neglected begin to isolate themselves by responding less positively to overtures by friendly adults and avoiding peers (George and Main, 1979). As adults, these individuals might make contacts rather than friends, have no meaningful interactions with neighbors and family members, and rarely join groups or organizations. They feel less than adequate in social situations and endure much loneliness. For parents, such isolation results in their having no outside outlets for tension and frustrations (Campbell, 1984).

If the dysfunctional family is geographically or emotionally separated from the extended family, support or help is usually minimal in times of stress and crisis. The lack of supportive relationships might serve further to alienate the family from its resources, although at times a dysfunctional family can benefit from its isolation, especially if members of the extended family have served as role models for dysfunctional parenting.

If the family is isolated from the community, the lack of belonging and acceptance places the family at further risk. Because a problem or stressor is often lessened by knowing that others have successfully mastered the problem, isolation deprives family members of common problem-solving techniques. Family members who do not profit by their mistakes also are unlikely to learn to solve problems. For example, sharing child-care skills and responsibilities is common in many cultures and communities and provides parents the opportunity to exchange both knowledge and services. An isolated family is denied this sharing and struggles alone to provide continual care.

If the dysfunctional family's limited use of resources in turn causes alienation from neighbors, children might not be welcomed or made to feel in any way that they are part of the community. This fosters feelings of inadequacy in the children and sets the stage for hostile responses such as vandalism and aggressiveness (see Chapters 24 and 25) (Pelton, 1981).

Because isolation is likely to be both physical and emotional, lack of social skills might be misinterpreted as disinterest or snobbery and usually sets off behaviors that add to the problem. Efforts at friendliness might be missed, and mistrust becomes pervasive. Individual needs for acceptance and belonging go unfulfilled. Nurses who identify family isolation therefore might need to teach parents to break the bonds of isolation and learn to use resources.

Risk Factors for Dysfunctional Parenting

The Parent's Experience as a Child The type of parenting that a parent received as a child directly affects current parenting skills. The single most significant and predictable factor in all research is that parents who were significantly deprived, neglected, or abused are more likely to show dysfunctional behaviors toward their own children (Steele, 1975; Kempe and Kempe, 1978). In some families dysfunctional patterns can be traced back three or four generations. Steele (1975) reported that this finding outranks all other data such as race, age, religion, culture, environment, education, family structure, socioeconomic status, and psychiatric state.

Steele further described a "lack of empathetic mothering" as a basic dynamic of dysfunctional parenting, suggesting that parents who were not properly nurtured do not have healthy norms as a frame of reference. Not having been reared to experience parenting as nurturing, these adults are unable to nurture their own children. The problem then becomes cyclic. Ounstead and Lynch (1976) described the concept of the "hostile pedigree," a notion that suggests that parents who were abused as children are now "bonded in hate" to their own parents. Ounstead and Lynch further suggested that women in particular often have angry, yet dependent, relationships with their mothers. Many parents extend their unresolved hostile attitudes to all authority figures thereby fueling these relationships with anger originating from unmet childhood needs, which results in their inability to form satisfying relationships.

If they were made to feel guilty and inadequate as children, dysfunctional parents lack confidence in their abilities to parent and are unable to identify the needs of their children. The parent's lack of secure feelings can result in a state of parental dependence, which then places the child

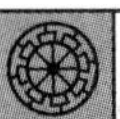

NURSING CARE GUIDE The Dysfunctional Family

Nursing diagnosis	Interventions	Evaluation
1. Inadequate parenting related to multiple family stressors	Document parental behaviors Listen actively to parents to identify needs and "cries for help" Encourage honest discussion of feelings through open-ended questions List problems and strengths as observed by staff and perceived by parents and share list with parents Identify behaviors that place the child at risk Establish contract that sets deadlines for behavioral changes Identify behaviors that must stop (eg, leaving children unattended, substance abuse) Identify resources to assist with family coping (eg, marital or personal counseling, employment counseling)	Problem areas are specifically identified to initiate change
2. Inability to trust professionals related to unmet personal needs	Demonstrate caring for parents by attending to their needs Discuss available resources for parental support as perceived by parents Establish a means of parental support (eg, "lifeline") and encourage its use Praise efforts toward positive parenting Obtain services needed by the family (eg, homemaker or child care assistance) Involve family members in the evaluation process	Nurse–client relationship conveys dignity to the client and improves the client's level of trust
3. Knowledge deficit related to inadequate information or experience with normal child development and positive methods of discipline	Teach normal process of growth and development (see Chapter 21) Refer parent to parenting classes or establish support for parent in the home (eg, parent aide); provide for any secondary needs (eg, transportation or child care needed to attend classes) Role model positive parenting behaviors such as proper feeding, bathing, or comforting Foster parent–child attachment by pointing out child's strengths and praising positive parenting behaviors Discuss appropriate role enactment behaviors; praise parent when nurturing behaviors are performed and child is allowed to be dependent according to developmental level	Parent can describe normal needs of children and positive parenting behaviors

continued on next page

NURSING CARE GUIDE The Dysfunctional Family (continued)

Nursing diagnosis	Interventions	Evaluation
	Discuss parent's childhood experience and its reflection in parenting skills and expectations; provide appropriate means (parent aide, lifeline visitor) to meet the parent's needs for attention and approval	
4. Diversional activity deficit related to family social isolation	Encourage expanded range of parent activities by suggesting possible child care alternatives (see Chapter 21)	Parental involvement in activities outside the home provides family with additional social contacts
	Introduce family members to local families with similar interests	
	Provide information about possible family activities (eg, school, church)	
	Teach the importance of family growth in the growth and development of children	
	Arrange "time out" for parent to develop personal interests and care for self as needed	
5. Alteration in family dynamics related to dependent needs of parent and child and nonsupportive environment	Identify situational stressors such as poverty, inadequate housing, financial strains, overcrowding, and multiple demands from dependent others	Family dynamics are supportive of individual and family growth, and adaptive coping strategies predominate
	Tap community resources to help the family to meet basic needs for shelter, food, and clothing	
	Discuss various adaptive coping strategies to replace maladaptive behaviors of withdrawal, anger, or substance abuse	
	Identify and reinforce the child's age-appropriate behaviors demonstrating independence	
	Identify and reinforce parental behaviors that demonstrate autonomy and self-confidence	
	Help parent and child learn how to verbalize their feelings and needs to each other and to resource personnel	

at further risk. The insecure parent has difficulty understanding a child's cues and might become impatient when the child does not respond in an expected manner. For example, an infant's cry is loud and annoying so that the dependent infant can communicate basic needs. To insecure parents crying might be interpreted to mean that their children are "bad" or "spoiled" or that the parents have "failed," attitudes that lead to more insecurity. In such instances the child's failure to live up to a parent's distorted view of love only serves to release more feelings of parental inadequacy. Lacking confidence, such parents do not derive much pleasure from their children, a subtle clue to family problems that the nurse needs to investigate further.

Many dysfunctional parents also have had childhood

experiences that taught them to mistrust others. For some parents, lack of nurturing or intermittent nurturing has resulted in feelings of insecurity at each developmental stage so that feelings often affect future relationships with persons in authority. Referring to Erikson's theory of development, when mistrust instead of trust characterizes initial parent–child relations, it has repercussions throughout the developmental process. Anxiety typifies the child's interactions with others, especially adults, because the child never knows if a particular behavior will be met with approval or disapproval. Repeated parental disapproval contributes to a subsequent sense of guilt and inferiority. As an adult, this inability to trust others for fear of being betrayed limits any ability to provide a trusting environment for the child. The parent who has not experienced a trusting relationship cannot provide one. As one mother blurted out during a counseling session, "How can I be consistent with him, I have never known the meaning of consistency in my life? My mother practiced inconsistency to keep us girls on our toes and not take her love for granted."

Difficulty with relationships might result from many other causes. The adult who has difficulty in relationships usually has a history of school adjustment problems and poor academic performance. Sometimes, the lack of academic achievement is the result of a limited intellectual capacity, but far more often it is caused by difficulties with authority figures and relationships in general. These difficulties are often carried into employment patterns, with sudden job changes and long periods of unemployment, placing the family's economic stability at risk. Frequent job changes therefore might indicate inadequate skills, difficulties with interpersonal relationships, and a high degree of impulsivity (Kempe and Kempe, 1978).

The gnawing fear of rejection and disapproval, the fragile bubble of self-esteem, and years of unsuccessful attempts to satisfy the desires of others often result in a personality that is shattered easily by a lack of recognition or reward for a job done well. The lack of meaningful attention in the parent's past coupled with the demands to fulfill another's needs contribute to the parent's constant need for reassurance. When the need is unmet or the fear of criticism becomes overwhelming, the parent might suddenly decide to move or find a new job more worthy of assumed talents. This behavior contributes to family instability and the modeling of ineffective coping strategies for handling stress. Often, boasting about competence belies the reality of inadequate self-esteem (Josten, 1978).

The parent with unmet needs is greatly handicapped in providing effective parenting because the unmet needs result in a dependence that is similar to the dependence of the child. When two parents in a family have unmet needs simultaneously, the family might be in crisis because both parents attempt to manipulate the child to satisfy their own needs. The child is unprotected and vulnerable because both parents expect but are unable or unwilling to provide nurturing. The child's failure to gratify the needs of one parent or the other or to show favoritism are likely to result in criticism, punishment, and even abuse, thus repeating the cycle the parents had experienced in their own childhood (Hurd, 1975).

Sometimes, assisting parents to identify available resources to meet some basic needs is the first step in altering dysfunctional parenting. "Parenting the parent" is one avenue of resolution. Parents often benefit from a temporary dependence on a multidisciplinary team member, someone who takes a special interest in the personal problems of childrearing, homemaking, or employment difficulties, who makes appointments and offers reminders and transportation to keep clinic appointments, who provides a phone number to call any time there is a question or concern, and who calls periodically to check on the parent's welfare.

Nurses need to know that dysfunctional parents often are not aware that their family life-styles are different or abnormal, although many dysfunctional parents do describe their own childhoods as chaotic and report deep feelings of rejection. Nurses also need to be mindful that an insecure parent seems to have a very low tolerance for criticism. Any advice or health teaching therefore should be stated positively, carefully, and slowly.

Parent–Child Role Reversal People who take responsibility for their own lives, make sound judgments, and occupy a useful place in society are said to be mature, but many dysfunctional parents would have difficulty in meeting even one of these criteria. According to psychodynamic theorists, "maturity is the process of adjusting to the demands and pressures of both the instincts and outside society" (Paul, 1980). Dysfunctional parents who are immature therefore have more difficulty providing for dependent children, just as parents who did not experience good parenting as children have a great deal of difficulty in adjusting to the role of parent. The norms that create a loving atmosphere are not part of their memories. They might view children as little adults and in so doing expect too much too soon from their children.

If the child is seen as a competitor for the nurturance and love that the parent is seeking, parent and child might reverse roles, and the parent then seeks gratification from the child. The child then is called on to assume inappropriate levels of responsibility and to provide emotionally for the dependent parent. These unrealistic expectations set the child up for failure, repeating the cycle of dysfunctional parenting. The child also might succeed as an adaptive parent but at high cost.

The interchanging of traditional roles between the parent and child results in difficulties for both. The parent tends to distort reality, have unrealistic expectations for the child, and expect the child to fulfill parental needs, while ignoring the child's need (Flanzraich and Dunsavage, 1977). A child targeted with parental responsibilities in the absence of a responsive parent becomes the source of authority, control, and decision making for the family. All members of the family suffer when roles become confused, but in the dysfunctional family, removal of the "parental child" only results in another child's being assigned the parenting role (Flanzraich and Dunsavage, 1977).

Parent–child role reversal also leads to much family disharmony. Children need to feel protected by someone in authority, and role reversal robs the child of childhood, introducing adult responsibilities and anxieties much too early in the child's development. The child quickly learns to adapt behavior to the external cues provided by the parent. For example, one 3-year-old became very solicitous of the parent's comfort, providing a pillow and blanket every afternoon after lunch and telling the parent to take a nap. While the parent slept, this child quietly picked up the toys and stacked the dirty dishes. When the parent awoke, the child got a glass of juice for both of them. The child was expected to conform and perform before being developmentally ready. Because of the parent's own unmet needs, the parent rushes the dependent child to a state of independence. For example, this parent soon decided that the child should wash and dry the dishes as well.

Parents with limited knowledge of parenting frequently demand adult responsibilities of their older children as well, thereby depriving them of their right to be children (Ruger and Wooten, 1982). They expect them to care for younger siblings after school, wash and fold clothes, prepare meals, and do the shopping instead of participating with peers in club or athletic activities.

Multiple Stressors High-risk families often are victims of accumulated stress and might be subjected to more than one stressor in a short period of time. Families do not exist in a vacuum; they are composed of subsystems and are part of much larger suprasystems. As such, they are influenced both from within and without by many factors beyond their control (Johnson, 1979.) Many families face continuous multiple stressors. Reactions to stress vary, but in the face of recurring pressures, family members experience a sense of powerlessness if the family simply cannot cope.

Stressors might be part of the family subsystems and include illness, conflicts, role confusion, and unrealistic expectations for family members. Other stresses are related to the family suprasystems and might include the effects of poverty, housing problems, unemployment, and racial conflicts. In dysfunctional families most reactions are out of proportion to the threat. Minor stressors are viewed as major crises, and the energy expended to resolve the stress can be devastating. For example, the simple breakdown of a vacuum cleaner is a source of irritation to a functional family but a full-blown crisis to a family with limited resources and coping abilities.

The high-risk family is usually unstable and has many internal and external problems. When faced with multiple stressors, family members usually demonstrate predictable patterns of dysfunction. Stages in a family's developmental cycle, such as birth, marriage, puberty, entrance into school, career changes, and retirement, also tend to create periods of stress. The nurse who understands the family's developmental stage and supports the family at risk during situational stresses can do much to prevent further dysfunction.

Marital Problems In two-parent families the relationship between the parents also is closely intertwined with their parenting style. Dissatisfaction with any aspects of marital life, including sex, influences the parenting ability. If the parent feels rejected by the spouse, the lost love might be sought from the child by excessive demands for companionship or minimal tolerance for uncooperative behavior. Luckey and Bain (1970) noted that because companionship between spouses was low in unhappy marriages, these parents sought compensation from their children and identified them as the most satisfying aspect of the marriage. The nurse therefore assesses parent–child relationships in the context of other relationships within the family (see Chapter 17).

Many people enter marriage or a similar relationship with unrealistic expectations as to a mate's ability to fulfill needs and desires. Young adults who are dependent often fantasize that their partner will care for them but have little insight into the partner's needs. Adults with strong needs for dependence often select mates impulsively following a whirlwind courtship. Some of them even seem to have an uncanny ability to select mates whose need for dependence is equally high. In such marriages each partner romanticizes the dependent role and emphasizes taking rather than giving. Star (1980), in identifying patterns in family violence, cited inappropriate marital expectations as a primary cause of family dysfunction and reported that most battered women entered into the marriage believing that it would solve most of their problems.

The unmet needs of two parents in a dysfunctional family can cause them to feel dissatisfied with their relationship and contribute further to an unhealthy family atmosphere. One partner can feel set up for failure as the other tries to remedy defects in a prior relationship, or the parents might blame each other for their current unhappiness, exaggerate each other's faults, and generally stagnate rather than try to improve. Such parents often maintain an unhealthy marriage, with the potential of resorting to verbal abuse or violence.

The emotional climate that marital strife creates is likely to have negative effects on children. Belsky, Robins, and Gamble (1984) noted that when the husband–wife relationship functioned well, it served as a buffer to mute the potential negative effects of a difficult child. When this buffer was nonexistent, as was likely to be the case when the marriage was evaluated as being low in marital satisfaction, the parent–child relationship was described as dysfunctional. Women who were criticized and blamed frequently by their husbands were found to have a negative orientation toward their infants (Pedersen, Anderson, and Cain, 1977). A cyclic phenomenon appears to occur that links marital relationships and infant development (Belsky and Tolan, 1981). Marital satisfaction also appears to be a factor in parental relationships with older children. Bandura and Walters (1959) observed a higher incidence of nagging and scolding and fewer displays of affection by mothers toward their 3- to 5-year-old sons when the families were characterized by cool and distant marital relations. Stepfathers committed to their marriage and parenting role had a more favorable relationship with their 6- to 11-year-old stepsons than biologic fathers did with their sons when the fathers were dissatisfied with their marriage or experiencing marital discord (Santrock, et al., 1982). The relationship between the emotional quality of the marriage and parenting style appears to be true also for adolescents. Mothers who expressed negative feelings toward their 13- to 16-year-old sons had conflictual marriages. In addition, Olweus (1980) noted that these sons then tended to be aggressive and have an antisocial orientation. The quality of the parental relationship thus influences the children as they establish relationships with others. If a parent remains in an unhappy, unhealthy relationship "for the children's sake," the emotional climate in that family ranges from neutral to explosive. Children perceive nonverbal cues and often know about parental strife and problems despite parental efforts at concealment.

In two-parent families the history of the parents' marriage, especially their age and the circumstances surrounding their decision to be married, is most helpful. If the parents married young to escape unhappy home situations or if the marriage was impulsive, each partner might have little knowledge of the other's strengths and weaknesses (Kempe and Kempe, 1978). For such families, the first interference or crisis usually results in turmoil and frustration, and the family is at risk if the partners do not have time to grow together and learn about each other. If the first child arrives soon after the relationship begins, the family faces further risks. Applying Duvall's theory of family development (see Chapter 4), these families must work simultaneously on the developmental tasks of several stages (family as a couple, childbearing family, and family with an infant). Unless each parent is secure with self, honest with and respectful of the other parent, and capable of drawing on available resources, attempting to accomplish so many family and personal developmental tasks at the same time produces much stress. These partners frequently have not had time to establish a close positive relationship that permits intuitive understanding and meeting of each other's needs. They therefore do not have that buffer to help them cope with a difficult infant or additional environmental strain such as an overcrowded apartment or tight finances.

In addition, the parents' own history of family life provides clues as to the potential coping strategies, internal strengths, and external resources available. If, as a child, the parent experienced many family changes through divorce, the pattern is often repeated. Marital expectations, like many other behaviors, are learned from childhood experience. Seeing one's parents give and take teaches a child what a marriage is all about.

Family dysfunction is seen more frequently when partners have stereotyped ideas of appropriate male or female and husband or wife roles and behaviors. A husband, believing that he should be the head of the household, for example, might make major decisions in an autocratic manner. He might consider housework and child care woman's work and of little importance (Star, 1980). Families that allow few deviations from expected roles have high degrees of dysfunction and even resort to violence. Dobash and Dobash (1979) noted that women who get married believing in patriarchy (that is, accepting traditional values of the male as the controlling head of the household) assume that their primary responsibility includes all the tasks related to homemaking and childrearing. The performance of these tasks is a service to the husband and a symbol of commitment to please and remain subservient to him. When this mind set prevails, poor or reluctant performance deserves punishment, thus justifying for both of them the husband's verbal and/or physical abuse. Unfortunately, many men who abuse their wives believe that they are enacting the standards promoted in western civilization and the general acceptance of cultural norms espousing "aggressiveness, male dominance and female subordination." Lester's (1980) cross-cultural study of wife abuse found that it occurred significantly more frequently in societies where women were regarded as inferior to men.

The nurse who identifies marital tensions and disharmony from family assessment data encourages the parent to seek marital counseling. Counseling is often the first step taken by a couple attempting to gain insight into their relationship with each other. The nurse's knowledge of community resources is valuable in such cases. Open communication between parents is a long-range goal, and a mediator might be able to guide the husband and wife to listen effectively and discuss feelings as an alternative to force.

Parental Separation If the parent who was the primary source of family disharmony chooses to leave the family, the remaining members might feel a sense of relief or a sense of guilt or anger. The remaining parent, however, must struggle to keep the family intact. Financial hardships, loneliness, sadness, denial, and detachment are only some of the risk factors associated with separation.

The longer a separation lasts, the greater the tendency for family members to become ingrained in their new roles and be unwilling to surrender them if the original member returns. For instance, in military families in which the father is absent for an extended period, family members adjust to the new roles in decision making and become self-sufficient with time. The father then often has difficulty reclaiming the role as head of the family and actually might resent the autonomous role of his wife.

Reactions to a separation vary just as each family varies and to a large extent depend on the reasons and preparation for the separation. Most common is a period of mourning as family members struggle to cope with loneliness and loss. If the child is not helped to identify what is happening, the alternative is self-blame, which increases the risks for low self-esteem and dysfunction in a future family. In early childhood, for example, the child might view the separation as a penalty for being bad and may act in a manner that invites punishment. (See Chapter 12 for a discussion of children's coping strategies and responses to separation.)

Chronically Ill Parents Chronic illness in a parent has a profound and prolonged impact on all aspects of daily living. Family functioning is usually affected because of changes and pressure brought on by the altered life-style and ability of the parent to provide care as before. Parents with chronic illness are doubly challenged in that they must try to manage their personal, social, and occupational activities while continuing to be parents. Sometimes, their treatment regimen involves periods of discomfort, immobility, or pain. The illness itself might necessitate modifications in daily activities and routines, rearrangement of environment, and revised patterns of interactions. Parents who have limited socioeconomic resources, limited health knowledge, and unfavorable attitudes toward health care are less likely to continue long-term health supervision, which then affects the course of the illness. Parents with limited coping strategies, poor self-images, and dysfunctional relationships face enormous challenges in parenting as their fragile self-esteem is further challenged.

Chronic illness often causes a breakdown in communication, especially if the illness is endured but not discussed. Parents, because of fatigue and pressure, might find themselves communicating superfically, with much conversation about their own illness. The lack of verbal communication causes children in the family to rely heavily on nonverbal communication, which is markedly affected by physical and emotional fatigue. Children often are expected to know intuitively that they should be more helpful with household tasks. Anger and frustration might build as the parent struggles to complete a formerly easy task while the child plays happily in the next room oblivious to the parent's plight. The anger and frustration increase if the effort is taken for granted and goes unnoticed. This sequence then contributes to the expression of inappropriate behavior such as physical or emotional abuse. Prevention of such behavior depends on the parent's ability to provide a clear message for help when needed.

Multiple stressors intensify the family's vulnerability for dysfunction. Financial responsibilities become a new burden if the illness affects a family wage earner. Overwhelming pressures can occur when the bills mount up and income decreases or disappears. Financial hardships place additional stress on all family members and might result in drastic changes in life-style. The family then might be forced to move to less expensive housing and leave familiar community support services and resources.

Children might resent ill parents who become the center of attention, or they may be so solicitous and concerned that they have little time for themselves. Some illnesses require frequent medical and clinic visits, expensive medicines, time-consuming treatments, and periodic hospitalizations, changes that might require an older child to assume additional family responsibilities and all the children to limit their requests for material possessions.

Behavior during illness is usually consistent with past behaviors during frustration or crises. If the family has limited coping stragegies and is without the resources of an extended family, the risk for dysfunction usually is compounded. If the family was cohesive prior to the illness, the risks for dysfunction are lessened. Children's behaviors reflect the tensions and discomforts of their parents. If there is anger in the family, the child might withdraw to avoid unleashing new problems. If a parent withdraws, the children might misbehave or become loud and boisterous in an attempt to regain lost attention.

Parental Substance Abuse The use of mood-altering substances is now evident in all socioeconomic classes, in all ages, and in both sexes. Adolescents (and in some instances younger children) use these substances for some of the same reasons adults do: to satisfy curiosity, foster peer acceptance, relax, escape from boredom and the realities of life, alleviate anxiety, enhance social situations, and produce pleasurable states of euphoria. (Substance abuse in children is discussed in Chapter 24.) "Parents whose cognitive functions are dulled by the overuse of alcohol and other drugs are obviously unable to care well for their children, inevitably disregard the children's needs, and produce a typical picture of neglect" (Steele, 1976).

Alcoholism is one of today's largest health and social problems. It is a progressive terminal illness characterized by uncontrollable drinking. It affects all aspects of family life, including parenting.

Excessive intake of alcohol leads to physical dependence, which affects all body systems and creates major health problems for the abuser. The physical symptoms caused by malnutrition or alterations in coordination created by alcoholism might lead family members to seek help because physical illness is perceived to be more acceptable.

The nurse completes a thorough family and personal assessment that includes family dynamics, nutritional history, somatic complaints, alcohol intake, employment record, behavior changes, and concurrent stressors. It is important to be alert for subtle cues of alcohol abuse because the client often minimizes the degree to which alcohol is used and the extent to which it controls the family. If alcohol is used in combination with depressants, the effects are synergistic (that is, each drug increases the effectiveness of the other). The combination can be dangerous and even lethal. The effects of chronic alcoholism on family life depend on the length and severity of the abuse. The nurse cannot assume that all alcoholic parents abuse or neglect their children, nor can a causal link be made between alcoholism and abuse or neglect in situations in which both factors are present.

Chronic alcoholism has been divided into four stages for purposes of identifying family dysfunction (Tapia, 1980). The first stage is always denial. Drinking episodes are intermittent, and parents attempt to explain away early symptoms of dependence as normal social drinking. Denial both allows the drinking to continue and delays treatment. The parent struggles to balance parenting and family responsibilities with increased drinking, attempting to maintain control. In the second stage the nonalcoholic parent attempts to solve the problem using available resources. Behaviors such as nagging, bargaining, threats to leave, hiding bottles of liquor, attempts to control money, and avoiding social situations involving drinking are all common (Tapia, 1980). In two-parent families "helping" the alcoholic often diminishes the energy left for parenting. Children instead might be called on to perform household tasks and care for younger siblings.

The third stage is disorganization and chaos. The family is disrupted because of the problem. The nonalcoholic parent begins to look for help outside the family and usually shows signs of marital problems, acute anxiety, severe financial hardships, and problems with the children. If children are caught in a struggle between parents, they become confused as the alcoholic parent alternately ignores, indulges, or abuses the children while the nonalcoholic parent becomes increasingly embarrassed and irritable. Either parent might be strict or liberal or vacillate between extremes. The same behavior might be both accepted and rejected in a single day so that children are never quite sure what response their behaviors will evoke. Communication usually is distorted, especially as parents supply half-truths and white lies regarding the behaviors connected with the alcoholism, but children soon learn that certain kinds of communication precipitate quarrels, anger, and irritability. The children might, in a sense, be victimized by both parents (Hecht, 1973) and eventually have much difficulty trusting others.

In the fourth stage the nonalcoholic parent assumes authority and responsibility for all family decisions and activities while the alcoholic parent takes on the role of the child. Families with parental alcoholism show much role confusion. Parents often are unaware of their children's needs so that poor school performance, nutritional problems, and health deviations might go undetected. Because of the basic inconsistencies in their lives, children in families with alcoholism have great difficulty learning rules and regulations. They act out their impulses, often imitating the alcoholic parent. Occasionally, the school or health officials might be the first to identify a problem.

In 1972 Kempe estimated that alcohol dependence was a factor in about one-third of all cases of child abuse (Kempe and Helfer, 1972). More recent studies have placed that figure considerably higher. According to the National Center on Child Abuse and Neglect, studies are now linking parental alcohol dependence to sexual abuse and incest. The generational nature of family violence is also well documented. Some researchers have found that over 60% of abused children had at least one grandparent who was alcoholic (Wheat, 1981). In instances of both spouse abuse and child abuse, 41% of the reported cases had one or both parents abused by an alcoholic parent (Wheat, 1980). Sullivan (1981) cited findings that show the abstaining parent to be the abusive parent. She also found that clients who suffered the most severe forms of abuse began drinking between 3 and 12 years of age and came from families in which one or both parents were alcoholics.

From all of the current literature on alcoholism and its effects on the family, three important aspects of treatment are repeatedly stressed:

1. The whole family, including children over 5 years of age, need treatment. Alcoholism is a family problem.
2. Regardless of whether the alcoholic parent can be persuaded to seek treatment, the rest of the family needs specific supportive therapy (such as Al-Anon, Ala-Teen, Ala-Tot, Parents Anonymous). Any child reared in a family troubled by alcoholism is, by definition, at risk for emotional abuse and neglect.
3. In families with violence and alcohol problems, the alcoholism needs to be treated first for other therapies to have maximum benefit (Wheat, 1980).

Like the parent who abuses alcohol, the parent who abuses drugs causes many of the same problems within the household and family. Children are often neglected, confused, and cast into adult roles and responsibilities prematurely. If reliance on drugs is the primary coping strategy used by a parent, other coping mechanisms rapidly will fall into disuse (Mitchell, 1979).

The mood swings that accompany drug use can be most uncomfortable for the drug abuser and family. Small children are especially vulnerable when parents are between the drugged and nondrugged states. Dependent children are most at risk because the family dynamics might focus on the drug problem rather than the children's needs. Difficulties with distorted reality might cause the drugged parent to separate from family responsibilities and become helpless. The role of incompetent parent might be assumed with a degree of ambivalence–relief, guilt, and hostility, calling for an increased use drugs to cope (Mitchell, 1979).

Whether the drug is legal or illegal adds a new dimension to family problems. Many parents are ignorant of the laws, fines, or punishments associated with the use of illegal drugs, whereas others openly defy legal jurisdiction. Marijuana, for instance, although illegal, is widely used among all segments of the population. If users are apprehended and prosecuted, additional family problems might be caused by separation and incarceration.

Family life with a substance-abusing parent often requires child-care responsibilities to be assumed by extended family members without advanced planning. Sometimes, young children are left to care for themselves. Alcohol and other drugs decrease the appetite and result in poor nutrition because meal preparation is sporadic and unplanned. Health problems related to nutritional deficiencies might prompt the family's entry into the health care facility. A careful physical and nutritional assessment is done to establish the approximate intake of nutrients, which is compared with the Recommended Daily Allowances. In addition, chaotic meal schedules place the children at risk for nutritional problems so that physical complaints often provide clues about the family disorganization.

Because a child's security needs are closely related to the stability of the environment, children of a substance-abusing parent must learn to expect unreliability, inconsistency, ineptitude, and general household disorganization as the norm and are unable to trust the environment. Nurses working with children need to recognize these clues and plan intervention with support services. For example, the school nurse assessing a student might be the first to identify the risk. Other public health agencies might provide additional data so that multidisciplinary management is made available to the family.

Young Parents With Many Children Close in Age Not all large families are at risk. Some large families have adequate resources, such as experience, motivation, and health, and effective external support systems. Family health can be affected by many factors, one of which is the size of the family. Before a child is born, parents should feel both physically and emotionally ready. When children are fewer than 15 months apart, the older child is still very dependent, and both infants therefore present many demanding but different needs. If the family is experiencing other stressors (such as poverty or unemployment) or is not emotionally ready for the multiple demands, the result might be diminished parental care to one or both infants.

In addition, nutritional deficits might be found in large families, especially if the family income falls below the poverty level and the family has difficulty navigating through the forms to apply for supplemental food or food stamps. Many small, dependent children place another burden on the parent as one mealtime runs into the next. The parent has no free time for personal care. The laundry for many children also might seem monumental, especially if the children are active and independent in feeding and play. Families without the resources of home laundry facilities are doubly stressed by being forced to trudge to the laundromat or try handwashing, which is an overwhelming task. The point at which resources become overtaxed and tolerable levels of stress surpassed is the line separating the family's ability to cope with adversity and the potential for dysfunction.

In large families that are at risk, the developmental needs of one child sometimes are compromised by the developmental needs of another. For example, the parent who is attempting to toilet train a 2-year-old often is intolerant of bed-wetting and normal regression in a 4- or 5-year-old. A child who feels displaced by a new sibling at an early age is forced to surrender babyhood early and might be pushed to reach developmental milestones or become independent before the appropriate time. A parent with many children might demand early toilet training in an attempt to decrease the work load and have minimal tolerance if the child does not cooperate, which might lead to physical punishment.

Fatigue is a factor for parents with many small children. All parents need time-out periods from the multiple demands of parenting. The most motivated parent will burn out and feel entrapped if not given any free time to cultivate adult interests and hobbies. Body language and behavioral clues often suggest the amount of fatigue and stress a parent feels. An active listener can assist the parent in analyzing feelings about parenting. The nurse also assesses the physical stamina of the parent. For example, the nurse might ask a parent to describe the extent of routine chores in a single day. The nurse then might review the tasks and carefully analyze the energy level required. The parent who reports no free time or enjoyment with children needs further evaluation and special attention because chronic fatigue might be a major factor in feelings of entrapment. Open-ended questions such as, "How do you unwind?" or "What do you like to do to relax?" can assist parents in coming to terms with their own needs and feelings.

The nurse might need to explain to parents the importance of time away from their children. Some parents require additional discussion time to analyze resources within the extended family and tap these resources. For some, a nursery school, day-care program, or other babysitting arrangements can give relief, even if only for 1 day a week. Families with limited resources might need greater assistance initially, including a homemaker, parent aide, or friendly visitor in addition to child-care relief. Initially, some parents also might need guidance in planning free time and assistance in discussing anxiety. The nurse can convey to the parent that time-out periods are vital to children because their parents must be protected and assisted to achieve maximum health.

Single Parents With Inadequate Supports Because single parents assume all responsibilities and decisions traditionally shared by two parents, such factors as age, security, personality, maturity level, emotional stability, financial status, and motivation all determine the potential degree of risk that single-parent families face. Single parents are confronted with many problems and constraints. Society generally is geared to couples and to two-parent families and is slow to acknowledge alternative life-styles. Some single parents feel their status to be a stigma, whereas others draw praise and recognition for their ability to function alone. The number of parents in the home is not a measure of successful childrearing; rather, the nurse assesses the emotional climate, level of family functioning, quality of child supervision, and family dynamics before formulating any nursing diagnoses.

Financial strain usually heads the list of problems for single parents, especially for women. A single income often is not enough to meet all the necessities of the family members, especially if day care is needed while the parent works. Finding and evaluating child care facilities is often a priority for single parents (see Chapter 21). Financial worries detract from a parent's ability to be a good parent; a single parent who draws income from welfare assistance, for example, remains at the poverty level and has long-range financial worries about housing, food, and clothing. The responsibility of providing for the physical, social, and emotional needs of a child then might become an awesome task with no other parent to share the burdens.

Single parents might need the opportunity to discuss normal stages of development and their children's behavior and responses with other single parents or a trusted nurse. Without another parent with whom to discuss their children's needs or another adult for the child to interact with, single parents can misinterpret behavior. Problems in childrearing are more likely to lead to self-blame, guilt, and a sense of failure. Occasionally, single parents attempt to compensate for their role by being overly permissive (hoping to secure the child's love) or overly strict (proving to the world it can be done) (Curto, 1983). Although for many single parents the basic need for income necessitates leaving children with other caregivers, separation caused by the parent's employment might lead to feelings of insecurity, loneliness, and despair in children. Children who feel neglected might misbehave just to get the attention that discipline requires. Single parents need to understand this phenomenon and also might need help to learn how to make the best use of time spent with children.

Loneliness can have a crippling effect on the single parent. Dialogue with children can be fun, but it is limiting if there are no other adult contacts in the home. Physical and emotional isolation, together with the frustrations and tensions of the household, can create a potentially explosive situation if the single parent has no outlets for the release of tension. The single parent might need assistance in identifying and cultivating new interests and friends with similar problems and life-styles, and the nurse therefore can refer clients to single-parent organizations, community groups, and church or school resources. The nurse often assumes the role of coordinator when making such referrals and might then be called on to provide follow-up counseling and evaluation (Tankson, 1979).

Developmental Implications of Dysfunctional Parenting

Developmental Delays Children who are nurtured sporadically make only sporadic developmental progress, leading to delays in the age-expected norms (see Chapter 16). Dysfunctional parenting therefore might result in delays in biophysical, cognitive, affective, and social development. Other causes of developmental delays might become evident as the nurse assesses a child's development (see Chapter 16). (Nursing care of the child with developmental disabilities is discussed in Chapter 23.) Problems with the parent–child relationship affect the child at each developmental stage. Typical behaviors to alert the nurse to attachment problems were first defined by Helfer and Kempe (1976). The infant usually first exhibits feeding difficulties and might be irritable, never satisfied, or apathetic to the feedings. The irritability usually is accompanied by an annoying cry. Further developmental delays are evident as the infant is slow to turn over, reach out for toys, or sit. Associated findings are poor muscle tone and a delay in social responses such as smiling and vocalizing (Helfer and Kempe, 1976).

As the infant matures, other delays become evident. The child might not show separation anxiety and may respond indiscriminately to new stimuli. The child might accept toys passively and not protest when they are removed, or the child might show little interest in exploring the environment. Infants who have been abused, for example, exhibit a state of "frozen watchfulness," in which the child appears immobile and passive but is acutely alert to what is happening (Helfer and Kempe, 1976).

Developmental delays during early childhood are evident as the child is at play. The child might use toys in a primitive way and with a lack of interest. Lack of eye contact and much passivity are common. The child might have poor coordination, indicating delayed progress in both gross and fine motor development and poor muscle tone. Speech is usually delayed, with poor enunciation and vocabulary, and the child usually is unable to express feeling or describe family members. The child with disturbed parent–child relationships usually has difficulty relating to people, shows a sense of mistrust, has a poor self-concept, and is preoccupied with many fears (Helfer and Kempe, 1976). The child who fails to meet the excessive expectations of the parent might be rejected verbally or physically abused. The long-range results will leave the child with a sense of failure, a low self-esteem, and limited problem-solving abilities.

The nurse collecting assessment data therefore includes the child's gross and fine motor skills, language capacity, and ability to use toys in an age-appropriate way (see Chapter 16). The nurse might be the primary health provider to assist parents in understanding children and their needs. Helfer and Kempe (1976) warned that teaching child development is not an adequate solution if a parent's high expectations of the child's performance is connected with the parent's own developmental concerns and tasks. If the parents' fulfillment of their own needs interferes with their making use of knowledge and parenting skills, the nurse might need to refer the family for counseling. Assessing readiness to learn and parental motivation therefore are essential first steps before sharing information about the normal strivings children have to master developmental tasks (see Chapter 21 for a discussion of anticipatory guidance and its role in child health maintenance).

Inorganic Failure to Thrive The term *failure to thrive* describes a syndrome characterized by a lack of normal growth and development in children. The child's height and weight usually falls below the 3rd percentile on standard growth charts and is accompanied by lags in social, motor, adaptive, and language development (Table 22-1).

"Failure to thrive is a symptom, not a diagnosis" (Stephenson, 1980). Etiology is often difficult to identify because the child might have an illness with such symptoms as vomiting and diarrhea along with characteristics of behavioral withdrawal. Failure to thrive is classified as organic or inorganic in origin. Children with organic failure to thrive have difficulty using nutrients because of neurogenic, metabolic, endocrine, enzymatic, or genetic disease. (Organic failure to thrive is discussed in Chapter 38.) Inorganic failure to thrive has an environmental or social cause and often is seen in children from dysfunctional families.

Children with failure to thrive are usually thin, frail, and undernourished. Evidence of improper physical care, such

TABLE 22-1 Common Findings in Infants With Inorganic Failure to Thrive

Age	Findings
0–6 months	Prematurity
	Neonatal illness or anomaly necessitating early separation
	Feeding difficulties (eg, anorexia)
	Height and weight below 3rd percentile
	Unresponsiveness and withdrawal
	Watchfulness, little smiling
	Delayed socialization and vocalization
	Irregular sleep patterns
	Developmental delays
6–12 months	Absence of stranger anxiety
	Rumination
	No displeasure at separation
	Apathy/passivity
	Delayed milestones as to sitting and standing
	Muscular hypotonia
12–18 months	Indifference to caregivers
	Small physical size
	Delayed dentition
	Little vocalization
	Little eye contact
	Intense watchfulness
	Repetitive self-stimulation behaviors (eg, rocking, head banging, rolling, intense sucking)

as seborrheic dermatitis (cradlecap) or severe diaper rash, can suggest failure to thrive because of improper nurturance and care. The nurse obtains a history of the feeding techniques and assesses the quality, quantity, and consistency of intake. Infants with failure to thrive frequently are hospitalized to document weight gain and rule out organic causes for growth failure. Children with inorganic failure to thrive might show a substantial weight gain while in the hospital and also show progress in developmental skills while receiving the consistent nurturance of hospital personnel. Serial growth measurements often assist in identifying the onset or chronicity of weight loss.

The behaviors of an infant and parent might provide clues to the cause of the disorder. Harrison (1976) stated, "failure to thrive is a process in which both mother and infant contribute reciprocally to the other's problem." The parent–child relationship is usually problematic and maladaptive for both parent and child, and the child's temperament also might affect the child's vulnerability to failure to thrive. For example, the infant who is irritable, resists cuddling, and is unresponsive to initial attempts at nurturing creates a response pattern in the parent that increases fears, anxiety, and avoidance behaviors. If the infant is improperly fed, irritability and crying increase because of hunger.

The parent who suffers from unmet needs and has multiple environmentally related stresses is likely to have problems with such an infant (Table 22-2). The new, inexperienced parent, the depressed parent, and the adolescent parent are especially at risk of having a child who fails to thrive. Failure to have parental needs gratified can trigger unconscious feelings of rejection; therefore, failure to thrive is rarely the result of willful neglect but is more frequently a symptom of family dysfunction. The infant at risk thus becomes the recipient of resentments, fears, conflicts, and stress. The parent in turn responds with anxiety and tension to the infant who reacts with irritability and rigidity, and a vicious cycle of unmet needs is set in motion.

Children with inorganic failure to thrive predictably prefer distant social encounters and inanimate objects, whereas children with failure to thrive caused by medical problems consistently respond more positively to close personal stimuli such as touching and holding. Children from dysfunctional families might be stiff and unyielding when cuddled or may be slow in smiling and cooing, demonstrating a lack of trust in the person who cares for them (Yoos, 1984). A sense of trust, which normally develops in the first year of life, is essential to a healthy personality (see Chapter 7). Basic trust is established when the infant's physical needs are met consistently.

The family dynamics that lead to failure to thrive are stagnant. Members do not communicate, and a general feeling of helplessness pervades the family. Family members cannot identify what is happening. In their troubled, isolated lives, dysfunctional behaviors keep them from experiencing joy in living. Stewart (1973) stated that inorganic failure to thrive is an indictment of society as the

TABLE 22-2 Common Findings in Families With Children With Inorganic Failure to Thrive

Family member	Findings
Child's caregiver (usually mother)	Depression
	Limited knowledge of child-care responsibilities
	Inexperienced
	Limited homemaking, organizational, or management skills
	Feeling of being overwhelmed
	History of difficult labor and delivery
	Separation of child following birth because of prematurity or other neonatal problems
	Unplanned or unwanted pregnancy
Parent or other adults	Frequent absences of father
	Single parenthood
	Poverty or severe financial strain
	Unemployment
	Inadequate housing
	Lack of transportation
	Social isolation with few community supports
	Marital discord

TABLE 22-3 Common Findings Related to Child Neglect

Child	Parent	Family
Height and weight below 3rd percentile on growth chart	History of inadequate parenting	Marital discord, often with periods of separation
Apathy—does not smile; appears solemn and watchful	Use of denial and projection as coping strategies	Erratic habits (eg, no scheduled mealtime; little planning for food, rest, or recreation)
Stiff body that resists being held	Poor performance in day-to-day activities	Chronically unstable home environment
Suspicious and inability to trust adults	Intense need to be cared for	Poverty
Unkempt appearance—foul odor; ground-in dirt; ill-fitting clothing; clothing inappropriate for weather	Limited ability to plan	Employment instability
Restless sleep patterns	Few external resources	Substance abuse
Frequent absences from school	Inability to use resources	Children left unattended or in care of strangers
Developmental delays	Inability to assess infant's needs	Isolation, with minimal participation in any community activities
Marginal communication skills	Need for concrete direction in providing child care	Unhygienic environment—foul odor caused by accumulated garbage; bedding with urine odor; broken furniture; spoiled food
Few coping skills	Diminished self-esteem	Nutritional deficits in all members (eg, obesity, malnutrition)
Poor hand–eye coordination	Passivity; lack of warmth and tenderness	Lack of motivation to change
Poor dental care	Dissatisfaction with parenting role	Lack of emotional bonds among members
Chronic malnutrition; excessive intake of junk food	Little awareness of normal growth and development	Inconsistent or sporadic discipline
Haphazard medical attention—late or missing immunizations	Little awareness or concern for child's progress or problems in school	Medical care only in emergencies
Lack of safety (eg, in cars; has many "mishaps")	Does not attend any school programs or participate in parent–teacher conferences	
Skin problems (eg, crusting, impetigo, scabies, rashes)	Minimal awareness of child's activities, interests, or friends	
Rumination		
Arrives early and stays at school late		
Tired and falls asleep in class		

complex cycle of inadequate parenting breeds a succeeding generation of inadequate parents. Early identification and interventions with high-risk families are therefore crucial. However, funding to accomplish this goal has never been adequate and vacillates with the prevailing economic philosophy. The interrelationships of the child, family, and community cannot be overlooked in planning interventions aimed at breaking the complex cycle (Belsky, Lerner, and Spanier, 1984).

Health-Threatening Parenting

Child Neglect

Child neglect is the failure to provide a child with the basic necessities of life: food, clothing, love, shelter, supervision, and medical care. Neglect usually is associated with parental acts of omission. The neglect can be deliberate or unintentional, but in either instance the caregiver fails to provide the supports necessary for developing a child's physical, intellectual, and emotional capacities. Neglect is more commonly found in infants and young children; however, older children are not exempt (Johnson, 1979).

Child neglect is not easy to define because standards of care and neglect are so variable (Table 22-3). Most authorities agree, however, that neglect is any form of substandard child care. Although professionals can reach some consensus about what constitutes minimally adequate child care, the right to intervene when parents neglect or provide poorly for their children is limited because laws protect families from intrusion. Child neglect is more prevalent than child abuse, and its emotional and physical sequelae have been demonstrated to be equally serious. "In 1982 there were

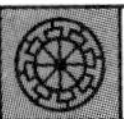

CASE STUDY Child Neglect

Assessment

A 5-month-old infant was brought into the emergency room by police after having been found alone in her crib in a small, dirty tenement. The baby's cries led neighbors to investigate and call for assistance. Neighbors reported having heard the infant cry in the past but were afraid to intervene.

Family

The 18-year-old mother, Beth, was located by police after they questioned various neighbors. The mother claimed that she had only stepped out for a few minutes but later admitted that she had met friends and had gone to a party. Background data revealed that Beth lived alone with her infant and that the infant's father, who lived across town with his wife and two children, visited inconsistently. (He subsequently stopped visiting and eventually left town after the publicity generated by this incident.)

Child

On admission, the infant was dirty and hungry but otherwise in good health. Her height and weight reached the 10th percentile on the growth curve. Her development in all areas was delayed. According to the Denver Developmental Screening Test, her behaviors and skills were more characteristic of a 3-month-old infant.

Following this incident, Beth became increasingly depressed over the loss of her boyfriend, the setback in her plans to return to school, and the demands of a young infant for whom she alone was responsible. She felt that she had to prove to herself and to her family that she was a good mother.

Nursing Diagnoses

1. Potential for further developmental delays in the infant related to inadequate parenting.
2. Dysfunctional parenting related to lack of support and lack of information about child care needs.
3. Disturbance in self-concept related to difficult transition to parenthood, limited opportunity to meet adolescent developmental tasks, and loss of accustomed supports.
4. Potential for growth related to motivation to learn parenting skills.

Plan for Interventions

Goals

1. Infant will evidence no further delays and will catch up in all developmental areas in response to positive parenting.
2. Beth will identify and attend available resources to learn about infant growth and development, appropriate expectations, and parenting behaviors and skills.
3. Beth will demonstrate self-confidence in decision making about returning to school, caring for her infant, and her living arrangements.
4. Beth will identify at least three ways in which her parenting skills have improved and how both she and her infant benefited.

Interventions

1. Report the case to Child Protective Services and identify a case coordinator for follow-up.
2. Discuss with Beth her feelings since the infant's birth and identify her current needs.
3. Suggest and role model ways to stimulate the infant to enhance parent–child bonding and manage the child's behavior.
4. Demonstrate infant care skills for feeding, changing, bathing, and holding and have Beth demonstrate these skills in return.
5. Demonstrate ways to play and interact with the infant and praise Beth for positive parenting behaviors that foster the infant's development.
6. Help Beth to identify the infant's cues and responses that demonstrate satisfaction and need fulfillment.
7. Test the infant's developmental level again in 3 months to note progress.
8. Refer Beth to possible child care providers to meet time-out needs.
9. Establish contract that lists goals and sets limits about keeping appointments.
10. Teach homemaking skills on practical matters, such as budgeting, using written material.
11. Refer Beth to a parental support group for contact with adolescent parents in similar situations.
12. Encourage Beth to use available child care and to plan for returning to school.

929,310 reports of child abuse and neglect nationwide . . . 26% of the reports involved abuse, 43% neglect, and 19% combined abuse and neglect" (Heins, 1984).

In some instances neglect has even been found to be lethal, such as an infant whom a parent "forgets" to feed for several days or young children who, when left alone in a house or apartment for extended times, fall out of windows or down stairs or ingest poisons.

Inadequate Physical Care Physical neglect might be evident in many ways. An infant, for instance, may be dirty or inadequately clothed, have evidence of diaper rash or seborrheic dermatitis (cradlecap), or appear unkempt, with a stale, urine odor. Nutritional neglect, which results either from lack of food or a bizarre diet, frequently is manifested by signs of malnutrition. The child often has little subcutaneous fat, decreased muscle mass, and an appearance of gauntness with prominent bones. An infant's height and weight often fall below the 3rd percentile, and physical assessment might reveal a bald spot on the back of the head from the infant's spending much time alone and unattended in the crib.

Infant behaviors, however, give the most valuable clues to the inadequacy of care. The neglected infant is often listless, makes few demands, and does not respond to the stimulation of voices or friendly faces. The infant prefers to turn away from people and engages in little eye contact. With prolonged and severe neglect, infants often arch their bodies when they are picked up.

Neurologic and neonatal examinations (using the Brazelton Neonatal Behavioral Assessment Scale [see Chapter 16]) at 1 month of age might show developmental progression but not the increased capacity for orientation, self-consolation, and social responses that are characteristic of the normal neonate (Greenspan, 1982). By 3 months of age, neglected infants show increased tendencies toward lability, muscle rigidity, and gaze aversion, and they lack organized sleep–wake and alert states and feeding patterns. Parental stimulation might be intense, chaotic, or intermittent (Greenspan, 1982).

As neglected children grow, developmental delays become more apparent. Physical size often suggests a much younger child; therefore, the nurse needs to identify the proper age and expected level of development for every child. Gross motor skills often are delayed because the child is reluctant to trust and interact with the environment. Nutritional neglect and failure to thrive also might cause the infant to lack the strength to explore the environment. Sitting, pulling to stand, cruising, and walking therefore are delayed. Delays in eye–hand coordination frequently affect reading and writing skills and ultimately affect the child's self-confidence and self-esteem (Haynes, 1980).

Language development is also frequently delayed in the neglected child because the infant needs to hear language to imitate it. Language skills are notably lacking from 2 years of age on, as children cannot name simple body parts or identify common objects within the home. (Chapter 8 discusses normal language development.) Their use of pronouns often does not begin until their early school years. Many neglected children speak only in phrases rather than in sentences and have limited vocabularies, although they frequently can repeat television commercials.

Interacting with strangers is especially difficult for neglected children because of their mistrust. They often have poor problem-solving and coping skills because these behaviors are learned from their parents. When supplied with toys, neglected children often need to learn how to use them because they simply have not learned how to play. A wide selection of toys, which might be evident in a hospital playroom, is often sensory overload to a neglected child.

In the older child poor physical care might be apparent by ill-fitting clothing or clothing that is inappropriate for the weather. The child might smell dirty and have multiple layers of dirt and grime, suggesting infrequent bathing. If the child or siblings have problems with enuresis, the stale odor of urine can be easily identified. Signs of a lack of nurturance can be both overt and covert. For example, the child might come to school with no lunch or money for food or may show signs of constant hunger. Fatigue is common because the child's sleep habits often are not supervised. Listlessness or falling asleep in class affects learning and leads to asocial behavior among peers.

Another sign of neglect might be a consistent lack of supervision, either in allowing children to engage in dangerous activities or in leaving small children unattended. Although leaving small children alone or in the care of another young child is considered acceptable among some parents, the parents might need to understand the dangers of such practices. Especially at risk for accidents when reared in neglectful families are young children because they require continuous supervision and protection. Unattended children are at risk for falls, causing fires, ingesting poisons or medicines, and playing with unsuitable companions. Children who favor extended stays at school (that is, arriving early or staying on the grounds after school) are often children who are unsupervised or neglected. Low-income parents often have no extra money for babysitters or day care and are forced to leave young children without supervision before and after school (Polansky, Hally, and Polansky, 1976).

Another form of physical neglect is inattention to medical needs. The child might have bad teeth, lice, various skin rashes, a sporadic, incomplete immunization record, and few follow-up visits for health problems. If much parental time and energy are spent on day-to-day survival, it is difficult to plan ahead to make and keep a health visit appointment; therefore, when the child does become ill, the illness is intensified because of poor nutrition, neglect, and multiple other problems within the family.

Children who do not see the same health care provider on a regular basis also are at risk for health care neglect. For example, the child who is seen only when acutely ill by a health care provider is at risk for developing complications from the acute illness when follow-up evaluations are omitted (such as some of the sequelae following streptococcal infections). In addition, chronic conditions or subtle indicators of other problems related to physical maturation or health often go unnoticed because attention is focused on the immediate and most obvious problem. For example, the child's laceration is sutured but the early, covert indicators of tuberculosis remain undetected because the reactivation of the grandparent's tuberculosis and the crowded, extended family living conditions of this child are unknown to the practitioner seeing the child for a single event in the emergency room.

Inadequate Emotional Care Emotional neglect is an act of omission on the part of the parent or caregiver. It frequently is the result of parental ignorance or indifference and often reflects a lack of motivation toward parenting. Lack of positive emotional support and stimulation is not necessarily accompanied by inadequate physical care but usually is evidenced by little attention to cognitive stimulation or few expressions of love and caring. Emotional neglect is difficult to identify early because only after the sequelae become apparent can help be directed toward the family.

The parent who emotionally neglects a child tends to respond only to such behavior as crying or misdeeds. The parent seldom looks at, touches, or talks to the child. Such parents show little interest in their children and often leave them unattended while the parents interact with other adults, leading to unsafe, dangerous situations. Limit setting is usually inconsistent because of lack of parental interest in the child. Any positive behaviors go unnoticed, and the child soon learns to increase the intensity of negative behaviors to get attention.

In the older child emotional neglect is evident in poor self-concept. The child might be distant or disruptive in the classroom but typically wants approval and affection from teachers. Young children develop "crushes" on their teachers but also might feel too afraid or deprived to trust teachers. Hostile, angry children also might alienate teachers just when they most need the teacher's care and affection (Howell, 1977).

Causes of Child Neglect Neglecting parents often were themselves victims of child abuse or neglect and might have had no positive role models for parenting. They often are not trying to hurt their children but merely are treating their children as they were treated. Neglectful parents also tend to report profound sadness over not having been loved or wanted by their own parents. Many of these parents are constantly under stress, which interferes with their ability to spend time to enjoy their children, or much of their time and energy is taken up with the basic necessities of life so that they have little time and energy left for child care. Inadequate knowledge about children, parenting, and normal development is also common.

Parents who often are unaware of the needs of children frequently have unrealistic expectations of their children and respond unfavorably when these expectations are not met. Their own low self-esteem prevents them from further attempts to meet their children's needs, and they frequently give up, leaving the children even more vulnerable to further neglect. A parent who displays a lack of affect, general apathy, or a lack of responsiveness to the child should alert any health care provider to investigate further.

Some cultures support what appears to be a pattern of neglect during the children's early years and only perceive value in the children once they are of an age to be useful within the home (Sung, 1978). Parents sometimes allow their children to live in foster homes during the dependent years but petition agencies to have the children returned once they can perform tasks around the house, babysit younger siblings, or earn money from various jobs. The unspoken message to these children is that they are valued only for what they can do for their parents. In reality the economic and social situation of these parents might have provided them no choice because of their unemployment, inadequate housing, and poverty (Pelton, 1981).

In severe instances of neglect, outright rejection of the child might have a number of complex causes related to the parent, child, and social environment. The child might be the "wrong" sex, unattractive, similar to a disliked family member, or similar to the rejecting parent. The parent describes feelings about the child with expressions such as, "that child has the soul of the devil in him; no way can he be good." Neglect is seen more frequently in economically deprived families where the mother is the primary caregiver and provider of the family's basic necessities.

Neglectful parents also tend to be impoverished, isolated, and involved in fewer relationships with others. They are less able to plan, less confident about the future, and more plagued by psychologic and psychosomatic problems (Polansky, Hally, and Polansky, 1976). Welfare families (who are paid on a monthly basis) are most at risk for malnutrition toward the end of the month when the money and food supplies are scanty or nonexistent. Living conditions might include inadequate laundry facilities, making it more convenient to neglect clothing, bedding, or body hygiene. Sleep patterns might be irregular, with little regard to the needs of the growing child. Children frequently do not have designated beds or areas for sleep but are allowed to fall asleep in front of the TV, on the sofa, or on the floor. Lack of heat in the household might contribute to sleeping in congested areas that are warm.

Child Abuse

Child abuse is "human-originated acts of commission or omission and human-created or tolerated conditions that inhibit or preclude unfolding and development of inherent potential of children" (Pelton, 1981). In the past 20 years, child abuse has been identified in epidemic proportions throughout the world. Abuse is always complex. It is not a diagnosis but is instead a symptom of family dysfunction. Data now indicate that the social environment as well as children and parents show many patterns of risk, but no single family configuration is most likely to cause child abuse (Table 22-4). Newberger and colleagues (1977) explored the relationship of historical and contemporaneous stress to the pediatric social diseases of accidents, child abuse, failure to thrive, and poisonings. They found that although certain attributes were more likely to be present in families of children with a pediatric social disease, there were no clear-cut similarities across the groups. In addition, it became evident that the critical issue was to disentangle the apparent causal associations from the extent of misclassification that was identified (that is, the poor were labeled as abused and the middle class as accidents). These researchers concluded that the focus for identification, treatment, and prevention had to include the child, family, and life setting and analyzed the contribution of both the stresses and strengths present in the abusive family. When child abuse occurs, each member of the family is in some way a victim and needs help if the family is to achieve any degree of positive functioning.

Estimates of the incidence of victimized children and families are only crude measures because of the lack of uniformity in defining the problem and the hesitancy in reporting it. Some authorities place the figure at over 2 million

TABLE 22-4 Parental Risk Factors for Child Abuse

Risk factor	Assessment findings
Lack of nurturing experience	Inadequate experience with parenting (eg, multiple foster homes)
	Parent neglected or abused as a child
	Parent expected to meet high demands of own parents as a child
Lack of knowledge of normal growth and development	Inability to read "cues" of child
	Impatience when child does not respond as expected; unreasonable discipline
	Unrealistically high expectations for the child
Isolation	Inadequate use of supports
	Inability to identify resources
	Unknown to others in community
Low self-esteem	Lack of trust, particularly of authority figures
	Expect rejection
High vulnerability to criticism	History of family violence in family of origin or in current family system (eg, spouse abuse)
	Low tolerance for frustration
	Impulsive
Many unmet needs	Feelings of being unloved or having unresponsive spouse, unstable marriage, or no marriage at all
	Youthful marriage, forced marriage, unwanted pregnancy
Multiple stressors	Poverty, unemployment, substandard housing, lack of job opportunities
	Inadequate clothing and insufficient food
Substance abuse	Abuse of alcohol or drugs
Role reversal	Emotional immaturity, lack of patience, inability to make judgments
	Preoccupied with self
	Depression
	Dependent on others

cases of child abuse annually in the United States, whereas other professionals estimate the incidence to be as high as 6 cases per 1000 live births (Heins, 1984). Abuse of adolescents is often not included in these data, usually because adolescent abuse is called something else (such as, adolescent–parent conflict, discipline problems, adolescent provocation, arrest, training for sports). Some data might classify all adolescents in a separate category. Statistics also give only part of the picture because most abusers are repeating child-care patterns from previous generations. About 6000 children die annually from child abuse or neglect, more than from any disease (Ten Bensel and Berdie, 1976).

History of Child Abuse The phenomenon of child abuse is not new. It appears in ancient records and as part of myths and legends. The Bible, for example, records murder (Cain and Abel), abandonment (Moses in the bullrushes), and sacrificial offerings of children (Isaac and Abraham). DeMayse (1974) found that history records a low level of child care and that in many cultures children were likely to be neglected, beaten, terrorized, abandoned, sexually abused, and murdered. Infanticide, for example, has been documented in almost every culture and in every era. It often was used to rid society of the weak and deformed, control the size of the family, and limit the number of females (Brodie, 1982).

Throughout history, children were considered the "property" of their parents; they had no rights and as possessions were sent into mines, factories, and sweatshops to work in unsafe and unsanitary conditions. Harsh treatment historically has been considered best for the child. Ownership of children also was transferable to others, as in child slavery or arranged marriages, and children could be abandoned or disposed of according to the whims of the parents. Under Roman law, for example, a father had the power of life and death over his children.

Whipping of children, especially boys, has been recorded since ancient times and was the prerogative of teachers and parents. In England and Colonial America, teachers are pictured with forms of birch whips. Discipline in the colonies often was severe, with little regard for its effects on children. Even today, many states allow the use of "reasonable" force, or corporal punishment, as a form of discipline in school (Humphreys, 1984).

The earliest recorded case of child abuse in the United States was the "Mary Ellen" case in 1874. This 9-year-old child was whipped daily, tied to a bed, and punished by being stabbed with scissors by her foster parents. Neighbors reported the case to Etta Wheeler, a church worker, who ultimately appealed to the Society for the Prevention of Cruelty to Animals on the premise that the child was a member of the animal kingdom. Public outcry then led to the formation of the Society for the Prevention of Cruelty to Children in New York in 1875.

In the medical literature Dr. John Caffey, in 1946, reported infants suffering multiple fractures in the long bones and chronic subdural hematomas. He associated the findings with trauma but did not connect the trauma to abuse. In 1960 Dr. C. Henry Kempe addressed the annual convention of the American Academy of Pediatrics, describing fractures and subdural hematomas that he found to be inflicted by parents. The first definition of child abuse was thus "any child who received nonaccidental physical injury (or injuries) as a result of acts or omissions on the part of his parents or guardians" (Kempe 1973; Kempe and Helfer, 1976).

In 1962 the Social Security Administration amended its regulations to require states to plan the protection of children. In 1963 the Department of Health, Education and Welfare (HEW) developed a model mandatory reporting law for states to follow in writing their own regulations. Within 5 years, every state had laws mandating certain professionals to report abuse and established state agencies to receive and investigate all such reports. In 1973 the federal government passed the Child Abuse Prevention and Treatment Act. Public Law 93-247, also known as the Mondale Act, provided financial assistance for projects for preventing, identifying, and treating abuse and neglect. It also established a national center on child abuse and neglect, provided an information clearinghouse, and published annual summaries of research into abuse and neglect.

During the 1960s, early efforts at treatment emphasized detection and the removal of abused children to foster homes. Initially, many families were lost to follow-up because few outreach programs were available. Trends revealed, however, that many dysfunctional parents who had more children repeated patterns of abuse. Clearly, society needed to assist the families in learning new parenting styles.

Some children who were removed from their parents fared well; other children experienced profound loss and grief, particularly if they did not feel loved or wanted in the foster family. Children who had learned only dysfunctional behaviors were sometimes more at risk for abuse in their new families. Some foster parents were selected merely because they were willing and available. Because they were not part of a carefully considered treatment plan, they were not helped to understand the loyalty, grieving, loss, and separation that children experienced. If the original family was reunified, the foster parents often were overlooked as valuable contributors to success. Some children remained in foster care permanently, whereas others moved often between foster families and their original families.

Patterns of Abuse Child abusers are found among all socioeconomic, religious, and ethnic groups. Some child abusers are irrational or even psychotic, but most are ordinary people who feel trapped in stressful life situations with which they cannot cope satisfactorily. Many abusive parents are simply confused and overwhelmed by parenthood or by life in general and often vent their frustrations on their children. Because all parents have negative feelings about their children at one time or another, the difference between parents who abuse and those who do not is often only a matter of degree. All parents are at risk occasionally, but most parents are able to channel their frustrations and anger appropriately.

The parent with a potential for abuse is one who feels isolated, is unable to trust others, has no spouse, is too passive to be able to give, or has very unrealistic expectations for children. Parents at risk for abuse tend to expect their children to perform for parental gratification, and they tend to use severe physical punishment to ensure a child's proper behavior (Kempe and Helfer, 1972). As mentioned earlier, parents who abuse their children are likely to have been abused as children. This multigenerational pattern of child abuse, although disturbing, does help in identifying families in need of prevention.

Many abusive parents also have unrealistic expectations for themselves and unknowingly contribute to their problems. For example, one parent waxed the kitchen floor during a snowstorm and then abused the child who tracked mud into the house. Clearly, the parent's behavior and expectations for the child contributed to the problem.

Parents with a potential for abuse often expect their children to meet parental needs and therefore are most likely to abuse a child who is viewed as "different." Young children are sometimes targets for abuse, as are high-risk infants, who are often unresponsive to parental attention. (Nursing care of the high-risk infant is discussed in Chapter 31).

Children most at risk also might be the result of difficult pregnancies or deliveries, born at inconvenient times, born out of wedlock, the "wrong" sex, or too active or too passive. Some children are abused because they are the result of a forced pregnancy with an unloved partner or the result of rape or incest. Others have characteristics, such as looks and mannerisms, that evoke negative associations in the abusing parent. Children who have been separated from their families because of prematurity or neonatal disease are more likely to be at risk for abuse. Children with congenital anomalies, mental retardation, hyperactivity, or chronic illness are also at risk. Children with abnormal sleep–wake patterns or feeding difficulties and those who are unresponsive to caregiving also might be at risk if they are living in a family with other risk factors (Steele, 1980). Only a small percentage of premature or difficult children, however, are abused, and for all abused children, it is the combination of parental deficiencies and characteristics of the child that create the problems leading to abuse.

Child abuse is most likely to occur during times of crisis. The parent's loss of a job, for example, might be just enough to make the crying of a fretful infant unbearable. Some families hover on the brink of perpetual crises by living with constant changes that contribute to feelings of inadequacy. The magnitude of the crisis is not always in proportion to the abuse. Instead, the parental perception of the crisis coupled with the lack of available resources often leads to an abusive episode. A relatively minor crisis might be viewed as the "last straw" in an unhappy life situation.

Solving a crisis for troubled families is not enough if new crises and stressors merely reestablish dysfunctional patterns. Instead, the nurse teaches parents to develop their own coping strategies and to identify when and how to seek help. Parents who learn the problems inherent in isolation, for example, will then seek assistance when under stress and will avoid the patterns of behavior that cause them to abuse their children.

Types of Abuse

Physical Abuse Physical injuries might resemble those caused by accidents, but child abuse should be suspected whenever a child's injury has no explanation or plausible reason (Table 22-5). Children who sustain many injuries should be considered possible victims of abuse. Fresh and old injuries together suggests a series of traumatic events rather than a single accident. Another important clue is the distance from the child's home to the treatment facility because parents might go to distant facilities to escape detection.

Physical abuse might be obvious if marks on the child's body are inconsistent with a traumatic injury. Some of the more common injuries include localized burns on the buttocks from being placed on a stove or radiator and circular extremity burns from immersion in hot water. The child might have slap marks resembling a handprint; welts from beatings with coat hangers, belts, or buckles; or circular abrasions on the wrists and ankles from being tied down. A particularly harmful practice is shaking the child vigorously, which can lead to a whiplash injury and even cause brain damage, especially in the young infant who has not developed good head control. Children who are thrown into a crib or against a wall might have signs of both fractures and dislocations. During infancy, the periosteum is less securely attached to the bone, which allows it to be stripped from the shaft by hemorrhage (Table 22-6). Sometimes, the abused child will have a "paradox of clothing," which is the parent's attempt to hide the abuse by dressing the child in clothing such as a baptismal dress.

Physical abuse might result from overdiscipline or from punishment that is too severe. Some children are punished for behavior that is perfectly appropriate for the child's developmental stage but is not perceived as appropriate by the parent. For example, crying in the infant or toilet training in the toddler might precipitate abuse. Most parents who abuse their children have good intentions and really care about the welfare of their children. They might be trying to change the behavior of the child but overreact to stressors. Many abusive parents know that they need help but are afraid to ask for fear of losing their children to foster care.

TABLE 22-5 Types of Child Abuse

	Definition	Characteristics
Physical abuse	Nonaccidental injury of a child	Physical injury at variance with history or explanation given; repeated pattern of physical punishment with short- or long-term effects
Emotional abuse	Nonphysical, often verbal, assault on a child—usually critical, demeaning, and emotionally devastating	Attack inflicted by parent or other adult, often as part of a continuing pattern
Sexual abuse	Use of a child for sexual purposes, including incest, rape, molestation, prostitution, or pornography	Nonabusing parent or other family members often aware of the abuse (and might be criminally liable if they do nothing to stop it)
Adolescent abuse	Physical, emotional, or sexual abuse inflicted on an adolescent	Adolescent who runs away from home (see Chapter 24); abusing parent often considers abuse justified

TABLE 22-6 Signs and Symptoms of Physical Abuse

Indication of abuse	Assessment findings
Bruises or welts on eyes, mouth, lips, torso, buttocks, genital areas, calves	Injuries might be in shape of object used to produce them (eg, sticks, belts, hairbrushes, buckles)
	Injuries located on parts of body not usually injured (normal bruises commonly appear on forehead, shins, knees, elbows)
	Injuries often in various stages of healing
Burns	Shape suggests type of burn
Immersion burns	Immersion burns have "socklike" or "glovelike" appearance
Pattern burns	Pattern suggests object used (eg, iron, stove grate, electric burner, heater); small, circular burns on feet, face, hands, chest, or buttocks suggest cigar or cigarette
Friction burns	Friction often caused by rope on legs, arms, neck, or torso and might be caused by child having been tied up
Fractures of skull, face, nose, long bones	Multiple or spiral fractures caused by twisting motion
	Evidence of epiphyseal separations and periosteal shearing
	Shaft fractures from direct blows
	Fractures might be in various stages of healing if earlier fractures went untreated
Lacerations or abrasions on mouth, lips, gums, eyes, genitals	Human bite marks, especially those of adult size, might be evident
Child's behaviors that indicate fear or apprehension	Extreme aggressiveness or withdrawal; wariness of adults; fear of going home; apprehension when other children cry
	Appears frightened of parents
	Vacant stare; no eye contact
	Surveys environment but remains motionless
	Stiffens when approached as if expecting punishment of a physical nature

Emotional Abuse Emotional abuse is most difficult to define and diagnose because its scars are hidden and because both the victim and abuser might not recognize the behavior as dysfunctional. Variations in parenting styles and cultural norms compound the problem of defining and documenting the abuse. In most instances the child is called foul names, ridiculed, and made to feel stupid, hated, ugly, unlovable, or unwanted. The parent might blatantly reject the child and demonstrate a consistent lack of concern for the child's welfare. Sometimes, siblings or other family members are invited to join in the abuse, and the abused child becomes the family scapegoat.

Emotional abuse causes suffering and lasting effects on the development of the child's self-concept. Emotional abuse ultimately affects the child's future relationships with others, but because the scars are not obvious, its effects tend to be diagnosed only years after the event. The adult who was emotionally abused as a child has many unmet needs and is often filled with self-doubt and anger. Adults who were emotionally abused as children generally display the following characteristics (Milner and Wimberly, 1979):

1. Are unable to trust others
2. Exist in isolation
3. Are unable to choose a good mate
4. Are unsupportive of a spouse
5. Are highly dependent on others
6. Are inclined to feel low self-esteem and self-blame
7. Are likely to have difficulty in making decisions or taking risks
8. Are dysfunctional parents

Most physical abuse is accompanied by some degree of emotional abuse, but the reverse is not always true. Some children receive only verbal abuse, but the sequelae can have far-reaching effects, especially if these children repeat the pattern when they become parents. The manifested results of emotional abuse typically are speech disorders, developmental delays, and apathetic or hostile behaviors or depression. Sucking, biting, rocking, or enuresis are common behaviors; also common are sleep disorders, unusual fearfulness, and play disturbances. Behaviors might vacillate between extremes so that the child may be both aggressive and apathetic (Heindl, et al., 1979). The legal definition of emotional abuse varies. Some judges refuse to offer legal intervention without tangible evidence of emotional abuse, and most judges require proof that the child's growth and development have been affected. Legal intervention is often possible only if psychologic damage can be demonstrated. Health professionals and agencies responsible for protecting children need to develop consistent, accepted legal criteria defining emotional abuse. In the process nurses and other health professionals can take the following steps:

1. Contact the juvenile court and reach agreement on terms and guidelines
2. Document the abuse and its impact
3. Use expert witnesses such as psychiatrists and psychologists
4. Evaluate previous interventions and results
5. Educate the public to recognize and report emotional abuse
6. Act as an advocate for children and intervene before a child's behavior becomes the issue
7. Establish a network of community services to provide counseling to families with emotional abuse (Dean, 1979)

Sexual Abuse *Sexual abuse* is the exploitation of a child for the sexual gratification of an adult. Statistics reflecting its incidence are not available. Because secrecy and social taboos prevent cases from being reported and recorded, a "conspiracy of silence" often keeps victimized children from telling adults about the abuse, and the denial of some adults further contributes to the secrecy. Sexual abuse of children is essentially a crime of power in which an adult exploits the child's vulnerability. The behaviors are sexual, but the intent is domination rather than intimacy (Table 22-7).

Sexual offenses against children fall into two general categories: (1) nontouching offenses and (2) touching offenses. Nontouching offenses include verbal sexual stimulation, obscene telephone calls, exhibitionism, voyeurism, and violations of privacy in which the child watches or hears an act of sexual intercourse. Touching offenses include fondling; vaginal, oral, or anal intercourse or attempted intercourse; touching of the genitals; incest; prostitution; and rape (Gorline and Ray, 1979). Some forms of sexual exploitation use children to enhance adult sexual pleasures for profit. "Kiddie pornography," for instance, is a lucrative, illegal business.

Incest is a form of sexual abuse of a child by a family member. The adult might be a parent, stepparent, extended family member (such as a grandparent, aunt, uncle), or surrogate parent figure (such as a foster parent or common-law spouse). Incest always occurs within the family system, but the presence or absence of a blood relationship is far less important than the parental role of the adult (Sgroi, 1982). Most victims of incest are girls who are abused by older male relatives. Adults who commit incest often are family members in whom children have placed trust, and the power of the adult over the child contributes to the enforced secrecy. In some families the mother unconsciously sanctions the incest and even condones it as a means of providing the man a younger, more attractive sexual partner within the family (Lustig, et al., 1966; Kempe, 1978).

Incest can have serious, long-term consequences for the child. The child usually feels guilty for participating and is afraid of disrupting the family by revealing the incestuous relationship, which further contributes to the child's anxiety (Meiselman, 1978). Incest contributes to delinquency, substance abuse, prostitution, sexually transmitted disease, and

TABLE 22-7 Myths and Reality of Sexual Abuse

Myth	Reality
The child seduces the adult	Blaming the child is blaming the victim. A child needs nurturance and closeness, not sex. Sex with children is always initiated to satisfy adult needs
Nonviolent intercourse is not emotionally traumatic because the child receives pleasure (some professionals tend to foster this belief)	Sex with a child is a violation of trust. The child feels both physical and emotional discomfort. The issue for the adult is power
Sexual abuse of children is done by "dirty old men" or "sex fiends." Children need to be aware of "stranger danger"	Offenders come from all walks of life. They usually are known to their victims. Many offenders are "good with children" and occupy responsible positions
Incest is less traumatic to the child than sexual assault by a stranger	The child feels betrayed by the person who should be protective. Strong sense of ambivalence to both parents results. Child exhibits high level of guilt, depression, and anxiety
Incest is limited to one or two incidents	Most incestuous relations continue for 3–5 years
Children are telling "stories"	Adults wish to deny

unwanted pregnancies. Seventy-five percent of runaway children are said to be running from incest, and research suggests that 60%–90% of prostitutes claim to have been sexually abused as children (Densen-Gerber and Hutchinson, 1978).

Incest most often is a symptom of severe problems in marriage, family relationship, and life adjustment (Lieske, 1981). Life changes that typically lead to incest are that the parents stop having sex, one parent is absent from the home, the father loses his parents, the daughter begins puberty, one parent becomes an alcoholic, the family has a multigenerational pattern of sexual abuse, or the family is isolated (Justice and Justice, 1979). Some studies have shown that other family members might be aware of the incest but allow it to continue (Poznanski and Blos, 1975). If nonabusing adults in the family are passive, however, the child essentially is victimized twice, first by the abuser and then by any other adult who refuses to protect the child.

Children do not always have the sophisticated vocabulary to explain what is happening. They might give subtle clues in statements such as, "Mr. Smith sure has funny underwear" or "I don't like Uncle Joe anymore." They might attempt to disclose the abuse by statements such as, "Daddy said it was our special secret, but . . ." If the child attempts to tell and is not believed, the child is unlikely to try to reveal the abuse again (Table 22-8).

When a child does reveal sexual abuse, definitive steps must be taken to protect the child. The child might be in immediate danger, and in some instances the child's life is even endangered. Either the child or the offender must be removed from the situation. Disclosure puts the family in crisis, which might then add to the victim's guilt. The child then needs reassurance about not having caused the crisis. The victim needs a complete history and physical assessment, with gentle questioning about the abuse. Encouraging the child to discuss the abuse can aid in working out feelings. If the examination is hurried or insensitive, the child might resort to silence and refuse to cooperate. The timing of the assessment therefore is crucial in winning the child's cooperation.

Ideas for Informing Children About Sexual Abuse and Preventive Measures

1. A "good touch" is nice, like a hug, whereas a "bad touch" makes a person uncomfortable. Children need to be told, "Your body belongs to you; you can decide who touches it. Private areas are those covered by a bathing suit. If you are touched by someone and you don't like it, tell the person to stop and tell someone else about it."

2. Secrets and surprises are not the same. Secrets sometimes are not fair to keep. Surprises are fun; secrets are not fun if they make you feel funny or uncomfortable.

3. Strangers can be dangerous. Never go with someone you don't know who says anything like, "Your mother is ill and sent me to get you," or "Will you help me look for my lost puppy in the woods?"

4. Do not let others undress you, even if they promise to give you something such as candy or new clothes.

5. Do not listen when an older person tells you that they are going to help you grow up by showing you what big people do.

6. If you feel uncomfortable with someone, do not allow yourself to be left alone with that person.

TABLE 22-8 Signs of Sexual Abuse

Physical signs	Behavior signs
Laceration of labia, vagina, or perineum	Discussion of or implied involvement in sexual activity
Irritation, pain, or injury to genital area	Expression of severe emotional conflict at home with fear of intervention
Hematomas in genital area	Reluctance to participate in sports, showers, changing of clothes
Vaginal or penile discharge	Sitting carefully because of injuries
Dysuria	Unusual interest in genital area (eg, "French kissing" or fondling of genitals)
Sexually transmitted disease in young child (on eyes, mouth, anus, or genitals)	Sleep disturbances (eg, nightmares, enuresis, fear of sleeping alone)
Pregnancy	Reluctance to participate in activities with a particular person or at a particular place
Itching, bruises, or bleeding in genital area	Increased number of new fears
Unexplained vaginal or rectal bleeding	Fear of being alone
	Poor peer relations
	Change in performance at school
	Vague somatic complaints

The primary goals of treatment are to prevent further sexual abuse and to overcome any harmful effects. For example, disclosure might result in publicity, which is likely to result in ostracism of the family and condemnation and imprisonment of the offender. The family needs intensive counseling, both as individuals and as a group. Kempe (1978) noted that the mother must be willing to protect the children and both parents must admit that a problem exists and commit to solve it. A program that reports a high success rate includes individual counseling plus father–daughter, family, and group counseling (Giarretto, 1976).

The reporting of sexual abuse always involves Child Protective Services and law enforcement agencies. Because sexual abuse is a crime, an investigation is mandatory. In some states the parent who fails to protect the child might be tried as an accomplice to the crime. Police, teachers, nurses, and physicians also might be held liable for not reporting sexual abuse.

Adolescent Abuse The abuse of adolescents is a major social problem that is often caused by conflict and difficulty in parental regulation of adolescent behavior. Conflict between parents and adolescents tends to involve the refusal to cooperate or the deliberate violation of parental values and cultural traditions in areas such as personal appearance (dress, hairstyle, and so forth); choice of friends; curfews; school performance; choice of books, television programs, movies, or music; sexual activity; choice of boyfriend or girlfriend; alcohol or drugs; and responsibilities within the family.

Disciplining adolescents is often problematic to parents. Many parents of adolescents are confronting their own mid-life crisis just as their children challenge their authority; a time-out period might be needed by all. Parents who discipline with physical force need to learn other methods of control. Because adolescent abuse might be part of a pattern of abuse throughout childhood, the nurse identifies the discipline methods used when the child was younger (discipline is discussed in Chapter 13.)

Behavior patterns are sometimes the only indications of abuse in adolescents. Some abused adolescents are identified only when they run away from home, thereby drawing the attention of teachers or other families in the community (see Chapter 24). Once abuse is identified, however, intervention by the interdisciplinary team is initiated. Available community resources are assessed, and families and adolescents are directed to those services that are best equipped to meet their needs for counseling, activities, and support. Sometimes, the adolescent's perceiving one professional as an advocate can lead to some family resolution. Teachers, nurses, guidance counselors, physicians, or social workers all might be suited to respond to the needs of an abused adolescent, but all professionals need to understand that parent–child conflict might mean that the adolescent and the parents both are victims requiring intervention (Lourie, et al., 1979) (Table 22-9).

Legal Aspects of Child Abuse Child abuse is against the law in most industrialized countries, and the reporting of child abuse and neglect is governed by federal standards and regulations, state laws, and local policies and procedures. Most state statutes define child abuse and neglect and specify who must report, the form and content of the report, and to whom the report is sent. Because of the

TABLE 22-9 Myths and Realities of Adolescent Abuse

Myth	Reality
Adolescents provoke their parents into abuse	Adolescents can be difficult, but the problem lies with the parents' problems, frustrations, and inadequacies
Adolescents usually deserve punishment	Who ever deserves abuse?
Adolescents can protect themselves and fight back	The vast majority of adolescents do not strike back. They usually submit to the assault or run away. Adolescents might still be emotionally and psychologically dependent on their parents
Adolescents are less likely to have serious injuries	Adolescents in the throes of identity crises are vulnerable, especially to emotional abuse. Rejection has far-reaching sequelae as the adolescent internalizes the blame for problems

diversity in laws and state statutes, the nurse needs a copy of the applicable reporting form, laws, or position papers. Many states do not record sexual abuse as a separate offense. Some state statutes do not cover sexual abuse, and definitions of terms vary from state to state.

The purpose of all child abuse legislation is to protect children and prevent further abuse or maltreatment; the purpose is not to punish parents. Inherent in all laws is the assumption that the best way to help most children is to help their families. In essence, everyone is a mandated reporter. State laws mandate that suspicions of abuse and neglect be reported. No state requires the reporter to have proof of neglect or abuse, but incidents must be reported as soon as they are noticed. Sound nursing practice therefore means being honest with the family and reporting findings promptly. It is not wise to attempt to work with the family independently or to give family members a warning or second chance (McKittrick, 1981) because this might cause valuable time to be lost and contribute to additional risks. There are times when the second chance results in multiple severe injuries to or even the death of the child.

A report is not an accusation but is instead a request for an investigation. All persons who report suspected abuse or neglect are given immunity from criminal prosecution and civil liability if the report is made in good faith. Mandated reporters who fail to report can be fined as much as $1000. At issue, however, is the cost of failing to protect children. Because anonymous reports are not as valuable as those that are signed, a reporter should give name, title, and reason for the report (Table 22-10).

If a report is made to a social work supervisor or school principal, the nurse verifies that an official report was made and not lost. The nurse also can ask for an update on the progress of the case and will want to do so in anticipation of future dealings with the family or child. The report cannot, however, violate family confidentiality. The only information needed is whether the family is receiving assistance and attempting to learn alternative methods of coping with stress. Personal or family problems revealed during counseling are not shared without the family's permission.

Despite all the publicity and concern, many cases of child abuse or neglect still go unreported. The reasons for not reporting abuse or neglect include the following:

1. Professional denial because the child or parent looks well or the nurse has known the family for a long time and refuses to believe abuse and neglect could happen
2. Professional doubt about the nurse's role

TABLE 22-10 Components of Report of Child Abuse or Neglect

Aspect of report	Example
Reason for suspicion or assessment of incident	Child's comments; nature or extent of injury
Behaviors observed and by whom	Teacher's report; circumstances of discovery (eg, "child found alone by police in car")
Quality of parent–child relationship (if observed)	Any comforting measure noted or lacking (eg, "father speaks in angry tones")
What family has been told (to assist in follow-up for all team members)	Purpose of Children's Protective Services (if family is unaware of report, explain rationale)
What protection team should do first	Possible interventions (eg, assess home and risks to siblings; investigate and enlist possible community supports)

3. Fear of retribution, perhaps because of a history of violence in the family
4. Lack of "belief in the system," especially if the family was previously reported but with no subsequent improvement
5. Professional neglect or failure to understand that the risk to the child is increased when abuse or neglect is not reported
6. Conflict between professionals over the importance of reporting

Documentation In situations of child abuse and neglect, documentation of evidence is vital. Records provide the legal basis for intervening on behalf of the child. Nursing history and daily notes need to reflect accuracy, timeliness, and objectivity. The goal of documentation is to provide a written account of each visit or contact. If the nursing records become part of a court proceeding, they need to portray a family by specifying behaviors that indicate progress or failure in providing a safe, nurturing environment for the child. In some neglect cases much of the evidence is intangible and difficult to prove; therefore, input from many professionals is necessary to convince the court that a child is actually at risk for abuse or neglect. Evidence of risk might include the doctor's and nurse's notes on the child, the school nurse's report, and the social worker's impressions during a home visit regarding the child's physical appearance, interactions with parents, peers, and other adults, ability to respond to questions, and general development. Evidence of neglect might include developmental delays, substance abuse, poor medical care, poor school attendance, or lack of supervision. Careful documentaion and recorded evidence is essential when presenting a case to the judicial system.

At the onset, the nurse is careful to record all data. For instance, pertinent data include physical trauma or neglect, a factual description of the appearance and emotional state of the child and family, and any interactions observed between the child and family members. Behaviors are described in detail (Table 22-11). For example, if the child is said to be hyperactive and clumsy, the nurse might note that the child was unable to sit still for more than a few minutes or that the child knocked over objects in the examining room. The nurse also records any of the child's attempts to play or any of the parent's attempts to assist the child. Any explanations by either the parent or child also should be recorded. If the child is out of parental care, either because of hospitalization or foster care, the nurse records the number of parental visits, the child's response, and the parent's behavior and attitudes (Helberg, 1983).

In follow-up visits medical treatment is recorded with notes about whether appointments were kept. The nurse clearly documents the purpose of each visit by listing goals. Also included in the notes are the names of family members present at the visit and any evidence of new members living in the household. Cooperation in meeting goals should be documented as well. Although such documentation might affect a family's welfare status, concealing data may lead to a loss of credibility if the record ever goes to court. If the parent has been complying with any prescribed medical treatment for the child, this too is noted.

Investigations An investigation is a fact-finding process undertaken to determine whether child abuse or neglect has occurred. Each state has a designated agency that provides services on a 24-hour basis. Within 72 hours (and in most instances within 48 hours), services must be initiated. Agencies receiving abuse reports might include Child Pro-

TABLE 22-11 Common Behaviors at the Time of Injury

Parental behaviors	Child's behaviors
Hesitation to give information	Withdrawal, extreme passivity, evidence of fear
Illogical explanation	Does not cry when approached by a stranger
Inability to report the history of the injury	Little reaction to separation
Irritability or evasiveness when requestioned	Unwillingness to talk about the injury (although reactions vary)
Reluctance to look at or handle the child	Seeks to console the parent
Inability to comfort the child during painful or invasive procedures	Might express concern for siblings
Blaming the child for the injury	Little reaction to examination, including painful procedures
Little concern for the child's condition or course of treatment	Monotone answer to questions
Physical distance between the parent and child maintained	
Evidence of role reversal	
Leaving as soon as possible, with or without the child	
Infrequent visits to the hospitalized child	
Not keeping appointments with health care professionals	

tective Services, law enforcement agencies, juvenile courts, county health departments, and state or central registries.

Parents have the right to know that someone has reported suspected abuse or neglect, although exceptions might be made if the family has a history of violence. In such instances the child or children must be moved to safety before confronting the family. The child also needs to know what is happening. The child often is frightened by the process, especially if the child has revealed the abuse.

The child needs to expect to be questioned, have a medical examination, have pictures taken, and perhaps experience police involvement (in cases of assault). The child needs gentle explanations, a private place for unhurried interviewing, and someone to act as an advocate. Discussions about guilt should be ongoing because overt and covert repercussions might occur from parents, siblings, peers, extended family members, or others. The initial investigation focuses on the risks involved, the family dynamics, the nature of the incident or injury, and the duration of dysfunctional parenting. The investigation entails data collection by gathering evidence and interviewing parents and children separately. Verification of abuse or neglect might occur through an admission by the parent or offender or through medical or other factual evidence. Supportive services might be provided to the family if abuse or neglect is verified, and court intervention might be necessary if the child has serious injuries, the parent refuses to allow an investigation, the child is in immediate danger, or the risks do not diminish over time (Munro, 1984).

Under criminal codes, abusive parents might be charged with violating a criminal law. If a child recovers from the injury, the customary charge is assault and battery; if the child dies, prosecution is generally for manslaughter rather than intentional homicide. Although most experts agree that the parents are more in need of therapy than imprisonment, jail sentences are common. Most child abuse cases, however, are referred to juvenile court or family court rather than to criminal court. Juvenile and family courts have the power to declare abused or neglected children dependent on the court for proper care and protection. They also might, if necessary, remove children from their parents until the home problems can be resolved and the family safely reunited. In a few situations in which the parents disappear or cannot be located for long periods of time, the court terminates parental rights. This extreme measure is a last resort taken only after repeated instances of severe abuse or long-term abandonment and no response to rehabilitative efforts (Munro, 1984).

Long-Term Legal Involvement After the investigation, legal interventions might require a program for treatment, which may be voluntary or involuntary.

Voluntary treatment is possible if (1) the parents are willing to work on problems; (2) the reported injuries are not serious; (3) there is no continual history of abuse; and (4) the prognosis is favorable. In such cases services are slowly withdrawn when the home environment stabilizes and the danger to the child subsides. Involuntary treatment is likely, however, if (1) the parents are uncooperative; (2) the reported injuries are severe; (3) there is a history of past abuse; (4) the prognosis is poor; or (5) foster care or a termination of parental rights is indicated. Action then remains under the supervision of the court.

The first court hearing is an adjudicatory hearing, at which only one issue is to be resolved. The question at this hearing is whether the injuries or parental behavior can be classified as child abuse under state law. If child abuse cannot be verified, all legal proceedings cease, and the option of involuntary intervention is lost. If child abuse is verified, the court retains jurisdiction and schedules a second hearing.

The second hearing is a dispositional hearing, at which two issues are resolved: (1) what treatment will be mandated for the child and (2) who shall have custody of the child or children. Questions of custody usually present the court with four options, as follows:

1. Leave the child with the parent but under court supervision
2. Place the child with relatives under court supervision
3. Place the child in foster care
4. Permanently sever the parent–child relationship

Interventions for Health-Threatening Parenting

By the nature of their work, nurses in a variety of settings are involved in the identification, treatment, and prevention of child abuse and neglect. Nurses who see medical problems that suggest abuse or neglect or who see children and parents whose behavior indicates the potential for abuse or neglect are called on to collaborate with members of other disciplines in protecting children at risk and advocating care for both children and families. Because each family is part of a community system, nurses also need to be aware of community resources. Early detection of child abuse and neglect is essential to intervene and provide services to the child and family.

The American Nurses' Association Call for Action (American Nurses' Association, 1980) and the ANA Division on Maternal and Child Health Nursing Practice have passed resolutions concerning child abuse and neglect that call for action on the part of the Association, other organizations, and the government. The ANA has thus recognized the magnitude of the problem of child abuse and neglect, the need for early identification of high-risk families, and the use of multidisciplinary case finding, diagnostic assessment, long-term follow-up, and treatment. The resolutions call for nurses to participate in ensuring that funding of programs and services for high-risk families is adequate and that preparation for nurses in this area is provided in nursing curricula. Further resolutions state that family planning, counseling, and prenatal and postpartum services be available to all people in need and that the ANA supports the participation of nurses in decision making and planning stages of child abuse and neglect programs.

Prevention Because early recognition and reporting are crucial to preventing child abuse, primary prevention must be the ultimate goal of all who are involved with the well-being of children. Children who are abused or suspected of being abused must be protected until a thorough investigation can be conducted. Usually, the child is admitted to the hospital for more definitive assessment of the family dynamics. An emergency, court-ordered 96-hour hold might have to be obtained by the multidisciplinary team, thereby granting the institution temporary custody of the child. Safety of the child must be the primary objective of any treatment plan.

Primary Prevention For the family at risk, primary prevention efforts are aimed at influencing parents before dysfunction occurs. The emphasis is on wellness and identifying societal forces that affect parenting. For example, child-care courses taught to high school students to orient them to the roles and pressures of parenting are primary prevention. These classes give adolescents direct access to information about the management of time, money, and resources to provide for the basic needs of shelter, food, clothing, and family maintenance. In addition, they learn basic child-care skills and confront through discussion and role play some of the predictable childrearing challenges. This exposure to the realities of parenting and available sources for information about growth and development provides them with additional internal and external supports to cope with various life stressors.

Prenatal parent classes provide an excellent opportunity for nurses to not only help parents to prepare for the birth experience but also to anticipate and prepare for life as a parent. Listening carefully to parents' comments and observing their behaviors provide clues that help identify those individuals who might be at risk for dysfunctional parenting. The nurse spends extra time with the potential high-risk parent in order to foster trust and give support, whether it be providing additional information or listening and responding to the parent's concerns, referring the individual to social services for assistance with supplying basic needs, or referring the parent to counseling or family therapy for assistance with marital or interactional needs.

Some of the behaviors identified as prenatal indicators are overconcern about the infant's gender, minimal support from the family, attempts to deny or terminate the pregnancy, maternal sadness or depression, the feeling that this pregnancy is "the last straw" of many stressors, isolated life-style, or multiple, unrealistic fears (Kempe, 1976).

Assessment of parent–neonate interactions following delivery and during postpartum hospitalization provides important information concerning the attachment process and the potential for dysfunction. (See Chapter 7 for a discussion of attachment.) Indicators that should alert the nurse to perform a more thorough assessment and validate suspicions include lack of interest in the neonate, extreme awkwardness holding the neonate (such as the parent uses stiff, outstretched arms or the neonate's head and neck are inadequately supported), few if any attempts to make eye contact, disappointment about the gender or appearance of the neonate, an ill or deformed neonate, enforced separation of the neonate and parent, minimal family support for the parent, little home preparation for the neonate's arrival, disgust expressed at changing diapers, or resentment about the time demands for feedings (Kempe, 1976). The use of assessment tools enables the nurse to focus observations, compare them with a reliable standard, and formulate a nursing diagnosis to guide plans for intervention. Tools such as the Neonatal Perception Inventory and Degree of Bother Index are discussed in Chapter 17, and the Brazelton Neonatal Behavior Assessment Scale and Adaptive–Maladaptive Parenting Behavior Guide are discussed in Chapter 16. A helpful guideline also has been adapted from a tool developed by Funke and Irby (1978) to assess the risk factor potential in relation to parenting ability. The nurse gathers information about parental attitudes and behaviors in 13 areas and rates them on a descriptive scale from 1 to 4 (Fig. 22-2). Adaptive characteristics are rated as 4, and maladaptive characteristics are rated as 1. Behavior or attitude rated as 1 in a single area is not predictive of later problems; however, when there are several ratings in the 1 category, their significance as indicators of dysfunctional parenting increases. Early identification of potential problems and referral to community resources, including the public health nurse or visiting nurse, are primary prevention.

Parenting concerns are ongoing. The nurse who includes a family assessment update (see Chapter 17) with every well-child visit is more likely to note characteristics that have the potential to become a risk factor and plan interventions to prevent such a potential from becoming reality. For example, one mother questioned when to begin toilet training her 2-year-old. Further questioning revealed that the mother wanted the child to be toilet trained because an elderly parent had recently moved in with the family and the mother was busy caring for two dependent individuals. The nurse discussed with the mother the normal responses young children have when parental attention has to be shared, that regression and increased demands for affection are common. The nurse also empathized with the mother's situation and energy-draining responsibilities. Together, they planned to delay the toilet training and wait until the child and mother were both more ready and to arrange time out for the mother several times a week. Being sensitive to cues that parents provide and following up on them immediately enables the nurse to institute primary prevention.

Anticipatory guidance (see Chapter 21) is another method the nurse employs to provide primary prevention. Time

	1	2	3	4
Pregnancy planning	Unplanned and did not want to be pregnant	Unplanned	Not really planned but wanted	Wanted and planned
Support systems	No friends or relatives nearby or poor relationship with parents	New in town, few friends or no phone	Relatives far away, has friends	Relatives nearby, has many friends
Adjustment to infant	Not important to change; no adjustment	Hasn't thought about changes	Must wait and see what changes needed	Made plans for rest, safety, child's room, babysitters
Marital status	Single or under 18	Has boyfriend or hopes infant will improve marriage	Happily married up to $1\frac{1}{2}$ years	Happily married over $1\frac{1}{2}$ years
Delivery style	Wanted to be asleep	Father does not want to participate	Wanted to be awake but could not be	Father present at birth
Infant's name	Unusual name or delay in naming	Name chosen for one sex only	Chose name; changed mind	Chose names ahead of time
Feeding	Finds breast-feeding distasteful/ too anxious to breast-feed successfully	Chose bottle-feeding	Undecided—will try breast-feeding	Breast-feeding successfully
Living arrangements	Unsure of living arrangements after discharge	Living with friend(s)	Living with parents	Has own home or apartment
Eye-to-eye contact	Never occurs	Only occurs one-third of time together	Occurs 35%–50% of time	Occurs 50%–100% of time
Acceptance	Expresses many frustrations—resentful	Occasional frustrations, disappointments with infant	Neither accepts nor rejects	Pleased and concerned about infant's progress
Physical closeness	Holds infant away from body or does not hold	Distorts or misses infant's cues	Somewhat aware of infant's needs	Notices and interprets infant's cues most of time
Touching	No affection, rough or little touching	Does necessary handling only	A little caressing of infant	Caresses and plays with infant
Vocalizing/ talking	Rude or demanding words to infant	Does not vocalize	Little vocalizing	Talks with inflection, coos

Figure 22-2 Parenting ability risk quotient. Many parenting behaviors and circumstances that correspond to the criteria in the first two columns indicate a need for further assessment and possible referral. (Adapted from Funke J, Irby M: An instrument to assess the quality of maternal behavior. *J Gynecol Nurs* 1978; p. 19–22.)

spent in helping parents to understand the unique qualities of their child and their role as parents in nurturing and protecting that childs is primary prevention.

Primary prevention also includes advocating changes that will benefit children. As previously noted, what happens within the family is influenced by the prevailing cultural norm. Society's general acceptance of and even finding humor in violence is appalling and needs to be decreased. Children are exposed to violence as a way of winning through many forms of media such as cartoons, movies, television, comic books, and newspapers. Many of the video games enjoyed by children involve capturing and consuming the opponent, conveying the subliminal acceptance of violence. Supporting organizations that lobby for less violence and more programming directed toward children's interests is consumer advocacy and a primary prevention strategy.

Gil (1974) stated that primary prevention includes a reaffirmation of the rights of children; elimination of poverty, isolation, and alienation; and a rejection of the use of force. These changes would indirectly influence and enhance psychologic well-being, thus fostering improved parent–child interactions throughout society. Despite skepticism, public and professional resources are increasingly invested in such preventive programs. By being aware of the community resources and social and environmental conditions that affect parents, the nurse is able to advocate needed changes. Advocating changes that influence parents and children is an important role for the nurse. School changes might include the introduction of parenting in the curriculum, whereas changes in the health care system might involve introducing birthing practices that facilitate parent–infant bonding. By involving lay groups and civic leaders, public awareness and resources for primary prevention will increase.

Secondary Prevention Secondary prevention for families at risk consists of services for individuals considered to be at risk for dysfunctional parenting. This type of prevention is more problem focused and identifies particular stressors. Because adolescent parents usually face multiple stressors, adolescent support groups are one example of secondary prevention. With support, the adolescent learns child-care skills and positive interactive behaviors. In secondary prevention nurses must readily identify those families most at risk for dysfunction because of their current practices, past life experiences, and societal problems. The nurse who knows the indicators that signal risks and the community services available to these families at risk can recommend support services to relieve stress (Heindl, et al., 1979).

Resources for secondary prevention include telephone "hotlines" for specific needs, whether it is a personal call for help when a parent feels about to lose control or a plea for funds to obtain the basic necessities of food or fuel; available, low-cost health care, including services for mental health; emergency and maintenance homemaker or child-care services; self-help groups; day-care programs; counseling and family or individual therapy programs; job retraining programs; welfare assistance; and before- and after-school child-care programs. The nurse's role varies according to education and experience. "Essentially, nursing interventions are focused at gaining trust, role modeling, teaching problem solving and limit setting, attending to the parent, and facilitating the development of extra family resources" (Humphreys, 1984; p. 302).

Before working with dysfunctional families, many nurses have to identify their own feelings about the family's practices. The culture, life-style, and experiences of the nurse all contribute to personal beliefs and values, and the nurse therefore takes into account the culture, ethnic group, values, and beliefs of the family. (For a discussion of values clarification, see Chapter 3.) Although the nurse's values might conflict with the family's, the nurse's goal is to facilitate open, honest sharing.

Establishing mutually agreed-on goals is mandatory at the start of any working relationship. Goals must be clear and concise, citing specific outcomes and realistic deadlines. The nurse discusses specific maladaptive behaviors targeted for change or elimination with the parents. By agreeing to these goals, the parent is essentially agreeing to a contract. The criteria for evaluation also will aid the family in knowing what changes are expected. Family motivation and cooperation are the key factors in changing a dysfunctional family into a thriving family. An early indicator of a desire to alter behavior might be the keeping of appointments; later indicators include a willingness to take some personal responsibility for the dysfunction and not project blame onto others. The parent who can identify a problem and seek help is usually the one who will achieve success in behavior changes.

Tertiary Prevention Tertiary prevention is offered to families after dysfunctional parenting has occurred. Tertiary prevention is essentially treatment of the child and family following the damage of abuse or neglect; however, it is preventive in that it seeks to stop future dysfunctional behaviors (Coolsen, 1980). Tertiary prevention for dysfunctional parenting should begin as soon as the dysfunction has been identified. The goal is to prevent further trauma by having the parents change their childrearing habits. Efforts to involve the family in rehabilitation can be the first step in breaking the bonds of isolation.

The first concern always is the safety of the child, but providing for the child's safety is often a dilemma. Temporary removal of the child from an unsafe home might be the beginning of a series of unsatisfactory foster home or state institution placements. Interventions therefore should be matched carefully to goals that reflect possible outcomes (Table 22-12). Christensen, Schommer, and Velasquez (1984) found that the incidence of abuse, neglect, and out-of-home placement for children at risk can be reduced through multidisciplinary prevention strategies.

A recorded history of dysfunctional behaviors and resistance to change present especially challenging situations to the nurse. Sometimes, pointing out past patterns of behavior can assist the parent to realize the need for change. Many parents report that making a contract to change specific behaviors is the first time anyone ever spelled out expectations. To provide ongoing evaluation, the nurse needs to see the family at regular intervals. Specific evidence of progress or failure is identified during these evaluative sessions. Informing the parents of the consequences of failure to meet expectations and deadlines is a delicate and crucial issue for the nurse because most nurses find it difficult to discuss removing children from the family. Parents must know, however, that children's safety and security are of primary importance. The parents' failure to meet goals indicates a need for more intervention; otherwise, trust in the system would be compromised because the nurse also would be breaking the contract.

With a parent who has a history of inflicting trauma in response to personal stress, the expected behaviors need to be defined immediately. Trauma must stop; therefore,

TABLE 22-12 Evaluation of Interventions to Alter Dysfunctional Parenting

Goals for parental behavior	Evaluation
Identifies problems in the family system	Parent develops insight into the emotional climate of the family
Identifies factors that contribute to potential or actual abusive behaviors	
Demonstrates ability to meet own needs	
Finds positive alternatives to present coping strategies by first identifying external stressors	
Describes feelings toward self and children	
Demonstrates alternative coping strategies in stressful situations	
Demonstrates realistic expectations of children by identifying age-appropriate behaviors	Parent improves parenting skills
Identifies methods of discipline	
Demonstrates some consistency and appropriate use of discipline	
Identifies a person or agency to contact in a crisis	
Provides a safe environment for children by identifying an adequate caregiver during parental absence, identifying and correcting environmental hazards, providing ongoing health care for children	
Identifies family members and friends available for support	Parent establishes and uses a positive support system
Indicates frequency of visits to family and friends	
Identifies ways in which family, friends, community supports (church, school, etc) can be helpful	
Identifies ways in which health care system can be helpful	
Demonstrates appropriate use of health care system and other agencies by keeping appointments	
Earns income above the poverty level or receives and manages public assistance optimally (eg, food stamps used to buy food that is then allocated appropriately among family members)	Parent has adequate income to maintain family
Manages budget to purchase appropriate low-cost clothing for family members	
Provides adequate housing that meets minimal requirements (heat, electricity, cooking and refrigeration facilities, some furnishings)	
Remains at same residence without frequent moves	

SOURCE: Adapted from Christensen ML, Schommer BL, Velasquez J: An interdisciplinary approach to preventing child abuse. Copyright © 1984 American Journal of Nursing Company. Reproduced with permission from *Matern/Child Nurs* (March/April); 84(2).

the nurse might first suggest alternative methods of coping. In two-parent families both parents might need to be seen so that the nurse can assess their relationship with each other and their expectations of their children (Kempe and Kempe, 1978). Destructive behaviors that can harm the child or others must be eliminated. Assessing a parent's capacity for change is a multidisciplinary effort, and an essential assessment criterion is parental commitment. Other criteria are parent–child interactions, willingness to learn, and specific nurturing behaviors (see Chapters 16 and 17). Correcting knowledge deficits is most successful if the family is willing to participate in planning care. For instance, the plan might involve role modeling of professionals, or it might involve patiently teaching parents about the long-range ramifications of neglect for normal growth and development. Families should not, however, feel urged but instead should feel worthy of assistance.

Clients also learn from observing and imitating the behavior, values, and attitudes of those they view as people of influence and prestige. The nurse demonstrates nurturing behaviors that also endorse the family's cultural or ethnic beliefs. In this way nurses serve as role models in providing health teaching and anticipatory guidance (see Chapter 21). The nurse's behavior toward children is thus a nonthreatening teaching method that allows parents to learn through imitation. In addition, nurses can demonstrate correct child-care techniques and provide practice sessions to reinforce learning and foster the parent's readiness to relax and enjoy the time spent with a child. For many clients, this is the first such positive experience.

Because family dynamics are so significant in parenting, nurses from emergency rooms, industrial health settings, hospital inpatient units, ambulatory care clinics, mental health clinics, schools, and community agencies are all vital to the prevention and treatment of family dysfunction. The goal is to intervene prior to the need for tertiary level prevention. The nurse who is alert to subtle indicators can initiate interventions at the primary or secondary level. Indicators might include observing younger children requesting assistance from an older sibling rather than their parent during a clinic visit or an older child offering conciliatory statements to other adults. For example, one 10-year-old quickly commented, "That's okay, I have problems with art too" when the nurse made a mistake drawing a stick figure.

Because educators have daily contact with children, they also play a major role in preventing child abuse and neglect. Next to the family, the school is the system that has the most influence on a child's life. Nurses who work in school settings play a key role in assisting teachers in identifying children whose behavior indicates problems or whose families are incapable of nurturance. The collaboration of educators is important. Teachers can listen for messages of neglect and abuse from both direct and indirect comments of children and from their behaviors in the classroom (Howell, 1977). Nurses can contribute further by educating teachers through workshops and seminars on issues relating to parenting, divorce, child care, and discipline.

Prevention of sexual abuse should begin in early childhood. Parents and teachers can help by defining acceptable adult behavior and teaching young children what to do if they are not comfortable with adult actions.

Community Supports Intervention at all levels is more effective when multiple resources are available and the family can help to choose which resources to use. Most families need to draw on a variety of resources to break the cycle of a dysfunctional life-style. Nurses and other health professionals therefore need to be cognizant of the services available within their community. They need to help clients avail themselves of those programs most geared to their needs and then coordinate the program goals and client's progress. The goals and philosophy of community outreach programs must be clearly defined for all concerned. Presenting prevention services positively increases the likelihood that they will be used. For example, "positive parenting" is a better term than "prevention of child abuse and neglect," which tends to stigmatize the client. Some parents are reluctant to participate in any program, no matter how appropriate for them, that uses the word "abuse."

Community Services Commonly Needed by Families Demonstrating Health-Threatening Parenting

- Public housing
- Welfare
- Mental health centers
- Emergency shelters
- Subsidized child care
- Homemaker services
- WIC program
- Food stamps
- Free medical or dental care
- Family and/or marital counseling
- Vocational rehabiliation, employment services
- Foster care
- Parents Anonymous
- Fuel assistance agencies
- Child guidance centers
- Child development clinics
- Housing authorities
- Alcoholics Anonymous, Al-Anon, Ala-Teen, Ala-Tot
- Visiting Nurse Association
- Juvenile authorities
- DCYS (Division of Child and Youth Services)
- Ambulatory care settings
- Occupational health settings
- Religious-affiliated groups

Child-Care Centers Child-care centers have been established by many communities in an effort to assist families. These centers provide child care for parents who need support services and time-out periods from their children. The philosophy of each center varies, but most centers encourage parents to use their respite time to attend to some of their own needs, thereby improving the quality of their relationships with their children. Some centers encourage or require parents to spend some portion of their time at the center learning child-care skills and seeing positive interaction with children. Participation is usually voluntary, although courts occasionally direct a parent to use these services. Most centers charge a minimal fee based on a sliding scale. Some centers even provide transportation services both to and from the center.

Most child-care centers provide for children of all ages and give special attention to children exhibiting dysfunctional behaviors as a result of inadequate parenting. Children usually are assigned to a child-care worker who supplies surrogate parenting and encourages children to seek attention for positive rather than negative behaviors. Children who are old enough are encouraged to perform such self-care tasks as dressing, feeding, and toileting, and their accomplishments are identified and reinforced. Children also might learn basic hygiene such as handwashing and the proper use of tissues as well as sound nutritional practices. Children with aggressive tendencies are encouraged to work out their aggression on suitable toys rather than on people, and they are educated in principles of sharing and cooperation.

Many centers conduct weekly group meetings for parents to discuss common problems and concerns. For many, the group fosters an identity as a parent and stresses the importance of adequate child care. The sharing and collaboration elevates self-esteem and identifies feelings that might have been denied or repressed. Assisting another parent to cope with a problem that has been successfully resolved is a growth-producing experience and, for some parents, is a first step out of isolation.

As with all support services, evaluation of progress and behaviors is ongoing. Goals need frequent confirmation and reestablishment. An important aspect of evaluation is identifying behaviors that are positive signs of progress.

Lifeline to Avoid Isolation Isolation and withdrawal, which prevent access to role models for child care, also foster lack of trust. For isolated families, an intervention program therefore needs to provide frequent home visits to foster parental maturity and encourage socialization. For many parents, such visits are the first attempts to remove the barrier of isolation.

Some communities have established "friendly visitor" programs to improve the health and quality of family life. From data identifying family strengths and weaknesses, families with the potential for change and growth are identified, and a care plan is devised. The goals vary depending on the specific needs of each family, but the overall goal is to improve family dynamics so that all members move toward wellness. Some specific areas of focus are (1) maintenance of a stable home environment; (2) fostering feelings of adequacy as parents; (3) development of parenting skills; (4) acquisition of effective ways to manage stress; (5) identifying ways of increasing self-esteem and self-acceptance; and (6) reducing social isolation.

The visitor or family friend should be a culturally sensitive individual with experience in parenting and a willingness to serve as a role model. Parenting behaviors are best demonstrated at home so that reinforcement occurs where the parent most needs it. The visitor must, however, be accepted by the family and use a slow, warm approach to initiate the program. Time with individual family members is an opportunity to provide positive feedback for any nurturing behaviors or progress. Parents need to be involved in the physical care of their children, but they also need time for their own enjoyment and play. Focusing on the importance of the parent to the child helps to build parental self-esteem.

To foster parental maturity, the visitor teaches problem-solving techniques and guides parents in solving immediate problems while pointing out alternatives and consequences. Once the parent and visitor have established a trusting relationship, efforts need to be directed at expanding a social network for the family. For some parents, finding a single friend is monumental progress, whereas others can safely enter a group and become involved in school or community projects.

Foster Grandparents Grandparents play a special role in families. They usually have had years of successful living and bring warmth, love, and a sense of continuity to a family. Foster grandparents aim to provide such a role to children and families who have been fragmented or troubled. They serve to nurture and strengthen the emotional well-being of family members at risk. In return, many foster grandparents report a sense of fulfillment and satisfaction and an elevation in their own emotional well-being.

Some foster grandparents are volunteers, whereas others are paid a minimum wage to augment their Social Security income. All are retired and usually donate time far in excess of the required hours. Many report an improvement in their physical health once they feel needed and have a defined purpose in living. Some are isolated from their own families and welcome the chance to interact socially with a new family or child. Foster grandparent programs are connected to social service agencies, community mental health groups, and in many pediatric institutions, especially those whose clients are far from home.

Children in institutions for long periods (such as in burn centers or institutions for the mentally retarded) often respond favorably to foster grandparents. Foster grandfathers play an especially important role in families with an absent father. For many children, a foster grandfather is their first interaction with a male figure. Children from ethnic minorities often respond more favorably to a foster grandparent from the same ethnic background.

Parent Aides Parent aides visit selected homes several times a week, providing transportation and social experiences for either parent of a dysfunctional family. As paraprofessionals, parent aides are supervised by the health team and primarily provide long-term nurturing to parents rather than children, although children ultimately benefit. Parent aides are parents themselves who have highly successful relationships and current support systems in their own lives. Proper selection and training are crucial to any parent aide program, and past family life experiences and parenting successes are the criteria for selecting parent aides. Many have experienced personal difficulties themselves; therefore, their problem-solving abilities and coping strategies are useful in working with troubled families. Experience has shown that parent aides with school-age children are most effective because dysfunctional parents can view them as peers or friends and accept nurturing from them (Hollen, Carroll, and Carpenter, 1980).

A parent aide's experiences are extremely useful with most neglectful and abusive families because they provide the supportive relationship that the parent needs. A parent aide might seem much less threatening to a family than many health professionals, and they frequently assist parents to improve their coping abilities and strengthen their relationships with their children. In times of crises parent aides have been instrumental in linking parents to such community resources as volunteer foster care and nursery school placement. In some instances the decision to relinquish children voluntarily for adoption was facilitated by a parent aide, who helped the parent to consider this option in an uncritical atmosphere (Ballard, 1975).

Parent aide involvement is contraindicated when the parent is psychotic, sociopathic, extremely violent, addicted, or so disturbed as to overwhelm the aide. Because of their lay status, parent aides have potential limitations, including an overidentification with the parent, taking sides in a marital conflict, inability to identify medical or psychologic problems with the children, and keeping the parent overdependent for personal gratification. Regular supportive consultation and progress reviews with the multidisciplinary team usually can prevent these problems.

The parent aide begins working with a family in consultation with a social worker, nurse, and psychiatrist. The parent aide also is integrated into the multidisciplinary team by attending group meetings, listening to audiovisual tapes and discussions about child abuse in specific families, and meeting with team members and staff. All the assigned families are assessed by a professional, usually a social worker, who generally provides ongoing consultation and is available by phone if needed. Parent aides usually are employed up to 20 hours per week, the maximum amount of time a person generally can give to such emotionally draining relationships. Involvement between the parent and parent aide often lasts between 18 months and 2 years and is followed by a gradual diminishing of contact, although the relationship never formally ends. Ideally, the relationship matures to one of mutual friendship, with the parent aide being available to the family if the need arises.

Multidisciplinary Management Because many complex factors must be assessed in evaluating suspected or known cases of child abuse or neglect, no single professional group can best render services to a child or family. A multidisciplinary team approach is therefore best to aid in diagnosis, planning, and interventions. Teams can pool expertise from various fields and provide integrated planning and delivery of services. A multidisciplinary team might be composed of a mental health worker, lawyer, nurse, social worker, police officer, physician, teacher, juvenile division worker, and hospital or ancillary personnel. Ancillary personnel might include receptionists, drivers, custodians, secretaries, nutritionists, homemakers, or child-care workers. Some are volunteers who might or might not have expertise and training. Most personnel working with abusive or neglectful families need orientation concerning typical behaviors that suggest mistrust of the system, lack of self-esteem, or hostility and anger.

Ancillary personnel can aid professionals in convincing dysfunctional families that change is worthwhile and that they are worth the team's efforts. Ancillary personnel also might provide additional insight and collaboration in a decision-making process. Because each team member brings a different range of experiences and knowledge of dysfunctional families and successful treatment, each is called on to define needs and, if necessary, find legal grounds for intervention. Team involvement offers planning coordination and a way to offset the frustration that professionals feel when nothing helpful can be done (Table 22-13).

Many American communities have formed citizen councils on child abuse that involve experts from many disciplines. Professionals might include pediatricians, nurses, health visitors, social workers, police, lawyers, and psychologists. Other community residents might be involved as well (Kempe and Kempe, 1978). The system of resources varies from state to state but usually includes family support services such as Parents Anonymous and similar self-help groups, child-care and family shelter programs, parent aides and homemaker programs, and agency supports such as case consultation teams, child welfare practice forums, clinical seminars, and individual case consultations. Because Child Protective Services often are equipped only to handle crisis management, parent aides and others might be needed. Because of their understanding of planned intervention and health care delivery, nurses are essential to this process.

Five hours per month (or 60 hours per year) for each family is a minimally acceptable amount of time, and as much as 50 hours per month might be needed in some cases (Kempe and Kempe, 1978). The three distinct phases in the management of child abuse are (1) crisis management, which includes diagnosing the family situation and developing a long-term treatment plan for each family member; (2) implementing the plan; and (3) evaluating the results.

Identifying Dysfunctional Families In all cases of suspected abuse or neglect, the nurse needs to ask the child and family members present the following questions:

1. How did the accident (or incident) happen?
2. When did the accident happen?
3. Where were the child and other family members at the time?
4. Who was caring for the child at the time?
5. Who saw the accident?
6. What did the child do after the accident?
7. What measures were taken by the parent?

After recording answers to these questions, the nurse proceeds with the physical assessment, noting the location, color, and characteristics of all cutaneous lesions. Photographs might be needed as legal evidence, and orthopedic, surgical, ophthalmologic, and gynecologic examinations also might be needed depending on the type of injuries.

Skeletal radiographs should be obtained for all children under 5 years of age who are suspected of having been

TABLE 22-13 Advantages and Disadvantages of Multidisciplinary Management

Advantages	Disadvantages
Information sharing—efficiency; larger data base; shared experiences	Investment in time
Shared responsibility in decision making	Need to counteract "territoriality" to share information
Support for feelings and frustrations of team members (might help to counteract "burnout")	Fewer opportunities for peer review
Role clarification—shared roles among disciplines; respect for others enhanced; opportunities for students and practicing professionals to learn skills	Cost of meeting time and time spent in group dynamics
Family benefits—consistent implementation of plan; ongoing evaluation; family can choose with whom to work most closely among the team members	Family disadvantages—too many points of view for some families; possible concerns about confidentiality
	Possibility of manipulation by family

abused or neglected to identify any treated or untreated fractures. If the child has unexplained bruising, tests for blood dyscrasias are needed (see Chapter 36). In cases of sexual abuse, evidence for legal proceedings must be gathered. This includes cultures for gonorrhea and other sexually transmitted diseases, microscopic examination for blood and sperm, pregnancy testing, and clothing examination for semen, blood, or pubic hairs. To have data the courts will accept, strict procedures must be followed in collecting evidence and specimens.

The most important determination to make is the risk of reinjury to the victim or injury to other children in the household. Assessment of family functioning, coping strategies, and current state of crisis provides valuable data for such determination. Sometimes, even when the injuries are not severe, hospitalization or foster home placement is necessary. Protection of the child (or children) is always the priority.

An interview is needed with parents or extended family members. Interviewing adult family members separately allows the interviewer to compare the facts and check the validity of the data. Determining who caused the injury might not be critical because the passivity of the other parent often contributes equally to the dynamics (Helfer, 1976). In cases of severe injuries, however, police need to identify the guilty person to intervene legally.

The gathering of data is sometimes best accomplished over the course of several interviews. If the child is hospitalized, the hospitalization can be used as a "cooling off" time, during which the child is protected from further injury and the parent is relieved from the responsibilities of care. A home visit also might be necessary in gathering data about family structure and concurrent environmental stressors.

In assessing neglected or abused children and their families, the nurse considers the long-term ramifications of neglect and their possible effects on family cooperation in meeting goals. Some considerations in planning interventions are the following:

1. The parents' emotional ability to accept services
2. Communication patterns within the family
3. The range and availability of services
4. The family's use of services
5. Supportive counseling for all family members
6. Children's growth and developmental patterns
7. The parents' attempts to diminish isolation
8. The parents' responses to expectations to change behaviors
9. The quality of nurturance within the family
10. Family dynamics and other risk factors such as substance abuse or violence
11. Environmental stressors such as inadequate housing, hygiene, or nutrition

If parents lack motivation, their apathy is assessed and monitored carefully, with special attention to specific behaviors and their duration. Dysfunctional behaviors are cited, documented, and addressed individually. The ego strength of each parent is an important criterion in predicting success for any plan of care because parents who feel self-confident about the prospects for change are more likely to cooperate with the multidisciplinary team.

Usually, the various disciplines and agencies represented on a team can provide data about the child and family, support, expertise, and knowledge of various community resources. Multiple assessments of the family help to determine the likelihood of parental capacity for change and the likely length of time that the family will need services.

Each team needs a coordinator, a designated professional who is responsible for planning therapy, setting deadlines, and arranging team meetings. Because some families are mobile, much communication is required among social service agencies so that they are not lost to therapy. The coordinator therefore might invest a significant amount of time in charting the family's progress.

Supporting Dysfunctional Parents Providing parental supports to marginally functioning parents is preferable to

(Text continues on p. 738)

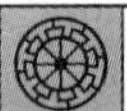

NURSING CARE GUIDE The Family and Child Following Abuse

Nursing diagnosis	Interventions	Evaluation
1. Ineffective parental coping related to stress	Discuss parent's usual pattern of coping with stress and assess whether parent shows a tendency to use force, power, or violence as a way to overcome frustration or settle arguments Discuss parent's perception of personal ability to control emotions such as anger; be alert for comments that indicate exceptions (eg, "I usually act responsibly but . . . ," "Sometimes I get so mad I lose it," or "I cannot tolerate being embarrassed publicly, otherwise I manage") Have parent explain what is meant by vague statements indicating exceptions (eg, "What happens when you 'lose it'?") Encourage parent to describe events, behaviors, or situations that present coping difficulties Have parent list stressors; as necessary, provide examples or verify whether some areas are or are not perceived as stressors (eg, employment, housing, fatigue, illness, irritability of child) Discuss with parent ways to facilitate coping (eg, talking oneself down; counting to 100; using time out for the child, self, or both; planning ahead to avoid certain events; obtaining additional resources for basic necessities) Have parent identify a plan for coping with stress that seems most compatible to personality; contract with parent to have parent practice it for 1 week and then return to discuss the results Discuss information with multidisciplinary team so that appropriate resources can be provided to alleviate stress	Parent demonstrates appropriate use of resources when stressed Parent copes adaptively to stress, using new behaviors that enhance personal and family growth
2. Alteration in parenting related to injury inflicted on the child	Help parent to identify factors leading to and resulting in the child's injury Attempt to establish whether such factors are chronic or acute Examine the child for evidence of bruises, healed fractures, burn sites, or scars Observe carefully the child's response to the parent, determining whether there is obvious fear or anxiety; docu-	Parent demonstrates positive parent–child interaction and is able to employ effective discipline without anger or violence

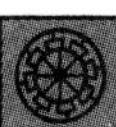

NURSING CARE GUIDE The Family and Child Following Abuse (continued)

Nursing diagnosis	Interventions	Evaluation
	ment all objective behaviors and responses, being conscious to omit personally subjective analyses Observe parent–child interaction; document behaviors such as noncommunication, oversolicitousness, further injury, or use of force Provide age–appropriate play for the child and note the child's use of materials; have available a variety of media, including clay, pencils, crayons, paper, a doll family, blocks, toy cars and trucks, and a dollhouse (see Chapter 28) Express interest and listen as the child talks about the pictures or plays with the toys; if beneficial, refer the child to a play therapist for a more extensive expression and an opportunity to work through feelings of anger, guilt, or betrayal	
3. Parental knowledge deficit regarding the normal process of growth and development of children	Determine what the parent knows about growth and development and temperamental differences, as well as what the parent's expectations are for the child's behavior Review the aspects of growth and development that normally occur, especially those resulting in changes in mobility, learning, and autonomy Have the parent discuss personal perceptions of the child's behavior and note any misconceptions; listen for phrases that indicate a loss of power or violation of expectations (eg, "I thought all babies were cuddly, but mine wants freedom," "She was so cute as an infant, but now she is a terror," or "He does that because he does not like me") Acknowledge the parent's frustration concerning the quantity and rapidity of changes that occur as the child develops Clarify the aspects of the child's behavior that the parent finds difficult; provide anticipatory guidance and model appropriate interactions (see Chapter 21) Discuss and demonstrate for the parent ways to promote development	Parent has a realistic perception of the child's abilities Parent's expectations of the child's skills and behaviors are age appropriate

continued on next page

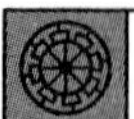

NURSING CARE GUIDE The Family and Child Following Abuse (continued)

Nursing diagnosis	Interventions	Evaluation
	through stimulation and realistic expectations Refer the parent to appropriate resources for additional information; if beneficial, review the age-related standard assessment form with the parent as a guide for revising expectations	
4. Parental knowledge deficit related to inexperience and inadequate role models for learning parenting skills	Observe parenting behaviors, noting whether the parent talks to the child and the tone of voice used, whether parent answers questions addressed to an older child, how the infant is held (eg, closely, stiffly, supported adequately or not), amount of eye contact sought and maintained, and parental response to cues and bids for attention Discuss with the parent the difficulty and demands of being a parent; note any comments that indicate disappointment or a deficit in personal need fulfillment Help the parent to compare expectations concerning parenting before the child's birth with the realities of parenting since that time Discuss the parent's experiences as a child and how parenting was role-modeled during childhood Provide guidance for the parent in identifying parenting behaviors to emulate, especially if the parent's childhood experience includes abuse Discuss the influence of the parent's culture together with personal ideas or philosophy about discipline and its purpose, form, and desired results (see Chapter 13) Provide anticipatory guidance for areas of parenting concern (eg, toilet training, self-feeding, tantrums, manipulative behaviors such as screaming in public, or threatening to run away) (see Chapter 21) Discuss alternative ways of disciplining that do not involve physical measures Discuss the parent's needs, noting a need for "parenting the parent" or befriending the parent temporarily Help the parent to express needs and discuss more appropriate ways of	Parent responds appropriately to the child's cues for attention or signals of distress Parent describes a realistic perspective of the positive and negative experiences of parenting

NURSING CARE GUIDE The Family and Child Following Abuse (continued)

Nursing diagnosis	Interventions	Evaluation
	meeting them (other than through the child) Work with health team members to find ways to assist the parent in meeting personal needs	
5. Disturbance in parent's self-concept related to low self-esteem	Point out and praise positive parenting behaviors and parent–child interactions Help the parent describe a sequence of events and analyze why specific interactions illustrate positive parenting behaviors Help the parent identify nurturing behaviors and support their continued practice Discuss parental expectations of the parenting role and the parent's performance; determine whether expectations are realistic Model positive, consistent parenting behaviors Teach the parent to identify positive feedback from the infant or child Help the parent to identify successful parenting actions; suggest keeping a diary of these examples for reference and positive feedback Discuss ways to ignore or not reinforce the child's negative behavior	Parent expresses pleasure and pride in role performance as a parent
6. Ineffective family coping related to inadequate support or ineffective role performance	Discuss with the parent the typical daily routine; have the parent identify ways to improve it or compare it with the personal ideal; note areas that are incongruous and suggest ways to compensate (eg, home health aide, day care, parent's group) Have the parent note significant people and discuss whether they are available for support; review the parent's history for recent losses by death, moves, or changes in commitment Discuss the parent's knowledge and use of community or religious resources Have the parent identify who in the family performs household chores, child-rearing tasks, and home management responsibilities; note whether distribution is a source of friction	Family members demonstrate satisfactory role performance and an ability to modify roles to help each other in times of need, thereby coping effectively with stress

continued on next page

NURSING CARE GUIDE The Family and Child Following Abuse (continued)

Nursing diagnosis	Interventions	Evaluation
	Discuss the parent's perception of personal role performance and (if applicable) the partner's role performance; have each family member identify who is blamed and who feels guilty for perceived incompetence Determine whether role performance meets the basic needs of the family; whether there is flexibility when needed; whether roles are ambiguous, overlapping, unfilled, or pejorative; whether role performers conflict or complement one another; and whether anyone occupies a dysfunctional role (eg, scapegoat) Share observations and information with a multidisciplinary team Encourage the parent to participate in family therapy or a parents' group, as recommended	
7. Alteration in family dynamics related to the arrival of a special child	Discuss with the parent the meaning attached to the child and why the child is special Help the parent identify ways in which family life has changed since the child's arrival Have the parent compare expectations for this child with those of other children Determine whether the parent is more or less patient, tender, demanding, or frustrated when interacting with the special child than with other children Help the parent identify realistic expectations for the child and acknowledge the need for personal assistance to accomplish parenting tasks	Family members demonstrate equal concern for each other without any favoritism or blame directed to a specific member
8. Developmental vulnerability related to dysfunctional parent–child interaction	Assess the child's developmental skills in physical, cognitive, affective, and social behaviors; compare with standard; note areas of delav (see Chapter 16) Provide child with a primary nurse Demonstrate acceptance of child, providing nurturing interactions and consistency in expectations Provide age-appropriate stimulation to foster development in all areas Assist the child in learning acceptable and unacceptable ways to gain attention; keep responses consistent and affirm positive behaviors	Child's development is within normal parameters Child and parent demonstrate adaptive changes in their interactions

NURSING CARE GUIDE The Family and Child Following Abuse (continued)

Nursing diagnosis	Interventions	Evaluation
	Suggest the use of age-appropriate facilities (eg, day care, nursery school, or YMCA program) to provide time out for parent and stimulation for child after discharge	
	Refer family to public health, visiting nurse, or social service for continued supervision and support after discharge	
9. Potential for disturtance in self-concept related to parental abuse	Observe the child's behavior and interaction with peers; note whether the child is overly aggressive or submissive; if the child is aggressive, provide time in a safe environment for the child to express feelings; discuss when aggression is appropriate and when it is not; provide guidelines and support the child in following them; offer positive feedback for evidence of control; if the child is submissive, support the child in gradual interaction with peers, beginning with one other child or small group in an activity that the child enjoys; provide positive feedback and affirm attempts at interaction	Child's behavior is age appropriate and demonstrates self-confidence in trying new skills and interacting with peers Parent demonstrates support and affirmation of child's abilities
	Observe the child's response to questions about injuries; encourage the child to talk about positive experiences and happy times with the parent; acknowledge the child's feelings for the parent and validate the importance of parental care	
	Observe the child's reaction to the hospital environment to identify unmet needs (see Chapter 27)	
	Prepare for discharge with age-appropriate teaching about the treatment plan (see Chapter 29)	
10. Potential for further injury	Monitor the home and family situation with respect to the likelihood for future injury to the child (or any siblings); use assessment tools as needed (see Chapter 17)	Child experiences no further injuries from parent
	Refer the family to assistance according to their perceived needs	
	Encourage parental cooperation in following through with family therapy; note any improvements in parent–child interactions	
	Discuss with the parent the commitment to learn and practice nonviolent coping strategies	

removing the child from the home. Removing children is first of all traumatic, and most communities lack adequate foster care homes. Foster care is more expensive than maintaining the family system. Dysfunctional parents also tend to continue the cycle of dysfunctional parenting with other children in the family.

Dysfunctional parents are often angry, argumentative, obstructive, rejecting, and evasive. If isolation has been prolonged, with little previous contact with agencies, parents are mistrusting and difficult to reach. They usually fear criticism, rejection, and ultimately punishment. For some, the initial contact is their first experience with supportive help.

Such parents have enormous needs for love, acceptance, and approval, and no treatment that seems rejecting, critical, or unreliable can be effective (Kempe and Kempe, 1978). Parents in need of treatment are extremely sensitive to rejection and often desperately need an accepting and friendly adult.

Although both professionals and nonprofessionals acknowledge intense feelings concerning child abuse and neglect, little concern usually is given to the abusive parents. Jolly K., a former abusive parent (and the founder of Parents Anonymous), described the needs of abused parents in this way:

> Child abusers are going through hell. We have a vision of how powerful our anger can be, a concept of where this anger will take us if we are pushed too far, and the constant dread that we will be pushed too far . . . We don't like being child abusers any more than society likes the problem of abuse. If a positive approach is offered to abusers, they will usually respond. We don't know how to listen—too many of us are afraid to go to agencies because of the fear that our children will be taken away (Reed, 1975).

Abusive parents are afraid. They are afraid of what they are doing, what will happen if they go for help, and what might happen if they do not go for help. Fontana described most abusive parents as "hurt, lonely, guilt-ridden, insufficiently mothered people who would like to do the right thing, but don't know how" (Fontana, 1973).

Working with neglectful and abusive parents is emotionally draining and disturbing for all people involved. Seeing a child victimized calls forth strong emotions, particularly among nurses, who might be required to provide nursing care during the time of the acute injury. The tendency is to protect the victim, the innocent child, and to punish the parent, who after all is the offender, but the nurse who perceives the family as a system understands that both the child and parent are victims (Smith, 1981). The etiology of abuse is complex and multifaceted. Parents "bring to the family and to their roles as parents developmental histories that may predispose them to treat their offspring in an abusive/neglectful manner. Stress-promoting social forces both within the family (e.g., handicapped child, marital conflict) and beyond (e.g., social isolation, unemployment) increase the likelihood that parent–child conflict will occur" (Belsky, Lerner, and Spanier, 1984, p. 175).

Nurses need to avoid "rescuer fantasies," which can stem from caring for a child and wanting to save that child from harm (Scharer, 1978). Unless recognized, these fantasies can blind the nurse to the real needs of the child and family. If the focus is the child's injuries, negative feelings toward the parent can multiply and ultimately affect interventions. Some nurses employ both overt (deliberately ignoring the parent or making accusatory remarks) and covert (supplying information in an offhand manner) behaviors toward abusive parents, thereby inhibiting rapport and parent teaching (Scharer, 1978). One approach to this problem might be to have two nursing teams, one to care for the child and one to interact with the parent. This might help to channel some negative feelings and maintain communication. Periodic discussions also can assist nurses to focus on the identified needs of both the parent and child and allow for the appropriate release of tension. Nurses need to recognize and affirm that child abuse is not simply the problem of a disturbed parent but is a social problem of vast dimensions.

Nurses can avoid judgmental attitudes by first examining their own thoughts, feelings, and beliefs about poverty, neglect, alternative life-styles, and different ethnic and cultural groups. Nurses need to understand the complex relationships among poverty, alienation, and neglect, not only to identify risk factors but also to recognize the social forces that keep some families locked in a cycle of dysfunction.

Approximately 10% of all parents who abuse or neglect their children cannot be treated or helped (Medical News, 1984). These parents are usually seriously mentally ill, and for them there is only one alternative—to sever the parent–child relationship. The child may be placed with relatives or in permanent foster care or may be placed for adoption after the formal termination of parental rights. The remaining 90% of parents might be helped, but of these, approximately 10% fail. The result is an overall rehabilitation rate of 80% (Kempe and Kempe, 1978). Because the sequelae of neglect are not always readily apparent, all data need to be reanalyzed periodically.

Helping Parents Cope With Stress A major task is helping dysfunctional parents to understand the impact of stress and crises in their lives and the appropriate responses to these crises.

In a family that is providing only marginal child care, any stress, however small, might create a crisis. Illness, separation of a family member, or problems with housing, heating, cooking, or laundry might trigger further neglect or apathy in an already fragile parent. The nurse who identifies stress in dysfunctional families therefore needs to assess coping strategies. A useful tool to facilitate assessing coping strategies is the Family Coping Index (see Chapter 17). Successful patterns of coping suggest growth and motivation. The nurse might be able to praise parents for positive coping behaviors or may need to teach appropriate ways to cope with stress. A family's reaction to stress is often a measure of the family's degree of strength as a system.

Most parents need support services as they learn to develop new coping techniques. Group therapy might assist abusive parents through peer support because finding others with similar problems minimizes isolation. Nurse therapists can address and help parents verbalize common fears and misconceptions about parenting. The first signs of dysfunctional parenting, however, must be discussed with the family because the nurse needs to guard against becoming so involved with the family that early indicators of serious parenting problems goes unrecognized. Progress might be slight at times but always must be identified, especially to the parent with low self-esteem.

Nurses and other professionals often need to make contracts and establish realistic deadlines in working with families. This in turn is good role modeling. Neglectul families need to be informed that the pattern of child care is inadequate and not acceptable to the community or school system. Facts of legal consequence, including removal of the children, need to be both verbalized and written out. These measures might seem drastic, but if they are handled in too gentle a manner, the family misinterprets the message and valuable time might be lost in mixed messages and conflicts.

Some parents appear to be docile, cooperative, and open but have merely learned responses that please. The nurse therefore is careful to identify concrete changes that indicate progress. Otherwise, the therapeutic contact might end too early for a family that appears to have changed. Periodic evaluation of family dynamics and interagency accomplishments and conflicts should ensure that the family does not manipulate workers or agencies and decrease the effectiveness of the plan. In some instances a child protective worker is needed to function as coordinator.

Support Services Various innovative programs have been developed specifically for the treatment of child abuse and neglect. One of the earliest of these programs is SCAN (Suspected Child Abuse and Neglect) Volunteer Service, Inc., which was organized in 1972. SCAN volunteers provide emergency intervention as well as long-term counseling and supportive services. Parents are offered the alternative of working with SCAN or facing law enforcement officials and possible foster placement of the child. Various other programs such as Homebuilders (Haapala and Kinney, 1979) are modeled after SCAN and are intended to rehabilitate both the child and parent and to hold the family together.

Many communities use public health nurses in the treatment of abusive parents so that care focuses on all family members and not just the abused child. Once the nurse and family have established goals, the nurse listens carefully to the parents and children and looks for signs of further risks of abuse.

In planning interventions long-term goals are usually to rehabilitate the dysfunctional family and to support and encourage normal development. Short-term goals are best planned together with family members, but the developmental needs of children must be the nurse's prime consideration.

Interventions may be accomplished both in and out of the child's home. If the child remains at home and the child's primary nurturing figure remains the natural parent, that parent also receives support. Treatment at home might include play therapy, recreational activities, homemaker services, Big Sisters or Big Brothers, and services for special needs such as dental, medical, nutritional, or remedial education. Other services might be provided outside the home while the child continues to live at home. The responsibility for care is then shared with the natural parent by crisis nurseries, day-care centers, respite care providers, and schools.

Homemaker services can provide cooking, cleaning, bed making, and laundry as a step toward improving the child's standard of living. The homemaker also might be a role model, the confidante, and "friend" of the parent. Other intermittent services include special education, health care, and "emergency parents" for short-term crises or stressors such as illness within the family.

If the child is removed from the care of the natural parent, nurturance becomes the sole responsibility of a substitute caregiver. Additional social services are then necessary, particularly if the child has special needs. These services might include shelters with temporary removal to a foster home or institution on a short-term basis, foster care, longer-term care oriented toward an ultimate return of the child to the original family, special care for physical disabilities or emotional disturbances, and guardianship or adoption, in which the child is permanently removed from the original home and custody is given to another caregiver.

Today, temporary foster care is intended to help rather than punish dysfunctional parents. Foster parents are taught about children's emotional needs so that children's feelings are incorporated into the treatment plan. When a child is in foster care, the focus of support to the foster family centers on helping the child understand the rationale for the change and facilitating the original parent's visits with the child. If the safety of the child might be threatened, the visit should be structured and monitored. If the original parents do not visit or contact the child, the child will feel rejected, and additional support will be needed to help the child comprehend the possible reasons for their absence. Studies have shown that if more than 2 years elapse without contact from the original family, the likelihood of reuniting the original family is less than 5% (Munro, 1984). The goal for all children should be a permanent home and the secure sense of belonging that accompanies it. Foster care is designed to be temporary and thus conveys a lack of continuity and permanence, even though extended placements are much too common.

Foster parents can play a key role in successfully uniting an original family when the birth parents come to visit. Sometimes, the amount of caring and nurturance given to the dysfunctional family serves as the model for future interactions between parents and children. In essence, the foster parents who can "parent the parents" and meet their needs for acceptance can promote self-esteem and self-worth.

Fanshel and Shinn (1978) conducted a longitudinal investigation of over 600 foster children over 5 years and concluded that even dysfunctional parents are important to their children and that efforts to preserve some kind of connection should be the goal of social service agencies. Other services for the original family center on assisting family members to identify their strengths and areas that need improvement. Discussion regarding the changes is needed before the family can be reunited.

In the evaluative process the input of all involved persons, including the children, should be sought. Professionals can express their views of the chances of family restoration; foster parents can report on behavioral changes, especially positive changes; original parents can report on progress or failure regarding the factors that led to the need for foster placement. A key behavior to evaluate is the way the original parent reacts to stress. Certain behavioral changes, such as moving from isolation to the ability to seek and use resources, are monitored in this way. The criteria for determining whether a home is safe for the child to return to need to be specific.

Providing health care to a foster child can be problematic. The nurse often is presented with a vague medical history and scanty information about early immunizations, serious accidents, illness, hospitalizations, allergies, or food dislikes. The child is often a poor historian because emphasis on health and maintenance behaviors has been lacking, and medical care usually has been episodic and crisis oriented.

Foster children who have been severely deprived frequently will have nutritional difficulties. They might experience extremes of lethargy and anorexia or hoarding and gorging of food. Many children have existed on peculiar diets, often consisting of junk food and empty calories, and they have difficulty accepting fruits, vegetables, and other nutritious foods because they are unfamiliar.

When a child is placed in foster care for whatever reason, all parties involved—the original parent or parents, the child, the foster parents, and the social worker—should have clear, behaviorally defined goals that everyone understands and agrees to. Realistic deadlines and periodic assessments should give all parties a time frame for evaluation. If the original parents fail to meet the preset goals within the specified time, the multidisciplinary team should discuss and evaluate the situation to ensure justice and then implement procedures to terminate parental rights, thus freeing the child for placement in a permanent adoptive home.

Termination of parental rights is a moral dilemma and must be balanced carefully between the parents' rights to have their children returned and children's rights to permanent homes and continuous relationships. It is never an easy decision, and each case must be evaluated separately because there are no black and white answers. The judicial system might be used as a continual or periodic reminder to parents of their minimal responsibilities. Courts view termination of parental rights as a last resort, however, and such judgments are always a multidisciplinary decision. The decision requires careful consideration of the long-range effects of unchanged dysfunctional parenting (such as mental illness, alcoholism, drug addiction) (Wiltze, 1978) and the likelihood of meeting the child's needs in a foster care family. The trend in foster care is now toward time-limited contracts so that the "professional foster child," who lacked a sense of security because of repeated moves, will no longer exist.

Child welfare agencies generally are involved in both the treatment and prevention of child abuse and neglect. Children's Protective Service also has a vested interest in the effectiveness and accessibility of a wide range of resources in the community and usually takes the lead in working with the family and mobilizing resources. A Children's Protective Service office generally is located in a department of social services and is administered by county, city, or state. Its prime functions include receiving, investigating, and evaluating reports of child abuse and neglect and providing necessary services, either directly or through referral. Its goals are to prevent injury to children, promote the development of healthy children, preserve and enhance family life, strengthen and support parents and families, and provide for children to remain in their own homes and communities whenever possible.

The Children's Protective Service usually coordinates fiscal and technical support to community-based child protection teams. Coordinated services are thus designed to accomplish the following:

1. Maintain and improve the availability of community resources for the prevention and treatment of child abuse and neglect.
2. Strengthen cooperative working relationships through interdisciplinary teams.
3. Integrate clinical knowledge with child welfare practice.
4. Educate the public and professionals about the prevention and treatment of child abuse and neglect.

Many communities have established "helplines" to help parents to cope with frustrations. These telephone hotlines for crisis intervention are available 24 hours a day, 7 days a week, and generally are staffed by trained volunteers, professionals, and paraprofessionals. The hotline reassures many parents who just need to know that someone is there if they are unable to cope and might lead others to seek help at an earlier stage of frustration.

Responding to a parent's cry for help frequently involves listening to the parent vent frustration and anger and identifying available resources. The empathetic, nonjudgmental attitude of a volunteer is sometimes enough to avert a crisis. If, however, the caller reports child abuse in progress, the volunteer attempts to identify the immediate risks and dangers involved. Response to the parent's distress might involve obtaining transportation to a treatment facility or shelter. The volunteer therefore needs to assess the level of crisis, presence of marital discord, provocative behaviors of the children, and actual or potential medical conditions. Data are then provided to a social services department for further follow-up. For life-threatening situations, most crisis lines provide for immediate intervention.

Parents Anonymous is a self-help group that is especially effective for both the prevention and treatment of child abuse. The organization was founded in 1972 in California by Jolly K., who was both an abusive parent and an abused child who had lived in 35 foster homes. Meetings of Parents Anonymous are led by a parent, and participants are invited to share their feelings, concerns, and problems, but meetings are neither therapy nor classes in parenting. Members are often able to confront one another about parenting behaviors, especially if they have experienced the same problems, and they also can share possible solutions to family dilemmas.

All members are parents who need a support group to meet family stresses. Most attendance is on a voluntary basis, but some members are ordered to attend by the court system. Meetings usually are held once a week for 2 hours in accessible locations in the community. Professional sponsors who are present during the meeting are there as consultants rather than authorities. Members often exchange phone numbers to contact each other between meetings because Parents Anonymous suggests, "Reach for your phone instead of your kid."

Two studies of Parents Anonymous have found that physical abuse usually stops within 1 month of the parent's joining and that verbal and emotional abuse decline significantly and continue to decline as long as the parent participates (Nix, 1980). Formerly abusive parents often report increased self-esteem as they assist other parents in distress. Some continue to attend meetings long after their initial needs are met, and many parents report pleasurable relationships with their children for the first time in their lives.

Supporting the Child If significant changes in the family are unavoidable, the child needs assistance in working through feelings of having caused the changes. Siblings also need to be included in the treatment plan of an abused or neglected child. If the child is hospitalized, fears of pain or violence are intensified by the unfamiliar surroundings and people. If a parent does visit, the parent often is unsupportive and might be angry with the child. The child is often confused, hurt, and frightened. Nurses and other hospital staff therefore can identify pain, fear, and confusion and assist the child in discussing feelings. The child needs to be told what will happen in developmentally appropriate terms and be reassured, as much as possible, that the parent will be back. The fewer the number of caregivers, the more likely it is that the child will establish trusting relationships.

Some children have never heard their names spoken in a gentle voice, and for them, a slow, gentle approach is essential in building any degree of trust. Children who withdraw from human contact must be allowed a reasonable period of time in which to grieve and appraise new people. If the child regresses, the regressive behavior needs to be accepted until the child can ease into a more appropriate developmental stage. (See Chapter 27 for a discussion of children's reactions to hospitalization.).

Younger children are likely to need nurturing in the form of rocking, cuddling, and soothing. The child initially might appear to reject any comforting, however, and children become aggressive in response to their overwhelming anxiety. The aggressive behaviors are learned responses to chaotic living and can become problematic if the child manages to manipulate many people. Team members therefore need to set consistent limits in a firm but kindly manner and assist the child in learning more acceptable behaviors. Aggressive children usually have feelings of deprivation, sadness, and loneliness and might believe themselves to be unworthy and bad. Such children have little faith in their ability to inspire approval and affection (Kempe and Kempe, 1978).

With individual therapy, aggressive children might be able to discuss the expectations their parents have for them and family dynamics. The therapeutic approach is to face reality honestly and not to arouse expectations in the child that the parent cannot or will not fulfill (Kempe and Kempe, 1978). Children who have been severely abused or who have witnessed severe abuse in a sibling also need much support in developing future relationships that are free of fears, guilt, and anxieties. Children facing loss of separation from their parents need therapeutic assistance to handle the loss and time to mourn the loss.

Long-term follow-up of dysfunctional families has no set time frame for completion. In some instances services are required until the children reach adulthood. Periodic evaluation of parental progress and family growth includes monitoring the behaviors of the children, who might exhibit anger, anxiety, intense loneliness, or apathy. The children's progress in school also must be assessed, together with their response to authority figures. Dysfunctional behaviors suggest that the child needs individual attention. Communication and caring, although time consuming for the team members, does assist both parents and children in coping with the normal stress of development.

Profiles of High-Risk Families

Adolescent Parents

The incidence of adolescent pregnancy has risen to epidemic proportions, especially among girls under 16 years of age. Young people are sexually active earlier but often lack information about the consequences and necessary precautions. About 20% of the total number of births in the United States today are to adolescent parents. Approximately 90% of these adolescent parents keep their infants, resulting in a double risk for both the infant and parent (Adolescent Perinatal Health, 1979).

Providing services and counseling to an adolescent parent requires a multidisciplinary team of health care providers, social service planners, and educators, with special emphasis on health care, nutrition, education, and the developmental needs of both the parent and child. A family centered approach is best to strengthen all possible resources. The family involved should be defined as broadly as possible to include all motivated persons. These people might be the father of the child, grandparents, siblings, aunts, uncles, and any significant others who might serve as family.

All adolescents are emotionally and intellectually immature and lack the physical, emotional, economic, educational, and social resources necessary for parenting. (Adolescent development is discussed in Chapter 11.) For most young women, the change from adolescent to parent is overwhelming. Most adolescent parents are faced with uncertainty, self-doubt, and inexperience, which are compounded by their immaturity. Although youthfulness gives them energy, their lack of experience and skills promotes maladaptive coping strategies.

An adolescent parent usually has a limited repertoire of coping skills, and the pregnancy itself might be both a symptom and cause of conflict. For some adolescents, pregnancy is sought as a means of escape from an intolerable family situation, as an unconscious wish to prove adulthood or punish parents for unmet needs, or as compensation for feelings of rejection and insecurity. Whatever the reason, the reality of the demands place the mother at risk for many problems and in greater need of family support.

Adolescent pregnancies occur at every social, economic, and intellectual level; however, adolescents from deprived backgrounds often complete rather than abort their pregnancies. Health care for the adolescent girl from a deprived socioeconomic background is apt to be episodic, crisis oriented, intermittent, or occur late in the pregnancy. These mothers usually are not accustomed to seeking or using health care as prevention, which adds another dimension of risk to parenting.

The child born to an adolescent parent is usually at risk. These infants are often preterm, small for gestational age (SGA), and face risks both during and after birth. The younger the mother, the greater the health risks of pregnancy, as the physiologically growing mother attempts to sustain the growth of the infant. The smaller the infant, the greater the potential health problems to be resolved and the longer the separation time while the infant is in intensive care. Lengthy separation from the infant is itself a risk factor for faulty parent–child attachment. The inexperienced parent also might misinterpret the constant demands of a dependent child. Knowledge about normal child development and care might be sketchy or poor, and mounting pressures may mean sporadic care and stimulation for the infant, which might then lead in the long term to developmental delays and an increased susceptibility to environmentally induced mental retardation (see Chapter 23).

At a time when the new mother needs the most emotional support, she often gets the least. Her boyfriend might be frightened of the awesome responsibilities and turn away from her; her family might voice disappointment or anger and restrict her activities by refusing to assist in child care, creating emotional detachment that serves to reinforce her feelings of unworthiness. Her peers are usually free from responsibility and still in school, leaving her without the support of family and friends. This emotional void is itself a crisis and often a sharp contrast to the adolescent's fantasies in which the infant provides love and affection to erase the confusion and conflicts of adolescence. The reality of the infant's demands places the infant at extreme risk for neglect or abuse.

Although the major impact of adolescent pregnancy is felt by the mother, the adolescent father's life is affected as well. He might deny his involvement with the mother, resulting in feelings of guilt and anxiety, or he might make emotional commitments and offer support and financial aid. In either case he must acknowledge his sexuality, which still might be an unresolved issue for him. Financial assistance usually has long-range effects on his educational and career plans. If he drops out of school to support the child, he often has to settle for jobs that pay poorly and might be unemployed and in need of financial assistance. All of these factors affect his ability to sustain a relationship with the infant's mother. Those who work with adolescent fathers have found that these boys feel more responsibility and concern than is sometimes assumed. They too need someone to assist them to sort out confused and troubled feelings.

Preparation for parenthood begins in childhood, but for the adolescent parent, the preparation time is abbreviated by the child's birth, and the younger the parent, the higher the degree of risk. Some adolescent parents willingly enter (or are forced to enter) into an early marriage, which also compounds the risks and delays important decisions. Teenage marriages are very fragile, prone to divorce, and often a crisis in themselves. If an adolescent parent comes from a dysfunctional family, the risks for successful parenting are compounded.

All mothers under 16 years of age need intense follow-up and nurturing for themselves and their infants. If the adolescent mother does not have a supportive family to assist her, a foster home with a surrogate family might be necessary. The older adolescent is better able to nurture an infant if her immediate family and friends are supportive. She often has enough maturity to place the infant's needs ahead of her own, but when children have children, society pays the price. Both parents and children require services to maintain their health. The responsibilities of parenthood might interrupt their education, limiting their skills and trapping them in low-income jobs or in need of still more social and financial assistance.

Developmental Needs of Adolescent Parents Adolescent parents face the developmental tasks of parenthood superimposed on the developmental tasks of adolescence. If the two sets of tasks become mutually exclusive, these parents are at high risk. The accomplishment of the developmental tasks of parenthood can be impeded by a lack of motivation or knowledge and by immaturity. Adolescence is itself a time of stress (see Chapter 11). A young girl's ability to accept the role of mother clearly is tied to her ability to accept herself as a woman. Parenting is markedly influenced by the extent to which adolescents attain some of their own developmental milestones.

Much family conflict usually precedes the birth of an infant to an adolescent parent. Attitudes in the extended family might range from overly strict to overly permissive, and family members might offer varying degrees of emotional and financial support, but one of the greatest conflicts for the pregnant adolescent is her independence. The young girl has probably tried, prior to the pregnancy, to prove her independence, both to herself and her parents. Pregnancy and parenthood, with all of the demands for change, only serve to increase her dependence. For the adolescent who has not achieved independence prior to parenthood, problem solving and decision making abilities will be minimal if not entirely lacking.

Because of strained or absent finances, young parents might be forced to rely more heavily on their own parents, thereby increasing their dependence when they were struggling to decrease it. The resulting conflicts might be expressed in many ways; substance abuse, depression, and anxiety are but a few reactions.

Adolescence is a time for establishing identity and ego strength. The pregnant adolescent might have attempted to solve identity problems through sexual behavior and frequently expresses feelings of being unloved. Sexual intimacy might have provided her the experience of being loved, and a strong wish for a child might be an expression of a need for an object toward which to direct her love. After birth, the child might be viewed as security against feeling unloved; therefore, much attention and a focus on fostering a positive self-concept will be necessary to alleviate further problems. Because adolescents find it difficult to focus on the needs of others, some feel intense conflicts between a wish to grow up and a wish to hold onto childhood security and dependence. Consequently, some adolescents literally turn their infants over to their own parents while they assume the role of sibling to the child.

Coping strategies in general are strained during adolescence, with normal inconsistencies in behavior and thought and many rapid mood fluctuations. Emotionally volatile adolescents tend to develop strained relationships with others; therefore, their children are most at risk if they are expected to conform to the moods of adolescent parents. Because acceptance by peers is an adolescent need, separation from peers, either physical or psychologic, denies the adolescent parent the emotional support of a peer group. Schools no longer require that a pregnant adolescent leave school, but many mothers choose to drop out rather than be unlike members of their peer groups. Without peer support, the risks for isolation intensify. The absence of a network of family and friends contributes to the probability of child abuse and neglect, depression, suicide, and marital stress.

Early adolescence is accompanied by a developmental need to accept the bodily changes associated with puberty. Pregnancy and motherhood bring about still greater bodily changes superimposed on the physical changes that might not have been resolved by the adolescent mother. Infants of young adolescents are most at risk if the mother perceives her pregnancy as a cause of changes in body image and consequently comes to resent the infant.

Supporting Adolescent Parents Adolescent parents need continual support services and much anticipatory guidance concerning their own needs, the needs of their children, and the relationship between these sets of needs. Support services and education for parenthood need to begin during pregnancy because if the mother emerges from pregnancy and birth with a feeling of dignity and self-worth, she will be better able to progress to motherhood. The type and extent of support services, however, vary with each adolescent parent.

Teaching Parenting and Homemaking Skills Classes in parenting skills are vital. Specific tasks of child care such as diapering, feeding, and burping an infant need to be discussed and practiced, especially with inexperienced parents. An infant rather than a doll during practice sessions is immensely valuable because an infant behaves spontaneously. Parents need to learn about infant stimulation and specific methods of accomplishing this. Emphasis should be placed on normal infant behavioral responses and concrete tasks to increase sensitivity to the infant's cues. The nurse then serves as a role model for adaptive parenting.

Normal growth and developmental stages need to be discussed along with realistic expectations for a child's abilities at each stage and level of development. Adolescent parents often have strong emotional needs that need to be addressed before they can assume child-care responsibilities. An empathetic listener can assist by discussing ambivalent feelings and attachment behaviors. Parents also need to know about negative responses and how these affect the relationship between the parent and child.

After the birth, most adolescent parents require careful follow-up and intensive community support to achieve success and wellness. Many schools, community health centers, and pediatric clinics provide home- and center-based intervention programs. The programs should extend well into early childhood, lasting a minimum of 3 years (Cannon-Bonventre and Kahn, 1979). Home-based services need to provide opportunities for parental involvement, enrichment, and reinforcement. Because specific concerns and questions usually arise at home, these programs can meet the need to monitor specific behaviors and provide explanations and rationales about positive parenting skills. Parents need attention to their role, and discussion usually helps to increase feelings of effectiveness, which eventually strengthen the parent's self-concept. Center-based programs also can offer day care, job training, discussion of homemaking skills, and financial incentives to enhance family life. Transportation might be needed for adolescent parents with limited resources. Group sessions can provide a new peer group for immature adolescents and access to common problem-solving techniques. A new peer group also serves to offset isolation and allows parents to share feelings, frustrations, and home management difficulties.

Discussions of basic homemaking skills need to be incorporated into support services for adolescent parents. Wise meal planning and budgetary hints are important topics because most adolescents have poor concepts of money and effective buying strategies. Many need to learn the pitfalls of time payments and charge accounts or how to balance a checkbook or plan a budget. Squabbles over money and bills are one of the largest factors in domestic quarrels, sometimes leading to violence, separation, or divorce. Knowledge of financial planning can do much to offset the risks.

Adolescent parents also need counseling and support services to complete their education. Most communities offer General Educational Development classes specifically geared to luring high school dropouts back into the educational system. Classes in skills, vocations, employment, and legal services are also valuable; child-care services and even transportation assistance might be required.

Contraceptive counseling and services should be made available to all young parents to prevent future unplanned pregnancies. Nurses cannot assume that these adolescents are informed about sexuality and contraception; many are hesitant to ask for information. Cost, availability, and acceptability are prime factors in contraception. Adolescents also need to know about their own physical and mental health, the value of exercise and nutrition in promoting healthy bodies, and the effective use of leisure time, including hobbies and personal interests. The danger of isolation—particularly of television viewing as a cause of isolation—needs to be addressed.

Ongoing Care of Adolescent Parents Nurses working with adolescent parents and children need as complete a data base as possible, including knowledge of past family risk factors. A thorough and complete assessment usually requires several appointments. Assessing the cognitive level of each adolescent parent allows the nurse to identify the level of maturity and ability to use resources. (Developmental assessment of the adolescent is discussed in Chapter 16.) For maturing adolescents, early interactions with the nurse are very important because the quality of these discussions frequently sets the tone by which the adolescent judges all authority and professional figures. The nurse needs to convey concern and caring while assisting the parent to sort out feelings and problems. This requires a nonjudgmental approach with active listening to fears and anxiety so the adolescent parents feel accepted and understood. Nonverbal communication is very important. The nurses's expression, the warmth of a smile, and the gentleness of touch all convey a special sort of caring.

Most adolescents have had little orientation to a health care system and are poorly able to describe physical problems. The nurse's first role is therefore to convey the importance of consistent, quality health care. A brief and simple explanation of the rationale of prevention and purpose of future health visits can assist in cooperation. The adolescent parent's prenatal care is also a predictor of future health-seeking behaviors. For example, if the parent understands why immunizations are necessary (rather than when they are scheduled), cooperation is enhanced. The parent should always be invited to ask questions and is likely to respond better when treated as an adult and not as a child. Whenever possible, adolescent parents should make their own choices rather than having decisions made for them.

Each adolescent parent needs a trusting relationship with a responsible adult, who might be a nurse. This relationship can establish a pattern of seeking resources for assistance. The nurse can be instrumental in fostering a special relationship by asking open-ended questions such as, "Who do you talk to when you feel troubled or anxious?" Because pregnancy has probably caused much family conflict and rejection, the adolescent mother might feel guilty, alone, and depressed. A nursing goal and a challenge is therefore to get the adolescent mother to express her feelings.

Nutrition is an important aspect of health and wellness, and sound nutritional practices need to be incorporated into every nursing care plan. The nurse assesses the parent's knowledge of specific food groups and daily requirements along with cultural variations in nutrition. (Nutritional assessment is discussed in Chapter 15.) The daily caloric requirements of both the mother and infant need to focus on the avoidance of "empty calories," but adolescent food fads might need to be incorporated into the nutritional plan. Specific foods, amounts, and exchanges need to be explained in a way that the adolescent can understand.

Support from the adolescent's family might affect the parenting role both financially and psychologically. Support should not, however, mean that the adolescent parent is barred from child care. If the parents of the adolescent are nonsupportive or show evidence of dysfunctional parenting in the past, family counseling is necessary to assist the adolescent in identifying family strengths and weaknesses and in learning how to cope. A substitute surrogate family also might be necessary for some adolescent parents.

Assisting the adolescent to develop communication skills also enhances parenting. Focusing on the positive expression of feelings and ways to improve relationships has longlasting benefits for any adolescent and is especially important for the adolescent from a dysfunctional family. A referral to mental health services might assist in offsetting problematic behavior. When focusing on parenting skills, the nurse stresses the adolescent parent's vital role in the care of the child and looks for and capitalizes on strengths in the parent's ability to care for the infant. For example, remarks such as, "You're doing a fine job; the baby's gaining weight nicely" will do much to enhance a parent's self-confidence. Helping the parent to elicit a social smile from the infant fosters bonding. If the infant is not gaining weight and is demonstrating signs of failure to thrive, parental assessment includes knowledge, motivation, and readiness to parent; supportive interventions are geared accordingly.

An important nursing role in working with adolescent parents is identifying positive behaviors and providing praise. All adolescents need recognition during the times of "troubled identity" and will respond to encouragement by trying to perform. Accomplishments might be small, but for a rebellious adolescent, the significance may be great. Cooperation with health care professionals, such as simply keeping appointments, might signal an early effort at maturity and responsibility.

Violence-Prone Families

A history of violent behavior places a family at risk for injury to family members, others, or the environment. Family violence means the threat or actual use of physical force between family members. Family violence includes spouse abuse, child abuse, incest, neglect, and abuse of the elderly. All forms of family violence are maladaptive responses to psychologic tensions, external stressors, or tension within the family. The problem is so widespread that abuse in some form occurs in more than half of all United States households.

Patterns of Family Violence Violent behavior is not limited to specific social classes, races, creeds, religions, or levels of education and income. Its cause is unknown but is certainly the result of biologic, psychologic, social, and cultural factors (Campbell, 1984). Alcoholism and drug abuse generally are present in families exhibiting abuse or violence, although research has not identified the exact causal relationship between substance abuse and violence. Steele (1975) reported that the most common element found in the lives of abusive or violent adults is the experience of abuse or neglect during their earliest years. Violence thus appears to be at least in part a learned behavior.

For some children, violence is a way of life. These children see adult family members behave aggressively and respond to frustrations and tensions by lashing out against anything or anyone within reach. Patterns of violence then become cyclic. Children who were neglected or abused grow up lacking trust in others and are unable to form close relationships. Once they have learned to use aggression as a means of problem solving, they have a decreased ability to cope with stress and often lack empathy toward others.

Violence affects every aspect of the family system. If a wife is abused, for example, the violence is likely to affect her self-image, her desire to have children, her sexual pleasure, and her physical well-being. Even when they themselves are not abused, children experience terror during violent episodes and fear of becoming victims. They might be treated as pawns in marital conflicts, moved among friends and relatives a great deal, and might in turn be neglected as a result of the parental distress (Finley, 1981).

A first step in planning care is to identify the victim of violence. The unusual combination of injuries coupled with timid and evasive behavior are often the initial clues that identify the victim. Multiple bruises in varying stages of resolution, for example, might indicate a series of violent episodes. Nurses must thoroughly assess any client who might have been battered. Open-ended questions such as, "Would you like to talk about what happened to you?" sometimes encourage a victim to share feelings and fears. Granting a victim time and privacy conveys a sense of dignity and concern. The best approach is nonthreatening so that the victim feels respected and protected and not rushed to make accusations, especially because the victim's ambivalence might prevent any cooperation if the approach is hurried or impersonal.

Many interventions can be offered to a victim of battering. Immediate referrals to provisional shelters allow victims to identify available options, but nurses should avoid counseling a family member to leave home before being ready. Many women hope that their marital relationship will improve, and it is this dream that gives them the energy to survive (Lieberknecht, 1978). Battered women, for example, must choose to leave home only when they have the internal strength to support the choice. Women often choose to remain in unhealthy relationships to protect their children. A woman might fear for the children's safety but knows that the family will lack financial support if she leaves with them (Iyer, 1980). In some instances the woman is legally guilty of abandonment if she leaves without her children, regardless of the circumstances, and in a court of law she might lose custody of the children for having left them in a dependent state.

In the past several years, temporary emergency shelters have been established for women seeking to leave dysfunctional families. Women with small, dependent children and minimal financial resources are especially at risk for becoming trapped in situations with abusive or alcoholic family members. Prior to the establishment of these shelters, such women had to endure the situation, risk sporadic violence, or be at the mercy of family and friends for assistance; many women and children were hopelessly locked in intolerable situations. Shelters offer a variety of services, including temporary safety for mothers and children. The locations are kept secret, giving the woman a brief respite and time to recover and think about her situation. During this time, she needs emotional and practical support as she sorts through her available options. The harsh reality is that whatever she decides, the immediate future will be difficult and her need for supportive resources great.

Death Caused by Family Violence The ultimate fear in a dysfunctional family is death caused by physical violence. When a death does occur, either because of neglect or trauma, the results are naturally devastating for all concerned. Family members compound their sorrow by identifying preventive measures they should have taken. Hindsight makes the awareness of dysfunction more acute and creates an overwhelming sense of guilt.

Nurses experience a sense of having failed the victim, family, and system and usually tend to evaluate and reevaluate the behavior responses to past methods of treatment. Those directly involved with the family can be rendered almost helpless as they struggle to exonerate themselves from feelings of responsibility. Newspaper headlines, reporters, and gossiping coworkers all serve to keep the tragedy very much alive for the nurse. Nurses associated with a troubled family often stop trying to assist the family further once trauma and death occur. At this time, however, services are even more essential if the emotional well-being of the surviving members is to be the nurse's concern.

As soon as the safety of the family members is assured, a period of neutrality, or time out, should follow. Just as the family needs time to mourn one of its members, likewise, the involved health care professionals need time to work through their grief and sense of loss. A period of adjustment and recognition is necessary to the grief response (even if the tragedy increases the need for services and therefore stretches health care resources).

Family responses to any death vary (see Chapter 32 for age-appropriate responses to death). Initially, fear, disbelief, numbness, and shock are obvious. Extreme reactions include manifestations of grief and no display of emotions of any kind. Because of the fragility of the family system, members usually have much difficulty in sharing sorrow or comforting each other. Each member might be left to face the reality of death alone.

If the victim was one of the parents, the children in essence suffer the loss of both parents and often are placed in foster care or in the care of relatives. In either instance the children need explanations and a great deal of assistance to face the tragedy, a need that often is lacking in the height of confusion and sorrow.

If the victim is a child, siblings are most anxious and confused. The scope of the tragedy often is erroneously thought to be beyond their comprehension, and they are given little support. Siblings have fears connected both with the trauma and with the parent's involvement. Physical symptoms are frequently their only ways of expressing anxiety and receiving help.

The parent involved in the death, either directly or indirectly, faces untold agony and little time for remorse or grief. Law enforcement officials hold repeated questioning sessions and tend to be none too gentle in dealing with the accused. The abuser reacts with sorrow, denial, depression, repentance, or anger, although the anger usually is directed at the victim for dying and causing the tragedy, especially if the trauma was not premeditated.

"Uninvolved" family members also might react predictably. They might face feelings of "guilt by association" from their remaining family and friends as they essentially suffer two losses, the death of the child and the loss of the mate. The task of holding together the remnants of the family falls on the uninvolved parent, who might be too passive to assume such a demanding role. Family disintegration frequently follows.

Multiproblem Families

Some families experience many problems at the same time. Each family member might have problems that impinge on the family system, but the sheer number of problems can seem overwhelming to both the family and nurses. Such families often are labeled "hard to reach" and "crisis oriented," and they might be shuffled from one health professional to another.

In many multiproblem families parents are psychiatrically unstable, experience many severe social and economic stressors, and generally lack adaptive coping skills. They usually have difficulties in judgment, planning for the future, and meeting daily responsibilities. Multiproblem families are at extreme risk for dysfunctional parenting because the parents are so overwhelmed by the immediacy of their own needs that the needs of their children frequently go unnoticed and unmet. Children are then at risk for developmental delays (Greenspan, 1982). They might in turn be hampered in behavior, mood, thought, controlling their impulses, and self-esteem.

Family members frequently appear apathetic, having conditioned themselves to tolerate problems without moving toward resolution. They often are living with much chaos and turmoil and usually are overwhelmed and unable to cope with the numerous problems without definitive help. Problems are usually complex because they are chronic and often have been partially resolved many times in the past. Individual needs usually add to the complexity of the family's problems. For example, substance abuse by a parent can result in problems of poor housing, nutrition, and safety for the children. The onset of family problems is often vague, as family members become accustomed to stressors and dysfunctional behaviors. Parents might be living with patterns they learned as children. Most often, they are living only for the present because most needs are immediate, and long-term goals are nonexistent. Parental immaturity or isolation further complicates family dysfunction.

The multiproblem family usually is known to many agencies. School officials, community workers, and health care professionals have often identified existing conditions that jeopardize the health and safety of children and parents. The family might be referred for a particular problem that seems foremost to the professional involved, although frequently not to the family. Only one or two family problems are usually addressed, however, and the rest remain dormant and unresolved until another agency becomes involved. The result is an intermittent community response in which only parts of the family system receive assistance. Multiple stressors mean that the family then always needs some agency support and community involvement, which makes the family system continually dependent on others.

The delivery of effective services to a multiproblem family often is hampered by the family itself. Many families provide incomplete or incorrect information, which makes follow-up very difficult. Appointments are not kept, calls are not returned, and the family generally appears to have little motivation to resolve problems. Mobility often impedes effectiveness because the family might move from one agency to another and automatically assume that the new agency will begin where the last agency left off. Over time, the multiproblem family "burns out" its resources and is left alone until a crisis such as overt neglect, physical abuse, or a runaway child requires further help. To a family with long-standing problems and dysfunctional roles, the loss of agency services further increases the feelings of mistrust. Only highly innovative and comprehensive services then succeed in achieving cooperation. One person or agency cannot, however, meet all the complex needs of multiproblem families, and many referrals might be needed so that various professionals can render assistance. A first step is for the nurse and family to list all the current services being used and the degree of family involvement. One agency or person is then designated as the coordinator, and control of the treatment plan then rests with the coordinator. Without a coordinator, efforts to assist the family are likely to be fragmented, thereby decreasing effectiveness and increasing the cost of services. The danger of multiple-agency involvement is fragmentation of care and the possibility of manipulation by family members.

Nurses often are best equipped to act as coordinators, although the coordinator of services need not be a nurse. Nurses are, however, always advised to recommend that a coordinator be named if this is not the usual procedure in a given setting. The family also should be consulted in the selection process to enhance compliance. The coordinator might decide on multidisciplinary management and plan a meeting for all involved or might determine that a one-to-one approach is best.

As the nurse assesses each family member's strengths and weaknesses along with the family system as a whole, family members usually benefit from having their strengths pointed out, especially if problems have always been the focus of attention. In analyzing problems the nurse and family together determine priorities and identify those that are most acute and those that might reasonably be resolved. Families often report that problems identified by health professionals are not those that they feel are important. A small success early on, however, will serve as the impetus for future attempts at resolution.

The history also includes past attempts at problem resolution and the family's reasons for any failures. A discussion of recurring problems and failures conveys to the family member that concerted efforts are being made to help and that they have a part in solving their own problems. Data are then analyzed to prevent future failures. Families who participate in the planning process also are given a sense of responsibility and accountability so that they learn to take responsibility for solving problems.

The nurse also assists the family to plan short-term goals with realistic deadlines and tasks. The family is asked to set the dates and times of meetings and needs to be confronted if these are not met. This in turn reinforces the family's responsibility. Frequent evaluation identifies both positive attempts and any nonparticipation in the treatment plan.

Providing professional services to the multiproblem family is one of the greatest challenges for health professionals. Professional burnout is high, and the support of colleagues is necessary because progress is slow and sometimes nonexistent. One advantage of multidisciplinary management of multiproblem families is therefore the support and assistance that team members can provide each other.

Key Concepts

- Risk factors are indicators of potential dysfunction; they are not predictors, althought their correlation with dysfunction is high.
- By knowing the factors that place a family at risk, the nurse is able to assess the potential for dysfunction and plan interventions to prevent dysfunction and its secondary effects from occurring.
- A family that is unable to provide for the physical or emotional needs of its members is said to be a dysfunctional family.
- Dysfunctional parenting characterizes the dysfunctional family and involves a disturbance in the parent–child relationship.
- Dysfunctional parenting is characterized by inadequate family communication, role confusion among family members, and isolation from community and other support systems.
- Risk factors that indicate a potential for dysfunctional parenting include the parent's experience as a child, parent–child role reversal, and multiple stressors, which might include marital problems, chronic illness in the family, or inadequate supports.
- The parent's experience as a child greatly influences parenting style and expectations of children.
- Dysfunctional parenting might lead to developmental delays and failure to thrive in the infant.
- Inorganic failure to thrive is a syndrome characterized by a lack of normal growth and development, physical symptoms that suggest malnutrition and lack of adequate care, and infant behaviors that show unresponsiveness and lack of trust.
- Child neglect is the failure to provide a child with the basic necessities of life, which might be physical or emotional.
- Indicators of child neglect include developmental delays, especially in social and language development; inattention to a child's safety, hygiene, or nutrition; and inadequate discipline and emotional support.
- Child abuse is physical violence or verbal assaults directed against a child.
- Parents who abuse their children often feel isolated, are unable to trust others, have few supports for coping with stress, or have unrealistic expectations for their children's behavior.
- Children who are abused might be the result of a difficult pregnancy and might have been high-risk infants whose care interfered with parent–child bonding, or they may have congenital anomalies, mental retardation, hyperactivity, or chronic illness.
- Indicators of physical abuse include a series of injuries in various stages of healing (especially a series of similar injuries), the family's delay in seeking treatment, use of multiple treatment facilities, and attempts to hide or minimize the abuse, sometimes with special clothing.
- Emotional abuse often is characterized by the parent's calling the child foul names, ridiculing the child, and making the child feel stupid, hated, ugly, unlovable, or unwanted.
- Sexual abuse is the exploitation of a child for the sexual gratification of an adult; incest is sexual abuse by a family member.
- When a child is sexually abused, the long-term goals are to prevent further abuse and help the child to overcome the psychologic effects of abuse.
- Children who in any way reveal that they have been sexually abused need to be taken seriously and helped to describe the experience with age-appropriate words.
- Adolescent abuse often is caused by conflicts in parental regulation of adolescent behavior.
- Prevention of child abuse and neglect involves early identification of risk factors and family dysfunction, teaching about parenting skills, and referral to appropriate community supports to improve family functioning and prevent further dysfunction.
- Child abuse is against the law, and suspected cases are mandated by law to be reported.
- The nurse documents evidence of child abuse by noting and describing specifically parent and child behaviors.

- When a child abuse or neglect case is heard in court and the court finds that abuse or neglect has occurred, legal interventions might require changes in the family system, although family therapy often can reestablish family functioning.
- Because a parent's childhood experiences are a strong influence and often an indicator of that parent's parenting style, the nurse teaches and models parenting behaviors, especially to new parents who are at risk.
- Cases of child abuse and neglect are best managed by a multidisciplinary team consisting of nurses, other professionals, ancillary workers, and volunteers.
- In cases of suspected abuse, the nurse questions the child and the family members present about the circumstances of the child's injury and collects data through physical assessment and parent–child interviews.
- Each multidisciplinary team needs a coordinator, who charts the family's progress and monitors interventions by all professionals and agencies.
- In supporting dysfunctional parents, the nurse assesses and teaches adaptive coping strategies and refers the family to appropriate support services, which might include help with household tasks, family therapy or self-help groups, or foster care.
- Termination of parental rights to care for a child is always court ordered, a complicated moral decision, and a choice of last resort.
- Abused and neglected children need assistance in understanding that they have not caused the abuse or the changes occurring in the family system, and they often need to learn adaptive coping strategies to avoid dysfunctional behaviors.
- Adolescent parents are at high risk because of the stress of their own developmental needs, the physical risks of pregnancy for both the mother and infant, and the need for support from both family members and peers.
- Nursing care for adolescent parents involves teaching parenting and homemaking skills, assessing risk factors, explaining health care needs, and providing emotional support.
- In the violence-prone family, all family members are affected by the violent behavior; therefore, interventions should be directed at both victims and abusers.
- Multiproblem families are those who have lived with chronic difficulties in meeting the needs of family members and usually are known to many agencies; generally, they have little or no history of effective problem solving.

References

Adolescent Perinatal Health. The American College of Obstetricians and Gynecologists Task Force on Adolescent Pregnancy. American College of Obstetricians and Gynecologists, 1979.

American Nurses Association. A call for action on behalf of children. ANA Division of Maternal and Child Health Nursing Practice. Clark, A. chairperson. Publication No. MCH-11 ZM (March) 1980.

Ballard C: Reaching out to the community: Unique program prevents child abuse/neglect. *Pediatric Nursing* (Sept/Oct) 1975; 1:31–33.

Bandura A, Walters RH: *Adolescent Aggression.* Ronald Press, 1959.

Barnard M: Early detection of child abuse. Pages 280–292 in: *Family Health Care.* Hymovich, DP Barnard, MU (editors). McGraw-Hill, 1979.

Belsky J, Tolan W: The infant as producer of his environment: An ecological analysis. In: *The Child as Producer of Its Own Development: A Life-Span Perspective.* Lerner R, Busch-Rossnagel N (editors). Academic Press, 1981.

Belsky J, Lerner RM, Spanier GB: *The Child in the Family.* Addison-Wesley, 1984.

Belsky J, Robins E, Gamble W: The determinants of parenting: Toward a contextual theory. In: *Beyond the Dyad: Social Connections.* Lewis M, Rosenblum L (editors). Plenum, 1984.

Brodie B: Children: A glance at the past. *Am J Matern Child Nurs* (July/Aug) 1982; 7:219–225.

Campbell J: Nursing Care of Families Using Violence. In: *Nursing Care of Victims of Family Violence.* Campbell J, Humphreys J (editors). Reston, 1984.

Campbell J: Theories of Violence. *Nursing Care of Victims of Family Violence.* Campbell J, Humphreys J (editors). Reston, 1984.

Cannon-Bonventre K, Kalm J: Interviews with adolescent parents: Looking at their needs. *Child Today* 1979; 8:17–20.

Christensen ML, Schommer BL, Velasquez J: An interdisciplinary approach to preventing child abuse. *Am J Matern Child Nurs* (March/April) 1984; 9(2):108–112.

Coolsen P: Community involvement in the prevention of child abuse and neglect. *Child Today* 1980; 9(5):6.

Curto JJ: *How to Become a Single Parent.* Prentice-Hall, 1983.

Dean D: Emotional Abuse of Children. *Child Today* 1979; 8(4):18–20.

DeMayse L (editor): *The History of Childhood.* Harper & Row, 1974.

Densen-Gerber J, Hutchinson SF: Medical–legal and societal problems involving children—child prostitution, child pornography and drug-related abuse: Recommended legislation. In: *The Maltreatment of Children.* Smith SM (editor). University Park Press, 1978.

Dobash RE, Dobash R: *Violence Against Wives.* The Free Press, 1979.

Fanshel D, Shinn EG: *Children in Foster Care: A Longitudinal Investigation.* Columbia University Press, 1978.

Finley B: Nursing process with the battered woman. *Nurse Pract* (July/Aug) 1981; 29:11–13.

Fontana VJ: The diagnosis of the maltreatment syndrome in children. Symposium on child abuse. *Pediatrics* 1973 (Suppl) 511:781–792.

Funke J, Irby M: An instrument to assess the quality of maternal behavior. *J Gynecol Nurs* (Sept/Oct) 1978; 7:19–22.

George C, Main M: Social interactions of young abused children: Approach, avoidance, and aggression. *Child Dev* 1979; 50:306–318.

Giarretto H: The treatment of father–daughter incest: A psychosocial approach. *Child Today* 1976; 5(4):2–5.

Gil DG: A holistic perspective on child abuse and its prevention. *J Sociol Soc Welfare* 1974; 2:110–125.

Gorline LL, Ray MM: Examining and Caring for the child who has been sexually assaulted. *Am J Matern Child Nurs* (March/April) 1979; 4(2):110–114.

Greenspan S: Developmental morbidity in infants in multi-risk–factor families: Clinical perspectives. *Public Health Rep* 1982; 97(1):16–23.

Harrison LL: Nursing intervention with the failure to thrive family. *Am J Matern Child Nurs* (March/April) 1976; 1:111–116.

Haapala D, Kinney J: Homebuilder's approach to the training of in-home therapists. In: *Home-based services for children and families: Policy, practice, and research.* Maybanks S, Bryce M (editors). Thomas, 1979.

Haynes U: *A Developmental Approach to Case Finding.* US Department of Health, Education, and Welfare. DHEW Publication no (USA) 77–5210. Government Printing Office, 1980.

Hecht M: Children of alcoholics are children of risk. *Am J Nurs* (Oct) 1973;1764–1766.

Heindl C, et al: *The Nurse's Role in the Prevention and Treatment of Child Abuse and Neglect.* US Department of Health, Education, and Welfare. DHEW Publication no (OHDS) 79–30202. Government Printing Office, 1979.

Heins M: The "battered child" revisited. *JAMA* 1984; 251(24):3295–3298.

Helberg JL: Documentation in child abuse. *Am J Nurs* (Feb) 1983; 83(2):236–239.

Helfer RE, Kempe CH: *Child Abuse and Neglect: The Family and the Community.* Ballinger, 1976.

Hollen P, Carroll JF, Carpenter C: The pediatric home liaison in a private practice. *Pediatr Nurs* (May/June) 1980; 6:25–27.

Howell DA: The sensitive teacher. In: *Children Alone.* Thomas MA (editor). Council for Exceptional Children, 1977.

Humphreys J: Child abuse. In: *Nursing Care of Victims of Family Violence.* Campbell J, Humphreys J (editors). Reston, 1984.

Humphreys J: Nursing care of abused children. In: *Nursing Care of Victims of Family Violence.* Campbell J, Humphreys J (editors). Reston, 1984.

Hurd J: Assessing maternal attachment. First step toward the prevention of child abuse. *J Gynecol Nurs* (July/Aug) 1975; 4:25–30.

Iyer PW: The battered wife. *Nursing '80* (July), 1980; 10(7):53–55.

Johnson SH: *High-Risk Parenting: Nursing Assessment and Strategies for the Family at Risk.* Lippincott, 1979.

Josten L: Out-of-hospital care for a pervasive family problem—child abuse. *Am J Matern Child Nurs* (March/April) 1978; 3(2):111–116.

Justice B, Justice R: *The Abusing Family.* Human Sciences Press, 1976.

Justice B, Justice R: *The Broken Taboo.* Human Sciences Press, 1979.

Kempe CH: A practical approach to the protection of the abused child and rehabilitation of the abusing parent. *Pediatrics* (April) 1973; 51(4):804–808.

Kempe CH: Sexual abuse, another hidden pediatric problem. *Pediatrics* (Sept) 1978; 62(3):382–389.

Kempe CH, Helfer RE (editors): *Child Abuse and Neglect. The Family and the Community.* Ballinger, 1976.

Kempe CH, Helfer RE: *Helping the Battered Child and His Family.* Lippincott, 1972.

Kempe RS, Kempe CH: *Child Abuse.* Harvard University Press, 1978.

Lester D: A cross-culture study of wife abuse. *Aggressive Behav* 1980; 6:361–364.

Liebnerknecht K: Helping the battered wife. *Am J Nurs* (April) 1978; 78(4):654–656.

Lieske AM: Incest: An overview. *Perspect Psychiatr Care* (March/April) 1981; 19(2):59–63.

Lourie IS, et al: Adolescent abuse and neglect: The role of runaway youth programs. *Child Today* 1979; 8(6):27–40.

Luckey EB, Bain JK: Children: A factor in marital satisfaction. *J Marriage Fam* 1970; 32:621–626.

Lustig N, et al: Incest: A family group survival pattern. *Arch Gen Psychiatry* 1966; 14:31–40.

McKittrick CA: Child abuse: Recognition and reporting by health professionals. *Nurs Clin North Am*(March) 1981; 16:103–115.

Medical News (editorial). *JAMA* 1984; 251(24):3201–3207.

Meiselman KC: Incest. In: *A Psychological Study of Causes and Effects with Treatment Recommendations.* Jossey-Bass, 1978.

Milner J, Wimberly R: An inventory for the identification of child abusers. *J Clin Psychol* 1979; 35(1):95–96.

Mitchell CE: The drug abusing parent. In: *High-Risk Parenting: Nursing Assessment and Strategies for the Family at Risk.* Johnson SH (editor). Lippincott, 1979.

Munro JU: The nurse and the legal system: Dealing with abused children. In: *Nursing Care of Victims of Family Violence.* Campbell J, Humphreys J (editors). Reston, 1984.

Newberger EN, et al: Pediatric social illness: Toward and etiologic classification. *Pediatrics* (Feb) 1977; 60(2):178–185.

Nix H: Why Parents Anonymous? *J Psychiatr Nurs* (Oct) 1980; 18:23–28.

Olweus D: Familial and temperamental determinants of aggressive behavior in adolescent boys: A causal analysis. *Dev Psychol* 1980; 16:644–660.

Ounstead C, Lynch M: Family pathology as seen in England. In: *Child Abuse and Neglect. The Family and the Community.* Helfer RE, Kempe CH (editors). Ballinger, 1976.

Pedersen F, Anderson B, Cain L: *An Approach to Understanding Linkages Between the Parent–Infant and Spouse Relationships.* Paper presented at the biennial meeting of the Society for Research in Child Development, New Orleans, March, 1977.

Pelton LN (editor): *The Social Context of Child Abuse and Neglect.* Human Sciences Press, 1981.

Polansky NA, Hally C, Polansky NF: *Profiles of Neglect: A Survey of the State of Knowledge of Child Neglect.* US Department of Health, Education, and Welfare. DHEW Publication no (SRS) 76–23037. Government Printing Office, 1976.

Poznanski E, Blos P: Incest. *Medical Aspects of Human Sexuality* (Oct) 1975; 9:46–76.

Reed J: Working with abusive parents—a parent's view. *Child Today* 1975; 4(3):6–9.

Ruger J, Wooten R: A developmental approach to helping families at risk. *Soc Casework* 1982; 63:3–14.

Santrock JW, et al: Children's and parent's observed social behavior in stepfather families. *Child Dev* 1982; 53:472–480.

Sgroi SM: *Handbook of Clinical Intervention in Child Sexual Abuse.* Lexington Books, 1982.

Smith JB: Care of the hospitalized abused child and family. *Nurs Clin North Am* (March) 1981; 16:127–137.

Star B: Patterns in family violence. *Soc Casework J Contemp Soc Work*

1980; 61:339–347.

Steele BF: Psychodynamic factors in child abuse. In: *The Battered Child.* Kempe CH, Helfer RE (editors). University of Chicago Press, 1980.

Steele BF: Violence within the family. In: *Child Abuse and Neglect. The Family and the Community.* Helfer RE, Kempe CH (editors). Ballinger, 1976.

Steele BF: Working with abusive parents—a psychiatrist's view. *Child Today* 1975; 4(3):3–6.

Stephenson C: Non-organic failure to thrive. *Nurse Pract* (May/June) 1980; 5:16–23.

Stewart R: The family that fails to thrive. In: *Family Health Care.* Hymovich DP, Barnard MU (editors). McGraw-Hill, 1973.

Sullivan C: *Child Abuse in Relation to Chemical Dependency and Antisocial Behavior—Study Presented at the Fifth National Conference on Child Abuse in Milwaukee.* Eden House, 1981.

Sung BL: Families without parents. In: *National Center for Child Abuse and Neglect.* Special Issue. *Child Abuse, Neglect and the Family Within a Cultural Context.* US Department of Health, Education, and Welfare. DHEW Publication no (OHDS) 78–30135. Government Printing Office, 1978.

Tankson EA: The single parent. In: *High-Risk Parenting: Nursing Assessment and Strategies for the Family at Risk.* Johnson SH (editor). Lippincott, 1979.

Tapia J: Fractionalization of the family. In: *The Process of Human Development: A Holistic Approach.* Schuster C (editor). Little, Brown, 1980.

Ten Bensel RW, Berdie J: The neglect and abuse of children and youth: The scope of the problem and the school's role. *J School Health* 1976; 46(8):453–461.

Wheat P: *The Standoffs—A Story About Touching.* Parents Anonymous Booklet, 1980.

Wiltse KT: Current issues and new directions in foster care. In: *Child Welfare strategy in the coming years.* DHEW Publication no (OHDS) 78–30158, 1978.

Yoos L: Taking another look at failure to thrive. *Am J Matern Child Nurs* (Jan/Feb) 1984; 9(1):32–36.

Additional Readings

Aguilera DD, Messick JM: *Crisis Intervention Theory and Methodology.* Mosby, 1982.

Ainsworth M: *Public Health Paper 14, The Effects of Maternal Deprivation.* World Health Organization, 1962.

Anderson G: Enhancing listening skills. For work with abusing parents. *Soc Casework J Contemp Soc Work* (Dec) 1979; 60:602–608.

Ayoub C, Pfeifer DR: An approach to primary prevention: The "At-Risk" Program. *Child Today* 1977; 6(3):14–17.

Bakan D: *Slaughter of the Innocents: A Study of the Battered Child Phenomenon.* Beacon Press, 1972.

Berdie J, Bauzerman M, Lourie I: Violence towards youth: Themes from a workshop. *Child Today* 1977; 6(2):7–35.

Berkan WA: Co-parenting: An outgrowth of a boarding home program for handicapped children. *Child Today* 1979; 8(4):10–12.

Besharov D: Building a community response to child abuse and maltreatment. *Child Today* 1975; 4(5):2–4.

Bishop B: A guide to assessing parenting capabilities. *Am J Nurs* (Nov) 1976; 76:1784–1787.

Bloch J: Impaired children. *Child Today* 1978; 7:3.

Bonney A, Rowe LH: FACES aids formerly abused young adults. *Caring* 1983; 8(3):3–5.

Braden JA: Adopting the abused child: Love is not enough. *Soc Casework J Contemp Soc Work* 1981; 62:362–367.

Brady K: *Father's Days. A True Story of Incest.* Dell Publishing, 1979.

Brazelton TB: Reaching out to new parents. *Child Today* 1978; 7(4):27.

Broadhurst D: Project protection: A school program to detect and prevent child abuse and neglect. *Child Today* 1975; 4(3):22–25.

Broadhurst D: Update—what schools are doing about child abuse and neglect. *Child Today* 1978; 7(1):22–36.

Broek E: Protecting the family: A California act. *Child Today* 1981; 10(1):7–11.

Brown MS, Hurlock JT: Mothering the mother. *Am J Nurs* (March) 1977; (77)3:439–441.

Bruckman P, Ferguson L: Two steps forward and one back—familial patterns of child abuse *Can Nurse* (May) 1981; 77:29–34.

Burgess AW, McCausland MP, Wolbert WA: Children's drawings as indicators of sexual trauma. *Perspect Psychiatr Care* 1981; 19(2):50–58.

Burgess AW, et al: *Sexual Assault of Children and Adolescents.* Lexington Books, 1982.

Butler S: *Conspiracy of Silence: The Trauma of Incest.* Bantam Books, 1979.

Caffey J: Multiple fractures in the long bones of infants suffering from chronic subdural hematoma. *Am J Roentgenol Radium Ther Nucl Med* 1946; 56:163–167.

Caffey J: On the theory and practice of shaking infants. *Am J Dis Child* 1972; 124:161–169.

Caffey J: The whiplash shaken infant syndrome. *Pediatrics* (Oct) 1974; 54:396–403.

Cain LP: Child abuse: Historical precedent and legal ramifications. *Health Soc Work* 1980; 5(3):61–67.

Calaway B: Contracting: A means of clarifying roles in foster family services. *Child Today* 1976; 5(4):20–23.

Cantwell H: Child Neglect. In: *The Battered Child.* Kempe CH, Helfer RE (editors). University of Chicago Press, 1980.

Carmody FJ, Lanier, D, Bardill DR: Prevention of child abuse and neglect in military families. *Child Today* 1979; 8:16–35.

The child-beaters: Sick, but curable. *The National Observer.* March 24, 1973.

Clark A: Recognizing discord between mother and child and changing it to harmony. *Matern Child Nurs J* (March/April) 1976; 1:100–106.

Cohn AH, Ridge S, Collignon FC: Evaluating innovative treatment programs in child abuse and neglect. *Child Today* 1975; 4(3):10–12.

Combs J: An information system that measures foster casework effectiveness. *Child Today* 1979; 8(3):15–36.

Copans S, et al: The stresses of treating child abuse. *Child Today* 1979; 8(1):22–25.

Corey E, Miller C, Widlak F: Factors contributing to child abuse. *Nurs Res* (July/Aug) 1975; 24(4):293–295.

Cornwell G: Scapegoating: A study in family dynamics *Am J Nurs* (Sept) 1967; 1862–1867.

Critchley DL: Therapeutic group work with abused preschool children. *Perspect Psychiatr Care* 1982; 20(2):79–85.

Daniel JH, Hyde J: Working with high-risk families: Family advocacy and the parent education program. *Child Today* 1975; 4:23–36.

Davidson HA: The guardian ad litem: An important approach to the protection of children. *Child Today* 1981; 10(2):20–23.

Davis DL, Johnson GH: A way of caring. *AORN J* (March) 1978; 27(4):631–635.

Davoreen E: Foster placement of abused children. *Child Today* 1975; 4(3):41.

Davoreen E: Working with abusive parents—a social worker's view. *Child Today* 1975; 4(3):2–8.

Drydyk J, Menerville B, Bender L: Foster parenting a retarded child. The Arizona story. *Child Today* 1980; 9:10–24.

Edelson E: It's the parent who needs help. *Fam Health* 1970; 2(7):15–17.

Elbow M: Children of violent marriages: The forgotten victims. *Soc Casework J Contemp Soc Work* 1982; 63:465–471.

Ferro F: Combating child abuse and neglect. *Child Today* 1975; 4:1.

Fitzpatrick L: A team approach to child abuse. *Can Nurse* (Jan) 1979; 75(1):36–41.

Flanzraich M, Dunsavage I: Role reversal in abused/neglected families: Implications for child welfare workers. *Child Today* 1977; 6(6):13–36.

Foster, PH, Lanier MW, Whitworth JM: Expanding the role of nurses in child abuse prevention and treatment. *J Psychiatr Nurs* 1980; 18(2):24–28.

Fox GL: The family's influence on adolescent sexual behavior. *Child Today* 1979; 8(3):21–36.

Fraley Y: The family support center: Early intervention for high-risk parents and children. *Child Today* 1983; 12:13–17.

Funke-Furber J, Roemar C: Failure to thrive, *Can Nurs* (Dec) 1978;30–34.

Gallaway B: Contracting: A means of clarifying roles in foster family services. *Child Today* 1976; 5(4):20–23.

Geiser R: *Hidden Victims*. Beacon Press, 1979.

Gelles RJ: Child abuse as psychopathology: A sociological critique and reformulation. *Am J Orthopsychiatry* 1973; 43(4):611–621.

Gentry R, Brisbane F: The solution for child abuse rests with the community. *Child Today* 1982; 11:22–25.

Gill D, Bogart K: Foster children speak out: A study of children's perceptions of foster care. *Child Today* 1982; 11:7–9.

Gillette E: Child abuse. *J Nurs Care* (Dec) 1978; 11:12–32.

Greany GD: Is she a battered woman? *Am J Nurs* 1984; 84(6):725–727.

Groth AN: Patterns of sexual assault against children and adolescents. In: *Sexual Assault of Children and Adolescents*. Burgess AW, et al (editors). Lexington Books, 1982.

Hall M, de la Cruz A, Russel P: Working with neglected families. *Child Today* 1982; 2(2):6–36.

Harling P, Haines J: Specialized foster homes for severely mistreated children. *Child Today* 1980; 9:16–18.

Hayes P: The long-term treatment of victims of child abuse. *Nurs Clin North Am* (March) 1981; 16:139–147.

Heindl MC (editor): Symposium on Child Abuse and Neglect—Foreward. *Nurs Clin North Am* (March) 1981; 16:101.

Heindl MC: Who is the victim? *Nurs Clin North Am* (March) 1981; 16:117–125.

Helfer RE: *Childhood Comes First: A Crash Course in Childhood for Adults*. R.E. Helfer, 1978.

Helfer RE: Why most physicians don't get involved in child abuse cases and what to do about it. *Child Today* 1975; 4(3):28–32.

Hendrix M: Home is where the hell is. *Fam Community Health* 1981; 4(2):54–63.

Hindman M: Child abuse and neglect: The alcohol connection. *Alcohol Health Res World* (Spring) 1977; 5:2–7.

Hornby H: Foster care and the power of the state. *Child Today* 1981; 10(2):2–31.

Horton TE: Conceptual basis for nursing intervention with human systems; Families. In: *Distributive Nursing Practice: A Systems Approach to Community Health*. Hall JE, Weaver BR (editors). Lippincott, 1977.

Howard J: *Families*. Simon & Schuster, 1978.

Hurwitz A: Child abuse: A program for intervention. *Nurs Outlook* (Sept) 1977; 25:575–577.

Jackson PL, Runyon N: Caring for children from divorced families. *Am J Matern Child Nurs* (March/April) 1983; 8(2)126–130.

Jacobson DS: Step-families. *Child Today* 1980; 9(1):2–6.

Johnson SH: The family in transition: A judicial overview of changing sex roles. *Child Today* 1980; 9(4):7–9.

Johnston K: Maintaining the family unit. In: *The Process of Human Development–A Holistic Approach*. Schuster CS, Ashburn SS (editors). Little, Brown, 1980.

Jones M: Finding permanent homes for children in foster care: A do-it-yourself approach. *Child Today* 1979; 8(2):8–36.

Jordan FB: Recognizing child maltreatment syndrome. *AORN J* (March) 1978; 27(4):636–641.

Kamerman SB: Eight countries: Cross-national perspectives on child abuse and neglect. *Child Today* 1975; 4(3):34–37.

Kauffman CK, Neill MK: The abusive parent. In: *High-Risk Parenting: Nursing Assessment and Strategies For the Family at Risk*. Johnson SH (editor). Lippincott, 1979.

Kempe CH: Approaches to preventing child abuse. The health visitors concept. *Am J Dis Child* 1976; 130:940–945.

Kempe CH, Helfer RS: *The Battered Child*. The University of Chicago Press, 1980.

Kinney J: Home builders: An in-home crisis intervention program. *Child Today* 1978; 15–35.

Kittrell E: In defense of children. *Child Today* 1977; 6(1):28–29.

Kline DA: The consequences of neglected cases. In: *Children Alone*. Thomas M (editor). Council for Exceptional Children, 1977.

Kufeldt K: Including natural parents in temporary foster care: An exploratory study. *Child Today* 1982; 11(5):14–16.

Leaman K: The sexually abused child. *Nursing '77* (May) 1977; 7:68–72.

Leaman K: Recognizing and helping the abused child. *Nursing '79* (Feb) 1979; 9:64–67.

Ledray L: Victims of incest. *Am J Nurs* 1984, 84(8):1010–1014.

Lende E, Gilmore E, Cavenaugh N: Vivamos! A summer program for teenage parents. *Child Today* (Sept/Oct) 1980; 9:9–12.

Levenson P, et al: Serving teenage mothers and their high-risk infants. *Child Today* 1978; 7:11–36.

Levy B, et al: Failure to thrive and subsequent child abuse. *Health Values* 1981; 5:187–191.

Ludwig S: A multidisciplinary approach to child abuse. *Nurs Clin North Am* (March) 1981; 16(1):162–165.

Marder J: Skills for helping others to redirect emotional response. *AORN J.* (Oct) 1981; 34(4):658–671.

Marland S: Education for parenthood. *Child Today* 1973; 2(2):3–7.

McFadden E: Fostering the battered and abused child. *Child Today* 1980; 2:13.

McKeel NL: Child abuse can be prevented. *Am J Nurs* (Sept) 1978; 78(9):1478–1482.

McPherson KS, Garcia L: Effects of social class and familiarity on pediatrician's responses to child abuse. *Child Welfare* 1983; 62(5):387–393.

Miller DL, Baird SL: Helping parents to be parents—a special center. *Matern Child Nurs J* (March/April) 1978; 3:117–120.

Millor GK: A theoretical framework for nursing research in child abuse and neglect. *Nurs Res* (March/April) 1981; 30(2):78–83.

Mira M, Cairns G: Intervention in the interaction of a mother and child with nonorganic failure to thrive. *Pediatr Nurs* (March/April) 1981; 7(2):41–45.

Moore DA, Hofferth SL, Wertheimer R: Teenage motherhood—its social and economic costs. *Child Today* 1979; 8(5):12–16.

Nage SZ: Child abuse and neglect programs: A national overview. *Child Today* 1975; 4(3):13–17.

Newberger EH (editor): *Child Abuse*. Little, Brown, 1982.

Newberger EH: When the injury is a symptom: Interrelations among the pediatric social illnesses. In: *Minimizing High-Risk Parenting*. Johnson & Johnson Baby Products, 1983.

Newberger EH, Daniel JH: Knowledge and epidemiology of child abuse: A critical review of concepts. *Pediatr Ann* 1976; 5(3):140–144.

Nover RA, Williams DW, Ward DB: Preventive Intervention with infants in multi-risk–factor families. *Child Today* 1981; 10:27–31.

Olson RJ: Index of suspicion: Screening for child abusers. *Am J Nurs* (Jan) 1976; 76:108–110.

Ortman E: Attachment Behaviors in Abused Children. *Pediatr Nurs* (July/August) 1979; 5:25–29.

Ory MG, Earp JL: Child maltreatment and the use of social services. *Public Health Rep* 1978; 96:238–245.

Papalia DE, Olds SW: *A Child's World: Infancy Through Adolescence.* McGraw-Hill, 1982.

Pavenstedt E: To help infants weather disorganized family life. *Am J Nurs* 1969; 69(8):1668–1673.

Pelton LH: Child abuse and neglect: The myth of classlessness. *Am J Orthopsychiatry* 1978; 48(4):608–617.

Perozzi W: Speaking out for their rights—the Illinois Foster Children's Association. *Child Today* 1977; 6:16–34.

Ramey C, Gowen J: Children at risk: Identification and intervention. *Child Today* 1980; 9:12–16.

Rogers DE: *Hear the Children Crying.* Fleming H. Revell, 1978.

Rosenfeld A, Newberger E: Compassion vs. control—conceptual and practical pitfalls in the broadened definition of child abuse. *JAMA* 1977; 237(19):2086–2088.

Rosenkrantz L, Joshua V: Children of incarcerated parents: A hidden population. *Child Today* 1982; 11:2–6.

Sahin S: Physically disabled child. In: *High-Risk Parenting: Nursing Assessment and Strategies for the Family at Risk.* Lippincott, 1979.

Salguero C: Adolescent pregnancy: A report on ACYF-funded research and demonstration projects. *Child Today* 1980; 9:10–35.

Scharer KM: Nursing therapy with abusive and neglectful families. *J Psychiatr Nurs* (Sept) 1979; 17:12–21.

Scharer KM: Rescue fantasies: Professional impediments in working with abused families. *Am J Nurs* (Sept) 1978; 78(9):1483–1484.

Schroeder E: The birth of a defective child: A cause for grieving. In: *Nursing of Families in Crisis.* Hall JE, Weaver BR (editors). Lippincott, 1974.

Schuster C: The family with a disabled child. In: *The Process of Human Development. A Holistic Approach.* Little, Brown, 1980.

Seefeldt C: Young and old together. *Child Today* 1977; 6(1):21–25.

Sherwen LN: Alternative parenting patterns: Clinical implications. *Top Clin Nurs* (Oct) 1984; 6(3) [Entire issue].

Shoop L: Education for parenthood—living laboratories. *Child Today* 1979; 6:23–26.

Shorkey CT: A review of methods used in the treatment of abusing parents. *Soc Casework J Contemp Soc Work* 1979; 60:360–367.

Star B: Comparing battered and non-battered women. *Victimology* 1978; 3:37–39.

Sugar M (editor): *Adolescent Parenthood.* SP Medical and Scientific Books, 1984.

Sussman MB: The family today—is it an endangered species? *Child Today* 1978; 2:32.

Sze WC, Lamar B: Causes of child abuse: A reexamination. *Health Soc Work* 1981; 6:19–25.

Tagg P: Nursing intervention for the abused child and his family. *Pediatr Nurs* (Sept/Oct) 1976; 2(5):36–39.

Thistleton KE: The abusive and neglectful parent: Treatment through parent education. *Nurs Clin North Am* (Sept) 1977; 12(3):513–523.

Thomas JN: Yes, you can help a sexually abused child. *RN* (August) 1980; 43:23–29.

Thomas JN, Rogers CM: Sexual abuse of children: Case findings and clinical assessment. *Nurs Clin North Am* (March) 1981; 16:179–188.

Velasquez J, Christensen ML, Schommer BL: Intensive services help prevent child abuse. *Am J Matern Child Nurs* (March/April) 1984; 9(2):113–117.

Weinbach R, Edwards M, Levy R: Innovations in group services to foster parents: A survey of agencies. *Child Today* 1977; 1:18–20.

Weissbourd B, Grimm C: Family focus—supporting families in the community. *Child Today* 1981; (2):6–11.

Whiting L: A community multidisciplinary child protection team. *Child Today* 1977; 6(1):10–12.

Whiting L: Defining emotional neglect. *Child Today* 1976; 5:2–5.

Williams GJ, Money J: *Traumatic Abuse and Neglect of Children At Home.* The Johns Hopkins University Press, 1980.

Nursing Care of the Child With a Mental Deficiency

23

Marva Mizell Price

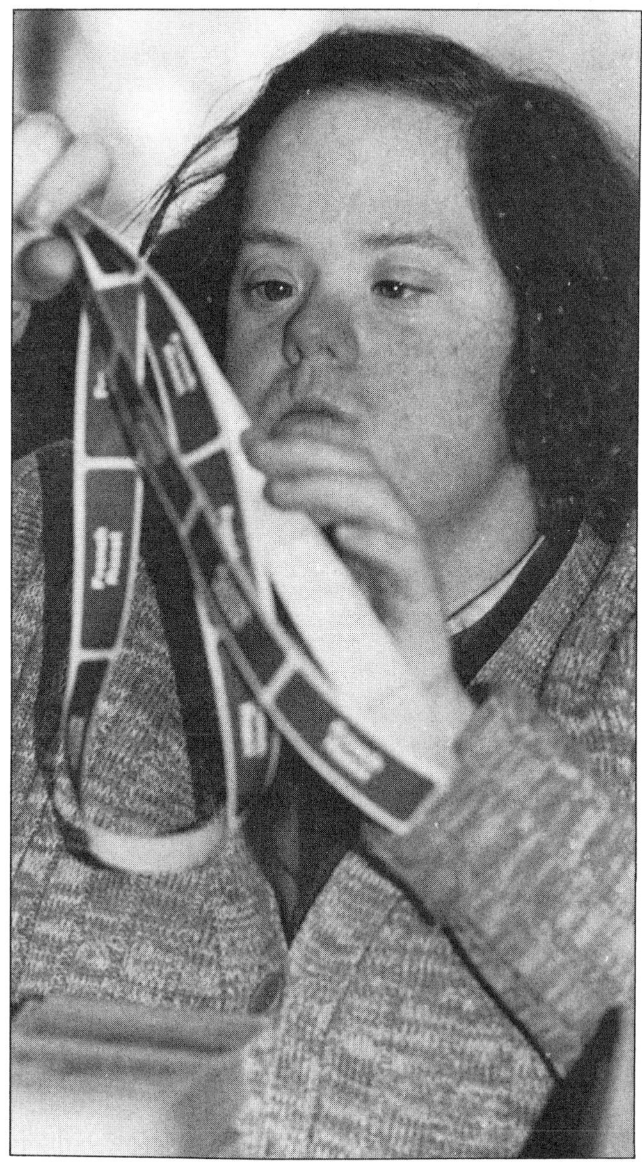

Chapter Outline

Objectives

- Distinguish between developmental disability and mental retardation.
- Define the terms used to classify retarded people.
- Describe the possible prenatal, perinatal, and postnatal causes of mental retardation.
- Describe methods used for diagnosing mental retardation.
- Describe common parental responses to a diagnosis of mental retardation in both infants and older children.
- Explain the effects of retardation on parent–infant attachment and on members of the family system.
- Explain the role of the nurse in both primary and secondary prevention of developmental disabilities.
- Delineate areas of concern that are likely to require parent teaching.
- List issues that are likely concerns in the care of mentally retarded children.
- Describe nursing goals related to nutrition, sexuality, toilet training, behavior and modification, health promotion, and independence, with regard to the developmentally disabled.
- Explain the role of the child health nurse in caring for the developmentally disabled child in the hospital and school settings.

To find these topics, see the following chapters

Hyperactivity	Chapter 42
Learning Disorders	Chapter 42
Neurologic Impairments	Chapter 42

Although mental retardation probably has been a concern in many societies throughout history, documented progress in addressing the needs of the developmentally disabled dates back only 200 years. Nursing, as a separate and unique profession, became recognized at about the same time that revolutionary trends occurred in diagnosing and treating the mentally retarded. Throughout the nineteenth century health care in the United States came to encompass institutions created to treat individuals with mental limitations. By the end of the nineteenth century, mental retardation was becoming differentiated from mental illness. Today our growing sophistication in nursing distinguishes our work on all levels of care for mentally retarded children.

In this chapter we describe the nurse's role in caring for the retarded child. Care for the child with any kind of developmental disability is often multidisciplinary and long-term. Specific nursing interventions vary according to the subsystems that determine the child's level of functioning. Mental retardation is often accompanied by neurologic impairment that interferes with the child's achieving independence in self-care. (Nursing care for the child with neurologic disorders is discussed in Chapter 42. Nursing care common to all chronic conditions is discussed in Chapter 30.)

Like other aspects of child health nursing, care for retarded children involves an analysis of the suprasystems that influence the child. For the retarded child these influences depend on the child's family, the setting in which the child lives, and the extent of the child's socialization.

Developmental Disabilities and Mental Retardation

At the end of the nineteenth century the definition for mental retardation was divided into categories based on defects occurring early in development, diseases of the nervous system, and the presence of low intelligence. Labels included moron, imbecile, idiot, feeble-mindedness, mental subnormality, mental deficiency, and oligophrenia (Scheerenberger, 1983). Current diagnostic criteria now delineate specific functional deficits in addition to mental functioning. Thus current trends include mental retardation as part of the larger category *developmental disabilities.*

The Developmentally Disabled Assistance and Bill of Rights Act of 1978 defined a developmental disability as a severe and chronic state that is

1. Attributable to a mental or physical impairment or combination of mental and physical impairments
2. Manifested before the age of 22
3. Likely to continue indefinitely
4. Evident in substantial functional limitations in three or more of the following areas of major life activities: (a) self-care; (b) receptive and expressive language; (c) learning; (d) mobility; (e) self-direction; (f) capacity for independent living; and (g) economic self-sufficiency
5. Reflected in the person's need for a combination and sequence of individually planned and coordinated multi-

disciplinary, or generic care; treatment; or other services of lifelong or extended duration (Payne and Patton, 1981).

Although some health and education professionals use developmental disability and mental retardation interchangeably, mental retardation actually is a part of the broad spectrum of developmental disability. The mental impairment associated with any compromised functioning, however, has come to be associated with mental retardation, but this is only a partial definition. The official definition published by the American Association of Mental Deficiency (AAMD) is

> Mental retardation refers to significantly subaverage, general intellectual functioning existing concurrently with deficits in adaptive behavior and manifested during the developmental period. The developmental period extends to approximately 18 years of age (Grossman, 1983).

Thus a diagnosis of mental retardation cannot be based on low intelligence alone but is also determined by the individual's capacity to adapt behaviorally to the environment (Fig. 23-1).

Thompson and O'Quinn (1979) make a further distinction between a developmental delay and a developmental deficit or disorder:

> When an aspect of functioning is not demonstrated by a child when the majority of children of similar age demonstrate it, the child is considered to exhibit a developmental delay or developmental disorder. If the system in question appears to be intact and not damaged, the discrepancy between functioning level and expectancy may reflect a slowness in rate of development (i.e., developmental delay). If the system is functioning appropriately, the discrepancy in functioning may reflect a developmental disorder. For example, an infant may be demonstrating a developmental delay in the motor area if he is not sitting at nine months of age. Later it may be determined that the motor problem is not a delay but a deficit or disorder such as cerebral palsy, which significantly hampers functioning throughout life and constitutes a developmental disability.

Adaptive behavior	Measured intellectual functioning: Retarded	Measured intellectual functioning: Not retarded
Retarded	Mentally Retarded	NOT mentally retarded
Not retarded	NOT mentally retarded	NOT mentally retarded

Figure 23-1 Classification based on measured intellectual functioning and adaptive behavior. A child is classified as retarded only if the level of intellectual functioning and degree of adaptive behavior are both impaired. (From Grossman HJ (Ed), (1983), *Classifications in Mental Retardation*. Washington, DC: American Association on Mental Deficiency, p. 12. Reprinted with permission.

Thomas and O'Quinn's conceptual scheme shows multiple interacting factors that may result in a developmental disability (Fig. 23-2).

Classification of Mental Retardation

A classification system for mental retardation was used in the eighteenth century by J. Langdon Down. It was a medical classification system that categorized idiots, the feebleminded, and imbeciles, together with ethnic subgroups, one of which was the "mongoloid," a label that lasted into the twentieth century. Mongolism, which was once a stigmatizing label, was eventually renamed Down's syndrome, and the classification system Down created is no longer used.

The 1983 AAMD classification system developed by the AAMD Committee on Terminology and Classification reflects current efforts in proper terminology to identify developmental disabilities and mental retardation. This system is consistent with the International Classification of Diseases-9 (ICD-9) of the World Health Organization and the American Psychiatric Association's Diagnostic and Statistical Manual III (DSM III). The categories and their corresponding ranges are as follows:

Term	*IQ Range*
Mild mental retardation	50–55 to approximately 70
Moderate mental retardation	35–40 to 50–55
Severe mental retardation	20–25 to 35–40
Profound mental retardation	Below 20 or 25

The category of borderline intelligence (a 70–84 IQ) was once included but has been eliminated to avoid classifying among the mentally retarded those individuals whose dysfunction might be caused by socioeconomic deprivation.

Children in the mild category are estimated to comprise 75%–90% of the retarded population and are termed "educable" in the educational system. They are expected to learn to read, write, and do basic computations up to a third- to sixth-grade level. Estimates of the number of moderately retarded people range from as low as 6% to as high as 17%–21% (Thain, 1980; Blackman, 1983) of the mentally retarded population. They can learn to care for themselves, develop social skills, and perform simple routine tasks. They rarely learn to read and write but can recognize important words and do basic counting. A program of training throughout childhood might enable a moderately retarded person to participate in structured employment such as a sheltered workshop. Moderately retarded adults

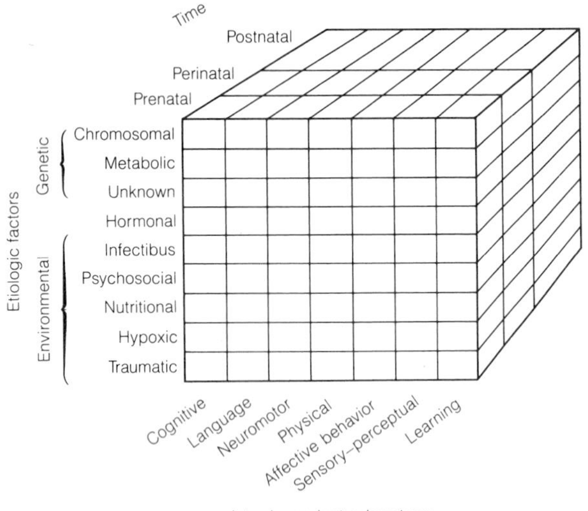

Figure 23-2 Interacting factors that can lead to developmental disabilities. Depicted as a cube, manifestations of developmental disabilities are a result of etiologic factors and developmental subsystems interacting during a period of time. (From Thompson RJ, O'Quinn AN: *Developmental Disabilities: Etiologies, Manifestations, Diagnoses, and Treatments.* Oxford University Press, 1979.)

might be able to live in communities in group homes, or individual households with varying degrees of supervision.

Severely retarded children frequently have detectable disabilities at birth, including physical handicaps. The nurse therefore is valuable in providing support to the parents at this time. (Chapter 30 describes the impact of the diagnosis of a chronic condition.) In addition to extremely low cognitive functioning, these children have minimal adaptive skills. Some learn to walk and acquire language skills. Most learn adaptive skills and are trainable to varying degrees.

Profoundly retarded children require ongoing nursing care to improve disabilities, prevent further difficulties, and maintain life. Many of these children develop life-threatening illnesses and die early in life from complicating illnesses. Profoundly retarded children acquire varying degrees of limited motor and self-help skills. They need general care as well as protection. The severely and profoundly retarded comprise about 4% of the retarded population.

Etiology of Mental Retardation

Factors related to mental retardation closely parallel the social, economic, and health status of a society and the resources available for education, development, and employment. The incidence of mental retardation therefore is higher in countries lacking mass immunization programs, proper nutrition, hygiene and safe environment, and public health services for pregnant women and children. The incidence of mental retardation in the United States is generally estimated at about 125,000 births per year. The most widely quoted figure is 3% of the general population, or more than 6 million people.

More than 200 causes of mental retardation are known, and new inborn errors of metabolism and other genetic diseases continue to be identified. For child health nurses, however, more than 75% of the retarded children with whom they work have no definitive medical diagnosis or defect. Current knowledge about the role of prenatal, perinatal, and postnatal influences on mental function therefore can assist in identifying children at risk and providing preventive health care.

Prenatal Causes Prenatal influences on the developing embryo start during the critical period, before a woman usually knows she is pregnant. Prenatal causes of mental retardation are largely genetic and environmental factors. (The role of genetics in development is discussed in Chapter 5.) During the first 12 weeks of pregnancy, the central nervous system undergoes morphogenesis. Some teratogens, such as the anticonvulsant phenytoin (Dilantin) or exposure of the fetus to excessively high temperatures from maternal infection or sauna baths have been associated with mental retardation.

During this postconceptual period a woman is susceptible to a small group of infections and hereditary influences. Early prenatal infections include pathogens such as toxoplasmosis, rubella, and cytomegalic inclusion disease, and herpes simplex type II, which causes damage around the time of birth. These are known as the TORCH infections and can cause multiple deformities. Toxoplasmosis, contracted from the feces of infected hunting cats, produces severe problems that are present at birth.

Therapeutic radiographs and exposure to severely high dosages of radiation are threats to the fetus in the prenatal period. Some maternal intoxicants, including street drugs and industrial and environmental chemicals, have been shown to have varying teratogenic effects on the fetus. A pregnant woman who works in a battery-manufacturing plant, for example, might receive excessive lead exposure leading to lead intoxication in the fetus. Recently, extensive research has been conducted on the effects of lysergic acid diethylamide (LSD), cigarettes, caffeine, and alcohol.

Little is known about the long-term effects of anorexia nervosa on the fetus. Emphasis is increasingly being placed on preconceptual nutrition, however, because critical periods of brain development occur before many women have their pregnancies diagnosed and begin prenatal care with improved diets.

Conditions occurring prenatally with no definite etiology are categorized as conditions of unknown prenatal influence. Among these are malformations of the cranium, cerebrum, cerebellum, and face. Well-known conditions in this category are anencephaly, primary microcephaly, macroencephaly, and congenital hydrocephalus. Meningoencephalocele and myelomeningocele are neural tube defects resulting from failure of fusion in development of the central nervous system (see Chapter 42). Neural tube defects are detectable through prenatal screening.

Metabolic Disorders Metabolic disorders are a complex group of inherited disorders resulting in abnormal central nervous system functioning. Among these are more than 50 varieties of neurolipid storage diseases. They include Hurler's disease, Sanfilippo's disease, mannosidosis, Niemann–Pick disease, and Fabry's disease. Defects in carbohydrate metabolism include galactosemia, glycogenosis, fructosemia (in which ingestion of fructose leads to abnormally elevated levels of fructose), and hypoglycemia, in which levels of glucose in the blood are abnormally low.

In galactosemia, the infant may be exposed to elevated levels of galactose in utero, before the pregnant woman is known to have a defective fetus. The infant is then already at risk for some degree of mental retardation at birth, but special dietary regimens can prevent further compounding effects. Galactosemia is detectable through amniocentesis, and a woman who has previously given birth to a child with the condition can undergo amniocentesis on succeeding pregnancies. If galactosemia is present in the fetus, the mother can go on a galactose-restricted diet during the latter part of the pregnancy. Children with galactosemia are treated with a galactose-free diet (see Chapter 38).

The best-studied amino acid deficiency is phenylketonuria (PKU), characterized by the body's inability to convert phenylalanine to tyrosine. Mental retardation in this condition is preventable through PKU screening in the first few days of life. (Screening and treatment for PKU is discussed in Chapter 38.) Normal phenylketonuric mothers may give birth to babies with mental retardation if the mother's diet was not restricted during pregnancy. When PKU is detected early and treated properly, children have normal intelligence or only mild symptoms of attention deficit disorders. Untreated infants are profoundly retarded.

Of the endocrine disorders, congenital hypothyroidism is the most common and is a preventable cause of mental retardation. Most states have laws requiring hypothyroid screening for neonates. Treatment with thyroid hormone is usually effective (see Chapter 40).

Severe hyperbilirubinemia, resulting from elevated serum bilirubin in the infant, produces kernicterus, which can cause mental retardation. (Neonatal hyperbilirubinemia is discussed in Chapter 31.)

Fetal Alcohol Syndrome Fetal alcohol syndrome (FAS) affects 1–2 infants per 1000 live births and is the leading preventable cause of congenital defects and mental retardation. Estimates suggest that there are 2.5 million female alcoholics of childbearing age in the United States. Studies indicate that a pregnant woman is at risk if she drinks 3 oz or more of absolute alcohol (100% alcohol) per day. This is equivalent to about six to eight average-size drinks. Intake of 10 drinks per week increases the risk of birthweight below the 10th percentile. (Care of infants who are small for gestational age is discussed in Chapter 31.) Infants of mothers who smoke and have only 5 drinks per week are also at increased risk for low birthweight.

Even when they do not show signs of FAS, infants of drinking mothers may be at high risk for neonatal respiratory depression, small stature, attention deficit disorders, and poor school performance. A small percentage of children are diagnosed with FAS in the nursery, while most are not identified until late infancy or early childhood. Some are not identified at all.

Infants with FAS have varying degrees of retardation and low birthweight. Anomalies include prenatal and postnatal growth deficiency, small head size, facial anomalies including droopy eyelids, a wide space between the nose and upper lip, a thin upper lip, and, occasionally, cleft palate and congenital heart disease.

Chromosomal Abnormalities Although new chromosomal aberrations are currently being researched and identified, some syndromes in this category are well understood (see Chapter 5). Klinefelter's syndrome, for example, is a

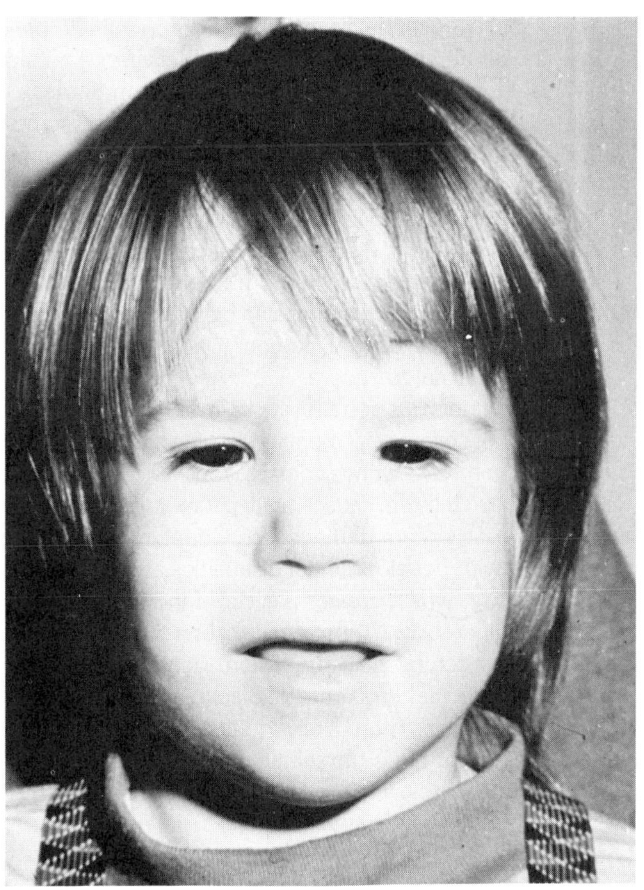

A child with fetal alcohol syndrome (FAS) has distinctive facial characteristics that will vary with the severity of the disability.

sex-linked chromosomal disorder and another cause of mental retardation.

Down's syndrome, also known as trisomy 21, is the most common chromosomal abnormality and is detectable through amniocentesis. Down's syndrome is estimated to affect 5%–10% of all retarded people. Children with Down's syndrome range in cognitive functioning from mild to severely retarded, although most are moderately retarded. With early intervention, many children with Down's syndrome are educable.

Classic clinical characteristics include inner epicanthal folds, simian palmar creases; a short, curved fifth digit; a short neck; and a thick tongue. Some have cardiac defects and other minor physical defects.

Perinatal and Postnatal Causes Encephalopathy, resulting from injuries to the fetus in utero, has been known to cause neurologic abnormalities resulting in developmental problems. Hypoxia during labor and delivery, which results from placenta problems or malpositions and malpresentations, is associated with varying degrees of neurologic complications in the young child. Severe premature birth and conditions having a negative influence on birth weight and fetal growth can cause mental retardation. Herpes simplex encephalitis, resulting from herpes simplex type II virus in the infected mother who delivers vaginally, is associated with severe central nervous system damage.

Nurses in the nursery are usually the first to detect symptoms of diseases that are often present prenatally but become evident only in the neonatal period. Brain diseases appear in the postnatal period, for instance, but originate from genetic influence. Gross brain diseases vary in degree of expressivity and time of appearance, from infancy to late childhood. These diseases are manifested by lesions and tumors of the skin and the central nervous system. Retardation ranges from normal to severe.

The central nervous system is vulnerable to infections in early life. For example, meningococcal meningitis and chickenpox can have serious complications. Excessively high lead levels in children causes lead poisoning, leading to central nervous system damage (see Chapter 20).

Children with developmental disabilities also are at risk for child abuse, which creates a cycle of increasing developmental vulnerability. Approximately one-third of abused children show central nervous system damage, and one-half have intellectual impairment. Blackman (1983) found that child abuse was more likely to occur in families under severe stress who have unrealistic expectations for a disabled child. (Nursing care of the family at risk for child abuse is discussed in Chapter 22.)

Diagnosis of Mental Retardation

The more retarded a child, the sooner that child will be noticed. If a child has definite physical abnormalities, particularly involving the face and head, evaluation usually takes place at a much earlier age. If a child fails to reach milestones in motor development, professional consultation is frequently obtained when the child is 2–3 years of age (Thain, 1980).

Intelligence Tests Diagnosis begins with testing. A diagnosis of mental retardation requires intelligence tests that have been standardized for large cross-sections of the population for which they are designed. The child then is assigned an intelligence quotient (IQ) computed by dividing the child's mental age by the chronologic age and multiplying the quotient by 100.

Mental age is the chronologic age for which performance is "average" or "normal." Determination of mental age is based on the child's ability to pass a battery of test items that are arranged from easiest to hardest and are representative of knowledge and skills expected of most children of a similar age. Intelligence tests must be administered by a well-trained psychologist who meets the certification standards of the profession. Among the tests that nurses caring for developmentally disabled children can expect are these:

- Stanford–Binet Intelligence Scale
- Gesell Developmental Schedules
- McCarthy Scales of Children's Abilities
- Weschler Intelligence Scale for Children—revised (WISC-R)
- Weschler Preschool and Primary Scale of Intelligence for Children 4–6 $\frac{1}{2}$ years (WPPSI)
- Slosson Intelligence Test
- Bayley Scales of Infant Development
- Catell Infant Intelligence Scale

Use of these intelligence tests is often limited for individuals with handicapping conditions, and other tests therefore have been devised especially for children with handicaps. A few of these tests are Nebraska Test of Learning Aptitude for the hearing-impaired child and the Arthur Adaptation of the Leiter International Performance Scale. This is a nonverbal test for children up to 12 years of age with hearing, speaking, or English language impairments. The Perkins–Binet Intelligence Scale can be used with the visually impaired. The Columbia Mental Maturity Scale was designed for those with motor and language impairments. The Merrill–Palmer Scale of Mental Tests are adapted for the speaking- and hearing-impaired. Neurometric specialists are researching the use of electroencephalographic readings as part of intelligence testing for children whose neuromotor handicaps rule out standard methods for cognitive testing.

In addition, cultural-free tests are designed to eliminate cultural factors that tend to favor one group over another. Inappropriate labeling of minority children as mentally retarded because of standard intelligence tests derived from the dominant culture has sparked the development of tests that are less likely to reflect cultural biases. Some of these are:

System of Multicultural Pluralistic Assessment (SOMPA)
Raven's Progressive Matrices
Catell's Cultural-Fair Intelligence Test
Porteus Mazes

Measurements of Adaptation To indicate mental retardation, behaviors must show significantly limited functioning. For example, an IQ test might show that a child is retarded, but an assessment of adaptive skills might show that the same child is normal. It is not unusual for some developmentally disabled children to exhibit impaired intellectual functioning but appropriate adaptive functioning. Such children may, however, be appropriately classified as mentally retarded if they exhibit functional limitations that require long-term intervention.

Child health nurses, who have a primary role in the overall assessment of the child, can use their knowledge of adaptive scales in providing guidance to parents and caregivers and in developing and evaluating programs. (Developmental assessment in a well-child setting is discussed in Chapter 16.) There are more than 29 published tests of adaptive behavior. Table 23-1 is a selected description of those that are widely used. Areas assessed in any adaptive scale might include independent functioning in activities of daily living such as dressing, toileting, and feeding; social skills with family and peer group; and responsible behavior.

According to Grossman (1983) there is a sequential manifestation of adaptive behavior deficits. During infancy and early childhood, sensorimotor, communication, self-help, and socialization skills ordinarily develop in a well-defined pattern that reflects the maturation process. Delays in acquiring these skills represent potential deficiencies in adaptive behavior and become the criteria for mental retardation.

The skills required for adaptation during childhood involve complex learning processes. Difficulties in learning usually are manifested in school, but the nurse's evaluation of adaptive behavior should focus on those skills essential for the child's coping with the environment, including concepts of time and money, self-directed behavior, social responsiveness, and interactive skills.

The nurse administers tests of adaptive behavior through direct observation, preferably in the child's home or school, through interviews with the primary caregivers, or through observation and interviews with the classroom teacher. The nurse then uses the identified deficits as a basis for working with parents and members of the health care team in designing programs for the developmentally disabled child.

TABLE 23-1 Assessment Tools for Measuring Adaptive Behavior

Test	Age group	Target population	Purpose	Components of self-care and social behavior
AAMD Adaptive Behavior Scale (110 items)	6 years and older	Developmentally disabled, mentally retarded, and all institutionalized children	Program development and evaluation, differentiation among levels and types of handicaps	Independent functioning; physical and language development; numbers and time; vocational, economic, and domestic activity; self-direction and responsibility; socialization; unacceptable and inappropriate behavior; use of medications
AAMD Adaptive Behavior Scale—School Edition (95 items)	7–13 years	Mentally retarded and learning-disabled children	To indicate areas of needed remediation in a school setting	Independent functioning; physical and language development; numbers and time; vocational and economic activity; self-direction and responsibility; socialization; unacceptable and inappropriate behavior; use of medications

continued on next page

TABLE 23-1 continued

Test	Age group	Target population	Purpose	Components of self-care and social behavior
Adaptive Functioning Index (274 items)	14 years and older	Mentally retarded individuals in community or rural settings	Group and individual needs assessment, program planning, evaluation of progress	Communication, time, community awareness, personal routines, social maturity
Camelot Behavior Checklist (399 items)	2 years and older	Mentally retarded children	Group program planning	Self-help, physical development, home duties, economic and social behavior, independent travel, responsibility
Cain-Levine Social Competency Scale (44 items)	5–13 years	Mentally retarded individuals who are "trainable"	Rapid assessment of relative standing of mentally retarded children	Self-help, initiative, social skills, communication
Balthazar Scales of Adaptive Behavior Scales of Functional Independence (132 items) Scales of Social Adaptation (84 items)	5–17 years	Severely to profoundly retarded individuals in institutional settings	Discrimination among component behaviors in eating, dressing, and toileting; program planning and evaluation	Eating, toileting, dressing; self-directed behavior; play
Adaptative Behavior Inventory for Children (242 items)	5 years to 11 years, 11 months	Children with mild to moderate mental retardation, normal children from cultures outside the norm	Descriptive data	Role performance in family and community, peer relations, nonacademic roles in school, self-maintenance
Fairview Self-Help Scale (34 items)	2–9 years	Mild to profoundly retarded children, institutionalized children	Screening, needs assessment, program planning	Self-help skills, communication, social interaction, self-direction
Fairview Developmental Scale (26 items)	Birth to 2 years	Severely and profoundly retarded children, institutionalized children	Screening, needs assessment, program planning	Self-help skills, communication, social interaction, self-direction
Fairview Social Skills Scale (36 items)	10 years and older	Mildly and moderately retarded children, institutionalized children	Screening, needs assessment, program planning	Self-help and occupational skills, communication, social interaction, self-direction
Minnesota Developmental Programming System—Behavioral Scales (360 items)	All ages	Mentally retarded individuals	Screening	Eating, dressing, grooming, toileting; social interaction; time, money, domestic behaviors; community orientation; recreation and leisure activities; vocational choices
O'Berry Developmental Tests—Behavior Maturity Checklist II (15 items)	All children	Institutionalized severely and profoundly retarded children	Screening, needs assessment, individual program development	Dressing, grooming, eating, toileting, social interaction

TABLE 23-1 continued

Test	Age group	Target population	Purpose	Components of self-care and social behavior
Progress Assessment Chart of Social and Personal Development (6 versions)	Birth to adulthood (each version targets a different age group)	Mentally retarded individuals, both institutionalized and noninstitutionalized	Individual assessment, evaluation of progress	Socialization, self-help and occupational skills
Vineland Social Maturity Scale	3 months to adulthood	All individuals with disabilities	Selection and planning of group-training programs	Socialization; self-help and self-direction; eating, dressing, and occupational skills

SOURCE: Data from Matson JL, Breuning SE: Pages 214–225 in: *Assessing the Mentally Retarded.* Grune & Stratton, 1983.

Impact of Developmental Disabilities on Families

Grief

To be told that one's child has a serious disability is one of the most painful events that a parent can experience. A first goal of nursing intervention therefore is to help the family resolve grief and avoid chronic sorrow so that family members can accept and adapt to the condition.

Grieving includes emotions such as ambivalence, denial, guilt, shame, self-pity, sorrow, depression, and a wish for the child's death. Mercer (1977) analyzes the phases of grief as a process that begins with numbness and progresses to reorganization and adaptation. The numbness and shock of the initial phase are time-limited and seldom observed beyond the 6th day of the child's life. Protest at a sense of loss and yearning for a normal infant were observed most frequently at 1 month. Despair, chaos, and depression, which characterize reorganization, were seen more often in the first 2 months but continued in varying degrees.

Professionals should not, however, expect grieving to be time-limited or circumscribed. Grief is not a one-time phenomenon. It may remain as part of the parent's emotional life. (The chronic sorrow associated with the diagnosis of a disability is discussed in Chapter 30.)

Most parents need the support of compassionate professionals who are honest and knowledgeable. Parents under stress usually cannot hear a great deal of information at once, so that the nurse needs to provide ample time for the parent to ask questions. Parents often ask the same questions over and over as they struggle with what has happened, why it has happened, their roles in causing the disability, and what they need to do. Nurses need to use caution in reassuring parents that they can "go on and have another child soon" or that "this could never happen again." The nurse therefore states only factual information about the disability, so that the parent has time to adapt to the diagnosis and its implications.

Effects on Parenting

Having a developmentally disabled child is a crisis that requires special coping abilities if the parent is to accept the child. Identification and acceptance of disabilities are difficult for many families, and developing ways to promote optimal development and include the child in the family requires joint adaptation by all family members. This process is assisted by nurses in contact with the infant and family at the time of delivery; in the nursery; during the postpartum period; and in the weeks, months, and years following the diagnosis.

Reactions of parents and other family members to the arrival of a retarded child vary according to religious orientation, the degree to which the child was wanted in the first place, the parent's previous experiences with crisis, the nature and degree of the problem, the parent's inner coping mechanisms and self-esteem, the family's socioeconomic resources, the child's similarity to other family members, and the quality of professional support.

Nurses can expect that a child represents an extension of the parent's self. A child who is less than perfect therefore can be shattering to a parent's ego. For example, Mr. Brown, an upwardly mobile businessman and the only son from a family of five sisters, was excited over the coming birth of his first child. The child was born with characteristics of Down's syndrome, poor tone, feeding difficulties, a heart murmur, and signs of cardiac disease. Before the defects were identified, the parents quickly were shown their son and told they had a baby boy. Shortly afterwards, the parents were told their baby needed to be seen by specialists and observed in the special-care nursery.

Meanwhile, Mr. and Mrs. Brown called their relatives to announce the birth of their perfect son, whom they had

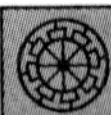

CASE STUDY Fetal Alcohol Syndrome

Assessment

Karena is an 8-month-old infant who is being seen in the clinic upon referral from the public health nurse. She is brought in by her mother. Mrs. M. tells the clinic nurse that Karena is a very difficult baby to care for. She cries all the time and feeds poorly, spitting up after almost every feeding. Mrs. M.'s other two children were not like this as babies. Mrs. M. appears quite impatient, disorganized, and expresses feelings of helplessness with this baby.

Family

The family consists of Mrs. M., 26 years old, Mr. M., 27 years old, and two other children, aged 3 and 5 years. They are in a preschool program. Mrs. M. did not work during the pregnancy, and her obstetric history reveals that she admitted to "only occasional alcohol intake." She consumed two 4-oz. glasses of dinner wine when she and her husband went out for their weekly Friday night dinner together. At her husband's office Christmas party, she recalled having drunk 3 mixed drinks and 2 glasses of wine, but was never intoxicated. She drank one 12-oz. can of beer each night with Mr. M. when he arrived home from work, and had 2 cans a day on weekends. Mrs. M. ate a balanced diet throughout the pregnancy. Mr. M. is a partner in an insurance business and works long hours.

Child

Karena was a full-term, small for gestational age infant, weighing only 4 lbs. 11 ozs. She stayed in the newborn nursery a total of 10 days for weight gain and observation. She was noticed to have jitteriness, dysmorphic features of microcephaly, small eyes, flat midface with a thin upper lip, hypoplastic nails on the 5th toes, and thick hair on the face and extremities, all signs being consistent with Fetal Alcohol Syndrome. Karena can get on her knees with her chest and arms on the floor. Karena occasionally will join in with siblings for pat-a-cake hand clapping, but does not like to be cuddled. Karena is on formula and a few strained foods. When a teething biscuit is placed in her hand she can take it to her mouth. Elimination patterns are normal. She sleeps through the night on most nights.

Environment

The family lives outside the city limits in a small neighborhood with six other families. Mr. and Mrs. M.'s extended families live several hundred miles away. Although Mr. M. has several friends in his office with whom he plays golf, Mrs. M. has no close friends and few social outlets.

Clinical Data

Karena is a small infant. She is sitting on her mother's lap, fretting and crying. She makes babbling sounds when not crying. Head size is at the 10th percentile. Weight and length remain at the 5th percentile. Physical examination revealed dysmorphic features consistent with those noted at birth. The clinic nurse assessed developmental milestones with the Developmental Profile. Findings were:

Holds head up without support

Rolls from back and stomach

Tries to get objects that are near

Grasps and holds an object for several seconds

Shows active interest in an object or person

Shows she wants attention paid to her

Babbles and uses vocal noises for play

Reacts by being more or less active to changes such as being picked up or having a person come into the room

Developmental milestones are at a 4-months level.

Nursing Diagnoses

1. Alterations in parenting due to the child's irritability and feeding problems secondary to Fetal Alcohol Syndrome.
2. Alterations in family process due to inability of family system to meet the needs of its members.
3. Developmental delay due to poor growth and delayed milestones.

Plan for Interventions

Goals

1. Support to Mrs. M. to help her deal with stressful life and family situations, particularly as they relate to alcohol consumption.
2. Mrs. M. will understand Karena's condition, developmental level, and learn ways to promote the child's growth and development.

Interventions

1. Thorough assessment of the marital relationship, parent–children interactions, and knowledge and perception of Karena's problems.
2. Assess health and adjustment of other two children.
3. Assess Mrs. M.'s present drinking patterns through a nonjudgmental attitude to avoid provoking guilt.
4. Strongly recommend to Mrs. M. that she be referred to an outpatient facility for counseling to reduce her alcohol consumption and to assist with social and emotional problems.
5. Help Mrs. M. arrange occasional childcare for Karena.
6. Observe Karena at feeding time and record intake for 3 days to compile assessment of nutritional status.
7. Collaborate with nutritionist to find ways to increase child's intake of nutrients.
8. Measure growth at frequent intervals.
9. Teach mother ways to attempt reducing Karena's spitting up.

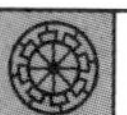

CASE STUDY Fetal Alcohol Syndrome (continued)

10. Discuss Mrs. M.'s interest in exploring employment counseling and job training if she lacks marketable skills.
11. Design infant stimulation program to teach Mrs. M. appropriate play activities that will decrease Karena's tactile defensiveness while promoting acquisition of new skills.
12. Evaluate family and child's progress at regular intervals.
13. Coordinate services to the family and discuss Karena's progress with her primary health care providers and other professionals who are closely involved in her care. Make a recommendation of referral for a comprehensive developmental evaluation of some specific time in the future.

named Thomas. Mr. Brown celebrated with coworkers, while his extended family brought a small celebration to Mrs. Brown's hospital room. This was the first grandson after five granddaughters for Mr. Brown's family.

Hours later, doctors came to explain the baby's problem and the possible need to do surgery in a few days. Programs that help parents foster their children's optimal development were explained, and they were given a list of resources and names of other parents who had children with Down's syndrome. Both parents were shocked and saddened. It was difficult for them to visit their baby in the nursery. Even when encouraged by the nursing staff, Mr. Brown was unable to touch the baby. Mr. Brown wondered how he would face his family and friends, and Mrs. Brown expressed guilt that she had caused the child's defects.

Nurses and other health professionals need to realize that parental expectations often mean that a child is socialized from the moment of birth. Furthermore, a child's gender often has special significance for one or both parents, even if parents do not express a preference for a boy or a girl. Any defect therefore is traumatic, especially when the defect affects the identity assumed of the child. The guilt that many parents express also might cause them to blame behaviors such as sexual intercourse during pregnancy, punishment from God, genetic background, or events, such as illness during pregnancy. Nursing interventions thus are planned to help parents resolve their feelings and to facilitate the normal process of parent–infant attachment.

Like Mrs. Brown, most parents feel guilty, even if they do not express their guilt. The nurse reassures parents with statements such as "the doctors do not feel that anything you did or did not do during your pregnancy caused this to happen." When parents express ambivalence, disappointment, or emotional upset, the nurse also can reassure them that these responses are normal.

The recognition of disability in a child has a profound impact on the family system and places that family at risk for dysfunction. In two-parent families, the birth of a disabled child also affects the parent's marriage. Many parents report that they are stronger and are drawn closer together in their crisis; others separate and divorce. Couples may face new marital difficulty after the diagnosis. For example, a grief-stricken husband might cope by becoming absorbed in his work; his wife might interpret this behavior as a lack of caring or concern about the child, which in turn may lead to anger and feelings of desertion. The husband might interpret his wife's response as being overemotional, overanxious, and too involved in the child's care. If this breakdown in communication is not resolved, the family is at risk and may become dysfunctional.

Keele (1983) indicates that marital problems tend to be slightly higher when children are severely or profoundly retarded. In these families, usual patterns of coping may not be sufficient to resolve conflicts. The nurse refers these family members to appropriate counseling. Through identifying family resources, the nurse can help the family use strengths to deal effectively with the situation (see Chapter 22).

Parent–Infant Attachment The complexities of parent–infant attachment have been researched and studied extensively, and although some factors influence bonding before birth, many factors contribute to attachment after birth (see Chapter 7). In the first few hours after birth, a mother's tactile exploration of her baby from head to toe enhances bonding. This exploration usually is followed by cradling and talking to the infant. Separation from the infant immediately after birth, at night, and for long periods during the day minimizes parent–infant interaction and negates this sensitive period (Johnson, 1979).

An infant with a defect is at risk during this period because the infant may not be able to interact with the parent. The infant might, for example, lack eye contact and cuddling responses. The nurse can reinforce parental caregiving by encouraging the parent to provide care to the baby immediately after birth. This acquaintance and early attachment process may be further altered when an infant requires special care. The nurse then encourages any degree of participation possible by the parent whether it be observing or participating in feeding, diapering, bathing, touching, and holding. Parental confidence is heightened by proper instructions and support while performing specific caregiving tasks.

The nurse's reaction to the child also has an impact on the parent. The infant's defect may, for instance, prevent the parent from noting normal features. The nurse can foster acceptance of the child by pointing out normal features, body processes, and temperament. Talking and reacting to the child as a person rather than as a "defect" or "condition" demonstrates acceptance of the child and provides a role model for parents.

Nursing interventions thus are planned to address the following areas:

1. Facilitating discussion of the pregnancy, labor and delivery, and condition of the infant
2. Listening empathetically
3. Reinforcing a positive self-image in the parents
4. Enhancing communication between parents and extended family by talking with them together
5. Allowing expressions of fear, ambivalent feelings, frustration, hopes, and aspirations
6. Facilitating adaptation to stress
7. Encouraging frequent interaction with the child and involvement in caregiving
8. Discussing availability of in-house or referral resources for genetic counseling (see Chapter 5)
9. Helping parents realistically plan for the immediate future (for example, purchasing special equipment and bringing the infant home)
10. Sharing knowledge of community resources for support systems

Health professionals cannot assume that mothers are most affected by the birth or the realization that the child has a serious disability or defect. Father–infant bonding also suffers when an infant is immediately and continuously separated from the parents after birth, as frequently occurs in infants with defects (Johnson, 1979). The nurse thus needs to be aware of specific fathering behaviors that influence early acquaintance with the infant and lead acceptance. In the first few days, these behaviors include touch, holding the baby close, talking to the infant, and eye contact.

The child health nurse's goals in working with fathers include the following:

1. Recognizing the father's role as an essential, contributing family member
2. Assessing adaptive and maladaptive behavior patterns
3. Assessing the effect of fathering behaviors on child response
4. Assessing the effect of the infant's behaviors on fathering response
5. Assisting the father in the development of adaptive behavior patterns
6. Reinforcing and supporting adaptive fathering behaviors
7. Providing feedback and alternatives to fathers who exhibit maladaptive behaviors
8. Fostering the growth of mutually satisfying father–child relationships and family interactions

Adaptations in the Family System Incorporating a disabled infant into the family system produces an unavoidable need to plan for the child in the home. Leaving the security of the hospital environment can be a frightening experience for many parents. This may be the first confrontation with family members, neighbors, and society as a whole. If the shock of the diagnosis has prevented family members from hearing about the details of the defect in the hospital, they often feel inadequate in caring for the child at home. If social supports dwindle, a referral and visits from the public health nurse can help the family identify needs for infant care and can provide ongoing support in the adaptation process. Parents need someone to listen. Talking with nurses provides parents with opportunities to express their feelings and allows nurses to identify new problems and areas of concern and to praise parents for problems successfully managed.

Blackwell (1979) confirms the unreadiness of family members to deal with an abnormal child in the home, even though they are faced with the child's daily care. Infants often are sent home before parents have passed through the initial shock of the diagnosis. For these parents, carrying out the tasks of the daily routine often produce ambivalence. Psychologic fatigue compounds physical exhaustion, so that many parents feel isolated and lonely. Internalized feelings surface as hostility toward the infant's demands. When parents fail to seek support services, they need others to act on their behalf. When a family is isolated from support, the nurse's assessment of family dynamics helps further in identifying the unmet needs of the child. (The process of family assessment is discussed in Chapter 17.)

Effects of Community Attitudes Having a baby is a social activity. When the baby has an obvious defect, defining one's role as parent can be frightening. Many parents feel alone and isolated, frustrated, and stigmatized or feel that their rights to be good parents have been challenged (Turnbull and Turnbull, 1978). Parental anxiety can be compounded by fear of rejection or fear of losing social standing in a community. Society tends to reject quickly those who have visible facial defects. A parent who perceives a child's facial appearance as a reflection of the parent is also likely to experience feelings of failure.

Although friends and neighbors might be awkward in attempts to talk about a retarded child, the parent might also contribute to the distance. Sometimes a parent's own questions and doubts make it difficult to talk about the child. At other times a parent might feel ambivalent about being a burden to others or arousing pity. Other parents worry that they will share too much information about the child, making others less able to accept and enjoy the child.

Some parents need to know that, in each situation, they must determine how much information they want to give. They are not obliged to answer rude and unthoughtful questions. When a parent relates that a total stranger asked an abrupt, tactless question, the nurse can suggest that the parent decide on a goal for similar encounters (for example, whether to educate the stranger about the child's disability or ignore the stranger entirely). If a parent wants to relate limited, factual information, the nurse can suggest that appropriate answers are "She is retarded" or "She can't walk" or some other brief explanation of the disability.

For some families this is the first time that family members experience social repugnance from strangers and feel a need to confront strangers to test their reactions. One mother who had an infant with Down's syndrome took him to shopping centers and amusement parks repeatedly while he was quite young and commented, "No one knew anything was wrong; they all said he was a pretty baby." Strangers' reactions seemed to comfort and assure her that she and infant would be accepted by society, at least temporarily (Mercer, 1977).

The nurse can help parents handle social situations by modeling responses to friends and strangers. For example, most people can appreciate a parent's honesty in saying, "There isn't much to be known right now. We can't do much more than wait. She will grow and learn like other children, but more slowly. I appreciate your asking." Some parents need to be reminded that they should continue their contacts and activities with friends, even securing a baby sitter when appropriate. Putting parents in contact with other parents or organized groups of parents of developmentally disabled children provides a good social outlet as well as a source of information. This helps parents realize that the social aspect of life should go on and that satisfying balances in their own lives are healthy.

Families also might find community support to meet their immediate needs. In one small mill town, two parents, both textile mill workers, told their neighbors and church members about a revolutionary implant that was available at a large medical center several states away. They had read that the implant possibly could stimulate their 6-year-old daughter's speech and gross motor abilities. She had cerebral palsy and neither talked nor walked. The town rallied around the family, raising several hundred thousand dollars to pay for medical bills for the implant.

Developmental Disabilities in Older Children For many parents, a diagnosis of a developmental disability does not come until the child is older and has passed such usual developmental milestones as walking, talking, and starting school. An infant who is retarded needs much the same care as any other infant, but when the infant reaches early childhood and cannot walk, talk, or be toilet-trained, the delays are much more apparent, and the impact is unavoidable. For example, a middle-class mother of three young boys, ages 5, 4, and $1\frac{1}{2}$ years held a birthday party for the 4-year-old. The mother was distraught by the end of the party when the boy did not seem to be aware that a special event was occurring and could not sing any of the words of "Happy Birthday." She went to her pediatrician with concern because her son's limitations had suddenly become obvious, although she and the pediatrician previously had agreed that the child should not be compared to his older brother, whose development was precocious. Until his delayed development become evident, both the mother and the physician had denied that the possibility existed, thinking that this boy was the middle child and would eventually catch up.

The typical mentally retarded child is seen in the physician's office after referral from school. Most of these children show significantly delayed educational development and progress more slowly than their peers (Thain, 1980). When developmental disabilities become apparent at this stage, denial is a common parental reaction. Parents might fail to keep appointments, "shop around" for other physicians, or hide facts about the child. Parental depression also is common and is manifested in social withdrawal, sad affect, deterioration in grooming, expressions of guilt, and marital tension.

Even when delayed development already was evident, an actual diagnosis of mental retardation can precipitate a crisis. For example, Mr. Smith, a hospital administrator, and his wife, a university admissions officer, had their $4\frac{1}{2}$-year-old daughter Penny referred to the local developmental pediatrician. Mrs. Smith related that she had been concerned about her daughter's development since infancy when the child fed poorly, was always irritable, and reached developmental milestones late, although not late enough to alarm her pediatrician. She was in an "open" preschool classroom with children ranging in ages from $2\frac{1}{2}$ to 4 years of age. Penny would be 5 years old and eligible for public school kindergarten in the fall.

Mr. and Mrs. Smith had discussed Penny's slow development with the preschool teacher, who suggested they see the developmental pediatrician. During the 6 months prior to the appointment, Mrs. Smith had read about children with certain nutritional intolerances that predisposed them to delayed development. She had consulted a nutritionist about a special diet, but the diet had not made any improvement in Penny's slow development.

After a genetic work-up, the developmental pediatrician diagnosed moderate mental retardation, cause unknown. A conference followed to discuss findings and possible treatment plans. At the conference, Mr. and Mrs. Smith were violently angry with disbelief and shock. They responded, "We cannot take Penny home. It would be impossible to fit a child with low mentality into our lives. Our daughter is expected to excel in private school. How could this be? We are both very intelligent people." For these parents, their expectations contributed to their reaction, and the diagnosis was thus a family crisis. Even when delayed development has been recognized, the diagnosis often precipitates grieving and requires the parent to adapt.

Crises also might occur throughout a child's development, as family members continue to compare the child's limitations with age-appropriate norms. Critical points that might precipitate crisis are these:

1. Separation of parent and child when the child first enters school
2. Riding to school on a special bus rather than the bus used by siblings or walking to school with other neighborhood children
3. Adolescence, when most children assume more independence in going places with other children and when parents are reminded of their earlier dreams for the child and their own aging
4. Family shopping trips, vacations, and outings, when the child's disability makes it difficult for the family to plan
5. Religious rituals such as first communion, confirmation or bar mitzvah
6. Holidays and family reunions
7. Conversations with other parents about normal children's successes and failures
8. Onset of puberty
9. Weddings of normal children in the family
10. Decisions concerning residential placement
11. Discussion of guardianship for a retarded child when parents are no longer able to provide care

The nurse can provide anticipatory guidance in helping parents prepare for expected stress, surges of anxiety, or the effects of chronic sorrow. Miezio (1983) points out that families of children with disabilities do not ordinarily seek professional help for their problems. Somehow, they think their troubles are unavoidable, and they know that the situation cannot be miraculously changed. They tend to forget that, while the child may not be able to have the "cure" they would like, they still can learn new strategies to cope with the stressors.

Effects on Siblings

In recent years, considerable attention has focused on the effect of the retarded child on the development of other children in the family (Grossman, 1972). Siblings observe their parents' grief and may be confused over the tension and worry. They may feel guilty that they were fortunate enough to be normal. Young children who are not given accurate information may fear that the disability is contagious or that it is a punishment for their own wrongdoing.

The nurse therefore suggests that parents reassure young children. If a disability is apparent at birth, the nurse guides parents in explaining this to the other children. Before leaving the hospital, parents should, as much as possible, explain what is expected of the baby at a level appropriate for each sibling's understanding. For siblings who are old enough, hospital visitation should be encouraged.

Siblings of severely retarded children show considerable variation in their degree of adaptation. Studies suggest that the more siblings understand about the condition, the better they adapt. If parents are able to help their children understand a retarded sibling's condition, to give all their children sufficient attention, and to set realistic expectations for each child, the mentally retarded child will benefit from the warmth, acceptance and positive influence received from the family (Payne and Patton, 1981).

Parents' Responses to Siblings Parents of younger children sometimes express concern that they are neglecting their other children because of the time required for the disabled child. Siblings too might feel a lack of adequate attention because the parent faces overwhelming responsibilities in caring for a retarded child. Parents might neglect their normal children because of guilt feelings and the seeming need to devote all available time to the handicapped child. Normal siblings might respond with anger toward the retarded child and might also display dysfunctional behavior to attract the attention of parents.

One large study of siblings of the retarded found that relationships between nonretarded siblings and the mother more often were affected adversely if the retarded child required a great deal of the mother's attention (Grossman, 1972). Another group of children suffered the effects of dysfunctional parenting, but this was only partially related to a sibling's disability. These parents had minimal parenting skills, and the disabled child only compounded an existing problem. These children are often in desperate need of attention. If they are unable to secure the attention at home, they may solicit it in socially unacceptable ways outside the home environment (Chinn, Clifford, and Logan, 1979).

Resentment might also ensue if the child's handicaps prevent normal family activities such as outings and vacations. Financial constraints as well as such responsibilities as baby sitting might also cause resentment. Shame and embarrassment are more common reactions when the retarded child is no longer small and "cute" and the normal sibling's social development brings friends in contact with the retarded child. One 14-year-old boy convinced his parents to remodel an unattached garage into a two-room apartment. He lived in the apartment, leaving from it for outings with friends, school, shopping, and meals with the family. He felt a sense of comfort, once he was free from the embarrassment of a retarded 10-year-old brother who was aggressive and occasionally destructive.

Siblings' Attitudes Toward Care Grossman (1972) found that older siblings adapt better than younger children. Older siblings are frequently expected to assume responsibility for the care of the retarded sibling, although this seems to be expected more of sisters than brothers. Normal siblings might find these expectations a positive result of the family situation. An older child might, for example, feel more responsible and competent when involved in helping to run the household, feelings that in turn can increase the sibling's self-esteem.

In one case, parents of two teenage daughters delivered a child with Down's syndrome. The parents were in their late 40s. The father worked in another town and was home only on weekends. The daughters were told of the diagnosis right away and were involved in discussion of the anticipated needs of their baby brother. Though saddened and disappointed, they welcomed the baby home and volunteered to help with the child's care. The mother was able to return to work. Her daughters took turns with her in providing for the daily needs of the child, including driving him to the baby sitter and developmental day school. When speech and language therapy was begun, one of the sisters quickly learned the therapist's home program and administered daily speech therapy sessions. The sister later went to college, majored in speech therapy; and now works with other developmentally disabled children.

Chinn, Clifford, and Logan (1979) suggest that a retarded child can influence vocation and marriage choices. Normal siblings who interact regularly with the retarded child tend to opt for more altruistic vocational choices, emphasizing "devotion to mankind" and "devotion to worthwhile causes." Normal siblings who maintain close relationships with their retarded brothers or sisters tend not to consider potential marriage partners who demonstrate little tolerance for the handicapped child.

The nurse works with parents to recognize the needs of normal children and to provide explanations about their parents' love for them. Parents might not be able to spend more time with normal children, but the quality of that time can demonstrate enough love and affection to reassure these children that their parents do love them (Johnson, 1979).

Researchers have found that adolescents have many questions and concerns, and benefit from short-term group sessions as a way to help them deal with their feelings. Group process can enable siblings to put their feelings into words, to identify problems, to analyze relationships, and to begin to think realistically about their own futures. Fear in older children may come from apprehension that they too will have handicapped children or that they will be responsible for their retarded siblings when their parents are no longer able to provide care. As time goes on, siblings who have had the benefit of group sessions seem to be able to look at the broader implications of mental retardation. Many can then recognize the needs of others who have retarded brothers and sisters (Wikler and Keenan, 1983).

Effects on the Extended Family

A new child is seen by grandparents as an extension of themselves. They hope for a healthy infant, a child who will enhance family life, make up for past disappointments, and help in conflicts with their own children. Grandparents want a grandchild to continue their beliefs, pursue higher education, surpass their own achievements, or practice a cherished profession (Wikler and Keenan, 1983).

When the child has a developmental disability, grandparents experience feelings of disappointment similar to feelings of pain and grief experienced by the parents. Family pride can be undermined by resentment, guilt, and embarrassment. Grandparents too will search for explanations for the calamity. They might look into the in-laws' family tree for evidence of other children with disabilities or retardation. Like parents and siblings, grandparents and other relatives need to mourn to resolve their grief. Grandparents and other relatives can, however, be a great influence in family life and can provide support, either emotional or financial, to the family system as a whole. If relatives can accept a disabled infant without horror or pity, parents have less fear of rejection.

Nursing interventions are directed toward restoring and maintaining a mutually supportive relationship of grandparents and parents who help each other accept new realities through understanding, compassion, and appropriate sharing of tasks.

Nurses can relieve some of a parent's burdens by explaining to relatives what has happened and what the family can expect, although such explanations are done only with the parent's permission and often in the parent's presence. Grandparents might have fears and anxieties, often about inheritance of the disorder. The nurse then can help the parents understand the extent to which the disability is inherited and can suggest books to read on the specific problem of the child. Realistic information often dispels fears and enables grandparents and relatives to interact normally with parent and child.

Role of Nursing in Care for the Mentally Retarded

The early to middle 1950s brought recognition of mental retardation as a major problem affecting American children. A special clinic was established for the retarded at Los Angeles Children's Hospital, and by 1958 most states had clinical services for retarded children living at home. Thousands of public health nurses were trained for evaluation and prevention. During the 1960s the President's Panel on Mental Retardation was established to improve residential care and services for the multiply handicapped and to establish comprehensive prevention programs. It soon became evident that the best approach was multidisciplinary management that included nurses to provide services to the mentally retarded and their families. Nurses then became involved in applying behavior modification to their teaching of activities of daily living.

In recent years nursing has extended involvement in the care of the mentally retarded to encompass nursing practice in the home, community, and institutions. Nursing goals generally include

1. Providing guidance to families in the areas of infant care and stimulation
2. Helping parents accept and adjust to the birth of retarded children
3. Screening for symptoms of developmental problems
4. Planning and implementing programs with other health and education professionals concerned with preventive health care (for example, exercise and weight reduction programs, sex and family life education, and maintenance of adaptive skills)
5. Providing family support for management of retarded children in the home and guidance in seeking respite care
6. Managing medical problems of children in acute-care hospital facilities and supervising daily care of retarded children in institutions and residential programs

Like other aspects of nursing, nursing care for the developmentally disabled involves collecting and analyzing data, making a diagnosis, and planning interventions. The overriding goals are ensuring optimal development and preventing further disability in the developmentally disabled child. Depending on educational preparation and experience, nurses are involved in providing direct care or acting as case coordinators to develop plans for treatment.

Nurses collaborate with physicians to provide follow-up for medical treatment, drug therapy (for example, in managing seizures or hyperactivity), and nutritional management (for example, in dietary counseling for PKU, galactosemia, and obesity). Nurses also support and coordinate with other health professionals, including social workers and mental health therapists to help parents cope with stress and use appropriate community resources. Community supports include agencies for health maintenance; child-care facilities; developmental programs; physical, occupational, and speech therapy; pediatric psychologists, early intervention programs; and organizations for respite care and planning for long-term placement.

Prevention

Primary Prevention Nurses engage in primary prevention by providing well-child care and immunization programs, which are effective ways to prevent mental retardation. Although national guidelines have been outlined to assure immunization in infancy and early childhood, immunization programs to protect the population from serious complications of childhood infectious diseases do not reach all of the target population. For example, between 5% and 10% of young women in their childbearing years are susceptible to rubella, which, along with Fetal Alcohol Syndrome, is a principal preventable cause of mental retardation.

An area of continuing concern in primary prevention of developmental disorders is the care of adolescent mothers. Early pregnancies often begin a cycle of poverty (see Chapter 22). In addition, adolescent pregnancies frequently are compounded by preterm deliveries, which are correlated with a higher incidence of complications that result in developmental disorders. Preventing adolescent pregnancies thus minimizes risk factors that predispose children and families to developmental disorders.

Parents of developmentally disabled children may be concerned about disorders in future children, and questions and anxieties concerning inheritance are often mentioned to the nurse caring for a disabled or retarded child. Amniocentesis now permits recognition of chromosomal abnormalities and some metabolic disorders. Many physicians offer amniocentesis to all women 35 years of age and older or women who are at risk in other ways for producing infants with defects and mental retardation. A vital nursing responsibility is referral of such women for genetic counseling (see Chapter 5). A new area of involvement for nurses is prevention through preconceptive health counseling, which might be provided by family-planning clinics. Counseling often includes education programs for women regarding the risks of such preconceptive health patterns as poor nutrition, smoking, or drinking alcohol. Through general health counseling, nurses are able to identify those needing more in-depth genetic counseling and to refer those who are at risk for having children with developmental disabilities.

Because acute and chronic diseases such as anemia, seizure disorders, hypertension, diabetes mellitus, and excessive maternal alcohol intake are potentially harmful to the fetus, the effects can be minimized when nurses help prospective mothers achieve a high state of wellness prior to conception.

Studies have shown a higher incidence of prematurity and complications in newborns whose mothers did not receive adequate prenatal care (US Department of Health, Education, and Welfare, 1978). Still disturbing in the 1980s is that 20%–40% of women in some low-income inner-city areas of the United States do not seek prenatal care prior to 20 weeks' gestation. Because the period of greatest environmental sensitivity for the developing fetus is between days 17 and 56 following conception, nurses who reach women early in pregnancy can teach them the necessity of early prenatal care and careful monitoring of maternal diseases during pregnancy.

Secondary Prevention Assessing risks, needs, and problems in the developmentally disabled child and the family is an ongoing process occurring throughout the child's developing years. Much of the assessment and long-term planning, however, occurs during infancy and early and middle childhood. Assessment of young children has two purposes: (1) identification of children whose developmental progress is already retarded and (2) identification of children who exhibit signs of developmental vulnerability, or potential for delayed development at a later time (Chinn, Clifford, and Logan, 1979). (Developmental assessment is discussed in Chapter 16.)

Early identification of the developmentally disabled child is highly desirable because the secondary effects of the condition might be substantially minimized through early intervention. For children who are developmentally vulnerable identification of risk factors helps to prevent permanent disabilities. Children whose disabilities are severe are more likely to require continuing nursing support.

Screening is the first step in identifying possible developmental problems. Screening tests are designed to be applied to large numbers of children and thus are usually short, objective, and easy to administer and score. They often are standardized and examined for their reliability and validity. When abnormal findings result, referral for diagnostic evaluation is necessary (Krajicek, and Tearney Tomlinson, 1983). Screening is often part of the nurse's assessment of the developmental status of normal infants and children (see Chapter 16).

Nurses in neonatal intensive care units, working with identified high-risk infants, do much of the initial screening. They might detect signs and symptoms indicating distress or other behavioral cues of concern. One tool used by nurses in early detection is the Brazelton Neonatal Behavioral Assessment Scale (see Chapter 16). This tool assists nurses and other health care professionals in making systematic behavioral observations for signs of neurologic impairment and brain damage. Many infants thus are identified as high risk although no specific impairment can be found.

Immediately after birth, the nurse assesses the infant's state by using the Apgar evaluation (see Chapter 7). Extremely low scores alert the nurse and medical staff that a problem may exist. According to Chinn, Clifford, and Logan (1979), infants at 1 year of age who had 5-minute scores of 3 or less have three times as many neurologic problems as infants of similar birth weight with Apgar scores of 7–10. Apgar scores of 6 or less are viewed with concern. Infants with such scores are usually monitored more closely for the first several days, and interventions are made as necessary.

During the first year of life, the Milani–Comparetti Motor Development Screening Test may be used by nurses at periodic intervals to identify children with motor delays and dysfunction. This screening test is practical, quick, and easy to score. It can be incorporated in the routine health assessment made by nurses in well-child clinics or used during home visits. Nurses use the screening information to identify a need for referral to a physical therapist or physician for a detailed developmental examination (Price, 1980).

Many hospitals use referral and tracking systems of community health programs to follow infants in high-risk categories because some of these infants later show developmental problems or signs of mental retardation. Nurses are often team members in such comprehensive tracking programs.

Nurses also promote and participate in case finding through screening programs to detect inborn errors of metabolism, usually in the nursery. For example, PKU screening is done by collecting a drop of blood from the infant's heel on filter paper after the infant has consumed milk. Public health nurses often find it necessary to visit infants discharged home early after delivery and before the usual time for screening. When an infant is discharged before 24 hours, the public health nurse may be requested to go into the home to perform the test, or the parents will be requested to take the infant to the pediatrician. If the blood test shows elevated levels of phenylalanine, the test is repeated by the nurse so that the laboratory can make certain that it is indeed positive. Treatment on a phenylalanine-restricted diet is started as quickly as possible to prevent severe mental retardation (see Chapter 38).

Screening opportunities for conditions such as congenital hypothyroidism are not freely used in the United States; only approximately 20 states have mass screening programs for hypothyroidism.

When a mass screening does not exist, the symptoms of congenital hypothyroidism during well-child visits should lead the nurse to suspect an affected infant. Hypothyroid infants show poor growth and poor appetite, sluggishness, constipation, large protruding tongue, and poor muscle tone likely to result in an umbilical hernia (see Chapter 40). When public health nurses are the only members of the health team to see infants consistently during the early months, these nurses observe for deviations from normal growth, provide follow-up assessment, and initiate referrals for medical evaluation. On well-child visits, the nurse measures and documents growth and conducts a thorough review of the child's health with the parent or primary caregiver. Severe mental impairment can be prevented by treatment with thyroid hormone before three months of age.

Care of the Family

The nurse's role with the developmentally disabled is focused primarily on the needs of the child, but like other aspects of child health nursing, the nurse's scope of practice includes the entire family system.

Family Assessment In assessing developmentally disabled children and their families, the nurse analyzes the suprasystems that affect the child and family. (Family assessment is discussed in Chapter 17.) Because sociocultural handicaps can cause delayed development, the nurse notes signs of poverty, child abuse, lack of emotional and social support by parents, and restrictive parenting styles that might conflict with dominant cultural norms. A longstanding lack of financial resources often brings poor living conditions that lack books and other materials for fostering child development. A lack of toys, books, and play equipment is in turn related to low performance on intelligence tests (Casey and Bradley, 1982). Parents who are economically destitute also tend not to have high regard for academic achievement (Menolascino, 1983). Because poverty seems to generate these negative parental attitudes, the nurse can expect to find developmental vulnerability associated with the family at risk (see Chapter 22).

Assessment tools can provide a preliminary means of planning an intervention program that allows measurement of progress. The Home Observation for Measurement of the Environment (HOME) is one such tool for analyzing data about the child and family (see Chapter 17 and Appendix D). Once a child's developmental problem has been identified, observing the child in the home environment helps the nurse to learn the family's concerns. A discussion of anxiety concerning the child's problems is more likely to be initiated by a family during a home assessment. Krajicek, and Tearney-Tomlinson (1983) provide a framework for assessing the home environment for a child who is developmentally delayed or disabled. Table 23-1 describes assessment tools that are useful in collecting data for specific age groups and needs.

Parent Teaching In establishing contact with the family, the nurse first clarifies the nursing role. A preliminary goal during this initial contact is to foster acceptance by the child and family. The nurse therefore views a client's behavior as a response to the nurse's actions and attitudes. If the nurse is to foster acceptance, nursing interventions need to communicate basic respect, or positive regard, for the client. Nursing care that is unqualified and unconditional in turn communicates respect for the client through concern for feelings, experiences, and human potential; through physical care; and through verbal and nonverbal responses to the client's expression of feelings and ideas. In establishing trust, the nurse also clearly defines the purpose of the nurse's interventions, when the nurse will be available, and how long the services will be available (O'Neil, 1976).

Another goal of nursing intervention is helping parents recognize the normal aspects of their defective children's development and behavior. Parents usually have to learn to distinguish behaviors that are healthy or expected from those that are real problems. The nurse therefore teaches parents to differentiate normal motor development from abnormal reflex activities. With careful explanations from the nurse and other health professionals most parents can become astute observers and managers of their child's special needs.

Many parents also need advice about handling problems of daily care, such as sleep, feeding, and temperament, that are common to all children (see Chapter 13). The special problems presented by the disabled child's vulnerability to acute illness might require more than the ordinary measures. The day-to-day responsibilities also can be taxing and stressful. Because nurses may be the most frequent contact person providing guidance and health supervision, they are likely to be alerted first to family stresses and crises that may cause a developmentally disabled child to be mistreated, neglected, or abused.

Parents of severely disabled children often are faced with such health problems as seizure disorders, abnormal reflex activity and abnormal body posturing, and episodes of acute illness. The nurse acting as coordinator might either provide care or provide access to specific programs for handling the child at home.

Assessment of the Hospitalized, Developmentally Disabled Child

1. Health history
   a) Pertinent prenatal and postnatal events
   b) Allergies to food or medication
   c) Number and length of previous hospital stays
   d) Child's reaction during and after hospital stays
2. Physical examination
   a) Muscle tone and skin turgor
   b) Height, weight, and head circumference
   c) Sensory function—visual, auditory, tactile, gustatory, olfactory, and kinesthetic responses
   d) Dentition and oral integrity
   e) Reflexes, postural patterns
3. Nutritional status
   a) Dietary intake (including calories and volume)
   b) Level of feeding skills
4. Health care history
   a) Availability of routine pediatric supervision
   b) Specialists (therapists, nurses, or others) who have evaluated, referred, or treated the child
5. Developmental assessment
   a) Milestones accomplished (gross and fine motor skills, toilet training, self-care abilities)
   b) Ability to understand and follow directions
   c) Methods of communication (sign language, special signs, speech)
   d) Ability to interact with others, especially strangers
   e) Comfort measures and routines used
   f) Necessity to continue special program of exercise or stimulation
6. Environmental assessment
   a) Place of residence
   b) Primary caregiver(s)
   c) Special equipment used
   d) Usual program of daily activities

Issues in Care of the Mentally Retarded

Nutrition and Feeding Nursing interventions related to nutrition for developmentally disabled children are planned to inform parents about appropriate developmental skills and feeding tasks, teach parents to feed children with motor impairment, and teach parents about maintaining adequate levels of nutrition. Children with developmental disabilities sometimes have brain damage that causes feeding problems, which in turn can cause alterations in nutritional status. Pipes (1981) lists several common problems reported by parents:

Slow growth in length and lack of appropriate weight gain

Excessive weight gain in relation to gains in length

Obesity

Iron-deficiency anemia

Refusal to consume specific foods and groups of foods

Pica and bizarre feeding patterns

Lack of appetite or excessive appetite

Gagging, vomiting, or rumination

Food allergies

Constipation

Abnormal motor patterns that affect a child's ability to consume food

Inability or unwillingness to eat finger food or to self-feed

Limited attention span at mealtime

Disruptive behavior at mealtime

Data from a collaborative study (Kozlowski, 1981) of the nutritional status of a group of developmentally disabled children showed dietary, clinical, biochemical, and social data indicating a general need for intervention. Forty percent of the children in this study were below the 5th percentile for weight and height measurements. Fifty-seven percent showed delayed feeding skills. Feeding problems therefore were correlated with short stature.

Dietary Planning Diets of many severely handicapped infants are deficient in calories, nutrients, bulk, and fluids. This presents a threat to adequate growth. Minimal ingestion of solids during the first year becomes an even greater problem later in life and contributes to other areas of health concerns, including dental hygiene, lower resistance to disease, and elimination problems (Zelle, 1983). According to Pipes (1981), dietary programs should include estimates of calories needed to support physical growth, and these should be based on kcal/cm of height rather than kcal/kg of body weight.

Calorie intake is affected by degree of severity and motor involvement. The developmentally disabled child whose condition reduces mobility tends to need fewer calories. Thus, mentally retarded children with motor impairment may need fewer calories and smaller quantities of most nutrients.

Some developmental conditions, such as Down's syndrome and Prader–Wili syndrome, are associated with weight gain and obesity, and some retarded children are sheltered by their parents and lead sedentary lives with fewer opportunities for active games and exercise. Obesity and fatigue then become established patterns. Parents who fail to see ways to express affection to their retarded children might overindulge their children with food, thus establishing a pattern leading to obesity. Nurses can suggest and demonstrate appropriate expressions of affection and can reinforce acceptable behavior that does not involve food.

Many developmentally disabled children have additional organ defects of the heart and neuromuscular system. Those children who have neuromuscular characteristics of fluctuating tone and athetosis need more calories to compensate for frequent and involuntary muscle activity. When abnormal oral motor problems involving tongue thrusting, muscle rigidity, and muscle tone severely interfere with feeding, there are increased risks to the child's health that can be life-threatening. Gavage or tube feeding then may be necessary (see Chapter 38). Because parents and health professionals necessarily are concerned about intake and weight gain in these children, weight gain can be a hopeful sign of progress, causing a tendency to overfeed the child.

The nurse's assessment of neurologic development, motor abilities, and feeding successes and problems is part of the collaboration with other health care therapists in the process of planning optimal dietary intake. (The process of nutritional assessment is discussed in Chapter 15.) Many children require numerous changes and trials before satisfactory intake is achieved, and collaboration therefore is important in setting priorities for feeding and nutritional programs. Pediatric physical therapists and occupational therapists can help in deciding correct positioning for abnormal tone and in assessing motor skills needed for feeding. Pediatric speech therapists can help by desensitizing children's resistance to different or new textures and can relate the feeding program to prespeech development. Pedodontists who are comfortable in working with developmentally disabled children should be consulted in cases of dental caries or gum disease, especially for children on anticonvulsants such as phenytoin. Other team members might include social workers, who can help families secure appropriate food, especially when resources for purchasing foods are inadequate. Nutritionists specializing in the nutritional needs of developmentally disabled children might also be available to train health care professionals in evaluating and managing nutritional treatment.

Infant Feeding Parents expect their infants to have pleasant feeding experiences, which are essential to the establishment of basic trust. Infants who show no interest in eating do not participate in the reciprocal process and so do not reinforce parenting behaviors.

Mothers who had planned to breast-feed their babies might automatically assume that a child with problems must be bottle-fed. Breast feeding, however, is a desirable choice for feeding developmentally disabled infants and can be encouraged by the nursing staff. Breast feeding disabled infants who have oral motor problems promotes development of the oral muscles. Infants with structural anomalies of the mouth and palate or with muscle tone abnormalities, however, do better with special nipples. For these infants nurses can guide parents in choosing among the commercially available nipples.

Zelle (1983) reports that several commercial nipples are especially difficult for the handicapped infant to manage. The nurse therefore can try the nipple with the infant before suggesting that a parent buy a particular type. Nipples with short shafts do not allow the infant to pull the nipple far enough into the mouth, and the too-short nipple then causes the infant to produce a clicking sound as the vacuum needed for proper sucking is broken. A high-arched palate increases the need for a nipple with a longer shaft. Some manufacturers claim that their nipple products simulate the action of drawing milk from the breast, thus stimulating development of oral musculature, although these nipples usually have short shafts. When increased volume is required, special nipples designed for this purpose should be tried, and parents should be discouraged from enlarging the holes of nipples because larger holes increase the risk of aspiration in infants who have poorly developed sucking, swallowing, and breathing patterns. Infant feeders should be used cautiously for the same reason, unless these are deemed most appropriate following a complete examination of oral motor ability.

When the mechanics of eating cause problems, parents need guidance in choosing the appropriate time in the child's development to offer solid foods. Poorly controlled tongue movements, abnormal posture and tone, and gagging and biting problems can present difficulties. Many parents feel pressured to offer solid foods early because of an infant's poor weight gain or fussiness related to neuromotor immaturity and dysfunction (Zelle, 1983).

Parents of developmentally disabled children sometimes subtly prevent their children from maturing, often because the child remains an infant and dependent in the parent's mind. Such children might be fed strained or junior foods even when the cues indicating readiness for unstrained are present. Because of a child's oral hypersensitivity to textures, the transition from strained to unstrained foods can be upsetting. The child might refuse to eat, and weight loss might result. A program of desensitization often increases a child's tolerance of textures.

Feeding Skills The mentally retarded child learns feeding skills in much the same way as the normal child but at an unpredictable and slower pace. Nevertheless, parents can identify times to promote progress by teaching more advanced feeding skills.

A primary goal is to help developmentally disabled children become as independent in their feeding skills as possible. Self-feeding, however, depends largely on the degree of motor impairment. When the developmentally disabled child has a motor dysfunction in addition to retardation, the ability to follow the normal sequence of feeding behaviors may be altered. For some children only very low levels of self-feeding are achieved. Because it is much less time consuming for a parent to feed the child, parents need much encouragement in remaining patient as their children learn. Children also must not be left to struggle unaided for too long, or they become discouraged by failure. The nurse teaches the parent to show the task to the child and then help the child to perform the movements. After a number of trials the child might be able to imitate the parent's behavior or at least to offer minimal resistance. At this point the parent should gradually withdraw effort, particularly at the end of a sequence, so that the child completes the feeding task independently (Finnie, 1975). The challenge of learning to eat solid foods also encourages development of self-help skills and enhances the child's self-confidence. Feelings of self-worth also can help the child maintain a desired food intake and hence a desired weight.

Retarded children sometimes develop inappropriate, negative behaviors associated with feeding. Behaviors such as spitting, purposeful gagging, vomiting, ruminating, and throwing food can overwhelm parents. The nurse helps parents understand that disruptive behaviors should not be tolerated or reinforced. In such instances the nurse might teach behavior modification techniques, so that negative behaviors can be extinguished in favor of functional feeding patterns. (Behavior modification is discussed in Chapter 13.)

Various problems also might contribute to decreased appetite in the developmentally disabled infant; these include frequent illness, medications such as dextroamphetamine and methylphenidate, central nervous system damage, and abnormal muscle tone. For example, children with Down's syndrome and Hurler's syndrome often have nasal congestion due to structural changes. Breathing and tasting then are difficult; more energy is required for breathing; and eating produces fatigue. Nurses can help parents by devising feeding schedules and reminding the parent to feed the child who is not interested in eating. In some cases the nutritional concentration of food also will need to be increased.

Anxiety over feeding sufficient quantities of food can lead a parent to choose foods high in calories, carbohydrates, and fats but deficient in nutrients. Parents therefore should be advised to make good choices in the quality of food and to feed smaller amounts more frequently, rather than offering a nutritionally poor selection of foods that seem more pleasing to the child's taste.

Sexuality Sexuality comprises the ways in which people use gender as a part of their roles, relationships, values, and customs. Krajicek (1982) defines sexuality even more broadly as the physical, psychologic, social, emotional, and spiritual makeup of each person. For developmentally disabled children, sexuality involves understanding and enjoying one's body and gender in ways that are consistent with levels of understanding, function, responsibility for self-care, and cultural norms.

Nurses and other professionals working with the families of retarded children need to examine their own conscious and unconscious attitudes toward developmentally disabled persons as sexual beings. Misconceptions that retarded individuals were sexually aggressive, dangerous, and incapable of heterosexual relationships, whether sensual or platonic, were once commonly accepted assumptions. Nurses working with parents who are resolving sexual issues plan care to provide anticipatory guidance and education to dispel misinformation, show respect for parents' values and beliefs, help prevent problems related to sexuality or sexual behavior, and counsel or arrange counseling when the therapy required is beyond the scope of nursing. Above all, a parent needs reassurance that the quality of the child's life is the nurse's primary goal.

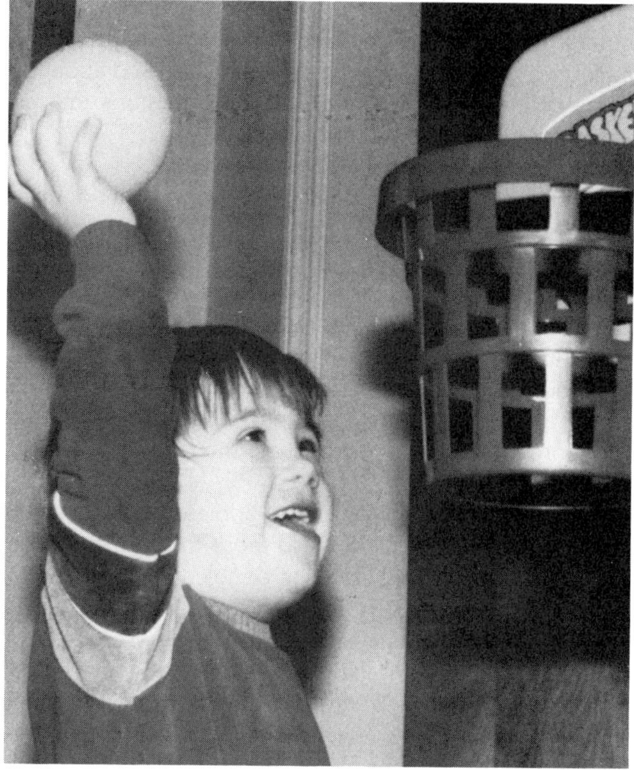

Like all children, those with developmental disabilities use play to promote psychomotor and social development.

Social Development In some families the sexual needs of a developmentally disabled child are ignored. Mentally retarded children are often raised in protective environments where they are deprived of many experiences and peer interactions that form the basis for healthy, fulfilling friendships in later years. Some parents of retarded children even tend unconsciously to deprive these children of sensory input and experiences in infancy that enhance normal sexual development. For example, many parents fail to hold, caress, or handle these infants as normal infants are usually handled. Curry and Peppe (1978) note that the earliest experiences of sexuality and pleasure through one's body begins in infancy, long before differentiation of self from others develops. Like the normal infant, the developmentally disabled infant learns that the body's senses produce good feelings about oneself through sensual experiences involving the eyes, ears, nose, mouth, and skin. Caressing, stroking, and other behaviors are a part of the bonding process that promotes this awareness.

In learning to discriminate among the sensory inputs children learn which body parts are most pleasurable and so learn that they can exert control to promote pleasant experiences with their bodies. Parents can facilitate children's sense of control by referring to body parts by name, just as they would for normal children. They also can provide sensory feedback through expressions of happiness, sadness, disappointment, embarrassment, or anger. For example, retarded children frequently are not taught or even permitted to learn physical skills that lead to a sense of mastery of the environment, and some children grow up lacking basic skills that lead to strategies for making choices or for expressing feelings of pleasure appropriately. Acknowledging feelings and modeling appropriate expressions of emotion are ways to teach control of sensory experiences.

Some parents fail to acknowledge that retarded children grow up, even when their children's levels of intelligence are adequate for some of the developmental tasks of normal children. When children are severely retarded, many parents and professionals contend that any attention to sex is inappropriate because these children are incapable of learning sexual behavior. When the severely retarded child masturbates, for example, the parent might be astounded and might want to know where the child learned the behavior. Such parents fail to recognize that natural and instinctive sexual needs are present from birth. A parent's denial of sexual maturation perpetuates attitudes that the retarded person is sexless and remains a child forever.

As with normal children, discussion of sexuality should occur prior to physical maturity and in the context of other body functions. Sexuality is not an isolated subject. Nurses can help parents understand that young developmentally disabled children should learn about their bodies and how to appreciate them. Parents often need to know that expressions of feeling promote a positive self-image and gender identity. Additionally, teaching about privacy to younger retarded children, often through role modeling, encourages the child to learn about sex roles and about the types of behaviors and expression of emotions that are acceptable in private but not in public.

Adolescence Although the physical development of many developmentally disabled adolescents is slower and secondary sex characteristics are acquired much later than normal, these adolescents and their parents have concerns about sexuality and sexual development. Many parents recognize the need to deal with sexual issues in their children but hold back because of insecurity and anxiety. To provide effective management of sexual issues, nurses therefore are required to anticipate the needs of the child and parent.

For developmentally disabled adolescents issues surrounding sexuality are similar to those for normal adolescents. The difference lies in the disabled person's lack of appropriate information about physical and emotional changes. Developmentally disabled adolescents need to be taught in simple terms about how male and female bodies work, how they are alike and different, how they grow and mature, how one becomes a mother or father, and how babies are made. When talking about their bodies, developmentally disabled children need to discuss and examine their own bodies, as they often have difficulty applying what they see in drawings and pictures. Nurses can help parents understand that what their developmentally disabled adolescent needs to know about sexuality can be taught in the context of differentiating self from others, learning about health and hygiene, and developing self-care skills. Sex education thus includes cultural mores, male and female roles, appropriate touching and showing of affection to family members and to others, and heterosexual friendships.

For retarded adolescents friendships with nonretarded adolescents also are extremely important. Such contact provides opportunities for mature role models with appropriate behavior patterns. The developmentally disabled adolescent who is physically handicapped also may have fewer opportunities for what other adolescents experience on their own. Warm, caring, nonintimate friendships enhance social development and help prevent loneliness for the retarded adult. Nurses can explore community groups such as churches, scouting, and civic groups such as the YMCA and YWCA where programs often are designed to integrate the retarded and normal peers in social activities. Helping parents recognize and accept signs of sexual maturity in developmentally disabled adolescents enables parents to dress, groom, and choose personal items appropriate for this developmental stage.

Retarded adolescents experience much of the internal conflict and turmoil of normal adolescents. One sign of this turmoil is moodiness. Retarded adolescents, however, usually lack the verbal skills to describe their emotions. For these children parents can model and label feelings; pointing out that other people are happy, unhappy, sad, or excited and then pointing out these same emotions when they are experienced by the retarded child.

As they mature physically, some mentally retarded adolescents experience erotic sensations that they do not understand. As a result they often act out these feelings with inappropriate public display of such behaviors as masturbation. Masturbation is normal, unharmful, and can be gratifying and fulfilling at any age. It is, however, a private matter and can be a problem at an inappropriate time or in the presence of others. Nurses often need to reassure parents that providing privacy does not encourage masturbation; privacy merely protects the feelings of others and should be ensured regardless of the child's age or functional level. Providing a private place can be difficult in institutional settings where the child's own bedroom is rarely available for privacy, but the masturbating adolescent can be taken to the bathroom and given time alone. For some adolescents excessive masturbation might be an indication of boredom and a need for other kinds of stimulation. Parents and caregivers then can provide recreational and enjoyable activities for the retarded child who lacks the ability to choose a variety of gratifying leisure activities.

Pubescent girls need preparation for the onset of menstruation so that they know that this is normal and unrelated to their developmental disability. Preparation prevents fear of menstruation and the tendency to try to hide its occurrence from parents or caregivers. Preparation includes teaching about the use of sanitary pads or tampons and special hygiene during the menses. Severely retarded girls may have trouble handling their own care, and in such instances, caregivers usually manage this along with other areas of personal care.

Parents may fear their child's interest in the opposite sex as a desire for a loving relationship that can lead to sexual intercourse. Nurses can reassure parents that, for the mentally retarded, sexual needs are often not synonymous with sexual intercourse. Retarded adolescents often attend school with normal children, however, and are not protected from the influence of peers, the media, and other environmental factors stressing sexual behavior. When they face peer pressure to engage in intimate relationships, retarded children are known to be compliant, which makes them vulnerable to promiscuity and sexual exploitation.

Reproduction Both parents and society in general often fear reproduction in retarded persons. For many developmentally disabled persons, reproduction is impossible because of hereditary defects associated with mental retardation or physical disabilities that make reproduction less likely. Infertility in retarded individuals is most common when the level of retardation is severe to moderate (Craft and

Craft, 1983). Males with Down's syndrome, for example, are rarely capable of reproduction. Nurses are often asked to refer parents to doctors who will perform hysterectomies or tubal ligation for sterilization. (Parents usually are more concerned about sterilization of retarded girls than boys.)

Blackwell (1979) suggests that nurses involved in sexual counseling of retarded clients or their parents be aware of the historical aspects of this concern. Early in this century, when retardation was thought to be caused solely by inferior genes, fear that mentally defective individuals would reproduce and destroy the genetic health of the nation led to a eugenics movement. Eugenics developed as a scientific and social cause for the purpose of protecting the population from "defective genes." Laws were passed at the state level permitting involuntary sterilization of all persons considered retarded. By 1975, most states had passed laws to stop involuntary sterilization of retarded persons, but in 13 states laws still permit the involuntary sterilization of mentally retarded persons living in institutions. Seven states also permit sterilization of mentally retarded persons living in the community (Krajicek, 1982).

Today parents can petition the courts for permission to have retarded children sterilized. Some parents believe they should have retarded girls sterilized when they are incapable of caring for their menses, cannot make responsible decisions concerning sexual behavior, and could not care for any children they might have. In these cases some states require that the medical opinions of more than one physician be obtained and that a legal guardian be appointed by the court to act in behalf of a retarded person. Laws governing criteria for deciding such cases, however, vary.

When sterilization is sought solely to prevent an unwanted pregnancy, nurses can inform parents of the various methods of contraception and clinics where contraceptive counseling may be obtained. Retarded persons require diverse solutions to their contraceptive needs. Many factors need consideration when helping retarded persons or their families choose the most appropriate contraceptive method. Some of these factors are individual needs; personality, including degree of motivation and amount of supervision required; other medication taken regularly; and convenience (Croft and Croft, 1983).

Although the nurse wants to be objective in providing information in this area, some contraceptive methods require more effort to use and more motivation than other methods. For example, barrier methods such as condoms, diaphragms, spermicidal foams, and sponges require planning and nearly normal motor ability. The nurse therefore can express reservations about these methods. A comparison of various contraceptive methods, with their advantages and disadvantages, is presented in Table 11-2. When used correctly, hormonal contraceptives, including oral contraceptive pills and long-acting progestin injections, offer the greatest protection against pregnancy. A major advantage of hormonal contraception is the predictability of the menses. For many retarded females, supervision by a parent, caregivers, or nurse is needed for correct administration of oral contraceptives.

Hormonal contraceptives do, however, have the potential to exacerbate preexisting conditions, such as emotional and neurologic disorders (Hatcher et al., 1984; Dickey, 1983). Nurses therefore need to alert parents to the necessity for close observation of danger signals when a retarded female is placed on birth control pills or given periodic contraceptive injections. A contraceptive injection, such as Depo-Provera, has an advantage of being long-acting and highly effective for 3–4 months. Despite its convenience and effectiveness, however, Depo-Provera produces major side effects including depression and weight gain, which are especially undesirable in retarded persons. It also has not been well accepted in the United States.

Other side effects might be caused by drug interactions. Nurses working with retarded individuals need to know that medications such as anticonvulsants, phenothiazines, antidepressants, and tranquilizers can produce side effects or interfere with the effectiveness of oral contraceptives.

Intrauterine devices (IUDs) are an effective and relatively safe alternative to hormonal contraceptives. All IUDs are contraindicated for individuals who have multiple sex partners because the device increases the risk of sexually transmitted diseases and pelvic inflammatory disease. If the retarded female or the caregiver cannot be taught to check for the presence of the IUD string, a nurse properly trained in vaginal examinations may do so.

Toilet Training Achievement of toileting is a step that parents of retarded children, like those of normal children, eagerly await. One study of incontinence services for 330 disabled children (Parker, 1984 a and b) found more than half of the families wanting more advice on management of toileting problems. These families suggested that nurses and other health professionals could be more helpful by volunteering advice early, providing practical help and advice about supplies and equipment, providing more accurate and detailed information about a child's condition and potential for continence, and providing more medical contact to investigate the reason for lack of toilet control.

Managing personal care is a demanding task for a parent. It is often unrewarding when the child is large and difficult to handle or when negative behaviors such as encopresis or smearing of feces are associated with elimination. Accomplishing toileting signals a major milestone in the retarded child's self-care.

Toilet training for the mentally retarded child requires patience and time. Rarely is it easy. Success, however, has been demonstrated with all levels of retarded children including the profoundly retarded. The age for management of toileting varies among retarded children. Some learn at the same age that normal children are toilet-trained, whereas others may never reach any degree of control in taking care of their own toileting needs. In some instances, neurologic impairments or organic conditions such as cerebral palsy, neural tube defects, and constipation make it more difficult to manage the smaller steps that make up the toileting task.

Parents are usually anxious to start working on toileting. (Toilet training for normal children is discussed in Chapter 13.) Nurses can help them recognize signs of readiness in the child by assessing the child's general developmental status in self-help, motor, and communication skills. Some maturity is necessary in those areas before the child indicates readiness. Bowel training is easier to initiate first because sphincter control is obtained earlier than bladder control. Generally, girls train more easily than boys, but no child should be compared to another. Seventy-five percent of retarded children achieve bowel control prior to bladder control, and daytime dryness is generally achieved 1 year ahead of nighttime dryness (O'Neil, 1977).

Observation of the child's defecating around the same time each day signals the parent to put the child on the training potty. The goal is to establish a schedule. Sitting on a potty can be a tense and upsetting experience for some children at first, and so this alone might be viewed as an achievement. Therefore, the nurse explains the need for preliminary steps in the toileting process. These might be getting the child to feel comfortable while sitting on the potty and gradually increasing the time until the child understands the purpose of the toilet and what is expected.

The parent can encourage cooperation by engaging the child in a pleasant, relaxing activity such as looking at a picture book or listening to a story or to music. Comfort is enhanced when the feet are flat on the floor or on an elevated box or stool, the trunk balanced, and the child has something to hold. Balance and support give a sense of security. Once the child is comfortable on the potty, toys and other play items need to be removed gradually so that the child is able to concentrate.

Parents should not be discouraged when the child produces as soon as he or she is removed from the potty. Regression too is common in the early stages of toilet training. This is frustrating for parents, nurses are often needed to lend a supportive ear and to offer hope and reassurance. Accidents are frequently mixed with successes. Mastering small steps therefore marks progress toward independence in self-care, and nurses need to help parents recognize small successes. The child's clean and dry periods should be rewarded with praise. Mentally retarded children look forward to pleasing their parents and are eager to receive praise following any success.

Nurses also are expected to guide families in selecting specific equipment, aids, and procedures that might be required. Some of the aids are disposable pads and sheets, waterproof pants, disposable bedding, mattress covers, urinals, raised commode seats, toiletries, and deodorants. For children with bladder dysfunction special equipment is helpful (Finnie, 1975). Pictures of devices and guidance about using adaptive equipment help parents determine what to purchase. Special potty seats and devices for children with cerebral palsy, for example, are commercially available. A little ingenuity, however, often can be used to improvise special equipment with household items when commercially designed devices are not comfortable or stable.

Behavior Modification Principles of behaviorism, although relatively new in nursing (O'Neil, 1977), are increasingly used for discipline and behavior change. Behavior modification is described in Chapter 13 as one of several methods of discipline. It is a method particularly appropriate for the mentally retarded.

The principal goals of behavior modification are to encourage behaviors that do not occur often enough and to weaken (or extinguish) behaviors that are excessive or undesirable. O'Neil (1977) lists the following seven areas to consider in the design and implementation of behavior modification programs:

1. Assisting the caregiver to identify major areas of concern
2. Assessing the situations in which the behavior occurs
3. Establishing the child's developmental level
4. Selecting target behaviors
5. Selecting consequent events
6. Implementing the program
7. Documenting behavioral changes

If behavior modification programs are to be successful, nurses need to believe that retarded individuals can be influenced to achieve positive behavioral outcomes. According to Strauss and Bumbalo (1979) nurses need a sound knowledge base and competence in initiating, maintaining, and evaluating behaviorally based interventions. Behavior programs that are improperly planned and carried out can result in little or no behavior change or in the addition of new and undesirable behaviors. Time to work with the child and caregiver is vital to observing the behavior in context. In such observations the nurse notes the behaviors that occur immediately before and after the behavior in question. The nurse is also needed to model positive reinforcement and to monitor progress.

Molding the behavior of retarded children makes care more rewarding for parents and is a way of teaching self-care. If basic self-care skills such as feeding, dressing, and bathing are not learned, the child does not attain greater independence and is less likely to engage in other activities inside and outside the home. Outside experiences in turn enhance learning. Retarded children often develop inappropriate behavior patterns simply because they are inactive, bored, or lacking in models of normal behavior. Even after the most carefully planned behavior modification program is executed by the most conscientious nurse, the child's family or caregiver must be able to carry out the program. The nurse collaborates with caregivers in analyzing the behavior and planning the program. Participation is essential. Program failure is unavoidable when caregivers are uncommitted or when family dysfunction prohibits adequate follow-through.

When behavior modification fails or is inappropriate for a particular family, the nurse assesses the availability of community support systems. Community resources can help the family cope with the child's day-to-day care and behavior problems.

Health Promotion Information about recurring health problems of developmentally disabled children serves as a basis for health teaching to parents and their children. Areas for the nurse to emphasize include basic nutrition, physical fitness, dental care, self-care and personal hygiene, safety, alcohol, and smoking. Decision-making processes also need discussion. Family-centered discussion and teaching allow all family members opportunities to promote health.

The nurse's method of teaching depends on the cognitive levels of both parents and children. The method differs from family to family. Visual aids or commercially available teaching aids can be valuable. Some of these are flip charts, dolls with realistic body parts, simple booklets, flannel boards, slide-tape programs, simulated items, and actual samples.

Theories of learning also differ between adults and children. Nurses thus need to consider ways to present information to increase motivation. For example, appropriate reinforcers for positive behaviors might be simple praise for the parent but tangible rewards are needed for the child. Positive feedback enhances both learning and cooperation. Jones (1980) suggests four instructional guidelines that are useful in teaching health promotion to mildly retarded children. They are (1) a high level of stimulation, (2) concrete directions for the child to follow, (3) decision-making opportunities, and (4) teaching the child to discriminate among alternatives when making a decision.

Independence For developmentally disabled adolescents who are functioning with a mild to moderate level of retardation and approaching adulthood, parents may express ambivalence that their children show readiness to live independently and are interested in dating and relationships that may lead to marriage. Nurses provide support to parents who are in turmoil about letting go of their children while providing information about supervised group living situations. In some communities, retarded young adults live together with relative independence and opportunities to visit individuals of the opposite sex who are in similar facilities. This allows greater chance to form heterosexual friendships that indeed may lead to marriage for those who are responsible enough to make decisions and support their families. In such instances retarded persons often prefer traditional and stereotypic roles because they are structured, clearly defined, and easy to understand.

Settings for Nursing Practice

Nurses care for developmentally disabled children in a variety of settings. These include the home, acute- and chronic-care facilities, and alternative living arrangements. Child health nurses are most likely to encounter mentally retarded children in the hospital, where the child might be admitted for acute care, or the school, where the school nurse might be involved in monitoring and coordinating a child's care plan.

Hospital

Mentally retarded children often are hospitalized for recurring infections and chronic illnesses. Common problems include immature immune response systems; failure to thrive; organically based behavior problems; and correction of neuromotor, metabolic, and nutritional problems.

Hospital staffs may be unprepared to meet the needs of the developmentally disabled child. When time permits, advance preparation for the family, child, and nursing staff is advantageous. Prior planning reduces the fear experienced by the child and the anxiety felt by the parent. A nurse familiar with the child can assist the parent in writing a description of the child's behavior. The parent should explain how the child makes needs known; how physical needs are provided; what routines are expected; any special adaptive equipment and chairs required for motor control, feeding, or toileting; and types of toys enjoyed. Portable items unavailable at the hospital but used at home should be taken when the child is admitted. Simple instructions about any special behavior management programs also should be included. All of this information can be incorporated in the nursing care plan for the child.

The child's admission process should document the child's level of functioning (Zelle, 1983). White (1983) found that learning-disabled children, those with problems understanding, interpreting, and expressing spoken language, have additional problems communicating with staff in an unfamiliar environment. Gestures and facial expressions help the child understand what is being said. Maintaining eye-to-eye contact, touching the child's arm or face, and calling the child by name helps to maintain the child's attention. Repeating information and having the child repeat it back to the nurse verifies that the child has understood.

Explanations of diagnostic procedures and surgery in simple terms reduce the child's anxiety when the child's developmental level permits an understanding of the information. Nurses can encourage parents to keep written records of notable components of the hospitalization, especially the name of special procedures and medications and the child's reactions to them. This information can be of great value when other health care providers are involved in the child's care in the future.

The nursing care plan should include structured plans for the child's free time; especially when the child has difficulty using long periods of unplanned time constructively. Close supervision is necessary, with a variety of carefully selected leisure activities based on the child's skill level in reading, counting, and fine motor control. Health teaching for both child and parents can occur during these unstructured time periods.

School

Because mentally retarded and developmentally disabled children who once were placed in separate schools and institutions are now integrated in educational settings with normal children, school nurses have an integral role on the educational team. As a consequence of Public Law 94-142, the Education for All Handicapped Children Act of 1975, school children include those with deafness, orthopedic and neuromuscular impairments, vision impairments, learning disabilities, mental retardation, emotional disturbances, and behavioral impairments. School nurses working with the developmentally disabled are involved in health promotion that is essentially primary prevention. School nurses assess the architectural and physical features of schools for barrier-free accessibility. They set policies for case finding, referral, and follow-up. If parents are unable to communicate pertinent medical data to school personnel, the school nurse assists the family in interpreting the information and in helping school administrators and teachers understand and incorporate the child's special needs into the child's educational plan. The nurse's knowledge of health problems allows the nurse to develop checklists and use screening tools for early identification of developmental vulnerability and to assess the health needs of children with developmental delays.

A specific activity of school nurses is appraisal of children in the Special Olympics program. Special Olympics is an international program of physical fitness and training for the mentally handicapped. It contributes positively to physical, social, and psychological development (Maxwell, 1984). Nurses assess the handicaps as well as the personal, social, and immediate health needs of children who want to participate, and make the necessary referrals to help them qualify for events.

Key Concepts

- Mental retardation is part of a broad spectrum of developmental disabilities and is distinguished by intellectual deficits and concurrent lack of adaptive behaviors.
- Mental retardation is classified according to degree, from mild to profound.
- Prenatal causes of retardation include environmental factors, such as maternal disease or exposure to teratogens, and genetic factors, such as chromosomal abnormalities or inborn errors of metabolism.
- Perinatal and postnatal causes of retardation include injuries and neonatal and maternal diseases.
- Diagnosis of mental retardation includes intelligence testing and measurements of adaptive behavior.
- Parental reactions to a diagnosis of a serious disability include ambivalence, denial, guilt, shame, self-pity, depression, and a wish for the child's death.
- Parental grieving when a child is mentally retarded often takes the form of chronic sorrow, a kind of unresolved grief that surfaces when the parent continues to recognize normal developmental milestones that the disabled child will not reach.
- After the initial diagnosis of mental retardation, nurses are often needed to answer a parent's questions, provide reassurance, and identify resources that the family is likely to need.
- Developmental disabilities can adversely affect parent–infant attachment and make the process of incorporating an infant into the family system difficult.
- Attitudes of friends, neighbors, relatives, and the community at large affect family members' perceptions of a child's disability and their abilities to cope with the child's needs.
- Some families report that the experience of adapting to and caring for a retarded child has enhanced family communication and family functioning.

- Nurses often need to teach parents effective ways to respond to inappropriate or unwelcome responses from strangers who comment about a child's disability.

- The effect of a disabled child on the child's siblings depends on the ages of the siblings and the extent to which they feel secure in their roles in the family system.

- Siblings might, at different stages in their own development, withdraw from the retarded child, resent the responsibilities that a retarded child creates, and welcome the opportunity to participate in the child's care.

- Like parents and siblings, members of the extended family system often require nursing support to help them maintain family functioning and adapt to the retarded child's special needs.

- Nursing care for developmentally disabled children is usually part of a multidisciplinary collaboration that might include physicians; social workers; mental health therapists; physical, speech, and occupational therapists; and community agencies.

- Primary prevention of developmental disabilities involves immunization programs, prevention of adolescent pregnancy, referral for genetic counseling, and preconceptive health counseling for women who plan to become pregnant.

- Secondary prevention of developmental disabilities focuses on preventing the secondary effects of existing conditions, which involves screening programs and planned follow-up for children at risk.

- Care of the family with a mentally retarded child involves ongoing family assessment and interventions to foster acceptance of the child and promote family functioning

- Developmental disabilities often cause feeding problems that can lead to alterations in nutritional status.

- Nursing interventions to promote nutrition are planned to prevent obesity or reduce weight, teach feeding skills to parents and children, and advise parents about children's nutritional needs.

- Mothers can choose to breast-feed retarded infants, although bottle feeding with special nipples may be necessary.

- Introducing solid foods is important for promoting feeding skills and adequate nutrition in the developmentally disabled child, but the parent might need advice about the child's readiness and about ways to teach feeding skills.

- Mentally retarded people have sexual needs and require personal contact and close relationships to promote development.

- Communication skills and the ability to respond to sensory stimuli are related to sexuality; acknowledging and modeling appropriate expressions of emotion are ways to teach control of sensory experiences.

- Retarded children need basic information about sex and body functions and are assisted if they are taught about body parts with simple and consistently used terms.

- Retarded adolescents need opportunities for peer contacts, privacy for such behaviors as masturbation, structured leisure activity, and assistance in achieving as much independence as possible.

- Nurses can teach parents and retarded adolescents about appropriate choices for contraception.

- Toilet training for retarded children requires patience and a series of steps that allow children to master toileting skills.

- Behavior modification is a form of teaching appropriate behaviors that is especially useful for nurses and parents of retarded children.

- Settings in which child health nurses are likely to be responsible for care of a retarded child are the hospital and school.

References

Azrin N, Fox R: *Toilet Training the Retarded: A Rapid Program for Day and Night Time Independent Toileting.* Research Press, 1973.

Blackman JA: *Medical Aspects of Developmental Disabilities in Children Birth to Three: A Resource for Special Service Providers in the Educational Setting.* The University of Iowa, 1983.

Blackwell MW: *Care of the Mentally Retarded.* Little, Brown, 1979.

Casey P, Bradley R: The impact of the home environment on children's development, *J Dev Behav Pediatr* 1982; 3:146–152.

Chinn PC, Clifford DJ, Logan DR: *Mental Retardation: A Life Cycle Approach.* 2nd ed. Mosby, 1979.

Craft A, Craft M: *Sex Education and Counseling for Mentally Handicapped People.* University Park Press, 1983.

Curry JB, Peppe KK: *Mental Retardation: Nursing Approaches to Care.* Mosby, 1978.

Dickey RP: *Managing Contraceptive Pill Patients.* 3rd ed. Creative Informatics, 1983.

Elder JO, Magrab PR: *Coordinating Services to Handicapped Children: A Handbook for Interagency Collaboration.* Brookes, 1980.

Finnie NR: *Handling the Young Cerebral Palsied Child at Home.* 2nd ed. E. P. Dutton, 1975.

Grossman HJ: *Classification in Mental Retardation.* American Association on Mental Deficiency, 1983.

Grossman FK: *Brothers and Sisters of Retarded Children: An Exploratory Study.* Syracuse University Press, 1972.

Hatcher RA et al: *Contraceptive Technology.* 12th revised ed. Irvington, 1984.

Johnson SH: *High-Risk Parenting: Nursing Assessment and Strategies for the Family at Risk.* Lippincott, 1979.

Jones B, Springer M: Teaching health education to the mildly handicapped child. *Health Values* (Nov–Dec) 1980; 4:262–265.

Keele DK: *The Developmentally Disabled Child: A Manual for Primary Physicians.* Medical Economics, 1983.

Kozlowski BW: *University Affiliated Facilities Collaborative Study of Nutritional Status of Developmentally Delayed Children.* University Research Foundation, 1981.

Krajicek MJ, Tearney Tomlinsin AI: *Detection of Developmental Problems in Children: Birth to Adolescence.* 2nd ed. University Park Press, 1983.

Krajicek MJ: Developmental disability and human sexuality. *Nurs Clin North Am* (Sept) 1982; 17:377–378.

Maxwell BM: The nursing role in the Special Olympics. *J Sch Health* (March) 1984; 54:131–133.

Menolascino FJ, Newman R, Stark JA: *Curative Aspects of Mental Retardation: Biomedical and Behavioral Advances. Paul H. Brookes, 1983.*

Mercer RT: *Nursing Care for Parents at Risk.* Charles B. Slack, 1977.

Miezio PM: *Parenting Children with Disabilities: A Professional Source for Physicians and Guide for Parents.* Marcel Dekker, 1983.

O'Neil SM, McLaughlin BN, Knapp MB: *Behavioral Approaches to Children with Developmental Delays.* Mosby, 1977.

O'Neil SM: The nursing process in mental retardation and developmental disabilities. Paper presented at International Association for the Scientific Study of Mental Deficiency, Washington, DC, 1976.

Parker G: Incontinence services for the disabled child. Part 1: The provision of aids and equipment. *Health Visitor* (Feb) 1984b; 57:44–45.

Parker G: Incontinence services for the disabled child. Part 2: The provision of information and advice. *Health Visitor* (March) 1984a; 57:86–88.

Payne JS, Patton JR: *Mental Retardation.* Merrill, 1981.

Pipes PL: *Nutrition in Infancy and Childhood.* Mosby, 1981.

Price MM: Critique of the Milani-Comparetti Motor Development Screening Test. *Phys Occup Ther Pediatrics* (Fall) 1980; 1:59–67.

Scheerenberger RC: *A History of Mental Retardation.* Brookes, 1983.

Strauss SS, Bumbalo JA: Factors influencing outcomes of behavioral home management programs. Pages 191–198 in: *Mental Retardation: Nursing Approaches to Care.* Curry JB, Peppe KK (editors). Mosby, 1978.

Thain WS, Casto G, Peterson A: *Normal and Handicapped Children: A Growth and Development Primer for Parents and Professionals.* PSG Publishing, 1980.

Thompson RJ, O'Quinn AN: *Developmental Disabilities: Etiologies, Manifestations, Diagnoses, and Treatments.* Oxford University Press, 1979.

Turnbull AP, Turnbull HR: *Parents Speak Out: Views from the Other Side of the Two-Way Mirror.* Charles E. Merrill, 1978.

US Department of Health, Education, and Welfare: *Health, United States.* National Center for Health Statistics, 1978.

White J: Special nursing needs of hospitalized children with learning disabilities. *Am J Matern Child Nurs* (May–June) 1983; 8:209–212.

Wikler L, Keenan MP: *Developmental Disabilities: No Longer a Private Tragedy.* National Association of Social Workers, 1983.

Zelle RS, Coyner AB: *Developmentally Disabled Infants and Toddlers: Assessment and Intervention.* Davis, 1983.

Additional Readings

Becker WC: *Parents Are Teachers.* Research Press, 1973.

Bobath B: *Abnormal Postural Reflex Activity Caused by Brain Lesions.* William Heinemann, 1976.

Bobath B, Bobath K: *Motor Development in the Different Types of Cerebral Palsy.* William Heinemann, 1976.

Bower FL: *The Process of Planning Nursing Care: A Model for Practice.* 2nd ed. Mosby, 1977.

Brady MA: Fragil-X syndrome: An overview. *Pediatr Nurs* (May/June) 1984; 10:210–211.

Christophersen ER: *Little People: Guidelines for Common Sense Child Rearing.* H and H Enterprises, 1977.

Coley IL: *Pediatric Assessment of Self-Care Activities.* Mosby, 1978.

Cook CL: Nursing services. In: *The Mentally Retarded Child and His Family.* Kock R, Dobson JC (editors). Brunner/Mazel, 1976.

de Leon Siantz ML: *The Nurse and the Developmentally Disabled Adolescent.* University Park Press, 1977.

Denhoff E, Feldman SA: *Developmental Disabilities: Management through Diet and Medication.* Marcel Dekker, 1981.

Erickson ML: *Assessment and Management of Developmental Changes in Children.* Mosby, 1976.

Gabel S, Erickson MT: *Child Development and Developmental Disabilities.* Little, Brown, 1980.

Gottilieb J, Strichart SS: *Developmental Theory and Research in Learning Disabilities.* University Park Press, 1981.

Haynes U: *A Developmental Approach to Casefinding Among Infants and Young Children.* US Department of Health, Education and Welfare, 1980.

Haynes U: *Holistic Health Care for Children with Developmental Disabilities With Special Reference to Young Children with Neuromotor Dysfunctions.* University Park Press, 1983.

Herr SS: *Rights and Advocacy for Retarded People.* Lexington Books, 1983.

Johnston RB, Magrab PR: *Developmental Disorders: Assessment, Treatment, Education.* University Park Press, 1976.

Knickerbocker B: *A Holistic Approach to the Treatment of Learning Disorders.* Charles B. Slack, 1980.

Kopelman L, Moskop JC: *Ethics and Mental Retardation.* D. Reidel, 1984.
Lewis M, Taft LT: *Developmental Disabilities: Theory, Assessment, and Intervention.* Spectrum Publications, 1979.
Matson JL, Breuning SE: *Assessing the Mentally Retarded.* Grune & Stratton, 1983.
McCormack MK: *Prevention of Mental Retardation and Other Developmental Disabilities.* Marcel Dekker, 1980.
McLean JE, Yoder DE, Schiefelbusch RL: *Language Intervention with the Retarded.* University Park Press, 1972.
Mira M, Cairns G: *Handbook of Positive Parenting.* Child Behavior and Development Associates, 1979.
Olshansky S: Chronic sorrow: A response to having a mentally defective child. *Social Casework* 1962, 43:190–193.
Patterson GR: *Living with Children.* Research Press, 1968.
Perske R: *New Directions for Parents of Persons Who Are Retarded.* Abingdon Press, 1973.
Robinson NM, Robinson HB: *The Mentally Retarded Child.* 2nd ed. McGraw-Hill, 1976.
Scheiner AP, Abroms IF: *The Practical Management of the Developmentally Disabled Child.* Mosby, 1980.
Smithells RW et al: Further experience of vitamin supplementation for prevention of neural tube defect recurrences. *Lancet* (May 7) 1983; 8332:1027–1031.
Stephens CJ: The fetal alcohol syndrome: Cause for concern. *Matern Child Nurs J* (July/Aug) 1981; 6(4):251–256.
Szymanski LS, Tanguay PE: *Emotional Disorders of Mentally Retarded Persons.* University Park Press, 1980.
White CS, Minor JW, Connolly B: *A Comprehensive Handbook for Management of Children with Developmental Disabilities.* University of Tennessee for the Health Sciences Child Development Center, 1977.
Williams JK: Evaluating the dysmorphic child. *Pediatr Nurs* (July/Aug) 1983; 241–248.

Nursing Care of the Child With Dysfunctional Behavior

24

Cathryn L. Glanville
Lyn Marshall
John F. Conley
Gretchen L. Kelly

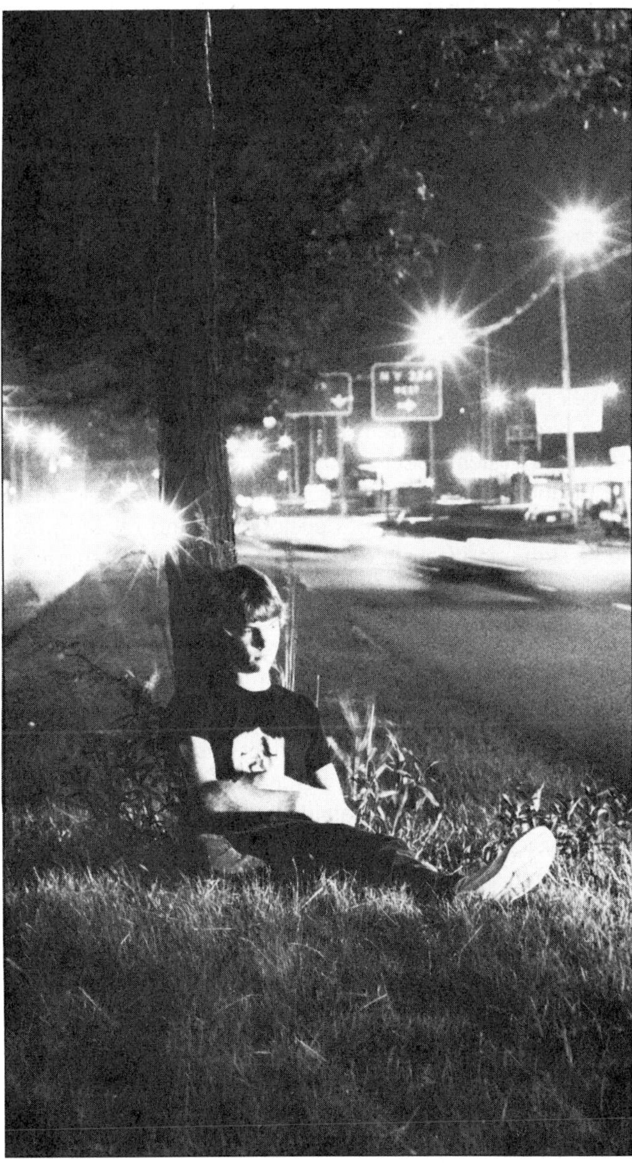

Chapter Outline

Objectives

- Describe dysfunctional behavior as a process of maladaptive coping.
- Explain the role of the child health nurse in identifying dysfunctional behaviors.
- Explain the types of substance abuse and their associated assessment criteria and nursing management.
- Describe the behaviors, likely assessment findings, and associated nursing management for obesity and for anorexia nervosa and bulimia.
- Describe the symptoms, assessment criteria, and nursing management associated with enuresis and encopresis.
- Describe the behaviors, likely assessment findings, and associated nursing management for the child with school phobia and for the child exhibiting runaway behavior.

As children undergo biophysical, affective, and cognitive development, they are expected to become integral parts of a larger social system that includes schools, churches, the legal system, peer groups and other social networks. Adjusting to these demands is one of the child's primary tasks, but complexities of development and related problems stemming from the influence of the child's suprasystems often make this task difficult to achieve.

As we discussed in Chapter 6, Maslow defined affective development in relation to a hierarchy of needs that every person experiences (Gable, 1970). Both real threats, such as the threat of physical harm, and perceived threats, such as the fear of the loss of love, affect this hierarchy in ways that also affect individual behavior. Some children ultimately require professional intervention for behaviors that are physically or psychologically dysfunctional.

Children's mental health therefore is one component of a developmental assessment. Emphasis on this aspect of development enables parents and others responsible for the well-being of children to seek early intervention for children at risk. With a projected increase in the number of children who enter the health care system each year, we can expect to find dysfunctional behaviors evident in a variety of child health care settings.

Because a child's repertoire of coping strategies is limited by biologic and social resources and by developmental stage, the nurse in a general pediatric setting can expect to encounter a variety of dysfunctional behaviors, as children's responses to threats take many forms. Not all of these responses are adaptive, although precise definitions of maladaptive coping strategies vary from setting to setting and depend on each family's cultural, socioeconomic, geographic, and educational background.

In this chapter, we define the relationship between dysfunctional behavior and children's coping strategies. We discuss substance abuse, eating disorders, specific problems of elimination and socialization. These behaviors are relatively common occurrences in both inpatient and outpatient settings and occur across socioeconomic boundaries. Various cultures have different definitions of functional and dysfunctional behaviors related to their specific beliefs about health (see Chapter 3). In this chapter we apply the nursing process to the needs of children who demonstrate patterns of behavior that are considered dysfunctional in most cultures.

Dysfunctional Behavior as Maladaptive Coping

Adaptive coping with real or perceived threats requires innate physical, psychologic, and cognitive strengths that facilitate successful problem solving. Individual strengths vary greatly and depend heavily on genetic, cultural, socioeconomic, and educational variables. For children, the ability to negotiate various threats successfully also depends on the child's developmental stage. A child's ability to perceive a threat grows in direct relation to developmental progress, and the child's repertoire of coping strategies also grows accordingly (see Chapter 12).

Coping strategies, however, offer only a temporary means of dealing with threats. When no progression toward effective problem solving is accomplished, however, the child becomes vulnerable to maladaptive coping. *Maladaptive coping strategies* are ineffective behaviors that a child uses over time to deal with perceived threats or stressors. Maladaptive coping thus results in dysfunctional behavior. Zeitlin (1980) further states that dysfunctional behavior increases the child's vulnerability and so generates more stress.

The child might attempt to reduce this stress through defensive or regressive behavior or through passive behavior, which places stress on the child's learning capacity and might also be viewed as dysfunctional. Wu (1970) and Byrne and Thompson (1971) suggest that dysfunctional behavior can also assist children in coping with crises, thus providing temporary stability. The child must, however, quickly replace maladaptive coping with adaptive coping strategies. For example, denial is a normal coping mechanism in the process of grief, but it becomes pathologic when no progression toward problem solving and resolution of grief occurs. Maladaptive coping thus prevents the child from experiencing interpersonal growth and often, though not always, results in problems related to social development.

Problem solving is the essential distinction between adaptive and maladaptive coping. Problem-solving steps involve the following:

1. Establishing a set—The child's orientation to the problem, which includes strengths, weaknesses, and innate and learned resources
2. Defining the problem—The child's ability to identify and prioritize the problem objectively
3. Identifying resources—The child's gathering all available information about resources that might be used to solve the problem
4. Generating solutions—The child's generating as many possible solutions to the problem as possible
5. Implementing solutions
6. Evaluating outcomes

Even small children employ rudimentary problem-solving skills in their activities of daily living. These are in turn refined and taught by parents and other role models. For example, the child who watches a parent cope with anxiety by eating often learns to solve problems through dysfunctional patterns of eating behavior, which might then lead to obesity or anorexia nervosa.

Child health nurses routinely encounter children and families exhibiting dysfunctional behavior that suggests deficient problem-solving skills and maladaptive coping strategies. The prevalence of dysfunctional childhood behavior varies according to the methodology of current research, but the bulk of data suggest that its incidence is throughout childhood. Pless (1974) reported that 1 child in 20 required some form of professional intervention for dysfunctional behavior, while Graham (1979) reported that 6–20 percent of children required such intervention. Earl's (1980) analysis of three epidemiologic studies in child psychiatry underscored the prevalence of widespread dysfunctional behavior in children, illustrating a substantial population at risk or in need of intervention.

As Chapter 16 explains, child health nurses assess behavior in children by comparing a child's affective and social development to normal ranges for each developmental stage. As Chapter 12 explains, coping behaviors are normal and expected responses to stress or transitions. Adaptive coping strategies, however, are age appropriate and assist the child in interacting with the environment. Maladaptive coping strategies threaten the child's mental health and therefore are an area for nursing intervention.

One component of the developmental assessment process is the nurse's analysis of data to identify any developmental vulnerability (see Chapter 16). Developmental vulnerability, which indicates lowered resistance to stress, may be evident in a child's behavior and may in turn suggest that adaptation to stress is maladaptive. A developmental assessment often provides the earliest indicators of potential behavioral dysfunction. The nurse analyzes data against expected norms for various areas of development and thus can identify deviations that need further assessment.

Information about identified developmental delays, developmental progress, childhood illnesses, immunizations, peer relations, parent-child interaction, school activities, temperament, and any significant losses, separations, or stressors all provide the nurse with data that might indicate vulnerability. The nurse can then analyze patterns of coping that compensate for the child's vulnerability. By identifying the stressor and the associated coping strategies, the nurse can determine the child's present level of functioning, understand potential problems, and plan interventions accordingly.

Before identifying dysfunctional behavior that suggests maladaptive coping, however, the nurse needs to conduct systematic assessments over a period of time. Developmental delays, such as enuresis after age 4 or inability to solve age-appropriate problems, may be either isolated incidents or emerging patterns. While child health nurses often intuitively suspect that a child is employing a maladaptive coping strategy to diminish a real or perceived threat, the assessment is needed to confirm the suspicion.

Dysfunctional behaviors such as substance abuse and obesity are more than maladaptive coping behaviors; they can be linked to stress and are direct physiologic threats to health, involving the nurse in health promotion and health education roles. These roles are discussed more fully in Chapter 18.

Substance Abuse

The abuse of mood-altering substances is a health issue that has been much researched and debated. A growing awareness of the extent and impact of the problem has created a new emphasis on limiting access to these substances and on treating abusers. Billions of dollars have been spent to fund research, education, and treatment programs, but the economic cost must also be calculated in lost productivity and in medical and criminal expenses.

The human cost is familiar to child health nurses. Conservative estimates are that over a quarter of all deaths in the United States are attributable to substance abuse and that cigarette smoking is the largest cause of substance-related illness and death, followed closely by alcohol and drugs (National Institute on Drug Abuse, 1979). The rapid increase in the use and abuse of these substances by chil-

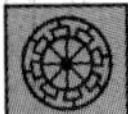

CASE STUDY A Substance-Abusing Adolescent

Assessment

Mary, a 17-year-old, was referred for assessment of substance abuse by local juvenile authorities after she was involved in an automobile accident while under the influence of drugs and alcohol.

The daughter of middle-class parents, and an average student, Mary is now in danger of failing four courses unless her grades improve substantially during the next quarter. Slightly overweight and concerned that she would not have a date for the prom, Mary took her friends' advice and began taking amphetamines regularly "to lose weight." She was found with six amphetamine capsules at the time of her arrest. She was discharged to her parents 4 days later with outpatient follow-up planned.

History of Substance Abuse

Mary first began smoking when she was 12 and became a pack-a-day smoker by the time she began drinking alcohol at age 14. She was introduced to marijuana at age 15 but insists that she only "smoked pot and drank on weekends." In the past 2 years, Mary claims to have used a variety of drugs for nonmedical reasons. She admits to amphetamine and barbiturate use but denies using narcotics or hallucinogens. "What do you think I am? A junkie or something?" she angrily asked during the admission interview.

Family

Both of Mary's parents smoke and drink socially. Her father admits to drinking "a daily cocktail or two to unwind after work," and her mother takes at least one diazepam a day for her "nerves" and flurazepam to aid in sleep. Both parents expressed surprise at Mary's being found with the amphetamines, but both were aware that she drank and smoked. "We trust that she won't go overboard with it; we have to since we both work, and no one's at home with her," reported Mary's mother. "She may have been a little drunk, but she's no alcoholic," her father flatly stated. Mary herself claimed that the accident was "a freak" and denied being intoxicated. "I had only two beers," she stated.

Clinical Data

At the time of her arrest, Mary's blood alcohol level was 0.2%. Her evaluation was uneventful; she had no major withdrawal symptoms except for a mildly elevated blood pressure and a fine hand tremor 24 hours after admission. Urine drug screening was positive for caffeine, nicotine, and dextroamphetamine (Dexedrine).

Nursing Diagnoses

1. Threatened self-concept related to potential loss of peer group
2. Potential dependence on nonmedical use of substances to cope with real or perceived stressors
3. Potential for dysfunctional parenting related to parents' lack of awareness of child's behavior and their own substance abuse

Plan for Interventions

Goals

1. Mary will identify specific peer pressures that cause her to ingest substances.
2. Mary will demonstrate adaptive techniques for refusing substances.
3. Mary will describe her own responses to stress.
4. Mary will demonstrate adaptive responses to stress.
5. Mary's parents will identify their own patterns of substance use.
6. Mary's parents will identify ways to enhance Mary's self-esteem to promote adaptive coping.

Interventions

1. Talk with Mary about peer group attitudes that promote substance abuse, pointing out areas that require exploration (for example, "I must smoke to be part of the gang. It's not habit forming anyway.").
2. Teach Mary to say "no" to offers of substances by role playing situations until Mary can express her refusal in ways that are comfortable for her.
3. Observe social behaviors to note extremes in interactional style, such as withdrawal or aggressiveness.
4. Use "distancing aids," such as games, third-person stories, or artwork with both Mary and her parents to facilitate expression of conflict and stress.
5. Discuss observations with parents to suggest ways to encourage more socially acceptable behavior and adaptation to stress.
6. Teach Mary a step-by-step method of problem solving (identifying the problem, generating solutions, implementing solutions, and evaluating the result).
7. Teach Mary relaxation techniques, such as slow breathing and tensing and relaxing of muscle groups.
8. Discuss patterns of substance use in the home, asking Mary's parents to list substances that they ingest and the circumstances that lead to substance ingestion.
9. Suggest referral to occupational therapy, family therapy, or recreational therapy, as needed.

dren poses a significant challenge to families, schools, and health care providers (Kropf, 1979).

Substance abuse represents the quintessential maladaptive coping strategy. It is a deliberate behavior based on a cognitive process, often in response to social expectation or stress. Substance abuse easily develops into a pattern of dysfunction that results in physiologic withdrawal or addiction. Use of alcohol, tobacco, and drugs has been considered an adult prerogative and is reinforced by legal statutes, social behaviors, and the media (Shopper, 1979). Normal experimentation with adultlike behaviors and the destructive, abusive use of these substances are two points on a continuum, but the point at which one leaves off and the other begins is most often very unclear even for professionals to decide.

Viewed as a point on a continuum of substance use, substance abuse is that stage in which the child establishes a pattern of abuse (Fig. 24-1). At this point, reduction in the number or intensity of abuse episodes becomes difficult without outside intervention. The nurse's interventions are therefore directed toward reversing the deficits in self-care that the child demonstrates.

Of children in various developmental stages, the adolescent demonstrates the most vulnerability to patterns of substance abuse. Because the peer group serves as both a learning source and a competitive arena, the adolescent's reliance on this social system creates anxiety and provides a stimulus for substance abuse. (Adolescence is generally discussed in Chapter 11.)

National Institute of Drug Abuse data further suggest that city-dwelling adolescent males are the most vulnerable group (National Institute of Drug Abuse, 1979). Pollin (1970) notes that most individuals who are involved in substance abuse are aware of the negative consequences but are unable to change their behavior even if they want to. Adolescents in particular are becoming increasingly well-informed about the health hazards of these substances, but their pharmacologic knowledge remains limited and idiosyncratic. The nurse's goal therefore is to guide the adolescent to responsible, informed decision making.

Because the adolescent is part of a larger family system, the adolescent substance abuser must be assessed and treated within the context of this system. Finley (1983) described this interdependence by stating, "When substance abuse is a reality for one family member, each member individually, as well as the entire unit, is involved in response to the abuse." (See Chapter 17 for a discussion of family assessment.) Accurate assessment of the family system may prove difficult because interactions and roles of family members may be substantially different and guarded outside the home. In clinical observations, the nurse therefore notes patterns and styles of interaction among members. Clues to family dysfunction may involve conflicts, themes, scapegoating, or other family issues. (Nursing care of families at risk is discussed in Chapter 22.)

Parents may initially express surprise when confronted with a substance-abusing child; some even deny the problem, and their cooperation in any further assessment or management may be minimal or nonexistent. Unfortunately, this is typically the first stage of a cycle that often delays needed treatment. Siblings, however, are often aware of patterns of substance abuse and may even be involved and in need of treatment themselves.

Tobacco

The most commonly used and abused substance by persons of all ages is tobacco. Most frequently smoked, tobacco has been identified as the "most addictive and dependence-producing form of self-administered gratification" (Pechacek, 1979). Lichtenstein (1979) suggests that many social elicitors of smoking behavior, along with the addictive properties of nicotine, encourage and support a smoking habit and that the failure of many treatment programs results from the emphasis on abstinence from smoking instead of maintaining lowered levels of smoking. Peer group pressure, identification with rebelliousness, and establishment of a self-concept all affect the adolescent's attraction to smoking behaviors. Although there is a steady decline in the proportion of smokers in general, there is a trend toward

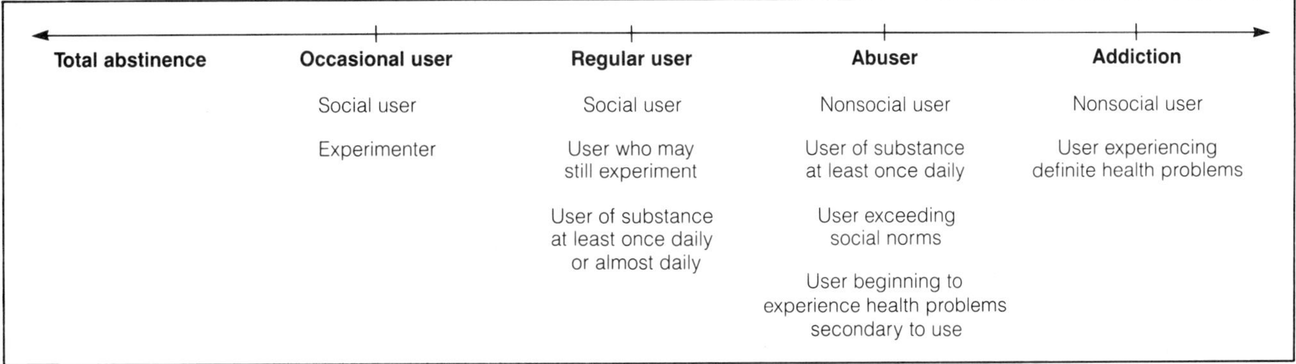

Figure 24-1 Intensity of abuse without interventions. The degree of abuse may be represented by a point on a continuum.

an increasing proportion of female smokers. As fewer social limitations are placed on smoking, the general popularity of tobacco remains high.

Assessment Assessing adolescent smoking behavior is relatively simple, as most adolescents readily provide information about their smoking habits. Objective data concerning the effects of smoking are obtained by a variety of laboratory procedures including blood gas studies, serum nicotine levels, and diagnostic spirometry. Nicotine stimulates smooth muscle, and so an elevated pulse, blood pressure, and other signs of smooth muscle contraction are common. Obvious smoking odors as well as tobacco-stained hands and oral cavity indicate heavy smoking.

Smokers and those who use oral tobacco preparations (for example, snuff, chewing tobacco) report an initial sense of alertness. In large doses, a "high" or a "buzz" is noted, partly because the binding of carbon monoxide molecules with hemoglobin creates a mild form of hypoxia in addition to the stimulating properties of nicotine.

Nursing Management Nursing management of the adolescent smoker should be directed at controlling rather than abstaining from smoking. Fad techniques designed to help the smoker cut down on smoking and the introduction of low-tar and nicotine cigarettes are of doubtful value. Most effective is behavior modification that pairs the act of smoking with an aversive stimulus and successive periods of abstinence with rewards. Mouth drops or gum activated by smoke to produce an unpleasant taste are among the available aversive stimuli. Pechacek (1979) reports research showing some promising results with nicotine gum although the precise role of nicotine in smoking behavior has not been clearly established. Fredericksen (1979) advocates a controlled smoking program emphasizing regulation.

Making smoking behavior contingent on some other behavior further reduces impulse smoking or smoking as a response to stress. The nurse therefore identifies sources of stress and teaches alternative methods of stress reduction with the goal of substituting smoking with a healthier behavior. For the adolescent, the nurse further helps in acquiring new skills to cope with having a restricted tobacco intake.

Alcohol

Widely used among adolescents, alcohol does not always result in abuse and personal trauma. Most people who use alcohol do so responsibly and with no malignant sequelae. Miller (1979), however, reports approximately 15 million "problem drinkers" in the United States, and that "one in eleven reports significant life problems related to alcohol use."

Bales (1969) hypothesizes that problem drinking is likely to be high in groups that (1) generate high levels of anxiety, (2) do not develop and value antialcohol attitudes among their members, and (3) have few or ineffectual coping strategies to relieve anxiety. These traits are all common among adolescents.

Social drinking is a behavior encouraged in American society, particularly among males, and patterns of alcohol use and abuse among adolescents are cause for concern. In dealing with adolescents with alcohol-related deficits in self-care, nurses need to assess their own values and attitudes toward alcohol. For example, condoning or tacitly accepting alcohol abuse among adolescent boys as a normal phenomenon of development blinds the nurse to the significance and scope of this health problem. Likewise, identifying an adolescent drinker as a problem drinker merely on the basis of age may inaccurately stigmatize the client.

Assessment The assessment of adolescent behaviors involves identifying not only the behavior, but also patterns of use and abuse, and resulting deficits in self-care. The adolescent is usually referred by parents, school, or juvenile courts and so may not share the view that a problem exists. Gathering subjective data about drinking patterns is a common but rarely reliable method. Some adolescents overstate their actual alcohol consumption to appear stronger or more mature, whereas others deny any alcohol abuse. The adolescent's emerging skill at rationalization may be evident in the reasons cited for excessive alcohol consumption. Memory deficits might also be caused by alcohol and might impair the adolescent's ability to report alcohol intake accurately. Alcohol abusers may also attempt frequent self-medication to help them cope with emerging anxiety or psychosis.

An essential first step is establishing when the adolescent last had a drink, as potentially life-threatening withdrawal symptoms are usually evident approximately 48 hours after the last drink and peak after 72 hours before finally subsiding after 4 or 5 days. Corroberative data are therefore essential in establishing a baseline. The nurse interviews family members, friends, teachers, and even employers about frequency of drinking behaviors, amount of alcohol consumed at one time, duration and intervals of drinking, and any behavioral changes noted. Family and peer group drinking patterns are assessed in the same manner. The nurse then identifies particular stressors in the adolescent's environment and assesses their impact.

Objective measurements for determining patterns of alcohol abuse can also validate the nurse's assessment data. The blood alcohol level (BAL) is the most direct measure of recent alcohol intake. Expressed as a percentage, the BAL measures the number of grams of alcohol in each 100 mL of blood. A balance of 0.1% suggests behavioral impairment; extreme intoxication is associated with balances greater than 0.3%–0.4%. Patterns of alcohol abuse are reflected in elevated serum glutamic-oxaloacetic transaminase (SGOT) and gamma-glutamyl transpeptidase (GGT) levels. Chronic alcohol abuse is suspected in those with these elevated liver function studies, a jaundiced appearance, and palpable hepatomegaly.

Nursing Management Unlike management for tobacco abuse, management of alcohol abuse is usually directed at stopping rather than regulating the behavior. Controlled drinking programs for alcoholics are not clearly effective. Therefore, in severe cases total abstinence is the desired adaptive behavior and therefore the goal of nursing management.

Severe Alcohol Abuse Detoxification is the first step and requires the withdrawal of alcohol for a period of time; depending on the extent of abuse. Detoxification is the most traumatic and potentially dangerous period of treatment. The body's physical response is widely variable and may be as mild as a headache or as dramatic as hallucinations, hypertensive crisis, and death. Supportive therapy depends on the severity of the withdrawal reaction and involves nutritional supplementation, administration of anxiolytic medications such as chlordiazepoxide (Librium) or diazepam (Valium), rest, and attendance to the safety needs of the adolescent. One goal of drug therapy is to minimize delirium tremens, which can persist after the initial phase of withdrawal.

Once detoxification has been achieved, therapy can begin. Establishing a trusting therapeutic relationship by demonstrating an attitude of caring for the person but disapproving the problem behavior is a crucial first step. The nurse who is prepared to deal with attempts by the adolescent to sabotage the relationship in its early stages expects attempts to test limits or place the nurse in a no-win situation.

Successfully weathering these challenges is crucial to a therapeutic outcome. The nurse's primary goal is to motivate the adolescent to change the behavior. Simply detoxifying the patient does not cure or inspire motivation, so the nurse guides the patient to the recognition of self-destructive tendencies inherent in alcohol abuse. Helping the adolescent substitute healthy activities for the unhealthy activity of alcohol abuse is a major teaching and role-modeling task. This may mean assisting the adolescent in acquiring a new and more supportive social network to replace the old alcohol-related network. Community resources such as Alcoholics Anonymous, the Salvation Army, church, or athletic teams can all serve this purpose (Hurd, Pattison, Llamas, 1981).

Stressors and stress reduction are analyzed according to the impact on drinking behavior. The adolescent may be without the means for stress reduction when the crutch of alcohol is removed. Discussing or role modeling stress-reducing skills and providing an arena to test these skills is critical. An external locus of control with an associated self-concept of helplessness and ineptness is linked to alcohol-abusing adolescents (Plumb, D'Amanda, and Taintor, 1975). Strategies toward improving self-concept and self-esteem while establishing an internal locus of control are therefore important nursing goals. Once the nurse has assessed the adolescent's strengths and attempts at self-care, these need to be reinforced.

A combination of group activity and one-to-one therapy works best when implementing these interventions. The peer group exerts primary influence over the adolescent, and so peer pressure to change dysfunctional behavior may be effective. One-to-one sessions and solitary activities also allow for privacy and intimacy.

Preventing Alcohol Abuse Educational efforts toward preventing alcohol abuse with the next generation include those run by student groups such as Students Against Drunk Driving, which uses peer influence to lead young people away from alcohol abuse. Other educational programs are oriented not toward fear and abstinence from alcohol and drugs, but toward controlled use with a strong injunction against combining chemical substances and driving (Shopper, 1979).

An important first step in intervening with substance-abusing young people is not to promise adolescents that nurses will keep their substance abuse secret. Rather, professionals should remember the self-destructive course that these adolescents are on and work with them to get the help they need. One study of the emergency department of a general hospital indicated that the hospital served a high-risk population and that the pattern of alcohol abuse could often be reversed through early identification and referral in an emergency setting (Stephenson et al. 1981).

Drugs

Although the prevalence of drug abuse and addiction is low for the general population, it is uniformly high for specific groups. Kandel (1978) reports patterns of drug involvement that most commonly begin in early adolescence and peak from 18 to 22 years of age. She asserts that medical involvement with a drug almost always precedes nonmedical involvement with other drugs and that a high proportion of adolescent marijuana users eventually experiment with other drugs. Crockett (1971) summarizes research indicating that 75% of all nonmedical drug users began using these drugs between the ages 16 and 21 and that some began drug use as young as 12 years of age. Many detoxification and drug rehabilitation programs established in the past decade, especially for adolescent abusers, are now admitting addicts as young as 12 years of age (Rice and Kibbee, 1983).

Bennett (1983) cites research showing an overall prevalence of marijuana use of 60%; stimulant use of 26%; cocaine and hallucinogen use of 16%; and sedative and tranquilizer use of 16% in the high school class of 1980. The dramatic increase in adolescent drug use in the late 1960s and 1970s seems to have been arrested, however, so that the daily use of marijuana, cigarettes, and alcohol is actually dropping (Bennett, 1983). Whether this is related to public health education or changing demographics is not clear.

The terms associated with drug use reflect the degrees of abuse and degrees of pharmacologic effects of long-term drug ingestion. The term *drug abuse* dates from the 1960s, when drug use among middle-class adolescents and young adults raised legal, social, and medical issues of popular concern (Williams, 1980b). Since then, a more complete vocabulary for describing drug use has developed.

Addiction is a metabolic response to regular drug ingestion. When a person is addicted, biologic processes adapt, so that the person develops a *physical dependence* on the drug. Abstinence from the drug then results in *withdrawal* symptoms, which may include fatigue, loss of appetite, chills, sweating, cramps, nausea, and elevated vital signs. *Habituation* is an emotional need, or *psychologic dependence,* in which the drug user feels driven to continue using a drug. For many drug users, habituation occurs because of the person's vulnerability to the drug's effects. Continued drug use does not necessarily lead to habituation, although all drugs may be habituating. The degree of dependence is related to the psychologic needs of the user.

Tolerance is a biologic response to regular administration of a given dose. With regular use some drugs become less effective, and larger doses are required. *Cross-tolerance* occurs when one drug is substituted for another to produce the same effects. This kind of substitution is the basis for detoxification with methadone in cases of heroin addiction.

Other factors contributing to a drug's effect are its purity and its method of administration. "Street drugs," or those that are obtained illegally, are usually "cut" with another substance (for example, starch, lactose, or talc), so that the amount of the psychoactive substance in a given dose often is not predictable. Some of the substances used to dilute the drug also may be contaminated or irritating to veins or mucosa. Drugs may be administered by almost any route; most common are subcutaneous injection, inhalation, smoking, sniffing, and oral administration. Intravenous injection usually produces the most notable effects; heroin and amphetamine injection are associated with an immediate "rush." Table 24-1 lists the major classifications of popular street drugs and nursing assessment and management considerations.

The environment in which the drug is ingested, together with the expectations and past experience of the user, can also affect the response (Hofmann, 1983). For many users the first few experiences with a drug tend to be unpleasant or disappointing. For the adolescent—and increasingly for younger children as well—the effect of the peer group is as significant as the effect of the drug.

For young people engaging in drug abuse the risks of such involvement are enormous and can be fatal. Meeks (1971) notes that some young abusers sacrifice their psychologic or emotional lives or the chance for full psychologic development. Others under the acute influence of drugs, alcohol, or both have tragically sacrificed everything through suicide or have suffered fatal injuries, often from driving while under the influence of drugs or alcohol. Still others, because of chronic drug or alcohol use, have destroyed their health by neglecting their bodies' basic needs. And some young people have, because of withdrawal resulting from substance abuse, given up any opportunity to be freely involved in the world.

Additional risks include increased susceptibility to disease, particularly to hepatitis or Acquired Immune Deficiency Syndrome (AIDS) if adolescents are injecting drugs. Drug sensitivities may develop with resulting organ damage, seizures, and so forth. Drug abuse often results in increased risk-taking behavior, changes in perception, disturbances in judgments and decision making, and poor impulse control. Of special concern are the growing number of "polyabusers," those who are dependent on a combination of alcohol and drugs or on more than one chemical substance.

Assessment Child health nurses in all settings eventually deal with children who are experiencing a condition or trauma directly related to nonmedical drug use, although nurses working in urban settings tend to find adolescent drug abuse a more common occurrence than those in rural settings. Poverty or low economic status has been correlated with drug abuse (Crockett, 1971; Kandel, 1978; Bennett, 1983), and biologic factors such as genetic predispositions to drug abuse, have been suggested but not substantiated (Bennett, 1983). Psychosocial factors contributing to abuse include a diminished sense of well-being, low self-esteem, poor school performance, and conduct disorders.

Drug abuse is usually only one of a variety of dysfunctional behaviors exhibited during a given time. Substance abusers are also often involved in truancy, runaway behavior, promiscuous sexual activity, or conduct disorders (see Chapter 25). In general, the adolescent who exhibits some of these behaviors is also at risk for drug abuse (Hofmann, 1983).

The nurse may encounter a drug abuser during a routine health assessment or may be called on to respond to the suspicions of parents or school personnel. Although nurses and physicians are sometimes expected to act as police and identify children who are ingesting drugs illegally, health care professionals cannot gain a child's confidence by promising to report illegal behavior. Instead the nurse assesses risk factors and notes any physical signs that might indicate drug use.

Physical examination sometimes reveals puncture sites, needle tracks, or skin-popping ulcers, but these are only evident among regular users and are relatively uncommon in young drug abusers (Hofmann, 1983). Reddened con-

TABLE 24-1 Commonly Abused Substances

Drug name	Effect and use	Assessment	Nursing management
Central nervous system depressants—barbiturates			
Amobarbital sodium (Amytal Sodium, blue birds, blue devils, truth serum) Butabarbital sodium (Butabell HMB, Quibron Plus, Tedral-25) Sodium pentobarbital (Nembutal, yellow jackets) Phenobarbital (Luminal, Antrocol, Bronkolixir, Quadrinal) Secobarbital sodium (Seconal; Tuinal, tooeys, reds, rainbows)	Depresses all areas of the central nervous system although many enhance pain sensation; used as hypnotics, sedatives, anesthetics, and anticonvulsants	Observe for decreased level of consciousness, drowsiness, ataxic gait. Barbiturates depress respirations so observe for shallow breathing or even respiratory arrest Pulse and blood pressure may drop, and circulatory insufficiency may occur in cases of overdose. Pupils are usually constricted	Monitor neurologic status for level of consciousness Monitor cardiopulmonary function to assess quality of circulation and respirations Death may result from pulmonary edema and renal failure
Central nervous system depressants—miscellaneous			
Antihistamines: Actifed, Benadryl, Chlor-Trimeton, Comtrex, Dimetap, Isochlor, Nyquil, Phenergan, Rondec, Sudafed, Triaminic	Used in prescription and nonprescription cold preparations for upper-respiratory symptoms, also found in sleep aids. Antihistamines exert an anticholinergic effect that results in drying of mucous membranes and sedation. These medications are also used for the treatment of motion sickness and parkinsonism and frequently are used in the management of allergic reactions	Observe for drowsiness and lethargy. Patient may also have photosensitivity, dry mouth, throat, and nose in addition to dizziness and blurred vision Sedation and dry mucous membranes are primary indicators of use Pupils usually appear dilated	Overdose should be treated by inducing vomiting These drugs are readily available to the general public and are easily abused, particularly by children (see Chapter 20)
Central nervous system stimulants—amphetamines			
Dextroamphetamine (Dexedrine) Methamphetamine (Desoxyn, speed, crystal, meth) Racemic amphetamine (Benzedrine, uppers, bennies) Amphetamine complex (Biphetamine, black beauties)	Stimulates the central nervous system and is commonly used in treatment for exogenous obesity and narcolepsy Those used in obesity treatment are called anorectics	Assess nutritional status, as long-term abuse can result in severe dietary deficiencies Note activity level, history of insomnia, and irritability Personality changes are common Cardiovascular and central nervous system overstimulation are most common. Therefore, note tachycardia, hypertension, palpitations, restlessness, euphoria, dysphoria, tremor, and occasional psychotic episodes	Abrupt cessation of amphetamines can result in depressive syndrome and extreme fatigue Nutritional supplementation may be indicated In acute amphetamine intoxication it is important to lower sensory input. Keep patient in a quiet room with no bright lights or moving objects
Amphetaminelike anorexics			
Methylphenidate (Ritalin)	Used with children as a treatment for hyperactivity and attention deficits		Abuse potential is relatively high with a more common prevalence as a street drug

continued on next page

TABLE 24-1 continued

Drug name	Effect and use	Assessment	Nursing management
Central nervous system stimulants—Miscellaneous			
Cocaine hydrochloride (cocaine, coke, blow, snow, lady, powder)	Cortical stimulant used to elevate mood, enhance alertness, and provide local anesthesia. Route of administration varies, but inhalation is most popular	Moderate doses stimulate central nervous system and cardiovascular activity. Therefore, note tachycardia, palpitations, hypertension, hyperalertness, constricted pupils, euphoria, and psychotic episodes in chronic users Note nasal mucosa for signs of cocaine powder, excoriation, and necrosis of the nasal septum	High doses and chronic cocaine use can result in a psychotic syndrome Extremely addicting with a high abuse potential
Caffeine (No-Doz, cola beverages, coffee, Anacin)	Central nervous system stimulant found in a variety of common over-the-counter products	High doses can result in caffeine toxicity. Therefore, note tachycardia, hypertension, tingling scalp, tinnitus, dizziness, irritability, and fine hand tremors Excessive use may suggest addictive personality, depression, or anxiety	Withdrawal should be initiated slowly Low-caffeine or caffeine-free products can be substituted
Opiates and synthetic opiates			
Morphine sulfate Oxycodone (Percodan) Hydromorphone (Dilaudid) Meperidine (Demerol) Methadone (Dolophine) Propoxyphene (Darvon) Pentazocine (Talwin) Butorphanol (Stadol) Heroin (smack, horse, junk, skag, zap, crank)	Affects the central nervous system, alters mood and provides analgesia, clinically used as an analgesia in postoperative and terminal conditions	Observe for signs of acute lethargy, drowsiness, blunted affect. Also observe for central nervous system depression, respiratory depression, hypotension In acute overdose, observe for signs of pyrexia, hypertension, hyperexcitability, and tachycardia As intravenous route of administration is most common, particularly for heroin, note antecubital area and other major vascular areas for signs of needle "tracks," scarring, cellutis, or other indications of needle use	Ensure availability of a narcotic antagonist (e.g., Narcan) to reverse symptoms of acute overdose Because heroin purity is rarely consistent, overdose is common. Complete resuscitative equipment should be available Patients may experience orthostatic hypotension, and so safety measures to prevent falls are important Heroin is frequently "cut" with foreign substances such as sugar or talc powder. Therefore, observe for complications created by these hyperglycemia or chemical sepsis
Hallucinogens			
Lysergic acid diethylamide (acid, blotter acid, crystal, microdot, windowpane) Psilocybin (mushrooms)	Alters mood, thought, behavior, perception, sensation, and often creates hallucinations Overt psychosis is common	Assess mental status noting orientation, quality, and content of thoughts; affect; mood; thought blocking; projection; or insertion	Behavior of the patient under the influence of hallucinogen is unpredictable "Flashback" phenomenon is common

TABLE 24-1 continued

Drug name	Effect and use	Assessment	Nursing management
Mescaline (mescalito, white line, peyote) Methoxyamphetamine (MDA) Phencyclidine (PCP, angel dust, horse tranquilizer) Cannabis (marijuana, grass, pot, tea, Acapulco gold, Maui wowie, Tai sticks, Colombian, hemp, weed) Hashish (knot, tar, oils)	Oral route of administration is most common although marijuana and its derivatives are typically inhaled	Note possible responses to hallucinations such as visual scanning, talking to self, abrupt head cocking Central nervous system effects vary from depressant to stimulant reactions. Therefore, close central nervous system monitoring is essential; prepare for reactions ranging from extreme agitation to coma and death	Large doses or synergistic reactions can be fatal Patient's response to hallucinations or delusions can be extreme and fatal (patients may believe they can fly or that people are out to hurt them) Suicide does occur in patients under the influence of these drugs

junctivae are sometimes associated with marijuana use. Slurred speech, decreased attention span, and inappropriate affect may indicate central nervous system depressants. Nasal and bronchial irritation may be seen with smoking or inhaling of any drug. Although these signs are indicators, they cannot alone confirm suspected drug abuse.

A better approach is to discuss patterns of drug use by beginning with nonthreatening questions. Adolescents are more likely to describe patterns of drug use among their peers than to report their own experiences. The nurse therefore might ask whether the child's friends use drugs, which drugs they use, and how much and how often they take drugs. Some children who describe drug problems in school or in their neighborhoods are indirectly asking for advice. The nurse then may use the opportunity to provide information about drugs or to refer the child to an agency or organization that works to prevent drug abuse.

Once the child has described the behavior of peers and has perceived that the nurse accepts the information without judgment, the child is more likely to report personal drug use or concerns related to it. If the child denies having a drug problem, the nurse can continue to establish a therapeutic relationship that might eventually lead the child to seek treatment. Blood and urine screening tests are seldom valuable, especially if they lead the nurse to confront the child and thus compromise the child's willingness to trust health care professionals.

The nurse can also question children about other daily activities and can question parents about behaviors that may be correlated with drug abuse. Hofmann (1983) notes that the following behaviors are indicators of existing or potential drug abuse:

1. Increasingly poor adjustment and deteriorating function at home or school or among peers
2. Emotional lability with rapid mood swings but with increasing depression, irritability, and restlessness
3. Secretive behavior, longer periods of time spent alone, longer periods of time away from home
4. Deterioration in personal hygiene or dress
5. Alterations in schedule (for example, sleeping longer, tardiness, truancy)
6. Existence of drug paraphernalia (for example, needles, syringes, pill containers, bottles)
7. Disappearance of family money or valuables, large amounts of money found in the child's possession
8. Bizarre behavior or behavior that seems inappropriate to a specific occasion or a particular context

Nursing Management Nursing care for drug abusers encompasses all three levels of prevention. School nurses

Risk Factors Associated With Drug Abuse

1. Peer group members who use drugs or alcohol excessively
2. Family history of alcoholism, drug abuse, or addiction
3. Dysfunctional family communication
4. Parental substance abuse
5. History of maladaptive coping with stressors or evidence of other dysfunctional behaviors
6. Inability to form close personal relationships
7. Poor self-esteem, sense of hopelessness, lack of planning for the future
8. Poverty, poor education, lack of job skills, poor prospects for future employment
9. Readily available drugs in the community

and community health nurses who are often involved in educational programs about drugs and their effects are engaged in primary prevention. Nurses in well-child or acute-care settings can also respond to questions and refer children and their families to appropriate resources when a child is at risk for drug abuse.

Secondary prevention occurs both in routine health assessment and in emergency settings. Tertiary prevention encompasses the variety of rehabilitation programs available to drug abusers. Any adolescent who seeks health care should be routinely asked about drug use, especially if an injury or medical condition might be associated with drug ingestion or intoxication. The nurse might first ask whether the child has taken any prescribed medications, has any allergies to medications, has ever had a bad reaction to a drug, or has ever had trouble stopping the use of a drug.

If the child who abuses drugs is willing to give honest answers, the nurse can act with other health care professionals to prevent the secondary effects of continued drug abuse. If the child is using drugs but has no significant risk factors, referral to a drug education program may be the most appropriate intervention. If assessment suggests risk factors coexisting with drug use, a more comprehensive plan of care is probably needed. Figure 24-2 depicts the decision making associated with management of drug abuse in adolescence. Hofmann (1983) notes that any plan of care must involve the following considerations:

1. The underlying psychologic problem(s) that gave rise to the abuse in the first place
2. The frequency with which the child denies the seriousness of the problem

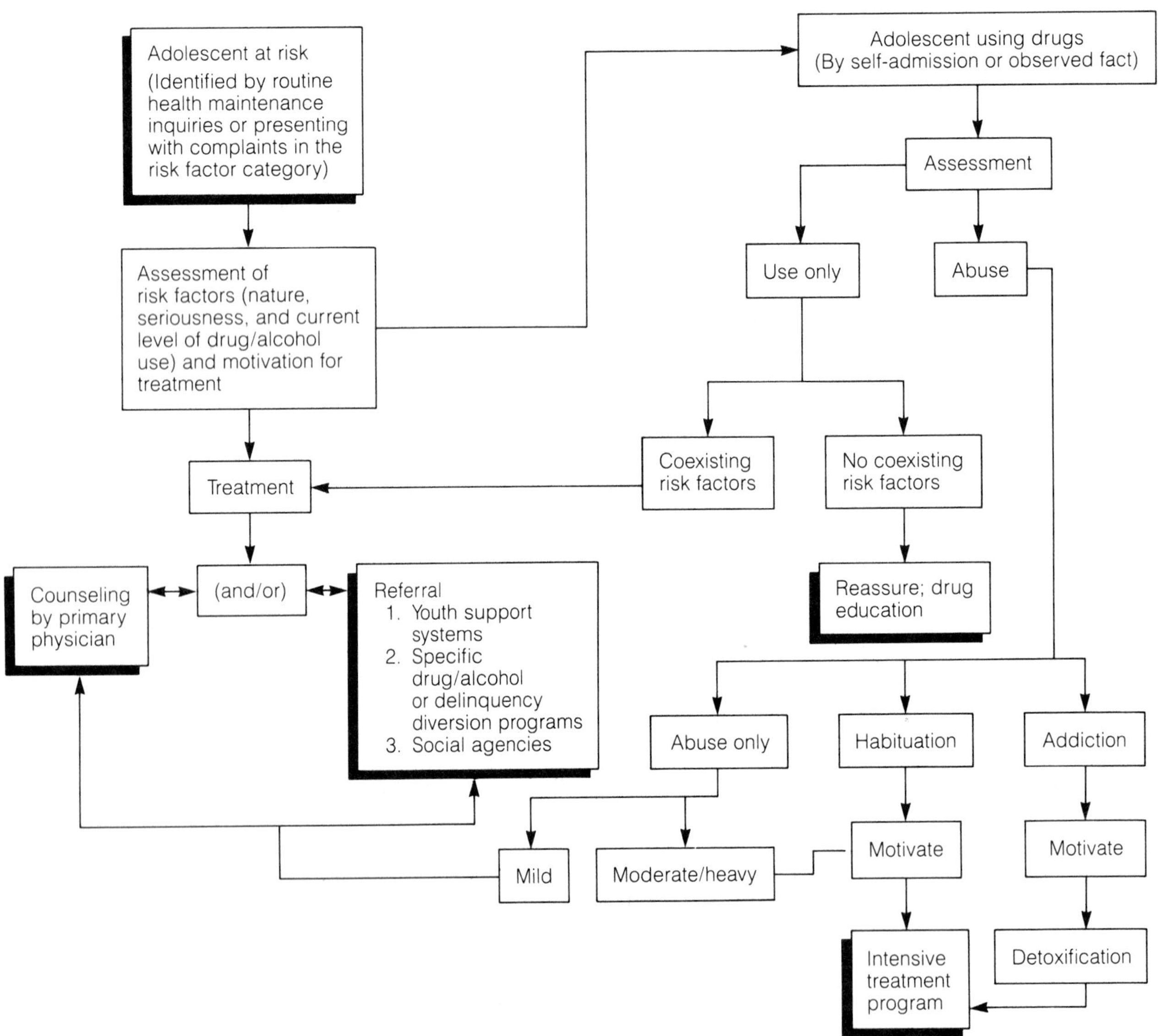

Figure 24-2 Decision making for the management of drug or alcohol abuse in adolescence. (From Hofmann AD: *Adolescent Medicine*. Addison-Wesley, 1983.)

3. The child's degree of motivation for treatment
4. The possible complications of addiction or habituation
5. The possible medical complications of drug therapy or routes of injection
6. The idiosyncratic responses common to strong hallucinogens (for example, "flashbacks" and "bad trips")

Emergency Care Drug abusers are sometimes seen in the emergency room with severe physical or psychologic symptoms characteristic of a "bad trip." The patient may be brought to the hospital by friends or by parents, and subjective data may indicate that the child is experiencing a drug reaction. Objective data include laboratory tests, especially thin-layer chromatography (TLC) and gas–liquid chromatography (GLC), which are used to detect drugs in blood and urine. Drug overdoses also cause central nervous system depression. If the child is disoriented or uncoordinated, the nurse monitors the child's state of consciousness. (Physical signs of drug overdose are summarized in Table 24-2.)

If the child is conscious but disoriented, the nurse intervenes to calm the patient and prevent panic. Controlling the environment and providing continual reassurance help to reduce stress and remind the child that the hospital environment is safe. The constant presence of one nurse adds to the child's sense of security. Clear directions in a calm tone of voice and accurate descriptions of what will happen enhance cooperation and reduce anxiety.

Long-Term Management For the habitual abuser or addict, management usually includes referral to one of a variety of programs or agencies. Addicts usually undergo a

TABLE 24-2 Acute Overdose Reactions: Physical Signs

Drug class	Mental status	Pulse rate	Respiratory rate	Blood pressure	Pupils	Temperature	Other
Narcotics	Lethargy → coma	↓	↓	No change	Pinpoint	No change	May have injection marks. Responsive to naloxone
Central nervous system depressants	"drunk" behavior → coma	↓	↓	No change	No change unless anoxic	No change	Nystagmus on lateral gaze. Characteristic odor with alcohol
Central nervous system stimulants	Agitation → paranoid psychosis	↑	↑	↑	Dilated (mild to moderate)	No change	Sometimes injection marks
Lysergic acid diethylamide	Detached → "bad trip"	↑	↑	↑	Dilated (mild to moderate)	No change	
Phencyclidine	Variable psychoses → coma	↑	↑ or ↓	↑; can be marked	Dilated (mild to moderate)	↑	Muscular rigidity, spasms; laryngeal stridor; rotatory nystagmus; ↓ perception of pain and touch; flushing; drooling
Atropinic drugs	Delirium → coma	↑	↓	No change or ↑	Dilated (marked)	↑	Marked flushing; dry hot skin; dry mucous membranes. Responsive to physostigmine

SOURCE: Hofmann AD: Page 347 in: *Adolescent Medicine*. Addison-Wesley, 1983.

two-step process that involves detoxification followed by rehabilitation. Drug maintenance programs, usually with a legally obtained drug substituted for the abused drug (for example, methadone for heroin), have been instituted for children 16–18 years of age, but such programs are controversial (Williams, 1980a).

Most children are advised to undergo withdrawal so that they can plan to live drug-free lives. The symptoms of the withdrawal syndrome depend on the drug. Some symptoms can be relieved with medications (for example, chlorale hydrate relieves insomnia associated with narcotic withdrawal). Other symptoms must be endured, sometimes by inducing sleep. In the hospital setting the nurse monitors vital signs and neurologic status during the withdrawal phase and provides quiet reassurance or stimulation with age-appropriate activities when distraction is possible.

Because adolescents often have difficulty with the commitment needed for long-term treatment, a rehabilitation program that involves peer support is usually advisable. The adolescent might remain at home, especially if the family is participating in therapy, or might be enrolled in a residential treatment program. Residential treatment programs are sometimes preferable when it is necessary to remove the adolescent from the environment that has contributed to the drug abuse. Common residential programs are halfway houses, which provide a structured, drug-free environment with some supervision, and therapeutic communities, which provide strict supervision and a carefully controlled environment.

Also available in some communities are self-help groups, which provide peer support, often in conjunction with psychotherapy, and counseling with both professionals and peers. Peer counseling also may be part of school drug abuse programs planned to prevent substance abuse and suggest alternative behaviors. Long-term counseling allows the child to learn and practice problem-solving skills and to take responsibility for drug-related behaviors.

Eating Disorders

While not necessarily indicative of depression, dysfunctional food consumption can be linked to anxiety and maladaptive coping in children. Obesity, anorexia nervosa, and bulimia are maladaptive responses involving self-image and self-control. All three present problems that require both child and family to learn new patterns of behavior and ways of managing stress.

Obesity

Obesity is a form of malnutrition commonly seen in infancy and early childhood (see Chapters 15 and 18). If untreated, it becomes a major threat to the child's health. During growth periods additional weight gain is an expected response to the growth spurt, so that any existing problem of overweight is compounded. Eighty-five percent of those who are obese in early childhood become obese adults (Abraham and Nondsieck, 1960). Obesity can begin in the first year of life but is often a health problem in older children and develops in response to a specific stressor or life event. Some children who exhibit obesity grow up among other family members who demonstrate maladaptive responses. The child decides, often unconsciously, to use food as a mechanism to meet emotional needs.

The psychosocial effects of obesity are cyclic. Overeating brings self-gratification along with increase in weight. Weight gain leads to low self-esteem, depression, and despair. The child may then withdraw, overeat, become inactive, gain more weight, and experience social isolation, all of which further diminish self-esteem.

Assessment Child and family history includes height, weight, duration of obesity, and the child's self-perceptions. The nurse assesses the family's attitude toward the child, roles assumed by the parent or parents, recent stressors encountered by the child, and the family's problem-solving skills. For example, the nurse may encounter a family that seldom visits a hospitalized child and attempts instead to placate the child with gifts of food. The nurse then needs to assess the extent of this behavior to identify any emerging patterns, whether or not the child's height and weight fit the definition of obesity.

Some children use food as a way of coping with stress, boredom, or loneliness. For others eating while engaged in other activities such as watching television becomes a habit and leads to excessive intake. The nurse therefore assesses the patterns of eating behavior for both the child and family. One family, for example, limited the child's diet during mealtimes but made potato chips, cookies, and other high-calorie snacks available at other times. Because the child was monitored only at the table, the family was unconsciously contributing to the problem.

In some families food is used as a reward for achievement or for good behavior and can eventually become a way of controlling a child's behavior. The nurse therefore assesses the family's attitude toward food before planning any behavior modification program. If food is generally used to punish or reward behavior, then the effect of the family system on the child is an important part of the nurse's assessment. Evidence suggesting a need for psychologic counseling or psychotherapy for the child and family includes severe depression, poor peer relationships, low self-esteem, and indicators of dysfunctional parenting (see Chapter 22).

Additional data include the child and family's physical activities and extent of physical exertion, physical assessment findings, and a nutritional assessment that includes a skinfold-thickness measurement. (Physical assessment is discussed in Chapter 14; nutritional assessment is explained in Chapter 15).

Nursing Management Nurses involved in well-child care and assessment are often involved in nutritional counseling for children and their families. Nutritional counseling is one way to prevent obesity (see Chapter 15). Nursing care for obese children usually involves a plan that combines nutritional and behavior management, sometimes in conjunction with individual or family counseling. Severe obesity requires medical management, which can include drug therapy and, in extreme cases, might involve surgical intervention.

Nursing management for obesity begins with realistic, mutual goal setting with both child and family. The nurse provides the structure for goal setting relative to weight reduction; long-term goals include modifying eating habits and enhancing the child's self-concept. After goals are set, the nurse assumes the role of teacher, counselor, and advocate, facilitating access to resources required by the child and family. Weight loss is slow and often difficult to maintain, particularly if changes in lifestyle do not accompany the loss. Therefore, the nurse continues to assess the balance between intake and activity and to refer the child and family to resources that might provide additional support.

Because adolescents are particularly concerned with peer group identity, providing a peer group, usually in a health care setting or through a commercial program, often motivates an obese adolescent to continue a weight reduction regimen. Sharing experiences and concerns with adolescents with similar problems also provides a forum for sharing accomplishments and for encouraging successful weight loss.

Behavior modification is one of several behavioral techniques used for successful weight reduction (see Chapter 13 for a general discussion of behavior modification). A system of rewards for changes in eating behavior or weight loss can provide positive reinforcement. For some children a new toy, record, or trip can serve as a motivator and reward. For others daily praise for adaptive eating behaviors, exercise, or small losses in weight is essential for continued success. If the child learns consciously to avoid the temptation to use food as a way of coping with stress or boredom, positive reinforcement will further support this adaptive behavior. Ongoing evaluation of progress toward goals is crucial for identifying necessary changes in the nursing care plan. Psychologic support, encouragement, and spoken praise can reinforce or sustain desired changes (see Chapter 18 for further discussion).

Anorexia Nervosa and Bulimia

Anorexia is a relatively common occurrence in inpatient pediatric settings. Children receiving medications or undergoing certain medical procedures are frequently nauseated, may vomit, and are transiently anorexic. This is particularly evident in children who are in the postoperative phase of hospitalization.

Anorexia nervosa, however, is a complex, disturbing, and sometimes life-threatening disorder that predominantly affects adolescent and young adult women. "Anorexia" is really a misnomer for this condition because these women do not experience a loss of appetite. Rather, they willfully limit their intake so that they eat drastically small amounts of food in a "relentless pursuit of thinness" (Bruch, 1973). The disorder can begin as a conscious effort to lose weight but then evolves into an obsessive preoccupation with food and weight reduction.

Anorexia nervosa should be distinguished from bulimia, bulimia nervosa (Russell, 1979), or bulimarexia (Boskind-White, 1983). The latter three are synonyms for a disorder characterized by cyclical binging on enormous quantities of food, followed by purging oneself with laxatives or by vomiting. Confusion may arise because some anorexic patients primarily restrict intake but also vomit, abuse laxatives, and occasionally engage in episodic binging. In addition, patients with bulimia (bulimarexics) often have histories of anorexia nervosa and prolonged periods of self-starvation.

A number of psychosocial theories and some biologic explanations have been proposed for the development of anorexia nervosa. Most experts agree that the onset of adolescence may trigger feelings that are overwhelming to these young people and lead to the symptomatic behaviors (Bruch, 1973; Crisp, 1980; Palazzoli, 1978; Garfinkel and Garner, 1982). Family dysfunction (Minuchin, 1978) or problems in the early mother–child interactions (Bruch, 1973) may contribute to personality factors that lend themselves to difficulty in the transitions of adolescence. In addition, the process of dieting itself is often rewarded by family members and friends who initially support and congratulate successful weight loss. For the vulnerable individual in need of external approval, this reinforcement tends to encourage further dieting and denial of more serious issues.

Because adolescents tend to be easily influenced by sociocultural norms, the current social emphasis on physique and thinness might be a factor in the increasing incidence of anorexia nervosa. Some researchers suggest that on a continuum of normal weight with diet-conscious adolescents on one end and hospitalized anorexic patients on the other, those who do develop anorexia nervosa have different degrees of underlying psychopathology as well (Swift and Stern, 1982). Still, not everyone who begins a diet develops anorexia. Although the mechanism is not fully understood, some researchers believe biologic factors such as changes in the hypothalamic-pituitary functions also contribute to the development or perpetuation of the starvation process (Garfinkel and Garner, 1982).

Assessment The overt clinical picture of anorexia nervosa is, however, similar among most individuals. Physical symptoms include weight loss to approximately 75% of original body weight as well as dehydration and electrolyte imbalances that might be secondary to vomiting or lack of fluid intake. Bradycardia, hypotension, and low body temperature are common, as is amenorrhea secondary to changes in the hypothalamic-pituitary functioning, weight loss, and loss of body fat. Other effects of starvation include dry skin, growth of lanugo hair, pallor, cold extremities and cyanosis of the feet and hands (Garfinkel and Garner, 1982).

Bruch (1979) points out that the anorexic adolescent thinks like a younger child, and she views this as a deficit in conceptual organization. She further suggests that anorexic adolescents show evidence of egocentricity and lack of progress beyond Piaget's concrete operational stage of cognitive development (see Chapter 6). Typically, the patient shows cognitive changes such as a decreased ability to concentrate and distortions in thinking, especially about body image. The nurse who hears the emaciated young individual complain of feeling "fat" might find this self-perception particularly startling. The distorted perception of body image, however, propels the anorexic patient to the extreme measures for achieving weight loss.

Body image and the self-image are closely intertwined concepts but for the patient with anorexia nervosa, self-image is often narrowly focused and limited to the ability to control weight. The patient may ignore or be unable to identify physical signals from within the body, such as hunger and fatigue, and also typically has difficulty recognizing emotional needs. Anorexic patients feel incompetent in most areas beyond weight control and often withdraw from interpersonal relationships. When they do interact with others, they tend to be oriented to the needs and wants of others and seek approval from others. Some anorexics describe cooking gourmet meals for other people but rarely eat more than a few bites of what they cook (Marks, 1984). This pattern of behavior often has been long-standing, so that these patients are often described as having been "model children" (Bruch, 1973).

While a definitive diagnosis of anorexia nervosa requires a psychiatric assessment, the child health nurse may suspect anorexia nervosa in the cachectic adolescent with no medical explanation for an emaciated appearance. The nurse may have difficulty obtaining accurate information regarding the amount of weight loss, psychosocial stressors, or the duration of weight loss because anorexic adolescents often attempt to deny or conceal the problem.

Objective data that can validate a nurse's suspicion include height and weight, which are compared with norms, aberrant lab values for serum electrolytes, complete blood count, and urinalysis. Of particular importance are urinalysis ketone levels that suggest a self-imposed "starvation" as fats are metabolized with a subsequent elevation in ketone bodies in the urine. Abnormally low glucose, sodium, or red blood count values also suggest a threatened nutritional status indicative of anorexia nervosa.

Observations of behavior such as hiding food (particularly high-carbohydrate foods), refusing food (either by turning down offers of food or by disposing of food secretly), or vomiting also suggest anorexia or bulimia. Anorexic patients tend to look frequently in mirrors, as if to make sure that they have not been gaining weight. They also tend to talk constantly about food, food preparation, and eating. Bulimic patients tend to exhibit fluctuations in weight. They also can exhibit poor impulse control comparable to their difficulty in controlling their eating behavior. For instance, some bulimics also abuse drugs or alcohol (Marks, 1984).

Nursing Management Anorexic patients who are severely emaciated (that is, 40% below their ideal weight) are usually hospitalized, often against their will. For the anorexic in an acute-care setting, sensitive and consistent nursing management is the most essential component in the plan of care (Rockwell et al., 1982).

The long-term goals of nursing care are to restore weight with adequate nutrition and to provide a supportive environment to help ensure cooperation. Included will be specific measures to monitor and reduce the physiologic effects of starvation, vomiting, and laxative abuse. The process of weight restoration should be initiated slowly, preferably with a balanced 1200-calorie, salt-limited diet. Calories should be gradually increased to promote a weight gain of approximately 2 pounds each week.

Weight is usually measured daily and should be measured at the same time with the patient wearing the same clothing. Patients should void before being weighed because they may attempt to increase weights by drinking large quantities of water. To promote weight gain, activity should be restricted to a minimum. In some cases, bedrest may be necessary initially.

Eating after prolonged periods of starvation can lead to edema, abdominal distension, and constipation. The nurse needs to monitor such potential problems, keeping in mind that anorexic patients frequently complain of feeling "bloated" after meals because of psychologic discomfort with eating. Gradually inviting more patient control over issues related to food and body image can reinforce positive eating behaviors.

In the acute-care setting, the nurse needs to be supportive but firm during mealtime to assure that a significant portion of the meal is consumed. While power struggles with patients are certainly not desirable and tend to limit their control over their own eating behavior, the first nursing goal is to decrease the potential for nutritional deficiency in the patient who is already nutritionally compromised. If the patient refuses food, liquid protein supplements with equivalent caloric amounts can supplement uneaten food portions. Ideally, the patient should be observed while eating and closely monitored after meals for at least 1 hour to ensure that food is not regurgitated. Refusal of all oral intake may necessitate nasogastric tube feeding or in extreme cases, hyperalimentation.

Care of an anorexic patient is not an easy process. Most patients resist treatment efforts after an initial sense of relief that the treatment team has assumed responsibility for their decisions. Although patients with anorexia nervosa are usually not engaging in conscious efforts at suicide, they are overwhelmed with fear of gaining weight. The anorexic patient experiences anxiety, guilt, and panic after eating because of the distorted belief that all food is "bad" and will lead to excessive weight gain. This belief leads to such desperate behavior as hiding food during meals or vomiting afterwards.

The difficulties that arise around eating may be surprising to the staff in light of the patient's pleasing, cooperative facade in other areas of interaction with the nurse. In some instances nurses begin to feel angry and come to avoid the patient because of the apparent refusal to accept treatment. The nurse thus needs to remember during this stressful time that anorexic patients are not malevolent in their attempts to sabotage efforts of the staff, but rather are clinging to the security of their symptoms.

If the nurse uses a firm, matter-of-fact approach about eating, power struggles with the patient about particular foods and portions are more easily avoided. The critical factor is a consistent approach from all staff members. Coordinated efforts, often with the consultation of a psychiatric nurse specialist, should ensure that one nurse is not identified as stricter or more lenient than another.

In general, firm limits coupled with genuine sensitivity and support are most helpful to the anorexic patient. Patients need encouragement to explore their feelings about eating, without being given false reassurances. Limits might be defined by using such behavior modification techniques as granting privileges (for example, reduced observation, increased activity) if the patient meets a weight requirement.

At the same time, the nurse needs to be aware that the parents of anorexic patients may inadvertently collude in halting treatment. For example, patients may complain that nurses are cruel and punitive and may lead the parents into taking their children home before home care is medically safe. Parents should be forewarned about this phenomenon and encouraged to discuss it with the nurse. Parents should also be told not to discuss eating and weight with their anorexic children but to let the staff handle this aspect of care.

While dysfunctional family interactions have been cited as contributing to the development of eating disorders, the nurse cannot sit in judgment of the families of these patients but needs to remain sensitive to problems of parents of anorexic patients. The parent may have been struggling for many months to force the child to eat, and the distress of watching one's child willfully starve may be enough to cause chaos in a household. The parent is likely to feel guilty, ineffective, and depressed about the situation and will need support from the nurse to address these feelings.

Recent research suggests that drug therapy might become an option for treating anorexia and bulimia (Marks, 1984). The goal of drug therapy is to stimulate the patient's appetite and diminish feelings of depression. Cyproheptadine, a serotonin and histamine antagonist, reportedly decreases a patient's preoccupation with food while enhancing sociability. Tranquilizers that promote weight gain also are sometimes given for anorexia. Bulimic patients are sometimes given phenelzine or imipramine, both antidepressants, but usually when the condition has not responded to psychotherapy.

Problems of Elimination

Enuresis and encopresis are the primary problems of elimination for which parents seek professional intervention. American culture places heavy emphasis upon cleanliness and personal hygiene, and failure to achieve or maintain bowel or bladder continence is a major stressor for both child and family. Failure to resolve this stress typically results in additional stressors and feelings of inadequacy.

Enuresis

Toilet-training practices vary, but most children master diurnal and nocturnal bladder control between 3 and $3\frac{1}{2}$ years of age (Brazelton, 1962). Powell (1981) reports findings that most children achieve daytime bladder control between 2 years and $2\frac{1}{2}$ years of age and that the average age of both bowel and bladder control is 33 months. (Toilet-training management is discussed in Chapter 13.) Because the age at which toilet training is accomplished varies, *enuresis,* or involuntary discharge of urine, is not defined by the age of onset, although researchers describe enuresis as appearing after ages three or four and without organic causes. Enuresis typically appears as one of several symptoms.

Knopf (1979) reports a clinical correlation between enuresis and such observable behaviors as moodiness, excitability, disobedience, temper tantrums, nail biting, fear reactions, and encopresis. Kanner (1972) reports that 25% of children have enuresis at some time, while Werry's research (1979) indicates an incidence of 20% by 7 years of age. Werry (1979) also reported that research linking enuresis with frequency of psychopathology is still inconclusive and that problems with research design and statistical evaluation render such etiologic links questionable and unclear. Although more common in boys, Shaffer (1973) reported a small but significant correlation between enuresis and psychopathology in girls.

Assessment A first step is to rule out organic causes of urinary incontinence and to identify psychogenic or learning-related enuresis. Urinary tract insufficiency or pathology such as malformations or infections can be identified by cystograms, cystoscopy, and various laboratory tests (see Chapter 39). Any defects in the adrenergic mechanisms controlling the sphincter and bladder muscle are also identified.

The family is usually the source of information concerning toilet training and incidence of enuresis. The nurse establishes baseline data for both the child and family, as complete assessment and successful intervention require their participation. Information about the age at which toilet training was begun and about techniques used provide clues about the family's expectations or the effectiveness of toilet-training techniques. Clues to psychogenic or organic causes of enuresis may be related to the age at which the child mastered toilet training (if ever) and any subsequent physical or psychosocial insults or stressors that the child has encountered.

Physical illnesses of any type frequently result in regressive behaviors by children as a normal part of coping with the illness or hospitalization. Situational enuresis may be caused by such stressful experiences as the birth of a sibling, family separations, family discord, or any other real or perceived threat to the child's sense of security and self-concept. Helping the family reestablish and foster this sense of physical and psychologic security in the child is one of the nurse's therapeutic goals.

Nursing Management A variety of techniques can be helpful in managing the enuretic child. Werry (1979) reports that enuresis is responsive to a wide range of non-specific interventions. Providing a nightlight or a stuffed animal, restricting nighttime fluid intake, and even scheduling bathroom trips at night are among the methods that can be effective. Incidence of spontaneous remission and subsequent relapse is high among enuretics, and so establishing exact causes of remission is useful, although difficult.

Behavior modification with operant-conditioning techniques have proved to be by far the most effective approach to enuresis. (Behavior modification is described in Chapter 13.) The nurse in the clinical setting can make use of an intensive procedure that achieves initial success in one day. The nurse requires the child to urinate in the toilet in order to receive a reinforcer (e.g., snacks, hugs, praises). The child might need to consume a large amount of liquids to ensure a successful number of trial episodes. In the process, the nurse teaches the child the sequence of going to the bathroom, removing clothing, voiding, cleaning, and redressing, and the nurse rewards the child for dryness. "Accidents" are treated without punishment or disapproval, but the child is required to attend to all self-cleaning by removing soiled clothes and linen, disposing of them properly, and replacing them.

Another frequently used conditioning technique is the buzzer or bell method. The technique involves a urine-sensing bed pad connected to an alarm system placed on the child's bed. When the child urinates, the alarm is activated because the urine acts as an electrolyte. The alarm then awakens the child, inhibiting urination. To avoid being awakened by the alarm, the child learns to delay urination or awaken to increased bladder tension. These pad and alarm units are available commercially and, combined with behavior modification, have proved effective.

Other methods include medication—such as tricyclic antidepressants, amphetamines, and anxiolytic agents—and psychotherapy, but these have not been proved useful as therapeutic adjuncts. Evidence suggests instead that results derived from medications are temporary at best and that side effects and complications render such drugs unpleasant or dangerous. Few studies describe the efficacy of psychotherapeutic techniques, although Werry (1979) reports two studies showing psychotherapy to be no more effective after 6 to 12 sessions than no treatment at all.

Encopresis

Fecal incontinence in any place but a toilet after the age of four years is considered *encopresis*. A generally uncommon occurrence, encopresis is more widely reported in boys and usually occurs prior to age eight. Werry (1979) points out that it is a function of age and generally resolves completely by the age of 16, and he reports a study showing the prevalence of encopresis at age 8 to be 2.3% among boys and 0.7% among girls. Encopresis, unlike enuresis, is a diurnal phenomenon and not generally associated with periods of sleep. Some encopretic children refuse toileting; others are constipated and willingly go to the toilet but cannot defecate (Berg and Jones, 1964).

Research does not clearly link encopresis with psychopathology, but Bellman (1966) suggests that encopretic children demonstrate increased anxiety, passive–aggressive behavior, withdrawal, and problems with social skills and family interactions than a matched control group of normal children and that behaviors are part of the etiology and not the results of encopresis. Knopf (1979) reports a clinical correlation between the encopretic child and temper tantrums, feeding problems, parental illness, separations, and the arrival of a new sibling. Passive–aggressive behavior was also noted to be a feature of retentive encopretics, those who have retained feces for so long as to have extinguished the normal urge to defecate and have distended their colons with hard, impacted feces. Seepage often results, and recurring episodes of constipation occur.

Assessment Assessment of the encopretic child begins with attempts to rule out organic causes such as gastrointestinal pathology or nutritional deficiencies and food intolerances (see Chapter 38). Endoscopy, proctoscopy, various radiographic procedures, and stool analysis are used to identify any parasites, ova, or other indicators. A nutritional history helps to identify any dietary factors (see Chapter 15). The nurse gathers information about how toilet training was conducted and at what age, if ever, the child mastered bowel control. Family expectations, knowledge, and any traumatic training techniques are identified in this way;

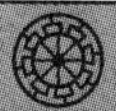

CASE STUDY An Encopretic 8-Year-Old

Assessment

Eight-year-old Carl was admitted for evaluation of a 6-month history of fecal soiling in his pants. Carl is now encopretic every day and regularly hides or throws his soiled underclothing away. He seems unconcerned about this, even though other children at school make fun of him.

Family

Carl is the next-to-youngest child in a family of seven and has a younger sister who is now 1 year old. Carl reached all developmental milestones within a normal period of time, and his mother reports that toilet training was uneventful and that Carl copied his older brothers ("They toilet-trained him").

Carl's mother is currently in the process of separating from her husband. She reports that she has regularly cleaned up after Carl and now plans to use disposable diapers to make the clean-up easier.

Hospitalization

On admission, Carl was neither anxious nor depressed and interacted readily with the other children. He adapted easily to the unit routine and participated in all activities. No organic reasons for the encopresis could be found, and no food intolerances were identified. Carl's stools were noted to be well-formed with no evidence of seepage or constipation.

Nursing Diagnoses

1. Threatened self-concept related to fecal soiling
2. Potential for dysfunctional parenting related to child's behavior and multiple stressors

Plan for Interventions

Goals

1. Carl will establish a consistent bowel-emptying pattern.
2. Carl's mother will cooperate with the bowel-training regimen and will encourage age-appropriate behavior.

Interventions

1. Arrange a schedule in which Carl goes to the bathroom and attempts to defecate (ideally at 30 minutes after each meal when the defecatory urge is usually greatest).
2. Establish a reward for defecating in the toilet.
3. Observe for evidence of fecal soiling, such as hiding soiled clothes.
4. If fecal soiling occurs, approach Carl in an unhurried, nonjudgmental manner and instruct him to clean himself.
5. Assist Carl in self-cleaning as necessary, taking care not to foster dependence with too much help.
6. Discuss with Carl's mother the child's history of behaviors during times of transition (for example, entry into school) and his attention-getting mechanisms to identify possible recurrence during current transitions (parental separation, birth of younger sibling).
7. Teach Carl's mother to follow the bowel-training regimen established in the hospital.
8. Suggest ways to encourage age-appropriate behavior, such as avoiding using diapers for an 8-year-old.
9. Suggest referral for occupational, recreational, play, or family therapy, as necessary.

---

and the nurse discusses stressors affecting the family, such as separations, deaths, illnesses, or births of siblings.

Like enuresis, encopresis is often a regressive symptom in the face of a real or perceived threat. Family interactions and parenting styles need close evaluation, for encopresis is often used by children as a means of defiance or passive–aggressive control of others. Parents usually are willing to provide information about the child but resistant to sharing information about their own behavior and methods of dealing with the problem. Clinical observations seem to indicate that parents often see themselves as innocuous "victims" of their children's behavior. Encopretic children often attempt to conceal their soiling by hiding stained linens, throwing soiled clothes away, or defecating into shoes, closets, or shower stalls. Supervision and observation are important in detecting episodes of encopresis.

Neutrally expressed acknowledgment of the impact of the problem on all concerned is most productive in eliciting an accurate assessment. Observing parent–child interaction in the clinical setting and monitoring the child's pattern of resistance or cooperation often sheds light on potential causes of difficulty.

Nursing Management Determining whether or not the encopretic child is a retentive encopretic and whether encopresis is caused by anxiety or failure to master bowel control during toilet training is important in planning interventions. The retentive encopretic is generally treated with laxatives, stool softeners, and enemas until the bowels are empty and bowel retraining can begin. Careful monitoring of the child's nutritional status and fluid and electrolyte balance are necessary during treatment with laxatives and enemas, as normal intestinal flora may be eliminated and thereby potentiate malabsorption syndromes or diarrhea. In small children, diarrhea can cause fluid and electrolyte imbalances and related complications. Bowel retraining involves gradually allowing the colon and anal vault to return to a more normal capacity and reestablishing the defecatory reflex.

Behavioral techniques similar to those used for enuresis are useful for facilitating toilet retraining. The nurse first fosters a sense of security in the child by removing the anxiety associated with toileting tasks and then teaches the family to foster this security by making the toileting behaviors both desirable and rewarding to the child.

Working through the young child's sense of anxiety and guilt over incontinence is best achieved through play. (Therapeutic play is discussed in Chapter 28.) Puppet or doll play with a relatively structured theme allows the child to express concerns. Mutual story telling and other story-telling techniques communicate in a nonthreatening way that the child's concerns are shared by others. Building trust is a major priority in dealing with such an emotional subject as elimination problems and is supported by all these methods of decreasing anxiety.

Problems in Socialization

School Phobia

Most children make the transition into the school setting without a great deal of trauma and difficulty, but some use maladaptive coping strategies much like the regressive behaviors associated with separation. *School phobia* evolves from the inability to make the transition into school. It is a disruptive condition marked by anxiety reactions and unwillingness or refusal to go to school. Knopf (1979) reports that school phobia occurs in 3 per 1000 school children and is most common in the 1st–5th grades.

The condition is evenly distributed between boys and girls, and affects children with average intelligence and relatively good academic performance. Hetherington and Martin (1979) report research indicating that school phobia is most prevalent among children who are generally overprotected, passive, and dependent and who have experienced less parental deprivation than those whose coping strategy is truancy. Also typical in these families is a higher incidence of neurosis and difficulty in parental separation and acceptance of the school's demands. Mothers often report that school-phobic children are more important to them than the children's fathers so that the overprotective mother and overdependent child comprise the most common dyad.

Clinical observations of school-phobic children reveal a high incidence of somatic complaints and crying and a low level of exploratory behavior and mastery of fears. Separation anxiety is usually acute and often dramatic. Families of children who are referred for a psychiatric evaluation of school phobia often abruptly terminate treatment before therapeutic interventions can be effective.

Assessment Graham (1979) reports that school phobia commonly occurs as a response to transitional periods in the child's schooling. Entering school is a primary transitional stage for children (see Chapter 9). Children who frequently miss school or voice somatic complaints need assessment to identify any stressors in the school setting. Failing classes, peer conflicts, and discipline and attention problems all pose significant threats to a child's self-concept. The nurse therefore collaborates with educational professionals familiar with the child by interviewing teachers or others involved in the child's development. Questionnaires about the child's school behavior and performance can also be useful in gathering data.

Complete psychological testing usually establishes objective baseline data and defines any learning disabilities (see Chapter 42). Clinical observations of parent–child interactions may indicate overprotection and mutual anxiety upon separation (see Chapter 16). Such observations might also show that parent and child have developed a pattern of behavior over time. In older children, patterns of withdrawal are assessed for any indications of a schizoid personality or emerging schizophrenic reaction.

Nursing Management Because school phobia usually involves both a parent–child dyad and the child's interaction with the school system, interventions are planned and implemented with parent, child, and teacher. Behavior modification is most helpful in managing the school-phobic child (see Chapter 13). A system of rewards is paired with the behavior of going to school, staying, and participating, and the reward, or reinforcer, is contingent on school attendance. Once school attendance becomes paired with the reward, the reinforcer can be eliminated. Reinforcers of the child's school attendance need to be discussed with both teacher and parent, along with the need for consistency and strict limits on school avoidance. At the same time, school avoidance behavior must be strictly aversive to the child; restriction of privileges, withdrawal of attention, and extra chores are among the possible aversive stimuli.

To be effective, any plan requires the consistent cooperation of both parent and teacher. A written contract with both the child and parent can be useful in achieving participation; contracting conveys a sense of mutual responsibility and formalizes the agreement. Concrete reminders of goals and rewards, such as star charts or other graphics, are especially useful for smaller children. Obtaining parental cooperation can be difficult because of the threat to the parent's dependence on the child's behavior. Substituting this dependence with concrete rewards such as free time to pursue other interests or goals helps the nurse to gain parental compliance. Parents might need help in developing new interests or goals, and the nurse is then called on to guide the family to appropriate resources.

Another technique is social imitation, in which the school-phobic child is exposed to nonfearful children interacting with the feared object or the feared environment. Play is particularly useful, as "playing school" is a direct but less

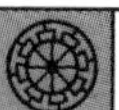

CASE STUDY A School-Phobic 7-Year-Old

Assessment

Bobby, a 7-year-old, was admitted to the hospital for evaluation after being referred for repeated refusal to attend school. Currently a first grader, Bobby missed an average of 3 school days a week with complaints of a stomachache. Bobby, the only child of a couple in their mid-twenties, was born after a much-wanted but highly complicated pregnancy.

Family

Bobby's father works as a mail carrier; Bobby's mother is a housewife. The family has recently moved to the city as the result of a job transfer and has developed few social supports. Neither parent actively pursues a hobby or similar interest.

Hospitalization

On admission, Bobby was a quiet, neatly dressed, well-mannered but passive boy who exhibited few spontaneous behaviors. Although very tentative in interactions, he obligingly cooperated in all aspects of the assessment, which included a gastrointestinal examination to evaluate his frequent complaints of stomach upset, as long as one of his parents was present. When his parents left for the evening, he cried uncontrollably until one of them returned. No physical basis for his complaint was established, and the frequency of these complaints decreased as the hospital stay progressed.

Bobby became involved in occupational and recreational therapy, play therapy involving various issues related to school, and some educational therapy, all with firm limits and clear behavioral expectations. Discharge preparation involved having Bobby immediately reenter the school in conjunction with a schedule of positive reinforcement to reward school attendance. Bobby was discharged and followed by the outpatient clinic in collaboration with the school nurse.

After 2 weeks, the school nurse reported that Bobby had missed a total of 6 school days and continued to complain of a variety of ailments while in school. Bobby was subsequently readmitted for further evaluation.

Nursing Diagnoses

1. Unresolved fear of going to school related to separation anxiety, inadequate coping skills, and avoidance behaviors
2. Potential for dysfunctional parenting related to inability to "let go" of child and to establish firm, consistent limits
3. Potential for family dysfunction related to family isolation

Plan for Interventions

Goals

1. Bobby and his parents will be able to identify stressors related to school.
2. Bobby will develop adaptive coping responses to fears of going to school.
3. Bobby's parents will facilitate Bobby's mastering fears of separation.
4. Bobby's parents will participate in discharge preparation.
5. The family will become involved in some aspect of the community to develop support systems.

Interventions

1. Involve Bobby in therapeutic play about separation situations.
2. Discuss with Bobby's parents his responses to therapeutic play activities.
3. Discuss with Bobby's parents his inability to separate from them when they attempt to leave the hospital.
4. Ask Bobby's parents whether he has had previous experiences with separation (for example, baby sitters, visits to relatives).
5. If Bobby has had experience with separation, ask the parents to describe Bobby's behavior.
6. Provide Bobby with opportunities for observation and interaction with peers during times of parental separation.
7. Work with Bobby's parents to develop a plan for behavior modification that does not reinforce Bobby's insisting on constant parental presence (a contract with the parents might help).
8. Plan with the parents for specific reinforcers when Bobby attends school for a full day (for example, his mother might promise to read a story to him immediately after school).
9. Discuss with Bobby's parents the possibility of involving Bobby in peer-related activities outside the home.
10. Suggest community supports that might assist the family in adapting to a new city (see Chapter 22).
11. Conduct a formal discharge conference that includes Bobby, both parents, Bobby's teacher, and the school nurse.
12. Suggest referral for family therapy or psychotherapy as necessary.

threatening way for the child to express fears about school and to work through them. Gradually introducing photographs, videotapes, or films of nonfearful children in a school setting prepares the child for actually observing and interacting with other schoolchildren. A process of desensitization then allows the child to overcome fears and rejoin the peer group.

Runaway Behavior

Children who run away from their families constitute a major problem that appears to be on the increase. Health prosionals need to know that runaway behavior in young people is a cry for help indicating serious trouble somewhere in their lives. Running away, however, poses dire, even fatal, risks until the child's safety is assured.

Runaway behavior has been defined a number of different ways. Engel and Lau (1983) define runaways as minors who leave home without the permission of their parents or guardians. Others define the behavior according to the time involved. Mirkin, Raskin, and Antognini (1984), for example, describe it as "staying away from home without parental permission for at least 24 hours."

Some runaway behavior is best viewed as a way of testing limits. Children who go to the homes of friends or relatives often return voluntarily. Other children are victims of dysfunctional parenting and have been abused or abandoned. Still others are adolescents who are unmotivated by traditional terms of achievement and choose to live in alternative, usually communal environments (Hofmann, 1983).

The incidence of runaway behavior in the United States is not precisely known. Two million children ran away in 1980, up from the "tens of thousands" quoted in a 1967 *Life* article (Engel and Lau, 1983). Runaways often head for large metropolitan areas, where many hope to find anonymity, others like themselves, or freedom from their problems. New York police estimate that at any given time there are 20,000 runaways 15 years of age or younger on the city's streets, and this figure does not include many homeless adolescents up to 21 years of age (Nerone, 1983).

The US Department of Health and Human Services estimates that the average age of runaway children is 15 years and that approximately 60% have never been in trouble before. About 67% are female; 70% are Caucasian (Jarvis, 1983). Runaways come from all socioeconomic classes, from all areas of the country, and from all ethnic groups (Nerone, 1983).

Assessment Young people who exhibit runaway behavior are often caught in conflicts between dependence and independence (Meeks, 1971). They are prone to feelings of helplessness and a desire to be dependent in a situation in which these feelings are dangerous, or shameful, or unable to be met. Those who run away may be trying to gain some control or self-sufficiency, to escape pain and danger, or to seek a kind helper. According to Meeks (1971, p. 212), runaways are running from something and toward something else.

> Most often, the runaway child is signaling a family disturbance which involves both himself and his parents. The running away serves both to discharge family tensions temporarily and to symbolize the conscious or unconscious wish of one or both parents to desert their family responsibility—to "walk off and leave it all."

Professionals increasingly report that runaways are escaping sexual, emotional, or physical abuse; parental scapegoating and family violence; friendlessness, isolation, and repression; neglect, lack of support, or outright rejection and hate (Engel and Lau, 1983; Gutierres and Reich, 1981; Mirkin, Raskin, and Antognini, 1984; Nerone, 1983). Low self-esteem and depression often result.

Runaway behavior and sexual abuse are increasingly correlated. The nurse who suspects sexual abuse can therefore also suspect that an abused child and sometimes the child's siblings are at risk for running away. (Sexual abuse is discussed in Chapter 22.) Kepler (1984, p. 205) states that adolescent victims of ongoing sexual abuse usually

> at some point in their childhood . . . gave up trying to fight the abuse. They stopped attempting to get someone to protect them or to intervene on their behalf—usually as a result of not being believed or supported the first time they spoke out. At this point . . . the child realizes she is more or less on her own. . . . The best she can hope for is to survive until she either reaches age 18, marries, or runs away.

Parental substance abuse (see Chapter 22) is also correlated with runaway behavior. An adolescent patient, Cheryl, described what happened in her family as follows (Kepler, 1984, p. 217).

> My Mom used to make me and my sisters support her drug habit. The three of us used to plan how we were all going to run away together or find someone that would raise us. We used to think Mom would get better and not make us do all that. But, those were all dreams. My youngest sister finally did run away. I haven't heard from her since. Lucy, my other sister, committed suicide when she was 14.

Children running away from dysfunctional families often are exploited and victimized again, particularly if they reach larger cities. Young runaways frequently are befriended, only to have their money and belongings stolen. What little self-assurance and self-sufficiency they did have becomes eroded, and problems of vulnerability and dependence become more serious. To survive the runaways are often forced into child prostitution, pornography, drug sales, panhandling, and theft; feelings of pain, shame, and worthlessness are then compounded.

If shelter is not available, the child literally might be forced to live on the streets. Accidental or purposeful injury can occur, and the child health nurse might therefore see the runaway child in the hospital emergency room. Runaways are at risk for a variety of physical and psychologic problems, including sexually transmitted disease; pregnancy; hepatitis; malnutrition; and continued physical, sexual, and emotional abuse (Nerone, 1983; Engel and Lau, 1983).

The nurse who suspects or knows that a child has run away therefore can incorporate these risk factors into the assessment process.

Meeks (1971) feels that most runaways wish to be found but that their pain, lack of trust, shame, and sense of worthlessness have reached the point that they feel unable to return home. Most have no legitimate job prospects to earn money or to pay for health care; many are ignorant of available resources and protection or are unable to use facilities that they do know about.

Nursing Management Nursing interventions need to address the complex situations that runaway behavior signals. Nurses who assess runaways cannot intervene effectively if they perceive these children as "bad kids" or criminals. The nurse needs to remember that

1. Runaways feel they have had no alternatives but to run away.
2. Runaways are legally still children who are immature and in need of help and protection (Engel and Lau, 1983).
3. Runaway behavior signals problems with the child's family or broader social systems.

The nurse also needs to be aware of resources that exist in the community. Many communities have shelters for runaways, most of which depend heavily on volunteer help. Engel and Lau (1983) describe resources at Covenant House in New York City, where nurses provide physical and psychologic assessments, document the runaways' stories and evidence of abuse, and work with other health professionals to obtain needed resources and support for the runaways. The overall goals of most shelters are to provide local, emergency resources for runaways by responding to their crises and preventing their running to more dangerous areas.

Nurses also might be involved in advising parents who seek help in finding a child who is missing and could have run away. Hofmann (1983) recommends the following steps:

1. Contact the child's friends, favored relatives, or other significant persons.
2. Call the police.
3. Call the National Runaway Switchboard (1-800-621-4000) and leave word that the child's family is interested in finding the child.
4. Leave word with nationally known centers for runaways, such as New York City's Covenant House. Begin with those in nearby cities.
5. Be prepared to become involved in family counseling and in some accommodations in the family system if the child returns.

Key Concepts

- Dysfunctional behaviors are often maladaptive coping strategies that the child uses to deal with perceived threats or stressors.
- Adaptive and maladaptive coping strategies are distinguished by the way in which the child uses the behavior to solve a perceived problem and promote social development.
- Child health nurses often identify dysfunctional behaviors in the process of developmental assessment.
- Dysfunctional behaviors may make the child vulnerable to delayed development and therefore require intervention.
- Substance abuse is a deliberate behavior that often develops into a pattern of dysfunction resulting in addiction.
- Adolescents are the population most vulnerable to substance abuse and need to be assessed in the context of the family system.
- Tobacco is the most commonly abused substance, is often readily identified, and is managed by finding ways to control smoking and reduce the stress associated with the behavior.
- Alcohol abuse, which often leads to serious self-care deficits, is managed by initial detoxification and by helping the child to find ways to reduce the need for alcohol and to establish an internal locus of control.
- Drug abuse can be correlated with low socioeconomic status, a diminished sense of well-being, low self-esteem, poor school performance, family dysfunctions, and other behavioral problems.
- Assessment for drug abuse involves observing physical signs and noting risk factors.
- Nursing management for drug abuse involves primary prevention, emergency and acute care, and referral for rehabilitation.
- Eating disorders are a maladaptive response to

problems of self-image and self-control and frequently require extensive family assessment in order to set goals and plan interventions.

- Obesity is often a cyclic phenomenon in which the child learns to use food to compensate for diminished self-esteem; management therefore involves ongoing support and planned changes in behavior patterns.
- Anorexia nervosa and bulimia are disorders that may be caused by fears and alterations in body image and may result in life-threatening syndromes.
- Nurses may suspect anorexia nervosa during routine health assessment; validating data can include cachexia, laboratory tests, and behaviors such as hiding or refusing food.
- When anorexia nervosa is managed by initial hospitalization, nursing goals include firm but supportive insistence on eating at prescribed times, preventing further nutritional deficiencies, and helping the patient to establish control over eating behaviors.
- Enuresis may be a temporary regressive behavior in response to stress, and is often managed by a variety of behavior modification techniques.
- Encopresis may be part of a pattern of behavior problems, is often a regressive behavior related to family stressors, and might be managed by initial bowel cleansing, behavior modification, and reducing anxiety through therapeutic play.
- Children often manifest school phobias through somatic complaints, crying, little exploratory behavior, and fear of separation.
- School phobias tend to occur at transitional times, require assessment of parent–child interaction to identify possible causes, and are usually managed by behavior modification that involves both child and parent.
- Runaway behavior is often correlated with child abuse, which is often sexual abuse and begins a pattern of emotional problems that leads to feelings of pain, shame, and worthlessness.
- The nurse who assesses runaway children needs to be aware of potential health problems that place these children at risk and needs to know about available community resources that can help address the child's needs.

References

Abraham S, Nondsieck M: Relationship of excess weight in children and adults. *Public Health Rep* 1960; 75:263–273.

Bales RF: Cultural differences in rates of alcoholism. Page 281 in: *Deviant Behavior and Social Process*. Rushing WA (editor). Rand McNally, 1969.

Bellman M: Studies on encopresis. *Acta Pediat Scand [Suppl]* 1966; 170.

Bennett G: Youthful substance abuse. Page 163 in: *Substance Abuse. Pharmacologic, Developmental, and Clinical Perspectives*. Bennett G, Vourakis C, Woolf D (editors). Wiley, 1983.

Berg I, Jones K: Functional fecal incontinence in children. *Arch Dis Child* 1964; 39:465–472.

Boskind-White M: *Bulimarexia: The Binge/Purge Cycle*. Norton, 1983.

Brazelton T: A child-oriented approach to toilet training. *Pediatrics* 1962; 29:121–128.

Bruch H: Anorexia nervosa. Pages 101–115 in: *Nutrition and the Brain*. Vol 3. Wurtman RS, and Wurtman JJ (editors). Raven Press, 1979.

Bruch H: *Eating Disorders: Obesity, Anorexia Nervosa, and the Person Within*. Basic Books, 1973.

Byrne M, Thompson H: *Key Concepts for the Study and Practice of Nursing*. Mosby, 1971.

Crisp AH: *Anorexia Nervosa: Let Me Be*. Academic Press, 1980.

Crockett R: *Drug Abuse and Personality in Young Offenders*. Appleton-Century-Crofts, 1971.

Earls F: Epidemiological child psychiatry: An American perspective. Pages 3–27 in: *Psychopathology of Children and Youth: A Cross-Cultural Perspective*. Purcell EF (editor). Josiah Mary, Jr., Foundation, 1980.

Engel NS, Lau Sr AD: Nursing care for the adolescent urban nomad. *Am J Mater Child Nurs* 1983; 8:74–77.

Finley B: The family and substance abuse. Pages 119–134 in: *Substance Abuse, Pharmacologic, Developmental, and Clinical Perspectives*. Bennett G, Vourakis C, Woolf D (editors). Wiley, 1983.

Frederiksen L: Controlled smoking. *Behavioral Analysis and Treatment of Substance Abuse*. Krasnegor N (editor). National Institute on Drug Abuse Research Monograph Series 25. DHEW Publication, 1979.

Goble F: *The Third Force: The Psychology of Abraham Maslow*. Grossman, 1970.

Garfinkel P, Garner D: *Anorexia Nervosa: A Multidimensional Perspective*. Brunner/Maazel, 1982.

Graham P: Epidemiological studies. Pages 185–209 in: *Psychopathological Disorders of Childhood*. Quay H, Werry T (editors). Wiley, 1979.

Gutierres SE, Reich JW: A developmental perspective on runaway behavior: Its relationship to child abuse. *Child Welfare* 1981; 60(2):89–94.

Hetherington E, Martin B: Family interaction and psychopathology in children. *Psychopathological Disorders of Childhood*. 2nd ed. Quay H, Werry J (editors). Wiley, 1979.

Hofmann AD: *Adolescent Medicine*. Addison-Wesley, 1983.

Hurd G, Pattison M, Llamas R: Models of social network intervention. *Int J Fam Ther* (Winter) 1981; 3(4):246–257.

Jarvis V: Runaway kids. *Imprint* 1983; 30(2):31.

Kandel D: *Longitudinal Research on Drug Use. Empirical Findings and Methodological Issues.* Hemisphere, 1978.

Kanner C: *Child Psychiatry.* 4th ed. Charles C Thomas, 1972.

Kepler V: *One In Four—Handling Child Sexual Abuse—What Every Professional Should Know.* Social Interest Press, 1984.

Knopf IT: *Childhood Psychopathology, A Developmental Approach.* Prentice-Hall, 1979.

Lichtenstein E: Social learning, smoking, and substance abuse. Pages 114–127 in: *Behavioral Analysis and Treatment of Substance Abuse.* Krasnegor N (editor). National Institute on Drug Abuse Research Monograph Series 25. DHEW Publication, 1979.

Marks RG: Anorexia and bulimia: Eating habits that can kill. *RN* (Jan) 1984; 47(1):44–47.

Meeks JE: The runaway. Pages 212–217 in: *The Fragile Alliance.* Williams & Wilkins, 1971.

Miller W: Problem drinking and substance abuse: Behavioral perspectives. In: *Behavioral Analysis and Treatment of Substance Abuse.* Krasnegor N (editor). National Institute on Drug Abuse Research Monograph Series 25. DHEW Publication, 1979.

Minuchin S, Rosman B, Baker L: *Psychosomatic Families.* Harvard University Press, 1978.

Mirkin MP, Raskin A, Antognini FG: Parenting, protecting, preserving: Mission of the adolescent female runaway. *Family Process* 1984; 23: 63–74.

National Institute on Drug Abuse. *Report to Congress on Drugs and Health,* 1979.

Nerone BJ: Throwaway children. *Imprint* 1983; 30(2):31–37.

Palazzoli S: *Self-Starvation.* Jason Aronson, 1978.

Pechacek T: An overview of smoking behavior and its modification. Pages 92–113 in: *Behavioral Analysis and Treatment of Substance Abuse.* Krasnegor N (editor). National Institute on Drug Abuse Research Monograph Series 25. DHEW Publication, 1979.

Pless I: The changing face of primary pediatrics. *Ped Clin North Am* 1974; 21:223–244.

Plumb M, D'Amanda C, Taintor Z: Chemical abuse and perceived locus of control. Pages 223–261 in: *Predicting Adolescent Drug Abuse: A Review of Issues, Methods, and Correlates.* Lettieri D (editor). National Institute on Drug Abuse Research Issue Series II. DHEW Publication, 1975.

Pollin W: Foreword. *Behavioral Analysis and Treatment of Substance Abuse.* Krasnegor N (editor). National Institute on Drug Abuse Research Monograph Series 25. DHEW Publication, 1979.

Powell M: *Assessment and Management of Developmental Changes and Problems in Children.* 2nd ed. Mosby, 1981.

Rice MA, Kibbee PE: Review: Identifying the adolescent substance abuser. *Am J Matern Child Nurs* 1983; 8:139–142.

Rockwell WJK et al: Anorexia nervosa: Review of current treatment practices. *South Med J* (Sept) 1982; 75:1101.

Russell G: Bulimia nervosa: An ominous variant of anorexia nervosa. *Psychol Med* 1979; 9:429–448.

Shaffer D: The association between enuresis and emotional disorder: A review of the literature. *Bladder Control in Enuresis. Clinics in Developmental Medicine.* Kolvin I, Mackeith R, Meadow S (editors). Heinemann, 1973.

Shopper M: Adolescent problems. Pages 214–221 in: J. Noshpitz *Basic Handbook of Child Psychiatry. Vol. 4.* Noshpitz J (editor). Basic Books, 1979.

Swift W, Stern S: The psychodynamic diversity of anorexia nervosa. *Int J Eating Disorders* 1982; 2(1):17–35.

Werry TS: Psychosomatic disorders, psychogenic symptoms, and hospitalization. Pages 160ff in: *Psychopathological Disorders of Childhood.* Quay H, Werry T (editors). Wiley, 1979.

Williams D: Substance abuse treatment settings. Chapter 17 in: *Nursing Care of Adolescents.* Howe J (editor). McGraw-Hill, 1980a.

Williams D: Substance use and abuse. Chapter 6 in: *Nursing Care of Adolescents.* Howe J (editor). McGraw-Hill, 1980b.

Wu R: *Behavior and Illness.* Prentice-Hall, 1970.

Zeitlin S: Assessing coping behavior. *Am J Orthopsychiatry* (Jan) 1980; 50(1):140.

Additional Readings

Abraham SF, Beumont PJ: How patients describe bulimia or binge eating. *Psychol Med* (Aug) 1982; 12(3):625–635.

Ballar WR: *Bed Wetting: Origins and Treatment.* Pergamon Press, 1975.

Blackford N: Drug dependency: A family matter *Nurs Mirror* (Sept 9) 1981; 153(11):28–29.

Boswell J: Helping children with their anger. *Elementary School Guidance and Counseling* 1982; 16(4):278–287.

Bruch H: Perils of behavior modification in the treatment of anorexia nervosa *JAMA* 1974; 230:1414–1422.

Casper RC et al: Bulimia, its incidence and clinical importance in patients with anorexia nervosa. *Arch Gen Psychiatry* 1980; 37:1030–1035.

Crisp AH, Bhat AV: Personality and anorexia nervosa—The public avoidance stance. Its origins and its symptomatology. *Psychother Psychosom* 1982; 38(1):178–200.

Epstein LH, Masek BJ, Marshall NR: A nutritionally based program for control of eating in obese children. *Behav Ther* 1978; 9:766–778.

Fagin C (editor): *Readings in Child and Adolescent Psychiatric Nursing.* Mosby, 1974.

Fond K, Brosnan J: School phobia: The school anxiety symptom. *Pediatr Nurs* 1980; 6(5):9–13.

Garfinkel PE, Moldofsky H, Garner DM: The heterogeneity of anorexia nervosa: Bulimia as a distinct subgroup. *Arch Gen Psychiatry* 1980; 37:1036–1040.

Lehmann A: Emancipation by emaciation. *Can Nurse* (Nov) 1982; 31–34.

MacDonald D, Newton M: The clinical syndrome of adolescent drug abuse. *Adv Pediatr* 1981; 28:1–25.

McKendry J, Steward D: Eneuresis. *Pediatr Clin North Am* 1974; 21:1019–1028.

Michael M, Sewall KS: Use of the adolescent peer group to increase the self care agency of adolescent alcohol abusers. *Nurs Clin North Am* (March) 1980; 15(1):157–176.

Mowrey BD: Family oriented approach to childhood obesity. *Pedriat Nurs* 1980; 6(2):40–44.

Nader PR, Bullock D, Caldwell B: School phobia. *Pediatr Clin North Am* 1975; 22:605–617.

Penning M, Barnes GE: Adolescent marijuana use: A review. *Int J Addict* (July) 1982; 17(5):749–791.

Rampling D: Abnormal mothering in the genesis of anorexia nervosa. *J Nerv Ment Dis* 1980; 168(8):501–504.

Rosenthal C et al: *Nurses, Patients and Families.* Springer, 1980.

Ruble J: Childhood nocturnal enuresis. *Am J Matern Child Nurs* 1981; 6(1):26–31.

Sanger E, Cassino T: Eating disorders: Avoiding the power struggle. *Am J Nurs* (Jan) 1984; 84:31–33.

Skuse D, Burrell S: A review of solvent abusers and their management by a child psychiatric out-patient service. *Hum Toxicol* (July) 1982; 1(3):321–329.

Smart RG, Murray G: A review of trends in alcohol and cannabis use among young people. *Bull Narc* 1981; 33(4):77–90.

Smith ME: Enuresis: Guidelines for nursing management. *Current Practice in Pediatric Nursing.* 3rd ed. Chinn P, Leonard KB (editors). Mosby, 1980.

Starfield B: Enuresis: Its pathogenesis and management *Clin Pediatr* 1971; 11:343.

Strober M et al: Validity of bulimia—restricted distinction in anorexia nervosa personality characteristics and family psychiatry mobility. *J Nerv Ment Dis* 1982; 120(6):345–351.

Sugarman A, Quinlan DN, Devenis L: Ego boundary disturbance in anorexia nervosa: Preliminary findings. *J Pers Assess* (Oct) 1982; 46(5):455–461.

Taitz LS: Obesity in pediatric practice: Infantile obesity. *Pediat Clin North Am* 1977; 24:107–115.

Tennant FS, LaCour J: Children at high risk for addiction and alcoholism: Identification and intervention. *Pediatr Nurs* 1980; 6(1):26–27.

White AJ: Outpatient treatment of oppositional non-eating in a deaf retarded boy. *J Behav Ther Exp Psychiatry* (Sept) 1982; 13(3):251–255.

Wilson CP, Mintz I: Abstaining and bulemic anorexics. Two sides of the same coin. *Primary Care* (Sept) 1982; 9(3):517–530.

Nursing Care of the Child With a Psychiatric or Social Disorder

25

Janet A. Grossman Christine Herrmann

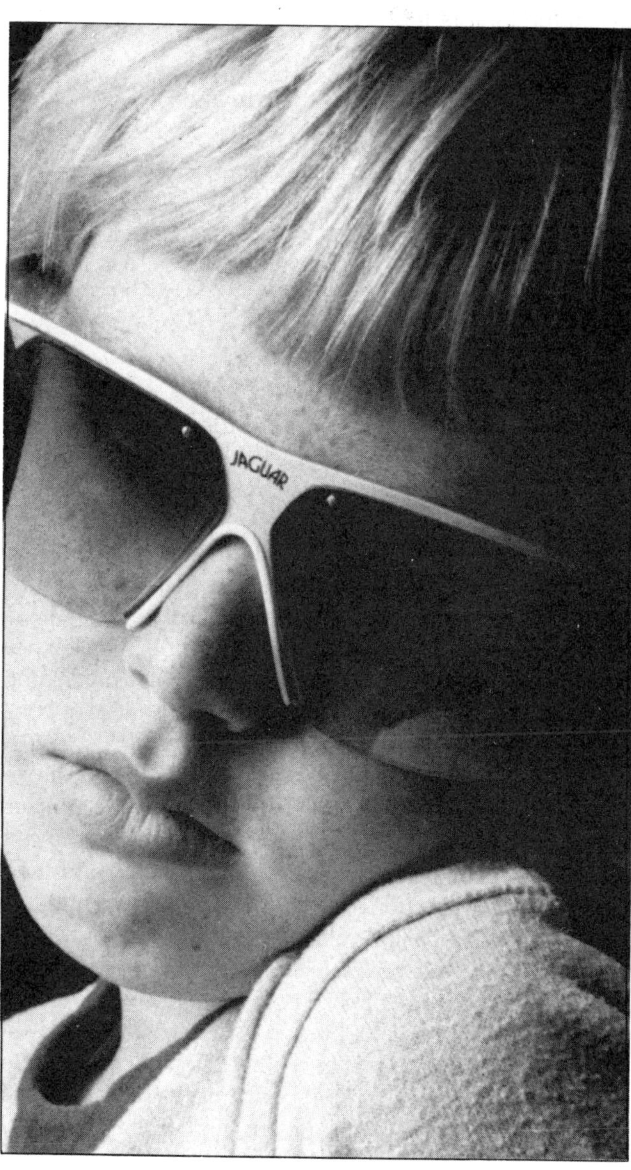

Chapter Outline

Objectives

- Describe the role of the nurse in identifying psychiatric disorders in children.
- List the factors that contribute to psychiatric disorders in children.
- Explain the DSM III classification and its applicability to nursing.
- Describe assessment criteria and nursing management with psychiatric and social disorders in children.
- Describe the clinical manifestations of autism, schizophrenia, depression, and conduct disorders in children.
- Explain the etiology, diagnostic methods, treatment, and nursing goals associated with autism, schizophrenia, depression, and conduct disorders in children.

Children with severe emotional disorders present a challenge that taxes the knowledge and resources of the child health nurse. Children with these disorders typically experience problems functioning in the family, school, and community. They tend to exhibit developmental delay, which causes them to lag behind their peers. Their parents or significant others complain about their behavior or are frustrated by their lack of response. These children might experience somatic problems typical of adults with psychiatric disorders and may have communication difficulties or confused perceptions of reality.

Nurses often encounter these children, particularly those who are undiagnosed or under-treated, but not all nurses understand psychiatric disorders, and some nurses find it difficult to plan interventions with these children and their families. Child psychopathology needs to be included in nursing curricula so that valuable opportunities for assessment, referral, guidance, and support are not missed. We believe that the study of child psychopathology should be a basic component of the nursing care of children.

Psychiatric disturbances in children range across a wide continuum. At one end of the spectrum are children whose everyday worries overwhelm them, and at the other end of the spectrum are the children who need constant supervision because they might hurt themselves or others or because their thought processes are disturbed. In Chapter 24 we focus on dysfunctional behaviors that the nurse might identify in a variety of settings. In this chapter we focus on the other end of the continuum, on children with a severely impaired ability to function, and we explore four major psychiatric and social disorders in children and adolescents. Although not the most common childhood disorders, they represent major disturbances in mood, thought processes, and social functioning. Nursing care for children with these disorders can serve as a model for nurses working with all disturbed children and their families.

The Child Health Nurse and Mental Health

Pediatrics, Child Psychiatry, and the Nurse

Pediatrics and child psychiatry had little relationship to each other prior to the 1930s. Until that time, pediatricians showed little interest in child psychiatry, and child psychiatrists did not fully use data concerning the physical development of children (Senn, 1948). In 1937 Kanner began to bridge the gap between the disciplines by developing a training program in child psychiatry for pediatricians at the Philadelphia Guidance Home. Pediatricians then began to make long-term observations of children to help fill the gaps in knowledge about childhood development.

Child psychiatrists in turn encouraged pediatricians to use child psychiatric theory for anticipatory guidance with parents (Hirschberg, 1980). These were the beginnings of collaboration, although acceptance and sharing of data between these fields continues to vary widely. A comprehensive diagnostic evaluation, however, often depends on such collaboration.

As the first professional to encounter a child who might need a differential diagnosis involving both pediatrics and child psychiatry, the child health nurse might be in a position to facilitate this collaboration. Ingestion of toxic levels of drugs and alcohol, for instance, can produce toxic psychosis in adolescents; lead poisoning can produce symptoms of an attention deficit. Children have been known to ingest toxic levels of bromides, which result in confusion, depression, or delirium; toxic levels of prochlorperazine (Compazine) suppositories also can result in confusion and delirium. (Substance abuse is discussed in Chapter 24.) Steroid treatment for adrenocortical dysfunction can produce steroid euphoria or psychotic behavior, and vitamin deficiency can produce symptoms of dementia. Chemotherapy and progressive degenerative brain disease can lead to intellectual deterioration and personality change, chronic subdural hematoma can result in intellectual deterioration, and acute porphyria can produce schizophrenic symptoms (Herskowitz and Rosman, 1982).

In 1980 an estimated 10 million children, or 15% of the 65 million children in this country, suffered from mental health disorders (Dumas, 1980). In tight economic times, psychiatric services, particularly those for children, are among the first services to be sacrificed. Many institutions also are cutting back their services, and health care benefits are being reduced. Contemporary society therefore carries a huge population of undiagnosed and untreated children with psychiatric problems.

Many of these children will be seen first by child health nurses in hospitals, schools, clinics, and homes. The nurse might be confronted with physical conditions associated with psychiatric symptoms, a child with an emotional or behavioral problem, or a high-risk family/parenting situation. These situations will require further interventions and assessment by the child health nurse or referrals to other health care professionals.

Nursing intervention in the form of primary prevention can start even before the birth of an infant in prenatal classes where the nurse will provide information on infant growth and development and assess parenting skills (see Chapter 22). Even as early as the first few days after birth, the nurse can assess any abnormal interaction between the parent and neonate. In the home the public health nurse is in a key position to reinforce information on growth and development and observe firsthand whether there are any problems in parenting.

Referring to or consulting with parent's groups is another method of primary prevention. As applied to mental health, primary prevention is "the process involved in reducing the risk that people in the community will fall ill with mental disorders" (Caplan, 1961). Common preventive activities at the primary level include observation, anticipatory guidance, and developmental education. The opportunity to work with parents in a group situation could be instrumental in reducing the risk that children and adolescents will develop emotional disorders. Many parents of children with emotional and behavioral problems and parents in general have remarked that they were never taught how to be parents or that all parents should be required to take classes on parenting. The nurse also can be involved in primary prevention by acting as a responsible citizen and change agent, taking an active interest in issues related to children on a local, state, and federal level.

Secondary prevention, as applied to mental health and defined by Caplan (1961), is the prevention of disability by case finding, early diagnosis, and effective treatment. Common preventive activities at the secondary level include observation, counseling for developmental and situational crises, and providing access to services and support systems. The child health nurse in a variety of settings might begin to notice mannerisms in the infant or toddler that could be cause for concern. For example, in autism these behavioral characteristics might include an infant who doesn't cuddle, a toddler who prefers inanimate objects to people, a preschooler who uses toys inappropriately in a stereotypic, repetitious manner, or a child who isn't developing language. Often, the parents of autistic children first begin to admit there might be a problem when language development does not occur, expressing concern about possible hearing problems. Whatever the presenting concerns, the nurse listens carefully to the parent, offers reassurance and guidance, carefully follows the infant or child at risk and the family, and refers the child and family for an extensive diagnostic workup. Early diagnosis and the institution of effective treatment can do much to help the family. An awareness of what to look for and how to interpret behaviors can assist the nurse in case finding, early diagnosis, and effective treatment or referral. The nurse also needs to be aware of family crises, particularly those related to loss and separation and family transitions between developmental stages. (Family assessment techniques are discussed in Chapter 17.)

The child health nurse is not likely to be involved in tertiary prevention for emotionally disturbed children. This level of nursing intervention is best performed by nurse specialists trained in child psychiatry. Common activities at the tertiary level include providing a therapeutic milieu, teaching, with specific reference to emotional and social development, conducting child, family, and group psychotherapy, and functioning as an advocate for children and adolescents. Nurse specialists in child psychiatry work with disturbed children and their families in residential settings, inpatient units, outpatient clinics, and day treatment programs.

Etiology of Psychiatric Disorders

Many factors contribute to the development of psychiatric disorders in children. The variables defined by researchers and clinicians depend on their theoretic framework, but nursing theorists view the etiology of psychiatric disorders as multidimensional. For child health nurses, etiologic factors generally fit the following four categories:

1. Genetic and biophysical factors
2. Social and cultural factors
3. Family system factors
4. Acquired illness and injury

Figure 25-1 shows the factors that comprise each of these categories. These variables are the components of suprasystems and subsystems that influence the mental health of the child.

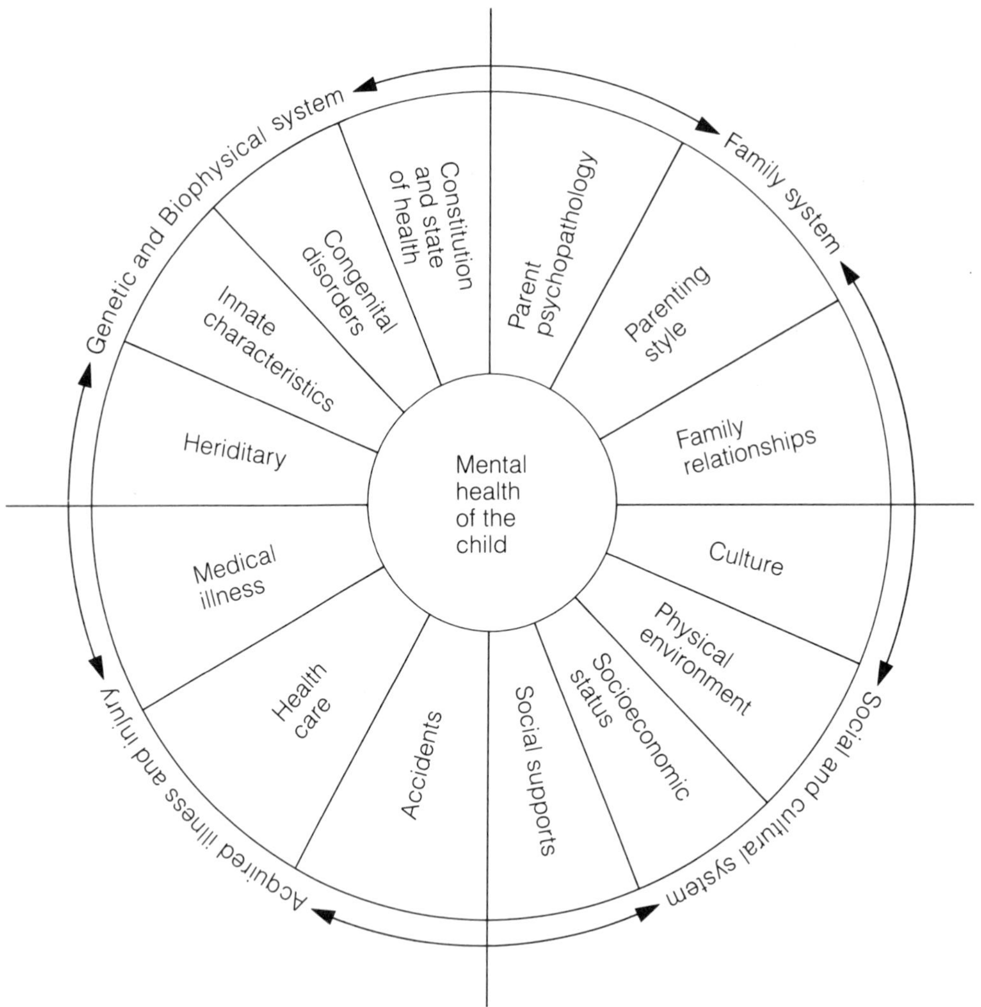

Figure 25-1 Factors that contribute to psychiatric disorders in children.

Hereditary variables include information transmitted by intact genes. For example, phenylketonuria, which is caused by recessive genes, can result in mental retardation (see Chapter 23). Constitutional factors, part of the child's biophysical structure, include physical appearance or other factors such as minimal brain damage resulting from birth injury. Innate factors refer to the "effects of mutation and regrouping of genes as they formed in the germ cells of parents and transferred to the gametes" (Achenbach, 1982) and occurs, for example, in children of alcoholic mothers who are born with fetal alcohol syndrome. Congenital factors are changes that occur between conception and birth; premature birth is one possible congenital variable affecting behavior and social adaptation (Phillips, 1983).

The role of social and cultural factors in the etiology of psychiatric disorders has been acknowledged in the last 20 years. Gerald Caplan, who has advocated primary prevention for psychiatric disorders in adults and children, viewed these psychiatric disorders as one of a set of intermediated social problems that must be handled at the community level. Viewing psychiatric disorders as dysfunction of the suprasystems as well as dysfunction in the child requires a revision of theory and practice (Caplan, 1961).

Social and cultural variables affecting the child's mental health are factors in the child's environment, which include the physical environment of the home and aspects of the community, the family's socioeconomic resources, and cultural and social supports. When the child's environment is inadequate, as is the case with poverty or deprivation, the child is at greater risk for developing psychiatric problems. For example, an adolescent from a family with few socioeconomic resources is more likely to join a delinquent gang and resort to stealing.

Aspects of the family system include parental psychopathology, parenting style, and intrafamilial relationships (such as marriage, siblings, and extended family networks) (see Chapter 4). Achenbach (1982) stated that "most children are dependent on their families, directly involved in their conflicts, and shaped by models, rewards, and punishments they provide." Ackerman (1968) believed that psychiatric disorders in children are often preceded by family conflict. For example, one 10-year-old girl became depressed after her parents divorced. The nurse's role in working with families requires that psychiatric problems in children must be understood in the context of the family.

Acquired illness and injury also contribute to psychiatric disorders in children. Children who become disabled because of accidents and illness might develop psychiatric disorders and are more vulnerable if they are not treated in the context of their families and other supports. The parents of these children are called on to provide additional warmth, acceptance, support, and resources. Poor health care practices might predispose the child to emotional and behavioral problems; for instance, children with poor nutrition tend to be lethargic, show impaired school performance, and be less interested in social activities.

Typically, it is not possible to isolate a specific etiologic factor resulting in a psychiatric disorder in an individual child. More often, professionals view etiology as an accumulation of or interaction of etiologic factors. When parents are counseled, references might be made to factors that have contributed to the child's disturbance (such as stress in the family, illness, or the child's constitution).

Assessment of the Child With a Psychiatric Disorder

Because nurses frequently encounter children with major psychiatric and social disorders or might suspect a psychiatric problem in a child, nurses need to assess psychologic functioning. Assessment in child health or mental health settings is distinct from the evaluation performed by the child psychiatrist, child psychologist, or clinical specialist in psychiatric nursing. Child health nurses in clinic or outpatient settings might do an initial assessment, but they do not diagnose, conduct psychologic testing, or carry out intensive psychiatric treatment. Their assessments and concerns, however, should be shared with mental health professionals who have extensive training in the area of childhood psychopathology. Table 25-1 presents a guide for

TABLE 25-1 Areas for the Assessment of Psychologic Functioning in Children

Child	Parent
General appearance	Developmental history
Grooming	Health history
Hygiene	Description of typical day in child's life
Orientation—time, place, person	Behavioral concerns—frequency, severity
Motor behavior—fine, gross	Digestion and elimination
Ability to relate/socialization	Sleep
Peers—best friend/ages	Appetite
Adults	Motor activity
Ability to separate from parents	Speech
Activities	Vision and hearing
Interests, hobbies	Mannerisms
Groups	Aggression—toward self and others
Chores	School history
Ability to have fun	Family
Speech/language	Structure
Expressive language	Developmental stage
Receptive language	Parent–child interaction—warmth, empathy, spontaneity, physical nurturing
Content	Activities
Mood (affect)	Discipline
Behavior—skills and activities of daily living	Social supports
Attitudes	History of psychotropic drugs
School—teacher, homework, performance	Dose
Hospitalization or other health care	Duration
Family—parents, siblings, significant extended family	Effect on mood, activity
Self-concept and body image	Side effects
Behavior	Child's extrafamily relationships
Aggression, fears, ability to follow limits	Peers
	School
	Antisocial behavior

nurses assessing psychologic functioning in the child. The assessment should be repeated with both the child and parent.

Cognitive functioning of children can best be assessed by the professional with advanced and specialized training in child psychiatry and child psychology. Thought disorders are difficult to assess in adults and are even more difficult to assess in children because of developmental issues associated with language and cognitive development. A well-trained and experienced clinician can differentiate between a child's hallucinations and delusions and normal childhood fantasies. Even the clinical specialist in child psychiatry collaborates with the psychiatrist whenever these symptoms are suspected or confirmed. Although psychiatric symptoms resulting from medication or hospitalization fall under medical practice, the nurse does not ignore them; rather, the nurse who suspects a psychiatric disorder carefully documents and reports observations.

Assessment of the disturbed child underscores the versatility required of nurses working with these children. In addition to understanding the wide spectrum of developmental issues that occur from infancy to adolescence, the nurse defines dysfunctional behavior in a developmental framework because behavior that is typical of one developmental stage might be considered maladaptive or severely dysfunctional at another stage. For example, one anxious 5-year-old on the pediatric unit drank only from a bottle, even though he had not used one in years. His dysfunction indicated regression to an earlier stage of development, a common response to hospitalization (see Chapter 27). More severely dysfunctional was a 9-year-old encopretic girl who, although previously bowel trained, had regressed to an earlier developmental stage to cope with family conflict and her feelings about the conflict.

Assessments and interventions made by child health nurses therefore must be based on an understanding of normal growth and development as well as the types of behaviors that one might expect to see in hospitalized children. The 5-year-old should return to a previous level of functioning when he feels less anxious. Certainly, once he is home with his parent or significant others and in familiar surroundings he will give up the bottle. If this behavior continues, it is cause for concern that the initiating conflict is unresolved, and this boy might need further intervention. The 9-year-old encopretic girl and her family, on the other hand, will require intensive psychiatric intervention to help her return to her age-appropriate level of developmental functioning.

Classification of Psychiatric Disorders in Children

Approaches to classify psychopathology in children include developmental, systems, and disease models. All of these models can be used as a framework from which to plan nursing care. A developmental model applies developmental theories and describes how symptoms and syndromes that develop during a stage interfere with developmental norms and tasks. Fagin (1974) used this model as a framework for understanding the normal child, identifying maladaptive coping, and providing a basis for nursing interventions. Shaffer and colleagues (1983) developed a children's global assessment scale, which is a systems approach.

The current and most commonly used method of classifying childhood psychopathology is the *Diagnostic and Statistical Manual of Mental Disorders* (third edition) (American Psychiatric Association, 1980), which generally is called the DSM III. This is a disease model for psychopathology and defines a mental disorder as "a clinically significant behavioral or psychological syndrome or pattern that occurs in an individual and that is typically associated with either a painful symptom (distress) or impairment in one or more important areas of functioning (disability)."

The DSM III method for classifying childhood disorders, outlined in a section entitled "Disorders First Evident in Infancy, Childhood and Adolescence," divides childhood disorders into five groups: (1) intellectual; (2) behavioral; (3) emotional; (4) physical; and (5) developmental (Table 25-2). Disorders not described in the childhood section of DSM III are considered the same as adult disorders, that is, affective disorders and schizophrenic disorders.

Problems that appear in children are not necessarily classified as psychiatric disorders. These conditions might be those for which appropriate diagnosis cannot be determined, for which no psychiatric disorder has been found, or for which a psychiatric diagnosis is not the current focus of treatment. For example, the child's problem might be rooted in parent–child difficulties and therefore is not a psychiatric disorder in the child.

Williams and Wilson (1982) suggested that the DSM III is useful to nursing because it accomplishes the following:

1. Provides a framework for interdisciplinary communication.
2. Bases subsequent revisions on a series of formative evaluations.
3. Represents a collaborative achievement.
4. Represents progress toward a more holistic view of mind–body relations.
5. Makes a provision for diagnostic uncertainty.
6. Incorporates, at least in part, biologic, psychologic, and social variables.
7. Has achieved positive results in extensive testing of its validity and reliability.
8. Considers adaptive strength as well as problems.
9. Provides for a comprehensive biopsychosocial approach.
10. Reflects a descriptive, phenomenologic perspective.

Within the framework of the DSM III, nurses can conceptualize major psychiatric and social disorders in children.

TABLE 25-2 Disorders First Evident in Infancy, Childhood, and Adolescence

Intellectual disorders	Behavioral disorders	Emotional disorders	Physical disorders	Developmental disorders
Mental retardation Mild Moderate Severe Profound	Attention deficit disorder With hyperactivity Without hyperactivity Conduct disorders Aggressive Nonaggressive Socialized Undersocialized	Anxiety disorders Separation anxiety disorders Avoidant disorder Overanxious disorders Reactive attachment disorder Schizoid disorder Elective disorder Oppositional disorder Identity disorder	Eating disorders Anorexia nervosa Bulimia Pica Rumination disorder Stereotyped movement disorders Chronic motor tic Transient tic Tourette's disease Disorders with physical manifestations Stuttering Functional enuresis Functional encopresis Sleepwalking disorder Sleep terror disorder	Pervasive developmental disorders Infantile autism Childhood-onset pervasive developmental disorder Specific developmental disorders Reading disorder Arithmetic disorder Language disorder Articulation disorder

SOURCE: Adapted from the American Psychiatric Association: *Diagnostic and Statistical Manual of Mental Disorders*. 3rd ed. The American Psychiatric Association, 1980.

Loomis (1983) suggested that the behaviors listed in the DSM III also provide the basis for making a nursing diagnosis. Nurses diagnose and treat human responses as they interact with people experiencing actual or potential health problems. Infantile autism, for example, is a health problem characterized primarily by gross deficits in language development. Thus, the human response is to the actual health problem (autism), and the nursing diagnosis is "impaired verbal communication." Nursing interventions are then based on communication and not on the medical diagnosis of infantile autism.

Nurse educators, clinicians, and researchers need to develop nursing diagnoses and interventions that address the emotional and behavioral problems of children.

Pervasive Developmental Disorders —Infantile Autism

Pervasive developmental disorder, although rare, is one of the most serious psychiatric disorders in childhood. It can be detected in the earliest developmental stages and is characterized by withdrawal, self-absorption, and unresponsiveness. Although the prognosis is guarded, early detection and treatment can enhance the family's abilities to cope and possibly increase the child's chances for a better prognosis.

Pervasive developmental disorders are divided into two categories: infantile autism and childhood-onset pervasive developmental disorder. Because infantile autism and childhood-onset pervasive developmental disorder are similar in symptomatology, it is necessary to delineate the features of only one in order to illustrate nursing care. Infantile autism presents a picture of a unique infant and is therefore the logical choice. What separates infantile autism from childhood-onset pervasive developmental disorder is primarily the age of onset. Infantile autism develops in the first 30 months of life, whereas childhood-onset pervasive developmental disorder develops after 30 months and before 12 years of age. Children diagnosed with childhood-onset pervasive developmental disorder have demonstrated a period of more normal development and a more appropriate use of language. Later, however, they begin to demonstrate much of the symptomatology seen in infantile autism.

The autistic child's perceptual dysfunctions severely distort personal experiences. Thus, the autistic child's behaviors can appear to be bizarre to individuals who do not share this unique reality.

One sensitive father's description of his autistic son provides some insight into the mannerisms and world of the autistic child:

> The rocking back and forth on the leverage of his own eternity. The soft and gentle retreat to the outside perimeter of our world. The spinning and fixed stare. His great agility and his hypnotic fascination with inanimate objects. The self-stimulating smile and repetitious motion of his fingers against his lips. The pushing away of people and the silent aloneness. When Raun turned to you, he turned through you as if you were transparent. And then there was the keen awareness that he did not use language. Not just a slow talker, he offered no communication by sound or gesture, no expression of wants, likes or dislikes. Almost one and a half years old, Raun, a new creature in a strange land (Kaufman, 1976).

The syndrome was first described by Leo Kanner in 1943, which he later labeled "early infantile autism." Since this initial description, many investigators have expanded and refined the characteristics of these children (DeMeyer, et al., 1971; Rutter, 1974; Ornitz and Ritvo, 1976). These researchers all suggest three characteristics common to all autistic children: (1) disturbances in social development; (2) disturbances in the development and use of language; (3) insistence on sameness or compulsive repetition. According to the DSM III, the current diagnostic criteria for infantile autism are as follows:

1. Onset before 30 months of age.
2. Pervasive lack of responsiveness to other people.
3. Gross deficits in language development.
4. If speech is present, peculiar speech patterns such as immediate and delayed echolalia, metaphoric language, and pronoun reversal.
5. Bizarre responses to various aspects of the environment (such as resistance to change or peculiar interest in or attachment to animate or inanimate objects).
6. Absence of delusions, hallucinations, loosening of associations, and incoherence such as in schizophrenia.

Etiology and Incidence

Although the incidence of autism is low, generally estimated at 2–4 cases per 10,000 children, research as to the cause has been abundant. Even so, no definitive cause for autism has been uncovered. Paluszny (1979) enumerated the following possible causes:

1. Psychogenic (Bettelheim, 1967; Tustin, 1973).
2. Biogenic: viral (Desmond, et al., 1970; Chess, 1971), genetic (Rimland, 1964), or Biochemical (Coleman, 1976).
3. Disturbances of modulation of perception (Ornitz and Ritvo, 1968).
4. Impairment in abstract memory (Hermelin, 1976).
5. Defects in processing information and responding to stimuli (DeMeyer, et al., 1971).
6. Language defect (Rutter, Bartak, and Newman, 1971; Rutter, 1974).
7. Lack of cerebral dominance (Tanguary, 1976).

The general consensus is that some type of organic problem causes autism. This problem frequently is present from birth, although it often goes undetected initially. Males are affected three times more often than females, and there is a wide range of IQs in these children. No correlation between autism and birth order has been established, although the DSM III states that "The prevalence of Infantile Autism is 50 times as great in siblings of children with the disorder than in the general population" (American Psychiatric Association, 1980). Thus, a familial pattern is seen.

Signs and Symptoms

Pervasive developmental disorders are characterized by distortions in multiple areas of development and affect many areas of behavior. An infant or child might demonstrate mild to severe degrees of the characteristic symptomatology.

In infancy the autistic child appears unresponsive to normal nurturing, does not cuddle, and might even stiffen when held. The child exhibits no anticipatory posturing when about to be picked up. On one end of a continuum, the infant might be very content for hours to be left alone and at the other end of the spectrum might be very irritable. As infants, autistic children might refuse the breast and often continue to be fussy eaters. Many autistic infants do not appear to respond to loud noises near them but might focus on distant sounds such as music in another room.

It has been hypothesized that the inability to perceive and process sensory stimuli presents the autistic infant and young child with an environment that appears to be constantly changing. The behaviors that develop are their attempt to cope with this situation. They demonstrate ritualistic and repetitive behaviors (such as spinning a favorite toy for hours), are resistant to change, often displaying tantrums, and develop self-stimulating behaviors (such as rocking), which often progress to self-mutilating behaviors (such as head banging).

The difficulty in screening visual and auditory stimuli causes these children to resort to behaviors such as covering their eyes and ears, shrieking, or producing repetitious, monotonous sounds (Harris, 1978). Perceptual problems can produce inadequate sensory awareness of body parts or boundaries. Thus, these children often walk or run on their toes while flapping their arms at their sides.

Autistic children usually have a high degree of receptive language but often lack expressive language. If they do develop any speech, it is inappropriate and abnormal. Autistic children who develop some language often reverse their pronouns, saying "you" when they mean "I." They demonstrate *echolalia,* which is repeating over and over the words they hear. For example, if the nurse asks, "John, do you want a cookie?", he will repeat "John, do you want a cookie? John, do you want a cookie?" The child's degree of receptive language and potential intelligence is illustrated by a child who can repeat verbatim a story or a television commercial. The speech that does develop, however, is not used to communicate in a way that helps others to understand the autistic child's wants and feelings.

As they grow older, autistic children continue to demonstrate impairment in social relationships. They often prefer inanimate objects to people and will use people as objects to have their needs met. An example of this is the autistic child who does not see his mother's hand as part of her but as the object that will give him a cookie. Autistic children are unable to control their behaviors appropriately, have poor reality testing, and need constant supervision.

Diagnosis

The diagnosis of infantile autism is difficult at best, especially because diagnosticians still disagree on which criteria should be used. The DSM III criteria are currently the most widely used for clinical practice. Autism is a developmental disorder diagnosed early in childhood, which means that the clinical picture can change as the child develops. Any child with features resembling those of autism can present with various combinations of symptoms that are difficult to sort out, adding to the diagnostic dilemma.

Other childhood disorders can be confused with pervasive developmental disorder. Children who are mentally retarded can present similar behavioral abnormalities but are very responsive to nurturing. Children who become schizophrenic also display some of the behavioral mannerisms seen in pervasive developmental disorders but have an initial period of normal development. Therefore, schizophrenia has a later onset and typically involves hallucinations, delusions, and loose associations, which are not present in pervasive developmental disorders. Blindness, hearing disorders, and speech and language disorders also must be ruled out in the process of differential diagnosis.

In childhood pervasive developmental disorder, the full syndrome of infantile autism is not present, and the age of onset is after 30 months and before 12 years of age. These children have demonstrated a period of normal development and a more appropriate use of language. They do begin, however, to demonstrate impairments in social relationships (such as inappropriate clinging or asocial behaviors). They might become excessively anxious, self-mutilating, and resistant to changes; they tend to show inappropriate affect, strange motor movements, a hypersensitivity or hyposensitivity to sensory stimuli, and speech abnormalities. Hallucinations and delusions are not evident; but the child frequently has bizzare ideas and fantasies or is preoccupied with morbid thoughts or interests.

Treatment

Such a complicated diagnosis requires a multidisciplinary approach. The disciplines usually involved in the treatment of infantile autism are audiology, speech and language, neurology, psychology, psychiatry, social work, pediatrics, and nursing. The staff nurse in an inpatient unit or a residential treatment setting or a master's-degree-level child psychiatric nurse is most likely to be a part of the diagnostic process, but child health nurses or nurse practitioners also might be members of multidisciplinary teams. Nurses have valuable information to contribute from observations made in public health, hospital, physician office, or school settings.

No "cure" has been found for infantile autism. In treating the child with infantile autism, Morgan (1981) stated, "You have to start with the basic elements of human responsiveness and try to gradually incorporate those into the child's behavioral repertoire . . . you have to build the person." A wide range of treatment modalities have been proposed, implemented, and researched. These include psychologic, behavioral, educational, and biochemical models, although current emphasis is on behavioral and educational treatment. The current thrust also is to involve parents in working with autistic children, a change from the previous tendency to blame and accuse parents for their children's problems and exclude them from direct treatment. Even though there is no cure, much can be done to help the child and family.

The prognosis for most autistic children is poor. Lotter (1978) reviewed all follow-up studies on autistic children and found that only 5%–17% achieve near-normal social development and satisfactory school and work performance and that 61%–74% are incapable of leading any kind of independent life. The best prognosis is for children with language development and near-normal IQs and for those whose initial symptoms are less severe. Early placement in educational programs increases the chances for a better outcome. The indications are that autistic children who can play appropriately with toys by around 5 years of age will do better and that those who have seizures and other signs of neurologic dysfunction will most likely have a poorer outcome. Whatever the initial symptoms and testing results might indicate, each child should be given the best possible treatment available to ensure optimal mental health.

Autistic children do grow up to become adolescents and adults. The problems they present at each developmental stage depend on the progress they have made to that point. In the past if no good developmental history were available, these children frequently were labeled as mentally retarded or schizophrenic. Today, with longitudinal follow-up studies of autistic children into adolescence and adulthood, there is more information available about the special needs and the appropriate interventions for this population (Schopler and Mesibov, 1983).

Nursing Management

Child health nurses are not involved in the intensive, extensive psychologic treatment of the autistic child and the child's family. The child health nurse might, however, encounter a child with autism in an acute care setting. Working with an autistic child presents many challenges to the nurse. The nurse needs a basic understanding of the autistic child's world.

When an autistic child is admitted to a pediatric unit, a comprehensive history is needed from the parent. This helps the nurse adhere to the child's routine as much as possible. The parent should be encouraged to bring familiar toys and to stay with the child. Stimulation should be kept to a minimum, and unfamiliar sounds and activities and routines should be labeled or explained in simple terms to the child.

Effective nursing interventions are facilitated by providing a safe, secure, consistent environment in which the autistic child can learn to trust. Interventions might include setting limits on behavior and providing appropriate alternatives while attempting to understand the reason for the child's behavior.

The autistic child does not respond to nurturing as other children do, and caring for these children usually provides little gratification. Many other feelings might be aroused in the nurse caring for these children, whose behaviors can be frustrating and confusing. The nurse needs the opportunity to share, discuss, and work through feelings of frustration, anger, disappointment, sadness, and helplessness, as well as elation when progress is made. The intensive treatment needed for autistic children arouses strong feelings, and continuous awareness and monitoring of feelings and reactions to the child are part of the nurse's interventions. This can be accomplished by one-to-one supervision with the head nurse, peer, or psychiatric clinical nurse specialist, as well as at patient care conferences.

One goal of working with parents is to help them deal with their guilt. In the past parents have been wrongly accused of causing their children's severe emotional problem and have been excluded from care. Even if the cause of autism is primarily organic, the diagnosis is difficult for parents to accept. Nursing interventions therefore focus on active empathetic listening and helping the parents to work through their feelings so that they are better able to help their children. Parents need continued guidance and support to help them deal with the frustrations that arise in dealing with an autistic child. (The psychosocial aspects of chronic childhood conditions are discussed in Chapter 30.)

The nursing care plan in this chapter illustrates interventions for an autistic child who has been admitted to a child psychiatric inpatient unit and also requires nursing care in an acute-care setting.

Schizophrenia in Adolescents

Schizophrenia is a severe psychotic disorder that most often becomes evident in late adolescence or adulthood. *Psychosis* is a term used to describe the condition of a person who is moderately to severely deviant in thought, language, behavior, and social adaptation (Cantor, 1982). Kraeplin (1919) introduced a classification of mental disorders with two major psychoses—manic-depressive psychosis and dementia praecox—and he wrote that similar disorders can develop in early childhood. Bleuler's (1950) description of the disturbance of affect and the concept of autism led to an emphasis on social relations rather than metabolism. Freud further defined schizophrenia as a process beginning in early childhood.

Schizophrenia in children is so rare that the child health nurse is unlikely to come in contact with such a child. The nurse is more likely to encounter an adolescent with schizophrenia who has been hospitalized for a pediatric condition. Adolescents who demonstrate a range of bizarre behaviors tend to tax the resources of the nursing staff just as they tax the resources of their parents and teachers.

Bleuler (1950) described three primary symptoms of schizophrenia: a disturbance of association, a disturbance of affect, and a disturbance of activity. He also described detachment from reality that resulted in autism and ambivalence. Bleuler's system is referred as to the four As. Bleuler derived the name of the disease from the concept of splitting of the person from reality. *Schizophrenia* is a term that means splitting of the mind.

The DSM III has a category for schizophrenic disorders, which is used for both adolescents and adults; occasionally, a younger child also meets these criteria. According to the DSM III, the essential features of a schizophrenic disorder are (1) the presence of psychotic features during an active phase of the illness; (2) characteristic symptoms involving multiple psychologic processes; (3) deterioration from a previous level of functioning; (4) onset before 45 years of age; and (5) duration of at least 6 months. Because schizophrenic disorders always involve delusions, hallucinations, or certain disturbances in the order of thoughts, family members and friends often describe the person in such words as "he just is not the same." Kaplan, Freedman, and Sadock (1980) provided an extensive discussion of this disorder.

Much has been written describing psychosis in children, using such labels as infantile psychosis, atypical development, symbiotic psychosis, and childhood schizophrenia. These categories are not used by the DSM III, but disorders involving delusions, hallucinations, and affective disorders are differentiated into the following three categories:

1. Affective disorders with psychotic features
2. Schizophrenic disorders
3. Schizoaffective disorders

Schizoaffective disorders are not well defined for adults or children, and in general, the DSM III classification of psychotic disorders in children often is criticized (Cantor, 1982).

Etiology and Incidence

The incidence of psychotic disorders in children is difficult to estimate because of the inconsistency of diagnostic measures. Studies agree that the disorder is rare, occurring in fewer than 1 out of every 1000 children (Werry, 1979). Psychosis in children is rare compared with adults (Achenbach, 1982). Males are more likely to develop schizophrenia prior to puberty, but the disorder is equally common in both sexes in adults. Schizophrenia is diagnosed more frequently in lower socioeconomic groups.

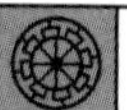

CASE STUDY Schizophrenic Adolescent

Assessment

Anna is a 14-year-old female transferred to a pediatric unit from a child psychiatry inpatient unit for treatment of infectious hepatitis.

Family

Anna's parents were both born in Mexico but came to the United States as adolescents and married and had their children here. Anna has two younger siblings who are functioning well. Several family members in the extended family have serious psychiatric problems, and the family therefore was quite tolerant of Anna's bizarre behavior. The mother is a housewife, and the father is a machinist. Anna reported that there are fights in the family. Anna was disciplined with a belt until 11 years of age. Her father continues to threaten this form of punishment but does not use it.

Child

Anna has been hospitalized for several weeks following her first psychotic episode. This was her first psychiatric hospitalization. Prior to her hospitalization, she was managed at home and in a therapeutic day school. Anna was placed in the school at 11 years of age because of severe social isolation and some bizarre behavior. At that time, Anna was diagnosed as having a possible schizoid disorder of childhood.

During the evaluation, Anna had a vacant stare and rarely smiled. Her motor activity was limited, and she sat on a chair with her arms around her knees. Her speech was slow and hesitant. She responded to questions in either a slow or hesitant manner or not at all. Her voice was soft. At times, Anna giggled to herself. She avoided eye contact and tended to look over the heads of the people who attempted to interact with her.

Anna had no friends on the child psychiatry unit and did not initiate any contact with her peers. Anna does not like boys and says they talk behind her back. The classroom teachers on the inpatient unit reported that Anna would suddenly get up and wander out of the classroom. Anna worries about such things as her studies, being in crowds, being hit with the belt, and the weather.

Clinical Data

Anna is tall, thin, and jaundiced, with dark circles under her eyes. She tends to be poorly groomed unless carefully supervised. Her shoulder-length hair was mussed up and hanging in her face. Anna's arms are covered with sores, which she caused by picking at her skin. Anna had menarche at 12 years of age and often worries about her periods, which are irregular.

Anna's inflamed liver was caused by the hepatitis, and her antipsychotic medication consequently was discontinued temporarily. Medically, the hepatitis indicated the need for isolation. Both the necessary isolation and discontinuation of the antipsychotic medication can result in an increase or recurrence of the psychotic symptoms and have implications for nursing interventions.

Nursing Diagnosis

1. Alteration in thought processes related to discontinuation of antipsychotic medication and the enforced isolation.

Plan for Interventions

Goals

1. Anna will become oriented to her surroundings.
2. Anna will understand that the isolation and medical procedures are not punishment.
3. Anna will not be overwhelmed by stimuli in the environment.
4. Anna will remain safe in her environment.

Interventions

1. Provide Anna with frequent data to orient her (such as a calendar, clock, references to time and place, the reason for her hospitalization, and introducing the staff to her).
2. Set up a structured routine for Anna's day. A chart of the routine could be drawn, with clocks and pictures representing the activities.
3. Discuss Anna's typical daily routine with the parents or staff from the psychiatric unit.
4. Explain repeatedly the reason for the physical isolation in a simple manner.
5. Keep painful and invasive procedures to a minimum.
6. Explain each procedure clearly and simply.
7. Keep communication direct, concrete, and simple.
8. Avoid the use of jokes and puns commonly used with children.
9. Provide a minimum of changes in nursing staff (that is, provide a nursing model for each shift).
10. Avoid the unnecessary use of stimuli (such as intercoms or whispering between staff in Anna's room).
11. Perform procedures in a consistent manner.
12. Facilitate contact with Anna's therapist or primary nurse from the psychiatric inpatient unit (that is, scheduling procedures during the visit).
13. Note and record disturbances in Anna's thought processes.
14. Supervise Anna frequently.
15. Remove dangerous materials from Anna's room.

The study of schizophrenia has generated volumes of literature and multiple research studies (Wohlman, 1972). Genetic research has demonstrated a biologically inherited pattern of schizophrenia (Kallmann, 1962), but questions about the pattern and nature of the inheritance still remain. Biochemical researchers have explored the contribution of such factors as vitamin and mineral deficiencies, cerebral circulation, encodrine function, levels of protein in cerebrospinal fluid, lag in embryonic maturation, energy metabolism, and sensory and response disorders (Wohlman, 1972). The findings in each of these areas are typically divergent. Somatopsychologic theorists also have considered biochemical deficits as a cause or consequence of schizophrenia.

Many patterns of family interactions have been identified with schizophrenia. It is difficult, however, to determine whether the family patterns or the condition developed first. In the 1940s and 1950s, researchers blamed mothers of schizophrenic individuals as "immature, narcissistic, overintellectual, and incapable of mature relationships" (Rank, 1949). The contribution of the family to schizophrenia is a controversial issue. The family as a primary pathologic agent has been proposed by Bateson and colleagues (1956), Lidz, Fleck, and Cornelison (1965), and Wynne and Singer (1963).

Life crises do not appear to be more common in persons with schizophrenia, although the timing of crises (for example, early parental death) might influence the timing of schizophrenic episodes (Rabkin, 1980).

Signs and Symptoms

Because schizophrenia is a complex disorder with a variety of severe and bizarre symptoms, it is difficult to diagnose. Cantor (1982) began to specify the developmental variations of this disorder in children and adolescents and has compiled a comprehensive physical description. Researchers have not, however, reached a general consensus regarding these characteristics and variations. Any adolescent with a schizophrenic disorder exhibits only some of the characteristic symptoms.

Both hallucinations and delusions are rare before adolescence. In addition, research has shown little agreement concerning what constitutes a childhood hallucination. Hallucinations typically are defined as "apparent perception of an external object when no such object is present" (Hinsie and Campbell, 1970). Hallucinations in children, however, can be confused with other mental phenomena, such as fantasies, obsessions, imaginary play objects and companions, and dreams. Researchers have tried to distinguish between these processes and hallucinations by describing characteristics of the hallucinations as bizarre and nonvolitional (Rothstein, 1981). Freeman and colleagues (in press) summarized some consistent findings regarding hallucinations and delusions in children.

Schizophrenic children exhibit developmental delays, particularly in speech. Speech might be monotonous, or the child may speak very little. They might have eating and sleeping disturbances, with such behaviors as pickiness, taking prolonged periods to complete meals, and wandering around during the night. Mannerisms include activities such as pacing, rocking, and head banging. Adolescents might be agitated or lethargic or awkward in gross motor activities. They might grimace or have a distorted facial expression, especially when concentrating on a difficult task. Regression often is observed in adolescents with schizophrenia. They might, for example, be poorly groomed or oblivious to their appearance.

In schizophrenic adolescents social relationships are severely impaired, and the schizophrenic adolescent is socially withdrawn (that is, avoids eye contact, might talk very little, and relates slowly). Adolescents often seem to focus their attention on a limited number of objects and rituals, which leaves very little energy for relating to others. The bizarre behavior of a schizophrenic adolescent also tends to make others uneasy. For instance, the adolescent might respond to requests by doing the opposite of what was requested or may appear perplexed or puzzled by any interaction.

The schizophrenic adolescent has a fragile identity and might fluctuate between grandiosity, overvaluation of the self, and an impoverished self-esteem. Ego boundaries, or the ability to distinguish self from others, is impaired. Affect might be blunted or inappropriate. An adolescent with blunted affect has a constricted range of feelings or is unable to express degrees of feelings. An adolescent with inappropriate affect expresses feelings that are inconsistent with the message expressed. Schizophrenic adolescents might be highly anxious, extremely fearful, or hypersensitive. They have difficulty regulating intense emotions. They are upset easily, and as a result, both nurses and parents find it difficult to anticipate when they might lose control (Cantor, 1982).

Autism in schizophrenic adolescents refers to "preoccupation with internal stimuli and subjective wishes" (Cantor, 1982). The adolescent with schizophrenia might exhibit a variety of thought disturbances, with hallucinations being the most characteristic symptom. Schizophrenic adolescents might talk to themselves or exhibit signs of paranoia. They might exhibit concrete thinking or the tendency to insist on literal and specific meanings of words, ideas, and feelings. Reality testing typically is impaired, so that schizophrenic adolescents lack the ability to evaluate what is occurring around them.

Twelve-year-old Doris, for example, described hearing the voice of her mother calling her name and yelling at her, although her mother was not present. At times, she heard her own voice telling her to do things such as chores for her mother. She experienced her mother's voice as coming from outside her head and her own voice as coming from inside her head. She reported seeing women who looked like her mother and she thought that they were her mother. She also believed that her mother was watching her. Doris described going to the bathroom in the morning and "daydreaming" that objects were weapons (for example, Q-tips were sticks to stab people, and washcloths were used to smother people). All of these experiences seemed real to Doris as they happened.

Doris also believed that the world was coming to an end. She described hearing on the news that a hole was breaking apart pieces of the earth, and she thought this was going to happen. She also expressed concern that a heat wave might result in there not being enough air to breathe.

Diagnosis

The diagnosis of schizophrenia requires an extensive multidisciplinary diagnostic evaluation with a child psychiatrist, child psychologist, and clinical nurse specialist. The evaluation includes clinical interviews and observations with the child, parent interviews, and psychologic testing. Psychologic testing is needed to rule out mental retardation because retarded children can demonstrate some of the same behaviors as psychotic children. The diagnostic team must consider the developmental aspects of the symptoms.

A complete pediatric and neurologic evaluation is indicated to rule out an organic process or drug intoxication. For example, an $8\frac{1}{2}$-year-old female was described by her teachers as being withdrawn and quiet. She had a flat affect and poor self-esteem. At home she was argumentative, dependent, unmotivated, and aggressive. The child psychiatrist who was evaluating her began to suspect there was an underlying organic process and referred her for a neurologic evaluation. A petit mal seizure disorder was diagnosed. The child began a regimen of anticonvulsant medication and her behavior improved considerably.

Two childhood disorders, avoidant disorder and schizoid disorder, might resemble the impaired social functioning of schizophrenia although these conditions are much less severe. Children with avoidant disorder of childhood or adolescence demonstrate excessive shrinking from contact with strangers, to the extent that their avoidance interferes with social functioning. These children do desire acceptance and affection, however, and have warm and satisfying relationships with their family and other familiar persons, unlike the child with schizophrenia. Children with schizoid disorder have no peer relationships and show no interest in their peers or peer and social activities. Both disorders are uncommon, and children with these conditions do not have the psychotic symptoms that are seen in children with schizophrenic disorders (American Psychiatric Association, 1980).

Some children have psychotic episodes that are brief and follow a significant psychologic stress. These disorders might qualify as schizophreniform disorder or brief reactive psychosis (American Psychiatric Association, 1980). Manic episodes can be confused with psychotic episodes. A differential diagnosis is important because the treatment of the two episodes is different.

Schizophrenic disorder is distinguished from pervasive developmental disorder by the presence of delusions, hallucinations, loosening of associations, and incoherence. Some clinicians use childhood-onset pervasive developmental disorder as a diagnosis for children who would have been labeled as schizophrenic prior to the DSM III.

Treatment

The schizophrenic adolescent is likely to require simultaneous treatment modalities or a series of modalities. Education is a key component of the treatment program for the child with schizophrenia. The therapeutic program focuses on activities of daily living, socialization, community activities, and parental education and counseling (Achenbach, 1982). Educational settings include therapeutic nurseries and day schools and classrooms for emotionally disturbed children in public schools. These children tend to do better clinically if they live at home, but the variables influencing the prognosis of each child and family have to be considered individually. Even children who remain at home might need to be hospitalized in inpatient units during acute episodes.

A carefully controlled environment that includes consistent relationships with staff is part of both inpatient and residential treatment programs. A controlled environment, or *milieu therapy*, typically is used in conjunction with therapies based on a specific theoretic framework. For example, psychodynamically oriented programs provide intense relationships to help the child deal with inner conflicts. Behavioral programs include such techniques as token economy systems, isolation, and modeling appropriate behavior.

Psychopharmacology in the treatment of psychotic children is limited because few controlled studies have been done on the effect of major tranquilizers on children (Campbell, et al., 1978). The psychopharmacologic treatment of the psychotic adolescent is similar to that used with adults.

Parents need ongoing counseling to deal with their feelings toward their children, understand their children's behavior and development, and plan management at home. Parents can be trained in behavioral management and assisted to develop a behavioral program for the home. Parents can be helped to assess and build on their children's strengths.

Adolescence presents special problems for parents and professionals (Cantor, 1982). Some clinicians believe individual psychotherapy should not be initiated during adolescence because the anxiety associated with puberty will make it difficult to initiate a therapeutic relationship. Parents need to avoid pressuring the adolescent for high achievement. Adolescents should be prepared for physical changes in puberty to avoid behavioral regression caused by anxiety over these changes.

The adolescent might need protection or support in dealing with the insensitivity of peers. For example, peers might misinterpret the schizophrenic problems as retardation and taunt the adolescent with names such as "retard." The adolescent might be helped to achieve a skill that will gain positive attention from peers. Schizophrenic adolescents might project negative feelings about themselves onto others or attempt to hurt others. For example, the parents of a 16-year-old schizophrenic boy sought treatment after their son had a burst of rage. The mother asked her son to do the dishes. The son, without any anticipatory indication, jumped at his mother and attacked her. He scratched her and yelled at her not to tell him what to do. He had never acted like this prior to this occasion. As adolescents grow older, interventions are geared toward group, community, and work activities.

Nursing Management

Consistency and structure are key elements in the care of the schizophrenic adolescent. It is not the responsibility of the child health nurse to interpret psychotic symptoms. Documentation of observations of symptoms by the nursing staff is, however, invaluable.

Schizophrenic adolescents tend to isolate themselves and when hospitalized for treatment of a medical condition may be further isolated because of it. The nurse might have to be persistent and somewhat intrusive to make contact with the child. This might be difficult for nurses who have been taught to respect another person's space (Scharer, 1983).

In addition, children with major psychiatric disorders are more vulnerable to life stresses. The stress of the illness could precipitate an acute episode of psychosis. Most child health nurses have never seen children in acute psychotic episodes. These children are management problems even in an inpatient psychiatric unit and are considered intensive psychiatric care patients. In the event that an acute psychotic episode occurs, the child's care on the pediatric unit should be carefully planned and managed through the collaboration of the pediatric and psychiatric nursing staff. Parents must be prepared and supported if the child regresses.

Childhood Depression

Childhood depression has become a popular topic in professional and lay literature in the 1980s because both professional and lay people are concerned about the increasing suicide rate in children and adolescents. Suicide is the third leading cause of death for American adolescents. Because most children and adolescents who are suicidal are also depressed, depression must be considered a major mental health problem of youth. Parents and professionals are now recognizing that children do get depressed in ways that are not normal developmental phenomena. Clinical work and research in the field of childhood depression, however, are far behind the work in adult depression, which was spurred on by findings in psychobiology and psychopharmacology. Psychiatric nurses need to become knowledgeable in this field and develop their roles in diagnosing and treating childhood depression. As members of interdisciplinary health care teams, child health nurses also might encounter children with undiagnosed depression in hospital and outpatient settings. These children might be receiving treatment for unrelated problems.

Childhood depression might be caused by grief. Grief reactions in children are not well understood. A prolonged grief reaction extending beyond 6 months generally is considered pathologic in adults, but the timing of extended grief that should be considered pathologic in children is not defined and might vary across the developmental stages. Children also might rework grief reactions when they enter new developmental stages. Some children with major life changes, such as parental divorce or a move to a new community, fail to make transitions within a reasonable amount of time. In addition to difficulties in adjustment (such as not making friends or a decrease in school performance), the child might be sad. These situations, however, usually are not viewed as primary depression because the sadness is secondary to adjustment problems.

Depression is an affective disorder. Under the DSM III classification, affective disorders are defined as mood disorders; the DSM III defines mood as "pronounced emotion that colors the whole psychiatric life and generally involves either depression or elation" (American Psychiatric Association, 1980). Affective disorders are divided into several categories (Table 25-3). The distinctions are basically between depressions and manic disorders and the major and minor disorders.

The DSM III classification system uses the same criteria for both adults and children and does not describe specific affective disorders in children. Child psychiatric clinicians and researchers are beginning to describe differences in children (Freeman, 1983) and are proposing alternative methods of classification (Poznanski, et al., in press).

The most common type of depression seen by the child health nurse is *secondary depression,* or reactive depression. This is the sadness that occurs in response to a particular situation or event. The situations include the trauma of hospitalization, surgery, or separation from a family event. Children might become depressed secondary to medical diseases, such as diabetes mellitus, asthma, and cardiac anomalies, or cognitive and behavioral problems. Children with learning disabilities frequently become depressed because of their frustration with school, particularly if the disorder is not recognized or special academic assistance is not provided. Depression that is not a response to the stress of an event is termed *primary depression.* Primary depres-

TABLE 25-3 Classification of Affective Disorders

Affective disorders	Examples
Bipolar disorders (mania)	Elevated mood and hyperactivity
Major depressions	
Major depression	Severe sadness or loss of pleasure
Depression with psychotic features	Depression with gross impairment in reality testing
Major depression with melancholia	Depression with biologic features
Other affective disorders	Minor disorders
Dysthymic disorder	Pattern of episodes of minor depressions
Cyclothymic disorder	Pattern of episodes of minor depressions and episodes of hypomania (mild manic symptoms)

SOURCE: Adapted from the American Psychiatric Association: *Diagnostic and Statistical Manual of Mental Disorders*. 3rd ed. American Psychiatric Association, 1980.

sion is a depressive syndrome with identifiable symptoms; its etiology, however, is not clearly understood.

An important distinction is the difference between the child who has depressive feelings and the child who has a depressive syndrome. Many children feel sad at some point during a day, but the sadness does not last all day or for several days. For example, in an interview with a nurse clinician, one 10-year-old girl described feeling sad but said that the sadness went away when she talked to her mother or when she woke up the next day. Unlike this child, depressed children have sad feelings that persist for 1–4 weeks. One depressed child reported to the nurse clinician that she could not remember the last time she felt happy or had a good time.

Etiology

Depression in children was first described in the 1920s and 1930s as infantile depression related to maternal deprivation. Researchers described a lack of responsiveness and difficulty forming attachments in children who had been separated from their parents (Levy, 1937). Spitz (1946) described anaclitic depression as a psychiatric syndrome rather than marasmus, or "wasting disease," which was the label given earlier to it by pediatricians. Depression occurred in infants who had satisfactory relationships with their mothers, and who, when separated, became weepy, sad, apathetic, distant, and inactive with poor appetites and sleep patterns. This syndrome also was referred to as "hospitalism" because children with these symptoms typically were seen in hospitals and institutions. This early work, which defined physical separation as deprivation, has been criticized because it is not universal and because intervening variables have not been acknowledged (Malmquist, 1972). (Separation anxiety and other reactions to hospitalization are discussed in Chapter 27.)

Psychodynamic theorists focused on the notion of early trauma that leaves the child vulnerable to depression as an adult. Some psychodynamic theorists claimed that children did not become depressed because depression was a phenomenon of the superego and the child's superego was not completely developed. Psychodynamic theories of depression in children were dominant for many decades, but theorists with other orientations also have contributed to the understanding of depression in children.

In the 1960s a group of clinicians developed the concept of depressive equivalents in children, suggesting that dysfunctional behaviors (such as enuresis, conduct disorders, aggressive behavior, phobias, and academic underachievement) emerged and masked depressive affect (Toolan, 1962). Poznanski and Zrull (1970) began describing overt and unmasked depression in children. The controversy over depression in prepubertal children continued throughout the 1970s, and the major view was that depression as a disorder did not exist. The syndrome is becoming more widely accepted in the 1980s, but it continues to be underrecognized, underdiagnosed, and untreated in a large proportion of prepubertal children who are depressed. Depression in adolescents is more widely accepted and more frequently diagnosed because it more closely resembles depression in adults.

No one biologic or genetic factor has been identified as a sole determinant of an affective disorder. Any factor or accumulation or interaction of factors might predispose a child to an affective disorder. So far, little work in this field has fully described the interaction among genetic–biologic and sociologic–psychiatric factors. Preliminary studies of the family histories of depressed children appear to show trends similar to those uncovered in adult studies. A higher incidence of affective disorders is found in the relatives of depressed children than is expected for a normal population (Grossman, et al., 1984).

Theories describing depression tend to define individuals outside their family and cultural systems. Furthermore, almost no research has examined the relationship of depression to developmental levels. Research on depression and families relates the incidence of depression to such factors as loss of a parent (Hill and Price, 1967), birth order (Grosz, 1968), age of the parents when the child is born (Dennehy, 1966), and family characteristics such as discipline (Ferranto, 1966).

Models for depression in families have not incorporated interaction as an essential factor (Akiskal and McKinney, 1975). Many theorists have tended to view the depressed individual as a closed system rather than to consider the effects of the depressed person's behavior on the family (Coyne, 1967). Although some theorists have developed systems approaches to depression, these have not been well integrated into research and clinical programs.

Some clinicians and researchers in affective disorders are interested in the relationship of psychosocial factors and depression. Durkheim (1951) first hypothesized that the more isolated a person is, the greater the danger that the person will commit suicide. Crisis theory, which developed in the 1960s, focused on the role of support systems in determining a person's vulnerability to crisis.

A child's support systems might be limited by the parent. Adequate support systems might not be available to the parent or the parent might not perceive the supports that are available. This occurs freqently in families where a parent is depressed. Some families operate as a closed system, limiting the opportunities for the family members to use external support systems. Some families who typically are open become closed systems in crises and operate under the myth that they should "do it themselves." Both situations sharply curtail the use of external resources (Grossman, Constantine, and Poznanski, 1981).

Depressed children and adolescents often are able to identify some of the causes of their depression. When asked about what makes them worry or feel sad, they bring up family problems, school problems, and lack of friendships. Although all known biopsychosocial factors should be identified, attention always should be given to what the child and adolescent identifies as distressing. A nursing perspective on depression must consider depression in youth as an interaction of biopsychosocial factors.

TABLE 25-4 Symptoms of Depression in Children

Type of symptom	Example
Mood	Depressed feelings (verbal) Depressed feelings (nonverbal) Irritability Weeping
Somatic symptoms	Appetite—increase or decrease Sleep—initial, middle, or terminal disturbance Excessive fatigue Psychomotor retardation—slow activity and/or tempo of speech Physical complaints (nonorganic)
Subjective symptoms	Decreased self-esteem Guilt Morbid ideation Suicidal ideation
Behavior	Anhedonia Social withdrawal Schoolwork impairment

SOURCE: Adapted from Poznanski, E, et al: Diagnostic criteria in childhood depression. *Arch Gen Psychiatry* (in press).

Signs and Symptoms

Children differ from adults in the biologic, developmental, and cognitive manifestations of depression, although depressive symptoms in adolescents are similar to depressive symptoms in adults.

Freeman (1983) described the differences in depression between children and adults, but little has been published on the developmental aspects of the clinical manifestations of childhood depression. The possibility of a depressive syndrome in infancy is beginning to be explored by a few researchers. The symptoms of depression in children are summarized in Table 25-4.

Depressed children exhibit depressed affect, or *dysphoria,* which generally lasts a minimum of 1–4 weeks. Poznanski (1982) described nonverbal signs of sadness such as fleeting smiles and a bland, frozen look. Even the most experienced nurses might be unable to identify sadness in the face of a child because they may be looking for characteristic adult features. Poznanski also distinguished between verbal and nonverbal sadness, because children might appear sad but verbally deny these feelings. Children use a variety of terms such as bad, gloomy, blue, empty, and not being able to stand it (Puig-Antich and Chambers, 1980) to describe sad feelings, and the nurse therefore needs to listen carefully to the child's description.

Anhedonia, or the inability to enjoy oneself or to have fun, is the most characteristic symptom of depression in children. Play is a primary experience in a child's day. Children who are questioned about their activities typically report several activities, whereas a depressed child might have difficulty thinking of something enjoyable. One depressed child, for example, spent many hours watching television but could not remember what he had watched. Children occasionally experience boredom, but a child who reports being bored 50%–90% of the time is probably anhedonic.

By middle childhood, children with a positive self-concept can describe their appearance, schoolwork, and friendships positively. A child with a poor self-concept is more likely to describe personal characteristics negatively and report the use of derogatory nicknames by other children as if they were accurate.

Social withdrawal is also characteristic of depressed children but must be distinguished from a child who has never developed good peer relationships. Many depressed children had good peer relationships at one time but now report that, "I have no friends" or "The kids don't like me." The withdrawn child might reject opportunities to play with other children or watch other children play.

Schoolwork often is impaired when a child is depressed, even though the child might previously have done well in school. The impaired schoolwork might be the result of the general apathy, an inability to concentrate, or distraction by internal stimuli.

Children who are depressed often are preoccupied with morbid thoughts, which typically are about themselves or others dying. For example, one child drew himself in a family drawing as if he were thinking of his grandmother who had died 2 years earlier. Suicidal thoughts, plans, or actions also are reported by depressed children. One 7-year-old girl tried to jump out of a car on a busy expressway. Her mother also had been depressed and suicidal following the imprisonment of the child's father, who had committed several violent crimes. Professionals and parents must acknowledge that children do think about and try to kill themselves. Nurses need to be aware of the factors that place children at risk for suicide, including the following:

1. Drug and alcohol abuse
2. Depression with prolonged helplessness
3. Conduct disorders, especially impulsive behavior
4. Emerging psychosis
5. Losses (particularly close peers with adolescents and dependency relationships with children)

Associated symptoms of depression include irritability, weeping, and somatic complaints. Irritable children are those who are easily bothered by the smallest event. Some depressed children cry more than their peers, feel like crying frequently, or appear to be about to cry. Depressed children might complain of minor aches and pains that have no organic cause.

Occasionally, a depressed child will have some symptoms of mania. Manic symptoms are difficult to diagnose in children, although in adolescents the symptoms resemble adult symptoms. Puig-Antich and Chambers (1980) identified the following manic symptoms in children:

1. *Elation*—feeling very good, cheerful, high, or terrific, feeling on top of the world.
2. *Decreased need for sleep*—needing less sleep than usual.
3. *Unusual energy*—nonstop activity, having more energy than usual.
4. *Increase in goal-directed activity*—more activity or involvement in more things than usual.

Diagnosis

The diagnosis of depression in children typically is made on the basis of an extensive psychiatric evaluation of both the child and parent. The essential feature of this evaluation is that the child is seen over a 1- to 3-week period so that the persistence of depressive affect can be evaluated. Ideally, the evaluation includes interviews with the child and parent, psychologic testing, a family psychiatric history, and reports from the school and pediatrician (Poznanski, et al., 1983). Multiple sources of data are considered, including the child, parent, and teacher. Children tend to be more accurate reporters of some symptoms, whereas parents more accurately report other symptoms. Clinical evaluations document not only the presence but also the severity of the depression (that is, mild, moderate, or severe).

Several physical disorders must be differentiated from mood disorders; therefore, the child must have a pediatric evaluation to rule out illness or disease. Children who have depressions associated with other life-threatening or incapacitating illnesses might have a major depression, but their depression is considered secondary to the illness or disease. Children with central nervous system disorders are not diagnosed as having a major depression because mood changes can be a secondary effect of structural changes in the neurologic system.

Affective disorders can coexist with other forms of child psychopathology (such as conduct disorders, attention deficits, or separation anxiety). Depression is difficult to diagnose in children with mental retardation because these children tend to be emotionally labile. Children who are schizophrenic might have considerable depressive symptoms, but the differential diagnosis is based on the predominant symptoms, family history of affective disorders, and the child's premorbid functioning. Children with schizophrenic episodes tend to exhibit a more chronic course than depressed children.

Treatment

The treatment of depression in children should always be preceded by a comprehensive diagnostic evaluation and thorough discussion of the disorder with the parent. Depression does not have the stigma of some other childhood psychotic disorders such as autism and schizophrenia, and the parent therefore is often able to accept the diagnosis. In fact, parents might suspect the diagnosis because of their own depression or a history of depression in the family.

Currently, the treatment of children with affective disorders tends to be carried out by child psychiatrists because of issues concerning psychopharmacology. Some drugs used to treat depression can cause severe side effects and children need to be monitored closely during any period of pharmacologic therapy for depression. It is recommended frequently that children with a major affective disorder receive individual psychotherapy with a professional who specializes in psychiatric disorders of children (such as the child psychiatrist, child psychiatric nurse, or child psychologist). The focus of treatment is to build a relationship with the child and to provide an opportunity for the child to deal with conflicts and feelings through play and verbalization.

For example, one 7-year-old girl with major depression spent almost 6 months in therapy with a psychiatric nurse. Play therapy stimulated the child to verbalize the violent threats her father had made to her mother, sibling rivalry, acting out in school, deliberate accidents, and role confusion. The nurse then worked with the mother to deal with the boundaries related to the child's role and with school personnel to help them understand the child's behavior in the context of her life situation.

Family or marital therapy might be recommended in conjunction with individual psychotherapy for the child or as the primary method of treatment. This method is indicated when the child's depression appears to be a manifestation of such family dysfunction as child abuse, neglect, intense sibling conflicts, and noninvolvement of a parent. Some psychodynamically oriented clinicians believe that family therapy is contraindicated when a family member is depressed, because the depressed member is thought to be unable to engage in family treatment and to need individual therapy. It has only been recently that clinicians have begun to realize the family's contribution to and maintenance of individual depression.

Social skills training is another approach used with depressed patients. Depressed persons are trained in the social skills they lack to receive more reinforcement from interaction with others (Coyne, 1976). Depressed children also might lack social skills as a result of withdrawal or a chronic disturbance in peer relationships. Inadequate socialization is best managed in a group situation, such as a social skills group, although programs of this type are uncommon.

Children who do not respond to psychotherapy in 2–3 months might be considered for psychopharmacology in conjunction with psychotherapy. The children with affective disorders who are the most likely candidates for medication include the following:

1. Children who are melancholic and therefore severely depressed.
2. Children with psychotic symptoms.
3. Children who are too withdrawn and sad to use psychotherapy.
4. Children who are exhibiting manic symptoms.
5. Children who have a family history of affective disorders, particularly relatives who have responded positively to the medication being considered.

The administration of antidepressants in prepubertal children is controlled by the Federal Drug Administration so that only a small number of physicians may prescribe them. Desipramine typically is administered to children because it is less cardiotoxic than other antidepressants. The dose is weight related, and a strict protocol is indicated to monitor laboratory values, electrocardiographic status, vital signs, and side effects. These medications provide a potential source of overdose, which can be extremely toxic. Suicidal children are at risk for the use of medication. Parent and child education is therefore essential, and a collaborative role for the nurse is indicated. Physicians and nurses need to agree about the nature of this collaborative role.

Children who have psychotic depression might show improvement in their psychotic symptoms following antidepressant treatment, but if the psychotic symptoms persist, the physician might consider the simultaneous use of an antipsychotic medication. On rare occasions, lithium carbonate is used with children who are exhibiting early symptoms of bipolar disorders, although it is more likely to be prescribed for an adolescent. Lithium is an antimanic agent, but controlled studies of lithium in children have not been done. Therefore, little is known about how lithium effects cognition in children, although adults on lithium complain of confusion and concentration problems (Judd, et al., 1977). Lithium treatment also can result in serious metabolic and endocrine side effects, which might be even more serious in children. Establishing baseline laboratory data and continuous monitoring are therefore part of care.

Hospitalization might be indicated for depressed children with psychotic symptoms or children who require psychopharmacologic treatment. Hospitalization for the child who is exhibiting suicidal ideation is critical to the child's safety. In the event that parents do not agree to this plan, suicide precautions should be planned for the home (such as constant supervision and the removal of medicines). Nurses have a role in facilitating the implementation of a suicide prevention plan in the hospital or home. Most pediatric units are not prepared to deal with suicidal preventions, but pediatric and psychiatric nursing collaboration can result in the implementation of a program for the prevention of suicide in a child.

Nursing Management

During a depressed child's hospitalization, it might be appropriate for the child health nurse to be involved in parent education and counseling. This should be done only in collaboration with the child's therapist. Education and counseling can include such areas as development, limit setting, discussion of symptoms, and ways to support the child when the child is feeling sad or bad about self. Parents can be encouraged to seek group activities for their child in the community because many depressed children are socially withdrawn. Depressed children typically are somewhat sedentary. Parents need to be educated about the mild antidepressant effect of exercise because they might tend to excuse the child from physical activities.

Children who have major depression and conduct disorders might become involved in serious delinquency as adolescents and require long-term inpatient hospitalization or residential treatment. The most effective treatment for

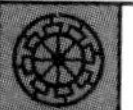

CASE STUDY Suicidal Behavior

Assessment

Ken, $8\frac{1}{2}$ years old, was admitted to the pediatric unit for observation of suicidal behavior and to begin a regimen of antidepressant medication. Ken's parents were resistant to a psychiatric hospitalization, so Ken was admitted to the pediatric unit through the collaborative efforts of the pediatrician and child psychiatrist.

Family

Ken lives with his parents and is their only child. The father has two jobs, and the mother works at a local store. The family is socially isolated, and the majority of their outside contacts are with extended family members. The parents are overprotective of Ken, anxious about his health, and somewhat suspicious of outsiders. The parents are extremely close to Ken.

Two months previously the maternal grandmother, with whom the family was very close, died after a long illness. Ken was frequently at the hospital and at the grandmother's house. Prior to the grandmother's illness, Ken would sleep in the grandmother's bed when he stayed over at her house. The family history revealed a history of alcoholism in the father and a severe grief reaction in the mother. It also was noted that the parents and several extended family members had hypochondriacal traits or psychosomatic illnesses.

Child

Ken's problem began 8 months prior to admission, when he had gone to emergency rooms several times with complaints of severe chest and stomach pains. He also had undergone a complete gastrointestinal and cardiology workup, both of which were negative. A radiologist suggested that the parents seek a child psychiatric evaluation.

Ken was evaluated extensively in an outpatient clinic and was diagnosed as having a major depression and separation anxiety disorder. Ken had no evidence of a developmental disorder but does have a history of asthma. Ken's depression was evident by the child's description of his sadness, sad appearance, inability to have fun, social withdrawal, impaired schoolwork, sleep difficulty, and morbid and suicidal ideation. Ken's depression was accompanied by somatization, a handwashing compulsion, severe anxiety, and refusal to go to school. He was constantly worried that something was happening to his body.

Clinical Data

Physical Assessment Data: Ken is a short, well-developed child. He is well groomed and well dressed, appearing more like a small adult than a child.

Laboratory Data: The premedication baseline laboratory workup was within normal limits. The electrocardiographic results also were normal.

Nursing Diagnosis

1. Alteration in mood related to severe stress (ie, loss).

Plan For Interventions

Goals

1. Ken's physical safety will be maintained.
2. Ken and his parents will understand the use and effects of antidepressant medication (at their cognitive level).
3. Ken will feel more hopeful about his world.

Interventions

1. Provide constant supervision of Ken.
2. Explain precautions to Ken and his parents.
3. Monitor Ken's room for potentially harmful medication.
4. Check Ken's mouth after administering medication.
5. Reinforce family and staff concern for Ken's safety.
6. Encourage Ken to share his wishes, fears, or thoughts about harming himself.
7. Note and record observations such as changes in mood or suicidal behavior.
8. Reinforce the seriousness of Ken's suicidal threats to his parents.
9. Attend the session between the physician and parents when medication is explained.
10. Provide ongoing medication teaching for Ken and his parents, including the name of the medication, reason for taking it, description of what the child can expect, frequency and dosage, list of side effects (including serious and annoying effects), and potential for overdose.
11. Provide support and education for Ken when he receives venipunctures to measure blood levels of antidepressant medication by preparing and educating Ken and his parents, comforting and reassuring Ken during the procedure, and providing play materials and experience to help him master the trauma.
12. Monitor Ken's vital signs daily, including one standing and two sitting blood pressures.
13. Report any abnormal vital signs or signs of illness (ie, dehydration or an elevated temperature can influence metabolism of the medication).
14. Plan for discharge—for example, storage and administration of medication, safety, danger of sudden withdrawal from medication, when and how to report problems and take vital signs. (Explain that plastic boxes are available in pharmacies with compartments for daily doses.)
15. Provide a model for Ken to express his feelings and worries.
16. Offer emphathetic statements about Ken's worries (ie, it must be hard to concentrate in school when you're worried about your mom).
17. Avoid pressuring Ken for verbal performance.
18. Offer activities that the nurse can engage in with Ken (ie, games, storytelling).

continued on next page

CASE STUDY Suicidal Behavior

19. Reinforce Ken's strengths and assets.
20. Note and record changes in Ken's mood (ie, Ken becomes sad when talking about his father).
21. Encourage physical activity within the restrictions of the unit (exercise is a mild antidepressant).
22. Support and encourage Ken's contact with his peers.

children with a mood disorder is generally a treatment plan that involves more than one method of intervention.

School nurses and other nurses in the community need to be aware that any threat of suicide in a child should be taken seriously and appropriate action initiated. The Samaritans are a nationwide group of volunteers specifically trained in suicide prevention. This group maintains local 24-hour telephone hot lines to talk with people who are considering suicide or with families or others who are concerned that a person may be considering suicide.

Conduct Disorders

Children with conduct disorders exhibit repeated and tenacious patterns of conduct that violate the basic rights of others or major age-appropriate societal norms and rules. The acting out that is demonstrated by these children is more than just mischievous pranks. These are the children who can be and often are labeled juvenile delinquents.

Juvenile delinquency is a term used freely to describe a variety of behaviors. Technically, however, it is a legal term applied to individuals under a certain age who violate the laws and ordinances of their communities and come to the attention of the legal system. A large proportion of children, however, exhibit similar behaviors but do not come to the attention of the legal system. They are treated in the mental health system and are more likely to receive psychiatric diagnoses. A third group of children do not come to the attention of either the legal system or the mental health system. They are deceptive, manipulative, and smart enough to avoid being caught, or their conduct disorders are more minor, and their parents or school systems attempt to deal with them.

Precise figures on the prevalence of conduct disorders are therefore unavailable. Statistics are available for children who display acting-out and antisocial behaviors, but these figures vary depending on the definitions used, geographic area studied, and population screened. However, it is clearly evident that conduct disorders are prevalent in modern American society. "Some general population surveys have suggested that 5 to 15 percent of all children show conduct problems serious enough to alarm some adults, although not all of these youngsters fit the diagnostic criteria of DSM III" (Meeks, 1980).

Conduct disorders, according to DSM III, are divided into four categories—undersocialized aggressive, undersocialized nonaggressive, socialized aggressive, and socialized nonaggressive—based on the presence or absence of social bonds and the presence or absence of aggressive antisocial behavior (Table 25-5).

Undersocialized children are unable to develop and maintain any lasting peer relationships and have no close friends. They might associate with much younger or much older children or have superficial relationships with other antisocial children. They use others to meet their own needs but show a lack of concern for others and appropriate feelings of guilt or remorse for their antisocial behaviors. These children will, for example, blame or "tell on" others to get themselves out of difficult situations.

Meeks (1980) described the socialized child as having developed age-appropriate relationships with peers and having close friends. Antisocial behaviors in these children

TABLE 25-5 Four Categories of Conduct Disorders

	Undersocialized	Socialized
Aggressive	Failure to establish social bonds Aggressive antisocial behaviors	Established social bonds Aggressive antisocial behaviors
Nonaggressive	Failure to establish social bonds Nonaggressive antisocial behaviors	Established social bonds Nonaggressive antisocial behaviors

Interventions for Suicidal Behavior in Children and Adolescents: A Guide For Professionals, Parents, and Peers

Step 1: **LISTEN.** A person in a mental crisis needs someone who will listen to what the person is saying. Every effort should be made to understand the problems behind the statements.

Step 2: **EVALUATE THE SERIOUSNESS** of the child's thoughts and feelings. If the child has made clear suicide plans, the problem is more acute than when the child's thinking is less definite.

Step 3: **EVALUATE THE INTENSITY OR SEVERITY OF THE EMOTIONAL DISTURBANCE.** The child might be extremely upset but not suicidal. A person who has been depressed and then becomes agitated and moves about restlessly is a possible cause for alarm.

Step 4: **TAKE SERIOUSLY EVERY COMPLAINT AND FEELING THE CHILD EXPRESSES.** Do not dismiss or undervalue what the child is saying. In some instances the child might minimize the difficulty, but beneath an apparent calm profoundly distressed feelings might be present.

Step 5: **DO NOT BE AFRAID TO ASK DIRECTLY IF THE CHILD HAS ENTERTAINED THOUGHTS OF SUICIDE.** Suicide might be suggested but not openly mentioned during the crisis period. Experience shows that harm is rarely done by inquiring directly about suicide at an appropriate time. As a matter of fact, the child frequently is glad to have the opportunity to open up and discuss it.

Step 6: **DO NOT BE MISLED BY THE CHILD'S SAYING THAT THE EMOTIONAL CRISIS HAS PASSED.** Often, the youth will feel initial relief after talking about suicide, but the same thinking might recur later. Follow-up is crucial.

Step 7: **BE AFFIRMATIVE BUT SUPPORTIVE.** Strong, stable supports are essential in the life of a distressed child. Provide emotional strength by giving the impression that you know what you are doing and that everything possible will be done to assist the child.

Step 8: **EVALUATE AVAILABLE RESOURCES.** The child might have inner resources, including various mechanisms for rationalization and intellectualization, which can be strengthened and supported, and other resources, such as ministers, relatives, and friends, who can be contacted. If these resources are absent, the problem might be more serious.

Step 9: **ACT SPECIFICALLY.** Do something tangible; that is, give the child something definite to hang on to such as arranging to see the child later or subsequently contacting another helpful person. Nothing is more frustrating to a child than to feel that nothing has been gained from the discussion.

Step 10: **OBTAIN APPROPRIATE ASSISTANCE AND CONSULTATION.** Do not try to handle the problem alone. Seek the advice of physicians, school specialists, mental health professionals, or other knowledgeable persons.

This list was prepared by Dr. Calvin Frederick, National Institute of Mental Health, and appears in *Trends in Mental Health: Self-Destructive Behavior Among Younger Age Groups*. US Department of Health, Education, and Welfare. DHEW Publication no (ADM) 76–365. Government Printing Office, 1976.

arise from a need for continued peer acceptance and hunger for excitement, companionship, and purpose. Such children might join delinquent gangs to fill a social vacuum not filled by family or community. The acceptance they get from gang members can help to avoid the pain of their failure according to conventional values.

Antisocial behaviors run the gamut from nonaggressive whining, demanding, or temper tantrums to severe aggressive destructiveness, stealing, and physical violence (Table 25-6). The seriousness of the behavior depends on the age of the child.

Etiology and Incidence

The causes of conduct disorders are multiple and interrelated. Undersocialized children might have suffered from

TABLE 25-6 Degrees of Aggressive Behaviors

Nonaggressive	Mildly aggressive	Moderately aggressive	Severely aggressive
Self-protective and manipulative lying	Bullying	Physical aggression	Serious, repeated physical aggression, mugging, beating, gang fighting
Whining, demanding, temper tantrums	Cruelty toward peers	Reckless driving	
Bed-wetting	Abusive language	Breaking and entering	
Stealing	Vandalism	Extortion	
Truancy		Car theft	

severe parental rejection and unusual frustration of dependency needs, whereas the more socialized children appear to have had emotionally healthier early family experiences, enabling them to develop a greater capacity for empathy, affection, and social skills.

Many variables can contribute to the development of antisocial behaviors. Discipline is usually inconsistent at some point during development; fathers are often absent from the home or are indifferent or abusive; marital problems between parents are common. In some instances one parent has been diagnosed as an antisocial personality or has demonstrated antisocial tendencies. Children with learning disorders or physical deformities also are more vulnerable and at risk for developing conduct disorders.

Sociologically, the increased incidence of conduct disorders might be a result of a changing social system, the affluence of twentieth-century life, and current challenges to traditional moral and ethical values. A weakened religious system and changes in the traditional nuclear family and educational systems all can contribute to "norm erosion." Without continued reinforcement of traditional sanctions and value structures, children today are left with neither strong internal nor external controls to guide them (Reckless and Dinitz, 1972). Poverty, poor living conditions, overcrowding, and lack of family status in a community because of cultural or ethnic differences also might be contributing factors.

Signs and Symptoms

Children who are diagnosed as having a conduct disorder are likely to demonstrate behavior difficulties in school. Girls tend to be less aggressive than boys but are more self-destructive, exhibiting runaway and sexual acting-out behaviors. Both sexes, however, frequently exhibit precocious sexual acting out that is either aggressive or submissive. Drinking, smoking, and other substance abuse is common (see Chapter 24). With the exception of the undersocialized nonaggressive category, which is equally common in both sexes, conduct disorders are more prevalent in boys than girls; the ratios indicating boy to girl incidence range from 4:1 to 12:1.

Most of these children have poor self-concepts. Beyond the negative, defiant, and frequently hostile behaviors, however, the nurse might observe fleeting glimpses of inner vulnerability expressed as self-hatred, depression, and hopelessness. This group of children, however, direct all feelings outward and act out against parents, school, community, and society in general.

Because anger is a normal emotion emerging in childhood, children need opportunities to express anger and to discover that this emotion is not bad and can be expressed in appropriate ways. Given this opportunity, they can develop emotionally healthy responses to frustration and learn effective problem-solving techniques. Many children, however, develop maladaptive ways of managing anger. These children might be taught that expressions of anger at any level are unacceptable, or they may learn to express anger aggressively. They soon learn to repress feelings, only to have them surface later in inappropriate and unhealthy ways, which often are learned by imitating. Social learning theorists suggest that role models teach children to express anger aggressively (Bandura, 1973).

Anger is the outward expression of inner feelings that might result from the accumulation of developmental experiences or a reaction to a particular situation. Dysfunctional expressions of anger can include psychosomatic illness, aggression, and escape into fantasy (Coffman, 1969). Children reacting in angry ways might be feeling helpless, anxious, or frustrated because of blocked goals and unmet needs, or they might be suffering from a loss of self-esteem.

Treatment

The earlier the problems in children with conduct disorders can be detected, the more likely it is that treatment attempts will be successful. Research has identified early indicators or predisposing factors that might show that a child is at risk for developing a conduct disorder and acting out in a delinquent manner (Hirschi, 1969; Glueck and Glueck, 1970, 1972).

Various treatment methods with this group of children have met with varying degrees of success. These methods include individual therapy, group therapy, family therapy,

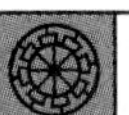

CASE STUDY Conduct Disorder

Assessment

Child History

Seth is a 14-year-old male who lives with his mother and six siblings. His family is poor, and his parents divorced when Seth was 8 years old. Seth's mother says that she is inconsistent in her disciplining of the children because she has to do it all by herself since their father has no contact with them. Seth has been displaying behavior problems since he was 10 years old. His mother feels that some of these problems are due to the peer group with whom Seth associates. She feels that he doesn't listen to her at all and is almost impossible to manage at home.

At school, Seth has been placed in a special education class for adolescents with learning and behavior problems, but he is frequently truant with his best friend. Seth has three close friends he has known since elementary school. On a recent dare from his friends and because he needed money to go to the movies, Seth attempted to steal money from a teacher's purse. He was caught, but the principal reported that he thought Seth felt genuinely sorry for what he had done. Seth told the principal that he had taken money from his mother's purse before so that he could do things with his friends.

Seth had been seen in a neighborhood mental health clinic and was diagnosed as having a socialized nonaggressive conduct disorder. He has been inconsistent in keeping his appointments with his therapist, stating that, "Only sissies talk about their feelings."

Current Behaviors

Seth was admitted to the orthopedic unit of a pediatric hospital by his mother for treatment of a compound fracture of his left tibia. Seth had been struck by a car while riding a go-cart in the street. When the accident occurred, Seth was disregarding stop signs and rolling through intersections yelling at pedestrians to get out of his way. The bone was stabilized with external fixation, and Seth's treatment involved dressing changes and bedrest.

Seth was verbally abusive and refused to cooperate with dressing changes. When approached for a dressing change after the procedure had been explained to him, Seth would begin yelling and calling the nurse names. It took three nurses to hold him still while a fourth changed the dressing. All of the nurses tried to ignore his sexually provocative language and name calling. During one dressing change, Seth spit in the face of a nurse.

The nurses were becoming very frustrated with the situation and angry at Seth. Everyone began to avoid going into his room except to do procedures. A patient care conference was called to develop a plan for dealing with Seth and his behaviors. The child psychiatric clinical nurse specialist was present.

Nursing Diagnoses

1. Ineffective coping related to Seth's anxiety about procedures.
2. Potential for acting out related to perceived loss of control.

Plan For Interventions

Goals

1. Seth will feel less anxious and more in control.
2. Seth will cooperate with dressing change by holding still, not yelling, and not being verbally abusive.

Interventions

1. Anger will be vented at Seth by focusing on the behavior and not on Seth (eg, "It makes me angry when you spit in my face and call me names. I don't want to spend time with you if you are going to do these things").
2. Give Seth some sense of control by negotiating with him, asking him what would be a good time to change his dressing.
3. Explain in detail the procedure of changing dressings to help decrease Seth's anxiety.
4. Communicate expected behaviors to Seth, state the limits firmly, and offer substitute behaviors (eg, "It is time for your dressing change; I expect you to hold still and not yell or call me names or spit. Why don't you yell into your pillow if you must").
5. Explain the consequences of unacceptable behaviors (eg, "If you move, this will hurt more").
6. State the reasons for the limit (eg, "The dressing needs to be changed; otherwise, your leg will become infected and you will become ill and need to stay in the hospital longer").
7. Present Seth with realistic and enforceable consequences if he tests the limits and continues inappropriate behaviors (eg, "Seth, if you do not hold still and it takes more than one nurse to change your dressing or if you yell and call me names, you will not be allowed to watch television until the next dressing change tomorrow").
8. Allow Seth to express his feelings about the limits.
9. Remain consistent about the limits and the consequences when Seth tests them.
10. Attempt to spend time with Seth (especially if his behavior improves). Find ways to give Seth positive reinforcement and attention as opposed to negative reinforcement and isolation.

and behavior modification. Children are treated in outpatient departments, school systems, day hospital programs, inpatient units, residential placements, juvenile detention homes, and the community.

Many prevention programs have been developed (Reckless and Dinitz, 1972). Selected case workers have infiltrated gangs in the hope that they can redirect delinquent acts and work toward changing group norms and values. Teachers have identified children at risk, who have been followed by counselors or placed in special classes. Community programs, such as those conducted by YMCAs and the Boy Scouts, also can be helpful.

The prognosis for undersocialized children is guarded. Treatment is difficult because of the inability of these children to develop trust and emotional attachments. The nonaggressive child is very skilled at manipulation and deception and is timid and socially inept; these children often are referred to as "born losers" and most often end up as sociopathic adults. Aggressive children are provocative, hostile, and defiant. They test the limits of the most caring, understanding, and consistent adults; therefore, they are very difficult to work with and are likely to become antisocial personalities as adults. Socialized children have a relatively favorable prognosis, probably because they are able to develop significant relationships. A large portion of this group might improve spontaneously. Factors facilitating spontaneous improvement might include an academic or athletic achievement, a romantic attachment, or the influence of one or more interested adults. These children also appear to settle down as they assume family responsibilities and secure employment (Meeks, 1980).

Nursing Management

Children with conduct disorders react toward others with anger and provoke anger in those who work with them. Nurses need basic knowledge concerning the developmental aspects of anger in children so that when confronted with an angry, acting-out, antisocial child, the nurse will understand the concept of anger, be aware of personal reactions and expressions of anger, and know the principles for managing these behaviors. Coffman (1969) based a discussion of the developmental aspects of anger on psychodynamic theory and examined expressions of anger in normal development and how these expressions can become dysfunctional and inappropriate.

Whatever the causes of anger, the provocative behaviors are very frustrating and test the limits of the nurse's patience. Nurses need opportunities to work out their own feelings toward these children to ensure that interventions will be appropriate and meet the children's needs. The nurse who deals with personal feelings of anger and frustration is better able to express feelings appropriately, explore the causes of behavior with the child, and present the child with appropriate expectations and limits. A psychiatric clinical nurse specialist can be of assistance in working through these feelings and developing a plan of care to deal effectively with children exhibiting conduct disorders.

Nurses need to be aware of behavior management techniques that will be helpful to them in caring for these children. Effective limit setting, for instance, is a technique all nurses should use in working with children because children need to have limits set on their acting-out or manipulative behaviors. They often are acting out because they are anxious or upset about something, and limits help to foster a sense of security. Children test these limits to check the predictability or safety of their surroundings. For these reasons, it is very important for the entire nursing staff to be consistent when setting limits with a particular child. Even the provocative behaviors of antisocial adolescents are often a plea for someone to show that they care. For example, one adolescent, named Mary, was admitted for a severe asthma attack. Whenever a nurse, doctor, or respiratory therapist entered her room, she began swearing at them; she was rude to all who came in contact with her. Her primary nurse decided to speak to Mary and set limits on her inappropriate behaviors. As the nurse stated firmly that Mary's behaviors were unacceptable, Mary began to cry. The nurse stayed with her as she cried, and Mary eventually was able to talk about her fear of dying.

"Limit setting is a process through which someone in authority determines temporary and artificial ego boundaries for another person. Determining for the patient the boundaries of acceptable behavior provides protection for the patient and others, provides security, decreases the patient's anxiety, and provides a reality contact between the person and his environment. The limit forms a framework within which the person is freer to function more adequately, to learn new behaviors, and is thus able to develop his self-identity and to raise his self-esteem" (Lyon, 1970).

Other behavior modification techniques can be implemented with various acting-out behaviors. Time-out (from positive reinforcement), for example, usually is successful with younger children (see Chapter 13). Behavioral contracting (Stuart, 1972) and other behavior modification techniques, such as the token economy, also can be implemented with the antisocial child; however, the physically aggressive child might need to be restrained. For these children, nurses need to be aware of appropriate techniques for holding and restraining to protect themselves, other persons, and the children from harm.

The child with a conduct disorder presents a challenge on many levels to nurses in various settings. Understanding the causes of these behaviors and how to manage them effectively is invaluable to the nurse in caring for these children and their families.

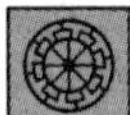

NURSING CARE PLAN An Autistic Child

Assessment Data

Ralph, age 5, is an attractive, blond-haired, blue-eyed child. His weight and height are both at the 50th percentile. He sits in a corner rocking back and forth in his chair or spinning a block with great skill on the table. Ralph carries the block in his pocket wherever he goes. He also is prone to episodes of head banging and similar self-mutilating behaviors. He makes no eye contact, and his only verbalization is a Burger King commercial, which he recites word for word.

Half running, half walking on his toes with his arms flapping out at his sides, Ralph follows his parents to his room to unpack. Ralph was transferred from the child psychiatric inpatient unit to the pediatric unit by his parents and psychiatric nurse. He needs a tonsillectomy, and his psychiatric nurse has developed a plan to ensure continuity of care while he is a pediatric patient.

Ralph's parents have been concerned about his behavior since the first few months of his life and have sought the opinion of multiple physicians. They have, however, just been given a diagnosis of infantile autism. They were shocked and overwhelmed by the magnitude of the diagnosis. After counseling and painful deliberation, they decided that Ralph needed to be admitted to an inpatient facility for further evaluation and treatment.

Ralph has three siblings, 8, 7, and 3 years of age. His father is an architect, and his mother is a housewife. Ralph's parents will try to stay with him as much as possible while he is on the pediatric unit. Staff from the psychiatric unit will come over and help if there are any major problems with Ralph's behaviors.

1. **Nursing diagnosis:** Increased level of anxiety associated with perceived threat to self and resistance to change.

   Long-term goal: Ralph will become acquainted with and feel comfortable in his new environment and realize that changes will not harm him.

   Short-term goals: (a) Ralph will adjust to this new environment with a minimum of anxiety and regressive behaviors (such as head banging, rocking, and extreme withdrawal). (b) Ralph will react to changes with decreased anxiety.

2. **Nursing diagnosis:** Impaired interpersonal relationships associated with difficulty with others intruding into his world.

   Long-term goal: Ralph will develop relationships with significant adults.

   Short-term goals: Ralph will begin to trust and form a significant relationship with at least one adult staff member.

3. **Nursing diagnosis:** Impaired verbal communication associated with developmental delays in perceptual and cognitive abilities.

   Long-term goal: Ralph will increase his language skills.

   Short-term goal: Ralph will be able to use language more appropriately to communicate with others.

4. **Nursing diagnosis:** Disturbance in body image and personal identity associated with inability to perceive self and surroundings appropriately.

   Long-term goal: Ralph will develop an appropriate body image and sense of self separate from others.

   Short-term goals: (a) Ralph will demonstrate a knowledge of body parts. (b) Ralph's bizarre mobility (walking on toes and flapping arms) will decrease.

5. **Nursing diagnosis:** Potential for acting out against self and others associated with a low tolerance for frustration.

   Long-term goal: Ralph will have fewer and shorter tantrums and not hurt himself or others.

   Short-term goals: (a) Ralph's tantrums will decrease in length and frequency. (b) Ralph's self-mutilating (head banging) behaviors will decrease. (c) Ralph will be less aggressive (hitting) with peers.

6. **Nursing diagnosis:** Disturbance in ability to socialize (play) at age-appropriate level associated with need for "sameness" and difficulty processing stimuli.

   Long-term goal: Ralph will develop appropriate play skills to aid him in socializing with his peer group.

   Short-term goals: (a) Ralph will use toys appropriately to play. (b) Ralph will begin to join in play activities with his peers more appropriately.

7. **Nursing diagnosis:** Self-care deficit (Level II); requires help from another person, assistance, supervision, and teaching because of perceptual and cognitive impairments.

   Long-term goal: Ralph will improve his self-care skills.

   Short-term goals: Ralph will learn to perform the basic activities of daily living: dressing, bathing, eating, brushing teeth, and combing hair.

8. **Nursing diagnosis:** Alteration in family coping and potential for growth associated with demands of helping and caring for Ralph.

   Long-term goal: Ralph's family members will develop a better understanding of Ralph's problems and ways to help him.

   Short-term goals: (a) Ralph's family will remain involved in his treatment. (b) Ralph's family will continue to identify the meanings of his behaviors and effective ways to promote Ralph's growth.

continued on next page

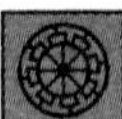

NURSING CARE PLAN continued An Autistic Child

Interventions	Rationale	Evaluation criteria
1. Prepare other children for Ralph's arrival and help them to understand Ralph and his special needs	Ralph will require 1:1 staff time, and other children might become jealous Ralph's behaviors and mannerisms might be disturbing to other children	Did Ralph adjust to the new environment with a minimum of anxiety and regressive behaviors?
Introduce Ralph gradually to new places and routines (see Chapter 29)	The autistic child's anxiety level can be maintained at a lower level if there is less stimulation	Did Ralph demonstrate decreasing amounts of anxiety to changes as he became more familiar with activities and routines?
Observe Ralph's different behaviors and mannerisms. Record the apparent meanings of various behaviors	This information will be useful in working with Ralph in the future. Understanding Ralph's behaviors also will help to decrease his anxiety and foster his growth To evaluate the success of nursing interventions, it will be necessary to obtain baseline information from parents, day-care program, and observations of his first days on the unit regarding the frequency of head banging and extreme withdrawal demonstrated by rocking behaviors. Once a baseline is obtained and a record of these activities is kept, the nurse can determine whether the incidents of regressive behaviors (eg, head banging and rocking) have decreased, indicating a decreased anxiety level	
Observe closely for Ralph's likes and dislikes and strengths and weaknesses. Record the data.	This information will be useful in getting Ralph to cooperate more easily and will decrease his level of anxiety	
Provide care with consistency and structure. Maintain a warm and understanding manner		
Prepare Ralph for all changes in routine, no matter how insignificant they might seem. Let him know what will happen next by using simple sentences; for example, "Ralph, it's time to eat, put the block in your pocket and go wash your hands"	Autistic children are extremely resistant to change and show a genuine lack of understanding	
Take the time to explain new things to Ralph. Allow some time for Ralph to express his frustration. Label his feelings for him; for example, "Ralph is sad (or angry or upset) because he has to stop playing with his block now and get ready to eat"	Autistic children have difficulty understanding and expressing their feelings appropriately	

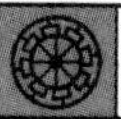 **NURSING CARE PLAN continued An Autistic Child**

Interventions	Rationale	Evaluation criteria
Record Ralph's responses to changes and interruptions in routine	This information will be helpful to others caring for Ralph. In anticipating Ralph's reactions, the nurse can plan interventions that will decrease his anxiety	
2. Give Ralph 1:1 supervision with a consistent staff	A few staff members working consistently with autistic children helps them to develop the trust necessary to form relationships	Did Ralph form at least one significant relationship with an adult?
When speaking with Ralph, have him make eye contact. Gently hold his head so that he is looking at you or request that he look at your nose or eyes	Autistic children need to become aware of people and how to interact with them appropriately	Does Ralph make eye contact when people speak to him?
At times, a staff member may join Ralph in his isolating behaviors (eg, rocking or spinning toys)	Autistic children need to know that people are trying to understand them	
Observe and record Ralph's attempts to reach out to others and how he reacts to others approaching him	This information will be helpful to others in approaching Ralph and in evaluating his progress in interpersonal relationships	
3. Have Ralph spend 30 minutes a day (9:30 to 10:00 A.M.), Monday through Friday, with a speech therapist	Speech therapy will improve Ralph's language skills	Was Ralph able to use language more appropriately to communicate with others?
Obtain baseline information to develop accurate outcome criteria		
Name the objects on the pediatric unit and encourage Ralph to repeat the words	Naming objects will increase Ralph's vocabulary	
Praise Ralph when he is able to ask for something using the correct words	Praise will increase the chances that the autistic child will use the word correctly again	
If Ralph points to an object and clearly wants it, give it to him but name it for him as well	Naming the object will increase Ralph's vocabulary and receiving the object decreases Ralph's level of frustration	
Use simple language and short phrases when speaking with Ralph	Simple language is easier for autistic children to imitate	
If Ralph knows the word for something he wants, expect him to use it	Autistic children need to be aware of expectations for their behavior	
When verbal or nonverbal communication is unclear, point this out to Ralph	Autistic children need to know when their communication is unclear	
Record the words used and context for their use. Note when Ralph tries to make his needs known and note his level of frustration	Records are helpful to others who work with an autistic child and will assist in setting reasonable goals and evaluating interventions	

continued on next page

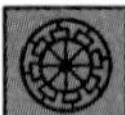

NURSING CARE PLAN continued An Autistic Child

Interventions	Retionale	Evaluation criteria
4. Play touching, feeling games; for example, identify and label body parts on Ralph and on staff members, using statements such as "Ralph, touch Ralph's nose; Ralph, touch Mary's nose; Mary, touch Ralph's nose"	Play helps autistic children become more aware that their bodies are their own and are separate from others	Was Ralph able to demonstrate a sense of self that is separate from others?
When Ralph is walking, remind him to walk "heel-to-toe" and make a game of this. Also remind him to keep his arms at his side	Such reminders help autistic children become more aware of the boundaries of their body and the space around them	Did Ralph's walking on his toes and flapping his arms decrease? Baseline data will be needed here as well
5. Ignore tantrums if possible and respond to Ralph positively when the tantrums stop. Label Ralph's feelings and restate requests	Ignoring tantrums will help to decrease their frequency and number. Labeling feelings helps Ralph to understand them	Have Ralph's tantrums decreased in length and frequency? Refer back to baseline data obtained
Praise Ralph when he follows through alone or with help but without a tantrum	Praise helps to teach autistic children the behavior that is expected of them	
Record the nature of the tantrum, the precipitating issues, and the length of the tantrum	Recorded observations help to determine whether the number and length of tantrums is decreasing	
When Ralph becomes frustrated and begins banging his head or becomes physically aggressive, restrain him physically until he is calm	Physically restraining autistic children protects them and others from harm	Have Ralph's self-mutilating behaviors decreased? Refer to baseline data obtained
Observe Ralph carefully	Self-mutilating behaviors can be subtle, and moods may change quickly	
Briefly and using simple language review with Ralph the reasons for his frustrations. Offer alternatives for his behaviors; for example, suggest that Ralph hit a pillow or say, "Let's tell Jack how that made you feel when he took your block"	Explanations help autistic children to understand their feelings and find ways to express their feelings more appropriately	Is Ralph less aggressive toward peers? Refer to baseline data obtained
6. Introduce one new activity at a time. Initially, Ralph should work one to one with staff to develop play skills. This can be done alone or parallel to a group activity	An autistic child's anxiety level increases if there is too much stimulation	Was Ralph able to play appropriately with toys?
Gradually introduce Ralph to group play activities. Always demonstrate appropriate use of a toy or play activity and take him through the motions	Expectations for Ralph should be raised	Was Ralph able to join in activities with peers appropriately?
Praise Ralph when he demonstrates appropriate play skills	Praise increases the chances that an autistic child will play appropriately in the future	
7. Show Ralph initially what is expected of him. Then expect him to do things such as dressing and washing his hands by himself	Autistic children initially need to be supervised and taught these skills; they also need to learn what is expected of them	Was Ralph able to learn the basic activities of daily living and do them by himself?
Raise expectations as Ralph improves	Raised expectations will lead to further improvement	

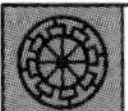

NURSING CARE PLAN continued An Autistic Child

Interventions	Rationale	Evaluation criteria
Allow Ralph enough time to accomplish these tasks	Adequate time decreases an autistic child's frustration level	
Praise Ralph matter-of-factly when he repeats tasks	Praise increases the chances that an autistic child will repeat appropriate behaviors	
8. During visits, demonstrate for Ralph's family techniques that succeed in modifying Ralph's behaviors	Family members will be able to carry on the therapeutic treatment begun on the pediatric unit when Ralph returns home	Did Ralph's family attend weekly family therapy sessions and visit regularly?
Keep Ralph's parents informed of Ralph's progress and aware of his daily activities	Information is helpful in keeping family members from feeling isolated from care and in keeping them involved	
Ralph's family will be involved in family therapy	Therapy will be helpful to family members in gaining insights for themselves and for Ralph so that both Ralph and his family can continue to grow	Did family members demonstrate an increased awareness of Ralph's problems and how to help him?

Key Concepts

- A knowledge of psychiatric symptoms allows the nurse to facilitate psychiatric referrals and intervene to prevent the manifestations of psychiatric disorders.
- Manifestations of psychiatric disorders vary according to the child's developmental stage.
- The etiology of psychiatric disorders is related to both suprasystems and subsystems, principally to biophysical, social and cultural, and family systems, and to the effects of acquired illnesses and injuries.
- The most common classification for psychiatric disorders is the *Diagnostic and Statistical Manual of Mental Disorders,* or DSM III, published by the American Psychiatric Association, which applies a disease model to psychopathology.
- Autism, a syndrome characterized by withdrawal, self-absorption, and unresponsiveness, is a developmental disorder that is difficult to diagnose.
- Nursing care for autistic children involves providing a safe, consistent environment, setting limits on the child's behaviors, and looking for ways to help the child learn.
- Schizophrenia in children is a severe psychotic disorder that involves moderately to severely deviant thought, language, behavior, and social adaptation; children often experience delusions and hallucinations.
- Nursing care for schizophrenic children requires a consistent, structured environment and concrete, direct communication.
- Childhood depression might be primary or secondary; secondary depression is a reaction to events or circumstances, and primary depression is not a response to a particular event or situation.
- Nursing assessment for depressed children involves an analysis of the family system, including family interactions and any family crises.
- Nursing care for depressed children might involve social skills training, family therapy, suicide precautions, and psychopharmacologic therapy.
- Children with conduct disorders exhibit repeated and tenacious patterns of conduct that violate the rights of others or age-appropriate societal or cultural norms.
- Nursing care for children with conduct disorders involves consistent limit setting and teaching appropriate ways to express feelings.

References

Achenbach T: *Developmental Psychopathology*, 2nd ed. Wiley, 1982.

Ackerman NW: The role of the family in the emergence of child disorders. In: *Foundations of Child Psychiatry*. Miller E (editor). Pergamon Press, 1968.

Akiskal H, McKinney W: Overview of recent research in depression. *Arch Gen Psychiatry* 1975; 32(3):285–305.

American Psychiatric Association: *Diagnostic and Statistical Manual of Mental Disorders* 3rd ed. The American Psychiatric Association, 1980.

Bandura A: *Aggression: A Social Learning Analysis*. Prentice-Hall, 1973.

Bateson G, et al: Toward a theory of schizophrenia. *Behav Sci* 1956; 1:151–264.

Bettelheim B: *The Empty Fortress—Infantile Autism and The Birth of Self*. Free Press, 1967.

Bleuler E: *Dementia Praecox or the Group of Schizophrenias*. International Universities Press, 1950.

Boatman MJ, Szurek SA: A clinical study of childhood schizophrenia. In: *The Etiology of Schizophrenia*. Jackson DO (editor). Basic Books, 1960.

Campbell M, et al: Childhood psychosis in perspective. A follow-up of 10 children. *Am Acad Child Psychiatry* (Winter) 1978; 17(1):14–28.

Cantor S: *The Schizophrenic Child*. Eden Press, 1982.

Caplan G: *Prevention of Mental Disorders in Children*. Basic Books, 1961.

Chess S: Autism in children with congenital rubella. *J Autism Child Schizophrenia* 1971; 1(1):33–48.

Coffman JA: Anger: Its significance for nurses who work with emotionally disturbed children. *Perspec Psychiatr Care* 1969; 7(3):104–111.

Coleman M: *The Autistic Syndromes*. Elsevier/North-Holland, 1976.

Coyne J: Toward an international description of depression. *Psychiatry* 1976; 39(2):28–40.

DeMeyer M, et al: A comparison of five demographic symptoms for childhood schizophrenia and infantile autism. *J Autism Child Schizophrenia* 1971; 1:175–189.

Dennehy CM: Childhood bereavement and psychiatric illness. *Br J Psychiatry* 1966; 112(491):1049–1069.

Desmond MM, et al: The early growth and development of infants with congenital rubella. *Adv Teratol* 1970; 4:39–65.

Drabman RS, Jarvie G: Counseling parents of children with behavior problems: The use of extinction and time-out techniques. *Pediatrics* 1977; 59(1):78–85.

Dumas RG: *Keynote Address—National Conference, Advocates for Child Psychiatric Nursing*. June 18, 1980.

Durkheim E: *Suicide*. Free Press, 1951.

Eggers C: Course and prognosis of childhood schizophrenia. *J Autism Child Schizophrenia* 1978; 8(8):21–36.

Fagin CM: *Readings in Child and Adolescent Psychiatric Nursing*. Mosby, 1974.

Ferranto SJ: Depressive illness in Jews and non-Jews. *Br J Psychiatry* 1966; 112(491):991–996.

Freeman L: Depression in children. How it differs from adult depression. *Medical Aspects of Human Sexuality* (in press).

Freeman L, et al: Psychotic and depressed children: A new entity. *J Acad Child Psychiatry* (in press).

Glueck S, Glueck E (editors): *Identification of Predelinquents*. Intercontinental Medical Book Corporation, 1972.

Glueck S, Glueck E: *Toward a Typology of Juvenile Offenders: Implications for Therapy and Prevention*. Grune & Stratton, 1970.

Grossman JA, et al: *Alcoholism in Family Histories of Prepubertal Probands with Affective Disorders*. Paper presented at the 34th meeting of the International Council of Alcoholism and Addiction. Athens, Greece, May, 1984.

Grossman JA, Constantine J, Poznanski, EO: *Family Models of Depression*. Paper presented at a National Meeting of the American Association of Psychiatric Services for Children, San Francisco, California, November, 1981.

Grosz HJ: The depression-prone and the depression-resistant sibling: A study of 650 three-sibling families. *Br J Psychiatry* 1968; 144(517): 1555–1558.

Harris M: Understanding the autistic child. *Am J Nurs* (October) 1978; 78(10):1683–1686.

Hermelin B: Coding and the sense modalities. In: *Early Childhood Autism*. Wing L (editor). Pergamon Press, 1976.

Herskowitz J, Rosman NP: *Pediatrics, Neurology, and Psychiatry—Common Ground: Behavioral, Cognitive, Affective, and Physical Disorders in Childhood and Adolescence*. Macmillan, 1982.

Hill OW, Price JS: Child bereavement and adult depression. *Br J Psychiatry* 1967; 113(500):743–751.

Hinsie LE, Campbell RJ: *Psychiatric Dictionary*. 4th ed. Oxford University Press, 1970.

Hirschi T: *Causes of Delinquency*. University of California Press, 1969.

Hirschberg JC: Child psychiatry. In: *Comprehensive Textbook of Psychiatry*. Vol 3. 3rd ed. Kaplan HI, Freedman AM, Sadock BJ (editors). Williams and Wilkins, 1980.

Judd LL, et al: The effect of lithium carbonate on affect, mood, and personality of normal subjects. *Arch Gen Psychiatry* 1977; 34: 346–351.

Kallmann, FJ (editor): *Expanding Goals of Genetics in Psychiatry*, Anniversary Symposium, 1961. Grune & Stratton, 1962.

Kaplan HI, Freedman AM, Sadock BJ: *Comprehensive Textbook of Psychiatry*. Vol 3. Williams and Wilkins, 1980.

Kaufman BN: *Son-Rise*. Harper & Row, 1976.

Kraeplin E: *Dementia Praecox and Paraphrenia*. Chicago Medical Books, 1919.

Levy D: Primary affect hunger. *Am J Psychiatry* 1937; 94:643–652.

Lidz T, Fleck S, Cornelison AR (editors): *Schizophrenia and the Family*. International Universities Press, 1965.

Loomis M: *Phenomena of Concern for Psychiatric and Mental Health Nursing Practice*. Paper presented at the American Nursing Association, New Knowledge for Nursing Practice Conference, Denver, Colorado, November 4, 1983.

Lotter V: Follow-up studies. In: *Autism: A Reappraisal of Concepts and Treatment*. Rutter M, Schopler E (editors). Plenum, 1978.

Lyon GG: Limit setting as a therapeutic tool. *J Psychiatr Nurs* (Nov/Dec) 1970; 8(6):17–24.

Malmquist C: Depressive phenomenon in childhood. In: *Manual of Child Psychopathology*. Wohlman B (editor). McGraw-Hill, 1972.

Meeks JE: Conduct disorders. In: *Comprehensive Textbook of Psychiatry* Vol 3. Kaplan HI, Freedman AM, Sadock BJ (editors). Williams and Wilkins, 1980.

Morgan S: *The Unreachable Child*. Memphis State University Press, 1981.

Ornitz E, Ritvo ER: Perceptual inconstancy in early infantile autism. *Arch Gen Psychiatry* 1968; 18:76–98.

Ornitz, E, Ritvo ER: The syndrome of autism: A critical review. *Am J Psychiatry* 1976; 133(6):609–621.

Paluszny MJ: *Autism: A Practical Guide for Parents and Professionals*. Syracuse University Press, 1979.

Phillips I: *Disastrous Beginnings and Favorable Outcomes: Psychosocial Adaptation of Distressed Infants*. Paper presented at the Institute of Juvenile Research, Chicago, Illinois, 1983.

Poznanski E: The clinical phenomenology of childhood depression. *Am J Orthopsychiatry* 1982; 52(4):308–313.

Poznanski E, Zrull J: Childhood depression: Clinical characteristics of overtly depressed children. *Arch Gen Psychiatry* 1976; 23(7):8–15.

Poznanski E, et al: Diagnostic criteria in childhood depression. *Arch Gen Psychiatry* (in press).

Puig-Antich J, Chambers W: *The Schedule for Affective Disorders and Schizophrenia for School-Age Children (Kiddie-Sads)*. New York State Psychiatric Institute, 1980.

Rabkin JG: Stressful life events and schizophrenia: A review of the research literature. *Psychol Bull* 1980; 87:408–425.

Rank B: Adaptation of the psychoanalytic technique for the treatment of young children with atypical development. *Am J Orthopsychiatry* 1949; 19:130–139.

Reckless WC, Dinitz S: *The Prevention of Juvenile Delinquency: An Experiment*. Ohio State University Press, 1972.

Rimland B: *Infantile Autism*. Appleton-Century-Crofts, 1964.

Rothstein A: Hallucinatory phenomena in children: A critique of the literature. *Am Acad Child Psychiatry* 1981; 20(3):623–635.

Rutter M, Bartak L, Newman S: Autism: A central disorder of cognition and language? In: *Infantile Autism: Concepts, Characteristics and Treatment*. Rutter M (editor). Churchill Livingstone, 1971.

Rutter M: The development of infantile autism. *Psychol Med* 1974; 4:147–164.

Scharer K: *Personal Communication: Medical Hospitalization of the Schizophrenic Child*. Children's Hospital, Chicago, 1983.

Schopler E, Mesibov GB (editors): *Autism in Adolescents and Adults*. Plenum, 1983.

Senn MJE: Pediatrics in orthopsychiatry. In: *Orthopsychiatry 1923–1948: Retrospect and Prospect*. Lowery L (editor). American Orthopsychiatric Association, 1948.

Shaffer D, et al: A children's global assessment scale (CGAS). *Arch Gen Psychiatry* 1983; 40:1228–1231.

Spitz R: Analytic depression. In: *The Psychoanalytic Study of the Child*. Vol 2. International Universities Press, 1946.

Stuart RB: Behavioral contracting within the families of delinquents. *J Behav Ther Exp Psychiatry* 1971; 2:1–11.

Tanguary PE: Clinical and electrophysiological research. In: *Autism: Diagnosis, Current Research, and Management*. Ritvo E (editor). Spectrum, 1976.

Toolan JM: Depression in children and adolescents. *Am J Orthopsychiatry* 1962; 32:404–415.

Tustin F: *Autism and Childhood Psychosis*. Jason Aronson, 1973.

Werry JS: An overview of pediatric psychopharmacology. *J Am Acad Child Psychiatry* 1982; 21(1):3–9.

Williams J, Wilson H: A nursing perspective on DSM-III. *J Psychiatr Nurs* (Apr) 1982; 20(4):14–20.

Wohlman B: Schizophrenia in childhood. In: *Manual of Child Psychopathology*. Wohlman B (editor). McGraw-Hill, 1972.

Wynne LC, Singer MT: Thought disorder and family relations of schizophrenics: A research strategy. *Arch Gen Psychiatry* 1963; 9:191–198.

Additional Readings

Arnold LE (editor): *Helping Parents Help Their Children*. Brunner/Mazel, 1978.

Babich K (editor): *A Workbook: Assessing The Mental Health Of Children*. Western Interstate Commission For Higher Education, 1982.

Barker, P: *Basic Child Psychiatry*. 2nd ed. University Park Press, 1976.

Beiser M: Etiology of mental disorders: Sociocultural aspects. In: *Manual of Child Psychopathology*. Wohlman B (editor). McGraw-Hill, 1972.

Beller EK, Nebauer PB: Sex differences and symptom patterns in early childhood. *J Am Acad Child Psychiatry* 1963; 2:417–433.

Bemporad JR: Adult recollections of a formerly autistic child. *J Autism Dev Disord* (Jun) 1979; 9(2):179–197.

Berlin IN, Critchley DL: The work of play for parents of schizophrenic children. *Child Psychiatry Hum Dev* (Winter) 1982; 13(2):111–119.

Bettelheim B: Joey: A "mechanical boy." *Sci Am* (March) 1959; 200: 116–127.

Blaik R, Genser SG: *Perceived Social Support and Risk of Depression*. Presented as new research at the American Psychiatry Association Meeting, San Francisco, California, May 4–9, 1980.

Bowlby J: Pathological mourning and childhood mournings. *J Am Psychoanal Assoc* 1963; 11:500–541.

Brink RE: How serious is the child's behavior problem? *MCN* (Jan/Feb) 1982; 7:33–36.

Cadoret RJ: Evidence for genetic inheritance of primary disorder in adoptees. *Am J Psychiatry* 1977; 135:463–466.

Campbell M, Small A: Chemotherapy. In: *Handbook of Treatment of Mental Disorders in Childhood and Adolescence*. Wohlman B, Eagan J, Ross A (editors). Prentice-Hall, 1978.

Campbell M, Geller B, Cohen IL: Current status of drug research and treatment with autistic children. *J Pediatr Psychol* 1977; 2:153–161.

Campbell M, et al: Psychopharmacological treatment of children with the syndrome of autism. *Pediatr Ann* 1984; 13(4):309–316.

Caplan G: *An Approach to Community Mental Health*. Grune & Stratton, 1961.

Capuzzi C: Hirschi's bond theory, juvenile delinquency and the school nurse. *J School Health* 1982; 52(5):280–282.

Christ A, et al: The role of the nurse in child psychiatry. In: *Readings in Child and Adolescent Psychiatric Nursing*. Fagin CM (editor). Mosby, 1974.

Clancy H, McBride J: The autistic process and its treatment. *J Child Psychol Psychiatry* 1969; 10:233–244.

DeMeyer M: Perceptual limitations in autistic children and their relation to social and intellectual deficits. In: *Infantile Autism: Concept, Characteristics, and Treatment*. Rutter M (editor). Churchill Livingstone, 1971.

DesLauriers AM, Carlson CF: *Your Child Is Asleep*. Dorsey Press, 1969.

Dizon MAB: Secure attachment—anxious attachment. *J Psychosoc Nurs* (Mar) 1984; 22(3):10–22.

Doane J: Family interaction and communication deviance in disturbed and normal families: A review of research. *Fam Process* 1978; 17: 357–376.

Dudziak D: Parenting the autistic child. *J Psychosoc Nurs* (Jan) 1982; 20(1):11–16.

Egeland J, Hosteiter A: Affective disorders among the Amish 1976–1980. *Am J Psychiatry* 1984; 141(1):56–61.

Feldman LB: Depression and marital interaction. *Fam Process* 1976; 15:389–395.

Frederick C: Interventions for suicidal behavior in children and adolescents. In: *Trends in Mental Health: Self-Destructive Behavior Among Younger Age Groups*. US Department of Health, Education, and Welfare. DHEW Publication no (ADM) 76-365, 1976.

Freeberg S: Anger in adolescence. *J Psychiatr Nurs* (Mar) 1982; 20(3):29–30.

Freeman BJ, Ritvo ER: The syndrome of autism: Establishing the diagnosis and principles of management. *Pediatr Ann* 1984; 13(4):284–296.

Freud A: *Normality and Pathology in Childhood*. International Universities Press, 1967.

Gillberg C, Schaumann H: Infantile autism and puberty. *J Autism Dev Disord* 1981; 11(4):356–371.

Gordon T: *P.E.T.: Parent Effectiveness Training*. New American Library, 1975.

Greenfield J: *A Child Called Noah*. Holt, Rinehart & Winston, 1972.

Hayden E, Godboot R: The child guidance center: Its contributions. In: *Readings in Child and Adolescent Psychiatric Nursing*. Mosby, 1974.

Kashani SH, et al: Current perspectives on child depression: An overview. *Am J Psychiatry* 1981; 138:143–153.

Killian S, McCarthy S: Hospitalization of the autistic child. Part I: Assessment and Part II: Autistic Children, Intervention. *MCN* (Nov/Dec) 1980; 5:413–427.

Klein M: *Contributions to Psychoanalysis 1921–1945*. McGraw-Hill, 1964.

Lefkowitz MM, Burton IN: Childhood depression: A critique of the concept. *Psychol Bull* 1978; 85:716–726.

Lovaas OI: *The Autistic Child: Language Development Through Behavior Modification.* Irvington Publishers, 1977.

Lovaas OI, Simmons JQ: Manipulation of self-destruction in three retarded children. *J Appl Behav Analysis* 1969; 2:143–157.

Lovaas OI, Screibman L, Loegel RL: A behavior modification approach to the treatment of autistic children. In: *Psychopathology and Child Development.* Schopler E, Reichler RJ (editors). Plenum Press, 1976.

Melichart MM: Using crisis theory to help parents cope with a child's temper tantrum. *MCN* (May/June) 1980; 5:181–185.

Middleton A, Pothier P: The nurse in child psychiatry: An overview. In: *Readings in Child and Adolescent Psychiatric Nursing.* Mosby, 1974.

Moss NG: Child therapy groups in the real world. *J Psychosoc Nurs* (March) 1984; 22(3):43–50.

Paluszny, MJ: *Autism: A Practical Guide for Parents and Professionals.* Syracuse University Press, 1979.

Pothier PC: Individual therapy with a mute autistic child. In: *Readings in Child and Adolescent Psychiatric Nursing.* Fagin CM (editor). Mosby, 1974.

Pothier PC: Child psychiatric nursing. *J Psychosoc Nurs* (March) 1984; 22(3):10–22.

Poznanski E, et al: The dexamethasone depression test in prepubertal depressed children. *Am J Psychiatry* 1982; 139(3):321–324.

Prange A, et al: L-tryptophan in mania: Contribution to a permissive hypothesis of affective disorders. *Arch Gen Psychiatry* 1974; 30: 56–62.

Price J: The genetics of depressive behavior. *Br J Psychiatry* (Special Publication) 1968; 2:37–54.

Puig-Antich J, Gittleman R: Depression in children and adolescence. In: *Handbook of Affective Disorders.* Paykl ES (editor). Goilford, 1982.

Puig-Antich J, et al: Sleep architecture and REM sleep measures in prepubertal children with major depression. *Arch Gen Psychiatry* 1983; 39:932–939.

Redl F, Wiseman D: *Controls from Within.* Free Press, 1952.

Ritvo ER, Freeman BJ: A medical model of autism: Etiology, pathology and treatment. *Pediatr Ann* 1984; 13(4):298–305.

Rosen BM, et al: Adolescent patients served in outpatient psychiatric clinics. *Am J Public Health* 1965; 55:1563–1577.

Russell A, Mattison R, Cantwell D: DSM III in the practice of child psychiatry. *J Clin Psychiatry* 1983; 44:86–90.

Rutter M, Graham P: Psychiatric disorder in 10- and 11-year-old children. *Proc R Soc Med* 1966; 59:382–387.

Schulman JL, Irwin M (editors). *Psychiatric Hospitalization of Children.* Thomas, 1982.

Shufer S: The pediatric mental health nurse clinician. *Nurs Outlook* 1971; 19(8):543–545.

Skoda CM, Skeels HM: A final follow-up study of one hundred adopted children. *J Genet Psychol* 1949; 75:85–125.

Spurgeon RK: Nursing the autistic child. *Am J Nurs* (July) 1967; 67(7):1416–1419.

Steiner P: The well child and the hospitalized disabled sibling. *J Psychosoc Nurs* (Mar) 1984; 22(3):23–26.

Stuart RB, Lott LA: Behavioral contracting with delinquents: A cautionary role. *J Behav Ther Exp Psychiatry* 1972; 3:161–169.

Thomas A, Chess S: *Temperament and Development.* Brunner-Mazel, 1977.

Wasow M: Parental perspectives on chronic schizophrenia. *J Chron Disord* 1983; 36(4):337–343.

Wilson H, Kneisl CP: *Psychiatric Nursing.* 2nd ed. Addison-Wesley, 1983.

Wing L: *Autistic Children: A Guide for Parents.* Redwood Burn, 1975.

Wohlman B, Eagan J, Ross A (editors): *Handbook of Treatment of Mental Disorders in Childhood and Adolescence.* Prentice-Hall, 1978.

HEALTH RESTORATION OF THE CHILD AND FAMILY

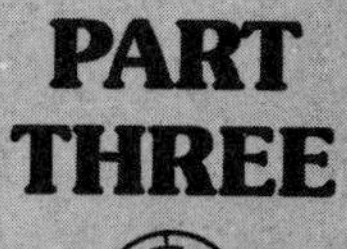

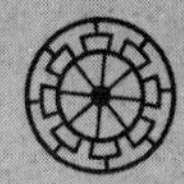

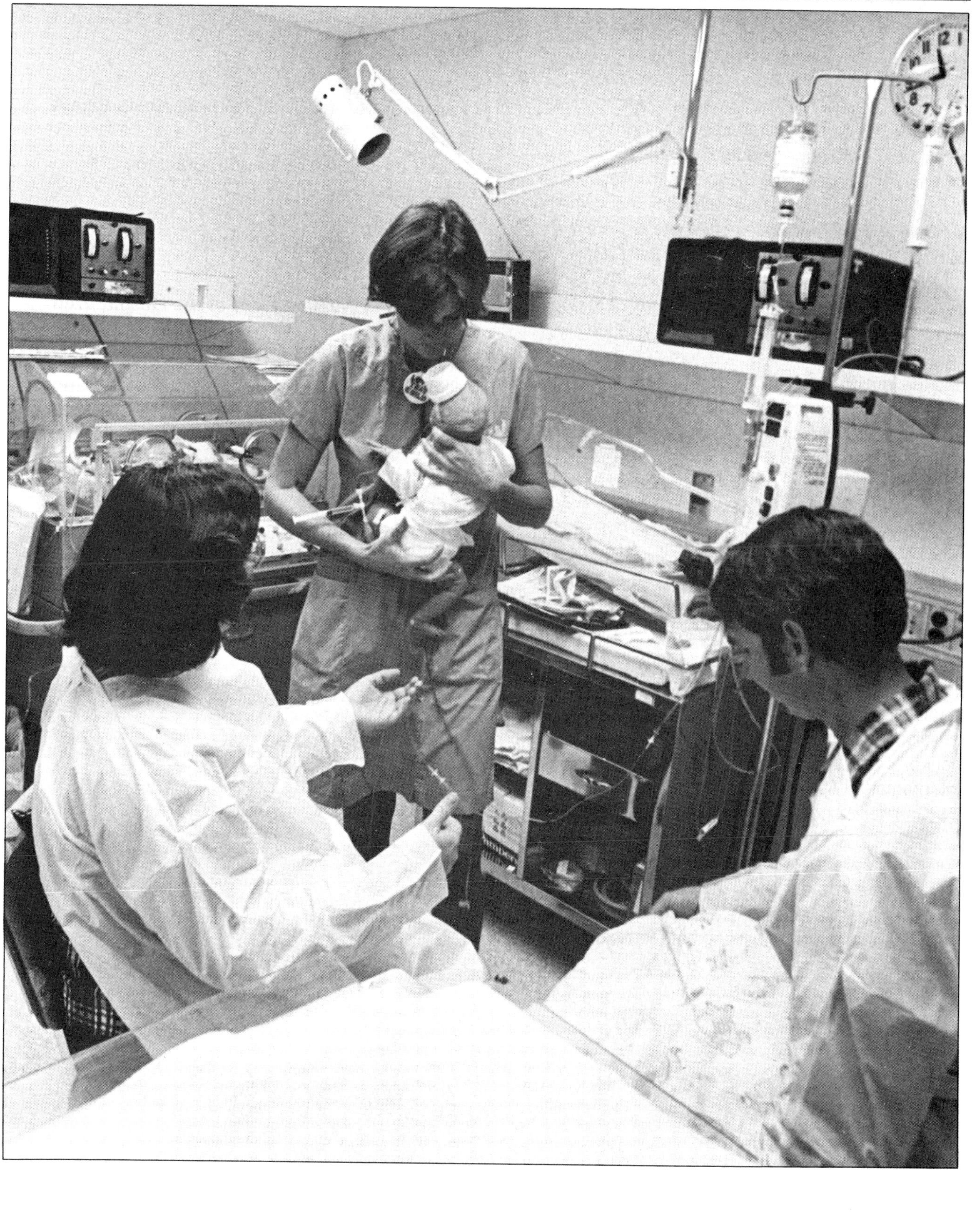

UNIT VII THE IMPACT OF ILLNESS ON THE CHILD AND FAMILY

Holistic child health nursing during illness is based on the psychologic as well as physiologic responses of children and families. A child's illness places stress on the entire family, stress that can stimulate growth or contribute to dysfunction.

In this unit we examine responses to illness and discuss the nursing process with ill children, whether at home or in the hospital, acutely or chronically ill, with mild, serious, life-threatening, or fatal illness. In Chapter 26 we detail criteria for deciding the possibility and desirability of home care for the child. The various considerations described include the nature of the child's illness, the home environment, and the family's cultural beliefs and health practices.

Chapter 27 addresses the reactions of children and their families to illness and hospitalization from both a cognitive and emotional standpoint. Play is an important aspect of communication, learning, and emotional care for children of all ages; adaptations of play for the ill child are thus presented in Chapter 28. Reactions of children and families to illness and hospitalization together with the value of therapeutic play are the basis for the principles of care of the hospitalized child brought together in Chapter 29.

Chapter 30 addresses the continuing need for the child and family to adapt to chronic conditions, promoting, as much as possible, healthy growth and development and appropriate independence and control. The immediate and ongoing considerations for the premature or ill neonate are discussed in Chapter 31. Chapter 32 covers the child's understanding of death; the reaction of child, family members, and nurse to the child's fatal illness or death; and the nursing care appropriate to meet these special needs. These chapters combine to lay a foundation for individualized, creative nursing care for ill children and their families.

Contents

Home Care of the Child With an Acute Illness

26

Mary Virginia Jacobs   Mary Walker

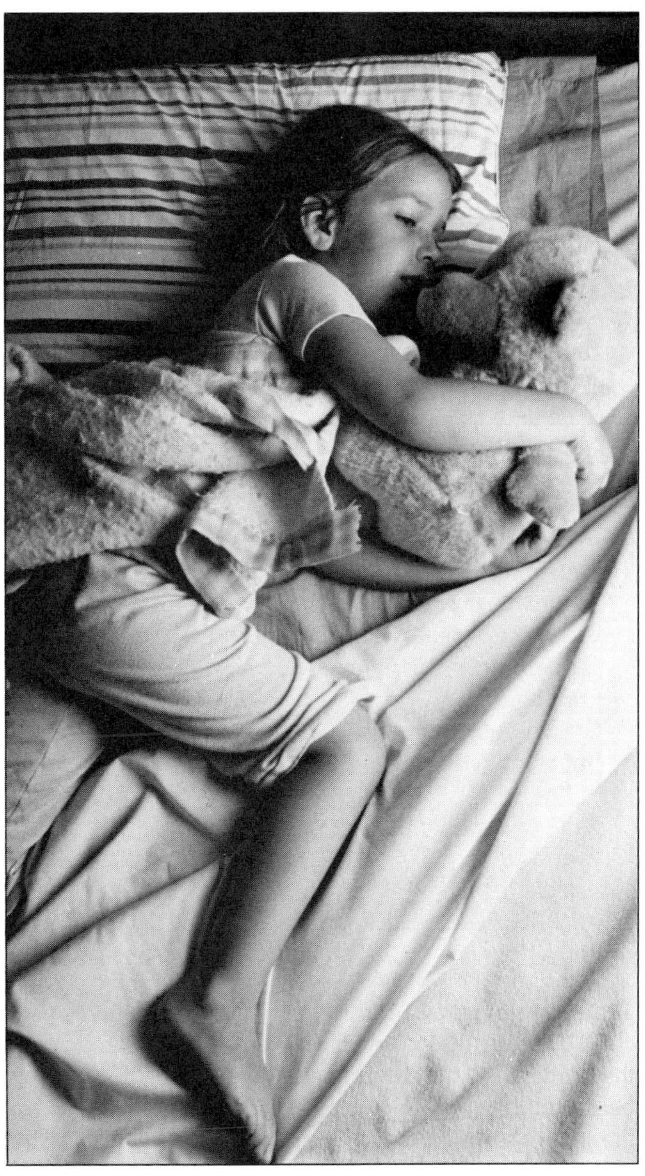

Chapter Outline

continued on next page

Disorders of the Skin
- *Pediculosis*
- *Scabies*
- *Allergic Reactions*

Emotional Disturbances

Minor Accidents and Emergencies
- *Epistaxis*
- *Contusions*
- *Lacerations*
- *Burns*
- *Exposure to Toxins*

Objectives

- Explain the rationale for the care of the acutely ill child at home.
- Describe the nursing process as it applies to home care.
- Assist parents to make decisions regarding their capabilities to provide appropriate care in the home.
- Provide parents with criteria to assist them in making decisions regarding medical consultation.
- Explain the home care involved with common acute illnesses.

To find these topics, see the following chapters

Acne vulgaris	Chapter 44
Atopic dermatitis	Chapter 44
Cradle cap (seborrheic dermatitis)	Chapter 7
Diaper dermatitis (diaper rash)	Chapter 7
Frostbite	Chapter 44
Gastrointestinal pathogens	Chapter 38
Impetigo	Chapter 44
Milia	Chapter 7
Miliaria (prickly heat)	Chapter 7
Psoriasis	Chapter 44
Warts	Chapter 44

The recent trend away from hospitalization of the acutely ill child means that many ill children are now cared for in the home. This trend has special implications for nursing because the nurse is likely to be the professional to whom the parent turns for advice in caring for an ill child. The physician also might depend on the nurse once the diagnosis has been made to help determine whether the child can be cared for at home, and the physician almost certainly will depend on the nurse to communicate instructions to the parent regarding home care of the child.

In this chapter we define and describe the role of the nurse in the home care of the acutely ill child, both when the child is to be cared for at home following an early hospital discharge and when the nurse is assisting the parents to determine the feasibility for home care in lieu of hospitalization. We illustrate decision criteria that nurses can use to assist parents to appropriately refer their children for medical consultation. The nursing process in all its phases is applied to the care of the child at home. Finally, we describe the approaches to the common childhood conditions that do not usually require hospitalization.

Rationale for Home Treatment

For most childhood illnesses, home care is preferable to hospitalization, although hospitalization is occasionally necessary for many chronic diseases and some acute illnesses. Major emergencies, life-threatening conditions, and potentially crippling illnesses necessitate hospitalization, and certain psychosocial situations in the home also might make it preferable to hospitalize the child. Hospitalization does, however, present additional risks, including the long- and short-term effects of separation, financial stress on the family and community, exposure of the ill child to the infections of other children or adults in the hospital, and undermining of the parents' confidence in their abilities as caregivers (Gardner and Charles, 1982; Schmitt, Duncan, and Riley, 1972). Health professionals must consider these risks and the potential that an acute illness will be further complicated when choosing how best to care for an ill child.

For the young child, the hospital is a strange, unfamiliar, and potentially frightening place. It is filled with strange people and unusual, confusing routines. The home, on the other hand, is a familiar place in which the child can be surrounded with personal possessions and where some of the child's normal routine can be maintained. The child who is cared for in the home does not have the stress of adjusting to an unfamiliar environment added to the stress of an acute illness.

Excellent guides are available to parents to assist them in providing home care for the ill child. Numerous books written for the lay person have been published on home care of the ill child and are available in most bookstores and libraries. Several books have comprehensive guides for home care, including appropriate home treatment methods as well as easy-to-understand instructions for determining when physician consultation is needed.

Nurses' Contact With Parents

Early discharge of children to the home is a direct result of the escalating costs of health care. Children might be sent home from the hospital requiring procedures such as complicated dressing changes, tube feedings or parenteral nutrition, and oxygen therapy, among others. Frequently, nurses are responsible for decision making regarding the feasibility of home care. Hospital home care coordinators, many of whom are nurses, work closely with local visiting nurses to assess the child's home as a potential setting for care. Both coordinators and visiting nurses plan for care and evaluate the child's progress toward recovery or achieving optimal status.

In rural areas, where physician involvement might be limited, nurse practitioners are primary providers of care. In many instances they are fully responsible for making recommendations regarding feasibility of home care or necessity for hospitalization of the ill child. These decisions are complex because in many rural homes, accessibility to appropriate water and sanitation facilities is a problem.

Nurses working in ambulatory settings, such as physician's offices, schools, camps, and clinics, are frequently the professionals who direct the parent initially regarding the care of common childhood illnesses and emergencies. From a purely social standpoint, any nurse is subject to questions from family, neighbors, and friends, and requests for assistance in deciding whether additional medical consultation is necessary are commonplace.

The Nurse's Role in Home Care

The nurse, through knowledge of pathophysiology, sociology, psychology, and family dynamics, is in a unique position to provide appropriate and accurate advice to parents and other health professionals. The nurse is capable of assessing the home setting to determine the family's ability to care for an ill child, and through the nursing process, the nurse helps the family to plan, implement, and evaluate home care. The nurse is also the one member of the health care team who is continually available to evaluate the effectiveness of home care.

The five steps of the nursing process are an integral part of home care of the acutely ill child (see Chapter 2). In the assessment phase the nurse appraises both the child and family to determine the potential for home care. This includes an assessment of the nature and seriousness of the illness as well as the interest and capability of the family to cope with the illness or disease and care for the child in the home. Once the assessment is complete, the nurse works with the family in formulating a care plan. In this phase the nurse integrates knowledge from the social and behavioral sciences with scientific knowledge in developing a plan of care that will be appropriate to the child, the pathophysiology of the disease or illness, and the cultural, social, and religious beliefs of the family. Implementation of the care plan is largely the responsibility of the family when the child is cared for in the home, but the thoroughness with which the nurse develops the plan will determine the potential effectiveness of its implementation.

Although the family implements the plan, the nurse is still responsible for evaluating and reassessing the child's response to treatment. It is the nurse who must decide whether the child is improving and whether continued care at home is feasible. This evaluation, although the last step of the nursing process, does not signal the end of the nurse's role. The nursing process is dynamic; evaluation leads to reassessment and possibly to a new care plan. It is this dynamic nature of the nursing process that establishes a format for caring for the ill child in the home.

Assessment

Assessment for home care is twofold. The nurse first needs to determine the particular needs of the individual child and family. The nurse then proceeds with a systematic assessment that provides the data needed to establish an individual plan of care. A detailed home assessment is performed when early discharge from a hospital is probable or when medical facilities are at a great distance from the home.

A major aspect of assessment for an acutely ill child is determining whether the family is able to care for the child. The nurse therefore assesses the seriousness of the illness, the home setting, and the family's support systems for each child to determine whether the child can be cared for at home. Table 26-1 outlines the criteria used to assess the home and family to determine whether home care is feasible.

How serious is the illness? The seriousness of the illness will have a direct bearing on the family's ability to care for the child at home. Is the illness self-limiting? Certain illnesses, including the common cold, *Salmonella* gastroenteritis, roseola, chickenpox, and such minor trauma as abrasions and contusions are generally self-limiting and can almost always be cared for in the home setting. Other illnesses, such as laryngotracheobronchitis or pneumonia, and such trauma as fractures and possible concussions might have potentially serious complications and consequently require that the home setting be assessed more carefully.

TABLE 26-1 Assessment Criteria for Home Care

Criteria	Assessment questions
Seriousness of the illness	Is the illness self-limiting?
	What are the potential complications? Are they life-threatening? Are they potentially debilitating?
	Have home remedies been used? Were they effective? Are they potentially helpful? Harmful?
	Is the child very young (less than 1 year)?
	Is the disease communicable?
	Is the child toxic? Is the oral temperature greater than 101° F? Has the child had a convulsion? Recently? Did the child have convulsions with a fever during a previous illness? Is the child dehydrated? Are complications present?
Support systems	Is there an adult available to stay with the child who knows the child and the home? A parent? A grandparent or aunt if both parents work? An older sister or brother? A neighbor or friend?
	Does the person who is to care for the child understand the instructions for care?
	Are resources available for Obtaining needed equipment? Appropriate nutrition? Transportation (private automobile; public transportation, taxi, or bus)?
	If needed, are visiting nurses and other support systems available in the community?
Potential for home care	Is the physical condition of the home appropriate for the care of an ill child? Is the source of water adequate? Acceptable? Are toilet facilities adequate? Indoor? Outdoor? City sewer system? Septic tank? Are bathing and washing facilities adequate? Hot water or heating facilities? Dishwashing facilities? Is a separate bed available for the ill child? Is heating adequate if the weather is cold? Are windows screened if the weather is hot? Can the child be isolated if the disease is communicable?
	Can the home be changed to make it appropriate for home care?
	Is the necessary equipment available? Thermometer—oral or rectal? Clean sheets and bedding? Soap? Hot water? Dishes and means for sterilizing (ie, dishwasher or pot and stove for boiling water)? Refrigeration for medications? Do the parents have adequate financial resources? To purchase the prescribed medication? To purchase analgesics? To purchase necessary equipment? Do the parents have the psychic energy necessary to care for an ill child at home? How many other family members live in the home? Is there a current family crisis, death, separation, or divorce? Do any other family members have a physical or emotional illness? Is there a special or handicapped child in the home? Is there reasonable assurance that the parent or designated caregiver will follow through in implementing a plan of care for the ill child? Are any cultural or religious beliefs likely to interfere with the care plan? Are these customs or beliefs a potential threat to the health of the child? Is there a history of noncompliance with prescribed treatment regimens?

How old is the child? Infants sometimes are more susceptible to developing complications from an illness that might be self-limiting in older children. Infants, because of their immaturity and greater proportion of body surface area to body weight, are likely to develop complications such as dehydration from simple diarrhea or pneumonia from a common cold. Because infants are unable to communicate their aches, pains, and needs, alert, capable people are needed to care for them during acute illnesses. Older children and teenagers are able to communicate their needs and usually understand reasonably well the need for health care. Thus, they require less constant supervision when ill.

Is the disease communicable? If so, the nurse must consider others in the home who might be harmed if they were to contract the disease. Very young infants, the elderly, and persons with an altered immunologic system are all particularly susceptible to communicable diseases. A susceptible person living in the home might preclude caring for an ill child in the home setting.

Is the child toxic? Is the child's temperature extremely high or has the child had convulsions? Has the child had previous convulsions with fever? Is the child already dehydrated? Are complications such as pneumonia already present? If any of these conditions are present, the feasibility of home care is reduced. In making the assessment the nurse identifies any complicating conditions and then determines whether the parent or designated caregiver is able to provide the necessary care.

Are support systems available and adequate? A good support system will greatly improve the potential of the family to care for an ill child at home. Can an adult stay with the ill child, monitor the progress of the disease, administer the appropriate medication, and provide needed rest, nutrition, and diversion? It is preferable for this person to be a parent or grandparent who is familiar to the child and familiar with the home setting, but another relative or close family friend might be an appropriate alternative if the parent cannot stay with the ill child. The person responsible for the child's care also must understand the nurse's instructions. The nurse therefore gives instructions directly to the person who will be caring for the child in a language that this person can understand. If necessary, a person who speaks the native language of the designated caregiver or an interpreter should be used for instructions. It is sometimes helpful to write out the instructions so that the caregiver can refer to them later.

Are resources available in the community to help the family meet the needs of the ill child? If the family does not have the necessary equipment at home to care for the ill child, can community resources supply this equipment? Perhaps the family can borrow the needed equipment from a friend or relative, or perhaps a health care rental agency can supply what is needed.

Is appropriate nutrition assured in the home setting? This is especially important if the illness or disease requires special dietary measures. Some gastrointestinal disorders, for example, require special oral electrolyte replacement solutions, and the nurse therefore determines the family's ability to provide the necessary nutrition before deciding the best place to care for the child.

Is transportation available? In many instances an ill child needs to return to the clinic or hospital so that the nurse can reassess the child's condition. Therefore, the family should have access to transportation. If the family does not have access to a car, is public transportation or taxi service available and will the family use this transportation? If transportation is not available, can alternative health care providers, such as visiting nurses or public health nurses, go to the patient's home to make the necessary assessments?

Is the home in good repair, and will the ill child be protected from the elements? If the roof leaks severely, there are no window panes, or screens are missing, the potential for adequate home care might be reduced. What is the source of drinking water? Is it city water or well water? Is the water a potential source of infection or disease? What are the bathroom facilities? Are they indoors or outdoors? Do they involve a city sewer, septic tank, or privy? Are the toilet facilities a potential source of infection? Are bathing facilities available? Is there a place for the child to sleep where adequate rest is assured and the potential for disease communicability is reduced? Does the child have a separate bed? If the weather is cold, is heating available? Can the child be isolated, if necessary, from other family members? The nurse also looks for solutions to problems. If there is some physical defect in the home, can changes be made to make the home an appropriate place for the care of the ill child?

In addition to determining the physical appropriateness of the home, the nurse also considers whether the equipment needed to care for the ill child is available. Is there a thermometer to assess fever? Are clean sheets and bedding available? Does the family have access to hot running water and soap for bathing and washing clothes? Can dishes be sterilized if necessary? (Either a dishwasher or a pot for water and a stove or hot plate for boiling water is essential.)

If any equipment is needed, are there financial resources available either in the family or community to purchase the necessary items? Will the family be able to obtain the prescribed medication and necessary analgesics, ointments, or bandages? It is sometimes just as important to determine whether the family will purchase the necessary medications, supplies, and equipment as it is to determine whether they can buy them. Occasionally, a family will not purchase the medication, even though family members are financially capable, and in these instances, alternative routes of administration must be considered. For example, the nurse who is aware that a family might not purchase an oral antibiotic for the child with pharyngitis can recommend a long-acting antibiotic administered by injection.

Another important consideration in assessing the feasibility of home care for the ill child is a determination of the parent's psychologic readiness for caring for the child. If a recent family crisis, such as divorce or death, has occurred or if the parent is physically ill or emotionally unstable, the nurse considers alternatives to home care. Certain children also pose a special problem for home care when they are ill. These are generally children who have such chronic conditions as muscular dystrophy or cerebral palsy or those who are emotionally disturbed or mentally retarded. Children with such conditions might have to be hospitalized when critically ill.

The nurse finally determines whether the parent or designated caregiver is likely to follow through in implementing the care plan for the ill child. The parent or designated caregiver must be willing to implement the care plan in the home setting and must agree to the plan of care before the nurse can be reasonably assured that the child will receive the needed care.

Occasionally, the family has cultural or religious beliefs that might interfere with the implementation of the care plan. For example, home remedies or methods for treating illness that have been handed down from generation to generation might preclude medical treatment. These remedies vary considerably among different cultures. When a family is using a home remedy, the nurse assesses whether the remedy is harmless, whether it could lead to complications compromising the child's health, and whether it will interfere with or complement the care plan. For example, in some cultures it is thought that cracking a raw egg into a bowl and placing it under the bed of a child with fever will "draw out" the fever and thus cure the illness. This practice is harmless as long as the parent understands that such measures as fluids, antibiotics, and analgesics might be needed in addition to the raw egg treatment. On the other hand, Hispanic people commonly tie a coin or amulet around the neck of a child who is teething. Because the child might put the coin or amulet in the mouth, with the possibility that it might be swallowed or become lodged in the trachea, this practice should be discouraged.

Consideration of cultural and religious beliefs is especially important if the caregiver has a past history of failure to cooperate with prescribed treatment regimens. Some cultural traditions cause parents to reject the germ theory of disease. A common belief is that because germs are not visible to the naked eye, they do not exist (Madsen, 1973). People who believe this tend to comply poorly with prescribed antibiotic regimens. If the nurse is aware of this attitude or suspects it might be present, long-term injectable antibiotics can be given to the ill child rather than oral antibiotics, which require parental cooperation.

In Chinese folk medicine the ill person receives a single dose of the prescribed medication for a cure; therefore, people of this culture might not understand why it is necessary to take a large number of medications over an extended period of time (Henderson and Primeaux, 1981). Cooperation with a prescribed treatment regimen therefore might be poor, and alternative treatment plans may need to be considered.

Native Americans will use both modern medicine and traditional folk medicine when the two systems are complementary, but they will not totally give up a traditional system of folk medicine that has worked for centuries in favor of what they view as fragmented health care (Henderson and Primeaux, 1981). In working with Native Americans, the nurse therefore might need to incorporate traditional folk beliefs into treatment plans to increase the potential for cooperation.

Other problems that might result from cultural or religious differences include an innate reserve which might prevent a family from asking questions about a treatment plan, the difficulty of distinguishing key family members in multigenerational families, and religious traditions that view illness as a punishment for wrongdoing or teach that illness is a mental phenomenon which can be cured through the power of the mind over the body. (See Chapter 3 for a further discussion of cultural influences on health practices.)

The nurse never questions the legitimacy of the patient's culture, religion, or beliefs and thus respects the patient's and family's rights to their beliefs. The nurse also keeps in mind the child's health status, beliefs, and traditions in planning care. This allows the nurse to determine whether home remedies can be incorporated into the treatment plan or whether they should be discouraged. The nurse making this determination also keeps in mind the pathophysiology of the disease process and psychosocial aspects of health and illness.

Nursing Diagnosis

Once the assessment data have been collected and analyzed, the nurse actively participates with other health professionals in determining a care plan that is best suited to the child. The nurse can determine whether secondary care or hospitalization is indicated and whether the severity of the illness or the potential for complications precludes primary or home care. Two levels of nursing diagnoses are related to the home care of the child. The first-level nursing diagnosis focuses on the potential risk that the child will develop complications. For example, a child with a very high fever and a previous history of febrile convulsions might be at greater risk for developing complications if cared for at home. The nursing diagnosis in this instance might be the potential risk of complications related to the difficulty of controlling fever.

Second-level nursing diagnoses obtained from the assessment data can support the nursing decision to recommend or reject home care for the child. These nursing diagnoses are related to the adequacy of environmental and personal factors uncovered in the assessment. The nursing diagnosis then provides a working basis for the construction of the home care plan if home care is chosen.

To illustrate how nursing diagnoses are constructed from assessment data, two situations are presented in Table 26-2. The background data are similar but differ in important areas that assist the nurse to make a judgment regarding the feasibility of home care for this particular child. In the first situation the risk of complications is slight because situational factors can be modified to provide adequate care for the patient at home. In the second situation the child is at much greater risk because of her family history and because the crowded conditions cannot be easily altered. Also, the family history of failure to cooperate with the medical reg-

TABLE 26-2 Construction of Nursing Diagnoses in Relation to Home Care

Patient data: Name: Susan Age: 8 Years Medical diagnosis: probable streptococcal pharyngitis

Situation 1

Assessment data	Nursing diagnosis
Self-limiting disease with potential complications	Potential cardiac complications from improper treatment or resistance to prescribed treatment regimen
Highly communicable problem, especially in crowded conditions	Potential for communicability to other family members
Oral temperature of 103° F. No signs of dehydration, convulsions, or other complications	Discomfort from fever and pain; potential dehydration caused by decreased fluid intake
Both parents work all day. Child is alone because older siblings attend school. No close family or friends nearby; however, the mother's employer is amenable to her taking sick time to care for child.	Potential for inadequate support for home care
Five people living in a three-bedroom, five-room apartment. Child shares a room with older sister. Child's brother has his own room. Bathing and toileting facilities are adequate. Family owns sleeping bags	Potential inability for the child to be isolated
Equipment necessary for home care is present. No dishwasher	Potential spread of disease through inadequate handling of dishes
Family is covered under a comprehensive health plan	
No history of failure to cooperate with medication regimen. Parents do not feel that once symptoms have disappeared, the medication can be discontinued	

Analysis leading to nursing diagnosis: Assessment factors indicate a strong probability that Susan can be cared for at home if the nursing diagnoses are addressed in the plan of care. For example, the isolation problem can be solved if the patient is put alone in the brother's room and the brother uses a sleeping bag on the floor of one of the living areas.

Situation 2

Assessment data	Nursing diagnoses
Self-limiting disease with potential complications. Patient's sister has history of rheumatic fever	Potential for complications is increased in patient because of sister's history of rheumatic fever. Potential for sister to become ill related to infectious characteristics of streptococcal pharyngitis and her own history of rheumatic fever
The disease is highly communicable in crowded conditions	Potential for communicability to other family members
Oral temperature of 103° F. No signs of dehydration, convulsions, or other complications	Discomfort from fever and pain; potential dehydration caused by decreased fluid intake
Mother will stay home to care for the child all day. Adequate supports	
Eight people living in a five-room apartment (three bedrooms). Patient shares a bedroom with two sisters	Inadequate rest; no way to isolate the patient
Equipment necessary for home care is present. No dishwasher	Potential spread of disease through inadequate handling of dishes
Family is covered under a comprehensive health care plan	
History of failure to cooperate with medication regimen. Parents discontinue the medication when the symptoms disappear	Knowledge deficit regarding germ theory leading to failure to cooperate with prescribed treatment regimen

Analysis leading to nursing diagnosis: Although the assessment data indicate similar problems to situation #1, home care in this situation might be contraindicated. The crowded living conditions are not easily modified, and the risk of the occurrence of rheumatic fever is increased because of inability to isolate the patient and the family history. The conclusive nursing diagnosis is that there is an increased risk for the development of complications because of personal and environmental factors.

imen in the second situation is a vital issue given the family history of rheumatic fever.

Planning

After problems are identified, the nurse determines the treatment setting most suited to the particular child. The care might involve referral to a hospital setting or a recommendation for home care. Planning then helps to determine priorities among the identified problems, identify or determine the person or persons responsible for resolving each problem, identify specific methods and steps to take in solving problems, and record information in a care plan (Yura and Walsh, 1978). A written care plan provides a comprehensive plan of action to care for the ill child in the home or hospital, and it provides a reasonable assurance that the needs of the patient will be met. It includes the identified problems and the stated goals to address those problems.

Once home care has been chosen as appropriate for an ill child, the nurse must begin immediately to develop a plan of care with the parent or designated caregiver. The plan must be developed with both the caregiver and the child if the child is old enough to participate. Including both the child and the caregiver in the development of the care plan increases the potential for cooperation with the prescribed regimen.

In planning care, the nurse considers all aspects of the child's illness: the causative agent, communicability, severity or seriousness, expected progress, and potential complications. The primary goals of care should be to promote recovery in the shortest possible period while preventing any complications. These goals can best be achieved when the nurse, caregiver, physician, and child all work together as a team in planning and implementing the care plan.

The resources that the caregiver has available are an important consideration in the development of a plan of care. If necessary equipment or supplies are not available, the parent might need assistance in developing alternatives. This might include borrowing, renting, or purchasing the needed equipment. If space in the home is a problem, the nurse can suggest viable alternative arrangements to create the necessary space for the patient. Physical problems in the home might be corrected with assistance from community resources. Family members might need assistance in budgeting their time to prevent fatigue while caring for the child at home. Table 26-3 carries the case presented in Table 26-2 into the planning phase of the nursing process.

Intervention

Once the plan of care has been developed and agreed on by the nurse and caregiver, it is time to put the plan into action through nursing interventions. This phase comprises the actions taken to achieve the goals established in the planning phase (Yura and Walsh, 1978). Assessment, planning, and evaluation do, however, continue while interventions are carried out (Yura and Walsh, 1978) because the child's response to treatment might require alterations in the nursing care plan. When the ill child is cared for in the home, the parent or designated caregiver is responsible for implementing the plan of care; the nurse's responsibility, however, does not end with planning. The nurse is still responsible for seeing that the plan is implemented properly. This can best be accomplished through teaching proper care, supporting the parent's efforts to provide care, coordinating the services of other health professionals, and, if necessary, referring the child to other health care providers or services.

Before sending the ill child home with a care plan, the nurse ascertains whether the parent fully understands the plan and knows how to implement it in the home setting. Instructions should be given, and, if necessary, correct procedures should be taught before the parent and child leave the office or clinic. If, for example, ear drops must be instilled at home, the parent should know the correct way to do this and might need to practice with supervision. If a special diet is needed, it should be given in writing and reviewed orally by the nurse with the parent or designated caregiver to ensure understanding. The nurse should be certain that the parent or caregiver has the information needed to care for the ill child at home, and information gaps should be filled with appropriate teaching. In teaching or explaining procedures to the caregiver or parent, the nurse applies the principles of teaching, gears the instructions to the parent's or caregiver's educational level, and avoids complicated medical terminology as much as possible. (Parent and child teaching is discussed in Chapter 29.)

Once the parent has taken the child home and the care plan has been implemented, it is important for the nurse to maintain contact with the family to provide support, encouragement, and any needed direction. This can be done either through a telephone call or a home visit. Many parents, unfamiliar with disease entities, need to be reassured that they are doing the right things and that the child is progressing satisfactorily. The nurse therefore calls the family or visits the home 48 hours after the initiation of the treatment plan.

More information can be gathered during a home visit, but this is not always economically possible or time efficient. During the call or visit, the nurse gathers sufficient information to determine whether the care plan is being properly implemented. By questioning the parent or caregiver with careful reference to the written care plan, the nurse can determine whether the nursing goals are being met, monitor the progress of the child, and identify any possible complications that might have developed. If the child is progressing satisfactorily, the parent needs positive reinforcement and encouragement to continue caring for the ill child as planned. If the child is not progressing satisfac-

TABLE 26-3 Planning Phase of the Nursing Process Related to Home Care

Nursing diagnoses	Plan
Potential cardiac complications from improper treatment or failure to cooperate with prescribed treatment regimen	Teach the parents the principles and importance of antibiotic therapy, effects of medication, and necessity to finish the prescription
Long-term goal: Susan's parents will provide appropriate home care to prevent the occurrence of complications	Teach the parents and/or caregiver to recognize the signs of complications—increased fever, fatigue, pain in one or more joints, tachycardia
Short-term goal: Susan will report any unusual fatigue or joint stiffness to her parent or caregiver	Recommend that caregivers administer antipyretics to control Susan's fever and reduce discomfort
Potential for communicability to other family members	Encourage the family to consider alternative sleeping arrangements, such as having the brother sleep in a sleeping bag in the living room, so that the child can temporarily have her own room; teach the family the importance of handwashing and the proper disposal of tissues
Long-term goal: No other family member will become ill from this current exposure	
Short-term goals: Susan will sleep in a room by herself	Recommend the use of paper plates and plastic cutlery if affordable, or make certain that all dishes and silverware are washed thoroughly with detergent and very hot water
Susan's dishes will be washed thoroughly and kept separate from other family member's dishes	Suggest using the same set of dishes for Susan at each meal
	Teach parent to provide moderate amounts of cool liquids frequently (including Jello and Popsicles)

torily or if complications have developed, the parent might need emotional support because guilt feelings or feelings of failure may interfere with care.

Evaluation

Evaluation is the final component of the nursing process and determines the patient's response to the treatment plan. It is implemented by assessing the extent to which the established goals have been achieved. The evaluation is helpful in identifying omissions during assessment, nursing diagnosis, planning, and intervention, and it provides direction for modification of the plan of care (Yura and Walsh, 1978).

Although evaluation is the last step in the nursing process, it does not necessarily occur only at the resolution of a problem or illness. Evaluation of the ill child's progress should occur periodically throughout the illness, and modifications of the care plan should be based on the results of the evaluation. In evaluating the progress of an ill child, the nurse thus determines whether the goals established in the plan are being or have been met. Have complications developed? Is the illness progressing as expected?

After determining whether the goals of care have been met, the nurse decides whether home care is still a viable option. (The assessment criteria described in Table 26-1 are useful as decision-making tools.) If the goals have not been met, the reasons must be explored, and the nurse therefore determines whether the parent or designated caregiver will be able to adapt to meet the goals of care. When the goals are not being met and the health of the child might be compromised, alternatives to home care are indicated.

Hospitalization is the most frequent alternative to home care, but many considerations are involved in deciding whether to hospitalize a child. The first consideration is the trauma of separation, and although most hospitals now allow a parent to stay with the hospitalized child, the hospital is still a strange and unfamiliar place. The expense of hospitalization to the family and the community is another consideration, as is the disruption to the family unit caused by hospitalization. The health and well-being of the child, however, should be the primary concern in determining whether hospitalization is needed.

Referral of the Ill Child

Occasionally, the parent of an ill child will consult the nurse for help in determining whether medical attention is needed. The child usually has been receiving some treatment at home and either is not improving or is getting worse. In addition to determining whether the home remedies and treatment being administered are appropriate (Fig. 26-1), the nurse determines whether additional treatment is needed. If the nurse can complete a history of the illness and an assessment of the child, objective data on which to base a decision are available. This might not be possible, however, because nurses often are asked these questions over the phone or in an informal setting such as the grocery store. In such cases it is usually best for legal and ethical reasons to recommend that the parent seek medical attention.

The nurse can assist the parents in determining when medical care is indicated for an ill child by assessing the status of the illness (Fig. 26-2). Did the illness occur sud-

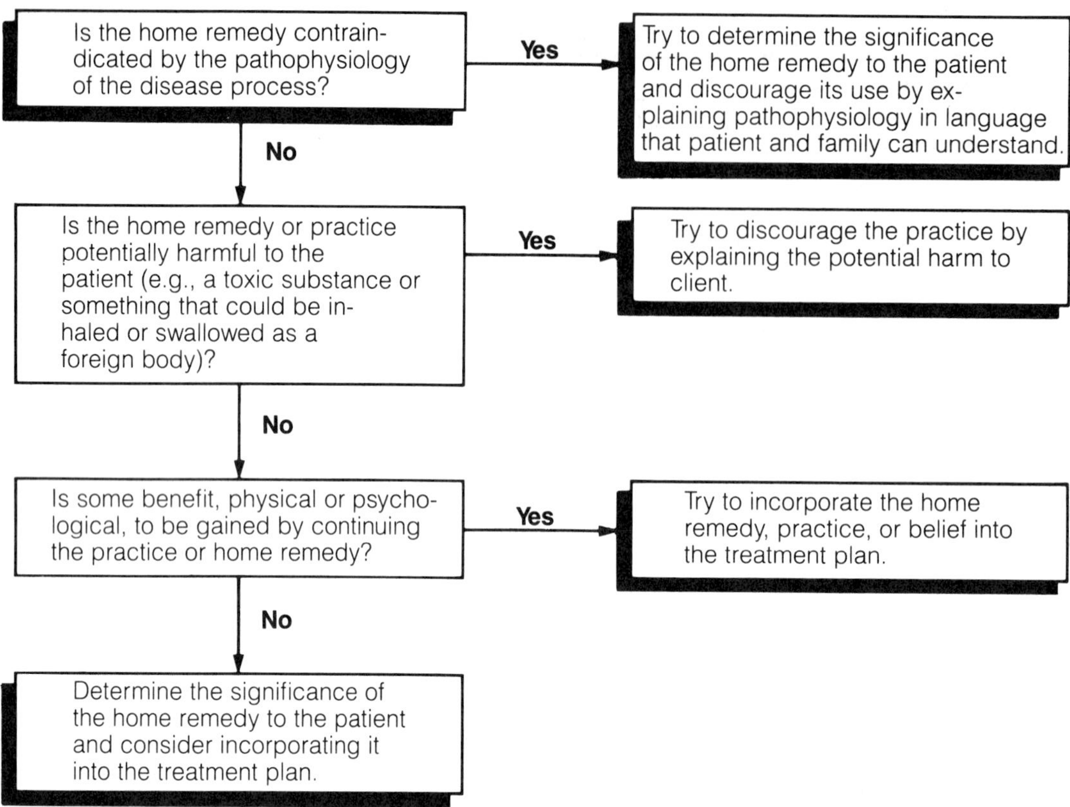

Figure 26-1 Home remedies and the nursing care plan.

denly? Many acute illnesses have a rather dramatic sudden onset of fever. Most illnesses that occur gradually over several days or weeks are less acute and usually do not require immediate referral to a health care provider. If the child had a sudden onset of high fever that has lasted for 24 hours and has not responded to antipyretic treatment, the child should be referred for medical attention. The age and general health of the child also should be considered when recommending to parents whether to seek medical care. A child with a chronic illness, such as diabetes mellitus, mus-

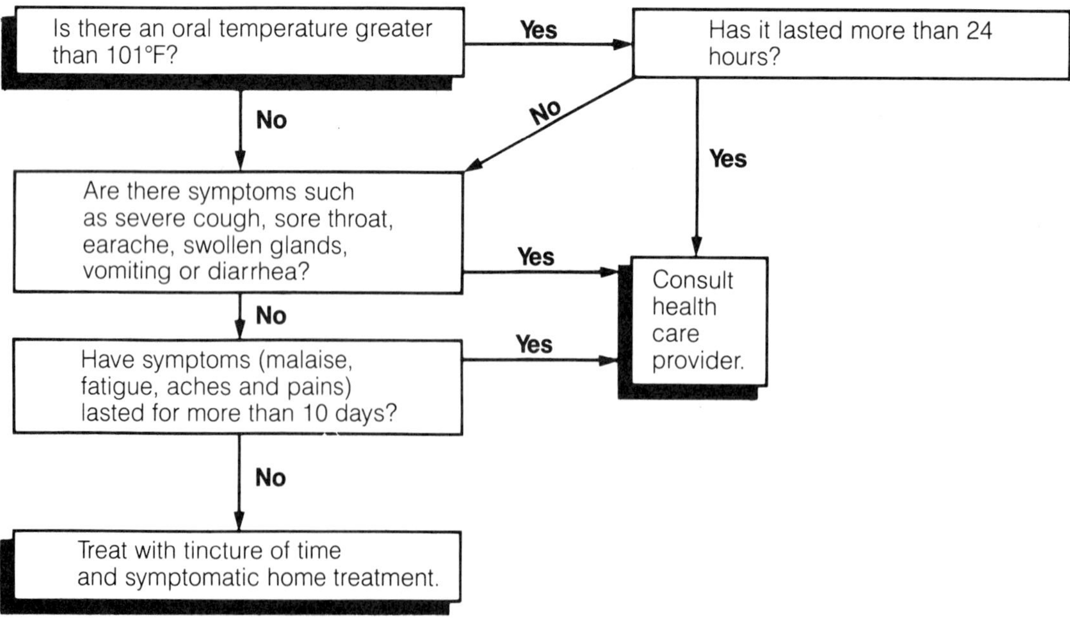

Figure 26-2 Parent decision: when to seek medical attention for an ill child.

cular dystrophy, or sickle cell disease, should seek medical attention early in the course of any illness to prevent possible complications. If a child has been ill for an extended period (over 10 days), a medical provider should be consulted. Only a thorough assessment can determine whether an extended illness is serious and if medical treatment is needed.

Acute Illnesses Amenable to Home Care

When the home is chosen as the care setting for an ill child, the parent or caregiver will need the support of the health care community until the illness resolves. Such questions as to when to seek additional medical attention are a prime concern in caring for the ill child at home. Figure 26-3 gives some guidelines to help the parent determine when further medical attention is needed after the initial treatment regimen has been started.

Disorders of the Respiratory System

Disorders of the respiratory system include those that affect the upper respiratory system—the ears, nose, and throat—and those that affect the lower respiratory system—the trachea, bronchial tubes, and lungs. Most disorders of the respiratory system are amenable to home care. Only the more severe, serious, or complicated cases require hospitalization. Children who might require hospitalization are those whose illnesses cause deprivation of air exchange, in which oxygenation of the tissues is jeopardized, and those who develop complications. An accurate assessment of the seriousness or severity of a respiratory disorder is essential to deciding the treatment setting.

The child with a respiratory disorder might demonstrate a variety of symptoms depending on the child's age and the pathophysiology of the disease. All children with respiratory complaints should receive thorough evaluations, including a history and assessment of the entire respiratory system. The nurse needs to be familiar with growth and development as well as the pathophysiology of each disease to assess the child with a respiratory disorder.

Otitis Externa Otitis externa, inflammation and infection of the external auditory canal, might be caused by an abrasion resulting from improper or overzealous cleaning (Harkess, 1982). Commonly called "swimmer's ear," the precipitating factor might be repeated removal of protective cerumen by water, which alters the pH of the ear canal, thus allowing for organism growth (Harkess, 1982). Organisms involved in the infectious process include bacteria, viruses, and fungi. The most common complaint is pain with movement of the aurical, decreased hearing, a feeling of fullness in the affected ear, purulent discharge from the

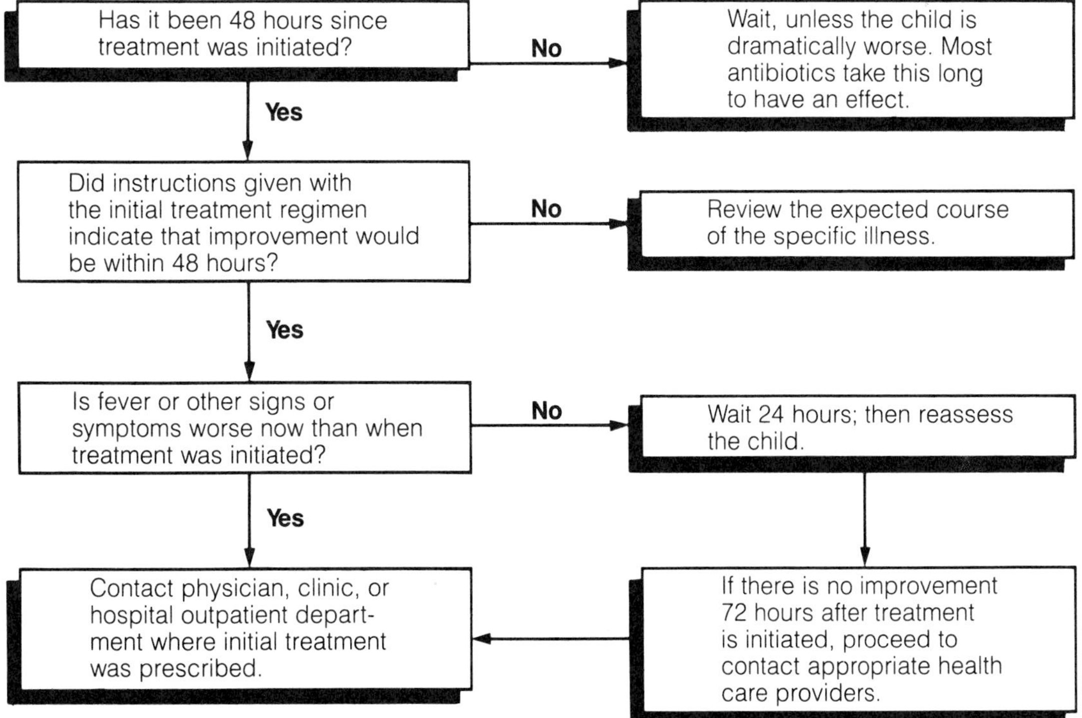

Figure 26-3 Parent decision: when to seek further medical attention for an ill child after initial treatment.

ear canal, and a low-grade fever. The usual treatment involves oral antibiotics and antibiotic ear drops with or without corticosteroids.

Home care of the child with otitis externa involves the administration of antibiotics and the instillation of the prescribed ear drops. In giving instructions to the parent for care of the child at home, the nurse emphasizes the importance of administering all of the prescribed medication, even though the child might begin to feel better after taking only a few doses. Furthermore, the parent should be cautioned not to use corticosteroid ear drops for longer than the prescribed period (usually 5 days) because of potential side effects. The parent should be taught to instill ear drops and should be instructed to keep the child's head tilted to one side after the drops are put in so that the medication is in contact with the affected ear for as long as possible.

The prevention of future infections of the external ear canal should be one of the goals of care. In this regard the nurse plays a major role in teaching the parent and child proper ear care. This includes avoiding cleaning the ears with bobby pins, cotton-tipped swabs, keys, and other objects. Recalling the physiology of the ear, the nurse can explain how the cilia, the small hairlike structures in the ear, normally keep the wax cleared from the canal. Very few people experience wax buildup of sufficient proportions to require professional ear cleaning. Because otitis externa sometimes masks otitis media due to exudates that occlude the ear canal, the importance of follow-up care must be stressed in child and parent teaching (Fig. 26-4).

Otitis Media Infections of the middle ear usually are caused by a bacteria; otitis media with effusion (serous), however, can result from eustachian tube blockage caused by allergies or congenital deformities (Adams, Evans, and Roberts, 1984). The symptoms include pain, with or without fever, and decreased hearing in the affected ear. The very young infant might simply become inexplicably irritable or might develop a fever. Infants might pull at the affected ear or bat that side of the head with their hands. Treatment of serous otitis media includes antibiotic therapy, usually orally, and might also include decongestant therapy to shrink swollen tissues in the eustachian tube. In addition, analgesic ear drops might be prescribed if the pain is severe. The parent should be instructed to give the child the antibiotic for the full prescribed period. If there is any doubt about whether the full prescription will be given, alternative routes, such as injection, should be considered.

Uncomplicated cases of otitis media usually can be cared for in the home. The nurse encourages the parent to increase the child's fluid intake and to relieve discomfort or fever with acetaminophen in appropriate doses. With very young children, it is sometimes necessary to find ingenious methods to encourage fluid intake. The parent should provide juices and drinks that the child likes along with ice cream, jello, and frozen drinks or Popsicles.

The parent or caregiver should be instructed to bring the child back to the clinic in 48 hours if there is no improvement. In addition, the parent should observe the child for a perforated eardrum, evidenced by sudden pain with bloody

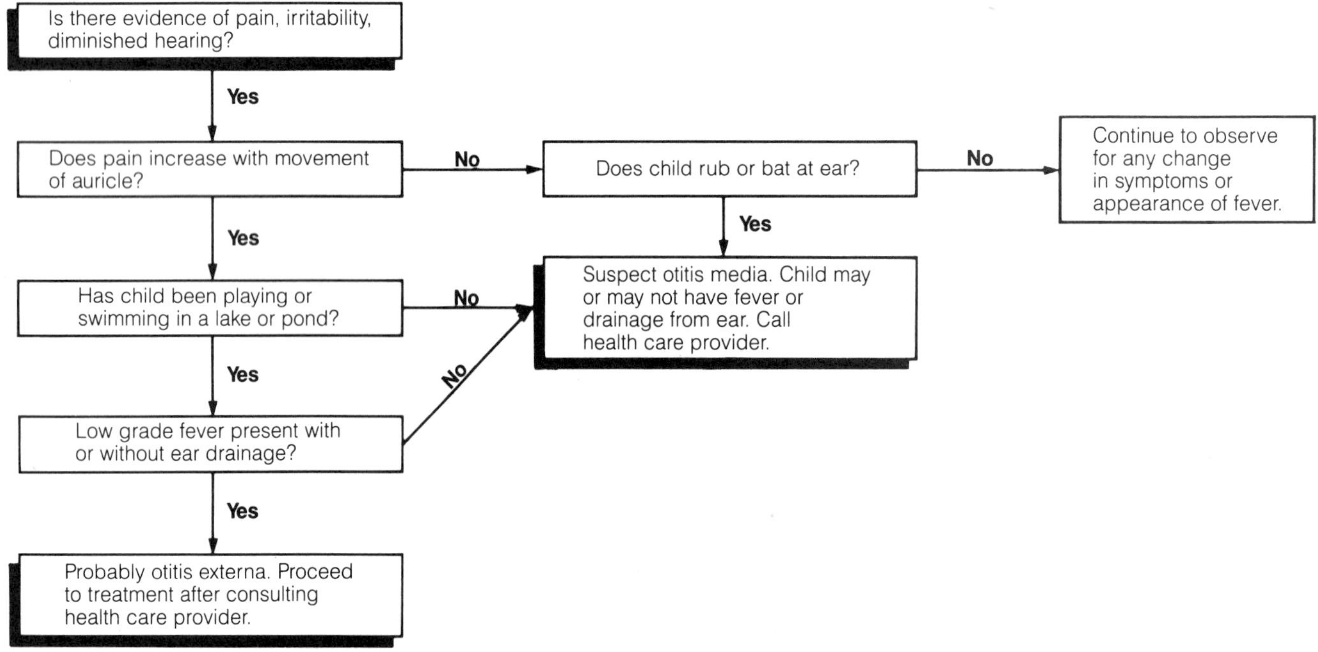

Figure 26-4 Parent decision: otitis.

drainage from the affected ear, and should bring the child back to the clinic should this occur. Because ear infections are sometimes difficult to cure, the nurse must stress the need to recheck the child when the antibiotics are completed, usually 10–14 days after treatment is initiated.

Allergic Rhinitis Allergic rhinitis (hay fever) occurs as a result of exposure to an allergen to which the child is sensitive. Symptoms include watery eyes, sneezing, runny nose, and occasionally a mild sore throat. Symptoms are similar to those of the common cold but differ in some respects (Fig. 26-5). The condition is usually self-limiting, and symptoms disappear as the pollen count decreases. Treatment is generally symptomatic and involves the use of an appropriate antihistamine. The nurse consults with the physician before recommending a particular medication to a parent because antihistamines can produce varied and annoying side effects. Parents might be bewildered by the number of over-the-counter antihistamines available and should be cautioned not to experiment with these medications without professional advice.

Many children have periodic episodes of allergic rhinitis. Most of these children will be cared for in the home without seeking professional health care advice. Frequently, however, the parent of a child with allergic rhinitis will contact the nurse for advice and help in deciding whether the child needs professional attention. Parents should be instructed to seek immediate medical attention if the child has difficulty breathing or swallowing. If the child develops an earache or fever or if rhinitis symptoms persist, medical consultation is indicated.

Acute Nasopharyngitis Most children will experience one or more episodes of acute nasopharyngitis (the common cold) each year. Very few of these children will ever seek medical attention. Acute nasopharyngitis might be caused by numerous viruses; it usually includes symptoms of nasal stuffiness, sneezing, sore throat, nonproductive cough, and low-grade fever. It is usually self-limiting and will resolve in 4–5 days without specific treatment. Parents need to have encouragement, information about the reasons antibiotics are not effective against viral illnesses, and information regarding the potential for developing antibiotic-resistant infections if antibiotics are not used judiciously.

The nurse encourages the parent to provide adequate rest, nutrition, and symptomatic treatment for the child with a cold. Acetaminophen might be given for fever, and fluids

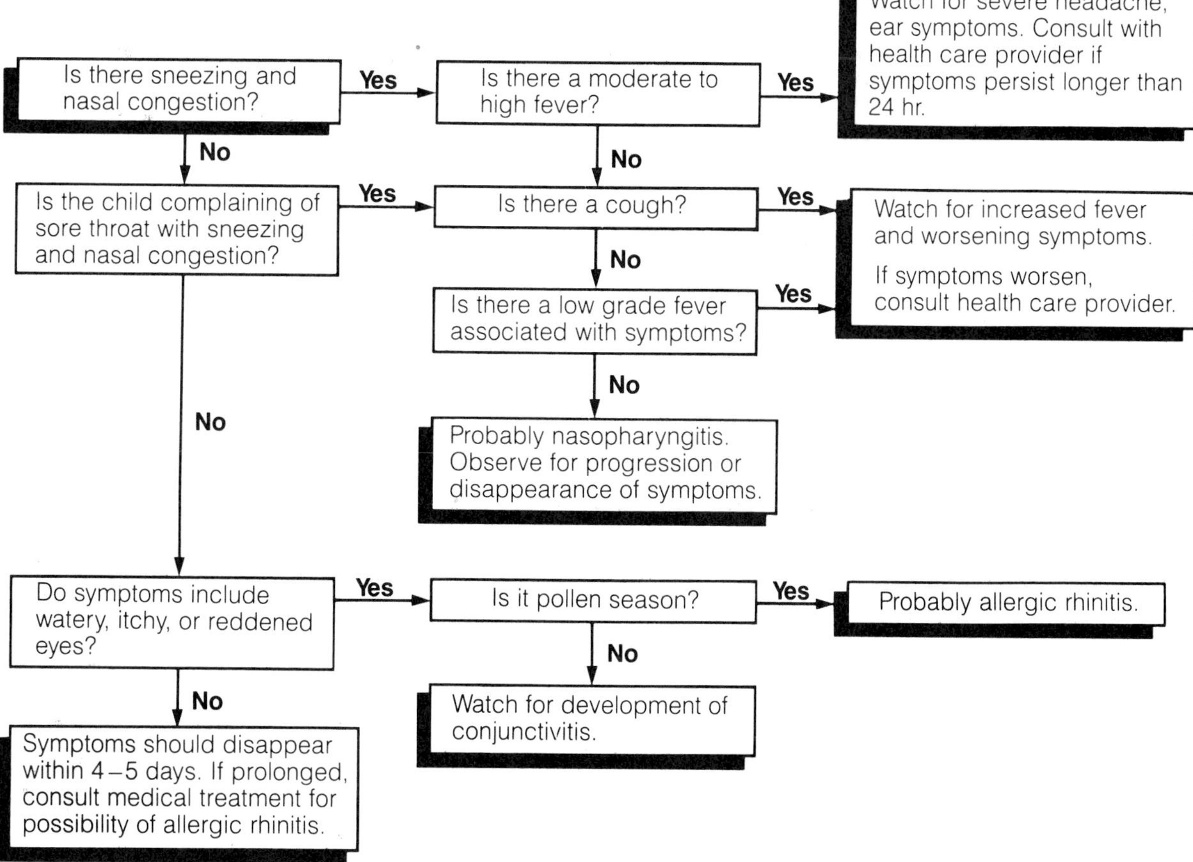

Figure 26-5 Parent decision: rhinitis.

such as fruit juice and cold drinks should be offered frequently to maintain adequate hydration. If nasal congestion is severe, the parent might want to consult the physician regarding the use of antihistamines for symptomatic relief. Great caution should be taken in the use of over-the-counter cold preparations because some of them contain aspirin, which has been implicated in the occurrence of Reyes' syndrome (see Chapter 42). Measures should be taken to prevent the spread of the cold to others by keeping the child home if possible, instructing the child to cover the mouth and nose when coughing or sneezing, and sterilizing dishes in a dishwasher or with very hot water. Parents should be advised that if complications such as ear involvement, high fever, or productive cough develop or if the cold persists for more than 1 week, medical attention should be obtained.

Asthma Asthma is an obstructive disease of the respiratory tract and is common in childhood. It is characterized by an audible, prolonged expiratory wheeze and is often associated with cough, congestion, dyspnea, and other signs of respiratory distress (see Chapter 34). It generally does not occur prior to 2 years of age, but it can be difficult to differentiate from other respiratory disorders and must be a consideration if the child has had previous episodes of allergic rhinitis or bronchitis. The initial asthmatic episode might occur in conjunction with an upper respiratory infection, further complicating the diagnosis (Chai, 1981).

Once the diagnosis has been made, the parents will need support and advice regarding the care of the asthmatic child at home. The child generally will have some type of bronchodilator—either oral, injectable, or inhaled. The nurse can help assess the proper route of administration for medication by evaluating the home setting, parental support system, and age and ability of the child to self-administer the medication. The parent and child will need to know when to administer the medication, how frequently, and how many times it can be repeated. They also need to be specifically instructed to get medical attention if the prescribed medication does not relieve the asthmatic symptoms.

Although it is impossible to rid most homes of all allergens, parents can be encouraged to remove the most common allergens from the child's environment (see Chapter 37). Because asthma might have emotional implications, nurses should be alert to the potential need for a psychologic referral. The parent should avoid overprotecting the child and should permit as normal a childhood as possible. The nurse encourages the parent to use community resources, including parental support groups and community mental health centers, if necessary.

Pharyngitis Pharyngitis (sore throat) is another common respiratory disease among children. It involves an inflammation of the pharynx, and its origin can be either viral or bacterial. Clinically, it is difficult to differentiate viral infections from bacterial infections because the symptoms are similar. Children with pharyngitis usually complain of a sore throat and have a fever and symptoms similar to the common cold. A throat culture is frequently necessary to identify the causative organism and to aid in selecting the appropriate antibiotic if one is indicated. The nurse will need to explain the process of obtaining a throat culture to both the parent and child. The parent also needs to know that it will be 24 hours before the results of the culture are known and that antibiotic therapy probably will not be started until then.

Occasionally, the physician will elect to begin antibiotic therapy immediately, a 2–5-day course of therapy being most commonly prescribed. Philosophies and empirical results concerning the use of antibiotic therapy differ. Some physicians advocate a 10-day course, even if the culture is negative, as this practice appears to protect the child from other organisms and promote a more rapid recovery. Once throat culture results are available, the physician will extend the dosage period for 10 days if the culture is positive for group A beta-hemolytic streptococci. Parents need to be aware of the possibility that the antibiotic course might be extended. The conditions under which physicians might prescribe antibiotics prior to the culture report include the following:

1. A patient or family history of rheumatic fever
2. If the goal is to minimize school absenteeism
3. If additional clinical signs indicate scarlet fever or if family or other intimate contacts have a positive throat culture
4. If the goal is the rapid relief of symptoms (Castiglia and Aquilina, 1982: 379)

Pharyngitis caused by group A beta-hemolytic streptococci may present a clinical picture of a sudden onset of moderate fever, fatigue, headache, abdominal discomfort, and anorexia, followed by the appearance of a sore throat. Some children might experience associated nausea and/or vomiting. The throat appears inflamed, with varying amounts of exudate (Castiglia and Aquilina, 1982). The incidence of streptococcal pharyngitis increases during the winter and spring, and the disease is more commonly found in children who live in crowded environments. The disease is self-limiting; however, if untreated, it can cause serious sequelae in children.

If not properly treated, streptococcal pharyngitis can lead to otitis media, peritonsillar abscess, sinusitis, mastoiditis, acute glomerulonephritis, or acute rheumatic fever (see Chapter 37). The antibiotic of choice is penicillin or one of its derivatives or erythromycin in penicillin-allergic children. It is important to assess the parent's understanding of the need to administer the entire amount of the prescribed medication. If failure to cooperate with the antibiotic regimen is a potential problem, intramuscular rather than oral medication should be considered. Intramuscular penicillin is effective in one dose, as opposed to the 10-day oral dosage schedule. However, because the injection is painful, the oral route is less traumatic and is the treatment of choice when cooperation is assured.

The nurse also stresses the importance of a follow-up visit to assess whether any sequelae have occurred and to obtain a repeat throat culture (Castiglia and Aquilina, 1982). The nurse instructs the parent to seek additional medical attention if the child develops a rash, swollen joints, stiff neck, periorbital edema, earache, or temperature above 101° F that cannot be controlled with acetaminophen.

A careful assessment of the home setting is important if the child with streptococcal pharyngitis is to be cared for at home; vigorous antibiotic therapy and measures to prevent sequelae and the spread of the disease must be instituted. Nursing management includes encouraging the parent to humidify the air; increase the child's fluid intake; relieve discomfort with gargles, lozenges, or hard candy; prevent the spread of infection to other family members; and observe the child for possible complications.

Laryngotracheobronchitis Laryngotracheobronchitis (LTB) is an inflammation of the laryngeal area of viral or bacterial origin that generally affects children under 3 years of age (Wilson, 1984). Laryngotracheobronchitis is similar to spasmodic croup, differing somewhat in the mode of onset and severity of symptoms (see Chapter 34).

Symptoms of laryngotracheobronchitis usually include fever, a persistent cough with a distinctive barking quality, and respiratory distress. The onset usually is preceded by an upper respiratory infection, and the cough commonly occurs at night. The child might appear listless and toxic, and immediate intervention may be essential; other conditions, such as foreign body obstruction, epiglottitis, and diphtheria, present with symptoms similar to laryngotracheobronchitis. The nurse therefore needs to be sure that the child who presents these symptoms is carefully assessed and diagnosed.

If the parent is capable of caring for the child in the home, hospitalization might be avoided, but a careful assessment of the home setting is necessary prior to choosing home care. The nurse carefully considers and assesses the age of the child, the severity of the illness, and the potential for cooperation with the treatment regimen. It will be necessary for the parent to humidify the child's air with cool mist. Sitting with the child in a bathroom with the shower running for steam is an acceptable alternative. Moist night air has been known to relieve symptoms by stimulating mechanoreceptors, which decrease the respiratory rate and facilitate airway opening (Wilson, 1984). The parent must maintain the child's hydration, and extra creativity will be needed to encourage fluids when the child is having difficulty breathing.

The most important consideration is that the parent know when to seek emergency care. Parents should be taught the signs of respiratory distress (see Chapter 34). If the symptoms worsen, if the child exhibits restlessness and anxiety and prefers a sitting rather than a reclining position, or if the child becomes febrile, emergency treatment is indicated. Immediate transportation should be available for this possibility. Parents should be discouraged from administering cough or cold preparations to the child because their drying effect might exacerbate symptoms (Wilson, 1984).

Pneumonia and Pneumonitis Pneumonia is an inflammation involving the lungs that generally is caused by a virus, although it occasionally might be caused by bacteria. Viral pneumonia is sometimes referred to as pneumonitis to differentiate it from bacterial pneumonia. The pathophysiology and treatment are similar regardless of the causative organism. Pneumonia might occur alone or as a complication of an upper respiratory infection. The child with pneumonia usually has a persistent cough, fever, rapid respiration, abdominal pain, and anorexia. Nausea, vomiting, and diarrhea also might be present (see Chapter 34).

Children with pneumonia frequently can be treated at home. The age of the child, the severity of the disorder, and the potential for cooperation with a treatment regimen are critical indicators of the potential for home care. The child might have to take antibiotics for 5–10 days depending on the cause of the pneumonia. In addition, rest and increased fluid intake will be necessary along with analgesics for fever. It might be helpful if the air in the child's room can be humidified with a cool-mist vaporizer. Parental understanding of the treatment regimen and cooperation are essential if the child is to be successfully treated at home. Respiratory complications or failure to improve within 24 hours after treatment is initiated indicate that hospitalization must be considered as an alternative to home care.

Infectious Mononucleosis Mononucleosis is a syndrome that occurs primarily in older children and adolescents. Although caused by the Epstein-Barr virus (De Angelis, 1979), its symptoms are seen in other diseases such as toxoplasmosis and cytomegalovirus (Kolff and Sanchez, 1979). Mononucleosis is characterized by lethargy, extreme fatigue, low-grade fever, mild pharyngitis, and generalized lymphadenopathy. More severe manifestations include splenic and/or liver enlargement. Laboratory tests reveal an elevated atypical lymphocyte count (greater than 10%). A heterophile antibody titer (see Chapter 37) becomes elevated approximately 2 weeks after the onset of the disease and is helpful in making a positive diagnosis (Kolff and Sanchez, 1979). Infectious mononucleosis is transmitted to a susceptible child through saliva. It is a self-limiting disease, usually resolving in several weeks. Relapses can occur if the child returns to vigorous activity before the condition is appropriately resolved.

Mononucleosis rarely requires hospitalization, although hospitalization might be indicated if signs of complications are evident. Peritonsillar abscess, upper airway obstruction, and potential splenic rupture are the complications most often seen. Abnormal liver function tests (see Chapter 38) might indicate impending difficulties.

Because mononucleosis can be associated with a streptococcal pharyngitis (De Angelis, 1979), a throat culture should be performed routinely. Treatment with appropriate antibiotics is indicated for a positive culture. Ampicillin, however, should be used with caution because an allergic-type rash can be seen in some children with mononucleosis who are receiving ampicillin. Corticosteroids might be prescribed for patients with potential airway obstruction or splenomegaly (De Angelis, 1979).

For individuals with mononucleosis, adherence to a home treatment regimen is essential. Because older children are most frequently affected, they should be included in the development of the treatment plan, which usually involves rest, adequate nutritional intake, and increased fluid intake. The nurse emphasizes the importance of diet and rest to both the child and the parent because these are absolutely necessary for optimal recovery. The required therapy is, however, atypical of the usual behavior of adolescents, and it might be difficult to enforce the regimen. The child and parent should understand that recovery might be gradual and that lack of adherence to the treatment plan may prolong the recovery period.

Occasionally, a child will not adhere to a treatment plan regardless of parental cooperation. In these instances hospitalization might be the only viable treatment modality. The parent should be encouraged to seek medical assistance if the child complains of excessive pain in the throat, exhibits any signs of respiratory distress, or complains of epigastric or abdominal pain.

Tuberculosis Active pulmonary tuberculosis occurs less frequently in the United States than it once did and is uncommon among young children (Grzybowski and Allen, 1981). However, immigration to the United States of persons from countries where tuberculosis is still common brings an occasional child with tuberculosis to the clinic or hospital. Tuberculosis is an infection caused by the acid-fast bacillus *Mycobacterium tuberculosis*, which is spread by droplet infection or by the handling of articles contaminated by a person who has the disease. The primary infection might be so mild that it goes unnoticed, but infants and very young children may develop a disseminated tuberculosis known as miliary tuberculosis (see Chapter 34).

If a child has good resistance to disease and is generally healthy, the primary lesion might cause only regional lymphadenopathy, after which the lesion becomes latent. The only sign of tuberculosis might be the conversion of the child's tuberculin test (see Chapter 18) to a positive reaction. These latent lesions might later become activated, usually in adolescence, and therefore children with a positive tuberculin reaction usually are treated with a 9-month to 1-year course of chemoprophylaxis with isoniazid (INH) and periodic chest radiographs to be certain that the disease remains quiescent (Grzybowski and Allen, 1981).

Active tuberculosis is treated by isoniazid (INH) in combination with streptomycin, aminosalicylate (PAS), or other medications such as rifampin (see Chapter 34). The child is no longer considered communicable when sputum and gastric secretions are free of the tuberculin bacillus.

Home care of a child with tuberculosis is a challenge for parents. The child must be isolated from others who are susceptible to tuberculosis, which requires that the child be given a single room. In the home setting parents must carefully dispose of tissues used by the ill child, preferably by incineration. The dishes the child uses must be disposable (burnable) or sterilized, and the child must have adequate rest, nutrition, and a place to sleep and play where exposure to other persons will be minimal.

If the parents want to care for the child at home, nurses can assist them to determine whether their family and home situation is conducive to the restraints placed on them by the care of the child with tuberculosis. If the physical aspect of the home is adequate for care, the potential stress on the family should then be weighed against the potential stress of hospitalization on the child.

It is rare for one member of a family to have active tuberculosis without other family members having at least a positive tuberculin test. Public health departments usually are involved in the follow-up care of families with children with active tuberculosis and will determine what family members might be at risk of developing the disease and therefore need chemoprophylaxis. Public health departments usually make some effort to identify the person from whom the child contracted tuberculosis and make certain that that person receives treatment. Laws vary from state to state, but in most states it is mandatory to report new cases of active tuberculosis to public health officials.

Disorders of the Gastrointestinal System

Disorders of the gastrointestinal system include those that affect the mouth, esophagus, stomach and intestines, colon, anus, and rectum. These disorders may be bacterial, viral, or parasitic in origin. In some instances disorders of the gastrointestinal system appear to be idiopathic, although emotional disturbances might predispose the patient to their development. Disorders of the gastrointestinal system occur in children almost as frequently as disorders of the respiratory system. Many disorders are amenable to home care if a competent parent or caregiver is available, if cooperation with a prescribed treatment regimen can be assured, and if the child is not exhibiting signs of dehydration or hemorrhage. (See Chapter 38 for a discussion of gastrointestinal disorders not covered here.)

Thrush Thrush, often referred to as oral moniliasis or oral candidiasis, is a superficial fungal infection involving the oral cavity. It is caused by *Candida albicans* and might be a result of overgrowth from antibiotic therapy, contamination from an infected person, or contact with infected objects. The incidence seems to be higher in infants, with neonates acquiring the condition from the mother during birth.

There are generally no symptoms of thrush, although if the infection is severe, the child might have pain with swallowing. The child usually is brought to the physician following the appearance of white, tenacious plaques on the oral mucosa. These plaques resemble milk curds but are difficult to remove, and bleed when removal is attempted.

Treatment is with an antifungal agent, such as nystatin oral suspension, which is instilled into the mouth three or four times daily for 1 week. The nurse needs to teach the parent to drop the suspension on the lesions and into the front of the mouth slowly so that the medication will be in contact with the lesions for as long as possible. Sterilization of baby bottles and nipples is recommended to prevent reinfection. If the infant is breast-fed, the mother is advised to wash her nipples with soap and water after each feeding (De Angelis, 1979).

The parent should be advised to bring the child back if the infection does not clear up or if it recurs. The nurse teaches the parent to recognize the signs of dehydration, particularly when oral discomfort prevents adequate fluid intake. A simple method for observing for dehydration includes having the parent watch for infrequent urination or a marked decrease in the number of wet diapers, dry skin, dry lips and tongue, and sunken fontanelles in an infant. Recurrent infection with *Candida albicans* warrants further investigation to rule out such underlying systemic diseases as diabetes mellitus and hypoparathyroidism.

Acute Gastroenteritis The child with acute gastroenteritis (inflammation of the stomach and intestines) usually experiences diarrhea or vomiting or both. Causes of gastroenteritis can be viral or bacterial (see Chapter 38), although in most cases the causative organism is unknown because of the rapid course of the disease.

Fever might or might not be present and, depending on the severity of the vomiting and diarrhea, the child may be dehydrated. Dehydration and the resultant electrolyte imbalance (see Chapter 33) might contraindicate home care for the very young infant with gastroenteritis.

If the origin of the acute gastroenteritis is nonspecific, it is generally treated with dietary restrictions. The parent should be instructed that no specific therapy other than dietary control is available, and because of the potential side effects, the nurse discourages parents from using antidiarrheal and antiemetic medications unless specifically prescribed by the physician. The child should be removed from the current diet and receive only sips of water or ginger ale, approximately 1–2 tbsp every half hour, for the first 12 hours. The health care provider might recommend that the very young infant receive an electrolyte solution such as Pedialyte by mouth. As the child improves, the amount of liquids should gradually be increased over the next 12 hours. If the diarrhea and vomiting continue to improve, easily digested foods such as jello, dry toast, and crackers can be added to the diet. After 48 hours, if improvement continues, the parent may give cereal without milk, bananas, and broiled meat to the child. Milk, eggs, cheese, and other milk products should not be included in the diet until the child has been asymptomatic for 24–48 hours, because temporary lactose intolerance frequently occurs following diarrhea. If the vomiting and diarrhea fail to improve within 24 hours after dietary restrictions are initiated or if the child shows signs of dehydration, additional medical consultation is indicated. The nurse should be certain that the parent understands and will follow the dietary instructions and that the parent knows how to observe for dehydration (Fig. 26-6). If the nurse has any doubts about parental cooperation, alternatives to home care might be indicated.

Acute gastroenteritis occasionally might be caused by a bacterial agent such as *Shigella* or *Salmonella*. The child with a bacterial disorder will have vomiting and diarrhea accompanied by fever, and the history might implicate the ingestion of contaminated food or water. Sources of *Salmonella* include ingestible foods, poultry and eggs for example, as well as certain pets such as turtles. *Shigella* is transmitted through human contact, either directly or through contaminated food or water. If the source of water for the family is a private well and if other members of the family are affected, only boiled water should be used for human consumption until the water supply can be checked by health officials.

Food handlers in the home should make certain that all food is properly covered and refrigerated and that they wash their hands thoroughly before preparing meals. Eating raw eggs and undercooked poultry should be discouraged.

Gastroenteritis caused by *Shigella* or *Salmonella* might be difficult to distinguish from other forms of gastroenteritis on the basis of symptoms. Isolation of the causative organism in stool cultures is the only method to determine the diagnosis positively. The treatment for *Salmonella* gastroenteritis is the same as for nonspecific gastroenteritis, but antibiotics might be indicated for the child with *Shigella* gastroenteritis. These diseases also need to be differentiated from more severe forms of gastroenteritis such as cholera and typhoid. Bacterial organisms as a cause of nausea

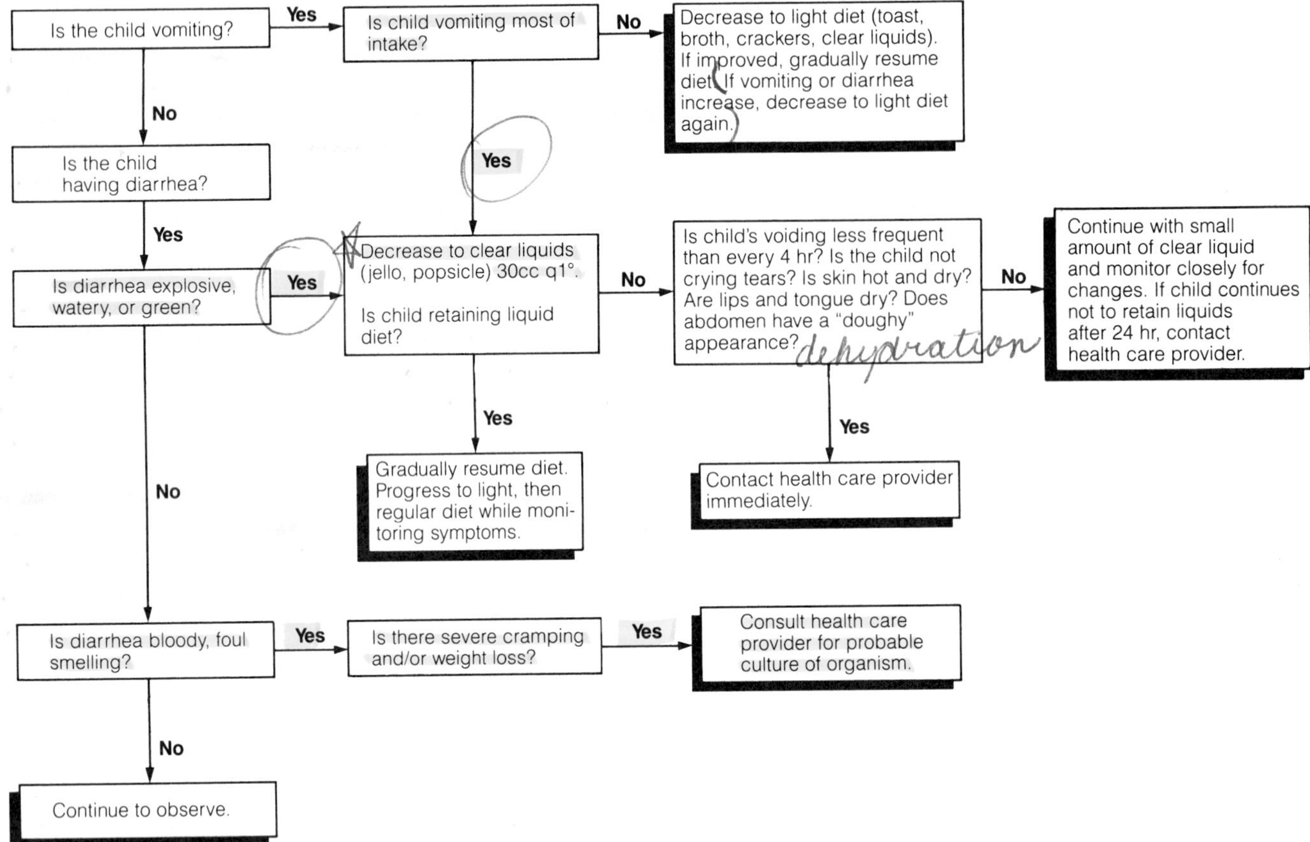

Figure 26-6 Parent decision: acute gastroenteritis.

and vomiting should be a consideration in any child with acute gastroenteritis who does not respond to dietary measures within 24–48 hours.

Intestinal Parasites Many children with intestinal parasites will be asymptomatic, but vague abdominal discomfort, rectal bleeding, anorexia, weight loss, or anemia might be present. Infestation with intestinal parasites is common among school-age children and should be a consideration in all children with vague abdominal complaints. Fortunately, intestinal parasites are easy to eradicate with antiparasitic agents. Frequently, however, it will be necessary to treat the entire family, and, unfortunately, because of the pathophysiology and life cycle of the parasite, reinfestation is likely.

Oxyuriasis (infestation by pinworms), the most common parasitic infection of children in the United States, is caused by *Enterobius vermicularis*. The child complains of rectal itching, although the parent occasionally might see the adult pinworm in the stool. The mature pinworm looks like a short piece of white thread. Diagnosis is made by the brief application of cellophane tape to the perianal region at night and subsequent examination of the tape for the presence of eggs. Infestation usually occurs as a result of the ingestion of eggs by the anus-to-mouth route from contaminated articles. If one member of a family is infested, it is likely that other members are also infested; therefore, all family members are treated simultaneously with an antiparasitic agent such as mebendazole or pyrantel pamoate.

In addition, it is necessary to launder thoroughly all underclothing, bed sheets, night clothes, and towels in hot water to destroy the eggs. The nurse explains to the parent the route of transmission of the parasite and explains the importance of cleaning the clothing and sheets and treating all family members simultaneously. The parent should be encouraged to use good hygiene, including handwashing before eating and after using the toilet, and see that the child does so as well.

Ascaris lumbricoides (roundworm) is a large, round worm, infestation which can be asymptomatic or produce only vague abdominal discomfort. This organism is more common in warm climates, where the egg from an infected person might survive for weeks in the soil before being ingested. The life cycle of the ascaris worm begins with the ingestion of the eggs from contaminated soil. The eggs develop into larvae in the intestine and penetrate the intestinal wall, eventually migrating to the liver, heart, and lungs. If many larvae are present, the child might develop symptoms of atypical pneumonia at this stage, although the child is usually asymptomatic until the larvae ascend to the glottis and are swallowed, thus becoming established in the small intestine, where they may produce symptoms of vague abdominal discomfort. Nausea, vomiting, and weight loss can occur with heavy infestation.

The treatment for ascariasis is the same as for oxyuriasis. All family members must be treated simultaneously, and the prevention of reinfestation requires good personal hygiene. As with oxyuriasis, the parent should launder towels, sheets, underclothing, and night clothing. The parent should scrub toilet facilities and should wash the hands thoroughly after using the toilet and before meals. Rarely do children with intestinal parasitic infestations need to be hospitalized, but extremely heavy infestations might result in partial bowel obstruction, necessitating hospitalization.

Nonspecific, or Functional, Abdominal Pain Children frequently will complain of vague abdominal pain for which no organic cause is apparent. These children should receive a complete and thorough evaluation to rule out all possible pathologic processes. If no pathologic condition is found, the child's environment, family, and progress in school should be evaluated. Functional abdominal pain often has a psychologic origin; therefore, a psychologic consult should be considered (Fig. 26-7).

Constipation Constipation is a disorder of a society that is overly concerned with bodily functions. The emphasis on a regular, daily bowel movement has led parents to interfere with their child's individual bowel schedule in a misguided attempt to prevent constipation.

True constipation is rare in a child. The truly constipated child has infrequent bowel movements that are hard and dry and usually painful to pass. Constipation is treated with dietary measures, including whole-grain cereals, fresh fruits and vegetables, and large quantities of fluids. Laxatives and enemas usually are not necessary and might be harmful. In severe cases a natural laxative or glycerine suppository might be given under the physician's direction.

Occasionally, a child withholds the bowel movement as a form of rebellion against the parent. This is especially likely if the parent has been overly concerned about early toilet training. The nurse can then assist the parent in developing a relaxed attitude toward toilet training and letting nature take its course (see Chapter 13). The parent can be sure the child receives an appropriate diet that is high in fresh fruits and vegetables, whole-grain cereals, and liquids

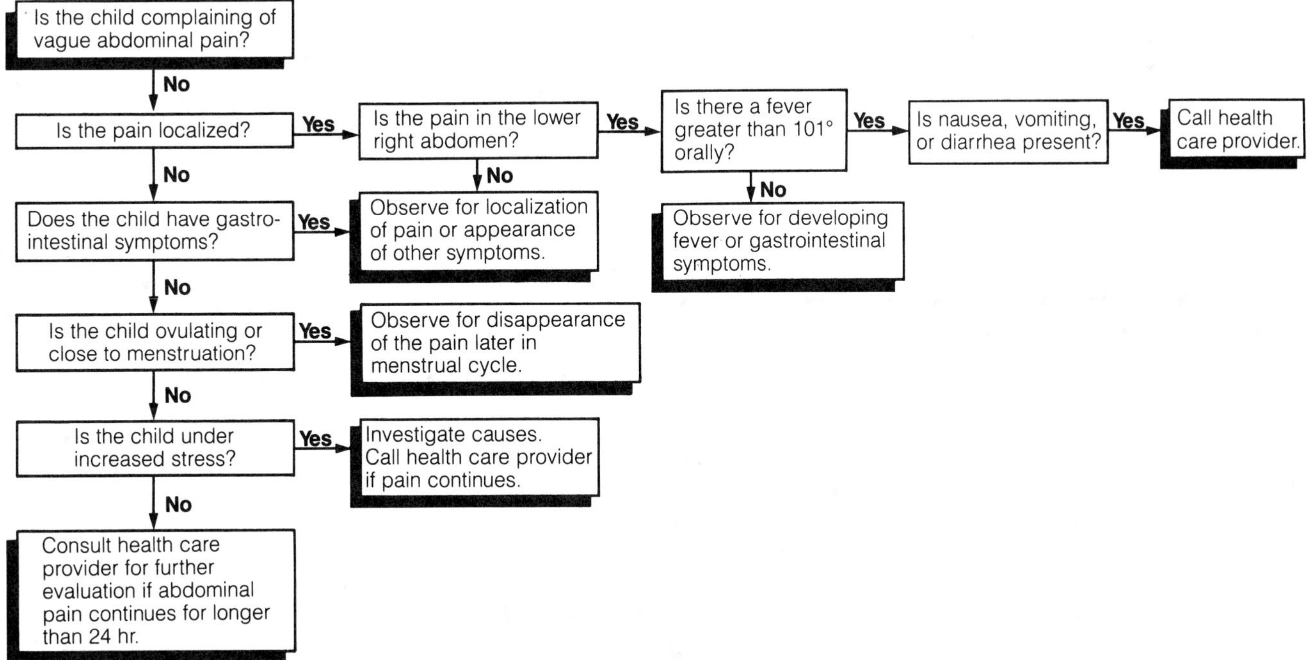

Figure 26-7 Parent decision: abdominal pain.

and low in sugar and starches. Breast-fed infants often might go several days without a bowel movement. Parents can be assured that this is normal so long as the stool appears soft.

Foreign Body Ingestion Infants and young children are constantly putting inappropriate materials in their mouths, most common of which are small objects such as buttons, coins, and marbles. Invariably, if a child puts foreign objects in the mouth, some of them will be swallowed. Smooth objects that reach the stomach without lodging in the esophagus usually will pass through the gastrointestinal tract without difficulty, but sharp objects such as open safety pins, hairpins, and straight needles or pins might perforate the gastrointestinal tract and must be removed either by gastroscope, if the object is in the stomach, or surgically if the object has passed out of the stomach. Occasionally, a smooth object might not pass the pylorus or will become lodged in the intestine, necessitating surgical intervention.

The physician initially will want to know what the child has swallowed and might want radiographs to locate the object in the gastrointestinal tract. If surgical intervention is not indicated, the child will be sent home to be cared for by the parent. No special care is indicated. The child should continue a regular diet, and the parent should examine the stools daily to determine whether the object has passed. Parents can accomplish this by macerating the stool with a tongue depressor if the object is not readily visible. If the child is 6–8 years old or older, helping to search the stool for the foreign object might be a deterrent for placing foreign objects in the mouth in the future.

Communicable Diseases

The development and widespread use of immunologic agents has greatly reduced the incidence of many communicable diseases once common in childhood. Immunizations are available for such childhood diseases as rubeola (measles), rubella (German measles), mumps, pertussis (whooping cough), diphtheria, and tetanus (see Chapter 18). In parts of the United States, immunizations are required for public school attendance. Parents should be urged, however, not to wait until a child is school age to begin the immunizations.

The nurse occasionally might be confronted with a child who has a preventable communicable disease. Such cases appear because most vaccines used for immunizations are about 90%–95% effective, leaving a margin of ineffectiveness, and because there is still a population of children who remain unimmunized, either because of religious beliefs, financial hardship, or lack of parental health education. One of the goals in caring for a child with a communicable disease is to prevent the spread of the disease to others. Therefore, the child usually is cared for at home. Another goal of care is preventing complications from the disease, and the nurse's responsibility is to assist the parent in planning and implementing nursing care to meet this goal.

Many communicable diseases produce a skin rash. Table 26-4 lists the characteristics of the common skin rashes and should help in differentiating one from another.

Rubeola Rubeola (measles) is an acute viral disease that begins as an upper respiratory disorder with fever, sore throat, and cough. The typical red, blotchy rash usually appears 4–5 days after the onset of symptoms. The diagnosis is based on the presence of Koplik's spots in the mouth. These spots have grayish centers with red, irregular outer rings; they are pathognomonic of measles.

Measles progresses in stages, from an incubation period that lasts for 7–14 days to a prodromal period that might last for 3–5 days before the rash appears. The child will be very ill during the prodromal stage, with a fever as high as 104° F, cough, coryza, and possibly conjunctivitis. Koplik's spots appear on the buccal mucosa toward the end of the prodromal stage, a few days before the rash appears. The eruptive stage begins with a dull reddish maculopapular rash on the face and neck, which descends progressively to the trunk, arms, and legs. The child is considered contagious and must be isolated from the onset of the prodromal period until 5 days after the eruptive stage begins. Convalescence usually requires 7–10 days depending on the severity of the illness and the development of complications.

Most children with measles are cared for in the home. The parent should understand that the child's symptoms might worsen through the prodromal stage but that once the eruptive stage is complete, usually on the sixth or seventh day, marked improvement will occur. Treatment is symptomatic. Acetaminophen is given for fever; the child should rest in a dimly lit room to prevent eye discomfort, and increased fluid intake is necessary to maintain hydration. If the child has a cough, it is helpful to humidify the air with a cool-mist vaporizer. The child should be isolated at home until 5 days after the rash appears, and parents should try to protect unimmunized persons from exposure.

The complications of measles include otitis media, pneumonia, myocarditis, or encephalitis. The parent should be told to contact the physician if earaches, productive cough, difficulty in breathing, chest pain, or a headache occur. The child should not be brought to the clinic or hospital without first checking with the physician to avoid exposing susceptible persons.

Parotitis Parotitis (mumps) is a viral disease that is characterized by painful enlargement of the parotid gland. The child with mumps usually will have fever, malaise, and pain behind the ear with chewing or swallowing. Orchitis (swelling of the testicles) occurs in 20%–30% of infected post-

TABLE 26-4 Rashes Associated With Communicable Diseases in Children

Communicable disease	Prodromal symptoms	Appearance of rash	Progression of rash	Supporting clinical data
Measles (rubeola)	Fever of 101–104° F (higher before rash erupts)	Irregular, macular erythema that coalesces into larger red patches; lasts 4–7 days	Begins on face and behind ears; spreads to trunk and extremities	Cold symptoms; Koplik's spots on buccal mucosa; light sensitivity
Rubella (German measles)	Fever rarely over 101° F; possible malaise	Discrete macular rash	Appears first on face, then on trunk and extremities	Posterior cervical lymphadenopathy
Chickenpox (varicella)	Minimal fever; may be preceded by headache, nausea, and/or vomiting	Crops of lesions progressing from macular to papular to vesicular to pustular	Begins on trunk and clusters there with some lesions on extremities; few lesions on face and scalp	Fever might be high in adolescents
Roseola	High fever (to 104° F) for 1–5 days before the rash appears	Diffuse macular rash appears when fever subsides	Primarily confined to trunk	Possible mild pharyngitis
Erythema infectiosum (Fifth disease)	Usually none	Red coalescent macules that are raised and warm	Appears first on cheeks, then spreads to extremities	Usually none
Scarlet fever	Fever of 102° F or higher	Diffuse erythematous rash that fades with pressure except in the antecubital area	First noticed in areas of warmth and pressure; spreads to trunk and extremities	Sore throat with exudative pharyngitis and lymphadenopathy; strawberry-colored tongue; desquamation of palms and soles of the feet as the disease resolves

pubertal males (Thomson, 1982). Treatment is symptomatic and involves analgesics to relieve pain, ice packs to reduce swelling, and rest. If orchitis is present, the physician might prescribe cortisone; because of the weight of the swollen testicle or testicles, it might be necessary to suspend the scrotum in a sling or suspensory to prevent discomfort. Because mumps is a contagious disease, the child should be isolated at home until the parotid swelling is gone, usually 7–10 days.

Encephalitis is the most severe potential complication that can occur with mumps. The parent should be advised to observe the child for any signs of mental confusion, sudden severe headache, projectile vomiting, stiffness in the neck or back, or a sudden dramatic increase in fever up to 105° F. The physician should be contacted or the child brought to the clinic or hospital if any of these symptoms develop.

Rubella Rubella (German measles), a viral infection, usually is manifested as a discrete macular rash beginning on the face and spreading rapidly to the trunk, arms, and legs. Symptoms include lethargy, anorexia, a slight temperature elevation, and general lymphadenopathy, but these symptoms might be mild and may not be recognized. Rubella is a mild disease that lasts only 3–5 days and requires no specific treatment. If contracted during pregnancy, the infection, can, however, affect the fetus, causing severe congenital anomalies such as cardiac defects and cataracts. Thus, the major goal of treatment is to isolate the child at home to prevent the possible exposure of pregnant women. A rubella titer to determine susceptibility to the disease might be advisable for preadolescent girls who have not been immunized. Nurses might need to advise parents of preadolescent girls to have their children immunized to prevent congenital anomalies should they be exposed to rubella when they are pregnant. (*See Color Plate.*)

Pertussis Pertussis (whooping cough) is a bacterial respiratory infection caused by the gram-negative bacillus *Bordetella pertussis*. Pertussis is transmitted from person to person by droplets or by contact with soiled articles from someone infected with the disease. The incubation period is from 7 to 10 days, and the child is considered communicable from 1 week before to 3 weeks after the onset of paroxysms of coughing. Although a vaccine against pertussis has been available since 1950, approximately 2000 cases are still reported each year in the United States. Half of these cases occur in children under 1 year old, and parents who delay in beginning immunizations for their infants leave them unprotected against the disease. The pertussis vaccine is not, however, as effective as some of the other vaccines, and the immunity it provides declines rapidly. Few adults, even those immunized in childhood, are immune to pertussis, and transplacental passage of the pertussis antibody to the fetus is uncommon (Baraff, 1981).

Pertussis begins with symptoms of an upper respiratory infection: fever, runny nose, sneezing, and cough. Within 2 weeks, however, the cough becomes paroxysmal with a series of coughs followed by a deep inspiration that produces the characteristic whoop from which the disease gets its name. Periods of cyanosis might occur as a result of severe paroxysms of coughing in the very young child. Coughing spasms might cause vomiting in infants and very young children, resulting in problems with nutrition and hydration. These problems might contraindicate home care for the very young child with pertussis, but when an appropriate caregiver is present, older children might be cared for at home.

Home care goals include symptomatic care and the prevention of complications. Although antibiotics probably do not affect the course of the disease, an antibiotic, usually erythromycin, may be prescribed, to be given by mouth for 10 days to prevent pulmonary complications. Because many children vomit with the paroxysmal coughing, the parent should offer frequent small feedings and observe the child for signs of dehydration. Aspiration of the emesis is also a concern, and the most common serious complication is pneumonia. The parent should be advised to maintain a quiet environment for the child because excitement might precipitate a coughing spasm (De Angelis, 1979). The parent should be advised to observe the child for symptoms of respiratory distress between the paroxysms of coughing; these symptoms include rapid respirations and retractions. If these occur or if the child develops a fever, further medical attention is necessary.

Diphtheria Diphtheria is an acute febrile upper respiratory infection caused by *Corynebacterium diphtheriae.* It is a rare disease, with only about 250 cases reported in the United States each year; the fatality rate, however, is approximately 10% (Fekety, 1981). It primarily affects unimmunized children under 15 years of age and is spread by droplets from a diseased person or carrier. The incubation period is from 1–7 days, with a short prodromal period of a mild sore throat that might interfere with breathing. The formation of a false membrane on the nasal or pharyngeal wall or the tonsils causes cyanosis and eventual respiratory obstruction. Diphtheria antitoxin must be given promptly, and respiratory and cardiac complications are common. Therefore, the child with diphtheria cannot be cared for in the home setting and must be hospitalized.

Tetanus Tetanus is an acute disease caused by the toxin of the bacillus. *Clostridium tetani,* which is introduced into the body through open wounds via contaminated soil. The incubation period varies from 5 days to 5 weeks depending on the amount of exposure, the speed with which the bacterium reproduces, and the amount of toxin produced. The fatality rate ranges from 35%–70% depending on the severity of the disease, the age of the patient, and the time lapse between initial exposure and the initiation of treatment.

Tetanus is a preventable disease, and immunization should begin at 2 months of age (see Chapter 18). Because tetanus can result from relatively minor wounds, children who receive any injury in which there is a laceration should receive tetanus prophylaxis according to their immunization status (see Chapter 44). All wounds should be thoroughly cleaned as a preventive measure.

The symptoms of tetanus primarily are painful muscular contractions of the neck and jaw but also of the trunk, leading to spastic rigidity. Intensive therapy is necessary because tetanus might affect the muscles of respiration. Thus, the person suspected of having tetanus is always hospitalized.

Chickenpox Chickenpox (varicella) is an acute communicable disease caused by the herpes zoster virus. The incubation period is from 11 to 21 days but may be as long as 25 days, the average being 15 days. The child is considered to be communicable from up to 5 days before the skin eruptions occur until the lesions are dry.

A slight prodrome of fever might precede the appearance of skin lesions, which tend to erupt in crops. The lesions begin on the neck or the trunk and spread to the face, scalp, mucous membranes, and extremities. The lesions first appear as small, flat, red blotches that progress to raised vesicles; crust formation occurs over a period of 2–4 days. Pruritus might be severe, and the prevention of secondary infection is a major goal of care. Isolation at home is necessary to prevent inadvertent exposure of nonimmune adults and persons with altered immunologic status. Prevention might be undesirable in children, however, because chickenpox in the adult is often more severe. Children receiving corticosteroid therapy should be referred to a physician immediately if exposed to chickenpox.

The goal of treatment is to prevent complications and relieve symptoms. The parent should be advised to cut the child's fingernails short and have the child wear gloves if necessary to prevent scratching and secondary infection. Antihistamines or antipruritic medications may be prescribed to be given orally to relieve pruritus. Also, calamine lotion or a mild anesthetic ointment may be applied to the lesions. Tepid sponge baths seem to relieve the pruritus, and an antiseptic soap reduces the risk of secondary infection. Complications from chickenpox include encephalitis and abscess of secondarily infected vesicles, but these complications are unusual, and the child usually can return to school in 1 week if there are no new lesions. Reye's syndrome (see Chapter 42) might possibly be linked to the occurrence of varicella, and the nurse should advise parents to be alert for signs of fever, severe vomiting, abrupt behavior change, and changes in the level of consciousness. (*See Color Plate.*)

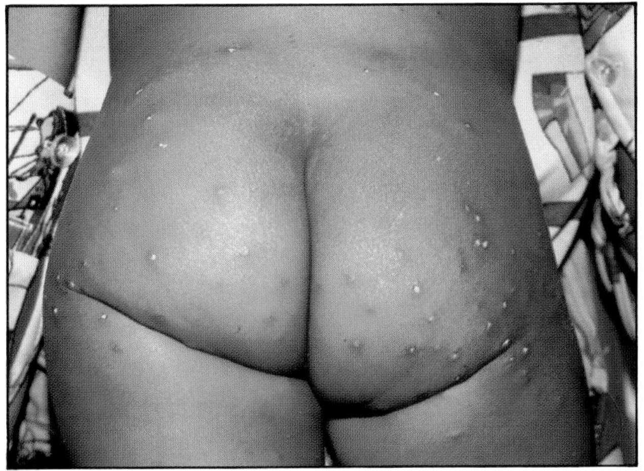

1 Varicella (see Chapter 26)

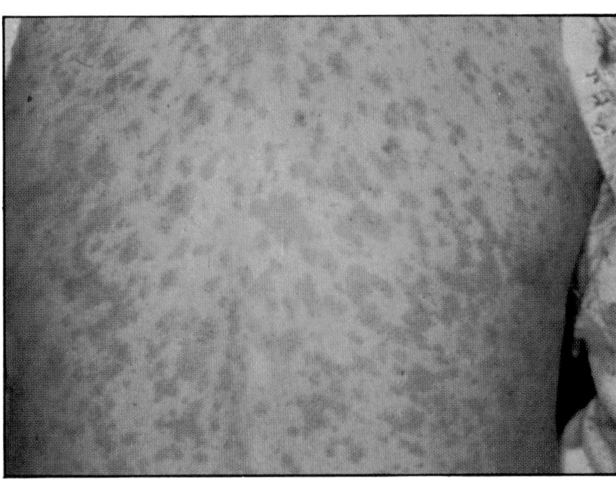

2 Rubeola (see Chapter 26)

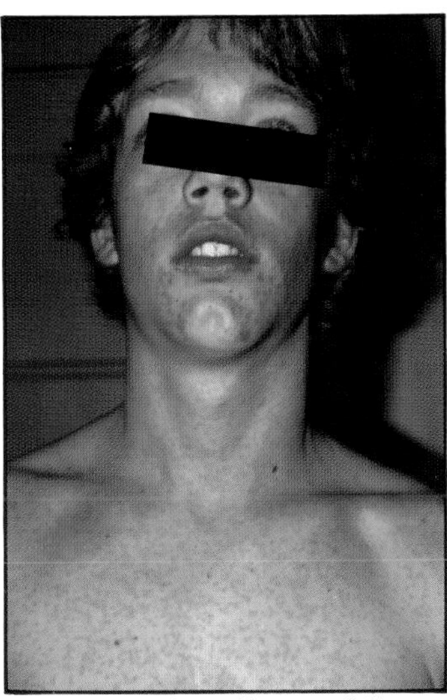

3 Rubella (see Chapter 26)

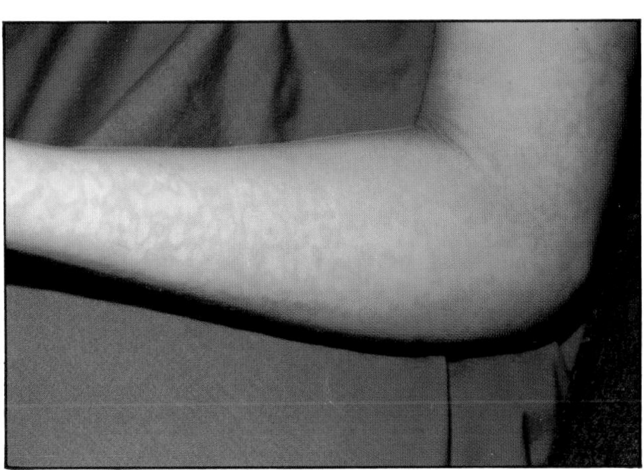

4 Erythema infectiosum (see Chapter 26)

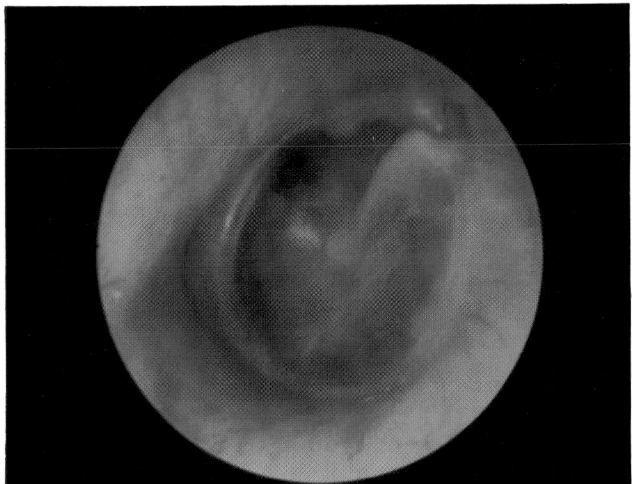

5 Normal tympanic membrane (see Chapter 26)

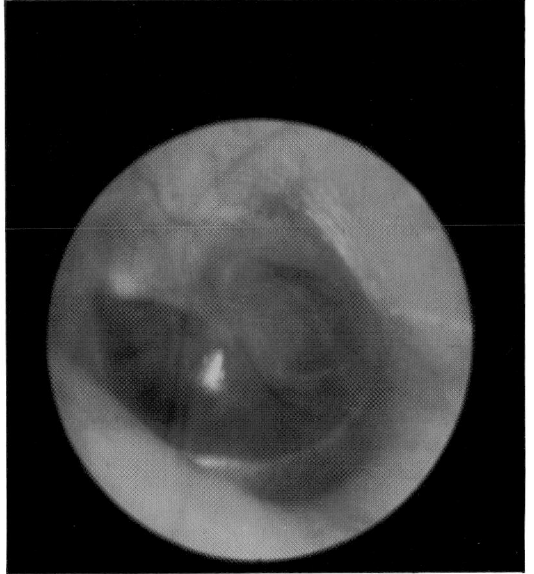

6 Serous otitis media (see Chapter 26)

Photos 1–4 courtesy of Steven Binnick, MD, PC.

Photos 5 and 6 courtesy of Terry L. Fry, MD and Benjamin Chen, PhD, Division of Otolaryngology, University of North Carolina School of Medicine.

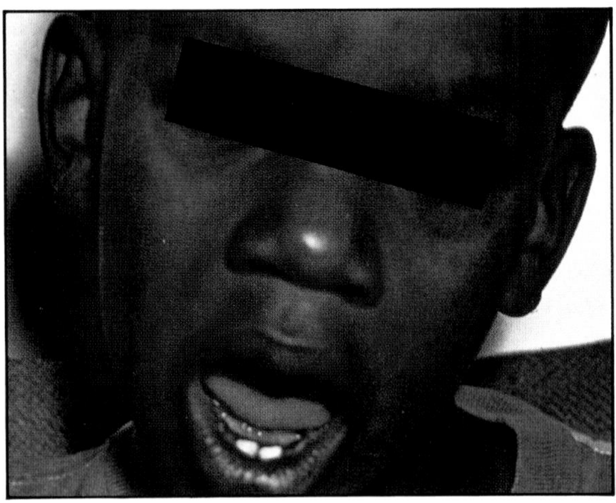

7 Cyanosis in pigmented skin (see Chapter 35)

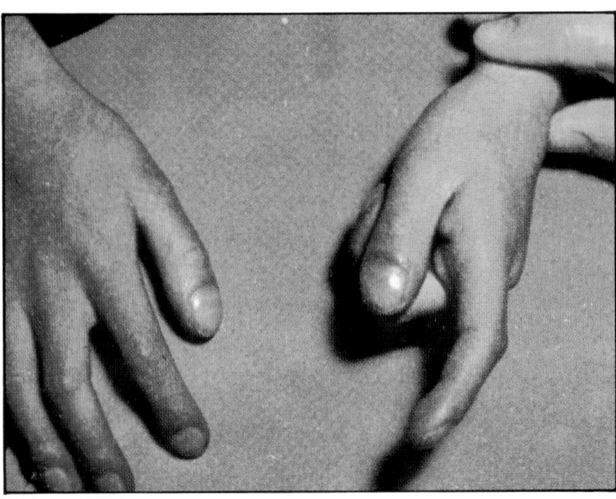

8 Clubbed fingers (see Chapter 34)

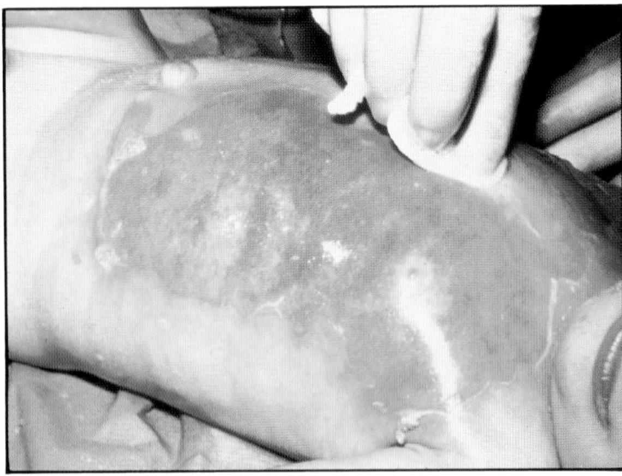

9 Partial thickness burn—child with a scald to chest and abdomen (see Chapter 44)

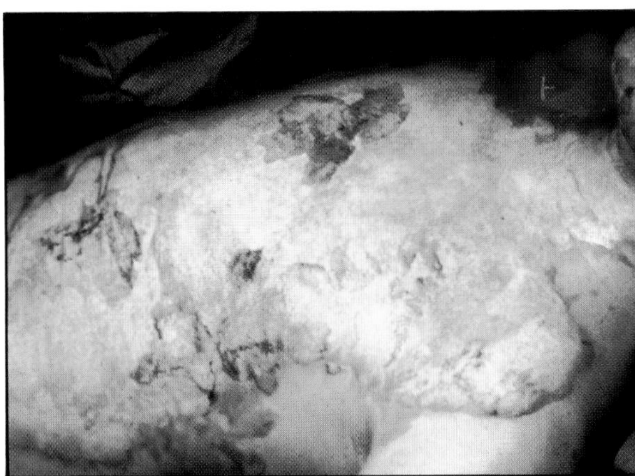

10 Full thickness burn—child burned from clothing ignition, a short time after the burn occurred (see Chapter 44)

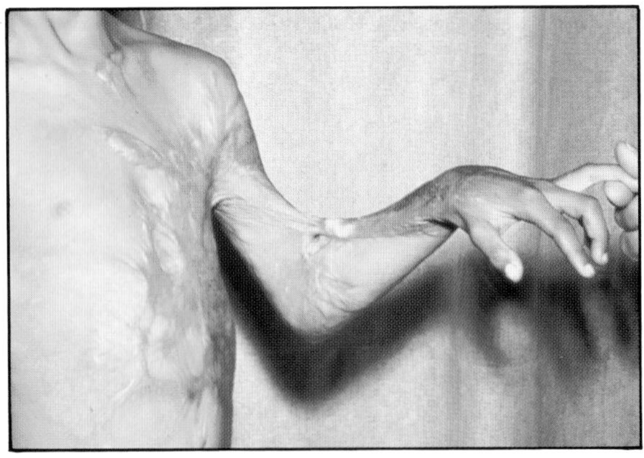

11 Scar band resulting in elbow joint contracture; splints not used after a full thickness burn (see Chapter 44)

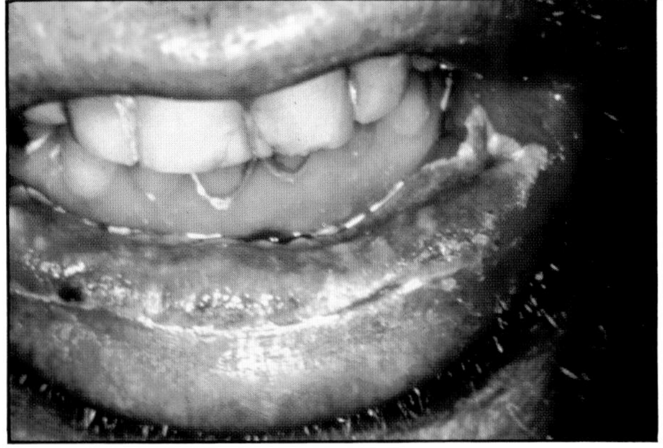

12 Mucositis (see Chapter 45)

Photo 8 courtesy of James Moller, MD, and Roy Anderson, MD, University of Minnesota Hospital.

Photos 9–11 courtesy of Shriners Burns Institute, Boston, Massachusetts.

Photo 12 used with permission, from Arthur T. Skarin, MD, Dana-Farber Cancer Institute, Boston, Massachusetts.

Roseola Roseola (exanthem subitum) is an acute febrile illness in infants and young children that is believed to be caused by a virus. The mode of transmission and incubation period are not known. It is characterized by a high fever of 101–104° F that lasts from 1 to 5 days and is followed by a faint rash as the fever subsides. The rash first appears on the chest and trunk and spreads to the face and extremities. It is a discrete maculopapular rash that might last from 2 to 48 hours. Roseola is a mild disease lasting only a few days and is always treated at home. The principal complication is febrile seizures. Treatment is usually symptomatic, with rest and acetaminophen for fever. Tepid sponge baths may be given if the fever is not controlled by acetaminophen. (*See Color Plate.*)

Erythema Infectiosum Erythema infectiosum (fifth disease) is a mild, contagious viral disease that is characterized by a rash similar to the rash seen with measles. The incubation period is from 7 to 14 days. The child is afebrile and might be asymptomatic. A rash appears first on the cheeks as red coalescent macules that are raised and warm. It spreads to the extensor surfaces of the extremities on the second day and over the next several days to the flexor surfaces and trunk. The palms and soles usually are not involved. The rash might last 3–7 days and may recur after 7–10 days. It tends to occur in epidemics and requires no special treatment, but a careful differential diagnosis is indicated to rule out other causes of childhood rashes. (*See Color Plate.*)

Scarlet Fever Scarlet fever involves a streptococcal pharyngitis plus a systemic reaction to the erythrogenic toxin of the *Streptococcus* bacterium. Scarlet fever is not communicable, but the streptococcal pharyngitis that causes it is communicable. It occurs most frequently in children under 10 years old and is characterized by a rash that appears 12–18 hours after the onset of fever.

The rash appears first in areas of pressure and warmth, such as the neck, axilla, and groin, and spreads to involve the trunk and limbs. It is a diffuse erythematous rash that fades with pressure, although transverse areas of rash at the antecubital area do not fade with pressure (Pastia's sign). The tongue might take on a beefy red, raspberry appearance with the papillae desquamated, enlarged, and erythematous. Desquamation of the skin might occur in the second week; peeling of the fingertips, palms of the hands, and soles of the feet is significant diagnostically. The treatment for scarlet fever is the same as for streptococcal pharyngitis, and the same complications might occur.

Vectorborne Diseases

Communicable diseases that are transmitted from humans to humans or from animals to humans by an arthropod intermediary such as mosquitos, fleas, or ticks are called vectorborne diseases. Many of the vectorborne diseases, such as yellow fever and malaria, are endemic to tropical countries and are seldom found in temperate climates. Examples of vectorborne diseases in the United States include Rocky Mountain spotted fever, equine encephalitis, babesiosis, and, in rare instances, plague.

Prevention of vectorborne diseases includes avoiding exposure to potentially hazardous arthropods and destroying any breeding grounds near inhabited areas.

Rocky Mountain Spotted Fever Rocky Mountain spotted fever (RMSF) is caused by a rickettsial organism that is transmitted to humans by infected ticks. It occurs most frequently in the spring and summer months in the southern United States, along the Atlantic coast, and in the Rocky Mountain region. It is characterized by a prodrome of nonspecific symptoms, including fever, restlessness, headache, and anorexia. One to five days later, a pale, discrete maculopapular rash appears, beginning first on the wrists, ankles, soles of the feet, or palms. Later symptoms include edema and central nervous system manifestations.

Treatment includes antibiotic therapy, which is most effective if begun early in the course of the disease. Tetracycline or chloramphenicol are the drugs of choice (Thompson, 1983). If treatment is delayed or if nausea and vomiting are present, intravenous antibiotic therapy will be necessary, which requires hospitalization of the ill child. If the disease is mild and therapy is initiated early, the child may be cared for in the home. The nurse should explain to the parents the importance of taking the prescribed medication and have them contact the physician or bring the child to the clinic should nausea or vomiting develop. Complications include pneumonia, otitis media, dehydration, myocarditis, and neurologic disorders; children with complications should receive immediate medical attention, possibly including hospitalization.

Because the infected tick must be imbedded in the child for 4–6 hours before the organism causing RMSF is transmitted (Thompson, 1983), frequent tick checks are an effective preventive measure. Ticks inhabit trees and long grass; therefore, the nurse should advise parents to check their children for ticks twice a day if they play in wooded or grassy areas. Removal of an imbedded tick can be a difficult task because complete removal, including the head, is essential. Methods for removal include the application of substances such as nail polish, petroleum jelly, or oil in an attempt to prompt the tick to loosen its grip. Because it takes approximately 30 minutes for the tick to relax, an alternative method of removal is to extract the tick by pulling with the fingers or preferably tweezers and turning the tick counterclockwise as close to the skin as possible. The fingers should be protected with paper towel or tissue because it is possible for rickettsiae to enter the body even when there is no opening in the skin.

Once the tick is removed, the wound and the parent's hands should be washed thoroughly, preferably with an antiseptic solution. Tick removal can be an unpleasant task for the parent and child. If the parent is unable to remove the tick, professional assistance should be sought.

Other Vectorborne Diseases Other diseases associated with ticks include tick toxicosis, an ascending paralysis that resolves after tick extraction, Lyme disease, a syndrome resembling arthritis that is caused by *Ixodes dammini,* and babesiosis, a disease transmitted by the smaller deer tick (Thompson, 1983). The severity of symptoms associated with equine encephalitis transmitted by mosquitoes from infected horses, and plague caused by *Yersinia pestis* infection and sometimes transmitted by lice, necessitate that the child be hospitalized.

Disorders of the Skin

Skin disorders usually are not acute illnesses. They are almost always cared for in the home setting. Many skin disorders, however, if not appropriately treated, can lead to complications, and it is therefore important for the parent or caregiver to have complete, accurate information regarding the appropriate prescribed treatment (see Chapter 44 for the nursing care of children with tinea infections and acne).

Pediculosis Pediculosis (head lice) causes intense pruritus, which is usually the first symptom. The nape of the neck is most frequently the site of the initial infestation of this easily transmitted infection. The lice are very difficult to find, but the eggs, or nits, are readily identifiable. They are small, translucent, white ovals attached to the base of the hair shaft approximately $\frac{1}{4}$ to $\frac{1}{2}$ in from the scalp. They are literally glued to the hair shaft by the female louse and are difficult to remove. Occasionally, secondary infection or excoriation might be caused by scratching.

Lice epidemics are becoming more prevalent among school-age children (McLaury, 1983), although they are not exclusive to this population. They are highly communicable from child to child, usually through sharing hats, combs, and articles of clothing that contact the head. If pediculosis is discovered by the school nurse, affected children will be sent home for treatment and not readmitted until they are appropriately cared for. The nurse's sensitivity to this issue is important because lice infestation historically has been associated with unsanitary conditions.

Nurses need to instruct parents carefully regarding the appropriate management of pediculosis. If a secondary infection is present, it should be cleared prior to initiating treatment for the infestation. A variety of pediculocide shampoos are presently available: gamma benzene hexachloride (lindane), malathion, and pyrethrin are most commonly used. Although lindane is more convenient to use because of its shorter time on the scalp, central nervous system and hematologic complications recently have been found to be associated with its use (Clore, 1983; McLaury, 1983). Lindane should not be applied to infants or pregnant women. Treatment involves applying the shampoo according to directions, being careful not to get the shampoo in the child's eyes. Should the shampoo accidentally contact the eyes, they should be rinsed with large amounts of water. After shampoo is rinsed from the hair, the nits must be combed out with a fine-tooth comb or removed individually by hand. This procedure is essential because the shampoo is not guaranteed to kill all the eggs. Parents should repeat the treatment in 7–10 days to kill any lice that might have hatched since the initial treatment.

Control of lice in the home includes laundering all contaminated articles with hot, soapy water or putting them through a 20-minute hot cycle in a clothes dryer (McLaury, 1983). Combs and brushes can be soaked in the pediculocide. Thorough vacuuming eliminates any lice harbored in furniture or carpets. Clothing or blankets that cannot be laundered or dry cleaned can be stored in a sealed plastic bag for 10 days (McLaury, 1983).

Parents should check their children's heads frequently by parting the hair with two Popsicle sticks or tongue depressors. Preventive measures include not sharing such objects as hats, combs, brushes, or scarves. The nurse therefore explains this to both the parent and the child.

Scabies The itch mite, *Sarcoptes scabiei,* is the causative agent of scabies. The mite burrows under the skin, causing a fine papular rash and intense pruritus that is sometimes worse at night. The mite leaves a telltale burrow under the skin, which is occasionally visible between the fingers and in the axillary and cubital regions. Lesions are rarely found on the face.

Burrows may be overlooked in young children because they may be distributed on the head, palms, and soles of the feet. Finger webs, nipples of females, and the penis and scrotum of males seem to be target areas. Most parts of the body, however, can be affected. Scabies appear as gray-white, very thin lines. The mite may appear as a tiny white dot at the end of the thin line. Papules, pustules, wheals, and bullae may also be present. These lesions do not contain mites. A burrow that has not been excoriated is likely to contain the mite.

Feces from the mites are thought to be the cause of the itching. Itching, which is worse at night, is the major complaint of a child infected with the scabies mite. Clean, hygienic persons, contrary to many people's thinking, may also have scabies. They probably will not have as many burrows and the burrows may not be as easily seen. Poor hygiene and close living quarters increase the susceptibility to the infection.

Treatment is with gamma benzene hexachloride lotion, applied at bedtime, left on for 12–24 hours, and then washed off. The lotion is applied over the entire body from the neck to the feet. Retreatment might be necessary after several days. Again, caution should be exercised to prevent complications from lindane. The bed linens and clothing should be washed in hot water at the time of treatment, and all affected family members should be treated simultaneously.

Secondary infections from scratching are common in children with scabies. If a secondary infection is present, it must be treated and cleaned prior to using the gamma benzene hexachloride lotion because open lesions will cause potentially harmful levels of the medication to be absorbed. If a secondary infection is not present, measures such as cutting the fingernails and scrubbing with soap and water should be employed to prevent this complication from developing.

Allergic Reactions Allergic reactions can be classified into two broad groups: those caused by exogenous agents and sometimes referred to as contact dermatitis and those caused by endogenous or systemic agents such as foods, medications, or inhalants. Depending on the agent, the amount, and the sensitivity of the individual, these reactions can range from mildly irritating to life-threatening. The nurse is frequently the person that the parent first contacts in trying to determine whether medical care is needed.

Systemic reactions are more likely life-threatening than localized reactions. They can be caused by injections of antibiotics or by other biologic sources such as immunizations to which the individual is sensitive, ingestion of medications, insect stings, or foods (see Chapter 37). The most severe reactions generally are caused by injected medications or by insect stings in a highly sensitive person. A systemic reaction that might result in anaphylaxis begins with a generalized flush, followed rapidly by welts, wheals, rash, and intense pruritus. Difficulty breathing or wheezing might precede the onset of shock and indicates that immediate medical attention is needed. The shorter the interval between the initiating event and the onset of symptoms, the more severe the reaction and the greater the possibility of anaphylaxis. Parental action depends on the symptoms involved (Fig. 26-8). (See Chapter 37 for a discussion of other allergic skin manifestations.)

Emotional Disturbances

Many emotionally disturbed children are cared for in the home. Most emotional disorders are chronic, but acute exacerbations might occur. A careful assessment of the home (Table 26-1) is as necessary before selecting a treatment setting for the emotionally disturbed child as it is for the child with a physical disorder. The nurse participates in decision making and treatment planning with the cooperation and participation of those who will be responsible for the child's care. The implications of chronic illness are covered in Chapter 30; the implications of dysfunctional behavior are discussed in Chapter 24.

Minor Accidents and Emergencies

Parents intervene in most minor accidents and emergencies in the home setting, and the child might never see a health professional. If the parent is in doubt about whether to seek professional care, however, the nurse might be consulted. The nurse therefore needs to know the accidents and emergencies that can safely be cared for at home, acceptable

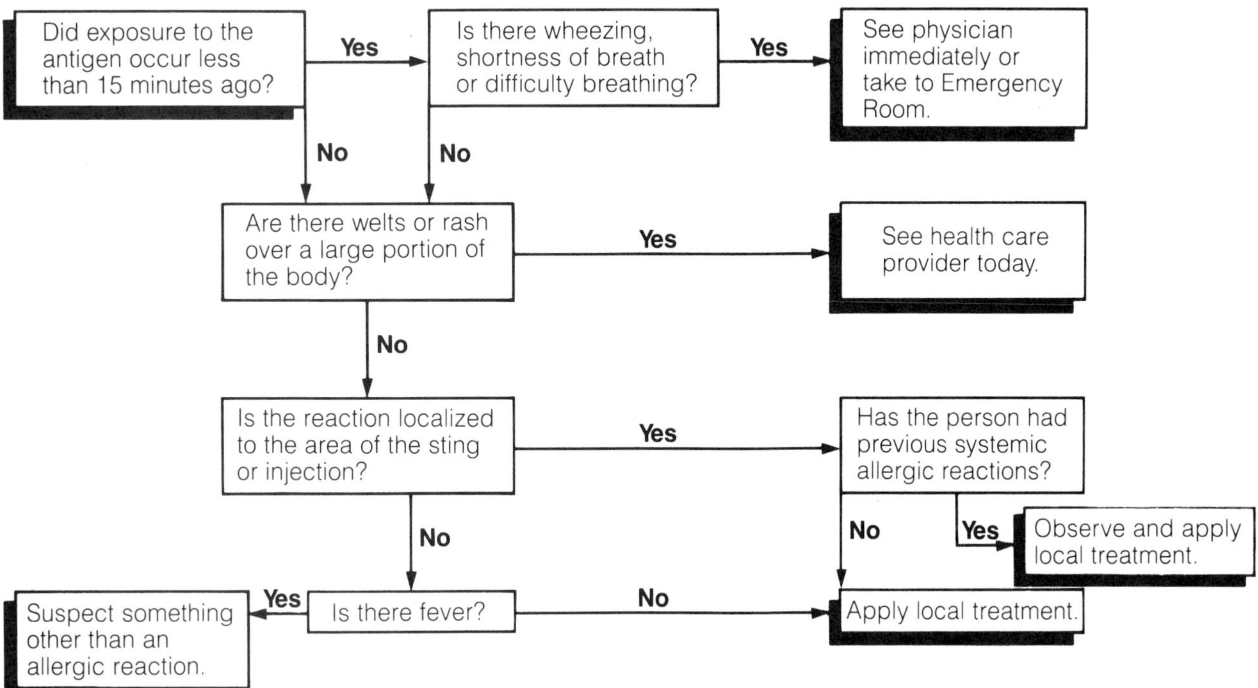

Figure 26-8 Parent decision: systemic allergic reactions.

home treatments, and parameters that indicate referral for further medical care.

Epistaxis Epistaxis is a spontaneous hemorrhage from the nose as a result of a ruptured blood vessel in the nares. It might be caused by a blow to the head or nose, picking the nose, or a foreign body or object inserted into the nares. It occurs most frequently in the winter months when the air is dry and home heating removes moisture from the air, which causes the nasal mucosa to become fragile and dry.

Treatment consists of applying pressure to the site of the bleeding by pressing the nares together. The child should be instructed to breathe through the mouth. Sitting upright and leaning slightly forward will prevent blood from going down the throat. Compression of the nostrils should be continued for 15 minutes, and the child should rest quietly for 15–20 minutes after the bleeding stops. If the bleeding cannot be controlled by compressing the nares together for 15 minutes, further medical consultation is indicated.

Children who have recurrent episodes of epistaxis should be instructed in preventive measures. A cool-mist humidifier should be used in the child's room during the winter months to humidify the air. The child should be discouraged from picking at the nares, and if the nares are dry, a water-soluble lubricant (such as K-Y jelly) can be rubbed on the septum two or three times a day. If episodes of epistaxis are frequent or difficult to control, an evaluation to rule out anemia or hemorrhagic disorders might be indicated.

Contusions A contusion is an injury caused by a blunt blow to the body in which the skin is not broken. A contusion causes the rupture of small blood vessels beneath the skin, which results in swelling and discoloration (bruise) at the site of the injury. The treatment for contusions is to apply ice for 48 hours to reduce swelling. Applications of heat are indicated in 48 hours if significant swelling is still present.

Parents should observe children with contusions of the head for cerebral concussion for 12–24 hours following the injury. A concussion should be suspected if there is any loss of consciousness, headache, apathy, irritability, or vomiting. Tense or bulging fontanelles in an infant might indicate increased intracranial pressure. If concussion is suspected, the parent should seek immediate medical attention for the child.

Lacerations A laceration is a regular or irregular cut or tear of the skin. Children who are active by nature seem to be forever falling, jumping, and bumping into objects that cause lacerations. Minor lacerations usually can be treated at home. Major lacerations, those that are deep or involve tendons or nerves, require medical attention. A minor laceration does not penetrate the subcutaneous tissue (Fig. 26-9).

Home treatment of lacerations includes cleansing the wound with soap and water, making certain that all dirt and foreign objects are removed, and bandaging the wound with a sterile dressing. The bandage should be kept clean and dry and should be changed if it becomes wet because bacteria multiply rapidly in warmth and dampness. Decisions about suturing lacerations need to be made within 6 hours of the injury because a longer time interval will jeopardize the success of the procedure.

The parent needs to be taught to watch for signs of infection. Any redness, heat, and purulent drainage in the wound indicates the need for medical consultation. Red streaking from the site is a dangerous manifestation. The nurse assesses the immunization status of any child with a laceration, and tetanus prophylaxis should be carried out if indicated (see Chapter 44).

Burns Burns usually are caused by exposure to heat. They also might result from exposure to electricity or chemicals, but burns caused by heat are the most common type of burn in children. Burns are classified according to how deeply they penetrate the skin layers (see Chapter 44 for discussion of degrees of burns).

Sunburn is a common complaint in young children, particularly at the beginning of the summer months when the skin is most sensitive because of lack of exposure to the sun. Mild sunburn can cause discomfort, whereas severe sunburn with blistering can result in additional complications. Treatment for sunburn involves the application of cool compresses and/or an anesthetic lotion or spray such as Solarcaine or Noxema. The child should be protected from further exposure to the sun. If blistering occurs over an extended area, the parent should be encouraged to call the physician.

Sunburn can be prevented by gradual exposure, avoidance of the midday sun, keeping sensitive areas covered with hat and clothing, and the use of sunscreens. The parent should remember to reapply the sunscreen after the child has been swimming. Some children exhibit allergic reactions to certain ingredients in sunscreens. Should this occur, the parent might try a sunscreen with alternate ingredients.

Exposure to Toxins Exposure to certain toxins can cause allergic reactions that might be severe in some children. Toxins might be from biologic sources, such as insect stings or *Rhus* resin, or they may be from chemical sources such as pesticides or herbicides. The severity of the reaction is directly related to the extent of the exposure, the method of exposure (contacted, inhaled, ingested, or injected), and the susceptibility of the individual. The reaction may be local or systemic, much like an allergic reaction, or it might be neurogenic (see Chapter 18). All children with suspected toxic chemical exposure and neurologic symptoms should receive immediate medical attention.

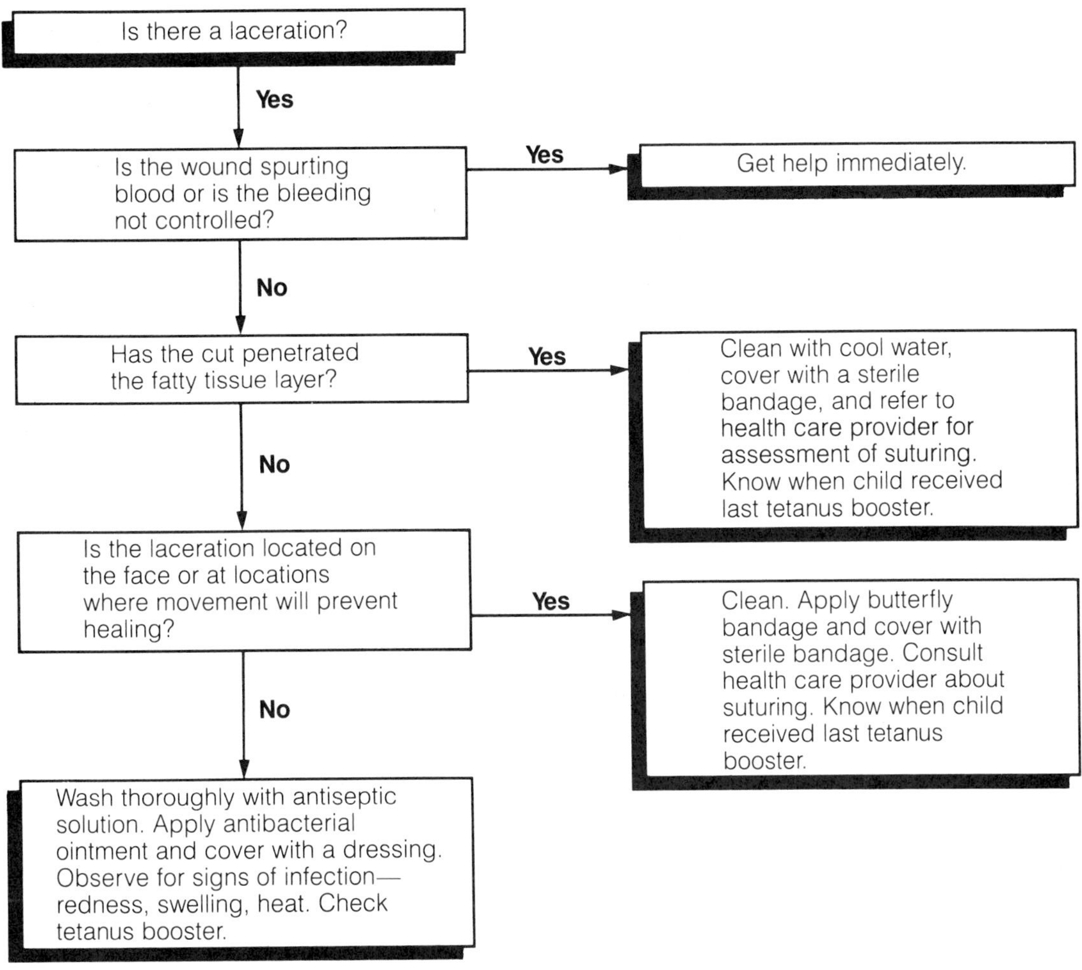

Figure 26-9 Parent decision: lacerations.

Key Concepts

- Many childhood illnesses can be treated successfully in the home.
- Given appropriate home conditions, home care of the child can pose fewer risks than hospitalization.
- Nurses in ambulatory care settings, rural areas, communities, and hospitals are uniquely suited to assess for and recommend home care.
- The nurse's role in home care includes the five steps of the nursing process.
- Nursing assessment provides data that enable the nurse and parent to decide whether home care is feasible, as well as data that provide a basis for the home care plan.
- Assessment is based on the physical, emotional, and social conditions of the home as well as on the conditions of the child's illness.
- Nursing diagnosis focuses on the potential risk for complications and the nursing care problems identified by the assessment.
- The written care plan provides a comprehensive plan of action to care for the ill child at home and involves providing reasonable assurances that the child's needs will be met.
- Although it is the parent's or caregiver's responsibility to implement the care plan in the home, the nurse is responsible for overseeing its proper implementation.
- Changing circumstances in the child or in the home require constant evaluation and restructuring of the home care plan.
- The nurse is an important resource for parents in deciding whether the child needs referral for medical evaluation.

- Disorders of the respiratory system that are amenable to home care include otitis, allergic rhinitis, nasopharyngitis, asthma, pharyngitis, laryngotracheobronchitis, pneumonia, mononucleosis, and tuberculosis, among others.
- Disorders of the gastrointestinal system that are amenable to home care include thrush, acute gastroenteritis, intestinal parasites, constipation, foreign body ingestion, and nonspecific abdominal pain.
- Communicable diseases that can be cared for at home include rubeola, parotitis, rubella, pertussis, varicella, exanthem subitum, erythema infectiosum, and scarlet fever.
- Many vectorborne diseases, such as Rocky Mountain spotted fever, are transmitted by infected ticks, mosquitos, and fleas.
- Disorders of the skin that are amenable to home care include pediculosis, scabies, and many allergic reactions, among others.
- Many emotionally disturbed children can be cared for successfully at home.
- The home is the appropriate care setting for minor lacerations and injuries.

References

Adams J, Evans G, Roberts J: Diagnosis and treatment of otitis media with effusion. *Am J Matern Child Nurs* (Jan/Feb) 1984; 9:22–28.

Baraff: Pertussis (whooping cough). In: *Current Therapy*. Conn H (editor). Saunders, 1981.

Castiglia A, Aquilina S: Streptococcal pharyngitis. *Pediatr Nurs* (Nov/Dec) 1982; 8:377–381.

Chai H: Asthma in children. In: *Current Therapy*. Conn H (editor). Saunders, 1981.

Clore E: Lice: Ancient pest with new resistance. *Pediatr Nurs* (Sept/Oct) 1983; 9:347–350.

De Angelis C: *Pediatric Primary Care*. Little, Brown, 1979.

Fekety R: Diphtheria. In: *Current Therapy*. Conn H (editor). Saunders, 1981.

Gardner P, Charles D: Infections acquired in a pediatric hospital. *J Pediatr* 1982; 81:1205–1210.

Grzybowski S, Allen E: Tuberculosis and other mycobacterial diseases. In: *Current Therapy*. Conn H (editor). Saunders, 1981.

Harkess C: Clearing the occluded auditory canal. *Pediatr Nurs* (Jan/Feb) 1982; 8:23–25.

Henderson G, Primeaux M: *Transcultural Health Care*. Addison-Wesley, 1981.

Kolff C, Sanchez R: *Handbook of Infectious Disease Management*. Addison-Wesley, 1979.

Madsen W: *Mexican-Americans of South Texas*. Holt, Rinehart & Winston, 1973.

McLaury P: Head lice: Pediatric social disease. *Am J Nurs* (Sept) 1983; 83:1300–1303.

Schmitt BD, Duncan BR, Riley CM: Ambulatory pediatrics. In: *Current Pediatric Diagnosis and Treatment*. 2nd ed. Kempe CH, et al (editors). Lange, 1972.

Thompson S: Summertime ticks. *Am J Nurs* (May) 1983; 83:768–769.

Thomson W: No need to report. *Nurs Mirror* (Sept) 1982; 155:49.

Wilson J: Pediatric emergency! Croup and epiglottitis. *Can Nurse* (March) 1984; 77:25–29.

Yura H, Walsh M: *The Nursing Process*. Appleton-Century-Crofts, 1978.

Additional Readings

Baylor K: Bacterial diseases of the skin. In: *Current Therapy*. Conn H (editor). Saunders, 1981.

Clinical News: Will chicken pox bite the dust? *Am J Nurs* (Aug) 1984; 84(8):978.

Furste W, Paulson G: Tetanus. In: *Current Therapy*. Conn H (editor). Saunders, 1981.

Grundfast K: Acute otitis media. In: *Current Therapy*. Conn H (editor). Saunders, 1981.

Hand J: Lice. *RN* (Nov) 1979; 42(11):27–29.

Holt SJ, Robinson TM: The school nurse's "family assessment tool." *Am J Nurs* (May) 1979; 79(5):950–953.

Hudgel DW, Madsen LA: Acute and chronic asthma. *Am J Nurs* (Oct) 1980; 80(10):1791–1795.

John RL: Giardiasis and amebiasis. *RN* (April) 1981; 44(4):52–57.

Morris E: Home care today. *Am J Nurs* (March) 1984; 84:340–345.

Muramoto N: *Healing Ourselves*. Avon Books, 1973.

Oill P: Streptococcal pharyngitis. In: *Current Therapy*. Conn H (editor). Saunders, 1981.

Pinney M: Pneumonia. *Am J Nurs* (March) 1981; 81(3):517–518.

Pohl ML: *The Teaching Function of the Nurse Practitioner*. Brown, 1968.

Reinhardt AM, Quinn MD: *Family Centered Community Nursing*. Mosby, 1973.

Sataloff RT, Colton CM: Otitis media: A common childhood infection. *Am J Nurs* (Aug) 1981; 81(8):1480–1483.

Selekman J: Immunization: What's it all about? *Am J Nurs* (Aug) 1980; 80(8):1440–1445.

Silver HK, Kempe HC, Bruyn HB: *Handbook of Pediatrics*. Lange, 1975.

Simkins R: Asthma: Reactive airways disease. *Am J Nurs* (March) 1981; 81(3):523–524.

Simkins R: Bronchiolitis. *Am J Nurs* (March) 1981; 81(3):514–515.

Simkins R: Croup and epiglottitis. *Am J Nurs* (March) 1981; 81(3):519–520.

Tinkham C, Voorhies E: *Community Health Nursing; Evolution and Process*. Appleton-Century-Crofts, 1972.

Todd B: Twenty-seven reasons why people don't take their meds. *RN* (March) 1981; 44(3):54–57.

Weiner M: *Earth Medicine, Earth Food*. Collier Books, 1972.

Wieczorek RR, Horner-Rosner B: The asthmatic child. *Am J Nurs* (Feb) 1979; 79(2):258–262.

Reactions of the Child and Family to Hospitalization

27

Joy Hinson Penticuff

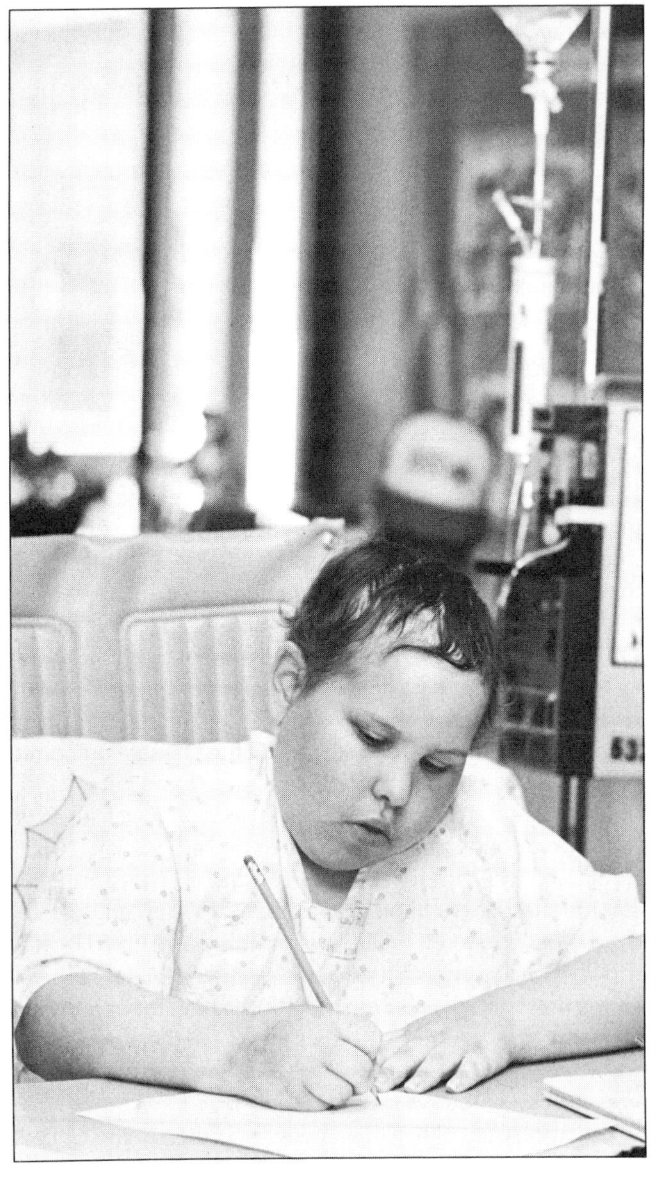

Chapter Outline

Objectives

- Define the components of both stress and crisis for families with hospitalized children.
- Relate coping behaviors to children's developmental stages.
- List the assessment criteria for identifying levels of stress and anxiety.
- Explain the developmental changes in the child's understanding of illness and its causes.
- Describe the common stressors related to hospitalization.
- Explain the developmental changes and age-appropriate needs for coping with the separation imposed by hospitalization.
- Explain the developmental changes in the child's experience of body image, function, and control.
- List the factors that affect the parent's perception of the child's illness.
- Describe the possible effects of the child's hospitalization on the family's day-to-day functioning.
- Compare the assessment criteria and possible interventions needed for the variety of family configurations.
- Describe the common needs of both the parents and siblings of hospitalized children.

Hospitalization during childhood is an experience with lasting effects that might be positive or negative. Approximately 4.5 million children are hospitalized annually; of these children, 90% are treated in general hospitals, which might or might not have pediatric units and specially trained staff (Azarnoff and Hargrove, 1981). Nurses therefore need to examine the events of hospitalization to predict its long-term effects for the child. Will the hospital stay result in physical and emotional health, or will the ultimate outcome be emotionally traumatic for the child and family?

The current trend to avoid hospitalization for children is based on a sound principle. Research findings (Prugh, 1953; Robertson, 1970; Triplett and Arneson, 1970; Kunzman, 1971; Johnson, Kirchhoff, and Endress, 1971; Meng, 1980; Azarnoff and Woody, 1981; Tesler and Savedra, 1981) have shown conclusively that children who are ill, frightened, fatigued, or in pain need the support of their primary caregiver (usually the mother and/or father) to make psychologically healthy adjustments to these stressors. The younger the child, the more true this principle.

The availability of health services to children in the United States varies. Among the factors affecting health care are the distribution of neighborhood "satellite" or public health well-child clinics, the ability to pay for private pediatric services, the existence of inpatient pediatric units with specially trained staff, the use of the local hospital emergency room for routine illnesses, the availability of physicians and child health nurse practitioners, and such cultural traditions as the *curanderos* (traditional Mexican healers).

In most instances the child is brought to a physician's office or to the hospital emergency room when the child's family becomes convinced that an illness will not respond to home cures or culturally derived healing methods (see Chapter 26). If they are admitted to acute care facilities, many of these children enter general hospitals that might not have pediatric units and whose staffs are not specially trained in either the physical or the emotional care of children.

In this chapter we examine the experience of illness and hospitalization for both the child and family. We analyze the coping strategies that the nurse can expect to see in hospitalized children, note the changes in coping behaviors that occur as the child matures, and examine the effect of cognitive development on the child's view of illness.

The hospitalized child remains an open system that is affected, to some extent, by the same suprasystems that affect the child when well. Therefore, we also examine the effects of hospitalization on the family. Family coping is an important part of the child's perception of illness. Nurses thus need to know the common needs of family members and should be prepared to identify disruption in family functioning, which might require nursing interventions.

Stress and Crisis for Children and Families

Hospitalization of a child might or might not be a crisis for the child and family depending on their perception of the seriousness of the illness and the amount of stress that hospitalization and treatment entails. A crisis is an event that cannot be handled or resolved by the child's or family's usual coping strategies and problem-solving techniques. Families and children experiencing a crisis are unable to deal with the threat and stress with which they are confronted without some assistance because the intensity of the stress overtaxes their abilities to cope. Responding to feelings of helplessness and anxiety in the face of great threat, families and children often exhibit behaviors that indicate that they are overwhelmed.

Crises present families with circumstances that can draw family members together or tear them apart. Much depends on the nature of family relationships before the crisis occurs and the amount and quality of support available to the family during the crisis.

In assessing the impact of stress and crisis on the family and child, the nurse determines whether the family's usual coping behaviors are adequate to meet the stress of illness and hospitalization. If the imbalance between the family's support system and the stress is critical, the nurse looks for those factors that make the family vulnerable to stress and increase the need for support.

Indicators of Stress and Coping

The indicators of stress are varied. Regression, for example, occurs to some extent in most ill children, and the child returns to usual functioning after recovering from the illness. Some children faced with prolonged illness and stress develop somatic complaints that might be unrelated to the original medical problem. Ulcerative colitis and stress ulcers of the stomach, for example, might develop in response to prolonged stress in children, even at very young ages. For these children, the nurse makes every effort to investigate the child's usual day-to-day experiences and identify stressors that can be modified or removed.

The effectiveness of the child's coping strategies depends on the adequacy of the child's internal and external sources of support, the child's problem-solving capacity, and the problem-solving capacities of the child's caregivers. Coping behaviors usually are a combination of four general styles of response: (1) direct expression of emotion (such as crying, anger, anxiety, sadness); (2) behavioral expression (for example, physical movement such as hitting, stamping the feet, withdrawal, delinquent behavior, overcompensation); (3) somatic complaints (such as ulcerative colitis or headaches); and (4) cognitive approaches (for example, talking about the stress and exploring alternatives).

In determining whether a child's coping is adaptive or maladaptive, the nurse notes whether the child's behavior is age appropriate. For example, the 10-year-old child who prefers to play with 6-year-olds, has no hobbies, is highly dependent on a parent, and protests about separation is behaving like a 6-year-old. Similarly, if such a child is able to pay attention to a description of a venipuncture but refuses to hold still during the procedure, the nurse probably would conclude that this child is behaving in an immature manner.

Because hospitalization and separation from usual friends and family normally produce regression in children of all ages, the nurse also determines whether a child's behavior is consistently immature. If this is the case, the nurse needs to find ways to help the child to cope constructively, usually by providing more support and lessening the stressors that the child faces. This process involves not only the nurse and health care team but also those family members who can be supportive to the child.

Assessing Stress Levels

The nurse in an acute care setting assesses the degree of stress on the child, the support available to the child and family, and the need for support from the health care team. The nurse then assesses the balance between the child's stress level and sources of support to determine whether the child's behavior is signaling too much stress. Questions that address this concern include the following:

1. Does the child have frequent visits from supportive, close relatives?
2. Does the child express emotions appropriately? (For example, does the 3-year-old protest the mother's leaving or appear apathetic?)
3. How frightened does the child become during required procedures or separations?
4. Does the child attempt to socialize with children of the same age in the hospital unit?
5. Does the child attempt to cooperate with health care staff?
6. Is the child's sleep seriously disrupted?
7. Does the child seem unusually irritable, anxious, or depressed?
8. Does the child continually test the limits imposed by the parent or staff?

If a number of behaviors indicate stress, the nurse notes that the child's ability to cope might be jeopardized and that a crisis may be developing.

In looking at the family's responses to stress, the nurse also assesses the relationships within the family to determine how much internal support is present. Questions to consider in this respect include the following:

1. To whom does the child turn for comfort when upset?
2. Who stays with the child in the hospital?
3. How does the child interact with this person?
4. Who is significant to the child?

Some young children develop particularly close relationships with caregivers other than their parents. In such instances, whoever has a close, enduring relationship with the child should be allowed to visit during the hospital stay, and plans for the child's care should reflect the importance of this relationship to the child.

To identify whether a family or child is becoming overwhelmed by stress and whether a crisis is developing or has already developed, the nurse assesses characteristic behaviors that reflect the loss of abilities to solve problems and cope with emotions. A nursing diagnosis of ineffective family coping indicates the need to plan interventions. (Fig-

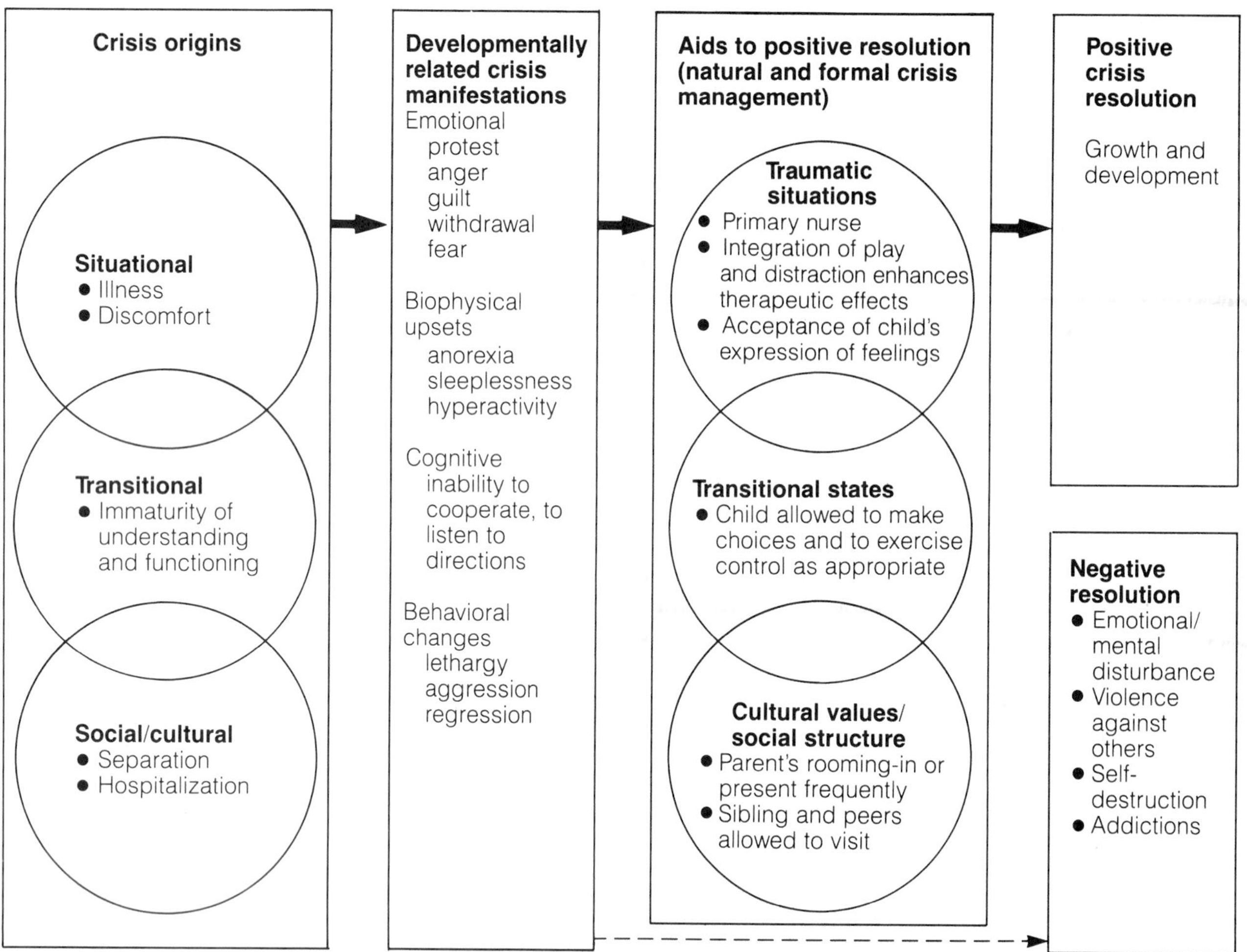

Figure 27-1 Crisis origins, manifestations, and outcomes relative to hospitalization.

ure 27-1 applies the paradigm illustrated in Figure 22-1 to the family's experience with hospitalization.)

Parents frequently are unable to talk with each other about their feelings, and family stability therefore can be threatened. High levels of anxiety, intense emotions, changes in appetite, insomnia, and lack of personal hygiene are indicators of disruption caused by a crisis.

Because the extent to which a person perceives a threat corresponds directly to that person's level of anxiety, assessment of the anxiety level of both the child and primary caregiver are most important. Anxiety should be most evident when the child faces the danger of loss or harm. If, for example, the nurse finds that family members or an older child do not show signs of anxiety when facing a threatening diagnosis or threatening information (such as that the child requires open heart surgery), the nurse might correctly conclude that the family or child does not recognize or allow themselves to recognize the threat in the situation.

This lack of recognition might be caused by denial, which may temporarily protect the child and family from the threatening reality. Denial and similar coping strategies are unconscious (see Chapter 12). A parent does not simply "decide" to deny that a child has terminal cancer but instead copes with the painful reality by refusing to face it for a time. Denial also is evident in the initial stages of grieving (see Chapter 32). Nurses might find that even after careful explanation of a child's condition, parents may not comprehend information that is too overwhelming to be accepted readily. Given support and consistent presentation of this reality, however, families and children usually can face painful facts and begin to use appropriate problem-solving strategies.

Families and children in a crisis usually show high levels of anxiety, emotion (commonly sadness or anger), somatic changes (especially changes in sleep patterns and appetite), and an impaired ability to manage the day-to-day tasks of living. For example, other children in the home might not attend school because the household is too disorganized for them to be fed, dressed, and transported as usual. Meals might not be prepared. Parents might not be able to sleep or may cry uncontrollably in the presence of their children.

Thus, the nurse assessing the crisis sees a family overwhelmed by emotion and the disorganization of usual family life. (Nursing care for families at risk is discussed in Chapter 22.)

The Child's Experience of Illness

To understand the child's and family's reactions to illness and hospitalization, the nurse views the experience of the illness and its treatment as the child and family see them. Nurses working in an acute care unit might become so familiar with the routines and the hospital environment that they gradually forget just how frightening the hospital can be to children and parents alike. Nursing assessment involves learning parents' and children's views of illness and treatment.

Increasing interest in finding out about children's understanding of illness dates from the 1930s when investigators found that children frequently associate illness with punishment, guilt, and self-blame. In an early study by Beverly (1936), 90% of children hospitalized with cardiac defects and diabetes answered the question, "Why do children get sick?" with, "Because they're bad"—an interpretation of illness common among children under 7 years of age.

Recent research has found a relationship between children's understanding of illness and their cognitive development. With increasing cognitive abilities, children can understand causation, treatment, and prevention in ways that parallel their intellectual growth. Children's levels of cognitive functioning also determine the ease with which they comprehend what has caused their illness and how they can maintain as much healthy functioning as possible (Bibace and Walsh, 1980).

Some researchers have hypothesized that the negative emotions experienced during a prolonged or severe illness might interfere with the cognitive development that leads to a mature understanding of illness. With hospitalized children, the emotional effects of separation from parents and other aspects of hospitalization often cloud their notions of illness and causality. For example, when healthy 6-, 8-, and 10-year-olds were asked about their understanding of illness, they did not see illness as punishment, but children of the same ages who had experienced repeated illness and hospitalization tended to perceive illness as punishment.

In general, children do not understand illness logically until 12 years of age. At approximately this age, children are able to understand the multiple interrelationships of factors, including host and agent, in causing disease. Bibace and Walsh (1980) studied 4-, 7-, and 11-year-olds to determine whether there is a relationship between the child's understanding of illness and the child's sense of control over becoming ill. They found that between 2 and 6 years of age, children do not feel that they can do anything to prevent becoming ill. They do not, for example, recognize that the body has internal parts as well as the visible external parts, so that the child conceives of the stomach as only the external surface of the abdomen. Bibace and Walsh (1980) also pointed out that with cognitive development the child is able to recognize some personal control over illness causality. They are not as much at the mercy of circumstances but can prevent some illnesses by staying away from people who are sick and by taking care of themselves.

In addition, repeatedly hospitalized children generally have more immature explanations of other phenomena than children who have not had repeated illnesses and hospitalization. The reasons for this difference have not been explored, but possible factors include cognitive regression caused by the stress and anxiety associated with acute illness or hospitalization and a limited exposure to general information.

Common Stressors Related to Hospitalization

Children's responses to the stressors faced during illness and hospitalization vary depending on their prior experiences, cognitive development, available emotional support, preparation for the experience, and temperament. Certain stressors are, however, common to illness and hospitalization for all children.

Fears Because of its unfamiliarity, the hospital environment is often frightening to children. Hospital routines are foreign to children who have not experienced hospital stays, and even for those who have been hospitalized before, each experience is unique and might evoke memories of prior experiences and unresolved fears. Children who are debilitated by fever, pain, or fatigue become anxious in unfamiliar environments.

Not knowing what will happen next is itself anxiety producing. Not understanding preoperative procedures such as being "put to sleep" and not feeling in control of events is stressful for children of all ages. Age-appropriate play is often therapeutic in helping children resolve their fears (play for hospitalized children is discussed in Chapter 28). Adequate preparation for the experience of hospitalization, when possible, and for specific procedures is therefore important in alleviating these fears (see Chapter 29).

Another common fear is the fear of death. Although in infancy and early childhood the concept of death is vague, children react to the emotional climate around them. If the parent fears that the child's illness is grave, even the young child senses the parent's anxiety. As children mature, they might ask directly whether they are going to die, even though they might have a limited understanding of death.

From early childhood through adolescence, children fear painful procedures and illnesses. Because their cognitive abilities for dealing with pain are less mature than an adult's, they might find pain overwhelming. Many children have difficulty concentrating and following instructions to relax and therefore miss opportunities to diminish their perception of pain. (Assessment and the nursing management of pain are discussed in Chapter 29.)

Isolation Isolation is difficult for children of all ages but affects children under 12 years of age severely. When children are placed in laminar-flow units because of an impaired ability to resist infection, for example, parents and siblings may visit only when they have been gowned, gloved, masked, and capped.

The child who is critically ill in such an isolation unit is then confronted with an additional number of stressors. First, visitors might be uncommon because gowning and other preparations to enter the isolation unit are frightening to them, complex, and time consuming. Nursing interaction with the child also might be limited because of the preparations required before entering the unit.

Second, family and nurses who do interact with the child do so while clothed in hospital gowns, masks, gloves, and head covers. For the young child, this might be frightening, and the child may have difficulty relating to caregivers who appear so different from usual. After a period of weeks or even days, many young children become so depressed and withdrawn within the isolation unit that they prefer to lie curled up on their beds than to interact with people (Kellerman, et al., 1977). Although isolation procedures are a necessary and significant portion of treatment, the effects of deprivation can be profound.

Invasion of Privacy The lack of privacy in hospitals often violates the child's sense of modesty, especially children in middle childhood through adolescence. Privacy is especially important to adolescents, who often are embarrassed by body changes and might feel that adults touching their bodies is a violation. Such nursing acts as palpating lymph nodes might cause acute embarrassment. The nurse should explain procedures that might cause embarrassment and allow children as much self-care as possible. Some children are able to treat the situation humorously, and the nurse can then encourage this type of adaptive coping.

Stressors in Infancy

Stress and coping behavior in infancy often is characterized by emotional expressions and physical activity that indicate anxiety, grief, and anger.

Separation Being separated from the people who are the child's usual sources of support causes the child to feel more anxious about the unfamiliar environment of the hospital. Separation from attachment figures during frightening or painful procedures deprives the child of needed comfort. Furthermore, the child's inability to understand that the separation is temporary and the reasons for the parent's absence frequently results in feelings of abandonment.

The relationship between the infant and parent during the first several months after birth is continually developing, and prolonged separation—especially when coupled with serious illness in the neonate—can inhibit the usual progress of the parent–infant relationship (see Chapter 31).

Separating infants from their caregivers and having them cared for in the hospital by many strangers is a far from optimal arrangement and might result in interactional deprivation and developmental delays. Separation further deprives the infant and the parent of the essential interactions that form the basis of the parent–infant attachment (see Chapter 7). Lack of contact with the primary caregiver who is sensitive to the child's cues and the care given by multiple caregivers in the hospital both interfere with the development of trust. If, however, the nurses who care for infants are sensitive to each infant's need for reciprocity in interactions and if they provide cuddling, rocking, and other soothing care, brief hospitalization usually is not overwhelmingly stressful.

In infancy and early childhood, children typically experience *separation anxiety,* a painful reaction to the threat of or actual separation from a loved one. Until they are able to understand that their parent will return, separation is equated with loss. As the notion of object permanence develops and the child's sense of self emerges, the stress of separation during illness and hospitalization becomes easier for the child to withstand.

For the infant who is old enough to differentiate the primary caregiver from others, the main response to hospitalization often is related to separation from the primary caregiver. By 9 months of age, developing attachment to the primary caregiver and the sense of dependence on the parent–child relation usually is evidenced by anxiety in the infant (see Chapter 7). Bowlby (1953) demonstrated that the separation of infants and young children from their primary caregivers usually first produces protest, followed by depression and withdrawal, and finally by apathy and disinterest in forming close relationships.

Protest In the stage of protest, the child cries, screams, and might hit and kick in apparent outrage, grief, or anger. This behavior occurs when the parent is leaving or has been away and then returns or when another adult approaches the child in the parent's absence. The nurse or parent might question this behavior in a child who previously was happy and playful in the parent's presence. To the child, the parent's leaving and absence, especially the nurturing parent on whom the child relies most, is devastating. Protest is a healthy response of the young child to separation from the all-important parent.

Despair Despair might begin within an hour to days following separation. Infants and children who despair feel that their loved ones have left and that no amount of protest will cause them to return. They then become sorrowful, uncharacteristically quiet, and seem to be grieving a loss.

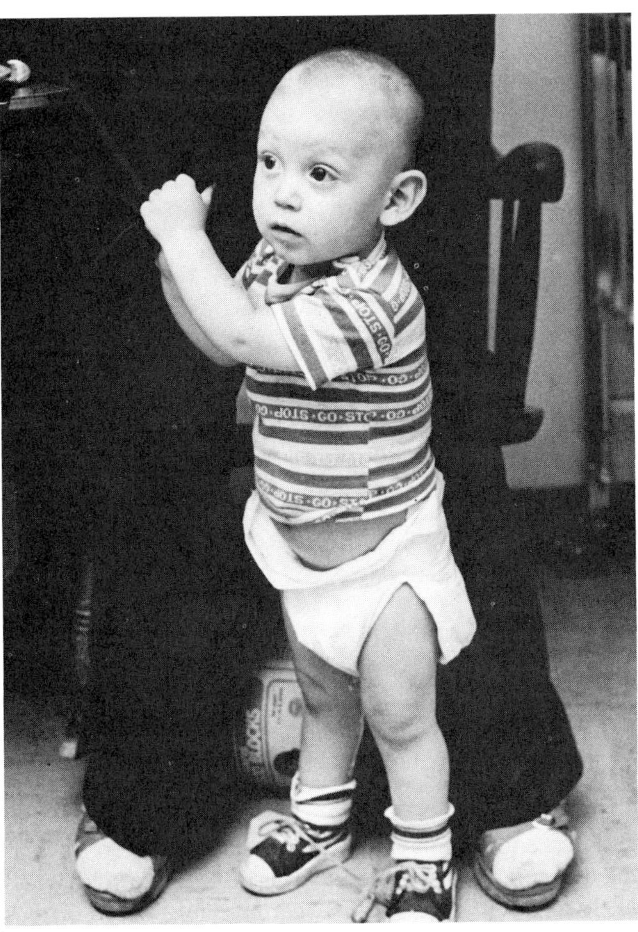

In infancy and early childhood, children typically express separation anxiety by clinging to parents.

These children are not interested to the usual degree in the activities and people around them. They might sit sucking their thumb, refuse to make eye contact, turn away from anyone approaching them, and fail to cuddle or reach for someone picking them up. They might not enter into play activities and sometimes will not eat. These children are literally grieving for the lost person.

The parent's return during this stage might be marked by the young child's return to the stage of protest. With protest, the child expresses grief and anger and regains faith in the possibility of the parent's return. This reaction is clearly healthier than depression.

Detachment In the phase of detachment or denial, the child has given up expecting the loved person to return. Children protect themselves from the pain of separation by denying the importance of the loved person and by pretending that being left by that person does not matter. In this stage children might seem to have recovered from the parent's absence. They relate to those around them, and their play can seem quite natural. When the parent visits, however, this same child, who previously seemed to have a close, warm relationship with the parent, protested the parent's leaving, and grieved in the absence, now ignores and might not even seem to recognize the parent's presence.

Some children do, however, become adjusted to the hospital setting. These children usually have the advantage of the parent's almost continual presence. They differ from children in the stage of detachment in the depth and warmth of their relationships, particularly their relationships with the parent.

The nurse might be relieved when the infant's or young child's protests or depression ceases because the child becomes much more pleasant and less demanding. Rather than indicating that the child is making a good adjustment to the separation, however, this response suggests the opposite. Repeated angry demands, irritability, inconsolable crying, and shrieks of rage are more typical and adaptive responses for infants and young children who are coping with separation. Lack of protest at separation also might indicate a tenuous relationship between the young child and the primary caregivers. Therefore, if the nurse notes that the child is indifferent to the coming and going of the parent and others with whom a close relationship should exist, the nurse makes a further assessment of the family to identify risk factors suggesting dysfunctional parenting (see Chapter 22).

Dealing with the signs of separation anxiety is difficult for the parent. Parents usually are very upset when their children cry. They might wish to avoid tears upon separation and can be devastated when their children cry when they return to the hospital. The lack of responsiveness evident during the stage of despair is no easier to withstand. The parents might feel that the children no longer care to have them near or might be so hurt by their children's reactions that they leave the children alone.

Even more difficult might be the stage of denial. The child's seeming to do quite well without the parent, particularly if the nursing staff does not see the behavior as a problem, might cause the parent to feel replaced and then to withdraw. After a period of separation, infants and young children tend either to cling to or reject the parent. These behaviors, too, are difficult for the parent to deal with.

Parents require explanations of their children's behavior. Nurses therefore need to discuss separation anxiety and the child's responses to it because it is helpful for the parent's understanding and acceptance of the child's behavior. This might require persistence on the nurse's part because some parents are so hurt by the separation and the child's behavior that they have difficulty listening. The parents also need to protect themselves, particularly when they are experiencing the stress of their children's illness and hospital stay, and might do this by talking about how much needs to be done at home, giving them an excuse to leave the hospital quickly.

Loss of Function and Control The lethargy that often accompanies illness increases the child's dependence on others. Until 9 months of age, this poses little threat to the

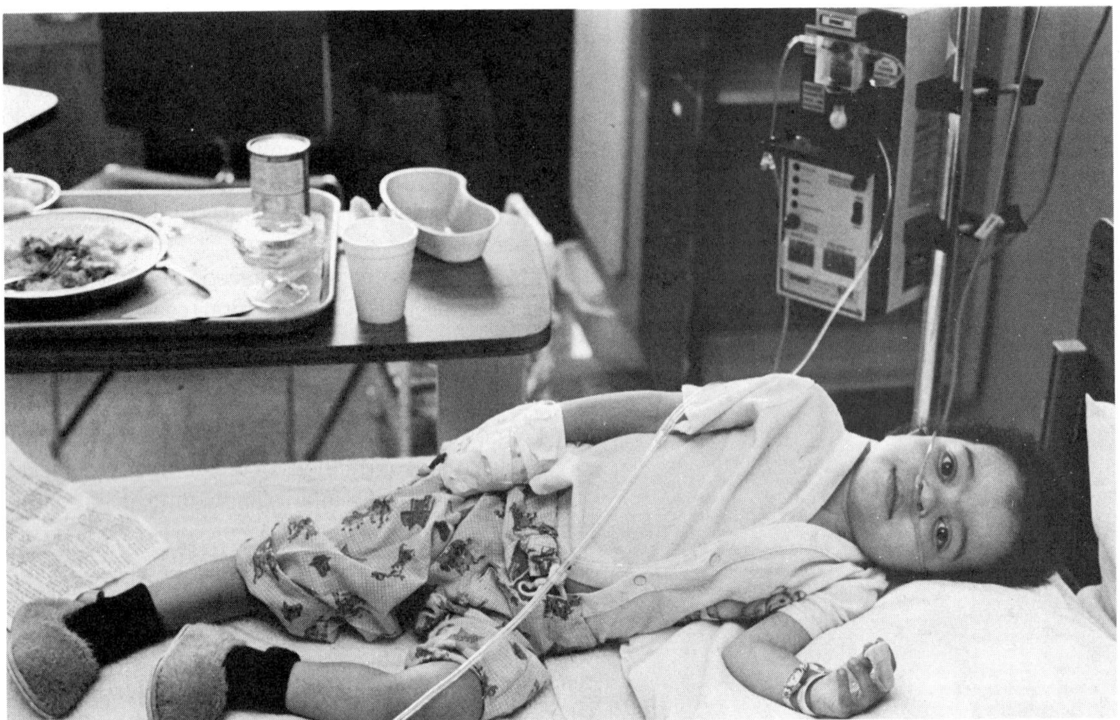

Children experiencing separation anxiety express despair through withdrawn behavior and lack of responsiveness.

child's development, but after the infant begins to sit and crawl, the loss of mobility can result in emotional distress. Restraints on the arms, legs, or hands or confinement to a crib or a small room can produce considerable stress.

The nurse thus keeps restraints to a minimum and encourages movement and activity. A mobile and other crib toys are stimulating to the infant and might offset some of the effects of limited mobility. Bringing the child to the playroom or placing him in the playpen, crib, or playtable outside the hospital room is very helpful. An infant can enjoy the change of scene and the activity of the surroundings in the playroom or hallway. Nurses also are more likely to smile and coo at, talk to, and hold the infant while the infant is more in the mainstream of activity.

Altered Body Image and Pain Infants have only a vague perception of body image, but with the development of motor skills such as crawling, the infant discovers body boundaries and forms a rudimentary knowledge of the body. As children become more aware of their bodies, they are concerned with changes in appearance such as scratches or a disfiguring trauma. Any lesion of the skin therefore might upset the child, especially if bleeding occurs. The child might look at the injury at first with a stunned expression. This quickly might develop into a quivering lower lip, wailing, and showing the injury to the parent.

Painful associations also add to the child's anxiety. In infancy, for example, the color of the nurse's uniform might become associated with the administration of painful procedures, and the infant may cry every time someone wearing that color comes into view. This response to color is less likely to occur when nurses wear colorful smocks or tops than when nurses wear uniforms that are all white. Children are seldom informed nor can they understand the scope of nursing. The nurse, at least initially, is feared as someone associated with painful procedures. A nurse who consistently provides care and spends time comforting the infant is beneficial to the child.

Psychodynamic theory holds that sensations in the mouth and genital areas are especially significant to the psychologic development of the infant. The infant might gain much comfort from sucking on a finger, bottle, or pacifier, thus helping to alleviate the stress caused by separation, loss of mobility, altered body image, or pain. Holding, cuddling, quiet talking, or singing to the infant also gives much comfort. The attention of the infant's primary caregiver is, however, usually the most important factor in comforting the hospitalized infant.

Stressors in Early Childhood

In early childhood the direct expression of emotion, such as crying, angry outbursts, and sadness, is a healthy coping strategy for children confronted with the stress of hospitalization. Because crying and other emotional expressions are a means by which children can express feelings and cope more readily with stress, the nurse acknowledges the child's emotions and avoids belittling or scolding the child for this behavior.

Understanding of Illness In early childhood the child begins to use magical explanations of illness as punishment for bad behavior. Children in this stage have a limited understanding of the world around them. Therefore, two events related only in time can become, in the child's mind, related by cause and effect. For example, a child who marks up the wall with crayons and becomes ill on the same day might think that the illness was caused by the misbehavior.

In early childhood children have difficulty understanding why they do not feel well, why they cannot play with other children, or why they are in pain or must go to the hospital. If treatment of the illness requires that they be separated from their primary attachment figures, they might feel that they have been abandoned and that this abandonment is a punishment for wrongdoing.

Children react in two ways to the belief that they are being punished. Some children will be unusually cooperative, helpful, and passive, as if atoning for their wrongdoing so that they can return to wellness and go home. Other children, perhaps not seeing any logic in their being "punished," punish the parent in return. These children will turn away when the parent enters the room and might show a superficial preference for the nurse or another child's parent. The child might be angry with the parent or be unable to risk the pain of reestablishing a relationship only to be left again.

The nurse might have to quickly educate parents who are receiving the cold shoulder from their children. Otherwise, the parents might take their children's rejection seriously and be very hurt, feel that they are not needed in the hospital, and even become angry with their children. Only if they understand their children's actions can the parents give needed support. All children need repeated reassurance that they are not to blame for their illness or hospitalization. They need understanding and support from their parents and help in expressing their feelings (see Chapter 28).

Another fairly frequent explanation for illness typical of the preconceptual level of thinking is that illness comes from outside sources. These sources can be as remote as the sky, the sun, trees, or God, or as close as people who get near the child. The child sees mere closeness or "magic" as causing the illness (Bibace and Walsh, 1980). Because these children often have active imaginations, their fantasy lives also might include believing that monsters and demons have entered their bodies to harm them. For young children, parents, and nurses can acknowledge and address the fear of having something unknown and frightening happen to them.

Because young children attempt to answer questions about the world through their experience and observations, they also tend to associate illness with external, observable events. Therefore, it is helpful to explain events by describing what the child sees, hears, smells, or feels. For instance, preoperative teaching with a 4-year-old focuses primarily on external, observable aspects of surgery such as the lighting in the operating room or the nurses' uniforms.

Separation In early childhood the most powerful force in the young child's life continues to be the parental relationship. The child derives security, comfort, and stability from the parent's presence while striving increasingly for independence and growth. Children fear separation and might not understand that they are not being abandoned when their parents leave the hospital. These children often have nightmares, and their vivid imaginations can cause them to be frightened by monsters, ghosts, and other aspects of the unknown. Consequently, they frequently are afraid of the dark, strangers, people in white clothes, and people who give bad-tasting medicines.

During early childhood, children continue to benefit from the reassuring presence of the parent, especially during painful or invasive procedures. Many facilities allow rooming-in when the parent is willing and able to stay with the child. In many instances the parent sits at the child's bedside where the child can see the parent doing some everyday activity such as reading or knitting. Even when there seems to be no interaction between the parent and child, the parent's presence gives the child needed support.

The child at this age has a limited memory; therefore, visits from and reminders of siblings also help to ease the pain of separation from home. Siblings sometimes can visit the child in the hospital. If they are not allowed in the child's room, the child might be able to meet siblings in the hospital

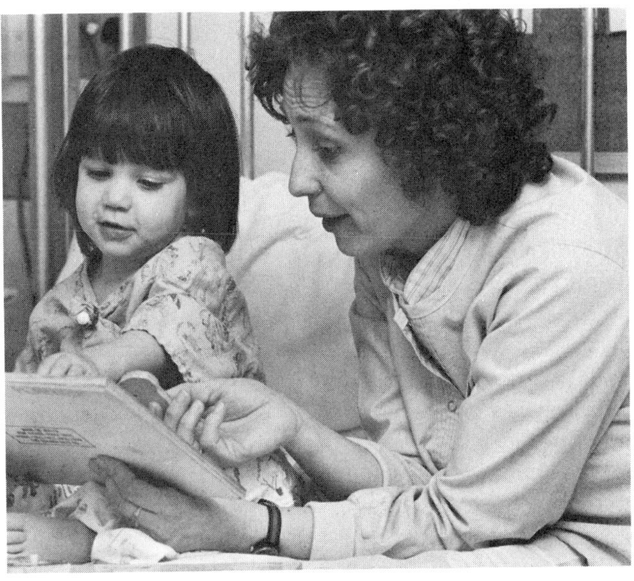

The presence of a parent and the parent's continued interaction with the child are ways to diminish separation anxiety in early childhood.

playroom, lobby, or cafeteria. Pictures at the child's bedside also serve as a reminder of those at home, and the nurse and parent can talk about brothers and sisters by name.

When the child is evidencing regression during hospitalization, the nurse encourages the parent to remain with the child in the hospital. The nurse also talks with the parent about ways to explain hospitalization to the child and encourage the child to master this unfamiliar environment. The parent might bring favorite toys to the hospitalized child and play familiar games. In early childhood family support in remaining with the child as much as possible, participating with the nurse in explaining procedures, and obtaining the child's cooperation are powerful means of combating hospital fears.

This is a particularly difficult age for coping with hospitalization because of ever-increasing awareness in the face of limited cognitive development and communication skills. When nurses must temporarily become primary caregivers, the child does best with a few consistent nurses who devote a great deal of time and attention to the child. The nurse must not be discouraged if the child screams when the nurse approaches. Children, especially between 18 months and 3 years of age, might need to observe the nurse for half an hour or more before feeling comfortable with the nurse's being in proximity or actually caring for the child. This time might be shortened considerably if the child becomes familiar with a nurse in the presence of the parent.

Parents must always say goodbye or tell their children when they are leaving. Despite the pain of tears, screams of protest, and pleading to stay, it is far better to acknowledge leaving than to sneak away. Confronting the issue conveys respect and faith in a child's ability to cope with separation.

Loss of Function and Control Because the rapid acquisition of motor and cognitive skills in early childhood is important to the child's emerging self-concept, the child might experience a sense of failure if newly mastered skills cannot be exercised. Children who are learning to run, talk, dress, and use the toilet need to practice these skills. Loss of function in these areas therefore can result in true lack of confidence. It can hinder the sense of autonomy and lead to feelings of shame and self-doubt.

In early childhood children usually are just mastering specific developmental tasks, and their mastery of these skills might be fragile. The child might, for example, be in the initial phases of toilet training. The stress of hospitalization often results in the loss of this newly gained skill, and this loss might be very upsetting to both the small child and the parent. Some children return to thumb sucking, whine, and become withdrawn or refuse to eat.

For young children, restraints can cause anxiety because gross motor activity is the primary means by which the child releases tension. Holding the child still for a procedure, such as a rectal temperature, or the application of four-point restraint to arms and legs causes anxiety and fear. If restraints must be applied (such as hand restraints for a child with an intravenous infusion), the nurse determines whether the benefit of restraints is worth the cost in terms of the child's anxiety. If the child must be held immobile for a procedure, the nurse should keep the time and extent of immobilization to a minimum. Perhaps the child's arms can remain free during a rectal temperature and the child be allowed to walk or run as soon as possible after the procedure.

Altered Body Image and Pain Children from early childhood on often feel uncomfortable about changes that treatment, injury, or disability cause in bodily appearance or function. They might fear facing others and may not wish to look at themselves. A $3\frac{1}{2}$-year-old boy, for example, whose head had been shaved for craniofacial surgery was outgoing and gregarious as long as he wore a baseball cap. He appeared embarrassed and became withdrawn the moment he took off his cap.

Invasive procedures are stressful for children of all ages. Invasive and painful procedures therefore require age-appropriate preparation to facilitate coping (see Chapter 29). During early childhood and thereafter, children quickly associate pain with specific procedures such as drawing blood samples, bone marrow aspiration, or dressing changes. Young children usually have very vague ideas of what nurses do and tend to associate the nurse with giving injections and medication and taking temperatures.

In early childhood such invasive procedures cause anxiety, and injections, especially if painful, cause anxiety for children of all ages. A 4-year-old child who receives repeated painful injections for lead poisoning, for example, might not be able to understand and may feel attacked by hurtful people. The child uses kicking and fighting to cope with this apparently purposeful injury. The experience can be very traumatic if some trusted person is not present to comfort and reassure the child.

Stressors in Middle Childhood

Middle childhood is a time when children tend to act out their stress if they are not so ill that their mobility is limited. Such behavior might include hitting, wheelchair racing, battling with the laboratory technician who wishes to draw a blood sample, and unwillingness to hold still. All of these behaviors are ways in which children diminish their anxiety. At this stage, as with younger children, restraints or immobilization can result in greater anxiety.

Understanding of Illness Children from about 5 to 7 years of age define themselves as ill only when they are told about or shown signs of illness such as, "You have to stay in bed." They believe they get sick because they performed or failed to perform certain actions. At this stage, children might think they can keep from getting sick by obeying a set of rigid rules associated with illness, and they might expect to recover from illness simply by adhering rigidly to another set of rules such as staying in bed and drinking chicken soup.

With developing cognitive skills, children begin to understand that illness might result from exposure to infection or trauma and that it is not the result of bad behavior. By about 7 years of age, they become better able to understand ideas and concepts, and the nurse is able to explain with the aid of concrete examples the reasons for illness and the various aspects of treatment.

Simeonsson, Buckley, and Monson (1979) explored the views of illness of 60 children 5, 7, and 9 years of age and identified their stages of understanding. These children showed considerable individuality in their understanding of illness, however, and some of the older children showed a relatively limited understanding of illness. In the first stage the children's responses reflected magical ideas about illness and its causes. In addition, the 5- and 7-year-old children believed, like younger children, that illness was the result of misbehavior.

In the second stage, which was more characteristic of the 7-year-olds, illness was attributed to a variety of specific acts or events associated with breaking rules such as walking barefoot in the rain or getting too close to people. The 7-year-olds often related breaking rules to becoming ill and following rules to getting well and, unlike older children, did not recognize that the body can fight infection and that an individual need not become ill, even after exposure to infection.

In this stage children's understanding of illness does lag behind their understanding of other phenomena, however, and this in turn can be very misleading to the nurse. For example, the nurse who is preparing the child for discharge and wishes to explain a chronic condition might find that by middle childhood the child has a somewhat sophisticated understanding of the world in general but a less advanced notion of the causes and effects of illness. The nurse therefore assesses what the child already knows about the condition and proceeds from that point. The nurse might first need to clarify the child's misconceptions about what caused the illness, exactly what body parts are affected, and how the child can help to keep the illness under control.

For example, the child might have an extensive vocabulary and be able to describe events, but in explaining diabetes mellitus, the nurse can expect that such a child will never have heard the word "diabetes" before and will likely have no comprehension of the location and function of the pancreas. Drawings of the human body therefore are useful with children at this stage and would help in explaining the disease and insulin's function. It is beneficial also to explain the disease and treatment in concrete terms that children understand and to use familiar illustrations that relate to their experiences. A child's cognitive functioning in this instance is highly significant. A child cannot be expected to cooperate with a treatment regimen without some understanding of how the treatment will help to control the disease and maintain health.

Children's previous experiences always influence their understanding of disease. A child might be quite familiar with a disease such as diabetes if someone close to the child has the same disease. The experiences of another family member, such as the child's mother or uncle, or even a neighbor or friend might have helped the child to form a concept of the disease. The child's understanding might, of course, be correct or incorrect, and will usually elicit either positive or negative emotions. These emotions might help the child feel comfortable with and able to control the disease or very fearful and anxious. The emotional aspects of disease management techniques, such as insulin injections, also affect the child's comprehension and acceptance, so that a thoughtful teaching program and acceptance of emotion expression are essential to gaining such a child's cooperation.

By about 7 years of age, children have additional cause and effect explanations for illness. They might, for instance, understand illness as contamination from persons, objects, or actions external to the body that have a quality that is "bad" or "harmful." Children infer that the body must physically touch the harmful person or object before contamination takes place. A 7-year-old, for example, was very indignant when she got chickenpox. She was certain that she had not touched anyone who had chickenpox and could not understand why she now had all these spots.

Another common explanation is that an illness is located inside the body, although its ultimate cause is external. The external cause, usually a person or object, is linked to the internal illness through a previously understood and experienced process such as swallowing or inhaling. Although the child views the illness as something within the body, the description is vague, thereby showing the child's lack of understanding of the body's organs and their functions (Bibace and Walsh, 1980).

Separation As children grow older, they are better able to understand why separations occur and can comprehend how long separations will be. Thus, from middle childhood on children can anticipate when they will see their loved ones again and have learned age-appropriate coping strategies (see Chapter 12). At this stage, it is meaningful for the parent to tell the child they will visit together after the child has had lunch. By middle childhood, the child is increasingly able to use developing cognitive skills to understand that a parent's leaving is sometimes necessary and that the parent will return.

At this stage, the child often is able to tolerate separation from parents for longer periods of time, but careful preparation of children requires that parents tell children when they will be coming back. These children might feel comfortable in the hospital without continual parental presence, but the stress of illness requires that parents and other supportive people in the child's life be present frequently.

Because children are increasingly influenced by systems outside the home during this stage, separation from school routines and from friends and teachers becomes important when children are hospitalized. Even children who claim not to like school express concern about missing school activities. The child facing a prolonged separation from school routines thus benefits from planned contact with peers and teachers.

Loss of Function and Control From middle childhood on a threat to the child's self-esteem is likely to result in feelings of frustration, anger, and even depression if the perceived loss relates to a valued skill or activity. Because these children often fear losing emotional control, they may be embarrassed if they cry during frightening procedures.

Children who are learning to be independent fear dependence on others and need to be able to control, to an appropriate extent, the events affecting them, although they also need to feel secure in knowing that the adults around them are powerful enough to impose limits for their protection. This delicate balance between allowing the child to make some choices, such as which juice to drink or whether an injection will be in the right or left thigh, and imposing limits on unacceptable behavior is difficult to maintain. For the nurse caring for hospitalized children, a principal nursing goal is to make the child feel secure by creating a predictable environment and to give the child opportunities to exercise control over that environment that are consistent with the child's abilities and developmental stage.

Giving the opportunity to make controlled choices enhances to a large degree the child's self-esteem. A major developmental task for the child at this age is the development of initiative. With the loss of function and control that accompanies illness and hospitalization, children might feel that the initiatives they took went too far. They then are likely to feel guilty for previous actions and might be unusually quiet and passive. Passivity in the child at this stage is rarely a sign of healthy adjustment and should alert the nurse to the need for further assessment.

The nurse who recognizes the child's level of cognitive development can make sense of the child's interpretation of illness and help to make it more accurate. Explanations of illness and treatment should diminish the child's fear and enhance the child's sense of control. For example, the nurse might explain what the child can do to make a procedure go well. The 5-year-old who is having an intravenous infusion started might be told, "If you will try to hold your arm still, that will help me to put the needle in exactly the right spot. You may say anything you like, and you may move any of the rest of your body the way you want to, but it is important for you to hold your arm still." The child's parent or some other person can assist the child by saying, "If you want me to help you to hold your arm still, I can put my hand right here to remind you to hold still." The nurse needs to remember to give the child choices whenever possible. The nurse also plans activities that encourage creativity and allow physical movements.

Altered Body Image and Pain By middle childhood, children might be able to find some diversion from pain through games and activities, although distraction might not work if the pain is severe. It is not unusual for a child on the first postoperative day to require no analgesic when playing games or being read to but need medication when left alone for adequate rest.

Even as children comprehend procedures and learn to cooperate in middle and late childhood, they dread body disfigurement. In middle childhood body mutilation is a major, although usually unspoken, fear. Children frequently cannot look at mutilated body parts and might, for instance, be afraid to view a Penrose drain or an incision. Surgery involving the genitals is particularly threatening. Nurses can first help children to learn about these changes and then encourage them to look at themselves by talking about changes, treatments, and the progress of recovery. The nurse can say something like, "Your incision looks wonderful. It's really healing well." Then saying, "It doesn't look good to you, perhaps" usually allows the child to loosen a grip on and sometimes express an inner thought or fear. The nurse might also ask the child to describe how something looks as a step toward helping the child adjust to tubes, traction, or injuries.

Stressors in Late Childhood

In late childhood growth and adaptive coping with illness and hospitalization are more apt to involve the child's increasing ability to understand the reasons for things. Understanding and problem solving are themselves coping strategies for older children, who are learning to cope with their fears as they strive for independence. Carefully planned patient teaching thus is increasingly important as the child grows older (see Chapter 29).

Understanding of Illness Throughout late childhood, children begin to view illness as caused by exposure to germs or other external factors. Not until they approach 12 years of age, however, can they begin to grasp the notion that illnesses might have multiple causes. With cognitive development comes the ability to recognize that illness is an interaction between a set of causes external to the body and the body's vulnerability to illness.

Because children at this stage can specify relationships among events or objects, classify them into categories, and recognize their effects on each other, 9- to 11-year-olds usually define illness according to a set of multiple concrete symptoms. They tend to believe illnesses are attributable only or primarily to germs, which have a predetermined and powerful effect on their bodies. They believe further that illness can be prevented simply by avoiding germs and thus are likely to see external phenomena impinging on the body and both causing and curing illness. Because they show a limited understanding of the role of the body in healing itself or resisting infection, children at this age might attempt to prevent illness with such maxims as not going anywhere near sick people.

Bibace and Walsh (1980) found that 11-year-olds had an increasingly more accurate understanding of illness and some sense of control over becoming ill. By this age, the child is able to understand illness according to the characteristics of the infecting agent or harmful events and the vulnerability of the host to the illness. Therefore, in late childhood some children are able to understand that they become ill not only because of exposure but also because of the body's vulnerability.

At about 11 or 12 years of age, children begin to understand that illness is triggered by external events but that the source and nature of the illness can be found in specific internal physiologic structures and functions. The cause usually is described as the nonfunctioning or malfunctioning of an internal organ or process and is explained as a step-by-step internal sequence of events that culminate in illness. Therefore, with an older child who can conceptualize the internal parts of the body as well as their functions, preoperative teaching can include both the details of anatomy and what is happening inside the body.

Separation In late childhood and for some children in adolescence, parental presence is crucial to the child's feeling of well-being. Parents must, however, give older children some distance and freedom to be independent while still listening to and guiding them.

Although children at this age might not wish to express their emotions openly, they need to have someone with whom they can discuss their feelings and concerns. By late childhood, coping behaviors are less likely to be aggressive and immediately obvious to the nurse. Older children might be withdrawn, unresponsive, or disinterested in social activities. Because they are striving for independence, they might not ask the nurse for help or support, and thus the nurse needs to monitor the older child's behavior to assess emotional needs.

As children become increasingly influenced by systems outside their families and less dependent on their parents for support, separation from peers and school activities is likely to be a major source of concern. The nurse's encouraging continued contact with friends and other important people helps support the child.

Children often fear the responses of friends or any person with whom they have temporarily lost contact to their illness. Suggesting some responses the child can give and simple answers to questions they might be asked therefore enhances their self-confidence. The nurse also can role-play these questions and answers so that the child has a more concrete idea of what might be encountered and can practice possible responses (see Chapter 28).

Loss of Function and Control As they attempt to become less dependent on parents and more "grown up," older children come to equate control of their emotions with adult behavior. Consequently, these children might fear loss of self-control as much as they fear treatment or pain. Older children are likely to grit their teeth, act brave, or pretend that a procedure does not hurt. They do not want to look frightened or childish to their peers and might feel embarrassed if they express their feelings. In fact, these children frequently are so brave that others assume that they are not upset by hospitalization and have no fears.

Nurses can help by giving these children opportunities to discuss their feelings and express their frustrations. If the child learns to view the nurse as a trustworthy and supportive person, the nurse can help the child to express emotions appropriately and maintain self-control.

Children who have been model patients with the staff and other children and their parents might unleash much anger and hostility when their own parents arrive. They sometimes blame their parents for all their difficulties, and the parents might wonder why they came to visit. This behavior is difficult to understand and manage. The child usually feels sure of parental love and thus feels free to express feelings and frustrations. Many people, including the parent, assume that this is negative coping and imma ture behavior. They might decide that the parent's presence is not very helpful to the child. It is, of course, immature behavior, but it is very necessary to the child's well-being. It is similar to the child at home selectively using tears to receive needed tender, loving care.

The parents might or might not be able to see beyond the specifics of a child's tirade to the child's deeper frustration and fears, and the nurse often can help the parent both to understand and to deal with the child. At home, parents have developed means for disciplining their children for inappropriate behavior. Although often imperfect, these means usually are adequate for meeting both the children's and parents' needs. In the hospital the child is both ill and outside the privacy of the home. Although verbal abuse must not be tolerated, the parent needs to listen through the words to hear the deeper meanings the child, often unknowingly, is trying to convey. Some parents can do this easily or can quickly be helped to listen to the child. Other parents err by being either permissive or inappropriately strict. Some parents allow their children's rudeness to go far beyond the level they would tolerate at home, which tends to breed resentment in the parents. It also incorrectly teaches the child that these behaviors, actually unacceptable in the family's culture, are tolerable. Other parents expect their children to be as polite and alert to the world around them as they would be if they were helping out at a parent's party. In any event the nurse can talk with parents about their children's needs for both discipline and loving attention. The parent can then feel less guilty for disciplining when needed or less embarrassed about the child's behavior.

The child regains control and self-esteem through knowledge about hospitalization and illness and through participating in the plan of care. Because children at this stage are better able to understand the details of the illness, procedures, and their bodies' needs, teaching can be quite sophisticated and intellectual. This is an excellent opportunity to involve the child in the care plan because the child can, when given limits, make many decisions concerning the mechanics of carrying out the care plan. The child might plan walks and activities to meet ambulation needs and may readily drink fluids when the goal for ingesting the type and quantity of fluids is clear. The child should be given as many choices in daily care as possible. This is also an appropriate time to teach the child about wellness and remaining as healthy as possible (see Chapter 18).

Altered Body Image With cognitive development comes an ability to understand the seriousness of an illness and the consequences of treatment. By late childhood, children are more likely to fear long-term disability or possible death than pain and invasion procedures. They usually want information, and it is important that procedures and their rationale be explained carefully. Unlike younger children, who fear the strange environment and apparatuses, they need to know what will happen, for example, during surgery and what they will find when they awaken.

Older children also are concerned about procedures that affect the genital area. As they approach adolescence, their awareness of sexual functioning makes them especially vulnerable to real or perceived threats to body image. Any procedure, including routine physical assessment of the genital area, also might violate the child's sense of privacy. Some children choose not to have their parents present during such procedures. Careful explanations and reassurance are important to these children.

Stressors in Adolescence

By adolescence, cognitive development allows children to understand abstract ideas and complex causes for illness and recovery, and adaptive coping is facilitated by the nurse's recognizing the child's individual preferences and interests. As adolescents grow increasingly independent from parents, they actually might achieve a sense of mastery when allowed to cope with procedures and treatments without much parental assistance.

Understanding of Illness At around 12 years of age, children are better able to reason like adults about the complex causes of illness, and they come to understand that they can contribute to their regaining health (see Table 29-6). The most advanced of all the means by which children cope with illness and hospitalization are therefore cognitive approaches, especially problem-solving behavior or talking about what is troubling them.

By the time children reach 13 or 14 years of age, they are able to think more hypothetically and can associate events with prior concrete experiences. They can understand that illness involves internal physiologic structures and systems and that possible dysfunctions are manifested by a variety of external symptoms. Older adolescents might learn to describe illness as a psychophysiologic phenomenon in which internal physiologic processes interact with additional or alternative psychologic causes. The child at this stage is aware that a person's emotions and stress can affect the way the body functions.

Younger adolescents typically define illness abstractly, emphasizing internal feelings independent of specific complaints or external signs. Children 13 or 14 years of age are likely to answer the question, "How do children know when they are sick?" with responses such as, "You don't have much energy," or "You just don't feel right." They understand that illness might be caused and cured by the complex interaction between the host and agent, but very few children understand the concept of prevention of illness in any real depth. Prevention is a more difficult concept to grasp than causation and treatment. The nurse involved in health teaching therefore continues to explain the relationship between prevention and illness by using concrete examples to illustrate the concept. Prevention of cavities might be explained, for example, by using a model of teeth and putting sugar and other foods on the teeth, brushing one side, and observing the chemical changes and residue formation on the unbrushed side.

Separation Adolescents, who are much influenced by their peers and might be concerned with prolonged separation from their friends, need to participate in planning day-to-day care that includes contact with peers. Some adolescents prefer to minimize contact with their friends outside the hospital, especially if disability is a threat to the adolescent's role in a particular peer group. Isolation from peers, however, might leave an adolescent without adequate support systems. For these patients, contacts within the hospital might be an important part of care.

For example, in one hospital adolescents with cystic fibrosis were grouped together. They were free to decorate their areas as they wished and often made close friends. The girls washed and set each other's hair and did each other's makeup, and the boys worked on model airplanes together. The group held meetings and established rules for their unit. Outside activities were planned periodically so that hospitalization was less boring.

Loss of Function and Control Illness for the adolescent poses special difficulties because independent func-

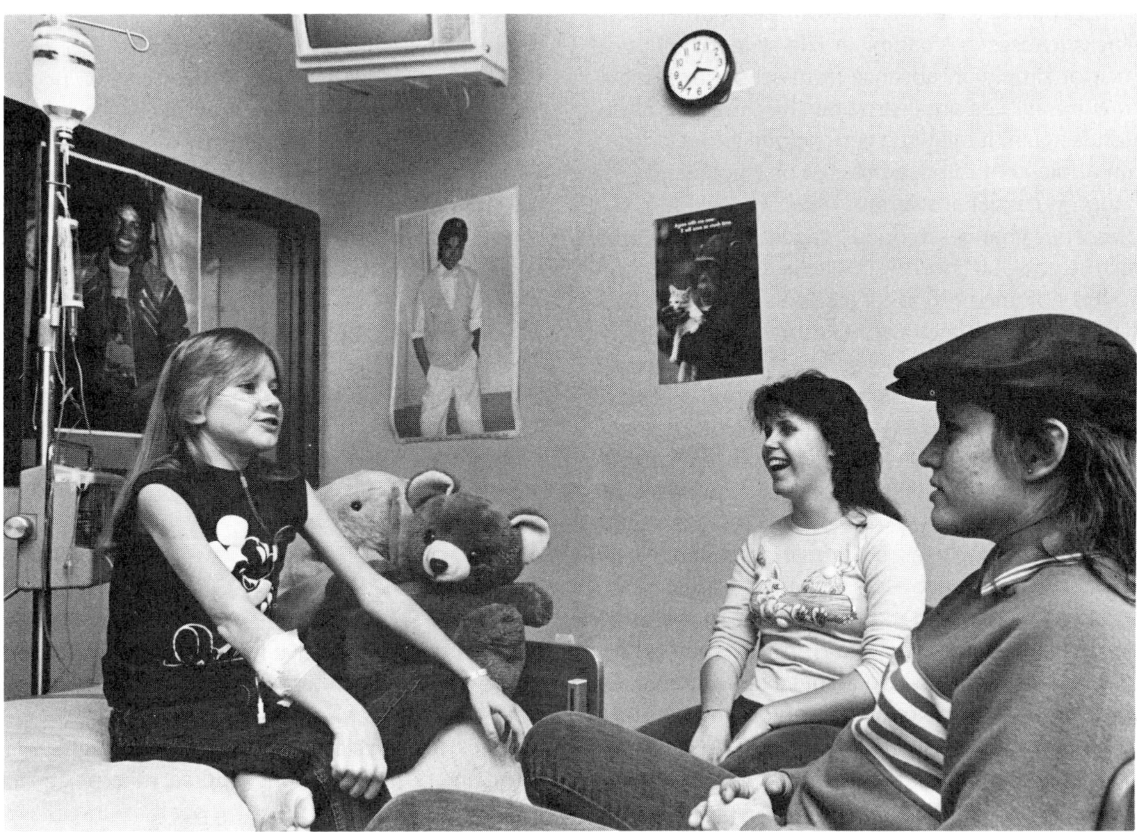

When adolescents are able to meet each other, they benefit from the support that interaction with peers provides.

tioning might be impaired at a time when psychologic independence from parents is highly significant. This often makes it hard for the adolescent to admit to needing assistance, either physical or emotional. Illness in adolescence, especially chronic illness or conditions that leave permanent scars or cause loss of function, threaten the adolescent's developing self-concept. Adolescents therefore need the nurse to listen and acknowledge their perceptions of illness and the limitations it brings.

Some adolescents respond to the threat of dependence with anger or frustration, whereas others react by withdrawing. If adolescents are to use appropriate problem-solving skills, they need to feel comfortable in talking about their problems with a supportive, accepting adult. The nurse therefore assesses the adolescent's sources of support and intervenes if there is no one to whom the adolescent can honestly express feelings about and perceptions of the illness. Adolescents often are better able to talk outside the hospital setting or at least outside of their rooms or units. The older the adolescents are, the more necessary it is that they feel comfortable in sharing. Talking with adolescents in a teen room, hospital cafeteria, on the grounds of the facility, or even in the unit hallway is more likely to facilitate conversations than talking in their rooms.

Adolescents who cannot leave their rooms need to maintain some control over and privacy in conversations. The nurse can look for cues that the child wishes to talk. Sometimes the child will ask several seemingly small questions or make minor requests. "Do you like this song?" (or television show, etc.) can be an invitation to sit down and talk. Many adolescents will find it easier to talk with props such as a game or other simultaneous activity because in this way they can maintain control over the intensity and direction of a conversation.

Because the adolescent is achieving more and more independence from parents and other adults and illness might be a threat to this independence, the hospitalized adolescent should be given as many options as possible. The nurse assists the adolescent by providing factual information about the disease and allowing the child as much decision making as possible in the plan of care.

Altered Body Image Because by late childhood the peer group has become an essential system in the child's socialization, illness that causes an adolescent to be viewed as different from peers might affect the adolescent's ability to cope with the stress of a changed body image. These children might fear the responses of others, are often self-conscious, and worry about being teased.

As with slightly younger children, role-playing is very

effective in preparing for questions from peers and others. When illness causes a change in life-style or physical appearance or simply an absence from school and activities, the nurse can listen and learn how the child feels about seeing friends again. It might be very helpful to the worried or hesitant adolescent to pose possible questions and help think through potential answers.

In adolescence changes in body image that deviate from the socially acceptable norm are likely to cause embarrassment. It is not uncommon for an adolescent to be hospitalized as a result of failure to take prescribed anticonvulsant medication or maintain a diabetic diet. Because sexual functioning and the attainment of adult roles are important to adolescents, illnesses or conditions that threaten the normal development of these roles also cause stress. A pelvic examination, for example, is stressful even for a well-prepared adolescent girl.

One 14-year-old boy was so embarrassed about his somewhat large breasts that he was unwilling to allow others to see his chest. He refused to go swimming and wore a sweat shirt even when playing tennis in hot weather. He and his family decided that he would have breast reduction surgery, and even at this point he told no one of the problem. The surgery was done in a neighboring state, although scheduling it in a hometown hospital was possible. To explain postoperative dressings and the temporary need to decrease his activities, he decided to tell his friends that he had had a cyst removed.

For the adolescent, threats to body image can be especially anxiety producing because the process of achieving independence from parents and other adults is a goal at this stage. Illness is often perceived as a threat because it inhibits independent functioning. The nurse or parent who supports the child's striving for independence, no matter how difficult or frustrating it might be, is enhancing learning and self-esteem by limiting regression, discouragement, and helplessness.

Although specific reactions and associated behaviors are typical of children at various ages, remnants of earlier thinking and behavior often occur during illness and hospitalization. Separation anxiety, although usually seen in children under 3 years of age, is possible in the older child. The parents' reassuring presence is still crucial to the child's comfort and reassurance despite the growing need for independence. Distress with physical restraint occurs well beyond early childhood, and something akin to mutilation fears from such intrusive procedures as injections often is seen in older children. One adult who was hospitalized at 10 years of age remembered feeling that the illness and hospital stay were a punishment for her thoughts and behavior.

One 14-year-old girl was very fearful about having a tuberculin test and having her finger pricked to obtain blood for a hematocrit. She listened intently as the nurse casually told her that younger children often were truly afraid that something dreadful might happen with a break in the skin such as their insides might come out. She repeatedly asked the nurse whether young children really thought that way. When reassured that they did and that they needed a bandage to keep themselves together, this girl smiled and relaxed. She was able to go through the procedures with only mild protest and obvious pride in her more mature responses. Another adolescent, an unusually polite boy, needed adult help to hold still for an injection of a needed postoperative analgesic. He was embarrassed about it and apologized for his behavior. He needed therapeutic play, actually handling a syringe and learning about injections, to gain a sense of control.

The nurse needs to be alert to each child's possible thoughts and fears because earlier thinking and possibly unresolved previous negative experiences can resurface in the older child undergoing the stress of hospitalization.

Psychosocial Development—Potential for Unmet Needs

Hospitalized children have the same needs to develop, learn, and grow as healthy children, but hospitalization places a great deal of stress on the child and limits many natural avenues for development. Despite children's uncertainty about and possible fear of the nurse, nurses need to address potential problems by planning goals for the effective management of psychosocial needs. A thorough knowledge of developmental norms for each age aids the nurse in understanding children's perceptions of the hospital (see Chapters 7–11).

Nursing interventions that are planned to enhance children's coping with hospitalization have the following long-term goals:

1. To nurture the child and family's self-esteem and hope
2. To allow the child and family to express their emotions and to facilitate their understanding of feelings
3. To help the child and family understand more fully the medical condition and options they have
4. To enhance communication among family members and encourage interactions with the health care team
5. To prepare the child and family for threatening events that they are likely to encounter during the hospitalization and illness

In communicating with a child, the nurse first builds a trusting relationship that will help the child work through some of the feelings that accompany hospitalization. The therapeutic relationship developed between the nurse and child aids in providing emotional care. The nurse might be one of the few people who is in frequent contact with the child and can talk about fears and answer questions. The nurse who is planning for all aspects of care therefore provides consistency, sensitivity, and individuality, all of which are essential in meeting emotional needs.

Nurses cannot underestimate the significance of communication because it is the key that unlocks the private world of fantasy, the feelings of guilt or helplessness, and the imagined purpose or results of treatment. Through age-appropriate communication, the nurse can help children to understand their feelings as well as the purpose of various treatments.

Children can be unable, for example, to look at skeletal traction, drainage tubes, or incisions because they are unattractive or frightening. Children need opportunities to express these feelings to someone who can sympathize with their concerns and answer their questions honestly. The nurse who is attentive to their concerns and willing to invest time and energy when they need it lays the foundation for a trusting relationship. Once trust is established, children are more willing to discuss their concerns and to learn about themselves, their treatments, their personal responses to treatment, and the need for treatment.

An important aspect of care is assisting the child to understand the reality of a situation. Although this is difficult and potentially alienating at first, it is more important to tell the child the truth than to obtain the child's cooperation through deception. Facts need to be reinforced, and the child must have consistently honest answers from all of the staff. This helps the child to accept reality and work through feelings.

Dependence and Independence The better children are able to manage their own care, the greater their sense of independence and self-confidence. Although nurses often find it easier to do things themselves than to teach, support, or even insist that children do the tasks for themselves, nurses should encourage independence by teaching about hospitalization and treatment.

Children need to understand what is happening to them and what their role is in the process. Nurses also can teach children the techniques that will aid in recovery. For example, a 9-year-old child might need to remain inactive and on bedrest after a particular eye injury to facilitate the recovery process. The nurse can then explain the purposes of these restrictions so that the child understands that they are temporary. Older children also can learn that getting up and about after surgery is necessary, despite their not wanting to do so. As treatment goals become clear, children are better able to cooperate and become independent within the limits imposed by their condition. Treatment goals should be presented clearly so that the child can follow them and will not misunderstand their intent.

Children and nurses need to agree about what is acceptable and unacceptable behavior. This understanding helps to prevent conflict, which is preferable to experiencing conflicts and then having to work through them. Specific expectations and discipline for the child help to encourage independence and feelings of security and self-worth. Children need to know what they must not do. They also need outlets for their energy through play and diversion. Consistency and good communication are essential among all those involved in care so that children receive consistent treatment and are not able to manipulate their caregivers. Nurses need to teach about the possibilities as well as the limitations. For example, a child who must get up and sit in a chair can use a wheelchair and gain some mobility and control.

The nurse's response to the child's illness also can influence the child's own perceptions of the threat to normal functioning. For example, if the nurse explains that the child's intravenous infusion can be placed on a mobile pole, the child will realize that illness will not mean remaining in bed throughout the hospitalization.

Sensory Needs Because of separation, hospitalization for the infant is generally stressful. The parent's voice is a source of stimulation to the infant. Parents characteristically raise the pitch of their voice when talking to infants, and their voices tend to have a singsong quality. The positioning of the infant in the parent's arms so that the infant's trunk is cuddled next to the parent's trunk is another characteristic behavior that provides appropriate tactile stimulation. The infant's contact with the caregiver's body actually might be one means by which infants establish early perceptions of their own body's boundaries. As the parent rocks the infant, this stimulation is thought to develop the infant's kinesthetic perceptions further.

By the time they reach early childhood, children learn by doing, by exploring their environments, and by experimenting with and manipulating objects. The hospital, regardless of whether the child is technically immobilized, places the child in a restricted environment in which sensory deficit or overload is likely. Nurses therefore need to be attuned to each child's need for stimulation. Toys need to be appropriate for the child's stage of development (see Chapter 28). Some toys should be challenging, but other toys should be old favorites. Crib sides (or any other apparatus on the bed) are useful for hanging toys and keeping them within easy reach for the young child. Changing them periodically maintains interest and curiosity.

The child needs a balance between activities with others and quiet, solitary activities. Nurses might easily overwhelm some children with too many stimulating toys or activities, which causes them either to habituate for self-protection or become irritable from the confusion of too many sights, sounds, and demands. Structuring the days with some degree of regularity benefits everyone. It gives the family a routine to follow and helps to prevent the child from being overstimulated and fatigued or understimulated and bored.

Television is frequently a favorite diversion, although parents and nurses need to use discretion in the amount and types of programs allowed. Children sometimes use television as a means of escape from reality, but more often they use it to escape boredom. In the long run the presence of a person, whether the person is a staff member, family member, or peer, is more stimulating to growth and more satisfying. The nurse, family, and child can use television wisely by identifying a few favorite programs and including them in the day's routine. Then, providing other activities and appropriate responsibilities will foster the child's development. Television should not be used as a "babysitter" or as an excuse for not spending time with a child.

Nurses can encourage sensory stimulation as well as links to family and friends by having the child decorate the bed and room area. Large bulletin boards by each bed are good areas to put up cards, pictures, and posters. Some facilities allow walls and windows to be decorated. Frames and parts of mist tents provide additional space for get-well messages and seasonal decorations. A frame can be used for some games with soft or fabric balls. Shelves, boxes, or lockers for toys, games, and possessions help to create a personal, homelike atmosphere, which lessens the trauma of separation from home. The older child and adolescent can use tables to help keep books, games, and activities within easy reach. The longer the hospital stay, the more homelike the child's area can become and the more significant the accumulated possessions become.

Auditory stimulation can be provided by radios, tapes, and records. These also keep the child in touch with the outside world. Tapes made by family members and friends become a new means of communication and are available whenever this communication is desired. Adolescents sometimes use records for emotional release or entry into a world of fantasy. Music sometimes provides an enjoyable socializing activity; at other times, headphones provide private enjoyment.

Learning Some children spend a considerable amount of time either in the hospital or recuperating at home; therefore, planning for children's general learning and schoolwork is best begun at the time of admission. As soon as the acute phase of illness and treatment is over, learning experiences should become part of the nursing care plan. To ensure their cooperation, older children should be included in the planning.

Children in school need some arrangement for continuing their education. Classroom or tutorial services are provided at some hospitals, but more often children have tutors from their school or community, or attempt to learn on their own with the help of available adults.

During illness, however, the child's attention span and concentration are decreased. Education activities and homework therefore are better done in short blocks of time. More time, support, and encouragement are needed to complete assignments and do them well because children often lack their usual drive and interest in the outside world when they are ill and hospitalized.

Nurses might be able to tap the child's current interests creatively and use them to satisfy academic requirements. For example, having a child calculate the amount of fluid or protein in the diet might be interesting and useful and may serve the same purpose as a regular math or health science project. A child might be able to write a story, a poem, or lyrics to a song about some aspect of hospitalization to fulfill an English or writing assignment.

The nurse assesses the child to determine the appropriateness of introducing hobbies. Particularly when illness and hospitalization are lengthy, the nurse might strongly encourage the child to become involved in an ongoing activity. Children whose minds and bodies are creatively active within the constraints of illness are more likely to maintain their pace of development.

Hobbies might be continued or introduced to provide a good learning experience. Children have opportunities to develop or improve skills, to make something for others or for profit, to learn about responsibility, or to entertain themselves and others. Planting seeds and caring for plants are good activities and can vary in size and involvement from a single plant to a window garden.

Learning to play a harmonica, guitar, or other musical instrument might be a challenge and one from which adolescents especially enjoy earning peer recognition and appreciation. Ideas for hobbies and collections are endless. Some activities might be temporary, whereas others can become lifelong interests.

Socialization Maintaining social contacts aids in meeting developmental tasks. From infancy through adolescence, children need opportunities to interact with peers and adults. Not only is companionship beneficial, but the encouragement and stimulation of companions help children to grow in all aspects of development. Companions help to provide the child with the impetus to keep striving toward health.

The infant's social behavior is learned from reciprocal interaction, first with the parents and later with siblings. Infants gradually learn to smile responsively, to seek the company of others, and to play such games as peek-a-boo. The attachment between the primary caregiver and infant is the most significant determinant in the socialization of the infant.

All children, unless critically ill, also benefit from changes in the environment. The use of the playroom or solarium and trips to other parts of the hospital are helpful. The area around the nursing station is also a gathering place on some hospital floors. The nurse, however, is often called on to keep friends, relatives, and visitors informed about a child's capabilities and restrictions so that they can reinforce treatment goals. Having parents and friends help with treatment assumes that they feel comfortable with both the treatment plan and the goals. Obviously, the children's fears and anxieties are made worse if their parents also are fearful.

The nurse can greatly increase comfort by talking with family and friends about the nature of treatment and the function of any apparatus or equipment. Many people are frightened, uncomfortable, and overwhelmed when they see medical equipment. Patiently explaining and demonstrating how a piece of apparatus benefits a child, what can or cannot be done because of the illness, or the nature of the equipment and then being present to answer questions will decrease apprehensiveness. The more at ease the family or visitor, the more frequent and extended the visits will be.

Children who are hospitalized make many new friends, some of whom recover quickly and return home, whereas others require extended time and therapy before being able to leave the hospital. Close attachments among these children are beneficial, and helpful relationships can form between children who are mobile or further along in therapy and those who are just beginning treatment or are immobilized. Peer support and explanations of approaching events help in preparation and the development of coping strategies that sometimes make illness and hospitalization tolerable. Children who have gone home often return to visit those friends still in the hospital. This contact with friends who have "made it through" is encouraging for children in various phases of treatment and recovery.

The realization that they are not alone is itself reassuring to children. Child-to-child teaching and support allow for the discussion of topics not possible when talking with an adult. Peer interaction and support become increasingly helpful to the older child and adolescent.

Cultural traditions and expectations frequently dictate how adults respond to the ill child. Knowledge of the family's roots and assessment of family dynamics allow nurses to adapt nursing approaches to mesh goals and expectations, thus encouraging cooperation (see Chapter 17).

The family and significant friends are best able to provide the hospitalized child with the support and continuity necessary to meet the child's emotional needs. Involving the family in the child's plan of care and in actual physical care when appropriate helps to create a mode for giving this support.

As much as possible, the child should remain a part of family activities. Celebrations such as birthdays should occur, at least in part, wherever the child receiving treatment is located. The closer the family ties, the more difficult it is for the hospitalized child not to be a part of family rituals and events. When plans are altered to accommodate the needs and limitations of one member, however, other members must not be inadvertently forgotten. For example, both siblings and parents need to be present for these events.

When family members continue to work and play together and a routine is established that encourages growth for both the child and family, normal development continues. The family becomes very important to the member who is separated either because of location or immobility. Nurses need to be sensitive to the needs of whole families as well as to individuals within a family; therefore, the nurse adapts approaches and routines accordingly.

The Family's Experience of Illness

Serious illness, whether acute or chronic, affects every member of the family and, to a greater or lesser extent, alters their roles, daily routine, and expectations of each other and the ill child. The emotional upheaval of acute illness, the financial pressures of hospitalization, and the individual grief of family members place the entire family under stress. If relief and help are not available, family members might cope by escaping into work, withdrawal, alcohol abuse, or separation and divorce. Other children in the family also might act out their hostility at having to sacrifice for the ill sibling.

A nurse's attitudes and expectations often can influence the family's ability to cope with the child's problems. In case of child abuse or neglect or fetal alcohol syndrome, for example, nurses might feel that the child's parents should feel guilty and have difficulty communicating and planning care with these parents. These parents, do, however, need assistance in changing the factors that have led to the child's disorder. Nurses therefore can assist parents in understanding their role in caring for their children. (Child abuse and neglect are discussed further in Chapter 22; fetal alcohol syndrome is discussed in Chapter 23.)

Impact of the Diagnosis

When children are diagnosed as having serious illnesses, their parents often feel an element of injustice. For many parents, it seems almost inconceivable that their children might become seriously ill and die or experience serious limitations. Parents often say that they would do anything in the world to change places with the child.

The impact of the diagnosis depends on several factors. One factor is the suddenness with which the child becomes ill. If a disease has a gradual onset, the family, through gradual recognition of the symptoms and their implications, might be better able to deal with the diagnosis. If the illness has a sudden, unexpected onset, however, families often are totally unprepared and might not be able to cope with the sudden development of a disorder.

The seriousness of the illness is another factor that affects the family's reaction. Obviously, if the child has a disease for which there is a well-known treatment and a high cure rate, the family usually will be less anxious than the family whose child is ill with a mysterious ailment for which there is no known treatment. The degree of seriousness is also defined by the family, and what the nurse deems serious therefore is not always viewed as serious by family members.

For example, the parents of a young child who appears physically normal but begins to tire easily might have difficulty accepting the diagnosis of a heart condition, even though health professionals are quite concerned. Family members might require more evidence of illness in the child before they can accept such a diagnosis and its seriousness. On the other hand, a family might view as very threatening an illness that health professionals consider minor. To nurses accustomed to caring for children undergoing renal dialysis and transplant, the diagnosis of undescended testicles (cryptorchidism) might seem insignificant. To the child, surgery on the genitals can be terrifying, and to the parents, it might seem major.

Parents frequently have intense emotional reactions to illnesses that permanently limit their children's potential and are usually less threatened by conditions, such as mild asthma or milk intolerance, that often are outgrown and do not permanently limit the child's growth and future capabilities.

The parent's views concerning a disease and its ultimate outcome are the factors that most influence the child's view of the disease and consequent use of adaptive coping strategies. For example, if a mother of a child who experiences hair loss during chemotherapy encourages the child to wear a wig or hat and attend a party, the child is less likely to view the illness as requiring separation from friends. The mother's acceptance of the hair loss and constructive management of the problem by encouraging wearing a wig or hat allows the child to continue important social interactions. This ability to help the child maintain friendships, adjust to changes in appearance, and continue sound development during illness indicates true acceptance of the child's condition, which most often is achieved by parents who have strong support systems. Parents who cannot deal realistically with the problems that result from their children's illness often are unable to support their children in remaining functional in areas such as school, friends, and hobbies.

Conditions or treatments that result in obvious deviation from expected physical appearance, such as cleft lip, amputation, and baldness resulting from chemotherapy, also usually produce some emotional response in the child's parent. Emotional responses cannot be hidden from children, even though they might not be old enough to realize that their appearance differs from the norm. As children grow older and become more aware of how they should look, however, they usually view illness or treatments that produce alterations, such as Cushing's syndrome produced by prolonged high-dose steroid therapy, as threatening.

Yet another factor related to the impact of the diagnosis is the course of the illness. Some families are better able to cope with diseases that are beyond their control than with diseases that were caused by events to which the parents might feel they contributed. For example, the family of a child with juvenile arthritis might feel sorry for the child but cope fairly well. On the other hand, if the child has a sepsis from an untreated injury that became infected, the family might be so overwhelmed with guilt at having failed to treat the injury promptly that family members are unable to deal with the problems arising from the child's illness. The family with a child injured in an accident in which a family member might have been at fault also may have difficulty in dealing with the illness because of the associated anger or guilt.

Feelings of guilt, anger, and blame often control the family's response. For example, the family whose adolescent daughter has become pregnant and is now suffering from preeclampsia might respond to her in a way that is very different from the family whose adolescent daughter has severe asthma. The parents of an infant born with Down's syndrome might feel ashamed of their baby and may feel that they did something wrong that resulted in the birth of a retarded child. On the other hand, parents of an infant with a congenital heart defect might not feel this sense of shame because the condition does not involve intellectual impairment, although concern for the child's physical well-being may be just as stressful.

These situations might be reversed. Many parents of children with Down's syndrome, neonates as well as older children, consider their children beautiful and special, mobilize quickly to deal with associated congenital difficulties, and become knowledgeable in infant stimulation measures. On the other hand, one mother whose 3-year-old child was diagnosed as having a congenital heart defect needed to place blame. She searched her family for a history of such defects and, finding none, concluded that the defect must have come from the father's side of the family. Families can thus view illness in different ways. For some families, mental retardation and physical deformity are among the most difficult conditions to cope with, whereas for other families, sexually transmitted disease or pregnancy is intolerable.

Effects on Family Functioning

Patterns of Communication The nurse determines whether family members are able to discuss their feelings and concerns openly and frankly with each other. If they are not able to do so, the nurse notes dysfunctional communication within the family and plans interventions accordingly. The nurse needs, for instance, to determine whether children are able to obtain needed support from parents and siblings.

The parent is concerned not only with the magnitude of the child's illness and the associated discomfort and pain but also with the wider impact of the illness on the entire family. The parent might be very concerned about their other children and their reactions to the child's hospitalization. The nurse therefore observes interaction among the family members and assesses the usual patterns of communication (see Chapter 17). The nurse frequently finds that family members are able to discuss their concerns, feelings, ideas about the illness, and beliefs about its causes as they come to recognize the need to participate in the child's treatment.

In some families, however, communication patterns are not effective, and such severe stressors as serious illness and prolonged hospitalization might result in uncontrollable emotional responses that disrupt communication and family relationships. One parent, for example, might blame the other for the child's illness, feeling that the child was supervised inadequately and that this caused the illness. In other cases the parent might be so unable to overcome the first emotional response to the child's hospitalization and illness that subsequent information cannot be grasped fully.

In the early phase of an illness, the family members might not have much information about the child's condition or treatment regimen or about the eventual outcome of the illness. This ambiguity produces anxiety, frustration, and a sense of helplessness because the family is unable to act and plan constructively in the absence of necessary information. As the illness progresses, more information becomes available, but it might be negative. A parent might learn, for example, that a child's treatment requires various resources that are not available or will drain the family financially, physically, and emotionally. Such demands might then produce further feelings of anger, desperation, helplessness, and guilt if necessary treatment cannot be obtained.

The child's adaptive capacity is related to the adaptive capacity of the parents or other significant persons. Thus, if family members are able to talk with and draw comfort from each other during the child's illness, if they are able to explain to and comfort the child and siblings, the ill child perceives that the illness can be managed and that loved ones will be available to help with the unknowns that the illness presents.

The emotional responses of each parent to the child's illness or limitations are individual; seldom do two parents progress through their emotions in concert. For example, if a 4-year-old were hit by a car, the mother might feel a deep sense of guilt that she chose an inadequate babysitter who did not supervise the child properly. The father, on the other hand, might be extremely angry at the driver of the car. The mother might be unable to express her depression and guilt because the father is ranting and raving about the car and driver. Therefore, although those close to the child need to express their feelings openly, they must at some point listen to and understand other people's feelings.

This difference in emotional experience might cause difficulty in communication between parents who may blame each other for the child's problem. Feelings can include guilt and anger and they also might center on the child's no longer being perfect (see Chapter 30). If the parents have great difficulty in resolving their feelings about their ill child's problems, these feelings might result in distortion of the parents' relationship with each other, with their other children, and with the ill child.

Anger about the "unfairness" of the child's illness is difficult to resolve because no logical explanation is available. Parents might question their religious beliefs or scrutinize their own behaviors and the behaviors of others in a painful search for an explanation. They might question another's being out of a room when an accident happened or not noticing symptoms quickly enough.

Parents' anger might spill over onto the nurses and physicians who deal with them, and family members may make angry accusations toward each other. Nurses often do not recognize that anger comes from parental pain and grieving. This is particularly true when it is directed at the nursing staff. For example, one father whose 10-year-old son had just had a biopsy for staging of Hodgkin's disease was furious with his son's nurse for not preventing his child's discomfort or immediately answering the call light. The nurse needed to recognize the father's inappropriately directed anger, listen to his concerns, and continue to care for the child.

Therefore, the nurse assesses the parents and others who are part of the child's support system and have enduring emotional ties to the child. Siblings, close friends, grandparents, a cherished aunt, the primary caregiver at the day-care center, or a favorite teacher at school all might be invited to give their support to the child and family in the hospital. The nurse also assesses the family's access to such supportive groups as church organizations, peer support groups, and extended family members. The nurse further assesses the family's acceptance of assistance from external persons and agencies and observes family members for signs of lost self-esteem or violation of privacy.

Family Roles Another factor affecting the family is the possible shift in family roles and functions caused by the child's illness. When the child faces a long hospital stay and recovery, the impact on family life is clearly serious. When a child is hospitalized, family members must change their ways of functioning so that the family can continue to operate smoothly despite one of the member's being ill. The child's illness might require that someone give up work temporarily. For example, the mother of a hospitalized infant might take a leave of absence from her job so that her child does not experience the emotional trauma of a long separation, or the expense of therapy might require family members to take on additional jobs to pay for the child's care.

Therefore, for all hospitalized children, the nurse identifies who in the family is most able to deal realistically with the problems presented by the child's illness. Who is most able to comfort the child? Who can understand and carry out the responsibilities entailed in the child's treatment? Who is most desperately in need of support? To what extent can the family allow nonfamily members to enter into the daily life of the family, invade family privacy, and request that the family change its usual functioning?

The nurse assesses the significant persons in the child's life to determine who in the family can alter their daily routine to care for the ill child. Are family members locked into their life-styles, preventing them from making the changes required for the full recovery or emotional support of the child? Are the adults in the family able to focus on the needs of the dependent child, or are they themselves so entangled and preoccupied with disharmonious relationships, financial pressures, work stress, or low self-esteem and depression that the ill child is given inadequate care?

Can the family sustain the effort required to treat and care for the child for the required period of time? If adequate diversions, recreations, and opportunities for self-fulfillment are continually denied family members because of the child's illness, exhaustion and treatment failure are likely to occur.

The nurse and family therefore need to form a plan based on information and consultation from health professionals, and the plan should take into account how each member will be able to change day-to-day activities and schedules to meet the specific goals for the ill child's therapy. If this can be accomplished, the whole family is on the road to coping successfully with problems. Chronic or life-threatening illness in a child quickly exhausts the family, however, and much outside support might be needed to relieve the family members of seemingly unending treatments and postponement of rest and recreation. (The effects of chronic illness are discussed in Chapter 30.)

Family Configurations

Nuclear Families The parents' relationship to each other is important. The nurse assesses the parents' relationship to determine the extent of support and to identify any stress the parents' marriage might have been under before the child's illness. For the most part, the nurse assesses how much emotional and practical support the parents are able to give each other during the crisis. Does one parent blame the other for the child's illness? For example, does one parent point to a history of birth defects or other problems on the other parent's side of the family? Are the parents able to talk about the child's condition and prognosis together?

Do they have similar or differing views about the long-term consequences of the child's illness? Is one parent able to comprehend the reality while the other denies it? Does one parent accept blame for the child's problems? If the parents are grieving for the child's lost potential, are they able to talk with and support each other? Nurses often find that in times of crisis parents have difficulty in communicating their fears and disappointments to each other and may indeed view a crisis in different ways.

Single-Parent Families Single parenting is the norm in approximately one-third of American households today, and in most instances the head of the household is a single mother or a grandmother. In single-parent families the stress of illness and hospitalization is greater than in two-parent families. Most single parents, however, are able to rise to the occasion and to cope successfully with the stress.

In assessing single-parent families, the nurse determines whether the level of stress is inordinately high. If stress and the need for support are critical, the nurse refers the parent to appropriate resources (see Chapter 22). Single parents sometimes feel guilty that the child is deprived of the company of the other parent, especially if the child becomes ill and longs for the other parent. This guilt, coupled with the guilt that parents frequently feel when their children are ill, makes the role of the single parent especially difficult.

Because approximately 60% of households headed by a female live at or below the poverty level, a problem for many single parents is a lack of financial resources. Furthermore, because most single parents are women and most women earn less than men, the child's hospitalization can place exceptional stress on finances and be very difficult to manage. The nurse therefore assesses the financial support that the parent receives. Supportive grandparents and other relatives sometimes can help, but a single parent's situation is difficult when the hospitalized child requires the parent's presence during most of the child's waking hours. If the single parent must work and no other adults are close to the child or are able to stay with the child in the hospital, the nurse might need to arrange for a hospital volunteer to spend time with the child. In some hospitals retired persons have served as parent surrogates when parents are unable to remain with small children. The parent surrogate should be introduced to the parents and parental permission received before the surrogate parent's visits to the child are instituted.

Divorced or Separated Parents Other difficulties might arise when the parents of the hospitalized child are divorced or separated. In such instances the nurse separately assesses the child's relationship with each parent. In families with marital disharmony, children often feel loyal to one parent or the other, or one parent might attempt to win the affection of the children away from the other parent. A parent might, for instance, bitterly point out the negative behaviors of the other parent, or the child might play one parent against the other by making demands such as, "If you loved me as much as mother does, you would come to see me more often or you would buy me what I want." These tensions add to the stress of illness and hospitalization for the child and for the family members involved.

When the parents are separated, the nurse also needs to assess the parents' interaction with each other. In the initial period of the child's illness and hospitalization, can the two parents discuss the situation realistically and work together toward the child's recovery? Is one parent going to assume the responsibility for the child's recovery while the other parent leaves the child alone? Are the parents able to agree on the child's treatment? How will visiting arrangements for both parents be handled? If both parents are present in the hospital, are they able to remain civil and polite to each other and to the staff? If stepparents are involved, how supportive are they, both to the parent and to the child?

Nurses might have to remind the parents that they should not raise the child's anxiety level further and that the child should not have to feel embarrassed by a parent's behavior. In times of illness the child should receive support from both parents, and both parents need access to a child with a serious illness. In many such families, members of the extended family (such as grandparents, aunts, or uncles) also are very important to the child and should be allowed unlimited visiting privileges. In hospitals with limited space, family and friends can schedule their visits so that rooms are not crowded and the child has adequate time for quiet and rest.

Common Needs of Parents

Because the parent of a hospitalized child sees that the child's well-being is seriously threatened, the parent is likely to be anxious, which frequently leads to misunderstandings in communication. Therefore, the nurse who notes that the family is in a high state of anxiety takes this into account in communicating with the family.

People who are under stress might manifest anxiety in physical ways. They might, for example, be unable to pay attention to and retain information. They might not be able to focus on the most relevant information but may instead focus on nonessential or trivial aspects of what they are told. For example, the parent of a child who has just been admitted to a pediatric intensive care unit because of near-drowning might not understand why a neurologist is being called in, even though the reasons are presented in detail. Because the anxiety level is so high, the parent is not able to grasp the essential aspects of the child's neurologic status and instead might ask repeatedly about the intravenous fluids or the condition of other children in the unit.

Long-term hospitalization also creates stress, and the parent faces constant reminders of the child's condition. The impact of an empty bed or a missed child at the dinner table is often an added source of stress. When a child is seriously ill and hospitalized, the family's daily activities become severely disrupted. Parents might spend large amounts of time at the hospital and thus may be unable to fulfill work commitments. Employers are not always understanding when a parent misses work because of a child's illness, and this places additional pressure on the parent. Some parents complain that they are unable to sleep because of worry and emotional upset. Sleep deprivation is common in families with hospitalized children, and it too increases irritability and limits the parents' abilities to comprehend information and solve problems effectively.

Parents need some diversion from the constant stress and anxiety caused by a child's illness and hospitalization. They need to deal with the tension, restlessness, and fear that high anxiety generates. Intense, prolonged anxiety can cause behavioral and emotional breakdown. Therefore, the nurse assesses the family's means of coping with stress. Do family members find time for some diversion from the hospital and work routine? Do they allow themselves some escape from their concerns and troubles? Is this escape constructive, as in playing a hard game of racquetball, or is it destructive, as in drug or alcohol abuse? Are they able to express their innermost feelings with a trusted, supportive person?

A person experiencing a high level of anxiety is usually restless and has elevated respiratory and heart rates. The nurse thus is often able to assess a parent's level of anxiety by observing physical signs. Communication and health teaching can then be tailored to the family's needs.

Multiple stressors compounded by the illness of a child can place parents at risk for dysfunctional parenting (see Chapter 22). Therefore, when family members are highly anxious, the nurse plans interventions to decrease unnecessary anxiety. For example, the nurse is either available to answer the family's questions or makes some other person available to the family, such as a social worker, who will be able to give family members the time they require.

Need for Support The ultimate impact of the child's hospitalization is related to the balance between the child's illness and the family's ability to use resources either from inside or outside the family. If disruption in usual family functioning inhibits problem solving, a constructive response to stress and adaptive coping strategies probably have not been learned. The family that has little problem-solving experience is in great need of support. The family is handicapped further in problem solving because of the emotional reaction caused by having a child in the family with a serious illness and because of a limited knowledge of options and effective behaviors to use in overcoming the crisis.

Support generally is demonstrated by practical assistance to parents, siblings, and ill children in families. People who are supportive typically help members of the family maintain emotional balance by encouraging them to express their emotions openly, helping them to find solutions to immediate problems, and assisting them to accomplish required tasks during the crisis. Does a family friend listen as the mother repeatedly talks about her concerns? Is someone tending siblings when the parent visits the ill child?

In some families the extended family (such as aunts, grandparents, or grown siblings) recognizes that the family is confronting stress and steps in to give assistance. In the best of situations, such family members provide uncritical emotional support and practical help with child care, transportation, meal preparation, and housekeeping chores. Today, however, many families do not live near their close relatives, and young families with small children who have moved away from their hometowns might be especially isolated.

Friends of children and friends of parents can play important supportive roles during times of stress and crisis, and their support also might prevent a stressful situation from becoming a crisis. The nurse therefore assesses the amount of constructive help provided by friends. Help during times of trouble includes acceptance of feelings, wishes, and hopes, and such concrete tasks as cooking, listening, and taking care of the other children.

It is essential for the health care team who perceives the child's illness as a crisis for the family to support the child and family. Because the nurse is one member of the team who is in frequent, direct contact with the child and family, the nurse's support can diminish family disorganization and help both the family and child to learn adaptive coping strategies and thus become even stronger than they were before the crisis.

Parents need to be able to express their emotional responses to their child's illness and hospitalization, but not all families need nursing or other health care professionals for this purpose. For instance, a mother and father who are close to their own parents or have friends available to them might choose not to discuss their emotional responses with the nurse. In fact, such families might appear to hold together very well. On the surface, they might appear calm, rational, and accepting of treatment; they might very well grasp the seriousness of the child's illness but can depend on an extended family and close friends.

As the nurse works closely with any family over a period of time, however, the nurse is likely to become an important family support. If family members begin to trust the nurse, they might begin to share their more private emotions and feelings about events surrounding the child's illness. Not all families, however, immediately expect the nurse to be supportive and thus do not volunteer their responses to the child's illness and hospitalization. One essential nursing responsibility therefore is to diagnose the family's immediate needs for support and to intervene as necessary.

Once the family has expressed uncertainty and fearfulness to supportive persons, family members are better able to deal realistically with the problems at hand. This is not to say that feelings that are expressed do not recur; parents might become quite depressed over the course of a long illness in which the outcome is in doubt and will require long-term supportive care from either close family and friends or from a few health care professionals to whom the parents feel close. For this reason, the nurse monitors the family's need for one person to be available throughout the child's illness.

In trying to be with both the hospitalized child and the siblings at home, who are also upset, parents might become exhausted. For these families, outside help is essential, and if the assistance of relatives or close friends is not available, the household can deteriorate rapidly. Some families are able to use outside services, whereas other might feel that contact with outside persons is an invasion of privacy. Some families are unable to accept outside help because this violates their feeling that families should be able to "take care of their own." The nurse needs to be sensitive to each family's beliefs and views and accept the parents' rights to their own opinions and goals.

Supports outside the family include community agencies for assistance, which range from food stamps to employment counseling, and groups of families who have experienced similar problems. Because community resources vary, the nurse provides up-to-date information about the appropriate supportive services available. Families also can be swamped by dealing with too many people from too many agencies; therefore, ideally, one nurse works continuously with the family and coordinates the contacts the family makes when many agencies are involved. The continuity provided by a single nurse in charge of care also minimizes inconsistencies in the care plan while easing the problem of the child's separation from familiar caregivers.

If, however, the care and ultimate recovery of the child is jeopardized by the family's inability either to recognize or deal effectively with problems arising from the child's illness, outside services might need to be consulted. In general, such cases are reviewed extensively by nursing personnel, medical staff, social workers, and possibly personnel from child protective services (see Chapter 22).

Need for Information Parents need information to begin problem solving. Once the family has an accurate grasp of the child's illness and treatment, the nurse presents the options available so that parents might choose the options that are consistent with family values. It is important that all members of the health care team present a consistent picture of the child's condition and treatment, but this is sometimes more easily said than done. Medical personnel might disagree about the best therapy for a particular child; nurses might have differing ideas about the best care plan. As much as possible, however, the nurse coordinates care by reminding health care professionals that the family needs a consistent and honest assessment.

The nurse's discussions with the family and child focus on their concerns because family members will not see the nurse as helpful if their concerns are not sought each time they interact with the nurse. When family members are informed about the child's illness and treatment, medical procedures, and hospital policies, the nurse provides this information at a level that the family is able to grasp. If family members are highly anxious, their ability to retain information is limited, and they might not be able to focus their attention while information is being given. For this reason, the nurse plans to review with family members their understanding of the child's situation and treatment and might need to repeat this information throughout the course of the child's hospitalization.

Because parents frequently are disorganized, confused, and unable to comprehend events, the nurse makes every effort to communicate clearly and to present to the family a coherent picture of the child's condition and treatment.

The nurse thus assesses the changing nature of the family's ability to understand both the broader picture of the child's illness and prognosis and the many details of therapy. Some families want to know only the broad aspects of the child's condition, whereas others tend to focus on minor details.

General information is initially better than giving many small details of the child's situation. For example, when a neonate is admitted to a neonatal intensive care unit (NICU), an abundance of laboratory data and technical information usually is available. Arterial blood gases might be measured every 4 hours and bilirubin levels measured every 8 hours; mechanical ventilator settings might change. If the nurse discusses every laboratory value and every oxygen and ventilator change within the first 24 hours, such a mass of data will overwhelm most anxiety-laden parents.

Even so, the nurse cannot apply a set of hard and fast rules about appropriate topics to discuss with parents. Some parents actually cope better when all their detailed questions are answered, even if the nurse thinks that they are focusing unduly on minute changes in laboratory values and technical information. Such parents actually might be seeking reassurance that the nurse understands their child's complex care, or they might be coping through intellectualization. If their questions are answered consistently and without defensiveness, the parents might begin to focus on larger matters after a time.

Family members often become anxious when the nurse withholds requested information. This is a good reason for the nurse to know what the entire health care team thinks about the child's condition and plan of care, so that communication can be open rather than guarded. For those families who focus almost exclusively on minute details, the nurse can repeat the broad picture of the child's condition as often as necessary. If the assessment indicates that the family really has a limited understanding of the child's illness, treatment, and prognosis, even after repeated explanations over several days, the nurse might need to arrange a conference involving those health care professionals who interact with the family so that plans can be made to present the family with a clear picture.

Further assessment might show that the family's needs for emotional support are not being met and that the family therefore continues to experience the disorganization and loss of function typical of families in crisis. The nurse then helps to reduce anxiety levels through supportive discussions in which the family's resources might be evaluated and the family might come to recognize the need to rely on others for a period of time.

Need for Participation Families need to continue to interact with their hospitalized child, both for the child's sake and for their own sense of security and need to see progress. Family members should be allowed to take part in the child's care to the extent that they are able. This process of caregiving by family members should be negotiated on a day-to-day basis, with initial and continued input from the family into the child's care plan.

As the child's condition changes, the nursing care plan is revised so that parental input and participation can be maximized. Some hospitals' pediatric units are designed to enable a family member to remain with the child day and night and to provide varying amounts of the child's care. The child—especially the young child—benefits greatly from the continual presence of parents or other family members.

The family's participation will depend, of course, on the child's illness. The family might participate in care simply by being present, talking, reading, singing, giving a bed bath, or feeding. The family might bring in treasured toys for the child so that the hospital seems more familiar. (In some units these toys will be sterilized before being placed in the child's room.)

A parent's involvement in care, which provides both a welcome continuity in routine and sense of close caring for the child, does not mean that the nurse turns over responsibilities to the parent. Even when a parent becomes adept at meeting an ill child's physical needs, the nurse needs to relieve the parent of the full responsibilities for care. Nurses also need to provide parents with the required rest time away from their children and a sympathetic ear for the parents to express their own needs. Many parents must be reminded that the nurse can and will stay with a child so that the parent can eat or relax without the constant pressure of meeting the child's needs.

In some hospitals visiting with a hospitalized child sometimes is limited to parents, grandparents, and siblings. Because hospitalization of a child is very stressful, however, nurses need to be flexible enough to consider exceptions to many rules. For example, an unmarried 14-year-old might need the support of her best friend rather than her brother or sister if her newborn infant is in the NICU. There is very little evidence that rules prohibiting the visitation of extended family members and close friends serve any useful purpose in the hospitalization of children. Where such rules exist, they should be reviewed and made to reflect an increasing understanding of the significance of social support and family support in the child's ability to cope with serious illness and hospitalization.

Common Needs of Siblings

As with the reactions of parents, the reactions of siblings depend on their experience of illness in the family and their developmental stages. Often, in the midst of worrying about the ill child, the adults in the family forget about the needs of the healthy children for attention, emotional sharing, explanation, and continuity of routine.

The children at home often are sent to neighbors or relatives who are not prepared to care for them. The healthy children's usual patterns of awakening, eating breakfast, dressing for school, playing with peers, interacting with parents, and going to bed may be seriously disrupted. The nurse inquires about the care of the other children in the family to determine whether they must leave home and visit other people's homes during a family crisis. If this is the case, the nurse might be able to assist the parents in planning to minimize the disruption of the healthy children's routines.

Even if the children remain at home, the home atmosphere often is seriously disrupted, and the children might worry that they somehow caused their sibling's illness. These children need to be reassured that they are not to blame and that their magical thoughts will not make the ill child's condition worse.

For example, one usually happy and well behaved 4-year-old girl became increasingly difficult to manage when her infant brother became ill. When she was quite out of control, spinning herself around and screaming, it occurred to her mother that the girl might feel she was responsible for her brother's illness. The mother stopped the girl's spinning, held her by the shoulders, looked straight in her eyes and said, "It's not your fault that the baby is sick." The child's behavior immediately changed. She visibly relaxed and went off to play by herself.

Siblings also might fear the ridicule of peers, who might taunt them with jeers such as, "Your sister is retarded." Siblings then might reject the ill child or become overprotective and not allow an ill or handicapped sibling to do things unaided.

A response common to children of all ages is jealousy. If the hospitalized child receives the lion's share of attention from parents and other family members, jealousy might be a way to demand attention. Behavioral problems in siblings often are bids for attention, but if the children at home misbehave more frequently than usual, this is yet another source of stress for the family.

The honest, open expression of such emotions as sadness, grief, despair, anxiety, anger, confusion, and depression that usually accompany serious illness and hospitalization of children are healthy and adaptive responses. If the adults and older siblings in the family can talk together about problems and express their feelings, acknowledging that it is all right to cry and feel angry, this is a step in the right direction. After the more mature family members have dealt with their own feelings, they can be more comforting to the younger children, whose verbal skills might not be sufficiently developed to allow them to comprehend the severity of the problem.

Key Concepts

- Illness and hospitalization are stressful for the child and family and might lead to a crisis in which previously learned coping strategies are not adequate for dealing with the perceived threat.
- The indicators of stress and coping in children include regression, somatic complaints, direct expression of emotion, expressive behaviors, and cognitive approaches.
- The extent to which a child's coping strategies are adaptive rather than maladaptive depends on the child's developmental stage, previous experience, and perception of the threat posed by the illness.
- The indicators of ineffective family coping include anxiety, family disorganization, inadequate communication, and inadequate support systems.
- Children progress from viewing illness as punishment in early and middle childhood to understanding infectious agents and exposure in late childhood to recognizing a variety of interrelated factors in adolescence.
- Stressors specific to hospitalization include fear of the unknown, isolation, and invasion of privacy.
- Separation anxiety is an extreme reaction to the perceived loss of a parent and is most common in infancy and early childhood, until the child learns that the parent will return.
- Without appropriate interventions, separation in infancy progresses through three distinct stages leading to withdrawn behaviors and lack of interest in human contact.
- Rooming-in of parents, especially when the hospitalized child is in infancy or early childhood, can help to offset the effects of separation.
- In later infancy and early childhood, the child's developing mobility and sense of autonomy are greatly threatened by restraints or confinement.
- Infants and young children fear painful procedures and associate people, colors, or surroundings with pain.
- In early childhood the child's mastery of new skills often is threatened by hospitalization and normal regression.
- In middle childhood children are uncomfortable with

changes in body function or appearance and often become anxious about invasive procedures and procedures involving the genital area.

- From middle childhood on, children learn to use developing cognitive skills to cope with separation from family, school, and peers.
- In middle to late childhood, children fear body disfigurement and might react with anger, frustration, or depression when faced with loss of control.
- In late childhood children use cognitive skills to control emotions and cope with separation and loss of function; therefore, nursing interventions focus on providing opportunities for discussion and problem solving.
- Older children and adolescents are especially fearful of long-term disabilities, possible death, and procedures that affect the genital area.
- Older children and adolescents might react to separation from peers as much as from parents and therefore might benefit from contact with friends outside the hospital and with other patients.
- The need for independence makes change of body image and function especially threatening for the adolescent, who often depends on the norms of a peer group to reinforce self-concept.
- Nursing interventions are planned to enhance coping by facilitating understanding and age-appropriate expression, enhancing family communication, and preparing the child and family for the real or perceived threats of illness.
- Nursing care for children of all ages involves providing as much independence as possible, monitoring sensory needs, planning opportunities for learning, and maintaining social contacts, both with family members and others.
- Parental perception of a child's illness depends on its onset, likely outcome, extent of long-term limitations for the child, and possible feelings of guilt or anger.
- In assessing the effect of a child's illness on the family, the nurse observes family interactions and communication, family roles, and changes in the family's usual level of functioning.
- The nurse assesses the parents' relationship with each other and adapts interventions to the assessment criteria and to the family configuration.
- Parents typically need support in the form of financial assistance, emotional support of other parents or professionals, and help with day-to-day tasks.
- Parents need accurate, consistent information and might need to hear it repeated until they are ready to comprehend it.
- Family participation in the care of an ill child helps to maintain family functioning and to provide siblings with as much involvement as possible, which helps to offset the jealousy that siblings often feel.

References

Azarnoff P, Hargrove C (editors): *The Family in Child Health Care.* Wiley, 1981.

Azarnoff P, Woody PD: Preparation of children for hospitalization in acute care hospitals in the United States. *Pediatrics* (Sept) 1981; 68(3): 361–368.

Beverly B: The effects of illness upon emotional development. *J Pediatr* 1936; 8:533–543.

Bibace R, Walsh ME: Development of children's concepts of illness. *Pediatrics* (Dec) 1980; 66(6):912–917.

Bowlby J: Some pathological processes set in train by early mother–child separation. *J Ment Sci* 1953; 99:265–272.

Johnson JE, Kirchhoff KT, Endress MP: Altering children's distress behavior during orthopedic cast removal. *Nurs Res* 1975; 24:404.

Kellerman J, et al: Disease-related communication and depression in pediatric cancer patients. *J Pediatr Psychol* 1977; 2(2):52–53.

Kunzman L: Some factors influencing a young child's mastery of hospitalization. *Nurs Clin North Am* 1971; 18:625.

Meng AL: Parents' and children's reactions toward impending hospitalization for surgery. *Matern Child Nurs J* (Summer) 1980; 9:83–98.

Prugh DG, et al: A study of the emotional reactions of children and families to hospitalization and illness. *Am J Orthopsychiatry* 1953; 23:70–106.

Robertson J: *Young Children in Hospital.* 2nd ed. Tavistock, 1970.

Simeonsson RJ, Buckley L, Monson L: Conceptions of illness causality in hospitalized children. *J Pediatr Psychol* 1979; 4(1):77–84.

Tesler M, Savedra M: Coping with hospitalization: A study of school-age children. *Pediatr Nurs* (March/April) 1981; 7:35–38.

Triplett J, Arneson S: The use of verbal and tactile comfort to alleviate distress in young hospitalized children. *Res Nurs Health* 1970; 2:17–23.

Additional Readings

Ack M: New perspectives in comprehensive health care for children. *J Pediatr Psychol* 1976; 1(4):9–11.

Arneson S, Triplett J: How children cope with disfiguring changes in their appearances. *Am J Matern Child Nurs* (Nov/Dec) 1978; 3:366–370.

Azarnoff P: The care of children in hospitals: An overview. *J Pediatr Psychol* 1976; 1(4):5–6.

Azarnoff P: Mediating the trauma of serious illness and hospitalization in childhood. *Child Today* 1974; 3(4):12–17.

Benoliel JQ: The concept of care for a child with leukemia. *Nurs Forum* 1972; 11:194.

Birchfield ME: Nursing care for the hospitalized child. *Am J Matern Child Nurs* (March/April) 1981; 6(2):47–52.

Brammer LM: *The Helping Relationship: Process and Skills*. Prentice-Hall, 1973.

Brill NI: *Working with People: The Helping Process*. Lippincott, 1973.

Burton L: *The Family Life of Sick Children: A Study of Families Coping with Chronic Childhood Disease*. Routledge & Kegan Paul, 1975.

Daniel WA: *The Adolescent Patient*. Mosby, 1970.

Davis A: The skills of communication. *Am J Nurs* 1963; 63:40.

Drotar D, et al: Psychosocial functioning of children with cystic fibrosis. *Pediatrics* (March) 1981; 67(3):338–353.

Dunlop D, Higgins L, Ling N: Crisis intervention in basic nursing education. *J Nurs Educ* 1978; 17:37–41.

Eland JM: Minimizing the hurt. Paper presented at the 17th Annual Conference of the Association for the Care of Children's Health. Seattle, Washington, June 2–5, 1982.

Erickson F: Helping the sick child maintain behavioral control. *Nurs Clin North Am* (Dec) 1967; 4:695–703.

Erickson F: Nurse specialist for children. *Nurs Outlook* 1968; 16:34.

Fagin CM, Nusbaum GC: Parental visiting privileges in pediatric units: A survey. *J Nurs Adm* 1978; 7:24–27.

Farrell M, Haley M, Magnasco J: Teaching interpersonal skills. *Nurs Outlook* 1977; 25:322–325.

Fletcher B: Rooming-in: A reassessment. *Matern Child Nurs J* (Summer) 1981; 10:85–98.

Freud A: The role of bodily illness in the mental life of children. *Psychoanal Study Child* 1952; 7:69–81.

Galligan AC: Using Roy's concept of adaptation to care for young children. *Am J Matern Child Nurs* 1979; 4(2):24–28.

Gratz RR, Piliavin JA: What makes kids sick: Children's beliefs about the causative factors of illness. *Child Health Care* (Spring) 1984; 12(4):156–162.

Hagemann V: Night sleep in children in a hospital. Part I: Sleep disruption. *Matern Child Nurs J* (Spring) 1981; 10:1–13.

Hagemann V: Night sleep in children in a hospital. Part II: Sleep disruption. *Matern Child Nurs J* (Summer) 1981; 10:127–142.

Hardgrove CB, Rutledge A: Parenting during hospitalization. *Am J Nurs* 1975; 25:836.

Hazzard ME, Thorndal ML: Patient anxiety: Teaching students to intervene effectively. *Nurse Educator* 1979; 4:19–21.

Hersh SP: A perspective on behavioral medicine and pediatric psychology. *J Pediatr Psychol* 1976; 1(4): 3–4.

Hodapp RM: Effects of hospitalization on young children: Implications of two theories. *Child Health Care* (Winter) 1982; 10:83–86.

Hoff LA: *People in Crisis: Understanding and Helping*. Addison-Wesley, 1978.

Hoffman AD, Becker RD, Gabriel HP: *The Hospitalized Adolescent*. The Free Press, 1976.

Hollenbeck AR, et al: Children with serious illness: Behavioral correlates of separation and isolation. *Child Psychiatry Hum Dev* (Fall) 1980; 11 (1):3–11.

Holmes S: The use of control by a hospitalized five year old girl. *Matern Child Nurs J* (Fall) 1976; 5:189–196.

Infante MS: *Crisis Theory: A Framework for Nursing Practice*. Prentice-Hall, 1982.

Kalish B: An experiment in the development of empathy in nursing students. *Nurs Res* 1971; 20:202–211.

Kalish B: Strategies for developing nurse empathy. *Nurs Outlook* 1971; 19:714–718.

Katz R, et al: School intervention with pediatric cancer patients. *J Pediatr Psychol* 1978; 2(2):72–76.

Kerr NJ: The effect of hospitalization on the developmental tasks of childhood. *Nurs Forum* 1980; 18:108–130.

King J, Ziegler S: The effects of hospitalization on children's behavior: A review of the literature. *Children's Health Care* (Summer) 1981; 10:20–28.

Kister MC, Patterson CJ: Children's conceptions of illness: Understanding of contagion and use of immanent justice. *Child Dev* 1980; 51:839–846.

Klinzing DR, Klinzing DG: *The Hospitalized Child: Communication Techniques for Health Personnel*. Prentice-Hall, 1977.

Lambert VA, Lambert CE Jr: *The Impact of Physical Illness and Related Mental Health Concepts*. Prentice-Hall, 1979.

Latimer E: Play is everybody's business in the children's ward. *Nurs Mirror* (Sept) 1978; 147:21–24.

Layton J: The use of modeling to teach empathy to nursing students. *Res Nurs Health* 1979; 2:163–75.

Luciano K: The who, when, where, what and how of preparing children for surgery. *Nursing '74* (Nov) 1974; 4(11):64–65.

McAnarney ER, Sahler OJ: *The Child from Three to Eighteen*. Mosby, 1981.

McCorkle R: Effects of touch on seriously ill patients. *Nurs Res* 1975; 23:125–132.

McGoran S: On developing empathy: Teaching students self-awareness. *Am J Nurs* 1978; 78:859–862.

Magrab PR, Bronheim S: The child-life model and pediatric hospitalization. *J Pediatr Psychol* 1976; 1(4):7–8.

Mathews B: Measurements of psychological aspects of the nurse–patient relationship. *Nurs Res* 1962; 11:154–162.

Meyers M: The effects of types of communications on patients' reactions to stress. *Nurs Res* 1964; 13:131.

Millerd EM: Health professionals as survivors. *J Psychiatric Nurs* 1977; 77:33–37.

Miya T: The child's perception of death. *Nurs Forum* 1972; 11:214.

Moss JR: Helping young children cope with the physical examination. *Pediatr Nurs* (March/April) 1981; 7:17–20.

O'Malley JE, Koocher GP: Psychological consultation to a pediatric oncology unit: Obstacles to effective intervention. *J Pediatr Psychol* 1977; 2(2):54–57.

Oremland EK, Oremland JD (editors): *The Effects of Hospitalization on Children*. Thomas, 1973.

Parad HJ, Caplan G: A framework for studying families in crisis. In: *Crisis Intervention: Selected Readings*. Parad HJ (editor). Family Service Association of America, 1965.

Peitchinis J: Therapeutic effectiveness of counseling by nursing personnel: Review of the literature. *Nurs Res* 1972; 21:138.

Perrin EC, Gerrity PS: There's a demon in your belly: Children's understanding of illness. *Pediatrics* (June) 1981; 67(6):841–849.

Peters BM: School-aged children's beliefs about causality of illness. *Matern Child Nurs J* (Fall) 1978; 7(3):143–154.

Petrillo M, Sanger D: *Emotional Care of Hospitalized Children: An Environmental Approach*. Lippincott, 1972.

Piaget J: *Play, Dreams, and Imitation in Childhood*. Norton, 1952.

Pidgeon J: Functions of preschool children's questions in coping with hospitalization. *Res Nurs Health* 1981; 4:229–235.

Plan E: *Working with Children in Hospitals*. Year Book, 1971.

Postner EC: Stress immunization: Techniques to help children cope with hospitalization. *Matern Child Nurs J* (Summer) 1983; 12:119–134.

Puskar K: Structure for the hospitalized adolescent. *J Psychiatr Nurs* (July) 1981; 19(7):13–16.

Rager PM, Vipperman JF: Childhood coping: How nurses can help. *Pediatr Nurs* (March/April) 1980; 6(2):11–18.

Rothenberg MB: The unique role of the child life worker in children's health care settings. *Child Health Care* 1982; 10(4):121–124.

Rumfelt JM: How five-year-old children perceive the nurse. *Matern Child Nurs J* (Spring) 1980; 9:13–24.

Schmeltz K, White G: A survey of parent groups: Prehospital admission. *Matern Child Nurs J* (Summer) 1982; 11(2):75–86.

Shamansky SL: Characteristics contributing to attachment behavior and its outcomes in student nurse–family relationships. *Nurs Educ* 1981; 20:26–31.

Smith EC, et al: Reestablishing a child's body image. *Am J Nurs* 1977; 77:445.

Stetler C: Relationship of perceived empathy to nurses' communication. *Nurs Res* 1977; 25:432–438.

Stinson N: *Chronic Illness and the Family: Coping and Support Systems.* (Thesis.) Graduate School of Nursing, University of Texas at Austin, 1981.

Sundeen SJ, et al: *Nurse–Client Interaction: Implementing the Nursing Process.* Mosby, 1976.

Terry G: A five-year-old-boy's aggressive and compensatory behavior in response to immobilization. *Matern Child Nurs J* (Spring) 1979; 8(1): 29–38.

Vipperman J, Roger P: Childhood coping: How nurses can help. *Pediatr Nurs* (March/April) 1980; 6:11–18.

Vulcan B: Major coping behaviors of a hospitalized three-year-old boy. *Matern Child Nurs J* (Summer) 1984; 13:113–123.

Waechter EH: Children's awareness of fatal illness. *Am J Nurs* 1971; 71:1168.

Youssef MHS: Self-control behaviors of school-age children who are hospitalized for cardiac diagnostic procedures. *Matern Child Nurs J* (Winter) 1981; 10(4):219–277.

Play for the Hospitalized Child

28

Sandra R. Mott   Betty M. Lovelace

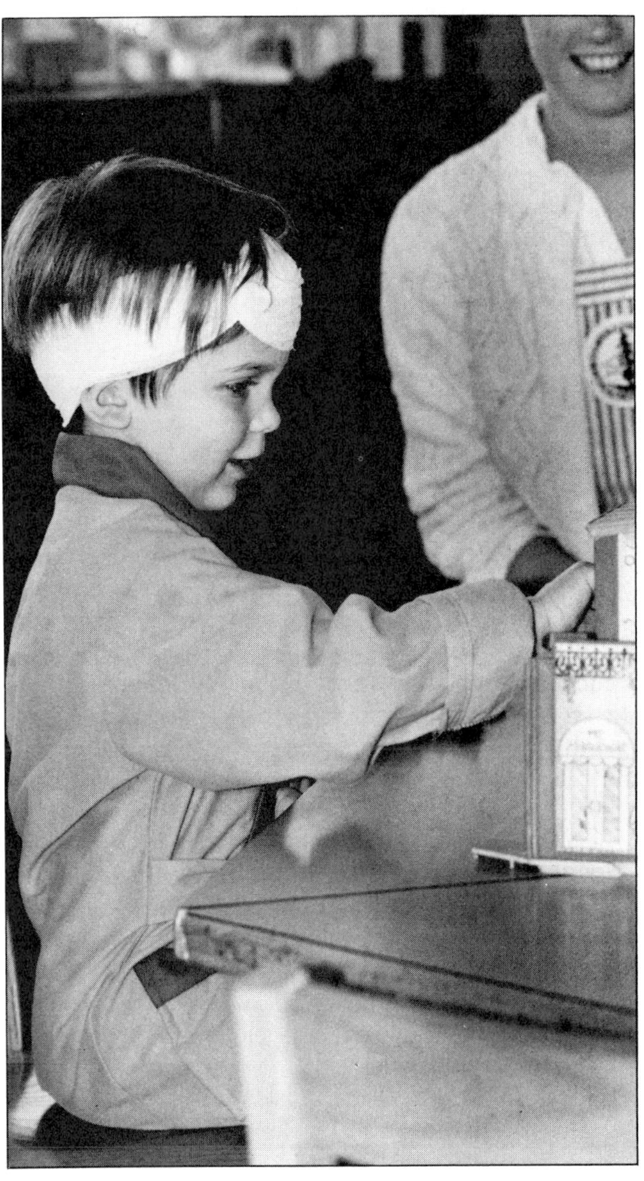

Chapter Outline

Objectives

- Explain the purpose of play for the hospitalized child.
- Distinguish between play therapy and therapeutic play.
- Relate the purpose of play in the hospital to each developmental stage.
- Define the role of the nurse and the play therapist in the hospital setting.
- Describe ways to provide play for the immobilized or isolated child.
- Explain the use of play as a means of developmental assessment.
- Explain the ways in which the child uses play to cope with the experience of hospitalization.
- Describe the nurse's role in facilitating the child's coping with and learning about the hospital environment.

As George Bernard Shaw wrote,

> All children should be tirelessly noisy, playful, grubby-handed except at meal-times, tearing such clothes as they need to wear, bringing not only the joy of childhood into the house but the mess as well; in short, everything that makes the quiet and order of sickness and nursing impossible.

It would be wonderful if all children could be as Shaw desires. But those children stricken by disease or injury serious enough to require hospitalization usually are restricted by their conditions, their treatments, or the hospital environment to a less-than-ideal existence. The challenge of the health care team is to adapt the hospital environment and the staff's goals to meet the hospitalized child's needs and to minimize the possible deleterious effects of hospitalization.

The goal of the members of the health team is to combine their efforts so that both medical and developmental objectives can be realized. One way of accomplishing this is to develop a care plan that incorporates play activities to provide hospitalized children with opportunities to accomplish the normal tasks of development as well as to deal with fears, anxiety, frustration, and anger concerning their hospitalization or illness.

In Chapter 27 we explore the child's and family's responses to hospitalization. In this chapter we examine how the nurse can use play activities for the purpose of assessment, teaching, and therapeutic play. We look at the various methods of play, the types of play relative to each developmental stage, the creation of an atmosphere conducive to play, and the role of the nurse and play therapist in the hospital setting.

What Is Play?

Meaning of Play for Children

Children engage in play during most of their waking hours, yet play is a most difficult concept to define. Numerous theorists have studied various aspects of play, defining sequential steps of content, structure, and themes as enacted in the process of play and then defining these steps according to their major focus of interest (see Chapters 7–11). Few of these theorists have attempted an inclusive definition. Participating in a symposium on play and development, Erik Erikson commented about some of the possible meanings evident in play: "True, the themes presented betray some repetitiveness such as we recognize as the 'working through' of a *traumatic* experience; but they also express a playful *renewal.* If they seem to be governed by some need to *communicate* or even *confess,* they certainly also seem to serve the *joy of self expression.* If they seem dedicated to the *exercise* of growing faculties they also seem to serve the *mastery* of a complex life situation. As I would not settle for any one of these explanations alone, I would not wish to do without any one of them" (Piers, 1972).

In other words, play is "a many-splendored thing," and the intricacies as well as the variety of themes in children's play should be respected and appreciated. Play is complex, and its specific values overlap the diverse themes, content, and forms of expression it takes throughout life. An educator during the early 1800s, Friedrich Froebel has been called the "apostle of play." He influenced Jean-Jacques Rousseau and others with his belief that play was essential to the full and harmonious development of the child and that the child learned best through spontaneous play (Lowenfeld, 1967). Lowenfeld's interesting commentary on play organizes play into four general categories: (1) play as a bodily activity in its earliest form; (2) play as a realization of experience gained in previous years; (3) play as an interpretation of fantasy—experience feeds fantasy and fantasy interprets experience; (4) play as a realization of the environment (Lowenfeld, 1967). Garvey inventoried the following descriptive characteristics of play:

1. Play is pleasurable and enjoyable. Even when not actually accompanied by signs of mirth, it is still positively valued by the player.
2. Play has no extrinsic goals. Its motivations are intrinsic and serve no other objectives. In fact, it is more an enjoy-

ment of means than an effort devoted to some particular end. In utilitarian terms it is inherently unproductive.
3. Play is spontaneous and voluntary. It is not obligatory but is freely chosen by the player.
4. Play involves some active engagement on the part of the player (Garvey, 1977).

These theoretic statements about play summarize and organize many of the commonalities concerning the process and content of play. Clearly, play serves many functions in the child's physical, emotional, and cognitive development.

Play is important to the child's development of all subsystems. (See Chapters 7–11 for discussions of the integrative function of play at each stage of development.) Children learn while playing as they actively construct, create, and reinvent meaning through playful interaction with objects and people. Play is the essence of childhood, the means by which time–space sequences are explored, problem-solving tasks accomplished, and mastery gained. It provides the means of expressing emotions such as joy and mirth; of reversing roles to cope with fear, anger, or disappointment; and of engaging in fantasy to express bewilderment, awe, or hilarity. Physical activity leads to the acquisition and refinement of gross and fine motor skills. Children appear to have endless energy as they move from one activity to another, exercising and perfecting muscular coordination while having fun. They are so preoccupied with the activities themselves that they are unaware of the learning and achievements that are occurring simultaneously.

Play is also a great socializer. Through play, children learn to interact, share, take turns, express ideas, compromise, and respect rules and each other. Sociodramatic play allows the child to play out various roles of significant people and in so doing to learn about the environment. The child's evolving social structure, degree of cooperation, and coordinated efforts toward a group goal all develop as the child matures.

A key characteristic of play in whatever form it takes is that play is fun. As Lois Barclay Murphy stated, "It seems that play is most fun and most playful, when it is spontaneous, evolving from an integration of impulse and ideas and providing expression, release, sometimes climax, often mastery, with a degree of exhilaration and refreshment" (Piers, 1972). Murphy indicated that play is intrinsic and that it comes from within the individual and is done for internal satisfaction, not for external rewards or as a means to an end. Play is spontaneous—taking place by the child's initiation and freely chosen from a variety of available possibilities. Play is fun; it results in feelings of happiness, the expression of satisfaction, and joy, peace, and tranquility.

At a Pediatric Round Table discussion in 1979, the topic "Play and Learning" was addressed by researchers in the area of child development and play. The discussion focused on the meaning and value of play, and although definitions still eluded this group, they concluded that attempted definitions reinforced the subtleties and intricate complexity of play. As one researcher wrote, "Play is like love, a complex phenomenon that deserves serious attention" (Chance, 1979).

Play for the Hospitalized Child Erik Erikson described play as a "function of the ego in an attempt to synchronize the bodily and social processes with self" (Erikson, 1950). According to Erikson, the ego needs to master the various areas of life, especially at those times when self-image, body integrity, or social role is at risk. Only in play can one feel superior to the limits of time, space, and social realities.

Yet what could be a more threatening or more limiting experience for a child than hospitalization? Separated from family, friends, and familiar community surroundings at a time when physical strength is low, the hospitalized child is assaulted physically and mentally by a myriad of real and imagined experiences. Surrounded by strangers and in unfamiliar surroundings, the child might suffer a loss of identity and become a "patient" instead of a person.

In a simplistic sense the reality of the hospital is two-sided: it is a place to seek relief, treatment, and care for sickness and injury, and it is also a place where people suffer and even die. To many adults, hospitalization means limited freedom, potential loss of control, pain, altered body integrity, and possible death. Children have the same fears, but for them there is the added dimension of the immaturity of their developing subsystems, especially the cognitive and affective subsystems. Children frequently are unable to differentiate between inner physical and psychologic events and external events or to distinguish reality from imagined fears.

Hospital play is a relatively new concept but one that has demonstrated enormous benefits. The Children's Memorial Hospital in Chicago was one of the early supporters of play and initiated a program in 1930 (Poston, 1982), but it was not until the 1960s that the significance of this concept was generally accepted. One of the reasons for the long delay seems to be the conservative economic and political climate that prevailed in the United States during that time. England, on the other hand, responded more quickly to children's needs as identified by psychologists, pediatricians, and psychiatrists. "In the late 1950s Parliament supported these research findings by passing a law permitting mothers of hospitalized children to room-in at government expense" (Petrillo and Sanger, 1980).

In the United States play programs were first organized in large children's hospitals or teaching hospitals. Since then, many community hospitals have come to believe in the positive results of play. Play increases the child's capacity for laughter and reduces the incidence of tears. It provides an opportunity for the child to work through questions, fears, and concerns about the injury, illness, treatment modalities, and environment. Play also has the potential to make the hospital stay a learning experience that results in more constructive parent–child interactions and more realistic perceptions of events and the meaning of the illness or injury.

For children, play is an extremely important way of coping with their fears and anxieties. It is a way of acting out feelings, escaping problems, and exerting control over life. To the hospitalized child subjected to unavoidable manipulation and possible discomfort during procedures or treatments, play and the play area provide the freedom to express emotion and a sanctuary from stress. Uninterrupted periods of play permit the child opportunities to continue behaving normally in the midst of coping with unpleasant experiences by attending to age-appropriate developmental tasks.

A longitudinal study by Douglas (1975) documented the long-term effects related to the stress of hospitalization. The data were significant enough to indicate that admissions exceeding 1 week or repeated admissions before 5 years of age had lasting implications for the child's affective development. These children were more likely to have poor reading scores, behavior problems, or unstable work habits than children who had not experienced such distress. The implications of such studies for hospitals and nurses are clear. It is imperative that everyone caring for children attempt to minimize the stress and create an atmosphere that is supportive, trusting, and as much like home as possible.

Play Facilitators Recognizing the complexities of child health care, many institutions employ a team approach, using the expertise of several health care specialists to avoid or at least minimize the negative effects that hospitalization might have on the child. The team includes nursing, medical, and social service personnel and diet therapists, physical therapists, play therapists, and hospital schoolteachers or tutors who are involved in specific aspects of the treatment plan. All members of the health care team need to be familiar with the techniques of instructional and therapeutic play to ensure an effective and positive hospital experience for the child and family.

The Play Therapist The role of the play therapist is to design, implement, and direct a play program. Depending on the institution, this program might be called such various names as child life, children's activities, or recreation therapy. The play therapist provides invaluable guidance to all members of the health care team regarding space for a play area, age-appropriate equipment, such as toys, books, games, and projects, and the most effective use of the space and equipment to promote the child's adaptation to the stressful hospital experience. Although some hospitals do not have play therapists as staff members, these professionals can make a great contribution to the child's adjustment to hospitalization and continued growth and development. A play therapist also might serve as a consultant to a group of hospitals, leaving volunteers to staff the playroom and organize activities.

The following are three major areas of care in which play therapists work:

1. Providing opportunities for normal growth and development in the stress-free environment of a play area as well as the bedside
2. Designing and using teaching tools that can be adapted to each child's level of comprehension to promote understanding of hospital events and procedures, to minimize anxiety, and to help each child meet the challenge of the experience
3. Assessing the child's psychosocial response to hospitalization and illness and providing guidance and support to other members of the team to maximize the child's ability to function during this period

The Nurse Nurses who work with children need a basic understanding of growth and development and age-appropriate play or recreational materials and activities. This understanding then should be incorporated automatically into their interactions. In addition, the knowledgeable nurse can be a valuable resource to children and their families by providing guidelines for the selection of materials and activities that promote a child's learning and self-esteem while offering safe outlets for the frustration and anger that can develop in the restrictive hospital setting.

Every child needs to play. The nurse adapts many procedures and motivates the child to participate in treatments through play. The nurse also ensures the child's comfort so that play can be enjoyed because even play is impossible when the child is in pain (see Chapter 29). The playing child becomes engrossed in the fun of the activity, the challenge of initiating or finishing a project, and the joy of being with other children. During play, the child is more active and uses muscle groups that might facilitate recovery. Friends are made and skills learned as the normal process of growth and development is continued.

Play also might be therapeutic. Children view illness and injury with much fear and anxiety, and the hospital experience further arouses many fantasies (see Chapter 27). Children need help in dealing with these fantasies, or their adverse effects might manifest themselves in later developmental or behavioral problems. The nurse's initiative and creativity are challenged to find the most appropriate medium that allows children to express themselves.

Play for children is also a regulating mechanism. Each child seeks to overcome traumatic anxieties by releasing aggression. Play is a permissible and acceptable medium that satisfies the child's very basic need to learn how to get along with the self and others.

Therapeutic Play Versus Play Therapy Therapeutic play and play therapy are not the same thing. *Play therapy* is a form of psychotherapy used by the psychiatrist, psychologist, or psychiatric nurse-practitioner to assist the child in gaining an understanding of self, acknowledging and accepting emotions, and using emotions positively to achieve an integrated ego. "The goal of play therapy is to promote the child's insight into his own behavior and feel-

Types of Therapeutic Play

Getting ready—Aprons, plastic sheets, newspapers, paper towels, sponges, and wise supervision are the crucial key to success with art materials. At first, some children cannot accept simple aprons, but as they see other children proceeding naturally within safe, practical limits, they also can do the same. An occasional paint-spotted johnnie is surely a simple problem in light of the gains made when a child first attempts an art experience. Often, the apron can be slipped on unobtrusively when painting is in progress if an earlier attempt fails.

Play-Doh or clay—Although clay has qualities that surpass Play-Doh, it also requires closer supervision and special storage. Play-Doh, therefore, is a nice substitute that is safe for bed play and table play. The wise adult resists making recognizable objects or makes them on request and then squashes them, opening the way for the children to spend long periods of time squeezing, pounding, rolling, and stretching the Play-Doh just for the fun of it.

Sand play—Sand play is not as free but affords the same quality of fun as Play-Doh. Cornmeal may be substituted for sand, poured in a plastic-lined box 4 ft by 4 ft and 6 in. deep. Cups, funnels, cars, and small blocks are useful accessories.

Water play, bubble blowing—This is a main activity. In the bath, the sink, the dishpan, or outdoors, water soothes, calms, engages, and lures children into undemanding, concentrated, therapeutic play. Soap or color added to the water enhances its interest. With a pitcher or funnel, it can be poured, and boats may be floated or sunk. Children of all ages love blowing bubbles and watching them float or pop.

Fingerpainting—Fingerpainting is not as simple as water play. It is somewhat more exciting, requiring skillful supervision, but is satisfying and therapeutic. Fingerpaint allows a freedom of expression, an important asset in the hospital world of many essential "do's" and "don'ts," and children might express strong feelings that require active outlets for their emotional balance.

Doctor play—By acting out situations, children come to understand them. By play-working about difficult life experiences, they gain a reassuring sense of control, and they master the situations for themselves. As they understand and act out what the doctor does, they control and lessen their fear of medical procedures and personnel.

Playthings with moving parts—Because physical activity is vital to growth, restricted movement blocks a basic need temporarily. A substitute for real activity is a game that children can operate and make move. In the child's mind, moving with the game temporarily fills a basic need to move and be active.

Crafts—A busy child is a happier child. During times of stress, children might be temporarily unable to socialize because the things on their minds are too frightening to talk about. If, however, they can be occupied with a simple craft and in the company of an understanding adult, they feel safer and comforted. During long periods of convalescence, crafts of all types are useful to help the hours pass happily while waiting for that special day when the child goes home.

Meal time—Sick children away from home often present eating problems. As an antidote for this, meals might be served in a play setting for a group of children. Music is helpful, or a story may create a relaxed atmosphere conducive to eating, a natural activity that happy children enjoy.

Board games, both simple and complex—Games extend from solitaire, checkers, and Parcheesi to Monopoly and even more complicated games. A simple game might act as a tool to help the shy, quiet child come to know the nurse. Undemanding, it serves as a focal point around which a more personal relationship can gradually develop. The sociability accompanying a game creates a warm, friendly occasion that is important to everyone. Some games have moving parts or springs that make cars run. Whether restricted simply by an intravenous line or almost totally by a body cast, moving games counteract frustration from physical limitations and contribute to emotional stability. Older convalescent children need longer, more complicated games to hold their interest. Contests for winners add to the fun. Video and computer games are popular with children of all ages whether played to win or for the fun of watching and moving the characters on the screen.

Creative art experiences—Voluntary art activity that is individual and personally expressive is therapeutic for children in stressful situations. Art materials will be so used by children. A knowledge of the materials, how to prepare them, and how to set the stage for free participation is important for the attending adult.

Dramatic play—Through pretending, acting, or playing dress-up, children accomplish many therapeutic ends. They can escape from the present and find relaxation in a happy make-believe world. One can be "mommy" and reinforce the fact that mommy is real although temporarily separated. Or,

continued on next page

they can play "nurse" and "doctor" and begin to understand what is happening to them while in the hospital, opening the door to relief from anxiety, to acceptance, and to appreciation.

Punching, pounding, cutting, breaking down—All of these activities provide safe outlets for pent-up feelings. It is important to supervise closely because few children can tell when they are getting overexcited, and hysteria might be too close to the surface for comfort. A hysterical child is a frightened child, out of control, and needing help. Activities that provide an emotional outlet, when well managed, contribute largely to a child's ability to handle the many mystifying hospital experiences. A 15-minute period of vigorous punching might determine whether a child can rest, eat, take the next medication, and cooperate with the many demands critical for recovery.

Throwing games—Throwing can be casual, friendly, forceful, angry, or skillful, serving many purposes in therapeutic play. Targets might vary from a companion to catch, a wall, a big box, a little hat, a round-numbered board, or a funny face. The child who is allowed to choose the target will find the game most therapeutic and might want to let off steam or make friends, using the game to do so.

Balloons—Anxiety and tension accompany new experiences, treatments, and restrictions. Balloons are children's delight, as they flaunt the balloon's bright colors and bounciness. Balloons can be freely thrown or punched, and bounce right back for more, delighting a child on bedrest who needs activity and fun. Ambulatory children also can toss or kick balloons safely. (Broken balloons must be removed as children may put the pieces in their mouths and inhale them.)

Cooking—Food is close to everyone's heart. It represents home, love, and parents. It is also essential to recovery and health. Sociable occasions where nurses, children, and parents cook and eat together are a great success. When children cook a favorite food such as pizza, hamburgers, or brownies, not only are they caught up in the fun, but they also enjoy generally improved appetites as well.

Trips in the hospital—The hospital setting can become static and heavy, causing unhappiness and depression. Planned events to anticipate help keep time in better perspective. Trips within the hospital fight boredom and depression because they can be talked about before, during, and after they occur. Surrounding patients benefit as a happier child returns refreshed and talkative.

Group activity—Children socialize among themselves, often relating to each other in ways that differ from their contacts with adults. Both are important, the one leading to the other as a child adjusts to new life experiences. Constructo straws encourage group activity and are fun for all ages. They can provide the base for colorful, eye-catching mobiles, which are a pleasure to watch as they slowly revolve.

Parties—Party occasions to celebrate, birthdays, holidays, and just for fun, bring children, parents, and nurses together into a happy group, providing a time of relaxation as well as a time to be remembered. Word games, guessing contests, and simple carnival stunts can lure children into happy participation.

Music—Music has many advantages, and nearly every child will respond to some type of music. With an easy experimental approach, the nurse usually can find a particular favorite that each child will enjoy and want to hear replayed many times. Strongly rhythmic songs often catch their interest. Rhythm instruments can be used for accompaniment. Many children who don't want to talk will join in with a rhythm band. Even teenagers join in the fun, especially if the adult in charge steers clear of teaching and sets a permissive, happy atmosphere. A community sing-along also can grow out of music. Simple song sheets with words of favorite songs encourage participation. The child in isolation particularly needs stimulation to help combat depression. Music can be used to advantage at these times along with brightly colored decorations and pictures.

Hairdressing—Young people in the hospital still care about their appearances. Hair styles have always been subject to discussion by everyone. Doctors, nurses, and patients become interested and enlivened at hair-dressing time. A shampoo and blow dry by a friendly nurse ranks high on the list of therapeutic activities.

Blocks—Building with blocks, either small or large, brings to a child a sense of skill and control, of particular importance while hospitalized and temporarily under enforced dependence and subject to many orders and unfamiliar events. Individually or in group play intricate constructions can be formed and destroyed and reformed in new designs. For that period of time, the child is master and thus maintains feelings of self-capability, self-control, and personal strength, which are so important during the hospital experience.

Bowling—Today, synthetic materials have provided opportunities for game construction that is light and safe. Bowling with a styrofoam set in a controlled area affords active children necessary physical play.

Busy box or picture books—A busy box with dials to turn, knobs to slide, and doors to open, can be used with younger children to provide movement, distraction, and learning. A loving story with lots of pictures also can help prevent depression and give the child a time of relaxed happiness.

ings" (Green, 1974). The play therapist works with the child over a period of several months or years. At times, play therapists are nondirective; at other times, they are directive, but either approach serves as the "catalyst for, and participant in, the healing play of the troubled child" (Hyde, 1971).

Therapeutic play, on the other hand, helps the nurse and other staff members to gain insight into the child's thoughts or feelings, likes or dislikes, wants or needs. "The main purpose of therapeutic play is to afford the child a comfortable means of telling you—verbally or nonverbally—about his fears and concerns" (Green, 1974). Therapeutic play only allows the nurse to reflect on what the child says. The nurse does not try to interpret or discuss with the child the meaning of nonverbal play. In other words, through play, the child tells the nurse what help is needed or where perceptions about illness and hospitalization are confused or lacking, and based on this information, the nurse provides additional explanations or extra time to explore fears or misconceptions further.

Time for therapeutic play can be planned or can occur spontaneously by taking time to chat with a child already working on a project. When play is planned, a variety of available toys is helpful; these toys might include hospital-related equipment, construction toys, art materials, props for sociodramatic play, and aggression-release toys. By offering several types of play, the nurse leaves the child free to pick and choose. Feelings and preferences differ widely, as do children's abilities to express their feelings and preferences. As always, safety and age appropriateness are major considerations when selecting toys (see Chapter 19).

It is more beneficial to have the child select and decide

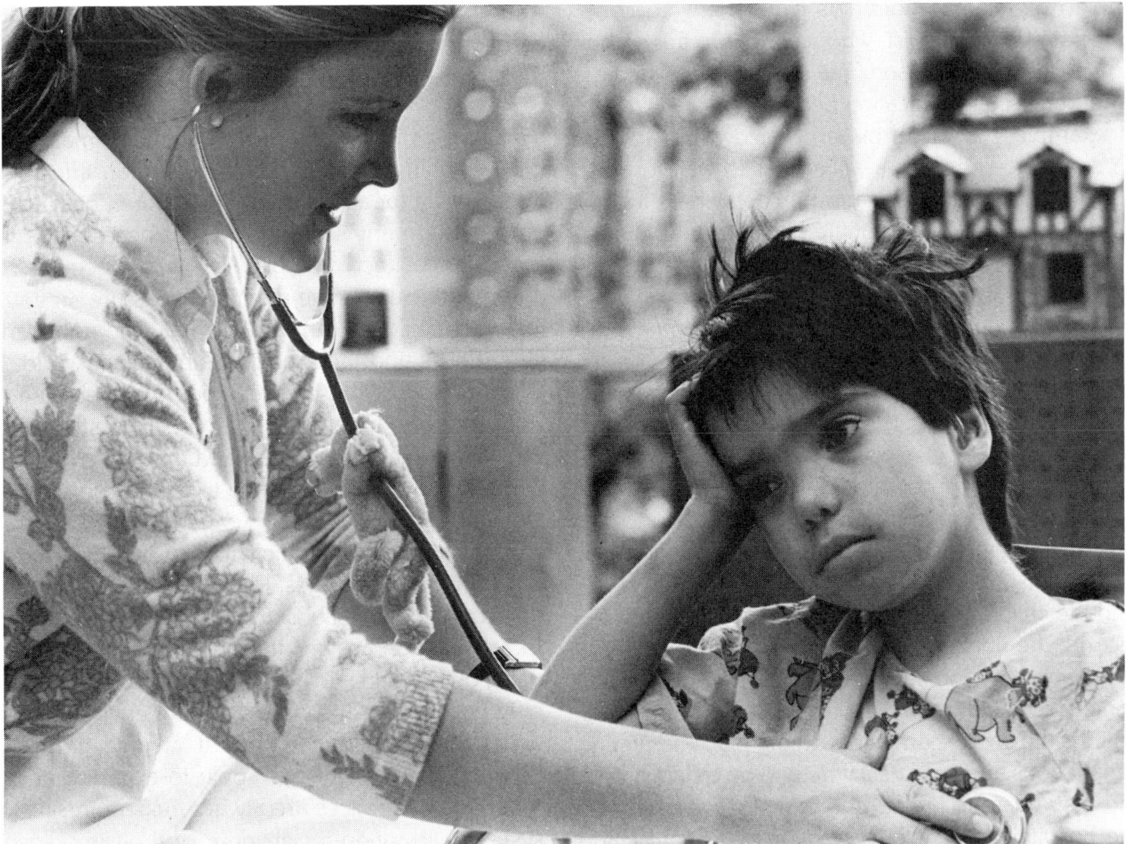

Performing procedures or treatments in a playroom can undermine the function of the play area as a child's sanctuary from stress.

how to play with the toys. In this way internalized fears, concerns, or questions can be expressed freely. If the nurse or play therapist tries to direct the play, the child might do or say what is expected rather than what is really felt. In all forms of therapeutic play, the facilitator is nondirective and ever watchful for the child's clues because the child's real concern might be very different from that supposed by the professional.

For example, a 12-year-old boy hospitalized because of a fractured leg was very withdrawn. He spent most of the day watching television. He passively complied with requests but seldom initiated any conversation. Thinking he was concerned about his leg, which was being treated by traction, or its implications for playing sports, the nurse casually left some hospital-related dolls and small pieces of rope and a pulley by his bedside. Initially, he ignored the articles, but later that week he was observed quietly playing out an entirely different event. The rope was being used by the adult male doll, identified as the father, on the child doll, identified as himself. Further exploration revealed that this boy's main concern was the punishment he feared he would receive from his father. His accident happened while he had been climbing a rock ledge he had been told repeatedly not to climb; in fact, the day before the accident his father had threatened to punish him severely if he ever went there again. This boy's feelings of guilt and fear of punishment so overwhelmed him that he was immobilized and unable to respond to his environment. His concerns were conveyed to the staff psychologist, who was able to intervene effectively with the father and son. The end result was greater respect and better communication between them.

In this example the child's play revealed a previously unknown concern. The nurse's willingness to wait for this boy to use the articles for play and perceptiveness to his clues afforded the family appropriate help. Had the nurse directed his play toward the supposed concern, his real fear might never have been revealed, and interventions to enhance the boy's and father's mental health would not have occurred.

As significant as involving the child in therapeutic play is the plan that follows. Green (1974) has suggested a seven-step process to use the clues provided by the child's play. First, the nurse observes how the child interacts with the materials, what objects are chosen, the length of concentration, the energy expended during the play episode, the feelings expressed, any facial expressions and body movements, and the child's distractability or intensity of involvement. Second, the nurse examines the who and what that comprise the play by looking for consistent or recurring themes and for repetitive or varied episodes. Third, the nurse analyzes the child's comments during play and when giving explanations and considers whether the child's statements and play relate to events and experiences endured during the hospitalization. These observations might lead to insight into the child's concerns or fears. Nurses also need to examine any relationships between their knowledge of the child's personality and history and the activities the child chooses. Fourth, the nurse's thoughts and conclusions concerning the first three steps are validated with those of a colleague. If there is congruence, the nurse might then proceed to intervene; if not, the nurse repeats the preceding steps.

Fifth, the nurse determines the child's needs and the person who is best qualified to intervene. Sometimes it is the nurse; at other times, it is the psychiatrist, psychologist, psychiatric nurse-clinician, or social worker. Sixth, the nurse plans interventions to meet the child's needs. This involves deciding what modifications in nursing care have to be made, what explanations need to be given, or how to involve the child in the care plan and increase the child's independence. The care plan might include additional therapeutic play or referral to other staff members who can support the child in gaining personal insight into behavior, emotions, and attitudes. Seventh, the nurse evaluates whether the plan is effective in reducing the child's concerns, answering questions, and clarifying misconceptions. The plan can only be effective if the child's needs were identified correctly. Correct identification and appropriate intervention is evidenced by a decrease or cessation of clue-giving behavior.

Therapeutic play affords the nurse valuable insight into a child's perception of self, the hospital stay, or events surrounding the current experience. Information conveyed through this medium and responsible follow-through intervention enhance the child's mental health and are a part of holistic nursing care.

Play and the Child Although the ultimate definition of play remains elusive, play is clearly an effective survival mechanism for all children. For children of all ages, all cultures, and in any setting, play is as necessary as love. The important aspect in all play is not so much the content as the mode. Supportive adults must assure an environment in which children can, through play, come to understand themselves and their relationship to their world. The hospitalized child, whose psychologic well-being and physical condition are threatened, will benefit greatly from interacting with nurses who understand this powerful tool and use it to help each child continue to develop into a joyful, total human being.

Ideas for games and activities should be appropriate for children of various ages. Play facilitates the child's learning about objects, relationships, plus the child's own abilities. In selecting an activity, the nurse should take the individuality of the child into account. Children do develop at their own paces and reflect their cultural environments, so that although generalizations about an age group might be accurate, they might not apply to a particular child. Tremendous differences are always evident in skills and subsystem maturation for children of the same age. Physical maturation shows the idiosyncratic nature of this phenomenon in that the span of months for acceptable ages for walking, riding a bike, or the correct use of scissors suggests that children of the same age might have different skill levels, which in turn influence the choice of activities.

Play in the hospital should be fun, similar to that engaged in at home, and related to the ability of the child. A child's attention span usually decreases in the hospital, and children regress in their ability to perform or accept losing. The nurse is therefore better off choosing familiar activities that hospitalized children can accomplish and master than activities that provide too great a challenge. Children might request the same game because they know they can win and might refuse to play a game they previously lost or refuse to learn a new one because they do not like to expend that much effort in concentration.

Children also have different preferences, or as Gardner described it, different "cognitive styles" (Chance, 1979). Gardner discussed children's use of blocks as play objects. Some children seemed fascinated with the properties of the blocks, how they compared with each other, and what could be constructed from them. Other children used the blocks symbolically and designated different blocks as certain characters and played "house," "school," or whatever. He concluded that these differences did not indicate that "one child is functioning at a higher level than the other, they just function differently" (Chance, 1979). The child need not play "correctly" with blocks or clay, make something, or draw with some definite idea or purpose in mind. The form of art need not be refined, nor does the child need to make "a pretty picture." Play is a way in which children express themselves, and any direction given by another person will make their play an expression and extension of that other person, thereby negating its value.

The child's gender and cultural background play a role in maturation and play preferences. Girls tend to mature at a faster rate in all subsystems than boys until approximately 11 years of age. After that, boys catch up and overtake them, especially in the biophysical and cognitive subsystems. Cultural variations and adult expectations affect some of these differences. The child's ability to play with and relate to certain toys is influenced by the social milieu in which the child lives. The play of the affluent child who has access to various lessons, clubs, and equipment is very different from that of the child from a low-income family, who has learned to play with whatever could be found and to create the desired article from boxes or broken toys. Creativity, imagination, and toy manipulation reflect prior experiences and responses to various needs. These differences also affect how the child relates to other children and adults.

Play is fun but only if it suits the individual child. Nurses need to adapt play activities to each child so that play is consistent with the child's growth and development. Thus, the nurse needs to know each child's idiosyncracies and how they affect what is or is not play for that child. The nurse's initial attempts to obtain this information are directed by the guidelines for choosing toys and activities combined with the nursing assessment. As nurses provide play materials for children, they also can learn each child's preferences, temperament, and style by observing how the objects are used. This in turn provides clues for relating to the child and determining the types of activities to offer later on.

Play as a Part of Growth and Development in the Hospital Setting

Erikson's classification of the developmental challenges for each stage of development (see Chapter 6) establishes general qualifications for appropriate play for infants, children, and adolescents who are hospitalized (Table 28-1).

Infancy The first challenge with an infant is to develop a sense of trust, which the parent achieves by meeting the infant's needs for food, warmth, sleep, relief from discomfort, social contact, and sensory stimulation. The first stage of play thus is categorized as autocosmic (Erickson, 1950), sensorimotor (Piaget and Inhelder, 1969), or play that develops muscular control and bodily skills.

Through an active exchange of signals, the infant receives feedback from significant persons within the environment. In the hospital this significant person often is the infant's nurse. The hospitalized infant is particularly vulnerable to sensory deprivation. Most hospitals now recognize the importance of early maternal–child bonding and encourage rooming-in and parental involvement. Minimal rotation of caregivers also assures a continuity of care because by 1 month of age, the infant identifies the human voice and responds to it. Multiple sounds and sights, however, are present in the average hospital nursery; therefore, nurses need to limit extraneous stimulation and provide infants with quiet time to sleep as well as "one-to-one" interaction. An infant's developing a sense of trust during hospitalization is almost impossible in view of the limitations caused by treatments, restrictions, and the inability of the infant's body to function optimally. The challenge is to focus sensory input appropriately and to use every opportunity to rebuild the infant's trust in self and parent.

The sense of touch can be encouraged by using different textures for bed coverings. Nurses can help infants explore objects that are held in the nurses' hands. They can incorporate stroking and massage into such daily care as bathing to facilitate the infant's awareness of the sensation of touch and body. The human face is a favorite visual stimulation. Because color discrimination is not developed early in infancy, patterns provide a better visual focus at the bedside. If the crib can be placed near a window, the infant will be fascinated by changing shadows, clouds, or the movement of birds. The great danger of auditory overstimulation in the hospital nursery requires the infant to develop discriminatory hearing. The human voice, when accompanied by

TABLE 28-1 Age-Appropriate Playroom Activities

Age group	Play activities
Infants under 18 months	Toys that are bright, clean, and too large to be swallowed (everything the child holds is tasted) Dropping toys to be retrieved may be tied to the side of the bed, chair, or stroller so that the child can pull them back People watching Constant mobility and investigation requires close supervision
Two- and three-year-olds	Blocks Stacking toys Push and pull toys Balls Soft toys Stories Music Simple puzzles (fewer than six parts) Free play
Older three- and four-year-olds	Real-life play Puzzles Play-Doh Bubbles Imitative play Music Stories Simple games Group play with adult supervision
Four-and five-year-olds	Real-life play Games (with an adult to help follow rules) Tearing and pasting (with difficulty handling scissors) Plain paper to color (coloring books require a separate page for each child) Paper bag puppets Paper bag masks Paper plate crafts
Five- to ten-year-olds	Structured games Group play (but with adult attention) Games or crafts Puppet shows Wooden construction sets Musical instruments (e.g, rhythm bands) Magic tricks Video games
Ten-year-olds through adolescence	Games Crafts Conversation Music Complicated models Sewing Long-term or group projects Video games Ping pong or pool

eye-to-eye contact with the infant, yields an optimal response. Audiotapes made by parents also are effective in the parents' absence. Musical mobiles or music boxes will provide repetitious tunes to soothe the child.

By 1 month of age, the infant can follow an object to midline and can grasp an object. The choice of toys is not as important in early infancy because infants need first to know themselves, absorb the surrounding world through the senses, and develop trust. Sights, sounds, and touch that help the infant identify and relate to significant people, specific aspects of the environment, and the self are actually the first forms of play.

By 4 months of age, toys may be introduced. It should be kept in mind that the infant's mouth is the primary tool of exploration. Large, colorful, washable objects that are lightweight and varied in texture and shape are best. The nurse can hang these toys above the crib but within reach. Placing the infant in a car seat or chalasia chair will expand both the infant's view of and accessibility to the world. An infant bouncer or swing and being transported in strollers or wagons provide vestibular stimulation. Mirrors (unbreakable) that reflect the child's own movements and facial expressions furnish hours of fascination.

The older infant needs opportunities to develop normal physical skills as the body matures. The nurse thus encourages sitting, crawling, and standing within the limits of the infant's illness or disability. Children often develop innovative ways to compensate for restrictions. Feet might grasp articles if the arms are restrained; therefore, the nurse should be alert for this possibility and encourage the child by placing "play tools" for maximum stimulation. Familiar toys are more beneficial than a great variety of toys. Infants enjoy repetitive use and soon recognize familiar objects. A small box or pail in which objects or toys can be stored also serves as a stimulus for such varied purposes as dumping things out, putting things in, sitting on or in, or banging.

The hospitalized infant's developmental age might vary considerably from the norm for the infant's chronologic age. The nurse therefore is perceptive of the developmental level and provides appropriate play materials for the individual infant as needs change.

Early Childhood According to Erikson, the challenge of early childhood is first to develop a sense of autonomy and mastery over certain aspects of life and then to become comfortable and confident in initiating new experiences. Play at this state is identified as the microsphere (Erikson, 1950), the world of manageable small toys in which the child can create and learn in miniature the events of real life. An active imagination allows the child to enter the world of make-believe and thus cope with feelings, longings, fears, or experiences by enacting certain wishes or events to achieve a positive end result. For example, a 4-year-old girl worked through her fear of getting lost by enacting, with the help of her family of dolls, her version of the fairy tale "Hansel and Gretel." She eliminated the wicked stepmother and had the children wandering off to pick berries and then getting lost. She included the candy house and the witch who lived there who enticed and captured the children, but she had the parents find the children quickly and destroy the witch. Her expression, communication, and actions during the play demonstrated total involvement and a belief that these events were really happening, yet she controlled the sequence of events so that the ending was happy, with lots of hugs and kisses.

Children in this stage also engage in fantasy play, which is where ideas develop and find expression. "Play is in a sense artistic creation" (Lowenfeld, 1967). Parents provide children with examples of the external reality and its relationship to the child, and through play, the child expresses aspects of personality and the development of an integrated ego. For hospitalized children, miniature replicas of the family and meaningful characters in their lives can help them to create, through doll play, the events that are unmanageable. This make-believe offers children opportunities to express feelings and fears that they are unable to express in other ways because their verbal skills are primitive.

Because anxiety inhibits a child's exploration of environment, the reassuring presence of family and a playroom

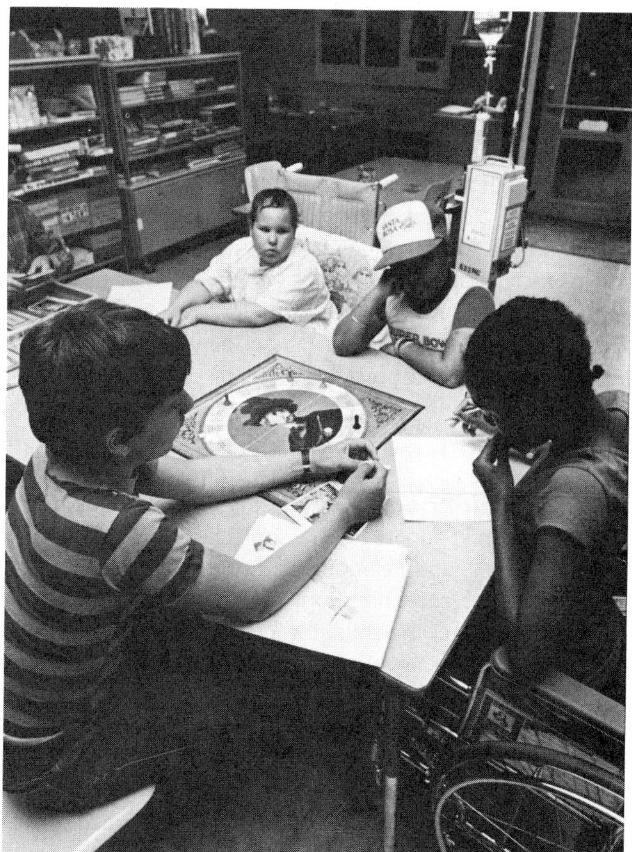

The playroom can be a stimulating environment, allowing hospitalized children the chance to meet and interact with each other.

sanctuary provide opportunities to exercise physical skills and natural curiosity. Ambulation is encouraged through push or pull toys, wagons, tricycles, or doll carriages. The child might win approval by throwing balls or bean bags at targets instead of throwing objects out of bed or at other people. The child needs to be protected from negative behavior that would lead to the sense of shame and doubt that Erikson described (see Chapter 6). For instance, if movement is limited by body casts, placing the child in a wagon, on a body scooter, or perhaps simply moving the bed to another room increases the child's sense of mobility. Toys on pulleys will suggest ideas for manipulation to the child. Young children enjoy play materials on which they can have a direct impact; these include clay, sand or cornmeal, wood, and water. The child who can build a tower of blocks, knock it down, and then rebuild it acquires a sense of control. Puzzles also offer opportunities to reconstruct materials successfully. For the young child, play and the adult response to play are important for language development. As the adult talks to the child about play activities, names animals or objects in the environment, or sings songs or reads stories, the child learns about the symbols that constitute language. The nurse therefore spends time talking and listening to the young child. Early efforts at mastering language thus can be enhanced through play and adult participation, whether this involves describing or naming interesting aspects of the hospital surroundings or entering into the child's pretend world and participating as the child directs.

The nurse can help sad or lonely children to gain a sense of familiarity and comfort by going on a walk through the unit and having the nurse identify and talk about the colors or objects in pictures on the wall, the location of the playroom and the special things that occur there, and the location of the child's room with reference to other rooms or ward fixtures. Young children combine play and language to explore, try out new ideas, and cope with thoughts and feelings at their levels of understanding. Listening and talking to young children thus are part of their nursing care.

Middle Childhood Play during middle childhood reflects the child's increasingly sophisticated interactions. Using materials, understanding their properties, and working with both objects and people are elements of play during these years. For the child, the joy is in doing, in creating, and in gradually achieving a more realistic impression. The end product does not become the goal of the activity until the end of this phase.

Drawing and, later on, story writing provide more outlets for expression and play. "Kramer links the freedom of expression inherent in art to that found in imaginative play, where forbidden wishes and impulses can be expressed symbolically" (McLeavey, 1979). Luquet determined that "until about eight or nine a child's drawing is essentially realistic in intention, though the subject begins by drawing what he *knows* about a person or an object long before he can draw what he actually sees" (Piaget and Inhelder, 1969). These children draw what they understand or know from previous experience. Their drawings depict personal concepts of the image rather than what they see objectively in space. Important or feared objects therefore are disproportionately large. The new football, for example, might be as big as the boy in the drawing, or the feared syringe might be even larger than a frightened child huddled in a corner or lying flat on a bed. Thus, art provides a means of communicating, of expressing or sharing ideas or concerns and thereby coping with them.

Children at this stage thrive on recognition and praise for their endeavors. No matter how simple or crude the creation, honest, positive comments are essential to encourage self-esteem and continuation of the activity. When the nurse cannot identify the intent of a drawing or clay model, a comment on the use of colors, the presence of certain shapes, or the process of the activity in making the project is just as helpful. The nurse can then readily ask the child to talk about the project.

For example, one quiet, cooperative, but sad-appearing 7-year-old girl drew a picture of girls doing various gymnastic exercises, but instead of teachers, the picture showed doctors and nurses with the girls. Some girls had happy faces, whereas some girls were sad. The girls also looked alike, with the same color hair, eyes, and clothes. When questioned, the child explained that the girls were her. The happy girls had a nurse by them and were doing skills she could do well; the sad girls had a doctor by them and were doing things she found difficult. Further conversation revealed that this child was afraid and angry that her surgery and hospitalization would prevent her from participating in the gymnastics show planned for the next week. She felt sure that someone else would get her spot and that this was all the doctor's fault; therefore, she had made the girls sad, and she never smiled at the doctors. The drawing explained much of her behavior and her lack of enthusiasm for the playroom activities. The trauma for her was not so much the hospital experience, as the nurse had previously assumed, but the effect on her gymnastics activities. Later, this girl's mother added some significant information. An older sister was very talented and in some ways acted both as competition and as a role model for this child. This gymnastic show would have been the 7-year-old's first. She had practiced hard, and it had been the focus of her conversation until her hospitalization. As a result of the picture story, the nurses redirected their efforts, supported her in her disappointment, and reassured her that she could practice and perform her beloved gymnastics once she was fully recovered. The child and nurse made a calendar together and planned how and when she would resume practice, beginning with simple warm-ups and gradually extending the length and complexity of her practice sessions. The child could talk about her disappointment and became a happier, more outgoing girl.

Besides drawing and telling stories, other appropriate activities for children of this age are puzzles, simple board or card games, and crafts. These can be done with a special friend or a group of children, and they encourage socialization. Construction activities, such as making collages or puppets, building with blocks (such as Lego® blocks), or using wood and tools are good for creativity and the perfection of fine motor skills.

Sociodramatic activities are always popular and are another means of skill development. Having props or making props for the situation adds realism. Puppets are also useful, and children might put on simple puppet shows such as familiar fairy tales. Children also respond well to contests, competition, and awards. These contests might be group efforts or individual efforts between the nurse and the child or between the child and an inanimate object such as a clock. It is best not to have children competing against each other in the hospital because stress decreases competence, increases liabilities, and allows for feelings of inferiority.

Winning or achieving the goal is important, so tasks should be easily manageable for the child. Nurses might include awards in the form of stickers, stars, or even special privileges, but lots of praise is always important. Contests might be made up simply for their own sake or designed to complement the child's therapy by such means as increased movement of an extremity or increased fluid intake. Giving the child a booklet of papers or a piece of construction paper to serve as an award chart gives the child accomplishments to show to family and friends. The nurse or therapist needs to monitor these activities so that each child succeeds at something and receives appropriate recogni-

Board Games for Children

3 Years old and under

These children are too young for board games.

4–6 Years old

Candy Land®
Winnie the Pooh®
Win By A Wisker™
Cat's Eye®
Strawberry Shortcake in the Big Apple™
Care Bears Card Game®

6–10 Years old

Chutes and Ladders®
Uncle Wiggley®
Sorry®
Checkers®
The Fox and the Hound®
Jack Straw®
Hi-Q®
Husker-Du™
Mad Magazine Game®
Slide Five ™
Aggravation®
UNO®

10–12 Years old

Boggle®
Life®
Othello®
Racko®
Chain Lightning™
Backgammon™
Yahtzee®
Stratego®
Clue®
Inner Circle™
Superfection®
Mastermind®
Game of the States®
Kimbo®

Teens

All American Football Game®
Monopoly®
Scrabble®
Chess
Cribbage
Quiz Whiz™
Password™
Rook®
Mille Bornes™
Careers®
Pit®

tion. When winning becomes an all-consuming passion, the contest is no longer play but becomes work. This, of course, defeats the original purpose of this sort of play.

Children in middle childhood also like to collect things, and they will collect anything and everything. Having their own boxes or bags for such objects as pictures or projects made in the playroom provides each child with a personal collection of accomplishments. Cleaned-out medicine cups and other safe equipment such as a clean bandage, tongue depressor, or disposable tape measure also will provide "show and tell" items for when the child returns home.

Late Childhood Erikson (1950) identified the major challenge for children in late childhood as developing a sense of industry, and he asserted that failure to do so will result in a sense of inferiority. Play materials offer many opportunities for children at this stage to succeed in developing this sense of industry and achievement. Games provide a format for social interaction, an experience of adventure, and a structure with rules to follow that can lead to success and learning. The child who feels threatened might wish to play a game repeatedly to become assured of the ability to succeed. The child's intellectual curiosity provides further incentive for learning about the body, its functions, and health care. Models and crafts are teaching tools, diversions, and opportunities to learn new skills and share acquired skills.

Late childhood is a time of increased sociability, and recreation provides many nonthreatening tools for acquiring social skills, educational skills (such as math, reading, and spacial concepts), and physical skills without the stress of possible failure, which could lead to a sense of inferiority. The child who is successful in games will have more confidence during interactions with peers and adults in other aspects of life. The challenge for the nurse is to present the appropriate task and guide the child to a sense of achievement and a degree of mastery over both self and the environment.

Fantasy is still an important tool used in play to correct the perceived social injustices of life. Hospitalization and the injury or illness that necessitated it usually are perceived as injustices, and the child often fantasizes that the doctors and all others who inflict pain are in some way controlled or captured and that the child immediately becomes healthy and is victorious. The nurse provides the means and the uninterrupted time for such expressions. Nurses can encourage such play by having hand or finger puppets, art supplies, clay or Play-Doh™, and various types of blocks for the construction and transportation of objects available. Children might or might not discuss their fantasies with their nurses, but commenting on what the child is doing may open the way for an explanatory comment. "Instead of speaking about what the child is making, it might be helpful if you comment on what he is doing. 'We're having lots of fun, aren't we?' will strike a more responsive chord than 'What are you making?'" (Hartley, Frank, and Goldenson, 1952).

"Mastery, achievement and excellence are important themes throughout this phase. Recognition and popularity are gained through the acquisition of skills" (Petrillo and Sanger, 1980). This knowledge should guide the nurse in providing play and related experiences for children in late childhood. The nurse might teach younger children certain games or the use of tools and wood to make simple objects, or the nurse might demonstrate craft skills. Having an area or bulletin board by each bed for projects, posters, photos, and favorite cartoons or riddles helps to personalize each space and facilitates the gathering of peers to "check out" each other's interests.

Doing things together and being active is characteristic of this age. Organizing such activities as publishing a ward paper, compiling a photograph album or scrapbook to which everyone contributes, making a "clubhouse" from large boxes, or presenting a puppet show are ways to foster group participation. Conversation assumes added importance at this age as children learn and experiment with verbalizing their ideas, thoughts, favorite experiences, or jokes. "The hospital environment can capitalize on the school-age child's appetite for skills and knowledge. The play setting can be supplied with familiarizing educational materials such as slides, books, hospital maps and models about biological processes, hospital procedures, health and illness" (Riserchia, Bragg, and Alvarez, 1982).

Adolescence Regardless of whether hospitalized adolescents are housed in the pediatrics unit or in the adult section of the hospital, they have special needs. Illness and hospitalization might cause great stress on peer relationships and on adolescents' sense of what they are and what they will be. If bodily function and control have been affected severely, recreation might provide alternative skills. Games offer safe avenues for social interaction. Electronic games offer opportunities for manipulation and control for even the most severely handicapped adolescent. Most adolescents enjoy exploring new career models (that is, staff roles). Regression to earlier stages of behavior is common, but constant reinforcement of self-identity through shared concerns for individual interests can encourage growth.

For example, the adolescent who is a car enthusiast might participate in planning auto trips with maps and travel guides, car magazines, or making models. The adolescent who is fashion conscious might enjoy designing clothes or practicing interior decorating. Recreation, or literally the focusing on the individual's special interests and talents, is probably a more acceptable term than play when referring to the adolescent. Long-term projects that are challenging and can be done either alone or with others are valuable forms of recreation. Such things as 1000-piece jigsaw puzzles, complicated models, paint-by-number reproductions, knitting, and other craft projects provide a sense of accomplishment, independence, and self-worth.

Adolescents need space and the opportunity for both private times and group activities. A room or corner where they can go with their friends and listen to a stereo (sometimes using headphones for noise control) helps to decrease the unfamiliarity and sterility of the hospital environment. If someone plays a guitar or other musical instrument, that talent can serve as a focus for get-togethers. Allowing adolescents to have their personal radios enables them to have times for private listening.

Gab sessions and long telephone conversations are vital for adolescents, a fact of life that nurses need to respect. Adolescence is a time for bouncing thoughts and ideas off friends to evaluate their appropriateness. Adolescents enjoy such games as cards, pinball, and mind-stretching exercises. They also might communicate through art, stories, poems, or diaries. Some adolescents share their creations, thus providing an opening for conversation, validation, or the exploration of feelings. For other adolescents, their work is private and should be respected as such.

Play and the Movement-Restricted Child

Some children cannot be moved to the play area. They might be in isolation rooms or on bedrest that prohibits moving the bed. However, these children are beset by the same threats of illness common to all hospitalized children, and their stress is compounded by separation from peers, greater immobility, and increased sensory deprivation. For them, play must be adapted to the immediate environment at the bedside or in the room. Activities might include the following:

- Scrapbooks, cloth or vinyl books (for younger children)
- Tracing
- Card games (appropriate to age)
- Musical instruments
- Paints: water, finger, or felt-tip markers
- Pegboard and hammer
- Clay or Play-Doh™
- Puppets
- Puzzles
- "Explore" or "Sunshine" box
- Beading (size of beads depends on the age of the child)
- Art materials
- Camera (for older child)
- Tape recorder
- Aquarium
- Dolls (type depends on age but might include baby dolls or older dolls such as Barbie® and Ken® dolls)
- Stuffed animals
- Collections
- Sponge balls, blocks
- Velcro-related games
- Hospital-related toys and equipment
- Toys with wheels

Pictures, mobiles, posters, plants, and even pets (those confined to safe places) can change a hospital room into a personal space. Walkie-talkies, tape recorders, and telephones provide communication opportunities. A window in the isolation room might provide a play space for the isolated child and a peer to play games such as checkers or tic-tac-toe. Water-soluble markers often work well for this because the game can be drawn on the glass and later washed off without leaving permanent markings. Sharing in the planning of a playroom event or previewing a movie can transform the isolated child into a privileged individual. The child in an immovable traction bed will regain some sense of power and control if designated the starter or caller of such group activities as games of lotto or bingo. Such a child also might be the director of puppet shows put on within the room for other children to watch.

The nurse must use every opportunity to reinforce these children's sense of self-esteem and assure them that their developmental needs will be met. Creativity in adapting play materials provides alternatives for regressive behavior or for an aggressive reaction, which these children often exhibit in response to the deprivation inherent in restricted movement or isolation. A popular activity, which also involves various degrees of vigorous arm movements, are the Velcro-related games. Some of these games use darts, some use balls, and some involve characters; the object is to throw the Velcro-backed object toward a special board and score points or make a bull's-eye. "Nerf"® basketball is another safe and popular game that meets a variety of needs for the immobile child.

Play as a Tool for Nursing Management

The Play Setting

Because play facilitates the development of all subsystems, it is an ideal means to encourage the continuation of normal growth and development and to obtain a more accurate developmental assessment (see Chapter 16). For play to occur, a normal environment is necessary. Children need an area, preferably both indoors and outdoors, where they can gather to have fun, interact with objects and people, learn, and refine skills in play-related experiences. Play materials should do more than provide superficial diversion; they must enhance the child's development. Providing activities and supportive interventions that satisfy the needs of individuals at every age, from infancy through adolescence, is one way of translating caring feelings to caring behaviors. Materials that allow for gross and fine motor activities, multisensory stimulation, opportunities for exploration and experimentation, freedom to express feelings, and participation with others in social interchange provide a rich variety of play experiences from which children might choose what most effectively meets their needs.

Play as a Diagnostic Tool

Observing children at play enables the nurse to collect a wealth of data related to growth and development. Various assessment tools aid the nurse in planning appropriate nursing management, identifying realistic goals and expectations, and communicating with the child in play or in teaching episodes (see Chapter 16). As the nurse collects this information, it is shared with others through the written nursing care plan.

The nurse might first notice physical developmental delays or vulnerabilities while observing a child at play. The developmental delays or vulnerabilities might, for instance, be vision or hearing limitations evidenced by the child's behavior or responsiveness during play or a neuromuscular disease first noted because of the child's changing styles of play. In this case the consistent use of one hand and arm for pulling, pushing, and reaching might be more significant than a simple preference for that side over the other. Children with chronic or congenital problems might show considerable deviance between chronologic and developmental age, and the nurse who is aware of this can alter expectations and consider safety and stimulation. Through play, the child learns to master skills, but this mastery depends in part on the adequacy and functioning of the biophysical subsystem. Problems or inadequacies in the subsystem are reflected in the play abilities of the child.

Play, however, is not only physical skill and combinations of motor movements. "For many years play has been described as activity that involves reason, imagination and attention on one side and motivated feelings on the other. It is important to put these two together so that, when observing a child playing, one can see the status of his mental development interrelated with his emotional state" (Petrillo and Sanger, 1980). Piaget firmly believed that play is the child's avenue to learning. Once the work of accommodation and mastery are complete, assimilation through repetition of the activity is play. This repetition leads to perfection and a sense of power and control over the activity, whether it be motor, verbal, or symbolic, and to the ability to use the activity in new and different ways.

The playing child reveals the nature and quality of individual thought processes. The ways in which the child uses objects, relates to the environment, solves problems, identifies means-to-ends relationships, imitates others, and uses language all provide clues to cognitive development. An accurate assessment of cognitive abilities enables the nurse to adapt teaching methods to coincide with the individual's level of understanding.

Emotional development is reflected in the child's expression of self-esteem and self-control. Nurses often find it informative to observe how the child copes with frustration, disappointment, and stress. A good question to ask is who is in control, the child or the emotions. Evaluating the appropriateness of the child's play with reference to activity, use of toys and materials, and response to outcome is another method of determining ego development. The child who demonstrates delayed development of an integrated ego, whose impulse control is weak, or whose self-confidence is lacking requires supportive attention and the opportunity to achieve some degree of mastery in play. The child is particularly vulnerable to trauma caused by the hospital experience but is also responsive to intervention and can benefit from therapeutic play.

The nurse also might assess the development of the social subsystem by observing the child at play. Assessment criteria involve noting whether the child interacts with other children, and if so, which children, or whether the child interacts only with adults. Assessing peer interactions in this way demonstrates the child's need for adult support or comfort. The nurse also considers the type of play in which the child engages—solitary, onlooker, parallel, associative, or cooperative—and whether this play is age and situation appropriate. The child's ability to share, accept responsibility, and respond to rules indicates the level of social development.

Through play, children learn to interact with others, have their needs met, and meet the needs of others. They learn to achieve a balance between give and take and between submission and control. Children with limited peer or group experiences have difficulty when one child's egocentricity clashes with that of another; therefore, these children sometimes need help to learn how to play with others. They might find the playroom too confusing and noisy, or they might be overwhelmed by the requests of other children. Such children also might profit from a more gradual introduction to play activities. Some of these introductions might take place within a small, supervised group in a separate corner or section of the playroom.

Play thus is valuable for both the child and nurse. "Through play the child learns to manipulate and master his body, his mind, his emotions, and his relationships. Such mastery is essential to strong ego development and good mental health" (Schuster and Ashburn, 1980). Observation and analysis of the child's play are excellent means of obtaining a realistic assessment of the child's growth and development for use in providing nursing management.

Play as a Means of Coping with Hospitalization

One of the primary goals of nursing care of hospitalized children is to promote wellness by assisting the child to retain or develop the ability to deal with stresses in ways that contribute to physical and psychosocial growth. Care for the hospitalized child has become comprehensive. It requires the diverse expertise of many professionals. The nurse frequently is the person responsible for integrating and coordinating these interventions into a care plan to provide organized management that focuses on the child's return to health and self-care. Play is an integral part of this management. Time needs to be designated as "free time" for the child to play either in the playroom or at the bedside. During this time, the child should not be disturbed for treatments unless they are absolutely necessary. Although play therapists, play libraries, and puppet therapists are becoming recognized and important components of the pediatric unit, the nurse cannot assume that the nursing role does not include play and therapeutic play. The nurse needs to be active in the overall care of the child, and this means using play to its best advantage. Nurses should incorporate play into rounds and bedside care by talking with the children, supplying stimulating play materials, allowing for uninterrupted play time, permitting them to play at their own pace, and being as nondirective as possible. These activities serve to promote wellness.

Diversion and Creative Outlets Play in the hospital is partly diversional activity. During play, the child is safe from unpleasant experiences. The time goes faster, and the trauma of being in unfamiliar surroundings is not as acute when the child is having fun. The playroom also provides children with the opportunity of meeting others with whom to share experiences. Play encourages children to focus on something and someone other than themselves and why they are hospitalized. Play gives the child the opportunity to control a situation, make choices, and experience a sense of power.

Creative expression and the use of art materials or various types of construction toys enhance the child's sense of self-esteem and self-confidence. Children might be introduced to new experiences and responsibilities such as how to care for the fish or plants in the children's unit. They might discover new ways to be creative with paints, clay, or sand (or cornmeal). Craft skills such as sewing, paper and yarn projects, needlework, or leatherwork might be learned and useful personal projects completed (Table 28-2). The playroom also allows for the manipulation of familiar and new materials, freedom to explore and experiment, and time for conversation with new and old friends.

Expression of Feelings and Perceptions Play helps the child to cope with separation from home, family, and friends and to facilitate the child's reconstructing these familiar and cherished people and places during "pretend," or sociodramatic, activities. Children are comforted by playing house and reenacting family events. Sometimes, they even take on their own identities to enhance the similarity to home, and this play might become an exact replication of familiar events as the child recreates the longed-for home environment. The child occasionally takes on the role of an adult, usually in imitation of one of the parents. Home scenes acted out often provide the child with the authority to tell others—be they peers, dolls, or stuffed animals—what to do, where to go, or how to do it. The confusing hospital admission procedure often is the chosen scene. This type of play is partly imaginative and partly imitative as the child attempts to understand and cope with adult actions and surrounding events.

Children who do not easily express themselves in words often benefit from doll play or art activities such as painting and drawing. For example, the repetitive putting on and taking off of a "cast" on a doll or favorite stuffed animal might reassure the young child that the appearance or size of the arm or leg does not change while it is in the cast. A nurse talking with the child about this activity frequently might identify some fears and fantasies that the child needs to explore because simply reassuring the child that the arm or leg is okay is not adequate. The nurse might need to make it clear that no question is too trivial and no fear too ridiculous to be shared. The nurse can communicate this fact best by entering the child's role-play and having another doll or animal ask questions or talk about what it is like to have a cast.

From early childhood through adolescence, art is often an effective means of identifying the emotional needs of children. Art, both nondirected and directed, allows children to express feelings through clay, paper, or other media. As the nurse encourages the child to talk about drawings, the interaction helps the child to understand that the nurse is interested in the child's thinking and concerns. This interest alone often opens the door to more therapeutic conversation.

When children are more easily able to discuss their thoughts and feelings, having the child talk about the content and colors of the pictures or tell a story about the drawing might give the nurse some insight into the child's perception of the environment.

Dolls, stuffed animals, and puppets can be used for expressive play as well as for teaching and learning. Allowing children to manipulate equipment, either miniature equipment used for dolls or apparatuses similar to and the actual size of those being used in their treatment, reaps enormous benefits. Having older children write about their experiences and thoughts is another means of encouraging expression. These writings can be collected, printed, and distributed in the form of a hospital "newspaper." Sometimes, they are put in a scrapbook or on a bulletin board in the playroom for other children with similar problems

TABLE 28-2 Play Materials for Types of Play

Activity	Materials

Construction toys	Blocks
	  Sponge
	  Wood
	  Put-together (Lego®, Loc Blocks®)
	Tinker toys®
	Lincoln logs®
	Models

Sociodramatic play	Dolls Cars, trucks Dress-up clothes and props Kitchen set-up, dishes Doll beds, furniture Doll houses and family Cardboard boxes Stuffed animals Puppets
Aggression-release toys	Drums Styrofoam blocks Bean bags Hammer and nails Pegboard, pegbench Cymbals Xylophone
Art-related toys	Paper (various colored, construction, plain white) Pencils, crayons Markers Paints (water, tempera, finger) Glue Scissors Scraps of material, yarn ribbon Macaroni shapes for collage Cotton balls Popsicle sticks or tongue depressors
Hospital play	Stethoscope Blood pressure cuff Tongue depressor Reflex hammer Intravenous tubing and soluset Band-aids Tape, gauze Tape measure Syringe without needle Gown, mask, surgery cap and booties Dolls—nurse, doctor, children Other equipment appropriate to child's situation

and treatments to read. This activity helps individual children to work through their concerns and makes them feel that they are contributing to the understanding and mental health of other children.

Fantasy Playing out ideas and emotions also might be done through fantasy. An idea or event precipitates the initial form and direction of this play. However, as the play activity unfolds, the child adds associations from memory and from previous games and experiences and adds suggestions from other children or adults in the effort to externalize inner concepts of events so that these events eventually can be understood. Children of all ages use fantasy. Instead of play, older children and adolescents might daydream about what their lives would be like if they did not have certain illnesses or injuries, if they were the doctors and nurses instead of the patient, or if they won some contest and the prize was a glamorous vacation or new car. Fantasy play gives some insight into children's understanding or lack of understanding concerning ideas, perceptions, and events. Communicating in this manner, children effectively are telling the nurse about the personal significance of events. Being alert to what might be expressed in this way enables the nurse later to provide additional information and encourage the children to discuss their understanding of why they were hospitalized.

Lowenfeld noted that children move in and out of fantasy play. One moment they completely identify with the characters and happenings in the fantasy creation, and the next moment they are consciously imagining and are fully aware of the pretend nature of the play. Fantasy play "enables a child to realize the nature of his own preconceived ideas and spontaneous feelings and by doing so to bring them within reach of comparison with reality" (Lowenfeld, 1967).

Interpretation of Play The nurse who knows some of the accepted interpretations of play activities and who spends time observing children during uninterrupted play is able to incorporate this information into nursing management. For example, the nurse might see a child building enclosures with blocks while busily talking to the doll or stuffed animal about obeying or being punished if directions are not followed. These forms can be made with smaller blocks enclosing or surrounding a doll or some other object or with larger cardboard blocks arranged to form a "room" in which the child spends most of the play time with the doll. Enclosures have a variety of meanings. "When constructed only occasionally, enclosures have no deep significance, but when a child concentrates on them repeatedly, they may indicate a desire for control, since things put inside them are 'under the thumb' of the block builder" (Hartley, Frank, and Goldenson, 1952). The child participating in this activity might be expressing feelings of being controlled by others, of losing self-esteem and decision-making abilities, and of bewilderment. Modifying the nursing care plan to give this child allowable choices, areas of control, and opportunities for positive recognition will restore self-esteem and provide an opportunity to clarify misconceptions about the rationale behind certain procedures and treatments.

Children who are angry and frustrated by illness-related treatments and limitations might use play to vent the hostile feelings that rage inside. Building towers with cardboard, styrofoam, or sponge blocks (for safety measures), only to knock them down dramatically, rebuild, and destroy them again helps these children to express and thereby eradicate these feelings. Such towers sometimes are named for the people who are imposing the restrictions. The destruction of the "person" objectifies the rage and allows the child and nurse to deal with it. Play that involves gross motor activity benefits the angry child. Other types of activity include throwing sponge balls or bean bags at a wooden clown with basketlike pockets or through a hoop or into a box, pounding on a pegboard, or for older children, pounding nails into wood. Musical toys such as cymbals, drums, and xylophones afford constructive means of expressing feelings. Clay is another useful medium for expression as children roll, pound, squeeze, or punch it. It gives children the opportunity to create and destroy without guilt, in the process releasing their aggression.

Older children can use chalk, crayons, or paints effectively in expressing their feelings. For example, one 8-year-old boy walked from the treatment room to the playroom as fast as he could while tugging his intravenous pole behind him. He marched up to the chalk board, grabbed a piece of chalk, and wrote "I HATE IT" over and over again as fast as he could. The hated object was the intravenous infusion and the discomfort associated with having just had a new one inserted. Once his mission was completed, this boy joined another group of children and played happily. One 10-year-old girl who had considerable artistic talent once spent an entire day drawing a witch. This witch was extremely ugly with detailed pimples, bumps, and moles covering the face, long arthritic-appearing hands and fingers, a hunched posture, and ragged clothes. The girl said that the witch was her doctor, who was mean and ugly and whom she hated, but that now she felt better and was a little sorry she had made the witch so horrible. The effort expended in the project had released pent-up feelings of anger and helped her to understand herself better and to realize why she felt so angry.

The anxious or withdrawn child is common in hospitals and is often a child in early or middle childhood (see Chapter 27). These children are old enough to understand much of what is happening but are too young to have sufficient coping mechanisms on which to draw. They might not be able to "talk it out" the way an older child or adolescent might. "The preschool child does not have sufficient verbal, motor and social skills to deal with frightened feelings in a modulated and socialized way. Therefore, he may ventilate his angry feelings by behaving aggressively. Successful discharge of anger allows the child to get rid of resentment and associated guilt feelings so that he is free to achieve new and better coping techniques" (Rumfelt, 1980). "The school-aged child relies heavily on the use of fantasy to reduce tension, to resolve conflict and to fill gaps in his understanding of reality. It may require examination of the hospitalized child's fantasy expression through the use of projective techniques in order to reveal beliefs about illness which are not verbalized directly" (Peters, 1978).

The child's beginning and completion of a project are often very different. What might begin as a display of aggressive impulses in furious pounding or repetitive destruction changes at some point and becomes a constructive and creative endeavor. As others join an activity, a game might be devised, and the child who is once again in control of hostile feelings might become the leader or organizer. Initial drawings and paintings are often purely the demonstration of feelings, emotions, and attitudes and are not meant to be anything in particular. The child might be unable to talk about these efforts and will say instead that a piece is a "design." Successive pictures might reveal something about the child's perceptions, fears, wishes, or fantasies associated with hospitalization, treatment, or self-image.

The child also uses play as a subtle way of controlling adult intrusion, such as, "Don't bother me, I'm playing" or "Cars don't need medicine." These and similar statements are common as nurses attempt to interrupt play for necessary procedures. "Although it can progress to being resistive, initial attempts to control are the healthy response of individuals to monitor the amount of stress, pain, sensory input and demands made on them in a way that they can successfully cope. From this behavior they gain a sense of mastery and satisfaction and as such it needs to be recognized and supported" (Savedra and Tesler, 1981).

Play as a Means of Learning About the Hospital Environment

Children learn though play, through their own manipulation of objects and events, and through the exploration of materials and situations in their environment. In this way the unknown becomes known, and once known, it can be understood and used in a variety of ways. Play is the child's natural means of learning and communicating and is one of the most important aspects of a child's life. The hospitalized child needs time and the opportunity to learn about the new environment and the many instruments various staff members use to check this or that part of the body. To facilitate this learning, the child needs to have real and facsimile equipment available. Garvey (1977) noted that when novel objects are given to children, they first explore, manipulate, and practice with the object before they begin to play. This process of familiarization preceding play with unknown objects or persons or in new settings involves learning. Once the children develop ways of dealing with the properties or characteristics of the new object, they can engage it in their play. This activity whereby children transform an object into something that is part of their own imagination is quite literally the process of play.

Nurses need to provide frequent opportunities for children to participate in supervised hospital play sessions with commonly used equipment such as syringes without needles, intravenous apparatuses, blood pressure cuffs, stethoscopes, and other material. As children touch the equipment, pick it up, turn it, squeeze it, or take it apart, they discover its functions and learn about its uses. Once comfortable with an object, they might use it as part of a play sequence. The play action might imitate how the equipment has been used by adults, or it might be used in an entirely different manner.

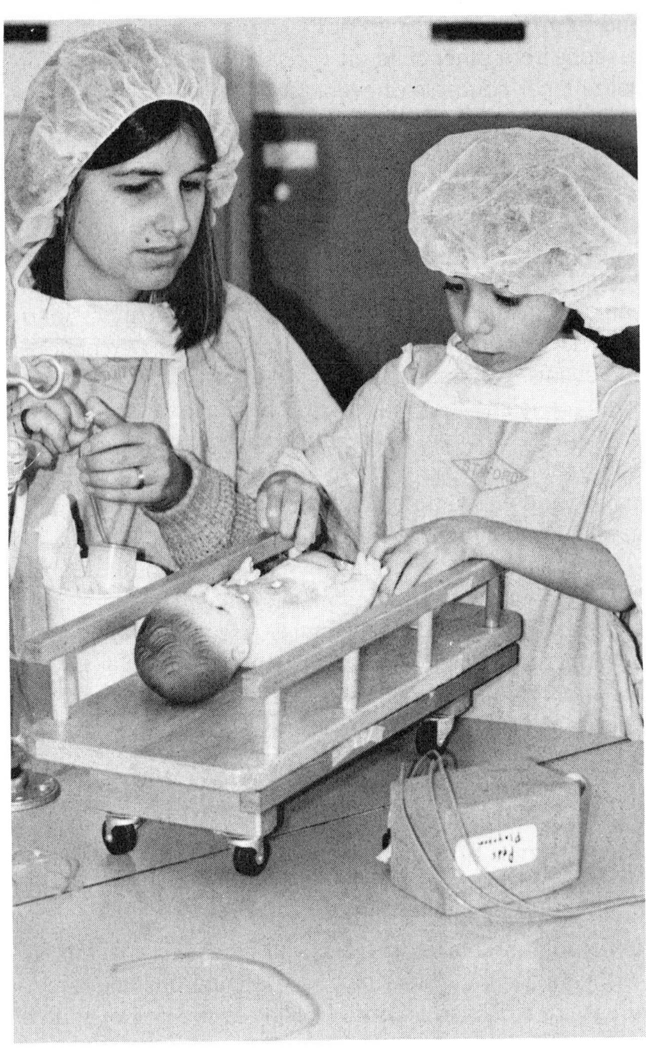

Play is a useful means of communication and teaching for the nurse and child and can help prepare the child for stressful procedures and treatments.

For example, 5-year-old Gigi required prolonged intravenous antibiotic therapy and had many intravenous needles inserted. When presented with the hospital equipment, she carefully explored each piece, then assembled the intravenous apparatus, and proceeded to "start an IV" in the doll's arm. She reenacted her experiences as she talked to the doll, telling it what she was doing, cleansing the arm, warning the doll to hold still while she looked for a vein, and then poking the tubing into the doll's arm and attaching tape to the tubing and all around the doll's arm. Periodically, she alternated her role between that of the intravenous therapist and that of the child. For instance, after telling the doll to hold still, she cried and whined as if she were the doll, then stated sternly, "You can cry, just don't move your arm," followed by a sobbing, "I'll try." Once the task was completed, she proudly showed it to her nurse, stating that the doll didn't like her anymore but that was okay because she made the doll well so it could go home.

In her play she communicated her understanding of the rationale for intravenous therapy as well as her desire to return home. She also expressed her dislike of those who caused her pain and her general unhappiness about her plight. As she continued to play the role of the intravenous therapist with the support of her nurse, she overcame some of her fears and resentment about the hospital. The nurse's support was provided by repeating or reflecting the child's statements, thus showing interest and encouraging further discussion. As trust grew, Gigi asked more questions about aspects of her therapy and environment and enacted other roles such as those of the doctor, nurse, x-ray technician, and laboratory technician.

Another child, Tommy, ignored all the equipment except the syringes, which he used in an entirely different manner. He pretended that they were guns, and he shot everyone. Tommy had had numerous injections and blood tests during this hospitalization, and each one was met with great protest, including kicking, screaming, and arm flinging. Although he offered no explanation for his choice of activity, the nurse might wonder whether his protests were related to his perceptions of injections as "shots" and these shots being perceived as similar to those from guns. He benefited from his play, and his resistance to blood tests and injections, although still present, was more controlled. He requested a clean, needleless syringe after each encounter and promptly "shot" the person who had given him the injection or drawn blood. Children who are exposed to needle play and who are able to act out the unpleasant experience are then able to tolerate the procedure with less apparent distress. Although they still protest when they must receive an injection, their behavior is less violent and lasts for a shorter time.

The adult supervising hospital play needs to monitor the children's aggressive use of equipment. It is important that the play not reinforce the belief that they are victims of aggressive rather than therapeutic action. Fear concerning injections and blood tests can dominate the child's consciousness and make it difficult to concentrate or become involved in other activities. The basis of this fear is related to the painful experience of the injections and an inability to understand why someone who is identified as a helping, caring person would hurt someone else deliberately (see Chapter 27).

The nurse can provide alternative opportunities to express aggressive feelings by intervening when equipment is being used nontherapeutically. A play project can be organized using syringes for water play, painting, or even cake frosting. The nurse must then emphasize the caring use of potentially painful procedures and must reiterate this frequently. By sharing these experiences in the safe environment of the play area and under the guidance of supportive adults, each child is given the opportunity to explore feelings and fears as well as express concerns or fantasies.

For example, Brian, who had sustained multiple internal injuries, including a broken leg, in a car accident, ignored the hospital play materials until he spied a roll of gauze. He then lined up as many dolls and stuffed animals as were available and wrapped each one's leg. He claimed that everyone's leg was broken and that no one could run and play. He guarded the dolls and animals lest someone else disturb their "casts" and free them. Later that day, he was given some plaster of Paris-impregnated gauze and shown how to make a cast for the doll just like his cast. Instead of making a cast, however, he experimented with the casting material by first making a rock and then a house. The next day, he requested that the cast made for the doll be removed so that he could check the doll's leg. He appeared very relieved to find that the leg still looked the same. This precipitated many questions about what was happening to his own leg under the cast.

Some exploration and use of equipment can be incorporated in nursing routines. Allowing children to listen to a teddy bear's heart, their own heart, or even the nurse's heart gives them experience with the stethoscope so that its purpose becomes familiar and less feared. The younger child pretends to be a nurse or doctor and might discuss the "patient's" condition, whereas the older child interested in anatomy might ask questions and learn about the location, function, and purpose of the heart. This also can be done with the blood pressure cuff, otoscope, or other instruments. The child who understands the equipment through personal experimentation with its qualities is more cooperative when it is actually used than the child who feels controlled by these unknown instruments that restrain and restrict desired activity periodically during the day.

Play as a Means of Communication

Play offers the child a nonverbal, or alternative, means of communication. The child with a limited vocabulary can play out feelings, master anxiety, or express aggression in a safe, acceptable way. Children continually demonstrate that play is their language and the means whereby they give expression to joy or sadness, eager anticipation, or anxious apprehension.

Hospitalized children might feel tension, frustration, insecurity, aggression, anger, hostility, loneliness, fear, bewilderment, and confusion; play is the best medium by which they can express these feelings. The nurse or play therapist thus allows each child to choose a play activity, the people involved, the length of time spent in the play, and the direction of the play. Play is the child's natural means of expressing and acquiring ways to cope with fears, fantasies, and conflicts. It affords children opportunities to demonstrate their personalities, interact with others, and learn about themselves by discovering new ways of handling problems or conflicts.

Therapeutic play, using the child's language to gain insight about the child's feelings, perceptions, and needs, communicates to the nurse information that the child could not otherwise give. Immaturity, inability to identify feelings, or basic apprehension and guilt about having such feelings or thoughts prevent more direct communication, even for older children. Play neutralizes and objectifies these fears and feelings and permits their expression. The nurse or play therapist then needs to analyze the possible meaning of the play activity and the child's statements to plan appropriate interventions. This form of communication is often subtle. It is related to the trusting relationship between the child and nurse, as well as the nurse's skill in observing and interpreting the child's play. Parents also are helpful in interpreting the child's play behavior. They are keenly aware of subtle changes in their child that might go unnoticed by someone else. Their concerns and questions are also clues about the child's total well-being.

Through therapeutic play, children share more information about what is really bothering them than they are able to provide through other means of communication. They reveal their concerns about their families not missing them, having fun without them, rival siblings taking their places, or being left in the hospital forever. For other children, fears focus on their treatments, worries about body image or body integrity, and anxiety that peers will no longer accept them. Each child is unique; each has different concerns based on previous experiences, knowledge, and personal maturity. Nurses never presume to know what is bothering a child but instead provide the means whereby the child can communicate these concerns.

Through play, children reveal aspects of their personalities and their physical and mental states of well-being. The nurse or play therapist notes behavioral changes that might be clues to the child's recovery or change in status. Children who usually cope with stress by active, aggressive, take-charge behavior but who suddenly want to be held, told a story, or listen to records might be saying indirectly that they are not feeling as well physically, are exhausted, need help coping, or want reassurance. The reverse is also significant. Children who become active, noisy, and uncooperative in contrast to their usual accepting, tolerant attitude about procedures are providing important clues concerning their health, and these clues should lead the nurse to further investigation.

The tired, acutely ill, or uncomfortable child cannot play because extra energy is not available for play. When these children begin to show an interest in their surroundings and play activities, it is often a sign of recovery. Initially, their interest and investment are necessarily brief, and the nurse needs to be sensitive about their energy limitations and not overinvolve and thus overextend them.

Play also stimulates communication with other children. Through play, friendships evolve and become an asset for coping during hospitalization. Children normally play with other children at home, in school, on the playground, during club activities, or at a play group. Bringing hospitalized children together for play thus simulates their home routine. "The hospitalized child needs to play with other children so that he maintains a sense of continuity in his life" (Klinzing and Klinzing, 1977).

The playroom might bring children together from opposite ends of the hall or even from different units, but their mutual involvement in projects provides a common ground for communication. Children discover others with similar interests or experiences, and they begin to seek each other out for companionship. As Klinzing and Klinzing (1977) noted, children discuss things with each other that they conceal from adults. Thus, it is sometimes the playmate who tells the nurse or doctor that a friend is not feeling well, has increased pain, or is scared about a procedure.

Play facilitates communication between parents and children. The involvement in a game or an activity reminds parents of similar experiences at home and diminishes their sense of helplessness or awkwardness in an unfamiliar environment. Watching and participating in play helps them to keep the hospital experience in perspective. The hospitalized child is the same child that was at home, with the same desires to laugh, play, sing, and run.

Some children communicate through quiet activities. They respond best to having a story read to them or by listening to story tapes or records. The comfort and reassurance of individual attention gives them the security needed to ask questions or talk about their experiences. Children might identify with the characters in the story who are in similar situations or express the same emotions they feel. They might ask their questions through the story by talking about how the character feels or might have felt in the situation. The nurse also can use this technique to encourage the child to talk about emotions. By distancing the discussion to the story, what might be threatening when applied to the child becomes a safe topic. As the child feels accepted and comes to trust the nurse, more concerns are expressed directly.

The enthusiasm of the nurses and their commitment to communication through play is essential. Nurses convey to children and parents their attitudes toward play. They show whether they think play is important by the time, materials, and space they devote to it. The nurse's understanding of the needs of children is evidenced by providing times to be noisy, messy, and rambunctious safely and engaging the children in quiet, relaxing, creative, expressive activities at other times. The compassionate nurse communicates a sensitivity to human concerns and a desire to create a healthy social and emotional climate. This atmosphere fosters communication among nurses, parents, and children.

Key Concepts

- Play is important to the child's development in all subsystems in that it provides opportunities to explore the environment, solve problems, exercise motor skills, and practice social interactions.
- For hospitalized children, play is a way of coping with fears and anxieties, exerting some control over the environment, learning about treatments and procedures, and communicating concerns to the staff.
- In the hospital setting play facilitators might include the play therapist, who is responsible for designing and directing a play program, as well as the nurse, who makes use of play in the process of nursing care.
- Therapeutic play is the means by which the child communicates fears and concerns; it is distinctly different from play therapy, which is a form of psychotherapy designed to promote the child's insight into behavior.
- In the process of therapeutic play, the nurse observes the child's use of materials, looks for recurring themes, analyzes the child's comments, validates conclusions, coordinates care, plans interventions, and evaluates results.
- Play activities during hospitalization should be fun, age appropriate, similar to play at home, and matched with the child's abilities during the hospital stay.
- Because infants in the hospital are vulnerable to sensory deprivation and sensory overload, they need stimulation appropriate to their developmental stage.
- In early childhood the hospitalized child needs opportunities for make-believe play with objects that allow physical skills to be practiced.
- In middle childhood play in the hospital should provide social interaction and opportunities for communication through developing language skills.
- In late childhood play in the hospital needs to be interactive and stimulating, reflecting the child's developing cognitive abilities and social skills.
- For the hospitalized adolescent, play requires much social interaction and opportunities for private reflection and accomplishment.
- For children who are immobilized, the nurse looks for opportunities to adapt play activities to provide the child with a sense of control.
- Play in the hospital setting provides the nurse with opportunities for developmental assessment.
- Play in the hospital should provide the child with diversion, creative outlets, expression of feelings, and opportunities to learn about procedures.
- In observing the child's choice and expression of play, the nurse can identify areas of concern and plan interventions to address the child's emotional needs.
- Expressing feelings about treatments, procedures, equipment, and hospital staff provides the child with a way of controlling the experience and resolving fears.

References

Chance P: *Learning Through Play.* Gardner Press, 1979.

Douglas JWB: Early hospital admissions and later disturbances of behavior and learning. *Dev Med Child Neurol* 1975; 17:456.

Erikson E: *Childhood and Society.* Norton, 1950.

Garvey C: *Play.* Harvard University Press, 1977.

Green CS: Understanding children's needs through play. *Nursing 74* (Oct) 1974; 4:31–32.

Hartley RE, Frank L, Goldenson RM: *Understanding Children's Play.* Columbia University Press, 1952.

Hyde ND: Play therapy: The troubled child's self-encounter. *Am J Nurs* (July) 1971; 71(7):1366–1370.

Klinzing DR, Klinzing DG: *The Hospitalized Child.* Prentice-Hall, 1977.

Lowenfeld M: *Play in Childhood.* Wiley, 1967.

McLeavey KA: Children's art as an assessment tool. *Pediatr Nurs* (March/April) 1979; 5(2):9–14.

Peters BM: School-aged children's beliefs about causality of illness. *Matern Child Nurs J* (Fall) 1978; 7(3):143–154.

Petrillo M, Sanger S: *Emotional Care of Hospitalized Children: An Environmental Approach.* Lippincott, 1980.

Piaget J, Inhelder B: *The Psychology of the Child.* Basic Books, 1969.

Piers MW (editor): *Play and Development.* Norton, 1972.

Poston LI: Finding time to play. *Am J Matern Child Nurs* (Jan/Feb) 1982; 7(1):19–20.

Riserchia EA, Bragg CF, Alvarez MM: Play and play areas for hospitalized children. *J Assoc Care Child Hosp* 1982; 10(4):135–138.
Rumfelt JJ: How five-year-old children perceive the role of the nurse. *Matern Child Nurs J* (Summer) 1980; 9(2):13–27.
Savedra M, Tesler M: Coping with hospitalized children. *Pediatr Nurs* (March/April) 1981; 7(2):35–38.
Schuster CS, Ashburn SS: *The Process of Human Development*. Little, Brown, 1980.

Additional Readings

Acord LT: One five-year-old boy's use of play. *Matern Child Nurs J.* (Spring) 1980; 9(1):29–32.
Azarnoff P, Flegal S: *A Pediatric Play Program*. Thomas, 1979.
Elkins PD, Roberts MC: A preliminary evaluation of hospital preparation for nonpatient children: Primary prevention in "let's pretend hospital." *Children's Health Care* (Summer) 1984; 13(1):31.
Elmassian J: A practical approach to communication with children through play. *Am J Matern Child Nurs* (July/Aug) 1979; 4(4):238–230.
Gelhard HL: Drawing and development. *Pediatr Nurs* (Nov/Dec) 1978; 4(6):23–26.
Goldman M, Sponseller D, Ream B: A play program in a community hospital. *Am J Matern Child Nurs* (Jan/Feb) 1978; 3(1):42–45.
Iveson-Iveson J: Toy libraries and play. *Nurs Mirror* (Sept) 1978; 147:38.
Matterson EM: *Play and Playthings for the Preschool Child*. Penguin Books, 1967.
Ostrenga MA: *Guidelines for Medical Play*. Booklet available from Dr. Victor C. Dye, Hospital Play Equipment, 1122 Judson, Evanston, IL 60202, 1980.
Schulz J, et al: The effects of a preoperational puppet show on anxiety levels of hospitalized children. *Child Health Care* 1981; 9(4):118–121.
Tizard B, Harvey D: *Biology of Play*. Lippincott, 1977.
Whitson BJ: The puppet treatment in pediatrics. *Am J Nurs* (Sept) 1972; 72(9):1612–1614.
Winnicott DW: *Playing and Reality*. Basic Books, 1971.

Principles of Nursing Care of the Hospitalized Child

29

Nancy Fiero Fazekas

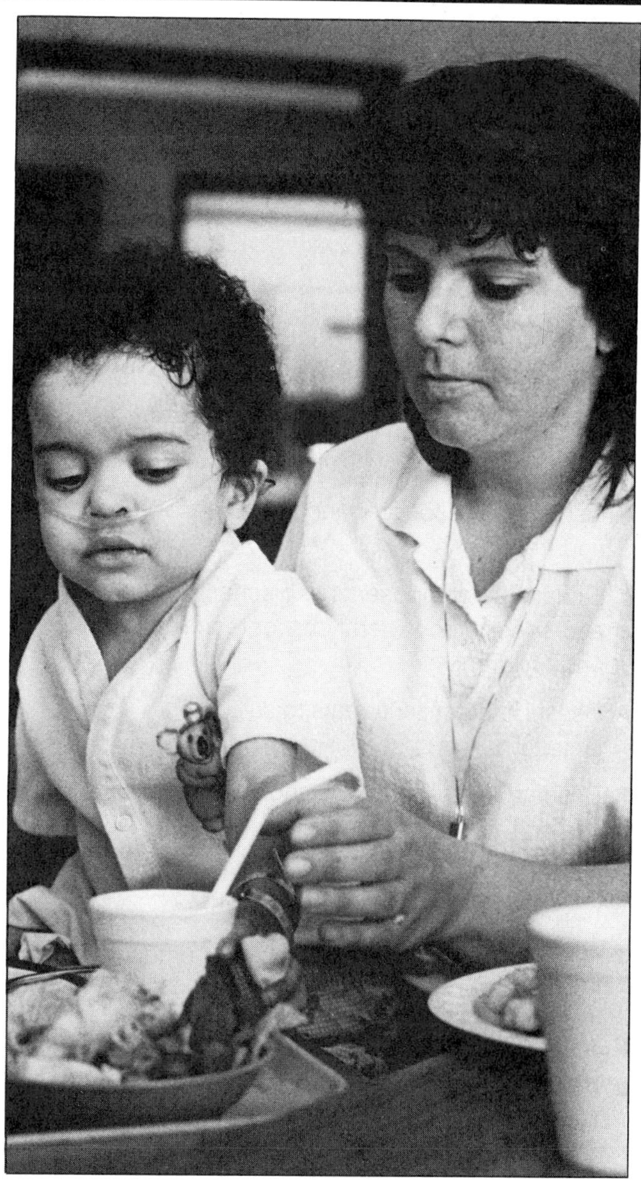

Chapter Outline

continued on next page

Objectives

- List guidelines for parent and child teaching.
- Describe specific methods for preparing the child and family for hospitalization.
- List principles for preparing children for procedures and treatments.
- Explain the components of discharge preparation and specific considerations for teaching families and children.
- Describe potential threats to safety that hospitalization poses for a child.
- Define types of restraints and indications for their use.
- Describe principles of nutritional management for hospitalized children.
- Describe nursing care appropriate for the child who has an order for nothing by mouth.
- Explain methods of feeding hospitalized infants.
- Describe methods of increasing and limiting fluid intake.
- Delineate potential difficulties in elimination posed by hospitalization and nursing interventions which address them.
- Describe nursing care to promote sleep and rest in the hospital.
- List potential complications of immobility and nursing interventions to prevent them.
- Explain criteria for assessing pain in a child.
- Describe nursing care for pain relief in children.
- List criteria assessing for color, sensation, and motion assessment.
- Describe methods of collecting urine and stool specimens with both continent and incontinent children.
- Compare the physiologic differences affecting dosage calculations in adults and children.
- Define dosage formulas used for medicating children.
- Describe methods of oral, topical, rectal, intramuscular, and intravenous administration of medications.
- Explain the components of psychosocial management in administering medications to children.
- Describe components of nursing care for children placed in isolation.
- Describe principles of postoperative care that are specific to children.

"... no greater gulf can be imagined than that existing between the practical, factual, and realistic approach of most medical and nursing personnel on the pediatric wards and the unrealistic, affective response of their patients" (Bergmann and Freud, 1965). The "gulf" that Bergmann defines could just as easily be applied today to the chasm between the feelings of nurses as we provide care for our patients and families and the feelings of these children and families experiencing illness and hospitalization. As a result of the study of the reactions of children and their families to hospitalization and of the cognitive and affective development of children, hospitals and medical and nursing personnel have made great strides in accommodating themselves to the increased understanding of the needs of hospitalized children and their families. Medical and nursing professionals now recognize play, for example, as an important tool for meeting the developmental needs of the ill child. Play also has educational and therapeutic value. Thus we attempt to gear explanations, treatments, and routines to the needs of hospitalized children and their families.

In caring for children and communicating with their families, however, it is all too easy for us to act as if others share our familiarity with procedures, equipment, and routines, and the same priorities and concepts of what is serious or minor. To children and often to their families, any illness or condition is major and any surgery is threatening. To a young child, hospitalization seems endless, regardless of its length.

Nursing and medical personnel often judge a condition as minor and insignificant if it is not permanent, deforming, or life threatening. A short hospital stay indeed does not seem very stressful to us. We can sympathize to an extent with children or families whose lives are disrupted by a medical or surgical emergency, but a scheduled admission may seem manageable, and we may assume that preoperative or preadmission preparation is adequate to meet the needs of children and families. If we view a hospital stay as short and insignificant when the child cannot see beyond it and finds it very stressful and if we believe teaching to be adequate when a child and family are not able to listen and learn, no wonder we may not recognize or accept a child's depth of feeling or despair and children and parents do not always cooperate fully with treatment plans and hospital routines.

When drawing up and executing our nursing care plans, we need to remember to listen to and to discern the perceptions and feelings of others, to teach them, to learn from them, to remain open-minded, and to communicate respect. In this way we can better bridge the gap between the feelings and thoughts of children and families and nursing plans and approaches. We can arrive at mutual goals—mutual plans of care—so that we are truly helping the child and family members regain control of their lives.

In this chapter we discuss the nursing care required to meet the physical and emotional needs of the hospitalized child; such care is continually included in the nursing process. All nursing care requires a careful assessment of what the child and family need to regain equilibrium and maximum independence. Care is based on a knowledge as thorough as possible of the child and family before hospitalization, the child's physiologic problem, and the child's and family's responses to hospitalization. This care is far more likely to meet the needs of the child and family than care routinized for a child of a particular age or with a particular diagnosis. There are, of course, general principles to consider in caring for the ill child, a thorough knowledge of which enables the nurse to proceed from a firm theoretical base and leaves the nurse free to assess the unique characteristics of individual children and their families. In this chapter we will discuss these principles and their application.

Parent–Child Teaching

Teaching is a major role and responsibility of the child health nurse and a necessity for helping the child adjust to the new and unusual environment of the hospital; for preparing the child for specific procedures, tests, and surgery; and for promoting the child's growth and development. Hospitalization can be a marvelous opportunity for ongoing extended interactions with the child and family. The nurse can establish a relationship of mutual respect and can use this for an assessment of the child's life at home. The nurse can then provide encouragement and support in the difficult areas of a child's and parent's growth and include anticipatory guidance, as needed, concerning the child's development (see Chapter 21). Teaching should not, however, follow a formula. Even when family members need to learn specific information, such as administering home hyperalimentation to a child, the teaching plan needs to be individually designed. Individualized teaching is most effective because the child and family learn more and then feel more in control of their lives and their medical and nursing care. Teaching is individualized when the approach, pace, and the content of the teaching plan are geared to the specific child and family.

Guidelines for Teaching

When preparing a child for admission, examinations, or procedures, it is often helpful to do so, at least in part, through play. In this way passive listening becomes active participation. Play usually increases the child's coping abilities and gives the child a sense of control, promoting cooperation in the process. (The importance of play for hospitalized children is further discussed in Chapter 28.) Some general guidelines for selecting teaching formats, play materials, and the vocabulary to use for explanations follow; more specific guidelines relative to specific developmental levels are included in Tables 29-1 through 29-6.

Establishing a Baseline First, and perhaps most importantly, the nurse finds out from the parents and the child what information they have received about the admission, examination, or procedure; what they understand; and what their response is to this information. Teaching plans have become so much a part of nursing practice that it may seem simplistic and obvious to say that teaching must be geared to what a child and family need to know. Yet many nurses proceed with a teaching plan without first obtaining this baseline information.

TABLE 29-1 Preparation for Children Under Age 2

Nursing management	Rationale
Prepare parents carefully with details of procedure	Parents are often deeply upset when an infant or small child undergoes procedures. Parents' feelings are communicated to child
Prepare child at the time of the event	Ability to understand explanations and understand event is very limited
When possible, encourage primary care giver to stay with child	The infant's sense of self is closely tied to the parents. The child derives comfort from their presence. Extreme distress results from separating the older infant from the parents
Approach child slowly and calmly. Have nurse familiar with child perform or assist with procedure	Stranger anxiety occurs during the first year of life. Young children may need 20 to 30 minutes in nurse's presence before accepting nurse
Use face-to-face position, from 1 to 2 feet, when talking to and touching infant before procedure	The very young infant shows a preference for the parent's face. The deliberate use of touch, voice, and *en face* position helps communicate the nurse's feelings and helps to identify the nurse as different from the parent
Talk calmly, quietly, and directly to child	Word repetition is calming to the younger child. Tone of voice is significant in communicating feelings and assisting the child in developing a sense of trust
Give simple explanations of procedures as events unfold. Use common words such as "ouch" or "owie" right before a painful aspect of procedure	Verbalization is beginning. Many older infants truly understand words and to a degree can anticipate events
Use gentle movements. Touch, hold, and cuddle child when possible	Child understands care giver's feelings through touch
Touch area where child will feel pain or discomfort (for instance at site of IV insertion or injection) in addition to words	The child may understand specific as well as general communication through touch
Use transitional object such as security blanket or favorite toy. Give to child during and/or after procedure	Child derives true comfort from these objects. They aid the child in coping with the procedure
Provide bottle or pacifier (if child uses these) during and/or after procedure	Sucking is a means of coping for young children. It helps them settle themselves and thus gain some control
Hold and cuddle child after procedure	Assists in child's coping with stress. Helps reestablish relationship and sense of trust
When surgery or painful procedures are anticipated, the older infant (over 9 months or 1 year) can play with the equipment to be used or playact before the event. Allow child to hold equipment. Play peek-a-boo with surgical mask	Tactile familiarity with equipment may help decrease fears. Peek-a-boo helps child deal with separation issues

The nurse therefore finds out what the child and family already know, or feel a need to know, and are ready to learn. The nurse listens carefully to their questions and acknowledges their anxieties and then clarifies these areas of concern first, even though these very same topics may be covered later. So often, unless these questions are answered first, the anxiety level is not reduced sufficiently for the family to hear any other information. A good rule to follow is to answer their questions first but then reiterate that same information in its usual sequence when teaching. Sometimes what concerns family members most may be a relatively insignificant aspect of a procedure. As this aspect is not minor to them, however, the nurse needs to give it the time and attention necessary to relieve their concerns.

Identifying Coping Strategies The nurse also identifies the child's and parent's usual patterns of coping and the effectiveness of these patterns. If the child has been given any prior information about the anticipated experience, the nurse discusses the child's response to the information, behavior changes, and questions asked. Children normally manifest anxiety when confronting a new experience, so nurses need to learn each child's expression of this anxiety. After being told that he would be going to the hospital so the doctor could help him not to have so many sore throats and high temperatures anymore, one little boy ritualistically played "doctor" with his stuffed animals. Immediately upon waking every morning, he took the animals to the "hospital," gave them medicine or operations, and sent them home. Only after completing this sequence was he willing to eat breakfast and get dressed for the day. Some accounts of children's reactions to impending hospitalization noted that all children experienced increasing anxiety that peaked on the admission day (Meng and Zastowny, 1982).

Children and parents often use denial as a coping behav-

TABLE 29-2 Preparation for Children Ages 2–3½

Nursing management	Rationale
Keep primary care giver near child especially during times of preparation for procedures, have care giver present and involved in procedures in comforting role, if possible. If procedure is done elsewhere, tell or show child where care givers will be waiting	Separation from primary care giver is even more a major trauma than the illness
Use play as means of explanation, either with puppets' telling what is to be done and a puppet telling what it will feel like and asking questions concerning the event; a story about a similar event; or dolls and hospital equipment that depict the event. Talk about how the puppet or doll might feel and what they might be thinking	Imagination and fantasies are intertwined with reality thinking
Have the child's support systems available, usually parents or primary care giver. Give the child specific things to do such as squeezing someone's hand, crying, or holding onto some object. Observe the child's rituals and maintain continuity with them. Have security objects such as stuffed animals, blankets, or pillows with the child during procedures or times when parents are not there	Coping skills are limited
Use single-meaning words in explanations. Avoid words that the child will not understand or have previous experience with; substitute simple words or use their definition	Interpretation of words is literal; child imitates words without understanding true meaning
Expect vague feelings of anxiety and anger, confusion and frustration. Use play to help child express these. Have aggressive toys such as blocks, soft balls, beanbags, punching balloons available for child's use	Expression of feelings is nonspecific
Allow child to be involved in play and explanations; leave props with child for further exploration and play	Child learns through trial and error, imitation, and play
Keep discussion short and use play and visual aids to encourage attention	Child's attention span is short
Use play to distract; when possible, have someone to play with the child while the second person does the procedure, such as taking vital signs. When lying still is required, distract the child with stories, puppets, talking, or books. Use restraints as minimally as possible; have child help by holding still while directing attention elsewhere. Be positive; explain to the child that the nurse will gently hold or touch the involved extremity as a reminder to hold still	Child protests strongly whenever something is disliked, especially when the child is being restrained
Emphasize the helping and healing purpose of procedures. Reassure child that there is no relation between procedures and punishment; it is often helpful for the doll or puppet to ask that question so the nurse can clarify any misconceptions	Child is unable to comprehend intentional pain

ior (see Chapter 12). The nurse therefore needs to determine what children and parents truly don't know and what information they may be denying. Nurses can do this by being specific and personal with questions. Rather than asking, "What do you know?" or "What have you been told?" a nurse might ask, "What do you think will happen to you?" or "What do you like or dislike about this?" For younger children, it is often helpful to discuss the situation using a story such as *Curious George Goes to the Hospital* or one of the other books about a child's hospital experience. In this manner, children can hear about what is or will be happening to them.

While conversing with them, the nurse can assess their responses, their acceptance or denial of information, any increased need for parental support, and any signs of regression or anger. Once the coping behaviors and their applications are known, the nurse can adapt teaching to the individual not only to include information but also to facilitate beneficial coping strategies. Play and personal information thus enhance children's mental health.

Providing Honest Explanations Honesty is an essential part of preparing a child for medical or nursing interventions. Nurses should be specific as to what will and what will not happen and what parts of the body will and will not be involved in such interventions. Children learn about and relate to events through their senses. They need to know what they will be hearing, seeing, feeling, touching, tasting, and smelling. For example, it is better for the child to know that an injection will hurt than to deceive and temporarily pacify the child by stating that it is like a mosquito bite. The child may perceive a big difference between the brief pain of an injection, which is often acute and burning, and the repeated itchiness of a mosquito bite.

Establishing Limits A nurse does not give choices when, in reality, there are no choices. For instance, it is not a good idea to ask whether the child is ready for the treatment. The answer may be "no," and it may continue to be "no," but the treatment still has to be done. Disregarding

TABLE 29-3 Preparation for Children Ages 3½–5

Nursing management	Rationale
Use play and help child to prepare for events by having doll or stuffed animal enact event with actual equipment or replicas of equipment. Have equipment proportional to size of doll or animal to lessen fears that equipment is overwhelming	Understands only what seen, unable to conceive of events logically. Thinking depends on perception
Allow child time to play and use equipment before actual procedure. To enhance understanding and clarify misconceptions, use role-playing where child can be the doctor, nurse, or patient	Child is involved in trial-and-error learning. Taking an active role encourages mastery of events
Give child complete explanations about what part of the body is and what parts are not involved. Have child point to the part that is involved. Specify whether the procedure takes place inside or outside the body and what the outside will look like when the procedure is over (eg, presence of bandage or tubing). Demonstrate event on doll or stuffed animal, including immediate appearance and later appearance when ready for discharge	Child's fears of body mutilation are common
Watch child play out events both before and after actual procedure to observe perceptions, beliefs, and feelings about what happened. Clarify and further explore as needed	Child vacillates between reality and fantasy in thinking because of vivid imagination, which is sometimes an asset and sometimes a deficit in understanding explanations. Fears may be increased because fantasy and imagination take over and exaggerate events
Answer questions simply and directly. Provide information at the child's level of understanding. Emphasize the helping, healing purpose of procedures and medical personnel	World is ordered by asking questions. Incessant questioning helps child to learn about the world and roles of people in the world. All questions must have an answer; child is not concerned about the logic or correctness of the answer but that the question has an answer
Have primary care givers present for stressful events and times. Follow child's rituals and provide continuity. Have security objects present and affirm their value. Familiarize the child with the event and equipment beforehand; encourage child to play with equipment to learn its properties	Coping behaviors are limited; child relies on primary care givers
Give the child specific directions on what can or cannot be done, eg, state that "crying is okay but hold the leg still." Have the child hold or squeeze a nurse's hand, hold tape or dressing package, count to ten, or recite the alphabet. Give honest praise for the child's performing the task; be specific and relate to the initial request with such statements as "You held your leg very still just as I requested; you really did a good job"	Child is becoming more social and wants to please others, especially adults
Incorporate time for play and expression of fears and feelings following explanations for procedures. Have available toys that facilitate expression of aggressive feelings	Expression of feelings is limited
Discuss events according to activities of daily living. Explain when an event will take place by relating it to meal time, bedtime, or another part of the routine	Understanding of time is limited

the child's decision while having offered a choice jeopardizes a trusting relationship. When not listened to earlier, why should the child trust the nurse at a later time? When the child is receiving an injection, for example, it is better for the nurse to say something like, "I am going to count to five; tell me at what number to start." That way, the child has a choice and can maintain some control. The treatment will begin when the chosen number is reached; the child is not given a choice whether or not to accept the treatment and stalling is limited.

Teaching for Understanding of Purpose The nurse reassures the child that an exam, procedure, treatment, or hospital admission is not punishment. Children often feel that they are to blame for their illnesses or that treatment is the result of some misdeed they committed (see Chapter 27). Parents and professionals need to increase their awareness of how children interpret certain admonitions. The child who had been told, "Wear your hat, boots, or jacket or else you will get sick" naturally concludes that any disobedience in this regard caused the current illness.

The nurse who tells the child to drink fluids or take medicine to get better is also conveying the message that if these orders are not followed, the child may become sicker. The nurse instead states why the child should drink and how fluids will help restore health. A better approach is therefore to tell the child to take the medicine so it can help the germ fighters in the body work better or that the germ fighters need supplies and the medicine provides the supplies. This helps the child understand why the medicine is important and how it works. Likewise, explaining to the child that fluids help to wash bad germs out of the body just like water

TABLE 29-4 Preparation for Children Ages 5–8

Nursing management	Rationale
Use simple medical terminology that is defined and illustrated during explanations	Child has improved language skills and is interested in new words and their meanings
Use anatomic drawings, dolls, or models to demonstrate procedures. Use these also to clarify thoughts about how the body functions, where organs are located in general	Child is beginning to understand body functions
Illustrate and give specific information about what body part or parts will be involved as well as what areas will not be involved	Child is concerned about body integrity and fears body mutilation or change in appearance
Give the child opportunity to play out experience both before and after its occurrence. Allow child to manipulate hospital-related equipment; use equipment or its facsimile on doll or stuffed animal	Child is helped to master situations through play
Provide child with a degree of control and give choice as much as possible. Allow child to help with procedure as much as possible by doing tasks such as holding dressing or tape package. If procedure is repeated, keep methodology the same	Coping behaviors are increased; child is more self-directive but parents are very important for support. Maintaining self-care is important to the child. Ritual behavior is a frequent coping mechanism
Reassure child that the experience is not a punishment for some misdeed. Relate events to body function and ways that procedures assist the body to recover or the doctors and nurses to identify the problem so the child can be helped and then return home	Child is beginning to sense right and wrong and needs reason to justify experience. Child tends to view hospitalization as punishment
Emphasize the helping, caring nature of the procedure. Spend time with child following the procedure doing a favorite activity such as playing a game or reading a story	Child is beginning to separate intent from conclusion

washes dirt off hands gives both a rationale for drinking and a concrete example of its benefits. The child may need repeated assurances that germs were the cause of an illness or that drinking fluids or taking medicine is not a punishment for becoming sick.

Choosing Words Carefully The nurse uses words the child understands. Nursing has a vocabulary all its own, and it is easy to mystify the child and parents with complex technical words. The nurse who takes time to explain what a phrase or word means whenever a quizzical or confused expression is observed will ease both the child's and the family's anxiety. For example, the family or child may not know the meaning of the sign "NPO after midnight" taped to the bed. They need to be told specifically that the child is not to eat or drink anything after midnight and that this means no breakfast because it is necessary for the stomach to be empty for a procedure. After it is over, the nurse then tells them when the child can start to drink and eat again.

Words that have multiple meanings are confusing for children and nurses therefore need to avoid using idioms. Pontious (1982, p. 115) lists the following words whose dual meaning may provoke unnecessary anxiety in children: cut, incision, take, fix, organs, test, and dye. It is less confusing for the child to hear "I want to listen to your heart and count how many times it makes a sound" than "I want to take your pulse"; it is better to hear "I want to count how many times you breathe when you are sitting quietly" than "I want to take your respirations."

Sometimes it is best to find out what a particular word means to the child before using it. In an effort to choose words carefully during preoperative teaching, the nurse told 6-year-old Susie that the doctor was going to repair her heart. She immediately asked whether the doctor planned to use glue, staples, tape, thread, or string for the repair. This question was followed by a long story of how her mom used these to repair her toys, clothes, and books and which products worked best for the type of repair that was needed. She then decided that the doctor should discuss this with her mom since her mom could repair everything and could tell the doctor just what to do. After that, the nurse wisely decided not to pursue what was going to be done but to focus on the results. Susie was reassured that the doctor and her mom would discuss how to do this repair so she could run and play as she wanted. The remainder of the preparation related to how this experience would help her to grow taller, to play relay games and tag, and to be more like her friends.

Children want to know how an event will affect them, what will change, and what will be the same. As they get older, their concerns change from body integrity to body image, but the emphasis is still the preservation of self. This needs to be the emphasis of preparation, not a technical explanation of the procedure but how it will affect the child and what the results will mean. Puppets and doll play are good ways to prepare a child for these changes (see Chapter 28).

Proceeding From Simple to Complex Material presented to the child should proceed from simpler ideas, facts, and concepts to those that are more complex and

TABLE 29-5 Preparation for Children Ages 8–11

Nursing management	Rationale
Prepare child for procedures on one-to-one basis when peers are not likely to be present. Reassure child of the appropriateness of asking questions, that questions will not be shared with others, and that it is okay to talk about fears and concerns and to cry. Praise the child's actions instead of the child so child can relate to the specific act when determining its appropriateness	Peer group and "being brave" in front of friends is important
Teach by demonstration on anatomic model or by diagram illustrating body parts and functions. Encourage child to participate in recalling the explanation and demonstration. Use art or writing as means of communication and working through experience	Child is concrete thinker and judges actions by logical effect. Intent is important and understood as separate from behavior
Give basic explanation, using and defining medical or technical terms. Discuss how to prevent certain illnesses and accidents	Child has increasing interest in body parts, functions, and relation of disease and health
Support coping behaviors. Facilitate expression of concerns, fears, and anger through appropriate play and equipment. Accept some regression and help child identify feelings; reassure their normalcy. Use of rituals and participation in procedures helpful	Increased coping skills and self-reliance but regression and overt expression of feelings common under stress
Prepare well in advance and include time involved for event and for recovery	Good concept of time relative to past and future
Include illustrations about body appearance after intrusive event, length of time in recovery, and final effects. Discuss implications of major change in appearance. Encourage daydreaming, writing, and playing out event with hospital-related characters and equipment	Child is concerned about body image, both immediate and future
Respect child's need to be independent and explain events with or without parents according to child's choice. Assist parents to accept and understand child's need to be independent	Child shows increased independence from parents yet needs their understanding and support
Discuss relation of events leading to hospitalization and the rationale for care. Reassure child that hospitalization is not punishment, that discomfort and pain are not inflicted as discipline but as efforts to achieve recovery	Child has strong sense of justice. Child still might interpret hospitalization as punishment
Spend time with child to develop trust. Discuss common fears and events while child is absorbed in other activities such as playing a game, working a puzzle, or doing a craft to allow think time and reflection as well as to decrease the stress of having to respond	Child is able to verbalize some fears; others are more difficult to conceptualize (eg, fear of death)

difficult to understand. In this way, the child can retain interest in the subject and can feel a sense of mastery over the material presented. The nurse obtains feedback from the child as the teaching progresses to make certain that the material is understood. When simpler material is mastered, the nurse can proceed. Presenting complicated material later helps avoid confusion and anxiety.

Spacing Teaching The nurse spaces information over several sessions, depending on its complexity, and needs to be sensitive to signs of restlessness and inattention, which indicate the child needs time to absorb what has been discussed. Interposing information with play allows expression of feelings. Allowing the child to play with the doll and props used for explanations diminishes the anxiety associated with the unknown. Repeating material willingly and as often as requested helps to establish trust. Questioning the child about information given previously helps the child to review and clarify ideas. Tables 29-1 through 29-6 provide specific guidelines to prepare children of different ages for procedures.

Adjusting Teaching to Developmental Level The nurse often faces a situation where assessment of developmental stage does not coincide with a child's chronologic age. Many children are anxious when hospitalized and may regress in their behaviors and in their abilities to learn. Other children, because of mental retardation or developmental delays, have not reached a mental or emotional level expected for their age (see Chapter 23). Whatever the cause of the discrepancy, nurses need to treat children as they present themselves.

So that a child understands, teaching is geared therefore to developmental stage rather than chronologic age. An anxious child will need a more concrete, slower, simpler explanation than would be necessary if the same child were relaxed. A retarded child or emotionally disturbed child also needs teaching that is understandable. When teaching, the nurse continually seeks evidence of understanding. Can the child repeat explanations? Does a child demonstrate through play an understanding of hospitalization and treatments?

When evaluating teaching effectiveness with children who are performing below their chronologic ages, the nurse uses criteria appropriate to each child's developmental stage to assess understanding. For example, perhaps a 16-year-old retarded girl will repeat preoperative teaching by demonstrating on a doll what she thinks will happen to her. She

TABLE 29-6 Preparation for Children Ages 12–18

Nursing management	Rationale
Respect need to be like peers and to maintain their respect. Do procedures in private so as not to restrict adolescent's expression of feelings in order to "save face." Sometimes, it is beneficial for experienced person to discuss procedure with the one anticipating it	Peer group is extremely important; child is dependent on peer group
Use anatomic drawings and illustrations to describe event. Discuss procedure and its purpose in correcting problem that necessitated hospitalization	Child basically understands body parts and functions
Include all aspects of changes in body image, both temporary and permanent, caused by the procedure. Discuss and illustrate how to cope or adapt to permanent ones. Anticipate expressions of anger and grief when discussing changes in body image	Child is concerned about body image and long-range implications of procedures
Provide opportunity to express feelings of anger, disappointment, and frustration through crafts and games. Anticipate regression and accept it without judging or inferring loss of respect. Encourage participation and asking of questions to clarify events; give choices whenever possible to aid in sense of mastery	Child's coping behaviors are well established, but regression is common when experiencing stress. Independence, growth, and mastery are encouraged by participation and increased control over events
Review what the individual thinks will happen so that misconceptions and fears can be corrected. Child often finds it helpful to talk with someone of similar age who has experienced the event positively and helpful to talk about feelings and sensations during the event	Child is able to conceptualize and think in abstract
Encourage discussion of fears. Explain roles of people involved in procedures. Respect fears; never belittle them	Child is better able to verbalize fears
Promote positive sense of self-esteem in achieving independence. Discuss procedures and perform them in private. Respect ability to make decisions and give options as appropriate	Child is in the process of becoming independent of adults and parents

might also enjoy reading *Curious George Goes to the Hospital.* Some children are not able to respond in ways that are easy for nurses to understand. Some cannot speak or do not have the organized thinking and motor control necessary for demonstrating what they learn. Many of these children, however, do understand and benefit from teaching. The nurse working with such children can plan simple teaching exercises with much repetition of facts and concepts. Often, someone accompanying the child is attuned to fine alterations in the child's behavior and can interpret the effects of teaching on the child.

Children often understand more than nurses think or can know. One 12-year-old comatose boy resisted a nurse's holding his arm. When she told him that she was going to give him a shot and it would hurt less if he held still, the child appeared to relax and did not move his arm. A child with cerebral palsy and limited speaking ability was given slow, careful preoperative teaching. His parents expressed tremendous gratitude. They felt that he understood what was taught and was more relaxed after the teaching. He had previously been hospitalized for extensive surgery requiring a postoperative stay in intensive care. Because he was not instructed before this previous operation, his parents felt that he had been unnecessarily frightened.

Some children are gifted. Nurses need to give truthful, accurate answers when such children ask seemingly endless questions. In following the rule of going from the simple to the complex, nurses may find themselves presenting very complex information indeed and can forget that they are talking to children. Nurses thus need to remember that, despite the intelligence of such children, their logical thinking and emotional development need time to mature. The 7-year-old who is self-taught and adept at long division and simple algebra is still only 7 years old. The child still has the fears and fantasies of a 7-year-old.

These children may already suffer from peer interaction problems, as their vocabularies, interests, and activities often do not match those of their age mates. They need protection from feeling a need to act as if they were adults. Nurses can help by speaking to their fears and anxieties as well as answering their questions.

Providing Reinforcement for Learning At times, rewards may be appropriate when a child cooperates with a teaching plan and with care and changes necessitated by hospitalization. For the child there are such natural rewards as feeling better and seeing progress in recovery. The nurse therefore should point out such rewards to a child and family. Many times, however, a child does not immediately seem better and may, in fact, not show signs of recovery from an illness. The nurse then tells both parent and child in what way they are contributing to recovery or health, as specifically as possible. When a parent follows the treatment plan and, for example, offers fluids very slowly to a postoperative child, despite the child's complaints of a dry mouth, the parent is told that this helps to ensure the child's comfort and to decrease the chance of nausea and vomiting in the early postoperative period. When other parents encourage necessary fluid intake despite their children's protests, the parent is told how much this is truly helping the child.

When children cooperate as necessary with their treatment plans, the nurse encourages such cooperation by offering such rewards as taking them to the hospital cafeteria or coffee shop, where the change of scene and different food may be very satisfying. Children often need rewards for appropriately participating in their treatment plans. These rewards may be anything safe and reasonable that serves to encourage children. A child may want something to keep, such as a sticker or star. A chart of a child's accomplishments may be a reward for which a child enjoys working. The nurse may give attention to a child by playing a game or reading a story. Attention may be withheld by leaving a child's room, or other appropriate limits may be established for deviant or negative behavior. With the goal of helping children to help themselves, nurses may use many approaches, all of which are similar to specific parenting strategies (see Chapter 13).

Preparation for Specific Procedures and Treatments

Most children who are properly prepared are cooperative during routine procedures. Many of these procedures—blood tests, radiographic examinations, and physical examinations—the children have experienced before or have observed while someone else experienced them. Blood tests nonetheless are disliked and feared by children of all ages. The child needs careful preparation before undergoing a test no matter how many times it has been done previously. In fact, the child's previous experiences with routine procedures are important factors in determining the current level of anxiety about a procedure. For example, discomfort from blood tests closely resembles that from injections or IV insertion. If a child has experienced either of these previously, the reaction to a blood test might be more severe. Because of a child's earlier traumatic experience, routine procedures, treatments, or tests often produce the most anxiety.

Radiographs are used frequently in medical diagnosis and follow-up of hospitalized children. All children, especially the younger child, need honest explanations and support before procedures. Large machinery and the experience of being left alone while a radiograph is taken may be very frightening. The nurse emphasizes that the child must hold still during the procedure; otherwise, the repeated attempts can become tiring and frustrating. Some children cooperate better if a parent or nurse wears a protective lead apron and stays with the child. The child should also be protected from radiation as much as possible, and gonads should be shielded.

For examinations involving the injection of contrast material, preparation includes explanations of the procedure for injecting the dye or air and the sensations this causes. The timing of the explanation depends on the child's developmental level and specific needs. Some children need more time to learn than others. Honesty must prevail in all discussions, so that the child learns to trust the nurse and has time to react with appropriate coping strategies. The parent also needs to feel comfortable about the procedure and its purpose. Parents then can communicate strength and reassurance to their children.

The preparation of children for specific tests or treatments constituting the diagnostic or therapeutic regimen should be individually designed. The most effective preparation involves several members of the health team. Information about the child, which has been gathered by team members, is combined with facts that relate to the specific procedure. The nurse, play therapist, and others can then determine how best to prepare the child. For all children, regardless of age, play is a component of the preparation plan. At times, play is used for the explanation of the procedure and at other times as a means of expression about the experience (see Chapter 28). No matter how benign or simple a procedure seems to the nurse, that same procedure may be awesome and feared by the child and family. The nurse thus uses the information obtained from the assessment process and adapts the explanation or teaching accordingly.

The teaching approach most likely to diminish anxiety focuses on the sensations the child will experience and the reasons for that particular experience. The way that something will feel, smell, sound, and look is crucial information for the child. Knowing that a medication stings when injected, hearing the sound of a cast saw before it is used, knowing a cleansing solution is brown and will feel cold on the skin—these bits of information help immeasurably in reducing the child's anxiety and helping the child successfully cope with an experience. The child also needs to know what will happen and when this will occur. Details concerning specific tests and ways in which to prepare children are included in Chapters 33–45.

Preparation for Hospital Experiences

Ideally, preparation for hospitalization begins well before hospital admission. When family members first know that a child needs to go to the hospital, they must be as fully informed as possible. Parents, along with the referring source and the hospital to which the child will go, need to plan what, how, and when to teach the child. Timing, words, and the complexity of teaching vary with a child's age, stage of development, personality characteristics, and plan of care expected in the hospital. By late childhood, most children benefit from several weeks of preparation. They need to know about, learn reasons for, obtain details about, talk about, and act out ideas and feelings concerning an upcoming hospital stay. This time can be well used to teach and work through the older child's feelings so that the child is mentally and emotionally ready for hospital admission. Children in middle childhood need less preparation time. From a few days to a week is ample time for introducing the idea of hospitalization and for allowing the child to play through feelings and fantasies. A child in early childhood may be introduced to the idea of hospitalization within a few days of admission, since the child's cognitive and verbal abilities do not allow for teaching about and playing out the experience until it is about to happen. A still-younger child can also be prepared when the experience is close at hand or is occurring.

Preparation begins with the referring source (doctor's office, clinic, emergency room). Nurses prepare parents of young children so that the parents in turn can prepare their children. With the older child the nurse prepares both the child and the parent. Often the parent is not ready to take on the responsibilities of preparing the child. A minor situation can seem very serious to a family, and anxiety might prevent the parents from supporting their children throughout the experience. Many parents fear surgery for their children, sometimes because of their own fear of anesthesia. Parents who have worked through fears, misconceptions and guilt feelings of their own, however, have less of a problem helping their children work through fears and misconceptions about an upcoming hospital stay.

Nursing care must help support both parents and child. Only after establishing a relationship that allows fears to be expressed are parents in need of support, free to receive it, and in turn able to support their children. If parents can receive this support before their children are admitted to the hospital, children may best learn about and ready themselves for the event. In the safety and security of their homes, they can express their concerns verbally, through art or through play.

Parents need to be emotionally ready to support and teach their children. They also must know what to teach and have some understanding of usual reactions to the anticipated experience for the age and developmental level of their child (see Chapter 27). To help parents know what to teach, many hospitals and referring physicians have teaching protocols they can give to parents before a child is admitted to the hospital. These are invaluable in assisting a parent and child to know what to expect from the hospital experience.

Play and parental reinforcement of teaching is a real aid to the child. A parent can, for example, allow a child to play with makeshift or actual hospital equipment. This may be introduced and used in a nondirective way, presenting hospital equipment and allowing the child to use it as the child wishes. Equipment can also be used to teach or demonstrate procedures. Puppet or doll play can be used to help a child talk through fears and concerns and ask questions (see Chapter 28).

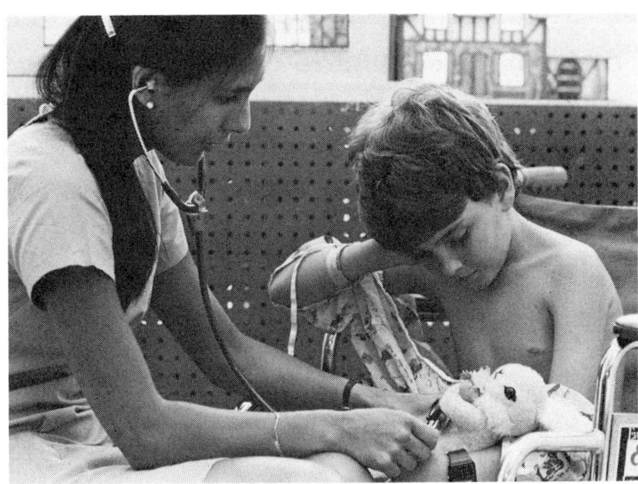

Play is an important part of a child's preparation for procedures.

The reality of the hospital environment might be different from the child's previous experiences or fantasies. Some hospitals have preadmission programs for children and their families. Some programs are elaborate; some are very simple. If an orientation is offered, it should honestly depict the admission process for that particular institution. The child's comfort after admission will reflect the correlation of the reality of the hospital to the orientation. For instance, if the hospital identification bands are green, this is what should be shown during orientation. If rooming-in of parents is permitted, the facilities and possible restrictions should be carefully described so that parent and child have realistic expectations.

Commercially produced films are available that depict the hospitalization experience. Some are filmed in a real-life setting; some use actors; some are in the form of cartoons. The child's health team should, however, review several of these before deciding which accurately portrays the institution's procedures.

Another alternative is to develop an individual orientation for the specific institution. Many hospitals have instructional media departments that cooperate with the staff in developing such tools. Possible media are videotapes, movie films, and slides. To acknowledge the ethnic variety of a community, children from different ethnic groups can be shown. Because children respond most favorably to similar-age models, a film should portray children of various ages or should feature ages similar to the audience.

Other audiovisual aids that may prove useful are dolls, puppets, models, and actual hospital equipment. Puppets can represent hospital personnel, patients, and families. Two approaches to puppetry are common. One method is to present a puppet show to demonstrate some event. This usually follows a script, should be well rehearsed, and should be presented in a manner that can hold the audience's attention while imparting information. The other approach

Bibliography of Children's Books for Hospital Preparation

So You're Going to the Hospital
Northfield Hospital
Northfield, Minn.

Paul in the Hospital
Jessel-Jolly
Metheun Children's Books

You and Your Child in the Hospital
Charing Cross Hospital
London, England

Fiona Goes to the Hospital
John McIndoem Ltd.
Dunedin, New Zealand

A Child in the Hospital
Lutheran General Hospital
Park Ridge, Ill.

Michael's Heart Test
Margaret's Heart Operation
Children's Hospital of Philadelphia, Pa.

A Hospital Story
Stein & Pinney

The Sunshine Book
Janet Bubar
Women's Graphic Center
Los Angeles, Calif.

Elizabeth Gets Well
A. Weber, MD
Thomas Y. Crowell

What Happens When You Go to the Hospital
Arthur Shay
Henry Regnery Co.

A Child's First Stay
Medic Media
New York, N.Y.

A Child's Visit to the Hospital
Core Communications in Health
Bryant Street, Palo Alto, Calif.

A Visit to the Hospital
Betty Lovelace–Joyce Delaney
Stanford University Hospital

No More Tonsils
Paullin, Deacon Press
Boston, Mass.

Nancy Plays Nurse
Sherman, Rand McNally

A Visit to the Hospital
Chase and Rossi, Grosset

Doctors and Nurses—
What Do They Do?
Greene and Kessler
Harper & Row

Curious George Goes to the Hospital
M. and H. Rey
Scholastic Book Services

Your Friend the Doctor
Sanders and Hinkelman
American Medical Assoc.

Johnny Visits the Doctor
Sever, Children's Medical Center
Boston, Mass.

Your Child Goes to the Hospital
Ross Laboratories

When a Child Goes to the Hospital
Moore, Dept. of Child Study, Tufts University
Medford, Mass.

Going to the Hospital
Children's Hospital
Oakland, Calif.

It's Your Body
Pat Azarnoff Dept. of Pediatrics
UCLA Medical Center

The Hospital Book
Johns Hopkins Hospital
Baltimore, Md.

Johnny and Jay at the Hospital
Blue Devil Book Div.
Salisbury, N.C.

Going to the Hospital
Arnold, Children's Hospital
Akron, Ohio

Melissa Has Her Heart Fixed
Children's Hospital Medical Center
Oakland, Calif.

My Hospital Coloring Book
Children's Hospital Medical Center
Oakland, Calif.

Pop-up Going to the Hospital
Random House

Nicky Goes to the Doctor
Richard Scarry
A Golden Book

to puppetry is to involve children in role-playing with puppets. A degree of skill and sensitivity is necessary to orchestrate the various roles represented in a puppet show and to interpret and respond to the needs of children as expressed through their puppets.

The choice of teaching tools will, of course, depend on the audience. A child with specific disabilities may benefit from a more individual presentation. Flexibility of the staff and the institution's programs are key ingredients to meeting the needs of these special children. Additionally, information obtained about the child and family gathered at the preadmission program can be invaluable to the staff in providing effective personal management during the hospital stay.

A preadmission program usually includes a simple description of the actual facility, the people a child usually meets, and common procedures a child may experience. Actually viewing the hospital is helpful. Coming to the hospital for the preadmission program is in itself a tour and benefits a child. A more elaborate tour can include the places a child will see, such as the admission area, the laboratory where blood samples are obtained, the pediatric unit, part of the surgical floor including any anesthesia waiting area, and the recovery room. Tours may be conducted by nurses, child life workers, or public relations personnel. The preadmission program and tour are generally geared to enhancing familiarity with the experience and thus diminishing anxiety.

Young children who attend the orientation, whether in the hospital or through a school program, can be given a certificate of attendance. Allowing children to choose the color of the certificate they prefer, writing their names on the certificates, and/or placing stars on certificates because they were good listeners are all measures that acknowledge their individuality and provide immediate reward for their participation. The appropriateness of this depends on the age and developmental stage of the child. The preadmission program might be designed for teaching the child in either middle or late childhood. In this way, experiences such as the manipulation of hospital equipment are age appropriate, and words and explanations used are clear to the child. An adolescent, either alone or with other adolescents, also benefits from a preparation program and tour.

Hospital Admission

Allaying Fears On the day of admission, the members of the staff who oriented the child to the hospital (for example, nurse, play therapist) should, ideally, greet the child and family within a few minutes of arrival. This reassures the child and family that continuity of care is important to the staff and that they do have a support person in the hospital.

Not every child and family can prepare for hospitalization, and preparation may not, in fact, lessen fears, concerns, and fantasies. It would be a mistake to assume that a family who has been through preadmission preparation has no remaining concerns. Parents and children may not have benefited from preadmission preparation; furthermore, many children come to the hospital on an emergency basis. The nurse is making a mistake in assuming that a child who has had preadmission teaching and a tour has had all questions answered and misconceptions clarified.

Familiarity does not always remove fear. For example, the child (or adult, for that matter) who has experienced multiple hospital admissions and multiple surgical procedures may bring unresolved fears to the new hospital stay. A child who is returning to the hospital may be more afraid than the child hospitalized for the first time. The child therefore may know what to expect and may fear and anticipate specific situations. Depending on the child's age and development, these fears may express themselves as fear of separation; fear of doctors, nurses, or all people in white; fear of anesthesia; or fear of pain. For instance, a 10-year-old boy admitted for one of a series of many minor surgical procedures asked, after the admission interview had been completed, whether he could leave the floor to go to one of his favorite areas of the hospital. He was told that he would have to wait for the anesthesiologist to see him. He immediately said with obvious feeling, "Anesthesia . . . they put you to sleep . . . *really* to sleep." This statement from a poised, hospitalwise child could have been ignored, but instead it alerted the nursing staff to his unresolved fears and allowed the nurses to listen carefully and give the child a means to express himself. Because of this open communication, he was better prepared to face surgery the next day.

Orienting Child and Family to the Environment

Many hospital admissions are due to acute illness or injury. Preadmission preparation is possible only in the general sense of the child's receiving health instruction, health promotion, and information about hospitalization given by school or children's organizations. Specific preparation occurs as the child is admitted, after admission, and after the acute phase of illness or recovery from surgery. Therefore, because children and parents may still be worried or even uninformed despite preparation and because some cannot be prepared, all children and their families need assessment for learning and emotional needs (see Chapter 27). All families and children then need plans of care established to meet their needs.

Whether or not a child first comes to the hospital ward from the admissions department or from the operating room through the recovery room, each child and family needs an introduction to the pediatric unit because the hospital environment is, of course, new to the child and family. They have left their familiar surroundings, where they have possessions, routines, security, and control, for an environment where nurses and physicians control and determine the routines, where they do not own anything except what they bring with them from home, and where they often cannot use what they have brought from home because of the child's condition or because of hospital policy. For example, they will probably have to relinquish medicines brought from home, and children may have to wear hospital clothing to accommodate physical needs and care.

As soon as possible after admission, the family and child need to have a space of their own. The child's bed or crib space and bedside table often comprise the extent of the family and child's "territory" in the hospital. They need to be shown this space, however, and anything else that will be theirs during the child's hospital stay needs to be "given" to them. There may be a chair that can remain at the child's bedside, and sometimes there is a locker or closet for clothes or a private bathroom. The family should also see the equipment that will remain in the bedside stand for the child's use.

In addition to creating a personal physical environment for the child and family, the nurse protects the small environment that the child and family have brought with them. Toys, clothing, and other possessions from home may not need much special attention if a child has enough space for them and if the possessions will remain at the bedside. But if a favorite blanket or toy will accompany a child to tests or surgery or if clothing or blankets could end up in the hospital laundry, these will have to be protected from loss. Nurses need to understand that these objects are the child's link to home and family, and perhaps provide the child with a sense of security (see Chapter 27). A hospital bracelet identifying the child and carrying a hospital number or a label with such information usually saves a stuffed animal or toy from loss, but great care needs to be taken with a security blanket or article of clothing. If these are inadvertently placed in the hospital laundry, they are frequently not recovered. New, brightly colored garments or blankets might find their way back to a child in time, but security blankets are usually well used and "well loved." Although worth their weight in gold, they may look like old rags, especially if only one blanket or one corner of one blanket provides comfort. The staff thus takes great care to protect these precious and often irreplaceable items. Not only should such objects be labeled but their existence also should be noted in a child's records so that all staff will know about and care for these objects.

By showing a child and family the space on the pediatric ward that belongs to them and by caring for their possessions, a nurse is giving them a small degree of control over their lives during the hospital stay. Nurses are in this way giving them the privacy, respect, and territory that are essential for their security and growth. As much as possible, this space must be respected. Nurses need to knock before entering a room, announce their presence before opening a curtain around a bed, and try not to disturb a child's belongings on a bed or bedside stand. These courtesies are often forgotten in caring for a child, but they help create an atmosphere for respect and cooperation—an atmosphere in which children can begin to take on as much responsibility as possible for their health and well being.

During admission the nurse also assesses and listens and learns as well as teaches. A formal written assessment needs to be a part of each child's hospital record. This includes the chief complaint, a history of the current illness, a description of the child's coping mechanisms, and emotional and developmental needs. Care is then based on this assessment. The nurse also obtains a physical and developmental history and does an appropriate examination. The nurse records as much as is known about the family's needs and their plans for participation during their child's hospital stay. A sample admission guide is shown in Appendix F.

The next part of the admission process is often the introduction of the child and family to the entire unit. If a tour is not possible because of the child's condition, it is postponed until the family and child are ready. A tour of the unit should include all areas that the family or child will use and those areas that will otherwise be important to them. Where are the children's bathrooms? Where is the kitchen, and can family members help themselves to food? Where is the playroom, and what are its guidelines for operation? Where can family members get linen if the child or parent wishes to participate in some aspects of care? What parts of the unit are noisy and might startle or disturb the family? (For example, the child might be shown an ice machine and told that it makes a good deal of noise when it is used.) How do bathroom fixtures work? When are meals served, and where can parents eat, use the bathroom, and make telephone calls? How can the child or family call for a nurse? How can they arrange to ask questions of the physician?

Preoperative Preparation

Parents—and sometimes other family members—need to be included in the teaching session regarding their children's surgery. Children need not only the security of parental support but also the assurance that their parents share their concerns and understand and approve of the activity. A nonthreatening presentation of a potentially frightening event provides an opportunity for parents to understand both the event and their child's response. At a time when their normal roles are altered, it is imperative to reassure parents of their importance to their children and members of the health care team.

Because surgery is a very personal event in one's life, teaching is at least partially done on a one-to-one basis. Group teaching is supportive for hospital admissions and perhaps for some aspects of surgery, but the child and family need the attention and support that can be given only when the nurse can spend undivided time with them. It is essential that they feel comfortable enough to voice any questions or concerns at any time during teaching sessions.

For children in the early and middle childhood years, an explanation of preoperative preparation and the rationale for it can be depicted through manipulation of dolls or puppets. Drawings, diagrams, and anatomic illustrations plus discussion are appropriate for older children and adolescents. The orientation should be given in the sequence in which the child will experience events, beginning with scrubs and cleansing procedures, nothing to eat or drink after a certain time, the preoperative medication, the ride to surgery, and the preanesthesia room. Children need to know where their parents will be waiting for them during surgery. When talking about the operation, it is important to reassure them that they will be asleep and not feel anything but that as soon as the doctor is finished, they will wake up again. They may wake up in a different room called the recovery room and soon after that will return to their rooms, where their parents will meet them again. When a child is to receive an injection preoperatively, it may be wise to present this information last. Some children become so anxious when learning they will have a shot they do not attend to further teaching.

Other teaching tools can be added to provide additional information relative to the particular child's experience. Real-to-life dolls that are anatomically correct assist in demonstrations. Creating or purchasing dolls or stuffed animals that can be used to demonstrate changes in body image can be especially beneficial for children anticipating such types of surgery. For example, a cast can be correctly applied to a doll in the same manner that a child will acquire one. This activity helps the child to understand the event and the subsequent limitations in mobility. If the child is informed ahead of time about tubes and appliances that will be present following surgery, these are not as frightening upon awaking.

The presentation of the information is important, but the nurse is also able to assess the child's and parents' response to the situation so that the nurse can provide support and understanding to lessen the trauma for them. When the child can deal with the potentially threatening experience of surgery, as indicated by the response to the simulation with dolls or puppets, that mastery can then be transferred to the child's experience.

Rehearsing an event can also lessen anxiety. Therefore, the teaching session might be followed with a tour of the surgical facilities. Encouraging children to operate the elevator controls on the way to surgery and allowing children to open the door to surgery and to meet some of the personnel who will be providing care (who will often give a child surgical hats, gloves, etc.) reassure children of their importance and the concern that the hospital staff shares for their ultimate recovery.

Postoperative Teaching and Play

Equally significant for the child's recovery and mental health is the opportunity to complete the experience with directed postoperative play. Children who are normally very active find the various constraints placed on them because of the surgery and recovery process difficult. For many, their coping behavior was some form of physical activity that is now denied. One therapeutic alternative is art in all its various forms. It may be necessary to protect such things as a cast or surgical dressing with a plastic cloth, but the child should then be allowed full expression of feelings with paints, clay (Play-Doh®), or crayons. Other forms of expressive and aggressive play can be used as well (see Chapter 28). Art may often be the only means of communication for the child concerned with the surgical experience. The child may discuss the picture drawn or figure created, but if that is too difficult, much can be conveyed nonverbally through using the materials that lend clues to the child's impressions and ability to handle this recent experience.

Even though the child is well prepared for surgery and the postoperative phase, the reality of the experience is often quite different from what was expected. Actually coping with the strange sights, smells, and noises, the pain and limitations, and alterations in body integrity is much more difficult than thinking about having these problems occur in the future. The younger the child, the fewer the coping strategies and the less able the child is to conceptualize the changes and what they will mean. Fantasies and fears increase, and the child's reality becomes increasingly distorted. Younger children become convinced that this experience can only be justified as retribution for some wrong they committed. As a result, they may become passive and compliant or angry and anxious.

It is essential that the nurse be sensitive to the behavioral changes of children following surgery and various procedures. (Therapeutic play is discussed in Chapter 28.) Behavior such as increased irritability, crying, regression, temper tantrums, nail biting, bed wetting, nightmares, passivity, withdrawal, and dependence are the child's way of asking for assistance to cope with the demands and traumas of hospitalization.

Parents need to be included in discussions about the child's behavior and possible reasons for the changes in response to surgery. The parent who understands why the child is expressing fears and concerns in certain behaviors and understands that the child's perception of these events is governed by developmental stage is able to be more supportive and can help the child cope. The nurse can offer suggestions on ways to incorporate play into daily activity that will give the child an opportunity to express the fears, concerns, feelings, and fantasies that were and often continue to be overwhelming. Nurses may initially need to serve as role models for the parents in using games, puppets, art, or other forms of expressive play to facilitate communication.

Children who are helped to cope with events after they happen and are prepared for them beforehand are less anxious and better able to mobilize their energies toward recovery. Postprocedural play and teaching sessions as well as preprocedural teaching should be a part of the child's hospital experience. Teaching sessions help to maximize growth by reducing stress and encouraging mastery of the experience.

Discharge Preparation

Preparation for returning home begins when the child is admitted. The initial assessment provides information about the family such as composition and roles, strengths, previous experiences with illness or hospitalization, understanding of the rationale for treatment, and fears and beliefs about health and illness. Using this as a guide, the nurse begins to plan the teaching and learning activities needed and begins to assess those who will need to be involved both as teachers and as learners.

Some of the teaching may be accomplished by discussing a treatment or procedure and its rationale with the family while giving care. For example, when changing a dressing that will need to be changed again after discharge, the nurse's talking about what is done and why it's done begins to involve everyone in this aspect of routine care. By including the family from the beginning, learning takes place gradually and at a pace more accommodating to the needs of the learner. This also creates an atmosphere conducive to asking questions. The family members feel more comfortable about mentioning their concerns or asking about some aspect of care. They have the opportunity to observe and to think through their management of care when the child returns home. The transition from hospital to home will be much smoother for all concerned if there is this time to anticipate the changes that will have to occur in daily routines.

Teaching Plan In addition to this informal teaching, the nurse needs a structured plan. Information needed by the family regarding the child's care should be identified, and someone, ideally the nurse responsible for planning care, organizes and coordinates the teaching. This teaching plan is adapted to the family and made specific to the family's situation and learning needs.

Included in the teaching plan are all of the physical, psychosocial, and developmental aspects of care the child requires. Beginning with observation, written information, and discussion of any procedure and then advancing through a step-by-step presentation and return demonstration, the family begins to assume responsibility for various aspects of care. When one procedure is well learned, another can be introduced. In this way, the family assumes more and more of the care for the child until family members feel confident and well prepared to continue at home. If family members have had previous experience with necessary procedures, they should be encouraged to continue doing them during hospitalization. The nurse assesses their performance, compliments them, and, if necessary, adds suggestions or corrections.

Physical Aspects of Discharge Preparation Physical aspects of discharge preparation might include dressing changes, cast care, and assessment of complications or recurrence of illness. Provision for changes in the activities of daily living is another aspect of physical care that has implications for teaching. Some children have an increased need for assistance in doing things formerly self-managed such as bathing, hair care, dental hygiene, and dressing. Safety factors and any adaptations according to activity restriction need to be taught. Sometimes the child's room needs to be changed if negotiating stairs or reaching a bathroom is a problem; at other times rearranging furniture and redirecting traffic flow are needed. The nurse guides the family in thinking through these details and thereby facilitates the transition from hospital to home and lessens potential frustrations, surprises, and aggravations. Some families need the help of outside resources to meet the child's physical needs. The nurse carefully assesses requirements and plans for referrals where outside help is needed after discharge.

The nurse also reminds the family to include the child in family activities once the child has returned home. Family members should eat together, if this is their pattern, and should spend some time socializing, whether it be playing a game or talking. If the child is unable to join family members where the family usually eats, the nurse might suggest that the family or a family member eat with the child wherever this is possible. If a child has dietary restrictions, all members of many families may wish to adopt, at least temporarily, the new diet. Discussing the child's nutritional needs and providing for them in a way compatible with the family life-style and individual food preferences is a nursing responsibility that should be first addressed as soon as these needs are known. It is, of course, very difficult for the family to insist on good nutrition at home if a child has been allowed to eat "junk" foods at the hospital.

Psychosocial Aspects of Discharge Preparation Providing for the child's needs presents a challenge if activity is restricted for a period of time. Sometimes special arrangements need to be made with the school for a home teacher. Some children need additional tutoring before reentering the classroom, and some are able to reenter without difficulty.

Immobilized children become bored easily, and planning activities and diversions for them at home demands forethought and creativity. Children who feel well but must refrain from usual activities present a special challenge.

Arranging for release of energy in constructive ways that include a child's hobbies and pastimes is essential for emotional health. Nurses need to discuss these facts with the family, to provide ideas compatible with the child's interest that can be managed by the family, and to give the family information about resources in the community such as transportation aids, bookmobile availability, or children's programs.

Arranging for peer group contact and activities is another area for which plans should be made before discharge. The family needs answers to questions about a child's restrictions and the feasibility of having friends and relatives visit. How many at a time, what time of day or evening, for how long are among the questions that should be discussed with the family and answered before discharge. In warm weather, it may be possible to have the child spend time outdoors, which facilitates peer group involvement. If restriction is minimal, the child may be able to join the activities of peers. Safety becomes a primary concern in determining what may or may not be an appropriate activity.

Developmental Aspects of Discharge Preparation After discharge, children often show reactions to their hospital stays (see Chapter 27). With pain, with such frightening experiences as invasive procedures and surgery, and with separation and possible misinterpretation of intentions and actions of staff and parents, children experience aftereffects of hospitalization. These reactions can be annoying, frightening, or confusing to parents. Children's reactions then need to be handled in a manner conducive to their growth.

Parents should understand that the infant's patterns of feeding, napping, and waking are often disrupted by hospital routines. The child who previously slept through the night is likely to awaken for a time following hospitalization. Stranger anxiety may be more pronounced, and separation fears can increase. A child may seem overly dependent and constantly seeking the reassurance of parental presence. Leaving the child with a sitter may meet with tremendous protest. Children may regress in toilet training or weaning from bottle to cup, behaviors that are upsetting to parents. A child's behavior tends to be either more negative and disruptive or quiet and withdrawn.

The child who interpreted hospitalization as punishment may feel wronged or afraid of again being "bad" and thus repunished. Children feeling wronged by their hospitalization tend to punish parents for causing or allowing the seemingly unjustified hardships of hospitalization. They may be aloof and hesitant to allow parental closeness and affection. They may seem angry and may talk back to parents. Parents need to understand these reactions so that they remain loving and available to the child. They can teach by their actions and words that hospitalization was not a punishment. They can try to reteach the reasons for the child's hospitalization. Such reassurances also help the children who thought they were "bad." When minor transgressions seem to evoke excessive fear of punishment, or when children are uncharacteristically weepy, hearing and understanding the real reasons for hospitalization will often have dramatic effects.

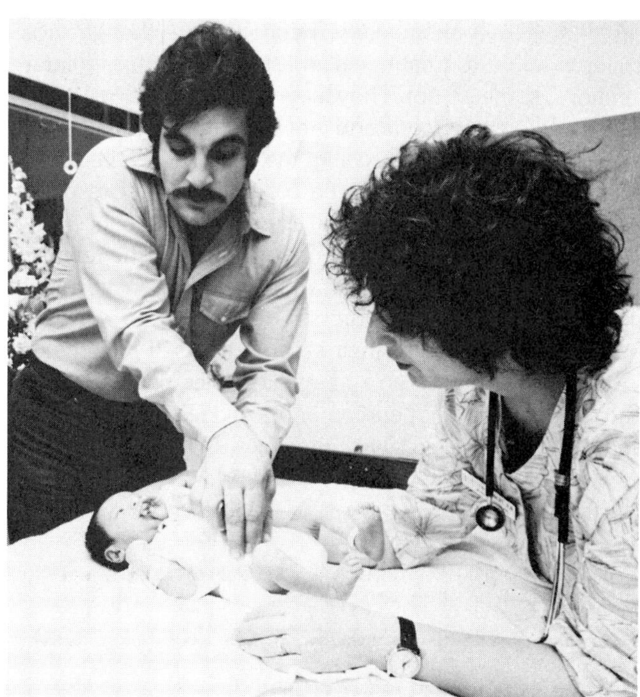

In supervising a return demonstration, the nurse teaches the primary caregiver to assume responsibility for the child.

Similar reactions occur with siblings of hospitalized children. Particularly vulnerable are children in early or middle childhood whose younger siblings have been hospitalized. These children often believe that thoughts cause events. They may have had less-than-loving thoughts about sharing their parents and home with the new baby, or they may have wished out of the way the younger sibling who disrupts their play and life. If this younger child then suffers illness or injury, older siblings may feel responsible and guilty. One 4-year-old girl whose infant brother was being assessed for vague signs, including poor growth, became agitated and disruptive. The girl's mother reported that she told her daughter clearly and directly, but only once, that the baby's illness was not her fault. The child was immediately more relaxed, and her negative behavior ceased.

The better prepared parents are for the reactions of children after hospitalization, the better they can deal with the situation. The family can avoid unnecessary tension and can help the child use hospitalization as an experience that leads to growth and development.

The family who knows the care plan and has anticipated and planned for possible events is well prepared for the child's discharge. The more confident the family is in knowledge and ability to provide for the child's needs, the fewer problems family members will encounter. Although most children adjust to treatments and supportive nursing interventions, some do not. They may require the help of counseling or therapy to cope and grow through the experience. In addition to careful teaching, the nurse gives the family several resources that may be contacted if a question or problem arises. Resources may also be needed concerning the purchases of any supplies or appliances or the rental of equipment. Providing families with written instructions and diagrams and telephone numbers of resources to use when questions arise adds to their security and self-confidence. Including the child, when appropriate, in the plans for home care also aids in cooperation and provides a healthy perspective about recovery.

Physiologic Needs of Hospitalized Children

Safety—Potential Alterations

General Guidelines Although safety is always important for adults who are responsible for children, the hospital presents special considerations. Whenever children are hospitalized, they are, by definition, removed from their familiar, usually comforting environment and are exposed to stress. These two factors alone make the child susceptible to accidents. The hospital environment also adds several obvious hazards for the child. Beds are usually higher than they are at home. A young child able to climb out of the crib at home may have had the crib side rails left down so that climbing out is relatively safer or may have graduated to a bed. In the hospital this child may have to be placed in a crib with the side rails up to prevent roaming within or even out of the hospital. The child may be frustrated by the unaccustomed restraint to mobility and may try to climb over the raised side rails. A resulting fall onto the hard hospital floor could cause considerable injury. Children whose axillae come above the top of the side rail can pull up and tip themselves over the side of the crib. These children need to be protected from falls.

Infants learn to roll over suddenly, although within a predictable time period. Even when a parent seems certain that the infant is safe with the crib side left down, the nurse acts on the premise that the child could choose that moment to roll over for the first time. Even very young infants move about in their cribs. The nurse therefore protects the child by raising the crib rail to a stable position high enough to prevent the child from falling. The most careful of parents have had their children roll off a surface when the parent either thought the child could not yet roll over or assumed that the child was too far from the edge to fall. For example, two parents were standing so as to block the open side of their child's crib and turned to talk to the nurses wheeling another crib into their child's hospital room. The child chose that moment to roll, rolled off the crib right between the parents, and landed head first on the floor. The child was immediately seen by a physician, had radiographs taken, and was carefully observed by the nursing staff. She was unharmed, but other children have not been as lucky.

Beds on pediatric wards are often high off the floor to facilitate nursing care and are frequently nonadjustable, preventing children playing with their beds and incurring injury. A child either has a very big step when getting out of bed or has the use of a stool or chair as an aid. Either of these options is a new experience for the child. A child may forget when getting out of bed unassisted that it is necessary to take a large step or to step in the middle of the chair or stool. In either case, many children are prone to accidents at points in their hospital stays unless they accept help in an activity that is totally independent for them at home. They need to be carefully taught to keep themselves safe in the hospital. They also need to be assured of their independence in other areas and need to feel that the assistance is temporary.

Medications and equipment present special hazards in the hospital. Anything left on or in a bedside stand should be considered within reach of a child. Medications or small objects left in a bedside stand can be taken out and left within reach of a child by other staff members, parents, other children, or the child. In one instance, a hospitalized 4-year-old was given a dime, and the dime was put away safely in the bedside stand. The next time the dime was seen, it was wedged between two of the child's back teeth. Luckily, the dime was not lodged in the child's throat, and with considerable effort it was safely removed. In another instance, a semicomatose adolescent had a box of chocolates on his bedside stand. The stand was several feet from his bed and seemingly out of reach, the bed rails were raised, and the boy couldn't walk. A night nurse found him with the box, loose chocolates, and wrappers on his bed. A 20-month-old child was having wound care with povidone–iodine (Betadine). A bottle of the solution was inadvertently left on her bedside stand, and, again, the stand seemed to be well out of reach of the child. The child was in a crib with the side rails up, but a nurse found her happily squirting the solution on the walls of her room.

The reach of children is much longer than it seems to be, and nurses cannot assume that something is safely out of reach merely because the child appears to be a safe distance away. Whenever introducing a child to an area and especially when leaving a child unattended, the nurse thoroughly checks the hospital environment for all the elements of safety. The same principles apply whether the child is in bed for a nap or in bed for the night.

When a child is out of bed, the nurse needs to be aware of all safety hazards in the general environment. Making a pediatric unit "child-proof" is difficult enough, but many children are hospitalized in locations with no specific unit for children. A few additional questions are then in order. Are all external and cleansing solutions out of reach? Are medications, syringes, and needles either locked away or constantly supervised? Are electrical outlets covered when not in use? Anything that must be left plugged in should ideally be locked in so that little fingers cannot unplug equipment. Are laundry chutes supervised or locked? Are treatment rooms accessible? Can the child open doors, such as bathroom doors, when necessary?

Children with IVs pose special problems. With the fear and fascination that IVs hold for children, and with their precarious positioning, IVs are prone to failure and require further safety considerations. Both infants and older children have been found changing the flow rates of their IVs. In one case, as an evening nurse was giving a report on one of her charges, stating that he was sleeping and that his IV was infusing well, he was then seen running down the hall of the unit without his IV. Older children, after they have become accustomed to their IVs, sometimes try to use their portable IV poles as skate boards in the hospital corridors.

To prevent a child's reregulating an IV, the clamp can be slid up on the tubing so that it is far away from the child but still within reach of the nurse. Infusion pumps should be placed out of the child's reach. An IV must be secured against direct interference by the child so that it has as little positional variation in flow rate as possible. The amount of taping and restraint needed to protect a child's IV will vary with the site of the IV, the age and development of the child, and the child's ability to understand and cooperate with the treatment. An explanation of the need for and care of the IV and the nurse's help as the child learns to be mobile with an IV are enough for many children from age 4 and older. A younger child and the child who cannot cooperate may need to be restrained when not under one-to-one supervision.

One important safety measure is the prevention of sparks and resulting fire when oxygen equipment is in use. A pediatric unit usually has a rule prohibiting smoking in the rooms. When a child is admitted to an adult division, where smoking is usually permitted, the usual practice is to place a sign on the door of the room advising people not to smoke. This and reminders are all the deterrence most people need to keep matches or lit cigarettes away from the equipment. Children's toys, however, can also give off sparks. Any toy with a movement or mechanism that works by way of friction can produce a spark. These should be removed from the bedside and from the hospital to prevent children using them and endangering themselves and others. The child's own radio or stereo may need to be checked by hospital maintenance before use to be sure it is compatible with the hospital electrical system.

Restraints Many different kinds of restraints are used to help ensure the maintenance of necessary therapy and the safety of children. Although restraints interfere with a child's freedom, mobility, and independence, they are sometimes necessary. Most nurses and parents intensely dislike restraining a child, and young children often find the loss of control stressful (see Chapter 27). As long as the child's safety can be maintained without restraint, this is preferable by far. If a child leaves an IV or nasogastric tube alone as long as a parent or nurse is by the crib or bed or if a child will not try to climb out of bed when someone is nearby, then the child can play and rest unrestrained for part or all of the hospital stay. Unfortunately, there are times when a child is in danger if mobility is unrestricted. In these instances, some kind of restraint is needed. Table 29-7 summarizes the characteristics of various restraints.

Mummy Restraint Neonates and very young infants derive security and comfort from being swaddled. This need can be used to the child's advantage for comfort and positioning and also for the safety of a nasogastric tube or an IV in a scalp vein. The method is called the *mummy restraint.* A child is placed on a small sheet or, more commonly, a receiving blanket. With a small blanket, the child is placed with the head on one folded-down corner. One side of the blanket is tucked around one shoulder and arm and then around the child's opposite side and behind the child's back. Then, the lower corner of the receiving blanket is tucked over the feet. The nurse allows enough room for full extension of the child's legs and a bit of kicking room by folding the blanket the width of the nurse's hand beyond the point to which the legs extend. With the remaining corner of the blanket, the other shoulder and arm are secured. With a larger blanket or sheet, the arms and shoulders can be secured first and then the lower end of the restraint can be folded up and around both sides and to the back of the child (Fig. 29-1).

When an IV is in a scalp vein, the child will frequently need to be positioned carefully so that head movements on the sheet will not dislodge the IV. A small receiving blanket can be rolled and placed against the child's back to keep a child on one side. Blanket rolls along each side can keep a child lying on the back. Sand bags are also very effective in supporting the infant. A child who is a few weeks or months of age, however, often becomes impatient and uncomfortable with the mummy restraint. Kicking and wriggling will loosen it, and the nurse must find another method.

Bubble-Top or Net-Top Crib To protect a child from falling out of a crib, many hospitals have clear-plastic bubble tops that can be secured to the top of each end of the crib. When the crib rails are raised securely, the child cannot fall from the crib, as the crib is totally enclosed. The child may have unrestricted mobility within the crib and has full visibility. The top of the crib may also be made secure with a net top. The net is spread over the top and secured around

TABLE 29-7 Principles for Using Restraints for Children

Restraint	Use	Principles	Rationale
Mummy	Infants For comfort, scalp vein IV, NG tube	Arms in anatomic position as blanket/ sheet is wrapped around each shoulder and arm, lower portion allows for leg extension, position on side allows for oral drainage	Prevents undue discomfort and strain on arms and joints Maximizes mobility within the restraint while still providing comfort of close wrapping Secretions or vomitus could be aspirated if child's position prevents drainage
Clove hitch	Child of any age For restraining one or more extremities; for IVs, NG tubes, and other tubes; for prevention of self-injury	Extremity must be padded under each restraint Knot used must be a clove hitch Nurse checks to see whether the knot will tighten with a child's resistance or pulling Restraint attached to frame of crib or bed with a slip knot Limb distal to the restraint checked every 15 minutes Restraint released frequently—all at once or one extremity at a time	Restraint could irritate skin without padding Knot will not tighten as the child pulls against the restraint (other knots could tighten and reduce circulation) Nurse needs to be certain the knot is correct In emergency, nurse must be able to release the restraint quickly with one hand No pressure applied when side rail is lowered
Jacket	Child of any age Keeps child in crib or bed Can be used to prevent sitting or standing	Must fit child well. Ties in back Attached to bed frame with a slip knot Child must be checked every 15 minutes or be continually observed Restraint released as much as possible	Child can slip out of a poorly fitting restraint Airway can be totally occluded if a child wriggles to get out of tight but poorly fitting restraint
Elbow	Child of any age Prevents flexion of elbows and thus the touching of face, scalp, IV, other tubes, cleft lip or palate repair, skin conditions of face and upper trunk	Sleeves must fit well Restraint must be secured with pins or straps Color, sensation, and motion of fingers must be checked frequently Restraints must be removed frequently for range of motion	This prevents flexion of elbow Keeps restraint in place Nerve damage is possible from pressure of restraint on the brachial area
Bubble top and net-top crib	Older infant and young child Prevents falling and climbing out of crib	Bubble secured to ends of crib with clamps Net tight and secured to frame and legs of crib Side rails all the way up and secure	Firm attachment to frame of the crib allows child mobility and play without danger of dislodging the crib top With crib rails up and crib top tightly in place, child cannot climb out under the restraint
Bed cradle	Older infant and older child Protects lower part of the body from pressure of bedding and from child's hands	Cradle padded with a sheet or bath blanket secured with pins Hospital gown may be spread over the cradle and pinned to cover	Protects child from metal of bed cradle and provides some privacy Keeps gown off the child's body, provides privacy Pinning gown may be enough to keep child's hands from touching surgical site or from scratching irritated skin

TABLE 29-7 continued

Restraint	Use	Principles	Rationale
Safety straps	Child of any age Prevents child's falling from a cart, chair, or frame	Folded sheet or strap firmly secured Large hospital gown may be used over clothes Ends of straps tied in back of a chair (high chair or stroller) Child checked very frequently	Child may climb or fall from go-carts, guerneys, high chairs, infant seats, feeding tables, orthopedic frames Child may slip within the restraint, endangering airway or circulation Child may fall

the frame and legs of the crib. If this net is tight, the child cannot either fall or climb over the top of the side rails. The net does not give the child as much standing room as does the bubble top and may seem more confining to the child (Fig. 29-2).

Jacket Restraint Another means of preventing a child from falling or climbing over the crib or bed rails is the *jacket restraint.* Jackets come in various sizes, go around the torso, and tie in the back. Long, thick straps extend from the restraint and tie to the frame of the crib or bed in such a way that the side rails may be raised or lowered without interfering with the restraint. This restraint must fit the child closely so that the child cannot slip down into the restraint and obstruct the airway. This is usually a restraint of last resort. The child should preferably be under continual observation or, at the very least, checked frequently to assess for airway compromise, as children have suffered airway obstruction and severe anoxia from the use of this restraint. At best, the jacket restraint is very confining to the child, as it allows very little mobility.

Clove Hitch It is sometimes necessary to restrain one or more limbs to protect children from touching equipment or an area of the body undergoing treatment. Restraining each limb as necessary must be done with a well-padded knotted tie that does not become tighter as the child pulls against it. Stockinette or cotton tape of the kind used to make tracheostomy ties can be used. It should be padded with stockinette, cotton webril, or a bulky bandage such as Kerlex so that the tape does not cut into the skin. The knot used is the clove hitch (Fig. 29-3). Some facilities have specially manufactured extremity restraints. Whenever an extremity is restrained, the color, sensation, and motion of the body part distal to restraint must be checked frequently. The restraint should be released to allow for passive or active range of motion at least every 2 hours.

Whenever a restraint ties to the bed, two criteria must be met. First, the restraint must be tied to the bed so that the nurse may release the restraint with one hand in case of an emergency such as a fire or the child's poor condition. A

Figure 29-1 Mummy restraint.

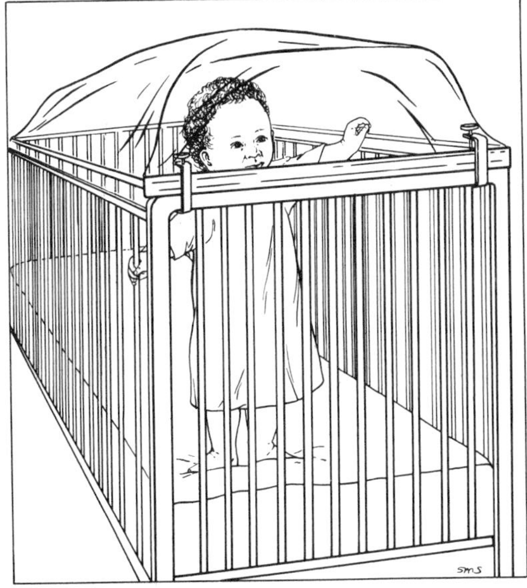

Figure 29-2 Bubble-top crib.

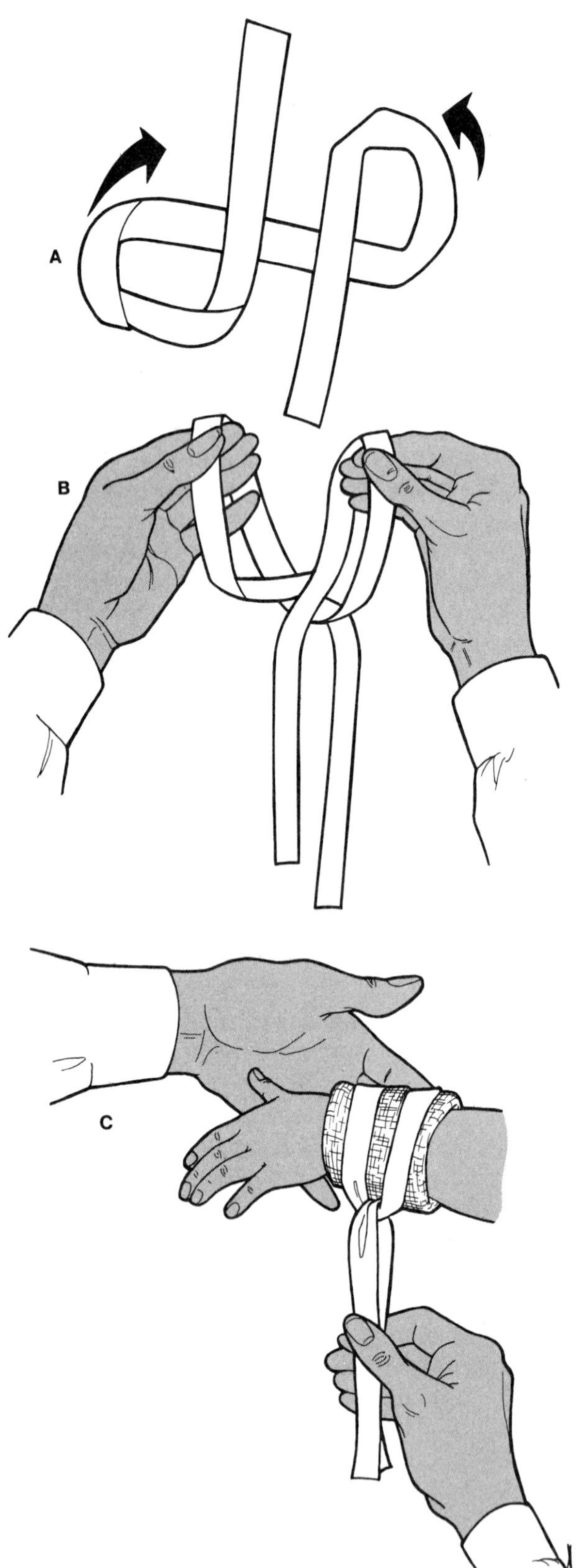

Figure 29-3 Clove hitch restraint. *A*. Make a figure-eight. *B*. Pick up the loops. *C*. Put the limb through the loops and secure it. (From Kozier B, Erb G: *Fundamentals of Nursing*. 2nd ed. Addison-Wesley, 1983.)

restraint attached to the bed frame with a slip knot or a bow can be released instantly with one hand. Second, the restraint must be tied to the frame of the bed or crib, and not to the side rail. The side rail must be free to move completely up or down without pulling or putting any pressure on the restraint and consequently on the child.

Elbow Restraint *Elbow restraints*, also called "welcome sleeves," prevent the child from bending the elbow yet leave the child with mobility of the arms and hands. These are used whenever it is imperative that a child not touch the face or neck area. These restraints are useful when the child has undergone cleft lip or cleft palate surgery, when nasogastric tubes or scalp vein IVs are in place, and sometimes when a child must refrain from scratching. A tubular sleeve in a size that will fit the child has wooden slats or tongue blades inserted into pockets in the sleeve. These make the sleeve unbendable. The proximal end of the restraint is either pinned to the child's clothing or has a string or ties that fasten under the opposite axilla (Fig. 29-4).

These restraints must be removed for skin care and range of motion, either one at a time or together, with care that the child remain safe, every few hours. The color, sensation, and motion distal to the restraint should be checked very frequently. The restraint must fit the child well so that the tongue blades or wooden slats do not jab the child. Because restraints might be tight under the child's axillae, they must be checked carefully and removed often to prevent any damage to skin or nerves.

Bed Cradle A *bed cradle* is used to ease the pressure of the top sheet on the child and/or to prevent a child from touching the lower part of the body. The cradle is covered with a sheet or bath blanket as padding. If it is necessary, as in some forms of genitourinary surgery, to remind children not to touch themselves under the bed cradle, the hospital gown can be pinned to the covering of the bed cradle.

Safety Straps When a child is in a wheelchair, a high chair, an infant seat or go-cart, or is at a feeding table, the child must be prevented from falling out by the use of a safety strap. A sheet can be used as a strap, as can a large hospital gown reaching under the tray or arms of the chair and being tied in back of the chair.

Nutrition—Potential for Unmet Needs

General Considerations Many factors make eating and mealtimes difficult for hospitalized children. The first is the lack of routine and familiarity, which are critical to the young child's comfort. The food may also be quite different from food at home, either because of cultural variations or because preparation and selection differ. Children hospitalized for illness and surgery often do not feel well enough to eat or drink what they need. They are frequently upset by hospital procedures and tests, and their feelings interfere with appetite and eating. Children who are ill or hospitalized lose control of much of their environment and lives. A child may need to control food intake as a means of feeling more whole and healthy even when desire and refusal interfere with physical well-being.

For these reasons, nursing care for the nutritional well-being of the hospitalized child is many directional and multifaceted. Meeting the needs of the whole child and family in areas seemingly unrelated to food can help to ensure optimal food and fluid intake during a child's hospital stay.

The nurse first needs to obtain a thorough history of a child's and family's eating habits and preferences. In this way, nurses can better duplicate, whenever possible, a child's familiar and comfortable routine (see Chapter 15). Mealtime itself provides an opportunity for assessment. The nurse can observe the child's eating habits, the foods the parent encourages, and the degree to which a parent allows a child developmentally appropriate independence. A child may regress when ill and in the hospital, but may, on the other hand, be ready and anxious to help with self-feeding. A parent sometimes does not recognize or allow this development. The family's culture may allow or even encourage dependence of the ill child on others, and the nurse therefore talks with the parent to understand more fully the child and family and thus the reasons for feeding methods. If families need and are ready to learn about children's capabilities, nurses can demonstrate these and encourage the parents to allow the children to develop further.

Nurses strive for optimal nutrition of the hospitalized child both for health and healing and as a way of teaching sound nutritional practices to children and their families (see Chapter 15). Hospitalization can be a time to demonstrate principles of good nutrition and meal planning. Many times, however, diets of hospitalized children must be altered to ensure that food and fluids are easily assimilated or to encourage an increased fluid intake. A child may be on a diet to meet short-term goals that would be unacceptable for growth and nutrition in the long run. A diet rich in juices, carbonated beverages, Popsicles, gelatin desserts, and ice cream may be easy for a child to accept and digest. It may also serve as a stepping stone from going without food and fluids to ingesting a regular diet, and it may be used to increase fluid intake in a child who needs a large-volume fluid intake. The reasons for the "unbalanced" diet must be explained to the child and family lest they learn a negative lesson about the proper diet for a child.

The Child Who Has Nothing by Mouth Mealtimes in the hospital are particularly significant and uncomfortable for one group of children, those who cannot eat. Some children have nothing by mouth (NPO) for a short period of time, as when they are awaiting surgery. Other children remain NPO for days or months while they are in the hospital. Watching, hearing, and smelling the preparation of food and the pleasant aspects of mealtime can be extremely painful for these children.

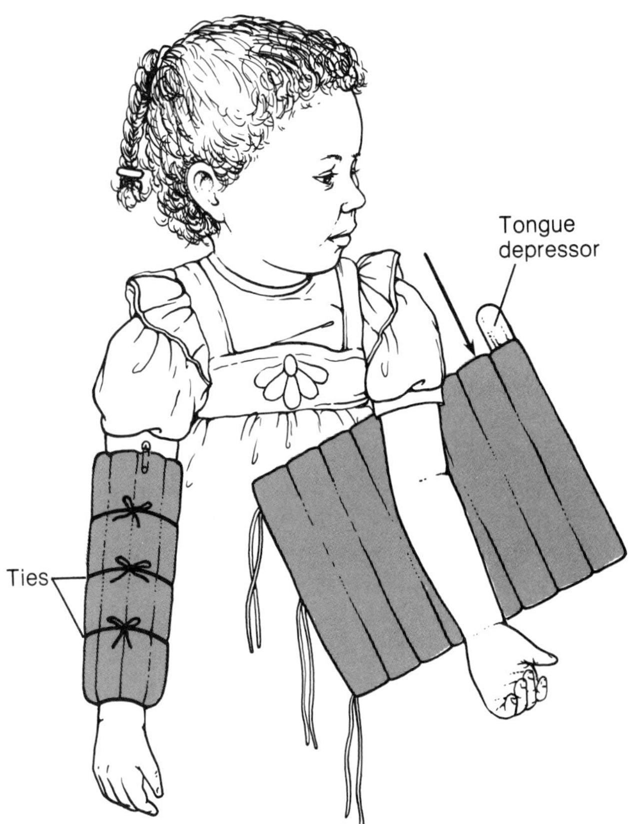

Figure 29-4 Elbow restraint.

The child missing a meal because of impending surgery may be at least as upset as a child remaining NPO for an extended period of time. Many children have IVs started after anesthesia is induced, and so thirst- and hunger-relieving fluid is withheld prior to surgery. A child on the pediatric unit waiting for surgery until 2 or 3 o'clock in the afternoon has truly suffered while surrounded by children, parents, and even staff eating and discussing food. Many worries about impending surgery can become displaced on food. Although it may occasionally be helpful to distract children's attention from their upcoming surgery, it is usually preferable to deal directly with worries about surgery and distract attention from the discomforts of going without food.

Whether or not a child remains NPO for a morning or for months, the nurse assesses the effect of going without food on a child's physical and mental well-being. Children who are NPO need good mouth care. Some children can be trusted to brush their teeth and rinse their mouths without swallowing water. Others will need to have their mouths swabbed by the nurse with a damp washcloth or a prepackaged swab to ensure their not drinking any fluid.

Many children are upset when watching others eat. Some can be taken from their hospital rooms or even from their floors during mealtime. A nurse can wheel a bed to a playroom and engage a child in an art project or game or take a child for a walk in the hospital. For children who telephone out of the hospital to speak with family or friends, suggesting that they place a call during mealtime can help ease their discomfort.

For the infant who must remain NPO, a major pleasure source and coping mechanism is thwarted. These children can be helped by being held and stimulated at regular intervals no fewer than if they were being fed. The child should be allowed to suck on a pacifier unless there are medical contraindications to a pacifier. If a commercial pacifier is not available, one can be fashioned from a nipple stuffed with cotton or gauze and closed securely at the back with tape. Care must be taken to burp the NPO infant at intervals to allow the escape of any air sucked in from around the pacifier.

Feeding of Infants in the Hospital The hospitalized infant's diet and feeding regimen are usually very similar to those at home. Formula and solid foods, if any have been introduced, will remain the same unless changes are indicated for therapeutic purposes, as when a child is recovering from anesthesia, has a gastrointestinal problem, or is not tolerating formula. If a child has been growing well and has remained healthy on the home diet, hospitalization is not the time to make a change. A careful history shows what foods a child has been given and generally how the child has tolerated these foods. Because new foods should be introduced slowly and carefully during infancy so that parents can recognize allergies and ease the infant's adjustment to the change in taste or texture, no new foods should be introduced for taste or convenience when an infant is hospitalized. The nipple and bottle used should be the same type as that used at home. This enhances feelings of familiarity for the child, encourages fluid intake, and also reinforces a parent's choices for the child. A feeding period should not extend beyond 30 minutes, as after 30 minutes the child fatigues and fluid intake is minimal; and the time that the feeding ends should not approach too closely the beginning of the next feeding.

Encouraging the hospitalized infant's growth and development during feedings should mirror what would be done at home (see Chapter 15). An infant is much more likely to be successful in holding a plastic bottle than a glass bottle. Formula can therefore be transferred from a glass bottle to a disposable or sterilizable plastic bottle. When children can have some solid food, they may gain much pleasure in holding a biscuit or cracker during the feeding. They should never be left alone with the biscuit or cracker, however, because of the danger of choking. Older infants can sometimes use a spoon if they have considerable help.

After a feeding, an infant may, unless contraindicated by the condition, be bundled and placed on the right side to facilitate the rising of any air in the stomach; the chance of having food above the air is therefore minimized. Infants may also be placed in infant seats or chalasia chairs. The chair is helpful to the child who remains awake after feedings and can benefit from stimuli in the environment. It is also helpful and indicated for the child who regurgitates or vomits after a feeding. A child may at times be placed on the stomach after feedings; but to prevent aspiration in case of vomiting, a child should not be left on the back.

The Breast-Fed Infant Hospitalization can threaten the continuation of breast-feeding. Feedings may be missed, routines interrupted, and stress and fatigue may result in the mother's inconsistent eating and drinking. If a mother is planning to continue breast-feeding, the nurse can play a major role in its success. First, a mother needs to recognize and express her true feelings about breast-feeding. A nurse can sit with and listen to the mother as she talks about what the child's illness and hospitalization mean to her, what breast-feeding has meant to her, and what her plans for breast-feeding were before the child became ill. The mother may wish to stop breast-feeding, and in most instances this will not adversely affect the child. Sometimes, however, a child needs to continue with breast-feeding if at all possible because of difficulty tolerating various formulas or the need for security of minimal changes in routine. Often, mothers wish to continue breast-feeding but may think this is difficult or impossible. A mother may need special provisions for privacy, ranging from assurance that she can nurse behind a curtain without being interrupted to the privacy of a special room in which to nurse. Although privacy is a rare commodity in the hospital, a suitable arrangement can usually be found.

Hospitalization of an infant, because it frequently shakes parental confidence and often leads to parental guilt (see Chapter 27), may undermine the assurance and ease crucial to successful breast-feeding. Helping the mother regain confidence facilitates breast-feeding. A nurse can assist the parent to resume care of the child. Showing parents how to pick up children who have scalp vein IVs, helping a parent hold a child with a burn, teaching about the reasons for and method of packing a wound, and pointing out the child's attachment to and recognition of the parent can all help with the continuation of breast-feeding.

The mechanics of breast-feeding are, however, difficult to maintain when a child is ill. A mother needs to drink, eat, and be rested, and the child needs to suck enough to maintain a somewhat-steady demand for milk production. These criteria are rarely met when a child is hospitalized. The nurse can help a mother recognize whether or not she is tired, hungry, or thirsty. The nurse can offer to keep a child close by or look in on a child more frequently so that the mother can take a break for the rest, food, and fluids she needs. It is helpful to ask a mother whether or not she has eaten, how much she is drinking, and whether she is rested. The mother may talk about any concerns with lowered milk production and, often for the first time, really may make the connection between her health practices and production of milk. This realization tends dramatically to decrease worry and concern over her ability to produce enough milk for her baby.

When a child cannot suck to ensure continued milk production, the nurse can teach and/or provide the equipment for the mother to pump her breasts. Most women find an electric breast pump easier to use than a nonelectric model. One or more electric pumps may be in the hospital, especially if the hospital has a neonatal intensive care unit or a maternity division. The nurse can tell nursing mothers where these pumps are located and when the mother may use them. For mothers who are unable to be at the hospital for every feeding but who wish their children to receive breast milk, an electric pump can be rented. Milk is pumped at home, frozen, and kept in the hospital for feedings when the mother is unable to be there. With lowered anxiety and such aids for expressing milk, most mothers who wish to continue breast-feeding their children can do so.

Women who choose to stop breast-feeding should do so gradually whenever possible, phasing out one feeding for a few days or longer before stopping other feedings. Thus breast engorgement is kept to a minimum, and both mother and child have an opportunity to adjust. Ending breast-feeding is, for some women, a difficult emotional transition. Anything that the nurse can do to help breast-feeding continue during hospitalization can help reduce the stress of hospitalization for most mothers and children.

The Bottle-Fed Infant The bottle-fed child also requires some special considerations when hospitalized. Some children, when at home, are left in their cribs with their bottles. This is an established pattern in certain households, although it is a questionable health practice, as it encourages dental caries (see Chapters 7 and 15). Children in the hospital who are without the security of home and routine frequently do not receive sustained attention from their usual care givers. For these reasons, children should be held whenever possible while they are being fed through a bottle. Children can also be held when they are fed solid foods, though older infants may benefit from being placed in a high chair or at a feeding table for the satisfactions that go with their customary attempts at self-feeding.

Burping the hospitalized infant should be done with the child sitting on the nurse's lap. In this way, the child can be continually observed. As the infant is held on the lap, the chin and trunk are carefully supported with one hand and arm and the nurse runs two fingers along either side of the spine with the other hand. This support of the chin and trunk allows a clear passage of air from the stomach. The fingers rubbing slowly but firmly up either side of the spine tend to make even very young infants' trunks straighten, thus encouraging the escape of air. An infant should be burped frequently, at least once midway through the feeding and again after the feeding.

Nutrition and the Older Hospitalized Child The more similar mealtime in the hospital is to mealtime at home, the more likely is a child to perform as independently as possible and to eat the optimal quality and quantity of food. Appropriate independence and proper nutrition aid the child's physical and emotional well-being, the child's emotional and physical growth, and the child's physical healing.

Managing the Mealtime Environment The physical environment should resemble a natural situation as much as possible. Children can, for example, eat at a table instead of in bed whenever their conditions allow. Some facilities have tables and chairs sized appropriately to the usual age of the child on the unit. A young child may sit at a full-sized table and chair when closely supervised for safety. Feeding tables may be available. For reasons of safety, young children usually need to be strapped into the chair of a feeding table with safety straps as a restraint or by having full-sized hospital gowns put on them with the tails of the gown tied in back of the chair. When a playroom is available, children may prefer to eat there instead of in their hospital rooms.

Whatever the facilities, the environment for meals should be emotionally safe for the child. Areas where painful treatments or tests are performed are frightening and are not conducive to a child's feeling comfortable enough to eat well. These areas should not be used for meals. Some children may not leave their beds or rooms for any reason. When a special room is in use for a child, as with a fog room for children with respiratory problems or a laminar-flow area for children who need to be protected from infection, the nurse does not have the freedom to alter the environment. Treatments and meals then occur in the same physical area. In these situations, the nurse must be aware of the emotional strain that remaining in the same area puts on the child and must try to encourage the child's eating in ways other than changing the scene for the meal.

Encouraging Children to Eat Children are more likely to eat foods that coincide with food preferences and choices. Just as hospitalization is a poor time to introduce new foods to the infant, as illness can mask adverse reactions or allergies to new foods, it is a poor time to introduce new foods to older children because they are not likely to be well accepted. Many hospitals allow children to select their meals from menus. Others will allow long-term patients or children on special diets to have choices. Sometimes, canned foods, soups, or peanut butter and jelly are available on the unit for the child who does not like the food served. When a child is using food to control the hospital experience, it may be helpful to fix special meals for the child only after the child eats some or all of the food served on the meal tray. It may be acceptable, however, simply to serve requested food to a child who is restricted in some ways by illness and hospitalization. If the food is on the child's diet and is reasonably nutritious, it does not always matter whether the child first eats what is on the meal tray. Careful assessment of the child's needs can guide the nurse in granting requests or setting limits. Generally, children eat better when they are given some choices in food and mealtime environment.

Companionship during meals is one of the most effective measures for encouraging children to eat. Arranging a child's food at a table where other children are eating; pulling some beds close together so that children on bedrest have company; or having parents, friends, or a nurse sitting with a child can bring dramatic changes in the child's attitude towards meals and food consumption. Talking with a child and creating a pleasant atmosphere with children and parents can help to diminish a family's and thus a child's anxiety. Creating a more homelike atmosphere thus helps a child to eat. Sometimes, a child will eat better if there is a promise of an enjoyable activity after the meal. "We'll read a story after you finish" or "We'll play that game (or do a puzzle or draw a picture or go to the playroom) after you eat" are specific promises that may encourage the child.

Since the nurse controls the appearance and convenience of the food on the tray, the nurse is responsible for the presentation of the child's food. The meal should be appropriate to the developmental level and physical condition of the child. It should be easily reached and presented in appropriate portions, and all containers should be opened. The nurse needs to ensure that the food given to the child corresponds to any dietary restrictions or developmental considerations.

A seemingly obvious but frequently omitted intervention is making the food and tray physically attractive. A picture on a place mat or napkin, a decorated cup, a tea party with doll dishes, a picture on the bottom of a bowl or plate that is visible when the food or fluid is gone can all make mealtimes more fun and thus encourage the child to eat. A small toy placed near the plate may help make the meal pleasant. Food can also be cut into decorative shapes.

Portions that are too large for a particular child may encourage a child's playing with the food instead of eating it. Children usually benefit from small portions, which encourage eating. Children who are just starting to take liquids or solid foods following surgery are often able to eat small portions without difficulty but may suffer from distention and discomfort or even nausea and vomiting if they eat large amounts of food. Children who don't feel well and have poor appetites may be discouraged or repulsed by the sight of what appears to them to be large amounts of food or fluid. Some children use food as a means of attention or control and will tend to be less manipulative with smaller portions. The nurse can then put small portions of food on a medium-sized or small plate or bowl. This can easily be refilled as the child eats and needs more food.

Large amounts of liquids cause a child to feel satisfied and thus discourage solid food intake. For the child having difficulty with solid food intake, small amounts of fluids can be put in a cup or glass. This encourages food intake and discourages a young child's play or spilling. A bottle-fed child should usually have access to a bottle only after completing solid food intake.

One extremely common deterrent to sound nutritional intake is presenting dessert along with the meal. Some children will be encouraged to eat nutritious, unsweetened foods if a dessert is a reward. Other children may temporarily not feel well enough to eat vegetables and meat (the more difficult-to-digest foods) and may need the calories of sugary foods. For these children, showing or giving the dessert along with the meal may be beneficial, but for many children looking at the dessert will make the meal unacceptable or, at best, establish a battleground for the child's attempt at control. In these situations, it is best to keep the dessert off the meal tray until the child has eaten as much of the regular meal as possible, thus encouraging healthier and more homelike eating habits.

Young children who are beginning to feed themselves are generally very proud of their budding independence. They will better accept any needed help from the nurse if they are allowed to help feed themselves with spoons, cups, small glasses, or finger foods. Such a child can usually hold a cracker or a piece of soft food such as a hot dog. Older children also can have difficulty feeding themselves; acceptable finger foods for the older child include raw vegetables, fruit, bread, a hamburger or hot dog on a bun, cookies and even cake, cold fluids in a glass, and certain warm fluids in a cup.

An older child may be too tired to eat well unassisted but will rarely ask for assistance. The child may not feel the need for or even want assistance from the nurse. The nurse's unsolicited assistance may be welcomed if introduced in a matter-of-fact, informal way. Nurses and parents naturally cut food for the young child without being asked, but a child may need this same assistance through late childhood and adolescence when illness interferes with self-help abilities. Asking, "Do you need anything?" will usually be answered, "No." When the nurse sees that a child is eating very little, eating slowly, or avoiding difficult-to-manage foods such as meat, assistance can be offered. Simply saying, "I'm going to cut your meat. It's hard to do it with an IV" as the nurse picks up the knife and fork allows the child to accept needed help without feeling embarrassed, infantile, or dependent. This child also has the choice of refusing help and maintaining independence. Children who have mastered the task of self-feeding despite such impediments as IV, cast, or bedrest will then tell the nurse they can do it by themselves.

Managing Fluid Intake Some children need additional encouragement and management to meet nutritional and fluid needs, and occasionally the nurse needs to limit food or fluids. In either situation, cooperation among the child, family, and nurse is necessary in meeting the child's needs. As with any medical treatment, the child and family needs to understand medical and nursing goals, and the nurse needs to understand the goals of the child and family.

Increasing Fluid Intake In many instances, as in the postoperative phase and particularly after certain types of genitourinary surgery, children need to drink a lot of fluid and must be strongly encouraged to do so. "Force fluids," so familiar as a directive for nursing management, can be very difficult to accomplish.

In general, the nurse uses the same guidelines that are designed to encourage children to eat. Fluids offered should be familiar and acceptable to the child. Parents and children need to understand the importance of the fluids. Many initially cannot see the need for encouraging sweet, less-nutritious fluids such as soft drinks, ice cream, puddings, or gelatin. If they understand why a large volume of fluid is needed, the child's drinking and the parents' encouragement are more likely. Frequent, small glasses or bottles of a variety of fluids usually accomplish the goal. Some children feel well enough to drink but suffer from enforced dependence, bedrest, loneliness, or boredom. For these children, large, less-frequent servings intermingled with care to meet their other needs may best encourage fluid intake.

Generally, fluid intake will be much higher when the nurse brings the child a variety of fluids at spaced intervals without first asking whether the child wants a drink. This helps sidestep the ever-present "no" of early childhood, the "no" and stalling of middle childhood, and the late childhood and adolescent need to control the environment and gain some independence, all of which will occur at the expense of needed fluids. The nursing plan should therefore include bringing unsolicited fluids to the child, and the nurse plans to offer fluids at the times a child feels relatively well and is likely to accept them. Times when children are enjoying themselves with company, during a game, or doing a project may be very good times to bring in a glass of fluid and encourage the child to drink. At these times, the child is somewhat distracted from physical problems and unhappiness with hospitalization and illness and may more readily accept fluids.

Timing fluid administration to coincide with periods of relief from pain can also improve fluid acceptance, since the diminished pain allows the child to be interested in other things. Some children may have their IVs removed if they have an adequate fluid intake. In this circumstance the nurse may have the freedom to reduce the IV rate to below fluid maintenance level, so that the child becomes thirsty and increases oral intake.

The child and family need to know the consequences of a child's drinking or not drinking. If it is honest to say that an IV will remain in or that a child will not be discharged from the hospital until oral intake reaches a certain level, then the child and family should be told this. Such statements are not threats or punishments if they are honest and presented without anger. Intravenous fluids are sometimes continued or restarted when a child's oral fluid intake is low. Children, especially after throat surgery, may not be discharged until they demonstrate that they can drink enough to meet their fluid needs. Child and family deserve to know the importance of fluid intake.

Limiting Fluid Intake For some children, the nurse helps restrict, rather than increase, fluids. Children starting fluids after surgery usually start with small amounts and progress to optimal fluid and calorie intake as their physical conditions allow. Some children cannot mobilize fluids well. The child with cardiac or renal problems, for example, may have a restricted fluid intake. Some children's gastrointestinal systems are unable to handle large amounts or even maintenance amounts of fluids. (See Chapters 35, 38, and 39 for a discussion of children with cardiac, gastrointestinal, or renal problems.)

Nursing management for these children will vary with the developmental level of the child. Despite a child's and family's understanding, accepting, and participating in the treatment plan, this aspect of the plan may be difficult to follow. The nurse can plan with the child and family when and how the child will be allowed fluids. The family then must not offer more than the child should have at a particular time.

Infants who are limited to 1 oz of fluids should be given a bottle containing only 1 oz of fluid. If more fluid is in a bottle or cup, a vigorous suck or momentary inattention to the amount consumed could mean that the child obtains too much fluid. This will risk overloading the gastrointestinal, renal, or cardiac system. In the same way, an older child should be offered no more than the child is allowed to drink. To offer more is tempting the child to rebel against the treatment plan and is truly unkind. It would emphasize what the child cannot have, while offering fluids that the child can finish emphasizes the positive aspects of following the plan. Children in late childhood and adolescence can usually plan their own fluid intake when they are given specific guidelines. Many will enjoy making charts outlining how they hope to meet their fluid goals.

Rewards for a child's appropriate restriction of oral intake are many. A child may notice feeling better, having increased activity tolerance, or exhibiting less edema, as the case may be, if fluids are appropriately restricted. Some children will find cooperation easier with additional rewards. Spoken praise for a job well done, a star for reaching each small goal, a special food, or a special time with the nurse may all encourage a child. Sometimes, withholding something is also appropriate. One nurse caring for an adolescent boy who was struggling to finish a liquid meal through wired jaws intercepted his mail and then gave him a letter for each significant amount he drank. It was effective in this particular situation in turning a pleading session into a joke and game for both child and nurse.

Elimination—Potential Difficulties

The elimination patterns of children may be altered during hospitalization; the change may be related either to the stress of hospitalization or to the child's illness. Nursing care for these alterations reflects what is appropriate for the child's developmental stage and physical condition.

Needs of the Younger Child Many hospitals now supply disposable diapers for the infant, and most infants can use these without difficulty. Children who have developed rashes when disposable diapers have been used will, however, need cloth diapers. Usually these children will have no difficulty if the nurse uses a cloth diaper to line a disposable diaper, making sure that the disposable diaper does not touch the child's skin. This practice protects the child's skin and also the outer plastic of the disposable diaper helps keep the child's bed from being changed as frequently as would be necessary if a cloth diaper were used alone.

Diaper rash is a common difficulty for any infant, hospitalized or not hospitalized. The nurse may use treatment measures that the child's parents have found helpful or can institute new practices when necessary (see Chapter 7). The nurse keeps the child as dry and as clean as possible, by frequently checking and changing the diaper and by carefully cleaning fecal matter from the child's skin. The child may also benefit from having the affected area exposed to air when possible. This is easily done by putting the child in the prone position and placing the child on an open diaper. When the anterior perineal area is irritated, the open-to-air method can still be used with a girl placed supine on an open diaper and a boy placed on his side with the diaper draped so that it will be likely to intercept urine.

Children are sometimes admitted to the hospital when they are in the process of being toilet trained or when bowel or bladder control have recently been achieved. The stresses of hospitalization cause many children to regress and temporarily to lose any recently acquired skill (see Chapter 27). A child who was previously dry and clean may, for example, begin to wet and soil. Because toilet training is an important milestone to both child and parent, any regression is usually very upsetting to the entire family. The nurse can help the family by supporting the child in maintaining as much continence as possible and by reassuring the child and teaching the parent that regression is common in such a situation.

Supporting a child's skills requires a good assessment and prior detailed knowledge about the skills. A child wearing diapers and a child wearing pants on admission may both be in the process of toilet training. Any child accustomed to using a toilet or a potty chair should know where these are located in the hospital and should know how to ask to use them. Because the child's verbal skills and vocabulary are usually quite limited at the age of toilet training, the nurse learns from the parent and records on the nursing care plan the words the child uses to express toileting needs. Many parents help children in toileting by placing a child on the toilet or potty chair at specific times or after special cues from the child. If nursing staff can continue the parental practices, they will help to prevent unnecessary regression with its guilt and frustration for children and families.

Many children, despite support in toileting from family and nurses, do regress during hospitalization. The family needs to know that children frequently regress in skill levels when they are sick and hospitalized. After hospitalization, children will resume training when physically and emotionally ready. The child also needs to understand this problem. The nurse avoids scolding and making an issue of incontinence. Children needing diapers may be told that diapers are all right for now and that they will wear pants again when they are able.

Needs of the Older Child Older children, secure in their urinary or bowel continence, also have difficulties with toileting during hospitalization. In various stages of development, children are very modest about toileting needs, words, and actions and are resistant to any exposure of their genitals. Many children in the hospital have their urine measured, need to give specimens of urine or feces, need to use a bedpan, or are asked whether they have had a bowel movement and to describe it. Those who can use a bathroom unassisted have some privacy, although on many pediatric units the bathroom is off the main hall and may even have a door that remains open. Many children cannot, for medical or safety reasons, use a bathroom independently. Some are too unsteady or groggy because of illness, medication, or recovery from anesthetic, and these children need the nurse's or family's assistance to ambulate to the bathroom. Asking for, waiting for, and accepting help can all be difficult. Once in the bathroom, some children need help to remain safely seated on the toilet.

Assisting while giving the child all possible privacy is a difficult task for the nurse. Nurses can physically support but look away from children; they can tell children that they are looking elsewhere; they can chat while assisting, which serves to distract a child and to assure with actions that the nurse is not concentrating exclusively on the child's toileting.

Many children are unable to get out of bed and use a toilet, and learning to use a urinal and bedpan is not always easy or natural for them. One 15-year-old boy had to remain in bed on the day of surgery and had not yet voided postoperatively. He told his nurse he did not need to void, but when he was asked to tell the nurse how to use the urinal, it was obvious that he did not know, was embarrassed to ask, and was afraid of wetting his bed. Repeated, simple, careful teaching about positioning the urinal and reassurance of privacy during voiding enabled this boy to void. For whatever reason—fatigue, effect of medication, pain, embarrassment—the child had not learned from previous teaching. Modesty, discomfort, or illness can interfere with any child's learning how to use a bedpan or urinal. The nurse thus individualizes teaching and support for each child and evaluates the child's understanding and acceptance of this means of toileting.

Some hospitalized children require catheterization or enemas. (Catheterization of the child is discussed in Chapter 39, and the procedures for enemas are discussed in Chapter 38.)

Sleep and Rest—Potential Deficits

The hospitalized child has an obvious need for sleep to promote growth and restore health. For equally obvious reasons, it is difficult for these children to obtain needed sleep and rest. The hospital environment is new, different, often noisy, and without the usual security of home and routine. Most hospitalized children feel physically drained and uncomfortable even if they are not in actual pain, and sleep and rest are thus more difficult than usual. Children may be anxious or afraid and may find it difficult to trust the hospital environment. The very inactivity of most hospitalized children is a dramatic contrast to their normal routines. A child used to burning off energy through vigorous physical activity rarely has the ability or opportunity to be as active in the hospital. Sleep may come slowly and sporadically to the child who is not physically tired.

Nurses may actually overlook some simple areas for nursing management when planning care. One helpful intervention is to follow the child's bedtime routine as closely as possible, but several factors can interfere with this. For instance, nurses may find themselves ready to put children to sleep for the night and realize that they do not know the child's routine. A careful nursing history is thus crucial on admission. The nurse may also find that the home routine is in some way contraindicated in the hospital. A child may be accustomed to having a bottle before going to sleep, and this may be impossible when the child has had oral surgery, is to receive limited fluids, or is NPO. A nurse may not feel it is possible to spend the time and energy needed to follow a child's bedtime routine. Many children are put to bed at home with a quiet story read or told to them or with a private conversation with someone they love. The nurse may feel far too busy to stop for any of these activities, but it is often more efficient to stop and read a short story than to quiet fretful, crying children who keep themselves and many other children awake. Furthermore, if a child has felt somewhat secure at bedtime, obtains adequate rest, and feels more trusting of the hospital environment, he or she is likely to be more cooperative with nursing care.

The easiest and usually most satisfactory way to ensure close adherence to the child's bedtime routine is to have a parent available to the child. With young children, rooming-in is very beneficial (see Chapter 27). For the older child and when rooming-in is not possible because of hospital policy and facilities or other demands on the parent, having the parent available to the child up to bedtime can provide the continuity that a child needs to relax and obtain needed rest. In middle childhood, children often appreciate the parent's presence, perhaps a kiss and being tucked in, and a story before going to sleep. Even in late childhood and adolescence, a child often appreciates the parent's being nearby.

To prevent injury from hard or sharp objects, only soft toys should remain in a child's bed or crib at bedtime. All objects purposefully removed from a child's bed must, of course, be truly out of reach. A child should be as comfortable as possible before going to sleep for the night. A high temperature or pain would ideally be relieved before bedtime. It may be possible to time an analgesic so that it will reach its peak when a child needs to sleep. Although nursing care does not mean withholding medication, a child may find adequate relief from noninvasive pain relief measures during waking hours, and it may be possible to time a medication for its effect at bedtime or naptime.

A child's feeling trustful rather than fearful is crucial to adequate rest. Nursing management to assist the child includes much that goes on at times other than bedtime. A child's preparation for procedures and ability to play out fears and fantasies aid the child's ability to rest. Keeping the child's sleeping area as nonthreatening as possible is also important to a child's being able to use the space for rest. Painful or frightening procedures should, whenever possible, be done away from the child's bed. Finally, the nurse can attempt to plan the child's waking activities so that the child is tired at bedtime. This involves a creative use of play for the hospitalized child (see Chapter 28).

Immobility—Potential Complications

Immobility has multiple effects, both physiologic and psychologic, on a child. One of the most prominent characteristics of immobilized children, however, is their mobility. Many children confined to bed are hardly immobile. They scoot and slither, bounce and jump. Children asked to rest quietly can frequently be seen running, playing, and shouting with total abandon. Children in leg casts, for example, have climbed trees. Unless extremely developmentally delayed or paralyzed either physically or emotionally, the immobilized child is to some degree mobile.

The general antidote for immobility is, within the confines of medical treatment plans and safety, mobility. Participation in self-care is one of the best ways to encourage increased activity. The activity is purposeful and physically therapeutic, and it encourages and stimulates self-respect. It encourages movement with a decrease of pressure on the skin, increased muscle tone, increased lung expansion and venous return, and improved gastrointestinal and genitourinary function. These contribute to better health and faster recovery. Play, whether it be for fun and pleasure or expression and learning, also provides activity and growth.

Skin Complications The skin shows the effects of immobility and requires careful nursing management. Pressure sores and the more-frequent skin irritation from treatment apparatus, bandages, or friction of bed sheets can develop in the child. Warning signs of adverse effects on the skin include lingering redness over a bony prominence following turning and massaging. Complaint of discomfort is another clue. A young child may complain indirectly of discomfort with increased irritability and restlessness when in a particular position. Skin irritation in the child on bedrest often stems from a child's restlessness and increased mobility of nonimmobilized parts, which causes friction on bedsheets. Elbows, ears, knees, and heels are particularly vulnerable to irritation, and a paralyzed or unconscious child or a child lacking usual sensation has a greater risk of skin breakdown.

The general condition of the skin contributes to its ability to withstand stress. Unrelieved pressure on the skin over bony prominences decreases circulation to this skin and leads, if the process is uninterrupted, to skin breakdown. Predisposing factors to skin breakdown include skin that is not healthy or intact, the presence of a chronic or debilitating condition, and poor nutritional status. Soft, thin, or fragile skin is less able to withstand pressure or irritation. A child who is obese tends to have more difficulties with moisture remaining in skin folds.

Skin breakdown is much more easily prevented than it is treated. Therefore the immobilized child's position is changed every 2–4 hours, the skin condition is assessed, and the skin (especially over bony prominences) massaged. Massaging the skin stimulates circulation. If lotion is used in skin care, any excess should be removed with a towel, as remaining moisture leads to softening and maceration of the skin and thus increases the risk of skin breakdown. Any redness should start to disappear after massaging and should disappear completely within several hours when there is no pressure on the affected area. If redness is still apparent, more frequent skin care—as often as every hour—should be given, and the child should be positioned off the reddened area as much as possible.

Many devices to reduce pressure on any one area, reduce friction, and maintain desired positions are available. Sheepskins, gel or foam pads, and alternating-pressure air or water mattresses equalize pressure. Extra pillows, blankets, and trochanter rolls can be of great benefit in maintaining positions for the child. Many children do not make specific complaints, do not ask to be turned, and rarely ask for a back rub from the nurse. The child may, however, be in just as great need of these measures as an adult. Despite the mobility of most children, the healthy nature of most children's skin, and the child's not specifically requesting skin care, this remains part of the nurse's repertoire when working with children. Preventive measures and, when necessary, treatment measures begin with a child's immobilization and continue until the threat of skin breakdown is eliminated.

Muscle and Tendon Complications Immobility can also result in the loss of muscle tone leading to tissue atrophy. The general health status of the child and the length, extent, and cause of the immobility all contribute to the degree of tissue atrophy. The normally continuous renewal of collagen fibers does not continue effectively during immobilization. Instead, the fibers become thick, fibrous, and resistant to stretching. Unused muscles become weak. Limiting the extent of this atrophy and preventing any contractures depend to a large degree on nursing management.

For the most part, adequate management consists of engaging children at frequent intervals in play activities that do not interfere with the treatment plan or the child's safety. Previously healthy and mobile children, in bed for a week to 10 days for postoperative recuperation or respiratory conditions, will regain mobility and muscle strength soon after they are up out of bed and resume their normal activities. Considerations for these children center around adequate stimulation to combat their feelings of immobility, helplessness, and isolation (see Chapter 27).

For children immobilized for a prolonged period of time and for those particularly prone to tissue atrophy or contractures (for example, those children with cerebral palsy or severe burns), a more intensive management strategy is needed. A program of joint and muscle exercises done either actively by the child or passively by the family or nurse is an integral part of the care plan. Range-of-motion and isometric exercises; weight lifting with dumbbells; or pull-ups using an overbed trapeze are examples of exercises to include.

Cardiovascular Complications Activity and exercise also help prevent the ill effects of immobility on the cardiovascular system. Muscle tone is important to facilitate the venous return of blood to the heart. Poor muscle tone allows some of the blood to pool in dependent parts. Although immobilized children are unlikely to experience thrombi, venous stasis is one of the factors that contributes to thrombus formation. Another factor involved is venous pressure related to a child's position. Therefore, any position that restricts circulation by causing pressure at a joint or on another body part should be avoided. Dependent parts often appear edematous. Shifting position helps to relieve the swelling.

Respiratory Complications Impairment of respiratory function due to immobility is a very real threat to the child. Decrease in lung expansion occurs with immobility and is furthered by a child's pain, fear, and the pressure of some treatment devices. The decrease in lung expansion and resulting decrease in movement of air during inspiration and expiration tends to discourage adequate movement of secretions. Stasis and pooling of secretions make the child more susceptible to infection.

Nursing care can help prevent respiratory complications. Adequate lung expansion can be accomplished by coughing and deep breathing several times every few hours. For a young child, blowing games such as blowing a paper tissue, a party favor, or a mobile can be effective motivators for adequate lung expansion. An older child can make good use of an incentive spirometer or blow bottles.

With any type of blowing activity, however, the nurse keeps firmly in mind that the goal is lung expansion—deep breathing—and not blowing. Children are capable of excessively blowing to accomplish the perceived goal and can actually cause atelectasis. The nurse observes a child's inspiration as carefully as the expiration and teaches the child who can understand the true goal of the therapy.

The upright position encourages lung expansion, and changes of position help prevent pooling of secretions. Lung expansion is also caused by the movement in the changing of positions. The nurse frequently assesses an immobilized child's respiratory status and initiates nursing interventions to deal with any inadequate air exchange or adventitious breath sounds.

Gastrointestinal Complications The gastrointestinal tract is sluggish with decreased mobility. Accelerated catabolism incurred with inactivity over a long period of time causes negative nitrogen balance. This state, along with lowered energy needs and some children's feelings during inactivity, contributes to decreased appetite and food intake. Mass peristaltic waves in the colon are stimulated when the stomach and duodenum fill with food. Thus decreased appetite and irregularity of food intake interfere with regularly timed peristaltic activity. If a child cannot sit when attempting to defecate, the usual aids of thigh pressure on the abdomen and downward pressure on the rectum are lacking. Because of positioning and possible embarrassment in using the bedpan, a child may ignore the defecation reflex or attempt to inhibit defecation. Feces thus remain in the rectum, and the child becomes constipated.

Increased fluid and roughage help combat these effects and aid normal bowel evacuation. The child also needs sources of protein and calories. The older child can and should be taught the connection between immobility and the temporary need for changes in dietary pattern. Children who are immobilized often use food as a means of maintaining independence and control of the environment. Without an understanding of the rationale for their diets, they are usually not particularly eager to eat nutritious foods, drink extra fluids, and consume roughage such as fresh fruits and prune juice. One immobilized 10-year-old child who refused most fluids and all fruits and vegetables required an enema. When he understood why he did not need enemas at home, what was different about his activity now, and what effect this had on his gastrointestinal tract, he was most accepting of preventive measures.

Genitourinary Complications The genitourinary system is also affected by immobility. Without upright positioning, a child has a tendency toward urinary stasis in the renal pelvis. In addition, urinary retention may result from failure of perineal muscles to relax and from reduced muscle tone of the bladder. Stagnation of urine promotes infection. This tendency is furthered by alkaline urine associated with increased calcium excretion that occurs during immobilization and inactivity. With stasis and increased excretion of minerals, renal calculi may form, but this is not common in children.

Increased fluid intake is again helpful, as it flushes the kidney and stimulates its normal physiologic activity. Increased fluids flush the bladder, helping remove contaminants and thus prevent infection. Fruit juices and water are good sources of liquid, and the nurse therefore encourages plenty of each. Fruit juices, especially cranberry juice, have the additional advantage of providing vitamin C and helping to maintain the acidity of urine. Frequent assessment of urine pH guides the nurse in determining the type of fluid to offer. If the urine pH is consistently borderline or high (alkaline), the prescription of daily ascorbic acid tablets has sometimes been used to correct the problem.

The amount of calcium to include in the diet is controversial. Some authorities recommend a diet low in calcium as a possible way to decrease the formation of renal calculi. Other authorities recommend calcium intake normal for the child's age and weight (Hilt, 1975). It is important for the nurse to know the calcium requirements for each child. With a lengthy immobilization or a child prone to renal calculi development, the nurse can keep an accurate flow sheet of calcium intake. The nurse also involves the dietary department in monitoring calcium in the diet. It is often beneficial to involve the child in this task, as total calcium intake and the amount of calcium present in a fluid or snack determine whether or not the food is a good choice. In this way, the child gains a sense of control from being able to make decisions within established guidelines.

Checks of specific gravity will guide the nurse in deciding on the amount of fluid intake needed. Children without renal or cardiac problems should consume more than their

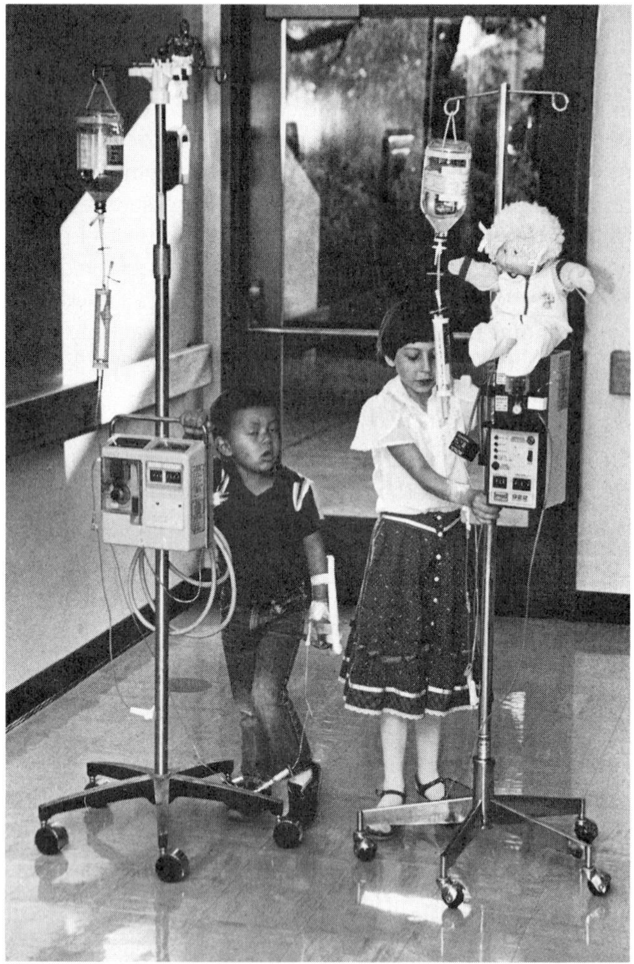

Mobile IV poles minimize children's feelings of frustration and sense of dependence.

daily requirements of fluid. When the urine specific gravity for these children is high, they need to be encouraged to drink additional fluids.

Psychosocial Complications Immobilization places a person in a very unnatural psychologic state. Movement means independence, and particularly to the young child, movement is the essence of life. Through mobility the child discovers the environment and the self. Children thus find immobility very hard to accept, especially when not in pain and feeling relatively well. One 7-year-old, describing a hospital stay several years earlier, said, "I really wasn't sick, but I had to stay in bed." Young children often interpret these restrictions as punishment, and these feelings grow when additions or changes are made in the treatment regimen. This same child then continued, "There was something wrong with my testicle." He could remember the reason for his restrictions, and he did not seem to interpret these restrictions as punishment. It is critical for their healthy development that nurses prepare children for restrictions in mobility.

Mobility is involved in many coping behaviors. Restricted mobility sometimes compounds the emotional needs of the child. The person who deals with disappointment or frustration by leaving the scene in which these feelings occur is usually deprived of major means of coping and has to develop new coping strategies. Because mobility is often needed to participate in peer activities, those immobilized may feel left out or rejected. The child may be humiliated by enforced dependence in activities of daily living.

In short, immobility may not be well tolerated. Children react in different ways to these restrictions and may take several days or weeks to make a transition and adjust to a specific type of confinement. Their coping resources, support systems, and interpretation of the restrictions are critical factors during the adjustment phase (see Chapter 27). An immobilized child has an environment confined to what can be seen, reached, or manipulated. For such a child to learn and advance in development, it is essential that caregivers compensate for these limitations.

As much as possible, the environment needs to be changed. Changes in surroundings include stimulation, opportunities for learning, and socializing experiences. Just being near someone else is reassuring and comforting for the confined child and also allows for natural communication with the child. A change of environment decreases sensory deprivation or the sensory overload of being unable to escape unpleasant or excessive stimuli. Most children on bedrest can be moved either in their beds or on stretchers or in wheelchairs or go-carts to the unit's playroom, solarium, or other gathering place so they can participate in conversation and activities. Older children particularly benefit from time spent in or on wheeled devices of which they can control the direction and movement. This returns some needed feelings of independence and well-being. If a child cannot be moved without disrupting treatment apparatus or necessary therapy, activities can be organized in the room so that the child can feel a part of a group.

Games and other play activities can be adapted to individual limitations. Table games, card games, memory games, and puzzles provide both group and individual involvement. Some of these can be played more easily with the use of prism glasses or when the child is prone. To accommodate mobility restrictions, more active games may be modified by creating special roles for the immobilized child. Being a scorekeeper or rules keeper, for example, involves one in the game. It has the additional benefit of helping the child learn a game better through increased knowledge of the rules and observation of skills used.

Pain—Alteration in Comfort

Any parent who has inadvertently jabbed a healthy infant with a diaper pin can attest to the child's squalling and apparent outrage. Children indeed do feel pain, but research has shown, unfortunately, that nurses do not always medicate infants and children as frequently as they would adults (McGuire and Dizard, 1982; Eland and Anderson, 1977). For example, a postoperative infant's crying may be attributed to hunger instead of pain. Nurses may find themselves waiting for children to articulate clearly the need for pain medication. Some nurses decide that children should not have analgesics, usually because of misguided concern about causing addiction or because many children can be distracted from their pain.

Distraction is a powerful pain relief measure, and children's reactions to it can confuse nurses. The effectiveness of distraction ceases, however, when the distraction is over. Those children who can play wholeheartedly, even when experiencing postoperative or other pain, do attain temporary pain relief in this way, but nurses might forget that the child needs additional pain relief measures when the child is not distracted.

Another source of confusion stems from children's relying on and deriving true comfort from their parents. A large percentage of children reported that parental presence helped them most when they were in pain (*AJN*, 1984). Therefore a child's being upset around the time a parent leaves may be related to an increased perception of pain and a need for nursing intervention. Nurses who might attribute complaints or crying to a parent's absence and not to pain need to recognize this correlation.

Children may actually be less able than adults to tolerate pain. The pain threshold increases slightly throughout childhood. Children do suffer, and the younger the child, the more the child might experience pain with the same stimulus (Eland and Anderson, 1977). Children's pain certainly has emotional as well as physical components. Fear, anxiety, and deeply missing home and family all add to physical stressors and in turn increase the sensation of pain. Children often see pain as harmful or negative, and they may fear bodily harm. Their thinking about pain tends to be immature, and they are often unable to see pain as a helpful signal that something is wrong (*AJN*, 1984). The child's experiences then contribute to pain, and pain then affects the whole child.

Pain in the child, as in the adult, is subjective and fully appreciated only by the one in pain. When pain is suspected to be primarily psychogenic, it is less likely to evoke sympathy and concern from the nurse. Psychogenic pain is nevertheless real pain, and it too causes suffering and requires intervention.

When the nurse cannot identify a cause for pain, the pain might have physiologic origins. Children sometimes have pinpointed pain where there is no discernible pathology, only to have pathology, which might be a serious infection or a tumor, discovered in the exact location at a later date. Therefore, both for children's psychologic and physiologic health, nurses need to take complaints and signs of pain seriously.

Assessment of Pain Assessment of pain in the child requires looking at all aspects of behavior. The nurse looks for such general signs as irritability, restlessness, withdrawal, personality change, pallor, a drawn appearance, and failure to eat, drink, or play. A child might be unusually inactive and quiet. The pulse and respiratory rates typically increase with pain but infrequently may decrease with failure to maintain homeostasis and impending collapse from deep, visceral, or prolonged pain.

Children may exhibit specific signs of pain, such as pulling at or favoring a part of the body. One mother, for example, knew to take her 11-month-old infant to the doctor to have an ear infection diagnosed because the child pulled at his ear. Children with leg or hip pain will often limp, thus reducing the time that the leg in pain carries the body's weight. A parent is frequently more aware of a child's subtle behavior change and may know when the child is in pain better than health professionals caring for the child.

Pain, which is often hard for adults to describe, is even harder for children. With young children and those lacking good verbal skills, the nurse relies most heavily on a general assessment of the child. The nurse can often assist older children's describing pain first by demonstrating interest in them and their complaints. The nurse–patient relationship then improves, and the child is more willing to share. The nurse can also convey interest by sitting with and listening to the child. Supplying descriptive words helps a child to describe pain. Children, like adults, usually reject incorrect words and search for accurate descriptors, and many children are capable of graphically describing pain. Understanding a child's complaints requires skillful listening, as children's use of words may be different from that of adults and believing complaints is not the same as taking words at face value. The nurse needs to question and requestion until understanding is assured. This understanding is usually a tremendous relief for the child (unless the child fears an injection).

Play can help in the expression and description of pain. A young child may respond to a story of a child or animal who goes to the hospital. The nurse can start the story describing circumstances that parallel the child's. The child can fill in some details as the nurse asks what happened to the character in the story. "What did it feel like? Did it hurt?" Some children share their feelings when the nurse tells a story in which the main character has pain. Such questions as "Does this sound right? What do you think is happening?" may elicit responses from the child and help in pain diagnosis.

Many children can speak through art. Both younger and older children are able to fill in an outline of a person. The child's color choice and the markings on particular parts of the picture have been accurately correlated with pathology (Eland and Anderson, 1977). A child may also draw a picture that helps communicate about pain; such pictures are sometimes obvious and sometimes obscure. A child may have to tell the nurse what the picture means, but even when the nurse cannot discern the meaning, the child has the benefit of expression and perhaps increased insight into the self (see Chapter 28).

As with the adult, much information is needed about pain so that the nurse can truly help the child. The intensity, type, location, time, and duration of occurrence; events surrounding occurrence; and what worsens or lessens the pain are all questions that need to be answered before the nurse can decide how to relieve the pain. Assessment should, whenever possible, occur separately from painful remedies for pain. At times, however, the nurse cannot avoid verifying the existence of pain and then appearing with a syringe in hand. The problem with this sequence is that after one such experience, a child is not likely to admit to pain when asked the next time. Even so, for a child who will have few injections, either because oral analgesics will soon be an alternative or because the pain is an isolated experience, this association of injections with a confession of pain need not greatly undermine future nurse–patient communication. For such children, the nurse specifically reassures the child that soon injections will not be necessary.

Even though nurses attempt to dissociate the nursing history from resulting intervention, children may still hide their pain. They may fear a shot. They may feel a need to act bravely in front of nurse, peers, or parents. Boys in particular often have been conditioned to "act like a man," deny their pain, and not cry or confess to such weaknesses (see Chapter 27). The nurse then has to rely on assessment of nonverbal behaviors.

Nursing Management of Pain Remembering children's responses to painful procedures helps guide the nurse in choosing appropriate pain relief measures and in individualizing an approach for the child. Children try to avoid pain. They ask the nurse to be gentle, not to hurt. They want to postpone or avoid the procedure. "Maybe I'll have it later. Let me just finish watching this television show." They may go off the unit when a dressing change is needed. They may hit or kick the nurse. Maintaining a stream of conversation tends to postpone procedures for a short time. A nurse may go into a child's room, find the child "napping," and be tempted to leave the sleeping child alone.

In view of these tactics and the child's understandable reluctance to experience pain, nurses need to stand firm in their assessment. If analgesia would help a child perform necessary activities such as postoperative ambulation, coughing, and deep breathing, if it would free the child to interact with others and to play, and if it would allow the child to sleep soundly instead of intermittently, then it is needed. Because not every pain relief measure is invasive, the least intrusive measures are used whenever possible. Medication, whether by mouth, rectal suppository, or injection, is not always necessary.

Noninvasive Measures for Pain Relief Because anxiety works with physical stimuli to intensify the sensation of pain, any measure to diminish anxiety will help make the child more comfortable. General teaching to increase a child's understanding will help. To the best of their abilities, nurses also need to teach children about their pain and about what they are experiencing and why.

Knowledge is power in this case, power over the unknown. In the same way that preparation for childbirth can lessen the discomfort of contractions, children can benefit from knowing what sensations mean. Nurses can emphasize that postoperative pain is temporary. They can remind the child that the skin itches as it heals. Other pain relief measures include involving the family and other significant people in a child's care. Familiar objects from home make the child feel comfortable. Telephone calls from family and friends help. A child's assisting, when possible, in a treatment or procedure helps return control to the child and can reduce the sensation of pain. For example, a child may help remove tape securing an IV or a dressing. Some children want to watch painful dressing changes or scrubs; others can be involved extensively in this care. All the measures that nurses use to decrease anxiety and enhance development also help to decrease pain (see Chapter 27).

Specific noninvasive techniques for children are the same as those used for adults. With children, however, nurses have an advantage not applicable to adults in that children will willingly participate in many games and new ideas. Much of nursing care with children involves distraction, and this is a powerful pain relief measure for the period in which it is used. Play for entertainment purposes distracts the child from fears, from focus on the self, and from pain. Nurses can talk to children and can change a child's environment by bringing a child to the playroom, to another part of the hospital, or simply out into the hallway. Children often play together when encouraged and will then distract each other. The nurse can also help distract the child during specific painful experiences. Holding the child's hand and talking during an injection or dressing change is one example of the use of distraction.

Some children can easily be helped to relax by using imagery. They can think of themselves doing some enjoyable, restful activity such as floating on their backs in the water. Although the nurse frequently uses distraction or imagery at the spur of the moment, the nurse and child can plan to use these during painful experiences of relatively short duration. Children are more likely to feel supported and in control of themselves when interventions are planned.

Cutaneous stimulation is another noninvasive measure. Nurses frequently hug and rock an infant or a young child; the older child might receive a back rub. Other measures can be used, usually with the child's knowledge of their purpose. Rubbing an injection site or rubbing the side opposite the part of the body that hurts may help some children.

Medications for Pain Relief Any pain relief measure will be enhanced if it is initiated before pain is severe and if the nurse "sells" its effectiveness to the child and family. Explaining the purpose of specific distraction techniques, mental images and relaxation, or even a back rub will help in gaining the child's full cooperation and trust. Medication effectiveness is also enhanced when the nurse raises the child's confidence in it and thus in the entire treatment plan.

The nurse does not, however, minimize the discomfort that the child will experience. If a medication has a very bitter taste, the nurse should not say that it tastes good. If the nurse is not honest, the child will not be able to trust the nurse in later explanations of procedures and treatments. When medications are needed, the nurse explains their purpose and emphasizes their effectiveness. The nurse tries to give an oral medication when possible. The next preference is a suppository, as it is essentially not painful, and the least preferable is an injection, as it is always the most painful. When an injection is necessary, the nurse needs to build the child's confidence, both in the medication and in the nurse. The nurse always uses the most careful, least painful techniques and says this to the child. Nurses can emphasize that giving an injection is a skill. Confidence in one's skill is contagious, makes the child feel secure, aids the child's relaxation and cooperation, and enhances the chance of success for both the nurse and the medication.

A combination of pain relief measures is often very helpful to the child. A nurse administering a medication cannot forget to include noninvasive pain relief measures in the plan of care.

Pediatric Adaptations of Common Procedures

Color, Sensation, and Motion Assessment

The nurse obtains baseline data for color, sensation, and motion for a body part to ascertain the status of innervation and vascularity. This is a necessary assessment in pediatric conditions in which surgery or tissue swelling may impair innervation or vascularity, a cast or splint is used, an extremity is bandaged and suspended, or restraints are used.

The nurse notes the color, warmth, or coolness of a body part. Coolness and lack of color, in comparing one part to the same body part on the child's other side, may be related to impaired circulation. When a portion of the skin is lightly squeezed and released, the skin should blanch and normal color should then return immediately. A rapid return of color indicates tissue perfusion, while delayed or slow capillary refill would mean restricted circulation.

The nurse assesses sensation to determine whether pressure or edema is interfering with normal nerve pathways. The nurse can assess sensation in a child over age 10 with normal emotional and cognitive development by asking whether the child feels a body part and whether there are any unusual feelings in that particular part of the body. The nurse touches a toe or finger and asks the child to state which toe or finger was touched. The nurse notes how much pressure had to be applied before the child felt the sensation. Assessment of sensation is a critical observation, and children who are below age 10 or delayed in development are not necessarily reliable enough as historians (Hilt, 1975). Therefore, in a younger or developmentally delayed child, a nurse proves sensation by observing the child's facial or withdrawal reaction to a light pinch or a prick.

Motion can be assessed by watching the child's physical reaction to being touched or by asking a child capable of responding to try to move an affected part.

Urine and Stool Specimen Collection

Collecting urine and stool specimens from a child, while frequently more difficult than collecting them from an adult, is a routine aspect of nursing care. Urine specimens are obtained on the admission of a child to the hospital. They are also needed when there is suspicion of infection, when assessing urine specific gravity or pH, when the child is to undergo surgery, and in various other situations. Among other purposes, stool specimens are needed when testing for occult blood, culture, ova and parasite identification, and in assessing products of digestion.

General Considerations Although reasons differ among children of various ages, most feel private and embarrassed about their bodies' excrements. A 15-year-old boy, when handing a cup containing his admission urine sample to a young, attractive female nurse, did not meet her eyes and refused to talk with her for hours after the admission. Many children state that the urine specimen container feels wet, despite the fact that it is dry. The temperature of the sample combined with the child's embarrassment probably account for this sensation. The nurse's reassuring the child that the container is dry, if it is, or that it is perfectly all right and easily remedied if it is wet, will help the child feel more comfortable in the hospital setting.

A child may need more assistance with giving a urine or stool sample than that needed for basic toileting. A toilet-trained 2-year-old cannot hold a cup in place to obtain a specimen. This child can sit on a toilet where a container for collecting urine has been placed under the seat. A boy may wish to stand while voiding but may not be able to hold a cup or specimen container. In this instance use of a urinal may be indicated.

Clean-Catch Specimens Children are in particular need of help for obtaining clean-catch specimens. Before adolescence, they can rarely clean the meatus, hold back labia or foreskin, or hold a sterile specimen cup and void simultaneously. A parent or nurse can help these children. For the child's feelings of increased dependence or modesty, the nurse must explain in a matter-of-fact way the need for the specimen and additional assistance. For a routine urine specimen, the child's perineal area should be clean and washed with soap and water if necessary. Cleansing for a clean-catch specimen is done by holding apart the labia on a girl and cleansing with separate applicators (cotton or wipes), going from outside to inside and from front to back. The specimen must be obtained before releasing the labia. A boy has the foreskin retracted and the penile area cleansed before voiding. Solutions for cleansing vary with facilities. They range from liquid soap and water to an iodine solution. A clean-catch specimen must be collected in a sterile container and sent to the laboratory as soon as possible.

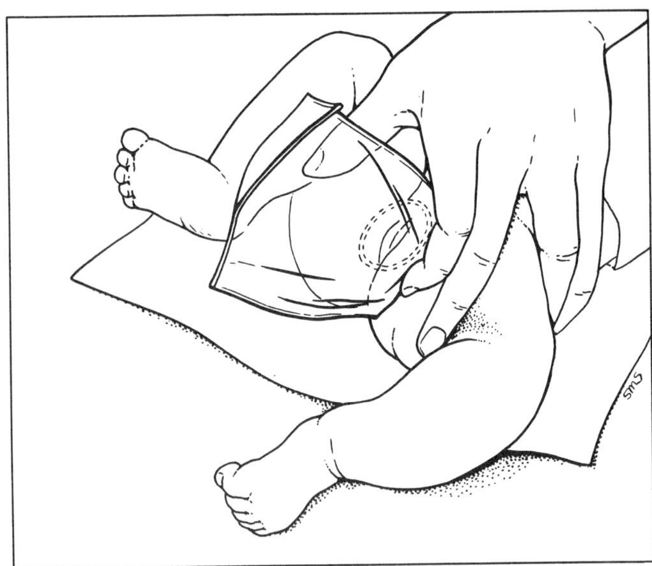

Figure 29-5 Application of a pediatric urine collector.

Urine Collection With the Incontinent Child A specimen can be obtained in various ways from an infant or an incontinent child. In some facilities, plastic wrap may be used as a diaper, especially for premature infants. The urine is collected easily in the plastic, and the nurse can quickly determine whether the infant has voided. The plastic should not remain too long in place, however, as it could contribute to skin breakdown. The crib mattress is placed in Fowler's position to aid the collection of urine in the loose part of the diaper. After the child voids, the diaper is removed and the specimen collected.

Collection Bag Application A pediatric urine-collecting device that fits over the perineal area of the child commonly is used (Fig. 29-5). The open end has an adhesive backing that adheres to the skin. In the most experienced of hands, however, the collective device sometimes fails to adhere adequately, and the desired urine specimen is found in the child's diaper. Unless the skin in the perineal area is broken down, the bag may be reapplied. Several steps and precautions will help prevent the trauma to the skin and the child of any unnecessary reapplications. These are described in Table 29-8.

Urine collectors are available in various sizes in clean or sterile packaging. For collecting a 24-hour urine specimen, they come with tubes extending from the collectors. The tube may either be drained at intervals or, when urine flow is moderate to large, they may be connected to a closed-drainage system.

Specific Gravity Determination To test for specific gravity on an incontinent child, the nurse can use a sample obtained from a pediatric urine-collecting bag. Some nurses have use of a refractometer on their units, and only a few drops of urine are needed for the test. Withdrawing urine from a wet diaper by using a syringe without a needle has been found to give an accurate specific gravity value in tests with a specific brand of diaper (Pampers) (Strohbach and Kratina, 1982). Nurses can repeat the study on the brand of diaper used in their facility. Aspirating urine from a child's diaper for specific gravity determinations saves the child the discomfort of urine bag applications and relieves the nurse of a time-consuming procedure.

Urine Collection With the Continent Child For a continent child, the nurse works in a more cooperative way with the child or parent in obtaining a specimen. The child needs an age-appropriate explanation concerning the purpose and method of obtaining the needed sample. Some children can voluntarily give a urine sample, even when only partially toilet trained. One mother, upon learning that a urine sample was needed from her 18-month-old hospitalized child, asked the child to "tinkle" in a specimen container. The child had been wearing a diaper in the hospital, but within a minute and with no tears or protest, the child was able to give the sample.

Stool Specimens A stool specimen is usually easy to obtain from an incontinent child. Scraping a soiled diaper with a tongue blade to obtain a specimen is all that is needed in most cases. When a stool specimen cannot be contaminated with urine, the nurse will have to observe the diaper carefully to determine whether or not the specimen can be used. A continent child can use a bedpan placed either on a bed or a toilet seat. A child will usually be embarrassed about giving the sample to the nurse or telling the nurse about the sample. Children need to understand, as well as they are able, the rationale for collection of the specimen. They may need help dealing with their feelings about the

TABLE 29-8 Application of Pediatric Urine-Collecting Bag

Procedure	Rationale
Clean and dry the skin before application	Aids adherence of device
Place child supine with hips abducted	Provides clear access to perineal area. Stretches skin and helps eliminate skin folds
With girl, position lower center of opening in perineal area below urinary meatus. With boy, position penis inside collecting device	Proper positioning helps ensure collection of specimen and comfort of child
Remove paper backing from lower portion of bag and apply smoothly from back to front	Smooth application helps prevent wrinkles through which urine can leak
Remove paper backing from upper portion of collecting device and continue to apply without wrinkles	(See above)
Inspect for any loose areas	Reinforcement or immediate reapplication can save discomfort and delay
Tape may be used to reinforce bag if necessary	Pressure of urine filling the bag may loosen adherence
Diaper, if applied at all, should either be loose around the device or should have a hole made with the bag extended through the hole	Tight diapering will encourage the bag's overfilling at the upper portion and coming loose from the skin. When diapering is loose, it is exposed to less pressure from the diaper. When bag extends through the diaper, the child's voiding can be observed and the bag removed immediately

odor and about viewing the shape and color of the stool. The nurse's casual, straightforward handling of the situation will help the child accept the procedure as a necessary but minor part of the hospital care.

Medicating a Child

Medicating children differs from medicating adults in many ways. First are the physical differences beyond the obvious difference in height and weight between the small child and the adult. Second, the mechanics of administering medications must be adapted to the child's changing characteristics and capabilities. Third, in teaching and other measures, the nurse takes into account the child's cognitive level and emotional needs. Although variations among adults mean that medication administration must always be painstakingly individualized, the variations between adults and children are still more pronounced.

Physiologic Differences Between Adults and Children If children were simply small but with the body composition and function of adults, pediatric dosages could be converted from adult dosages based on a child's weight. Although dosages are often estimated in this manner, the differences between child and adult are far more complex.

Physiologic differences are many. Particularly in the neonatal period, the immaturity of body systems renders the effects of medication administration less predictable and riskier for the child. This is less true of the child over 2, as many body systems then function at close to adult levels.

Diluting Effect The young child's body mass is less than an adult's since the body surface area is greater in relation to weight and a far greater proportion of the child's body weight is water. A substantially greater proportion of this water is extracellular fluid, while most of an adult's fluid is within body cells. The child's metabolic rate is higher, and the by-products of metabolism are excreted with the aid of the kidneys. This, in addition to the infant's inability to concentrate urine efficiently, leads to a high turnover of body fluids (see Chapter 33). These three factors have a diluting effect on some medications and may mean that the dosage required is higher than would be expected from calculating the medication dosage by using the child's weight.

Permeability of Membranes The child's kidneys are not the only immature body organ or system. The permeability of membranes affecting the skin and the blood–brain barrier is also increased. Thus such topical medications as corticosteroids are more likely to be absorbed by the infant or young child, leading to the possibility of systemic effects and drug toxicity. The nurse must be especially careful to rinse off cleansing or other solutions that do not need to remain on the young child's skin. Topical medications should be applied in a very thin layer and to as few areas of the child's body as necessary. Certain medications such as lipid-soluble anesthetics and analgesics are more likely to be absorbed by the brain, yielding an increase of central nervous system effects and possible toxicity.

Absorption of Oral Medication Gastrointestinal immaturity affects use of oral medications. Ingested substances have a decreased transit time through the intestines of the small child. The neonate lacks the gastric acid, intestinal flora, and enzymatic function needed in medication digestion; the infant gradually acquires these functions. For these reasons, absorption of oral medications is less efficient in the infant and young child.

Binding to Plasma Proteins and Drug Receptors Some drugs bind with plasma proteins. Binding is lower in the infant, especially in the neonate, leaving more of the circulating drug available for systemic effects. Other drugs act by combining with an enzyme or cellular component. Certain receptors in the young child have an increased affinity for drugs while others have a decreased affinity. This may explain the child's need for a lower-than-expected dose for some drugs and a higher-than-expected dose for others. For instance, the child often needs a higher dose of digoxin per unit of body weight than does the adult.

Medicating a child, particularly a neonate, requires extreme care. Drug dosages, given for therapeutic purposes without untoward effects, may need to be higher or lower than a proportion of an adult dose, which has been based on the proportion of the child's weight to the weight of an average adult. Illness accompanied by dehydration, acid–base, or electrolyte imbalance can further complicate the expected effect of a medication on a child. The nurse therefore constantly assesses the child for desired and undesired effects of any medication.

Dosage Formulas Information about recommended medication dosages, for a child of a particular age and weight, should be available to the nurse. Most pediatric medications are prescribed in milligrams per kilogram of body weight per 24 hours. A hospital formulary or other pharmacologic reference is a reliable source of information to aid the nurse in evaluating the safety of a dose. The hospital pharmacy can help clarify questions of dose and medication compatibility. With the stated qualifications and precautions, the nurse also should be familiar with formulas for calculating pediatric dosages. No formula, however, can accurately and consistently determine safe and effective medication dosage for the child, but the following methods give the nurse a rough guide to the safety of a dose. These formulas are for use with the child over age 2.

1. *Clark's rule.* Clark's rule for young children uses body weight of a child in comparison with the recommended adult dosage and the average adult weight (assumed to be 150 pounds).

$$\text{Estimated child's dosage} = \frac{\text{weight (lb) of child}}{150\text{ lb}} \times \text{adult dosage}$$

2. *Body surface calculation.* Body surface area is considered to be a more accurate means of calculating pediatric dosages. Body surface area is estimated when the child's height and weight are plotted on nomogram (Fig. 29-6). Nomograms are found in most standard pediatric medical and nursing texts. The average adult is considered to have a body surface area of 1.7 square meters.

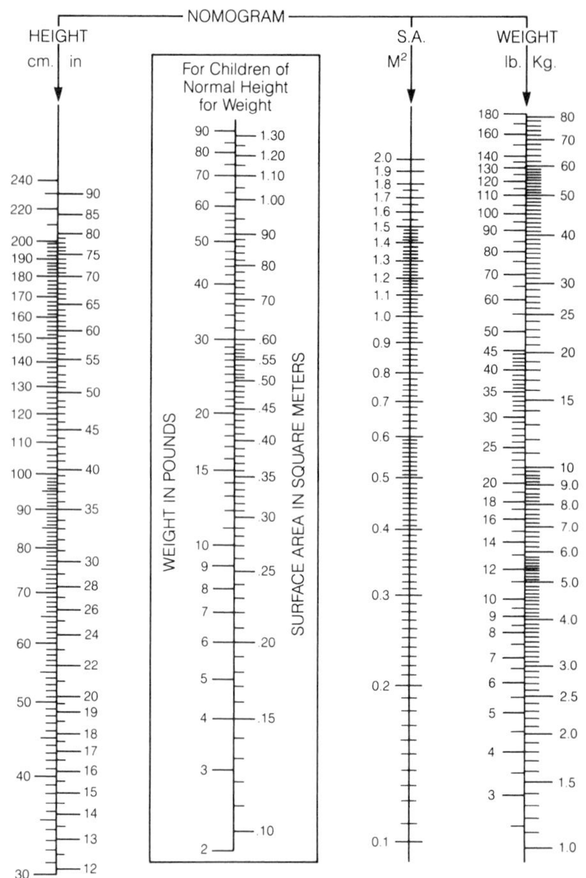

Figure 29-6 Nomogram with estimated body surface area. A straight line is drawn between the child's height and weight. The point at which the line intersects the surface area column is the estimated body surface area. (Courtesy of the Commonwealth Fund and Harvard University.)

$$\text{Estimated child's dosage} = \frac{\text{surface area of child (m}^2\text{)}}{1.7\text{ m}^2} \times \text{adult dosage}$$

Oral Medication Administration Special considerations for oral medications center around the child's abilities to suck, drink, and swallow and around the small measurements necessary for liquid medications. Some children may take liquid medications from a small cup or spoon. Many infants and children need to have a medication placed directly into the mouth. This can often be accomplished with a syringe. The medication is drawn up in a syringe without a needle. The tip of the syringe should be placed midway back at the side of the child's mouth. By using this position, the child is less likely to gag when the medication is administered or to expel the medication from the mouth with a syringe. The medication is drawn up in a syringe without a needle. The tip of the syringe should be placed easily and is not in danger of aspirating. When an infant will suck from a nipple, the nipple can be placed in the child's mouth, and as the child begins to suck, the liquid medication can be placed into the nipple from a needleless syringe. This is a very simple, pleasant way to administer liquid medication to an infant. Despite the convenience, however, another method should be used for unpleasant tasting medication, so the infant will not associate the unpleasant taste with the nipple.

Measurement of liquid medications must be accurate and performed with a standard measurement source. A graduated medicine cup is acceptable if the markings match the amount of medication needed and no estimation is necessary. Measurement of small amounts of liquid medications can be accurately performed with some graduated cylinders or with a syringe. Some facilities have use of less expensive, nonsterile oral syringes for this purpose. Measuring spoons specifically made for accurate medication measurement and administration are commercially available, and many parents find these useful. The nurse does not use a household tableware teaspoon or tablespoon and so instructs parents to follow the same principle. These household spoons vary in their actual size, and their use could lead to overmedication or undermedication of a child. Standard measuring spoons are appropriate for medication administration in the home.

Some oral medications do not come in a liquid but are instead in tablet or capsule form. Some very young children can and will swallow pills while many older children and adolescents have not mastered the skill. A careful history usually determines the children who can safely swallow pills and capsules. If such a history is not available, the nurse can show the medication to the child and ask the child whether swallowing it is possible. Liquid medication may be available for the child who needs it, but often the nurse can alter the form of a pill or capsule so that a child can swallow it. Some medications have an enteric coating to prevent irritation to or deterioration in the child's stomach. These medications must be swallowed whole. The nurse needs to request another form of the medication for the child unable to swallow them. If the medication does not have an enteric coating, a child may choose to chew or the nurse may crush or dissolve the medication. Crushed medication may be placed in food or drink with which it does not adversely react.

Medication is mixed with the smallest possible amount of food or fluid to help ensure the child's taking the entire dose. Despite attempts to make the mixture palatable, it is likely to retain some of the medication's taste, and even a hungry or thirsty child would have difficulty consuming a moderate or large amount. The altered medication must be presented to the child honestly and not as food or a treat.

Topical Medication Administration When any medication is administered from a dropper or tube, the nurse must be careful not to touch the child with the applicator. Such contact could cause injury or contamination to the child or applicator.

Ophthalmic Instillations Eye drops are administered to children as they are to adults. The child is positioned so that the head is back. The child should look up while the nurse gently retracts the lower conjunctival sac. Moving the dropper from the outside below the child's line of vision may help prevent the child's blinking. As the drops are instilled, the dropper is held 1–2 cm above the middle to outer portion of the conjunctival sac. The nurse applies pressure for several seconds to the nasolacrimal duct to prevent medication from being lost through the nose. Absorption is increased if the child's eyes remain closed, and the child doesn't blink. After the medication has bathed the eye, the child can resume activities. Ophthalmic ointment is applied in the same manner with 2 cm of ointment squeezed from the tube onto the conjunctival sac. The child may then close the eyes and in so doing will spread the medication. When a child will not hold the eyes open, the nurse can place a liquid medication on the inner corner of the closed eye. Then when the eyes are opened, the medication spreads across the eyes.

Otic Instillations Solutions for the ear are administered with the child's head on the side so that the affected ear is uppermost. For the child under the age of 3, the pinna is gently pulled down and back, thus straightening the external auditory canal. With a child over the age of 3, as with the adult, the pinna is pulled up and back. The child remains with the head to the side for several minutes after the instillation of medication to help ensure the medication's bathing the entire external canal and reaching the eardrum. To aid in the spread of the medication, the nurse can apply gentle pressure and massage the outer ear after medication is instilled.

Nasal Instillations Before nasal instillations, the nasal passages should be cleared by the child's blowing the nose or the nurse's using a bulb syringe. The head is hyperextended. With an infant or young child, the child's head can be positioned over one of the nurse's arms, with the arm and hand also used to restrain the child as necessary. Holding the infant's or young child's head in a lateral, though lowered, position can help prevent swallowing, with resulting increased absorption of the medication. After nasal drops are instilled, the child should keep the head back for 5–10 minutes for the medication to be effective.

Dermatologic Medication Administration Dermatologic medication administration is similar with children and adults. Since the young child's skin is more permeable, there is increased risk for medication absorption and resultant systemic effects. The nurse is especially careful to apply a thin layer of medication and confine it to those portions of skin where it is essential. The nurse assesses the child for signs and symptoms of systemic effects of the medication.

Rectal Medication Administration The rectal route of medication administration is very useful in children, often avoiding subjecting a child to an injection and providing needed medication when fluids are not well tolerated as is the case preoperatively, postoperatively, or when a child is vomiting. Medication blood levels subsequent to rectal administration may vary somewhat from those after other routes. Blood levels could be higher, it is thought, because medication absorbed into the venous system of the rectum does not pass through the liver before entering the systemic circulation (Hahn et al., 1982). A medication's absorption could be inhibited if it is embedded in feces in the rectum or expelled before being absorbed.

The child needs to be well prepared emotionally as well as physically. The rectal route is invasive and often embarrassing to the child. The nurse focuses on the purpose of the medication to decrease fantasies and increase understanding; how the medication will feel when being inserted; and what the child can do to facilitate the procedure and increase personal comfort. If the child knows the sensation of a suppository's insertion resembles a bowel movement and realizes relaxation will decrease discomfort, the child has increased control over and opportunity for mastery of the situation.

For insertion of a suppository, the child assumes a side-lying position with the upper leg flexed. A very young child may be supine with both legs flexed. With a gloved finger, the nurse inserts the lubricated rounded end of the suppository past the rectal sphincter and positions it along the wall of the rectum. The suppository is inserted to a depth of 5 cm (2 in) or less for a small child and as much as 10 cm (4 in) for a fully grown child. The finger can then be removed and the child's buttocks gently held together until the child no longer strains or claims the urge to expel the medication. Suppositories may need to be divided to administer a child's correct dose. To increase precision, the nurse may longitudinally split the suppository.

Intravenous Medication Administration The intravenous route has definite advantages for medication administration in children. The intravenous administration of antibiotics, for instance, allows therapy free from repeated painful intramuscular injections. Medication effects can be very rapid and serum levels high.

The route is not without difficulties, however. Many children fear any manipulation of their IVs. Although the child will generally not experience any altered sensation when a medication is given intravenously, the nurse needs to prepare the child for the experience. Some children do mention having a sensation, such as a slight burning, when there is a change in the IV solution, for instance, when medications are added or the maintenance IV is continued after a medication. Children's IVs are often delicate, and placement may be close to the small vein wall. Any movement can dislodge the needle or vary the flow rate of the IV (see Chapter 33). The initial IV insertion is painful and traumatic to most children, and if the IV fails during the course of treatment, the child may have to have another. It is possible, from medication infusing directly into tissues instead of the vein, to cause tissue damage that can be extensive and result in deformity. The nurse assesses carefully for inflammation, infiltration, and patency of the IV before administering any intravenous medication.

There are various methods of intravenous medication administration. Some medications, such as vitamins and electrolytes (for example, potassium), may be added to the child's IV bottle or bag. Frequently, medication is directly added to the child's maintenance IV Soluset. The medication must, in this case, be compatible with the child's maintenance IV solution. The nurse also needs to be aware of how much a medication should be diluted and at what rate it can be safely infused.

Medication generally will need to be infused over time of an hour or less, thus ensuring the medication's administration at the hour required and at its greatest potency. Some medications are supplied in powder form since they are unstable in solution. Ampicillin in solution and at room temperature, for example, begins to decompose within an hour. Such medications must be infused within an hour after reconstitution for the child to receive full therapeutic effect.

For medication to infuse, it must clear both the Soluset (or other calibrated burette) and IV tubing. The tubing contains at least 10 mL of fluid and, with extensions, may contain 15 mL or more. When the Soluset functionally empties (some solution usually remains after solution ceases to drip), fluid must be added to the Soluset and then infused to flush the medication from the tubing. This fluid must be added and begin to flow immediately to prevent clotting of the IV needle at the infusing site. The amount of fluid added depends on the length of the IV tubing and generally ranges from 10–15 mL. The major principle is for the child to receive the full dose of medication at the appropriate time. If a child receives two or more medications consecutively, each medication may need to be flushed before the next is added. This creates a buffer of solution between medications.

When a medication is incompatible with the child's maintenance IV, a compatible solution with its own Soluset and tubing may be piggybacked into a portal in the maintenance IV. After the new IV is attached, it is started and the maintenance solution stopped during the entire course of the medication administration. The tubing must be flushed with the new solution before and after medication, so as to avoid incompatibility of medication and solution.

Sometimes a child receives such a small amount of intravenous fluid, as with a neonate or a child with cardiac or renal disease, that a medication added to a Soluset would not infuse for an hour or more. For these children to receive timely medications, the medication in solution might be injected retrograde into an IV portal close to the child. The medication is injected back up into the tubing with the tubing proximal to the child momentarily clamped. The medication is allowed to mix with the solution in the IV tubing and then to infuse. Thus medication is diluted and infuses more slowly than if it were injected toward the vein or if the tubing were not clamped.

Intramuscular Medication Administration Although the actual technique used with children receiving intramuscular medication is the same as with adults, variations are needed depending on the child's size and muscle development. Because of children's smaller size, an intramuscular injection is often done with a shorter needle; a 1-in needle is a common choice. Because of underdevelopment of the posterior gluteal muscle in a child who has been walking for less than a year, this site is usually avoided in the infant and young child; its use risks injury to the sciatic nerve. It should not be used in the child under the age of 2 and is preferably avoided until the child is over age 4.

Preferred injection sites in the young child are the thigh and the deltoid muscle. The vastus lateralis on the lateral aspect of the thigh or the rectus femoris on the anterior aspect are the usual choices. These are large muscles, and medication is generally well absorbed. Using the thigh as an injection site is not, however, without controversy. Multiple injections in the quadriceps group of the thigh have been linked to quadriceps contracture (Drehobl, 1980). Sites should always be rotated when a child needs repeated injections, and the nurse carefully assesses the tissue perfusion and general condition of the skin.

The deltoid muscle is small but its use has some advantages. Children will sometimes feel it is less invasive than the thigh, and medication is absorbed most quickly from this site. This makes it ideal for giving medication in an emergency or analgesics for the child who is already feeling a high degree of pain. Medication is absorbed somewhat less quickly from the quadriceps of the thigh, and most slowly from the buttocks. Site identification is reviewed in Figure 29-7.

Because of vast differences in size, muscle mass, and subcutaneous tissue, it is especially important to note bony prominences as landmarks for intramuscular injections in children. The muscle mass of the deltoid can be used for aqueous, nonirritating medications; the vastus lateralis for medications except those that stain or are particularly irritating; and the dorsogluteal for any intramuscular medication as long as the child has a well-developed gluteal muscle. If the muscle mass chosen for an injection is small, either the needle used must be 1 in or less or the muscle mass is supported and lifted slightly with one hand during needle insertion. Often it is necessary to both use a short needle and lift the muscle gently to ensure the needle's adequately penetrating the muscle while not striking bone.

The injection and any restraint necessary are first explained to the child. The child is gently but firmly restrained. The injection site is carefully chosen and the area cleansed. Allowing the alcohol to dry helps slightly to minimize the pain of the injection both by eliminating the sting of alcohol as the skin is pierced and reassuring the child the nurse's goal is to make the injection as painless as possible. The skin is quickly pierced with the needle at 90° for an intramuscular injection. The nurse aspirates to clear the needle (0.2 mL when a 1½-in needle is used) to rule out the needle's having entered a blood vessel. Medication is injected at a moderate rate, and then the needle is withdrawn. Except when contraindicated, as with an irritating or anticoagulant medication, the skin should be massaged after the injection. This encourages absorption of the medication and distracts and reassures the child. The nurse and/or parent then must provide appropriate comfort measures.

The entire injection procedure should be as rapid as possible so as to minimize fear, anxiety, and restraint of the child. The nurse, however, must not sacrifice technique for speed. The nurse carefully teaches and explains, selects the appropriate site, and utilizes such necessary methods as the Z track with irritating medications. Some of the most important nursing measures are then comforting, reestablishing a relationship with the child, and providing a means for the child's working through the experience.

Psychosocial Management of Administering Medications Preparing children and adolescents for medications requires the same concepts that the nurse applies to parent and child education. The nurse first needs to be honest in explaining the purpose and necessity of medications. Will the medicine help control infection? Will it reduce pain or fever? The nurse then describes, as accurately as possible, any sensations the child might experience. Does the drug leave a bitter taste in the mouth? Does it hurt and sting as it is injected? An ophthalmic ointment, for example, makes vision blurry for a while. A rectal suppository's insertion feels somewhat as if a bowel movement is taking place. A child prepared for blurry vision will not be as frightened by it. A child prepared for the sensations of having a suppository can relax more during and after its insertion. Children prepared for a bitter taste can gain an appropriate mental set before drinking a medicine, and it is less likely that a child will spit out or refuse to finish a dose and the child can be ready to wash away the taste with a pleasant-tasting food or drink. Children understanding that a medication stings but that an injection itself hurts very little have more mastery over the situation and may better cooperate.

The timing and complexity of preparation depend on the situation as well as the developmental stage of the child. With injections, for example, most older children can learn

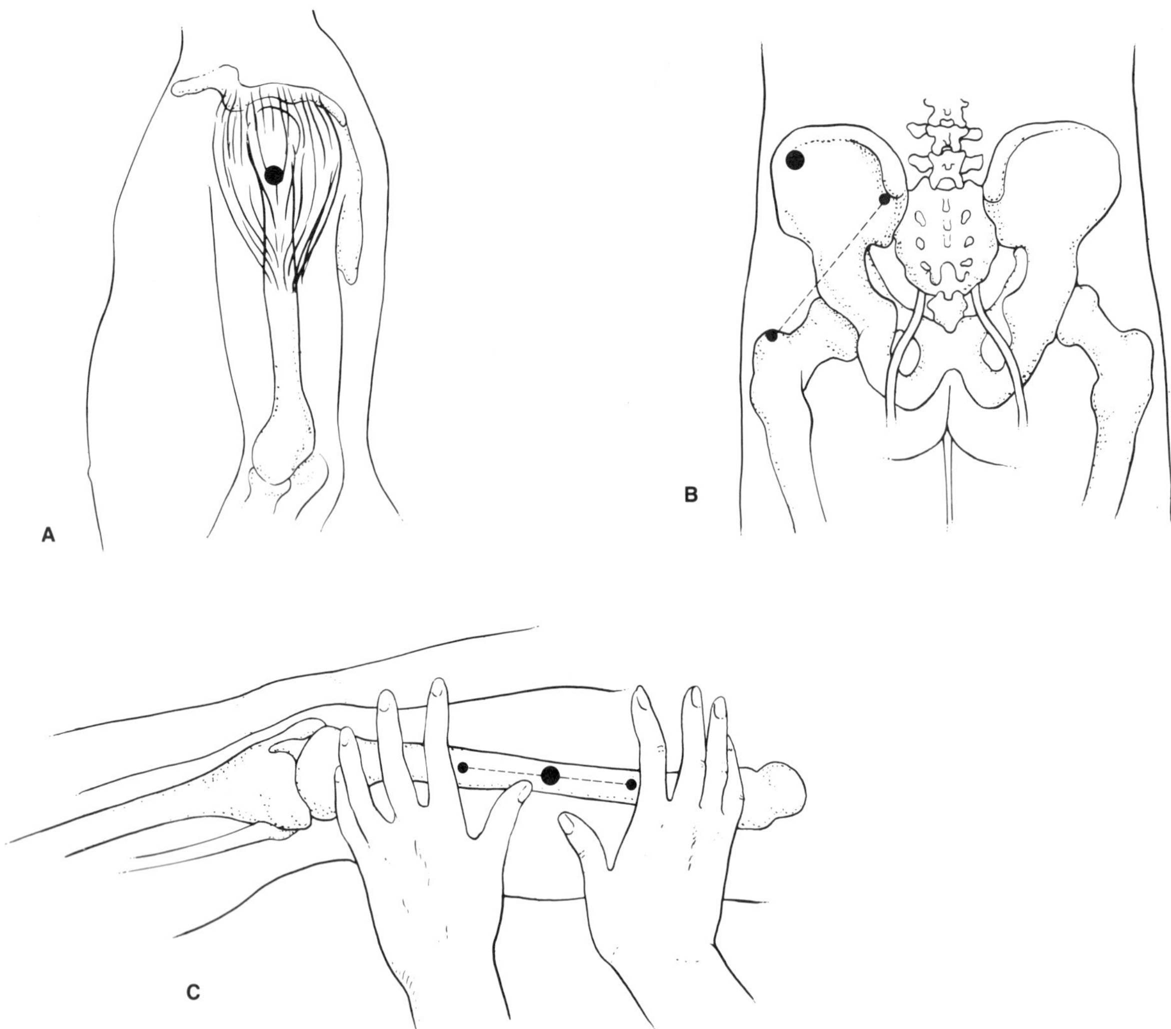

Figure 29-7 Sites for intramuscular injection. *A.* Deltoid muscle. *B.* Dorsogluteal muscle. *C.* Vastus lateralis.

the night before a test or surgery that an injection will be part of the premedication. This knowledge should come at the end of preparatory instruction as it often raises a child's anxiety to a point that prevents understanding of subsequent information. Some children are best prepared immediately before an injection; this is best for the child whose developmental level is below age 3. This is also the case when PRN medications are needed. A child's fears and fantasies then do not have much time to develop. If the child asks whether or not a shot will be given, however, the nurse should always give an honest answer.

The nurse uses historical information and current behavioral assessments to decide when and how to prepare a child. When a child is to learn about an injection right before its occurrence, the nurse needs to guard against inadvertent preparation. The child should not overhear discussions with the family concerning the injection, should not witness the injection's preparation, or see the syringe in the nurse's hand before hearing the nurse's explanation. The child should, however, have a chance to see and touch the syringe before the injection actually takes place, as this is a part of the preparation.

Mastery and cooperation during the medication administration increase when children know what is expected of them, exactly what they are supposed to do, and what the nurse's role is. A child needs to know that holding still and trying to relax can make an injection less painful. The child also needs to know that the nurse wants no movement during an injection or expects the child to hold the head back and look up for instillation of ophthalmic ointment. When the child understands the nurse's purpose, misinterpretation of nursing actions is less likely. It is helpful to describe actions in ways such as, "I'm going to put my hand on your leg to help you hold still. Now I'm cleaning the skin with alcohol. I'll let it dry so that the shot will hurt less."

Even an infant can be prepared for a medication. The nurse automatically looks at, talks to, and touches an infant when giving an oral or topical medication; for an injection, the nurse also needs to remember to talk to and touch an infant. Going through a very simple verbal explanation, such as saying the infant is going to get a shot and that it will hurt, as the skin is cleansed will do no harm, and this kind of intervention may in fact help the child relax.

When time allows, a child benefits from age-appropriate therapeutic play before the experience (see Chapter 28). Adolescents too need to "play" by seeing, touching, and manipulating such equipment as syringes. When therapeutic play is not possible prior to the injection, it is needed afterward so that the child can work out feelings and is able to clarify thoughts about a medication. Playing and talking through the experience also can improve a child's coping skills by allowing expression of fears and feelings, thus turning a passive situation into an active one. The nurse can use these sessions to teach children more effective coping mechanisms. A child can then practice positive coping behaviors such as squeezing a hand instead of hitting the nurse or such as saying "ouch" rather than screaming.

For some children, medication is a way of life, and very little is demanded of the nurse either in preparation or in setting limits. For other children, even drinking an oral medication is traumatic. After an appropriate explanation, the nurse may need to set firm, though gentle, limits on the child. The 2-year-old almost always offers the proverbial "no" to any suggested activity. The child around age 4 is particularly adept at offering countless, seemingly plausible excuses to delay or prevent medication, such as, "It doesn't hurt at all now. I need to go to the bathroom. Right now!" Although an anxiety-raising experience may cause a child to feel the need to void and there may be rare occasions when a nurse should allow the child to do so before being medicated, a child can almost always be medicated first. Delay simply serves to raise a child's anxiety level even further. Preparation time then becomes lengthy, and the confusion causes the child to question who is the adult. The nurse's setting appropriate limits helps control the child's fears as well as the situation.

Children need a role in the medication process, and they can have a degree of independence and make decisions. The 4-year-old who shouldn't be allowed to use the bathroom before receiving an injection can choose, within appropriate limits, the injection site. A child can tell a nurse to give a shot on the count of 3 and can do the counting. A child can hold a medication cup or have a parent actually give an oral or dermatologic medication. An older child or adolescent may be able to help plan the timing of medications so as not to interfere with rest or activities.

Sometimes a nurse will need to provide physical limits for a child. With an infant, the nurse can cradle the child's head while administering oral medications. An older infant or young child may need to have the head held firmly and can be encouraged to open the mouth with the gentle pressure of one hand. Medication is administered slowly, and the child's head is somewhat elevated to prevent choking. Oral medication should not be forced on the totally uncooperative child. This is prohibited because of dangers of aspiration. It is also harmful to the child's relationship with the nurse and encourages feelings of helplessness and rebellion. The nurse can reteach and prepare the child and can search for new, creative nursing approaches. Perhaps a child will take medication if it is offered by a parent or if the nurse will read a story afterward. As a last resort, the nurse can attempt to have the route of administration changed.

When restraint is needed for topical administration, the methods used are similar to those used for oral administrations. When additional assistance is needed for eye, ear, or nose instillations in the infant or young child, the nurse can place the child in a mummy restraint. Unless the child is an infant comforted by the restraint, it is released as soon as the child is allowed to move freely.

For parenteral administration of medications, the nurse frequently needs the assistance of another person or other persons to restrain the child safely. The child needs to remain still, with hands not interfering, and the injection site must be immobilized. So as not to be overwhelming, as few people as necessary should approach the child. A child's parent or other visitor should never be asked to restrain a child. Many are very upset seeing their child receive an injection or any treatment causing pain. Some do not wish to stay in the room and watch, and some will even leave the unit during painful procedures. Asking to restrain and thus help with the injection unnecessarily exposes them to anxiety and a guilt-producing experience. If parents or other visitors wish to stay with a child and if the child so desires, they can stay near the child's head, hold a hand, and comfort the child. Many will repeat the nurse's teaching, encouraging the child to hold still and reassuring the child that the injection is necessary and will soon be over.

The last and perhaps most important nursing measures in medicating a child are comforting, building self-esteem, and establishing or reestablishing a trusting relationship after medication administration. In a developmentally appropriate way, the nurse comforts the child. This is very important following all pain-causing interventions. The nurse picks up, hugs, talks to, and perhaps rocks the infant and young child. Even an adolescent may need and enjoy a hug. Holding the child's hand and perhaps expressing unhappiness at causing pain can help. Despite the importance of specific teaching and play techniques, it is the relationship between the child and nurse that to a large degree determines the child's acceptance of and cooperation with necessary medications and treatments. The nurse's expressing personal feelings, learning about the child's feelings, and spending time with the child, time beyond that needed for physical nursing care, forms a basis for a healthy relationship.

Isolation Procedures

Pediatric adaptations for isolation techniques center around variations in children's developmental levels, their abilities to understand and cooperate with isolation procedures, and the feelings, fears, fantasies, and needs brought about by these procedures. Young children tend to touch anything and everything within reach. When enteric precautions are necessary for young children, the nurse considers the child's general environment contaminated and should wear gloves for direct patient care. Table 29-9 outlines basic isolation procedures.

When isolation is prescribed, a child is likely to experience, and in fact suffer from, extremes of sensory alteration. Most common is sensory deprivation. Children often cannot leave their rooms or beds and so cannot join in group activities or natural socialization available to them on the unit. The difficulties, time, and energy involved in gowning and gloving are not great, but they tend to discourage frequent, short visits from nurses and thus reduce opportunities for talk and play. Nurses need to guard against appearing at the child's bedside only for treatments, procedures, and necessary hygienic care. They need to plan time for other aspects of a child's care and allow time for reading, playing, or simply being near the child.

For isolation practices, children need explanations geared to their developmental levels. Particularly in middle childhood, the child can interpret such practices as punishment and proof of "badness." The nurse needs to avoid use of words that feed these fantasies by seeing to it that children hear encouragement for cooperation with treatments without hearing the expressions "good girl" or "good boy." These reinforce the idea the child is bad. (Stressors associated with isolation are discussed in Chapter 27.)

As children grow, they do separate their individual actions from their concepts of self. A "good job" is not the same as a good boy or girl, and so this expression may be used. There are very fine lines between these expressions. Rather than telling children that cooperation with the treatment plan will make them "better," they can hear that such actions will make them well so that they can go home and play as they did before. Ultimately, nurses need to rely on the overall relationship with a child to reassure, comfort, and clarify that illness is not a punishment. The nurse first observes the child's general behavior as well as specific responses to words, explanations, and teaching. Play can then greatly assist the nurse in understanding the impact of isolation on the child and in teaching the true meaning of isolation (see Chapter 28).

Both visitors and children need appropriate explanations. Many parents resist the imposed barriers of gown, gloves, or mask between them and their children, as they are accustomed to and often highly value close physical contact and directly touching the child. When a child has a medical condition or treatment that the parent considers serious (for example, a bone marrow transplant or an extensive burn), the parent may freely and eagerly cooperate with these restrictions. When a child has a condition the parent does not consider serious, cooperation may be less complete. The nurse attempts to learn the parent's perceptions of the child's illness and isolation. Denial and guilt may be contributing to a parent's lack of cooperation with isolation measures. Teaching the necessary components of and reasons for isolation may need to be repeated frequently.

Postoperative Care

The adaptations of postoperative care for children depend on psychologic as well as physical differences. An operation, regardless of its extent, alters a child's body image. An incision exists; a child moves from a relatively independent to a dependent condition. The nurse focuses on increasing a child's independence and expressing feelings.

Many children do not fully understand preoperative teaching until they are required to participate in postoperative nursing interventions. The child needs a repetition of preoperative teaching and preoperative play opportunities. Postoperatively, the nurse may need to reteach the purposes of the IV, coughing and deep breathing, catheters, tubes, and other postoperative care measures. The nurse needs to reemphasize their use and thereby defuse feelings of punishment, anger, helplessness, and dependence.

Children's postoperative play is adjusted to individual feelings, responses to suggestions, and opportunities for play. Many children in the early postoperative period need rest and quiet companionship. Play then centers around entertainment and activities familiar to the child. Soon many children are ready for expressive, creative play. Paints and clay are usually well accepted, as these give a child opportunities to work out frustrations and anger. Many children do not draw in the postoperative phase of hospitalization, but they can be encouraged to express themselves through other art media, and also stories and dramatic play. Many of these same children express themselves through drawing when they are seen for follow-up care.

Some hospitalized children do make good use of drawing. For instance, a 5-year-old girl was unavoidably not visited by her family from the day of surgery until discharged from the hospital after her tonsillectomy and adenoidectomy. The day after surgery, she was very withdrawn and expressed little emotion. She was not able to talk about her surgery and didn't seem to listen to reassurances. She did not play and would not accept oral fluids. Her nurse asked her to draw a picture with available materials, a tray, place mat, and pen. The child drew her family, and she left herself out of the picture. Nursing reassurances could then be focused. She was assured that her parents missed her and would soon come to take her home. The child was then better able to play and drink, and when her parents did arrive, she cried and eventually laughed and smiled.

Physical care for the child after surgery includes the same optimal care measures used for the adult. Several considerations specific to children's physiologic immaturities are outlined in Table 29-10.

TABLE 29-9 Recommended Types of Isolation and Precautions

Type of isolation	Purpose	Private room	Gowns	Masks	Gloves	Articles
Strict	To prevent the transmission of pathogens spread both by contact and by airborne sources	Necessary; door must be kept closed	Must be worn by all persons entering room	Must be worn by all persons entering room	Must be worn by all persons entering room	Discard or wrap before sending to central supply for disinfection or sterilization
Respiratory	To prevent airborne infection and contaminated articles (eg, tissues) from respiratory droplets that are coughed, sneezed, or exhaled	Necessary; door must be kept closed	Not necessary	Must be worn by all persons entering room	Not necessary	Discard or disinfect articles contaminated with secretions
Protective (Reverse Isolation or Barrier Technique)	To protect an uninfected patient with lowered resistance from any pathogens in the environment	Necessary; door must be kept closed	Must be worn by all persons entering room	Must be worn by all persons entering room	Must be worn by all persons having direct contact with the patient; use sterile gloves for burn patients	Sterilize some articles that come in direct contact with the patient prior to use, eg, linen for a burn patient
Enteric	To prevent the transmission of pathogens in the feces	Necessary for children only	Must be worn by all persons having direct contact with the patient	Not necessary	Must be worn by all persons having direct contact with infected area or articles contaminated by fecal material	Disinfect or discard articles contaminated with urine and feces using special precautions
Wound and Skin	To prevent the transmission of pathogens transmitted by direct contact with wounds or articles contaminated by wounds (eg, dressings or linen)	Desirable	Must be worn by all persons having direct contact with the patient	Not necessary except during dressing changes	Must be worn by all persons having direct contact with the infected area	Special precautions are necessary for instruments, dressings, and linen
Blood	To prevent the transmission of organisms carried by blood or blood products	Depends on disease entity	Depends on disease entity	Not necessary	Depends on disease entity	Dispose of all needles in a box clearly labeled as precaution. Extreme caution needed to prevent accidental skin puncture. Label specimens for laboratory
Secretions	To prevent the spread of organisms transmitted through saliva and mucous secretions	Depends on disease entity	Not necessary	Depends on disease entity	Necessary when handling linen, dishes, tissues and other contaminated articles	Use disposable dishes or wrap and send for sterilization. Special precaution necessary for all tissues, linens, and other articles that come in contact with body secretions

NOTE: For all types of isolation the hands must be washed on entering and leaving the room.

SOURCE: Adapted from Kozier B, Erb G: *Fundamentals of Nursing*. 2nd ed. Addison-Wesley, 1983.

TABLE 29-10 Postoperative Checklist for Physiologic Needs

Body system	Assessment/management	Rationale
Respiratory	Assess airway patency	Child may show signs of a deepened anesthesia effect even after return from the recovery room; aspiration after vomiting is possible
	Assess quality of respirations for adventitious sounds and for depth and symmetry	Pooling of secretions can lead to pneumonia; inadequate air exchange is possible because of pain and inactivity; atelectasis may occur
	Assess vital signs	Increased respiratory rate can indicate respiratory distress or infection; increased temperature in the first few days after surgery usually indicates respiratory infection
	Encourage adequate deep breathing and, if not contraindicated by the surgical procedure, coughing. Use play as appropriate to encourage child; time pain relief measures so that child is as comfortable as possible before attempting deep breathing and coughing	Encourages adequate air exchange and loosens secretions; a slightly elevated temperature will often decrease after adequate coughing and deep breathing; coughing after certain ear, nose, throat and plastic surgeries could cause stress to the surgical repair
Circulatory	Check incisional site or dressing for bleeding	Observable bleeding may be first indication of hemorrhage
	After ear, nose and throat surgery, observe for oozing of blood from the nose; examine the back of child's throat for bleeding; observe for frequent swallowing	
	After genitourinary surgery, observe for clots and obvious or occult blood in the urine	Bleeding is expected after certain GU surgeries but should decrease in time as healing takes place (see Chapter 39)
	After gastrointestinal surgery, observe for blood in stool or vomitus	Blood in the stool is expected during the healing phase after certain surgeries (see Chapter 38)
	After orthopedic surgery, observe for bleeding on cast, dressing, or splint; outline any staining on cast, date and mark time	Some oozing may occur after surgery (see Chapter 41); a rapid increase in staining can indicate hemorrhage
	After neurologic surgery, observe neurologic signs and checks (see Chapter 42)	Increased intracranial pressure can be a sign of internal bleeding
	After gynecologic surgery, observe for vaginal bleeding	Abnormal vaginal bleeding can occur while abdominal dressings remain dry and intact
	Monitor vital signs	An increase followed by a decrease in blood pressure occurs with hemorrhage; the pulse rate increases as a compensation for decreased circulating blood volume
	Provide optimal oral or parenteral fluid intake (see Chapter 33) by monitoring the IV, encouraging oral fluids when the child is taking p.o.s, monitoring specific gravity of urine, monitoring volume of urine output, assessing for signs of overhydration such as puffiness around the eyes or moist rales (see Chapter 33), and assessing for electrolyte imbalances and monitor laboratory values (see Chapter 33)	Fluid needs vary with age and weight of child; because of postoperative sequestering and diuresis of fluids and immaturities in newborn and infant body systems, postoperative fluid needs for the infant may be considered to be 100 mL/kg body weight for 24 hours; in the absence of cardiac or renal disease, specific gravity is an excellent indicator of hydration status; urine output, in the absence of cardiac and renal disease or urinary retention, mirrors circulating blood volume and hydration status, and lowered output can be an early indicator of impending shock. A child may become overhydrated from parenteral or oral fluids, and the infant is especially prone to fluid and electrolyte imbalances; children are prone to imbalances, particularly to metabolic acidosis, and close, careful assessment is necessary
Gastrointestinal	Assess for returning motility by monitoring bowel sounds, flatus, absence of nausea or vomiting, first bowel movement after surgery, and frequency, quality, and quantity of stools	Depending on the individual child, intraoperative manipulation, and actual procedures done on the gastrointestinal tract, motility can return postoperatively at varying times; giving oral fluids before they can be assimilated leads to distention

TABLE 29-10 continued

Body system	Assessment/management	Rationale
	Measure abdominal girth and note or place a mark on the anatomic location of this measure	When abdominal distention is suspected or anticipated, nursing assessment of abdominal girth must be consistent
	Monitor status of nasogastric tube, if in place (see Chapter 38)	Nasogastric tube prevents distention when gastrointestinal motility is impaired
	When oral fluids can be started, begin them very slowly. Start with easily assimilated fluids, such as water followed by bland clear fluids (flat carbonated beverages, ice pops)	Slow introduction of fluids may prevent or lessen postoperative nausea or vomiting
	After abdominal surgery hold apple juice or strained orange juice until fluid intake is well established. Assess acceptance of fluids by monitoring for nausea, vomiting, abdominal distention, or diarrhea. With adverse signs or symptoms, return child to NPO status or to a more bland diet	These may not be well accepted with some children and may lead to cramping or diarrhea
Genitourinary	Measure first voiding after surgery; monitor total output; monitor voiding pattern. Observe for patency of drainage tubes (see Chapter 39)	Anesthesia and other medications may lead to retention of urine; inadequate volume of void can be a sign of urinary retention with overflow
Musculoskeletal	Turn every 2–4 hours, have the child ambulate as soon as possible, encourage increasing ambulation and mobility; provide range-of-motion exercises and other activity within medical restrictions	Helps prevent skin breakdown and pooling of respiratory secretions, promotes gastrointestinal and genitourinary mobility, muscle strength, and venous return. Formal range-of-motion exercises are not always needed with temporary immobility
	Assess skin in general. Assess wound area for redness, quantity and nature of drainage, excessive warmth dehiscence, or evisceration. Correlate with vital signs	The child, as well as the adult, may have red, irritated areas, and skin breakdown may occur. Wound infections or complications must be evaluated as quickly as possible. An increase in temperature after the first few postoperative days is usually indicative of a wound infection

Key Concepts

- Child and family teaching need to be individually planned to facilitate adjustment to hospitalization and to promote health after discharge.
- The first steps in child and family teaching are assessing what the child and family know and determining what they need to know, discussing what most concerns them, and identifying usual coping strategies.
- Teaching for both parents and children requires honest explanations, appropriate limits, a stated purpose, carefully chosen words, time between sessions, adjustment for developmental stage, and reinforcement of learning.
- Preparation for specific procedures or treatments should be individually designed, include opportunities for play, and describe the sensations the child will experience.
- The timing and content of preadmission teaching should be age appropriate and specific to the hospital and should involve as much parental participation as possible.
- Because preadmission teaching does not always bring reassurance, nurses need to assess anxiety levels and identify specific needs for additional preparation and emotional care.
- Hospital orientation includes touring the facilities on the unit, acquainting the child and family with the space allotted to them, and respecting their needs for personal possessions and privacy.
- Parents should always be included in preoperative preparation and postoperative care and may choose to take part in preoperative play and age-appropriate explanations of procedures and anticipated bodily changes.
- Discharge preparation requires assessment of physical, psychosocial, and developmental needs.

- In preparing the child and family for discharge, the nurse's teaching plan may include step-by-step demonstrations, recommended changes in the home environment, and adjustments in nutrition, behavioral expectations, and activity patterns.
- Hospitalization may provide an opportunity for a thorough nutritional assessment and appropriate child and family teaching, which may be accompanied by explanations about temporary changes in nutritional needs.
- Children who have nothing by mouth require special nursing attention during mealtimes.
- Feeding patterns for a hospitalized infant should, as much as possible, approximate feeding patterns at home.
- Mothers may need encouragement and assistance to continue breast-feeding hospitalized infants.
- The mealtime environment should be as homelike as possible and is best located away from rooms and equipment associated with painful procedures.
- Small portions of food, special utensils, and mealtime companionship encourage children to eat and help to avoid a child's tendency to use food as a means of control.
- Fluid intake is best managed with the cooperation of both the family and the child and with fluid given at planned intervals to encourage or limit intake, as required.
- For young children who are learning toileting skills, the nurse supports the child and family's efforts and explains that any regression is normal and temporary.
- Older children who need assistance with toileting may require special attention to their needs for privacy and modesty.
- The nurse may help a child to sleep by following the child's accustomed bedtime rituals, when possible, and by managing pain relief and activity to promote comfort and rest.
- Preventive measures to promote skin integrity and activity help to avoid complications of immobility that involve the skin, muscles, tendons, cardiovascular, and respiratory systems.
- Additional intake of fluids and fruits and monitored intake of calcium help to prevent gastrointestinal and genitourinary complications of immobility.
- Immobilized children need an environment that allows them some measure of control and feelings of independence.
- Management of pain is essential in caring for children, whether the origin of the pain is primarily physical or psychological.
- Assessment of pain includes observing behaviors that indicate discomfort, encouraging the child to discuss pain, and using play to help the child describe painful experiences.
- Nurses cannot allow children to avoid necessary painful procedures, including injections for pain relief.
- Diminishing anxiety, explaining the cause and temporary nature of a pain, and planning activities that distract children from attention to their pain are all possible noninvasive measures for pain relief.
- Medication for pain relief is best tolerated if the child knows what sensations to expect when the medication is administered.
- Color, sensation, and motion assessment are necessary in determining the vascularity and innervation of body parts.
- In providing urine and stool samples during hospitalization, children often need nursing assistance that includes matter-of-fact, age-appropriate explanations with words they understand.
- For the incontinent child, urine may be collected by means of a collecting bag or by properly withdrawing urine from a wet diaper.
- Medicating a child requires painstaking attention to dosages because of the diluting effect of the child's higher proportion of body fluids, the permeability of membranes, and rates of absorption.
- Oral medications require careful measurement and may require combining the medicine with food or drink if the child finds swallowing a pill or capsule difficult.
- Intramuscular administration of medication for a child is similar to that for an adult, although the size of the needle and preferred sites of injection vary depending on the child's size and muscle development.

- Playing and talking about unpleasant procedures and sensations are effective in helping children to cope with these experiences.
- Parents may choose to leave the room when their children must undergo painful procedures, although some parents are willing or able to assist the nurse in restraining or consoling their children.
- Children who are placed in isolation need age-appropriate explanations to assure them that the treatment is not a punishment and that they will eventually rejoin normal activities.
- Postoperative play is extremely valuable in helping children express and resolve their feelings of anger, helplessness, and violation of body integrity.

References

Bergmann T, Freud A: *Children in the Hospital.* International Universities Press, 1965.

Children in pain. (Pain consult.) *Am J Nurs* (Feb) 1984; 84:247.

Drehobl P: Quadriceps contracture. *Am J Nurs* (Sept) 1980; 80:1650–1651.

Eland JM, Anderson JE: The experience of pain in children. Pages 453–473 in: *Pain: A Sourcebook for Nurses and Other Health Professionals.* Jacox A (editor). Little, Brown, 1977.

Hahn AB, Barkin RL, Oestreich SJK: *Pharmacology in Nursing.* 15th ed. Mosby, 1982.

Hilt N, Schmitt E: *Pediatric Orthopedic Nursing.* Mosby, 1975.

Kozier B, Erb G: *Fundamentals of Nursing.* 2nd ed. Addison-Wesley, 1983.

McGuire L, Dizard S: Managing pain in the young patient. *Nursing* (Aug) 1982; 12:52–55.

Meng A, Zastowny T: Preparing for hospitalization: A stress inoculation training program for parents and children. *Matern-Child Nurs J* 1982; 11:87–94.

Pontious SL: Practical Piaget: Helping children understand. *Am J Nurs* (Jan) 1982; 82:114–117.

Strohbach ME, Kratina SH: Diaper versus bag specimens: A comparison of urine specific gravity values. *Am J Matern Child Nurs* (May/June) 1982; 7:198–201.

Additional Readings

Abbott NC, Hansen P, Lewis K: Dress rehearsal for the hospital. *Am J Nurs* 1970; 70(11): 2360–2362.

Adom D, Wright A: Dissonance in nurse and patient evaluations of the effectiveness of a patient-teaching program. *Nurs Outlook* (Feb) 1982; 30:132–136.

Apley J: Pain in childhood. *J Psychosom Res* 1976; 20:383–389.

Atkins DM: Evaluation of a preadmission preparation program: Goals clarification as the first step. *Child Health Care* 1981; 10(2):48–52.

Beckemeyer P, Bahr JE: Helping toddlers and preschoolers cope while suturing their minor lacerations. *Am J Matern Child Nurs* (Sept/Oct) 1980; 5:326–330.

Betz CL: After the operation—postprocedural sessions to allay anxiety. *Am J Matern Child Nurs* 1982; 7(4):260–263.

Beyerman K: Flawed perceptions about pain. *Am J Nurs* (Feb) 1982; 82:302–304.

Birchfield ME: Nursing care for hospitalized children based on different stages of illness. *Am J Matern Child Nurs* (Jan/Feb) 1981; 6:46–51.

Black CD, Popovich NG, Black MC: Drug interactions in the GI tract. *Am J Nurs* (Sept) 1977; 77:1426–1429.

Crowshore TM: Postoperative assessment: The key to avoiding most common nursing mistakes. *Nurs 79* (April) 1979; 9:47–51.

D'Apolito K: The neonate's response to pain. *Am J Matern Child Nurs* (July/Aug) 1984; 9:256–257.

Evans ML, Hansen BD: Administering injections to different-aged children. *Am J Matern Child Nurs* (May/June) 1981; 6:194–199.

Fernald CD, Corry JJ: Empathic versus directive preparation of children for needles. *Child Health Care* 1981; 10(2):44–46.

Galligan AC: Using Roy's concept of adaptation to care for young children. *Am J Matern Child Nurs* (Jan/Feb) 1979; 4:24–28.

Gohsman B, Yunck M: Dealing with the threats of hospitalization. *Pediatr Nurs* (Sept/Oct) 1979; 5:32–35.

Hansen BD, Evans ML: Preparing a child for procedures. *Am J Matern Child Nurs* (Nov/Dec) 1981; 6:392–397.

Hawley DD: Postoperative pain in children: Misconceptions, descriptions and interventions. *Pediatr Nurs* (Jan/Feb) 1984; 10:20–23.

Hardgrove CB, Dawson RB: *Parents and Children in the Hospital.* Little, Brown, 1972.

Hymovich DP: Parents of sick children, their needs and tasks. *Pediatr Nurs* (Sept/Oct) 1976; 2:9–13.

Jacox AK: *Pain: A Source Book for Nurses and Other Health Professionals.* Little, Brown, 1977.

Johnson JE et al: Altering children's distress behavior during orthopedic cast removal. *Nurs Res* (Nov/Dec) 1975; 24:404–410.

Klein C: Going home. *Pediatr Nurs* (Sept/Oct) 1980; 6:59–60.

Kline J: Recovery room care for the child in pain. *Am J Matern Child Nurs* (July/Aug) 1984; 9:261–264.

Leifer G: *Principles and Techniques in Pediatric Nursing.* 4th ed. Saunders, 1982.

Lentz M: Selected aspects of deconditioning secondary to immobilization. *Nurs Clin North Am* (Dec) 1981; 16:729–737.

Huth MM: Guidelines for conducting hospital tours with early school-age children. *Pediatr Nurs* (Nov/Dec) 1983; 9:414–415.

McCaffery M: Patients don't have to suffer: How to relieve pain with injectable narcotics. *Nursing 80* (Oct) 1980; 10:34–39.

McCaffrey M: Relieving pain with noninvasive techniques. *Nursing 80* (Dec) 1980; 10:55–57.

McCaffrey M: Understanding your patient's pain. *Nursing 80* (Sept) 1980; 10:26–31.

McCaffrey M: When your patient's still in pain don't just do something: Sit there. *Nursing 81* (June) 1981; 11:58–61.

McGuire M, Shepherd R, Greco A: Hospitalized children in confinement. *Pediatr Nurs* (Nov/Dec) 1978; 4:31–35.

Malseed RT: *Pharmacology: Drug Therapy and Nursing Considerations.* Lippincott, 1982.

Nelson M: Identifying the emotional needs of the hospitalized child. *Am J Modern Child Nurs* (May/Jun) 1981; 6:181–183.

Petrillo M, Sanger S: *Emotional Care of Hospitalized Children.* 2nd ed. Lippincott, 1980.

Pidgeon VA: Characteristics of children's thinking and implications for health teaching. *Matern Child Nurs J* (Spring) 1977; 6:1–8.

Poston LI: Finding time to play. *Am J Matern Child Nurs* (Jan/Feb) 7:19–20.

Russell H: *Pediatric Drugs and Nursing Intervention*. McGraw-Hill, 1980.

Schumann D: How to help wound healing in your abdominal surgery patient. *Nursing 80* (April) 1980; 10:34–40.

Sciarillo WG: Using Hymovich's framework in the family-oriented approach to nursing care. *Am J Matern Child Nurs* (July/Aug) 1980; 5:242–248.

Schmeltz K, White G: A survey of parent groups: Prehospital admission. *Matern-Child Nurs J* (Summer) 1982; 11:75–85.

Schults NV: How children perceive pain. *Nurs Outlook* (Oct) 1971; 19:670–673.

Scott JG, Rigney-Radford K: Factors affecting the management of pain. *Am J Matern Child Nurs* (July/Aug) 1984; 9:253–255.

Shepherd MJ, Swearington P: Z-track. *Am J Nurs* (June) 1984; 84:746–747.

Sheredy C: Factors to consider when assessing responses to pain. *Am J Matern Child Nurs* (July/Aug) 1984; 9:250–252.

Tesler M, Savedra M: Coping with hospitalization: A study of school-age children. *Pediatr Nurs* 1981; 7:35–38.

Treloar DM: Ready, set—no: Something is missing from pediatric pre-op preparation. *Am J Matern-Child Health* 1978; 3(1):50–51.

Vipperman JF, Rager PM: Childhood coping: How nurses can help. *Pediatr Nurs* (March/April) 1980; 6:11–18.

Weeks HF: Administering medication to children. *Am J Matern Child Nurs* (Jan/Feb) 1980; 5:63.

White JE: Special nursing needs of hospitalized children with learning disabilities. *Am J Matern Child Nurs* (May/June) 1983; 8:209–212.

Zollo M: Management of pain in critically ill children. *Am J Matern Child Nurs* (July/Aug) 1984; 9:258–261.

Psychosocial Dimensions of Chronic Conditions in Childhood

30

Barbara J. Leonard

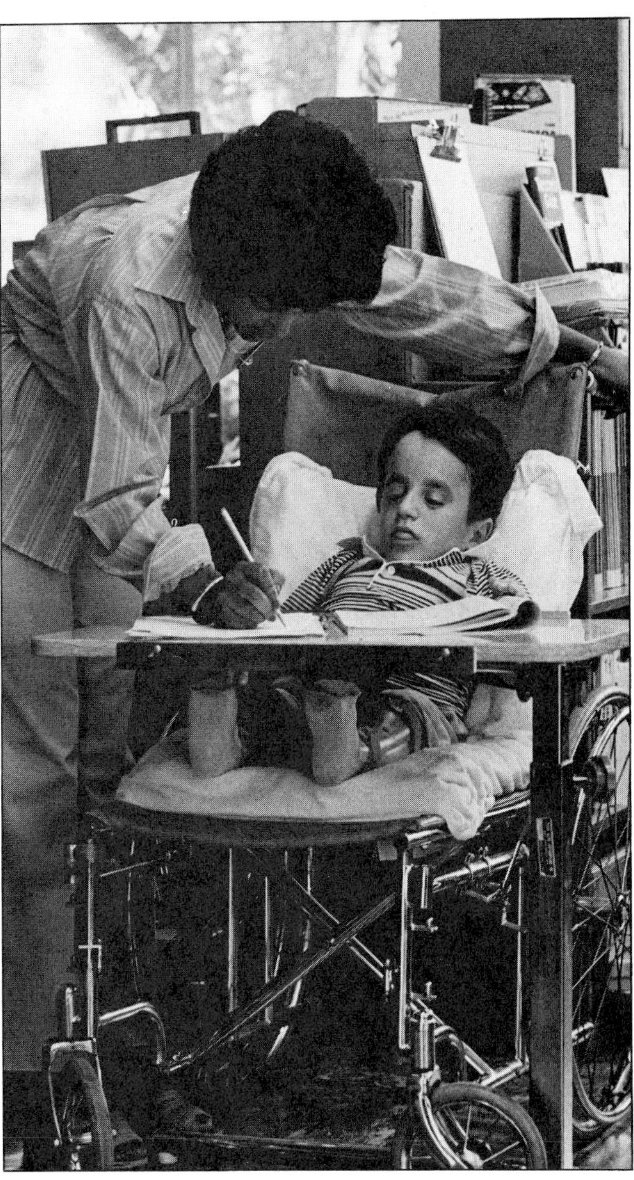

Chapter Outline

Objectives

- List the factors that affect a family's response to the diagnosis of a child's chronic illness.
- Explain the need for community resources in supporting the family with a chronically ill child.
- List common needs of parents with chronically ill children.
- Describe developmental changes in children's responses to chronic conditions and their limitations.
- Explain how temperament and social development affect the child's response to chronic illness.
- List the factors affecting siblings' responses to chronic illness in a child.
- Delineate principles of care and nursing goals common to chronically ill children.
- Present assessment criteria for both the family and the child with chronic illness.
- Compare the purpose of the evaluation in chronic care with evaluation in acute, short-term care.

Chronically ill children comprise 10%–20% of all children who are hospitalized. They are hospitalized not only for problems related to their chronic illness but also diagnostic studies or treatment of acute problems. All treatments and illnesses affect and are affected by the disease or handicap. Chronically ill children also have the same needs and developmental concerns of well children. Children with chronic illness have a continuing need for more frequent and more comprehensive health care than their healthy peers. For these children, contact with the nurse is not an isolated event but one in a series of contacts, each having potential to enhance or inhibit the development and optimal health of the child and family. Nursing care of a child during an acute episode or for routine primary care therefore requires planning for continuity of care including not only the child's acute or wellness needs but also special needs related to the chronic illness.

Pless and Roughmann's 1971 study of childhood chronic illness identified three factors associated with chronic physical disease or disability that correlate with the development of secondary problems. These are

1. The age of onset of the condition. The earlier a physical disability is acquired, the more likely secondary problems will develop. Although his conclusions are not universally accepted, Pless contends that early disability not only interferes with ongoing development over a long period of time but also disturbs fundamental developmental processes such as social relationships and language acquisition.
2. The permanence of the disability. Children who understand the nature of their handicap and recognize that their disabilities are permanent may be depressed as a result. Such is the case with children who have progressive degenerative diseases such as cystic fibrosis.
3. The severity of the disease or handicap. The more severe a condition, the more it interferes with development progress and day-to-day living.

Pless asserts that approximately one-third of children with chronic disease will develop secondary emotional, psychologic, learning problems, or all three. Experts in this area of study agree that the specific disease or handicap is less important in predicting psychosocial outcomes than are the factors that Pless identifies.

In this chapter we consider the role of nursing in the care of chronically ill children, their parents, and their siblings. Chronically ill children require continuous nursing care by nurses possessing the requisite knowledge of and skills for the complex task of coordinating health care from the time of diagnosis and providing nursing care during hospitalizations. Nursing is a health discipline appropriate to coordinate health care for chronically ill children.

Impact of Chronic Illness on Children and Families

The Parent

Parents expect their children to grow and develop free of physical and emotional problems. When a child acquires a chronic illness or is born with a physical handicap, this expectation is directly challenged. Although parental responses to learning the diagnosis of a chronic illness in a child vary from severe emotional upheaval to a more moderate reaction, most parents suffer some sense of disequilibrium in the initial phases of the child's disease. Long-term reaction to the diagnosis cannot, however, be predicted from the initial reaction; but parents of chronically ill or handicapped children may well be at increased risk for development problems such as incomplete bonding and maladaptive copying mechanisms. (Families at risk are discussed in Chapter 22.)

Initial Response to the Diagnosis Parents who experience the diagnosis of chronic illness in their children describe learning of it as a crisis during which the first few hours and days are filled with anxiety, fear, and emotional upset, although expression of feelings varies. Some parents tend to block their feelings; others become overtly angry; still others cry. Regardless of their observable responses, these parents, siblings, and sometimes grandparents are in the midst of a crisis, and consequently, their usual individual and emotional equilibria are affected.

The parental grieving and guilt associated with the birth of a premature infant and with a diagnosis of mental retardation (Solnit and Stark, 1961; Olshansky, 1962) are responses that are also evident with the diagnosis of chronic illnesses. Responses always vary both between and within families, however, as grieving is not a steady progression through the various phases with no return to those already experienced. (See Chapter 32 for a discussion of grieving.) For example, the families of two 12-year-old girls diagnosed as having diabetes reacted in far different ways. One was interested and ready to learn about the condition, whereas for the other family the diagnosis was a tremendous blow. The child spent much of her time in bed as the family gathered around the bedside and spoke in low voices, openly grieving. Another family had been so upset when their son was born with a cleft lip that they told the boy when he was older that his surgical scar was related to an accidental fall he had had as an infant and were unable to talk with him about the defect.

Leonard (1983) found in a study of 49 families that parents experiencing the diagnosis of cancer, cystic fibrosis, diabetes, or epilepsy in a child unanimously described their initial response as shocking. For example, upon receiving the diagnosis that his son had epilepsy, one father reported that he was thoroughly heartbroken, and all parents studied recounted significant disruption of family life at first. Some were unable to share their feelings, as the family seemed to be on an emotional teeter-totter; when one parent was down, the other was up. Yet as early as a few months from the time of the initial diagnosis, most of the parents reported that the initial family disorganization and emotional upheaval did not persist. Most said that while the child's diagnosis was the worst family problem they had ever faced, their families were doing well, although all recognized that they had made many adjustments in a short period of time. Objective measures of family cohesion such as expression of feelings and commitment were also all within normal limits; so were measures of each parents' emotional health. Additional research published in the late 1970s and early 1980s confirms these findings. Therefore, while the diagnosis of chronic disease in childhood is very upsetting and stressful, it may not be as devastating as earlier researchers described (Lavigne and Ryan, 1979).

In determining the family's definition of the diagnosis and its significance, the nurse considers not only verbal messages but also family member's nonverbal cues. For example, the nurse notes whether the behavior of family members is congruent with what they say. Incongruence between their verbal expressions and physical appearance and behavior was illustrated by a father who sat quietly while listening to the doctor describe his child's diagnosis of cancer. As the conference ended, the distraught man assaulted the unsuspecting physician.

While most people do not react so violently to hearing distressing news, the nurse often needs to help family members express their feelings, as getting past the frightening feelings can facilitate better communication among all family members. The father who can admit to his son that he is scared of the diagnosis and that he is going to try to help in any way he can has, by example, permitted his son to talk about fears. Handled in this way, feelings become a topic, and family members can begin to communicate about the many issues they face.

Families Under Chronic Stress In discussing families under stress and families approaching crisis, Hill (1965) emphasized that the family's response is not so much a product of the event itself as it is a particular family's definition or perception of the event and the family's available resources to help deal with stress. Some families regrieve as children enter new stages, such as starting school or entering adolescence, but most achieve a level of acceptance which results in a child's healthy emotional growth and a family's basic satisfaction in child care. Hill further suggested that physical social and emotional resources affect family members' perceptions of the impact of chronic illness. For example, a family with an unemployed father could perceive the child's chronic illness as extremely stressful, since financial resources are limited. A family in a better financial situation might not have that added stress. The literature further substantiates the crisis-producing effects of childhood chronic illness for most families (Hewett, 1976; Spinetta and Deasy-Spinetta, 1981), but nurses need to be careful not to attempt to predict which families and children are headed for trouble and which are going to do well. The overall outcome or impact of chronic illness on a child and family is, for all involved, the result of a complex set of interactions among three systems: community, family, and child.

The community in which a family lives reflects the shared values and attitudes of its members toward the institutions serving families. Providing health care and education for the handicapped and chronically ill for example is a manifestation of a community's positive attitudes toward disability. Families are influenced both directly and indirectly by the community, and the child in turn is affected by the family–community interaction.

For instance, the health care system and educational institutions in the community have a direct impact on the child and family. Lack of such resources as early intervention programs might, for example, allow secondary effects of disability to become more severe. The family's position in the community and its political affiliations can also affect the impact of chronic illness on the child. The relative ease with which the family can influence the community to provide needed resources, for example, increases or decreases the degree of stress that family members experience. The family that feels powerless and incapable of influencing positive change in the community experiences additional stress. These direct and indirect factors also affect family members' perceptions of available options and thus affect family dynamics, so that the outcome for any child is much more than a direct result of the disease. It is instead a complex interplay among the child, family, and community.

Fortunate indeed is the child who, in spite of disability, lives in a community that can support both family and child; less lucky is the child born into a marginally functional family with minimal resources in an impoverished community (Fig. 30-1). For example, 7-year-old John has parents and siblings who are able to travel 2,000 miles to accompany him for a bone marrow transplant and remain with him during several months of hospitalization. Eight-year-old Robert, on the other hand, needs a bone marrow transplant, but his mother must work to support him and his 3-year-old brother and can visit the hospital only on weekends.

The first family, while away from extended family and friends, is together, not concerned about finances, and able to focus attention on caring for John and for each other. In contrast, Robert's mother struggles to provide the basic necessities, is able to be with Robert a short time each week during his hospital stay, and has few supports on which to rely. As a single-parent family facing additional stress, Robert's family is at greater risk for dysfunctional parenting (see Chapter 22).

In families with handicapped children, dysfunction may appear as the child grows older. Parents may cope successfully with a handicapped child during infancy and early childhood, when all children are dependent, but find that

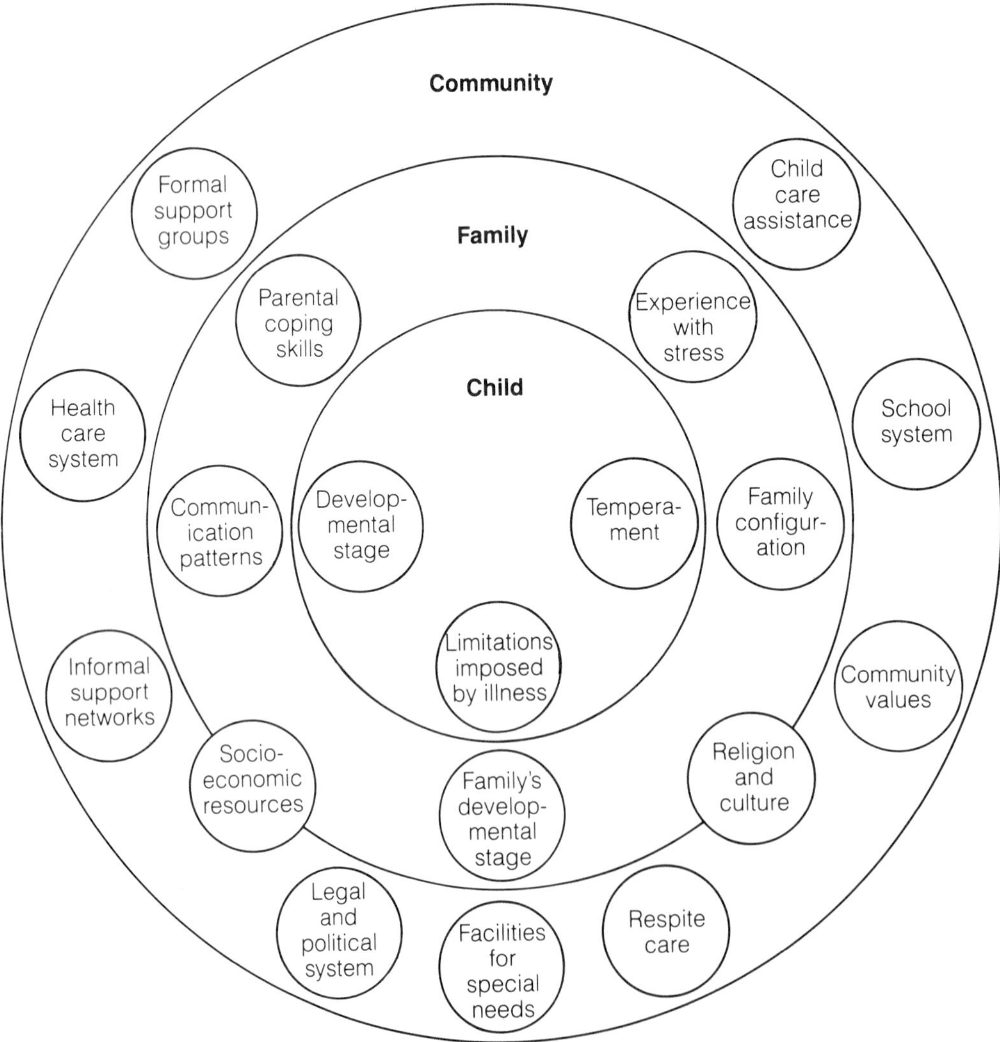

Figure 30-1 Factors affecting family and child adjustment to chronic illness.

the physical and emotional exhaustion that comes with chronic care eventually taxes their resources. A child's normal growth and development may also be restricted by a treatment regimen or by physically restrictive equipment such as prosthetic devices for orthopedic problems. As the child must learn to adapt to physical and developmental differences from peers and siblings, the stress of adaptation may negatively affect the family's normal course of growth and development as well.

The nurse therefore watches closely for behavioral clues to dysfunction and maladaptive coping. Even if interpersonal communication between parents is relatively poor, they may maintain the appropriate social roles and may continue to show a united front to others. As stress builds for such families, nurses might need to help parents identify additional sources of support. Doing so serves to take the "spotlight" off the ill member and to create a more normal situation for all. Knowing about the many stresses and concerns these families must face, nurses can guide them in this process of normalization.

In spite of the extraordinary burdens of chronic illness, some families express heightened excitement about living and ascribe high value to interpersonal relationships because they are acutely aware of the transitory nature of life. For instance, a family with four children, one of whom was an adolescent with cystic fibrosis, derived great pleasure from each other's accomplishments and company. As the boy's illness progressed, the family seemed to draw closer together, not in a way that restricted the boy's contacts with peers but in a way that actually drew in supporting people in the environment. They simply enjoyed the minute-by-minute activities of each day together.

Factors Affecting Parental Response

Child's Health Status The child's general development and health prior to the diagnosis are among the many contributing factors influencing a parent's reaction and adjustment to the child's diagnosis. A previously healthy child diagnosed with an incurable disease can be a psychologic blow, but the parent of a chronically ill child may experience a sense of relief when the medical diagnosis is finally determined. Some diagnoses are ironically relieving to parents.

For example, the parents of an adolescent boy who was subsequently diagnosed with cancer spent 9 months trying to convince health care providers and other authorities that a black-and-blue spot was not self-inflicted or the result of parental abuse. Needless to say, the diagnosis was a significant relief even though the sadness of cancer was itself nearly overwhelming. Developmental and health histories therefore provide critical information which the nurse uses to assess a family's response to the diagnosis of a child with chronic disease.

The family members must often alter their expectations for the child. In some cases, this involves coping with grief, a form of psychologic work that does not go unnoticed by the affected child, and siblings may cause changes in children's relationships with their parents.

Gender and Birth Order The child's gender can place the parent at a particularly high risk for the development of secondary psychologic problems. One father said his hopes were dashed when his infant and only daughter developed epilepsy. The fact that he had three healthy sons did not relieve his pain. He had hoped for a daughter but was crushed by her potentially significant health problems. Another father was withdrawn and was described as depressed by other family members and neighbors. He had a diabetic first-born son but eventually realized that his hopes and aspirations for his son were only moderately altered and was able to talk about the disease with his son. If the father had not been able to accept his son's illness, both the family and the son's development would have been affected. An adolescent boy, cut off from effective communication with his father, might have blamed himself for causing his father's problems and the family's as well.

Parents of children who are at greater risk for developing a sex-linked disease, such as hemophilia, may have psychologic problems at the birth of a male child. Feelings of anxiety about the child can interfere with appropriate bonding and thus distort the parent–child relationship at its beginning.

The number of children in the family can often affect parental reactions. In one- and two-child families, the intensity of the reaction may be greater than that in larger families. The father who described his hopes as "dashed" by the diagnosis of his daughter's epilepsy might not have had such an intense reaction to an infant son's diagnosis of the same condition. The father of the diabetic adolescent boy may have had an entirely different reaction to the diagnosis in one of his daughters. Later-born children with chronic illnesses may not threaten a family as seriously as earlier-born children. A younger child with cystic fibrosis who has several older siblings, none of whom has the disease, may receive special attention from these older siblings. Their participation in the ill child's daily care not only takes pressure off the parents but may also give the siblings the pleasure of participating.

Religion and Culture Parents may be helped to cope with chronic childhood illness by using religious supports. Religion plays a role in several ways. First, family members feel assisted when care and empathy are expressed by people in the religious community. Second, religion may help the family gain perspective on the situation by focusing attention toward new priorities that are more humanistic than materialistic. Some parents describe the child's illness as a kind of blessing that requires a redefinition of what is really important in their lives. Many describe themselves as living a day at a time and trying to get the most out of each day. They mention a heightened sense of the meaning of life and feel that they are not in control of life but that life itself is a gift. Many parents faced with a child's impending death may use religious beliefs to come to terms with the child's shortened life span. Nurses might well remember that parents whose children are dying need to find some sense of purpose in the child's suffering and reduced life span. (Nursing care of the dying child is covered in Chapter 32.)

Nurses also need to recognize that not all families use organized religion to work through the difficulties of chronic illness. Some who have drifted away from a religious orientation come back to it during times of stress; others do not. Furthermore, the research on this issue is scarce so that generalizations are at best cautious. What is not known is why families who have religious persuasions seem to do better, overall, than those who do not. This may be due not only to the perspective that religion can bring to the child's illness but also to the cultural benefits of family involvement and community support.

A family's cultural values will also influence the family's response to the diagnosis of chronic illness. For instance, in cultures that value education highly, a mentally retarded child might be a serious threat (see Chapter 23). In those that prize athletics, the birth of a child with mild cerebral palsy but with no mental retardation will be hard to accept. As with religious values, the nurse needs to ascertain the ways in which cultural differences are likely to influence a particular family's acceptance of a child's disability.

Experience With Stress and Crisis Other family resources include the parents' previous experience with resolving crisis and handling stress. Older families, that is, those in which the parents have been married for several years, may have had the advantage of working through problems as a couple. Together, they may have experienced the illness of their own parents, perhaps even the death of a loved one. While the death of one's parents is not equated with the loss of a child, the experience, if faced and dealt with adequately, will provide a measure of maturity that those who have not had the experience will lack. Yet even parents who have encountered many problems and have handled them well describe the diagnosis of fatal disease in a child as the most serious problem they have ever faced (see Chapter 32).

In general, parents who have experienced and have coped well with problems prior to a child's diagnosis have the experience with stress that may protect them from family disruption. Nurses might therefore expect families that have experienced problems to accept a serious diagnosis better than a less experienced family learning of a less serious condition. Even "experienced" parents can, however, be overwhelmed by the specific problems they face. Previously successful coping strategies, which are part of the psychologic repertoire for any individual or family, are not invincible. For example, a middle-aged mother of a teenage daughter described her reaction to the daughter's diabetes as "not too upsetting." Comparing her daughter's diagnosis of diabetes to the learning and behavioral problems of her teenage son and the severe asthma of her young son, she said that the problem was minimal, albeit serious. Hill (1965) stresses that it is not the event itself that causes disequilibrium; it is instead the family's response to it.

Another important factor in predicting family disruption in the face of stress or crisis is the developmental stage of the family's life cycle. The family with the diabetic girl was a family with children in the process of leaving home. The diabetic daughter was leaving the family to attend college within a few months. Family members did not have to be intimately involved in helping her manage her condition. Instead, they were left free to carry on with their own developmental tasks. In contrast to this family, a young parent with an infant who has diabetes requiring constant supervision of a life-threatening condition is faced with both a serious disruption in family life and perhaps a profound disappointment.

The vast differences in the abilities of families to deal with a child's illness are based on the life experiences of these families. Young parents trying to establish families are particularly vulnerable to stress and crisis because family members have little experience worrying together and are most often greatly burdened with expenses (Litman, 1974). For example, a young father may have to take a second job in order to allow his wife to stay at home with a child who has a chronic illness. Lack of available resources often compounds the problem. Adequate child care for a child with a serious chronic illness is very difficult to find. Even if a place is located, the staff of the center is often untrained to deal with the child's needs. One family in which the mother took an evening position so that her husband could be at home with the child was fairly typical in that she found her marital relationship strained and her other children relatively ignored.

One type of service available to families to reduce the stress of caring for a chronically ill child is respite care. *Respite care* is a type of care developed specifically to reduce family stress of caring for a person who is chronically ill. Respite programs train workers to enter homes and care for the ill person in order to provide a break for the family. If the family needs to get away for a few hours or even a weekend, respite care provides relief.

Child's Prognosis While the specific disease does not generally determine a family's unity or dissolution, different diseases require different resources from families. A fatal disease, such as cystic fibrosis, is manageable in the child's early years, but if the disease advances, the demands on parents increase exponentially. Hospital stays become more frequent, home treatments intensify, restriction of the child's and often the family's activities increase dramatically, and family members are allowed little personal time for themselves. Even cancer, so threatening to so many, may also be relatively easy to live with in its early stages.

Static, nonprogressive conditions may be least difficult for a family to live with, even when the condition is relatively severe. For example, spina bifida in a young child requires maximum parental involvement from the time of diagnosis. As children with spina bifida grow and develop, however, they are able to manage their own disease, and parental involvement is reduced.

The predictability of a condition together with the assumption of a nonfatal outcome ease the psychologic burdens common to parents with children having nonprogressive diseases. The child with cerebral palsy, for instance, will encounter problems due to the condition, but the family can look forward to a relatively predictable future, especially after the child reaches maturity. Children with rheumatoid arthritis may experience long periods without any change in the condition, and so their families may plan for the future and attend to other developmental tasks.

When a child's illness is degenerative, however, the increasing demands of chronic care may lead to increasing stress and family disharmony. Nurses therefore need to consider parental age and vitality when helping a family care for a child with a chronic degenerative condition. Duchenne's muscular dystrophy, for example, poses incredibly difficult problems when the child or adult loses significant bodily functions. Parents in their late forties who are still caring for children now in their twenties may be less enthusiastic about their tasks than they were when they were younger. Alternative care arrangements, such as respite care or residential care, permit these parents to maintain involvement with their children but also free them for other important issues in their lives.

Chronic illnesses vary considerably in the amount of interference they impose on the lives and development of children. Although very little research has specified these differences, nurses do find that fatal illnesses are generally disruptive to families, producing fear in both parents and children. Living with a fatal illness further places all family members "on emotional hold." As one mother of a child with cancer said, "When my daughter was in crisis, family living was in moratorium; when the crisis was past, all of us could go on living." Having a child with a life-threatening illness makes a family highly vulnerable and creates long-term implications for the family as a unit and for family members as individuals. Recognizing this vulnerability is a first step in planning nursing interventions, and it ensures consideration of the needs of all family members in the care plan. Parental adjustment is the keystone to the children's response and must be central in the plan.

Common Needs of Parents Following the diagnosis, the family makes crucial psychologic and environmental adjustments in family living. The prior level of functioning is the foundation on which the family accommodates the chronic illness. Therefore, a family that has been marginally meeting its physical and emotional needs prior to the child's treatment may be at greater risk for family dysfunction and dissolution than one that has previously functioned at a high level of integration. (Nursing care for families at risk is discussed in Chapter 22.)

Although families with chronically ill children differ in a multitude of ways, they do share common basic problems and needs that form a framework for nursing management. Because the availability of financial resources or of an adequate support system varies widely among families, these issues need to be addressed as the nurse tailors the care plan to the needs peculiar to a particular family.

Financial Needs The impact of increased financial demands varies among families. Financial concerns constitute a serious threat for some families and minimal problems for others, depending on both the family's resources and the expenses of a particular condition. Over time, however, many chronic illnesses impose heavy financial burdens on families regardless of their financial stability. Concerns include insurance benefits, entitlement programs, and actual out-of-pocket expenditures. Many families may have insurance to cover doctor and hospital charges but have many indirect expenses not covered by insurance.

For example, families coming to a tertiary care center must pay for transportation, lodging, and food, and provide child care services for their other children. Often, these expenses are not covered by insurance or entitlement programs. Changes in US government policies regarding financial assistance for medical problems are resulting in higher and more direct costs to families. For some families the availability or decreased availability of these resources may well influence their ability to carry out recommended treatments.

Need for Support Systems Although some families tend to be isolated from kin and neighbors and are therefore more vulnerable to the disruption of chronic disease, families experiencing childhood chronic illness may well be part of supportive networks, extended families, surrogate families, or friendships. Such a family is fortunate because the support of family and friends is critical to preventing the physical, psychologic, and even financial stresses occurring from a child's chronic illness. The nurse therefore assesses the family's actual or potential support systems because the resolution of a particular family's experience of stress or crisis is influenced by cultural and socioeconomic background (Hill, 1965). For example, a family that has recently moved into an area may have to rely more on professional services than one that has lived in an area for many years with an extended family available, an extensive number of friendships, or both.

The nurse needs to be cautious here, however, for even though a family may be well integrated into a community, the diagnosis of chronic illness might change family patterns if not immediately then eventually. For example, the more restrictive the child's handicap, the less time, energy, and money are available for the family to maintain friendships. Much depends on a particular family's creativity in dealing with the circumstances of the illness. For instance, not to be denied a community camping trip, the ingenious parents of a child with cystic fibrosis rigged a generator to the child's mist tent so that he could have the prescribed therapy while they all enjoyed their outing. These enterprising parents also arranged to have medical backup available should their child need it. Anticipation of the problems they might encounter allowed them to be both part of the group and relatively worry free. Other families, lacking their ingenuity and resources, might have given up activities with friends and other families to protect the affected child and to conserve finances.

Parents often form new friendships to replace those that cannot be maintained. Support groups composed of families experiencing similar problems are often effective because the issues faced in rearing a child with chronic disease are better understood by those directly involved. A health professional, however, needs to be available to these groups because parents may often be so overwhelmed with their own problems that they are incapable of reaching out and supporting others. As one mother commented about an encounter with another similarly affected parent, "I knew what she was going through. I felt terribly guilty not getting involved, but I knew I just couldn't do it."

Thus the nurse might best direct parents to groups that include professionals who listen and guide discussion as appropriate to the situation. A sensitive health professional is often helpful to parents by relieving their guilt and providing them with needed emotional support.

Need for Time Away From Care Chronic illness involves a constant and ever-present regimen of care that must be maintained, and many medical routines are time-consuming and inflexible. A child needing dialysis, for example, must literally live by the clock. Parents may become resentful because the regimen impinges on their personal time.

These families usually experience increased stress from the day-to-day burden of caring for the ill child. Depending upon the disease, parental involvement in care can range from an additional 15–20 minutes per day to an extra 5 to 6 hours. Parents describe feeling frustrated and fatigued at being on call 24 hours a day, 7 days a week, year in and year out. A mother of an epileptic 4-year-old, for example, said she never had a waking moment when she was free from thinking about her child's safety. Another mother, one with a diabetic 4-year-old, said that diabetes affects everything in her life and in the functioning of her family.

The Child

The emotional impact of the diagnosis of chronic illness on a child is a highly complicated phenomenon. Just as each family has its unique strengths with which to meet stress and crisis, children have their own personal resources. Developmental stage, temperament, effect of the illness on social roles, and the nature of the illness itself determine a child's response to a chronic condition.

Developmental Stage The child receiving a diagnosis of chronic disease responds to the information in a way appropriate for both the child's age and developmental level. Inasmuch as age and development are correlated, the nurse can anticipate a child's response on the basis of age, but the nurse cannot presume to do this in individuals whose development has been compromised by earlier problems. Nurses thus need to remember that children with chronic illness react to a diagnosis appropriately for a given developmental stage and that the disease in turn interferes with development. The younger the child, the greater potential impact the disease will have on critical developmental stages.

Infancy Lacking the cognitive capacity to comprehend the need for invasive procedures and treatments or having to be handled by strangers, an infant may well show signs of developmental delay and stranger wariness. The infants may be highly irritable, may not sleep deeply, or may have basic physical rhythms disrupted. For example, because the infant with retinoblastoma requires immediate treatment, the attachment process may be disrupted by repeated hospitalizations and separations from parents. Reciprocal parental interaction may also be affected by parental feelings about the disease, especially its genetic implications. Blind infants may then be slower to develop cognitively if their caregivers do not learn to communicate effectively with them using the tactile and auditory routes. Infants with sensory and central nervous system handicaps are therefore vulnerable to delays in cognitive, social, and affective development.

Early Childhood The young child who develops a chronic illness or acquires a disability has difficulty understanding and accepting treatment and its limitations. For example, the $2\frac{1}{2}$-year-old insulin-dependent diabetic child, who is typically establishing autonomy, often refuses to eat on parental demand and does not understand the need for injections. The child may also perceive injections as punishment for bad behavior (see Chapter 27). Parental understanding of child development, patience, and a positive attitude are essential qualities to help the young child through this difficult period.

Although children of this age group are developing language skills rapidly, they may demonstrate protest against procedures by shutting down communication, or simply not talking. They demonstrate their frustration in the extreme by becoming either rebellious against or totally compliant with adult requests. In early childhood, the younger the child at the time of diagnosis, the more the disease process interferes with critical foundations of development. As young children attempt to comprehend their situations, they piece together available verbal and nonverbal cues from significant people in their lives. One 4-year-old told an interviewer that she could tell how serious her condition was by watching her mother's eyes as the mother talked to the doctors. The young child's conclusions are often accurate so that children whose parents have not discussed the seriousness or fatal nature of a disease with the child find that the child often learns of possible death anyway because of overhearing a parent discussing the issues with a sensitive and interested listener. An inherent danger, however, is that children may possess misinformation or reach the wrong conclusions with the correct information.

Middle Childhood By middle childhood cognitive development allows the child to grasp the reasons for treatment so that the child is less likely to see treatment as punishment for real or imagined misdeeds. Because these children still have problems separating fantasy and reality, however, parents need to be aware of their children's perceptions of illness, treatment, and limitations.

Because the child's attitudes toward school, learning, and social relationships are in a state of transition during the middle childhood years, chronic problems that interfere with developmental changes may, if poorly handled, have long-term consequences for the child. School requires increasing cognitive skills and greater application of learned principles. Social relationships are formed in school and in the many extracurricular activities offered to children of this age. Inability to function appropriately in a learning environmnt might therefore cause social isolation. Not only does the nature of the condition itself interfere with the developmental tasks, but long hospitalizations and lost contact with peers might also exacerbate the problem. For example, a 6-year-old boy demonstrated learning problems secondary to epilepsy as a result of incorrect classroom placement rather than from decreased learning potential. Educators need to know that control of seizures allows a child to function normally so that there is no need for most children to be placed with learning disabled children. If control of seizures is not entirely possible, the teacher and school administrators should educate classmates about the condition and express a positive attitude about the child and the disease. The quality of both academic and social environments thus affect the child's developing initiative, academic competence, industry, and social skills. An environment that promotes attainment of greatest learning potential and promotes positive continuing relationships with peers gives the child confidence to adapt to the upper grades, which require greater academic application and more intense social relationships.

Late Childhood By late childhood, appropriate cognitive development and a healthy self-esteem allow the child to understand chronic illness and accept responsibility for much of its treatment. At this stage the child is characteristically emotionally stable, so that the diagnosis of chronic illness or disability, while traumatic, is not as upsetting as it may be for the early adolescent.

Because a child in this stage faces many demands for academic and athletic achievement and peer group involvement, intense competition develops, and peer groups often include or exclude others on the basis of their physical attributes. Children who are chronically ill or handicapped, who may be already developmentally delayed because of their condition, tend to fall behind their peers during the late childhood years. The child who is unable to sit still and listen in class now faces increasing classroom discipline and more homework. Although chronically ill and handicapped, children should be encouraged to participate in activities as much as possible. The child who cannot fully participate because of such physically limiting conditions as arthritis, spina bifida, or cerebral palsy has to develop a sense of industry and worth that is independent of the resources available to peers.

Because athletics and academic achievement foster a sense of industriousness and self-esteem, they also keep children in the mainstream with peers. The child lacking in both intellectual and athletic ability is in serious jeopardy for forming and maintaining needed friendships. Children who are separated from peers repeatedly or extensively for hospitalization or home care are also in danger of being excluded. Organizations outside school and sports, such as scouting and church groups, can help such children achieve at their own level and stay in contact with peers.

Adolescence Because early adolescence is characterized by bodily and emotional changes that disrupt the child's social roles, this period is especially troublesome to children who are different from their peers. Being shunned by intolerant peers is devastating to adolescents because peers are the suprasystem on whom they rely for self-acceptance and emotional separation from parents. Older children, while better able to comprehend the disease and its therapy, might become anxious and depressed. Handicapped younger adolescents might handle developmental tasks by denying them or by putting off required demands until later. Others rebel against the disease, either through denial or through inconsistent self-care. Some adolescents develop illness-related problems because of self-inflicted neglect.

The impact of the disease is modified by the extent to which the illness interferes with an adolescent's life-style. Adolescents with diabetes, for instance, may neglect to carry out their diabetic therapeutic regimen to show that they are truly able to live without insulin or to prove that they are actually just like their peers. While these assumptions are not at all accurate, adolescent cognitive development may interfere with reality testing, so that a perception of invincibility allows the adolescent to challenge reality by denying what is obvious to anxious parents and health providers. The adolescent may possess sufficient knowledge of the disease to write a quality term paper on the subject and at the same time behave in ways that contradict this knowledge. Adolescents undergoing chemotherapy, for example, have been known to discontinue treatment that promised cure in order to have a normal head of hair. The loss of hair and its concomitant social isolation, real or imagined, prevailed for these patients even over the longer-term goal of staying alive.

When ignoring the disease becomes the means by which the adolescent expresses emancipation from parents, the family interactions may become strained. Parents who have invested much of themselves in the care of their children over the years find this seemingly destructive behavior intolerable. Some parents overreact, which makes the situation worse. For example, Jenny, a 15-year-old with temporal lobe epilepsy, rebelled against her domineering mother by using alcohol and street drugs. Multidisciplinary treatment for chemical abuse involved the family and helped Jenny's mother develop parenting behaviors appropriate for an adolescent daughter. As the adolescent comes to terms with the illness and comes to be accepted by peers, however, better self-care is evident. This can take several years, however, so that the adolescent's health is sometimes compromised.

Later adolescence requires not only emotional emancipation from parents but also financial and social independence. During late adolescence, developmental tasks include clarifying career or job decisions and establishing satisfying relationships with members of the opposite sex. Chronically ill adolescents and those with disabilities may be at a disadvantage in accomplishing these tasks. Society is beginning to recognize the capabilities of the disabled and chronically ill, but while public policy supports education and employment of the handicapped, strong disincentives impede such progress (Bowe, 1978). For example, Marty, a bright 19-year-old with cystic fibrosis, found that a month-long hospital stay forced her to drop out of vocational school for 6 months and that when she was readmitted, she was required to retake the courses that she had so nearly completed. As a result of the additional amount of time she had to remain in school, she was forced to depend on her parents for support in order to receive health insurance coverage. The nurse who works with adolescents therefore needs to be aware of the many barriers they face in completing developmental tasks.

Temperament The child's temperament, like the child's developmental stage, affects the process of adaptation to illness. Children respond to their diseases and their consequences much as they do to other stressors. Placid, easygoing infants may continue to make good developmental progress socially and emotionally just because they are low-keyed and adaptable, but a basically irritable infant who is quick to respond to any environmental change has more difficulty with the stress of chronic illness. Easy-going children generally remain so, while irritable children exhibit additional psychological and behavioral problems.

The nurse thus assesses a child's temperament to establish a baseline, since subtle changes in behavior may later indicate shifts in either the disease process or in the child's response to it. (Assessment of temperament is discussed for each developmental stage in Chapter 16.) For example, a child with diabetes who is beginning to have an insulin reaction is described as being irrational, irritable, and generally different from the norm. Adolescents with diabetes may have the same changes in temperament, but they may be due instead to the adolescent's rebellion against the disease. Likewise, children who have seizures may demonstrate seizure phenomena by subtle shifts in temperament. Regression to wetting in a previously trained young child with epilepsy may indicate that the seizure disorder is worsening, that the anticonvulsant dosage is incorrect, or that the child is expressing an emotional reaction to the disease. Temperament is thus an important variable in determining an individual's response to the diagnosis and subsequent treatment of chronic illness.

Effect on Social Roles The disruption of the child's social roles also influences overall adjustment; severe discontinuity in social roles has a negative effect on adjustment. Helping a child continue actual participation with peers is critical. This is especially important for children in late childhood and adolescence. These children need to maintain contact with friends during episodes of illness or hospitalization so that their emotional investment can be sustained.

While all responsible adults should encourage such contacts, the child's social interactions remain the immediate responsibility of the child's parents. Teachers can encourage schoolmates to write to or visit the child, if appropriate, since a class visit to the hospital could mean a great deal to the child. In addition, teachers might spend some time with classmates explaining the nature of the disease and its usual therapy, thereby preparing them for the child's return to the classroom. The child and family's preference in this matter should, however, determine the extent to which the illness is discussed, as some families do choose to protect the child by keeping information about the disease confidential. Physicians and nurses can facilitate the child's peer contact by stressing to the parents that it is an important aspect of treatment.

The Siblings

When a brother or sister is diagnosed with a chronic illness, the lives of siblings are changed. As with both parents and ill children themselves, the initial impact of the diagnosis on the child's siblings is determined by several of the following factors. To plan care that addresses the needs of the entire family, the nurse assesses siblings' responses to a child's illness and its effect on family functioning.

Parental Behavior Toward Siblings Among the most important factors is the parent's ability to recognize the siblings' psychologic needs. Although parents usually tell siblings about the disease and its probable implications for their brother or sister, parents sometimes fail to determine their level of comprehension. In addition, a common assumption is that if parents are secure in their roles as parents and as individuals, and if they are receiving support from family and friends, they will have energy not only to care for the ill child but also to care for their other children.

Spinetta's longitudinal study of children with cancer and their siblings (1981), however, reported that parents met the emotional needs of their healthy children less well than they met the needs of the child who was ill. Even when the child with cancer was in remission, the sibling's needs were a low priority because other long-neglected family concerns had to be taken care of. Spinetta then found that these children had more emotional difficulties than the ill child (Spinetta and Deasy-Spinetta, 1981). For example, one family of four children included a youngest child with cystic fibrosis. The three siblings, twin girls 6 years of age and an older brother 10 years of age, believed that they were susceptible to the disease. They could not explain how they might contract the disease, but they all admitted to worrying about it. Their brother had been diagnosed 2 months earlier, and shortly thereafter they were tested and all found to be normal. An explanation of these tests and results, however, did not prevent their continued concern, which they could not express to their parents.

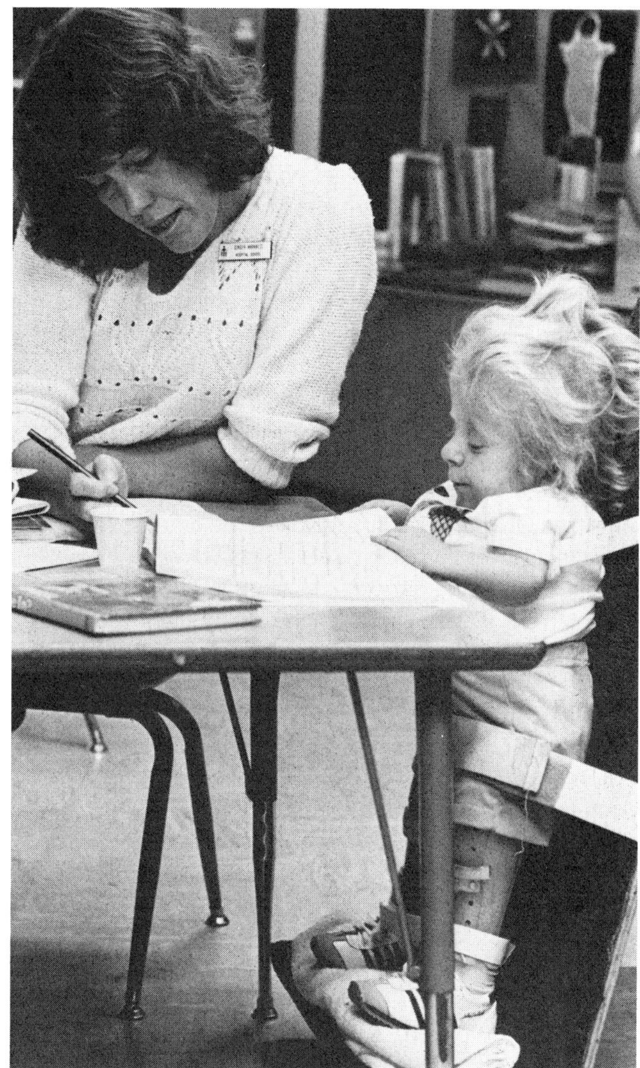

Children with chronic conditions require special attention, adaptation, and assistance from educators.

Parents are thus not entirely to blame for communication difficulties. Children also sometimes withhold their feelings and questions because they do not want to bring up a sensitive issue, fear their parents' display of feelings, and perhaps fear their own feelings.

Like adults, children are able to cope with only a limited amount of anxiety-producing information at a time. Parents may therefore misinterpret a child's hesitation to ask for further information, thinking that the child has completely understood the issue or that there is a lack of interest. A parent, especially one who is emotionally distraught, may not sense a child's need to discuss problems. Because parents are dealing with their own intense emotional needs as well as those of the affected child, they may block out the needs and concerns of the other children.

A similar pattern of parental response was found in families undergoing divorce (Heatherington, 1979; Wallerstein and Kelly, 1980). During this time of emotional upheaval in a family, the parents, who are essential to providing reassurance and support for the children, are frequently unable to do so because their emotional energy is depleted. Frightened and emotionally labile, parents required to protect ill children often feel as if they've lost control to the professionals and thus feel they are emotionally unable to meet the needs of the other children, especially those in crisis. Frequently, such parents are surprised by a healthy child's negative behavior toward them and toward the ill child. For example, a mother of 4-year-old twin daughters, one of whom was critically ill with neuroblastoma, was completely dismayed by the normal twin's regressive behavior. The ill sibling displayed maturity beyond her years while the healthy sibling rejected her mother's attempts to correct her behavior. The mother, college-educated and employed as an elementary school teacher, could not understand this child's rebellion. During an interview, she discussed, concurrently, plans for her daughter's funeral as well as the possibility of taking the child to a foreign country for a bone marrow transplant. She discussed the need she would have for time to get her life in order after her daughter's death. This mother's tremendous needs superseded her ability to recognize her other daughter's needs, let alone to begin to meet them. Her husband and son were also peripheral to her thinking.

Sibling's Responses The greater the number of demands placed on parents caring for ill children, the less likely they are able to provide physical or emotional care to the other children. This reality is intensified when parents must stay in an urban medical center many miles from their home. The siblings, who are also psychologically vulnerable, often find themselves without parental attention and must therefore cope with the stress of separation from parents (see Chapter 12), in addition to the other stresses they have incurred as a result of a sibling's illness.

When assessing siblings' reactions and adjustments to having a chronically ill child in the family, the nurse considers age, temperament, gender, and birth order. Younger children are more cognitively deficient as well as more emotionally vulnerable than older children. They are less able to understand a situation and less able to delay their own emotional needs. The other 4-year-old twin, whose mother's attention was focused on her ill sister, fantasized that her mother and sister were off at the hospital having a good time and not including her. She was accustomed to having her sister and mother available, and the hospital was a major barrier to contact during frequent hospital stays. This child responded by acting out her anger and frustration with her mother through wetting the bed and being generally noncompliant, ornery, and rebellious, much to her mother's consternation. Siblings, like the child with the disease, react to situations according to the developmental stage they are in and thus with the emotional and cognitive faculties associated with this stage. Therefore the 4-year-old who has become used to constant companionship with a sister and whose temperament may be a bit irritable will behave in a manner consistent with her usual reaction to stress.

Some children, keenly aware of parental discomfort but not understanding it, react by becoming overly anxious and withdrawn. Siblings express feelings of jealousy and anger toward the child with the illness and feelings of anger toward parents. They also report being very lonely and scared. Very young children are unable to accept their parents giving extra attention to the ill sibling. Their feelings are expressed in many ways, from being aggressive toward the parent, to meeting parental demands unconditionally, to developing symptoms of the illness in an effort to gain attention. Children in middle to late childhood are able to rationalize their parents' attention to the sick sibling, but they find it difficult to tell their parents how they are feeling. They "read" the situation quite well and try to cooperate even when it means putting their own needs aside. Adolescents appear to be less troubled by parental involvement with an ill sibling, but they may resent being expected to provide services at home that interfere with their social activities.

Relationships among siblings can also affect and be affected by the family's response to a childhood illness. One adolescent boy related that he did not share his problems with his sister, who was 2 years his senior, because, as he put it, "It's a long, boring story, and who's interested anyway? She's got her life, and she's not much interested." He may have been right in assessing his sister's reaction, but on the other hand she may not have known how to approach him. Neither party could help the other or share other facets of their lives as long as the communication barrier remained.

Nursing Care for Children With Chronic Illness

The Health Care System for Chronic Care

Nurses care for chronically ill children in a health care system designed for treatment of acute, short-term problems of adults and for medical cures rather than extended care. Chronically ill children have needs that contrast sharply with those of children who are temporarily ill (Table 30-1), and the health care system, with its advanced technology, is ill-suited to deal with such special needs. When a cure is not possible, the long-term goal of nursing care is to maintain physical function and the adverse physical, social, and emotional effects of the disease process.

Health care services also are needed to accommodate the child's long-term requirement for medical intervention. Nurses working within the health care system are therefore pivotal in adapting the system to accommodate the needs of the child and the family. Some health care providers and families may become so well acquainted that they may be able to use the telephone to consult on simple, recurrent problems or for anticipatory guidance, which otherwise would require the family's visiting the facility. This can decrease the burden and stress of a chronic condition on the family. Such an approach enables the family and child to live without unnecessary intrusion from health care providers.

Principles of Care for Chronically Ill Children

The nurse considers the following principles in planning specific care for any child with a chronic illness:

1. Care is based on the child's cognitive, affective, and social development.

TABLE 30-1 Usual Characteristics of Acute and Chronic Childhood Illness

Factor	Acute Illness	Chronic Illness
Causative agent	Single	Multiple
Diagnosis	Usually easily made	Often complicated, time consuming
Treatment	Specific, not pervasive, short duration	Difficult, trial and error, pervasive, ongoing
Organ systems	One or two	Many
Psychosocial implications	Minimal	Extensive
Participation in care	Minimal, short term	Full, long term
Prognosis	Highly predictable, no residual losses	Ambiguous, often poor, many residual losses
Health care system involvement	Minimal	Extensive
Other social systems involved	Usually none	Extensive usually education and vocational rehabilitation
Parental involvement	Minimal	Extensive, every aspect of life affected

2. Procedures and treatments allow as much mobility and comfort as possible, so that the child and family have maximum control.
3. Separation from the family is minimized.
4. Both child and family are prepared for procedures to maximize cooperation and minimize trauma.
5. The child's dignity is respected at all times and in all situations.
6. Both child and family are included in planning care, so that medical treatment is carried out in the context of an overall care plan for the child.

Such a strategy requires that the nurse thoroughly know the child's developmental level, personality characteristics, and needs, so that nursing care can be adapted to fit the needs of the child and family.

Home-Centered Care Whenever possible, children should be cared for in their own environments but with careful monitoring of the family's capabilities (see Chapter 26). The advantages of home care include avoiding the separation of family members and allowing parents to carry on essential family routines for maintenance of the family unit.

Some families, however, may not be able to cope with sick members without respite care, especially when the emotional and physical drain proves overwhelming. The nursing management approach therefore includes both an ongoing assessment of family dynamics (see Chapter 17) and careful observation for signs of unmet needs and potentially dysfunctional parenting (see Chapter 22).

Provider Continuity Continuity of care is essential in chronic illness, and although advocated by both physicians and nurses, it is often ignored in favor of short-term expediency. Continuity assures coordination of care. When many professional people are involved in a child's care, a typical situation for chronically ill children, one person needs to serve as the family's and child's "quarterback," or, if the professional is a nurse, the primary nurse. This arrangement is especially important for multihandicapped children who are served by a variety of health care and other providers, such as educators and vocational and psychological counselors. Multidisciplinary management necessitates a designated coordinator who can identify needs and assure that services are not duplicated. The nurse is, with the family's permission, well-suited to assume the role of coordinator. The continuity that a coordinator can bring thus compensates for an otherwise-fragmented system of care.

A positive, mutually respectful relationship among provider, patient, and family is essential to quality long-term care. Children who are able to communicate effectively with their providers are more likely to comply with therapy. This directly affects the extent to which the child's illness is controlled. A well-established pattern of honest communication also means that as children develop and new problems and concerns arise, such difficult topics as alcohol and drug abuse can be openly discussed.

Family-Centered Care The needs of families with chronically ill children must be paramount. The family is the unit of care, and the younger the child, the more critical this unit becomes. Unlike chronically ill older adolescents and adults, the development of infants and young children depends directly on family resources. Parents of these children therefore must acquire and develop skills as parents that far exceed normal expectations for parenting roles. Parents need help to accommodate family life for the chronically ill child and to provide for their own needs and those of their other children. This is an extraordinarily difficult task and invariably needs the nurse's attention.

Because the family is the unit of care, nursing responsibilities include family assessment, mutually determined treatment plans, provision for home care, and advocacy for multidisciplinary collaboration. For parents with chronically ill children, needs for family education and anticipatory guidance require special attention. Like other parents, parents of chronically ill children need to understand the normal process of growth and development along with the special needs of the ill child. (Anticipatory guidance is discussed in Chapter 21.)

Child Participation The chronically ill child and the family might need encouragement to be as independent in the management of the condition as possible. This often involves teaching both the child and family to use equipment designed for the child's needs (Fig. 30-2). The nurse works with other health care providers and parents to facilitate independence, while recognizing dependence as appropriate during periods of extreme stress or crises. Nurses might encourage families and ill children to act as members of the health team, although this role cannot develop unless health care providers insist on it, create an atmosphere in which it is fostered, and reinforce it when the family and child demonstrate participation and self-care.

This begins at as simple a level as encouraging the child and parent to talk about their responses to treatment regimens. Many will give their opinions, thinking that health care personnel know what is best and must be aware of their problems. The child and family, on the other hand, may even withhold information important in planning further treatment. With an ongoing illness or condition, family participation in planning care is crucial. For example, a juvenile diabetic failing to report incidents of hypoglycemia actually hinders appropriate insulin, diet, and exercise regulation. Some families become so involved in their children's care they form support groups, or institute legislation to aid their children's cause.

From the beginning the nurse should invite the child to participate as much as possible in self-care. By requiring the child to participate, the nurse not only conveys respect for the child's ability but also implies that the child's participation is essential to recovery. A child must come to understand that neither parents nor health professionals "own" the disease and that the child can be an agent in or an obstacle to recovery. Using the child's responses to guide further conversation, the nurse then learns the child's perception of the illness and can use this initial contact to gather information on the child's psychologic as well as physical status.

Parent and child education is the means by which family members become part of the health care team. Family and child education is thus an essential component of any nursing care plan, and the nurse needs to view education as an intervention equivalent in importance to medical care.

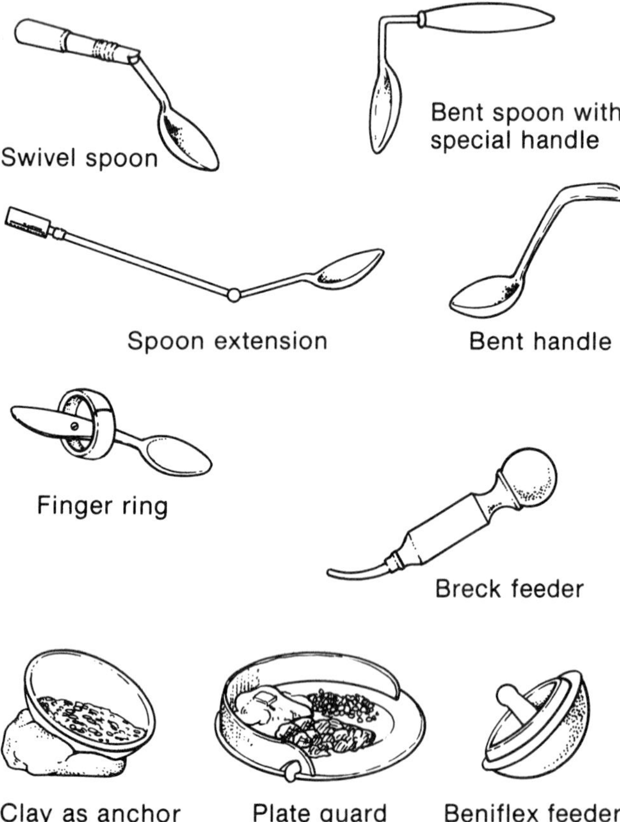

Figure 30-2 Eating utensils for handicapped children.

Assessment

The Family Assessment includes both the family and the ill child. Parents, the family "executives," are strategic in the treatment process. Before meeting with a parent, the nurse reviews the child's medical and hospital records because knowledge of the family's background and the medical problem guides the assessment process. The nurse creates a "family tree" diagram, or genogram, and uses the one in the medical history if it is available (see Fig. 5-10).

Psychologic turmoil typically accompanies the family's learning the diagnosis of chronic disease. Therefore, to establish rapport, gain trust, and obtain baseline data, the nurse needs to be sensitive to the family's immediate concerns. Both nurse and family should expect more than one interview to gather the essential information. A useful division of assessment criteria is to analyze both internal and external factors affecting the family as a system; in other words, to consider both the family's subsystems and suprasystems.

Family Subsystems Part of a family assessment focuses on the family's configuration and communication patterns (see Chapter 17). For the family coping with chronic illness, areas for discussion include the emotional impact of the diagnosis on the child and the parents, their feelings, their day-to-day level of functioning, the affected chld's role in the family, and how the diagnosis may have changed family life. Possible questions might include these:

How are family members dealing with their feelings?

Are any family members experiencing eating or sleeping disturbances?

Are the parents preoccupied and unable to attend to tasks within the home or at work?

Are the parents able to share the care of the affected child and the other children?

In addition, the nurse explores how the healthy children are responding to the sibling's illness. What have they been told? What provisions have been made for their care? Siblings inadvertently excluded from the activity around a newly diagnosed child generally receive little information or emotional support. By inquiring about the other children, the nurse subtly alerts the parent to their needs and pulls the siblings back toward the center of care planning and assessment activities. This subtle, albeit deliberate, effort may help to enhance family communication.

The assessment includes not only interview data but also unstructured observations of family behavior. Observations of family communication may include noting who is most verbal and who expresses feelings. The behavior of siblings and the family's attitude toward the health care team are also important to note. The nurse needs to determine how disruptive the child's condition is to ongoing family functioning in order to plan both short-term and long-term care. For instance, a two-parent family in which the parents are unable to talk with each other about their feelings will need help to express their concerns.

With two-parent families, the nurse assesses the child's parents together to determine their commitment to the family, their ability to communicate, and their individual strengths and limitations. How well the parents communicate with their children is a key factor, for parents who have difficulty in doing this well need more assistance than those who do so readily. Parental roles and needs also require review. In a two-parent family, how have the parents viewed their parental responsibilities? Are they shared equally? Or are the roles of these parents more traditionally structured so that the mother is principally responsible for child care? What kinds of adjustments will the parents have to make to accommodate the child's problems in the family?

The genogram is the nurse's reference for the siblings' ages, sex, and health status. Using this as a starting point, the nurse inquires about the reaction of siblings to the child's illness. Direct observation of siblings supplements the parental interpretation of their behavior. The nurse might observe siblings during the ill child's clinic visit or hospital stay, or while making a home visit. Home visits usually provide the most accurate assessment of the siblings' responses.

Talking with the siblings privately or with their parents affords an excellent opportunity not only for nursing assessment but also for education about the illness and its implications for them. The nurse is concerned primarily with the psychosocial health of the ill child's siblings, which is evident in their behavior toward adults, peers, and school.

Family Suprasystems An analysis of the suprasystems that influence the family includes the extended family's role, the family's social network, and the community's attitudes and resources.

In assessing the extended family, the nurse considers the health and ability of all those who may play a role in care. Grandparents, for example, may have their own health problems and needs and may not be counted on to help with day-to-day child care or other household tasks, although they may be able to contribute financially. The nurse needs to address these questions with sensitivity. Even in families who have been estranged, illness in one of the members can facilitate reconciliation. If the potential to resolve old grievances is enhanced, reconciliation may be one of the positive outcomes of chronic childhood disease.

The family's social network of community organizations, which might include religious and secular associations, may provide services or support to the family on both an immediate and ongoing basis. The nurse needs to investigate prevailing attitudes toward sick children in the family's community and, more important, the expression of these values in the availability of services and programs. A community that provides early intervention programs for multihandicapped children, for example, is one motivated to prevent secondary sequelae for these vulnerable community members. The existence of such a program speaks to the high value placed on the weakest members of the community and the concern for them and their families.

By contrast, a community that offers minimal services places a family with a disabled child at a disadvantage in acquiring assistance. One family with a hearing-impaired child lived in a sparsely inhabited rural state and was forced to relocate so that needed services could be procured for the child. Even so, the child was under the age for mandated services and was ineligible to receive the necessary care. This unusually persistent family was able to persuade the state legislature to change its age requirements, but many families would not be willing to pursue a cause with such tenacity.

The Child The nurse who is organizing care, guided by a knowledge of the child's family, age, and developmental status, begins the assessment by trying to establish a trusting relationship with the child. The goal is to build the child's confidence in the nurse as caregiver and advocate. Asking the child for a personal introduction and giving a brief description of the nursing role is therefore helpful in establishing a working relationship.

The nurse can obtain data about such personal matters

as sleeping, eating, and elimination habits either from parents or from the child, but older children and adolescents feel respected if they are asked these questions themselves. Even very young children can respond to simple questions and describe reasons for visiting the doctor or for hospitalization. Their responses are congruent with their knowledge and their ability to communicate about their illnesses and needs for care.

A complete physical assessment is necessary at the time of diagnosis (see Chapter 14). Without disturbing the child, who may be very ill, the nurse can perform most of the assessment through careful history taking. Gentleness coupled with honest discussion about the circumstances of the illness help to establish trust.

The nurse assesses the child's developmental status gradually. Knowing that the child reacts to the diagnosis and management of chronic illness according to developmental stage, the nurse compares the child's abilities, both affectively and cognitively, with age-appropriate norms. (Developmental assessment is discussed in Chapter 16.)

Standard assessment tools may also be indicated for screening. Observations are then specifically directed toward identifying coping strategies and current needs. With older children, the nurse also inquires about peer relationships and family interactions. Analysis of assessment data may indicate a potential for developmental problems related to the illness. Assisting the child with normal developmental progress may therefore need to be a goal of nursing care.

Multidisciplinary Management

Planning Following a complete assessment and the formulation of nursing diagnoses, the nurse and other members of the health care team meet with the family to review the medical protocol and plan for the child's care. Unless the parents are health care providers themselves, they may feel at a disadvantage in such company unless the professional health care providers insist, encourage, and demand their participation. Children and adolescents have a double disadvantage in participating as they, like their parents, lack knowledge of the disease and are not adults. Thus health care providers need to encourage their participation in the team and the nurse monitors interventions to see that this goal is accomplished.

Family members involved in the care plan include the parents, any affected child over age 9 or 10, and any siblings of a similar age. Younger children are involved at their appropriate level of understanding. This does not mean that the nurse withholds information, but rather that information should be comprehensible to the child. Young children readily grasp the seriousness of a problem, and the nurse therefore helps the parent explain the child's illness and the plan of care in an effective, open manner so that the child is not frightened.

Unfortunately, siblings are often forced into the background during periods of extreme stress in the course of the illness. As a result, siblings often learn of a brother or sister's illness under less-than-desirable circumstances. If the siblings cannot be part of the conferences, the nurse alerts the parents about discussing the affected child's care with other children in the family. The nurse organizing care can set up a time to talk with the brothers and sisters separately if this is best for both parents and children. When available, peer groups can also be used for sibling support; one highly successful support group for brothers and sisters of children with cancer was one in which a nurse and a child life worker set aside one evening a month to talk with siblings. Over a period of several months, the real concerns of these children surfaced and were handled in the group. As the children learned to trust one another and their leaders, each child resolved feelings of uniqueness and isolation, and these children were better able to deal with their parents and with their own developmental needs.

The entire family benefits when given ample opportunity to ask questions and make suggestions. Family members should be encouraged to voice their concerns and hesitations regarding the care plan. Even though they are forced to delegate decision making to their doctors, they must be told that they are indeed delegating, and are not at the mercy of the staff's decisions. Except in the most urgent situations, families must be provided sufficient time to review the medical and nursing plans privately. Even in a serious life-threatening situation, the nurse can provide the family with a few minutes or even an hour for private discussion.

Nurses can also work with the family to determine the goals of intervention. The goals should reflect the family's values and beliefs, be realistic and achievable, and seek to return the child to a maximum level of functioning. Short-term goals might include learning the medical and nursing care regimens, creating a support network, and finding ways to permit family members to fulfill their normal commitments.

Interventions Interventions for the child with chronic illness involve both direct and indirect nursing care. Direct care includes physical and developmental monitoring together with emotional support. Laboratory tests specific to the disease augment the findings of the history and physical examination. Additionally, the nurse continually intervenes to monitor the child's responses to living with the disease. Self-esteem, relationships with adults, peers, and siblings, and academic progress constitute critical areas for monitoring.

Education of the child about the disease and its treatment is also updated regularly. The balance among health team, parents, and child in health planning shifts continually as a child grows with the child gradually assuming more and more responsibility for self-care. The relationship between the nurse and the child forms the basis for the support so needed by both child and family.

Indirect nursing services are necessitated by the complexity of care of chronically ill children. Beginning with establishing communication among members of the health care team, the nurse coordinates care with the family, the school, and other institutions. This may involve education of family members about the disease and about the necessary support in caring for the ill child. Conferences with school personnel are a frequent form of indirect nursing care. A child with a seizure disorder, for example, might need careful monitoring during the school day. Teachers and other school personnel involved in data collection regarding the disease and its treatment usually require extensive education.

Preventing Secondary Effects The nurse who is organizing care for a child and family sets long-term goals congruent with the child's situation and disease condition. The first of these goals is to prevent long-term disability through rehabilitation. If the child has lost physical function because of illness, the nurse, in concert with the medical and health care team, attempts to restore the lost function.

The second goal is to prevent secondary emotional and learning problems. Approximately one-third of children with chronic illness develop problems secondary to their chronic conditions (Pless and Roughmann, 1971; Pless, 1975; Wallace, et al., 1982). Many of the secondary problems can be prevented by careful planning of the child's care. Fostering normal development, for example, enables the child to continue to grow in areas unaffected directly by the disease. One adolescent with epilepsy needed to develop social skills, which required interacting with peers. The nurse discussed with the adolescent the issues surrounding anticonvulsant therapy, such as confiding in others about the condition and experimentation with alcohol and street drugs. By addressing such sensitive issues honestly, the nurse helped this adolescent come to terms with both the epilepsy and the need to be part of a peer group.

The third goal is to prevent physical sequelae. The nurse monitors the medical therapy closely to detect signs of iatrogenic pathology. The child who requires long-term steroid therapy, for example, requires careful monitoring for signs of hemorrhage or superinfection and thus needs frequent general physical examinations.

Helping Parents Become Advocates The role of the parent as advocate is critical for both the child's and the family's well-being, but most parents learn this role in an environment that all too frequently fails to support their efforts. They learn, for example, to be advocates of their children's medical care and education in ways that parents of healthy children are almost never required to do (Gliedman and Roth, 1980). They are forced to learn about the disease process and its care and management in order to make crucial decisions regarding their child's care.

Most parents are unprepared for this role, and most learn it by trial and error, in chance discussions with other parents and all too infrequently through organized educational efforts. Parental advocacy is necessary when the family deals with the health care system and with other institutions, including the educational system. Nurses often need to inform parents of their rights. These are explicitly stated in many hospitals as a "Patient Bill of Rights" and under PL 94-142, Education for All Handicapped (Wallace, et al., 1982).

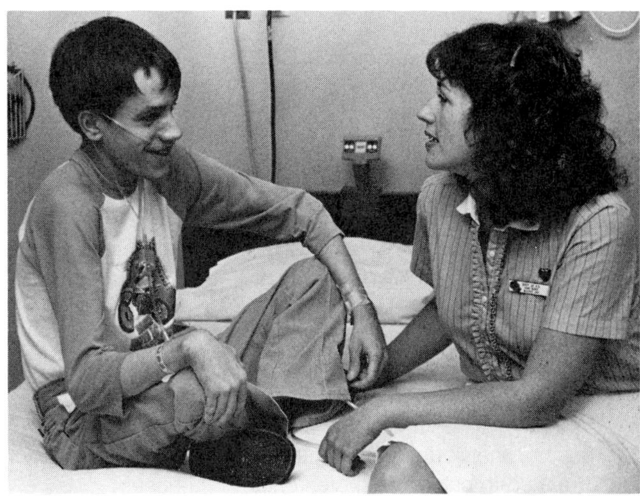

Emotional support is an important component of nursing care for the chronically ill adolescent.

After making family members aware of their rights under these and other rules and policies, the nurse can be helpful to the family in applying them. For example, a family of a child with a degenerative chronic illness such as Duchenne's muscular dystrophy is entitled to free and appropriate education in the least restrictive environment, even if the child lives in a rural area with sparse resources. Families need encouragement to secure services in spite of the all-too-frequently encountered community resistance. For example, children who have cerebral palsy or mental retardation are entitled to have developmental services from birth or from the time the problem is identified (Wallace, et al., 1982). Nurses therefore need to be informed of these services and urge parents to secure them.

Teaching Self-Care Families with chronically ill children share a need for education in their roles as caregivers and advocates. These are generally roles that they did not expect when they became parents, and few feel prepared.

Child and parent teaching regarding the illness and its management includes guidelines for parent–child responsibilities. The family first needs to learn about the illness, and the parent and affected child are initially the focus of the nurse's efforts. A child who can comprehend the disease and its treatment sufficiently should be educated along with the parent; otherwise, the child will need education about the condition geared to the appropriate cognitive ability and developmental stage.

NURSING CARE GUIDE The Child With a Chronic Condition

Nursing Diagnosis	Interventions	Evaluation
1. Potential for adverse emotional response in the child related to the problems of chronic illness: poor self-concept, fear, denial, depressed affect	Observe the child's solitary play, art, interactions with others, and ability for and interest in self-care Encourage child to express feelings about self and the effects of illness on the child's life Provide realistic reassurance through verbal communication, or role play the child's actions in response to siblings', peers', and adults' questions about the illness Encourage family and peer support Observe the child for more severe psychologic alterations (see Chapter 24)	Child's affect is appropriate Child's responses, play, drawings, are within normal limits Child has positive and realistic self-concept and body image Child indicates ability to manage personal concerns and disappointments Child indicates readiness to rejoin some previous activities Child has support of family and peers
2. Possible knowledge deficit in the child related to causes of the chronic condition	Ask child to describe the illness and its causes Clarify misconceptions Determine child's goals for learning Set mutual long- and short-term goals for learning Implement teaching plan at child's functional developmental level, making use of drawings, stories, and games when possible Share teaching plan with other nursing staff members Repeat and augment teaching as needed if evaluation indicates incomplete comprehension	Child listens to and participates appropriately in teaching sessions Child can either correctly repeat teaching or can pick correct information out of several choices Child shows interest in self-care
3. Potential self-care deficit related to the treatment regimen	Observe the child's level of self-care Set mutual goals with the child for increasing participation in self-care Teach the child the appropriate skills, with sensitivity to the child's need to participate, observe, practice, and withdraw Demonstrate enthusiasm and encouragement for any progress Repeat and augment as needed if evaluation indicates incomprehension or reluctance to perform skills Plan any further learning necessary for proper care of condition (eg, special hygiene, medications, activity recommendations, or diet) Facilitate referral to community resources if needed	As appropriate for developmental level, child is knowledgeable, skilled, and motivated concerning self-care Any follow-up necessary for child's learning is planned
4. Potential for adverse emotional responses in the parent related to the diagnosis of the child's chronic condition	Observe the parent for overt signs of anger, fear, depression, denial or guilt Listen to and note any verbally expressed psychologic needs of family members Actively elicit verbal expression of feelings from parent Observe family interactions and parental behavior for indications of maladaptive coping related to adjustment to the child's condition	Parental response is within normal limits for the duration of the child's condition, the seriousness of the condition, and the child's current health status Family interactions seem mutually supportive Parent expresses interest in community support group

Nursing Diagnosis	Interventions	Evaluation
	Support parent and provide reassurance Reassess parental response before a hospitalized child is discharged Facilitate referral to community resources or support services as parental needs and readiness indicate	
5. Potential parental knowledge deficit concerning child's condition	Elicit parental perception of the child's illness and observe for factors indicating readiness to learn: decreased anxiety, increased interest in and attention to the child's case, increase in appropriate questions Design education plan for all aspects of physical care regimen Using books, diagrams, and participation in care, as appropriate, provide teaching based on parental readiness Discuss changes in home routine or environment that might benefit child and family Communicate teaching plan to other members of the nursing staff Repeat and augment if necessary Facilitate referral to outside resources as needed for appropriate follow-up and further teaching	Parent listens to teaching Parent explains care accurately Parent properly carries out all physical care necessary for child Parent describes home changes needed because of child's condition
6. Potential deficit in parental ability to raise child with a chronic condition	Initiate discussion of the effects of the chronic condition on parental perceptions of child and child's needs Help parents decide appropriate parental behavior toward child in relation to normal development, discipline, independence, involvement in child's health care, school, and peer activities Plan for multiple follow-up discussions as child grows Monitor for overt behavior indicating overprotection, resentment, overpermissiveness Facilitate referral to counseling if problems arise	Parent sees the child as growing, maturing, and needing the security of limits and the freedom of appropriate independence Parent provides for alterations and special considerations necessitated by the child's condition Parent expresses basic satisfaction in care of the child
7. Potential adverse sibling reactions to the child, the child's condition and to alterations in family life	Monitor siblings' reactions through direct observation and conversations and through active listening to parent and child Observe for fears, feelings of guilt, and jealousy; unmet needs; difficulty in coping Note siblings' reactions toward the ill child, particularly expressions of pity and anger Observe for withdrawal, unhappiness, or acting-out behavior Clarify any misconceptions for sibling Support sibling Assist sibling and parent in plans to meet siblings' needs Facilitate referral to outside resources or counseling if needed	Siblings' feelings and concerns are within normal limits Siblings' basic needs are met Siblings have no major misconceptions concerning the child's condition

The nurse's teaching necessarily begins when the child is first diagnosed and continues as the child lives with the illness. The education for both the child and parent is anticipatory, geared to the readiness and learning styles of both the child and family. Through education and living with the child, the parent's knowledge of the child's specific condition often supersedes that of the professionals.

Parents often become aware of subtle changes in a child's condition before health professionals become concerned. For instance, the mother of a young child with insulin-dependent diabetes was able, through careful observation, to regulate the child's insulin so carefully that reactions were extremely infrequent. The physician, after a bit of convincing, worked with this parent to achieve a level of control higher than is generally thought possible. The nurse's initial teaching plan had, in this case, helped the parent to become an informed member of the health care team and a partner in the child's treatment.

Facilitating Family Communication The family needs to help incorporate the ill member into the family system, where communication among family members becomes critical. The nurse therefore works with family members to foster communication and may also help directly as parents attempt to explain illness and its limitations to siblings. The nurse can role-play with family members to give them the courage to discuss important matters with each other and thus enable family members to anticipate feelings and to find ways of dealing with them. For instance, older adolescents often avoid discussing emotionally labile issues because they are afraid of both their own and others' reactions. One young man wanted desperately to talk with his dying brother about his feelings, but refused because of the emotions such communication would evoke. Fear of expressing feelings prevented the necessary communication.

Unfortunately, this is an all-too-frequent occurrence between dying children and their parents (see Chapter 32). Binger (1973) described poignantly the emotional distance that grew between a 9-year-old boy and his mother as the boy was dying. The mother's avoidance of her son's dying became a barrier. They could not discuss the boy's concerns, creating a superficial and distant relationship at a time when emotional empathy and closeness was crucial. Eventually, it was the boy who forced his mother to face his dying and, in so doing, helped his family to cope with his problems.

Bluebond-Langer (1978) notes that children, regardless of the state of the disease, need to feel loved, supported, and able to communicate with parents and siblings. Chronically ill children are at risk for developing communication problems for the following several reasons: (a) they may receive special treatment from well-meaning but errant parents; (b) they may become distanced from friends because of hospitalizations and physical incapacity that prevent them from keeping up with peers; and (c) siblings, unsure about dealing with the ill child's problems, limit communication. Thus the nurse's working with the entire family to maintain good communication patterns is vitally important.

Developing Family Support Systems Facilitating the family's ability to build and use support networks is important to prevent the damaging secondary effects of isolation. Families come to the diagnosis of chronic illness generally ignorant of the problems and issues they will face in caring for the child and the implications of the child's illness to the family. Nurses need to help families not only to use their networks of friends and relatives but also to develop relationships with families who have similar problems.

Families will benefit from both networks for support. While the extended family and old friends are needed, friendship with families experiencing similar problems provides companionship with those who understand exactly the relevant issues and problems. The parents of a child with cystic fibrosis maintained relationships with family and friends at church but also met regularly with a cystic fibrosis parents' group. Because many of these families spend many hours in the care of their children, they are often unable to maintain reciprocal relationships with friends who are not so encumbered. For many families, this is a part of the difficult but realistic sequelae of chronic childhood disease. Isolation from previous friends and even a way of life is all too easy. The nurse therefore talks with family members about the problem and encourages them to find ways to maintain friendships.

Parents must also maintain their responsibilities as parents of their children. The nurse, aware of the parents' readiness to assume aspects of their child's care, can support their efforts directly or through community health nurses. Parents should be encouraged to tell nurses that they feel overwhelmed by their child's care. For example, at a parent's request, one nurse arranged for the community health nurse to assist the mother of a neonate and an older child with cystic fibrosis.

Supporting Parenting Skills While planning intervention for families, the nurse also addresses the problems of emphasizing the continuation of normal parenting behaviors. The child's illness can cause parental feelings of guilt, anger, and frustration, which parents often repress because they feel these feelings are unacceptable. An inherent danger in this situation is that these repressed feelings can affect what would be otherwise normal parenting. For example, a parent who would normally establish firm limits for their child's behavior might tend to relax discipline and allow the child to manipulate family members. Some parents, often mothers who are overburdened with the care of the ill child, become overprotective and encourage the child's dependence rather than promote the child's self-care. These parents might then become resentful of the child's inappropriate behavior and become subsequently more angry, guilty, or depressed. This cyclical pattern affects not only the ill child but also the parental relationships with other children. Children then who become more demanding might in turn be pampered by both parents and siblings. Again this leads to parents' and siblings' feelings of resentment, which may be communicated unconsciously to the ill child. The end result is a child with poor self-esteem in addition to the problems associated with the chronic condition.

This pattern can be avoided by helping parents understand how they can cope with their children's demands. Parents of children with chronic illnesses may have special needs for information about methods of discipline (see Chapter 13). The nurse helps parents differentiate between appropriate illness-related behavior and children's nuisance behavior. To do this, the nurse needs a child's developmental history from the parents and, if possible, from the child's teachers. In addition, the nurse might use an assessment tool in order to quantify the severity of a behavioral problem (see Chapters 16 and 17). If the child's behavior proves to be dysfunctional or not age-appropriate, the nurse seeks help from a child psychologist in further assessing the problem. (Age-appropriate discipline is discussed in Chapter 13; nursing management of dysfunctional behavior is discussed in Chapter 24.)

If a child's behavior is considered to be outside the limits for the appropriate age group and condition, the nurse can work both with parent and child to achieve more satisfactory behavior. The nurse who has educated parents to be good observers of their children will have enabled them to determine whether a child's behavior is due to the stress of the physical condition or the stress of the environment and whether the child is merely seeking parental attention or attempting to take control. If the child's behavior is an attempt to control, the nurse can help the parent find constructive ways to discipline the child.

By helping parents identify appropriate and inappropriate demands and by teaching them to respond appropriately, the cycle of dependence can be averted. Should it develop, it can be more easily broken when the appropriate behavior is facilitated. Nurses might need to remind parents that their roles as socializers and shapers of their children continue even though their children have special problems.

Evaluation Finally, the evaluation component of the nursing process, which serves as assessment for the next phase of care, is especially important for children with chronic illness. The goals established for both the family and the ill child are the criteria with which progress is measured. Because nurse and family participate in defining goals, both participate in evaluation, and a specified time should be set aside for this function.

For example, if the goal is to acquire skills to administer insulin safely, evaluation would require gathering information either by direct observation of the technique or by report of the family. If the goal is to secure appropriate monitoring of seizure activity by the school, then by checking school reports against those that parents recorded on weekends is a means of evaluation. The evaluation process requires that goals specify behaviors as the bases for evaluation. The nurse therefore does not simply accept a parent's casual statement that something is "going along all right," but instead asks for specific examples supporting this statement.

Since the course of a chronic illness is not static, constant evaluation is required for optimal nursing care. Evaluation and reevaluation facilitate the process of setting new goals and thus improving the quality of life for the chronically ill child.

Key Concepts

- Parents view a child's diagnosis of chronic illness as a crisis that initially causes family disorganization and emotional upset.
- A family's perception of a chronic illness is affected by the child's condition, the child's gender, the family's religious and cultural background, the family's experience with stress and crisis, and the child's prognosis.
- The overall impact of chronic illness on a child and family is a result of interactions among three systems: community, family, and child.
- Families need to make psychological and environmental adjustments for children with chronic illness, which in turn place a family with marginal coping skills at risk for dysfunction.
- Parents of chronically ill children commonly need assistance with financial burdens, resources for support, and ways of finding time away from the demands of constant care.
- The impact of the diagnosis on the child depends on the child's developmental stage, temperament, and current social roles.
- Adolescents are especially likely to rebel against the limitations of illness and treatment and need support in accomplishing developmental tasks.

- Siblings of children with chronic illness are affected by changes in family dynamics and communication patterns, by parental behavior toward them, and by fears of the illness.
- Because the health care system is designed for acute, short-term needs, nurses need to plan specific long-term interventions that provide continuity of care and participation for the child and family.
- Health care for the child with a chronic illness should be home- and family-centered so that family functioning can be maintained as much as possible.
- The nurse's assessment of the family involves analysis of both the family subsystems (parent, child, siblings) and the family suprasystems (social contacts, relatives, community).
- All family members should be as involved as possible in planning care for the child with chronic illness, and the ill child and siblings should be involved at their appropriate levels of understanding.
- Nursing goals for a child with chronic illness include preventing secondary effects, helping parents act as advocates for their children, teaching self-care and parenting skills, and facilitating communication within and support for the family.
- Evaluation is an essential component of nursing care for chronic illness and serves as the assessment phase for reviewing and revising nursing diagnoses and goals.

References

Binger CM: Childhood leukemia: Emotional impact on the sibling. In *The Child and His Family: Impact of Disease and Death.* Anthony EJ, Kouperinck E, (editors), 2nd ed. Wiley, 1973.

Bluebond-Langner M: *The Private Worlds of Dying Children.* Princeton, 1976.

Bowe F: *Handicapping America: Barriers to Disabled People.* Harper & Row, 1978.

Gliedman J, Roth W: *The Unexpected Minority: Handicapped Children in America.* Harcourt, 1980.

Heatherington E M: Play and social interaction in children following divorce. *J Soc Iss,* 1979; 35:26–49.

Hewett S: Research on families with handicapped children—an aid or an impediment to understanding? Pages 46–53 in *Birth Defects: Original Article in Series. 17th ed. The National Foundation, 1976.*

Hill R: Generic features of families under stress. In: *Crisis Intervention.* Family Service Association of America, 1965.

Leonard B: *Impact of Chronic Illness on the Siblings of an Affected Child.* University of Minnesota, unpublished.

Litman T: The family as a basic unit in health and medical care: A social behavioral overview. *Soc Sci Med* 1974; 6:495–519.

Olshansky S: Chronic sorrow: A response to having a mentally defective child. *Soc Casework* 1962; 43:190–193.

Pless IB, Roghmann K J: Chronic illness and its consequences: Observations based on three epidemiologic surveys. *J Pediatr* 1971; 79:351–359.

Solut AT, Stark MH: Mourning and the birth of a defective child. *PsychoStu Child* 1961; 16:523–537.

Spinetta J, Deasy-Spinetta P: *Living With Childhood Cancer.* Mosby, 1981.

Wallace H, Gold E, Oglesby A: *Maternal and Child Health Practices.* Wiley, 1982.

Wallerstein J, Kelly J: *Surviving the Breakup.* Basic, 1980.

Additional Readings

Allmond B, Gofman: *The Family Is the Patient.* Mosby, 1979.

Anderson S, Bauwens EE: *Chronic Health Problems.* Mosby, 1981.

Bradshaw J, Lawtonb D: Tracing the causes of stress in families with handicapped children. *Br J Soc Work* 1978; 8:181–192.

Burr W et al: *Contemporary Theories About the Family.* 1st ed. Free Press, 1979.

Burton L: *Care of the Child Facing Death.* Routledge & Kegan Paul, 1974.

Debuskey M (Editor): *The Chronically Ill Child and His Family.* Charles C. Thomas, 1970.

French A, Berlin IN: *Depression in Children and Adolescents.* Human Sciences, 1979.

Gaspard NJ: The family of the patient with long-term illness. *Nurs Clin North Am* (March) 1970; 5(1):77–84.

Holaday B J: Achievement behavior in chronically ill children. *Nurs Res* (Jan/Feb) 1974; 23:25–30.

Harvard Child Health Project: Children's medical care, needs and treatments. *I, II, III.* Ballinger, 1977.

Hymovich DP: Asssessing the impact of chronic childhood illness on the family and parent coping. *Image* (Oct) 1981; 13:71–74.

Ireys H: Health care for chronically disabled children and their families. In: *Better Health for Our Children: A National Strategy.* US Department of Public Health, 1981.

Johnson B H, Steele BB: Community networking for improved services to children with chronic illnesses and their families. *Child Health Care* (Fall) 1983; 12(2):98–102.

Kempe H et al: *Pediatric Diagnosis and Treatment.* 4th ed. Lange Medical, 1976.

Kleinberg SB: *Educating the Chronically Ill Child.* Aspen, 1982.

Koocher G, O'Malley J: *The Damocles Syndrome: The Psychosocial Consequences of Surviving Childhood Cancer.* McGraw-Hill, 1981.

Lewis C et al: *A Right to Health: The Problem of Access to Primary Medical Care.* Wiley, 1976.

McKeever PT: Fathering the chronically ill child. *Am J Matern Child Nurs* (Mar/Apr) 1981; 6:126–128.

Minuchin et al: *Psychosomatic Families.* Harvard, 1980.

Montague JP, Rheba A: Use of parents' suggestions in evaluating a long-term care program for disabled children. *Child Health Care* (Summer) 1984; 13(1):24. (Fall) 1983; 11(2):74–77.

Pierce PM, Freedman SA: The REACH project: An innovative health delivery model for medically dependent children. *Child Health Care* (Fall) 1983; 12(2):86–89.

Pierce PM, Giovinco G: REACH: Self-care for the chronically ill child. *Pediatr Nurs* (Jan/Feb) 1983; 37–39.

Pless IB: The care of children with chronic illness. *Report of the 67th Ross Conference on Pediatric Research.* Moore, T. (editor). Ross Laboratories, 1975.

Reiss I: *Family Systems in America.* 3rd ed. Holt, 1980.

Rodgers et al: Depression in the chronically ill or handicapped school-aged child. *Am J Matern Child Nurs* (July/Aug) 1981; 6:266–273.

Rutter M: *Changing Youth in a Changing Society.* Harvard, 1980.

Rutter M: *Helping Troubled Children.* Plenum, 1975.

Schilling R, Gilchrist L, Schinke S: Coping and social support in families of developmentally disabled children. *Family Relations* 1984; 33:47–54.

Schwartz H, Kart CS: *Dominant Issues in Medical Sociology.* Addison-Wesley, 1978.

Steele S: *Nursing Care of the Child With Long-term Illness.* Appleton-Century-Crofts, 1977.

Stein R: A home care program for children with chronic illness. *Child Health Care* (Fall) 1983; 12(2):90–92.

Steiner P: The wall child and the hospitalized disabled sibling. *J Psychosoc Nurs* (Mar) 1984; 22(3):

Talbot N: *Raising Children in Modern America.* Little, Brown, 1976.

Travis G: *Chronic Illness in Children.* Stanford University, 1976.

Yancy WS: Approaches to emotional management of the child with a chronic illness. *Clin Pediatr* (Feb) 1972; 11:64–67.

Ongoing Nursing Care of the High-Risk Infant

31

Diane Holditch Davis

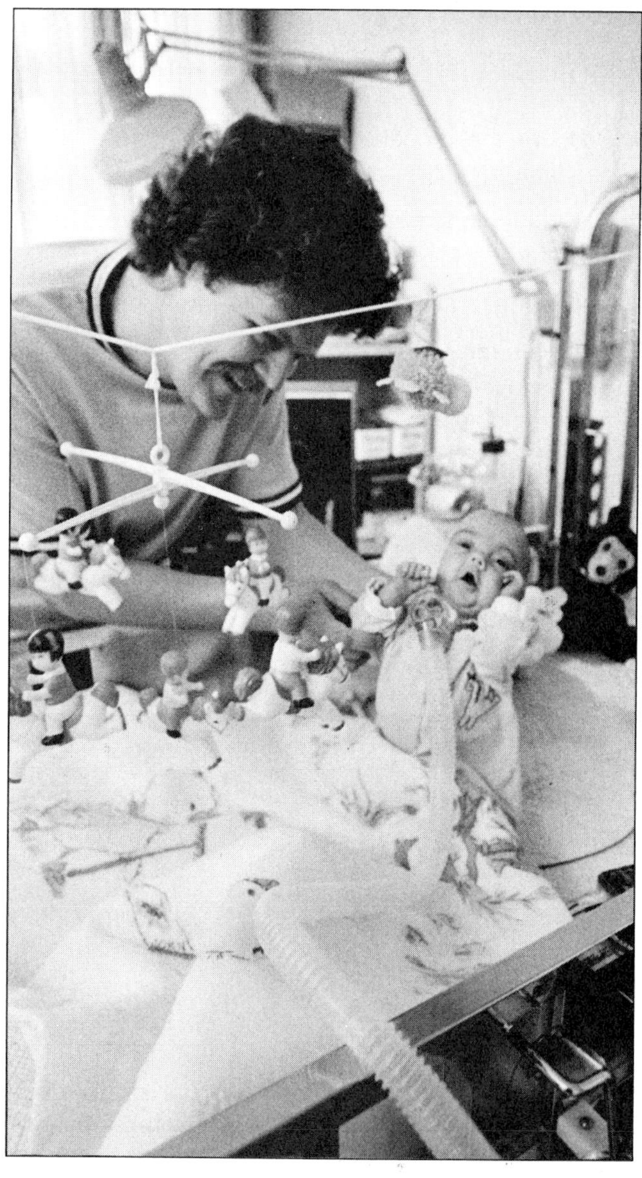

Chapter Outline

continued on next page

Objectives

- Explain the history and current regionalization of health care for high-risk infants.
- Describe the impact of high-risk infants and neonatal intensive care on the infants' families.
- List risk factors associated with the birth of a high-risk infant.
- Define the terms used to classify high-risk infants.
- Compare the growth and development of premature infants to the growth and development of normal full-term infants.
- List the special problems of high-risk infants.
- Describe the assessment criteria, nursing goals, and nursing management associated with heat regulation, metabolic imbalances, and neonatal hyperbilirubinemia in high-risk infants.
- Explain the implications of the immaturity of the immunologic, respiratory, circulatory, and neurologic systems for the premature infant's physiologic state.
- Describe the assessment criteria, nursing goals, and nursing management associated with immunologic, respiratory, nutritional, circulatory, and neurologic disorders in high-risk infants.
- Describe the causes, assessment criteria, nursing goals, and nursing management associated with developmental delays.
- List the causes of alterations in parenting for high-risk infants.
- Describe the assessment criteria, nursing goals, and nursing management associated with both parenting problems and neonatal death.

To find these topics, see the following chapters

Child abuse	Chapter 22
Inorganic failure to thrive	Chapter 22
Neonatal assessment	Chapter 7
Organic failure to thrive	Chapter 38
Sudden infant death syndrome	Chapter 32

Although infant mortality has decreased significantly in the past 100 years, early infancy remains a high-risk period. The death rate for the first year of life exceeds the death rate of the next 64 years, and two-thirds of these deaths occur in the first month of life, the neonatal period (Babson et al., 1975). More than one-fifth of all infants require medical treatment after birth, often in neonatal intensive care units.

Because society views pregnancy as a happy event that results in a healthy infant, parents are unprepared to deal with an infant who requires medical care. Nurses working with high-risk infants provide not only skilled care to assist infants in their adaptation to extrauterine life but also support and information for the parents.

A high-risk infant is any infant who is at risk for medical, developmental, or psychologic problems persisting into later years. Identification and treatment of these infants can prevent many of these problems, but the needs of high-risk infants and their families do not end with hospital discharge. Thus nurses will come into contact with high-risk infants in many different settings.

In this chapter we describe strategies for meeting the needs of high-risk infants and their families throughout childhood. We concentrate on the nursing care of infants who are biologically at risk, particularly those with conditions unique to the neonatal period and due to physiologic immaturity or to the stresses of labor and delivery. Because the birth of a high-risk infant affects the entire family, we discuss the emotional reaction of parents, siblings, and other family members and the ways in which the high-risk infant may become part of the family system. Finally, we discuss the effect of neonatal death on the family and the nursing care needed when families are grieving.

The Health Care System for High-Risk Infants

History of Neonatal Intensive Care

Although today seriously ill infants are treated in neonatal intensive care units (NICUs), these are rather recent developments. Prior to the twentieth century, premature and

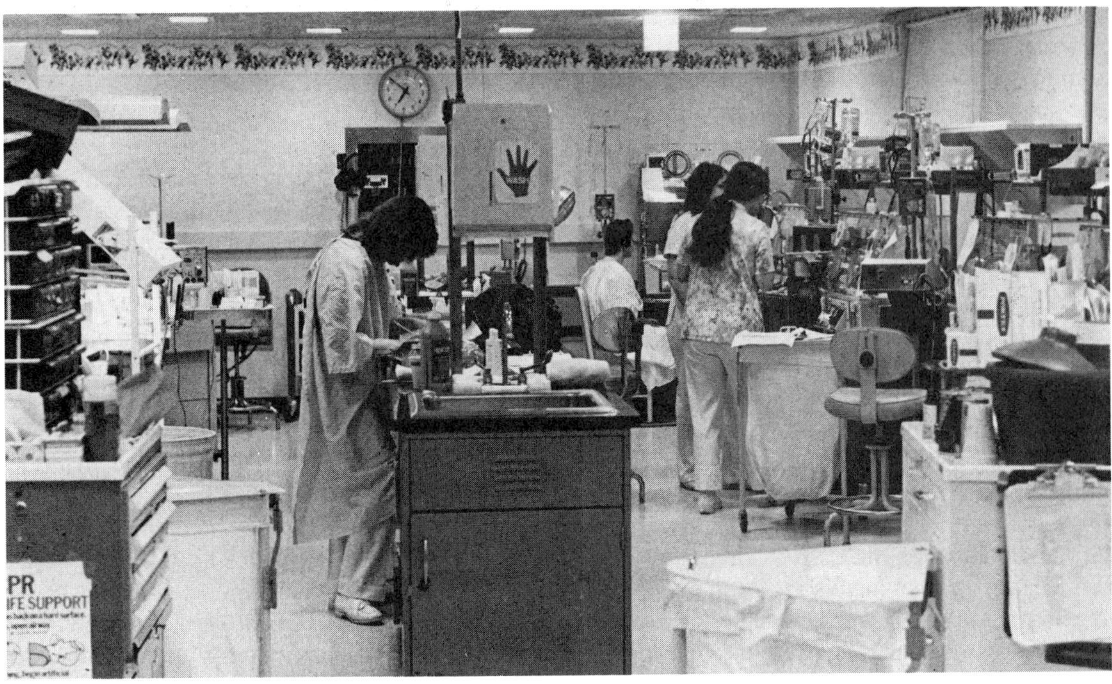

A neonatal intensive care unit (NICU) (Christine Acebo, photographer).

other high-risk infants had little chance of survival and so received only minimal care after birth. Interest in the medical and nursing care of these infants began with Pierre-Constant Budin's development of incubators and gavage feeding techniques. Martin Couney, a student of Budin, popularized premature care by exhibiting preterm infants in incubators at various fairs from 1920 to 1940, thus beginning the tradition of excluding parents from the care of premature infants. Couney gave his mothers free admission to the exhibits, but they could only look.

Most of Couney's premature infants survived, and so hospitals gradually emulated his methods. The emphasis in these new hospital-based nurseries was on providing supportive care, primarily warmth, and nutrition. By the late 1950s, the care of preterm infants had expanded to include the treatment of a variety of disorders among which were elevated bilirubin levels and respiratory problems.

Neonatal intensive care began in 1965 with the first reported use of mechanical ventilation to treat respiratory distress syndrome (RDS). Since then, the emphasis has been on developing treatment programs that meet the special needs of newborn infants rather than on merely adapting existing treatments developed for adults. For example, respiratory support for neonates has been aided by the development of continuous positive airway pressure and pressure ventilators. Because infants have small blood volumes, microtechniques that require only small samples of blood for laboratory testing have been developed. Transcutaneous oxygen monitoring allows continuous monitoring of oxygenation without blood samples. In addition, perinatology, a special field of obstetrics concerned with the management of high-risk pregnancies and treatment of the fetus, has reduced the number of medical problems that begin before birth.

Neonatology, or the management and treatment of the newborn infant, is a new field, and it is continuing to change rapidly. Researchers now find it impossible to make predictions about the outcome of care for a high-risk infant because by the time that the long-term outcome of a group of infants is determined, the medical care has changed. Thus nurses who concentrate solely on the technical aspects of neonatal care find that their knowledge rapidly becomes obsolete. The skills involved with meeting the emotional needs of parents and the developmental needs of infants, on the other hand, remain necessary both in the hospital and after discharge.

Regionalization of Perinatal Care

The development of modern NICUs has resulted in the regionalization of perinatal and neonatal care. Because the equipment required for neonatal intensive care is expensive and NICU personnel—neonatologists, nurses, laboratory technicians, and respiratory therapists—require special training, it is not economically feasible for all hospitals to provide this care. Instead, a three-tiered system of perinatal care has evolved.

Level I consists of small, and usually rural, community

hospitals providing primary obstetric and neonatal care to essentially normal maternity patients. Patients who develop problems during pregnancy are referred to other hospitals.

Level II, or intermediate care, consists of larger hospitals with facilities to care for moderate-risk pregnant women and moderately ill infants as well as normal patients. Some of these hospitals accept infants who require intermediate care and are referred from Level I hospitals. In addition, infants who improve during intensive care are often transferred back to Level II hospitals until they are well enough to go home.

The final level of perinatal care is Level III, or intensive care. Level III hospitals are usually teaching hospitals. They serve a large geographic area and accept referrals from all Level I and Level II hospitals in their regions. Individual units often treat infants with particular problems, such as premature birth, respiratory problems, congenital heart disease, or surgical problems, as NICUs in children's hospitals usually have facilities to treat infants requiring major surgery. Level III general hospitals frequently have referral obstetric units as well as NICUs, so that high-risk infants can receive special care even before birth.

This current regionalization has generally functioned well and has resulted in a number of beneficial effects, although it creates some problems. Studies have demonstrated improved care and reduction in mortality of high-risk infants treated in regional intensive care units (Lucey, 1973). A recent study (Clark et al., 1981) showed that the incidence of intraventricular hemorrhage was significantly reduced in those infants for whom the mother was transported to a regional perinatal center prior to the infant's birth. Regionalization has also prevented a financially unfeasible duplication of services. NICUs are, however, usually profit-making areas of the hospital that are subject to periodic low censuses (Shearer, 1980). Thus the availability of special care may tempt some physicians to admit infants to NICUs to maintain a full unit even though the infants need a lower level of care (Richards, 1980).

Another problem is that the infants are geographically separated from their parents and communities. This problem is exacerbated by the lack of equal distribution of NICUs. Some urban areas are overserved while other areas are not served at all (Lucey, 1973). For example, Boston has four neonatal intensive care units, whereas the rest of Massachusetts has only one. Therefore, some parents have to travel long distances to visit and may be unable to visit frequently. Pediatricians, nurse practitioners, and public health nurses in some communities may not understand the expected risks of neonatal intensive care or recognize its complications. They are often unable to improve their level of knowledge because in-service programs tend to be centered at Level III hospitals. Neonatal intensive units are attempting to provide this education through outreach programs, but more needs to be done (Hawkins, 1980).

Impact of High-Risk Infants on Families

Although family systems vary greatly, a family environment of some kind is probably best suited to meet the physical and psychologic needs of infants. Studies of healthy infants raised in institutions show that these infants exhibited delays in both physical and mental growth (Provence and Lipton, 1962).

High-risk infants also spend the first weeks of life in an environment very different from a normal home. The neonatal intensive care unit emphasizes meeting medical needs over all others. These infants are more vulnerable to environmental insults than were the healthy infants in the institutional studies. Yet even when well, high-risk infants do not return to normal home environments because in each home the family system has been altered by the stresses involved with neonatal intensive care.

Understanding the needs of high-risk infants and their families therefore first requires understanding the normal process by which the infant is incorporated into the family system at birth. This system is diagrammed for a traditionally structured two-parent nuclear family in Figure 31-1. Similar roles occur with other family configurations, but different members may fill them. All members of the family engage in reciprocal interactions with the infant. The basic interaction occurs in the relationship with a primary caregiver, usually the mother. This interaction centers around feeding and other basic care-giving functions but also incorporates an emerging social relationship. The other family members provide social stimuli for the infant. Secondary caregivers, usually fathers, play more games with infants than primary caregivers generally do (Field, 1978), and they provide support for the primary caregivers. Siblings affect infants through play and through limitations on the time parents have available for infants. Significant others, including friends, relatives, and some professionals, also affect the family system although the amount of influence varies greatly among families. Other acquaintances have less impact. The final layer in Figure 31-1 thus represents the effects that general society has on the family.

High-risk infants do not enter this family system. Instead, they are incorporated into the neonatal intensive care system, which is diagrammed in Figure 31-2. The basic system consists of the infant, nurses, physicians, and other patients. Most of the interactions are unidirectional: from the professionals to the patients. The infant's behavioral cues are usually ignored. The infant's parents are outside the basic system, so they are removed to the first environmental layer on the diagram. Siblings have even less influence on the infant, as they are often unable even to visit a hospitalized infant. Thus, the NICU not only denies the infant an opportunity to take part in reciprocal social interactions but also disrupts the family system.

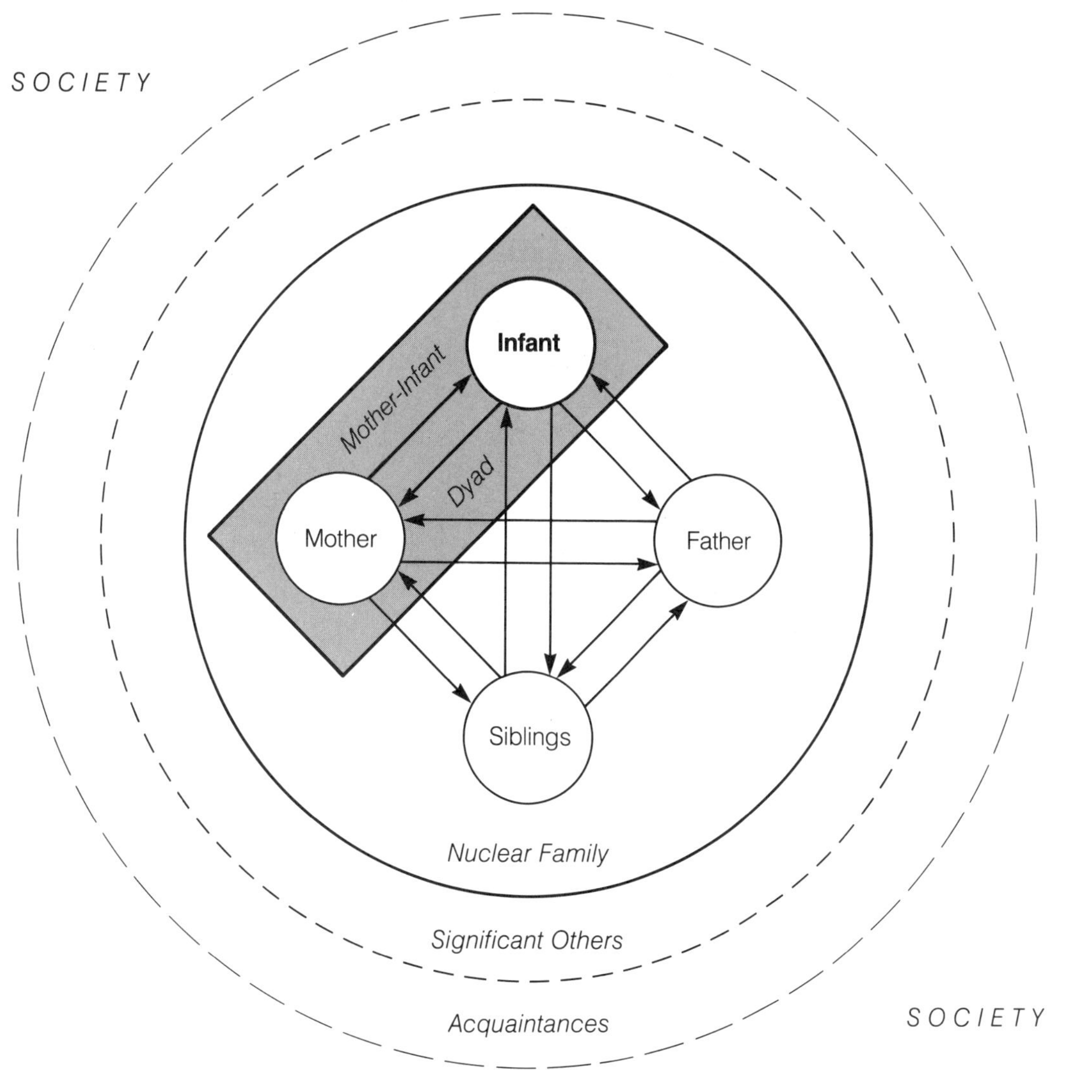

Figure 31-1 A systems diagram for a traditional American family. Arrows represent interactions between members. The solid line represents the boundary of the family. Broken lines separate outside influences on the family; the more effect an outside influence has on the family, the closer to the center it is located on the diagram.

Each member contributes to the disruption of the family system and is affected by its breakdown. The infant's inability to provide social cues in the form of cries, visual attention, or smiles severely limits the attachment process. The neurologic immaturity of premature infants further restricts their abilities and causes faint cries, poor sucking, tremulousness, and weak grasp reflexes (Johnson and Grubbs, 1975). The physical environment of the NICU does not promote the development of social skills. Infants receive little affectionate handling. Instead, they are exposed to bright fluorescent lights, a loud noise level, and stressful procedures, such as heelsticks, suctioning, and lumbar punctures. Because the pattern of these stimuli does not vary consistently throughout the day, the infant is unable to develop a circadian activity cycle (Lawson et al., 1977). Finally, because several different nurses care for the same infant and because parental visiting is infrequent, hospitalized neonates seldom have the opportunity to learn one-to-one interaction.

For the parents, the birth of a high-risk infant represents a crisis that disturbs the ability of the family system to function (Caplan, 1960). Kaplan and Mason (1960) described four tasks that parents of premature infants must accomplish in order to establish relationships with their infants: (a) preparing for the possible death of the infant, (b) overcoming the guilt caused by the failure to deliver a normal infant, (c) resuming the process of relating to the infant, and (d) developing an understanding of the infant's special needs. (These tasks are equally relevant to the parents of other high-risk infants.)

A parent's emotional reaction also may be out of proportion to the severity of the infant's illness (Benfield et al.,

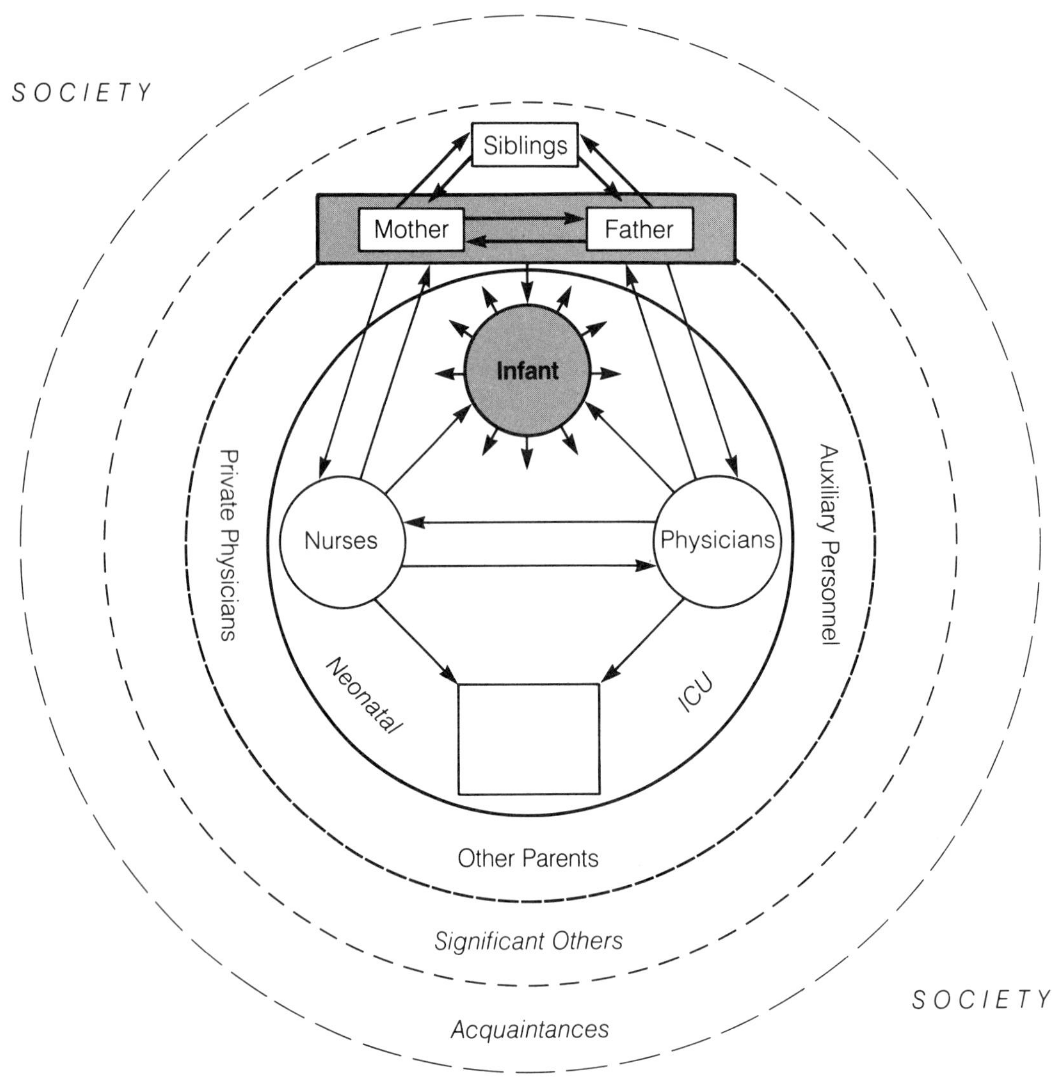

Figure 31-2 A systems diagram for an infant in an NICU. Arrows represent interactions between members. The solid line represents the boundary of the NICU system. Broken lines separate various outside influences on this system; the greater the effect an outside influence has on the infant, the closer it is located to the infant on the diagram.

1976; Jeffcoate et al., 1979b), but the stresses involved with having a seriously ill infant also can cause emotional problems for the parents. The costs of neonatal intensive care, for example, can average as high as $50,000 for surviving infants with serious illnesses, which places additional stress on parents (Phibbs et al., 1981; Pomerance et al., 1978).

Parents of high-risk infants must overcome their isolation from their infants and their feelings that these infants belong to the unit personnel (Klaus and Kennell, 1982). This is often difficult, as parents may be unable to visit frequently because of distance; studies have shown that the average parent may visit as infrequently as once every 6 days (Barnett et al., 1970; Rosenfeld, 1980). When parents do visit, they exhibit decreased tactile and social behaviors (Klaus et al., 1970; Leifer et al., 1972; Minde et al., 1978).

An infant's siblings also contribute to the disruption of the family system. They are seldom allowed to see the infant prior to discharge because nursery personnel are concerned about infection and about upsetting the siblings. Yet children's fantasies are usually far worse than the realities of an NICU. If their fears and fantasies are not addressed, siblings may develop behavioral problems to attract parental attention. The "magical thinking" characteristic of early childhood may cause a child to believe that a new baby's illness is due to the child's desire to eliminate the baby, or these children may believe that the parent's emotional upset is due to their own misbehavior.

Characteristics of High-Risk Infants

Risk Factors

Although most of the infants admitted to NICUs are born prematurely, a large number of infants at risk are full-term births. Table 31-1 lists the common perinatal complications associated with biologic risks. The listed risk factors are interrelated; most high-risk infants experience more than one. In fact, a high-risk infant is usually the result of a high-risk pregnancy. The risk factors can be divided into two general categories—biologic and psychosocial.

The psychosocial risk factors include adolescent parenting, parental psychiatric problems, multistressed parent, single parenting, and low socioeconomic status (see Chapter 22). Nurses working with infants medically at risk also need to understand the psychosocial risk factors because many of these factors are associated with biologic risks. For example, a premature infant may have an unwed adolescent mother or a woman may develop complications during her pregnancy because she lacked the money to obtain adequate prenatal care. In addition, apparently normal infants with psychosocial risk factors may develop subtle biologic problems at later ages. For example, the children of adolescent mothers have average lower intelligence quotients than the children of more mature mothers (Record et al., 1969). Therefore, these infants often benefit from follow-up programs similar to those provided for infants at biologic risk.

Classification of High-Risk Infants

High-risk infants do not constitute a homogeneous group (Fig. 31-3). They are classified on the basis of gestational age (GA) at birth and body size, and studies have demonstrated that these variables affect mortality and morbidity rates (Lubchenco et al., 1972; Philip et al., 1981). Moreover, medical treatments differ among infants of varying GAs and body sizes.

The *gestational age* of an infant is usually somewhat uncertain. It is defined as the number of weeks of fetal development but is calculated from the first day of the mother's last menstrual period. Therefore, at 38 weeks from the date of conception, or 40 weeks from the date of the mother's last menstrual period, the infant is considered to have a GA of 40 weeks. Many mothers, however, are uncertain of the date of the last menstrual period, and very few mothers know the date of conception. Therefore, ultrasound examinations may be performed in the second trimester to estimate GA, but because this method is based on head growth, it is not accurate when there is early intrauterine growth retardation.

Dubowitz et al. (1970) developed a method of assessing GA after birth by using 10 neurologic criteria (Fig. 31-3A) and 11 physical or external criteria (Fig. 31-3B). The Dubowitz examination is accurate within 1 to 2 weeks of the actual GA when the assessment is performed within 24 hours after birth. This assessment can be administered in 10 minutes and is easily learned, but some of the neurologic criteria, such as the ventral suspension, cannot be safely performed on seriously ill infants. Therefore, Ballard et al. (1977) developed an abbreviated version of the Dubowitz assessment and eliminated the difficult items while

TABLE 31-1 Perinatal Complications Associated With Infants at Biologic Risk

Prenatal complications	
Maternal chronic disease	Maternal drug addiction
Diabetes/endocrine diseases	Maternal infections
Hypertension	Multiple birth
Gynecologic problems	Maternal age
Cancer	Less than 20
Renal disease	More than 35
Immunologic disease	Infertility
Heart/lung disease	Maternal or paternal exposure
Thyroid disease	to teratogens
Neurologic disease	Medications
Others	Smoking
Toxemia	Alcohol
Blood group incompatibilities	X-rays
Maternal malnutrition	Others
Obesity	Polyhydramnios
Anemia	Maternal stress
Hyperemesis	Maternal trauma
Lack of nutrients/calories	Grand multiparity
Bleeding after 12 weeks	Father older than 40
Intrapartal complications	
Asphyxia	Prolonged rupture of
Placental abnormalities	membranes
Breech/transverse presentation	Maternal medication or
Prolonged labor	anesthetic
Difficult delivery	Cord prolapse
Forceps delivery	Cephalopelvic disproportion
Premature labor	Cesarean section
	Delivery trauma
	Meconium staining
Neonatal complications	
Dysmaturity	Prematurity
Small for gestational age	Postmaturity
Large for gestational age	Cold stress
Anemia/polycythemia	Hyperbilirubinemia
Congenital infections	Sepsis
Surgery	Heart disease
Respiratory problems	Apnea and bradycardia
Gastrointestinal problems	Metabolic disturbances
Malnutrition	Neurologic abnormalities
Necrotizing enterocolitis	Meningitis
Medication	Seizures
Congenital anomalies	Intracranial hemorrhage

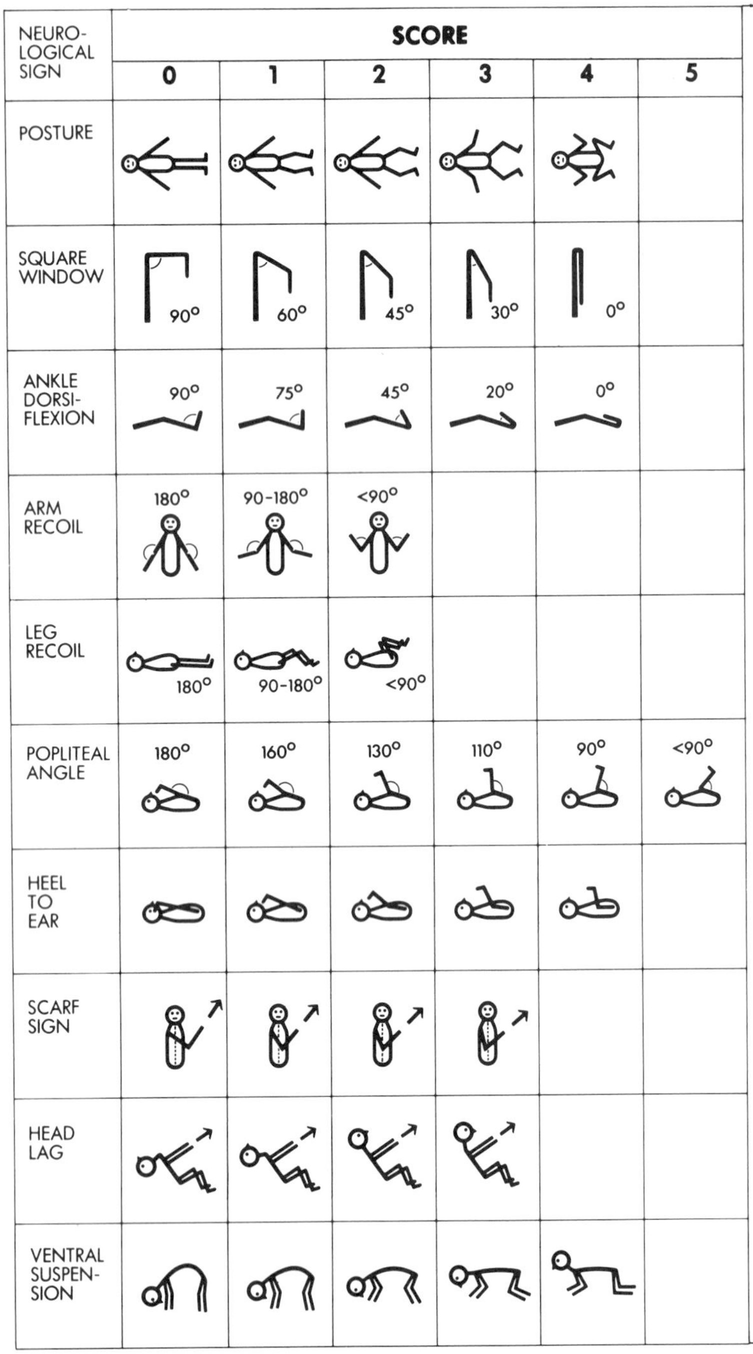

NEURO-LOGICAL SIGN	SCORE 0	1	2	3	4	5
POSTURE						
SQUARE WINDOW	90°	60°	45°	30°	0°	
ANKLE DORSI-FLEXION	90°	75°	45°	20°	0°	
ARM RECOIL	180°	90-180°	<90°			
LEG RECOIL	180°	90-180°	<90°			
POPLITEAL ANGLE	180°	160°	130°	110°	90°	<90°
HEEL TO EAR						
SCARF SIGN						
HEAD LAG						
VENTRAL SUSPEN-SION						

Some Notes on Techniques of Assessment of Neurologic Criteria

If score differs on the two sides, take the mean.

Posture: Observed with infant quiet and in supine position. Score 0: Arms legs extended; 1: beginning of flexion of hips and knees, arms extended; 2: stronger flexion of legs, arms extended; 3: arms slightly flexed, legs flexed and abducted; 4: full flexion of arms and legs.

Square window: The hand is flexed on the forearm between the thumb and index finger of the examiner. Enough pressure is applied to get to get as full a flexion as possible, and the angle between the hypothenar eminence and the ventral aspect of the forearm is measured and graded according to diagram. (Care is taken not to rotate the infant's wrist while doing this manuever.)

Ankle dorsiflexion: The foot is dorsiflexed onto the anterior aspect of the leg, with the examiner's thumb on the sole of the foot and other fingers behind the leg. Enough pressure is applied to get as full flexion as possible, and the angle between the dorsum of the foot and the anterior aspect of the leg is measured.

Arm recoil: With the infant in the supine position the forearms are first flexed for 5 seconds, then fully extended by pulling on the hands, and then released. The sign is fully positive if the arms return briskly to full flexion (Score 2). If the arms return to incomplete flexion or the response is sluggish it is graded as Score 1. If they remain extended or are only followed by random movements the score is 0.

Leg recoil: With the infant supine, the hips and knees are fully flexed for 5 seconds, then extended by traction on the feet, and released. A maximal response is one of full flexion of the hips and knees (Score 2). A partial flexion scores 1, and minimal or no movement scores 0.

Popliteal angle: With the infant supine and his pelvis flat on the examining couch, the thigh is held in the knee-chest position by the examiner's left index finger and thumb supporting the knee. The leg is then extended by gentle pressure from the examiner's right index finger behind the ankle and the popliteal angle is measured.

Heel to ear maneuver: With the baby supine, draw the baby's foot as near to the head as it will go without forcing it. Observe the distance between the foot and the head as well as the degree of extension at the knee. Grade according to diagram. Note that the knee is left free and may draw down alongside the abdomen.

Scarf sign: With the baby supine, take the infant's hand and try to put it around the neck and as far posteriorly as possible around the opposite shoulder. Assist the maneuver by lifting the elbow across the body. See how far the elbow will go across and grade according to illustrations. Score 0: Elbow reaches opposite axillary line; 1: Elbow between midline and opposite axillary line; 2: Elbow reaches midline; 3: Elbow will not reach midline.

Head lag: With the baby lying supine, grasp the hands (or the arms if a very small infant) and pull him slowly towards the sitting position. Observe the position of the head in relation to the trunk and grade accordingly. In a small infant the head may initially be supported by one hand. Score 0: Complete lag; 1: Partial head control; 2: Able to maintain head in line with body; 3: Brings head anterior to body.

Ventral suspension: The infant is suspended in the prone position, with examiner's hand under the infant's chest (one hand in a small infant, two in a large infant). Observe the degree of extension of the back and the amount of flexion of the arms and legs. Also note the relation of the head to the trunk. Grade according to diagrams.

A

Figure 31-3 The Dubowitz assessment of gestational age. *A*. Neurologic criteria. *B*. Physical or external criteria. (From Dubowitz LMS, Dubowitz V, Goldberg C: Clinical assessment of gestational age in the newborn infant. *J Pediatr* 1970; 77:1–10.)

maintaining a reliable estimate of GA. The Ballard version is the assessment most commonly used in neonatal intensive care units today.

The three gestational age divisions are (a) *full-term,* (b) *premature,* and (c) *postterm.* More than 80% of infants are born between 38 and 42 weeks GA. They are called full-term. The 7%–10% of infants born prior to 38 weeks GA are considered premature or preterm (Babson et al., 1975). The remaining 7% of births occur after 42 weeks' GA and are called postterm (Creighton, 1978). The term postmature is used only when a postterm infant exhibits the *postmature syndrome* caused by a prolonged pregnancy and placental insufficiency.

Four terms are used to classify infants on the basis of

External sign	*Score**				
	0	*1*	*2*	*3*	*4*
Edema	Obvious edema of hands and feet; pitting over tibia	No obvious edema of hands and feet; pitting over tibia	No edema		
Skin texture	Very thin, gelatinous	Thin and smooth	Smooth; medium thickness. Rash or superficial peeling	Slight thickening. Superficial cracking and peeling especially of hands and feet	Thick, and parchment-like superficial or deep cracking
Skin color	Dark red	Uniformly pink	Pale pink; variable over body	Pale; only pink over ears, lips, palms, or soles	
Skin opacity (trunk)	Numerous veins and venules clearly seen, especially over abdomen	Veins and tributaries seen	A few large vessels clearly seen over abdomen	A few large vessels seen indistinctly over abdomen	No blood vessels seen
Lanugo (over back)	No lanugo	Abundant; long and thick over whole back	Hair thinning especially over lower back	Small amount of lanugo and bald areas	At least ½ of back devoid of lanugo
Plantar creases	No skin creases	Faint red marks over anterior half of sole	Definite red marks over > anterior ½; indentations over < anterior ⅓	Indentations over > anterior ⅓	Definite deep indentations over > anterior ⅓
Nipple formation	Nipple barely visible; no areola	Nipple well defined; areola smooth and flat, diameter < 0.75 cm.	Areola stippled, edge not raised, diameter < 0.75 cm.	Areola stippled, edge raised, diameter < 0.75 cm.	
Breast size	No breast tissue palpable	Breast tissue on one or both sides, < 0.5 cm. diameter	Breast tissue both sides; one or both 0.5–1.0 cm.	Breast tissue both sides; one or both > 1 cm.	
Ear form	Pinna flat and shapeless, little or no incurving of edge	Incurving of part of edge of pinna	Partial incurving whole of upper pinna	Well-defined incurving whole of upper pinna	
Ear firmness	Pinna soft, easily folded, no recoil	Pinna soft, easily folded, slow recoil	Cartilage to edge of pinna, but soft in places, ready recoil	Pinna firm, cartilage to edge; instant recoil	
Genitals Male	Neither testis in scrotum	At least one testis high in scrotum	At least one testis right down		
Female (with hip ½ abducted)	Labia majora widely separated, labia minora protruding	Labia majora almost cover labia minora	Labia majora completely cover labia minora		

*If score differs on two sides, take the mean.

SOURCE: Adapted from Farr V et al.: The definition of some external characteristics used in the assessment of gestational age in the newborn infant. *Devel Med Child Neurol* 1966; 8:507.

B

Figure 31-3 continued

body size: *low birth weight, average for gestational age* (AGA), *small for gestational age* (SGA), and *large for gestational age* (LGA). Each of these terms may be used with each gestational age classification so that it is possible to have a low-birth-weight full-term infant or an LGA preterm infant.

Any infant with a birth weight of less than 2500 g (5½ lb) is considered to be of low birth weight. Most low-birth-weight infants are premature, and in the past, the two terms were used interchangeably, even though some premature infants weigh more than 2500 g and one-third of low-birth-weight infants are full-term or postterm (Sweet, 1979). Most infants, however, are average for gestational age and have birth weights between the 10th and 90th percentiles for

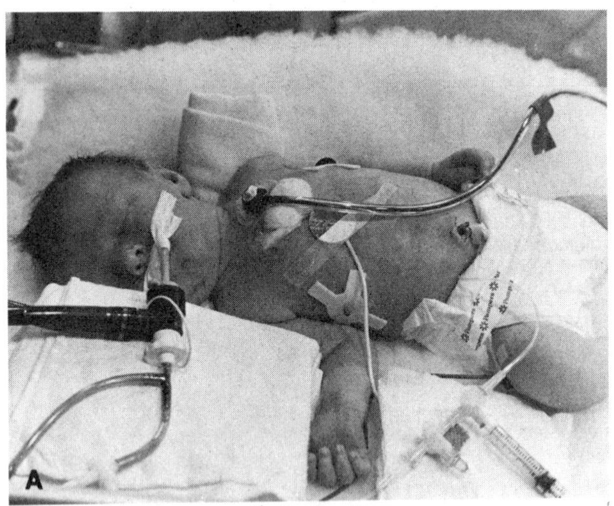
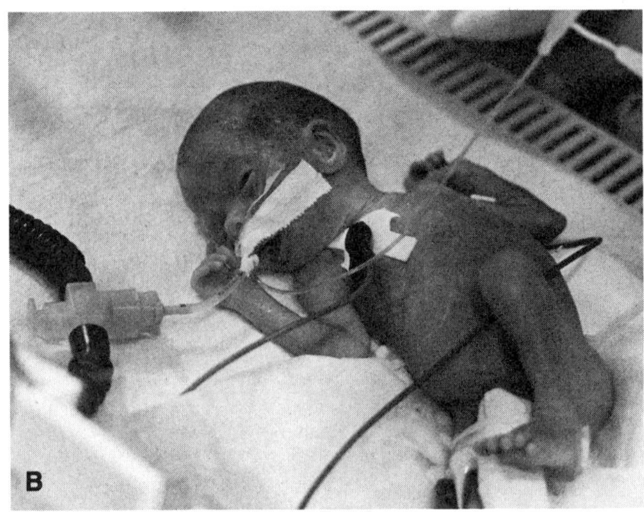

Differing appearances of two high-risk infants requiring mechanical ventilation. *A.* A newborn, full-term infant. *B.* A 2-week-old premature infant born at 26 weeks' GA. (Christine Acebo, photographer.)

their GAs. Small-for-gestational-age infants weigh less than those in the 10th percentile for GA, and large-for-gestational-age infants weigh more than those in the 90th percentile. Intrauterine growth retardation is a common cause of SGA infants; infants of diabetic mothers are usually LGA.

Classifications of body size are generally made using percentiles calculated at the University of Colorado from a sample of white, black, and Hispanic infants (Battaglia and Lubchenco, 1967) (Fig. 31-4). The body weights of infants from ethnic groups not included in the standardization sample may, however, deviate significantly from these values. For example, an Indo-Chinese infant can be below the 10th percentile and still be within the normal size range for Indo-Chinese infants. In addition, this classification system does not differentiate between those infants who are small because of their genetic background and those infants who have experienced intrauterine growth retardation. To identify growth retardation, the relationship between body length and body weight must be known. Miller (1972) used the ponderal index (weight in grams × 100 divided by body length in centimeters cubed) to determine whether infants were growth retarded, but because growth retardation can also be diagnosed with clinical signs, this statistic is more commonly used in research than in clinical practice.

Growth and Development of High-Risk Infants

The capabilities of infants change rapidly during the first year of life. These developmental changes are particularly dramatic during the preterm and early postterm periods, so that nurses working with high-risk infants need to know the normal course of growth and development during infancy (see Chapter 7). In general, high-risk infants without major handicaps show a pattern of growth and development that is similar to that of normal full-term infants. Severe illness or prolonged hospitalization may alter this course. Thus infants born more than 2 months prematurely frequently exhibit changes in development. Specific handicaps also alter an infant's developmental pattern.

Biophysical and cognitive development depend on *biologic age,* or the age from conception. Affective and social development depend on experience as well as biologic age. Therefore, when assessing the development of a premature infant, the infant's age should be corrected by subtracting the amount of prematurity from the birth age. A premature infant develops at the same rate as a full-term infant with the same biologic age. Therefore, an infant born 2 months prematurely never "catches up" with a full-term infant born at the same time because the central nervous system of the preterm infant is always 2 months less mature. A study by Hunt and Rhodes (1977) confirmed that the cognitive development of a premature infant is consistent with biologic age, rather than age since birth. Clinicians frequently stop correcting for prematurity sometime between 1 and 5 years, however, because the rate of development slows after 1 year and 2 months and no longer has as much impact on development.

Although biologic age cannot be altered, the social experiences necessary for development may be. Therefore, an infant who exhibits developmental delays after prolonged hospitalization or severe illness may experience rapid development once the problem is resolved. These rapid changes often continue until the infant's development is normal. In addition, premature infants occasionally exhibit small accelerations in learning social skills.

Biophysical Development When high-risk infants receive adequate nutrition, body weight and length grow at generally the same rate as normal full-term infants of the same biologic age (see Chapter 7). Small premature infants, however, usually experience some malnutrition due to feeding difficulties, and thus they often remain somewhat

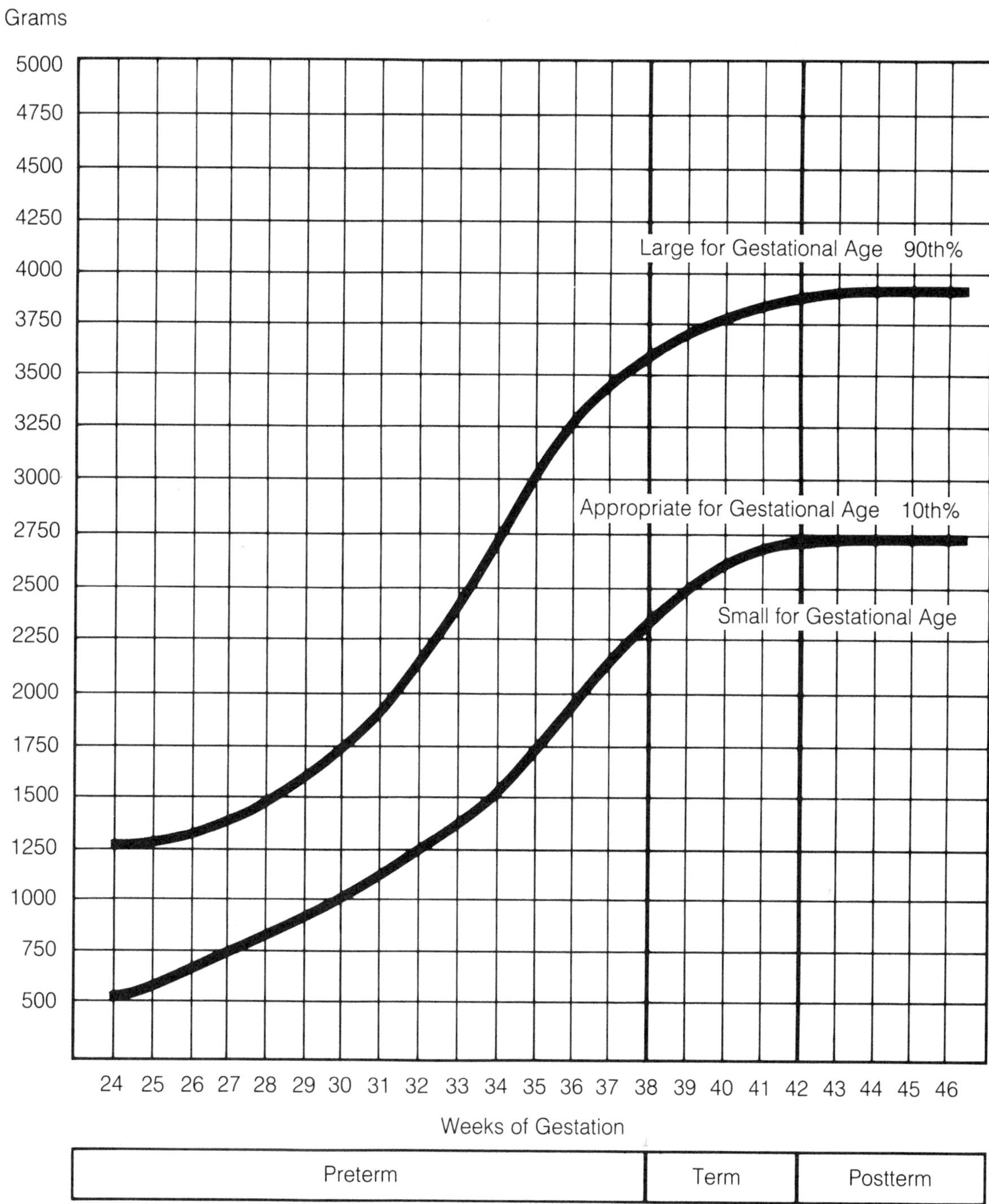

Figure 31-4 Classification of newborns by birth weight and GA. (From Battaglia FC, Lubchenco LO: A practical classification of newborn infants by weight and gestational age. *J Pediatr* 1967; 71:159–163.)

light for length throughout life (Desmond et al., 1980; Kimble et al., 1982). Infants who are SGA who experienced intrauterine malnutrition may remain below the 10th percentile in both length and weight (Desmond et al., 1980).

The head growth of premature infants and normal full-term infants differs dramatically. This difference is more pronounced for infants at a greater degree of prematurity. Premature infants tend to have large, thin heads. The sides of the head are flatter, and the distance between the temples is narrower than that in full-term infants; but the volume of the skull remains the same (Largo and Duc, 1977). This tall, thin head may persist for several years or even into adulthood (Desmond et al., 1980).

Neuromuscular Development The central nervous system develops rapidly during the preterm and neonatal periods, but unless there is neurologic damage, the neuromuscular development of high-risk infants remains very similar to that of healthy infants. Again, the differences most affect the very premature infant. These central nervous system effects can be seen in reflex and state behaviors.

The development of muscle tone and reflexes during infancy parallels central nervous system development. During the preterm period, the infant becomes more hypertonic and develops stronger reflexes (Amiel-Tison, 1968). This pattern can be seen in the Dubowitz examination (Dubowitz et al., 1970) (Fig. 31-3), which indicates that the infant's posture has become increasingly flexed with age and that there is a greater resistance to moving the extremities. Preterm infants never become as hypertonic as normal full-term infants (Amiel-Tison, 1968), and at term, they exhibit weaker and more asymmetric reflexes (Howard et al., 1976). In addition, improper positioning during hospitalization may cause the infant to develop external rotation of hips, knees, and ankles or increased abduction tone in the shoulders, which will interfere with later efforts to bring the hands to the midline (Desmond et al., 1980). After term, muscle tone and reflex strength gradually decrease so that voluntary movements can begin. Persistence of infantile reflexes beyond their normal age of disappearance may indicate neurologic damage.

Sleep–wake states are patterns of behavior that occur together and determine the infant's ability to respond to stimulation (see Chapter 16). The ways these behaviors are grouped into separate states is somewhat arbitrary; thus different researchers have developed slightly different state classification systems. A six-state system is used by Brazelton (1973) for clinical assessments of predominant state, quality of alertness, and frequency of state changes. Anders et al. (1971) have described an eight-state system to be used with electroencephalographic recordings, and Thoman (1975; 1983) has developed a ten-state system for continuous behavioral observations.

The sleeping and waking states of high-risk infants have a developmental course similar to that of normal full-term infants. At 1 month postterm, infants sleep about 17 hours a day (Erickson, 1976). Approximately two-thirds of sleep is spent in active sleep, which is rapid-eye-movements (REM) sleep, or light sleep, and the rest in quiet sleep, which is non-REM sleep, or deep sleep. By 1 year postterm, they are sleeping about 14 hours a day (Erickson, 1976). Active sleep decreases more rapidly than quiet sleep, so that by 2 years infants exhibit the adult pattern of about 80% quiet sleep and 20% active sleep. The increase in waking time as infants mature results from a dramatic increase in the amount of alertness. The nonalert waking states and the transitional states decrease with age.

A number of factors may alter sleeping and waking state patterns during the neonatal period. A variety of stresses or conditions, such as Down's syndrome, asphyxia, and fetal distress, decrease active sleep and increase waking (Prechtl et al., 1973). Infants with hyperbilirubinemia show an increased amount of sleep and long periods of active sleep (Prechtl et al., 1973). Drug treatment also affects sleep–wake states. For instance, phenobarbitol decreases active sleep and increases quiet sleep (Gabriel and Albani, 1977); theophylline increases waking (Demarquez et al., 1978; Guilleminault and Souquet, 1979). The effects of theophylline persist for at least 8 weeks after it is discontinued (Denenberg et al., 1982; Thoman et al., 1984). The stability of the infant's sleep–wake states is also predictive of developmental outcome: infants who exhibit erratic patterns in the early weeks are more likely to develop later problems (Thoman et al., 1981).

Prematurity also affects sleep–wake states. During the preterm period, infants exhibit increased amounts of active sleep and transitional states and decreased amounts of waking (Dreyfus-Brisac, 1970; Parmelee, 1975; Parmelee et al., 1967). During the postterm period, premature infants exhibit irregular state development with increased amounts of time in transitional states and a greater amount of waking (Davis and Thoman, 1983; Dreyfus-Brisac, 1970; Parmelee, 1975). In sleep, they exhibit longer bouts of quiet sleep and greater regularity of respiratory patterns (Booth et al., 1980).

Social Development The social skills of young infants include both inborn reflex behaviors (such as sucking, smiling, and grasping) and learned behaviors. The reflexes mature at the same rate for both normal and high-risk infants and are fully developed at term. During the preterm period, all reflexes are weak. The grasping reflex is absent before 30 weeks' GA, and the sucking and swallowing reflexes are not coordinated well enough to permit oral feedings before 32 to 34 weeks' GA (Amiel-Tison, 1968; Johnson and Grubbs, 1975). In addition, infants during the preterm period exhibit only short periods of alertness, so they are unable to maintain prolonged visual contact with adults. The nurse who counsels parents can prevent them from interpreting this lack of social responsiveness as rejection or mental retardation.

During the postterm period, infants develop social skills with learned components, but to develop these skills the infant must have the opportunity for reciprocal interactions with nurturing adults. Thus the appearance of social skills, such as social (responsive) smiling, laughing, responsive vocalization, and visual following of parents, will be delayed in infants who experience prolonged hospital stays. Some differences in social development may also be the result of biologic insults. At term, SGA and preterm infants exhibit deficits on the Brazelton Neonatal Behavior Assessment Scale (Als et al., 1976; Field, 1977). In addition, for the first 4 months postterm, premature infants visually fixate longer and are less attentive to facial patterns than are normal full-term infants (Field 1979b; Kopp et al., 1975; Sigman et al., 1975; Sigman and Parmelee, 1974).

The extent of these differences can be reduced if parents and nurses provide an appropriate environment for social growth. In fact, evidence now shows that healthy preterm infants who receive adequate nurturing begin social smiling at an earlier postterm age than do normal full-term infants (Foley, 1977).

Mortality and Morbidity of High-Risk Infants

The mortality risk of infants depends on both GA and birth weight. Lubchenco et al. (1972) outlined the mortality risk for various GA and birth weight groups (Fig. 31-5). Recent improvements in perinatal care have also improved the survival rates of all infants. Table 31-2 compares the mortality rates of infants born in the late 1970s (Philip et al., 1981) with infants from the 1960s (Lubchenco et al., 1972). As the table shows, the largest improvements have occurred for the smallest and youngest infants.

A common concern is that this decrease in mortality is associated with an increase in morbidity but, fortunately, this concern is unwarranted. A continuing study in one NICU showed that as survival increased, the percentage of survivors with significant handicaps decreased (Hunt, 1976; Tooley, 1981). Recent studies of infants with birth weights under 1500 g (3½ lb) have shown morbidity rates ranging from 10% (Kumar et al., 1980) to 30% (Pape et al., 1978). This rate is comparable with morbidity rates of larger premature infants born in the 1960s (Caputo and Mandell, 1970). Mechanical ventilation, perinatal asphyxia, and intraventricular hemorrhage, however, do increase the risk of significant neurologic handicaps or developmental delays (Driscoll et al., 1982; Saigal et al., 1982; Trotter et al., 1982).

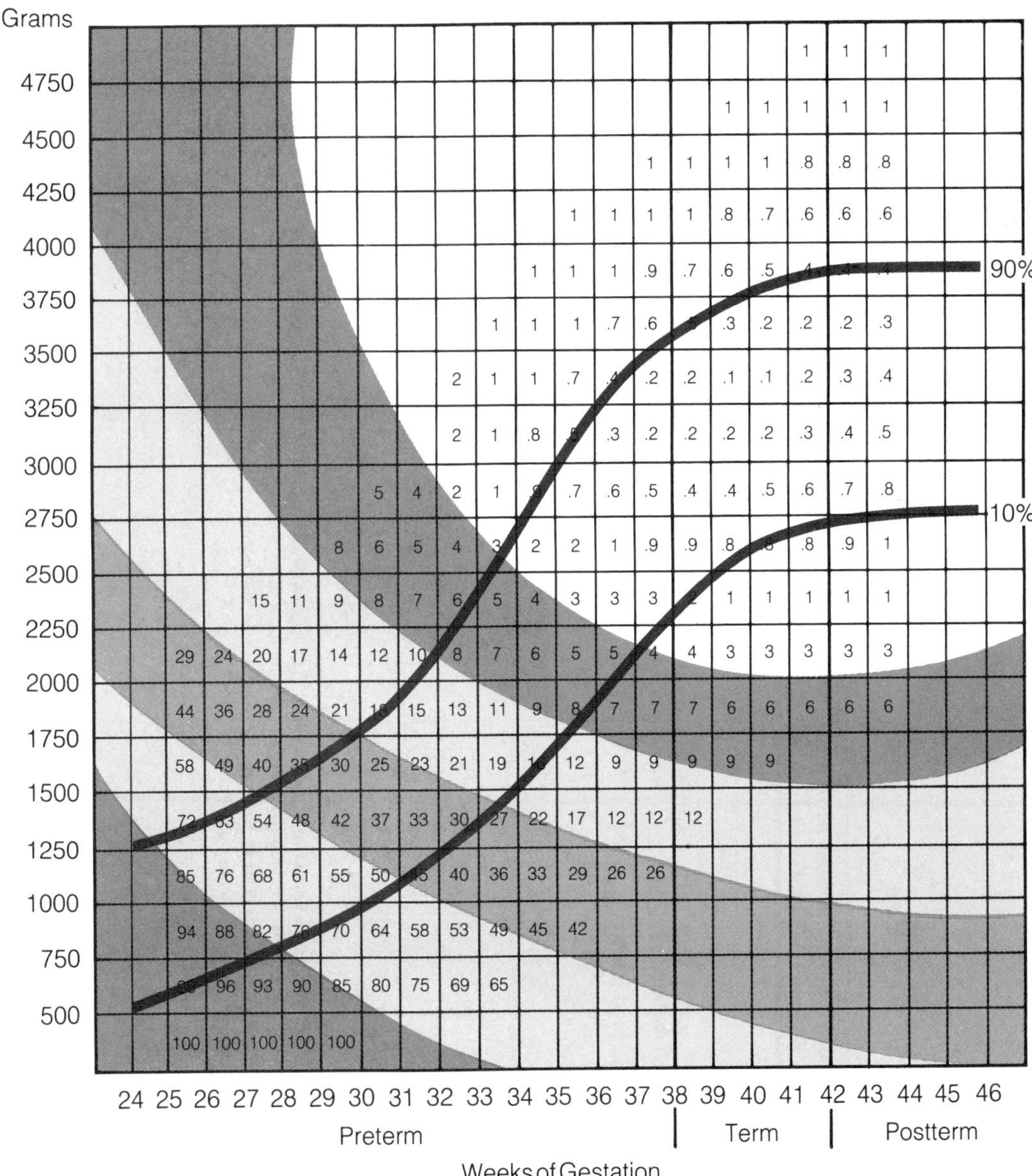

Figure 31-5 Newborn classification and neonatal mortality risk by birth weight and GA. (From Lubchenco, LO, Searls DT, Brazie, JV: Neonatal mortality rate: relationship to birth weight and gestational age. *J Pediatr* 1972; 81:814–822.)

TABLE 31-2 Percent Mortality for Vermont/New Hampshire (1976–1979) Compared to the University of Colorado (1958–1969) by 250-g—1-Week Groups

	Gestational age (week)																						
	≤25		26		27		28		29		30		31		32		33		34		35		>35
Birth weight (g)	VT/NH	Col	VT/NH	Col	VT/NH	Col	VT/NH	Col	VT/NH	Col	VT/NH	Col	VT/NH	Col	VT/NH	Col	VT/NH	Col	VT/NH	Col	VT/NH	Col	VT/NH
2250–2499											—				—		8	5	2	4	0	3	2 (2/111)
2000–2249													—		7	8	3	7	0	6	8	5	5 (7/151)
1750–1999													0	15	5	13	0	11	1	9	3	8	2 (4/210)
1500–1749					—		—				0	25	9	23	8	21	5	19	3	16	0	12	6 (13/205)
1250–1499					—		25	48	33	42	26	37	5	33	11	30	0	27	0	22	—		13 (22/168)
1000–1249	60	85	—		30	68	26	61	19	55	16	50	12	45	11	40	0	36	17	33			20 (33/168)
750–999	90	94	67	88	58	82	64	76	25	70	56	64	—		17	53			—		—		57 (54/95)
500–749	96	99	67	96	—		—		—		—				—				—				77 (37/48)
≤2499 g	89 (34/38)†		64 (18/28)		53 (19/36)		38 (26/69)		27 (13/48)		24 (22/93)		8 (9/107)		8 (16/199)		2 (4/161)		2 (5/220)		4 (6/158)		

*—Denominator less than five. Boxes highlight the Vermont/New Hampshire data.

†Values in parentheses indicate number of deaths/number of live births in each birth weight and gestational age group.

SOURCE: Philips AGS et al: Neonatal mortality risk for the eighties: The importance of birth weight/gestational age groups. *Pediatr* 1981; 68:122–130.

Special Problems of High-Risk Infants

Immaturity of Heat Regulation Mechanisms

An infant should maintain a core body temperature of approximately 37 C (98.6 F). When core temperature is significantly lower or higher than 37 C, metabolic rate and oxygen and glucose consumption increase. A lowered core body temperature, or *cold stress,* is often due to exposure to a cold environment; an elevated core temperature is due to exposure to a hot environment, or overheating. Overheating occurs when the core temperature is above 37.5 C (99.6 F) and the infant's high temperature is not related to illness. The increased metabolic rate in both of these conditions leads to acidosis, hypoxia, and hypoglycemia. These problems are worsened by vasoconstriction caused by cold stress, which decreases blood flow to peripheral tissues. Overheating, on the other hand, causes vasodilation, which may lead to shock.

Neonates have limited abilities to regulate their body temperatures. They become overheated in excessively warm environments because they are unable to sweat adequately. In cool environments, infants lose heat more readily than older children because they have less subcutaneous fat to act as insulation and they have large surface areas for their body volumes. Infants are also unable to shiver effectively in response to cold and must instead rely on increasing activity.

Unlike older children, however, neonates are able to produce heat through *brown fat metabolism.* Brown fat is distributed in several areas on the trunks of infants. When temperature sensors in the skin cause norepinephrine release in response to cold, the norepinephrine stimulates the brown fat to release heat. This mechanism enables healthy full-term infants to maintain their body temperatures in moderately cold environments. Persistent cold stress, however, can exhaust an infant's brown fat supply. Neurologic damage may interfere with the ability of the skin sensors to stimulate norepinephrine release. In addition, the free fatty acids released by brown fat metabolism interfere with bilirubin binding and may increase the likelihood of kernicterus, or indirect bilirubin in the blood.

Premature infants have even less ability to regulate their body temperatures than do full-term infants. They have higher surface-to-volume ratios than full-term infants and less subcutaneous fat, so they lose heat more rapidly. Moreover, they have less brown fat and poorer defenses to overheating, as their sweating mechanisms are particularly ineffective (Harpin and Rutter, 1982).

Assessment Principal criteria for assessing heat regulation are physical signs of cold stress such as overheating and body temperatures. The nurse assesses the body temperatures of each hospitalized infant at least every 4 hours to determine whether core temperature is between 36.5 C and 37.5 C (97.6 F and 99.6 F) and skin temperature is between 35.8 C and 36.7 C (96.5 F and 98 F).

Core temperatures are obtained by taking axillary or rectal temperatures. The values of these two temperatures do not differ significantly in neonates although axillary temperatures take about 1 minute longer to stabilize in larger infants (Torrance, 1968) and may take even longer to stabilize in small infants. Axillary temperatures are preferred, however, because of the danger of bowel perforation if a rectal thermometer is inserted too far (Centers for Disease Control, 1977).

Skin temperatures can be obtained from skin probes on incubators and radiant warmers or, more crudely, by comparing the temperature of the extremities and abdomen. If the abdomen feels significantly warmer than the legs, cold stress is probably causing vasoconstriction in the legs, which in turn causes peripheral cyanosis.

When the infant is in an incubator, the environmental temperature is also recorded because it affects the nursing diagnosis concerning the infant's temperature regulation. When the incubator temperature and the infant's temperature are both falling, the infant is experiencing cold stress, whereas if the infant's temperature is falling while the incubator's temperature is rising, the infant is experiencing hypothermia, which signals a serious insult such as sepsis.

Infants experiencing early cold stress increase their activity levels and appear restless and irritable. Severe cold stress causes respiratory problems with symptoms of rapid breathing, difficult breathing, pallor, and hypoactivity. The vasodilation of overheating, on the other hand, causes infants to appear flushed. Their skin feels warm, and they may be sweating.

Large fluctuations in core temperature or environmental temperature are also stressful, and so graphs of the infant's temperature are analyzed to make certain that the infant is in a neutral thermal environment. In addition, infants who fail to gain weight despite adequate calorie intake may be experiencing mild cold stress.

The nursing diagnosis for an infant experiencing cold stress is generally ineffective temperature regulation. The factors related to the nursing diagnosis, however, depend on the specific assessment data gathered for each infant.

Nursing Management The goal of nursing care for infants with problems in heat regulation is to maintain the infant in a neutral thermal environment. This requires an environmental temperature at which metabolic rate and oxygen consumption are minimized and the infant's core body temperature is between 36.5 C and 37.5 C. A neutral thermal environment also minimizes the following four sources of heat loss:

1. *Evaporation* from vaporization of moisture from lungs and body surface, as occurs when an infant is wet from bathing
2. *Conduction* through direct contact with cooler surfaces, as occurs when an infant is placed on cold scales

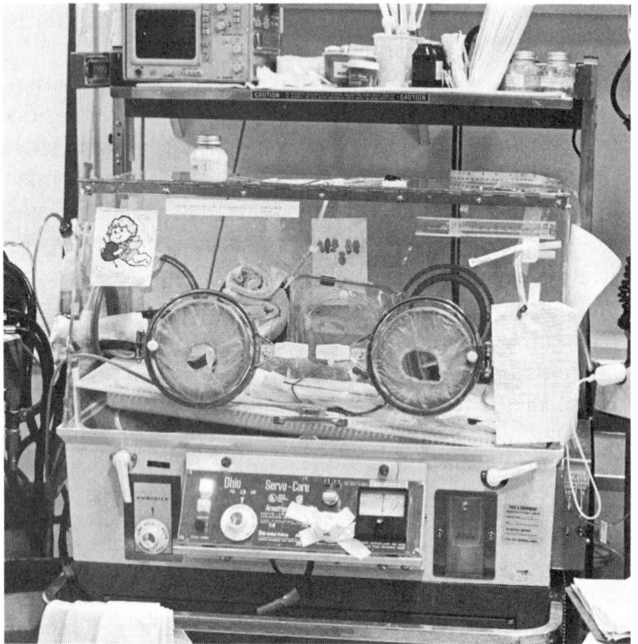

An incubator. (Christine Acebo, photographer.)

3. *Convection* to cool air currents passing over the infant, as occurs when an infant is in a drafty room
4. *Radiation* to cooler areas not in direct contact with the infant, as occurs when an infant loses heat to a cooler nursery

Various methods minimize heat loss and provide a neutral thermal environment. Most high-risk infants are initially placed in incubators in which the air is heated to maintain either a constant air temperature or a constant skin temperature. When the portholes are closed, convection and conduction are minimized. Evaporation is reduced by humidifying the air in the incubator, but humidified air is sometimes not done to prevent bacterial colonization of the water, which might in turn cause infection. Some radiant heat loss to the walls of the incubator does occur, but these walls are warmer than the walls of the room. For small infants, the radiant heat loss can be further reduced by placing a clear plastic heat shield over the infant.

Infants who require frequent assessment are placed in radiant warmers with a radiant heat supply located above the infant and used to maintain a constant skin temperature. Because the infant in such a warmer is open to the air, convective heat loss to air currents in the NICU and radiant losses to the walls of the room occur, causing the infant's metabolic rate to increase. Thus infants in warmers usually have higher metabolic rates than infants in incubators (LeBlanc, 1982).

Full-term infants and recuperating high-risk infants are placed in open bassinets. Infants in bassinets are exposed to all four types of heat loss, but the nurse minimizes this process by clothing and covering the infant. Covering the head with a hat also reduces heat loss, because the brain is a major heat-producing organ and the head has a proportionately large surface area.

If the infant is showing signs of cold stress or overheating, the environmental temperature should be changed, although temperature changes should not be excessive. The temperature settings on warmers and incubators can be adjusted, and clothing and blankets can be added or removed for infants in bassinets. Rapid reheating after cold stress is not recommended because it may result in apneic spells (Stern, 1970). Overheating while correcting a low core temperature is also possible. To prevent this, the nurse warms the infant slowly, while monitoring temperature. Metabolic rate returns to normal as soon as skin temperature is normal even though core temperature is still low. Thus once skin temperature is normal or core temperature begins to rise rapidly, the temperature in the incubator or warmer is returned to that of a neutral thermal environment.

Complications Uncorrected cold stress can lead to hypoxia, acidemia, respiratory failure, and death. A number of infants have been placed on mechanical ventilators because of severe cold stress.

Improper use of incubators and radiant warmers can also cause complications. Incorrect temperature settings can lead to either cold stress or overheating. Using radiant warmers without skin probes may cause burns.

Considerations for Follow-up Because infants may experience cold stress after discharge, the nurse teaches parents to recognize the symptoms of cold stress (cold hands and feet, peripheral cyanosis, and irritability) and to minimize heat loss by clothing and covering the infant and by preventing exposure to cold surfaces. This education is especially important for parents of premature infants, who may be discharged from the hospital weighing as little as 2000 g (4½ lb).

The nurse also needs to teach parents to recognize overheating. One infant was brought to the emergency room with a temperature of 40 C (104 F), admitted to the NICU, and subjected to an expensive and painful septic workup. No evidence of infection was found, and the fever disappeared within a couple of hours. The source of the fever was determined to be overheating; the parents had wrapped the infant in several blankets and placed him by a radiator on a warm day.

Immaturity of the Immunologic System

Because of the immaturity of their immunologic systems, all infants, especially premature infants and those undergoing invasive procedures, are susceptible to infections. Their leukocytes are less efficient in migrating to the sites of infections and engulfing pathogens than those of older children. Neonates have very few actively acquired antibodies because antibody production depends on exposure to specific infective agents. Therefore, their immunologic systems depend on short-lived maternal antibodies that cross the placenta, especially during the third trimester. Not until 3 months postterm has the infant produced enough antibodies to replace the rapidly declining supply of maternal antibodies. Premature infants are even more vulnerable to infections because they are not in the uterus for the entire third trimester and thus receive fewer antibodies.

Immaturity of the immunologic system also leaves the infant susceptible to infections caused by organisms that are not ordinarily pathogenic in older children. For example, one nursery experienced an outbreak of diarrhea caused by *Staphylococcus epidermidis,* a normally harmless bacterium found on the skin of adults. In addition, infections of infants are more often generalized, involving meningitis, septicemia, or pneumonia. (The immune system is more generally discussed in Chapter 37.)

Assessment The symptoms of infections in infants are seldom specific. Because of the immaturity of their heat regulation mechanisms, infants rarely develop fevers, and hypothermia in an adequately warm environment instead indicates sepsis (systemic infection). Other symptoms include poor feeding, jitteriness, hyperbilirubinemia, apnea, diarrhea, abdominal distension, respiratory distress, lethargy, cyanosis, irregular or rapid respirations, vomiting, edema, bleeding, pallor, hypotension, jaundice, and rapid heart rate.

Because sepsis can mimic a number of other conditions, the nurse needs to know that an infant has been exposed to an infection. Infants contract illnesses from their mothers during pregnancy or birth and from other patients or staff during the neonatal period. Infection should be suspected whenever the mother develops an illness during the perinatal period or the amniotic membranes are ruptured more than 24 hours prior to birth.

The nursing diagnosis in such cases is potential for altered health state related to introduction of bacteria. Exposure to bacteria may be secondary to invasive procedures, maternal infection, or other environmental factors. The specific nursing diagnosis thus depends on the assessment of each client.

Nursing Management The goals of nursing care are to prevent infection whenever possible and to identify infections in the early stages. Because prevention of infection is always the best intervention, all nurseries should practice preventive measures that include

1. Good hand washing with an antibiotic soap on entering the nursery and between handling infants
2. Wearing scrub suits or gowns over street clothes when in the nursery
3. Wearing a different gown for directly handling each infant
4. Placing particularly vulnerable infants in incubators
5. Isolating all infants with infections

Another essential aspect of prevention is determining whether an infection is hospital acquired and was thus preventable. In most hospitals, an infection control nurse routinely cultures surfaces to determine whether possible infective agents are present. Some nurseries also routinely culture high-risk infants. Also important is determining how well the nursery staff is conducting the infection control measures.

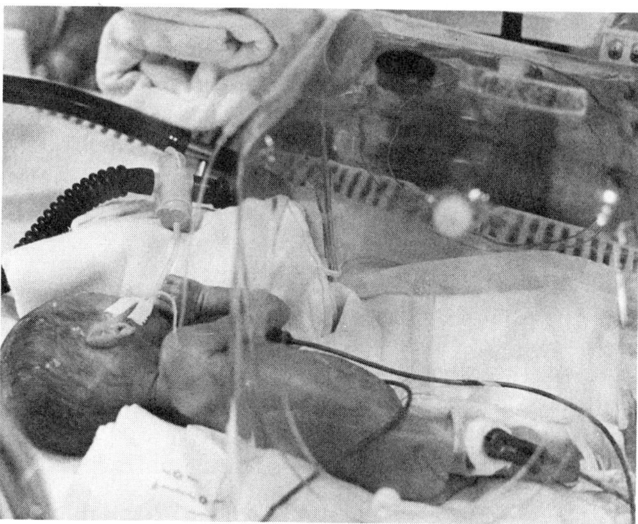

A small, premature infant (weight = 760 g) under a heat shield in an incubator. (Christine Acebo, photographer.)

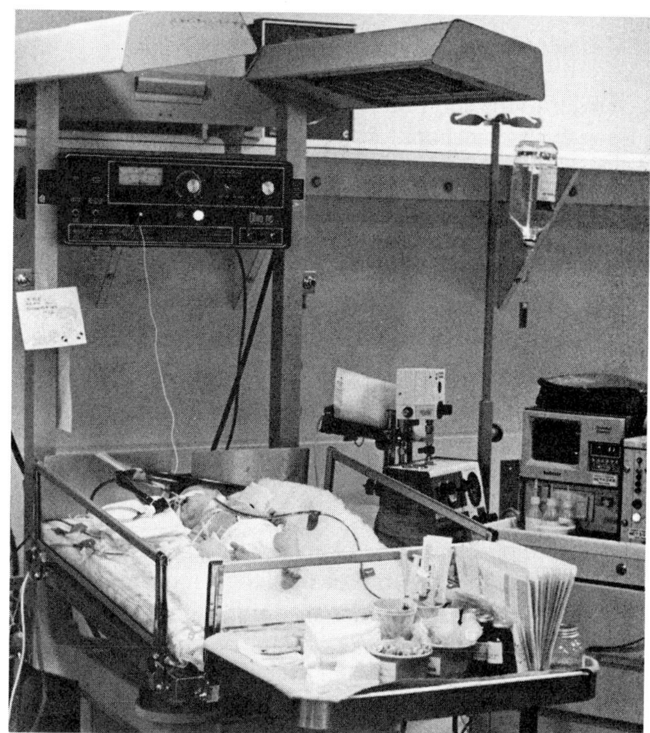

A radiant warmer. (Christine Acebo, photographer.)

Definitive diagnosis of infections can only be made from bacterial cultures. Because the sites of serious infection in neonates are the central nervous system, urinary tract, lungs, and circulatory systems, cultures of spinal fluid, urine, tracheal aspirations, and blood are included in the usual septic work-up. Cultures are also often repeated to determine whether the infection is resolving.

A serious infection is treated with antibiotics and determination of antibiotics depends on the culture. Therefore, until results of cultures are available, infants are treated for both gram-positive and gram-negative bacteria and are thus given both a penicillin (ampicillin, oxacillin, or penicillin) and an aminoglycoside (kanamycin or gentamicin). If the pathogen is resistant to these drugs, cephalosporins or chloramphenicol may be given.

Complications Both the infection and the antibiotics used to treat it may cause complications. For example, meningitis, septicemia, and pneumonia can cause death, and the mortality rate from sepsis caused by group B streptococcus has been reported to be as high as 50% (Speck et al., 1979). Meningitis can also cause significant neurologic damage.

Prolonged antibiotic use may lead to superinfection from fungus or yeast. Localized superinfections are treatable, but generalized superinfections often cause death because the antifungal drugs are toxic to infants. Prolonged use of the aminoglycosides may lead to deafness due to nerve damage; chloramphenicol may cause aplastic anemia.

Considerations for Follow-up High-risk infants remain susceptible to infections for at least 3 months postterm. One study showed that premature infants had more respiratory infections throughout the first year than did normal full-term infants (Goodman, 1973). Therefore, all high-risk infants need close nursing follow-up. In addition, nurses need to instruct parents to avoid crowds and people who are obviously ill; many parents of high-risk infants have spent up to a year confined to their houses for fear of infections. In addition, all infants treated with aminoglycosides should have their hearing tested.

Alterations in Respiration

Respiratory problems are common in the neonatal period because of the immaturity of the lungs and the cerebral respiratory centers. The lungs are among the last organs to develop in the fetus; the alveoli are not fully developed until 26–28 weeks' GA. Surfactants, chemicals that reduce the surface tension in the alveoli and allow a small amount of air to remain in them after expiration, develop in the second and third trimesters. Synthesis of surfactant begins at 22–24 weeks' GA and is present in fairly adequate amounts by 35 weeks' GA (Korones, 1976).

Pulmonary circulation does not assume the adult pattern until the infant's first breath (see Chapter 7). In the uterus, fetal circulation has a right-to-left shunt, and oxygenated blood from the placenta is shunted away from the nonfunctioning lungs and into the peripheral circulation. In the first seconds after birth, the umbilical arteries begin to constrict and the infant receives less oxygenated blood from the placenta. The stimulation from the cold environment and from handling along with the decreased arterial oxygenation and increased acidosis cause the infant to breathe. Changes in blood pressure and the increased oxygenation from this breath result in the closing of the shunt and increased blood flow to the lungs.

The cerebral controls on breathing are also immature in the early months after birth. Brief respiratory pauses of less than 10 seconds are common during this period.

Assessment Assessment of the respiratory system involves taking vital signs, observing physical symptoms, and obtaining blood gases. Vital signs are taken for all hospitalized infants at least every 4 hours. A respiratory rate above 60 breaths per minute (tachypnea) and a cardiac rate above 160 beats per minute (tachycardia) are common signs of respiratory distress. A heart rate less than 100 beats per minute (bradycardia) and apnea may result in hypoxia or respiratory failure.

The physical signs of respiratory distress include cyanosis or pallor, nasal flaring, retractions of the chest wall, and expiratory grunts. Severely ill infants are usually flaccid, hypoactive, and edemic. In addition, respiratory problems alter the breath sounds heard on auscultation. The specific changes depend on the problem.

Blood gases should be monitored in all infants suspected of having respiratory problems. Normal arterial PO_2 in infants ranges from 60–80 mm Hg, which is lower than the level in older children; PCO_2 and pH levels are similar to those of older children. The three types of blood gases obtained are: (a) capillary, (b) arterial, and (c) transcutaneous.

Capillary blood gases are obtained from a finger or heel that has been warmed to promote vasodilation. Arterial blood gases are obtained either by an arterial stick or from an indwelling arterial catheter, usually in the umbilical artery. Oxygen levels are lower in capillary than arterial samples, but because both capillary and arterial blood gases are obtained intermittently, the level of oxygenation between sampling times is not known. Intense crying during the procedure also lowers the oxygen and carbon dioxide levels. Continuous monitoring of an infant's oxygen and carbon dioxide levels is possible with a transcutaneous oxygen monitor. A heated electrode continuously measures the oxygen and carbon dioxide levels in the capillaries so that the effect of stimulation on oxygenation can be determined. Blood samples are still necessary, however, to monitor pH.

Vital signs are taken at least every 4 hours and more often if respiratory symptoms are present. The nurse then records descriptions of the infant's color, degree of respiratory distress, and breath sounds at the same time. The assessment data determine the specific nursing diagnosis. Respiratory dysfunction suggests ineffective airway clearance, ineffective breathing pattern, or impaired gas exchange.

Nursing Management The goal of nursing care for high-risk infants with respiratory problems is to maintain adequate oxygenation by modifying the environment and by treating the underlying problem. The nurse also moni-

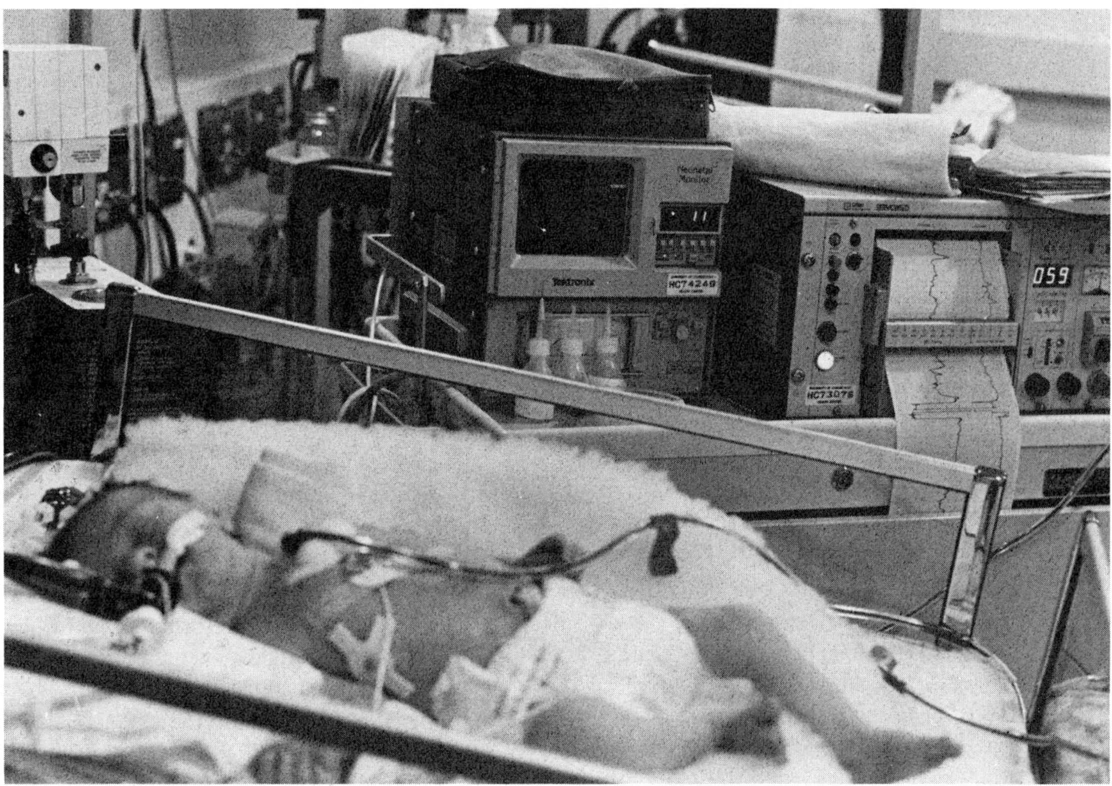

A transcutaneous oxygen monitor attached to a full-term infant receiving mechanical ventilation. (Christine Acebo, photographer.)

tors the infant's status to identify complications of treatment as early as possible.

Supportive interventions to treat respiratory problems include reducing cold stress, metabolic disturbances, and the stress of infections. During the acute phase, however, excessive handling may cause hypoxia, although infants should be repositioned every 2 to 4 hours to prevent pooling of secretions. Elevating the head slightly tends to increase oxygenation (Ennis and Harris, 1978). A diaper roll placed behind the neck helps keep the airway patent, but overextending the neck, which tends to close off the trachea, should be avoided.

In addition, chest physiotherapy and suctioning may eliminate excess secretions. Chest physiotherapy consists of positioning to promote drainage of congested lobes and percussion and vibration to loosen secretions. This treatment can cause hypoxia, and so it should be done with caution in severely ill infants (Dingle et al., 1980). The nose and mouth of each infant with respiratory dysfunction are suctioned to remove secretions that might block the upper airway. Endotracheal tubes require suctioning every 1 to 4 hours (depending on the amount of secretions) to maintain the patency of the tube.

Respiratory support is provided in one of four ways: (a) environmental oxygen, (b) continuous positive airway pressure (CPAP), (c) continuous negative chest wall pressure, and (d) mechanical ventilation. Environmental oxygen is extra oxygen mixed with the air the infant is breathing. Low concentrations of oxygen can be supplied directly to the incubator, but higher concentrations must be administered through an oxygen hood, which is a small, clear plastic box that covers the infant's head. Oxygen is administered to older infants by nasal cannula or oxygen tent. Whenever oxygen is administered it must be humidified and warmed to prevent cold stress; the nurse monitors its concentration at least once every hour.

Continuous positive airway pressure provides oxygen and continuous pressure on the distending airway to prevent alveolar collapse without overdistending the alveoli. By maintaining positive pressure at the end of expiration, alveolar air is retained representing the functional residual capacity necessary for continued diffusion of oxygen into the blood and less airway resistance, thereby lessening the work of breathing. The infant breathes unaided. The oxygen is administered by endotracheal tube to the lower airways or by nasal prongs to the upper airways. A head hood or face mask might be used, but these devices restrict accessibility for nursing care. Both oxygen concentration and pressure level are monitored closely. Local irritation may occur to the infant's nares or lips at the site of the delivery system.

For continuous negative chest wall pressure, an infrequently used treatment, the infant is placed in a specially designed incubator that supplies negative pressure to the infant's chest wall to prevent the alveoli from collapsing.

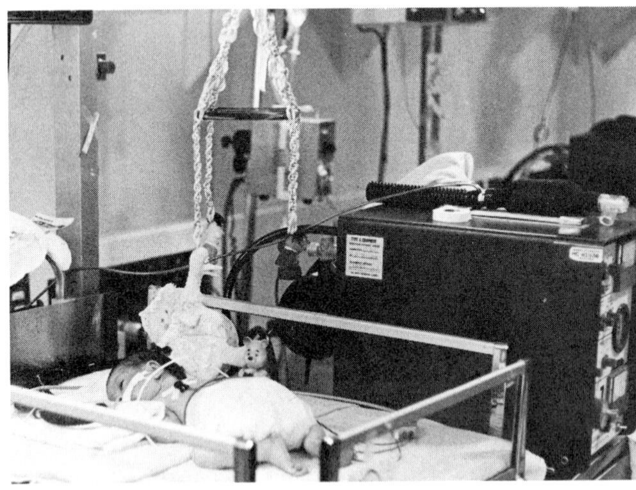

A premature infant at 36 weeks' GA receiving mechanical ventilation. The ventilator is the large box behind the infant. (Christine Acebo, photographer.)

Oxygen is administered through a hood, and the infant breathes unaided. Pressure level and oxygen concentration are monitored. When the portholes are open, cool air is sucked into the incubator and the nurse therefore needs to intervene to prevent cold stress.

Severe respiratory problems must be treated with mechanical ventilators, which provide breaths of oxygen for the infants. Some ventilators are time cycled, whereas others are volume cycled. The ventilator is set to provide a given volume of oxygen with each breath at a given pressure. The settings vary, but the criterion is normalization of arterial oxygen and carbon dioxide. The breathing rate of the ventilator can be varied and is sometimes set fast enough that the machine does all the breathing. At a slow rate (below 20 breaths per minute), the infant is able to breathe between the ventilator breaths. A small positive pressure is usually maintained at the end of a breath so that the alveoli do not collapse.

Drugs given to treat respiratory problems include sodium bicarbonate to correct acidosis that does not improve after adequate oxygenation, theophylline, and caffeine. The last two are closely related drugs given to treat apnea. Theophylline reduces the frequency of apneic spells and hypoxia (Peabody et al., 1978) but can also cause tachycardia, digestive difficulties, and wakefulness.

Specific Respiratory Problems Treatment of a respiratory problem depends on its cause. In infants with RDS (hyaline membrane disease), a respiratory problem caused by a deficiency of surfactant in the immature lungs of premature infants, alveolar collapse is the cause of inadequate ventilation. RDS occurs primarily in infants with birth weights between 1000 and 1500 g (2¼ and 3½ lb) and is the major cause of mortality in the neonatal period (Klaus et al., 1979). Alveolar collapse results from surfactant deficiency and can lead to the collapse of segments of the lungs (atelectasis).

Symptoms of RDS include expiratory grunting, retractions, nasal flaring, cyanosis, tachypnea, and diminished breath sounds. This syndrome begins within a few hours after birth, progressively worsens for about 2 days, and usually improves within 5 days. Severity of symptoms varies. Some infants require only a small amount of supplemental oxygen to recover; others die despite mechanical ventilation and intensive nursing care.

Mechanical obstruction of the upper or lower airways is another cause of respiratory distress. Upper airway blockage occurs in Pierre-Robin syndrome, a syndrome of related congenital anomalies including a small mandible, large tongue, and cleft palate. The large tongue may fall backward and block the airway. Positioning the infant and suturing the tongue to the floor of the mouth prevent this problem until the jaw grows large enough to contain the tongue.

Lower airway blockage occurs in transient tachypnea, in meconium aspiration, and in pneumonia. Transient tachypnea is a mild disease that occurs in full-term infants and older preterm infants, particularly those born by cesarean section or depressed by obstetric drugs. Delayed clearing of fluid from the alveoli after birth interferes with gas exchange. Infants with transient tachypnea recover within 48 hours after birth and rarely require more treatment than environmental oxygen. Symptoms are similar to mild RDS.

Meconium aspiration and pneumonia may occur in both premature and full-term infants. In meconium aspiration, the infant aspirates meconium-contaminated amniotic fluid, and the foreign material in the lungs then interferes with gas exchange in the alveoli and may cause atelectasis. Pneumonia, an infection of the lungs, occurs as either a congenital infection or a complication of other dysfunctions or procedures. Endotracheal intubation, for example, allows bacteria to enter the lungs, so that when atelectasis is present the collapsed areas provide excellent sites for bacterial growth. The increased secretions caused by pneumonia also interfere with air exchange. Symptoms of meconium aspiration and pneumonia include cyanosis, mild retractions, tachypnea, and hypoactivity. Breath sounds are diminished over areas of atelectasis, and crepitant rales may be heard in other areas. Both diseases cause increased pulmonary secretions, but in the early stages of meconium aspiration, the secretions are meconium tinged.

Apnea caused by prematurity occurs as an extension of normal periodic breathing in about one-third of infants with GAs less than 32 weeks (Babson et al., 1975). Instead of respiratory pauses, these infants have prolonged apneic episodes that cause hypoxia and bradycardia. The duration of an apneic pause that makes it pathologic is uncertain, but episodes longer than 20 seconds are considered abnormal, and bradycardia can occur with episodes briefer than 10 seconds (Deuel, 1973). Severe apnea can lead to respiratory arrest and death. Because this problem is caused by the immaturity of the central nervous system, it improves as the infant matures. Other conditions that can cause prolonged apnea include sepsis, hypoglycemia, dehydration, hypocalcemia, cardiac abnormalities, and neurologic damage. Apnea caused by these conditions improves only when the underlying problem is treated.

Impaired gas exchange is the cause of respiratory problems in bronchopulmonary dysplasia (BPD) and Wilson-Mikity syndrome. BPD occurs in infants with RDS who have been treated with mechanical ventilation. It is apparently caused by oxygen toxicity and pressure damage in the lungs. Wilson-Mikity syndrome occurs after the first week of life in infants with birth weights less than 1000 g and is not related to oxygen therapy. In both conditions, chronic changes in the lungs, including thickening and necrosis of alveolar walls and bronchiolar linings, impair the diffusion of oxygen from the alveoli to the capillaries. These infants require respiratory support—additional oxygen and often mechanical ventilation—for weeks or months.

Complications Complications can result either from the initial respiratory problems or from their treatment. Inadequate or ineffective treatment may result in respiratory failure or right-to-left shunting. Respiratory failure occurs when the PCO_2 level is above 60 mm Hg, PO_2 is below 45 mm Hg, and pH is below 7.2. Clinical signs include severe apnea and bradycardia, which, if untreated, will result in death. Infants are usually placed on cardiac and respiratory monitors to detect episodes of bradycardia and apnea.

Shunting of blood occurs because the circulatory areas involved in fetal right-to-left shunting—the foramen ovale, ductus arteriosus, and ductus venosus—reopen as a result of significant hypoxia, elevated carbon dioxide levels, or acidosis. These areas are not permanently closed by fibrosis for several weeks to months after birth, so impaired gas exchange, hypoxia, hypocapnia, and acidosis lead to pulmonary vasoconstriction and pulmonary hypertension whereby unoxygenated blood is shunted into the peripheral circulation and hypoxia is worsened.

Significant complications may also result from treatment, such as CPAP and mechanical ventilation, which may cause pneumothorax. A pneumothorax occurs when alveoli are ruptured, allowing air to escape into the pleural spaces. The negative pressure between the lungs and the chest wall is thus disrupted, and part of the lung collapses, causing hypoxia. Pneumothorax occurs in 10% of infants receiving CPAP and in 33% of infants receiving mechanical ventilation; only 3% of infants receiving only environmental oxygen develop it (Stavis and Krauss, 1980). Evidence also indicates that pneumothorax is a precursor to intraventricular hemorrhage (Hill et al., 1982).

Endotracheal intubation also can cause complications. It provides a route for bacterial infection because repeated suctioning through the endotracheal tube causes irritation of the trachea and bronchial tubes, which predisposes the lungs to infection. Improper placement of the tube, accidental extubation, and plugging of the tube with mucus result in hypoventilation and hypoxia and are major causes of mortality and morbidity among high-risk infants (Stavis and Krauss, 1980).

Umbilical artery catheters also may cause significant complications. Thromboemboli form at the end of a large percentage of umbilical catheters (Stavis and Krauss, 1980). Small emboli break away from the catheters frequently, and occasionally large emboli are formed resulting in major damage or death. Transient blanching of one or both legs occurs frequently, probably because of arterial spasm or emboli. Bacterial colonization of umbilical catheters is also common and may result in serious infections.

The supplemental oxygen used to treat respiratory problems also causes complications, as oxygen toxicity is related to the development of BPD. In addition, oxygen toxicity causes retrolental fibroplasia (RLF), an eye condition in some infants that may result in blindness. The etiology of RLF is the high level of oxygen that creates changes in the retinal vasculature, which in turn lead to scarring and retinal detachment. The elevated oxygen levels do not have to be prolonged; RLF may result from brief elevations, as when extra oxygen is given an infant after an apneic attack. The very immature infant is more vulnerable to this problem. Generally, RLF is associated with PO_2 levels above 100 mm Hg, but it sometimes occurs at lower levels, especially in infants with GAs less than 30 weeks.

Considerations for Follow-up Most infants recover completely from respiratory problems. Nevertheless, they should be followed closely during the first year after discharge because of the increased risk of pulmonary infections. In addition, all premature infants receiving oxygen therapy should be examined by an ophthalmologist. Although RLF cannot be cured, it can be treated and retinal detachment prevented.

Infants who develop chronic lung disease (BPD or Wilson-Mikity syndrome) require long-term hospital treatment and their parents therefore need support in developing positive relationships with their infants. Parents should be encouraged to participate in caregiving and in specific respiratory treatments so that they can learn the needs and capabilities of their infants. A few infants with chronic lung disease require continued respiratory support for months, or even years. These infants should be managed at home, where they can experience normal family stimulation. (These aspects of chronic illness are discussed in Chapter 30.)

For chronically ill infants, oxygen can be administered by nasal catheter or nasal cannula during the day and by an oxygen tent at night. Some of these infants require tracheostomies either with or without a ventilator. Their parents can be taught tracheostomy care, chest physiotherapy, and suctioning (see Chapter 34). The physical and psychological development of infants with chronic lung disease is as important as their respiratory care. Because infancy is marked by development of locomotion and speech, infant jumpers and walkers can enable infants with chronic lung disease to practice their gross motor skills despite the restrictions posed by oxygen equipment (Schraeder, 1979). Parents should be encouraged to talk and sing to their infants to stimulate their speech capabilities. Young children with tracheostomies learn to make noises by covering the tracheostomy opening briefly (Kennedy et al., 1982).

A small percentage of infants with apnea do not improve by term age. Others develop prolonged apnea, which is confirmed by a pneumogram, a 12- to 24-hour recording of an infant's respiratory pattern. These infants often have chronic lung disease, chronic neurologic disabilities, cardiac defects, or siblings who died from sudden infant death syndrome (SIDS) (see Chapter 32). These infants may be treated with theophylline, a bronchodilator, to decrease bronchospasms that may occlude the airway. Infants with prolonged apnea are sent home with apnea monitors to be used during sleep because of the danger that a prolonged apneic episode might lead to respiratory arrest. If breathing ceases for 15 to 20 seconds, the alarm sounds and summons the parent.

Parents need to learn to manage the monitor and to stimulate infant breathing. They need support in dealing with their anxiety about their infants, their knowledge that they are responsible for their infants' survival, and their isolation from other parents (Dimaggio and Sheetz, 1983). Thus these parents often benefit from joining support groups with other parents of infants with prolonged apnea.

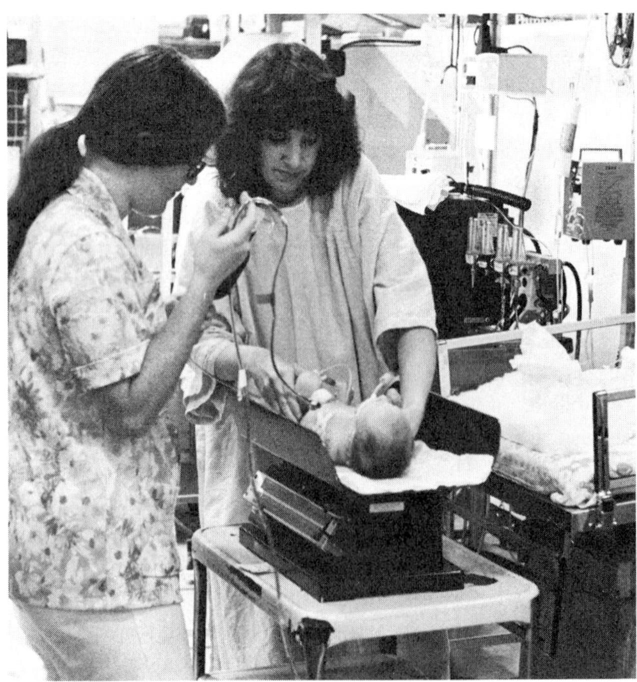

Two nurses weighing a ventilator-dependent infant. (Christine Acebo, photographer.)

Few infants exhibit prolonged apnea after 1 year of age, so most monitors are discontinued at that time. The exact relationship between SIDS and prolonged apnea is unclear. SIDS can be diagnosed only on autopsy, whereas infants with prolonged apnea can be resuscitated (Bakke and Dougherty, 1981). In addition, not all SIDS infants exhibit prolonged apnea in the early weeks of life (Thoman et al., 1977).

Alterations in Nutrition

The nutritional needs of high-risk infants are difficult to meet. Serious illness can impair an infant's ability to suck; calorie and nutrient needs are increased by the stress of illness; and after oral or gastric feedings, high-risk infants tend to regurgitate milk into the lower half of the esophagus, which causes an increased respiratory rate (Fanaroff and Klaus, 1979).

Premature infants are even more vulnerable to nutritional problems because they have less subcutaneous fat and diminished stores of glycogen, calcium, and iron. Their ability to digest protein, fats, and lactose (milk sugar) is impaired because gastric acidity and the amount of some digestive enzymes are decreased. Moreover, the stomach capacity of premature infants is very small and the sucking reflex is not fully developed and coordinated with swallowing until 35–36 weeks' GA (Boettcher and Pereira, 1983). (Gastrointestinal disorders are further covered in Chapter 38.)

Assessment The nurse assesses the nutritional status of every high-risk infant on a daily basis. The nutrition available to an infant for growth equals the calories consumed minus the calories expended and excreted (Boettcher and Pereira, 1983). Infants receiving and using adequate calories and nutrients show adequate growth. Therefore, repeated measurements of length, weight, and head circumference are used to assess the nutritional status of high-risk infants (see Appendix A).

Every high-risk infant should be weighed daily, and length and head circumference should be recorded once a week. All infants lose weight for the first few days after birth and continue to lose weight until feedings are well established and they are receiving 100–120 calories per kilogram (Fanaroff and Klaus, 1979). SGA infants and stressed infants may require more calories.

The adequacy of an infant's growth is determined by comparing it with a standard growth chart. Research has not yet determined the exact rate of growth necessary to maximize intelligence, length, and quality of survival (Fanaroff and Klaus, 1979), but adequate growth is probably occurring if head circumference, weight, and length remain at or above the percentiles they reached at birth and all three measurements are at approximately the same percentile.

Assessment also determines how well infants are tolerating feedings. Symptoms of feeding intolerance or gastrointestinal disease include gastric aspirate larger than half the hourly food intake (Boettcher and Pereira, 1983), bile-tinged aspirate or emesis, large emesis, abdominal distension, and occult blood in the stool. Some premature infants have difficulty absorbing sugar and thus excrete it in the stool.

Assessment of feeding tolerance therefore involves estimating the amount of any residual. Before each tube feeding, the contents of the stomach are aspirated and measured. The abdomens of all small premature infants and all infants with severe illnesses should be measured at least once every 8 hours and their stools checked for occult blood and sugar. (See Chapter 38 for discussion of procedure for tube feedings.)

Generally, the nursing diagnosis for infants with nutritional deficiencies is alteration in nutrition (less than body requirements). In order to provide adequate nutrition, however, it is important to determine not only whether an infant's growth is adequate but also the cause of any inadequacy. The cause of the inadequacy completes the nursing diagnosis and defines the circumstances that result in fewer nutrients than the body's requirements. Excess expenditure of calories occurs because of cold stress or serious illness, so that environmental stresses should be minimized and seriously ill infants should be given additional calories. When an infant is receiving inadequate calories or nutrients for growth, dietary supplementation will improve nutritional status. Some infants excrete excess calories through vomiting or in the stool, and nutrients must therefore be provided by another route until absorption improves. Other infants, because of congenital enzyme deficiencies, are unable to use nutrients even though they are provided with adequate nutrition and can absorb it. (These disorders are discussed in Chapter 40.)

Nursing Management The long-term goal of nursing care is to provide an adequate balance of calories and nutrients for brain and body growth and to prevent diseases caused by deficiencies of specific nutrients. High-risk infants receiving adequate nutrition maintain adequate growth in weight, length, and head circumference.

The selection of the type of food and its delivery route is important to providing each infant with adequate nutrition. The route of administration for feeding should progress from parenteral fluids, to continuous tube feedings, to gavage feedings, and finally to oral feedings.

Ideally, infants should be given their mothers' milk, which is easily digested and contains maternal antibodies to protect against infections. Several studies have demonstrated that breast-fed full-term infants experience fewer infections (Grams, 1978; Young et al., 1982). Breast milk is believed also to provide protection from necrotizing enterocolitis (Gennaro, 1982). In addition, breast-feeding enables the mother of a high-risk infant to play a unique role in the infant's recovery. The breast milk of mothers of preterm infants contains extra protein necessary to meet their increased needs (Pittard, 1981), but breast-fed premature infants still require nutrient supplements, particularly of phosphorus, copper, vitamins B_{12}, D, and E, and folic acid, for ideal growth (Boettcher and Pereira, 1983).

Even so, fewer mothers of high-risk infants breast-feed than mothers of healthy infants, usually because these mothers are separated from their infants because of the infants' hospitalization and often have had difficult pregnancies and deliveries. The mothers of these infants must also pump their breasts to provide breast milk. In order to initiate a milk supply, each breast must be pumped for about 10 minutes every 2–3 hours during the day (Boggs and Rau, 1983). Not every mother is willing or able to make that large a commitment to breast-feeding. Another concern is that many drugs are excreted in breast milk (Anderson, 1977; Bertino, 1981), and ill mothers take a number of medications.

If the infant's mother is unable to breast-feed, the infant may be fed donated breast milk. This provides adequate nutrition but no protection from infection because milk from a breast milk bank must be pasteurized to destroy pathogenic bacteria that may have contaminated it (Lemons, 1981).

Most high-risk infants are instead fed commercial formulas that are universally available and have assured nutrient contents. Special formulas have recently been developed, and these contain the types of proteins, carbohydrates, and fats that are easily digested and meet the nutritional needs of premature infants. Extra vitamins and nutrients are also included in these formulas.

High-risk infants not receiving these special formulas require dietary supplements to meet their nutritional needs, and multivitamins are therefore given with feedings. Premature infants in particular require additional amounts of liposoluble vitamins during the first 2 months of life. Vitamin D supplementation prevents rickets, and vitamin E is given to prevent hemolytic anemia. Medium-chain triglyceride oil (MCT oil) is sometimes given to provide extra calories for infants who have difficulty gaining weight or who are on fluid restrictions.

Feedings can be provided in several ways. Ideally, infants should be allowed to suck from a bottle or breast. Feedings can be given by the parents and thus promote closeness between parents and infants, but many high-risk infants are unable to suck well enough to receive oral feedings. Instead, they receive tube feedings, usually by gavage, in which a tube is inserted through the nose or mouth and passed into the stomach and feedings of formula, breast milk, or sugar water are given every 2–4 hours and allowed to drain into the stomach by gravity. The tube is usually inserted just before the feeding and removed when it is completed, although in some nurseries the tube is left in place for 24–72 hours (Zieman and Carroll, 1978).

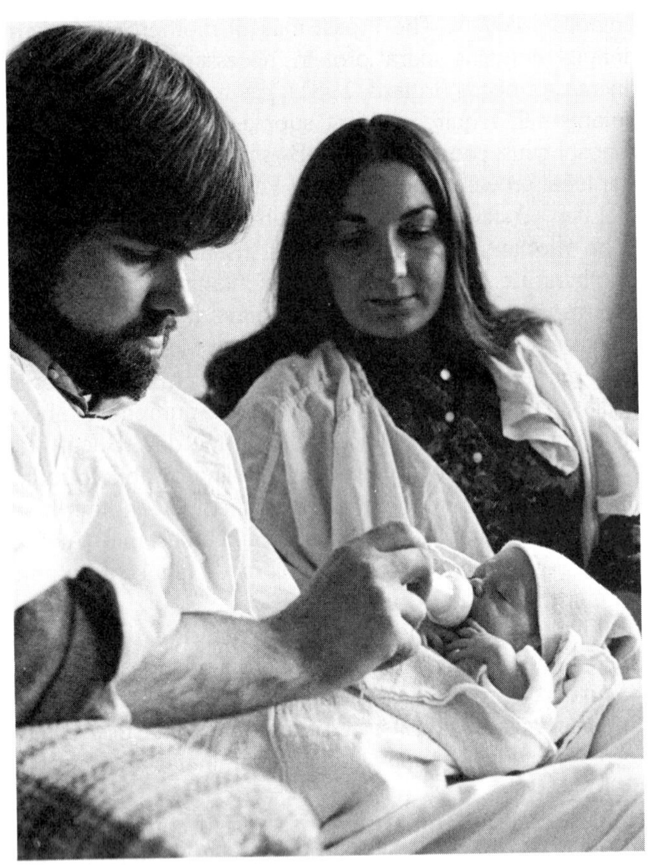

Parents feeding their premature infant shortly before discharge. (Christine Acebo, photographer.)

Continuous tube feedings are also given by placing the feeding tube in the stomach, duodenum, or jejunum and pumping feedings through the tube by an infusion pump at a slow, constant rate. Placement of the tube creates certain risks. Locating the tube in the stomach occasionally causes regurgitation. This problem is avoided by intestinal placement, but digestion and absorption are less complete, and intestinal perforation and intussusception may occur, particularly if the tube is placed in the jejunum.

When infants are unable to tolerate gastrointestinal feedings, they must receive fluids and nutrients parenterally. Immediately after birth, parenteral fluids (usually 10% dextrose in water) are given to prevent dehydration and hypoglycemia until a feeding regimen can be established. If infants have difficulty tolerating feedings, they are given parenteral fluids in addition to feedings for several weeks. Because of extreme prematurity or surgical problems, some infants are unable to tolerate gastrointestinal feedings for long periods and are instead given parenteral nutrition. This is either in the form of intralipids, a high-calorie solution of fats, or hyperalimentation, a concentrated solution of dextrose, proteins, electrolytes, and vitamins. Both intralipids and hyperalimentation with a low sugar content (no more than 10% dextrose) are infused through peripheral veins, but hyperalimentation with higher concentrations of sugar must be infused into the superior vena cava through a cutdown of the internal or external jugular vein (Colley and Wilson, 1979). Because of the risk of infection with hyperalimentation, it should never be infused through an umbilical catheter.

No matter how they receive their feedings, all infants need opportunities for sucking. In the uterus, fetuses develop this ability by sucking on their fingers, but because infants receiving tube feedings or hyperalimentation may be restrained or otherwise prevented from sucking their fingers, they should be offered pacifiers frequently. Sucking on a pacifier calms an infant and raises the oxygen level (Anderson et al., 1980). Evidence also suggests that sucking aids digestion. One study showed that preterm infants who were given pacifiers during tube feedings were ready for bottle feeding sooner and were discharged earlier than infants who had not had this experience (Measel and Anderson, 1979).

Complications Inadequate nutrition can lead to serious complications. Severe malnutrition can result in inadequate brain growth and permanent mental retardation. Fortunately, however, the brain receives nutrition in preference to other parts of the body so inadequate brain growth occurs only after prolonged nutritional deficiency.

Inorganic failure-to-thrive syndrome is another serious consequence of inadequate nutrition and can occur when inappropriate nurturing and stimulation are accompanied by improper feeding techniques or inadequate calories and nutrients. The syndrome occurs in both institutionalized infants and home-reared infants, but infants who are hospitalized for long periods and whose parents fail to establish adequate relationships with them are particularly vulnerable for inorganic failure-to-thrive syndrome after discharge. For these infants, assessment of parenting and family environment are essential parts of nursing care. (Families at risk are further discussed in Chapter 22.)

The feeding techniques used with high-risk infants may also cause complications. Regurgitation after oral or tube feeding may cause aspiration of formula or breast milk. Positioning the infant on the right side or on the abdomen increases the rate of gastric emptying and thus decreases the risk of aspiration (Fanaroff and Klaus, 1979). Perforation of the stomach, esophagus, or intestine occurs, although rarely, during the insertion of tubes for gavage or continuous feedings (Stavis and Krauss, 1980).

Hyperalimentation and intralipids cause other complications. The high glucose content of central hyperalimentation may cause hyperglycemia if the infusion rate is too rapid. Using an infusion pump therefore helps to maintain a constant infusion rate. This high sugar content is also an excellent medium for bacterial growth. Intralipids cause hyperlipidemia (elevated fats in the blood), and so serum lipids should be checked daily. Hyperlipidemia can interfere with the binding of bilirubin to albumin and intralipids may rarely cause fat emboli. Symptoms of this condition include dyspnea, cyanosis, and bradycardia or tachycardia. Because of these potential problems, intralipids are not given when the infant has hyperbilirubinemia or lung disease.

A life-threatening complication is necrotizing enterocolitis (NEC), which strikes some high-risk infants, particularly those who are premature. It is characterized by necrosis of the mucosa of the large and small bowel. The necrotic areas are localized at first but spread rapidly and cause bowel perforation or infarction. An episode of hypoxia in the prenatal period predisposes an infant to NEC by causing the blood to be shunted away from the gut. This decrease in tissue perfusion makes the bowel susceptible to infection so infants with immature or compromised immunologic systems are particularly at risk for NEC (Smith, 1981). The carbohydrates of feedings allow the bacteria to proliferate; thus high-calorie formulas (with more than 20–24 calories per ounce) are particularly associated with NEC.

Early symptoms include increases in gastric aspirates, abdominal distension, occult blood in the stool, bile-stained emesis, lethargy, temperature instability, and hypotension. If not treated early, this condition worsens rapidly. Medical treatment is supportive: resting the bowel by discontinuing feedings and providing hyperalimentation, administering antibiotics to treat the infection, ensuring adequate intravenous fluids for hydration, and closely monitoring the infant's vital signs and general condition. If the infant's condition deteriorates, surgery is performed to remove the necrotic bowel. Despite the best treatment, 25%–75% of affected infants die (Gennaro, 1980). Early treatment improves the survival rate.

Considerations for Follow-up High-risk infants continue to have greater-than-normal nutritional needs after hospital discharge. They need vitamin supplementation. Iron supplementation is begun at 4 months for full-term infants but, because of their decreased iron reserves, it is begun at term for premature infants. Those weighing less than 3200 g (7 lb) at discharge and those with weak sucking reflexes may require feedings at least every 3 hours. Because of neurologic or surgical problems, a few infants are unable to take oral feeding at home but can be managed at home with gastrostomy feedings or hyperalimentation (see Chapter 38).

Mothers who choose to breast-feed their infants require support, for high-risk infants often are unable to breast-feed exclusively by the time of discharge. These infants need adequate nutrition to complete their recovery from perinatal insults, and they need more fluid intake than full-term neonates to avoid dehydration. Some mothers choose to supplement their breast-feeding with bottle feedings and gradually decrease the amount of fluids given by bottle. Sometimes sucking on the softer rubber nipple interferes with the infant's learning to nurse from the breast.

The Lact-Aid system is another method of supplementing breast-feeding. A small bag containing formula is hung around the mother's neck, and a tube connected to the bag is placed in the infant's mouth. The infant then sucks on the tube and the breast simultaneously. As more breast milk is produced, the amount of formula is decreased. Even if the infants are not able to be breast-fed exclusively using either supplementation method, they still experience the closeness of breast-feeding and receive protection from infection.

Special problems occur if the breast-fed high-risk infant is rehospitalized. Nursing attention in such situations includes support for the mother. If possible, she should be allowed to room-in and feed the infant. When this is not possible, expressed breast milk should be fed.

Metabolic Imbalances

High-risk infants cannot maintain metabolic homeostatis as well as healthy full-term infants, as the stress of a difficult delivery or a serious illness often leads to metabolic imbalance. The lungs and kidneys of neonates have limited abilities to compensate for excess hydrogen, and so metabolic and respiratory acidosis is common. Many of the enzyme systems necessary to maintain equilibrium are not fully mature in preterm infants. In addition, some infants have congenital abnormalities of enzyme systems affecting metabolic balance (for example, hyperinsulinism and congenital adrenal hypertrophy) (see Chapter 40). Table 31-3 presents the common metabolic imbalances of high-risk infants.

Approximately 50% of infants with diabetic mothers (IDM) develop hypoglycemia in the early postnatal period (Babson et al., 1975). This problem occurs both in the infants of women with gestational diabetes and those with insulin-dependent diabetes. In the uterus the infant is exposed to excess blood sugar, and the infant's pancreas produces large amounts of insulin to metabolize this sugar. Thus the infant develops large stores of subcutaneous fat and is large for GA.

After birth the infant no longer receives maternal glucose but continues to produce excess insulin for several hours. Hypoglycemia results. When maternal glucose levels are maintained in the normal range for the last 2 months of pregnancy, infants have a lower incidence of hypoglycemia (Babson et al., 1975; Jovanic et al., 1981). Greater survival rates have been attained by monitoring the maternal uterine estriol levels during the third trimester and terminating the pregnancy either by inducing labor or by performing a cesarean section when the estriol level starts to fall. Declining estriol levels indicate placental insufficiency, which places the fetus at risk. Hypoglycemia seldom occurs in the infants whose mothers have diabetes-caused vascular problems because these problems affect the placental vessels and reduce the circulation between mother and infant. Other problems common in the IDM include late third-trimester

TABLE 31-3 Metabolic Imbalances Common During the Neonatal Period

Imbalance	Cause	Symptoms	Treatment
Acidosis (excess hydrogen)	Anaerobic metabolism (lactic acid) caused by hypoxia or cold stress	Pallor Tachypnea	Improve oxygenation Neutral thermal environment If acidosis persists, sodium bicarbonate or Tham
Hypoglycemia (deficient blood sugar)	Increased rate of glucose use due to stress (eg, asphyxia, hypothermia, or RDS) Decreased rate of glucose intake Excess insulin (eg, IDM)	Apnea Jitteriness Convulsions Apathy Hypotonia Poor feeding Cyanosis High-pitched cry Temperature instability	Extra glucose intake Reduce energy needs, place in neutral thermal environment Treat sepsis if present, correct acidosis Use of steroids
Hyperglycemia (excess blood sugar)	Excess glucose intake	Brain swelling and intraventricular hemorrhage Dehydration	Decrease glucose intake
Hyponatremia (deficient sodium)	Inadequate sodium intake Excess sodium excretion (eg, inappropriate ADH, CAH, or diarrhea) Excess fluid intake or CHF	Apnea Hypotonia Lethargy Convulsions	Increase sodium intake or decrease fluid intake
Hypernatremia (excess sodium)	Excessive sodium intake Dehydration	Tremors Lethargy Hypotonia Convulsions	Correct dehydration Decrease sodium intake
Hypocalcemia (deficient calcium)	Deficient calcium intake Stress Treatment of acidosis with bicarbonate Infusion of citrated blood Immaturity of parathyroid gland due to prematurity	Twitching Increased tone Jitteriness Convulsions Prolonged Q-T segment on ECG High-pitched cry Cyanosis Vomiting	Increase calcium intake
Hypokalemia (deficient potassium)	Excess potassium excretion due to diuretics or diarrhea	Low, broad T wave RS-7 deviations Rapid, irregular pulse Malaise	Increase potassium intake
Hyperkalemia (excess potassium)	Infusion of old blood Salt-losing CAH Renal failure	Tent shaped T wave on ECG	Decrease potassium intake Kayexalate enemas Partial exchange transfusions in life-threatening situations
Hypomagnesemia (deficient magnesium)	Fetal malnutrition IDM Exchange transfusion	Tetany Jitteriness Convulsions S-T depression and T inversion on ECG	Increase magnesium intake
Hypermagnesemia (excess magnesium)	Treatment of mothers with preeclampsia with $MgSO_4$	Cyanosis during feedings Hypotonia Lethargy Poor feeding Rarely—inadequate respiration	Usually none Partial exchange transfusions in cases of respiratory depression

fetal death, prematurity, RDS due to delayed lung maturation, hyperbilirubinemia, hypocalcemia, hypomagnesemia, hyperkalemia, and elevated phosphate levels.

Assessment A variety of different techniques are used in the assessment of metabolic equilibrium. Vital signs and blood pressure are taken at least every 2–4 hours, as many metabolic imbalances cause disturbances in vital signs. Cardiac and apnea monitors are needed because metabolic problems cause apnea and bradycardia, and infants are observed closely for the physical symptoms of metabolic disturbances (see Table 31-3).

Because infants with mild metabolic imbalances usually are asymptomatic and the symptoms that do occur are not specific, laboratory tests are necessary for definitive diagnoses. The levels of each electrolyte and of glucose in the blood are monitored closely. Urinalysis may also be performed to determine whether there is an excess of electrolytes or glucose being excreted.

Several tests can be performed by nurses in the nursery. The blood glucose level is monitored by using Dextrostix, an inexpensive 1-minute test that estimates blood glucose level from one drop of blood. Thus frequent samples can be obtained from infants at risk for hypoglycemia or hyperglycemia, and the results known immediately. Urine testing is also conducted in the nursery. Specific gravity and urine glucose level are monitored every 8 hours. Specific gravity is monitored to test for low levels of antidiuretic hormone (which result in renal failure to concentrate urine) and potential dehydration. Glucose is normally present in the urine only when the infant is hyperglycemic, but some small premature infants, because of their immature kidneys, spill sugar in their urine even when their blood sugar is normal. Samples may be collected from a urine bag, aspirated from a cotton ball placed below the meatus, or aspirated from a disposable diaper. All methods are equally accurate if tested within 15 minutes of voiding (Hutton and Schreiner, 1980; Strohbach and Kratina, 1982), although repeated application and removal of urine bags may damage the skin.

Not all cases of gestational diabetes are diagnosed, and so all LGA infants should be screened for IDM. Beginning at birth, Dextrostix blood sugar levels should be monitored hourly for 8 hours or until hypoglycemia resolves and then every 4 hours for 24 hours. If the Dextrostix reading is below 45 mg/100 mL, blood sugar levels should be drawn. Blood sugar levels are frequently elevated immediately after birth in the IDM, and so a single elevated reading is not definitive and blood levels need to be redrawn in about 15–30 minutes. In addition, laboratory tests to check the levels of bilirubin, calcium, magnesium, potassium, and phosphate are performed because these infants are at risk for imbalances.

Nursing Management The goal of nursing care is the early detection and correction of metabolic imbalances, which may require treatment of the underlying problems. The treatments for common metabolic imbalances of the neonatal period are given in Table 31-3. In deficiency states, the intake of the metabolite is usually increased, and in situations of excess, intake is decreased. Active attempts to remove excess electrolytes, such as by exchange transfusion, are limited to life-threatening conditions.

After the metabolic disturbance is corrected, the electrolytes and glucose levels continue to be monitored closely for as long as and whenever the infant is at risk for further metabolic problems. The times of risk for metabolic disturbances include the early postnatal period for all high-risk infants, the periods of serious illnesses for infants with other medical problems, and from several months to entire lifetimes for infants with congenital metabolic abnormalities.

Nursing interventions for the IDM include providing a neutral thermal environment, supporting respiration, and monitoring bilirubin levels. Feedings should be started at 2 hours of age with 10% glucose in water and be given every 2 hours until blood glucose level stabilizes. Earlier feedings are sometimes given when early hypoglycemia is present. Infants who cannot tolerate feedings or have blood sugar levels below 30 mg/100 mL are given parenteral infusions of 10% glucose. Because the symptoms of electrolyte imbalance are similar to those of hypoglycemia, the nurse also monitors electrolyte levels.

Complications If untreated, metabolic imbalances can lead to serious complications and death (see Chapter 33). Acidosis can result in respiratory failure and arrest. Severe respiratory depression in hypermagnesemia might cause respiratory failure. Hyponatremia might cause apnea or shock. Cardiac arrhythmias and cardiac arrest might result from hypocalcemia, hypomagnesemia, or hyperkalemia. Osmotic changes from hyperglycemia increase renal electrolyte and water loss and lead to dehydration. Brain damage can be caused by metabolic imbalances in any of the following ways: during seizures from hypoglycemia, hypocalcemia, hypomagnesemia, hypernatremia, or hyponatremia; by generalized swelling of the brain from osmotic changes in hyperglycemia causing fluid shifts and increased brain volume and sometimes intraventricular hemorrhage; or by intraventricular hemorrhaging in preterm infants as a result of anoxia and hypernatremia.

Considerations for Follow-up Most metabolic disturbances are resolved prior to discharge, so that the only intervention necessary on follow-up is to reassure parents that the problems will not recur. Infants with severe or persistent imbalances associated with brain damage should be evaluated by a developmental specialist so that planning can be done to assist the infant and family attain realistic goals. Those infants with congenital metabolic disturbances require long-term follow-up (see Chapter 40).

Immaturity of the Circulatory System

The immaturity of a neonate's circulatory system can lead to significant problems. Occasionally, as a result of hypoxia, the circulatory areas involved in the fetal right-to-left shunt reopen. A patent ductus arteriosus (PDA) is the most common result and occurs primarily in premature infants. Because of increased aortic pressure and decreased pulmonary vascular pressure after birth, however, the blood is often shunted from the aorta to the pulmonary artery (left-to-right shunt). A PDA should be suspected whenever recovery from respiratory problems is prolonged or the infant's condition deteriorates suddenly (Liebman et al., 1979). PDAs occur in 32% of infants born prior to 36 weeks' GA (Stahler-Miller and Gewitz, 1983) and account for 10% of the congenital heart disease found in full-term infants (Leykauf, 1981).

Congestive heart failure results from the inability of the heart to pump all of the blood returned to it from the peripheral circulation and the lungs. Heart failure occurs as a result of fluid overload, left-to-right shunting from a PDA, or a pulmonary disease causing increased vascular resistance (RDS or pneumonia).

Prior to heart failure, physiologic compensatory mechanisms attempt to improve the efficiency of the heart's pumping by increasing heart rate and the strength of each contraction. As the heart fails, blood pools in the peripheral circulation, causing impaired perfusion of nutrients and oxygen. Thus the body depends on anaerobic metabolism, and metabolic acidosis results. The pooling of blood in the lungs decreases the capacity of the lungs and stimulates neuroreceptors, which cause dyspnea and tachypnea. Apnea may occur. Decreased cardiac output also causes decreased perfusion of the brain, digestive system, and kidneys. Therefore, alterations in the level of consciousness and feeding problems are common. Excretion of urine is reduced, and specific gravity is high. This conservation of fluid further contributes to the excess circulatory volume. Congestive heart failure can also be caused by congenital cardiac anomalies (see Chapter 35).

Diagnosis consists of determining whether a PDA or congestive heart failure is responsible for the infant's symptoms. Many different conditions, including respiratory problems, metabolic imbalances, and sepsis, can cause similar symptoms, and an infant might develop more than one of these.

Cardiac problems related to fluid excess are significant because of the relatively small fluid capacity of the infant's circulatory system, less than 100 mL per kilogram. Thus it is relatively easy to cause fluid overload in high-risk infants.

Assessment The circulatory status of high-risk infants is assessed to identify the early stages of PDA and congestive heart failure and to monitor their progression. Vital signs are taken frequently, as tachypnea and tachycardia are common signs of PDA and heart failure. Blood pressure elevations may occur in heart failure, and infants with PDAs usually have wide pulse pressures. Cardiac and apnea monitors should be used, as apnea is often worsened by these conditions and the drugs used to treat heart failure may also cause arrhythmias and bradycardia.

Heart sounds and breath sounds should be auscultated whenever vital signs are taken. A PDA murmur is often intermittent; it is usually systolic in the early stages and becomes a loud continuous murmur later (Philip, 1977). Pulmonary rales or rhonchi are common with congestive heart failure, and a galloping rhythm occasionally occurs.

Physical signs are also part of the assessment of cardiac problems. Bounding peripheral pulses indicate a PDA. Cyanosis may occur with a PDA or heart failure but is of little value in assessment because these infants often have respiratory illnesses as well. Other signs of heart failure include fatigue or difficulty during feedings, peripheral edema, especially periorbital, an enlarged liver (3–5 cm below costal margin), and chest wall retractions. Infants with heart failure or a large PDA have difficulty growing. Rapid weight gain (more than 30 g a day) often is caused by fluid retention and congestive heart failure. Therefore, infants with heart failure are weighed every 8–12 hours.

Laboratory tests are used to validate assessment findings. An echocardiogram may indicate the presence of a significant left-to-right shunt across a PDA or may show hypertrophy of one or more of the heart chambers, which is caused by heart failure. The hypertrophy improves as the heart failure responds to therapy. The chest radiograph of an infant with congestive heart failure may show an enlarged heart, changes in the contours of the heart, or changes in the pulmonary vasculature. More extensive tests, such as cardiac catheterization, are performed when congenital cardiac anomalies are suspected (see Chapter 35).

The nurse also monitors electrolyte and glucose levels in all infants suspected of cardiac problems because metabolic imbalances can mimic the symptoms of cardiac problems. Moreover, the fluid retention in congestive heart failure and the drugs used to treat it can cause electrolyte imbalances.

The nursing diagnosis for the infant with cardiac dysfunction is alteration in cardiac output (decreased). Furthermore, because these infants are at risk for fluid overload, nursing care is also based on the potential for alteration in fluid volume.

Nursing Management The goals of nursing care are to prevent fluid overload and to detect circulatory problems as early as possible. While a circulatory problem is being treated, nursing care focuses on maintaining adequate oxygenation of tissues and reducing the workload of the heart.

Interventions depend on the severity of the underlying cardiac problem. An infant with a mild PDA without congestive heart failure or significant respiratory disease requires only supportive care because this PDA usually closes spontaneously. The nurse then observes for signs of hypoxia and acidosis, both of which are to be avoided, thereby preventing further opening of the ductus. Occasionally, fluids are restricted to prevent congestive heart failure.

A large PDA with a significant left-to-right shunt, congestive heart failure, or severe respiratory disease requires intense nursing care and concentrated efforts to reduce cardiac workload. If the PDA does not constrict or if the infant requires prolonged mechanical ventilation, the PDA should be closed. Indomethacin, a drug that inhibits prostaglandin synthesis, is given during the first 2 weeks of life to close the PDA. This drug can cause a transient decrease in renal function or mild upper gastrointestinal bleeding, and so it is contraindicated in infants with kidney or gastrointestinal disease (Foster, 1982). When indomethacin fails to close the ductus or the infant is unable to receive the drug, surgical closure is performed (see Chapter 35).

Interventions for infants with congestive heart failure are planned to reduce the workload of the heart and to strengthen the heart's ability to pump. Fluids and sometimes sodium are restricted to reduce fluid retention. Diuretics, such as furosemide (Lasix), are given to increase urine output, and therefore urine output and specific gravity are monitored. Electrolytes are also monitored because hypernatremia and hypokalemia may result from diuresis. Supplemental oxygen is supplied to prevent hypoxia. The infant's head is elevated 20°–30° to cause pooling of blood in the peripheral circulation and thus to decrease the amount of blood returning to the heart.

Digoxin is given to slow the heart rate and to strengthen each contraction. Infants receiving digoxin must be monitored closely with a cardiac monitor and serial digoxin serum levels must be taken because of the narrow range between the therapeutic and toxic levels of this drug. Digoxin also is excreted very slowly through the kidneys, especially in premature infants. The toxic level of digoxin is even lower when the infant's serum potassium level is low. Signs of toxicity include lethargy, cardiac arrhythmias, bradycardia due to heart block, and vomiting.

Complications The complications of PDA and congestive heart failure are frequently fatal. When cardiac output is very low, tissue perfusion is inadequate which can lead to cardiogenic shock. Symptoms of shock are similar to those of severe heart failure, with the addition of hypotension (less than 35 mm Hg in a full-term infant).

Pulmonary edema occurs when large amounts of blood pool in the lungs. Fluid enters the interstitial spaces and interferes with the diffusion of oxygen through the alveoli. Symptoms include dyspnea, tachypnea, and pink-tinged mucus. Treatment of both conditions involves treating the underlying cardiac failure, supporting respiration (often mechanical ventilation), restricting fluids, and providing diuretic therapy. Occasionally, rotating tourniquets or leg wraps are used to decrease the volume of blood returning to the heart. Infants with pulmonary edema also require frequent suctioning.

Toxic reactions to digoxin also can occur and occasionally cause cardiac arrest, so that all infants receiving this drug should be closely monitored.

Considerations for Follow-up Most cardiac problems due to circulatory system immaturity have resolved prior to discharge. A PDA generally has closed either spontaneously or because of medical or surgical intervention. Cardiac failure due to a PDA, fluid overload, or pulmonary problems resolves when these problems improve. Therefore, parents need reassurance that the circulatory problems, no matter how severe during hospitalization, are cured and that there is no reason to restrict the infant's activities. Most of these infants have other problems, such as prematurity, neurologic insults, or respiratory dysfunction, which require additional follow-up.

Occasionally, the PDA of a high-risk infant fails to close prior to hospital discharge. Usually, PDAs close spontaneously during the first year, but until then parents need support and instruction. The nurse teaches parents about any fluid or diet restrictions and about the signs of congestive heart failure and encourages parents to treat their infants as normally as possible. When an infant has chronic congestive heart failure, digoxin is given at home, and the parent needs to learn to give the proper dosage at the right time, to identify the symptoms of digitalis toxicity, and to store the medicine safely to avoid accidental poisoning (see Chapter 20) (Jackson, 1979). Additional information on the home management of the chronic cardiac infant is given in Chapter 35.

Neonatal Hyperbilirubinemia

Hyperbilirubinemia is an extremely common condition in the neonatal period. The condition is characterized by jaundice, which is caused by an excess of indirect bilirubin in the blood. The major source of indirect bilirubin is free hemoglobin formed during the breakdown of red blood cells. Indirect bilirubin in the bloodstream is bound to albumin until the liver converts it to direct bilirubin, a water-soluble form, which is excreted in the feces.

The immature neonatal liver, however, has limited capacity to metabolize indirect bilirubin and thus may not be able to compensate for any increase in its formation. Moreover, within the intestines, some of the direct bilirubin is changed back to indirect bilirubin by the action of the enzyme β-glucuronidase and reabsorbed into the bloodstream. When excess indirect bilirubin is produced, all of the albumin-binding sites become filled and unbound bilirubin is present in the blood. This unbound indirect bilirubin easily enters tissues with high lipid content and interferes with the metabolism of the cells. Hyperbilirubinemia also results from the breakdown of red blood cells in areas bruised during a traumatic delivery. Permanent brain damage can result from indirect bilirubin in the brain, a condition called kernicterus.

A variety of factors cause the breakdown of red blood cells in neonates thus increasing the formation of bilirubin. High-risk infants may experience several of these problems. Fetal red blood cells mature and die every 70–80 days (Pearson, 1976). Because of the low arterial oxygen level experienced in the uterus, fetuses require more red blood cells than do infants. Physiologic jaundice then results from the breakdown of excess mature fetal red blood cells.

Another cause of red blood cell breakdown is hemolysis, the destruction of both mature and immature red blood cells. Hemolysis usually is caused by blood group incompatibility between the mother and fetus. When incompatibility is present, maternal antibodies cross the placenta and destroy fetal red blood cells; these antibodies continue to destroy the infant's red blood cells after delivery. ABO-hemolytic disease is usually a mild and self-limiting condition that occurs in about one-seventh of the cases in which the mother is blood group O and the fetus is A or B (Clarke, 1972). Rh-hemolytic disease (erythroblastosis fetalis) is more serious and can result in the death of the infant. It occurs only when a previously sensitized Rh-negative mother carries an Rh-positive fetus. Sensitization occurs when Rh-positive blood enters the mother's circulation during a previous pregnancy, abortion, or blood transfusion. Fortunately, this disease is now rare because Rh_o (D) immune globulin (RhoGAM) is given to all Rh-negative women within 3 days after each birth or abortion to prevent sensitization.

A number of other factors interfere with the conversion of indirect bilirubin to direct bilirubin. Drugs, such as morphine, sedatives, some tranquilizers, vitamin K, and oxytocin given to the mother during pregnancy, can interfere with the liver's ability to metabolize indirect bilirubin. About 1% of breast-fed infants develop hyperbilirubinemia as a result of breast-feeding (Simkin et al., 1979). Breast milk jaundice develops slowly and often is not apparent until the second week of life; it is believed to be caused by a chemical in the breast milk that interferes with the enzyme activity of the liver.

There are other factors that can interfere with the binding of indirect bilirubin to albumin and thus increase the risk of kernicterus without increasing the amount of indirect bilirubin. When the level of albumin is low, as is common with premature infants, less indirect bilirubin can be bound. Hematin, an organic compound released by hemolysis, displaces bilirubin from albumin. Acidosis, cold stress, and a number of drugs (including sulfanilamides, diazepam, salicylates, heparin, caffeine, hydrocortisone, gentamicin, and sulfadiazine) interfere with the ability of albumin to bind bilirubin.

Diagnosis of neonatal jaundice depends on differentiating between it and other conditions that can cause jaundice. Hemolytic disease should also be identified because it is more likely to cause kernicterus.

Assessment Physical signs and laboratory tests are used to assess infants suspected of hyperbilirubinemia. Jaundice, the major symptom of neonatal hyperbilirubinemia, becomes apparent at an indirect bilirubin level of 4–8 mg/100 mL (Schuman, 1976). Thus the nurse observes the neonate's skin color at least once every 8 hours and monitors bilirubin levels once jaundice appears. Normally, physiologic jaundice appears 24–72 hours after birth and lasts for 3 to 7 days.

Jaundice appearing in the first day of life often is due to hemolytic disease, and jaundice that appears after 1 week usually is due to breast-feeding or gastrointestinal diseases. Mild behavioral changes, such as lethargy and poor feeding, might accompany hyperbilirubinemia, and infants with hyperbilirubinemia do less well on the orienting items of the Brazelton Neonatal Behavior Assessment (Telzrow et al., 1980) (see Chapter 16).

Laboratory tests are used to determine the severity of hyperbilirubinemia. Because there is no easy test to determine the amount of unbound indirect bilirubin, most laboratories report the total amount of indirect bilirubin. Kernicterus usually does not occur unless the indirect bilirubin level is above 20 mg/100 mL, but it can occur at lower levels in infants with increased albumin binding (for example, premature infants, asphyxiated infants, and infants with hemolytic disease), so for these infants treatment is begun sooner. Because hemolytic jaundice can cause severe anemia, all infants and mothers should be blood-typed. When a blood group incompatibility is identified, a complete blood count and a direct Coombs' test should be performed on the infant. The Coombs' test is positive in the presence of Rh-hemolytic disease, although it may or may not be positive in cases of ABO disease.

Other conditions also can cause hyperbilirubinemia and jaundice. Elevation of the direct bilirubin occurs in a number of gastrointestinal problems including biliary atresia and hepatitis. Although these conditions often require surgical correction (see Chapter 38), direct bilirubin does not cause kernicterus. Sepsis and congenital thyroid deficiency also cause jaundice, which disappears when the underlying disease is treated.

Nursing Management Because neonatal hyperbilirubinemia cannot be prevented, the goal of nursing care is early identification and prevention of kernicterus and complications caused by treatment.

The initial interventions for infants with neonatal hyperbilirubinemia are supportive: closely observing vital signs and neurologic behavior, providing a neutral thermal environment, and nutrition. Early feedings (prior to 6 hours of age) can reduce the amount of bilirubin reabsorbed from the intestines (Ostler, 1979), but many high-risk infants cannot tolerate early feedings. Adequate fluid intake is important because dehydration may worsen jaundice. If breast milk jaundice is suspected, breast-feeding should be stopped. The bilirubin level usually falls to near normal within 2–4 days, and breast-feeding can be resumed.

The nurse also monitors the serum bilirubin levels of all infants with jaundice until a definite decline is evident. Bilirubin levels take 3–4 days to peak before there is any decline. If the serum bilirubin level is greater than 15 mg/100 mL in a full-term infant or greater than 10 mg in an infant with decreased albumin-binding capacity (for example, a premature or asphyxiated infant) or if jaundice appears in the first 24 hours of life, attempts should be made to lower the indirect bilirubin level (Babson et al., 1975). *Phototherapy* is the most common treatment. The unclothed infant is exposed to fluorescent lights, which change the indirect bilirubin into a water-soluble form that is excreted in the bile and urine. The infant's eyes are covered with a mask to prevent retinal damage from the light source. Phototherapy provides radiant heat as well as light so that incubator and warmer temperatures should be adjusted to maintain a neutral thermal environment. Phototherapy increases insensible water loss, so fluid intake must be increased. While the infant is receiving phototherapy, the nurse monitors bilirubin levels every 12 hours and again 12 hours after therapy is discontinued to check for a rebound effect.

Phenobarbitol is used on rare occasions to decrease the indirect bilirubin level, but its action is slow (about 2 weeks), and its long-term effects are unknown (Babson et al., 1975).

Exchange transfusions are used to lower indirect bilirubin levels in severe hyperbilirubinemia—that is, in cases occurring prior to 24 hours of age, hyperbilirubinemia with anemia, and indirect bilirubin levels in excess of 20 mg/100 mL in full-term infants or 15 mg in premature infants (Babson et al., 1975). An exchange transfusion is performed by withdrawing a small amount of the infant's blood and infusing the same amount of warmed, fresh or partially packed blood through an umbilical vein catheter. The procedure is repeated until about 170 mL of blood for each kilogram of body weight has been infused. The bilirubin level is usually lowered about 20%–30% (Babson et al., 1975). The nurse monitors the infant's blood pressure by Doppler method throughout the transfusion to avoid fluid overload.

During and following the procedure, the nurse observes the heart rate and ECG closely because this treatment can cause arrhythmias. Electrolytes, especially calcium and sodium bicarbonate, are given to counteract metabolic imbalances present in the transfused blood. Phototherapy is used both before and after exchange transfusions to lower the bilirubin level and thus to decrease the number of exchange transfusions needed.

Complications The most serious form of neonatal hyperbilirubinemia is Rh-hemolytic disease, and because it can be prevented by preventing maternal sensitization, any occurrence should be considered a complication. Rh-hemolytic disease begins during pregnancy, when maternal antibodies cross the placenta and destroy fetal red blood cells. When sensitization occurs, each subsequent Rh-positive pregnancy will be more seriously affected.

Symptoms include severe anemia, an enlarged liver, and jaundice. Hypoglycemia, petechiae, and purpuric spots also often occur. In the most severe cases (hydrops fetalis), the infant has such a severe deficiency of protein in the blood that edema, a distended abdomen, and respiratory distress result. The death rate of hydrops fetalis is as high as 90% (Babson et al., 1975). The disease often causes fetal death or premature birth. Rh-hemolytic disease is treated with exchange transfusions and phototherapy. Severely affected fetuses require intrauterine exchange transfusions. Because the best treatment is prevention, all women with Rh-negative blood should receive Rh_o (D) immune globulin (RhoGAM) after each Rh-positive delivery or abortion. Community nurses need to make a special effort to identify women who plan home deliveries. Their blood can be typed prior to delivery, and if they are Rh negative, they can receive the injections as outpatients.

Kernicterus is another complication of neonatal hyperbilirubinemia. Early symptoms include refusal of feedings, vomiting, hypoactive reflexes, and increased muscle tone. Later symptoms include internal rotation and adduction of arms, apnea, cyanosis, and seizures. The survivors exhibit hypotonia, mental retardation, impaired eye movements, and hearing loss. Neurologic damage can sometimes be prevented by performing an emergency exchange transfusion when the infant's behavior indicates early kernicterus, but even early kernicterus is preventable by close monitoring of bilirubin levels and the use of phototherapy and exchange transfusions.

The treatment of neonatal jaundice also causes complications. Phototherapy causes dehydration, temperature instability, and metabolic imbalances. Occasionally, the skin turns a bronze color, or "flea bite" dermatitis occurs. The eye patches used to protect the infant's eyes occasionally slip down and block the nose causing upper-airway obstruction and apnea (Stavis and Krauss, 1980). Therefore, an infant receiving phototherapy should never be left unattended in the nursery and ideally should be placed on an apnea monitor. Phototherapy also interrupts the early attachment process because infants are separated from their parents and their eyes are patched so they cannot interact visually. Loose green stools are common in infants receiving phototherapy (Simkin et al., 1979) because this treatment increases bowel motility and decreases the activity of the enzyme that aids the digestion of lactose (Donlen and Budd, 1983). Changing to a lactose-free formula helps to prevent this problem.

The complications of an exchange transfusion are more serious. Heart failure may occur because of either fluid overload or rapid loss of blood volume. Serious electrolyte imbalances can cause bradycardia or cardiac arrest. Air or thrombotic emboli may occur, and the venous catheter may be a source of infection. Hypothermia is possible if the blood is not adequately warmed.

Considerations for Follow-up Most infants with neonatal hyperbilirubinemia are completely cured at the time of discharge. Occasionally, an otherwise-healthy full-term infant is sent home with mild hyperbilirubinemia (less than 15 mg/100 mL). The nurse therefore instructs parents to return to the hospital for follow-up bilirubin tests as ordered by the physician and encourages patients to expose infants to the sun as much as possible, as sunlight has the same effects as phototherapy. Neurologic and developmental follow-up also are required for all infants with kernicterus or Rh-hemolytic disease.

Alterations in Neurologic Function

The last trimester of pregnancy and the period of early infancy are times of rapid brain growth. The gray and white matter in the brains of neonates is poorly differentiated, and most of the neurons are immature in form and function. The central nervous system of a premature infant is even less developed. Little myelination has occurred, and many synapses are not fully formed (Horwitz and Amiel-Tison, 1979). Therefore, any insult that occurs during this period can cause extensive brain damage. On the other hand, the central nervous systems of infants can compensate in order to minimize some types of brain damage. For example, damage to the speech centers in the brain does not affect language acquisition even though damage to these areas in adults causes aphasia.

Additional factors, such as other health problems and the home environment, affect neurologic outcome, so that the nature and extent of handicaps from the size and location of brain damage are not predictable. Although, generally, the larger the lesion, the more disabled an infant will be, many individuals are exceptions. For instance, although positive outcomes are more common after mild intraventricular hemorrhages (IVH), all possible outcomes, ranging from normal development to death, can occur at any level of severity (Krishnamoorthy et al., 1979; Papile et al., 1978).

The four main causes of neurologic damage in the neonatal period are hypoxia, birth trauma, hemorrhage, and infection. Episodes of hypoxia caused by birth asphyxia or by cardiac or respiratory abnormalities can damage neural tissues directly or cause brain edema. Tissue compression caused by edema leads to further brain damage. Birth trauma causes brain damage through tissue compression and tearing.

Several different types of hemorrhage can occur. Intracranial hemorrhage is caused by both trauma and hypoxia. Subdural hemorrhage occurs in full-term infants because of tearing of dura, falx, or tentorium during birth trauma. Symptoms vary from mild to severe. Intraventricular hemorrhage (IVH) occurs in premature infants as a result of hypoxia, anoxia and subsequent hypernatremia or hyperglycemia. Approximately 40% of preterm infants with birth weights below 1500 g (3½ lb) experience at least a mild IVH (Papile et al., 1978). Tissue damage occurs at the site of the hemorrhage. In severe IVH, blood fills the ventricle, causing dilation, tissue compression, and further brain damage. Subarachnoid hemorrhage occurs in both full-term and preterm infants as a result of trauma or hypoxia. Infants with small hemorrhages have symptoms of hypotonia and irritability, which resolve within the first week of life. In more severe hemorrhages, the blood in the subarachnoid space causes tissue compression.

Meningitis can also cause significant neurologic damage and is more common in the neonatal period than at any other age. Premature infants are 4 times as susceptible to this disease as full-term infants (Babson et al., 1975). The mortality rate for meningitis in infancy is 30%, and over half the survivors have residual neurologic damage (Babson et al., 1975).

Assessment Physical symptoms, behavioral changes, and laboratory tests are used to assess infants for possible neurologic problems. The diagnosis of neurologic problems has two parts: (a) identifying the cause of the problem—hypoxia, trauma, hemorrhage, metabolic imbalance, or infection—and (b) determining the extent of neurologic disabilities. Disabilities that can be diagnosed in the neonatal period include alterations in muscle tone, weakness or paralysis of an extremity, abnormal sleep–wake state patterns, and seizure activity. These disabilities may resolve prior to hospital discharge, may continue for several months, or may last throughout the infant's life. Other neurologic disabilities, such as mental retardation and cerebral palsy, might not appear until the infant is older. Nursing care therefore is based on a general nursing diagnosis of potential neurologic impairment, while the specific factors depend on the assessment data gathered for each infant.

Signs and Symptoms Abnormalities in vital signs—especially bradycardia and hypotension—may be symptoms of intracranial hemorrhage. Any episode of hypoxia, which might occur during prolonged apnea or bradycardia, can cause brain damage. Because rapid head growth is a sign of hydrocephalus, daily measurements of head circumference are performed on all infants suspected of neurologic problems. The fontanels of infants also are palpated when vital signs are performed, as bulging or full fontanels are signs of hydrocephalus. In subdural hemorrhage, only the anterior fontanel feels full.

A number of behavioral changes signal neurologic problems. Neurologic damage causes weak, asymmetric, or hypoactive reflexes. Muscle tone also is frequently affected and becomes either hypotonic or hypertonic. Because premature infants have less muscle tone than full-term infants, their muscle tone should be compared with that of normal preterm infants rather than the muscle tone of a full-term infant. If muscle tone is weaker on one side, hemiparesis may be present. Optimal performance on muscle tone and reflexes are best obtained when the infant is in an alert state. Neurologic problems may diminish spontaneous activity, and so the nurse assesses the infant's activity level. Because mild abnormalities of tone, reflexes, or activity level are often transient in high-risk infants, all infants with any of these problems should be reassessed.

The infant's state organization can be altered by neurologic problems. Frequently, infants with neurologic problems appear irritable or lethargic. Their cries may be abnormal; active sleep may be depressed; and waking increased (Prechtl et al., 1973). When in the alert state, infants with neurologic insults may appear unresponsive, although prematurity alone can have a similar effect on the quality of alertness.

Seizures and jitteriness are other signs of neurologic problems, and nurses therefore need to be able to distinguish between them. According to Gale (1981), these phenomena are differentiated by three criteria: (a) jitteriness is not accompanied by abnormal eye movements or gaze abnormalities; (b) episodes of jitteriness can be affected by stimulation; (c) jittery movements are of equal amplitude and rate, whereas the movements of seizures have fast and slow components.

A number of different problems, including neurologic damage, metabolic imbalance, and drugs, can cause jitteriness or tremulousness in neonates. Jitteriness may also occur in healthy infants during the first 24–48 hours of life (Horwitz and Amiel-Tison, 1979). Cerebral irritability due to narcotics withdrawal is a common cause of jitteriness. Narcotics readily cross the placenta causing the fetus of narcotics-addicted mothers to become addicted. After delivery the neonates no longer receive the drug, and thus manifest signs of withdrawal. Additional signs and symptoms of withdrawal include restlessness, irritability, hyperactivity, high-pitched cries, increased muscle tone, nasal stuffiness, and sneezing (Finnegan and Macnew, 1974).

Seizures are more ominous symptoms than jitteriness. The overall mortality of infants with seizures is 30%, and more than half of the survivors have permanent neurologic disabilities (Babson et al., 1975). Seizures are caused by neurologic damage, by severe metabolic disturbances, and rarely by withdrawal in the narcotics-addicted infant. Neonates do not exhibit the generalized tonic–clonic seizures typical of adults and older children. Instead, neonatal seizures involve intermittent periods of hypertonia with deviation of the eyes and jerking of one or more extremities.

Occasionally, the only symptoms of seizures are eye blinking, repetitive mouthing, apnea, and circumoral cyanosis. In infants, the size or location of neurologic damage is not indicated by the symptoms of the seizure. A seizure involving jerking of all four extremities might be localized in only one hemisphere, whereas extensive brain damage involving both hemispheres might result in a small seizure involving only one limb (Horwitz and Amiel-Tison, 1979). During active sleep, small jerks normally accompany rapid eye movements in the neonate, but these jerks should not be confused with seizures.

Clinical symptoms, however, cannot be used to identify all neurologic problems. One study, for example, found that only 54% of infants with IVH could be distinguished clinically (Lazzara et al., 1980). A number of medical tests therefore are used to diagnose neurologic problems.

Diagnostic Tests An electroencephalogram (EEG) is performed to diagnose and locate seizure activity in the brain. The only preparation necessary is to sedate the infant. This test can be performed in the nursery, but because of electrical interference from cardiac monitors and mechanical ventilators, it is more accurate when performed in a separate room. The EEG has only limited value in diagnosing mild seizures, as clinical symptoms may be accompanied by minimal, brief, or no electric discharges (Horwitz and Amiel-Tison, 1979).

A CT (computed tomography) scan is the most common test used to diagnose intracranial hemorrhages. Horizontal sections of the brain are examined by narrow x-ray beams that detect the site of bleeding. These pictures are clearer than standard radiographs and the multiple views of the brain obtained by CT scan indicate the extent of bleeding in all three dimensions. Because IVH can worsen for at least 2 weeks (Shankaran et al., 1982) and ventricular dilation occurs as late as several months after the hemorrhage (Levene and Starte, 1981), the CT scan should be repeated, even though the infant receives repeated exposures to radiation. A sedative is usually given prior to the scan because a half hour is needed to take the multiple pictures.

Ultrasonography has been used recently to diagnose intracranial hemorrhages. The extent of the hemorrhage and the presence of hydrocephalus can be determined effectively with this test (Levene, 1981; Levene and Starte, 1981; Shankaran et al., 1982), and repeated ultrasound examinations appear to be safe and can be performed in the nursery.

The lumbar puncture is used to diagnose meningitis and IVH. Small samples of cerebrospinal fluid (CSF) are obtained and examined for color, cellular content, protein, sugar, and bacteria. Meningitis is indicated by the presence of bacteria or white blood cells in the CSF; red blood cells indicate intraventricular hemorrhage. No special preparations are necessary for this test, and it can be performed in the NICU with the infant properly held. Transient decrease in PO_2 and instability of heart rate or respiration are frequent complications. If the needle breaks a small blood vessel, causing a traumatic puncture, fresh blood is present in the sample and it is difficult to determine whether a hemorrhage has occurred.

Attempts at lumbar puncture often fail to provide CSF samples. In one study, 20 of 48 attempts were unsuccessful (Silverboard et al., 1980). Intraventricular hemorrhages continue to spread for several days, and so lumbar punctures may need to be repeated. Recent research also has questioned the reliability of lumbar punctures in diagnosing

IVH. One study found that only 8 of 15 cases of IVH were diagnosed by the initial lumbar puncture, and 3 cases were never diagnosed (Silverboard et al., 1980).

Nursing Management Nursing care focuses on identifying neurologic problems as early as possible and minimizing residual handicaps. Unfortunately, however, neurologic damage cannot be repaired. Therefore, interventions are supportive.

Because hypoxia can damage brain tissue, infants with suspected neurologic problems should be well oxygenated and placed on cardiac and apnea monitors with vital signs monitored closely. Apnea and bradycardia, which always indicate hypoxic episodes, may also be symptoms of seizure activity. Hypertension or hypotension can be signs of intracranial hemorrhage.

Adequate nutrients and calories are needed to promote brain growth. Infants with neurologic damage may require tube feedings because they frequently have weak sucking reflexes. Metabolic imbalances should be avoided because they can cause brain damage. The nurse also monitors body temperature closely because severe neurologic damage can cause temperature instability. Repeated subdural taps may be done to remove blood in cases of severe subdural hemorrhages.

Neonatal seizures are treated with medication, usually phenobarbitol. The duration of therapy depends on the causes and severity of the seizures (Horwitz and Amiel-Tison, 1979). Individual requirements vary, and so the nurse monitors blood levels to maintain a level of about 20 μg/mL. Phenobarbitol affects the infant's state organization causing more quiet sleep and less active sleep (Prechtl et al., 1973).

If the infant exhibits abnormal state organization, the nurse can use the infant's brief alert periods for interaction. Interventions are clustered during waking periods so that infants have opportunities for rest. Parents also need support so that they do not interpret the infant's abnormal state organization as personal rejection.

Other interventions are planned to minimize neurologic handicaps. Abnormalities of movement, such as paralysis, weakness, and abnormal tone, can be minimized by maintaining flexibility and movement through range-of-motion exercises and positioning. Nurses need to continue to hold infants and to provide opportunities for brief interactions, even if the infant appears lethargic and hypotonic. All infants with these problems also should be referred to occupational and physical therapists.

Complications Hydrocephalus is the major complication of intracranial hemorrhage. The bleeding interferes with the circulation of CSF, and the CSF accumulates, causing swelling of the head, increased intracranial pressure, and tissue compression. The infant's head circumference increases rapidly, and the fontanels bulge, although these symptoms may not appear immediately. In the case of IVH, the ventricles may be dilated for weeks before clinical symptoms are apparent (Volpe, 1978).

In general, the risk of hydrocephalus increases with the severity of the hemorrhage (Ahmann et al., 1980). Early diagnosis and treatment therefore minimize brain damage. One-third of the cases of hydrocephalus resolve spontaneously (Ahmann et al., 1980), and another third can be managed medically. Serial lumbar punctures are performed to drain excess CSF; diuretics may be given to decrease CSF production (Chaplin et al., 1980). In the rest of the cases, progressive hydrocephalus develops and must be managed by shunting the excess fluid away from the brain to another site (Ahmann et al., 1980; Shankaran et al., 1982) (see Chapter 42).

Permanent neurologic disability and mental retardation also may result from any neurologic problem. For example, more than half the infants with IVH or meningitis experience permanent neurologic handicaps (Babson et al., 1975; Chaplin et al., 1980; Krishnamoorthy et al., 1979). The degree to which hypoxia causes permanent damage is unclear, but data from animal studies indicate that significant hypoxia must exist for 20 minutes for permanent brain damage to occur (Nelson and Ellenberg, 1981), and the longer that infants experienced birth asphyxia, the more likely they were to develop residual disabilities (Nelson and Ellenberg, 1981). The extent to which brief hypoxic episodes cause permanent disabilities is therefore unknown, but because high-risk infants experience a large number of hypoxic episodes from birth asphyxia, respiratory problems, apnea, malnutrition, anemia, and cardiac problems, hypoxia is probably also a major cause of neurologic problems.

Considerations for Follow-up Because of the risk of permanent neurologic disabilities, all infants with neurologic problems need to be monitored for neurologic and developmental problems. Neurologic and developmental follow-up consists of complete neurologic and developmental examinations conducted every 4 months during the first year and at least yearly thereafter until about age 6.

Most high-risk infants are followed by pediatricians or nurse practitioners, but those at risk for permanent disabilities because of IVH, meningitis, hydrocephalus, seizures, or abnormalities detected on neurologic follow-up should be followed by a neurologist. Infants with significant tone or posture abnormalities also require continuing treatment from physical and occupational therapists. Many of these motor problems are transitory, but because they interfere with the infant's development of locomotion and the ability to manipulate objects, they should not be ignored.

Two common neurologic problems seen on follow-up are epilepsy and cerebral palsy (see Chapter 42). Usually, seizure disorders in infants begin during hospitalization. Many episodes of seizures resolve prior to discharge, but those infants who continue to have seizures are discharged on anticonvulsants—usually phenobarbitol although phenytoin (Dilantin) is given when the seizures are refractory. Parents should be instructed on the importance of giving medications as ordered and on the value on neurologic and developmental follow-up. Some of the infants are able to discontinue medication at later ages, whereas others require treatment throughout their lives. Infants whose seizure disorders begin after discharge should be examined by a neurologist. The symptoms of many cerebral insults, including subdural hematomas, may not become evident for several weeks after birth (Horwitz and Amiel-Tison, 1979). Occasionally, apnea may be the only symptom of neonatal seizures; thus all infants with symptoms of prolonged apnea require assessment for neurologic problems.

Cerebral palsy is any aberration in motor function due to pathology in the motor centers in the brain. It affects speech, locomotion, and the ability to manipulate objects. The three principal abnormalities are spasticity (tight muscles and stiff movements), athetosis (uncontrolled movements of body parts), and ataxia (poor coordination). Paralysis and muscle weakness also occur. Possible signs of cerebral palsy in the neonatal period include poor suck, decreased activity level, weak cry, seizures, and asymmetric movements, but these signs are unreliable. Only 1 of 14 infants with abnormal neurologic examinations at 4 months postterm develops cerebral palsy. These infants, however, do run a greater risk than infants with normal (1 in 1000) or suspect (1 in 100) examinations (Ellenberg and Nelson, 1981).

Because the motor problems of early infancy are often transitory, definitive diagnosis of cerebral palsy cannot be made until late infancy. Symptoms seen at this age include abnormal postures or reflexes, persistence of neonatal reflexes, limitations of movements, tone abnormalities, extension of head when ventrally suspended, resistance to dorsiflexion of feet, difficulty in sitting alone, adductor spasm on abduction of legs, toe-walking, hyperreflexia with sustained clonus, and hypotonia (Babson et al., 1975). Treatment consists of therapy to maximize the child's motor abilities.

The parents of infants with neurologic problems need emotional support. These infants sometimes show behavioral abnormalities such as hyperresponsivity or irritability, which make caring for them unrewarding. When an infant has experienced a serious neurologic insult, such as meningitis or intracranial hemorrhage, most parents are aware of the possibility of permanent brain damage. If health professionals also raise this possibility, parents may interpret the possibility as a certainty, even though predicting whether an individual infant will develop a permanent disability is impossible. Klaus and Kennell (1982) therefore recommend that the possibility of permanent brain damage not be raised and that nurses can instead encourage parents to express their concerns, can discuss these concerns realistically, and can explain the impossibility of making accurate predictions in the early months.

Parents need support in dealing with this uncertainty. If the infant develops normally, the parent can be reassured that there is no longer any reason to worry. When permanent disabilities occur, parents need assistance in dealing with them. The severely affected infant or child may require institutional care, and the nurse thus assists in making this decision and provides support to help deal with any guilt this decision causes.

Prevention and Detection of Developmental Delays

Developmental disabilities in young children are severe physical or mental disabilities that substantially limit the child's self-care, receptive or expressive language, learning, or locomotion (Denhoff, 1981). The term is usually limited to impairments that slow the course of development and the acquisition of skills.

High-risk infants are more likely to exhibit developmental delays than are normal full-term infants because a variety of risk factors, including prematurity, low birth weight, asphyxia, severe illness, and neurologic insult, are associated with developmental delays. Generally, the more risk factors an infant experiences, the greater the likelihood of developmental delays (Littman and Parmelee, 1978; Michelsson et al., 1981).

Accurate predictions of developmental delays are not possible in the neonatal period, essentially for four reasons. First, brain development is immature, and so reorganization of the brain can compensate for some insults. Second, the risk factors that actually cause developmental delays are unknown. Prematurity, for example, probably does not directly cause delays, but premature infants are more likely than full-term infants to experience a number of causative factors, such as hypoxia and IVH. Because the frequency with which preterm infants experience insults has decreased as medical care has improved, premature infants born in the 1970s and 1980s are less likely to be developmentally delayed than those born in the 1950s, even though a higher percentage of very small and severely ill infants survive (Caputo and Mandell, 1970; Knobloch et al., 1982; Pape et al., 1978; Stewart et al., 1977; Trotter et al., 1982).

The third difficulty in predicting developmental delays is that delays become apparent at different ages, and thus only through long-term follow-up can the actual incidence be determined. Infants born within the past 5 years are not old enough for predictions to be made about their developmental outcome. Fourth, parents and home environments have a large impact on the development of high-risk infants. Studies have shown that the nature of the family environment, rather than the number of medical risk factors, is the best predictor of developmental outcome (Barnard, 1975; Sameroff, 1975). High-risk infants are vulnerable to environmental insults, and multistressed or dysfunctional families are less able to provide physical and intellectual stimulation, adequate nutrition, and appropriate nurturing (see Chapter 22).

Assessment Because developmental delays manifest themselves at different ages, assessment is an ongoing process. (Developmental assessment is covered in Chapter 16.) Figure 31-6 outlines the ages at which different developmental problems become apparent in premature infants; a similar pattern occurs in other high-risk infants. Because most areas of development depend on biologic age, assessment data are always corrected for prematurity.

Developmental delays can occur in physical growth, reflexes, state behaviors, cognitive skills, social interaction, language, and motor skills. A developmental assessment therefore includes examination of all of these areas (see Chapter 16). Neurologic and developmental assessments are conducted together.

The nurse assesses physical growth as a part of assessments for all children at risk for delays. One high-risk infant, for example, ceased physical growth as well as social interaction and language development when her mother became depressed after separation from her father; the infant's growth resumed when the mother obtained counseling. If the nurse had limited the assessment to the infant's motor and cognitive skills, the fact that the infant was reacting to a catastrophic event that required urgent intervention might not have been discovered.

Several standard tools can be used in developmental assessments. The Brazelton Neonatal Behavior Assessment Scale, a tool that examines the interactive abilities, state organization, and neurologic competence of newborn infants, should be performed on all high-risk infants prior to hospital discharge (Brazelton, 1978) (see Chapter 7). It can also be performed on hospitalized infants when their medical conditions are stable and they have reached 36 weeks' GA, but before this age, this assessment is too long, and some of the items are of no value because all infants fail them, although assessment of reflex and orientation can be performed. Planning the assessment so that the parent can watch allows the parent the opportunity to recognize the abilities of the infant and provides the nurse with time to reinforce positive parental responses.

The Denver Developmental Screening Test (DDST) (see Appendix C and Chapter 16) is conducted as part of the regular follow-up of high-risk infants (Frankenberg et al., 1975). Because the DDST is a screening test and not diagnostic, all infants who are rated as suspect or questionable should be referred for developmental evaluation. The DDST can also be used to demonstrate the capabilities of infants for their parents.

Other assessments are also used. Tools, such as the Home Observation for Measurement of Environment (HOME) (see Chapter 17 and Appendix D), Carey Temperament Questionnaire (see Chapter 16), and Erickson's Parent–Infant Care Record (Erickson, 1976), are useful in determining sources of infant–parent difficulties. Developmental follow-up often includes infant developmental tests, such as the Bayley Mental and Motor Development Test, which can be helpful in identifying infants whose cognitive development is clearly delayed, although none of the tests is predictive of future intelligence.

Because learning disabilities and hyperactivity are more common in children who experienced perinatal problems, the nurse assessing an older child who was a high-risk infant questions the parent about school performance and discipline problems. The activity level and behavior of these children should be observed during routine follow-up visits.

Nursing Management The goals of nursing care are to prevent developmental delays whenever possible, to identify existing delays as early as possible, and to minimize disabilities.

Interventions during the initial hospitalization are first planned to prevent developmental delays. One study demonstrated that the developmental outcome of infants is related to the developmental expectations of mothers (Snyder et al., 1979). Therefore, parents need to be well informed about infant development. If repeated developmental assessments are performed in the presence of the parent, the parent then learns about the infant's specific capabilities. Even young premature infants are capable of grasping a parent's finger and of achieving eye-to-eye contact (Johnson and Grubbs, 1975).

Developmental assessments of ill or preterm infants should be brief to avoid tiring the infant. The infant's optimal performance can be best obtained if the same person (usually the primary nurse) performs the assessment, and the parent comes to view this nurse as a role model in interactions with the infant and as a source of information about the infant's development (Brazelton, 1981). Prior to discharge, the parent also can be taught to administer the MABI (Mother's Assessment of Behavior of the Infant) scales, which contain items from the Neonatal Behavioral Assessment Scale. Weekly administration of the MABI scales during the first month after discharge has been shown to increase parental awareness of infant development and to improve the rate of infant development throughout the first year (Widmayer and Field, 1981).

Infant stimulation programs are hospital-based interventions designed to prevent developmental delays; however, studies of their effectiveness have had contradictory results (Brown et al., 1980; Kramer et al., 1975; Leib et al., 1980; Scarr-Salapetek and Williams, 1973; Solkoff et al., 1969; White and Labarba, 1976). Such studies are based on the assumption that infants exhibit developmental delays because they are deprived of stimulation in the NICU (Cornell and

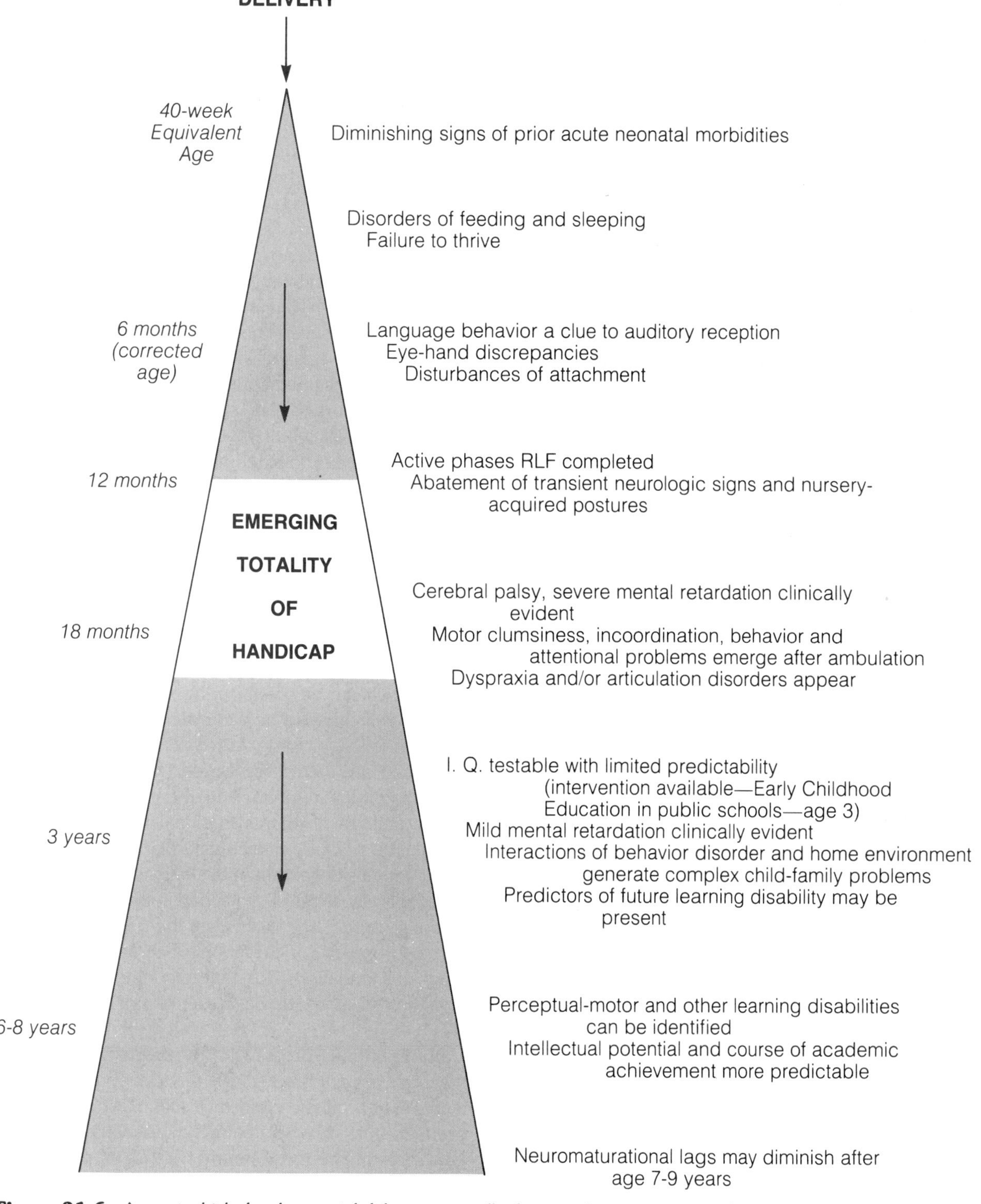

Figure 31-6 Ages at which developmental delays are usually diagnosed in premature and other high-risk infants. [Reproduced with permission from Desmond, MM, et al: The very low birth weight infant after discharge from intensive care: Anticipatory health care and developmental course. In *Current Problems in Pediatrics*. Gluck L, et al (editors). Copyright © 1980 by Year Book Medical Publishers, Inc., Chicago.]

Gottfried, 1976), and do not account for the fact that many developmental delays are due to neurologic damage that cannot be repaired. Other researchers have questioned the notion that NICUs are stimulation deficient, suggesting that high-risk infants are actually exposed to much light and sound and are handled too frequently (Lawson et al., 1977), especially since most handling involves routine nursing care or painful medical interventions rather than affectionate touching (Barnard and Blackburn, 1981).

High-risk infants do experience less kinesthetic and vestibular stimulation (movement and position change) than either normal full-term infants or fetuses, but providing extra stimulation is not a benign procedure. Too much stimulation causes healthy full-term infants to withdraw into quiet sleep (Brackbill, 1971) and can lower the oxygen levels of preterm infants (Gorski et al., 1981). Sick and preterm infants are particularly sensitive to stimulation; for example, Bench and Parker (1971) showed that premature infants were hyperresponsive to sounds. Another disadvantage is that parents are usually not included in standard infant stimulation programs.

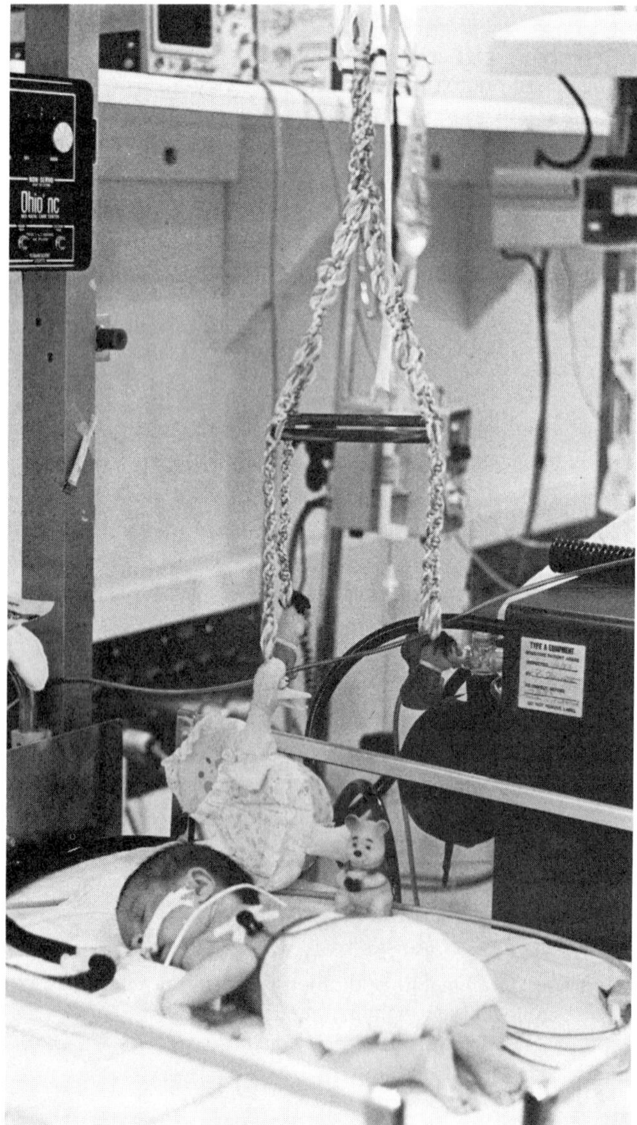

Mobiles and toys hung on a radiant warmer so that a ventilator-dependent infant can see them. (Christine Acebo, photographer.)

Any infant stimulation program therefore should not be planned merely to provide extra stimulation several times a day. Instead, routine nursing care should be modified to provide for the infant's developmental needs. All infants have a need for rest. Whenever possible, interventions should be grouped so that infants have periods of undisturbed rest. The lights in the NICU should be dimmed, and the sound level decreased several times a day to encourage sleeping. During the early stage of illness, the nurse needs to decrease the amount of stimulation that the infant experiences, as even routine nursing care, such as taking vital signs, can be stressful for a sick infant. Infants may actually recover more quickly if they are touched no more frequently than every 4 hours for the first few days of an illness and are instead assessed visually and from monitors. (Suspected deterioration, however, requires interventions that involve touching.)

As the infant's condition improves, the nurse incorporates stimulation lacking in routine NICU care into routine nursing care. Kinesthetic stimulation can be provided with water beds, by holding and rocking the infant, or by changing the elevation of the infant's head. Affectionate touches and strokes can be given during routine care, and eye-to-eye contact can also be achieved for brief periods. Interesting mobiles, pictures, or toys can be placed where the infant can see them. Responses to infant behaviors, such as picking infants up when they cry, aid the development of the abilities of infants to signal needs, although such stimulation must be individually planned and appropriate to the infant's developmental status.

Parents also are easily included in this type of infant stimulation program and often help the nurse choose stimulation appropriate for the infant (Schraeder, 1980). Some types of stimulation—for example, holding the infant during feedings—may be best reserved for the parents.

Complications Most high-risk infants develop normally, but they have a greater risk of developmental problems than children without perinatal insults. Developmental delays occur despite optimal treatment, but some problems can be avoided. The most common cause of problems is the failure to diagnose a developmental delay and to refer the child to appropriate specialists. Occasionally, pediatricians or nurse practitioners fail to identify a developmental delay because of desire for a positive outcome. Some practitioners also avoid referral in attempts to manage problems on their own. Multidisciplinary intervention can improve the developmental status of most children; primary care physicians and nurses seldom have the expertise to plan exercises and games that foster development and coordination of specific muscle groups but should continue to follow these children and provide support for parents.

Overstimulation, a major complication of infant stimulation programs, may be avoided by reducing extraneous stimulation. For instance, one mother of an easily overstimulated premature infant was able to achieve much eye-to-eye contact by placing the infant in an infant seat. Apparently, eye contact while being held was too intense a form of stimulation for this infant (Davis, 1980). Infants attempt to reduce stimulation by gaze aversion or by going into quiet sleep. If excess stimulation continues, oxygen level falls and the infant may react physiologically by vomiting (Gorski et al., 1981).

Considerations for Follow-up All high-risk infants need developmental follow-up. Most can be followed by their nurse practitioners or pediatricians. Infants with neurologic insults, extreme prematurity (less than 30 weeks' GA), or developmental delays need follow-up by a multidisciplinary developmental clinic. Because parental expectations are important to the ultimate outcome of infants, routine follow-up visits provide an opportunity for nurses to instruct parents about both normal infant development and the capabilities of their infants.

Infants with developmental delays also need referral to early intervention programs, which are multidisciplinary and involve physicians, nurses, psychologists, social workers, educators, and physical and occupational therapists. These professionals work with parents to provide educational experiences and physical therapies appropriate to the infant's developmental status, along with emotional support and developmental guidance for the parents. Interventions to assist parents are important because most of the therapy for these children is provided by the parents.

Parents should not have unrealistic expectations for intervention programs. Exaggerated expectations may lead to parental depression when a child fails to be cured of the developmental delay. Children can be helped to maximize their potential and avoid complications, but early intervention programs cannot repair neurologic damage (Ferry, 1981).

Alterations in Parenting

Because the birth of a high-risk infant is a crisis for a family (Caplan, 1960), the degree of parental distress may bear no relation to the severity of the infant's illness (Benfield et al., 1976). Emotional distress does, however, interfere with a parent's ability to nurture an infant.

Other psychological factors also interfere with parenting. The early adjustment to parenting begins during pregnancy when the mother first incorporates the fetus into her body image and then prepares to accept the infant as a separate individual. Women with high-risk pregnancies are often so concerned with maintaining the pregnancy that they are unable to deal with the infant as a separate individual (Floyd, 1981). Pregnant women use fantasy to cope with their concerns. In the third trimester, these fantasies are often associated with negative emotions and subjects, such as being attacked or unprepared or experiencing dangerous intrusions from the world (Rubin, 1967; Sherwen, 1981). The birth of a high-risk infant can confirm the worst of these fantasies. In addition, when the infant is premature, the parents do not have enough time to complete the tasks of pregnancy and to prepare for the infant.

After birth, parents must relinquish their fantasies about the infant and become acquainted with the characteristics of the actual infant. This process is easier when the expected infant and the actual one are similar. Parents often expect an infant that looks and acts like a 3-month-old, so that the appearance and behavior of a normal neonate may be disappointing. High-risk infants who are even less similar to the expected child are even more disappointing (Mercer, 1981). Premature infants, with their large heads, skinny bodies, and lack of muscle tone, are particularly different from the expected infant; even at term age they do not look like full-term infants.

The guilt that a parent feels after the birth of a high-risk infant interferes with the ability to form a relationship with that infant. Parents worry that they or their partners were responsible for the problems of their infants. All parents experience some degree of ambivalence about a pregnancy. This ambivalence may be particularly pronounced when a high-risk pregnancy restricts a woman's activities, requires many expensive medical interventions, and disrupts family life. Other factors that increase ambivalence include an unplanned pregnancy, financial or emotional problems, and negative feelings about the pregnancy from other family members or friends. When the infant is born with a problem, parents may believe that their negative feelings contributed to the problem. Finally, because the actions of parents can cause problems for the infant, parents may worry that their actions were responsible for the high-risk birth. Fathers may worry about their exposure to hazardous chemicals, and mothers may feel guilty about drinking or smoking during the pregnancy. These feelings, whether rational or irrational, need to be resolved in order to develop an appropriate relationship with the infant.

The NICU is a poor environment in which to build such a relationship. Nurses and physicians provide inadequate role models for parenting because their actions are often based on immediate medical, rather than long-term psychologic, needs. For example, an infant should be held so that the infant is cuddled close to the body and the adult is looking directly at the infant's face, but NICU nurses generally hold infants on their knees so that they can clearly see the entire infant (Klaus and Kennell, 1982). Occasionally, physicians and nurses can become so involved with a particular infant that they actually compete with the parents (Kachoris, 1977).

In addition, parents usually have limited contact with their infants while they are in the NICU. The long distances between the NICU and home, family and work responsibilities, and the reluctance of parents to see a sick infant all contribute to this problem. Some researchers have speculated that this separation is a major cause of interactional problems between high-risk infants and their parents (Klaus and Kennell, 1982) since other studies indicate that extra contact between normal full-term infants and their mothers facilitates bonding (De Chateau and Wiberg, 1977; Kennell et al., 1974).

Because of illness or prematurity, however, high-risk infants are not as responsive as normal full-term infants and thus are unable to participate in reciprocal interactions during the early part of their hospitalizations. One study of high-risk infants indicated that interactional difficulties are due to problems with the infants' abilities rather than the amount of separation (Field, 1977). Seeing the infant early in the hospitalization also draws parental attention to the infant's problems and may actually increase anxiety in some cases (Ross, 1980). Therefore, contact between parent and infant should be encouraged but never forced. Even when parents have spent a great deal of time with their infants, interactional difficulties may occur.

Assessment Because parenting is a process, the relationship between a parent and an infant continues to grow and change. Repeated assessments therefore are necessary to determine both the degree of parental involvement with the infant and the infant's interactional abilities.

Because psychological disturbances can interfere with parental abilities to relate to the infant, parents should be encouraged to discuss their feelings. Potential parenting problems are indicated by the inability to express guilt or responsibility, apparent lack of anxiety about the infant's condition, lack of interest in information about the infant, consistent misinterpretation or exaggeration of information, failure to communicate with spouse or partner, and inability to accept or use help (DuBois, 1975).

Discussions enable the nurse to determine how well the parents are dealing with the following four psychological tasks: (a) preparing for the possible death of the infant, (b) dealing with the failure to produce a healthy infant, (c) establishing a relationship with the infant, and (d) understanding the special needs of the infant (Kaplan and Mason, 1960). Parents who are still preparing for the possible loss of the infant are not ready to begin a nurturing relationship. The parents' abilities to accomplish these psychological tasks depends on their own developmental stage. Adolescent, young adult, and middle-aged parents approach these tasks differently. Supportive family and friends aid in this process while lack of support interferes with the process.

Family members and friends involved in the care of the infant also need an opportunity to discuss their feelings, as they too experience emotional difficulties in dealing with a high-risk infant. The nurse thus assesses the degree of involvement, level of tension, and interest in learning infant care exhibited by parents and other caregivers. Parents should visit or phone frequently; failure to do so is a sign of potential problems. One study showed that parents who visited less frequently than 3 times in 2 weeks were more likely to develop parenting problems (Fanaroff et al., 1972).

The behavior of parents with their infants should be observed. Touching during the early acquaintance period follows a normal progression: first touching the extremities with the finger tips, then stroking the infant's trunk with the palms, and then finally encircling the infant with the entire arm and holding the infant (Klaus et al., 1970). Mothers of normal full-term infants complete this progression in a few minutes; parents of high-risk infants take much longer (as much as several weeks), but no matter how hesitant parents are to touch their infants at first, they should gradually progress through the various phases of touching and begin to assume some aspects of care.

Because the infant's ability to respond to the parent influences interactions, infant interaction is also assessed. Items from the Newborn Behavioral Assessment Scale (Brazelton, 1973) can be performed for the parent. If the infant exhibits interactional difficulties, the parent can be reassured that the parent is not responsible for the infant's lack of responsivity. The parent should be encouraged to find ways of eliciting at least brief responses from the infant. The infant's low tolerance for stimulation limits the number and type of stimulation to which a response is possible. The infant may respond more to the parent's face than to a noisy toy.

Nursing Management The general goals to promote parenting remain constant: providing support for parents in resolving their feelings of disappointment, anger, guilt, and responsibility and in progressing through their developmental and psychologic tasks of parenting, helping them to view their infant as an individual with unique characteristics, and promoting positive interactions between parents and infants (Fig. 31-7).

Interventions to promote healthy parenting begin at birth. If desired, the father should be present in the delivery room. In any case, both parents should have an opportunity to see and touch the infant before transfer to the nursery, and they should be allowed to hold the infant if the infant's condition permits. When the mother has received a general anesthetic and is unable to see the infant immediately after delivery, she should be allowed to see and touch the infant as soon as possible.

Moderately ill infants can sometimes remain with their mothers and be cared for by the recovery room nurse. For example, the blood glucose level and vital signs of a full-term infant of a well-controlled diabetic mother can be monitored by the recovery room nurse, thus reassuring the mother and facilitating bonding. More seriously ill infants

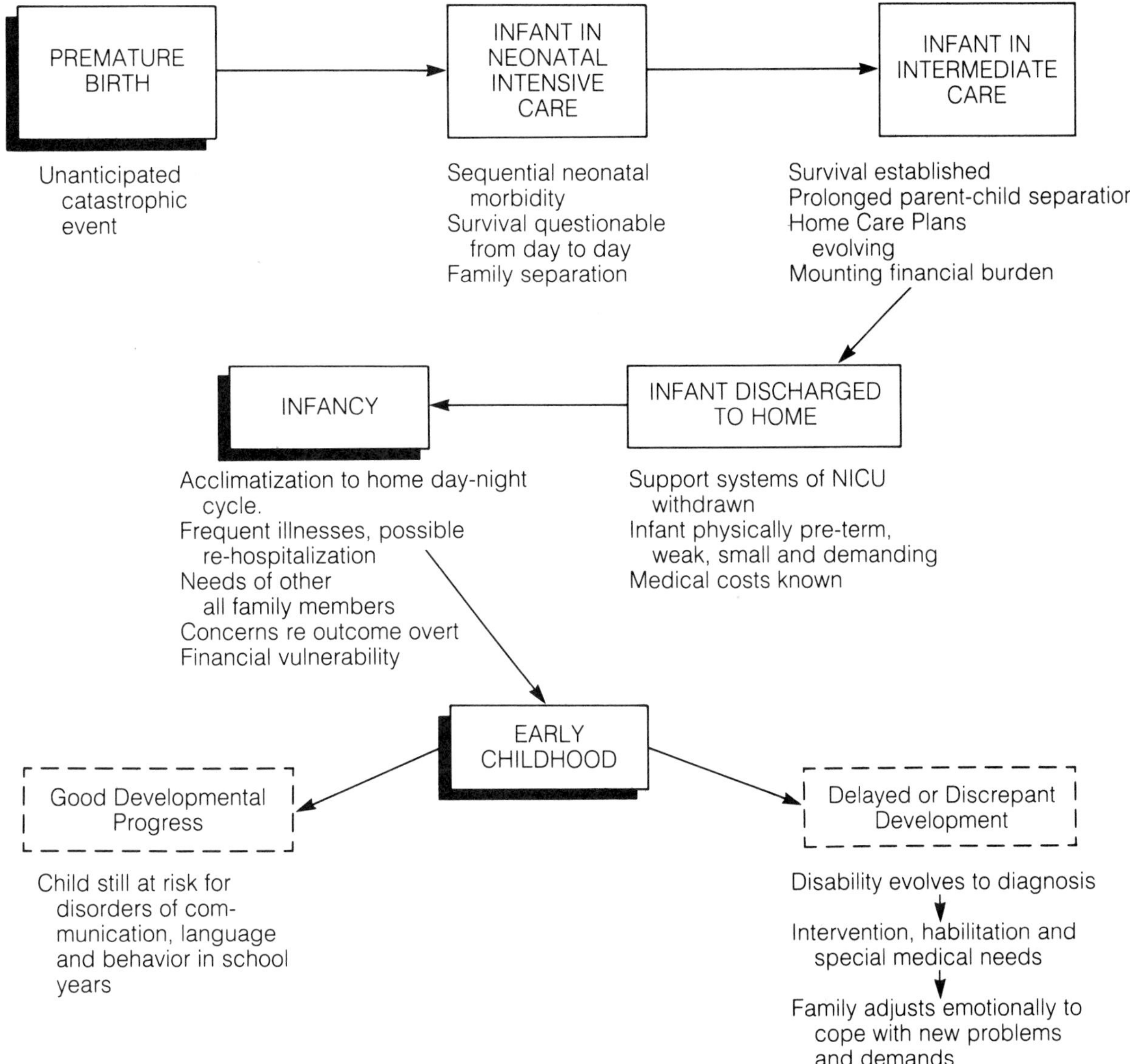

Figure 31-7 The sequential developmental course of premature infants and the adjustments required of parents. [Reproduced with permission from Desmond, MM, et al: The very low birth weight infant after discharge from intensive care: Anticipatory health care and developmental course. In *Current Problems in Pediatrics.* Gluck L, et al (editors). Copyright © 1980 by Year Book Medical Publishers, Inc., Chicago.]

need to be transferred to the nursery, but their parents can still participate in their care. One father bottle-fed his hypoglycemic baby shortly after birth. Later, he was able to reassure his wife that the infant ate well and was not as sick as she had thought.

Some critically ill infants must be transferred to NICUs located in other hospitals. A transport team consisting of a physician and one or more nurses then accompanies the infant, and as this team is usually from the referral hospital, team members can inform the parents about the unit's policies, and consent forms can be signed. Both parents should be allowed to see and touch the infant prior to departure. When the father accompanies the infant, he should be given an opportunity to see the infant as soon as the admission procedures are complete. In addition, the admitting nurse should phone the mother to give her a progress report. A photograph of the infant can be sent to the mother (Guy, 1978). Because infant transport involves medical risks to the infant and separation from the mother, many perinatal centers are accepting transports of high-risk mothers prior to delivery. Maternal transports involve less risk, and the infant gets optimal care from birth (Giles et al., 1977).

A variety of interventions are used in the NICU to promote healthy parenting. Supportive counseling assists parents in resolving the crisis. Ideally, this support should be provided by the infant's nurse, as parents find it easier to deal with only a small number of people (Bell, 1976). The nurse develops a plan for parental support and teaching (Bresadola, 1977), which includes teaching parents about the infant's capabilities, demonstrating these abilities for parents, and serving as a role model for interactions. The nurse can also promote self-esteem in the parents by emphasizing their essential role in the infant's recovery.

The nurse provides parents with frequent reports about the infant. Even if frequent visits are impossible, parents can begin to relate to their infant if given information about individual activities and developmental accomplishments, such as, "She sleeps best on her right side" or "He looked at your picture today." Letters from the infant can be sent to the parent outlining the infant's condition and desire to see the parent (Eager, 1977; Fuller and Petering, 1979). Incubators can be decorated for special occasions; for example, one group of parents was delighted to find Valentine's Day cards, addressed to them from their infants, on the incubators.

The nurse also encourages parents to obtain and use other sources of support, such as family and friends, remembering however that family members and friends occasionally might work against the best interests of parents and infants. For example, one maternal grandmother, who had only seen pictures of the infant, fostered unrealistic expectations in the mother and thus increased parental concern (Zimmerman et al., 1978).

Referral for counseling may involve psychologists and psychiatrists who work with parents who have unresolved emotional problems. Social workers assist families with financial difficulties, housing problems, and family problems. Clergy provide assistance with spiritual problems, which is particularly important, as some parents view the birth of a high-risk infant as a punishment from God.

Peer counseling can also help parents in resolving their emotional disturbances. Parents of high-risk infants experience similar anxieties and stresses and thus can provide support for each other. Two different frameworks are used to provide this parent-to-parent support. In some programs, experienced parents whose infants have been discharged from the NICU talk with individual couples whose infants are currently in the NICU. After discharge, the experienced parents continue to provide information about community resources and hints for home care (Eager and Exoo, 1980; Mangurten et al., 1979). Other hospitals conduct group meetings for all parents whose infants are currently in the NICU. These meetings allow the parents to interact and to express their concerns. In addition, the staff can present basic information about the NICU and the needs of high-risk infants (Houser, 1980; Elsas, 1981; Erdman, 1977). These parents often continue to interact when they meet while visiting their infants.

The nurse also encourages parental involvement in infant care and provides individually planned care for infants and parents as well as goals that can be accomplished together. Schraeder (1980) outlines three stages of parenting behaviors: (a) initial touching and acquaintance, (b) caregiving, and (c) incorporating the infant into the family. Nurses thus assist parents in moving through these stages by demonstrating nurturing behaviors and by encouraging parents to perform activities appropriate to their stage of parenting.

In the acquaintance stage, nurses encourage parents to visit and phone frequently. Most NICUs allow 24-hour visiting for parents, and studies have shown that parents value this opportunity. Parents believe that the infants feel loved when visited (Yu et al., 1981), and even those parents whose anxiety is increased by visiting do not want it restricted (Harper et al., 1976). Other caregivers also need opportunities to visit; grandparents and siblings, for instance, should see the infant even if only through a viewing window. When the mother is in another hospital, the nurse maintains frequent phone contact and provides photographs or videotapes of the infant.

In the second stage of parenting behavior, parents begin to assume caregiving responsibilities. As the infant's condition permits, they should be encouraged to hold, feed, and change the infant. The nurse also includes parents in decisions about infant care, such as when to feed or bathe the infant. Parents can help the nurse in planning an appropriate infant stimulation program (Schraeder, 1980) and can provide clothes, toys, and photographs of the family to decorate the incubator or warmer. Siblings often feel more involved with the infant when they provide drawings for the baby.

This parental involvement can actually alter attitudes. One study conducted in an NICU in Italy found that although no father of a healthy full-term infant participated in infant care, one-third of the fathers of NICU patients continued to be involved in care after discharge (Paludetto et al., 1981).

In the final stage, as parents incorporate the infant into the family, they need to assume control over infant care in preparation for discharge and to learn to perform any necessary medical procedures. The nurse plans individual care for the infant, parent, and other caregivers during all three stages.

The period just prior to hospital discharge requires special interventions because the parents are losing the familiar supports of the NICU. Approximately half of the infants are transferred back to the referring hospital prior to discharge, which allows them to complete recovery and to grow in an intermediate care setting, which is closer to their parents' homes. The nurse therefore contacts the other hospital to familiarize the nurses there with the infant's nursing care plan, the degree of parental involvement, and the ongoing teaching plan (Abbey et al., 1977). The parent is informed about the policies of the new nursery, such as the visiting hours for family and friends and whether rooming-in is possible. After transfer, the nurse can ease the transition by remaining available for phone consultations with the new nursery and the parent.

Discharge is an even more important step, for suddenly the parent is faced with providing all of the infant's care. Additional interventions thus assist the parent in making the transition from the NICU or community hospital to home. The parent needs competence in performing routine infant care and any special medical treatments that the infant requires. To identify parental concerns about discharge and to plan additional teaching, a predischarge conference is held with the parent, any other caregivers, the nurse, the neonatologist, and other interested staff members (Waddell and Fresholtz, 1978). The parent often benefits from rooming-in with the infant for a day or two prior to discharge so that help from experienced professionals is available as the parent begins to provide total infant care (Klaus and Kennell, 1982; Varner et al., 1980).

Families are referred to public health nurses so that they can continue to receive support. In addition, the nurse phones the parent within a few days after discharge to learn how the infant is doing. All parents experience a dramatic change in their lives after an infant comes home, but high-risk infants are particularly disruptive. If the infant has been hospitalized for several weeks, the parent has adjusted to life without an infant. The mother has often returned to work to help pay medical bills and with the infant's arrival home must adjust to being a full-time mother.

High-risk infants often are unresponsive or irritable in the early weeks; thus they do not provide many rewards for their parents. As a result, parents may experience mild depression. If parents do not have nursing support available, they may exhibit strange behaviors in an effort to obtain it. One mother of a premature infant refused all help, but in a few days after her infant's discharge, she called the NICU and stated that she felt like abusing the infant. Investigation showed that the mother was very good with the infant and that they had many positive interactions. A public health nurse then spent long hours talking with the mother. Although the mother continued to insist that she did not need help, she no longer worried about hurting the infant.

Additional interventions are needed for multiple births. The parents must be helped to view the infants as individuals so that they can develop special feelings for each one (Gromada, 1981; Klaus and Kennell, 1982). Specific parental behaviors, such as giving the infants rhyming names or calling them "the twins," may be signs that parents are having difficulty in seeing the infants as individuals (Sater, 1979). Sometimes, one infant is more seriously ill than the other(s), and parents then may experience difficulty in developing a relationship with one infant while worrying about the survival of another. If the parent takes one infant home while another remains in the hospital, a stronger attachment to the infant at home might develop (Gromada, 1981). Therefore, Klaus and Kennell (1982) recommend that all infants in a multiple birth be discharged at the same time. Unfortunately, this is not always possible; for example, one infant of twins may require several months of hospitalization while the other one is well. The greatest problem arises, however, when one infant dies and another lives. The parent must grieve for the loss of one infant while trying to form a relationship with another infant. Because these two activities are usually mutually exclusive, the parent needs a great deal of support (Klaus and Kennell, 1982).

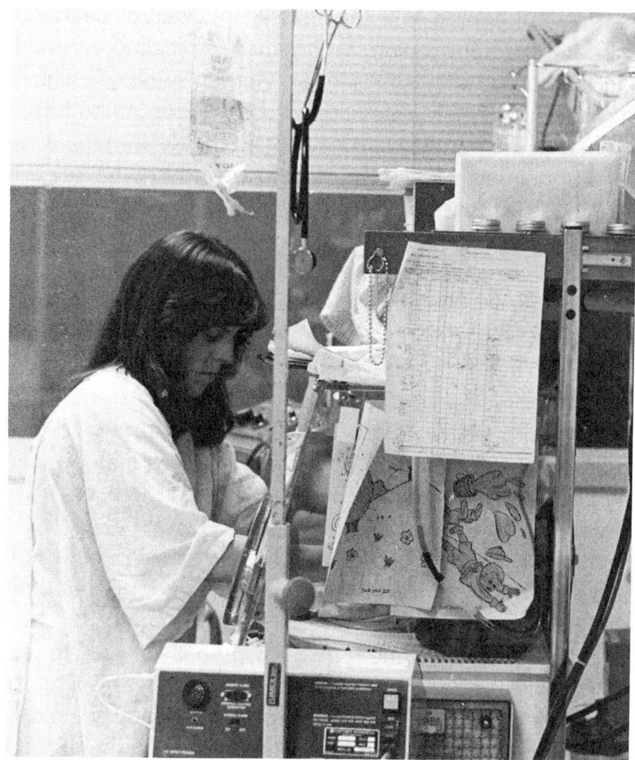

Drawings from siblings have been placed on the incubator of a high-risk infant. (Christine Acebo, photographer.)

Complications The development of a healthy relationship between parents and high-risk infants may be complicated by several factors. Occasionally, nurses become attached to infants and compete with the parents for the infant's affection (Kachoris, 1977). For example, one nurse gave a name to an infant when his parents were slow to select one. When the parents eventually did name their son, it was a different name from the one the nurse had selected. She refused to call the infant anything but her name and generally avoided the parents. Needless to say, this type of competition prevents nurses from working effectively with families. Nurses develop these attachments as a way of coping with the stresses involved in neonatal intensive care and obtain gratification by feeling parental affection for the infants. (A primary nursing system, in which the nurse immediately develops a commitment to both the infant and the parents, can help avoid the development of this competition, while still providing rewards for the nurse.)

Family disruption is another complication in the early progress of parenting high-risk infants. Parents are more likely to relinquish high-risk infants to foster care or adoption than they are healthy full-term infants (Klaus and Kennell, 1982). In addition, the stresses involved with having a high-risk infant can lead to other dysfunctional behaviors. Siblings may develop behavioral problems or parents may fail to communicate with each other except through arguments. Not surprisingly, the divorce and separation rate is higher for parents of high-risk infants than for parents of healthy infants (Klaus and Kennell, 1982; Leifer et al., 1972). The infant may also become a source of tension between parents and other family members. One grandmother repeatedly commanded her adolescent daughter to care for the infant in the same tone of voice that she used to tell this daughter to clean up the room. The daughter responded by stalling and minimizing contact with the infant. (Families at risk for dysfunctional or health-threatening parenting are further discussed in Chapter 22.)

Most studies indicate that high-risk infants are more likely to be victims of child abuse and neglect than are healthy full-term infants (Corey et al., 1975; Hunter et al., 1978; Jeffcoate et al., 1979a; Klein and Stern, 1971). Child abuse occurs more often when the potential for abuse is present, such as a special child and a crisis situation (McKeel, 1978).

Consideration for Follow-up Nursing follow-up should continue after discharge. Parenting problems may not become evident until the parents have cared for the infant. Depending on the desires and needs of the parents, this follow-up can be provided from a variety of sources. The nurses at the hospital can maintain phone contact with the parents, or other support may be available from child health nurses and those at developmental follow-up clinics. Public health nurses are usually the major source of support and should visit at least twice in the first 2 weeks after discharge and then three additional times during the first year (Noga, 1982).

These visits should include assessments of the home environment, the family's interactional status, the infant's medical and developmental condition, and the relationship between the infant and parents. In addition, the nurse discusses the infant's activities, the parents' feelings about the infant, their concerns, and their follow-up plans (Noga, 1982). (Family assessment is discussed in Chapter 17.) These discussions provide an opportunity for parents to obtain answers to their questions and for nurses to conduct parent teaching (see Chapter 21).

Assessments of the degree to which the infant has been incorporated into the family system and the amount of parental involvement with the infant should be included in all follow-up contacts with the family. Sometimes, parents fail to develop feelings of affection for the infant, but more often they have these feelings but are unable to translate them into appropriate parenting behaviors. Studies have shown that high-risk infants and their parents appear to have less successful interactions and to enjoy each other less than do normal full-term infants and their parents (Bakeman and Brown, 1980; Field, 1977, 1979a; Leifer et al., 1972). Many of these interactional problems probably are due to the infant's limited energy available for interaction. Nurses assessing these interactions should not expect them to be the same as those of normal full-term infants and their parents. For instance, parents of high-risk infants may need to engage in shorter interactions and to be more sensitive to infant cues.

Whenever a high-risk infant is rehospitalized, the parents need emotional support, as they often relive the emotional disturbances that they experienced during the first hospitalization. For example, one mother of a premature infant could not understand why she was so upset when her infant was hospitalized at 6 months of age for a relatively minor infection. She stated that she felt more upset than she had during the initial hospitalization. Child health nurses need to discuss this resurgence of painful memories with parents whenever a high-risk infant is rehospitalized.

Parental Knowledge Deficit

Parents of high-risk infants have a special need for education about infant care. Parents usually make their preparations for the infant in the last trimester of pregnancy. At this point, they read child care books and talk with friends and relatives to learn about feeding methods, routine care, and infant development. During a high-risk pregnancy, however, parents may be afraid to become too involved with the infant, and parents of premature infants have not had this preparation period. Even if the parents did prepare for the infant during pregnancy, their anxiety over the infant's condition may cause them to forget much of what they had learned. In addition, high-risk infants often require medical treatment after discharge, and parents of high-risk infants therefore need education about the infant's special needs along with the information about infant care and normal growth and development.

Information about development is especially important for the parents of premature infants. Unless they are taught about the importance of age correction, for example, they expect the infant to develop at the same rate as a full-term infant born at the same time. Thus they may come to believe the infant is delayed when the infant is instead developing as expected for the corrected age.

Assessment The nurse assesses the parents' level of knowledge about infant care, infant development, and the special needs of their own infant. The parents' and other caregivers' abilities to understand explanations and their readiness to learn also are determined. Information about development is of little value if given to the mother, for instance, when the grandmother will be caring for the baby.

Nursing Management The goals of nursing care are to determine the level of knowledge about infant care of all potential caregivers and to provide any additional information they need to be effective. Anticipatory guidance that includes information about infant needs generally is part of child health nursing (see Chapter 21), but parents of high-risk infants often need special assistance. Parents are unable to make preparations for the infant's care until they believe the baby will survive, and so the nurse plans parent teaching after the critical stage of illness has passed.

Specific topics that may need to be covered include infant development up to 3 months of age, feeding methods, bathing, diapering, identifying childhood illnesses, giving medications, taking temperatures, and performing any special medical treatments. The nurse also discusses the importance of affection and appropriate stimulation to an infant. Many parents appreciate being referred to appropriate child care books.

Information about caregiving techniques and medical treatments is explained and then demonstrated by the nurse. Parents then need opportunities to practice these skills so that prior to discharge they are performing much of the infant's care. Spending a day or two rooming-in with the infant gives the parents a final opportunity to consult with nurses and experience success in providing care to foster their confidence as parents.

The rooming-in period is the ideal point to assess parental skills and evaluate the success of parent teaching. If the parents choose not to room in or if rooming-in is not available for them, this evaluation can be part of routine health care visits. The nurse may need to encourage parents to discuss any questions they have about infant care so that if parents continue to exhibit knowledge deficits, the nurse can use different teaching strategies.

Additional information should be provided as part of nursing follow-up after discharge. Public health nurses and nurses in developmental follow-up clinics need to plan ongoing teaching to inform parents about developmental changes, types of stimulation that infants need at different ages, changes in medical treatments, and care of older infants and children.

Neonatal Death

Despite recent improvement in perinatal care, infant mortality remains a major problem. All nurses working with high-risk infants will thus at some time need to help parents accept the death of a newborn. Parents who have lost an infant experience the same stages of grief as anyone experiencing a major loss (Bliss, 1976; Elliot, 1978; Elliot and Hein, 1978). (The death of a child and the process of grieving are further discussed in Chapter 32.) Some factors, however, are unique to a neonatal death. Parental guilt may be prolonged when the parent feels or is partially responsible for the death (for example, a diabetic mother who did not control her blood sugar level). Parents who lose a newborn must grieve for their fantasy baby as well as the real one; mothers also mourn the loss of their pregnancies (Lewis, 1979).

The death of an infant affects other family members as well. Grandparents grieve not only because of the loss of a grandchild but also because of the pain experienced by their children. Siblings are affected. They may feel isolated from parental communications (Hardgrove and Warrick, 1974), yet parents are often too involved with their own grief to help their children. Young children may feel that their jealousy and fantasies about harming the baby are responsible for the death (Hardgrove and Warrick, 1974; Zelauskas, 1981). Older children fear that they too will die (Oehler, 1981), and their feelings may result in behavior problems.

Unfortunately, few community supports are available for the grieving family. Generally, a newborn infant who dies is not recognized as a person. Thus mothers and fathers of first-born infants who die lose their status as parents (Borg and Lasker, 1981). Parents are often comforted with such statements as, "It's for the best," "The baby would have been brain-damaged," or "You can always have another baby," which deny the reality of the parents' grief. Funerals are often not held for infants, especially those who were premature. Therefore, helping the parents to work through their grief is an important nursing role, especially as the degree to which they resolve their grief will influence their relationships with their other children and each other.

Assessment Two aspects of the assessment of families experiencing neonatal death are, first, determining each person's stage of grieving and, second, identifying family and community supports. The nurse also assesses the quality of the relationships among family members to determine whether communication and support is adequate. The need for outside support depends on the nursing diagnosis and associated risk factors. If grieving is dysfunctional or family coping is ineffective or potentially disabling, nursing care should include referrals to provide adequate support. Isolated families or adolescent parents require extra support (see Chapter 22).

Nursing Management The goal of nursing care is to help parents and other family members work through their grief and eventually accept the infant's death. For most people this process takes about 6 months, although they will continue to have periods of depression and sadness when reminded of the infant's death.

Most families do resolve their grief, but nursing interventions can make this process easier. Interventions should begin prior to death and are planned first to individualize the infant for the parent, which helps to resolve the grief for the expected infant. Memories of touching, holding, and caring for the infant comfort the parent because the parent knows that the infant felt loved. Photographs provide tangible reminders that the infant lived.

When death becomes inevitable, parents need to participate in decisions about infant care. One study showed that when parents participated in the decision to withdraw respiratory support, they did not experience increased guilt or pathologic grieving (Benfield et al., 1978). When parents desire, baptisms can be performed by the clergy or, in the case of sudden deterioration, by the infant's nurse. Parental preferences in this area should therefore be discussed early in the hospital stay. Parents should have the opportunity to be with their infant at the time of death and to hold the infant if desired (Wooten, 1981). Other family members, such as grandparents, should also be present if this is what the parents want.

In the early period after death, interventions focus on helping the parents to accept the reality of the death. They and other family members should be allowed to spend time with the infant's body in private, to take pictures of the body, and to bathe the body (Wooten, 1981). If parents choose not to see the body or if the mother is still hospitalized, photographs of the infant's body should be placed in the records so that the parents can see them later if they desire (Borg and Lasker, 1981). The nurse encourages parents to express their feelings to their partners and other family members and should also feel free to display their own grief to the families. Funeral arrangements should be discussed, and parents encouraged to have a funeral; this may be an appropriate time for the nurse to contact clergy for the parents.

Complications Family members who do not eventually accept the infant's death develop dysfunctional grief reactions, which are distortions of normal grieving or delayed grief reactions (Lindemann, 1944). Symptoms include inappropriate cheerfulness or anger, severe or prolonged depression, or psychosomatic illness (Elliot and Hein, 1978). People who have exhibited poor emotional adjustment prior to the death are more prone to this problem.

The need to become attached to another infant interferes with normal grief work. Thus parents with a surviving twin or an immediate pregnancy are at higher risk of developing a prolonged grief reaction (Rowe et al., 1978). To prevent this problem, parents should be advised to delay a subsequent pregnancy for at least 6 months after the death. The desire for an immediate pregnancy to replace the infant is often a sign that grief has not been resolved (Poznanski, 1972).

Dysfunctional grieving can lead to family disruptions. Parents who lose a child are more likely to separate or divorce than are parents without a loss. Older children may develop behavior problems, including discipline problems, sleep disturbances, and school failure as a result of dysfunctional grieving. Any family member with pathologic grief reactions requires professional counseling.

Considerations for Follow-up Follow-up is needed after a neonatal death. Although this contact can be maintained by phone, research indicates that mothers who had in-person follow-up were more satisfied with the information they received (Rowe et al., 1978). An initial follow-up interview should be scheduled in the first month after the death to discuss parental concerns and answer questions (Elliot and Hein, 1978). The nurse asks parents about how they and other family members are handling their grief and encourages open expression of emotion and communication between family members. Books about death often provide an opening for this discussion (Berg et al., 1980; Oehler, 1981). Parents also need to know about the stages of grieving and the feelings of anger, guilt, and depression that they will experience.

Subsequent interviews should be scheduled at approximately monthly intervals. These allow parents to express their feelings and help the nurse monitor the grieving process in order to intervene as necessary. Parents may find participation in a group with other parents who have lost infants to be particularly helpful at this point (Cordell and Apolito, 1981). If parents are concerned that their children are having difficulty in dealing with grief, the children can be referred for counseling or play therapy (Zelauskas, 1981). Once the family has accepted the death, the regular interviews can be discontinued.

Nurses cannot expect families to "get over" their grief readily within 6 months. Bouts of depression are common in situations that strongly remind parents of the infant or on anniversaries of the birth or death. Subsequent pregnancies and illnesses of the other children may cause parents to relive some of the emotion they felt on losing the infant. Nurses need to be sensitive to these feelings and begin a discussion of grief if parents are reluctant to do so.

Key Concepts

- The development of neonatal intensive care has improved the prognosis for high-risk infants and has created a nursing and medical field of specialization.
- NICUs are often regionally based, providing optimal care but causing difficulties for families located far from a regional center.
- Both an infant's social development and the process by which the infant is incorporated into the family system are greatly altered by serious illness and the environment of the NICU.
- Risk factors associated with the birth of a high-risk infant are both biologic and psychosocial.
- High-risk infants are classified on the basis of gestational age at birth and body size.
- Developmental assessment for high-risk infants requires correction for prematurity when comparing the assessment data to norms for growth and development.
- Neuromuscular development—including muscle tone, reflexes, and sleep–wake states—is affected by neurologic damage and prematurity.
- Immaturity of the subsystems of biophysical development creates specific special problems for premature infants.
- Inadequate heat regulation in high-risk infants may lead to cold stress, which requires nursing interventions to control environmental temperature and prevent complications.
- Immaturity of the immunologic systems in high-risk infants leaves the infants susceptible to infection and thus requires interventions planned to prevent exposure to bacteria.
- Respiratory assessment for high-risk infants involves monitoring vital signs, observing physical symptoms, and taking blood gases.
- Nursing management for respiratory dysfunction in high-risk infants involves supportive interventions to maintain adequate oxygenation and prevent complications.
- Specific respiratory problems in high-risk infants include respiratory distress syndrome, mechanical obstruction, meconium aspiration, pneumonia, apnea, bronchopulmonary dysplasia, and Wilson-Mikity syndrome.
- Nutritional deficiencies in high-risk infants may be caused by impaired ability to suck, increased calorie requirements due to serious illness, diminished stomach capacity, or impaired digestion.
- Lack of adequate growth is the principal indicator of nutritional deficiency.
- Feedings for high-risk infants may be supplied with breast milk, which is preferable, or formula; feedings may be given orally or through gavage, continuous tube feedings, or parenteral fluids.
- Maintaining metabolic homeostasis requires early detection and correction of metabolic imbalances.
- Infants of diabetic mothers require assessment for hypoglycemia in the early postnatal period.
- Immaturity of an infant's circulatory system may lead to a patent ductus arteriosus, congestive heart failure, or fluid overload.
- Physical signs, laboratory tests, and electrolyte and glucose levels are used to assess circulatory status.
- Nursing management for circulatory problems is planned to maintain oxygenation, reduce the workload of the heart, and prevent fluid overload and complications.
- Neonatal hyperbilirubinemia is caused by the immature neonatal liver and hemolytic disease and, if untreated, may lead to kernicterus.
- Assessment for hyperbilirubinemia includes physical signs (especially jaundice) and laboratory tests.
- Nursing management for neonatal hyperbilirubinemia includes early detection and prevention of complications, especially kernicterus and Rh-hemolytic disease.
- Neurologic damage in the neonatal period is usually caused by hypoxia, birth trauma, hemorrhage, or infection.
- Assessment for neurologic dysfunction includes physical symptoms, behavioral changes, and laboratory tests.
- Nursing management for neurologic problems focuses on minimizing disabilities, which may

include alterations in muscle tone, weakness or paralysis of an extremity, abnormal sleep–wake state patterns, and seizure activity.

- High-risk infants are more likely to exhibit developmental delays than are normal full-term infants.
- Accurate predictions of developmental delays are not possible in the neonatal period, and so developmental assessment to identify problems is an ongoing process.
- Infant stimulation programs need to be individually planned with attention to preventing overstimulation.
- Nurses can promote positive parenting by assisting parents in resolving their emotional reactions to their infants' status and in helping them to view their infants as individuals capable of positive interactions.
- Parents of high-risk infants have special needs for health teaching to care for their infants.
- Parents should be encouraged to assume as much responsibility as possible for care of their infants before hospital discharge.
- In the event of neonatal death, parents and other family members may need assistance in working through their grief and accepting the infant's death.

References

Abbey BL et al: Nursing responsibility in referring the convalescent newborn. *Am J Matern Child Nurs* 1977; 2:295–297.

Ahmann PA et al: Intraventricular hemorrhage in the high-risk pre-term infant: Incidence and outcome. *Ann Neurol* 1980; 7:118–124.

Als H et al: The behavior of the full-term but underweight newborn infant. *Dev Med Child Neurol* 1976; 18:590–602.

Amiel-Tison C: Neurological evaluation of the maturity of newborn infants. *Arch Dis Child* 1968; 43:89–93.

Anders T, Emde R, Parmelee A: *A Manual of Standardized Terminology, Techniques and Criteria for Scoring States of Sleep and Wakefulness in Newborn Infants.* UCLA Brain Info. Serv./BRI Public. Off., 1971.

Anderson CC et al: *Nonnutritive Sucking Opportunities: A Safe and Effective Treatment for Premature Infants.* Presented at Int. Conf. on Infant Studies, New Haven, Conn., March 1980.

Anderson PO: Drugs and breast feeding—a review. *Drug Intell Clin Phar* 1977; 11:208–223.

Babson SG et al: *Management of High-risk Pregnancy and Intensive Care of the Neonate.* 3rd ed. Mosby, 1975.

Bakeman R, Brown JV: Early interaction: Consequences for social and mental development at three years. *Child Dev* 1980; 51:437–447.

Bakke K, Dougherty J: Sudden infant death syndrome and infant apnea: Current questions, clinical management, and research directions. *Iss Compr Pediatr Nurs* 1981; 5:77–88.

Ballard JL, Kazmaier K, Driver M: A simplified assessment of gestational age, abstracted. *Pediatr Res* 1977; 11:374.

Barnard K: Trends in the care and prevention of developmental disabilities. *Am J Nurs* 1975; 75:1700–1704.

Barnard KE, Blackburn S: Features of the premature infant's animate and inanimate environment in relation to adult activity. In: *Caregiver–Infant Interactions and Stimulation Characteristics of Intensive Care Nurseries.* JL Gaiter (chair). Symposium presented at the biennial meeting of the Society for Research in Child Development, Boston, Mass. April 1981.

Barnett CR et al: Neonatal separation: The maternal side of interaction deprivation. *Pediatr* 1970; 45:197–205.

Battaglia FC, Lubchenco LO: A practical classification of newborn infants by weight and gestational age. *J Pediatr* 1967; 71:159–163.

Bell GJ: Moths and butterflies. *Pediatr Nurs* (May/June) 1976; 2:37–41.

Bench J, Parker A: Hyper-responsivity to sounds in the short-gestation baby. *Dev Med Child Neurol* 1971; 13:15–19.

Benfield DG, Leib SA, Reuter J: Grief response of parents after referral of the critically ill newborn to a regional center. *N Engl J Med* 1976; 294:974–978.

Benfield DG, Leib SA, Vollman JH: Grief response of parents to neonatal death and parent participation in deciding care. *Pediatrics* 1978; 62:171–177.

Berg PJ, Devlin MK, Gedaly-Duff V: Bibliotherapy with children experiencing loss. *Iss Compr Pediatr Nurs* 1980; 4:37–50.

Bertino JS: The pharmacology of human milk. *Birth and the Family J* 1981; 8:237–243.

Bliss VJ: Sharing another's death. *Nursing 76* (Apr) 1976; 6:30.

Boettcher MD, Pereira GR: Nutritional management of the critically ill neonate. In: *Neonatal and Pediatric Critical Care Nursing.* Stahler-Miller K (editor). Churchill Livingstone.

Boggs KR, Rau PK: Breastfeeding the premature infant. *Am J Nurs* 1983; 83:1436–1444.

Booth CL, Leonard HL, Thoman EB: Sleep states and behavior patterns in preterm and full-term infants. *Neuropediatr* 1980; 11:354–364.

Borg S, Lasker J: *When Pregnancy Fails.* Beacon Press, 1981.

Brackbill Y: Cumulative effects of continuous stimulation on arousal level in infants. *Child Devel* 1971; 42:17–26.

Brazelton TB: *Neonatal Behavior Assessment Scale.* Spastics International Medical Publications, in association with Heinemann Medical Books and Lippincott.

Brazelton TB: Assessment as a method for enhancing infant development. *Zero to Three.* (Sept 1981); 2:1–8.

Bresadola C: One infant/one nurse/one objective: Quality care. *Am J Matern Child Nurs* 1977; 2:287–290.

Brown JV et al: Nursery-based intervention with prematurely born babies and their mothers: Are there effects? *J Pediatr* 1980; 97:487–491.

Caplan G: Patterns of parental response to the crisis of premature birth. *Psychiatry* 1960; 23:365–374.

Caputo DV, Mandell W: Consequences of low birth weight. *Dev Psychol* 1970; 3:362–383.

Centers for Disease Control: *CDC National Nosocomial Infections Study Report,* HEW publication No. (CDC) 78-8257. US Government Printing Office, 1977.

Chaplin ER et al: Posthemorrhagic hydrocephalus in the preterm infant. *Pediatrics* 1980; 65:901–909.

Clark CE et al: Risk factor analysis of intraventricular hemorrhage in low-birth-weight infants. *J Pediatr* 1981; 99:625–628.

Clarke CA: Practical effects of blood group incompatibility between mother and fetus. *Br Med J* 1972; 2:90–95.

Colley R, Wilson J: Meeting patients' nutritional needs with hyperalimentation: Providing hyperalimentation for infants and children. *Nursing 79* (July) 1979; 9:50–53.

Cordell AS, Apolito R: Family support in infant death. *J Obstet Gynecol Neonatal Nurs* 1981; 10:281–285.

Corey EJB, Miller CL, Widlak FW: Factors contributing to child abuse. *Nurs Res* 1975; 24:293–295.

Cornell EH, Gottfried AW: Intervention with premature human infants. *Child Dev* 1976; 47:32–39.

Creighton D: Postmaturity. *Iss Health Care Women* 1978; 1:21–27.

Davis DH: *The Social Competency of Premature Infants Discharged From the Hospital Prior to Forty Weeks Conceptional Age,* Master's degree thesis. University of Connecticut.

Davis DH, Thoman EB: *The Organization of Behavioral States in Premature and Full-term Infants.* Paper presented at the biennial meeting of the Society for Research in Child Development, Detroit, Mich., April 1983.

De Chateau P, Wiberg B: Long-term effect on mother-infant behaviour of extra contact during the first hour post partum. *Acta Paediatr Scand* 1977; 66:137–151.

Demarquez JL et al: Traitement préventif des apnées du prématuré par la théophylline. *Arch Fr Pediatr* 1978; 35:793–805.

Denenberg VH et al: Effects of theophylline upon behavioral state development in the newborn rabbit. *J Pharmacol Exp Ther* 1982; 221:604–608.

Denhoff E: Current status of infant stimulation or enrichment programs for children with developmental disabilities. *Pediatrics* 1981; 67:32–37.

Desmond MM et al: The very low birth weight infant after discharge from intensive care: Anticipatory health care and developmental course. *Curr Prob Pediatr* (Apr) 1980; 10:1–59.

Deuel RK: Polygraphic monitoring of apneic spells. *Arch Neurol* 1973; 28:71–76.

Dimaggio GT, Sheetz AH: The concerns of mothers caring for an infant on an apnea monitor. *Am J Matern Child Nurs* 1983; 8:294–297.

Dingle RE et al: Continuous transcutaneous O_2 monitoring in the neonate. *Am J Nurs* 1980; 80:890–893.

Donlen JM, Budd RA: The low-birth-weight infant: A nursing perspective. In: *Neonatal and Pediatric Critical Care Nursing.* Stahler-Miller K (editor). Churchill Livingstone.

Dreyfus-Brisac C: Ontogenesis of sleep in human prematures after 32 weeks of conceptional age. *Dev Psychobiol* 1970; 3:92–121.

Driscoll JM et al: Mortality and morbidity in infants less than 1,001 grams birth weight. *Pediatrics* 1982; 69:21–26.

DuBois DR: Indications of an unhealthy relationship between parents and premature infant. *J Obstet Gynecol Neonatal Nurs* (May/June) 1975; 4:21–24.

Dubowitz LMS, Dubowitz V, Goldberg C: Clinical assessment of gestational age in the newborn infant. *J Pediatr* 1970; 77:1–10.

Eager M: Long-distance nurturing of the family bond. *Am J Matern Child Nurs* 1977; 2:293–294.

Eager M, Exoo R: Parents visiting parents for unequaled support. *Am J Matern Child Nurs* 1980; 5:35–36.

Ellenberg JH, Nelson KB: Early recognition of infants at high risk for cerebral palsy: Examination at age four months. *Dev Med Child Neurol* 1981; 23:705 –716.

Elliot BA: Neonatal death: Reflections for parents. *Pediatrics* 1978; 62:100–102.

Elliott BA, Hein HA: Neonatal death: Reflections for physicians. *Pediatrics* 1978; 62:96–100.

Elsas TL: Family mental health care in the neonatal intensive care unit. *J Obstet Gynecol Neonatal Nurs* 1981; 10:204–206.

Ennis S, Harris TR: Positioning infants with hyaline membrane disease. *Am J Nurs* 1978; 78:398–401.

Erdman D: Parent-to-parent support: The best for those with sick newborns. *Am J Matern Child Nurs* 1977; 2:291–292.

Erickson ML: *Assessment and management of developmental changes in children.* Mosby, 1976.

Fanaroff AA, Kennell JH, Klaus MH: Follow-up of low birth weight infants—the predictive value of maternal visiting patterns. *Pediatrics* 1972; 49:287–290.

Fanaroff AA, Klaus MH: The gastrointestinal tract—feeding and selected disorders. Pages 113–145 in: *Care of the High Risk Infants.* 2nd ed. Klaus MH, Fanaroff AA (editors). Saunders, 1979.

Ferry PC: On growing new neurons: Are early intervention programs effective. *Pediatrics* 1981; 67:38–41.

Field TM: Effects of early separation, interactive deficits, and experimental manipulations on infant-mother face-to-face interaction. *Child Dev* 1977; 48:763–777.

Field T: Interaction behaviors of primary versus secondary caretaker fathers. *Dev Psychology* 1978; 14:183–184.

Field T: Games parents play with normal and high-risk infants. *Child Psychiatry Human Dev* 1979; 10:41–48. (a)

Field TM: Visual and cardiac responses to animate and inanimate faces by young term and preterm infants. *Child Dev* 1979; 50:188–194. (b)

Finnegan LP, Macnew GA: Care of the addicted infant. *Am J Nurs* 1974; 74:685–693.

Floyd CC: Pregnancy after reproductive failure. *Am J Nurs* 1981; 81: 2048–2050.

Foley H: When do pre-term and light-for-date babies smile? *Dev Med Child Neurol* 1977; 19:757–760.

Foster S: Indomethacin: Pharmacologic closure of the ductus arteriosus. *Am J Matern Child Nurs* 1982; 7:171.

Frankenburg WK et al: *Denver developmental screening test: Reference manual.* Revised 1975 ed. University of Colorado Medical Center. Copyright © W. K. Frankenburg.

Fuller R, Petering M: A letter from Tommy. *Nursing 79* (Nov) 1979; 9:54–56.

Gabriel M, Albani M: Rapid eye movement sleep, apnea, and cardiac slowing influenced by phenobarbital administration in the neonate. *Pediatrics* 1977; 60:426–430.

Gale E: Neonatal seizures. In: *Protocols for Perinatal Nursing Practice.* Perez RH (editor). Mosby, 1981.

Gennaro S: Necrotizing enterocolitis: Detecting it and treating it. *Nursing 80* (Jan) 1980; 10:52–55.

Giles HR et al: The Arizona high-risk maternal transport system: An initial view. *Am J Obstet Gynecol* 1977; 128:400–407.

Goodman MB: Incidence of respiratory infections in full-term and premature infants during their first year. *Nurs Res* 1973; 22:160–164.

Gorski PA, Hole WT, Leonard CH: Behavioral and physiological observations of infants and their caregivers in an intensive care nursery. In: *Care giver–infant interactions and stimulation characteristics of intensive care nurseries.* Gaiter JL (chair). Symposium presented at the biennial meeting of the Society for Research in Child Development, Boston, Mass., April 1981.

Grams KE: Breast-feeding: A means of imparting immunity? *Am J Matern Child Nurs* 1978; 3:340–344.

Gromada K: Maternal-infants attachment: The first step toward individualizing twins. *Am J Matern Child Nurs* 1981; 6:129–134.

Guilleminault C, Souquet M: Sleep states and related pathology. In: *Advances in Perinatal Neurology.* Vol. I. Korobin R, Guilleminault C (editors). Spectrum, 1979.

Guy M: Neonatal transport. *Nurs Clin North Am* (March) 1978; 13:3–11.

Hardgrove C, Warrick LH: "How shall we tell the children?" *Am J Nurs* 1974; 74:448–450.

Harper R et al: Observations on unrestricted parental contact with infants in the neonatal intensive care unit. *J Pediatr* 1976; 89:441–445.

Harpin VA, Rutter N: Sweating in preterm babies. *J Pediatr* 1982; 100:614–618.

Hawkins MM: Nursing and regionalization of perinatal services. *J Obstet Gynecol Neonatal Nurs* 1980; 9:215–217.

Hill A, Perlman JM, Volpe JJ: Relationship of pneumothorax to occurrence of intraventricular hemorrhage in the premature newborn. *Pediatrics* 1982; 69:144–149.

Horwitz SJ, Amiel-Tison C: Neurologic problems. Pages 360–381 in: *Care of the High-risk Infant.* 2nd ed. Klaus MH, Fanaroff AA (editors). Saunders, 1979.

Houser J: Therapeutic groups for parents of high-risk infants. *Iss Compr Pediatr Nurs* 1980; 4:31–35.

Howard J et al: A neurologic comparison of pre-term and full-term infants at term conceptional age. *J Pediatr* 1976; 88:995–1002.

Hunt JV: Mental development of the survivors of neonatal intensive care. In: *Ethics of Newborn Intensive Care.* Jousen AR, Garland MJ (editors). Health Policy Program, Berkeley: Institute of Government Studies.

Hunt JV, Rhodes L: Mental development of preterm infants during the first year. *Child Dev* 1977; 48:204–210.

Hunter RS et al: Antecedents of child abuse and neglect in premature infants: A prospective study in a newborn intensive care unit. *Pediatrics* 1978; 61:629–635.

Hutton NM, Schreiner RL: Urine collection in the neonate: Effect of different methods on volume, specific gravity, and glucose. *J Obstet Gynecol Neonatal Nurs* 1980; 9:165–169.

Jackson PL: Congenital heart disease: Digoxin therapy at home: Keeping the child safe. *Am J Matern Child Nurs* 1979; 4:105–109.

Jeffcoate JA, Humphrey ME, Lloyd JK: Disturbance in parent-child relationship following preterm delivery. *Dev Med Child Neurol* 1979; 21:344–352. (a)

Jeffcoate JA, Humphrey ME, Lloyd JK: Role perception and response to stress in fathers and mothers following preterm delivery. *Soc Sci Med* 1979; 13A:139–145. (b)

Johnson SH, Grubbs JP: The premature infant's reflex behaviors: Effect on the maternal-child relationship. *J Obstet Gynecol Neonatal Nurs* (May/June 1975); 4:15–21.

Jovanic L, Druzin M, Peterson C: Effect of euglycemia on the outcome of pregnancy in insulin-dependent diabetic women as compared with normal control subjects. *Am J Med* 1981; 71:921–927.

Kachoris PJ: Psychodynamic considerations in the neonatal ICU. *Crit Care Med* 1977; 5:62–65.

Kaplan DM, Mason EA: Maternal reactions to premature birth viewed as an acute emotional disorder. *Am J Orthopsychiatry* 1960; 30:539–552.

Kennedy AH, Johnson WG, Sturdevant EW: An educational program for families of children with tracheostomies. *Am J Matern Child Nurs* 1982; 7:42–49.

Kennell JH et al: Maternal behavior one year after early and extended post-partum contact. *Dev Med Child Neurol* 1974; 16:172–179.

Kimble KJ et al: Growth to age 3 years among very low-birth-weight sequelae-free survivors of modern neonatal intensive care. *J Pediatr* 1982; 100:622–624.

Klaus M, Fanaroff A, Martin RJ: Respiratory problems. Pages 173–204 in: *Care of the High-risk Infant.* 2nd ed. Klaus MH, Fanaroff AA (editors). Saunders, 1979.

Klaus MH, Kennell JH: *Parent–Infant Bonding.* 2nd ed. Mosby, 1982.

Klaus MH et al: Human maternal behavior at the first contact with her young. *Pediatrics* 1970; 46:187–192.

Klein M, Stern L: Low birth weight and the battered child syndrome. *Am J Dis Child* 1971; 122:15–18.

Knobloch H et al: Considerations in evaluating changes in outcome for infants weighing less than 1,501 grams. *Pediatrics* 1982; 69:285–295.

Kopp CB et al: Neurological organization and visual fixation in infants at 40 weeks conceptional age. *Dev Psychobiol* 1975; 8:165–170.

Korones SB: *High-risk Newborn Infants: The Basis for Intensive Nursing Care.* 2nd ed. Mosby, 1976.

Kramer M et al: Extra tactile stimulation of the premature infant. *Nurs Res* 1975; 24:324–333.

Krishnamoorthy KS et al: Neurologic sequelae in the survivors of neonatal intraventricular hemorrhage. *Pediatrics* 1979; 64:233–237.

Kumar SP et al: Follow-up studies of very low birth weight infants (1,250 grams or less) born and treated within a perinatal center. *Pediatrics* 1980; 66:438–443.

Largo RH, Duc G: Head growth and changes in head configuration in healthy preterm and term infants during the first six months of life. *Helv Paediatr Acta* 1977; 32:431–442.

Lawson K, Daum D, Turkewitz G: Environmental characteristics of a neonatal intensive-care unit. *Child Dev* 1977; 48:1633–1639.

Lazzara A et al: Clinical predictability of intraventricular hemorrhage in preterm infants. *Pediatrics* 1980; 65:30–34.

LeBlanc MH: Relative efficacy of an incubator and an open warmer in producing thermoneutrality for the small premature infant. *Pediatrics* 1982; 69:439–445.

Leib SA, Benfield DG, Guidubaldi J: Effects of early intervention and stimulation on the preterm infant. *Pediatrics* 1980; 66:83–90.

Leifer AD et al: Effects of mother–infant separation on maternal attachment behavior. *Child Dev* 1972; 43:1203–1218.

Lemons PK: Hospital use of expressed breast milk. *Iss Compr Pediatr Nurs* 1981; 5:195–203.

Levene MI: Measurement of the growth of the lateral ventricles in preterm infants with real-time ultrasound. *Arch Dis Child* 1981; 56:900–904.

Levene MI, Starte DR: A longitudinal study of post-haemorrhagic ventricular dilatation in the newborn. *Arch Dis Child* 1981; 56:905–910.

Lewis E: Mourning by the family after a stillbirth or neonatal death. *Arch Dis Child* 1979; 54:303–306.

Leykauf C: Congenital heart disease. In: *Protocols for Perinatal Nursing Practice.* Perez RH (editor). Mosby, 1981.

Liebman J, Borkat G, Hirschfeld S: The heart. In: *Care of the High-risk Infant.* 2nd ed. Klaus MH, Fanaroff AA (editors). Saunders, 1979.

Lindemann E: Symptomatology and management of acute grief. *Am J Psychiatry* 1944; 101:141–148.

Littman B, Parmelee AH Jr.: Medical correlates of infant development. *Pediatrics* 1978; 61:470–474.

Lubchenco LO, Searls DT, Brazie JV: Neonatal mortality rate: Relationship to birth weight and gestational age. *J Pediatr* 1972; 81:814–822.

Lucey JF: Why we regionalize perinatal care. *Pediatrics* 1973; 52:488–489.

Mangurten HH, Slade C, Fitzsimons D: Parent–parent support in the care of high-risk newborns. *J Obstet Gynecol Neonatal Nurs* 1979; 8:275–277.

McKeel NL: Child abuse can be prevented. *Am J Nurs* 1978; 78:1478–1482.

Measel CP, Anderson GC: Nonnutritive sucking during tube feedings: Effect on clinical course in premature infants. *J Obstet Gynecol Neonatal Nurs* 1979; 8:265–272.

Mercer RT: The nurse and maternal tasks of early postpartum. *Am J Matern Child Nurs* 1981; 6:341–345.

Michelsson K, Ylinen A, Donner M: Neurodevelopmental screening at five years of children who were at risk neonatally. *Dev Med Child Neurol* 1981; 23:427–433.

Miller HC: Fetal growth and neonatal mortality. *Pediatrics* 1972; 49:392–399.

Minde K et al: Mother–child relationships in the premature nursery: An observational study. *Pediatrics* 1978; 61:373–379.

Nelson KB, Ellenberg JH: Apgar scores as predictors of chronic neurologic disability. *Pediatrics* 1981; 68:36–43.

Noga KM: High-risk infants: The need for nursing follow-up. *J Obstet Gynecol Neonatal Nurs* 1982; 11:112–115.

Oehler J: The fun family books: Color the pictures "sad" or "glad." *Am J Matern Child Nurs* 1981; 6:281–283.

Ostler CW: Initial feeding time of newborn infants: Effect upon first meconium passage and serum indirect bilirubin levels. *Iss Health Care Women* 1979; 1:1–23.

Paludetto R et al: Reactions of sixty parents allowed unrestricted contact with infants in a neonatal intensive care unit. *Early Hum Dev* 1981; 5:401–409.

Pape KE et al: The status at two years of low-birth-weight infants born in 1974 with birth weights less than 1,001 gm. *J Pediatr* 1978; 92:253–260.

Papile LA et al: Incidence and evolution of subependymal and intraventricular hemorrhage: A study of infants with birth weights less than 1,500 gm. *J Pediatr* 1978; 92:529–534.
Parmelee AH: Neurophysiological and behavioral organization of premature infants in the first months of life. *Biol Psychiatry* 1975; 10:501–512.
Parmelee AH Jr et al: Sleep states in premature infants. *Dev Med Child Neurol* 1967; 9:70–77.
Peabody JL et al: Transcutaneous oxygen monitoring in aminophylline-treated apneic infants. *Pediatrics* 1978; 62:698–701.
Pearson HA: The blood. In: *The Physiology of the Newborn Infant.* 4th ed. Smith CA, Nelson NM (editors). Thomas, 1976.
Phibbs CS, Williams RL, Phibbs RH: Newborn risk factors and costs of neonatal intensive care. *Pediatrics* 1981; 68:313–321.
Philip AGS: *Neonatology: A practical guide.* Medical Examination, 1977.
Philip AGS et al: Neonatal mortality risk for the eighties: The importance of birth weight/gestational age groups. *Pediatrics* 1981; 68:122–130.
Pittard WB III: Special properties of human milk. *Birth and the Family J* 1981; 8:229–235.
Pomerance JJ et al: Cost of living for infants weighing 1,000 grams or less at birth. *Pediatrics* 1978; 61:908–910.
Poznanski EO: The "replacement child": A saga of unresolved parental grief. *J Pediatrics* 1972; 81:1190–1193.
Prechtl HFR, Theorell K, Blair A W: Behavioral state cycles in abnormal infants. *Dev Med Child Neurol* 1973; 15:606–615.
Provence S, Lipton RC: *Infants in Institutions: A Comparison of Their Development With Family-Reared Infants During the First Year of Life.* International Universities Press, 1962.
Record RG, McKeown T, Edwards JH: The relation of measured intelligence to birth order and maternal age. *Ann Hum Genet* 1969; 33:61–69.
Richards MPM: Is neonatal intensive care overused? *Birth and the Family J* 1980; 7:225–233.
Rosenfeld AG: Visiting in the intensive care nursery. *Child Dev* 1980; 51:939–941.
Ross GS: Parental responses to infants in intensive care: The separation issue reevaluated. *Clin Perinatal* (March) 1980; 7:47–60.
Rowe J et al: Follow-up of families who experience a perinatal death. *Pediatrics* 1978; 62:166–170.
Rubin R: Attainment of the maternal role. Part 1. Processes. *Nurs Res* 1967; 16:237–245.
Saigal S et al: Follow-up of infants 501 to 1,500 gm birth weight delivered to residents of a geographically defined region with perinatal intensive care facilities. *J Pediatr* 1982; 100:606–613.
Sameroff AJ: Early influences on development: Fact or fancy? *Merrill-Palmer Quarterly* 1975; 61:267–294.
Sater J: Appraising and promoting a sense of self in twins. *Am J Matern Child Nurs* 1979; 4:218–221.
Scarr-Salapetek S, Williams ML: The effects of early stimulation on low-birth-weight infants. *Child Dev* 1973; 44:94–101.
Schraeder BD: A creative approach to caring for the ventilator-dependent child. *Am J Matern Child Nurs* 1979; 4:165–170.
Schraeder BD: Attachment and parenting despite lengthy intensive care. *Am J Matern Child Nurs* 1980; 5:37–41.
Schuman H: Understanding neonatal jaundice: "That darn yellow baby." *Pediatr Nurs* (July/Aug) 1976; 2:38–40.
Shankaran S et al: Sonographic classification of intracranial hemorrhage. A prognostic indicator of mortality, morbidity, and short-term neurologic outcome. *J Pediatr* 1982; 100:469–475.
Shearer MH: The economics of intensive care for the full-term newborn. *Birth and the Family J* 1980; 7:234–241.
Sherwen LN: Fantasies during the third trimester of pregnancy. *Am J Matern Child Nurs* 1981; 6:398–401.
Sigman M, Parmelee AH: Visual preferences of four-month-old premature and full-term infants. *Child Dev* 1974; 45:959–965.
Sigman M et al: *Infant Visual Attentiveness in Relation to Birth Condition.* Presented at the biennial meeting of the Society for Research in Child Development, 1975.
Silverboard G et al: Comparison of lumbar puncture with computed tomography scan as an indicator of intracerebral hemorrhage in the preterm infant. *Pediatrics* 1980; 66:432–437.
Simkin P, Simkin PA, Edwards M: "Physiologic" jaundice of the newborn. *Birth and the Family J* 1979; 6:23–41.
Smith N: Necrotizing enterocolitis. In: *Protocols for Perinatal Nursing Practice.* Perez RH (editor). Mosby, 1981.
Snyder C, Eyres SJ, Barnard K: New findings about mothers' antenatal expectations and their relationship to infant development. *Am J Matern Child Nurs* 1979; 4:354–357.
Solkoff N et al: Effects of handling on the subsequent development of premature infants. *Dev Psychology* 1969; 1:765–768.
Speck WT, Fanaroff A, Klaus M: Neonatal infections. Pages 267–293 in: *Care of the High-risk Infant.* 2nd ed. Klaus MH, Fanaroff AA (editors). Saunders, 1979.
Stahler-Miller K, Gewitz MH: Current considerations for patent ductus arteriosus in the critically ill newborn. In: *Neonatal and Pediatric Critical Care Nursing.* Stahler-Miller K (editor). Churchill Livingstone, 1983.
Stavis RL, Krauss AN: Complications of neonatal intensive care. *Clin Perinatol* (March) 1980; 7:107–124.
Stern L: The newborn infant and his thermal environment. *Curr Prob Pediatr* (Nov) 1970; 1:1–32.
Stewart AL et al: Prognosis for infants weighing 1000 grams or less at birth. *Arch Dis Child* 1977; 52:97–104.
Strohbach ME, Kratina SH: Diaper versus bag specimens: A comparison of urine specific gravity values. *Am J Matern Child Nurs* 1982; 7:198–201.
Sweet AY: Classification of the low-birth-weight infant. Pages 66–93 in: *Care of the High-risk Infant.* 2nd ed. Klaus MH, Fanaroff AA (editors). Saunders, 1979.
Telzrow RW et al: The behavior of jaundiced infants undergoing phototherapy. *Dev Med Child Neurol* 1980; 22:317–326.
Thoman EB: Early development of sleeping behaviors in infants. In: *Aberrant Development in Infancy: Human and Animal Studies.* Ellis NR (editor). Wiley & Sons, 1975.
Thoman EB: *States of Sleep and Wakefulness in Infants.* Unpublished manuscript. (Available from E. B. Thoman, Box U-154, The Department of Biobehavioral Sciences, University of Connecticut, Storrs, Connecticut 06268 USA.)
Thoman EB et al: Theophylline affects behavioral state development in premature infants. *Neuropediatrics* 1984. In press.
Thoman EB et al: Behavioral state profiles in infancy are predictive of later medical or behavioral dysfunction. *Neuropediatrics* 1981; 12:45–54.
Thoman EB, Miano VN; and Freese MP: The role of respiratory instability in the sudden infant death syndrome. *Dev Med Child Neurol* 1977; 19:729–738.
Tooley W: *Neonatology.* Presented at the biennial meeting of the Society for Research in Child Development, Boston, Massachusetts, April 1981.
Torrance JT: Temperature reading of premature infants. *Nurs Res* 1968; 17:312–320.
Trotter CW, Chang PN, Thompson T: Perinatal factors and the developmental outcome of premature infants. *J Obstet Gynecol Neonatal Nurs* 1982; 11:83–90.
Varner B, Ossenkop D, Lyon J: Prematures, too, need rooming-in and care-by-parent programs. *Am J Matern Child Nurs* 1980; 5:431–432.
Volpe JJ: Neonatal periventricular hemorrhage: Past, present, and future. *J Pediatr* 1978; 92:693–696.
Waddell CS, Fresholtz M: Discharge of the premature infant. *Nurs Clin North Am* (March) 1978; 13:63–71.
White JL, Labarba R: The effects of tactile and kinesthetic stimulation on neonatal development in the premature infant. *Dev Psychobiol* 1976; 9:569–577.

Widmayer SM, Field TM: Effects of Brazelton demonstrations on the development of preterm infants. *Pediatrics* 1981; 67:711–714.

Wooten B: Death of an infant. *Am J Matern Child Nurs* 1981; 6:257–260.

Young HB et al: Milk and lactation: Some social and developmental correlates among 1,000 infants. *Pediatrics* 1981; 69:169–175.

Yu VYH, Jamieson J, Astbury J: Parents' reactions to unrestricted parental contact with infants in the intensive care nursery. *Med J Aust* 1981; 1:294–296.

Zelauskas B: Siblings: The forgotten grievers. *Iss Compr Pediatr Nurs* 1981; 5:45–52.

Zieman M, Carroll JS: Infant gavage reconsidered. *Am J Nurs* 1978; 78:1543–1544.

Zimmerman M et al: Nursing grand rounds: Meeting long-term needs in an acute-care nursery. *Nursing 78* (Sept) 1978; 8:81–84.

Additional Readings

Affonso D, Harris T: Continuous positive airway pressure. *Am J Nurs* 1976; 76:570–573.

Agarwala B, Baffes T: Congestive heart failure in the infant. *Heart Lung* 1976; 5:62–70.

Aladjem S, Brown AK, Sureau C (editors): *Clinical Perinatology*. Mosby, 1980.

Belko DP, Menard S: The pediatric intensive care unit. *Nurs Management* (Apr) 1983; 14(4):36–37.

Brown RSK, Valman HB: *Practical Neonatal Pediatrics*. 4th ed. Mosby, 1980.

Chase BA, Ludington-Hoe SM: Sensory stimulation in the NICU. *Am J Nurs* (Jan) 1984; 84(1):68–71.

Chernick V, Vidyasager D: Continuous negative chest wall pressure in hyaline membrane disease: One year experience. *Pediatrics* 1972; 49:753–760.

Choi MW: Breast milk for infants who can't breast-feed. *Am J Nurs* 1978; 78:852–855.

Duxbury ML, Broz LJ, Wachdorf CM: Caregiver disruptions and sleep of high-risk infants. *Heart Lung* (March)1984; 13(2):141–147.

Editorial: Knowing what to do for seriously ill newborns. *Nursing Life*. March/April, 1984, pages 46–47.

Fanaroff AA, Martin RJ (editors): *Behrman's Neonatal-Perinatal Medicine: Diseases of the Fetus and Infant*. 3rd ed. Mosby, 1983.

Glassandos MR: Infants who are oxygen dependent—sending them home. *Am J Matern Child Nurs* 1980; 5:42–45.

Hazinski MF: *Nursing Care of the Critically Ill Child*. Mosby, 1984.

Hutchinson SA: Creating meaning out of horror. *Nursing Outlook* (March/Apr) 1984; 32(2):86–90.

James FW, Love E: Congestive heart failure in infants and children. *Heart Lung* 1974; 3:396–400.

Johnson SH (editor): *High-risk Parenting: Nursing Assessment and Strategies for the Family at Risk*. Lippincott, 1979.

Johnson SH: Avoiding communication blocks with high risk parents. *Iss Compr Pediatr Nurs* 1980; 4:61–72.

Korones SB: *High-Risk Newborn Infants: The Basis for Intensive Nursing Care*. 3rd ed. Mosby, 1981.

Lyon J: New treatments, new choices. *Nursing Life*. March/April, 1984, pages 48–52.

Nalepka CD: The oxygen hood for newborns in respiratory distress. *Am J Nurs* 1975; 75:2185–2187.

Nelson N: *Current Therapy in Neonatal-Perinatal Medicine 1984–85*. Mosby, 1984.

Penfold KM: Supporting mother love. *Am J Nurs* 1974; 74:464–467.

Perez RH (editor): *Protocols for Perinatal Nursing Practice*. Mosby, 1981.

Plapp PR: Nursing implications in the early recognition of necrotizing enterocolitis. *Iss Compr Pediatr Nurs* 1980; 4:77–81.

Price E, Gyotoku S: Using the nasojejunal feeding technique in a neonatal intensive care unit. *Am J Matern Child Nurs* 1978; 3:361–365.

Rasch D et al: Neurobehavioral effects of neonatal hypermagnesemia. *J Pediatr* 1982; 100:272–276.

Roper KE et al: Failure to thrive: An opportunity for innovative nursing. *Pediatr Nurs* (Sept/Oct) 1976; 2:43–45.

Rothfeder B, Tiedeman M: Feeding the low-birth-weight neonate. *Nursing 77* (Oct) 1977; 7:58–59.

Schraeder BD: Attachment and parenting despite lengthy intensive care. *Matern Child Nurs J* (Jan/Feb) 1980; 5:37–41.

Slade CI, Reidl CJ, Mangurten HH: Working with parents of high-risk newborns. *J Obstet Gynecol Neonatal Nurs* (March/Apr) 1977; 6:21–26.

Smith KM: Congenital heart disease: Recognizing cardiac failure in neonates. *Am J Matern Child Nurs* 1979; 4:98–100.

Voyles JB: Bronchopulmonary dysplasia. *Am J Nurs* 1981; 81:510–514.

The Dying Child

Thomas Eoyang Robert R. Riedel Deanna Edwards

32

Chapter Outline

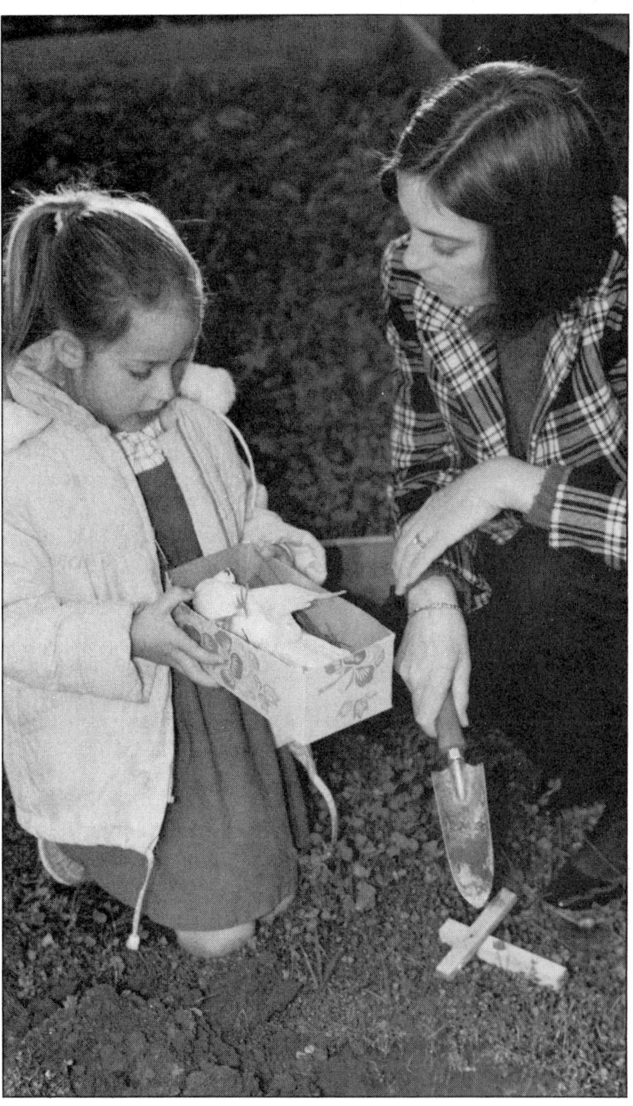

A Child's View of Death

A Child's Experience of Death

Self-Concept and Perception of Illness
Trajectories of Death
Critical Junctures
Time and Certainty
Awareness of Death
The Child's Reactions to Dying
- *Intellectualization*
- *Fear*
- *Regression*
- *Denial*
- *Anger*
- *Guilt*
- *Shame*
- *Grief*
- *Active Preparation*

Reactions of Others to a Child's Dying

Parents
- *Disruption*
- *Isolation*

Siblings
The Nurse
- *Being Overwhelmed*
- *Overidentification*
- *Avoidance*
- *Personal Growth*

Influence of Culture

Elements of Nursing Care

Assessment
Communication
Assisting Grief
Peer Support
Home Care
Hospice
Evaluation and Follow-Up

Sudden Infant Death Syndrome

Proposed Causes
Nurse's Role

Objectives

- Explain why it is necessary for nurses to prepare both cognitively and emotionally for the experience of dealing with dying children and their families.
- Distinguish the characteristic perceptions of and responses to death of children at various developmental levels.
- Discuss the factors of timing, degree of certainty, and level of awareness that affect a child's experience of death.
- Identify the most common coping mechanisms and emotional responses used by the dying child.
- Discuss the additional effects of the child's dying on the family.
- Anticipate the nurse's possible responses to the experience of caring for dying children and their families.
- List the main elements of nursing care that specifically apply to the dying child and family.
- Discuss the special challenges of nursing support of the family in the aftermath of a SIDS (sudden infant death syndrome) incident.

One day in Chagrin Falls, Ohio, Jerry Kocheff, a bright-eyed, curly headed boy who had been playing in his yard, complained to his mother, Jay, about a sore throat. Hours later, Jerry died of epiglottitis.

The morning of Jerry's funeral, Jay, numb with grief, found words surfacing in her mind and wrote them down as they came to her. The poem became a song, which was used in a multimedia presentation, "Playclothes." Both the song and the presentation are used extensively today in grief counseling.

The death of a child is an intense emotional experience. Health care professionals need to prepare themselves to handle this experience, and the most important preparation takes place in the affective realm. For this reason, this chapter refers often to the personal experiences of dying children and those who survive them. Poems and songs—attempts to translate the vivid feelings of those who experience a child's dying—are included to present these feelings to the reader in an immediate way. Nurses thus can begin to get acquainted with the personal feelings that are triggered by this experience and to identify the feelings that help and those that hinder the process of nursing care.

The death of a child is a traumatic event for health care providers not only because of a child's young age but for other important reasons as well. One reason is the relative infrequency with which children die today. As discussed in Chapter 1, mortality rates for children have decreased dramatically in the twentieth century, dropping from a rate of 62 deaths per 1000 children in 1900 to a rate of 4.1 deaths per 1000 children in 1982 (see Fig. 1-2). Because it is comparatively rare today, the death of a child causes more intense emotional reactions than the death of an adult. It is important to note that a nurse working on a unit with dying children does not necessarily escape this emotional involvement because of more frequent contact with death.

Survivor guilt is a second factor that can intensify the emotional reactions to a child's death. Survivor guilt can occur when any person experiences the death of a loved one, but it is a particularly common adult response to the loss of a child, whose life seemed filled with promise, vitality, and hope. Survivor guilt is greater when a child dies because the adults have experienced more of life, and they regret the child's unactualized potential.

This chapter examines the feelings and reactions surrounding the experience of a child's death, first from the child's point of view and then from the perspective of others, including the nurse. Although implications for the nurse will be evident throughout, the chapter also deals with the nurse's specific role in caring for the dying child and the surviving family.

A Child's View of Death

A child's level of cognitive development plays a major role in that child's perception of death. A 3- or 4-year-old child, for instance, has a very different concept of death than an older child or adult. Whatever the child's age, however, questions about death and dying should be answered frankly and in a manner appropriate to the child's level of understanding. The adult should respond to what the child asks and not simply talk about what the adult thinks the child ought to know.

The work of Nagy (1948) is central to an understanding of the child's developmental views on death. This research, reported in 1948, was completed in Hungary right after the end of World War II and is a classic research study investigating children's reactions to death. At the time, authorities questioned whether one could generalize from such a study in light of the extraordinary horror witnessed at close range by the children studied; however, her findings have proved to be consistent with those of subsequent researchers.

The child's developmental view of death, particularly regarding common coping strategies, is presented in Chapter 12. The key points are summarized in Table 32-1, together with communication guidelines for the nurse. It should be remembered, however, that a child's behavior and responses are influenced by more than chronologic age. Grollman (1967) has suggested that consideration be given to all the relevant variables in the child's background with respect to ideas about death. Perhaps nobody is more of an expert on death than the dying child or the siblings experiencing the situation and its moment-to-moment ramifications. They can be the nurse's greatest teachers and most valuable sources of information for assessment.

A Child's Experience of Death

It will be helpful to present various theories concerning the child's experience of death to pinpoint the significant elements of the dying process. The work of Bluebond-Langner (1975a; 1975b; 1976; 1977) has great significance in understanding the child's experience of death. Bluebond-Langner's study of terminally ill children and their perceptions of death led her to describe five different stages, which can be applied to children of all ages beyond infancy, depending on their developmental level.

The first stage is the acceptance and understanding of the diagnosis, that is, that "it" is a serious illness. The child realizes that something is wrong, that the doctor is involved, that the family is worried, and that something bad is happening to the child.

The second stage is when the child begins to understand the names of drugs, their effects, and their side effects. The child understands that drug X causes a feeling of nausea or drug Y results in hair loss. The child can paint exquisite pictures of what the drug's effects are on the body and can remember even the long name of the most complex drug.

The third stage is when the child begins to understand and is able to talk about the purposes of treatments and procedures. The child understands the purpose of drug therapy, irradiation, and other treatments. In the work of Achterberg and Lawlis (1978), Leshan and Worthington (1965), and Simonton and Simonton (1975), children who reached this stage were asked to visualize the drug and personalize its effects, and some evidence suggests that this potentiated the treatment effects.

The fourth stage is when the disease is seen as a series of relapses and remissions but not yet with the concept that death is the final outcome of the disease. At this stage, children realize that they will experience some pain and discomfort and perhaps a hospital stay with medication, but that they will get better and eventually be able to go home. They see the future as a string of relapses and remissions.

Playclothes

You lie here so still my little son,
With long dark curls and your playclothes on.
How I wish I could watch you run—
Your soft hair shining in the sun.

How many times I prayed you'd sleep
For one more hour in my busy week
So I could wash, or clean, or bake
A pie, some cookies, or a cake.

How many times did I get upset
When you spilled your milk upon the step
Or scattered your crumbs on my clean floor,
Or left those smudges on the door?

If only you'd wake in my bad dream
And scatter your toys over everything.
If only I could see you smile
And hold you close for a little while.

Oh, God, please forgive all those bad days I had
When I got so upset with this sweet little lad.
Take care of his love while we are apart
And leave his footprints in my heart.

With his curls and smiles, his laughter and fun
Who lies here so still with his playclothes on.

SOURCE: Goveia, B: "Playclothes," an Order of the Golden Rule presentation.

In the fifth and final stage, it becomes inescapably clear that the disease is not only a series of relapses and remissions but that eventually a time will come when there are no more remissions and death becomes imminent. The nurse's support is particularly critical at this stage to reinforce the child's own coping mechanisms.

Self-Concept and Perception of Illness

Bluebond-Langner went beyond this description of the dying child and cognitive knowledge and looked at how the child views the self in relation to the illness. She proposed that there are also five stages in self-concept, which are intertwined with the child's developmental concept of death and dying. The health care worker should know these stages to interact appropriately with the child and to understand and be able to meet the child's needs.

The first stage is after diagnosis, when children realize that they are seriously ill. Children in the second stage realize that they are seriously ill but believe they will get better. In the third stage, children are always ill but feel that they eventually will get better. In the fourth stage, children are

TABLE 32-1 The Child's View of Death: Implications for Communication

Age	Common concepts of death	Representative behaviors and responses	Implications for communication
Infancy	No concept of death. Reacts to all separation in a similar way	Experiments with object permanence and separation with "throwaway" and "peek-a-boo" behaviors	Understand the strategies appropriate to deal with separation anxiety (see Chapter 12). Focus communication on other family members
Early childhood	Concept of death begins to form. The child responds to other people's reactions to death. Death is viewed as temporary, gradual, and reversible (that is, as a kind of sleep or absence). Popular media (for example, television) and magical thinking reinforce the child's belief in the reversibility of death	The child retains a sense of the dead person's being; might be concerned that the corpse can sense cold or discomfort or may worry about how it goes to the bathroom; might look forward to the dead person's return or to a visit from the dead person; might carry on imaginary conversations with the dead person	Assess the need to correct the child's misconceptions, which might be either functional or dysfunctional depending on the circumstances
Middle childhood	Begins to understand that death is permanent. Uses fantasy to personify death. The child is likely to believe that wishes, misbehavior, or unrelated actions can be responsible for death	Imagines death as a skeleton, bogeyman, or grim reaper. Might engage in burial rites or other enactments of death with dolls or small pets. Might want to touch the corpse to see what it feels like	Use fantasy figures, pets, or other elements of the child's experience as points of reference in achieving an understanding appropriate to the child's developmental level
Late childhood	Understands that all people die eventually. Begins to understand the mortality of self. Might show an interest in questions of an afterlife. Fear of death also might surface	Uses rituals to decrease anxiety; reckless behavior to demonstrate invulnerability; and humorous or tough demeanor to hide fearfulness	Allow the child to verbalize fears and help the child to accept them as normal. Discuss the realistic consequences of reckless activity
Adolescence	Reaches an "adult" perception of death but might be emotionally unable to accept it (Waechter, 1979). Might still hold over concepts from previous developmental stages, depending on actual experiences with death in childhood. Might still view death, for instance, as the result of mere intention, punishment for wrongdoing, or confirmation of evil character	Anxiety on the subject of death might be particularly acute because body image and emerging self-concept are threatened. Withdrawal might be the preferred coping strategy	Avoid assumptions of an adult understanding by assessing the adolescent's specific perceptions. Reactions might resemble those of an adult's, but the nurse should be alert to additional feelings of guilt or hostility associated with confusion of wishes, wrongdoing, or bad character with the actual cause of death

always ill and feel that they will always be ill. The fifth stage is when children realize that they are dying.

Obviously, these stages will be affected by the child's cognitive abilities, socioeconomic background, age level, and type of illness. They also will be affected by the so-called "trajectory of death."

Trajectories of Death

The concept of the trajectory of death comes from the work of Glaser and Strauss (1968). Glaser and Strauss postulated that there were several different courses that death could take. They identified six forms of trajectory: (1) abrupt surprise; (2) expected swift; (3) expected lingering; (4) short-term reprieve; (5) suspended sentence; and (6) entry–reentry. These different forms influence both the child's experience of dying and the reactions of the family and health care providers to that experience.

In association with the death of children, the abrupt surprise trajectory is usually either by accident or the sudden infant death syndrome (SIDS). With this trajectory, the shock potential is the greatest, as is the potential for personal guilt among the survivors. The child has little time to become anxious, ask questions, or deepen understanding. Support and counseling by the nurse will be most needed by the survivors. (SIDS will be discussed in more detail later in the chapter.) The second type of trajectory, the *expected swift* death, is seen only in some units of the hospital—the emergency room, recovery room, and intensive care unit being the most common. This type of death occurs to the child who has become suddenly ill by severe illness or accident and whose death is not immediate. *Expected lingering* occurs most often in chronic illness. (See Chapter 30 for a fuller discussion of this trajectory.) Often, the *short-term reprieve* is associated with medical technology's ability to forestall but not alter the inevitable. Certain diseases might be put into partial or even complete remission but will certainly recur. Parents and children will need to be gently coaxed into accepting the temporary nature of the remission and the need to follow any prescribed medical regimen. The nurse must walk a tightrope between supporting this necessary reality orientation while simultaneously supporting hope.

The *suspended sentence* trajectory is subtly different from the short-term reprieve. In the suspended sentence trajectory, the child is expected to die, but the disease unexpectedly is considered to be cured. An example would be a cure resulting from an extraordinary medical measure, such as an organ transplant, or a treatment that had been given a low probability of success in an otherwise hopeless situation.

The entry–reentry trajectory is actually an extended form of a short-term reprieve in which the person goes in and out of the hospital. The nurse facing this kind of trajectory is aware of the likely length of stay outside the hospital, the treatments that will best support the person's health, the need for individualized and updated discharge planning, and the interdisciplinary collaboration and support needed for home care.

Critical Junctures

Glaser and Strauss (1968) hypothesized that any trajectory has certain critical junctures. The first juncture is when the patient is defined as dying. In hospitals with a traditional philosophy, such a definitive statement often was not made, but simply implied.

The second juncture is when the hospital staff or family make preparations for the child's death; the child who is aware of impending death also might begin to make preparations.

The final juncture is reached when intervention procedures are withdrawn or considerably curtailed. This final phase is ended only by the child's death. Although certain junctures might be anticipated, some may take the child and family by surprise. The nurse provides as much information as possible about the child's condition and what to expect, and supports the family when the dying process does not follow the expected course.

Time and Certainty

In relation to death, the definition of time and certainty are very important. For example, if there is a definition of the expected time when the death will occur, this is useful information and might be demanded by the family. In many cases, however, the time of death cannot be predicted with any accuracy; many patients have surprised the medical world by living longer than anticipated. There is also a point at which any uncertainty about the course of the dying process is resolved; it is known whether the child will have any more remissions, whether the child will improve, or whether the child is going to die.

In looking at the relationship between certainty and time, four types of death expectations can be identified. The first type is certain death at a predictable time. For example, it is known that this child will die within the hour. The second type is a certain death at an unknown time. For example, it is known that the child has a particular form of cancer and will die, but death can occur in hours or months. In the third type, there is an unknown death but a known time when certainty will be established; for example, it is not known whether the child is actually dying until the laboratory results have been processed and analyzed. In the fourth type, there is both uncertain death and an unknown time for certainty to be established. This often happens when the diagnosis and laboratory results are uncertain. The nurse's behavior is, to a certain extent, influenced by these factors of certainty and uncertainty, because concrete support might be more difficult to offer in the face of many unknowns but no less essential for the child and family.

Awareness of Death

Not only are the trajectory of death, critical junctures, and level of certainty important factors, but so also is the awareness context, another concept put forth by Glaser and Strauss (1965). They identified four different types of awareness concepts which have to do with how aware the players in the drama of the dying are of the impending death. Most traditional hospital units have a closed awareness of death. People do not speak of death, and health care professionals do not define death, even though people are dying around them.

The second type of awareness is mutual pretense, in which, to spare the feelings of others, the dying child, family, and health care professionals pretend that the child is not dying and talk about everything but that which is most important for them to share. With her typically incisive candor, Kubler-Ross stated that it is such a shame to see a couple who have been married for decades end their lives together playing a game rather than relating directly to each other at a time when they need each other's support so much (Kubler-Ross, 1969). This would seem to be equally true for children and their families.

A third type of awareness is suspected awareness, in which the nurse might suspect that the child is dying, but the physician has not confirmed such a judgment or made enough information available to confirm the suspicion. This is a particularly anxiety-provoking situation. Children are able to understand and deal with what is happening to them. They have the right to believe that their nurses, phy-

Factors Influencing *Collective* Response	
Awareness context	**Level of certainty**
• Open awareness	• Death certain/time known
• Suspected awareness	• Death certain/time unknown
• Mutual pretense	• Death uncertain/time of certainty known
• Closed awareness	• Death uncertain/time of certainty unknown

sicians, and parents are being honest with them so that they will not have to worry that their caregivers will withdraw from them in a time of extreme need.

The final type is open awareness, a concept that is best exemplified by the hospice setting. In this atmosphere it is appropriate to talk about death and deal with feelings and thoughts about death. Although sometimes uncomfortable or unpleasant, such discussions can be conducted in an open and easy atmosphere, giving nurses and other caregivers the opportunity to deal with the child's problems directly, competently, and compassionately.

Although individuals might sense their impending death long before the medical certainty has been established, the communication of the diagnosis can be considered the starting point of the awareness process. The physician either does or does not give the child and family the diagnosis, and this, of course, affects whether the process is accelerated or decelerated and whether the process is infused with extreme anxiety. When a child or parent knows the diagnosis, it can either be accepted or rejected, or, with what might be called "incomplete understanding," it might be partially accepted and partially rejected. Although they initially reject the idea that they are dying, most children ultimately will realize and begin to accept that they are dying. It is also possible to revert from acceptance back to rejection, in which the child or family suppresses the awareness that the illness is terminal and goes back to believing that everything will be all right.

The Child's Reactions to Dying

Whereas the work of Bluebond-Langner and Glaser and Strauss dealt with the variability in the timing of death and the level of awareness in the child and others, Kubler-Ross (1969) described five stages of the individual's grieving reactions to the process of dying: denial, anger, bargaining, depression, and acceptance. Although Kubler-Ross's theory of stages is widely known, Schneidman (1973) and other prominent scholars in the field have expressed concern about the use of the word "stage." One concern is that the concept of stages might be restrictive.

For example, one of the authors of this chapter, Deanna Edwards, was on her way to northern California to conduct a workshop when she read in the newspaper that some close friends in the area had been murdered in their homes. She remarked to one of the workshop participants, "When I read the article, my eyes wanted to erase their names from the newspaper," to which the participant replied, "Oh, you're in the stage of denial. Everybody goes through that."

The insensitivity of this remark points up the danger of taking the stages of grieving as a curriculum that a patient, with the help of the nurse, must get through. Moving from denial through anger, bargaining, depression, and eventually to acceptance, which is "graduation," might be seen as the only correct and inevitable way for everybody to proceed. It might, on the other hand, be preferable to view these not as stages but as "states" that might be present during the same day, hour, or even in the same sentence. The patient and family might experience these conflicting emotions all at the same time, with any one of these feelings dominant at a particular moment, or they may move back and forth through various emotions without demonstrating any "progression." The nurse recognizes all of these possibilities as normal. Using the word state instead of stage enables the nurse to apply the insights of Kubler-Ross without the pitfalls of viewing the five emotions as steps through which the patient and family must be guided in sequence. The nurse should remember that each of these reactions can be an adaptive coping strategy and that a key priority should be to relate to the child and family according to their particular state of mind.

The types of coping mechanisms employed by the dying child and the family tend to be those used in other life situations. Unless there are unusual circumstances, it is usually inappropriate for health care providers or family members to attempt to break down defenses or move the person to a different level or state than the one they are in. Rather, it is more appropriate for them to acknowledge the pain, offer assistance, and deal with the child and family as they are. It could be that the person has no defenses in reserve that can be applied with any skill; therefore, removing the coping mechanisms being used leaves the individual completely vulnerable.

Intellectualization Although one would not expect *intellectualization,* or the focus on facts and reason at the expense of emotion, to be a child's coping strategy, older children, adolescents, and parents might well use this method to skirt or deny the painful feelings they must face. This might be true regardless of whether the child has been raised in an intellectual environment. One form of intellectualization is to learn as much as possible about the illness and treatment. Indeed, many dying children and family members become mini-experts on the disease from which the children are suffering. This might lead to hostile interactions with the nurse, physician, or other health care staff if they do not demonstrate a similar expertise with this specific malady. The nurse should be particularly sensitive to some people's need for information and others' need to protect themselves from information. By far the biggest complaint received from children and families, however, is that they are not given enough information about the disease entity and its progress.

Fear Brantner (1970) has described three fears related to dying: darkness, pain, and the fear of being alone. Nurses can help to alleviate and in some cases eliminate these fears if they are sensitive to them. For example, a 9-year-old girl who was dying asked her sister to do a special favor for her. She had always been afraid of a darkened room, and her concern had been transferred to fear of a dark casket. She asked the sister if she would put a nightlight in her casket after her death. It was unimportant that the nightlight could not be plugged into the casket. It was an honor for the sister to pick out a nightlight and place it in the dead girl's casket.

The fear of dying alone is a universal fear for old and young alike. For example, one little boy whose father died of a heart attack was concerned about his father being all alone in the casket, so he found a wallet-sized picture of himself that had been taken at school and wrote on the back, "You're not alone, Daddy, I'm with you." He tucked it between his father's hands when he thought no one was looking. Nurses should be alert for specific ways in which young children can care for the dying family member.

The fear of pain is also universal. Sensitive pain management and comfort measures are primary priorities for the nurse, and are discussed in Chapter 29.

Kastenbaum and Aisenberg (1972) discussed fear both in relationship to death of self and the deaths of loved ones. Fears have been expressed concerning the process of dying, afterlife, and the basic fear of the unknown, extinction, or nothingness. One person said, "I am not afraid of death itself. But I am afraid of dying." Fear of personal suffering and indignity in relation to one's own death can carry over into experiencing suffering and a sense of disintegration when others are terminally ill. It is this latter part that nurses need to be aware of, not only in themselves but also in the parents and siblings of the dying child.

Belief in an afterlife is determined not only by religious faith but also by the level of cognitive development. The child who fears punishment or rejection after death or feels that the illness is a punishment will have a seriously impaired ability to cope. Siblings in particular but also parents might fear retaliation from the dead person because of some imagined culpability related to death, pain, or disfigurement.

Factors of *Individual* Awareness and Response

Stages of understanding	Stages of self-concept and perception of illness	Coping rections (can occur in any order)
1. Accepts and understands diagnosis	1. Realizes seriousness of illness	• Intellectualization • Grief • Anger
2. Understands drug names and effects	2. Believes in possibility of recovery	• Active preparation • Denial
3. Understands treatments and procedures	3. Always ill but believes in eventual recovery	• Shame • Fear • Regression
4. Sees disease as relapse/ remission	4. Always ill and will stay ill	
5. Realizes death inevitable as outcome of illness		

Finally, the basic death anxiety and all of the fears of death-related objects affect the nurse's reaction to the dying child. Death terrifies most people. The first step to overcoming that terror is to define and examine the fears that surround it. The imagination is almost always worse than the reality, and with knowledge and understanding, nurses can do a great deal to help dying children and their families to cope with their own fears.

Regression Regression usually means becoming dependent and childlike regarding the activities of daily life. Children might retreat to much earlier levels of development and become even more helpless. Although this might appear to be a poor adaptive measure to many caregivers, regression may be an extremely appropriate method of coping for some children and might even be the only one possible. The nurse assists the child to become more independent in ways that do not threaten the child's self-esteem and supports the child during the search for effective coping mechanisms at whatever developmental level.

Many children fear regression. Adolescents in particular might fear the surrender of autonomy and the return to a former, more childlike state. Lonely and in need of understanding, the adolescent might simultaneously seek the care and concern of others, especially parents, and resent and reject this support when it is offered. Perhaps because older adolescents have a more mature concept of death on both

Don't Be Afraid

Don't be afraid of what you don't understand—
There's always a reason.
Don't be afraid when your neighbor takes your hand—
Love is always in season.
If someone's lonely outside your door
Say "Come on in, we have room for more."
Don't be afraid to let love come into your life.

Walkin' along, walkin' along the street.
There's people all over.
Singin' a song, singin' a song so sweet.
You're lookin' them over.
For all God's children there's room to grow.
A stranger is a friend that you don't know.
Walkin' along, singin' a song of love.

Don't be afraid of the feeling in your heart—
Be willing to wear it.
Love is so warm you will want to pass it on
Knowing others can share it.
The world is waiting to hear your song
So sing out loud and we'll sing along!
Don't be afraid to let love come into your life!

SOURCE: From the album, *Music, Laughter and Tears*, by Deanna Edwards. Reprinted by permission of Epoch Universal Publications, 10802 N. 23 Ave., Phoenix, Arizona 85029 © 1978.

a cognitive and emotional level, they might not fear the threat of regression as acutely as the younger teenager. More secure in their self-image and less fearful of a childlike dependence, they might not need to struggle against parental love and comfort.

Denial Denial also is a useful coping strategy when the child feels overwhelmed by what is happening. When a child has shown full awareness and openness and then slips back into denial, health care personnel and the family might feel that they should discourage this retreat. Nurses should be sensitive to children's need for periodic retreats from the dying process and allow them to use denial as a coping strategy when the need arises.

In addition to various styles of coping, there are also emotional reactions to the dying process that occur both in the child and family. The reactions of anger, fear, anxiety, guilt, shame, and overt grief are common.

Anger Most children feel at least some anger against God or fate for having selected them to die young. This anger might be coupled with resentment toward others whose very lives are a reminder of the child's own imminent demise. Anger might be expressed toward nurses and health care personnel for their power and importance in dealing with the life-threatening condition.

Anger can be a common reaction among children in late childhood and adolescence because these children have begun to appreciate more concretely the possibilities of their thwarted adulthood. Teenagers in midadolescence, for instance, have just developed new self-confidence and a sense of mastery over life. A life-threatening illness can provoke anger and rage as the fulfillment of their life's promise is taken from them.

Guilt Guilt is a natural reaction to dying for many children and families. It might occur in the form of survivor guilt—why did this happen to this person I loved and not me? The dying child might look on the illness as a punishment. Parents also might feel somehow responsible for the death. Many adolescents do in fact die as a result of some transgression of society's rules regarding drugs, alcohol, and automobiles. Their behavior might have stemmed from a wish to test limits and explore their power. To them, the resulting injury and emotional trauma for themselves and their families might well seem to be deserved punishment and lead to feelings of intense guilt.

Parents also can feel guilty about not having given the child "enough"—love, understanding, material things, attention, and the like—during the short lifetime allotted. If unresolved conflicts exist between the parents and child, the burden of guilt becomes compounded.

Regardless of whether the feelings of guilt are reasonable or have any basis in fact, they should be acknowledged and worked through. Parents and children need to be told that such feelings are normal. In helping families acknowledge and deal with such feelings, the nurse can help to identify adaptive coping strategies to handle the grief process.

Shame Shame is another common reaction to dying. Bodily exposure, incontinence, and the inability to care for oneself often cause the child to feel shame, warranted or unwarranted. Adolescents in particular are concerned with body image and peer approval. They have been in the process of disengaging from parents and family and identifying more closely with their peer group. A life-threatening condition, especially if there are drastic alterations in physical appearance, might seem to be an insurmountable barrier to continuing participation in the peer group. The teenager's peers might in fact feel threatened by the dying person's situation—because death negates their own feelings of vitality, hope, and potential—and may not be available for emotional support, thus reinforcing the teenager's sense of rejection, isolation, and shame. Caregivers should be alert for shame, which is a common reaction, and be careful that their behavior and attitudes, as shown by facial expressions and gestures of withdrawal, do not increase the child's sense of shame. They also can help to alleviate the sense of shame by actively providing acceptance and support.

Grief Grief is an inevitable emotion for the dying child and the family. The dying child grieves over the loss of the future, and the family and caregivers grieve over the loss of the child. Regardless of the child's developmental level, the child will focus feelings of loss and grief on particular aspects of life. For younger children it might be a favorite activity or, more often, the relationship with family and friends; for the older child and adolescent, the focus of grief might be future plans and goals that must now be given up.

Children and parents undergo anticipatory grief in response to impending death. Fulton and Fulton (1971) discussed anticipatory grief in a poignant essay. Some grief counselors feel that anticipatory or "preparatory" grief must be handled with care. They believe that when a grieving parent experiences this emotion, the parent will be "all grieved out" when death finally occurs. Death almost always comes as a surprise, however, and the family will have a great deal more grief work to do when death actually occurs. As long as the parent and child remain open to each other, the danger of a premature leave-taking can be avoided. On the other hand, the benefit of participating in the grief experience with the child while still alive can be a more fulfilling and satisfactory resolution of the parent–child relationship, one that includes the child's own perspective and feelings and leaves fewer sources of doubt and reproach for the survivors.

It should be emphasized that whatever the specific emotions that constitute the child's reaction, it is certain that the child perceives the seriousness of the disease. Through the experience of dying, the child develops a more defined and accurate concept of death than would seem normal for the child's stage of cognitive development. Caregivers and parents will notice this development as an extremely rapid maturing process on the part of the dying child. Nurses are open to this wisdom and help parents appreciate these changes. This acceleration in development affects the communication and caregiving process and makes it imperative that the nurse be able to assess and keep pace with the child's growing understanding and interpret it to the family if needed.

Active Preparation Although children do not often have financial affairs to settle before they die, there can still be a good deal of emotional "business" to attend to. Relationships with family members or friends might contain problems that need resolution. A child can demonstrate an acceptance of impending death by actively preparing in such ways as giving away a favorite toy, writing letters to loved ones, planning the funeral arrangements, or talking about the afterlife. The reactions of others will affect the atmosphere of open communication that can make this active preparation a successful growth experience for the child.

Reactions of Others to a Child's Dying

Almost all the emotions that normally can be experienced by the dying child—fear, denial, anger, guilt, shame, and grief—are also part of the normal spectrum of reactions for those around the child. Parents, siblings, and nurses, however, often will have different reasons for experiencing these emotions. For instance, where the dying child might feel shame about an alteration in physical appearance or exclusion from the peer group, a parent might feel shame over a perceived failure in parenting, and a nurse might be ashamed of the apparent failure to provide effective care as the child's condition declines and the family's grief intensifies. It is important that the nurse not only identify the emotions felt by those around the dying child but also explore the specific bases that underlie these emotions for each individual.

Parents

"Guilt is the feeling experienced most intensely by parents" (Waechter, 1979). Parents might feel that the illness was their fault—through insufficient love, attention, or understanding. Guilt might be particularly strong if a genetic component is suspected in the child's illness. Denial is also common, a means to protect the parent from overwhelming anxiety. As a means to limit the emotional burden to what the parent can bear, denial can be an adaptive coping mechanism, but if the parent persists in denial long into the course of the child's illness, important lines of communication will break down even as the need for clear and honest communication increases.

Anger is another common reaction for the parent of a dying child. Parents might be angry at the injustice of the tragedy, at their own helplessness, at the threat to their future plans for the child, or at the disruption in their lives caused by the illness. Very often, this anger might be directed at the staff, who must recognize the roots of the parents' emotions and not get caught up in responding as if to a personal attack. Instead, health care providers accept the parents' rage and help them to deal with the feelings of impotence underlying the anger.

Guilt, denial, and anger can be particularly acute and felt for a longer time in cases of the abrupt surprise trajectory (such as the death of a teenager in a motor vehicle accident). This is related partly to the parents' feeling that they should have offered more protection or guidance. The greater intensity of these reactions also is related to "the fact that there is simply more with which to cope in a relatively shorter period. Problems also derive from the absence of the opportunity of anticipatory grief" (Gonda and Ruark, 1984).

Disruption Immeasurably more than hospitalization and chronic illness alone (see Chapters 27 and 30), a child's dying severely disrupts normal family functioning. "In many instances, the pattern of family life will be changed from the initial period of diagnosis until some time after the [child's] death, when a reorganization of family roles takes place. In some cases, the family may be completely and permanently disrupted through divorce or separation of the parents" (Waechter, 1979). The emotional, physical, and financial strain of long-term hospitalization, emergency measures, or life-support systems can be staggering and, in the absence of community or other outside resources, can increase the family's vulnerability to other problems. Even if no visible disruption takes place, the family will be altered permanently by the empty space created by the lost child.

Many clinicians have focused on the particular disruptive effects on the mother. Wong (1980) coined the phrase "empty mother syndrome" to depict the particularly disruptive effects the child's death has on the mother. While the child is dying, the mother might have severed many social relationships; postponed her career; grown somewhat apart from older children who are less dependent on her; and seen her husband withdraw into work to avoid prolonging the pain of the loss. All of this can result in a sense of having lost the mothering role, particularly for those mothers without additional, career-oriented roles outside the home. "While the other family members picked up their lives as they were before the child's death, the mother was left in the lonely, empty house without her sick child to care for, or to visit, if he had been in the hospital" (Wong, 1980).

Isolation One of the results of a child's illness and death can be a sense of isolation, both for the family as a whole with respect to the community and for each individual family member with respect to each other. Isolation from the community is a natural result of the time and energy devoted exclusively to the care of the dying child. Friends and neighbors, even if they wish to be supportive, might not be sure how best to express their concern and may fear that their efforts to help will be considered intrusions. Community members also might fear the pain that emotional involvement in the family's crisis may bring and refrain from offering the support that would lead to that involvement.

Parents also might drift apart from each other in the face of the child's dying. The intense grief that each parent feels individually can obscure the fact that the other parent is also in great pain. If the parent's coping strategy is to avoid sources of pain as much as possible, withdrawal from the other partner might be an important, albeit unconscious, need. Finally, the ongoing stress of the family's crisis can throw up barriers, such as overloaded schedules, emotional turmoil, fear of another pregnancy, guilt about feeling pleasure, or simple fatigue, to the couple's sexual intimacy, thereby reinforcing each parent's sense of isolation. In fact, for parents, "the ability to again enjoy intimate relations seems to be one milestone in resolving grief" (Wong, 1980).

Siblings

It is important to be aware of the reactions of siblings to a child's death. The nurse must deal not only with the dying child's feelings but also must be aware of vital interactions with all members of the family.

Children frequently see death on television as a result of guns, bombs, or other forms of violence. A sense of unreality sets in, however, because the aftermath of death and its effect on the family rarely are shown on television. Children get used to seeing their favorite actors and actresses or cartoon characters "die" and instantly reappear or show up in other programs. Consequently, they develop a sense of unreality about death and cannot believe that it will strike them personally or strike someone they love.

Just like the dying child, the sibling understands death in a way that is related to the level of cognitive development. The dying child, however, can quickly gain a fuller and more mature concept of death. Even children who are not told about the nature and extent of their illness gain an awareness they are reluctant to share in the presence of adult fears. Without this firsthand experience, siblings of the dying child are more likely to continue understanding in ways appropriate to their cognitive level. It is important for the nurse to keep this disparity in mind in adjusting the style and content of communication to the needs and understanding of the various children regarding counseling, comfort, and care.

Siblings also might experience a deprivation of parental time and may be aware of economic and other pressures that have resulted from a brother's or sister's illness. Siblings might be left in the care of extended family members. In their preoccupation with the sick child, parents might neglect the routine needs of the siblings. Older children might be assigned additional household tasks, or the dying child might be granted a special request, such as a trip, which the siblings also might desire. All of these possible reactions often cause jealousy and resentment in siblings, which would seem natural but also could cause guilt feelings in the surviving siblings if they feel their own destructive wishes are selfish or contribute to the dying child's death. As mentioned earlier, even older, seemingly mature children are capable of believing their wishes or actions in some way contributed to the death of another. In addition to feelings of guilt and jealousy, siblings might respond to parental deprivation in many other ways, including hostility toward the ill child, acting out in ways that cause discipline and performance problems at home or in school, and other dysfunctional behaviors. Nurses who are sensitive to these possibilities can gain insight into the sibling's problems, help the sibling express and accept the feelings, and work with others, such as the school nurse or teacher, to develop a support system for the sibling.

Another reaction common to the siblings of the dying child is to feel left out, vulnerable, and caught up in their own grief experiences. Often, they are home attempting to live as normally as possible with one or both parents absent. Both their routines and emotions are in turmoil, however, and they need a great deal of support from parents and the health care team.

It should be recognized that siblings, too, can play a supportive role in the child's dying. Especially if the trajectory of death is sudden, the siblings should be given time together with the child before death occurs. Siblings should not be made to feel helpless but should be encouraged to develop feelings of strength and support and should be given the opportunity to participate in the process of the child's dying and to help ease the child's death in whatever ways they are capable of. Nurses can work with parents to help siblings keep their connection to the dying child by creating vehicles to collect memories while the child is still alive—a photo album or other collaborative project, for instance. Siblings also should be allowed to participate in funeral arrangements and the service itself, if they wish to. The nurse can make an invaluable contribution by helping siblings to find their own way of saying good-bye.

A Sibling's Grief

Deanna Edwards conducted a MAKE TODAY COUNT workshop in Council Bluffs, Iowa. The panel consisted of children who were there to teach the participants what it was like to lose a brother or sister. At the end of the table sat a freckled-faced, sandy-haired boy about 8 years old. When the microphone came to him, he picked it up and tried to speak but the tears cascaded down his cheeks. She took him into the sunshine for a walk, and as soon as they walked outside he blurted, "It's my fault my brother died. I killed him!"

Thinking that was a heavy burden for such a young child to carry, she asked him how his brother died. He told her he died of leukemia. When she asked why he felt he had killed his brother, he said, "Because I used to fight with him a lot and I used to wish bad things would happen to him."

Deanna told him she had little boys who fought so much she couldn't get a word in edgewise and that he should be proud that he treated his brother like "one of the guys." She said, "Your brother would not want to be treated differently because he was sick."

The little boy explained that no one at home seemed to want to talk about his brother. Deanna told him that might change because his mother was in the audience.

He suddenly turned to Deanna and said, "There is something I have to say to the audience."

Returning to the workshop, he marched up in front of the audience alone, picked up the microphone, and in a loud voice said, "I just wanted to say I loved my brother."

After this short but beautiful sermon, the participants in the workshop became the boy's substitute brothers, and he was able to let them know that, in spite of fights and quarrels, he had loved his brother very much.

The Nurse

Nurses are not exempted from being human by their training and experience. The nurse's reactions to the death of a child are influenced by cultural background, professional training, and personal and religious philosophies. The cultural background will affect both the manner of response and the ability to express emotional reactions. Although cultural groups differ in their emotional responses to crisis and loss, all cultures share the same feelings of grief and love.

Adams (1984) suggested six variables that play an important part in how nurses react to a dying patient:

- The length of hospitalization
- The frequency of admissions
- The role of the family
- The condition of the child when admitted
- The child's coping style
- The role of the nurse's subconscious

Any one of these factors can affect the way a nurse feels about the dying child and family. The nurse whose feelings seem to block effective communication and nursing care therefore might find it helpful to examine any or all of these variables as possible sources of the problem.

The child's trajectory of death also can affect the nurse's reaction and in particular the intensity of the nurse's grief. Extended involvement with a terminally ill child might make the nurse's grieving more intense than a quick death in an emergency room or a death caused by SIDS. This more intense grief might allow the nurse, on the one hand, to empathize more fully with the family members, or it may be so self-absorbing as to block the nurse's emotional availability to the survivors in need of care.

Mandel (1981) identified some concerns that nurses felt most strongly in dealing with dying patients, including being overwhelmed, overidentification, and avoidance.

Being Overwhelmed Just as one cannot look at the sun all the time, one cannot look at death all the time. In areas of hospital care where death and severe illness are a part of the daily care pattern, particularly the intensive care unit, an oncology unit, a medical research unit, and emergency rooms, nurses can find themselves victims of emotional depletion. In these surroundings great human and

The Surrogate Sufferer

We are tempted in all areas of the helping professions to become surrogate sufferers, attempting to alleviate the victims' suffering by shouldering some of the pain. A pervasive pattern in caregiving among professionals and nonprofessionals alike, it encompasses all attempts to shield persons subject to care from painful or otherwise difficult experiences. An attempt to run interference on pain, it is a well-intentioned strategy; tragically, however, the intention is seldom, perhaps never, realized. Can one cry the tears for another? Do the grief work for another? Solve the problems for another? True professionals do not solve the problems of others. They assist others in solving their own problems.

The "surrogate suffering syndrome" is rooted in feelings of helplessness. Both those in need and those trying to help are subject to such feelings. Both struggle with what to say and do. Both seek ways of functioning meaningfully in the face of tragedy. Both are groping for control. By saying, "Let me do this for you," we mitigate our own sense of helplessness. We feel better having "helped." Those needing help are left passive, uninvolved spectators to the drama of life, and their feelings of helplessness are not addressed.

The alternative mode in caregiving is to help sufferers to function for themselves. Such an approach mitigates the helplessness of both the sufferer and the caregiver. The result is increased feelings of competence and satisfaction among caregivers as they succeed in helping those in their care to function meaningfully. . . . True professionals do not solve problems for others, nor do they protect and shield from truth. They assist others as others solve their own problems.

SOURCE: Adapted from Dr. Glen Davidson, Roy Nichols and Tom Attig, The Pastor's Letter 4(1) (Nov) 1982; Watts RG (editor).

technologic resources are being devoted to keeping the child alive. The nurse can very easily take the child's death as a personal loss and individual failure (Woods, 1984). Those nurses who have not become familiar with their own fears and feelings might find themselves changing to a new area of nursing or leaving the profession altogether. Others might stay but find themselves terribly unhappy in their careers. Some nurses feel that nursing shifts should be shortened in these areas of care to help prevent the consequences to any individual who is feeling overwhelmed.

Overidentification Faced with the immense physical pain and emotional suffering associated with a child's dying, the nurse might be tempted to do more than supply the necessary palliative care, attempting to shoulder some of the child's and family's burden of grief as well. This reaction, called the *surrogate sufferer syndrome,* runs counter to optimal self-care goals for the child and family because it further deprives them of autonomy in a setting in which little autonomy is left them to begin with. The natural tendency to identify strongly with the dying child, especially if the nurse is close in age to a dying adolescent, might in part be responsible for the surrogate sufferer reaction.

Avoidance Another response to death is an attempt to become immune to personal feelings and reactions. Nurses frequently hide behind technology and focus on children who are cured, thus blocking the pain of involvement with those who die. Pain is inherent in any meaningful relationship. There are times when it is necessary to build temporary walls of protection, but when those walls become impenetrable, the nurse loses some of the sensitivity needed to deal with dying patients. Patients might become objects rather than persons. A great deal of emotional risk is involved in letting patients know that nurses care about them as well as for them.

The most effective building material for emotional walls is fear. A nurse who is simply afraid to become involved might label any human response to the dying patient "unprofessional" or "inappropriate." Although objectivity is vital in terminal care, the nurse who suppresses feelings might find emotional hardness blocking successful interaction with the dying patient. Patients might not be interested in how much the nurse will do for them until they know how much the nurse cares. Nurses can also tend to avoid another nurse who is grieving for a dying or deceased child. Busy nursing units do not stop or slow down to facilitate the sharing of grief, and it is easy to leave a crying or intensely sad nurse alone. The caring nurse might feel lonely indeed despite the presence of well-meaning coworkers.

Personal Growth A more positive response to working with dying children is the powerful and rewarding sense of personal growth. Through working with dying children, nurses might restructure their priorities and develop stronger value systems. Human relationships can become more precious, and the nurse's ability to communicate honestly can be enhanced. In addition to the care, feeding, and administration of medication, the nurse becomes more committed to friendship, trust, and interaction. For a dying child, the spiritual, emotional, and physical touch of another person can make the journey into the unknown more bearable. For nurses who work with dying children, facilitating that journey becomes a special privilege, and their own lives might become enriched rather than depleted by the process.

The death of a child can make nurses aware of their own mortality and vulnerability. It is impossible to deny this awareness when touched by the death of a young child, who is supposed to be strong, beautiful, and healthy. Denying this awareness might push it to a subconscious level that hampers the nurse's response to dying children.

If the nurse has hidden fears and unresolved feelings, they usually will be picked up by the child. Some nurses who are afraid of their own mortality might view death as "contagious" in some way and may be repulsed by the dying child. This repulsion and withdrawal will affect the nurse–child relationship adversely and damage the child's self-concept. Nurses who look at beauty from the inside out and who have faced their own fears can help the child who has experienced dramatic physical changes to feel beautiful and whole. Hugs and smiles are reassuring to a frightened child. Weight loss, loss of hair, physical disfigurement, or swelling of tissues can be dealt with better by a child who has been made to feel beautiful by a caring and sensitive nurse.

Influence of Culture

How others react to a child's dying will depend on a great many factors, including the child's own experiences in the process of dying. Culture is one vitally important factor that affects both the process of death and grieving and the care that the nurse is able to give. "Competent nursing care demands a commitment to helping clients and their families as they try to realize life and death experiences that are in accordance with their personal and cultural values" (Ross, 1981).

A variety of cultural factors can affect the nurse's interactions with the dying child and the family. Perhaps the most important factor is the extreme emphasis that American culture places on youth, as evidenced, for instance, in advertising. A seriously ill or dying child is something of a contradiction in an environment where vigor, success, and physical attractiveness are identified so exclusively with the young.

Consistent with the emphasis on youth is the American uneasiness about death, especially where children are concerned. Whereas the mainstream of American culture tends to shield children from the realities of death, some cultures, such as the Samoan, Amish, Native American, and Mexican-American cultures, allow children to participate actively in terminal care, funerals, and mourning practices (Ross, 1981).

As with the child's and family's response to care in nonterminal situations, failure to cooperate with medical and nursing treatments might reflect the family's cultural realities rather than willfulness or perversity. Attention to the family's cultural views of health and illness is an important nursing concern. (See Chapter 3 for an overview of various cultural perspectives and particularly Table 3-1 for specific details of different cultural perceptions of death.)

Culture also will affect the nurse's and family's expressions of grief. Cultural traditions might specify quite precisely not only the length and program of the grieving process but also the intensity of grief expressed. Some ethnic communities support the family by helping family members to control their bereavement and forget the loss, whereas others might try to help the family to express and experience its grief more fully (Ross, 1981). If the nurse has trouble understanding or responding to the family's expression of grief, talking to staff members more informed about different cultural styles can be beneficial (Adams, 1984).

In applying cultural knowledge to an individual family, however, the nurse should be wary of relying on cultural stereotypes and remain sensitive to uniqueness and variability. Not all people from a given ethnic group will subscribe to that group's cultural standards with the same intensity or commitment.

Elements of Nursing Care

As with other facets of the care of children, the nurse may assume a variety of roles in terminal care, including primary care provider, child and family advocate, patient teacher, and counselor. The nurse might be of increasing assistance to the child and family, in fact, as medicine and technology have less to offer. One physician remarked, "Nurses not only may be more vital to the quality of care received by terminally ill patients, but also may be more likely than physicians to possess the expertise to be authoritative" (Gonda and Ruark, 1984). The nurse is also in an excellent position to make referrals for the family and identify community resources such as support groups and community-based health services.

With a child who is expected to die, as opposed to one who is expected to recover, the nurse's goals shift in focus from the restoration of health to the promotion of comfort, with the first priority being attention to the child's physical needs. If the nurse cannot adjust to this modification of goals, feelings of helplessness, frustration, anger, and guilt can result. Recognizing and overcoming these feelings can free the nurse to pursue the primary goals of providing comfort and hope for the dying child and the family.

Assessment

The nursing assessment of the dying child and the family covers many of the concerns already discussed in this chapter, including:

1. *The child's understanding of the illness, treatment, and prognosis as well as the child's concept of death.* These parameters are established as a baseline that underlies all other assessments. Information may come from the child or family or both.

2. *The normal coping mechanisms and support systems of the child and family.* Discussing feelings surrounding difficult procedures affords an opportunity to explore the family's ability to cope with the larger crisis posed by the child's severe illness.

3. *The specific details of family functioning and any special risk factors, as well as the effects of the child's condition on the family.* Examples of additional risk factors include single parents, families who live elsewhere, families with another ill member, and families with other young children or infants (Williams, Rivara, and Rothenberg, 1981). The initial nursing assessment of the family therefore should include attention to these points:

- financial resources of the family, measured against the costs of the child's illness
- marital stress
- medical or psychosocial problems in family members other than the dying child
- the family's usual support system in other crises and its effectiveness
- the community resources used by the family
- the potential resources and supports available to the family
- the openness of communication between parents or between parents and other family members
- the parent's predominant reactions such as denial, anger, or guilt
- whether the parent tends to become isolated from other family members, social support systems, or other potential sources of help. (Additional information regarding family assessment and special risk factors is presented in Chapters 17 and 22.)

4. *The family's cultural perspective.* Any religious and moral beliefs that might affect the family's experience of illness, death, and grief should be assessed and taken into account so that the comfort, guidance, and support offered by the nurse can be presented in a way that is most likely to be accepted.

Communication

The complex and intense emotions that surround the dying child and family can make communication difficult among all the people involved—child, family members, and health care workers. It is precisely in this situation, however, where honest and sensitive communication skills are most needed. The hospital setting can be rushed, chaotic, and distracting, causing the child and family to feel more bewildered and fearful than they are already. Nurses and other health care workers can help to create a relatively relaxed and unpressured atmosphere when dealing with patients, thus reducing the stress on children and families and allowing them calm moments in which to come to grips with their situation and resolve unfinished emotional business.

Especially in the limited amount of time imposed by a terminal illness, poor communication between the child and family can delay the necessary resolution of family problems and relationships until it is literally too late. Over and above the normal grief that survivors can expect to feel, an added burden of guilt and regret can result from unexpressed feelings or unresolved conflicts. Poor communication between the nurse and child or between the nurse and family also can have the following undesirable consequences (Gonda and Ruark, 1984):

- Mistrust
- A sense of powerlessness
- Anger
- Feelings of isolation and abandonment
- Failure to attend to important business

Sometimes the failure to communicate fully, openly, and honestly might stem from a wish to protect the child. Children should not be sheltered more than necessary, however, from either the fact of death or the feelings of grief that surround it. Although the clinical facts may be difficult for the nurse to communicate or for the child to bear, it is important to reassure the child who must deal with these feelings that the emotional security and physical care the child looks for from the parent or other caregiver will not cease because of the crisis. Attempts to protect clients from the truth may in any case be ineffective because children and parents both will very likely sense the nurse's true feelings, even if the nurse wishes to disguise them. Honesty is thus an important component of effective communication for both nurses and parents.

In communicating with the child about death, Gonda and Ruark (1984) proposed three guiding principles: (1) avoid lying; (2) let the child determine how much to say at a particular moment; and (3) tailor the content of the communication as closely as possible to an accurate assessment of the child's concept of death. Nurses also can provide parents with guidelines for discussing death with children. Two specific guidelines to stress are (1) do not say death was the will of God or some other superior being because this might engender hostile feelings toward the deity; and (2) do not associate death with sleep because children may learn to fear going to bed and falling asleep (Sheer, 1977; Hutton, 1981).

In all interactions that the nurse might have with the child and family members, reflecting feelings "is perhaps the communication skill that is most specific to the care of the terminally ill" (Gonda and Ruark, 1984). *Reflecting feelings* is a kind of paraphrase of the client's emotion as expressed in word or deed. Judicious use of this communication skill can (1) validate and support the child's feelings; (2) clarify the feeling, which the child might have denied or failed to identify; and (3) encourage the child to explore the feeling, its bases, and its consequences without fear that the nurse is sitting in judgment. The paraphrase should be based on

Children's Books About Death

Bach A: Mollie Make-Believe. Harper & Row, 1974
Bartoli J: Nonna. Harvey House, 1975
Beckman G: Admission to the Feast. Holt, Rinehart, 1979
Bond N: The String in the Harp. Atheneum, 1976
Caines JF: Abby. Harper & Row, 1973
Carner C: Tawny. Macmillan, 1978
Carrick C: The Accident. Seabury, 1976
Center for Attitudinal Healing: There is a Rainbow Behind Every Cloud. Celestial Arts, 1978
Cleaver V, Cleaver B: Grover. Lippincott, 1970
Cohen B: Thank You, Jackie Robinson. Lothrop, 1974
Coutant H: The First Snow. Knopf, 1974
Craven M: I Heard the Owl Call My Name. Doubleday, 1973
DePaola T: Nana Upstairs and Nana Downstairs. Putnam, 1973
Donovan J: Wild in the World. Harper & Row, 1971
Farley C: The Garden is Doing Fine. Atheneum, 1975
Fassler J: The Boy with a Problem. Behavioral Publications, 1971
Fassler J: My Grandpa Died Today. Gerontology Series, Behavioral Publications, 1971
Frederick RW: Charlie's Moment of Truth. Angel Creations, 1980
George JC: Julie of the Wolves. Harper & Row, 1972
Greene C: Beat the Turtle Drum. Viking, 1976
Grollman EA: Talking About Death. Beacon Press, 1971
Guest J: Ordinary People. Viking, 1976
Hall L: Shadows. Follett, 1977
Harris A: Why Did He Die? Lerner Press, 1970
Hunter M: The Sound of Chariots. Harper & Row, 1972
Jones R: The Acorn People. Bantam Books, 1977
Kaplan B: The Empty Chair. Harper, 1978
Klein N: Sunshine. Avon, 1974
Lee, M: Fog. Seabury, 1972
Lorenzo CL: Mama's Ghosts. Harper & Row, 1974
Lund D: Eric. Lippincott, 1974
Mann P: There Are Two Kinds of Terrible. Doubleday, 1977
Mathis S: The Hundred Penny Box. Viking, 1975
Miles M: Annie and the Old One. Little, Brown, 1971
Moe B: Pickles and Prunes. McGraw-Hill, 1976
Mohr N: Nilda. Harper & Row, 1973
Morris J: Brian Piccolo: A Short Season. Random House, 1971
Parks, G: The Learning Tree. Norton, 1978
Paulus T: Hope for the Flowers. Paulist Press, 1972
Peck, R: Dreamland Lake. Holt, Rinehart, 1973
Rabin G: Changes. Harper & Row, 1973
Rinaldo CL: Dark Dreams. Harper & Row, 1974
Rock G: The Thanksgiving Treasure. Knopf, 1974
Scopperttone S: Trying Hard to Hear You. Harper & Row, 1974
Smith D: A Taste of Blackberries. Crowell, 1973
Stanek M: I Won't Go Without a Father. Albert Whitman, 1972
Steig W: Amos and Boris. Farrar, Straus & Giroux, 1971, and Penguin Books, 1977
Stolz M: The Edge of New Year. Harper & Row, 1974
Tobias T: Petey. Putnam, 1978
Vavra R: The Lion & Blue. Reynal, 1974
Viorst J: The Tenth Good Thing About Barney. Atheneum, 1971
Waber B: Ira Sleeps Over. Houghton Mifflin, 1972
Warburg SS: Growing Time. Houghton Mifflin, 1969
Windsor P: The Summer Before. Harper & Row, 1973
Winthrop E: Walking Away. Harper & Row, 1973
Zolotow C: A Father Like That. Harper & Row, 1971

specific verbal and nonverbal cues and not simply a wild guess. The nurse should in any case phrase the reflected feelings in such a way as to allow the child room to clarify or correct the nurse's interpretation.

Conversation is not the only useful medium of communication, especially with younger children, whose cognitive development might not support verbal skills equal to the complexity of the experience through which they are living. Various activities, including play and reading aloud, can provide the context and direction for an open exploration of the child's feelings and concerns. Reading and discussing a book together can be an excellent means of broaching the subject of death with the child and assessing the child's level of understanding (Sheer, 1977).

Music can be another way of expressing emotions and communication for the child. Because our society tends to deny death and pain, popular music does not often deal with the problems of dying. If the nurse is uncertain about a child's readiness to accept or understand the illness, a tape can be given to the child containing a variety of songs, including songs about dying. The songs the child listens to often and comments on will most likely reflect that child's readiness. Dying children who have strong adult support systems usually cultivate lively senses of humor and startlingly candid outlooks. Experiences in music therapy can help a child feel free to express laughter and tears.

Art is another invaluable mode of communication in working with dying children. In her books and lectures,

Kubler-Ross reported the insights gained by dying children who were given the opportunity to express their feelings through art (Kubler-Ross, 1969). One funeral director, for instance, makes sure he has crayons and paper in his funeral home for grieving children to explore their feelings. Dying children should be given frequent opportunities through painting, drawing, and sculpting to express their feelings. As the child develops art into a form of communication, the nurse or therapist might need to respond to the child in the same language. The sensitive pictures nurses draw for children can be a very helpful form of communication.

Assisting Grief

Especially when death is known to be the inevitable outcome for the child, assisting the child and family "with the resolution of emotional issues may constitute the most concrete help that professionals have to offer" (Gonda and Ruark, 1984). Nurses can facilitate the grieving process by providing opportunities for the expression of emotions, helping children and parents to anticipate and master these emotions, and providing an objective presence when these emotions become overwhelming.

Nurses have feelings of their own that they need to accept and work through before attempting to respond to the intense grief of others. When they understand their own emotions and the normal emotions inherent in a situation, nurses will be better able to reassure the child and family and handle aggressive feelings, such as anger, when they are misdirected at the health care staff. In response to the anger of the ill child, the nurse can provide outlets for the child's rage and reaffirm the child's self-control and sense of worth.

Once nurses have explored and understood their own emotions, they can begin to help others take command of theirs. The nurse should not judge feelings or attempt to console by saying, "You shouldn't feel guilty." This will simply add the weight of self-judgment to the child's or family's already heavy emotional burden. Rather, the nurse offers reassurance that such feelings are a normal part of the grief process and will become manageable with the passage of time and with their verbal expression, and encourages the child and family to focus on needs and specific problems in the present.

At critical moments, grief might become especially acute, and the hospital can provide a special room where feelings can be expressed without restraint. Particularly at the time of the child's death, the nurse should help ensure the family's privacy "to protect them while they absorb the shock, and to facilitate emotional closure" (Williams, Rivara, and Rothenberg, 1981). It should be remembered, however, that grief is a lifelong process. Although families do regain their equilibrium and precrisis level of functioning, they never cease to miss the dead child or mourn the loss in some way.

The death of an infant can pose special problems for the grieving process because the family might feel a vacuum as a result of not completing attachment. Detachment from the dead infant might be problematic when the attachment process was incomplete. Nurses can encourage the family to have as much contact as possible with the infant both while alive and after death. "Having had some opportunity for direct involvement and being certain of what their baby was actually like, parents may then be better able to cope with the pain of their loss" (Thomas and Cordell, 1983). Wooten (1981) suggested that parents of terminally ill infants be given a chance to do the following:

- Touch and hold the infant while alive
- Photograph the infant before or after death
- Discuss funeral arrangements
- Be present at the time of the infant's death
- Touch, hold, and even bathe the infant after death

Peer Support

For all those involved in a child's dying—the child, family members, and health professionals—support by other people who are experiencing or have experienced similar situations can provide a kind of emotional assistance that cannot be obtained from any other source.

Support groups of parents who have lost their children can help newly bereaved parents express their grief, share it with others who will understand, and eventually to put it in perspective. Nurses can be instrumental in referring parents to these support groups. "The goal of parents who attend the group meetings is to come to terms with the pain of their loss and to gain mastery over the difficult feelings involved, as they cherish memories of their baby and their parenthood" (Thomas and Cordell, 1983).

Parents should not assume that their friends and neighbors are unwilling to help or incapable of doing so. Some friends and relatives may in fact be too uneasy around the circumstances of dying to offer any real help, but others might only be waiting for a signal that an offer of help will not be perceived as an intrusion on the family's grief. Some people may go so far as to ask the advice of health professionals who are in a position to notice what the family's special needs might be. The nurse thus might be able to suggest to a concerned neighbor, for instance, the need for an afternoon of child care for a young sibling of the dying child or for assistance with housekeeping or cooking. Such concrete assistance often might be a welcome substitute for the awkwardness of "not knowing what to say" and can bolster parents by letting them know that their friends, relatives, and neighbors are there for them.

Support for siblings and other peers of the dying child is an important nursing concern. Especially in cases of remission, the dying child might continue to interact with healthy children, perhaps even with classmates in the school

Support Resources for Children, Parents, and Nurses*

American Cancer Society: 777 Third Avenue, New York, NY 10019; (212) 371–2900.
The Candlelighters Foundation: Suite 1011, 2025 Eye Street NW, Washington, DC 20006; (202) 659–5136.
The Compassionate Friends, Inc.: PO Box 1347, Oak Brook, IL 60521; (312) 323–5010.
Concern for Dying: 250 West 57th Street, New York, NY 10019; (212) 246–6962.
Council of Guilds for Infant Survival: 923 Central Park Avenue, Davenport, IA 52804; (319) 322-4870.
Make Today Count: National Office, PO Box 303, Burlington, IA 52601; (319) 753–6521.
National Hospice Organization: 1901 North Fort Mier Drive, Suite 402, Arlington, VA 22209; (703) 243–5900.
National Sudden Infant Death Syndrome Foundation: Two Metro Plaza, Suite 205, 8240 Professional Place, Landover, MD 20785; (301) 459–3388.
Parents of Murdered Children: 1739 Bella Vista, Cincinnati, OH 45237; (513) 242–8025.
Resolve, Inc.: PO Box 474, Belmont, MA 02178; (617) 484–2424.
SHARE: St. John's Hospital, 800 East Carpenter Street, Springfield, IL 62769; (217) 544–6464.

*For a directory that describes organizations that help bereaved families, please consult Part II of Donnelly KF: *Recovering From the Loss of a Child*. Macmillan, 1982.

setting. It is essential that these healthy children be informed and supported as they watch their friend die. Helping them learn to support each other is a primary goal. Coordination with the school nurse or community health nurse is an obvious strategy to achieve this kind of peer support.

The dying child also can benefit from interacting with other seriously ill children. A child's socialization needs do not cease upon admission to the hospital or confinement to a bed at home. Roommates of similar ages and interests can help meet each other's social needs. Children with the same disease can develop close bonds based on their common experiences, fears, and frustrations. Nurses will wish to monitor such relationships as they develop, not only to measure the psychosocial benefits to each child but also to watch for any health risks such as possible exposure to respiratory and other infections.

Two girls, 9 and 10 years of age, shared a room in the hospital. Both were scheduled to have heart surgery on the same morning. Both surgeries were considered high risk. As the 9-year-old girl left for the operating room, she said to the other child, "Well, if I don't see you tonight, I'll see you in heaven." Both giggled nervously at the comment. The 10-year-old girl died during her surgery. As far as the parents or nurses knew, the girls had not spoken to anyone of their fear of surgery. However, the 9-year-old later confided that on the night before the surgery, the two had talked of their fear of dying and promised to "look for each other in heaven" if they did die. (Example supplied by Gayle Olsen.)

The nurse can be instrumental in promoting friendships between individual children and should recognize the potential benefits of such associations.

Peer Support for the Dying Child

Deanna Edwards was asked to visit with Doug, a little boy of great strength and humor, who had been diagnosed as having a malignant brain tumor.

Doug had been transferred to a hospital far from home where a physician's research seemed to hold out new hope. Because of the tumor's rapid growth and spread, however, Doug was not selected for treatment. Doug understood the implications of this decision, but instead of despairing, he directed his attention to the unit's other dying children, in particular to a little boy named Jimmy, who spent his days in bed, curled up in a fetal position, and waiting for death to come. His parents were divorced and rarely came to see him. Jimmy refused to eat, speak to staff members or visitors, or smile. Living with a life-threatening illness had become too great a burden for Jimmy, who was in effect dying alone.

Doug crept into Jimmy's room one day, and after he emerged, Jimmy was smiling again. Emerging from his shell of isolation, Jimmy began to ask for food, communicate with the staff, and become more physically active.

Deanna asked Doug if he could remember what he had said to Jimmy that made such a difference.

Doug blinked long lashes over blue eyes and said modestly, "Oh, nothing much. I told him I had a brain tumor just like his and that if he had any unfinished business to take care of—any special things he wanted to do—that I would be happy to help him. I told him I had lots of candy bars in my room, and if he was ever hungry, he could have some of my candy bars. I also said, 'Jimmy, if you ever feel like crying, why don't you come into my room and we'll cry together.' The last thing I told him was, 'Don't be afraid to die, Jimmy. I'm not afraid.' "

But Doug's voice hesitated as he confessed, "To tell you the truth, Deanna, I am kind of scared because I've never had any experience!"

Lastly, nurses should not neglect their own self-care needs. In addition to the individual coping strategies that each nurse develops to deal with the highly stressful atmosphere of death and dying, mutual support and collaboration among health professionals are essential for maintaining an appropriate level of emotional involvement without losing sensitivity. Such support can be formalized into regular group meetings of concerned staff members to discuss the various issues, frustrations, and problems that they face. Regular peer support can lead to greater awareness, reassurance, and emotional resiliency for the nurse. Professional relationships based on mutual trust and support also will help to keep channels of communication open among the various health care team members, resulting in more organized and effective care for the child and family. "Coordination is one key and compassion the other to optimal care and support for the family of the dying child" (Williams, Rivara, and Rothenberg, 1981).

Home Care

One option for terminal care that parents might wish to consider is caring for the child at home. Martinson and colleagues (1977; 1978) pioneered nursing research in this area. Although there are undoubtedly many advantages to home care, the choice might not be for everyone, and the nurse will have to help each family to make the best decision for them. This in turn means giving the family as much information about home care as possible and supporting whatever decision is reached.

Many of the advantages of home care stem from having the family physically in one place rather than dividing them between the hospital and the home. The isolation and separation that this division causes are thus diminished. Siblings can have more of their normal needs taken care of by parents instead of others, and their responses to the situation can be observed and discussed more frequently, which helps to prevent normal feelings of resentment or guilt from becoming destructive. The entire family can participate more fully in the care of the ill child, thus lessening the physical burden on any one individual. Most importantly, perhaps, the greater amount of time spent together in the familiar environment of home will give family members more opportunities to resolve unfinished emotional business, to deepen their relationship with the child, and to adjust their role relationships in response to the child's illness and eventual death.

Home care also allows the child and family a greater sense of independence and responsibility, thereby reducing feelings of helplessness. While parents and other family members can reassert their control over their disrupted routines and environment, thus creating a more normal atmosphere, the ill child can assume a greater role in self-care activities such as feeding and administering medications. This sense of self-reliance can be particularly important for adolescents.

In addition, home care can significantly affect the family's readjustment following the child's death. One study (Lauer, et al., 1983) suggested that parents who provide home care for the child are less likely to need professional mental health services or maintain feelings of denial or guilt to the point of developing pathologic grief reactions. Parents who care for the child at home appear better able to confront the realities of the situation and work through their guilt feelings as a result of being more fully involved in the child's care. Marital relations, instead of deteriorating, often are enhanced by the experience of caring for the child together because many parents find that the home care experience "deepened their respect for each other, facilitated communication by causing fewer separations, and enabled them to recognize each others' strengths more fully" (Lauer, et al., 1983).

Many factors can influence the decision to care for the child at home, and the nurse has an important responsibility to help the family make the most informed choice possible and the one most suited to their physical and emotional resources. The family might not even have considered home care as a possibility, so it may be up to the health professional to broach the subject. In helping the family to decide, the nurse needs to make sure that they understand what to expect in the way of symptoms—such as vomiting, choking, or diarrhea—and that they feel capable of handling the care of such symptoms. Parents and nurses together need to assess the family's readiness to shoulder the physical, mental, and emotional weight of providing the needed comfort and physical care to the dying child while maintaining the household and normal family function. If parents and other family members have been participating in the care given in the hospital, this might indicate their readiness to do the same at home.

Home care does not mean an end to professional involvement in the child's care. On the contrary, home care requires careful coordination among community and hospital-based professionals to provide the backup, consultation, and additional personnel needed to implement a plan of care at home. Full medical support, 24-hour access to nursing services, spiritual counseling, and lay support from relatives, friends, or hospice volunteers are all important components of a viable home care program. The parents must be clear about exactly what services they can rely on so that they can pursue the tasks of caring with as much confidence as possible. They also need to be aware of the option of rehospitalization should the physical or emotional stress, especially in the final stages of the child's life, prove too much to bear. Every nurse has the opportunity to encourage home care for those families who find it appropriate. (See Chapter 26 for a further discussion of home care.) Although home care and hospice are by no means synonymous, they share a humanistic, supportive philosophy.

Hospice

There is some question whether hospice refers to a group of people, a place, or an idea. For the purposes of this discussion, it is useful to concur with Dobihal (1980) that "it is possible to apply hospice principles and philosophy wherever someone is dying." In the minds of some authorities, hospice may be associated exclusively with the terminally ill adult and not with the dying child. "Hospices are unfortunately not getting referrals of children, because many health care professionals believe that any child who has parents needs no other help. . . . [N]othing could be further from the truth" (Kubler-Ross, 1983). In fact, there is nothing inherent in the hospice philosophy that makes it incompatible with the care of the dying child, and actual pediatric hospice programs have shown that the principles can be applied in a structured way to the terminal care of children (Miller, 1982; Burne, 1984).

The hospice concept has much in common with the goals of nursing. In both settings the patient is seen as a complete person with spiritual, emotional, and social needs and as part of a family whose other members are also the nurse's charge (MacElveen-Hoehn and McIntosh, 1981). The primary features of hospice care reveal much that is similar to the goals of home care:

1. Both the family and patient constitute the unit of care and caregiving.
2. Comfort, referring to the alleviation of physical, emotional, psychologic, and spiritual pain, is a primary goal.
3. An interdisciplinary team that includes the child and family plans and implements care. Medical backup is particularly important because the psychosocial care offered to the client might be ineffective if physical care needs are not attended to first.
4. Support is made available to the client at all times.
5. Trained volunteers may assist in achieving hospice goals.
6. Bereavement and follow-up care are provided.
7. Support for care providers themselves is an important part of the concept (MacElveen-Hoehn and McIntosh, 1981).

A hospice program can take a variety of forms, one of which is a physical place, with a staff, that offers inpatient residential care (Burne, 1984). Other programs offer home care exclusively to terminally ill patients and might include nurses as part of an interdisciplinary staff or may contract for nursing personnel through home health agencies. Hospitals might develop their own hospice programs and choose to designate a unit or a number of beds for this purpose or to form an interdisciplinary team that functions as a resource for terminally ill patients throughout the hospital (MacElveen-Hoehn and McIntosh, 1981).

Hospice can be a way of making home care possible. Especially when the family is subject to other stresses, such as single parenthood, other young children, or other ill family members, the support provided by a hospice program can extend the family's physical, emotional, and spiritual resources to meet the demands of terminal care. Even if only providing respite care for the parents—managing household responsibilities so that the parents can run other errands or attend to their own self-care needs—hospice can render a vital service to the entire family.

> Hospice volunteers will come in and do housework, cook meals ahead for the family, or just pick and arrange a bouquet of flowers to make the home more cheerful. They allow the mother more time for the sick child and her other children, who are so often ignored and neglected during this time of crisis.
>
> The hospice counselor can become available to the parents who may have difficulties in communicating openly with each other or with the child. A less emotionally involved outsider can function as a marvelous catalyst in times like this and also be available to siblings, who have problems sharing their pain with the already bereaved parents.
>
> The hospice nurse is available twenty-four hours a day for anxious parents, to minister to the medical needs in the home and to answer questions and explain things that the family did not comprehend when they were explained in the formal language of physicians (Kubler-Ross, 1983).

Evaluation and Follow-Up

Nursing care does not end with the death of the child. The surviving family members will continue to grieve and, in the absence of the ill child as a focus for their attention, might begin to manifest this pain in new ways that are dysfunctional.

After the child has died, the family will feel the need to begin reestablishing normal routines and resume their former activities, both at home and in the workplace. Picking up on interrupted social contacts might be one of the most difficult aspects of this effort. Well-meaning expressions of sympathy, sometimes accompanied by such presumptive statements as, "I know how you feel," might prove irksome to parents wishing to resume their normal lives and even cause them further anguish and anger.

Families need time not only to work through their grief but also just to become accustomed to the child's absence. Parents might continue to sense the child's presence for a period of time after death has occurred by mistaking strange children on the street for their own child or by hearing doors slam, the teenager's record player, or the infant's cry. Parents should be reassured that this is normal and not a sign of insanity or some other pathologic process.

Family relationships, particularly marital bonds, which are already strained by the child's illness might suffer further disruption after the child's death. Some studies have shown a 50%–70% incidence of marital problems and divorce in families in which a child died from cancer (Lauer, et al., 1983). Parents might feel that they no longer have a common bond. They might project their own feelings of guilt on to each other to give the death a cause, however unfounded. Each parent might feel that the other is a reminder of grief and not a consoling presence and begin to engage more intensely in activities that exclude the other parent such as career or solitary interests. An inability to understand the other parent's grieving style or a need to "be strong" for the spouse also can reinforce each parents' individual isolation. As with other aspects of the grieving process, open and honest communication is the best preventive care individuals can provide for themselves and their family.

Various changes in parent–child interactions might take place with the surviving siblings after the death of a child. The surviving siblings might become scapegoats, the objects of projected guilt and idealization of the dead child. The parents might overprotect the surviving siblings in the hope of preventing a similar fate, or they may place the siblings in the role of substitute for the dead child. They might feel incapable of making decisions regarding the care of the siblings if their confidence in their parenting ability has been shattered by the child's death. Grieving parents also might try to seek relief by deciding to have another child immediately. Such a decision, made in an intensely emotional climate, might be predominantly the wish of one parent; the nurse should encourage the parents to ensure that a mutual decision is reached and to realize that no other child can truly fill the void left by the dead child.

How well survivors cope depends on the strengths of the family's normal support systems, the support they feel from extended family members, friends, and neighbors, the role the dead child played in family function while alive, the parents' relationship with each other and with the other children, and the ability of each family member to readjust and learn new role functions. Readjustment also can be affected by the family's degree of involvement in the terminal care of the child, whether in the hospital or at home. Greater involvement with the child's care can assist the resolution of guilt feelings and enhance family relationships strained by the crisis of losing a family member.

The nurse can assist the family's adjustment by promoting a climate of full and open communication both to identify individual feelings and problems and to reveal any changes in family role relationships that have taken place silently. Feelings of helplessness on the part of all family members can be addressed by encouraging them to engage in activities that renew their sense of purpose and usefulness. These are as likely to be new activities as they are those that occupied the person before the bereavement.

Most importantly, the nurse should make sure that the primary health caregiver, whether primary nurse or physician, contacts the family at some interval after the child's death. The period of time may range from 10 days to 1 month and will depend on the family's own needs, desires, and religious mourning practices. "At this time the family can be observed for such normal grief reactions as somatic complaints, anger, preoccupation with the dead image, depression, guilt, and changes in normal daily patterns" (Williams, Rivara, and Rothenberg, 1981). Nurses also take this opportunity to extend themselves in offering sympathy, sharing their own memories of the child, and assuring the family that the support of the health care team remains available to them.

The aftermath of a child's death is a critical time for the family, one in which nursing evaluation, follow-up, and collaboration with other health professionals such as the community health nurse will be key factors in the family's ability to return to their normal state of functioning. In one circumstance, however, the aftermath is virtually the entire focus of the nurse's interventions, that is, the sudden infant death syndrome.

Sudden Infant Death Syndrome

Sudden infant death syndrome (SIDS) is currently the leading cause of postneonatal death in the United States, claiming 7000–10,000 lives each year and accounting for about one-third of all deaths in infants aged 1 week to 1 year (Beckwith, 1978; DeFrain and Ernst, 1978; Khoury, Erickson, and Adams, 1984). A great deal of research, debate, and uncertainty surrounds this phenomenon, which can not only intensify a parent's bewilderment and grief but also can cloud the health professional's ability to give care.

Also called "crib death" or "cot death," SIDS refers to the sudden and unexpected death of an infant who has been previously healthy, with the cause of death being still unexplained after a thorough postmortem examination; it is thus a "diagnosis of exclusion" (Bakke and Dougherty, 1981). Sudden infant death syndrome is characterized by at least two features: (1) it has a very specific age distribution, with a peak incidence between 2 and 4 months of age and rarely occurring in the first month of life or after the first year; and (2) it almost always occurs during sleep (Beckwith, 1978).

The relationship between SIDS and infant apnea has been the focus of much clinical attention and some debate. When an infant is discovered to have stopped breathing for a long period of time (20 seconds or more) but later recovers (frequently in the emergency room), the situation often is termed a case of "aborted" or "near-miss" SIDS. Many hospitals now have home-monitoring programs to allow home care for the infant with apneic spells. Some clinicians, however, feel that the term "near-miss SIDS" is inappropriate and that infant apnea and SIDS are two distinct syndromes, with the latter being confirmed only by an autopsy and therefore unpreventable (Bakke and Dougherty, 1981; Sperhac, 1982). Other authorities feel that the two syndromes are related, with infant apnea being "a symptom as well as a cause" of SIDS, and that home apnea monitoring is in fact a measure to prevent SIDS (Favorito, Pernice, and Ruggiero, 1979; Ariagno, 1984). Further research and debate are needed to resolve this controversy. (Infant apnea and home monitoring programs are discussed in Chapter 31.)

Proposed Causes

In dealing with the survivors of the SIDS infant, the abrupt trajectory of death and the lack of an identifiable cause are the main features that make the grief process particularly difficult. Beckwith (1978) listed over 70 proposed theories of causation, observing that "new ideas are being published almost weekly." Although no definitive answer has yet been found, two explanations that seem to occur immediately to parents and cause them intense guilt—suffocation and allergy to cow's milk—have been all but refuted. The nurse is in a key position to help alleviate the parents' guilt by eliminating these ideas as explanations. Understanding some of the arguments against these theories might help nurses to convince parents that they do not explain the causes of SIDS (Table 32-2).

One promising direction of research is in the area of neurology (Beckwith, 1978). Researchers have found elevated levels of the neurotransmitter dopamine in the carotid bodies of SIDS infants, which would tie in to one current theory that SIDS is the result of a neurological learning deficit (Greenberg, 1984). Although such evidence might suggest that some of the causal factors of SIDS are congenital, it is important to reassure parents that research has not substantiated a genetic basis for the disease (Beckwith, 1978; Sperhac, 1982). Although siblings of SIDS infants seem to have a higher incidence of SIDS than the general population, a theory of hereditary causation also would need support from a higher incidence among such family members as first cousins, and this has not been reported. The distinction between a congenital and hereditary condition can be important for the nurse to make because a genetic cause of death often can be an added source of guilt for the parents of a dead child.

Nurse's Role

Although studies have drawn attention to the reactions of family members in cases of SIDS and the appropriate nursing interventions (Mandell, McAnulty, and Reece, 1980; Nikolaisen, 1981; Mandell, McAnulty, and Carlson, 1983), these reactions are virtually all identical in kind to those felt by survivors of children who died of other causes—guilt, denial, intellectualization, anger, and so forth. In cases of SIDS, however, the nurse can be instrumental in helping the family deal with the shock caused by the unanticipated nature of the event, the bewilderment resulting from the still unanswered questions concerning the cause, and, most importantly, the parents' own guilt, which stems from their assumption that they somehow must have been the cause.

TABLE 32-2 Reasons Invalidating Suffocation and Anaphylaxis Theories as Causes for Sudden Infant Death Syndrome

Suffocation—parents might feel that the infant was suffocated by bedclothes and thus died as a result of parental carelessness. This reasoning is unfounded because:

1. The very young infant would be at least as susceptible to accidental suffocation but is relatively spared according to epidemiologic data on SIDS
2. Infants found with their faces free are clinically and pathologically identical to those found with covered faces
3. Ordinary bedding is probably insufficient to suffocate the infant

Anaphylaxis—an allergy to cow's milk as the cause of death might be related in the parent's mind with a decision not to breast-feed the infant. This reasoning is unfounded because:

1. Sudden infant death syndrome cannot be correlated with infant feeding patterns
2. Personal and family allergy histories have been found to be identical for SIDS cases and matched controls
3. Levels of antibodies to cow's milk proteins and of the cells that produce these antibodies are not increased in SIDS infants
4. The age spectrum of SIDS cases is not compatible with the age spectrum of hypersensitivity diseases

SOURCE: Adapted from Beckwith JB: The sudden infant death syndrome. US Department of Health, Education, and Welfare. DHEW Publication No (HSA) 78–5251. Government Printing Office, 1978.

These feelings can complicate and intensify the grief process. Another by-product of the lack of a definitive explanation can be a tragic withdrawal of the family's social support because friends, neighbors, grandparents, and even health care providers who are uninformed about SIDS might hold the parents responsible and shun them. The nurse plays an important role in explaining to parents and those around them that SIDS is a specific, identified condition but one that is poorly understood as yet.

With SIDS cases, the nurse's task might be more complex, but it is essentially the same as in other cases of pediatric death. Supporting the family by decreasing feelings of isolation and rejection becomes particularly important (Smialek, 1978). Aiding parents in the detachment process by letting them hold and spend time with the dead infant is another useful intervention. Making sure that the lines of communication among all family members, especially surviving siblings, remain as open as possible is just as important in SIDS as in other cases of childhood death. Parents should be encouraged to explain the circumstances of the infant's death to the siblings. Families of SIDS infants might be more prone to react to their grief by moving away or breaking up the family, and so the nurse should be especially careful to make early intervention after the death of

To Deanna With Love From Doug

Deanna my friend, so sweet and dear
She helps me to get by when I am in fear.
When they are near there is no need to shed a tear
For there is no fear.

My sister Megan, Deanna and I travel when we can.
We run through the grass and play in the sand—
Sing and rejoice
And have fun again.

We travel over the mountains and across the land
Chasing skunks in the Grand Canyon.
Climbing mountains in Utah
We roast weinies around the campfire
And then we make smores
And end up just wanting more and more.

When we have a chance to go see our Hero play.
He is the number one quarterback to us
And there is no fuss.
He plays for the Cowboys and we win, win, win.
His name is Roger Staubach, and that is the end.

an infant a high priority (DeFrain and Ernst, 1978). Encouraging referral and coordination with other health care professionals such as the visiting nurse association is essential to ensure that adequate follow-up is maintained during this critical time. The nurse gives the family the address and phone number of the local chapter of the national SIDS support group and explains the kind of support the group can offer.

The emotional and clinical complexities that surround the dying child can lead to feelings of helplessness on the nurse's part. One tempting coping strategy is to look for "things to do"—to seek new nursing interventions, find reasons to consult with other health professionals, or do any little task simply to engage in some positive activity. "Professionals' willingness to provide safe passage through this difficult time by abiding peacefully and responsively with their patients may be the greatest service they can offer. Very often, the golden rule in terminal care may be *Don't just do something, sit there!*" (Gonda and Ruark, 1984).

Difficult as it might be to believe, there are joys in caring for the dying child. One of the most important nursing tasks is helping the child to discover the joys in the short period of life that remains. Nurses who feel continuously drained, depleted, and hurt when working with dying patients might decide that they are temperamentally unsuited to their role or may wish to deepen their insight into their own feelings and expectations. For everyone, life is in many ways nothing more than preparing for death. The nurse who works with the dying child is one of the most significant persons in that child's life. Not only do nurses have one of the most clearly defined opportunities to serve and give, they also have one of the most significant opportunities to receive. To minimize the pain and maximize the comfort in death are the ultimate privileges in the nursing experience. Nurses who take joy in their work will grieve at the loss of every single patient but also will feel a great fulfillment in being able to help others achieve the final goal of their lives.

Key Concepts

- Nursing care of the dying child is an intense emotional experience, requiring personal preparation in both the affective and cognitive realms.
- Although a child's responses to death and dying are influenced by more than chronologic age, it is important for the nurse to understand the child's developmental view of death as a baseline for assessment.
- To understand the child's experience of dying, the nurse considers several factors, including the child's progressive understanding of the illness, the child's progressive self-concept in relation to the illness, the trajectory of death and the occurrence of the critical junctures along the trajectory, the level of certainty as to when death will occur, and the atmosphere of awareness in the health care environment.
- The behavioral and emotional reactions to the dying process do not occur in a progressive sequence of stages but can be used as coping mechanisms in any order. The nurse refrains from imposing an agenda on the child or family member to move them through stages but rather recognizes these common reactions as states that can affect the nurse's role in communication, education, and therapeutic or palliative interventions.
- The nurse and the dying child's family also can experience the common coping reactions of the dying child, although usually for different reasons.

- In addition to the common coping reactions, parents often experience disruption of their personal and marital lives and isolation from the society of friends and neighbors as a result of the child's dying.
- The reactions of the dying child's siblings are too often ignored and can include jealousy and hostility toward the ill child, as well as the other reactions of grief. As with the dying child, the nursing assessment of the sibling's reactions is based on an understanding of that child's developmental level and perception of death.
- In addition to other normal grieving reactions, nurses should be aware of other responses that they themselves often experience such as feeling overwhelmed, overidentifying with the dying child and/or family, and avoiding emotional involvement with the dying process. Nurses also should be open to the possibilities of personal growth as a result of the intense experience of caring for dying children.
- Cultural differences influence both the perception of death and the expression of grief and should therefore be taken into account as the nurse interacts with the dying child and family.
- Nursing assessment of the dying child and family will cover the child's understanding of death and illness, the normal coping mechanisms of the child and family, the specific details of family functioning (including special risk factors), and the family's cultural perspective.
- Communication skills and fostering an open atmosphere for communication are perhaps the most important contributions the nurse can make to the care of the dying child, family, and fellow health care professionals.
- The nurse is also instrumental in supporting feelings of grief and initiating and promoting peer support for the child, family members, and other nurses.
- Home care is a terminal care option that can strengthen the bonds between the child and family, minimize family disruption, and positively affect the family's readjustment after the child's death. It does not, however, reduce the involvement of the nurse, who continues to play a strong role in support, counseling, and the coordination of services.
- The hospice concept has much in common with the goals of nursing and of home care, with its focus on the family as the unit of care and caregiving.
- Follow-up and evaluation, especially with the family after the child has died, is an essential nursing role.
- Sudden infant death syndrome (SIDS) presents special challenges to the nurse in addition to the problems commonly encountered in other cases of childhood death.

References

Achterberg J, Lawlis GF: *Imagery of Cancer.* Institute for Personality and Ability Testing, 1978.

Adams FE: Six very good reasons why we react differently to various dying patients. *Nursing 84* (June) 1984; 14(6):41–43.

Ariagno RL: Evaluation and management of infantile apnea. *Pediatr Ann* (March) 1984; 13(3):210–213.

Bakke, K, Dougherty J: Sudden infant death syndrome and infant apnea: Current questions, clinical management, and research directions. *Issues Compr Pediatr Nurs* 1981; 5:77–88.

Beckwith JB: The sudden infant death syndrome. US Department of Health, Education, and Welfare. DHEW Publication No (HSA) 78–5251. Government Printing Office, 1978.

Bluebond-Langner M: *Awareness and Communication in Terminally Ill Children: Pattern, Process, and Pretense.* Unpublished doctoral dissertation, University of Illinois, 1975a.

Bluebond-Langner M: *Field Research on Children's and Adult's Views of Death.* Field Notes, 1975b.

Bluebond-Langner M: *Field Research on Children's and Adult's Views of Death.* Field Notes, 1976.

Bluebond-Langner M: Meanings of death to children. In: *New Meanings of Death.* Feifel H (editor). McGraw-Hill, 1977.

Brantner J: *Death and the Self* (Audiotape). University of Minnesota Center for Death Education and Research, 1970.

Burne SR: A hospice for children in England. *Pediatrics* (Jan) 1984; 73(1):97–98.

DeFrain JD, Ernst L: The psychological effects of sudden infant death syndrome on surviving family members. *J Fam Pract* 1978; 6(5):985–989.

Dobihal SV: Hospice: Enabling a patient to die at home. *Am J Nurs* (Aug) 1980; 80(8):1448–1451.

Favorito J, Pernice JMO, Ruggiero P: Beyond the hospital: Apnea monitoring to prevent SIDS. *Am J Nurs* (Jan) 1979; 79:101–104.

Fulton R, Fulton J: A psychosocial aspect of terminal care: Anticipatory grief. *Omega* 1971; 2:91–99.

Glaser BG, Strauss AL: *Awareness of Dying.* Aldine, 1965.

Glaser BG, Strauss AL: *Time for Dying.* Aldine, 1968.

Gonda T, Ruark J: *Dying Dignified: The Health Professional's Guide to Care.* Addison-Wesley, 1984.

Greenberg J: Infant death tied to dopamine excess. *Science News* (Sept 15) 1984; 126(11):165.

Grollman EA (editor): *Explaining Death to Children.* Beacon Press, 1967.

Hutton LM: Annie is alone: The bereaved child. *Am J Matern Child Nurs* (July/Aug) 1981; 6:274–277.

Kastenbaum R, Aisenberg R: *The Psychology of Death.* Springer, 1972.

Khoury MJ, Erickson JD, Adams MJ: Trends in postneonatal mortality in the United States. *JAMA* 1984; 252(3):367–372.

Kubler-Ross E: *On Children and Death.* Macmillan, 1983.

Kubler-Ross E: *On Death and Dying.* Macmillan, 1969.

Lauer ME, et al: A comparison study of parental adaptation following a child's death at home or in the hospital. *Pediatrics* (Jan) 1983; 71(1):107–112.

Leshan L, Worthington RE: Some recurrent life-history patterns observed in patients with malignant disease. *J Nerv Ment Dis* 1965; 124:460.

MacElveen-Hoehn P, McIntosh EG: The hospice movement: Growing pains and promises. *Top Clin Nurs* (Oct) 1981; 3(3):29–38.

Mandel HR: Nurses' feelings about working with the dying. *Am J Nurs* (June) 1981; 81(6):1194–1197.

Mandell F, McAnulty E, Reece RM: Observations of paternal response to sudden unanticipated infant death. *Pediatrics* (Feb) 1980; 65(2):221–225.

Mandell F, McAnulty EH, Carlson A: Unexpected death of an infant sibling. *Pediatrics* (Nov) 1983; 72(5):652–657.

Martinson IM, et al.: Home care for children dying of cancer. *Pediatrics* (July) 1978; 62(1):106–113.

Martinson IM, et al: When the patient is dying: Home care for the child. *Am J Nurs* (Nov) 1977; 77(11):1815–1817.

Miller, JK: Pediatric hospice program. *Kentucky Nurses Assoc Newsletter* (Feb/March) 1982; 30:26–27.

Nagy MH: The child's view of death. *J Genet Psychol* 1948; 73:3–27.

Nikolaisen S: The impact of sudden infant death on the family: Nursing intervention. *Top Clin Nurs* (Oct) 1981; 3(3):45–53.

Ross HM: Societal/cultural views regarding death and dying. *Top Clin Nurs* (Oct) 1981; 3(3):1–16.

Schneidman ES: *Deaths of Man.* Quadrangle, New York Times Book Co., 1973.

Sheer BL: Help for the parents in a difficult job—broaching the subject of death. *Am J Matern Child Nurs* (Sept/Oct) 1977; 2(5):320–324.

Simonton OC, Simonton S: Belief systems and the management of the emotional aspects of malignancy. *J Transpersonal Psychol* 1975; 7:29–47.

Smialek Z: Observations on immediate reactions of families to sudden infant death. *Pediatrics* (Aug) 1978; 62(2):160–165.

Sperhac AM: Sudden infant death syndrome. *Nurse Pract* (Sept) 1982; 7:38–40, 44.

Thomas N, Cordell AS: The dying infant: Aiding parents in the detachment process. *Pediatr Nurs* (Sept/Oct) 1983; 9(5):355–357.

Waechter EH: The adolescent with a handicapping, chronic, or life-threatening illness. In: *Perspectives on Adolescent Health Care.* Mercer RT (editor). Lippincott, 1979.

Williams HA, Rivara FP, Rothenberg MB: The child is dying: Who helps the family? *Am J Matern Child Nurs* (July/Aug) 1981; 6:261–265.

Wong DL: Bereavement: The empty mother syndrome. *Am J Matern Child Nurs* (Nov/Dec) 1980; 15:385–389.

Woods JR: Death on a daily basis. *Focus Crit Care* (June) 1984; 11(3):50–51.

Wooten B: Death of an infant. *Am J Matern Child Nurs* (July/Aug) 1981; 6:257–260.

Additional Readings

Anthony S: *The Discovery of Death in Childhood and After.* Basic Books, 1972.

Arnold JH, Gemma PB: *A Child Dies: A Portrait of Family Grief.* Aspen, 1983.

Chitwood L: A lesson in living. *Nursing 84* (Jan) 1984; 14(1):55–56.

Clayton PJ, Halikes JA, Maurice W: The bereavement of the widowed. *Dis Nerv System* 1971; 32:597–604.

Cook SS, et al: *Children and Dying: An Exploration and Selective Bibliographies.* Expanded edition. Health Sciences, 1974.

Cushing M: Whose best interest? Parents vs. child rights. *Am J Nurs* (Feb) 1982; 82(2):313–314.

Davis AJ: A newborn's right to life vs. death. *Am J Nurs* (May) 1981; 81(5):1035.

Edwardson SR: The choice between hospital and home care for terminally ill children. *Nurs Res* (Jan/Feb) 1983; 32(1):29–34.

Gyulay JE: *The Dying Child.* McGraw-Hill, 1978.

Henretta CB, Van Brunt PF: Sudden pediatric death: Meeting the needs of family and staff. *Nurse Educ* (Winter) 1982; 7:13–16.

Jackson EN: *Telling a Child About Death.* Channel Press, 1965.

Johnson-Soderberg S: The development of a child's concept of death. *Oncol Nurs Forum* (Winter) 1981; 8:23–26.

Klimin G: *Psychological Emergencies of Childhood.* Grune & Stratton, 1968.

Lacasse CM: A dying adolescent. *Am J Nurs* (March) 1975; 75(3):433–434.

Lauer ME, et al: Home care for dying children: A nursing model. *J Pediatr* 1980; 97:1032–1035.

McIntire M, Angle C, Struempler L: Concept of death of midwestern children in youth. *Am J Dis Child* 1972; 123:527–532.

Piaget J: *The Child's Conception of the World.* Routledge and Kegan Paul, 1929.

Piaget J: *The Child and Reality: Problems of Genetic Psychology.* Rosin A (translator). Grossman, 1973.

Putnam ST, et al: Home as a place to die. *Am J Nurs* (Aug) 1980; 80(8):1451–1453.

Schowalter JE: The adolescent patient's decision to die. *Pediatrics* (Jan) 1973; 51(1):97–103.

Singher LJ: The slowly dying child. *Clin Pediatr* (Oct) 1974; 13(10):861–867.

Smith ML: When a child dies at home. *Nursing 82* (Aug) 1982; 12(8):66–67.

Zeligs R: *Children's Experiences With Death.* Thomas, 1974.

UNIT VIII NURSING CARE OF THE ILL CHILD

Theorists have made many recommendations regarding the most effective method of learning. Underlying most learning theories, however, is the idea that successful learning proceeds from the simple to the complex, or from the general to the specific. Inherent in this principle is the concept that the student need not learn every detail of every situation to function but can learn general concepts that relate to a variety of new situations. In Unit VIII, our final unit, this basic framework of learning, combined with our holistic systems approach, helps the student apply nursing principles to the care of any specific child.

In each Unit VIII chapter we begin with the basic information needed to provide comprehensive nursing care for children experiencing alterations in functioning of a particular body system. We introduce each chapter with a concise discussion of the anatomy and physiology of the system, including pertinent aspects of embryonic development. An extensive section follows describing the nursing assessment of a child with a disorder of that system, including appropriate diagnostic tests and the meaning of alterations in normal results. We follow the assessment section with a discussion of nursing care principles that includes preparation for diagnostic tests; principles of acute nursing care; and exploration of the physical, nutritional, emotional, developmental, and health maintenance needs of children with alterations in the particular system under discussion.

Finally, we conclude with the application of the general principles to the care of children with specific disease entities related to the system. Throughout these Unit VIII chapters are assessment guides, nursing care guides, and nursing care plans, which help the student synthesize data and apply the nursing process.

Contents

Fluid and Electrolytes
Implications of Imbalance

Frances Ward Quinless

33

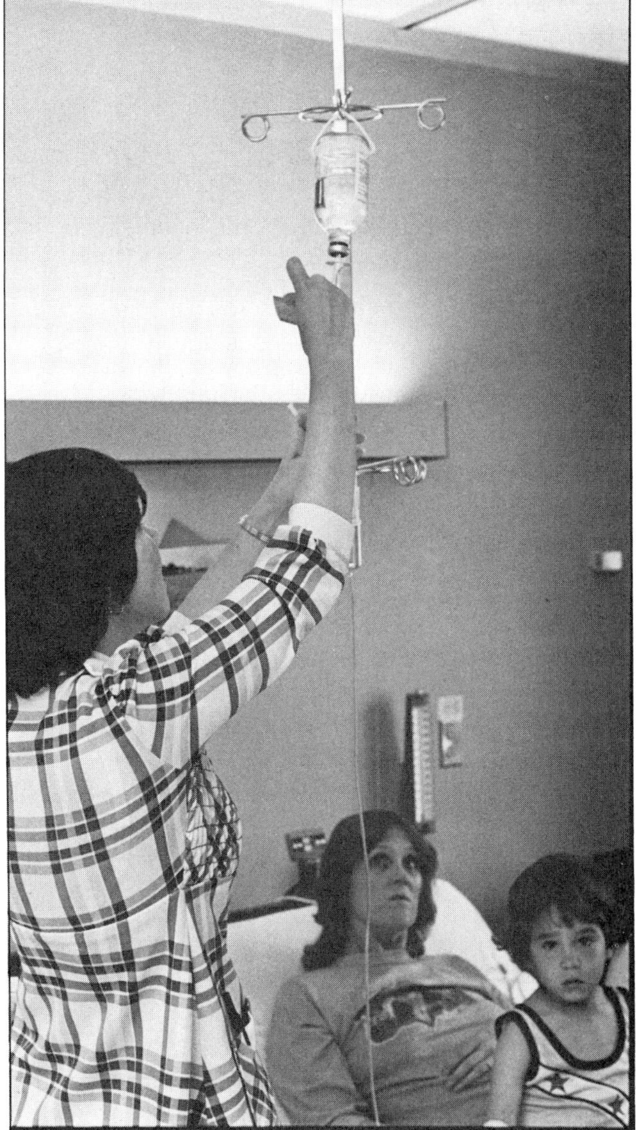

Chapter Outline

continued on next page

Objectives

- Identify the components of extracellular and intracellular fluid.
- List the factors that affect water balance.
- Define the regulatory mechanisms that maintain fluid and electrolyte balance.
- Explain the nursing care measures associated with oral fluid therapy and intravenous administration.
- Describe methods of output measurement associated with monitoring fluid balance.
- Identify principal sites for intravenous administration.
- Describe the physiologic dysfunction, assessment criteria, and nursing care associated with imbalances of major electrolytes.
- Explain the physiologic processes that control acid-base balance.
- Describe the physiologic dysfunction, assessment criteria, and nursing care associated with acid-base abnormalities.

To find these topics, see the following chapters

Burns	Chapter 44
Gastroenteritis	Chapter 38
Hyperalimentation	Chapter 38
Nephrosis	Chapter 39
Pyloric Stenosis	Chapter 38
Salicylate Poisoning	Chapter 20
Toxic Shock Syndrome	Chapter 39

Clinical symptoms rapidly become apparent in the child suffering from an imbalance of fluid and electrolytes. Body water, electrolytes, and acid-base balance (for example, pH) must be regulated within narrow limits to maintain proper physiologic functioning. Because of the high proportion of water contained in the child's body, the child is particularly vulnerable, even to slight shifts in body fluid electrolytes and arterial pH.

Knowledge of the physiologic processes involved in maintaining fluid and electrolyte balance is vital to a complete assessment of a child's health status. Because of the child's vulnerability to dehydration, the nurse needs to be cognizant of both the subjective and objective signs of fluid and electrolyte imbalance.

In this chapter we focus on two major aspects of fluid and electrolyte balance: (a) assessment factors in ascertaining the status of body fluid, electrolytes, and acid-base balance and (b) nursing management of the child exhibiting imbalance.

Body Fluid Composition of the Child

The percentage of total body water (TBW) varies among individuals according to age and amount of adipose tissue. Fat is essentially water-free, being approximately 10% water; thus adult and some adolescent females have significantly less TBW than males with the same weight, and obese children have less TBW than nonobese children of the same weight. The infant's TBW is markedly higher than that of the adult (approximately 77% rather than the adult average of 45%–60%). The child's TBW reaches the adult percentage at approximately 2 years of age.

Water Distribution

Body fluid is contained in two compartments: intracellular and extracellular. In the healthy child, a state of dynamic equilibrium exists between these two compartments. Considering TBW as 60% of the older child's total body weight, the intracellular fluid (ICF) comprises 40% of body weight while the extracellular fluid (ECF) is 20%. The infant, on the other hand, has a higher volume of water in comparison to that of the older child and this increased body water is located in the extracellular compartment. Thus, if the infant's TBW is 77%, ECF is 37% since ICF remains constant at approximately 40% of total body weight during growth. Because a greater proportion of water in the infant is ECF, and it is the ECF which depletes most rapidly during disease, the infant is subject to more severe consequences of fluid volume shifts.

The ICF provides the medium for physiochemical functioning of the cell. Potassium and magnesium are the major cations (positively charged ions) of the ICF; proteins and organic phosphates are the major anions (negatively charged ions).

The ECF is the transport mechanism for delivering such nutrients as water, oxygen, and electrolytes to and removing waste products from the cells. The major cation in ECF is sodium; the major anion is chloride. Electrolyte composition of both ICF and ECF is illustrated in Figure 33-1.

The ECF is further composed of three major components: (a) interstitial fluid, (b) plasma, and (c) transcellular fluid. The interstitial fluid (approximately 15% of body weight) is the fluid outside the vascular space and the cells and contains mainly crystalloids. The plasma (approximately 5% of body weight) is the fluid of the blood and contains colloids in the form of proteins. Plasma is essential for maintaining normal intravascular volume. Plasma proteins are important in regulating fluid volume between the intracellular compartment and the extracellular compartment. The transcellular fluids are the liquids secreted or excreted from cells. These include saliva, sweat, hepatobiliary tract secretions, gastrointestinal juices, and urine.

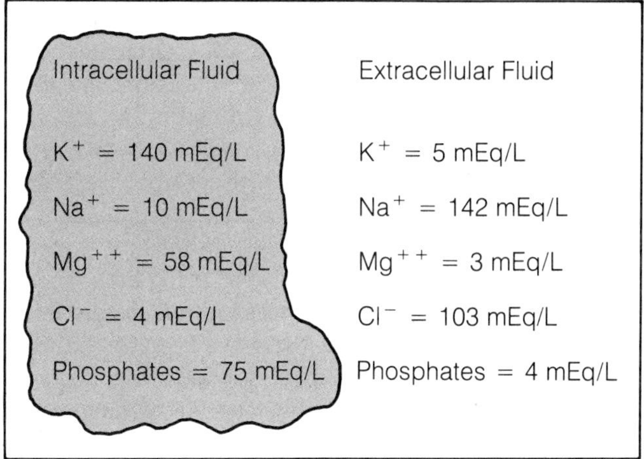

Figure 33-1 Electrolyte composition of the intracellular fluid and extracellular fluid. (Adapted from Guyton A: *Textbook of Medical Physiology*. 6th ed. Saunders, 1981, p. 41.)

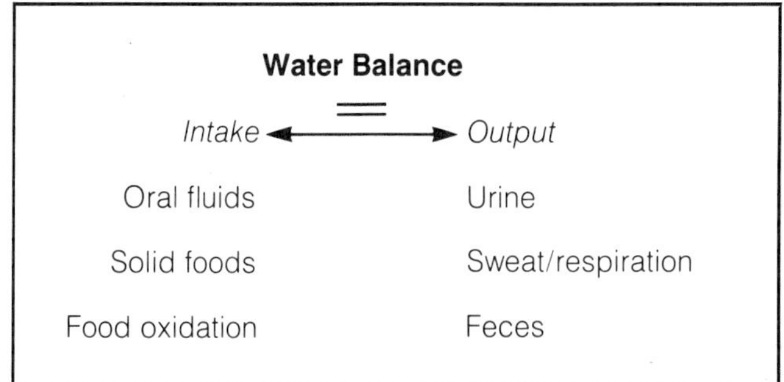

Figure 33-2 Factors affecting water balance.

Factors Affecting Water Balance

To maintain a state of body fluid balance, water intake must closely approximate water output over a 24-hour period. The major sources of water are (a) oral fluids, (b) water contained in solid foods, and (c) oxidation of food substances (carbohydrate, fat, and protein) (Fig. 33-2). People normally obtain 50% of their water from oral fluids and the remaining 50% from solid food and food metabolism. Water production from food oxidation varies. For example, oxidation of 100 g of fat produces 100 mL of water; 100 g of carbohydrate produces 60 mL of water; and 100 g of protein produces 45 mL of water. Urea, the principal end product of protein metabolism, also requires water for excretion.

The greatest factor in water output is water volume and solute regulation by the kidneys. The ability of the kidneys to concentrate or dilute the glomerular filtrate is of prime importance in maintaining water balance (see Chapter 39).

Water is also lost from the gastrointestinal tract and, through insensible loss, from the skin and lungs. Conditions causing an elevated metabolic rate (for example, fever) increase the amount of water eliminated. Basal metabolism increases approximately 10% for each degree Celsius above normal body temperature, yielding a comparable increase in fluid requirements.

Infants and young children are at risk for fluid and electrolyte imbalance because of the immaturity of their kidneys, their high metabolic rate, and their high ratio of body surface area to weight. Young children, particularly neonates, cannot concentrate or excrete urine as efficiently as adults and thus have difficulty regulating fluids, electrolytes, and pH. They also use more fluid for the excretion of waste products. The kidneys mature quite rapidly, beginning to concentrate urine more efficiently even within the first few weeks of life, and are relatively mature by age 1 year.

Metabolic rate and thus caloric needs are higher in the young child. With higher metabolic rates come both increased heat production and increased by-products of metabolism. Greater heat production yields increased insensible fluid losses from the skin and lungs, and the increased by-products of metabolism are relatively greater in proportion to body weight and require dilution with water and excretion by the kidneys. The young child has a far greater body surface area in relation to body weight than does the adult and thus loses relatively more fluid through the skin and lungs.

Thus immaturity of the kidneys, high metabolic rate, and relatively large ratio of body surface area to weight contribute to the child's needing more fluid in relation to body weight than does the adult and also to being more at risk for fluid and electrolyte imbalances. Where adults need approximately 40 mL of fluid intake per kilogram of body weight per day, infants from 1–3 months of age need up to 150 mL/kg/24 h. Appendix E shows fluid requirements under normal conditions for children of various ages and weights. Because of the ratio of body surface area to weight, metabolic rate, and kidney maturation, the total volume of water needed by the child per day increases only gradually as the child's weight increases.

Mechanisms of Fluid and Electrolyte Balance

Water Transport Mechanisms

Water performs a major role in the physiologic functioning of any cell. It is the transport medium for cellular nutrients and waste products. It regulates body temperature and is essential in the maintenance of intravascular volume. As a solvent, water contains many of the solutes (electrolytes) needed for cellular activity.

Five physiologic processes enable water to move between the intracellular fluid and the extracellular fluid. These are diffusion, osmotic pressure, hydrostatic pressure, active transport, and vesicular transport.

Diffusion Diffusion is the free, random movement of substances caused by the normal kinetic motion of matter. Factors affecting the diffusion rate of a substance from one area to another are

1. The greater the concentration difference, the greater the diffusion rate.
2. The smaller the molecular size, the greater the diffusion rate.
3. The shorter the distance, the greater the diffusion rate.
4. The greater the metabolic rate, the greater the diffusion rate.
5. The greater the electric charge difference, the greater the diffusion rate of opposite-charged ions.

Potassium and sodium do not diffuse readily across the cell membrane as they are both positively charged and cell membrane pores are also lined with positively charged ions.

Facilitated diffusion is the process by which some substances, large molecules such as amino acids and sugars, diffuse through a cell membrane when combined with a carrier substance within the membrane. Glucose, for example, is thought to enter the cell only in the presence of a specific carrier substance.

Osmotic Pressure Osmosis is the transfer of water across a semipermeable membrane when a solute concentration difference exists on either side of the membrane. Water osmosis is created by the application of pressure across the semipermeable membrane in the direction opposite to the osmosis. Osmotic pressure is the amount of pressure needed to oppose the osmosis.

Colloid osmotic pressure, or oncotic pressure, is the osmotic pressure due to colloid substances. The capillary membrane is permeable to plasma substances, with the exception of plasma proteins. The plasma proteins (albumin and globulin) act to hold water within the capillary space. Thus plasma protein concentration is extremely important in maintaining normal blood volume.

Osmolarity, or tonicity (the osmotic concentration per liter of solution, expressed as osmoles per liter [osm/L]), is an important phenomenon regulating fluid movement across the cell membrane (Table 33-1). The tonicity of a solution introduced into the body fluids thus determines the solution's effect on the amount of water within the cells.

An isotonic solution has the same tonicity as body fluids. A hypertonic solution contains a higher concentration of solutes than plasma. A hypotonic solution contains a lower concentration of solutes than plasma. A hypertonic solution introduced into the body fluids thus causes rapid loss of water from the cells and cellular crenation, or shrinking. The introduction of a hypotonic solution causes water movement into the cells, and cells therefore become edematous, and then hemolysis may occur.

Hydrostatic Pressure Hydrostatic pressure causes the movement of water and solutes through a permeable membrane from an area of high pressure to an area of lower pressure. It's caused by the pumping action of the heart. The degree of hydrostatic pressure varies according to the blood pressure, capillary flow rate, and venous pressure.

Hydrostatic pressure is the force that transfers fluid from the glomerular capillaries into the collecting tubules. As the capillary hydrostatic pressure increases, fluid transudes out of the capillary network into the interstitial compartment. This pressure is counteracted by the force of plasma proteins, which tend to maintain intravascular volume.

Active Transport Unlike passive mechanisms, active transport requires energy (in the form of adenosine triphosphate, or ATP) to accomplish the movement of solutes against a concentration gradient. The mechanism respon-

TABLE 33-1 Osmolarity (Tonicity) and Physiologic Consequences

Tonicity of solution	Examples	Consequence
Isotonic	0.9% saline 5% dextrose in water	No cellular changes
Hypotonic	0.45% saline Water	Cellular edema (hemolysis)
Hypertonic	3% saline 10% dextrose in water	Cellular crenation (shrinking)

sible for active transport is as yet unknown. Sodium, potassium, chloride, hydrogen, calcium, urea, amino acids, and sugars all use active transport to cross cell membranes.

Vesicular Transport Vesicular transport is the physiologic process by which large molecules transverse cell membranes. Such molecules (for example, large protein molecules) enter cells by the process of pinocytosis, in which the cell membrane engulfs some of the extracellular fluid and the molecules contained in it. Molecules then leave the cell by the process of exocytosis, in which the cell membrane allows some of the intracellular contents to exit from the cell.

Regulatory Mechanisms

Thirst is essential in regulating fluid intake and thus in maintaining extracellular fluid volume. When the osmolarity of the extracellular fluid increases, which means that cellular dehydration exists, the thirst center of the hypothalamus is stimulated. Higher cerebral centers then receive impulses that produce the subjective sensation of thirst.

Extracellular fluid volume is further maintained by a number of important physiologic mechanisms. Chief among these are the action of specific hormones (antidiuretic hormone and aldosterone) and the renin–angiotensin mechanism of the renal system (Fig. 33-3).

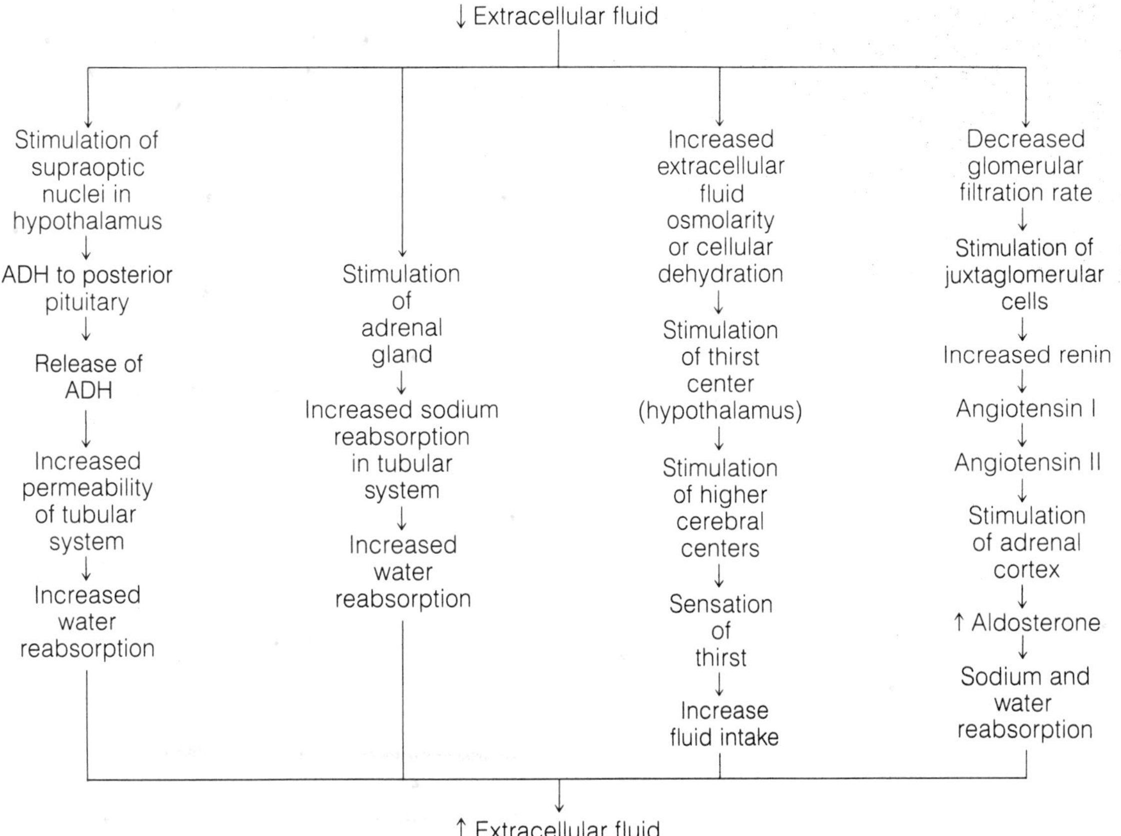

Figure 33-3 Mechanisms that maintain extracellular fluid volume.

Antidiuretic Hormone Antidiuretic hormone (ADH) is formed in the supraoptic nuclei of the hypothalamus. It accumulates in the posterior pituitary gland (or neurohypophysis) and is released into surrounding capillaries. Secretion of ADH increases the permeability of the nephron's collecting ducts and distal tubules and thus permits a significant amount of water in the tubular fluid to be reabsorbed. This reabsorbed water therefore increases the extracellular fluid.

When the concentration of the extracellular fluid compartment increases, the supraoptic nuclei are stimulated and ADH is released from the hypothalamus and transported to the posterior pituitary. Loss of blood volume and resulting hypotension relax atrial stretch receptors, thus stimulating ADH secretion from the posterior pituitary into the capillaries. The ultimate result of ADH secretion is thus to expand the intravascular blood volume.

Aldosterone Aldosterone is the principal mineralocorticoid secreted by the adrenal cortex. The primary physiologic effect of aldosterone is to increase the reabsorption of sodium in the ascending limb of the loop of Henle, in the distal tubule, and in the collecting tubule. By reabsorbing sodium, aldosterone also enhances water reabsorption in the tubular system. Thus aldosterone results in an expansion of the intravascular volume.

Renin–Angiotensin Mechanism The juxtaglomerular cells lining the walls of the juxtaglomerular apparatus, that point of contact between the ascending limb of the loop of Henle and the afferent arteriole, contain the enzyme renin. When the extracellular fluid volume is depleted, the glomerular filtration rate (GFR) decreases. A low GFR decreases sodium concentration in the tubular system; which in turn stimulates renin release. Renin is reduced to angiotensin I in the blood, which is further split into angiotensin II in the lungs. Angiotensin II also stimulates the adrenal cortex to increase aldosterone secretion. The aldosterone released then causes sodium and water reabsorption in the renal tubular system.

Nursing Principles for the Child With a Fluid Imbalance

Nursing care of the child with an imbalance of fluid regulatory mechanisms is geared toward restoring balance and preventing further disequilibrium. Generally, nursing interventions include ongoing observation of the child's status, accurate recording and reporting, and facilitating medical interventions.

For any child with suspected imbalance, observations need to include the following areas for abnormalities and impending failure of regulatory mechanisms:

Vital signs
Respiratory rate and quality
Intake, output, and urine specific gravity
Weight
Skin color, turgor, moistness, edema
Changes in laboratory data—sodium, potassium, chloride, hematocrit, blood gases, bicarbonate
Changes in orientation and sensorium
Symptoms of the underlying condition precipitating the imbalance

In addition to the general observations for signs of imbalance the nurse assesses fluid status by keeping accurate records of fluid intake and output. Because many children receive parenteral fluid therapy, accurate regulation and frequent recording of intravenous fluid administration is essential. Hospitals differ as to recording procedures, but generally the nurse checks every 15–30 minutes to ensure an accurate flow rate, and then makes hourly recording of intake on a flow sheet.

Oral Fluid Therapy

In addition to parenteral therapy, children may be receiving oral fluids at a prescribed rate. The child who is dehydrated, for example, may have oral fluids initiated after a period of parenteral therapy. An oral electrolyte solution (for example, Lytrin or Pedialyte) might be prescribed, or other clear fluids might be introduced gradually. An accurate record of oral intake is as important for fluid assessment as recording intravenous fluids. Fluids are administered initially in small doses, often as small as 30 mL (or 1 oz) an hour. If no vomiting occurs, amounts are gradually increased. When the child is tolerating fluids well, the physician might decide to discontinue parenteral therapy. (Interventions for managing fluid intake are discussed in Chapter 29.)

All children whose oral intake is restricted or who have nasogastric tubes need special mouth care for comfort. Frequent brushing of teeth and use of water or mouthwash for rinsing the mouth is helpful for the older child. Lemon and glycerine swabs frequently are used for younger children. If the child is allowed ice chips, this minimal amount of fluid should be recorded.

Output Measurement

An accurate record of output is equally important as a record of intake. Major fluid loss can occur through urinary excretion, liquid bowel excretion, emesis, and nasogastric tube drainage. In cases of fluid imbalance, all of these need to be measured and recorded accurately.

In an older child who can use the bathroom, measurement of urinary output presents little difficulty, although the nurse needs to encourage cooperation with the procedure (see Chapter 29). The child should use either a urinal or bedpan or a plastic "hat" that fits tightly under the seat of the toilet.

Output measurement for the child who has not been toilet trained becomes more of a problem, as accuracy can be compromised. The use of pediatric urine collectors is common practice in many institutions, but their accuracy depends on correct application and constant vigilance to detect voiding. Repeated use of collecting bags can cause skin breakdown; therefore, use of a skin protector such as tincture of benzoin is necessary. For greater accuracy in urine measurement, a 24-hour collecting bag can be used. This facilitates measurement without bag removal, but the extra tubing is bulky and may be uncomfortable for the child. Depending on the type of receptacle used, hourly measurements or single voiding measurements are possible. For the active child, the tubing may be cut and the end plugged to lessen the bulkiness, but this adaptation means that the free flow of urine into a receptacle during the night is no longer possible without changing the collecting bag.

A much less traumatic method for the young child is simply to weigh the wet diaper. Weight in grams corresponds to the volume voided. The dry diaper weight is subtracted from the wet diaper, and the difference equals the volume in milliliters voided. Many of the disposable diapers have fairly standard weights for each of the types and sizes manufactured by the company. This method is acceptable when approximate rather than strictly accurate output records provide the necessary information concerning fluid balance. Urine aspirated through a syringe from the diaper can also be used for testing and measuring specific gravity. (See Chapter 29 for a discussion of specimen collection.)

If possible, emesis and liquid stools should be measured and recorded. If the nurse cannot obtain an accurate measurement, an estimate should be made as closely as possible. Again, diapers can be weighed for liquid stool measurement. Because nasogastric drainage itself can alter electrolyte balance, careful monitoring of drainage amounts and quality is necessary. Some physicians replace gastric drainage loss by increasing the amount of parenteral electrolyte solution.

Daily weight measurements indicate total fluid loss or gain. The nurse weighs the child at the same time each day, usually before breakfast or before a feeding. The child should always be undressed or in standard hospital pajamas. Infants should be weighed without a diaper on an infant scale.

Intravenous Infusions

Intravenous Sites The site used for an intravenous infusion in the child should allow for both protection of the IV and maximum mobility of the child. Figure 33-4 illustrates the most commonly used intravenous sites in children. Infusion sites frequently used for children include the back of the hand, the forearm, the dorsum of the foot, and the scalp for infants. These sites offer some natural restraint for protection of the IV as they are not usually very close to points of flexion, and so additional restraint of the child can be minimized.

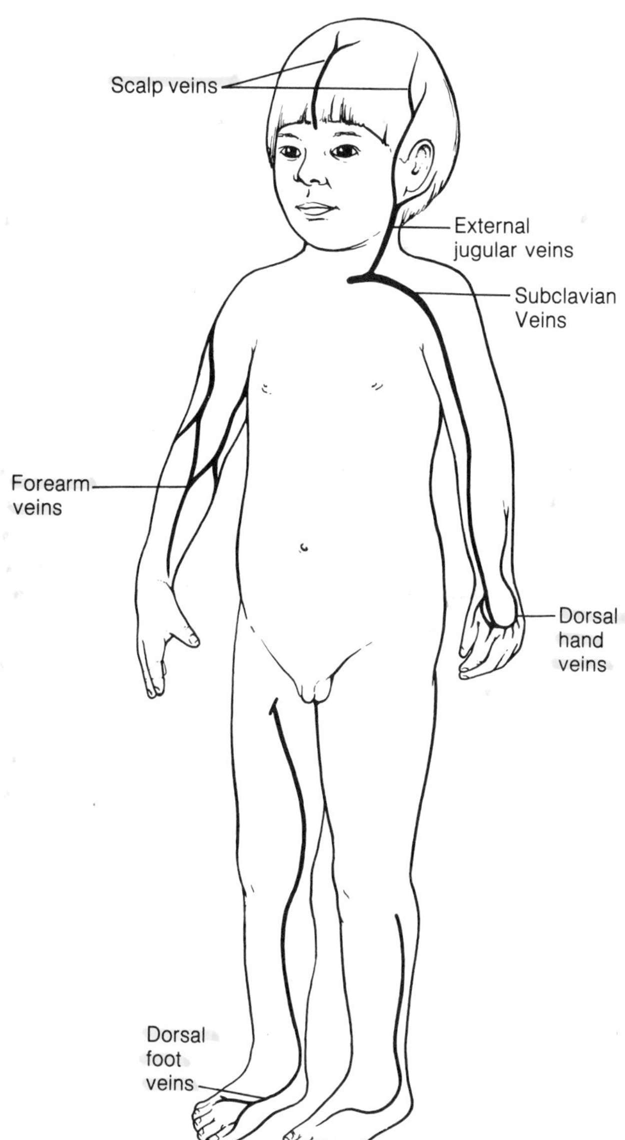

Figure 33-4 Common sites for intravenous infusions in children.

With the hand or forearm, the nondominant side of the body should be used since even the infant can be highly dependent on sucking one particular thumb. The dorsum of the foot is a less desirable site for an ambulatory child as the child must not walk on the affected foot. It can be an adequate site for the infant and sometimes must be utilized with the older child. Scalp veins are often used with infants. Many young infants derive pleasure from being bundled, which is the preferred method of restraint when the infusion site is a scalp vein. Some infants require additional restraints to protect their IVs. For a discussion of restraints for infants and older children, see Chapter 29.

The antecubital fossa and neck veins are sometimes used as a last resort for a peripheral IV. Either site is difficult to immobilize in the child, and the immobilization is restrictive. Both sites demand close nursing observation for signs of infiltration or phlebitis. The child has relatively good use of the arm when a forearm or hand vein is used but does not when the elbow is extended and restrained. Although a neck vein may be used for a peripheral IV during surgery, it is difficult to maintain when a child regains consciousness and becomes somewhat active.

Intravenous Equipment Drip control chambers, or burettes, are used with children's IVs for various reasons. They permit very accurate determinations of fluid infused since they are marked in 1-mL gradations. They have a mechanism for preventing air from entering the IV tubing and thus the child. They also help prevent fluid overload in the child by limiting the amount of fluid to the amount in the burette. If the flow rate inadvertently increases, as it might with position changes, the fluid infused is limited to that in the burette instead of the entire IV bottle. To prevent fluid overload effectively, the burettes themselves must not contain excess fluid. The burette should contain a maximum of 2 hours worth of fluid and even less with infants or children at risk for imbalance. Lastly, burettes facilitate intravenous medication administration. (For a discussion of intravenous medication administration, see Chapter 29.)

Most intravenous administration sets used for children are calibrated to flow at 60 drops per milliliter (60 gtt/mL), and since there are 60 minutes in an hour, the number of drops per minute (gtt/min) equals the number of milliliters to be delivered per hour.

In addition to gravity administration sets, infusion pumps and syringe pumps are used to deliver a specified amount of fluid in a given period of time. The syringe pump is useful for small amounts of fluid. Either pump delivers fluid at a standard infusion flow rate despite changes in a child's activities or other resistance, such as a needle or IV catheter resting against the wall of a vein.

Infusion pumps are usually accurate to within 2%, but this very accuracy can give the nurse a false sense of security. Pumps do malfunction, and the nurse therefore determines the amount of fluid actually infused in a given period of time. Also, as pumps continue to work against pressure, they can pump fluid into the tissues when an IV is infiltrated (although with different pumps an alarm will sound if flow is actually obstructed). Thus an infusion pump, if not care-

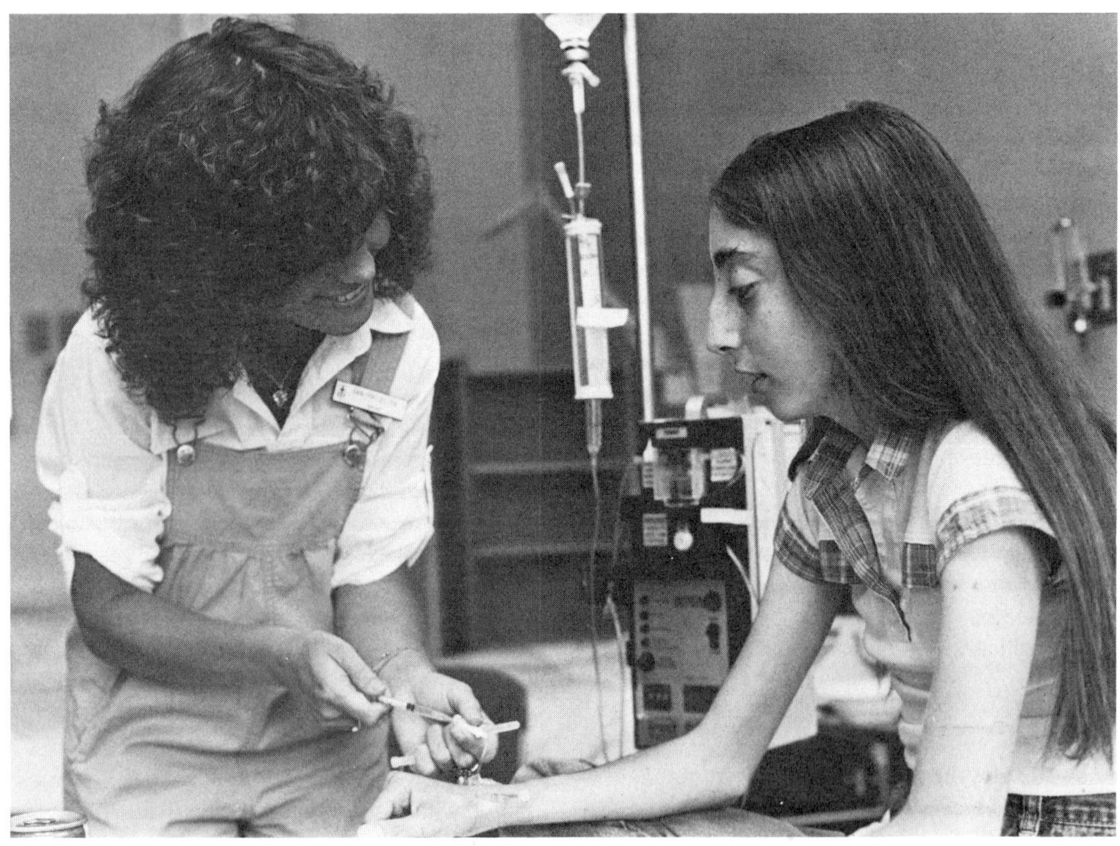

Intravenous administration by means of an infusion pump with a heparin lock.

fully monitored, could produce a serious infiltration with potential for tissue damage. In a gravity administration set the flow rate would slow or stop with the increased resistance to fluid entering the tissues instead of the vein. Even with controlled infusion, the nurse's hourly observations of drip rates and amount of fluid infused are essential.

Nursing Management for Intravenous Infusion

Three major aspects in the nursing care of the child with an intravenous infusion are (a) preventing complications, (b) maintaining safety, and (c) providing for developmental needs.

Complications of Intravenous Infusions The most common complications of intravenous therapy are listed in Table 33-2. Nursing interventions to prevent such complications center on frequent, thorough checks of the IV insertion site and entire administration set. The less the site is encumbered by tape, dressings, or protective devices such as trimmed-to-fit-the-area cups, the more easily the nurse can make observations and the earlier an infiltration might be determined. Some compromise must be struck, however, between ease of observation and protection of the IV. If the site is difficult to observe, the nurse looks for other indicators of infiltration such as whether the tape over the IV site appears tight, whether there is puffiness in the general area of insertion, whether there is a difference between the body part into which the IV is inserted and the corresponding part on the child's opposite side, or whether the skin at the infiltration site is cool or cold to touch.

When it is difficult to maintain as rapid an intravenous flow rate as the child needs, the nurse should assess the site for indications of infiltration. As a final check the IV bottle may be lowered to ascertain adequate backflow and thus IV patency. If this step is necessary, it should be done as a last check, for blood backflow through the small-lumen needles used with some children could contribute to increased slowing of the fluid flow or actual clot formation.

To decrease the risk of inflammation, strict aseptic technique is necessary when the IV is inserted or if IV dressings are changed. Policies concerning dressings, the length of time a needle or IV catheter remains in place, the frequency with which IV tubing is changed, and the routine for changing solution bottles or bags vary with the facility. Because of the emotional trauma and physical difficulties of IV insertion in children, some facilities do not change IV needles

TABLE 33-2 Common Complications of Intravenous Therapy

Complication	Objective sign(s)	Nursing intervention
Infiltration	Swelling around site (possibly extending further up from site) Poor or absent flow rate Poor blood backflow Cool to cold skin at site	Discontinue infusion Remove angiocatheter or needle Apply warm, wet compresses to site
Thrombophlebitis	Tenderness or pain at site Warm or red site Fever, leukocytosis Possible hardness of vein Possible swelling at site Poor or absent blood flow	Discontinue infusion Remove angiocatheter or needle Apply warm, wet compresses to site
Fluid overload	Increased blood pressure Increased urinary output Tachycardia Possible neck vein distention Respiratory signs—tachypnea, dyspnea, orthopnea, rales Edema, particularly periorbital Bulging, tense fontanelles in infant	Slow infusion to keep vein open (KVO) rate Place child in semi-Fowler's or Fowler's position Monitor vital signs as needed Give oxygen as needed Monitor edema, intake, output and urine specific gravity Monitor fontanelles in infants
Air embolism	Signs of shock—tachycardia, hypotension, loss of consciousness	Turn child on left side Give oxygen if needed Inspect IV system for disconnections

or dressings for a peripheral IV. The IV is removed when it is no longer needed or when there are signs of infiltration or phlebitis. The IV solution and often the tubing are changed every 24 hours.

With thrombophlebitis the IV site is characteristically tender, warm, and red. The vein may feel hardened and appear somewhat swollen. There can be swelling at the site, and blood return might be poor.

For both infiltration and thrombophlebitis, the IV is discontinued and the angiocatheter or needle removed. Warm, wet compresses encourage fluid absorption for infiltration and give comfort and increase the blood flow to the site for relief of an inflammation.

Fluid therapy, even when administered at the prescribed rate, may be excessive or inadequate for a particular child's needs. Conditions affecting fluid needs as well as signs and symptoms of dehydration and overhydration will be discussed later in this chapter. The nurse carefully monitors the infusion for rate and the child for both adequate therapeutic effect and possible fluid overload. To maximize therapeutic effect, the nurse checks the IV at frequent intervals, every 15–30 minutes, to determine whether or not the gravity system or pump is delivering the proper amount of fluid. When too little or too much fluid is infusing, the IV rate should be adjusted appropriately. If the incorrect rate has been infusing for more than 1 hour, some adjustment often can be made. With too rapid an infusion, it is necessary to slow the rate, perhaps so that it is just enough to *keep* the *vein open* (KVO). If the rate has been too slow, the nurse carefully evaluates the child's needs and the method and desirability of "catching up." When a child is not a neonate and is free from cardiac, renal, or other fluid utilization difficulty, the IV rate can be increased slightly for a number of hours until the child's intake meets fluid requirements.

The nurse must always be aware that fluid overload is a possible complication of intravenous therapy. With an infant whose fontanelle is open, fluid overload will cause the fontanelle to bulge. Other signs of fluid overload include increased urinary output, increased blood pressure, pulse and respirations, dyspnea, and bilateral rales. In addition, the child's neck veins may become distended and periorbital edema may be present. For fluid overload, the nurse slows the IV rate to a KVO rate. The child may benefit from being placed in a semi-Fowler's or Fowler's position and may need oxygen. The nurse carefully monitors vital signs and observes for the resolution of the overload.

Air embolism is an uncommon but very serious complication of IV therapy. The child may show signs of shock with rapid pulse and low blood pressure and may lose consciousness. The nurse turns the child to the left side, assesses need for oxygen, and inspects the IV system for the source of the problem. The physician should be notified if the nurse suspects overload or air embolism.

Safety and Intravenous Infusions The child's physiologic need for fluids or electrolytes requires the nurse's being concerned for the IV's safety and possibly restraining the child. Use of a scalp vein for an infant allows some limb mobility, but the child still must be positioned so that head and limb movements are not likely to disrupt the IV. When the child is not being held, mummy or extremity restraints may be necessary. The young child with an IV in any site may, when unattended, need to have extremities restrained. Some children can be helped to understand the importance of the IV and may not need restraints. Any restraints should be periodically removed and the infant or child held in order to provide comfort, security, and tactile stimulation (see Chapter 29).

Other aspects of safety include knowledge of compatibility of medications and maintenance infusions. An infusion line may need to be flushed before and after a medication with a solution compatible with the medication and maintenance solution. The medication can then be "piggybacked" and infused with the compatible solution. The nurse monitors urine output and sugar content when a child receives parenteral hyperalimentation. (For a discussion of intravenous hyperalimentation, see Chapter 38.) Insulin is administered as ordered if osmotic diuresis due to the hypertonic glucose infusion occurs.

Developmental Needs During Intravenous Infusions Play and the active manipulation of the environment are paramount for the cognitive and motor development of the child. Intravenous therapy restricts the child's mobility so that the nurse needs to consider the restrictions imposed when a vein is selected for intravenous therapy. The dominant hand, need to ambulate, and convenience of the scalp vein for the infant were discussed earlier. The older child may maximize mobility and control of restrictions by choosing within acceptable limits, the IV site. The child needs emotional support during IV insertion and removal and needs help in expressing feelings. Activities from holding and rocking the infant to facilitating games and peer interaction for the adolescent are an integral part of nursing care. Explanations for child and family need to be realistic and understandable. (Chapter 29 describes principles of nursing care to meet developmental needs.)

Assessing Signs of Fluid and Electrolyte Imbalance Interpreting certain signs of fluid and electrolyte imbalances requires extra caution. For example, the character and frequency of the child's stools may directly reflect a fluid volume deficit with the child becoming more constipated as dehydration increases. The child's dehydration might, however, be related to diarrhea. Stools are then loose, tend to be frequent, and might have noticeable free water, seen easily in the diapered child as a ring of liquid feces surrounding any solid stool.

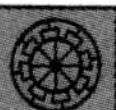

ASSESSMENT GUIDE The Child With a Fluid or Electrolyte Imbalance

System	Subjective data	Objective data	Validating data	Nursing management
EENT	Thirst	Dark circles around eyes Sunken eyeballs Tearless cry Dry mucous membranes and tongue—check membranes between cheek and gum	Blood chemistry Urine specific gravity	Question recent fluid loss related to illness, severe injury, or hemorrhage Note whether longitudinal furrows are present on tongue
	No thirst	Periorbital edema		Question recent fluid gain secondary to underlying illness (cardiac or renal) or excess intake
Head		Depressed fontanelle Bulging, tense fontanelle		Monitor for changes Access for evidence of head injury or other signs of cerebral edema if fontanelles are bulging
Integumentary		Pallor, grayish color Skin cold or warm to touch Skin doughy or rubbery to touch Clammy skin Tenting of skin	Blood chemistry	Identify signs of poor skin turgor related to fluid loss and hypotonicity Careful replacement of fluid by monitoring IV therapy or small amounts of oral fluids
Cardiovascular	Palpitations	Arrhythmias—bradycardia; tachycardia A B	Blood chemistry ECG	For electrolyte imbalance, most serious of which is K^+, monitor serum K^+ and place child on cardiac monitor Observe for hyperkalemia evidenced by tall, peaked T wave and flat P wave **(A)** Observe for ventricular fibrillation and cardiac arrest Hypokalemia evidenced by flat T wave, possible U wave, and prolonged S-T segment **(B)**

continued on next page

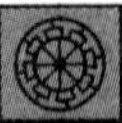

ASSESSMENT GUIDE The Child With a Fluid or Electrolyte Imbalance (continued)

System	Subjective data	Objective data	Validating data	Nursing management
Cardiovascular (cont.)	Palpitations (cont.)	Weak, rapid, thready pulse Hypotension Increase in blood pressure Generalized edema		Observe for further signs of shock Monitor fluid replacement Observe for evidence of overhydration or other cause of fluid retention Restrict fluid intake; slow IV infusion rate
Gastrointestinal	Anorexia Nausea Abdominal cramps Constipation Diarrhea Polydipsia	Vomiting Abdominal distention Liquid, loose, or hard and dry stools	Blood chemistry Urine test for electrolytes	Determine whether symptoms are part of underlying disease or response to imbalance (hypokalemia in paralytic ileus, hypercalcemia in gastrointestinal atony, hyponatremia in vomiting and abdominal cramps without diarrhea) Provide ordered fluid and electrolyte replacement
Respiratory	Dizziness Anxiousness, apprehensiveness	Hyperventilation Hypoventilation Restlessnesss Dyspnea Signs of respiratory paralysis	Blood chemistry Arterial blood gases	Facilitate respirations; position in Fowler's or semi-Fowler's; monitor fluid replacement for hydration; have child do breathing exercises (see Chapter 34) Remain calm to allay child's anxiety Provide oxygen therapy if PCO_2 is markedly elevated or cyanosis is present
		Deep rapid breathing Fruity odor to breath	Blood chemistry Blood and urine glucose tests	Give insulin as ordered (see Chapter 40) Replace fluid and provide carbohydrate source
		Larynogospasms, bronchospasms	Blood chemistry	Provide for calcium replacement (must infuse with 5% dextrose as saline increases loss of Ca^{2+})
Genitourinary	Infrequent voiding	Oliguria, anuria	Urine electrolytes Urine specific gravity Blood chemistry	Measure accurately intake and output Monitor urine specific gravity Withhold K^+ until voiding is established
	Frequent voiding	Polyuria, signs of renal damage Hematuria		Restrict or increase fluid intake as indicated
Neuromuscular	Muscle weakness Exhaustion	Hypotonicity or hypertonicity Diminished reflexes	Blood chemistry	Provide rest Provide fluid and replacement therapy as indicated

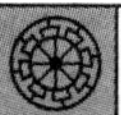

ASSESSMENT GUIDE The Child With a Fluid or Electrolyte Imbalance (continued)

System	Subjective data	Objective data	Validating data	Nursing management
	Confusion Muscle cramps Numbness of fingers	Muscle weakness Facial grimacing, spasms Tetany, carpopedal spasm Positive Chvostek's sign Tremors		Observe for signs of increased neuromuscular irritability leading to convulsions (pad siderails and have airway at bedside) Observe for signs of increased lethargy leading to coma Check neurologic signs, muscle tone with vital signs
Skeletal	Skeletal pain	Skeletal changes, rickets, osteoporosis, pathologic fractures	Blood chemistry	Provide comfort measures and rest

The child's skin characteristically becomes cool and dry as fluid deficit increases, but if a deficit is related to fever, the skin would be warm and tend to be moist with perspiration. Skin turgor can reflect fluid loss with tenting, the skin remaining elevated for several fractions of a second to a few seconds when a small portion (usually from the abdomen) is gently lifted between two fingers and then released. Without fluid deficit, the skin should immediately return to its normal position. In many instances tenting is not a reliable sign. When a child has a fluid loss in excess of a sodium loss, some fluid leaves the cells and enters the extracellular spaces in an attempt to maintain a balance in osmotic pressure. The skin then is rubbery or leathery to touch and tenting is less apparent than would be expected for the child's fluid loss.

Skin turgor also will suggest underestimated fluid loss in the obese child or the child with abdominal distention. With the malnourished child, loose skin is related to loss of subcutaneous tissue as well as acute fluid loss and thus may be too sensitive a sign for the child's actual fluid loss. Under normal circumstances skin shows some signs of tenting with a mild loss of approximately 3%–5% of body weight.

The nurse inspects the mouth to evaluate the moistness of a child's mucous membranes. This inspection, too, can be deceptive, for mouth breathing causes the tongue and mouth to become dry with or without fluid volume deficit. The area where the gums and cheek meet, however, provides a differential assessment site as it remains moist during mouth breathing. The nurse therefore inspects this area to be certain a dry mouth is related to fluid volume deficit. Longitudinal wrinkles on the tongue are an excellent indication of dehydration. Thirst is a good indication of fluid deficit, but the nauseous child may not wish to drink, despite fluid loss.

Urine output and specific gravity are reliable signs of hydration status in most instances. Decreased volume, however, may not be a reflection of dehydration but rather a sign of fluid retention in the child with cardiac or renal disease. The child under considerable stress may have decreased output in response to stress. Urine specific gravity, in most instances an excellent sign, can be dramatically increased with protein or glucose in the urine. With a child at risk for severe deficit or shock, however, urine output is important enough that an indwelling catheter may be inserted to allow for close monitoring of output.

Other signs of fluid electrolyte imbalance are discussed in relation to specific imbalances.

Fluid and Electrolyte Imbalances

Although certain signs and symptoms characterize individual fluid and electrolyte imbalances, there is a large variation in the clinical picture for any one child. Because of the disease process underlying the imbalance, a child's other conditions, and the age and size of the child, various signs may show (Table 33-3). Seldom is an imbalance one pure imbalance but is instead a mixture. For example, chloride is usually gained or lost with sodium, while serum potassium is usually increased in acidosis as the kidneys selectively rid the body of H^+ and save K^+.

Signs also vary with a condition's rapidity of onset. The more rapid the onslaught of an excess or deficit, the more dramatic the signs may be and the more serious the imbalance for the child. A baby experiencing explosive diarrhea, for example, tends to show signs of extracellular fluid volume deficit quickly but might not show as serious signs if

TABLE 33-3 Clincial Manifestations of Specific Fluid and Electrolyte Imbalances

Imbalance	Blood chemistry	Clinical manifestations
Hyperkalemia	$K^+ > 5.5$ mEq/L	Bradycardia, arrhythmias, ventricular fibrillation, cardiac arrest Oliguria, anuria Muscle weakness, irritability General flaccid paralysis, respiratory paralysis; nausea, intestinal colic
Hypokalemia	$K^+ < 3.5$ mEq/L	Arrhythmia, tachycardia or bradycardia Drop in diastolic blood pressure Polyuria, persistent dilute urine, impaired renal function Polydipsia Abdominal distention, paralytic ileus Muscle weakness or irritability Diminished reflexes
Hypernatremia—Fluid deficit or sodium excess (hypertonic dehydration)	$Na^+ > 150$ mEq/L	Sunken eyes with dark circles Rapid pulse, low blood pressure Doughy consistency to skin, fair turgor Very dry mucous membranes Sunken fontanelles in infant Oliguria, tearless cry, thirst Reflex hyperirritability Lethargy, coma
Hyponatremia—fluid retention or sodium deficit (hypotonic dehydration)	$Na^+ < 130$ mEq/L	Potential for shock, rapid, thready pulse, low blood pressure Clammy skin, poor turgor Absence of thirst Nausea, vomiting, abdominal cramps Muscular weakness, twitching, irritability Oliguria, slightly dry mucous membranes Weight gain, cerebral edema, disorientation, coma
Extracellular fluid volume deficit (isotonic dehydration)	Na^+ within normal range Hemoconcentration	Thirst, fatigue Dry mucous membranes, poor skin turgor Dry skin, absence of tears Sunken and soft eyeball Oliguria, anuria Longitudinal furrows on tongue
Extracellular fluid volume excess (isotonic overhydration)	Na^+ within normal range Hemodilution	No thirst Increase in pulse and blood pressure Acute weight gain, polyuria Signs of congestive heart failure—periorbital edema, diaphoresis

TABLE 33-3 continued

Imbalance	Blood chemistry	Clinical manifestations
		Signs of pulmonary edema—rales, dyspnea, cough
		Signs of cerebral edema—bulging, tense fontanelle in infant, convulsions, coma
Hypercalcemia	$Ca^{2+} > 5.7$ mEq/L	Hypotonicity and muscle weakness
		Lethargy
		Anorexia, nausea, vomiting
		Constipation
		Polyuria, polydipsia
		Weight loss
		Impaired renal function
		Osseous changes, growth failure
Hypocalcemia	$Ca^{2+} < 4.5$ mEq/L	Generalized neuromuscular irritability
		Facial spasms, grimacing
		Laryngospasms
		Tetany, positive Chvostek's sign
		Convulsions
		Arrhythmias, cardiac arrest
Hypermagnesemia	$Mg^{2+} > 2.1$ mEq/L	Drop in blood pressure, weak pulse
		Nausea, vomiting
		Diminished reflexes, drowsiness
		Heart block, cardiac arrest
		Muscle weakness, flaccid paralysis, coma
		Respiratory depression
Hypomagnesemia	$Mg^{2+} < 1.2$ mEq/L	Insomnia
		Cardiac arrhythmias
		Muscle weakness, twitching
		Seizures, tetany

the same actual degree of dehydration had resulted from a gradual loss of fluid. Also, a young child is more able to handle a deficit than an excess. For example, hypernatremia may be caused by either excess sodium intake or fluid loss in excess of sodium loss. The young child's kidneys are better equipped to handle the deficit than the excess, and thus the excess produces more severe signs and has more serious implications for the child.

The nurse needs to check and recheck the child's laboratory values. Compensatory mechanisms such as fluid shifts and the movement of potassium between extracellular and intracellular fluids can create rapid changes in the laboratory values as the underlying illness is treated. As one problem is corrected, another may arise, and any imbalance may need to be treated. For example, an elevated serum potassium level in acidosis may become a serum deficit as acidosis is treated and potassium returns to the intracellular fluids.

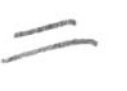

Potassium

Potassium, the dominant cation of the intracellular fluid, is critical to several physiologic functions: (a) regulation of intracellular osmolarity and electroneutrality; (b) conduction of nerve impulses; (c) energy production by means of enzyme systems used in cellular work; (d) cellular growth; and (e) myocardial and skeletal muscle activity.

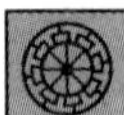

NURSING CARE GUIDE The Child With a Fluid Imbalance

Nursing diagnosis	Interventions	Evaluation
1. Potential for fluid volume deficit related to loss of body fluids	Monitor vital signs Compare current weight to preillness weight; weigh daily Maintain accurate intake and output Monitor urine specific gravity with each voiding Describe quantity and character of stool and vomitus Test skin for turgor; note color and temperature of skin In infants, observe fontanelles for depression Observe for sunken eyeballs and dark circles around eyes Describe condition of mucous membranes and degree of dryness Describe child's neurologic state—drowsiness and irritability, restlessness and tremors Note presence or absence of thirst or tears Monitor blood chemistry and laboratory reports Replace fluid loss as directed Monitor IV therapy Begin clear oral fluids gradually and monitor child's response and ability to retain Gradually advance diet as tolerated and reduce rate of IV therapy	Child's state of hydration returns to normal and fluid loss ceases
2. Potential for fluid volume excess related to overhydration	Monitor vital signs In infants, observe fontanelle for bulging or tenseness Maintain accurate intake and output Monitor urine specific gravity Monitor laboratory values Note evidence of hemodilution Observe for edema, both periorbital and generalized Observe for signs of circulatory overload, pulmonary edema, and cerebral edema Restrict fluids as directed	Child's hydration status returns to normal with no evidence of edema or impaired function

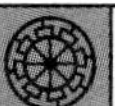

NURSING CARE GUIDE The Child With a Fluid Imbalance (continued)

Nursing diagnosis	Interventions	Evaluation
3. Potential for electrolyte imbalance related to fluid imbalance	Monitor laboratory reports of serum electrolytes Monitor vital signs; take apical pulse; note any arrhythmias Note changes in blood pressure, especially hypotension Place on cardiac monitor if indicated by changes in vital signs Document renal function prior to administration of K^+ replacement Monitor progressive changes in muscle weakness and any evidence of paralysis Describe muscle tone and evidence of hyperirritability and tetany Monitor child's sensorium and any evidence of convulsions or progressive drowsiness and coma	Child's sensorium remains intact; vital signs and muscle tonicity are normal for age
4. Potential for altered breathing pattern related to compensatory mechanism	Observe rate and quality of respirations Monitor laboratory values of blood gases and serum pH Describe changes in sensorium	Child has normal respiratory pattern
5. Potential for altered skin integrity related to loss of body fluids	Observe child's skin for evidence of redness or breakdown Apply protective ointment to perineal area if diarrhea is present Provide mouth care and oral hygiene Lubricate dry lips with ointment	Child's skin is intact, and color is normal

Potassium is easily absorbed from the gastrointestinal tract. Normally, 10%–20% of ingested potassium is excreted in the feces, and almost 90% is excreted in the urine. Because the body does not have a sophisticated means of conserving potassium, daily consumption of potassium must approximate the daily amount excreted in the urine.

Hyperkalemia Hyperkalemia, an excess of potassium in the blood, is a medical emergency. The most common causes of hyperkalemia are (a) conditions that cause inadequate excretion of potassium ions and subsequent retention in body fluids (for example, acute renal failure, chronic renal insufficiency, and adrenocortical insufficiency); (b) potassium ion release from the intracellular compartment (for example, crushing injuries, extensive surgery, early burns, dehydration, and severe infection); (c) intravenous potassium administration (either excess amount or infused too rapidly); and (d) acidosis.

Hypokalemia Common causative factors in the development of hypokalemia are (a) low potassium intake (which may be caused by severe dieting or parenteral feedings deficient in potassium); (b) gastrointestinal tract losses (which may be caused by vomiting, diarrhea, excessive nasogastric suctioning, fistulas, or frequent enemas); (c) excessive renal loss (which may be caused by Cushing's syndrome, chronic pyelonephritis, renal tubular acidosis, diuresis due to diuretics or the diuretic phase of renal failure, burn healing, or corticosteroid therapy); and (d) alkalosis.

Nursing Management for Potassium Imbalance Nursing management of the hyperkalemic child varies with the severity of the disturbance and the causative factor(s). In severe hyperkalemia, the amount of excess potassium is most effectively reduced through increasing urinary output.

If renal failure is a factor, urinary output is promoted by peritoneal dialysis or hemodialysis (Chapter 39). In addition, sodium polystyrene sulfonate (Kayexalate) or insulin may be administered. Sodium polystyrene sulfonate is an ion-exchange resin that removes potassium ions from the gastrointestinal tract by binding with them. It is given orally or as a retention enema. Small doses of intravenous insulin and glucose promote the movement of glucose and potassium into the intracellular compartment. Limitation of protein catabolism through an adequate balanced diet decreases tissue wasting. Intravenous potassium infusions are stopped. Foods high in potassium content must be eliminated from the diet. Potassium is found in many foods, including meat, fish, bananas, citrus fruit, dried fruit, many vegetables, and milk. Finally, controlling infection and remaining cognizant of the causes of hyperkalemia are of paramount importance.

Nursing management of the hypokalemic child includes replacing the potassium loss and treating the primary physiologic imbalance. A nursing care plan might include (a) oral or parenteral potassium replacement, (b) careful monitoring of flow rate of potassium infusions, (c) intake and output recordings, (d) accurate measurement of nasogastric tube output when one is present, and (e) evaluation of diagnostic tests such as serum potassium level and a 12-lead electrocardiogram (ECG).

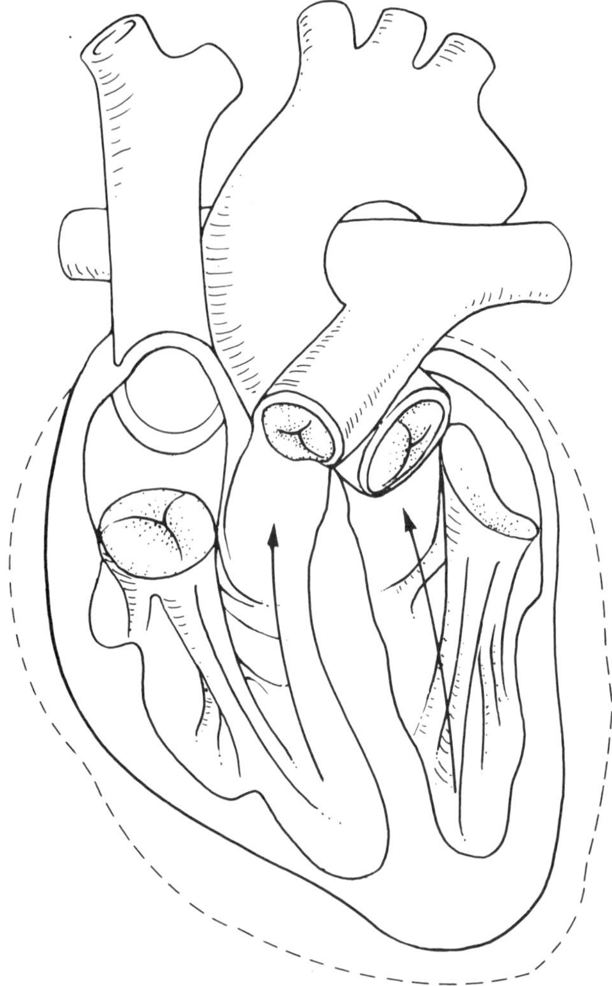

Figure 33-5 Calcium, a positive inotropic agent, increases the strength of myocardial contractility.

Calcium

Ninety-nine percent of calcium is concentrated in bone. The rest is distributed in other tissues and extracellular fluids. The cardiac, the skeletal, and the neuromuscular systems depend on calcium. Calcium is a positive inotropic agent; that is, it increases the strength of muscular contractions. Calcium therefore enhances myocardial contractility, decreases neuromuscular irritability and capillary permeability, and is essential for growth of bones and teeth, normal muscle contractility, and normal coagulation (Fig. 33-5). It is also important for the proper transmission of nerve impulses.

The normal serum calcium level is 4.5–5.7 mEq/L. A normal serum calcium level depends on the availability of vitamin D, the intake of calcium in the diet, the serum phosphorus level, and the functioning of the parathyroid glands. Calcium is excreted in the urine.

Hypercalcemia Hypercalcemia results from (a) excessive intake of calcium or vitamin D, (b) immobilization, (c) hyperparathyroidism, (d) decreased calcium excretion by the kidneys, and (e) miscellaneous conditions (for example, some children with leukemia or other tumors; thyrotoxicosis; prolonged milk intake with alkali; and with the infant, excessive maternal intake of vitamin D during pregnancy leading to mental retardation, elfin facies, and other congenital defects).

Hypocalcemia Hypocalcemia is an extremely life-threatening electrolyte imbalance that may be caused by (a) low dietary intake of calcium, (b) excessive loss with diarrhea, (c) inadequate vitamin D intake, (d) chronic renal insufficiency, (e) use of cow's milk formula in some infants, (f) hypoparathyroidism, and (g) excessive transfusion with stored citrated blood. Severe hypocalcemia results in tetany.

Other objective indications of hypocalcemia are laboratory findings, ECG changes, and a positive Chvostek's sign. Blood chemistry reports illustrate a decreased calcium level and an elevated phosphorus level. Hypocalcemia causes the cardiac muscle to dilate, leading to cardiac arrest. Hypocalcemia causes irritability of the seventh cranial nerve (facial nerve) as demonstrated by a positive Chvostek's sign (the child's lip, nose, or entire side of the face will contract when the area below the temple is tapped). A positive Chvostek's sign is indicative of tetany.

Nursing Management for Calcium Imbalance For the hypercalcemic child, the goal of management is to correct the physiologic dysfunction causing the hypercalcemia. Specific therapies to decrease serum calcium include administering corticosteroids or isotonic saline infusion or decreasing calcium intake. High-calcium foods are primarily milk and cheese. Some green, leafy vegetables and dried beans and peas are also good sources of calcium.

A child with a documented mild hypocalcemia or a child with potential for hypocalcemia must be closely monitored for respiratory function. Tetany is a medical emergency. A tracheostomy set and a syringe of calcium gluconate should be near the child's bedside. Calcium deficit is treated by administering calcium salts orally, intramuscularly, or intravenously. In addition, vitamin D may also be administered to assist in the absorption of calcium.

Chloride

Chloride is an anion located primarily in the extracellular fluid compartment. Chloride is highly concentrated in the stomach because it is essential to the production of hydrochloric acid. The normal serum value of chloride is approximately 100 mEq/L.

In addition to being a major component of hydrochloric acid, chloride is also important in maintaining the arterial pH. Chloride is excreted by the kidney in the form of sodium chloride.

Because chloride combines with sodium in the fluid compartments, a deficiency or excess of chloride essentially mimics the status of sodium. Hyperchloremia, due to decreased excretion or excess ingestion of chloride, results in metabolic acidosis. The kidneys excrete the base bicarbonate when excess chloride is present, yielding a deficit in bicarbonate and therefore acidosis. Chloride out of proportion to sodium is reflected in an acid-base imbalance.

Hypochloremia may occur as a result of excessive loss of hydrochloric acid through vomiting, resulting in alkalosis, or through the chloride shift occurring as a compensatory mechanism with acidosis. In these situations, control of the vomiting or correction of the acid–base imbalance should return the serum chloride value to normal.

Sodium

Sodium is the major cation within the extracellular fluid, which contains approximately 140 mEq/L of sodium. Its most important function is to maintain water distribution through the fluid compartments of the body. Sodium controls water balance by maintaining osmotic equilibrium between the intracellular and the extracellular fluid. Other functions of sodium include (a) maintaining intravascular volume, (b) controlling muscle contractility (especially cardiac contractility), (c) assisting in nerve impulse conduction, (d) maintaining neuromuscular irritability, (e) acting as a buffer base, and (f) increasing cell membrane permeability.

Because water imbalance affects sodium balance and sodium imbalance in turn affects water balance, the relationship between these two constituents must always be considered in the child with fluid and electrolyte imbalance. The two types of sodium and water imbalances are osmolar imbalances and volume imbalances. When body fluid osmolarity is disturbed, water moves from an area of lesser osmolarity to an area of greater osmolarity. Thus water distribution between fluid compartments changes. If water and sodium levels change together, causing isotonic imbalances, volume disturbances will develop. Osmolar imbalances result in cellular changes while volume imbalances do not.

Hyperosmolarity Hyperosmolar disturbances are caused by a water decrease or an extracellular sodium excess (hypernatremia), which may be created by a variety of conditions. The following list outlines the conditions that may cause hyperosmolarity.

Water Decrease	*Hypernatremia*
Decreased intake—cerebral injury, dysphagia; anorexia	Increased dietary intake, saltwater intake, near-drowning
Increased output—diarrhea, diabetes insipidus, polyuria, fever, hyperventilation	Excessive solute loads—tube feedings (protein), intravenous infusions of saline

When a hyperosmolar imbalance exists, the serum sodium level rises and water leaves the cells, causing cells to shrink. Assessment of the child thus reveals many subjective and objective signs of dehydration, and the child is closely observed for evidence of any of the following:

- Changes in vital signs—decreased blood pressure, decreased central venous pressure, increased temperature, tachycardia, tachypnea
- Skin changes—flushed appearance, rubbery skin, dry sticky mucous membranes
- Dry tongue
- Thirst
- Soft, sunken eyeballs
- Oliguria, increased specific gravity
- Cerebral changes—irritability, restlessness, eventual coma
- Depressed fontanelles in infants

As the water is reduced in all fluid compartments, the viscosity of the blood increases and the hemoglobin value rises. The nurse is particularly observant for central nervous system signs, as damage can follow intracellular fluid losses and intracranial hemorrhage.

Hypo-osmolarity Hypo-osmolar imbalances are caused by a water increase or an extracellular sodium decrease. In hypo-osmolar disturbances the serum sodium level decreases, causing hyponatremia. Hypo-osmolar imbalances may be caused by a variety of conditions. The following list outlines the conditions that may cause hypo-osmolarity.

Water Intoxication	*Hyponatremia*
Increased intake—fluid overload without corresponding electrolytes, tapwater enemas, freshwater near-drowning	Decreased intake
Decreased output—renal injury, brain injury	Increased output—diuretics, cystic fibrosis

A hypo-osmolar imbalance causes the serum sodium level to decrease and water to enter the cells, causing cellular swelling, or edema. The brain is most severely affected by cellular edema. Thus the child with an actual or potential hypo-osmolar imbalance must be observed closely for signs of neuromuscular irritability. Since water enters the cells, the extracellular fluid volume decreases. Urine output may decrease due to the body's attempt to conserve sodium, and concurrently chloride and water, by secreting aldosterone. Urine specific gravity can increase. Shock is a threat particularly in hypotonic dehydration. Subjective and objective signs include

Neuromuscular changes—muscle fatigue, weakness, twitching, irritability, headache, disorientation, confusion, convulsions, coma (increased intracranial pressure)

Bulging fontanelles in infants

Gastrointestinal changes—anorexia, nausea, vomiting

Absence of thirst

Shock is particularly a threat in hypotonic dehydration, as extracellular fluid deficit can be severe with fluid shift into the cells.

Volume Disturbances The term *volume disturbance,* or *isotonic disturbance,* implies that sodium and water increase or decrease proportionately. Because this does not disturb osmolarity, cellular changes do not occur.

Circulatory overload with resultant edema, however, occurs in conditions causing an increase in extracellular volume. Such conditions include congestive heart failure, renal disease, and hepatic failure. Decreases in the extracellular fluid volume create circulatory collapse with resultant dehydration. Such decreases are caused by hemorrhage, burn edema, fever, and excessive vomiting. Isotonic dehydration is the most common type of dehydration in children.

Table 33-4 compares the subjective and objective findings occurring in extracellular fluid volume excess and extracellular fluid volume deficit.

Nursing Management for Sodium and Water Imbalances The management of the child with a hyperosmolar imbalance involves replacing fluid losses (reversing dehydration) and preventing or treating the effects of hypertonic dehydration (fever, hypovolemic shock, and acute tubular necrosis).

Physiologic criteria used to evaluate the effect of fluid replacement include (a) intake and output recording; (b) daily weight measurement; (c) vital sign trends (for example, stabilization of blood pressure, pulse, respirations, and temperature); (d) improvement of skin characteristics, such as color or temperature; and (e) laboratory values within normal limits.

Treatment for the child exhibiting a hypo-osmolar imbalance involves restricting fluids and possibly administering a hypertonic solution. The success of the medical therapy is determined by the clinical improvement of the child: normalization of neuromuscular status, absence of nausea and vomiting, improvement in mental state, and the return of the serum sodium level to normal.

Management of volume disturbances primarily involves fluid and sodium therapy. The child with an extracellular fluid volume depletion is treated with infusions of isotonic solution; the child with an extracellular fluid volume excess is treated with fluid restriction, diuretic therapy, or sodium restriction, or all three. Specific data recorded for such children include

Vital sign trends

Daily weight and hourly intake and output measurements

Respiratory status—rate, quality, abnormal breath sounds, thoracic excursion

Cardiac status—heart rate, quality of pulse, peripheral pulses, extra heart sounds

Skin color, temperature, turgor

Laboratory findings—hematocrit, serum protein and serum sodium levels, urine specific gravity

Acid–Base Balance

Nursing care of the child requires a thorough understanding of the physiologic processes involved in maintaining normal arterial blood gases. Disturbances of acid–base equilibrium can be life-threatening to a child.

TABLE 33-4 Comparison of Objective Findings in Extracellular Fluid Volume Excess and Extracellular Fluid Volume Deficit

	Extracellular fluid volume excess	Extracellular fluid volume deficit
Cardiac	Congestive heart failure	Blood pressure decrease
	Blood pressure increase	Weight loss
	Weight gain	
Pulmonary	Pulmonary edema	No severe changes
	Dyspnea	
	Cough	
	Rales	
Renal	Increased output	Oliguria
	Eventual decrease in output as congestive heart failure progresses	Anuria
		Acute tubular necrosis
Skin	Diaphoresis	Poor turgor
	Edema (periorbital)	Dry mucous membranes
Laboratory data	Normal Na^+	Normal Na^+
	Decreased hematocrit	Increased hematocrit
	Decreased protein	Increased protein
	Decreased urine specific gravity	Increased urine specific gravity

When hydrogen ion concentration increases, arterial pH decreases, and the child is in a state of acidosis. When the hydrogen ion concentration decreases, the arterial pH increases, and the child is said to be in a state of alkalosis. Both severe acidosis and severe alkalosis disturb physiologic stability, so that the body initiates compensatory mechanisms to convert arterial pH to a normal range, which is 7.35–7.45. Three physiologic mechanisms assist in the regulation of the pH; these are blood buffers, pulmonary compensation, and renal compensation.

Mechanisms of Acid–Base Control

Buffers In essence, a buffer is a mechanism that acts as a shock absorber; it lessens the force of any drastic change in the pH. A buffer is a solution of the salt of a weak acid or a weak base. The presence of the buffer prevents severe changes in pH when a stronger acid or a stronger base is mixed in the solution. Specific buffer pairs include (a) carbonic acid and sodium bicarbonate, (b) hemoglobin and oxyhemoglobin, (c) organic and inorganic phosphates, and (d) plasma proteins and intracellular proteins.

The major blood buffer is the carbonic acid–sodium bicarbonate system. Carbonic acid is a weak acid that dissociates into hydrogen ions and bicarbonate ions, which are excreted by the kidneys, and water and carbon dioxide, which are excreted by the lungs. Thus if a strong acid or a strong base is added to a solution containing the carbonic acid–sodium bicarbonate buffer pair, the substance is quickly neutralized and the end products are excreted by the kidneys and the lungs. The reaction is

$$CO_2 + H_2O \rightleftharpoons H_2CO_3 \rightleftharpoons HCO_3^- + H^+$$

Carbon dioxide then diffuses into red blood cells.

Hemoglobin molecules are also important in buffering hydrogen ions. The isohydric reaction in red blood cells is a process whereby an increase in hydrogen ion concentration is accompanied by a reduction of oxyhemoglobin to form a weak acid. The chemical reaction is

$$H^+ + HbO_2 \rightleftharpoons HHb + O_2$$

(HHb is reduced Hb.) Oxygen then diffuses into the cells.

The bicarbonate ions (HCO_3^-), which resulted from the previous dissociation of carbonic acid, are buffered by another hemoglobin buffer, potassium hemoglobin (KHb).

$$HCO_3 + KHb \rightleftharpoons KHCO_3 + HHb \qquad KCl \text{ (in cell)}$$
$$KHCO_3 \rightleftharpoons K^+ + HCO_3 \qquad NaCl \rightleftharpoons Na^+ + Cl^-$$
$$NaHCO_3 \text{ (in plasma)}$$

The diffusion of chloride ions into the cell allows potassium chloride to form. The union of sodium ions and bicarbonate ions in the plasma then forms sodium bicarbonate. This process is called the *chloride shift*. Thus a child in a state of acidosis might evidence a lowered serum chloride value.

Arterial pH can be conceived of simplistically as the relationship between the base and the acid content of the blood. The normal ratio of base to acid is 20:1.

The value of the pH remains in the normal range as long as the base to acid ratio is maintained at 20:1. Therefore the pH would be normal, even if the body contained twice the usual amount of both acid and base. It is the relative amount of each component that is vital in determining the arterial pH.

Thus the buffer system can achieve normal acid–base balance, but excess acid or base are not excreted from the body. The lungs and kidneys perform this function necessary for maintaining normal acid–base balance for a prolonged period of time.

Pulmonary Compensation The most important chemical in the pulmonary control of arterial pH is the partial pressure of carbon dioxide (PCO_2). The normal PCO_2 in the child is 35–45 mm Hg.

When the child's arterial PCO_2 increases, the arterial pH decreases because of an increase in the hydrogen ion concentration. Thus the child will be in a state of acidosis, and the following sequence will be initiated:

Hypercapnia, or PCO_2 greater than 45 mm Hg

Increased H^+ in blood and cerebrospinal fluid and decreased pH

Stimulation of respiratory chemoreceptors

Hyperventilation

Decreased PCO_2

Decreased H^+ concentration and increased pH

If the child's nonvolatile (or fixed) acids increase, the hydrogen ion concentration will increase as it does with hypercapnia. Mechanisms of pH increase and decrease are thus

Increased pH	Decreased pH
Decreased PCO_2	Increased PCO_2
Decreased nonvolatile acids	Increased nonvolatile acids

A metabolic disturbance (such as diabetic ketoacidosis, lactic acidosis, or renal or hepatic failure) increases the hydrogen ion concentration in the cerebrospinal fluid. This in turn causes hyperventilation, a respiratory mechanism that functions to rid the body of volatile acid (CO_2). This process ultimately produces a base-to-acid ratio of 20:1. Thus the lungs quickly begin to compensate for a metabolic disturbance and attempt to return the pH value to normal.

Renal Compensation The renal system compensates for an acid–base imbalance resulting from a pulmonary or metabolic disturbance. It is responsible for the actual loss of hydrogen ions from the body. When a child's PCO_2 increases, the hydrogen ion concentration increases and the pH decreases. If a hypercapnic state continues, the kidneys begin to respond by excreting hydrogen ions and reabsorbing bicarbonate ions. The normal bicarbonate value in a child is 22–25 mEq/L. Thus the bicarbonate content (in mEq/L) rises to compensate for the elevated PCO_2 level. This proportionate increase in both components returns the base-to-acid ratio to 20:1, with the following chemical reaction:

$$CO_2 + H_2O \rightleftharpoons H_2CO_3 \rightleftharpoons HCO_3^- + H^+$$

Bicarbonate is then reabsorbed in the renal tubules, and hydrogen is excreted by the renal tubules. The renal system compensates in a like manner with a metabolic cause for acid–base disturbance.

Potassium ions are also excreted through the kidneys, although with a large loss of hydrogen ions, fewer potassium ions are excreted. Thus potassium retention may occur when the child is in a state of acidemia. This ability of the kidneys to compensate for a respiratory or metabolic disturbance is a slow process. Therefore, compensation for metabolic disturbances can be faster than for respiratory disturbances. Mechanisms of compensation are summarized as follows:

Primary Disturbance	*Compensation*
PCO_2	HCO_3^-
HCO_3^-	PCO_2

Acid–Base Abnormalities

Causes and clinical manifestations of acid–base imbalances are summarized in Table 33-5.

Respiratory Acidosis Alveolar hypoventilation is the primary cause of respiratory acidosis. Hypoventilation results in an increased PCO_2, which in turn elevates the hydrogen ion concentration. Thus the pH decreases, and the child is in a state of acidosis.

Many conditions produce alveolar hypoventilation and subsequent respiratory acidosis. Among these are

Obstructive pulmonary diseases such as asthma, emphysema, chronic bronchitis, cystic fibrosis

Restrictive pulmonary diseases such as obesity, voluntary restriction of thoracic expansion due to chest trauma or pain (for example, following thoracic surgery), neuromuscular diseases (for example, poliomyelitis, muscular dystrophy)

Atelectasis

Central nervous system depression that may be caused by head trauma, anesthesia, or drugs

Central nervous system infection

TABLE 33-5 Causes and Clinical Manifestations of Acid–Base Imbalance

Imbalance	Causes	Blood chemistry	Clinical manifestations
Respiratory acidosis	Hypoventilation Retention of CO_2 Ineffective	pH < 7.35 PCO_2 > 46 mm Hg	Restlessness, apprehensiveness leading to disorientation, coma Rapid pulse Diaphoresis Cyanosis, if critical
Respiratory alkalosis	Hyperventilation Loss of CO_2	pH > 7.45 PCO_2 < 34 mm Hg	Deep, rapid breathing Anxiousness, fearfulness Tingling of hands and face Dizziness
Metabolic alkalosis	Loss of acid through vomiting Retention of base Hypokalemia	pH > 7.45 CO_2 > 32 mEq/L HCO_3^- > 30 mEq/L	Confusion, irritability Hypertonicity of muscles Tetany, tremors Restlessness Nausea, vomiting, diarrhea Depressed respirations
Metabolic acidosis	Loss of base through diarrhea Increased acids, excessive catabolism of fats (diabetes) Hypoxia resulting in lactic acid accumulation	pH < 7.35 CO_2 < 22 mEq/L HCO_3^- < 25 mEq/L	Lethargy leading to drowsiness, stupor, coma Fruity odor to breath Anorexia, nausea, vomiting Diarrhea Hyperventilation

The effects of acidemia on the central nervous system provide objective evidence that a child is experiencing acute respiratory acidosis. The child may initially be lethargic and slow to respond to verbal stimuli, such as spoken commands. As the acidemia progresses, the central nervous system becomes more severely affected and the child may appear disoriented, confused, and eventually delirious. At its most severe level, acidemia is manifested by a stuporous state, convulsions, and coma.

Because acute respiratory acidosis is a pulmonary disorder, compensatory mechanisms to restore the pH to a normal level occur through the buffers and the kidneys (Table 33-6). The kidneys selectively reabsorb bicarbonate ions and excrete hydrogen ions, thus attempting to return the ratio of base to acid to 20:1.

Correcting the primary physiologic problem constitutes the major treatment goal in the management of the child in respiratory acidosis. Nursing measures therefore are directed to increasing alveolar ventilation (for example, breathing exercises, chest percussion and vibration, and

TABLE 33-6 Acute vs. Compensated Respiratory Acidosis and Alkalosis

	Respiratory acidosis		Respiratory alkalosis	
	Acute	*Compensated*	*Acute*	*Compensated*
pH	↓	Normal	↑	Normal
PCO_2	↑	↑	↓	↓
HCO_3	Normal	↑	Normal	↓

postural drainage) and to alleviating the cause of hypoventilation (for example, reducing pain or identifying and reporting a tight body cast) (see Chapter 34).

Respiratory Alkalosis Alveolar hyperventilation is the primary cause of respiratory alkalosis. Hyperventilation is defined as an increase in the rate and depth of respiration, and occurs with anxiety. It also occurs with salicylate intoxication (early), encephalitis or meningitis, or hyperventilation related to overstimulation of the respiratory center. Respiratory alkalosis is a change that "washes" carbon dioxide out of the lungs. Thus respiratory alkalosis decreases PCO_2, which in turn decreases the hydrogen ion concentration and elevates the pH (Table 33-6). Because carbon dioxide can be considered an acid (because of its affinity for water and the resultant production of carbonic acid), a decreased PCO_2 produces a relative excess of bicarbonate. The body compensates for respiratory alkalosis by selectively excreting bicarbonate ions, sodium ions, and potassium ions and reabsorbing hydrogen ions.

Respiratory alkalosis is treated by correcting the physiologic problem resulting in alveolar hyperventilation. The voluntary slowing of respirations or inhaling of carbon dioxide, however, may relieve symptoms and cause the pH to return to normal.

Metabolic Acidosis A serum elevation of nonvolatile, or fixed, acids or a decrease of base bicarbonate causes the hydrogen ion concentration to increase and the arterial pH to decrease. The resulting condition is called *metabolic acidosis* (Table 33-7).

The most common pathologic processes creating metabolic acidosis are (a) elevation of nonvolatile, or fixed, acids as in diabetic ketoacidosis, lactic acidosis (for example, circulatory failure), renal failure, and acid ingestion including salicylism and (b) a decrease in bicarbonate as in excessive bicarbonate excretion and loss of gastrointestinal fluids, especially severe diarrhea.

The child in acute metabolic acidosis appears lethargic, disoriented, and slow to respond to verbal stimuli. Respirations are stimulated. Urine pH will eventually be decreased as kidneys compensate for the imbalance. Eventually, the child becomes stuporous and subject to convulsions and coma.

Metabolic acidosis is a disorder of nonvolatile acids, and compensation occurs as acids are buffered and also through the pulmonary and renal systems. Pulmonary compensation begins following the onset of metabolic problems. As bicarbonate decreases, the compensatory response is hyperventilation in an effort to "blow off" carbon dioxide, which is a volatile acid. If the renal system is intact, the kidneys excrete excess hydrogen ion and retain bicarbonate.

Clinical management of metabolic acidosis requires correcting the primary physiologic problem. Intravenous administration of sodium bicarbonate temporarily increases the bicarbonate level and results in an increase in pH. Intravenous sodium bicarbonate administration must be carefully monitored by means of blood gases. Examples of direct correction for conditions causing metabolic acidosis are

Condition	*Correction*
Diabetic ketoacidosis	Insulin
Circulatory failure (lactic acidosis)	Improve cardiac action
Renal failure	Dialysis

Metabolic Alkalosis Metabolic alkalosis results from either a loss of nonvolatile acids or an excess of bicarbonate, which reduces the hydrogen ion concentration and thus increases arterial pH (Table 33-5).

Metabolic alkalosis is caused by (a) loss of nonvolatile, or fixed, acids, which occurs with persistent vomiting and excessive loss of hydrochloric acid, and excessive nasogastric tube drainage, and (b) elevation of bicarbonate, as in bicarbonate ingestion.

The child in metabolic alkalosis may exhibit the following objective signs: restlessness, irritability, malaise, numbness and tingling of the extremities, carpopedal spasm, weak muscles, depressed respirations, and elevated urine pH. The body compensates for metabolic alkalosis through the respiratory and renal systems. The child's reduced respiratory rate thus causes hypoventilation, carbon dioxide retention, and an elevation in the hydrogen ion concentration. The kidneys excrete bicarbonate.

Metabolic alkalosis is managed by correcting the physiologic imbalance, which might mean replacing lost fluid and electrolytes, correcting pyloric stenosis, or reducing diuretic therapy.

TABLE 33-7 Acute vs. Compensated Metabolic Acidosis and Alkalosis

	Metabolic acidosis		**Metabolic alkalosis**	
	Acute	*Compensated*	*Acute*	*Compensated*
pH	↓	Normal	↑	Normal
PCO_2	Normal	↓	Normal	↑
HCO_3	↓	↓	↑	↑

Key Concepts

- Body fluid is contained in two compartments: intracellular and extracellular.
- Major sources of water are oral fluids, water contained in solid foods, and oxidation of food substances.
- Water output is determined by the solute regulation of the kidneys and by water loss through the skin, lungs, and gastrointestinal tract.
- Water is transported between the intracellular fluid and the extracellular fluid by the processes of diffusion, osmotic pressure, hydrostatic pressure, active transport, and vesicular transport.
- Fluid and electrolyte balance is regulated by thirst and by antidiuretic hormone (ADH), aldosterone, and the renin–angiotensin mechanism of the renal system.
- Nursing care for the child with a fluid imbalance is directed toward restoring the balance and preventing further disequilibrium.
- Assessment of a child's fluid status involves observation of signs of dehydration or fluid overload and accurate recording of intake and output.
- The choice of a site for intravenous infusion is determined by accessibility, type of solution, likely duration of the infusion, and the age and condition of the child.
- Intravenous fluids may be delivered by gravity administration and by infusion and syringe pumps, all of which need to be carefully monitored for accuracy.
- Nursing care for the child receiving an intravenous infusion is planned to prevent complications, provide for developmental needs, and maintain safety.
- Nursing management for the child with hyperkalemia involves increasing potassium output and decreasing intake.
- Nursing management for the child with hypokalemia involves recording potassium replacement and evaluating diagnostic tests.
- Nursing management for the child with hypercalcemia is directed toward correcting the physiologic dysfunction causing the imbalance and administering corticosteroids or isotonic saline.
- Nursing management for the child with hypocalcemia requires close monitoring for respiratory dysfunction, calcium administration, and preparation for possible emergency tracheostomy.
- Chloride combines with sodium in body fluids, so that a deficiency or excess of chloride is accompanied by a comparable level of sodium.
- Sodium functions to maintain water distribution throughout the fluid compartments.
- The two types of sodium and water imbalances are osmolar imbalances and volume imbalances.
- Hyperosmolar imbalances are managed by replacing fluid losses and preventing or treating the effects of dehydration.
- Hypo-osmolar imbalances are managed by restricting fluids and by administering hypertonic solutions.
- Volume disturbances are managed by fluid and sodium therapy, which may be infusions of isotonic solution or diuretics with sodium restriction, depending on the specific imbalance.
- A child with increased hydrogen ion concentration and decreased arterial pH is in a state of acidosis; a child with decreased hydrogen ion concentration and increased arterial pH is in a state of alkalosis.
- A buffer is a solution that prevents drastic changes in pH when a strong acid or base is mixed in the solution.
- Both pulmonary compensation and renal compensation are mechanisms that function to control acid–base imbalance by altering the partial pressure of carbon dioxide or the concentration of hydrogen ions.
- Respiratory acidosis, which is principally caused by alveolar hypoventilation, is managed by correcting the physiologic dysfunction so that kidneys reabsorb bicarbonate and excrete hydrogen ions.
- Respiratory alkalosis, which is principally caused by hyperventilation, is managed by correcting the physiologic dysfunction and administering carbon dioxide, so that the body reabsorbs hydrogen and potassium and excretes bicarbonate and sodium ions.

- Metabolic acidosis is managed by administration of sodium bicarbonate to increase the bicarbonate level and the pH. Pulmonary compensation causes a reduction in carbon dioxide, which acts as a volatile acid.
- Metabolic alkalosis is managed by replacing lost fluid and electrolytes so that nonvolatile acids are replaced and hydrogen ion concentration is increased, thus reducing arterial pH.

Additional Readings

Anand SK et al: Neonatal hypernatremia associated with elevated sodium concentration of breast milk. *J Pediatr* (Jan) 1980; 96(1):66–68.

Aperia A: Salt and water homeostasis during oral rehydration therapy. *J Pediatr* (Sept) 1983; 103(3):364–369.

Arant BS, Jr: Fluid therapy in the neonate—concepts in transition. *J Pediatr* (Sept) 1982; 101(3):387–389.

Boh DM, VanSon AR: The water load test. *Am J Nurs* (Jan) 1982; 82(1):112–113.

Burke SR: *The Composition and Function of Body Fluids*. Mosby, 1976.

Caffee HH: Skin necrosis from extravasation of intravenous fluids in children. *Plast Reconstr Surg* (Feb) 1980; 65(2):244.

Callery P: Nursing care study—hypocalcaemia: Mother and child reunion. *Nurs Mirror* (Feb) 1982; 154(6):38–39.

Cohen S: Metabolic acid-base disorders. Programmed instruction in three parts. *Am J Nurs* (Oct) 1977, (Jan/March) 1978.

Driggers DA: Managing the dehydrated child. *Am Fam Phys* (Nov) 1982; 26(5):189–194.

Dutcher IE, Fielo SB: *Water and Electrolytes: Implications for Nursing Practice*. MacMillan, 1967.

Felver L: Understanding the electrolyte maze. *Am J Nurs* (Sept) 1980; 1591–1595.

Filston HC et al: Estimation of postoperative fluid requirements in infants and children. *Am Surg* (July) 1982; 196(1):76–81.

Finberg L: The role of oral electrolyte-glucose solutions in hydration for children: International and domestic aspects. *J Pediatr* (Jan) 1980; 96(1):51–54.

Finberg L et al: *Water and Electrolytes in Pediatrics: Physiology, Pathophysiology, and Treatment*. Saunders, 1982.

Ghishan FK, Roloff JS: Malnutrition and hypernatremic dehydration in two breast-fed infants. *Clin Pediatr (Phila)* (Aug) 1983; 22(8): 592–594.

Golden SM, Steenbarger J, Monaghan WP: Osmolality and oncotic pressure of volume-expanding fluids for newborn administration. *Crit Care Med* (Dec) 1982; 10(2):863–864.

Grant MM, Kubo WM: Assessing a patient's hydration status. *Am J Nurs* (Aug) 1975; 1306–1311.

Greco A: Fluids, Electrolytes, and Nutrition. In *Pediatric Critical Care Nursing*. Vestal KW (editor). Wiley & Sons, 1981.

Kahn A, Blum D: Hyperkalemia and UNICEF-type rehydration solutions. *Lancet* (May) 1980; 1(8177):1082.

Kahn A et al: Controlled fall in natremia in hypertonic dehydration: Possible avoidance of rehydration seizures. *Eur J Pediatr* (Feb) 1981; 135(3):293–296.

Kerpel-Fronius E: Evolution of knowledge on infantile dehydration. *Contrib Nephrol* 1980; 21:62–67.

Keyes JL: Basic mechanisms involved in acid-base homeostasis. *Heart and Lung* 1976; 5:239.

McFadden EA, Zaloga GP, Chernow B: Hypocalcemia: A medical emergency. *Am J Nurs* (Feb) 1983; 83(2):227–230.

McGrath BJ: Fluids, electrolytes, and replacement therapy in pediatric nursing. *Matern Child Nurs J* (Jan/Feb) 1980; 5(1):58–62.

Meeuwisse GW: High sugar worse than high sodium in oral rehydration solutions. *Acta Paediatr Scand* (March) 1983; 72(2):161–166.

Millam DA, Cohen S, Morris ME: Intravenous therapy; A special feature. *Am J Nurs* (July) 1979; 1268–1296.

Nalin DR et al: Comparison of low and high sodium and potassium content in oral rehydration solutions. *J Pediatr* (Nov) 1980; 97(5): 848–853.

Nash MA: The management of fluid and electrolyte disorders in the neonate. *Clin Perinatol* (June) 1981; 8(2):251–262.

Nursing 80 Books: *Monitoring Fluids and Electrolytes Precisely*. Intermed, 1979.

Nursing 81 Books: *Managing I.V. Therapy*. Intermed, 1981.

Okstein CJ: Patient tampering with electronic intravenous fluid regulators. *Pediatr* (Feb) 1984; 73(2):250–251.

Perkin RM, Levin DL: Common fluid and electrolyte problems in the pediatric intensive care unit. *Pediatr Clin North Am* (Aug) 1980; 27(3):567–586.

Press S, Setzer N: Profound acidosis in infancy. *South Med J* (Aug) 1983; 76(8):1070.

Rando JT: A review of past and current thinking in pediatric fluid therapy. *AAANA J* (Oct) 1980; 48(5):437–440.

Ree GH, Clezy JK: Simple guide to fluid balance. *Trop Doct* (Oct) 1982; 12(4, Part 1):155–159.

Sack DA et al: Risk of hypernatremia with oral rehydration. *J Pediatr* (July) 1982; 101(1):154–155.

Santosham M et al: Storing oral rehydration solution. *Lancet* (April) 1982; 1(8275):797.

Santosham M, Carrera E, Sack RB: Oral rehydration therapy in well-nourished ambulatory children. *Am J Trop Med Hyg* (July) 1983; 32(4):804–808.

Sinclair HC: Babies and children: Fluids in balance. *Nursing 80* (May) 1980; 10(4):574–575.

Snyder JD: From Pedialyte to popsicles: A look at oral rehydration therapy used in the United States and Canada. *Am J Clin Nutr* (Jan) 1982; 35(1):157–161.

Sugijanto, Abbas N: Edema in oral rehydration. *Paediatr Indones* (Nov/Dec) 1981; 21(11–12):229–234.

Suh, KK: Care of infants and children. *Int Anesthesiol Clin* (Spring) 1983; 21(1):117–125.

Tejani A, Dobias B, Mahadevan, R: Osmolar relationships in infantile dehydration. *Am J Dis Child* (Nov) 1981; 135(11):1000–1005.

Vaughan A: *Nelson Textbook of Pediatrics*. Saunders, 1983.

Vick RL (editor): *Contemporary Medical Physiology*. Addison-Wesley, 1984.

Wink DM: Fluid-induced hyponatremia in infancy: A preventable problem. *Am J Nurs* (May) 1983; 83(5):765–767.

Winters RW (editor): *The Body Fluids in Pediatrics*. Little, Brown, 1973.

Oxygenation
Implications of Airway Obstruction and Infection

Margaret I. Marusek-Dozois
Margo Ann Pinney
Rosemary A. Simkins
Annette Calvi

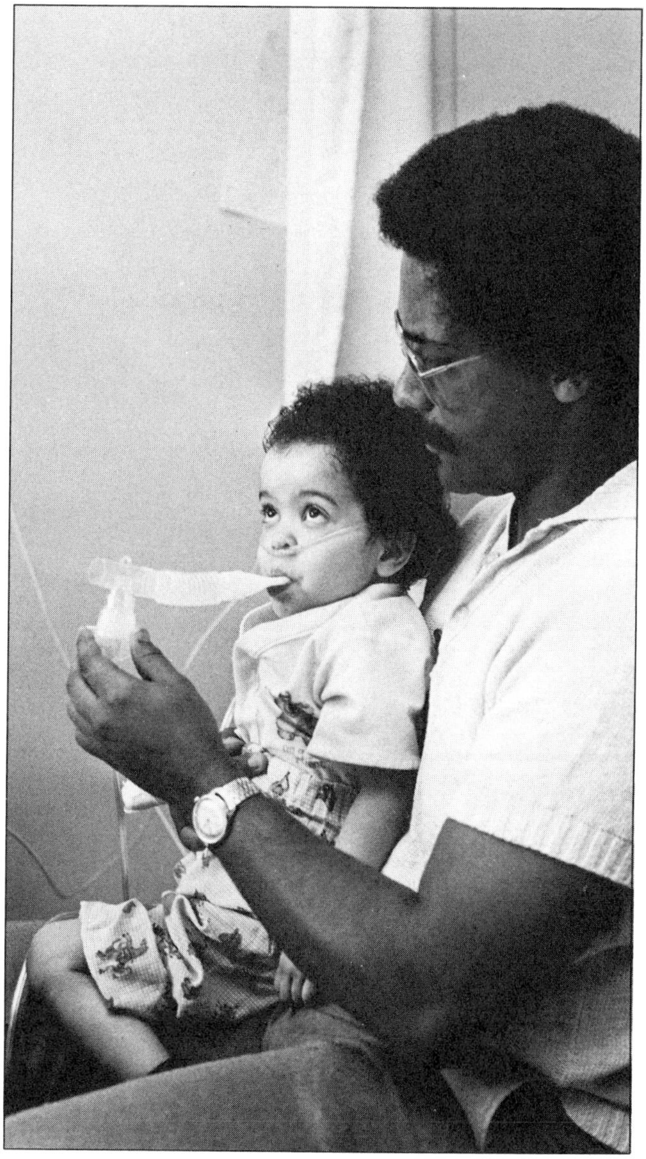

34

Chapter Outline

continued on next page

Objectives

- Describe the embryonic development, postnatal development, and function of the respiratory system.
- Describe the history, physical examination, and associated clinical findings for a child with suspected respiratory dysfunction.
- Describe the purpose and nursing roles associated with diagnostic tests for respiratory dysfunction.
- Describe the nursing care required in providing oxygen therapy and chest physiotherapy.
- State the purpose of inhalation therapy, intermittent positive pressure breathing, and transcutaneous oxygen monitoring.
- Describe nursing responsibilities relative to care for the child with pharyngeal airways, endotracheal or orotracheal intubation, and tracheostomy.
- State nursing diagnoses applicable to obstructive lung disease, restrictive lung disease, inefficient gas transfer, and respiratory failure.
- State the chief nutritional deficit likely in the child with respiratory dysfunction.
- Describe the developmental, emotional, and health maintenance needs related to the child with respiratory dysfunction.
- Identify common viral and bacterial respiratory tract infections and classes of drugs used to treat them.
- Compare the cause, onset, clinical manifestations, treatment, and usual outcome of acute spasmodic croup, laryngotracheobronchitis, and epiglottitis.
- Describe nursing management for the infant with bronchiolitis.
- Describe the diagnosis and treatment of mycoplasmal pneumonia and aspiration pneumonia.
- List nursing responsibilities related to the diagnosis and treatment of tuberculosis.
- Explain procedures for removal of a foreign body lodged below the trachea.

- Describe nursing care for the child who is recovering from near-drowning.
- Describe precipitating factors and nursing management for the child with mild, moderate, and severe asthma.
- Explain the respiratory effects of and the goals of nursing management for the child with cystic fibrosis.
- List nursing interventions to prevent further damage to the lungs of an infant with bronchopulmonary dysplasia.
- Describe emergency treatment and nursing management for the child with hydrocarbon inhalation.
- Describe the process by which alpha$_1$-antitrypsin deficiency impairs lung function.

To find these topics, see the following chapters

Acute nasopharyngitis	Chapter 26
Cardiopulmonary resuscitation (CPR)	Chapter 19
Heimlich maneuver	Chapter 19
Infant apnea	Chapter 31
Pneumonitis	Chapter 26
Respiratory distress syndrome (RDS)	Chapter 31
Sudden Infant Death Syndrome (SIDS)	Chapter 32

All the cells and organs of the body rely on the respiratory system for their supply of oxygen and for removal of carbon dioxide. Anything that interferes with the functioning of this system threatens life itself. Obstruction of airflow, restriction of normal lung mechanics, and impaired gas exchange can result from infection, trauma, or physical abnormality. Any of these disturbances alone or in combination interfere with respiratory function.

In this chapter we review the normal structure and function of the respiratory system. We describe specific disturbances in function, and we discuss the nursing care for the child with a respiratory disorder.

Anatomy and Physiology of the Respiratory System

Embryonic Development of the Respiratory Tract

The first indication of intrauterine growth of the respiratory tract and development of the lung is the appearance of the laryngotracheal groove at about the fourth week of gestation. The three succeeding stages are the pseudoglandular (weeks 5–17), canalicular (weeks 16–24), and terminal sac phases (week 24–birth).

Structures develop in an orderly, gradual manner. During the fourth week, the larynx develops from the endodermal lining of the laryngotracheal groove. Simultaneously, the laryngeal cartilages begin to form, and the vocal cords develop from laryngeal mucous membranes. The trachea is formed similarly.

The endodermal lining of the middle segment of the laryngotracheal tube develops into the epithelium and glands of the trachea. Tracheal cartilage, connective tissue, and muscle are derived from surrounding mesenchyme.

The caudal end of the laryngotracheal groove develops into two lung buds. Each bud grows laterally and divides into two bronchopulmonary buds, which differentiate into the bronchi, saccules, and primitive pleural cavities. The right bud is larger than the left and is directed less sharply to the side. Subsequently, three lobes develop on the right side and two develop on the left.

The development of the bronchial tree occurs predominantly during the pseudoglandular phase. By the sixteenth week of gestation, all bronchial generations are intact, from the trachea to the terminal bronchioles. The canalicular period is characterized by luminal and blood vessel growth in the bronchi and bronchioles. At the end of the canalicular period, the epithelium thins and capillaries form.

When the terminal sac phase begins at week 24 of gestation, the walls of alveolar ducts and capillaries are thin enough to permit diffusion of gases across membranes. The production of surfactant in the alveolar cells begins during the terminal sac period. *Surfactant* is a phospholipid–protein complex that reduces the surface tension of the alveoli, thus stabilizing the air sacs and preventing closure at the end of expiration.

The neonate is at risk if the upper and middle airways fail to develop normally. For example, the lumina of the nose, pharynx, and larynx, which are occluded in the early weeks of gestation, normally open prior to birth. If the lumen of the nose fails to open prior to birth, *choanal atresia* results. This is a potentially life-threatening event, since most infants are obligatory nose breathers. *Choanal stenosis* is the partial, though usually inadequate, opening of the nasal lumen. Partial or complete closure of the larynx or pharynx by a *web* (tissue or membrane) prevents the action of respiration and requires immediate relief in the delivery room.

Postnatal Development of the Respiratory Tract

Lung growth and development continue from birth through young adulthood. Airways and blood vessels increase in length and diameter, and the number of alveoli increases tenfold by age 3. During infancy and childhood, the narrowest part of the upper airway is the cricoid, or subglottic, area. By the end of late childhood, the larynx has become the narrowest area and remains so through adulthood. The pharynx is proportionately smaller in the neonate and infant than in the adult because the maxilla and mandible of the infant are short, while the soft palate is proportionately large. The relatively short mandible and maxilla begin to grow forward within months of birth. Significant elongation of both, however, does not occur until late childhood. In conjunction with the narrow posterior nasooropharynx, the neonate or young infant's tongue is large and may occlude the pharynx, particularly during sleep.

The trachea extends from the lower edge of the larynx to the *carina*, where the airway bifurcates into the right and left main stem bronchi. The upper half of the trachea lies in the neck and the remainder in the thorax. At birth, the trachea is covered by minimal amounts of smooth muscle. By age 4, muscles are in the same proportion to airway size as in an adult. Cartilaginous plates totally circumscribe the airway by adolescence.

All lower airways are present at birth, although they are asymmetric. There is wide variation in the size and number of branches, ranging from 10 to 25 generations. As bronchi branch and decrease in size, cartilage disappears and they become bronchioles, which terminate in respiratory units. The airways are lined with ciliated epithelial cells that propel mucus from peripheral airways to the pharynx.

The *respiratory unit* consists of terminal bronchioles, alveolar ducts, and alveoli. True alveoli are not present until 2 months of age. Collateral ventilation between alveoli develops after birth by means of the pores of Kohn and canals of Lambert. The alveoli are lined by type I and II epithelial cells. Type II cells produce pulmonary surfactant.

The principle muscle of respiration is the *diaphragm*, which separates the thoracic and abdominal contents. Several types of muscle fibers make up the diaphragm. Type I fibers, which are relatively resistant to fatigue, increase with age from 20% of the diaphragmatic muscle in the neonate to 55% in the adult. Type I fibers are also found in intercostal muscles and increase proportionately with age.

Lung Mechanics

The lung is an elastic structure whose mechanical function is measured as elastance and compliance. *Elastance* (elastic recoil) is the pressure generated at a given lung volume. *Compliance* is the change in lung volume per unit of pressure. Dynamic lung compliance is considered in assessing airway obstruction.

Physiology of the Respiratory Tract

Gas Exchange The function of the respiratory system is to oxygenate arterial blood and remove carbon dioxide from venous blood. Oxygenation is achieved by movement of air from the atmosphere to the alveoli, diffusion of oxygen across the alveolocapillary membrane, and oxygen's combination with hemoglobin, which is carried by red blood cells (see Chapter 36). Carbon dioxide is removed in a reverse process.

Normal respiratory function depends on adequate ventilation, diffusion, and perfusion. *Ventilation* is the movement of gases from the atmosphere to the alveoli and the removal of carbon dioxide from the alveoli. It takes place in the lungs. Adequate ventilation depends on movement of the diaphragm and chest wall muscles, elastic properties of the lung and chest wall, and the unobstructed flow of gas through the airways. A change in any of these three components affects the other two and compromises ventilation.

Diffusion is the transfer of inhaled gases across the alveolocapillary membrane to the lung capillaries. It is a passive process caused by pressure differences. In the healthy child, the alveolar gas tension is approximately 100 mm Hg. This is higher than the approximately 40 mm Hg of mixed venous blood. The difference in alveolar and arterial gas tensions results in a driving pressure of approximately 60 mm Hg across the alveolocapillary membrane, causing rapid movement of oxygen from alveoli to capillary blood. Once in a capillary, oxygen diffuses through capillary plasma and across the erythrocyte (red blood cell) membrane. Then the slowest part of the process occurs. The oxygen combines chemically with hemoglobin molecules carried by red blood cells. During times of increased pulmonary blood flow, there is less time for diffusion, and *hypoxemia* (deficient oxygenation of the blood) occurs. Carbon dioxide is very soluble and diffuses 21 times faster than oxygen in a gaseous state. Therefore, carbon dioxide diffusion is rarely disturbed in disease. The extent to which oxygen combines with hemoglobin depends on blood pH, temperature, and the partial pressure of oxygen (oxygen tension) in the blood.

Perfusion is the transport of oxygen from the pulmonary capillary to the body tissues. Oxygen is transported in two ways. A very small portion (3%) is dissolved and carried in plasma. Most oxygen is carried by hemoglobin molecules (as oxyhemoglobin). In rare conditions in which little or no hemoglobin is available, hyperbaric oxygen (oxygen under high pressures) is administered. This treatment causes approximately 180% more oxygen to be dissolved and delivered in the plasma, thus meeting the body's resting oxygen requirements.

Control of Respiration The body guards against hypoxia and *hypercapnia* (excess of carbon dioxide in the blood) through the respiratory control center. The two main systems involved in the regulatory process are a neural system and a chemical system. The neural system is composed of four parts located in the pons, medulla, and spinal cord. This system coordinates the rhythm of the respiratory cycle and regulates the depth of respiration. Proprioceptive vagal impulses from impulses in the lung (Hering-Breuer reflex) control maximal inspiration. At slow respiratory rates, inspiration is increased. With rapid respiratory rates, inspiration is inhibited slightly.

The chemical system (neurohumoral system) is primarily concerned with regulation of alveolar ventilation and maintaining normal blood gas tensions. Central chemoreceptors and chromatin tissue along the great vessels sense changes in pH, carbon dioxide partial pressure (PCO_2), and oxygen partial pressure (PO_2). An increase in PCO_2 stimulates an increase in ventilation, and a decrease in PCO_2 stimulates a decrease in ventilation. Blood bicarbonate also influences this system, but in a much slower manner.

Two chemoreceptors of great importance are carotid bodies and aortic bodies. Both are specifically responsive to arterial oxygen partial pressure (PaO_2) rather than to arterial carbon dioxide partial pressure ($PaCO_2$). PaO_2 affects these receptors primarily when significant fluctuations are present. Thus peripheral chemoreceptors maintain respiration primarily through their sensitivity to *hypoxia* (reduction in tissue oxygenation caused by decreased PaO_2).

Assessment of the Child With Respiratory Dysfunction

History

The history provides valuable data for assessment and nursing diagnoses related to present or potential respiratory dysfunction. The nurse adapts interviewing techniques to the child's developmental level and the severity of the chief complaint (see Chapter 14). It is important to encourage the child to supply as much information as possible. If the parent of an adolescent supplies most of the health history, the nurse should be alert to the child's possible inappropriate dependence on the parent. The parent may have assumed too much responsibility for the child's illness, particularly if the illness is a chronic and life-threatening one, such as cystic fibrosis. Because any pulmonary disease can be life threatening, the nurse may decide to defer taking the history until the child's condition is more stable.

The family's health history is important for several reasons. Some diseases of the lungs, such as cystic fibrosis, are inherited. Such diseases as asthma, bronchitis, and bronchiectasis have both genetic and environmental causes. For example, it is believed that certain individuals are genetically predisposed to asthma, particularly if they have a family history of atopy. *Atopy* is the inherited tendency to produce antibodies to environmental antigens and is manifested by asthma, rhinitis, hay fever, infantile eczema, urticaria, and angioedema. Viral infection can also precede the onset of asthma symptoms. Reviewing the health status of family members can also help identify pulmonary disease caused by common exposure to infectious or physical agents in the environment. A particular microorganism may cause gastrointestinal symptoms in a parent or older sibling and upper or middle respiratory tract infection in an infant. Smoking in the home can cause symptoms of respiratory dysfunction in the patient and other family members.

Neonatal History Information about the child's neonatal health and health during early infancy can help differentiate among disease processes. Infants who had neonatal respiratory distress syndrome (RDS) frequently have bronchopulmonary dysplasia, chronic bronchitis, or asthma later (see Chapter 31). Recurrent symptoms of upper, middle, or lower tract infections require further assessment. If the child has had chest radiographs in the past, they can be compared with current radiographs to evaluate the chronicity and progression of disease. It is also helpful to elicit information from the family about both successful and unsuccessful prior treatments.

History of the Present Illness The history of the present illness includes information about the child's cough, mucus production, *dyspnea* (difficult breathing, or "air hunger"), fatigue, exercise tolerance, *orthopnea* (difficult breathing except in an upright position), wheezing, pain, exposure to irritants or infection, weight gain, growth, gastrointestinal status, and stools.

Coughing is a protective reflex of the respiratory system. The nurse records information about the onset, frequency, duration, pattern of recurrence, sound, and productivity of the cough. Information about when the child or parent first remembers hearing the cough can provide clues to its cause. The nurse asks the parent and child what precipitates the cough, and whether it is intermittent, sporadic, recurrent, and increasing or decreasing in frequency. What time of day does the cough typically occur? A child with asthma or cystic fibrosis typically coughs more in the early morning

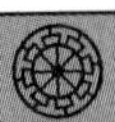

ASSESSMENT GUIDE Child With a Respiratory Problem

System	Subjective data	Objective data	Validating data	Nursing management
Head, eyes, ears, nose, throat	Hoarseness, aphonia, sore throat; difficulty breathing; runny nose	Crowing sound on inspiration or associated with cough, croupy cough, stridor. Signs of increased respiratory effort indicating occluded airway. Dark circles under eyes, eyes wide open with anxious appearance. Flaring of nostrils. Difficulty handling secretions, drooling	Laryngoscopy, radiography of neck	Place child in a cool, humidified environment. Administer oxygen therapy if ordered. Encourage fluids if airway occlusion does not appear to be imminent. Position in semi- or high-Fowler's position. Observe for signs of increased airway occlusion such as refusal to swallow
Integumentary	Thirst. Complaints of feeling hot	Generalized or circumoral cyanosis; poor skin turgor, sunken fontanelles in infant	Serum electrolytes. Arterial blood gases—PaO_2, $PaCO_2$	Treat for dehydration (See Chapter 33)
Respiratory	Family history of respiratory problems; exposure to tuberculosis or immigration from a foreign country. Recurrent respiratory infections; history of respiratory distress syndrome (RDS) or foreign body aspiration. Cough, difficulty breathing, fatigue and decreased exercise tolerance, chest pain. Anxiety and restlessness; crying, irritability, disinterest in play activities	Presence of adventitious breath sounds (rales, ronchi, wheezing); diminished or altered breath sounds; pleural friction rub; changes in mucus amount or quality. Signs of increasing respiratory distress (tachypnea, retractions, nasal flare, expiratory grunt); abnormal respiratory patterns (Cheyne Stokes respiration, Kussmaul's respirations, hypoventilation or hyperventilation). Orthopnea; asymmetrical chest movements; observable chest mass; apnea and respiratory failure	Arterial blood gases, O_2 saturation, complete blood count, throat and sputum cultures, immunoglobulins, chest radiographic studies, pulmonary function tests, bronchoscopy, tissue studies (see Table 34-2)	Maintain a patent airway through positioning and encouraging effective coughing and deep breathing. Provide adequate humidity and hydration. Give chest physiotherapy and suction when indicated. Provide for sufficient oxygenation. Observe respiratory pattern and auscultate breath sounds for changes in respiratory status. Relieve the child's anxiety Organize nursing care to provide periods of rest. Inquire about methods used to treat the child's respiratory problem at home. Have endotracheal or tracheostomy set at bedside
Cardiovascular	History of congenital heart defects or chronic pulmonary obstructive disease. Fever	Clubbing of fingers; changes in vital signs—increased pulse, alteration in blood pressure; cyanosis	Pulmonary function tests (see Table 34-2), chest radiography to detect cardiac enlargement and congestive heart failure	Prepare the child to undergo testing. Inquire about changes in exercise tolerance

ASSESSMENT GUIDE Child With a Respiratory Problem (continued)

System	Subjective data	Objective data	Validating data	Nursing management
Gastrointestinal	Nausea, anorexia, lethargy, abdominal pain, failure to gain weight or weight loss	Vomiting. Frequent foul-smelling, bulky gray stools	Sweat chloride test (pilocarpine iontophoresis test), stool test for fat and reducing substances, barium swallow, theophylline levels	Discourage child from swallowing mucus. Observe for additional signs of cystic fibrosis. Inquire about family history of cystic fibrosis. Note characteristics of stool. Ask whether the child is taking theophylline in any form
Musculoskeletal		Increased anterior or posterior diameter of chest; alterations in skeletal structure—kyphosis, scoliosis, pectus carinatum or pectus excavatum	Chest and spine radiography	Monitor height and weight and compare with norms and individual growth curve. Note degree of skeletal deformity. Observe for symmetry of chest expansion
Neuroendocrine	Lethargy, confusion, drowsiness, numbness and tingling, stupor, coma	Signs and symptoms of hypoxemia	Arterial blood gases	Administer O_2 as ordered. Contact physician if signs of hypoxemia appear

and upon awakening. Some children have no cough symptoms at all during the night but awake coughing and cough continuously for several hours thereafter. It is sometimes helpful to have the parent fill out a daily report sheet to keep track of the times of day when the cough occurs, how long the coughing episodes last, and the number of coughing episodes a child is having. The parent can also note the child's activity prior to a coughing episode. Information about the sound of the child's cough and its productivity also indicates possible causes. For example, infection is more likely in a child whose parent reports a loose-sounding cough productive of yellowish-white mucus than in a child having a dry, nonproductive cough.

The nurse asks the child and parent to describe the consistency of sputum as viscous (thick) or nonviscous; its color as green, yellow, white, or blood-tinged; and the amount expectorated as small, moderate, or large. Some mucus also has an odor. Very viscous, greenish mucus suggests infection by *Pseudomonas aeruginosa,* which is common in children with cystic fibrosis.

Very young children are not able to describe dyspnea, and so the nurse looks for clues in the history. The parent may report the child's decreased exercise tolerance or shortness of breath with exercise, orthopnea, retractions, grunting, or nasal flaring, which are all signs of dyspnea. A child experiencing some dyspnea might be described as quiet, inactive, and lacking interest and enthusiasm for normal play. A child who is uncomfortable breathing except in a semisitting or standing position has orthopnea. Children with pulmonary edema or asthma may demonstrate orthopnea by propping themselves up and resting their weight on their arms, which they extend behind them. Retractions are commonly seen in children with airway obstruction due to such disorders as laryngotracheobronchitis, bronchiolitis, asthma, or cystic fibrosis. *Retractions* are caused by the pulling in of the soft tissues surrounding the middle and upper intercostal spaces and the sternum, and in the jugular notch, supraclavicular, and infraclavicular spaces.

Grunting and nasal flaring are most frequently seen in respiratory distress syndrome or hyaline membrane disease in the neonate (see Chapter 31). Grunting usually suggests pulmonary edema or problems with alveolar compliance. *Grunting* is an expiratory grunt heard as the child strives to force air past a partially closed glottis. This maneuver helps to maintain some pressure at the alveolar level and prevents complete collapse of alveoli with each expiration. *Nasal flaring* is enlargement of both nares (nostrils) during inspiration. It is a sign that the accessory muscles of respiration are needed to breath.

Wheezing, which may occur on inspiration or expiration, is also noted in the history of the present illness. Wheezing is caused by air passing through edematous mucous membranes, over thick secretions and through contracted bronchioles, all of which create a partial obstruction in the bronchi or bronchioles. The vibration of the edematous membranes or secretions causes the characteristic high-pitched whistle (sibilant sound) or low-pitched snore (sonorous sound). Wheezing occurs most commonly in the child with bronchiolitis, asthma, foreign body aspiration, or cystic fibrosis. The nurse gathers information about its onset, duration, and severity.

Chest pain is frightening at any age, and it may be the chief complaint. The neonate or infant may react to chest pain with crying, irritability, withdrawal, changes in vital signs, and loss of interest in food, fluid, and play. Very young children are apt to indicate their discomfort in general terms (for example, "It hurts"), but they are seldom able to give more specific information about the location, intensity, nature, duration, frequency, and events surrounding the occurrence and relief of the pain. (See Chapter 29 for a discussion of pain assessment techniques adapted to the child's developmental level.)

The history of the present illness includes information about possible exposure to infectious microorganisms and irritants. If infection is suspected, the nurse seeks data about possible contributing factors, such as inadequate nutrition, unsanitary living conditions, or delays in obtaining routine immunizations. If tuberculosis is suspected, the nurse discovers whether the child has been exposed to active bacilli and obtains records pertaining to immunization and results of tuberculin skin tests. If the child lives on or has traveled to the Western Appalachian slope, histoplasmosis must be ruled out. The lesions and clinical pictures of histoplasmosis and tuberculosis are similar, and so it is important to verify whether the child has been in an area where *Histoplasma capsulatum* is endemic. The nurse always asks about recent cold or influenza symptoms of other family members, because many agents that produce respiratory infections are airborne and easily passed throughout the household. The same microorganism usually has a more profound effect on the infant and small child than on parents and older siblings, who may report only minor symptoms.

If the child is being assessed for asthma, the nurse seeks information about possible irritants in the child's home environment that may be exacerbating asthma symptoms. The nurse also inquires about local industrial pollutants, air quality, pets and animals at home, the type of vegetation in the area and home, toys and bedding in the child's room, and heating and cooling systems used in the home. It is also important to ask whether anyone smokes in the home. Adolescents are questioned in private about smoking, because they may be hiding this behavior from their parents.

Often, one of the earliest indications of chronic lung disease is the failure to gain weight. If the disease continues unchecked, weight loss and subsequent failure to gain height follow. If the child's weight and height have been recorded since birth, the nurse plots these measurements on a standard growth chart to help determine when the altered growth pattern began.

The nurse also questions the child and family about the onset, severity, frequency, and duration of gastrointestinal symptoms and signs of fatigue. Acute or chronic infection invariably produces lethargy, anorexia, vomiting, and abdominal pain, which further interfere with growth. Nausea, vomiting, and resultant poor intake of food can be problems for children who swallow mucus. The nurse also questions the child and family about the child's stools. A history of frequent, foul-smelling, bulky gray stools and associated abdominal pain may indicate a malabsorptive problem or cystic fibrosis (see Chapter 38 for information about the gastrointestinal effects of cystic fibrosis).

Physical Examination

Respiratory arrest or the inability of the respiratory system to oxygenate the blood and remove carbon dioxide may result from acute or chronic dysfunction. In either case, the child's life may depend on the nurse's rapid and accurate clinical assessment and ability to initiate emergency interventions within moments. Table 34-1 lists the clinical signs and symptoms most often associated with impending or frank respiratory failure.

Although cyanosis is listed in Table 34-1 as a sign of respiratory failure, it is not always a reliable sign. In order for cyanosis to be observed, there must be approximately 5 g of reduced hemoglobin per 100 mL of blood. Anemia masks cyanosis, and children with vasoconstriction or polycythemia, or the chilled neonate, may have cyanosis despite adequate oxygenation. If cyanosis persists despite oxygen administration, the child may have multiple right-to-left cardiac shunts.

While inspecting the nail beds for cyanosis, the nurse also looks for clubbing (see color plate). *Clubbing* of the fingers and toes is evidenced by the lateral and longitudinal spreading of the nail base by tissue proliferation on the dorsal surface of the terminal phalanx. The fingernails and toenails appear shiny and bulbous. The exact cause of clubbing is unknown, but it is always significant. It usually is associated with diseases involving some degree of hypoxemia such as cystic fibrosis and bronchiectasis. It becomes more pronounced in a child with cystic fibrosis as the child's condition deteriorates. Clubbing can be reversed if the disease process is reversed.

TABLE 34-1 Criteria for Diagnosis of Respiratory Failure in Infants and Children With Acute Pulmonary Disease

Clinical	Physiologic
Decreased or absent inspiratory breath sounds	$PaCO_2 \geq 75$ mm Hg
Severe inspiratory retractions and use of accessory muscles	$PaO_2 \leq 100$ mm Hg in 100% oxygen
Cyanosis in 40% ambient oxygen	
Depressed level of consciousness and response to pain	
Poor skeletal muscle tone	

NOTE: Three clinical symptoms and one physiologic symptom must be present to confirm the diagnosis of acute respiratory failure.

SOURCE: Downs JJ et al: Acute respiratory failure in infants and children. *Pediatr Clin North Am* (May) 1972; 19(2):429.

A change in the shape of the thorax is another indication of chronic disease. Children who have chronic respiratory diseases, such as cystic fibrosis or severe asthma, may have *pectus profundum,* or barrel chest. This is caused by chronic obstruction. A nurse following a child with chronic obstructive lung disease in a clinic might plot measurements of chest diameter serially on a graph at each visit to help assess response to therapy or the course of the disease.

Assessment of other skeletal deformities is discussed in Chapters 14 and 41. Deformities of the sternum, ribs, or spine can interfere with respiration. The nurse observes for symmetry of thoracic expansion during inspiration. If one side of the thorax does not expand as fully as the other, or lags behind, the child may have a fractured rib, chest trauma, pneumothorax, or a skeletal deformity.

The physical examination includes obtaining baseline vital signs (see Chapter 14). Alterations in vital signs provide significant data concerning the child's response to the disease process or its treatment. Temperature may be significantly elevated with a bacterial infection, but only slightly elevated or normal with a viral infection. Hypoxia causes an increased pulse rate and increased blood pressure. Hypercapnia causes decreased blood pressure. Any of the medications given to children with asthma or cystic fibrosis can cause changes in pulse and blood pressure. Side effects of the theophyllines and the B_2 sympathomimetic bronchodilators include increased pulse and hypotension. Steroids, sometimes given to children with asthma or cystic fibrosis, also elevate blood pressure.

Four aspects of the child's respirations are assessed: rate, depth, ease, and rhythm. The nurse counts the child's resting respiratory rate for 1 minute for two reasons. First, normal respirations do not occur at a consistent, regular rate. Both depth and interval can vary. Periodic deep breaths are normal and help prevent *atelectasis* (incomplete expansion) of small airways. Second, the margin of error increases proportionally with a decrease in the length of time respirations are counted. (Normal resting respiratory rates for children are listed in Appendix B. Abnormal respirations are defined in Chapter 14—see Table 14-8. Temporary *apnea* (cessation of breathing) in the neonate and infant is discussed in Chapter 31.)

After an initial assessment of the child's ability to sustain respiration and a general assessment of the child's color, thoracic movements, vital signs, and character of respirations, the nurse begins the "hands on" part of the physical examination: palpation, percussion, and auscultation (see Chapter 14).

Validating Diagnostic Tests

Table 34-2 summarizes the diagnostic tests used in assessing respiratory status. Normal values, alterations, and possible causes also are given.

Nursing Management for Procedures and Treatments

Preparation for Diagnostic Tests

The nurse needs an understanding of the many diagnostic tests used to assess the respiratory system to prepare the child physically, cognitively, and emotionally. Some test procedures are carried out independently by the nurse; others may require the nurse's presence or assistance.

Laboratory Tests

Blood Gases Arterial blood gas studies are done to assess oxygenation and the acid–base balance (pH) of the body. Arterial gas determination is preferred to venous sampling in infants and children because it assesses lung function separately from circulatory factors and is not affected by metabolic functions of the body part. The blood sample usually is obtained from the radial artery by means of a single percutaneous stick or an indwelling catheter. In premature infants requiring frequent sampling, specimens are usually drawn from an umbilical artery catheter. A heparinized syringe is used to prevent clotting. Although only a small amount of blood is withdrawn, the amount is recorded on the intake and output record. If blood is withdrawn percutaneously, the nurse applies pressure to the site for at least 5 minutes after the needle is withdrawn.

Immunoglobulins and Alpha$_1$-Antitrypsin Serum immunoglobulin levels are obtained to rule out immune deficiency disease. The child who has a deficiency of one or

TABLE 34-2 Diagnostic Tests for Respiratory Dysfunction

Test	Normal value	Alteration	Significance
Blood gases			
PaO_2	Sea level: 80%–100% Altitude > 5,000 feet: 65%–75%	Increased	Excessive administration of oxygen
		Decreased	Hypoxemia from pulmonary or cardiac disease
$PaCO_2$	Sea level: 35%–45% Altitude > 5,000 feet: 32%–38%	Increased	Respiratory acidosis (asthma, upper or lower airway obstruction, respiratory depressants)
		Decreased	Respiratory alkalosis (incorrect ventilator settings, anxiety, high altitude, mild hypoxia)
pH	7.35–7.45	Increased Decreased	Alkalemia Acidemia
Base excess	Sea level: −2–+2 Altitude > 5,000 feet: −4–+2	Increased	Metabolic alkalosis (vomiting, gastric drainage to high suction, rapid infusion of $NaHCO_3$, ingestion of alkali)
		Decreased	Metabolic acidosis (ketoacidosis, salicylate poisoning, renal failure, hypoxia, diarrhea)
Blood bicarbonate (HCO_3)	Sea level: 22–26 mEq/L Altitude > 5,000 feet: 18–26 mEq/L	Increased Decreased	Metabolic alkalosis Metabolic acidosis
Oxygen saturation	Sea level: 95% Altitude > 5,000 feet:	Increased	Excessive administration of oxygen
		Decreased	Hypoxemia from pulmonary or cardiac disease
Immunoglobulins	IgG: 639–1,349 mg/dL	Decreased	Immune deficiency disease, increased susceptibility to respiratory infections
	IgA: 70–312 mg/dL	Decreased	Immune deficiency disease, increased susceptibility to respiratory infections
	IgM: 56–356 mg/dL	Decreased	Immune deficiency disease, increased susceptibility to respiratory infections
	IgE: 100–200 IU/mL	Increased	Hypersensitivity
	IgD: 0–6 mg/dL	Decreased	Immune deficiency disease, increased susceptibility to respiratory infections
$Alpha_1$-antitrypsin	130–238 mg/dL	Decreased	$Alpha_1$-antitrypsin deficiency
Complete blood count (CBC)			
Hemoglobin Hematocrit	Varies with child's age (see Chapter 36)	Increased	Transient exposure to high altitude
		Decreased	Decreased oxygen-carrying capacity

TABLE 34-2 continued

Test	Normal value	Alteration	Significance
White cells	Varies with child's age (see Chapter 36)	Increased	Infection (see Chapter 36)
Circulating eosinophils	0–450/mm^3	Increased	hypersensitivity reaction
Pilocarpine iontophoresis (sweat chloride test)	Sodium < 70 mEq/L	Increased	Cystic fibrosis
	Chloride < 60 mEq/L	Increased	
	Potassium < 60 mEq/L	Increased	
Cultures			
Throat		Growth of pathogens	Upper or lower respiratory tract infection or contamination of specimen
Sputum			
Radiologic examinations			
Anterior–posterior lateral views	Normal appearance	Abnormal appearance	Congenital or acquired defects of rib, spine, thoracic cavity, sternum; abnormalities of diaphragm; chest expansion; pneumothorax; mediastinal shift; certain cardiac abnormalities; abnormal density of lung tissue; hyperinflation; atelectasis
Assisted inspiratory–expiratory radiograph	Normal and equal lung expansion on both sides	Hyperexpansion of one side of chest	Foreign body aspiration
Barium swallow	No evidence of reflux	Reflux of barium from stomach into esophagus	Gastroesophageal reflux
Pulmonary function			
Tidal volume	Varies with age, sex, height, weight	Decreased	Restrictive lung disease
Expiratory reserve volume		Decreased	Restrictive lung disease
Inspiratory reserve volume		Decreased	Restrictive lung disease
Residual volume		Increased	Obstructive lung disease
Capacities		Decreased	Obstructive or restrictive lung disease
Flow rates		Decreased	Obstructive lung disease
Diffusion		Decreased	Alveolocapillary membrane defect

more of the immunoglobulins may have a recurrent respiratory infection. An immune deficiency can complicate an underlying pulmonary disorder (see Chapter 37).

Serum determination of alpha$_1$-antitrypsin, a protease inhibitor, is done to rule out alpha$_1$-antitrypsin deficiency.

Complete Blood Count A complete blood count (CBC) includes the white blood cell count, differential count, hematocrit, and eosinophil count (see Table 36-1). The total number of white blood cells per 100 mL of blood is elevated when a child has an infection, and the differential count of white blood cell types can provide important information about the nature of the infection. A low hematocrit indicates a reduction in the oxygen-carrying capacity of the blood. The number of eosinophils increases dramatically when an allergic reaction has occurred.

Sweat Chloride Test The sweat chloride test, or pilocarpine iontophoresis sweat test, is the only reliable method of diagnosing cystic fibrosis. It is usually performed in large medical centers or cystic fibrosis centers. The child's sweat glands are stimulated painlessly with pilocarpine nitrate, sodium nitrate, and electrodes. The sweat produced over a 30-minute period is collected onto a preweighed gauze pad. The sample is then analyzed for sodium (or chloride) and potassium content. The test is positive for cystic fibrosis if the sodium content of a 50-mg sample exceeds 70 mEq/L and chloride or potassium exceeds 60 mEq/L. A diagnosis of cystic fibrosis is made if the results of two separate tests are positive.

Cultures Throat cultures are done to isolate and identify pathogens from the throat, and blood cultures are done to isolate pathogens causing generalized infections. Sputum cultures are difficult to obtain from children. It may be helpful to have the child rinse the mouth with a warm saline solution before the nurse performs percussion and postural drainage to stimulate the child to expectorate sputum. The child's posterior pharynx also may be aspirated. Sputum is always collected in a sterile container and taken to the laboratory immediately for analysis.

Radiographic Studies It is frequently appropriate for the nurse to accompany a child during a radiographic examination. Normally, adequate diagnostic information can be obtained through an anterior–posterior view and a lateral view. If the child is too young to sit or stand unsupported for several seconds, both views are taken with the child in the recumbent position. The nurse ensures that the child's immature gonads are protected with a lead shield.

The inspiratory–expiratory radiograph is taken from an anterior–posterior view at the end of expiration. It is used to demonstrate air trapping in children with suspected foreign body aspiration. The barium esophagram is taken to detect mediastinal masses, swallowing disorders, and such malformations as tracheoesophageal fistulas (see Chapter 38).

Assisted Forced-Expiratory Radiographs Foreign body aspiration into the lower airways frequently results in atelectasis or air trapping due to partial airway obstruction. Upon inspiration, air flows beyond the object, commonly a seed, nut, or small toy, as it lifts away from the bronchial wall. During expiration, however, the object blocks the airway, causing air to be trapped distally. This is referred to as "ball-valving."

An assisted forced-expiratory radiograph is used to diagnose foreign body aspiration because children are not able to cooperate with the technique voluntarily. The technician places a gloved fist against the epigastrum and applies pressure as the child exhales, maximizing expiration. Hyperexpansion of the involved airway is seen if ball-valving is occurring. This radiograph is compared with the inspiratory radiograph, which often shows no pathologic change.

Barium Swallow The barium swallow fluoroscopic study is used routinely to diagnose gastroesophageal reflux (see Chapter 38). The child (usually an infant) is bottle- or tube-fed barium. Serial fluoroscopic views are taken throughout the ingestion process, from swallowing to early emptying of the barium from the stomach into the duodenum. Pressure may be put upon the child's epigastrum to challenge the competency of the distal esophogeal sphincter (DES). Radiographs are taken in the prone and supine positions. In the supine view, the DES is below the level of the barium. Reflux is more likely to occur in this position.

The barium swallow not only documents the degree of gastroesophageal reflux, but furnishes information about other pertinent problems as well. The child undergoing the study for example may have experienced an episode of apnea, choking, or color change during feedings. Abnormal suck–swallow coordination, aspiration during swallowing, and vascular ring can also be detected. The barium swallow request form should state all the problems considered to be possible diagnoses, particularly if the suspected problem is a swallowing disorder.

Lung Scan A lung scan can be done to pinpoint an area of pathology in the lungs. A radioactive gas, such as xeon (^{133}Xe), is used to visualize and measure regional distribution of ventilation. The child is asked to take a normal, quiet inhalation of the xeon and then to hold the breath for 10–20 seconds while photoscintograms are made. This maneuver may be repeated several times over a 10- to 15-minute period.

Pulmonary Function Tests Pulmonary function tests indicate the lungs' ability to perform mechanical ventilation, deliver oxygen to the cardiovascular system, and remove carbon dioxide from venous blood. Pulmonary function tests and the significance of alterations are listed in Table 34-2.

Nurses are often responsible for helping children learn to perform the maneuvers required for pulmonary function testing. Many of these maneuvers are difficult for children to perform. It is helpful for children under 5 years of age to attempt the maneuvers even if they cannot do them well enough to provide data. With practice, praise, and rewards, some children under 5 can learn to perform the maneuvers correctly. Children with cystic fibrosis, for which pulmonary function data are critical, may start practicing as early as 3 years of age.

The most common basic test maneuver that children learn is the forced-vital-capacity maneuver. The child inspires slowly to maximal lung volume, holds the breath briefly, expires suddenly, and then sustains maximal expiratory effort for at least 3 seconds. To help young children learn this

Indicators of Pulmonary Function

Tidal volume (TV) The volume of gas inhaled or exhaled during each respiratory cycle.

Expiratory reserve volume (ERV) The maximum volume of gas that can be exhaled following a normal, quiet expiration.

Inspiratory reserve volume (IRV) The maximum volume of gas that can be inhaled following a normal quiet inspiration.

Residual volume (RV) The volume of gas remaining in the lungs at the end of a maximum expiration.

Vital capacity (VC) The maximum volume of gas that can be forcefully exhaled from the lungs following a maximum inspiration. (*VC = TV + ERV + IRV*)

Functional residual capacity (FRC) The volume of gas remaining in the lungs following a quiet resting expiration. (*FRC = ERV + RV*)

Inspiratory capacity (IC) The maximum volume of gas that can be inhaled following a quiet resting expiration. (*IC = TV + IRV*)

Total lung capacity (TLC) The amount of gas contained in the lungs following a maximum inspiration. The maximum amount of gas the lungs hold (*TLC = TV + ERV + IRV + RV*)

Forced expiratory volume in one second (FEV_1) The volume of gas forcefully exhaled from the lungs during the first second of a forced vital capacity maneuver.

Forced expiratory flow 25%–75% ($FEF_{25-75\%}$) also termed *maximal midexpiratory flow* The mean flow rate calculated over the midportion of the forced expiratory curve—ie., after the first 25% of the vital capacity has been forcefully exhaled and before the last 25% of the forced vital capacity has been exhaled.

Peak expiratory flow rate (PEFR or PF) The greatest flow that can be obtained during a forced expiratory maneuver.

skill, the nurse can ask them to "blow out all the candles" or have them practice by blowing bubbles or blowing a Ping-Pong ball across a table.

Although it is difficult to teach children to perform pulmonary function testing maneuvers, these maneuvers are important and are often the only means of identifying early changes that might lead to worsening pulmonary function. Pulmonary function testing has the following uses:

1. *Screening for disease.* Often, a slight change in one of the parameters of pulmonary function can be identified before any changes in the child's daily functioning become apparent. For a disease such as cystic fibrosis, early detection and intervention can add years to the child's life.

2. *Determining the diagnosis.* Pulmonary function testing can help differentiate obstructive disease from restrictive disease.

3. *Evaluating response to treatment.* Improvement, stabilization, or deterioration of the child's condition can be assessed to evaluate treatment regimens if pulmonary function tests are done serially.

4. *Following the course and progression of the disease.* Pulmonary function tests are often more indicative of subtle physiologic changes than reports of symptoms and other signs.

Normal values for lung volume, capacity, and flow vary according to the child's age, sex, and height. The spirograph of Figure 34-1 shows normal relative volumes. Generally, volume and capacity diminish with lung disease. Flow usually diminishes in obstructive lung disease and is normal in restrictive lung disease. A sudden change or decline in any of these values is noted and reported by the nurse.

Diffusion Test Pulmonary function tests are used to assess the mechanical and ventilatory properties of the lungs. Diffusion tests are used to assess the alveolocapillary membrane's capacity for gas exchange, or diffusion. The test is based on the capacity of carbon monoxide to combine with hemoglobin about 210 times more readily than does oxygen (Fischbach, 1984). If the amount of hemoglobin in the blood is normal but the alveoli are damaged by pulmonary disease, diffusion across the alveolocapillary membrane is compromised.

The child sits in a chair and expires as fully as possible. Following complete expiration, the child takes a deep breath of a gas mixture containing low concentrations of helium and carbon monoxide. After holding the breath for 10 seconds, the child expires fully, then inspires air containing low concentrations of carbon monoxide, and holds the breath

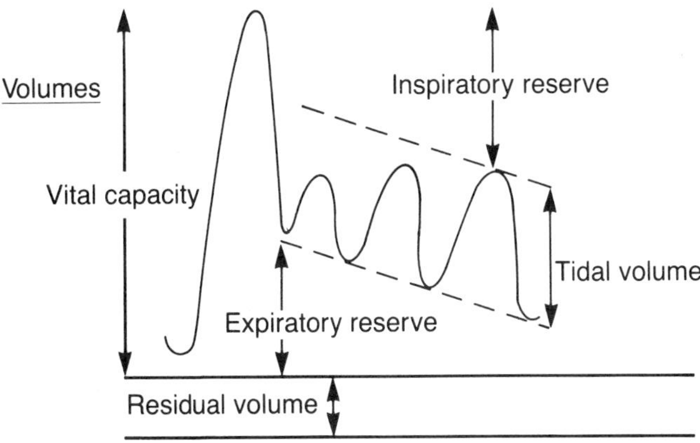

Figure 34-1 Normal spirograph.

for 10 seconds. The concentration of carbon monoxide in the expired air is then a measure of carbon monoxide uptake, and the difference between the two expirations of alveolar gas is analyzed to determine the diffusion rate of the carbon monoxide. Diffusion rates below certain levels indicate pulmonary disease.

Exercise Tests Exercise testing is used to assess overall respiratory function. Riding a stationary bicycle or running on a treadmill might demand more of a child's respiratory system than daily play and school activities. For example, a child with slight impairment might choose less strenuous activities and therefore be unaware of a respiratory impairment. Many children with asthma experience exercise-induced bronchospasm. Exercise testing reproduces the symptoms of exercise-induced bronchospasm in the clinic or hospital and assesses the ability of the child's respiratory system to function above usual levels. First, various pulmonary function values are obtained to serve as baseline data. Next, the child rides a stationary bicycle or runs on a treadmill while the pulse is monitored. After the target heart rate is reached and maintained for a predetermined amount of time, the child stops exercising and pulmonary function is retested. Significant changes from baseline pulmonary function data indicate disease or, in the case of asthma, exercise-induced bronchospasm.

Esophageal pH Monitoring Gastroesophageal reflux (see Chapter 38) commonly causes respiratory signs and symptoms. Esophageal pH monitoring is used to diagnose gastroesophageal reflux, particularly in the infant with a history of failure to thrive, episodes of sudden color change, brief periods of apnea, and aspiration pneumonia, but no history of spitting up or vomiting.

The procedure for testing for the presence of reflux is as follows. A pressure manometer catheter is inserted to determine the level of the distal esophageal sphincter prior to positioning the esophageal pH probe. Usually, a triple-lumen catheter is used. One lumen is for instillation of dilute hydrochloric acid and water; one is for pressure monitoring; and one is for a micro-pH probe assembly. The triple-lumen catheter is passed into the stomach and pulled back slowly through the gastroesophageal junction 3 times while pressure at midrespiration is measured. Peak pressure occurs at the level of the distal gastroesophageal sphincter.

Once the level of the distal esophageal sphincter has been determined, the catheter is returned to the stomach, and acid is instilled through one of the lumina. Next, the catheter is withdrawn to 2 cm above the level of the distal esophageal sphincter, where pH measurements are obtained for 0–24 hours, depending on protocol. If pH measured at 2 cm is high, the catheter is raised to 5 cm, and monitoring continues for another 10 hours. Spontaneous reflux is diagnosed if the pH drops to less than 4 on two occasions while the infant is lying in the supine or lateral positions.

During esophageal pH monitoring, the nurse continues feeding and routine nursing care. All activity is recorded on the monitoring chart. The nurse observes and records episodes of coughing, crying, and Valsalva's maneuver because these actions induce increased esophageal pressure. Events recorded on the chart are compared with pH values.

Tracheal Aspiration Tracheal aspiration is done to obtain specimens of secretions for bacterial and viral cultures or smears. The aspirate is obtained through laryngoscopy or, if the child is intubated, through a suction catheter inserted into the tube to withdraw secretions. Tracheal aspiration is a sterile procedure. The nurse uses aseptic technique and ensures that the child is well oxygenated before and after the procedure.

Bronchoscopy Visualization and manipulation of the larger branches of the tracheobronchial tree are possible through bronchoscopy. This procedure is ideal for the removal of aspirated foreign bodies; the aspiration of thick, tenacious mucus (relief of atelectasis); biopsy; culture; and direct observation.

Rigid bronchoscopy is usually performed under general anesthesia. Fiberoptic flexible bronchoscopy is now preferred because it can be performed on a sedated or awake, cooperative patient. The flexible, fiberoptic bronchoscope makes observation of bronchi branching off at angles possible.

Both rigid and fiberoptic bronchoscopy pose the risk of partial airway obstruction. The patient can be mechanically ventilated through the rigid bronchoscope, but this is not possible with the fiberoptic bronchoscope. On the other hand, the fiberoptic bronchoscope can be passed through the endotracheal tube of a mechanically ventilated patient without interrupting ventilation. This depends, however, on the size of the endotracheal tube and fiberoptic catheter. The flexible fiberoptic bronchoscope permits observation of more normal airway function, since the patient is not anesthetized. This is especially important in diagnosing malacias of the larynx, trachea, and bronchi.

The nurse monitors the child's pulse, respirations, and color continuously during the procedure and administers supplemental oxygen.

Prior to either rigid or flexible bronchoscopy, the child is given nothing by mouth to avoid vomiting and potential aspiration. After the procedure, mist is helpful in reducing laryngeal swelling caused by the insertion and withdrawal of the bronchoscope. Until swelling is reduced, the child must be observed closely for airway obstruction.

Lung Biopsy When prolonged serious lung disease cannot be diagnosed by less invasive means, open lung biopsy is performed. Lung biopsy may also be used to determine the degree of pulmonary hypertension in children with congenital heart disease.

While the child is under general anesthesia, an incision is made at the site of known disease. Tissue and vascular samples are obtained for pathologic study. Cultures can also be obtained. Percutaneous needle biopsy is not often used in pediatrics.

Postoperatively, the child might be placed in an intensive care unit. After open thoracic surgery, a chest tube is inserted and connected to suction to clear blood and oozing secretions. Vigorous chest physiotherapy is recommended. It must be remembered that the child who has undergone biopsy usually has serious underlying pulmonary disease.

Tuberculin Skin Test Any child who has a history of contact with someone actively infected with the tubercle bacillus should have a tuberculin skin test 2–10 weeks following contact. A positive reaction to the tuberculin skin test indicates the presence of the bacillus, but it does not indicate whether it is active or encapsulated. Purified protein derivative (PPD) is the recommended solution used for testing. In individual testing, the Mantoux test is done by injecting 0.1 mL of solution into the volar surface of the forearm. A wheal must be formed if the test is to be valid. The injection site is observed at 48–72 hours. The test is considered positive if the induration is more than 9 mm in diameter. An induration 5–9 mm across is inconclusive, and the test should be repeated. The test is negative if the induration is less than 5 mm in diameter. If the test is positive, the child should have a chest radiograph to identify extent of disease, and all subsequent evaluations should be done with radiographs. For mass screening, several types of puncture tests are available (for example, Tine, Sterneedle, Mono-Vac). In all cases, careful attention to application of the test procedures is mandatory. All children should be tested at 1 year of age and every 1–2 years thereafter.

Oximetry Oximetry is a noninvasive means of assessing hypoxemia. An oximeter is a photoelectric device used to determine oxygen saturation of the blood. The oximeter is placed on the ear lobe or, for the neonate, on the hand or foot.

Oxygen Therapy

Indications The indication for administration of supplemental oxygen is arterial hypoxemia, which leads to tissue hypoxia. Hypoxemia is evidenced by an increased respiratory rate, pallor, headache, tachycardia, and cyanosis. Severe hypoxemia causes mental confusion. The degree of hypoxemia is assessed through arterial blood gas studies, transcutaneous skin monitoring, or ear oximetry.

Acute hypoxemia is far more serious than chronic hypoxemia, because it is accompanied by acidosis. Acute hypoxemia may be due to asphyxia from near-drowning, aspiration, or airway constriction (for example, status asthmaticus). Chronic hypoxemia may be due to cystic fibrosis, chronic obstructive pulmonary disease (COPD), or congenital heart defects. The body compensates for the acid–base imbalance that occurs with chronic hypoxemia, and so it is not as life-threatening as acute hypoxemia.

Administration Equipment used to give supplemental oxygen includes hoods, isolettes, masks, cannulas, and catheters. The mode of delivery depends on the child's age and the percentage (concentration) of supplemental oxygen required.

The delivery of high concentrations of oxygen (above 40%) requires an isolette with ports blocked, hood, a face tent, or a nonrebreathing mask. For lesser concentrations, nasal cannulas are the most efficient and best-tolerated mode. Cannulas are now available for infants as young as 6 months of age. Oxygen delivery to younger infants requires some ingenuity. A small catheter with several distal holes or a cannula with the prongs cut off can be secured under the infant's nose. Placing squares of stoma adhesive on each cheek and then taping the cannula or catheter to the adhesive works well and prevents skin breakdown, as the stoma adhesive is not removed until it falls off and the cannula tape can be replaced as needed. An oxygen tent is seldom used for infants or children unless they are being treated for croup, in which case the tent's primary purpose is to deliver mist, not oxygen.

The nurse can use a number of oxygen-concentration analyzers continuously or intermittently to monitor supplemental oxygen delivery by hood, isolette, or mask. It is most difficult to measure the oxygen concentration delivered by cannula or catheter. Oxygen delivery by these means is best monitored through blood gas values or transcutaneous oxygen monitoring. There is usually a desired PaO_2 value for any infant or child receiving supplemental oxygen. The oxygen concentration needed to achieve that PaO_2 is prescribed by the physician. In acute conditions, PaO_2 may be determined as frequently as every 15 minutes. Continuous, long-term administration of oxygen generally is low-flow and is monitored much less frequently. For example, an infant receiving oxygen therapy at home may be assessed monthly.

Complications Like drug administration, oxygen administration must be monitored. Administration of too much or too little oxygen can cause deleterious effects. Retrolental fibroplasia (see Chapter 31) can occur in preterm infants if PaO_2 reaches 100 mm Hg or more at sea level, or 60 mm Hg or more at high altitudes. Another complication for infants needing prolonged high-concentration oxygen delivery and positive airway pressures is bronchopulmonary dysplasia, or chronic lung disease of infancy. Delivery of insufficient concentrations of oxygen can lead to pulmonary vascular constriction, airway constriction, tissue hypoxia, heart damage, and ultimate death.

Whenever the long-term delivery of high concentrations of supplemental oxygen is needed, it can cause interstitial fibrosis. Little is known about why this complication occurs, but it often follows several days of high-concentration (80%–100%) oxygen therapy, usually in conjunction with artificial ventilation. The prognosis of interstitial fibrosis in adults is poor, but children can survive it because the formation of new alveoli continues into adolescence.

Inhalation Therapy and Humidification

In inhalation therapy, drugs in liquid form are atomized by a nebulizer into a mist of fine particles, which are inhaled by the child. Drug solutions prepared for delivery by nebulizers are called *aerosols*. The three types of drugs most commonly given as aerosols are bronchodilators, antibiotics, and mucolytics. Ultrasonic nebulizers are capable of delivering very small particles. Nebulizers that are driven by compressed air or oxygen have varying particle-size ranges. Prefilled, hand-held, freon-propelled units (for example, Medihalers) are used at home. The device chosen for a particular child depends on the medication to be delivered and the ability of the child to cooperate with treatment.

An aerosol must be inhaled deeply for maximum benefit, and so patient education is important. It has been well documented in the literature that aerosol therapy must be administered correctly to be effective (Sexton, 1981). Any nebulizers may be used with children, but the nurse's close observation and stimulation is required to encourage deep breathing.

Because dry air irritates the airways, humidity (moisture) is added to dry air. Humidification is not used to deliver aerosols. A humidifier is merely a source of moisture through which air passes. Whenever the natural pathway of ventilation is bypassed, as with an artificial airway, humidity must be provided. The moisture source may need to be heated as well, because the energy required for the body to heat cold air is significant. Humidity is also needed when supplemental oxygen is given, since oxygen is a dry gas and can irritate the nasopharynx.

Combination nebulizer–humidifier units are available, making the choice of humidification equipment confusing. The nurse and respiratory therapist decide the purpose for delivering moisture to the airway and then choose the most appropriate equipment to do the job.

Intermittent Positive Pressure Breathing

Intermittent positive pressure breathing (IPPB), usually referred to as intermittent positive pressure ventilation, can be done in conjunction with artificial ventilation or as a treatment for a child capable of breathing independently. In IPPB, a pressure source (for example, a Bennett or Bird machine or a hand-held device, such as a Hand-i-vent) inflates the lungs during inspiration. The device must be capable of delivering 10–20 cm of water pressure. Either a tight-fitting mask or a mouthpiece is used. The purpose of IPPB is to deliver a prescribed aerosol or to enhance deep breathing.

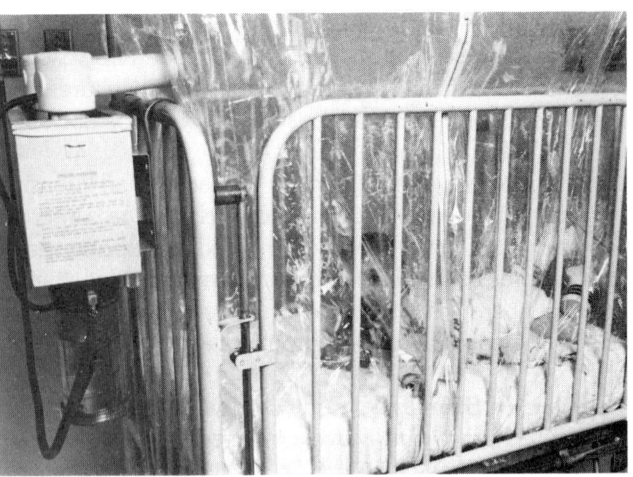

Pneumatically powered system for delivery of oxygen and humidity in a temperature-controlled environment. (From Swearingen PL: *The Addison-Wesley Photo-Atlas of Nursing Procedures*. Addison-Wesley, 1984, p. 339.)

For years, IPPB has been a controversial treatment for both adults and children, partly because of its complications, such as overdistention of the stomach due to air swallowing, hyperinflation, and pneumothorax. These complications may result from poor patient teaching and a lack of patient cooperation, especially with children. Studies have shown that the administration of an aerosol through a powered nebulizer with active deep breathing is as effective as the administration of an aerosol with IPPB and much less dangerous (Wade, 1982). If IPPB is used, a great deal of patient education and monitoring of delivered volumes is necessary. Sometimes IPPB is used for children with largngotracheobronchitis to deliver racemic epinephrine. This medication is intended for the upper airway, and so the child's cooperation is not as critical. The primary difference between IPPB and inhalation therapy with a nebulizer is that in IPPB the aerosol is delivered under pressure.

Transcutaneous Oxygen Monitoring

Transcutaneous monitoring (TCM) of oxygenation, a technique widely used in neonatal intensive care units, is becoming an accepted technique for children as well. A monitoring transducer probe is secured to the skin so that air cannot leak into the area of skin-probe contact. A heating element warms the small area of skin to 43–44.5 C (preset and age-dependent). As the skin temperature rises, the capillary bed in the skin dilates and arterializes. Oxygen molecules diffuse across to the probe membrane. The pressure of the oxygen is then measured and recorded.

Monitoring can be done continuously for patients with tenuous oxygenation or intermittently during diagnostic procedures or manipulation. It also may be used as a "spot check" on oxygenation in lieu of drawing an arterial sample for determining blood gas values.

In a well-perfused child, transcutaneous measurements may correlate very closely with actual arterial oxygenation. With underperfusion, however, the transcutaneous values may indicate only trends, not accurate oxygenation status. As long as it is known that trends are being monitored, transcutaneous monitoring is very helpful.

The reliability of transcutaneous recordings generally depends on consistent use and upkeep of the equipment and consistent, frequent, and accurate calibrations. Operators must either know how to calibrate the machine accurately or designate a group of individuals to assume this responsibility. Casual use of this expensive equipment usually leads to mistrust and premature disregard for valuable data.

To obtain a transcutaneous reading, the operator checks calibration and selects an appropriate site. The anterior chest and abdominal walls are most often used. The back, especially in the costal vertebral arch over the kidneys, is also appropriate. The skin is cleansed of oils, lotions, and powders with an alcohol swab. An appropriate amount of distilled water is inserted between the skin and the probe to form an airtight seal. Probe temperature is set according to skin thickness. A premature infant may require only 43 C. An older infant may require 44–45.5 C. If monitoring is to be done continuously, the probe site must be changed every 3–4 hours to prevent burning of the skin. Heating takes between 12–15 minutes. A heat-output monitoring display indicates when the set temperature has been reached and shows the pressure of transmembranous oxygen.

Transcutaneous monitoring is very helpful during weaning from oxygen therapy. A reading is obtained while the child breathes the prescribed supplemental oxygen. If this reading is within or above the normal oxygenation range (adjusted for higher altitudes), the concentration or flow of oxygen is gradually reduced. A transcutaneous recording is made following each adjustment of oxygen concentration or flow.

If the child's oxygenation remains within normal limits with minute flows of 1/4–1/8 L or concentrations of 22%–23%, room air may be tried. In some protocols, the nurse decides the appropriate amount of supplemental oxygen to be administered. If there is no set protocol, the physician orders the desired oxygen concentration or flow rate.

In some small infants, hypoxemia causes diminished cardiac output and perfusion, and the transcutaneous monitoring may suddenly drop to the 20–30 range without obvious clinical signs of cyanosis and tachypnea. This drop is an important indirect reflection of oxygenation and must not be disregarded. It is a dramatic demonstration of the cardiovascular response to even brief hypoxemia in young infants.

Artificial Airways

Pharyngeal Airways Oropharyngeal airways are used in adults to stabilize the airway for bag-to-mask ventilation. They are rarely used for children because of the danger that they may block rather than stabilize the child's small airway. For children, a nasopharyngeal tube ("nasal trumpet") may be inserted into the nose and aimed posteriorly to maintain a patent airway. The nasopharyngeal tube is used if the infant or child has a poorly supported airway that obstructs during sleep, such as in Pierre Robin syndrome.

Endotracheal or Orotracheal Tubes Nasal or oral intubation ensures airway patency and provides a means for artificial ventilation. If artificial ventilation is required, a cuffed tube is used. A noncuffed tube is used if the purpose of intubation is solely to maintain airway patency. Noncuffed tubes are used for both purposes in infants and children up to 8 years of age.

There are several formulas for determining tube size and length. If the patient is an infant, tube length may be determined by the formula, $0.21 \times \text{body length} + 1.25$. For the older infant or child, tube length should equal the distance (by way of the ear) from the tip of the nose to just below the sternal notch. Tube diameter should be the largest that will pass through the nares, except in the child with croup, where a tube one size smaller is used to avoid further irritation. Most tubes are of plastic or silicone, are disposable, and are cut to size.

If a cuffed tube is required, the nurse selects one with a permanent cuff that cannot be detached. The cuff should be of a soft material that inflates to high volume but exerts little pressure on the trachea. To prevent tracheal irritation, the nurse checks cuff pressure periodically (every 3–4 hours). The cuff need not be inflated sufficiently to prevent all leaks. A small leak does not interfere with ventilation and lessens chances of pressure necrosis. Following placement of the tube, a radiograph is taken to note the location of its distal end.

Tracheostomy Tubes A tracheostomy is usually done if an artificial airway is going to be required long-term for ventilation or for removal of secretions. It is a surgical procedure done under controlled circumstances. The most commonly used tube is the Shiley tube, which comes with or without an inflatable cuff. Tube size depends on age and size of the child and the reason for placement. The tube is cut to the appropriate size.

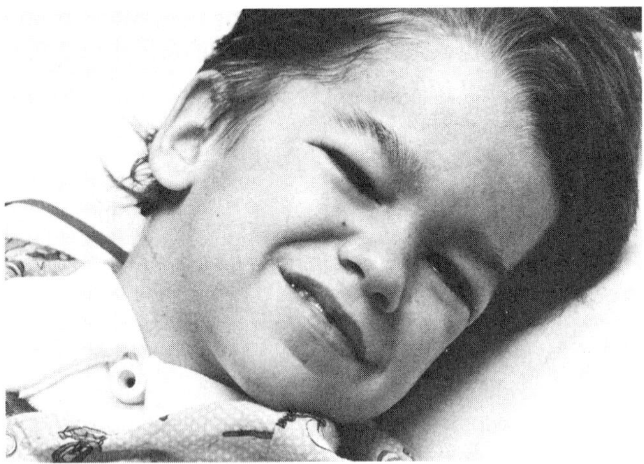

Tracheostomy tube secured in place.

Nursing Considerations The nurse's main responsibilities in caring for the child with an artificial airway are

1. Making sure the tube does not inadvertently come out. The child might have to be restrained.
2. Monitoring cuff pressure, if a cuffed tube is used.
3. Suctioning accumulated secretions through the tube as necessary to maintain a patent airway and providing extra breaths of oxygen both before and after suctioning.
4. Providing skin and stoma care to prevent breakdown and infection.
5. Changing the tape on the tube as needed to keep it dry and secure. If the child has a tracheostomy, the nurse changes wet ties to prevent neck irritation or dislodgment of the tube. Gauze is not placed under the flange of the tube, because it prevents observation of the site and does not allow the skin to dry.
6. Relieving the child's anxiety. The intubated child is unable to talk or cry audibly, which is very frightening.

Chest Physiotherapy

Postural Drainage, Percussion, and Vibration To perform postural drainage, the nurse or physiotherapist positions the child so that gravity enhances removal of secretions from specific lobes of the lungs. Postural drainage is usually done in conjunction with percussion and vibration. The purpose of all three procedures is to stimulate productive coughing. The nurse schedules postural drainage procedures before feedings or meals to avoid inducing vomiting.

Percussion is done by clapping a cupped hand over the area to be percussed. The wrist and arm remain relaxed, while the cupped hand is clapped on the child's body firmly enough to cause a popping sound. If the patient is a premature or very small infant, the nurse can use an infant-sized mask, rather than the cupped hand. Percussion should not be done over bare skin, the sternum, spine, stomach,

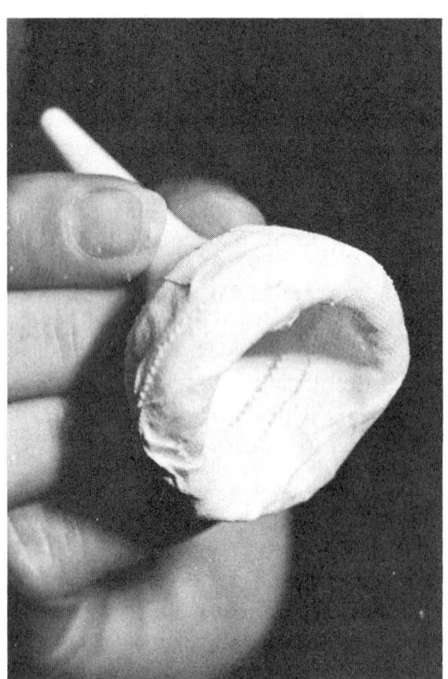

A. Bulb syringe adapted for an infant too small for hand percussion. The bulb is cut in half and the edges padded with tape. The nurse percusses while holding the nozzle of the syringe.

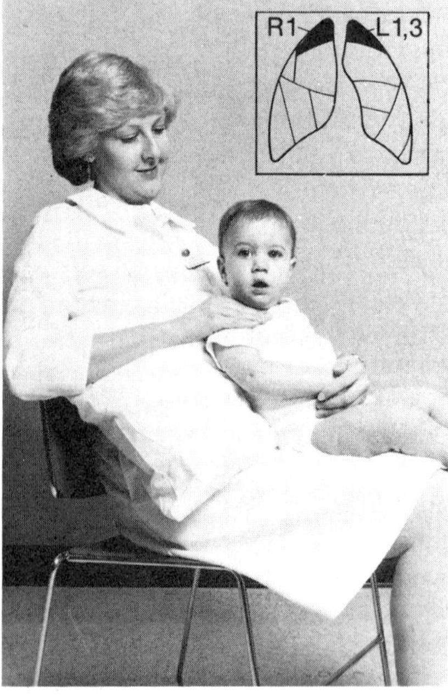

B. Drainage apical segments of upper lobes. The child reclines at a 30° angle while the nurse percusses and vibrates segments between clavicles and scapulae.

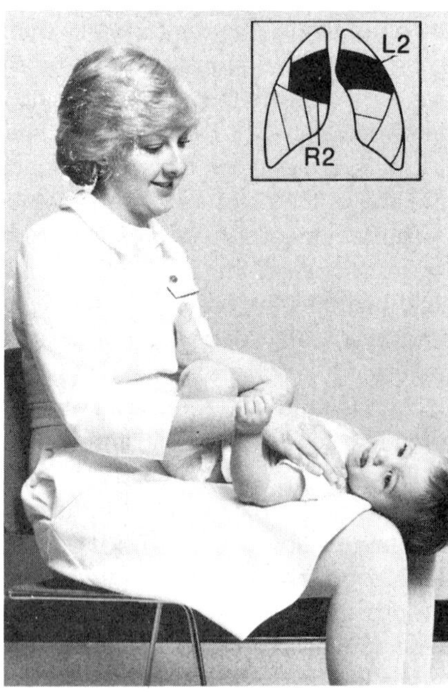

C. Draining anterior segments of the upper lobes. The child lies supine while the nurse percusses and vibrates segments between clavicles and nipples.

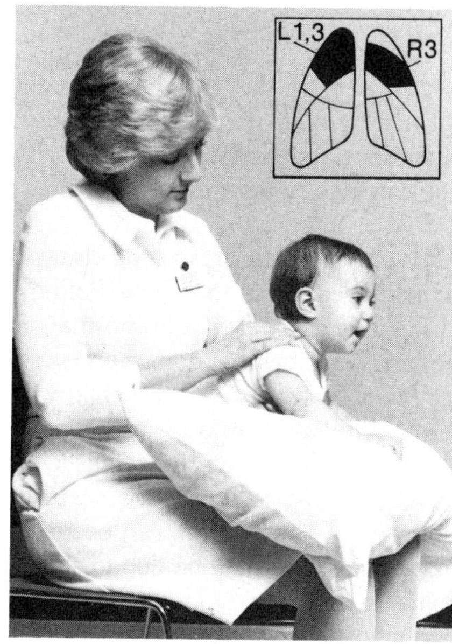

D. Draining posterior segments of upper lobes. The child is propped at a 30° angle while the nurse percusses and vibrates the upper back on both sides of the spine.

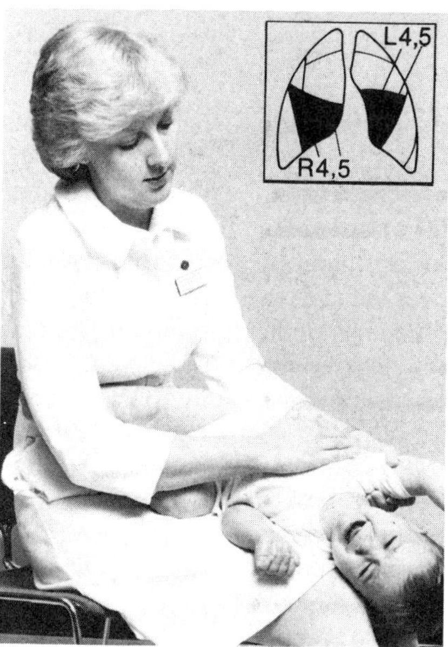

E. Draining lateral and medial segments of the right middle lobe. The child lies on the side with head down 30°. The nurse rotates the child a quarter turn to the back and percusses and vibrates over the uppermost nipple. To drain lingular segments of the left upper lobe, the nurse turns the child to the corresponding position on the opposite side and repeats over the uppermost nipple.

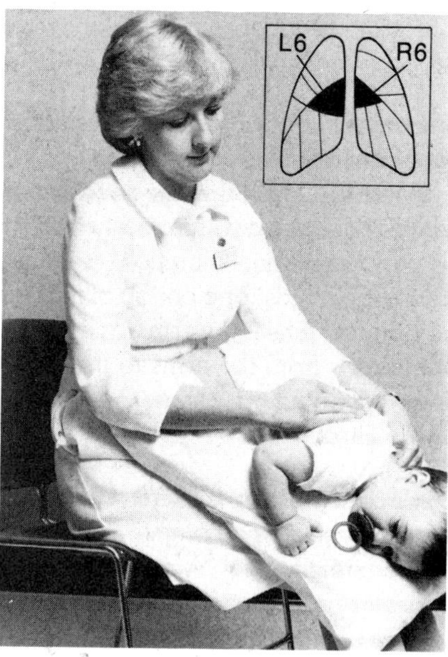

F. Draining the superior segments of the lower lobes. The child lies prone with head down 15° while the nurse percusses and vibrates on both sides of the spine, below the tips of the scapulae.

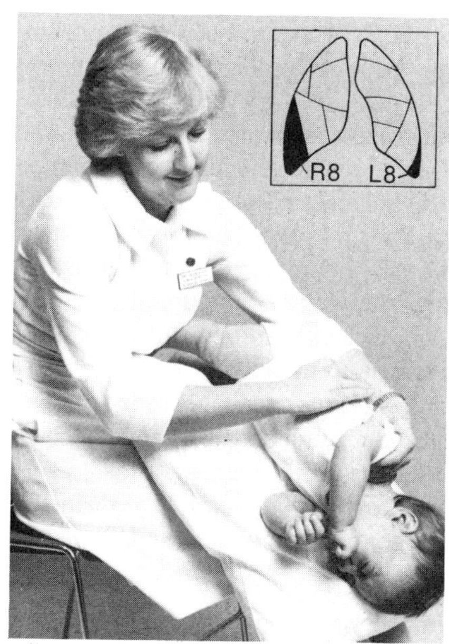

G. Draining anterior basal segments of lower lobes. The child lies on the side with head down 30° on the nurse's extended legs. The nurse percusses and vibrates over the lower ribs beneath the axillae, then turns the child and repeats on the opposite side.

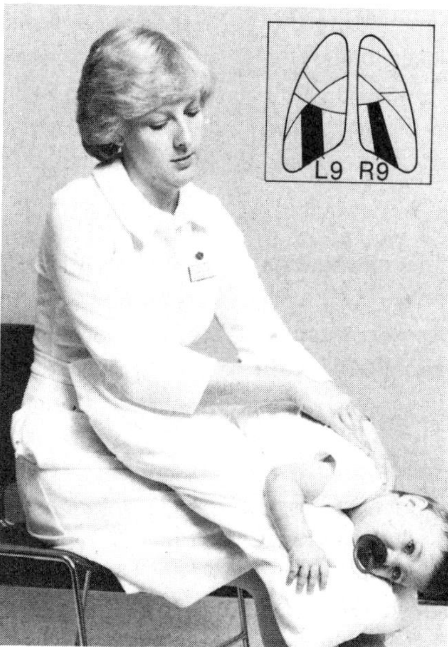

H. Draining the lateral basal segments of the lower lobes. The child lies prone with head down 30°. The nurse rotates the upper half of the child's body a quarter turn toward the side and percusses and vibrates over the lower ribs, then turns the child to the opposite side and repeats.

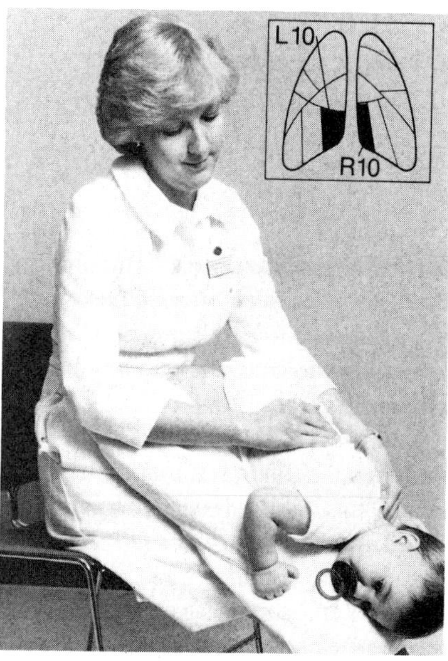

I. Draining the posterior basal segments of the lower lobes. The child lies prone with head down 30° while the nurse percusses and vibrates over the lower ribs on both sides of the spine, avoiding the area over the kidneys.

Postural drainage procedures for an infant. (From Swearingen PL: *The Addison-Wesley Photo-Atlas of Nursing Procedures*. Addison-Wesley, 1984, pp. 364–366).

or kidneys. Usually, percussion is done for 1–2 minutes in each postural drainage position.

Vibration, which is often done in addition to percussion, can be performed with a mechanical vibrator or manually. To perform manual vibration, the nurse or physiotherapist places the hands, one on top of the other, over the area to be vibrated, tenses the arms, and creates a vibrating motion that travels from the arms to the child's body. Vibration is done only during expiration, to enhance the child's respiratory effort.

Breathing Deeply and Coughing A deep breath usually generates a cough in a child with excess mucus in the respiratory tract. A deep breath followed by a forced expiratory movement greatly enhances mucus clearance. A deep breath also opens up areas of atelectasis, so breathing deeply is critical postoperatively (see Chapter 29). If coughing irritates the airway, resulting in airway constriction, the physician may prescribe an aerosol bronchodilator for administration prior to cough stimulation.

Incentive Spirometry *Spirometry* is measurement of the breathing capacity of the lungs. Incentive spirometry is used to encourage the child to fill the lungs to capacity. The child must inspire fully so that, a small, plastic ball that the child can see is forced upward through the device. The goal is to encourage maximal inspiration. This is accomplished by gradually increasing the resistance, thus increasing the inspiratory effort required to move the plastic ball. The nurse can devise games to achieve the same purpose, such as having the child inspire through a straw to pick up small pieces of paper or inspire through a tube to move water between two connected bottles.

Breathing Exercises Breathing exercises strengthen respiratory muscles and increase lung capacity. They also enhance deep breathing and coughing. The child inspires to capacity, holds the breath briefly, and then expires slowly and completely.

Huffing Huffing is a maneuver that aids in mucus clearance. The child exhales in a series of four to five short, forced, expiratory breaths repeatedly over a minute or two. The expiratory huffs "milk" mucus up through the airway so that it can be expectorated with one good effective cough. Huffing helps prevent the prolonged coughing spells that children with asthma or cystic fibrosis often experience.

Principles of Nursing Care

Acute Care Needs

The acute care needs of the child with respiratory dysfunction depend on whether the dysfunction is obstructive, restrictive, or caused by inefficient gas transfer. Any of these dysfunctions can lead to development of one or both of the others, and all three can lead to respiratory failure.

Obstructive Lung Disease Obstructive lung disease is characterized by increased resistance to airflow. Pulmonary function tests indicate decreased flow, with normal or slightly decreased volumes. Blood gases are normal unless the obstruction is prominent, in which case the child will have respiratory acidosis. Wheezing, rhonchi, retractions, coughing, tachypnea, and dyspnea are all characteristic of obstructive lung disease. Clubbing and cyanosis occur if obstruction is chronic or severe. Obstruction can occur at any level of the respiratory tract and may be due to structural or functional anomalies, aspiration of foreign bodies, infection, tumors, or bronchospasm caused by allergens or irritants.

Acute care is based on a nursing diagnosis of ineffective airway clearance. Gordon (1982) defines this as the "inability to effectively clear secretions or obstruction from the respiratory tract." Interventions related to airway clearance are discussed in the sections on asthma and cystic fibrosis.

Restrictive Lung Disease Restrictive lung disease is characterized by impaired lung expansion related to loss of lung volume, decreased distensibility, or a chest wall disturbance. A typical cluster of signs and symptoms might include decreased lung volumes demonstrated by pulmonary function testing, poor exercise tolerance, chest deformity, altered chest excursion, shallow respirations, and nasal flaring. The site of disturbance may be the lung parenchyma, the chest wall, or nearby skeletal structures. Restrictive disorders include atelectasis from hyaline membrane disease or Wilson-Mikity syndrome, pneumonia or other infections, such anomalies as congenital cysts, or pneumothorax due to alveolar rupture. Also included are chest disturbances due to diaphragmatic hernia, muscular dystrophy, kyphoscoliosis, thoracic dystrophy, or congenital absence of ribs.

Acute care is based on a nursing diagnosis of ineffective breathing patterns. Gordon (1982) defines this as "respiration (respiratory compensations) inadequate to maintain sufficient oxygen supply for cellular requirements."

Inefficient Gas Transfer Inadequate alveolar ventilation or any defect that impairs diffusion across the alveolocapillary membrane results in inefficient gas transfer. Inadequate ventilation may be the result of a defect in the respiratory control mechanism. Inefficient gas transfer from this cause is manifested by signs of central nervous system depression.

Inefficient gas transfer related to a defect in diffusion causes signs and symptoms of dyspnea, cyanosis, dullness on percussion, bronchial breath sounds heard on ascultation of the peripheral airway, and blood gas values that indicate

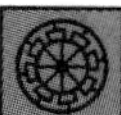

NURSING CARE GUIDE Child With a Respiratory Problem

Nursing Diagnosis	Interventions	Evaluation
1. Ineffective airway clearance related to accumulation of mucus in the respiratory passages	Assist child to cough productively. Tell child not to suppress cough or waste energy on weak coughing	Child clears respiratory passages of mucus and breathes through nose without difficulty
	Monitor fluid intake, measure and record intake and output accurately, maintain intravenous flow at appropriate rate	
	Offer small amounts of favorite fluids frequently. Avoid ice-cold fluids because they may cause bronchospasm	
	Monitor hydration status, check urine specific gravity every shift. Note skin turgor, presence of tears, moistness of mucous membranes	
	Provide humidity. Keep child in mist tent or room with vaporizer	
	Change child's position at least every 2 hours and encourage activity as tolerated	
	Note presence and character of nasal discharge	
	Note quantity and quality of sputum or presence of mucus in vomitus	
	Help child to cooperate in inhalation therapy. Administer aerosol as ordered	
	Provide chest physiotherapy (percussion, vibration, and postural drainage) as indicated. Use games or diversion to encourage child to cooperate	
	Listen to breath sounds before and after chest physiotherapy to assess effectiveness	
	Suction nasopharyngeal area to remove thick secretions or vomitus. (Remember that too-frequent suctioning stimulates mucus production)	
2. Impaired gas exchange related to inadequate oxygenation	Observe for signs of hypoxia, tachypnea, tachycardia, elevated blood pressure, restlessness, anxiety	Child's respiratory rate, skin color, and activity tolerance return to child's normal or preillness level
	Observe for cyanosis: note mucus membranes, nail beds, periorbital area. Monitor arterial blood gases	
	Monitor vital signs and listen to breath sounds every 30–60 minutes	
	Provide oxygen therapy as ordered	
	Provide rest to reduce oxygen requirements. Plan periods of undisturbed rest, group scheduled procedures together, observe closely for signs of fatigue	
	Observe anterior–posterior dimension of chest for signs of hyperinflation	

continued on next page

NURSING CARE GUIDE Child With a Respiratory Problem (continued)

Nursing Diagnosis	Interventions	Evaluation
	Observe and report evidence of increasing hypoxia, fatigue, lethargy, bradycardia, bradypnea, decreasing blood pressure, coma Administer medications as ordered to relieve bronchospasm and dilate bronchi	
3. Ineffective breathing pattern related to difficulty getting air into or out of the lungs	Observe for retractions. Identify retractions as intercostal, substernal, supraclavicular. Note depth of retractions Describe use of accessory muscles of breathing, abdominal breathing, flaring of nares Observe chest for symmetry of movements during respirations Note length and character of inspiratory and expiratory phases of respiration	Child is able to inspire and expire sufficient amounts of air without difficulty
4. Potential upper airway obstruction	Observe for orthopnea and hyperextension of the neck in efforts to inspire more air Note inspiratory stridor, barky cough, hoarseness, drooling, refusal to swallow Support child in upright position and monitor closely for signs of upper airway obstruction Prepare child and family for possible intubation or tracheostomy Remain calm and offer reassurance to child and family	Child is able to inspire and expire sufficient amounts of air without difficulty
5. Potential lower airway obstruction	Observe for expiratory grunt, rapid shallow breathing, hyperinflated lungs Teach and practice breathing exercises with child, use of incentive spirometer, paper bag breathing, games with straws, or blowing that require maximal inspiration Provide continuity of care and anticipate child's needs so as to conserve energy and decrease respiratory effort	Child is able to inspire and expire sufficient amounts of air without difficulty
6. Alteration in comfort related to chest pain	Observe for signs of dyspnea, such as shallow breathing, chest splinting Listen to breath sounds to detect areas of absent or greatly diminished ventilation Observe child's posture in lying, sitting, and standing positions for signs of painful respiration Ask child to describe pain: when it began or first occurred, whether it is sharp or dull, episodic or continuous Demonstrate to child how to support or hold painful area with pillow or hand Administer analgesics as ordered	Child breathes without discomfort

respiratory acidosis and hypoxemia. Restlessness, confusion, and other signs of hypoxia and hypercapnia may also be present. Disorders that impair gas transfer include pulmonary edema, pulmonary embolism, anemia, hemorrhage, cerebral trauma (birth injuries), meningitis, maternal oversedation, and tetanus.

Acute care is based on a nursing diagnosis of impaired gas exchange, which Gordon (1982) defines as "disturbance in oxygen or carbon dioxide exchange in lungs or at a cellular level." Medical treatment is focused on maintaining the alveolocapillary surface area, maintaining red blood cell and hemoglobin levels (see Chapter 36), and maintaining an intact respiratory control center (see Chapter 42). Nursing interventions are supportive. Nursing goals are to help conserve the child's energy, prevent infection, preserve pulmonary function, and prevent pulmonary crippling by maintaining an optimum level of activity.

Respiratory Failure Respiratory failure can be related to obstructive disease, restrictive disease, or inefficient gas transfer. Respiratory failure may have an abrupt or an insidious onset, and the cause may be an acute or chronic dysfunction. For example, a child with cystic fibrosis, a chronic disease, may suddenly become very ill with an infection that causes the child's condition to deteriorate rapidly. Whatever the cause, respiratory failure results in hypoxemia and hypercapnia.

Hypoxemia and acidemia lead to pulmonary capillary and arteriolar constriction, which may cause thrombi or emboli or both to form as blood flow through these vessels is restricted. Pulmonary hypertension occurs, which leads to right ventricular hypertrophy and finally to right ventricular failure.

The nurse who is caring for a child with respiratory dysfunction watches for early signs of respiratory failure and is prepared to intervene. (The clinical signs of respiratory failure are listed in Table 34-1.) Acute care for the child with respiratory failure is the rapid initiation of cardiopulmonary resuscitation (CPR), which is discussed in Chapter 19. Immediate intervention is mandatory because cardiac function continues only a few minutes after breathing stops.

Nutritional Needs

The nature of body fluid composition and metabolism in infants and young children makes them much more susceptible than adults to rapid depletion of body stores of water and electrolytes (see Chapter 33). Anorexia, vomiting, diarrhea, and fever are characteristic of acute infections of the respiratory system, and so dehydration is always a risk. Dehydration also results from an increased respiratory rate. Approximately two-thirds of the child's total daily water loss normally occurs through the respiratory tract lining. The amount lost increases in direct proportion to increases in the respiratory rate. To prevent dehydration, the nurse offers small amounts of the child's favorite fluids at frequent intervals. Unless the respiratory illness is chronic, it does not compromise the child's nutritional status. The nurse offers favorite foods as much as possible. High-calorie liquids, such as soda pop or fruit juices, can provide calories and prevent dehydration for the child who is having difficulty swallowing solid foods. If the child has had vomiting or diarrhea, the nurse may offer commercially prepared fluids that contain electrolytes (see Chapter 33). Dehydration can cause mucus to become too dry or too vicous and difficult for the child to expectorate. Therefore, adequate hydration is a priority for a child whose disorder causes mucus production. Inhalation therapy also may be employed to enhance hydration and prevent mucus plugs from becoming viscous.

If fever is the cause of dehydration, the nurse employs measures to reduce the fever. Acetaminophen is the antipyretic of choice, as aspirin has more side effects including possible association with Reye's syndrome, especially when given during an infection (see Chapter 42).

Developmental Needs

The developmental and psychosocial needs of the child who is chronically ill or hospitalized are discussed in Chapters 27–30. Specific needs relative to respiratory disorders are covered in this section.

Children with chronic lung disease, particularly asthma, need to exercise at a level consistent with endurance. Medications can be taken before exercise to prevent exercise-induced bronchospasm. If the child has become increasingly sedentary to avoid dyspnea or bronchospasm, a carefully planned exercise program is needed to increase stamina and muscle mass. If the child has cystic fibrosis, exercise can stimulate coughing and help the child to raise and expectorate sputum. Swimming is excellent exercise for children with chronic lung disorders because it requires breath control and exercises several muscle groups.

Children who have been bedridden for extended periods or who have been mechanically ventilated also benefit from appropriate exercise training. Infants with bronchopulmonary dysplasia, who often are born prematurely and who are developmentally immature, need therapeutic play and a graded exercise program to compensate for developmental delays (see Chapter 31).

Emotional Needs

The Child With an Acute Respiratory Illness A child who is admitted to the hospital with acute spasmodic croup, epiglottitis, or foreign body aspiration has had little or no preparation for admission. The nurse can use principles of crisis intervention to help the child and family cope with the experience in a positive way (see Chapter 27). For example, Nancy is 2 years old. Her health was normal until

3 days ago, when she developed an upper respiratory tract infection. She became progressively more ill over the next 3 days, with increasing hoarseness, a brassy cough, general malaise, and a low-grade fever. About 8 o'clock this evening, Nancy's mother called her pediatrician because Nancy was beginning to have inspiratory stridor, retractions, and tachypnea. Nancy was admitted to the hospital at 9:00 PM.

Nancy's mother appears anxious and refuses to leave her daughter's bedside. She talks continuously and keeps asking the same questions about the purpose of the oxygen and mist tent. Nancy is crying hysterically and needs her mother's support to help calm her down and provide the rest she needs. After talking with the nurse, Nancy's mother explains that she is afraid that Nancy will die "just like her grandfather did of asthma." The nurse carefully explains the difference between asthma and *laryngotracheobronchitis* (inflammation of the larynx, trachea, and bronchi), a common infectious condition in children.

Further assessment leads to a nursing diagnosis of compromised family coping, as Nancy's mother temporarily is unable to provide effective support, comfort, and assistance. Instead, she is preoccupied with her own reactions of guilt and anger. Nursing interventions include helping Nancy's mother express her feelings of guilt and anger, reducing her anxiety, and helping her to gain a better understanding of laryngotracheobronchitis, its usual treatment, and the prognosis. Nancy recovers from acute laryngotracheobronchitis in a few days and is discharged. The experience in the hospital has been positive for Nancy and her mother.

The Child With a Chronic Respiratory Illness

Chronic illness creates chronic stress and often a series of crises that occur throughout the child's life (see Chapter 30). The first crisis occurs when the child and family learn the diagnosis. The immediate response is intense anxiety. Information given to the family at this time is kept brief, and any instructions are written out, since high levels of anxiety interfere with learning. The nurse helps the family to express feelings and handles the situation as an acute crisis.

The nurse's assessment of the family's strengths, prior experiences in coping with crisis, and concurrent stressors begins with this initial contact with the family. The child's developmental level, sex, and prior coping abilities also affect the family's and child's ability to cope emotionally with chronic illness.

A child's fear of dying is one of the most difficult emotions for parents and health professionals to deal with (see Chapter 32).

Health Maintenance Needs

The child who is hospitalized for treatment of an acute or chronic respiratory dysfunction usually requires home care or follow-up after discharge. (Home care for the child with an acute illness is discussed in Chapter 26.) Home care for the child with a respiratory disorder frequently involves home administration of oxygen, inhalation therapy, and physiotherapy aimed at mucus clearance. A prescribed exercise regimen or breathing exercises also may be continued at home.

The parents of children who are sent home with inhalation therapy or oxygen therapy equipment should practice using the equipment with the nurse several times before the child's discharge. The parent learns proper techniques for cleaning nebulizers, which can harbor infectious microorganisms. The nebulizer and mask are washed daily with soap and water and soaked twice weekly in a weak solution of vinegar and water. The nurse gives the parent detailed written instructions about aerosol treatment schedules, doses, and precautions. If oxygen equipment is to be used at home, rental of oxygen tanks and regulators is arranged before the child is discharged. The nurse teaches the parent how to use the equipment and reviews the safety measures listed in Table 34-3.

Even if the child is being discharged on the same home care regimen that was carried out before admission, the nurse reviews all aspects of home care with the child and family to be sure that incorrect procedures have not inadvertently become habitual. The nurse also can use this opportunity to increase the child's and parent's understanding of the disorder and its treatment.

If the child has been admitted for foreign body aspiration or near-drowning, the nurse discusses safety and well-child issues with the parent, being careful not to add to any guilt that the parent already might feel. If it is possible to make a home visit after discharge, the nurse works with the parent to identify safety hazards in the home. The nurse also recommends that the parent learn CPR and emergency maneuvers for managing airway obstruction by foreign bodies (see Chapter 19). If the child has been admitted for an acute infection or inflammation, such as acute spasmodic croup or laryngotracheobronchitis, the nurse reviews with the parent the signs and symptoms that indicate the need for immediate medical attention.

It is extremely important for the child, parent, and nurse to plan details of emergency care before discharge. All children who are old enough to use the telephone should learn who and how to call for help in an emergency. The emergency care number should be placed on the telephone, and each child should practice dialing the number and stating the nature of the emergency and his or her name, address, and telephone number.

Most parents appreciate knowing when the next follow-up contact will occur. It is helpful to arrange the time of the next visit before discharge, so that parents have plenty of time to arrange their schedules to keep the appointment.

The nurse prepares the parent for any changes or deterioration in the child's condition that are expected. For ex-

TABLE 34-3 Safe Use of Oxygen at Home

Safety guidelines	Rationale
Secure oxygen tank in upright position	Oxygen tanks are highly explosive. If a horizontally positioned tank explodes, the rapid release of oxygen can catapult it through walls and into people
Keep oxygen tanks at least 5 feet from heat source and electrical devices (that is, space heaters, heating vents, fireplaces, radios, vaporizers and humidifiers)	Heat can increase pressure inside the tank, causing it to explode
Ensure that no one smokes in the room or area of the oxygen tank	Smoking increases the risk of fire, which could cause the tank to explode. Escaped oxygen would feed the fire
Use lemon–glycerin swabs to relieve dryness around the child's mouth. Avoid oil- or alcohol-based substances (for example, petroleum jelly, vitamin A and D ointment, baby oil)	Alcohol and oil are both flammable and increase the risk of fire
Have the child wear cotton garments	Silk, wool, and synthetics can generate static electricity and cause fire
Keep a fire extinguisher readily available	It is necessary to put out fire immediately
Turn off both volume regulator and flow regulator whenever oxygen is not in use	If the volume regulator is on when oxygen is turned on, the child may receive a rapid, forceful flow of oxygen in the face that could be frightening and uncomfortable
	Oxygen leakage, which might not be detected because oxygen is odorless, can cause fire

ample, the parent of a child with asthma might be warned that the upcoming cold weather could predispose the child to more frequent infections and therefore to exacerbations of asthma. The nurse also discusses age-appropriate reactions to stress with the parent. The nurse might say, "It is common for young children to lose interest in taking their respiratory treatments correctly after they return home. You will need to set firm limits." This helps prepare the parent for "posthospital syndrome." The longer the child has been hospitalized, the more difficult it will be to return to the home care routine. The nurse can test the child's behavior relative to medicine or postural drainage and advise the parent to remain firm about the need for treatment but be flexible about other issues.

The nurse identifies sources of parental support in the community, such as mental health workers, psychiatrists, psychologists, social workers, community health nurses, and clergy. Other parents who have had similar problems with chronic illness can provide the unique support that comes through experience. There are many cystic fibrosis and asthmatic parents' groups throughout the country. The American Lung Association and the Cystic Fibrosis Foundation are good sources for information about these groups.

The Child With an Acute Respiratory Infection

Rhinitis

Rhinitis is inflammation of the mucous membrane of the nose. It is manifested by a nasal discharge and is almost always associated with an underlying disturbance. The most common causes of rhinitis are allergy, the common cold, infected adenoids, chronic sinusitis, foreign body aspiration, and various congenital anomalies. Besides nasal discharge, symptoms may include foul breath and disturbances of taste and smell. In allergic rhinitis, mucous membranes are pale and boggy; nasal obstruction is common and often cyclic.

Rhinitis is treated by correcting the underlying problem. Emphasis is placed on eradicating any foci of infection. Medications that provide symptomatic relief are used with mixed results. Short-term inhalation therapy with aerosol steroids is moderately successful in treating allergic rhinitis. (See Chapter 26 for a discussion of home care.)

Tonsillitis and Pharyngitis

Infections of the tonsils and throat (pharynx) can be viral or bacterial. Nonbacterial exudative tonsillitis is generally a mild disease requiring little medical intervention. The onset is gradual and is typified by low-grade fever, mild headache, and loss of appetite. Sore throat, hoarse voice, and a productive cough are common symptoms. Treatment includes comfort measures, acetaminophen for pain, and oral fluids. Complications are rare.

The symptoms of bacterial tonsillitis and pharyngitis may be dramatic. Group A beta-hemolytic streptococcus is the most common bacterial cause. Fever (38–40 C) usually is the first symptom. Generalized symptoms of muscle aches, headache, and vomiting develop within 18–24 hours. The severity of pharyngeal pain varies. In its early stages, bacterial infection is often difficult to diagnose, and a second throat culture might be needed to determine whether the causative agent is viral or bacterial.

The sequelae of streptococcal infection sometimes include skin rashes and extension of the disease resulting in peritonsillar abscess, sinusitis, middle ear infection (otitis media), and involvement of the mastoids or meninges. Late sequelae might include rheumatic fever and acute glomerulonephritis.

A throat culture is done, and an appropriate antibiotic is prescribed, generally penicillin or, if pencillin is contraindicated, erythromycin. Comfort measures include bed rest, fluids, acetaminophen, and warm saline gargles for throat pain.

Many upper respiratory infections can be prevented if the child avoids close contact with infected individuals, washes the hands correctly, and disposes of upper airway secretions carefully. In the hospital or group living settings, children with viral or inadequately treated bacterial respiratory infections must be kept in strict respiratory isolation (see Chapter 29).

A group of children may require a tonsillectomy or adenoidectomy or both because of "recurrent symptomatic hypertrophy associated with signs and symptoms of obstruction and chronic infection" (Behrman and Vaughan, 1983). These children have chronic enlargement of the tonsils or adenoids, which interferes with swallowing or breathing, a history of four or more documented episodes of Group A β-hemolytic streptococcal infections, recurrent otitis, media, peritonsillar abscess, retropharyngeal abscess, or in rare instances a tonsillar tumor. Although tonsillectomy and adenoidectomy (T and A) were done frequently in the past, surgeons and pediatricians are more selective about performing the procedure now. The lymphoid tissue of which tonsils and adenoids are composed is one of the body's lines of defense against infection. Also, a normal shrinking of the lymphoid tissue occurs during middle childhood that resolves many of the problems related to hypertrophy.

If the procedure is necessary it is rarely done before the child's own immune system is functioning at around two years of age. The surgery is never performed during times of acute infection or if the child has a bleeding disorder or cleft palate.

Parents need to be cautioned that the procedure will not guarantee fewer infections, increased appetite, or increased growth. It may lessen snoring during sleep and improve nasal speech.

Preoperative nursing care for a child undergoing a T and A includes routine preparation and use of play discussed in Chapters 28 and 29. In addition, the nurse must know the results and implications of the bleeding and clotting studies done. The child also needs to understand, either through doll play or verbal instructions, that although the throat will be very sore postoperatively, it is necessary to drink plenty of fluids. Children sometimes have a difficult time understanding how the tonsils can be removed when there is no incision. Often their anxiety is relieved when told that the doctor uses a special instrument that can take the tonsils and adenoids out through the mouth. Some children also need reassurance that nothing will happen to their voice and they will be able to talk after surgery.

Postoperatively, these children require close observation for bleeding during the first 24 hours. The child should lie prone with head slightly lower than chest to decrease the likelihood of swallowing blood from any active bleeding sites during initial postoperative phase. Frequent throat and nasal checks with a flashlight are done to note the location of clots and to check for any signs of bleeding, such as bright red blood trickling down the back of the mouth from the nose. Any increase in the frequency of swallowing is investigated because often it is an indicator of active bleeding. Vital signs, including blood pressure, are monitored frequently. An increase in pulse rate or restlessness that might or might not be accompanied by decreased pulse quality or lowering blood pressure also indicates active bleeding. Since sutures seldom are used and needed hemostasis is obtained by pressure, there is a risk for bleeding until the clot is well formed. In many hospitals, routine postoperative care for a child following a T and A includes vital signs and throat checks every hour for the first four hours and then every 2 to 4 hours for the next 24 hours or duration of hospitalization.

Other nursing care measures include ensuring an adequate fluid intake to promote healing of the operation site and to maintain hydration. Ice chips should be offered as soon as the child is fully awake. If tolerated, tepid water is offered and then other clear liquids. Hot or very cold fluids should be avoided, and it is best to withhold full liquids until the next day. Because the child's throat is sore, considerable nursing ingenuity may be required to convince the child that drinking is imporant. Hydration status is monitored by accurate records of intake, output, and urine specific gravity. If a potential for dehydration exists, intravenous therapy might be necessary.

Measures to prevent bleeding need to be observed such as no straws, forks, or sharp-pointed toys available to be placed in the mouth. Aspirin in any form, including the gum, should not be given as it prolongs bleeding time.

Pain control measures are utilized as needed. An ice collar applied postoperatively is an effective pain reliever. Mild analgesics such as acetaminophen or mouth sprays also provide relief. The child usually is more willing to drink fluid following an analgesic.

It is not unusual for the child to vomit once or twice and sometimes even more often as a result of having swallowed blood during surgery. There is little concern as long as the emesis contains old, dark red, or brown colored blood. If an appreciable amount of bright red blood appears it probably is a indicator of the presence of active bleeding. Since vomiting is distressful and the retching painful, antiemetics are given for comfort as well as reduction of emesis. Oral rinses with tepid water may be helpful in ridding the mouth

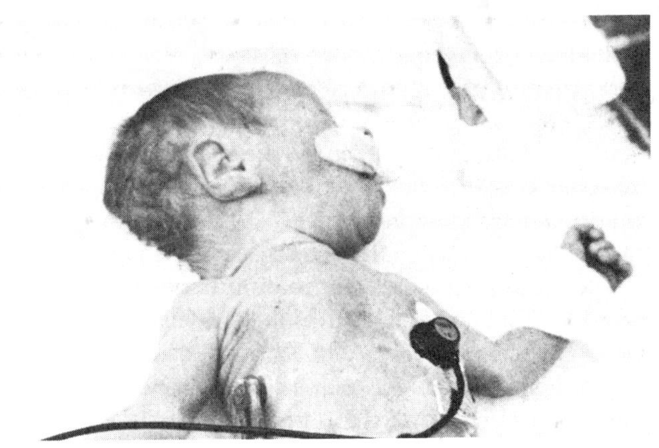

Child with substernal and intercostal retraction.

of the bad taste after vomiting. The child should be cautioned not to gargle but only swish the water around in the mouth.

Most children are discharged the day after or even the evening of surgery. The parents are given discharge instructions, which include

- Quiet activity for the first week
- Soft diet—bread but no toast, eggs but no bacon, mashed potatoes but no french fries—no spicy, rough, or coarse foods in general for the first 7–10 days
- Plenty of fluids—1 to 1½ quarts a day as a minimum; tepid fluids or slow-melting fluids (ice chips, frozen fruit juices) are usually tolerated best
- Do not give child any straws, forks, or sharp-pointed toys because putting them into the mouth may injure the operative site
- Use acetaminophen for pain relief; do not use any form of aspirin
- Halitosis is common for 10–14 days and may be relieved with mouth rinses
- Call physician if any bleeding, fever, or complaint of earache (potential for bleeding 5–7 days postoperatively when operative site membrane begins to slough)
- For 1–2 weeks after surgery, avoid crowds or contact with anyone known to be ill
- May return to school 1–2 weeks postoperatively
- Surgical followup appointment usually 2 weeks after operation

Acute Spasmodic Croup

Acute spasmodic croup, commonly known as croup, is an obstructive narrowing of the larynx thought to be due to viral infection, genetic predisposition, or emotional upsets. Its chief symptom is stridor (see Table 14-10). Acute spasmodic croup is common in young children. Its onset is sudden, usually during the night. Symptoms are relieved by humidity and cool air. The parent is instructed to take the child into a steamy bathroom or out into cooler and more humid night air. If these measures are unsuccessful, the child is seen in the emergency room. Acute spasmodic croup usually occurs in an otherwise healthy child and is resolved quickly (see Fig. 34-2).

Laryngotracheobronchitis

The signs of obstruction caused by laryngotracheobronchitis (LTB) are similar to signs of acute spasmodic croup,

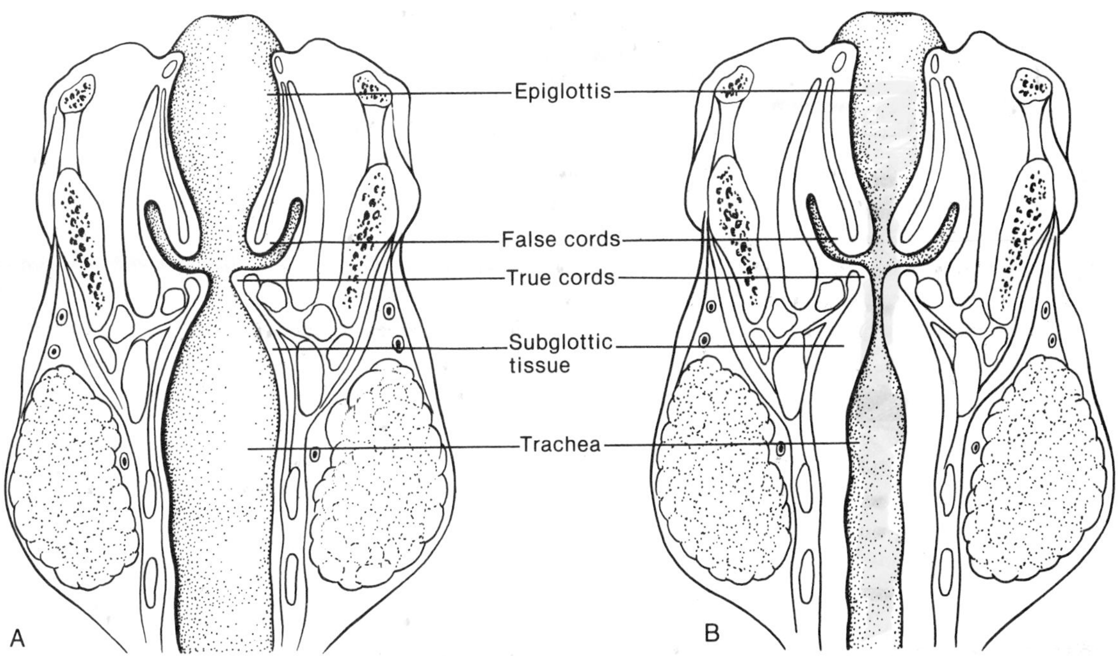

Figure 34-2 *A.* Normal larynx. *B.* Obstruction and narrowing caused by the edema of croup.

but LTB develops more slowly and is less quickly resolved than acute spasmodic croup (Table 34-4). LTB is a viral infection of the larynx, trachea, and bronchi. Inflammatory edema of the mucosa and submucosa of the airway causes narrowing. In severe cases, vocal cord spasm may cause airway obstruction. Because of the infant's small airway size, particularly in the subglottic area, any narrowing is significant, and respiratory distress may result.

Parainfluenza 1, 2, and 3 viruses; respiratory syncytial virus; and rhinoviruses are the most common causes of LTB. Rarely, primary or secondary bacterial infections are the cause. The disease occurs throughout childhood, but incidence peaks at 18 months. The typical age range is 6 months–4 years. Like many other respiratory diseases, LTB is more common in boys than in girls.

The onset of LTB is gradual. Typically, it develops over several days in conjunction with upper respiratory infection and rhinorrhea. Initial symptoms of LTB include a harsh, croupy or barky cough, hoarse voice, inspiratory stridor on exertion, low-grade fever, and continuing cold symptoms. The signs of increasing obstruction that require hospitalization and close observation include stridor and retractions at rest, tachypnea (respiratory rate greater than 60 breaths/min at rest), tachycardia (pulse rate greater than 140 beats/min at rest), restlessness, and circumoral and circumorbital cyanosis. Late signs of obstruction that require immediate intubation are listlessness, decrease in stridor, bradycardia, cyanosis, and retractions without clinical improvement.

Treatment Inhalation therapy with an aerosol preparation of racemic epinephrine is presently the treatment of choice for LTB. Epinephrine may be given with a hand-held nebulizer or in conjunction with IPPB. Racemic epinephrine is not used in outpatient therapy since close observation and repeated treatments are required. Antibiotics are not prescribed unless the child has a secondary bacterial infection, such as otitis media. Treatment with steroids is still controversial (Behrman, Vaughan, McKay, 1984).

Low concentrations of oxygen (less than 30%) may be given to relieve mild hypoxia. Greater concentrations of oxygen may mask signs of obstruction and therefore are avoided. Because adequate hydration is important to decrease the viscosity of secretions, fluid intake may be maintained by intravenous infusion.

If signs of moderate hypoxia develop, intubation is carried out immediately. A tube one size smaller than usual is chosen to decrease the risk of subglottic stenosis. Either oral or nasotracheal intubation is acceptable, but the latter is often more comfortable for the child. Generally, the nasotracheal tube remains in place for 3–5 days. It is removed when the child can breathe and cough around the tube and is afebrile.

Nursing Management Nursing management for a child with LTB includes conservation of energy, humidification with cool mist, monitoring vital signs, intake and output, making frequent observations of color, respiratory effort, and evidence of fatigue, administration of medications and fluids, and measures related to possible intubation for respiratory failure or obstruction. Through all phases of nursing management, explanations and a reassuring manner are needed to reduce the anxiety of parent and child. (Home care of the child with LTB is discussed in Chapter 26).

The nurse plans care so as to disturb the child as little as possible. Anything that disturbs the child causes hyperventilation, which increases airway obstruction and oxygen consumption. Hands-on nursing care and examination is minimal. Direct examination of the epiglottis should only be done by skilled personnel in a facility where immediate intubation can be done, since examination may precipitate spasm and total obstruction. Throat cultures should not be taken by the nurse if the child is acutely ill.

Cool, large-particle mist is the mainstay of treatment for LTB, because cool mist decreases edema in the subglottic area. In the home, hot water vaporizers are not used because of the risk of spilling the water and burning the child. In the hospital, croup rooms or large, clear plastic tents that envelop the whole bed are best because the child need not be restrained.

Close observation by skilled nursing personnel is essential. Knowledge of normal growth and development and responses to illness are keys because the downward course of LTB is often subtle and rapid. The nurse frequently checks pulse rate, respiratory rate, color, activity, and quality of stridor and retractions to detect early signs of hypoxia.

The adequacy of oral fluid intake is assessed through urine specific gravity, which should be maintained between 1.008–1.015. Both overhydration and dehydration should be avoided. Intravenous fluids are given only if adequate oral intake is not possible.

Epiglottitis

Epiglottitis is a bacterial infection of the epiglottis and arytenoepiglottic folds that obstructs the airway. It is less common than LTB, but its course is rapid. Without prompt diagnosis and treatment, mortality from epiglottitis is high (Molteni, 1976). The causative microorganism is *Hemophilus influenzae* type B or, rarely, a beta-hemolytic streptococcus. The incidence of epiglottitis has little seasonal variation. The patient's usual age range is 3–7 years and peaks at 3.1 years.

The clinical picture is typified by sudden onset of fever (generally above 38.5 C) and lethargy. The parent often reports that the child has had a minor upper respiratory infection for a day or so. During the next 2–4 hours, difficulty in breathing increases. The child's voice has a muffled quality, but rarely is there a cough. Drooling and refusing to eat or drink because of an intensely sore throat are classic signs of epiglottitis.

TABLE 34-4 Characteristics of Acute Infections Resulting in Croup Syndromes

Acute spasmodic croup	Laryngotracheobronchitis (LTB)	Acute epiglottitis
Age of child		
1–3 years	6 months–4 years	3–7 years
History of present illness		
Sudden symptoms in otherwise healthy child, usually at night	Preceded by acute upper respiratory tract infection; respiratory distress frequent at night	Preceded by mild upper respiratory tract infection
History of repeated episodes		Severe, sudden onset of respiratory distress
Clinical manifestations		
Laryngospasm	Edema and inflammation of vocal cords and tissue below vocal cords, including bronchi	Edema and inflammation of epiglottis and surrounding area above vocal cords, large red epiglottis
Mucosal edema in subglottic area		
	Laryngospasm	
Anxiety, restlessness	Anxiety, fatigue, apprehension, restlessness	Anxiety, restlessness, fear
Dyspnea	Dyspnea	Dyspnea
Inspiratory stridor	Inspiratory stridor, prolonged inspiratory phase	Deliberate inspiratory stridor, mouth breathing with hyperextended neck
Hoarseness	Hoarseness	Sore throat
Barky, metallic cough	Barky cough	Muffled voice, dysphagia (difficulty swallowing), drooling of saliva
No fever	Fever, usually low-grade	Fever greater than 38.5 C
Mild or moderate supraclavicular, suprasternal, substernal retractions	Moderate to severe supraclavicular, suprasternal, substernal retractions	Mild to moderate suprasternal and substernal
		Retractions, use of accessory muscles of respiration
Respiratory rate 45–55	Respiratory rate 45–60	Respiratory rate 45–50
Pulse 140–160	Pulse 140–160	Pulse less than 160
No adventitious breath sounds	Rhonchi, coarse rales	Usually wheezy breath sounds
	Nasal congestion	Paleness, sallowness, or cyanosis
Occasional mild cyanosis	Paleness or cyanosis	Rapid, progressive worsening of distress
Etiology		
Unknown, but thought to be viral, emotional, or familial predisposition	Usually viral, but occasionally bacterial	Bacterial, usually *Hemophilus influenzae*

The signs of increasing obstruction are restlessness, tachycardia, thready pulse, and orthopnea manifested as the desire to sit up and breathe through the mouth. The characteristic breath sounds are wheezy inspiratory stridor and a snoring expiratory sound, depending on the degree of obstruction. Some children have a "crouplike" appearance on initial assessment. Late signs of hypoxia due to obstruction are listlessness, cyanosis, bradycardia, bradypnea, and decreased inspiratory and expiratory sounds.

The history of the illness and the clinical appearance of the child enable the physician to make a tentative diagnosis. To confirm the diagnosis, a visual examination of the epiglottis can be done. This is dangerous, however, because it can precipitate obstruction. Visual examination must be done in a controlled situation where intubation, oxygen, and suction equipment is available. If visual inspection is deemed inadvisable and the diagnosis is in doubt, the physician may order neck radiographs. Lateral neck views are preferred to visual inspection of the epiglottis by many physicians. The physician or nurse must remain with the child and parent during the radiographic examination, since the procedure is disturbing to the child and may cause total obstruction.

Treatment for acute obstructive epiglottitis is relief of obstruction with a nasotracheal tube and intravenous administration of antibiotics. Prior to intubation, the nurse helps the child to sit up and position the head comfortably. This position is often referred to as the "sniff" position.

Oxygen may be given through a face mask a few minutes prior to intubation as a safety measure. The nasotracheal tube can often be removed after 24 hours. In general, the more rapid the onset of the disease, the more rapid its remission.

Appropriate antibiotics are started as soon as intubation is done and an intravenous line is in place. Large doses of ampicillin or, if resistance is a problem, of chloramphenicol, are effective. Steroids may also be efficacious.

Bronchiolitis

Bronchiolitis is a widespread inflammation and obstruction of the bronchioles that is sometimes difficult to distinguish from acute asthma of infancy and bronchopneumonia (see Table 34-5). Bronchiolitis usually occurs in infants between 1–6 months of age and occasionally is seen in children up to 2 years of age. Boys are about 60% more susceptible than girls. Occurrence increases during the winter (Sminkins, 1981).

The prognosis of bronchiolitis is generally good, although several studies have shown that 50% of infected infants develop subsequent episodes of wheezing associated with allergies. Some researchers think that infants with a strong family history of allergy are susceptible to bronchiolitis in infancy or that bronchiolitis may trigger the development of asthma (Behrman, Vaughan, and McKay, 1984).

Respiratory syncytial virus is the most common cause of bronchiolitis, but it is also caused by parainfluenza virus and rhinovirus. Bronchiolitis is characterized by inflammation of the small airways or bronchioles. The ciliated epithelial cells lining the bronchioles become necrosed because of viral colonization. Edema and increased mucus production contribute further to nonuniform obstruction of the bronchiolar lumina. Plugs of mucus and cell debris cause atelectasis and collapse of alveoli. Partly obstructed bronchioles trap air distal to the plug, causing hyperinflation. The alveoli are poorly ventilated but well perfused, a situation that results in hypoxemia or shunting.

The parent usually reports that the infant had an upper respiratory infection for several days, causing eating difficulties, a barky harsh cough, low-grade fever, and wheezing with activity. Physical examination of the moderately or acutely ill infant reveals barrel chest due to hyperinflation, and radiographs show evidence of air trapping. The infant demonstrates the signs of increased work of breathing, rapid shallow respirations, tachycardia, nasal flaring, and mild to severe intercostal and subcostal retractions at rest. Crying, eating, and activity exaggerate these signs. Wheezing and rales may or may not be present, depending on the degree of obstruction. As obstruction increases and airflow decreases, wheezing diminishes. Usually, respiratory distress becomes more severe during the first 24–72 hours of hospitalization. Cyanosis, pallor, listlessness, and sudden diminution or absence of breath sounds indicate impending respiratory failure.

Treatment Medical treatment consists of oxygen therapy, fluid and electrolyte replacement, and antibiotic therapy if a secondary bacterial infection is identified. Bronchodilators are only rarely beneficial. Infants who have not responded to epinephrine may respond to aminophylline. Sedatives are avoided because they are respiratory depressants. In 1% of infants with bronchiolitis, respiratory failure develops. Intubation and ventilatory assistance may be required for several days.

Nursing Management Nursing management consists of measures relative to oxygen therapy, hydration, and chest physiotherapy. Humidified oxygen is given through a hood, face mask, tent, or nasal catheter. Supplemental oxygen concentrations are based on arterial blood gas values. Any infant receiving oxygen concentrations greater than 40% requires arterial blood gas or transcutaneous oxygen monitoring. Mist is not beneficial, and may make some infants worse.

Nursing care includes frequent observations of respiratory status, particularly observations for respiratory failure during early hospitalization. Respiratory isolation is maintained throughout hospitalization, since the mode of transmission of respiratory syncytial virus is by droplet.

Dehydration due to increased insensible losses and feeding difficulties is assessed early in the child's care. Oral feedings and unnecessary handling tire the acutely ill infant and increase the risk of aspiration. Intravenous therapy to replace fluids and electrolytes is initiated early if there is any feeding difficulty. Initially, the nurse checks the infant's hydration status, including urine specific gravity every time the infant voids. As the infant recovers, specific gravity is checked every 8 hours. The urine specific gravity is maintained between 1.008 and 1.015, since fluid overload may increase the work of the cardiovascular system and cause pulmonary edema.

Elevation of the head of the bed decreases compression of the diaphragm and aids in ventilation. An infant seat is used if the infant can maintain the head in the midline. Any extreme flexion or hyperextension of the neck must be avoided because the infant's poorly supported large airways become compressed very easily, increasing the work of breathing.

The infant with moist-sounding rales and minimal hypoxia might benefit from percussion with postural drainage. The moderately to acutely ill infant often cannot tolerate this procedure, and extra handling is kept to a minimum to prevent tiring. Postural drainage is postponed until toleration is improved and moist rales are present.

TABLE 34-5 Characteristics of Bronchiolitis and Pneumonia

Bronchiolitis	Pneumonia
Age of child	
2 years or less	Any age, higher incidence during first 5 years of life
Etiology	
Viral infection, usually respiratory syncytial virus	Viral, bacterial (for example, *Klebsiella, H. influenzae,* staphylococcal, streptococcal, pneumococcal, or *Mycoplasma pneumoniae* infections)
	Aspiration of food, fluid, medication, poisonous substances (for example, hydrocarbons), powders
	Hypostatic (related to immobility, or postoperative accumulation of secretions)
History of present illness	
Accompanies or follows upper respiratory tract infection	Follows upper respiratory tract infection
Gradual onset over 1–3 days	Acute or gradual onset
Clinical manifestations	
Fatigue, anxiety, irritability	Fatigue, irritability, anxiety, lethargy
Dyspnea, shallow respirations	Dyspnea, shallow respirations
Paroxysmal, dry, harsh cough	Productive or congested harsh cough
Clinical manfestations (cont.)	
Mild to moderate intercostal, subcostal retractions	Mild to moderate intercostal retractions
Fever (low grade) or hypothermia	Fever
Respiratory rate 60–80	Tachypnea
Cardiac rate 180–200	Tachycardia
Rales, expiratory wheeze, expiratory grunt	Rales, rhonchi, wheeze, expiratory grunt, pleural friction rub (sometimes heard)
Prolonged expiratory phase	Respiratory lag on affected side
Increased anterior–posterior dimensions of the chest (barrel chest)	
Nasal flaring	Moderate respiratory distress with pneumococcal pneumonia
Cyanosis	Circumoral cyanosis with pneumococcal pneumonia
Obstruction present from trapped air	Pain with respirations
Barely audible breath sounds if very severe	Decreased breath sounds
Diminished appetite	Diminished appetite, vomiting (in young children)
	Great variation in signs and symptoms among patients

Bronchitis

In childhood, bronchitis often occurs in conjunction with other respiratory diseases. It is a transient inflammation involving the trachea and large bronchi. The primary symptom is a productive or dry cough. Rhinovirus is the most frequent cause of acute bronchitis, though parainfluenza adenovirus and respiratory syncytial virus have also been isolated.

The onset is usually gradual, with such cold symptoms as a runny nose and a productive cough developing over 3–4 days. Rales and wheezing are frequently present. Symptoms usually subside in 7–10 days. Chest radiographs are usually normal. If symptoms persist, secondary infection should be suspected.

Treatment consists of adequate fluid intake and rest. Antibiotics are not necessary unless a secondary bacterial infection develops. Sedation and cough suppressants are contraindicated for bronchitis, as they are for most respiratory diseases in children.

Pneumonia

Pneumonia, a relatively common condition of childhood, is caused by a variety of infectious agents, such as bacteria, viruses, mycotics, and others (for example, mycoplasmas, chlamydiae). Pneumonia is defined as an inflammation of the parychema of the lung. Most childhood pneumonia is described as bronchopneumonia; that is, a combination of disseminated lobular pneumonia (patchy areas of infiltrates in both lung fields and surrounding the bronchi) and interstitial pneumonia (diffuse bronchiolitis with exudate evident in alveolar walls but not alveolar spaces). Bacterial pneumonias more often cause lobular involvement and sometimes even lobular consolidation whereas viral pneumonias cause inflammation of interstitial tissue.

Clinical manifestations of pneumonias are diverse (see

Table 34-5). Young infants, and children with chronic respiratory conditions are more likely to be severely affected. Because of wide variations in infectious agents, treatment depends on the causative organism. Differentiation among causes, however, is often difficult because of the lack of correlation between nose and throat cultures and pathogens in the lungs. When it is important to identify the pathogen, counterimmunoelectrophoresis is used to detect specific bacterial antigens. Most often, however, therapy is based on the clinical picture, symptoms, and history.

Pneumonococcal pneumonia, the prototype of bacterial pneumonias, appears among all age groups but more frequently in children under 4 years of age. Occasionally, it occurs as a primary infection, but more often it follows as a complication of some other infectious disease. Chest radiographs may demonstrate a pleural effusion or consolidation of a lobe or segment.

Streptococcal pneumonia usually follows either an upper respiratory infection or a communicable disease such as measles or epidemic influenza. *Hemophilus influenzae* occasionally causes pneumonia, usually following illnesses such as acute bronchitis, laryngotracheobronchitis, or bacteremia. Chest radiographs may show pleural effusion. Group B beta-hemolytic streptococcus is a cause of infant mortality and morbidity, especially during the neonatal period. Group A beta-hemolytic streptococcus is the more prevalent strain infecting children between 3 and 5 years of age (Pinney, 1981).

Staphylococcal pneumonia occurs most often among infants during the first year of life and usually is severe (Shinefield, 1966). Chest radiographs may demonstrate the presence of pneumatoceles. Evidence of empyema may be found as well. It follows a mild upper respiratory infection and may progress rapidly from bronchopneumonia to consolidation of an entire lobe and increased respiratory distress. Pyopneumothorax or pneumatocele are also possible complications.

Treatment Treatment of pneumonia is related to causative organism and presenting symptoms. If a bacterial agent is suspected, either intravenous or oral antibiotic therapy is instituted. Oxygen is ordered as needed to maintain normal arterial blood gas levels. Fluids are provided to meet daily requirements and to compensate for the additional fluid lost through rapid, shallow, difficult breathing. In addition, vigorous pulmonary hygiene measures are ordered. Progress is monitored by chest radiographs and the patient's response to therapy. Rarely, an infant requires intubation or chest tube insertion to treat pneumothorax.

Nursing Management Nursing management includes close observation of the child's respiratory status, color, required effort, and cardiovascular status. Vital signs including auscultation of breath sounds are monitored frequently (every 1–2 hours initially). Hydration status is assessed, and the child is encouraged to drink fluids. If fluid intake is inadequate, intravenous infusion will be necessary, as fluids prevent secretions from becoming too viscous. An environment that provides ultrasonic mist therapy either by means of a mist tent or a face mask also helps to loosen secretions. This increased humidity is combined with frequent position changes and chest physiotherapy to loosen and remove secretions further.

Percussion, vibration, and postural drainage are done every 4–6 hours, with particular attention to areas of consolidation as noted on chest radiographs. Oxygen therapy is used as indicated. When oxygen is used, the nurse monitors the concentration of the oxygen in the tent or hood as well as the child's arterial blood gases.

Oropharyngeal suctioning sometimes is needed when the infant or young child is unable to remove secretions effectively. Suctioning should be done carefully and with discrimination; too-frequent suctioning irritates the mucosa and causes increased mucus production.

Fever control measures are instituted whenever the child's temperature is elevated. Good skin care and frequent linen changes are needed to keep the child dry in the high-humidity environment. Changing the child's position every 2 hours, while maintaining a semi-Fowler's position, facilitates respiration and pulmonary drainage.

Whenever possible, the parent should be involved in the child's care. It is not unusual to observe a parent sitting inside a mist tent reading stories or playing games with the child.

Mycoplasmal Pneumonia

Mycoplasmal pneumonia is a disease of middle and late childhood. Occurrence peaks at 10–15 years of age. Onset is gradual, often with nonspecific symptoms, such as headache, malaise, low-grade fever, and cough. Auscultation of the chest reveals rales. Dullness on percussion and sputum production are also common signs. Radiographic findings often reveal interstitial involvement or bronchopneumonic inflammation, particularly of the lower lobes. Diagnosis is confirmed by throat culture.

Treatment includes a 7- to 10-day course of erythromycin and such comfort measures as bed rest, acetaminophen, and fluids. The prognosis is generally excellent. Although mycoplasmal pneumonia is not highly communicable, careful handwashing and other good hygiene measures are important to protect other family members. Even so, susceptible persons might become infected over a period of weeks. (Home care for the child with pneumonia is described in Chapter 26.)

The Child With Tuberculosis

Tuberculosis in children has decreased dramatically in many

countries but remains a significant problem in the world today. The causative agent is *Mycobacterium tuberculosis*, an acid-fast, red rod. Tubercle bacilli may survive and remain virulent for many months if kept in the dark, but die if they are exposed to ultraviolet rays (for example, direct sunlight) or are boiled for 1 minute.

The most common mode of transmission of tubercle bacilli is by droplet. Consequently, the most common site of primary lesions is the lung. The body's response to primary pulmonary tuberculosis is healing, but lesions may spread to and involve surrounding tissue and an expanding, residual cavity results. In acute miliary tuberculosis, tubercle bacilli are disseminated to various organs of the body through the bloodstream or by way of regional lymph nodes and the thoracic duct. Complications of primary tuberculosis usually occur within the first year of infection.

In its early stages, tuberculosis usually causes few if any symptoms. Consequently, any child who has a history of contact is tested 2–10 days after the contact. If a tuberculin skin test is positive, chest radiographs are taken. Tuberculosis is confirmed by cultures of gastric contents obtained by repeated gastric lavage. Acid-fast tubercle bacilli are found in gastric washings from a child with tuberculosis because the child swallows some sputum rather than expectorating it.

Medical treatment and nursing management involve early detection, vigorous chemotherapy, isolation of the patient, and serial radiographs to monitor the course of infection. Attention is also given to nutrition, vitamin supplements, rest, and protection from other infections, particularly measles. Tuberculosis of the lungs is treated with isoniazid, streptomycin, para-aminosalicylic acid (PAS), ethambutol, or rifampin. For older children, the usual regimen consists of 1 year of isoniazid and rifampin therapy. A third drug is added if immediate response to treatment is inadequate. Home care for the child with tuberculosis is discussed in Chapter 26.

Prevention of tuberculosis is the goal of most public health officials. Basic principles of prevention include isolation of adults with infectious tuberculosis and the administration of isoniazid for 1 year to household contacts of tuberculosis patients. Bacille Calmette-Guérin (BCG) vaccination increases resistance in children living with an adult who has infectious tuberculosis. BCG vaccine is also recommended for children who live where the incidence of tuberculosis is high.

The Child With an Acute Noninfectious Respiratory Problem

Foreign Body Aspiration

Aspiration of foreign material is most common in children from 6 months–6 years of age and results in more than 2,000 deaths per year. Aspiration may not be witnessed, so awareness of its potential in the identified age group and knowledge of the common symptoms are crucial to diagnosis. Symptoms depend on the material aspirated and where in the respiratory tract the object lodges. A large object is likely to lodge in the trachea, resulting in complete obstruction. A smaller object could lodge in a mainstem bronchus, causing obstruction to one lung. A very small object could merely obstruct one segment of a lung.

A foreign body aspirated into a mainstem bronchus or smaller airway causes immediate severe coughing, which usually subsides in minutes. Therefore, if aspiration is not observed or reported, it can be missed for hours, days, or even months. Eventually, such secondary symptoms as wheezing or chronic coughing occur. These symptoms might accompany infection, which is likely to develop if the foreign body has been lodged in an airway for a significant period. Other complications include atelectasis, bronchiectasis, and, rarely, erosion of the airway.

It is not difficult to recognize the signs of complete obstruction caused by aspiration of a large object. Emergency measures must be performed immediately, since complete obstruction can cause death within minutes. (These measures are described in Chapter 19.) If obstruction is not complete, and if aspiration was not witnessed, the diagnosis is based on a well-taken history, physical examination of the chest for signs of uneven excursion or inspiration, and an inspiration–expiration radiograph. Even if assessment provides no evidence of foreign body aspiration, it should not be ruled out if the child is in the typical age range and has the classic symptoms.

Treatment If an object is thought to be lodged beyond the trachea, bronchoscopy is performed to locate and remove it. Bronchoscopy is done by a physician with special training. This may mean transferring the child and delaying removal of the object. Since a foreign body lodged beyond the carina is not life threatening, delay in removal of the object is reasonable and probably wise. After removal of the foreign body, treatment consists of inhalation therapy with an aerosol bronchodilator and chest physiotherapy.

In some circumstances it is reasonable to attempt postural drainage and percussion to dislodge a foreign body. If aspiration is suspected but the history and initial examination are negative, then a limited trial of percussion and postural drainage at home or in the hospital is warranted to attempt dislodging the object before performing a bronchoscopy.

Nursing Management Nursing care following the removal of a foreign body from the airway involves keeping the child NPO until the gag reflex returns and then providing sips of water while observing the child's ability to swallow. Once satisfied that the child can manage fluids, the nurse gradually advances the diet. Nursing care also includes administering an inhaled bronchodilator and performing percussion and postural drainage every few hours for the first 12 hours or so. The child who is doing well after 24 hours is usually discharged. The nurse instructs the parent to carry out postural drainage procedures 2–3 times daily for a specified number of days. The nurse also instructs the parent about measures that can be taken to prevent foreign body aspiration in the future (see Chapter 19).

Near-Drowning

Hypoxemia is the major concern in near-drowning. The degree and duration of hypoxemia depends on the length of time the child has been submerged, whether the child has aspirated water, and water temperature. The child who is submerged in cold water can survive longer because cold reduces the metabolic rate, which in turn decreases oxygen demand. Water is generally swallowed, but aspiration may be prevented (until death occurs) by reflex laryngospasm. Blood volume is altered in both fresh- and salt-water drowning, but by different mechanisms. This is not what kills. Death occurs from severe hypoxemia and acidosis. Therefore, the primary goal at the site of near-drowning is to oxygenate the victim. The quickest and most effective way to oxygenate the child is by CPR (see Chapter 19), which must be started immediately and continued until the child revives or a physician determines that death has occurred. The stomach is evacuated as soon as it is possible and safe to do so. This prevents vomiting and aspiration. Complications of near-drowning include hypoxic brain damage, pulmonary edema, aspiration of gastric contents, and infection.

Care of the child who is recovering from near-drowning includes monitoring arterial blood gases to determine the need for artificial ventilation in addition to supplemental oxygen, and monitoring and correcting blood pH and electrolytes. Bronchospasm, which can occur due to the irritation of aspiration, is treated with bronchodilators. The nurse also observes for signs of infection. Appropriate antibiotics are prescribed once the infection is identified. The child is hospitalized and observed for a minimum of 28 hours after the event so that treatment can be given if untoward reactions occur. Prior to discharge, methods of preventing such an accident are discussed with the whole family (see Chapter 19).

The Child With a Chronic or Noninfectious Respiratory Disorder

Asthma

Asthma is a reversible obstructive respiratory disease that occurs in about 26 of 1,000 children. Although seldom fatal, asthma is the most common chronic respiratory illness in children and causes more school absences than any other chronic disorder (Shiffer and Hunt, 1963).

In the child with asthma, attacks may be precipitated by physical or emotional factors. During an asthma attack, bronchospasm causes air trapping in the bronchioles. Bronchial narrowing increases as the mucosa lining the bronchial lumina becomes edematous and produces increasing amounts of thick mucus (see Figure 34-3). The child has difficulty breathing, particularly on expiration.

Researchers theorize that asthma is caused by abnormal neuromuscular function, altered immunologic function (see Chapter 37), or viral insult coupled with genetic predisposition (Sexton, 1981). This discussion will focus on asthma caused by altered immunologic function, that is, extrinsic or allergic asthma. Allergic asthma is most commonly triggered by inhaled irritants. Rarely, it is triggered by a food allergy.

Initial symptoms of an impending attack may be a feeling of tightness in the chest, and an expiratory wheeze. As bronchial smooth muscles contract, airway wall edema and mucus production progress, and as wheezing and chest tightness continue, they may be accompanied by fatigue, tachypnea, coughing, dyspnea, retractions, cyanosis, and diaphoresis (excessive sweating). If the child is not treated promptly, status asthmaticus may result. *Status asthmaticus* is asthma that does not respond to the usual treatment within a certain period, usually several hours. It is an indication for hospital admission and treatment because prolonged attacks can lead to increased respiratory distress and possible respiratory failure. Other complications of asthma include pneumonia and cor pulmonale.

Diagnostic tests for asthma include radiographs, immunologic assays, the alpha$_1$-antitrypsin test, a complete blood count (including an eosinophil count), a sweat chloride test, and pulmonary function tests. The child's response to an aerosol bronchodilator may be assessed through pulmonary function testing. If the bronchodilator improves pulmonary function, asthma is the likely diagnosis. Following diagnosis, skin sensitivity tests may be performed to identify the causative allergen.

Treatment Treatment depends on whether the asthma is mild, moderate, or severe. In mild asthma, attacks are episodic (no more than once a week) and of short duration if treated with bronchodilators. Between attacks, the child carries on a normal life free from medication. If the attack begins at home, the child is placed in a humidified environment. The parent encourages the child to drink fluids, promotes rest, and helps the child to use relaxation techniques. If the child has prescribed medications, they are taken (see Table 34-6). Usually, these methods reverse the attack.

In moderate asthma, attacks occur more frequently than once a week. Between episodes, the child may have a chronic

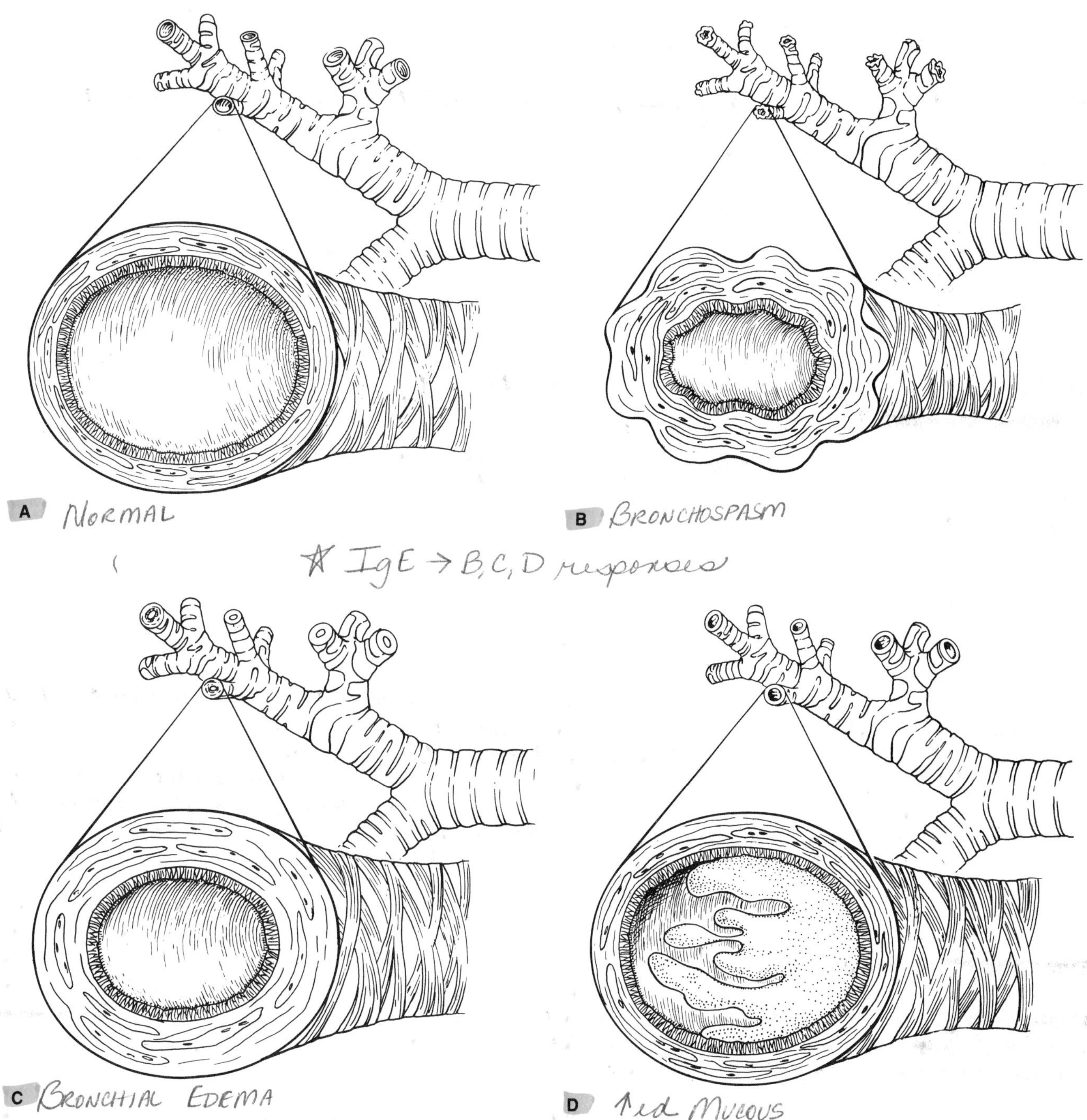

Figure 34-3 Bronchia changes that decrease lumen size occur during an asthma attack. *A.* Cross-section of a normal bronchial tube. *B.* Bronchospasm. Smooth muscle surrounding the bronchus contracts. *C.* Bronchial edema. *D.* Increased mucus production.

cough or wheeze, especially at night. The child may miss school or other activities due to illness and require constant bronchodilator therapy. Children with severe asthma demonstrate continuous wheezing punctuated by more severe attacks. Attacks frequently need to be treated in the hospital. The child usually requires steroid therapy in addition to routine medications. Respiratory difficulties and airway obstruction are more difficult to reverse with conventional treatment.

Whether the child has mild, moderate, or severe asthma, if the usual measures fail to alleviate an attack, the child is treated in the emergency room. Initially, the child is given epinephrine injections at 20-minute intervals for an hour (Table 34-7). An intravenous line is started if epinephrine

TABLE 34-6 Drugs Used to Control Asthma

Generic name (brand name)	Action	Side effects
Theophyllines	Relax bronchial smooth muscles, opening the airways	Stomachache, nausea and vomiting, loss of appetite, abdominal cramps, headache, dizziness, nervousness, tachycardia, pounding in chest, trouble sleeping
Theophylline (Theo-Dur, Slo-Phyllin, Somophyllin, Theolair, Aminophylline, Quibron, Theospan, Choledyl)		
Adrenergics	Relax bronchial smooth muscles	Tachycardia, pounding in chest, nervousness, tremors, nausea and vomiting, drowsiness, bad taste in mouth
Metaproterenol (Metaprel, Alupent)		
Isoetharine (Bronkosol, Bronkometer)		
Albuterol (Proventil, Ventolin)		
Terbutaline (Brethine, Bricanyl)		
Antihistimines	Prevent release of histamine, lessening response of the lungs to allergenic triggers of asthma. Blocks exercise-induced asthma	Coughing, wheezing
Cromolyn sodium (Intal, Aarane)		
Glucocorticoids	Reduce edema, inflammation, and mucus production in bronchial tubes	Thrush, hoarseness, dry mouth, weight gain, interference with growth, increased appetite, chemical and electrolyte imbalances, cushingoid signs, acne, delayed sexual development, hirsutism, gum infections, dental caries, adrenal gland suppression, cataracts
Beclomethasone (Beclovent, Vanceril)		
Prednisone (Deltasone, Prednisone)		
Prednisolone (Delta-Cortef, Prednisolone)		
Methylprednisolone (Medrol)		

fails to resolve the attack. The physician administers an initial dose of theophylline, which is followed by a constant infusion. If the child has severe respiratory distress, theophylline administration may be augmented by the administration of a steroid. Oxygen is administered if indicated. If the physician fears respiratory failure is imminent, intubation and mechanical ventilation may be necessary until drugs alleviate symptoms. This child is admitted to the hospital, often to the intensive care unit.

Nursing Management During the acute phase of an asthma attack, the nurse assists with oxygen administration, subcutaneous or intravenous injections of bronchodilators or corticosteroids, aerosal therapy, and postural drainage to provide immediate relief of the child's symptoms. Oxygen may be given by nasal cannula or mask, depending on the child's preference. The nurse should be prepared to assist with intubation if the child is in severe respiratory distress. Rapid-acting bronchodilators are commonly given (see Table 34-7), and the nurse observes the child for adverse effects. A child receiving intravenous theophylline is observed carefully for signs of toxicity. The intravenous rate must be accurate. With children, a mechanical drip regulator should be used to ensure accuracy. Signs of toxicity are reported to the physician immediately.

The nurse notes and reports any signs of increasing respiratory distress, including alterations in blood gases or changes of consciousness. Vital signs are monitored frequently.

The nurse assesses the child's hydration status and encourages the child who is alert and can cooperate to drink clear fluids. Milk is avoided, since it can thicken secretions. Comfort measures include positioning the child for optimum ventilation and maintaining a comfortable room temperature. All nursing interventions are carried out in a calm, reassuring manner to promote rest and allay the child's anxiety.

When the child is in the recovery phase, the medication schedule is changed from intravenous to oral. The nurse assesses the continued effectiveness of medications by observing improvements in respiratory status and noting episodes of wheezing and the resolution of signs of respiratory distress. If the physician orders chest physiotherapy, the nurse either remains with the child or performs the procedure.

Before the child is discharged from the hospital, the nurse discusses prevention and early intervention measures with the child and parent. Once precipitating factors are identified, the child can learn to avoid them. Allergens can be identified by subcutaneous or intradermal skin tests. If the history of the attack shows that it may have been triggered by emotional upset or exercise, the child and family should learn how to minimize recurrence. The nurse teaches the child and family to watch for the early warning signs of asthma attack and to intervene immediately to minimize the severity of the attack. At the first sign of an impending attack, the child should slow down, rest, relax, and do abdominal breathing. Sometimes this can prevent an attack.

TABLE 34-7 Rapid-Acting Bronchodilators Used in Acute Asthma Attacks

Bronchodilator	Route of administration	Side effects
Epinephrine (Adrenalin)	Subcutaneous injection; dose may be repeated every 20 minutes, up to 3 times	Palpitations, tachycardia, increased blood pressure, tremors, nausea and vomiting, headache, pallor
Epinephrine (Sus-Phrine) Contains both rapid-acting and slow-release epinephrine preparations. Immediate action and sustained release up to 8 hours	Subcutaneous injection	Same as for adrenalin
Isoetharine (Bronkosol, Bronkometer) Effective up to 3–4 hours	Inhaled via nebulizer, Medihaler, or IPPB	Tachycardia, palpitations, nervousness, nausea and vomiting, loss of appetite, stomachache, trouble sleeping, headache, dizziness
Metaproterenol (Metaprel, Alupent) Effective up to 3–4 hours	Inhaled via nebulizer, Medihaler, or IPPB	Same as for isoetharine
Albuterol (Proventil, Ventolin) Effective up to 4–6 hours	Inhaled via nebulizer, Medihaler, or IPPB	Same as for isoetharine
Terbutaline (Brethine) Effective up to 3–7 hours	Inhaled via nebulizer or IPPB; subcutaneous injection	Same as for isoetharine
Theophylline (Aminophylline) Wide variation in duration of effect	Intravenous infusion, intramuscular injection, or rectal suppository	Same as for isoetharine

Even if it does not, it provides the child with some energy reserves (see Chapter 37).

Patient teaching also includes instructions related to medications the child will be taking at home to prevent attacks. The nurse discusses compliance and teaches methods of administration. In addition, expected side effects and signs of toxicity are explained to the family.

Cystic Fibrosis

Cystic fibrosis is a syndrome characterized by widespread dysfunction of the exocrine glands. It occurs in from 1 of 1,600 to 1 of 2,500 live Caucasian births (Cystic Fibrosis Foundation, 1978). The incidence of cystic fibrosis in other racial groups is considerably less. The disease is transmitted to the child as an autosomal recessive trait, and the carrier rate is estimated as 1 in 20 white Americans (O'Neill, 1981). Carriers have no symptoms and cannot be identified by any reliable test. If both parents are carriers, there is a 25% chance with each pregnancy that the infant will have cystic fibrosis, a 50% chance that the infant will be a carrier, and a 25% chance that the infant will be neither victim nor carrier. Cystic fibrosis cannot be diagnosed by amniocentesis.

The severity of symptoms varies greatly. Some children have minimal involvement, although others have extensive involvement resulting in limited growth and development and death before adolescence. Median age at death is 18–20 years, though some patients die in infancy.

All exocrine glands are affected to some extent, but 95% of deaths from cystic fibrosis are due to abnormal mucus secretion and fibrosis in the lungs. Mucus secreted by the mucous glands of children with cystic fibrosis is abnormally viscous, sticky, and tenacious. It adheres to the walls of the glandular ducts and eventually obstructs them entirely. Obstruction causes fibrosis of the glands themselves. This

Early Warning Signs of Asthma Attack

"Funny feeling" in the chest
Headache
Dry mouth
Itchy chin
Itchy throat
Changes in breathing pattern
Moodiness
Fatigue
Paleness
Glassy eyes
Sadness
Nervousness
Runny nose
Dark circles under the eyes

process occurs in many parts of the body. Most affected are the respiratory and gastrointestinal tracts. In the gastrointestinal tract, the pancreas, small intestine, and biliary system are especially affected (see Chapter 38). The reproductive system becomes involved at puberty. Integumentary involvement causes the sweat glands to produce sweat containing four times the normal concentration of sodium chloride. This fact makes pilocarpine iontophoresis (the sweat chloride test) important in confirming the diagnosis.

The child is born with healthy lungs. Early symptoms in infancy are failure to thrive; frequent, foul-smelling stools; and voracious appetite. More rarely, the child presents with meconium ileus (see Chapter 38), hypoproteinemia, and pulmonary symptoms. Usually, pulmonary evidence of cystic fibrosis appears gradually as the bronchi become hypertrophied in response to abnormal mucus production. As mucus clogs the bronchi and bronchioles, the child becomes increasingly susceptible to such respiratory infections as bronchitis, bronchiolitis, and bronchiectasis, which often become chronic. Susceptibility to infection is thought to be related to altered immunity at the alveolar level (O'Neill, 1981). *Pseudomonas* and *Aspergillus* are the most common causes of infection. Except in the lungs, the child's general immunity and ability to produce antibodies are within normal ranges.

Cough, which may be dry and hacky or loose and productive, is often the first sign of pulmonary involvement. This usually occurs during infancy and is intermittent at first. The cough becomes progressively worse, especially during periods of illness, when dyspnea makes excessive secretions more difficult to manage. Over time, the child develops clubbing of the fingers, and a barrel chest results from hyperinflation of the lungs. Pulmonary complications include cor pulmonale, portal hypertension, hemoptysis, pneumothorax, and polyps. Increased flatus, thin stature, cough, and delayed puberty may present psychosocial problems for the child.

Treatment The goals of medical treatment are to maintain airway patency and control lung infection. Airway patency is maintained by chest physiotherapy (percussion and postural drainage), inhalation therapy with aerosol bronchodilators, breathing exercises, and an appropriate exercise program. Mucolytics are rarely used. Infection is treated with appropriate antibiotics, particularly the aminoglycosides (amikacin, gentamicin, and tobramycin) and the semisynthetic antipseudomonal penicillins (carbenicillin, ticarcillin, azlocillin, and piperacillin). Increased salt intake is prescribed during prolonged hot weather or febrile periods, because children with cystic fibrosis are prone to electrolyte imbalances that, if not corrected, can lead to heat prostration and circulatory collapse.

Nursing Management Nursing management for the child with pulmonary effects of cystic fibrosis includes maintaining airway patency by administering aerosol bronchodilators and performing or supervising chest physiotherapy. Chest physiotherapy, breathing exercises, and inhalation therapy (with aerosols) are done 2–3 times daily and more frequently during acute illness. If these treatments are carried out at home, the nurse instructs the child and family about correct procedures. The nurse also instructs and encourages the child in appropriate breathing exercises and advises the child and family about the positive results of participation in physical activity and certain sports. The child with cystic fibrosis can benefit from activities such as swimming, which requires breathing control and enhances correct posture. Activity promotes coughing which, if done effectively, helps to clear the respiratory passages. The nurse advises the child and family about measures to prevent pulmonary infection. If infection occurs, the nurse administers prescribed antibiotics or instructs the child and family about their use at home. Oxygen therapy may also be part of hospital or home care. Close follow-up in a recognized cystic fibrosis center is very important in the early detection of lung changes that require hospitalization for a thorough pulmonary clean-out and reassessment of maintenance regimen to be continued at home.

Cystic fibrosis is a chronic disease that causes many physical and psychosocial problems throughout the child's life. The primary role of the nurse is that of educator. The more parent and child know about the disease and its treatment, the better they can cope (see Chapter 30). The nurse plans teaching by gauging how much and what information the child and family are ready to hear at any given time. As the disease progresses and pulmonary symptoms worsen, the nurse and all other members of the health team must be supportive, honest, and available. (See Chapter 32 for a discussion about the dying child.)

Brochopulmonary Dysplasia

Bronchopulmonary dysplasia occurs in 10%–15% of premature or ill infants who have been treated with supplemental oxygen and mechanical ventilation, usually for hyaline membrane disease. It is progressive and potentially fatal. It is thought that positive inspiratory pressures and high concentrations of oxygen injure the alveolar saccules and epithelium of the small airways, causing fibrosis of these structures. Cystic, nonventilating areas form throughout the lung parenchyma. These changes result in poor lung compliance, chronic respiratory distress, and the need for long-term oxygen therapy.

Northway et al. described bronchopulmonary dysplasia in 1967 after reviewing outcomes for 32 mechanically ventilated infants. All the infants had had hyaline membrane disease. All had received high concentrations of oxygen during mechanical ventilation and all had developed progressive lung injury. These authors also described the phases of injury related to age and duration of treatment. These phases and the potential clinical course of the disorder are identified in Table 34-8. Since the early days of its recognition, bronchopulmonary dysplasia has been diagnosed in infants suffering from diseases other than hyaline membrane disease. Any immature infant who is mechanically ventilated and receiving high concentrations of inspired oxygen is now considered to be at risk for bronchopulmonary dysplasia.

The prognosis for survival has improved as the management of bronchopulmonary dysplasia has improved. Cor pulmonale is the leading cause of death. Promoting oxygenation and reducing pulmonary hypertension reduce the risks of cor pulmonale. Follow-up studies no not agree on the prognosis for eventual normal pulmonary function. Some researchers report long-term functional abnormalities (Voyles, 1981). Others report nearly normal to normal function by the time the child is 6–8 years of age. If the damage is to only the alveolar ducts and alveoli, then the generation of healthy alveoli, which continues into early adolescence, may compensate for earlier destruction. Normal function is compromised, however, if respiratory viral infections, to which chronically ill infants are particularly susceptible, have permanently damaged the small airways.

Treatment Medical treatment for the infant suffering from the acute stage of hyaline membrane disease and early stage of bronchopulmonary dysplasia is geared primarily toward life support, but efforts are made to limit the extent of bronchopulmonary dysplasia. Oxygen concentrations, peak inspiratory pressures, and mechanical ventilation rates are lowered as quickly as possible. Newer modes of high-frequency ventilation, which allow for lower pressures, are being used in an effort to prevent lung injury. Care is taken not to overhydrate the infant, because an increase in interstitial lung water compresses the tiny airways and causes necrosis in the epithelial lining.

TABLE 34-8 Stages and Clinical Manifestations of Bronchopulmonary Dysplasia

Stage	Characteristic	Age of child	Clinical manifestations
Stage I	Acute respiratory distress	2–3 days	Tachypnea, grunting, retractions, cyanosis in room air
Stage II	Pulmonary regeneration Healing and recovery course Low lung compliance, increasing respiratory insufficiency	4–10 days	Slow improvement, weaning from FiO_2, peak inspiratory pressure; child may be weaned to a hood Drop in lung compliance more difficult to ventilate; FiO_2 increased; child may die
Stage III	Transition to chronic lung disease	10–30 days	Stable oxygen and ventilator requirements; child may slowly improve or deteriorate
Stage IV	Chronic lung disease	Beyond 1 month	Oxygen dependence; child may need months of supplemental oxygen; slow improvement; ventilated child may remain stable with slow improvement; right heart failure, pulmonary hypertension may develop; child may die from cor pulmonale

Nursing Management Nursing management for the infant with bronchopulmonary dysplasia is related to respiratory support, nutrition, and protection of the injured lungs from further damage due to infection, overhydration (interstitial fluid), hypoperfusion, shock, pneumothorax, or interstitial air.

Respiratory support may include continuous mechanical ventilation or prolonged administration of supplemental oxygen via hood, nasal catheter, or cannula. If long-term mechanical ventilation is prescribed, the infant is weaned to the lowest possible oxygen, peak inspiratory pressure, positive end expiratory pressure, and ventilatory rate settings. If mechanical ventilation is not required, the child is weaned to the lowest tolerated inspired oxygen concentrations or liter flow. Criteria used to assess safe weaning include (a) maintenance of normal to low normal arterial blood gases or transcutaneous oxygen and carbon dioxide levels, (b) no increase in the work of breathing, and (c) normal growth and physical development.

Chest physiotherapy is an integral part of the infant's care. Postural drainage with percussion and vibration is essential but very stressful to the infant. If the infant is very small or acutely ill, the nurse reads transcutaneous oxygen monitoring levels during each position change. If the infant becomes hypoxic or takes a long time to return to pretreatment oxygen levels, the nurse consults with the physician to design a more appropriate and less stressful chest physiotherapy routine.

Small premature infants and those with indwelling feeding tubes cannot be placed in the head-down position because of the risk of aspiration. Therefore, positions for draining the right middle lobe, the left lingular lobe, and the lower lobes cannot be used.

Changing the infant's position from side to side and front to back improves bronchial drainage and promotes expansion of different lung areas in turn, ensuring ventilation of all lung areas.

Nursing care for the infant with bronchopulmonary dysplasia also involves providing optimal nutrition without overhydration and protection from infection. (These and other aspects of nursing management of the high-risk infant are discussed in Chapter 31.)

Aspiration Pneumonia

Swallowing disorders and gastroesophageal reflux are the primary causes of aspiration pneumonia in infants. Severely retarded children continually aspirate oropharyngeal secretions, causing irritant and bacterial pneumonias. Other causes of aspiration pneumonia are accidental aspiration of liquids or solid food and near-drowning.

Swallowing disorders during infancy may be related to general neuromuscular disease and *dyskinesia* (lack of coordination) of the tongue, soft palate, pharynx, or hypopharynx. Laryngeal stridor, nonclosure of the larynx, or absence of the cough reflex may also predispose the infant to aspiration pneumonia.

Tracheoesophageal fistulas not diagnosed in the neonatal period often are recognized after a persistent cough develops (see Chapter 38). The H type fistula is usually not identified until respiratory symptoms caused by aspiration occur.

Gastroesophageal reflux (see Chapter 38) also causes aspiration pneumonia. Laryngospasm occurs as the aspirated food or fluid (usually formula) reaches the larynx, thus stimulating a protective spasm. Apnea may occur as the acid formula stimulates nerve receptors at the base of the tongue. This stimulus causes centrally mediated, rather than obstructive, apnea.

In most young infants, some reflux occurs into the lower esophagus after feedings because of immature cardiac sphincter tone. Aspiration can occur if reflux reaches the hypopharynx, which it may do in some infants when they are in a supine position.

The degree of lung response to aspirated substances is related to the concentration of the substance, rather than its volume. Very highly concentrated fluids may cause fulminating pulmonary edema. Most commonly, though, alveolar macrophages ingest aspirated matter, forming granulomatous lesions that infiltrate the interstitium. The aspiration of large volumes of liquid or boluses of food causes immediate life-threatening airway obstruction (see Chapter 19).

Diagnosis of aspiration pneumonia is made with chest radiographs and a history of episodes of sudden coughing and color change. More important, however, is diagnosis and correction of the disorder that caused aspiration.

Swallowing disorders are identified by direct observation of the infant during a feeding session. Unusual swallowing noises, stridor, cough, or gurgling indicate oropharyngeal dyskinesia. A speech pathologist may assess palate movement or abnormal tongue thrusting. Electromyography enables the physician to determine which of the oropharyngeal muscles are affected and recommend corrective therapies.

The barium swallow provides a dynamic view of the infant's swallowing coordination. When requesting the barium swallow, it is extremely important to indicate on the request form that swallowing is to be observed. If this is not stated, the radiologist may omit information about swallowing in the report, since the more common reason for the test is to assess gastrointestinal dysfunction. Coughing after feedings, frequent spitting up, or clearing of the throat are signs of gastroesophageal reflux. The barium swallow can demonstrate the presence of reflux and the level in the esophagus to which the formula rises or the formula's presence in the airway.

Esophageal pH monitoring is employed more often than the barium swallow to determine level of reflux. Studies using this diagnostic technique have demonstrated that reflux and subtle aspiration of gastric contents occur in some patients with severe asthma. These children have a history of nighttime wheezing not related to inappropriate serum theophylline levels. Reflux and aspiration occur during sleep, and wheezing follows episodes of aspiration. In more severe cases of reflux, manometric measurements of esophageal pressure changes are made. This information is correlated with the pH of the esophageal contents and the child's oxygenation status.

Medical treatment consists of correcting the cause of aspiration. Special feeding techniques, prefeeding oral stimulation, and external manipulation of the tongue and jaw often dramatically reduce dyskinesia. Specific maneuvers are recommended by the speech pathologist. Reflux is prevented by thoroughly burping the infant after each feeding and then placing the infant prone for 2–3 hours (see Chapter 38). If these measures fail and reflux is severe, surgery (fundoplication) may be performed.

Hydrocarbon Inhalation

Inhalation or aspiration of hydrocarbons accounts for between 4%–10% of all childhood poisonings. It usually occurs in children under 5 years of age. Pneumonitis is the most common symptom. Rarely do children drink the volume necessary to cause systemic problems and central nervous system manifestations. Small amounts cause an immediate burning sensation in the mouth and throat, gagging, choking, and coughing.

The type of hydrocarbon and the presence of additives such as camphor, naphthalene, heavy metals, nitrobenzene, or trichloroethane affect the degree of toxicity and injury. Hydrocarbon's low surface tension, low viscosity, and high volatility cause it to move rapidly over tissue and migrate into distal airways. The higher volatility of hydrocarbon makes it easy to inhale.

Respiratory symptoms usually occur within 30 minutes after inhalation. A nonproductive cough, tachypnea, dyspnea, grunting, retractions, and cyanosis are typical early signs. Continuation of the nonproductive cough usually indicates severe involvement.

Severe inhalation may cause rapid development of hemoptysis and pulmonary edema. The short time between inhalation and onset of symptoms strongly suggests that injury is due to inhalation rather than to ingestion and absorption of the hydrocarbon through the gastrointestinal tract and its excretion through the lungs.

The ventilation–perfusion defects of hypoxemia and hypocarbia reflect the destruction of epithelium in the airways and irritative bronchospasm. Alveolar stability is lost with the loss of surfactant. Oil absorption by the lung causes parenchymal damage. Defenses against secondary infection may be altered by the injury.

Generally, pulmonary effects peak by 24 hours, remain severe for several days, and start to subside within 2–5 days. Respiratory symptoms may persist for several weeks. Severely affected survivors of hydrocarbon inhalation may have persistent wheezing and frequent lower respiratory tract illnesses. Follow-up pulmonary function testing of asymptomatic children 6–14 years after injury has demonstrated residual damage to the small airways.

Diagnosis is made by the history of hydrocarbon ingestion and rapid onset of respiratory symptoms. Abnormal arterial blood gases and radiographic evidence of chemical pneumonitis confirm that inhalation injury has occurred.

Treatment Emergency treatment is controversial. Some clinicians prefer to use ipecac and induce vomiting, provided that the substance is not corrosive and the child is conscious and alert. This treatment is based upon the belief that the neurologically intact child will not aspirate during emesis. The parent is never advised to give the child ipecac, however. It is given only in the hospital and never to a child who is comatose or convulsing or who has signs of central nervous system depression. Some clinicians prefer not to initiate vomiting unless there is a toxic additive or heavy metal mixed with the hydrocarbon. If central nervous system depression is evident, an endotracheal tube is inserted first, and the poison then is lavaged from the stomach.

If possible, the child is cared for at a facility that can provide the best respiratory support available. Immediate stabilization may be necessary at one facility, but early referral to an appropriate critical care facility is preferable.

Supportive care of the child starts with immediate attention to hypoxemia. Mechanical ventilation may be necessary if pulmonary edema or respiratory failure occurs. Because of poor lung compliance secondary to injury, a volume respirator is preferable to a pressure respirator. The addition of positive end expiratory pressure (PEEP) helps support the unstable alveoli and control pulmonary edema. Although steroids have not proved to be effective in treating the lung injury directly, they are used frequently in serious inhalation injury because they stabilize the pulmonary capillary membrane, which helps to control pulmonary edema and leakage from the capillary.

Nursing Management Nursing care of the child and family starts in the emergency room. The rapidity with which symptoms occur is frightening to the child and family, and rapid assessment and treatment is critical. One care provider, usually a nurse, acts as the informational liaison between other members of the emergency team and the family. A liaison also is needed in the intensive care unit. As more and more personnel, equipment, invasive procedures, and treatments are added, family anxieties rise. Consistent updating of the family may help ameliorate stress.

Nursing care for the child with serious inhalation and lung injury is complex. An endotracheal tube is inserted, and the child is mechanically ventilated. With severe hypoxemia, restlessness and struggling may interfere with the ventilator efficiency. Muscle paralysis and sedation may be necessary to achieve and maintain adequate ventilation and oxygenation.

Multiple intravenous and intraarterial catheters are used to monitor blood gases, pulmonary artery pressure, pulmonary wedge pressure, arterial blood pressure, and perhaps even central venous pressure. Maintenance fluids are given intravenously, as well as any medications. A nasogastric or orogastric tube is in place, as is a Foley catheter. Accurate monitoring of input and output is critical. The nurse uses aseptic technique during invasive procedures, such as suctioning, because the lung injury increases the child's susceptibility to secondary pulmonary infection.

Counseling and safety education related to prevention of hydrocarbon ingestion is delayed until the child is out of danger, but if there are other children in the family who might be at risk for the same accident, the parent is advised immediately to remedy the situation. During family turmoil, children are more likely to become victims of accidents. (See Chapter 20 for a discussion about the prevention of poisoning.)

Alpha$_1$-Antitrypsin Deficiency

Alpha$_1$-antitrypsin is an antiprotease that limits the proteolytic action of certain enzymes. It is produced in the liver and transported with alpha$_1$ globulins. Alpha$_1$-antitrypsin contributes 90% of the trypsin-inhibitory capacity of the serum. It is found in many body fluids and tissues, in the cytoplasm of pulmonary alveolar macrophages, on the surface of polymorphonuclear leukocytes, along the walls of adult human terminal bronchioles, and in platelet granules.

Serum alpha$_1$-antitrypsin volume may double or triple in response to acute inflammatory processes that occur, for example, in the immediate postoperative period, during pregnancy, and with estrogen treatment. Its major function is thought to be the inhibition of one or more elastases that, when normally released by the polymorphonuclear leukocytes, attack and damage tissue, particularly elastin-containing connective tissue. Damage is prevented by alpha$_1$-antitrypsin as it diffuses into interstitial spaces and body fluids. Alpha$_1$-antitrypsin may also act as a "shuttle protein," bringing enzymes released in tissue back into the circulation. This enables other serum protease-inhibitory actions to occur and facilitates the ultimate disposal of the enzymes in the reticuloendothelial system.

Alpha$_1$-antitrypsin deficiency is genetically determined. Most individuals inherit the protease-inhibitor allele from both parents. This homozygous pairing is normal. About 10% of the United States population is born with abnormal pairings of the protease-inhibitor allele. A heterozygous paring (in which only one allele is abnormal) results in partial alpha$_1$-antitrypsin deficiency and may produce mild symptoms. A homozygous pairing in which both alleles are abnormal results in severe symptoms of alpha$_1$-antitrypsin deficiency. The abnormal homozygous pairing is very rare, affecting less than 0.1% of the United States population.

Degradation of elastin by elastase is the prominent pathologic process in alpha$_1$-antitrypsin deficiency. The alveolar septae are destroyed, which leads eventually to panacinar emphysema. Infectious diseases and toxic injury increase the damage because inflammation increases the number of granulocytes or pulmonary macrophages in pulmonary tissue. This process releases elastase and accelerates elastin and tissue damage.

Clinically, the patient with alpha$_1$-antitrypsin deficiency has few problems until the third or fourth decade, when a subtle progression of dyspnea and wheezing is noted. Basilar hyperinflation is seen on chest radiographs. Chronic, progressive, and irreversible obstructive disease develops. Emphysema may be complicated or exacerbated by infection, bronchiectasis, and smoking. Emphysematous disease is not common in children with alpha$_1$-antitrypsin deficiency. In children who are affected, such symptoms as chronic cough, dyspnea, wheezing, and clubbing of the fingers develop when they are between 18 months and 6 years of age. Pulmonary disease can also develop in heterozygous children. They tend to have recurrent bronchitis, pneumonia, asthma, bronchiectasis, and lung abscess, and to be at risk for developing mild emphysema as adults.

Liver disease is the most common manifestation of alpha$_1$-antitrypsin deficiency during childhood. Cirrhosis develops during childhood (see Chapter 38), and survivors almost always have emphysema as adults.

Diagnosis of this deficiency is made by either radioimmune or electroimmune diffusion assay of alpha$_1$-antitrypsin. Electrophoresis can indicate decreasing levels of alpha$_1$-antitrypsin. A full genetic history of the family may be necessary.

Infants and children with a history of chronic cough, dyspnea, and wheezing of unknown origin, with or without a family history of chronic lung disease, should be evaluated for the deficiency. Children who have chronic liver and respiratory problems should also be evaluated.

Medical treatment and nursing management consist of relieving symptoms and preventing exacerbation. Infections are treated early and aggressively with antibiotics to limit tissue damage. Bronchodilators alleviate dyspnea. Supplemental oxygen may be given during acute infections and as damage progresses. Chest physiotherapy and breathing exercises are crucial for children with bronchiectasis and recurrent infection. Immunizations against influenza and measles are recommended.

Avoidance of smoking by the child and others in the home is extremely important because smoke inhalation worsens emphysema. Exposure to polluted air and noxious fumes must also be avoided to prevent acceleration of elastin damage.

Nursing management is most often related to the chronicity of the disease and its impact upon the child and family (see Chapter 30). A degenerative course is expected if emphysema develops during childhood. Support, counseling, and education for parent and child are critical to the child's quality of life. Children with the heterozygous trait and homozygous children who develop the less destructive form of the disease are instructed to avoid cigarette smoking and polluted air. The child and family are advised of the high risk of emphysema development during adulthood, especially if the patient smokes.

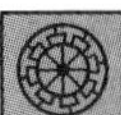

NURSING CARE PLAN A Child With Severe Asthma

Assessment Data

Chad is a 5-year-old male accompanied to the emergency room by his mother. Chad's mother appears very anxious and keeps repeating, "My baby can't breathe; someone help him before he dies."

Chad weighs 20 kg (44 lb), and he is 114 cm (44.5 in) tall. He is diaphoretic and has circumoral and nail bed cyanosis. Inspection of Chad's chest reveals substernal and intercostal retractions. Ascultation reveals audible wheezing on inspiration and expiration, with prolonged expiration.

Nursing Diagnoses and Goals

1. **Nursing diagnosis:** Ineffective airway clearance related to increased mucus production and narrowed respiratory passages indicated by audible wheeze.

   Long-term goal: Chad will inspire and expire freely and be able to remove excess pulmonary secretions.

   Short-term goals: (a) Chad will relax and practice his breathing exercises. (b) Chad will cooperate with aerosol treatments and breathe deeply. (c) Chad will report any feelings of tightness or difficulty in breathing. (d) Chad will practice effective coughing. (e) Chad will breathe without having to use accessory muscles.

2. **Nursing diagnosis:** Potential for fluid volume deficit related to tachypnea and dyspnea.

   Long-term goal: Chad's hydration status will be normal.

   Short-term goals: (a) Chad and his mother will participate in keeping an accurate intake and output record. (b) Chad's fluid intake will increase to a minimum of 2,000 mL daily.

3. **Nursing diagnosis:** Anxiety related to strange environment.

   Long-term goal: Chad will cope with his anxiety about the hospitalization and cooperate with necessary treatments.

   Short-term goals: (a) Chad will appear calm and relaxed. (b) Chad will become less restless. (c) Chad will verbalize or play out his fears.

4. **Nursing diagnosis:** Knowledge deficit related to immediate and continued treatment of asthma attack.

   Long-term goal: Chad and his mother will have a basic understanding of asthma and its treatment with inhalation therapy with aerosol bronchodilator, epinephrine injections, and oxygen therapy.

   Short-term goals: (a) Chad and his mother will describe early signs and symptoms of an attack. (b) Chad and his mother will list the steps to be taken to treat an impending attack. (c) Chad will point out and identify equipment used for treatments to nurse or mother. (d) Chad will demonstrate anatomic location of lungs on a doll and his own body.

5. **Nursing diagnosis:** Alterations in family functioning related to Chad's illness.

   Long-term goal: Chad and his family will return to normal, effective functioning after asthma attack is over.

   Short-term goals: (a) Chad and his mother will express their fears to the nurse. (b) Chad's mother will participate in his care. (c) Chad's mother will support and reassure her child. (d) Chad's mother will ask appropriate questions about his care.

Interventions	Rationale	Evaluation criteria
1. Identify factors that contribute to ineffective airway clearance (for example, anxiety, allergic reactions, infection)	This information is needed to initiate appropriate treatment	Did Chad's breathing become easier? Was he able to raise and expectorate excess mucus? Did Chad's respiratory rate fall to less than 25? Did signs of cyanosis disappear from nail beds and mucous membranes? Did auscultation demonstrate normal breath sounds and adequate air exchange bilaterally? Did Chad cooperate with breathing exercises and aerosol therapy?

continued on next page

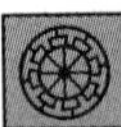

NURSING CARE PLAN A Child With Severe Asthma (continued)

Interventions	Rationale	Evaluation criteria
Eliminate contributing factors, particularly parental anxiety	A calm parent will have a calming effect on an anxious child	
Assist Chad to sit upright, relax shoulders, maintain good posture, and use accessory abdominal muscles of breathing	Position, posture, and correct use of muscles will improve ventilation. Use of abdominal muscles forces trapped air from lungs	
Help Chad to relax and concentrate on one aspect of breathing by doing breathing exercises with the nurse	Bronchospasm is less likely to worsen in a relaxed child who is concentrating on moving trapped air from lungs	
Encourage Chad to practice these exercises by devising a game for them	Children are more cooperative and results more apparent if children enjoy the exercises	
Offer Chad sips of clear fluids or engage him in another type of diversional activity	Sipping is a simple diversion that will help the child to relax	
Administer epinephrine, bronchodilators, as ordered	Timely and correct administration of medications will relieve asthma symptoms	
Monitor effects of medications, particularly epinephrine and theophylline, by monitoring vital signs, especially pulse and blood pressure	Dosage may need to be adjusted if signs of ineffectiveness or toxicity such as hyperalertness, agitation, tachycardia, arrhythmias, hypotension occur	
Auscultate breath sounds when doing vital signs (initially every ½–1 hour)	Auscultating breath sounds helps to define air movements and restrictions as evidenced by wheezing and rhonchi	
Observe mucous membranes for signs of cyanosis	Mucous membranes provide best indicator of cyanosis in children of color	
Administer aerosol treatments with a bronchodilator as necessary when wheezing or dyspnea increase	Direct inhalation of bronchodilator is an effective means to reduce bronchospasm and dilate airways	
Teach Chad proper use of aerosol therapy and the importance of taking deep breaths	Aerosol therapy is effective only when the child inhales deeply to bring medication into the lungs	
Monitor vital signs carefully during and following treatment; discontinue if untoward signs become evident	Bronchodilators have toxic side effects of tachycardia and hypotension	
Explain to Chad the importance of telling his mother or the nurse whenever breathing becomes difficult, his chest feels tight, or he has to take many little breaths and is unable to take a deep breath	Early reporting of breathing difficulty enables prompt intervention and avoidance of further distress	
Teach Chad how to cough effectively and raise mucus from lungs; note whether he swallows mucus or expectorates it	Removal of secretions from lungs permits better movement of air; children have difficulty expectorating mucus and tend to swallow it instead	

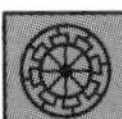

NURSING CARE PLAN A Child With Severe Asthma (continued)

Interventions	Rationale	Evaluation criteria
Monitor arterial blood gases to determine response to treatment and pulmonary mechanics	Arterial blood gases provide accurate, objective measurement of ventilation and diffusion	
Monitor Chad's response to therapy and evidence of return to normal respiratory pattern	The child's ability to breathe at a normal rate without using accessory muscles is a subjective indicator that therapy is effective and pulmonary mechanics are improved	
2. Observe Chad for signs of dehydration evidenced by changes in vital signs, skin turgor, mucosa, sunken eyes, dark circles, urine output, urine specific gravity	Insensible fluid loss increases during an asthma attack. Adequate hydration makes respiratory secretions less viscous and easier to clear	Did Chad remain adequately hydrated? Is urine output adequate and specific gravity between 1.008 and 1.015?
Offer Chad frequent small amounts of his favorite clear fluids; set goal of 150 mL of fluid each hour	Small amounts are more likely to be consumed by the child; goal is compatible with total fluid requirement	
If signs of dehydration are present, prepare Chad for intravenous infusion	Intravenous infusion will provide for the child's fluid needs and restore deficits	
Monitor intake and output	Accurate recording is necessary to determine fluid demands and adequacy of intake	
3. Maintain a calm and relaxed manner	The nurse's manner will have a calming effect on the child	Did Chad relax sufficiently to enhance rather than hinder treatment?
Give Chad a doll with mask and nebulizer, stethoscope, syringe, and other equipment to play with and examine (see Chapter 28)	Observing the child's play enables the nurse to assess child's feelings about therapy. Play gives the child an opportunity to express fears	
Give Chad choices, if possible, about modes of treatment (for example, oxygen therapy with mask or cannula)	Participation in self-care fosters feelings of control, which make the child less anxious	
Calm Chad's mother and encourage her to stay with him	The presence of a calm, reassuring parent is the most successful measure of all to reduce the child's anxiety	
4. Review with Chad and his mother the signs and symptoms of an asthma attack (chest tightness, wheezing, dyspnea, cough, anxiety, diaphoresis)	Understanding and knowing the early signs and symptoms of an attack will enable the parent and child to take appropriate action and not to panic	Did Chad and his mother demonstrate an appropriate understanding of the acute asthma attack and its treatment?
Discuss with and provide written instructions for Chad and his mother concerning the immediate treatment and steps to be taken when an attack occurs (medication to be given, breathing exercises, position for breathing, hospitalization)	Knowing what to do and having written directions helps the parent remain calm and initiate appropriate action. Following prescribed medication plan is important to avoid overdose of potent bronchodilator	
Explain to Chad and his mother the purpose of each procedure, using age-appropriate terms for Chad and more detailed explanations for his mother	Knowing reasons for procedures helps the child to cooperate and the parent to support and emphasize the need for each procedure	

continued on next page

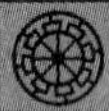

NURSING CARE PLAN A Child With Severe Asthma (continued)

Interventions	Rationale	Evaluation criteria
Use a doll or puppet with exposed lungs to teach Chad and his mother about lungs and what happens during an asthma attack	This will help the child and mother to understand the disorder and the body parts affected	
Have Chad point to his own lungs and listen to them with stethoscope	This will help the child to apply knowledge gained in playing with a doll or puppet to his or her own body	
Supervise Chad in therapeutic play with respiratory equipment and ask Chad to describe equipment he is playing with and to state its purpose (see interventions for nursing diagnosis 3)	Play enhances the child's knowledge and gives the nurse opportunities to answer the child's questions and clear up misconceptions	
5. Help Chad to use play (clay, balls, pounding toys, art) to express feelings about his illness (for example, fear, anger, guilt, anxiety, helplessness)	Knowing how the child is feeling helps the nurse to act as liaison between parent and child. The nurse might be a more constructive listener than the already-anxious parent	Are mother and child able to express feelings? Did mother participate in child's care? Is mother able to offer support? Are mother's questions about home care answered?
Explain Chad's feelings and coping mechanisms to his mother	Explanations help the parent to respond positively to a child who may be exhibiting negative behavior	
Assist Chad's mother to verbalize her feelings of fear, helplessness	The parent also needs opportunity to verbalize feelings about the experience and be reassured that these feelings are a normal response when frightened	
Encourage Chad's mother to assist with his care and support him	The opportunity to do something useful for the child helps the parent to overcome fears and feelings of helplessness	
Prepare Chad and his mother for discharge by reviewing medication regimen, activity limitations, diet, and health maintenance routines. Encourage Chad's mother to ask questions; provide phone number to call if questions arise	Patient, thorough discharge preparation facilitates ability to carry out plan when child and parent are home. Answering questions helps the parent to make the plan a reality and to prepare for home care; providing a phone number reassures the parent that someone is available to assist when questions arise	

Key Concepts

- Embryonic development of the respiratory tract begins with development of the laryngotracheal groove at about the fourth week of gestation and continues through three stages, the pseudoglandular, canalicular, and terminal sac stages.
- Ventilation of the lungs, diffusion of gases to and from capillary blood, and perfusion of body tissues by capillaries are necessary for adequate respiratory function.
- Physical examination of a child with a suspected

respiratory dysfunction includes observation for signs of hypoxia and dyspnea; assessment of the rate, depth, ease, and rhythm of respiration; palpation; percussion; and auscultation.

- Pulmonary function tests are done to measure the volume of air normally inspired and expired, the capacity of the lungs to inspire and expire more than the usual volume, and the rate of flow in and out of the lungs.
- Diffusion tests are done to assess gas exchange of the alveolocapillary membrane; exercise tests are done to assess overall respiratory function.
- Esophageal pH monitoring, which is done to determine whether respiratory symptoms are due to gastroesophageal reflux, requires careful observation and recording of events that could stimulate reflux, as well as routine nursing care.
- Tracheal aspiration is a sterile procedure used to obtain specimens of secretions for cultures or smears.
- Nursing responsibilities related to invasive diagnostic procedures are to monitor pulse, respirations, and skin color during the procedure; to administer supplemental oxygen; and to ensure that the child is adequately oxygenated before, during, and after the procedure.
- Supplemental oxygen is administered to correct hypoxemia (insufficient oxygenation of arterial blood), which is assessed by arterial blood gas studies and manifested clinically as tachypnea, tachycardia, headache, pallor, cyanosis, and mental confusion.
- In inhalation therapy, aerosols are atomized into fine mist by a nebulizer and inspired by the patient.
- Humidity is added to air inspired through an artificial airway and to supplemental oxygen to prevent drying and irritation of the respiratory mucosa.
- Postural drainage, percussion, and vibration are done by the nurse or physiotherapist to enhance clearance of respiratory secretions or an aspirated foreign body.
- Huffing, deep breathing, and coughing are clearance measures the nurse or physiotherapist teaches the child to perform.
- Incentive spirometry and breathing exercises help the child to increase capacity, ventilation, and control of respirations.
- For the child with obstructive lung disease, in which resistance to airflow is increased, acute care is based on a nursing diagnosis of ineffective airway clearance.
- For the child with restrictive lung disease, in which lung expansion is impaired, acute care is based on a nursing diagnosis of ineffective breathing patterns.
- Nutritional needs of the child with a respiratory disorder involve careful attention to hydration status.
- The developmental needs of the child with a respiratory disorder involve maintenance of optimal exercise tolerance and activity levels.
- Health maintenance needs of the child with a respiratory disorder may include teaching related to home therapy involving oxygen equipment, nebulizer-delivered aerosols, chest physiotherapy, exercise regimens, prevention and management of emergencies, and follow-up care.
- Nursing care for the child with rhinitis, tonsillitis, or pharyngitis involves comfort measures, adequate fluid intake, acetaminophen administration, careful handwashing, and monitoring for symptoms of bacterial infection.
- For the child with acute spasmodic croup, nursing care involves humidification of inspired air and monitoring for increasing obstruction that requires emergency treatment.
- Nursing care for the child with laryngotracheobronchitis (LTB) requires interventions and assessment relative to inhalation therapy, oxygen therapy, humidification, hydration, conservation of energy, careful observation for signs of respiratory failure, and possible intubation.
- Nursing care for the child with epiglottitis includes assessment for signs of obstruction, assistance during radiographic or direct inspection of the epiglottis, potential need for intubation, and the administration of intravenous antibiotics.
- For the infant with bronchiolitis, nursing management includes frequent observations of respiratory status and measures related to hydration, humidification, oxygen therapy,

respiratory isolation, positioning and chest physiotherapy to improve ventilation.

- Nursing care for the child with bronchitis includes the provision of adequate fluids and rest and observation for signs and symptoms of secondary infection.
- Childhood pneumonia is described as bronchopneumonia; has multiple causes; and varies greatly in number, type, and severity of signs and symptoms.
- For the child with pneumonia, nursing responsibilities include monitoring respiratory status, vital signs, and hydration status, and providing fluids, fever control measures, mist therapy, chest physiotherapy, oxygen therapy, and antibiotic therapy when indicated.
- Nursing care relative to suspected tuberculosis may involve administering and evaluating the tuberculin skin test, instructing the family about immunization of contacts, and assisting with such diagnostic procedures as radiographic examination and gastric lavage.
- For the child with tuberculosis, nursing care involves isolation measures, administration of medications, patient teaching about compliance with the drug regimen, and monitoring the course of infection.
- Nursing care for the child with a foreign body lodged beyond the trachea includes measures relative to bronchoscopy, aerosol bronchodilator therapy, and chest physiotherapy.
- Nursing care for the child recovering from near-drowning involves monitoring blood gases, oxygen therapy, artificial ventilation; monitoring and correcting pH and electrolyte status; and observing for signs of bronchospasm and infection.
- Nursing care for the child with severe asthma includes emergency administration of epinephrine, theophylline, or a steroid, as ordered; assistance with intubation and mechanical ventilation; and oxygen therapy.
- Nursing care for the child with chronic asthma is related to administering the aerosol bronchodilator, teaching the child and family how to avoid precipitating factors, and instructing the child and family about early warning signs of asthma attack and measures that can be taken to alleviate or prevent severe attacks.
- Nursing care for the child with pulmonary disease due to cystic fibrosis involves maintaining airway patency by administering aerosol bronchodilators and performing or supervising chest physiotherapy, administering antibiotics for infection, providing emotional support, and educating the child and family about the disease and its treatment.
- For the infant with bronchopulmonary dysplasia, nursing care involves weaning the infant to the lowest possible oxygen concentrations and inspiratory pressures, protecting the child from infection, preventing further injury to the child from overhydration and chest physiotherapy.
- Treatment for aspiration pneumonia is correction of the cause, which is commonly a swallowing defect.
- Nursing care for the child with hydrocarbon inhalation involves correcting hypoxemia and stabilizing the alveolocapillary membrane by mechanical ventilation and steroid administration, as appropriate.
- Treatment for alpha$_1$-antitrypsin deficiency is supportive and includes prevention and treatment of infections, chest physiotherapy, and avoidance of irritants, such as cigarette smoke and polluted air.

References

Behrman RE, Vaughn VC, McKay RE: *Nelson Textbook of Pediatrics.* Saunders, 1984.

Cherniack RM: *Pulmonary Function Testing.* Saunders, 1977.

Cohen S, Boyce B, King TKC: Programmed instruction: Pulmonary function tests in patient care. *Am J Nurs* (June) 1980; 80:1135–1161.

Cystic Fibrosis Foundation: Cystic fibrosis: A plea for a future. Vol 2. The Foundation, 1978.

Fischbach FT: *A Manual for Laboratory Diagnostic Tests.* 2nd ed. Lippincott, 1984.

Gordon M: *Nursing Diagnosis: Process and Application.* McGraw-Hill, 1982.

Molteni RA: Epiglottitis: Incidence of extraepiglottic infection: Report of 72 cases and review of the literature. *Pediatrics* 1976; 58:526–532.

Northway WH, Rosan RC, Porter DY: Pulmonary disease following respiratory therapy of hyaline membrane disease: Bronchopulmonary dysplasia. *N Eng J Med* (Feb) 1967; pp. 357–368.

O'Neill E: Cystic fibrosis. Pages 58–83 in: *Chronic Obstructive Pulmonary Disease.* Sexton DL (editor). Mosby, 1981.

Pinney M: Pneumonia. *Am J Nurs* (March) 1981; 81:517–518.

Rarey KP, Youtsey JW: *Respiratory Patient Care*. Prentice-Hall, 1981.
Schiffer CG, Hunt EP: *Illness Among Children*. Children's Bureau Publication no 405, Department of Health, Education and Welfare, 1963.
Sexton DL: *Chronic Obstructive Pulmonary Disease*. Mosby, 1981.
Shinefield HR: Pneumonia. Pages 141–144 in: *Current Pediatric Therapy 1966–1967*. Gellis SS, Kagan BM (editors). Saunders, 1966.
Simkins R: The crises of bronchiolitis. *Am J Nurs* (March) 1981; 81:514–516.
Traver, GA (editor): *Respiratory Nursing: The Science and the Art*. Wiley, 1982.
Voyles JB: Bronchopulmonary dysplasia. *Am J Nurs* (March) 1981; 81:510–514.
Wade JF: *Respiratory Nursing Care: Physiology and Technique*. Mosby, 1982.

Additional Readings

Adair JC et al: Ten-year experience with IPPB in the treatment of acute laryngotracheobronchitis. *Anesth Analg* (July-Aug) 1971; 50(4):650–655.
Bates B: *A Guide to Physical Examination*. Lippincott, 1974.
Brandeburg J: Inhalation injury: Carbon monoxide poisoning. *Am J Nurs* (Jan) 1980; 80:97–100.
Castiglia PT, Aguilina S: Streptococcal pharyngitis: A persistent challenge. *Pediatr Nurs* (Nov/Dec) 1982; 377–381.
Cotton EK et al: Removal of aspirated foreign bodies by inhalation and postural drainage. *Clin Pediatr* (May) 1973; 12:270–278.
Cotton E, Altman M, Eigen H: Aspiration of foreign bodies in children. *Am Thorac Soc*, 1981.
Curran CL, Kachoyeanos MK: The effects on neonates of two methods of physical therapy. *Am J Matern Child Nurs* (Sept/Oct) 1979; 4:309–313.
Dean JM, Kaufman ND: Prognostic indicators in pediatric near-drowning: The Glasgow coma scale. *Crit Care Med* (July) 1981; 9:536–539.
Do day-care centers pose excessive health risks to children? *Pediatr Alert* 1983; 8(2):5–6.
Educational Design, Inc: Respiratory tract aspiration: Programmed instruction. *Am J Nurs* (Nov) 1966; 66(11):2483–2510.
Ellmyer P, Thomas NJ: A guide to your patients safe home use of oxygen. *Nursing 82* (Jan) 1982; 12:56–57.
Emami CL, Delbianco LM: an improved technique for securing nasoendotracheal tubes. *Am J Matern Child Nurs* (Sept/Oct) 1981; 6:337–340.
Ennis S, Harris TR: Positioning infants with hyaline membrane disease. *Am J Nurs* (March) 1978; 78:398–401.
Fuchs P: Understanding continuous mechanical ventilation. *Nursing 79* (Dec) 1979; 9(12):26–33.
Garvey J: Infant respiratory distress syndrome. *Am J Nurs* (April) 1975; 75(4):614–617.
Gaston SF, Schumann LL: Inhalation injury. *Am J Nurs* (Jan) 1980; 80:93–97.
Geis DP, Lambertz SE: Acute respiratory infections in young children. *Am J Nurs* (Feb) 1968; 68(2):294–297.
Gordon M: *Manual of Nursing Diagnosis*. McGraw-Hill, 1982.
Helming MG: Nursing in respiratory diseases: A symposium. *Nurs Clin North Am* (Sept) 1968. Reprinted for National Tuberculosis and Respiratory Disease Association.
Huhit E et al: Association of viral and mycoplasm infections with exacerbations of asthma. *Ann Allergy* (Sept) 1974; pp. 145–149.
Hymovich DP: Parents of sick children: Their needs and tasks. *Pediat Nurs* (Sept/Oct) 1976; 2:9–13.
Jennings C: An alternative: Nasal cannula oxygen therapy for infants who are oxygen dependent. *Am J Matern Child Nurs* (March/April) 1982; 7:89–92.
Kendig EL, Chernick V (editors): *Disorders of the Respiratory Tract in Children*. 4th ed. Saunders, 1983.
Kennedy AH, Johnson WG, Sturdevant EW: An educational program for families of children with tracheostomies. *Am J Matern Child Nurs* (Jan/Feb) 1982; 7:42–49.
Larter N: Cystic fibrosis. *Am J Nurs* (March) 1981; 81:527–532.
Lehnert BE, Schacter EN: *The Pharmacology of Respiratory Care*. Mosby, 1980.
McCollum A: *The Chronically Ill Child: A Guide For Parents and Professionals*. Yale University Press, 1981.
McFadden R: Decreasing respiratory compromise during infant suctioning. *Am J Nurs* (Dec) 1981; 81:2158–2161.
McIntosh R et al: The association of viral and bacterial respiratory infections with exacerbations of wheezing in young asthmatic children. *J Pediatr* (April) 1973; 82:578–590.
McPherson SP: *Respiratory Therapy Equipment*. 2nd ed. Mosby, 1981.
Metaproterenol (Alupent) now available without prescription. *Pediatr Alert* 1983; 8(7):25–26.
Moozam F, Talbert JL, Rogers BM: Foreign bodies in the pediatric tracheobronchial tree. *Clin Pediatr* 1983; 22:148–150.
Murphy RLH, Holford SK: Lung sounds. *Am Thorac Soc News* (Spring) 1980; pp. 24–28.
Nalepka CD: The oxygen hood for newborns in respiratory distress. *Am J Nurs* (Dec) 1975; 75(12):2185–2187.
New formulations and devices for administering asthma medications. *Pediat Alert* 1983; 8(2):7–8.
Ng L, McCormick KA: Position changes and their physiological consequences. *Adv Nurs Sci* (July) 1982; 4(4):13–25.
Nielsen L: Mechanical ventilation: Patient assessment and nursing care. *Am J Nurs* (Dec) 1980; 80:2191–2217.
Petty L (editor): *Intensive and Rehabilitative Respiratory Care*. 3rd ed. Lea and Febiger, 1982.
Pinney M: Foreign body aspiration. *Am J Nurs* (March) 1981; 81:521–522.
Rachelefsky GS: Asthma self-management programs for children. *Child Care Newsletter* 1984; 3(2):5–8.
Rau J, Rau M: To breathe or be breathed: Understanding IPPB. *Am J Nurs* (April) 1977; 77:613–617.
Reeves KR: Acute epiglottitis—Pediatric emergency. *Am J Nurs* (Aug) 1971; 71(8):1539–1542.
Scarpelli EM, Auld PAM, Goldman HS (editors): *Pulmonary Disease of the Fetus, Newborn and Child*. Lea and Febiger, 1978.
Schuler PM, Cloutier MM: Chronic cough in children. Pages 10–14 in: *Pediatric Basics #38*; 1984.
Simkins R: Asthma: Reactive airways disease. *Am J Nurs* (March) 1981; 81:522–526.
Simkins R: Croup and epiglottitis. *Am J Nurs* (March) 1981; 81:519–520.
Stepdesign Inc: Blood-gas and acid-base concepts in respiratory care. *Am J Nurs* (June) 1976; 76(6).
Stepdesign Inc: Pulmonary function tests in patient care. *Am J Nurs* (June) 1981; 80:1135–1161.
Sweetwood H: Acute respiratory insufficiency: How to recognize this emergency . . . How to treat it. *Nursing 77* (Dec) 1977; 7(12):24–32.
Sweetwood H: Bedside assessment of respirations. *Nursing 73* (Sept) 1973; 3:50–51.
Tecklin JS: Positioning, percussing, and vibrating patients for effective bronchial drainage. *Nursing 79* (March) 1979; 64–71.
Thompson SW: How to use the Heimlich maneuver on choking infants and children. *Pediatr Nurs* (Jan/Feb) 1983; 13–16.
VanArsdel PP, Motulsky AG: Frequency and hereditability of asthma and allergic rhinitis in college students. *Acta Genet* (Sept) 1959.
Waring WW, Jeansonne LO: *Practical Manual of Pediatrics*. Mosby, 1975.
Webber-Jones JE, Bryant MK: Over-the-counter bronchodilators. *Nursing 80* (Jan) 1980:34–39.
Wotring KE: Adult respiratory distress syndrome as a complication of pregnancy. *Am J Matern Child Nurs* (Sept/Oct) 1979; 4:314.

Circulation
Implications of Abnormalities in Structure and Pressure

Gayle P. Olsen David Driscoll

35

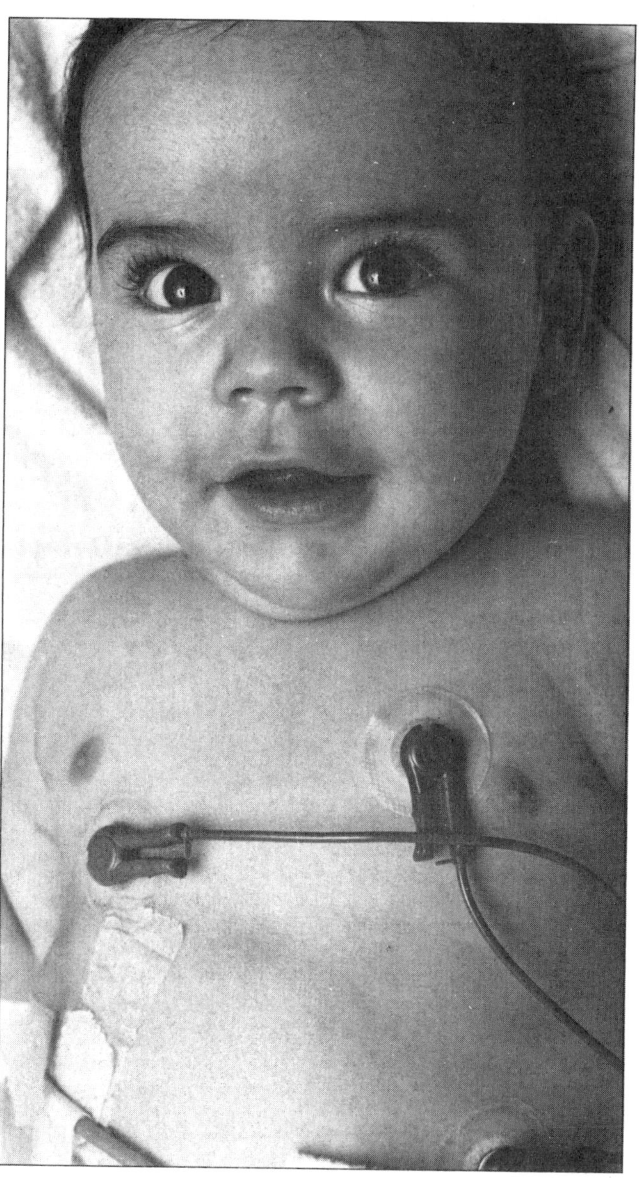

Chapter Outline

continued on next page

Objectives

- Describe the anatomy and physiology of the heart, arteries, veins, and cardiac conduction system.
- Explain how prenatal circulation differs from postnatal circulation.
- Explain the physiologic effects and changes in circulation caused by left-to-right shunts, right-to-left shunts, and obstruction defects.
- Identify assessment criteria and diagnostic tests pertinent to history talking and physical examination of the child with suspected or diagnosed cardiac disease.
- Explain nursing care common to procedures and treatments that involve the cardiovascular system.
- Describe the acute-care, nutritional, developmental, emotional, and health maintenance needs of the child with cardiac disease.
- Describe nursing management and parent teaching involved in the administration of diuretics, digoxin, and prophylactic antibiotics.
- Identify the causes, signs, and symptoms of congestive heart failure.
- Describe the major acyanotic cardiac defects and their general clinical manifestations.
- Describe the major cyanotic cardiac defects and their general clinical manifestations.
- Describe nursing management for the child undergoing cardiac surgery.
- Describe assessment and nursing management for the child with subacute bacterial endocarditis, the child with hypertension, and the child with hyperlipidemia.

To find these topics, see the following chapters	
Cardiopulmonary Resuscitation (CPR)	Chapter 19
Rheumatic Fever	Chapter 37

The cardiovascular system consists of a pump (the heart) and a series of conduits (arteries and veins) that move blood to and from organs for the purpose of supplying the metabolic needs of the organs and removing metabolic products. Because its function is essential to life, any dysfunction of the cardiovascular system is serious and often life threatening.

Treatment for cardiovascular disorders often requires surgery, extended periods of hospitalization, and long-term follow-up care. The stress of a child's cardiac condition can also place the family system at risk for dysfunction. (The implications of chronic childhood conditions are discussed in Chapter 30.)

In this chapter, we discuss nursing care specific to children with cardiovascular disorders. We review the structure and function of the heart and the circulation of blood; we describe the assessment criteria and procedures associated with cardiac conditions; and we discuss nursing management for cardiovascular disorders that occur in children.

Anatomy and Physiology of the Cardiovascular System

Embryonic Development of the Cardiovascular System

The heart is one of the first organs formed, and the cardiovascular system is the first system to function. Its developmental sequence is important, for it allows the embryo to receive an adequate supply of nutrients and to dispose of wastes, thus facilitating rapid growth. The primitive heart is a fairly straight tube consisting of only two chambers. Between the second and tenth week of gestation, however, this tube undergoes a series of rotations, invaginations, and partitionings, thereby creating a four-chamber heart and its great arteries.

At approximately the twenty-first day after conception, the blood begins circulating and the heart begins beating. The lungs cannot exchange gas in utero, and so gas exchange takes place in the placenta. Deoxygenated blood is carried to the placenta by two umbilical arteries, which are branches of the fetal iliac arteries. Oxygenated blood returns to the fetus through the umbilical vein, which is a tributary of the fetal inferior vena cava. The umbilical vein connects to the inferior vena cava through the ductus venosus. Maternal and fetal blood remain separate in the placenta, which functions as an interface for gas, nutrient, and waste exchange between the two separate circulatory systems.

Fetal circulation differs from adult circulation in several ways. In the fetus, oxygenated blood returns from the placenta to the umbilical vein. Approximately half of this blood goes directly to the inferior vena cava through the ductus venosus, thereby bypassing the liver. The remainder perfuses the liver and then enters the inferior vena cava. In the vena cava the oxygenated blood mixes with some deoxygenated blood returning from the lower extremities. From the vena cava the blood enters the right atrium, where most of it passes through the *foramen ovale* (a valvelike opening in the interatrial septum) into the left atrium.

The blood in the left atrium then mixes with some deoxygenated blood from the pulmonary veins. Because the lungs are not functional, the amount of blood from the pulmonary circulation is relatively small. The oxygen content of the blood remains fairly high as it passes into the left ventricle and then into the ascending aorta to supply the vessels of the head, neck, and upper extremities.

Most of the deoxygenated blood returning via the superior vena cava enters the right atrium and traverses the tricuspid valve to enter the right ventricle. Thus, in the fetus, the oxygen content of blood in the left ventricle is higher than the oxygen content of blood in the right ventricle. From the right ventricle blood is ejected into the main pulmonary artery, but because the lungs are collapsed and pulmonary resistance is high, only a small amount of the blood (approximately 8% of the combined ventricular cardiac output) goes into the right and left pulmonary arteries. Most of the blood travels through the *ductus arteriosus* (a descending thoracic aorta) and enters the connection between the main pulmonary artery and the proximal descending aorta.

The oxygen content of the blood ejected into the head is greater than the oxygen content of the blood traversing the patent ductus arteriosus and perfusing the lower portion of the body. As the blood traverses the descending aorta, some of it enters the umbilical arteries and returns to the placenta, where it is reoxygenated (see Fig. 7-3).

After birth, the lungs expand, and the umbilical arteries and veins are severed. At this time the neonate's lungs take over the role of oxygenating the blood. Now blood from the right ventricle that, in utero, had passed through the patent ductus arteriosus perfuses the lungs. The ductus arteriosus is no longer necessary, and it closes functionally by 48 hours of age and structurally by 6 weeks of age. The ductus venosus likewise obliterates, becoming the ligamentum venosum. The foramen ovale is no longer necessary, and it closes as a result of the decreased pulmonary resistance, lowering right atrial pressure and creating a corresponding increase in left atrial pressure that presses the valvelike opening so that it closes.

Changes in pressure and resistance also occur in pulmonary and systemic circulation after birth. Prior to delivery the lungs are collapsed, and pulmonary vascular resistance is high. Systemic vascular resistance is quite low. These differences in resistance to blood flow explain why most of the blood in the fetal circulation bypasses the lungs and shunts directly to the systemic circulation through the foramen ovale and the ductus arteriosus.

After delivery, as the neonate's lungs expand, oxygen in the precapillary vessels causes dilatation of the pulmonary vasculature, and pulmonary resistance to blood flow drops markedly. Simultaneously, as the umbilical cord is cut and serum pH drops briefly, systemic vascular resistance increases. Thus as blood from the right ventricle flows to the pulmonary system, shunting across the foramen ovale and ductus arteriosus decreases. These structures begin to close, partly in response to oxygen partial pressure (PO_2).

Pulmonary vascular resistance drops rapidly in the first hour of life and more gradually for the next 4–6 weeks. By 6 weeks, pulmonary vascular resistance approaches adult levels, although a slight drop continues throughout the first year.

These postnatal changes in resistance and blood flow explain why some types of heart disease may not be recognized in the neonatal period. For example, if the fetus has ventricular septal defect, blood shunts across the defect from right to left, just as it shunts across the foramen ovale and ductus arteriosus. After delivery, as pulmonary resistance drops, blood from the right ventricle is ejected into the pulmonary artery. Because pulmonary vascular resistance is still relatively elevated, however, there may be minimal left-to-right shunting and few symptoms of heart disease. During the first month, as pulmonary vascular resistance continues to decline, pressure in the left ventricle predominates, and left-to-right shunting increases to the point that symptoms of ventricular septal defect become evident.

Under certain conditions, such as hypoxia and acidosis, pulmonary vasoconstriction occurs, and pulmonary vascular resistance remains high after birth. Blood continues to shunt through the ductus arteriosus from right to left. This occasionally happens in premature infants, especially those with respiratory distress syndrome (see Chapter 31). As the hypoxia, acidosis, or lung disease lessen and pulmonary vascular resistance falls, systemic pressure exceeds pulmonary pressure, and shunting through the ductus arteriosus reverses from right to left to left to right. This reversal may cause congestive heart failure.

Physiology of the Cardiovascular System

The Heart, Arteries, and Veins The heart is a muscular organ consisting of two atria (receiving chambers), two ventricles (pumping chambers), and four valves (tricuspid, pulmonic, mitral, and aortic valves) (Fig. 35-1). Deoxygenated blood returns to the heart from the organs of the body through the superior and inferior vena cavae. The superior vena cava enters the cephalad portion of the right atrium and conducts venous drainage from the head, neck, arms, and cephalad portions of the thorax. The inferior vena cava enters the caudal portion of the right atrium and conducts blood returning from the organs below the diaphragm and from caudal portions of the thorax.

Besides the superior and inferior vena cavae, the coronary veins enter the right atrium. The coronary veins conduct blood returning from the heart muscle itself. The opening of the coronary veins into the right atrium is called the *coronary sinus*. The right atrium is a thin-walled muscular structure suited to its function of receiving rather than forcefully pumping blood. From the right atrium, the deoxygenated blood passes through the tricuspid valve and enters the right ventricle. The tricuspid valve, like all four valves of the heart, can be likened to a one-way door. It allows blood to flow forward (prograde) but not backward (antegrade). Unlike the right atrium, the right ventricle is composed of thick muscle that forcefully ejects blood through the pulmonic valve into the main pulmonary artery.

The main pulmonary artery divides into the right and left pulmonary arteries, which conduct blood into the right and left lungs. In the lungs, the blood enters pulmonary capillaries that surround the alveoli, where gas exchange occurs. Carbon dioxide is released from the blood, passes into the alveoli, and is expired. Inspired oxygen travels to the alveoli,

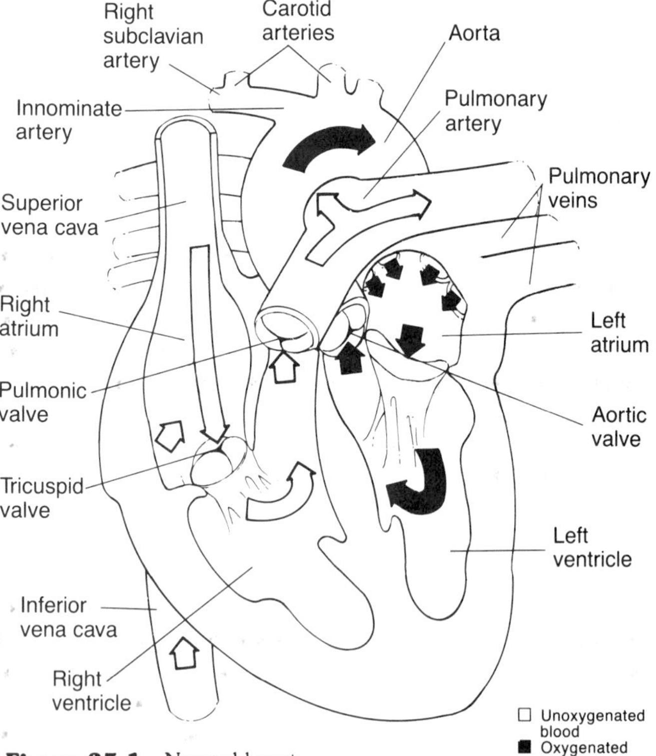

Figure 35-1 Normal heart.

where it enters the blood. Oxygen combines with hemoglobin in the blood to form oxyhemoglobin, which gives oxygenated blood its red color. The oxygenated blood returns to the left atrium of the heart through four (there may be three to five) pulmonary veins.

Oxygenated blood collects in the left atrium, which, like the right atrium, is a thin-walled structure. From the left atrium the blood travels through the mitral valve to the left ventricle. The left ventricle is the major pumping chamber of the heart. Consequently, it is the chamber with the thickest muscular walls. The left ventricle pumps oxygenated blood under relatively high pressure through the aortic valve and into the aorta, which conducts the blood from the heart to the organs of the body.

The aorta originates in the left ventricle, extends cranially (the ascending aorta), curves posteriorly (the aortic arch), and then extends caudally (the descending aorta) through the thoracic cavity, traverses the diaphragm, and continues through the abdomen until it bifurcates into the iliac arteries, which supply blood to the pelvis and legs. The first branches of the aorta are the coronary arteries, which arise just distal to the aortic valve leaflets and supply blood to the heart muscle itself. The next branch of the aorta is the innominate artery, which subdivides into a subclavian artery (supplying blood to an arm) and a carotid artery (supplying blood to the head). After the origin of the innominate artery, a second carotid artery arises followed by a second subclavian artery that supplies the other arm. Along the course of the aorta other branches occur that supply organs in the thoracic and abdominal cavities.

The amount of oxygen in the blood can be quantified either by measuring the partial pressure of oxygen in arterial blood (PaO_2) or the percentage of hemoglobin that is combined with oxygen (that is, the oxygen saturation). Normally, the deoxygenated blood returning to the heart from the body has an oxygen saturation of about 65%–70%. The oxygen saturation remains at 65%–70% as the blood traverses the right ventricle and pulmonary artery. Because the blood "picks up" oxygen in the lungs, the blood that returns to the left atrium and circulates through the body has an oxygen saturation of 95%–98%. The level of oxygen saturation of the blood in the various chambers of the heart is abnormal in certain types of congenital cardiac defects, and the extent of the abnormal levels of oxygen saturation aids the diagnosis and assessment of the severity of the congenital defect.

Because the heart is a pump intended to propel blood in one direction, the movement of blood by the heart obeys the laws of hemodynamics. In essence, blood (or fluid) flows from a high-pressure to a low-pressure area. Systemic venous blood returns to the right atrium propelled by the force of gravity (from the head and neck) or assisted by the pumping action of skeletal muscles, especially in the legs and one-way valves in the veins. Blood pressure in the right atrium is 0–5 mm Hg. During *diastole* (relaxation), pressure in the right ventricle is slightly lower than pressure in the right atrium, so blood flows from the right atrium through the tricuspid valve and into the right ventricle. During ventricular *systole* (contraction), pressure in the right ventricle increases to 15–25 mm Hg and blood is ejected into the pulmonary artery, where the pressure is 15–25 mm Hg during systole and 5–10 mm Hg during diastole. The pressure in the left atrium is similar to that in the right atrium (0–8 mm Hg), and during ventricular diastole blood flows from the left atrium to the left ventricle, where the diastolic pressure is 0–5 mm Hg. During systole the left ventricle generates pressures of 90–140 mm Hg and ejects blood into the aorta, where blood pressure is approximately 120/75 (Fig. 35-2). Pressure in the aorta is reflected in the blood pressure measurement obtained in the arm using a conventional sphygmomanometer. Blood pressure in the aorta varies considerably from person to person and with age (see Appendix B).

Basic measurements of cardiovascular function include heart rate, blood pressure, cardiac output, stroke volume, and vascular resistance. (Normal values for heart rate and blood pressure are summarized in Appendix B.) *Cardiac output* is the volume of blood ejected by the left ventricle and is expressed as liters of blood per minute. Because cardiac output varies with body size, it is customary to convert cardiac output to *cardiac index*, which is cardiac output divided by the body surface area (in square meters). *Stroke volume* is the volume of blood ejected by the left ventricle during each heart beat and is expressed as liters per beat. Cardiac output equals heart rate times stroke volume.

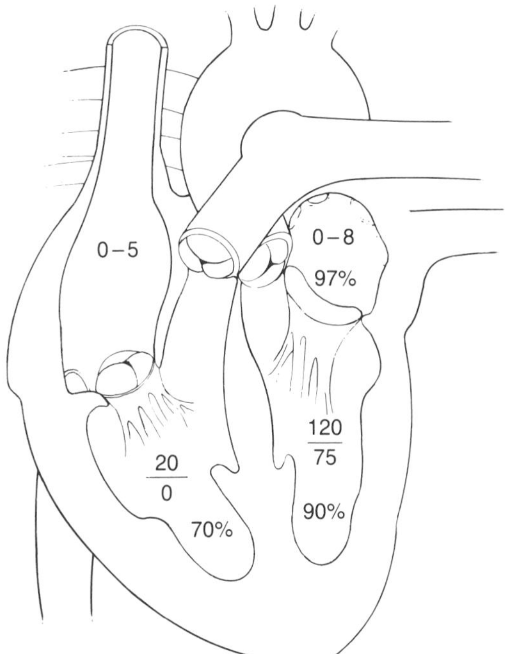

Figure 35-2 Oxygen saturation (percentages) and pressures during systole.

The tremendous length of the vascular system, together with the properties of blood and vessel walls that resist blood flow, make a certain degree of force necessary to propel blood through the vascular system. Resistance to blood flow in the aorta and its branches is called *systemic resistance.* Resistance in the pulmonary artery and its branches is called *pulmonary resistance.* The degree of resistance to blood flow is very important, as the higher the resistance, the more work the heart must do to pump blood. Resistance is calculated by dividing the blood pressure difference across a vascular bed by the cardiac index. Therefore, systemic vascular resistance is the difference between mean aortic blood pressure and mean right atrial blood pressure divided by cardiac index, and pulmonary vascular resistance is equal to the difference between mean pulmonary artery pressure and mean left atrial pressure divided by cardiac index.

The Electrical Conduction System The heart contracts when it is stimulated by rhythmic electrical impulses that originate in the sinus node. The sinus node, the normal pacemaker of the heart, is a microscopic collection of specialized myocardial tissues located in the region of the superior vena cava and right atrial junction (Fig. 35-3). Impulses originating in the sinus node alter the permeability of myocardial cell membranes, allowing potassium, sodium, chloride, and calcium ions to cross into the cells. This causes the myocardial fibers to contract.

From the sinus node the electrical impulse travels in concentric waves throughout the left and right atria until the impulse reaches a second group of specialized conducting tissue located near the coronary sinus entrance and on the right side of the interarterial septum, the atrioventricular node. The atrioventricular node is the bundle of His, the collection of Purkinje fibers prior to their passing through the atrioventricular junction and bifurcating. One branch of the bundle travels on each side of the septum, one to the left ventricle and one to the right. Both bundle branches become a network of Purkinje fibers distributed throughout the inner surface of both ventricles.

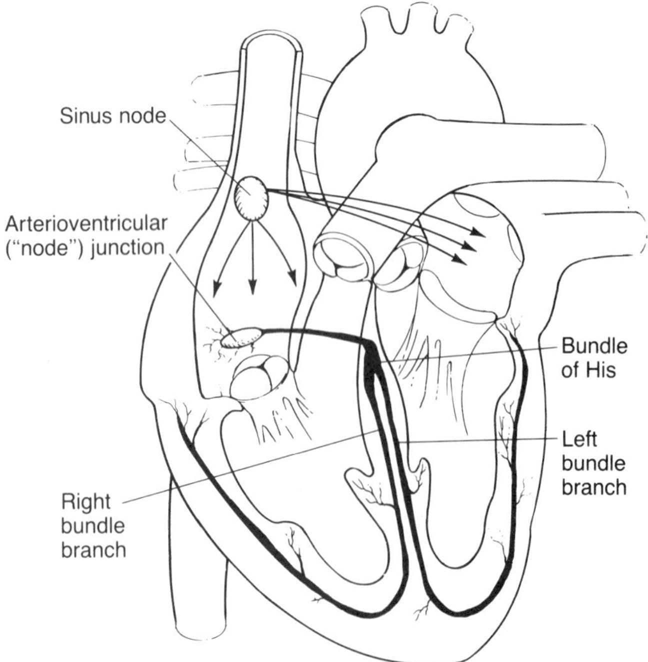

Figure 35-3 Cardiac conduction system.

Physiologic Effects of Cardiac Defects and Disease To understand the acute-care needs of the child with cardiovascular problems, the nurse needs to understand the physiologic effects that occur most commonly. Not all of these effects occur with each type of cardiac problem. In general, cardiac defects are defined as alterations in blood flow and pressure related to the presence of shunts or obstructions.

Shunts Blood always flows from an area of high pressure to an area of low pressure and takes the path of least resistance. Blood flow through an abnormal communication between the right and left sides of the heart is called a *shunt.*

Left-to-Right Shunts Normally, pressures in the left side of the heart are significantly higher than the pressures on the right side of the heart. Therefore, if there is an abnormal opening in the septum between the right and left sides, blood flows from the left to the right. If the abnormal opening (septal defect) is small, only a small amount of blood flows or shunts through it. If the defect is large, a large volume of blood flows left to right, creating a left-to-right shunt.

The shunt does not usually cause significant hypoxemia and cyanosis. The workload of the right side of the heart is increased because the right ventricle must pump its normal volume of blood plus the extra volume shunting from the left side. The heart responds by pumping at a faster rate (causing tachycardia) and by pumping more blood with each contraction. This increased workload causes the myocardial fibers to enlarge and the right ventricle to dilatate, resulting in *cardiomegaly* (cardiac enlargement).

The lungs normally receive blood from the right ventricle under relatively low pressure. With a left-to-right shunt, the lungs are exposed to an increased volume of blood under high pressure. Tachypnea, dyspnea, and pulmonary edema may result. Blood pools in the lungs and creates conditions that promote bacterial proliferation. Recurrent respiratory infections occur. In an attempt to protect the lungs from the increased volume and pressure, *hypertrophy* (thickening) of pulmonary arterial walls develops. Hypertrophy increases the resistance of blood flow to the lungs, causing pulmonary arterial hypertension. While this is a helpful short-term response, severe restriction of pulmonary blood flow may occur over time. If not treated, the changes become irreversible. Because they do not directly cause hypoxemia and cyanosis, defects that result in left-to-right shunting are among the *acyanotic heart diseases.*

Under certain circumstances, a left-to-right shunt may reverse direction so that blood flows from right to left. This usually occurs when pressure in the pulmonary vasculature increases. It may occur in conjunction with hypoxia or acidosis, which can cause marked pulmonary vasoconstriction and reversal of a left-to-right shunt. It may also occur as the lungs are subjected to high volumes and pressure from a left-to-right shunt over time, causing pulmonary hypertension, which may reach a point at which the pressure in the right ventricle exceeds pressure in the left ventricle, so that the shunt reverses.

Right-to-Left Shunts In some types of defects, the pressure in the right side of the heart may be greater than in the left side of the heart. This might occur if resistance in the lungs is abnormally high or if the pulmonary artery is constricted. If a septal defect is present, deoxygenated blood from the right side of the heart shunts to the left side and out into the body (blood from the right side normally goes to the lungs). Significant right-to-left shunting may be due to any of a number of defects known collectively as *cyanotic heart disease.*

Decreased arterial oxygen saturation *(hypoxemia)* in the systemic circulation results in *hypoxia* (decreased tissue oxygenation). Secondary polycythemia develops as the body attempts to compensate for hypoxemia by producing more red blood cells. Although secondary polycythemia enables the blood to carry more oxygen, it has important negative effects. The viscosity of the blood increases significantly, thus creating resistance to the blood flow, making the heart pump harder to overcome the resistance. Circulation becomes sluggish, and the risk of thrombus formation increases.

A right-to-left shunt also causes a portion of the blood to bypass the filtering system of the lungs. Bacteria or emboli may pass through the shunt and go to the brain, causing a stroke or brain abscess.

Chronic hypoxia might also result in metabolic acidosis, which may be partially compensated. In normal metabolism, pyruvic acid is converted into carbon dioxide, water, and energy in the Krebs cycle. This process requires oxygen. If sufficient oxygen is not available, pyruvic acid is anaerobically converted to lactic acid, which collects in the tissues and causes acidosis. The body can compensate for mild acidosis, but severe acidosis, if not promptly treated, leads to death.

Obstruction Defects In obstruction defects the forward progress of the blood is impeded by a narrowing or blockage in the valves or great vessels. Obstructive lesions generally create elevated pressure proximally and decreased pressure distally. Congestive heart failure may occur as a result of obstructive lesions.

Assessment of the Child With Cardiovascular Dysfunction

History

Children with heart disease often have histories of decreased tolerance for exercise. They may become excessively fatigued or short of breath with normal activity because of hypoxemia, inadequate myocardial function, or obstruction to cardiac outflow. The parent might first become aware of this when the infant becomes fatigued and breathless during feedings, taking only limited quantities of milk before needing to rest. Infants with heart disease also may have weak cries and hypotonic or flaccid postures. The older child might be unable to keep up with siblings and peers, may need to stop and rest at intervals or might consciously select quiet, more sedentary activities.

The nurse inquires about changes in the child's skin color because children with heart disease often have unusually pale or mottled skin, or varying degrees of cyanosis, ranging from a mild blue tinge of the lips during exercise to severe cyanosis at rest. The nurse asks the parent whether the child has experienced dizziness, syncope, diaphoresis, congested cough, edema, rapid respirations, or repeated respiratory infections. A tendency to assume a squatting posture might also be a sign of heart disease.

Hypoxic spells are assessed for frequency, severity, precipitating factors, and family management. In addition, the nurse refers to the child's medical record or asks the parent about any delays in physical growth and development.

Any of the child's symptoms are then further assessed according to severity, frequency, chronology, aggravating and alleviating factors, setting, associated symptoms and changes, and impact on the child and family. If the child is known to have heart disease, the nurse documents when the diagnosis was made, the course of the disease, and the management thus far.

The nurse also explores the health of the mother during pregnancy. Any illness, particularly infectious illness, should be noted. Several viral infections (rubella and infections due to cytomegalovirus, coxsackie, and herpes hominis B viruses) are known to be associated with congenital heart disease. Maternal diabetes, alcoholism, and poor nutrition also have been associated with heart disease in the infant. Any medications taken by the mother should be noted. Folic acid antagonists, anticonvulsants, and possibly lithium, progesterone, estrogen, and warfarin are thought to be related to heart defects. Exposure to radiation also may be a cause of congenital defects.

The nurse ascertains whether any intrapartum or postpartum complications were present. Low birthweight, prematurity, congenital infections, cyanosis, respiratory problems (respiratory distress syndrome, apneic spells, hypoxic

(text continued on p. 1164)

ASSESSMENT GUIDE Child With Cardiovascular Problems

System	Subjective data	Objective data	Validating data	Nursing management
Head, eyes, ears, nose, throat	History of sore throat	Injected conjunctivae (may accompany cyanotic disease). Cyanosis of mucous membranes of mouth and pharynx	Throat culture. ASO titer	Teach importance of prevention and early treatment of streptococcus infections
Integumentary	History of cyanosis with exertion or stress. History of easy bruising. History of rashes, Kawasaki disease, scarlet fever	Cyanosis. Pallor, mottling. Bruising. Ruddy appearance of face and fingers. Diaphoresis. Edema (often a late sign of congestive heart failure). In infants and young children periorbital and sacral edema are more common than extremity, but edema of the extremities and ascites may be seen in older children	Blood gases. Complete blood count. Urine specific gravity. ASO titer, erythrocyte sedimentation rate	Monitor changes in cyanosis including extent of cyanosis, effect of activity on degree of cyanosis, effect of supplemental oxygen. Observe for decreased peripheral perfusion by noting capillary refill, blood pressure, peripheral pulses, temperature of extremities. Monitor intake and output and urine specific gravity; provide skin care; and administer diuretics if ordered, position the child in semi-Fowler's, and follow dietary modifications as ordered
Respiratory	History of repeated respiratory infections or pneumonia. Difficulty in breathing. Cough	Tachypnea. Hacking or congested cough. Rales, rhonchi, wheezing. Dyspnea. Expiratory grunt. Nasal flaring. Asymmetric thoracic expansion. Costal retractions	Chest radiographs. Blood gases Hemoglobin concentration. Red blood cell indices (see Chapter 36)	Monitor respirations carefully. Minimize oxygen needs by providing rest, minimizing activity, preventing hyper- or hypothermia. Place child in semi-Fowler's position. Avoid pressure on chest wall. Administer supplemental oxygen as ordered. Provide chest physiotherapy as ordered. Prevent exposure to respiratory infections. Teach child and parent about importance of prompt treatment of infections

ASSESSMENT GUIDE Child With Cardiovascular Problems (continued)

System	Subjective data	Objective data	Validating data	Nursing management
Cardiovascular	History of known heart disease. Family history of hypertension, atherosclerosis, hyperlipidemia, stroke, myocardial infarction, or arrhythmia. History of exercise intolerance. History of squatting posture with exercise or fatigue. History of hypoxic spells	Cyanosis. Polycythemia. Tachycardia. Arrhythmia. Hypertension. Lower blood pressure in legs than in arms or difference in pressure between arms. Distention of jugular veins. Precordial bulge. Clubbing of fingers and toes. Displacement of apical beat and/or point of maximal impulse. Palpable thrill or heave. Murmur, click, snap, friction rub, gallop rhythm, fixed split of S_2. Change in the sound of a murmur. Decreased peripheral pulses, delayed capillary refill, coolness, pallor, or mottling of extremities	Complete blood count. Blood gases. Serum electrolytes. Electrocardiography. Phonocardiogram. Echocardiogram. Chest radiograph. Cardiac scan. Cardiac catheterization	Monitor vital signs and cardiovascular status. Observe for change in symptoms. Prepare child and family for diagnostic tests. Minimize cardiac workload by providing rest, organizing care, anticipating needs, minimizing anxiety, monitoring activity, and preventing hyper- and hypothermia. Maintain fluid balance by avoiding over-underhydration, monitoring intake and output, administering diuretics as ordered, checking urine specific gravity, measuring weight daily or more often, accurately administering intravenous fluids. Administer cardiotonic and blood pressure medications as ordered, and observe for therapeutic or side effects. Teach subacute bacterial endocarditis prophylaxis
Gastrointestinal	History of feeding difficulties. Fatigue during feeding. Weak suck during infancy. Anorexia. Abdominal pain. Vomiting and nausea. Diarrhea	Poor weight gain. Abdominal tenderness on palpation. Ascites. Hepatomegaly	Strict calorie count. Serum digoxin level. Serum electrolytes, hemoglobin, hematocrit	Provide high-calorie diet. Ensure adequate intake by allowing rest periods during feeding, providing frequent small feedings, feeding hungry child immediately, enlarging nipple hole, holding infant in knee–chest position during feeding. Administer iron supplement as ordered. Restrict dietary sodium as ordered. Weigh child

continued on next page

ASSESSMENT GUIDE Child With Cardiovascular Problems (continued)

System	Subjective data	Objective data	Validating data	Nursing management
				daily or more often. Monitor intake and output
Genitourinary	History of change in amount of urine output, concentrated urine	Oliguria or polyuria. Alterations in urine specific gravity	Blood urea nitrogen. Serum creatinine. Urine specific gravity	Monitor intake and output. Weigh child daily. Monitor urine specific gravity
Musculoskeletal	Poor growth pattern. Developmental delay, particularly in gross motor skills. Decreased exercise tolerance, excessive fatigue. Anxiety, irritability	Inadequate weight and height gain. Shortness of breath with activity. Weak cry. Restlessness or lethargy. Poor muscle development. Thin extremities	Denver Developmental Screening Test or more comprehensive developmental assessment. Testing with bicycle treadmill	Explore feelings about body image. Discover child's or parent's feelings about child's development, including family's perceptions and expectations. Explore impact of exercise intolerance on child's daily activities
Neuroendocrine	History of syncope, lethargy, anxiety, restlessness	Restlessness, irritability. Lethargy. Confusion, change in level of consciousness. Focal neurologic finding. Seizure activity. Hypotonia	Brain scan for emboli or abscess	Monitor level of consciousness and neurologic signs. Monitor for hypoxia. Report episodes of fever, seizures, or syncope immediately

spells), and heart murmur may all indicate an increased risk of heart problems.

The nurse inquires about previous or concurrent conditions that may be associated with cardiac disease. Many genetic syndromes, such as mental retardation, blindness, deafness, and renal disease, have congenital heart disease as one manifestation. Streptococcal pharyngitis is an antecedent to rheumatic fever and rheumatic heart disease. Repeated respiratory infections may be related to congestive heart failure. Subacute bacterial endocarditis and Kawasaki disease may lead to chronic cardiac disease. Myocarditis is a rare complication of certain viral diseases.

The nurse further inquires about congenital heart disease or genetic disorders in any blood relative (see Fig. 5-10). A history of atherosclerosis, hyperlipidemia, hypertension, stroke, myocardial infarction, or arrhythmia in a family member may indicate the child is at increased risk for acquired heart disease.

Although most children with heart disease have normal intelligence, children with certain genetic defects or histories of severe hypoxia may be mentally disabled. A thorough developmental assessment of all children with cardiac disease thus is essential (see Chapter 16). Even the child with cardiac disease and normal cognitive development might show significant physical developmental delays, and delay in one area of development potentially affects performance in other developmental areas.

Because cardiac disease might have an impact on the child's nutritional status, the nurse explores the child's feeding behavior and diet history (see Chapter 15). Exercise intolerance may limit the amount of nutrients an infant is able to ingest. Anorexia may be a side effect of medications or congestive heart failure caused by liver and bowel edema. The nurse also notes the occurrence of fatigue, dyspnea, cyanosis, or diaphoresis during feeding. If the child is to be hospitalized, specific feeding routines used at home should be recorded and integrated into the plan of care (see Chapter 29). If the child is on a special diet (for example, a high-calorie or low-sodium diet), the nurse determines how the family has managed this.

Physical Examination

Measurement Measurement of vital signs provides information that is essential to the assessment of the cardiac system. An elevated temperature may be evidence of an infection and also causes an increase in heart and respiratory rates. Because the cardiac and respiratory systems function together, cardiac disease may be manifested by respiratory symptoms. The nurse therefore notes any grunting, respiratory retractions, nasal flaring, or dyspnea (see Chapter 34).

In a child with suspected heart disease, blood pressure should be measured in all four extremities. Pressure in one arm and one leg should be measured simultaneously. This can be done by attaching two cuffs to the sphygmomanometer with a Y connector. In young infants, blood pressure in the arms and legs is usually equal. In older infants and children, pressure in the legs is usually 10–30 mm Hg higher than in the arms. A lower pressure in the legs or a difference between arms may indicate coarctation of the aorta. During blood pressure measurement, it is essential that the child be at rest for the nurse to obtain accurate readings. The values obtained should be compared with normal values for the child's age (see Appendix B).

The *pulse pressure* is the difference between the systolic and diastolic pressures and is usually 20–50 mm Hg. A greater pulse pressure might occur with hypertension, patent ductus arteriosus, anemia, fever, and aortic regurgitation. A lower pulse pressure occurs with heart failure, tachycardia, aortic stenosis, and pericardial effusion. (The techniques and equipment for obtaining blood pressure in children are described in Chapter 14.)

Because children with heart disease often have associated delays in growth, measurement of height and weight are important. Fluid retention, however, is manifested by an increase in weight and is thus an important parameter to assess and note on the record during acute episodes.

Inspection The nurse observes the child by noting alertness, activity level, posture, and any obvious deviations from normal. Anxiety, restlessness, lethargy, and irritability might be signs of hypoxia. In assessing the neonate,the nurse might be the first to note initial signs of impending distress related to cardiac malfunction (Gillon, 1973).

During inspection, the nurse assesses the child's skin color. Pallor and mottling might be signs of vasomotor instability or decreased peripheral perfusion. Cyanosis occurs when approximately 5 g/100 mL of hemoglobin is reduced. Reduced hemoglobin imparts a bluish color, especially in areas with concentrated capillary networks, such as the lips and mucosa. Cyanosis may be as mild as a slight bluish tinge of the lips or as severe as a dark blue discoloration of all skin and mucous membranes. Cyanosis is usually most evident in the lips, nail beds, and mucous membranes. *Acrocyanosis* is blueness of the hands and feet that occurs in normal neonates. This is not indicative of heart disease in an otherwise-normal infant.

Cyanosis might be difficult to detect in children of color (see Color Plate). It is most evident in persons with dark skin in the mucous membranes of the mouth, which may have a violet hue. If cyanosis is detected, the nurse notes (1) the extent of the cyanosis and (2) the effect that activity has on the cyanosis (that is, does it worsen with crying and activity?). The physician may order oxygen, and the nurse then notes whether the cyanosis is reduced or unchanged with the oxygen.

Some children with cyanotic heart disease have ruddy faces and fingers. Some also have injected conjunctivas. During inspection, the nurse observes the neck veins for evidence of distention or pulsation, which may indicate elevated right atrial pressure or congestive heart failure. The nurse carefully observes the precordium from the side and the front, noting any bulge over the area of the heart, which may indicate cardiomegaly. In some children, the point of maximal impulse may be apparent as a pulsation over the apex of the heart.

The nurse then assesses for clubbing of the fingers and toes, which is indicative of chronic hypoxia. With clubbing, the ends of the fingers and toes are widened and thickened. Wrinkles and creases normally present are obliterated, and the digits may have a shiny appearance (see Color Plate).

Palpation Pulses commonly assessed are summarized in Table 14-12. The femoral pulse is particularly significant. This is usually a strong and easily palpable pulse in infants and children. A weak femoral pulse may suggest coarctation of the aorta. Table 35-1 defines various abnormal pulse patterns. In general, a strong pulse is associated with a widened pulse pressure. Weak pulses are usually associated with partial occlusion of the artery or decreased cardiac output.

TABLE 35-1 Abnormal Pulse Patterns

Pulse	Characteristics
Thready pulse	Weak, difficult to palpate, seems to appear and disappear
Water-hammer (Corrigan's) pulse	Very forceful and jerky, associated with wide pulse pressure
Pulsus alternans	Alterations of weak and strong beats without changes in cycle length
Paradoxical pulse	Force weaker with inspiration and stronger with expiration
Sinus arrhythmia pulse	Rate increases with inspiration and decreases with expiration
Bigeminal pulse	Beats occur in pairs because of premature beats

The nurse assesses capillary refill by compressing the tip of a finger or toe to cause blanching, then noting how long (in seconds) it takes for usual color to return. With normal circulatory function, color returns immediately. Pale, cool extremities and delayed capillary refill might indicate decreased peripheral perfusion.

Edema sometimes occurs in children with heart disease, although overt peripheral edema is not usually evident in infants. Edema is most evident in the periorbital and dependent areas of the body and would most likely be seen in the feet, ankles, and legs in a child who is ambulatory. In a bedridden child, edema is more likely to be evident in the sacral region.

Because hepatomegaly is one of the cardinal signs of congestive heart failure, it is important to assess liver size in a child with cardiac problems. Since an enlarged liver may extend far down into the abdomen, the nurse begins palpation in the lower right quadrant by the iliac crest, then proceeds upward until the lower edge of the liver is felt. The nurse then measures in centimeters the distance between the right costal margin in the midclavicular line and the lower edge of the liver. The liver is normally not more than 1–2 cm below the costal margin. It may not be palpable at all or palpable only on deep inspiration. The nurse assesses the consistency of the liver. An enlarged, congested liver feels hard.

Auscultation The nurse uses a stethoscope with a diaphragm and a bell to auscultate the heart. The diaphragm detects high-pitched sounds and is pressed firmly over the skin. The bell detects low-pitched sounds and is placed lightly over the skin. The nurse systematically listens to the heart sounds.

Heart sounds are produced by the opening and closing of the heart valves and by the action of blood against the walls of the heart and vessels. Two sounds normally are heard, S_1 and S_2. S_1 is caused by the closure of the mitral and tricuspid valves. S_2 is caused by the closure of the aortic and pulmonic valves (see Fig. 14-18). S_3 is sometimes heard in early diastole (just after S_2) and is caused by blood flowing from the atria to the ventricles. S_1, S_2, and S_3 combined produce a triple sound that resembles the sound of a galloping horse and is often referred to as a gallop rhythm, or ventricular gallop. S_3 may be normal but because it is associated with congestive heart failure, its presence potentially is significant. S_3 is heard best near the apex with the bell of the stethoscope in the left lateral decubitus position. S_4 is heard in late diastole, just before S_1. Although it may be a normal sound, it is often abnormal in children (see Tables 14-13 and 14-14).

Two additional heart sounds that are always abnormal are ejection clicks, which occur in systole, and opening snaps, which occur early in diastole. Both clicks and snaps indicate diseased heart valves. Pericardial friction rubs occur when the pericardial sac becomes inflamed and the two surfaces rub together. This characteristic scraping sound always is abnormal.

Murmurs can occur at various points in the cardiac cycle and are caused by the turbulence of blood as it passes between cardiac chambers or into major vessels. Murmurs are classified as innocent (also functional or benign), meaning that there is no cardiac pathology, or organic, meaning that there is cardiac pathology.

Murmurs are described according to six criteria:

1. *Timing in the cardiac cycle.* Murmurs can occur in systole (between S_1 and S_2) or during diastole (between S_2 and S_1). The timing may be broken down more specifically within systole or diastole. For example, a systolic murmur may be described as early systolic, midsystolic, late systolic, or holosystolic (pansystolic, or occurring throughout systole). Similar descriptions are used for diastolic murmurs. A continuous murmur is one heard throughout systole and diastole.
2. *Frequency.* Frequency refers to the sound of the murmur, which may be high-pitched, low-pitched, or medium-pitched.
3. *Location.* This is the anatomic location where the murmur is heard best (for example, the left sternal border in the fourth intercostal space).
4. *Radiation.* Radiation indicates where, besides the location, the murmur is heard.
5. *Intensity.* The intensity, or loudness, of murmurs is graded on a scale from I to VI, with I being the softest and VI the loudest (Table 35-2). Intensity may have variations. Crescendo murmurs begin softly but become louder. Decrescendo murmurs begin loudly and become soft. Crescendo–decrescendo murmurs start softly, become louder, and then become soft again.
6. *Effect of respiration and position.* The nurse notes whether the murmur increases, decreases, or remains the same during inspiration, expiration, and position changes.

Usually, the nurse attempts to describe murmurs that are present. Occasionally, it is important to document that a murmur is absent. If a child with heart disease has a documented murmur that diminishes or disappears, this may represent a significant pathologic change.

Validating Diagnostic Tests

Hematology and Blood Chemistry Studies One of the major functions of the cardiovascular system is to transport oxygen to the organs. In the blood, oxygen is bound to hemoglobin. While small amounts of oxygen can be transported dissolved in plasma, hemoglobin is necessary for transport of adequate amounts of oxygen. With congenital cyanotic heart disease, the body compensates for chronic hypoxia by producing increasing amounts of hemoglobin. Hemoglobin concentration is therefore an

TABLE 35-2 Scale of Intensity of Heart Murmurs

Murmur	Characteristics
Grade I	Faint, requires careful listening
Grade II	Quiet but readily heard
Grade III	Moderately loud, no thrill
Grade IV	Loud, usually associated with thrill
Grade V	Very loud, thrill present, may be heard with only partial contact of stethoscope and chest
Grade VI	Loud, thrill present, may be heard with stethoscope off chest wall

important indicator of the degree of hypoxia. Hemoglobin concentration and red blood cell indices should be determined in all children with significant cardiac defects.

Basic tests of blood clotting (prothrombin and partial thromboplastin times and platelet count) should be done prior to cardiac operations. Cyanotic children who have polycythemia might have thrombocytopenia.

Serum sodium, potassium, carbon dioxide, and chloride levels can be affected by some forms of congenital heart disease and by some medications. Children with congestive heart failure and fluid retention can have abnormally low serum sodium levels. This is a "dilutional" form of hyponatremia that usually results from water retention, not sodium deficiency. In fact, total-body sodium is usually normal or above normal, so sodium administration is contraindicated. Instead, a diuretic may be given to eliminate excess body water. Some diuretics deplete body stores of potassium, so the child receiving diuretics, especially in high doses, requires careful monitoring of serum potassium levels. If the child is receiving digitalis, its toxic effects can be accentuated by low serum potassium levels. Chloride levels are monitored in children on long-term diuretic therapy, as such therapy might cause uncompensated hypochloremic alkalosis, which may be manifested by reduced serum chloride levels.

Serum creatinine and blood urea nitrogen are measured to assess renal function before beginning treatment with drugs that are excreted by the kidneys. These values also are determined prior to cardiac operations.

Arterial blood gases and hydrogen ion concentration (PaO_2, $PaCO_2$, pH, and O_2 saturation) are helpful in assessing hypoxemia, acidosis, and the extent of pulmonary insufficiency complicating or accompanying a cardiac disease. Blood gas values are particularly helpful in postoperative management.

Cardiographic Studies Cardiographic studies are summarized in Table 35-3. The *electrocardiogram* is a measurement of the electrical activity of the heart. It is used to detect cardiac rhythm and cardiac chamber thickness (hypertrophy). The normal electrocardiogram consists of a P-wave; a P–Q interval; Q-, R-, and S-waves; an S–T interval; and a T-wave. The P-wave reflects electrical activation of the left and right atria (Fig. 35-4). The P–Q interval reflects a pause during which the electrical impulse travels from the atria to the ventricles through the atrioventricular junction and bundle of His. The QRS deflection indicates ventricular electrical activity. The S–T interval reflects the delay between depolarization and repolarization. The T-wave results from ventricular repolarization.

Because electrical activity begins in the sinus node and progresses through the atria and then the ventricles, the normal electrocardiogram is characterized by a P-wave followed by a QRS complex and then a T-wave. If the atria and ventricles are beating (contracting) asynchronously (as in complete atrioventricular block) the P-wave and QRS complexes are dissociated.

The morphology of the P-wave and QRS complex is affected by the thickness of the respective chambers and by the exact route by which myocardial depolarization occurs. Thus the electrocardiogram is useful for detecting enlargement of cardiac chambers and determining whether the sequence of electrical conduction through the heart is normal. Interpretation of electrocardiograms is complex and requires special training and experience. A few common arrythmias are presented in Fig. 35-5.

Because the heart is a three-dimensional structure, its electrical activation is also three-dimensional. Unlike the electrocardiogram, which reflects electrical activity in only one physical plane (plus time), the *vectorcardiogram* reflects electrical activation of the heart in three dimensions (plus time). The vectorcardiogram can reflect cardiac chamber enlargement in instances when the electrocardiographic assessment is indefinite.

The *phonocardiogram* (Fig. 35-6) is recorded using a microphone placed on the child's chest. The heart sounds are recorded on a strip-chart recorder. Combined with a simultaneously obtained electrocardiogram and carotid pulse

Normal Electrocardiographic Findings

Rate The number of beats per minute depends on oxygen needs and electrophysiologic function. The normal range varies with age.

Regularity The interval between beats (R–R interval) should be consistent.

Association between P-wave and QRS complex The P-wave should precede each QRS complex, and the P–R interval should be consistent.

Configuration of P-wave, QRS complex, and T-wave Configuration should be consistent for each.

TABLE 35-3 Cardiographic Studies

Study	Purpose	Procedure	Nursing management
Electrocardiogram (ECG)	Measure electrical activity of heart in one dimension (plus time) to detect arrhythmias, cardiomegaly, myocardial hypertrophy	Electrodes attached to arms, legs, chest. Electrical activity recorded on graph	Explain procedure to the child. Instruct child to remain still during procedure. Allow child to "play ECG" with doll. Clean off electrode jelly after procedure
Vectorcardiogram	Measure electrical activity of heart in three dimensions (plus time) to detect changes relative to altered conduction (arrhythmias, cardiomegaly)	Same as for ECG	Same as for ECG
Phonocardiogram	Obtain visual image of heart sounds and, in combination with ECG, timing of cardiac events	Microphone or transducer moved over chest. Pattern of heart sounds recorded on strip-chart graph	Explain procedure to child. Instruct child to remain still and quiet during procedure. Allow child to "play phonocardiogram" with doll. Practice procedure ahead of time
Echocardiogram	Visualize cardiac structures by recording sound waves bounced off of them	Same as for phonocardiogram	Same as for phonocardiogram
Radiography	See cardiac structures to detect abnormalities and distinguish cardiac from pulmonary disease. Assess volume of pulmonary blood flow. Detect (with barium) aberrant blood vessels around esophagus	Standard anteroposterior and lateral views taken of chest Barium esophagogram	Describe room and equipment to child. Explain procedure to child. Remain with child if appropriate (see Chapter 29). Instruct child to remain still while radiographs taken. Explain use of barium and need to drink special liquid, lie on table that will tilt, probability of white bowel movements due to barium
Radioisotope scanning	Visualize anatomy and hemodynamics in cardiac structures. Measure left ventricular ejection and chamber volume	Isotope injected intravenously. Scanner detects and records isotope distribution on chart	Explain procedure and equipment to child. Prepare child for insertion of intravenous line
Cardiac catheterization	Measure oxygen saturation and pressures in cardiac chambers and major vessels. Measure direction and volume of blood flow. Assess anatomy of cardiac structures. Assess electrophysiologic function of the heart	Cardiac catheter introduced into femoral or brachial vessel and advanced to the heart. Catheter guided into cardiac chambers and major vessels (visualized by fluoroscopy). Pressure and oxygen saturation measured at various points. Radiopaque dye injected into catheter. Blood flow visualized by fluoroscopy; radiographs taken at selected times. Balloon septostomy may be done during procedure	Obtain history and perform physical assessment prior to procedure. Explain procedure to child and parent. Obtain baseline vital signs. Document pulses distal to catheter site. Keep child NPO 4–6 hours prior to procedure. Withhold digoxin, as ordered. After procedure, monitor for signs of complications (arrhythmias, hemorrhage, infection, impaired circulation, adverse reaction to dye or medication, dehydration) Encourage fluids once fully awake (about 1–2 hours after procedure). Keep involved extremity straight and relatively immobile for approximately 6 hours. Prepare the child and family for discharge, if appropriate

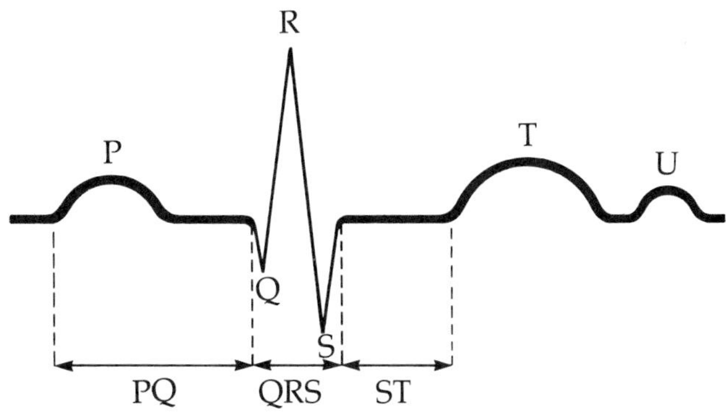

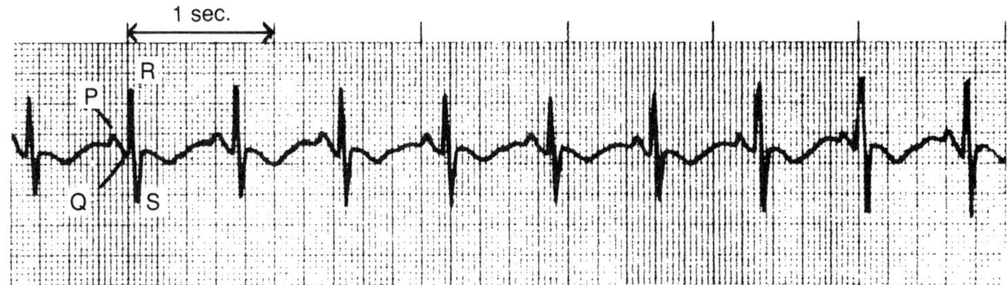

Figure 35-4 Normal electrocardiogram.

tracing, a phonocardiogram can measure time intervals between important cardiac events.

Echocardiography is a technique of visualizing cardiac anatomy by recording sound waves reflected from cardiac structures. Sound is beamed through the heart, and sound beams reflected from cardiac structures are recorded. There are two basic types of echocardiography: (1) M-mode and (2) two-dimensional (sector) echocardiography. M-mode echocardiography records only a very narrow beam of sound activity, which limits the structures that can be visualized. Two-dimensional (sector) echocardiography, as the term implies, allows the clinician to visualize cardiac structures in two dimensions (plus time). This technique provides much better definition of intracardiac structures than M-mode echocardiography.

Radiography of the chest is an important part of the assessment of infants and children with heart disease. In some cases the chest radiograph enables the physician to distinguish between primary pulmonary disease and heart disease. The radiograph is a relatively accurate and reproducible representation of cardiac size and configuration. An assessment of the volume of pulmonary blood flow can be made from the appearance of pulmonary vessels in a standard anteroposterior chest radiograph. A radiograph, combined with a barium esophagogram, can be used to detect any aberrant vascular structures that impinge on the esophagus.

Radioactive tracers use radioisotope techniques to define intracardiac anatomy, including shunts and anatomic details, and cardiac function such as hemodynamic measurements. Left ventricular ejection-fraction and chamber volume can be determined relatively easily and reproducibly by using these techniques. In addition, pulmonary blood flow can be mapped and alterations detected.

Cardiac catheterization is an invasive procedure. A cardiac catheter is introduced into a large vessel and advanced into the heart. The catheter may be inserted into a vein (usually femoral), advanced to the inferior vena cava for right heart examination or into an artery (femoral or brachial) and then advanced into the descending aorta or subclavian artery for left heart examination. The catheter may be inserted through a small incision in the vessel (cutdown) or through a large-bore needle inserted in the vessel through the skin. The procedure is done in a room equipped for fluoroscopic visualization. If the child has a septal defect, the catheter may be passed through the defect from the right ventricle to the left or vice versa. A radiopaque dye injected through the catheter aids in fluoroscopic visualization of cardiac structure and direction of blood flow. Cardiac catheterization provides data about

- Oxygen saturation in various cardiac chambers and major vessels
- Pressure levels in cardiac chambers and major vessels
- Direction and volume of blood flow
- Anatomy of the heart and vessels
- Electrophysiologic function of the heart

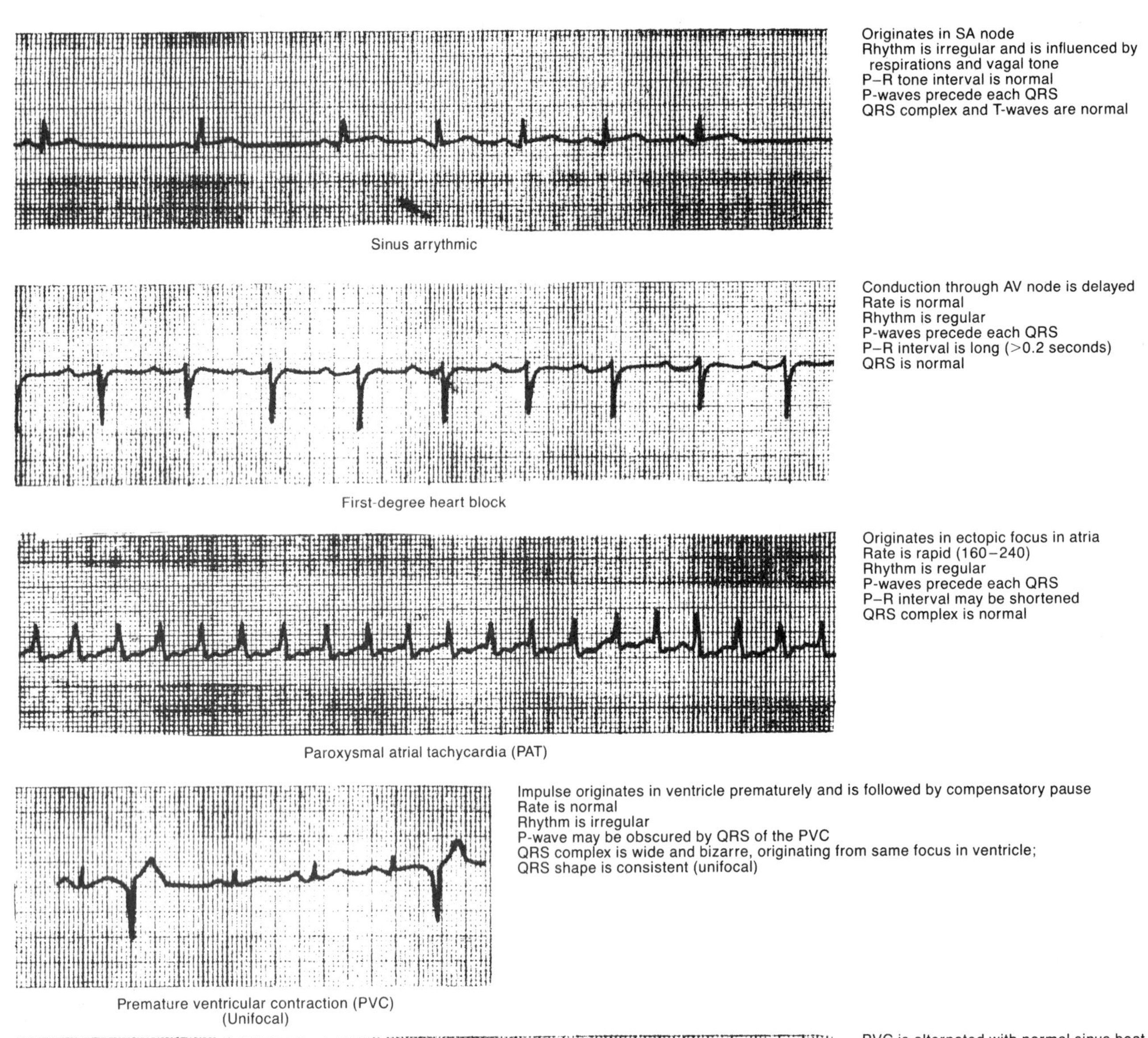

Figure 35-5 Abnormal electrocardiograms.

The cardiologist synthesizes this information in assessing cardiac structure and function. Other special procedures, some of which may be life-saving (for example, Rashkind balloon septostomy), may be performed during catheterization.

Cardiac catheterization is necessary to diagnose accurately many types of congenital cardiac defects. With the availability of echocardiography, however, the role of cardiac catheterization is diminishing.Cardiac catheterization involves risks. Occasionally, the blood vessel used to introduce the catheter becomes occluded. If a blood clot (embolus) forms on the tip of a catheter and dislodges, it can travel to the brain, causing a stroke. The incidence mortality associated with cardiac catheterization is about 0.5%. The cardiologist therefore weighs the risks of cardiac catheterization against its benefits before proceeding.

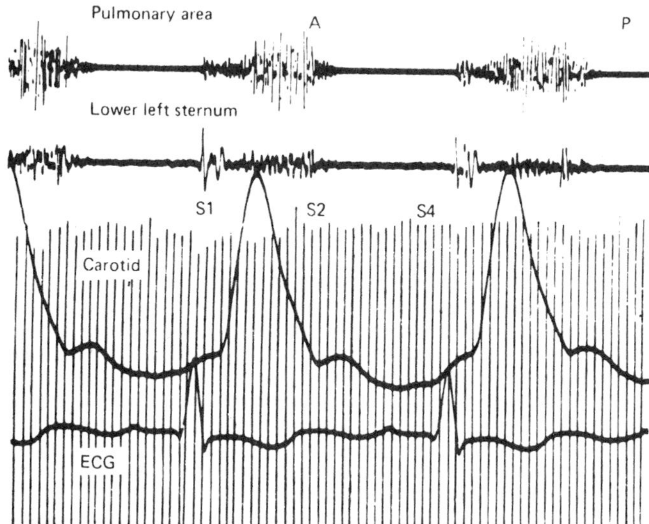

Figure 35-6 Phonocardiogram.

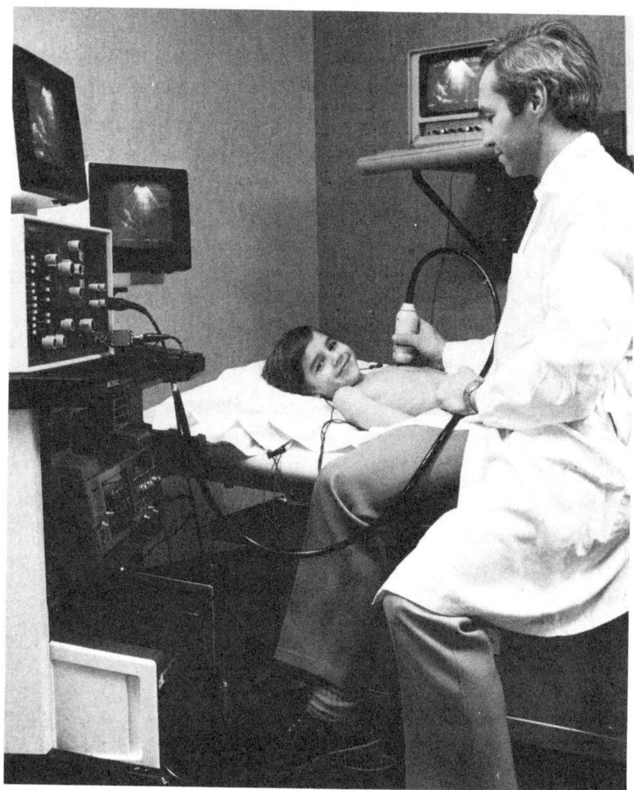

Echocardiography. (Photograph courtesy of the Mayo Clinic, Rochester, Minnesota.)

Nursing Management for Procedures and Treatments

Preparation for Diagnostic Tests

Children with heart disease are subjected to many laboratory studies. The experience may be new or familiar to the child, but either way, it frequently creates considerable anxiety. The procedures and equipment often are frightening, so that preparation of the child for the procedure and support during and after the procedure are primary nursing responsibilities (see Chapter 29).

Blood Tests The nurse observes for bleeding or bruising after blood is withdrawn. If an arterial sample is obtained, the nurse applies direct pressure to the site for at least 5 minutes, and longer if bleeding persists. To prevent the trauma of repeated tests, the nurse handles specimens carefully and exactly according to instructions (for example, protected from exposure to air, packed in ice). If blood gases are to be measured from a capillary sample, the nurse applies a warm compress to the site for 10 minutes before collecting the sample. This procedure increases the reliability of results. Providing a syringe and a doll and letting the child perform tests on the doll may help the child to work through the experience. It also gives the nurse an opportunity to assess the child's perception of the event.

Cardiographic Studies Cardiographic studies are painless, but the equipment may be frightening to the child. The nurse informs child that

> The test will show the doctors and nurses how the heart is working. Older children may be interested in more details.
>
> The top clothing will be removed, and the helper will place jelly on the chest. This will feel cool and wet.
>
> Small round disks will be placed on the child's arms and legs. These will be connected to wires that go to the machine.
>
> A small suction cup will be placed on the chest over the jelly.
>
> The machine will make a soft noise, but it will not hurt.
>
> It is very important that the child remain still and quiet.

Practicing with the equipment ahead of time helps to diminish the child's fear during the procedure. After the procedure the jelly is cleaned off. If possible, the child should be given a chance to "play ECG" with a doll.

Preparation for a phonocardiogram and echocardiogram is similar to preparation for an electrocardiogram. In addition, a microphone or transducer is moved over the chest. It is important that the child hold still. Practicing holding still and using a pretend transducer ahead of time may alleviate anxiety and enhance cooperation.

Cardiac Catheterization A history and physical examination should be completed before cardiac catheterization. This provides baseline data and allows recognition of changes that might occur as a result of the procedure. Any sign of infection (for example, fever, cough, nasal discharge, sore throat) is reported to the physician. Infection increases the risk of the procedure considerably and is a contraindication except in an emergency.

It is often helpful to mark with ink the exact location of pulses distal to the proposed catheter-insertion site. If a femoral vessel is to be used, the posterior tibial and dorsal pedal pulses are marked. The quality and strength of the pulse also is documented, as this information makes the critical assessment of pulses after the procedure more accurate.

Usually, a complete blood count and urinalysis are done before the procedure. Clotting studies may also be indicated. To prevent aspiration, the child is generally kept NPO for 4 to 6 hours before the procedure. Digoxin is usually withheld before the procedure, although this should be clarified with the physician. The nurse also inquires about allergies to medications, especially reactions to medication or dye that may have occurred during previous catheterizations.

Cardiac catheterization is often a stressful and frightening procedure for children, and careful preparation therefore is essential (Uzark, 1978). Family members may also fear the diagnosis and prognosis that will be revealed, and this adds to their anxiety. The following important points are adapted to the situation in preparing the child and family for the procedure:

1. Assessing the child's perception of cardiac function, symptoms, reason for hospitalization, and procedures. The nurse may clarify and reinforce the child's perceptions by discussing normal cardiac function at a level appropriate to the child's cognitive level, explaining how the child's symptoms are indicators to the doctor that the heart might not be working as well as it should, explaining how the test will help the doctor know how to make the heart work better, and reassuring the child that the heart problem and the test are not anyone's fault.
2. Explaining that the child will not be able to eat or drink before the test.
3. Describing the appearance of the room where the test will be performed. Many institutions allow children and parents to visit the catheterization laboratory the day before a procedure. If this is not possible, photographs of the room are helpful. The nurse also explains how the child will get to the room.
4. Informing the child where the parent will wait during the procedure and assuring the child that the parent will return right after the test.
5. Describing how the people will be dressed. Gowns and masks can be used to demonstrate to young children that "real" people are present under the surgical clothing.
6. Explaining that the child will be on a special table that moves, that electrocardiogram leads will be placed on the arms and legs, and that, because it is very important to lie still, restraints will be placed on the arms and legs. Using a doll at this point helps to demonstrate the leads and the restraints.
7. Explaining that a cutaneous or rectal temperature probe will be used and demonstrating on a doll.
8. Demonstrating on a doll that the doctor will wash the arm or groin with special soap and will give some medicine with a small needle and that the needle will hurt a little but then there will be no more pain. It is best to save this information until the end, since anxiety about the needle may inhibit further learning.
9. Explaining that the doctor will make a small opening and will put a little tube into the arm or leg. The tube will not hurt, but the child may feel pressure as the tube is advanced. The nurse demonstrates taping of a tube to the doll's "catheter site."
10. Describing that the machine will take pictures similar to radiographs of the tube and the heart, will make noises, but will not hurt or touch the child. (As some machines take pictures, the pictures fall into a box, and this makes a loud banging noise.) When the pictures are being taken, the doctor might turn off the lights, but the room will not be completely dark. Sometimes the people go out of the room while the pictures are being taken, but they come right back in again.
11. Explaining that during the test the doctor will put some special medicine into the body. Avoid using the word *dye*, as the child may confuse this with *die*. This medicine will make the child feel hot for a short time. The child might not like this feeling, but it goes away quickly.
12. Telling the child that it is all right to go to sleep during the test and that it is OK to ask questions and talk to people when awake.
13. Demonstrating on the doll that at the end of the test the tube will be removed and a bandage placed on the site.
14. Informing the child that after the test the child will return to the hospital room and that the nurses will check pulses, blood pressure, and the bandage. An hour or so after the test, the child may have something to drink. The child will need to remain in bed for several hours (depending on the physician's order).
15. Explaining that the premedication will make the child sleepy. The nurse honestly explains that an injection is required but saves this information until shortly before the actual administration to minimize anxiety. Older children may be told ahead of time that an injection is needed.
16. Asking whether the child would like to listen to stories or music during the procedure.

Possible complications following cardiac catheterization include cardiac arrhythmias, hemorrhage (from catheter site or from cardiac perforation), infection, swelling and inflammation at the site, phlebitis, thrombus, adverse reactions to dye, and dehydration. Skilled nursing care is essential if these complications are to be recognized or avoided. Vital signs are monitored frequently, usually every 15 min-

NURSING CARE GUIDE Child After Cardiac Catheterization

Nursing diagnosis	Interventions	Evaluation
1. Potential for altered cardiac output related to cardiac arrhythmias	Monitor vital signs every 15 minutes until stable, then every 2–4 hours Observe oscilloscope of cardiac monitor Auscultate apical pulses to detect irregularities Report arrhythmias to physician	Cardiac arrhythmias do not occur. Vital signs are stable
2. Potential for altered tissue perfusion related to hemorrhage	Monitor vital signs as scheduled above Maintain pressure dressing over catheter site for 24 hours (or as ordered). Observe catheter site frequently for signs of bleeding Minimize movement of affected extremity Auscultate heart frequently, noting muffled heart sounds (i.e., tamponade) Compare 6-hour postcatheterization hematocrit with the value of the precatheterization hematocrit to determine degree of possible blood loss	Vital signs, especially pulse and blood pressure are stable. Dressing is clean, dry, and intact. Values for precatheterization and postcatheterization hematocrits are similar
3. Potential for altered skin integrity related to infection at catheter site	Protect catheter site from contamination For infants with femoral catheter site, protect pressure dressing from urine and stool with plastic tape. Change diapers often. Change dressing if contaminated with feces	Skin at catheter site remains intact and not inflamed
4. Potential for altered circulation related to obstruction	To detect weak or absent pulses, palpate pulses distal to catheter site at same frequency schedule as vital signs. Use opposite extremity for comparison If pulses weak or not palpable, use Doppler or other, similar device Assess warmth, color, and capillary refill of extremity	Involved extremity is warm; distal pulses are equal to preprocedural quality
5. Potential for fluid volume deficit	Monitor intake and output Encourage child to drink fluids once fully awake Observe for signs of dehydration (poor skin turgor, dry mucous membranes, absence of tears, sunken fontanelle) Observe and report vomiting or fluid refusal. Intravenous fluids may be required if oral intake not adequate Adjust intravenous infusion rate according to fluid intake for children with polycythemia, for whom adequate hydration is critical	Hydration status is adequate
6. Potential for discomfort	Observe for signs of pain at site (usually mild discomfort) and ask child to report pain Administer analgesics Provide comfort measures (rocking, holding, gentle touch, position change, diversion)	Pain or discomfort is minimal and relieved

continued on next page

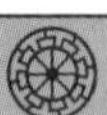

NURSING CARE GUIDE Child After Cardiac Catheterization (continued)

Nursing diagnosis	Interventions	Evaluation
7. Potential for altered functioning related to adverse reaction to dye	Monitor for adverse reactions to dye, such as increased temperature, urticaria, wheezing, edema, dyspnea, headache, tremor, nausea, vomiting	Child shows no evidence of adverse reaction
8. Potential for emotional trauma relative to catheterization	Identify fears and misperceptions Encourage child to talk about the procedure Encourage therapeutic play (see Chapter 28)	Child is able to cope positively with experience of cardiac catheterization through play or discussion
9. Potential for knowledge deficit related to home care	Teach child and family how to care for catheter site at home Allow older child to shower; give infant and young child a sponge bath for 3 days, then give tub bath Change small bandage over catheterization site daily (or more frequently as needed) for 3 days. Observe for signs of inflammation or excessive tenderness; if these are present, report to physician	Child and family demonstrate ability to care for catheter site at home

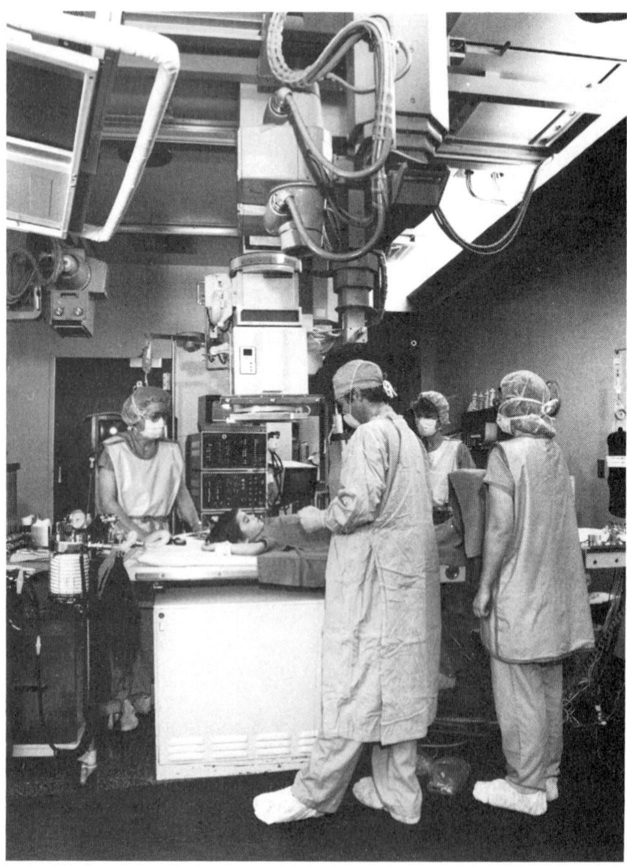

Cardiac catheterization laboratory. (Photograph courtesy of the Mayo Clinic, Rochester, Minnesota.)

utes for the first few hours then less frequently if signs are stable. Blood pressure measurements are not made on the extremity used for catheterization. Often, the child is placed on a cardiac monitor with an oscilloscope so that heart rhythm can be closely watched. Any evidence of arrhythmia (including tachycardia or bradycardia) or blood pressure change is reported to the physician immediately.

When checking vital signs, the nurse also carefully assesses circulation in the extremity used for the catheterization. Arterial spasm, thrombus formation, phlebitis, or excessive swelling at the site all may obstruct blood flow into the extremity. The nurse palpates pulses distal to the catheter site. Marking pulse sites prior to catheterization makes this easier. The opposite extremity can be used for comparison. If the pulses are not easily palpable, a Doppler device may be used to locate them. A weak or absent pulse is reported to the physician immediately. The nurse also assesses temperature, color, and capillary refill of the affected extremity. Coolness, pallor, cyanosis, swelling, and delayed capillary refill might be further indications of compromised circulation and should be reported. Wrapping the unaffected leg in a warm pack causes vasodilatation in both legs and may increase blood flow to the affected extremity. The affected extremity is not warmed, as the application of heat would increase metabolic demands at a time when circulation is already compromised. If a thrombus is present, heparin therapy, surgery, or both might be needed.

The child usually is kept in bed for several hours after the procedure to reduce the risk of bleeding or trauma at the catheter site. A pressure dressing usually is in place.

The nurse checks the site frequently for signs of bleeding, hematoma, or infection and protects the site from contamination, which can be difficult if the child with a femoral insertion wears diapers. Waterproof, clear plastic tape might be placed over the dressing to protect it from urine and feces, but the tape must not interfere with observation.

Dehydration may occur after cardiac catheterization. Not only is the child NPO before and during the procedure, but also nausea and vomiting are common side effects of both the premedication and the dye, which may further limit intake and increase fluid loss. Additionally, the dye used is hyperosmotic and might cause hyperosmotic diuresis because large amounts of urine are needed to excrete the solute contained in the dye. Following catheterization, the nurse assesses the child's hydration status carefully. Intake, output, skin turgor, moistness of mucous membranes, and weight are monitored. Specific gravity of the urine is not useful, as abnormally high specific gravities are common because of the excretion of the dye. As soon as the child is fully awake, oral fluids are encouraged to maintain hydration and aid in the excretion of the dye. If the child is unable to tolerate oral fluids, intravenous therapy may be indicated.

Adverse reactions to the dye include elevated temperature, urticaria, wheezing, edema, dyspnea, headache, tremor, nausea, and vomiting. These are reported to the physician. Anaphylaxis, flushing, dizziness, and hypotension generally occur shortly after the dye is administered and are problems during but not after the procedure.

Children are often frightened after cardiac catheterization. They are awake but often groggy during the procedure. They hear comments by the staff that they may not understand. The sounds, sights, and somatic sensations might be scary, and misperceptions are common. After the procedure, nurses need to provide opportunities for children to talk about their perceptions of the procedure. Therapeutic play in the presence of a familiar and trusted nurse therefore should be a routine postprocedure intervention (see Chapter 28).

Monitoring Devices

Cardiac Monitor Cardiac monitors are often used for ongoing assessment of cardiac rhythm and rate. Monitors vary in type from those that simply measure heart rate to those that provide a continuous visual electrocardiographic display on an oscilloscope. If cardiac arrhythmias are an actual or potential problem, a monitor with continuous oscilloscope display and printout capabilities is most helpful. The printout provides a permanent record of the arrythmia. It is essential that any electrical equipment be properly grounded.

Electrode pads are applied for a specific lead pattern. Right arm, right leg, and left leg is a commonly used lead II pattern. The electrodes must be applied carefully to ensure a clear tracing of cardiac rhythm. Electrode pads are changed every 1–2 days or more often if necessary to prevent skin irritation and breakdown. Some electrode pads are premoistened with jelly, and others require that electrode jelly be applied directly. If the oscilloscope picture is unclear, the electrode pads and all connections should be rechecked. Upper and lower pulse limits should be set according to the child's age and condition. If the child's pulse exceeds the upper limit or drops below the lower limit, an alarm sounds. With some monitors, a printout is obtained automatically if the alarm is triggered. It is essential that the alarm be set at all times unless a professional is actually at the bedside evaluating the child directly.

When an alarm sounds, the nurse quickly observes the rhythm tracing on the oscilloscope and assesses the child directly. Often, the alarm results from a mechanical problem, such as a loose electrode pad or loose wire, rather than an arrhythmia, but it is important to assess the child directly to make this determination. If an arrhythmia is present, a permanent tracing is obtained and the nurse assesses the child's color, respiratory rate and effort, changes in sensorium, position, activity, precipitating factors, and anxiety. Depending on the child's condition and the nature of the arrythmia, the physician might have to be notified.

The child and family should receive an explanation of the monitor's basic function and sounds. It is important that they know what the alarm sounds like before it goes off unexpectedly. They should understand that the alarm does not necessarily mean that the child is in danger and that a nurse will always respond immediately if the alarm sounds.

Occasionally, anxious children or parents may focus all concerns on the monitor and feel that they must personally

Procedure for Evaluating an Electrocardiogram

1. Calculate ventricular rate. Count the number of R-waves in a 6-inch strip and multiply by 10.
2. Note regularity of R-waves (R–R interval). If they occur regularly, with variance less than 0.12 seconds (3 small squares), the ventricular rhythm is normal.
3. Examine P-waves. Calculate atrial rate. If P with consistent contour waves precede each QRS complex, then a sinus rhythm probably exists.
4. Measure P–R interval. Normally P–R interval is 0.08–0.20 seconds. A longer P–R interval indicates a delay in conduction between the atria and ventricles.
5. Measure QRS complex. It is normally less than 0.12 seconds. Wider QRS complexes may indicate an intraventricular conduction defect.
6. Examine T-waves. Tall, tented T-waves may indicate hyperkalemia.

observe the rate and rhythm. In some cases, this represents a lack of trust in the staff. More often, however, it is an attempt by parents to alleviate a feeling of powerlessness by "doing something." The nurse who recognizes monitor watching as symptomatic of a deeper issue, such as lack of trust or a sense of powerlessness, can address that issue.

Sometimes a child or parent becomes somewhat dependent on the monitor. The continuous audible pulse provides a certain sense of reassurance, as does the prompt response of the staff to the alarm. Anxiety may result when the monitoring is discontinued, and the parent may fear that an arrythmia will be missed. A thorough discussion of the rationale for discontinuation usually reduces such worries.

Holter Monitor A Holter monitor, which is worn by the child, provides a continuous electroradiographic recording for 12–24 hours. Sporadic arrhythmias that might not be detected during a regular electrocardiogram may be identified as the child proceeds with usual activities. Electrode leads are placed on the child's chest and arms and connected to the small recorder or transmitter, which is held in place by a harness the child wears.

Principles of Nursing Care

Acute-Care Needs

Children with heart disease need careful ongoing assessment. The condition of a child with serious heart disease can change rapidly, and the nurse therefore needs to recognize such changes quickly.

Minimizing Cardiac Workload The body's demands for oxygen directly affect cardiac workload. Therefore, a major nursing goal in caring for a child with cardiac disease is to minimize the oxygen needs of the body (Pidgeon, 1967).

Providing Adequate Rest Since oxygen consumption is generally lowest when the body is at rest, nursing care is organized so that the child's rest is disturbed as little as possible. Each time the child is stressed by interventions and procedures (that is, bath, turning, and assessment of vital signs), oxygen needs increase. Care is organized after careful assessment of the child's tolerance of procedures. Some children can tolerate several interventions or procedures at one time. This allows longer periods of uninterrupted rest. Other children show signs of distress (increased pulse and respiration, dyspnea, increased cyanosis) with even brief disruptions of rest. For these critically ill children, each activity (for example, turning, eating, voiding) is alternated with rest periods to allow time for recovery. Optional activities, such as complete baths and changes of linen, may be deferred until the child's condition improves. Besides tolerance, the nurse determines the child's usual wake-sleep pattern. Scheduling meals, naps, and procedures to coincide with the child's usual sleep pattern reduces stress and facilitates rest.

Interruption of rest periods should be avoided. The nurse might need to remind other members of the health care team of the child's need for undisturbed rest, and often works with them to plan necessary activities accordingly.

If the child's rest is disturbed by irritability and restlessness not relieved by comfort measures, the physician might prescribe a sedative. Morphine sulfate is usually the drug of choice. Before administering the sedative, the nurse rules out hypoxia as the cause of the child's restlessness and irritability. Once the sedative is administered, it will mask these symptoms, so the nurse needs to be alert for other signs of hypoxia in the sedated child. The nurse also assesses respiratory rate, as respiratory depression is an adverse effect of sedation.

Anticipating the Child's Needs Anticipating the child's needs prevents unnecessary crying and frustration. The stress of crying increases oxygen demands and wastes limited energy. While it is probably impossible to prevent crying entirely in infancy or early childhood, the frequency and intensity of crying episodes can be reduced by careful attention to the child's needs for food, water, comfort, holding, and stimulation. For example, an infant is fed as soon as hunger cues (such as sucking on fists or restlessness) are noted. For older children, the nurse can place items they are likely to need within easy reach. This prevents exertion and frustration on the part of the child. Call lights are answered promptly. This approach is helpful in reducing the energy expenditure in an acutely ill child but must be tapered as the child's condition improves.

Minimizing Anxiety Anxiety stimulates the sympathetic nervous system and results in increased cardiac work. While elimination of all anxiety is neither possible nor desirable, reduction of excessive and unnecessary anxiety is important in the care of the child with heart disease. The nurse needs to be alert for both verbal and nonverbal signs of anxiety. Careful assessment as to the cause of anxiety is necessary if anxiety is to be reduced. (Reactions to hospitalization are discussed in Chapter 27. Parent–child teaching to minimize anxiety is discussed in Chapter 29.)

The nurse needs to be sensitive to spoken and unspoken concerns and answer questions that the child or parents have as clearly and honestly as possible. For questions that are best answered by the physician, the nurse can help the family to formulate and present these questions.

Monitoring Activity Level and Exercise Tolerance Because exercise tolerance is an important measurement in assessment of cardiac function, the nurse monitors the child's activity level to assess the physiologic and psychologic response to activity or its limitation. Many children with heart disease do well at regulating their own activities. These children are sensitive to internal cues that indicate the need to rest. Such children usually do not need external restrictions on activity, but the nurse continues to monitor their response to activity and notes evidence of exercise intolerance.

Other children do need external controls to limit activity. In some types of heart disease, there are medical indications for restricted activity even though activity does not produce symptoms, and it may be hard for the child to understand the importance of rest if play activities cause no distress. Other children might persist in activity to the point of distress and beyond. They seem unable to regulate activity in response to internal cues. In an older child, persistent activity might be a form of denial or an effort to prove that "everything is OK."

Children who are unable to follow activity restrictions need a clear, age-appropriate explanation of why restrictions are necessary. They also need to be told exactly what their limits are, and these limits need to be enforced consistently. Allowing the child to express or "play out" frustration and anxiety related to activity restrictions is helpful. (Therapeutic play is discussed in Chapter 28.) If the child seems to be using persistent activity as a form of denial, basic anxiety about the physical condition must be addressed. It is important to plan quiet activities with children to keep them occupied and stimulated while at rest. It also is important to remember that the imposition of activity restrictions on a child who is normally active does not necessarily reduce cardiac workload. Sometimes the frustration of imposed bed rest creates more work for the heart than limited out-of-bed activity. Therefore, the nurse assesses each child individually and discusses appropriate activity limitations with the physician.

Preventing Hyperthermia and Hypothermia Both hyperthermia and hypothermia increase the body's need for oxygen. If the child is in an insufficiently warm environment, metabolic rate increases to produce heat and maintain body temperature. Increased metabolism requires increased oxygen, and the heart must work harder to meet this demand. If the heart and lungs are unable to provide the additional oxygen, anaerobic metabolism with resultant metabolic acidosis might occur.

Infants are particularly susceptible to heat loss. (Temperature regulation in high-risk infants is discussed in Chapter 31.) Changes in temperature may be subtle and may occur undetected over an extended period. Young infants are best placed in isolettes, where they may be kept warm yet closely observed. Older infants and children should be appropriately dressed, and their rooms should be kept warm. The child's bed or play area should not be near cold external walls or windows. Heat loss by evaporation can be minimized by uncovering only one body part at a time during the bath and drying it thoroughly. Wet linen must be changed promptly.

Fever also increases metabolic rate and the need for oxygen. As a rule of thumb, the heart rate increases 10 beats per minute for each degree of temperature over 99. Therefore, fever can have a significant impact on a circulatory system that already is compromised. The child's temperature therefore should be monitored on a regular basis, and in cases of fever, antipyretics, such as acetaminophen, are used. Sponge baths with tepid water may be helpful, but it is important to avoid chilling.

Facilitating Elimination of Excess Fluid and Sodium *Preload reduction* refers to reducing the workload of the heart by eliminating excess sodium and fluid, which increase the circulating blood volume. This most commonly is accomplished with diuretics. Intake of excessive sodium (salty foods) is avoided, and a low-sodium diet may be necessary. Restrictions on oral intake of fluid usually are not needed, except for severe heart failure. Dehydration must be avoided, especially in children with polycythemia.

Diuretics vary in their action, therapeutic effects, side effects, and adverse reactions. The nurse therefore needs to be familiar with specific types of diuretics to monitor their effects and the child's tolerance. Excessive fluid loss and electrolyte imbalances are possible consequences of diuretic therapy. Furosemide and the thiazides promote the excretion of potassium and potassium supplements often are indicated. Spironolactone, which spares potassium from excretion, may be used in conjunction with thiazide. Excessive potassium loss is a particularly serious problem in children who take digitalis, because hypokalemia enhances the effect of digitalis and may cause toxicity. The most commonly used diuretics are summarized in Table 35-4.

Minimizing Resistance to Cardiac Outflow *Afterload reduction* refers to reducing the work of the heart by decreasing resistance in the systemic circulation. This is accomplished by administering vasodilators and antihypertensives. Commonly used agents are summarized in Table 35-5. These are potent medications, and the nurse needs to be alert for serious side effects, especially hypotension. Blood pressure is monitored closely (every 30 minutes) after administration of the drug. Expected therapeutic effects are decreased pulse and decreased respiratory rate and effort.

Facilitating Cardiac Function Myocardial function is enhanced by digitalis, a cardiac glycoside that increases myocardial contractility, decreases the rate of contractions, slows conduction through the atrioventricular node, and promotes diuresis because of increased blood flow through the kidneys. Effective digitalis therapy results in an increase

TABLE 35-4 Diuretics Used in Congenital Heart Disease

Drug	Side effects	Nursing implications
Furosemide (Lasix) Potent, rapid-acting	Electrolyte imbalance (especially hypokalemia), dehydration, hypotension, nausea, vomiting, diarrhea, dermatitis, ototoxicity	Monitor blood pressure. Monitor fluid intake and output. Weigh child daily. Encourage foods high in potassium or give potassium supplements
Chlorothiazide sodium (Diuril) Inhibits sodium and potassium reabsorption in renal tubule	Nausea, weakness, dizziness, paresthesias, cramps, rash, hypokalemia, metabolic alkalosis, thrombocytopenia	Encourage foods high in potassium. Monitor fluid intake and output. Schedule doses to avoid nocturia. Inspect skin and mucous membranes for petechiae. Discontinue 48 hours before surgery
Spironolactone (Aldactone) Potassium-sparing, promotes sodium excretion Often used in conjunction with thiazides	Lethargy, headache, drowsiness, cramps, nausea, vomiting, hyperkalemia, rash, ataxia, impotence, hyponatremia	Monitor intake and output. Monitor for hyponatremia and hyperkalemia

TABLE 35-5 Medications for Afterload Reduction: Vasodilators

Drug	Side effects	Nursing implications
Tolazoline hydrochloride (Priscoline)	Nausea, vomiting, gastric irritation, hypotension, hypertension, tachycardia, other cardiac arrhythmias, tingling	Give with meals or with milk to reduce gastric irritation. Check pulse and blood pressure regularly, $\frac{1}{2}$–$1\frac{1}{2}$ hr after oral administration. Check pulse and blood pressure more frequently with IV administration, starting 15 min after dose is given. Caution child about postural hypotension and assist child as needed
Prazosin hydrochloride (Minipress)	Dizziness, headache, drowsiness, tachycardia, syncope, hypotension, vomiting, diarrhea, constipation, rash, urinary frequency, impotence	Monitor pulse and blood pressure carefully after administration (peak action 2–4 hr). Caution child to change positions slowly and avoid situations where injury could occur due to syncope. Assist child as needed
Sodium nitroprusside (Nipride)	Hypotension, mild decrease in cardiac output, nausea, retching, increase or decrease in pulse rate, restlessness, agitation, muscle twitching, rash	Give by IV route only. Use infusion pump to ensure precise control of rate. Monitor pulse and blood pressure vigilantly. Monitor intake and output

in cardiac output and a reduction in heart size, venous pressure, edema, and liver size (Meissner and Gever, 1980).

There are two commonly used preparations, digoxin and digitoxin. Digoxin is used almost exclusively in children because its onset of action is more rapid than that of digitoxin, and its rapid rate of excretion reduces the risk of toxicity. Digoxin may be given orally, intravenously, or intramuscularly. Oral preparations include a sweet-flavored elixir for infants and younger children and tablets for older children and adolescents.

Initiation of therapy is termed *digitalization*. Loading doses of the drug are given at 6- to 8-hour intervals to achieve therapeutic levels. After therapeutic levels have been reached, a maintenance dose is given every 12 hours (Table 35-6). Serum levels are checked, and the range of serum levels considered to be therapeutic is 1.7–2.0 mg/mL.

Digoxin is a potent medication with a relatively narrow therapeutic range. Fisch (1971) states that "The margin of safety between the therapeutic and toxic and the toxic and lethal dose is relatively narrow. It has been estimated that when the desired therapeutic response is attained, 60 percent of the toxic dose has been administered; and when toxic reaction is manifested, approximately 50 percent of the lethal dose is ingested." For this reason, the utmost care is required when calculating and preparing dosages. An error in decimal placement could result in administration of a lethal dose. Institutions often have special policies for safe administration of the drug.

TABLE 35-6 Digoxin Dosages

Objective	Oral administration	Intravenous or Intramuscular administration	Schedule
Digitalization (dose per 24 hr)	0.06–0.08 mg/kg	0.03–0.06 mg/kg	Initial dose: 50% of 24-hr total Second dose: 25% 6–8 hr later* Third dose: 25% 6–8 hr after second dose
Maintenance (dose per 24 hr)	20–25% of digitalization dose	10–20% of digitalization dose	Divided equally into two doses: one dose given every 12 hr

*Electrocardiograph is assessed before each dose is given. Ideally, cardiac monitor is in place during entire procedure.

Digitalis toxicity is a serious complication. Careful observation for signs of digitalis toxicity is important for all children on this drug. Toxicity may occur at any time during therapy, but it is most likely to occur during digitalization, when dosage is being adjusted, or in the presence of hypokalemia.

Signs of digitalis toxicity may be manifested in different organ systems. Cardiac manifestations include bradycardia, pulse deficit (apical pulse by auscultation greater than palpated radial pulse), and arrhythmias. The nurse checks both apical and radial pulses for a full minute prior to administration of the drug. If the apical pulse is abnormally slow or if a pulse deficit is present, the drug is withheld, and the physician is notified. The apical rate requiring that the drug be withheld is not absolute, but varies according to the child's age and apical rate prior to digitalization. If the pulse rate is significantly lower than previous rates or if there is a progressive downward trend over time, the dose is withheld pending specific orders from the physician. Usually, the child is on a cardiac monitor when therapy is initiated. A prolonged P–R interval (signaling first-degree heart block) and sinus bradycardia are both early signs of toxicity. Premature ventricular contractions, varying degrees of heart block, and ventricular tachycardia are other electrocardiographic changes associated with toxicity.

Anorexia, nausea, and vomiting are among the earliest manifestations of toxicity. Although vomiting for other reasons is not uncommon in children, especially infants, its occurrence should always raise suspicion of toxicity and be reported to the physician.

Neurologic manifestations of toxicity include headache, drowsiness, insomnia, dizziness, and confusion. Such visual disturbances as halos around objects, glittering spots, variations in color perception, and reading difficulty may occur. Young children have difficulty describing these symptoms; hence, they may go undetected. Older children are usually more reliable in their descriptions.

Hypokalemia enhances the effect of digitalis and increases the risk of toxicity. A dose that is correct in normal circumstances can cause toxicity in the presence of hypokalemia. Potassium depletion occurs as a result of the following:

1. Inadequate intake—administration of an intravenous fluid that does not contain added potassium, limited intake of nutrients
2. Excessive losses—diuretic therapy, diarrhea, vomiting, nasogastric suction without potassium replacement, hyperglycemic diuresis, corticosteroid therapy
3. Shift of intracellular fluid (K^+) to replace extracellular fluid (Na^+) loss—metabolic alkalosis

If the child is receiving a potassium supplement, the nurse ensures that it is taken as prescribed. Serum potassium levels are checked; the physician is notified; and digoxin is withheld if there is laboratory evidence of hypokalemia. Clinical signs of potassium depletion include muscle weakness, hyporeflexia, ileus, apathy, drowsiness, irritability, and fatigue. Electrocardiographic changes include prolonged Q–T interval, a widening and lowering of T-waves, and depression of the S–T segment.

Facilitating Effective Respiration Alveolar gas exchange is often impaired in children with heart disease because of alterations in pulmonary blood flow, pulmonary congestion, or both. A major nursing goal is to facilitate optimal gas exchange (see Chapter 34).

Positioning Placing the child in a semi-Fowler's position prevents abdominal organs from exerting pressure on the diaphragm and allows greater expansion of the lungs. An infant seat or car seat may be used to maintain an infant in this position. If the infant is in an isolette, one end of the platform can be raised. A padded sandbag placed under the buttocks and thighs helps to maintain the child in position when the platform is slanted.

Pressure on the chest wall is avoided. Clothing should be loose and nonrestrictive. Arms should be placed at the child's side and not over the chest. Restrictive or binding chest dressings should be avoided.

Oxygen Therapy Supplemental oxygen may be used to improve tissue oxygenation. The oxygen is warmed to prevent chilling and humidified to prevent drying of the mucous membranes. Oxygen concentration is monitored carefully. Supplemental oxygen is not always beneficial for the child with heart disease. If it is given for a trial period, the nurse carefully documents its effect on the child's color, vital signs, respiratory effort, and comfort.

Humidification Humidification without oxygen may help liquify secretions. When using mist therapy, the nurse keeps clothing and bedding dry to prevent chilling.

Suctioning Suctioning may be necessary to keep the airway clear, especially if there is pulmonary edema. Additional oxygen is administered before and after tracheal suctioning. Suctioning is stressful for the child and causes discomfort, hypoxia, fatigue, and irritation to the mucosa. Stimulation of the vagus nerve during suctioning can cause bradycardia. Careful auscultation of breath sounds before and after suctioning is important in assessing the effectiveness of the procedure. Excessive suctioning should be avoided. The nurse judges in each instance whether the benefit of suctioning is worth the disadvantages.

Chest Physiotherapy Chest physiotherapy may be helpful to the child with pulmonary complications of cardiac disease (see Chapter 34). The full procedure, which includes postural drainage, percussion, and vibration, is very exhausting. In children with heart disease, only a few positions usually are used per session, and to prevent fatigue, postural drainage might not be included. The nurse uses data from auscultation of the lungs and recent radiographic reports in deciding which areas of the lung to percuss. The nurse also carefully monitors the child's tolerance of the procedure and discusses signs of distress with the physician. The benefits of chest physiotherapy must be weighed against the stress it causes. Modifications, such as more frequent but shorter sessions, might be needed.

Bronchodilators Bronchodilators (mainly xanthines, such as aminophylline) may be prescribed to improve ventilation of the lungs. The nurse needs to be familiar with these powerful drugs and monitors their effects on the cardiac, pulmonary, and central nervous systems. Cardiovascular effects of the xanthines include myocardial stimulation, tachycardia, hypotension, palpitations, and arrhythmias (extrasystoles). In addition, xanthines can increase the potential toxicity of digitalis preparations. For these reasons, bronchodilators are used cautiously and with careful monitoring in children with heart disease.

Maintaining Fluid Balance Proper fluid balance is of critical importance to the child with heart disease. Excess fluid causes additional work for the heart. Dehydration is a serious condition for all children, but it is especially serious for children with cyanotic heart disease. If the child also has polycythemia, dehydration further increases the viscosity of the blood and increases the risk of thrombus formation and stroke.

Fluid intake and output are accurately measured and recorded for all children hospitalized with cardiac disease (see Chapter 29). Parents and children must be instructed in the importance of notifying the nurse or self-recording all intake and output.

The nurse carefully compares the intake and output at regular intervals and notes excessive or inadequate fluid intake. Disparity between fluid ingested and urine excreted is reported to the physician. Decreased urine output (in relation to intake) might indicate fluid retention. Increased urine output might be a positive response to diuretic therapy but, if excessive, can cause dehydration.

Weight is one of the most reliable indicators of fluid balance and is measured at least daily for all children hospitalized with heart disease. Increased weight may indicate fluid retention, worsening of congestive heart failure, and poor perfusion of the kidneys. Decreased weight may indicate inadequate intake or diuresis in response to therapy.

Other clinical indicators of fluid balance are assessed on a regular basis. The nurse observes for moistness of the mucous membranes, tension of the fontanelle, the presence of edema or ascites, and the presence or absence of tears in infants older than 6 weeks.

Fluid restrictions may be required in congestive heart failure. (Interventions related to oral fluid restriction are discussed in Chapter 29). Intravenous fluids also must be administered carefully (see Chapter 33). Infusion pumps or burettes should be used for accurate measurement of fluids. Great caution must be taken to prevent excess fluid administration, which may cause circulatory overload.

It is critical to avoid introducing air emboli and particulate matter intravenously in a child with a right-to-left shunt. In a right-to-left shunt, a portion of the venous blood shunts directly to the left heart and systemic circulation without passing through the lungs, where air emboli normally are absorbed and particulate matter is filtered. Therefore, air emboli clots, bacteria, and particulate matter may travel directly to the brain or other organ, causing infarction, infection, and tissue damage.

Preventing Infection Children with heart disease are at special risk for respiratory infections and bacterial endocarditis. Nursing goals related to infection include preventing exposure to and early detection of infections.

Respiratory Infections Altered pulmonary blood flow and pulmonary congestion make the child with some forms of heart disease more susceptible to lower respiratory infections. Recurrent pneumonia is one of the common symptoms of congenital heart disease (see Chapter 34). Respiratory syncytial virus (RSV) is one of the more frequent causes of acute lower respiratory infections in infants and young children. Research by MacDonald (1982) and associates compared the effect of RSV infection on infants with congenital heart disease to infants without heart disease. Results indicate that infants with congenital heart disease had significantly more severe disease than infants without heart disease and require intensive care and assisted ventilation more frequently.

When RSV infection is prevalent in the community, elective admission of children with heart disease therefore should be avoided. Hospital personnel must be aware of the significant risks that respiratory infection presents to these children. When in the hospital, exposure to staff, patients, or visitors with respiratory infections must be avoided. Clearly, children with heart disease cannot share rooms with children who have respiratory infections. Correct hand washing is essential, as contaminated hands are one of the major sources of inoculation. If children with active respiratory infections are present, strict isolation procedures must be employed according to hospital policy.

The nurse needs to be alert for early signs and symptoms of respiratory infection. Rhinorrhea, cough, fever, sore throat, rales, and rhonchi should be reported to the physician promptly so that appropriate evaluation and therapy may be initiated. When antibiotics are used for treatment of bacterial infection or prevention of secondary bacterial invasion, they are administered at equally divided intervals to ensure constant therapeutic serum levels.

Bacterial Endocarditis Children with congenital heart disease and rheumatic heart disease are at risk for developing bacterial endocarditis, an infection of the valves and inner lining (endocardium) of the heart. Endocarditis occurs most frequently in children with bicuspid aortic valve, patent ductus arteriosus, coarctation of the aorta, ventricular septal defects, tetralogy of Fallot, and aortic stenosis. Endocarditis usually occurs as a sequela to bacteremia, which may result from dental work; any manipulation of the genitourinary tract (including catheterization), gastrointestinal, or respiratory tracts; prolonged intravenous infusion; cardiac catheterization and surgery; and childbirth. It is also associated with infectious disease such as tonsillitis, pneumonia, and pyoderma.

Susceptible children generally are treated with prophylactic antibiotics before and after invasive procedures and during febrile illness. Parents must be educated about the importance of prophylaxis and the necessity of informing dentists and other health professionals of the child's increased risk status.

Signs and symptoms of bacterial endocarditis include unexplained fever, chills, lethargy, petechiae, splenomegaly, and congestive heart failure and are reported to the physician promptly. Early treatment is important if cardiac damage is to be minimized and complications (for example, emboli to various organs, brain abscess) prevented.

Managing Hypoxic Spells Hypoxic spells, also called hypercyanotic episodes or "tet" spells, occur with some forms of cyanotic heart disease, most often tetralogy of Fallot or other defects causing right ventricular obstruction. Hypoxic spells usually result from an abrupt reduction in pulmonary blood flow. During the episode, the child becomes agitated, dyspneic, limp, and develops severe cyanosis. The child may rub the hands over the chest as if experiencing pain. The onset usually is sudden and unpredictable. Disappearance of a systolic murmur might be noted. Severe spells may progress to unconsciousness, seizure, and death.

Hypoxic spells require immediate treatment. The child is soothed and held in a side-lying, knee–chest position with the head and thorax slightly elevated. If the spell does not resolve, morphine sulfate (0.01–0.05 mg/kg subcutaneously) is administered, and oxygen may be given. If the child is known to have such episodes, it is helpful to have a syringe containing the correct dose of morphine available for immediate use. Increased frequency or severity of hypoxic spells is an indicator for surgical intervention.

Metabolic acidosis results if the spell does not resolve quickly. Intravenous sodium bicarbonate might be required for a prolonged spell. Intravenous phenylephrine hydrochloride (Neo-Synephrine) sometimes is used to increase systemic resistance and thereby reduce the right-to-left shunt. Occasionally, an episode continues despite interventions, and emergency surgery is necessary.

The nurse teaches the parent to manage hypoxic spells, in case a spell occurs at home. The parent is taught to place the child in a knee–chest position and provide oxygen if it is available. The physician should be contacted if a spell does not resolve quickly, and the child should be taken to the hospital immediately. The most effective way for parents to learn management of hypoxic spells is to observe competent professionals calmly and skillfully manage a spell in the hospital. Instead of ushering the parent out of the room during a spell, the nurse can encourage the parent to observe and even participate in the child's care. After the episode, both parent and child should be given an opportunity to discuss the anxiety engendered by the spell and review steps in its emergency management.

Nutritional Needs

Children with heart disease often have special nutritional needs. Growth retardation is common in children with congenital heart disease (Linde et al., 1971; Feldt et al., 1969*b*; Ehlers, 1978). Factors that play a role in growth failure include these:

- Inadequate intake of nutrients related to fatigue
- Chronic hypoxia that affects the use of nutrients at the cellular level
- Hypermetabolism

Malabsorption of nutrients

Anorexia secondary to medications

Adequate Intake A major nursing goal is to provide adequate intake of nutrients and calories. Sucking requires a significant expenditure of energy, and infants with heart disease often become exhausted and dyspneic before they can consume an adequate volume of formula. Such infants are likely to suck and pant alternately through the feeding until they become fatigued and give up. Holding the infant in a semiupright knee–chest position helps (D'Antonio, 1979) to prevent fatigue and enables the infant to eat more. Using a soft nipple designed for premature infants reduces the work of sucking. The hole in the nipple might be enlarged slightly, although if the hole is too large, the infant might become overwhelmed by the volume of formula and aspirate some of it. The infant is allowed to pause and rest as needed and should not be forced to eat when fatigued. If at all possible, the infant should be held during feedings. If the infant is receiving oxygen, it must be continued during the feeding. Infants should be fed at the first sign of hunger and not allowed to tire themselves by crying. Other procedures should be scheduled so that the child receives adequate rest prior to the feeding and is not disturbed after the feeding. Small feedings should be offered frequently, such as every 2–3 hours around the clock. Smaller feedings minimize fatigue, and the small volume of food exerts less pressure on the diaphragm (Cloutier and Measel, 1982).

Parents need to be warned that infants with heart disease will not sleep through the night at the same age as normal children and that night feedings may continue for several months. Nurses can help the parents see the importance of sharing this task and enlisting the help of others as much as possible. After feedings, the infant is placed in a semiupright position (such as in an infant seat) to reduce the risk of vomiting and to facilitate respirations.

Breast feeding may require more energy than bottle feeding, but this is not a contraindication for breast feeding if the infant is able to obtain enough milk without undue effort. If the infant does become fatigued and the mother remains committed to breast feeding, breast milk may be expressed and fed by bottle or gavage (see Chapter 38). Some infants are placed on a schedule that alternates bottle and gavage feedings. If gavage or gastrostomy feedings are necessary, the infant should be provided with a pacifier during the feeding. In a few cases of severe heart disease, parenteral nutrition may be required (see Chapter 38).

High-Calorie Diets To provide as many calories as possible, special formulas containing 24–30 calories per ounce may be used. These formulas have additional carbohydrates, making them concentrated. Therefore they must be introduced gradually, or diarrhea may result. It is also important to ensure that the child receives an adequate amount of free water to prevent dehydration.

Solid foods provide additional calories with limited expenditure of energy and often are introduced early for children with heart disease. It is important to ensure that the child continues to receive adequate fluid. Self-feeding and use of a cup should be encouraged at the usual ages for the child to maintain an adequate intake. If the child's own intake is inadequate, the parent can let the child handle food and self-feed while continuing to feed the child.

Children should be offered a choice of high-calorie, nutritious foods at mealtimes and as snacks. While high-calorie, nutritious snacks, such as milkshakes, are encouraged, empty-calorie snacks are avoided, as they require energy to ingest and digest but do not provide essential nutrients. (Interventions to encourage children to eat are discussed in Chapter 29.)

Iron Supplementation Because avoiding iron-deficiency anemia is especially important for children with cyanotic heart disease and polycythemia, supplemental iron might be prescribed to prevent this conditon. Research by Linderkamp and associates (1979) indicated that viscosity of the blood increases in the presence of microcytosis associated with iron-deficiency anemia. The increased viscosity increases the risk of thrombus formation and cerebrovascular accident.

If an iron supplement is prescribed, parents need to be taught the correct procedure for giving the medication and the importance of preventing accidental overdose.

Sodium Restriction A low-sodium diet may be advisable for some children with heart disease, especially for those with congestive heart failure. Sodium restriction is usually accomplished by not adding salt to the food and avoiding heavily salted foods (potato chips, bacon, pickles). Low-sodium milk formulas are available. Infants often accept these well, but older children may find them unpalatable. Breast milk is low in sodium and is acceptable for infants on low-sodium diets.

Consultation with a nutritionist is helpful in planning for the nutritional needs of a child on sodium-restricted diets. Both parents and children need to understand the importance of minimizing the intake of salt and need to know how to accomplish this on a day-to-day basis. Parents need to know which foods are high or low in sodium, how to read labels for sodium content, how to modify recipes to reduce sodium, and how to order low-salt foods in a restaurant. The nurse also teaches parents that table salt should never be used.

Developmental Needs

Most children with heart disease are intellectually and developmentally normal. Some children, however, particularly those with cyanotic heart disease, are at risk for developmental delays. Chronic heart failure or chronic hypoxia limit strength and endurance, delaying the development of gross motor skills. Perceptual motor function and motor coordination are decreased in children with cyanotic heart disease. Linde and associates (1971) found that children with cyanotic heart disease had lower mean IQ scores (but within the normal range) than children with acyanotic heart disease or no disease. Newburger and colleagues (1984) studied the effects of chronic hypoxemia on cognitive function. Their study indicated a correlation between cognitive impairment and increased age of repair in children with cyanotic heart disease. This lag was in part related to physical incapacity, and gains in IQ scores were seen after surgery.

Congenital heart defects may occur in association with other abnormalities. For example, 40% of children with Down's syndrome also have congenital heart defects (Scoggin and Patterson, 1982). Severe hypoxic episodes and cerebrovascular accidents may also impair neurologic function.

Parental attitudes can affect the child's development. If a parent thinks the child is less capable than normal, this attitude is communicated to the child, who begins to feel inadequate in meeting developmental challenges. A parent might fear that increased motor activity will be harmful to the child and therefore not encourage the child to try new skills. Occasionally a parent may actually prohibit developmental progress. (The emotional effects and coping responses associated with chronic conditions in childhood are discussed in Chapter 30.)

Dependence and Independence Because independence is an important determinant of self-concept, children need to be encouraged to assume as much independence as they are able. This often is difficult for children with cardiac disease. It frequently is easier and faster to do something for the child than to let the child spend the time and exert the effort to do it alone, particularly if the child's efforts result in increasingly apparent symptoms. Often, a well-intentioned but mistaken parent prevents the child from doing things independently.

Activity Restrictions For a small number of children, increased physical activity does not produce obvious symptoms but carries a risk of myocardial ischemia, arrhythmia, and death. It is often difficult for these children to understand why vigorous physical activity must be avoided when it seems to cause them no problem.

A second group of children whose activity must be limited includes those with heart failure and certain other diseases, such as rheumatic fever. Bed rest may be ordered for an extended period of time. During the acute phase of the illness, such children feel ill and want to rest. During the recovery phase, however, they may feel well enough for active play, although it continues to be contraindicated medically.

In assisting a child to adapt to restricted activity, the nurse assesses the child's perception of the restrictions. Young children may feel that restriction is a form of punishment. Older children may feel that they are being "babied." Once the nurse understands the child's perception, it is possible to explain the rationale for restrictions in an honest and age-appropriate way and to correct any unrealistic expectations or worries the child may have.

The nurse also keeps in mind that the overall goal of activity restrictions is to reduce strain on the heart. If a particular restriction, such as confinement to bed, creates undue frustration and tension in the child, the restriction might actually increase the work of the heart. The nurse therefore works with the parent and physician to find ways of limiting activity while avoiding unnecessary frustration. One young child, for example, rejected the notion of staying in her crib, but she was content to play quietly in a high chair or playpen.

For many children with heart disease, limitations on physical activity are related to exercise intolerance. These children generally regulate their own activity in response to the symptoms they experience. Most of these children need few external controls to limit physical activity. Because increased activity may lead to worsening of symptoms, however, a parent may tend to inhibit the child's activity more than necessary (Condon, 1973). It usually is neither necessary nor desirable for parents to impose limits on the child, although there are important exceptions to this generalization. With certain defects (for example, critical aortic stenosis) vigorous activity can be dangerous for the child, even in the absence of symptoms.

Parent Participation Parents need help from the start to understand the hazards of overdependence. The parent who feels guilty, angry, or inadequate, may do extra things for the child to compensate for these feelings. To counteract this natural tendency, the nurse helps the parent to focus on the child's capabilities rather than the child's limitations. It is also helpful to encourage the parent to identify personal adequacies as a parent. A parent who feels adequate most of the time is less likely to try to compensate for occasional feelings of inadequacy by doing too much for the child (Gottesfeld, 1979).

As children develop, parents should encourage them to assume increasing responsibility for their own care. Older children can be responsible for taking their own medication, observing appropriate limits, and observing dietary restrictions.

An infant or child with heart disease needs but may not receive the same type of developmental stimulation as a normal child. For example, children with heart disease may not have the physical capacity to explore the environment to the same extent as a normal child and may not receive the same type of encouragement from adults. Instead of being told to "Go on—try harder," the child with cardiac disease may be told, "Don't try so hard—be careful." Intervention may be needed if the child is to receive appropriate experiences that foster learning.

The nurse can work with the parent to develop strategies to help the child experience some normal activities while preventing undue cardiac stress. For example, the normal infant crawls from room to room, but the infant with cardiac disease might need to be moved from room to room to experience new sights and sounds. A normal infant might be able to sit alone at 6 months of age. The 6-month-old infant with cardiac disease might need to be propped or held so that the world is seen from an upright position and the hands are free for manipulation of objects. A young child with heart disease might not have the stamina to walk alone but can experience the sensation of moving in an upright position if an adult provides support while the child moves the feet and legs. With a mobility aid, such as a walker, the child can move about easily with limited expenditure of energy. Parents should understand that children with cardiac disease need to have stimulating experiences brought to them.

Because children with heart disease may be small for their ages and may be passive rather than active, parents may think of them as younger than they actually are and often underestimate their capabilities. Nurses need to be alert for these assumptions and need to help parents see that appropriate activities will foster normal development.

Because the child with heart disease may have limited energy, it is important to avoid overstimulation and fatigue. A regular routine that includes play times and rest times is beneficial and aids in integrating the child's developmental activities into the family's day (Roberts, 1972).

The nurse assesses the parent's understanding of the child's heart disease. Many people have limited knowledge of normal cardiac structure and function. Therefore, an explanation of the normal circulatory system often must precede a description of the child's problem, if the parent is to understand the significance of the defect, its symptoms, and its treatment.

Simple, two-dimensional drawings of cardiac structures are useful teaching tools. The parent should learn about the four chambers of the heart and how they work, the major vessels, normal blood flow through the heart, and the importance of adequate cardiac output. This basic knowledge equips the parent to understand the nature of the child's defect and how it affects circulatory function.

The nurse also teaches the parent what the child's defect is *not*. The parent may be unnecessarily fearful that, for example, the child with heart disease will have a sudden heart attack and die, as adults with heart disease do. Whereas this is a risk for a small number of children with some defects, most parents can be reassured that the child is not at risk for a "heart attack." It is important to discuss the parent's fears and to help the parent to distinguish unrealistic fears from realistic concerns.

Discipline Discipline is a special issue for children with some forms of cardiac disease. If symptoms worsen when the child becomes upset or cries, the parent may go to extremes to appease the child and prevent such episodes. Although this meets the short-term goal of preventing hypoxemia and dyspnea, it is not consistent with the long-term goal of raising a well-adjusted child who can delay gratification. Reasonable efforts to meet the child's needs help to prevent unnecessary frustration, but parents cannot and should not try to prevent all crying. Most children with cardiac disease stop crying on their own when crying becomes too tiring. Unless specifically advised otherwise by the physician, the parent can assume that normal episodes of crying are not harmful to the child, even though symptoms may worsen. The parent needs to learn early to prevent manipulative behavior by the child (for example, "If you don't let me have a cookie, I'll cry and turn blue!"). This is accomplished by attending to positive behaviors in the child and ignoring negative behaviors as much as possible. When the child learns that the parent is not upset by negative behaviors, the child will be less likely to use symptoms to manipulate the parent.

The parent also needs guidance and support in management of day-to-day issues in raising a special child. The child needs to develop an understanding of the disease and an increasing responsibility for self-care. The child should be treated as much like siblings as possible with respect to household tasks, discipline, and responsibilities, although modifications may be necessary, depending on the child's physical status. A child with heart disease might not be able to do yard work but could be responsible for folding laundry and other less physically demanding jobs. Parents must understand the hazards of overprotection, overindulgence, and undue restrictions at home or school. The cardiologist is responsible for determining what restrictions, if any, are needed for the child, but the parents might then need assistance in applying these restrictions to particular situations. Unless there are contraindications, the child should attend school regularly and participate in permitted activities with peers. Parents should be encouraged to consult with the doctor or nurse if they are unsure about whether a certain activity should be restricted. It is better to check than to impose an unnecessary restriction on the child.

Emotional Needs

Children with congenital heart disease have an incidence of psychologic maladjustment similar to that of children with other chronic disease (see Chapter 30). Garson and colleagues (1978) estimate that 30%–60% of children with chronic disease suffer from emotional problems, a rate two to three times that of the general population. Psychosocial problems may lead to emotional disability, which is more serious than the physical disability caused by the heart disease. Clearly, attention to the emotional needs of children and families is of paramount importance. Nurses and other health professionals need to promote realistic and appropriate parenting if the child is to develop as a socially competent and productive individual.

Effect on Families Many children with heart defects, especially acyanotic defects, do not have obvious symptoms. It is often difficult for parents of these children to believe that an infant has a serious, perhaps life-threatening condition. A parent might "shop around" for other physicians who will reassure the parent that the infant is healthy. Heart disease is often not apparent at birth, and symptoms may not appear for several weeks. The parent typically is delighted and relieved initially to hear that the infant is normal, only to be told a few weeks later that the infant is ill. To accept the infant as healthy and then to find that the infant is ill make the parental adjustment particularly difficult. A parent often does not understand the rationale for the lapse between the birth of the child and the diagnosis and may fear that the physician "missed" the diagnosis or tried to hide the truth. A loss of trust in health care providers may result.

Anxiety and fear are common reactions when a parent learns of the child's heart disease. The term *heart* has metaphysical as well as biologic connotations, and the heart has a special significance not associated with other organs. The diagnosis of heart disease is frightening, and the parent often fears for the survival of the child. The symptom of cyanosis is especially anxiety-provoking, and it is very frightening for a parent to watch the child turn blue during feedings or other activities. Impending surgery also creates tremendous conflict and ambivalence in many parents. The parent might realize that surgery may significantly improve the child's condition, but the threat of death is also present, and the parent faces the pain of deciding whether to let the child live with present impairments or to risk the loss of the child.

Misconceptions are common. People are very aware of the occurrence of heart attacks. The parent might assume that because the child has a heart defect, a "heart attack" and sudden death may occur. (This fear is realistic for some children.) The well-known association between exercise and heart attacks leads some parents to limit their children's activity unnecessarily. Careful and repeated explanations of the child's defect or disease and its relation to any activity restrictions are necessary.

The parent might experience feelings of anger because the child is not normal. This anger might be directed at themselves, the sick child, the spouse, the healthy siblings, God, or the professional involved in the care of the child. Professionals must recognize the source of the anger and allow the parent time to deal with it. Reacting angrily to the parent's anger, unrealistic restrictions on the child, or demands on the staff only intensifies the problem. Nurses can assist the parents to deal with these feelings by helping parents understand how vital their love and concern is to the child's care. While the technology of health care may be impressive, the child's confidence in the parent's love and protection is truly central to the child's well-being. Parents should be encouraged to participate as fully as possible in the care of their children. Initially, parents might feel threatened and hesitant, but as they become more confident, their participation benefits children, parents, and professionals.

Caring for children with serious heart disease on a day-to-day basis can be demanding and stressful. Frequent feedings, special medications, and constant vigilance lead to tensions and exhaustion. Parents often feel inadequate in dealing with children's complex needs. The parent might see the child's symptoms (for example, poor feeding, irritability) as proof of parental failure. Activities, such as feeding, which are ordinarily pleasurable, are often times of high anxiety when the child has heart problems. (Alterations in parenting related to the high-risk infant are discussed in Chapter 31.)

Anxiety is more likely if the child has had critical episodes from which the parents feared the child would not recover. The excessive fears of the parent are often transferred to the child, who feels vulnerable and fearful. Parents with exaggerated fears often have misperceptions about the cardiac disorder despite repeated explanations from professionals. Anxious parents often hear explanations that are quite different from what a professional actually said. For example, professionals often tell parents to treat the child as normally as possible. Parents, however, may interpret "normal" in ways different from professionals. For example, one mother had repeatedly been told by the cardiologist that her son had no need for activity restrictions and should be treated like any other 14-year-old boy. At one clinic visit, the mother stated that she always had treated him absolutely normally—this said as she tucked in his shirt and bent to tie his shoe. Clearly, her anxiety influenced how she interpreted "normal" in the case of her son. Nurses need to assist parents to distinguish realistic fears from unfounded anxiety.

When the child and family are unable to accept the fact of heart disease, cooperation with the therapeutic regimen is jeopardized. For example, a 7-month-old infant with chronic congestive heart failure related to a congenital defect was well-stabilized on digitalis. For no apparent reason, the child's condition deteriorated abruptly, and he needed emergency intervention. The mother later confided that the child seemed to be doing so well that she was sure his heart was better and that he no longer needed his medicine; she therefore did not give the digitalis. In this situation, the mother's inability to accept the reality of the child's defect was life-threatening.

Garson and associates (1978) held discussions with the parents of 260 children with congenital heart disease. Certain groups of parents seemed to share common concerns and behaviors depending on the stage and seriousness of their child's disease. Five patterns were identified:

1. Symptomatic child, preoperative. Children in this group had serious heart disease that would require surgery. The children appeared ill and were treated as such. Parents in this group tended to focus on the surgery as providing relief from the present condition. Much time and energy was devoted to getting the child ready for surgery (for example, promoting weight gain). Parents expressed anger at symptoms and medical procedures.
2. Asymptomatic child, preoperative. Children in this group had a heart defect that would require surgery but did not cause obvious symptoms. Parents expressed a strong wish to avoid surgery and continued to hope that the defect would go away. Parents felt guilty about inflicting pain and suffering on their apparently healthy child.
3. Nonoperative, serious. Children in this group had obvious symptoms of serious disease that was not surgically correctable. Parents expressed feelings of helplessness and anger about the hopelessness of the situation. Some in this group were unable to "hear" the prognosis. Others withdrew from the child in anticipation of the child's death.
4. Nonoperative, benign. Children in this group had heart lesions that were not serious and for which surgery was not needed. The children were asymptomatic, and parents were told to "treat them normally." Parents stated that it was not possible to treat them normally because "something is wrong with the heart." The parents tended to overprotect the children, who were made to feel sick.
5. Postoperative. These children may or may not have had symptoms preoperatively. All had undergone surgery. Garson noted two patterns of response. In the first pattern, the parents continued to relate to the child as if the heart lesion had not been corrected and the child was still "defective." In the second pattern, the parent's attitude changed and the parent tended to treat the child more normally. A "second mourning" response was noted in some parents whose children were dramatically improved by surgery. At birth the parent had mourned the loss of the normal child the parent had fantasized about prenatally. After surgery, the parent mourned the loss of the "sick" child and accepted the healthier child. Parents noted they missed the special closeness the preoperative condition had allowed.

Effect on the Child Several factors determine the effect that the heart problem has on the child's self-image. A major factor is the child's perception of the heart disease. This depends in part on the child's concept of the heart. Reif's (1972) studies of how children of different ages conceptualize the heart indicate that children between 4 and 6 years of age have a general idea of the heart's anatomic position. They characterize it as having a valentine shape and making tick-tock sounds. Children between 7 and 10 years of age realize the heart is not shaped like a valentine, and they recognize that the heart plays a vital role in body functions, although they are not generally sure what that role is. By 10–11 years of age, children have a basic understanding of how the heart works and why cardiac function is necessary to life.

Older children are more likely to have a realistic perception of their illness because of their better understanding of the circulatory system. Children under 8–10 years of age, particularly those in early and middle childhood, are likely to have misperceptions regarding the meaning and cause of their illness. For example, one 6-year-old believed her heart became "sick" because she "ran too much." Their inaccurate cause-and-effect reasoning might lead children to believe that their parents, siblings, or they themselves are responsible for the defect. Children may feel guilty or angry depending on who they believe "caused" the disease. (Children's developing perceptions of illness are generally discussed in Chapter 27.)

Health Maintenance Needs

Observing for Symptoms Once the parent understands the basics of the child's heart disease, the parent can better appreciate why certain signs and symptoms might occur. The parent therefore needs to know which signs and symptoms to watch for and what to do if these become evident. The specific symptoms that are taught depend on the nature of the child's disease, but in general the parent should observe and report fever, decreased intake, increased respiratory rate or pulse rate, difficult breathing (shortness of breath, congestion, grunting, retractions, cough), edema, increase in cyanosis, pallor, decreased urine output, and vomiting or diarrhea.

The child's hospital stay is an important opportunity to teach parents about monitoring the child at home. For example, during hospitalization, parents might practice counting respirations (and pulse if indicated) under the guidance of the nurse. Parents need to know how to use a thermometer safely and to read it accurately. The nurse also can evaluate parental awareness of symptoms. When a parent accurately assesses symptoms, the nurse can validate and reinforce the parent's judgment. Some parents, however, miss important symptoms, whereas other parents overreact to minor findings. The nurse therefore identifies patterns of over- or underreaction prior to the child's discharge, as errors in judgment might have serious consequences for the child's health. If parents over- or underreact, the nurse can give corrective feedback. Underreaction to symptoms might be a form of denial (a maladaptive behavior in cases of chronic illness); overreaction might be a manifestation of anxiety. In either case, the underlying issues must be addressed.

Administering Medications One of the major parental responsibilities is the administration of medications. Parents need careful explanations about why the drugs are given, how they affect the body, what the side effects are, and what precautions are necessary. Parent education should begin when the medication is started. Attempting to teach about drugs just before discharge increases the risk of misunderstandings and mistakes. Parents can begin by observing the nurse measure and administer the medication. After parents understand the procedure, they need supervised practice in measuring the medication and giving it to the child. The nurse can offer suggestions that will make the task easier and enhance the parent's confidence. The child gets used to the parent's methods before going home, and if problems arise (vomiting, refusal) the parent can handle these with guidance from the nurse. (Parent teaching is generally discussed in Chapter 29.)

Some people have difficulty reading and using the dosage scales on syringes or droppers. Enlarged visual aids may be helpful. Parents should be taught to place a liquid medication slowly in the side of the child's mouth about halfway back while the child's head is slightly elevated. If the medication is mixed with food, only a small amount of food should be used. If the child fails to finish the food, there is no way of knowing how much medication was taken. Parents also need to be aware of the risk of accidental overdose and the importance of safe storage of the drug. Written information on the drug container is valuable. Drugs vary considerably with respect to action, dosage, and side effects, and it is often difficult for parents to keep the drugs straight, especially if the child is taking several.

Digoxin Jackson (1979) surveyed parents whose children received digoxin to evaluate their knowledge of the drug. Results of the survey revealed frightening gaps in the parents' knowledge, particularly in regard to symptoms of digoxin toxicity. With a drug as potent and potentially dangerous as digoxin, it is essential that parents receive careful instruction regarding dosage, administration, signs of toxicity, and management of common problems.

Jackson (1979) notes that the following points should be included in teaching family members about digoxin:

1. Digoxin is a very effective but very potent medication. It enables the heart to pump more effectively with a slower and more regular rhythm.

2. The major danger is digoxin toxicity. This is caused by too much digoxin in the body. Usually no problems develop, but it is important to recognize signs of toxicity as early as possible. Signs of toxicity include loss of appetite, vomiting, slow or irregular pulse, and visual disturbances. Digoxin toxicity is most likely to occur when digoxin is first begun, when the dosage is increased, when other medications are changed, and when the child is ill, especially with vomiting and/or diarrhea. If any signs of digoxin toxicity occur, the physician should be notified.

3. Digoxin should be given exactly as prescribed. It is dangerous to give more or less than prescribed.

4. It is important to give the medicine every 12 hours. This helps establish a routine and also results in stable levels of digoxin in the body. It may be helpful to record doses, as they are given, on a small calendar.

5. Digoxin should be given 1 hour before or 2 hours after a meal. The drug is absorbed better this way. If digoxin is given with the meal and the infant vomits after eating (as infants often do), then an undetermined amount of digoxin will also be lost.

6. If a dose is forgotten and 4 hours or less have elapsed since the dose was due, the dose may be given and the next dose given at the regular time. If more than 4 hours have elapsed, it is best to skip the dose entirely. The subsequent dose should never be doubled or increased to make up for the forgotten dose.

7. If for any reason two doses are missed, the physician should be notified.

8. Most children like the taste of digoxin. If, however, the child spits out the medicine, the dose should *not* be repeated unless the parents are sure none of the medication was swallowed.

9. If the child vomits within 15 minutes of receiving the digoxin and it seems that all or most of the digoxin was lost, all or part of the dose may be repeated. If the child vomits more than 15 minutes after the dose, it should *not* be repeated, as part of the digoxin will already be in the bloodstream. The normal dose should be given the next regular time. If the child vomits all or part of two doses of digoxin, the physician should be notified.

10. If the child becomes ill and has loss of appetite, vomiting, diarrhea, difficulty breathing, or a slow or irregular pulse, the physician should be notified. A normal level of potassium in the body is necessary for digoxin to be effective. If the potassium level is too low, digoxin toxicity may result. Potassium levels may become low if the child has vomiting or diarrhea, if the child fails to ingest sufficient potassium or if too much is lost through the urine (the result of some diuretics). Foods that are high in potassium (for example, oranges, potatoes, bananas, peaches, milk) should be encouraged. Occasional vomiting or diarrhea is not unusual in children, but if the child seems ill or if the problem continues for more than 24 hours, the physician should be notified.

11. Digoxin must be stored in a place that is safe from all children. Accidental overdose may be fatal. Because it is pleasant-tasting, children may ingest a large amount. A locked cabinet is preferred for storage. Cupboards, counter tops, unlocked medicine chests, and the like are not safe.

12. If accidental overdose should occur, the child should be taken immediately to the nearest emergency room. Ipecac should be given before transport if the child is conscious. The medicine bottle should be brought along also.

Recommendations vary, depending on institutional policy and the physician's preference, about whether the parent should take the child's pulse before giving digoxin and at what point (pulse rate) the drug should be withheld.

Diuretics Diuretics are used frequently in children with heart disease. Instructions for parents vary according to the specific diuretic agent prescribed. When potassium-excreting diuretics are used, the parent must understand the risk of hypokalemia. If the child also is receiving digoxin, the parent should be aware that low potassium levels may precipitate digoxin toxicity. Signs of hypokalemia include anorexia, nausea, vomiting, numbness, confusion, irritability, and weakness. Parents should know which foods are high in potassium; these include bananas, oranges, grapefruit, prune juice, canned apricots, milk, carrots and potatoes. If potassium supplements are ordered, the parent is instructed in their use. Illnesses that result in decreased appetite, vomiting, or diarrhea increase the risk of hypokalemia. The parent therefore is encouraged to notify the physician if this occurs.

Doses should be scheduled so that diuresis does not occur at night in children who are toilet-trained. If diuretics are given in the late afternoon or evening, enuresis might occur. It may not be possible to avoid late-day administration for children with serious disease, however, as the uppermost consideration is to maintain a steady serum level. Parents should understand that increased urine output is an expected effect. Decreased output, edema, and respiratory distress might indicate that the diuretic is ineffective and that the physician should be notified.

Skin and mucous membranes should be inspected daily for petechiae and other signs of bleeding if the child is receiving large doses or prolonged therapy with thiazide diuretics. Complete blood count, serum electrolytes, blood urea nitrogen, creatinine, uric acid, and blood sugar should be checked periodically for children receiving thiazide diuretics.

A potassium-sparing diuretic, such as spironolactone (Aldactone), may be used in conjunction with another diuretic such as one of the thiazides (Diuril). Because this drug prevents the excretion of potassium, it helps to counteract the potassium-loosing effect of other diuretics, but hyperkalemia is a risk, particularly if this drug is used alone.

Preventing Infection Parents must also be informed if their children are at special risk for infection. Generally, parents must avoid exposing their children to persons who might have communicable diseases. This is not easy to do, since social contact is desirable for children, and infectious diseases are common in children. Siblings also bring illnesses home from school, and casual contacts at public places, such as stores and places of worship, might lead to infection. Common-sense precautions are indicated. Correct and frequent hand washing by everyone in the home is of primary importance. Isolating sick individuals from the child provides some protection. Use of common drinking glasses should be avoided. Infants should not be taken to crowded places where exposure cannot be controlled. If the child attends a day-care center or school, teachers must be told about the risk from infectious disease. The child may need to remain home in order to prevent exposure to diseases "going around" at school.

Parents should not, however, be so frightened by the risk of infection that their children are never allowed to leave the house or play with other children. The goal is to strike a balance between avoiding unnecessary exposure and providing social contact. If signs of an infectious disease do occur, the physician should be notified.

Virtually all children with organic heart disease require prophylactic treatment with antibiotics to reduce the risk of endocarditis associated with dental work, minor surgery, and illnesses. The nurse therefore instructs parents to tell others involved in the care of their children about the presence of heart disease. For example, doctors, dentists, and emergency room personnel who evaluate and treat the child must be informed. Early symptoms of subacute bacterial endocarditis include fever, chills, and lethargy. These should be reported to the physician.

In addition to the special care related to the cardiac disease, the child needs routine health care. Regular assessments, immunization, recommended laboratory studies (urinalysis, hemoglobin), vision and hearing screening, developmental screening, and anticipatory guidance are especially important for the child with heart disease.

Regulating Temperature Because both hyperthermia and hypothermia increase the child's (and especially the infant's) need for oxygen, it is important that the parent understand the need to prevent chilling or overheating. Young infants are most susceptible to temperature variations in response to environmental conditions, and special precautions might be necessary. Diaphoresis, which may occur in infants with heart failure, can increase the risk of chilling. During baths, only one body part should be washed at a time and then thoroughly dried before another part is exposed. The rest of the infant should be kept covered. The infant's room should be kept warm, and blankets should be used according to the infant's thermal state.

The Child With Congestive Heart Failure

Congestive heart failure is a condition in which the blood supply to the body is insufficient to meet the metabolic requirements of the organs. Congestive heart failure is a manifestation of an underlying disease rather than a disease in itself. It can be due to reduced myocardial function or abnormally increased demands placed on the heart.

Prior to the development of congestive heart failure, compensatory mechanisms are activated in attempts to maintain adequate cardiac output. Several compensatory mechanisms are brought into play by the sympathetic nervous system. Decreased blood pressure stimulates vascular stretch receptors and baroreceptors in the aorta and carotid arteries, which in turn trigger the sympathetic nervous system. Catecholamine release and beta receptor stimulation increase the rate and force of myocardial contraction. Catecholamines also increase venous tone, so that blood is returned to the heart more effectively. Circulation to the skin, extremities, splanchnic bed, and kidneys is decreased to maximize blood flow to the heart, lungs, and brain. Decreased urine output, pallor, cool extremities, and weak peripheral pulses might be present. In addition, decreased renal blood flow stimulates the release of renin angiotensin and aldosterone. The resultant retention of sodium and fluid causes *hypervolemia* which increases the workload of an already stressed myocardium. Stimulation of sympathetic cholinergic receptors in the skin might produce sweating.

Other compensatory mechanisms are mechanical. Heart muscle thickens in an attempt to maintain cardiac output by increasing pressure in the ventricles. Myocardial hypertrophy is effective temporarily, but as muscle mass increases, compliance decreases, and greater filling pressure is required to achieve an adequate diastolic volume. Also, the increasing muscle mass might outgrow its blood supply, resulting in myocardial ischemia.

Ventricular dilatation results as myocardial fibers stretch during diastole to accommodate increased ventricular volume. A mild-to-moderate stretch increases the force of the contraction, but beyond a certain point contractility does not increase.

Causes of Congestive Heart Failure

Causes of congestive heart failure can be classified as (a) increased volume, (b) obstruction to outflow, (c) ineffective myocardial function, (d) arrhythmias, or (e) excessive demand for cardiac output. In congestive heart failure due to increased volume, myocardial function is normal, but the heart is called on to pump an excessive volume of blood. Excessive volume might be due to hypervolemia, which could be caused by excessive fluid intake or retention. Fluid retention alone usually does not cause congestive heart failure, but it might complicate failure from other causes. In children, the demand for the heart to pump an increased volume most often is caused by congenital defects and altered hemodynamics. For example, with patent ductus arteriosus, a certain volume of blood ejected from the left ventricle returns to the heart by way of the patent ductus arteriosus but without perfusing any organ. The heart must pump this recirculated blood in addition to the normal volume it ejects into the systemic circulation. Compensatory mechanisms that enable the heart to pump the increased total volume of blood include increased heart rate (tachycardia) and increased size of the pumping chambers (myocardial hypertrophy and dilatation). Despite the tachycardia, cardiomegaly, and diagnosis of congestive heart failure, the heart muscle is functioning normally. Other congenital abnormalities that cause chronic congestive heart failure due to increased volume include ventricular septal defect, atrial septal defect, endocardial cushion defect, and aortic, pulmonic, tricuspid, or mitral valve insufficiency.

Congestive heart failure due to obstruction to outflow may occur if the normal myocardium is expected to pump against increased resistance. Structural defects, such as valvular stenosis or coarctation of the aorta, may cause obstruction to outflow. Pulmonary disease and pulmonary arterial hypertension are two conditions that increase the resistance in the lungs and the work of the right ventricle. Congestive heart failure that occurs as a result of pulmonary pathology is termed *cor pulmonale.* Severe systemic hypertension also increases systemic resistance to outflow and can cause congestive heart failure.

Although congestive heart failure in children usually is due to abnormal stresses placed on the heart, sometimes it is due to a primary heart muscle disorder. Causes of primary myocardial dysfunction include rheumatic fever, infectious myocarditis, idiopathic congestive cardiomyopathy, mucocutaneous lymph node syndrome (Kawasaki disease), beriberi, anomalous origin of the left coronary artery from the pulmonary artery, Pompe's disease, endocarditis, polyarteritis nodosa, and metabolic disorders. Electrolyte imbalances, acidosis, and myocardial ischemia also adversely affect myocardial function.

Congestive heart failure can accompany certain arrhythmias. Complete atrioventricular block, which results in an abnormally slow heart rate, or sustained primary tachycardia can lead to congestive heart failure. With tachycardia, there is insufficient time for ventricular filling, and cardiac output is therefore decreased.

Congestive heart failure due to excessive demand for cardiac output can occur with severe anemia. Because anemia reduces the oxygen-carrying capacity of the blood, the heart must pump more blood per minute to supply the tissues adequately. If the volume of blood required by the tissues is greater than the pumping capacity of the heart, congestive heart failure occurs.

Congestive heart failure thus is a poor term, as the signs and symptoms of congestive heart failure can occur when the heart is not truly "failing." In many instances, the heart meets increased demands and functions normally, perhaps supernormally. In addition to its inaccuracy, the term *congestive heart failure* is frightening to patients and families, as *failure* implies cessation of function.

Signs and Symptoms of Congestive Heart Failure

Signs and symptoms of congestive heart failure are summarized in Table 35-7. Children with compensated congestive heart failure might show no symptoms during daily activities. The presence of compensated failure can be demonstrated, however, by measuring the child's total working capacity using a bicycle ergometer or treadmill. Patients with compensated congestive heart failure have reduced working capacity when the cardiovascular system is stressed.

As the degree of congestive heart failure increases, the cardiovascular system can no longer compensate adequately, and symptoms of cardiovascular insufficiency occur at rest or with minimal stress. Tachycardia, a cardinal symptom of congestive heart failure, develops as the heart attempts to compensate for decreased stroke volume with an increased rate. This compensatory mechanism has disadvantages. Tachycardia decreases diastolic filling time, which results in reduced ventricular filling and reduced coronary blood flow (coronary blood flow occurs during diastole). In addition, tachycardia increases the oxygen needs of the myocardium. A gallop rhythm (S_3) may also occur with failure. Cardiomegaly due to hypertrophy and ventricular dilatation is a second cardinal sign of congestive heart failure.

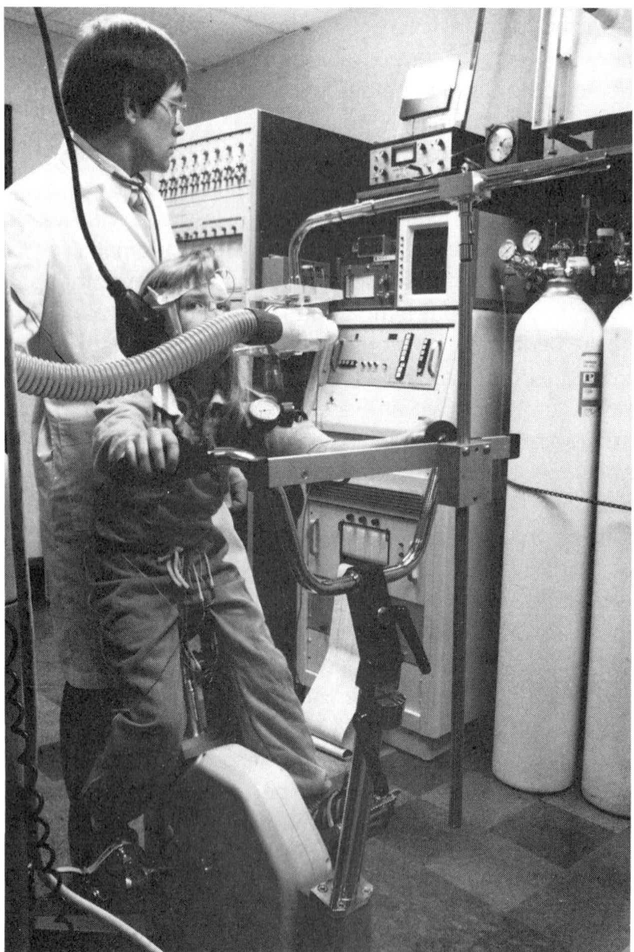

Exercise tolerance test. (Photograph courtesy of the Mayo Clinic, Rochester, Minnesota.)

Congestive heart failure can be classified as right-sided or left-sided failure. Each has specific clinical manifestations. Because each side depends on the effective function of the other, failure of one side usually results in reciprocal failure in the other side. In children, clinical right- and left-sided failure usually occur together.

Because the left ventricle is unable to empty completely during systole, end-diastolic pressure and volume increase. The left atrium is unable to expel blood into the left ventricle. Pressure in the left atrium rises, and blood returning from the pulmonary circulation is unable to enter the left atrium. As pressure in the pulmonary veins increases, hydrostatic pressure exceeds osmotic pressure in the capillaries, and fluid leaks from the capillaries to the interstitial spaces. When the amount of leaked fluid exceeds the capacity of the lymphatics to remove it, pulmonary edema results. Tachypnea is a cardinal sign of congestive heart failure. Dyspnea, retractions, nasal flaring, expiratory grunt, cough, rales, rhonchi, and orthopnea are all manifestations of left-sided heart failure.

When pressure in the pulmonary vasculature is elevated, the right ventricle is unable completely to eject the blood into the pulmonary artery. The resultant increase in right ventricular end-diastolic pressure prevents emptying of the right atrium. Elevated atrial pressure inhibits the return of blood from the superior and inferior vena cavae. Elevation of pressures in the systemic venous circulation results in systemic congestion.

Hepatomegaly is another cardinal sign of congestive heart failure and results from elevated pressure in the inferior vena cava. Elevation of pressure in the superior vena cava may result in distention of jugular veins. Because venous pressure in infants is generally lower than in adults and older children, distention generally is not observed in young infants. As hydrostatic pressure in the venous system rises, edema occurs. This usually is not observed in infants. If present, it is most commonly seen in the periorbital and sacral areas. In older children, dependent edema in the legs and sacrum is observed. Pitting edema and ascites also might be noted. Weight gain is an indication of fluid retention in both infants and older children.

The nursing care of children with congestive heart failure is directed toward reducing the cardiac workload and enhancing cardiac output as previously discussed.

TABLE 35-7 Signs and Symptoms of Congestive Heart Failure

Infants	Older children and adults
Tachycardia	Tachycardia
Tachypnea	Tachypnea
Hepatomegaly	Hepatomegaly
Cardiomegaly	Cardiomegaly
Gallop rhythm	Gallop rhythm
Oliguria	Oliguria
Diaphoresis	Diaphoresis
Rales, gasping, and grunting expirations are late signs	Rales
Poor feeding, slow growth pattern, fatigue	—
Hypotonia, flaccidity	Exercise intolerance
Dyspnea, costal retractions (if severe), subcostal retractions	Dyspnea, shortness of breath; orthopnea, noctural dyspnea
Periorbital edema	Edema, weight gain
Pallor and mottling of skin, transient duskiness	Pallor, mottling of skin
Persistent, hacking cough	Dry, hacking cough
Poor peripheral circulation, cold extremities	Poor peripheral circulation, cold extremities
Hypotension	Hypotension

The Child With an Acyanotic Cardiac Defect

Patent Ductus Arteriosus

The *ductus arteriosus* is a blood vessel that connects the pulmonary artery to the proximal descending thoracic aorta. Because the lungs are unexpanded in the fetus, most blood entering the pulmonary artery traverses the ductus arteriosus into the aorta. At birth, with expansion of the lungs, blood entering the pulmonary artery perfuses the lungs, and the ductus arteriosus is no longer needed. Normally, the patent ductus arteriosus contracts, and its lumen is obliterated 10–15 hours after birth (Moss, Adams, and Emmanouilides, 1977). Persistent patent ductus arteriosus occurs if the lumen fails to obliterate (Fig. 35-7).

In full-term infants, persistent patency of the ductus arteriosus occurs in approximately 1 of 2000 live births and accounts for 10% of all types of congenital heart disease. The occurrence of persistent patent ductus arteriosus is higher

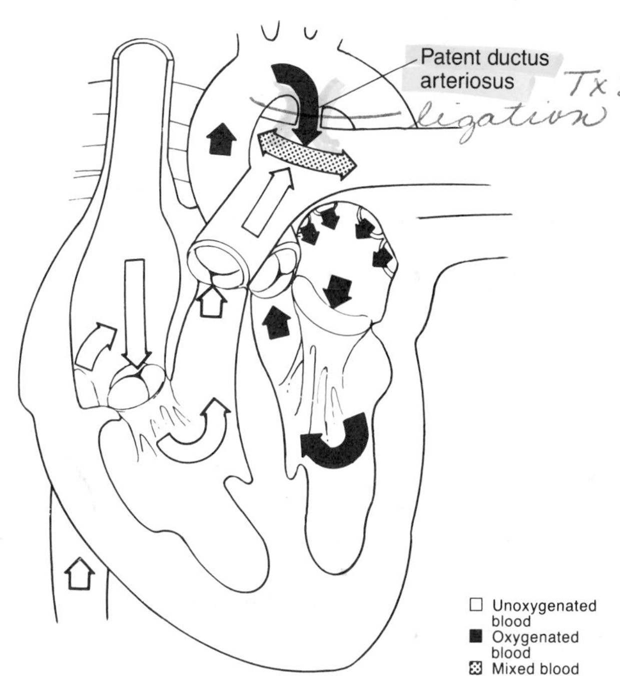

Figure 35-7 Patent ductus arteriosus.

in premature infants and infants born at high altitudes than in infants born at term or at sea level.

Persistence of a patent ductus arteriosus allows oxygenated blood that has been ejected from the left ventricle into the aorta to return to the lungs. Because this blood is already oxygenated, its recirculation through the lungs serves no useful purpose. Instead, it creates volume overload in the lungs and left cardiac structures. Overload can result in left atrial and left ventricular enlargement as well as pulmonary edema and congestive heart failure. If the volume of blood traversing the persistent patent ductus arteriosus is small, these effects are minimal, but if the volume is large, significant congestive heart failure can occur.

The clinical manifestations of persistent patent ductus arteriosus depend on the size of the patent ductus arteriosus and the age of the child. In full-term infants and in older children and adolescents a small patent ductus arteriosus is asymptomatic. The sole clinical manifestation might be a continuous murmur best heard at the upper left sternal border or across the back. A moderate-to-large patent ductus arteriosus might be associated with congestive heart failure and failure to thrive. In addition to a continuous murmur, the child might have cardiomegaly, left ventricular hypertrophy, left atrial enlargement, increased pulse pressure, and bounding peripheral pulses. A premature infant with moderate to large patent ductus arteriosus might have congestive heart failure, cardiomegaly, and increased pulse pressure. In a premature infant with associated respiratory distress syndrome, a patent ductus arteriosus can cause continued respiratory insufficiency.

Treatment consists of operative ligation or division of the structure. This can be done relatively safely in patients of all ages. In premature infants, the ductus arteriosus sometimes can be closed using prostaglandin synthetase inhibitors, such as indomethacin (Cohen, 1983) (Table 35-8). In adults, calcification of the patent ductus arteriosus also can occur, increasing the operative risk due to rupture of the ductus arteriosus at the time of operation. The general nursing care of children with this and the following cardiac defects has been discussed previously. See The Child Undergoing Cardiac Surgery (p. 1201) for further nursing interventions.

Coarctation of the Aorta

Coarctation of the aorta (Fig. 35-8) consists of a shelflike projection of tissue into the lumen of the aorta and most commonly occurs just distal to the origin of the left subclavian artery and immediately opposite the insertion of the ligamentum arteriosum into the descending thoracic aorta. Other locations are possible. This results in narrowing of the aortic lumen. Coarctation of the aorta occurs in 1 of 13,000 children (Moss, Adams and Emmanouilides, 1977). The condition might be an isolated defect or might be associated with other cardiac abnormalities, such as bicuspid aortic valve, minor or major abnormalities of the mitral valve and its support apparatus, or ventricular septal defects.

Narrowing of the aorta causes increased systolic blood pressure proximal to the area of coarctation and decreased systolic blood pressure distally. Pulse in the legs also may be less prominent than the pulse in the arms. Because the left ventricle must generate abnormally increased systolic pressure, left ventricular failure can occur, resulting in pulmonary edema and congestive heart failure. In some patients, collateral blood flow develops, bypassing the area of coarctation.

The clinical manifestations of coarctation of the aorta depend on the degree of narrowing, the presence or absence of associated congenital cardiac abnormalities, and the extent of collateral flow around the area of coarctation. The child with isolated coarctation of the aorta might have upper extremity hypertension. Severe isolated coarctation of the aorta may be present, particularly in infants, as congestive heart failure with cardiovascular collapse. Congestive heart failure is more likely to occur when coarctation of the aorta is associated with other intracardiac abnormalities than when it is an isolated malformation.

Coarctation of the aorta should be suspected in any child with systemic hypertension or congestive heart failure. Diminished pulses in the lower extremities, but normal-to-increased pulses in the upper extremities suggest the diagnosis, and a measured discrepancy between upper and lower extremity blood pressure confirms the diagnosis. Because abnormalities of the origin of the subclavian arteries can occur, it is essential to measure blood pressure in both arms and a leg if coarctation of the aorta is suspected.

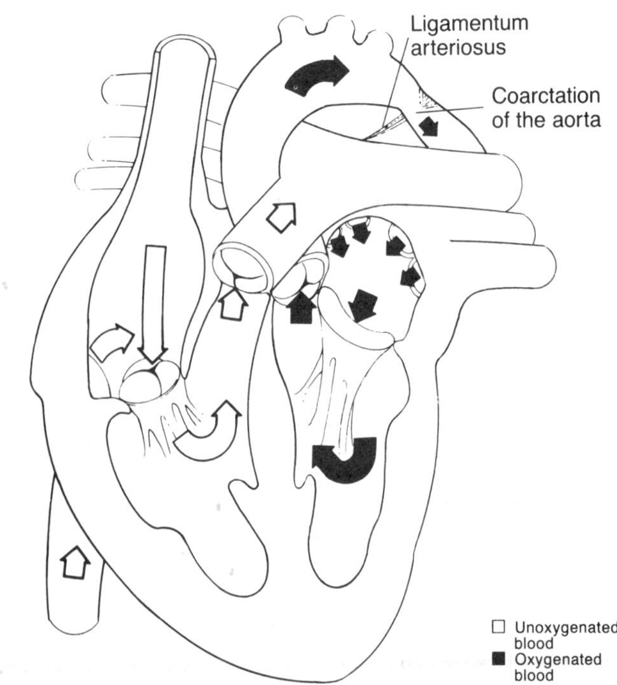

Figure 35-8 Coarctation of the aorta.

TABLE 35-8 Drugs That Affect the Patency of the Ductus Arteriosus

Prostaglandin synthetase inhibitors (indomethacin)	Prostaglandin E (PGE)
Indications	
Patent ductus arteriosus	Tricuspid atresia, severe tetralogy of Fallot, pulmonic valve stenosis, juxaductal coarctation of the aorta, transposition of the great arteries, hypoplastic left heart syndrome
Action and therapeutic effects	
Constricts patent ductus arteriosus by stimulating smooth muscle in vessel walls to contract	Prevents postnatal closure of patent ductus arteriosus by relaxing smooth muscle in vessel walls, may increase pulmonary flow by reversing initial vasoconstriction, thereby increasing P_aO_2
Alternative to surgical ligation of ductus arteriosus	Keeps ductus arteriosus patent until permanent shunt or correction provided surgically
Side effects	
Oliguria, gastrointestinal bleeding, platelet dysfunction, possibly bilirubinemia	Fever, apnea, bradycardia, seizures, muscle twitching, irritability, hypotension, flushing
Nursing implications	
Obtain baseline values: blood urea nitrogen (BUN), serum creatinine, serum bilirubin, clotting function, vital signs	Obtain baseline values (blood gases, vital signs). Maintain continuous infusion and constant infusion rate. Monitor blood gases frequently. Monitor vital signs and ventilatory status
Monitor cardiovascular status to detect evidence of patent ductus arteriosus (heart murmur, wide pulse pressure, bounding pulses, congestive heart failure)	Monitor cardiovascular status to detect improvement or deterioration. As pulmonary blood flow increases, the foramen ovale may close and P_aO_2 may fall
Monitor urine output and check urine for blood and protein	
Monitor BUN and serium creatinine levels	
Observe for signs of gastrointestinal bleeding in stools, gastric aspirate	
Monitor platelet count, prothrombin time, partial thromboplastin time	

Significant coarctation of the aorta is treated by surgically removing the area of aortic obstruction. This can be done by excising the area of coarctation and then sewing the aorta together in an end-to-end fashion. Alternatively, the aorta can be incised, the obstructing shelflike membrane removed, and the aorta enlarged with a gusset, patch, or subclavian flap. Children with congestive heart failure can be treated with digitalis and diuretics until surgical repair can be done. In some children, particularly those undergoing surgery before 1 year of age, coarctation can recur. In most children, operative repair of coarctation of the aorta relieves upper body hypertension.

Ventricular Septal Defect

A ventricular septal defect is a hole in the septum between the left and right ventricles (Fig. 35-9). The size of the ventricular septal defect and its location in the ventricular septum are quite variable. Ventricular septal defect, which is the most common congenital cardiac abnormality, occurs in 1.5–2.5 of 1000 live births and comprises 20% of all

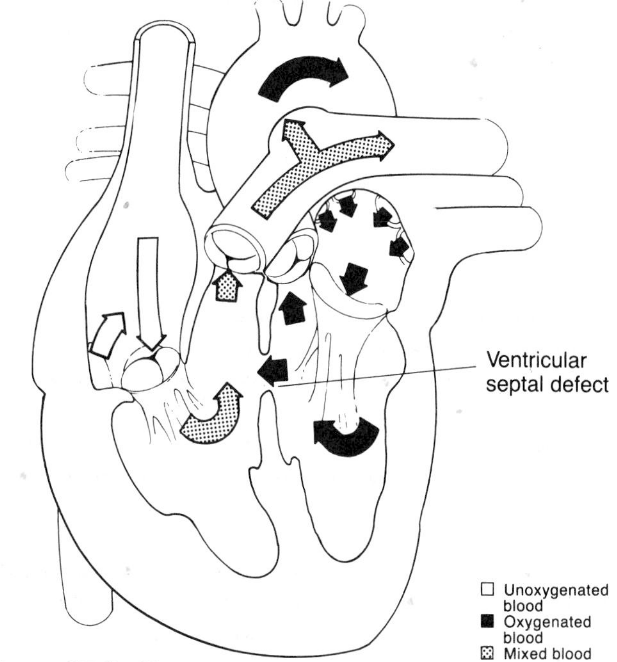

Figure 35-9 Ventricular septal defect.

forms of congenital heart disease (Krovetz, Gessner, and Schiebler, 1979). Most defects are located in the upper membranous portion of the septum, but some occur in the lower muscular portion of the septum. Occasionally, there are multiple small-to-medium defects throughout the septum, resembling the appearance of Swiss cheese. Ventricular septal defect may occur as an isolated malformation or it may be associated with other congenital cardiac defects.

A ventricular septal defect allows systemic venous and oxygenated arterial blood to mix. In uncomplicated ventricular septal defect, some of the oxygenated blood from the left ventricle is ejected through the ventricular septal defect into the right ventricle rather than into the aorta. This blood mixes with the blood in the right ventricle and is ejected with it into the pulmonary artery. Thus, an abnormally increased volume of blood flows to the lungs and returns to the left atrium and ventricle. This might result in pulmonary edema and enlargement of the left atrium, left ventricle, and sometimes the right ventricle. If the ventricular septal defect is large, pressure in the right ventricle and pulmonary artery is increased. If pulmonary artery pressure remains elevated for a number of years, it can damage the blood vessels of the lung, resulting in obstructive pulmonary vascular disease.

The clinical manifestations of a ventricular septal defect depend on its size. Small ventricular septal defects (0.1–0.6 cm) are asymptomatic and usually are diagnosed because of a characteristic heart murmur. Children with moderately large (0.8–1.5 cm) and large (1.5–3.0 cm) ventricular septal defects might have congestive heart failure and pulmonary edema (Krovetz, Gessner, and Schiebler, 1979).

Small, hemodynamically insignificant ventricular septal defects require no specific treatment, and most close spontaneously. Moderately large and large ventricular septal defects can be closed surgically by sewing a Dacron patch over the hole. This operation, which has a mortality rate of less than 5%, requires a cardiopulmonary bypass. In some patients, the ventricular septal defect recurs postoperatively, usually because of dehiscence of the sutures. In rare instances, the conduction system is damaged during the operation, resulting in atrioventricular block. Medium and large ventricular septal defects have 40%–65% of the pulmonary blood flow originating from the left-to-right shunt. They are repaired as early as possible because of the risk of becoming inoperable once pulmonary vascular obstructive disease develops. Congestive heart failure and pulmonary edema associated with the ventricular septal defect can be treated with digitalis and diuretics until surgical closure can be performed or spontaneous closure occurs.

Although a complete repair is preferred in young infants, the risks of surgery are higher than in older children. Therefore, if the infant is a poor surgical candidate, a palliative surgical procedure, in which a small constricting band is placed around the pulmonary artery to reduce blood flow to the lungs, may be performed. The procedure, known as pulmonary artery banding (PAB), does not require cardiopulmonary bypass.

Atrial Septal Defect

An atrial septal defect consists of an abnormal hole in the wall separating the left and right atria (Fig. 35-10). The types of atrial septal defects are defined by their location in the atrial septum and their embryonic origin: (a) ostium secundum defect, (b) ostium primum defect, (c) sinus venosus defect, and (d) coronary sinus defect (also called inferior vena cava defect). The ostium primum defect is an endocardial cushion defect. Coronary sinus defects are quite rare. They are located in the dorsocaudal aspect of the atrial septum. The sinus venosus defect is located in the dorsocranial aspect of the atrial septum and frequently is associated with anomalous pulmonary venous return of the right upper pulmonary vein. Secundum defects are the most common type and are located in the central portion of the atrial septum in the region of the fossa ovale. Secundum atrial septal defects comprise 9%–10% of all congenital cardiac malformations (Huntington, 1981) and occur twice as often in girls than in boys.

An atrial septal defect allows oxygenated blood returning from the lungs to the left atrium to pass into the right atrium. From the right atrium the blood enters the right ventricle and returns to the lungs, causing the lungs to receive all systemic venous return plus oxygenated blood that traverses the atrial septal defect. An abnormally increased vol-

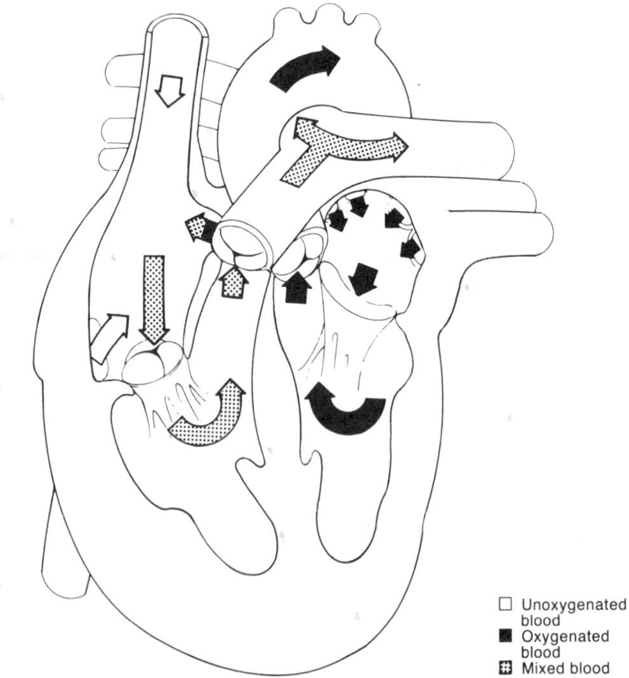

Figure 35-10 Atrial septal defect: ostium secondum.

ume of blood must be pumped by the right atrium and right ventricle, which can result in right atrial and right ventricular enlargement. The added volume of blood being pumped to the lungs can result in mild or moderate pulmonary edema.

In complicated forms of atrial septal defect associated with other cardiac malformations, movement of deoxygenated blood from the right to the left atrium can occur as well. In patients with uncomplicated atrial septal defects, however, the predominant movement of blood is from the left to the right atrium, and little if any blood shunts from right to left. This results from relative differences in the compliance of the right and the left ventricles.

The child with an uncomplicated atrial septal defect usually is asymptomatic, and the defect is detected by the presence of a cardiac murmur in an otherwise-healthy child. Frequently, however, the nurse can elicit a history of exercise intolerance. The murmur of an atrial septal defect is a systolic ejection murmur heard best at the left upper sternal border. The murmur is not due to blood passing through the atrial septal defect, but is instead due to an abnormally increased volume of blood traveling through the pulmonic valve. Thus, the murmur is similar to that heard in children with mild pulmonic valve stenosis or a functional pulmonary flow murmur. The atrial septal defect is distinguished by an abnormal second heart sound. Normally, S_2 is single during expiration but split during inspiration. In children with atrial septal defect, S_2 is widely split throughout the respiratory cycle.

The chest radiograph of the child with an atrial septal defect reveals mild-to-moderate cardiomegaly and prominent pulmonary vascular markings. The electrocardiogram might reveal mild right ventricular enlargement. The atrial septal defect can be visualized with echocardiography.

In males, atrial septal defects of significant size are repaired surgically. In females, all atrial septal defects are repaired, regardless of size. Even hemodynamically insignificant atrial septal defects are closed in females to eliminate the risk of paradoxical emboli during pregnancy. Operative closure requires cardiopulmonary bypass, and the risk of death due to operation is less than 1%. The operation is performed when the child is about 4–6 years of age. Left untreated, the atrial septal defect can cause heart failure and atrial arrhythmias to develop.

Endocardial Cushion Defects

Defects in the embryonic formation of the endocardial cushions result in a spectrum of congenital cardiac malformations, ranging from an isolated cleft in the septal leaflet of the mitral valve to atrioventricular canal defects. Endocardial cushion defects are classified as complete or incomplete atrioventricular canal.

A *complete atrioventricular canal* consists of a ventricular septal defect located relatively posteriorly in the ventricular septum, an atrial septal defect located caudally in the atrial septum, and incomplete formation of the mitral and tricuspid valves, such that there is one common atrioventricular valve rather than two separate atrioventricular valves (Fig. 35-11). In essence, the central portion of the heart is missing, as the left ventricle and left atrium and right ventricle and right atrium all communicate.

Endocardial cushion defects are the most common cardiac defects in children with Down's syndrome. The major physiologic consequences of endocardial cushion defects are increased pulmonary blood flow and volume overload in the left and right ventricles. The severity of symptoms depends on the specific defect, but in general a complete atrioventricular canal is more symptomatic and more difficult to treat than an incomplete atrioventricular canal. Because both interatrial and intraventricular septal defects are present in complete atrioventricular canal, a considerable amount of oxygenated blood returning to the left atrium and left ventricle shunts to the right atrium and right ventricle and recirculates to the lungs, resulting in abnormally increased pulmonary blood flow and pulmonary edema. If the child also has atrioventricular valve insufficiency, atrial pressures elevate, increasing pulmonary congestion and pulmonary edema. This combination produces pulmonary edema and congestive heart failure, which, in infants, can be serious enough to result in growth failure.

The optimal treatment for endocardial cushion defect is surgical repair. The risk of surgical repair increases proportionately with the severity of the defect and inversely with

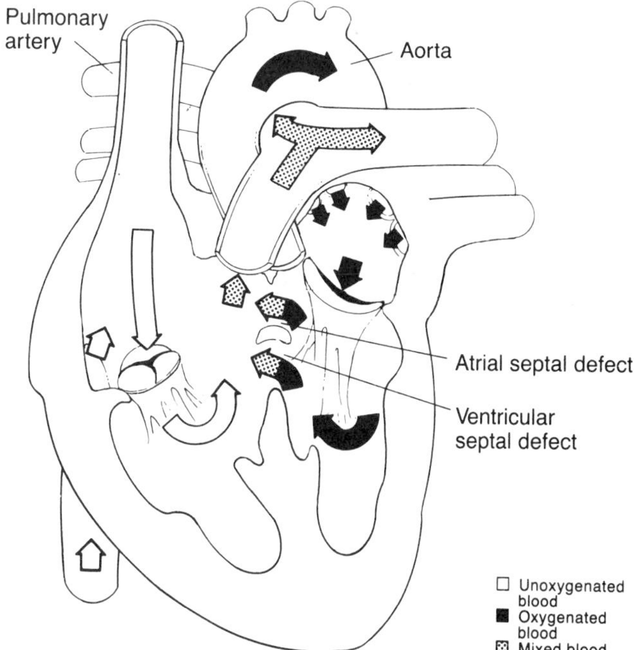

Figure 35-11 Complete atrioventricular canal.

the age of the child. In general, the repair of incomplete forms of endocardial cushion defects is safer and more successful than repair of complete atrioventricular canals. In infants less than 3 months of age, repair of a complete atrioventricular canal carries a 20%–30% risk of death (Feldt, 1976). In older children the risk is considerably less. Surgical repair consists of closure of the atrial and ventricular septal defects and creation of separate mitral and tricuspid valves.

Prior to the operation, the child can be treated with digitalis and diuretics to reduce the degree of congestive heart failure and pulmonary edema. A pulmonary artery band may be placed to decrease blood flow to the lungs. Attempts are made to maximize caloric intake in infants with growth failure. The child requires subacute bacterial endocarditis prophylaxis before and after surgical correction. Most children with complete atrioventricular canal have considerable pulmonary hypertension, so correction of the intracardiac defect should be performed before the onset of significant pulmonary vascular obstructive disease.

Pulmonic Valve Stenosis

The defect in pulmonic valve stenosis is an abnormally small valvular orifice caused by thickened, relatively immobile valve leaflets with fused commissures (Fig. 35-12). The etiology of pulmonic valve stenosis is unknown. This abnormality constitutes 7%–9% (Huntington, 1981) of all congenital cardiac defects.

Normally, the systolic pressure of the right ventricle and pulmonary artery are equal, about 20 mm Hg. In the presence of pulmonic valve stenosis, right ventricular systolic pressure is abnormally elevated, while pulmonary artery pressure remains normal. This difference occurs because greater pressure is required to pump a normal amount of blood through the stenotic pulmonic valve. The narrower the pulmonic valve, the higher the right ventricular pressure will be.

Children with mild to moderate degrees of pulmonic valve stenosis usually are asymptomatic, and the lesion is detected by the presence of a cardiac murmur. Severe pulmonic valve stenosis can result in right ventricular failure, tricuspid insufficiency, and low cardiac output. In infants, severe pulmonic valve stenosis associated with a patent foramen ovale can result in cyanosis as a result of right-to-left atrial shunting.

Mild pulmonic valve stenosis (right ventricular pressure less than 20 mm Hg greater than pulmonary artery pressure) requires no specific treatment. Severe stenosis (right ventricular pressure equal to or slightly less than left ventricular pressure) requires valvotomy. There is some difference of opinion about the advisability of surgery for moderate pulmonic valve stenosis (right ventricular pressure 40 mm Hg greater than pulmonary artery pressure). Except in the neonate, the operative risk for pulmonic valve stenosis is less than 5%. In neonates with severe stenosis, the surgical risk is 5%–15%.

Aortic Stenosis

In aortic stenosis, the orifice of the aortic valve is abnormally small (Fig. 35–13). Frequently, the valve is bicuspid rather than tricuspid, and leaflets are thickened and relatively noncompliant. Aortic stenosis forces the left ventricle to generate abnormally high systolic pressure to pump a

Stenotic pulmonic valve

☐ Unoxygenated blood
■ Oxygenated blood

Figure 35-12 Pulmonic valve stenosis.

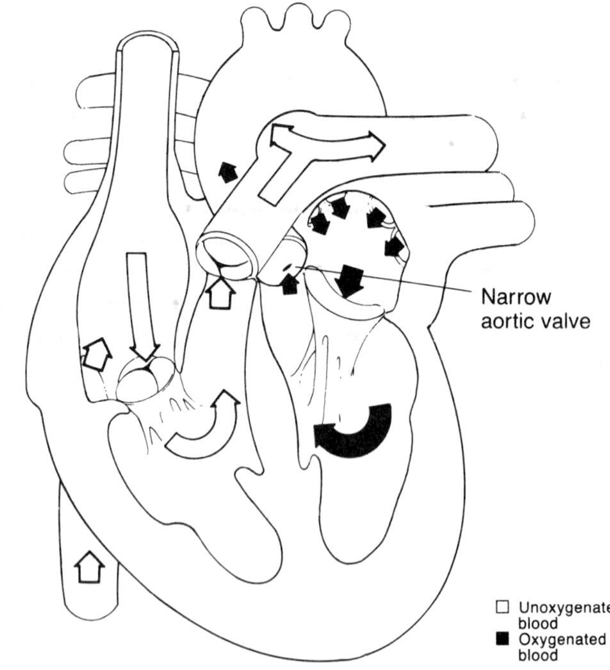

Figure 35-13 Aortic stenosis.

normal amount of blood, which results in left ventricular hypertrophy.

The clinical manifestations of aortic stenosis depend on its severity. In mild or moderately severe aortic stenosis (left ventricular pressure less than 20 mm Hg greater than aortic pressure or 20–60 mm Hg greater, respectively) the child is asymptomatic, and aortic stenosis is detected through cardiac murmur. Severe aortic stenosis can be associated with syncope, reduced exercise tolerance, and fatigue. In infants, severe aortic stenosis can cause congestive heart failure.

Mild aortic stenosis requires no treatment, but the condition is progressive and requires ongoing assessment. Moderate and severe aortic stenosis require operative relief. Aortic valvotomy is the preferred procedure for children, although aortic valve replacement may be necessary in childhood or later in life. Aortic incompetence is a potential complication of valvotomy.

Mitral Valve Dysfunction

The most common forms of mitral valve dysfunction are mitral valve prolapse, mitral stenosis, and mitral insufficiency. Mitral valve prolapse is a condition in which one or both of the mitral valve leaflets "buckle" toward the left atrium during ventricular systole. It can be associated with mitral valve insufficiency. Prolapse can be seen on echocardiograms.

Mitral valve stenosis can be congenital or acquired. The most common cause of acquired mitral stenosis is rheumatic fever (see Chapter 37). If congenital, mitral stenosis usually is associated with other cardiac malformations, such as coarctation of the aorta and aortic stenosis. Mitral valve insufficiency also can be congenital or acquired, and its most common acquired cause is rheumatic fever. Congenital mitral insufficiency may be due to poorly formed valve leaflets or to a cleft in one of them (a form of endocardial cushion defect).

Mitral valve prolapse usually is asymptomatic. It can, however, be associated with cardiac arrhythmias and palpitations. Mitral valve prolapse itself requires no treatment, but associated arrhythmias may require treatment if they are serious or symptomatic.

The clinical manifestations of mitral stenosis or insufficiency depend on the severity of the lesion. Both defects cause pulmonary edema, congestive heart failure, and fatigue. Severe mitral stenosis can be associated with hemoptysis. Congestive heart failure associated with mitral stenosis or insufficiency can be treated with digitalis preparations and diuretics; moderately severe and severe defects require surgical treatment. In some cases mitral stenosis can be treated by commissurotomy, but mitral valve replacement is often necessary. Mitral insufficiency can be treated by mitral valvuloplasty or mitral valve replacement.

The Child With a Cyanotic Cardiac Defect

Tetralogy of Fallot

The child with tetralogy of Fallot has a ventricular septal defect; right ventricular outflow obstruction from pulmonic valve stenosis (infundibulum, subpulmonic valve stenosis, or frequently both); an aorta that overrides the ventricular septal defect; and right ventricular hypertrophy (Fig. 35-14). Because of the shunt and displaced aorta, the right ventricle hypertrophies in response to the added workload of pumping blood to the systemic circulation. Tetralogy of Fallot comprises about 10% of congenital cardiac malformations and is the most common cyanotic defect (Krovetz, Gessner, and Schiebler, 1979).

The principal clinical manifestation of tetralogy of Fallot is cyanosis, which varies in degree, depending on the severity of pulmonary stenosis. The infant with minimal pulmonary stenosis has mild right ventricular outflow obstruction. The infant consequently has a left-to-right shunt and is acyanotic, as the right ventricular pressure is not raised significantly. As the infant grows, however, the degree of stenosis increases proportionately, and the direction of the shunt changes, resulting in cyanosis.

Tetralogy of Fallot may cause hypoxic spells. Hypoxic spells are unusual before two months of age and occur most commonly in the morning, 1–2 hours after the child awakens.

Children with tetralogy of Fallot, especially those with infundibular stenosis, may squat, particularly after exertion. A squatting posture effectively changes the relationship

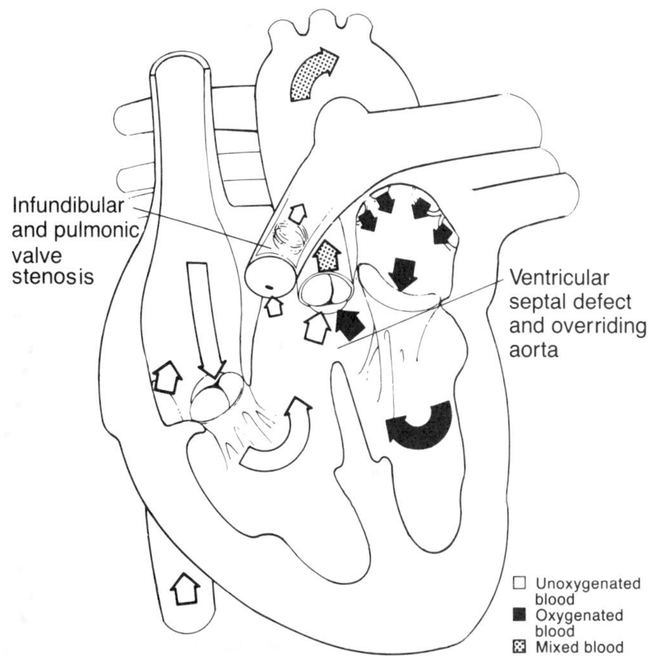

Figure 35-14 Tetralogy of Fallot.

between the systemic and pulmonary vascular resistances, resulting in increased pulmonary blood flow. Besides cyanosis, hypoxic spells, and squatting, the child with tetralogy of Fallot is underweight, has a systolic murmur and prominent ejection click, and is polycythemic and therefore at risk for central nervous system emboli, thromboses, and abscesses.

Definitive treatment for tetralogy of Fallot is surgical closure of the ventricular septal defect and relief of right ventricular outflow obstruction. The success of this procedure depends to a large extent on the size and distribution of the pulmonary arteries and the size of the left ventricle. In small infants and children with markedly underdeveloped pulmonary arteries, total surgical correction might not be feasible, and a systemic-to-pulmonary arterial shunt might be created. The original shunt procedure for tetralogy of Fallot is the Blalock-Taussig operation, in which the subclavian artery is anastomosed to the pulmonary artery. Alternatively, the ascending aorta can be anastomosed to the right pulmonary artery (Waterston shunt) or the descending aorta to the left pulmonary artery (Potts anastomosis). Another approach to the correction of tetralogy of Fallot associated with small pulmonary arteries is a staged correction. Initially, the pulmonary artery stenosis is relieved, but the ventricular septal defect is not repaired. In many infants the pulmonary arteries grow at an increased rate following this procedure because of the increase in pulmonary blood flow. At a later date, the ventricular septal defect is closed.

Results are often unsatisfactory following the creation of a shunt and its later repair at the time of corrective surgery. Some cardiac centers have had good results with total corrective surgery during infancy by using deep hypothermia (core cooling) and limited cardiopulmonary bypass. Palliative shunting is reserved for those infants with pulmonary atresia or severe hypoplasia of pulmonary arteries and descending coronary artery malplacement (Castaneda et al., 1976).

Transposition of the Great Arteries

Transposition of the great arteries is a condition in which the aorta arises from the right ventricle and the pulmonary artery arises from the left ventricle (Fig. 35-15). Deoxygenated blood returning from the body to the right atrium traverses the right ventricle and then, instead of traveling to the lungs to become oxygenated, is directed back to the body through the aorta. Oxygenated blood returning from the lungs to the left atrium traverses the mitral valve, enters the left ventricle, and is returned to the lungs through the pulmonary artery. Thus, in the absence of associated defects, the body receives no oxygenated blood, and death occurs.

Most infants with simple transposition of the great arteries have a patent foramen ovale that allows some oxygenated blood from the left atrium to shunt into the right atrium

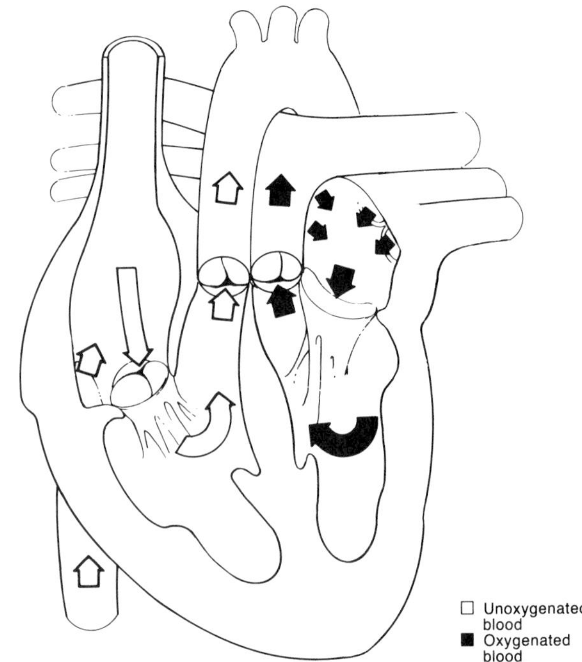

Figure 35-15 Transposition of the great arteries.

and vice versa. Others may have a patent ductus arteriosis or ventricular septal defect, which allows oxygenated and deoxygenated blood to mix. In general, the more abnormal communications that exist between the two circuits, the less cyanotic the infant will be.

Patients with transposition of the great arteries usually are cyanotic neonates. In general, they appear to be otherwise healthy. The detection of cyanosis at birth is critical. If the only cardiac defect is transposition of the great arteries, the untreated neonate will become more hypoxic and acidotic as the foramen ovale and ductus arteriosus obliterate. It is critical to identify these neonates so that interventions can be initiated to improve mixing of oxygenated and deoxygenated blood.

Transposition of the great arteries causes an abnormal increase in pulmonary blood flow, resulting in pulmonary edema and congestive heart failure. Like all children with cyanotic congenital heart disease, infants with transposition of the great arteries are at risk for polycythemia and right-to-left intracardiac shunts, with secondary complications of stroke, brain abscess, and severe headache. The infant with transposition of the great arteries and a large ventricular septal defect might develop severe congestive heart failure and also is at risk for pulmonary vascular obstructive disease.

The neonate with transposition of the great arteries requires emergency treatment. Cardiac catheterization is done, and balloon atrial septostomy (Rashkind procedure) is performed to increase interatrial mixing of oxygenated and deoxygenated blood. A specially designed catheter with an inflatable balloon at its tip is advanced from the right atrium through the foramen ovale to the left atrium. The balloon is inflated in the left atrium, and the catheter rapidly is withdrawn into the right atrium, thus enlarging the foramen ovale. This frequently is a life-saving procedure. A neonate with transposition of the great arteries and a large ventricular septal defect might require banding of the pulmonary artery to prevent the development of pulmonary vascular obstructive disease. A neonate with congestive heart failure also might benefit from digitalis and diuretics.

Ultimately, surgical correction is required to direct all the deoxygenated blood to the pulmonary artery and the oxygenated blood to the aorta. A number of surgical procedures have been described to accomplish this. In Senning's and Mustard's operation, a baffle is connected to redirect the flow of oxygenated and deoxygenated blood in the atria such that deoxygenated blood returning from the superior and inferior vena cavae is directed by way of the baffle through the mitral valve to the left ventricle and then to the lungs. The oxygenated blood returning from the lungs through the pulmonary veins is directed (through the baffle) through the tricuspid valve into the right ventricle and into the aorta. When a ventricular septal defect is present, it is closed at the time of the procedure.

If the child with transposition of the great arteries has a ventricular septal defect, Rastelli's operation can be performed. This consists of closing the ventricular septal defect such that the left ventricle ejects blood through the ventricular septal defect and into the aorta. The pulmonary artery is divided, and a synthetic conduit is interposed between the right ventricle and the pulmonary artery. A more recent operative approach to transposition of the great arteries involves switching the aorta and pulmonary artery and connecting the coronary artery to the newly transposed aorta, which now receives blood from the left ventricle.

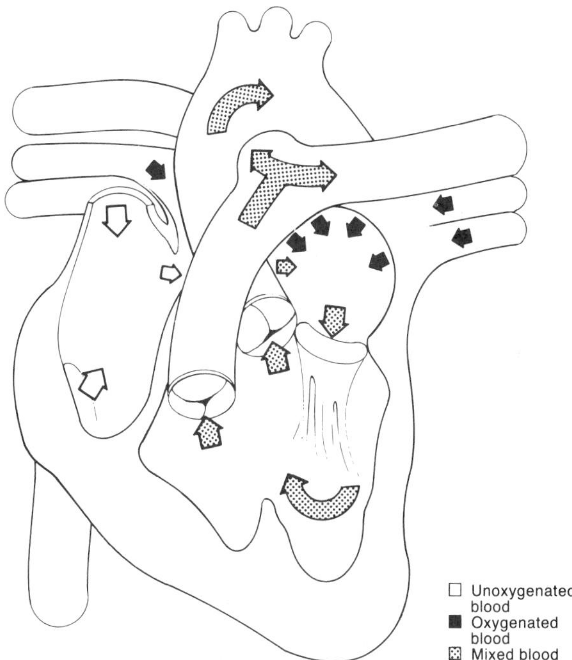

Figure 35-16 Tricuspid atresia.

Tricuspid Atresia

Tricuspid atresia is a condition in which the tricuspid valve did not form (Fig. 35-16). Thus, there is no direct communication between the right atrium and right ventricles. Survival is not possible unless an interatrial communication or its physiologic equivalent is present. Usually, the right ventricle is hypoplastic, and a ventricular septal defect is present. The aorta and pulmonary artery might be normally related or transposed such that the aorta arises from the hypoplastic right ventricle and the pulmonary artery arises from the left ventricle. Tricuspid atresia constitutes 2% of congenital cardiac defects (Krovetz, Gessner, and Schiebler, 1979).

In tricuspid atresia, systemic venous blood returns to the right atrium. From the right atrium, the deoxygenated blood passes through an interatrial communication, enters the left atrium, and mixes with oxygenated pulmonary venous blood returning from the lungs. The blood traverses the mitral valve, enters the left ventricle, and leaves the left ventricle through the aorta and the pulmonary artery. The relative amount of blood entering the pulmonary artery and aorta depends on the position of the great arteries (that is, whether they are normal or transposed), the absence or presence and severity of pulmonic valve stenosis, and the size of the intraventricular defect. Tricuspid atresia is a cyanotic form of congenital heart disease, and in general, the degree of cyanosis is inversely proportional to the volume of pulmonary blood flow.

The principal manifestation of tricuspid atresia is cyanosis. The excess amount of blood the left ventricle must pump eventually leads to left ventricular failure. If the interatrial communication is small, right atrial enlargement, significant hepatomegaly, and signs and symptoms of low cardiac output can occur.

Because of left ventricular volume overload, many children with tricuspid atresia benefit from digitalis therapy. At one time only palliative operations were available for patients with tricuspid atresia: pulmonary artery banding for excessive pulmonary blood flow, a systemic-to-pulmonary artery shunt if pulmonary blood flow was deficient, an atrial septectomy–septostomy if interatrial communication was inadequate. A more definitive or "physiologic" surgical procedure has since been developed by Fontan and colleagues (Fontan and Bandet, 1971). This operation consists of closure of the interatrial communication, connection of the right atrium to the pulmonary artery by a synthetic conduit, and isolation of the pulmonary artery from the ventricle. Thus, systemic venous (deoxygenated) blood is directed exclusively to the lungs, and pulmonary venous (oxygenated) blood to the aorta. Mixture of oxygenated and deoxygenated blood is eliminated, as is cyanosis. In addition, the volume of blood pumped out of the left ventricle is reduced to normal.

The chief negative result of this operation is that blood must flow into the pulmonary artery without benefit of a ventricular pump. Many children are markedly improved with this operation, but others have chronic fluid retention and reduced exercise tolerance. Not all children with tricuspid atresia are candidates for the Fontan operation. Its success depends on a relatively normal pulmonary vascular bed, adequate left ventricular function, and absence of significant mitral regurgitation.

Total Anomalous Pulmonary Venous Return

Total anomalous pulmonary venous return is a condition in which all the pulmonary venous blood returns to the heart but does not initially enter the left atrium (Fig. 35-17). The condition can be described as supracardiac, cardiac, infracardiac, or mixed, depending on how the pulmonary venous blood returns to the heart. In supracardiac total anomalous pulmonary venous return, the pulmonary veins coalesce behind the left atrium, but instead of connecting to the left atrium, they drain into a left vertical vein that connects to the anomalous vein or directly to the superior vena cava. In the cardiac type of condition, the common pulmonary venous chamber drains directly into the right atrium or into the coronary sinus. In the infracardiac type of condition, the common pulmonary venous chamber drains through a blood vessel that descends through the diaphragm and empties into the portal venous system. Mixed total anomalous pulmonary venous return is a combination of the other types of conditions. Survival with total anomalous pulmonary venous return is not possible unless an interatrial communication or its equivalent is present.

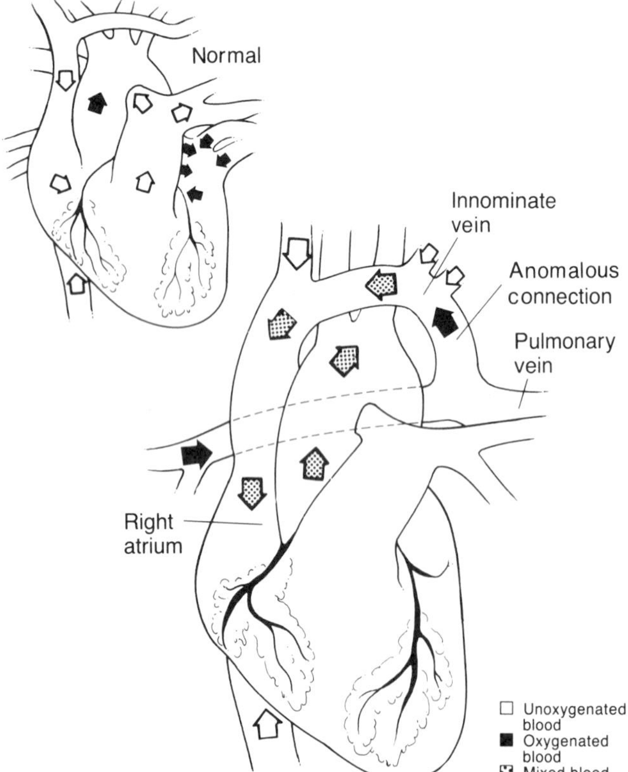

Figure 35-17 Total anomalous pulmonary venous return.

The physiologic effect of total anomalous pulmonary venous return depends on whether or not the communication connecting the common pulmonary venous chamber and the heart or the interatrial septum is obstructed. If unobstructed, total anomalous pulmonary venous return results in excess blood flow circulating to the right atrium, right ventricle, and pulmonary artery. In addition, because oxygenated blood returning from the lungs and deoxygenated blood returning from the body are mixed, systemic arterial hypoxemia and cyanosis can occur. If the return of pulmonary venous blood is obstructed, significant pulmonary venous hypertension occurs, and if the obstruction is unrelieved, death might result.

The clinical presentation of neonates with total anomalous pulmonary venous return depends on the presence or absence and degree of obstruction of pulmonary venous return to the heart. Usually, infracardiac total anomalous pulmonary venous return is associated with severe obstruction. Neonates with this lesion usually have cyanosis and severe respiratory distress. This represents a true emergency requiring immediate diagnosis and surgical treatment.

Treatment of total anomalous pulmonary venous return is surgical and consists of directing the pulmonary venous blood into the left atrium. The manner in which this is done depends on the type of defects. If pulmonary venous return is obstructed, surgery is urgent. If there is no significant obstruction, the timing of the operation depends on the clinical situation. Preoperatively, the child with obstructed total anomalous pulmonary venous return but significantly increased pulmonary blood flow might benefit from digitalis and diuretic therapy.

Truncus Arteriosus

Truncus arteriosus is a condition in which one artery (the truncus) rather than two arteries (the aorta and pulmonary artery) arises from the ventricles (Fig. 35-18). After arising from the heart, the truncus divides into the pulmonary artery and aorta. The pulmonary artery might arise from the truncus as a single blood vessel that subsequently divides into the left and right pulmonary arteries (truncus I). Alternatively, the right and left pulmonary arteries may arise as separate branches from the side (truncus II) or from the posterior aspect (truncus III). Truncus arteriosus always is associated with a large intraventricular septal defect positioned immediately below the origin of the truncus arteriosus.

Unless the pulmonary arteries are abnormally small, children with truncus arteriosus have abnormally increased pulmonary blood flow resulting in pulmonary edema and congestive heart failure. Because of the excessive pulmonary blood flow and high pressure of that flow, these children are susceptible to pulmonary vascular obstructive disease at a relatively early age. If the pulmonary arteries are abnormally small, such children might have relatively reduced pulmonary blood flow and cyanosis.

Neonates with truncus arteriosus might appear normal or cyanotic at birth or might have severe pulmonary edema and congestive heart failure, depending on the size of the pulmonary arteries and the pulmonary vascular resistance. As pulmonary vascular resistance declines, congestive heart failure increases, and pulmonary edema occurs. Most infants with truncus arteriosus have significant pulmonary edema and congestive heart failure, at times poorly controlled by digitalis and diuretic therapy. If growth failure occurs despite optimum medical management, surgical intervention is necessary.

Until recently, the only surgical option available for infants with truncus arteriosus was banding of the pulmonary artery. The mortality for this operation was high, and the outcome for survivors often was poor. Presently, surgeons at many large medical centers perform a "corrective" operation for infants with truncus arteriosus. This operation involves closing the ventricular septal defect, removing the pulmonary arteries from the truncus arteriosus, and interposing a valve-containing conduit between the right ventricle and distal pulmonary artery. Because the lumen of the conduit usually is too small to accommodate the pulmonary blood flow of an adult, it must be replaced as the child grows. In general, truncus arteriosus should be corrected before the child is 2 years of age. If the operation is delayed, severe pulmonary vascular obstructive disease can occur, precluding complete intracardiac repair at a later date.

Hypoplastic Left Heart Syndrome

Hypoplastic left heart syndrome consists of an abnormally small mitral valve, left ventricle, aortic valve, and ascending aorta. It is a lethal cardiac malformation, and few neonates survive beyond 6 weeks of age. Survival is possible while the ductus arteriosus remains patent. In this situation, most of the blood returning from the body to the right atrium passes through the tricuspid valve and right ventricle into the pulmonary artery. Some of the blood continues to the lungs, while some of it traverses the patent ductus arteriosus and perfuses the body. As pulmonary vascular resistance declines or the ductus arteriosus closes, pulmonary edema and low cardiac output occur, leading to hypoxemia, acidosis, and death.

Infants with the hypoplastic left heart syndrome usually look quite well at birth but within a few hours or days develop signs of congestive heart failure, cyanosis, or both. The diagnosis of hypoplastic left heart syndrome can be made with echocardiography, obviating the need for cardiac catheterization in most cases. Medical management is

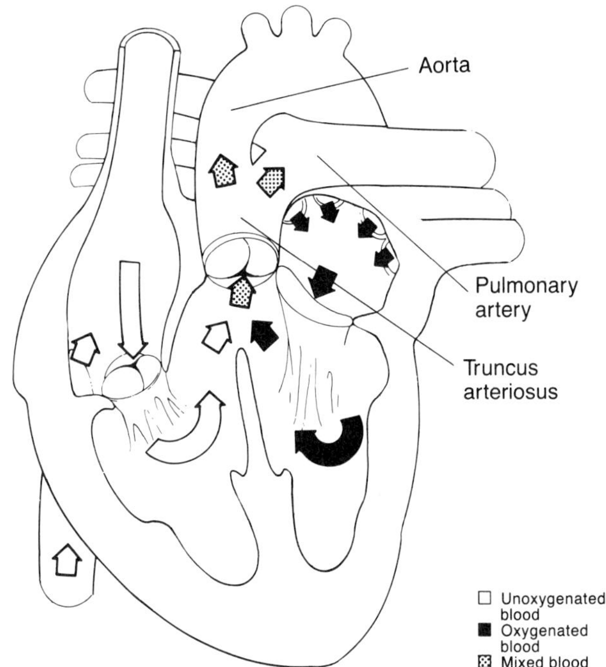

Figure 35-18 Truncus arteriosus.

symptomatic, and results are temporary. Initial attempts at surgically correcting the lesion have been developed (Norwood, Kirlin, and Sanders, 1980), although results have had limited success. Currently, extensive research is being done to develop a satisfactory approach to correcting this lesion.

The Child Undergoing Cardiac Surgery

Cardiac surgery is a stressful experience for both the child and family, and the quality of nursing care in the perioperative period is a critical factor in the child's recovery. While excellent physical care is of primary importance, promotion of the child's psychologic adjustment is an integral part of nursing care (Peterson, 1979).

Cardiac surgery may be done on an emergency or elective basis. "Closed-heart" surgery involves structures related to the heart but not the heart muscle itself and can be done without cardiopulmonary bypass. "Open-heart" surgery involves structures within the heart, necessitates an incision into the myocardium, and requires cardiopulmonary bypass. Palliative surgery provides a temporary or partial correction, whereas corrective surgery provides a permanent and total correction of the defect. Unfortunately, only palliative surgery is possible for some defects. Generally, the younger the child, the higher the surgical risk. In the past, palliative surgery was usually all that was available for infants and young children. Corrective surgery, because of its complexity was reserved until the child was older and the surgical risks lower. With technologic advances, however, corrective surgery is now available for infants and even for neonates with certain types of defects.

Preoperative Management

The child is generally admitted to the hospital 1–2 days before elective cardiac surgery. During this time the child's readiness for surgery is evaluated, and preoperative preparations are performed (Pelletier, 1982). (Principles of care related to preoperative preparation are discussed in Chapter 29.) Preoperative assessment data include the following:

1. *Laboratory data.* Tests that are routinely done before surgery include chest radiographs, electrocardiogram, complete blood count, serum electrolytes, clotting studies, and urinalysis. Other studies, such as echocardiogram and cardiac catheterization, are done if necessary.
2. *Vital signs.* Temperature, pulse, respiration, and blood pressure are monitored prior to surgery.
3. *Sleep–wake patterns.* The nurse notes the child's usual pattern of sleep and activity. This information can be used postoperatively to plan periods of rest that coincide with the child's usual pattern. Stressful procedures can be scheduled during normal waking times when hydrocortisone secretion is likely to be highest.
4. *Height and weight.* These must be accurately measured and recorded, as they will be used in calculation of medication doses and fluid orders.
5. *Intake patterns.* Fluids and foods that the child particularly enjoys are documented. Information about the usual amount and times of intake can be used to plan progressive introduction of oral intake postoperatively. For example, a young child who is used to a bottle early in the morning might obtain some comfort by receiving a portion of the day's fluid allotment at that time.
6. *Elimination patterns.* The nurse needs to understand the words the child uses for bowel and bladder functions. Information on the usual pattern of urination and defecation will be useful in helping the child resume these functions as soon as possible after surgery.
7. *Signs of infection.* Any sign that might indicate the presence of an infection is reported to the physician. Infection is usually a contradiction to surgery.

Preoperative skin preparation, which may include bacteriocidal cleansing and shaving, is usually ordered, although this varies depending on the surgeon and institution.

The nurse also needs to check all medication orders carefully. Generally, digitalis is withheld for the 24 hours before surgery. Other medications may be initiated, discontinued, or modified. Any order that is unclear is reviewed and verified with the physician.

Parent Preparation Parent preparation usually begins at the time of diagnosis. At that time the nature of the defect is described and the possibility of surgery often is introduced. Parents face the prospect of surgery with emotions that are different and sometimes are conflicting. For some, the operation represents a resolution of the child's problem and a hope for a normal life. For others, surgery represents the threat of losing the child through death. Most parents feel a painful ambivalence—hope for improvement in the health of the child and fear of the loss of the child.

Parents must be prepared for both the preoperative and postoperative experience the child will face. The nurse can use a diagram or doll to explain the incision. The nurse also describes or shows parents the equipment they will see, such as arterial and venous catheters, chest tubes, nasogastric tubes, pacemaker wires, urinary catheters, respirator, and electrocardiographic monitor. The nurse needs to warn parents that children are unable to speak while endotracheal tubes are in place. The nurse explains alarm systems, so that parents will not become unduly frightened when an alarm sounds in their presence. Parents are also forewarned that blood in the chest tubes is normal. Unless the parents understand the reasons for such postoperative procedures as suctioning, turning, and chest physiotherapy, these procedures may be perceived as unnecessary or cruel.

The parents are in need of special support at the time the child leaves them for the operating room. Although the parent may appear calm and composed, the fear of never seeing the child alive again is often just below the surface. Remaining with the parent for a time in the waiting area is therefore an appropriate intervention. The long wait during surgery can be agonizing. Parents should be informed that operating room schedules are never exact and that the surgery that is not over at the anticipated time does not mean problems have occurred. Parents tremendously appreciate periodic progress reports, however simple.

Despite careful preparation, a parent is often shocked to see the child postoperatively in the intensive care unit. The shock is less severe if the parent has visited the intensive care unit ahead of time and has been exposed to its myriad sights and sounds.

Preparation for Intensive Care At each point in the preoperative discussion, the nurse emphasizes what the child will see, hear, and feel, as these sensations are of primary importance, particularly to the young child. Older children are more interested in the rationale for various procedures.

Many children benefit from seeing where their parents will wait during the surgery, visiting the intensive care unit, and meeting the nurses there. This is anxiety-producing, but the experience allows children to prepare themselves. It is not a desirable experience for all children, however, as the child who is very anxious may not be able to tolerate the stress of seeing the intensive care unit ahead of time.

Most children, however, benefit from an introduction to certain kinds of postoperative apparatus. These include

1. *Endotracheal tube.* The nurse explains that the child will not be able to talk while the tube is in place but will be able to talk after the doctor takes it out, although the throat might be a little sore.
2. *Nasogastric tube.*
3. *Chest tube.* The nurse can connect the chest tube to a small saline bottle with red water in it to demonstrate the bloody drainage that is normal.
4. *Intravenous and intra-arterial catheters.* The nurse connects these to small saline-filled bottles to demonstrate how the child will get "drinks" of water, since the child will not be able to drink by mouth for a couple of days.
5. *Electrocardiographic leads and monitor.*
6. *Urinary catheter.* The nurse explains that the child will not have to go to the bathroom because the catheter will collect the urine.

It is important to reassure the child that these apparatus are not permanent and will be removed in the first few days after surgery.

Age-appropriate explanations are another vital aspect of preoperative preparation. The nurse tells the child that there will be pain and that medicine is available to relieve the pain. Usually, narcotics are given intravenously in the intensive care unit; however, if injections will be required, the child is informed. The nurse can explain that the little hurt of the needle will make the bigger hurt of the incision go away. The nurse explains postoperative procedures, such as coughing, deep breathing, and turning, which can be practiced.

The child is reassured that all the doctors and nurses understand that children feel like crying when they feel scared or if something hurts and that it is all right for the child to cry or tell them when something is wrong. The doctors and nurses then will try to help the child to feel better.

Using the doll, the nurse demonstrates placement and removal of the tubes. The nurse explains that after a time in the intensive care unit, the child will stay in a regular hospital room for a few days and then can go home. The doll should then be changed to street clothes to emphasize this important point. Near the end of the teaching session, the nurse tells the child that the medicine that is given before the operation will involve an injection. It is helpful to allow the child to practice giving injections to the doll.

Intraoperative Management

Repair of intracardiac lesions requires the use of cardiopulmonary bypass. This is accomplished by use of a pump oxygenator with a high-efficiency heat exchanger. A cannula collects the venous blood at the right atrium and diverts it to the machine, where carbon dioxide is removed and oxygen added. The oxygenated blood is returned to the circulation through a cannula that enters the ascending aorta and is circulated through the body, perfusing the organs and body tissues.

Hypothermia reduces the metabolic demands of the heart and other organs and is usually used in conjunction with cardiopulmonary bypass. The child's temperature is reduced to 20–32° C to compensate for reduced blood flow during bypass. For small children with complex intracardiac lesions, profound hypothermia may be required. The child is initially cooled to a core temperature of 28° C, is placed on cardiopulmonary bypass, and is then rapidly cooled to 15° C. At that point bypass circulation is terminated. This provides a bloodless operative field and a motionless heart. After the lesion is repaired, bypass is resumed, and the child is rewarmed. Children are able to tolerate up to 60 minutes of profound hypothermia with total circulatory arrest.

During surgery there is constant monitoring of blood volume, arterial blood gases, blood pressure, and other indices of cardiac output.

Postoperative Management

Care of the child who has had cardiac surgery is complex and challenging. After surgery, the child is transferred directly to the intensive care unit and remains there until stable, generally for 1–3 days. Although cardiovascular function is of primary concern, virtually every organ can be affected by cardiac surgery. Therefore, assessment must be constant and comprehensive. The nurse therefore makes astute observations so that subtle signs of potential problems are to be identified early and complications prevented. The goals of nursing care in the early postoperative period include

- Prevention of complications (Table 35-9)
- Early detection of potential problems
- Minimizing the psychologic trauma of the surgical and intensive care unit experiences

Monitoring Vital Signs Vital signs are measured and recorded frequently in the early postoperative period. An apical pulse is taken for a measured minute. Any of the following signs are reported immediately:

- Change in heart rate or rhythm
- Muffled or distant heart sounds
- Presence of S_3 or S_4
- Development of (or change in) a heart murmur

A cuff blood pressure may be taken on the arm or leg, although the peripheral vasoconstriction that occurs with hypothermia or low cardiac output might make interpretation difficult. Intra-arterial monitoring of blood pressure is routinely used after cardiac surgery.

Respirations are measured for a measured minute. Tachypnea is an early sign of both cardiac and respiratory compromise.

TABLE 35-9 Postoperative Complications of Cardiac Surgery

System	Complications
Cardiovascular	Decreased cardiac output Congestive heart failure Tamponade Arrhythmias Shock
Renal	Acute tubular necrosis
Respiratory	Atelectasis Pneumonia Pneumothorax Emboli
Neurologic	Emboli (air or particulate) Decreased cerebral blood flow
Infection	Wound Mediastinal Endocarditis Sepsis
Fluid and electrolyte	Hypervolemia/hypovolemia Acidosis Hypokalemia/hyperkalemia Hypocalcemia
Hematologic	Surgical bleeding Thrombocytopenia Disseminated intravascular coagulopathy Bypass related coagulopathy Anemia

Temperature is monitored frequently. Generally, the child is cold because of hypothermia induced during the operation. Warming lights may be needed to prevent cold stress, especially for infants. A mild elevation of temperature is common in the first 24–48 hours after surgery because of the normal inflammatory response. Marked or prolonged elevations of temperature are indications of atelectasis, retained pulmonary secretions, infection, or neurologic damage.

Observing for Hemorrhage Blood loss after cardiac operations is relatively common. An anticoagulant (heparin) is administered during cardiopulmonary bypass. Protamine is given near the end of the operation to neutralize the effect of heparin. During hypothermia, however, heparin may be deposited in the adipose tissue and then gradually released as the child is rewarmed, causing postoperative bleeding. In addition, platelets may be damaged as they circulate through the tubes and filters of the bypass machine, and blood-clotting factors may be diluted by fluids used to prime the machine. Preexisting coagulopathies, such as the relative thrombocytopenia common in children with cyanotic heart disease, may make them especially vulnerable to blood loss. Disseminated intravascular coagulation (DIC) might occur as a result of shock, hypoxia, or infection.

Vital signs are monitored frequently to detect signs of shock. Excessive bleeding from the chest tubes or incision is reported immediately, and might necessitate transfusions of whole blood or platelets.

Monitoring Cardiovascular Status Continuous electrocardiographic monitoring is done routinely. Changes in cardiac rhythm are reported immediately, and a printout of the rhythm is placed in the child's record. Twelve-lead electrocardiograms are obtained immediately after surgery and whenever a change in rhythm occurs. Pacemaker wires are usually inserted so that an external pacemaker can be used if serious arrhythmias develop. Arrhythmias that occur following heart surgery may be due to acid–base or electrolyte imbalances, hypoxia, or surgical disruption of cardiac conduction pathways.

Because peripheral vasoconstriction might render cuff blood pressures inaccurate, systemic artery pressure can be measured directly. A catheter is placed in the artery and connected to a transducer. This provides a continuous display of the pressure wave on an oscilloscope. The nurse compares the pressures obtained by the arterial catheter to the pressures obtained by sphygmomanometer. A discrepancy between the two may indicate a change in peripheral vascular resistance or a malfunction in the catheter or electronic equipment.

Pulmonary artery pressure also may be monitored by an arterial catheter that is inserted during the operation. This procedure is particularly useful in children with increased pulmonary vascular resistance who are at risk for decreased pulmonary blood flow. Hypoxia, acidosis, and hypercapnia can cause an increase in pulmonary vascular resistance.

A left atrial pressure catheter can be used to measure the pressure in the left atrium, which is normally 0–8 mm Hg, but after surgery is maintained at 10–11 mm Hg. Hypovolemia or inadequate left ventricular filling are both manifested by a low left atrial pressure. Resistance to left ventricular outflow is manifested by increased left atrial pressure.

An arterial line can be used to obtain arterial samples for blood gases, but it is never used to administer blood, fluid, or medications. Arterial catheters are kept open with a continuous, slow infusion of heparinized saline (approximately 3 mL per hour). An infusion pump, which creates a pressure greater than that in the arteries, is necessary to prevent backflow of blood into the line. If the catheter becomes disconnected or develops a crack, rapid blood loss may occur. A clamp should always be available at the bedside in case bleeding from the catheter does occur.

The major complications of atrial catheters are air or particulate emboli, which may travel to the brain or coronary arteries. Arrhythmias may also occur as a result of the cath-

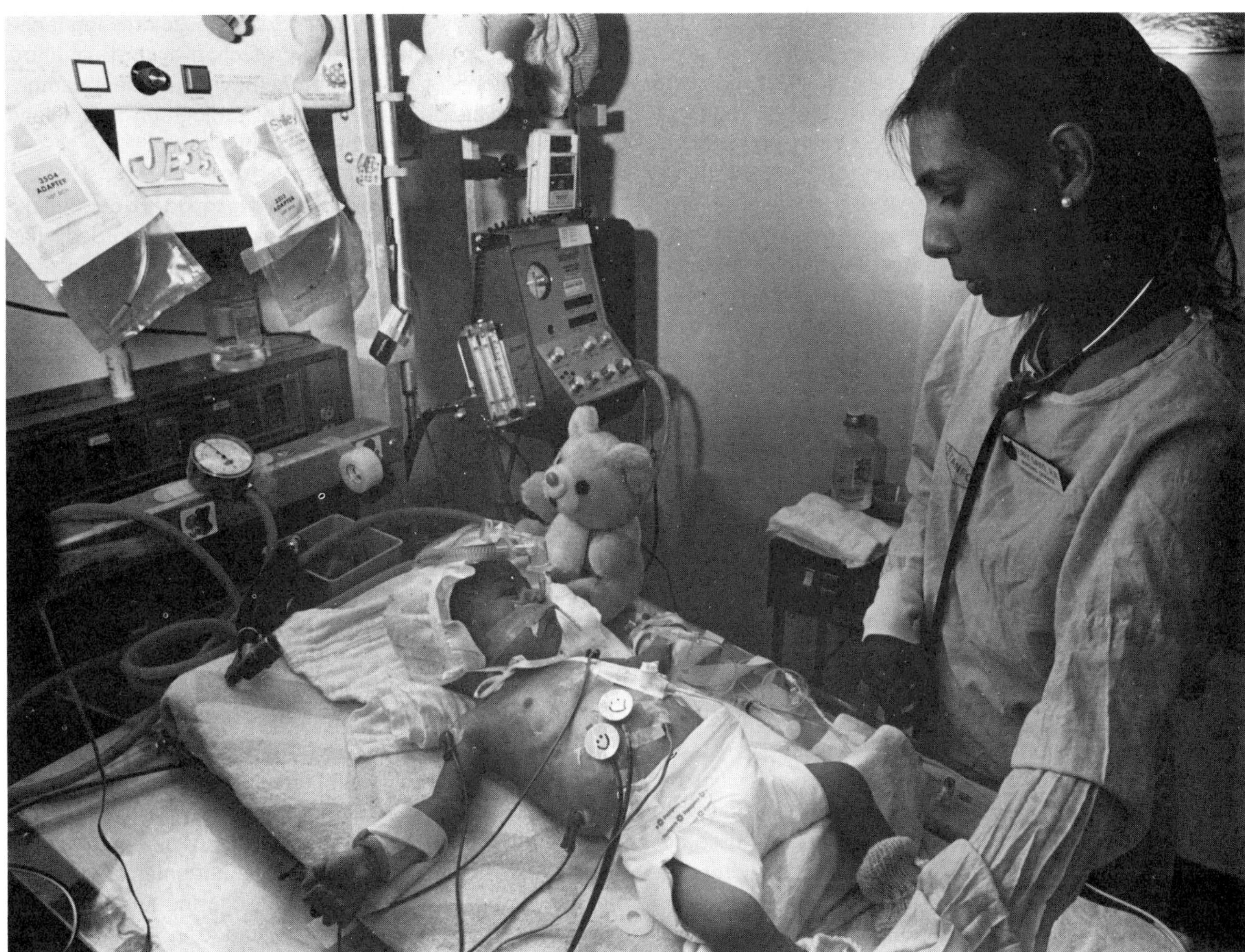

Child in intensive care unit after cardiac surgery.

eter's presence in the cardiac structures. Another potential complication is infection. Blanching or cyanosis distal to the arterial line is reported immediately, as are signs of inflammation.

A central venous pressure catheter is placed in the right atrium and attached to a monitor. Normally, central venous pressure is 0–5 mm Hg. Elevations might indicate hypervolemia, congestive heart failure, or cardiac tamponade. A low reading might indicate hypovolemia or shock. Complications of central venous pressure catheters include emboli, arrhythmia, pneumothorax, and infection.

The position of the catheter is checked by means of radiographs. Malpositioning might result in serious ventricular arrhythmias. Mild fluctuations in pressure readings with respiration indicate a patent catheter. Vigorous fluctuations, however, may indicate placement in the right ventricle, and the physician should be notified.

While all of these techniques are useful in assessing the child's cardiovascular status, they cannot take the place of standard nursing observations. Clinical signs of low cardiac output and poor tissue perfusion include pale, cool extremities; cyanosis or mottled skin; delayed capillary refill; weak, thready pulses; oliguria; and alterations in level of consciousness.

Maintaining Effective Respirations Mechanical ventilation often is used after cardiac surgery, and the child therefore has an endotracheal tube in place. When the child awakens after surgery, the nurse explains that talking will not be possible until the tube is removed. Humidified air or supplemental oxygen (by mask, nasal cannula, or hood) is given when mechanical ventilation is discontinued.

Breath sounds are auscultated frequently. Absent or diminished breath sounds, which may represent atelectasis, pneumothorax, or malposition of the endotracheal tube, require assessment by the physician. Auscultation also helps the nurse determine the need for suctioning and the lobes most in need of chest physiotherapy. In small infants breath sounds can be referred throughout the chest. The nurse therefore also observes chest expansion and symmetry when assessing adequacy of ventilation.

Retention of secretions is a common complication following heart surgery, and interventions to promote clearance are of primary importance. The child is turned every 1–2 hours. Suctioning is performed while the endotracheal tube is in place. High (100%) concentrations of oxygen are administered before, during, and after endotracheal suctioning to prevent episodes of hypoxia. The heart rate is monitored closely, as suctioning may cause vagal stimulation. After the tube is removed, suctioning might be necessary to stimulate coughing. If the child is able to cough effectively unaided, however, the unpleasant experience of suctioning can be avoided. Judicious use of pain medication and splinting of the incision will make turning, coughing, and deep breathing more effective.

Chest physiotherapy is done on a regular basis to mobilize secretions and to improve ventilation. Chest physiotherapy consists of postural drainage (positioning the child so that gravity assists the flow of secretions into a larger airway), percussion, vibration, and coughing (see Chapter 34). These procedures may be used therapeutically or prophylactically. Auscultation of the chest precedes chest physiotherapy and may identify areas that need particular attention. Breath sounds are assessed after each treatment to determine effectiveness. Chest physiotherapy might be fatiguing for the child, and not all lobes must be percussed with each treatment. Trendelenberg's position and vigorous percussion are contraindicated for recent surgical patients, as vigorous percussion might disrupt the incision, dislodge drains, or cause bleeding. Percussion might be interpreted by children as hitting or punishment, so the nurse explains to the child and parent the importance of chest physiotherapy in loosening secretions and hastening recovery.

Chest tubes are placed in the pleural or mediastinal spaces or both to remove blood, fluid, and air. The chest tubes are connected to an underwater seal drainage system to prevent the entry of air into the thoracic cavity. Suction (usually up to 20 mm of water) is applied to facilitate drainage. Chest tubes are stripped (or milked) by firmly stroking the tube toward the drainage container. This is done to prevent clot formation in the tubes and to promote removal of blood and fluids.

Tube drainage is checked hourly during the first 24 hours and every 4 hours thereafter if it is not excessive. In the first few hours after surgery, the drainage is bright red, gradually becoming serosanguineous. If drainage exceeds 2mL/kg/hour for 3 hours or more it is considered excessive and should be reported to the physician (Mills, et al., 1979).

Chest tubes are usually removed between 36 and 48 hours postoperatively if drainage is serous in nature and minimal in volume. Because of the risk of bleeding at the time of removal, chest tubes are always left in place until after the left atrial pressure catheter is removed. Removal of the chest tubes is painful, and premedication is beneficial. As the tube is removed, purse-string sutures that surround the site are quickly pulled tight to prevent entry of air into the chest cavity. A petroleum gauze dressing taped on all sides provides further protection against air entry. Complications of chest tube removal include pneumothorax and hemorrhage. A chest radiograph is obtained after removal to detect these complications.

Monitoring Fluid and Electrolyte Balance Intake and output are accurately calculated and recorded. The nurse measures all intake, including fluids used to flush intravascular catheters, and monitors urine output hourly. Foley catheters are usually in place so that urine measurements can be precise. Urine specific gravity is also checked. Output from nasogastric tubes and chest tubes is measured, and nasogastric replacement fluids are usually ordered. Weight is measured daily and more often, if indicated.

Fluids are generally restricted in the immediate postoperative period to prevent hypervolemia, which would place additional stress on the heart, possibly contributing to congestive heart failure. The cardiopulmonary bypass pump is primed with large volumes of electrolyte solution, which dilutes the circulating blood. Some of this fluid may diffuse into the tissues and then, postoperatively, diffuse back into the vascular space, contributing to hypervolemia. Decreased perfusion of the kidneys during bypass might stimulate the secretion of aldosterone and the retention of sodium and water. Increased secretion of antidiuretic hormone also can cause resorption of additional water.

The nurse auscultates for bowel sounds and palpates the abdomen for distention. When the abdomen is soft and bowel sounds are present, the nasogastric tube is pulled, and clear liquids are introduced. Fluid restrictions may continue for several postoperative days. The nurse schedules the administration of oral fluids permitted during the child's waking hours.

Renal failure might result from inadequate perfusion during or after surgery. Decreased urine output, and elevations of blood urea nitrogen and serum creatinine levels are the most common signs of renal failure (see Chapter 39).

Potassium imbalance also might occur postoperatively. Intracellular potassium is released as cell destruction occurs from surgical trauma and the destruction of blood cells by the pump. If this potassium is excreted in the urine (as it should be) hypokalemia can develop if the potassium is not replaced. If, however, the potassium is not excreted (as in renal failure) hyperkalemia may result.

Calcium might be depleted if citrated blood is transfused. Citrate binds with the calcium, which is then excreted, resulting in hypocalcemia. Because acid–base disturbances often occur after heart surgery, blood gases, electrolytes, and arterial blood are monitored frequently.

Maintaining Normal Body Temperature Hyperthermia increases the oxygen needs of the body and consequently the work of the heart. Since fevers are an important sign of infection, it is not desirable to suppress temperature elevations entirely. Because a fever does increase the work of the heart, however, it is important to control the degree of elevation. Often the physician will order antipyretics to be used when the child's temperature reaches a certain point.

While major reductions in body temperature result in slowing of body functions and decreased oxygen consumption, mild to moderate degrees of hypothermia increase oxygen consumption, therefore, chilling and temperature loss also should be avoided.

Managing Pain Pain is expected after heart surgery. The nurse must be alert for signs of pain, since young children and children with endotracheal tubes will be unable to cry or verbalize their pain. Some children hesitate to complain of pain because they fear an injection. The judicious use of pain medication provides comfort for the child, facilitates effective coughing, and encourages movement and ambulation.

Narcotics are generally used postoperatively and usually are given intravenously in the intensive care unit, where careful monitoring is possible. When the child is transferred to the regular pediatric unit, oral, subcutaneous, or intramuscular analgesics are used.

The nurse needs to be aware that pain medications can mask important symptoms, such as decreased level of consciousness, anxiety, confusion, restlessness, and irritability. Narcotics, especially morphine, can cause smooth muscle relaxation, which may cause a slight fall in blood pressure.

Preventing Infection Prophylactic antibiotics are used routinely after open-heart surgery. These are started preoperatively and continued postoperatively for several days. Despite prophylaxis, infections might occur. Infections of intracardiac prosthetic valves or conduits are particularly serious and have high mortality rates.

Meticulous aseptic technique is critical in all phases of care. Intravenous and intra-arterial catheters, central venous pressure catheters, temporary pacemaker wires, and chest tubes all provide access for bacteria. The need for each catheter should be assessed frequently, and the catheter should be removed as soon as possible. All intravenous tubing is changed every 24–48 hours, and entry sites for all catheters are cleansed daily with an iodine solution.

The nurse assesses the incision frequently, and reports any sign of infection immediately. The child's temperature is taken at least every 4 hours, and any elevation is reported. White blood counts are obtained daily.

Monitoring Neurologic Status Neurologic impairment can occur as a result of hypoxia or decreased cerebral blood flow during or after surgery. Emboli of air, thrombus, or particulate matter also can cause damage.

The nurse assesses neurologic function routinely and reports signs of focal or diffuse impairment. Level of consciousness, pupillary responses to light, bilateral equality of musculoskeletal strength and movement, and responses to pain are all indicators of neurologic function. The nurse needs to be alert for focal or generalized seizures, which may result from electrolyte imbalances or insult to the central nervous system. If the child's level of consciousness is impaired or other neurologic deficit is present (for example, paralysis, abnormal posturing), special nursing care is needed. (Care of the neurologically impaired child is discussed in Chapter 42.)

Postpericardiotomy Syndrome Postpericardiotomy syndrome can occur in some children after cardiac surgery. It typically appears 7–21 days after surgery but might appear earlier or later. Manifestations include fever, pericardial friction rub, chest pain over the heart, and possibly congestive heart failure. It results from the production of heart antibodies, an autoimmune response to the surgery, and it is treated with aspirin and activity restriction. The problem is usually self-limiting but may require intervention if pericardial effusion becomes significant.

Managing Activity Restrictions Major nursing goals are to prevent unnecessary stress and promote rest. Because there are many postoperative procedures, these goals are accomplished through careful organization of nursing care. Periods of rest should be clearly identified, and the child should not be disturbed at all during rest time unless absolutely necessary. As much as possible, special procedures are scheduled for times when the child is normally awake and hydrocortisol secretion is likely to be highest. During the child's usual sleep times, lights should be low and stimulation kept to a minimum.

Movement is necessarily limited immediately after surgery by the number of catheters and tubes. Nevertheless, turning is begun, and passive range-of-motion exercises may be performed. The nurse assesses the extremities for signs of thrombophlebitis.

Progressive activity is begun soon after surgery. Initially the child is able to sit on the bed, then is able to transfer to a chair, and finally is able to walk. The nurse monitors the child's tolerance of activity, which should be scheduled when the child is well rested and comfortable. A rest period should follow each activity period.

Providing Emotional Support The intensive care unit is a most frightening and stressful place for both children and parents, and the nurse therefore needs to be sensitive to their spoken and unspoken concerns. Parents should be allowed to be with their children as much as possible. Their presence makes the children feel more secure and helps the parents feel as if they are contributing to the children's well-being. The sense of powerlessness and uncertainty parents experience in the waiting area is very difficult for most of them to endure.

The nurse can remain with parents when they first see their children in the intensive care unit. Short, simple explanations of the equipment are appropriate at this time. More detailed explanations can follow later. Parents may participate in caring for their children as they feel able, but the nurse remains alert for signs of anxiety and fatigue. Even parents who seem to be coping well need encouragement to take breaks from their children and the intensive care unit to meet their own needs.

All procedures are explained to the child before they are done, with an emphasis on what the child will feel. Explanations of the necessity of surgery and treatment in the intensive care unit should be repeated to dispel misperceptions. Therapeutic play is begun as soon as the child is able (see Chapter 28). If the child is hesitant to play, the nurse can play through some of the experiences the child has had.

Occasionally, a child exhibits angry or rejecting behavior toward a parent. This is very difficult for most parents to handle, although this behavior often is a positive comment on the parent–child relationship. The child may be angry that the parent has failed to provide protection and has allowed all the surgery to occur. Children who are sure of their parents' love, however, know that the anger will be accepted and that their parents will continue to love them. Parents often need to have this behavior interpreted for them, and they may need help in understanding the importance of remaining with the child and providing consistent support.

Managing Convalescence Once the child is physiologically stable and is transferred out of intensive care, nursing goals include helping the child gradually resume normal activity and responsibilities and preparing the family for discharge.

The nurse monitors the child for signs of complications, encourages coughing, provides chest physiotherapy, and measures intake, output, and vital signs. As the child becomes more active, periods of activity are alternated with quiet times until the child regains strength.

The nurse assesses the child's readiness to relinquish the "sick role" and assume more healthy behavior. The nurse also is alert for signs that the child is seeking secondary gain from symptoms or surgery. The nurse can promote the child's adjustment in this area by gradually expecting more independence and more self-care from the child.

A parent might need help in adjusting to the child's condition after surgery. The physician and nurse therefore address directly the importance of allowing the child appropriate independence, with its privileges and responsibilities. In preparation for discharge the parents should learn to provide care in the hospital. They should have experience in giving medications and performing treatments. The family needs instructions regarding medications, diet, activity restrictions, return to school, care of the incisions, and signs and symptoms to report. Follow-up appointments and the name and number of people to call with questions should also be provided.

Behavior disturbances in children after discharge are relatively common and include nightmares, sleep problems, overdependence, and separation anxiety. The nurse can discuss with parents how to handle these problems if they occur. Parents should encourage their children to continue to talk about the hospitalization and surgery. In play, a toy doctor or nurse kit is very helpful, as are pictures of the hospital and visits to the hospital. While it is important to compliment children on how well the experience was handled and how brave they were, praise should not be emphasized unduly. Rather, the child should be encouraged to seek gratification from normal, healthy experiences (Rogers et al., 1984).

The Child With Subacute Bacterial Endocarditis

Subacute bacterial endocarditis is an infectious disease that usually involves abnormal portions of endocardium or endothelium associated with a cardiac or vascular malformation. Subacute bacterial endocarditis can complicate even hemodynamically insignificant lesions, such as a small ventricular septal defect or mitral valve prolapse. The microorganism, commonly an alpha streptococcus, gains entry to the circulation through an interruption of the skin or mucous membranes. Because the alpha streptococcus is a natural inhabitant of the mouth, its entry into the vascular system can occur during dental manipulation. This is why subacute bacterial endocarditis prophylaxis is indicated for dental procedures.

The child with subacute bacterial endocarditis usually has an unexplained fever and an underlying cardiovascular malformation. Frequently, subacute bacterial endocarditis is associated with anemia, fatigue, splenomegaly, petechiae, splinter hemorrhages under the nails, and raw spots on palms and soles. Tender areas of inflammation may develop on the finger pads. The diagnosis of subacute bacterial endocarditis is confirmed by blood cultures.

Untreated subacute bacterial endocarditis is uniformly fatal. With antibiotic treatment, however, the infection can be eradicated. Treatment must be continued 3–6 weeks. Although curable, subacute bacterial endocarditis can cause further damage to infected heart structures while it lasts. If, for example, an abnormal aortic valve is infected, valve function can be diminished further by the infection. Antibiotic therapy may be less effective in the presence of prosthetic material, such as an artificial valve. Occasionally, the infection cannot be eradicated with antibiotics until the prosthetic material is removed.

The risk of developing subacute bacterial endocarditis can be reduced in susceptible children if antibiotics are administered before and after the skin or mucous membranes are violated, particularly during dental work. Penicillin is the drug of choice if the child is not already receiving penicillin and is not allergic to it.

The nurse plays an important role in the prevention of subacute bacterial endocarditis by

- Reinforcing teaching about the importance of prophylaxis
- Teaching parents and children when and how antibiotics are to be administered
- Emphasizing the importance of oral health maintenance to reduce the chance of bacterial invasion
- Instructing parents to notify the physician if symptoms of subacute bacterial endocarditis occur

All those involved in the child's care (dentists, emergency room personnel, school nurse, and others) should be informed of the child's susceptibility.

Treatment of subacute bacterial endocarditis requires hospitalization for a prolonged period. Children need careful preparation for intravenous therapy and blood cultures. The nurse discusses with the child the need for hospitalization and activity restrictions and helps the child cope with these aspects of care.

Intravenous antibiotics must be administered on schedule to maintain therapeutic serum levels. The nurse monitors carefully for side effects. Prolonged use of high doses of intravenous antibiotics can cause inflammation of the vein. The nurse also observes closely for signs of complications, namely congestive heart failure and embolism.

The Child With Hypertension

Systemic arterial hypertension is much less common in children than in adults. Because blood pressure increases during childhood, blood pressure norms must be related to the patient's age or other indices, such as size or stage of maturation. For example, a blood pressure of 120/70 is normal for a 16-year-old boy but is abnormally elevated for a 4-year-old boy. (Normal blood pressure measurements are listed in Appendix B.)

Usually, blood pressure is determined using a sphygmomanometer. Using the proper-size cuff is important when measuring blood pressure in children. The width of the cuff should be at least two-thirds of the length of the upper arm and the bladder of the cuff sufficiently long to encircle the entire upper arm. During blood pressure measurement the child must be relaxed and comfortable.

Hypertension can be primary or secondary. Primary, or essential, hypertension has no known cause and is the most common form of hypertension in adults and probably in children. Numerous causes of secondary hypertension are known; the most common are renal disease and coarctation of the aorta. Renal diseases that can cause secondary hypertension include pyelonephritis, glomerulonephritis, hydronephrosis, renal artery disease, renal dysplasia, and polycystic kidney disease. Rarer causes of secondary hypertension include pheochromocytoma, hyperaldosteronism, hyperthyroidism, Cushing's syndrome, and ingestion of amphetamines or licorice.

All children should have their blood pressure measured at some time during childhood and adolescence (see Chapter 21). Children with elevated blood pressure should be referred for appropriate evaluation, and if necessary, treatment. Treatment varies but generally consists of weight reduction (if needed), a low-sodium diet, diuretic therapy, and stress reduction. (Prevention of primary hypertension is discussed in Chapter 19.)

The Child With Hyperlipidemia

Hyperlipidemia is an abnormal increase in serum lipids such as cholesterol. Increased serum cholesterol is a risk factor for coronary artery disease, and identifying children with abnormal elevations of serum cholesterol is therefore important so that appropriate treatment regimens can be initiated. Ultracentrifugation techniques are used to separate and analyze serum lipids and to determine levels of triglycerides, chylomicrons, low-density lipoproteins (LDL), very-low-density lipoproteins (VLDL), intermittent-density lipoproteins (IDL), and high-density lipoproteins (HDL). The risk for atherosclerosis depends on which type of lipoprotein predominates. LDL are most atherogenic, while HDL have a protective effect.

There are five types of hyperlipoproteinemia due to increased serum cholesterol or triglyceride levels. They are defined by the specific lipoprotein fraction that is elevated. Type I hyperlipoproteinemia is characterized by increased levels of chylomicrons and triglycerides and is usually diagnosed in infancy or early childhood. These children develop pancreatitis, abdominal pain, and xanthomas, but are not at increased risk for vascular disease. Type II hyperlipoproteinemia can be subdivided into types IIa and IIb. Type IIa is characterized by increased levels of LDL cholesterol, and type IIb is characterized by increases of both IDL and LDL cholesterol. Children with type II hyperlipoproteinemia are at increased risk for atherosclerosis. Type III hyperlipoproteinemia is characterized by increased IDL, type IV by increased VLDL, and type V by increased VLDL and chylomicrons.

Dietary regulation is prescribed to lower cholesterol levels. Occasionally, drug therapy is also necessary. Colestipol, cholestyramine, clofibrate, nicotinic acid, para-aminosalicylic acid, dextrothyroxine sodium, and probucol can be used to lower cholesterol levels. The specific drug prescribed depends on the type of hyperlipoproteinemia, response to therapy, and the child's age.

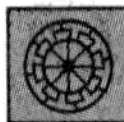

NURSING CARE PLAN Child With a Ventricular Septal Defect

Assessment Data

Matthew A. is an 8-month-old infant who was diagnosed as having a large ventricular septal defect at 2 weeks of age. He was hospitalized at that time with mild-to-moderate congestive heart failure (CHF). Diagnosis was confirmed by cardiac catheterization, and he was stabilized on digoxin and discharged at $3\frac{1}{2}$ weeks of age. He did well at home until 1 month ago, when he developed a cough and respiratory congestion. He became short of breath, pale, and diaphoretic while feeding and has not gained weight in the last $1\frac{1}{2}$ months. Matthew was taking a 6–7-oz bottle of formula 4–5 times a day, but since becoming sick he has been taking 3–4 oz every 3–4 hours. He also eats strained baby food three times a day. He is currently being admitted to the hospital for evaluation of worsening CHF.

Matthew is the third child in the family, which consists of his mother, father, and two older sisters, aged 2 and 3. Matthew's mother, who plans to stay with him in the hospital, reports that he usually smiles and babbles but that for the last few days he has been "too sick." She says, "It would have been terrible if we had lost him before, but if anything happened now, I know we couldn't take it."

Nursing Diagnoses and Goals

1. **Nursing diagnosis:** Alteration in cardiac function related to congestive heart failure.

   Long-term goal: Matthew will respond positively to treatment and be less uncomfortable.

   Short-term goals: (a) Matthew will experience less diaphoresis, tachypnea, and tachycardia when active. (b) Matthew will take his digoxin regularly and have no vomiting. (c) Matthew will sleep quietly in an upright position for 2-hour intervals or longer. (d) Matthew will have increased urinary output in response to diuretic therapy. (e) Matthew will not appear anxious but will be alert and responsive.

2. **Nursing diagnosis:** Alteration in respiratory effectiveness related to increased pulmonary congestion.

   Long-term goal: Matthew will breathe without excessive effort and at preillness rate.

   Short-term goals: (a) Matthew will expend less effort and not have to use accessory muscles for respiration. (b) Matthew will no longer have a cough.

3. **Nursing diagnosis:** Alteration in fluid balance related to retention of fluid.

   Long-term goal: Matthew will have no fluid retention.

   Short-term goals: (a) Matthew will void in amounts consistent with intake. (b) Matthew will not have any evidence of edema.

4. **Nursing diagnosis:** Decreased exercise tolerance related to impaired cardiac and respiratory function.

   Long-term goal: Matthew will feed and play without distress.

   Short-term goals: (a) Matthew will play for longer periods of time before tiring. (b) Matthew will be more interested in activities, less irritable.

5. **Nursing diagnosis:** Inadequate caloric intake related to fatigue with feeding.

   Long-term goal: Matthew will gain in weight and length steadily.

   Short-term goals: (a) Matthew will ingest adequate calories for growth (at least 700 calories per day). (b) Matthew will require fewer rest periods during feeding. (c) Matthew will ingest greater quantity (preillness amounts) at a feeding.

6. **Nursing diagnosis:** Potential for developmental delay in gross motor skills related to decreased exercise tolerance.

   Long-term goal: Matthew will reach normal developmental milestones at or near expected time.

   Short-term goals: (a) As condition improves, Matthew will practice age-appropriate developmental activities. (b) Parents will express perceptions of Matthew's development. (c) Parents will describe appropriate ways to promote Matthew's development.

7. **Nursing diagnosis:** Potential for emotional trauma related to hospitalization.

   Long-term goal: Matthew will adjust to hospital routine and procedures with a minimum of disruption.

   Short-term goals: (a) Matthew's parents will participate in his care. (b) Matthew will accept care from primary nurses.

8. **Nursing diagnosis:** Parental anxiety related to illness of infant.

   Long-term goal: Parents will cope adequately and experience growth in family relationships.

   Short-term goals: (a) Parents will express anxiety and questions. (b) Parents will discuss their needs with each other and family members. (c) Parents will use previously helpful coping strategies. (d) Parents will describe needs

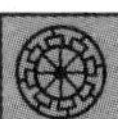

NURSING CARE PLAN Child With a Ventricular Septal Defect (continued)

of healthy siblings at home and will identify ways to minimize fantasies and fears in siblings.

9. Nursing diagnosis: Potential for infection related to pulmonary congestion.

Long-term goal: Matthew will remain free of infection during and after hospitalization.

Short-term goals: Matthew's parents will learn how to prevent and detect infection.

Interventions	Rationale	Evaluation criteria
1. Organize nursing care to provide periods of uninterrupted rest. Eliminate unnecessary interruptions in acute phase of illness	Oxygen needs are lowest when child is at rest. Each episode of stress increases oxygen needs and therefore increases the work of an already stressed myocardium	Did Matthew become hemodynamically stable in response to treatment? Was cardiac workload minimized? Did Matthew become less uncomfortable?
Plan meals, rest, and procedures to coincide with child's usual sleep–wake cycle	Hydrocortisol secretion is likely to be highest at times child is normally awake	
Coordinate procedures with other members of health care team	Although nursing care may be well planned, interruptions by other team members may interrupt child's rest and must be avoided	
Attend to child's needs promptly to reduce crying and frustration	Crying increases oxygen needs and wastes limited energy	
Avoid chilling by dressing child appropriately for ambient temperature, keeping child warm during bath, changing wet linen promptly. Report temperature elevations promptly	Both hypothermia and hyperthermia increase metabolic rate and oxygen needs. With exposure to cold, metabolic rate may increase to maintain temperature in normal range	
Monitor vital signs every 30 min–1 hour during acute phase. Monitor cardiovascular status, including heart sounds, liver size, and peripheral perfusion frequently	Signs of improvement or deterioration may require prompt, appropriate action	
Administer digoxin as ordered Observe for toxic effects	Digoxin is a highly toxic drug that must be given cautiously	
Administer diuretics as ordered	Diuretics are given to promote diuresis and reverse fluid retention	
Monitor serum electrolyte values; prevent hypokalemia by administering potassium supplement as ordered and encouraging foods high in potassium	Digoxin toxicity is more likely to occur in presence of hypokalemia	
Monitor for signs of hypokalemia, particularly if child is receiving diuretic for CHF	Some diuretics promote excretion of potassium	
2. Monitor respiratory rate, characteristics of respiration, and breath sounds frequently	Changes in condition require prompt treatment	Did Matthew's respiratory function become stable and effective?
Position in semi-Fowler's and alternate use of infant seat with elevation of head of bed to maintain semi-Fowler's position while allowing position changes	Elevation prevents abdominal organs from pressing on diaphragm and allows for greater expansion of lungs Without position changes, skin breakdown may occur	

continued on next page

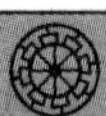

NURSING CARE PLAN Child With a Ventricular Septal Defect (continued)

Interventions	Rationale	Evaluation criteria
Dress child in loose, nonrestrictive clothing	Tight clothing limits thoracic expansion	
Administer oxygen as ordered and monitor effect	Supplemental oxygen improves tissue oxygenation and decreases cardiac workload	
Provide humidification as ordered. Keep clothing and bedding dry	Humidity helps to liquify respiratory secretions	
Use face mask instead of tent for oxygen and mist, if feasible, to minimize child's stress	Face masks provide adequate oxygen and humidity levels in most situations and are less frightening and isolating than tents	
Have suction available at bedside in case child unable to cough up secretions	Suctioning may be necessary to keep airway clear	
Provide chest physiotherapy as ordered. Monitor breath sounds before and after treatments. Concentrate on areas most in need of drainage. Modify procedure if needed to reduce stress to infant	Postural drainage and percussion help mobilize and remove secretions from the lungs. If the procedure increases the child's distress, modifications may be needed	
3. Administer diuretics as ordered. Check serum electrolytes prior to giving Furosemide (lasix) and withhold if hypokalemia is present. Monitor for side effects, especially hypokalemia	Diuretics promote the excretion of excess fluid, sodium chloride, and, with some drugs, potassium. Hypokalemia increases risk of digitalis toxicity	Was fluid balance achieved? Was diuresis effective? Did edema and congestion lessen?
Weigh child b.i.d. on same scale. Monitor intake and output. Check urine specific gravity of each voiding	Weight is one of the most sensitive indicators of fluid balance	
Assess hydration status frequently	Diuretics can cause dehydration	
4. Monitor child's physiologic responses to nursing care activities, such as feeding, chest physiotherapy, bathing	Exercise tolerance is an important parameter in the assessment of cardiac function. Decreased tolerance indicates decreased cardiac function	Did Matthew's exercise tolerance improve?
Modify procedures to decrease stress if necessary	Modification may be needed to minimize oxygen needs and conserve energy	
If confinement in bed or infant seat causes undue frustration, modify plan to include more holding, walking (portable oxygen), and quiet stimulation while in bed or infant seat	Frustration of imposed inactivity may create more work for the heart than limited out-of-bed activity	
5. Feed infant in semiupright, knee–chest position	This position prevents fatigue and minimizes abdominal pressure on diaphragm	Was Matthew's caloric intake adequate? Wash he able to eat with fewer episodes of fatigue? Did he start to gain weight?
Use soft nipple and enlarge hole in nipple if needed	This allows child to obtain more milk with less energy expenditure	

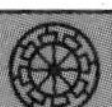

NURSING CARE PLAN Child With a Ventricular Septal Defect (continued)

Interventions	Rationale	Evaluation criteria
Allow infant to pause and rest as needed		
Feed infant at first sign of hunger. Do not allow infant to tire self by crying	Crying wastes valuable energy needed for sucking	
Provide adequate rest before and after feeding	If fatigued, infant will be unable to ingest and digest an adequate amount of formula	
Provide frequent, small feedings, for example, 4–5 oz of 20-calorie/oz formula every 3 hours	Smaller feedings minimize fatigue and exert less pressure on diaphragm	
Feed infant cereal and strained foods at usual times and in manner used at home	Maintenance of homelike routine that infant is familiar with will facilitate intake	
Weigh infant twice a day	If adequate calories are consumed, slow, steady growth is reflected by weight gain	
6. Provide quiet types of stimulation during acute phase (for example, colorful mobile, small objects to hold and manipulate, peek-a-boo, music, soft toys to hold)	Quiet stimulation prevents boredom and frustration while maintaining infant's interest in environment and conserving energy	Were developmental delays minimized? Were parents' expectations realistic of child's abilities?
As condition improves, provide for more vigorous activity (for example, blanket on floor for play, bouncing chair, sitting with pillow support)	Child may lack the energy and motor skills to obtain own stimulation, so stimulating experiences should be provided	
Change scenery and toys frequently throughout day		
Engage Matthew in verbal games		
Explore parents' feelings and perceptions about Matthew's development	Parents may fear that child is retarded or that delays are due to inadequate parenting	
Point out areas of developmental success that parents may not recognize (for example, verbal, cognitive, social)	Parents may need help in seeing subtle but important signs of progress	
Teach parents about Matthew's need for age-appropriate stimulation	Parents may underestimate infant's developmental level because of small size and gross motor delays	
Assure parents that Matthew will limit his own activity, and they do not need to inhibit his activity except during acute periods	Parents may inappropriately inhibit child's physical activity to prevent "strain on heart"	
7. Encourage parents to participate actively in all phases of Matthew's care	Presence of parents helps alleviate stress of strange environment for infant	Did Matthew remain free of emotional trauma during hospitalization? Did parents participate in his care?
Arrange to have Matthew cared for by two or three primary nurses	Care is less stressful for infant if he develops relationship with familiar nurses	

continued on next page

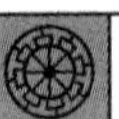

NURSING CARE PLAN Child With a Ventricular Septal Defect (continued)

Interventions	Rationale	Evaluation criteria
Ask parents to bring familiar toys and objects from home	Familiar objects, people, and routines make hospital seem less strange	
Allow siblings to visit frequently		
Make hospital routine as homelike as possible		
Provide for periods of holding, rocking, and play by nurses, separate from procedures	This promotes trust and prevents perception of nurses as people who only bring discomfort and stress	
Acknowledge and respond to signs of distress and discomfort	This promotes trust between infant and nurses	
8. Accept parents' expressions of anxiety and explain them to other staff members as needed	Interpretation of parents' negative behavior to other staff members may prevent conflicts	Did Matthew's parents remain free of undue anxiety? Did parents identify and use methods of coping with anxiety that have helped previously?
Encourage parents to ask questions and talk about feelings and fears	Accurate information and expression of fears lessen anxiety	
Encourage parents to participate in Matthew's care and decision making about his care	Participation in care minimizes feelings of powerlessness and helplessness	
Assist parents in identifying methods of managing stress and anxiety that have been helpful before (time alone with spouse, walks, exercise, prayer)	Previous methods of coping may be helpful in current stressful situation	
Assist parents in obtaining support in the community (chaplain, parent support group, etc.)	Parents may be unaware of resources or need help in contacting them	
Encourage parents to spend time together each day. Provide care for Matthew during that time	It is important for parents to maintain their own relationship during periods of stress	Did Matthew's family cope adequately with stress caused by his heart condition?
Determine parents' awareness of the needs of siblings at home	Parents are often so focused on needs of sick child that they are unaware of needs of siblings	
Assist parents to identify common fears and fantasies in siblings of hospitalized child and how to deal with these	Siblings frequently have many fears and fantasies, including guilt, fear for own health, and jealousy. These are often expressed indirectly and are hard for parents to recognize	
Encourage siblings to visit and take time to observe their reactions during visits	It may be necessary to discuss siblings' reactions with parents	
9. Isolate Matthew from persons with respiratory infections	Children with CHF are particularly susceptible to respiratory infections	Did Matthew remain free of respiratory infection?
Monitor Matthew closely for signs of infection and notify physician promptly if any occur	Respiratory infections in children with CHF tend to be serious	
Teach Matthew's parents how to recognize signs of respiratory infection. Instruct them to report signs to the physician promptly	Infection may develop after Matthew is discharged from the hospital	

Key Concepts

- The heart is a muscular organ consisting of two atria (receiving chambers), two ventricles (pumping chambers), four valves (the tricuspid, pulmonic, mitral, and aortic valves), and an electrical conduction system (sinus and atrioventricular nodes, bundle of His, and Purkinje's fibers).
- Normally, there is no communication (opening) between the right heart, which receives deoxygenated blood from the systemic circulation and pumps it to the lungs, and the left heart, which receives oxygenated blood from the lungs and pumps it into the systemic circulation.
- Before birth, the fetal lungs are collapsed, and gas exchange takes place in the placenta, where the maternal and fetal circulatory systems meet but do not mix, and blood bypasses the collapsed lungs by means of the ductus arteriosus and the foramen ovale.
- Cardiac rhythm is determined by electrical impulses that originate in the sinus node, travel to the atrioventricular node, the common bundle and then through the bundle branches, and cause impulses throughout the ventricals.
- A shunt is an abnormal communication between the left and right sides of the heart.
- In a left-to-right shunt, the right ventricle pumps an increased volume of blood at increased pressure into the pulmonary arteries and lungs, causing dilatation and hypertrophy of the right ventricle, eventual hypertrophy of pulmonary arterial walls, pulmonary edema, susceptibility to respiratory infection, tachypnea, and dyspnea.
- In a right-to-left shunt, deoxygenated blood flows into the aorta instead of the pulmonary arteries, resulting in hypoxemia and cyanotic heart disease.
- An obstruction defect is a lesion or malformation in the heart valves or great vessels that impedes the forward flow of blood.
- Assessment history for the child with cardiovascular dysfunction includes data about exercise intolerance, cyanosis, diaphoresis, feeding difficulties, respiratory distress (particularly hypoxic episodes), growth and development, past health history, and family health history.
- Physical examination of the child with cardiovascular dysfunction includes measurement of vital signs, height, and weight; and inspection of the skin for pallor or cyanosis, of the neck veins for distention, of the chest for convexity, and of the fingers and toes for clubbing.
- Diagnostic tests used in assessment are hematologic and blood chemistry studies and cardiographic studies, including electrocardiography, vectorcardiography, phonocardiography, echocardiography, radiography, heart scans, and cardiac catheterization.
- Care of the child undergoing blood tests includes monitoring the puncture site for bleeding and bruising, careful handling of withdrawn blood samples, explaining the procedure to the child, and following procedures carefully to avoid the need for repeated tests.
- Preparation of the child for noninvasive cardiographic studies involves explaining the procedure to the child; describing the equipment, the room where the procedure will be done, and how the child will get to and from the room; practicing the procedure; and, if appropriate, doll play.
- Care of the child undergoing cardiac catheterization involves preoperative physical, cognitive, and emotional preparation and postoperative assessment for complications, including arrhythmias, hemorrhage, infection, edema and inflammation, phlebitis, thrombus formation, adverse reactions to dye, and dehydration.
- Nursing care for the child on a cardiac monitor, which is used to detect arrhythmias, includes thorough preparation of the child and family, the application and maintenance of electrode pads, monitoring of the oscilloscope, and assessment of the child's and family's dependence on the monitor.
- In caring for the child with cardiac disease, the nurse can minimize cardiac workload by providing adequate rest, anticipating the child's needs, minimizing anxiety, limiting activity to tolerated levels, preventing hyperthermia and hypothermia, eliminating excess sodium and fluid from the body,

and administering drugs that reduce systemic resistance to cardiac outflow.

- Cardiac function is enhanced by the administration of digitalis (usually digoxin).
- Fluid balance is important in the child with cardiac disease because fluid overload increases cardiac workload, and dehydration (particularly in cyanotic disease with polycythemia) increases the risk of thrombus formation.
- Children with heart disease are at risk for respiratory infections and bacterial endocarditis, an infection of the valves and inner lining (endocardium) of the heart.
- Hypoxic spells, which are usually due to an abrupt reduction of pulmonary blood flow, are managed by placing the child in a side-lying, knee–chest position; administering oxygen; administering morphine and sometimes intravenous sodium bicarbonate and phenylephrine hydrochloride; and, if these measures fail, performing emergency surgery.
- Nursing care for the child with cyanotic heart disease, particularly tetralogy of Fallot, involves teaching the child and family how to manage hypoxic spells at home and emphasizing the need to obtain medical attention immediately.
- Besides adequate intake, the nutritional needs of the child with cardiac disease may require high-calorie diets, low-sodium diets, and iron supplementation.
- Physical development of children with cardiac disease may be delayed if hypoxia limits strength and endurance, if severe hypoxic spells or cerebrovascular accidents impair neurologic function, or if parents do not encourage maximal activity.
- The nurse helps parents to promote the child's normal growth and development by instructing them about the child's need for exercise, activity, stimuli, discipline, realistic limits on activity, and as much independence as possible.
- Emotional problems of parents may be related to difficulty in accepting the diagnosis, misconceptions about the child's condition, realistic or unrealistic fears that the child will die, and the stresses of caring for a chronically ill child.
- Children's emotional reactions to cardiac disease depend on their age, developmental level, and perceptions about what caused the disease.
- In addressing the health maintenance needs of children with cardiac disease, the nurse teaches parents to observe for symptoms, administer medications, prevent infections, and regulate temperature.
- Symptoms that parents should report to the physician include fever, decreased intake, increased respiratory or pulse rate, respiratory difficulties, edema, increased cyanosis, pallor, decreased urine output, vomiting, and diarrhea.
- The nurse teaches parents how to administer digoxin, emphasizing that careful attention to exact dosage and schedule, avoidance of overdose, and recognition of symptoms of toxicity are of paramount importance.
- The nurse informs parents of children with organic heart disease about the need for prophylactic antibiotic administration at the time of any dental work, minor surgery, or illness, to reduce the risk of bacterial endocarditis.
- Congestive heart failure can be due to hypovolemia, obstruction to cardiac outflow, ineffective myocardial function, arrhythmias, or excessive demand for cardiac output; signs and symptoms include tachycardia, cardiomegaly, tachypnea, dyspnea, hepatomegaly, and weight gain from edema.
- The physiologic effects of most acyanotic defects have to do with volume overload in the right ventricle and pulmonary circulation, with resultant congestive heart failure and pulmonary edema.
- The cardinal signs of cyanotic cardiac defects are the signs of hypoxia, which include cyanosis, respiratory symptoms, poor growth, and exercise intolerance.
- Nursing care for the child undergoing cardiac surgery involves thorough preoperative assessment, obtaining of baseline data, and preparation of parent and child, particularly for intensive care.
- Postoperative care involves monitoring vital signs, observing for hemorrhage, monitoring cardiovascular status, maintaining effective respirations, monitoring fluid and electrolyte

balance, maintaining normal body temperature, managing pain, preventing infection, monitoring neurologic status, and observing for postpericardiotomy syndrome.

- The nurse organizes postoperative care so as to disturb the child's rest as little as possible.
- In assessing the child with hypertension, it is important to remember that blood pressure increases during childhood and must be compared with norms for the child's age, size, and stage of maturation.
- Nursing care for the child with hyperlipidemia involves dietary restrictions and, occasionally, administration of drugs.

References

Castaneda AR et al: Tetralogy of Fallot: Primary repair in infancy. Pages 63–69 in: *The Child With Congenital Heart Disease After Surgery*. Kidd BSL, Rowe RD (editors). Futura, 1976.

Cloutier J, Measel CP: Home care for the infant with congenital heart disease. *Am J Nurs* (Jan)1982; 82:100–103.

Cohen MA: The use of prostaglandins and prostaglandin inhibitors in critically ill neonates. *Am J Matern Child Nurs* (May/June)1983; 8:194–199.

Condon MR: The cardiac child: What his parents need to know. *Nursing '73* (Oct)1973; 60–61.

D'Antonio IG: Cardiac infant's feeding difficulties. *West J Nurs Res* 1979; 1(1):53–55.

Ehlers KH: Growth failure in association with congenital heart disease. *Pediatr Ann* (Nov)1979; 750.

Feldt RH (editor): *Atrioventricular Canal Defects*. Saunders, 1976.

Feldt RH et al: Children with congenital heart disease, motor development, and intelligence. *Am J Dis Child* (March)1969; 281*a*.

Feldt RH et al: Growth of children with congenital heart disease. *Am J Dis Child* (May)1969; 573*b*.

Fisch C: Digitalis intoxication. *JAMA* (June)1971; 216:1770–1773.

Fontan F, Bandet E: Surgical repair of tricuspid atresia. *Thorax* 1971; 26:240–248.

Fyler DC, Silbert AR, Rothman KJ: Five-year followup of infant cardiacs: Intelligence quotient. Pages 409–419 in: *The Child With Congenital Heart Disease After Surgery*. Kidd BSL, Rowe RD (editors). Futura, 1976.

Garson A et al: Parental reactions to children with congenital heart disease. *Child Psychiatry Hum Dev* (Feb)1978; 86.

Gillon, J: Behavior of newborns with cardiac distress, *Am J Nurs* (Feb)1973; 73.

Gottesfeld IB: The family of the child with congenital heart disease. *Am J Matern Child Nurs* (March/April)1979; 101–104.

Huntington J: Care of the child with a disorder of the cardiovascular system. Pages 97–150 in: *Critical Care Nursing of Children and Adolescents*. Oakes AR (editor). Saunders, 1981.

Jackson PL: Digoxin therapy at home: Keeping the child safe. *Am J Matern Child Nurs* (March/April)1979; 105–110.

Krovetz LJ, Gessner IH, Schiebler GL: *Handbook of Pediatric Cardiology*. University Park Press, 1979.

Linde LM et al: Physical and emotional aspects of congenital heart disease in children. *Am J Cardiol* (June)1971; 721.

Linde LM, Rasof B, Dunn OJ: Mental development in congenital heart disease. *N Engl J Med* 1967; 263:65.

Linderkamp P: Increased blood viscosity in patients with cyanotic congenital heart disease and iron deficiency. *J Pediatr* (Oct)1979; 95(4): 567–569.

MacDonald NE: Respiratory syncytial viral infection in infants with congenital heart disease. *N Engl J Med* (Aug) 1983; 307:397–400.

Meissner JE, Gever LN: Reducing the risks of toxicity. *Nursing '80* (Sept)1980; 29–38.

Mills LJ et al: Cardiothoracic surgery: Perioperative principles. In: *A Practical Guide to Pediatric Intensive Care*. Levin DL, Morriss FC, Moore GC (editors). Mosby, 1979.

Moss AJ, Adams FH, Emmanouilides GC: *Heart Disease in Infants, Children and Adolescents*. Williams & Wilkins, 1977.

Newburger JW et al: Cognitive function and age at repair of transposition of the great arteries in children. *N Engl J Med* (June) 1984; 310: 1495–99.

Norwood WI, Kirlin JK, Sanders SP: Hypoplastic left heart syndrome: Experience with palliative surgery. *Am J Cardiol* (Jan)1980; 45: 87–91.

Pelletier L: Collecting information: A way to cope with cardiac surgery. *Matern Child Nurs J* 1982; 143–154.

Peterson MC: Preparation of the cardiac child and the family for surgery. *Issues Compr Pediatr Nurs* (Dec)1979; 3(7):61–71.

Pidgeon V: The infant with congenital heart disease. *Am J Nurs* (Feb)1967; 67:290–293.

Reif K: A heart makes you live: What children believe about their hearts. *Am J Nurs* (June)1972; 72(6):1085.

Roberts FB: The child with heart disease. *Am J Nurs* (June)1972; 72(6):1080–1084.

Rogers TR et al: Heart surgery in infants: A preliminary assessment of maternal adaptation. *Child Health Care* (Fall)1984; 13(2):52.

Scoggin C, Patterson D: Down's syndrome as a model disease. *Arch Intern Med* 1982; 142: 462–64.

Silbert AR et al: Cyanotic heart disease and psychosocial development. *Pediatrics* 1969; 43:192.

Uzark K: A child's cardiac catheterization—Avoiding the potential risks. *Am J Matern Child Nurs* (May/June)1978; 151–161.

Additional Readings

AJN Self Study. Congenital cardiac defects. *Am J Nurs* (Feb)1978; 78: 255–278.

Anderson DJ, Thibault J: Nursing management of the pediatric patient with Kawasaki's disease. *Issues Compr Pediatr Nurs* (Jan-Feb)1981; 5(1):1–10.

Barnes CM: Levels of consciousness indicated by responses of children to phenomena in the intensive care unit. *Matern Child Nurs J* (Winter)1975; 4(4):215–290.

Barnes CM: Working with parents of children undergoing heart surgery. *Nurs Clin North Am* (March)1969; 4:11–18.

Boll TJ, Dimino E, Mattsson AE: Parenting attitudes: The role of personality style and childhood long-term illness. *J Psychosom Res* 1978; 22(3):209–213.

Brantigan CO: Hemodynamic monitoring: Interpreting values. *Am J Nurs* (Jan)1982; 82:86–89.

Broda D: Extending the role of the coronary care nurse. *Superv Nurse* (June)1981; 12(6):48–50.

Campbell C: Careers—Cardiothoracic nursing: Heart and soul. *Nurs Mirror* (Feb 10)1982; 154(6):44.

Cavanaugh AL, Mancini RE: Drug interactions and digitalis toxicity. *Am J Nurs* (Dec)1980; 80:2170–2171.

Chameides L: Congenital heart disease—Its effect on the school-age child. *J Sch Health* (April)1979; 49(4):205–209.

Coats K: Noninvasive cardiac diagnostic procedures. *Am J Nurs* (Nov)1975; 75(11):1980–1984.

Cook D, Morch J, Noble E: Improving attendance at follow-up clinics. *Dimens Health Serv* (Sept)1976; 53(9):46–49.

Engle MA: Management of the child after cardiac surgery. *Pediatr Ann* (April)1981; 10(4):53–60.

Evans J: Nursing care study: Fallot's tetralogy. *Nurs Times* (June 1)1978; 74(22):917–920.

Foster SB: Pump failure. *Am J Nurs* (Oct)1974; 74(10):830–834.

Foster SD: MCN pharmacopoeia. Indomethacin: Pharmacologic closure of the ductus arteriosus. *Am J Matern Child Nurs* (May/June)1982; 7: 171–172.

Freis PC: Sounds of a healthy heart. *Issues Compr Pediatr Nurs* (Dec)1979; 3(7):1–4.

Friedberg DZ, Caldart L: A center for pediatric cardiovascular patients. *Am J Nurs* (Sept)1975; 75(9):1480–1482.

Gersony WM, Bierman FZ: Cardiac catheterization in the pediatric patient. *Pediatrics* (May)1981; 67(5):738–740.

Gersony WM, Hordof AJ: Infective endocarditis and diseases of the pericardium. *Pediatr Clin North Am* (Nov)1978; 25(4):831–846.

Gillon JE: Behavior of newborns with cardiac distress. *Am J Nurs* (Feb)1973; 73(2):257.

Guntheroth WG: Initial evaluation of the child for heart disease. *Pediatr Clin North Am* (Nov)1978; 25(4):657–675.

Hall RK: Oral and dental changes and management of children with cardiac disease. *J Int Assoc Dent Child* (June)1980; 11(1):19–28.

Hazinski MF: Critical care of the pediatric cardiovascular patient. *Nurs Clin North Am* (Dec)1981; 16(4):671–697.

Hencz P et al: Hyperuricemia of infants and children: a complication of open heart surgery. *J Pediatr* (May)1979; 94(5):774–776.

Hoops EJ: Cardiopulmonary resuscitation of children. *Nurs Clin North Am* (Dec)1981; 16(4):623–634.

Johnson DL: Pediatric arrhythmias: A nursing approach. *Dimens Crit Care Nurs* (May-June)1983; 2(3):147–157.

Ladyshewsky A: Increased intracranial pressure: When assessment counts. *Can Nurse* (Oct)1980; 76(10):34–37.

Lavigne JV, Ryan M: Psychologic adjustment of siblings of children with chronic illness. *Pediatrics* (April)1979; 63(4):616–627.

Liebman J, Barkat G, Hirschfeld S: The heart. Pages 294–323 in: Klaws MH, Fanaroff AA (editors). *Care of the High-Risk Neonate.* Saunders, 1979.

Lloyd JK: Dietary problems associated with the care of chronically sick children. *J Hum Nutr* (April)1979; 33(2):135–139.

Lloyd P: Post-operative nursing care following open heart surgery in children. *Nurs Clin North Am* (Sept)1970; 5:399–409.

Longo A: Teaching parents CPR. *Pediatr Nurs* (Nov/Dec)1983; 9(6): 445–447.

L'Orange C, Werner-McCullough M: Kawasaki disease: A new threat to children. *Am J Nurs* (April)1983; 83(4):558–562.

Manning C: WPW syndrome: A case study. *Can Nurse* (Dec)1979; 75(11):34–37.

McElnea J: Spotlight on children. Childhood hypertension. *Nurs Times* (Sep 29–Oct 5)1982; 78(39 Suppl):5–6.

McEvoy M: Functional heart murmurs. *Nurse Pract* (March-April)1981; 6:34–36.

McNeal GJ: Twenty-four hours ambulatory monitoring: A new electrocardiographic tool. *Nurs Clin North Am* (Sept)1978; 13(3):437–448.

Moss, AJ: What every primary physician should know about the postoperative cardiac patient. *Pediatrics* (Feb)1979; 63(2):320–330.

Nadas AS: Update on congenital heart disease. *Pediatr Clin North Am* (Feb)1984; 31(1):153–164.

Ng L: Nursing aspects of the surgical treatment of idiopathic hypertrophic subaortic stenosis. *Heart Lung* (Jul-Aug)1982; 11(4):364–375.

Noonan JA: Association of congenital heart disease with syndromes or other defects. *Pediatr Clin North Am* (Nov)1978; 25(4):797–816.

Norwood WI et al: Experience with operations for hypoplastic left heart syndrome. *J Thorac Cardiovasc Surg* 1981; 82:511–519.

Norwood WI, Lang P, Hansen DD: Physiologic repair of aortic atresia—Hypoplastic left heart syndrome. *N Engl J Med* (Jan 6)1983; 308(1): 23–26.

Pasternack SB: Hypertension in children and adolescents. *Issues Compr Pediatr Nurs* (Dec)1979; 3(7):23–57.

Pless IB: Chronic disease in children: Current controversies and technical advances. *Pediatr Clin North Am* (Feb)1984; 31(1):259–273.

Powers D: Nursing care study: Subacute bacterial endocarditis. *Nurs Times* (April 20–26)1983; 79(16):50–53.

Pyles SH, Stern PN: Discovery of nursing gestalt in critical care nursing: The importance of the gray gorilla syndrome. *Image* (Spring)1983; 15(2):51–57.

Ramirez B: When you're faced with a neuro patient. *RN* (Jan)1979; 42(1):67–76.

Rehm RS: Teaching cardiopulmonary resuscitation to parents. *Am J Matern Child Nurs* (Nov/Dec)1983; 8(6):411–414.

Reid TJ: Newborn cyanosis. *Am J Nurs* (Aug)1982; 82:1230–1234.

Rice V: Shock, a clinical syndrome. Part I: Definition, etiology, and pathophysiology. *Crit Care Nurse* (March–April)1981; 1(3):44–50.

Richard K et al: Care of children with conditions characterized by high nutritional risks. *J Am Diet Assoc* (Jun)1976; 68(6):546–550.

Rushton CH: Preparing children and families for cardiac surgery: Nursing interventions. *Issues Compr Pediatr Nurs* (July–Aug)1983; 6(4): 235–248.

Sasso SC: MCN pharmacopoeia. Prostaglandin E_1 for infants with congenital heart disease. *Am J Matern Child Nurs* (Jan/Feb)1983; 8(1):29.

Saul L: Heart sounds and common murmurs. *Am J Nurs* (Dec)1983; 83:1680–1689.

Scordo KA: Taming the cardiac monitor. Part 2. Understanding what the monitor's telling you. *Nursing '82* (Sept)1982; 12(9):61–67.

Slota MC: Cardiac pacemakers in children. *Crit Care Nurse* (Nov-Dec)1981; 1(7):35–41.

Slota MC: Congestive heart failure. Part II: Medical and nursing management. *Crit Care Nurse* (Nov-Dec)1982; 2(6):58–63.

Slota M: Pediatric cardiac catheterization: Complications and interventions. *Crit Care Nurse* (May–June)1982; 2(3):22–26.

Smith BC: Congestive heart failure. *Am J Nurs* (Feb)1969; 69(2): 278–292.

Smith KM: Recognizing cardiac failure in neonates. *Am J Matern Child Nurs* (March/April)1979; 79:98–99.

Stevenson JG: Acyanotic lesions with increased pulmonary blood flow. *Pediatr Clin North Am* (Nov)1978; 25(4):743–758.

Stevenson JG: Acyanotic lesions with normal pulmonary blood flow. *Pediatr Clin North Am* (Nov)1978; 25(4):725–742.

Stewart P: The young cardiac patient: Management considerations. *Pediatr Nurs* (Jan–Feb)1980; 6(1):E–F.

Strangway A et al: Diet and growth in congenital heart disease. *Pediatrics* (Jan)1976; 57(1):75–86.

Stroud ET: Acquired, chronic aortic insufficiency in the child. *Nurse Pract* (Nov–Dec)1980; 80:26–27.

Umansky R, Hauck AJ: Factors in the growth of children with patent ductus arteriosus. *Pediatrics* (Oct)1962; 30(4):540–551.

Uzark K et al: Primary preventive health care in children with heart disease. *Pediatr Cardiol* (Oct–Dec)1983; 4(4):259–263.

Hematologic Composition
Implications of Altered Blood Elements

Mary Jo Eoff

36

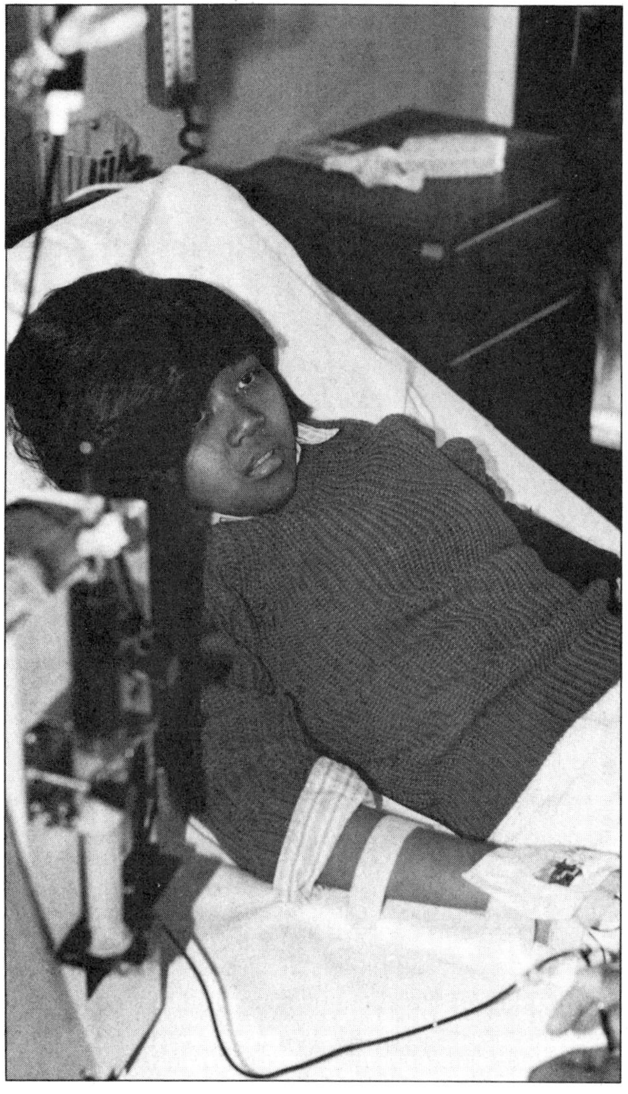

Chapter Outline

continued on next page

Objectives

- Describe the chief function of red blood cells, white blood cells, and platelets.
- Identify the laboratory tests (hematologic studies) used in the diagnosis of (1) anemias, (2) sickle cell disease and trait, and (3) clotting disturbances.
- List the topics most relevant to the history of a child with a hematopoietic disorder
- Describe by body system the signs and symptoms that might be found in the physical examination of a child with (1) an anemic disorder and (2) a clotting disturbance.
- Describe the nurse's responsibilities regarding preparation for diagnostic tests, administration of blood transfusions, bone marrow aspiration, and bone marrow transplantation.
- Explain how the following transfusion reactions occur: hemolytic reaction, pyrogenic reaction, allergic reaction, circulatory overload, and embolic reaction.
- Compare and contrast the acute-care needs of children with red blood cell disorders (the anemias) and platelet disorders (clotting disturbances).
- Describe the principles of nursing care related to infection control and nutrition for the child with hematopoietic dysfunction.
- Identify the nursing interventions appropriate for the child with iron deficiency anemia.
- Explain why splenectomy is used in the treatment of (1) spherocytosis, (2) sickle cell disease, (3) β-thalassemia, and (4) idiopathic thrombocytopenic purpura (ITP).
- Describe nursing management for the child with aplastic anemia.
- Describe the nursing interventions appropriate for vaso-occlusive, sequestration, and aplastic sickle cell crises.
- List the methods the child can learn to prevent hypoxia.
- Describe the signs and symptoms of β-thalassemia (Cooley's anemia, or thalassemia major).
- Describe the clinical manifestations of hemophilia A, in which coagulation Factor VIII is deficient.
- Describe the nursing interventions used to control internal and external bleeding.
- Identify the health maintenance needs of a child with hemophilia.
- Describe nursing management for the patient with idiopathic thrombocytopenic purpura (ITP).
- List the common predisposing factors for disseminated intravascular coagulation (DIC).

To find these topics, see the following chapters:

Leukemia	Chapter 45
Autoimmune disorders	Chapter 37
Epistaxis	Chapter 26
Hemorrhage	Chapter 19
Bone Marrow Aspiration	Chapter 45

Disorders associated with alterations of blood elements affect the erythrocytes (red blood cells), thrombocytes (platelets), or leukocytes (white blood cells). In this chapter we discuss alterations of erythrocytes and thrombocytes and their effects on the child. Alterations affecting erythrocytes reduce the oxygen-carrying capacity of the blood, causing anemia and its associated manifestations in the child. Conditions such as iron deficiency anemia and aplastic anemia are associated with the decreased production of red blood cells in the bone marrow, while the hemolytic anemias are caused by accelerated destruction of red blood cells.

Disorders of coagulation cause bleeding in the child which, if severe enough, can result in anemia, bone and joint degeneration, and psychologic complications. Hemophilia is a coagulation disorder caused by a deficiency in clotting factor, usually Factor VIII or IX. Alterations in the thrombocytes also can result in bleeding, either through a decrease in circulating platelets, as seen in ideopathic thrombocytopenic purpura, or through diminished platelet adhesiveness, as in Von Willebrand's disease.

Regardless of the disease, children affected by disorders of hematalogic composition require comprehensive nursing care that focuses on preventing complications and maintaining an optimal level of health. Disorders caused by alterations in white blood cells are discussed in Chapters 37 and 45.

Physiology of the Blood Cells

Blood consists of two components. The first component is the liquid, or plasma portion, which contains proteins, carbohydrates, lipids, electrolytes, pigments, clotting factors, immunoglobulins, and many other substances. The second component is the cellular portion, which includes erythrocytes, leukocytes, and thrombocytes. These three types of cells evolve from undifferentiated stem cells in the bone marrow.

Erythrocytes

The erythrocytes, or red blood cells, give blood its color and comprise the primary cellular component of the blood. Red blood cells are biconcave, non-nucleated disks whose principal function is to transport oxygen to and carbon dioxide away from body tissues. These gases are carried by hemoglobin molecules attached to the red blood cells. As many as 300 million hemoglobin molecules can be attached to one red blood cell. The uptake of carbon dioxide by hemoglobin affects the regulation of blood pH.

The red blood cells are produced in the marrow of short, flat bones, such as the bones of the hands, feet, ribs, sternum, iliac crest, and vertebrae, and in the spleen and liver of the fetus and neonate. The body produces 200 billion red blood cells each day and is capable of producing six to eight times that amount. The rate of red blood cell production is determined by the oxygen tension of the blood. Tissue *anoxia* (absence of oxygen) or *hypoxia* (deficiency of oxygen) stimulate red blood cell production. Erythropoietin, a substance thought to be produced in the kidney, is released in response to the body's need for tissue oxygenation. Erythropoietin release increases red blood cell production. The red blood cells live approximately 120 days. Old and abnormal red blood cells are destroyed and removed from the bloodstream by the spleen.

Laboratory tests are used to detect the amount, size, and oxygen-carrying capacity of red blood cells. Table 36-1 lists and defines these tests and shows the normal values for different age groups.

Leukocytes

The leuckocytes, or white blood cells, are nucleated cells whose primary function is to protect the body against infection. There are three types of leukocytes: (1) the granulocytes, which include the neutrophils, eosinophils, and basophils; (2) the monocytes; and (3) the lymphocytes.

Granulocytes, also called polymorphonuclear leukocytes, are produced in the bone marrow. They evolve from myeloblasts into myelocytes and finally into mature granulocytes. The types of granulocytes are distinguished by cell staining. Neutrophils can leave the bloodstream and enter the tissues, where they ingest foreign substances and bacteria through a process called phagocytosis. These cells that ingest microorganisms, other cells, or foreign particles are called *phagocytes*. Eosinophils are also phagocytes because they can ingest and destroy antigen–antibody complexes. The function of the basophils is not certain, although they appear to act like the mast cells found in connective tissue and as such they release histamine (a broncho-constrictor) and heparin (an anticoagulant).

Monocytes originate from the bone marrow and develop into macrophages, which are phagocytic. Monocytes ingest foreign particles and fragmented cells.

Lymphocytes originate in such lymphogenous sites as bone marrow, lymph nodes, spleen, liver, thymus, subepithelial lymphoid tissue, and connective tissue. Lymphocytes develop from lymphoblasts or other lymphocytes. They are involved in cell immunity and antibody formation (see Chapter 37). There are two different types of lymphocytes. T-lymphocytes are responsible for cell-mediated immunity, and B-lymphocytes produce antibodies. Infections stimulate the increased production and maturation of lymphocytes.

The number of white blood cells formed depends on the body's need for them. Infection, tissue damage, or viral agents promote the production and circulation of leukocytes. Table 36-1 gives the average normal values for total and differential white blood cell counts. Table 36-2 breaks these normal counts down by white blood cell type.

Thrombocytes

Thrombocytes, or platelets, are small, colorless bodies that contain the blood coagulation factors. The life span of a platelet is approximately 1 week.

When a blood vessel is damaged, hemostasis is maintained by a sequence of events called the coagulation process, or clotting mechanism (Fig. 36-1). The first event, vasoconstriction, occurs from platelet release of serotonin. The platelets then adhere to the exposed site of injury, forming

(text continued on page 1224)

TABLE 36-1 Average Range of Normal Blood Values

Test	Description	Age	Normal value
			(M/μL)
Red blood cell count (RBC)	Number of RBC in 1 μL (mm^3) of blood	Newborn (1–3 d)	4.0–6.6
		Neonate (1–4 wk)	3.0–6.3
		Infant (1–18 mo)	2.7–5.4
		Child (2–12 y)	3.9–5.3
		Adolescent	
		Male	4.5–5.3
		Female	4.1–5.1
			(g/dL)
Hemoglobin (Hgb)	Amount of hemoglobin in a given volume of blood	Newborn (1–3 d)	14.5–22.5
		Infant (2 mo)	9.0–14.0
		Child (6–12 y)	11.5–15.5
		Adolescent	
		Male	13.0–16.0
		Female	12.0–16.0
			(%)
Hematocrit (Hct)	Percentage of blood that is composed of RBC	Newborn (1–3 d)	44–75
		Infant (2 mo)	28–42
		Child (6–12 y)	35–45
		Adolescent	
		Male	37–49
		Female	36–46
Erythrocyte indices	*Calculations that characterize the size and hemoglobin content in individual red blood cells*		
			(μm^3)
Mean corpuscular volume (MCV)	Average or mean volume of a single RBC $MCV = \frac{Hct}{RBC}$	Newborn (1–3 d)	95–121
		Infant (0.5–2 y)	70–86
		Child (6–12 y)	77–95
		Adolescent	
		Male	78–98
		Female	78–102
			(pg/cell)
Mean corpuscular hemoglobin (MCH)	Average or mean quantity, by weight, of Hgb in a single RBC $MCH = \frac{Hgb}{RBC}$	Newborn (1–3 d)	31–37
		Neonate (1–4 wk)	28–40
		Infant (2–24 mo)	23–35
		Child (2–12 y)	24–33
		Adolescent	25–35
			(%Hb/cell)
Mean corpuscular hemoglobin concentration (MCHC)	Average concentration of Hgb in a single RBC $MCHC = \frac{Hgb}{Hct}$	Newborn (1–3 d)	29–37
		Neonate (1–2 wk)	28–38
		Infant (1–24 mo)	29–37
		Child/Adolescent	31–37

TABLE 36-1 continued

Test	Description	Age	Normal value
			(%)
Reticulocyte count	Percentage of young RBCs that stain positively for basophil reticulin with a supravital stain	Newborn (1 d)	3.2 ± 1.4
		Neonate (1–4 wk)	0.6 ± 0.3
		Infant (5–12 wk)	0.3–2.2
		Adults	0.5–1.5
			(× 1000 cells/μL)
White blood cell count (WBC)	Number of WBC in 1 μL (mm^3) of blood	Newborn	9.0–30.0
		Neonate (1 mo)	5.0–19.5
		Infant (1–3 y)	6.0–17.5
		Child (4–13 y)	4.5–15.5
		Adult	4.5–11.0
Differential white count	Percentage of various types of WBC seen on examination of a slide of peripheral blood		
			(%)
Neutrophils		Newborn	32–62
		Infant (1 y)	23
		Child (10 y)	31–61
		Adult	54–75
Basophils		Newborn	0.5–1.0
		Infant (1 y)	0.4
		Child (10 y)	0.5
		Adult	0–1
Eosinophils		Newborn	2–2.5
		Infant (1 y)	2.6
		Child (10 y)	2–2.5
		Adult	1–4
Lymphocytes		Newborn	26–36
		Infant (1 y)	61
		Child (10 y)	28–48
		Adult	25–40
Monocytes		Newborn	5–6
		Infant (1 y)	5
		Child (10 y)	4–4.5
		Adult	2–8
Platelet count	Number of platelets in 1 μL (mm^3) of blood	Newborn	84,000–478,000
		Thereafter	150,000–400,000
Bleeding time	Amount of time it takes for bleeding from small superficial wound to stop	Newborn	1–8 min
		Thereafter	1–6 min
Whole blood clotting time	Amount of time it takes for blood to clot in a glass tube	All ages	5–8 min
Prothrombin time (PT)	Amount of time it takes for blood to clot after thromboplastin and calcium chloride are added to blood plasma. Detects deficiencies of Factors V, VII, and X, fibrinogen, and prothrombin	Newborn	< 17 s
		Thereafter	11–15 s
Partial thromboplastin time (PTT)	A clotting test that measures activity of thromboplastin. Detects various factor deficiencies.	Newborn	< 90 s
		Thereafter	
		Nonactivated	60–85 s
		Activated	25–35 s
Thromboplastin generation time	Measures the blood's ability to generate thromboplastin. Distinguishes between Factor VIII and IX deficiencies.	Newborn	8–20 s
		Thereafter	8–16 s

continued on next page

TABLE 36-1 continued

Test	Description	Age	Normal value
Prothrombin consumption	Measures thromboplastin generation and prothrombin response	Almost complete consumption is indicated by a clotting time of greater than 20 seconds	
Fibrinogen level	Measures fibrinogen levels in the blood	Newborn Thereafter	125–300 mg/dL 200–400 mg/dL

Data compiled from Behrman RE, Vaughan VC: *Nelson Textbook of Pediatrics*, 12th ed., Saunders, 1983; and Byrne CJ, et al: *Laboratory Tests: Implications for Nurses and Allied Health Professionals*, Addison-Wesley, 1981. Normal values may vary significantly with different laboratory methods.

TABLE 36-2 Normal White Blood Cell Counts

White blood cells	Counts per mm^3
Granulocytes	
Neutrophils	3000–7000
Eosinophils	50–400
Basophils	0–50
Monocytes	100–600
Lymphocytes	1000–3000
Total	5000–10,000

a temporary clot, or plug. The third event is the release of various blood coagulation factors. The end product of coagulation is a fibrin clot.

Assessment of the Child With Hematopoietic Dysfunction

In assessing the child with *hematopoietic dysfunction* (alteration in the formation of blood cells), the nurse seeks data relevant to the suspected or diagnosed disorder. In anemia, for example, the nurse assesses the clinical manifestations of hypoxia. In clotting disorders, such as hemophilia, the nurse assesses the causes and effects of bleeding episodes. Assessment of the child with white blood cell disorders is described in Chapters 37 and 45.

History

A comprehensive history of the child and family is essential to determine nursing diagnoses and interventions for children with hematopoietic alterations. The nurse obtains the physical, psychologic, and social history of the child since birth (see Chapter 14). The nurse also gathers data regarding the causes and symptoms of common anemias and interferences in blood coagulation. Special emphasis is given to (1) a familial history of hereditary diseases; (2) adequacy of the child's diet, including dietary patterns; (3) history of chronic or recurring infections; (4) possible exposure to insecticides or any other toxic agents; and (5) physical activity and exercise tolerance. The family's cultural background and socioeconomic level are also noted. Some blood disorders are linked to heredity (spherocytosis, hemophilia), race (sickle cell disease), or place of birth (thalassemia).

Physical Examination

The Child With Anemia Anemia results in a wide range of symptoms depending on its severity and duration. Typ-

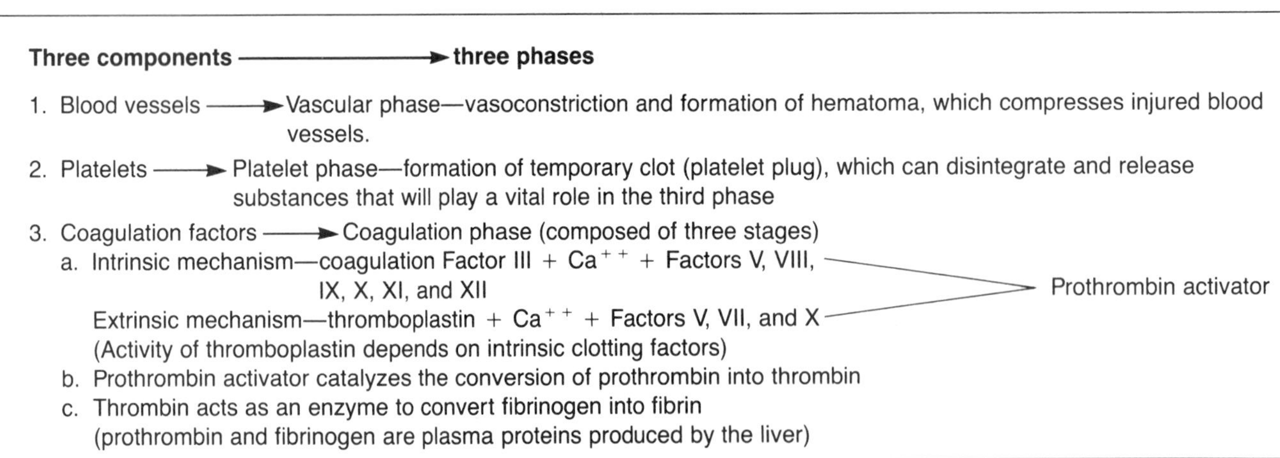

Figure 36-1. The coagulation process.

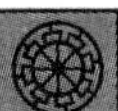

ASSESSMENT GUIDE Hematologic Composition

System	Subjective data	Objective data	Validating data	Nursing management
Head	Family history of thalassemia or Fanconi's syndrome	Craniofacial anomalies, particularly maxillary hyperplasia, broad prominent forehead or microcephaly	Complete blood count, erythrocyte indices, hemoglobin and hematocrit, skull radiography	Explore self-image through art, play, discussion. Refer family for genetic counseling.
Eyes, ears, nose and throat	Family history of anemias	Yellow sclera, pale conjunctiva, abnormalities of eyes or ears	Sickle cell slide prep, serum bilirubin, bone marrow aspiration	Observe for additional signs of anemia. Inquire about family hereditary patterns. Elicit information about dietary habits
	Family history of coagulation disorders; history of recent exposure to drugs, radiation, chemicals; or severe systemic disease such as Lupus Erythematosus	Epistaxis, oral ulcerations	White blood cell count and differential, platelet count, coagulation factor levels, PT, PTT, bleeding time, thromboplastin generation time, prothrombin consumption, fibrinogen level, reticulocyte count	Give meticulous mouth care (see Chapter 29). Give first aid to control epistaxis. Observe child for purpura or other manifestations of Von Willebrand's disease or aplastic anemia
Integumentary	Fatigue, lethargy	Waxy, pale appearance. Pallor noted on palms of hands, mucous membranes, and conjunctiva of dark skinned child. Jaundice indicating increased bilirubin or hemachromatosis (excess iron deposits in tissue). Discolorations of skin—petechiae, ecchymoses, hematomas, purpura. Cyanosis. Ulcerations on lower extremities		Monitor changes in pigmentation. Note location and size of any skin discolorations. Give meticulous skin care (see Chapter 29). Provide a safe, trauma-free environment. Teach prevention of injury to parent (see Chapter 19). Elicit any history of drug, chemical, or radiation exposure, or history of underlying disease
Respiratory	Fatigue, dizziness, anxiety, decreased exercise tolerance	Tachypnea (compensatory from hypoxia), dyspnea, signs of increasing respiratory distress (see Chapter 34)	Arterial blood gases	Inquire about exercise tolerance and physical activity. Facilitate adequate respiratory function (see Chapter 34). Monitor respiratory status. Promote adequate hydration

continued on next page

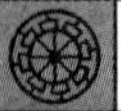

ASSESSMENT GUIDE Hematologic Composition (continued)

System	Subjective data	Objective data	Validating data	Nursing management
Cardiovascular	Tingling and numbness in extremities, pain, prolonged bleeding after trauma or surgery	Tachycardia, eventual cardiomegaly and congestive heart failure. Circulatory collapse. Signs of hemorrhage (decreased blood pressure, increased pulse, pallor, thirst)	Hematologic values (see Table 36-1), chest radiography	Inquire about family history of hereditary diseases and include information about sociocultural background. Elicit information about precipitators of bleeding episodes. Closely monitor vital signs and observe for signs of shock. Treat bleeding episodes promptly. Monitor transfusions and observe for transfusion reactions (see Table 36-3)
Gastrointestinal	Discomfort, pain, indigestion, anorexia, diarrhea, constipation	Protruding abdomen, splenomegaly, cholelithiasis (gallstones). Occult blood in stool	Stool for occult blood	Measure abdominal girth. Inquire about dietary habits particularly in relation to iron consumption. Give pain relief wih non-aspirin analgesics
Genitourinary	Enuresis	Hematuria. Signs of progressive renal impairment (see Chapter 39)	Urine for blood	Monitor renal status (see Chapter 39)
Neuroendocrine	Headache, dizziness, numbness, tingling	Hemiplegia or other signs of central nervous system involvement (see Chapter 42). Delayed puberty		Monitor neurologic signs. Elicit information about precipitators of sickle crisis. Observe for presence of secondary sex characteristics. Allow verbal expressions regarding self-image. Monitor for signs of associated endocrine problems in children with thalassemia (see Chapter 40)
Musculoskeletal	Weakness, pain in joints	Impaired growth. Decreased range of motion from bleeding into joints or muscles. Swelling of hands and feet (sickle cell crisis). Bone or joint degeneration. Pathologic fractures	Radiography	Monitor hypoxia and bleeding episodes. Use active and passive range of motion. Encourage exercises that build muscles but are free from injury potential. Administer non-aspirin analgesics for pain

ically, the child's skin looks waxy and pale. As more red blood cells are destroyed, bilirubin levels in the blood rise, giving the skin a yellow cast. In assessing patients with dark skin, the nurse looks for pallor of the palms of the hands, mucous membranes, conjunctivas, and scleras.

Anemic hypoxia has cardiac and respiratory effects. Insufficient tissue oxygenation stimulates a compensatory increase in respiratory and heart rates. Eventually, *cardiomegaly* (enlargement of the heart) and *dyspnea* (difficult or labored breathing) occur. If abnormally high heart and respiratory rates continue, congestive heart failure develops.

As red blood cells die and are removed by the spleen, the spleen enlarges, causing the child's abdomen to protrude. As the spleen invades the abdominal cavity, it pushes against other organs. The patient might experience dyspnea. Gastrointestinal symptoms of splenic enlargement include *anorexia* (loss of appetite), indigestion, pain, and frequently recurring diarrhea or constipation.

Most children with anemia experience weakness and become fatigued easily. Hypoxia might cause dizziness, headache, and tingling of the fingers and toes.

The Child With Clotting Disturbances Discolorations of the skin are characteristic signs of an alteration in the normal clotting mechanism. The nurse observes the skin for *petechiae* (small, purplish, hemorrhagic spots that resemble flea bites); *ecchymoses* (extravasations of blood into the skin or mucous membranes, which form bruises); and *hematomas* (tumors or swollen areas that contain blood).

If the child is bleeding at the time of the nursing assessment, blood pressure, heart rate, and respiratory status are monitored. Prompt treatment is necessary during active bleeding episodes to avoid a life-threatening situation.

The nurse assesses the range of motion of all extremities. Loss of joint mobility might result from bleeding into joints and muscles or from disuse due to fatigue (as in anemia). The nurse notes how well the child is able to move each joint through its full range of motion and determines the need for assessment by a physical therapist.

Nursing Management for Procedures and Treatments

Preparation for Diagnostic Tests

The child undergoing diagnosis and treatment for specific diseases endures a multitude of tests and procedures. The nurse should explain each procedure completely to the child beforehand at the child's level of understanding. This helps to alleviate fears of the unknown and clear up misconceptions. It is essential that the nurse or someone not involved in carrying out the procedure be with the child to provide emotional support. Holding the young child during and after the procedure increases comfort and security. The nurse might only need to hold the older child's hand to give emotional support. Older children should participate in the procedure, if possible. This helps them to feel involved in their own care. Allowing the child to handle the equipment to be used in the procedure also decreases fear and anxiety. See Chapter 29 for a more complete discussion about preparing a child for diagnostic tests.

Administration of Blood and Blood Products

Medical therapy for hematopoietic dysfunction might include transfusions of whole blood or blood products to replace deficient blood components. No transfusion is without risk. The nurse caring for a child receiving a transfusion should be alert for the signs and symptoms of a reaction. Table 36-3 summarizes six major tranfusion reactions.

Hemolytic Reaction Before transfusions are given, the patient's blood and the donor's blood are cross-matched as to group (A, B, AB, or O) and Rh factor (positive or negative). Blood typing determines the antigens present in the patient's and donor's red blood cells. Cross-matching of the donor's blood with the patient's blood lessens the chances that the patient's blood will contain antibodies against the donor's blood. Typing for HLA (histocompatibility locus antigen, which is present in lymphocytes) also might be done, especially if the patient requires repeated transfusions.

If blood is mismatched, red blood cells clump together and might occlude the blood vessels. Eventually, *hemolysis*, the destruction of red blood cells, decreases blood volume and causes the patient to go into shock. The patient then requires treatment to replace blood volume and avoid kidney shutdown caused by renal vasoconstriction.

The symptoms of a hemolytic reaction can occur within a few minutes of the start of the transfusion or hours later. Symptoms of a hemolytic reaction include headache, lumbar pain, chills, nausea and vomiting, hemoglobinuria (hemoglobin in urine caused by the liberation of hemoglobin from the destroyed red blood cells), and symptoms of shock and congestive heart failure.

Pyrogenic Reaction Pyrogenic (febrile) reaction is caused by the introduction of foreign material (antigen) into the recipient's blood, causing a febrile response from the antigen-antibody response (see Chapter 37). This type of reaction is common in children with thalassemia. Prophylactic antihistamines may be administered prior to the transfusion in patients who require frequent transfusions.

Allergic Reactions Allergic reactions usually occur when an allergen in the donor's blood is transmitted to a recipient who is allergic to that foreign antigen. The patient might respond with acute respiratory distress, urticaria (hives),

TABLE 36-3 Transfusion Reactions and Nursing Interventions

Reaction	Cause	Symptoms	Nursing interventions
Hemolytic (incompatible)	Mixing of incompatible blood or blood typing error	Reactions may occur within 10 minutes of transfusion Fever Headache Sharp lumbar (flank) pain Shaking Chills Nausea/vomiting Red or black urine Symptoms of impending shock Hemoglobinuria	Type and cross-match blood prior to the transfusion Make a positive identification of the patient and blood to be transfused; verify with another nurse or physician Start the infusion slowly for 15–20 minutes or the first 50 mL of blood Monitor the patient closely—stay with the patient for the first 15 minutes If a reaction occurs, (1) stop the infusion of blood and keep the intravenous line open at a keep-open rate; (2) return blood to the blood bank to cross-match again; (3) monitor the patient's vital signs every 5–15 minutes; (4) monitor the patient's urinary output hourly and insert a Foley catheter; (5) watch for signs of intravascular coagulation; and (6) treat for shock using supportive medical therapies
Pyrogenic (febrile)	Introduction of foreign material into the patient's blood, which produces an antigen–antibody reaction	Chills Fever Headache Nausea/vomiting	Use aseptic technique in administration Monitor the patient's vital signs at least every 30 minutes to 1 hour during infusion May give antihistamines prior to infusion to alleviate a potential reaction although effectiveness is questionable If reaction occurs, (1) stop infusion; (2) report data to physician for evaluation
Allergic (hypersensitivity)	Introduction of donor's allergens into recipient's blood (recipient allergic to the allergen)	Flushing Urticaria Wheezing Laryngeal edema Tightness in chest	Assess the patient for allergies Administer antihistamines or steroids prior to the infusion, as ordered Infuse blood slowly If reaction occurs, (1) stop infusion; (2) have epinephrine available to treat respiratory distress or anaphylaxis
Circulatory overload (hypervolemia)	Administration of too large a volume of blood or too rapid a transfusion	Dyspnea Precordial pain Cyanosis Distended neck veins Dry cough Pink-tinged secretions	Transfuse slowly—use infusion pump if necessary; assess flow rate frequently Use specific blood product needed by patient rather than whole blood whenever possible If reaction occurs, (1) stop infusion and keep intravenous line open at the slowest rate using an infusion pump; (2) place the patient in an upright position to increase venous return; (3) administer oxygen; (4) administer digitalis, as ordered
Embolic	Air enters bloodstream	Sudden respiratory distress Chest pain Dyspnea Apprehension	If administering blood under pressure, make sure pressure is normalized before container is empty Clear tubing of all air bubbles and keep tubing free of air bubbles If reaction occurs, (1) stop infusion and keep intravenous line open at keep-open rate; (2) position patient on left side with slight Trendelenburg's position to divert air from pulmonary area
Hypothermia	Administration of blood that has not been warmed to body temperature	Chills Decreased body temperature Irregular heart rate Bradycardia Possible cardiac arrest	Allow blood to warm to room temperature before administering

wheezing, chest tightness, bronchospasm, or laryngeal edema. Epinephrine should be available to treat possible anaphylactic shock. Allergic reactions occur most frequently in children who have a history of asthma, allergies, or repeated transfusions.

Circulatory Overload Circulatory overload can occur if the blood transfusion increases the circulating blood volume above the level that can be tolerated by the patient. Careful regulation of the transfusion can prevent this type of reaction. Particular attention should be paid to the rate of transfusion in infants and individuals with cardiac disease because circulatory overload in these patients can cause congestive heart failure or pulmonary edema.

Embolic Reaction The introduction of air emboli (air bubbles) during transfusion is rare. To prevent air emboli, the nurse clears the tubing of air bubbles and makes sure the tubing remains free of them. Air bubbles can also occur in infusion pumps, which are commonly used to administer blood to children.

Nursing Considerations The nurse who is administering transfusions has many responsibilities besides watching for signs and symptoms of a reaction. Before beginning the transfusion, the nurse obtains baseline vital signs. Medication that is ordered to prevent reaction is given at least 30 minutes before the transfusion. The nurse and another health team member together verify the identification of the recipient's and donor's blood type and group. When the blood or blood product is ready to be given, the nurse flushes the intravenous line with normal saline. Dextrose solution should not come in contact with the blood because it causes hemolysis of blood cells. The transfusion is administered through a filter to eliminate particles in the blood.

Reactions usually occur within the first 15–20 minutes of transfusion or while the first 50 mL of blood is being transfused. The nurse stays with the patient during this time and assesses the patient for signs and symptoms of reactions. Vital signs are monitored every 5–15 minutes for the first 30 minutes and every 30 minutes to 1 hour during the remainder of the transfusion. If a reaction is suspected, the nurse stops the transfusion, begins appropriate interventions, and notifies the physician. The remainder of the blood is returned to the laboratory for examination (along with a urine sample) if the patient has had a hemolytic reaction.

Blood decomposes if it is exposed to room temperature for more than 4 hours, so the nurse stores it in a blood-storage refrigerator until it is needed. Drugs are not administered during the transfusion. If it is necessary to give a medication, the nurse stops the transfusion, flushes the intravenous line with normal saline, administers the medication, flushes the line again with normal saline, and then resumes the transfusion.

Bone Marrow Aspiration

Bone marrow aspiration might be done to establish a diagnosis and is necessary when leukemia or aplastic anemia is suspected. In most red blood cell dysfunctions, only the initial aspiration is necessary. In leukemia or aplastic anemia, repeated aspirations must be done.

There are three types of bone marrow tests: (1) aspiration, in which marrow is aspirated from a bone by means of a large-gauge needle; (2) biopsy, in which a piece of bone is removed by means of a special needle; and (3) trephining, in which a section of bone is removed surgically. Bone marrow aspiration is done most frequently and is preferred. The iliac crest is the most common aspiration site in young children. The sternum may be used in older children but should be avoided in young children because it is a fragile bone that is not fused, and vital organs are in close proximity to it. (See Chapter 45 for a description of bone marrow aspiration.)

Bone Marrow Transplantation

Bone marrow transplantation is becoming a common treatment for patients with leukemia (see Chapter 45) and for aplastic anemia. At present, there are two types of bone marrow transplants. In *allogenic transplantation* several bone marrow specimens are aspirated from a matched donor, usually a sibling, and implanted in the recipient intravenously. In *autologous transplantation* the patient's own marrow is collected from disease-free tissue and frozen for future implantation. If transplantation is successful, the transplanted marrow cells begin to produce functioning blood cells in the patient.

Prior to bone marrow transplantation, drugs are given to induce immunosuppression, and all blood production is suppressed. These measures help to prevent rejection of the transplanted tissue. The patient's body also should be free of cancer.

The nurse assesses the child's and family's understanding of the procedure and offers explanations, as needed. The patient and family should have a clear picture of what to expect after the transplantation.

After the procedure, the patient undergoes chemotherapy to eliminate the patient's own bone marrow function and allow the donor's marrow to produce functioning blood cells. Infection, hemorrhage, toxic effects of drugs, and rejection are the major complications. Eradicated blood products, such as platelets, red blood cells, and white blood cells, might need to be replaced. Infection is the major complication of bone marrow transplantation. Strict aseptic technique must be maintained before and after transplantation. Initially, the child is isolated in a germ-free environment (a specially designed hospital unit with laminar air flow), and sterile linen and clothing are used. The child must be kept in this unit for 10–20 days. (See Chapter 37 for a discussion of laminar air flow units.) After discharge from the unit, the child continues to be protected from infection. The child, family, and health team members should be alert to any indication of infection so that aggresive antibiotic therapy can be initiated immediately.

Rejection of a bone marrow transplant can create a stressful situation for the family, especially if the condition fails to respond to treatment. The donor might feel like a "failure," and everyone involved needs an opportunity to express their feelings and help to accept the rejection.

Principles of Nursing Care

Acute-Care Needs

Prevention of Injury Disturbances in coagulation result in hemorrhage of varying severity. The child should be protected from any type of injury that could result in bleeding. In the hospital the bedrails should be up and the bed placed in the low position to prevent accidental falls. Bedrails should be padded or bumper pads used to prevent injury during sleep. The nurse alerts all health team members to the special need to protect the child from injury. It might be necessary for the nurse to supervise play and monitor the selection of toys. The child's nails are cut short to prevent scratching of the skin. Adolescents who need to shave are advised to use an electric razor rather than a straight-edge razor. Intramuscular injection should be avoided. If it is required, the nurse applies prolonged pressure to the site. Mucous membranes in patients with clotting disturbances are prone to bleeding, so good oral care is necessary. A soft toothbrush provides good hygiene while preventing injury.

When active bleeding occurs, prompt treatment is required to stop the bleeding. The child is immobilized until the bleeding is under control, and the nurse keeps the child calm as a means of decreasing the pulse. The nurse reduces bleeding by applying cold compresses, which cause vasoconstriction, and direct pressure. The child's extremities are kept elevated higher than the heart. Nasal packing might be necessary for nosebleeds. During all these interventions, the nurse carefully assesses the child and is prepared to treat the child for shock. Whole blood or blood products might be required to aid in clotting or replace blood the child has lost.

Bleeding into a joint might lead to joint degeneration and altered mobility. Once active bleeding has ceased, the nurse moves each joint through its passive range of motion as far as possible without causing pain. Physical therapy might be indicated.

Facilitation of Oxygenation Decreasing the oxygen needs of the child's body helps to prevent hypoxia. The nurse can accomplish this by providing a restful environment for the child and helping the child to avoid stressful activities. Generally, the anemic child does not feel well and is fatigued easily, so it is fairly easy to limit the child's activities. Nursing activities and medical therapies are scheduled to maintain optimum rest. Disturbing noises are avoided, and regular nap or rest periods are scheduled. Procedures and stressful situations are avoided prior to meals so that the child is rested enough to eat a well-balanced diet.

Promoting good respiratory function enhances oxygenation. The nurse helps the child to maintain an upright position, which decreases pressure on the diaphragm and allows greater lung expansion. A chalasia chair or infant seat can be used to keep an infant upright. The nurse also promotes good hydration to liquify secretions. Mobility and position changes prevent pooling of secretions and improve the oxygenation of blood in the lungs.

Control of Infection Patients with anemia have a decreased resistance to infection. Some anemias (such as aplastic anemia) and bone marrow damage decrease the white blood cell count, which predisposes the patient to infection (see Chapter 37).

The best way to prevent infection is to protect the child from exposure to it. Aseptic technique should be practiced by everyone who has contact with the child. When hospitalized, the child should be in a private room or have a noninfectious roommate. No one with an active infection should come in contact with the child. This not only includes family and friends but also members of the health care team. The child is encouraged to eat a well-balanced diet to maintain resistance against infection. Oral hygiene and skin care can prevent skin breakdown and eventual infection (see Chapter 44). The nurse assesses the child continually so that if an infection occurs, cultures can be done and antibiotics started promptly.

Outside the hospital environment, the child should avoid sources of infection. The child usually is allowed to return to school because developmental and social needs also need to be met. The family should be alert for signs and symptoms of infection so that immediate medical intervention can be initiated if an infection occurs. Routine immunizations and health care examinations should be maintained.

Nutritional Needs

A continuous supply of nutrients is needed to maintain and nourish all the cells in the body. Adequate hydration maintains homeostasis between cellular and extracellular fluids (see Chapter 33). Children with red blood cell disturbances might require one and one-half to two times their normal fluid requirements. To promote fluid intake, the nurse offers oral fluids at frequent intervals (such as every hour). Attempts are made to meet the fluid requirement during the child's waking hours so that rest is not interrupted. Foods that are liquid at room temperature, such as ice cream, flavored gelatin, or Popsicles, can be used as fluid sources. (See Chapter 29 for a discussion about managing fluid intake.)

A nutritious, well-balanced diet is necessary to maintain a healthy body (see Chapter 15). Some nutritional anemias, such as iron deficiency anemia, might even be avoided with a nutritious diet rich in iron and vitamins. Foods high in iron include meat, fish, poultry, eggs, green leafy vegetables, potatoes, dried fruit, beans, bread, and cereal. Multivitamins may be prescribed along with the well-balanced diet. Vitamin C often is recommended because it enhances absorption of iron, or iron supplements can be given with citrus juice. Poor eating habits or inadequate absorption might cause folic acid and vitamin B_{12} deficiencies. These vitamins play a role in the formation of red blood cells; therefore, a deficiency in either or both of these substances can cause anemia. The child's diet should include foods rich in the deficient vitamin, and oral supplements might be needed to replenish the body's stores.

Infants over 6 months of age should be limited to 1 quart or liter of milk per day so that they will become hungry enough to eat solid foods rich in iron. New, unfamiliar foods should be offered one at a time so that the child can change food preferences and eating preferences gradually. Older children, particularly adolescent girls, are also at risk of developing iron deficiency anemia as a result of fad or starvation diets, which are usually low in iron.

Whenever dietary restrictions are necessary, the nurse provides diet counseling for the child and family. They should be taught why dietary changes and good nutrition are essential.

Developmental, Emotional, and Health Maintenance Needs

Children affected by disorders of the hematopoietic system often manifest the struggle between dependence and independence. Throughout their lives, many of them are dependent upon others for assistance with, for instance, transfusions, sickle crises, or other consequences of their disease. Since the developing child derives emotional satisfaction from self-care and acquiring independence, every effort should be made to encourage the child's active participation in care. As the child matures, increasing responsibility can be given in regard to diet, exercise tolerance, and safety. Parents are encouraged to allow the child freedom to explore while setting reasonable limits for safety. Parental overprotectiveness is a trap to be avoided so as not to stifle the child's emotional development.

Activity restriction may make these children seem different to their peers, thus undermining their self-esteem and decreasing the satisfaction gained from social contact. Non-contact, but competitive, sports can provide team participation and a network of social interactions.The child's interest also can be directed toward other extracurricular activities or clubs.

The child should be allowed to express any feelings regarding alteration in body image, and the nurse encourages parents to facilitate this process.

The Child With Anemia

Iron Deficiency Anemia

Iron deficiency anemia is caused by an inadequate supply, intake, or absorption of iron (see Chapter 15). Iron is essential for the formation of red blood cells. Lack of iron results in smaller red blood cells and, in turn, decreased hemoglobin synthesis. Adequate daily ingestion of iron and iron released from disintegrating red blood cells supply iron for red blood cell production (*erythropoiesis*). Iron is absorbed primarily in the duodenum. When iron intake is inadequate, the body uses stored iron. Eventually, the stored iron is depleted, and symptoms of anemia develop.

Iron deficiency is the most common cause of anemia in children. Possible causes of iron deficiency anemia are (1) inadequate dietary intake of iron, such as might occur in bottle- or breast-fed infants who do not receive supplemental iron; (2) malabsorption of iron, such as occurs in chronic diarrhea, malabsorption syndromes (celiac disease), or gastrectomy; (3) blood loss caused by gastrointestinal bleeding, heavy menstruation, or hemorrhage; (4) excessive demands caused by periods of stress or rapid growth; and (5) intravascular hemolysis, resulting in hemoglobinuria.

Clinical findings of pallor, fatigue, and irritability, combined with a history of an iron-deficient diet, suggest anemia. Because iron deficiency anemia occurs gradually, most patients do not seek medical attention until it has progressed to an advanced stage. The actual medical diagnosis is made following laboratory tests. The red blood cell count might be normal or slightly reduced. Hemoglobin is below the normal range for the child's age. The *hematocrit* (percentage of blood that is made up of red blood cells) is below normal. The red blood (erythrocyte) indices are important in diagnosis because they demonstrate any decrease in size and concentration of hemoglobin in a single red blood cell. The reticulocyte count is usually low (see Table 36-1 for laboratory tests and normal values).

Treatment Treatment for iron deficiency anemia involves iron replacement therapy and diet counseling. An oral preparation of ferrous sulfate is given or a combination of iron and ascorbic acid, which enhances the absorption of iron. If the patient is uncooperative or if the gastrointestinal tract cannot absorb iron, the iron is administered parenterally.

Blood transfusions are rarely necessary in the management of iron deficiency anemia. If the anemia is profound or if infection is present, transfusions of packed red blood cells may be prescribed.

Nursing Management Nursing management of the child with iron deficiency anemia focuses on nutrition and cooperation with the medical regimen. The nurse informs the child and family that both dietary changes and supplemental iron therapy are needed to cure iron deficiency anemia.

The nurse teaches the child and family about the side effects of iron therapy, which include nausea, vomiting, and diarrhea or constipation. These symptoms might indicate a need to change the dosage. If the child is taking an oral iron preparation, it should not be consumed with milk or antacids because they interfere with iron absorption. If a liquid iron preparation is being used, the child should drink it from a straw to prevent staining the teeth. Children who have not had ascorbic acid prescribed with the iron should take iron with a high vitamin C content juice. The nurse also should warn the patient and family that the patient's stools will become darker.

If intramuscular injections of Imferon are prescribed, the Z-track injection method should be used to prevent the accidental deposition of iron in the skin, which could lead to a change in skin color or scarring.

Dietary modifications are necessary indefinitely to keep the anemia from recurring, and oral iron supplements must be taken until the prescription runs out. After the anemia subsides, the nurse encourages the parent to seek routine medical examinations for the child. Hemoglobin levels should be checked every 6 months to detect recurrences.

Aplastic Anemia

In aplastic anemia the formation of red blood cells, white blood cells, and platelets is depressed, resulting in profound anemia, leukopenia, and thrombocytopenia. Aplastic anemia is caused by injury or destruction of stem cells in the bone marrow. The disease may be primary (congenital) or secondary (acquired). There are two forms of the congenital type: congenital hypoplastic anemia and Fanconi's syndrome.

Hypoplastic anemia (Blackfan–Diamond syndrome) is a rare disease characterized by the destruction of red blood cells and a slight decrease in white blood cells and platelets. The disease develops as a profound anemia in infants between 2 and 3 months of age and is treated with transfusion, splenectomy, and the administration of corticosteroids. Treatment is similar to that for other profound anemias such as thalassemia. If remission is achieved the prognosis is usually very good, and long-term survival is likely. Remissions occur in approximately one-fourth to one-third of patients with hypoplastic anemia. Death usually is caused by overwhelming sepsis, hepatitis from repeated transfusions, or cardiac failure.

In Fanconi's syndrome *cytopenia* (deficiency of all cellular elements of the blood) is associated with multiple congenital anomalies such as dwarfism, *hypoplasia* (underdevelopment) of the kidneys and spleen, *microcephaly* (abnormal smallness of the head), abnormalities of the eyes and ears, and mental retardation. Fanconi's syndrome appears as an autosomal recessive trait, but the penetrance varies. Affected children might have several different combinations of defects.

Approximately one-half of the aplastic anemias have an acquired or secondary cause. The most common causes of acquired aplastic anemia are (1) drugs such as chloramphenicol (an antibiotic); (2) irradiation; (3) toxic agents such as household dyes, paint removers, insecticides, and compounds with benzene; (4) severe diseases such as hepatitis or sepsis; and (5) immunologic deficiencies such as in leukemia.

The symptoms of aplastic anemia include progressive weakness, fatigue, *tachycardia* (rapid heart rate), *tachypnea* (rapid breathing), and pallor. Thrombocytopenia is evidenced by ecchymosis, petechiae, and hemorrhage. Leukopenia may result in infection.

Bone marrow aspiration is necessary for diagnosis. The normally red marrow is yellow and fatty in patients with aplastic anemia. The prognosis in aplastic anemia is poor. The mortality rate is over 70%, and about 50% of patients die within 6 months to 1 year of diagnosis.

Medical and Surgical Treatment Blood products, such as red blood cells, white blood cells, and platelets, and antibiotics are administered as supportive therapies. Drug therapy is used to stimulate *erythropoiesis*. Androgenic steroids (such as testosterone) in combination with corticosteroids, which enhance the effects of testosterone, are somewhat effective. It is unknown exactly how testosterone stimulates erythropoiesis, but it is thought that the drug affects the erythroid elements, which stimulate erythroid hyperplasia in the fatty, hypocellular bone marrow. Response to drug therapy is gradual. It might be 2–6 months before any change is seen in the patient.

Early bone marrow transplantation can improve survival. One study (Camitta, 1979) showed that transplantation produces 60% survival in about half of the patients who undergo marrow transplantation. Another approach to treatment is the administration of antithymocyte globulin (ATG). This treatment is recommended for children who are not candidates for bone marrow transplantation. The basis for this treatment lies in the theory that some aplastic anemias may be the result of an autoimmune response (see Chapter 37). This autoimmune response either destroys bone marrow stem cells, or prevents the cellular differentiation that allows for eventual bone marrow repopulation (Goldstein, 1980). Antithymocyte globulin suppresses the T-cell-dependent autoimmune response. Antithymocyte globulin has many severe side effects, including fever, chills, rash, serum sickness, severe thrombocytopenia, anaphylaxis, and death (Gale et al., 1981).

Nursing Management Nursing care for patients with aplastic anemia focuses on (1) preventing complications from the anemia—infection and bleeding; (2) preparing the child and family for diagnostic and therapeutic procedures; (3) giving emotional support to the child and family during terminal illness; and (4) giving nursing care related to transfusions, therapy with androgenic steroids, and/or bone marrow transplantation. Nursing management is similar to that for patients with leukemia (see Chapter 45).

The decreased number of platelets in the blood makes the child susceptible to bleeding. The nurse protects the child from injury and carefully assesses the skin, urine, and stool for blood. Bleeding problems must be detected early so that prompt treatment can be initiated.

The side effects of drug treatment result in changes in self-image. Testosterone causes deepening of the voice, growth of pubic hair, hirsutism, enlargement of the penis in males, flushing of the skin, acne, and growth retardation. These side effects, combined with the side effects of corticosteroids, which include the formation of fat pads on the upper back (buffalo hump) and on the face (moon face), acne, and hirsutism, are difficult for the child to understand and accept. It is important for the nurse to approach the child in a positive manner and inform the child and family about the possible side effects before they develop.

The nurse protects the child from infection, giving special attention to the care of the skin and mucous membranes. Skin care and comfort measures appropriate for the child with leukemia (see Chapter 45) are also appropriate for the child with aplastic anemia.

If the child does not require hospital care, the nurse encourages the parent to make the child's life at home as normal as possible (see Chapter 26). Nursing care for the dying child is discussed in Chapter 32.

Anemia Caused by Corpuscular Defects

Hemolytic anemias are anemias which result from *hemolysis* of the erythrocytes (destruction of red blood cells with subsequent separation of hemoglobin). The two major categories of hemolytic anemia caused by corpuscular defects are (1) those caused by an enzyme deficiency (such as glucose-6-phosphate dehydrogenase [G6PD] deficiency) and (2) those caused by membrane deficiencies (such as spherocytosis). These anemias are generally inherited.

Glucose 6 Phosphate Dehydrogenase Deficiency Most people who have G6PD deficiency have episodes of hemolysis after exposure to infectious microorganisms or certain drugs such as analgesics, sulfonamides, antipyretics, nitrofurans, or synthetic vitamin K. The disease is characterized by a mild anemia because only older red blood cells are affected. The production of young red blood cells increases in response to the hemolytic process, elevating the reticulocyte count. Treatment for anemia caused by G6PD deficiency is primarily supportive. The causative agent is removed, and transfusions are given as needed.

Spherocytosis Spherocytosis is characterized by the production of small, spheroidal red blood cells and chronic hemolysis, which results in anemia, splenomegaly, and hyperbilirubinemia. Gallstones are frequent complications of spherocytosis. Treatment is by splenectomy, which generally eliminates the anemia. Because splenectomy in infants predisposes them to sepsis and meningitis, the operation generally is not done until the patient is 2 years of age.

Anemias From Altered Hemoglobin

Sickle Cell Disease Sickle cell disease is a common genetic disease found predominately in blacks. Sickle cell disease, which is associated with the presence of hemoglobin S (Hgb S), may be manifested as active sickle cell disease (homozygous gene Hgb SS) or as the sickle cell trait (heterozygous gene Hgb AS). In sickle cell disease and trait, Hgb S (the abnormal hemoglobin) replaces all or part of the normal hemoglobin. This causes the red blood cells to sickle, or change from round to crescent-shaped disks (sickles) when oxygen is released to the tissues. See Table 36-4 for other characteristics of sickled cells.

Parents with sickle cell disease or trait can pass the condition on to their children. Approximately 1 out of every 10 black Americans has sickle cell disease or trait (Jenkins, 1983). Sickle cell disease (homozygous) is an inherited autosomal recessive disorder that follows Mendelian law. Because the person who has the sickle cell trait (heterozygous) can exhibit symptoms under certain conditions, the inheritance pattern for the sickle trait is autosomal dominant (see Chapter 5). Figure 36-2 illustrates the genetic transfer of sickle cell disease and trait.

TABLE 36-4 Comparison of Normal and Sickled Red Blood Cells

Characteristics	Normal cells	Sickled cells
Shape of RBC	Round	Crescent, or sickle
Life span of RBC	120 days	30–40 days
Oxygen-carrying capacity of Hgb	Normal	Decreased
Hgb per milliliter	12–14 g	6–9 g
Type of Hgb	Hgb A	Hgb S
Destruction rate of RBC	Normal	Greatly increased

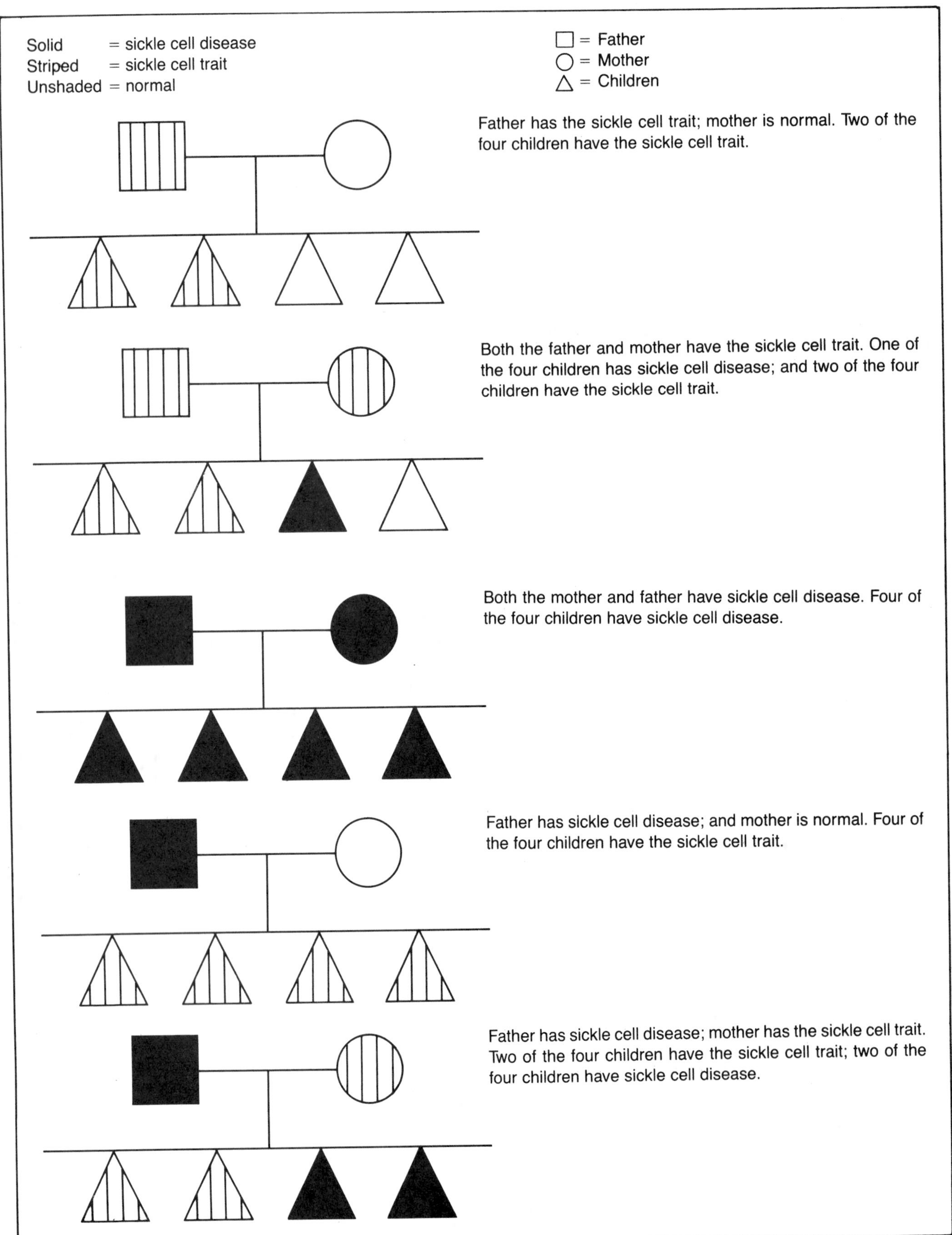

Figure 36-2. Genetic transfer of sickle cell disease.

All black persons should be screened for the presence of Hgb S, which is detected by blood tests called sickling tests. Two common sickling tests are the Sickledex Test and the Sickle Cell Slide Prep Test. If a sickling test is positive, the patient is tested further for the presence of active disease. Positive findings in such tests as stained blood smears or hemoglobin electrophoresis indicate sickle cell disease.

People with the sickle cell trait usually do not have active disease. Although about 25%–45% of their hemoglobin is Hgb S, normal hemoglobin predominates, and the red blood cells do not sickle but continue to function normally. Persons with the sickle cell trait might, however, be affected by the following:

1. Decreased ability to withstand extreme physical stresses such as hard physical labor or exercise.
2. Greater difficulty with pregnancy and an increase in the infant mortality rate.
3. Inability to withstand atmospheric conditions of low oxygen content (such as high altitudes or nonpressurized airplanes).
4. The need for supplemental oxygen during surgical procedures.

Persons living in climates where malaria is prevalent have an advantage if they are carrying the sickle cell trait because the malarial parasite is incapable of invading the cells carrying Hgb S (Jenkins, 1983). Since many black Americans are descendants of equatorial Africans it might be assumed that the presence of the sickle trait in black Americans has evolved from their protective mechanism against malaria. Under ordinary circumstances persons with sickle cell trait never develop or require treatment for sickle cell disease.

Sickle cell disease is a chronic anemic condition marked by physiologic crises. Complications of sickle cell disease can be recognized, predicted, and treated, but they cannot totally be prevented.

In the child with sickle cell disease, Hgb S is present from the time of conception, but significant amounts of fetal hemoglobin tend to inhibit sickling and anemia until the infant is about 6 months of age. After 6 months of age, red blood cells with Hgb S begin to outnumber cells with normal hemoglobin, and signs of a progressive, lifelong anemia begin to develop (Vichinsky and Lubin, 1980). Frequently, the first signs of sickle cell disease are lack of appetite, irritability, and an increased susceptibility to infection. The child might be small for age and gain weight poorly. The mucous membranes are pale, and scleral icterus is evident. In the older child the trunk usually is short, the extremities long, the hips and shoulders narrow, and the hands and feet slender. Changes in the bone might be found radiographically as early as 6 months of age. Sexual maturation might be delayed or absent. The spleen might be palpable during the first decade of life. Later, the liver might be palpable, and cardiac complications might develop.

Complications of sickle cell disease are frequent severe infections, chronic leg ulcers, problems in pregnancy, and bone weakness. Patients with sickle cell disease also might have a lowered resistance to pneumococcal and salmonella microorganisms.

For variable periods, a child with sickle cell disease might have no complaints other than chronic anemia. Then, with the occurrence of a common childhood illness, such as tonsillitis or an upper respiratory infection, or for no apparent reason, the child becomes acutely ill. This sudden change in health is termed *sickle cell crisis.* Sickle cell crises may be of the vaso-occlusive (thrombocytic), sequestration, or aplastic type. Crisis occurs when physiologic stress reduces hydration or deprives the Hgb S of oxygen. Once it begins, the sickling process is self-sustaining because its anoxic effects cause further sickling. The sickling process and its physiologic effects are shown in Figure 36-3.

Vaso-occlusive (thrombocytic) crisis, the most common type of sickle cell crisis, is sometimes called "painful crisis" because of its painful symptoms. In *vaso-occlusive crisis,* red blood cells clump and block small blood vessels, causing distal *ischemia* (deficiency of blood). Ischemia may lead to *infarction* (death of tissue cells) in various body sites. Vaso-occlusive crisis can result in a group of skeletal prob-

Types of Sickle Cell Crises KNOW

1. Vaso-occlusive, or thrombocytic, crisis. Occlusion of small blood vessels causes the following:
   - Pain
   - Distal ischemia
   - Infarction in the following:
     - Bones and joints, causing swelling and pain
     - The spleen, causing acute abdomen, with symptoms of rigidity, distention, pain, and fever; and fibrosis and scarring
     - The brain, causing stroke, hemiplegia, and death
     - The lungs, causing fever, respiratory distress
2. Sequestration crisis. Pooled blood in the spleen and impaired blood flow to the liver cause the following:
   - Enlargement of the spleen
   - Liver failure and necrosis
   - Circulatory collapse (shock)
3. Aplastic crisis. Bone marrow failure causes the following:
   - Cessation of red blood cell production
   - Life-threatening anemia

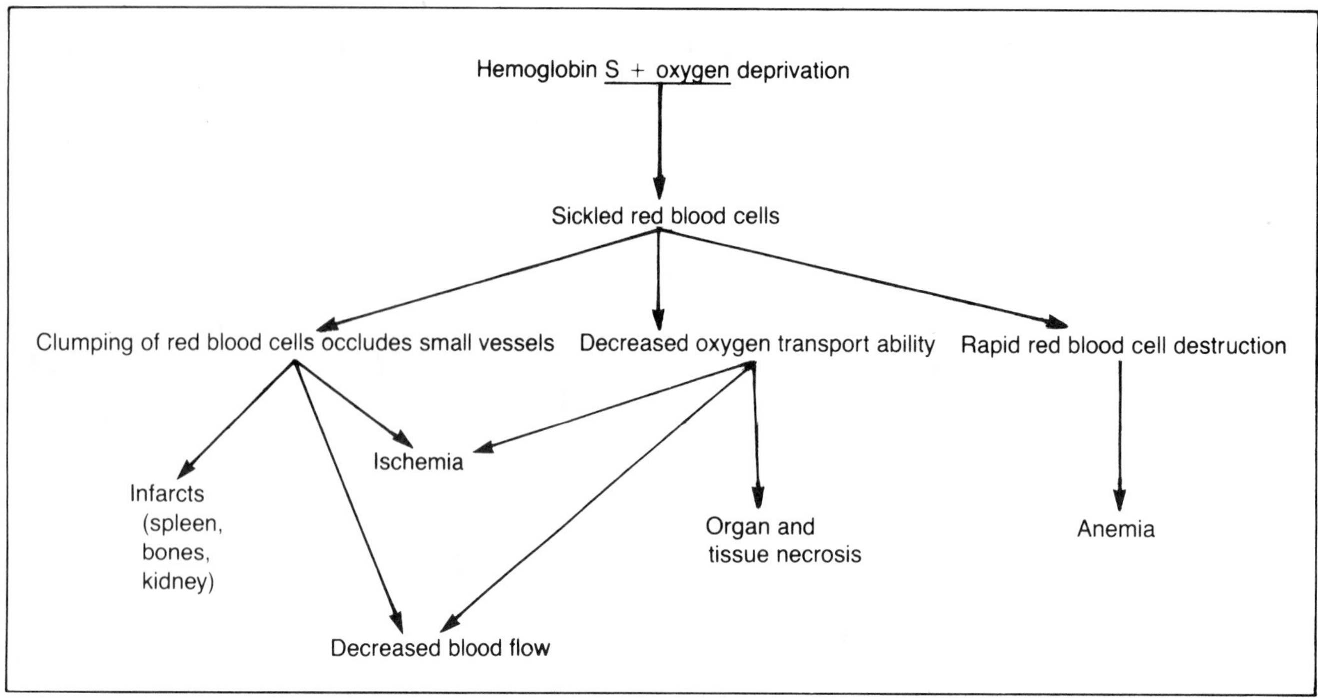

Figure 36-3. The sickling process and its physiologic effects.

lems known as hand–foot syndrome. Painful swelling occurs in the hands and feet, with a decrease in the range of motion of the extremities involved. These symptoms are frequently confused with those of rheumatic fever or osteomyelitis. There is no high fever. Pain is not relieved with mild analgesics (aspirin or acetaminophen). Occlusion of blood vessels in the abdomen causes distention and pain, symptoms resembling acute abdomen. Bowel sounds are normal. These symptoms last 3–4 days. Chronic leg ulcers are common effects of decreased peripheral circulation. Occlusion of blood vessels serving the central nervous system might result in hemiplegia or other neurologic findings resembling symptoms of stroke. Vaso-occlusive crisis in the lungs frequently is initiated by pneumococcal infection, and it is difficult to determine whether the patient's respiratory distress results from infarction or infection.

The second type of sickle cell crisis is *sequestration crisis*, in which sickling causes sudden pooling of blood in the spleen. Sequestration crisis usually is seen in infants and children under 5 years of age. The liver and spleen become enlarged. This is the most dangerous of the sickle cell crises because it results in shock and even death. The symptoms are sudden weakness, pallor, shortness of breath, tachycardia, and a distended abdomen. With prompt treatment, sequestration crisis is reversible.

In *aplastic crisis* red blood cell production accelerates, but the body destroys the new red blood cells faster than they are produced. Red blood cell production stops for 10–14 days, resulting in profound anemia that can become life threatening. The child is weak and listless and has tachycardia and tachypnea. Aplastic crisis usually ends spontaneously.

The prognosis of sickle cell anemia is affected significantly by the quality of medical care and nursing management and the child's and family's response to the disease, which lasts for life. The cause of mortality during the first years of life is usually from overwhelming sepsis and sequestration crisis. As the child grows older, sickle cell crises occur less frequently.

Treatment Therapy consists of treating the crisis symptoms and giving supportive care. Treatments and their objectives are as follows:

1. *Hydration.* Fluids are given orally or intravenously to produce *hemodilution* (an increase in the fluid volume of the blood), which helps to prevent sickling and thrombosis.
2. *Electrolyte replacement.* This counters the acidosis caused by hypoxia.
3. *Analgesic administration.* Acetaminophen is given for mild pain. Meperidine and morphine are reserved for extreme pain. Aspirin (in large doses) is avoided

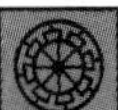

NURSING CARE GUIDE: The Child With Sickle Cell Crisis

Nursing diagnosis	Interventions	Evaluation
1. Pain	Determine location of pain (joints, bones, or abdomen) Determine degree of warmth of affected extremity	Pain tolerance is increased Child doesn't require narcotics for pain Pain is minimized
2. Respiratory distress	Observe respiratory patterns to determine need for further assessment Observe child for signs of cyanosis Administer oxygen by tent, mask, or nasal cannula Elevate head of bed to facilitate breathing Maintain calm atmosphere to decrease child's anxiety	Child is not in respiratory distress as evidenced by stable vital signs, minimal respiratory effort, pink skin and mucous membranes, and decreased need for oxygen (see Chapter 34 for further evaluation)
3. Alteration in fluid balance	Observe for signs of fluid imbalance (see Chapter 33) Record intake and output Maintain ordered intravenous fluid rate Encourage child to drink fluids (see Chapter 29)	Child receives one and one-half to two times maintenance fluid requirements daily; child appears well hydrated
4. Potential infection due to lowered resistance	Observe for signs of infection: increased temperature, irritability or lethargy, decreased appetite, redness or swelling of tissue, pain Protect child from known sources of infection Administer antibiotics as ordered	Child remains free of infection
5. Weakness and fatigue	Organize nursing care to provide optimum rest by providing bedrest and scheduling rest periods as needed Encourage age-appropriate nonstrenuous activities	Child's weakness and fatigue diminish
6. Potential complication of shock	Observe child for signs of shock (check vital signs frequently, report change in child's condition promptly) Maintain hydration by intravenous therapy Measure and record intake and output accurately Provide routine shock therapy (flat position, elevated legs, warmth, fluid volume restoration, vital signs, and level of consciousness)	Child shows no evidence of shock; vital signs are stable

because it can worsen metabolic acidosis and cause bleeding.

4. *Bedrest.* This conserves the child's energy.
5. *Antibiotic administration.* Antibiotics are used to treat or prevent infections. All patients over 2 years of age are given Pneumovax pneumococcal vaccine because of their susceptibility to infection.
6. *Oxygen therapy.* Reduced pulmonary oxygenation due to infiltrates and infarcts can lead to hypoxia. Oxygen therapy may also be used to treat the anemia.
7. *Transfusion.* Packed red blood cells are administered to treat the anemia and reduce the number of circulating sickle cells. Exchange transfusions are reserved for life-threatening situations and are not employed routinely in painful crisis.

In children with splenic sequestration crisis, *hypovolemia* (reduced blood volume) is corrected promptly with volume expanders, and whole blood transfusions are required. Splenectomy is considered if the child has one or more severe crises because the spleen is one of the major sites of sickling, sequestration, and destruction of red blood cells.

Priapism, or persistent erection of the penis, is an occasional and painful effect of sickling. The usual treatment for priapism includes hypotonic fluids and warm baths. The errection should be relieved within several hours because of the danger of ischemia to the penile tissue. It might be necessary to aspirate the corpora cavernosa to relieve the erection.

Nursing Management Helping the child and family adjust to a lifelong disease and preventing the sickling process are the two key factors in nursing management for the child with sickle cell disease. The nurse explains the disease and its effects to the child and family and informs and guides them in periods of crisis. Genetic counseling is strongly encouraged (see Chapter 5).

Tissue hypoxia can initiate the sickling process, so it is essential that the child avoid factors that increase cellular requirements for oxygen. The nurse helps to avert hypoxia by the following:

1. Teaching the child to refrain from strenuous physical activities, such as contact sports, encouraging the child to participate in activities that are tolerated, and teaching the child to set realistic limits independently.
2. Teaching the child to avoid environments that are low in oxygen concentration such as high altitudes, unpressurized airplanes, and deep-sea diving.
3. Helping the child to minimize and deal with emotional stress.
4. Protecting the child from known sources of infection and ensuring prompt treatment of any current infection.
5. Encouraging the child to drink one and one-half to two times the usual fluid requirement to facilitate hemodilution (see Chapter 29).

Enuresis (bed-wetting) should be considered a complication of sickle cell disease. Nursing management of elimination for the hospitalized child is covered in Chapter 29. If the child is being cared for at home, the nurse explains to the child and family that enuresis is likely to occur. Fluids should continue to be encouraged, but the parent might want to make sure that the child empties the bladder before going to bed. The nurse encourages the parent not to awaken the child during the night to empty the bladder because disruption in the normal sleep pattern alters the child's ability to conserve energy.

During a sickle cell crisis, intravenous fluid therapy may be combined with oral hydration because the child is less likely to eat and drink. The nurse carefully regulates the fluid intake and monitors the fluid and electrolyte balance. Accurate measurements of intake and output, specific gravity of the urine, and the child's daily weight enable the nurse to assess and manage hydration.

Pain during a crisis can be managed with analgesics. If narcotic analgesics are prescribed, the nurse should be alert for signs of drug abuse (see Chapter 24). Pain also is managed with comfort measures such as repositioning the child, immobilizing or elevating the painful part, or applying heat. Cold is not applied because it causes vasoconstriction, which extends the sickling process. Diversional activities usually are effective in taking the child's mind off the pain.

The nurse assesses the child's respiratory status so that proper interventions can be initiated in the event of respiratory distress. If oxygen is required, the nurse administers it by tent, mask, or nasal cannula, as appropriate for the child.

The child usually is fatigued and weakened during a sickle cell crisis, so it is fairly easy to provide bedrest. The nurse arranges nursing care, medical tests, and therapy so that the child receives maximum rest. Rest periods are scheduled before mealtimes so that the child will have the energy to eat. Play activities, which should not be strenuous, are essential for the child's development (see Chapter 28). The nurse also might be responsible for coordinating the daily visits of an occupational therapist.

Children with sickle cell anemia are not prone to infection, but infection can precipitate a sickle cell crisis, so well-balanced meals, protection from sources of infection, frequent medical supervision, and adequate rest are necessary.

Vascular collapse and shock might occur as a result of a sickle cell crisis. The nurse observes the child for signs of shock: vital signs, blood pressure, and level of consciousness are closely monitored. Changes are reported to the physician immediately so that prompt treatment can be initiated.

β-Thalassemia (Cooley's Anemia) Thalassemia is a group of hereditary hemolytic anemias that are caused by a deficiency in the normal synthesis of hemoglobin polypeptide chains. Subcategories of thalassemia are named according to the polypeptide chain affected, that is, as alpha-, beta-, gamma-, or delta-thalassemia. In β-thalassemia the basic defect is a deficiency in the synthesis of β-chain hemoglobin molecules, which results in defective hemoglobin formation. Stimulated by inadequate supplies of hemoglobin, the bone marrow becomes *hyperplastic* (overproductive), forming red blood cells that are fragile and easily destroyed. The body attempts to compensate for the decrease in hemoglobin by producing fetal hemoglobin, which does not contain β chains.

There are two forms of β-thalassemia: thalassemia minor, the heterozygous form, and thalassemia major, the homozygous form, also known as Cooley's anemia. If the patient inherits only one thalassemia gene (which combines with a normal gene), mild to moderate anemia develops, and the patient is classified as having the heterozygous trait, or thalassemia minor. If two thalassemia genes are inherited (homozygous), the patient is born with the severe, life-threatening form (thalassemia major).

Thalassemia major is an autosomal recessive disorder. People whose ancestors lived near the Mediterranean Sea or in the Mediterranean Desert have the highest incidence of the disease, but it also can occur as a result of spontaneous mutations.

β-thalassemia (homozygous) is suspected in patients who are severely anemic, have a Mediterranean background, and have the classic appearance of patients with the disease (thickened cranial bones, flat nose, and malocclusions of the teeth). Hematologic tests reveal *hypochromic* (lacking in hemoglobin), abnormally small red blood cells that are distorted in shape, numerous target cells, and numerous nucleated red blood cells. There is also a predominance of fetal hemoglobin and decreased amounts of normal adult hemoglobin.

Thalassemia major causes severe, progressive, hemolytic anemia that begins in affected infants at about 6 months of age, when the protective effect of fetal hemoglobin diminishes. The child's spleen enlarges, causing an enlarged abdomen. As the bone marrow becomes hyperplastic, it expands the marrow cavities of the bones, causing skeletal changes. The head enlarges, and facial features change to resemble those characteristic of patients with Down's syndrome. Chronic anemia causes growth retardation, so children with β-thalassemia commonly have small bodies. Bone cartilage thins with age, making the child susceptible to spontaneous fractures. *Hemochromatosis,* in which excess iron is deposited in the tissues, can cause changes in the heart such as fibrosis or hypertrophy of cardiac muscle fibers. Cardiac changes increase the heart's work load and can eventually cause congestive heart failure.

Progressive hemochromatosis also affects the spleen, liver, and gallbladder. As the spleen enlarges, it causes the abdomen to protrude and might push against other abdominal organs and the lungs, interfering with their function. Splenectomy might be necessary. Signs of cirrhosis of the liver eventually occur, and gallstones are common. *Cholecystectomy* (gallbladder removal) might be done at the time of splenectomy if gallstones are present.

Cardiac complications, such as cardiomegaly, heart failure, or *arrhythmias* (abnormal heart rhythms), are associated with β-thalassemia and are related to a condition called hemosiderosis. *Hemosiderosis* is an accumulation of the iron-containing substance, hemosiderin, which results from the rapid destruction of defective red blood cells. The frequent blood transfusions that are required to maintain hemoglobin levels replenish the supply of red blood cells which, when destroyed, add to excess iron deposits, resulting in cellular damage.

The child's skin is a muddy-yellow color. This is a result of jaundice caused by increased bilirubin, hemosiderosis, and pallor from the anemia.

Medical and Surgical Treatment There is no cure for β-thalassemia. Therapy consists of maintaining adequate hemoglobin levels to prevent tissue hypoxia. Frequent blood transfusions are required, so the effects of resultant iron overload have to be considered. If abnormal sequestration of red blood cells in the spleen increases the need for transfusions, splenectomy might be necessary. The major complication of splenectomy is infection, so prophylactic antibiotics and pneumococcal and meningococcal vaccines are given. Research is in progress on the use of bone marrow transplantation, but its effectiveness as a treatment for β-thalassemia has not yet been confirmed.

The prognosis of the disease depends on its severity. Children with thalassemia major seldom live to adulthood. Children with thalassemia minor require no treatment and can have a normal life span.

Nursing Management Nursing care for children with thalassemia major is supportive. Red blood cell transfusions are required to combat the anemia. The nurse administers blood transfusions and observes the child for signs of transfusion reactions (see Table 36-3). The nurse also observes the child for signs and symptoms of hepatitis and iron overload.

As children with thalassemia major grow older, they might have difficulty adjusting to the body changes caused by the disease. They look different from their peers and usually cannot keep up during physical activities. These children need opportunities to express their feelings and guidance in handling the problems that might arise.

As many procedures as possible are done on an outpatient basis. Home care treatments can be arranged if the family is comfortable with them. The nurse arranges contact with community agencies that can give the child and family additional support. Thalassemia major eventually results in death. The children and their families need much support in dealing with crisis periods and the eventual death of the child. See Chapter 32 for methods of helping children and families through the death and dying process.

Because parents might have questions regarding the possibility of future offspring having thalassemia, genetic counseling should be made available (see Chapter 5). Patients with thalassemia minor, which is asymptomatic, should be informed that they can transmit thalassemia major to their children if their spouse or partner also has either thalassemia minor or thalassemia major. They can transmit thalassemia minor even when their partner is free of the trait.

The Child With Coagulation Dysfunction

Hemophilia

Hemophilia is a lifelong, hereditary disorder that is characterized by a disturbance of blood clotting factors. The disease almost always occurs in males, but it is transmitted by females. It is a sex-linked recessive trait that follows the mendelian law of genetic transfer (Fig. 36-4). The gene that causes hemophilia is carried on the X chromosome. A woman is considered a carrier if she carries the abnormal gene on one of her two X chromosomes. She will not have the disease, because the other X chromosome is normal. A male has one X and one Y chromosome. Therefore, if a male inherits an X chromosome carrying the hemophilia gene, he will have the disease.

Genetic counseling should be made available to families with hemophilia to educate them about genetic transfer (see Chapter 5). If a pregnant woman is a carrier or if the father has hemophilia, amniocentesis might be performed early in the pregnancy to determine the sex of the fetus. A woman who is a carrier has a 25% chance of having a child with hemophilia each time she becomes pregnant. If the child is a male, he has a 50% chance of having hemophilia. If the child is female, she has a 50% chance of being a carrier. If the parents know that their unborn child is male, they might begin to prepare themselve emotionally for the chance that the child might have the disease. Some choose to terminate the pregnancy.

Recently, fetal blood sampling has been developed to determine whether the male fetus has hemophilia. This test is still experimental, and the risks have not been fully determined.

It is possible for the hemophilia gene to be hidden for several generations, that is, without any males being born with hemophilia. Then, when a male is born with hemophilia, there is no apparent family history of the disease. Hemophilia also can result from spontaneous genetic mutation. Over one-third of patients with hemophilia have no family history of the disease.

Classic hemophilia A affects about 75% of the patients with hemophilia. In hemophilia A the patient's plasma is deficient in Factor VIII (antihemolytic factor [AHF] or antihemolytic globulin [AHG]). Table 36-5 lists the normal blood clotting factors. The degree to which a patient is deficient in Factor VIII tends to be familial. Relatives with hemophilia have similar factor levels and symptoms. Normal individuals have Factor VIII at levels that vary from 50% to 200%. Table 36-6 illustrates how the level of Factor VIII affects the hemophiliac. The second most common type of hemophilia is hemophilia B, or Christmas disease. It is caused by a deficiency of Factor IX, also known as plasma thromboplastin component (PTC).

A smaller number of patients have hemophilia C, caused by a deficiency of Factor XI, or plasma thromboplastin antecedent (PTA). Hemophilia A and B are very similar in symptomatology and inheritance. Hemophilia C is an autosomal recessive trait that affects both males and females.

The clinical manifestations of hemophilia A, B, and C are similiar. Hemophilia is seldom diagnosed in infancy unless there is excessive bleeding from circumcision, the umbilical cord, or birth trauma. Hemorrhage indicates the need to assess clotting functions. Usually, bleeding episodes do not occur until early childhood, when the child becomes more active. Hematomas develop from minor bumps and falls or after immunization. Hemophilia can cause prolonged bleeding anywhere in the body. The child might bleed from the gums or from the loss of deciduous teeth.

Diagnosis usually is made on the basis of a prolonged bleeding episode following trauma, or from a family history of hemophilia. Petechiae are not seen because hemophilia does not interfere with platelet function. Bleeding time is normal. Blood coagulation studies are done to determine which clotting factor is deficient. These tests include the prothrombin time (PT), partial thromboplastin time (PTT), thromboplastin generation test (TGT), and prothrombin consumption tests (see Table 36-1).

Hemarthrosis, the oozing of blood into a joint cavity, such as the knee, elbow, or ankle, can cause the joint to become swollen, tender, and painful. Repeated hemorrhage into a joint results in damage to the synovial membrane, degeneration of articular cartilage, and formation of subchondral cysts. Long-range consequences, such as contractures, ankylosis, and severe crippling, might develop.

Internal bleeding might cause severe physical complications. For example, bleeding into the neck or pharynx can cause airway obstruction; bleeding into the eyes or ears can destroy vision or hearing; and bleeding into the spinal column can cause paralysis. Spontaneous *hematuria* (blood in the urine) may occur two to three times per year.

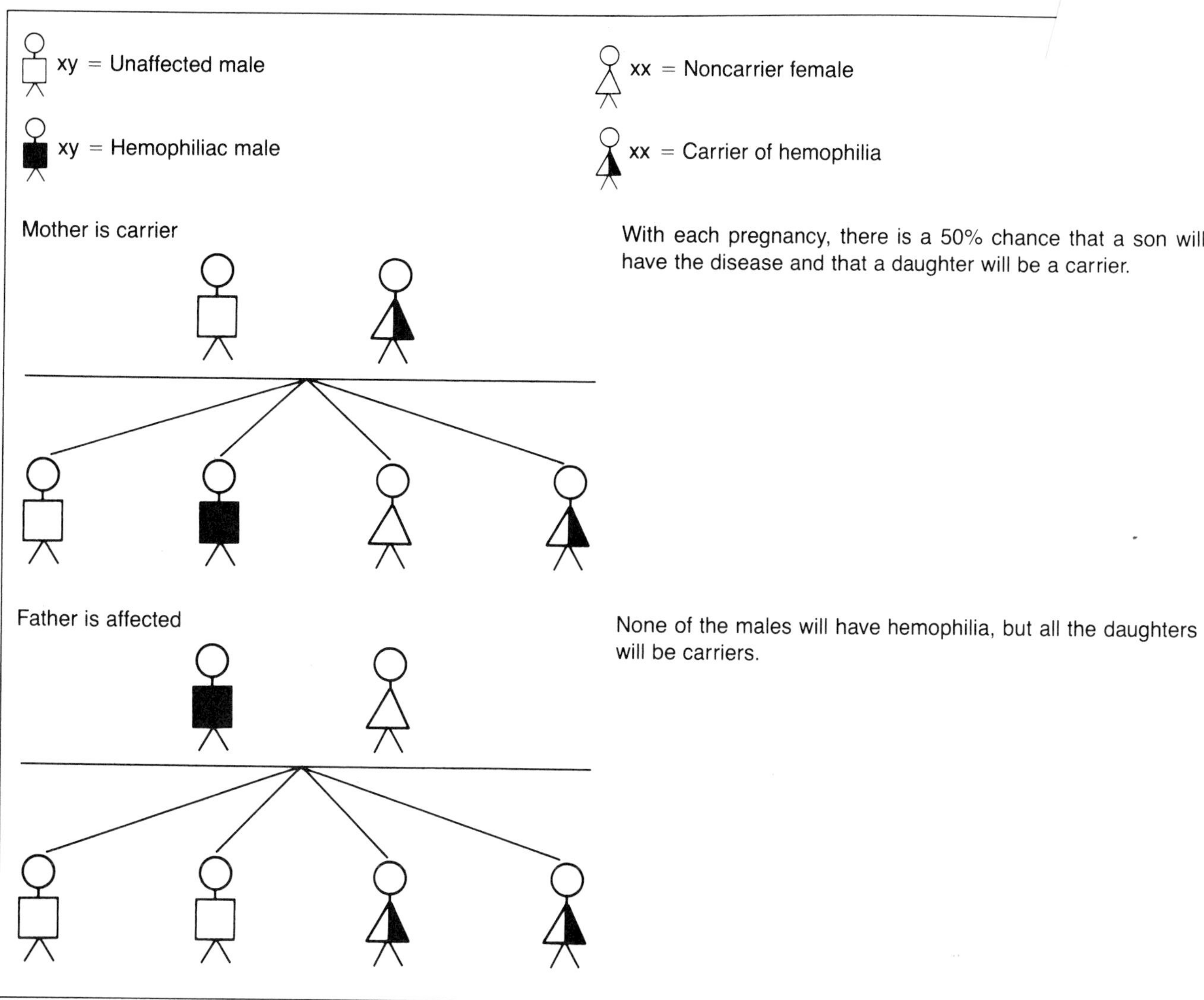

Figure 36-4. Examples of sex-linked hereditary patterns in hemophilia.

TABLE 36-5 Clotting Factors Present in Normal Blood

Factor number	Alternate names
I	Fibrinogen
II	Prothrombin
III	Thromboplastin
IV	Calcium
V	Labile factor, proaccelerin
VI	Accelerator globulin (AG)
VII	Serum prothrombin conversion accelerator (SPCA), proconvertin, autoprothrombin I
VIII	Antihemolytic factor (AHF), antihemolytic globulin (AHG)
IX	Plasma thromboplastin component (PTC), Christmas factor, autoprothrombin II
X	Stuart-Prower factor, Stuart factor, Prower factor
XI	Plasma thromboplastin antecedent (PTA)
XII	Hageman factor
XIII	Fibrin (protein) stabilizing factor (FSF)

TABLE 36-6 Effects of Factor Deficiencies in Hemophilia A and B

Severity of hemophilia	Percentage of factor VIII or IX present	Characteristics
Mild	5–50	Bleeding only after severe insult Coagulation screening tests normal or low normal
Moderately severe	2–5	Infrequent spontaneous hemorrhages Significant hemorrhage after minor trauma Prolonged partial thromboplastin times Coagulation screening tests rarely passed
Severe	Less than 1	Frequent spontaneous hemorrhages throughout lifetime Coagulation screening tests always abnormal

Medical and Surgical Treatment Minor, external hemorrhage responds well to prolonged pressure and the application of cold. For more extensive bleeding episodes, the missing clotting factor is administered. It is essential to stop the bleeding quickly to prevent damage to tissue, nerves, and joints.

The three types of plasma products available for the treatment of hemophilia A are fresh-frozen plasma, cryoprecipitated Factor VIII, and lyophilized Factor VIII concentrate. Fresh-frozen plasma is obtained from fresh whole blood. It is then frozen and stored until needed. It is necessary to infuse the thawed plasma promptly because Factor VIII deteriorates at room temperature. The amount of Factor VIII in the plasma depends on the donor's level of Factor VIII. Cryoprecipitate of Factor VIII is prepared from slow-thawing, fresh-frozen plasma. Lyophilized concentrates of Factor VIII are prepared by pharmaceutical companies from pools of plasma. Once lyophilized Factor VIII is obtained, it is stored in vials at room temperature until needed. Commercially prepared concentrates of Factor VIII include Profilate, Koāte, Hemofil, Humafac, and Antihemophilic Factor. The dosage of Factor VIII is based on the plasma volume desired and the patient's weight.

Costs of the products vary from area to area, but because they are derived from whole blood, they are all extremely expensive. Blood donors usually are paid for the blood they give, and the cost increases as the product is refined. Accessibility, ease of handling and storage, and cost are considered in selecting the product to be given.

A very small number of patients develop an inhibitor or antibody to the factor. The inhibitor or antibody inactivates the factor, preventing it from assisting in coagulation. Alternative approaches to treatment are being investigated. Success has been achieved with giving larger doses of Factor IX to a patient with Factor VIII deficiency when inhibitors are present.

Therapy for hemophilia B is similar to that for hemophilia A, except that fresh-frozen plasma or lyophilized Factor IX concentrate is administered. Konȳne and Proplex are examples of concentrates containing Factor IX. No concentrate is available for Factor XI (PTA) deficiency, so fresh-frozen plasma is given.

Because all of the substances used to treat hemophilia are blood products, the patient is at risk for serum hepatitis. Allergic reactions might occur from the infusion of fresh-frozen plasma but are rare with cryoprecipitate or the concentrates. Blood typing and cross-matching are not necessary for the administration of plasma, cryoprecipitate, or the concentrates. Within the last few years hemophiliacs have been listed among the high-risk groups for contracting acquired immune deficiency disease (AIDS) (see Chapter 37). AIDS can be transmitted through blood products to unaffected recipients. Because hemophiliacs receive so many transfusions, they are at greater risk of contracting the disease. Although blood donors are screened carefully for possible exposure to AIDS, no reliable method exists for identifying contaminated blood, which concerns many hemophiliacs and their families.

Non-narcotic or narcotic analgesics are prescribed to control pain, depending on its severity. Steroids have been used to decrease the inflammatory process in affected joints. Casts, traction, and joint aspiration might be necessary to preserve joint function. Surgical replacement of joints is considered in the event of total disability.

Nursing Management A nursing care plan for the child with classic hemophilia A is included at the end of the chapter. The most important aspect of care for the child with hemophilia is control of active bleeding episodes. This is accomplished by administering the missing factor and taking nursing measures to stop the bleeding. External bleeding from a wound or mucous membrane can be controlled by applying pressure to allow clot formation and applying cold to promote vasoconstriction. The nurse instructs the parent to keep ice packs in the freezer for emergencies. Plastic bags of ice or a wet sponge placed in a plastic bag can be kept in the freezer, or commercially prepared cold packs can be obtained.

Joint hemorrhage and hemarthrosis occur most commonly in the knees, ankles, and elbows. When bleeding occurs, the child experiences discomfort and is unable to move the affected joint. Swelling occurs, and local skin temperature increases. The nurse administers the deficient factor and immobilizes the affected extremity during the acute bleeding episode. Immobilization controls pain and prevents further bleeding.

Pain from a joint hemorrhage is caused by pressure or muscle spasm. Cold packs alleviate the pain of acute hemorrhage. If pain persists, appropriate analgesics, such as acetaminophen, should be considered. Aspirin or any salicylate-containing compound is contraindicated because of its depressive effects on platelet function, which can last up to 10 days. The nurse cautions parents of patients with hemophilia to read the labels of all medications (such as cold tablets) for possible aspirin content. The parent can obtain a list of aspirin-containing drugs from the local pharmacy and, when in doubt, ask the pharmacist to select an appropriate over-the-counter analgesic.

Mild pain is treated with acetaminophen or propoxyphene compounds. For more severe pain, the physician may prescribe codeine, meperidine (Demerol), or morphine. The nurse helps to prevent drug abuse or dependence by administering the more potent analgesics promptly and instructing the child and family to set firm limits on the amount that may be taken at home. Chronic pain may occur as a result of bone and joint degeneration. The nurse helps the child and family to accept the possibility that the drug might not alleviate all the pain and discomfort.

When active bleeding into a joint has stopped, exercise begins. Physical therapy promotes maximum function of the affected joints and maintains range of motion and tone of unaffected body parts. It might be necessary to continue the exercise program at home, in which case the nurse refers the patient to a visiting nurse or physical therapist for continuity of care.

Preventing Injury The nurse teaches the families of children with hemophilia how to protect the child from injury without being overprotective. While the patient is in infancy, the parent should pad the crib and use nonbreakable feeding utensils. The home should have wall-to-wall carpeting to cushion falls. Toys should not have rough edges or sharp surfaces. Approved car seats should be used routinely. As the child becomes more active and begins to walk, play areas must be supervised. Knee and elbow pads and a helmet can help prevent injury while the child is mastering walking. The child should play on a fenced lawn rather than a concrete yard or driveway.

The nurse informs the parent that because strong muscles help to protect the joints from bleeding, exercise should be encouraged. Swimming and tricycle riding are ideal for young children. Older children should not take part in contact sports, such as football, because of the obvious dangers. Snow skiing and tennis are not suitable because they place a great deal of strain on the knees and ankles, which could cause bleeding. Swimming and golf are safe physical activities which can satisfy the child's competitive interests. It is generally felt that active hemophiliac children bleed less than sedentary hemophiliac children.

Discipline is important for the safety of young children with hemophilia. As young children, they must learn to obey safety rules and, as early as possible, they must become responsible for their own safety. The nurse reminds parents that teaching their children self-discipline and instilling a sense of responsibility may well be the most important thing they can do to prevent injuries.

Routine Health Care Needs Comprehensive management of the child with hemophilia should consist of a team approach that provides for the physical and psychologic needs of the child. The team should consist of the pediatrician, hematologist, orthopedist, dentist, social worker, physical therapist, psychologist, and nurse.

Hemophilia is a lifelong condition requiring continuity of care. All people who care for the hemophiliac child should be informed about the disorder and know what to do in the event of a bleeding episode. The dentist selected to care for the child must understand the disease and be aware of the need to administer the factor promptly when bleeding occurs. The child with hemophilia should wear medical identification jewelry and should be taught to recognize the earliest symptoms of bleeding so that prompt treatment can be instituted. The National Hemophilia Foundation has more than 50 chapters across the country to help families of hemophiliacs with financial, psychologic, and medical care. The child's reaction to the disease or disability depends upon how well the family responds to the problems that arise. It is essential that the family members demonstrate a positive attitude toward the child with hemophilia to foster a safe environment and to increase the child's self-esteem.

Home Care The development and widespread use of cryoprecipitate and factor concentrates have prompted changes in the philosophy of care and the development of home management programs. Home transfusions are a critical part of home care. Patients are taught to recognize early symptoms of bleeding. They or a family member infuse the deficient factor and initiate treatment whenever a bleeding episode develops. Some patients with severe spontaneous bleeding problems undergo prophylactic transfusions. Routine infusions of the factor are given every other day by the child or a family member. Prophylactic transfusions maintain adequate blood levels of the clotting factor, preventing bleeding and enabling the child to lead a more normal life. Home therapy promotes independence by enabling hemophiliac children to take part in their own care (Sergis and Hilgarten, 1972). See Chapter 26 for a general discussion of home care.

Von Willebrand's Disease

Von Willebrand's disease is a common inherited (autosomal dominant) disease that causes exessive bleeding, usually from the skin or mucous membranes. Both males and females are affected. The severity of the bleeding varies from patient to patient and from time to time, and symptoms tend to diminish in adulthood. The disease is far less severe than hemophilia. Hemarthrosis is rare. Bruises occur over bony prominences such as the shins or the iliac crest. About one-fourth of the patients develop *purpura,* a purplish or brownish discoloration caused by hemorrhage into the tissues. Common sites of spontaneous mucosal bleeding are the lining of the nose and the gastrointestinal tract. Female patients who have reached puberty experience *menorrhagia* (excessive menstrual bleeding). Extensive bleeding may follow dental extractions, surgery, or trauma and is usually stopped by pressure or suturing.

Blood tests reveal prolonged bleeding time and decreased levels of Factor VIII. There is a marked reduction of platelet adhesiveness.

Medical therapy and nursing interventions are similar to those for the child with hemophilia. Mangement of acute hemorrhages may include the administration of fresh-frozen plasma or cryoprecipitate. Bleeding from the nose and mouth are treated with the application of cold, pressure, or nasal packing. If the patient is to have surgery or any dental extraction, plasma is given before the procedure and might be necessary afterward. Pain is managed with acetaminophen. Aspirin is contraindicated because of its effects on platelet function.

Menorrhagia sometimes is alleviated by a transfusion given prior to menstruation. If severe blood loss occurs during menstruation, anemia might develop, and whole blood transfusions may be necessary.

Idiopathic Thrombocytopenic Purpura

Idiopathic thrombocytopenic purpura, commonly known as ITP, is characterized by a reduction in the number of circulating platelets, causing purpura, or bleeding into the tissues. In ITP the thrombocytopenia is caused by an antiplatelet antibody produced in the spleen (see Chapter 37 for discussion of the autoimmune response). Secondary causes of thrombocytopenia include systemic lupus erythematosus, past transfusions, drug sensitivities, and hemolytic anemia.

The platelet count in ITP is always below 50,000/mm^3 and can plunge way below this level. Bone marrow examination is necessary to rule out aplastic anemia or leukemia. A diagnosis of ITP is made if red and white blood cells in bone marrow are normal, the platelet count is decreased, and the bleeding time is prolonged. The most common clinical signs of ITP are petechiae and areas of ecchymosis. Bleeding from mucous membranes in the mouth or nose, hematuria, bloody stools, and menorrhagia are other manifestations of ITP.

Medical and Surgical Treatment Corticosteroids, such as prednisone, are given to stimulate platelet formation and promote vascular integrity. Steroid therapy is used for severe bleeding. It also is used prior to a splenectomy (to decrease the risk of surgical bleeding) and sometimes to treat chronic ITP. The transfusion of platelets is only beneficial after the platelet count has begun to rise in reponse to steroid therapy.

In recurrent or chronic ITP, a splenectomy is done to remove the major site of antiplatelet antibody production. Within 1–2 weeks after splenectomy, platelet values are normal. Splenectomy frees 70%–90% of patients from the effects of ITP. The prognosis for ITP is excellent. Approximately 80% of patients recover within 6 months of treatment.

Nursing Management Families need a great deal of emotional support, especially during diagnostic procedures, because they might fear that their child has some form of cancer. Acute care focuses on controlling bleeding and preventing hemorrhage (see the section on hemophilia). Pain is controlled with analgesics that do not contain aspirin. If steroids are prescribed, the nurse explains to the child and family that such side effects as moon face, increased appetite, behavioral changes, and weight gain might occur. They also are instructed never to stop the drug abruptly.

If splenectomy is indicated, the children and families need preoperative teaching (see Chapter 29). Because of the hazards of overwhelming infection after a splenectomy, patients are placed on prophylactic antibiotic therapy. The nurse instructs the child and family about preventing infections and seeking prompt medical attention if the child contracts any infectious disease.

Petechiae, purpura, and the side effects of steroid therapy change the physical appearance of the child. The nurse offers emotional support and reassures the child and family that recovery is likely to occur within 6 months, after which steroid therapy will end and the child's appearance will return to normal.

Disseminated Intravascular Coagulation

Disseminated intravascular coagulation (DIC) is characterized by abnormal overstimulation of the coagulation process. Massive fibrin formation occurs, which causes widespread thrombi. Eventually, all the platelets and clotting factors are depleted, and the fibrinolytic mechanism is stimulated to dissolve the clots. Clinically, manifestations of DIC include (1) a tendency toward generalized bleeding; (2) ischemia of organs and tissue from vaso-occlusion; and (3) secondary anemia.

Disseminated intravascular coagulation is not a primary disease but rather is secondary to any number of acute pathologic processes. Common predisposing factors are respiratory distress syndrome, abruptio placentae, shock, acidosis, trauma, sepsis, and surgical procedures involving extracorporeal bypass. It is unknown exactly how these acute conditions cause DIC.

Petechiae, ecchymoses, and hemorrhage, combined with evidence of thrombosis or vaso-occlusion, are indicative of DIC. Thrombosis in a blood vessel serving the central nervous system causes changes in mental status. Thrombosis in a peripheral blood vessel might cause coolness and cyanosis of an extremity. Hematuria is a sign of renal system involvement. Hematologic findings include decreased platelet and fibrinogen levels and prolonged prothrombin time (PT) and partial thromboplastin time (PTT) (see Table 36-1 for normal levels).

Treatment Resolving the underlying disease process is the primary treatment for DIC. Heparin, an antagonist to thrombin, is given to inhibit further clot formation. When the platelet count rises and clinical findings suggest that DIC has ceased, heparin therapy is terminated. Replacement of platelets is seldom necessary, but platelets may be transfused after heparin therapy has begun. Whole blood or blood products can be given to replace the depleted clotting factor, but this treatment carries the risk of stimulating more clotting.

Nursing Management Nursing care for children with DIC depends on the underlying cause of the condition. The nurse protects the child with DIC from any unnecessary bleeding episodes and is alert for signs and symptoms of vaso-occlusion and bleeding in the child who is at risk for DIC.

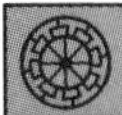

NURSING CARE PLAN Child With Classic Hemophilia A

Ryan is an 8-year-old boy with severe Factor VIII deficiency. He was hospitalized for left elbow and proximal forearm soft tissue bleeding that occurred 2 days previously. He presently is being treated with a soft tissue splint and cryoprecipitate transfusion. Ryan is to wear the splint at all times, except during range-of-motion exercises four times a day.

Ryan has had no other recent joint bleeding episodes, blood in the stool, or hematuria. His last hemarthrosis occurred 8 months previously in the left elbow. All Ryan's previous bleeding episodes have been stopped promptly with factor replacement therapy. He has no known allergies and does not have any history of reactions to replacement therapy.

Physical examination reveals a child of average height and below average weight. Vital signs are within normal limits. Laboratory studies reveal normal range blood values on CBC. His Factor VIII assay is less than 1%. Resolving bruises are noted, primarily on the lower extremities. The soft tissue splint is in place on his left arm and elbow. The fingers are warm and pink, and the nails have good capillary refill. Ryan complains of pain and stiffness of the left elbow upon movement. Discoloration and swelling occur around the elbow joint. Ryan has full range of motion of all other joints.

Ryan was diagnosed as having hemophilia when he was 9 months old. His father was diagnosed at 36 years of age with less than 1% hemophilia. Ryan lives at home with his parents and a 5-year-old sister. Developmentally, Ryan is within normal limits. This is Ryan's third hospitalization. For all other bleeding episodes, Ryan has been treated with factor replacement as an outpatient.

Nursing Diagnoses and Goals

1. **Nursing diagnosis:** Alteration in comfort, pain.

   Long-term goal: Ryan will be free of pain.

   Short-term goal: Ryan will state that he is more comfortable.

2. **Nursing diagnosis:** Potential for injury and bleeding.

   Long-term goal: Ryan will develop a life-style that will decrease the risk of injury.

   Short-term goals: (a) Ryan and his family will be aware of potential sources of injury that can result in bleeding. (b) Ryan and his family will be able to recognize signs of bleeding. (c) Ryan and his family will know how to initiate appropriate care when bleeding occurs.

3. **Nursing diagnosis:** Potential for joint degeneration.

   Long-term goal: Ryan will maintain function of all joints through a regular exercise regimen.

   Short-term goals: (a) Ryan and his family will learn measures to maintain joint function and prevent degeneration.

4. **Nursing diagnosis:** Potential for ineffective coping of child and family.

   Long-term goal: Ryan and his family will adjust to the limitations imposed by hemophilia.

   Short-term goals: (a) Ryan and his family will be able to express their feelings regarding the disease and its treatment.

continued on next page

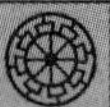

NURSING CARE PLAN Child With Classic Hemophilia A (continued)

(b) Ryan will begin to show signs of independence in his self-care. (c) Ryan's family will learn about the resources available to them. (d) Ryan and his family will demonstrate adaptive coping styles.

5. **Nursing diagnosis:** Potential for knowledge deficit about the disease and its complications.

Long-term goal: Ryan and his family will understand hemophilia and its long-term effects.

Short-term goals: (a) Ryan and his family will increase their understanding of hemophilia. (b) Ryan's family will understand the genetic implications of hemophilia.

Interventions	Rationale	Evaluation criteria
1. Observe Ryan for signs of pain	Baseline data is useful in determining future needs for intervention	Is pain relieved? What measures resulted in pain reduction?
Position and support the affected joint	Minimizing stress on the joint promotes comfort	
Provide a restful, quiet, supportive environment	A soothing environment relieves tension	
Provide diversional activities and psychologic support	Diversion focuses the child's attention on stimuli other than pain	
Immobilize the affected joint	Immobilization minimizes stress on the joint	
Place a bed cradle over the affected joint	Keeping the weight of bedclothes off the painful part reduces pain	
Administer aspirin-free analgesics or narcotic analgesics, as ordered	Aspirin-free, non-narcotic analgesics reduce mild pain not relieved by comfort measures. Narcotic analgesics relieve severe pain	
Explain to Ryan why he feels pain	Information reduces fear	
2. Instruct Ryan to avoid activities, such as contact sports, that increase the possibility of trauma	These activities are potential sources of trauma	Is the potential for injury reduced?
Foster Ryan's interest in intellectual, creative activities as he matures	These activities do not cause trauma, yet stimulate the child's mind	Do Ryan and his family know how to protect him from sources of injury? Do Ryan and his family know what to do when bleeding occurs?
Encourage Ryan to participate in physical activities (bike riding, swimming, bowling) that are not likely to cause trauma	Strong muscles protect the joints from bleeding. Active children are less likely to bleed than sedentary children	
Teach Ryan about good health habits, including adequate rest and nutrition	These habits improve health status	
Plan Ryan's physical education program with school personnel	Awareness of the child's limitations helps school personnel to provide a safe and appropriate exercise program	
Instruct Ryan's family that he must avoid all aspirin-containing drugs	Aspirin and drugs containing aspirin interfere with platelet function, which could cause bleeding	
Instruct Ryan and his family that he must wear the medical-alert tag and carry the medical-alert card at all times	If bleeding should occur, prompt treatment can be given	

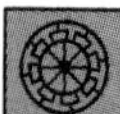

NURSING CARE PLAN Child With Classic Hemophilia A (continued)

Interventions	Rationale	Evaluation criteria
Teach Ryan and his family that special precautions should be taken during such procedures as dental work	It might be necessary to give Factor VIII prior to some procedures to minimize the effects of bleeding	
Teach Ryan and his family to recognize the following signs of bleeding: blood in stools or urine, nosebleeds, tachycardia, faintness, confusion, and feeling of fullness in affected area	Recognizing the early signs of internal or external bleeding enables the child to obtain prompt treatment, which can minimize complications	
Explain to Ryan and his family medical methods used to control bleeding: administration of blood factor; transfusion of whole blood or packed red blood cells when Hgb level falls	Information about the medical regimen gives the family a better understanding of the child's need for care	
Teach Ryan and his family emergency measures to control bleeding: application of pressure for 10–15 minutes, immobilization of the joint, elevation of the joint above the heart, and application of cold	Prompt treatment with emergency measures minimizes bleeding by aiding in clot formation, decreasing blood flow to the extremity, and producing vasoconstriction	
Instruct Ryan's family to seek medical assistance if bleeding is not stopped by usual measures	It is essential to prevent complications of excessive bleeding	
Protect Ryan from trauma in the hospital by padding bed rails, keeping bed in low position, assisting with ambulation and activities when necessary, rotating injection sites, and applying direct pressure over puncture sites	These measures will minimize the risk of injury or bleeding	
Establish routine good oral hygiene by referring Ryan to a dentist who is aware of Ryan's special needs and teaching Ryan to use a soft toothbrush that has been soaked in water	The dentist must be knowledgeable about hemophilia so that precautions can be taken when treating the child. Gentle cleaning of the teeth prevents mucosal bleeding	
3. Maintain range of motion of unaffected joints and muscles by providing range-of-motion exercises while Ryan is on bedrest and encouraging early ambulation and activity	Exercise minimizes the loss of muscle tone, promotes circulation, and prevents contractures	Are Ryan and his family able to identify measures to prevent joint degeneration?
Move the affected joint through passive range of motion, as ordered by the physician	Passive range-of-motion exercises help prevent degeneration of the affected joint	Are Ryan and his family aware of the effect of hemarthrosis?
Immobilize the joint during active bleeding	Immobilization helps control bleeding into the joint and promotes absorption	Is Ryan doing active and passive exercises?
Administer aspirin-free analgesics prior to range-of-motion exercises or physical therapy	Reduction of pain enables the patient to better tolerate exercise and maximizes its effects	
Encourage Ryan's family to participate in his exercise program	Participation promotes the family's involvement in the child's care	

continued on next page

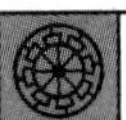

NURSING CARE PLAN Child With Classic Hemophilia A (continued)

Interventions	Rationale	Evaluation criteria
Refer Ryan to a public health nurse and/or physical therapist for aid with his home care program	Follow-up is needed to ensure that home care measures are being carried out	
Provide a diet that is nutritious but does not allow for weight gain	Obesity places additional pressure on weight-bearing joints	
Encourage Ryan to participate in sports that maintain joint function but are not potential sources of injury	Exercise helps maintain joint function	
Educate Ryan and his family about the long-term consequences of hemarthrosis	Knowledge about the effects motivates the child and family to follow the plan of care	
4. Encourage Ryan and his family to discuss their feelings about hemophilia	The child and family need to express their feelings and ask questions	Does Ryan feel comfortable with himself?
Provide opportunities for Ryan's parents, especially his mother, to talk about the genetic component of the disease	The child's mother might feel guilty that she passed this disorder on to her child	Do Ryan and his family use healthy coping measures? Is the family aware of the resources that are available?
Find out how hemophilia has affected Ryan's parents' childrearing practices, for example, imposing discipline, setting limits, and fostering independence	Parents need opportunities to learn what childrearing practices can best benefit a child with hemophilia. These measures promote self-esteem, a sense of control, a more positive attitude regarding the disease, and the opporunity to socialize with peers	
Foster Ryan's independence by allowing him to help make decisions about his care, focusing his attention on the things he can do, supporting his ego strengths, and fostering a positive self-image, encouraging him in self-care during hospitalization, and introducing him to other children with hemophilia who are adjusting well to the disease		
Help Ryan and his family to identify factors that help them to cope well in crises, for example, previous coping patterns, the ability to seek out and use the help of others, and family stability	Recognition of positive coping patterns prepares the patient and family to use them during future crises	
Encourage Ryan's family to join the National Hemophilia Foundation	The family needs an opportunity to communicate with other families having the same problem	
Inform Ryan's family about possible sources of financial aid such as the local chapter of the National Hemophilia Foundation and social service agencies	Treatments for hemophilia can be very costly, and the family might need financial assistance	
Encourage Ryan to participate in age-appropriate activities	The hemophiliac child needs to participate in activities with peers	

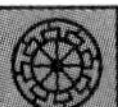

NURSING CARE PLAN Child With Classic Hemophilia A (continued)

Interventions	Rationale	Evaluation criteria
Encourage Ryan's parents to promote a sense of independence and responsibility as he grows older	Th child with hemophilia must learn to assume responsibility for self-care and should not be discouraged in this endeavor	
Determine whether a home-care program would be suitable for Ryan	A home-care program would allow the hemophiliac child and family greater participation in treatment	
5. Discuss with Ryan and his family the long-term effects of hemophilia	Discussion increases cognitive knowledge	Is there a change in attitude regarding the effects of Ryan's disease?
Explain to Ryan and his family all aspects of care and procedures involved in the treatment of hemophilia	Knowing what to expect decreases fear of the unknown	Do Ryan and his family recognize Ryan's health needs? Are the parents aware of the implications of genetic transfer and its effects on future children?
Teach Ryan and his family the importance of preventive measures in the treatment of hemophilia	Knowledge helps the child and family to understand and comply with preventive aspects of treatment	
Discuss with Ryan's family the genetic components of hemophilia	The family needs to know that subsequent offspring could have hemophilia	
Refer Ryan's family to a genetic counselor	A genetic counselor will be able to give the parents specific infomation about the genetic transmission of hemophilia in their own family	

Key Concepts

- Blood consists of two components, a liquid, or plasma, component and a cellular component.
- The cellular component of blood is made up of erythrocytes (red blood cells), which carry oxygen; leukocytes (white blood cells), which protect the body from infection; and thrombocytes (platelets), which aid in coagulation and clotting.
- The red blood cells transport oxygen by means of hemoglobin molecules, hundreds of which may be attached to one red blood cell.
- Red blood cells are produced in the marrow of short flat bones and are removed and destroyed by the spleen after about 120 days in the bloodstream.
- Abnormal red blood cells are removed and destroyed by the spleen as fast as the spleen can absorb them.
- Leukocytes, which may be granulocytes, monocytes, or lymphocytes, are produced in lymphogenous tissues.
- Granulocytes and monocytes can ingest and destroy foreign particles, cells, and microorganisms by a process known as phagocytosis.
- Lymphocytes are involved in cell-mediated immunity and antibody formation.
- Platelets aid in blood clotting and coagulation by adhering to the exposed site of injury, forming a temporary clot, and stimulating the release of the blood coagulation factors, whose mechanism of action produces coagulation and cessation of bleeding.
- Assessment of the child with suspected or diagnosed hematopoietic dysfunction includes a

complete history that focuses on familial hereditary diseases, nutrition, infection, possible exposure to toxic substances, and exercise tolerance.

- In the physical examination part of the assessment, the nurse gathers and assesses subjective and objective data relevant to the anemias or clotting disturbances.
- The child with anemia is likely to be pale, fatigued, and listless, and to have signs of hypoxia and splenic enlargement.
- The child with clotting disturbances is likely to have painful joints, skin discolorations, and other signs of internal or external hemorrhage.
- Diagnostic procedures and tests for blood disorders include hematologic studies and bone marrow aspiration, all of which are invasive or painful, necessitating careful preparation of the child and emotional support.
- Nursing responsibilities related to blood transfusions include explaining the procedure to the patient, verifying correct blood-typing and cross-matching between patient and donor, administering the transfusion, observing the patient for signs and symptoms of transfusion reaction, and beginning treatment if a transfusion reaction occurs.
- Nursing responsibilities related to bone marrow transplantation include standard preoperative and postoperative measures (see Chapter 29), careful monitoring for signs of infection or rejection, and providing emotional support to the child, family, and donor.
- The acute care needs of the child with clotting disturbances involve protecting the child from injury, detecting and controlling hemorrhage, administering analgesics, administering blood products, and helping the child to maintain maximum function of joints and muscles by beginning passive exercises as soon as bleeding stops.
- Aspirin and aspirin-containing drugs should never be given to patients with blood disorders because aspirin inhibits platelet function.
- The acute care needs of the child with anemia involve promoting rest and good respiratory function to alleviate hypoxia, administering blood or blood products, protecting the child from infection, administering antibiotics as appropriate, providing a nonstressful environment, and encouraging the child to eat nutritious meals.
- The nutritional needs of children with red blood cell disorders include a diet rich in iron and vitamins, particularly vitamin C, and an increase in fluid intake to one and one-half to two times the normal daily requirement.
- Nursing care for the child with iron deficiency anemia focuses on dietary teaching and promoting cooperation with the regimen of iron supplementation.
- For the child with aplastic anemia, nursing care involves preventing complications from anemia, infection, and bleeding; preparing the child and family for diagnostic and therapeutic procedures; giving emotional support; and providing appropriate care associated with transfusions, steroid therapy, and bone marrow transplantation.
- Hemolysis is the destruction of red blood cells with subsequent separation of oxygen-carrying hemoglobin.
- Corpuscular defects that cause hemolytic anemia are glucose-6-phosphate dehydrogenase (G6PD) deficiency and spherocytosis.
- Sickle cell disease and the sickle cell trait are inherited disorders that affect about 1 in 10 black Americans and are detected by screening tests for the presence of abnormal hemoglobin (Hgb S) in the blood.
- The sickle cell trait is usually asymptomatic, while sickle cell disease is a lifelong anemic condition marked by severe symptoms and crises.
- The three types of sickle cell crisis are vaso-occlusive crisis, in which thrombi obstruct small blood vessels; sequestration crisis, in which circulation is jeopardized by sudden pooling of blood in the spleen; and aplastic crisis, in which red blood cell production ceases, causing profound anemia.
- Nursing care for the child with sickle cell disease involves recommending genetic counseling for the family, giving explanations and emotional support, preventing crises by teaching the child how to avoid hypoxia, and assessing and treating crisis symptoms when they occur.
- β-thalassemia, an inherited disorder that occurs most commonly in people from Mediterranean

areas or of Mediterranean descent, may be asymptomatic (thalassemia minor) or severe and fatal (thalassemia major).

- For the child with thalassemia major, nursing care is supportive, involving administering blood transfusions; assessing the child for transfusion reactions, signs and symptoms of hepatitis, and iron overload; providing emotional support; assessing the family's ability to care for the child at home; and recommending genetic counseling for the family.
- Hemophilia, which is caused by a deficiency in a blood clotting factor, is transmitted genetically from females to their male offspring, who develop active disease, or to their female offspring, who become carriers.
- Supportive nursing care for the child with hemophilia includes protecting the child from injury; teaching the child and family measures to prevent injury at home; recommending appropriate exercises, age-appropriate group activities, and physical therapy; teaching the child and family home care procedures; and recommending genetic counseling for the family.
- Acute care for the child with hemophilia consists of detecting and stopping active bleeding; administering the deficient factor; using comfort measures and analgesics to control pain; and minimizing the long-term effects of bleeding into joints by beginning passive exercises as soon as the bleeding ceases.
- External bleeding is stopped by applying pressure (or nasal packing), which promotes clot formation, and cold, which promotes vaso-constriction.
- Bleeding into joints is controlled by immobilizing the extremity and raising it above the level of the heart.
- Von Willebrand's disease is an inherited clotting disorder that affects both sexes and is characterized by excessive bleeding from the skin and mucous membranes, necessitating nursing measures similar to those for hemophilia.
- In idiopathic thrombocytopenic purpura (ITP), an abnormally low number of circulating platelets results in bleeding into tissues.
- Nursing care for the child with ITP includes providing emotional support; administering corticosteroids and platelets; explaining the side effects of drug therapy; carrying out preoperative and postoperative measures associated with splenectomy, and emphasizing the necessity for prophylactic antibiotic therapy after splenectomy.
- For the child with disseminated intravascular coagulation (DIC), nursing care includes assessing the child for signs of vaso-occlusion or bleeding and administering heparin.

References

Camitta BM, et al: A prospective study of androgens and bone marrow transplantations for treatment of severe aplastic anemia. *Blood* (March) 1979; 53:504–514.

Gale PR, et al: Aplastic anemia: Biology and treatment. *Ann Intern Med* 1981; 94(4):477–494.

Goldstein M: The aplastic anemias. *Hosp Pract* (May) 1980; 15:84–94.

Sergis E, Hilgarten M: Hemophilia. *Am J Nurs* (Nov) 1972; 72:2011–2017.

Vaughn VC, McKay RJ, Behrman RE (editors): *Nelson Textbook of Pediatrics.* Saunders, 1979.

Vichinsky EP, Lubin BH: Sickle cell anemia and related hemoglobinopathies. *Pediatr Clin North Am* (May) 1980; 27(2):429–447.

Additional Readings

Agle D, et al: *Home Therapy for Hemophilia.* The National Hemophilia Foundation, 1977.

Aledort L: *The Treatment of Hemophilia—Current Management: A Physician's Manual.* The National Hemophilia Foundation, 1978.

Aledort L, Levine P: *The Treatment of Hemophilia—Surgery in Hemophilia.* The National Hemophilia Foundation, 1977.

Alter BP: Bone marrow failure in children. *Pediatr Ann* 1979; 8(7): 53–70.

Bonner SE: Nursing care of a child with sickle cell disease. In: *Current Practice in Pediatric Nursing.* Vol 1. Brandt P, Chinn P, Smith ME (editors). Mosby, 1976.

Boone D: *Comprehensive Management of Hemophilia.* Davis, 1976.

Boone D, Spence C: *The Treatment of Hemophilia—Physical Therapy in Hemophilia.* The National Hemophilia Foundation, 1976.

Boutaugh M, Patterson PC: Summer camps for hemophiliacs. *Am J Nurs* (Aug) 1977; 77(8):1288–1289.

Brittner E: *Your Child and Hemophilia—a Manual for Parents.* The National Hemophilia Foundation, 1976.

Buchanan GR: Disseminated intravascular coagulation. In: *A Practical Guide to Pediatric Intensive Care.* Levin B, Morris F (editors). Mosby, 1983.

Byrnes JJ: Thrombotic thrombocytopenia purpura. *Adv Intern Med* 1980; 26:131–157.

Child J, et al: Blood transfusions. *Am J Nurs* (Sept) 1972; 79(9):1602–1605.

Calbreath D: Serum iron and iron-building capacity. *J Nurs Care* (Sept) 1979; 12(9):30.

Dallman PR, Siimes MA, Stekel A: Iron deficiency in infants and childhood. *Am J Clin Nutr* (June) 1980; 33:86–118.

Desforges JR, et al: Sickle cell anemia: Improving the odds for the young patient. *Patient Care* 1972; 6:116.

Dietrich S: *The Treatment of Hemophilia—Comprehensive Care for the Person With Hemophilia*. The National Hemophilia Foundation, 1977.

Diseases. Nursing '81 Books. Intermed Communications, 1981.

Doenges, Jeffries, Moorhouse: *Nursing Care Plans: Nursing Diagnosis in Planning Patient Care*. Davis, 1984.

Doswell W: Sickle cell disease: How it influences preoperative and postoperative care. *Nursing '74* (June) 1974; 4(6):19–22.

Dressler D: Understanding and treating hemophilia. *Nursing '80* (Aug) 1980; 10(8):72–73.

Evans B: *The Treatment of Hemophilia—Dental Care in Hemophilia*. The National Hemophilia Foundation, 1977.

Fischback FT: *A Manual of Laboratory Diagnostic Tests*. Lippincott, 1980.

Foster S: Sickle cell anemia: Closing the gap between theory and therapy. *Am J Nurs* (Oct) 1971; 71(10):1952–1956.

Gilbert M: *The Treatment of Hemophilia—Orthopedics*. The National Hemophilia Foundation, 1975.

Greene P: Teaching aid for children with sickle cell disease. *Am J Nurs* (Dec) 1977; 77(12):1953.

Hallock JA, David E, Marshall L: Pneumococcal infections in sickle cell anemia. *JAMA* ((Apr. 27) 1970; 212:629.

Hathaway WE: Care of the critically ill child: The problem of disseminated intravascular coagulation. *Pediatrics* (May) 1970; 46(5):767–773.

Jackson DE: Sickle cell disease: Meeting a need. *Nurs Clin North Am* (Dec) 1972; 72(4):727–742.

Joyce B, Reid C: *Sickle Cell Anemia—a Programmed Instruction*. Unpublished manuscript, 1972.

Kneut C: Sickle cell anemia. *Issues Compr Pediatr Nurs* (Sept–Dec) 1980; 4:19–27.

Lanzkowsky P: *Pediatric Hematology—Oncology—a Treatise for the Clinician*. McGraw-Hill, 1980.

Levine P: *The Treatment of Hemophilia—Control of Pain in Hemophilia*. The National Hemophilia Foundation, 1975.

Lightsey AL Jr: Thrombocytopenia in children. *Pediatr Clin North Am* 1980; 27:293–308.

Mangrum R: *Manual of Hematology*. Reston, 1975.

Mauer A: *Pediatric Hematology*. McGraw-Hill, 1969.

Mayer GG: Disseminated intravascular coagulation. *Am J Nurs* (Dec) 1973; 73:2067–2069.

McClure PD: Idiopathic thrombocytopenic purpura in children. *Am J Dis Child* 1977; 131:357.

McFarlane JM: Everyday care of the child with sickle cell anemia. *Pediatr Nurs* (Jan/Feb) 1972; 2(1):9–11.

Miller C, Lubs M: *The Inheritance of Hemophilia*. The National Hemophilia Foundation, 1977.

Nathan D, Oski F: *Hematology in Infancy and Childhood*. Vol II. 2nd ed. Saunders, 1981.

Necheles T, Allen D, Fenkew H: *Clinical Disorders of Hemoglobin Structure and Synthesis*. Appleton-Century-Crofts, 1969.

Nuscher R: Bone marrow transplantation. *Am J Nurs* (June) 1984; 84:764–772.

O'Brian B, Woods S: The paradox of DIC. *Am J Nurs* (Nov) 1978; 78:1878–1880.

Oski FA, Stockman JA: Anemia due to inadequate iron sources or poor iron utilization. *Pediatr Clin North Am* 1980; 27(2):237–252.

Price S, Wilson LM: *Pathophysiology—Clinical Concepts of Disease Processes*. McGraw-Hill, 1978.

Prochedly C: Fanconi anemia: Clues to early recognition. *Clin Pediatr* (Jan) 1972; 11(1):20–24.

Prochedly C: Sickle cell anemia: Recognition and management. *Am J Nurs* (Oct) 1971; 71(19):1948–1951.

Reindorf CA: Sickle cell anemia. *Curr Concepts Pediatr Nurs* (Mar/Apr) 1980; 6(2):E to G.

Selkurt E (editor): *Physiology*. 3rd ed. Little, Brown, 1971.

Selkurt E: Sickle cell anemia. *Med World News* 1971; 36–50.

Smith C: *Smith's Blood Diseases in Infancy and Childhood*. 4th ed. Mosby, 1978.

Smith L: Reactions to blood transfusions. *Am J Nurs* (Sept) 1984; 84:1096–1101.

Strauss H: *Diagnosis and Treatment of Hemophilia*. 3rd ed. Albany Medical College, 1972.

Tetrick AP: Ambulatory care of the hemophiliac. *J Assoc Care Child Hosp* 1978; 7(2):19–27.

Vaz DD: The common anemias: Nursing approaches. *Nurs Clin North Am* (Dec) 1972; 7(4):711–726.

Widmann F: *Clinical Interpretation of Laboratory Tests*. Davis, 1980.

Willoughby M: *Pediatric Hematology*. Churchill Livingstone, 1977.

Zimmerman S, et al: Bone marrow transplantation. *Am J Nurs* (Aug) 1977; 77(8):1311–1315.

Defense
Implications of Impaired Immunity

Susan Rowen James

37

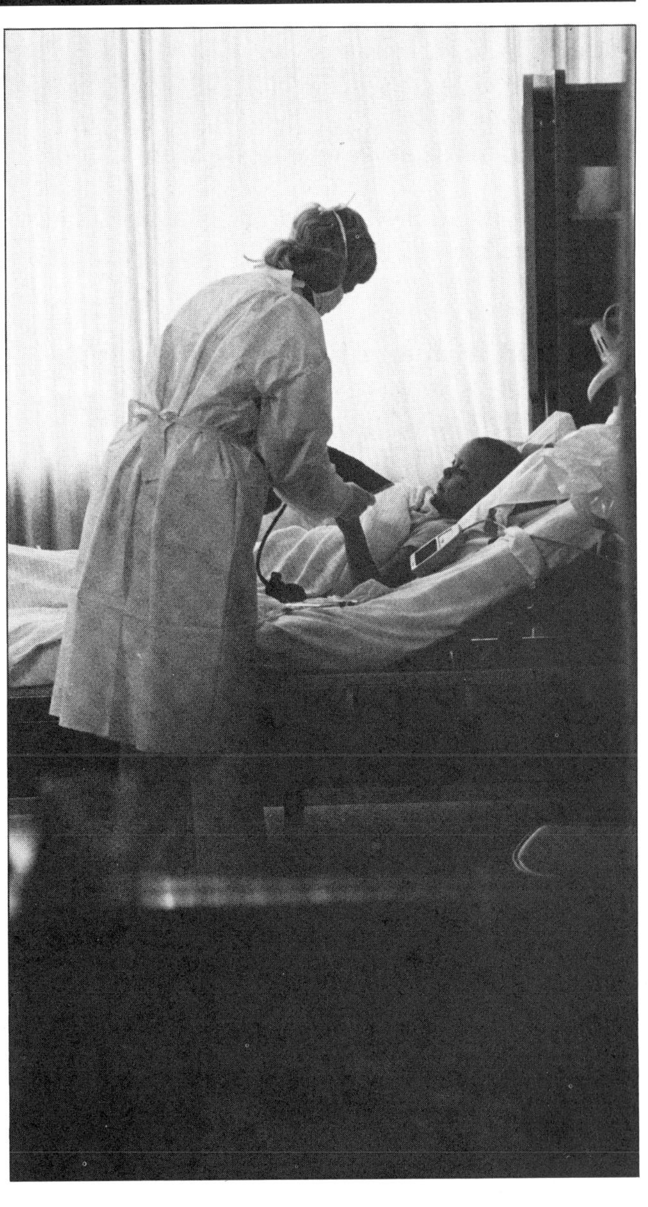

continued on next page

Objectives

- Define the components of the immune system.
- Define types of immune response.
- Explain the disease processes associated with altered immune system function.
- Describe the assessment process related to immune system dysfunction.
- Describe the essential acute-care, developmental, emotional, nutritional, and health-maintenance needs of children with immune dysfunction.
- Explain the physiologic processes, common medical treatments, and principles of nursing management for immune deficiencies.
- List the principal autoimmune and immune complex diseases.
- Describe the common manifestations of allergic reactions.
- List the common irritants that cause allergic reactions.
- Describe the assessment process specific to allergic reactions.
- Describe the essential acute-care, nutritional, developmental, emotional, and health-maintenance needs for the child with an allergy.
- List the signs and symptoms for specific allergic manifestations.

To find these topics, see the following chapters

Allergic Rhinitis	Chapter 26
Asthma	Chapter 34
Cancer	Chapter 45
Eczema	Chapter 44
Diabetes	Chapter 40

The human body has a network of defenses to keep it intact and free from disease. Chapter 44 discusses the protective functions of the skin, one of the body's first lines of defense against invasion by pathogens. In this chapter we examine both the nonspecific and specific protective functions of the immune system, the body's response to an immunologic alteration, and treatment and nursing care of children with immunologic dysfunction.

The major functions of the immune system are to defend the body against invasion by such pathogenic agents as bacteria, viruses, parasites, and toxins and to protect the body systems from abnormal cell proliferation (cancer) (Hood et al., 1984). Defense is accomplished through the unique qualities of the system, which include

1. The ability to distinguish "self" from "nonself," then activating a response against pathogens ("nonself") or suppressing a response against one's own cells ("self")
2. Surveillance capability to detect and eliminate abnormal cells
3. Long-term memory
4. Capability for extensive diversity and elaborate specificity against an infinite variety of pathogens

The actions of a properly functioning immune system are continuously effective barring any trauma or insult to the system itself that alters the immune response.

Problems resulting from alterations of the immune system can affect persons at any point in the life cycle and many of the diseases affect children younger than age 20. Immune system diseases can be physically debilitating as well as emotionally overwhelming and they provide a challenge for effective nursing care. Immunologic research has made much progress in uncovering causes and treatments for these often-bewildering diseases; however, this rapidly expanding field promises even more successful approaches for the future as more sophisticated techniques are developed and become widely available.

Conditions that affect the system can be grouped into the following four major categories: (a) immune deficiency diseases, (b) autoimmune diseases, (c) allergic manifestations, and (d) cancer. (Cancer is discussed in detail in Chapter 45.)

Anatomy and Physiology of the Immune System

Antigens

Antigens are substances such as organisms, toxins, or foreign tissues capable of eliciting an immune response. There are unique configurations on the surface of antigens—antigenic determinant sites—that cause the immune system to recognize them as foreign to the body. Most antigens have more than one antigenic determinant site, and the majority of antigens have multiple sites (Fig. 37-1*A*).

Antibodies

Antibodies are proteins produced by the immune system in response to the introduction of an antigen. Each antibody produced is specific for a particular antigen and has combining sites that are the complement in configuration to the antigenic determinant sites (Fig. 37-1*B*). Thus the antigen and antibody fit together like a lock and key (Fig. 37-1*C*). This combination of antigen and antibody is called the *antigen–antibody complex* or *immune complex*. Once

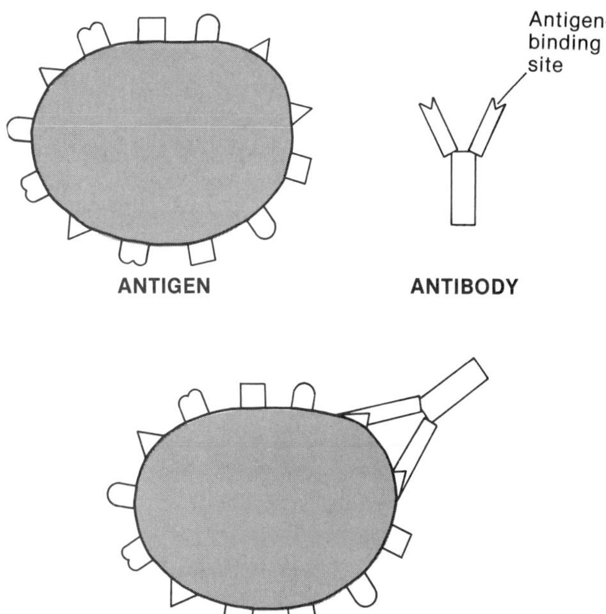

Figure 37-1 Antigens and antibodies. *A*. The majority of antigens have multiple determinant sites, causing the immune system to recognize the antigens as foreign bodies. *B*. Each antibody protein has combining sites that makes it specific for a particular antigen. *C*. The lock-and-key combination of antigen and antibody is known as the immune complex.

the antigen has combined with the antibody, the complex can be eliminated by the immune system. Antibodies act to destroy antigen by coating the antigen surface in such a way as to attract phagocytes, by disabling bacterial toxins, and by preventing viral entry into cells (US Department of Health and Human Services, 1983).

Antibodies are also known as immunoglobulins. Each antibody has a combining site specific for a particular antigenic determinant site, and each antibody has a basic molecular structure characteristic of one of the five major classes of immunoglobulins (Table 37-1).

The recognition of antigens as "nonself" and the combining of antigen and antibody for elimination from the body is facilitated by various components of the lymphatic and circulatory systems. Table 37-2 lists the organs of the immune system. These organs are connected to one another by both the circulatory system and a network of vessels carrying lymph. Lymph is a fluid composed of lymphocytes, antigens, and other molecules that drain from body tissues into the lymphatic network. There, it is filtered by lymphoid organs and eventually enters the bloodstream. Thus lymphocytes, the primary effectors of the immune response, are constantly circulating throughout the body, and the multiple locations of lymphoid tissue can trap foreign invaders before they can do great damage to body systems.

Mature *lymphocytes* are immunologic-competent leukocytes, which means that they have the capability of reacting in specific ways to antigens. The following major classes of lymphocytes are involved in the immune response: (a) T-lymphocytes, which mature in the thymus during the late prenatal and early neonatal period, can react specifically to viruses, fungi, foreign tissue, and other antigens by immediate destruction. Receptor sites on their cell surfaces allow the T cell to discriminate between "self" and "nonself." (b) B cells, which mature in the bone marrow, become antibody-producing plasma cells. Both types of lymphocytes descend from stem cells that are located in the liver before birth and the bone marrow after birth and that then migrate to the thymus (T cells) and other lymphoid tissue, where they become immunologically competent.

Both T cells and B cells respond specifically to antigens. A third type of lymphocyte, natural killer cells, can destroy foreign substances without any prior exposure to antigens. Cells most susceptible to killer cell action include cells infected by viruses and tumor cells (US Department of Health and Human Services, 1983).

Although lymphocytes are the primary leukocytes of the immune system, they only comprise 25%–30% of the total white blood cell count after age 12 (Groenwald, 1980). In younger children the leukocyte count varies from 53%–57% during the first year and then gradually decreases to adult levels around 12 years of age (Behrman and Vaughan, 1983). The other leukocytes that function in the immune system are illustrated in Table 37-3.

The Immune Response

Nonspecific Defense In order for antigens to produce disease in the body, they must first breach the front-line defenses. As mentioned previously, intact skin and mucous membranes provide primary protection against foreign substances. Other protection barriers include *chemical barriers*—bacteriocidal and fungicidal substances and enzymes in body secretions; *interferon*—a protein pro-

TABLE 37-1 Immunoglobulins

Class	Normal serum levels	Structure	Associated characteristics
IgG	0.8–1.6 g/dL	T-shaped, becomes Y-shaped after binding with antigen, probably to expose other parts of the structure to additional immune functions	Most common antibody found in blood and body tissues. Can cross the placenta into fetal circulation, thus giving the fetus the ability to resist infection. Coats microorganisms allowing for faster recognition and elimination by phagocytes. When combined with an antigen, can activate the complement system, which helps destroy foreign substances and mediates the inflammatory response
IgM	0.06–0.2 g/dL	Star-shaped with five antigen-binding sites. The largest of all the immunoglobulin molecules	First antibody produced in an immune response. Present mainly in the blood and too large to cross the placenta. Effective against microorganisms because of its multiple antigen-binding sites. Can activate the complement system
IgA	0.15–0.4 g/dL	Y-shaped. Structure can also consist of two Ys joined together by a chemical bond	Found in body secretions such as saliva, tears, and sweat. Is present on mucosal surfaces of the gastrointestinal and respiratory tracts, where it protects mucosal surfaces from antigen invasion. Is passed to the infant via breast milk, thus conferring immunity to certain diseases
IgE	Trace	Y-shaped structure	Serves a protective function on mucosal surfaces. Attaches to the surfaces of certain cells, causing them to release chemical substances, such as histamine, which can result in an allergic response
IgD	Trace	Y-shaped structure	Present in only trace amounts in the blood. Functions are generally unknown

TABLE 37-2 Organs of the Immune System

Organ	Location	Composition	Major functions
Primary organs			
Thymus	In the thoracic region behind the sternum	Multiple lobes containing lymphocytes and a plentiful blood supply	Contains precursor lymphocyte cells that mature into immunocompetent T lymphocytes. T-cell precursors, stem cells are collected by the thymus during embryonic development, although some stem cells migrate to the thymus from the bone marrow throughout life. Controls cellular immunity
Bone marrow	Soft tissue of long bones	Hematopoietic tissue	Contains stem cells for B lymphocytes, which mature into immunocompetent B cells capable of producing antibodies
Secondary organs			
Lymph nodes	Located throughout the body. Chains of nodes are found in the cervical, axillary, inguinal, and abdominal areas	Zones where classes of lymphocytes are stored. Has a high concentration of macrophages, allowing for interactions between lymphocytes and antigens. Contains a blood supply that facilitates lymphocyte entry from the circulatory system	Initiate the immune response by filtering out antigens and allowing them to come into contact with the lymphocytes. Site of antibody production
Spleen	Below the stomach in the abdomen	Has separate areas for T and B lymphocytes. Similar to lymph nodes. Is connected directly to the circulatory system to allow for increased circulation of lymphocytes	Hematopoietic—elimination of aging or defective red blood cells Immunologic—initiates the immune response by filtering antigen in a similar fashion as lymph nodes
Other			
Tonsils and adenoids	Throat		Close proximity to antigens entering the gastrointestinal and respiratory tracts allows for direct filtering by lymphoid tissue in these organs
Peyer's patches	Small intestine		
Appendix	Large intestine		

TABLE 37-3 Immune Function of Secondary Leukocytes

Secondary leukocytes	Functions
Agranulocytes	
Monocytes (macrophages)	Phagocytic function—digest antigens and cellular by-products of an inflammatory response Present antigens to lymphocytes for recognition and elimination Secrete chemical substances that help mediate the immune response
Granulocytes	
Neutrophils	Phagocytosis—particularly of bacteria. Contain enzymes that destroy antigens
Eosinophils	Phagocytosis and lysing of cells. Less rapid in action than neutrophils. Level increases in allergies
Basophils	Phagocytosis. Can release chemical substances when combined with an antigen that causes allergic manifestations

duced in response to viral invasion that inhibits viral proliferation and stimulates destructive actions of phagocytes and lymphocytes; and the *inflammatory response*, which includes the release of chemical mediators resulting in increased capillary permeability, vasodilatation, phagocytosis, and clearance of cell by-products (Groenwald, 1980). These protection measures are activated in the presence of an antigen but are nonspecific in response to the antigen. They represent the body's attempt to destroy the foreign substance without necessitating a specific immune response.

Entrance of an antigen through a compromised barrier can result in an inflammatory reaction at the site of the entry. Tissue damaged by an antigen releases chemicals that cause vasodilatation and increased capillary permeability at the invasion site. Vasodilatation and the attraction effects of these chemical substances draw phagocytes to the area. At the site the phagocytes engulf and digest the antigen and then either die or survive (Groenwald, 1980).

When phagocytes die, they release additional chemical mediators, which lure more phagocytes to the area. Clinically, vasodilatation and increased capillary permeability result in redness and edema at the site of the invasion.

By-products of phagocyte and antigen death include toxins that can produce fever, pain, and purulence (pus). Tissue damage at the site activates coagulation factors that barricade the site from other tissue areas and prevent the infection from spreading. As the antigen is eliminated, by-products are cleared by the regional lymph nodes, which may become enlarged in response. If the response has been successful in eliminating the antigen, the inflammatory response subsides. The prodromal signs that precede a communicable disease, for example, are due to the nonspecific immune response (see Chapter 26).

Specific Immune Responses

Humoral Response If the antigen remains alive within the phagocyte, it can cause further harm to body tissue. Under these circumstances the body activates its specific immune responses, humoral and cellular. These responses are mediated by B-cell and T-cell activity in the lymphoid tissue. Both the humoral and the cellular immune response are initiated by the macrophages, which carry antigen markers on their surface and expose the markers to the lymphocytes.

The mechanisms of humoral response are presented in Figure 37-2. A measurement of the amount of circulating antibody in the blood is called a *blood titer*. Initial exposure to an antigen yields a low titer. Circulating IgM appears first, followed by IgG. The appearance of these antibodies occurs after a lapse period of several days, when no detectable antibody is found in the blood. This low antibody measurement is referred to as the primary antibody response. Subsequent exposures to the same antigen will activate memory cells and a rapid, strong antibody response—the secondary antibody response—will ensue. The high titer from this response may last several months or years (Groenwald, 1980). Mechanisms of humoral response are:

- Stem cells in the bone marrow migrate to B-cell zones in the lymphoid tissue, where the cells become ready to be activated by an antigen. Each B cell is preprogrammed to react to a specific antigen and displays the type of antibody it can produce on its cell surface (receptor sites).
- When an antigen is introduced to the circulatory system, it is ingested by macrophages, which then display the antigenic determinant sites on their own cell surfaces.
- Macrophages present the antigen to the B lymphocytes, and B cells with specific receptors for that antigen are activated.
- B cells mature and differentiate into plasma cells, which then develop antibodies specific for the antigens.
- Antibodies are released into the circulation, where they can combine directly with the antigen, resulting in antigen–antibody complexes.
- The antibody can kill the microorganism directly or activate accessory systems to kill the antigen.
- Memory cells are produced that will immediately recognize and act against the subsequent invasion by the antigen.
- When the antigen is eliminated, suppressor elements in the immune system reduce the production of antibody (Tortora, Funke, and Case, 1982).

Cellular Response Some antigens such as viruses, parasites, fungi, graft tissue, and tumor cells have no appropriate sites on their cell surfaces for antibody binding. These cells must be destroyed directly by the T lymphocyte.

- Stem cells in the thymus migrate to the T-cell zones in lymphoid tissue, where the cells are ready to be activated by an antigen. Each T lymphocyte is programmed to react to a specific antigen and contains antigen-binding receptors on its cell surface.
- The antigen is presented to the T cell by the macrophage, resulting in sensitization of the T cell.
- Sensitized T cells replicate themselves and migrate to the site of the antigen invasion.
- Killer T cells bind to the antigen and release chemical substances (lymphokines) that act in the following ways: to destroy organisms directly, to attract phagocytes to the area and to increase phagocytic response, to stimulate nonsensitized T cells in the area to perform killer functions.
- Memory T cells remain in lymphoid tissue and mount a swift response to a subsequent antigen invasion (Tortora, Funke, and Case, 1982).

The mechanisms for this cellular response, listed below, are shown in Figure 37-3.

Not all of the T lymphocytes become killer cells or memory cells. Some T cells have cooperative functions with the humoral immune response. These cells are referred to as *helper* and *suppressor* T lymphocytes. Helper T cells interact with B lymphocytes and assist in antibody production. Suppressor T cells can inhibit the humoral response and assist in the shutdown of antibody production as the antigen level decreases.

Complement When antibodies combine with antigens, the molecular shape of the antibodies changes to expose additional areas (Tortora, 1982). One area exposed in this process is the complement fixation site. The complement system is a series of proteins labeled C1 through C9 that circulate in the blood. Certain antibodies (IgM and IgG) can activate this system when bound with antigen. Activation of the initiator component triggers the activation of

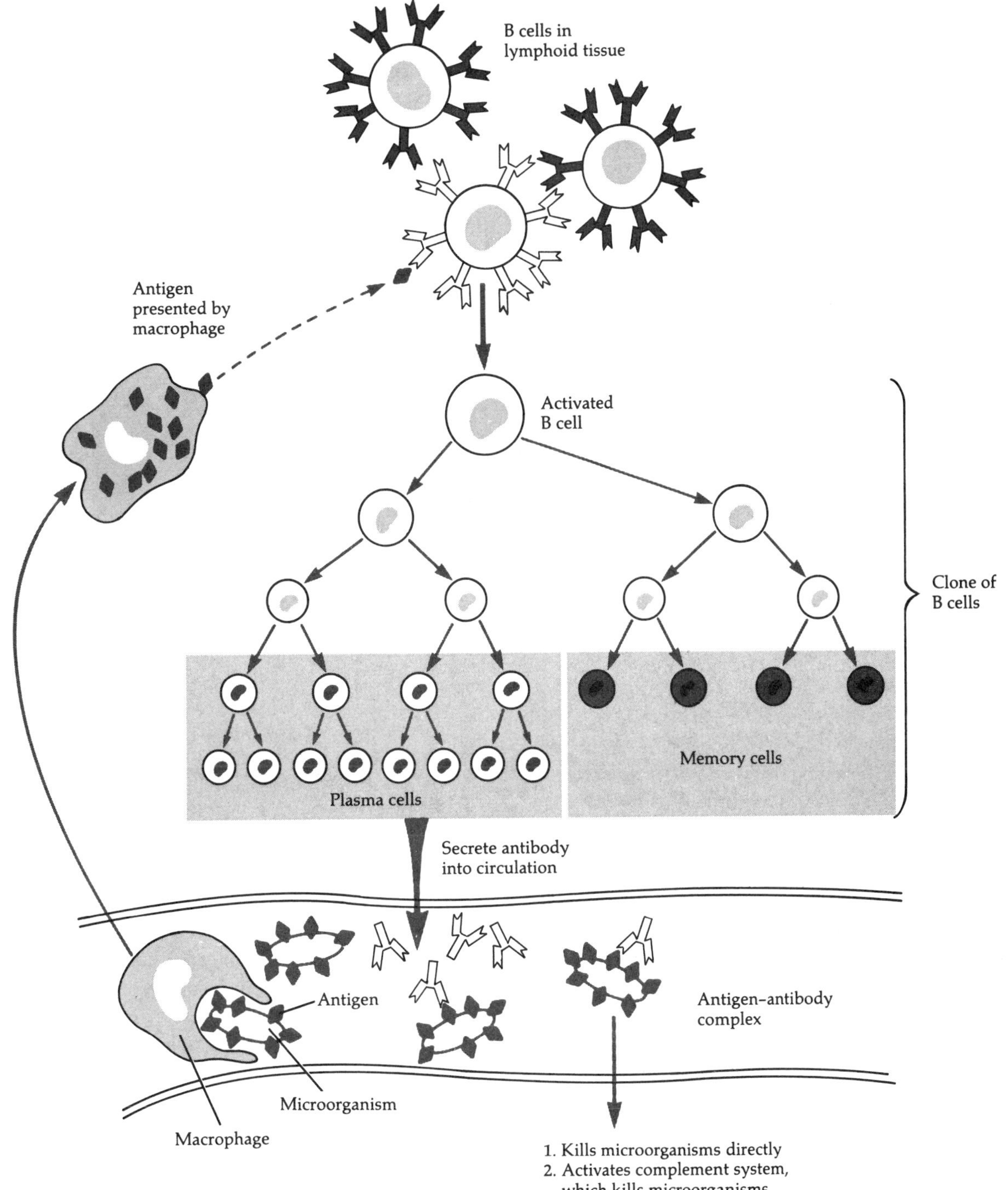

Figure 37-2 Role of B cells in humoral response. (From Tortora GL, Funke BR, Case CL: *Microbiology: An Introduction.* Benjamin/Cummings, 1982, p 406.)

each of the others in the series in a predictable sequence known as the complement cascade (US Department of Health and Human Services, 1983). Complement assists the antibody with antigen destruction, enhances the inflammatory response by releasing chemicals leading to vasodilation and capillary permeability, and attaches to the antigen to enhance phagocytosis (Vick, 1984). Complement also can be destructive to antigen without the presence of antibodies by an alternate pathway.

Developmental Considerations of the Immune System

During fetal development stem cells for both B and T lymphocytes are found in the liver. Shortly before birth and

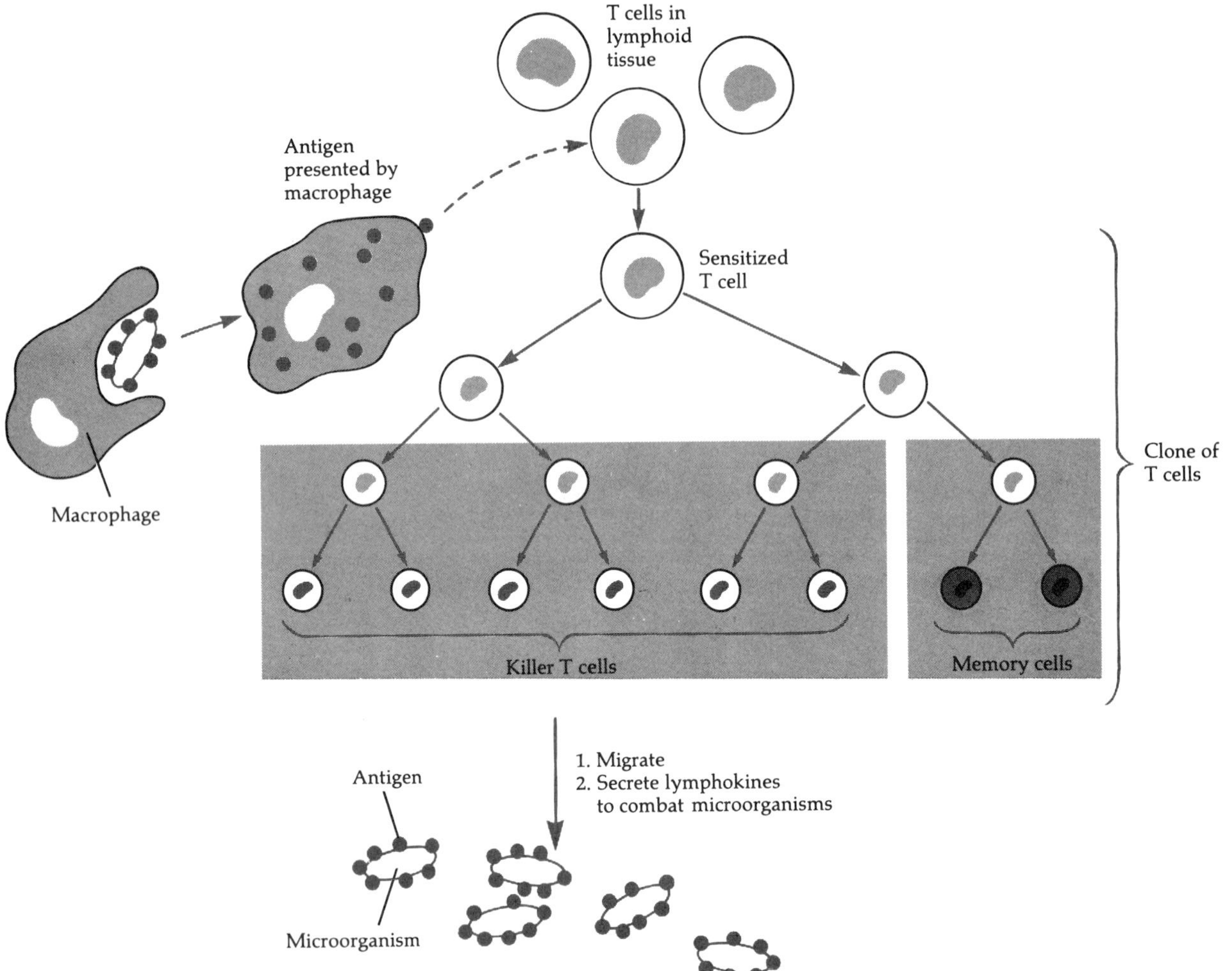

Figure 37-3 Role of T cells in cellular response. (From Tortora GL, Funke BR, Case CL: *Microbiology: An Introduction*. Benjamin/Cummings, 1982, p. 407.)

for several months after, T cells migrate to the thymus, where they become immunologically competent. B cells become competent in the bone marrow and lymphoid tissue. The neonate, then, has potential for developing intact immune responses but needs exposure to antigens to stimulate the development of these responses and to build a repertoire of antigen-specific cells. Protection from infection in the first few months of life comes from maternal IgG, which crosses the placenta. Breast-fed babies receive IgA via breast milk, which provides additional disease-fighting capabilities. At approximately 6 months of age (see Chapter 7) IgG levels decrease and the child's own immune system assumes its defensive role. By puberty the thymus reduces in size but continues to produce competent T lymphocytes.

Children acquire immunity naturally and artificially, passively and actively. Prenatally acquired IgG is an example of *naturally acquired passive immunity*. The process occurs under natural conditions and does not require active participation of the child's own immune system. Passively acquired immunity is short-lived since the supply of antibody is not replenished.

Artifically acquired passive immunity results from the injection of antibodies from a source other than the child, and given to the child for immediate protection against disease. An example of this is administration of gamma globulin to prevent hepatitis.

Naturally acquired active immunity occurs when the child's own immune system produces antibodies against antigens. Active immunity can last many years, and often confers lifelong immunity, as in many of the communicable diseases of childhood (see Chapter 26).

Artificially acquired active immunity also induces the immune system to produce antibodies against antigens and develop memory cells to maintain the immunity. Artificially acquired immunity occurs when a vaccine is given to the child, such as in childhood immunizations against communicable diseases (see Chapter 18). Organisms or toxins in a weakened or inactive state will not produce symptoms of disease but will stimulate a specific immune response. Occasionally, immunizations will have side effects that reflect the inflammatory reaction to the altered antigen. Immunizations activate the primary immune response, thereby protecting the child against illness from subsequent exposures. Booster doses of vaccine such as tetanus elicit a secondary response that protects the child for years and sometimes confers lifelong protection.

Altered Immune System Function

Alterations in immune system functioning can be manifested in many forms. Disease entities fall into several general categories—deficiency diseases, autoimmune diseases, immune complex diseases, allergy, and cancer—but other immune system conditions may be due to incomplete clearing of immune complexes.

Immune Deficiency Diseases

Immune deficiency diseases may affect the cellular or humoral immune response, or both. They can be partial or complete, chronic or self-limiting, mild or severe, depending on the cause and the immune system components involved. Children born with defects in the humoral system are unable or only partially capable of producing antibodies, thus making them particularly susceptible to bacterial infections (Hood et al., 1984). Some children are born with an abnormal thymus, which affects T-cell production. These children are more susceptible to viral and parasitic infections, as well as certain forms of cancer, since the surveillance capabilities of the system are altered (Hood et al., 1984). Rarely, children demonstrate a congenital deficiency in both classes of lymphocytes—severe combined immunodeficiency disease (SCID). Lymphoid tissue in these children is incompetent and lacking both classes of lymphocytes. The occurrence of SCID is genetically based and the disease can be inherited through a sex-linked or autosomal recessive mode (Hood et al., 1984). Children with SCID are unable to combat any antigens and must live in an antigen-free environment such as a germ-free room or "bubble" in order to survive. Recent success with bone marrow transplants promises hope for these children.

Mild or transient deficiencies of the immune system can occur in connection with certain diseases or medication effects.

Autoimmune Diseases

Relatively recent advances in the science of immunology have recognized that some diseases, particularly those affecting connective tissue, are the result of the body's attack on itself (autoimmunity). The lack of recognition of "self" by the immune system results in activation of antibodies (autoantibodies) against body tissues that have assumed antigenic properties, or activation of the cellular response against "self." The autoimmune response is exacerbated by malfunction in helper or suppressor T lymphocytes, that is, an overabundance of helpers and an inhibition of suppressors (Hood et al., 1984). Autoimmunity may be activated in the following ways:

1. Some body tissue is normally antigenic, but during fetal development the immune system incorporates these antigens as natural. Autoimmunity occurs in individuals who for some unknown reason had these natural tissue antigens masked during development, so tolerance to them never developed. Upon later contact with them, the immune system recognizes them as foreign and destroys them.
2. It is felt that some viruses or tissue injuries alter normal tissue constituents causing the body to reject and destroy them as foreign. These tissues may be functioning normally until the time of tissue injury.
3. Certain organisms or antigens closely resemble the structure of normal body cells and in recognizing the antigen as foreign the normal cells are also considered to be foreign (US Task Force on Immunity and Disease, 1980).

Autoimmune diseases are both long-term and self-limiting. The long-term diseases are often marked with exacerbations and remissions. Therapy has generally been experimental. Remissions are often spontaneous, without any effectively proven intervention.

Autoimmune diseases in children include acute rheumatic fever, juvenile rheumatoid arthritis, systemic lupus erythematosus (SLE), and juvenile-onset diabetes mellitus among others. Recent evidence has suggested that diabetes may be the result of an autoimmune response against the B cells in the islet of Langerhans. The autoimmune response may be activated by certain viruses that cause tissue damage to the islet cells and alter their composition (Hood et al., 1984). See Chapter 40 for further discussion of diabetes mellitus.

Immune Complex Diseases

Immune complex diseases result from inefficient clearing of antigen–antibody complexes from the body systems. These complexes remain in the circulation until they become caught in the small blood vessels of various body systems. There they initiate an inflammatory response that results in tissue damage. Immune complex diseases may be self-limiting, such as acute glomerulonephritis, or they may be influential in the course of chronic autoimmune diseases such as SLE or juvenile-onset rheumatoid arthritis. Table 37-4 lists some classifications of immune system dysfunctions.

Hypersensitivity—Allergy

Hypersensitivity reactions are detrimental inflammatory responses in body tissues secondary to tissue injury from either the humoral or cellular immune responses. Since first exposure to an antigen does not elicit the specific immune responses, hypersensitivity reactions occur as a result of a second exposure to an antigen. Depending upon the specific response elicited by the antigen, hypersensitivity reactions can be immediate or delayed.

Immediate hypersensitivity reactions occur from antigens causing inflammation and tissue injury as a result of a humoral response. Allergy (class I hypersensitivity) is an immediate reaction to the introduction of an allergen (antigen) such as pollen, dust, foods, drugs, and other environmental substances. Upon first exposure to an allergen, the body manufactures IgE. The IgE binds to "mast" cells (granulocytes). Upon second exposure to the allergen, the allergen binds with the IgE on the mast cells and causes rupture of the cell membranes and release of cell contents. The cell contents include such chemical substances as histamine, bradykinin, and slow-reacting substances of anaphylaxis (SRS-A), all having adverse effects on various body systems (Fig. 37-4).

In class II hypersensitivity antigen–antibody stimulation of the complement cascade causes release of chemicals that are harmful to antigens, but can also be harmful to normal cells in the area, such as erythrocytes. This process is the cause of some blood transfusion reactions (see chapter 36).

Immediate hypersensitivity reactions usually occur within minutes to hours after exposure to the antigen. They subside quickly, often within 48 hours (Hood et al., 1984).

Delayed hypersensitivity is a response to activation of the cellular immune response. It appears from 24–48 hours after the T-cell response is initiated and lasts at least 72 hours before subsiding (Hood et al., 1984). Contact dermatitis such as poison ivy is a delayed hypersensitivity reaction. This reaction occurs when an antigen (chemical, viral, foreign tissue, etc.) stimulates T-cell destructive action resulting in a proliferation of sensitized lymphocytes that increase the destruction of normal cells in the vicinity of the response. Delayed hypersensitivity is the mechanism for graft rejection; it also is the basis for tuberculosis skin tests.

Assessment of the Child With Immune System Dysfunction

History

A child who presents with a suspected immune system disorder can exhibit symptoms that are often bewildering as well as frightening. Because many of these disorders mimic one another, a careful nursing history is essential to assist in establishing a differential diagnosis.

In addition to the routine information about the child, the nurse should first obtain a description of the course of the disease up to the time of the interview. Relevant data include the age of the child, occurrence and pattern of fever, the appearance of any type of rash, and a description of colds or infections experienced during the past year and any medications used to treat them. Particularly important when inquiring about recent infections is to document any history of a sore throat, especially in conjunction with a fever. The nurse should also note any recent history of "flu" symptoms and any occurrence of injuries.

Since some of the immune system diseases may be triggered by exposure to a drug or toxic chemical, it is essential for the nurse to determine what medications, if any, the child had received prior to onset of symptoms. Some antibiotics and sulfa drugs have been associated with the onset of some of the self-limiting immunologic diseases such as *Stevens–Johnson* syndrome and H.S. purpura. Procainamide (Pronestyl) and hydralazine (Apresoline) have been known to produce lupus-like symptoms in sensitive individuals (Koffler, 1979). Also, the nurse should note any unusual environmental factors, particularly exposure to toxic chemicals.

TABLE 37-4 Common Immune System Dysfunction in Children

Deficiency	Thymic—Di George's syndrome Cancer (see Chapter 45) Acquired Immune Deficiency Syndrome (AIDS)
	Humoral—Agammaglobulinemia Hypogammaglobulinemia
	Combination—Wiskoff-Aldrich syndrome SCID
Autoimmune	Acute rheumatic fever Juvenile rheumatoid arthritis Systemic lupus erythematosus Erythema multiforme Juvenile diabetes mellitus (see Chapter 40) Acute glumerulonephritis
Immune complex	Henoch-Schönlein's purpura Mucocutaneous lymph node syndrome—Kawasaki disease
Allergy	

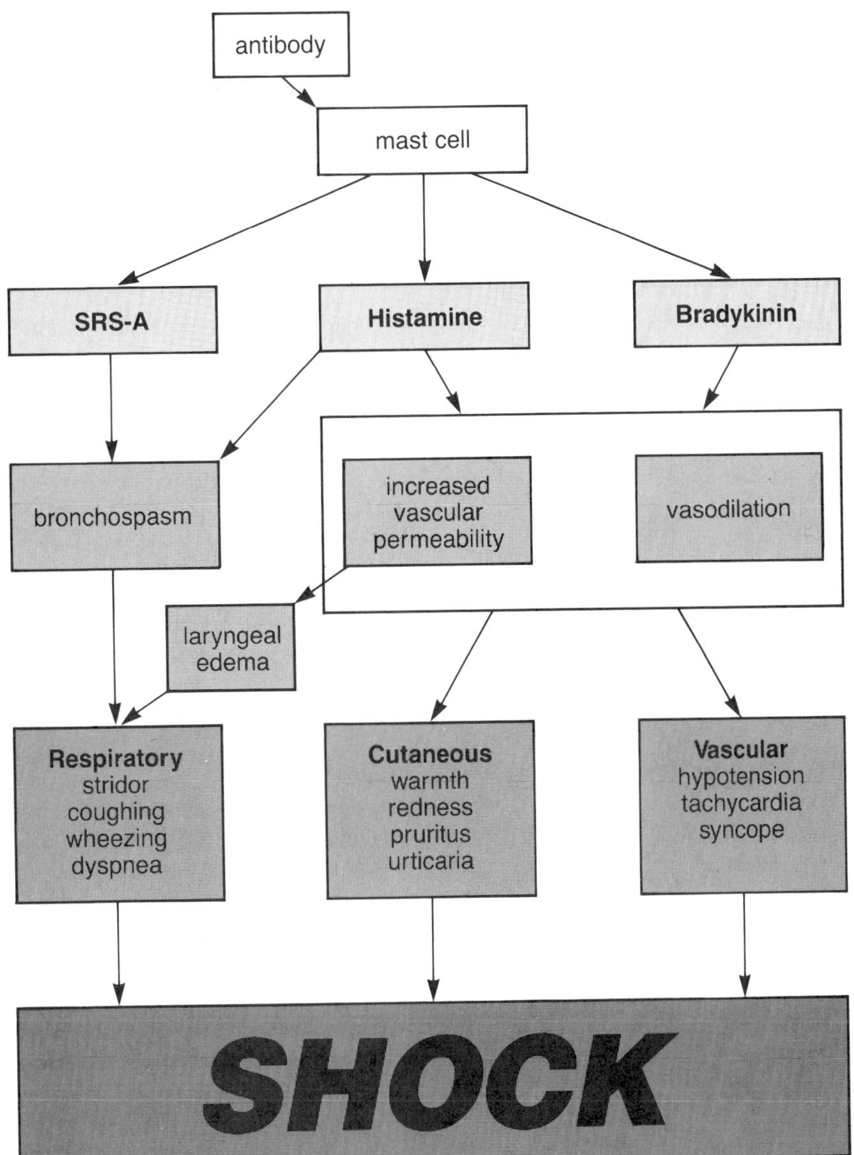

Figure 37-4 Mechanisms of anaphylaxis. Anaphylaxis is initiated by antigens interacting with antibodies on the surfaces of mast cells and basophils, which then release certain chemical mediators, such as SRS-A, histamine, and bradykinin. These mediators have profound effects on the pulmonary and vascular systems, resulting in brochospasm, increased vascular permeability, and laryngeal edema. These physiologic changes in turn produce a variety of respiratory, cutaneous, and vascular signs and symptoms that can be precursors to shock. (From Harmon A, Harmon D: Anaphylaxis—sudden death anytime. *Nursing80* (Oct 1980; 8:43).

A history of joint pain necessitates questions directed toward the pattern of the pain, for example, the time of day it occurs, the joints involved, and the transiency of the pain. It is also important to note any recent disappearance of joint pain. The immune system disorders that affect joint function differ according to the number and location of joint involvement.

Allergies of any type should be documented as well as any hypersensitivity reactions (Lind, 1980). A history of persistent rhinitis, headaches, or respiratory congestion may be indicative of allergic manifestation of which the child's family may be unaware. The nurse should record any allergy desensitization regimen.

The child's immunization status is important to determine, not only to see whether the child is appropriately immunized but also to indicate any reactions to the immunizations. For instance, certain vaccines such as the MMR (see Chapter 18) are grown on fibroblast tissue cultures of chickens and ducks and can cause an allergic reaction in children who are allergic to eggs and feathers.

Finally, since some immune disorders have a hereditary pattern, it might be necessary for the parents to delve into the family records or talk to relatives about family incidence. Often, however, no known hereditary pattern will be evident.

Nursing assessment of a child with an immune system dysfunction is presented in the Assessment Guide.

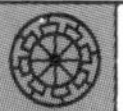

ASSESSMENT GUIDE Child With an Immune System Dysfunction

System	Subjective data	Objective data	Validating data *Diagnostic tests*	Nursing management
EENT	Sore throat, fever, cherry red tongue	Throat red, inflamed; exudate present	Throat culture for β-hemolytic *Streptococcus* ASO titer CBC ESR ECG	Question exposure to streptococcal pharyngitis or scarlet fever. Ask about family history of rheumatic fever. Observe for desquamation of hands and feet
	History of frequent respiratory infections	Thin, pale skin, hair appears lifeless	Immunoglobulin levels, bone marrow aspiration for presence of plasma cells	Discourage parents from exposing the child to other ill children. Encourage them to avoid taking the child out in crowds
	Altered and inadequate vision, eye irritation	Noticeable corneal ulcerations, inflammation of eye, dark circles under eyes	Slit-lamp examination for iridocyclitis Possible allergy testing	Darken room to combat photophobia with corneal ulceration. Dark circles under eyes may be indicative of allergy
		Irregularities in facial features—slanted eyes, abnormal ears, protruding upper lip	Serum electrolytes Skin testing to demonstrate T-cell immune function	May indicate Di George's syndrome—watch for occurrence of tetany and overwhelming infections
		Enlarged regional lymph nodes	CBC, WBC and differential	Indicative of infectious process in body's first line of defense. Observe for worsening symptoms in other body systems
Integumentary	Pruritis	Eczematous rash, urticaria, weeping lesions, particularly in areas of contact to an allergen (arms and legs for plant allergens, chest and abdomen for detergent allergen)	RAST, skin tests WBC for increased eosinophil count Immunoglobulin levels for increased IgE	Assess history of other associated allergic manifestations. See Chapter 44 for nursing management of pruritis
	Painful lesions	Bullous lesions of mucous membranes, particularly oral, spreading to other integumentary surfaces		Check history of sulfa or antibiotic treatment course. Meticulous mouth care. See Chapter 44 for management of child with burns

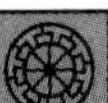

ASSESSMENT GUIDE Child With an Immune System Dysfunction (continued)

System	Subjective data	Objective data	Validating data: Diagnostic tests	Nursing management
		Vesicular and crusted lesions on face, buttocks, or other skin surface	ASO titer	Educate parents regarding signs of acute glomerulonephritis. See Chapter 44 for skin care
		Butterfly pattern rash on cheeks and over nasal bridge	ANA Le-cell serum complement levels, IVP for kidney involvement	Elicit history of exacerbation during exposure to the sun. Observe for other signs and symptoms consistent with systemic lupus erythematosus
		Erythema—generalized or over joints	ANA RF ASO titer ESR Throat culture for β-hemolytic *Streptococcus* ECG CBC—including platelet count Radiograph of joints	Observe for cardiac irregularities, excessive fatigue, high fever, enlargement of cervical lymph nodes. Plan care for optimal rest
		Purpura—especially of thighs and buttocks	ESR Immunoglobulins for elevated IgA CBC—focus on platelet count Bleeding/clotting times Urinalysis	Elicit history of medication exposure. Observe for kidney or gastrointestinal involvement
Cardiovascular	Weakness, fatigue	Abnormal ECG Presence of heart murmurs Alterations in pulse or blood pressure Edema Raynaud's phenomenon	ECG	Nursing care to provide maximum rest, antihypertensives if ordered. Rapid fall in BP may indicate anaphylactic shock. Keep child's hands and feet warm. Encourage relaxation techniques
Gastrointestinal	Pain in abdomen or epigastric region	Enlargement of liver or spleen, Tense abdominal area	Hematocrit CBC Stool for occult blood SGOT, SGPT	Careful monitoring of vital signs. Observe for jaundice. Auscultate for absence of bowel sounds, thus indicating obstruction. See Chapter 38

continued on next page

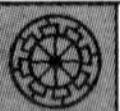

ASSESSMENT GUIDE Child With an Immune System Dysfunction (continued)

System	Subjective data	Objective data	Validating data *Diagnostic tests*	Nursing management
Respiratory	Fatigue, sneezing, coughing	Wheezing, congestion, dyspnea, retractions, barrel-shaped chest, cyanosis	RAST Skin tests Chest radiograph	See Chapter 34. Careful monitoring of respiratory rate and breath sounds for increased dyspnea, obstruction, respiratory fatigue
Musculoskeletal	Joint pain and tenderness	Edema and joint effusion, limited range of motion, pain worst in early morning	Synovial fluid aspiration for culture ESR RF ANA Radiograph of joints	See Chapter 41. Observe pattern of pain. Encourage range-of-motion and self-care activities
Genitourinary	Infrequent voiding	Decreased urine output, hematuria, proteinuria	Urinalysis IVP	See Chapter 39. Accurate intake and output. Test each voiding for specific gravity, presence of blood, protein, pH
Neurologic		Seizure activity, chorea, tetany	Serum electrolytes	Provide safety precautions for seizures—see Chapter 42

Diagnostic Tests

Much of the laboratory work performed for diagnostic workup of immune diseases involves serologic studies (Table 37-5). It is important for the nurse to remember that children of various age groups are affected differently by the blood withdrawal procedure. The nurse must explain the procedure to the child as carefully as possible to minimize traumatic effects. See Chapter 29 for further discussion of nursing interventions during stressful procedures.

Principles of Nursing Care

Although immune system disorders differ widely as to etiologies and symptoms, there are some common features. For this reason then much of the nursing care of children with these problems can be applied to a variety of situations. However, immune disorders can affect multiple body systems. Nursing interventions then are similar to those for children with specific system disorders.

Acute-Care Needs

Pain Relief Some of the immune system diseases involve pain and partial limitation in one or more joints. Nursing care then must be directed toward pain relief and prevention of joint contractures (see Chapter 41).

A physical therapy program may be established for the child. This program may encompass not only exercises to maintain mobility, but also other treatments such as whirlpool, heat application, and instructions for promoting self-care activities. It is imperative that the nurse and physical therapist communicate carefully for a coordinated, consistent approach. A timetable for exercises should be posted in such a way that nurses on all shifts can continue the therapy. The nurse performs range-of-motion exercises of both affected and unaffected joints (see Chapter 41). The child should perform active exercises when possible, and the nurse should encourage this by using play to stimulate this activity. The use of nerf balls, trapezes, modeling clay, and any other tools for facilitating pleasant activity is beneficial. Games between similarly affected children not only

TABLE 37-5 Diagnostic Studies Related to the Immune System

Study	Normal values	Alterations	Significance
Humoral response			
Measurement of serum immunoglobulins	See Table 37-1	Decrease—IgG, IgM, IgA	Increased susceptibility to infection. Levels decreased in some immune deficiency diseases
		Increase in IgE	Implicates an ongoing allergic response or is a predictor for development of allergy
Radioimmunoassays—radioactive antigen is combined in a sample with unknown antigen. Antibody is added. Antigen–antibody complexes are separated and radioactivity of the mixture is measured		High-level reactivity indicates more of the known antigen combined with the antibody; therefore the unknown antigen is probably not the same Low-level reactivity indicates antigen the same as the known antigen	Measure the amount of circulating antigen. Helps to identify the presence of an unknown antigen. The level of measured radioactivity indicates the relative amount of circulating antigen
Example: Rheumatoid Factor (RF)	0	Presence of rheumatoid factor	RF is present in many autoimmune diseases, especially juvenile rheumatoid arthritis
Immunofluorescent techniques—antibodies from serum are combined with fluorescent dye. Pathogenic organisms are presented to the fluoresced antibody. If the organs are specific for the antibody, they will also fluoresce.			
Example: Antinuclear Antibodies (ANA)	0	Presence of ANA. Antibody to specific nuclear component (DNA, RNA) is determined by the fluorescent pattern	Implicated in autoimmune diseases such as systemic lupus erythematosus, juvenile rheumatic fever
Precipitation tests—antigens combined with antibodies in solution form heavy lattice, which precipitates out of solution and can be measured		Determine the amount of antigen or antibody in specimen Either positive or negative test depending on the combination of antigen and antibody	Used to detect the presence or absence of a particular antigen
Agglutination tests—antigens combined with antibodies cause cell clumping		Determines the presence of antibodies to a particular antigen. If no antigen is present, cells will not agglutinate. The concentration of antibodies is the titer	
Example: ASO titer	150 μ/mL	Elevation	Increased ASO titer indicative of recent or current streptococcal infection. Implicated in acute rheumatic fever and acute glomerulonephritis
Complement tests—complement is added to solution of antigen–antibody complexes. If it fixes to the complexes, it will lyse them, causing destruction		Amount of cell lysis is measured. Lysis will be high if the antibody is appropriate for the antigen. Measures individual components of complement cascade	This test only valid with antibodies of the IgG or IgM class since they are the only ones who can bind complement Decrease in C_2 implicated in systemic lupus erythematosus
Skin tests for allergy	No reaction	Presence of wheals—immediate hypersensitivity	Indicates reaction to a specific allergen
Cellular response			
Skin tests—intradermal (vaccine injection)	Presence of a wheal after 48 hours		Indicates actively functioning T cells; delayed hypersensitivity
		No reaction	May indicate T-cell deficiency
Other studies			
Erythrocyte sedimentation rate—the rate that erythrocytes precipitate out of solution	12 mL/h	Elevation	Inflammation alters blood protein allowing red cells to clump and therefore fall faster. Elevated in inflammatory diseases—acute rheumatic fever, acute glomerulonephritis, Kawasaki's disease

continued on next page

TABLE 37-5 continued

Study	Normal values	Alterations	Significance
LE cell—artificially created cell formed by combining serum of suspected child's with normal leukocytes. Cell is antigen–antibody complex	0	Presence	Present in children with SLE but may also be present with other autoimmune diseases
CBC, WBC, and differential		Elevated WBC	See Chapters 36 and 45
		Elevated eosinophils	Infection
		Elevated lymphocytes	Allergy
			Immune response

promote physical health but also answer a need for social contacts among peers.

Hazards of Immobility In addition to joint contractures, some immune system disorders may result in severe complications to the heart and kidney if measures are not taken to prevent their occurrence. For this reason, complete bed rest or severely limited activity may be required until the danger of complications recedes. Complete bed rest, however, can also be hazardous. Therefore, the nurse addresses the prevention of the hazards of immobility, which can affect body systems, and takes regular measures to prevent them (see Chapter 29).

Integumentary Alterations Of particular importance in preventing the hazards of immobility is the promotion of skin integrity. As discussed earlier, children with immune diseases often manifest peculiar skin manifestations (such as in SLE or allergy). These vary from the butterfly rash of lupus to the severe bullous skin lesions of Stevens–Johnson syndrome. Because of these inherent skin sensitivities the nurse must be more vigorous than usual with efforts to prevent skin breakdown during periods of immobility. Care of skin lesions depends upon the type of lesions involved (see Chapter 44).

Protection from Infection Because some alterations in the immune system can result in severe, overwhelming infections for the child, protection from infection is a primary nursing responsibility. Children with immune deficiencies such as agammaglobulinemia, Wiskott–Aldrich syndrome, and SCID need scrupulous protection from infection while in the hospital. Children with Stevens–Johnson syndrome also benefit from protective techniques since the massive skin lesions can result in secondary infections similar to a child with burns.

Protective isolation, or reverse precaution, varies somewhat according to hospital policy and the physical arrangements available. The nursing goal is to maintain an environment as free from pathogens as possible. The child should be placed in a private room with the doors to the corridors closed at all times. Entry and exit from the room should ideally be via a clean anteroom large enough to allow for dressing in the appropriate sterile clothing. Nursing care of the child in protective isolation is presented in the Nursing Care Guide.

Some hospitals, particularly if they are set up for bone marrow transplants, attempt to maintain a germ-free environment for their children through the use of a laminar airflow system. This may be a series of rooms joined by a separate corridor in which everything is decontaminated before entry. Every patient room has a laminar airflow unit, which consists of a fan blowing air at a constant speed through two filters into the child's room. The filters remove not only dust particles but also extremely small contaminants, resulting in almost 100% sterile air. Every item entering the room must be sterilized appropriately, or disinfected. This includes such items as equipment, food, medications, toys, and linens. Care for a child in any type of protective environment presents a nursing challenge. The balance between adequately meeting the child's social and emotional needs without jeopardizing the physical is a delicate one requiring creative nursing approaches.

Special Medication Regimens

High-Dose Salicylates Since some immune system disorders cause pain and inflammation in one or more joints, high doses of salicylates are given for their anti-inflammatory and analgesic actions. Aspirin is given in doses high enough to relieve symptoms without causing toxicity. This balance is a difficult one to maintain and requires accurate nursing observation as well as frequent measurement of blood salicylate levels. The level at which toxicity is unlikely to occur is 25 mg/100 mL of blood. The nurse must be alert for the first signs of toxicity—tinnitus, headache, dizziness, dimness of vision, confusion, and hyperventilation (Govoni and Hayes, 1982). If aspirin is not reduced or discontinued, toxicity may lead to coma and eventual death. The side effects of aspirin can be annoying. Gastric discomfort may be relieved by giving doses with meals, or by using

NURSING CARE GUIDE Child in Protective Isolation

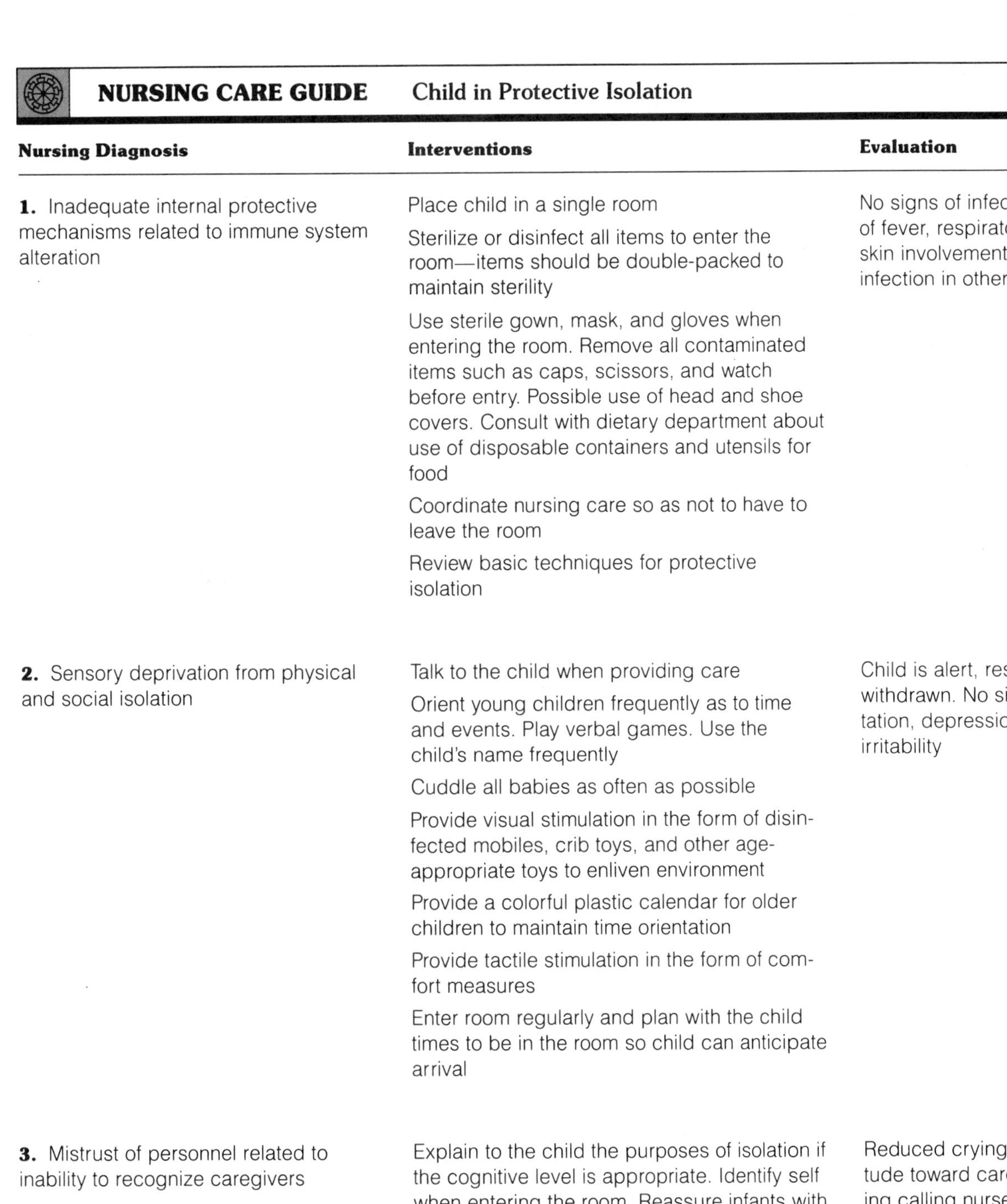

Nursing Diagnosis	Interventions	Evaluation
1. Inadequate internal protective mechanisms related to immune system alteration	Place child in a single room Sterilize or disinfect all items to enter the room—items should be double-packed to maintain sterility Use sterile gown, mask, and gloves when entering the room. Remove all contaminated items such as caps, scissors, and watch before entry. Possible use of head and shoe covers. Consult with dietary department about use of disposable containers and utensils for food Coordinate nursing care so as not to have to leave the room Review basic techniques for protective isolation	No signs of infection—absence of fever, respiratory involvement, skin involvement or signs of infection in other body systems
2. Sensory deprivation from physical and social isolation	Talk to the child when providing care Orient young children frequently as to time and events. Play verbal games. Use the child's name frequently Cuddle all babies as often as possible Provide visual stimulation in the form of disinfected mobiles, crib toys, and other age-appropriate toys to enliven environment Provide a colorful plastic calendar for older children to maintain time orientation Provide tactile stimulation in the form of comfort measures Enter room regularly and plan with the child times to be in the room so child can anticipate arrival	Child is alert, responsive, not withdrawn. No signs of disorientation, depression, or extreme irritability
3. Mistrust of personnel related to inability to recognize caregivers	Explain to the child the purposes of isolation if the cognitive level is appropriate. Identify self when entering the room. Reassure infants with a calm, soothing voice and plenty of cuddling. Use primary nursing whenever possible	Reduced crying. Trusting attitude toward caregivers, including calling nurse by name. Cooperation with care
4. Feelings of isolation related to separation from family	Encourage parental visits Teach parents precaution techniques Include parents in child's care Talk about family when family is absent. Discuss what family may be doing at home Support child when parents leave	Protest reaction when family leaves. Child expresses interest in hearing about family events

buffered preparations. Aspirin can increase bleeding tendencies and nosebleeds are not uncommon. Frequent monitoring of vital signs can alert the nurse to signs of internal bleeding. Epistaxis can be frightening to a child so nurses need to be calm in their approach. Laying the child flat and cleaning the face with a cool cloth, followed by gentle, steady pressure for 5 minutes above the nares tends to resolve the problem.

Antihistamines Antihistamines are given to children suffering from symptoms brought on by the release of histamine such as in allergic reactions—pruritis, sneezing, urticaria, and edema of mucous membranes. They are used to ameliorate the symptoms of hay fever, urticaria, and contact dermatitis. Antihistamines are usually given orally, although they may be given intramuscularly or intravenously in emergencies. Diphenhydramine (Benadryl) is most often prescribed. Others include chlorpheniramine (Chlor-Trimeton), dimenhydrinate (Dramamine), brompheniramine (Dimetane), and promethazine (Phenergan). Nurses should be aware that children can react in two distinct fashions to these drugs. Their usual side effect is drowsiness. Children experiencing drowsiness should be watched carefully so they don't injure themselves. Side rails should be up when in bed, and the child should be supervised when out. Other children experience the opposite side effect and experience restlessness, insomnia, euphoria, and nervousness.

Corticosteroids Children suffering from allergies may receive corticosteroids in either topical or systemic form depending upon the condition being treated. Corticosteroids applied to the skin function as anti-inflammatory agents. By reducing inflammation, they also counteract pruritis. Topical steroids are prescribed for allergic skin conditions and usually in ointment form. However, if the affected skin demonstrates a generalized allergy, the steroid may be mixed with a lotion for easier application. In many cases, there is a potential for absorption of the medication through the skin. In such instances the nurse should observe for systemic side effects. There is also a possibility that a secondary inflammation may occur at the contact site. In these cases, the drug may be discontinued or changed. Examples of topical steroids include Hydrocortisone, triamcinolone (Aristocort), triamcinolone acetonide (Kenalog), and betamethasone valerate (Valisone).

Systemic steroids are prescribed to reduce the inflammatory symptoms of generalized allergic disease. They are given most often for asthma, generalized urticaria, and severe cases of contact dermatitis. These drugs have serious side effects and should always be used with caution. Because they affect the body's own production of ACTH, they can cause inhibition of the adrenal cortex's abilities to produce hormones, resulting in atrophy (Govoni and Hayes, 1982). Therefore, when discontinuing the drug, it should be tapered off slowly rather than withdrawn abruptly so as to allow for return function of the adrenal cortex.

Additionally, steroids can affect the fluid and electrolyte balance to create retention of sodium and fluid. Children receiving these drugs over a long period of time may exhibit signs of edema, particularly in the face. These medications also may be irritating to the gastric and intestinal mucosa, causing bleeding. Because anti-inflammatory agents suppress the body's normal immune response to an invading organism, children may acquire infections more easily. These infections may go unrecognized because of immune suppression.

Nursing care of the child receiving steroids is directed toward observation for adverse effects and support of the child with an alteration in body image. The child should be observed for signs of fluid retention, that is, weight gain, edema, and reduced urinary output. Blood pressure should be monitored frequently for symptoms of internal bleeding. To prevent gastric irritation, medications should be given with meals or milk. Nurses should encourage children receiving steroids to avoid situations where they may be in contact with someone who is ill to prevent acquiring an underlying infection. The nurse can support the child and allow expressions of feelings about altered body image. The edema and other effects will disappear once the drug is withdrawn.

Nutritional Needs

Generally speaking, children with immune system disorders should maintain their usual diet if that diet contains adequate nutrients for growth and development. Since most products of the immune system are proteins, increased protein consumption may be advised. Children with food allergies have unique dietary problems that will be discussed in the section about nursing management of the child with allergies.

Kidney complications are a threat inherent in some immune disorders. Assessment of hydration status is essential in order to recognize signs of renal problems. The nurse needs to maintain an accurate record of intake and output since a decreased urinary output may be one of the first signs of renal problems (see Chapter 39).

Developmental Needs

Children with immune system disorders, like other hospitalized children, need to continue their normal developmental progression within the hospital setting. Some children with immune system disorders require hospitalization only during a short, acute phase of a self-limiting disease. Others can expect long hospital stays, or repeated hospitalizations. Those children in the hospital who are acutely ill will have most of their developmental needs met secondarily to physical needs. Children hospitalized on a longer-term basis and those who are repeat admissions have unique developmental problems because of interruption in normal routine. See Chapter 30 for further discussion of the child with a chronic condition. Allowing the older child to telephone friends to maintain peer relationships is helpful. If visiting is impractical,as it may be for the isolated child, some effort should be made for the child to receive letters or tapes from friends. As with any child, children should be allowed to make some decisions about their care and to have some control over their environment.

Emotional Needs

Children who suffer from immune system disorders and their families have a variety of emotional needs. Nurses first of all need to support the child and family during the acute, somewhat frightening phase of illness. If the disease is self-limiting, the nurse needs to give reassurances that, as ill as the child may appear, with precautions, the child may recover with no permanent aftereffects. Because some of these conditions affect vital body organs such as the kidney and the heart, reassurance may be difficult. The nurse can help the family verbalize fears and view the condition realistically. The reassurance, combined with nursing efforts to prevent complications, presents a nursing care challenge.

Children with immune deficiency disorders may be in more of a life-threatening situation than those with other kinds of illnesses. A normally simple infectious process could be fatal. Parents, and the child if capable of understanding, need vigorous support They need encouragement to develop a positive attitude for living as well as needing help with the adjustment to the possibility of death. The nurse should intervene to facilitate the anticipatory grieving process (see Chapter 32).

Children with certain immune system disorders experience a chronic disease course of exacerbations and remissions. Exacerbations are usually discouraging to both child and family. Nursing care of the child with a chronic illness is discussed in Chapter 30.

Health Maintenance Needs

When preparing a child with an immune system disorder for discharge, the nurse must acquaint the family with plans for follow-up care. Disease complications may not appear for several months to years after recovery. The child and family should be alerted to symptoms of complications or of disease exacerbation. Regular examinations will probably be required.

Some children may be discharged with joint limitation, necessitating regular physical therapy. The therapist should demonstrate and explain any home care therapy regimen including range-of-motion exercises and prevention of joint contractures. The nurse should assist the parents to plan for this at home. If the child is to return to school, therapy may be needed during the school day. The nurse should communicate with the school nurse, both verbally and in writing, about exactly what needs to be done to maintain continuity of care.

One additional note: if a child is suffering from an inherited immune system disorder, the nurse or physician may recommend that the parents receive genetic counseling.

The Child With an Immune Deficiency

Deficiency in the Cellular Immune Response

Children who have deficiencies in cellular immunity exhibit signs of repeated infections from viruses, fungi, and parasites. Because there is diminished T-cell activity, discrimination between "self" and "nonself" is impaired, resulting in an increased potential for developing malignancies. T-cell deficiencies can be demonstrated through the delayed hypersensitivity responses to various skin tests. Antigens used in skin testing include vaccines in inactive form such as diphtheria, tetanus, pertussis (DPT) and dinitrochlorobenzene (DNCB) among others. Absence of response may be indicative of a T-lymphocyte deficiency. It is important to remember that when caring for infants with any T-cell deficiency immunization with live viruses, such as polio or measles, mumps, rubella (MMR), is contraindicated because of the chance of the child developing an overwhelming infection by these viruses (*Pediatric Currents,* 1971).

Thymic Deficiency—DiGeorge's Syndrome Di George's syndrome is a relatively rare disease of unknown etiology that occurs as a result of a defect in embryonic development. It results in failure of the development of the thymus and the parathyroid glands. Because associated organs are developing concurrently, other anomalies such as cardiac anomalies may also be present. The thymic defect results in a below-normal or absent production of T lymphocytes that affects the body's ability to fight infection via cellular immunity. Abnormalities of the parathyroids cause neonatal hypocalcemia with resulting tetany.

The first symptom of DiGeorge's syndrome in infants is the appearance of tetany (muscle spasms). Sensitivity to infections usually is delayed, probably because of protection. The baby often has a distinctive appearance—a shortened upper lip, small receding mandible, and low-set ears. Signs of congenital cardiac anomalies such as abnormalities of the great vessels and tetralogy of Fallot also may be evident.

Laboratory studies usually reveal normal immunoglobulin levels (humoral immunity), but the child will not react to skin testing designed to prove the efficiency of cell-mediated immunity. Serum values indicate hypocalcemia and elevated phosphorus. Cardiac anomalies usually involve defects of the great vessels, particularly the aortic arch. Tetany can cause neurologic deficits resulting in mental retardation.

Immediate treatment of a child with DiGeorge's syndrome is directed toward resolving hypocalcemia. Intravenous solutions with calcium gluconate are administered, concurrently with vitamin D. Calcium is given until serum calcium levels reach normal limits (Behrman and Vaughan, 1983). Life-threatening cardiac anomalies may be treated surgically. Thymic tissue transplants have been successful in some cases for establishing cell-mediated immunity.

The prognosis for these infants is grave. They die at a young age (usually before age 2) usually from overwhelming viral or fungal infection.

Because the child is particularly susceptible to yeast and fungal infections, the nurse must be scrupulous about handwashing and the use of clean equipment, especially for feeding. Visitors with viral syndromes are prohibited. The child may be placed in protective isolation. The nurse encourages the parents to participate in the infant's care as much as possible by teaching isolation technique and emphasizing cleanliness.

Nursing interventions are geared toward assessment of neurologic and cardiac status and prevention of injury from seizure (tetany) activity. Seizure precautions for the child with tetany should be initiated, including frequent vital signs. Intravenous solutions for calcium replacement need to be monitored carefully. Any evidence of cardiac arrhythmia should be brought immediately to the physician's attention as high concentrations of serum calcium prevent relaxation of the heart muscle.

In situations where the infant is allowed to go home from the hospital, discharge instructions are necessary. Discharge planning should include education about infection prevention and methods to facilitate normal development within medical restrictions.

Parents may need additional counseling to cope with their feelings toward the child as well as their own feelings of guilt. Repeated hospital admissions are a certainty, possibly causing financial difficulties. Under these circumstances, referral to social services should be considered.

Acquired Immune Deficiency Syndrome Acquired immune deficiency syndrome (AIDS) is a fatal immune disorder that primarily affects the cellular immune response, causing an inverted ratio between helper T cells and suppressor T cells. There are normally twice as many helper cells as suppressor cells in the blood, and in AIDS patients this ratio is reversed (Thomas et al., 1984). This increase in suppressor cells "turns off" the cellular immune response so that the patient is subject to unusual overwhelming infections of a type not ordinarily seen—opportunistic infections. These opportunistic infections include severe manifestations of herpes, cytomegalovirus, and fungal infections; protozoan pneumonias; and a rare type of skin cancer, Kaposi's sarcoma.

Although a relatively rare disease that affects members of certain high-risk groups, AIDS has increased dramatically between its recognition in 1979 and the present. The groups most prone to developing AIDS include male homosexuals, addicts of intravenous drugs such as heroin, hemophiliacs receiving transfusions of factor VIII, Haitian people living in the United States, sexual partners of those affected with AIDS, and infants and children of these risk groups (Thomas et al., 1984).

A diagnosis of AIDS in an infant is related to the following factors:

1. Membership in an at-risk population, recipients of multiple transfusions, absence of any other cause of immune deficiency or suppression
2. The presence of any of the following: failure to thrive, persistent lung infiltrates or oral candidiasis, enlargement of liver or spleen, prolonged diarrhea
3. Laboratory evidence of an abnormal helper–suppressor ratio and hypergammaglobulinemia (Scott and Parker, 1984).

Although the cause of AIDS has not been definitively established, strong evidence points to a virus—human T-lymphoma virus (HTLV). The mechanism of AIDS transmission to infants has not yet been established. The possibility of placental transfer has been raised. The other possibility is related to the infant's immature immune system being unable to resist environmental exposure to the disease (Shearer, 1984).

Treatment for AIDS is directed toward ameliorating the opportunistic infections. The administration of interferon to alter the immunologic status has been attempted with variable results.

Nursing care is supportive and similar to that for any child with an immune deficiency. AIDS patients usually are on blood, needle, enteric, urine, and secretion precautions. Gloves should be worn when handling any of these sources of possible transmission of the disorder.

Humoral Deficiency—Agammaglobulinemia

One of the primary manifestations of a deficiency in humoral immunity is agammaglobulinemia. This disease has a sex-linked hereditary pattern, with female carriers passing the defect on to their sons. The disease is seen mainly in young boys, although symptoms usually don't appear until 9 months to 2 years of age probably because of the effect of maternal antibodies. The child demonstrates high susceptibility to bacterial infections, particularly common bacteria—staphylococcus, streptococcus, and *Hemophilus influenzae*. Unless the disease is recognized early, death may occur from infection. When recognized, this disease can be successfully treated.

In addition to X-linked agammaglobulinemia, an acquired form has been identified. Children of either sex may acquire this disease of unknown etiology. Symptoms and treatment are the same as for the hereditary form.

Children who have repeated bouts with pneumonia or skin infections should be tested for agammaglobulinemia. Laboratory results will demonstrate low or nearly absent levels of IgG. Gamma-A globulin and gamma-M globulin will also be significantly lower than normal. Examination of lymph nodes or bone marrow will reveal a deficiency of plasma cells. Levels of T-lymphocytes are normal. Children often appear thin and ill-looking. Their hair appears lifeless and dull.

Treatment Antibodies are administered to treat infections and injections of gamma globulin are given on a monthly basis. An initial three doses, each of 100 mg per kilogram of body weight, are administered followed by a monthly maintenance. A blood IgG level of 200 mg/100 mL is maintained.

Nursing Management The nurse should teach the parents about preventing infections. Cleanliness, avoidance of crowds, and prompt treatment for the earliest signs of infection should be emphasized.

Careful administration of gamma globulin is essential. Injections are given intramuscularly and, depending on the size of the child, may need to be given in divided doses. The nurse and parents must give extra support to the child at the time of injections, since they can be a frightening as well as painful experience.

Very often, prophylactic chest physical therapy is ordered to prevent the occurrence of pneumonia. The nurse needs to demonstrate this procedure to the parents and ask for return demonstrations until the parents appear to be competent (see Chapter 34). Although chest percussion and postural drainage appear painful, it must be emphasized that in actuality the treatment can be very relaxing for the child.

Upon hospital discharge, a visiting nurse referral would be helpful in most instances. The nurse can assist parents with preventive measures as well as reinforce the chest therapy technique.

Some children experience hypogammaglobulinemia that is a much milder form of immune deficiency resulting from a decrease rather than an absence of immunoglobulins. These children typically manifest frequent, recurrent infections, particularly when they reach school age, and are exposed to pathogens in school. Treatment may also involve gamma globulin injections to boost immune system function.

Mixed Immune Deficiency—Wiskott–Aldrich Syndrome

Young boys are most commonly affected by Wiskott–Aldrich syndrome, a sex-linked recessive disease. The syndrome is classified as a mixed immune deficiency disease since it affects both the cellular as well as the humoral systems. The body has an inability to produce antibodies and there appears to be an associated loss of cellular immunity. The immune system appears to function normally, initially, and symptoms do not appear until about 1 year of age. This disease is usually fatal with death occurring before age 6 as a result of hemorrhage or overwhelming infection. These children are also susceptible to malignancy.

The child presents with eczema, thrombocytopenia, and repeated infections. Bleeding is the most common clinical sign that brings the child for diagnosis. Infections can be bacterial or viral in origin. Serum IgG levels are normal, but IgM is greatly reduced. There is also a decrease in T lymphocytes. Blood work reveals decreased and abnormal platelets, although this can be corrected by platelet transfusions.

Treatment Topical steroids are applied to eczematous skin and antibiotics are administered prophylactically for infections. Platelet transfusions are successful in temporarily correcting the thrombocytopenia. Gamma globulin is given to provide increased resistance to infection. No one treatment is known to cure or completely correct the disease. Recently, bone marrow transplantation has been attempted and has been successful in curing the disease (Nuscher et al., 1984). With early treatment, the prognosis for these children is optimistic.

Nursing Management Again, nursing interventions are directed toward prevention of infection. Parents are taught to apply topical steroids and to observe the child for adverse effects. The nurse should carefully monitor transfusions, particularly observing for reactions. The parents should be encouraged to protect the child from bruising, while still allowing development to proceed as normally as possible. Guidance similar to that given to parents whose children have hemophilia, regarding the use of padded clothing and protective helmets, is helpful when the child is learning to stand or walk (see Chapter 36). Because this disease is sometimes fatal, the nurse should intervene to facilitate the grieving process.

The Child With an Autoimmune Disease

Acute Rheumatic Fever

Acute rheumatic fever (ARF) is an autoimmune disease that occurs as a result of invasion by group A beta-hemolytic streptococcus. It is not a contagious disease, although the precipitating factors—strep pharyngitis, scarlet fever—are. There are two major theories for this disease:

1. The streptococcus has similar antigen determinant sites as normal collagen tissue cells. When targeting the streptococci for destruction, the immune system also destroys the normal cells, resulting in an inflammatory response at the site of tissue destruction—myocardium, and the connective tissue portions of the heart, joints, and eyes, particularly.
2. Antistreptolysin O (antibody) is toxic and is itself an antigen. As an antigen it is destructive to normal cells (Kaplan, 1978).

ARF can affect children of all ages, but primarily school children. Close contact in a classroom can enhance the transmission of streptococcal diseases, as can any overcrowded living conditions. It is a self-limiting disease, usually resolving in 3 weeks.

Because of the overuse of penicillin, occasionally organisms have become resistant. Physicians may not prescribe antibiotics unless absolutely necessary. Since symptoms of ARF do not usually appear before 10 days after invasion of an untreated strep, it is safe to wait the 48 hours for a positive throat culture before initiating antibiotic therapy.

The incidence of strep-related immune diseases has decreased dramatically since the discovery of penicillin. Prompt attention to identification and treatment of strep throats will continue to decrease the disease incidence and prevent cardiac complications.

Criteria for a positive diagnosis of rheumatic fever have been established. Because overuse of the criteria have, at times, led to misdiagnosis, the criteria have been revised to recommend that positive history of strep is essential to conclude ARF (Kaplan, 1978).

Major Criteria:	Polyarthritis
	Carditis
	Erythema Marginatum
	Chorea
	Subcutaneous nodules
Minor Criteria:	Fever
	Arthralgia
	Alteration in ECG
	Previous history of ARF
	Leukocytosis
	Elevated ESR
	Positive C-reactive protein

For a diagnosis, two major criteria *or* one major and two minor plus a history of previous strep infection must be present.

Arthralgia can be in one or more joints, although it usually occurs in major joints. It is transient and does not produce contractures. Carditis is detected by murmurs as well as ECG changes. Laboratory work reveals an elevated ASO titer—above 330 in a child (DiSciascio and Taranta, 1980) (norm. 150 U/mL). A highly elevated erythrocyte sedimentation rate is secondary to the inflammatory autoimmune process.

Treatment Treatment of ARF is directed toward preventing cardiac complications. Aspirin is prescribed for pain, and prednisone is also given if carditis is present. Complete bed rest is maintained until the ESR drops to within normal limits. A throat culture is performed, and if it is positive, the child is treated with antibiotics.

The American Heart Association emphasizes that adequate prevention will reduce the incidence of ARF. Children with fevers and sore throats should be cultured and any positive culture should be treated with a 10-day course of oral penicillin, penicillin G preferred. Once a child has been diagnosed as having rheumatic fever, prophylactic penicillin is administered to prevent future occurrences. Penicillin is not effective in treating the cardiac problems; its use is to prevent recurrence by preventing streptococcal infection. Recommended schedules are

1. Intramuscular penicillin injections every 4 weeks or,
2. Oral penicillin, 250 mg tablets four times a day (American Heart Association, 1977)
3. Erythromycin for children sensitive to penicillin

Penicillin prophylaxis continues until the child is 20 years old or 5 years after the attack, whichever is longer. At any other time in life when exposure to streptococcus infection is likely (family incidence of strep throat, dental procedures), prophylaxis should be initiated.

Nursing Management Maintenance of bed rest to prevent cardiac complications is a major nursing intervention for a child with ARF. Cardiac involvement may lead to mitral valve disease in later life. Because exercise is strictly limited, the nurse must use ingenuity to present diversional activities that are interesting, age appropriate, and quiet. School work should be continued and the child should maintain contacts with family and peers. For some children, strict bed rest is extremely anxiety provoking, placing undue stress on the heart. Occasionally limited activity will be allowed in order to minimize anxiety.

Because this disease can result in cardiac damage, parents and children may have undue anxiety. Contact between the nurse and family should encourage verbal expressions of concern. With prompt treatment and proper rest, complications can be minimized.

If the child is suffering from chorea, seizure precautions are necessary (see Chapter 42). Children may be disturbed by jerky muscular movements and need extra support and reassurance that these symptoms will disappear.

Arthritic joints can be painful and swollen, limiting movement. Nursing interventions include pain assessment and relief. Limited range-of-motion exercises may be performed if allowed and they should be incorporated into diversional activities.

Prolonged bed rest leads to development of the hazards of immobility and nursing interventions need to consider this. Lack of activity and boredom might contribute to weight gain, necessitating diet reduction.

Discharge planning should include teaching about the signs and symptoms of strep as well as measures to prevent it. The child should avoid direct contact with susceptible persons and keep away from crowds. The importance of cooperating with the antibiotic regimen should be emphasized and the dangers of noncooperation explained. The older child should assume some responsibility for taking medications. Prompt treatment of any sore throat is essential.

Camp and school nurses need to be informed of any history of rheumatic fever in order to ensure prompt treatment. Some state health departments provide free strep culture kits. Any child presenting with a persistent fever and sore throat should be cultured. Accompanying symptoms may include headache and nausea.

Acute Glomerulonephritis

Acute glomerulonephritis like ARF is an autoimmune disease occurring in response to a previous streptococcal invasion. Unlike ARF, it is not necessary to have an upper respiratory infection, since the disease can occur as a result of organisms entering through the skin, as in streptococcal impetigo. It mainly affects young boys and can occur as close as 3 days after development of an untreated streptococcal infection. Again, theories about causes of AGN differ, but it is generally suspected that immune complexes lodge in the Bowman's capsule of the kidney, leading to inflammation and obstruction. This process causes decreased glomerular filtration. Consequently, less sodium and water are passed to the tubules for reabsorption and excretion. The kidneys enlarge and sodium and water are retained, leading to edema. Because of the fluid overload, the child can develop congestive heart failure. The kidneys may eventually shut down if the disease isn't treated.

Along with the edema, the child may experience hematuria, hypertension, decreased urinary output, and possibly congestive difficulties. Laboratory tests reveal a high ASO titer, leukocytosis, anemia, increased blood urea nitrogen (BUN), and decreased creatinine. Urinalysis yields increased blood, leukocytes, protein, and cells (see Chapter 39 for nursing care).

Erythema Multiforme—Stevens–Johnson Syndrome

Stevens–Johnson syndrome occurs mainly in boys of any age. Current theories of causative factors indicate that it may be the result of an autoimmune skin reaction to either drug ingestion or a common viral agent. Drugs which have been implicated include sulfonamides, co-trimoxazole (Bactrim, Septra), antibiotics, and barbiturates. This syndrome is generally considered to be self-limiting, with the active disease process subsiding after 2–6 weeks. However, the mortality may be as high as 10% and 20% of these children develop the disease again with subsequent exposure to the same antigen (Behrman and Vaughan, 1983).

Symptoms occur suddenly. They are preceded by fever, fatigue, headache, and possible sore throat. Lesions appear on the mucosal surfaces and spread to most areas of the body. They are bullous in nature and round with a vesicular center. Lesions in the mouth and in and around the eyes can be exceedingly painful. Lesions are apt to bleed and crust and as outer skin layers peel, underlying tissue appears bright red similar to that seen in second degree burns (see Chapter 44). The child appears acutely ill and may exhibit signs of pneumonia. Photophobia is common from eye involvement.

Treatment Intravenous fluid and electrolyte replacement is usually a necessity because of exudation of lesions. Treatment is similar to that of a child with extensive burns. Topical silver sulfadiazine can be applied to the lesions (Stevens–Johnson Syndrome, 1978). Medications may be ordered for pain. If there is extensive eye ulceration, an ophthalmologist should be consulted to prevent corneal scarring. Antibiotic administration will treat the symptoms of pneumonia. Care must be exercised to avoid any class of drugs suspected to have precipitated the disease.

Nursing Management The child with Stevens–Johnson syndrome provides a challenge for nursing intervention. Nursing care is similar to that of the child with burns (see Chapter 44). For purposes of preventing secondary infection, protective isolation is usually ordered. Extreme cleanliness must be maintained, particularly of the bed linens. The nurse should perform frequent special mouth care, including mouth rinses for comfort.

These children have diminished appetites, and if they eat at all, they will limit themselves to liquids. Because of precarious fluid and electrolyte balance, nutritious liquids should be encouraged and accurate measurement of intake and output recorded. The nurse should offer liquids high in protein and calories.

Application of topical ointments may be painful for children with this problem. In this case, the nurse may request an analgesic for them, to be given a half hour prior to any treatments.

Because the child's skin eruptions appear so severe, both parents and child may be extremely frightened about permanent scarring. The nurse can offer reassurance that skin manifestations will disappear. As stated in general nursing management for children with immune disorders, care must be taken to prevent sensory deprivation.

When considering discharge planning, the nurse needs to inform parents about the possibility of recurrence. If a medication has been implicated, parents should be warned that the child should avoid it in the future.

Discharge planning should also include a recommendation for frequent ophthalmologic examinations to detect the presence of corneal scarring.

Juvenile Rheumatoid Arthritis

Juvenile Rheumatoid Arthritis (JRA) is a relatively common long-term autoimmune disease of the connective tissue consisting of spontaneous exacerbations and remissions. It is theorized that tissue injury in the joint causes changes in normal immunoglobulins that cause them to become antigenic. Autoantibodies develop in response and are referred to as rheumatoid factors (RF) (Irby, 1978). The resulting antigen–antibody complexes cause joint inflammation, which can lead to joint limitation and subsequent bone destruction. In some cases, circulating immune complexes can result in tissue injury in other body systems that contain connective tissue.

This disease can affect children of all ages and affects girls approximately 5 times as often as boys. It affects children differently but disease patterns usually have the following three general pathways:

1. Monoarticular, 40% of cases
   a. Fewer than four joints are affected. Girls tend to develop iridocyclitis. Arthritic symptoms are generally mild.
   b. Boys demonstrate arthritis in lower extremities. They can develop spondylitis (Fink, 1979).

2. Polyarticular—40%—Greater than four joints are affected. The presence of the RF for IgM indicates a poorer prognosis in this type. Disability can be mild to severe.

3. Systemic—20%—Begins with high fever, rash, anorexia, and weight loss. Multiple joint involvement occurs later in the disease process. Additionally, there may be carditis, pleurisy, and enlargement of the liver. Disability ranges from mild to severe (Koffler, 1979; Fink, 1979).

The joints most commonly affected are the knees, wrists, ankles, elbow, and neck. Joint stiffness is usually worse in the morning. The prognosis is variable and seems to be related to the level of rheumatoid factor. Many children experience spontaneous remissions within 1–2 years. Others, approximately 30%, continue to have the disease, creating permanent disabilities. Children with these disabilities often have physical growth retardation because of destruction of bone epiphyses.

The symptoms of JRA are somewhat dependent upon the number of joints involved and the disease progression. Some children initially experience high fever with transitory rash, while others complain of vague symptoms of malaise, low-grade fever, anorexia, and joint pain.

Hematologic tests are performed to establish the diagnosis. Serum usually reveals leukocytosis and positive ANA. In many cases there is an elevated ESR and ASO titer, which can occasionally confuse the diagnosis with ARF. Rheumatoid factor, antibodies reacting with gamma globulin IgM, is present in most cases but it is not specific for rheumatoid arthritis as positive results usually are associated with most polyarticular disease.

Very often a joint aspiration and examination of synovial fluid is performed. The fluid will be thick and may demonstrate leukocytes from increased lymphocyte response as well as RF. Radiographs of the joints reveal joint effusion and possible degeneration.

Approximately one child in ten will develop iridocyclitis. This is diagnosed by slit-lamp eye examination.

Treatment Treatment of JRA is geared toward pain relief, reduction of inflammation, and prevention of joint contractures. Anti-inflammatory agents such as tolmetin sodium (Tolectin) and indomethacin (Indocin) are frequently prescribed. Aspirin, however, is the most common. Aspirin is given in doses of 75–100 mg/kg/day (Fink, 1979). This is high enough to decrease inflammation and provide analgesic effect, but low enough to avoid toxicity. Salycilate levels are monitored constantly.

Gold salts are sometimes given, although their therapeutic value in children is questionable. They are given in weekly injections over a period of several months before their therapeutic effects become evident.

Corticosteroids are not ordinarily prescribed because of their serious side effects and also because of their tendency to mask other infections. If prescribed, it is usually because of carditis or the fact that other treatment has failed and there is a massive effort to reduce the inflammatory process.

In addition to drug therapy, a regular program of physical therapy and exercise is ordered. This may include not only exercise of the joints, but also applications of heat in various forms including wax treatments, hot packs, and whirlpool. In some cases immobility of an affected joint is desired. This may be accomplished with either traction or a splint, depending upon the joint involved.

Because JRA can be aggravated by stress, physicians must treat the child holistically. Children are usually hospitalized during the diagnostic period or during acute flare-ups. Many physicians believe it is less stressful for the child to be at home participating in as many activities as possible. Parents can be taught the physical therapy and heat treatments, or the physical therapy can be done through a community nursing agency.

Because of the long-term nature of the disease, the family may experience an overwhelming financial burden. If this happens, they may become more susceptible to claims of miraculous cures. Quackery has become a thriving business that directs itself to making money for so-called cures of arthritis. It is the health team's responsibility, and a necessary part of the treatment scheme, to be educated and to educate patients and parents to avoid quick cures. Pamphlets published by the US Government Printing Office and the Arthritis Foundation give objective viewpoints about legitimate treatments, as well as listing those treatments that are questionable.

It is worth mentioning that researchers are accumulating data constantly about the etiology and treatments of JRA. Recently a new treatment called plasmaphoresis has been attempted for JRA and SLE, another autoimmune disease; its value is still questionable. Based on a principle similar to kidney dialysis, the treatment calls for blood to be removed from the client. The blood is then filtered to remove antibody–antigen complexes and replaced along with donated plasma. The treatment is necessary several times a week and is very expensive. Plasmaphoresis as an aid in the care of clients with arthritis is too new to be considered effective, although preliminary results are promising. When data collection is complete, it may be a treatment of choice in the future (Colen, 1981).

Nursing Management Nursing care of the child with JRA is multifaceted and challenging. It provides nurses with the opportunity of giving holistic care while excelling in their function as team coordinators. Since this condition may result in repeated hospitalizations for the child, continuity of care is vitally important. The primary goal of nursing intervention is to prevent complications without restricting the child's normal development. Additionally, the nurse needs to encourage the parent to strike a healthy balance between protection and overprotection.

While the child is hospitalized, interventions are directed toward preventing joint contractures, alleviating pain, observing for complications, and providing emotional support.

Nursing observations include recognition of signs of salycilism, notations about disease progression, and comments about the child's emotional status. If synovial fluid aspiration is necessary, the nurse should explain the procedure to child and family and provide support during it. This can be a threatening experience, but fear can be minimized by a step-by-step realistic explanation.

Dr Elizabeth McAnarney and Barry Pless, MD (1975) in an article titled "Psychological Problems of JRA Patients" give several situations the nurse may encounter while caring for a child with JRA. In addition to psychologic problems related to normal development, children have problems according to the severity of their disease and the family's ability to cope.

Children in early childhood whose primary focus is mobility experience developmental deprivation when activity is limited. They have a narrowed view of their environment and can become fearful when forced to expand. Conversely, if they derive emotional gain from voluntarily limiting their horizons, they will demonstrate decreased independence (McAnarney and Pless, 1975).

Children in middle childhood, embarrassed by their limitation, may become passive about activity for fear of failing to keep up with peers. At other times, they may act out their anger and frustration at the situation (McAnarney and Pless, 1975).

One of the major developmental tasks of adolescents is the development of independence. When limited by disease to dependence on others, they react with anger and depression (McAnarney and Pless, 1975).

Nurses must identify and work with these psychologic problems but, more importantly, should assist parents to recognize them and intervene. It is difficult for parents to let go and encourage the child to perform at an appropriate developmental level. The concern is that the child will become overtired and precipitate an exacerbation. The other side of the coin, however, is an overprotectiveness that stifles normal development. The nurse then should work with parents and children and teach them how to recognize fatigue and limit activity accordingly. The child should be encouraged to exercise moderately, with exercise such as biking, swimming, and playing tennis, as exercise is good for joint mobility. Contact sports should be avoided. Attention should be focused on adequate rest and good nutritional habits.

In preparing for discharge, the nurse should refer the child to a visiting nurse for continuity of care in the home. Parents are taught heat application and physical therapy routines. The Visiting Nurse Association (VNA) may be able to help obtain any needed equipment.

Parents should be encouraged to explain to the school teacher what can realistically be expected from the child. The disease has an unpredictable course and severity of symptoms can vary from day to day. Flexibility is required from all concerned.

The Arthritis Foundation has local chapters in every state and is available as a resource to the public. Parents should be encouraged to contact the Foundation for further information about the disease and its implications for home care.

Systemic Lupus Erythematosus

Systemic lupus erythematosus (SLE) is the last of the autoimmune diseases to be discussed, although it is by far the most complex. It generally affects women of childbearing age although it is seen frequently in younger girls. The disease is not rare and 20% of cases are in girls over age 8 (Behrman and Vaughan, 1983). The disease rarely affects boys, the female-to-male ratio being approximately 5 to 1. Less than 30 years ago, SLE was considered to be a fatal disease. Now, with improved approaches, the disease may not be curable, but approximately 90% of those affected can achieve a remission of 10 years or longer.

Lupus affects nearly all body systems and thus increases its complexity as an immune system disease. The cause is unknown although several precipitating factors are acknowledged. Disease onset may be triggered by exposure to ultraviolet light, drugs, pregnancy, or stress.

The immune mechanisms are little understood. There is a possibility that any of the precipitating factors can alter cell structure as to allow for escape of nuclear contents—DNA, RNA, ribosomes (Muir, 1980). These nuclear elements function as antigens, causing production of autoantibodies. Complexes of DNA antibody–antigens lodge in multiple body tissues—skin, joints, heart, lungs, kidneys, brain, and circulatory vessels—and produce onsite inflammatory reactions. Because there is an increased incidence in families, it is theorized that there may be a genetic influence. Many women with the disease have been found to have diminished complement levels, particularly C_2. Since the production of complement is influenced by heredity, this may account for the familial occurrence (Gavaghan, 1980). Finally, it is theorized that in the patient with SLE, antibodies bind to T suppressor cells, making them less effective. Because of this suppression of suppressor cells, B cells become overactive, causing overproduction of antibodies and autoantibodies (Gerhold).

The American Rheumatism Association has established 14 criteria (Figure 37-5) for purposes of diagnosing SLE. Presence of four or more is strongly suggestive of a positive diagnosis. The prognosis of clients with SLE is good and improving as more research is conducted to determine the nature of the disease. The prognosis is, however, related to the involvement of vital organs, particularly the kidneys. Depending upon the location of immune complexes in the kidneys, they may be more or less responsive to therapy. Fatalities would be due to renal failure.

Initial clinical manifestations include fatigue, weight loss, fever, and joint tenderness. These may be accompanied by mental or emotional alterations, including headaches and seizures. Erythematous rashes appear. The classic symptom is the butterfly rash that affects both cheeks and the nasal bridge. The symptoms may seem worse after exposure to the sun. A small percentage of clients experience ongoing Raynaud's phenomenon, which is peripheral vasospasm causing pallor and numbness in fingers and toes in response to exposure to cold or emotional stress.

Because of its similarity to many of the other immune system disorders, the disease may be difficult to diagnose. Laboratory studies indicate a positive LE cell, decreased complement levels, positive C-reactive protein, and positive test for syphilis. Any or all of these can be present in other immune system disorders. The definitive test for a

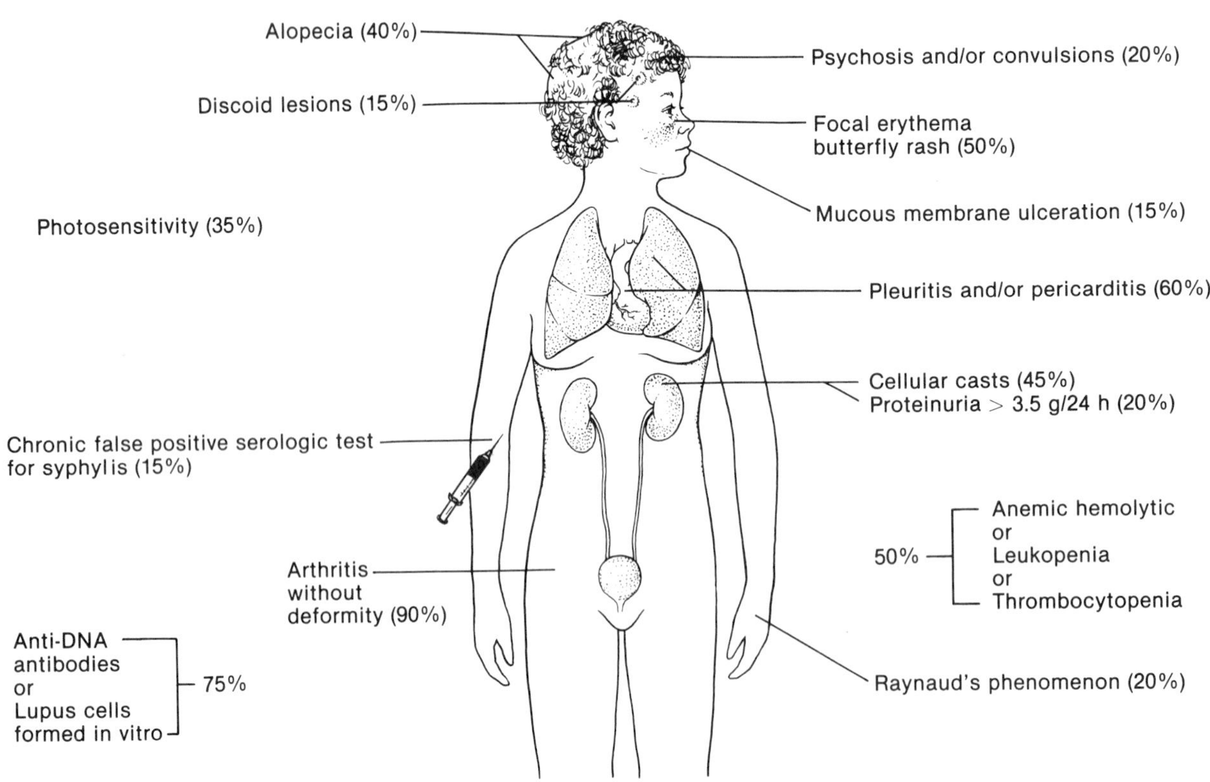

Figure 37-5 Major diagnostic criteria of systemic lupus erythematosus (SLE). At least four criteria should be present for diagnosis. (Modified from American Rheumatism Association criteria.)

positive diagnosis of SLE is the presence of ANA and, more specifically, the anti-DNA antibodies. The synovial fluid contains fewer leukocytes than in JRA and may exhibit the presence of LE cells.

As the disease progresses, there may be an increase in systemic involvement. Proteinuria is one of the first signs of immune complexes in the kidney. Complexes in the lungs cause pleurisy and cardiac inflammation is detected by ECG or audible sounds. There may be anemia, leukopenia, and a decrease in platelets.

Treatment Since disease exacerbation tends to increase during times of sun exposure or stress, treatment is initially directed toward avoiding trigger mechanisms. Girls are encouraged to avoid the sun or to apply an effective sunscreen during exposure. The holistic approach encourages plenty of rest, good nutritional habits, and a positive outlook on life. Infections are treated vigorously.

If arthritis occurs, salycilates are ordered both as anti-inflammatory agents and for pain relief. The dosage is regulated so serum levels are maintained at the upper limit of the therapeutic range. Other medications commonly used to treat SLE are antimalarial agents and corticosteroids. Antimalarials such as chloroquine are prescribed for their anti-inflammatory action. They are often given in conjunction with steroids to enhance effectiveness, as well as allow for a reduced steroid dosage. Chloroquine can cause gastrointestinal disturbances and must be used with caution because of the incidence of visual disturbances (Govoni and Hayes, 1982).

More recently researchers have attempted treatment with immunosuppressive therapy—nitrogen mustard and methotrexate, and methotrexate being most often used. This mode of treatment is still in experimental phases and is used with extreme caution because of undesirable side effects.

Finally, the physician must be aware of the role of stress in the disease process. Clients should be encouraged to verbalize feelings about having a long-term illness and the physician needs to emphasize the positive prognosis. Careful monitoring of levels of complement, anti-DNA antibody, and immune complexes can prevent serious complications by ensuring prompt treatment. A referral for mental health and emotional counseling is indicated for obvious problems.

Nursing Management Nursing care is directed toward maintaining open lines of communication between nurse, client, and family. Because many clients are adolescents, they are concerned about appearance. Alopecia may be distressful. The nurse might encourage use of a wig and other aids to improve or maintain appearance. As mentioned earlier, adolescents are attempting to achieve independence. Nurses need to recognize this developmental need by promoting independence and allowing clients control over part of their therapy. Medication schedules should be planned to coordinate as much as possible with the client's life-style. Clients need to administer their own medicines and should be taught to recognize undesirable side effects. Unfortunately, some parental control is needed because adolescents may skip doses in the normal spirit of rebellion.

If Raynaud's phenomenon presents a problem, measures to prevent its occurrence should be discussed. When the child expects to be exposed to the cold, layered clothing is the dress of choice. The air space between layers insulates. Mittens are preferable to gloves, and wide-toed boots allow for freedom of toe movement. Mylar or silk gloves and sock liners help retain warmth.

Raynaud's phenomenon occurs in summer as well as winter, and so the child should avoid swimming in cold water. Something as simple as holding an ice cream cone can trigger vasospasm. Simple measures like wrapping the cone or ice cream stick with paper napkins will alleviate the problem.

If the child cannot participate in normal activities, the nurse should attempt to discover an area in which the child can excel while not overextending. This will foster improved self-image and a more positive outlook on life.

The Lupus Erythematosus Foundation has chapters in many cities and states. It is a helpful resource as it offers support to clients and families and disseminates information to the public for increased public awareness.

The Child With an Immune Complex Disease

Mucocutaneous Lymph Node Syndrome—Kawasaki Disease

In 1961 Dr Tomisaku Kawasaki identified a collection of symptoms occurring with increasing frequency among Japanese children. Since then the disease has affected children in other parts of the world and has become more frequent in the United States. The Centers for Disease Control has been keeping accurate records of children with suspected Kawasaki Disease since 1974 and has been able to identify epidemiologic trends in the United States (Morens and Nahmias, 1978). The disease affects children of both sexes, although boys predominate. Average age of onset is 4 years. The disease is not contagious and its precipitating factor is unknown. Studies investigating possible viral or rickettsial origins or environmental antigens have so far proved inconclusive. Increase in the erythrocyte sedimentation rate and circulating immunoglobulin levels, along with a markedly elevated white blood count ($15-40 \times 10^3$) and platelet count (above 500,000), may point to an inflammatory response of an immune complex disease.

Because the disease incidence has risen dramatically since 1960, environmental factors probably provide the closest link. However, this increase may actually be due to better identification and reporting methods.

Kawasaki disease affects multiple body systems, predominantly the skin, mucous membranes of the respiratory tract, lymph nodes, and heart. Fatality rate is low, with death being the result of cardiac difficulties, particularly aneurysms. It is felt that the fatality chance is greater in boys under 1 year of age.

The syndrome is self-limiting and usually resolves after 3 to 4 weeks. Approximately 2% of the children contracting the disease are left with cardiac damage, particularly aortic aneurysm, and need close postrecovery supervision. This damage can appear even years after recovery (Morens and Nahmias, 1978).

Careful studies of children with this disease have contributed to the delineation of criteria for diagnosis. Because the symptoms mimic other diseases, physicians have established that five of six criteria are necessary for disease diagnosis (Table 37-6). The disease begins with a high fever, followed by generalized rash, conjunctivitis, oral and peripheral changes, and enlarged nodes. The children are extremely irritable, reminiscent of central nervous system pressure. They appear acutely ill.

As the disease progresses, they may experience symptoms of arthritis. Cardiac changes appear on ECG. Blood work reveals a highly elevated white blood count ($15-40 \times 10^3$). Platelets are increased above 500,000 after the second week. The increase in platelets causes obstruction of the digital capillaries, resulting in peripheral stasis and necrosis of the digits. The ESR is usually elevated and immunoglobulins are also in some cases. Blood tests are negative for ANA and LE cell. ECG monitoring is performed regularly and usually indicates cardiac changes during the acute stage. Desquamation of the skin on the fingers, palms, and plantar surfaces occurs during the second week. The ECG will usually revert to normal upon disease resolution. The ESR decreases within 6 to 8 weeks (Lynch and Gray, 1982).

Treatment is symptomatic. There is no known drug that will enhance recovery or prevent complications. There is a possibility that excessively high doses of aspirin (140 mg per kilogram of body weight) may speed recovery and prevent the occurrence of aneurysm.

Nursing interventions during the acute phase of the disease are directed toward maintaining comfort. Tepid sponge baths decrease the fever and relieve the discomfort from skin manifestations (Lynch and Gray, 1982). The nurse should maintain adequate hydration. Since the inflammatory process affects the mucous membranes, clear, cool liquids may provide relief as well as fluid volume (Lynch and Gray, 1982). Environmental stimuli are reduced to minimize irritability. Parental support is essential, particularly since the child appears so acutely ill and there is a danger of cardiac complications. The nurse must observe for changes in vital signs and report the occurrence of tachycardia or arrhythmias to the physician.

Parents must be allowed to express their concerns but can be assured of the child's spontaneous recovery. Discharge planning should emphasize the need for regular cardiac testing for early recognition of cardiac complications.

TABLE 37-6 Diagnostic Criteria for Kawasaki Disease

1. Fever of five or more days*
2. Bilateral congestion of ocular conjunctivae
3. Changes of the mucous membranes of the upper respiratory tract:**
   Injected pharynx
   Red, dry, fissured lips
   Protuberance of tongue papillae (strawberry-tongue)
4. Changes of the peripheral extremities:**
   Peripheral edema
   Peripheral erythema
   Desquamation
   Periungual desquamation
5. Rash, primarily truncal and polymorphous
6. Cervical lymph node swelling (nonpurulent)

*The diagnosis of KD is considered confirmed by fever and four of the remaining five criteria.

**One or more of these findings is sufficient to establish the criterion

From Lynch M, Gray J: Kawasaki disease. *Pediatr Nurs* (March/April) 1982; 8:96–101. Reprinted with permission of the publisher, Anthony J. Jannetti, Inc. from *Pediatr Nurs.*

Henoch–Shöenlein (H.S.) Purpura

Henoch–Shöenlein (H.S.) purpura is a disease that can be precipitated by exposure to medications, infection, or insect bites. It is a relatively common condition affecting children 2–8 years old with boys being affected twice as often as girls (Behrman and Vaughan, 1983). The immune insult causes increased circulatory immune complexes of IgG, which effuse into skin, mucous membranes, joints, and other body systems (*Nursing Mirror,* 1983).

H.S. purpura is a self-limiting disease that usually resolves in approximately 6 weeks. Full recovery is expected, although the child may experience sudden gastrointestinal complications, intussusception being the most common. Occasionally, acute or chronic renal problems develop that mimic glomerulonephritis.

The onset of H.S. purpura can be sudden or gradual. The child may complain of abdominal cramping or nausea. Arthritis-like symptoms affect various joints, usually of the lower extremities. Purpuric lesions most often appear on the buttocks and legs, although they can also be elsewhere. Over the course of the disease the lesions change color from pink to purple, then fade to yellowish brown before disappearing. The child may be febrile. Blood studies reveal leukocytosis, elevated ESR, and elevated IgA concentrations. Bleeding and clotting times are generally normal as are platelet counts. Unless there is internal bleeding from gastrointestinal or renal complications, hematocrit and hemoglobin will also be within normal range. Urinalysis will demonstrate increased leukocytes and erythrocytes if there is kidney involvement. The stool should be examined for presence of occult blood.

Treatment Treatment is symptomatic. Salycilates are prescribed for pain. The child is observed for gastrointestinal complications and signs of nephritis. Renal involvement usually resolves but may recur later in life as chronic renal disease. Rarely, the child may exhibit signs of central nervous system involvement. Treatment with steroids seems to alleviate this condition.

Nursing Management Primary nursing interventions include observation for internal organ involvement. Vital signs, particularly blood pressure, should be performed on a regular basis to detect indications of internal bleeding. The nurse should keep accurate records of intake and output and should observe or test urine and stools for presence of frank or occult blood. A markedly decreased urine output may be indicative of impending renal failure. A careful description of pain will assist the physician to diagnose problems.

If the child experiences any transient arthritis, it should be stressed to the child and parents that this is temporary and will resolve itself. Diversional activities must be presented that include range-of-motion activities to exercise joints. If the child is confined to bed, the nurse must take precautions to prevent complications from immobility.

Discharge planning includes instructions to parents for recognizing signs of renal difficulty. The nurse should caution them that kidney problems may not appear for many years and that, when old enough, the child should be advised of symptoms. If a drug has been implicated as a possible cause, it should be avoided in the future. Any sign of frank blood in the urine or stool should be immediately reported to the physician. Parents should be encouraged to keep follow-up appointments.

The Child With an Allergic Manifestation

As was previously discussed, an allergic reaction is a result of a hypersensitive immune system response. Immediate hypersensitivity reactions are mediated by IgE response to an allergen, resulting in a release of chemicals that may have adverse effects on the body, including such symptoms as respiratory distress, skin manifestations, and vascular hypotension. Delayed hypersensitivity is caused by a T-lymphocyte response to certain allergens.

Allergic reactions can be local or generalized and they can be immediate or delayed. Initial contact with an allergen does not usually evoke an histamine response. However, subsequent exposures will activate histamine release.

Localized Allergic Reactions

Integument Allergic skin manifestations include a variety of rashes, most common of which are eczema, urticaria (hives), and lesions from contact allergens. Pruritis (itching) from any of these can be severe and cause the child extreme discomfort.

An eczematous rash may be initially dry and red, followed by scaling. If the eczema becomes chronic, skin thickening can occur, causing a leathery appearance. Itching is constant and can be exacerbated by dryness.

Urticaria (hives) is caused by the release of histamine. Capillaries in the skin dilate and allow exudation of fluid. This results in a raised, plaquelike wheal that can be intensely itchy. Urticaria can differ in size from pinpoint to extremely large. Hives are transitory in nature, appearing, disappearing, and reappearing in various body locations. They can be acute or chronic and are caused by a wide variety of environmental factors including pressure, heat, cold, food, drugs, and stress. Often, there is no observable cause and the urticaria resolves spontaneously. Antihistamines are given to reduce the pruritis by decreasing the histamine action.

Contact dermatitis most commonly consists of erythema followed by the appearance of vesicles that, upon rupture, form yellowish crusts. In severe cases, there may be a constant weeping of fluid with subsequent loss of the surface skin layer. Pruritis can be intense.

Allergic skin manifestations can occur singly or in combination with one another, depending upon the irritant and the magnitude of the response. Urticaria is also a symptom in systemic allergic responses.

Mucous Membranes Allergens can affect the mucous membranes of the eyes and upper respiratory tracts. The membranes become red, edematous, and itchy. There may be an increase in clear mucous discharge. Rhinitis and conjunctivitis are common examples of eye and upper respiratory allergic manifestations. They often occur together as a result of seasonal pollen and are referred to as hay fever. Frequent sneezing is an initial symptom, followed by itchiness and rhinorrhea. Some children have dark circles under their eyes that do not disappear. This may be an indication that the child is suffering from an inhalant allergy. Edema of nasal passages can cause a sinus headache.

Systemic Allergic Reactions

Gastrointestinal Tract Histamine causes spasm of the smooth muscles, resulting in gastrointestinal symptoms on contact with an allergen—usually food. Symptoms include abdominal cramping, nausea, vomiting, and diarrhea. In infants, colic is the predominant manifestation.

Respiratory System Lower respiratory tract allergies are complicated by histamine's effect on smooth muscles. Smooth muscle spasm of the bronchioles can cause bronchospasm. Bronchospasm leads to air trapping in the lungs, with a resulting disturbance in oxygenation (asthma). Asthma may be precipitated by a number of irritants, including pollens, foods, and stress.

Vascular System Vasodilatation in the brain can cause migraine headaches. These headaches are severe and are often accompanied by nausea, vomiting, and light sensitivity. Foods have been implicated as precipitating factors, particularly those containing amines such as chocolate, cheese, alcohol, and citrus fruits (Grant, 1979). Avoidance of a known precipitator will reduce the attacks. Ergotamine, a drug that promotes vasoconstriction, has been effective when given at the onset of an attack of migraine.

Anaphylaxis Anaphylaxis is a systemic allergic response to an excessive release of histamine. It may occur suddenly in response to an allergen that has not previously evoked a reaction. In addition to histamine, two other chemical mediators affect the magnitude of the response—SRS-A and bradykinin (see Fig. 37-4). Because these do not respond to the administration of antihistamines, the reaction is severe and life-threatening (Harmon, 1980).

Initial symptoms of impending anaphylaxis include sneezing, generalized urticaria, weakness, and restlessness. These symptoms may be followed by laryngeal spasms and edema, gastrointestinal symptoms, dyspnea, and signs of circulatory collapse. If untreated, death occurs from blocked airway and vascular shutdown. Anaphylaxis can occur from seconds to approximately 30 minutes after exposure to an allergen. The most common precipitating factors are insect stings, penicillin (particularly when administered intravenously), and foods.

Irritant Allergens

Allergic reactions occur after exposure to many allergens. Not everyone will develop allergies, although allergic tendencies appear to be familial. As our environment becomes more complex, and new chemical compounds are synthesized and used in industry, our chances for developing allergies increase. Allergic irritants fall under four distinct categories—environmental, food, insects, and medications.

Environmental Irritants There are a multitude of environmental factors related to development of allergic response. Whether the irritants are inhaled, applied, or intrinsic usually determines the type of allergic manifestation. Inhalants usually result in upper or lower respiratory problems, while applied irritants cause dermatitis in various forms. Intrinsic factors of stress and emotional upset affect the whole spectrum of allergic disease.

Inhalants include pollens, dust, molds and mildew, fungi, and animal dander. The most common pollen allergen is ragweed, with goldenrod being a close second. Pollen allergies tend to be seasonal, occurring primarily in the spring or the fall or whenever the plants are flourishing.

Dust, mold, and mildew inhalants occur in many older homes, particularly those that are damp. Mildew may develop beneath wall coverings, in bathrooms, and in furniture as well as other household locations. In this case, the allergic response is chronic and will not disappear until the child is removed from the environment.

Animal dander (scales from animal hair) is a common inhalant allergen, made more irritating because a child can react not only by direct contact with the animal, but also by contact with clothes or furnishing the animal has touched. Down bird feathers react similarly. In a study by Murray (1983) it was found that cats were more likely to produce allergies than dogs in sensitive children.

Applied irritants usually include allergens that come in direct contact with the skin. They include items like heat and cold, as well as various forms of clothing and cosmetics. Wool clothing can be highly irritating, particularly if damp. In addition, a child who experiences any type of contact dermatitis would do well to use hypoallergenic cosmetics. Permanents and hair coloring kits should be skin tested before use. Sunscreens containing para-aminobenzoic acid (PABA) are also irritants.

Another class of applied irritants are plant oils. Poison ivy, oak, and sumac along with some less well-known plants can cause dermatitis. The dermatitis varies in degree of severity, depending upon the time lapse involved between contacts.

Food Any food can be allergenic to a specific individual. Frequently seen food irritants include milk, wheat, eggs, citrus fruits, chocolate, nuts, and shellfish. It is recommended that all common food allergens be withheld from a baby's diet until after 6 months of age. Since cow's milk is a common irritant, mothers who have a known allergic history or a familial history of allergies should breast feed exclusively for at least 6 months before adding foods or milk products (Hamburger, 1979). Foods should be added to the baby's diet one at a time and spaced several days apart to observe for an allergic response. Food allergies take many forms, including rashes, irritation of the gastrointestinal tract, respiratory manifestations, and irritation of the neurologic system (headache, irritability) (White and

Owsley, 1983). Known food allergens such as orange juice and tomatoes may be mixed into commercial baby food preparations either to flavor or preserve. Parents should be taught to read labels prior to giving their children commercial baby food. Estimates of the risk of food allergies to infants with allergic parents are as follows (Hamburger, 1979):

Both parents with allergy	40% chance for child
One parent with allergy	29%
Neither parent	13%

Insects Hymenoptera are insects of the bee, wasp, and hornet variety. Stinging insects, aside from causing local inflammation at the sting site, can cause generalized anaphylaxis. Unless the stinger is removed carefully, the toxin can remain active at the site, increasing the severity of the reaction.

Medications Antibiotics, specifically penicillin and its derivatives, can cause general urticaria or anaphylaxis, or both. Some drugs like cephalexin (Keflex) are chemically related to penicillin and should be given with extreme caution to known allergic children. Occasionally, medication preparations, especially some immunizations like measles vaccine, are prepared or grown in egg white. For this reason, they should be administered with caution to children allergic to eggs.

Assessment Specific to Allergic Reactions

History

In addition to routine history taking, the nurse needs to concentrate on eliciting detailed information about allergic manifestations and precipitating factors. Depending upon the age of the child and the type of allergy manifested, certain areas will need greater emphasis. An allergy survey can be conducted in the hospital upon admission or, even better, in the home if the child is being treated as an outpatient. A home assessment will allow the nurse to construct a more detailed data base for later intervention. See Figure 37-6 for the allergy survey sheet. This survey should be completed by the nurse, not by the parent, since questions may need to be explained or information expanded upon.

Validating Diagnostic Tests

The child presenting with severe allergic manifestations will undergo a variety of tests designed to document the allergic reaction and determine the precipitators. Routine blood work, radiographs, and urine studies are performed. Special attention is given to an increased eosinophil count in the differential. Elevated eosinophils seem to be a compensatory reaction in response to histamine release. Blood work also includes immunoglobulin levels. Children who are allergic demonstrate higher levels of IgE than the general population. Elevated IgE levels, particularly in infants, tend to predict future allergic occurrences (Hamburger, 1979).

Skin Tests In order to determine a specific allergen, the allergist may elect to perform skin tests. There are three different approaches to skin testing—the scratch, the prick, and injections. All work on the same principle; that is, a specific allergen is introduced and will cause a small localized reaction if the client is sensitive. Tests are done on either the forearm or back. Usually, allergens of a class are tested at the same time. For the *scratch test,* a small scratch is made with a sterile tool after allergens have been placed on the skin. The scratches are usually done in a pattern to facilitate identification of the allergen. The *prick test* is a similar method using a needle and solution; *injections* are intercutaneous. The test chosen depends upon the physician's preference. After a time period, reactions are noted. If the child is sensitive, a raised wheal will be evident. The size of the wheal determines the degree of the sensitivity (Patterson, 1980). It is important to note that certain medications such as epinephrine, aminophylline, and antihistamines may alter the accuracy of the tests and should not be taken prior to testing.

Radioallergosorbent Test There are two major drawbacks to skin testing. First, at any time a child could experience a massive allergic reaction to one of the allergens used in testing. Second, in circumstances where allergic dermatitis is the sensitivity response, there can be enough alteration in the skin to make testing unreliable. In these cases, allergists prefer to use the radioallergosorbent test (RAST) method.

The RAST method involves in vitro blood testing, that is, combining antigen with antibody in a laboratory. Allergens are introduced to the sample to see if they will activate IgE specific to the allergen. This will indicate whether the allergen has previously provoked an antibody response. Because the test is done in vitro, it poses no danger to the client. It is particularly useful to test allergic reactions to stings, penicillin, and certain foods.

Provocation Tests Food allergies can be so confusing because of the number and variety of foods available that provocation tests are conducted to determine specific allergens. First, a food diary is kept for several days to record everything eaten and whether reactions occur. The child then may be placed on a diet free from known allergens. After several days on a diet without an allergic reaction,

ALLERGY SURVEY SHEET

Name ______ Age ______ Sex ______ Date ______

Chief complaint

Present illness

Associated allergic symptoms

Eyes: Pruritis______ Burning______ Tearing______
Swelling______ Infection______ Discharge______

Ears: Pruritis______ Fullness______ Popping______
Frequent infections______

Nose: Sneezing______ Rhinorrhea______ Obstruction______
Pruritis______ Mouth breathing______
Prurulent discharge______

Throat: Soreness______ Postnasal discharge______ Mucus in A.M.______
Palatal pruritis______

Chest: Sputum______ Dyspnea______ Wheezing______
Color______ Rest______
Amount______ Exertion______

Skin: Dermatitis______ Eczema______ Urticaria______

Family allergies

Previous allergic treatment or testing

Skin testing

Drugs taken		Improved	Unimproved
	Antihistamines	______	______
	Bronchodilators	______	______
	Nose drops	______	______
	Hyposensitization	______	______
	Antibiotics	______	______
	Steroids	______	______

Physical agents and habits. Are you bothered by

Cigarette smoke______ Heat______ Air conditioner______
Cold______ Muggy weather______ Weather changes______
Perfume______ Paints______ Insecticides______
Cosmetics______ Chemicals______ Hairspray______
Pollens______ Clothing______ Sun______
Animals/feathers______ Dust______ Adhesive tape______

Food agents. Describe reaction to

Formula______ Cereals______ Fruits______
Vegetables______ Meats______ Juices______
Cheese______ Milk______ Eggs______
Soda______ Fish______ Nuts______
Citrus______

In infants: How and when were foods introduced?

Figure 37-6 Allergy survey sheet. This survey should be filled out by the nurse, not the parent, because questions may need clarification or information may need expansion. (Adapted from Patterson R: *Allergic Diseases—Diagnosis and Management.* Lippincott, 1980, pp 78–79.)

Where symptoms occur

Place of residence at onset
Place of residence since onset
Symptoms better indoors or out
Effect of school
Effect of staying elsewhere nearby
Effect of hospitalization
Do symptoms occur around

Old leaves______	Hay______	Lakeside______
Barns______	Summer homes______	Damp basement______
Dry attic______	Lawn mowing______	Animals______
Other______		

Home: City______ Rural______
House______ Age______
Apartment______ Basement______ damp______ dry______
Heating system______
Pets______ dog______ cat______ hamster______ bird______

Bedroom: Type	Age	Living: Type	Age
Pillow______	______	Rug______	______
Mattress______	______	Furniture______	______
Blankets______	______	Curtains______	______
Furniture______	______	Stuffed animals______	______
		Security blanket______	______

Are symptoms worse anywhere else in home?

When symptoms occur

Time and circmstances of first episode
Prior health
Course of illness over time
Time of year Perennial______
Seasonal______
Seasonally exacerbated______
Time of week (weekends vs weekdays)
Time of day or night
After insect stings

What does child or family think makes the child worse?

Is the child ever free of symptoms?

Other comments

Figure 37-6 continued

foods are introduced one at a time at 6-hour intervals (Parker, 1980). Reactions are noted. In this way, specific foods can be identified for avoidance. It must be kept in mind, however, that many foods are combined with preservatives or use artificial flavors and colors. The child may not be allergic to the food itself, but to the artificial ingredients.

Other types of provocation tests are tried in the hospital setting. An example of this would be the hymenoptera challenge test. After the child has been desensitized (received allergy shots), the allergist may wish to test the efficiency of the desensitization. The child is stung under controlled conditions and observed for reactions. Of course, the obstacle to this type of challenge is the life-threatening reaction that can occur from the sting.

Nursing Management for Treatments and Procedures

Acute-Care Needs

Preparation for Diagnostic Tests Children should be prepared for blood withdrawal as mentioned earlier in this chapter. Because skin testing can be equally as frightening to the child, the explanation of the procedure should be similar to that for an injection. The nurse should approach the explanation with the child's cognitive level in mind. It is possible that there will be pruritis during the skin testing. The child should be aware of this and encouraged not to scratch. If itching occurs, the nurse should attempt distraction techniques, particularly the introduction of toys involving use of the hands. For a young child this might be a puzzle; the older child might enjoy a computer game.

Diet challenge tests can be most annoying to a child, and adolescents may be particularly difficult to control in this area. The diet may be boring. The adolescent who is free to wander in the hospital may be tempted to cheat. A complete explanation of the purpose of this test should be given in order to ensure cooperation. It should be explained that any variation from the prescribed regimen will prolong the test as well as the hospitalization. Older children can participate in their care by recording reactions themselves or reporting them to the nurse as they occur. Families also need to be informed about the test so they won't bring foods from home for the child to eat. All unauthorized food must be removed from the child's environment.

Emergency Care for Anaphylaxis Anaphylactic reactions can occur both in and out of the hospital. They most often occur as the result of an insect sting but can follow administration of certain medications, or following desensitization injections. Supportive therapy must be administered immediately, since it may be only a matter of minutes before the child goes into shock.

In case of an insect sting, a tourniquet should be applied just proximal to the sting site if possible. It should be tight, but not tight enough to cut off the circulation to the limb. Immediately after, the child should receive 0.2–0.5 mL of 1:1000 aqueous epinephrine subcutaneously, depending on body weight (0.01 mL/kg of body weight). The injection should be repeated at 20-minute intervals until help is obtained. The child should also be treated for shock by being kept warm and lying flat or with feet slightly elevated. If the child is conscious, administer nonalcoholic liquids slowly.

In a controlled setting such as a physician's office or hospital, the epinephrine should be followed by diphenhydramine (Benadryl) given intravenously or intramuscularly. An IV should be started to maintain a line for fluid replacement in case of shock. The nurse should maintain an adequate airway and keep a tracheostomy kit and laryngoscope available at the bedside. The nurse must take frequent vital signs, especially blood pressure, and observe for signs of shock. Should the client appear to have signs of impending circulatory collapse, extra fluids and plasma expanders would be given intravenously.

Epinephrine is a drug that causes vasoconstriction. Its effect is rapid but lasts for only a short time. It is given to prevent circulatory collapse and effects this by causing vasoconstriction and resulting increase in cardiac output. Children receiving this drug experience tachycardia and possible heart palpitations. For this reason, they may be extremely frightened and experience a high degree of anxiety. The nurse can reassure them that these effects are normal and will eventually disappear.

Desensitization Under some circumstances, allergen desensitization may be indicated. Desensitization may be seasonal or year round depending on the allergens involved. The procedure involves injecting minute amounts of the allergen subcutaneously to trick the immune system into accepting the allergen. The underlying principle is that by introducing allergens in extremely small quantities the immune system will develop tolerance to it. Injections are usually given weekly, with gradually increasing allergen concentrations until tolerance is reached. Monthly maintenance doses are then administered. If the child develops a local or systemic reaction, the schedule reverts to the previous concentration that did not produce a reaction. If the procedure provides allergy relief, it is usually discontinued after 2 years.

The child and family need to know about the injections and the fact that the child must remain in the physician's office for at least 20 minutes after each injection to be observed for reactions. The nurse in the office must always be alert for signs of anaphylaxis, and epinephrine should be available at all times.

Nutritional Needs

Since food is a common source of allergens, it may be necessary for the nurse to assist the child and family with identification of allergens and dietary management.

If the mother is unable or unwilling to breast-feed her baby, hypoallergenic formulas may be advised. These are usually soybean preparations such as Isomil or Prosobee. In extreme cases, meat-based formula may be recommended.

The child may be older, however, before an allergy is evident. Pinpointing the foods responsible is time consuming and requires much patience and strict adherence to a prescribed dietary regimen. The physician may elect to try food challenges or elimination diets.

Elimination diets are the reversal of food challenges. The child or parent keeps a diet record for an established time period, noting any reactions. After that, suspected allergens are eliminated one at a time from the diet, each for a period of several days. If reactions subside, that food is implicated as an allergen. Elimination diets are often followed by food challenges. The allergen is reintroduced to confirm the allergic response.

Elimination diets are often done at home. It is the nurse's responsibility to make certain both child and family understand what is expected. The child's cooperation should be enlisted whenever possible. Because there are so many sources outside the home where the child may have access to food, the child's active participation is essential for a successful test.

Once specific allergens have been identified, the general treatment is avoidance. All foods containing the allergen should be eliminated from the diet. Parents need to become label watchers. So many foods are combined with others, either as preservatives, flavoring, or coloring, that it is well to avoid some packaged foods. Food preparation then may place an added burden on the parent who prepares the foods. Children need to be taught which foods to avoid, including hidden ingredients in common foods. A dietary consultant can assist the parent to adapt to specific diet constraints. Children need to be supported in the adjustment to a new dietary regimen. Even older children tend to cooperate with dietary restrictions, since they know they may experience reactions if they don't.

Aside from allergy to cow's milk, common special diets may be gluten-free, wheat-free, egg-free, or a combination of all. The dietician will have resources to recommend for meal planning, and books containing recipes. In order to minimize the "difference" for a child, as much dietary planning as possible should include foods children generally enjoy. Many recipes can be adapted to fit dietary restrictions. For instance, some recipes can be made without eggs by increasing the amount of baking powder and soda used and adding other spices and flavorings. If recipes call for small amounts of milk, substitute water or juice or soybean baby formulas (White and Owsley, 1983). There are many other grain flours that can be substituted for wheat flour in recipes and that may actually add to the flavor.

Developmental Needs

Adjustment to Chronicity As with children suffering from other immune system disorders, children suffering from chronic allergic conditions need to make the adjustment of coping with a long-term illness (see Chapter 30). Some children appear to outgrow their allergies, while others can keep them controlled only with vigorous therapy. The nurse needs to give both the child and family support in coping with the problems. There are two major difficulties apparent here—interruptions in schooling and curtailment of activities.

All children need to participate in activities appropriate to their age level. Problems occur when the strenuousness of an activity precipitates an attack of a respiratory allergy, such as asthma. Participation in athletics should not be discouraged for asthmatic children. However, activities involving sudden physical exertion, such as short running dashes and other bursts of activity, should be avoided. Slower, sustained activity, such as swimming, should be encouraged, because it not only allows children to participate with their peers, but also facilitates lung expansion. If a child continues to have problems with athletics, the physician might allow the child to take prescribed medication prior to participating. It cannot be emphasized enough that the child should have as normal a life as possible for complete and healthy development.

Another obstacle to normal development is the frequent interruptions in schooling that can occur in children with asthma or chronic allergic disease. Naturally, prevention and prompt treatment of episodes will cut down on absenteeism. As part of the responsibility for their own care children should be encouraged to keep up with school work even when their problems prohibit classroom attendance. Keeping up with the work will increase the child's sense of self-esteem and prevent the failure of being held back and removed from the peer group.

Development of Independence The development of independence and responsibility for one's self is a process spanning several developmental stages. Children are normally encouraged to assert themselves and assume responsibility for self-care while adhering to limits set by the parents. Unfortunately, it is easy to shelter a child suffering from a chronic illness whether out of guilt or from a sense of overprotectiveness. To a child with a chronic allergic disease, limiting independence and responsibility, regardless of age, can be destructive. The feelings evoked in the child not only retard normal development, but result in anger and frustration, both of which are detrimental to disease control.

A primary nursing intervention in the care of a child with an allergic problem is the encouragement of the parents to let go and treat the child as normally as possible. This requires great effort on the part of parents, because in actuality they must maintain control until the child is old enough to assume responsibility for self-medication. Nursing intervention toward this goal must be initiated on first contact with the family and reinforced consistently thereafter.

Children at an early age recognize overprotection and fast learn to manipulate parents accordingly. The nurse can assist parents to break the cycle by being firm and recognizing and limiting manipulative behavior. Parents need support to break the cycle, but the results will be worth the effort. To this end, the American Lung Association has developed a program for elementary-school-age children with asthma called *Superstuff*. It is a packet of play activities designed to teach asthmatic children to know the symptoms of their disease, recognize the precipitators, initiate their own treatment, and practice tension-reduction techniques. Developing responsibility for one's disease is the underlying principle. Although the packet is directed toward the child with asthma, its visual and participatory teaching method would be applicable to any child with an allergic disease. A creative nurse could devise a similar program for other allergic children.

Included in this packet is advice and assistance for parents. Situations are presented that promote parental decision making and teach the parents how to break the overprotectiveness cycle. Perhaps the most important fact emphasized is that rewards should be given for progress in assuming responsibility and independence. Rewards given for illness only encourage manipulative behavior (American Lung Association, 1981).

Emotional Needs

Stress Many allergic diseases have an emotional, psychologic component. It is often uncertain whether the disease triggers the emotional problem or whether the emotional problem triggers the disease. It is a fact, however, that stress may contribute to an enhanced antibody response. In addition, stress can activate the autonomic nervous system, resulting in the "fight or flight" mechanism. This can cause bronchospasm that will exacerbate an asthma attack or eczema. There may be a sense of depression from the chronic nature of the disease or fear that symptoms will appear suddenly (Patterson, 1980).

The family life may be disrupted when the child is diagnosed. There may be financial burdens. Allergens need to be eliminated from the environment, including cigarettes and possibly a favorite pet. Attention is focused on the identified patient, perhaps to the exclusion of the other children.

Causes of stress are both internal and external. In addition to the feelings of stress from within due to handling the adjustment to chronic disease, the child is affected by external stress in the environment. Since we have said that stress can exacerbate allergic disease, it is important for the nurse to attempt to reduce internal and external sources of stress.

Nursing interventions consist of assisting the parents to recognize and cope with the external causes of stress. This may include referrals to a visiting nurse association for allergy evaluation of the home or to a social service agency for assistance with the financial burden. It may involve encouraging the parents to take time off for themselves or for special attention to other children in the family.

Relaxation techniques should be taught to both parents and child. If parents are able to control their feelings of stress during an attack, the child will be calmer and complications may be avoided.

Techniques may be as simple as counting to ten or as complicated as meditation. Usually, the relatively simple technique of slow, deep breathing combined with complete muscle relaxation will ease feelings of stress. Children should be encouraged to practice relaxation for several minutes daily. The nurse should also encourage a technique specific for an impending attack. The "Ease Up Relaxation" record from the *Superstuff* is an example. The poem is easy to remember and, combined with slow respirations, may help the child avoid an attack.

Ease up . . .
Ease up . . .
You can be cool and so free
Let the worries go by
Let the tensions all fly
Relax, it's the best way to be . . .

Ease up, ease up
Let breathing be gentle and deep
Don't be uptight
Just relax and feel right
And you'll put your fears
all to sleep . . .

Ease up . . .
Ease up . . .
Help your worries slip past
You're breathing with ease
Just relaxed as you please
You're breathing the smart way
at last . . .

From *Superstuff,* "Ease Up Relaxation Record," American Lung Association. Reproduced with permission.

Alterations in Body Image Any number of body changes can result from allergic disease. Some, like the effects of steroids, are temporary, while others are more permanent. Eczema causes an obvious rash or a thickening of the skin, or both. Children with asthma may be smaller and more sickly in appearance than peers. Because of the destructive action of stress, teasing from peers may exacerbate the condition.

In addition to the support ordinarily given for an alteration in body image, the nurse needs to teach the child and parents how to cope with teasing. In some instances, it may involve having the child teach peers about the allergy; it may involve teaching the child a quick comeback; or it may involve suggesting methods of minimizing the appearance change. The more comfortable children feel with their peers, the more responsive they'll be with any restrictions imposed by the disease.

Parents also need to be taught how to assist the child to cope with the inevitable uncomfortable situation. The nurse can present some common situations to parent and child, depending upon the child's age level. Discussing how each would handle the situation will allow the nurse to intervene. Above all, good communication between parents and child is essential for optimum emotional health.

There have been many theories concerning the relationship between psychologic problems and chronic allergic disease. Current theories discount the early emotional trauma theories, although they admit to a definite correlation between emotional states and disease control. With early intervention and adequate attention to all family members, emotional contributors can be minimized.

Health Maintenance Needs

Parents and children need to be informed about all medications, dosages, effects, and side effects. Any inhalant medications should be carefully demonstrated. In the case of a sting allergy, both child and family members should be taught proper application of a tourniquet as well as how to administer the epinephrine. Proper timing of medications is important, particularly when steroids are required and must be given with food.

In addition to information about medications, the child and family may need information about other treatment measures. All children with sting allergies need to know how to recognize stinging insects in order to avoid them. They should be required to carry a sting kit with them when they are in areas where they may be stung. Sting kits are produced by a variety of manufacturers, and all include a tourniquet, injectible epinephrine, and an antihistamine or sublingual isoproterenol hydrochloride (Isuprel).

The parents need to be taught how to allergy-proof their home and should be referred for dietary consultation if needed. If special bath preparations are required for skin disorders, these should be explained. Children should wear Medic Alert tags if anaphylaxis is a possibility.

ALLERGY-PROOFING CHECKLIST

Routine

______	Nylon or acrylic fabrics for furniture upholstery, carpets, blankets, sweaters, and other articles of clothing. No wool
______	Cushions, pillows, and jackets filled with foam rubber or polyfill synthetic rather than feathers
______	Frequent vacuuming, daily if necessary
______	No pets with dander, particularly cats and dogs
______	Mold and mildew removed from moist surfaces, particularly in bathroom
______	Frequent dusting to remove plant pollen
______	Spray irritants (perfume, hairspray) not used in children's areas
______	Humidification and dehumidification when necessary

Special

______	Artificial Christmas tree
______	Old wallpaper removed and walls cleaned to remove spores found in old houses

The Child With a Specific Allergic Manifestation

Atopic Dermatitis—Eczema

Eczema is an allergic disease that affects the skin, particularly areas of frequent perspiration: the bend of the elbow, the back of the knees, and the hands. It is a disease of allergic origin that can be aggravated by stress. Common causes of the disease are food allergies, hair, feathers, and certain fabrics. It is more frequent in girls, most frequently in infants and toddlers, and can be associated with asthma or rhinitis. Atopic dermatitis (no known cause) occurs as a result of elevated levels of IgE specific for certain allergens eliciting an inflammatory response in the skin. Sensitivity to the allergens may occur gradually as the child is repeatedly exposed. There tends to be a familial pattern with the occurrence of this disease and it is theorized that high levels of IgE production in certain children are genetically controlled through multifactorial inheritance (Rocklin, 1984). Eczema may occur as a single episode resolving after the allergen is removed, or it may become chronic with remissions and exacerbations.

The child may initially experience localized or generalized "erythema, papules, vesiculation, oozing, crusting, and intense itching" (Stiehm, 1973). If the condition becomes chronic, the skin may thicken and take on a leathery appearance. The child is particularly susceptible to skin infections from the breakdown in the skin barrier. Laboratory results demonstrate an increase in IgE and eosinophils. See Chapter 44 for nursing management of eczema.

Asthma

Asthma is probably the most common chronic disease of childhood. It affects children of all ages and both sexes with boys in a slight majority. It is classified as extrinsic or intrinsic, intermittent or chronic, and mild, moderate, or severe. It is a complex disease process, affected by a multitude of factors, both physical and emotional. Asthma is an obstructive respiratory disease, usually with reversible respiratory insults. It is characterized by bronchospasm with subsequent air trapping in the bronchioles. This results in difficulty in breathing, particularly on expiration, thick mucous secretions, and edema of the respiratory mucosa.

Asthma can be precipitated by a variety of stimuli. Physical factors include allergic responses, hormonal alterations, and exercise. Emotional stress can also precipitate an attack. It is important to note, however, that although asthma may occur initially in response to an allergen, subsequent attacks are not usually without other influences.

Inhalant irritants are most commonly implicated in asthma. Rarely is asthma caused by a food allergy. The allergic theory presents the allergen as directly irritating the respiratory mucosa. This triggers the immune response resulting in the production of IgE. The antibody attaches to basophilic mast cells and causes destruction and subsequent release of the chemical mediators. These chemicals cause bronchospasm, edema, and increased mucous production (Leffert, 1978). Like eczema, asthma occurrence appears to be a result of multifactorial inherited predisposition for producing IgE. Laboratory values reveal eosinophilia, elevated IgE, and alterations in arterial blood gases. Nursing management for asthma is presented in Chapter 34.

Contact Dermatitis

Contact dermatitis is a delayed hypersensitivity reaction that usually doesn't appear until 12–48 hours after exposure to the allergen. It is usually a localized reaction but may be systemic, as seen in contact with plant irritants. Generally, allergens implicated in contact dermatitis are detergents, clothing, cosmetics, and such plants as poison ivy, oak, and sumac. The immune response to a contact allergen can diminish over the years as long as contact is avoided. Subsequent accidental contact may yield a milder response.

The type of rash in contact dermatitis is similar to eczema. Weeping and crusting may be more severe, however, and can result in sloughing of the surface skin layer. Poison plant irritants such as ivy, oak, and sumac can also cause severe systemic reactions. The episode usually begins with mild erythema and fluid-filled vesicles at contact sites. Eventually all of the exposed body areas may become involved. As the reaction continues, the child may exhibit generalized erythema, edema, urticaria, and fluid seepage. Itching is intense. Particularly, if the oil has been carried by smoke, the face may be extensively involved, causing periorbital edema. The child may be unable to open the eyes and will be excessively uncomfortable.

Treatment Treatment for mild cases of contact dermatitis involve the administration of antihistamines to control itching and the histaminic release. Additionally, topical drying lotions such as calamine are recommended. Corn starch or baking soda baths may relieve pruritis.

There are some over-the-counter preparations of ½% hydrocortisone cream that people may use for the treatment of contact dermatitis. Pharmacists discourage their use with open skin, however, because of the danger of absorbing the steroid.

Severe and systemic manifestations of dermatitis may be treated with an adrenocortical steroid (glucocorticoid). An initial injection of prednisolone will be followed by oral medication in a tapered-dose schedule, taking approximately 6–7 days to complete. For weeping skin, Burow's compresses are recommended several times a day. The solution should not be used on the eyes, however. Again, allergen avoidance is recommended.

Nursing Management Nursing management for mild cases is similar to that for eczema (see Chapter 44). Children with severe manifestations should be observed for alterations in fluid balance as well as for an impending anaphylaxis. Antihistamines are given for itching. The nurse must observe for side effects of steroid administration. Supportive measures are required if the child has severe manifestations. Reassurance should be given that the reaction is self-limiting and usually disappears within 2 weeks. Children treated by systemic steroids demonstrate marked improvement within 48 hours.

Allergy to Bites and Stings

Reactions to stinging insects range from mild to severe depending on the allergic tendency of the child and the frequency of prior exposure. Reactions can become progressively more severe with each sting. Insects most often implicated in allergic reactions are those of the hymenoptera class—bees, yellow jackets, wasps, and hornets. The first leaves a stinger, the rest bite.

Symptoms of allergic sting reactions can range from mild to severe. Normal response to a sting includes erythema, the presence of a small wheal, and itching. The reaction would subside in a matter of hours. A more severe reaction would include localized swelling and erythema extending out from the sting site. Systemic reactions of urticaria, bronchospasm, and angioedema can lead to anaphylactic shock (Bonner, 1978). Some children might also experience a delayed reaction causing generalized inflammation and possible encephalitis (Bonner, 1978).

The pain from stings can be relieved with applications of meat tenderizer. The nurse should observe the child for manifestations of systemic reaction and institute measures to treat anaphylaxis if necessary.

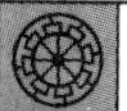

NURSING CARE PLAN Child With Juvenile Rheumatoid Arthritis

Assessment

Nancy is a 13-year-old girl diagnosed as having juvenile onset of rheumatoid arthritis. At age 10 she was visiting friends when she suddenly developed headache and joint stiffness. The joint pain was worse in the morning. Both eyes were pink and irritated. After many visits to a variety of phsyicians, the diagnosis was established. She was placed on aspirin therapy and entered a remission. She is now complaining of pain in the knees and ankles with limited joint mobility. She has just moved to a new home in New Hampshire and had been looking forward to learning how to ski.

Nursing Diagnoses and Goals

1. **Nursing diagnosis:** Potential for joint contractures related to joint limitation in knees and ankles.

   Long-term goal: Nancy's symptoms will subside and she will enter another remission.

   Short-term goals: (a) Nancy will cooperate with exercise regime. (b) Nancy will assume self-care responsibilities for exercise regime. (c) Nancy will be able to judge her activity tolerance level.

2. **Nursing diagnosis:** Potential for side effects of aspirin.

   Long-term goal: Nancy will be able to remain on appropriate salicylate therapy until remission is achieved.

   Short-term goal: Nancy will report any signs of aspirin toxicity.

3. **Nursing diagnosis:** Potential for ineffective coping related to inability to achieve personal goal of learning how to ski.

   Long-term goal: Nancy will adjust appropriately to the limitations of her disease during its exacerbation.

   Short-term goals: (a) Nancy will discuss that limitations may be temporary. (b) Nancy will find another activity of interest until her condition improves.

Interventions	Rationale	Evaluation Criteria
1. Administer buffered aspirin as ordered	ASA decreases the inflammatory response and alleviates joint pain	Does return demonstration from Nancy indicate adequate knowledge of exercise regimen? Does she appear to be interested in assuming responsibility for care as evidenced by self-initiation of regimen at appropriate time?
Demonstrate exercise regimen: 1. 2-lb weights strapped to ankles 2. Circular ankle motion exercises 3. Leg lifts—20 times	Demonstration of exercises teaches proper procedure and is the first step toward promoting self-care	
Apply hot packs to ankle and knees prior to exercise	Heat reduces the level of pain to ease movement of the joints during exercise	
2. Assess for signs of aspirin toxicity—headache, dizziness, tinnitus, and confusion	High doses of ASA necessary for treating JRA can cause serious side effects	Are vital signs stable with no signs of aspirin toxicity or abnormal bleeding?
Give aspirin with meals or directly after meals with milk	Aspirin can cause gastric irritation—buffered aspirin reduces its incidence	
Observe carefully for any signs of external hemorrhage, epistaxis, or internal bleeding—decreased blood pressure, increased pulse, restlessness, thirst	Aspirin alters bleeding time and nosebleeds are common. Gastric bleeding is more severe manifestation and may lead to massive hemorrhage	
Check blood salicylate levels	Should be below 25 mg/100 mL	
3. Reassure Nancy that she may be able to ski once symptoms are relieved	Skiing is a noncontact sport that would be permissible when ankles and knees are more flexible	Does Nancy discuss her disappointment and read about skiing during this exacerbation? Does she also participate in a swimming club at school?
Suggest swimming as an alternative if a pool is available	Swimming places less strain on joints and connective tissue	
Encourage Nancy to express any feelings of anger or depression	Verbalization facilitates resolution of a problem	

Key Concepts

- The human body has a network of defenses to keep it intact and free from disease.
- The major functions of the immune system are to defend the body against invasion by pathogenic agents such as bacteria, viruses, parasites, and toxins.
- Antigens are substances capable of eliciting an immune response because the immune system recognizes them as foreign and attempts to eliminate them.
- Antibodies are proteins that are produced by the immune system and that bind to antigens as part of the immune response.
- Lymphocytes are primary effectors of the immune response and are constantly circulating throughout the body as well as remaining in lymphoid tissue to be exposed to antigens.
- There are two types of lymphocytes: B lymphocytes and T lymphocytes.
- The inflammatory response is a nonspecific defense in response to an antigen.
- Specific immune responses include cellular and humoral responses.
- The complement system is an accessory system to the humoral response and mediates the inflammatory reaction.
- Protection from infections in the first few months of life is conferred on the child by maternal antibodies.
- Children acquire immunity naturally and artificially, actively and passively.
- Alterations in immune system function include immune deficiency diseases, autoimmune diseases, immune complex diseases, allergy, and cancer.
- Immune deficiency diseases affect both cellular and humoral response, causing decreased resistance to infection and malignancy.
- Autoimmune diseases involve a lack of recognition of "self," and overproduction of antibodies destructive to normal tissue.
- Immune complex diseases result from trapping of immune complexes in body systems and subsequent inflammatory response.
- Allergy is the immune response to an allergen that causes hypersensitivity reaction in various body systems.
- Nursing assessment of the child with an immune system dysfunction includes history taking, physical assessment, and laboratory studies.
- Acute-care needs of the child with immune system dysfunction include pain relief, prevention of the hazards of immobility, maintaining intact integument, and protection from infection.
- Medications common to children with immune system disorders include salycilates, antihistamines, and corticosteroids.
- Children with immune system disorders may need a diet with increased protein or a special allergy diet.
- Emotional needs include adjustment to disease chronicity and adjustment to the life-threatening nature of some conditions.
- Some complications of immune system disorders do not manifest themselves until years later, and parents should be encouraged to provide regular medical care.
- Immune deficiency diseases include DiGeorge's syndrome, AIDS, agammaglobulinemia, and Wiskott–Aldrich syndrome.
- Autoimmune diseases include acute rheumatic fever, acute glomerulonephritis, erythema multiforme, juvenile rheumatoid arthritis, and systemic lupus.
- Immune complex diseases include Kawasaki disease and H.S. purpura.
- Allergic reactions can be local or generalized, immediate or delayed.
- Local reactions affect skin and mucous membranes. Systemic reactions affect most other body systems.
- Anaphylaxis is a sudden occurrence of vascular collapse due to a massive release of histamine.
- Allergic irritants include environmental, food, insects, and medications.
- Common diagnostic tests for children with allergies are skin tests, RAST, and provocation tests.

- Desensitization involves injecting small amounts of allergen to develop immune tolerance.
- Common food allergies are to milk, eggs, and wheat and dietary modifications may be made for each.
- Stress reduction and relaxation techniques can alleviate and prevent the allergic response.
- Specific allergic manifestations in children include eczema, asthma, contact dermatitis, and sting allergy.

References

American Heart Association Committee Report; Prevention of rheumatic fever. *Circulation* (Jan) 1977; 55:1–3.

American Lung Association: *Superstuff,* 1981.

Baltzer R et al: Bone marrow transplantation. *Am J Nurs* (Jun) 1984; 84(6):764–772.

Behrman RE, Vaughan BC: *Nelson Textbook of Pediatrics,* 12th ed. Saunders, 1983.

Bonner J: Stinging insect allergy—what to do for the patient. *Consultant* (Sep) 1978; 18:49–50.

Colen BD: New therapy gives disease 'the needle.' *Cape Cod Times,* May 12, 1981, p. 13.

DiSciascio G, Taranta A: Rheumatic fever in children. *Am Heart J* (May) 1980; 99:635–655.

Donley D: Nursing the patient who is immunosuppressed. *Am J Nurs* 1976; 76:1619–1625.

Fink C: Predicting the outcome of JRA. *Consultant* (Oct) 1979; 19:40–46.

Gavaghan J: Learning to live with lupus. *AHC News:* Affiliated Hospitals Center, Spring, 1980.

Gerhold S: Research gives hope to patient with lupus. Information from the Lupus Erythematosus Foundation. No date.

Govoni LE, Hayes JE: *Drugs and Nursing Implications,* 4th ed. Appleton-Century-Crofts, 1982.

Grant E: Food allergies and migraine. *Lancet* (May) 1979; 1:966–969.

Groenwald S: Physiology of the immune system. *Heart Lung* 1980; 9:645–650.

Hamburger R: Allergies in infants—perhaps they can be prevented. *Consultant* (Oct) 1979; 19:23–29.

Harmon A, Harmon D: Anaphylaxis—sudden death anytime. *Nurs 80* (Oct) 1980; 10:40–43.

Hood L et al: *Immunology,* 2nd ed. Benjamin/Cummings, 1984.

Irby R: Diagnostic tests that identify connective tissue disease. *Consultant* (Oct) 1978; 18:157–164.

Kaplan E: Acute rheumatic fever. *Pediatr Clin North Am* (Nov) 1978; 25:817–829.

Kawasaki disease in childhood. *Emergency Med* (May) 1979; 11:55–56.

Koffler D: The immunology of rheumatoid disease. *Clin Symp* 1979; 4:2–36.

Leffert F: Asthma—a modern perspective. *Pediatrics* (Dec) 1978; 62:1061–1069.

Lind M: The immunologic assessment: A nursing focus. *Heart Lung* 1980; 9(4):658–661.

Lynch M, Gray J: Kawasaki disease. *Pediatr Nurs* (Mar/Apr) 1982; 8:96–101.

McAnarney E, Pless B: Psychological problems of JRA patients. *INFLO* 1975; 8:1–2.

Matthay R: Practical management of pediatric asthma. *Update: Asthma Therapy Symposium Proceedings.* KPR Infor/Media, May 1979.

Morens D, Anderson L, Hurwitz E: National surveillance of Kawasaki disease. *Pediatrics* (Jan) 1980; 65:21–15.

Morens D, Nahmias A: Kawasaki disease: A 'new' pediatric enigma. *Hosp Prac* (Sep) 1978; 13(9):109–120.

Muir B: *Pathophysiology—An Introduction to the Mechanisms of Disease.* Wiley, 1980.

Murray A et al: Allergies to cats *vs* dogs. *Allergy Clin Immunol* (Aug) 1983; 72:145–149.

Nursing Mirror, May 25, 1983. (Inside back cover.)

Nuscher R et al: Bone marrow transplantation. *Am J Nurs* (Jun) 1984; 84:764–772.

Parker C: Food allergies. *Am J Nurs* (Feb) 1980; 80:262–265.

Patterson R: *Allergic Diseases—Diagnosis and Management.* Lippincott, 1980.

Pediatr Curr (Nov/Dec) 1971; 20:57–64. Ross Laboratories.

Rajka E, Korosay S: *Immunological Aspects of Allergy and Allergic Diseases,* Vol 7: *Allergic Diseases of the Skin.* Plenum, 1976.

Rocklin R: Immunologic diseases—a conference at Children's Hospital Medical Center, Boston, March 20, 1984.

Rosen F: Wiscott-Aldrich syndrome. In: *Immunological Diseases.* Talmage D et al (editors). Little, Brown, 1978.

Scott G, Parks W: Letter to the editor. *N Engl J Med* (Jul 19) 1984; 190.

Shearer G: Letter to the editor. *N Engl J Med* (Jul 19) 1984; 189.

Sherlock M et al: Caring for the AIDS patient fearlessly. *Nurs 83* (Sep) 1983; 13(9):50–55.

Stiehm R, Fulginity V: *Immunologic Disorders in Infants and Children.* Saunders, 1973.

Stevens-Johnson syndrome. *Consultant* (Sep) 1978; 18:156–157.

Thomas PA et al: Unexplained immunodeficiency in children. *JAMA* (Aug 3) 1984; 252:639–644.

Tilkian S, Conover M, Tilkian A: *Clinical Implications of Laboratory Tests,* 3rd ed. Mosby, 1983.

Treating patients with AIDS. *Health Affairs* 1984; 16:16–18.

Tortora GJ, Funke BR, Case CL: Specific defenses of the host: Immunology. Pages 396–433 in: Tortora GJ, Funke BR, Case CL: *Microbiology: An Introduction.* Benjamin/Cummings, 1982.

US Task Force on Immunity and Disease: *Immunology.* US Department of Health and Human Services; NIH 80–940, 1980.

US Department of Health and Human Services: *Understanding the Immune System.* NIH 84–529, 1983.

Vick R: *Contemporary Medical Physiology.* Addison-Wesley, 1984.

White J, Owsley V: Helping families to cope with milk, wheat, and soy allergies. *Matern Child Nurs* (Nov/Dec) 1983; 8(6):423–428.

Additional Readings

Abeles M et al: Systemic lupus erythematosus in the younger patient: Survival studies. *J Rheumatol* (Jul/Aug) 1980; 7:515–522.

Buckley R: Immunodeficiency diseases. In: *Textbook of Rheumatology.* Kelley W et al (editors). Saunders, 1981.

Chipps B et al: Diagnosis and treatment of anaphylactic reactions to hymenoptera stings in children. *J Pediatr* (Aug) 1980; 97:177–184.

Conley ME et al: The spectrum of DiGeorge's syndrome. *J Pediatr* 1979; 94:883–890.

Davis S: X-linked agammaglobulinemia. In: *Immunological Disorders in Infants and Children.* Stiehm R, Fulginity V (editors). Saunders, 1973.

Fischbach F: *A Manual of Laboratory Diagnostic Tests.* Lippincott, 1980.

Hedlin A: The immune system. *Can Nurse* (Jul/Aug) 1979; 75:29–31.

Hitzig W: DiGeorge's syndrome. In: *Immunological Disorders of Infants and Children.* Stiehm R, Fulginity V (editors). Saunders, 1973.

Lewis E, Roberts J: Is autoimmunity a common denominator in immune complex diseases? *Lancet* (Jan 26) 1980; 1:178–180.

L'Orange C, Werner-McCullough M: Kawasaki disease: New threat to children. *Am J Nurs* (Apr) 1983; 83(4):558–562.

National Institutes of Health: Outlook for SLE patients. . . . *JAMA* (Jan) 1979; 241:23–24.

Steinberg A: Management of SLE. In: *Textbook of Rheumatology.* Kelley W et al (editors). Saunders, 1981.

Taylor DL: Immune response. *Nurs 84* (May) 1984; 14:52–54.

Taylor DL: Anaphylaxis. *Nurs 84* (Jun) 1984; 14:44–45.

Wieczorek R, Horner-Rosner B: The asthmatic child—preventing and controlling attacks. *Am J Nurs* (Feb) 1979; 79:258–262.

Winkelstein A: An overview of immune deficiency disorders. *Consultant* (Oct) 1978; 18:118–134.

Zvaifler N: Etiology and pathogenesis of SLE. In: *Textbook of Rheumatology.* Kelley W et al (editors). Saunders, 1981.

Ingestion, Digestion, and Elimination
Implications of Inflammation and Obstruction

38

Jean Marie Rockenhaus

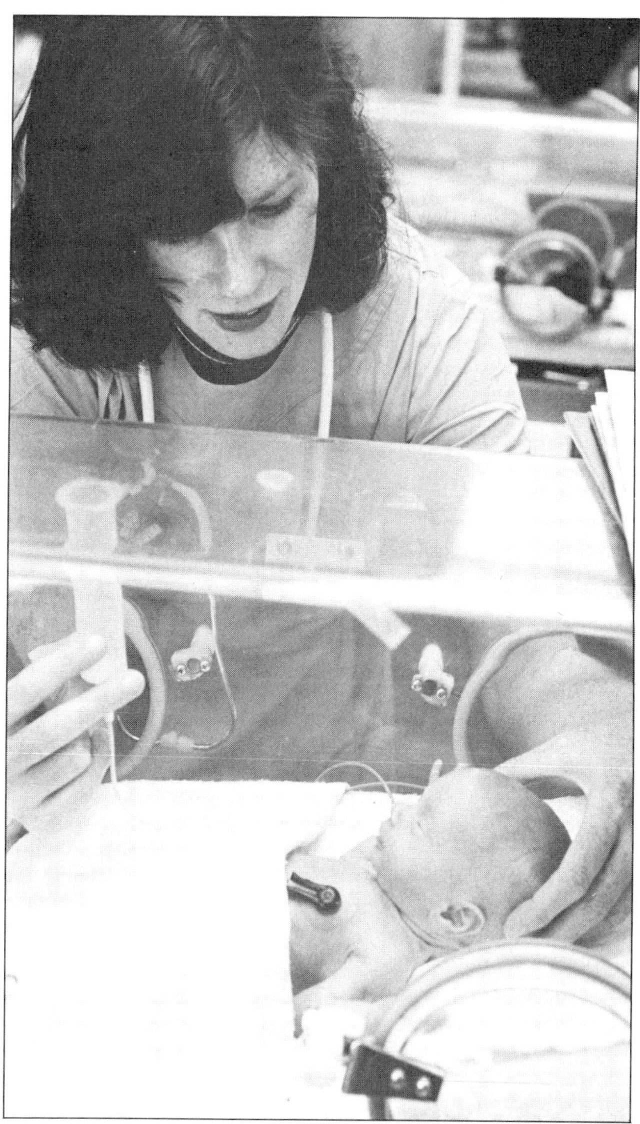

continued on next page

Objectives

- Describe the anatomy, physiology, and embryonic development of the gastrointestinal system
- Describe the assessment criteria and diagnostic tests specific to assessment of the gastrointestinal system
- Explain the principles of nursing care common to procedures and treatments involving the gastrointestinal tract
- Define methods of feeding used for children with feeding problems
- Explain the principles of nursing care for children undergoing abdominal surgery
- Describe the essential developmental, emotional, and health maintenance needs of children with gastrointestinal dysfunction

- Explain the physiologic processes, common medical treatments, and principles of nursing management for conditions hampering or preventing ingestion or digestion
- Explain the physiologic processes, common medical treatments, and principles of nursing management for conditions interfering with the absorption or use of nutrients
- Explain the physiologic processes, common medical treatments, and principles of nursing management for conditions characterizing inflammation of the digestive tract
- Explain the physiologic processes, common medical treatments, and principles of nursing management for conditions affecting hepatic functioning
- List major bacterial, protozoal, and viral causes of diarrhea in children
- Describe interventions commonly used for children with diarrhea or severe constipation

To find these topics, see the following chapters.

Abdominal pain	Chapter 26
Foreign body ingestion	Chapter 26
Intestinal parasites	Chapter 26
Neonatal hyperbilirubinemia	Chapter 31
Thrush	Chapter 26

Disorders of the gastrointestinal system vary greatly in their impact on the lives of the affected child and family. Minor illnesses may cause inconvenience or disrupt the child or family's life for only a brief period. Many disorders (for example, intestinal obstruction, severe dehydration) are life-threatening unless emergency treatment, often surgery, is instituted quickly. Other acute gastrointestinal conditions can assume life-threatening proportions. For example, parents are usually unaware of the potentially drastic effects of something as simple as vomiting or diarrhea in infants and small children.

Other gastrointestinal defects (for example, cystic fibrosis, ulcerative colitis) may be more chronic and can severely affect the child's growth and development. Any chronic disorder that disrupts the child's ability to eat and grow normally can also have serious effects on the parent–child relationship. If the child fails to thrive, the parent may view this as a deliberate rejection of parental love and nurturance and thus needs nursing assistance to refocus energies on helping the child and family to accept and manage the disorder.

In Chapters 29 and 30, we presented principles of nursing care for children hospitalized with acute illnesses and for children and families coping with chronic conditions. In this chapter we apply these principles to disorders of the gastrointestinal system. The nurse caring for a child with a condition that affects ingestion, digestion, or elimination also needs to know the anatomy, physiology, and pathophysiology of the digestive tract. The nurse who is cognizant of the profound psychological effects of illness, surgery, or hospitalization on children at each developmental age can plan care to meet each child's needs (see Chapter 27). In this chapter we therefore cover nursing care common to children with gastrointestinal disorders, and we summarize the anatomy and physiology of the gastrointestinal tract.

Anatomy and Physiology of the Gastrointestinal System

Embryonic Development of the Digestive Tract

The primitive gut is formed during the third week of gestation and consists of the foregut, midgut, and hindgut. Each section then contributes to the development of specific anatomic features of the gastrointestinal tract.

Foregut The foregut is the precursor of the pharynx, esophagus, lower respiratory tract, stomach, a portion of the duodenum, and the liver, pancreas, and biliary tree. The esophagus arises from the embryonic tracheoesophageal septum. The esophagus normally separates from the trachea during the third to sixth week of intrauterine life. If the esophagus and trachea are not differentiated, anomalies such as tracheoesophageal fistulas or esophageal atresia may result.

The stomach arises from the base, or caudal portion, of the foregut, as does the beginning portion of the duodenum. If these structures are not differentiated, the result may be duodenal atresia or stenosis.

The liver, gallbladder, and biliary tree are formed from the most caudal portion of the foregut. The cystic and common bile ducts develop into distinct entities and are recanalized, at which time bile is introduced into the duodenum. This occurs during the thirteenth to sixteenth weeks of gestation. Failure of these structures to differentiate at this point may contribute to such anomalies as biliary atresia or choledochal cysts.

Midgut The midgut develops into the small intestine, the cecum, the appendix, the ascending colon, and the initial portion of the transverse colon. During the early weeks of life, the embryonic ileum and colon are herniated into the umbilical cord. This intestinal loop rotates 90° counterclockwise around the superior mesenteric artery. During the tenth week of gestation, the intestines return to the abdominal cavity after undergoing another 180° counterclockwise rotation. The bowel has then assumed its standard anatomic position. Failure to differentiate or rotate correctly can lead to the development of intestinal atresias, malrotation, volvulus, omphalocele, and other defects.

Hindgut The final portion of the transverse colon, the descending colon, the sigmoid colon, the rectum, and the anal canal are derived from the embryonic hindgut. The blind end of the hindgut develops into a common cloaca (genitourinary and anorectal structures). Lateral tissue folds then arise and separate these structures. Failure of these segments to differentiate or develop may cause colonic atresias or anorectal malformations. Failure in the development of embryonic innervation may contribute to aganglionic megacolon.

Physiology of the Digestive Tract

The digestive tract functions to ingest, digest, and absorb nutrients. Each portion of the gastrointestinal system is responsible for specific digestive functions (see Fig. 38-1).

The digestive process begins in the mouth, where chewing breaks the ingested food into smaller portions. Salivary mucin and amylase are mixed with the food particles. Complex carbohydrates are initially catabolized by the salivary enzyme amylase before swallowing. Once the food is swallowed, the food bolus passes into the esophagus. Peristaltic waves propel the bolus past the cardiac valve and into the stomach.

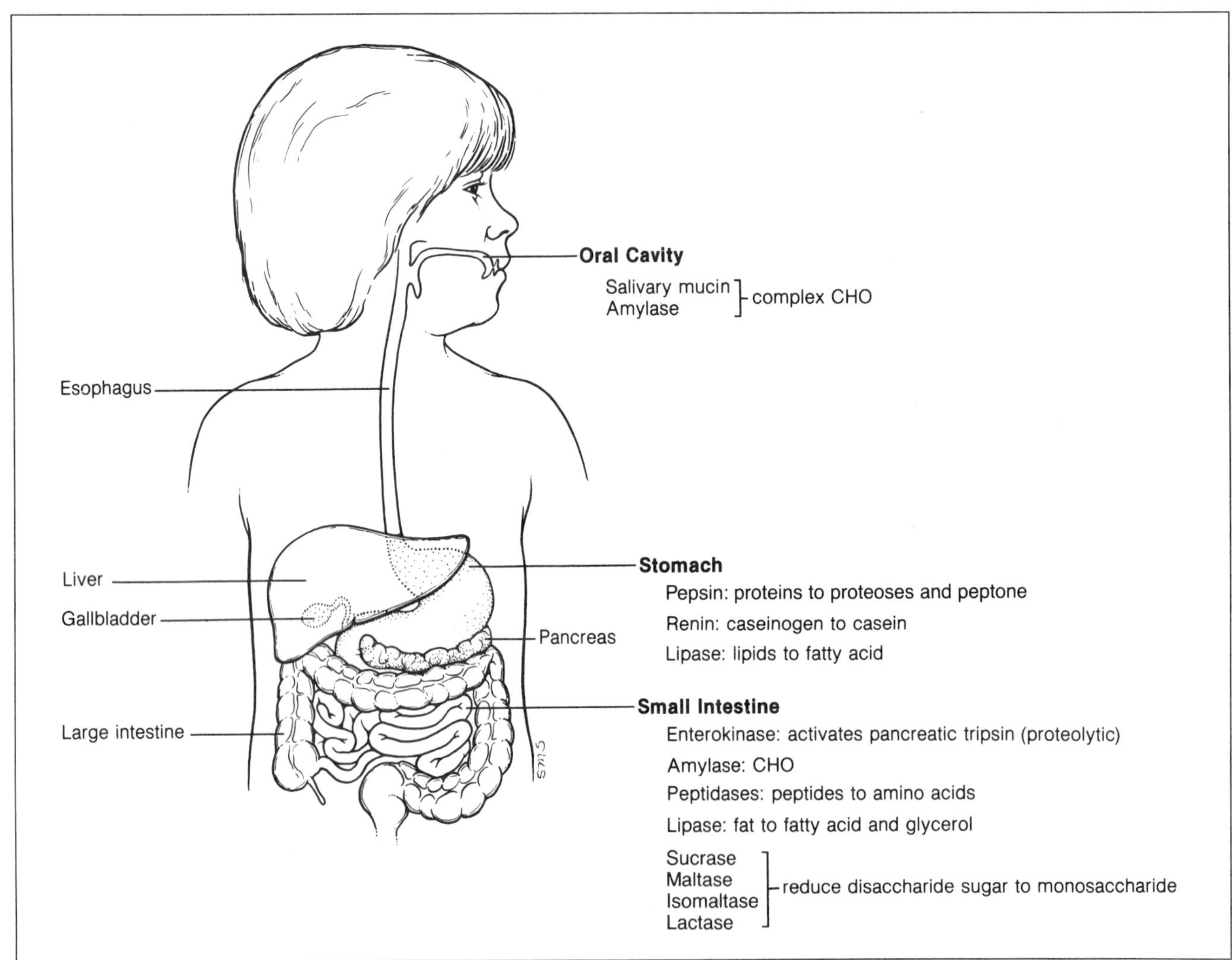

Figure 38-1 Structures of the digestive system showing major enzyme locations.

The stomach is responsible for breaking the food into even smaller portions and for mixing these with gastric juice. This gastric juice consists of mucus, water, hydrochloric acid, and the digestive enzymes pepsin, rennin, and lipase. Pepsin converts proteins to proteoses and peptones. Rennin is a coagulating enzyme that converts the principal protein in milk (caseinogen) into casein. Gastric lipase acts to split lipids into fatty acids. The mucus within the digestive tract is thought to protect the mucosa from the digestive enzymes and secretion.

The food (now called *chyme*) passes through the pylorus and into the small intestine. The inner mucosa of the small intestine contains many folds and ridges, which allow more surface area for absorption of nutrients. In addition, small fingerlike projections (villi) protrude from the surface of the folds, further expanding the absorptive surfaces. Microvilli cover the surface of each villus, again multiplying the absorptive surface many times over.

The crypts of Lieberkühn are located at the base of each of the villi and are responsible for the regeneration of mucosal absorptive cells, which secrete intestinal juice containing enterokinase and amylase. Enterokinase activates the pancreatic proteolytic enzyme trypsin, and amylase breaks down complex carbohydrates. In addition, the epithelial cells contain peptidases, sucrase, maltase, isomaltase, lactase, and lipase. The peptidases are responsible for splitting peptides into amino acids, and lipase is needed to convert fats into fatty acids and glycerol. The other enzymes are responsible for converting certain disaccharides into such usable monosaccharides as glucose, fructose, and galactose.

Absorption of water, carbohydrates, proteins, fats, vitamins and mineral salts occurs throughout the small intestine. Monosaccharides are absorbed directly into the intestinal capillaries. Most protein digestion occurs in the proximal small intestine, and therefore the greatest absorption of amino acids occurs in the duodenum and jejunum. These nutrients are then returned to the portal circulation for further metabolism or storage. Water, mineral salts, and water-soluble vitamins are absorbed primarily in the small intestine, although water and electrolytes continue to be absorbed in the colon. Fatty acids and glycerol are converted to triglycerides within the intestinal cells. These triglycerides, in combination with bile salts and fat-soluble vitamins, are absorbed into the lymphatic capillaries of the intestinal villi and are returned to the circulation through the thoracic duct.

The liver and pancreas are responsible for secreting other digestive enzymes and fluids. The liver produces bile, storing it in the gallbladder. The presence of fat within the digestive tract triggers the release of bile from the gallbladder into the duodenum through the common bile duct. Bile lowers the surface tension of fat and allows for the formation of a fat emulsion. This enables pancreatic lipase to act effectively on the smaller particles of fat.

The pancreas produces trypsin, lipase, and amylase. These enzymes become activated in the small intestine in order to prevent autodigestion of the pancreas. The pancreas also produces insulin and glucagon. (These metabolic agents are discussed in Chapter 40.)

By the time the ingested food reaches the terminal ileum, the digestive process is almost completed. The rest of the intestinal contents is propelled through the cecum and into the large intestine, ultimately to be excreted as feces.

Assessment of the Child With Digestive Dysfunction

Children suspected of having a gastrointestinal problem require a complete physical assessment (see Chapter 14). In addition, particular attention should be paid to the functioning of the organs and processes of the gastrointestinal tract. Tests used to diagnose gastrointestinal disorders are summarized in Tables 38-1 and 38-2.

In addition to obtaining a standard history (see Chapter 14), the nurse questions parents of children with suspected gastrointestinal disorders about past events or behaviors that might point toward a diagnosis. These questions are general but provide an overall view of the functioning of the child's intestinal tract. Not all areas of questioning are appropriate for all suspected problems, and nurses therefore need to choose questions that direct attention to the suspected problem.

A review of the child's prenatal history yields information that may aid in the diagnosis of a gastrointestinal disorder. This includes the child's estimated gestation and birth weight. Any incidence of maternal polyhydramnios may indicate intestinal atresias or other proximal defects of the intestinal tract. In addition, any family history of gastrointestinal anomalies may prove very important in establishing a working diagnosis (see Fig. 5-10).

Relevant data about the neonate include any obvious anomalies such as abdominal wall defects (gastroschisis, omphalocele, hernias), facial defects (cleft lip or palate), or imperforate anus. More subtle indicators of intestinal problems may include difficulty with initial feedings, episodes of aspiration, frequent vomiting or regurgitation, neonatal diarrhea, prolonged jaundice (neonatal hepatitis, biliary tree anomalies), gastric distension, respiratory distress (diaphragmatic hernia), or failure to pass meconium.

A history of subsequent events includes specific information about any of these and questioning about growth patterns, weight gains or losses (particularly in relation to time involved), feeding history (breast or bottle feeding, vomiting, ability to suck), and the presence of diarrhea or constipation. A history of bowel habits may be helpful in older children suspected of having Hirschsprung's disease, malabsorption problems, anorectal malformations, or enterocolitis. These conditions may produce stools that are

TABLE 38-1 Diagnostic Tests Used in Gastroenterology

Tests	Elevated in	Decreased in	Comments
Blood tests			
Bilirubin	Obstructive jaundice, hepatitis, cirrhosis	—	—
Ammonia	Hepatocellular failure, Reye's syndrome	—	Used as an indicator of hepatic protein metabolism
Amylase	Pancreatic duct obstruction	Hepatitis, cirrhosis	—
Serum glutamic-oxaloacetic transaminase (SGOT)	Cirrhosis, hepatitis, acute pancreatitis	—	—
Serum glutamic-pyruvic transaminase (SGPT)	Hepatocellular failure, cirrhosis, hepatitis, obstructive jaundice	—	—
Alkaline phosphatase	Obstructive jaundice	—	—
Stool tests			
pH	Base–protein breakdown	Acid–carbohydrate fermentation or disaccharide intolerance	Normal pH = 7–7.5
Ova and parasites	Amoebae, *giardia*, helminths	—	Stool tests for ova and parasites should be body temperature and examined within 30 minutes
Stool culture	Elevation of pathogenic organisms in certain forms of diarrhea	—	—
Stool electrolytes	Sodium and chloride loss excessive in certain forms of diarrhea	—	Can be used as an indicator for electrolyte therapy
Fecal fat	Idiopathic steatorrhea, ulcerative colitis, Crohn's disease, cystic fibrosis, malabsorptive syndromes, short-bowel syndrome, others	—	Fecal fat can be determined from one specimen or may require a 72-hour collection with a charcoal marker and dietary fat determination. Stool collection begins when charcoal is noted in stool, and ends 72 hours later
Trypsin	—	Some pancreatic diseases, may be absent in cystic fibrosis	—
Reducing substances	Present in disaccharidase deficiencies	—	Clinitest of liquid stool is positive

constipated, ribbonlike, or diarrheic. The nurse also questions the parent about the presence of any undigested food particles in the stool, or the presence of greasy, foul-smelling stools. An in-depth dietary history is necessary for children with suspected food allergies or malabsorption syndromes (see Chapter 15).

A history of the current concern includes questions regarding the length of the problem and any outstanding signs and symptoms such as vomiting, diarrhea, altered eating patterns, pain, or jaundice.

Previous episodes of vomiting should be assessed for frequency, quantity, quality (digested or undigested foods, blood, mucus), color, force (that is, projectile or regurgitation), and relationship to last feeding. The odor of the emesis may also be important if intestinal obstruction is suspected, as a fecal odor may be present on occasion.

A history of diarrhea is also documented as to frequency, quantity, quality (pus, mucus, blood, undigested food), color, and odor. The nurse also questions the parent and child regarding any abdominal discomfort with diarrhea, as the presence of pain requires more in-depth questioning. Frequency, intensity (severe, mild), nature (cramping, colicky), and location are assessed, and the nurse questions the parent about the location of any pain early in the course of

TABLE 38-2 Radiologic Tests Used in Gastroenterology

Test	Comments
^{131}I rose bengal	Hepatic retention of radioactive iodine is increased in obstructive jaundice. A diffuse nodular scan pattern indicates cirrhosis or hepatitis. A cystic scan pattern indicates choledochal cysts. Precautions must be taken because the isotope is excreted in the urine and stool of the child. All waste is considered radioactive, and no pregnant women are allowed to care for the child. A urinary catheter may be placed in young children to avoid contamination of linen with radioactive urine. Observe for allergy to iodine dye
Abdominal flat-plate and upright abdominal x-rays	Often used to diagnose or rule out pneumatosis intestinalis, free peritoneal air, organ displacement, subphrenic abscesses, intestinal obstructions
Upper-GI series	Used to diagnose esophageal abnormalities, gastric ulcers, bezoars
Small bowel follow through (SBFT)	Used to diagnose duodenal and jejunal ulcers, perforation, Crohn's disease, ileal stenosis or atresia, Meckel's diverticulum
Barium enema	Used to diagnose anal and rectal stenosis, rectal polyps, diverticulum, ulcerative colitis, Crohn's disease, Hirschsprung's disease, fistulas, intussusception
Intravenous cholangiography	Used to diagnose biliary tree anomalies (atresias, choledochal cysts, cholestasis)
Duodenal and jejunal biopsy or aspirate	Biopsies used for celiac disease, Crohn's disease, disaccharidase deficiencies. Aspirates used for pancreatic enzyme deficiencies, ova or helminths, *Giardia lamblia*
Rectal and colon biopsy	Used to diagnose Crohn's disease or ulcerative colitis, Hirschsprung's disease
Liver biopsy	Used to diagnose hepatitis, cirrhosis, other liver disease
Endoscopy	Fiberoptic examination for diagnosis of esophagitis, gastritis, ulcers, foreign bodies
Colonoscopy or proctosigmoidoscopy	Visualization of rectum and colon used to diagnose ulcerative colitis, Crohn's disease, anomalies, cause of bleeding, diverticulitis

the illness. (In appendicitis, for example, pain is frequently periumbilical before localizing in the right lower quadrant.) Timing of the pain may also be significant and may, for example, occur before or after eating, defecating, or intense activity.

Eating habits are part of a complete dietary history, and may be important in identifying problems that alter eating patterns. For instance, children who normally have good appetites may exhibit sudden anorexia or nausea when eating. Reactions to ingested foods (for example, diarrhea, abdominal distension) may also be important.

The nurse questions the parent closely regarding the onset of any jaundice, its duration, and any changes in its degree. The presence of dark urine should be confirmed. A report of clay-colored stools might indicate biliary obstruction. A parent may report that a child is jaundiced when the child is actually carotenemic. Carotenemia is the benign storage of the pigment carotene in the subcutaneous tissues of the body. Sclera remain anicteric, and urine and stools are usually normal in color. The palms and soles of the feet may appear orange, as may the tip of the nose. The dietary history usually reveals recent, frequent feedings of yellow or green vegetables or fruits. Return to a balanced diet will eliminate the yellow coloring.

Nursing Management for Procedures and Treatments

Preparation for Diagnostic Tests

Children with gastrointestinal disorders undergo a variety of diagnostic procedures. These may be invasive or noninvasive, and the child's need for preparation varies accordingly.

Noninvasive tests that may be used in the diagnosis of gastrointestinal disorders include flat-plate radiographs, stool tests, and barium swallow radiographs. Blood tests are frequently considered noninvasive, even though a venipuncture or fingerstick is necessary, and the child may perceive

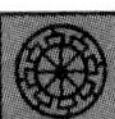

ASSESSMENT GUIDE The Child With a Gastrointestinal Problem

			Validating Data		
System	**Subjective Data**	**Objective Data**	*Laboratory Data*	*Radiographs or Biopsy*	**Nursing Management**
Head, eyes, ears, nose, throat	Burning sensation or pain in lips, mouth, esophagus History of toxic ingestion (for example, lye)	Presence of clefts, anomalies Presence or absence of gag reflex, sucking and swallowing capabilities Regurgitation or rumination Bleeding varices	Esophageal pH	Radiographs for esophageal anomalies Esophagoscopy	Elicit and document history of chief complaint Raise head of bed if esophageal anomaly is suspected Suction excess secretions
Gastrointestinal					
Stomach	Pain, nausea, emesis, anorexia, pica	Location and intensity of pain Hematemesis, distension, tympany Visible peristalsis Emesis: (a) force (for example, projectile, regurgitative); (b) color (green = bile; clear = gastric; coffee = blood; red = blood); (c) odor (fecal odor = obstruction); (d) amount; (e) timing in relation to last meal (note presence or absence of food)	Serum electrolytes Occult blood	Upper-GI series Endoscopy	Document all relevant data that may aid in final diagnosis Strictly monitor intake and output Position to prevent aspiration if patient is vomiting
Abdomen (liver, colon, small intestine)	Diarrhea or constipation Pain, discomfort Jaundice History of food allergy Nausea/vomiting History of foreign travel	Location and intensity of pain Abdominal distension Absent, hypoactive, or hyperactive bowel sounds Hepatosplenomegaly, masses, anemia Stool: (a) consistency (formed, pasty, liquid); (b) quality (slimy, tarry, frothy, curdlike); (c) color (brown, black, green, yellow, white/clay, clear);	Serum bilirubin Hepatitis antigen Amylase, serum glutamic-oxaloacetic transaminase (SGOT), serum glutamic pyruvic transaminase (SGPT) Alkaline phosphatase Serum ammonia Serum electrolytes Complete blood count Stool pH and reducing substances Stool culture and	Flat-plate or upright abdominal radiograph Upper-GI series with small bowel follow through Duodenal/jejunal biopsy or aspirate Cholangiography Liver biopsy ^{131}I rose bengal Sonogram/CT scan Endoscopy/colonoscopy	Document all relevant data that may aid in final diagnosis Record intake and output; monitor vital signs Maintain adequate hydration and caloric intake Begin stool record

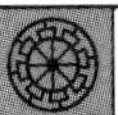

ASSESSMENT GUIDE The Child With a Gastrointestinal Problem (continued)

			Validating Data		
System	**Subjective Data**	**Objective Data**	*Laboratory Data*	*Radiographs or Biopsy*	**Nursing Management**
		(d) presence of mucus, blood, pus	ova or parasites Stool electrolytes Fecal fat, occult blood Stool trypsin		
Rectum/anus	Difficult defecation, encopresis, constipation	Patency of anus, presence of fissures, fistulas, abscesses Tone of anal sphincter, tenesmus, bleeding Rectal prolapse	Pinworm preparation	Barium enema Tonometry Rectal biopsy for ganglia	Document stool pattern and characteristics Teach bowel regimen if indicated Begin colostomy teaching if indicated
General	Fatigue, malaise	Icteric skin or sclera, distribution of body fat Cachexia, hydration status			Document child's general condition Document dietary and gastrointestinal history

the test as threatening. Preparation for these tests varies according to the developmental age and emotional needs of the child, which should be determined during the initial assessment.

Invasive tests that may be used in the diagnosis of gastrointestinal disorders include barium enema, intestinal biopsy, endoscopy, colonoscopy, duodenal aspirates, and intravenous cholangiography. Preparation for these should be more extensive than for noninvasive tests. The child is more likely to fear the test and to fantasize about the experience. The child's concerns depend, however, on the child's developmental stage and previous experience with procedures or hospitalization. The nurse therefore plans according to the needs of the child and family. (Chapter 29 discusses principles of care for both invasive and noninvasive procedures.)

Certain tests also require specific preparation. For example, the nurse needs to be aware that the rose bengal study often requires bladder catheterization in order to collect the radioactive urine. In early childhood, this can cause great problems in mobility and interference with toilet training; for older children, the same procedure may cause body image problems.

Several pretest procedures are also specific to gastroenterology. These include enemas, certain medications, and special dietary restrictions.

Enemas Many children require an enema or other bowel-cleansing routine before undergoing gastrointestinal procedures. Infants and young children require careful administration of enemas because of the small size of the rectal vault and the increased possibility of iatrogenic fluid and electrolyte imbalances associated with repeated enemas in small children. The enema solution should be isotonic (usually normal saline), as plain tap water, which is hypotonic, or some hypertonic commercial enema solutions can cause rapid fluid shifts leading to hypervolemia or hypovolemia and concomitant electrolyte imbalances. In small children, the usual procedure for "enemas until clear" may need to be modified to prevent these problems. The catheter used to administer the solution should also be flexible, well lubricated, and inserted no farther than 2–4 in.

Administration of enemas in children is similar to the procedure for adults. The solution should be at body temperature and should be administered slowly to prevent rapid expansion of the rectal vault. The nurse determines the amount of solution according to the child's body size, not just the child's age, but suggested volumes corresponding to age ranges are

Age	Volume
0–18 months	50–200 mL
18 months–5 years	200–300 mL
5–12 years	300–500 mL
12 years and older	500–800 mL

Infants and young children who do not exhibit sphincter control must be assisted in retaining the enema. The nurse firmly presses the buttocks together to prevent the immediate expulsion of the solution. Children who are still in diapers may be allowed to expel the solution into a diaper. The older child needs an explanation about retaining the solution. Most children age 3 and older can retain the enema for at least a brief period. A bedpan should be available, or the child may be allowed to expel the enema in the toilet. The nurse then notes the quantity and character of the returned solution.

Medications The principal medications used before gastrointestinal procedures are antibiotics and anticholinergics. Kanamycin, neomycin, colistin, and other gut-specific antibiotics may be used to decrease the bacterial flora prior to surgery. Atropine, scopolamine, and other anticholinergic drugs may be administered in preoperative injections in order to inhibit the production of saliva and mucus. These medications are commonly used in such procedures as cleft lip and cleft palate repairs, esophagoscopy, and gastroscopy. The parent and child should be aware that anticholinergics may cause flushing and dryness of mouth.

Dietary Modifications The child undergoing gastrointestinal diagnostic tests may be placed on a restricted diet. The most common dietary change is to allow nothing by mouth (NPO). The nurse then assesses the child's fluid status once the child has been NPO for more than 4–6 hours. Other diet regimens may include clear liquids, full liquids, high- or low-fat diets, or exclusionary diets for certain disaccharides. Clear liquids include apple juice, Gatorade, Pedialyte, some kinds of soda pop (for example, 7-Up), Popsicles, gelatin, and broth. Full liquids contain milk or pulp and include orange juice, milk, ice cream, puddings, custards, cream soups, and commercially prepared diets (for example, Sustacal). Most hospitals maintain lists of foods that may be served for each type of diet. The nurse can often encourage cooperation with dietary restrictions by offering the child a choice of foods or by allowing substitutions whenever possible. (Principles of managing a child's food intake are discussed in Chapter 29.) If dietary restrictions are to be maintained for longer then 24 hours, the nurse may need to assess the child's intake for caloric and dietary sufficiency (Chapter 15 discusses nutritional assessment).

Gastric Decompression

Many kinds of gastrointestinal dysfunction require placement of a nasogastric (NG) tube for gastric decompression. Children with diarrhea, pancreatitis, or other inflammatory conditions may be placed on NG suction in order to rest the stomach and bowel. Children with an intussusception, obstruction, or postoperative ileus require drainage of gastric juices until normal bowel function returns. For these children, certain principles of nursing care can prevent complications.

The first principle is to choose the correct tube. The person who places the initial tube should choose the smallest possible sump tube that will still allow proper suctioning. Children with gastric bleeding or those swallowing large amounts of mucus may require a tube with a large lumen. A tube of appropriate size can prevent necrosis of nasal tissues due to pressure, minimize postplacement tissue damage, and limit the stimulation of the gag reflex. The tube should be measured correctly and be well lubricated before placement. It is then securely taped to the child's nose or upper lip in a way that prevents traction against the nares.

Once gastric decompression has been started, the nurse observes the tube for proper functioning. When connected to suction, the tube should drain freely. Drainage should be clear to yellow-green. The presence of blood may indicate gastric wall irritation or trauma. Children undergoing prolonged gastric suctioning are also prone to mechanical irritation and development of ulcers, so that many physicians prescribe prophylactic antacids in conjunction with intubation.

Nurses frequently encounter problems with NG tube function. Placement of the tube is checked by aspirating gastric contents or by injecting a small amount of air while listening with a stethoscope over the fundus of the stomach. If the tube is properly placed but no drainage returns, it may be necessary to irrigate the tube with saline. If the tube is occluded, the gastric pressure is elevated, or the air vent is lower than the stomach (thereby creating a siphon effect), the gastric contents may drain through the air vent. If this occurs, the vent may be irrigated with a small amount of saline followed by enough air to clear the vent of saline. The nurse then secures the vent at a level higher than the patient's stomach to prevent further siphoning. This may be accomplished by pinning the vent to the pillow or with older children, by taping the suction tubing to an IV pole. Taping, however, requires close observation to prevent their dislodging the tube. If these measures fail or the child continues to vomit around the tube, the nurse replaces the tube in order to ensure adequate gastric decompression.

Children who are receiving gastric decompression through gastrostomy (a procedure in which a tube is surgically placed and secured in the stomach) are ordinarily not connected to suction. Instead, the open tube is placed to dependent drainage. Some physicians prefer clamping the tube but removing gastric fluid every hour or so if gastric output is limited.

The nurse records all gastric output in the intake and output record and reports any unusual color, odor, or substance. Because children lose large amounts of fluid and electrolytes during gastric suctioning, these are replaced intravenously. The nurse therefore observes for signs and symptoms of electrolyte imbalances (see Chapter 33).

Ostomy Care

Children undergo placement of ostomies for many reasons. Colostomies and ileostomies are most commonly performed because of congenital anomalies (for example, gastroschisis, intestinal atresias), or because of bowel ischemia (for example, volvulus, necrotizing enterocolitis). Trauma or chronic inflammatory bowel disease may also necessitate ostomy placement.

The child who requires an ostomy requires age-appropriate patient teaching. Psychologic preparation of both child and parent is vital to their acceptance of the stoma as a condition allowing a normal life.

The nurse may be able to provide the parent and child with some measure of control during preoperative procedures by involving them in selection of the stoma site (Beyers and Dudas, 1984). This is also a good opportunity for both parent and child to see and handle ostomy appliances, although several types of appliances may be tried before one is found to provide adequate skin protection, a reasonable wearing time, comfort, and easy availability. The appliance will need to fit well while the child sits or bends, so that selecting a site is best done when the child is awake and can participate as much as possible.

Ostomy care varies depending on the placement site and the location of the opening along the bowel. Ostomy supplies include a variety of protective agents and appliance sizes. Disposable rather than reusable appliances have also become more common now that the wide choice of disposable equipment allows for more efficient odor control and ease of application. When teaching a new ostomate and family, the nurse considers economic, physical, and psychologic needs. For example, parents with limited funds may prefer a reusable appliance. Parents may need to be made aware that they are able to choose equipment other than the brand used by the hospital. Several companies supply pediatric ostomy appliances and parents may wish to try several brands before making a choice. They also need to be informed that a growing child is likely to need frequent readjustments of a permanent appliance.

Principles of Nursing Care

Acute-Care Needs

A child with a suspected gastrointestinal disorder requires close observation of functions related to the digestive tract. Nursing principles that are particularly important to these children include intake and output records, stool records, emesis records, daily weight measurements, infection control, and continued assessment for complications that may arise from the disease process.

Intake and output records are vitally important in monitoring any gastrointestinal dysfunction. Besides providing an indicator of fluid status, these records also help in identifying changes in stool patterns, nutritional patterns, or recurring emesis. Intake and output records of hospitalized children should include the following:

1. *Intravenous fluids*—type of solution, rate of infusion, amount infused, blood products
2. *Oral intake*—type and amount of oral liquids and solid intake if calorie count or dietary estimates are needed
3. *Emesis, Levine tube/pump output*—quantity, quality, color, and presence of blood (if any)
4. *Urine*—color, quantity, pH, and glucose (if needed)
5. *Stool*—quantity, quality, consistency, color, texture, presence or absence of blood, pus, mucus, unusual odors, glucose, or reducing substances

Children receiving hyperalimentation or constant-drip fluids also require infusion pumps for more accurate delivery of these fluids. For infants, infusion pumps for intravenous fluids whenever possible are a safety measure and may prevent fluid overload or rapid administration of intravenous fluids. (Safety measures associated with intravenous administration are discussed in Chapter 29.)

Accurate stool records are essential in childhood diarrhea and allow the nurse to evaluate the results of the nursing or medical interventions. In addition, infants receiving total parenteral nutrition require continuous monitoring of all urine and stool output to indicate the child's response to the hyperalimentation. Children with severe constipation or encopresis (see Chapter 24) also require stool records to document the problem.

Children with gastrointestinal disorders causing chronic or severe weight loss, failure to thrive, or fluid retention (ascites) require frequent weight measurements. Although daily measurements are usually sufficient, certain children may need to be weighed more frequently. Those with severe diarrhea or those with liver damage resulting in ascites may need to be weighed as often as two to three times per day. Each child should also be weighed on the same scale each day, as differences between scales can vary significantly enough to alter treatment regimens. Metabolic or bed scales may be needed for comatose children.

The child should be weighed in similar clothing each day. Infants are weighed without diapers, and older children should remove excess clothing or slippers. Only clothing necessary for the child's sense of modesty should remain. The presence of an armboard or bulky bandage should also be noted in the weight records and the weight of the board recorded, if known.

Abdominal Surgery in Children Children undergoing abdominal surgery require many of the same preoperative preparations as adults, but for the child, age-appropriate explanations of the impending surgery are also important (see Chapter 29).

(text continued on p. 1308)

NURSING CARE GUIDE The Child Undergoing Colostomy or Ileostomy

Nursing Diagnosis	Interventions	Evaluation
Preoperative		
1. Potential for infection from inadequately or improperly cleansed bowel	Administer oral or intravenous medications and saline or antibiotic enemas as required Maintain gastric suction or restricted diet if needed	Bowel is cleansed preoperatively
2. Potential for dehydration	Assess need for intravenous fluids if child is NPO Record intake and output, including emesis, enema return, and retained enema solution	Adequate hydration status is maintained
3. Potential for complications related to preoperative preparation or presenting condition	Observe for signs of sepsis or shock due to perforation or peritonitis (decreasing blood pressure, tachycardia, hyperthermia or hypothermia, behavioral changes) Observe for signs of obstruction (gastric distention, emesis, abdominal discomfort)	There are no preoperative complications
4. Potential knowledge deficit related to preoperative procedures and operative environment	Explain all preoperative procedures with age-appropriate terms; answer questions honestly, frankly, and concretely (see Chapter 29) Take child on tour of recovery room and ICU, if possible	Child is appropriately prepared for impending surgery and postoperative care
5. Potential knowledge deficit related to operative procedure and changes in body image	For young child, teach child with concrete terms and drawings or ostomy doll showing ostomy at corresponding body part (urine collection bag may be used to illustrate appliance); describe all dressings and drains accurately (see Chapter 29) For older child, begin teaching several weeks before surgery, if possible, using drawings, dolls, or other models showing placement of ostomy and appliance; answer questions frankly and honestly; encourage child to express anxieties, ask questions, and perform self-care Involve enterostomal therapist, if possible	Child explains ostomy surgery in language appropriate to developmental stage
6. Potential parental knowledge deficit related to need for surgery and postoperative care	Review need for ostomy Encourage questions Use doll or pictures to show stoma placement Explain future closure procedure if ostomy is temporary Begin explaining stoma care, familiarizing parent with basic equipment	Parent describes the need for and impact of the child's surgery and postoperative care
Postoperative		
1. Potential for postoperative complications related to abdominal surgery	Perform necessary procedures related to gastric decompression, hydration status, respiratory function, prevention of infection, and immobility	Child experiences no postoperative complications

NURSING CARE GUIDE The Child Undergoing Colostomy or Ileostomy (continued)

Nursing Diagnosis	Interventions	Evaluation
2. Potential for complications related to stoma	Note color of mucosa, which should be red; pale or livid mucosa may indicate circulatory compromise, although stoma is normally edematous for several days after surgery	Stoma maintains normal function
	Record drainage from stoma, which should begin to drain mucus or liquid stool after bowel sounds are heard	
	Observe for any herniation of the bowel through the stoma site	
	Observe for fresh bleeding from the base of the stoma	
3. Potential for skin breakdown at stoma site	Change dressings frequently, using Telfa; transverse, descending, or sigmoid colostomy may be left open to air	There are no signs of skin breakdown at stoma site
	Apply occlusive ointment to skin around stoma site if ostomy has begen to drain and stoma appliance is not applied	
	Apply ostomy bag to prevent maceration if drainage is extensive or excoriating (which is common in ileostomy)	
	Clean skin thoroughly at stoma site before applying new appliance; use skin barrier (for example, karaya, Skin Prep, Stomadhesive) to protect skin from drainage (karaya and Stomadhesive should be placed as close to the stoma edge as possible to prevent leakage of fecal material)	
	Observe for excoriation, weeping skin, maceration, infection, and ulceration at the stoma site	
	Empty ostomy bag frequently to prevent the weight of the contents from placing traction on the skin	
4. Potential knowledge deficit related to stoma care	Have parent and child observe nurse during stoma care and appliance change; explain all steps in these procedures	Child and parent are appropriately prepared for discharge
	Supervise parent and child as they perform ostomy care; verify that they are capable of performing care without assistance	
	For older child, encourage as much self-care as possible	
5. Potential for fears related to alteration in body image	Allow both parent and child to express fears, perceptions, and psychological distress; observe both parent and child for signs of extreme distress	Parent and child recognize fears and stress of altered body image and use appropriate means of expression
	For older child, encourage visit from another ostomate	

continued on next page

NURSING CARE GUIDE The Child Undergoing Colostomy or Ileostomy (continued)

Nursing Diagnosis	Interventions	Evaluation
6. Potential parental knowledge deficit related to specific dietary needs	Explain any dietary restrictions or limitations (for example, limiting gas-causing foods such as cabbage or spices) Explain need for increased fluid intake, especially following ileostomy	Parent can explain any dietary needs and limitations
7. Need for appropriate activity levels related to degree of healing at surgical site	Explain all activity limitations, noting that child may resume all normal activities except contact sports once the site is healed Explain to the parent that a child who resumes normal activities begins accepting the ostomy	Parent and child can explain any limitations in activity and their rationale
8. Potential need for support related to ongoing management of changes in body image and activities of daily living	Provide parent with written instructions about care and return appointments Provide a contact person (for example, public health nurse or enterostomal therapist) for questions that arise after discharge Provide parent and child any available helpful hints for ostomy care, as needed Inform parent about national organization of ostomates and any local community support groups that are available	Parent and child can explain the need for follow-up care and are aware of additional support systems

Because a large percentage of abdominal operations in children are emergency interventions, preoperative teaching is often extremely limited. The nurse attempts to explain to the child and family as much of what is taking place as is possible, but the nurse also plans postoperative discussions with the child to minimize the effects of having been unprepared for surgery. The parent usually requires more intensive psychologic support if emergency surgery is necessary, so that the nurse often needs to make a concerted effort to keep the parents informed of what is happening to the child.

Control of Infection and Complications Because of the organisms involved, infection control is particularly important in gastrointestinal disorders. Diarrhea and hepatitis, for example, can be highly contagious, and it has been hypothesized that an infectious agent is responsible in multiple outbreaks of necrotizing enterocolitis in neonatal nurseries. Nurses therefore need to be cognizant of routine infection control methods. Hands should be washed before entering a room, before caring for a patient, and before leaving the room in order to prevent cross-contamination between patients and to protect the nurse. Parents, family members, and patients should be reminded of the importance of hand washing, and nurses need to insist on compliance. Children with diarrhea or hepatitis also require enteric isolation precautions; those with wound infections or ruptured appendices require wound and skin isolation precautions. Isolation procedures vary from institution to institution, but some basic guidelines are presented in Table 38-3.

Children with gastrointestinal problems may experience complications related to either the disease or the treatment. Nurses therefore need to observe children for changes that may indicate the onset of complications. Sepsis may occur in necrotizing entercolitis and toxic megacolon; shock may occur with perforation or acute gastrointestinal bleeding; obstruction may occur in the small or large bowel (Table 38-4). Complications related to treatment can include stress ulcers, wound infections, obstruction due to prolonged constipation or retained barium, skin breakdown due to inappropriate positioning, insufficient perineal care, or ineffective ostomy care. Children receiving drip feedings or tube feedings are prone to aspiration. Children who are at nutritional risk should be observed for signs of iatrogenic malnutrition due to prolonged intravenous glucose solutions; these children may require hyperalimentation. Those children currently receiving hyperalimentation should be observed for problems relating to fluid overload, hyperglycemia, or catheter contamination.

NURSING CARE GUIDE The Child Undergoing Abdominal Surgery

Nursing Diagnosis	Interventions	Evaluation
1. Potential knowledge deficit related to preoperative procedures and operative events	Explain purpose of surgery in language that the child can understand For young child, reinforce teaching that surgery is not a punishment but must be done to fix a problem Inform parent and child about preoperative procedures and reasons for them; include routine preoperative procedures such as blood tests, enemas, and injections with age-appropriate explanations (see Chapter 29) Discuss specific postoperative preparation as indicated by nature and severity of problem	Child and parent are appropriately prepared for surgery
2. Potential alteration in fluid volume, excess or deficit	Maintain NPO status, intravenous administration, or special diet as required	Appropriate fluid volume is maintained
3. Potential for infection related to altered health status and surgery	Administer oral and intravenous antibiotics as required Administer antibiotic enemas or nasogastric instillations as indicated	Child has no signs of infection prior to surgery
4. Potential alteration in nutrition, less than body requirements, related to altered health status	Maintain special diet as required	Child is physically prepared for surgery
5. Potential alteration in comfort related to preoperative procedures	Provide age-appropriate teaching about preoperative routines (see Chapter 29) Minimize discomfort during procedures	Child experiences minimal discomfort and cooperates with preoperative procedures and routines
6. Potential for complications related to presenting condition	Observe for increasing abdominal distension or emesis, absence of bowel sounds, or acute pain, which may indicate intestinal obstruction Observe for changes in vital signs (tachycardia, tachypnea, hypotension, hypothermia), which may indicate sepsis or shock	Child experiences no preoperative complications related to existing gastrointestinal problem
7. Potential for postoperative complications related to inadequate gastric drainage from NG intubation	Monitor vital signs Maintain child NPO with NG tube Check frequently for patency and proper functioning Irrigate NG tube (as indicated) if tube becomes blocked by mucus or will not drain well Use suction (as indicated) to prevent gastric irritation Observe for blood in gastric drainage, which may indicate early irritation or ulceration	Child exhibits no signs of immediate postoperative complications Adequate drainage is maintained while bowel sounds are absent
8. Potential postoperative complications related to healing of surgical site	Observe for signs of unusual bleeding or drainage and report amount and characteristics Observe for signs and symptoms of wound infection (redness, edema, purulent, or foul-smelling discharge) Change dressings as indicated, using sterile technique	Child does not develop complications related to healing of surgical site

continued on next page

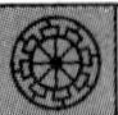

NURSING CARE GUIDE The Child Undergoing Abdominal Surgery (continued)

Nursing Diagnosis	Interventions	Evaluation
9. Potential for ineffective breathing pattern related to postoperative status	Have child turn, cough, and deep-breathe at least once every 2 hours Have child ambulate as soon as possible Auscultate lung fields for breath sounds when taking vital signs to assess for signs that might indicate early impaired pulmonary function	Child does not develop complications of postoperative pulmonary status
10. Impaired physical mobility related to postoperative status	Turn child at least once every 2 hours Have child ambulate as soon as possible Perform range-of-motion exercise if child is confined to bed	Child does not develop complications related to immobility
11. Potential alteration in fluid volume related to postoperative status	Maintain intravenous fluids until oral fluid intake is adequate Record intake and output Record first postoperative urine sample in order to verify kidney function Assess intravenous site frequently for phlebitis or infiltration	Hydration status is maintained
12. Potential for postoperative ileus related to surgical procedure	Maintain child NPO with NG suction until intestinal function returns Assess for bowel sounds and the passage of flatus Record amount and characteristics of first postoperative stool	There are no signs of postoperative ileus
13. Alteration in comfort related to surgical procedures	Encourage parent to hold infant or young child Allow child to assume comfortable position unless otherwise indicated Turn and reposition child every 2 hours Provide frequent mouth care with petroleum jelly to dry lips Position NG tube to prevent tension on tape or tissue necrosis of nares Administer analgesics as needed Record child's reaction to pain and need for medication (see Chapter 29)	Child remains as comfortable as possible
14. Potential knowledge deficit related to postoperative condition and home care	Review any necessary wound care, dressing changes, and similar procedures Provide both written and oral instructions with return demonstrations Inform parent about any necessary supplies that may be needed on child's return home Inform parent and child about diet, activity limitations, and return appointments Inform parent and child about any possible complications (for example, increased tem-	Child and parent are appropriately prepared for discharge

NURSING CARE GUIDE The Child Undergoing Abdominal Surgery (continued)

Nursing Diagnosis	Interventions	Evaluation
	perature, nausea, vomiting) that they should report Provide parent with a contact person in case of questions or problems regarding dressing changes, diet, or similar procedures (contact person might be physician, public health nurse, primary care nurse, or enterostomal therapist) Remind parent that sleep problems and behavior problems, including regressive behaviors, are common reactions to hospitalization (see Chapter 27) Encourage parent to discuss hospitalization with the child and to seek help if child exhibits prolonged problems	

TABLE 38-3 Isolation Precautions

	Enteric precautions	Contact precautions
Room	Child requires private room	Child requires private room
Gown and gloves	Gowns and gloves worn by all persons having direct contact with excreta (urine, stool, emesis, saliva) or having contact with soiled linen, instruments, or other articles	Gowns and gloves worn by all persons having direct contact with contaminated dressings or linens
Masks	Not necessary	Not necessary
Hand washing	All persons must wash hands before entering and after leaving room	All persons must wash hands before entering room and after caring for child
Other precautions	All instruments or materials contaminated by urine, stool, emesis, or saliva must be double-bagged and labeled for sterilization	All dressings and disposable instruments must be double-bagged, labeled, and discarded; all linens and reusable items must be double-bagged and labeled for sterilization

TABLE 38-4 Symptoms of Obstruction in the Small and Large Bowels

Symptom	Small bowel	Large bowel
Vomiting	Profuse, frequent, may or may not be bile-stained	Little or no vomiting Bile-stained
Dehydration	Occurs quickly	Little or none
Distention	Minimal	Occurs early, is often severe
Onset of symptoms	Rapid, acute	Slow, progressive
Pain	Severe, cramping, intermittent	Mild, steady rather than intermittent
Shock	Onset may be rapid because of massive loss of fluid into gut or because of sepsis	Less common unless colon ruptures
Stool	Stool and flatus remaining in colon may be passed initially	No stools

Nutritional Needs

Children experiencing a change or disruption in gastrointestinal function require continued assessment of fluid or caloric intake. Fluid supplementation is important when the child cannot maintain oral fluid intake (for example, when the child is NPO) or when the child is losing large amounts of fluid and electrolytes (for example, in vomiting, diarrhea, or short-bowel syndrome). Adequate caloric intake is necessary to maintain normal growth and development. Caloric supplementation is begun when oral intake is restricted or insufficient to prevent negative nitrogen balance. Children with malabsorption syndromes or severely restricted diets also require caloric supplementation in order to provide for normal growth.

Fluid requirements are calculated on the basis of the child's age and weight. The degree of dehydration often determines the type of fluids and the speed at which fluids are delivered. Such conditions as diaphoresis, diabetes insipidus, and renal disorders require alterations in fluid replacement therapy.

Caloric requirements are calculated according to body weight, age, and physical activity. (Chapter 15 discusses caloric and nutritional needs in relation to these variables.) Children who cannot maintain an adequate caloric intake require enteral or parenteral supplementation. Enteral alimentation may include special formulas or diets and special techniques for providing these supplements (for example, continuous NG drip or gavage). Parenteral alimentation may include standard intravenous glucose and electrolyte solutions or may encompass total parenteral nutrition (TPN).

Table 38-5 lists standard and special infant formulas or supplements. The more common indications for these also provide a guide to caloric supplementation or dietary therapy. Children who are unable to take these oral formulas may require tube feeding or special feeding nipples, cups, or spoons.

Enteral Nutrition The two most common forms of tube feedings are gavage and gastrostomy feedings. Gavage feedings are usually temporary and are used when the child is unable to suck or swallow, when the child has respiratory or cardiac distress associated with nipple feedings, or when the child is unconscious. A gastrostomy tube may be placed for children with anatomic anomalies of the oropharynx, esophagus, or cardiac sphincter. Children who are dysphagic or who are severely mentally and physically handicapped may also require gastrostomy placement.

Gavage feeding involves intermittent placement of a feeding tube into the stomach through the nostril or mouth (Fig. 38-2). The tube is usually removed after each feeding, and a new tube is placed for each successive feeding. Tubes left in place for several feedings require replacement every

TABLE 38-5 Special Formulas and Formula Supplements

	Product	Manufacturer	Indications and comments
Electrolyte solutions	Pedialyte	Ross	Clear liquid diet for use in diarrhea and oral rehydration
	Lytren	Mead Johnson	Clear liquid diet for use in diarrhea and oral rehydration
Soy based formulas	Neo-Mull-Soy	Syntex	Allergy to milk protein
	Prosobee	Mead Johnson	Allergy to milk protein
	Isomil	Ross	Allergy to milk protein
Elemental diets	Vivonex	Eaton	Dietary supplement or total diet
	Flexical	Mead Johnson	Contains soy and medium-chain triglycerides
Diets for malabsorptive conditions	Portagen	Mead Johnson	Used for short-bowel syndrome and fat malabsorption; fat is in form of medium-chain triglycerides and safflower oils
	Nutramigen	Mead Johnson	Enzymatic hydrolysate of casein frequently used in children with cystic fibrosis or any difficulty absorbing food proteins
	Pregestimil	Mead Johnson	Used for various malabsorption syndromes, contains medium-chain triglycerides
	CHO-Free	Syntex	Carbohydrate free (specific carbohydrates must be added as tolerated), often used in short-bowel syndrome
	Meat Base	Gerber	For allergy to milk protein and for children requiring a lower osmolality in formula
Low-phenylalanine formulas	Lofenalac	Mead Johnson	For children with phenylketonuria
	Albumaid XP	Ross	Used primarily for older children with phenylketonuria

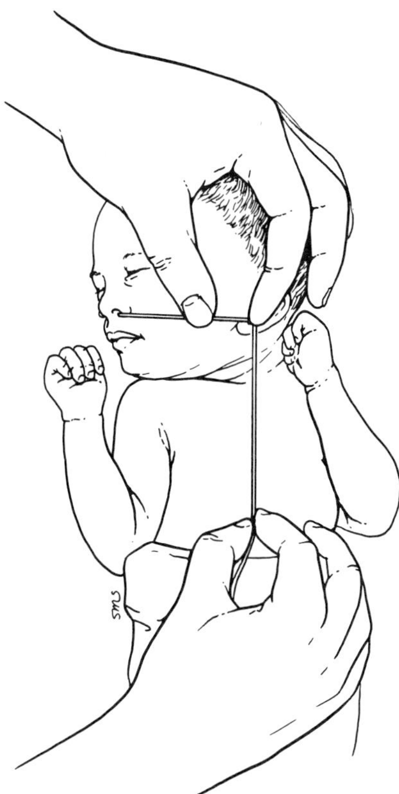

Figure 38-2 A gastrostomy tube for gavage feeding is measured from the tip of the nose to the earlobe and then to a point midway between the tip of the sternum and the umbilicus.

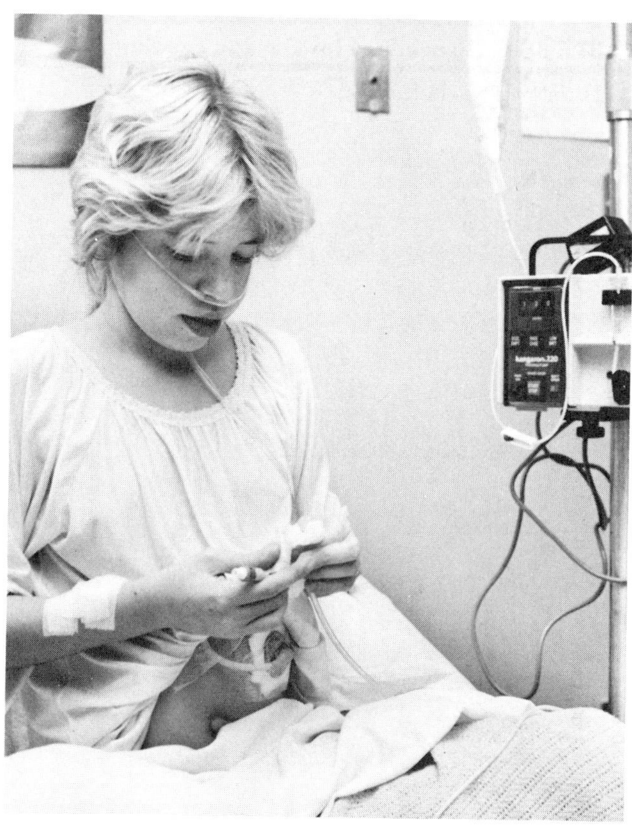

Child with gastrostomy feeding.

24–72 hours. Older children, particularly those with chronic disabilities requiring long-term tube feedings may only require tube changes every 3–7 days. Those requiring continuous drip feedings require frequent bottle changes to prevent bacterial contamination of formula that is at room temperature. Children receiving blender-prepared tube feedings may experience more problems with blockage of the tube than those receiving commercial formulas. Table 38-6 describes the steps and precautions involved in gavage feedings.

A *gastrostomy* involves operative placement of a tube through the abdominal wall and into the greater curvature of the stomach. The stomach is sutured to the peritoneal wall at the ostomy site in order to prevent the leakage of gastric contents into the abdominal cavity. The tube is a large-lumen retention catheter which facilitates holding it in place in the stomach. The site is kept clean and dry, and no dressing is required once healing has occurred. The nurse needs to prevent tension on the catheter, as this may cause bleeding or damage to the ostomy site. Table 38-7 describes the steps and precautions involved in gastrostomy feedings.

The child with neurologic or anatomic anomalies may require other feeding methods, which may include special nipples, spoons, or cups. Cleft palate nipples, lamb's nipples, or special cleft palate feeding systems (for example, Beniflex) may be required for children with cleft lips or palates. All of these methods allow the child to maintain adequate caloric intake orally.

Vitamin and Mineral Supplementation Children with increased metabolic needs or impaired gastrointestinal absorption may require vitamin and mineral supplementation. These supplements are given orally, intramuscularly, or intravenously. For example, children with steatorrhea, pancreatitis, or hepatic damage may require oral supplementation with water-soluble forms of the fat-soluble vitamins A, D, E, and K. Vitamin B_{12}, if indicated, may be given intramuscularly.

Children at general nutritional risk for other reasons may require supplementation of all vitamins and some minerals. (Nutritional assessment and vitamin requirements are discussed in Chapter 15.)

Parenteral Nutrition When oral intake is restricted, inadequate, or impossible, parenteral nutritional supplementation may be necessary. Parenteral supplementation can consist of carbohydrates, protein, lipids, or any combination. In addition, certain vitamins, electrolytes, and trace minerals can be given intravenously if therapy is prolonged.

TABLE 38-6 Procedure for Gavage Feeding

Assemble needed materials	Appropriately sized feeding tube: 5–8 French for infants, 10–14 French for older children, and thicker formulas Syringes: one large (20–50 mL) and one small (3–5 mL) Lubricant: water or water-soluble jelly Tape: to secure tube to child's face Stethoscope: to check placement
Position and restrain child	Slightly right side–lying or with chest elevated If child is able to resist, swaddle wrap child, obtain assistance to hold child's arms, or hold child in lap
Measure correct length of feeding tube	Measure from mouth to earlobe for oral insertion, or from tip of nose to earlobe for nasal insertion, and then to a point midway between the distal xyphoid process and the umbilicus Mark this length with a small piece of tape
Insert lubricated tube	Insert tube with firm, steady motion but do not force. If difficulty is encountered, try other nostril; pass to designated tape mark
Verify proper positioning of tube	Aspirate stomach contents into attached small syringe or inject 2–5 mL of air into tube while listening with a stethoscope over the stomach (bubbling or gurgling indicates proper positions), withdraw air
Secure tube with tape	Wrap strip of one-half-inch tape around tube and secure to child's nose. Bring tube to side of face and secure with tape again.
Instill feeding	Pour formula at room temperature into large syringe barrel attached to tube Allow formula to flow by gravity (initial plunger pressure may be needed to begin flow) A tube feeding should take approximately as long as a normal bottle feeding (15–20 min) Allow child to suck on pacifier while instilling formula
Flush tube with sterile water or air	
Remove tube	Pinch or crimp tube before removing to prevent leakage of formula
Burp and reposition infant	Gastric air intake is limited during gavage feedings. If child has been allowed a pacifier during feeding, it is very important to burp infant well to prevent retention of swallowed air

Total parenteral nutrition is commonly used for bowel atresias, prolonged ileus, intractable diarrhea, short-bowel syndrome, or obstruction and can be used to provide bowel rest in cases of Crohn's disease or ulcerative colitis.

The standard hyperalimentation fluid consists of a high concentration of glucose and amino acids. Glucose concentrations greater than 12% are irritating to peripheral vein walls and are usually delivered through a central venous catheter, which can be placed through either the external jugular or the subclavian veins. These catheters can be short term or long term (for example, Broviac or Hickman). Because the central line is placed in a large vein and reflux of blood into the line is common, the fluid needs to be placed on an infusion pump. This allows for continuous, regulated administration of fluid and prevents clot or embolus formation. An in-line filter is used to prevent introduction of bacteria or air into the central circulation. Medications are not usually given through a central line during hyperalimentation and should never be given through the in-line filter because the filter screens out the medication and may become blocked. A Y-connection or Y-vent may therefore be needed if central line medications are necessary and no peripheral line is possible. If medications are to be given through the central line during hyperalimentation, the nurse checks with the pharmacist about the compatibility of the solution and the drug, as it may be necessary to discontinue

TABLE 38-7 Procedure for Gastrostomy Feeding

Assemble needed materials	Syringe (20–50 mL) Formula (room temperature)
Check for gastric residue	Attach syringe to gastrostomy and aspirate residue. If amount of residue is large (5–10 mL for premature infants, 10–25 mL for newborn), replace residue and decrease present feeding by equal amount. If residue continues or increases, report to physician
Instill formula while allowing child to suck on pacifier	Formula is poured into barrel of attached syringe and allowed to flow by gravity Formula should flow easily. Feeding should take same amount of time as regular bottle feeding (15–20 min)
Clamp tubing or suspend open end to allow for escape of trapped air	Most children's tubes are clamped or plugged between feedings. Observe for gastric distention. If distention occurs, tube may be suspended to open air to allow for escape of trapped air
Reposition child	Place child in right side-lying or Fowler's position to promote gastric emptying

the TPN solution until the medication has been infused. If TPN must be temporarily discontinued, the nurse infuses a high-glucose solution (for example, 10% dextrose in water) in order to prevent hypoglycemia. If additional calories are needed or if prolonged therapy is expected, it may become necessary to augment the glucose and protein solution. Emulsified lipid solutions can be delivered through peripheral veins or central lines.

Complications Complications of hyperalimentation are related to the protein and glucose concentration, the rate of administration, the possibility of fat or air emboli, and infection related to contamination of the fluid, tubing, or insertion site. These complications can be life-threatening, and children undergoing TPN require close monitoring.

Complications related to fluid strength can be prevented by gradually introducing the child to more concentrated glucose solutions. Starter-strength TPN solution is usually 10% glucose, and the concentration can be slowly increased until the child is receiving at least 20% glucose through the central catheter. During hyperalimentation, frequent blood tests are needed to determine glucose, electrolyte, mineral, and protein levels, and laboratory tests are carried out to determine renal and hepatic function. All urine should be tested for glucose and protein, and stools for glucose and pH. An increase in urine glucose may indicate that the child is not tolerating the increased solute load or that a fluid overload has occurred. Insulin may need to be added to the fluid to aid the child in metabolizing high-glucose concentrations. Infusion pumps set to a prescribed flow rate can prevent underinfusion or overinfusion, but increases in the infusion rate in order to make up for underinfusion are contraindicated, as they may lead to hyperglycemia and osmotic diuresis. Furthermore, decreasing the infusion rate to compensate for overinfusion may lead to hypoglycemia. Any marked change in the infusion rate is therefore reported to the child's physician.

Air emboli can be prevented by using an in-line micropore filter, which prevents large quantities of air from entering central circulation. Rapid tubing changes and removal of air bubbles introduced during tubing changes can also limit the introduction of extraneous air. Infusion pumps that monitor the presence of in-line air are also useful in preventing large air boluses caused by accidently disconnected tubing. Fat emboli can be prevented by making sure that lipid solutions are fully emulsified (no evidence of separation). Continuous-infusion pumps ensure that lipids are delivered at the slow rate that has been ordered.

Infection leading to septicemia is a life-threatening complication. Bacterial or fungal contamination may occur in the bottle, the tubing, at the catheter insertion site, or at the catheter tip. Hyperalimentation fluid is prepared under the laminar-flow hood in the pharmacy. Multiple-line or multiple-filter tubing may also be prepared under the hood in order to limit the possibility of contamination on the unit during tubing setups. Contamination of the tubing during tubing changes can be prevented by using appropriate aseptic technique. Many hospitals have developed special procedures related to hyperalimentation, which vary from very clean techniques to entirely sterile technique.

Infection at the catheter insertion site is minimized by performing sterile dressing changes every 24 to 48 hours. The nurse then examines the site for erythema, induration, or suppuration. The skin surrounding the insertion site is then cleansed with an antiseptic solution (usually providone-iodine). An antibiotic ointment may also be applied to the site before a sterile, occlusive dressing is applied.

Formation of a thrombus at the catheter tip is a frequent complication in children undergoing long-term hyperalimentation. This thrombus may embolize or may become the site of an infection. If infection of the tip is suspected, the physician may wish to perform blood cultures. The tip of the catheter should also be cultured if a suspected infection necessitates the removal of the central line.

Home Hyperalimentation Home hyperalimentation is feasible for children who require long-term TPN. With home care, the adverse effects of prolonged hospitalization can be diminished and the cost of administration minimized while allowing the family to function without dividing attention between home and hospital. Assessment of the home environment and the feasibility of home care are discussed in Chapter 26.

In addition to family resources and capabilities, the nurse needs to ask whether the family's insurance company or another agency is willing to continue coverage once the child begins TPN at home. Many companies have agreed to extend coverage to home care once they have determined the 25%–35% possible savings. Once the child and family are deemed candidates for home hyperalimentation, the nurse begins parent education. Parent and child teaching needs to be planned to minimize exposing the parent to a variety of contradictory or confusing techniques. Performing procedures in a consistent manner should avoid confusion.

The parent needs to learn the concepts, principles, and possible complications involved in the administration of TPN at home. Parents need both explanations and demonstrations of the necessary skills and should participate in their children's care at the hospital while supervised by the nurse. The parent should also practice 24-hour TPN care at the hospital before the child is discharged. This may be accomplished by having the family provide total care for 48–72 hours in the hospital or at a motel or a friend's home near the hospital. This level of responsibility allows the family to become familiar with the home care routine and to work out any "bugs" while the nurse is readily available.

Once the child has been discharged, the hospital nurse or a local public health nurse maintains close contact with the family. This provides a local resource person in the event that any problems arise. The local physician should also know about home hyperalimentation and should be responsible for the necessary monitoring the child requires.

Long-term hyperalimentation has been associated with many physical and emotional difficulties. Possible physical complications include sepsis, thrombus, embolus, fluid overload, electrolyte imbalances, growth disturbances, and osteopenia. Emotional complications may include problems with body image, peer relationships, behavior disturbances, depression, and those associated with any chronic illness (see Chapter 30). The nurse evaluating the child receiving long-term TPN thus continually assesses the child and family for physical and psychological complications of therapy.

Developmental Needs

Children with gastrointestinal disorders may experience difficulty in meeting normal developmental needs. Prolonged gastrointestinal disorders frequently result in failure to grow and gain weight. Intellectual, musculoskeletal, and neurologic abnormalities resulting from chronic malnutrition or malabsorption may thus directly affect the child's ability to achieve developmental milestones.

Developmental needs of infancy and early childhood, which include oral gratification and locomotion, may be compromised by cleft lip or cleft palate. These children are unable to suck well. Frequent surgical repairs and special feeding methods may also prevent infants from receiving adequate oral stimulation. Malabsorption syndromes with resulting intestinal discomfort may lead children to refuse nipple feedings; many children with failure to thrive or rumination syndromes develop alternative, inappropriate means of meeting oral needs, such as constant sucking of their hands, a specific pacifier, a piece of cloth or blanket, or their tongues.

Children undergoing long-term hyperalimentation or medical therapy may also experience restricted mobility and impaired motor development. Arm or leg restraints needed during intravenous therapy, together with the limitations of tubing length, may prevent the infant from learning to roll over, creep, crawl, or walk. Children with long-term malnutrition may not even have the muscle strength needed to elevate their heads or to sit without assistance. Older malnourished children may be unable to develop such motor skills as skipping or running. In addition, older children with aganglionic megacolon, colostomies, anorectal malformations, and some malabsorption syndromes may be unable to attain adequate bowel control.

Emotional Needs

Families of children with chronic gastrointestinal disorders experience a variety of reactions to the diagnosis and its implications (see Chapter 30). Families of children with acute gastrointestinal disorders also experience emotional reactions associated with any acute illness (see Chapter 27). Parents may feel incapable of caring for their children, thereby compounding the stresses of hospitalization. Nurses therefore need to involve families of ill children in planning and contributing to care. Parents may need encouragement to ask questions and share perceptions of their children's responses to illness.

Families of children born with congenital anomalies of the gastrointestinal tract need support while learning to cope with the implications of the defect. Families of children with very obvious anomalies (for example, cleft lip or palate, gastroschisis), or marked failure to thrive are at high risk for attachment problems because their expectations for a healthy, normal infant have been so quickly destroyed. (Nursing care for families of high-risk infants is discussed in Chapter 31.)

Health Maintenance Needs

Parents of children discharged from the hospital require specific information about home care. The nurse provides both spoken and written instructions in order to prevent misunderstandings and may provide a contact person or telephone contact in case the parent encounters difficulties. (Principles of discharge preparation are discussed in Chapter 29.)

Parents need instructions about medications, dietary restrictions, and feeding techniques. The nurse may identify commercially prepared formulas that are available at supermarkets and those that may be specially ordered from pharmacies. If special formulas or diets are to be prepared at home, the parent requires teaching by the nurse or by a nutritionist. Parents may need lists of acceptable foods or lists of specifically banned foods. A nutritionist may be able to provide recipe hints or guidelines to prevent a restrictive diet from becoming boring and repetitious.

The nurse explains any restrictions in activity with reference to the child's normal activities. The ultimate goal is for the child to return to optimal functioning as soon as possible.

Children with Hirschsprung's disease, anorectal malformations, or chronic severe constipation may require additional home teaching regarding bowel training or a bowel regimen. Most bowel-training regimens are based on adequate fluid and dietary fiber intake. Stool softeners or bulk agents may initially be needed to regain normal bowel activity. In addition to softening the stool, most regimens also suggest that the child be required to attempt defecation at the same time every day. Younger children may require toileting after each meal to prevent soiling. The daily routine encourages the child to develop a regular defecation schedule and prevents further stool retention. Those children with neuromuscular anomalies of the pelvis may also require daily enemas or cathartics to prevent the development of an impaction.

The Child With Problems Involving Ingestion

Cleft Lip and Cleft Palate

Clefts of the lip or palate are relatively common, occurring in about 1 in 1000 births in white Americans and less frequently in American blacks. Cleft palate alone occurs in about 1 of every 2500 births (Rudolph, 1982). Transmission of these defects appears to be multifactorial, and affected infants may have close relatives with the defect. Teratogens have also been implicated in certain isolated occurrences.

Cleft lip and cleft palate are facial defects that result from failure of fusion of the primary or secondary palates during gestation. The primary palate is responsible for the development of the lip and anterior maxilla. If closure is not completed by the seventh to eighth week of gestation, the infant is born with a cleft lip. Unilateral cleft lips are usually left sided; bilateral cleft lips are more commonly associated with cleft palates and vary in degree from a simple notch in the vermillion border to a separation that extends into the floor of the nose. The hard and soft palates arise from the secondary palate. If the palatine processes fail to fuse before the twelfth week of gestation, a cleft of the hard or soft palate results. These clefts also vary in severity from a bifid uvula to a complete cleft of the hard and soft palates and may be unilateral, bilateral, or midline.

Cleft lip and cleft palate may occur separately, or may combine to produce a complete unilateral or bilateral cleft from the lip through the soft palate. Cleft lip, either alone or in combination with cleft palate, is more common in males; cleft palate alone is more common in females. Clefts of the lip and palate are more common among those with chromosomal anomalies, and infants with either cleft lip or cleft palate should therefore be examined closely for other congenital anomalies, hearing defects, or mental impairment.

Diagnosis includes classification of the type and severity of the defect as well as a thorough physical examination to rule out related birth defects. An assessment of internal clefts should be done both visually and manually. Visual examination reveals obvious hard palate defects or more subtle defects such as soft palate irregularities or bifid uvula. Digital examination allows for an assessment of the depth and degree of hard palate anomalies as well as for assessment of the infant's sucking capabilities.

Medical and Surgical Treatment Initial medical management of the child with a cleft lip or palate focuses on preventing aspiration of secretions and providing adequate nutrition. The child is usually unable to suck adequately on a standard nipple. Soft nipples with larger holes are used to provide formula while encouraging the child to develop the muscles used for sucking, swallowing, and speech. A cleft palate allows for the escape of formula through the nose. Because the infant is unable to suck and swallow normally, secretions pool in the nasopharynx and may then be aspirated, so that frequent suctioning and careful feedings are important in the prevention of complications.

Surgical correction of the lip defect is usually accomplished at 1 or 2 months of age, although surgery may be performed at any age. Z-plasty, a type of closure consisting of a staggered incision line that minimizes retraction of the

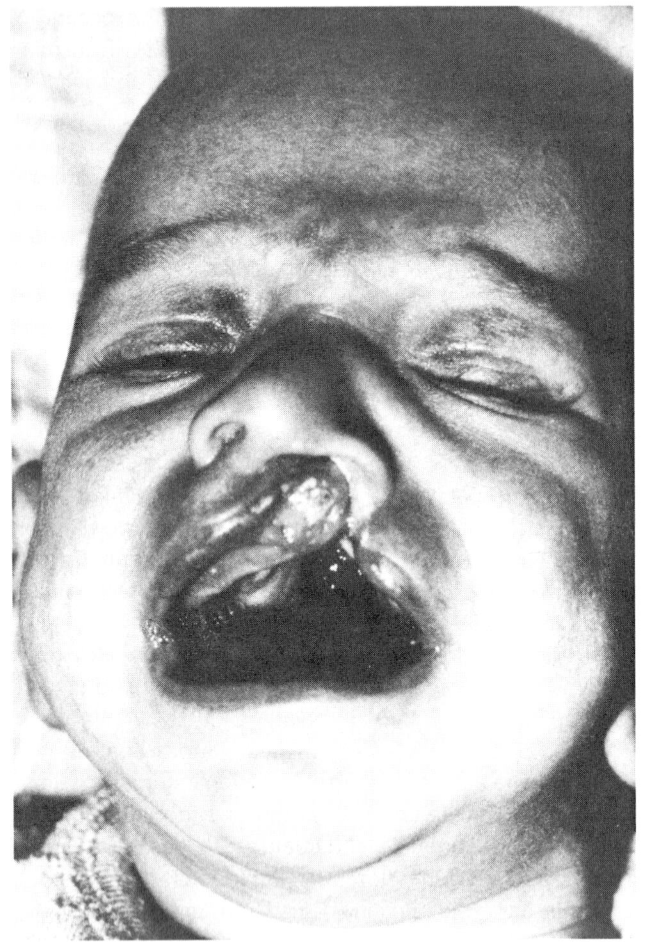

A

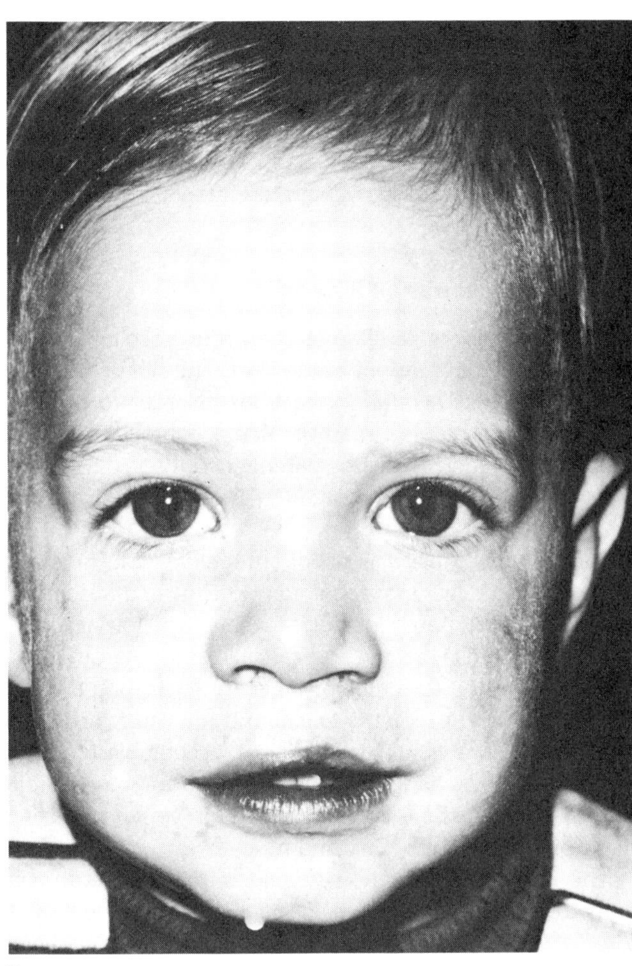

B

Child with cleft lip and palate, before and after repair. (Courtesy David F. Sloan, M.D.)

lip due to scar tissue, is the preferred procedure and allows for a natural-looking closure of the defect. After surgery, a Logan bow (a metal wire arch) may be attached to the cheeks with adhesive tape. This prevents tension on the upper lip and promotes healing with less chance of noticeable scarring.

The timing for surgical correction of cleft palate is based on the severity of the defect. It is usually accomplished between 6 and 18 months of age but may continue in stages until the child is 4 or 5 years of age if the defect is severe. Early correction allows for development of more normal speech patterns, and delayed closure or large defects may require the use of prosthodontic appliances in addition to intensive speech therapy.

Long-term considerations are focused on promoting acceptable speech, preventing or correcting dentition abnormalities, preventing and treating chronic ear infection, and providing psychological support to the child. Speech therapy should begin early in life and may continue through adolescence. Orthodontia is also necessary throughout childhood to correct such problems as extra, malformed, or absent teeth. A myringotomy with tubes may be necessary to prevent recurring ear infections due to improper drainage of the middle ear. The child may require counseling in order to cope with feelings relating to multiple surgeries, residual scarring, or noticeable speech defects.

Nursing Management Immediate nursing care covers three essential areas: (a) maintaining a clear and adequate airway, (b) maintaining fluid and caloric intake, and (c) providing emotional support to the parents. Because cleft lip is an immediately noticeable defect and most parents are unaware of the advances in plastic surgery that now allow for a normal appearance, parents may require repeated reassurance from medical and nursing personnel. The nurse may also act as a role model by treating these infants like any others. Speaking to and cuddling these infants while feeding them allows parents to see that their children are indeed lovable human beings. Most plastic surgeons are willing to provide pictures of children before and after cleft lip repairs. Parents are usually relieved to see that good results even with severe defects.

Nutrition: Potential for Fluid and Calorie Deficit
Nutritional intake may be limited because the infant has trouble sealing the nipple well enough to create effective suction. The size of the defect may preclude breast feeding, but mothers may express milk for bottle feedings if they wish. Special feeding systems and soft nipples with enlarged holes have been developed to aid in easier and safer nipple feedings. Some of these nipples are attached to soft plastic reservoirs that allow slow expression of the formula and limit the need for the child to create suction. Slower delivery of formula also prevents excess milk from escaping through the nose in infants with cleft palates.

Infants should be held upright during feedings. This may be accomplished by holding the child's head while the child is in a seated position or by cradling the infant in the arm. A pillow propped between the nurse or parent's hand or arm and the chair arm can help hold the infant in a more upright position. Because these infants do not "seal" the nipple well, they are prone to swallowing excessive amounts of air and require frequent burping. If the child with a cleft palate vomits, oropharynx and nasal passages require thorough bulb suctioning. The nurse encourages parents to feed their infants as often as possible before discharge and may use these opportunities to teach any special feeding techniques and assess parental knowledge and capabilities. The nurse often needs to reassure parents that it is normal for their infants to make loud noises while eating and that their infants may appear to choke more frequently than normal infants. With practice, the parent becomes familiar with the method and rate of feeding suited to the child.

Children who are incapable of nipple feeding may require tube or dropper feedings. Plastic medicine droppers may be used initially but are tedious and time consuming. Asepto or bulb syringes may then be used, or a homemade feeding system may be created. For this, a 12 or 14 French red rubber catheter is shortened, leaving the distal vents intact. A 10- or 20-mL Luer-lock syringe is then attached to the tubing. The result is a system that allows regulated delivery of very small amounts of formula. The flexible catheter can be placed so as to deposit formula at the back or lateral back of the tongue. This method may also be used after the initial surgery in order to avoid harming the suture line.

Preoperative Preparation Immediate preoperative nursing care is directed toward instructing parents in the care of their children after surgery. The parent should be aware that the child will have both arms restrained in order to prevent damage to the suture line. Children who have had cleft lip repairs are required to remain on their backs or sides and are not allowed to sleep in a prone position, although children with palate closures only may sleep in any position. The child is cup-fed or syringe-fed during the immediate postoperative period. Parental anxiety and infant's reactions to changes in routine can be alleviated somewhat by practicing postoperative measures before surgery. Infants should be able to sleep comfortably in supine or side-lying positions. Occasional cup feedings at home may encourage more ready acceptance of this feeding method after successful surgery. If atropine is given preoperatively, parents should be aware that their children may appear flushed and warm after surgery.

Postoperative Care Postoperative nursing care is focused on care of the surgical site. The nurse cleanses lip suture lines frequently with dilute hydrogen peroxide and cotton-tipped applicators and removes all crusts or exudate thoroughly. Antibiotic ointment may be prescribed to prevent infection, maintain a supple incision line, and promote softening of any sanguineous crusts.

Feedings are usually begun with clear liquids once the child is fully awake, and are followed by full liquids as tolerated. Because of possibe trauma to the incision line, children with palate repairs are never tube-, syringe-, or fork-fed. As in any surgery, vomiting may occur during the initial feedings, and parents should be aware that this is common. The infant who is cup-fed also requires frequent burping to prevent vomiting or abdominal discomfort.

Several types of restraints are available; the type used depends on the age of the child. Small infants may require only elbow restraints, while the older child may require elbow or wrist restraints. Children undergoing lip repairs may need jacket or wrist restraints to prevent them from turning onto their abdomens. Restraints may be removed when the parent is holding or comforting the child but are best removed only one at a time. The nurse needs to caution the parent who removes restraints that the child's fingers should be kept away from the mouth. Extremely restless children may require diphenhydramine hydrochloride (Benadryl) or chloral hydrate sedation. Parents should know that their infants may be extremely restless, may appear uncomfortable, may cry more than usual, and may not be as easily comforted as before.

Children undergoing cleft palate repair have copious serosanguineous nasal discharge. Positioning of the child can facilitate drainage of secretions and decrease risk of aspiration. Preoperative medications may cause oral secretions to be thick and sticky. Children with cleft lip repairs should be placed on their sides, and children with only cleft palate repairs may lie prone. If oral suctioning is necessary to prevent aspiration, it should be done as gently as possible and directed toward the sides of the mouth and the lateral back side of the tongue. Following formula feedings with several sips of water helps prevent formation of sticky oral secretions. Adequate hydration also allows for the production of adequate saliva.

Surgery may be necessary to revise lip scars, perform nasal realignment, or complete the palate later in early childhood. A velopharyngeal flap repair may be necessary to allow for a more competent soft palate, and speech therapy may become more effective after this surgery. Further surgery requires age-appropriate preoperative teaching (see Chapter 29) and parental involvement in planning and postoperative care. (The nursing care plan at the end of this chapter illustrates care for a child undergoing cleft lip repair.)

Esophageal Atresia and Tracheoesophageal Fistula

Esophageal atresia occurs when the cells of the embryonic foregut fail to develop, leaving a blind pouch. Tracheoesophageal fistula (TEF) arises when the foregut fails to differentiate into a totally separate esophagus and trachea, resulting in a patent fistula between the two structures. Although esophageal atresia or tracheoesophageal fistula may occur separately, the most common anomaly is a combination of both defects.

Esophageal atresia occurs in approximately 1 of every 3000–4000 live births. A high percentage of these infants are premature or of low birth weight (Rudolph, 1982). More than three-fourths of affected infants have defects consisting of a blind upper esophageal pouch with a fistula between the trachea and the lower esophagus (type C) (Fig. 38-3). Figure 38-3 also indicates the less common forms of TEF, along with their relative frequency of occurrence. More than 25% of all infants with esophageal atresia or TEF also have other congenital anomalies. Cardiovascular anomalies are most prevalent, but pulmonary, intestinal, genitourinary, and neurologic defects may also occur.

Infants with esophageal atresia or TEF may present a variety of symptoms depending on the severity of the defect and the location of the fistula. They may develop cyanotic episodes and are usually unable to handle oral secretions. Copious oral and nasal secretions requiring frequent suctioning may be noted in the delivery room or nursery. The infant may cough or choke on secretions or may become cyanotic because of laryngospasms. Suctioning the infant or attempting to perform gastric lavage indicates that the catheter cannot be passed into the stomach. All or any of these problems should lead to suspicion of esophageal atresia or TEF.

A history of maternal polyhydramnios is also common in infants with atresias. This is due to the inability of the infant to adequately swallow and excrete amniotic fluid in utero. Less dramatic symptomology may result in a missed diagnosis and further complications, when the diagnosis

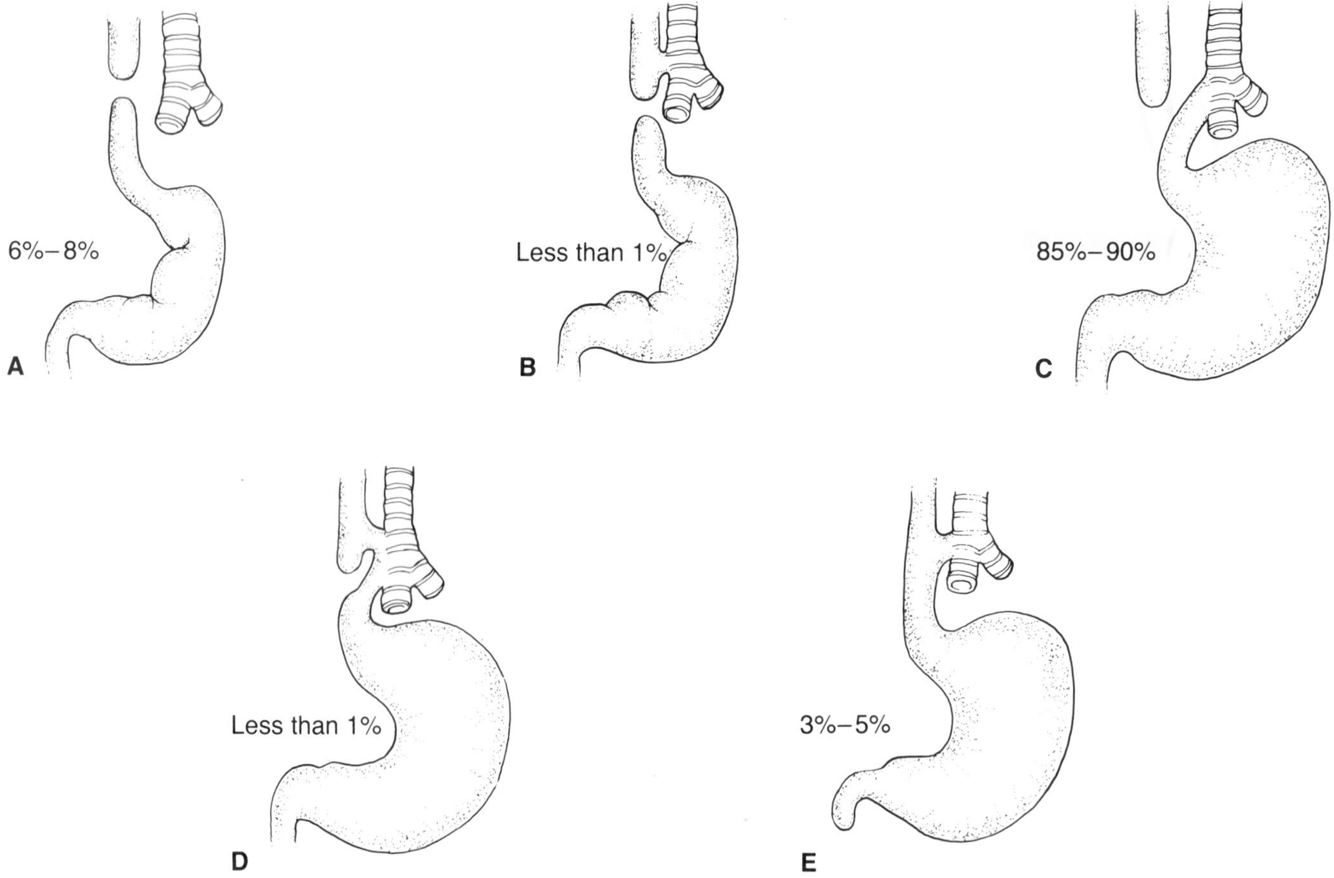

Figure 38-3 The five most common forms of tracheoesophageal fistulas and esophageal atresias, with their frequencies of occurrence.

becomes apparent with feeding. Feeding infants with esophageotracheal fistulas (Fig. 38-3, types B and D) leads to aspiration. Those with lower esophageotracheal fistulas (Fig. 38-3, types C and D) may develop tympanic abdomens due to trapping of air. Infants with no connection to the distal esophagus (Fig. 38-3, types A and B) have flattened, scaphoid abdomens. The only indicators of the H-type defect (Fig. 38-3, type E) may be recurrent aspiration pneumonia or chemical pneumonitis (due to reflux of gastric secretions into the trachea).

Fluoroscopic studies and bronchoscopy are needed to determine the extent of the defect as well as the location of fistulas. If contrast material is used, it should be administered slowly and should be removed to prevent chemical pneumonitis. All contrast studies are dangerous because of potential aspiration or difficulty removing contrast medium and are only performed if safer tests are not effective. In H-type defects, bronchoscopy may reveal a fistula (Fig. 38-3, type E). An abdominal radiograph revealing an absence of air in the stomach is indicative of a blind pouch at the gastric end (Fig. 38-3, types A and B).

Medical and Surgical Treatment Esophageal atresia is considered a surgical emergency. Initial medical care is focused on preventing aspiration. Placement of a drainage tube through the nose and into the esophageal pouch allows frequent intermittent suctioning of pooled secretions. Infants then remain in a high-Fowler's position to prevent reflux of gastric acid into the lungs. For infants exhibiting gastric distention, a gastrostomy may be necessary to allow escape of trapped air. This also helps to prevent reflux of gastric acids into the trachea. Antibiotic therapy may also be instituted as a prophylactic measure in instances where aspiration pneumonia may have occurred.

Repair may be accomplished in single- or multiple-stage operation. In the single-stage procedure, all fistulas are ligated, and an end-to-end anastomosis of the esophageal pouches is performed. If, however, the ends of the esophagus are separated by a wide margin or the child cannot tolerate extensive surgery, an alternative operation is performed. The fistulas are ligated as before, but the proximal esophagus is exteriorized in a cervical esophagostomy. This ostomy is usually located at the left base of the neck, and allows free drainage of swallowed secretions. A gastrostomy is necessary to provide feedings until a final reconstruction is performed at 18–24 months of age. At that time, a segment of colon is transplanted to create a continuous esophageal passage and is implanted to provide the same proximodistal peristalsis as a normal esophagus. The esophagostomy and gastrostomy are then closed.

The principal long-term complication of either type of surgery is esophageal stricture formation. Frequent dilatations often are necessary to prevent obstruction of the trachea by scar tissue. Some surgeons perform dilatations at routine intervals as a preventive measure. Surgical revision of esophageal strictures may also be necessary. Colon transplants might become necessary for children who have frequent strictures and do not respond favorably to dilatations.

Nursing Management The goals of preoperative nursing care for the infant with esophageal atresia or TEF are detection of the defect and prevention of aspiration. Nurses in the delivery room and newborn nurseries therefore suspect altered esophageal structure in any infant who is experiencing difficulty handling secretions. Although an infant may have other problems causing respiratory distress (for example, respiratory anomalies, brain damage, or cleft palate), the possibility of an atresia or fistula is much better discovered before feeding than after. Unfortunately, many infants are not diagnosed until after they have aspirated their first feeding. (This is why many institutions require the first feeding to be sterile water.)

Laryngospasm, a protective reflex to prevent aspiration, may cause the infant to become cyanotic. The nurse therefore suspects cyanotic infants with no known cardiac or respiratory anomalies of having anomalous formation of the esophagus and a possible conduit between the esophagus and the trachea.

Because most infants have distal esophageotracheal fistula (Fig. 38.3), affected infants should be placed in a head-up position in an isolette or radiant warmer. This prevents reflux of damaging gastric secretions into the trachea. Suctioning of the esophageal pouch may be intermittent or continuous. Continuous suctioning prevents frequent blockage of the tube by mucus and prevents a sudden build-up of secretions. Low-pressure, continuous suctioning is therefore often preferred, although this may cause ulceration of the mucosa if used for an extended period of time. The nurse also observes secretions for any evidence of fresh bleeding. These infants are placed NPO, and a gastrostomy may be placed to gravity drainage to decompress the stomach. Gastrostomy feedings are not given before ligation of the fistula because of the possible reflux of stomach contents into the trachea. Infants receive intravenous fluid and electrolytes and may require hyperalimentation if surgery is postponed for more than 24–48 hours.

Postoperative Care Surgical correction of esophageal atresia or tracheoesophageal fistula frequently involves a transthoracic approach. Immediate postoperative care thus includes care of the thoracotomy site, chest tubes, and maintenance of ventilatory support when necessary. (See Chapter 35 for recommended care of the child who has undergone thoracic surgery.)

Infants who have undergone ligature of fistula or reanastomosis of esophageal pouches are prone to pulmonary infections. The nurse therefore monitors the child closely for signs of atelectasis or pneumonia. Decreased breath sounds, increased respiratory rate, increased temperature, pallor, or cyanosis may indicate pulmonary infections or pneumothorax.

The infant usually returns with a gastrostomy, which serves several purposes. It allows initial gastric decompression after surgery, prevents mechanical irritation of the esophageal reanastomosis site, and allows early reintroduction of feeding without harming the surgical sites. The gastrostomy tube is often left to gravity drainage to allow gastric decompression. When bowel sounds return, the gastrostomy tube may be elevated above the level of the stomach. This allows gastric secretions to pass through the pylorus yet allows escape of swallowed air through the open tube. Eventually, the tube is clamped or plugged between feedings.

Infants who have undergone this type of surgery are susceptible to fluid and electrolyte imbalances and nutritional deficits. Loss of electrolytes through gastrostomy drainage during the first 48–72 hours may be significant. Many infants are placed on additional intravenous replacement therapy to prevent electrolyte disturbances. Accurate records of intake and output including gastric drainage are necessary.

The infant remains NPO until bowel sounds return and until there is no danger of disrupting the surgical site. Intravenous therapy provides hydration but often does not provide adequate calories. Infants who remain NPO for longer than 48–72 hours may require parenteral nutritional support. Infants who are gastrostomy-fed are given initial feedings of water or glucose and water. If these feedings are tolerated, the diet is advanced to include standard formulas that provide adequate calories for the infant's weight. Gastrostomy feedings are continued until the esophageal anastomosis has healed (10–14 days). Oral feedings are then begun. Nursing care should include time to allow the child to learn to swallow.

In infants undergoing multiple-stage surgery, the gastrostomy is left intact, and feedings progress as tolerated. The open end of the gastrostomy tubing should initially be elevated above the child's stomach to help prevent backflow of stomach contents and to allow for the escape of trapped air. These infants also return from surgery with a cervical esophagostomy. Because constant drainage of enzyme-rich saliva can cause excoriation of neck tissues, frequent, meticulous skin care is needed, and a thin layer of an occlusive ointment should be applied. If excoriation is severe, a collection bag may be necessary although this presents great difficulty because of location of the esophagostomy and the nature of the secretions. These infants are also able to swallow saliva but quickly lose the coordination needed to suck and swallow if they are not allowed to practice. A pacifier and "sham" feedings are therefore encouraged. Sham feedings consist of small amounts of glucose water for infants and may later include juices or pureed fruits. The feeding is taken orally and is expelled from the esophagostomy. This allows the infant to experience varying taste and texture sensations and makes the child less likely to experience feeding difficulties after reconstruction is completed.

Needs of Parents The nurse is concerned not only with the physical care of the infant but also with the emotional and educational needs of the family. Parents of children with congenital defects require intensive emotional support, but the emotional needs of parents are even greater when immediate surgery is needed for the infant to survive. (The needs of parents with high-risk infants is discussed in Chapter 31.) Quiet, calm discussions about the infant's condition offer the parent a chance to ask questions and can help alleviate some of the stress. Ideally, these parents should receive as much preoperative information as possible and continued postoperative information and family advocacy.

Discharge Preparation Parents of children undergoing multiple-stage surgery should be capable of caring for their children before discharge. The nurse provides both oral and written instructions along with actual demonstrations of gastrostomy feedings and esophagostomy care. The parent should then return the demonstration. If sham feedings are to be used, the parent should be aware of the frequency and amount of each feeding. Gastrostomy feeding supplies are often available through the hospital or may be provided by public health or Crippled Children's Services.

Nurses may need to encourage these parents to hold and cuddle their infants frequently. Because the normal attachment experienced during feeding has been disrupted, parents should understand that alternative contact is needed. Tube feeding while holding the infant is sometimes awkward, and the parent may feel more at ease with the child lying down or in an infant seat during feedings. Parents should then make concerted efforts to cuddle after feeding or to provide frequent, close, eye-to-eye contact throughout the day.

Infants who have the single-stage repair need to be observed for signs of stricture formation. The nurse explains and provides a written list of signs that indicate possible stricture formation and instructs the parent to contact the physician if any one of these signs occurs. Signs of stricture formation include choking or gagging on solid foods while tolerating pureed or liquid foods, refusing food and sometimes even liquids, dysphagia, increased drooling, and frequent coughing and choking that appear to be related to swallowing.

Parents also need to be informed that stricture formation resulting from contraction of scar tissue and dilatations are common occurrences after surgery involving anastomosis of the esophagus. Prompt reporting of signs of stricture facilitates treatment, which usually is mechanical dilatation.

The Child With Existing or Potential Obstruction

Diaphragmatic Hernia

Diaphragmatic hernias occur when the abdominal contents are displaced upward into the thoracic cavity through a defect in the diaphragm. The defect occurs most frequently in the posterolateral portion of the diaphragm; 85%–90% are found to be left-sided. This defect is the result of the failure of the foramen of Bochdalek to close correctly. This leaves a patent pleuroperitoneal canal. Peritoneal contents are then able to enter the thoracic cavity.

Diaphragmatic hernia constitutes a medical-surgical emergency, and immediate surgery is usually necessary to prevent death. Mortality is related to age at onset of symptoms, with those exhibiting symptoms during the first 48 hours of life having the poorest prognosis. The mortality rate for these infants is approximately 50%–65% (Rudolph, 1982).

Infants present with a wide variety of symptoms depending upon the location and severity of the defect. If the defect is small or herniation is limited, the infant may exhibit only mild respiratory distress. These marginal hernias are often discovered later in life when the child develops frequent indigestion, hiatal hernia, or esophagitis due to displacement of the stomach and distal esophagus. The most dramatic and most common clinical presentation occurs when most of the abdominal contents have been displaced into the thoracic cavity, leaving the child with a flattened (scaphoid) abdomen.

Hypoplasia of the left lung is possible if herniation has been present during much of fetal life. The increased pressure within the thoracic cavity causes the mediastinum to shift toward the right, thereby impeding expansion of the right lung. These infants therefore experience acute respiratory distress with tachypnea, dyspnea, and cyanosis. Air swallowed during crying adds to gastrointestinal distention, thereby decreasing thoracic volume even more. Fatalities are usually the result of severe respiratory compromise, acid–base alterations, cardiovascular anomalies, or infection. Other factors such as prematurity or birth defects also contribute to the high mortality.

Surgical Treatment Immediate respiratory support and resuscitation may be necessary while the infant is still in the delivery room. A diagnosis of diaphragmatic hernia may be suspected if lung sounds are unilaterally absent or if the infant has a scaphoid abdomen. Confirmation of the diagnosis is reached through radiologic studies showing air-filled loops of bowel or a gastric bubble within the thoracic cavity. A radiopaque NG tube during radiographic studies may show the esophagus to be displaced to the right. Emergency corrective surgery involves the return of all herniated contents to the abdominal cavity and closure of the diaphragmatic defect.

Nursing Management The maternity or child health nurse is often the first to notice these infants' increasing respiratory distress and scaphoid abdomens. If a diaphragmatic hernia is suspected, the nurse places the infant with the head and chest above the abdomen. This helps to reduce the intrathoracic pressure and allows downward displacement of the herniated abdominal contents. An NG tube is passed and connected to intermittent suction thereby preventing the infant from swallowing air, which only increases respiratory distress. Keeping the infant as quiet as possible also prevents the swallowing of air that occurs normally during crying.

Postoperative care is similar to that following most surgeries. The nurse is especially alert to signs and symptoms of respiratory problems resulting from mediastinal shift, impaired pulmonary circulation, or underdeveloped and sometimes hypoplastic lung on the affected side.

Gastroschisis and Omphalocele

Gastroschisis is a congenital defect in the abdominal wall that allows evisceration of the abdominal contents. This defect is approximately 2–5 cm in diameter and is most often located to the right of an intact umbilicus. The degree of herniation varies and may include not only intestines but also other organs. Because there is no covering sac, the intestines are usually edematous, leathery, shortened, and malrotated. Malrotation is due to an incomplete rotation of the fetal intestine when reentering the abdominal cavity. In addition, the mesentery of the small intestine is not attached appropriately, and a volvulus (twisting of intestine) may occur. In infants with gastroschisis, the intestines fail to reenter the abdomen, thereby resulting in a malrotation. Edema, malrotation, or volvulus can cause infarction and gangrene of the bowel. Intestinal atresia may also be present at single or multiple sites. Although the mortality rate has decreased to 10%–15%, recent studies have shown an increase in the incidence of gastroschisis (Mayer et al., 1980).

An *omphalocele* is an embryonic defect that occurs when the intestines fail to return to the abdominal cavity during the 10th week of gestation. Abdominal contents remain herniated into the umbilical cord, and because they are within the cord itself, they remain covered by the fetal amniotic membrane. The degree of herniation varies and may be slightly larger than an umbilical hernia to large enough to contain intestines and liver. Rupture of the sac may lead to further herniation, infection, or complete intestinal obstruction due to rotation of the intestines during rupture. Associated anomalies are found in more than one-half of all infants with omphalocele because of the defect's early gestational occurrence, whereas concomitant anomalies are rare in cases of gastroschisis. These concomitant anomalies contribute to the high mortality rate (30%–35%) noted in infants with omphalocele (Mayer et al., 1980).

Surgical Treatment Because of the extent of exposed bowel, infants with either gastroschisis or omphalocele may encounter complications involving massive heat and fluid losses, increased caloric requirements, intestinal obstruction or infarction, and infection of the site with resultant septicemia.

Initial treatment of the infant focuses on closure of the defect. If a large amount of the bowel has remained outside the abdominal cavity during fetal development, the cavity may be too small to allow primary closure of the defect without compromising intestinal circulation. In these cases, a prosthetic sac (or silo) of synthetic material (for example, Silastic), may be constructed to contain excess viscera. This pouch is then suspended over the infant to allow gradual return of the viscera to the abdominal cavity. The sac may be gently compressed over a period of 5–10 days as bowel wall edema resolves and abdominal musculature expands. Contents of the pouch are never forced into the abdominal cavity as this can cause obstruction of the intestinal blood flow, severe hypotension due to compression of the inferior vena cava, and compromised respiratory function due to pressure on the diaphragm.

Once all contents have returned to the abdominal cavity, closure of skin and muscle layers can be completed. If gravity fails to return the intestines to the abdomen, additional surgery may be necessary to identify other anomalies.

Nursing Management Preoperative assessment of the infant for signs of circulatory compromise, intestinal obstruction, and septicemia is an important nursing responsibility. Nasogastric suction is begun to prevent harmful distension of the bowel. The nurse needs to take great care to prevent infection when handling the exposed intestines in gastroschisis or the ruptured omphalic sac in omphalocele. The sac is kept moist in cases of omphalocele in order to prevent rupture of the sac due to dry, friable tissue.

Until surgery can be performed, the omphalocele or the open intestines of gastroschisis are wrapped in sterile, warm, moist dressings and are covered with plastic to prevent evaporation. Some sources suggest that only a sterile, dry dressing is needed to prevent hypothermia (Hrabovsky et

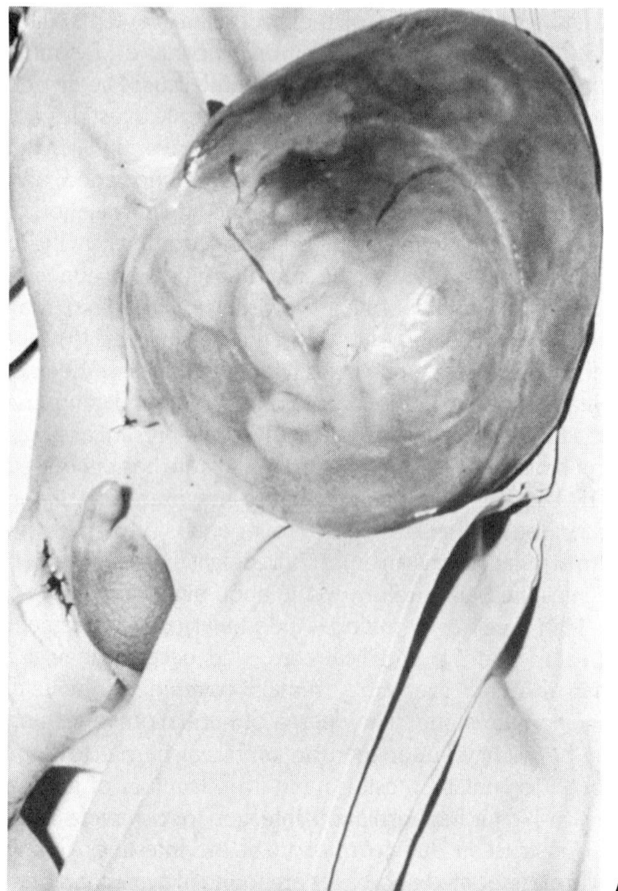

A

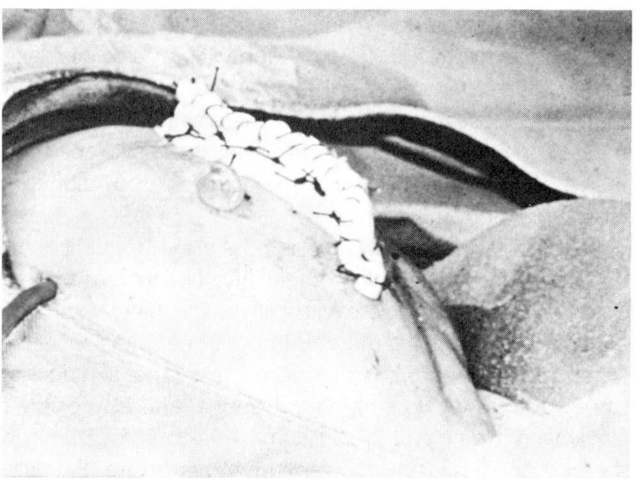

B

Infant with omphalocele. *A.* An omphalocele sac is lying to the right of the abdomen. *B.* A Silastic mesh bag covers the abdominal contents. Sutures in the bag decrease its size and move the abdominal organs back into the abdominal cavity. (Courtesy Paul Winchester, M.D.)

al., 1980). Movement of the infant should be minimized. The nurse may need to restrain all four of the infant's extremities to prevent further damage. Heat loss should be minimized to prevent hypothermia and unnecessary expenditure of calories.

An infant with a large defect may have an infarcted, malrotated, or atresic bowel. Resection may be accomplished by removal of the affected bowel with subsequent end-to-end anastomosis or ostomy placement. Resection of large amounts of small intestine may result in short-bowel syndrome causing chronic malabsorption of nutrients due to decreased intestinal length. Prolonged TPN may therefore be necessary until either the remaining bowel can compensate or some special formula can be tolerated.

Nasogastric suction is continued postoperatively until active bowel sounds are heard. Because these infants have increased metabolic needs, short-term hyperalimentation may be necessary until the child can return to formula or breast milk. If the mother wishes to breastfeed her infant, the nurse assists her in planning to retain an adequate milk supply.

Because these infants are frequently confined to intensive care units for extended periods and have visibly severe defects with long-term hospitalization, parents may encounter difficulties in the attachment process. The nurse may need to encourage parents to visit frequently and to talk to and cuddle these infants. Parents may become anxious if continued nutritional risk causes delayed physical growth or social development and may need reassurance that physical growth will accelerate if normal nutrition can be maintained. Social skills can also be enhanced through such stimulation as frequent eye-to-eye and voice contact and environmental stimuli such as mobiles, music, and age-appropriate toys.

Intestinal Atresias

Intestinal atresia is a complete obstruction of the intestinal tract due to the lack of development of the embryonic intestinal lumen. These atresic sections may be singular or multiple and are thought to be secondary to insufficient vascular supply to the affected regions during fetal development. Atresia is classified as duodenal, jejunal, ileal, or colonic according to the location of the lesion. Duodenal and ileal atresias are by far the more common (1:3,500 and 1:4,000, respectively) and appear more frequently in infants with Down's syndrome (Rudolph, 1982). Jejunal (1:5,000) and colonic (1:20,000) atresias are less common. Maternal polyhydramnios may indicate the presence of intestinal atresia in the fetus because the fetus with atresia is unable to ingest amniotic fluid in utero.

Surgical Treatment Initial presenting symptoms are usually those of intestinal obstruction (see Table 38-2). Obstructive lesions distal to the ampulla of Vater often cause development of bile-stained vomitus shortly after birth. Peristaltic waves may be visible across the epigastrium. Upright radiographs often reveal a "double-bubble" effect due to swallowed air and gastric fluids forming a fluid-air interface line in the stomach and duodenum. Gastric decompression is then begun, and the infant is prepared for surgery. If loss of electrolytes through vomiting has been severe, surgery should be postponed until fluid and electrolyte imbalances have been corrected.

Distal atresias (ilieal-colonic) present symptoms of low intestinal obstruction. Gastric distention is evident, and radiographs reveal patterns of trapped air with dilated bowel loops. Vomiting may or may not be present and is often a late sign of lower-intestinal obstruction.

Surgery is directed toward reconstruction of normal intestinal functioning. Resection of atresic segments with end-to-end anastomosis may be done if the intestine that is proximal to the lesion is not severely dilated. Because portions of bowel that were unused during fetal life remain relatively small, infants with ileal or colonic atresia may require placement of a "chimney" ostomy until bowel size approaches normal. The "chimney" is a single ostomy in which the end of the atresic segment is brought to the surface. The small portion of unused bowel is then anastomosed to the side of the atresic segment. This allows decompression of the bowel if large amounts of feces cannot be accommodated by the microcolon. If resection of multiple atresic sections is necessary, the infant may develop short-bowel syndrome.

Nursing Management Preoperative nursing responsibilities include close monitoring of the infant for signs and symptoms of obstruction or fluid and electrolyte imbalance. Infants are NPO with intravenous fluids and gastric decompression.

Postoperative nursing care involves NG suctioning until active bowel sounds are heard and the infant passes flatus and stool. Feedings are begun when appropriate function of the gastrointestinal tract has been ascertained. Infants with multiple atresic segments may require hyperalimentation if short-bowel syndrome develops.

Meconium Ileus

Meconium ileus is an obstruction of the ileum with meconium and occurs in 5%–10% of infants with cystic fibrosis, although the presence of an ileus is not an indicator of the severity of the disease. The defect in the exocrine glands in children with cystic fibrosis contributes to the production of thick, gluey, tenacious meconium. This meconium usually occludes the area just proximal to the ileocecal valve, giving rise to signs and symptoms of lower-intestinal obstruction.

Medical and Surgical Treatment If radiologic contrast studies support the diagnosis of meconium ileus, an attempt may be made to reduce the obstruction using a

Gastrografin or Hypaque enema. This procedure is successful in about half of affected infants, but if it is not successful, surgery must be performed to relieve the obstruction. Initially, these infants may be left with temporary ileostomies with permanent closure planned for a future procedure.

Occasionally, the meconium plug is found within the rectal vault and it may be removed by careful digital exploration or through enemas. In such cases, care must be taken to prevent perforation of the rectal wall.

Nursing Management Preoperative nursing responsibilities are much like those for any infant with intestinal obstruction. Nasogastric suctioning, monitoring of vital signs, and accurate intake and output records are all important.

Postoperative nursing care depends on the type of surgery. For children with ostomies, nurses may begin instructing parents in care of the site and application of appliances. The nursing care plan should also address needs for parental education for the care of a child with cystic fibrosis, as the child now has both an acute and a chronic problem (see Chapter 34). Sharing information about the child's surgery, allowing the parent to participate in daily care, and encouraging active participation in seeking answers to questions help a parent become familiar with the infant and the disease. Long-range educational and home management plans should begin during this initial hospitalization.

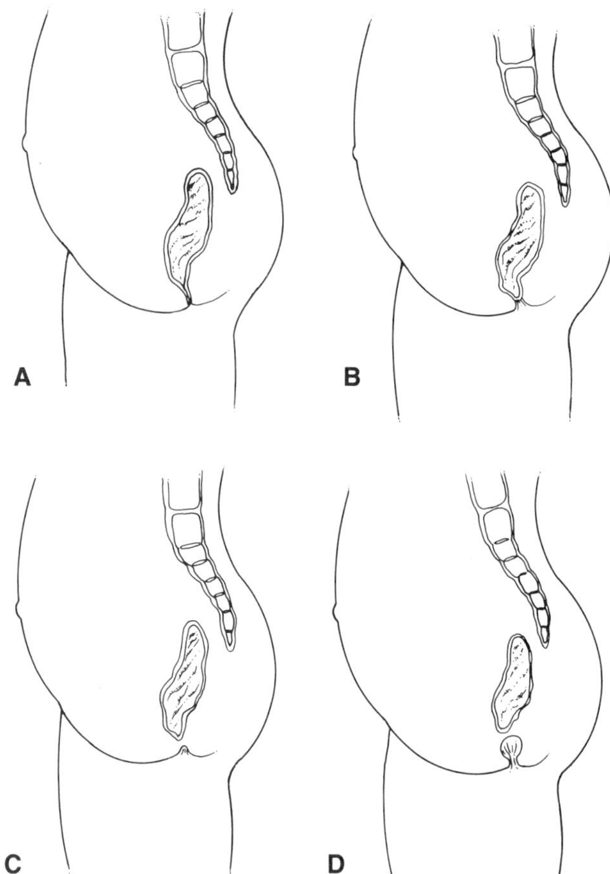

Figure 38-4 Anorectal malformations. *A*. Anal stenosis. *B*. Membranous atresia. *C*. Anal agenesis. *D*. Rectal atresia.

Imperforate Anus

Imperforate anus is a term describing a group of anorectal malformations. Anomalies of this type occur in about 1 of every 5000 live births (Rudolph, 1982) and are clinically classified as "high" or "low" anomalies depending on whether or not the rectum passes through the puborectalis sling of the levator ani muscle (see Fig. 38-4).

The anus and rectum develop from the embryonic hindgut. The blind end of the hindgut develops to form the cloaca, the precursor of genitourinary and anorectal structures. Lateral tissue folds develop and separate this cloacal chamber into the genitourinary sinus anteriorly and the anorectal sinus posteriorly. By the eighth week of gestation, the membrane ruptures, creating the anal canal. Anything that impedes the development of the necessary structures results in an anorectal malformation. The shared embryonic genitourinary structures may also be affected, leading to fistulas or the persistence of a cloaca.

In anal stenosis (Fig. 38-4*A*), the anal opening is present but constricted. This may be noticed early in infancy during a digital exam or may only become apparent later, when the child encounters problems with chronic constipation, ribbonlike stools, and difficulty in toilet training. Anal membrane atresia (Fig. 38-4*B*) occurs when the embryonic anal membrane fails to rupture by the eighth week of gestation. Anal and rectal structures may appear normal except for the presence of a shiny, translucent membrane. In anal agenesis (Fig. 38-4*C*), the rectum terminates in a blind pouch, either above or below the levator ani muscle. This defect in development accounts for approximately 80% of all anorectal malformations. Rectal atresia (Fig. 38-4*D*) occurs when the anal canal is appropriately developed but does not communicate with the rectum. The distance between the two structures may be significant, or they may be divided by only a membranous tissue. Fistulas connecting with the perineum, urethra, bladder, or vagina may be present in a large number of anorectal malformations.

Medical and Surgical Treatment Infants suspected of having anorectal malformations should be evaluated in depth in order to determine the level of the defect and the presence or location of any fistula. Frequent abdominal radiographs are performed with the child in an inverted position. This allows air to fill the blind colonic pouch and permits clearer identification of the level of the defect. Another diagnostic tool is catheterization of any external fistulae, injection of contrast material, and subsequent radiographs to provide a more exact classification of the defect.

Anal stenosis is most often managed with repeated manual dilatations of the anus. These dilatations are begun soon after birth and are continued by the parents once the child is discharged. Parents need information regarding the proper technique of manual anal dilatation in order to prevent accidental perforation.

The type of surgical intervention is determined by the position of the defect. Low defects may be corrected by an abdominoperineal pull-through procedure with anoplasty or, in the case of anal membrane atresia, by anoplasty alone. High defects necessitate a temporary colostomy for at least 6–12 months. Surgery is then performed to correct any remaining fistulas and to position the bowel within the puborectalis sling.

Bowel control depends on location of the defect. When repaired, low defects usually allow the child to achieve continence without problems. The higher the defect, the less successful a bowel control regimen may be. Many children with high defects also have other pelvic anomalies, including vertebral defects and pelvic neurologic anomalies. Because of the anomalies, complete bowel continence may be extremely difficult or impossible to achieve. If innervation is affected, the child may lack the sensation of stool within the rectum and should be encouraged to defecate at the same time daily rather than waiting for the urge. Enemas or suppositories may be required if constipation is severe. If effective bowel control is not achieved before the child enters school or if chronic impaction is a problem, the child may be reassessed for placement of a permanent colostomy.

Nursing Management The nurse is often the person who first identifies an anorectal malformation in a neonate, often when attempting to take the initial rectal temperature. Other observations important in establishing a diagnosis are whether the child has passed meconium in the first 24 hours and whether meconium appears in an inappropriate place. Meconium in the urine or meconium appearing from the perineum or vagina are indicators of external fistulas.

Postoperative nursing care depends on the degree of surgery necessary to repair the defect. If an abdominoperineal pull-through is performed, nursing care includes prevention of infection of the perineal or anal surgical site. The site should be kept very clean and observed for signs of infection. The use of a heat lamp or exposure to open air can promote healing of the site. When a colostomy is necessary, the nursing care plan incorporates postoperative colostomy care and instruction for the parents. Although these colostomies are present for only 6–12 months, appropriate care also needs to include prevention of skin breakdown or appliance leakage.

Information about bowel training becomes important in early childhood, and the nurse needs to explain that children with anorectal malformations may encounter difficulty in toilet training. Parents should be encouraged to use patience and persistence and should establish a daily routine when attempting bowel training.

Hirschsprung's Disease (Aganglionic Megacolon)

Hirschsprung's disease occurs when there is an absence of autonomic parasympathetic ganglion cells of the myenteric and submucous plexuses, leading to the term "aganglionic" colon. Because of the absence of these ganglions, there is a lack of peristalsis within that segment of the colon. The defect in innervation extends upward from the anus, and the severity of the condition is determined by the level at which active ganglia can be found. Approximately 80% of patients have an aganglionic segment that is limited to the rectosigmoid only. The rest vary upward to the hepatic flexure and in rare cases include the entire colon.

Lack of peristalsis results in constipation and signs of functional intestinal obstruction. Presenting symptoms vary from acute obstruction to chronic constipation, depending on the age of the child. Infants might fail to pass meconium or might have vomiting and abdominal distention. Emesis might be bile-stained and in severe cases might have the odor or texture of feces. Older infants might have histories of chronic constipation alternating with diarrhea or histories of failure to thrive. Occasional bouts of constipation or diarrhea may develop into an enterocolitis with explosive diarrhea, fever, and severe dehydration. Fatalities may occur if enterocolitis is not treated immediately.

Older children exhibit increasing constipation and abdominal distention. Occasionally, a fecal mass might be present in the lower left quadrant, but the rectal vault is often empty of stool. These children often appear chronically malnourished, are often anemic, and exhibit malabsorptive hypoproteinemia.

Diagnosis of aganglionic megacolon usually involves performance of a rectal biopsy to determine whether ganglion cells are present. In small neonates, anorectal manometry may be preferred. In this test, a balloon is placed just beyond the external sphincter, while the other balloon is placed at the internal sphincter. In normal individuals, distention of the balloons mimics presence of stool within the rectum, causing relaxation of the internal sphincter with contraction of the external sphincter. Children with megacolon exhibit contraction of the external sphincter without relaxation of the internal sphincter.

Barium enemas may be used to define the transition point between the narrow aganglionic and the distended megacolon segments. Because this marked difference may not be apparent for a month or more, the credibility of barium studies as a sole diagnostic tool in neonates is somewhat limited.

Medical and Surgical Treatment Treatment of Hirschsprung's disease in the older child might be limited to medical intervention with enemas, stool softeners, and low-residue diets. Such treatment is only palliative.

Surgical intervention is performed to remove the aganglionic bowel. Initially, a temporary loop or double-barrel colostomy is performed. A pull-through procedure involving removal of the aganglionic colon with reanastomosis of normal colon may be done during the initial colostomy or in a staged operation (colostomy followed by the pull-through, then colostomy closure). The timing of the colostomy closure is determined by the condition of the child and the response to initial surgery but is usually accomplished within 3–12 months. Only rarely is it necessary to maintain a permanent colostomy. In these instances, the extent of aganglionic colon is severe, and a permanent ileostomy may be necessary.

Nursing Management Preoperative nursing care focuses on observation and assessment of the infant. Once the diagnosis has been established and surgery is indicated, nursing care also involves preparing the child and parent for impending surgery. Physical care involves bowel preparation. In neonates with bowels that are still sterile, no preparation is needed. In older infants and children, preparation may begin several days prior to the surgery.

If low-residue or liquid diets are required at home before admission for surgery, parents need both oral and written instructions. If enemas are required at home, parents need instructions in preparing and performing an isotonic saline enema. The nurse then emphasizes the dangers of tap water, soap, and commercial phosphate enemas. Isotonic saline solutions may be obtained without a prescription at pharmacies, or the parent can mix one teaspoon of noniodized table salt with one pint of lukewarm tap water. Return demonstrations by the parent are helpful in identifying needs for further instructions.

In addition to preparation through diet and enemas, systemic antibiotics may be given to reduce intestinal flora. Frequent oral administration of antibiotics may be used in conjunction with antibiotic enemas. Close monitoring of fluid status is necessary for children who are NPO and receiving repeated enemas. Small infants may require intravenous fluids if oral liquids are withheld for any length of time.

Postoperative nursing care involves routine postabdominal surgery care as well as ostomy care. Children return from surgery and remain NPO with NG suctioning until peristalsis returns. Intravenous fluids are used to provide fluids, electrolytes, and calories. The nurse records the amount of ostomy drainage as well as NG drainage. Accurate intake and output is especially essential in small infants. When the stoma is less edematous, the enterostomal therapist or nurse fits the appliance.

Postoperative colostomy care instruction should include both parent and older child. The family should be able to care for the child's stoma completely before the child is discharged from the hospital. Parents should also be given a contact person to call if they encounter problems with the appliance or stoma. A community health nurse, primary care nurse, or enterostomal therapist may provide home care follow-up if needed.

Pyloric Stenosis

Pyloric stenosis occurs because the circular muscle of the pylorus becomes progressively more hypertrophic and hyperplastic (Fig. 38-5*A*). This narrowing, or "stenosis," of the pylorus can cause the muscle to enlarge to almost twice its normal size. The thickened and cartilaginous muscle leads to an obstruction of the pyloric outlet with subsequent gastric distention, dilatation, and hypertrophy.

Although the causative agent is unknown, heredity may play an important role. The higher incidence of this lesion in monozygotic rather than dizygotic twins as well as the higher incidence in infants with previous family histories of pyloric stenosis all suggest genetic influence. The disorder also occurs more commonly in males (1:150) than females (1:750) and appears to be more common among first-born males.

Infants with pyloric stenosis have a variety of signs and symptoms. Because of the progressive nature of the obstruction, the infant may appear normal in the first week or two of life, but regurgitation, or nonprojectile vomiting may begin in the second and third week of life. Projectile vomiting may develop suddenly, becoming quite forceful and startling, within 1–2 weeks of the initial onset. Projectile vomiting is sometimes forced 2 or 3 ft from the child. It may occur during or immediately after feeding or may be delayed for an hour or more. Because the obstruction is proximal to the ampulla of Vater, the emesis is not bile-stained but will contain gastric secretions and undigested formula. Emesis may occasionally contain flecks of blood due to continual gastric irritation.

After vomiting, the infant appears voraciously hungry and usually takes another feeding immediately. Observation after feeding may show visible peristaltic waves moving from left to right towards the pylorus. Abdominal palpation may reveal a mass (approximately the size of an olive) in the epigastrium to the right of midline. This "olive" is present in an infant with a severely hypertrophic pylorus and is a classic indicator of pyloric stenosis.

Because of the incessant vomiting, the child will lose large quantities of chloride, sodium, and potassium and may present a clinical picture of failure to thrive and dehydration. Weight loss is common, and the infant may have marked loss of subcutaneous fat. Weight loss and dehydration are sometimes so rapid and severe that infants may present in critical condition with marked hypochloremic alkalosis.

Diagnostic studies include observation of the emesis pattern, palpation of the abdomen for presence of an "olive," and contrast studies. If contrast studies are necessary, the child is fed contrast material and radiographs are taken to determine the obstruction. If pyloric stenosis is present ra-

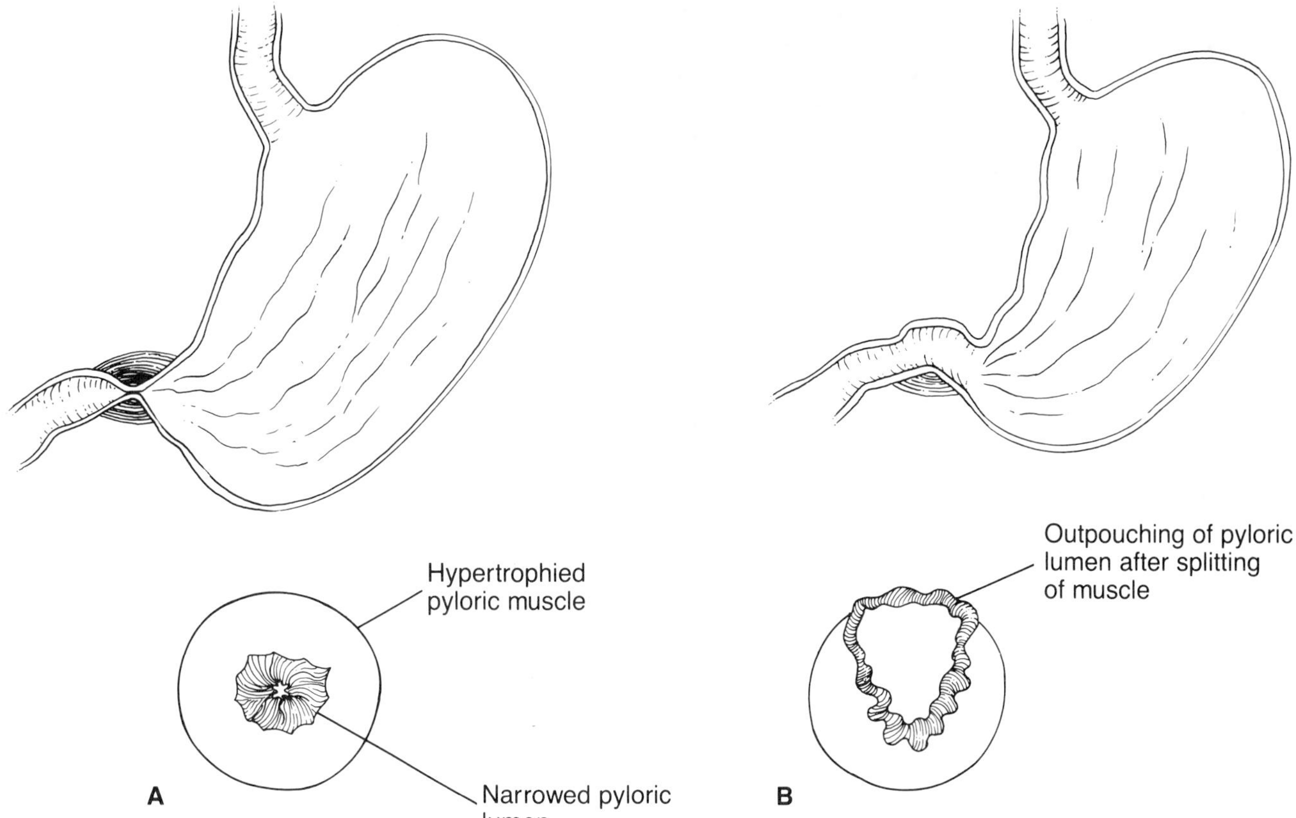

Figure 38-5 Pyloric stenosis. *A*. Obstruction of pyloric lumen by hypertrophied muscle layers. *B*. Release of submucosal layer after pyloromyotomy.

diographs will show delayed or absent gastric emptying with the pylorus appearing as a narrow channel (commonly termed the "string sign").

Surgical Treatment Pyloromyotomy is the standard surgical treatment for pyloric stenosis. Although nonsurgical treatment was once common, the efficacy and safety of the present surgical procedure far outweighs the slow and lengthy medical treatment.

Surgery is usually performed as soon as fluid and eletrolyte imbalances have been corrected. Infants who appear well hydrated and whose electrolytes are balanced may undergo the procedure as soon as is feasible. Surgery of an infant with hypochloremic alkalosis, however, may need to be postponed for as long as 2 or 3 days in order to restore metabolic balance prior to surgery.

Infants are NPO prior to surgery; gastric lavage is occasionally employed to ensure that the stomach is totally empty at the time of surgery. Entry to the abdomen is through a small incision in the right upper quadrant. The seromuscular layer of the pylorus is incised, and the muscle is separated with a blunt instrument until the submucosa is encountered. This allows the mucosa to bulge between the split muscle, thus enlarging the lumen of the pylorus (Fig. 38-5B).

The infant remains NPO for 4–6 hours after surgery. At that time, small feedings (approximately 5mL every hour) of glucose water or glucose and electrolyte solutions are begun. If these first feedings are retained, the volume of the feedings is increased. Dilute formula or breast milk are then introduced in small quantities. If tolerated, volume and concentration are increased until the child is tolerating full-strength feedings at 3- to 4-hour intervals.

Intravenous fluids administration continues until the child has shown the capability to retain adequate amounts of fluids by mouth, as these infants often experience some vomiting during the first 24 hours after surgery. If this occurs more than once, feedings may be withheld for several hours or may begin again with the first feeding of the regimen. Depending on the infant's ability to tolerate formula and retain feedings, a complete formula or breast milk diet may be reached within 24–36 hours. Many infants are discharged within 36–48 hours of surgery.

Nursing Management Preoperative nursing care includes observation of the infant for signs and symptoms that facilitate the diagnosis of pyloric stenosis. Strict intake and output records are essential, and documentation should include not only the amount of emesis, but the character, quantity, and timing in relation to the last feeding. Frequent measurement of urine specific gravity may be done to monitor the infant's state of hydration. Dehydrated infants require continued assessment for level of dehydration as well as for signs that might indicate an electrolyte imbalance (see Chapter 33). The nurse proceeds with rehydration of severely dehydrated infants slowly in order to prevent hyponatremia, vascular overload, or other complications. Gastric lavage, if prescribed, is performed using isotonic saline irrigations in small amounts.

After surgery, care includes routine postoperative measures with continued observations for fluid and electrolyte imbalances. The operative site may be covered with collodian or with a small dressing. The nurse then keeps the site clean and dry to avoid infection and observes the infant for signs of inflammation.

The nurse monitors the feeding regimen as feedings are gradually increased in volume and feeding intervals are increased. Some hospitals have adopted standard post-pyloromyotomy feeding schedules that list feeding intervals as well as concentrations of formula or milk to be used, although some surgeons prefer to individualize postoperative feeding schedules.

Occasional emesis is common after surgery so that nurses need to inform parents that individual reactions to anesthetics as well as residual gastric irritation may cause intermittent vomiting during the initial 24–36 hours. Frequent or continued vomiting needs to be reported, and adjustments in the feeding schedule are then made. Infants may be placed in any position after surgery, but positioning in a right side-lying or Fowler's position promotes gastric emptying.

During preoperative and postoperative periods, the nurse encourages the parent to hold and cuddle the infant. Parental participation in feedings is also important when these are resumed postoperatively. Many of these parents may feel that the child's problem was a result of something they did or did not do. "Helpful" friends and relatives may have only nurtured this sense of guilt. The nurse's explanation of the physical nature of the condition should therefore reassure parents that the problem does not reflect their parenting capabilities.

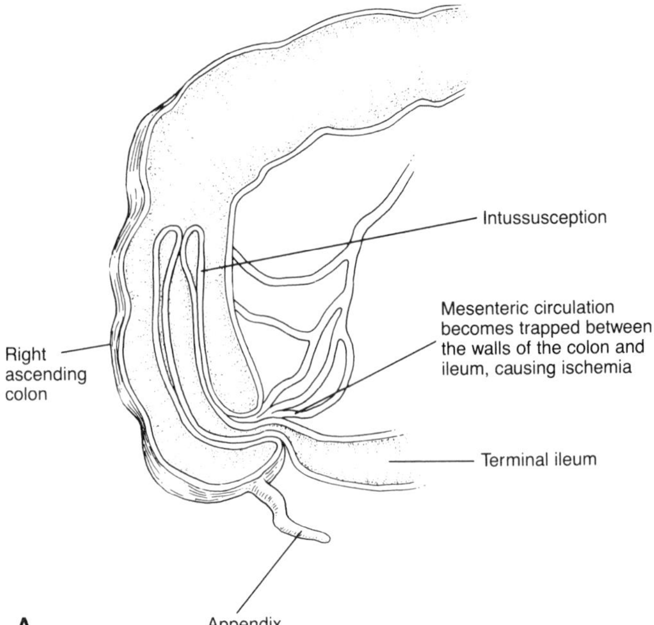

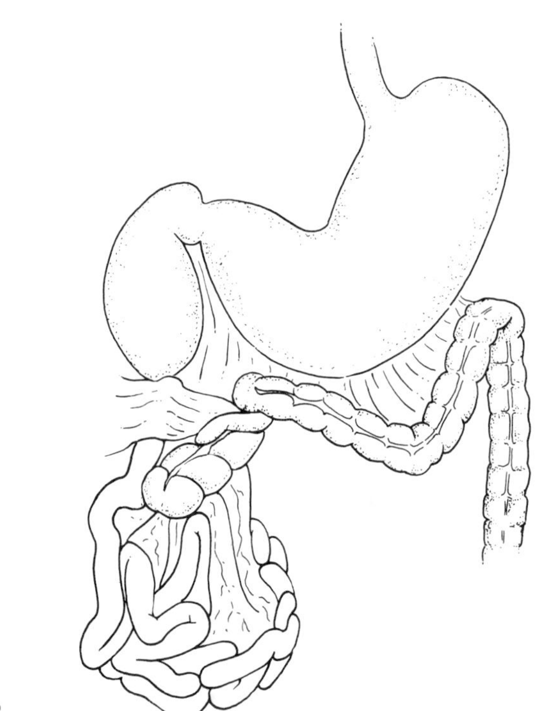

Figure 38-6 *A.* Intussusception of the terminal ileum and ascending colon. *B.* Malrotation and volvulus.

Intussusception

Intussusception occurs when there is a telescoping or invagination of one portion of the intestine into another (Fig. 38-6). It is the most common cause of intestinal obstruction in infants and young children. It is more common in males than females and may occur more frequently in patients with gastroenteritis, cystic fibrosis, or celiac disease. Identifiable causes for intussusceptions may be found in only 5% of the patients. These include lesions such as Meckel's diverticulum, intestinal polyps, or tumors, all of which may intensify peristalsis in an attempt to rid the intestine of the mass.

Intussusceptions are classified according to the involved segments of the intestine. Most are ileocolic and occur at the ileocecal valve. The terminal portion of the ileum telescopes into the cecum and colon, thereby obstructing the passage of intestinal contents. Other classifications include colocolic, with the telescoped sections consisting only of colon, and ileoileal, an extremely uncommon invagination of ileum into ileum.

Because of the constriction of the blood supply that occurs during the invagination, the involved bowel becomes edematous and friable. This leads to bleeding within the intestines, and resulting stools may contain red blood and mucus. These stools are described as "currant jelly" stools and occur in over half the affected children.

The classical presenting symptoms include severe paroxysmal abdominal pain in a previously healthy child. Children may scream and draw their knees upward during the spasms but appear to be comfortable between episodes and may even make attempts to play. Vomiting might occur and the child might initially pass a normal stool. The longer the obstruction is present, however, the more lethargic and weak the child becomes. Continued obstruction leads to bile-stained emesis, currant-jelly stools, a shock-like syndrome with severe prostration and eventual death.

Examination of the infant may show distention of the abdomen, tenderness, and some guarding of the affected site. A sausage-shaped mass may be felt in the right upper quadrant or may appear in the epigastrium if the transverse colon is involved. A rectal examination often reveals the presence of bloody mucus.

Diagnosis of intussusception is often made with a combination of subjective and objective findings. The classic symptoms of intermittent intense abdominal pain, currant-jelly stools, and vomiting allow for an initial diagnosis. A barium enema may reveal the presence of an obstruction as well as the "coil-spring" appearance of barium within the intussusception itself.

Medical and Surgical Treatment If the diagnosis has been made within the initial 24 hours of obstruction or if there are no signs of shock or peritonitis, hydrostatic reduction by barium enema may be attempted. A Foley catheter is placed in the rectum and inflated. The buttocks are taped firmly together to prevent leakage of barium, and barium is then allowed to flow into the colon by gravity. Repeat or serial radiographs show free filling of the small intestine if the procedure has been successful. With early diagnosis, this procedure is successful in approximatly 75% of cases.

If the procedure is not successful or if signs of sepsis or peritonitis exist, the child must undergo open surgical reduction of the intussusception. It may then be necessary to resect necrotic bowel in order to reinstate intestinal continuity.

Nursing Management Documentation of severe intermittent abdominal pain, vomiting, or passage of currant-jelly stools help to establish an early diagnosis. Attention must be given to parent's interpretations of the child's behavior. Because parents are more familiar with their children's reactions to pain or discomfort, they may provide an excellent history of the sudden onset of the obstruction.

For the child undergoing surgery, preoperative nursing care includes close monitoring of the child for signs of intestinal obstruction. Parental preparation includes not only a description of intussusception but also an explanation of reduction by hydrostatic pressure. If parents understand that hydrostatic reduction is not always successful, they can understand why surgery may then become necessary. Explanations should be accompanied by drawings or visual aids. A visual aid can be created by telescoping a section of Penrose drain. If the distal end is then clamped or tied and slowly filled with water, parents can see the principle of hydrostatic reduction in action.

Nasogastric suctioning and intravenous fluids are begun for any child for whom surgery may be necessary. Children exhibiting signs of shock or peritonitis may also require blood, plasma, and antibiotics prior to surgery. All stools are recorded with the presence or amount of fecal blood described. The passage of more than the initial normal stool may indicate spontaneous resolution of the obstruction.

The nurse observes children who have undergone hydrostatic reduction for passage of stool and barium, keeping in mind that a few children (less than 10%) who have undergone hydrostatic reduction have a recurrence of the intussusception and that this usually occurs within the first 36 to 48 hours of the initial reduction.

Congenital Inguinal Hernia and Hydrocele

Inguinal hernias and hydroceles are due to a defect in the closure of the lumen of the processus vaginalis during the eighth month of gestation. This pouch of peritoneum exits the inguinal canal at the external ring, and precedes the testicle into the scrotum. Normally, the upper lumen atrophies and the lower lumen (tunica vaginalis) encases the testicles. When the upper lumen fails to close, however, peritoneal fluid or intestines may be forced down the inguinal canal, through the external ring, and into the scrotum. Varying degrees of closure defects are possible. Large defects allow segments of small intestine to enter the canal, while small defects may only allow the entrance of peritoneal fluid. Presence of intestine within the canal indicates a hernia, while entrapment of fluid within the canal or scrotum describes a hydrocele.

Congenital hernias occur overwhelmingly in males but approximately 10% do occur in females. The inguinal swelling is painless unless strangulation of intestines occurs. The mass is usually easily reduced by gentle compression or may disappear when the infant is resting or feeding quietly. The defect becomes more noticeable during coughing, straining, or crying. In older children, hernias may appear more noticeable at the end of the day.

Strangulation (incarcerated hernia) occurs when the herniated loops of small bowel are trapped within the defect and cannot be reduced into the abdominal cavity. Symptoms of intestinal obstruction become evident, and the site may appear swollen, reddened, or warm. Gangrene of the intestine occurs if the hernia is left unreduced.

The hydrocele also appears as an asymptomatic bulge in the inguinal and scrotal area, but, unlike the hernia, the hydrocele cannot be reduced, nor can it be produced by coughing or crying. Scrotal edema may appear greater at the end of the day because of gravity filling of the defect. Many totally encapsulated hydroceles in young infants resolve spontaneously when the trapped fluid is reabsorbed by the body. The continued presence of a hydrocele, however, may predispose the child to traumatic hernias later in life.

Medical and Surgical Treatment Surgery for repair of hydroceles involves closure of the connecting defect to prevent further collection of fluid within the scrotum. Treatment of choice for nonincarcerated hernias is the prompt surgical closure of the defect to prevent future incarceration. If incarceration has occurred, however, closed reduction may be attempted first. If successful, surgery may be delayed to allow healing of any damaged intestinal tissues. The infant awaiting surgery for incarcerated hernias may be placed in a Trendelenburg's position to prevent further edema and damage of the affected intestine.

Nursing Management Most noncomplicated herniorrhaphies (repair of hernia) and hydrocele repairs are now done on an outpatient basis. The wound is frequently covered with collodion or left open to the air to promote healing and allow thorough cleansing of the site. The nurse therefore informs parents of infants undergoing herniorrhaphies that these children require frequent diaper changes to prevent infection. Activity is not limited, and older children are encouraged to ambulate.

The nurse carefully observes children requiring surgical reduction of incarcerated hernias for signs and symptoms of peritonitis or complete bowel obstruction. Postoperative care for these children includes NG suctioning and intravenous fluids, which are continued until normal bowel function returns.

The Child With a Problem of Use of Food

Children are frequently admitted for a hospital work-up because of failure to thrive, which is often used as a catchall admitting diagnosis for infants or young children who fail to grow and gain weight normally. Technically, failure to thrive is characterized by a persistent deviation from the child's previous growth curve, so that any child who is more than two standard deviations below the mean weight may fit the definition. The classic picture of failure to thrive includes extreme thinness, weight loss or failure to gain weight, loss of subcutaneous fat, and muscle wasting. Many of the children are also socially or developmentally delayed. The multiple etiologies of failure to thrive include both organic and nonorganic causes. Inorganic failure to thrive is discussed in Chapter 22.

Organic causes of failure to thrive include a variety of disorders that interfere with the child's nutritional status. Specific causes may include renal disturbances, gastrointestinal disorders, neurologic problems, cardiovascular anomalies, and general malnutrition or protein deficiencies. Only 10% of all cases of failure to thrive are found to have no organic cause.

Another general cause of failure to thrive is mutations within the genetic information codes of the cell that in turn leads to errors in body metabolism. These are called *inborn errors of metabolism* and they cause defects in the metabolism of amino acids, carbohydrates, lipids, minerals, vitamins, and other chemical processes. These defects can cause clinical effects that range from mild to severe. Because these disorders are genetic, they may be classified as dominant, recessive, or mixed. (Genetic transmission is discussed in Chapter 5.) These errors of metabolism may affect any body system and frequently affect several systems. Some of these disorders (lactose intolerance and phenylketonuria) are discussed in this chapter.

Gastroesophageal Reflux (Chalasia)

Gastroesophageal reflux is a process that occurs when the cardiac valve at the distal end of the esophagus is relaxed or incompetent. This allows frequent reflux of gastric contents into the esophagus. A hiatal hernia may or may not be present.

Presenting symptoms might include a history of excessive vomiting during the first week or two of life. In severe cases, children who have been fed and then placed in a prone position in bed may regurgitate or vomit a large portion of their formula. Other problems encountered include esophagitis due to constant exposure to gastric acidity, aspiration pneumonia, weight loss, and esophageal hemorrhage.

The presence of reflux can be confirmed through a history of signs and symptoms or through the use of a barium esophagogram. The child receives a bolus of barium and is then placed in a head-down position with the abdomen compressed. The presence of refluxed material that is not quickly cleared from the esophagus or repeated reflux of contrast material is indicative of gastroesophageal reflux. Esophageal pH monitoring (see Chapter 34) is another diagnostic test that aids in evaluating the presence of gastric acidity in the esophagus.

Medical and Surgical Treatment Medical management is often effective in handling reflux in infants but is less successful with older children. The routine approach includes careful and frequent burping followed by propping the infant in an upright position for an hour after each feeding. Recent research, however, suggests that the child who is propped upright may experience more reflux episodes or that these episodes may last longer (Orenstein, et al., 1983). Clinical implications of this research indicate that infants may have less reflux and be less irritable if they are burped thoroughly during and after each feeding and then placed on their abdomens for 2–3 hours. This routine is recommended until the disorder is outgrown sometime between 4 and 6 months of age (Balistreri and Farrell, 1983).

When infants are positioned upright to prevent severe reflux, however, they often remain upright for a full 24 hours throughout the day. A chalasia chair or slant board is recommended in this case. Formulas may be thickened with infant cereals to help prevent reflux. Antacids between feedings may be needed if esophagitis is present. More than half of these children respond well to therapy before age 2.

If infants do not respond well to positional therapy or thickened feedings, then surgery may be indicated to prevent the possible occurrence of aspiration pneumonia. A Nissen fundoplication or Boerema anterior gastropexy resolves reflux in over 90% of these intractable cases. These surgeries create a mechanically competent cardiac sphincter and prevent further reflux.

Nursing Management The goals of nursing care in gastroesophageal reflux are to decrease the frequency of reflux, maintain adequate nutrition, promote parent–infant bonding, and provide adequate infant stimulation if prolonged positional therapy is indicated. Treatment for reflux traditionally has involved frequent small feedings of formula or formula with cereal, careful burping, and propping of the infant with chest and head higher than the stomach for at least an hour after feeding. If a chalasia chair or slant board is used, the nurse checks for adequate padding of the board and straddle bar and provides restraints that prevent the infant from slipping off the board. Minimal movement after feedings also helps decrease the incidence of vomiting.

If vomiting occurs, the character, frequency, amount, and timing since the last feeding are documented. Accurate intake and output records are important. Infants who regurgitate large quantities of formula should be refed an amount equivalent to the lost formula.

Parents of infants with gastroesophageal reflux often feel inadequate in their parenting skills. They may, for example, have been told by well-meaning relatives that they are not feeding or burping their infants correctly. The frequent vomiting of feedings with resultant weight loss only contributes more to parents' feelings of guilt. Because of this, parent–infant bonding may be impaired or delayed. An explanation of the physiologic cause of the infant's reflux helps parents realize that they are not to blame for their child's condition. Efforts to involve the parent in the child's feeding and physical care help facilitate attachment. The nurse encourages the parent to feed the child as often as possible during hospitalization so that the parent feels comfortable with the procedure upon discharge.

Adequate stimulation becomes vitally important for infants confined to a chalasia chair or slant board. Bright and colorful objects placed within reach, wrist rattles, and mobiles offer the infant a variety of stimulation. Talking to the infant with direct eye contact is important during feeding and diapering. Touching and stroking the infant provides tactile stimulation. Parents may also cuddle their infants upright on their shoulders, or with the child's head and chest higher than the stomach while held in the parent's arms. Care should be taken that the child is not held in such a way as to compress the abdomen.

If vomiting occurs, the child should be refed. The nurse can also inform the parents that reflux is not uncommon and that it frequently resolves as the child begins eating thicker foods or table foods.

Cystic Fibrosis

Cystic fibrosis is a disease affecting the exocrine glands, which include the mucus-producing glands of the respiratory and digestive tracts, the pancreas, the sweat glands, and the salivary glands. The disease is thought to be autosomal recessive, but spontaneous mutations do occur. The respiratory pathophysiology, treatment, and prognosis of cystic fibrosis is discussed in Chapter 34.

The gastrointestinal manifestations of cystic fibrosis are related to the secretion of thick, tenacious mucus. The earliest complication is meconium ileus, which occurs most frequently at the ileocecal valve and may be seen in approximately 5% to 10% of infants with cystic fibrosis. The equivalent of meconium ileus, due to hardened, inspissated stool obstructing the intestine, may be seen in older patients. Many infants and older children with cystic fibrosis develop rectal prolapse, which occurs most commonly when the children have been passing large quantities of bulky stool or have been straining at stool. If reduced quickly, it poses no hazard to the child.

The dysfunction of the mucus-producing glands contributes to the development of multiple gastrointestinal absorption problems. The thick mucoidal secretions block the pancreatic ducts, leading to formation of cysts within the pancreas. These cysts are later replaced by fibrotic tissue. This ductal obstruction and continued fibrosis prevents the secretion of the digestive enzymes. The absence of trypsin, lipase, and amylase in duodenal fluid causes the malabsorption of fats and proteins. The dietary fats remain undigested, and the fat-soluble vitamins, A, D, E, and K, are not absorbed efficiently. Unabsorbed food fractions are then excreted in the stool, resulting in steatorrhea and high-nitrogen stools, which are bulky and foul smelling, may appear greasy, or may float in the toilet. The loss of vital nutrients and fat-soluble vitamins contributes to the classic picture of failure to thrive. Poor skin healing and easy bruising may result from the malabsorption of fat-soluble vitamins. The islet cells of the pancreas may be affected, and glucose intolerance may develop as the child grows older. Insulin supplementation is rarely needed, and ketoacidosis does not occur.

Cystic fibrosis can also contribute to the development of biliary obstruction and fibrosis. In marked or prolonged instances, a multilobular biliary cirrhosis may develop. When this type of cirrhosis is present, the child may exhibit signs of portal hypertension (hepatosplenomegaly, esophageal varices, and caput mudusae). Rarely do these children exhibit signs or symptoms of hepatic failure until liver damage is severe.

Diagnostic tests for cystic fibrosis include the sweat test, fecal fat determination, and fecal trypsin levels. Two sweat chloride test results should exceed 50–60 mEq/L before cystic fibrosis can truly be documented. Fecal fat output is also elevated, and fecal trypsin is absent or decreased.

Medical Treatment Medical management of gastrointestinal involvement in cystic fibrosis is directed toward promoting absorption of nutrients. The infant is given predigested protein formula (Pre-gestimil), and medium-chain triglycerides (MCT) may be used as a calorie supplement. Older children may require a high-protein or a low- or limited-fat diet, although some can tolerate a normal diet. Individual response to a regular diet should be determined before automatically limiting a child's diet. Those children requiring a low-fat diet may use MCT oil as a supplement for cooking oil. Foods that are high in salt or additional salting of foods may be necessary in warm weather.

Pancreatic enzyme supplementation is based on the individual response to diet therapy. Supplementation may not be needed for those with early-stage disease or those with limited pancreatic involvement. If needed, however, enzyme capsules, tablets, or powders (for example, Pancrease, Cotazym, Viokase) are given with all meals or snacks.

In addition to enzyme supplementation, water-soluble supplements of vitamins A, D, and E are necessary. Vitamin K supplements are indicated if hypoprothrombinemia occurs. Anabolic steroids may be used on a short-term basis to increase appetite and facilitate weight gain.

Other complications are treated symptomatically. Intussusception or obstruction may require surgery. A prolapsed rectum may be reduced by exerting gentle pressure against the everted portion with a lubricated glove finger. The child's buttocks are then taped together to prevent immediate reprolapse.

Nursing Management The goal of nursing care for the child with gastrointestinal manifestations of cystic fibrosis is parent and patient education and support for the chronically ill child and family (see Chapter 30).

Parent education should begin immediately after the diagnosis is confirmed. Initial information should include a discussion of the genetics of cystic fibrosis as well as an explanation of the pathology of the disease. This enables the parent to understand the child's chronic illness and its long-term implications.

Parent and child teaching also includes dietary information. The nurse or nutritionist provides the parent with information regarding the preparation of a high-protein, low-fat diet. The nutritionist might provide appropriate meal plans, snack suggestions, and helpful hints to assist the family and child to adjust to the sudden changes in diet. In any foods requiring cooking oil, MCT oil may be used, or it may be used as a calorie supplement in infant formulas.

The parent also needs to learn the appropriate use and type of supplemental enzymes that the child will be using. If the infant requires enzymes, a powdered form may be mixed in pureed fruit, or the pancrease capsule may be opened and mixed with pureed fruit. The parent needs to clean the face and lips of the child after feeding enzymes in this manner in order to prevent excoriation. Older children can use capsules or tablets, and should remember to take enzymes with all meals and snacks. Vitamin supplementation is usually necessary and usually includes vitamins A and E and often vitamins D or K as well. Some children also require iron supplementation.

Another nursing goal is to provide ongoing emotional support to the family and child. Parents of a newly diagnosed infant might express feelings of guilt or might attempt to blame each other for causing the disease. Genetic counseling may identify problems that will affect future pregnancies or might alter parental expectations for their intended family. Because of the limitations forced on the family, stress may become overwhelming for parents, siblings, or the affected child. Families may find they are unable to dine out or travel as before because of dietary restrictions or the need for frequent respiratory therapy. Siblings may encounter many questions from peers regarding their "sick" brother or sister.

The affected child may also encounter continual questions, or may become an object of ridicule by peers because of the marked delay in growth and development. Adolescents with cystic fibrosis usually experience delayed sexual development, and girls may be amenorrheic or lack breast development, delays that may cause emotional distress. The cachectic appearance together with a chronic cough may also cause problems with peer relationships. Older children or adolescents may fear that the disease is contagious or may be repelled by the continual coughing and expectoration of mucus encountered in children with pulmonary involvement.

The nurse therefore provides psychologic support necessary to deal with these chronic problems as they affect both the child and the family (see Chapter 30). In addition, family support groups consisting of families of children with cystic fibrosis are a great help to parents of a newly diagnosed child because group members are familiar with the stress and practical concerns and difficulties encountered by affected children and their families. They can offer information for meeting day-to-day needs and are of great help when parents must cope with an acute illness or approaching death.

Celiac Disease

Celiac disease is a malabsorption syndrome characterized by a permanent intolerance of gluten, a protein component found in wheat, rye, barley, and oats. It has also been called celiac sprue, nontropical sprue, or gluten-induced enteropathy. Although the mode of genetic transmission is not known, a small number of children with celiac disease also have relatives with the disorder. Theories of the etiology of the gluten intolerance include the presence of an inborn error of metabolism and an impairment of the immunologic function.

Duodenal and jejunal biopsies provide a clue to the pathology of the disease. These biopsies show a flat mucosal surface, absence or atrophy of the villi, and the presence of deep crypts. Changes within the mucosa begin in the proximal small intestine and continue distally if the disease remains untreated. Initially, the reduced absorptive surface due to atrophy of the villi causes a marked decrease in fat absorption, resulting in the production of large quantities of fatty, frothy, foul-smelling stools (steatorrhea). As the disease progresses, the absorption of proteins, carbohydrates, calcium, iron, and vitamins D, K, B_{12}, and B_9 (folic acid) is also impaired. These deficiencies can lead to hypoproteinemia, osteoporosis, osteomalacia, and hypoprothrombinemia.

Symptoms of the disease can appear at any time after gluten-containing foods have been introduced into the diet. Although most of these children develop problems before age 2, symptoms can be delayed for many years. Early symptoms of the disease are subtle and include behavioral changes (such as apathy or irritability) as well as the physical symptoms of weight loss, abdominal distension, and diarrhea. Signs of progressive disease include colicky abdominal pain, vomiting, protuberant abdomen, subcutaneous fat loss, muscle wasting, and dependent edema of the lower extremities secondary to hypoproteinemia. Children are pale because of anemia, and bruising may develop secondary to inadequate vitamin K absorption. Late signs might include severe growth retardation osteoporosis, and osteomalacia.

Diagnostic procedures may include analysis of a 72-hour quantitative fecal fat level to determine the degree of steatorrhea, as well as assessment of serum protein, clotting factors, and electrolytes. A sweat chloride test is frequently performed to rule out the possibility of cystic fibrosis. A duodenal and jejunal biopsy should be performed in order to ensure a definitive diagnosis.

Medical Treatment The dietary management is the principal intervention in early or chronic celiac disease. The child is prescribed a gluten-free or gluten-restricted diet. Foods containing grains such as wheat, rye, oats, and barley are eliminated, and rice and corn are used as substitutes. Temporary parenteral hyperalimentation may be necessary for children who are severely malnourished. Supplemental vitamins, calcium, and iron may be needed if malabsorption is severe. Behavioral improvement is often noticed within the first few days of dietary treatment, with weight gain, increased appetite, and a decrease in soapy stools noticed several weeks later. Repair of diseased intestine proceeds proximally, and function may return to normal within months of beginning the new diet. The intolerance for gluten is permanent, and lack of adherence to a gluten-restricted diet can cause a relapse.

A severe crisis may develop when the child exhibits profuse, watery diarrhea and vomiting. This results in severe dehydration and metabolic acidosis. These crises may be triggered by any intestinal infection, by fasting, or by ingestion of gluten-containing foods. Treatment is symptomatic and consists of gastric decompression and replacement of fluid and electrolytes.

Nursing Management The long-term goal of nursing care is to provide dietary education and supervision. The nurse explains the disease and the rationale behind the gluten-free diet to the parent. A nutritionist is an excellent resource for nutrition education and dietary planning and is often able to provide special recipes for gluten-free foods. The nurse emphasizes the importance of screening the labels of all commercial foods for the presence of gluten or gluten-containing products. For example, such terms as *cereal fillers* or *hydrolyzed vegetable protein* indicate the presence of gluten. Many nutritionists can provide a list of "safe" commercial foods as well as a list of ingredients that may indicate the presence of gluten in the product.

Initial dietary restrictions depend on the degree of inflammation present in the bowel. Children who exhibit lactose intolerance due to atrophy of the intestinal villi may be further restricted from milk-containing foods. Raw vegetables, gas-producing vegetables, raw fruits, and nuts may initially be restricted until inflammation subsides. Although most celiac patients can tolerate small amounts of gluten, the diet is always continued for life. Older children and adolescents are often tempted to compromise their diets because the disease has been asymptomatic for long periods and they feel "different" from other children because they are unable to eat spaghetti, hamburgers, hot dogs, or pizza.

Because occasional dietary transgressions may not cause significant problems, these may only reinforce the child's view that the disease has been "cured." Research has shown, however, that a significant number of these people suffer relapse if dietary restrictions are not maintained.

Parental cooperation may also waver as the child continues to appear healthy on the restricted diet. Parents may also need to be reminded of the child's appearance before dietary therapy and of the permanent growth retardation that is possible if dietary restrictions are not followed. Chronic illness and fatigue may also be subtler indicators of dietary transgression. Boredom with a repetitive, bland diet may also lead to dietary mismanagement. Children and parents should therefore learn to cook a variety of acceptable foods. The nurse might encourage older children and teenagers to discover foods or recipes that are acceptable and to begin developing a sense of responsibility toward their own dietary management.

Parents need to be cognizant of those factors that can lead to problems. Avoiding exposure to infections is important, and the development of diarrhea or vomiting warrants close observation if a crisis is to be prevented. Anticholinergics have also been implicated in the development of crises. Because these drugs are often prescribed as antihistaminics, mild sedatives, or preoperative medications, the parent or child needs to remind any physician or dentist of the child's intolerance before such drugs are prescribed.

Because the disease is chronic, many children or families develop emotional problems. The child's cooperation with dietary restrictions may change dramatically with age, and parents may find that normal childhood disciplinary problems are exacerbated by the restrictions required. Manipulative behaviors on the part of parent or child may develop. Siblings may demonstrate behavior problems due to the extra attention given the affected child. The family may require outside counseling or long-term therapy. (The impact of chronic illness on the child and family is discussed in more depth in Chapter 30.)

Lactose Intolerance: Congenital and Acquired

Congenital lactose intolerance is classified as an inborn error of metabolism. It occurs least frequently in people of northern European ancestry but may affect up to 70% of American blacks (Hug, 1979). It is characterized by a deficiency or absence of the enzyme lactase within the border of the intestinal villi. Lactase is necessary to hydrolyze (or reduce) the sugar lactose. Because lactose is not hydrolyzed, it can cause excessive fermentation by intestinal bacteria. Therefore, the ingestion of lactose by affected individuals may lead to abdominal cramps, distention, and severe diarrhea. The build-up of a fermentation by-product (lactic acid) leads to a low-pH stool. Watery diarrhea results because of the irritation of the acid build-up as well as the increase in intraluminal intestinal osmolality.

A transient, or acquired, lactose intolerance may develop after an infant has undergone a protracted seige of diarrhea or has had a large segment of small bowel removed. Damage to the intestinal villi results in an insufficient quantity of lactase. This can cause a vicious cycle of malabsorption and diarrhea. These children should be placed on alternative, nonmilk, nonlactose formulas for several weeks. Slow reintroduction of lactose-containing formula is begun after this. Acquired forms of lactose intolerance are usually transitory and are easily remedied within a short period of time.

Medical Treatment Congenital lactose intolerance should not be confused with milk allergy (see Chapter 15). The latter condition is caused by a sensitization to one of the many milk protein fractions. A differentiation may be made by administering a lactose challenge. The child receives clear, lactose-free liquids until the child is diarrhea-free for at least 24 hours. The stool should have a pH greater than 6, and there should be no reducing substances present in the stool specimen. Lactose is then administered orally. The child is observed for the onset of diarrhea, gastric distension, vomiting, or acidic stool. These signs indicate true lactose intolerance. In affected individuals, the serum level of lactose does not change after administration of large doses of oral lactose because of the child's inability to metabolize lactose efficiently.

Nursing Management Infants who have a suspected intolerance of lactose may develop severe diarrhea leading to severe dehydration. All stool samples should be tested for pH to identify acids released during fermentation of unabsorbed carbohydrates. Clinitest tablets may be used to identify the presence of reducing substances in the stool. Because of the acid and enzyme content of these diarrhea stools, meticulous perineal skin care is indicated.

Once a diagnosis of lactose intolerance has been confirmed, the nurse begins dietary teaching. Parents need to understand the rationale behind a lactose-free diet. A nutritionist can provide counseling regarding a lactose-free diet for older children, who require a diet more varied than formula. Older children may be able to tolerate small amounts of dietary lactose without experiencing severe discomfort.

Short-Bowel Syndrome

One form of acquired malabsorption is commonly referred to as the short-bowel syndrome. This usually occurs after massive resection of the small intestine resulting from multiple intestinal atresias, necrotizing enterocolitis, gastroschisis, or other gastrointestinal disorders of early infancy. Although infants are capable of adapting to limited intestinal resection without problems, a resection of 25% or more of the small intestine can cause severe malabsorption. Any adaptation of remaining intestines usually takes place within the first 12 months after surgery (Jewett and Lebenthal, 1978).

The location of the resection is important in determining both the ultimate prognosis and the nature of the malabsorption. Loss of proximal bowel may lead to a "stagnant loop syndrome" caused by bacterial contamination of the lumen. This causes an overgrowth of bacterial flora, overproduction of intestinal gas, and diarrhea. Resection of the jejunum may lead to malabsorption of iron, calcium, and folic acid and decreases the production of lactase, sucrase, and maltase. Distal resections cause more dramatic problems such as malabsorptions of bile salts, Vitamin B_{12}, and fat-soluble vitamins. Fluid and electrolyte imbalances are common after major resections, and may present a difficult management problem.

Medical Treatment Treatment of infants with short-bowel syndrome is focused upon maintaining nutritional status until normal intake is possible. Infants are frequently placed on long-term TPN and need adequate supplementation of trace elements and necessary vitamins until a normal diet can be resumed. Vitamin and mineral levels are measured to determine any deficiencies.

Infants usually receive small amounts of sterile water or isotonic electrolyte solutions. As the infant continues on the diet, isotonicity and osmolality of the formula can be adjusted according to the child's malabsorptive problem. Special hospital formulas are frequently used until the child's bowel can accommodate elemental diets or dilute standard formulas. (See Table 38-5 for special formulas.)

These infants are at high risk for many reasons. Hyperalimentation exposes them to systemic infections and certain nutrient deficiencies if they are not monitored closely. Frequent diarrhea can cause rapid dehydration, electrolyte imbalances, and excoriation of perineal skin due to nonabsorbed bile acids and enzymes. Circulating immunoglobulins may be decreased after massive resections, and frequent infections may cause major clinical setbacks.

With the advent of TPN, more of these infants are surviving than ever before, but physical, emotional, and social development may be affected because of prolonged hyperalimentation, chronic illness, and length of hospitalization. Many of these infants have remained on hyperalimentation for 6–12 months or longer.

Nursing Management Nursing management is primarily symptomatic, and continued assessment of the child is important for planning care. Because of the prolonged hospitalization of these infants, the nurse takes care to avoid overlooking signs or symptoms that require immediate attention.

Children on chronic hyperalimentation must be monitored closely for signs and symptoms of infection, both at the site of the line insertion and systemically. Hypothermia or hyperthermia may indicate infection, as might sudden development of diarrhea. Irritability, lethargy, mottling, or apnea might indicate sepsis. Erythema and purulent discharge at the central line insertion site are indicators of infection. Children undergoing TPN also are observed for unusual rashes, bruising, bleeding, muscle twitching, seizures, or other neurologic changes that might indicate mineral or vitamin deficiencies.

The nurse observes infants given oral feedings for signs of formula intolerance. A sudden change in stool frequency or character is the most common problem, but vomiting and gastric retention also might occur. These infants should be NPO with intravenous fluids until dietary changes can be tolerated.

Diarrhea is common in these infants. The nurse therefore monitors frequency, character, color, and volume of all stools. Tests for stool pH are also performed, and Clinitest may be used to identify the presence of reducing substances in the stool and urine. Testape may be used to indicate glucose in the stool or urine. Strict intake and output records are important, whether the child is receiving hyperalimentation or oral feedings. Measurement of urine specific gravity may be done to determine fluid status, and daily weight measurements are necessary.

Skin rashes or skin breakdown are common. Rashes may indicate trace element or vitamin deficiencies. Candidal rashes may cause severe skin breakdown in the perineal region, as may malabsorption of bile acids and enzymes. Antifungal creams are used to combat candidal infection, and exposure to air or a heat lamp might speed healing. Cholestyramine may be used if bile acid malabsorption is suspected. This medication is often given orally in feedings but has also been used in mixture with a topical agent to prevent further perineal excoriation. Frequent skin care and thorough cleansings after each stool and voiding help prevent skin breakdown.

Although the many physical problems appear to be overwhelming, emotional concerns also are vitally important. Parents of these children have not only been faced with the necessity of immediate surgery for their infants, but also have had to face long-term hospitalization and complex care regimens. Nurses need to encourage family participation in the infant's care. These parents usually welcome the opportunity to learn about the nursing care needs of their infants and frequently become quite knowledgeable about their infant's condition and about hyperalimentation.

Family dynamics are often strained because of prolonged hospitalization, and the extended family may play an important role in supporting the parents during these times. Young siblings should be allowed to visit if possible and should be offered a chance to discuss their feelings regarding their mother's or father's prolonged absences. Support groups of affected parents and siblings may be formed by the nursing staff as an organized approach to aid these families, or families may develop individual support groups among themselves.

Family members should be encouraged to bring the infant mobiles or stuffed toys and should talk to and cuddle the infant whenever possible. This helps facilitate parental attachment and contributes to the infant growth and development. Some parents feel that infant clothes brought from home make their children more like individuals. The nurse therefore encourages all these activities. (Nursing care of high-risk infants is generally discussed in Chapter 31.)

Phenylketonuria

Phenylketonuria (PKU) is one of the few inborn errors of metabolism that is treated exclusively through dietary management. Phenylketonuria occurs because a genetic defect results in the ability of the body to metabolize phenylalanine, an essential amino acid. The absence of an hepatic enzyme (phenylalanine hydroxylase) prevents the conversion of phenylalanine to tyrosine. Instead, the phenylalanine is transaminated to phenylpyruvic acid or decarboxylated to phenylethelamine. These abnormal by-products of phenylalanine accummulate in the bloodstream and are excreted in the urine and sweat. They may also be stored in the cerebrospinal fluid or body tissues.

Untreated infants develop a typical picture of moderate to severe mental retardation due to degeneration of the brain and defective myelination of the nerves. Eczema or seborrhea may be present, and there is a musty or mousey odor to the urine and sweat. They may develop seizures, hyperactivity, a bizarre or schizoid personality, and marked behavior problems. These children are characteristically blond and blue eyed with fair skin because their bodies do not convert phenylalanine to tyrosine and tyrosine is necessary for the production of the pigment melanin.

Phenylketonuria screening is mandatory in most states. The most frequently used method of testing involves a bacterial inhibition assay in which a drop of blood is placed in a culture medium with an organism known to require a particular amount of phenylalanine in order to survive. If the bacteria grow, then an abnormal blood level of phenylalanine is suspected. The accuracy of this test is predicated on adequate ingestion of protein for 24–48 hours. Vomiting, NPO status, or early testing can lead to false-negative results, and many states require retesting of infants at 14–28 days of age.

Other tests are based on the presence of abnormal metabolic by-products that are present in the urine of affected infants, although it may take 2–4 weeks before the by-products are present in sufficient quantities for the test to be performed with any accuracy and brain damage may already have occurred during this time. Experience has shown that children who begin dietary treatment within the first 2 to 3 weeks of life stand a greater chance of incurring no brain damage. For this reason, early blood tests using the bacterial inhibition method are preferred.

Medical Treatment Medical management is directed toward minimizing intake of dietary phenylalanine. Because phenylalanine is an essential amino acid, minimum intake of this substance is necessary, and because tyrosine is not being formed, an adequate amount of this amino acid is necessary also.

Infants are begun on a formula consisting of an enzymatic hydrolysate of casein (Lofenalac), which lowers the phenylalanine concentration from the normal 5% to approximately 0.4%. The diet is expanded to include low-phenylalanine foods as the child grows older. It is important to monitor serum levels of phenylalanine as an indicator of dietary control. Blood levels between 2 and 7 mg/100 mL appear to provide adequate growth without mental impairment.

It is suggested that the diet be maintained until the child is at least 7–9 years old, at which time at least 90% of brain growth has occurred. Individuals of childbearing age should receive genetic counseling. Affected women considering pregnancy should know that high levels of phenylalanine in the maternal bloodstream can cause mental retardation or congenital malformations in the fetus. Women of childbearing age may thus consider returning to a phenylalanine-restricted diet.

Nursing Management The long-term goals of nursing care are dietary education and emotional support. Because parents must first become familiar with dietary requirements, nurses need to provide both oral and written information on phenylketonuria. Parents then must face the importance of long-term dietary management and the problems it usually creates. Special formulas are expensive; children dislike the taste of these formulas, and low-phenylalanine foods (vegetables, fruit juices, limited cereals) can become restrictive and repetitive. Parents may encounter problems with dietary control when children become old enough to visit with friends or go to school. Peer pressure is difficult to handle and might cause the child to transgress on the diet.

Monitoring of serum phenylalanine levels is an important part of follow-up care. The nurse also observes the child for signs of hypophenylalinemia. Metabolic acidosis and recurrence of skin rashes may indicate a deficiency. Height and weight growth patterns also may be adversely affected if intake of phenylalanine is cut too drastically.

The Child With a Problem of Inflammation

Necrotizing Enterocolitis

Necrotizing enterocolitis (NEC) is an idiopathic ischemic disorder of the intestine that occurs predominantly in premature infants but may also be seen in any highly stressed neonates. Although the exact cause of the disorder is not known a triad of factors has been identified as possibly contributing to the development of NEC. These factors are hypoxia, presence of bacteria, early feedings. Perinatal asphyxia, respiratory distress syndrome, exchange transfusions, or umbilical artery or vein catheterization may all contribute to ischemia of the bowel.

One hypothesis is that a vascular reflex causes shunting of the circulation away from the gut toward the heart, brain, and kidneys during hypoxic episodes (the diving reflex). This allows for the development of intestinal ischemia resulting in NEC. Other factors that may contribute in the development of NEC are early feedings of hyperosmolar formulas (high-calorie formulas for premature infants), polycythemia, and infections. Contrary to previous assumptions, however, NEC has occurred in infants who have been totally breast fed.

The ischemic sites usually occur within the small intestine, but may also affect the proximal colon. The bowel becomes distended, edematous, and hemorrhagic. Pneumatosis intestinalis (air within the walls of the intestine) is caused by the invasion of gas-producing bacteria. The necrosis may involve only the surface or may penetrate the entire thickness of the wall.

The signs and symptoms of NEC may be essentially those caused by endotoxins. Also, the insult to the intestinal wall allows for systemic endotoxemia. Clinically, the affected infant develops abdominal distention with gastric retention and vomiting at any time from 1–10 days following the supposed triggering event. The abdominal skin may become taut and shiny. Signs of sepsis (lethargy, hypothermia, acidosis, apnea, and cardiovascular collapse) develop rapidly. Stools may be guiac positive, indicating the presence of occult blood. Perforation of the intestine leads to peritonitis, and anterior wall cellulitis causes the skin of the abdomen to become reddened and indurated. Disseminated intravascular coagulopathy may develop secondary to intestinal hemorrhage or sepsis.

Flat-plate and upright abdominal x-rays reveal dilated bowel, and pneumatosis intestinalis can be seen in many of the affected infants. Pneumoperitoneum, or subphrenic air, indicates perforation of the intestine. Barium studies are contraindicated because the excess bulk and high osmolality may contribute to perforation of weakened bowel walls. Blood and spinal fluid cultures may be done to diagnose sepsis. The mortality rate varies from 25%–40% (Brown and Sweet, 1978).

Medical and Surgical Treatment Early diagnosis and treatment of NEC may significantly decrease the high morbidity and mortality rates. Therefore, many neonatal intensive care units screen all infants for signs and symptoms that might indicate the development of the disease. Treatment involves discontinuing any oral feedings, instituting NG suction, maintaining fluid and electrolyte balance with intravenous fluids, and administering appropriate antibiotics.

Surgery is indicated only if clinical symptoms or radiographic studies show widespread necrosis or perforation. Resection of large amounts of necrotic bowel can lead to development of short-bowel syndrome. A temporary ileostomy or colostomy may also be necessary in order to ensure surgical success. Oral feedings, if indicated, are reintroduced slowly after 1–2 weeks. Infants require some form of hyperalimentation or TPN until oral intake is adequate.

Nursing Management Nurses who care for neonates or premature infants need to be aware of the warning signs of NEC. Any infant with gastric distention, increasing gastric residuals, vomiting, or signs of sepsis should be assessed for possible NEC. These infants are placed NPO, and NG suctioning is begun. The nurse then measures abdominal girth at least every 8 hours at the same level on the abdomen each time. Marking the infant's abdomen immediately above and below the tape measure helps guide subsequent measurements. In addition, all gastric drainage and stools are tested for occult blood. Accurate intake and output is essential and should include hourly records of intravenous fluids, NG drainage, vomiting, and stools. The nurse monitors vital signs closely; septic or severely ill infants also might need to be placed on cardiac-respiratory monitors. Infants are observed for signs of perforation or advanced necrosis (rapid abdominal distention, abdominal wall cellulitis). Infants requiring prolonged NPO status (more than 48–72 hours) should receive nutritional support through hyperalimentation. If a central line is placed, the infant needs meticulous site and line care to avoid infection and sepsis.

Ostomies are frequently necessary because of perforation, and adequate skin care is needed to prevent maceration of abdominal skin. Parents of these infants need repeated explanations, information, updates, and emotional support. The nurse encourages families to participate in their infant's care and allows parents to bathe, cuddle, or feed their infants whenever possible.

A number of these infants develop intestinal strictures as they grow older. Children who did not require initial surgery appear to be more likely to develop strictures than those who underwent surgery. The nurse therefore instructs parents about the signs that indicate possible obstruction and explains that they should return to the physician immediately if such signs occur. Infants who develop short-bowel syndrome due to massive resection of the ileum require additional care and may remain hospitalized for a greater length of time.

Appendicitis

Appendicitis occurs when the vermiform appendix becomes inflamed. This may be caused by a physical obstruction of the lumen by fecaliths (hardened feces) or by anatomic defects within the cecum itself. It is one of the most common diseases requiring abdominal surgery in childhood. Although cases of appendicitis have been documented in infants under the age of 2, it occurs most frequently in later childhood and young adulthood.

The symptoms of appendicitis are diverse, and many cases therefore go unrecognized in children until rupture has occurred. The child may originally complain of a generalized periumbilical pain, with this pain later localizing in the right lower quandrant. Fever and vomiting are usually present, and the child may complain of either diarrhea or constipation. Children often remain lying on their sides with their legs drawn upward. A normally active child may voluntarily remain quietly in bed.

Examination of the child reveals a rigid abdomen, rebound tenderness, and decreased or absent bowel sounds. The child may complain of right lower quadrant pain when the body is moved or when the right leg is flexed and straightened. A rectal exam is necessary to rule out other conditions and may be quite painful in a child with appendicitis. Laboratory tests usually reveal an elevated white blood cell count, although it is seldom higher than 20,000/mm^3. Abdominal radiographs reveal a fecalith or some other cause of obstruction, although these rarely confirm the diagnosis.

The child whose appendix ruptures may indicate a sudden lessening of pain, but if rupture has occurred with peritonitis following, the abdomen becomes more rigid, and the child exhibits obvious guarding of the abdomen. The fever may elevate dramatically, as may the white blood cell count. A shocklike syndrome with tachypnea, tachycardia, pallor, and restlessness may be the result of rapid chest breathing or an indicator of incipient septic shock.

Several conditions may mimic appendicitis and should always be considered in a differential diagnosis. The two most common are Meckel's diverticulum and mesenteric lymphadenitis; in the young child another possible diagnosis is intussusception. A rectal examination that reveals blood should cause the examiner to consider intussusception or a diverticulum as alternative diagnoses. Treatment of a diverticulum is confined to surgical excision of the lesion.

Meckel's diverticulum occurs when the omphalomesenteric duct connecting the embryonic midgut to the yolk sac fails to disappear. Resulting cysts, fistulas, and fibrous bands can cause bleeding, ulceration, infection, and volvulus of the small intestine. Volvulus results when the small intestine becomes looped around the remaining fibrous band. The presenting symptoms of a diverticulum may include painless rectal bleeding and occasional abdominal pain. It is this pain that may mimic appendicitis.

Mesenteric lymphadenitis is an enlargement or inflammation of the mesenteric lymph nodes. It is often associated with viral upper respiratory tract infections. Symptoms include fever, abdominal pain, and vomiting. The pain is cramping and may occasionally be located in the right lower quadrant. The area of tenderness in mesenteric lymphadenitis may shift when the patient is rolled from side to side, whereas it remains the same with appendicitis. The white blood cell count may exceed 20,000/mm^3. Treatment is symptomatic, and surgery is unnecessary unless appendicitis cannot be completely ruled out.

Surgical Treatment An appendectomy (surgical removal of the vermiform appendix) is performed as soon as is feasible. The rationale is that it is much easier and safer to remove an intact appendix than it is to treat the resultant peritonitis if the appendix were to rupture. Children in shock or those exhibiting fluid or electrolyte imbalances should be treated medically prior to surgery. Fluid replacements, NG suctioning, and antibiotics may be required initially to stabilize the child. Children with a suspected perforation should be positioned in a high-Fowler's position. This promotes pelvic pooling of any fecal leakage and might prevent the development of a subphrenic abscess.

Nursing Management The goals of preoperative nursing care are to help establish a diagnosis and to prepare the child and parent for impending surgery. The first may be accomplished through continued assessment of the child's condition. Changes in behavior, location, or duration of pain; increase in vomiting; or any signs of shock or septicemia can become essential data when trying to diagnose appendicitis. Nurses functioning in a community or referral capacity need to remind parents that, because of the possibility of perforation, enemas, cathartics, or suppositories are contraindicated if appendicitis is suspected.

Preparation of the child and parents for imminent surgery involves interventions that are both physical and psychological. Physically, the child usually requires rehydration or replacement of lost electrolytes. An NG tube may be placed and intermittent suctioning begun. Antibiotics may be required if a perforation is suspected.

The child is usually fearful and extremely anxious. This is often the child's first hospital stay, and the child may arrive with many preconceived notions of doctors, nurses, and hospitals. Children should receive concise, age-appropriate explanations of what will take place before surgery whenever possible. Because of the brevity of preoperative preparation and emergency nature of the experience, these children need detailed explanations following surgery. They benefit from age-appropriate therapeutic play that provides them with opportunities to express their fears and concerns (see Chapter 28). (Preoperative teaching is discussed in Chapter 29; children's reactions to hospitalization are discussed in Chapter 27).

Psychologic support is important because of the emergency that appendicitis presents. Parents may offer recriminations for not having sought treatment earlier, or they may become hostile or anxious when surgery is not done immediately. They require patient and calm explanations of what is to be done and why. They need to be reassured that a well-hydrated, metabolically balanced child is a much safer surgical risk and that, for this reason, surgery is often postponed.

Postoperative nursing care of a child with simple appendectomy is basic care following any abdominal surgery. The surgical site is frequently covered only with collodian, Steri-strips, or a small gauze dressing. The hospital stay is usually only 2–5 days, and the child may resume normal activities quickly. Rough contact sports, abdominal muscle exercises, and heavy lifting are discouraged in the immediate postoperative period.

If a rupture of the appendix has occurred, Penrose drains are placed in the abscess site. The child should remain in a semi- or high-Fowler's position or may lay on the right side. Dressings are usually bulky in order to absorb copious drainage, which is extremely foul-smelling and irritating to abdominal skin. Frequent dressing changes are needed in order to prevent excoriation. These children may have to be placed on wound and skin precautions in order to prevent cross-contamination of other patients (see Table 38-1). Intravenous antibiotics are administered for 7–10 days and may be continued orally after discharge. The hospital stay may vary from 1–3 weeks depending upon the need for antibiotics. The surgical site is often allowed to granulate inward once the drain has been removed. Children may resume normal activities, but excessive activities as listed previously should be postponed.

Ulcerative Colitis

Ulcerative colitis is characterized by extensive inflammation of the mucosa and submucosa of the colon. It occurs predominantly in young adults but may be seen in children of all ages. Peak onset time is during the second decade of life. The disease is more common in whites than in American blacks or native Americans; incidence is also greater in upper socioeconomic groups; and Jewish populations experience a 3–4 times greater incidence than does the general population (Rudolph, 1982). Approximately 10%–20% of affected individuals have other family members with inflammatory bowel disease (Price and Wilson, 1982), suggesting that predisposition to the disease may be inherited.

Although several theories about the etiology of ulcerative colitis have been suggested, the exact cause remains unknown. One such theory is that the disease is an extreme response to certain intestinal bacteria; a second theory proposes an autoimmune reaction or other immunologic defect; and others address the common combination of physical and emotional problems. Until the exact cause is discovered, the presumption is that ulcerative colitis is an organic disease that may be exacerbated by emotional stress.

The inflammatory lesions found in ulcerative colitis begin in the rectum, proceed proximally through the colon, and may include the terminal ileum. Biopsy reveals abscesses of the intestinal crypts, ulceration, and large numbers of lymphocytes and polymorphonuclear leukocytes. The submucosa is highly vascular but does not appear edematous. Granulated tissue may be present in prolonged disease.

The child may show failure to grow, abdominal pain, and frequent liquid stools. The diarrhea may occur ten to twelve times per day and contains large numbers of leukocytes. Pus and blood may be evident without microscopic examination. Prolonged disease may result in frequent or severe hematochezia (red blood in the stool). Rectal examination reveals local tenderness; left lower quadrant discomfort is present on palpation. Children with severe disease may exhibit abdominal cramps, fever, anemia, hypoproteinmia, weight loss, and growth retardation with delayed sexual development. These children may also exhibit tenesmus (the persistent urge to defecate when little or no stool is present in the rectal vault).

Systemic symptoms may include leukocytosis, low-grade fever (particularly in late evening), arthritis, erythema nodosum (a red nodular rash), and mouth ulcers. Arthritis and erythema nodosum are rarely severe, and seldom cause permanent damage. Mouth ulcers may combine with existing anorexia to cause nutritional problems.

Diagnostic tests include barium enema and rectosigmoidoscopy. Children with ulcerative colitis may have normal barium enemas, and children with severe disease may reveal a "lead-pipe" appearance of the bowel. This occurs when there is shortening and decreased distensibility of the colon with marked loss of haustration. (Haustra are the sacculations of the colon that give it the normal scalloped appearance.) Microulcerations and pseudopolyps may be present. The bowel wall is inflamed and bleeding, and friability may be documented by wiping the mucosa with a cotton-tipped applicator. Fissures, fistulas, or anal ulcerations are uncommon in ulcerative colitis and may indicate the presence of Crohn's disease.

Medical and Surgical Treatment Mild cases may respond to topical application of steroids in the form of enemas. Moderate or severe cases may respond to systemic steroid therapy. The response to therapy is related to the severity and chronicity of the disease. If the disease is in remission, steroids are tapered, and sulfasalazine (Azulfidine) is begun. Children with *acute remitting* forms of ulcerative colitis usually respond well to medication during acute exacerbations. Those with *chronic continuous* colitis rarely obtain a true remission, and chronic malnutrition becomes evident. Children may develop toxic megacolon with scarring, adhesions, or strictures causing abdominal distension and ileus. If unrecognized or untreated, perforation and sepsis occur.

If medications are ineffective in attaining remission, TPN for total bowel rest while maintaining adequate protein and carbohydrate intake or surgical intervention may become necessary. Steroids are usually continued during this therapy, and antibiotics may be given to decrease colonic infection.

Surgical intervention involves a total colectomy with ileostomy. This procedure may be performed when growth retardation is severe or when there is profuse hemorrhage, toxic megacolon, perforation, or malignancy. When the colectomy is performed before epiphyseal closure, growth retardation may be reversed as the nutritional and metabolic status improves.

Ulcerative colitis is a severely disabling disease and poses long-term risks. Besides the obvious risks of chronic malnutrition, anemia, and hemorrhage, the affected child runs a great risk of developing cancer of the colon. This risk is increased with the length and severity of illness. Estimates are that there is a 3% risk of developing colon cancer in persons whose disease is of less than 10 years' duration. The risk increases by 20% for each successive decade of illness. For this reason, total colectomy is advised for those patients who have had chronic ulcerative colitis for more than 10 years (Price and Wilson, 1982).

Nursing Management Children who have been diagnosed as having ulcerative colitis require long-term medical and nursing follow-up. Teaching regarding dietary therapy, use of medications, and methods of reducing daily stress is important in the overall approach to care. The nurse also provides appropriate emotional support for families and children experiencing a chronic illness (see Chaper 30) and for those who are to undergo a total colectomy.

Dietary therapy involves a high-protein, high-calorie diet. In addition, foods should be low in residue to minimize the irritation of the gut. New approaches to dietary therapy are being developed, and many children are able to eat a normal diet. Foods that cause pain or diarrhea are eliminated, and high-protein foods are encouraged.

If children experience anorexia, small, frequent, snacks or meals are necessary and should include such protein and calorie-rich foods as milkshakes, puddings, ice cream, eggnog, or cream soups. Low-residue elemental diets that provide extra protein and caloric supplementation are available.

The child may develop aphthous stomatitis. These may be brought on by the emotional distress, immunologic toxicity to the oral epithelial cells, or in response to medications being taken. When mouth ulcers contribute to the anorexia, local applications of magnesium and aluminum hydroxides (Maalox) or lidocaine (viscous Xylocaine) may provide temporary relief and allows the child to eat or drink with minimal discomfort.

Steroid medications may initially increase the child's appetite, but will also cause Cushing-like symptoms if used over long periods of time. Sulfasalazine may cause gastric distress with nausea and vomiting. Dividing the dose throughout the day or providing enteric-coated tablets may lessen or eliminate these symptoms. (Younger children should not be allowed to chew these tablets; as this can damage tooth enamel.) Children taking sulfasalazine over long periods of time should be observed for possible blood dyscrasias. Adequate fluid intake is necessary to prevent crystalluria. The child is encouraged to drink a full glass of water with each medication dose. The nurse also cautions parents that the child's urine may be orange from the medication.

Stress can exacerbate the symptoms of colitis. The nurse therefore minimizes the stress encountered by the hospitalized child by explaining all invasive procedures and providing the child with opportunities to cope with stress through therapeutic play (see Chapter 28). Children who are not hospitalized may benefit from learning relaxation techniques or exercises. Families may require assistance in determining the activities or circumstances that contribute to stress in their children. Nurses may need to help parents recognize common manipulative behavior in chronically ill children. Multidisciplinary management may also include family counseling to assist parents in providing the discipline and structure that all children require (see Chapter 30).

Those children undergoing colectomy with ileostomy require specific preoperative preparation. The nurse or enterostomal therapist may begin ileostomy teaching or may introduce the child to another ostomate. The child should be prepared for imminent changes in body appearance. The nurse provides written and verbal instructions in ostomy care, and public health follow-up may be necessary. Many older adolescents and young adults willingly accept the colectomy because it reduces pain and diarrhea and virtually eliminates the risk of colon cancer. All patients undergoing a colectomy should understand that they can expect to lead normal lives.

Crohn's Disease

Crohn's disease (regional enteritis) is an inflammatory condition of the digestive tract. It may affect any area from the mouth to the anus but is most commonly found in the anus and terminal ileum. This disease affects males and females in equal proportions, approximately 1 person in every 100,000. Whites are more often affected than blacks, and the Jewish population is affected three to six times more often than the general population. A familial tendency toward some form of inflammatory bowel disease also has been identified (Price and Wilson, 1982).

Inflammation of the bowel affects all layers of the intestinal wall. Lymphocytes and plasma cells are present within the mucosal and submucosal layers. Crypt abscesses are apparent on biopsy, and granulomata is often visible. Ulceration of the walls is evident, and internal or enterocutaneous fistulas may develop. Regional lymph nodes may contain granulomas. Edema of the submucosa is present, whereas it is absent in ulcerative colitis. Table 38-8 compares Crohn's disease and ulcerative colitis.

Crohn's disease is more common in children than was previously known. The persistent inflammation seldom responds to current therapies. This chronic inflammation may cause mucosal atrophy, scarring, and formation of constricting fibrotic tissue. Bleeding may occur from ulcerated sites and may be chronic or acute. Intestinal obstruction is a major cause of surgical intervention in these children.

Manifestations of Crohn's disease vary greatly. Although its onset is usually gradual, Crohn's disease may also present symptoms mimicking an acute abdomen. General symptoms may include chronic fatigue, anorexia, or occult bleeding. There may be a generalized abdominal tenderness if a large segment of the bowel is affected. This pain may be periumbilical but is more commonly localized in the right lower quadrant. A mass may be felt in the lower right quadrant if the terminal ileum is involved. Frequent watery diarrhea is present in an overwhelming majority of patients, and fresh blood may become apparent. Fever occurring with Crohn's disease may be more persistent than that found in ulcerative colitis and may peak to higher levels during acute inflammatory episodes. Weight loss, anemia, growth retardation, delayed sexual development, and mouth ulcers may be seen. Failure to grow is a classic symptom of Crohn's disease and is more pronounced in children with colorectal involvement. Delayed sexual development will occur if the disease begins in prepubescent children. Arthritis may also be present but rarely causes permanent damage.

Children suspected of having Crohn's disease require anal and proctosigmoidoscopic examinations as well as barium enemas and biopsies of lesions. Tissue for biopsy may also be taken from apparently healthy tissue in order to detect subclinical disease in the absence of overt lesions. The effects of Crohn's disease are segmented, although the affected segments vary and the duodenum and jejunum may be included. A barium swallow is necessary to identify involvement of the jejunum and duodenum. Fissures or fistulas are a classic finding. A barium enema may show irregular lumen, fistulas, and ulcerations. It may also show more clearly those segments that are affected.

Medical Treatment Medical treatment of Crohn's disease is rarely effective over long periods of time. The treatment is essentially the same as for ulcerative colitis, except that surgery is seldom performed because the patchy, segmental occurrence of the lesions does not lend itself to surgical resection. Even when large segments of affected bowel are removed, it does not prevent recurrence of the disease in previously unaffected bowel.

Children who can attain temporary remission on steroids and sulfasalazine do so within the first week of therapy. Those who do not respond may require long-term TPN in order to achieve even a temporary remission. Continual NG feedings of elemental diets (residue-free preparations such as Vivonex) have been attempted with some success (Morin et al., 1980). Because the course of the disease is progressive and relentless and resection of the bowel is not effective, these patients are at a risk approximately 20 times greater than in unaffected individuals for developing intestinal cancer.

Nursing Management Although the pathologic process involved in Crohn's disease varies slightly from ulcerative colitis, the nursing goals are approximately the same. Children with Crohn's disease also are prone to the development of enterocutaneous fistulas and anal fissures. Fistulas occur most commonly in the perirectal area and may contribute to the development of perirectal abscesses, which

TABLE 38-8 Characteristics of Ulcerative Colitis and Crohn's Disease

Characteristics	Ulcerative colitis	Crohn's disease
Tissue involved	Mucosa and submucosa	All layers of submucosa
Area of involvement		
Rectum	Almost always	Approximately 50%
Right colon	Occasionally	Often
Small bowel	Rare	Always
Range of disease	Throughout colon	Segmental
Rectal bleeding	Very common	Rare
Anal abscesses	Uncommon	Very common
Enterocutaneous fistulas	Uncommon	Very common
Granuloma of tissues	Uncommon	Common
Cancer risk	Greatly increased after 10 years of active disease	Increased but less than in ulcerative colitis

require systemic antibiotics. Both fissures and fistulas may become infected or may bleed. They are intensely painful, and perirectal ulceration and excoriation may become severe. Frequent sitz baths may relieve some of the edema and discomfort, and meticulous skin care is needed. Drainage of perirectal abscesses is seldom curative, and proctocolectomy may be indicated in severe cases of colorectal Crohn's disease (Fonkalsrud et al., 1979).

Peptic Ulcer

Peptic ulcer is a broad classification for any erosion of the mucosa of the stomach, pylorus, or jejunum. More specific terminology includes gastric ulcer (ulceration within the stomach) and duodenal ulcer (ulceration of the pylorus or duodenum). The causative agent of peptic ulcers is unknown, but hypersecretion of gastric acid and peptin is considered a primary contributor to the development of these lesions. Another theory is that the protective mechanism of the stomach lining is in some way dysfunctional. Decreased mucus secretion, slow regeneration of damaged cells, and chronic irritation or inflammation may all be significant contributing causes.

The incidence of peptic ulcers in children varies widely from study to study. Males are affected more often than females, and children having close relatives with ulcer disease are also at greater risk. Young children may have either duodenal or gastric ulcers, while duodenal ulcers predominate in older children and adolescents.

Children also vary dramatically in the clinical symptoms that develop. Adolescents tend to describe the adult cycle of symptoms of pain-food/antacid-relief. They may complain of a gnawing, burning pain in the epigastrium (heartburn), which develops several hours after meals, and they may not experience vomiting or chronic abdominal pain. Young children, however, rarely have any standard group of symptoms. They may complain of general intermittent abdominal pain, late night or early morning abdominal pain, preprandial or postprandial pain, vomiting, or painless melena. The diagnosis of peptic ulcer therefore may be easily overlooked in a child exhibiting only intermittent abdominal pain.

Clinically, affected children may exhibit hematemesis, melena, or anemia. Endoscopy confirms the presence of an eroded site, and contrast studies may be necessary if a duodenal ulcer is suspected. Abdominal tenderness is noted during deep palpation of the epigastrium.

Medical and Surgical Treatment Medical treatment of peptic ulcer is the first and safest choice. Dietary management may be instituted in order to limit foods that stimulate hyperacidity. Although bland diets and diets containing large amounts of milk and cream have been used in the past, they are less common now that they have been indicated in the development of rebound hyperacidity. Bland diets are also difficult to maintain and may not offer the nutritional variety needed for growing children. Therefore, the diet is relatively free, but such items as tea, coffee, carbonated beverages, high-acid foods, and fried foods are restricted.

Frequent administration of antacids, as frequently as once an hour during the initial recovery period, is another component of treatment. Antacids containing magnesium hydroxide or magnesium trisilicate are preferred, although they may cause diarrhea and then need to be alternated with aluminum hydroxide antacids. The indiscriminate use of sodium bicarbonate is discouraged because of the high sodium load as well as the marked alkalinity. Chronic use of sodium bicarbonate also may lead to hyperacid rebound and severe electrolyte imbalances in children. Other drugs that contribute to the formation of ulcers are restricted. These include aspirin and corticosteroids. Cigarette smoking is also prohibited as it has been shown to contribute to gastric hyperacidity.

In addition to antacids, anticholinergic drugs or hydrogen ion blockers may be used. Preparations of propantheline bromide (Pro-Banthine), an effective anticholinergic, may be used to alleviate late night and early morning abdominal pain. Cimetidine (Tagamet) is one of the most commonly prescribed drugs in ulcer therapy. As an effective hydrogen ion blocker, it not only limits peak acid secretions but also lowers basal acid secretion levels.

In cases of hematemesis, NG drainage should begin immediately in order to determine the rate of bleeding. Irrigations with cold saline may aid vasoconstriction and slow or stop the hemorrhage. Blood transfusions, plasma expanders, oxygen, and fluid replacements may be necessary if the blood loss is massive or acute.

Surgery may be indicated in cases of chronic ulceration that does not respond to dietary or drug therapy, or in instances with repeated and severe hemorrhage. In these cases, subtotal gastrectomy (removal of a large portion of the lower stomach) is performed to prevent hypersecretion of acids. An alternative surgery is a vagotomy, in which the appropriate branch of the vagus nerve is cut. This prevents any secretions to the stomach for a period of time. Neither of these procedures is currently used for children, but either may be necessary treatment for intractable ulcers.

Nursing Management When the diagnosis of gastric or duodenal ulcer is confirmed in a child, the nurse formulates a coordinated plan of parent and child education to involve dietary and drug therapies as well as methods of stress reduction. Dietary education may be done by the nurse or nutritionist and includes oral descriptions and written lists of restricted foods together with the rationale for limiting acid-causing foods. The nurse encourages parents to serve nutritionally balanced foods but to avoid serving coffee, tea, spicy foods, fried foods, or carbonated drinks to these children. Parents should anticipate the difficulty in maintaining a strict diet in older children, who are exposed to peer pressure and the easy availability of "junk foods." Snacks between meals and at bedtime may prevent postprandial and nighttime epigastric pain.

Parents and older children need verbal and written directions regarding the administration of antacids, anticholinergics, or cimetidine. Cimetidine is most effective if taken prior to meals and at bedtime. Because of its ulcer-preventing effects, it is often continued for a longer period of time than other medications. Parents should also know that antacids inhibit the action of certain drugs (for example, tetracycline) and that any consulting physicians need to know that a child is taking antacids. Anticholinergics may cause drowsiness, so that children may sleep more frequently or for longer periods or may have difficulty concentrating on schoolwork. Adolescents should be cautioned about driving while drowsy or about drinking alcoholic beverages while taking any medication.

Because stress has been indicated as a possible contributor to hyperacidity, families usually need instruction in reducing physical and emotional stress. Adequate sleep, small frequent meals, and regular exercise can aid in the reduction of physical stress, but disturbed family relationships may require counseling before emotional stress can be alleviated. Because children may use illness in a manipulative manner at home or school, difficulties with these relationships also may require psychological counseling.

The Child With a Problem Related to Liver Function

Anomalies of the Biliary Tree

Biliary atresia and choledochal cysts are the two most common anatomic disorders of the biliary system. These may be two different manifestations of the same prenatal disease and constitute an acquired disease rather than a genetic anomaly. Fetal or neonatal hepatitis may also contribute to the obliteration of the extrahepatic biliary ducts (Anderson, 1978).

Biliary atresia may occur because of a failure in the development of the bile duct lumens, a defect that is classified as intrahepatic or extrahepatic. Intrahepatic atresia is very rare and may involve only the intrahepatic bile ducts or also may include defects in the production or synthesis of bile salts or bilirubin. The onset of symptoms is slow, and cirrhosis may become evident only in later stages of the disease. Extrahepatic ductal atresias are more common in females than males and are rarely found in premature or stillborn infants. (This last finding seems to lend evidence to the theory that atresias may be the result of a postnatal infectious process.) Because the disease is totally obstructive, signs and symptoms of liver damage become evident soon after birth. Early jaundice with elevated direct and indirect bilirubin levels is common, along with clay-colored stools and dark urine. Hepatosplenomegaly is evident, and portal hypertension, ascites, and esophageal varices may develop by late infancy.

Choledochal cysts may occur at any place along the biliary tree. Theories about their origin vary but the cause remains unknown. One hypothesis is that they consist of weakened "outpouchings" of the biliary tree. Choledochal cysts are four times more common in females than in males, are usually very thickwalled, and cause abdominal pain and jaundice. A mass is usually felt in the right upper quadrant, and liver enzymes and bilirubin levels are elevated. The cysts are thought to be present at birth, and early obstructive jaundice is often the initial clinical manifestation. The disease may progress to include symptoms of severe liver damage or hepatic failure.

Medical and Surgical Treatment Medical treatment of biliary atresia and choledochal cysts involves palliative treament of cirrhosis, portal hypertension, esophageal varices, and hepatic coma. Liver function tests are monitored closely, and the child is observed for any signs of possible liver failure.

Surgical correction for external biliary atresia may involve the use of the Kasai procedure in which the atresic ducts are exercised and a y-shaped portion of the jejunum is anastomosed to the porta hepatis at the base of the liver. The success of this surgery depends on the child's age when the procedure is performed. If done before 60 days of age, an initial success rate of 30%–50% has been noted (Kasai et al., 1978), although sustained bile drainage is present in only 20%–30% of these cases (Odièure, 1978). This surgery therefore is considered only marginally successful, and progressive liver disease is still quite common. Present research involving total liver transplantation may offer a more successful treatment in the future. Children who survive the surgery appear to be healthy and have normal liver function. Results of longitudinal research, however, are not available yet.

Surgery for choledochal cysts involves the removal of the cysts. If necessary, a Roux-en-Y choledochojejunostomy may be performed in order to maintain an intact biliary tree. The success of this surgery is also marginal, and liver transplantation is being researched as a possible corrective surgery for this anomaly.

Nursing Management Nursing care of nonsurgical patients with biliary atresia or choledochal cysts is essentially the same as for children with cirrhosis or liver failure. Postoperative care of children undergoing Roux-en-Y or Kasai procedures is like that for children undergoing abdominal surgery. Nurses need to be aware that surgery is rarely curative and that these children are frequently readmitted for complications of recurring liver damage or liver failure. The nurse may need to prepare the family and child for dealing with a chronic, potentially fatal disease (see Chapters 30 and 32).

Hepatitis

Although *hepatitis* is technically any inflammation of the liver, the term has come to indicate the infectious process caused by specific viruses. These viruses have been labeled hepatitis A and hepatitis B. They often produce the same clinical symptomology but their epidemiologic characteristics are distinctly different. Other viruses can cause non-A, non-B hepatitis, and these should be considered until diagnostic tests can determine the causative virus. Other viruses, such as cytomegalovirus, and coxsackie viruses, may produce incidental hepatitis.

Hepatitis A was previously called "infectious" hepatitis because it is highly contagious. The incubation period varies between 2 and 6 weeks from the initial exposure to the appearance of jaundice. The onset is acute and often includes a prodromal, anicteric stage of 5–7 days. During this period, the child exhibits the classical complaints of fever, malaise, and gastric disturbances. The latter may include nausea, vomiting, anorexia, and dull epigastric or right upper quadrant pain. This pain is due to the enlargement of the inflamed liver. The end of this stage is characterized by the onset of jaundice. Sclerae and mucosa become icteric; urine becomes dark; and stools may appear clay or putty colored. Children tire easily and may choose to remain in bed or at rest for long periods of time. They may exhibit irritability or possible emotional lability and depression. Many children may also develop a subclinical hepatitis with milder and more ambiguous symptomology. Children may begin feeling better even while extremely jaundiced. Although the clinical manifestations of hepatitis vary dramatically, the mortality rate of hepatitis A is actually quite low.

Hepatitis B was formerly called serum hepatitis because of its originally presumed mode of transmission. The onset of hepatitis B is less rapid or acute. Symptomatology is similar to hepatitis A but appears slowly and may include dermatologic phenomena (for example, rashes, urticaria) and arthralgia. The incubation period is 2–5 months, and the course of the disease lasts somewhat longer than hepatitis A. A subclinical, asymptomatic type of illness may also occur.

In either type of hepatitis, icterus is usually present for 1–4 weeks, and a complete recovery with normal liver function, appropriate levels of physical endurance, and less emotional lability occurs within 1–3 months in most individuals. Two types of complications, however, may produce chronic, progressive liver changes or even death. The first is *acute fulminating hepatitis* and is characterized by an extremely rapid onset with rapidly rising serum bilirubin. Encephalopathy, a hemorrhagic diathesis, edema, and ascites may develop rapidly into hepatic coma. The mortality rate exceeds 33%, with the majority of deaths occurring within the first 1–2 weeks. The second complication is *chronic active hepatitis* and is characterized by an insidious onset. It occurs more frequently in older girls. Chronic evidence of hepatic dysfunction and cirrhosis of the liver may occur.

The primary mode of transmission varies between the two forms. Hepatitis A is most commonly transmitted through oral-fecal contamination but may also be transmitted parenterally. Food, water, and fomites are the primary sources of contamination. Hepatitis B is often transmitted parenterally, through contaminated blood product transfusions or contaminated needles. The latter is often responsible for the occurrence of the disease in many drug abusers. Employees working with contaminated needles, blood, or blood products (for example, hemodialysis or blood bank personnel) are also at a higher risk than other people. Hepatitis B may also be transmitted during sexual contact by contaminated semen and vaginal or menstrual secretions. A higher incidence of hepatitis B has been found among homosexuals, paticularly homosexual men. Institutionalized individuals are also at greater risk for hepatitis B through contaminated feces and saliva. Both forms may be transmitted in utero or at the time of delivery. Exposure to hepatitis A confers immunity only for that type; exposure to hepatitis B confers immunity only for type B.

Pathologically, the parenchymal cells are edematous or necrotic, with infiltration by lymphocytes and macrophages. Cellular damage and edema may cause blockage of the biliary flow, which results in even more extensive damage. The damaged cells and blocked biliary flow are thought to cause the alternations noted in liver function tests. Elevations in serum glutamic oxaloacetic transaminase (SGOT), serum glutamic pyruvic transaminase (SGPT), alkaline phosphatase, and lactic dehydrogenase (LDH) levels indicate acute liver damage. Because of the severe destruction of the parenchymal cells, transaminase levels may fall below normal in cases of fulminant hepatitis. In addition, SGOT and SGPT levels remain elevated for a longer period in hepatitis B than in hepatitis A. Obstruction of the biliary flow causes malabsorption of fat-soluble vitamin K and may result in a prolonged prothrombin time. Decreased albumin production, resulting from severe liver damage, causes reduced serum protein levels, which in turn contributes to generalized edema and ascites. Indirect bilirubin levels indicate the degree of biliary obstruction. Urobilinogen is usually present in the urine. The sedimentation rate is increased in hepatitis A but not in hepatitis B.

Specific tests for hepatitis include hemagglutination tests and radioimmunoassay. These relatively new tests are based on the presence of the antigen-antibody complex. The hepatitis-associated antigen (HAA/Australian antigen) is present in 80% hepatitis B cases but is absent in cases of hepatitis A.

Medical Treatment Treatment of uncomplicated hepatitis is palliative and directed toward management of symptoms: nausea, vomiting, anorexia, and easy fatigability. Some degree of obstruction of biliary flow is present in almost all hepatitis patients, and because bile acids are necessary for the digestion of fats, hepatitis patients may find that low-fat foods are tolerated better than those with a high fat content. Foods that are high in carbohydrates should be provided, and high-protein foods may be given unless there are indications of severe liver damage or impending liver failure.

Nausea and vomiting may be triggered by high-fat foods or by odors such as tobacco smoke or cooking odors. Antiemetics are usually contraindicated because they are primarily metabolized in the liver. If vomiting is severe, extremely small doses of antiemetics may be attempted. If antiemetics are withheld, or persistent vomiting leads to dehydration, intravenous fluids may be necessary.

All medications, especially those metabolized by or possibly toxic to the liver, should be limited. Steroids may be used in chronic active hepatitis but do not appear to be of much benefit in cases of acute hepatitis.

Treatment of acute fulminant hepatitis is also symptomatic but focuses on the acute areas of encephalopathy, hemorrhagic diathesis, ascites, negative nitrogen balance, and severe electrolyte imbalances. (Treatment of these symptoms is comparable to treatment for hepatic coma.)

There is no immunization available against viral hepatitis. Although much less effective in hepatitis B, administration of serum immune globulin (SIG) has been shown to be effective in modifying the course of hepatitis A. The clinical course of the disease is thus averted, but the recipients may experience a transient rise in some of the liver function tests.

Nursing Management A large number of children with subclinical or uncomplicated hepatitis are cared for at home. (See Chapter 26 for guidelines in assessing the feasibility of home care.) The goals for nursing care of these children are therefore support measures and the prevention of further spread of the disease within the family.

Support measures include small, frequent meals or snacks that are high in carbohydrates and proteins but relatively low in fat. Parents must understand that their children have a physiologic reason for being anorexic and that they should not force these children to eat. The child's appetite may be better early in the morning, and the parent may find that a balanced breakfast is consumed more readily than lunch or dinner.

Parents should also understand that their children tire easily. These children frequently limit their own activities initially. Later in the illness, however, the child may begin feeling much more energetic and may wish to return to school or play, even though they are still quite jaundiced. Parents should know that this is quite common and is a sign of beginning recovery. Children are no longer considered infectious 7–10 days after the onset of jaundice and may therefore return to normal activities if they so desire.

Although the onset of fulminant hepatitis usually is severely acute, cases have occurred in children with presumed benign hepatitis. The nurse therefore instructs parents to report immediately any signs or symptoms that may indicate severely impaired liver function. These include confusion, increasing lethargy, restlessness, sudden behavioral changes or inappropriate behavior, tremors of hand or feet, difficulty speaking, or unusual eye movements such as nystagmus. In cases of fulminant hepatitis or hepatic coma, nursing care is directed toward the acute needs of the child.

When caring for children with hepatitis at home, infection control measures include (a) strict hand washing after using the toilet or changing diapers and before eating or drinking; (b) washing the child's eating utensils in extremely hot, soapy water or in a dishwasher; (c) washing clothing or bedding contaminated with stool or blood in hot, soapy water; (d) covering bleeding lesions and discarding bandages in plastic sacks; (e) discarding used tampons or sanitary napkins in plastic sacks; (f) not sharing drinking glasses, toothbrushes, or food; and (g) no intimate contact such as kissing with the affected individual.

Care of the hospitalized child also includes (a) private room and private bath, if possible, (b) enteric isolation, including gowns and gloves for patient contact or linen changes, and (c) appropriate disposal of all used syringes, medication cups, dressings, or examination equipment such as tongue blades or speculums. All laboratory blood tests are labeled "possible hepatitis", and all used equipment is double-bagged and labeled "isolation" or "possible hepatitis." The nurse reminds parents and visitors to wash their hands after toileting and before eating or leaving the hospital room. They should continue these practices once the child has been discharged. After discharge, all hospital room surfaces are thoroughly cleaned according to hospital policy, and linen is double bagged and labeled "isolation."

Cirrhosis

Cirrhosis is a widespread destructive and regenerative process involving the parenchymal cells of the liver. The creation of fibrous bands of scar tissue causes an abnormal increase in connective tissue growth, as well as an abnormal lobular structure of the liver. Cirrhosis is the result of liver damage or dysfunction and may be caused by a variety of diseases. Hepatitis, biliary atresia, choledochal cysts, and drug or alcohol abuse are frequent causative agents. Cirrhosis in children may also be caused by cystic fibrosis, genetic metabolic syndromes, congenital viral infections, or chronic malnutrition.

Damage to the parenchymal cells of the liver causes activation of fibroblasts. Collagen or fibrous connective tissue is then formed at the site of damage. In long-standing, chronic forms of cirrhosis, the cycle of destruction and regeneration may be balanced in such a way as to cause a subclinical form of cirrhosis. Symptoms become evident only when destruction and scarring exceed cell regeneration. The greater the discrepancy between these processes, the more severe the symptoms become. Initially mild symptoms such as jaundice, failure-to-thrive, pruritus, or steatorrhea may come to include severe anemia, coagulation disorders, portal hypertension, ascites, encephalopathy, and hepatic failure. Jaundice may vary in degree, may be present from soon after birth (biliary atresia, choledochal cysts), or may only become evident after a long-standing history of cirrhosis (cystic fibrosis, hepatolenticular degeneration). Pruritus may vary in intensity, with excoriation of the skin or xanthomas occurring in severe cases.

Children with severe liver damage may develop ascites, portal hypertension, or hepatic failure with encephalopathy and hepatic coma. Portal hypertension occurs in cirrhosis when intrahepatic scarring or portal vein scarring raises vascular resistance. The blood supply to the liver is not sufficient because the portal vein resistance is much greater than standard vascular pressures. Collateral circulation evolves, and dilated abdominal wall veins or spider angiomata may become evident over the chests or backs of affected children. Esophageal varices and hypersplenism may also occur. Portal hypertension, ascites, and esophageal varices are signs of end-stage liver disease.

Ascites occurs when the vascular osmotic pressure is decreased because of hypoalbuminemia, the vascular hydrostatic pressure is increased because of portal hypertension, and the hepatic venous drainage is obstructed by scarring. High pressures within the vascular system in conjunction with the low albumin levels cause leakage of serous fluid into the abdominal cavity. This fluid collects within the peritoneal cavity and causes severe abdominal distension. Respiratory distress may develop because of pressure on the diaphragm. The child is also more prone to the development of bacterial peritonitis. Encephalopathy or coma are thought to result from the increasing serum ammonia levels due to progressive hepatocellular failure.

Medical Treatment Medical treatment is symptomatic for most cirrhosis cases. Dietary management includes a high-carbohydrate, low-fat, moderate-protein diet. Water-miscible vitamin supplements are given for the fat-soluble vitamins (A, D, E, and K), and vitamin B_{12} may be given by injection if necessary. Pruritis is very common and is frequently treated by giving cholestyramine (Questran) by mouth. This helps prevent reabsorption of bile salts and promotes fecal elimination of these salts, but cholestyramine may cause decreased fat and fat-soluble vitamin absorption and may also exacerbate low folic acid levels. Phenobarbital may be given to reduce cholestasis if cholestatic jaundice is suspected.

More severe complications, such as portal hypertension or ascites, may be treated medically. These treatments, however, are rarely successful over long periods of time, although splenorenal or portacaval shunts have been performed with some success in children. Treatment of ascites includes a salt-restricted diet and the administration of spironolactone (Aldactone). Furosemide (Lasix) may be used if necessary and has been administered as a furosemide-albumin-furosemide regimen. The administration of albumin temporarily corrects systemic hypoalbuminemia and helps to retain fluid within the vascular system. The second dose of furosemide then flushes out the additional intravascular fluid but this treatment may cause hypervolemia if the albumin is given too quickly or hypovolemia if furosemide is administered too soon after the albumin. Ascitic fluid may also be removed by paracentesis if respiratory distress is severe. This is only done in severe cases and may lead to hypotensive shock, ascites rebound, or peritonitis.

Nursing Management Long-term goals of nursing care are physical and emotional support. Physical symptoms may include pruritus, a bleeding problem, and peripheral edema. Emotional problems are those common to children with a chronic or potentially fatal illness (see Chapter 30).

Pruritis is caused by the build-up of bile salts within body tissues. Mild pruritus may be managed by frequent cool soda baths, but this is seldom effective over a long period. Severe pruritus may require medication. Infants who scratch frequently may require mittens to prevent excoriation of skin.

Hypoprothrombinemia or the presence of esophageal varices may cause the child with cirrhosis to bleed severely. Nurses should observe for melenic stools or frank hematemesis. All blood tests should be performed during one venipuncture, if possible, and pressure should be applied on the site for a longer period than is normal. A pressure dressing may prevent severe bruising after venipuncture.

Peripheral edema is caused by hypoproteinemia. Children should be discouraged from dangling their legs or wearing restrictive clothing. Scrotal edema may become quite severe, and a scrotal support may be necessary to prevent damage to the delicate skin. A salt-restricted diet may help but only slightly.

Evidence of severe cirrhosis indicates a poor prognosis. Although liver transplantation is being researched and performed, its success in this situation still is marginal, and the availability of this procedure is limited. Nurses caring for children with end-stage hepatic failure therefore need to provide emotional support to the family and child. (Care of the child with a terminal illness is discussed in Chapter 32.)

Portal Hypertension and Esophageal Varices

Portal hypertension may occur whenever there is portal venous obstruction. Cirrhosis, biliary atresia infection, thrombus, trauma, and pancreatitis may contribute to portal venous obstruction, although the true cause of obstruction frequently is not known.

Normally, most of the blood leaving the stomach and intestines is routed through the portal circulation. Obstruction of the portal vein causes the blood to back up, and collateral circulations are formed. Dilated abdominal wall vessels (caput medusae) become evident, and spider angiomata may appear on the chest or back. Backwash of blood within the digestive system causes distension of the esophageal veins. These varices become severely dilated and friable, and they may rupture, causing an acute hemorrhage. Hematemesis or melena may thus indicate bleeding esophageal varices.

Medical Treatment Children who are known to have esophageal varices are instructed to eat soft, nonspicy foods and frequently are given antacids to prevent ulceration of varices by refluxed gastric secretions. They should avoid any activity involving Valsalva's maneuver (sudden coughing or straining at stool) and should learn to initiate bowel movements while mouth-breathing to prevent straining. Stool softeners or dietary fiber may be indicated if constipation is a problem.

Many children have acute hemorrhage, and treatment is directed toward stopping the hemorrhage and replacing lost blood volume. An NG tube often is placed to monitor the amount of bleeding. This also allows decompression of the stomach to prevent vomiting or reflux and cool saline irrigations until a Sengstaken-Blakemore tube can be placed. This triple-lumen tube consists of a distal gastric balloon and an esophageal balloon. Each may be inflated separately to produce a local tamponade of bleeding vessels. Vasopressin, which decreases blood flow to the digestive tract, may be given if bleeding continues. Vasopressin, however, may cause hypertension, bradycardia, cardiac arrhythmias, or facial pallor.

The plasma protein in the swallowed blood is acted on by intestinal bacteria, forming excess ammonia. Intestinal antibiotics such as neomycin or kanamycin may be given to prevent bacterial growth and thus decrease ammonia production. Lactulose, a nonmetabolizable polysaccharide, may be given to prevent absorption of ammonia, and spironolactone may be prescribed to reduce ascites.

Blood tranfusions may be given cautiously and only if blood loss is severe. These children often are chronically anemic, but the goal of therapy is *not* to attain a normal hematocrit level, because the additional intravascular volume may cause hypervolemia or may increase esophageal bleeding.

Surgery is rarely indicated in children with bleeding esophageal varices, unless bleeding is severe and continuous. Ligation of the varices is possible but rarely totally effective. An esophagogastrectomy (removal of esophagus and proximal stomach with replacement by colonic section) may also be done, but bleeding may then occur elsewhere. Splenorenal, portacaval, and mesocaval shunts have been performed to bypass the obstructed portal circulation. These may provide the best long-term effects in preventing repeat variceal bleeding.

Nursing Management The nurse teaches preventive measures to both parents and children. Dietary planning may also include a nutritionist.

In acute hemorrhagic episodes, nursing care is directed toward controlling and monitoring bleeding and assessing and managing signs of impending shock. Bleeding might be decreased initially by cool saline lavage, but this seldom is totally effective, so that a Sengstaken-Blakemore tube needs to be inserted. The nurse then monitors traction on the tube, which is needed to keep the tube in the appropriate position. This may be accomplished by pulling the tube taut and taping it to the cheek or by taping the tube to the mouth guard of a football helmet. Traction should not be so great as to dislodge the balloons. The nurse then suctions saliva from the esophagus because secretions cannot bypass the balloons. Alert, cooperative children may spit out secretions rather than swallowing. Unconscious, uncooperative, or extremely young children may require frequent esophageal suctioning or may need to have a small NG tube inserted to the level of the esophageal balloons to allow for intermittent suctioning. The balloons of the Sengstaken-Blakemore tube should be deflated every 6–8 hours for 5–10 minutes to prevent local tissue necrosis or ulceration. The nurse also monitors inflated balloons for appropriate pressure by attaching a manometer to the lumen to prevent overinflation, underinflation, or an unnoticed deflation.

Accurate intake and output records are necessary in order to monitor blood loss. Nasogastric drainage is observed for new or continued bleeding and stools are observed for melena. Chronic, slow blood loss may require stool tests for occult blood. Removal of the tubes may stimulate vomiting, and emesis is then observed for renewed bleeding. The nurse monitors vital signs frequently, as frequently as every 10–15 minutes during acute bleeding episodes.

Acute hemorrhage is frightening to both children and parents. Nurses therefore need to explain all procedures and provide emotional support to the child and family during emergency treatment. Parents of children with histories of hepatic damage or cirrhosis may need support when facing the child's imminent death. (Chapter 32 discusses the needs of the family of a terminally ill child.)

Liver Failure With Hepatic Coma

Hepatic coma, or hepatic encephalopathy, occurs when the liver can no longer convert ammonia to urea because of extensive hepatic damage. Ammonia begins collecting in the systemic circulation, and ammonia intoxication occurs.

High blood ammonia levels have an adverse effect on the brain and central nervous system, causing a wide array of changes in the level of consciousness and muscular coordination. These include confusion, disorientation, lethargy, restlessness, sudden behavior changes, stupor, and coma. The child may exhibit a lack of coordination, tremors of the extremities, asterixis (flapping of hands when stimulated), nystagmus, and changes in deep tendon reflexes (Davidson and Gabuzda, 1975). Hepatic coma is classified according to degree of severity. (Table 38-9 describes the stages of hepatic coma.) The level of hepatic coma may vary greatly during any 24-hour period. Those with insidious onset or extended duration seem to be associated with the highest mortality rates.

Although the combination of severe liver damage, cirrhosis, and portal hypertension appears to be the primary cause of hepatic coma, other factors may contribute to high blood ammonia levels. These include high-protein diets in conjunction with some degree of liver damage, conversion of ingested blood proteins to ammonia following gastric or esophageal bleeding, renal failure, and severe fluid and electrolyte imbalances.

Medical Treatment Hepatic coma is usually the end-stage of progressive liver disease or acute hepatic failure, and treatment is rarely more than symptomatic or palliative. Impending hepatic failure may be managed by low-protein diets and reduction of other sources of ammonia. Gastrointestinal or esophageal bleeding should be prevented, and intestinal tract antibiotics (neomycin, kanamycin) should be given to prevent production of ammonia if bleeding does occur. Lactulose (a nonmetabolizable disaccharide) reduces the intestinal pH, thereby trapping excess ammonia within the intestinal lumen. Acid-base balance should be monitored closely, and electrolyte balance should be maintained. A high degree of metabolic instability is common in hepatic coma.

Heroic measures such as total-body "wash-outs," exchange transfusions, or dialysis are only indicated in cases of acute, unexpected hepatic failure in which regeneration of parenchymal cells may still be possible. Children with chronically severe liver disease rarely profit from these measures, and any improvement is strictly temporary.

Nursing Management The goal of nursing care is detection of impending hepatic coma. Continued observation for changes in the level of consciousness or neuromuscular status is vitally important. Early recognition of impending hepatic coma may allow for initiation of treatment before permanent damage occurs. Parents are usually excellent judges of changes in their children's behavior and therefore should share their impressions. Asterixis may be assessed by requesting the child to extend both arms or legs without support so that the nurse notes any rapid flapping or jerking motions of the hands or feet. These tremors should be reported, and a serial record of neurologic signs should be maintained. In the older child, the nurse might also establish a record of serial samplings of the older child's handwriting to document neuromuscular degeneration.

Because of the marked metabolic instability, strict intake and output records are necessary. The nurse records emesis, urine, and stool volumes and performs serial measurements of urine specific gravity and morning and evening weight to provide a closer estimate of fluid status. Frequent blood studies include liver function tests and electrolyte, glucose, and hematocrit levels.

Dietary management includes low-protein, high-carbohydrate foods. Most children like foods that are high in carbohydrates, but progressive liver failure may contribute to severe anorexia. Intravenous fluids may become necessary, and a high concentration of intravenous glucose may be used to prevent protein breakdown.

Progressive hepatic coma is usually fatal, and the nurse therefore provides the family with the emotional support

TABLE 38-9 Four Stages of Hepatic Coma

Stage	Mental status	Tremor or asterixis
Prodromal stage	Confusion minimal or absent May be disorganized or may experience difficulty in concentrating	May be slight or absent
Precoma or impending coma	Confusion, disorientation Sleepy and inactive Inappropriate behaviors	Usually present or is easily elicited
Stupor	Extremely sleepy and lethargic Can be aroused Marked confusion and disorientation	Present but may be difficult to elicit because of uncooperativeness
Coma	Unconscious but may respond to noxious stimuli when in early coma; no response when in deep coma	Flaccid muscle tone, usually no tremor

necessary to deal with the child's impending death. The family may also be required to make decisions about continuing extraordinary treatment that offers little hope of success. If the family asks the nurse for advice, this is limited to an honest appraisal of the child's condition. The nurse also might help these parents by encouraging them to consider all alternatives in greater depth before arriving at a final decision, which in turn may help parents feel more comfortable with their decision to discontinue treatment. (Chapter 32 discusses the care of the terminally ill child and ways to provide emotional support to these families.)

The Child With a Problem Related to Elimination

Gastroenteritis

Gastroenteritis is a common problem during infancy and childhood and is characterized by varying degrees of diarrhea, vomiting and abdominal cramping. Mild gastroenteritis associated with colds or gastrointestinal viruses is easily managed at home. (Nursing management associated with home care is discussed in Chapter 26.)

Children who are more than 5%–8% dehydrated have moderate dehydration due to acute diarrhea and should be hospitalized for management of the dehydration. Children who are 12%–15% dehydrated may require intensive care, although this depends on age, cause of diarrhea, and type of dehydration (isonatremic, hyponatremic, hypernatremic). Causative agents of severe diarrhea in children are classified as bacterial, viral, and protozoal; these are listed in Table 38-10, together with their clinical features and medical treatments.

Medical Treatment Gastroenteritis caused by certain bacteria and parasites are amenable to drug therapy (see Table 38-10). A greater number of cases of acute childhood diarrhea, are viral and self-limiting, requiring treatment for dehydration and electrolyte imbalances.

Treatment for severe gastroenteritis is directed toward (a) restoration of body fluid volume (both intracellular fluid and extracellular fluid), (b) restoration of electrolyte balance, and (c) restoration of normal renal function. Fluid and electrolyte solutions are infused intravenously to replace losses. In cases of extreme intravascular depletion and circulatory collapse, protein solutions (for example, plasma or serum albumin) are administered as plasma volume expanders. (Nursing principles in the management of fluid and electrolyte imbalances are discussed in Chapter 33.)

Nursing Management Assessment findings for the child with gastroenteritis vary with the severity of the diarrhea and vomiting. The nurse observes and records the following signs and symptoms:

Change in sensorium. The child may appear tired, listless, lethargic, irritable, drowsy, or possibly confused.

Change in gastrointestinal functioning. The amount of loose watery stools varies with severity, and the characteristics of stools vary with infecting organism. Other changes are vomiting, possible abdominal cramping and abdominal tenderness on palpation, and tenesmus.

Fever.

Change in cardiovascular status. The child may have decreased blood pressure, tachycardia (due to dehydration and deficient intravascular volume), or signs of dehydration (poor tissue turgor, sunken eyeballs, dry tongue and mucous membranes).

Change in renal functioning. Oliguria is common as dehydration progresses. Acute renal failure may occur with anuria, hyperkalemia, azotemia, acidosis, anasarca, and cardiopulmonary overload.

Changes in laboratory values. The child may have metabolic acidosis, elevated hematocrit (due to volume loss), normal serum sodium levels (because the loss is usually isotonic), normal serum potassium levels, which may rise gradually as the glomerular filtration rate decreases, increased BUN as the glomerular filtration rate decreases, and leukocytosis.

Nursing goals are those principles of care related to severe dehydration or electrolyte imbalances. Continued assessment of vital signs, monitoring of laboratory reports, and accurate intake, output, stool, and emesis records are essential nursing interventions. Perineal skin care should be meticulous to prevent perineal excoriation due to enzyme- and acid-rich stools. Infection control measures for diarrhea are instituted according to the suspected causative agent. The nurse explains infection control procedures to families to prevent the spread of diarrhea among family members. Families of children with *Shigella* and amoeba infections will need to submit stool specimens so infected individuals can be treated in a subclinical carrier state.

Infants who remain NPO for long periods should be provided a pacifier if the parents are agreeable. This allows the infant self-comfort through sucking. Older children require frequent mouth care. Mouthwashes can aid in dislodging thick oral secretions, and petroleum jelly can be applied to the lips to prevent drying or cracking.

Severe Constipation

Mild constipation is a frequent, easily managed, problem in children. If constipation becomes severe, however, it can lead to intestinal obstruction or obstipation, which is characterized by abdominal cramping and distention and may

(text continued on p. 1354)

TABLE 38-10 Causative Agents of Diarrhea in Children

	Causative agent	Incubation period	Clinical symptomatology: Fever	Nausea and vomiting	Abdominal pain	H/A	Other	Site and mechanism of action	Stool characteristics: Color	Odor & consistency	Pus	Mucus	Blood	Medical treatment	Comments
Bacterial causes	*Shigella* *S. sonnei* *S. flexneri* *S. dysenteriae*	24–72 hours	Yes	Rare	Crampy	Yes	Seizures Rectal prolapse	Colon, sigmoid colon, rectum Produces an exotoxin that kills tissue and causes massive fluid loss	Yellow green or colorless	Watery	Yes	Yes	Yes	Usually self-limiting; stools clear in 7–10 days without antibiotics Antibiotics—ampicillin or chloramphenicol (Chloromycetin)—used only in cases of severe disability, or in high-risk children, or in infants or young children who are dehydrated	Seizures most common in young infants Toxicity more common in infants than in older children Bacteria may survive on linen for up to several weeks *Stool precautions necessary*
	Salmonella *S. paratyphi* *S. typhi*	8–72 hours	Occasionally low grade	Yes	Colicky	—	Septicemia Osteomylitis in children with sickle cell disease	Small bowel and cecum Causes local inflammation with high fluid, sodium, and chloride loss in stools	Green	Rotten egg odor Slimy Watery	No	Rare	Rare	Children are treated only if they are immune suppressed. Antibiotic therapy appears to prolong excretion of the organism in the stool; ampicillin is the drug of choice	Severe cases may lead to septicemia Debilitated children and children with certain chronic diseases may develop osteomyelitis, abscesses, or meningitis Often found in contaminated foods and water, especially eggs, poultry, milk, and shellfish; transmitted by animals
	Staphylococcus aureus	1–5 hours	Rare	Severe	Acute, crampy	—	Acute onset	Invasion of small bowel wall Produces an enterotoxin	Varies	Watery	No	Yes	Yes	Treatment is symptomatic; symptoms usually self-limiting within 24 hours	Severe dehydration may occur in infants; most often transmitted through contaminated foods
	Enteropathic *Escherichia coli*	24–72 hours	Rare	Vomiting in infant	Occasionally	—	More common in children under 2 years of age	Produces possible enterotoxin Causes loss of fluid and electrolytes	Green	Slimy Watery Foul odor	No	Yes	No	Treatment is symptomatic, but antibiotics often used in young children (neomycin, colistin, and ampicillin)	Transmitted through contaminated foods, or through contaminated fomites; most common in young infants

	Cholera (*Vibrio cholerae*)	6–60 hours	Occasionally low grade	Yes	Crampy Periumbilical	—	Rapid dehydration and circulatory collapse	Small intestine, particularly the jejunum Enterotoxin causes loss of fluid and electrolytes	Yellow or clear "rice water stool"	Fishy Profuse Watery	No	Yes	No	Immediate replacement of fluid and electrolytes Close monitoring of fluid and electrolyte status Oral tetracycline	Transmitted through contaminated food and water, shellfish Not transmitted person to person except in rare instances *Does not require strict isolation*
	Yersinia enterocolitica	7–10 days	Yes	Yes	Severe	Yes	Other family members might be carriers	Unknown; site of action thought to be small bowel	Green	Watery	No	Yes	No	Self-limiting but persists for 1–3 weeks: tetracycline or chloramphenicol (Chloromycetin) may be used	Transmission thought to be familial, and secondary to poor sanitation and hygiene, usually affects children under 3 years of age
Viral causes	Parvo-like virus Rotavirus Others	Varies	Yes	Occasionally	Occasionally	—	Child may have upper respiratory tract infection simultaneously	Small bowel?	Green	Watery	No	Rare	Rare	Treatment is symptomatic; child maintained NPO with fluid and electrolyte replacement	Often highly contagious, particularly in newborn nurseries, hospitals, and day-care centers; often occurs in conjunction with upper respiratory tract infection *Stool precautions necessary if the child is hospitalized*
Protozoal causes	Amoebae *Entamoeba histolytica*	Varies; may be present in nonsymptomatic carrier state	Rare	Varies greatly in children			Liver abscess Brain abscess	Deep invasion of the large bowel wall Can invade ileum, liver, lungs, brain	Varies	Varies	No	Clear mucus	Occasionally in infants	Antiprotozoals such as diiodohydroxyquin, paromomycin, metronidazole (Flagyl) Repeat stool examinations until clear	Transmitted person to person or through contaminated food and water Family members should be tested to allow for treatment of asymptomatic carriers
	Giardia lamblia	Varies	Varies greatly and may be asymptomatic				Intermittent diarrhea Malabsorption syndrome	Duodenum and jejunum	Varies	Varies but may be watery in infants		Varies greatly		Quinacrine, metronidazole (Flagyl)	Often transmitted through contaminated water supplies or foods Family members should be tested to allow for treatment of asymptomatic carriers

be accompanied by vomiting, anorexia, and passage of extremely liquid diarrhea. This last occurs only when the hardened feces are bypassed by liquid stool.

Severe constipation is usually a symptom of underlying disease. Several disorders that may involve severe constipation are intestinal obstruction, cystic fibrosis, malnutrition, pica, iron ingestion, chemotherapy (particularly vincristine therapy), chronic tube feedings, pyloric stenosis, anal stenosis, pelvic deformities or masses, spina bifida, paraplegia, and other neurologic disorders. These children may develop impaction, or blockage of the lower colon due to a hardened mass of fecal material.

Medical Treatment The primary focus of medical care is to determine the etiology of the problem. If an impaction is present, it may be removed during digital examination. Cathartics should not be used until the impaction has been removed. Chronic, severe constipation may be treated through regular use of stool softeners, mineral oil, bulk agents, dietary therapy, or saline enemas if necessary.

Nursing Management Most children with severe constipation have significant physical or neurologic disorders. Children with problems of mobility (for example, cerebral palsy, paraplegia, spina bifida) are particularly susceptible. Preventing impaction in these children requires standard bowel care, and the nurse therefore teaches parents to modify any regimen according to the needs of the child. Whenever possible, these children should be encouraged to attempt defecation each day at a set time in order to develop a regular elimination pattern.

Long-term management includes dietary management with high-fiber foods. Stool softeners, bulk agents, or mineral oils are usually effective if given regularly; supplemental cathartics, suppositories, or enemas also may be required.

Intrusive procedures, such as enemas or disimpactions, are carried out as safely as possible to prevent perforation of the rectal wall. The lubricated enema tube should be flexible and should be inserted to a depth proportional to the size of the child. Disimpaction should be accomplished with the smallest gloved finger possible, and long nails should be clipped before attempting to dislodge an impaction. This prevents rupture of the glove and limits possible trauma to the bowel wall. The nurse teaches parents of children who are prone to impactions to perform digital examinations for impaction before giving cathartics or enemas.

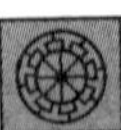

NURSING CARE PLAN The Child With Cleft Lip and Cleft Palate

Assessment Data

Michael is a 2-month-old with a left-sided cleft lip and palate. He was the product of an uneventful first pregnancy and weighed 7 lb 12 oz at birth. His parents were initially very upset that Michael was born with a defect. They received in-depth teaching and nursing support during his admission period and were able to speak to the pediatric plastic surgeon about repair options. They decided to wait until Michael weighed at least 10 lb. Their primary nurse encouraged them to feed Michael while she was there to offer support and suggestions, and they were able to decide on a feeding technique that was comfortable and provided adequate intake. Michael's mother chose to express breast milk for feedings and has not needed to offer formula supplementation. Michael now weighs well over 10 lb and has been admitted to the pediatric floor following his initial Z-plasty closure of his cleft lip. Repair of the cleft palate will be undertaken when he reaches 18–24 months of age.

On admission to the floor, the nurse notes that Steri strips are intact over the surgical site; there is an intravenous line in his foot; and elbow restraints are in place. He is crying and flailing his arms. His parents state that they are very pleased with the repair but are somewhat hesitant to handle him so soon after surgery.

Nursing Diagnoses and Goals

1. **Nursing diagnosis:** Potential for injury related to disruption of surgical site.

   Long-term goal: Surgical site will heal without disruption and with minimal scarring.

   Short-term goal: Suture line will remain uninfected and intact until healed.

2. **Nursing diagnosis:** Potential respiratory distress related to surgery.

   Long-term goal: Michael will experience no respiratory distress.

   Short-term goal: Nares will remain clear with no aspiration of fluids during feedings.

3. **Nursing diagnosis:** Potential for fluid or nutritional deficit.

   Long-term goal: Michael will return to normal diet for age before discharge.

   Short-term goal: Michael will make successful transition from "NPO with IV" to adequate clear liquid intake within 12 hours of surgery.

4. **Nursing diagnosis:** Alteration in comfort: pain and discomfort.

   Long-term goal: Michael's pain and discomfort will be relieved or minimized.

   Short-term goals: (a) Michael will receive oral pain medication prn. (b) Michael's parents or caretaker will respond to his crying with appropriate comfort measures.

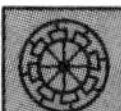

NURSING CARE PLAN The Child With Cleft Lip and Cleft Palate (continued)

5. Nursing diagnosis: Impaired mobility related to restraints.

Long-term goal: Michael will resume normal activities for age.

Short-term goal: Michael's arms will be exercised at least once every 4 hours.

6. Nursing diagnosis: Parental anxiety related to Michael's current condition.

Long-term goal: Parents will feel comfortable in caring for Michael at home.

Short-term goals: (a) Parental anxiety related to Michael's postoperative care will be diminished. (b) Parents will assume much of Michael's postoperative care.

7. Nursing diagnosis: Need for parental education and support regarding Michael's future care.

Long-term goal: Parents will state that they have sufficient information and guidance to enable them to continue caring for Michael.

Short-term goal: Parents will repeat instructions related to Michael's need for future care.

Interventions	Rationale	Evaluation criteria
1. Maintain Steri strips dressing to keep lip intact (Logan bow may be used)	Strips or Logan bow prevent lateral separation of suture line	At discharge, did Michael's surgical site appear to be healing well with no signs of infection?
Maintain elbow restraints in place unless Michael is being directly supervised	Elbow restraints prevent child from picking at surgical site yet leaves hands free	
Position Michael on back or side only (with palate repair *only*, child may be placed on abdomen)	Positioning prevents child from rubbing surgical site on bed linen	
Perform lip and nostril care frequently. Use cotton-tipped swab and hydrogen peroxide diluted with normal saline (or water as ordered)	Care for suture line, initially every ½–1 hour limits crusting, limits inflammation, and allows closer observation of site for infection	
Allow no bottle or pacifier. Use nontraumatic feeding techniques (Asepto or bulb syringe, syringe with rubber tubing, soft-edged cup, etc.)	Sucking on nipple places undue pressure on site. Limiting trauma to site speeds healing and prevents scarring	
2. Clean nares gently with swabs and saline. Use suction equipment if acute respiratory obstruction occurs	Patent airway ensures adequate respiration. Limiting suctioning limits trauma to site	Did Michael exhibit any signs or symptoms of respiratory distress?
Feed Michael slowly with frequent rests. Burp well; position on right side after meals	Small frequent feedings allow child adequate time to swallow completely, limit regurgitation, and prevent aspiration. Positioning aids gastric emptying and prevents aspiration	
3. Progress slowly from NPO status to adequate oral fluid intake	Fluid intake ensures adequate hydration status during postoperative period. Slow progression limits vomiting.	Were Michael's fluid and calorie needs met? Did Michael's weight remain stable? Was Michael able to tolerate a normal diet?
Progress from clear to full liquids until Michael is taking normal diet (breast milk)	Clear liquids are more easily tolerated in initial postoperative period. Breast milk provides balanced diet with sufficient calories and fluid	
4. Observe Michael frequently for pain and discomfort. Offer comfort measures (holding, rocking, music, talking, position changes, toys). Medicate prn	Limiting discomfort decreases anxiety and prevents trauma to site due to crying	Were Michael's comfort needs met in timely fashion? Was he able to sleep undisturbed?

continued on next page

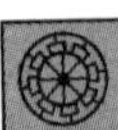

NURSING CARE PLAN The Child With Cleft Lip and Cleft Palate (continued)

Interventions	Rationale	Evaluation criteria
5. Remove restraints when Michael is directly supervised. Remove restraints and give skin care every 4 hours. Change positions frequently	Frequent position changes and release of restraints prevents harmful effects of limited mobility	Is Michael's skin intact under elbow restraints? Do his parents understand and practice adequate restraint care?
Encourage parents to hold Michael frequently. Use this time to instruct parents in restraint care at home	Demonstration of appropriate restraint care allows parents to practice this skill before discharge	
6. Explain and demonstrate all facets of Michael's care to parents	Adequate education, preparation, and support allow parents to reassume caregiving tasks with minimal anxiety	Did Michael's parents provide caregiving activities? Are Michael's parents capable of providing adequate home care (feeding, suture line care, restraint care)?
Encourage parents to assume many caregiving tasks while nurse is available for guidance and support. Begin home care instructions on return from surgery		
Allow Michael's parents to discuss their feelings related to Michael's surgery and condition	After initial surgery is over, parents begin to look forward to future surgery and care	
7. Allow Michael's parents to discuss their concerns regarding need for continued follow-up, further surgery, and rehabilitative therapy	Correction of cleft lip and cleft palate is long-term and requires considerable follow-up care. Parents who are able to discuss and plan for follow-up can understand that correction is possible but will take coordinated effort over extended period of time	Have parents discussed plans for follow-up care? Do parents speak of long-range care (e.g., palate repair, speech therapy, orthodontia)? Are parents aware of appropriate support groups in their area?
Include parents in planning follow-up therapy for Michael		
Encourage parents to seek support from outside groups	Contact with support group or other parents of children with cleft lip and cleft palate helps parents understand long-term nature of care and helps them cope	

Key Concepts

- During embryonic development, the foregut, midgut, and hindgut differentiate and develop into specific anatomic structures of the gastrointestinal tract.
- The gastrointestinal system functions to ingest, digest, and absorb nutrients; digestion of food begins in the mouth and progresses through the esophagus to the stomach and intestines, where enzymes break down food substances for absorption.
- Assessment of the child with a suspected gastrointestinal disorder includes a complete history and physical assessment, together with relevant data about dietary history, gastrointestinal symptoms, and eating and bowel habits.
- Diagnostic tests for gastrointestinal disorders may require enemas, medications, or dietary modifications in preparation for the diagnostic test; each of these procedures needs to be adapted to the age of the child and the developmental needs of both child and family.
- Gastric decompression for children requires choosing a tube of correct size, monitoring function and placement of the tube, observing drainage, and monitoring fluid and electrolyte status.

- Ostomy care involves extensive preoperative teaching for both child and family, which in turn involves selection of a stoma site and discussions about ostomy appliances and adaptations in daily living that allow normal functioning.
- Acute care needs for children with gastrointestinal disorders may specifically require precise intake and output records, accurate delivery of prescribed fluids, and frequent and consistent weight measurements.
- Children undergoing abdominal surgery require extensive preoperative teaching and postoperative attention to hydration status and comfort.
- Infection control may require enteric precautions or wound and skin precautions, which involve attention to hand washing; masks, gowns, and gloves; and handling of instruments, linens, and other articles.
- Complications of gastrointestinal disorders may be related to either the disease or the treatment; children therefore need careful observation to prevent complications.
- Nutritional needs for children with gastrointestinal disorders involve assessment of caloric intake, which may be provided through gavage or gastrostomy feedings, vitamin and mineral supplementation, or total parenteral nutrition through hyperalimentation.
- Total parenteral nutrition may consist of glucose, proteins, and lipids; complications of hyperalimentation are usually related to the concentration of the fluid, to fat or air emboli, or to infection caused by contamination of the apparatus.
- If a child and family are deemed candidates for home hyperalimentation, extensive discharge preparation is needed to teach appropriate family members about the concepts, principles, and complications associated with the procedure.
- Developmental needs for children with gastrointestinal disorders may be related to malnutrition, lack of oral gratification, or impaired mobility.
- Health maintenance for the child with a gastrointestinal disorder may involve ongoing medication, dietary modification, activity restrictions, and bowel-training regimens.
- Nursing care for the child with cleft lip or cleft palate involves adaptations in feeding to provide adequate nutrition and preoperative and postoperative care, which may include planning for further corrective surgery.
- For infants with esophageal atresia or tracheoesophageal fistula, the goals of nursing care include early detection and prevention of aspiration and adaptations in feeding methods that allow infants to practice feeding and to interact normally with parents.
- Nursing goals for the infant with a diaphragmatic hernia include early detection, prevention of respiratory complications, nutritional support, and parental education.
- For the infant with gastroschisis or omphalocele, nursing care involves prevention of circulatory compromise, intestinal obstruction, and septicemia; prevention of infection and heat loss; and nutritional support.
- For the infant with an intestinal atresia, nursing care includes nutritional support, monitoring for fluid and electrolyte imbalance, and assessment of postoperative gastrointestinal function.
- Nursing care for the infant with meconium ileus depends on the underlying cause and method of treatment but generally includes nasogastric suctioning, monitoring of vital signs, and recording of intake and output.
- For the infant with an anorectal malformation, nursing goals include early detection, nutritional support, general postoperative care measures, and parental education.
- For the child with Hirschsprung's disease, nursing care involves preoperative assessment and bowel preparation, dietary modifications, and postoperative ostomy care.
- Nursing care for the child with pyloric stenosis involves early detection of signs and symptoms, assessment and management of fluid and electrolyte imbalances, monitoring of nutritional status, and parental support.
- For the child with intussusception, nursing care includes assessment of signs and symptoms of intestinal obstruction, parental education, and preoperative preparation as necessary.
- Nursing care for the child with congenital inguinal hernia or hydrocele includes prevention of

postoperative infection and bowel obstruction and assessment and management of fluid status.

- Failure to thrive is characterized by extreme thinness, failure to gain weight, loss of subcutaneous fat, and muscle wasting; organic failure to thrive may be caused by a variety of gastrointestinal, metabolic, cardiovascular, and neurologic disorders.
- Inborn errors of metabolism are mutations within the genetic codes of a cell that in turn lead to errors in body metabolism and inadequate use of nutrients.
- Nursing goals for the infant with gastroesophageal reflux are prevention of frequent reflux, maintenance of adequate nutrition, and adequate infant stimulation through parental contact.
- For the child with cystic fibrosis, nursing goals include education for both the child and the family, support for health maintenance with a chronic condition, and planning and teaching for dietary modifications.
- Nursing care for the child with celiac disease involves planning for long-term dietary modifications, nutrition education, and anticipatory guidance related to complications of infection, side effects of specific drugs, and problems with compliance.
- For children with lactose intolerance, nursing care includes monitoring pH of stools, perineal skin care, and education of both child and parent concerning the child's dietary needs.
- Nursing care for the child with short-bowel syndrome involves monitoring signs and symptoms of infection, skin breakdown, and neurologic changes; nutritional support; assessment of stool changes and fluid status; and family support.
- Nursing goals for the child with phenylketonuria include education for long-term dietary management and anticipatory guidance related to problems with compliance in older children.
- For the infant with necrotizing enterocolitis, nursing goals include early detection, monitoring of fluid and electrolyte status and vital signs, observation for signs of complications, and emotional support for family members.
- Nursing care for the child with appendicitis includes monitoring of signs and symptoms to confirm the diagnosis, preoperative preparation, and postoperative wound and skin precautions.
- Nursing care for the child with ulcerative colitis involves teaching about dietary therapy, use of medications, reduction of stress, and management of a chronic condition.
- For the child with Crohn's disease, nursing goals include teaching about medications and dietary management and care of secondary symptoms.
- For the child with a peptic ulcer, nursing goals are directed toward teaching about dietary and drug therapies and stress reduction.
- For the child with biliary atresia or choledochal cysts nursing care is directed toward monitoring signs and symptoms and providing emotional support; if the condition is corrected surgically, the child also requires preoperative and postoperative care.
- Nursing care for the child with hepatitis is directed toward teaching about dietary needs, activity limitations, infection control, and signs and symptoms of severely impaired liver function.
- For the child with cirrhosis, nursing goals include management of symptoms, observation for signs of severe bleeding, and emotional support related to a chronic and potentially fatal condition.
- Nursing care for the child with portal hypertension and esophageal varices involves dietary planning, controlling and monitoring bleeding, monitoring fluid status and vital signs, and providing emotional support.
- For the child with impending hepatic coma, nursing goals include early detection, assessment of signs and symptoms, dietary management, and emotional support related to a progressively fatal disease.
- Nursing care for the child with acute diarrhea includes assessment of fluid and electrolyte status, perineal skin care, infection control measures, and mouth care if the child is severely dehydrated.
- For the child with severe constipation, nursing care is directed toward maintaining a regular elimination pattern, dietary management, and preventing impaction, especially in children with impaired mobility.

References

Anderson KD: Symposium on Neonatal Surgery: Biliary Atresia. *Clinics in Perinatology* (March)1978; 5(1):19–27.

Balistreri W, Farrell M: Gastroesophageal reflux in infants. *New Engl J Med* (Sept) 1983; 309:790–792.

Beyers M, Dudas S: *The Clinical Practice of Medical-Surgical Nursing.* Little, Brown, 1984.

Brown EG, Sweet AY: Preventing necrotizing enterocolitis in neonates. *JAMA* (Nov) 1978; 240(22):2452–2454.

Davidson CS, Gabuzda GJ: Hepatic coma. In: *Diseases of the Liver.* Schiff L (editor). Lippincott, 1975.

Fonkalsrud EW et al: Surgical management of Crohn's disease in children. *Am J Surg* (July) 1979; 138(7):15–20.

Hrabovsky EE et al: Advances in the management of gastroschisis. *Ann Sur* (Aug) 1980; 192(2):244–248.

Hug G: Defects in metabolism of carbohydrates. Pages 520–547 in Vaughan VC, McKay RJ, Behrman RE (editors). *Nelson's Textbook of Pediatrics.* Saunders, 1979.

Jewett TC, Lebenthal E: Recent advances in gastrointestinal tract surgery in children: The pathophysiology of the short bowel syndrome. *Curr Prob Pediatr* (Dec) 1978; 9(2):11–14.

Kasai M et al: Technique and results of operative management of biliary atresia. *World J Surg* (Sep) 1978; 2(5):571–578.

Mayer T et al: Gastroschisis and omphalocele: An eight-year review. *Ann Surg* (Dec) 1980; 192(6):783–787.

Morin CL et al: Continuous elemental enteral alimentation in children with Crohn's disease and growth failure. *Gastroenter* (Dec) 1980; 79(6):1205–1210.

Odièure M: Long-term results of surgical treatment of biliary atresia. *World J Surgery* (Sept) 1978; 2(5):589–594.

Orenstein S et al: The infant seat as treatment of gastroesophageal reflux. *N Engl J Med* (Sept) 1983; 309:760–763.

Price SA, McCarty Wilson L: *Pathophysiology: Clinical Concepts of Disease Process.* 2nd edition. McGraw-Hill, 1982.

Rudolph AM (editor): *Pediatrics.* Appleton-Century Crofts, 1982.

Additional Readings

Barkin RM, Lilly JR: Biliary atresia and the Kasai operation: Continuing care. *J Pediatr* (June) 1980; 96(6):1015–1019.

Bishop WS, Head JJ: Care of the infant with a stoma. *MCN* (Sept/Oct) 1976; 1(5):315–319.

Bjeletich J, Hickman RO: The Hickman indwelling catheter, *Am J Nurs* (Jan) 1980; 80(1):62–65.

Boyd CW: Postural therapy at home for infants with gastroesophageal reflux. *Pediatr Nurs* (Nov/Dec) 1982; 82(6):395–398.

Brueggemeyer A: Omphalocele: Coping with a surgical emergency. *Pediatr Nurs* (July/Aug) 1979; 5(4):54–56.

Burkle WS: What you should know about Tagamet: New drug therapy for peptic ulcers. *Nurs 80* (Apr) 1980; 10(4):86–87.

Campbell DL: Congenital abdominal wall defects: Gastroschisis and omphalocele. *Neonatal Network* (Aug) 1982; 18–23.

Chattriwalla Y et al: The use of cimetidine in the newborn. *Pediatr* (Feb) 1980; 62(2):301–302.

Christopherson ER, Berman R: Encopresis treatment. *Issues in Comprehensive Pediatr Nurs* (Oct) 1978; 3(4):51–55.

Colley R, Wilson J: How to begin hyperalimentation therapy. *Nursing 79* (May) 1979; 9(5):76–83.

Colley R, Wilson J: Managing the patient on hyperalimentation. *Nursing 79* (June) 1979; 9(6):57–61.

Colley R, Wilson J: Providing hyperalimentation for infants and children. *Nursing 79* (July) 1979; 9(7):50–53.

Corcoran MM: Nursing role and management of failure-to-thrive clients. *Issues in Comprehensive Pediatr Nurs* (Oct) 1978; 3(4):29–40.

Cupoli JM et al: Failure-to-thrive. *Current Problems in Pediatr* (Sept) 1980; 10(11):1–16.

Dickinson RJ et al: Controlled trial of intravenous hyperalimentation and total bowel rest as an adjunct to the routine therapy of acute colitis. *Gastroenterol* (Dec) 1980; 79(6):1199–1204.

Gatch G: Gastroschisis and omphalocele. *Today's OR Nurse* (Jan) 1980; 1(1):9–15.

Goldberg JH et al: A home program of long-term total parenteral nutrition in children. *J Pediatr* (Feb) 1979; 94(2):325–328.

Hazle N: An infant who survived gastroschisis. *MCN* (Jan/Feb) 1981; 6(1):35–40.

Jewett TC, Lebenthal E: The improved outlook in biliary atresia. *Current Problems Pediatr* (Dec) 1978; 9(2):45–50.

Kadner IJ: Inflammatory bowel disease. *Clinical Symposia* 1982; 34(1): 3–32.

Kadowaki H et al: Full-thickness punch biopsy for the diagnosis of Hirschsprung's disease. *J Pediatr Surg* (Apr) 1979; 14(2):162–164.

Kneut C: Acute stress ulcers in childhood. *Issues in Comprehensive Pediatr Nurs* (Oct) 1978; 3(4):41–50.

Kroner K: Are you prepared for your ulcerative colitis patient? *Nursing 80* (Apr) 1980; 10(4):43–45.

Kurfiss-Daniels D: Positioning as treatment for infant gastroesophageal reflux. *Am J Nurs* (Oct) 1982; 82(10):1535–1537.

Lander JD: Nursing care of children with fluid and electrolyte disorders. *Issues in Comprehensive Pediatr Nursing* (Apr) 1980; 4(2): 41–52.

Lee E et al: Proctocolectomy for ulcerative colitis. *World J Surg* (March) 1980; 4(2):195–201.

Ling L, McCamman SP: Dietary treatment of diarrhea and constipation in infants and children. *Issues in Comprehensive Pediatr Nursing* (Oct) 1978; 3(4):17–28.

Mabel DE et al: Practical problems in pediatric TPN—total parenteral nutrition. *Am J Intravenous Therapy* (Oct/Nov) 1978; 5:13–17.

McConnell EA: Ten problems with NG tubes . . . and how to solve them. *Nursing 79* (Apr) 1979; 9(4):78–81.

McGrath BJ: Fluids, electrolytes and replacement therapy in pediatric nursing. *MCN* (Jan/Feb) 1980; 5(1):58–62.

Mahoney JM: *Guide to Ostomy Nursing Care.* Little, Brown, 1976.

Mowat AP: Viral hepatitis in infancy and childhood. *Clinical Gastroenterology* (Jan) 1980; 9(1):191–212.

Page-Goertz S, Stewart DR: Is the baby just spitting? Consideration of the gastrointestinal reflux. *Issues in Comprehensive Pediatr Nurs*; (Apr) 1980; 4(2):53–66.

Parfitt DM, Thompson VD: Pediatric home hyperalimentation—educating the family. *MCN* (May/June) 1980; 5(3):196–202.

Perry SE et al: Gastrostomy and the neonate *Am J Nurs* (July) 1983; 83(7): 1030–1033.

Plapp PR: Nursing implications in the early recognition of necrotizing enterocolitis. *Issues in Comprehensive Pediatr Nurs* (Apr) 1980; 4(2): 77–81.

Raffensperger JG, Luck SR: Gastrointestinal bleeding in children. *Surg Clin N Am* (April) 1976; 56(2):373–377.

Salinas CF et al: Familial occurrence of gastroschisis. *Am J Diseases of Children* (May) 1979; 133:514–517.

Sanchez CL: Nursing care of the infant and child with cleft lip and palate. *Point of View* (Jan) 1980; 17(1):14–15.

Schaeffer CE: *Childhood Encopresis and Enuresis: Causes and Therapy.* Van Nostrand Reinhold, 1979.

Seashore JH: Congenital abdominal wall defects. *Clinics in Perinatology* (March) 1978; 5(1):61–78.

Shaw LM: A teaching plan for Nissen fundoplication . . . information your patient needs to know. *AORN Journal* (July) 1981; 34(7):47–55.

Spenner D: When the baby is sick and the mother's concerns are ignored—pyloric stenosis. *Am J Nurs* (Dec) 1980; 80(12):2222–2224.

Strauch B et al: Caring enough to give your patient control—Crohn's disease: Chronic, recurrent, and unpredictable. *Nursing 80* (Aug) 1980; 10(8):54–59.

Strobel CT et al: Home parenteral nutrition in children with Crohn's disease: An effective management alternative. *Gastroenterology* (Aug) 1979; 77(2):272–279.

Tanner MS, Stocks RJ: *Neonatal Gastroenterology: Contemporary Issues.* Intercept, 1984.

Vukovich VC, Grubb RD: *Care of the Ostomy Patient.* Mosby, 1977.

Walker RM: Surgery for the child ostomate. *J Enterostomal Therapy* (Jul/Aug) 1982; 9(4):18–20.

Walker-Smith J: Massive resection of the small intestine. In *Diseases of the Small Intestine.* John Wiley, 1975.

Weil WB, Bailie MD: *Fluid and Electrolyte Metabolism in Infants and Children: A Unified Approach.* Grune and Stratton, 1977.

Williams R: Congenital diaphragmatic hernia. *Heart and Lung* (Nov/Dec) 1982; 11(6):532–540.

Genitourinary Transport
Implications of Inflammation, Obstruction, and Structural Abnormalities

39

Carole C. Arenge Karen Mitchell Susan Rowen James

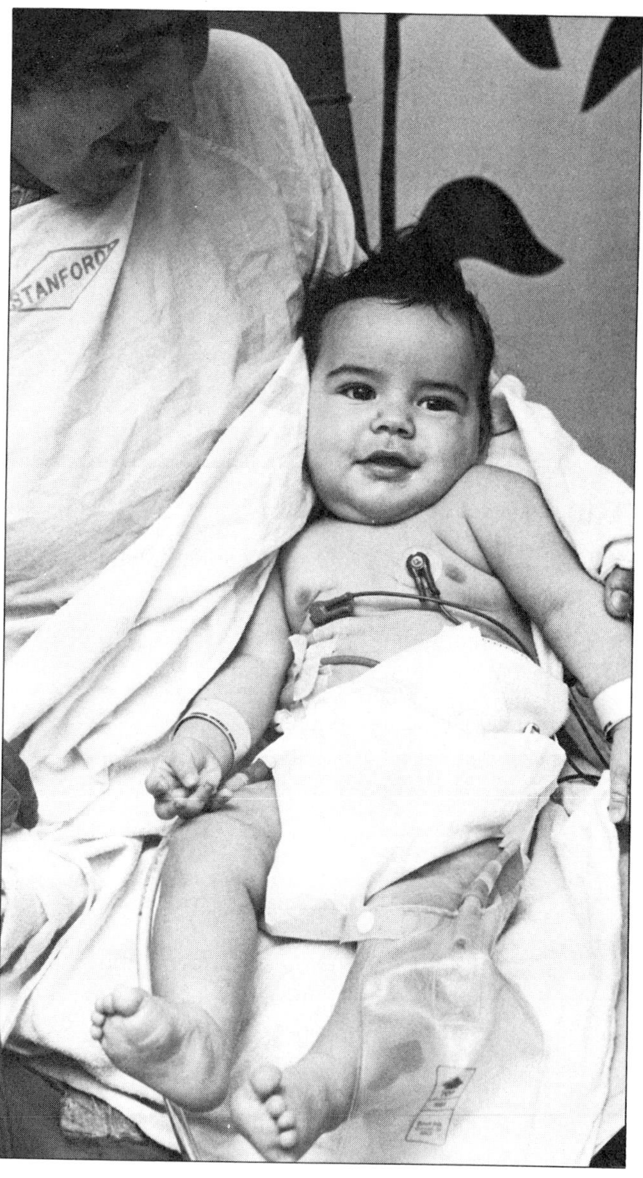

Chapter Outline

continued on next page

Objectives

- Describe the anatomy and physiology of the genitourinary system.
- List the criteria used in the assessment of a child with a genitourinary dysfunction.
- Describe principles of nursing interventions applicable to the child with a genitourinary condition.
- Explain the major treatment modalities used for the child with problems related to filtration of end products.
- Delineate nursing interventions to promote self-care in a child with a long-term genitourinary dysfunction.
- Summarize the principles of preoperative and postoperative nursing care of the child undergoing genitourinary surgery.

The state of the genitourinary system contributes to the general good health and homeostasis of the child. Organs of the system interact and impact upon other body systems to promote the constant composition and volume of body fluids through fluid regulation and elimination of wastes. Additionally, the system affects hormonal regulation, circulation, and reproductive function. Early diagnosis of pathology and appropriate interventions are critical for the optimal health of the child. Complex genitourinary dysfunction may lead to a state of chronic illness having serious effects on the child's growth and development.

Other concerns related to the system include adjustments to alterations in body image, fears of mutilation, and sexual/reproductive issues. Care of the child with a genitourinary problem is complicated by cultural factors related to privacy as well as confusion resulting from the wide variety of terms used to describe the organs and functions involved. Embarrassment and difficulty verbalizing concerns are typical problems encountered with children and families affected by disorders of the system.

Anatomy and Physiology of the Genitourinary System

Gross Anatomy of the Genitourinary System

The genitourinary system includes the body's vital filtration units (kidneys) and a comparatively simple collection system of ureters and bladder that transport waste products from the body. The kidneys are paired, bean-shaped structures lying in a retroperitoneal position just above the waist. The position of the right kidney is slightly lower than the left because of the position of the liver. The size of the normal kidney varies with the age and size of the child. Children's kidneys are larger in relation to body size than adults' and thus are more susceptible to injury from trauma (Kearney and Finn, 1981). Adrenal glands, located at the top of each kidney, affect endocrine system function by producing hormones that affect fluid and electrolyte regulation.

Ureters exit the kidney from a position just below the renal hilus. Ureters are long tubelike structures, consisting of three functional layers, which convey urine from kidneys to the bladder by peristaltic movement. At their bladder entrance points, their distal orifices are covered by the membranous bladder lining. This, along with muscular closure of these openings, assists in preventing urine reflux during micturation (Fig. 39-1).

The bladder is a muscular structure that collects urine for excretion via the ureters. An infant has a capacity of 15–20 mL, while an adult capacity reaches 600–800 mL of urine. Approximately 300 mL in the adult will cause the sensory nerves to stimulate bladder contraction, effecting micturation by concurrent relaxation of the urethral sphincter. Obviously, a much smaller volume will stimulate the stretch receptors in an infant or young child. The male and female urethra, the tubelike structure that conveys urine from the bladder, differ in length, with the adult female urethra 4 cm long and the male's five times that length. The female urethra exits the body at the urinary meatus, which lies between the clitoris and the vagina (Fig. 14-20). There is a close link between the male urethra and the reproductive system in that the urethra is a vehicle for both urine and semen (Fig. 14-21). The terminal meatus is located at the tip of the penis. During sexual stimulation, engorgement of blood and muscular contraction result in a closure of the connection to the bladder and allow for the movement of stored sperm in preparation for ejaculation.

Embryonic Development of the Reproductive System

Each embryo contains equipment for the development of either male or female characteristics. The genetic sex type eventually influences the development of organs of a particular sex and regression of organs of the opposite one.

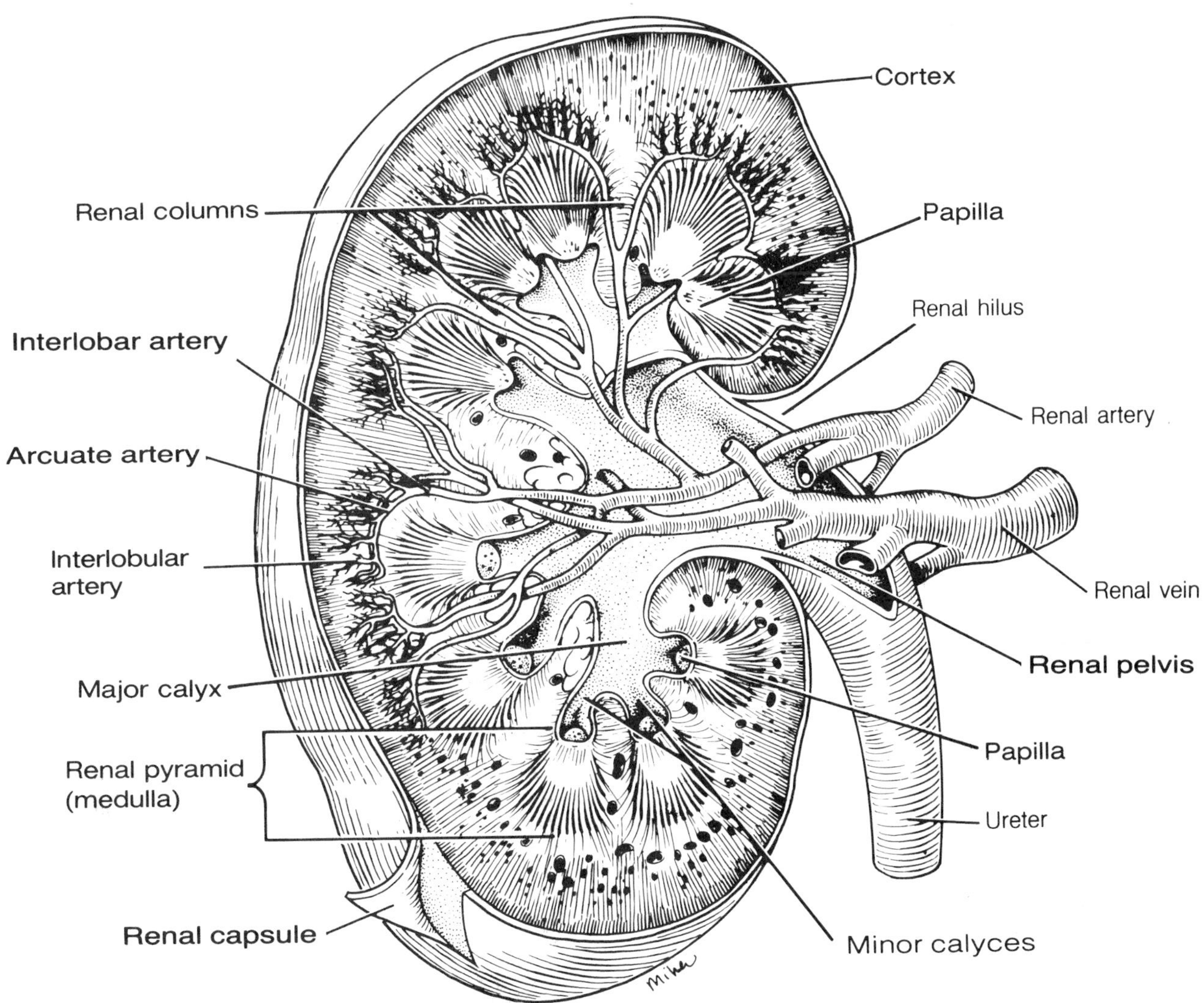

Figure 39-1 Longitudinal section of the kidney. (From Spence AP, Mason EB: *Human Anatomy and Physiology*, 2nd ed. Benjamin/Cummings, 1983, p. 685.)

The internal sex organs begin to differentiate at the end of the second month of fetal development. The testes develop earlier than ovaries and seem to control the development of external genitalia by producing a hormone that results in the appearance of male genitals. Absence of this hormone results in female external organs. Portions of the internal organs develop from duct systems. Wolffian ducts become the male genital duct; Mullerian ducts become the

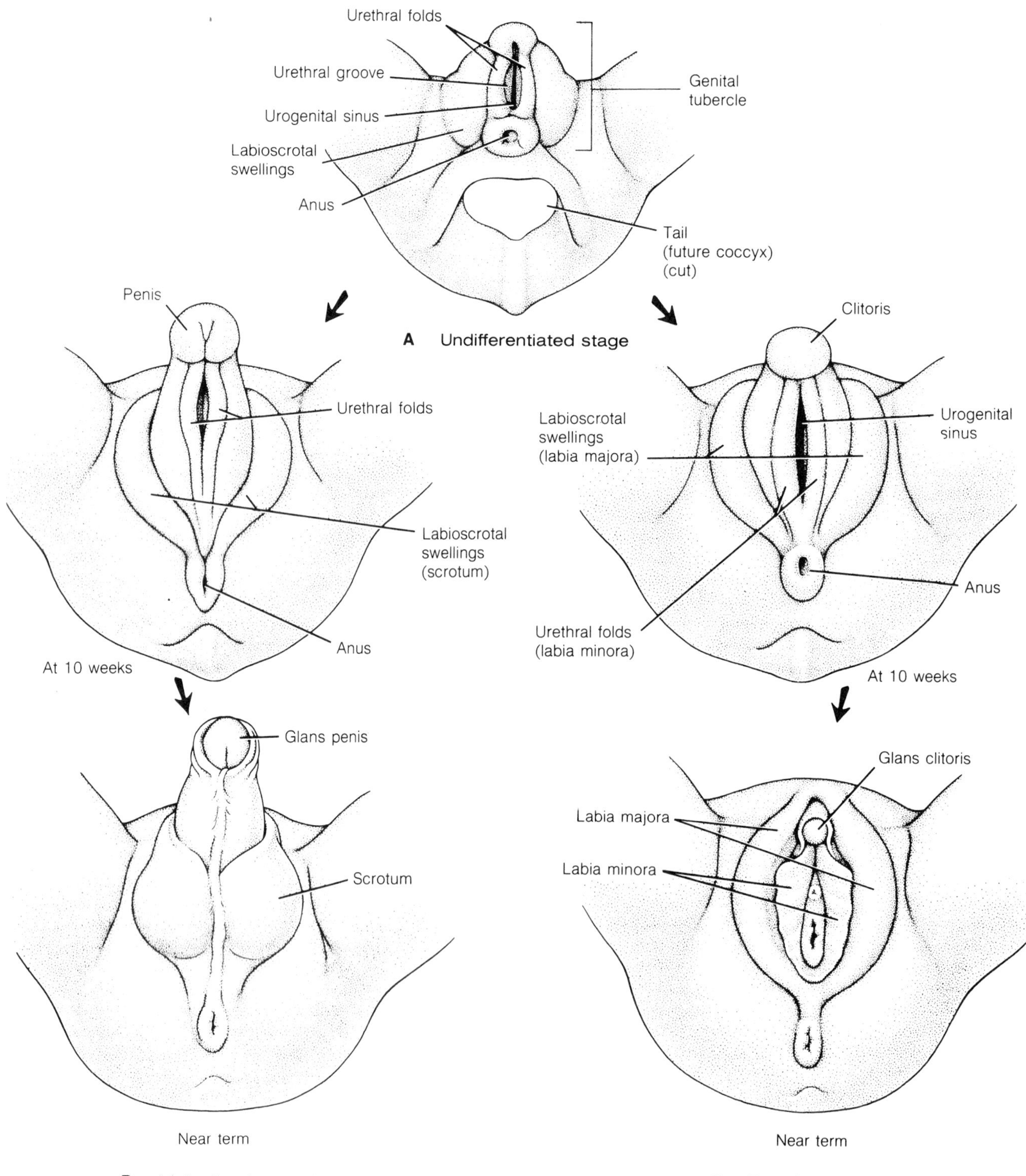

Figure 39-2 Embryonic development of male and female external reproductive structures. (From Spence AP, Mason EB: *Human Anatomy and Physiology*, 2nd ed. Benjamin/Cummings, 1983, p. 730.)

fallopian tubes; and the urogenital duct becomes the vagina and uterus (Allan, 1969).

By the seventh week of development external differentiation begins. Primitive structures become the genital tubercle, urogenital fold, urogenital groove, and genital swellings (Fig. 39-2A). In a male child, enlargement of all parts and the process of fusion complete the development. The tubercle enlarges to form the penis. Urogenital folds fuse and with the urogenital groove create the urethra. Finally, the genital swellings increase in size and fuse at the midline to become the scrotal sacs. The testes descend into these sacs by birth (Fig. 39-2B) (Allan, 1969).

Development of female genitalia is a longer process. Instead of enlarging, the tubercle shrinks to become the clitoris. The urogenital folds do not fuse and result in the labia minora. The groove forms the vestibule between the urethral meatus and vagina. Genital swellings fuse only below the vestibule to comprise the labia majora (Fig. 39-2C) (Allan, 1969).

The end result of embryonic development is a separate urinary and reproductive system for the female. Internal organs of the female reproductive system include the cervix, uterus, fallopian tubes, and ovaries (Fig. 39-3).

Physiology of the Renal System

Kidneys regulate and maintain the volume and composition of body fluids and excrete soluble wastes. They achieve homeostasis by acting on plasma through the mechanisms of glomerular filtration, tubular reabsorption, and tubular secretion. These mechanisms occur in the nephron—the functional unit of the kidney (Fig. 39-4). Sections of the nephron include Bowman's capsule, proximal and distal tubules, loop of Henle, glomerulus, and associated capillaries and venules. Nephrons are located primarily in the renal cortex (see Fig. 39-1), although juxtamedullary nephrons extend into the medulla. Microscopic drops of urine enter the collecting tubule and are transported into the renal pyramids (medulla). Urine drips through pores located in the pyramid apex (papillae) into the minor calyx. Subsequently, it collects in the major calyx and renal pelvis. The renal pelvis becomes the proximal end of the ureter.

Blood enters the kidney through the renal artery located at the renal hilus. The artery divides to become interlobar arteries that pass through the renal columns. These columns are extensions of cortical substance. Further division into arcuate arteries and capillaries results in direct contact of the circulation with the tubular system.

Unlike other body structures, where capillaries become venules, the kidney contains two sets of capillaries. Afferent arteries form capillaries that become the glomerulus. These then coalesce to become efferent arteries leading from the glomerulus to a capillary network surrounding the tubule. The tubular capillaries then become venules, arcuate veins, interlobar veins, and renal veins exiting from the kidney. Each of the capillary networks has a specific function for fluid regulation and maintenance of appropriate blood pressure for the proper functioning of the nephron.

Fluid, electrolyte, and acid–base balance depend on consistent high-quality performance of unimpaired kidneys. Beyond this, kidneys also help maintain the body's hormone balance and blood pressure.

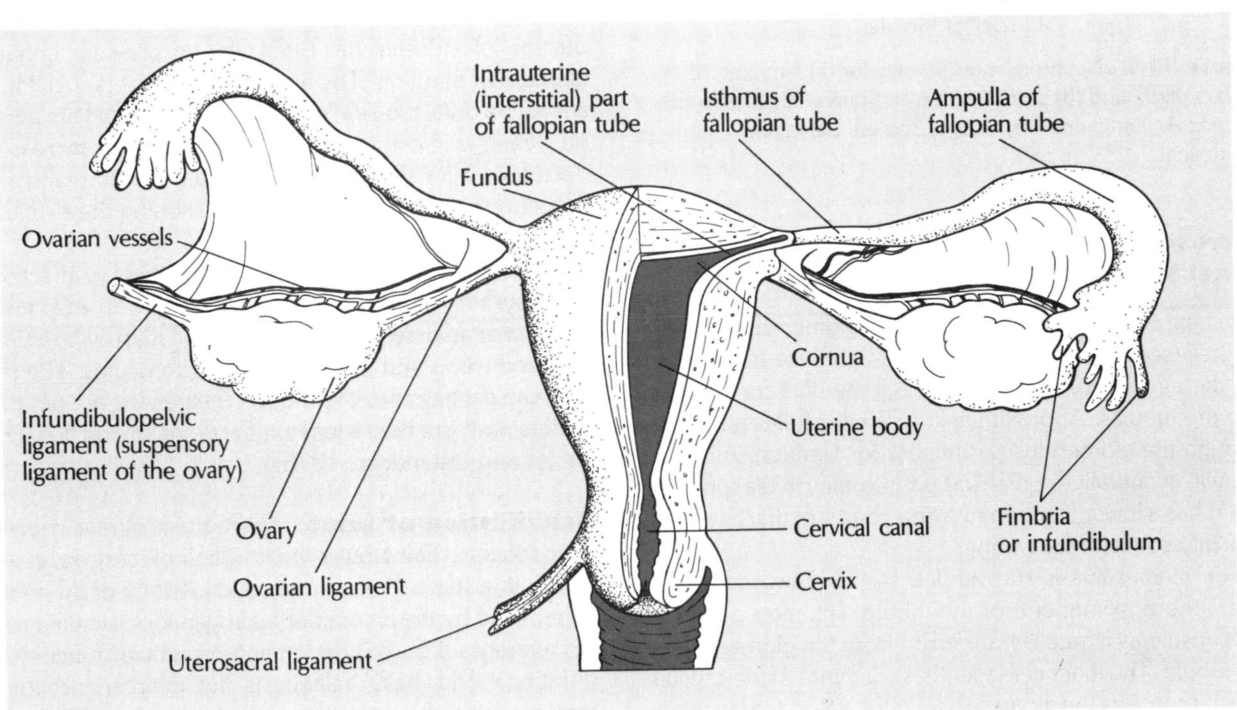

Figure 39-3 Organs of the female reproductive system. (From Olds SB et al: *Maternal-Newborn Nursing*, 2nd ed. Addison-Wesley, 1984, p. 82.)

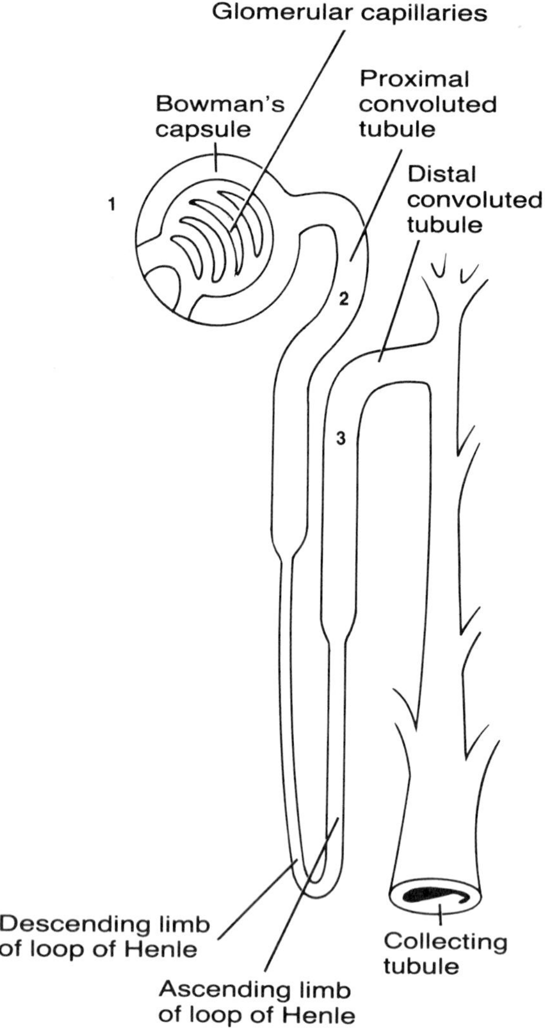

Figure 39-4 Nephron, showing sites for (1) filtration, (2) reabsorption, and (3) secretion. (From Spence AP, Mason EB: *Human Anatomy and Physiology*, 2nd ed. Benjamin/ Cummings, 1983, p. 689.)

Microscopic Anatomy and Physiology of the Renal System

The nephron is subdivided into the glomerulus and the tubules (see Fig. 39-4). Body constituents are transported via the circulatory system to the glomerulus for filtration into the tubules. Approximately 120 mL of plasma passes through the glomerulus per minute for filtration. All but 1 mL will eventually be reabsorbed into the circulation. The infant has a lower filtration rate and consequently has more difficulty concentrating urine.

The glomerulus is surrounded by the Bowman's capsule—the proximal end of the tubule. Filtration occurs in the capsule as filtrate is transferred from the glomerulus to the tubule. The inner cell layer (basal lamina) of the capsule directly contacts the glomerulus. Podocytes in the layer surround the capillaries in a network of folds or filtration slits. The endothelium of the glomerular capillaries is thin and contains microscopic pores (fenestrated epithelium). The contact point between the fenestrations and the filtration slits is the location of substances leaving the blood to enter the tubule. At this location, however, only substances smaller than blood cells are permitted to pass. This passage of water and soluble wastes is filtration—the first step in urine formation. Glomerular filtrate is isotonic at this point and proceeds from the capsule into the proximal convoluted tubule.

The second step of urine formation is tubular reabsorption—the reabsorption into the circulation of substances essential to the body. Approximately 90% of water and some solutes are reabsorbed by the cells comprising the convoluted tubules and the loop of Henle. Elements essential to metabolic homeostasis such as sodium (Na^+), chloride (Cl^-), bicarbonate (HCO_3^-), and glucose, among others, pass from the tubules into interstitial fluid, where they are absorbed into the circulation through the peritubular capillaries. The process is facilitated by active and passive transport (see Chapter 33).

Tubular secretion occurs at the distal tubule. Particles too large to be filtered by the glomerulus enter the tubule at this site for excretion. Additionally, there is interaction between a portion of the distal tubule and the afferent arterioles—the juxtaglomerular complex. Aldosterone, a hormone produced by the adrenal cortex, acts upon the juxtaglomerular cells to control reabsorption of sodium and water, thus affecting both blood volume and blood pressure. Maintenance of internal blood pressure is affected by renin, a substance secreted by juxtaglomerular cells. Renin stimulates liver production of angiotensin, a plasma protein, which increases blood pressure by stimulating adrenal production of aldosterone. Stable blood pressure enhances glomerular filtration. The antidiuretic hormone (ADH) also affects the distal tubule's function. Levels of ADH are affected by a change in osmotic pressure of the blood. Increases or decreases alter the amount of water that is reabsorbed, therefore becoming a factor in determining the dilution or concentration of urine.

Two other hormones produced by the kidney affect other body systems. Erythropoietin is produced in response to hypoxia or anemia. It prompts the bone marrow to increase the production and maturation of erythrocytes. The medulla manufactures prostaglandins. Their effects are not totally understood, but they seem to affect renal blood flow (Hekelman and Ostendorp, 1975).

Acidification of Urine Glomerular filtrate is an isotonic solution. The tubular reabsorption of solutes and water results in a hypertonic end product. Acidity of the urine is determined by the amount of hydrogen ions excreted. Urine pH averages 4.5–8.0 depending on tubular function and nutrition. Acid–base balance is the maintenance of the hydrogen-ion concentration of the body's fluid. The kidney serves as a final line of defense in the maintenance of acid–

base balance (see Chapter 33). The process of acidifying urine by excreting excess hydrogen and retaining bicarbonate is complex. A brief outline follows:

1. *Bicarbonate buffer system (proximal tubule).* Carbonic acid (H_2CO_3) in the tubular cells dissociates into hydrogen (H^+) and bicarbonate (HCO_3^-). The HCO_3^- is reabsorbed into the circulation, and the free H^+ diffuses into the glomerular filtrate. There the H^+ combines with the filtered HCO_3^- (originally from plasma) to form carbonic acid (H_2CO_3). This carbonic acid breaks down into carbon dioxide (CO_2) and water (H_2O). The water is eventually excreted or reabsorbed and the CO_2 diffuses back into the tubular cells to reinitiate the process.

2. *Phosphate system (distal tubule).* Electronically neutral acids in the filtrate (for example, Na_2HPO_4) accept the free hydrogen from carbonic acid breakdown to become acid salts (NaH_2PO_4). The acid salt is excreted and the freely released sodium is returned to the tubular cell. The reaction is

$$Na_2HPO_4 + H^+ \qquad Na\ H_2PO_4 + Na^+$$

3. *Ammonia excretion.* Ammonia (NH_3) is produced by all of the tubular cells and enters the filtrate. There it combines with free hydrogen to form ammonium (NH_4^+) and is excreted with associated negative ions. The neutralization of ammonia is the major vehicle for hydrogen-ion excretion.

Clearance Since some tests used to assess kidney function employ the concept of clearance, the nurse needs to understand this term. *Clearance* is defined as "the rate at which a substance is excreted in terms of its plasma concentration" (Brundage, 1980). Because the kidneys remove waste products from the plasma, the function of effective glomerular filtration is measured by the clearance of measurable substances, such as creatinine, which are produced by the body but not reabsorbed in the tubules.

Assessment of the Child With a Genitourinary Dysfunction

History

A detailed nursing assessment often begins with the prenatal history. Information regarding prenatal events such as maternal injuries, medications, or exposure to toxins might elicit helpful data. Relevant birth data includes the presence of oligohydramnios or polyhydramnios and the number of cord vessels, if known. Parental contact with any type of sexually transmitted disease is also important to note along with the treatment method employed.

Since heredity affects the occurrence of some genitourinary diseases, a family history is essential. In addition to the usual information solicited (see Chapter 14) familial occurrences of hypospadias, polycystic kidney disease, or other genitourinary pathology may have bearing on the child's present problem. When developing a rapport with child and family during the history-taking process, the nurse is sensitive to any expressions of parental guilt. Fears about mistakes made during pregnancy that may have affected the child might be expressed at this time. Fears and expressions of guilt should be identified in the nursing care plan. Allowance for the expression of guilt is appropriate when obtaining a history, and nurses thus provide a reassuring climate for this to occur.

Essential to obtaining a history for the assessment of a child with a genitourinary problem is information about toilet training and normal urinary habits. Unusual delays in achieving urinary control may be significant, although placing delays in a familial perspective, that is, time of control in relation to siblings' achievements of control, may diminish the importance of the delays. Generally, complete control is achieved by the end of early childhood (see Chapter 8). Close supervision by the child's primary medical-care provider is necessary if urinary control is not achieved by that stage. Regression to wetting after control is attained may be related to psychologic factors, but persistent wetting requires medical attention.

While the nurse is compiling a history, specific terms used by the child and family for urinary functions and organs should be recorded. Future ease of communication with the child is enhanced if personal terms are used. Terms may vary widely according to cultural and intellectual background. They range from those that are anatomically and physiologically correct to those that are completely unrelated to the system. Some of the words may be seemingly appropriate to the child's culture but may be considered vulgar in other contexts. Use of terms will change as the child matures, and the older child, while embarrassed to use a given word, may fully understand correct terminology.

History of past infections; pain; undiagnosed febrile episodes; urine of unusual color, odor, or volume assist in the assessment of the child's genitourinary status. Also, any history of vaginal or penile discharge or itching, or gastrointestinal complaints, can help establish that a problem exists. If sexually transmitted disease is suspected, adolescents need to be asked about sexual contacts with possible carriers. Recent changes in voiding patterns, alterations in the urinary stream, and changes in output are additional important factors to determine.

If the child demonstrates a history of previous or repeated urinary tract infections, the nurse obtains information about the causative organism, if known, duration of the infection, and any successful treatments or medications. A history of previous surgical procedures or diagnostic studies helps the nurse clarify the integrity of the urinary system. Finally, before beginning the physical assessment, it is important for the nurse to obtain a history of the presenting problem including precipitating factors, duration of symptoms, and home methods of treatment.

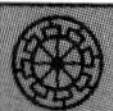

ASSESSMENT GUIDE Child With a Genitourinary Problem

System	Subjective data	Objective data	Validating data: Dx. tests	Validating data: Radiographs	Nursing management
Head		Abnormal position of ears (developing simultaneously with kidneys in fetus)			Question history of genitourinary problems
Eyes, ears, nose throat		Edema—periorbital	Glomerular filtration rate, ASO titer, ESR, blood chemistry		Accurate intake and output measurement, urine for protein and specific gravity; positioning; dietary modification
	Sore throat or recent sore throat	Injected throat, lymphadenopathy, fever	Throat culture for streptococcus, ASO titer, complete blood count, ESR		Teach methods of preventing strep, relationship between strep and AGN
Integumentary	Recent impetigo or other lesions, rashes, itching	Pallor, bruising, jaundice, excessive moisture, cold sores, previous incisions, abnormal openings (ostomies), skin lesions	Skin culture lesions, VDRL test, gonococcal culture		Skin care for maintaining integrity and prevention of infection; teach prevention of communicable disease; validate home management of ostomies; monitor signs of renal trauma
	Thirst, dry mouth	Poor skin turgor, absence of tears, sunken fontanelle, weight loss			Observe for signs of fluid and electrolyte imbalance; monitor intake and output;
Cardiovascular	Fever, generalized swelling	Elevated BP, anemia, lymphadenopathy, edema	Complete blood count, hemoglobin, hematocrit		Monitor vital signs; observe for signs of cardiac complications
Gastrointestinal	Abdominal pain, nausea, vomiting, anorexia	Lower quadrant tenseness, other abdominal rigidity, ascites	Urine culture and sensitivity tests, bladder tap, cystoscopy, urinalysis, serum values, gonococcal culture	KUB	

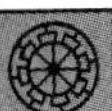

ASSESSMENT GUIDE Child With a Genitourinary Problem (continued)

System	Subjective data	Objective data	Validating data: Dx. tests	Validating data: Radiographs	Nursing management
Respiratory	Difficulty breathing, cough, fatigue	Respiratory distress, congestion, edema		Chest film	Positioning for optimum ventilation; organization of care to promote adequate rest
Genitourinary	Flank pain, frequency and urgency of urination, decreased urine, fever, chills	Palpable kidneys, hematuria, flank bruising, oliguria	Urinalysis, urine culture and sensitivity tests, cystoscopy	KUB, IVP, VCUG, renal angiography, renal ultrasound	Pain relief, fever control; accurate intake and output measurements; IV maintenance; explanation of workup
		Decreased output, intermittent voiding, pain in bladder area	Urine culture and sensitivity tests	Cystourethrogram	Encourage complete bladder emptying; teach prevention of UTIs
	Decreased urination, forced urination	Abnormal placement of meatus, chordee, inguinal bulge, absent testes, scrotal edema			
	Itching, pain on urination	Perineal inflammation, lesions, warts, abnormal discharge, vaginal plaques (*Candida*), malformations	Cultures from cervix, urethra, rectum, pharynx, VDRL tests, titer for herpes antibody, vaginal smears		Explanation of tests; support during pelvic exam; STD education and reporting; check location of female urethra in relation to vagina
Musculoskeletal		Short stature—usually in children with chronic renal insufficiency			Explore feelings about body image

Physical Assessment

Prior to completing an assessment, nurses need to carefully consider the approach to each child. Because genitourinary problems may involve a thorough examination of intimate body parts, children can be extremely threatened by the physical examination. Fear of the examination can alter other body responses—vital signs and abdominal reflexes. A calm, reassuring approach and verbal expressions of encouragement promote relaxation. Distraction techniques are particularly useful with the younger child (see Chapter 29). Explanations to the older child and reassurance that privacy will be protected ensure cooperation. The examination should proceed from the least to the most threatening system (see Chapter 14). See the Assessment Guide for the child with a genitourinary dysfunction.

Privacy is of paramount importance during the assessment process. The child should be properly draped at all times, and bedside curtains should be closed. The older child should decide whether parental presence is required. Because certain families emphasize modesty considerably, the child's embarrassment may be increased with the parent present.

Two aspects of the physical examination are important. The first is that retraction of the testes occurs frequently during physical examination and need not establish a diagnosis of undescended testicle. The nurse can observe for presence of the testes before proceeding with the scrotal examination. The second is that a vaginal examination is not usually necessary in the young child. If the adolescent girl will be seen by a physician who will perform a vaginal examination, the nurse need not do so.

Preparation for Diagnostic Tests

A diagnostic workup for a child with a genitourinary problem can be quite complex. Some of the procedures involved are uncomfortable as well as embarrassing. The age of the child must be considered when doing pretest teaching as some children will react more strongly against tests involving the genitalia than others. Fears of mutilation, which are common in the early childhood period, can result in an extremely uncooperative child. Careful explanation and reassurance that no change will occur as a result of the test may improve the situation. The presence of a familiar person or transition object during the procedure may assist to calm fears (see Chapter 29).

Noninvasive Tests Routine blood and urine testing including urinalysis, complete blood count (CBC), and serum values assist in the assessment process. Normal values and the significance of abnormalities are summarized in Tables 39-1 and 39-2. (See Chapter 29 for nursing management during these tests.) Despite advances in diagnostic technology, urinalysis remains the most important aspect of the initial evaluation of the genitourinary tract. If possible, a

TABLE 39-1 Urinalysis in Renal Disease

Component	Normal value*	Alteration	Significance
Color	Clear, amber	Colored	Some drugs, ie, methylene blue, preparations of phenazopyridine hydrochloride (eg, Pyridium)
		Red	Blood
Turbidity	Clear	Cloudy	Sediment, possible bacteria
Specific gravity—ratio of density of urine to density of water	1.016–1.022	Increased	Dehydration, nephrosis
		Decreased	Inability to concentrate urine, glomerulonephritis, severe renal damage
pH	4.6–8.0	Increased—alkaline	Persistent vomiting, alkalosis
	Average 6.0	Decreased—acidic	Acidosis, nephritis
Protein	0	Increased	Present in renal diseases involving glomeruli and tubules, infections of kidneys, and other noninfectious processes
Glucose	0	Increased	Diabetes mellitus
Ketones	0	Increased	Acidosis
Cells	Few	Increased	Can indicate kidney, ureter, bladder pathology depending on type
Erythrocytes (RBC)	0	Increased	Menstrual, glomerulonephritis, trauma, pyelonephritis, tumors
Leukocytes	Few	Increased	Urinary tract infection
Casts	0	Increased in conditions of low pH	Present in variety of kidney pathologies
Crystals	Some	Increased	Calculi

SOURCE: Byrne J et al: *Laboratory Tests: Implications for Nurses and Allied Health Professionals*. Addison-Wesley, 1981.
*NOTE: Values vary slightly depending upon source used.

TABLE 39-2 Alterations in Serum Values in Renal Disease

Component	Normal value*	Alteration	Significance
Sodium	135–148 mEq/L	Increased or stable	Decreased renal blood flow through glomeruli yields sodium and water reabsorption and retention, edema
Potassium	3.6–5.0 mEq/L	Increased	Renal failure, reabsorption of potassium and excretion of hydrogen ions
Chloride	95–108 mEq/L	Increased	Associated with some renal disorders
Phosphorus	2.3–4.1 mEq/L	Increased	Associated with kidney dysfunction, uremia, particularly tubular damage
Blood urea nitrogen	6–20 mg/dL	Increased	Inadequate excretion of urea due to obstruction or renal disease
Creatinine	0.6–1.5 mg/dL	Increased	Impaired renal function or urinary obstruction
Glucose	80–120 mg/dL	Increased or stable	Possibly indicative of diabetes mellitus
Hematocrit	Male: 40%–54% Female: 37%–47%	Decreased	Response to bleeding in acute glomerulonephritis, trauma
Hemoglobin	Male: 14–18 g/dL Female: 12–16 g/dL	Decreased	Response to bleeding in acute glomerulonephritis, trauma

SOURCE: Byrne J et al: *Laboratory Tests: Implications for Nurses and Allied Health Professionals.* Addison-Wesley, 1981.

*NOTE: Values vary slightly depending upon source used.

morning specimen should be sent for analysis since the concentration and acidity change as the day progresses. If possible a clean-catch urine sample should be obtained.

Twenty-Four-Hour Collection Twenty-four-hour urine collections are commonly required for urologic diagnosis. The creatinine clearance test (normal: male—107–141mL/min; female—87–132 mL/min) measures glomerular filtration efficiency plus tubular excretion. A decrease in urine creatinine clearance indicates impaired renal function. A blood level for creatinine is usually done at some point during the 24-hour collection time and normally shows elevated creatinine if the clearance level is low. The container for a 24-hour collection is labeled with the time the collection is initiated. All urine samples are stored in the container. The collection begins after the child has voided and ends the following day with a final void just prior to completion time.

Parent and child must be cautioned to inform the nurse each time the child voids. Boys should use the urinal, and girls should either use a bedpan or a plastic "hat" that fits into the toilet. Older children and adolescents can share the responsibility for obtaining specimens if given adequate instruction and equipment.

Twenty-four-hour collection poses a problem for the untrained or incontinent child. Special collection bags with long polyethylene tubing are applied to the perineal area (see Chapter 29). The bag stays in place for the collection period and is emptied into the container via the tube. A sign attached to the bed, sink, or bedpan flusher may prevent a well-meaning colleague or parent from accidentally discarding the urine.

Urine for Culture and Sensitivity (Clean-catch Urine) A diagnosis of urinary tract infection is based on the detection of significant bacteriuria. The finding of at least 100,000 (10^5) organisms per milliliter of urine in a clean-voided midstream specimen is considered indicative of an active urinary tract infection. Normal urine is sterile. Contamination is a significant problem in obtaining satisfactory urine specimens for culture from children, especially girls. Urine specimens contaminated during collection generally have counts of fewer than 10,000 bacteria per milliliter. Counts of between 10,000 and 100,000 per milliliter should indicate a repeat culture (American Academy of Pediatrics, 1977).

The nurse follows institutional procedure for procuring urine culture specimens. A midstream of clean-catch void is collected from toilet-trained children after a thorough cleansing of the perineum. Girls should be instructed to separate the labia and clean either side and the middle with three different wipes. Cleaning proceeds from front to back so as not to contaminate the cleaned area. After cleaning, the child should void a small amount into the toilet and the remainder into the specimen receptacle. After being labeled correctly, the specimen should be transported immediately to the laboratory. Any delay could result in multiplication of bacteria, leading to a false reading. Nurses follow a similar cleaning procedure with untrained children. The cleaning is followed by the application of a sterile urine-collecting bag (see Chapter 29).

Bladder catheterization may be ordered by the physician if the midstream technique is unacceptable. Some physicians prefer the bladder tap procedure. Both are considered to be invasive.

Abdominal Flat Plate Radiograph A simple flat plate of the abdomen allows visualization of the kidneys, ureters, and bladder (KUB). This radiograph is helpful when evaluating gross anatomic conditions (that is, hydronephrosis). The child may need reassurances that, unlike many urologic radiographic studies, the KUB is painless.

Sexually Transmitted Disease Diagnosis Diagnostic tests for sexually transmitted diseases are generally painless with the exception of serologic studies, which require a blood sample. Cultures for gonorrhea are essential for confirming diagnosis. Cultures are obtained from the cervix, urethra, rectum, and pharynx and are incubated on a Thayer-Martin plate. A suspicion of gonorrhea in boys is confirmed by the presence of gram-negative intracellular diplococci on a urethral smear (Martin, 1978).

Vaginal smears on a potassium hydroxide (KOH) slide may indicate presence of *Candida*. The KOH lyses other organisms and keeps the yeast intact (Martin, 1978).

Serologic studies are done to detect syphilis. During the first week after the chancre appears, serologic studies will be negative because of insufficient time for the antibody titer to rise. Within 1–3 weeks after the appearance of the chancre (4–6 weeks after initial infection), the serologic tests become positive. They attain high titer levels during secondary syphilis. The Venereal Disease Research Laboratory (VDRL) slide flocculation test is a standard test for syphilis. It is not absolutely specific or sensitive for syphilis and can be falsely positive in other disease conditions (Chow et al., 1979; Martin, 1978). Treponemal tests detect the specific treponemal antibody and are done to confirm the presence of syphilis after the VDRL returns positive. The Fluorescent Treponemal Antibody Absorption Test (FTA-ABS) is considered to be the most sensitive test for diagnosis of syphilis in all stages (Martin, 1978).

Blood titer levels of herpes antibody can be done when genital herpes is suspected. (Nursing responsibilities involved with serologic tests are covered in Chapter 29.) If a pelvic examination must be done to obtain cervical smears, the nurse gives a thorough explanation to the adolescent and practices relaxation and breathing techniques with her to facilitate the examination.

Invasive Procedures Adequate, honest preparation is most supportive to the child undergoing stressful procedures. When describing each test or procedure, the nurse carefully selects terms the child and family will understand. Often parents and their children are reluctant to ask for clarification of details or unfamiliar terminology when particularly stressed. Timing of the preparation should be geared to the age of the child. An in-depth discussion of the preparation of the child for procedures necessary during hospitalization may be found in Chapter 29.

Catheterization Bladder catheterization is a nursing intervention that the child with a genitourinary problem may face repeatedly. For young children this can be an unpleasant anxiety-provoking procedure. A successful initial experience facilitates subsequent catheterization. The purpose of the procedure should be explained, and an estimate of the time the catheter is to remain in place should be given. The use of dolls to demonstrate and explain the procedure is helpful, particularly with younger children (see Chapter 28).

The nurse explains to the child that there might be a feeling of pressure similar to the urge to urinate while the catheter is being inserted. The child should understand that, once inserted, the catheter presents no discomfort. Very young children may fear losing their insides through the tube, particularly if they see urine outflow. The sensitive nurse can anticipate this and give a realistic picture of what is happening.

Catheterization may be performed to empty the bladder prior to diagnostic tests, to obtain a sterile urine specimen, to measure residual volumes in the bladder, or to empty the bladder when the child is unable to void. The nurse needs to be familiar with the institution's procedure for bladder catheterization. Strict aseptic technique is essential as the urinary tract is most vulnerable to introduction of infection by catheterization. The technique for cleaning the perineal area is similar to the technique used for clean-catch specimens.

The catheter is inserted only until urine flow is observed (Fig. 39-5). If the catheter is to be indwelling, the balloon must be inflated, with care not to inflate it in the internal urethral sphincter. Indwelling catheters are connected to collection bags. If the bladder is particularly full, the nurse clamps the catheter at intervals to prevent a sudden rush of urine output. Infants and young children are customarily catheterized with a size-8 catheter. As the child grows, catheters with larger lumens are used. The lumen should be small enough for easy insertion but large enough to prevent leakage of urine.

An honest explanation with age-appropriate terminology will assist the anxious child. Discomfort during catheterization arises in response to tense musculature. Even the very young child can practice breathing exercises before the procedure to assist muscle relaxation. As the young child will need physical and emotional support, a parent or familiar staff member should also be present during the procedure.

Bladder Tap Because a sterile urine specimen is difficult to obtain from infants, the physician may elect to perform a bladder tap. The technique requires the puncture of the

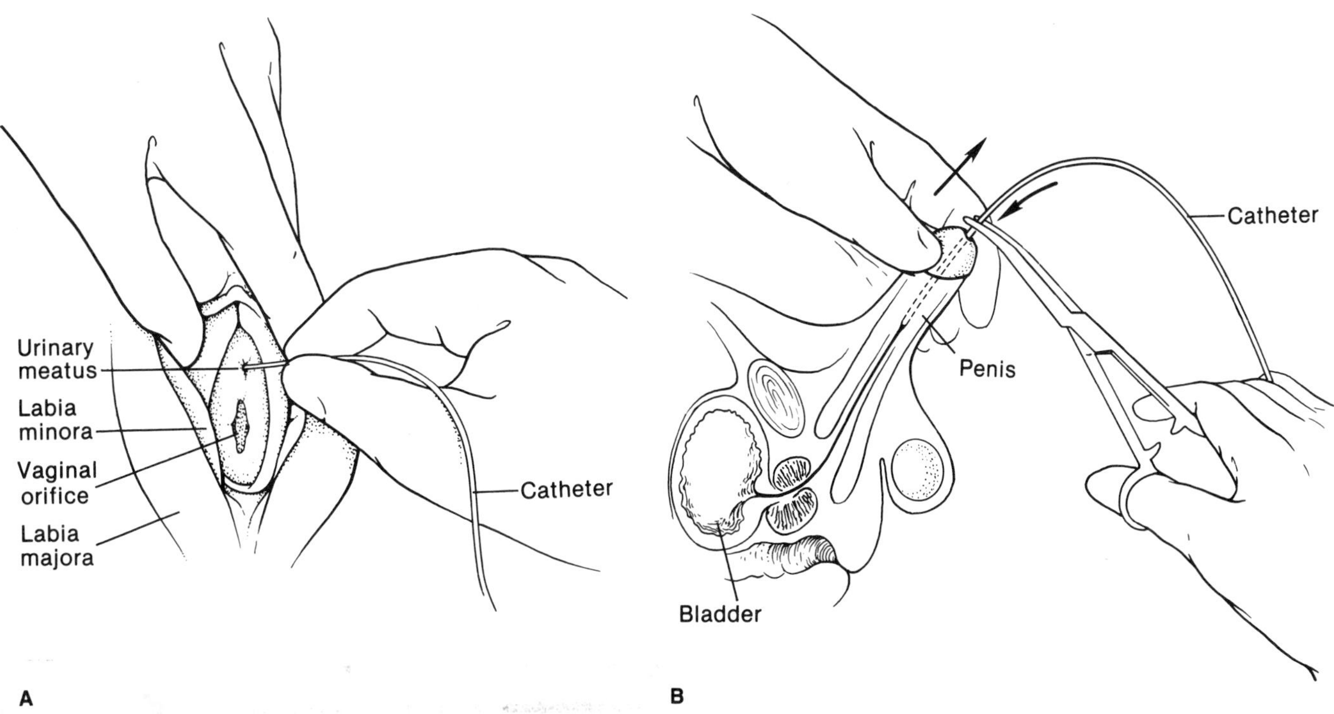

Figure 39-5 Bladder catherization. *A*. Female. *B*. Male.

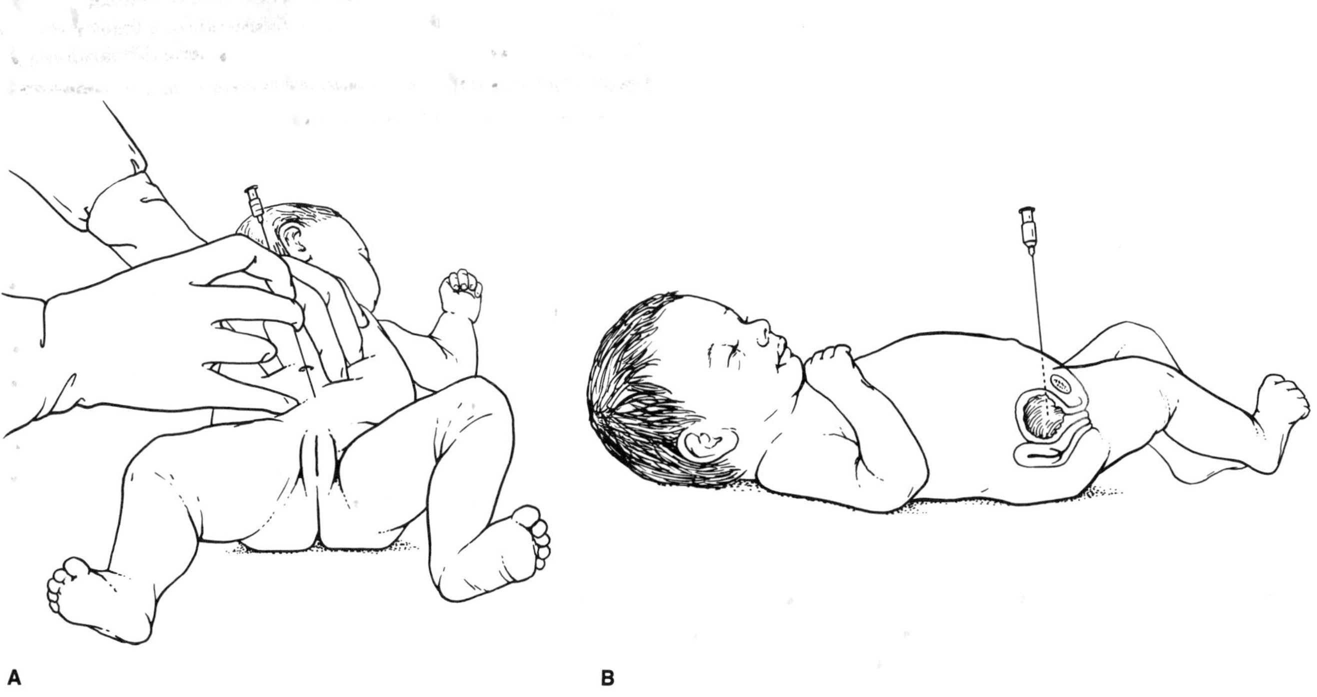

Figure 39-6 Bladder tap. *A*. Percutaneous bladder tap. The needle in position before insertion. *B*. Position of needle after entry into bladder.

Urinary Catheter Guidelines

1. Maintain closed sterile drainage system for children with indwelling catheters. Open the system only when irrigating the catheter by physician's order. Change to a new sterile collecting system only for signs of obstruction, leakage, contamination, or large amounts of sediment in the tube.

2. Use strict handwashing before and after doing catheter care.

3. Prevent movement of the catheter. Tape the catheter to the child's thigh and anchor the tube to prevent kinks or loops. Allow some slack to prevent tension on the catheter.

4. Position the child so that the drainage bag is below the catheter exit site and gravity drainage is facilitated.

5. Provide perineal hygiene and catheter care according to institution policy. Do not pull on the catheter when cleaning the perineum. Inspect the catheter site regularly for signs of irritation or leakage.

6. Use a sterile irrigation kit for each irrigation if irrigations are ordered.

7. Prevent entrance of organisms when obtaining a urine specimen. Clamp the catheter below the in-line porthole (rubber injection site). Disinfect the site and aspirate the urine with a 25-gauge needle and syringe. Disinfect the porthole again after needle removal. Remove the needle from the syringe before depositing urine in the sterile specimen container.

8. Prevent the entrance of organisms while measuring urine and emptying the drainage bag. Use gloves when handling the drainage spigot. Clean the spigot with povidone iodine; empty the urine into the child's own receptacle. Disinfect the spigot again when the bag is empty.

9. Observe for changes in urine output or for alterations in the color or turbidity of the urine.

10. Encourage increased fluid intake. Monitor intake and output as often as hourly for the first 8 hours after catheterization.

SOURCE: Information from Killion A: Reducing the risk of infection from indwelling urethral catheters. *Nursing '82* (May) 1982; 12:84–88.

skin and underlying bladder. A needle is inserted into the skin just above the symphysis pubis, and a specimen is obtained directly from within the bladder (Fig. 39-6). The procedure is considered to be low-risk (*Kidney and Urinary Tract Infections*, 1971). The nurse properly positions or restrains the child for the procedure and maintains the position throughout the procedure, to prevent unnecessary movement.

Cystoscopy The cystoscopic examination is used to detect malformations of the bladder, ureters, and urethra. It should be done under anesthesia for infants and children to ensure their cooperation (see Chapter 29 for preoperative preparation). Cystoscopy allows visualization of the urethra and bladder by means of a lighted tubular lens. It allows visualization of ureteral orifices, removal of small calculi, and insertion of ureteral catheters if necessary.

Nursing preparation in addition to preoperative teaching includes explaining the postoperative course. When voiding for the first time after a cystoscopy, the child may experience pain and burning. The child should be prepared for this discomfort and told that intake of extra fluid will alleviate the symptoms. The child should be observed closely for postprocedural urinary retention. If this is not the child's first experience, the retention may be intentional. Assurances can be given that with continued voids, discomfort lessens considerably. Often a warm sitz bath will relax the child, decrease bladder irritability, and encourage spontaneous voiding.

Radiographic Studies Several radiographic studies may be used to assess the function and structure of the renal system. They are summarized in Table 39-3. Some of these studies require intravenous injections of a radiopaque contrast material. Whenever children are prepared to experience studies involving the use of a dye, the nurse explains how they will feel while the dye is being injected. The dye often causes a general feeling of warmth, particularly in the face. There may be a burning sensation at the injection site, radiating up the extremity. The child may also feel nauseous. Nurses can reassure the children that these symptoms will soon disappear. Young children may feel particularly apprehensive, and the presence of a parent or sympathetic nurse might ensure cooperation during the dye injection.

A major nursing responsibility concerned with these radiographic studies is to obtain a history of any previous allergic response. In rare cases, the contrast material can precipitate an anaphylactic reaction. Parents will usually need to sign a special consent form for procedures such as an intravenous pyelogram because of this possibility, but they should be assured that the occurrence is rare. At the completion of the test, the child should be observed for any local irritation or allergic response.

Principles of Nursing Care

Acute-Care Needs

Maintenance of fluid and electrolyte balance is of extreme importance in the management of the child with a genitourinary condition. Children recovering from genitourinary surgery present an additional challenge as their fluid

TABLE 39-3 Radiographic Studies

Study	Organs	Procedure	Nursing management	Implications
Cystourethrography/ voiding cystourethrogram (VCUG)	Urethra, bladder	Urinary catheterization Insertion of dye Radiographs Voiding with radiographs	Prepare for catheterization and radiographic studies Relieve anxiety	Can spot disturbances in voiding patterns, vesicoureteral reflux, and structural defects
Intravenous pyelogram (IVP)	Kidney, ureters, bladder	IV injection of radiopaque dye—antecubital vein Radiograph films at established time intervals One postvoid radiograph	Restrict diet according to institution Assess previous allergic reactions Prepare for IV and radiographs Explain effects of dye Encourage fluids after tests Observe for reactions	Assures renal function and structural abnormalities. Can visualize calculi and certain kidney diseases
Renal angiography	Renal arteries and kidney circulation	Injection of dye through femoral or axillary arteries Radiography	Administer sedation Explain procedure and effects of dye Assess injection site posttest Maintain immobility of site to reduce edema and potential hematoma Check circulatory status in extremity distal to injection site for signs of obstruction	Differentiates types of renal masses
Renal scan	Kidney	Injection of isotope IV Radioscanner detects presence of isotope and records pattern on a chart	Encourage fluids prior to test Explain procedure and equipment	Detects hypertension, failure, obstruction, and other kidney disease

needs correspond to their size and the manipulation of their urinary tracts. The physician will consider the unique fluid management requirements of the child in prescribing intravenous fluid therapy and oral intake. The nurse then plays a major role in the successful implementation of the physician's plan by monitoring the child's intake and output carefully. Hourly checking and recording of intake and output is essential if the child is to remain adequately hydrated.

Many children experience postoperative diuresis caused by urinary tract manipulation. This condition necessitates even more careful assessment of the child's fluid balance. The nurse needs to be quickly able to recognize an intravenous infusion that is less than the prescribed volume or an inadequate oral intake and needs to correct the situation promptly to prevent dehydration. In an attempt to control the infusion more adequately, the nurse may elect to use an IV pump. This is particularly effective with infants and very young children. The pump does, however, somewhat limit mobility although, since it can be temporarily battery operated, it allows for limited freedom. The nurse checks the pump frequently for effective function and responds immediately to the warning alarm.

Despite improved methods of preventing and treating infections, the genitourinary tract remains quite vulnerable. Predisposing factors such as structural abnormalities or stasis of urine and foreign bodies (such as catheters and stents) add additional risk. There are several approaches the nurse can use to minimize infection. Good handwashing procedure is essential when dealing with all patients. Adequate handwashing prior to and after contact with each patient will lessen incidence of cross-contamination. A careful technique when inserting catheters or performing perineal care is a nursing measure that reduces the occurrence of infection.

The use of aseptic technique when contacting the child's wound or intravenous site is essential. Contaminated urine must be contained and disposed of properly to prevent nosocomial (hospital-acquired) infection. Routine cultures of urine assist in the assessment of infection. Any sign of infection (wound inflammation, intravenous-site phlebitis, etc.) must be reported to the physician. Changes in the appearance of the child's urine (for example, sediment or odor) are indicative of infectious processes. Fever, flank pain, and urinary frequency are also common indicators of genitourinary inflammation.

Frequent monitoring of vital signs, particularly the child's temperature, is necessary for the assessment of physiologic homeostasis. Any alteration in signs should be reported to the physician.

Preoperative Preparation for Genitourinary Surgery

Often the preoperative preparation for the child facing genitourinary surgery begins shortly after admission to the nursing unit. A detailed assessment is important at this time as the nurse plans an individualized teaching approach to the child and family. It is important that the nurse assess what the child and the parent understand about the anticipated surgical procedure.

There are many ways to communicate with children, even the very young, that convey the message and attempt to alleviate anxiety. As discussed in Chapters 28 and 29, the use of dolls to demonstrate the positions of tubes, dressings, and catheters can be particularly effective. Familiarity with the postoperative equipment such as catheters, drainage bags, mist tents, or other equipment will reduce tension.

The nurse gives a narrative description of the surgical experience including what is to happen postoperatively and how the child will feel. If a recovering child with a similar surgical experience is available, the nurse encourages a sharing of experiences. Such a sharing experience would be particularly helpful to a boy having genital surgery, as it helps to alleviate fears of castration or mutilation.

If immobility will be necessary in the postoperative period, the nurse prepares the child. Accurate information regarding the reason for immobility and the expected length of time involved will be helpful to the older child. The younger child may need reassurance that resuming appropriate physical activity is possible when the restriction is no longer necessary. A description of immobilizing devices such as testicular traction, bed cradles, and dressings will ease the postoperative course.

The discussion of pain must always be as truthful as possible. The responsibility for inflicting pain upon a child is often extremely distasteful to the nurse; nonetheless, the nurse does not lie to the child in a misguided attempt to make the inevitable easier. Using age-appropriate terms, the nurse should attempt to describe as truthfully as possible the pain the child will experience (see Chapter 29).

Maintenance of fluid and electrolyte balance is a postoperative nursing challenge that can be facilitated during the preoperative period. Methods of drinking (bottle, cup) and the child's fluid preferences should be included in the plan. Because normal voiding patterns may be interrupted, the child should be prepared for this. This may be particularly stressful for recently toilet-trained children, and parents should be cautioned to expect regressive behavior patterns.

Postoperative Care

Any child experiencing genitourinary surgical procedures might expect to have one or more urinary drainage tubes as well as the usual postoperative dressings, IVs, and routines. Postoperative nursing assessment is directed toward the areas of

- Physiologic homeostasis
- Fluid and electrolyte balance
- Patency of drainage tubes
- Infection potential
- Nutritional status
- Pain
- Injury or trauma
- Other postoperative complications
- Psychologic trauma of child and family
- Readiness for discharge.

See the Nursing Care Guide for a general plan for postoperative care of the child following genitourinary surgery.

Nutritional Needs The child with impaired renal function immediately becomes involved in the intricacies of fluid balance. Children with urinary drainage devices (such as catheters and stents) may need to be encouraged to drink large amounts of fluids; however, the child with filtration problems (nephrosis, chronic renal failure) may be severely restricted to a few hundred milliliters a day. The child with severe genitourinary problems must deal with the frustrations of alternating severe restriction with the need to drink large amounts.

Often young children faced with the stresses of immobilization or regression feel they have lost all control of their bodies. The one control remaining is the refusal to eat or drink. This reaction is common in children who perceive every other aspect of their lives to be beyond their control. A detailed assessment can be helpful in describing dietary likes and dislikes. Familiar foods and fluids offered by family members are usually more acceptable to the young child. Control is assisted by offering children choices about types of food and fluid within their dietary limits.

Increased fluid intake is recommended to prevent renal calculi and to potentiate many urologic drugs. Fruit juices, particularly cranberry juice, are usually acceptable to chil-

NURSING CARE GUIDE Child Following Genitourinary Surgery

Nursing diagnosis	Interventions	Evaluation
1. Potential for postoperative complications—hemorrhage, respiratory distress, pneumonia	(See Chapter 29)	
2. Alteration in fluid and electrolyte balance	Maintain ordered intravenous rate Offer oral fluids when indicated according to the child's preference Measure output accurately every hour to the eighth hour as output stabilizes Measure output from each catheter and record separately	Child shows no signs of dehydration or fluid overload—adequate urinary drainage Child shows effective resumption of oral intake
3. Pain	Observe for pain at incision site Observe for restlessness, rigidity, altered facial expression Provide physical measures for pain relief—position change, back rub, releasing catheter tension Administer analgesics (See Chapter 29)	(See Chapter 29.)
4. Potential trauma to catheters	Tape catheters securely at exit site and to leg whenever possible Apply tape so that catheter does not kink, twist, or rise against gravity Observe for patency Follow instructions for irrigation, instillation, and dressing changes	Catheters are secured effectively and are draining appropriately
5. Potential infection of urinary tract	Maintain sterile drainage system Use aseptic technique for dressing changes Give Foley catheter care if applicable See Chapter 29 for other infection control methods	Child shows no signs of infection such as fever, redness, pain at site, or bacteriuria
6. Potential hazards of immobility	(See Chapter 29)	Child shows no signs of muscle atrophy, constipation, urinary stasis, respiratory difficulties, skin breakdown
7. Potential emotional complications	Allow for expression of feelings Refer to other support for severe disturbances, especially regarding body image alteration	Child appears emotionally stable, demonstrates interest in surroundings
8. Knowledge deficit	Provide for continuation of schooling Provide discharge preparation to facilitate home care, catheter care, dressing changes, diet, fluid balances	Child and family are effectively prepared to maintain health at home and to follow home care routine adequately

dren and are a convenient source of vitamin C. Vitamin C acidifies the urine, thereby lessening the opportunity for calculi to form or for infection to develop. (Nursing measures to encourage food and fluid intake are described in Chapter 29.)

Urine pH measurements assist the nurse in the assessment of the child's fluid needs while attempting to adjust the acidity. The goal of increasing or decreasing the type and amount of fluid is to maintain an optimal pH of 5.

Most of the genitourinary problems described in this

chapter require adjustments in nutrition necessary for recovery and health maintenance only (see Chapter 15). Unique situations and the potential for long-term dietary adjustment are discussed when appropriate for specific conditions.

Developmental Needs The child experiencing urologic interventions is often physically incapacitated by the presence of urinary appliances for varying lengths of time. An infant learning to walk with the added burden of a bulky dressing over an exstrophied bladder is unaware of the situation. The preadolescent female returning to school with a catheter draining into a leg bag must face a much more challenging adjustment. Circumcision has entirely different implications for an infant than for an older boy. External appearance has a different significance to children of various age levels. Nurses therefore need to consider the developmental stage when assessing the disease impact.

Although the goal is to potentiate the child's ability to "be like the other kids," the reality of the genitourinary problem makes this very difficult. Acceptance by family and peers is vital to the child. Unfortunately, the child's peers are often cruel without cognitive sense of the damage being done to the affected child. This is often a very difficult period for the parent and child. Expression of feelings by the use of play or art facilitates adjustment. The nurse allows parent and child to express fears, feelings, and frustrations as they begin to process this difficult adjustment. A parent must be comfortable with personal feelings about the situation before being able to assist the child.

Many children with genitourologic problems require frequent, and often lengthy, hospitalizations. Multiple surgical interventions are often necessary. It is not uncommon for these children to be forced to miss weeks or months of school. Whenever possible, attempts should be made to continue the child's education while still hospitalized and the parent needs to be aware that although the child is ill, as normal a routine as possible should be encouraged. Tutors may be available from the local school department for long periods of confinement either in the hospital or at home. Peers should be encouraged to visit (see Chapter 29). Problems of immobilization frustrate a child's independence, resulting in potential disciplinary problems during hospitalization.

As nurses plan for the child's care, they should anticipate the need for independence. Often even young children can assume responsibility for some part of their care. The integration of children into their physical care may be continued at a later date with discharge teaching.

Emotional Needs

Alteration in Body Image Alteration in body image is the major emotional adjustment the child suffering from a disease of the genitourinary system may encounter. Infants and young children are not generally aware of body image in detail but are acutely aware of any gesture or motion that they perceive as threatening.

Children in early childhood are intensely aware of their body image. They may spend much time examining and exploring their bodies and those of their cooperative playmates. Children of this age with urologic problems often have their curiosity stimulated by the physical attention of professionals. The nurse is therefore aware of this natural inquisitiveness.

Because fantasy is also part of the young child's life at this time, a routine procedure such as suture removal can become a major crisis for the young child who fears that after suture removal, "my insides may all fall out."

The child in middle and late childhood views body image differently. For them the mere thought of "looking different" is extremely anxiety-provoking. Because fads, styles, and group activities control the world of these children, being different as the result of a genitourologic procedure is a major stressor. Strange dietary restrictions, inability to participate in sports, and fear of embarrassment plague many of these children. Often these present problems that the child perceives to be as serious as the illness itself.

The nurse thus attempts to prepare the child and family for the child's return to peer group with as little stress as possible. Often imaginative clothing designed to conceal drainage setups and creative approaches to difficult treatments evolve from discussion as concerned families and staff explore possibilities. For instance, a girl who must wear a urine-collecting appliance on her leg would profit from wearing loosely gathered knickers or slacks with banded bottoms, rather than conventional jeans. Manufacturers have produced pants similar to training pants for incontinent adults. Children who have problems with continence also benefit from this arrangement, possibly with the current fashionable underwear sewn over.

Body image is paramount in adolescence, and any disturbance is perceived as being of major significance. Rapid changes and surgical interventions are most difficult in this age group. Unfortunately, the response of adolescents experiencing such stress appears to be laden with negativism, unwillingness to communicate, and hostility. Sexual changes common to adolescence interfere with the adolescent's perception of illness and often intensify fantasies.

The mere nature of the illness means that fears of mutilation haunt many children with genitourinary problems. To minimize fears, surgical intervention must be explained by all involved with carefully chosen terms. Any manipulation of the penis or testes at this time gives rise to anxieties about future fertility or potency. Adolescent girls may be experiencing their first pelvic examination. Depending on what they have heard about the procedure, they also may fear loss of fertility or virginity, or harm to internal organs as a result of manipulation.

Careful preparation and ample opportunity for children

to express fears will enhance all necessary procedures. Reassurance that as little manipulation and trauma as necessary will be done is often reassuring to the young child. Nurses encourage the older, perhaps more articulate, child to express concerns and fantasies, if possible, so that they may attempt to allay fears and offer as much support as possible.

Other Emotional Needs Adolescents who have been positively diagnosed as having sexually transmitted disease have more complicated needs. Counseling them is a nursing challenge since, in addition to problems caused by the disease, the nurse may encounter knowledge deficits concerning the reproductive system itself. Most public health departments mandate the reporting of sexually transmitted diseases. The problem of reporting the disease and identifying contacts can result in lack of cooperation as well as embarrassment on the part of the adolescent. Issues such as appropriate reactions to peer pressure, decision making, and questions about future protection should be discussed, if not by the nurse, then by an appropriate other.

Girls particularly may have many questions about the effects of sexually transmitted disease on their childbearing potential. Realistic explanations by the physician and nurse are essential for the health of future children. This problem is especially pertinent when there is a diagnosis of genital herpes, since a normal vaginal delivery is unlikely during an exacerbation of the condition. Nurses need to remember that these problems will surface again as decisions about marriage and family are made, and the nurse might therefore provide a list of resources for subsequent reference.

Home Care and Health Maintenance Needs Certain aspects of urinary tract conditions require special attention as the child prepares to go home. (For detailed discussion of general discharge teaching see Chapter 29.)

The physical care of urologic equipment at home requires understanding of simple aseptic technique and infection control. Procedures for dressings or irrigations at home should be taught early in the hospitalization so that all learners will have ample opportunity to return the demonstration and gain confidence by repetition. For example, a young child discharged with home catheterization can eventually be taught to do the procedure alone. Meanwhile, both parents should be taught catheterization technique, which in the home is perhaps simpler than with hospital equipment.

Recently physicians have not been requiring aseptic technique for catheterizations performed at home. The procedure then merely involves a clean technique requiring no gloves, clean equipment (catheter and collection container), and thorough handwashing. After cleaning the area an extra application of povidone–iodine preparation is recommended before inserting the catheter. Expensive equipment is not required. Water-based diaper wipes can be used for cleaning with a clean plastic cup for collection. Catheters can be ordered through most medical supply stores.

To keep a routine check on urinary tract infections, home urine culture kits are available. They give results in 24 hours and, if positive, should be followed by a laboratory test for culture and sensitivity.

Older children and adolescents should be encouraged to participate fully in their own care. There is no reason why self-catheterization cannot be performed at school, thus allowing for full school participation without being singled out as different. Although ureterostomies and ileal loop conduits are not commonly seen, children can be responsible for their own cleanliness and appliance changes. Prevention of skin breakdown is important, and the child should demonstrate competence in skin care.

Children with genitourinary problems are often at risk because of the nature of the illness. Precautions necessary to protect the child's fragile renal function often include restrictions from vigorous play and from active sports. The nurse can suggest alternate activities that are suited to the child's personality and offer less physical risk. Life sports, such as tennis or swimming, allow for both aerobic exercise and team participation (see Chapter 19).

Because some genitourinary diseases require long-term care such as conditions necessitating dialysis, consideration should be given to the effects on the child's schooling and peer relationships. To ease adjustments, the school nurse and teachers need to be aware of the difficulties. Visiting nurse referrals are most beneficial for support and supervision after discharge from hospital care.

The Child With a Structural Defect Involving the Genitourinary System

Hydronephrosis

Any obstruction of urine outflow causes urine to collect in the renal pelvis and calices, producing a condition known as hydronephrosis. If the obstruction is allowed to continue, intrarenal pressure rises, causing diminished circulation to the kidney. Eventually, there is atrophy of renal tissue leading to renal insufficiency. Obstructions can occur anywhere in the urinary tract but are most common at the ureteral–pelvic junction. Obstruction occurs when an abnormal muscle function within the ureter impairs the flow of urine from the kidney. Pelvic dilatation follows, and further mechanical obstruction occurs. A definite tendency for the left side to be affected exists, but bilateral involvement is often seen (Harrison et al, 1979). Other causes of obstruction include calculi and scar tissue or adhesions from inflammation. A ureterocele, which is an enlarged sac formed by the ureter from stenosis at the bladder–ureter junction, may also be obstructive. Occasionally, the ureter is congenitally obstructed, or there is an ectopic ureter that joins abnormally with the primary ureter, resulting in blockage at the site.

Hydronephrosis can be unilateral or bilateral. The prognosis is directly related to the timing of diagnosis and intervention. If substantial irreparable damage is done to the renal tissue before intervention, chronic renal insufficiency persists. Since many cases of hydronephrosis occur in newborns, advances have been made in prenatal diagnosis with ultrasound. As technology advances and fetal diagnostic studies improve, neonatal hydronephrosis will undoubtedly occur less frequently.

Hydronephrosis is manifested by a variety of clinical symptoms. There may be a decreased urine flow alternating with a sudden outrush as the rising pressure temporarily forces the obstruction aside. A history of repeated urinary tract infections with or without the upper-tract symptoms of flank pain, fever, and chills should indicate follow-up for the occurrence of hydronephrosis. In addition to flank pain, there may be abdominal pain, or a sudden severe pain in the area of the kidney.

Young children may be completely asymptomatic except for a failure to thrive. Failure to thrive without any known or suspected cause should indicate the need for a thorough series of urologic tests. Often the kidneys are large enough to be easily palpable. Such tools as an intravenous pyelogram (IVP), ultrasound, and voiding cystourethrogram (VCUG) assist in locating the obstruction.

Treatment The goal of treatment is to preserve remaining renal function. The surgeon may excise the cause of obstruction (calculi, stricture) or reconstruct structural abnormalities (ectopic ureter, malformed ureter). Urinary diversion may be a temporary measure to decrease intrarenal pressure; it is accomplished by inserting a nephrostomy tube to drain the renal pelvis while awaiting surgery.

Several complex surgical approaches are available to correct ureteropelvic obstruction, including pyeloplasty and ureteropyeloplasty. If these are not feasible, nephrectomy may be considered.

Ureteroceles may be released surgically using an approach through a cystoscope. If this is unsuccessful, an incision may be made directly into the bladder (Scott, 1975).

Nursing Management The child with hydronephrosis may be asymptomatic; however, if the nurse's physical assessment reveals mild discomfort, pain in the abdomen or flank, or diminished urine output, the nurse may suspect the presence of this condition. An accurate history from observant parents may indicate a gradual decrease in the number of voids if the child is still in diapers, but once the child is toilet-trained, this observation is unlikely.

Nursing care for the child with hydronephrosis supports medical interventions that focus on identifying and relieving the urinary stasis. If the child is discharged with a nephrostomy, parents should be adept at care and should be taught to prevent and recognize signs of infection. Postoperative care after surgical reconstruction or excision has been previously discussed. Long-term follow-up is essential.

Exstrophy of the Bladder

Exstrophy of the bladder is a congenital malformation in which the lower portion of the abdominal wall and anterior wall of the bladder fail to fuse during fetal development. Along with this is a separation of the symphysis pubis. The bladder is everted through the abdominal opening, revealing bladder mucosa and observable ureteral orifices. Associated with this in boys is a short penis and epispadias. Other reproductive and/or bowel abnormalities may also be present.

Because of the open bladder, there is constant drainage of urine. The fragility of the mucosa as well as the direct access to the upper urinary tract through the open ureters predisposes the child to frequent infections.

The occurrence of bladder exstrophy is rare with the incidence being 1:30,000 births. The male-to-female ratio is 2:1 (Kelalis and King, 1976). Children with exstrophy of the bladder are unlikely to attain normal urologic status. Simple closure is most often unsuccessful. Achievement of continence without further diversion is unlikely.

Treatment Complete bladder turn-in may be attempted but is rarely successful. Its success usually depends on the amount of exposed bladder and more than one reconstructive procedure. Urinary diversion is the treatment of choice. Ureterosigmoidostomies (anastomosis of the ureters to the sigmoid to allow urinary excretion through the bowel) have generally been replaced by the ileal loop conduit. In this procedure the surgeon resects a small portion of the ileum, anastomoses it to the ureters, and creates an ileostomy. Urine drains through the ostomy into a collecting appliance. Ileal conduit is favored over ureterostomies because it results in a single opening rather than bilateral openings. Reconstructive surgery is performed on the genitals, and cystectomy may be included in the long-range plan.

Nursing Management Exstrophy of the bladder is immediately noticeable at birth. During the newborn assessment the nurse notes the size and extent of the defect, the condition of the mucosa, and the appearance of the surrounding skin (that is, color, amount, and turgor). Nursing interventions are directed toward preserving the integrity of the bladder mucosa and preventing an ascending infection. Frequent dressing or diaper changes will prevent skin breakdown and opportunity for infection. The dressing may consist of a light petrolatum (Vaseline) gauze or a piece of cloth diaper covered with petrolatum. Petrolatum prevents adherence of the dressing to the fragile mucosa.

Dressings should be removed carefully so as to cause minimal bleeding.

Another major nursing intervention during the neonatal period is to support the parents during their grieving process and their adjustment to their child's defect. Many questions and anxieties will surface, not only about urinary functions but also about appearance and the child's future reproductive capabilities.

The child will probably be discharged before any reconstruction is attempted. Discharge teaching will include proper dressing changes, infection control methods, and recognition of signs of infection or altered urinary function. Home care should be adapted from that received during hospitalization. Every attempt should be made to provide a plan of care that is as uncomplicated as possible for the ease of the child and family.

Prevention of trauma to the bladder is of extreme importance as the infant learns to walk. Extra padding in the diaper is helpful if the child is apt to fall. The bladder mucosa is very sensitive, and mild trauma may cause some minor bleeding. Parents of a neonate with exstrophy of the bladder should be alerted to this normal occurrence.

Fluid balance is important to the well-being of any child with a genitourinary problem and the child with this defect is no exception. Extra fluids will be needed in response to high temperature, infection, or hot weather.

After urinary diversion, the parents need to learn proper application and removal of the collection appliance. Because urine is extremely acidic, skin breakdown is a potential threat. Keeping the stoma clean and completely dry before appliance application reduces the chance of leakage. Preparations to toughen the skin may be helpful. A tight, leakproof appliance will not only preserve the skin but also reduce odor, which is a particular embarrassment to the older child. Infection is an ever-present potential.

Parents should be encouraged to promote normal development while protecting the bladder from trauma. They need to be prepared to help their children deal with functional or cosmetic problems. Counseling may be advisable for families having difficulties in this area.

Obstructive Anomalies of the Collecting System

Most anomalies of the urinary collecting system lead to restriction of urinary flow. Although the causes may vary, treatment and nursing management are similar. The most common causes of flow restriction are urethral stricture and posterior urethral valves.

Urethral stricture is a tightening or spasm of the urethral muscle causing restriction of urinary flow. The incidence of urethral stricture is unknown because some cases are so mild that they go undetected. The pathophysiology may be idiopathic or the result of recurrent infections. Prognosis for the child with urethral stricture is determined by the severity, repair, and response of the condition.

Posterior urethral valves are anomalous folds of mucosal tissue in the male urethra opening; their proximity to the bladder may obstruct the flow of urine. Like urethral stricture, the incidence of this condition is unknown because of varying severity. Pathophysiology reveals a congenital defect, possibly the result of the persistent urogenital membrane in utero. The prognosis depends on the severity of the obstruction and the resultant renal damage from the urine reflux.

Treatment The most common intervention for mild stricture is urethral dilatation. Circumcision may also be indicated. Catheterization may be necessary if the condition is acute or if dilatation is initially unsuccessful. Treatment for posterior urethral valves usually requires a long-term indwelling catheterization or surgical excision. The surgical approach usually destroys the extraneous tissue.

Nursing Management Assessment of voiding patterns and observation of the urinary stream is helpful in determining the extent of the flow obstruction. The plan of care is designed to assist in the restoration of urine flow and to prevent urinary stasis and the subsequent development of urinary tract infection. Close supervision of intake and output is essential along with observations of signs of retention (decreased output, bladder distension). If catheter drainage is to be instituted after the child's discharge, teaching should begin as soon as possible. The child should become accustomed to the collecting device, and clothing should be adapted to minimize its appearance.

Reflux Anomalies of the Collecting System

Reflux is a backflow of urine into either ureters or bladder depending upon the anomaly involved. Vesicoureteral reflux (Fig. 39-7) is the reflux of urine from the bladder into the ureters. The cause is a defect in the bladder implantation junctions at the distal portion of the ureters. The result is incomplete closure of the orifices during micturition. After urination the refluxed urine flows back into the bladder. If the amount is large, the child will shortly feel the urge to void again. If the amount is small, it may remain in the bladder and cause stasis, which predisposes the child to the development of urinary tract infection. The ratio of affected girls to boys has been estimated to be 8–10:1 (Kelalis and King, 1976). Black children have a much lower incidence of vesicoureteral reflux without apparent cause.

Urethrovesical reflux occurs when the pressure of a full bladder forces urine into the upper urethra. As pressure is decreased, the urine refluxes into the bladder, bringing with it bacteria from the urethra. Bacteria multiply and result in urinary tract infection. Causes vary, but it is felt that the

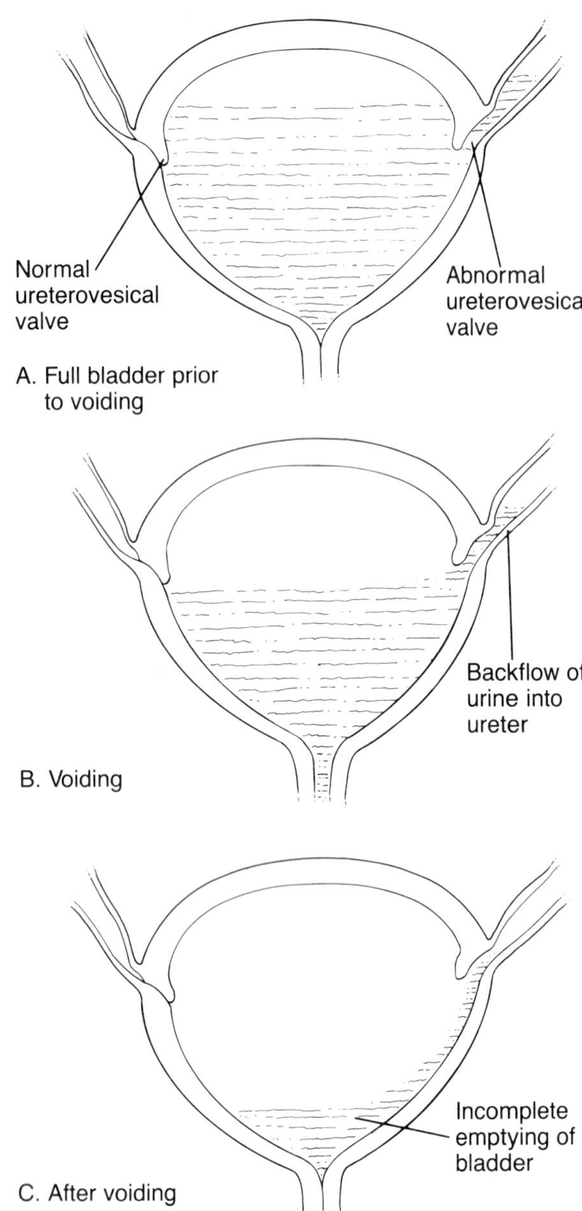

Figure 39-7 Vesicoureteral reflux.

reflux may be due to a disturbance at the inner bladder–urethral junction. Intermittent voiding strongly correlates with this type of reflux (*Kidney and Urinary Tract Infections,* 1971).

Duplication of ureters also may cause reflux in two ways:

1. If both enter the bladder, the upper entry tends toward reflux because of the thinness of bladder musculature at that point.
2. If the two ureters join, there may be reflux at the juncture (Scott, 1975).

The prognosis for reflux is favorable with early detection.

Persistent and repeated urinary tract infections are the most common indicator of reflux. Abnormalities can be detected with IVP, VCUG, and cystoscopy. Assessment of hydronephrosis is necessary since persistent reflux can result in this condition.

Treatment Antibiotics are administered to treat the urinary tract infection. If the child does not respond to several months of medication, surgery may be recommended. Surgical reimplantation of the ureters in vesicoureteral reflux is the procedure of choice. Because it is impractical to describe the many varieties of ureteral reimplantation here, reference to a pediatric urology test is advisable.

Nursing Management Most ureteral reimplantation procedures involve the use of ureteral catheters, or stents, during the postoperative course. The stents are covered by sterile dressings and drain into a collecting apparatus. Initially there will be gross hematuria, but the urine will gradually clear as the postoperative period progresses. In addition to the stents the child will have either a suprapubic or straight catheter. Before discharge all catheters are removed. The child should be followed closely by a urologist after discharge.

Urethrovesical reflux can be minimized by attention to voiding patterns. The child should be encouraged to void in a continuous stream and completely empty the bladder. Nurses need to urge parents to observe for this. School teachers can be warned to allow the child sufficient time and opportunity for voiding during the school day.

Anomalies of the External Structures

Phimosis Phimosis is a condition in which the prepuce is nonretractable from the glans penis. The foreskin contracts over the meatus, creating a diminished opening. Urine stream is obstructed and urination occurs only by force. The condition occurs mainly in uncircumcised boys.

A decreased urinary stream is the first sign. The pressure exerted on the area during urination causes inflammation of the foreskin with an infectious process leading to scarring and further adhesion of the foreskin to the glans.

Circumcision is the treatment of choice. This procedure involves excision of the foreskin to release the glans. Routine preoperative and postoperative nursing care is required. Older boys need careful explanation and demonstration of the procedure. They will need reassurance that the circumcision not only will relieve the problem but also will not destroy the function of the penis, although adjustment will have to be made to the alteration in its appearance. Postoperatively the penis will be covered with a petrolatum gauze. The site will be tender for several days. The child should be encouraged to void despite the burning that may be felt at the operative site.

Phimosis can be easily prevented with good nursing intervention. Neonatal circumcision usually prevents its occurrence but is by no means obligatory. Parents need to be taught to clean an uncircumcised penis properly. The foreskin need not be forcibly retracted for effective cleaning. Forcible retraction can cause inflammation leading to phimosis; thus the foreskin should be retracted gently and only to the point of resistance (Wayland and Higgins, 1982).

There has been much controversy over circumcision. In 1975 the American Academy of Pediatrics upheld an earlier recommendation that circumcision should not be routine (Wayland and Higgins, 1982). Many parental decisions about circumcision are related to sexual perceptions, that is, whether other male members of the family have been circumcised and future similarity to peers. The decision to circumcise may be based on religious custom. Contrary to popular belief, there is inconclusive evidence linking cancer and the uncircumcised male. Nurses therefore encourage prospective parents to decide about circumcision after weighing the evidence and examining their own feelings. The decision should be made before the child is born so as to reduce the pressure of decision making in the hospital setting (Wayland and Higgins, 1982).

Epispadias and Hypospadias Other anomalies of the penis include epispadias and hypospadias. Both of these involve abnormal placement of the urethral meatus. Epispadias also includes an abnormal fusion of the anterior abdominal wall, pubis, and bladder.

The urinary meatus in the child with hypospadias is commonly located on the ventral surface of the penis on the shaft or near the glans. A less common site for the urethral opening is the scrotum or perineum. Chordee, a fibrous line of tissue causing a downward curve of the penis, is associated with this condition. The extent of the chordee depends upon the location of the meatus; that is, the more retrograde the meatus, the greater the amount of chordee.

Epispadias results in a urinary meatus on the dorsum of the penis. Incidence is 1:50,000 births (Harrison et al, 1979). Urinary continence varies with the severity of the deformity. Urethral inadequacy is directly related to penile deformity. Epispadias may be associated with a dorsal chordee.

Urinary diversion is often necessary to achieve continence with epispadias. Management is like that for exstrophy of the bladder.

The incidence of hypospadias is 5:1000 births (Harrison et al., 1979). Genetic predisposition to the development of hypospadias appears to occur in families, sometimes affecting more than one family member. The condition results from incomplete closure of the embryonic tract (Fig. 39-8). A complete genitourinary workup is indicated to rule out associated anomalies.

A satisfactory hypospadias repair straightens the penis; the child is then able to void while standing and ultimately will have the ability to inseminate directly. The single-stage repair is usually more successful than multistaged repairs, although it is not always feasible. In the one-stage repair, a skin graft or flap is used to extend the urethra to the tip of the penis. The chordee is released at the same time.

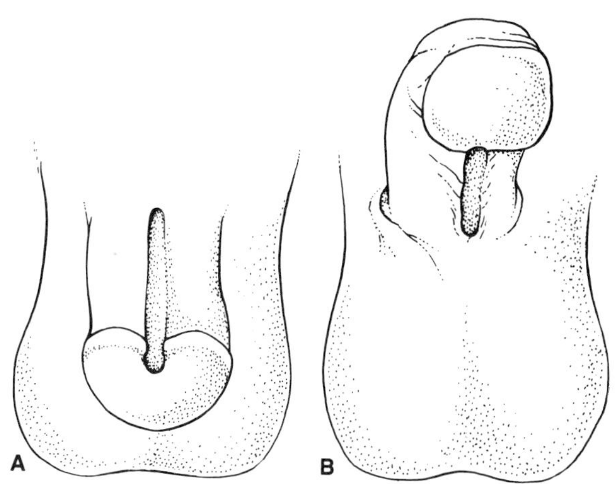

Figure 39-8 Anomalies of the penis. *A.* Penile epispadias with dorsal chordee. *B.* Penile hypospadias with chordee.

If the urethra lies near the scrotum or in the perineum, a multistage repair is best. The chordee is released initially. Subsequently, urethroplasty is performed in stages. This involves removing a flap of penile skin and creating an extended urethra with it. The meatus is then constructed as close to the tip of the glans as possible.

Hypospadias is discovered in the nursery by an alert nurse. Neonatal assessment involves examining the perineum and documenting the location of the meatus. Notation of any alteration in voiding is helpful to support the diagnosis. It is important for the nurse to assess the parent's understanding of the anomaly and the proposed plan for reconstruction. Neonatal circumcision is usually delayed as the prepuce may be needed for corrective tissue.

Because reconstruction takes place during early childhood, fears of mutilation are prominent. The child's developmental, emotional, and psychologic needs are important concerns, as are questions concerning genital manipulation and castration anxiety.

Catheter drainage is common following corrective surgery for hypospadias. Dressing changes must specifically be ordered by the surgeon, as considerable damage can be done if dressing changes are handled improperly. Frequently the dressing is left untouched for several days as the skin graft flap heals.

Hypospadias repairs often involve many stages and repeated surgical procedures may be necessary. It is beneficial to encourage diversional activities within the limits of immobilization. A normally active 3- to 5-year-old will present a particular nursing challenge (see Chapters 28 and 29). The child and family should be well informed, prepared, and involved in the decisions about timing of admissions, or other aspects, whenever feasible.

Cryptorchidism Cryptorchidism, or undescended testicle, is the failure of one or both of the testes to descend into the scrotum. At full-term birth, less than 3% of the male population is affected (Kelalis and King, 1976).

In utero, the movement of testes is initiated by androgenous hormones. Failure to descend may be related to hormonal deficiency or mechanical problems such as a narrow inguinal canal, a short spermatic cord, or adhesions (Saxton, 1983). Since proper function of the testes depends upon a temperature cooler than 98.6 F, failure to descend leads to decreased function and eventual atrophy of the gonad. Undescended testicles may be associated in some cases with an inguinal hernia on the involved side.

Orchiopexy is the preferred treatment. The testis is surgically brought down into the scrotal sac and kept in position by any number of different traction devices such as a button on the outer scrotal surface or an elastic band attached to the thigh. Choice of device is up to the surgeon. If the testis cannot be positioned correctly, the surgeon may elect to remove it to minimize the risk of malignancy. Recently some surgeons have been inserting a prosthetic "ping-pong ball" into the scrotal sac after excision of the testis. This is done purely for cosmetic reasons and may alleviate embarrassment for the older child. The prognosis varies with the timing of the repair. If cryptorchidism persists into adolescence, sterility may result. Risk of malignancy is elevated if atrophy occurs.

Preoperative assessment reveals an empty scrotum with unilateral or bilateral testes palpable in the inguinal canal. Preoperative teaching needs to include a description of the tension device. Postoperatively, the nurse checks the device for proper tautness. Bed rest is maintained until the tension suture is removed, usually in a few days. In conjunction with analgesics, ice packs are often indicated to relieve pain and thus enable the child to tolerate keeping his leg extended.

The Child With Calculi

Calculi are "stones" or any abnormal concretion within the urinary tract and are usually composed of mineral salts. Although renal calculi occur in people throughout the world, the condition is less common in children in the United States. Children living in Asia show a higher incidence, but available data do not explain this phenomenon (Kelalis and King, 1976).

Most renal calculi consist of calcium and are caused by hyperparathyroidism, increased ingestion of vitamin D, and acute osteoporosis—all of which are associated with hypercalcemia. Other causes include immobilization and renal tubular acidosis. Calculi are associated with increased blood calcium levels and can be detected by radiographic studies. The prognosis depends on the severity, location, and success of treatment.

If the child does not have signs of hydronephrosis, calculi may be suspected whenever there is an occurrence of severe radiating flank pain, or renal colic. The pain is associated with nausea, vomiting, pallor, and diaphoresis. There is usually gross or microscopic hematuria.

The noninvasive treatment for renal calculi consists of inserting a Foley catheter, administering analgesics, and "flushing" the urinary tract with large volumes of fluid. If the patient is unable to pass the stone spontaneously following the noninvasive approach, surgical intervention is indicated.

The surgical approach chosen depends on the location of the calculus. Calculi too large to pass through the urethra require surgical removal to prevent deterioration of renal function or infection. If calculi lodge in the ureter, visualization with a cystoscope may permit retrieval. Calculi located in the renal pelvis or calyx must be removed through a flank or lower-abdominal incision.

Assessment of altered voiding patterns may reveal decreased urination indicative of obstruction in the urinary tract. Notation of the location, character, and intensity of the pain assists in the identification of the location of the stone. Occasionally the pain may be radiating; referred pain can lead to confusion of diagnosis since the pain may mimic that of appendicitis or other lower-abdominal conditions. A history of infection combined with altered serum calcium levels and hematuria indicate calculi.

Nursing management is planned to identify and relieve the pain and anxiety caused by the condition. Antibiotics are administered to control infection. Renal colic is so severe that high doses of analgesics may be required.

A major nursing intervention is to strain all urine for stones. A piece of fine-mesh gauze stretched over the top of the urine-collecting bottle and secured with a rubber band will provide adequate straining. Frequent measurements of specific gravity help assess the state of hydration and renal function.

Large amounts of fluid used to flush the system should be encouraged and recorded if ordered. Encouraging fluids will require nursing creativity (see Chapter 29).

Depending on the type, composition, and cause of the stone, a low-calcium diet may be prescribed. Dietary restrictions may be implemented during the child's hospitalization and continued after discharge.

The Child With a Problem of Infection

Acute Urinary Tract Infection

Bacteriuria (the growth of bacteria in uncontaminated urine) indicates the presence of urinary tract infection even if no signs or symptoms of inflammation exist anywhere in the urinary tract. After respiratory infections, urinary tract infections (UTIs) are the most common type of childhood infection. The location of the UTI determines the characteristics of manifestations, which range from relatively mild asymptomatic infections in the lower tract to the more dangerous involvement of the renal parenchyma. Urethritis, cystitis, pyelonephritis, and prostatitis are among the types of UTIs (James, 1976; Kempe et al., 1976).

Except during the neonatal period UTIs occur predominantly in females. During the neonatal period, about 1% of children evidence bacteriuria with about 66% of these cases occurring in boys. This higher incidence correlates with the higher incidence of serious congenital anomalies in boys. In general, girls appear to have UTIs at a rate 30 times higher than boys (Kempe et al., 1976; Kunin, 1977). Because asymptomatic untreated UTIs during pregnancy increase the incidence of acute pyelonephritis, girls with persistent UTIs should be especially careful if they become pregnant (Gillenwater et al., 1979).

Urinary tract infections occur because of factors predisposing the entry of bacteria into the urinary system through upward passage into the urethra or, in infancy, through the bloodstream. Major factors facilitating bacterial invasion through the urethra in children include

1. The shorter urethra in girls vs. boys
2. Proximity of female anus and external genitalia to urinary system
3. Obstructive anomalies of the urinary tract
4. Vesicoureteral reflux with incomplete bladder emptying
5. Chemical irritants such as bubble baths
6. Voluntary retention of urine
7. Catheterization

Adolescents may be prone to UTIs for the following additional reasons:

1. Intercourse or masturbation enhancing transfer of bacteria from genital or anal area to urinary tract
2. Pregnancy
3. Wearing of nylon underwear or pantyhose

Escherichia coli (gram-negative) is the most common infecting organism, causing over 80% of initial infections and 70% of recurrences. Less common agents are *Klebsiella, Enterobacter, Pseudomonas,* and *Proteus.* These tend to be associated with more complex infections such as those related to obstructive anomalies. Gram-positive organisms such as *Staphylococcus aureus* and enterococci account for 5%–10% of UTIs (Chow et al., 1979; Kempe et al., 1976; Kunin, 1977).

Most UTIs are limited to the lower tract. Presenting clinical signs and symptoms vary markedly with gradual or acute onsets, and significant number of children, especially girls, may have asymptomatic bacteriuria.

Infants with urinary tract infections may exhibit signs of sepsis such as vomiting, poor sucking and feeding, lethargy or irritability, fever, jaundice, abdominal distention, and general failure to thrive. Gross hematuria may occur in 5%–10% of infants with acute UTIs (Stickler, 1979).

Young children may have symptoms related to the gastrointestinal tract such as anorexia, vomiting, diarrhea, and lower-abdominal pain. Symptoms also may include foul-smelling urine, urgency, frequency, dysuria (pain on urination), dribbling, and recurrent enuresis (bed-wetting) following a previously controlled dry state. Older children have the more classical picture of lower-tract infection: dysuria, frequency, urgency, and lower-abdominal pain (Chow et al., 1979; Kempe et al., 1976; Stickler, 1979).

Infection in the upper urinary tract (acute pyelonephritis) is evidenced by the signs and symptoms of fever, chills, vomiting, and lower-back pain in the costovertebral angle. Chronic pyelonephritis is actual renal disease resulting from bacterial infection in the kidney, either past or current, the clinical differentiation between pyelonephritis (upper-tract involvement) and cystitis (lower-tract involvement) is frequently difficult in young infants and children (Lorentz and Resnick, 1979).

In addition to urine tests for culture and sensitivity, routine urinalysis is performed. Urinalysis may demonstrate hematuria in cystitis and trace or 1+ proteinuria in pyelonephritis. Pyuria (white blood cells in the urine) may also be present. A consistently alkaline urine may indicate a urea-splitting bacteria such as *Proteus* (Kempe et al., 1976). A first morning specimen is preferred because of greater concentration, and if the specimen is to be transported from home, it should be placed in ice.

Further urologic studies, such as IVP and VCUG, are usually performed on all boys with urinary tract infections. In girls such urologic studies are generally deferred until the second or third episode of urinary tract infection. All cases suggesting pyelonephritis are evaluated with these radiologic studies (American Academy of Pediatrics, 1977).

Treatment Treatment of a urinary tract infection includes the following goals: eradication of the current infection, prevention and treatment of recurrent infections, and identification and correction of structural anomalies (Margileth et al., 1976).

To eradicate the current infection, an appropriate antibiotic must be selected. The choice depends on the infecting organisms, the age and weight of the child, and whether the infection is acute or chronic. Initial acute infections are generally treated for 2 weeks, with long-term treatments reserved for infections recurring within 2 months of the last treatment. Pyelonephritis is treated for a minimum of 6–8 weeks with possible long-term use of a urinary antiseptic following (American Academy of Pediatrics, 1977; Kempe, 1976).

Usually a sulfonamide such as sulfisoxazole (Gantrisin) or ampicillin is the drug of choice in UTIs. Other drugs also commonly used are nitrofurantoin (Furadantin) and cephalexin (Keflex). In nosocomial infections, however, such as those following catheterization, an aminoglycoside antibiotic such as gentamycin or tobramycin may be selected (American Academy of Pediatrics, 1977; Chow et al., 1979). More recently cefaclor (Ceclor) has been used to treat UTIs that are resistant to other antibiotics. Although effective, cefaclor is very expensive.

Presenting symptoms of the urinary tract infection should disappear within 48–72 hours after antibiotics are begun. Many sources recommend a repeat urine culture at this time to determine if the antibiotic chosen is effective. If the antibiotic is effective against this infection, the urine will be sterile. If bacteria are still present in the urine, a new antibiotic must be selected.

One to two weeks following completion of the antibiotic therapy, another urine culture should be obtained. If this culture is negative, the infection is classified as cured. Recurrence is a major problem in girls, however, with 80% having a recurrence within a year. Therefore, a follow-up program is generally recommended. Kunin (1977) recommends this follow-up schedule: once per month for 3 months, then at 3-month intervals for the next 9 months until the first year following the infection. Parental follow-up is essential. Depending on the cause of recurrent UTIs, the child may be placed on a prophylactic regimen of trimethoprim and sulfamethoxazole (Bactrim or Septra).

Nursing Management Supportive care during the infection involves encouraging the child to increase fluid intake and to increase the frequency of voiding. Additional rest may be desired. The nurse also plays a critical role in the collection of urine specimens. Proper procedure for the aseptic collection of clean-voided urine specimens must be followed (see Chapter 29).

If radiologic procedures such as IVPs or VCUGs are required, the nurse prepares the child and family for these intrusive procedures. Considerations of the child's developmental stage, general guidelines for teaching children, and methods for alleviating the stress of intrusive procedures are all noted.

The child hospitalized for pyelonephritis may appear acutely ill. Management of high fever is an important nursing goal. Intravenous therapy and provision for rest assist in the child's recovery. Nurses should have the following information about the antibiotic to be used: dosages, time schedules (that is, daily schedule and relation of medicine to mealtimes), organisms against which the drug is effective, contraindications, and side effects. The nurse strongly emphasizes to the parents the importance of taking all the medicine, even in the absence of symptoms.

Parent teaching should occur in the areas of possible causes for UTIs. Proper perineal care techniques of wiping from front to back should be noted. Children should be encouraged to drink fluids and void regularly. Baths should be avoided for girls, as bacteria easily enter the urinary tract during this process. Harsh detergents or bubble baths serve as chemical irritants to the perineal and urethral areas as well as altering the surface tension of the water, thus facilitating bacterial entry. Sexually active adolescents should be encouraged to urinate both before and immediately after intercourse.

Although the issue of routine urinalysis for children is still argued, routine screening is generally recommended for young children as early as 1–2 years of age with retesting later in early childhood (see Chapters 18 and 21). Dipslides or dip-strip culture methods might be used by the parent in testing first-voided specimens (Kunin, 1977).

Toxic Shock Syndrome

Toxic shock syndrome (TSS), which affects postpubescent young women, was first described in 1978 by a Denver pediatrician who had seen it in several of his pediatric clients. It is a fulminating illness with sudden onset, severe multisystem involvement, and a relatively high fatality rate (8.4%) (Brown, 1981). The disease incidence is rare—6 per 100,000 population in 1981 (Pope, 1981), but the greatest percentage of cases occur in young women or adolescents during their menstrual cycles. Incidence of TSS has also been associated with the use of tampons, particularly those with superabsorbency.

Although a causative organism has not been firmly established, strong evidence suggests that the symptoms and effects are caused by toxins of phage group I *Staphylococcus aureus*. Theories suggest that tampons themselves do not carry the organism but do provide a medium for organism growth. *Staphylococcus aureus* can be cultured from the cervix or vagina.

At some point during the menstrual cycle the patient with TSS demonstrates nausea, vomiting, profuse liquid diarrhea, high fever (above 102° F), severe abdominal pain, and signs of central nervous system alterations—disorientation, irritability, and combativeness. Upon admission to the hospital, signs of hypovolemia with extensive peripheral edema, severe hypotension, and a diffuse erythematous rash are apparent. Laboratory values are altered and reveal elevated levels of blood urea nitrogen, serum creatinine, bilirubin, and creatin phosphokinase (Wroblewski, 1981). Platelet levels become elevated after an initial thrombocy topenia, and leukocytosis with a shift to the left indicates severe bacterial infection (Brown, 1981). Other signs include conjunctivitis, cardiac and respiratory involvement, and acute renal dysfunction. Skin manifestations are followed approximately 10 days later by desquamation similar to that seen in scarlet fever (see Chapter 37). To establish a definite diagnosis of TSS, multisystem involvement must be documented.

Treatment Treatment for TSS is supportive. Massive volume replacement with intravenous colloids is essential to reverse the effects of shock. Pulmonary therapy for lung

Toxic Shock Syndrome Case Definition

1. Fever (temperature above 102 F)
2. Rash (diffuse macular erythroderma)
3. Desquamation (1–2 weeks after onset of illness, particularly of the palms and soles)
4. Hypotension (systolic B/P below 90 mm Hg for adults or below 5th percentile by age for children under 16 years of age, or orthostatic syncope)
5. Involvement of three or more of the following organ systems:
  a. Gastrointestinal (vomiting or diarrhea at onset of illness)
  b. Muscular (severe myalgia or creatine phosphokinase level above 2 × ULN [upper limits of normal])
  c. Mucous membranes (vaginal, oropharyngeal, or conjunctival hyperemia)
  d. Renal (BUN or Cr above 2 × ULN or above 5 white blood cells per high-power field in the absence of a urinary tract infection)
  e. Hepatic (total bilirubin, SGOT, or SGPT above 2 × ULN)
  f. Hematologic (platelets below 100,000/mm)
  g. CNS (disorientation or alterations in consciousness without focal neurologic signs when fever and hypotension are absent)
6. Negative results on the following tests, if obtained:
  a. Blood, throat, or cerebrospinal fluid cultures
  b. Serologic tests for Rocky Mountain spotted fever, leptospirosis, or measles

SOURCE: *Morbidity and Mortality Weekly Report* 29:442, Sept 19, 1980.

involvement, heparin administration in conjunction with blood replacement for platelet and clotting alterations, and dialysis to restore fluid and electrolyte balance may be employed, depending on the seriousness of the patient's condition (Wroblewski, 1981). A course of antibiotic therapy, while it does not appear to alter the clinical course, is believed to prevent recurrences. The use of tampons during menstruation should be strongly discouraged in patients who have experienced toxic shock syndrome. Although most patients recover, some may be left with residual damage to lungs or the peripheral vascular system.

Nursing Management Careful nursing observation is essential during the acute stages of TSS to recognize any deterioration in the patient's condition. Nursing care includes frequent monitoring of vital signs, accurate recording of intake and output, and assessment of signs of impending renal failure or respiratory distress (Wroblewski, 1981).

Toxic shock syndrome in adolescents, as in adult women, can be life-threatening and requires critical-care nursing. The nurse needs to be aware of family anxiety and should be available to answer questions. Information about the treatment should be provided and reassurance given when appropriate.

Discharge preparation includes teaching about perineal hygiene. Education regarding tampon use is an important nursing responsibility and a preventive measure. Girls who have not had TSS can use tampons but should follow these recommendations:

1. Alternate tampons with sanitary pads
2. Do not leave tampons in the vagina longer than 4 hours
3. Avoid tampon use at night
4. Wash hands thoroughly prior to inserting the tampon
5. Contact a physician immediately if sudden fever, vomiting, and diarrhea occur during the menstrual period and immediately remove the tampon

Sexually Transmitted Diseases

Overview Sexually transmitted diseases (STDs), formerly referred to as venereal disease (VD), are defined as those diseases transmitted primarily through sexual contact. These diseases may involve anal–genital, oral, ocular, and other body regions and may be caused by a variety of bacteria, viruses, fungi, and other organisms. Some STDs common within the United States include gonorrhea, syphilis, herpes simplex virus type 2, nongonococcal urethritis, cytomegalovirus, and trichomoniasis (Table 39-4 describes some common STDs).

The traditional name "venereal disease" was derived from Venus, the Roman goddess of love. Since STDs occur as a result of a behavior that is heavily value-laden, psychosocial and legal ramifications are paramount in the health care of people with these problems (Noble, 1979; Yarber, 1978).

The phenomenal increase in STDs since the 1960s has been attributed to many factors. Increased sexual freedom as a result of more permissive morals and social relationships has been noted, along with the opportunity for sexual expression without the continuous possibility of pregnancy because of oral contraceptive distribution has been of key importance. Regardless of the reasons, STDs are occurring at significant levels in all strata of society.

Of primary concern is the extremely high incidence in people 15–24 years of age. The 15- to 19-year-olds in particular pose a difficult problem in that they may have restricted access to health-care facilities acceptable to them and therefore may delay or avoid treatment. The nurse's role in reaching these adolescents and structuring health care environments receptive to their needs is essential (see Chapter 18). Nursing care of adolescents with STDs involves teaching effective methods for prevention.

TABLE 39-4 Sexually Transmitted Diseases

Disease	Causative organism	Epidemiology	Treatment	Specific nursing implications
Condylomata acuminata (genital warts)	Human wart virus	Occurs in sexually active people, transmitted by sexual contact; small papillary structures that enlarge to cauliflower-like masses in genital and perianal area, generally painless unless infected or irritated by friction	Podophyllin ointment or liquid applied directly to warts to dry them; causes sloughing of warts in 2 to 4 days; may need 3 or more treatments; cryosurgery or cautery may be indicated for large masses	Podophyllin must be washed off after 4–6 hours to prevent chemical burns to skin, not to be used with pregnant patients (Martin, 1978; Stewart et al, 1979)
Nongonococcal urethritis	*Chlamydia trachomatis* in 25%–50% of all cases in males (Ripa et al., 1978); 60% unknown etiology (Noble, 1979). T-strain mycoplasma also implicated (Noble, 1979)	Transmitted by sexual contact; small amount of mucoid, watery discharge noted in morning, dysuria, urinary frequency	Tetracycline therapy to both partners	Negative gonorrhea culture indicates nongonococcal infection; if tetracycline therapy is unsuccessful, trichomonas should be suspected; adolescent girls (under 25 years) using contraceptives have higher incidence of chlamydial infections than nonusers (Ripa et al, 1978)
Vaginitis	Foreign bodies, nonspecific organisms, intestinal parasites, UTIs, *Candida albicans*, inadequate perineal hygiene	Common in females of all age groups; allergic vaginitis results from allergen or irritant in vagina such as vaginal sprays, douches, soaps, perfumes, powders; recent change in sexual partner can introduce new flora; intense itching may be associated with a thick white discharge (*Candida*)	Removal of allergen or foreign body; application of topical antifungal agents for 7–14 days to treat *Candida*—mycostatin is most commonly used	Sitz baths may relieve itching and inflammation; *Candida* can be precipitated by antibiotic therapy and those antibiotics associated with it should be avoided; tampons should be removed frequently and attention sought if tampon becomes impossible to remove
Trichomonas vaginalis	Protozoa	Transmitted by sexual contact and possibly indirectly by bathing articles; highest incidence in females age 16–35 years (Noble, 1979); appearance of frothy, yellow-green foul-smelling discharge in copious amounts; severe itching and excoriation of vulva and perineum; asymptomatic in males	Metronidazole (Flagyl) to both partners after positive wet prep	Persons receiving metronidazole should not drink alcohol because of side effects of nausea and vomiting; not to be given during pregnancy
Hemophilus vaginalis	Hemophilus or Corynebacterium	Is present in about 33% of normal females (Noble, 1979); presence of symptoms depends on concentration of organism; scant amount of gray malodorous vaginal discharge; some complaints of itching and burning	Ampicillin 500 mg orally four times a day for 7 days after positive wet prep for organisms	

Preventive Teaching Guidelines for Reproductive Infections

Health teaching in the area of reproductive health is a primary responsibility of the nurse. Some guidelines for discussion include these:

1. Perineal hygiene should be practiced by both partners. Daily baths or showers with particular washing of the genital area may be helpful. Washing after intercourse may be advisable.
2. Both partners should urinate after sexual intercourse.
3. Adolescent girls should practice healthy urinary habits such as wiping from front to back, drinking fluids, and voiding regularly.
4. In order to avoid vaginal irritation, girls should wear cotton, loose-fitting underwear and should avoid bubble baths, hygiene sprays, and douching.
5. If using additional lubrication for intercourse, use contraceptive foams, creams, or jellies. These may provide some protection against sexually transmitted diseases. Petrolatum lubricants like Vaseline should be avoided as they tend to remain in the vagina and may promote infection.
6. Those who are sexually active with more than one partner should try to discriminate carefully and use condoms if at all possible.

Gonorrhea Gonorrhea is the most frequently reported communicable disease in the United States with approximately 550,000 civilian cases reported in 1983 (Centers for Disease Control, 1983). In contrast, there were only approximately 259,000 cases reported in 1960. From 1966 to 1973 reported cases of gonorrhea increased about 12% annually. This phenomenal increase during this period is considered to represent an actual increase in cases in addition to improved detection and reporting. Following 1973, when federally assisted state and local control programs were implemented, the reported case numbers leveled off at less than 1 million cases per year (Centers for Disease Control, 1980).

A large proportion of cases of gonorrhea each year are among teenagers (15–19 years). Gonorrhea has greater reported rates for males than for females, possibly because it is a much more insidious process in females. The incidence of gonorrhea is higher for blacks than whites. The estimated risk of acquiring gonorrhea from a single sexual encounter with an infected partner is less than 25%.

One difficulty in controlling gonorrhea is its rapid incubation period of about 3–5 days. Another problem is the large number of infected individuals who are asymptomatic. An estimate is that 80% of women and 50% of men with gonorrhea are essentially asymptomatic. An additional control problem stems from the development of penicillinase-producing gonococci first noted in 1976 in the United States. There is no immunity to gonorrhea (Noble, 1979).

Gonorrhea is caused by *Neisseria gonorrhoeae,* a gram-negative diplococcus. The gonococcus is a relatively fragile organism that is easily destroyed by heat, drying, or antiseptic application; therefore indirect spread through bedsheets or toilet seats is generally disputed. Gonorrhea is transmitted primarily through sexual contact with an infected partner, and in the neonate it is acquired by passage through an infected birth canal.

The organism can invade any mucosal area but commonly enters the urethra in males and the urethra, endocervix, and Skene's and Bartholin's ducts or glands in females. As many as 60% of girls with genital gonorrhea also have rectal gonorrhea, gonococcal proctitis. Persons engaging in oral–genital intercourse may develop gonococcal pharyngitis.

After exposure, the gonococcus produces an endotoxin, resulting in erythema and edema at the invasion site. A purulent exudate frequently develops. The infection may remain localized or disseminate through tissue extension or blood stream invasion.

The clinical picture varies in postpubescent boys, girls, and prepubescent children. Boys become symptomatic within several days following exposure, exhibiting symptoms of burning and purulent discharge from the urethra. Disseminate gonorrhea can occur but is more common in girls (Noble, 1979).

In postpubescent girls, gonococcal urethritis is rarely the sole manifestation, but girls with gonorrhea may complain of dysuria. Because gonococcal cervicitis is asymptomatic in about 80% of females, detection in adolescent girls is difficult. It may be discovered after a report of an infected contact. Routine cultures or pelvic examinations are unusual for this age group, thus limiting identification for prompt treatment.

Girls may have signs of pelvic inflammatory disease—dysuria, vaginal discharge, lower-abdominal pain, fever, lethargy, and abnormal uterine bleeding. Symptoms of pelvic inflammatory disease generally occur either during or after the menstrual period because menstrual blood is an excellent growth medium for the gonococcus (Martin, 1978; Noble, 1979). Rarely, a disseminated gonococcal infection presents as an arthritis–dermatitis syndrome. Onset of symptoms commonly follows menstruation with fever, chills, and migratory polyarthralgia. Joint stiffness, swelling, and tenderness may occur gradually. Skin lesions appear in conjunction with the arthralgia and occur as a painless, nonpruritic rash on the trunk and extremities.

In children, prepubescent gonorrhea must be investigated for the possibility of sexual abuse although indirect infection is sometimes considered a potential source. Gonorrhea in girls may cause vulvovaginitis, which is an uncommon primary disease in prepubescent girls. Symptoms may include itching or burning on urination, or a stain on the underpants from vaginal discharge may be noted. Ophthalmia neonatorum (gonococcal ophthalmia) is relatively uncommon today because of the instillation of 1% silver nitrate solution into the neonate's eyes. If infection occurs, however, symptoms occur from 48 hours postdelivery until the end of the first week. The affected eye exhibits pus between the lids, which are edematous and erythmatous on the inner surfaces. The conjunctiva becomes infected.

All persons tested for gonorrhea should have VDRL tests also. Incubating syphilis occurs in 3%–10% of all persons with gonorrhea (Martin, 1978).

Following confirmation of the diagnosis through cultures from the infection sites, treatment is initiated. Treatment for uncomplicated gonorrhea in both sexes is administration of a large single dose of penicillin (that is, 4.8 million units of aqueous procaine penicillin G intramuscularly or 3.5 g ampicillin orally). If the gonorrhea is penicillin-resistant, treatment includes tetracycline or another broad-spectrum antibiotic. Probenecid, a renal tubular blocking agent, is also given to increase effectiveness by delaying urinary excretion. Follow-up cultures are done in males 7 days after treatment and 7–14 days after treatment in females.

Gonorrhea in young girls can lead to chronic pelvic inflammatory disease and subsequent adhesions of the fallopian tubes. The incidence of infertility from tubal adhesions is relatively high. When counseling young adolescent girls about STDs, nurses need to explain the risks involved with repeated episodes. Prevention is accomplished by thorough education (see Chapter 18).

Herpes Genitalis Herpes simplex type II virus (HSV-2) is the second most common STD in the United States. Herpes simplex type 2 is the virus responsible for most genital herpes lesions; type 1 is responsible for most herpes lesions above the waist. Crossover between these viruses, however, does occur (Nahmias, 1973). Because genital herpes is not yet a reportable disease, accurate incidence statistics are difficult to obtain. The incidence of asymptomatic genital herpes may range as high as 45%.

The human herpes viruses are divided into the following four categories: (a) HSV-1 and HSV-2; (b) cytomegalovirus; (c) Epstein-Barr virus; and (d) varicella-zoster virus. All herpesviruses possess the ability to remain latent within the host, thus causing recurrences throughout life (Edwards, 1978).

Genital herpes is transmitted by direct contact with active virus; therefore, the infection can be spread as long as lesions are in the healing process (Martin, 1978). Genital herpesvirus infections have been linked with carcinoma of the cervix through three areas of research although more research needs to be done to confirm a definite correlation. First, about 80%–100% of persons with invasive cervical cancer have antibodies to herpes simplex virus type 2. Also, significant numbers of women with cervical dysplasia and carcinoma in situ have these antibodies. Second, a correlation between high herpes antibody titers and early onset of sexual activity and multiplicity of sexual partners has been noted. Third, viral nucleic acids and proteins have been obtained from persons with invasive carcinoma and carcinoma in situ. Herpesvirus also has been noted to be carcinogenic in vitro. Therefore, genital herpes appears frighteningly dangerous in its possible initiation of a process resulting in cancer following several years of latency (Martin, 1978; Noble, 1979).

If genital herpes infection occurs within the first 20 weeks of pregnancy, about 50% of pregnancies will result in spontaneous abortion. If an infection occurs after 20 weeks, prematurity is a significant risk. After 32 weeks' gestation, there is a 60% risk of neonatal herpes if a vaginal delivery occurs or if more than 4 hours after membrane rupture, a cesarean is performed. Neonatal herpes is extremely dangerous as it is often fatal or responsible for severe brain damage and other serious congenital anomalies (Martin, 1979; Noble, 1979).

Herpes genitalis may be primary, latent, or recurrent. Primary infections tend to be the most severe and often occur in adolescents and young adults. Within 3–7 days after exposure, the person experiences fever, malaise, anorexia, and a burning sensation or paresthesia (numbness) in the genital area prior to eruption of lesions. The lesions in primary herpes may involve the penis, scrotum, vulva, perineum, vagina, cervix, and perianal area. Initially, vesicles appear but rupture quickly to create shallow painful ulcerations. These lesions may coalesce to form extensive ulcerated areas of the vulva and perianal areas. As the vesicles appear, pain and tenderness become primary symptoms. Other manifestations include inguinal lymphadenopathy, leukorrhea, cervicitis, and dysuria or urinary retention. The primary lesions last 3–6 weeks (peaking at 10–14 days) and are followed by spontaneous healing without residual scarring or ulceration (Martin, 1978; Noble, 1979).

Some persons are fortunate enough to experience a latent form of the virus with no recurrence. However, there appears to be at least a 60% recurrence in the first 6 months after a primary infection with over 75% of persons experiencing a recurrence within 1 year afterward (Corey et al., 1976). An average is about four recurrent episodes per year at uneven intervals (Lukacs and Corey, 1977). Recurrences tend to occur 1–3 months after the primary infection and are milder infections usually affecting the same areas as the initial infection. Before a recurrence, the person notes a tingling or burning sensation in the affected area. Vesicles from 1–5 mm then appear, again progress to ulcerated form within 3 days, and resolve completely in 7–10 days. Unlike primary infections, recurrences rarely exhibit systemic symptoms or regional adenopathy. Recurrences are thought to be triggered by such factors as fever, emotional stress, premenstrual tension, systemic infectious disease, or neurologic manipulation of the trigeminal nerve. A common explanation of these recurrences is that the herpesvirus lies dormant within the sacral ganglia and travels down the nerve fibers to the affected genital area when infection recurs.

A particular transmission problem is in the often asymptomatic infected female with herpetic cervicitis. She unknowingly transmits the infection to her sexual partners. Infected males, however, usually avoid intercourse because of the pain and visibility of the lesions (Edwards, 1978).

Diagnosis of genital herpes is generally made upon the basis of clinical findings, although the Tzanck test may be performed. Unfortunately, there can be no distinction between varicella-zoster and genital herpesviruses. If needed, virologic cultures or blood titer levels of herpes antibody can be done to confirm the diagnosis.

There is no cure at present, and therefore treatment is designed to relieve symptoms. The most effective treatment aims to reduce pain and fever while promoting lesion healing through drying. Acetaminophen and aspirin may reduce fever and pain. Sitz baths and heat lamp usage may promote comfort and drying. Topical creams tend to delay healing (Lukacs and Corey, 1977).

Photoinactivation of the virus with a tricyclic dye such as neutral red or proflavine has been used to reduce pain and lengths of attack. The potential carcinogenicity of this treatment, however, has discouraged use (Martin, 1978; Noble, 1979). A variety of other treatments have been attempted; these include antiviral agents and immunotherapy.

Pregnant women with genital herpes should have cesarean deliveries to reduce risk to their infants. Adolescent girls must be made aware of the need for cesarean deliveries.

Girls with genital herpes should be advised to have Papanicolaou smears done every 6 months because of the potential for cervical cancer. Persons with herpes also should be counseled to reevaluate their sexual activity patterns and avoid intercourse during recurrences. Because the incidence of herpes in increasing, and widespread publicity has brought it to public attention, greater efforts have been directed toward emotional support of the person with herpes. Herpes support groups are common. Because of its incurable nature and lifelong course, problems relating to decisions about marriage and family are inevitable. Sympathetic nurses can allow affected adolescents to express their feelings and can assist them to clarify their thoughts regarding these important issues.

Syphilis Syphilis is the third most frequently reported communicable disease in the United States. There were 24,874 reported cases of primary and secondary syphilis in 1979 with approximately 40% of these cases occurring among 15- to 24-year-olds (Centers for Disease Control, 1980). In 1983, 19,733 cases were reported (Centers for Disease Control, 1983). The ratio of frequency between males and females is 2:1. Syphilis is a hazard to contacts of prostitutes, homosexuals, and bisexuals and their partners (Noble, 1979).

Syphilis is a systemic infectious disease caused by *Treponema pallidum,* a spirochete. Acquired syphilis is disseminated by sexual contact between a site of infection and a break in the mucous membrane or skin of any body area, particularly in the genitalia, anus, or pharynx. Congenital syphilis occurs via transplacental infection after the fourth month of pregnancy (Chow et al., 1979; Noble, 1979).

A single chancre generally appears at the site of contact about 3 weeks (range of 10–90 days) following exposure. As long as moist lesions are present or the disease is untreated during the primary, secondary, or latent stages, the disease is communicable. All ages are at risk, and no immunity is granted after infection. An estimate is that an uninfected sexual partner has a 30% chance of acquiring syphilis following a single exposure (Chow et al., 1979; Noble, 1979).

Syphilis is one of the more difficult to recognize of the STDs because of its variety of presentation in its different stages. The first clinical stage is primary syphilis, which is primarily characterized by the chancre. The chancre is a painless indurated ulcer often having a raised border. It may occur at any point of infectious contact; therefore it may be clinically unapparent if located in the pharynx, vagina, or anus (Chow et al., 1979; Noble, 1979).

The chancre is frequently accompanied by enlarged firm and painless regional lymph nodes (bubo). With or without treatment, the chancre resolves within 3–5 weeks and, if untreated, secondary syphilis results from 6 weeks to 6 months following initial infection. Secondary syphilis presents a varied picture and lasts 2–6 weeks in an untreated person. Recurrences of secondary syphilis during a 2-year period occur in 25% of cases. Persons are infectious during this secondary clinical stage (Chow et al., 1979; Noble, 1979).

The most common symptom of secondary syphilis is a nonpruritic, dry, symmetric rash associated with generalized nontender lymphadenopathy. Other symptoms include a flulike syndrome of malaise, fever, anorexia, and headache; patchy alopecia; condyloma latum (moist papules) in the anogenital area; mucous patches in the oropharynx; and iritis (Martin, 1978; Noble, 1979).

The disease is considered latent when the clinical manifestations of secondary syphilis disappear. Outcomes of this stage are extremely variable with about one-third of persons with latent disease developing late, or tertiary, syphilis. The latent stage is diagnosed on the basis of reactive serologic tests. The latent disease is considered infectious to sexual partners and to the fetus of an infected woman (Martin, 1978; Noble, 1979).

Late, or tertiary, syphilis may occur within 2–30 years after the initial infection in approximately one-third of all persons with untreated syphilis. The forms of late syphilis include (a) benign (with gummas); (b) neurosyphilis (including general paresis, tabes dorsalis, blindness, psychosis); and (c) cardiovascular (that is, aortic dilatation, saccular aneurysms).

Congenital syphilis is thought to be acquired through placental transfer after the eighteenth week of pregnancy. Women with latent syphilis may deliver infected infants with no clinical manifestations. Therefore, the key management tools in pregnant patients are quantitative serologic tests for syphilis (Noble, 1979). A VDRL test is commonly done during the sixth or seventh month of pregnancy.

Early congenital syphilis appears before 2 years of age. Following delivery, bullous skin lesions may occur. Later, a diffuse symmetric maculopapular rash primarily found on the face, palms, and soles occurs. Rhinitis may present in the first week with a mucoid discharge often hemorrhagic, which is highly infectious. After 1 month of age, the most common single finding is osteochondritis of the long bones noted by radiographic examination. About two-thirds of these infants evidence hepatosplenomegaly and most experience a self-limited hemolytic anemia. Abnormal cerebrospinal fluid examinations will be noted in about 50% of these infants (Chow et al., 1979; Noble, 1979). The VDRL and fluorescent treponemal antibody absorption tests provide positive diagnosis of syphilis.

Penicillin is the drug of choice in all stages of syphilis. Following treatment of primary and secondary syphilis, VDRL tests should be done at 3-, 6-, and 12-month intervals. The VDRL test becomes negative 6–12 months after treatment of primary syphilis and 1–2 years after treatment of secondary syphilis.

Nursing management includes encouraging adolescents to avoid sexual relations with unknown partners. If there is any question of exposure, a VDRL test should be performed.

The Child With a Problem With Filtration of Wastes

Acute Glomerulonephritis

Acute glomerulonephritis (AGN) is an immune complex disease that occurs in response to a previous invasion of group A beta-hemolytic streptococcus. The precipitating streptococcal infection is commonly in the upper respiratory tract or skin (impetigo). Theories about causes of AGN differ, but the prevalent theory indicates that AGN may involve an autoimmune response (see Chapter 37).

The antigen is similar to that of the membrane of renal glomeruli. Autoimmune complexes lodge in the glomerulus and Bowman's capsule, leading to inflammation and obstruction. This process causes decreased glomerular filtration and tissue injury at the site. Consequently, less sodium and water are passed to the tubules for reabsorption and excretion; red blood cells and casts are excreted. The kidneys enlarge, and sodium and water are retained, leading to edema. Because of the increase in extracellular plasma volume, protein is excreted in the urine.

The incidence varies with the environmental prevalence of streptococcal strains. For instance, because more children are affected by respiratory streptococcal infections in the winter, disease incidence rates are elevated at that time. The disease also is more common in boys in early childhood. The prognosis for children with AGN is generally favorable with the disease resolving spontaneously after a period of several weeks.

Hematuria and mild periorbital edema may be the first clinical manifestations. The urine may appear grossly bloody or be a dark brownish color (cola colored). Urinalysis reveals white blood cells, red blood cells, protein, and cellular casts. There is an associated increase in urine specific gravity. Blood chemistries are elevated, especially blood urea nitrogen and serum creatinine. There is also an elevated erythrocyte sedimentation rate (ESR), and antistreptolysin titer (ASO); hemoglobin and hematocrit are decreased. As the disease progresses, the child may experience mild generalized edema (often evidenced only by weight gain), oliguria, fever, anorexia, hypertension and, rarely, central nervous system symptoms (headache, seizures). The child is at high risk for developing pulmonary edema or renal insufficiency. Occasionally there may be evidence of a transient nephrotic syndrome.

Treatment Treatment necessitates hospitalization to monitor the disease progress and for recognition and prompt treatment of complications. Antibiotics are prescribed to treat any existing streptococcal infection. Careful and frequent monitoring of urinary output, weight, blood pressure, and blood chemistries helps to determine the fluid requirements. It is important to monitor carefully the fluid and electrolyte balance to reduce the risks of cardiac or renal failure. The child may be confined to bed, although some activity is allowed. Children tend to modify their activities according to their own tolerance. Children manifesting hypertension of over 100 mm Hg diastolic pressure may need antihypertensives; digitalis may be prescribed for circulatory overload (Behrman and Vaughan, 1983).

If renal insufficiency is present, the child's fluid intake is generally restricted. Peritoneal dialysis may be used in cases of severe renal or cardiopulmonary problems.

Increased caloric intake is necessary to decrease tissue breakdown. If renal insufficiency is demonstrated, a low-potassium diet is recommended. Other dietary restrictions, such as low-protein or low-salt diets, vary but are generally deemed unnecessary. Sensible limitation of protein and sodium is desirable. Diuresis usually begins after several days and is indicative of a resolving disease process.

Nursing Management The nurse assesses the family's awareness of the precipitating streptococcal infection. Physical examination identifies any clinical manifestations such as edema, weight gain, hematuria, and elevated blood pressure.

The goal of nursing management is to preserve renal integrity and prevent congestive problems. Strict monitoring of intake and output is essential, as is daily weight measurement. Vital signs, serum electrolyte values, and urine examination results are all good indicators of the status of renal function. The child should be observed for signs of further renal deterioration such as diminished output or a change in laboratory values. Additionally, anxiety relief measures and diversional therapy assist in the child's acceptance of the disease.

Discharge preparation includes teaching child and family to take blood pressures. Follow-up pressures are needed to confirm renal integrity. Parents may need to strip-test the urine for blood, although hematuria may be present to some degree for several weeks after other symptoms have disappeared.

Prevention of infection is important during the recovery period, as any infectious process will create excess strain on the kidneys. The parent must be cautioned to notify the physician prior to any dental or oral procedures since streptococcal infections are a danger with these procedures. Although recurrences are rare, they are possible, and oral antibiotics are prescribed as a precautionary measure for oral procedures.

Acute glomerulonephritis is usually a self-limiting disease resolving in approximately 14 days. Although further renal difficulties are uncommon, the child and family need to be alert to signs of renal complications. Long-term follow-up to assess renal status is necessary.

Nephrosis—Nephrotic Syndrome

Nephrosis is a syndrome, a group of conditions, characterized by proteinuria, hypoproteinemia, hyperlipemia, edema, ascites, and decreased urine output. Although its etiology is obscure, it is felt to be a result of an alteration of the glomerular membrane making the membrane more permeable to the passage of protein. Plasma proteins (particularly albumin), which ordinarily are too large to pass through the glomerular capillary walls, enter the tubule and are excreted in the urine (causing proteinuria). The altered oncotic pressure from the protein shift causes lowered plasma volume (hypovolemia). This hypovolemia activates the production of renin and angiotensin to stimulate adrenal secretion of aldosterone. Aldosterone in turn increases the reabsorption of sodium and water in the distal tubule. Additionally, lowered osmotic pressure of the blood triggers the production of ADH, thus further increasing the reabsorption of water in an attempt to counter the hypovolemia. These factors along with a generalized movement of plasma into the interstitial spaces result in edema.

Theories of the cause of hyperlipemia vary. The increase in blood lipids, especially cholesterol, may be due to metabolic error or may be an increase in production secondary to lowered serum albumin.

The course of the disease consists of exacerbations and remissions over a period of weeks to years. Treatment effectively shortens exacerbations. Nephrotic syndrome is occasionally seen in neonates as a manifestation of an inherited trait, but it is rapidly fatal. The disease also occurs secondarily to other disease entities such as glomerulonephritis, lupus erythematosus, diabetes mellitus, and allergic responses. In the large majority of children with nephrosis, however, the cause is ideopathic. The prognosis is somewhat unpredictable, as the disease may recur, although not always with increased renal damage.

Insidious or fulminating edema is usually the first sign of nephrosis. Edema may be periorbital but is worse in the scrotum and abdomen (where it causes ascites). Affected children have such severe generalized edema that they experience dramatic weight gain. In addition to edema the child is pale, fatigued, and anorexic. Gastrointestinal symptoms may be present, and the ascitic abdomen demonstrates visible networks of blood vessels.

Urinary output is decreased. The urine may be frothy from increased fat excretion and has an elevated specific gravity. Urinalysis reveals elevated protein excretion, as much as 30–40 g of plasma protein per day (Vick, 1984). Serum levels of blood urea nitrogen and creatinine are usually normal unless there is associated renal disease. The longer the edema lasts, the greater the chance of permanent renal damage. Blood cholesterol levels are increased because of the increase in circulating blood lipids. The ESR is elevated.

Children with nephrosis often experience respiratory distress from the fluid overload, and they demonstrate an increased susceptibility to infection probably secondary to the decrease in plasma protein. Exacerbations of edema are often subsequent to a recent infection. Malnutrition and muscle wasting can occur as a result of protein depletion but may not be noticed until the edema disappears.

Treatment Treatment is directed toward decreasing the excretion of urinary protein and controlling edema. Additional goals include infection prevention, restoration of metabolic balance, prevention of renal damage, and correction of malnutrition. The treatment is effected by the initiation of corticosteroid therapy to resolve the edema quickly. The child is maintained on steroids up to 12 months at the physician's discretion. Other pharmacologic therapy includes antibiotics for bacterial infections and thiazide diuretics during the edematous stage. Immunosuppressive drugs may be prescribed alone or in conjunction with steroids for children who do not respond well to steroids alone. In some instances anticancer drugs such as cyclophosphamide (Cytoxan) are effective in initiating remission.

To prevent or control malnutrition, a diet high in protein is desirable. Salt should be avoided. A decrease in the serum cholesterol level and a drop in the ESR are indicative of remission (Behrman and Vaughan, 1983).

Nursing Management The nursing care for the child with nephrosis is similar to care for the child with glomerulonephritis, for much of the emphasis is on supportive measures. Unfortunately, nephrosis can be a much lengthier process and the child may experience the realities of chronic illness (see Chapter 30).

The classical physical appearance of the child with nephrosis is one of lethargy, edema, pallor, and fatigue. Nursing management of these children therefore emphasizes rest and comfort measures with conservation of energy.

An accurate intake and output record along with careful and frequent weight monitoring assist in the assessment of the progress of the disease. Frequent urine checks for the presence of protein are essential. Measurements of abdominal girth correlate with the relative amount of edema. Significant changes must be assessed and reported to the physician.

The child with nephrosis requires scrupulous skin care because a break in skin integrity can easily cause infection. Frequent position changes are essential. Untrained children need meticulous perineal care because urine acidity predisposes the skin to breakdown. Diapers, whether worn or used as pads, must be changed as soon as they are wet. Some of the newer plastic disposable diapers have extra layers to keep moisture from contacting the perineal area. Because of severe scrotal edema, pressure from a diaper may be extremely uncomfortable. In such cases, alternatives can be explored that allow for containing urine without the constriction. The skin around the scrotum should be gently cleaned and allowed to dry thoroughly to minimize skin breakdown. In some circumstances a scrotal support may be necessary.

Diversional activities and school work may be encouraged while the child remains in bed. If the course of the illness becomes prolonged, more creative approaches to deal with the problems of long-term immobility are required.

As steroid therapy is indicated in the management of the child with nephrosis, the child must be monitored for drug side effects. Unfortunately, many of the side effects of steroid therapy are unpleasant and make the child more uncomfortable. (See Chapter 37 for discussion of steroid therapy.) The weight gain associated with this therapy is often localized in the trunk and face, causing noticeable changes in body contour and a feeling of self-consciousness in the child. The nurse therefore allows ventilation of feelings about altered body image and about the chronicity of the disease (see Chapter 30).

The potential for ulcers and gastrointestinal bleeding also warrants close surveillance in the child receiving steroids. Antacids administered in conjunction with the steroids help to lessen gastrointestinal irritation. Stools and vomitus should be tested for the presence of blood. Frequent blood pressure checks enable the nurse to recognize bleeding. It is beneficial to the child and family to know that the side effects of steroid therapy will subside when the therapy is discontinued.

Masked infection can best be detected by regular monitoring of the child's vital signs with close supervision of the child's temperature.

Dietary recommendations present a nursing challenge since it is difficult to encourage an anorexic child to eat the amount of protein required to prevent malnutrition. Small frequent feedings or liquids may be more palatable than larger meals; that is, an ice cream frappe can easily conceal a raw egg for extra protein.

Discharge preparation includes information about medications and their effects and about dietary maintenance. The parent may wish to speak to a dietician to learn about incorporating the high amount of protein required into a palatable menu. Urine monitoring for protein is essential, although the method will vary according to the physician. It is important to emphasize protection from infection, while encouraging normal activities.

Acute Renal Failure

Acute renal failure is a "sudden deterioration in renal functioning that results in abnormalities in body homeostasis" (Rielly, 1983). Contributing factors to the occurrence of acute renal failure in children include history of acute glomerulonephritis, diseases affecting the vascular system, allergic conditions, obstructions, hypovolemia, nephrotic syndrome, toxic drug or chemical exposure, and trauma. The three classes of acute renal failure (Table 39-5) have different causes and resolutions; accurate differential diagnosis therefore is most important.

Presenting symptoms in the child with acute renal failure include sudden oliguria and alterations in blood chemistries, particularly elevation of the blood urea nitrogen. Other symptoms include fluid and electrolyte imbalances, particularly hyperkalemia; gastrointestinal disturbances; anemia; increased susceptibility to infection from a depressed immune system; problems due to fluid retention; and urine with a specific gravity of 1.010 or less (Gralton, 1981).

Treatment Treatment of a child with acute renal failure depends on the underlying cause and contributing diseases. Interventions may be directed toward fluid and electrolyte replacement, removal of obstructions, management of hypertension, and treatment of infection. Specific treatment measures include fluid restriction (unless the cause is hypovolemia), surgical removal of obstructions, dialysis to promote more efficient urinary excretion and to correct electrolyte imbalances, and nutritional therapy—diet high

TABLE 39-5 Causes of Acute Renal Failure

Classification	Pathophysiology and manifestations	Nursing implications
Prerenal	Occurs as a result of massive extracellular fluid loss or loss of circulating blood volume from such conditions as hemorrhage, vomiting, and diarrhea; fluid volume depletion activates the renin-angiotensin-aldosterone mechanisms to conserve water and sodium from the tubules; decreased glomerular filtration rate from fluid loss causes decrease in urinary output (oliguria); compensatory constriction of renal blood vessels can result in tissue damage to renal cortex	Can be differentiated from renal failure by intravenous administration of 0.9% saline solution, 10–20 mL/kg of body weight over 20–60 min. If child voids 6–10 mL/kg/h within 1–2 hours, test results are positive for prerenal disease (Rielly, 1983). *Caution:* not to be attempted in children suffering from congestive heart failure, hypertension, sodium-related edema, and respiratory distress. One differential laboratory test includes measurement of fractional excretion of sodium—the measure of tubular sodium-ion reabsorption. Value of less than 1 indicates prerenal disease (Rielly, 1983). This classification is reversible with fluid and electrolyte replacement
Postrenal	Caused by an obstruction distal to the tubules that decreases urine flow; symptoms include complete cessation of urinary flow or variations in urinary output; there may be difficulty initiating or terminating urination	Reversible with correction of obstruction
Renal—Acute Tubular Necrosis	Acute ischemic injury—occurs as a result of fluid volume deficits, hemolysis, and infections that affect intravascular coagulation. Alterations in coagulation result in hypoxia and tissue death to renal tissue and subsequent necrosis of the tubule	Amount of damage to renal tubules and basement membrane determines prognosis
	Acute nephrotoxic injury—renal tubular insult follows exposure to drugs, and toxic chemicals; injury to proximal tubules from lesions caused by toxins results in tubular necrosis	Condition of the tubular basement membrane determines prognosis

in carbohydrate and low in protein, since the kidney's ability to manage proteins is impaired.

There are three distinct recovery phases. The *oliguric phase* shows a marked decrease in urinary output over a 24- to 48-hour period lasting for approximately 7–14 days. The child's blood urea nitrogen and serum creatinine levels increase. The blood urea nitrogen level rises 10–20 mg/100 mL/24 hours and the creatinine 0.5–1.0 mg/100 mL/24 hours (Rielly, 1983). If the cause of the acute renal failure is not hypovolemia, hypervolemia is a common clinical manifestation. The major complications from fluid overload are congestive heart failure and pulmonary edema (their treatment and nursing management are discussed in Chapter 35). Hyperkalemia may cause cardiac irregularities; dietary potassium is usually restricted. The child may also experience metabolic acidosis (see Chapter 33). Because of the alteration in the kidney's production of erythropoietin, a substance that stimulates bone marrow production of red blood cells, the child may experience anemia as evidenced by lowered hematocrit and hemoglobin. The elevated blood urea nitrogen can also alter other blood components, resulting in hemorrhage and further contributing to anemia. Children with acute renal failure can have a decrease in T-lymphocyte production, which makes them more susceptible to infection (see Chapter 37). Antibiotics may be prescribed but, unfortunately, they increase the work of an already compromised kidney.

The second phase of acute renal failure, the *diuretic phase,* is marked by a sudden increase in urinary output followed by 4–7 days of further, more gradual output increases. The blood urea nitrogen level continues to rise. Late in this phase the large amount of urine excretion is associated with excessive excretion of sodium and potassium, resulting in electrolyte imbalance, the major complication of this phase. A decrease in the blood urea nitrogen level signals beginning resolution.

The *recovery phase* lasts 2–3 months or for as long as a year. Tubular function returns, and all laboratory values return to normal. Some children are left with residual kidney damage, and complete recovery depends on resolution of the problem that originally triggered the acute renal failure. The child with acute renal failure is usually cared for in a critical care unit until into the recovery phase.

Dialysis Some children with acute renal failure require dialysis to restore homeostasis and correct electrolyte and acid–base imbalances. Indications for treatment by dialysis are

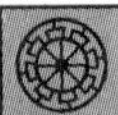

NURSING CARE GUIDE Child With Acute Renal Failure

Nursing diagnosis	Interventions	Evaluation
1. Cardiac irregularities subsequent to hyperkalemia	Monitor ECG and observe for prolonged P-R interval and tall, peaked T waves	Child's potassium values are within normal limits, with no signs of hyperkalemia
	Check laboratory electrolyte values (therapy begins when potassium is 5.5–6 mEq/L)	
	Observe for other signs—muscle weakness, numbness, and tingling, decreased blood pressure	
	Restrict dietary potassium (see Chapter 33)	
2. Alteration in fluid balance—hypervolemia	Observe for signs of congestive heart failure and pulmonary edema (see Chapter 35)	
	Take frequent vital signs, particularly blood pressure, as often as every 15 minutes during periods of acute hypertension	Child's vital signs are stable with blood pressure within normal limits
	Accurately observe and record intake and output; measure urine pH and specific gravity every hour	Child has diuresis; urine pH and specific gravity and within normal limits
	Weigh frequently—need to be extremely accurate, so same scale and clothing should be used	Weight loss of 0.5%–1% per day indicates successful treatment during oliguric phase (Rielly, 1983)
	Severely restrict fluid intake; this may be followed by encouragement of fluids during diuretic phase	Daily fluid intake is based on estimation of child's weight and fluid output (Rielly, 1983)
	Explain reasons for fluid restriction using age-appropriate terminology	Sudden increase in urinary output indicates diuresis and causes for reevaluation
	Give frequent mouth care	
	Use distraction techniques where necessary to divert child's attention from fluid restriction	
3. Associated electrolyte imbalances—hypocalcemia and metabolic acidosis	(See Chapter 33)	(See Chapter 33)
4. Energy depletion related to anemia	Conserve child's energy with organized nursing care	Hemoglobin and hematocrit are within normal limits; vital signs are stable
	Allow for maximum rest	
	Monitor blood pressure; examine stool for occult blood and other signs of internal bleeding	
5. Potential for infection	Administer antibiotics if prescribed	Child shows no signs of infection (such as elevated temperature)
	Use strict aseptic technique for dressing changes and catheter care	
	Wash hands frequently	

NURSING CARE GUIDE Child With Acute Renal Failure (continued)

Nursing diagnosis	Interventions	Evaluation
6. Nutritional deficit—decreased carbohydrates and increased metabolic processes leading to protein catabolism	Plan that 25%–40% of nutritional intake should be carbohydrate and fat (Rielly, 1983) Suggest total parenteral nutrition (see Chapter 38) if child is experiencing anorexia, nausea, or vomiting	Child shows no signs of protein catabolism, malnutrition, increased fluid retention
7. Deterioration in renal status as evidenced by anxiety, irritability, seizures, hallucinations, anorexia, nausea, vomiting—uremia	Report any signs of deterioration immediately Use seizure precautions (see Chapter 42)	Child shows no signs of central nervous system involvement
8. Anxiety in child and family	Give frequent explanations of procedures Allow for ventilation of feelings Give reassurance when appropriate Provide for child's developmental needs whenever possible	Family feels that nursing staff is accessible and that all questions will be answered honestly—decrease in anxiety levels
9. Potential for residual kidney damage	Teach family signs and symptoms of recurring kidney problems Encourage family to follow recommendations of physician for follow-up care	Parents understand what to look for and when to contact physician

Unresponsive hyperkalemia
Severe metabolic acidosis
Hypervolemia
Severe uremia
Blood urea nitrogen > 150 mg/100 mL
Congestive heart failure
Serum creatinine > 10–15 mg/dL (Rielly, 1983).

Dialysis is an artificial, mechanical process for removing body wastes and maintaining fluid and electrolyte balance. The underlying principle of dialysis involves the transport of water and other substances through a semipermeable membrane by the mechanisms of diffusion, osmosis, and hydrostatic pressure (see Chapter 33). The semipermeable membrane may be natural, such as the peritoneum, or artificial. Removal of wastes is accomplished by introducing a solution of fluid and electrolytes (dialysate) to one side of the membrane while the other side contacts the child's vascular system. The composition of the dialysate determines the substances that are to be removed. "Dialysate is essentially void of substances that must be removed . . . contains high concentrations of those that must be added . . . and has the same concentration as plasma for substances that will remain at the same concentration" (Rielly, 1983).

There are two major types of dialysis that are used to treat acute renal failure in children—peritoneal dialysis and hemodialysis. The advantages and disadvantages of each are presented in Table 39-6.

Peritoneal Dialysis Peritoneal dialysis is the physical movement of low-molecular-weight substances (such as glucose, electrolytes, and urea) through the semipermeable membrane of the peritoneum, where it comes in contact with the vascular supply of the area. The physician inserts a catheter and trocar into the peritoneal cavity through a small incision midway between the umbilicus and the symphysis pubis. When catheter and trocar have entered the cavity, the trocar is removed, and the catheter is positioned properly and sutured in place. A dry sterile dressing is applied. The procedure can be accomplished under local anesthesia, depending on the age and temperament of the child. The Tenckhoff catheter is commonly used for peritoneal dialysis. It is a Silastic tube with either one or two cuffs that hold the catheter in position. The one-cuff catheter is used for acute dialysis procedures as it is easier to insert and remove (Sorrels, 1981).

TABLE 39-6 Comparison of Hemodialysis and Peritoneal Dialysis

	Hemodialysis	Peritoneal dialysis
Speed	Rapid—up to 8 hours per treatment	Slow—up to 72 hours initially, up to 12 hours per treatment thereafter. Can be advantage in patients who cannot tolerate rapid fluid and electrolyte changes.
Cost	Expensive	Manual—relatively inexpensive; automated—expensive
Equipment	Complex	Manual—simple and readily available; automated—complex
Vascular access	Required	Not necessary, so suitable for patients with vascular problems
Heparinization	Required; systemic or regional	Little or no heparin necessary, so suitable for patients with bleeding problems
Technical nursing skill necessary	High degree	Manual—moderate degree; automated—high degree
Complications (other than fluid and electrolyte imbalances common to both)	Dialysis disequilibrium syndrome (preventable) Mechanical dysfunctions of dialyzer	Peritonitis Protein loss (0.5 g/L of dialysate) Bowel or bladder perforation

SOURCE: Holloway NM: *Nursing the Critically Ill Adult*, 2nd ed. Addison-Wesley, 1984, p. 295.

The dialysis procedure is effected in three stages:

Inflow—gravity infusion of the dialysate into the peritoneal cavity (approximately 10 minutes)

Dwell time—dialysis and equilibration occurs (15–30 minutes or longer according to type and amount of substances to be removed)

Outflow—peritoneal cavity empties and the cycle is ready to begin again if necessary (20 minutes)

Peritoneal dialysis can be accomplished manually (Fig. 39-9) or by machine. Because dialysis is continuous during early stages of acute renal failure, machine dialysis, which automatically cycles dialysate, may be more efficient because it requires less nursing time. As the child's condition progresses, dialysis may be required for a 24- to 48-hour period 3 times a week—intermittent peritoneal dialysis (Rielly, 1983).

Nursing interventions start before dialysis begins with reassurance and support for the child and family. Simple, honest explanations are essential before any and all interventions. A predialysis weight is desirable, and children should empty their bladders before the procedure begins, if possible.

The nurse may be asked to assist with the insertion of the trocar under strict aseptic technique. After insertion of the trocar, the nurse may connect the dialysate bottles (one or two) to it and begin infusion through gravity. After the prescribed length of time for the dialysate to remain in the abdomen has passed, the nurse removes the fluid by placing the bottles lower than the level of the abdomen.

While the dialysis procedure is in progress, it is important that the nurse watch for any evidence of blood or purulence in the dialysate fluid. The nurse also maintains and records an accurate measurement of the intake and output of dialysate. The child's vital signs are generally taken every 15 minutes to hourly, when stable. Any major changes should be assessed and reported to the physician, particularly complaints of abdominal pain, signs of respiratory distress, and any increase or decrease in blood pressure.

The child's weight and serum electrolytes are monitored closely as well as hemoglobin and hematocrit. If the child voids, the nurse measures the urine specimen for glucose, specific gravity, and presence of blood. The child should be observed for signs of hyperglycemia, hypotension, or hypertension. Risks of peritoneal dialysis include infection, perforation of the bowel by the trocar, and pulmonary edema.

The dressing at the trocar site should be changed, under aseptic technique, every 8 hours, or as necessary. The dialysate should be warmed before instillation (to 37 C) to approximate body temperature. Careful attention to and recording of the dialysis time cycle as well as the type and amounts of solution are essential.

With the child lying flat during peritoneal dialysis, nursing interventions should be directed toward comfort measures and providing distraction.

Hemodialysis In hemodialysis, the semipermeable membrane is a sheet of treated cellophane located in a dialysis machine. Blood leaves the body through an artery, circulates through the machine where it contacts the dialysate, and reenters the body through a vein. In a child suffering from acute renal failure, where access to circulation need not be permanent, an external shunt is often used (Fig. 39-10). The ends of the Silastic catheter are sutured into an artery and vein, while opposite ends are brought to the surface of the site (usually the leg in young children). The surface ends are connected to each other by a Teflon connector, and the continuous flow of blood between artery and vein assists in maintaining shunt patency (Saxton et al., 1983). When the child is ready to be dialyzed, the shunt ends are clamped, the connector removed, and the shunt connected to the dialyzer. The shunt is covered by a dry sterile dressing and careful technique is needed when handling the shunt to prevent infection.

The shunt cannulae are to be protected from trauma at all times. The clear cannulae allow visualization of the vascular flow. A bruit may be heard by auscultation directly over the site.

A nonrestrictive but secure dry sterile dressing must cover the shunt. Two bulldog clamps are to be kept attached to the dressing at all times. These are to be available to control hemorrhage if the shunt cannulae should become disconnected. These are essential, as the child may succumb if no means of catheter occlusion is available.

Hemodialysis in children is an extremely delicate metabolic process. The nursing management of the child undergoing dialysis demands an understanding of the biochemical, metabolic, and technical intricacies of the artificial kidney. The nurse functioning in a hemodialysis unit therefore receives extensive orientation and education according to institution protocol.

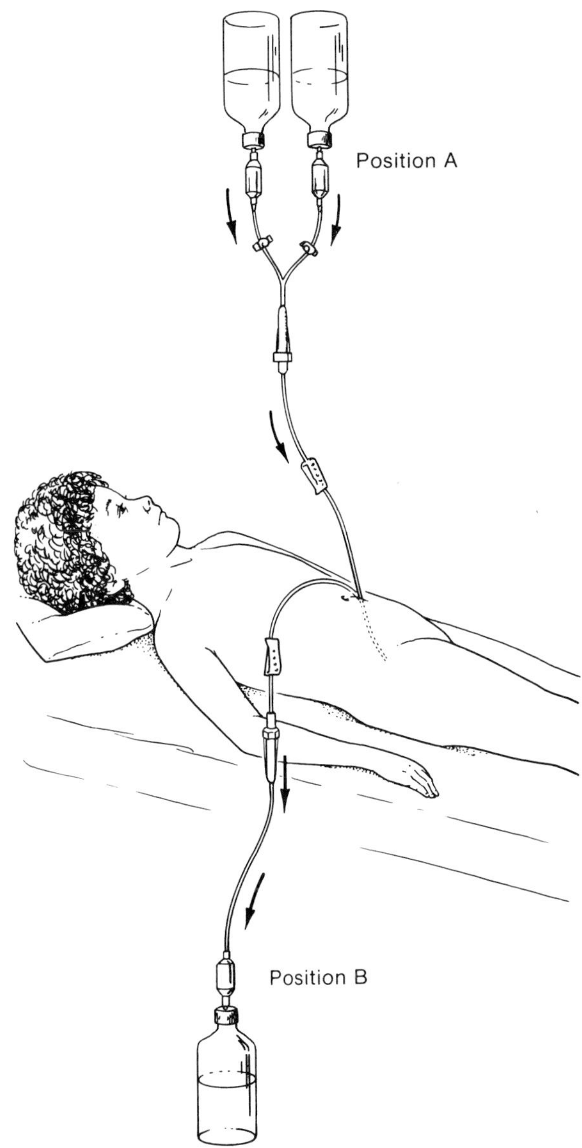

Figure 39-9 Child undergoing manual peritoneal dialysis.

The Child With Chronic Renal Failure

Chronic renal failure occurs as a result of progressive deterioration of the kidneys over a prolonged period of time. It is said to exist when the kidneys are no longer capable of balancing the composition of body fluids. Approximately 80% renal impairment must be present in order for symptoms to become apparent (Lewis, 1981). Symptoms of chronic renal failure are similar to those of acute failure, with elevated blood urea nitrogen levels and associated difficulties; however, since the disease is insidious in onset, the body develops a tolerance to adverse effects of imbalance until such time as kidney damage is severe.

Causes of chronic renal failure are varied and include glomerulonephritis, diabetes mellitus, kidney infections, immune system disorders (particularly autoimmune disorders), metabolic disorders, and obstructions (Lewis, 1981). Several hundred children are affected annually with some type of chronic renal disease; two to three children per million are candidates for dialysis or transplantation.

Chronic renal failure is best divided into three stages. The first stage presents as decreased renal reserve with slightly impaired function, but blood chemistries are not affected. In the second stage, renal insufficiency is noted, and the glomerular filtration rate is less than 50% of normal. At this point blood chemistries are affected with slight elevations of blood urea nitrogen and serum creatinine. In the third stage of chronic renal failure, known as end-stage renal disease, or uremia, the child suffers from azotemia (elevated blood urea nitrogen) and uremia. Renal function

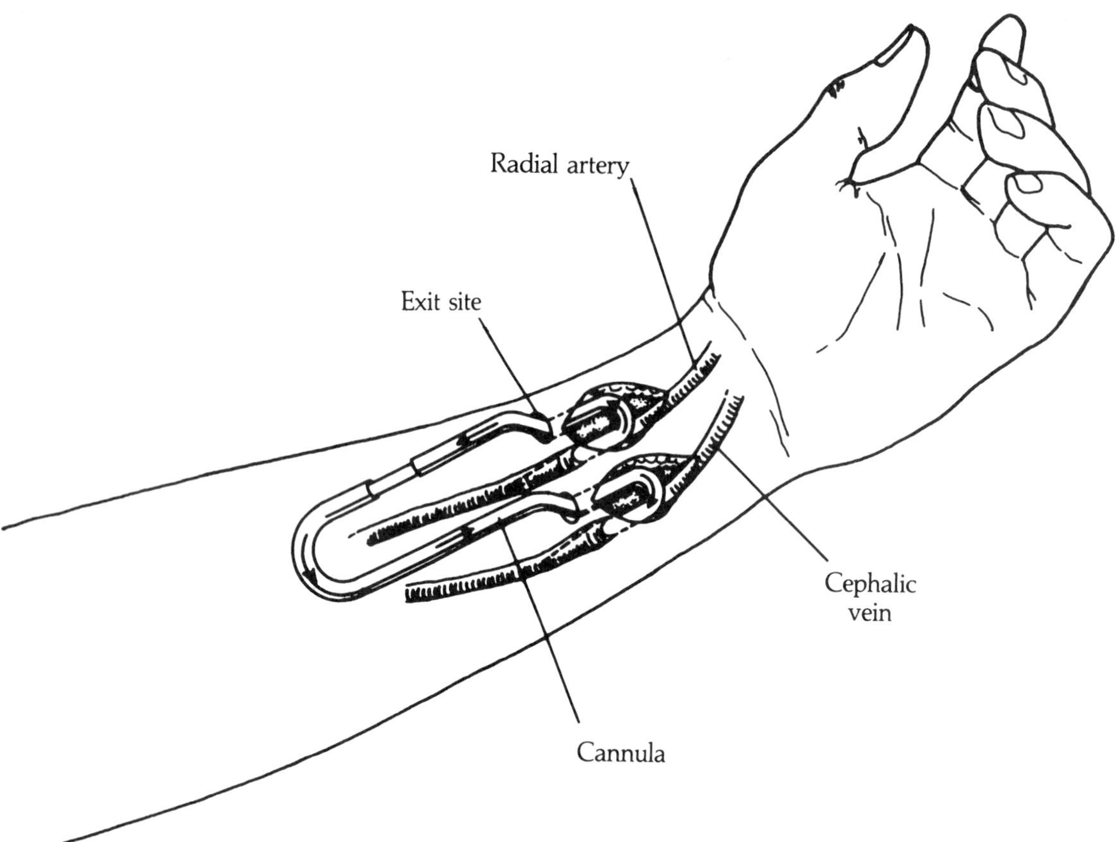

Figure 39-10 Arteriovenous shunt (cannula). (From Holloway NM: *Nursing the Critically Ill Adult.* 2nd ed. Addison-Wesley, 1984, p. 246.)

is minimal or absent, and blood chemistries are abnormal.

The pathophysiology of chronic renal failure is extremely complex. It is important to note that the accumulation of nitrogenous wastes in uremia, along with the associated fluid and electrolyte imbalances, adversely affect every body system. The impaired kidneys are unable to excrete normal acid load produced by normal metabolic process. Distal tubule ammonia production is reduced and the reabsorption of bicarbonate is impaired, resulting in metabolic acidosis (see Chapter 33).

Nitrogenous waste retention is caused by progressive nephron destruction and diminished function. The blood urea nitrogen level is affected by protein intake, but serum creatinine is not, and creatinine level therefore is a more reliable measure of renal function. In chronic renal failure the serum creatinine level is elevated. The corresponding anemia is proportional to the decline in renal function. Anemia is caused by diminished or absent renal erythropoietin function, impaired release of iron from stores, and iron deficiencies.

Renal osteodystrophy is a collective term for a variety of bony anomalies such as osteoporosis and rickets. This becomes a serious threat to the skeletal system of the child. This is caused by the kidney's inability to excrete phosphate and decreased ability to synthesize the active form of vitamin D.

If renal dysplasia or obstruction is involved as an underlying cause of the disease, large amounts of dilute urine with low sodium content are produced. If glomerular disease is present, sodium and fluid are retained, since glomerular filtration is reduced while tubular reabsorption continues. Retention of these substances leads to edema and vascular congestion in the end stages of the disease.

Potassium retention occurs when kidneys are no longer able to handle potassium ingestion and excretion time is seriously delayed. Hyperkalemia is apparent in end-stage renal disease.

The treatment for chronic renal failure is extremely complex. The goal of the conservative management of chronic renal failure is maintenance of metabolic homeostasis, which is achieved by maintaining a delicate balance between nutritional and pharmacologic alterations. As chronic renal failure progresses, biochemical manipulations become necessary and a dialysis program is initiated.

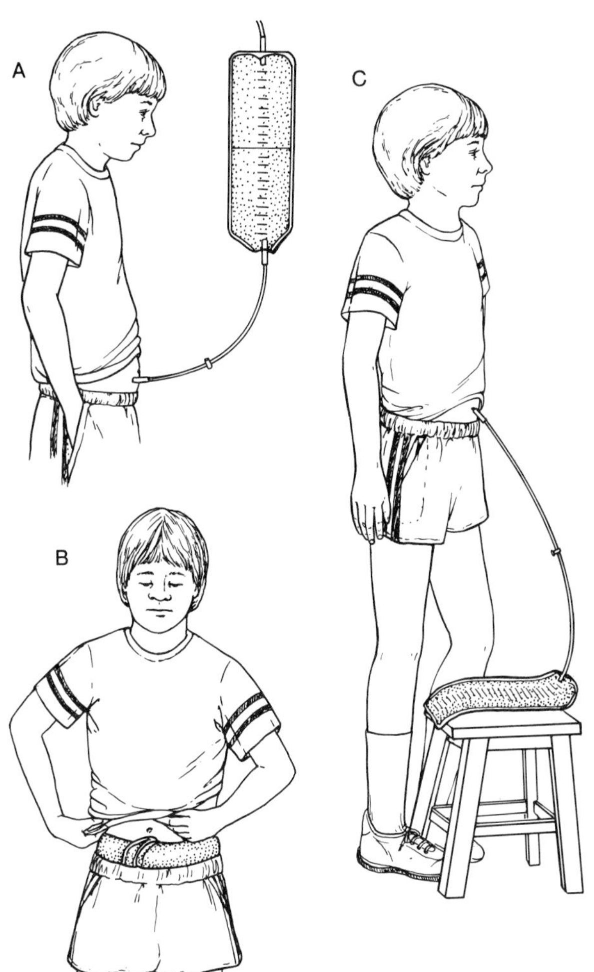

Figure 39-11 Child undergoing continuous ambulatory peritoneal dialysis. *A*. Tenckhoff tube is surgically implanted in abdomen, below umbilicus. Dialysate bag is aseptically attached to tube, and fluid is allowed to flow into peritoneal cavity. *B*. Dialysate remains in peritoneal cavity about 4–6 hours. Bag may be rolled up and tucked under clothing, allowing child to pursue normal activities during dialysis. *C*. Fluid is drained out of peritoneal cavity by unrolling the bag and suspending it below the pelvis, allowing gravity to drain fluid into the bag. After drainage, child aseptically attaches new bag of dialysate and refills the peritoneal cavity. Procedure is repeated 4–6 times per day.

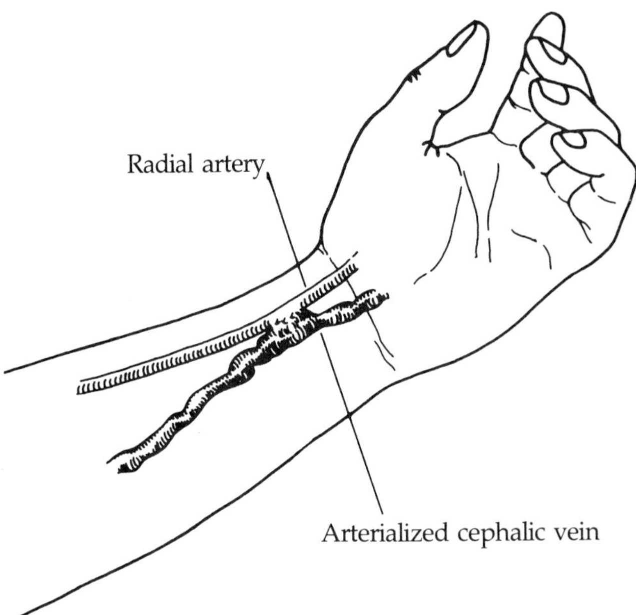

Figure 39-12 Hemodialysis. The arteriovenous fistula. (From Holloway NM: *Nursing the Critically Ill Adult*. 2nd ed. Addison-Wesley, 1984, p. 299.)

Medical Management With Dialysis

Treatment Continuous ambulatory peritoneal dialysis is a relatively new alternative to hemodialysis for ambulatory patients. Its major advantages are the freedom of movement that it allows the child and the capability for management.

A double-cuff Tenckhoff catheter is surgically implanted into the abdomen for instillation of the dialysate. The procedure then involves attaching a bag of dialysate to an indwelling catheter, infusing the dialysate for 10–15 minutes, rolling the bag, and securing the bag and catheter to the abdomen. The child is then allowed normal activity for 4–6 hours (8–10 hours at night). After allotted time, the dialysate is drained from the abdomen by hanging the bag lower than the pelvis. A fresh bag of dialysate is then attached and the process repeated. The cycle is performed three to five times a day, depending on the child's needs.

As the Tenckhoff catheter admits direct access to the peritoneum, the child and family must be comfortable with strict aseptic technique for use whenever the catheter is manipulated (Fig. 39-11). In addition, a thorough understanding of the procedure must be followed by repeated return demonstrations, so that the child and family may gain confidence.

Hemodialysis in the child with end-stage renal disease usually requires a more permanent circulatory access than the shunt. In these children an arteriovenus (AV) fistula is created (Fig. 39-12). This fistula is created surgically by anastomosing an artery and vein. It results in some arterial blood entering the venus circulation, which causes enlargement of the fistula because of the higher pressure in the arterial circulation (Saxon et al., 1983). When dialysis is desired, needles are inserted close to the fistula, providing access to the circulation.

The arteriovenous fistula is essentially hidden from view,

and after initial healing occurs, no dressing is necessary. A thrill is palpable over fistula site and a bruit may be heard on auscultation.

If the child's vascular system is poor, a venous graft may be considered to create the fistula. The graft vein is anastomosed with an appropriate artery and the connected to the child's venous system.

Hemodialysis treatment for children usually lasts 3–4 hours, three times a week. For some, the hours involved seem endless and a diversion is necessary.

Nursing Management The nursing mangement of the child with chronic renal failure is as complex as its medical counterpart and will offer the nurses one of their most significant challenges. An effective plan for management of these children demands not only understanding of the highly complex physiologic disturbances, but, equally important, an awareness of and sensitivity in dealing with the overwhelming impact that this chronic illness has on the children and their families.

Unlike many other chronic states, end-stage renal disease challenges the medical and nursing professions to join their collective talents in an attempt to minimize the suffering of the children and families involved. A total team effort, communication, and support are demanded by this progressively destructive disease. As nurses make their initial assessment of the child, they often see what is commonly described as the "chronically ill child." General signs of metabolic imbalance such as pallor, lethargy, anorexia, and headache afflict these children.

Hypertension is another major problem for the child with chronic renal failure. Blood pressure measurements should be taken regularly and signs and symptoms of increasing hypertension (such as headache and nosebleed) should be assessed immediately. Antihypertensives, in conjunction with dietary and fluid restrictions, are often effective in preventing extreme hypertension.

Seizures commonly affect the child with a metabolic imbalance. Anticonvulsant therapy greatly minimizes the frequency of seizures, but the nurse needs to be aware of the potential for the occurrence of seizures. Emergency equipment such as a padded tongue blade, suction, and oxygen must be available to the child at all times. Knowledge of nursing management of the child with seizures is essential for all nurses involved in the child's care (see Chapter 42).

Fluid and Dietary Management Accurate measurement of urine output is essential for assessment and maintenance of fluid balance. Fluid restriction, one of the most difficult aspects of care for the child and family, may be ordered to diminish the burden on the compromised kidneys. The need to deprive a loved one of desired fluids is often an intolerable demand put on families. The nurse caring for the fluid-restricted child therefore supports the child and family as they bear this hardship.

Often fluids become the focus of the child's need to control the environment. Manipulation, negativism, and hostility may develop as the child struggles with fluid restriction. A consistent approach to the child must be used by all members of the health team in conjunction with the family.

Dietary restrictions are not unlike those pertaining to fluids. An imaginative approach by the dietary staff may alleviate some of the unpleasantness of the protein- sodium-, and potassium-restricted diet. The protein-restricted diet is based on reduction of foods known as complete proteins—those containing all of the essential amino acids. Proteins in this group include eggs, milk, cheese, and meats. While necessary, the protein-restricted diet can cause growth retardation in young children. High-calorie foods are provided to the child to prevent protein catabolism and to supply energy. Because children with renal failure are sometimes anorexic, the number of calories they require can be given in a commercial calorie supplement such as Hycal.

Children on sodium-restricted diets should use no added salt. Depending on the severity of the restriction, salt also may be eliminated from cooking. Foods high in sodium are sodas, salted crackers or snacks, some processed and instant cereals, smoked meats, noodles and rice, and commercially prepared soups and bouillions.

Foods high in potassium are first—especially bananas, nectarines, peaches and prunes, and vegetables—squash, artichokes, and potatoes in skins. For children on dietary restriction of protein, sodium, and potassium, a dietary consultation is strongly recommended to provide the child with nutritional foods that also will appeal to the child's palate.

Coordination of Care To facilitate a consistent approach to the care of a child with chronic renal failure, the nurse often must assume responsibility for coordinating efforts and activities of other health professionals, particularly regarding dialysis and dietary restriction. As this is a progressively destructive disease, a long-range plan must be developed as soon as feasible, and this information must be shared with all involved. Family participation is crucial for the successful implementation of any plan, and parental input is essential.

The dialysis process quickly becomes a major part of the life of the child and family. The impact is such that many previous priorities now require reassessment. Often the child and family must travel a considerable distance to reach the dialysis unit. Although dialysis units for adults are numerous, units dedicated to the treatment of pediatric renal failure are relatively few. Dialysis centers designed to treat adults often are not appropriate for the treatment of children.

Home care of this child is often a continuation of the care

designed to meet the child's needs in the hospital setting. Parental involvement in the early days of the hospitalization will facilitate discharge teaching. Optimally, two members of the family should be taught to take the child's blood pressure. Often older children can learn to take their own blood pressure with little or no assistance. Return demonstration by all learners is essential before discharge, and the child and family must be comfortable with the demands and feasibility of care prior to discharge.

Research into the psychologic effects of long-term renal disease and dialysis delineates the adaptive processes of children. In a longitudinal study of five school-age children (Neff, 1978) it was found that children expressed anger and resentment toward their dependence on dialysis. Rebellion against fluid and dietary restrictions was common. These children requested information about illness, treatment, body changes, and about other children's reaction to themselves. The extent of their ability to be mobile and to participate in motor activity seemed important to their self-esteem. The grieving process was evident as they sought to cope with altered body image. Nurses need to be aware of these facts and other implications of long-term illness (see Chapter 30) to care most effectively for children with chronic renal failure.

Parent support groups can be extremely helpful with childhood catastrophic illnesses. The parents of children with chronic renal failure are no exception, and referral to such a group should be made whenever the resource is available. The traditional support systems such as psychiatry, psychology, social service, and the clergy are also important as the child and family deal with the illness.

While the child is hospitalized, health professionals associated with these children should use this time to its maximum potential. Family support groups, teaching sessions, discussion groups for the children, and the like allow exchange of ideas and support. Children suffering from end-stage renal disease deal with realities of life that are, for many, far beyond their chronologic years. Like other children suffering from a catastrophic illness, their needs for support are innumerable. Beyond the traditional supports, these children need each other. A peer group that encourages comparison, exchange of feelings, and simple companionship is essential. (Nursing care for the dying child is discussed in Chapter 32.)

Renal Transplantation

Renal transplantation is the surgical transfer of a human kidney (living, relative, or cadaver) from one individual to another. The transplanted kidney is usually placed in the right retroperitoneum. This site is optimal in children because of their size and vascular access.

The multidisciplinary approach necessary for renal transplantation may be exhausting. Consultations with specialists in orthopedics or internal medicine are usually requested, along with last-minute reviews of the child's status by infectious disease and hematology groups.

For the child receiving a living relative graft, the multitude of consultations and last-minute tests should be carefully scheduled over the few days before the procedure so the child can rest, have meals without unnecessary interruption, and prepare emotionally as well as physically for the surgery.

Children receiving cadaveric grafts have little or no time to prepare. Often they are called from school or home to come to the hospital as soon as possible. Much of the same preparation is necessary, but time is a more crucial factor because the cadaveric kidney is being perfused mechanically. Most children require a dialysis treatment before leaving for the operating suite.

Fear, anxiety, and expectations are all brought precipitously to the surface when the child and family prepare for transplantation. The nurse therefore joins other health professionals as they strive to reassure and support the child and family during this stressful period. Preoperative preparation thus is extremely important for the child anticipating such a major surgical procedure (see Chapter 29 for a discussion of teaching methods).

The nursing management of the child after renal transplantation is complex and challenging because the child experiences striking metabolic changes. Accurate assessment and maintenance of the child's fluid and electrolyte balance are essential for the child's recovery and the viability of the graft. (See Chapter 33 for discussion of fluid and electrolyte balance.) Prescribed intravenous rates and expected minimums for urinary output per hour establish limits within which the nurse maintains the child's fluid balance.

Acute tubular necrosis often occurs within the early postoperative period, and may cause extremely high or low outputs. The nurse aids in the diagnosis and management of acute tubular necrosis and other complications by assessing and communicating unusual findings from measurements and tests of urinary output. The results of urine tests for electrolyte content, specific gravity, and presence of blood or sugar, among others, assist the physician in managing the child's metabolic state. Nursing documentation of these values is best done on a flow sheet that shows hourly data for ease of comparison.

The child's weight must be measured at least daily. The nurse needs to be sure that the child's dressings, clothing, and diapers are the same with each weighing, so that accurate comparisons may be made.

To decrease incidence of rejection the posttransplantation child receives immunosuppressive therapy. Like anyone experiencing chronic renal failure, the posttransplant child must take a multitude of medications on a daily basis. These may include antihypertensives, diuretics, anticonvulsants, and antibiotics.

In the immediate postoperative period catheter drainage is essential to facilitate ease and accuracy of urinary output measurement. The catheter site must be watched carefully for infection in this immunosuppressed child; aseptic technique is warranted with any intervention (see the Urinary Catheter Guidelines).

In the immediate posttransplantation period (24–48 hours) many hourly assessments and interventions are necessary. Intake, output, and vital signs are often measured at least hourly until stable.

The nurse plans the physical care for the child with minimal interruption of the child's rest periods. Older children describe the first few days after such surgery as a "nightmare," during which time they have difficulty with time orientation. Planned periods during which the child may sleep without interruption are necessary if sleep deprivation and its associated problems are to be avoided. A simple gesture, such as leaving the blood pressure cuff loosly on the child's arm between measurements, often avoids interrupting a brief nap.

Nutrition and fluid management after renal transplantation remains a challenge. The difficulty for the child is amplified by what might appropriately be called the "Drink, Don't Drink . . . Eat, Don't Eat" dilemma. As the children's metabolic states fluctuate, so does their nutritional status, and they are alternately restricted or allowed food and fluid. Prior to the transplantation, the child has suffered with severe fluid restriction and a diet almost free of sodium, phosphorus, and potassium. Following transplantation, the child is allowed, often encouraged, to eat and drink almost anything. Many young children are totally confused by this phenomenon and often rebel. For the child who uses eating and drinking as control issues, the stress increases. Older children may continue to deal with previously "forbidden" foods and fluids with great uncertainty, even after adequate explanation.

Because transplanted kidneys often function erratically during the early postoperative period, the nurse needs to be ever-observant for signs and symptoms of rejection. A most common early sign of kidney rejection is fever, but since fever may be present for a variety of reasons, it is not to be viewed as a sole indicator of rejection.

Tenderness over the graft is of concern in the posttransplantation patient. Elevations in the white blood cell count, creatinine, and blood pressure all suggest difficulties. Unusual weight gain, edema, and decreased urine output are also indicators of rejection. The observant nurse may detect any of these deviations, and prompt communication to the physician may aid in the early detection and treatment of rejection episodes. Transplant rejection is usually treated according to institution protocol.

The Child With Renal Trauma

By far the most common cause of renal trauma in children is injury from automobiles. Motorcycle accidents and sports injuries with trauma to the genitourinary tract also are implicated in adolescents. Genitourinary trauma may cause blunt or penetrating injuries and should be suspected whenever there is injury to the flank, chest, abdomen, or pelvic area. Fractures of the ribs or pelvis indicate follow-up for renal injury.

Because the kidney is protected by muscles, most renal trauma results in minor injuries. In children, however, injuries may be more extensive because of less developed musculature and decreased body fat.

Assessment for genitourinary trauma includes inspecting the child for obvious contusions, abrasions, skin discolorations, and palpable masses. Gross or microscopic hematuria is present in children with renal damage and, depending on the extent of the injury, hemorrhage is a constant danger. The child may complain of pain in the flank, abdomen, or lower rib area. Radiographic examination may or may not reveal abnormalities. A sudden decrease in urinary output along with elevations in blood urea nitrogen and serum creatinine levels may indicate impending renal failure, particularly if the child is hypovolemic from hemorrhage.

Treatment for renal injury is conservative in most cases. If physical examination and radiographic studies are normal and the child demonstrates only microscopic hematuria, discharge with home observation may be indicated (Kearny and Finn, 1981). Children with abnormal findings usually are observed in the hospital to recognize quickly any deterioration in renal status. Kidney dialysis may be necessary for renal failure. Nephrectomy may be performed if conservative treatment is unsuccessful (Cook, 1983). Trauma to the ureters, urethra, or genitals usually is handled surgically.

Accurate observation of the child with genitourinary injury is essential to effective nursing management. Frequent monitoring and recording of intake and output, vital signs, serum electrolytes, hemoglobin and hematocrit, and hematuria gives clues to the child's renal status. The nurse measures abdominal girth daily to assess the size of any mass. Urinary catheter guidelines should be followed if the child has been catheterized. Quiet diversional activities occupy the child who is confined to bed. Discharge preparation needs to include information regarding signs of hemorrhage or renal damage, as complications can occur for up to 2 years after the injury (Cook, 1983).

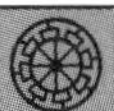

NURSING CARE PLAN Child With a Neurogenic Bladder

Assessment Data

Marguerite is a 2½-month-old infant who has been hospitalized since birth while awaiting adoption. A product of a full-term pregnancy, she was delivered by cesarean section because of cephalopelvic disproportion. An ultrasound performed during labor revealed that she had an extremely large, full bladder. Observation and diagnostic workup during the neonatal period indicated a neurogenic bladder of unknown origin and uncertain prognosis for urinary control. Because of repeated urinary tract infections, the baby has been catheterized 4 times a day to remove residual urine from the bladder and has been placed on prophylactic trimethoprim and sulfamethoxazole (Bactrim). A couple has been found that is interested in adopting her, but is uncertain about being able to care for her bladder problem.

Nursing Diagnoses and Goals

1. **Nursing diagnosis:** Potential for urinary tract infection as a result of urine retention.

   Long-term goal: Marguerite will remain free from infection as a result of proper management.

   Short-term goals: (a) Marguerite will demonstrate reduced amount of residual urine to decrease potential for organism growth. (b) Marguerite will have adequate fluid intake.

2. **Nursing diagnosis:** Knowledge deficit of prospective adoptive parents.

   Long-term goal: Prospective adoptive parents will feel confident in their abilities to care successfully for Marguerite at home.

   Short-term goals: (a) The parents will demonstrate understanding of the issues involved with the baby's care. (b) Both parents will participate in Marguerite's care.

Intervention	Rationale	Evaluation criteria
1. Catheterize qid using size 8 straight catheter	Regular removal of residual urine in the bladder removes potential for organism growth	Is there any sign of fever, irritability, anorexia, or changes in urine output. Is the infant taking fluids well? Is there any bladder distention? Has the post-void residual urine decreased? Are the weekly urine cultures remaining negative?
Demonstrate catheterization to prospective parents using clean technique	Organism growth in the bladder is not appreciably increased with use of clean rather than sterile equipment; procedure is less complicated and more easily managed at home, thus resulting in better compliance	
Encourage fluids—Enfamil 6 oz 5 times a day. Water between feedings as the child will take. Feed infant with Playtex nurser	Extra fluid decreases urine concentration and promotes more frequent micturation. If the infant refuses water, diluted fruit juice may be given, which also increases urine acidity, thereby decreasing potential for organism growth	
Urine for culture and sensitivity weekly	Close monitoring of infection status is necessary to prevent complications from untreated UTI	

continued on next page

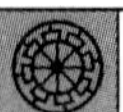

NURSING CARE PLAN Child With a Neurogenic Bladder (continued)

Intervention	Rationale	Evaluation criteria
Administer trimethoprim and sulfamethoxozole (Bactrim), ½ tsp twice a day, followed by sips of water	Prophylactic administration of antibiotic reduces incidence of UTI; Bactrim syrup is high in sucrose and should be rinsed from mouth even in an infant this young to reduce incidence of damage to erupting teeth	
2. Clarify information regarding the infant's medical diagnosis and its impact on the prospective family	Prospective parents need to know that the infant may never be toilet trained, but eventually will be able to learn self-catheterization if necessary; infections need prompt treatment, and constant vigilance is essential	Are both prospective parents interested in participating? Do both demonstrate skill in return demonstrations? Does the father express any embarrassment or uncertainty regarding catheterization? Do both prospective parents seem confident and knowledgeable regarding well-child care? Do prospective parents report that the home is conducive to set-up of catheterization?
Allow time to answer prospective parents' questions	This gives the nurse the opportunity to validate parents' understanding of the situation	
Realistically explain the time commitment involved with the infant's care and problems they will encounter in addition to normal care	Both prospective parents need to be involved in the infant's care—with both learning to catheterize. This allows greater freedom—one parent should not be tied down with care. Parents should explore resource people in their family or neighborhood who could catheterize the child when they need a vacation	
Assess parental knowledge of well-child care	Adoptive parents may have had little or no experience with infants	
Explore with the prospective father any feelings he may have about catheterizing the infant	Men and women both may have conflicting feelings about manipulating the genital area of opposite-sex children; allowing them to express their feelings provides a more realistic perspective	
Teach both prospective parents how to catheterize the infant; observe return demonstration	Parents must be confident and capable of assuming care before baby can be discharged	
Explain adaptations for home management: cleanliness and maintenance of catheters; use of home urine culture kits; how to obtain supplies; sterile urine collection for laboratory culture; positioning and restraint (if necessary) of baby	Catheterization area at home should be preferably close to a bathroom for easy disposal; infant should be catheterized on a flat surface at comfortable height for the parent; no restraint is necessary while infant is young, but this may need reconsideration when the infant is larger and rolls over frequently; sterile urine lab culture kits should be provided for follow-up of a positive home urine culture; catheters should be washed with soap and water, dried with clean cloth and stored in a covered clean container—no need to sterilize	

Key Concepts

- The state of the genitourinary system contributes to the general good health and homeostasis of the child.
- Concerns related to the system include maintenance of health and homeostasis, adjustments related to altered body image, and fears of mutilation or of sexual and reproductive deficits.
- Organs of the genitourinary system include kidneys, the collection system of ureters and bladder, and internal and external organs of reproduction.
- Physiology of the renal system is concerned with regulation and maintenance of the composition and volume of body fluids and the excretion of soluble wastes.
- The nephron is the functioning unit that facilitates renal physiology.
- Assessment of the child with a genitourinary dysfunction includes data gathering and assessment of all body systems, as alteration in the genitourinary system can have adverse effects on the whole body.
- Some diagnostic tests for genitourinary function are embarrassing and invasive and the child's privacy should be strictly respected.
- Urinary catheterization may be performed to empty the bladder prior to diagnostic tests, to obtain a sterile specimen, to measure residual volumes in the bladder, or to empty the bladder when the child is unable to void.
- Acute nursing care involves assessment of fluid and electrolyte balance, prevention of infection, assessment of physiologic function, and preoperative preparation and postoperative management if indicated.
- Emotional needs of children with genitourinary dysfunction include attention to problems resulting from life-style restrictions, alterations in body image, and questions regarding sexual and reproductive function.
- Special home care problems may include home catheterization or dialysis.
- Structural defects affecting the genitourinary system include hydronephrosis, exstrophy of the bladder, obstructive anomalies of the collecting system, reflux anomalies of the collecting system, and anomalies of external structures such as phimosis, hypospadias, epispadias, and cryptorchidism.
- Most structural anomalies require surgical intervention including preoperative and postoperative nursing management.
- Infections of the genitourinary system include upper and lower urinary tract infections, toxic shock syndrome, and sexually transmitted diseases.
- Nursing interventions for the child with a genitourinary infection are directed toward careful assessment and supportive care during acute episodes, and preventive education and counseling.
- Acute glomerulonephritis and nephrosis are two renal dysfunctions that affect the filtration of wastes.
- Assessment and nursing management of these dysfunctions address imbalances of fluid and electrolytes.
- Acute and chronic renal failure have devastating effects on multiple body systems in the affected child and require meticulous assessment and critical-care management.
- Kidney dialysis—peritoneal dialysis or hemodialysis—may be used to treat renal failure by allowing the body to excrete wastes and correct fluid and electrolyte imbalance.
- Renal transplantation can allow the child recovery from end-stage renal disease, but transplantation is not without the potential for severe complications.
- Care of the child who has sustained genitourinary trauma requires accurate observation to recognize quickly signs of deteriorating renal function.

References

Allan FD: *Essentials of Human Embryology*. Oxford, 1969.

American Academy of Pediatrics: Urinary tract infections. Pages 301–304 in: *Report of the Committee on Infectious Diseases*, 1977.

Behrman RE, Vaughan VC: *Nelson Textbook of Pediatrics*. 12th ed, Saunders, 1983.

Brown L: Toxic shock syndrome. *Am J Matern Child Nurs* (Jan/Feb) 1981; 6:57–59.

Brundage D: *Nursing Management of Renal Problems*. Mosby, 1980.

Centers for Disease Control: Annual summary 1979: Reported morbidity and mortality in the United States. *Morbidity and Mortality Weekly Report* 1980; 28(54).

Centers for Disease Control: *Morbidity and Mortality Weekly Report* (Aug 17) 1984; 33:461–463.

Chow M et al: *Handbook of Pediatric Primary Care*. Wiley, 1979.

Cook L: Renal trauma. *RN* (Feb) 1983; 46:58–63.

Corey LJ, Reeves WC, Vontver L: Controlled trial of BCG vaccine in genital herpes. Abstracted, XVIX ICAAC Meeting, 1976.

Edwards MS: Venereal herpes: A nursing overview. *J Obstet Gynecol Neonatal Nurs* (Sept/Oct) 1978; 7:7–15.

Gillenwater JY, Harrison RB, Kunin CM: Natural history of bacteriuria in schoolgirls. *N Engl J Med* (Aug) 1979; 301:396–399.

Gralton KS: Renal, endocrine, and metabolic crises. Pages 376–386 in: *Pediatric Critical Care Nursing*. Vestal K (editor). Wiley, 1981.

Harrison et al (editors): *Campbell's Urology*. Saunders, 1979.

Hekelman F, Ostendorp C: Nursing approaches to conservative management of renal disease. *Nurs Clin North Am* (Sept) 1975; 10:431–448.

James JA: *Renal Disease in Childhood*. Mosby, 1976.

Kearney G, Finn D: Trauma to the genitourinary tract. *Emergency Med* (Aug) 1981; 13:69–79.

Kelalis, King: *Clinical Pediatric Urology*. Saunders, 1976.

Kempe CH, Silver K, O'Brien D: *Current Pediatric Diagnosis and Treatment*. Lange, 1976.

Kory M, Waife SO (editors): *Kidney and Urinary Tract Infections*. Lilly Research Lab, 1976.

Kunin CM: Urinary tract infections. in: *Ambulatory Pediatrics II*. Green M, Haggerty RJ (editors). Saunders, 1977.

Lewis SM: Pathophysiology of chronic renal failure. *Nurs Clin North Am* (Sept) 1981; 16(3):501–513.

Lorentz WB, Jr, Resnick MI: Comparison of urinary lactic dehydrogenase with antibody-coated bacteria in the urine sediment as means of localizing the site of urinary tract infection. *Pediatrics* (Nov) 1979; 64(5): 672–677.

Lukacs J, Corey L: Genital herpes simplex virus infection: An overview. *Nurs Pract* (May/June) 1977; 2(5):7–10.

Margileth AM et al: Urinary tract bacterial infections: Office diagnosis and management. *Pediatr Clin North Am* (Nov) 1976; 23(4):721–734.

Martin L: *Health Care of Women*. Lippincott, 1978.

Nahmias AJ, Jasey WE, Naib ZN: Venereal herpes simplex virus infections. In: *Sexually Transmitted Diseases*. Nicholas L (editor). Charles C Thomas, 1973.

Neff EJA: Orienting, resistive, and adaptive responses of children undergoing hemodialysis for kidney failure. *Matern Child Nurs J* (Winter) 1978; 7:195–254.

Nelson WE et al: *Textbook of Pediatrics*. 12th ed. Saunders, 1983.

Noble RC: *Sexually Transmitted Diseases*. Medical Examination, 1979.

Pope T: Toxic shock syndrome. *Nurse Pract* (Sept/Oct) 1981; 6:31–32.

Rielly M: The renal system. Pages 387–408 in: *Pediatric Critical Care*. Bloedel-Smith J (editor). Wiley, 1983.

Ripa KT et al: *Chlamydia trachomatis* cervicitis in gynecologic outpatients. *Obstet Gyneco* (Dec) 1978; 52(6):698–702.

Saxton D et al: *The Addison-Wesley Manual of Nursing Practice*. Addison-Wesley, 1983.

Scott R, Deane RF, Callander R: *Urology Illustrated*. Longman, 1975.

Smith C et al: *The Critically Ill Child*. Saunders, 1977.

Sorrels AJ: Peritoneal dialysis: A rediscovery. *Nurs Clin North Am* (Sept) 1981; 16(3):515–528.

Stewart FH et al: *My Body My Health*. Wiley, 1979.

Stickler GB: Urinary tract infection in children: Diagnosis and treatment. *Postgrad Med* (Oct) 1979; 66(4):159–162, 164–165.

Vick R: *Contemporary Medical Physiology*. Addison-Wesley, 1984.

Wayland JR, Higgins PG: Neonatal circumcision: A teaching plan to better inform parents. *Nurs Pract* (June) 1982; 6:26–27.

Wayland JR, Higgins PG: Newborn circumcision: Father's involvement. *Pediatr Nurs* (Jan/Feb) 1983; 9:41–42.

Yarber WL: Preventing venereal disease infection: Approaches for the sexually active. *Health Values: Achieving High-Level Wellness* (March/April) 1978; 2(2):61–67.

Wroblewski S: Toxic shock syndrome. *Am J Nurs* (Jan) 1981; 81:82–85.

Additional Readings

Adatto K et al: Behavioral factors and urinary tract infections. *JAMA* (June) 1979; 241:2525–2526.

Albert M: Acid–base disorders in pediatrics. *Pediatr Clin North Am* (Nov) 1976; 23(4):639–650.

Belman AB. The clinical significance of vesicoureteral reflux. *Pediatr Clin North Am* (Nov) 1976; 23(4):707–720.

Brunner et al: *The Lippincott Manual of Nursing Practice*. Lippincott, 1978.

Byrne J et al: *Laboratory Tests: Implications for Nurses and Allied Health Professionals*. Addison-Wesley, 1981.

Ceccarelli CM: Hemodialytic therapy for the patient with chronic renal failure. *Nurs Clin North Am* (Sept) 1981; 16(3):531–549.

Charlton CAC: *The Urological System*. Penguin Education, 1973.

Fischbach FT: *A Manual of Laboratory Diagnostic Tests*. Lippincott, 1980.

Fochtman D, Raffensberger J: *Principles of Nursing Care for the Pediatric Surgery Patient*. Little, Brown, 1968.

Frommell GT et al: *Chlamydial* infection of mothers and their infants. *J Pediatr* (July) 1979; 95:28–32.

Guyton: *Textbook of Medical Physiology*. Saunders, 1976.

Hekelman F, Ostendorp C: *Nephrology Nursing*. McGraw-Hill, 1979.

Hoarsley J, Crane J, Reynolds M: *Clean Intermittent Catheterization*. Harcourt, Brace, 1982.

Malekzadeh et al: Current issues in pediatric renal transplantation. *Pediatr Clin North Am* (Nov) 1976;23(4):857–872.

Muir B: *Pathophysiology*. Wiley, 1980.

Murphy LM et al: Renal disease: Nutritional implications. *Nurs Clin North Am* (March) 1983; 18:57–70.

Price SA, Wilson LM: *Pathophysiology*. McGraw-Hill, 1978.

Rodrigues RD, Hunter RD: Nutritional intervention in the treatment of chronic renal failure. *Nurs Clin N Am* (Sept) 1981; 16:573–585.

Steiner KL: Teaching parents of renal transplant patients. *Nephrol Nurs* (Nov/Dec) 1980; 2:25–26.

Topor M: Chronic renal disease in children. *Nur Clin North Am* (Sept) 1981; 16:587–597.

Metabolism
Implications of Altered Hormonal Regulation

40

Beverly Giordano

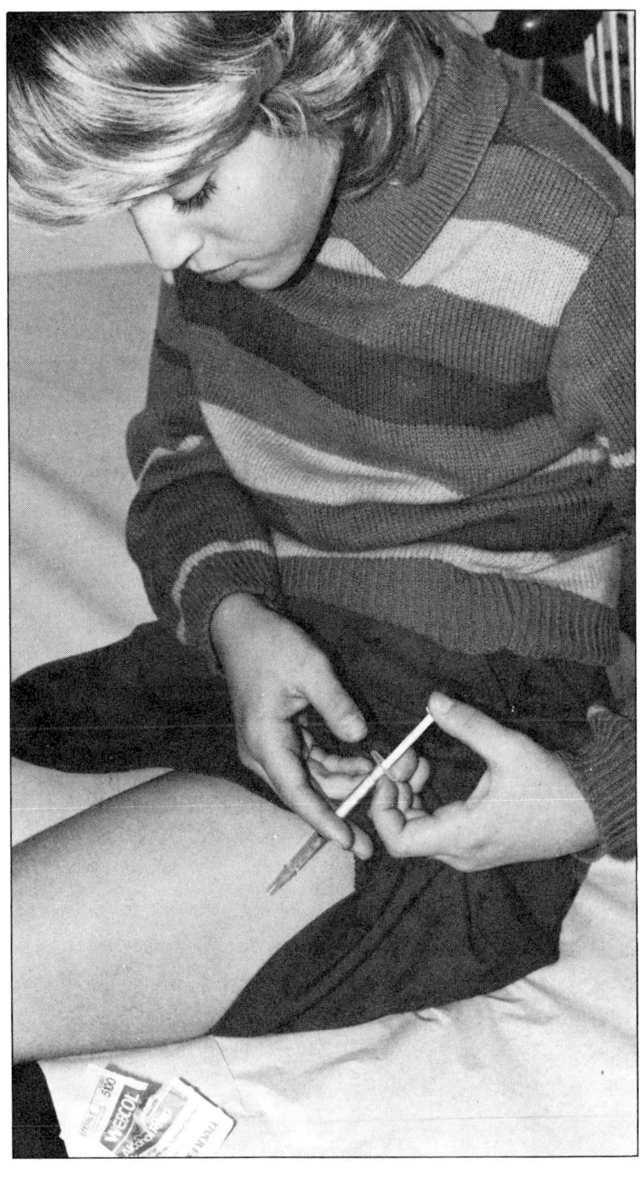

Chapter Outline

continued on next page

Objectives

- Describe the anatomy, embryonic development, and physiology of the endocrine system.
- Describe the assessment criteria for and physical examination of the child with endocrine dysfunction.
- Define the nurse's role in the procedures and treatments that involve the endocrine system.
- Outline the acute care, nutritional, developmental, socialization, emotional, and health maintenance needs of the child with endocrine dysfunction.
- Explain the clinical manifestations and medical treatment of diabetes mellitus.
- Describe the administration, measurement, dose adjustment, and storage of insulin.
- Outline the principles of nursing management for the child with diabetes mellitus.
- Explain the physiologic processes, medical treatments, and principles of nursing management for conditions involving the inappropriate hormonal secretions from the pituitary gland.
- Distinguish between diabetes mellitus and diabetes insipidus.
- Explain the physiologic processes, medical treatments, and principles of nursing management for conditions involving the inappropriate secretions from the adrenal glands.
- Explain the physiologic processes, medical treatments, and principles of nursing management for conditions involving the inappropriate secretions from the thyroid gland.
- Explain the physiologic processes, medical treatments, and principles of nursing management for conditions involving the inappropriate secretions from the parathyroid glands.
- Describe the physiologic processes, medical treatments, and principles of nursing management for children with hyperfunction of the ovaries or testes.
- Describe the physiologic processes, medical treatments, and principles of nursing management for children with delayed sexual maturity.

Hormonal imbalances that develop during gestation, childhood, or adolescence have pronounced effects on children's physical health, growth, pubertal development, and body image. Parents' perceptions of and expectations for children with hormonal dysfunctions might be affected by the serious nature of the problems and the demands placed on the families by the management of the disorders.

The most common hormonal problem in children is diabetes mellitus, which occurs in 1 out of every 500 children under 21 years of age (Sperling, 1982). Other common hormonal problems of childhood are hypothyroidism, congenital adrenal hyperplasia, short stature, and precocious puberty. Nursing care of children with hormonal dysfunction is based on a recognition of the age and developmental level of the child; cultural, ethnic, and religious factors; socioeconomic status of the family; meaning of the illness to the child and family; structure of the family and roles of the family members; and an assessment of family strengths.

Anatomy and Physiology of the Endocrine System

Gross Anatomy

The endocrine system is composed of glands which produce hormones that affect the functions of specifically receptive organs or tissues throughout the body. The glands of the endocrine system include the hypothalamus, pituitary, thyroid, parathyroid, adrenal, gonads (ovaries and testes), and the endocrine pancreas (Fig. 40–1).

The *hypothalamus* is located at the base of the brain, surrounded by the optic chiasm and the temporal lobe sulci. The pituitary stalk descends from the central region of the base of the hypothalamus.

The *pituitary gland* is located in a bony cavity, the sella turcica. It is a small organ, weighing approximately 0.5 g (Daughaday, 1981). The pituitary is divided into the anterior lobe (adenohypophysis), the intermediate lobe, and the posterior lobe (neurohypophysis). The anterior lobe constitutes 75% of the total weight of the gland. The anterior lobe contains five cell types, four of which synthesize and secrete specific hormones. The somatotroph cells secrete prolactin and growth hormone (somatotropin). Thyrotroph cells secrete thyrotropin (thyroid-stimulating hormone, or TSH). Gonadotroph cells secrete luteinizing hormone (LH), follicle-stimulating hormone (FSH), and human chorionic gonadotropin (HCG). Corticotroph cells release corticotropin (adrenocorticotropic hormone, or ACTH) and melanocyte-stimulating hormone (MSH). The fifth type of cell composes 25% of the pituitary but is nonsecretory (Daughaday, 1981). The posterior lobe synthesizes and transports two peptide hormones, antidiuretic hormone (ADH) and oxytocin. These two hormones are manufactured by the neurosecretory cells of the hypothalamic area.

The hypothalamic–pituitary unit is illustrated in Figure 40–2. Because of its location in the midbrain, this unit is susceptible to disease, damage, and malformation, which affect this portion of the central nervous system.

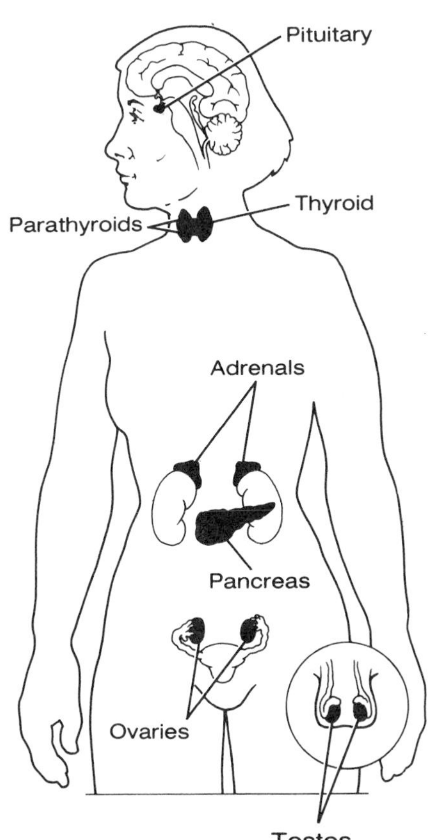

Figure 40-1 Glands composing the endocrine system. (From Spence AP, Mason EB: *Human Anatomy and Physiology*. 2nd ed. Benjamin/Cummings, 1983; p. 428.)

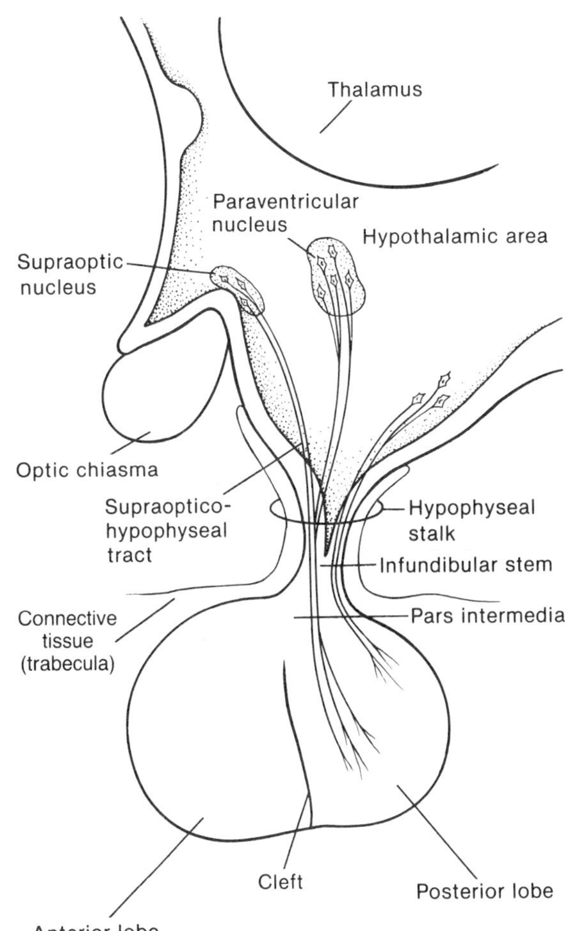

Figure 40-2 The hypothalamic–pituitary unit.

The *thyroid gland* is normally one of the largest of the endocrine organs and has tremendous growth potential. The thyroid is composed of two lobes joined by the isthmus, a thin band of tissue. Each lobe is approximately 2.0–2.5 cm in thickness and width and 4.0 cm in length. The thyroid is attached to the anterior and lateral aspects of the trachea; the upper margin of the isthmus lies just beneath the cricoid cartilage. Closely packed sacs, or follicles, fill the thyroid gland and synthesize thyroxine via the enzymatically controlled oxidation of iodide (Ingbar and Woebar, 1981).

The four *parathyroid glands* are located adjacent to, or embedded within, thyroid tissue. The parathyroids increase in weight throughout the first two decades of life; the average total weight of the four glands is 120 mg in adult males and 140 mg in adult females (Aurbach, Marx, and Spiegel, 1981). The cells of the parathyroid glands synthesize and secrete parathyroid hormone (parathormone, or PTH).

The *adrenal glands* sit atop the kidneys and are composed of an outer portion (cortex) and an inner portion (medulla). Normally, each adrenal gland weighs approximately 5 g; they become smaller in individuals with a deficiency in ACTH and enlarge dramatically in the presence of chronic excessive ACTH (Liddle, 1981). The adrenal cortex converts cholesterol to steroid hormones via a complicated biosynthetic pathway mediated by nine enzymatic steps. The adrenal medulla is a minor source of catecholamines (epinephrine, norepinephrine, and dopamine). Tumors in the adrenal medulla produce distinct clinical syndromes; however, there are no diseases known to be caused by adrenal medullary insufficiency (Melmon, 1981).

The *ovaries* are located in the pelvis and are attached to the broad ligaments. They are composed of follicles in varying stages of maturation or degeneration, supportive tissues, blood vessels, and lymphatic vessels. The follicles undergo morphologic changes during maturation, beginning as primordial follicles and culminating as graafian follicles just prior to ovulation. Beginning with *menarche* (the onset of the first menstrual period) and continuing until menopause, one (or, in rare cases, more than one) of the maturing follicles enlarges rapidly and ruptures, releasing an oocyte (Ross, Vande Wiele, and Frantz, 1981). The ovaries produce and secrete estradiol, estrone, progesterone, androstenedione, testosterone, dehydroisoandrosterone, and hydroxyprogesterone.

The *testes* secrete androgens and produce sperm. Testicles have descended from the pelvic cavity into the scrotal sac by birth in approximately 90% of males. During the first year of life, previously undescended testicles will descend in another 7%–8% of males, and in the majority of the remaining cases, descent into the scrotal sac occurs prior to puberty (Bardin and Paulsen, 1981). Testosterone synthesis occurs in the Leydig cells of the testes. Spermatogenesis begins in the average male at approximately 16 years of age (Jones and Scott, 1971).

The exocrine pancreas plays an important role in gastrointestinal function, but it is the endocrine islets that influence body metabolism through the effects of insulin and glucagon. Most of the islets of Langerhans are located in the tail portion of the pancreas. Glucagon-secreting alpha cells generally are present by the ninth week of gestation, and beta cells are identifiable by the eleventh gestational week (Porte and Halter, 1981).

Embryonic Development

Most of the glands and structures of the endocrine system develop within the first trimester of pregnancy. Maternal illness and exposure to toxins during this crucial time of development might contribute to lifelong endocrine dysfunction in the offspring.

The hypothalamus and pituitary glands appear as the brain develops flexures early in gestation; both glands arise from the diencephalon portion of the brain. The hypothalamus arises from the floor of the diencephalon by the time the embryo is approximately 15 mm in length (Hamilton, Body, and Mossman, 1972).

The pituitary gland's two lobes (adenohypophysis and neurohypophysis) arise from different embryonic structures. The neurohypophysis, or posterior lobe, develops as a downward growth from the ventral diencephalon and has a microscopic structure composed of nervous tissue. The adenohypophysis, or anterior lobe, develops as an upward projection of the pharynx and has the microscopic structure of an endocrine gland (Fig. 40–3).

The thyroid gland develops in three stages between the seventh and fourteenth weeks of gestation. It first appears as a thickening of the endoderm of the floor of the pharynx in the midline and is attached to the buccal cavity by the thyroglossal duct (Hamilton, Body, and Mossman, 1972). At the seventh week of gestation, the thyroid completes its migration to its location anterior to the first six tracheal cartilages. When the thyroglossal duct and pharyngobranchial duct become obliterated at 6–8 weeks of gestation, the thyroid loses its attachment to the pharynx (Hamilton, Body, and Mossman, 1972).

Parathyroid tissue becomes recognizable in the endodermal walls of the pharyngeal pouches when the embryo is 8 mm long at about 5–7 weeks of gestation. The parathyroid tissue separates from the pharyngeal pouches and becomes fully differentiated during the second half of gestation (Hamilton, Body, and Mossman, 1972).

The adrenal medulla arises from the ectoderm via the neural crest. The adrenal cortex develops from the lateral plate of the embryonic mesoderm (mesenchyma) (Hamilton, Body, and Mossman, 1972). The adrenal glands are large structures during fetal life and rapidly decrease in size during the first few months following birth.

The gonads (ovaries and testes) are identical in appearance prior to the seventh week of gestation. At about this

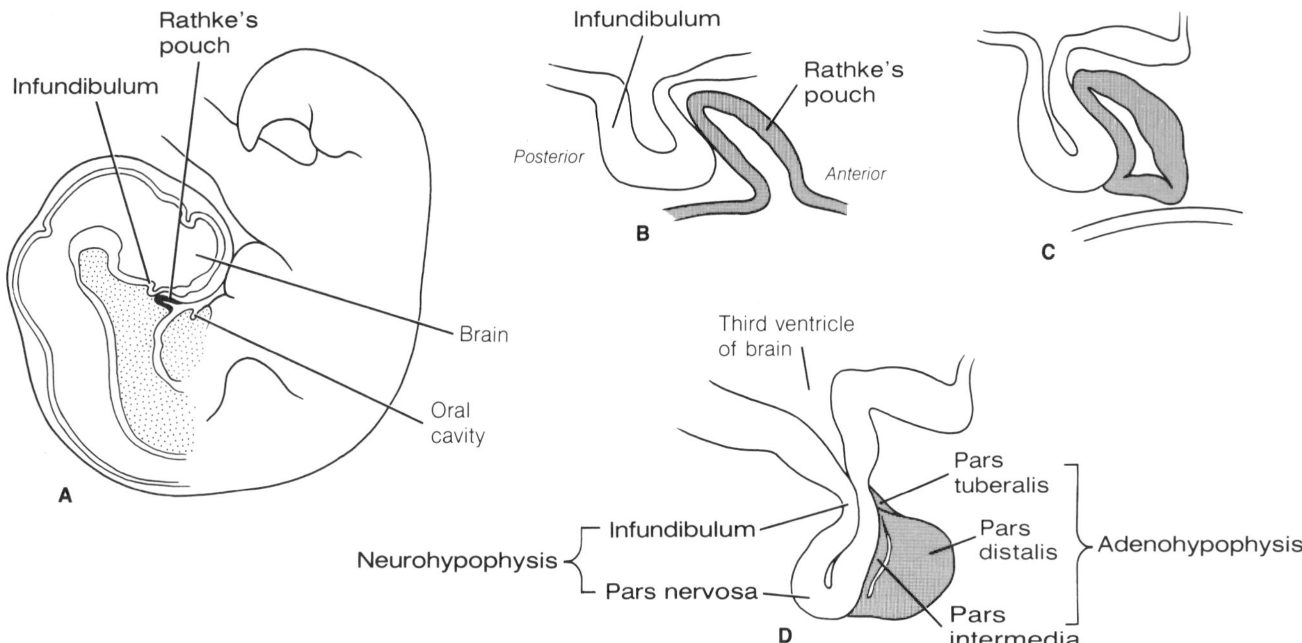

Figure 40-3 Stages in the embryonic development of the pituitary gland. *A.* Embryo. *B.* Outpouching (Rathke's pouch) grows toward the neurohypophysis. *C.* Rathke's pouch becomes the adenohypophysis. *D.* Pituitary includes the neurohypophysis and adenohypophysis. (From Spence AP, Mason EB: *Human Anatomy and Physiology.* 2nd ed. Benjamin/Cummings, 1983; p. 430.)

time, the testes begin to differentiate under the influence of a substance called the H-Y antigen. Testosterone synthesis begins at the ninth week of gestation; lack of testosterone at this time results in ambiguous genitals (Bardin and Paulsen, 1981).

In the absence of the H-Y antigen, the gonadal primordial cells develop into an ovary, provided that germ cells are present and survive. The epithelium and germ cells gradually enlarge and become oogonia, which give rise to oocytes at approximately the eleventh week of gestation (Grumbach and Conte, 1981). The first primary follicles are formed and the gonad has characteristics of an ovary by the twentieth to twenty-fifth week of gestation.

The pancreas develops from two separate types of primordial cells that arise from the duodenal endoderm and fuse to form a single organ at approximately the seventh week of gestation (Hamilton, Body, and Mossman, 1972). Several weeks later, the islets of Langerhans develop and insulin can be detected in the beta cells.

The end result of fetal development of the endocrine system is the ability to regulate metabolism, growth, puberty, and reproduction.

Physiology

The neuroendocrine system, composed of the endocrine system and the nervous system, functions to achieve and maintain internal homeostasis. The endocrine system functions by circulating very small amounts of specific chemicals (hormones). The nervous system functions by sending nerve impulses throughout the body. Together, these systems regulate homeostasis, metabolism, growth, and reproduction.

Endocrine glands synthesize hormones that are proteins or compounds made from proteins or steroids. The endocrine glands are ductless; that is, they secrete the hormones directly into the bloodstream. Hormones circulate widely throughout the body but are highly specific in their action on target cells. Hormones serve as messengers, providing communication between endocrine and target gland cells. Cyclic adenosine monophosphate (cyclic AMP) acts as the second mediator, influencing cellular function within a hormone's target cells (Fig. 40–4).

The hypothalamus controls pituitary function by secreting small peptides that reach the anterior pituitary gland via the hypophyseal portal system. The neurons in the supraoptic and paraventricular nuclei of the hypothalamus synthesize hormones secreted by the posterior pituitary; an example of this process is vasopressin, or antidiuretic hormone (ADH). Some hypothalamic neurons secrete releasing hormones, which act on the anterior pituitary lobe; examples of these releasing hormones are TRH (thyrotropin-releasing hormone) and LRH (luteinizing-releasing hormone). The hypothalamus also is involved in regulating appetite, sugar and fat metabolism, body temperature, maintenance of water balance, and secretion of inhibiting hormones, such as somatostatin, which inhibits release of growth hormone.

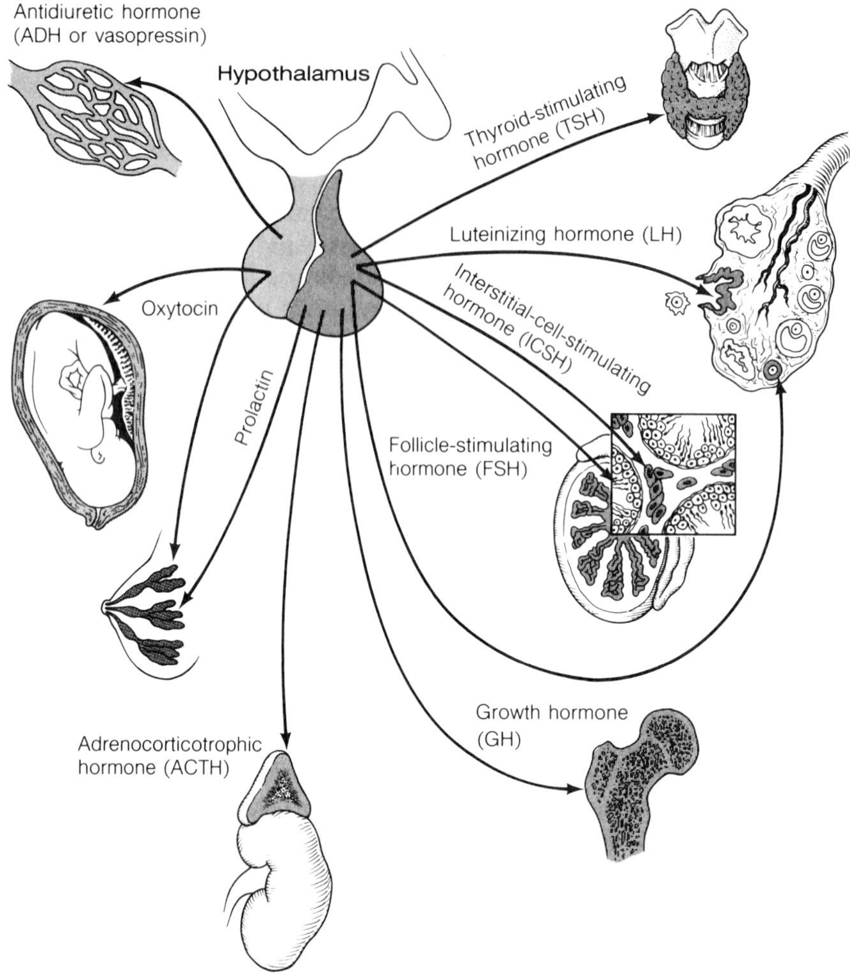

Figure 40-4 Functions of the pituitary gland: secretion of releasing hormones. (From Spence AP: *Basic Human Anatomy*. 1st ed. Benjamin/Cummings, 1982; p. 485.)

Negative feedback mechanisms control the pituitary gland's secretion of the tropic hormones somatotropin, ACTH, TSH, FSH, LH, and ADH. The principle of negative feedback is that high levels of tropic hormones stimulate target glands to increase hormone secretion. The resulting high blood level of hormone feeds back via the blood to the pituitary gland, inhibiting further secretion of the tropic hormones. An example of this negative feedback system is illustrated in Figure 40–5 for the ACTH–adrenal cortex system. This negative feedback mechanism applies to the regulation of adrenal, thyroid, and testicular function. The relationship between the hypothalamic–pituitary unit and the ovaries is more complex, as shown in Figure 40–6.

Parathyroid and pancreatic islet cell function are not directly regulated by the hypothalamic–pituitary unit. Parathormone (PTH) secretion is regulated by the blood calcium concentration. The release of insulin and glucagon from pancreatic islet cells is in response to the blood glucose concentration.

Hormonal secretion by the endocrine glands has specific, pronounced effects on the functioning of the human body. These hormonal effects are summarized in Table 40-1.

Assessment of the Child With Endocrine Dysfunction

The endocrine system regulates metabolism, growth, pubertal development, reproduction, fluid and electrolyte balance, and response to stress. In obtaining the history associated with the endocrine system, the nurse is sensitive to the important effects that endocrine function and dysfunction have on the child and family.

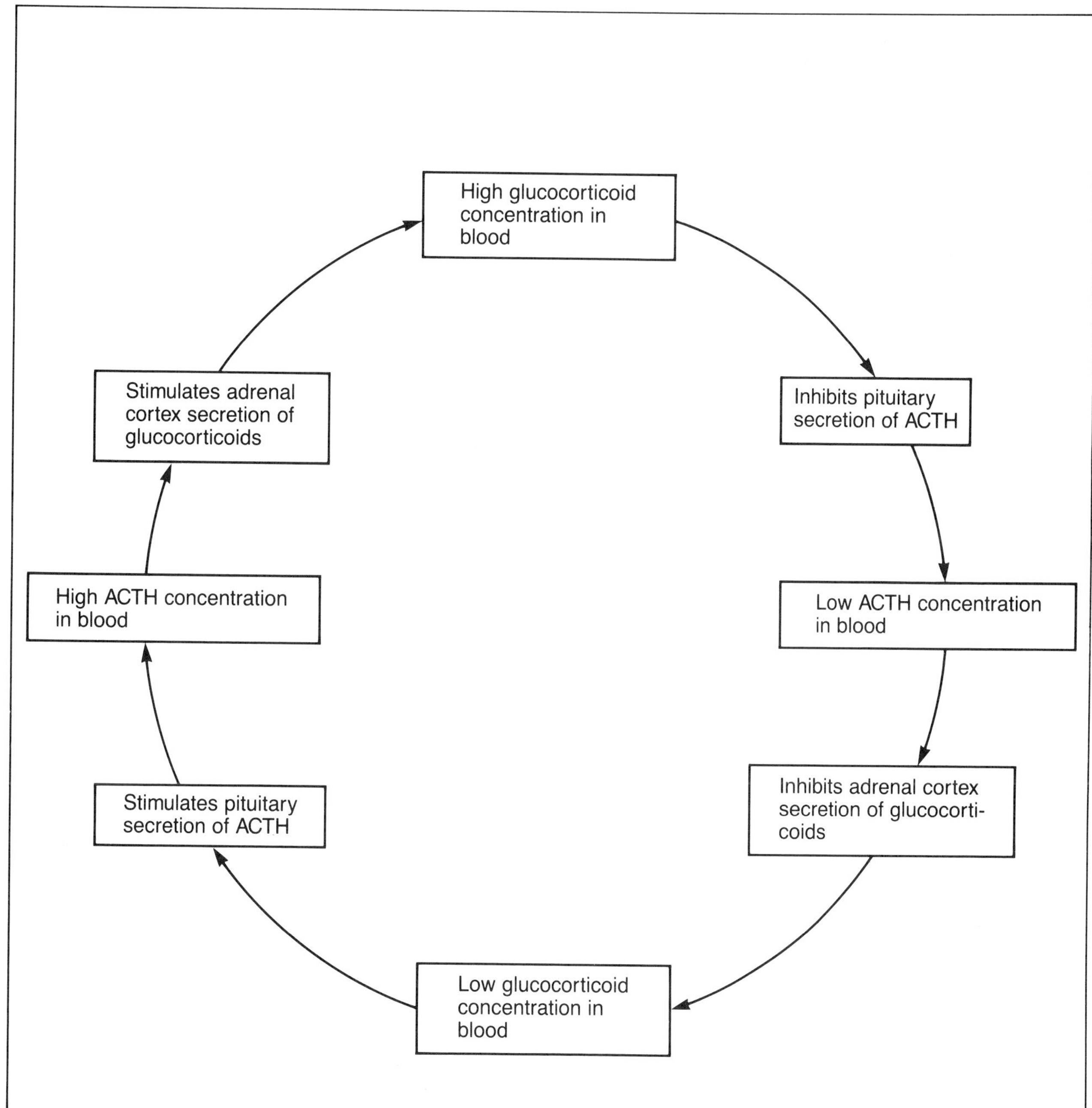

Figure 40-5 Negative feedback regulation of adrenocorticotropic hormone (ACTH) and adrenal hormones.

History

The prenatal history might reveal maternal endocrine dysfunction, which can affect fetal development. Maternal hyperthyroidism can cause either neonatal hyperthyroidism or congenital hypothyroidism. Maternal hyperparathyroidism can cause neonatal hypocalcemia. Diabetes during pregnancy is associated with both fetal macrosomia and small-for-gestation infants, as well as hypoglycemia, respiratory distress, and congenital anomalies of the cardiac, musculoskeletal, renal, and gastrointestinal systems. Because the mother might feel guilty about possibly causing her offspring to have health problems, the nurse needs to phrase questions tactfully to minimize further trauma.

Because some endocrine disorders are of genetic origin, a family history is essential. Nephrogenic diabetes insipidus, hypoparathyroidism, hyperparathyroidism, vitamin D-resistant rickets, familial thyroid enlargement (goiters),

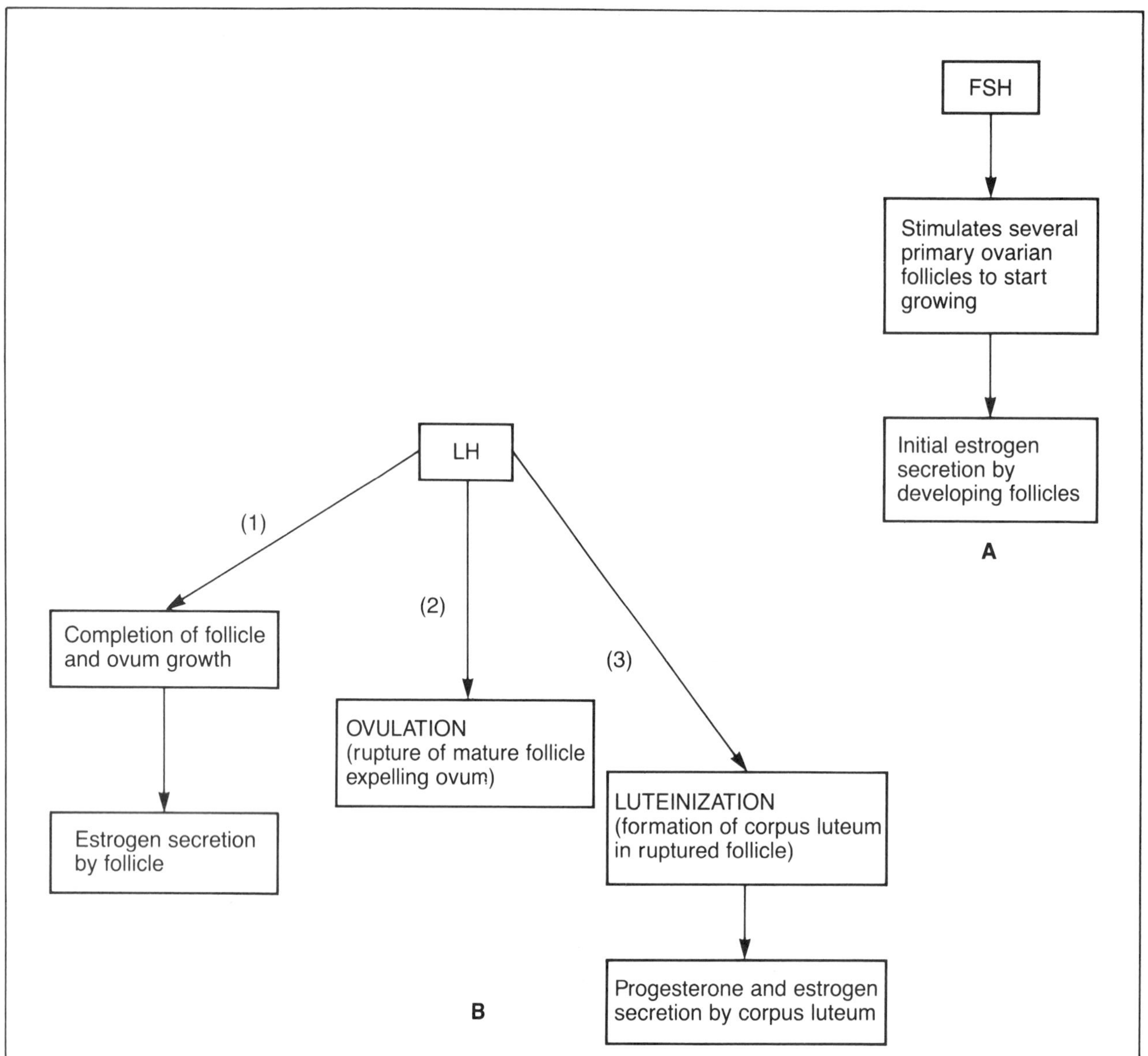

Figure 40-6 Regulation of ovarian function. *A.* A Folicle-stimulating hormone's principal effects on ovaries. *B.* Luteinizing hormone's effects on ovaries: (1) Luteinizing hormone (LH) acts as a synergist to follicle-stimulating hormone (FSH) to enhance its effects on follicular development and secretion. (2) Luteinizing hormone presumably triggers ovulation—hence, it is called "the ovulating hormone." (3) There is a luteinizing effect of LH (for which the hormone was named); recent evidence shows that FSH is also necessary for luteinization.

adrenogenital syndromes, and aldosterone deficiency are all thought to be heritable by X-linked or autosomal modes of transmission. The genetics of childhood diabetes mellitus are currently being defined, as are the growth characteristics of the X chromosome. The family history should include all blood relatives in the child's extended family (see Fig. 5–10).

Obtaining a history of the child's growth and attainment of developmental milestones is important because endocrine dysfunctions can alter growth and neurologic development. The nurse assesses the child's growth record, plotting the heights, weights, and head circumference measurements on standard growth charts (Appendix A). The average child will grow and gain weight at rates similar to those listed in Table 40-2.

Thyroid disorders, diabetes mellitus, and diabetes insipidus all produce changes in the child's daily habits that can affect behavior. The nurse therefore asks about changes in school performance, constipation or diarrhea, heat or cold intolerance, changes in appetite or food preferences, and

TABLE 40-1 Effects of Hormonal Action, Excess, and Deficiency

Hormone	Effect	Result of deficiency	Result of excess
Thyroxine	Regulates metabolic rate, growth, and tissue development	Hypothyroidism: Low metabolic rate Delayed growth Myxedema Thickened, dry skin Constipation Cold intolerance Fatigue Mental retardation in infants (cretinism)	Hyperthyroidism: High metabolic rate Accelerated growth Weight loss Increased appetite Smooth, moist skin Diarrhea Heat intolerance Nervousness, tremors Emotional lability Exophthalmus
Thyrotropin-releasing hormone (TRH)	Stimulates the pituitary gland to release TSH (thyroid stimulating hormone)	Tertiary hypothyroidism	—
Thyroid stimulating hormone (TSH)	Stimulates the thyroid gland to synthesize and release thyroxine	Secondary hypothyroidism	(Might be elevated in primary hypothyroidism)
Parathormone (PTH)	Maintains blood calcium concentration by promoting bone breakdown and absorption from the intestine and reabsorption of calcium and excretion of phosphate by the renal tubules	Hypocalcemia: Tetany Convulsions Muscle spasms	Hypercalcemia: Osteoporosis Bone masses Renal calculi Polyuria
Cortisol (hydrocortisone, glucocorticoid)	Maintains blood glucose concentration via protein breakdown and mobilization of fat for gluconeogenesis. Maintains normal blood pressure by assisting epinephrine and norepinephrine with vasoconstriction. Has antiinflammatory effect and helps body fight stress	Adrenal insufficiency: Addison's disease Congenital adrenal hyperplasia Hypotension, shock Hyperpigmentation Increased muscle mass Accelerated bone maturation	Cushing's syndrome Hypertension Fat redistribution Muscle wasting Glucose intolerance Weight gain and striae
Aldosterone (mineralocorticoid)	Maintains blood sodium concentration by causing distal renal tubules to reabsorb sodium and water. Helps to maintain blood potassium level and pH	Hypotension Dehydration Shock Often coexists with glucocorticoid deficiency in Addison's disease and congenital adrenal hyperplasia	Hypertension Edema
Adrenal sex steroids (androgens, estrogens)	Development of pubic and axillary hair	—	Virilization Advanced bone maturation
Adrenocorticotropic hormone (ACTH)	Stimulates the adrenal cortex to convert cholesterol into adrenal steroids	Adrenal insufficiency	Might be increased in adrenal enzyme deficiencies—congenital hyperplasia Cushing's disease (same symptoms as listed above in Cushing's syndrome)
Insulin	Storage of glucose, amino acids, and fatty acids from blood into cells	Diabetes mellitus	Hypoglycemia
Glucagon	Increases blood glucose concentration by promoting glycogenolysis by liver	Hypoglycemia	Hyperglycemia

continued on next page

TABLE 40-1 (continued)

Hormone	Effect	Result of deficiency	Result of excess
Estrogen	Promotes secondary sexual characteristics and promotes endometrial proliferation	Lack of secondary sexual development Amenorrhea	Precocious puberty Short stature
Progesterone	Prepares endometrium to nurture fertilized ovum; maintains pregnancy	Dysmenorrhea and functional bleeding Spontaneous abortion	—
Testosterone	Promotes male secondary sexual characteristics. Anabolic steroid—stimulates protein anabolism and skeletal growth	Failure to develop male secondary sexual characteristics Late closure of epiphyses—tall stature	—
Follicle-stimulating hormone (FSH)	Stimulates seminiferous tubules to produce sperm in males; stimulates the secretion of estrogen and progesterone in females	Low sperm count in males Lack of secondary sexual development in females	Early pubertal development Might also be elevated in primary gonadal failure
Luteinizing hormone (LH)	Stimulates ovulation in females; stimulates secretion of testosterone in males; also called ICSH (interstitial cell-stimulating hormone in males)	Failure to ovulate in females Low testosterone levels in males	Early pubertal development in males Might be elevated in primary gonadal failure
Luteinizing-releasing hormone (LRH)	Stimulates the release of FSH and LH by the pituitary gland	As above	—
Antidiuretic hormone (ADH, also called vasopressin)	Stimulates distal loop of kidney to reabsorb water and sodium	Diabetes insipidus: Hypernatremia Dehydration	Water intoxication: Edema Hyponatremia
Somatotropin (growth hormone)	Converted by the liver to somatomedin, which promotes somatic growth and maintains blood glucose level	Poor growth Hypoglycemia	Gigantism or acromegaly, depending on the age at which it develops

TABLE 40-2 Average Height and Weight Gain Per Year of Life

Age	Linear growth per year	Weight gain per year
0–12 months	10 in (25 cm)	13–18 lb (6–8 kg)
13–24 months	5 in (12.5 cm)	5–8 lb (2.5 kg)
25–36 months	4 in (10 cm)	4–6 lb (2 kg)
37–48 months	3 in (8 cm)	3–5 lb (1–2 kg)
4 years to puberty	2.0–2.5 in (5.0–6.5 cm)	4–6 lb (2–3 kg)

changes in sleeping habits. During the history-taking session, the nurse observes the child's behavior and requests for food, drink, and trips to the bathroom.

Physical Examination

Careful measurement is important for accuracy (see Chapter 14) and the nurse questions whether the current measurements are believable and whether they reflect a marked deviation from previous measurements.

In assessing the child's general appearance, the nurse observes the child's body proportions to determine whether the limbs appear to be proportional to the trunk, that is, whether the arms and legs appear too long or too short. Changes in the ratio of upper and lower skeletal segments

(text continued on p. 1422)

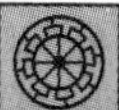

ASSESSMENT GUIDE Child With Altered Hormonal Regulation

System	Subjective data	Objective data	Validating data	Nursing management
Eyes, ears, nose, and throat	Blurred vision, impaired peripheral vision, seeing halos around lights, dryness of eyes in morning	Abnormal facies; flattened nasal bridge; small jaw and crowded teeth; large jaw, broad face, large tongue, high arched palate, coarse or immature features. Fasciculation of tongue. Exophthalmus. Lens opacity evident. Funduscopic examination reveals displaced lens, "cotton wool spots" (occlusion of retinal artery), dilatation, tortuosity, or irregularities of vessels. Cervical mass. Firm enlargement of thyroid.	Serum hormonal levels, blood glucose level. Tonometry; CT scan. Vision tests (see Chapter 43). Thyroid studies (See Tables 40-3, 40-4, and 40-5)	Obtain family history of any endocrine abnormalities. Teach parent to instill methyl-cellulose eyedrops at night to protect cornea. Discuss safety precautions necessitated by diminished vision, especially peripheral limitations. Emphasize importance of frequent eye examinations to monitor visual changes. Compare facial features of parent and child; note similarities and differences for potential diagnostic data.
Integumentary	Hands frequently wet and sweaty, increased or decreased perspiration. Hair loss. Excessive pigmentation. Puffy hands or feet. Heat and cold intolerance	Dry, cold, thick skin. Pallor, decreased skin turgor. Excess or lack of perspiration. Thin, velvety, moist skin. Purple–red striae and thin skin. Flushing, hyperpigmentation of scars and skin folds, café-au-lait spots, mottling of skin. Acne. Webbing of neck and low hairline. Brittle nails and fragile hair. Atropic areas or skin lesions	Serum electrolyte levels, serum hormonal levels, and blood glucose level	Observe for signs of dehydration and electrolyte imbalance. Provide fluid replacement. Monitor intake and output. Provide skin care. Monitor environmental temperature and protect child from sudden changes. Review method and rotation of injection sites for administration of insulin
Respiratory	Difficulty in breathing	Fruity odor of breath. Apneic episodes, nasal obstruction, noisy respirations. Laryngeal stridor. Kussmaul's respirations. Dyspnea, wheezing, tachypnea	(See Tables 40-4 and 40-5)	Monitor intravenous administration of insulin. Position patient so that large tongue does not obstruct airway. Observe for signs of adrenal crisis (cyanosis; cold skin; weak, rapid pulse; rapid, labored respirations). Monitor respiratory status. Note any family history of asthma because beta-adrenergic blocking

continued on next page

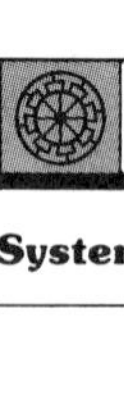

ASSESSMENT GUIDE Child With Altered Hormonal Regulation (continued)

System	Subjective data	Objective data	Validating data	Nursing management
				agent may trigger asthma attack in susceptible child
Cardiovascular	Faintness, dizziness. Palpitations. Easy bruising	Tachycardia, bradycardia. Hypertension or hypotension. Absent femoral pulses; signs of capillary fragility, weak, thready pulse, cardiomegaly, cardiac murmur. Signs of hypokalemia or hyperkalemia, hyponatremia or hypernatremia.	Serum electrolytes and hormonal levels. Radiograph of chest, electrocardiography. (See Tables 40-3, 40-4, and 40-5)	Monitor pulse, blood pressure, heart sounds. Observe for signs of dehydration or electrolyte imbalance. Observe for other signs of hypoglycemia or adrenal insufficiency. Observe for lethargy, dull expression, large tongue, puffy face. Inquire about changes in behavior, appetite, weight. Monitor intravenous infusion and child's response to replacement therapy. Observe cardiac monitor for electrocardiographic changes relative to electrolyte imbalance. Verify that child is receiving steroids and review dangers of suddenly discontinuing medication, even if child is ill
Gastrointestinal	Increased thirst and appetite. Anorexia, nausea, abdominal pain. Change in food preferences, craving for salt	Failure to gain weight or weight loss. Vomiting. Infant feeding difficulties such as sleepiness, slowness, lack of interest, choking. Constipation or diarrhea	Serum glucose, electrolyte levels. Urine testing for glucose and acetone levels. Serum calcium level. (See Tables 40-3, 40-4, and 40-5)	Obtain 24-hour dietary recall and compare with prescribed diet. Note frequency of child's requests for food and drink. Observe for other signs of ketoacidosis. Monitor intake and output. Keep record of character and number of stools. Teach or review dietary modifications relative to hormonal disorder. Discuss methods of feeding infant to increase intake and prevent aspiration

ASSESSMENT GUIDE Child With Altered Hormonal Regulation (continued)

System	Subjective data	Objective data	Validating data	Nursing management
Genitourinary	History of nocturia, nocturnal enuresis in previously continent child. Frequent urination. Early or delayed appearance of secondary sex characteristics. Difficulty in deciding whether child is male or female. Dysuria, history of recurrent urinary tract infections	Polyuria. Increased or decreased pubic hair. Overdeveloped or underdeveloped genitals for child's age. Abnormal or ambiguous genitals: fused labia, enlarged clitoris, undescended testes (cryptorchidism), hypospadius, decreased length and/or diameter of penis. Cloudy urine, elevated specific gravity, small frequent voids. Polyuria with decreased specific gravity	Radiographic studies for bone age. Serum and urinary hormone levels, urine culture, chromosomal studies, tissue biopsy (See Tables 40-3, 40-4, and 40-5)	Note excessive requests to use bathroom. Monitor intake and output and specific gravity of urine. Monitor growth on standard growth chart. Record signs of sexual precocity, provide for privacy during examination. Describe abnormalities of genitals. Observe for hyperpigmentation of tissues. Support the family and child during diagnostic testing, decision making, and treatment. Support adolescent experiencing delayed or absent secondary sex characteristics; refer for counseling if appropriate
Neuroendocrine	Family history of X-linked or autosomally transmitted traits: nephrogenic hypoglycemia, diabetes insipidus, hypoparathyroidism, hyperparathyroidism, vitamin D-resistant rickets, familial thyroid enlargement (goiters), aldosterone deficiency. History of delay in developmental milestones. Changes in behavior, school performance, sleep patterns, heat or cold intolerance. Faintness, nervousness, irritability, headache, confusion, fatigue. Numbness, tingling, prickling sensation in hands and feet	Small for gestational age, fetal macrosomia. Sluggish or brisk deep tendon reflexes. Excessive mobility or sluggishness. Altered balance and coordination. Labile mood, lethargy, somnolence, coma. Tremulousness, shaky handwriting, slurred speech. Developmental disability, mental retardation. Eyelid lag, restlessness. Signs of increased intracranial pressure. Tetany, convulsions	Electrocardiography. Serum calcium level and hormonal levels (see Tables 40-3, 40-4, and 40-5)	Validate family history of any metabolic disorders. Observe child's behavior, attention span, balance, and coordination. Monitor fluid and electrolyte balance and note child's response to replacement therapy. Assist family and child in managing diet, exercise, and medication. Provide easily assimilated carbohydrates for hypoglycemic episodes such as orange juice with sugar added, nondiet soft drinks, candy and administer glucagon as ordered. Teach the child and family the importance of cooperation with the medical plan to prevent further retardation or delayed development. Observe for signs of increased

continued on next page

ASSESSMENT GUIDE Child With Altered Hormonal Regulation (continued)

System	Subjective data	Objective data	Validating data	Nursing management
				intracranial pressure. Institute seizure precautions. Inquire about any paresthesia
Musculoskeletal	History of weight loss or gain, altered growth patterns. Muscle pain and cramps, numbness. Pain in back and extremities. Weakness, fatigue, listlessness, lethargy. Increased bruising. Hand tremors. Change in body proportions	Birthweight might be low, normal, or increased. Growth disturbance, growth retardation, short stature, with variable age of onset. Early closure of epiphyses, excessive growth, acromegaly, increased size of facial features, advanced or delayed osseous development, excess linear growth. Muscular wasting, hypotonia, or increased muscular development. Positive Chvostek's sign, positive Trousseau's sign. Evidence of frequent fractures from minimal stress, altered gait. Truncal obesity with thin extremities, "buffalo hump" on back	Radiography for bone age, fractures. Serum calcium levels (see Tables 40-3, 40-4, and 40-5)	Measure and plot on growth chart height, weight, head circumference. Note body proportions, measure arm span. Note muscle strength and evidence of muscle wasting. Explore child's feelings about body stature, proportions, weight. Monitor treatment of osseous deformities and fractures. Monitor treatment for altered calcium levels (intravenous infusion of calcium)

occur throughout childhood until they approach the adult ratio of 1:1. Assessment of arm span is accomplished by measuring the distance between the fingertips with the arms extended straight out from the shoulders. The nurse also observes the child's facial features for any of the following findings associated with endocrine dysfunction: flattened nasal bridge, small jaw and crowded teeth, bowing of the frontal bones of the skull, and the presence of a high, arched palate.

The eye examination includes checking for displaced lenses, cataracts, exophthalmos, and retinal hemorrhages, as well as careful assessment of visual acuity and visual fields.

The amount of testosterone to which the fetus is exposed during development affects the appearance of the newborn's external genitals. Insufficient testosterone alters the male genitals and excessive testosterone alters the female genitals thus resulting in abnormalities or ambiguous genitals. The female infant's external genitals are examined for enlargement of the clitoris, fusion of the labia, and hyperpigmentation of the tissue. The male infant's external genitals are examined for the presence of testes in the scrotum, hyperpigmentation, hypospadias, and length and diameter of the penis. The length of the penis is measured by using a short, stiff ruler that is pressed gently into the symphysis pubis as the penile length is noted.

When assessing the sexual development of the adolescent or older child, the nurse evaluates whether the parent should stay or leave the room. The nurse provides the patient with a gown and cover sheet and requests that all clothing be removed. Examination of breast development and axillary hair can be accomplished while assessing the heart and lungs, and pubic hair can be assessed when evaluating femoral pulses.

Secondary sexual characteristics (pubic and axillary hair in both sexes, facial hair in males, and breast development in females) are the external markers that distinguish the sexes from each other but play no direct role in reproduction. Secondary sexual development is described by a

TABLE 40-3 Evaluation of Endocrine Function: Diagnostic Tests

Procedure	Purpose	Invasive	Noninvasive	Preparation of patient
Thyroid functions: Triiodothyronine (T_3) Thyroxine (T_4) Triiodothyronine (T_3UR) uptake ratio Triiodothyronine by radioimmunoassay (T_3-RIA) Free thyroxine Thyroid-stimulating hormone (TSH)	Assess thyroid hormone regulation	Yes	No	The child who is taking thyroxine must take it regularly for 14 days prior to the test
Thyroid scan (Image)	Assess size and character of the thyroid gland	Yes	No	If the scan is to determine the presence of thyroid cancer, the patient must stop taking thyroxine for 4–6 weeks and triiodothyronine 10–14 days prior to the scan
Pelvic/abdominal ultrasound	Assess ovaries and adrenal glands for size, masses, cysts	No	Yes	Encouage oral fluids to fill the bladder prior to the sonogram
Bone age radiograph of hand and wrist	Assess skeletal maturation	No	Yes	Might require a hemiskeletal survey for a very young child
CT scan of head	Examine head for masses near pituitary gland	Yes	No	Sedation might be required. Child who needs sedation might be allowed nothing by mouth prior to the scan
Glucose tolerance test, intravenous or oral	Evaluate glucose tolerance and insulin secretion in response to carbohydrate intake	Yes	No	Child must have had an adequate carbohydrate intake (at least 50% of calories as carbohydrates for the previous 3 days. Nothing except water is allowed by mouth for 12 hours prior to the test. This test should not be performed on a child with an elevated fasting blood glucose level
Luteinizing releasing hormone (LRH, or luteinizing hormone releasing hormone, LHRH) stimulation test	Evaluate pituitary gland's ability to release luteinizing hormone (LH) and follicle-stimulating hormone (FSH)	Yes	No	Patient might be allowed nothing by mouth several hours prior to the test
Thyrotropin-releasing hormone (TRH) stimulation test	Evaluate pituitary TSH reserve	Yes	No	The test is performed in the morning after an overnight fast. Blood pressure and pulse are monitored. Thyroxine is stopped for 14–28 days prior to the test
Adrenocorticotropic hormone (ACTH) stimulation test	Evaluate ability of adrenal cortex to synthesize adrenocortical hormones	Yes	No	Nothing by mouth allowed for 12 hours prior to the test
Human chorionic gonadotropin (HCG) test	Assess ability of testes to secrete testosterone	Yes	No	Serum testosterone level is measured before and after a series of HCG injections
Metyrapone test	Assess ACTH and cortisol production	No	Yes	Baseline 24-hour urine specimens are collected for 1–2 days, then metyrapone is given every 4 hours

continued on next page

TABLE 40-3 continued

Procedure	Purpose	Invasive	Noninvasive	Preparation of patient
				for six doses, after which urine specimens are collected for 24 hours. The patient cannot be taking diphenylhydantoin (Dilantin). If the patient is on cortisone, this medication must be stopped, which places the patient at risk for adrenal insufficiency
Dexamethasone suppression test	Study cortisol suppression in Cushing's syndrome	Yes	No	Dexamethasone is given every 6 hours for 2 days, then the serum cortisol level is measured and urine is collected. The patient might develop adrenal insufficiency during this test

TABLE 40-4 Urine Studies in Endocrine Dysfunction

Substance studied	Endocrine dysfunction	Effect observed
Urinary 17-ketosteroids	Adrenal cortex dysfunction	Increased in enzymatic deficiency
Urinary 17-hydroxycorticosteroids	Adrenal cortex dysfunction causing early adrenarche	Increased
Urinary free cortisol	Adrenal cortex dysfunction	Increased in Cushing's syndrome; decreased in Addison's disease and enzyme deficiency
Urinary calcium	Parathyroid dysfunction	Decreased in hypoparathyroidism; increased in hyperparathyroidism
Urinary sodium	Adrenal cortex dysfunction	Increased in enzymatic deficiencies and Addison's disease
	Diabetes insipidus	Increased
Urinary glucose	Diabetes mellitus; Cushing's syndrome	Present in measurable quantities
Urinary Vanillylmandelic Acid (VMA)	Tumors of the adrenal gland	Increased

General considerations in collecting urine are to avoid catheterization; check on requirements for preservatives or refrigeration of urine; check on dietary restrictions; monitor the timing of collection carefully; and ensure collection of all urine.

"staging process" developed by Tanner (1971) and is described and illustrated in Chapter 11 (see Figs. 11-2 and 11-3).

Endocrine disorders might affect skin texture, temperature, turgor, and pigmentation. The nurse observes the skin for the following characteristics: thickness, coarseness, doughy feel, dryness, sallow color, moistness, warmth, hyperpigmentation of scars and skin folds, flushing, café-au-lait spots, pigmented nevi, and striae.

The child's respiratory status is assessed, noting the character and rate of respirations. The child's breath is assessed for the presence of a fruity odor (a sign of ketoacidosis) by requesting the child to repeat a sentence.

Because thyroid disorders affect the child's neurologic status, the nurse performs a thorough neurologic examination. Deep tendon reflexes are assessed for sluggishness, briskness, and speed of return, the tongue for fasciculations, the hands for tremors, and the eyelids for lag. The child's level of consciousness, orientation, balance, and coordination also are described.

The nurse assesses blood pressure, pulse, and patency of peripheral circulation because these parameters are affected by some endocrine dysfunctions. Any increase in muscle mass and muscle strength is noted because adrenal disorders can affect muscle tone.

While making objective observations during the physical examination, the nurse converses with the child and family, thereby obtaining additional subjective data. These data are then validated by the use of diagnostic laboratory and radiologic tests, when appropriate.

TABLE 40-5 Alterations in Serum Values in Endocrine Disease

Component	Normal Value*	Alteration	Significance
Sodium (Na^+)	135–145 mEq/L	Decreased	Sodium ions are bound by free fatty acids in diabetic ketoacidosis; excessive vasopressin dosage causes water retention; diluting the concentration of sodium in the blood; adrenal crisis with aldosterone deficiency causes sodium loss into the urine
		Increased	Hypernatremic dehydration in untreated diabetes insipidus
Potassium (K^+)	3.5–5.0 mEq/L	Decreased	Potassium loss into the urine with hyperglycemia and Cushing's syndrome
		Increased	Adrenal insufficiency with aldosterone deficiency
Calcium (Ca^{++})	8.8–10.1 mg/dL	Increased	Hyperparathyroidism; thyrotoxicosis
		Decreased	Hypoparathyroidism; vitamin D-resistant rickets
Phosphorus (P)	2.0–4.5 mg/dL	Increased	Hypoparathyroidism
		Decreased	Diabetic ketoacidosis; hyperparathyroidism
Glucose	70–100 mg/dL	Increased	Diabetes mellitus; Cushing's syndrome
		Decreased	Hyperinsulinism; hypopituitarism; adrenal insufficiency
pH	7.32–7.45	Decreased	Diabetic ketoacidosis
Hematocrit	12–16 g/dL	Increased	Cushing's syndrome
Glycosolated hemoglobin (HbA_{1c})	2.2%–4.8% of total hemoglobin: HbA_{1c}	Increased	Poorly controlled or newly diagnosed diabetes

*Values vary slightly depending on the source used.

Nursing Management for Procedures and Tests

Preparation for Diagnostic Tests

Children with suspected endocrine dysfunction undergo fairly extensive and sometimes invasive diagnostic workups. The nurse's role in the diagnostic workup might consist of coordinating the various procedures, teaching children and parents how to collect urine specimens, explaining procedures to children and parents, providing emotional support to children during procedures, and ultimately teaching children and parents how to administer medications required for management of the endocrine dysfunction. (See Chapter 29 for teaching/learning principles and age-appropriate methods of preparing children for diagnostic procedures.) Parents need to be included in the preparation for their own comfort and to assist the child in dealing with the new situation. The nurse is generous with time estimates because children and parents will become apprehensive in the face of unexpected delays. The nurse explains clearly what meals must be omitted before certain procedures.

For example, one 4-year-old girl was referred to an endocrine clinic because her mother had noticed pubic hair development, acceleration in linear growth, and body odor in her daughter for approximately 2 months. No symptoms of intracranial pressure were reported by the mother, but the mother did report emotional lability and pubic hair growth in the child. Physical examination by the nurse revealed the following objective data that are abnormal for a 4-year-old child: axillary sweating and odor, Tanner Stage II pubic hair, and a height/weight plot on the 90th percentile for age compared with previous growth parameters along the 50th percentile. Further diagnostic tests were ordered by the physician. The nurse explained the test procedures and accompanied the child and her family to the test locations. A radiograph of the girl's left hand and wrist was obtained to examine the degree of skeletal maturation. An ultrasonic study of her pelvis and abdomen was performed to examine the size and character of her adrenal glands and ovaries. A 24-hour urine specimen was requested to measure her 17-ketosteroid excretion. Blood was obtained by venipuncture to measure the levels of 17-hydroxyprogesterone, FSH, LH, and estradiol. The nurse explained to the child and her parents such details as the importance of having the bladder filled prior to the ultrasonic study and how to collect the 24-hour urine specimen and provided comfort during the venipuncture.

Care of a Child Receiving Steroid Therapy

Children with adrenal disorders take replacement (physiologic) amounts of cortisone. The dosage is prescribed for the child and on this amount of steroid, the child is not at risk for complications (infections, hypertension) that might occur when larger (pharmacologic) doses of steroids are used to treat renal disease, asthma, juvenile rheumatoid arthritis, and cancer. The most important aspect of steroid therapy for children with adrenal disease is ensuring regular (two to three times a day) administration of the medication. Without this daily steroid replacement, the children are in a state of adrenal insufficiency and at risk for developing adrenal crisis should a significant stress (trauma, illness) occur. The nurse explains to the child and family the importance of administering the medication every day at the appropriate time, watching for signs and symptoms of adrenal insufficiency and obtaining emergency treatment for adrenal insufficiency, and suggests ways to remember the daily medication. The nurse also reminds the family that the steroid dose must be continued and increased during illnesses characterized by fever or anorexia. The family must not allow any medical personnel to discontinue the steroids during an illness on the basis that steroids and infectious diseases are incompatible; to do so could lead to death from adrenal insufficiency.

Principles of Nursing Care

Acute-Care Needs

Acute nursing care of the child with endocrine dysfunction involves prompt, skilled observation and intervention. These children might present with or develop electrolyte abnormalities during treatment. A potassium deficit should be suspected if the child complains of muscle weakness and has a weak pulse, absent reflexes, hypotension, or arrhythmias; this problem must be recognized and treated promptly to prevent death from apnea and cardiac arrest (Burgess, 1979). The nurse also is alert for irritability, diarrhea, and oliguria, which are signs of hyperkalemia. Because excessive potassium levels slow or prevent the transmission of stimuli through the cardiac muscles, the child can experience intraventricular conduction disturbances (Burgess, 1979). Children who are hypocalcemic will report a tingling sensation in the fingers and around the mouth, muscle cramps in the abdomen, and carpopedal spasms or have convulsions. The child who is hypercalcemic has flaccid muscles, reports flank or deep thigh pain, has nausea and vomiting, or is stuporous. The child with hyponatremia will appear very apprehensive, complain of abdominal cramps and have diarrhea, be hypotensive with a rapid, thready pulse, have cold clammy skin, and possibly be cyanotic; seizures also might occur. With hypernatremia, the child may be agitated and appear flushed and have dry, sticky mucous membranes, a firm, rubbery turgor to the skin, and very little urine output (Burgess, 1979).

In addition to the previously mentioned electrolyte abnormalities, children with endocrine dysfunction also develop hypoglycemia, respiratory distress, and acidosis—all potentially fatal conditions that require intensive nursing care.

Endocrine dysfunction complicates the nursing care of the child undergoing surgery. The stress of surgery frequently changes the child's hormonal requirements. When the nurse plans preoperative and postoperative care of the child with an endocrine dysfunction, the assessment must include (1) when the child received the most recent dose of hormone (insulin, hydrocortisone, vasopressin, propylthiouracil); (2) how long the child will be unable to eat and take oral medication; (3) the current measurements of blood pressure, pulse, blood glucose level, and serum electrolyte levels; and (4) the medical plan for the administration of hormones during surgery and recovery.

For example, a 16-year-old with poorly controlled diabetes mellitus required emergency surgery for appendicitis. Preoperative interventions included (1) determining the exact time, dosage, and type of insulin that was last taken and recording this information clearly on the chart; (2) obtaining a history of recent food and fluid intake, vomiting, diarrhea and most recent voiding; (3) measuring vital signs and noting the odor of the breath; (4) assessing skin turgor and mucous membranes for hydration; and (5) careful explanation of events to allay the adolescent's anxiety. In addition to routine postoperative care, as discussed in Chapters 29 and 38, the nurse monitored blood glucose levels and performed dipstick urine tests for the presence of ketones.

Nutritional Needs

Certain endocrine disorders alter children's appetites, fluid requirements, and appetite control. Diabetes mellitus, hyperthyroidism, and Cushing's syndrome increase the child's appetite tremendously. Hypercalcemia, diabetes insipidus, diabetes mellitus, and adrenal insufficiency cause the child to be thirsty and require an increased fluid intake. For example, one 14-year-old female came to the endocrine clinic wanting help in controlling her weight gain. Over the past 6 months, she had gained 50 lb. She reported that she would get up at night to raid the refrigerator for food and that her intake of food at meals exceeded that of her father and older brother combined. The nurse inquired about the past health history and learned that this adolescent had had a pituitary abscess aspirated 3 years earlier. Her signs and symptoms indicated that her hypothalamus had lost its ability to control her appetite and that she had no sense of satiety. Diagnostic tests ordered included a CT (computerized tomographic) scan of the head, which demonstrated a mass in the hypothalamic–pituitary region.

Other endocrine disorders cause unusual or uncontrollable cravings. For example, one 11-year-old male presented with complaints of weakness and nausea. Assessment of his food intake revealed a preference for salty foods such as pretzels and dill pickles; he even reported drinking the liquid from the pickle jars. On physical examination, the nurse noted that the child had hyperpigmentation in his skin creases. Diagnostic testing confirmed that the salt craving was due to Addison's disease.

A 24-hour dietary recall or a written 3-day dietary history (see Chapter 15) provides for nutritional assessment, planning, and teaching in endocrine-related disorders. Children with diabetes require some dietary modifications to avoid hypoglycemia and hyperglycemia. These special needs will be addressed in the section on the management of diabetes in children.

Developmental Needs

Several endocrine disorders might cause neurologic impairment and learning difficulties in children who develop these problems during infancy and the early childhood years, when the brain is still developing. Congenital hypothyroidism, if not recognized within 1 or 2 months after birth, can cause serious mental retardation (cretinism). Severe or frequent hypoglycemia in young children with diabetes, panhypopituitarism, adrenal insufficiency, hyperinsulinism, and ketotic hypoglycemia has been associated with varying degrees of mental retardation and developmental delays. Girls with Turner's syndrome frequently have difficulty with problems involving spatial relationships, so the nurse considers carefully when a short, prepubertal female reports that she has problems in geometry but does well in other subjects at school.

Socialization Needs

Chronic health disorders might cause school absences, lack of participation in peer group activities, and an overprotection-dependence relationship between parents and children. All of these factors can interfere with the child's socialization. Most endocrine disorders have few visible stigmas. This is a mixed blessing for children, being positive in that the disorder is not visibly handicapping but negative in that some people might not believe that the children have serious health problems which can legitimately interfere with activities and responsibilities.

The nurse assists children in meeting their needs for socialization through education and role playing, and by providing emotional support through listening.

For example, one 13-year-old female who had recently moved to another state elected not to tell her new classmates that she had diabetes for fear of being ostracized, yet she hesitated to join in activities with her new acquaintances because she feared having an insulin reaction (hypoglycemia). The nurse worked with this young adolescent for 6 months, teaching her to manage her diabetes with the goal of gaining self-confidence in meeting new people and interacting in new situations. They practiced role playing in telling new friends about the diabetes. The nurse realized the goal was achieved when this adolescent called one night from a slumber party with her new friends requesting advice on what to eat for a midnight snack following a vigorous game of volleyball. The happy sound of her new friends could be heard in the background.

Emotional Needs

The child's ability to deal with a chronic endocrine dysfunction depends to a great extent on several variables: cultural influences, the child's age and developmental level, family's perception of the health problem, and strengths of the family system. (These variables are discussed in Chapter 30 in relation to chronic conditions in children.)

The child's cultural background contributes to the ways in which the endocrine disorder is perceived (see Chapter 3). The nurse adapts the method of and approach to teaching children and families to their unique cultural features.

The age at which children develop endocrine disorders can affect how they and their families perceive the seriousness of the disorder. Parents of infants and young children with diabetes mellitus might be so overprotective that they feel they cannot leave their children with babysitters and are reluctant to let their children enter school at the appropriate age.

Families perceive health problems in different ways. Some of the variance in perceptions depends on how seriously ill the child is when the disorder is diagnosed or how physically abnormal the child looks because of the disorder. Parents of newborn females with congenital adrenal hyperplasia generally are quite distraught initially because of the virilization of the external genitals. These families often continue to be very apprehensive about their daughters because the children can develop adrenal insufficiency quickly with intercurrent illnesses. Newborn boys with this condition generally are not diagnosed until they are 10–14 days of age, at which time they usually are quite ill; in fact, some newborn males nearly die before the diagnosis is made and treatment initiated. Girls with Turner's syndrome and their families must cope with the emotional burden of infertility and short stature. Children who develop Cushing's syndrome have altered body images, emotional lability, and limitation of activity, to which they must adjust until the symptoms are relieved. Children with deficiencies in growth hormone frequently are treated as younger children, and parents, peers, and schoolteachers either limit their participation in activities or have unrealistic expectations of their physical capabilities.

In assessing family strengths, the nurse might wish to use one of the family assessment tools discussed in Chapter 17. Parental support is the key to both good management of any health disorder and the child's having a healthy self-image. The nurse provides support, objective observations, and information concerning child development as it relates to the child's needs for parental support with a given task. Parents who can develop realistic and responsible attitudes toward their children's health problems, incorporate the children's health needs into the family's life-style, and maintain intact generational boundaries are the most supportive of their children. At times, health professionals might need to take over some aspects of parenting, both to give the parents respite and to serve as role models for the parents.

Health Maintenance Needs

Most endocrine disorders are chronic in nature and must be evaluated regularly by a health care team. The nurse has the opportunity to build rapport with the child and family and provide ongoing education in the areas of health maintenance, parenting, and child development. This can be a distinct advantage over the acute-care setting, in which the nurse has less time for teaching on such topics.

The nurse assesses the family's beliefs about health maintenance and makes plans for ongoing education accordingly. Families who use health care facilities only for acute, episodic care might have difficulty comprehending the need for regular well-child checkups. For example, one mother commented when reminded about her daughter's appointment at the diabetes clinic that she had not planned to keep the appointment because her daughter was not sick that day.

Children over 6 years of age and their parents must learn the basic survival skills associated with their endocrine disorder at the time of diagnosis. They must feel comfortable assuming the responsibility for home management of the problem and demonstrate competence in management and basic knowledge before the children are discharged. Survival skills include (1) understanding the action of the medication or medications to be administered; (2) knowing how to administer the medication and how to prevent, recognize, and treat any side effects of the medication; (3) knowing how to contact the health care team for both follow-up and emergency care; and (4) being able to explain the child's health problem to family, friends, and school personnel. With time, the family will acquire a more thorough understanding of the disorder and its treatment as a result of practical experience, self-education, and continued teaching by health professionals. The nurse does not attempt to teach the child and family everything at the initial contact because most people learn poorly under stressful conditions. The nurse identifies and concentrates on the basic skills and knowledge needed immediately by the family and teaches these facts slowly and patiently.

Children with endocrine disorders have the same basic requirements for rest and stimulation as other normal, healthy children, although extra rest might be required by children with untreated hypothyroidism, poorly controlled diabetes, Cushing's syndrome, and adrenal insufficiency. Children with hyperthyroidism frequently have difficulty sleeping because of their nervousness, tachycardia, and heat intolerance.

The family often finds a visiting or public health nurse helpful during the first few days or weeks at home to provide assistance in setting up home care. In many settings the nurse initiates the visiting nurse referral as part of the discharge planning. The nurse also can refer the family to community lay organizations such as Little People of America or the American Diabetes Association.

Frequently, a parent of another child with the same endocrine disorder can offer practical guidance to the parent of a newly diagnosed child on coping with everyday situations, where to obtain supplies, and the emotional stages experienced by children with chronic illnesses and their parents. The nurse might wish to be present during such a parent visit to gain personal insight into the reality of dealing with chronic illnesses in children.

At regular return visits, the nurse continues to provide anticipatory guidance and divides long-term goals (such as, "Johnny will be giving all his own shots by next summer") into smaller, more tangible steps (such as "by the end of the month, Johnny will be selecting the sites for injections and mixing the insulins"). It is often advisable to schedule checkups just prior to potentially stressful events, such as the beginning of the new school term or vacation, or anticipated developmental changes such as the onset of puberty. Children also need anticipatory guidance. The nurse rehearses with children situations they will encounter such as, "What will you do about taking your afternoon dose of medicine when you go to play at a friend's house after school?" or "What do you want your friends to know about your condition?"

The Child With Altered Secretion of Insulin

Diabetes Mellitus

Diabetes mellitus is a disorder of carbohydrate metabolism that affects 1 out of every 500–800 children under 21 years of age. As such, diabetes mellitus is a common health disorder of children and adolescents.

Diabetes mellitus is classified as *Type I* (juvenile-onset, insulin-dependent) and *Type II* (maturity-onset, usually noninsulin-dependent). Most children with diabetes have the Type I disorder. Recent research has demonstrated a genetic difference in the two types of diabetes; that is, a young child's diabetes probably is unrelated to the fact that an elderly relative has Type II diabetes.

Type I diabetes is associated with an increased frequency of certain histocompatibility antigens (HLA). The HLA system is the major histocompatibility complex, located on chromosome six, consisting of a cluster of genes that code for transplantation antigens and play a central role in the immune response (Sperling, 1982). Type I diabetes is associated with the presence of HLA-B8, B15, DW3, and DW4. Inheritance of HLA-B8 or HLA-B15 appears to confer a twofold to threefold relative risk for developing the disease. When both HLA-B8 and HLA-B15 are inherited together, the relative risk for developing diabetes increases sevenfold to tenfold, suggesting that HLA-B8 and HLA-B15 are additive in their effect of conferring relative risk (Sperling, 1982).

If a child develops diabetes, the risk of siblings developing Type I diabetes is probably 2%–6% as compared with a 0.2% risk for children who have no diabetic siblings. If a parent has Type I diabetes, the risk of offspring developing Type I diabetes is 1%–5% (Rotter and Hodge, 1980). The risk of developing diabetes increases slightly when several family members are diabetic. In the future HLA typing of families in which diabetes exists might estimate more precisely the risk for diabetes; at present, because no preventive therapy is available to at-risk siblings, HLA typing is used mainly for research purposes. Siblings might have periodic blood glucose testing, glucose tolerance tests, islet cell antibodies tests or glycohemoglobin measurements in an attempt to detect the disorder in its early stages.

For food to be metabolized correctly, insulin must be released in adequate quantities from the pancreas when the blood glucose level is rising. Any disruption in the release or effectiveness of insulin can lead to hyperglycemia. Within the broad category of diabetes are several subtypes: Type I, Type II, and MODY (Maturity-onset diabetes of youth). Type I diabetes might or might not be associated with high levels of islet-cell antibodies at the time of diagnosis. Children who have islet-cell antibodies are at risk for developing thyroiditis and Addison's disease, whereas children without islet-cell antibodies do not appear to be at increased risk for the other autoimmune endocrine disorders (Guthrie and Guthrie, 1983). Individuals with Type I diabetes require insulin therapy to live. Type II diabetes is subgrouped into obese and nonobese individuals, and multiple causes have been proposed. Individuals with Type II diabetes might require insulin to prevent hyperglycemia but will not die from lack of insulin therapy (Guthrie and Guthrie, 1983). Maturity-onset diabetes of youth (MODY) occurs most often in adolescents with strong family histories of Type II diabetes; these adolescents have impaired glucose tolerance but generally do not develop ketosis and have characteristics of Type II diabetes (Sperling, 1982). Children frequently ask why they must have insulin injections when their older relatives are able to take oral hypoglycemic agents, and most children secretly hope that their diabetes will convert to Type II diabetes when they become adults. The nurse must kindly but firmly explain the difference between the types of diabetes so that children's and parents' expectations about the course of the disease are realistic.

The histocompatibility complex (HLA) is thought to direct the body's response to various antigens, including viral infections. Some investigators (Nemchik, 1982) believe that children develop diabetes in response to the combination of having a genetic predisposition and HLA-directed response to viral infections, which culminates in the destruction of beta cells. The Coxsackie B4 virus is one virus that has been implicated in the development of diabetes (Nemchik, 1982).

The onset of diabetes mellitus in children and adolescents is generally fairly rapid, with the symptoms and signs appearing over a course of days to weeks. Children of all ages can develop diabetes, even very young children. Often, infants and young children are very ill and in ketoacidosis when diagnosed. Health care providers and parents do not think of very young children as having diabetes and attribute their symptoms initially to gastroenteritis. A quick check of a urine specimen for glucose and the discovery of *glucosuria* (presence of glucose in the urine) leads to the diagnosis of diabetes in the young child.

The classic symptoms of diabetes mellitus are *polyuria, polydipsia, polyphagia,* and weight loss. Polyuria is caused by the spillage of glucose into the urine when the renal threshold for the maximal reabsorption of glucose (160–200 mg/dL in most children) is exceeded. A resultant obligate water loss occurs because of osmotic diuresis. Dehydration and an increase in serum osmolality result, which triggers compensatory polydipsia. Water losses can lead to intravascular volume depletion, decreased perfusion to the kidneys, and decreased glucose clearance by the kidneys, leading ultimately to an increased plasma glucose level. The hyperosmosis pulls water from the cells to the intravascular compartment to minimize intravascular hypertonicity (Moorman, 1983). Insulin deficiency triggers the process of catabolism, in which fat and protein are used for energy; this state of starvation signals the hypothalamus that body stores are being used, and the appetite will then increase (polyphagia), unless significant nausea is present (Fig. 40–7). Despite the increased food intake, catabolism causes weight loss.

As fat is used for energy, the level of free fatty acids in the blood increases. The liver converts free fatty acids to the ketone bodies beta-hydroxybutyrate, acetoacetic acid, and acetone. The plasma concentration of counterregulatory hormones (epinephrine, growth hormone, cortisol, and glucagon) increase in the absence of adequate insulin, magnifying the metabolic derangement and further impairing insulin secretion and action (Sperling, 1982). The rate of

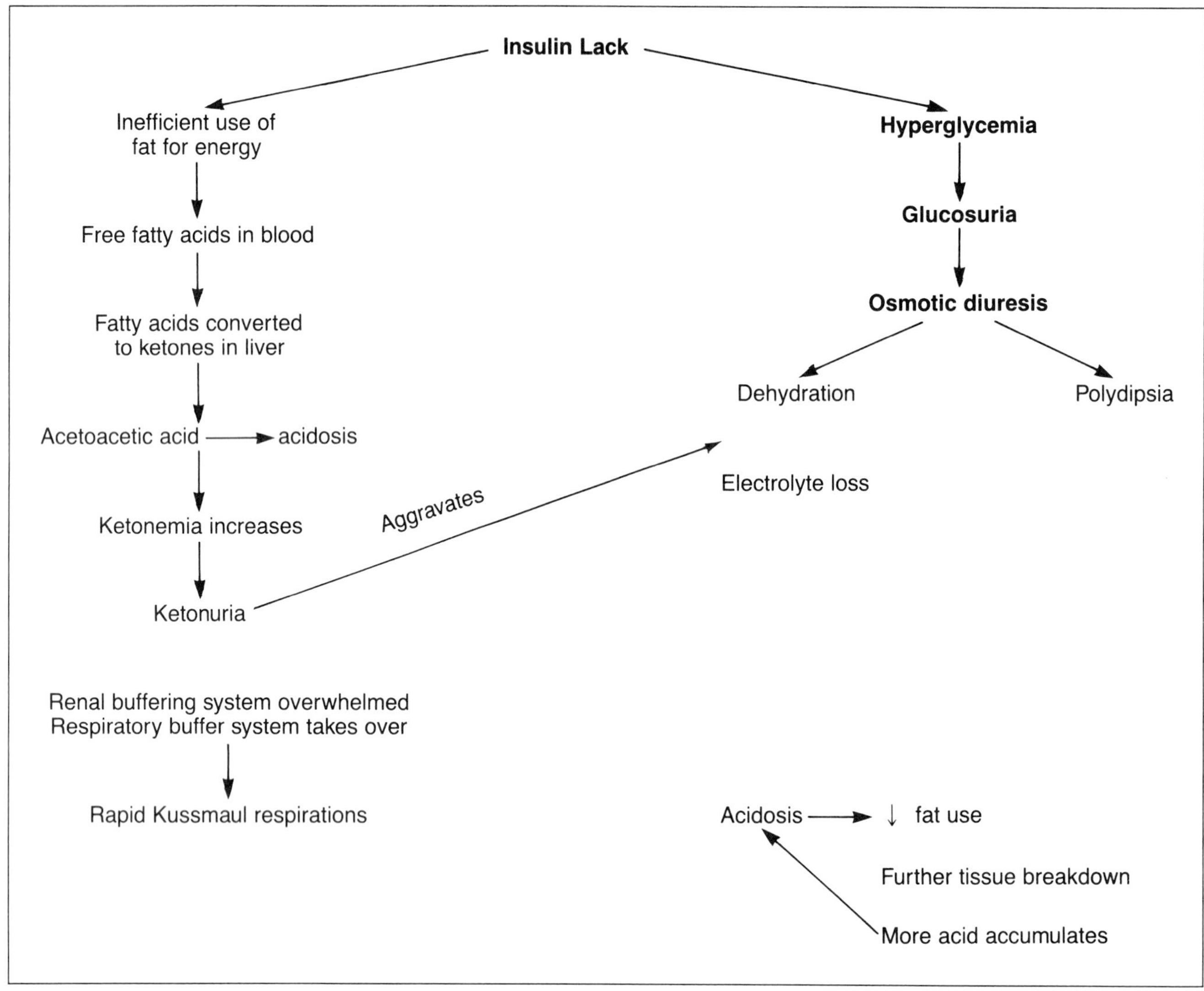

Figure 40-7 Insulin lack.

ketone formation exceeds the capacity for peripheral utilization, leading to an accumulation of ketoacids and metabolic acidosis. Compensatory deep breathing develops in an attempt to excrete excess carbon dioxide. The presence of acetone is responsible for the fruity breath sometimes observed in children with ketoacidosis. Diabetic *ketoacidosis* is defined by Sperling (1982) as a glucose level of over 300 mg/dL, ketonemia at a level greater that 1:2 dilution of the serum, a venous pH less than 7.3, a bicarbonate level less than 15 mEq/dL, glucosuria, and ketonuria. The individual's level of consciousness is affected by the progressive dehydration, acidosis, hyperosmolality, and diminished cerebral oxygen utilization.

Medical Treatment Prior to the discovery of insulin in the 1920s, few people with diabetes survived more than a few years after diagnosis. Insulin functions in a somewhat poorly defined manner. It is known that insulin binds to insulin receptors on cell surfaces, allowing glucose to be taken up by the cell. Factors such as obesity and hypercortisolism inhibit the action of insulin, whereas exercise promotes the action of insulin.

Insulin preparations are derived by several techniques. The oldest method is extraction of insulin from pork and beef glands. Biosynthetic insulin became available in the early 1980s; this insulin is made by a recombinant DNA technique in which genes are inserted into separate strains of *Escherichia coli* to produce A and B insulin chains, which are then chemically combined to make the human insulin molecule. Semisynthetic insulin also became available in the early-1980s; semisynthetic human insulin is produced by the enzymatic transformation of porcine insulin. One goal of the research involved in developing human insulin was to decrease the immunologic problems encountered when beef and pork insulin preparations were used. Early clinical trials of human and purified porcine insulin, however, appear to result in similar effects of hypoglycemia and the antibody response to injected insulin (Etzwiler and Karam, 1983).

The purification of insulin took place in the late 1970s and early 1980s with refinements in manufacturing that resulted in less contamination by other pancreatic hormones such as proinsulin, glucagon, pancreatic polypeptides, and somatostatin (Etzwiler and Karam, 1983). Table 40–6 lists the commercially available insulin preparations.

Insulin pumps became available in the 1970s, providing individuals with a new method of insulin administration. As of the mid-1980s, all pumps used by ambulatory persons are open-loop devices that do not contain a glucose sensor. Individuals must monitor their blood glucose levels regu-

TABLE 40-6 Insulin Preparations

Name of insulin	Manufacturer	Onset of action	Peak of action	Duration of action	Comments
Regular	Lilly; Squibb–Novo	30–60 minutes	2–3 hours	4–6 hours	Pork, beef, beef–pork, and human; clear solution; may be given intravenously; may be mixed with any other insulin
Velosulin	Nordisk	30–60 minutes	2–3 hours	4–6 hours	Purified pork only
Actrapid	Squibb–Novo	30–60 minutes	2–3 hours	4–6 hours	Purified pork and human only
Semi Lente	Lilly; Squibb–Novo	1–2 hours	3–4 hours	4–8 hours	Beef–pork and pork; cloudy suspension; may be mixed with Lente and Ultra Lente
NPH	Lilly; Squibb–Novo	4–6 hours	8–10 hours	12–16 hours	Pork, beef–pork, and human; cloudy suspension; may be mixed with Regular insulin
Insulatard NPH	Nordisk	4–6 hours	8–10 hours	12–16 hours	Purified pork
Protaphane NPH	Squibb–Novo	4–6 hours	8–10 hours	12–16 hours	Purified pork and human
Mixtard (Is 30% Velosulin, 70% Insulatard)	Nordisk	4–6 hours	8–10 hours	12–16 hours	Purified pork
Lente (Is 30% Semi Lente, 70% Ultra Lente)	Lilly; Squibb–Novo	6 hours	8–16 hours	12–30 hours	Beef, pork, and beef–pork; cloudy suspension; may be mixed with Regular and Semi Lente insulins. Peak time may be variable
Monotard	Squibb–Novo	6 hours	8–16 hours	12–30 hours	Purified pork
Ultra Lente	Lilly; Squibb–Novo	8–10 hours	None	36–48 hours	Beef–pork, pork, and beef; cloudy suspension; may be mixed with Semi Lente and Regular insulins

larly by capillary puncture and adjust their food intake and insulin administration by the pump accordingly. The portable pumps are not widely accepted by children and adolescents because of the "hassles" associated with frequent blood testing, visibility of the pump, and presence of the subcutaneous needle, which is part of the pumped insulin system.

Insulin is measured in units. At one time, there were three commonly used concentrations of insulin available to the individual with diabetes, and each concentration of insulin had a special syringe that could not be used with the other concentrations. In the late 1970s most patients converted to using U-100 insulin (100 units of insulin per milliliter of fluid), and the other concentrations of insulin (U-40 and U-80) were phased out of the market. The conversion of a patient's dose from U-40 or U-80 to U-100 insulin was simple because a unit of U-40 insulin was the same as a unit of U-100 insulin; only the volume of fluid used to dilute the insulin was changed. The nurse, however, might still encounter patients using U-40 and U-80 insulin.

A reliable index of long–term glucose control can be obtained from a blood test that determines the glucose concentration in the erythrocytes. Hemoglobin A_{1c}, or glycosylated hemoglobin, is hemoglobin to which glucose has been nonenzymatically coupled. Because the reaction is slow (proportional to the prevailing blood glucose concentration) and continues irreversibly throughout the 120-day life span of the red blood cell, the level of glycosylated hemoglobin is a reflection of the integrated "time-averaged" blood glucose concentration over the preceding 2–3 months. This test is not subject to variations in diet, exercise, stress, or time of day as are urine test results. The measurement of glycosylated hemoglobin in the blood is a valuable tool in the assessment of diabetes control (Sperling, 1982).

When glucose control is not maintained or stress or illness cause blood glucose levels to rise, ketoacidosis (diabetic coma) results. Treatment of the child in ketoacidosis consists of careful assessment of the level of consciousness; state of hydration, including skin turgor, mucous membranes, neck veins, and blood pressure; assessment of cardiac status; and a thorough but brief history of the events leading to ketoacidosis. Treatment is planned to monitor the child's rehydration, return to metabolic normality, and prevention of the complications of ketoacidosis (hypoglycemia, hypokalemia, and cerebral edema). Children in ketoacidosis have deficits in their water, sodium, potassium, chloride, magnesium, and phosphate chemistry; the degree of deficit depends on the length of time in ketoacidosis and their ability to maintain adequate fluid and electrolyte intake (Porte and Nalter, 1981).

Bicarbonate replacement is used cautiously and sparingly, if at all, because indiscriminate use of bicarbonate might reverse the acidosis too quickly and result in severe hypokalemia, leading to fatal cardiac arrhythmias (Moorman, 1983). In addition, large amounts of bicarbonate could exacerbate the cerebral acidosis because bicarbonate and hydrogen ions combine to make carbon dioxide and water. The carbon dioxide crosses the blood–brain barrier and redissolves in the spinal fluid. The resulting elevated level of carbonic acid prolongs the diabetic coma (Sperling, 1982). Metabolic acidosis generally is self-limiting with adequate rehydration and insulin therapy.

Nursing Management

Care for Ketoacidosis Most of the hospitalizations for diabetic children are related to episodes of ketoacidosis either at the time of diagnosis or during acute illnesses which alter blood glucose control. Nursing care of the child in ketoacidosis involves intensive measures. Nursing interventions include hourly recording of the child's total fluid intake and urine output. If the child cannot void, a urinary catheter might be needed, although catheterization is avoided because of the possibility of inducing a urinary tract infection. The goal of fluid therapy should be a gradual decline in osmolality because too rapid a decline predisposes the child to cerebral edema (Porte and Halter, 1981).

Because potassium deficit generally is the most pronounced electrolyte imbalance in ketoacidosis, the child's cardiac cycle should be monitored. The nurse checks the cardiac monitor for signs of hypokalemia (prolonged Q-T interval, low T waves, presence of U-V waves, and depressed S-T segments) and, in rare cases, hyperkalemia (widened QRS complex and high-peaked T waves) (Moorman, 1983).

Several methods exist for administering insulin during ketoacidosis such as intramuscular, intravenous, or some combination of these routes. The most popular method in the 1970s and early 1980s has been the intravenous continuous-insulin, low-dose infusion at a standard dose of 0.1–0.2 units per kilogram of body weight per hour (Lillo and Mastellar, 1982). This method provides a constant concentration that permits steady metabolic response without the fluctuations in concentration that occur with intermittent insulin injections. With this method, the blood glucose level declines gradually and in a linear fashion so that the time at which glucose will be needed to prevent hypoglycemia can be predicted (Sperling, 1982). Regular insulin is the only insulin that can be given intravenously. Insulin has a tendency to cling to the sides of the glass and plastic tubing used for intravenous administration. Priming the infusion set by running 50 mL of the insulin-prepared solution through the tubing and connectors before attaching it to the child helps to prevent the loss of insulin that would otherwise occur during the first few hours. The intravenous fluid is administered by a mechanical infusion pump to ensure a steady, safe flow.

In addition to the direct care outlined in the previous paragraphs, the nurse offers support to the child's parents and keeps them informed about all aspects of the treatment plan.

Insulin Therapy Parents and most children over 12 years of age must learn to administer insulin at the time of diagnosis. Some children younger than age 12 years also can be taught injection technique. Some health care teams insist that the child not leave the hospital until each parent has given the child at least one injection. The nurse teaching families to inject insulin makes certain the family (1) knows the correct insulin to use; (2) knows how to draw up the insulin doses correctly; (3) has a plan for the rotation of injection sites; (4) can give the injection comfortably; and (5) has a place to record the insulin dose and site used. Figure 40–8 demonstrates one plan for the rotation of injection sites. Site rotation occurs both among areas of the body and within specific areas. Most children do not use the abdominal sites until adolescence; even then, the abdomen often is a difficult area to use psychologically. For very young children, the buttocks are often the easiest site to use.

The nurse teaches and practices consistency in the order of drawing and mixing insulin preparations in a syringe. Most practitioners recommend drawing the short-acting (Regular) insulin into the syringe before the longer-acting insulin to prevent contamination of the short-acting insulin by the longer-acting preparation.

Insulin does not require refrigeration as long as it is not exposed to temperatures under 32°F or over 90°F. Extra, unopened bottles of insulin may be stored under refrigeration to prolong their shelf-life. The advantages of using nonrefrigerated insulin are that (1) insulin injections hurt less when the insulin is at room temperature; (2) there may be less tissue damage from insulin at room temperature than from chilled insulin; and (3) insulin suspensions (NPH and Lente) settle less out of suspension at room temperature than when refrigerated.

Insulin dose adjustment is a skill that many children with diabetes and their parents have learned in conjunction with regular home blood glucose monitoring. Table 40–7 presents guidelines for self-management and insulin adjustment based on premeal blood glucose levels. Prior to the advent of home blood glucose testing, individuals with diabetes relied on the assessment of urine glucose spillage to evaluate insulin therapy. The lag time between the blood glucose increase and urine spillage of glucose can vary between 20 minutes and 2 hours (Burns, 1983). Relying solely on urine testing for self-assessment is less safe and less accurate because adjustments in the insulin dose are based on a urine test that is outdated and qualitative rather than quantitative.

A Nursing Care Plan for the child with diabetes mellitus is included at the end of this chapter.

Diet Regulation All growing children require a balanced diet to provide adequate calories and nutrients, and children with diabetes are no exception. Regardless of the philosophy of the health care team toward dietary management, the goal is to provide a balance of nutrients aimed at sustaining growth and minimizing both hypoglycemia and hyperglycemia. The caloric level recommended for most children is based on age and weight.

Two approaches to teaching children about food management are the exchange lists and the free diet. Both systems restrict the types and amounts of simple sugars that are allowed. The *exchange lists* (Table 40–8) use six food groups to provide a framework for both qualitative and

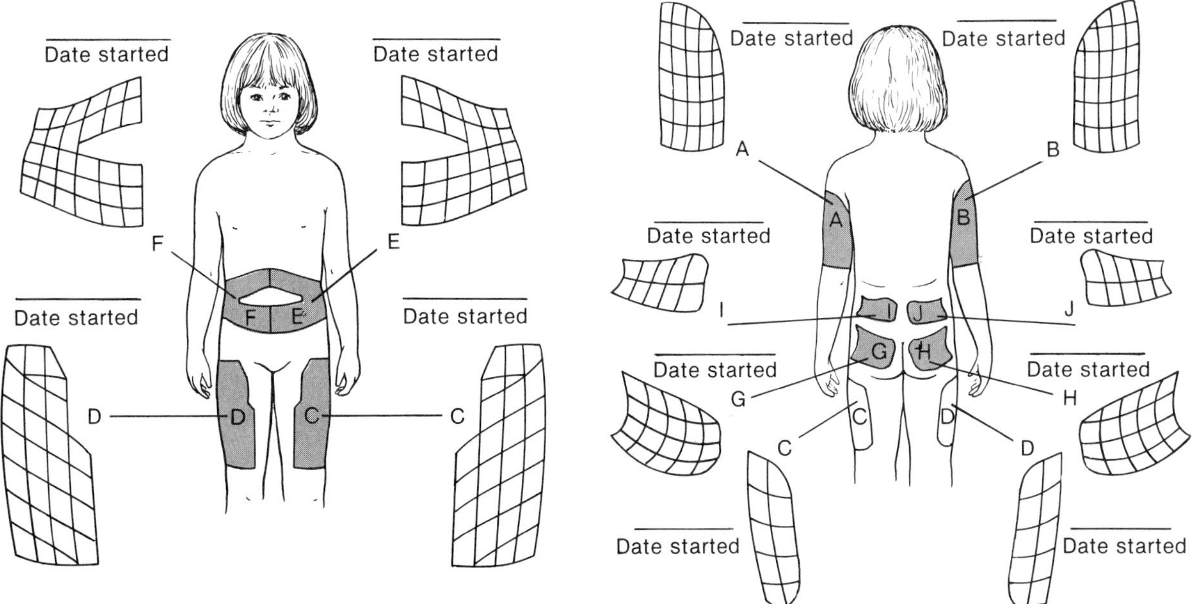

Figure 40-8 Sites for the rotation of insulin injections; rotation occurs within and among body areas.

TABLE 40-7 Guidelines for the Self-Management of Diabetes

	Before breakfast	Before lunch	Late afternoon	Before-bed-time snack	During the night
If blood glucose level is	*Too low*	*Too high*	*Too low*	*Too high*	*Too high*
Actions to take:					
First	Increase the protein in the bedtime snack	Omit the midmorning snack	Increase the carbohydrate in the midafternoon snack	Increase the evening short-acting insulin	Add or increase the long-acting insulin before the evening meal
Second	Reduce the evening long-acting insulin	Increase the morning short-acting insulin	Decrease the morning long-acting insulin	Add exercise after the evening meal	Check the blood glucose level at 3:00–4:00 A.M.
Third	Check the blood glucose level at 3:00–4:00 A.M.	Add exercise in the morning		Decrease the carbohydrate in the evening meal	Add exercise in the evening

TABLE 40-8 Exchange Lists for the Diabetic Diet

Exchange	Composition
Milk	Includes nonfat, low-fat, and whole milk. One exchange of milk contains 12 g of carbohydrate, 8 g of protein, a trace of fat, and 80 calories
Vegetable	One exchange of vegetables contains about 5 g of carbohydrate, 2 g of protein, and 25 calories
Fruit	One exchange of fruit contains 10 g of carbohydrate and 40 calories
Bread	Includes bread, cereal, and starchy vegetables. One exchange of bread contains 15 g of carbohydrate, 2 g of protein, and 70 calories
Meat	Lean meat: one exchange of lean meat (1 oz) contains 7 g of protein, 3 g of fat, and 55 calories
	Medium-fat meat: for each exchange of medium-fat meat, omit one-half fat exchange
	High-fat meat: for each exchange of high-fat meat, omit one fat exchange
	Fat: One exchange of fat contains 5 g of fat and 45 calories

quantitative control of the diet. The *free diet,* a qualitative approach, strives to avoid a rigid structuring of food patterns. It does not define specific types and amounts of food. The rationale for the free diet stems from the concern that calorically controlled diets do not provide the necessary allowances for normal growth and development, and the strict monitoring of food intake has the potential for emotional harm (Heins, 1983). Children and their families also benefit from information about fast-food restaurants so that the child might eat with peers.

Self-Testing Whether control is measured using blood or urine testing, the child and family must learn the proper technique, when to do the testing, how to record the results, and how to interpret the test results. Generally, the more often testing is performed, the more information is available on which to make decisions about diabetes management. Most children test in the morning before insulin and breakfast, in the late afternoon before insulin and dinner, and prior to the bedtime snack. Occasionally, tests are performed before lunch and during the night (2:00–4:00 A.M.). Some children also test before and after exercise to determine any necessary adjustments in insulin or food intake.

Timed collections of urine specimens can help to assess the total glucose spilled into the urine during specific times of the day or night. The child must begin and end a collection period with an empty bladder. All urine is then saved and measured at the end of the collection period. The urine is tested for glucose, and the amount of glucose spilled is calculated by multiplying the volume of the urine collected (in milliliters) by the grams per deciliter present in the tested collection. For example, the urine collected from breakfast until lunch measured 300 mL and tested at 5 g/dL; therefore, 15 g of sugar were spilled. This information indicates a need to increase the morning Regular insulin.

Fast Food Exchanges for Children with Diabetes

	Serving size	Calories (1 serving)	Carb. (g)	Pro. (g)	Fat (g)	Sodium (mg)	Exchanges (1 serving)
Kentucky Fried Chicken							
(edible portion of Original Recipe Chicken)							
Wing (one piece)	1.5 oz	136	4	10	9	302	$1\frac{1}{2}$ Med.-Fat meat
Drumstick	1.6 oz	117	3	12	7	207	2 Lean Meat
Side Breast	2.4 oz	199	7	16	12	558	$\frac{1}{2}$ Bread, 2 Med.-Fat Meat
Thigh	3 oz	257	7	18	18	556	$\frac{1}{2}$ Bread, $2\frac{1}{2}$ Med.-Fat Meat, 1 Fat
Chicken Breast Sandwich	5.5 oz	436	32	25	23	1,093	2 Bread, 3 Med.-Fat Meat, $1\frac{1}{2}$ Fat
Kentucky Fries	3.4 oz	184	28	3	7	174	2 Bread, 1 Fat
McDonald's							
Hamburger	3.5 oz	255	30	12	10	520	2 Bread, 1 Med.-Fat Meat, 1 Fat
Cheeseburger	4 oz	307	30	15	14	767	2 Bread, $1\frac{1}{2}$ Med.-Fat Meat, 1 Fat
Big Mac	7 oz	563	41	26	33	1,010	3 Bread, 3 Med.-Fat Meat, 3 Fat
Quarter Pounder	5.8 oz	424	33	24	22	735	2 Bread, 3 Med.-Fat Meat, 1 Fat
Filet-O-Fish	4.8 oz	432	37	14	25	781	$2\frac{1}{2}$ Bread, 1 Med.-Fat Meat, 4 Fat
French Fries (Regular)	2.4 oz	220	26	3	12	109	2 Bread, 2 Fat
Pizza Hut							
(Thin 'N Crispy)	½ 10" Pizza (3 slices)						
Beef	"	490	51	29	19	NA	3 Bread, 3 Med.-Fat Meat, 1 Fat
Pork	"	520	51	27	23	NA	3 Bread, 3 Med.-Fat Meat, 2 Fat
Cheese	"	450	54	25	15	NA	$\frac{1}{2}$ Bread, 3 Med.-Fat Meat
Pepperoni	"	430	45	23	17	NA	3 Bread, $2\frac{1}{2}$ Med.-Fat Meat, 1 Fat
Supreme	"	510	51	27	21	NA	3 Bread, 3 Med.-Fat Meat, 2 Fat
Taco Bell							
Beef Burrito	6.5 oz	466	37	30	21	327	$2\frac{1}{2}$ Bread, 3 Med.-Fat Meat, 1 Fat
Beefy Tostada	6.5 oz	291	21	19	15	138	$1\frac{1}{2}$ Bread, 2 Med.-Fat Meat, 1 Fat
Enchirito	7 oz	454	42	25	21	1,175	3 Bread, 3 Med.-Fat Meat, 1 Fat
Taco	3 oz	186	14	15	8	79	1 Bread, 2 Med.-Fat Meat

Exerpted from Franz M: Fast food: How to bypass the booby traps. *Diabetes Forecast.* Copyright © 1983 by the American Diabetes Association, Inc. Reprinted from *Diabetes Forecast* with permission. A more extensive version of this table is published in *Fast Food Facts* by the Diabetes Education Center, 4959 Excelsior Blvd., Minneapolis, MN 55416.

Exercise Planning When helping a diabetic child plan an exercise program, the nurse assesses the child's previous activity level and uses it as a guide for planning the type, intensity, duration, and frequency of exercise. The nurse then helps the child to establish short-term goals and identify bodily responses to exercise and the relationship of exercise, diet, and insulin (Cunningham and Barr, 1982).

Glucose for the exercising muscle comes primarily from the liver. Cortisol, epinephrine, growth hormone, and glucagon ensure the delivery of glucose to the exercising muscle, which acts like a "sink," rapidly draining available glucose. The metabolic effects of frequent exercise include the reduction of insulin requirements, increased storage and utilization of glucose, and less extreme fluctuations in the diabetic's blood glucose level over a 24-hour period. Other benefits of exercise are increased cardiac output, more effective stroke volume, and vascular conductance and decreased blood pressure (Cunningham and Barr, 1982).

Individuals with diabetes are encouraged to exercise; however, exercise is not without potential problems. Children and adolescents with diabetes might experience hypoglycemia during or after exercise because muscle and liver glycogen become depleted and the continued presence of injected insulin suppresses the hepatic output of glucose. Body tissues become more sensitive to insulin with exercise because of the increased affinity of the insulin-binding receptors. The nurse and the child with diabetes can rehearse exercise situations and plan changes in food intake or insulin dosage to prevent the occurrence of hypoglycemia. The opposite problem (hyperglycemia and ketonuria) also might occur when a person with diabetes exercises. Hyperglycemia occurs when insufficient insulin is available in the face of an overabundance of the counterregulatory hormones that stimulate the overproduction of glucose (Somogyi's reflex). Phillip Felig, in an address to the American Association of Diabetes Educators (1982), compared the hepatic glucose output of normal subjects with that of persons with diabetes during exercise, noting that the person with diabetes derives 20% more glucose from gluconeogenesis than does the nondiabetic person. The hepatic production of glucose lags behind muscle utilization, and the liver continues to produce glucose after exercise has ceased, causing an "overshoot of glucose." Based on this knowledge, the current recommendation is to exercise if the blood glucose level is under 200 mg/dL and there are no ketones present in the urine.

Skin Care Parents often have questions about skin care (use of topical ointments, care of blisters, permitting children to go without shoes) because of the skin and circulatory problems older individuals with diabetes experience. Children with well-controlled diabetes have good white blood cell function and patent blood vessels so that the healing of skin injuries is generally uncomplicated. The nurse advises children and families to file toenails straight across and even with the end of the toe; to wear comfortable shoes; to care for blisters, cuts, or abrasions by cleansing with soap and water; and to go without shoes only where there is no danger of injuring the feet.

Pubescent females and enuretic or pretoilet-trained young children with diabetes are susceptible to vaginal and perineal fungal infections. Fungi are present in these areas and thrive in the carbohydrate-rich environment characteristic of diabetes (Novak, Jones, and Jones, 1965). These infections can be minimized by maintaining good blood glucose control, keeping the perineal area as dry as possible, practicing good hygiene, and allowing air to reach the perineum by avoiding nylon underwear and tight-fitting garments.

Hypoglycemia Hypoglycemia must be treated promptly whenever it is suspected; severe hypoglycemia leads to seizures, possible brain damage, and death. Table 40–9 lists the signs and symptoms of hypoglycemia according to the body systems affected. Children over 5 years of age and parents, siblings, babysitters, athletic coaches, and school personnel should be familiar with the signs of hypoglycemia and know how to treat the condition when it occurs. Most children with diabetes experience mild hypoglycemia at least once a month because of the difficulty of balancing food, exercise, and insulin dosage.

TABLE 40-9 Signs and Symptoms of Hypoglycemia

Cerebral symptoms	Adrenal signs/symptoms
Dizziness	Shakiness, trembling
Headache	Sweating
Stomachache/nausea	Pallor
Drowsiness	Dilatation of pupils, causing blurred vision
Irritability	
Personality change	
Poor coordination	

Mild hypoglycemia can be managed with an oral feeding of a rapidly acting sugar such as fruit juices, table sugar, hard candy, or regular soda pop. Generally, 10 g of carbohydrate (40 calories) is sufficient to bring the blood glucose level back to normal, although the symptoms of shakiness and headache might persist for hours after the blood glucose level has been normalized. The immediate treatment is followed with a meal or snack. If the child is in the hospital or clinic when hypoglycemia is suspected, it is informative to determine the blood glucose level prior to initiating treatment. Each child's tolerance of a low blood glucose level is different and knowing the level at which symptoms occur assists in regulating daily diet, insulin and activity, and planning for special events for that child.

When the blood glucose has fallen to a very low level, the child might be semiconscious, combative, or unable to swallow and thus unable to take an oral feeding. Glucose pastes or gels can be squeezed into the pouches of the child's cheeks and the cheeks and neck massaged to speed up absorption of the glucose through the mucous membranes. If the child does not respond to this treatment in 5–10 minutes, glucagon may be given as an intramuscular injection. Glucagon is a hormone made by the alpha cells of the pancreas, and when injected, it raises the blood glucose level by releasing glucose from glycogen stores in the liver and muscles. The dose of glucagon is 0.5–1.0 mg (Sperling, 1982). The child generally will awaken within 10–15 minutes, and a snack or meal is then taken to sustain the blood glucose level. The rapid rise in glucose following the administration of glucagon might cause nausea and vomiting, and the blood glucose level might remain elevated for as long as 24 hours after the episode of hypoglycemia. With severe hypoglycemia, the child might lose consciousness and/or exhibit seizure activity. If this occurs at home, the parents can give glucagon; however, the child also might require intravenous glucose (1 mL/kg over 5 minutes) to correct the problem (Sperling, 1982). Caution must be taken with the concentration of glucose used and the rate at which it is administered. If the child remains in a postictal state following severe hypoglycemia, continuous slow-drip intravenous glucose might be required for several hours to maintain blood glucose levels until the child is able to eat. Because hypoglycemia may occur at any time, the nurse advises the child to wear a medical identification necklace or bracelet; adolescents also should mark their drivers' licenses and carry food in the car when driving. Most children keep snacks in their desks, school lockers, purses, or bookbags. After an episode of hypoglycemia has occurred and been successfully treated, parents, children, and health professionals need to discuss the cause of the hypoglycemia and take steps to prevent its recurrence.

Strategies for Special Problems Three special problems faced by the diabetic child are *illness, growth spurts,* and *difficulties during puberty.* The nurse can offer strategies for coping with each of these problems.

When a child with diabetes becomes ill, the family might encounter blood glucose levels that are above or below the child's usual level; in addition, ketones often develop. The usual diet might be unpalatable, and the insulin dose might need to be adjusted. Frequent testing of blood and urine is needed to determine how well the diabetes is being controlled. The parent also needs to be aware of the child's state of hydration because potassium imbalance is a special concern with dehydration. Parents often question the use of over-the-counter medications (cough suppressants, cold remedies, and so on). These drugs must be used with care because many contain concentrated sugar. Health care professionals provide emotional support for the child and family during the illness and help them to make any needed insulin adjustments. On sick days, the meal plan emphasizes easily digested carbohydrates. If food intake is problematic (because of anorexia, vomiting, or nausea), insulin may be given in small, frequent doses to avoid potential hypoglycemia. Most illnesses can be managed at home with careful monitoring by the parent in consultation with the health care team. If repeated vomiting occurs, the child will require emergency room evaluation and treatment with intravenous fluids. If this occurs, the nurse might encounter a parent who is very fatigued and discouraged bacause the child's condition did not improve despite all the efforts of home care. The nurse needs to recognize and praise the parent's efforts, thereby reassuring the parent that everything was done that could be done but that this time medical intervention was needed to restore balance. After the child's condition is stable, it is mutually beneficial for the nurse to spend time with the parent and review the events preceding the emergency treatment. This discussion will facilitate planning for management of the diabetes during future illnesses.

All children require insulin to promote growth; the amount of insulin needed increases with growth. Children with diabetes therefore, require periodic (three to four times per year) medical evaluations of their insulin requirements. Most prepubertal diabetic children require approximately 0.5–0.75 U/kg/day (Sperling, p. 143). During major growth spurts, the requirements generally will increase to 1.0–1.5 U/kg/day, which is then decreased to 0.5 U/kg/day after growth is completed.

Additional calories are required during a time of increased growth whether the child is a diabetic or a nondiabetic. Sporadic growth spurts, a characteristic of children, are accompanied by a marked change in appetite and demand for additional food. Parents describe these periods as a time when their children consume enormous quantities of food during a week and then return to their usual eating patterns. The following week these parents often note an increase in their child's weight, height, or both.

When the nondiabetic child goes through a growth spurt, the pancreas is able to produce additional insulin to facilitate the metabolic process of carbohydrates and provide a supply of glucose required by most for cells' energy expenditure. The diabetic child is unable to tolerate the extra carbohydrates. When additional insulin is not available to utilize the increased glucose produced and to convert it to energy, the kidneys waste it. Thus, when the child who has diabetes eats additional food to satisfy hunger, glucose spillage occurs as evidenced by polyuria, polydipsia, and polyphagia, glucosuria, and elevated blood glucose levels.

The nurse advises parents concerning growth spurts and encourages them to provide additional, nutritionally adequate, well-balanced proportions of proteins, carbohydrates and fats for their growing children and to adjust the insulin dosage accordingly so glucose is available for cell energy and growth. For optimal growth, the child requires flexibility in diet and insulin requirements to allow for these sporadic episodes of increased need. Parents who are prepared for these episodes can make the necessary adjustments and prevent potential conflict between hunger and glucose control. Understanding their children's unique needs within normal growth and development will help parents to enhance their children's sense of self-esteem rather than foster a sense of failure whenever glucose spillage occurs.

If the diabetes is adequately controlled, most children will enter and progress through puberty at the expected times (10–14 years of age for females and 11–16 years of age for males). Menstrual periods might be associated with hyperglycemia and ketonuria because of estrogen and progesterone changes, and the dosage of insulin might need to be adjusted during this time. The developmental tasks of adolescence might interfere with good glucose control and cause much friction between the parent and adolescent. The nurse can intercede, acting as an interested third party when the parents or adolescents need to talk about their frustrations.

Prevention of Complications Approximately 50% of individuals with diabetes develop microvascular disease of the retina and kidney, macrovascular disease (coronary artery disease and poor peripheral circulation), and neuropathy. The debate regarding the cause of this process has raged for years; some authorities feel that the vascular complications are directly related to hyperglycemia (and therefore that careful glucose control might prevent or minimize the problems), whereas other experts feel that there may be various subtypes of diabetes, with some people being more susceptible to the development of complications. Previously, no methods were available to control the blood glucose perfectly by the physiologic delivery of insulin; therefore, the question was unanswerable. With the advent of home blood glucose monitoring and portable insulin pumps, the questions might be resolved; however, because most individuals do not develop complications until at least 15 years after diagnosis, a generation of children using these latest management tools will have to be studied around the turn of the twenty-first century to assess the impact of improved control on the development of complications.

Macrovascular disease involves endothelial damage, smooth muscle proliferation, lipid and lipoprotein metabolic abnormalities, and hypercoagulability (Spies, 1983). Microvascular disease consists of thickening of the capillary basement membranes, tissue hypoxia, venous dilatation, red blood cell aggregation, and decreased red blood cell deformability. Neuropathy occurs as a result of microangiopathy. Peripheral vascular disease is a combination of macrovascular and microvascular disease.

When the filtering system of the kidney is affected, the result is decreased renal function. The first sign of kidney disease is proteinuria, which is followed by hypertension; therefore, the nurse checks the urine for protein and carefully monitors the child's blood pressure at each clinic visit. The nurse also teaches the child and adolescent about the benefits of frequent voiding to prevent urine retention and voiding after sexual intercourse to prevent cystitis. If antihypertensive medication is prescribed, the nurse explains its action, administration, and potential side effects. There is some evidence that excellent glucose control might retard renal disease (Spies, 1983), so the nurse also might teach about new methods of improving control.

Visual problems occur when the capillaries in the retina become friable, break, and bleed into the vitreous. It takes the body a long time to reabsorb the blood, and scarring possibly occurs. New capillaries that are weak and poorly supported then appear (neovascularization). Hemorrhages that involve the center of vision (the macula) put traction on the retina, leading to retinal detachment. Children with diabetes should see an ophthalmologist every year after the onset of puberty or after they have had diabetes for 10 years (Laws, et al., 1966). Canadian reports suggest that adolescents with puberty-onset diabetes develop retinopathy more rapidly and more severely than children who develop diabetes in the prepubertal years. Many of the puberty-onset group develop the first signs of retinopathy as early as 4 years following diagnosis (Laws, et al., 1966). Barta and Molnar (1971) noted that retinopathy in the early phase of diabetes seems to occur more frequently among rapidly growing children, suggesting that rapid growth is a significant stressor. There is debate about the efficacy of strict glucose control in halting the progression of retinal disease, however, because hypoglycemia can cause hypoxia to the retinal tissue and exacerbate the damage. The nurse's role when vision is altered is one of support and referral to vocational rehabilitation and occupational therapy for assistance in performing activities of daily living.

Cataracts might develop in the lenses of even young children's eyes if glucose control is poor. The accumulation of fructose and sorbitol results in swelling of the lens, deterioration of the fibers, and subsequent proteinaceous substances filling up the spaces created by the deteriorating fibers. The opaque lens is seen as gray against the black pupil with the light of a flashlight or as gray or black against the red reflex with ophthalmoscopic examination. The nurse and physician examine the diabetic child's eyes carefully at routine follow-up visits.

When the blood supply to the peripheral nerves is decreased, nerve dysfunction becomes apparent. Careful examination might reveal decreased sensation in the extremities, problems with proprioception, diminished deep tendon reflexes, and a history of diarrhea, pain in the legs and feet, injuries to the feet and hands of which the person is unaware, and complaints of *hyperhidrosis* (excessive sweating) in the trunk and face.

Diabetic mortality is caused primarily by macrovascular disease (Spies, 1983). Factors that predispose the diabetic child to such problems include hyperglycemia, hyperlipidemia, and hypertension. The nurse encourages the child and family to follow dietary recommendations that restrict the amount and types of fat in the diet and promote the intake of fiber. Most children have their blood lipid levels checked once a year. The nurse also encourages exercise, monitors blood pressure, and discourages smoking. Most of the complications of diabetes do not become apparent until the person has had diabetes for at least 15 years; therefore, adolescents with long-standing diabetes are at risk, and the nurse assesses them carefully for evidence of complications.

Coping and Acceptance Strategies Because their age, cognitive and developmental levels, and life experiences differ, children and adults (parents and health professionals) have different concerns about diabetes. Children do not have the cognitive or emotional capacity to consider or plan for the future nor the maturity to perform tasks consistently to ensure good health in later years. Children are concrete thinkers who function in the present (Bibace and Walsh, 1978). It is therefore unwise, impractical, and unsuccessful to use scare tactics (threats of possible vascular disease) to convince children to test more often, remember their injections, or eat appropriately.

Young children also have a difficult time accepting the fact that their parents have to hurt them purposefully to help them. Children at this level of moral development believe that the hurt is punishment for wrongdoing. The nurse and parent need to provide careful explanations for the child using age-appropriate terms and make a clear distinction between treating the disease and disciplining the child.

Children with diabetes might have difficulty understanding why they have to be different from their peers (see the discussion of chronic illness in Chapter 30). They are reminded constantly about the consequences of their disease because they have to eat certain foods according to a schedule, interrupt play for a snack or premeal testing and insulin, forego spontaneous trips for ice cream treats, and abstain from or limit their intake of sweets at birthday and school parties. The daily insulin injections are not only bothersome but also the source of fearful fantasies. Many children have latent fears of self-injury or body mutilation related to the daily insulin injections. For example, one 8-year-old girl was unable to give herself the insulin injection because of a fear that she would either hit her bone, causing it to break, or cause her leg to split wide open.

In late adolescence individuals develop the ability for abstract thinking and can begin to perceive what life at 30 or 40 years of age might be like; however, peer activities of the present might still be more important than doing tasks to ensure optimal glucose control (Hoffman, et al., 1982). As one adolescent candidly said, "If I have two minutes in the morning before school and a choice of putting on my eye makeup or doing a blood test, you know I'll choose to do the makeup!" Adolescents might react to information about potential vascular complications in any one of several ways. They might become depressed, feeling as if a "big cloud" were hanging over them and that they are doomed no matter how hard they try to control the diabetes. The depression might be manifested in behavior such as total denial of the diabetes, refusal to take injections, eating inappropriately, and a general disregard for all preventive measures or early warning signs. Another adolescent might develop an all-consuming concern about the future and feel that "if only I work hard enough to keep my blood glucose normal, this won't happen to me." This person may be quite compulsive about glucose testing and elect to use an insulin pump or take multiple insulin injections every day in search of normoglycemia and be angry and frustrated when these hoped-for results are not achieved.

Parents also deal with concerns about diabetes in a variety of ways. They might attend compulsively to every facet of the child's diabetes management, or they might expect the child to assume total responsibility for the management (denial). Parents of young children might feel guilty about inflicting the pain of injections and blood testing. Parents of older children might have mixed feelings of apprehension and relief as the children take over management tasks and become more independent. Parents of adolescents often have difficulty sorting out normal adolescent behaviors from problems related to diabetes.

Nurses and other professionals help children and parents set short-term and long-term goals for diabetes management by teaching them the concepts and skills needed to reach the goals, helping them to break down large goals into easily achieved smaller steps, and readily providing reinforcement and support (Table 40–10). The nurse can negotiate behavioral contracts with children and parents

TABLE 40-10 Guidelines for Diabetes Management Goals According to Age-Appropriate Steps

Age	Diet	Insulin	Testing
4–5 years	Helps pick foods based on likes and dislikes	Helps pick injection sites; pinches up skin; wipes skin	Collects blood or urine; watches parent do testing; colors test results on records
6–7 years	Can tell if food has no sugar, some sugar, or lots of sugar	Pushes plunger in after parent gives shot	Performs blood or urine test; records results; might need reminding; will need supervision
8–9 years	Selects foods based on exchanges	Gives own shots (at least once a day)	Does own blood test
10–13 years	Knows diet plan	Rotates sites; measures insulin	Looks for patterns in test results
14+ years	Plans meals and snacks	Mixes two insulins in one syringe (if needed)	Suggests insulin changes based on test patterns

SOURCE: *My Child Has Diabetes: A Book of Questions and Feelings.* Becton Dickinson Consumer Products, 1983, p. 7. Reprinted by permission.

and thus achieve shared responsibility for the diabetes management, as well as either teaching a new behavior or modifying an ineffective one (Hall and Hall, 1982).

Nurses must be alert to the types of parenting known to place the child at risk for problems in adjusting to diabetes. The four types of parenting behaviors that have been identified as dysfunctional for aiding the child's coping with diabetes are the overprotective/overanxious parent, overindulgent/overpermissive parent, the perfectionist/controlling parent, or the indifferent/rejecting parent (Johnson and Rosenbloom, 1982). (See Chapter 22 for a discussion of dysfunctional parenting and nursing interventions.)

The following example illustrates some of the common problems experienced by a family with a diabetic child. The family of a 13-year-old girl with diabetes had difficulty adjusting to the loss of flexibility in their life-style, which favored irregular mealtimes, keeping concentrated sweets in the home, and minimal parental supervision of the children. They were not accustomed to health maintenance activities and found relating to a diabetes care team difficult on all but the most superficial matters. Although the nurse on the diabetes team tried discussing child development with the parents in terms of what was appropriate to expect their daughter to do regarding diabetes management, the parents steadfastly insisted that at 13 years of age she had to be responsible for her own care.

The young adolescent had numerous hospital admissions while in junior high school for ketoacidosis from taking insulin irregularly and eating inappropriately. At one time, the diabetes team suspected she was actually overinsulinized and experiencing rebound hyperglycemia following hypoglycemia (Somogyi reaction). Finally, when she developed inflammation of the iris of her eyes on several occasions, a decision was made to have her learn blood glucose monitoring and use the portable insulin pump. Her control improved during the short time she used the pump, but what helped her the most was conferring with the team psychologist and nurse on a weekly basis. The psychologist worked with her mother on parenting skills, knowledge of child development, and realistic expectations of the mother–child relationship. As this adolescent's diabetes control gradually improved, so did her school attendance. At 17 years of age, she is now making plans for post-high school education and is able to adjust her insulin according to blood test results, planned exercise, and occasional eating "binges."

Families with a diabetic child mourn their loss of flexibility, mourn the loss of a "healthy child," resent the work involved on a daily basis, have difficulty sharing the work of managing the diabetes, and encounter financial hardships associated with hospitalizations, supplies, and physicians' fees. The nurse helps the family to assess their strengths and to have realistic expectations of the child's ability for self-management and provides continuing education to facilitate the ultimate goal of total self-management.

Lay groups composed of families and individuals with diabetes can be important resources for children and parents. Common concerns, fears, and problems as well as possible solutions are shared and discussed. Social group activities such as fundraising to support research offer both hope and an opportunity for action. Diabetes camps are another resource and one viewed by many parents and professionals as the most important learning experience for children. In camp skills are learned in an atmosphere of mutual support and peer acceptance while physical activity and wellness are stressed and experienced.

Diabetes is a challenging condition to manage. The nurse, working in a team with the physician, dietitian, psychologist, social worker, and other significant people, can offer vital support and education to the children and families who must live with this disorder.

The Child With Inappropriate Secretion From the Pituitary Gland

Anterior Lobe Hyperfunction

The anterior lobe of the pituitary gland secretes *somatotropin*, or *growth hormone*, which is then converted by the liver into somatomedin, the hormone that stimulates somatic growth. The height of an individual is determined by skeletal length, the growth of which is determined largely by the lengthening of the diaphysis. In bones with normal structure, the growth potential of the diaphysis depends on the progression of ossification within the epiphysis (Kaplan, 1982). Once the epiphyses have ossified, very little linear growth occurs.

Growth hormone excess is rare in children; when it occurs in childhood, a tumor often is present in the hypothalamic–pituitary unit. These tumors increase the secretion of the growth hormone. If this process occurs prior to epiphyseal closure, linear growth might be considerable. A child with excessive growth hormone secretion frequently will have visual impairment, carbohydrate intolerance, thickened bones, joint pains, osteoporosis, delayed sexual development because of decreased FSH, LH, and ACTH levels, hypertension, possible heart failure, and generalized visceral enlargement (Kaplan, 1982).

If excessive growth hormone secretion develops after epiphyseal closure, further linear growth does not occur and the individual does not achieve abnormally tall stature. The excessive growth hormone levels, however, do promote elongation of the mandible, causing malocclusion of the jaws and teeth; bony overgrowth of joints in the extremities, causing disabling arthritis; an increased quantity of soft tissue at the heels, increasing shoe size; and high levels of plasma growth hormone that is unresponsive to the presence of hyperglycemia (Kaplan, 1982).

Another disorder associated with tall stature, and which must be differentiated from growth hormone excess, is cerebral gigantism. In this condition, however, growth hormone levels are normal, as are other endocrine functions. Children with this disorder have prominent foreheads, high arched palates, hypertelorism, macrocephaly, mental retardation, and advanced skeletal maturation, which often results in mature height that is more normal than excessive (Kaplan, 1982). The cause of this condition is attributed to a cerebral defect rather than pituitary dysfunction.

Gonadotropin Hypersecretion One of the factors involved in the onset of puberty is the increased secretion of the gonadotropin hormones (LH and FSH), which results from the decreased sensitivity (a change in the set point for the negative feedback relationship) of the pituitary and/or hypothalamus to the levels of circulating testosterone and estrogen (Penney, 1982). The onset of puberty is considered *precocious* (early) in girls younger than 9 years of age and in boys younger than 10 years of age. In girls this process of early pubertal development is most frequently idiopathic, whereas in boys intracranial tumors more often stimulate the early pubertal development.

Girls with precocious puberty generally present with premature *thelarche* (breast development), which is sometimes unilateral but frequently is bilateral. Pubic hair might or might not be present along with the early breast development. Pubic hair grows in response to androgens from the adrenal cortex, whereas breasts develop in response to estrogen from the ovaries. Examination of the vaginal introitus might reveal evidence of increased estrogen secretion; that is, the vaginal mucosa thins and becomes reddened. Menstruation might occur.

Boys with precocious puberty generally present with pubic hair. They also might have accelerated linear growth, increased muscle mass, testicular enlargement, and penile growth.

When a child develops precocious puberty, the history and examination focus on discovering the cause of the early pubertal development. Possible etiologies for precocious development of secondary sexual characteristics include an intracranial mass (central precocious puberty), an adrenal mass or enzyme defect causing excessive secretion of adrenal testosterone, or an ovarian cyst or tumor secreting excessive estrogens. To assess the possibility that the pubertal development is caused by an intracranial mass, the nurse carefully checks the child's neurologic status. The child is questioned about the presence of any headaches or visual disturbances. An ophthalmologic examination is done to assess the child's visual fields and determine whether any papilledema exists. A CT scan of the child's head might be done to examine the hypothalamic–pituitary region for evidence of a mass. Pituitary gonadotropins are measured; these hormones (LH and FSH) are normally low in the prepubertal child but might be in the pubertal range in a child with precocious puberty (Bacon, Spencer, and Kelch, 1975). Further information regarding the evaluation of the child with precocious puberty is found in the section on alterations in ovarian and testicular function later in this chapter. The child who is discovered to have an intracranial lesion is referred to a neurosurgeon, who assesses the feasibility and necessity of surgically removing the mass. Nursing care throughout this initial assessment phase includes obtaining a careful history of the pubertal development, coordinating the diagnostic evaluation, supporting the child and parent through radiologic and laboratory procedures, explaining puberty to the child, and being present for support and teaching when the method of treatment is discussed.

Adrenocorticotropin Hypersecretion—Cushing's Disease *Cushing's disease* (ACTH hypersecretion) is rare in children. When present, it usually is caused by an intracranial mass in the hypothalamic–pituitary unit. Chronic ACTH oversecretion stimulates the adrenal cortex to produce excessive amounts of cortisol, which leads to the development of Cushing's syndrome (hypercortisolism). The features of hypercortisolism are discussed in the section on adrenal gland hyperfunction later in this chapter. Children with Cushing's disease generally undergo surgical removal of the intracranial tumor and/or have cranial irradiation. Before, during, and after surgery, these patients require stress (increased) dosages of steroid hormones (cortisone derivatives). Nursing care of these individuals includes a careful history of the progression of the symptoms, with close attention to symptoms of intracranial pressure from the mass, and support during the diagnostic procedures and surgery. Excessive ACTH secretion in conditions of adrenal insufficiency is discussed in the section on adrenal gland hypofunction later in this chapter.

Thyroid-Stimulating Hormone Hypersecretion Thyroid-stimulating hormone (TSH) is secreted in excessively large quantities when the thyroid gland is unable to secrete sufficient amounts of thyroxine; the amount of TSH increases because of stimulation via the negative feedback system described earlier in the chapter. Elevation of TSH is discussed in the section on thyroid gland dysfunction later in this chapter.

Melanocyte-Stimulating Hormone Hypersecretion Melanocyte-stimulating hormone (MSH) is secreted by some of the same cells that secrete ACTH. Melanocyte-stimulating hormone and ACTH also cross-react in the blood. When there is excessive ACTH secretion, MSH secretion also might increase, causing hyperpigmentation of the skin. This finding is seen frequently in children who develop Addison's disease.

Anterior Lobe Hypofunction

Growth hormone, which is secreted by the pituitary gland and has systemic growth-promoting effects, also plays a role in glucose homeostasis, preventing hypoglycemia by decreasing glucose uptake by muscles and promoting lipolysis.

Growth hormone deficiency is suspected in a child who is growing at a subnormal rate (less than 1.5 in/yr); who has hypoglycemia; who has small, infantile facial features, crowding of the teeth and chubby cheeks, a high arched palate, and a single central incisor (teeth); who has had an insult to the area of the pituitary gland (brain tumor, cranial irradiation, hydrocephalus, or encephalitis); or who has other pituitary deficiencies such as diabetes insipidus, ACTH deficiency, thyrotropin deficiency, or gonadotropin deficiency.

Some children have deficiencies in several or all of the anterior and posterior pituitary stimulating hormones. This condition is known as *panhypopituitarism*. Many of these children have congenital anomalies of the midbrain that did not permit the proper development of the hypothalamus and pituitary glands. Deficiency of ACTH leaves the child with adrenal insufficiency, which is discussed in the section on adrenal gland hypofunction later in this chapter. Deficiency of LH and FSH will make pubertal development impossible without the administration of exogenous estrogen or testosterone. Thyroid-stimulating hormone (TSH) deficiency causes secondary hypothyroidism, which is treated with thyroxine replacement (see the section entitled "The Child With Inappropriate Secretion From the Thyroid Gland"). If the posterior pituitary lobe is also affected by the process that causes anterior pituitary hypofunction, the child might have antidiuretic hormone (ADH, also called vasopressin) deficiency, which is discussed in the following section on posterior lobe hypofunction.

Medical treatment To document growth hormone deficiency, the health care team generally observes the child's growth rate for 6–12 months and then selects validating diagnostic tests designed to evaluate the child's ability to release growth hormone in response to provocative agents (levodopa, insulin, clonidine, and exercise).

Treatment of growth hormone deficiency involves intramuscular or subcutaneous injections of human growth hormone, which is obtained during autopsy procedures. These injections generally are given three to six times per week. Periodic outpatient visits are scheduled to evaluate the child's response to therapy. Very few children can administer these injections themselves, but their parents can learn to carefully mix and administer the growth hormone.

Nursing Management The nurse's role during diagnostic testing is to explain the tests to the child and family, to ensure the child has nothing by mouth (NPO) and remains on bedrest prior to and during the testing, to ensure the timely collection and proper handling of blood specimens (correct tubes, labels, and icing of specimens), to observe for signs of hypoglycemia during the tests, and to give the child a snack following completion of the tests. Other evaluation procedures might include radiographs of the hand to determine skeletal maturation and CT scans of the head to examine the area of the hypothalamus and pituitary glands for the presence of lesions.

Nursing care might involve referring the child for evaluation, assisting in the testing procedures, teaching parents to give the growth hormone injections, counseling the child about self-image, and assessing the growth response to therapy. If the child is prone to hypoglycemia, the nurse instructs the family to increase both the dose of growth hormone and the frequency of administration during illnesses and to have glucose pastes or gels on hand to give orally if hypoglycemia occurs.

Many children are quite short or grow very slowly but are not deficient in the growth hormone. In fact, it is more common to encounter this type of child than a child with a documented growth hormone deficiency. Some children are small in stature for genetic reasons; their parents might seek evaluation of their children's growth in the hope that their children will be spared the trauma they themselves might have experienced because of small stature. Some of these children have been treated with human growth hormone, but most children do not receive hormonal therapy. Nursing care for them and their families consists of counseling about appropriate clothing, physical activities, and the importance of tailoring expectations to the child's age rather than stature.

Another large group of children with small stature have constitutional delay of growth. These children generally grow at a normal rate, but they are at or below the 5th percentile for their age. Although most of these children eventually attain an average adult height, their entrance into puberty generally is delayed by 1–2 years as compared with their age-mates. Nursing care of children with constitutional delay of growth and puberty is similar to that for children with genetic short stature, except that the constitutionally delayed children generally can be reassured that they will attain average size by the time they are through growing.

Posterior Lobe Hypofunction

To conserve the water needed for cellular function and the maintenance of blood volume, the hypothalamus produces ADH, which is stored and released from the posterior pituitary gland. The distal renal tubules respond to ADH stimulation by conserving water.

Children with symptoms of polydipsia, polyuria, preference for ice water, the need to drink water during the night, decreased appetite, and weight loss are evaluated initially for the presence of diabetes mellitus. When no elevation in blood glucose or glucosuria is documented, these thirsty children often are discovered to have the "other" kind of diabetes—*diabetes insipidus*. Diabetes insipidus can occur

NURSING CARE GUIDE Child With Diabetes Insipidus

Nursing diagnosis	Interventions	Evaluation
1. Potential for dehydration and hypovolemic shock related to high volume urine loss.	Observe child closely for signs of dehydration (see Chapter 33). Monitor IV vasopressin administration carefully. Report immediately any signs of hypertension, hyponatremia, or water intoxication (see Chapter 33)	Child responds well to vasopressin therapy and side effects are reported immediately
2. Potential parental knowledge deficit related to the administration of the correct dosage of intranasal aqueous vasopressin and recognition of signs of incorrect dosage	Demonstrate to the parents the administration of nasal vasopressin. Have them practice the technique using saline and then administer the scheduled dose. Discuss the signs of incorrect dosage and refer the parents to appropriate literature	Parents are prepared to administer vasopressin correctly and can recognize the signs of underdosage or overdosage
3. Potential for grieving related to lifethreatening but invisible health problems and loss of normality	Encourage the child and parents to talk about their feelings. Facilitate expression of anger, guilt, and fear. Discuss lifestyle adaptations and how to monitor child's hydration status and diet	Family is able to verbally express feelings about child's illness; appears to be coping adequately
4. Potential for growth in family coping related to the use of community support systems	Introduce the parents to parents of other similarly ill children	Coping skills appear adequate; family appears less anxious as a result of talking with others with similar problems
5. Potential need for coordinating health care program and obtaining access to specialists	Help the parents to identify a primary health care provider to coordinate program	Parents consult with primary health care provider and find appropriate specialists

for several reasons. Central diabetes insipidus is caused by a lack of ADH. Nephrogenic diabetes insipidus is caused by renal unresponsiveness to ADH and is an X-linked recessive genetic defect. The treatment for nephrogenic diabetes insipidus is a diet low in sodium and protein and chlorothiazide to increase the urinary sodium loss and promote increased reabsorption of fluid from the glomerular filtrate (Bode, 1981). Psychogenic (compulsive) water drinking is rare in children. An individual with this emotional disorder will continue to drink excessively after being given vasopressin and will become water intoxicated.

Central diabetes insipidus (ADH deficiency) may be caused by incomplete formation of the pituitary gland. It might occur following brain surgery or other central nervous system insult and be transient in nature. Diabetes insipidus occasionally might be the presenting complaint when a child has developed an intracranial lesion.

Medical Treatment The presenting clinical picture for both types of diabetes insipidis is similar, with the child demonstrating polydipsia, polyuria, failure to thrive or weight loss, irritability, fever, dehydration, or even hypovolemic shock. The child's 24-hour fluid intake and output are increased, the urine specific gravity is very low, the serum osmolality is high, the serum sodium level is elevated, and the serum vasopressin level is low (in central diabetes insipidus). If the child has nephrogenic diabetes insipidus, the symptoms will not reverse with the administration of vasopressin. If the problem is central diabetes insipidus, however, the polyruia, thirst, and other abnormalities will resolve with vasopressin therapy. The diagnosis is made by a water deprivation test, which is a potentially dangerous test that should be done with the child in the hospital. The nurse and physician carefully monitor the child's blood pressure, pulse, urine specific gravity, weight, urine output, serum osmolality, and clinical status. It is critical that the child is not allowed to become severely dehydrated during the test.

Acute treatment of dehydration caused by diabetes insipidus includes the administration of free water to correct the fluid deficit and use of an intravenous drip of aqueous vasopressin, which is titrated to the child's urine output (Bode, 1981). Excessive vasopressin causes hypertension, hyponatremia, and water intoxication. Chronic management of central diabetes insipidus requires the administration of vasopressin, given either as an intramuscular preparation of Pitressin Tannate In Oil or as an intranasal spray of DDAVP (demopressin acetate). The injectable Pitressin is given every 1–2 days but is difficult to mix and painful to receive. The DDAVP nasal spray is used every 12–24 hours.

Nursing Management The nurse refers the child who has polydipsia and polyuria for evaluation. The nurse observes the child during the water deprivation test and teaches the child and family how to administer either vasopressin (for central diabetes insipidus) or diuretics (for nephrogenic diabetes insipidus). (See the Nursing Care Guide For the Child with Diabetes Insipidus.)

The Child With Inappropriate Secretion From the Adrenal Glands

Hyperfunction

Excessive Cortisol Secretion The adrenal cortex may synthesize and secrete excessive amounts of cortisol for several reasons. As previously discussed, Cushing's disease (excessive ACTH secretion) will stimulate the adrenal glands to secrete large amounts of cortisol. The adrenal cortex is also capable of functioning autonomously (independent of pituitary ACTH regulation) in the presence of an adrenal adenoma or adrenal carcinoma, nodular adrenal hyperplasia, or an ectopic ACTH-producing tumor that stimulates the adrenal cortex to overproduce cortisol. The result of chronic hypercortisolism is Cushing's syndrome.

Individuals with Cushing's syndrome have facial rounding, growth failure, truncal obesity, thinning of the extremities, muscle wasting, weakness and fatigue, thinning of the skin with purplish-red striae, bruising caused by increased capillary fragility, personality changes, buffalo hump on the back, hypertension, hyperglycemia, osteoporosis, and occasionally acne and other evidence of virilization.

Evaluation of the child with suspected hypercortisolism includes examination of the blood and urine cortisol and ACTH levels, special suppression tests (metyrapone and dexamethasone), ultrasonography of the abdomen, CT scans of the head, and skeletal radiographs to look for evidence of osteoporosis. The nurse's responsibilities during this extensive diagnostic workup include instructing the child and parents about the procedure for 24-hour urine collection, providing support to an emotionally labile child, carefully timing the administration of medications and drawing of blood for the special diagnostic tests, and giving skilled nursing care to the child who requires surgery for the removal of adrenal tumors, ectopic ACTH-producing tumors, or brain surgery for removal of a tumor in the pituitary region.

Hypercortisolism also might result from exogenous steroid therapy for treatment of asthma, renal disease, or as part of chemotherapy for cancer.

Excessive Aldosterone Secretion Aldosterone is the major mineralocorticoid synthesized by the adrenal cortex. Aldosterone secretion increases with hyperkalemia and decreases with hypokalemia. Serum sodium concentration also regulates aldosterone secretion, with hyponatremia stimulating aldosterone secretion. The major function of aldosterone is to cause the distal renal tubules in the kidney to retain sodium and chloride and excrete potassium and hydrogen ions. Aldosterone release is also influenced by ACTH secretion.

Excessive aldosterone causes hypertension and hypokalemia, which results in fatigue, muscle weakness, paresthesias, poor growth, poor weight gain, polyuria, polydipsia, tetany, and metabolic alkalosis (Bacon, Spencer, and Kelch, 1975).

Nursing care of the child with suspected hyperaldosteronism includes supervising the child's eating during testing (because the amount of sodium in the diet must be controlled), collecting 24-hour urine specimens, and monitoring the child's blood pressure. The child's adrenal glands might need to be removed surgically. Following diagnosis, nursing care focuses on teaching and supporting the parents. The nurse explains the importance of a diet high in potassium and the need for potassium supplements as well as describing and providing a list of signs for hypokalemia and hyperkalemia. If the child is treated with diuretics, they are given in the morning to prevent bedwetting. The nurse discusses the child's need for special lavatory privileges with the school personnel. In addition, frequent check-ups are needed to monitor the blood pressure.

Excessive Adrenal Sex Steroid Secretion Adrenal androgens increase linear growth, stimulate growth of pubic and axillary hair, and increase the maturation of the epiphyses (growth centers) of the bones. The adrenal androgens are androstenedione, dehydroepiandrosterone (DHEA), and DHEA-sulfate. These hormones are excreted in the urine as 17-ketosteroids.

Excessive production of adrenal sex steroids might be caused by the presence of tumors or enzyme deficiencies. Virilizing adrenal tumors may be either adenomas or carcinomas. The child with a virilizing adrenal adenoma might present with clitoromegaly in females or penile enlargement (with concomitantly small testicles) in males, pubic and axillary hair growth, increased linear growth rate, increased muscle development, and acne. Urine and blood measurement of adrenal androgens are elevated in the presence of adrenal tumors. The treatment is adrenalectomy, followed by irradiation and/or chemotherapy if the tumor is malignant. Male virility is unaffected by adrenalectomy because most testosterone is produced by the testes.

Enzyme deficiencies in the metabolic pathways of cortisol and aldosterone bring about excessive formation of adrenal sex steroids. When the adrenal cortex is unable to synthesize cortisol and aldosterone, the feedback message to the pituitary is that more cortisol and aldosterone are needed. The pituitary then releases more ACTH to stimulate the adrenal cortex. Under constant ACTH stimulation, the adrenal gland hypertrophies in an effort to make cortisol and aldosterone. When the adrenal gland is unable to fulfill this function, all the precursors of aldosterone and cortisol accumulate and are shunted along the pathway to the production of adrenal androgens. Thus, the adrenal gland secretes large amounts of testosterone and some estrogen.

Excessive androgen production in utero has little effect on the male fetus, other than possibly causing the penis to be slightly larger than average and causing some pigmentation of the scrotum. However, when the female fetus is exposed to excessive adrenal androgens, the external genitals become virilized (the internal sex structures are unaffected). The clitoris enlarges, and the labia partially or completely fuses to form what might appear to be a scrotum; however, there are no testicles present in the "scrotum." The enzyme deficiency that causes congenital adrenal hyperplasia is the most common cause of the ambiguous genitals observed in the neonatal period. Congenital adrenal hyperplasia is an autosomal recessive disorder. This genetic defect causes an enzyme deficiency in the pathway of cortisol and aldosterone formation; the enzyme most commonly missing is the 21-hydroxylase enzyme. The female child with this adrenal disorder will have a normal female karyotype (XX) and positive Barr bodies on the buccal smear.

The nurse supports the parents of an infant with ambiguous genitals by emphasizing the general health of the infant and accepting the infant as a female, by suggesting a delay in naming the infant and announcing the birth until the sex is confirmed, and by explaining the physiology of adrenal androgens. Treatment of this disorder is surgical correction of the female's external virilization.

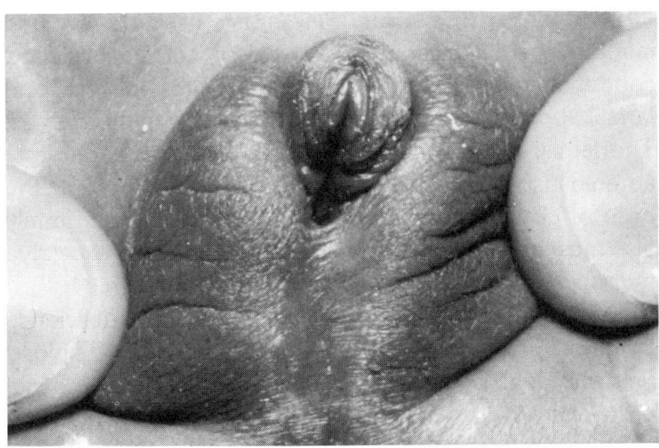

Partially masculinized external genitals of a child with congenital adrenal hyperplasia caused by adrenally produced androgen. (From Smith DW: *Growth and Its Disorders: Basics and Standards, Approach and Classifications, Growth Deficiency Disorders, Growth Excess Disorders, Obesity*. Saunders, 1977, p. 132. Reprinted by permission.)

The affected females are generally recognized at birth because of their ambiguous external genitals. Corrective surgery generally is performed before the infant is 3 months old. At puberty, these females might need to have their vaginas lengthened to permit intercourse. The affected male generally appears normal at birth and is often not diagnosed until 7–14 days of age when he presents with vomiting, dehydration, failure to thrive, and abnormal serum electrolyte levels.

Adrenal Cortex Hypofunction

Glucocorticoid insufficiency may be caused by congenital absence of enzymes in the cortisol production pathway, idiopathic atrophy of the adrenal glands, ACTH deficiency, or autoimmune destruction of the adrenal cortex. The child who develops glucocorticoid insufficiency might experience hypoglycemia, hypotension, and shock when significantly stressed by illness.

Aldosterone is the major mineralocorticoid. Isolated hypoaldosteronism is an uncommon childhood disorder. Children affected by this disorder crave salt, have intermittent fevers and dehydration, and gain weight poorly. This syndrome may be associated with diabetes mellitus. Frequently, a child with glucocorticoid deficiency also will have mineralocorticoid deficiency.

Enzymatic deficiencies in the adrenal cortex cause glucocorticoid deficiency, accompanied by mineralocorticoid deficiency in many of the affected children. The most common enzymatic deficiency is the 21-hydroxylase deficiency. These enzyme blocks are grouped together under the terms *congenital adrenal hyperplasia* or *adrenogenital syndrome*.

Medical Treatment Evaluation for glucocorticoid insufficiency generally includes a morning serum cortisol level measurement, which will be low, a 24-hour urine specimen measurement for free cortisol, which also will be low, serum sodium and potassium level determinations, and a blood urea nitrogen (BUN) measurement. An ACTH stimulation test might be used to demonstrate adrenal unresponsiveness to ACTH. Chronic treatment includes replacement therapy using hydrocortisone, given two to three times a day in a dose of 15–20 mg/m^2/day (Bacon, Spencer, and Kelch, 1975). Acute treatment consists of giving intravenous glucose and hydrocortisone and monitoring the child's recovery from shock and hypoglycemia.

Treatment for mineralocorticoid deficiency is replacement therapy with 9-alpha-fluorocortisol or desoxycorticosterone acetate (DOCA). Carefully regulated amounts of salt might be added to an affected infant's formula. These bottles must be obviously marked because salt potentially is lethal for healthy infants.

Treatment of enzymatic deficiencies consists of hydrocortisone replacement therapy, which lasts for life. The usual dose is 15–20 mg/m^2/day, given every 8 hours (Bacon, Spencer, and Kelch, 1975). Many of these children also have a mineralocorticoid deficiency, which is treated with 9-alpha-fluorocortisol or DOCA.

Nursing Management The nurse might be involved in referring a child with signs of glucocorticoid insufficiency, coordinating testing procedures, and teaching the child and family about the administration of replacement hormones. The family must know the signs and symptoms of acute adrenal insufficiency and understand the need to triple the dose of glucocorticoid during stress or illness. The family also must be aware of the signs and symptoms of excessive hydrocortisone therapy, namely, hypercortisolism.

Side effects of therapy for mineralocorticoid deficiency include hypertension, so the nurse monitors the child's blood pressure at follow-up appointments. A salt-losing crisis might occur with the stress of surgery. The acute nursing management of this condition involves monitoring blood pressure, keeping an accurate record of the child's fluid intake and urine output, and observing the recovery process from dehydration and shock.

Children with enzymatic deficiencies need close follow-up during their growing years so that dosages can be adjusted to allow for normal growth. Acute adrenal insufficiency can develop during times of significant illness. The parent is taught to increase the hydrocortisone dosage during febrile illnesses or when the child refuses to eat the normal diet. Acute nursing care during adrenal insufficiency includes close monitoring of vital signs especially blood pressure; prompt recognition and treatment for shock; instituting seizure precautions; continual assessment of child's hydration status and response to fluid replacement; and observation for potential electrolyte imbalance.

Adrenal Medulla Hyperfunction

Chromaffin tissue cells (found in the adrenal glands) synthesize, store, and secrete catecholamines (epinephrine and norepinephrine). *Pheochromocytomas* are tumors that arise in chromaffin tissues. This type of tumor is relatively rare in children but is twice as common in boys as in girls. Children with pheochromocytoma, or adrenal medulla hyperfunction, experience hypertension, headaches, sweating, nausea and vomiting, weight loss, and visual disturbances, all related to excessive catecholamine production by the adrenal medulla. Evaluation of the child with suspected adrenal medulla hyperfunction includes studies of urinary and blood catecholamines and their metabolites. Treatment is surgical removal of the tumor. Prior to surgery, the excessive catecholamines must be blocked by alpha-adrenergic agents. The side effects of these medications include hypotension, gastrointestinal irritation, and nasal congestion. The child might require glucocorticoids prior to surgery if a bilateral adrenalectomy is anticipated. Postoperatively, urinary catecholamines are measured to assess the effectiveness of the surgery and to observe for tumor recurrence (Vorhees, 1982).

The Child With Inappropriate Secretion From the Thyroid Gland

Hyperfunction

Excessive production of thyroxine (tetraiodothyronine, or T_4) appears to be caused by an autoimmune process and is more common in girls than in boys. It may appear at any age during childhood, but the incidence seems to peak during adolescence (Ingbar and Woeber, 1981). The child with hyperthyroidism might have tachycardia; personality changes, including irritability, nervousness, and emotional lability; tremors of the hands and poor handwriting; fasciculations of the tongue; exophthalmos and stare (Graves' disease); diffuse, firm enlargement of the thyroid gland (goiter); thin, velvety, moist skin; diarrhea; heat intolerance and sweating; weight loss and polyphagia; growth acceleration; hypertension; sleep disturbances; and weakness. The individual with hyperthyroidism generally feels miserable.

Laboratory findings will include an elevated thyroxine level, free thyroxine and triiodothyronine (T_3), and suppressed TSH levels. CT scans of the thyroid generally will demonstrate diffuse enlargement of the gland. In addition, the tests for thyroid gland function involving uptake of the radioactive isotope of iodine (^{131}I) by the thyroid as measured during a 24-hour period will be elevated.

Medical and Surgical Treatment Treatment goals are normalization of the thyroxine levels, reduction in the size of the thyroid gland, resolution of the exophthalmos, and resolution of the symptoms. Some of these improvements might not be evident for many months. The treatment of hyperthyroidism might involve surgical removal of the thyroid gland, ablation of the thyroid tissue using radioactive iodine, or conservative medical management using medication. The last approach generally is chosen for children because it has the least risk (Bacon, Spencer, and Kelch, 1975).

With medical management, agents are used to block thyroid hormone synthesis, allowing the thyroid gland to "rest." These medications, which in effect block the action of TSH, are propylthiouracil (PTU) and methimazole. They must be taken every 8 hours for maximal effect. Propylthiouracil generally is given as 100–150 mg/day; the dose of methimazole is 10–15 mg/day (Bacon, Spencer, and Kelch, 1975). Methimazole and PTU have potentially serious side effects, including leukopenia, agranulocytosis, rashes, arthritis, and hemolytic anemia. Complete blood counts are obtained routinely in children taking these medications. Whenever such a child has an infection, mouth sore, or unexplained fever, the medications are stopped and a blood count is obtained. Should a child develop these serious side

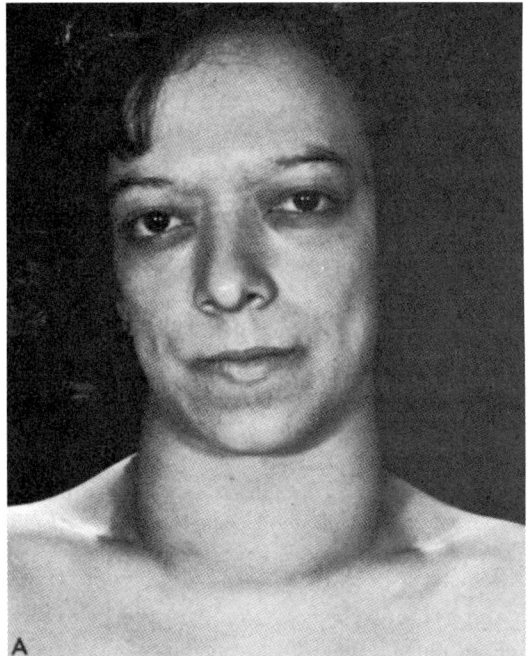
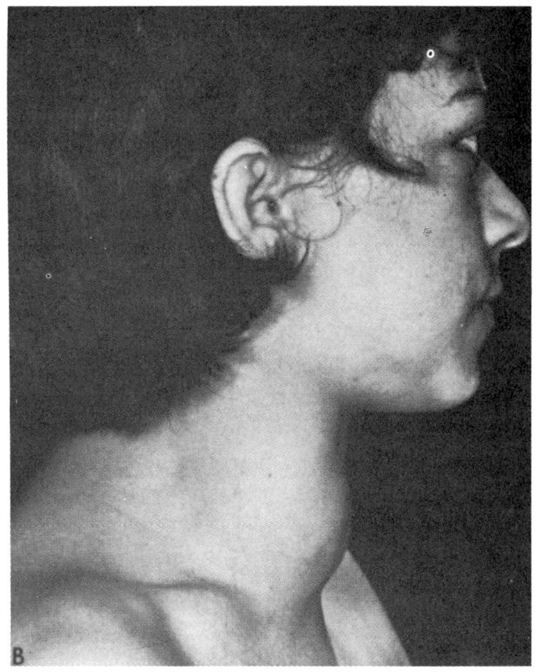

Hyperthyroidism. Note the sulcus between the thyroid and the lateral aspect of the neck, as well as the dilated veins overlying the thyroid gland. The only ocular abnormality was slight widening of the right palpebral fissure, without true exophthalmos. (From Williams RH: *Textbook of Endocrinology*. 6th ed. Saunders, 1981, p. 188. Reprinted by permission.)

effects of medical therapy, surgery or ^{131}I ablation of the thyroid must be considered.

If the child can take PTU or methimazole without side effects, this therapy generally continues for 2 years, after which the medication is tapered gradually while the child is observed for a recurrence of the hyperthyroidism. The main disadvantages of the medical treatment are the side effects, need for the child and family to cooperate with the frequent medication administration, and lengthy treatment regimen.

In addition to initiating treatment to block thyroid hormone synthesis, a short course of a beta-adrenergic blocking agent such as propranolol might be prescribed at the time of diagnosis to decrease tachycardia until the thyroxine level decreases. Propranolol is contraindicated for children whose history includes asthma or heart block because of the drug's potential side effects.

Regardless of the course of treatment chosen (irradiation, surgery, or medical management), the child eventually will have subnormal thyroid hormone levels and require daily thyroid hormone replacement. Synthetic thyroxine is the usual form of medication given; the dose is 100 $\mu g/m^2$/day (Bacon, Spencer, and Kelch, 1975). There are virtually no side effects of this thyroxine preparation, which is chemically identical to human thyroxine.

Nursing Management Nursing management of the child with hyperthyroidism might include referral for definitive diagnosis. The severely symptomatic child might require hospitalization for the treatment of tachycardia, hyperthermia, and exhaustion. The nurse designs a supportive, flexible care plan for this child, who literally might be unable

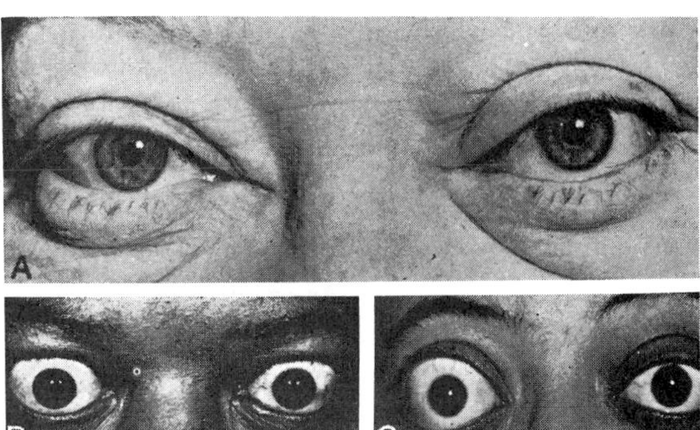

Exophthalmos. *A*. Palpebral edema. Swelling of the eyelids masks the protruding eyeballs. *B*. Marked widening of palpebral fissures; slight palpebral swelling. *C*. Unequal degrees of ophthalmopathy. (From Williams RH: *Textbook of Endocrinology*. 6th ed. Saunders, 1981, p. 190. Reprinted by permission.)

to sit down or sleep. Exophthalmos might prevent the eyelids from closing completely in sleep; the child and parent need to learn how to instill artificial tears at bedtime and understand the importance of this medication in preventing corneal ulceration. The nurse also instructs the parent and child about the action of all medications prescribed, the importance of adhering to the medication routine, and how to observe for side effects of the medications. If surgery is elected, the nurse plans and provides appropriate care before, during, and following surgery.

The child with hyperthyroidism is usually quite uncomfortable, nervous, and emotionally labile. After the onset of symptoms and prior to treatment, school performance and peer relationships generally suffer. The parents often become frustrated with the child's behavior and their attempts to deal with it. At the time of diagnosis, the child might be placed on three forms of medication: PTU or methimazole, propranolol, and eye drops. Until the thyroxine level returns to normal, the child is unable to help the parent remember the medication schedule.

The nurse might need to contact the child's school to explain the hyperthyroidism with regard to recent behavior and performance problems. The parent will need support in dealing with the child's behavior until the thyroxine level returns to normal.

Hypofunction

One neonate out of every 4000 live births has congenital hypothyroidism (La Franchi, 1982). Congenital hypothyroidism might be caused by nondevelopment of the thyroid gland during fetal life, the thyroid gland's being in an ectopic location (lingual), TRH or TSH deficiency, enzymatic defects within the thyroid gland, or the transplacental passage of antithyroid medications (PTU, methimazole, or ^{131}I).

Many states now require that neonates be screened for congenital hypothyroidism. This simple test can be done at the same time phenylketonuria (PKU), sickle cell, and other screening tests are performed. The neonate with hypothyroidism generally has a low thyroxine level and an elevated TSH level and might or might not have symptoms and signs of hypothyroidism. The symptomatic infant might have temperature regulation problems; sluggish reflexes; a large, protruding tongue; constipation or decreased stools; an umbilical hernia; a flattened nasal bridge; or mottling of the skin.

The earlier thyroxine therapy is begun, the better the chances that the infant will achieve normal intellectual capabilities (La Franchi, 1982). If the infant is not diagnosed until symptoms are evident, some intellectual impairment might have occurred already. Table 40–11 presents data on intellectual functioning related to the age at which thyroxine therapy was initiated.

Children might acquire hypothyroidism because of enzymatic defects; following an insult to the hypothalamic–pituitary area that causes a TSH or TRH deficiency; following surgical removal of the thyroid tissue; or because of an autoimmune process (for example, chronic lymphocytic thyroiditis).

Hypothyroidism frequently is discovered when the child experiences a significant slowing in linear growth. Figure 40–9 illustrates the growth pattern of a child with acquired hypothyroidism. The child with acquired hypothyroidism might have cold intolerance; constipation; lack of interest in normal peer activities; dry, thickened skin; coarse hair; and increased sleep requirements. School performance and behavior might be ideal because the child has just enough energy to do schoolwork and is not easily distracted by the desire to participate in other activities.

Laboratory evaluation generally will demonstrate a low thyroxine level, low level of free thyroxine, and high TSH level. A TRH stimulation test may be performed if there is a question of pituitary dysfunction.

Thyroid cancer does occur in children. The cancer may be papillary, follicular, medullary, or of an undifferentiated type (Bacon, Spencer, and Kelch, 1975).

TABLE 40-11 IQ in Relation to Age in 56 Cases

Age at diagnosis	Number of cases*	IQ Above 90	IQ Under 90
Before 4 months of age	40(19)	14	5
Between 4 and 7 months of age	23(12)	4	8
Between 7 and 25 months of age	78(25)	10	15
Total	141(56)	28	28

*Figures in brackets indicate the number of cases tested.

SOURCE: Raiti S, Newns GH: Cretinism: Early diagnosis and its relation to mental prognosis. *Arch Dis Child* 1971; 46:692. Reprinted by permission.

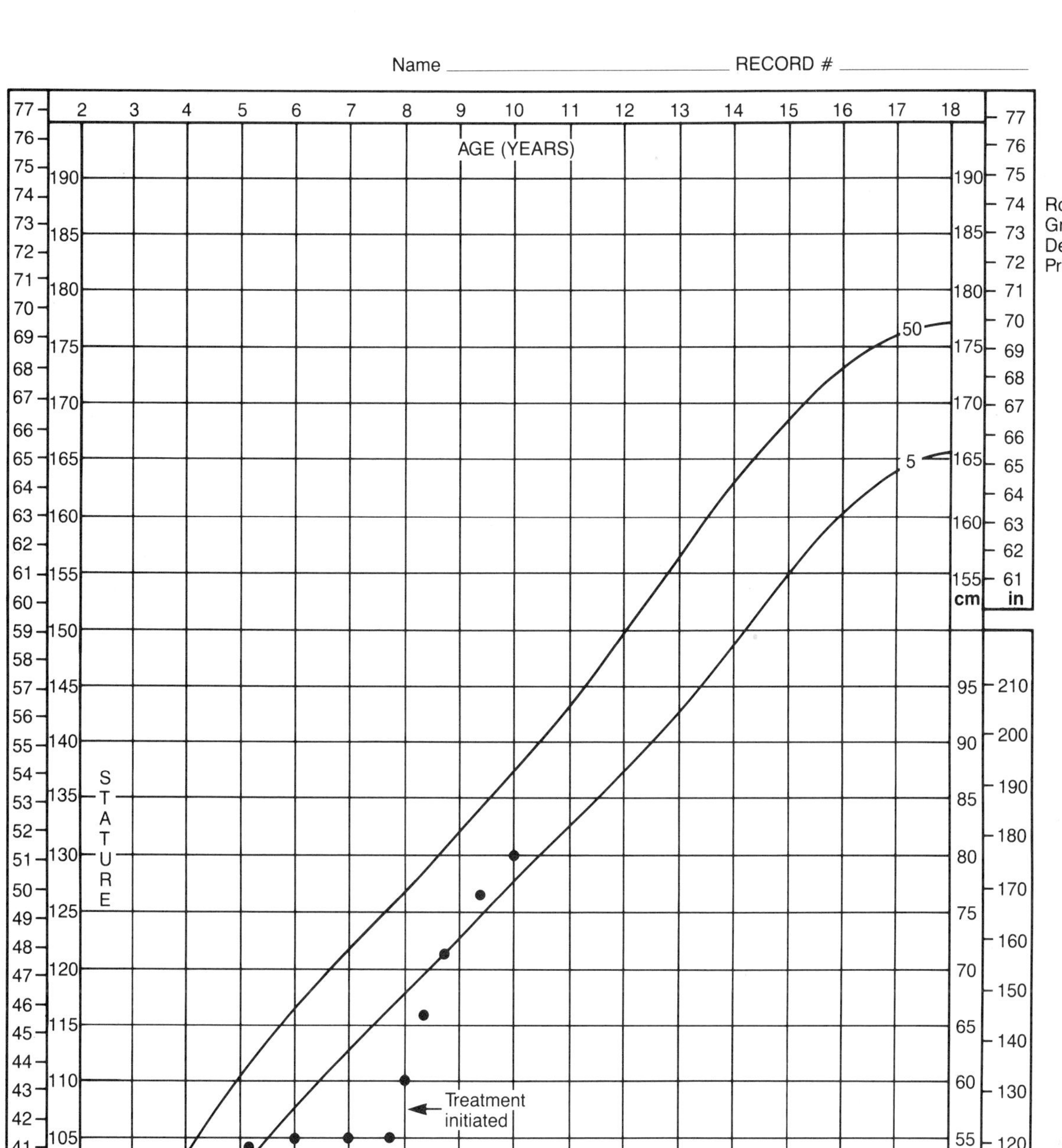

Figure 40-9 Growth chart illustrating significant slowing of linear growth with acquired hypothyroidism and rapid "catch-up" growth when therapy is instituted.

Medical and Surgical Treatment Treatment of congenital hypothyroidism consists of giving thyroxine daily; the dose is 100 $\mu g/m^2$/day. This pill can be crushed and given to the infant in a small amount of strained fruit. Treatment with thyroxine will be required throughout the individual's life. The amount of medication is adjusted for growth during childhood and adolescence. Follow-up consists of periodic assessment of the child's growth, weight gain, and attainment of developmental milestones. Psychometric testing prior to entering school might be indicated and helpful, particularly if the child was diagnosed after 2 months of age. Treatment of acquired hypothyroidism is identical to that for congenital hypothyroidism. The dosage of thyroxine is adjusted for growth during childhood and adolescence.

In the case of thyroid cancer, the child generally presents with one or more hard nodules in the neck. If thyroid cancer is suspected, a thyroid scan is ordered to examine thyroid tissue and lymph nodes in the neck and chest for cancerous involvement. A surgical biopsy might be performed as part of the initial evaluation. Blood studies are ordered, including calcitonin and thyroglobulin measurements. The usual treatment of thyroid cancer is surgical excision of the thyroid and surrounding lymph nodes, followed by ablative radioactive iodine therapy. Thyroxine therapy is then given to supply the necessary thyroid hormone and suppress any remaining thyroid tissue. Follow-up examinations, CT scans, and chest radiographs are done to identify any recurrence and metastases.

Nursing Management Nursing management of the infant with congenital hypothyroidism includes supporting and counseling the parents (see Chapter 31), explaining the function of thyroxine and the importance of administering the medication every day, and discussing infant stimulation. At follow-up visits, the nurse might assess the infant's development, using a standardized tool such as the Denver Developmental Screening Test (DDST). The DDST is designed to detect developmental delays during infancy and the preschool years (see Chapter 16).

In states where neonates are not screened for congenital hypothyroidism, nurses should carefully assess infants at well-child visits for symptoms of hypothyroidism.

Nursing management of the child with acquired hypothyroidism might involve referring a child who is growing poorly or who has other signs and symptoms of hypothyroidism. When thyroxine therapy is initiated, the nurse informs parents and teachers of the expected changes in the child's energy level and behavior; the child might appear to be hyperactive when compared with the previous hypothyroid demeanor. Nurses can help children and parents identify methods of remembering the daily medication.

The following example illustrates the change possible in a child and the adjustment required by the family. A 9-year-old boy was referred to the endocrine clinic for evaluation of short stature. Growth records indicated that his growth rate had begun to decelerate between 5 and 6 years of age. His parents had no complaints about his behavior or health; he was their "ideal child," always willing to sit quietly when asked and a model student at school. During the hour of interviewing his parents, he sat without saying a word or leaving his chair. When asked to climb up on the examination table, he took 3 minutes to cross the room, walking very slowly. His only spontaneous expression during the entire visit to the clinic was a smile when he was told he could take medicine (thyroxine) that would help him to grow. Physical examination revealed cold, dry, thickened skin and absent deep tendon reflexes. After consultation with the endocrinologist, the nurse ordered thyroid function blood tests and proceeded to teach the boy and his parents about thyroxine therapy. When blood tests confirmed the diagnosis of hypothyroidism, he began taking the prescribed thyroxine preparation. Two weeks later, his mother called the nurse to complain about the medication, stating that it was making her son "hyperactive" and that he had been in trouble at school for talking in class. In fact, this boy responded to therapy positively, displaying remarkable catch-up growth in the first year of taking thyroxine and enjoying age-appropriate activities for the first time in 3 years.

Nursing management of the child with thyroid cancer includes referral of any child with a nodule in the neck, preparation of the child for tests and surgery, instructing the family about the administration of thyroxine, and general emotional support of the child and family. Postoperative nursing care includes close observation for hemorrhage, vocal cord paralysis, and signs and symptoms of hypocalcemia because the parathyroid glands sometimes are damaged or inadvertently removed with thyroidectomy.

The Child With Inappropriate Secretion From the Parathyroid Glands

Hyperfunction

Hyperfunction of the parathyroids, or *hypercalcemia,* is a serious medical condition. Most cases of hypercalcemia occur in infants or adolescents with parathyroid adenomas. Hypercalcemia is defined as a serum calcium level over 11 mg/dL. Hypercalcemia can cause nephrocalcinosis, with hypertension and renal failure.

Signs and symptoms of hypercalcemia are polydipsia and polyuria, constipation, hypotonia and weakness, irritability, and listlessness. Laboratory evaluation will reveal normal or increased calcium levels, hypophosphatemia, an increased alkaline phosphate level, increased parathormone level, and increased urinary cyclic AMP excretion. Radiographs might demonstrate bone demineralization.

Medical and Surgical Treatment Acute treatment of severe hypercalcemia (serum calcium level greater than 15 mg/dL) consists of intravenous hydration, administration of diuretics, supplemental potassium and magnesium salts, and the use of corticosteriods. After the hypercalcemic crisis is resolved, measures are taken to decrease the serum calcium level, after which the parathyroids or parathyroid adenomas are removed surgically (Bacon, Spencer, and Kelch, 1975).

Nursing Management Nursing management of the child with hypercalcemia includes careful monitoring of fluid intake and output, monitoring serum electrolytes, collecting urine specimens to assess calcium excretion, and monitoring the child's cardiac status during acute treatment.

Hypofunction

Hypocalcemia is defined as a total serum calcium level of less than 7 mg/dL or an ionized calcium level of less than 2.5 mg/dL. Hypocalcemia can be a life-threatening condition because it can cause seizures and respiratory arrest.

Signs and symptoms of hypocalcemia are a tingling sensation of the hands and around the mouth; muscle cramps; muscle twitching; weakness; tetany and seizures; positive Chvostek's sign (seventh cranial nerve irritability); and positive Trousseau's sign (carpospasm when a blood pressure cuff is inflated). Some infants with hypocalcemia also might be lethargic, eat poorly, and vomit.

Premature infants who suffer birth asphyxia are likely to develop hypocalcemia in the first few days of life. Older children might develop hypoparathyroidism and hypocalcemia following thyroid surgery. Children with X-linked recessive or autosomal recessive hypoparathyroidism might have mild mental retardation, diarrhea, hyperreflexia, hypoplasia of dental enamel, brittle nails, and fragile hair, in addition to the other symptoms of hypocalcemia listed previously (Goldstein and Motulsky, 1981).

Treatment of acute, serious hypocalcemia includes the slow intravenous administration of calcium salts, with the nurse observing the cardiac monitor for bradycardia and the child's respiratory status closely because hypocalcemia can cause laryngeal stridor. A tracheotomy set should be at the child's bedside. The child with hypocalcemia might require the long-term administration of oral calcium gluconate, the dosage of which is adjusted to maintain a normal serum calcium level.

The Child With Inappropriate Secretion From the Gonads

Hyperfunction: Excessive Estrogen or Testosterone Production

Excessive estrogen production in the young female brings about early pubertal development and rapid bone maturation, with early closure of the epiphyseal growth centers and shortening of ultimate stature. Two causes of early puberty (gonadotropic hormone hyperfunction and adrenal tumors) are discussed earlier in the chapter. The third source of early estrogen production are ovarian tumors and cysts (Bacon, Spencer, and Kelch, 1975). Ovarian cysts might require surgical removal but generally regress spontaneously. Regression of puberty occurs following surgical removal of tumors in females under 8 years of age (Bacon, Spencer, and Kelch, 1975). If sufficient ovarian tissue remains, the child should enter puberty normally at the expected time. If all of the ovarian tissue is removed, estrogen and progesterone therapy will be required to complete secondary sexual development, and the female will be infertile.

Medical Treatment Assessment of the child with precocious puberty (male or female) includes a careful history to obtain information regarding how long the parents have been aware of the signs of early puberty; when pubertal development was first observed; and whether the child's linear growth has accelerated, the child has been complaining of headaches or visual disturbances (symptoms of an intracranial lesion), or the child has access to estrogens or androgens (oral contraceptives, estrogen-containing hand creams, or farm animal feed that is supplemented with androgens or estrogens). During the physical examination, the nurse assesses the amount of breast development, evidence of pubic hair, amount of axillary hair, presence of body odor, and evidence of estrogen effect on the vaginal mucosa in girls (or enlargement of the testicles and increase in penile length in boys). The child's pubertal development is compared with the Tanner standards (see Figs. 11–2 and 11–3). The nurse also assesses the child for impaired visual fields or evidence of papilledema.

Radiologic studies generally are ordered to assess the child's bone maturation and determine whether the skeletal maturation is advanced for the child's chronologic age. Pelvic and abdominal sonograms might be used to look for ovarian cysts or masses and adrenal hypertrophy or masses. A CT scan of the head might be ordered to look for intracranial masses, which could be the cause of the early pubertal development.

Laboratory assessment includes blood tests for the levels of LH, FSH, estradiol, and testosterone. The level of FSH is very low in children between 1 month of age and puberty; however, it might be in the pubertal range in a child with precocious puberty. The level of LH also is very low in children between 1 month of age and puberty but might be in the pubertal range in a child with precocious puberty (Bacon, Spencer, and Kelch, 1975). The level of estradiol (estrogen) is normally low until puberty but might be in the pubertal range in a child with precocious puberty. The level of testosterone is normally low in children between 1 month of age and puberty but might be elevated to the male pubertal range in a child with precocious puberty. If the testosterone level is elevated in a female, adrenal dysfunction is suspected. The level of plasma 17-hydroxyprogesterone might be measured. This substance is a precursor of cortisol and if elevated might suggest the presence of an enzyme deficiency in the adrenal cortex, which can cause the overproduction of testosterone. The level of urinary 17-ketosteroids, a by-product of adrenal steroid production, is measured to evaluate the possibility that an adrenal tumor is the cause of the precocious puberty.

At present, there is no ideal therapy for children with precocious puberty. Medroxyprogesterone has been the most widely used agent to treat this problem. It arrests the progression of secondary sexual characteristics by blocking the pituitary release of LH and FSH. Medroxyprogesterone generally is given by intramuscular injection on a monthly basis. Besides the discomfort of the injection, potential side effects include changes in testicular germ cells and suppression of the pituitary–adrenal axis, which could precipitate adrenal insufficiency if the child encounters stress or the medication is withdrawn suddenly. Often, this medication is not effective in halting the progression of puberty. It is used infrequently in females, mostly when menarche occurs at a very early age (Bacon, Spencer, and Kelch, 1975). Research is being conducted on the use of luteinizing releasing hormone (LRH) agonists and antagonists in the treatment of precocious puberty. Cyproterone acetate also has been used in Europe for this purpose.

Because precocious puberty is usually a process that waxes and wanes, many parents and physicians elect not to treat children with any medication but rather to observe the course of development and give the child guidance. Most parents agree with this philosophy of no treatment and ask for suggestions on how to deal with a large-for-age child in terms of peer relationships and parental expectations. The child with precocious puberty must deal with peer reactions to early breast development, menses, pubic hair, and penile growth and the emotional changes that accompany puberty.

Nursing Management Nursing intervention includes both the diagnostic procedures and counseling parents and children. The nurse always emphasizes that these pubertal developments are a normal process which merely are occurring at an early age.

Ovarian or Testicular Hypofunction: Delayed Sexual Maturation

Sexual maturation should begin prior to 15 years of age in girls and before 16 years of age in boys; most girls have breast budding by 12 years of age, and most boys will have beginning testicular enlargement by 14 years of age. If a child shows no signs of pubertal development by 14 years of age, the cause for the delay should be assessed.

Children with a history of insult to the hypothalamic–pituitary region might not have the ability to release LH and FSH and have hypogonadotropic delay of puberty. This problem is not very common in general pediatric practice but might be present in children with other pituitary gland dysfunction or following central nervous system irradiation. A more common cause of delayed pubertal development is constitutional delay of growth (see the section on anterior lobe hypofunction earlier in the chapter).

Puberty might be delayed in the female because of ovarian dysgenesis. The most common cause of ovarian dysfunction is *Turner's syndrome,* a chromosomal abnormality. The girl with Turner's syndrome most commonly has a 45XO karyotype rather than the normal 46XX female chromosome complement. Turner's syndrome may be suspected at birth if the female infant has webbing of the neck and a low hairline, absent femoral pulses, puffy hands and feet, and a high, arched palate. If Turner's syndrome is diagnosed in infancy, no specific treatment is recommended until approximately 7 years of age or until the growth rate decelerates.

More often, Turner's syndrome is not diagnosed until the girl's linear growth rate decelerates in late childhood and/or she fails to have secondary sexual development in her adolescent years. She might have some of the stigmas associated with classic Turner's syndrome such as neck webbing, broad chest, cubitus valgus, abnormal fingernails, high arched palate, hypertension, coarctation of the aorta, and a low posterior hairline.

Laboratory findings in the older girl with Turner's syndrome will include increased FSH and LH levels, decreased estrogen levels, delayed bone age, and the 45XO karyotype. Girls with Turner's syndrome might have single, rotated, or horseshoe-shaped kidneys. An intravenous pyelogram is needed to obtain this information. Girls with Turner's syndrome should be referred to a cardiologist for evaluation of hypertension because many girls with this condition have coarctation of the aorta or pulmonary stenosis.

Medical Treatment If the child cannot release LH and FSH and has hypogonadotrophic delay of puberty, regardless of whether the problem is with the hypothalamus (the hypothalamus cannot release LRH) or the pituitary (the pituitary cannot respond to LRH stimulation by releasing FSH and LH), the treatment is replacement therapy with estrogen and progesterone for girls and testosterone for boys.

When testicular function is questioned in a newborn male, a human chorionic gonadotropin (HCG) stimulation test is performed, which measures testosterone levels prior to and following a 5-day course of HCG injections (Bacon, Spencer, and Kelch, 1975). In the newborn with microphallus, a course of testosterone might be given and the penile response evaluated. Bilaterally undescended testicles (cryptorchidism) are associated more often with infertility than unilateral cryptorchidism. Young men with *anorchism* (congenital absence of the testes) will require exogenous testosterone therapy for secondary sexual development and usually elect to have prosthetic implants into the scrotum for cosmetic reasons. Enzymatic deficiencies can cause incomplete masculinization of the external genitals and cause gynecomastia at puberty. Chromosomal abnormalities such as Klinefelter's syndrome (XXY karotype) prevent secondary sexual development. The therapy for many of these disorders is intramuscular injections of testosterone on a 2- to 4-week schedule and support concerning issues of infertility (Bacon, Spencer, and Kelch, 1975).

Most children do not require hormonal therapy for the treatment of delayed puberty caused by constitutional delay. Satisfactory coping with the delay can be achieved if the young adolescent is reassured of general good health and is given some estimate of when puberty will begin. However, adolescents who are significantly smaller than their peers might elect hormonal treatment to initiate the natural process of puberty. Males can be given a 3-month course of testosterone; size and pubertal development are assessed 1 month after the last testosterone injection. Generally, one to two courses of testosterone therapy are sufficient to launch a male into puberty. Psychologically, adolescents might feel more assured of their sexual capacity if allowed to complete sexual maturation without further exogenous hormonal supplementation. Oral testosterone preparations are available but are less effective than the injectable forms and have been implicated in the development of hepatic dysfunction. Girls may be given estrogen and progesterone to hasten secondary sexual development. Prolonged therapy is contraindicated because of the risks of estrogen therapy (blood clots, uterine cancer, hypertension, and migraine headaches) and the possibility of accelerating epiphyseal closure, resulting in ultimate short stature. Before recommending estrogen therapy, however, a family history pertaining to blood clots, cerebral vascular accidents, and migraine headaches must be obtained and evaluated.

Understandably, parents are quite upset when the diagnosis of Turner's syndrome is made because these females are infertile. The child who is under 12 years of age generally is told that she requires medication to promote linear

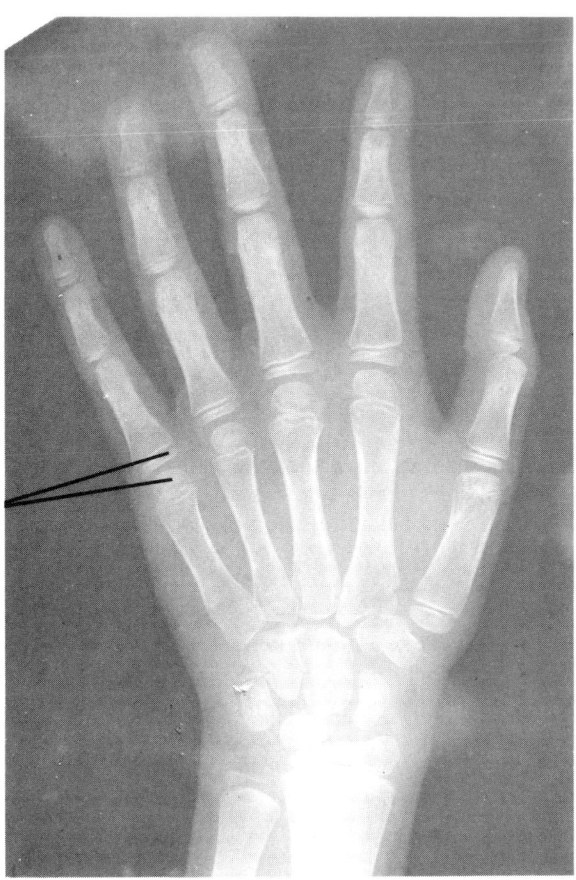

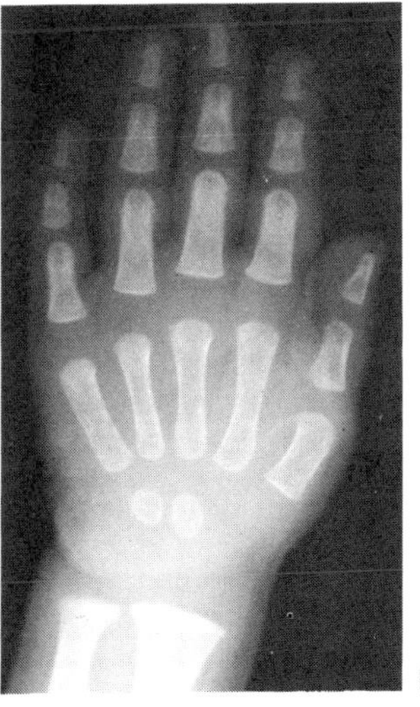

Radiographs of the right hands of (*A*) a 7-year-old child and (*B*) an 18-month-old child. The space between the bones are the cartilaginous epiphyses of the various bones. In the 7-year-old, the epiphyses have ossified, leaving thin epiphyseal plates. (From Spence AP, Mason EB: *Human Anatomy and Physiology*. 2nd ed. Benjamin/Cummings, 1983, p. 158. Reprinted by permission.)

growth. When she is old enough to be concerned about secondary sexual development and requires estrogen and progestrone therapy, the infertility problem is discussed. Current research with in vitro fertilization might allow females with Turner's syndrome to become pregnant at some point in the future.

Treatment of Turner's syndrome involves the administration of an anabolic steroid or growth hormone to promote linear growth. Anabolic steroids might mature the skeleton more rapidly than the height advances, so periodic bone age radiographs are required. Estrogen therapy, daily or every other day, is initiated when the girl becomes uncomfortable with her lack of pubertal development. Once she experiences breakthrough bleeding, progesterone is added to this therapy to cycle the bleeding. The side effects of estrogen therapy include potential endometrial cancer, blood clotting, hypertension, and headaches (Bacon, Spencer, and Kelch, 1975).

Nursing Management Nursing management of the child with delayed puberty might include referring the child for assessment, assisting in the initial assessment procedures, teaching the child and parent about testosterone or estrogen therapy, and counseling the child and parent about clothing appropriate for age and size.

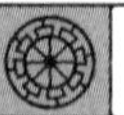

NURSING CARE PLAN Child With Diabetes Mellitus

Assessment Data

Teri, an 8-year-old black female, was diagnosed recently with Type I diabetes mellitus when she presented with a 2-week history of vaginitis, polydipsia, polyuria, and weight loss. Teri lives with her single mother, 6-year-old brother, and 4-year-old sister in an apartment in a low-income neighborhood near the hospital.

Nursing Diagnoses and Goals

1. **Nursing diagnosis:** Potential knowledge deficit related to diabetes management skills.

   Long-term goal: Teri and her mother will competently manage the tasks required for good control of Teri's diabetes.

   Short-term goals: (a) Teri and her mother will help to identify the most effective teaching techniques for learning diabetes management. (b) Teri and her mother will learn the technique for insulin administration. (c) Teri and her mother will learn additional management skills such as food planning, blood glucose testing, and prevention and treatment of hypoglycemia.

2. **Nursing diagnosis:** Potential alteration in health maintenance related to school staff's understanding of Teri's health needs.

   Long-term goal: School personnel will be able to monitor Teri for signs and symptoms of hypoglycemia.

   Short-term goal: Teri will identify the school staff member responsible for coordinating education and supervision of her diabetes care while in school.

3. **Nursing diagnosis:** Potential impaired gas exchange, fluid volume alteration, or impairment of skin integrity related to complications of acute diabetes.

   Long-term goal: Teri will have no episodes of vaginitis, diabetic ketoacidosis, or severe hypoglycemia in the first year after initial diagnosis and teaching.

   Short-term goals: (a) Teri and her mother will understand the importance of good blood glucose control and hygiene to prevent recurrences of vaginitis. (b) Teri and her mother will describe the initial treatment of symptoms of ketosis and hypoglycemia and when to refer when initial treatment is ineffective.

4. **Nursing diagnosis:** Potential disturbance in body image related to diabetes mellitus.

   Long-term goal: Teri and her family will exhibit minimal emotional and social effects from her adjustment to diabetes mellitus.

   Short-term goals: (a) Teri will receive support from her family to engage in normal peer group activities. (b) Teri will become acquainted with other children with diabetes mellitus. (c) Teri's family will find ways to decrease the financial burden caused by need of diabetic equipment and supplies.

Interventions	Rationale	Evaluation criteria
1. Discuss learning style preferences with Teri and her mother before teaching initial procedure and plan approach accordingly	Some people prefer oral communication, audiovisual materials, and demonstration/practice to reading educational materials. Learning occurs most easily when individual preferences are respected	Do Teri and her mother demonstrate ability to retain and utilize information taught about diabetes and its management?

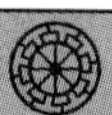

NURSING CARE PLAN Child With Diabetes Melliitus (continued)

Interventions	Rationale	Evaluation Criteria
Explain how the body responds to too much sugar (hyperglycemia) and provide family with list of related signs and symptoms Explain how the body responds to too much insulin (hypoglycemia) and provide family with list of related signs and symptoms	Knowing the signs and symptoms of hyperglycemia and hypoglycemia is necessary to maintain blood sugar control and to understand how the body responds to levels that are too high or too low	Are Teri and her mother able to list the signs and symptoms of hyperglycemia and hypoglycemia and tell how each might be precipitated?
Identify learning needs of Teri's mother and sources of greatest anxiety; patiently and thoroughly teach her one skill at a time beginning with administration of insulin to alleviate her anxiety about being unable to learn a complex procedure	High levels of anxiety interfere with learning; alleviating anxiety about giving injections will allow Teri's mother to focus on other teaching with more confidence	Can Teri's mother explain action and purpose of insulin and confidently give the injection of insulin to Teri?
Explain the function and need for insulin as well as the types of insulin, their onset, peak, and duration	Knowledge about insulin and its necessity for proper glucose usage is important to understanding and accepting the need for daily (and usually twice daily) insulin injections	
Demonstrate technique of drawing up insulin into syringe and have parent return demonstration Explain method of giving injection, have parent practice on doll before giving injection to child	Demonstration and practice at the person's own pace enhance learning	
Explain site rotation and demonstrate use of site rotation chart	Use of chart reinforces rotation of sites as concrete guide available and lessens potential for lipodystrophy	
Discuss care and storage of insulin and supplies	Proper care of supplies is important to ensure sterility of equipment and safety	
Teach Teri and her mother how to do blood glucose testing	Blood glucose testing provides a more accurate picture of diabetic control	Can Teri and her mother demonstrate the procedure for testing the blood glucose level; interpret the results of the test in terms of diabetes control; and keep an accurate record of blood glucose levels?
Explain how blood glucose results relate to diabetic control and the insulin, diet, exercise interrelationship Provide chart and demonstrate how to record results	Control of diabetes depends on how much the child and parent know about it; the separate parts of management need to be explained as being interrelated to provide better comprehension of condition and the importance of each phase of management	

continued on next page

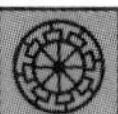

NURSING CARE PLAN Child With Diabetes Melliitus (continued)

Interventions	Rationale	Evaluation criteria
Review and reinforce dietary teaching done by nutritionist Discuss the role of diet in controlling blood glucose levels	A balanced diet consisting of proteins, carbohydrates, and fats is essential for growth and health. Consistent amount and pattern of food intake is necessary to maintain proper balance of insulin and sugar	Can Teri and her mother answer questions correctly about the effects of eating too much, too little, or inappropriate foods?
Discuss the specifics of Teri's diet and have Teri and her mother answer questions about kinds of food, amounts of food, and times of eating; emphasize importance of not skipping a meal or snack		
Have Teri and her mother plan a week's menu of meals and snacks	Actual meal planning defines options and reinforces dietary teaching	Can Teri and her mother plan a week's menu and compile a list of appropriate snacks?
Explain the effects of physical activity on the balance of sugar and insulin Discuss how to adjust insulin and food requirements for times of increased or decreased activity	Insulin dosage and diet are prescribed for normal activity. When activity level is increased, more food or less insulin is needed; when activity level is decreased, less food or more insulin is needed	Are Teri and her mother able to monitor activity and make the necessary adjustments to prevent episodes of hypoglycemia or hyperglycemia?
Provide the family with a telephone number of someone to call if questions arise	Having an available resource to answer questions helps the family plan for exceptions to routines and encourages participation in peer activities	Does Teri's mother know how to contact the resource person when questions arise?
Discuss with Teri and her mother how to adjust diet and insulin during times of illness or emotional stress Encourage Teri's mother to contact health care provider during times of stress so Teri's diabetes control will not be disrupted	Blood sugar increases during times of stress whether physical or emotional	Are Teri and her mother able to identify times of stress and learn how to adjust diet and insulin to maintain good control?
2. Contact school and identify school nurse who can teach other school personnel appropriate aspects of diabetes management. Designate school nurse as a member of Teri's diabetes education and management team. Staff education should stress the recognition of signs and symptoms of hypoglycemia and importance of Teri's nutritional and exercise regimen	School nurse can conduct staff education most efficiently because of familiarity with staff members and their levels of health-related knowledge	Is the school nurse available to communicate diabetes-related problems at school to the diabetes team at the hospital? Does Teri experience episodes of severe low blood sugar at school?
3. Teach Teri and her mother the importance of good skin care, wearing properly fitting shoes, prompt care of lacerations, good hygiene to prevent vaginitis, and the importance of regular well-child visits to monitor Teri's insulin requirements during puberty. Relate good self-care in the present to Teri's	Most endocrine disorders have few visible symptoms, so the family might not understand the seriousness of the disease and importance of adhering to prescribed regimen until they are related to a concrete experience such as the potential for normal childbearing	Can Teri explain how to prevent integumentary complications of diabetes? Are Teri's glycohemoglobin blood levels within appropriate limits?

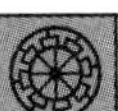

NURSING CARE PLAN Child With Diabetes Melliitus (continued)

Interventions	Rationale	Evaluation criteria
future health and ability to bear children without complications caused by diabetes		
Monitor Teri's glycohemoglobin levels to assess blood glucose control	Glycohemoglobin (Hb A_{1c}) is a blood test that demonstrates the quality of the individual's long-term blood glucose control	
Provide personal attention and interesting education during clinic visits	Quality of follow-up visits can motivate attendance at subsequent appointments	Does Teri regularly attend follow-up sessions?
Teach Teri and her mother simple treatments for ketosis and hypoglycemia and instruct them to go to the emergency room if the symptoms are not relieved. Have Teri obtain medical-alert identification to wear and carry some form of easily digested sugar with her	When early signs of acute diabetes complications are recognized promptly, simple treatment of symptoms is all that is necessary to reverse process of ketosis or hypoglycemia	Can Teri and her mother explain simple treatments for ketosis and hypoglycemia and criteria for emergency room care?
4. Refer Teri and her family to a visiting nurse association for home assessment of family functioning. Ask the social worker to assess the family's psychosocial adjustment to diabetes. Stay in touch with the school nurse for updates on Teri's reaction to diabetes	Networking and collaboration with other health professionals increase the contact and coverage for the child and family. Persons interacting in the home and school environment might be better able to assess the child's and family's reaction to illness	Do the visiting nurse, social worker, and school nurse periodically observe Teri and her family and report progress and any problems?
Encourage Teri and her family to attend lay diabetes meetings and explore any potential problems such as transportation. Refer Teri to a scholarship program for summer diabetes camp	The family might not be aware of the available resources for social support or how to contact other children and families who are dealing with diabetes also	Does the family demonstrate increased understanding and reduced anxiety related to diabetes? Does the family offer Teri support in leading a normal life and maintaining a positive body image?
Explore with the family and the social worker effective but least expensive diabetic equipment	Use of bottled alcohol and cotton balls is less expensive than prepackaged alcohol swabs; a glass syringe with disposable needles is less expensive than disposable syringes; however, the family must be competent with sterilizing the syringe	

Key Concepts

- The endocrine system is composed of glands, including the hypothalamus, pituitary gland, parathyroid glands, adrenal glands, gonads, and endocrine pancreas.
- Most of the endocrine system glands and structures develop within the first trimester of pregnancy.
- The endocrine system functions by circulating very small amounts of specific chemicals, called

hormones, which regulate metabolism, growth, puberty, and reproduction.

- Assessment of the child with possible endocrine dysfunction requires a complete history, including prenatal history and family history, and a physical examination, with special attention to appearance, vision, sexual development, and neurologic response.
- Because children with suspected endocrine disorders must undergo extensive diagnostic testing, the nurse coordinates the various procedures, teaches children and parents the correct methods, and offers emotional support to the family during testing.
- Acute care of children with endocrine dysfunctions might require prompt observation and intervention for children who present with electrolyte abnormalities or who develop hypoglycemia, respiratory distress, or acidosis—all of which are potentially fatal conditions.
- Because the stress of surgery frequently changes the child's hormonal requirements, preoperative and postoperative care involves monitoring the child's hormonal status and making adjustments, as needed.
- Nutritional interventions for children with endocrine disorders include assessment of children's appetites, fluid requirements, and appetite control and in some cases food plan modifications to avoid hypoglycemia and hyperglycemia.
- Although most endocrine disorders are not visibly handicapping, these children might be unable to participate in peer group activities, and therefore the nurse might need to assist them in meeting their socialization needs.
- The child's and family's ability to deal emotionally with a chronic endocrine disorder depends on the child's age and developmental level, seriousness of the condition, physical impairment to the child's appearance, and strengths of the family system.
- Because most endocrine disorders are of a chronic nature, children over 6 years of age and their parents must learn at the time of discharge from the hospital basic survival skills, including understanding the action of medications, knowing how to administer medications and prevent side effects, and knowing how to contact the health care team, as well as how to explain the disorder to family and friends.
- Diabetes mellitus, a disorder of carbohydrate metabolism, is the most common endocrine disorder, affecting 1 out of every 500–800 children under 21 years of age.
- The onset of diabetes mellitus in children is generally fairly rapid, and children often present with ketoacidosis, an acute form of insulin insufficiency; nursing interventions for ketoacidosis include hourly recording of fluid intake and urine output, cardiac monitoring, and insulin administration.
- At the time of diagnosis of diabetes mellitus, the nurse teaches children and their parents how to use the correct insulin, draw the dosage, plan to rotate injection sites, give an injection comfortably, and record the dose and site.
- Two methods of teaching diabetic children about food management are the exchange lists and the free diet.
- To assist diabetic children and their families in daily health care, the nurse helps them learn the proper technique for blood or urine testing.
- A long-term goal of nursing care for children with diabetes mellitus is teaching the care needed to prevent such complications as microvascular disease of the retina and kidney, macrovascular disease, and neuropathy.
- Working with a health care team, the nurse offers support and education to diabetic children and their families by providing thoughtful and age-appropriate explanations, allaying fears, setting goals for diabetes management, and arranging for contact with lay groups.
- For children with anterior lobe hyperfunction of the pituitary gland, or precocious puberty, nursing care involves collecting a careful history of pubertal development, coordinating the diagnostic testing, supporting the child and parents through radiologic and laboratory procedures, and being present for support and teaching.
- Nursing care for individuals with Cushing's disease incudes a history of the progression of the symptoms, with close attention to symptoms of intracranial pressure from the mass, and support through diagnostic procedures and surgery.

- The nurse's role in caring for a child with anterior lobe hypofunction of the pituitary gland, or growth hormone deficiency, is referring the child for assessment, assisting in test procedures, teaching parents to give growth hormone injections, counseling the child about self-image, and assessing the response to therapy.
- For the child with posterior lobe hypofunction of the pituitary gland, or diabetes insipidus, nursing care involves observing the child during a water deprivation test and teaching the child and family to administer vasopressin or diuretics.
- For the child with excessive cortisol secretion or excessive aldosterone secretion, nursing responsibilities include supervising the child's eating, collecting 24-hour urine specimens, monitoring blood pressure during testing, and offering skilled care if adrenalectomy is needed; in the case of excessive adrenal sex steroid secretion, the nurse supports the parents by emphasizing the general health of the infant and accepting the infant as a female.
- Nursing care for the child with adrenal cortex hypofunction involves teaching the child and family to administer replacement hormones and to recognize the signs of acute adrenal insufficiency.
- Nursing management of a child with hyperthyroidism might incude creating a supportive care program for the child who is very uncomfortable, helping to allay the child's fears, instructing the parent on medications, and providing appropriate care if surgery is elected.
- For an infant with congenital hypothyroidism, the nurse supports and counsels the parent, explains the function of thyroxine and the importance of daily medication, and discusses infant stimulation.
- The nurse's role in caring for a child with hyperfunction of the parathyroids, or hypercalcemia, includes careful monitoring of fluid intake and urinary output, monitoring serum electrolytes, collecting urine specimens to assess calcium excretion, and observing the child's cardiac monitor during acute treatment.
- For the child with excessive estrogen or testosterone production, or precocious puberty, nursing intervention consists of assisting in the assessment procedures and counseling the parent and child.
- Nursing management of the child with delayed puberty might incude referral for assessment, assisting in the initial assessment procedures, teaching the child and parent about testosterone or estrogen therapy, and counseling about clothing appropriate for the child's age and size.

References

Aurbach GS, Marx SJ, Spiegel AM: Parathyroid hormone, calcitonin and the calciferols. In: *Textbook of Endocrinology.* 6th ed. Williams RH (editor). Saunders, 1981.

Bacon GE, Spencer ML, Kelch RP: *A Practical Approach to Pediatric Endocrinology.* Year Book, 1975.

Bardin CW, Paulsen CA: The testes. In: *Textbook of Endocrinology.* 6th ed. Williams RH (editor). Saunders, 1981.

Barta L, Molnar M: Retinopathy in juvenile diabetics. *Acta Paediatri Acad Sci Hung* 1971; 12 (3): 239–244.

Bibace R, Walsh ME: Developmental conceptions in children's conceptions of illness. In: *Health Psychology: A Handbook.* Stone G (editor). Jossey-Bass, 1978.

Bode HH: Disorders of the posterior pituitary. In: *Textbook of Endocrinology.* 6th ed. Williams RH (editor). Saunders, 1981.

Burgess A: *The Nurse's Guide to Fluid and Electrolyte Balance.* McGraw-Hill, 1979.

Burns EM: Diabetes mellitus and pregnancy. *Nurs Clin North Am* (Dec) 1983; 18(4): 673–685.

Cunningham LN, Barr P: Developing an endurance exercise program for the diabetic patient. *Diabetes Educ* 1982; 8(3): 11–13.

Daughaday WH: The adenohypophysis. In: *Textbook of Endocrinology.* 6th ed. Williams RH (editor). Saunders, 1981.

Etzwiler DD, Karam JH: Human insulin: How it looks now. *Diabetes Today Tomorrow* 1983; 3(1): 1.

Felig P: *Exercise and Diabetes.* Address at the Tenth Annual Meeting of the American Association of Diabetes Educators. San Antonio, Texas, September, 1982.

Goldstein JL, Motulsky AG: Genetics and endocrinology. In: *Textbook of Endocrinology.* 6th Ed. Williams RH (editor). Saunders, 1981.

Grumbach MM, Conte FA: Disorders of sex differentiation. In: *Textbook of Endocrinology.* 6th Ed. Williams RH (editor). Saunders, 1981.

Guthrie D, Guthrie R: The disease process of diabetes mellitus. *Nurs Clin North Am* (Dec) 1983; 18(4): 617–630.

Hall RV, Hall MC: *How To Negotiate a Behavioral Contract.* H and H Enterprises, 1982.

Hamilton WJ, Body JD, Mossman HW: *Human Embryology.* 4th Ed. Williams & Wilkins, 1972.

Heins JM: Dietary management in diabetes mellitus. *Nurs Clin North Am* (Dec) 1983; 18(4): 631–643.

Hoffman RG, et al: Self-concept changes in diabetic adolescents. In: *Psychological Aspects of Diabetes in Children and Adolescents.* Laron Z, Galatzer A (editors). Karger, 1982.

Ingbar SH, Woeber KA: The thyroid gland. In: *Textbook of Endocrinology*. 6th ed. Williams RH (editor). Saunders, 1981.

Johnson S, Rosenbloom AL: Behavioral aspects of diabetes mellitus in childhood and adolescence. *Psychiatr Clin North Am* 1982; 5(2): 357.

Jones HW, Scott WW: *Hermaphroditism, Genital Anomalies and Related Endocrine Disorders*. Williams & Wilkins, 1971.

Kaplan SA: *Clinical Pediatrics and Adolescent Endocrinology*. Saunders, 1982.

LaFranchi S: Hypothyroidism: Congenital and acquired. In: *Clinical Pediatrics and Adolescent Endocrinology*. Saunders, 1982.

Laws HN, et al: A long-term study of retinal changes in the prepuberty and puberty-onset diabetic. *Can J Ophthalmol* 1966; I:104.

Liddle GW: The adrenals. In: *Textbook of Endocrinology*. 6th ed. Williams RH (editor). Saunders, 1981.

Lillo R, Masteller D: Outpatient management of children in diabetic ketoacidosis. *Pediatr Nurs* (Nov/Dec) 1982; 8:383–385.

Melmon KL: The endocrinologic function of selected autacoids. In: *Textbook of Endocrinology*. 6th ed. Williams RH (editor). Saunders, 1981.

Moorman NH: Acute complications of hyperglycemia and hypoglycemia. *Nurs Clin North Am* (Dec) 1983; 18(4): 708–713.

Nemchik R: Diabetes today: A whole new world. *RN* (Oct) 1982; 45(10): 31–36.

Novak ER, Jones GS, Jones HW: *Novak's Textbook of Gynecology*. Williams & Wilkins, 1965.

Penney R: Disorders of the testes. In: *Clinical Pediatrics and Adolescent Endocrinology*. Kaplan SA (editor). Saunders, 1982.

Porte D, Halter JB: The endocrine pancreas and diabetes mellitus. In: *Textbook of Endocrinology*. 6th ed. Williams RH (editor). Saunders, 1981.

Ross GT, Vande Wiele RL, Frantz AG: The ovaries and breasts. In: *Textbook of Endocrinology*. 6th ed. Williams RH (editor). Saunders, 1981.

Rotter J, Hodge SE: Racial differences in juvenile-type diabetes are consistent with more than one mode of inheritance. *Diabetes* 1980; 29(2): 115–118.

Sperling M: Diabetes mellitus. In: *Clinical Pediatrics and Adolescent Endocrinology*. Kaplan SA (editor). Saunders, 1982.

Spies ME: Vascular complications associated with diabetes mellitus. *Nurs Clin North Am* (Dec) 1983; 18(4): 721–733.

Tanner JM: Sequence, tempo and individual variation in the growth and development of boys and girls aged twelve to sixteen. *Daedalus* 1971, 100:907–930.

Vorhees ML: Disorders of the adrenal medulla—multiple endocrine adenomatosis syndromes. In: *Clinical Pediatrics and Adolescent Endocrinology*. Kaplan SA (editor). Saunders, 1982.

Additional Readings

Anthony CP, Thibodeau GA: *Textbook of Anatomy and Physiology*. 11th ed. Mosby, 1983.

Balodimos MC: Diabetic nephropathy. In: *Joslin's Diabetes Mellitus*. 11th ed. Marble A, et al (editors). Lea & Febiger, 1971.

Bradley RF, Ramos E: The eye and diabetes. In: *Joslin's Diabetes Mellitus*. 11th ed. Marble A, et al (editors). Lea & Febiger, 1971.

Curran D: *Traits of a Healthy Family*. Winston Press, 1983.

Faro B: Maintaining good control in children with diabetes. *Pediatr Nurs* (Sept/Oct) 1983; 9: 368–373.

Fow JM: Home blood glucose monitoring in children with insulin-dependent diabetes mellitus. *Pediatr Nurs* (Nov/Dec) 1983; 9:439–442.

Fredholm NZ: The insulin pump: New method of insulin delivery *Am J Nurs* (Nov) 1981; 81:2024–2034.

Guthrie DW: Exercise, diets and insulin for children with diabetes. *Nurs 77* (Feb) 1977; 7:48–54.

Harris CH: Assessment of children's behavior. In: *High-Risk Parenting: Nursing Assessment and Strategies For the Family at Risk*. Johnson SH (editor). Lippincott, 1979.

Loman D, Galgani C: Monitoring diabetic children's blood glucose levels at home. *MCN* (May/June) 1984; 9:192–196.

McCabe GS: Cultural influences on patient behavior. *Am J Nurs* (August) 1960; 60:1100–1103.

Metheny HM, Snively WD: *Nurses' Handbook of Fluid Balance*. 2nd ed. Lippincott, 1974.

Metzger MJ: A new blood test for blood sugar. *Am J Nurs* (May) 1983; 83:763–764.

Nathan SW, Goetz P: Psychosocial aspects of chronic illness: Group interactions in diabetic girls. *Children's Health Care* (Summer) 1984; 13(1):24–30.

Reichlin S: Neuroendocrinology. In: *Textbook of Endocrinology*. 6th ed. Williams RH (editor). Saunders, 1981.

Ory MG, Kronenfeld JJ: Living with juvenile diabetes mellitus. *Pediatr Nurs* (Sept/Oct) 1980; 6:47–50.

Petrokas JC: Common sense guidelines for controlling diabetes during illness. *Nurs '77* (Dec) 1977; 7:36–37.

Saucier CP: Self-concept and self-care management in school-age children with diabetes. *Pediatr Nurs* (March/April) 1984; 10:135–138.

Schumann D: Assessing the diabetic. *Nurs '76* (March) 1976; 6:62–67.

Simpson OW, Smith MA: Lightening the load for parents of children with diabetes. *MCN* (Sept/Oct) 1979; 4:293–296.

Skeletal Integrity and Mobility
Implications of Inflammation and Structural Abnormalities

41

Nancy Fiero Fazekas

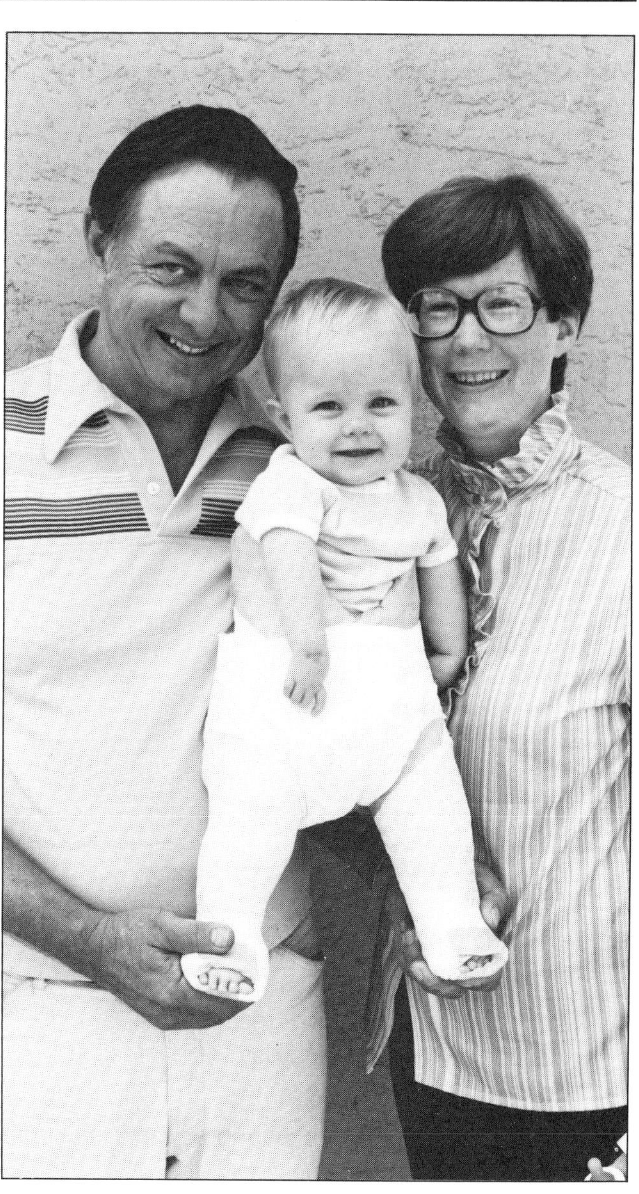

Chapter Outline

continued on next page

Objectives

- Identify the function of each component of the skeletal system.
- Describe how mechanical stress, trauma, circulation, nutrition, metabolism, and infection affect the development of bone.
- Describe procedures and diagnostic tests the nurse uses to assess skeletal function.
- Describe nursing management related to treatment with internal fixation and fusion, casts, traction, braces, continuous passive motion, Bradford frames, horizontal turning frames, and vertical turning frames.
- Identify nursing interventions used in preventing skin breakdown, controlling infection and complications, assessing and controlling neurologic and circulatory compromise, monitoring appliances and apparatus, and controlling pain.
- Describe preoperative and postoperative care of the child undergoing skeletal surgery.
- Identify the nutritional, developmental, emotional, and health maintenance needs specific to a child with a skeletal injury or disorder.
- Describe the chief abnormality, common medical treatments, and principles of nursing management of craniofacial defects, clubfoot, hip dysplasia, Legg–Calvé–Perthes disease, slipped capital femoral epiphysis, scoliosis, kyphosis, leg length discrepancy, and torsional deformity.
- Explain why fractures heal more quickly in children than in adults.
- Describe emergency and definitive medical treatments and principles of nursing management for fractures, sprains, strains, and contusions; and traumatic joint dislocations.

- Explain the physiologic processes, common medical treatments, and principles of nursing management for infections of bones and joints.
- Describe the usual causes, clinical manifestations, common medical treatments, and principles of nursing management of Osgood–Schlatter disease, osteogenesis imperfecta, and benign tumors of the bone.

The skeletal system contributes to the body's form and function. It supports the soft tissues and enables movement. Most muscles attach to a portion of the bony skeleton, many in such a way that their contraction causes movement at a movable joint. The bony skeleton of the body protects many organs: the skull protects the brain; the vertebrae, the spinal cord; the rib cage, the heart, lungs, liver, and spleen; and the pelvis, the reproductive organs. The bones are also a reservoir for storing minerals, primarily calcium and phosphorus. Although these minerals are quite stable, they can be mobilized and circulated by the blood to meet the body's needs. In addition, the bones' red marrow is responsible, under normal circumstances, for the production of blood cells (see Chapter 36).

In this chapter we describe the function of the skeletal system and the implications of its dysfunction. Nursing care for skeletal dysfunction often involves measures to offset the effects of immobility (see Chapter 29). The nursing care for the child with a skeletal disorder therefore is likely to involve teaching about adaptations needed for long-term care. (Nursing care of the child with a chronic condition is discussed in Chapter 30. The child with neurologic impairment is discussed in Chapter 42.)

Anatomy and Physiology of the Skeletal System

Gross Anatomy

Bones There are four basic shapes of bones: long, short, flat, and irregular. Long bones, which have a long axis, constitute most of the bones of the upper and lower extremities. Long bones carry the weight of the body and make ambulation possible. Short bones, such as the bones of the wrist (carpals) and ankle (tarsals), are in areas where strength and compactness are needed. Flat bones are thin and include the root of the cranial cavity, the sternum, and the ribs. Irregular bones cannot be categorized as long, short, or flat. Examples of irregular bones are the pelvic girdle, the vertebrae, and some of the bones of the skull.

Composition differs somewhat among bones with different shapes. In a long bone the shaft, called the *diaphysis,* ends in the proximal and distal *epiphyses* (Fig. 41-1). The diaphysis and epiphyses are separated in children by the cartilaginous *epiphyseal plate,* which also may be referred to as the *growth plate* because bone growth occurs at this place in the bone. In adults, the epiphyseal plate is called the epiphyseal line and can be seen on radiographs until late in life. The diaphysis consists of a hollow cylinder of compact bone. This cylinder surrounds the *medullary cavity,* also called the yellow bone marrow cavity, which is by adolescence a site for fat storage and has a yellow color. In the infant and young child, the medullary cavity is a site for hematopoiesis. By late adolescence, only the cranium, sternum, ribs, vertebrae, and pelvis are sites for hematopoiesis

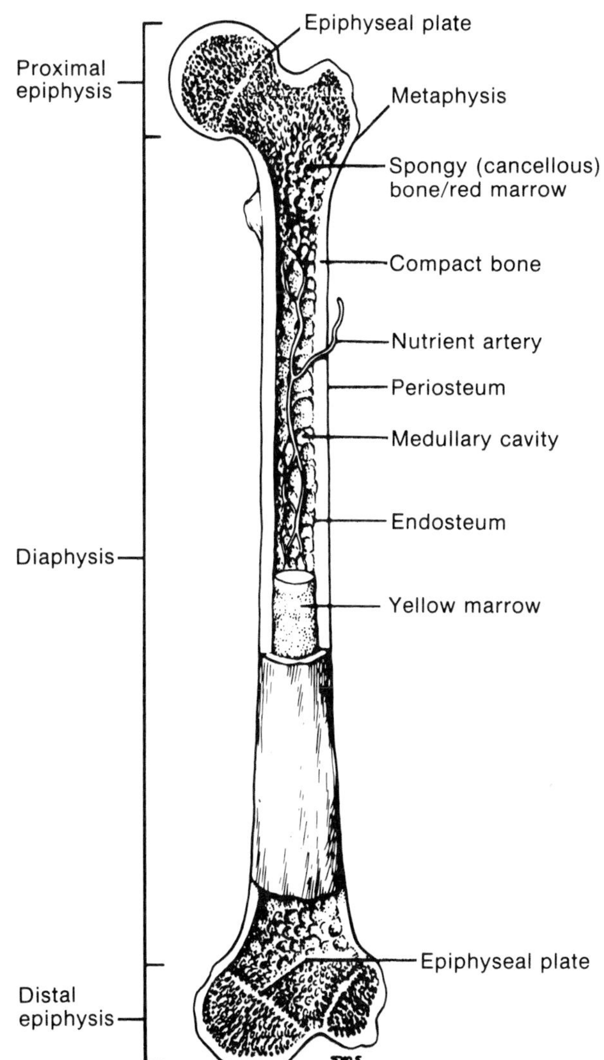

Figure 41-1 Parts of a long bone.

(Vick, 1984). A layer of connective tissue, the *endosteum,* lines the medullary cavity. The funnel-shaped end of the diaphysis adjacent to the epiphyseal plate is called the *metaphysis.*

Like the diaphysis, the epiphysis has an outer covering of compact bone. The central portion of the epiphysis contains cancellous bone, which consists of interconnecting plates of spongy bone. Flat bones contain red marrow; their outer bony surface is compact bone. Between layers of compact bone is spongy bone, where cellular components of the blood are formed.

A double layer of connective tissue, the *periosteum,* forms the outermost covering of the bones. In children, the periosteum is thick and very vascular, having an outer layer rich with blood vessels and nerves. Some of these enter the bone. The inner periosteal layer is attached to the bone, although less firmly in the child than in the adult, by collagenous bundles that penetrate the bone. The ends of bones within a joint are covered with articular cartilage instead of periosteum, and receive some of their nutrients from synovial fluid.

Joints Although some joints move very little or not at all, most are movable synovial joints. The degree of movement of individual joints is determined by ligaments, muscles, and tendons on the adjoining bones.

The *articular capsule,* made of dense, fibrous connective tissue, encloses the joint. The capsule is firmly joined to the periosteal layer of the bone. Capsule and ligaments hold the bones together and, along with muscles and the shape of the articular ends of the bones themselves, give the joint stability.

The knee and some other synovial joints, such as the sternoclavicular and distal radioulnar joints, have an *articular disk.* This dense, fibrous layer of connective tissue extends in from the articular capsule and separates the synovial cavity into two sections. The articular disk increases stability of the joint.

Lining the articular capsule is a thin layer of connective tissue, the *synovial membrane.* This membrane contains nerves and blood vessels and secretes synovial fluid, a highly viscous clear or straw-colored fluid that nourishes the avascular cartilage and lubricates the joint. The fluid is absorbed through the semipermeable membrane and is removed primarily via the vascular system.

In synovial joints the articular surfaces of bones are covered with a thin layer of cartilage. The viscous synovial fluid and the shape of the articular surfaces protect the cartilage from the pressures and stresses of body movement and weight bearing.

Muscles, Tendons, and Ligaments Muscles, with their muscle fibers and *fascia,* the thin connective tissue covering, may attach directly to bone. This frequently occurs at the proximal attachment of a muscle. A muscle may also be connected to bone by a tendon. *Tendons* are strong fibrous connectors that arise from the fascia as it extends past the end of the muscle. Tendon sheaths cover the tendons where they cross joints and help protect the tendons from constant friction. *Ligaments* are fibrous bands or sheets of connective tissue that support body organs, connect articular surfaces of bones or cartilage, and make movement possible in the various body parts.

Microscopic Anatomy and Chemical Composition of Bone

Bone is a living tissue supplied by blood vessels, lymph vessels, and nerves. Compact bone, such as that which surrounds the diaphysis, is composed of concentric layers of bone surrounding multiple, organized systems of interlocking longitudinal and horizontal canals and small cavities. *Osteocytes,* or bone cells, are located in these cavities. The longitudinal canals contain blood vessels, whereas horizontal canals contain blood vessels, lymph vessels, and nerves, which pass from the outer surface to the marrow cavity. Spongy bone also contains bone cells. Although spongy bone is comprised of cavities and canals, the surrounding bony layers are not concentric like compact bone but are arranged to withstand maximum pressure or tension. The small blood vessels within bone arise from larger vessels in the vascular layer of the periosteum or from within the marrow cavity. Blood generally flows from the medullary cavity outward (Salter, 1983).

In children the epiphyseal plate contains four zones. The first zone is made up of undifferentiated, or resting, cartilage cells that adhere to the epiphysis. As this zone is the germinal layer that supplies developing cartilage cells, injury to this layer causes cessation of growth. In the second zone, that of proliferating cartilage, cartilage cells grow, causing the bone to increase in length. The number of cells in the second zone varies with the activity and productivity of the epiphyseal plate. The cells become swollen as they mature in the third, or hypertrophic, cell zone, adding further to bone length. The fourth zone is the zone of cell degeneration, or provisional calcification. Here the cartilage cells die; their matrices calcify; and the dead cells are absorbed. Through this process, bone is formed around spurs of calcified intercellular substance in the metaphysis, thus firmly attaching the epiphyseal plate to the diaphysis.

The intercellular substance of bone has two major components: the inorganic salts and the organic framework. The inorganic salts of bone are highly insoluble crystals primarily of calcium and phosphorus. The organic framework consists of collagenous fibers similar to those in other connective tissue. Bone has great strength because the inorganic salts resist compression, and the collagen fibers resist twisting (torsion) and stretching.

Development of Bone

The skeleton arises from embryonic connective tissue of the mesodermal layer. Two different processes lead to bone of the same composition. Bone arising directly from undifferentiated mesoderm, or *mesenchyma,* develops by a process called intramembranous ossification, in which the bone is formed within membranes of the embryo. Some facial bones and the flat bones of the skull form in this simple manner. Other bones develop by a process called endochondral (intracartilaginous) ossification. This occurs in mesodermal cells that have first been transformed into cartilage. Most bones form by endochondral ossification from cartilage, which is present in the embryo early in gestation.

Intramembranous Ossification *Osteoblasts* (bone-forming cells) arise in fibrils (small fibers) of the embryonic membranes and begin to calcify the interstitial material between the fibrils. The osteoblasts produce small thread-like projections called *spicules,* which extend in all directions and unite to form the cavities of spongy bone. The osteoblasts eventually become trapped in these small cavities, or *lacunae,* and become osteocytes.

Additional thickening of spicules, bone deposition, and narrowing of spaces occur in areas that eventually become compact bone. The bones become covered with periosteum, which lays down new bone through further activity of osteoblasts. In this way bones thicken. Bones grow through bone deposition by osteoblasts and by a process called resorption. *Resorption* (removal) of bone is accomplished by bone-dissolving cells called *osteoclasts.* As bone is formed by osteoblasts, old bone is resorbed by osteoclasts.

Endochondral Ossification Some embryonic cartilage is similar in shape to future bone and thus is referred to as a *hyaline cartilage model.* Osteoblasts within the cartilage calcify the fibrous connective tissue surrounding the cartilage model, thus forming the periosteum. The diaphysis then becomes encased in compact bone. As deeper tissue (matrix) calcifies, cartilage cells are left without nourishment and therefore die. Their degeneration creates spaces in the matrix, and blood vessels enter and loop through the spaces. Osteoblasts transported from the periosteum through these blood vessels form the primary ossification center of the diaphysis. This occurs in most bones in the third month of embryonic development. The marrow cavity eventually forms as spongy bone is broken down by osteoclasts.

At birth, the ephiphyses of most bones are still made up of hyaline cartilage, whereas their diaphyses are composed of compact bone that surrounds spongy bone and a marrow cavity. Secondary ossification centers appear in the epiphyses soon after birth, but no marrow cavities form in the epiphyses. Eventually, the entire epiphysis ossifies except for a thin surface layer, the epiphyseal plate, which separates the epiphysis from the diaphysis.

Lengthening Bone increases in length by means of cartilage cell production, hypertrophy, and calcification at the epiphyseal plate. Growth and hypertrophy of cartilage cells increase bone length. As its matrix is calcified and bone is laid down, the size of the epiphyseal plate remains relatively constant, and the length of the diaphysis increases. When bone growth slows, usually in late adolescence, cartilage growth slows while calcification continues at the diaphyseal side of the epiphyseal plate. The epiphyseal plate is gradually replaced by bone until only the epiphyseal line remains. Once this happens, bone length cannot increase. Skeletal maturity is reached by age 25 in males and several years earlier in females.

Although bones do not grow longer after the epiphyseal plate disappears, they do increase in diameter and are altered in other ways. Bone diameter increases as new bone is deposited by osteoblasts on the inner layer of the periosteum. The marrow cavity also increases in diameter as osteoclasts cause bone resorption from the surface of the medullary cavity.

Factors Affecting Development

Mechanical Stress Prolonged mechanical stress can increase the number of collagen fibers and the amount of inorganic salts in bone, thus increasing its strength. Fibers align in relation to stress so that the bone withstands stress patterns. Gravity and muscular contractions both apply stress to the bones, so exercise influences skeletal development.

In the absence of stress, salts withdraw from the bone. With paralysis or immobilization, the bones do not grow and may degenerate, demineralize, and atrophy.

Trauma Fractures can cause bone to shorten if fracture fragments are overlapped and malpositioned. Shortening may not be significant in young children, however, since use and exercise mold and alter bone growth. In fact, injury stimulating additional blood supply to the epiphyseal area causes overgrowth. Metaphyseal injuries can also stimulate growth. Severe burns can retard growth.

Damage to the epiphyseal plate may disrupt or stop growth if it causes premature fusion of the epiphysis to the diaphysis. Growth disturbance relates to the extent and site of injury. An injury affecting the zone that replenishes cartilage affects bone development. Such an injury can cause bone bridges to form, fusing the epiphyseal plate to the metaphyseal region of the bone. Growth may be normal if the bone bridge is very small or retarded if the bridge is large and stable.

The weakest portion of the epiphyseal plate appears to be the third layer, the hypertrophic cartilage cell layer. Shearing, bending, or tension can cause epiphyseal separation at this layer. Separation leaves the zone of resting cartilage intact, however, so separation at the third layer can occur without disturbing growth.

Circulation Disruption of circulation can cause bone to die. If circulation to the epiphysis is disrupted, growth may be retarded. Abnormal increases in circulation, which may be due to trauma, arteriovenous shunts, or inflammation, tend to stimulate increases in bone length.

Depending on their location, blood vessels can be damaged by epiphyseal separation. Articular cartilage only partly covers the epiphyses of most bones, and blood vessels enter the epiphyses laterally. These vessels are not particularly vulnerable during epiphyseal separation. Articular cartilage surrounds the epiphyses of other bones, notably the proximal epiphysis of the femur, and blood vessels supplying the epiphysis enter at the periphery of the epiphyseal plate. These vessels are quite vulnerable to damage during epiphyseal separation. Damage to these vessels slows healing, and since the epiphyseal blood vessels supply the reproductive cells of the epiphyseal plate, damage to the vessels threatens growth in the length of the bone.

Nutrition Malnutrition and inadequate caloric intake inhibit skeletal aging and growth. A well-balanced diet is needed for normal bone growth. Protein, vitamins, calcium, and phosphorus are all necessary. Vitamin D is necessary for proper absorption of ingested calcium.

Metabolism Hormone production by parathyroid and thyroid glands affects bone growth. Bone resorption increases with increased production of the parathyroid hormone, parathormone. Parathyroid hormone stimulates osteoclasts, the cells that accomplish bone resorption. Resorption increases blood calcium levels, as calcium leaves the bone and enters the circulation. Thyroid hormones, on the other hand, stimulate formation of new bone and decrease the activity of osteoclasts. This lowers blood calcium levels.

Infection Infection can contribute to either increased or decreased bone growth. If infection damages the epiphyseal plate, bone growth is retarded. If infection stimulates circulation to the epiphyseal or metaphyseal region, the bone will overgrow.

Assessment of the Child With a Skeletal Condition

History

A child with a problem involving the skeletal system seeks medical attention because of various signs and symptoms. Common complaints include deformity, a limp, pain, general or local weakness, and swelling and stiffness in joints. In obtaining a history, the nurse seeks to establish how the complaint, its characteristics, and their cause are related.

The history of the child's delivery may be significant. The child may have experienced trauma or injury at birth, or asymmetry of the limbs or face may have been noted at that time. Breech delivery is associated with an increased incidence of dislocated hip and torticollis, or wryneck (unilateral contracture of the sternocleidomastoid muscle). Brachial palsy can be caused by traction on the shoulder in either vertex or breech delivery, and it may be suspected on seeing that one arm does not move when Moro reflex is stimulated.

A history of delayed or uneven achievement of developmental milestones occurs with certain skeletal conditions. If a child shows a clear hand preference before the age of 2, for example, there may be a defect in the other hand. Dislocated hip, if not diagnosed and treated in infancy, usually delays walking.

The nurse inquires about bone or joint disorders in other family members. This may elicit information about diseases, injuries, drugs, or exposures to toxins that have been or in the future may be linked to skeletal defects and disorders. For example, thalidomide, once believed to be an effective sedative and sleeping aid with few side effects, was found to cause serious birth defects when taken in early pregnancy.

By noting exactly how an injury happened and by putting the chief complaint in the child's or parent's own words, the nurse maintains some objectivity and facilitates identification of problems (see Chapter 14). It is important to know how a problem affects the child and family. Does the problem interfere with their life-style? Is the child's general health affected? Perhaps there are fears surrounding a problem or complaint. Exactly why was help sought?

Pain is associated with many orthopedic conditions in children. By remembering that many factors influence a child's perception of pain, the nurse can help interpret the complaint. For example, a young athlete might attempt to ignore or downplay pain in order to continue to engage in sports. Children in late childhood and adolescence likewise tend to minimize pain when around strangers so as to appear more grown up and strong. The nurse encourages the parent to confirm the accuracy of statements the child makes about pain. If pain is severe enough to prohibit activity, fear of loss of a function can greatly influence the child's description and expression of pain.

Injury is suspected if the child complains of sharp pain that worsens with activity and lessens with rest. Dull, boring pain that is constant, increases gradually, and awakens the child from sleep is likely to be due to infection or tumor growth. Table 41-1 lists conditions usually associated with sharp or dull pain.

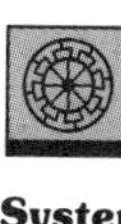

ASSESSMENT GUIDE Child With a Skeletal Condition

System	Subjective data	Objective data	Validating data	Nursing management
General	History of prenatal exposure to medications, illness, or alcohol. History of difficult delivery, or of infection or trauma. Pain that is dull, boring, or sharp and increasing with movement	Obvious deformity. Lack of symmetry of body parts. Muscle wasting. Swelling or enlarged areas of bones and joints. Abnormal prominence, thickening, malposition of bone in relation to landmarks	Hemoglobin and hematocrit. Serum calcium levels. Radiographs. White cell count and differential count	Explore feelings about body image; obtain history; monitor vital signs, explore circumstances surrounding any accident to determine need for teaching and to identify any possible abuse or neglect (see Chapter 22); examine for possible sprain or fracture; observe for signs of osteomyelitis or tumor
Integumentary	Pain, soreness. History of trauma, surgery	Reddened areas, contusions, cyanosis, pallor, scars, lacerations, sores, exudate or purulence	Complete blood count. Hemoglobin and hematocrit	Position to avoid pressure on bony prominences; monitor color, sensation, and motion; care for skin in contact with cast, splint, appliance, traction; provide skin care for immobilized child to help maintain integrity and prevent infection; inquire about scars and old injuries, surgeries; monitor for excessive blood loss, shock after trauma or surgery; carry out treatments and nursing care for infection
Respiratory	History of trauma, surgery. Decreased exercise tolerance. Anxiety	Pronounced degree of structural scoliosis, kyphosis. Shallow, painful respirations	Arterial blood gases	Monitor respiratory status; administer medications and carry out comfort measures for pain relief; encourage coughing and deep breathing postoperatively; reassure child
Cardiovascular	History of trauma, surgery. Feeling of coolness in extremity distal to injury or immobilizing apparatus	Frank bleeding. Increased pulse and blood pressure, followed by drop in blood pressure. Decreased strength or absence of peripheral pulses. Swelling distal to cast. Slow capillary refill	Hemoglobin and hematocrit	Observe wound areas frequently; monitor vital signs; compare serial laboratory values; monitor intravenous infusion; administer blood products as ordered; monitor peripheral pulses; notify physician of any impairment of circulation; draw a ring around any blood stain on cast; observe for signs of accompanying internal injury
Gastrointestinal	History of trauma, surgery. Nausea, distention. Discomfort, cramping, no recent bowel movement	Increased abdominal girth; tense, firm abdomen; vomiting. Abdomen somewhat distended, feces palpable as masses in area of colon		Care for nasogastric tube (see Chapter 38); measure abdominal girth frequently; listen for bowel sounds; carry out measures to treat

continued on next page

ASSESSMENT GUIDE Child With a Skeletal Condition (continued)

System	Subjective data	Objective data	Validating data	Nursing management
				vomiting, nausea (see Chapter 38). When beginning food and fluids, advance diet slowly. Increase fluid and roughage content of diet; encourage ambulation if child is ambulatory; teach child how to avoid constipation (see Chapter 29)
Genitourinary	History of trauma, surgery. Complaints of fullness, discomfort, pain, fever, frequency, urgency	Distension over symphysis pubis	Urine specific gravity. Urine for culture and sensitivity. Child unable to void adeqate amount	Care for Foley catheter; monitor intake and output; encourage fluids, particularly fruit juices
Neuroendocrine	Tingling, paresthesias	Decreased sensation and motion in affected body part. Decreased ability to identify area touched		Monitor color, sensation, and motion; loosen traction if possible; decrease weights of traction and notify physician immediately; observe for constriction of cast or other immobilizing device
Musculoskeletal				
Neck		Asymmetry, tendons prominent on one side	Radiographs of cervical spine	Review prenatal history and history of delivery; teach parent muscle-stretching exercises for congenital torticollis (wryneck)
Shoulders		One shoulder lower when standing or sitting; child can correct at will		Note any leg length discrepancy; teach parent and child about posture and appearance
Torso (viewed from behind)				
Standing		Uneven scapulae, lateral curvature of spine, one hip prominent, asymmetric flank folds, shoulders not over pelvis when plumb line dropped from occiput	Lateral and anterior–posterior radiographs	Provide support during multiple follow-up visits for diagnosis, monitoring, and treatment of scoliosis
Bending		Curvature, rotation of vertebrae toward convex side of curve, asymmetric prominence of ribs or scapulae		Inquire about functional problems or symptoms related to leg length discrepancy
		Rotation of vertebrae toward concave side of curve. Curve disappears if proper size block placed under foot of shorter leg		

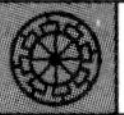

ASSESSMENT GUIDE Child With a Skeletal Condition (continued)

System	Subjective data	Objective data	Validating data	Nursing management
Hips				
Infant: standing, held from under axillae, or lying down		Asymmetric gluteal or thigh folds (see Fig. 41-2A)		Provide care related to brace, traction, cast, or surgery for congenital dislocated hip
Child: weight bearing on one foot	History of delayed walking	Opposite side of pelvis drops (see Fig. 41-3A)		Note additional signs of congenital dislocated hip
Child: walking		Lurching or waddling gait		Check for signs of bilateral dislocated hip: waddling gait, wide space between upper thighs, lordosis (see Fig. 41-3B)
Infant or child: supine				
Legs straight		Wide space between upper thighs		
Legs flexed at knees and hips		Galeazzis sign. Unequal abduction. Barlow's test positive. Ortolani's test positive		
Pain, especially on flexion and internal rotation. Chronic pain or acute limp, guarding of leg pain in hip or leg				Provide care related to treatment for Legg-Calvé-Perthes disease; provide care related to brace, traction, or surgery; provide care related to traction and surgery for slipped capital femoral epiphysis
Legs		Limp, apparent unequal leg length, Galeazzi's sign. Varus or valgus deformities of knee		Provide support during diagnosis and treatment of leg length discrepancy; compare findings with norms for age; teach parent about norms to decrease parent's anxiety; provide care related to surgical correction
Feet		Valgus or varus deformities of the forefoot; dorsi-flexion or plantar flexion		Provide care related to casts, splints, braces, special shoes, or surgery; teach parent prescribed passive stretching exercise for foot

Physical Examination

Physical examination for structural abnormalities includes assessment of clubfoot, hip dysplasia, Legg–Calvé–Perthes disease, slipped capital femoral epiphysis, scoliosis, kyphosis, leg length discrepancy, and torsional deformities. Hip inspection for the infant is illustrated in Figure 41-2. Instability or dislocation of the hip is evident from various signs.

The nurse first observes for any apparent shortening of the femur. This occurs on the affected side with congenital dislocation of the hip. The infant is placed in the supine position and the hips flexed at 90° while the knees are bent.

TABLE 41-1 Pain in Presenting Orthopedic Conditions

Type of pain	Musculoskeletal condition
Sharp	Bone injury with muscle spasm Bone injury with periosteal tear Fracture Dislocation Slipped capital femoral epiphysis Fragment of bone in joint Joint strain
Dull	Tumor Osteomyelitis Muscle strain Sprain

Galeazzi's sign is positive if the level of one knee on the affected side is lower than that of the other knee. Either thigh or gluteal folds or both are increased on the affected side when the two sides are compared. Abduction of the affected side is limited. Sometimes, Galeazzi's sign or limitation of abduction are not apparent in the neonate, as there may not yet be muscle spasms and contractures. After 4–6 weeks and some further shortening of adduction muscles, however, they become apparent. The greater trochanter is exaggerated and the buttock flattened on the affected side.

Ortolani's click is a reliable sign of hip dislocation in the neonate (see Chapter 14). Tendon and knee problems may also produce a click, so experience is needed to decipher

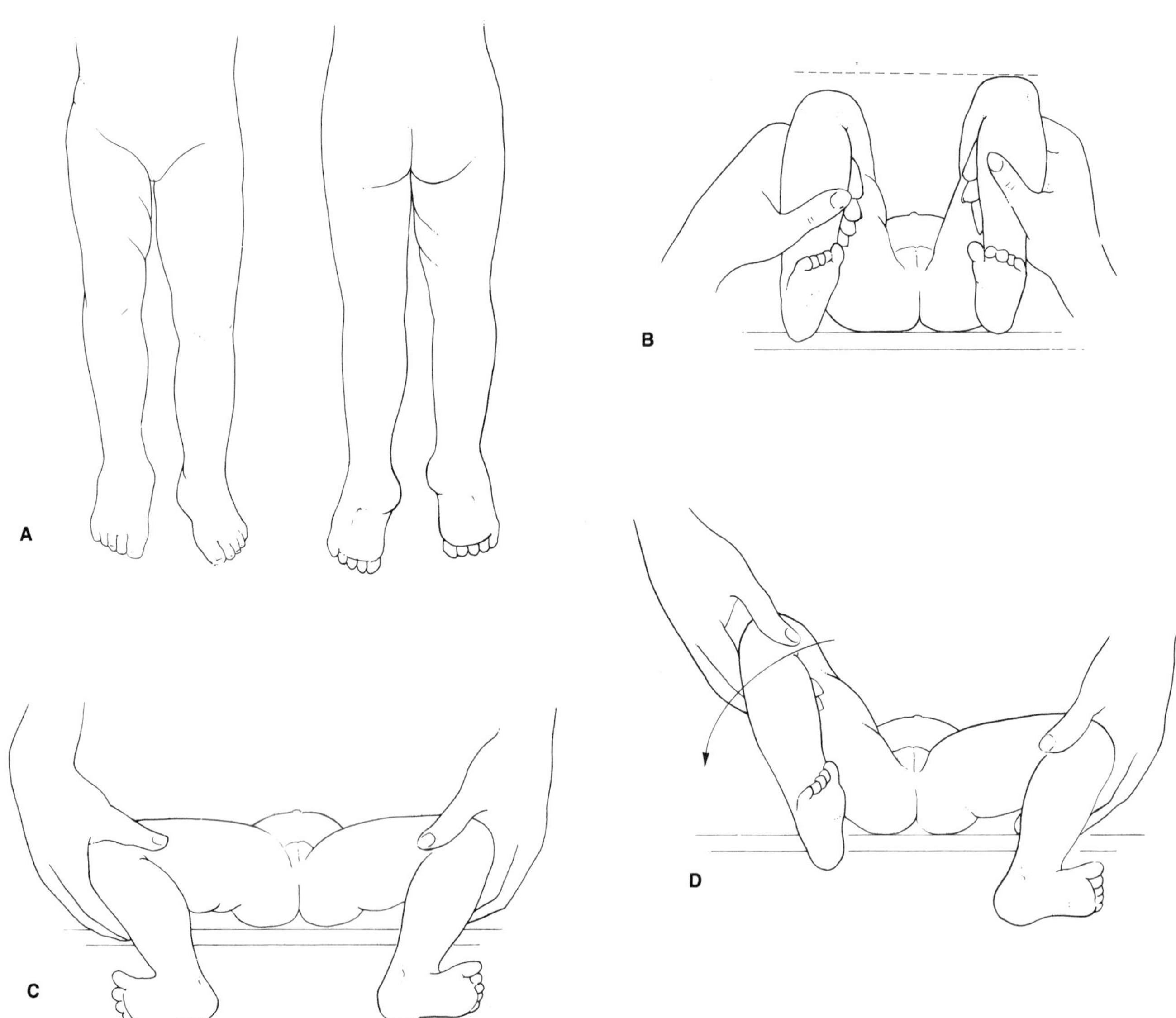

Figure 41-2 Signs of unilateral dislocated hip in an infant. *A.* Unequal thigh folds. *B.* Galeazzi's sign. *C.* Normal abduction of the thighs. *D.* Limited abduction of the thighs.

the true cause of the click. Barlow's test is used to identify an unstable, dislocatable hip in the neonate. The infant is relaxed and in a supine position with the hips flexed. The hip's instability can be felt and also seen as the hip is slightly adducted with downward pressure on the femoral shaft. Instability is evident again when the hip is slightly abducted while the femur is lifted upward and the nurse simultaneously puts forward pressure on the greater trochanter. If the hip is unstable, the femoral head actually exits and then reenters the acetabulum during the test. Both Ortolani's click and Barlow's test are important but should be performed on each neonate by a practitioner who is experienced in safely performing the maneuvers.

Another sign of displacement of the femoral head is the lack of the flexion contracture of the hip and knee normally present in the first few months of life. On the affected side, the abducted leg may be extended and the knee hyperextended. During passive, pistonlike manipulation, telescoping and abnormal mobility of the femoral head are felt.

The Trendelenburg test is used to assess hip dislocation in children who are old enough to stand and bear weight. When the child stands on the leg of the affected side, the opposite hip slants downward instead of remaining level (Fig. 41-3A). This is caused by the weakness of the hip abductor muscles. The downward slant of one hip is a positive sign of dislocation in the weight-bearing hip.

The child's learning to walk frequently is delayed with congenitally dislocated hip. When the child walks and bears weight, dislocation becomes evident. If one hip is dislocated, the child walks with a characteristic limp known as the Trendelenburg gait. Dislocation of both hips causes a waddling gait. With bilateral dislocation the perineal space also is widened, with both buttocks broad and flattened and both greater trochanters prominent (Fig. 41-3B). The pelvis is inclined forward, causing hyperlordosis.

Leg length is assessed by comparing the levels of the knees and both sides of the pelvis, and observing for functional curves of the spine. Although a degree of discrepancy between the length of the right and left legs is acceptable, any discrepancy greater than 1 cm may require referral. A significant leg length discrepancy, if untreated, may lead to degenerative problems in adult life. Gait is affected by leg length discrepancy, causing the head to bob excessively when the child walks. If weight bearing is painful for any reason, the stance phase on the affected side is shorter. A limp adopted in an attempt to reduce pain is called an *antalgic limp*.

The spine is inspected for lordosis, kyphosis, or scoliosis

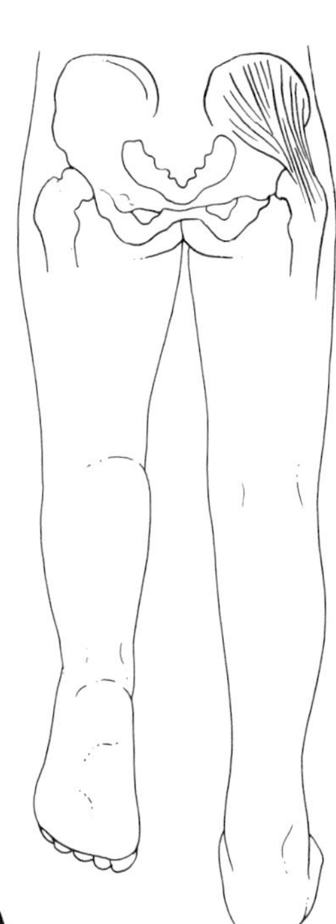

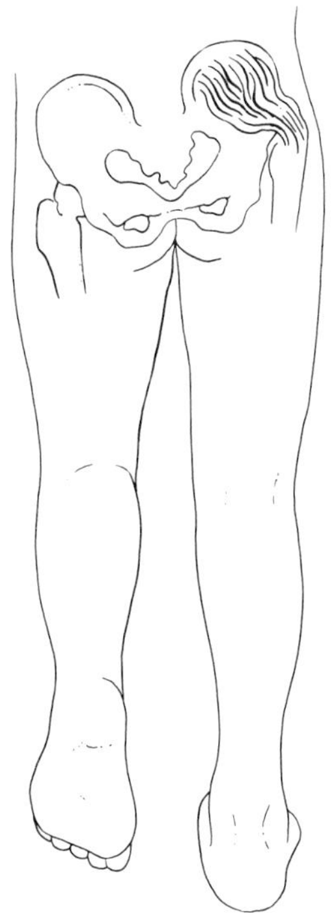

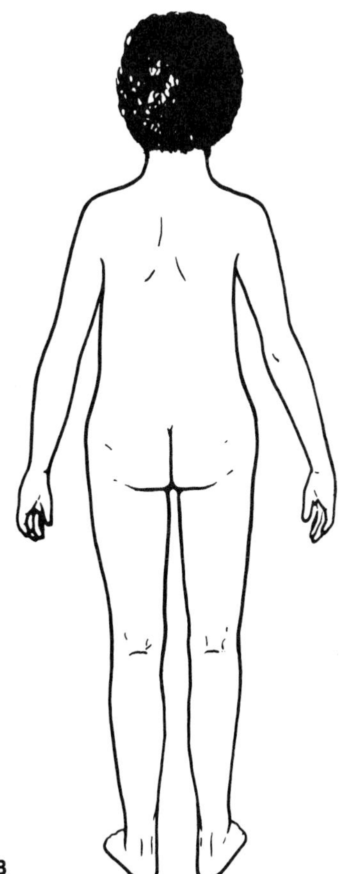

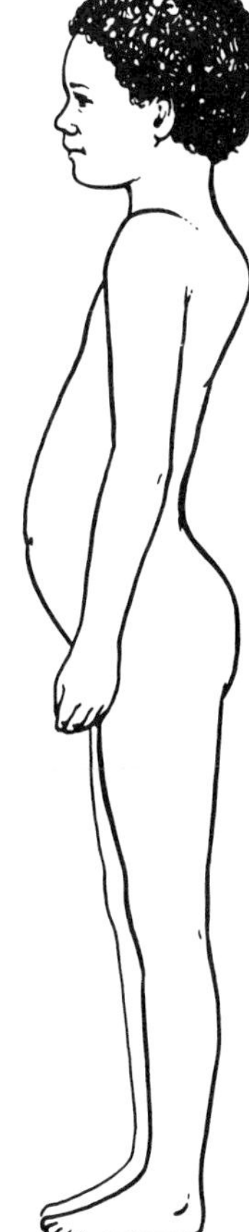

Figure 41-3 Signs of dislocated hip in a weight-bearing child. *A*. Trendelenburg test for unilateral dislocated hip. Drawing at left shows normal findings for the right hip. Drawing at right shows abnormal findings for the right hip: as the child bears weight on the right (affected) side, the opposite side of the pelvis drops. *B*. Signs of bilateral dislocated hips: flattened buttocks, widened space between thighs, lordosis.

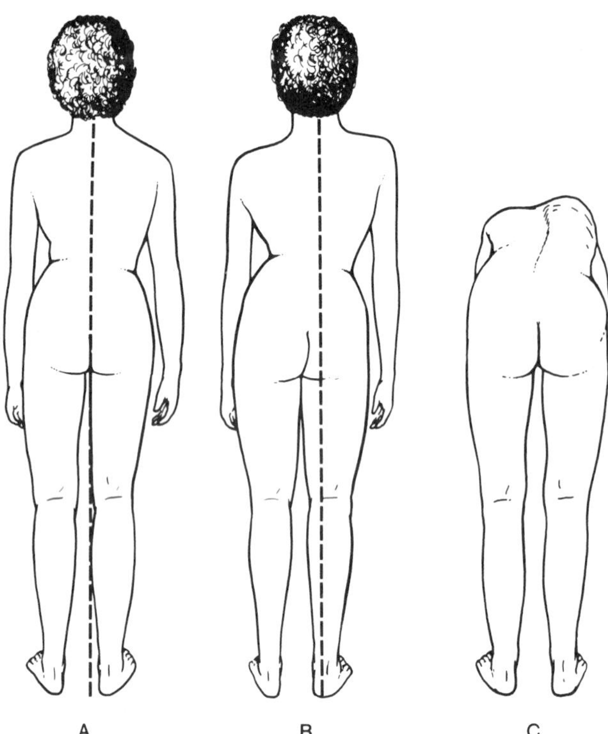

Figure 41-4 Lateral curvature of the spine. *A.* Mild, compensated scoliosis. *B.* Severe, decompensated scoliosis. *C.* Rotation of the vertebrae and ribs, visible when the child bends over.

(see Chapter 14). Postural changes caused by scoliosis are shown in Figure 41-4.

Physical examination of the child with suspected musculoskeletal injury or fracture includes assessment of pain and deformity of the painful part, and assessment of signs of injury, such as bruises, contusions, or wounds. The nurse palpates the outline and shape of the bones, noting any abnormal prominence, malpositioning in relation to landmarks, or thickening. Any scars indicative of old injury or surgery are noted.

Traumatic dislocation of the hip is not common in children; and its clinical appearance varies in relation to the position of the dislocation. In a posterior dislocation, in which the femoral head is displaced behind the acetabulum, the leg is held in flexion, adduction, and internal rotation so that the knee or foot rests on the opposite leg. The leg on the affected side appears shorter. In an anterior dislocation, the hip is held in abduction, external rotation, and a degree of flexion. The leg appears to be longer than the leg on the normal side. Central dislocation occurs with fractures of the acetabulum. The leg is not held in any characteristic position, but motion is very restricted.

Examination of the child with suspected infection or tumor growth includes assessment of the skin. The nurse palpates the skin to determine its texture, toughness, and temperature, and to detect lumps and swelling. Skin may be tender or reddened over an infected area. Warmth of the skin indicates increased vascularity and may be an indication of infection. Warmth may also occur over a rapidly growing tumor. Cyanotic or cool skin is a possible indication of impaired vascularity. The nurse obtains baseline data about color, sensation, and motion for a body part to use in later assessments of innervation and vascularity.

Validating Diagnostic Tests

Radiographic Studies In assessing a child with a condition involving the bone, radiographs are of primary value. They are used extensively for initial diagnosis and evaluation of treatment effectiveness and recovery. They show bone density in general and any local changes in density, breaks in the periosteum or surface of the bone, irregularities, and areas of new bone formation. The medulla of the bone may show changes in texture or areas of sclerosis or destruction. Radioigraphs of joints may show narrowing of cartilage space, changes in joint surfaces, loose or foreign bodies, and peripheral new bone. Skeletal age can be determined by comparing a child's radiographs to the norm. Skeletal age has implications for treatment and expected outcome with various conditions.

Radiographs do not necessarily show pathologic changes in the young child. When the child's epiphyses are still highly cartilaginous and when injury occurs at the epiphyseal plate, the history of the child's illness or accident, symptoms and signs, or special radiographic techniques may be necessary for diagnosis.

Usually, an anteroposterior or lateral radiograph of an area is sufficient for visualization and evaluation of a skeletal condition. At times, other techniques are needed. In a process called tomography, structures in a particular plane are shown more clearly by movement around the focal point during exposure of the film so as to blur structures in other planes. Tomography may show epiphyseal plate injury not apparent on a simple radiograph.

Another technique for showing an epiphyseal plate fracture is to apply stress or pressure to the body part during radiography. Contrast studies, in which air or radio-opaque dye is injected, can outline areas for diagnostic purposes. A myelogram aids in outlining spinal lesions. A sinus, arterial or venous network, or a joint may be filled with contrast material for more complete examination. Mobility of a joint may be recorded by obtaining a moving picture or videotape during radiography.

Arthroscopy is a technique for directly inspecting the interior of a joint, usually the knee, by means of a fine telescope introduced through a cannula. It is frequently carried out while the child is under a general anesthetic but may be done with local anesthetic. The joint is distended with fluid for visualization. Although it is a diagnostic tool, some corrective work may be done during arthroscopy.

Laboratory Tests Although history, physical examination, and radiographic studies are usually sufficient to identify a skeletal problem, laboratory tests may also be used in diagnosing and monitoring a condition. For instance, in osteomyelitis (infection of the bone) the white blood cell count may be as high as 15,000–25,000 cells or more (Behrman and Vaughn, 1983). The white count is used to monitor the resolution of infection and evaluate the effectiveness of treatment. Hemoglobin or hematocrit values help care providers to assess blood loss after injury or surgery. Blood calcium levels can be used to monitor bone growth, bone healing, and the general health of the musculoskeletal system. They correlate with the resorption of calcium from bone. Because blood calcium levels are altered in conjunction with alterations in parathyroid hormones, pathology that contributes to a change in the parathyroid hormone (see Chapter 37 for a discussion of DiGeorge's Disease) affects the blood calcium level. The normal blood calcium level during growth spurts and bone healing is elevated and can be as high as 12.0 mg/dL (Byrne et al., 1981).

Blood analysis is used in diagnosing or monitoring some skeletal defects and metabolic disorders that affect the bones. Serologic studies are used to detect congenital deficiency of thyroid hormone secretion, and chemical analysis of blood is used to identify rickets.

Nursing Management for Procedures and Treatments

Internal Fixation and Fusion

The child undergoing internal fixation or fusion requires standard preoperative and postoperative care (see Chapter 29).

Bony structures may be approximated in the most functional position possible through operative techniques of internal fixation and fusion. Plates and screws are sometimes used to approximate bone fragments after fractures or such procedures as leg lengthening. Screws may be driven carefully through bone to hold portions together. Bone grafting, with or without metal instrumentation, may be used to stabilize the spine in an inflexible but more functional position. Following either procedure, the repositioned bone usually is unable to support body weight until healing takes place. The child is immobilized following surgery and regains mobility gradually.

Casts

Types of Casts A wide variety of casts is used to immobilize and position body parts. Extremity casts may be long, short, or cylindrical (Fig. 41-5). A long leg cast surrounds the foot and extends to the groin, while a short cast includes the foot but ends below the knee. Some short or long leg

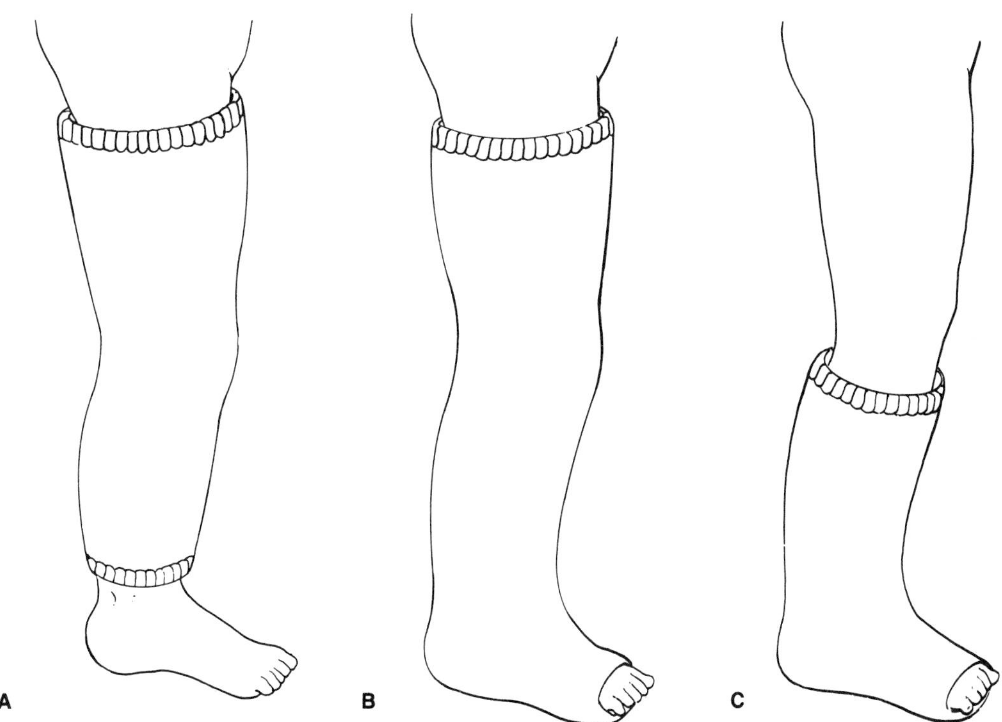

Figure 41-5 Leg casts. *A.* Cylinder. *B.* Long leg. *C.* Short leg.

casts have a built-up section under the foot. They are known as "walking casts." Arm casts are of the same three types. A cast from the hand to the upper arm is a long cast. A short arm cast encases the hand but ends at or just below the elbow. A cast covering only an arm or leg and not involving the hand or foot, is called a cylinder cast. Cylinder casts immobilize the elbow or knee.

There are also many special types of casts. A hinged cast has two sections connected by hinges to permit flexion of a joint. A cast applied to prevent or lessen contractures might consist of two long leg casts with a bar built between them to ensure abduction. A spica cast covers part of the torso and includes one or both extremities. A long cast might be used on one extremity and a short cast on the other. Spica casts often are used for hip or shoulder immobilization. A long leg spica cast may be used to immobilize femoral fractures (Fig. 41-6). Body casts, which cover part or all of the trunk, are used for correction or immobilization of curvatures of the spine and spinal injuries.

A cast may be bivalved, that is, cut into anterior and posterior sections. The two halves are held together by straps, which are secured in the bottom (posterior) half with additional casting material and fastened together on the top (anterior) half. Bivalved casts are ideal if continuous immobilization is not required but periodic splinting or positioning is desired.

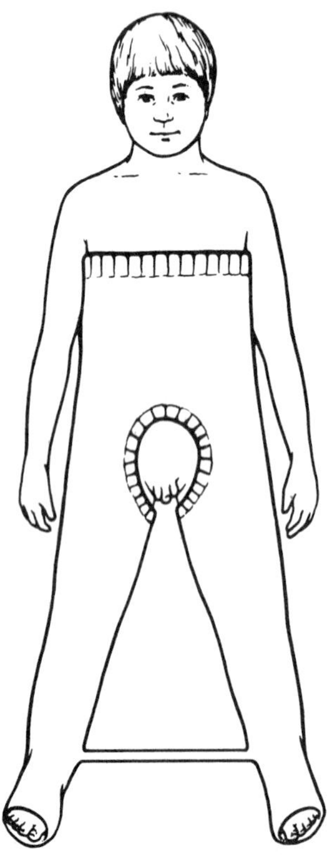

Figure 41-6 Bilateral, long leg, hip spica cast with abduction bar.

Cast Application and Removal Stockinet is applied to the area to be casted and is covered with cotton padding, or cotton padding alone is placed against the skin. Then rolls of wet plaster or fiberglass are wrapped around the body part to be immobilized. Because of the chemical reaction that takes place when rolls of casting material become wet, the cast feels quite warm when it is first applied. As the chemical reaction ceases and the cast dries, water evaporates. The cast and the child then feel cold. The nurse explains these sensations to the child to help the child feel less anxious and more in control.

Other nursing measures can increase the child's sense of control and comfort during cast application. For example, the nurse can help maintain the child's privacy. It may be possible to apply stockinet, especially for a body cast, in the child's hospital room instead of the often large and busy cast room. During cast application, the nurse can repeat teaching and, if appropriate, hold the child's hand or hold the body part being casted in the correct position. Humor and "small talk" can be used to lessen fears, decrease embarrassment, and promote feelings of self-worth.

The edges of the cast must be well padded and smooth to prevent skin irritation. If stockinet is used in a cast, it may be pulled out and over the edge of the cast and secured there with a layer of cast material. Adequate cotton padding between the stockinet and the cast provides a soft, smooth edge. When the cast is dry, the nurse can add more padding by slitting the stockinet, inserting padding, and reattaching the stockinet to the outside of the cast with tape. If a cast is made of cotton padding and fiberglass or plaster alone, tape is placed around the edge of the cast in the form of overlapping petals. "Petalling" is done when the cast is completely dry, and can be redone if necessary (Fig. 41-7). Fiberglass casts have particularly rough edges that may need to be smoothed with a file. Petalling with moleskin can further protect the skin from the sharp edges of fiberglass casts.

Removal of a cast by means of a cast saw can be very frightening for a child. As with cast application, the child and family need preparation for the experience. The cast saw is noisy, and many children are afraid of being cut by the saw. Careful demonstration of the saw can lessen fears. Before the cast is removed, the nurse describes to the child and parent how the skin under the cast will look. If a cast has been in place for a number of weeks, the skin will be flaky and brown because of the accumulation of dead skin. The body part will be stiff. Gentle coaching and exercise correct this problem.

If the child is in a bivalved cast, the nurse removes it to provide skin care, bathe the child, assist the child with range-of-motion exercises, or accustom the child gradually to cast removal. In reapplying a bivalved cast, the nurse checks to be sure that it has no wrinkles in the lining, no rough edges, and no damp areas that could cause irritation. Joints are carefully seated, since their bony prominences are most susceptible to pressure. To reapply a bivalved long-leg cast, the nurse positions the heel first and the knee second. For a bivalved arm cast, the wrist and hand are positioned first, and then the elbow. The nurse checks the edges of the posterior half of the cast to be sure that there is no overhanging skin that could be pinched when the anterior half is applied. Skin may be gently pushed inside the cast with a tongue blade. After the second half is in place, the two halves are fastened together securely with the straps. Bivalved casts used in treating neuromuscular disorders are discussed in Chapter 42.

Cast Maintenance After cast application, the nurse assesses color, sensation, and motion in the body part distal to the cast (see Chapter 29). Initially, checks are made as frequently as every 30–60 minutes, since edema from the injury or surgery may exert pressure against the cast. After 24 hours, the nurse assesses color, sensation, and motion at least every 4 hours until cast removal. The nurse handles the cast with care. While a plaster cast is drying, a child needs to be turned every hour so the cast dries and hardens on both sides. After the cast has cooled, the wet casted extremity may be supported by plastic-covered pillows.

After the cast has dried, the nurse turns and repositions the child every 2–4 hours. More frequent repositioning is necessary if areas of the skin are subjected to pressure. To position a child with a cast, the nurse follows the same principles used to position a child without a cast. The nurse uses pillows to prevent the cast edges from pressing the skin and to maintain body parts in functional positions. Some children need to be restrained to maintain proper positioning.

Protecting a cast from becoming soiled with food, urine, or feces can require a great deal of skill on the part of the nurse, especially if cast edges are near the perineal area. The nurse tucks plastic wrap under the edges of the cast. When a child in a spica cast or body cast uses a bedpan, the body needs to be slightly elevated so that urine and feces flow downhill into the bedpan and not up into the cast. An incontinent child should always be positioned so that the cast will not become soiled, and the incontinent child in a spica cast should be elevated on a frame, such as the Bradford frame, which has an opening for excreta. Plastic wrap can be secured to a completely dry cast with tape. The nurse removes and immediately replaces the plastic if it becomes soiled.

Traction

Traction is used to immobilize a fracture or body part, realign fracture fragments, and reduce muscle spasm, joint dislocation, or spinal curvature. Traction stretches and eventually relaxes tight muscles, and it maintains and stabilizes in proper alignment specific bones, joints, or body parts (Fig. 41-8). During traction maintenance a careful analysis of the child's radiograph may lead to alterations in the direction or amount of traction pull.

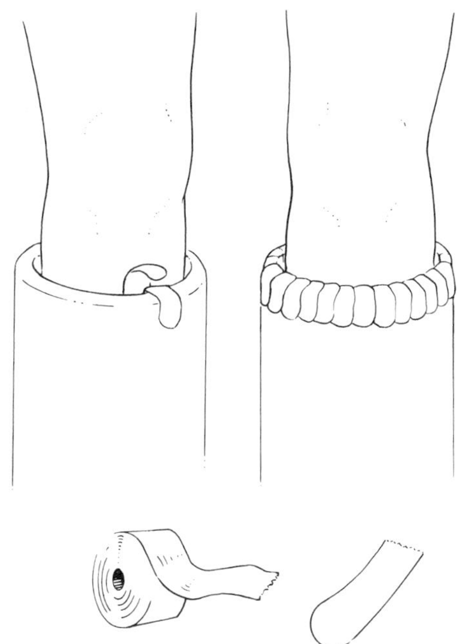

Figure 41-7 Petalling a cast. Tape edges are rounded to facilitate smooth application and prevent irritation and peeling from corners.

There are two basic kinds of traction: skin traction and skeletal traction. *Skin traction* achieves a pull on a body part by way of the skin. Its advantages include ease of application and removal. It is especially useful for the child who does not need continuous traction. The usefulness of skin traction is limited by the amount of pull that can be exerted on the skin. Skin traction is applied by placing foam-rubber straps against the body part and then wrapping the straps with elastic bandages. Sometimes, the straps are secured with adhesive. If this is done, the nurse protects the child's skin by first applying tincture of benzoin to any skin area that will contact the tape. Before applying skin traction, the nurse refers to the child's history to be sure that the child is not allergic to rubber or adhesive. If the child has a history of these allergies, an alternative method of treatment may be chosen.

The nurse assesses color, sensation, and motion distal to the traction at least every 4 hours. If the child's condition permits, the nurse removes the bandages securing skin traction to assess color, sensation, and motion further; to provide skin care; and temporarily to relieve pressure on the skin. The nurse then reapplies skin traction smoothly and securely. Adhesive-backed straps are not removed during skin care.

Skeletal traction is achieved by means of wires or pins inserted in the bones. Greater force can be exerted by skeletal traction, and it can be maintained longer than skin

(text continued on p. 1480)

NURSING CARE GUIDE Child With a Cast

Nursing diagnosis	Interventions	Evaluation
1. Potential for fear related to knowledge deficit regarding cast application and removal	Explain to child and parent procedures of cast application and sensations child will experience (for example, warmth of wet cast) Use model of cast and tools and materials to demonstrate cast application Let child handle tools and cast materials Explain procedure for cast removal; demonstrate use of cast saw	Child does not appear fearful during cast application and removal
2. Potential for alteration in tissue perfusion related to constriction of the cast	Check color, sensation, and motion of skin distal to the cast every 30 minutes for the first few hours after application and every 4 hours for the rest of the child's hospitalization Inquire about and observe for manifestations of pain with active or passive extension of fingers or toes of the affected extremity (do not encourage extension if it is medically contraindicated) Elevate casted extremity after cast application and if any swelling is evident Check perfusion status after cast has been elevated a while to allow for maximum venous return Check cast for tightness by slipping a finger under the edge; if this is not possible, cast is too tight Instruct child and parent in all these measures if child is discharged after cast application Ask parent and child to describe signs of inadequate perfusion and cast tightness; ensure that parent knows how to contact physician if these signs occur	Circulation to the affected extremity appears adequate—color is pink; capillary refill is rapid; there is no numbness or tingling; fingers or toes move freely Parent and child can describe signs of inadequate perfusion and can explain the importance of seeking immediate help if such signs occur
3. Potential for alteration in comfort; pain	Check color, sensation, and motion if child complains of pain When there are no signs of altered innervation or circulation, administer analgesics and provide comfort measures to relieve pain Relieve pruritis by blowing cool air between skin and cast with hair dryer Teach child and parent to identify and report sources of discomfort, such as muscle spasms, pressure sores, pruritis Check cast for discoloration and musty odor, which may indicate pressure sores or infection Ask parent and child to describe sources of discomfort; ensure that parent understands what to do about each and when to contact physician Instruct parent to notify physician if muscle spasms are frequent or severe	Child remains free of pain and discomfort as evidenced by resumption of normal activities and decrease in anxiety level

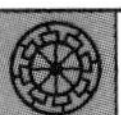

NURSING CARE GUIDE Child With a Cast (continued)

Nursing diagnosis	Interventions	Evaluation
4. Potential for alteration in skin integrity related to the cast	Handle wet cast carefully so as not to cause dents Elevate wet cast on pillows without plastic covering to prevent possible burns related to nondissipated heat of chemothermal reaction in setting cast Remove any plaster flakes from the skin; smooth rough cast edges; when cast is completely dry, petal cast edges with water-repellent tape or moleskin (see Fig. 41-7) Inspect skin under cast edges with a flashlight Instruct older child not to place objects between cast and skin; do not allow young child to play with small toys that could be inserted under cast Instruct child to report pain or discomfort under cast; determine whether pain or discomfort is related to skin breakdown, injury, or surgery Check cast for musty odor; ask child to report any warm areas that occur after cast is dry Support heavy cast with sling or pillows to decrease pressure of cast edges on skin Teach parent how to carry out these measures at home; ensure that parent knows when physician should be contacted; instruct parent not to let child get dirt or sand under the cast	Skin at or under cast edges is smooth and intact; there are no signs of infection at sites of incision or injury
5. Potential for knowledge deficit related to home care of child in a cast	Teach parent how to manage ambulation (for example, stair climbing); lift and move child safely, using correct body mechanics; restrain child in spica cast to prevent falling Instruct parent to avoid using a cross bar for moving child Instruct parent in measures to prevent physical and developmental deficits or complications related to immobility Teach parent and child how to keep child and cast clean with daily sponge baths of areas not covered by the cast, use of damp cloth and mild cleanser or mild solution of chlorine bleach to wipe cast daily, avoidance of lotions or powders around or under cast edges Instruct parent and child about the need for balanced diet, roughage, high fluid intake Instruct parent and child how to monitor elimination patterns, prevent constipation, keep cast sanitary and child's perineal area clean, prevent or correct cast wetness if child is diapered or incontinent Refer to a visiting nurse if appropriate	Parent can explain and demonstrate safe and appropriate home care

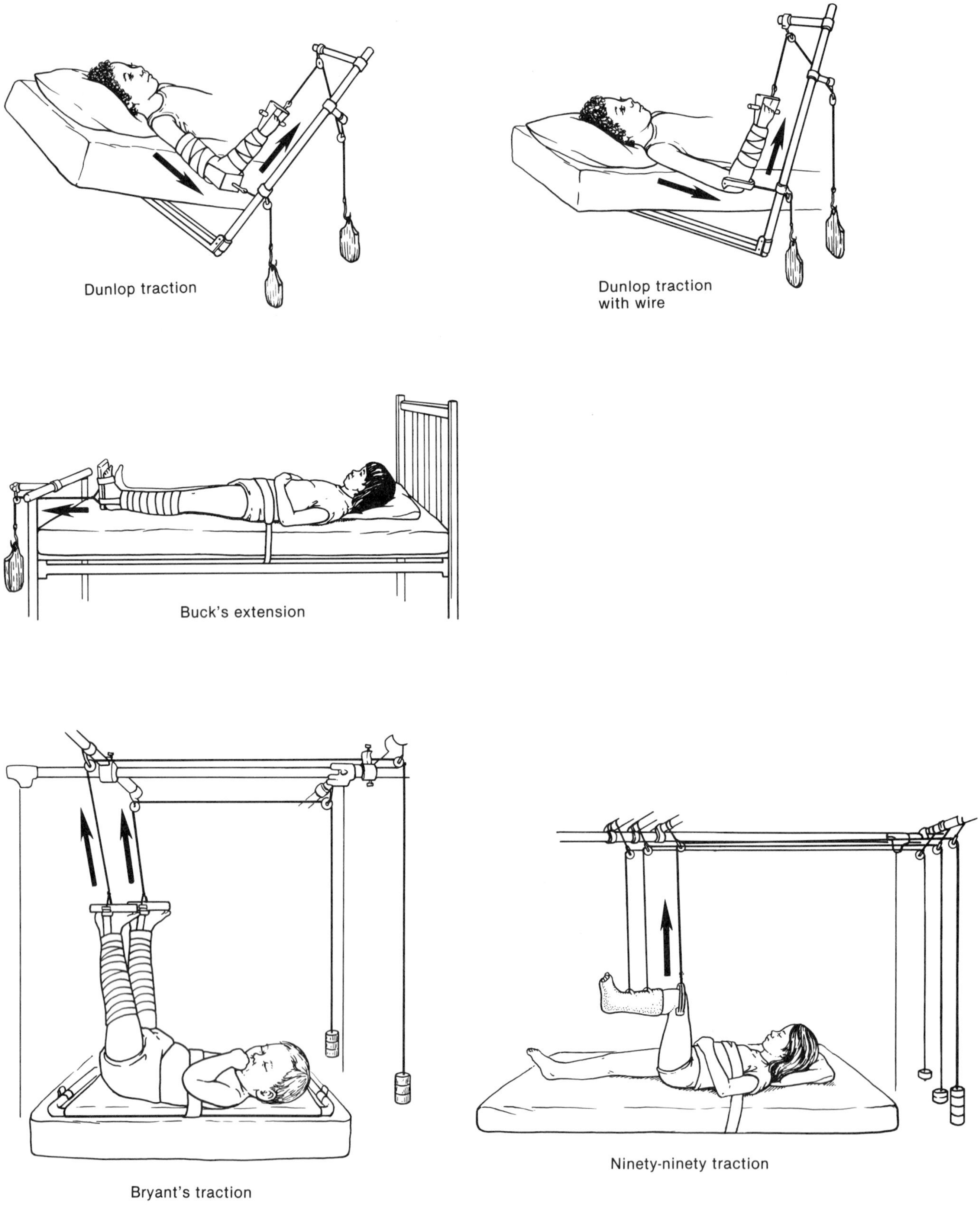

Dunlop traction

Dunlop traction with wire

Buck's extension

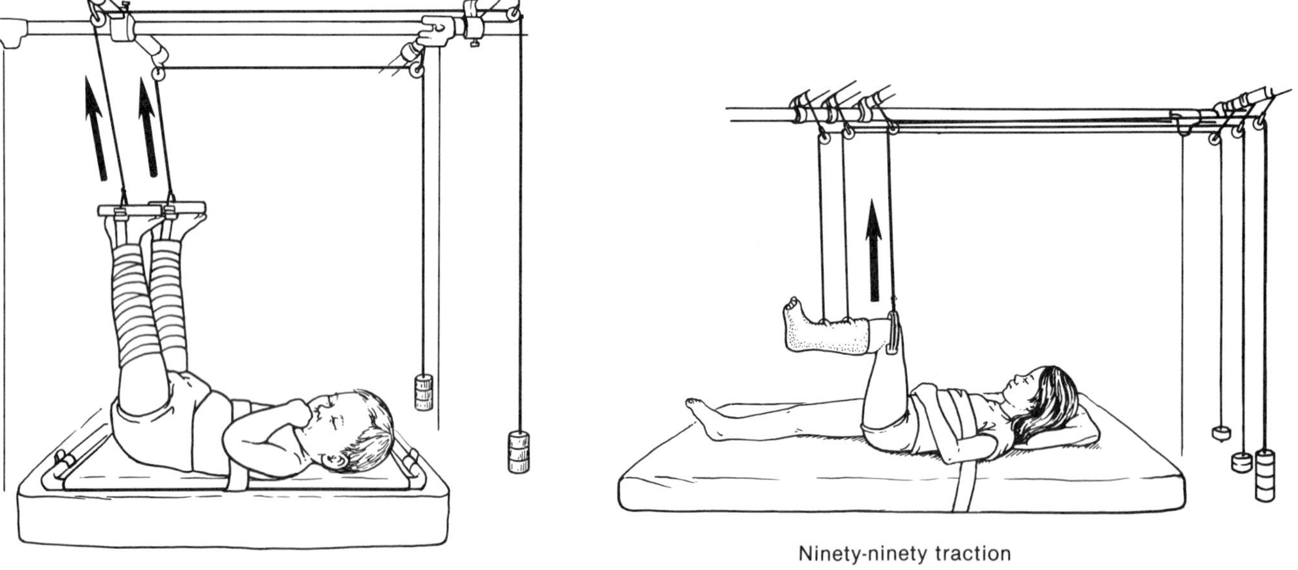

Figure 41-8 Traction devices used to treat musculoskeletal conditions in children. Arrows indicate direction of pull exerted by traction. Straps or jacket restraints and position of bed are sometimes used to keep the child positioned correctly and supplement countertraction exerted by the child's body weight.

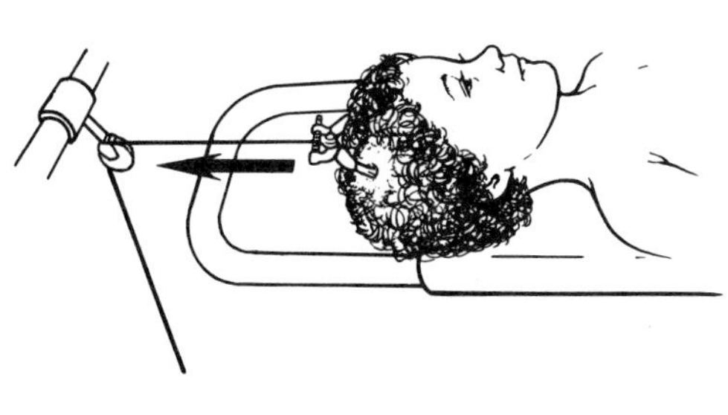
Crutchfield-tong traction

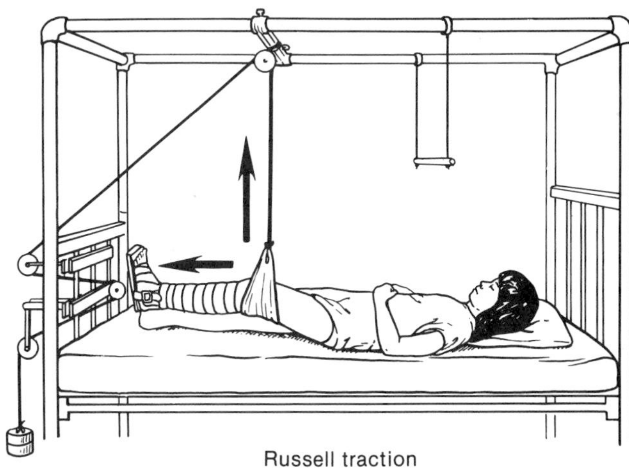
Russell traction

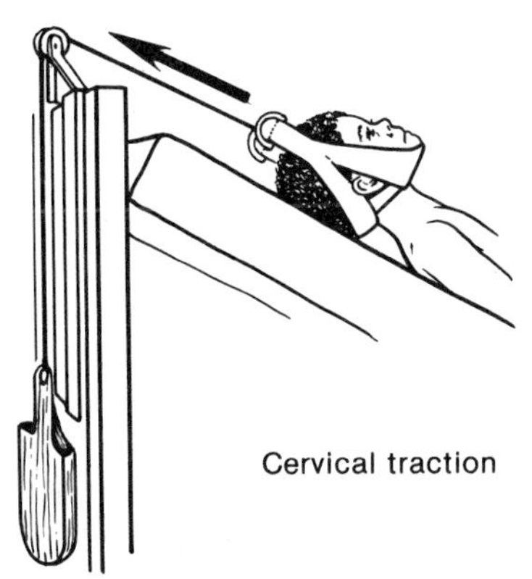
Cervical traction

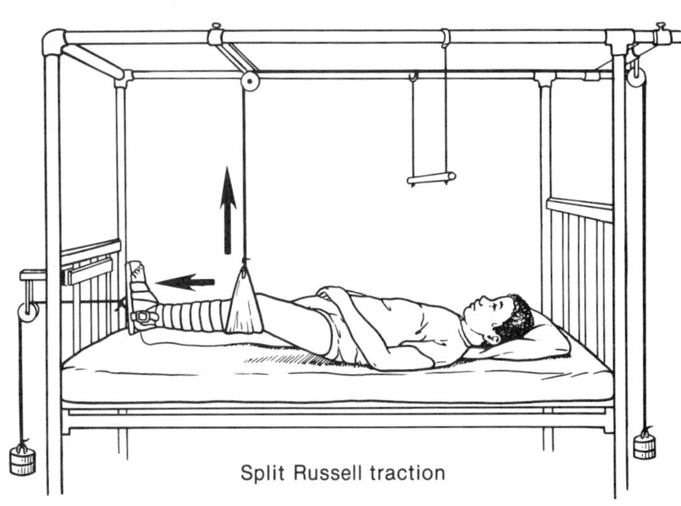
Split Russell traction

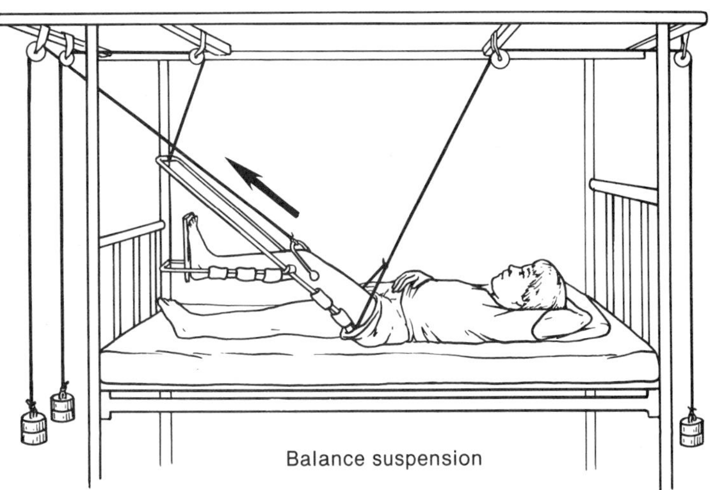
Balance suspension

traction. The wire pins or tongs used for skeletal traction are inserted by the physician. Some form of anesthetic may be used for the procedure. Skeletal traction is *never* removed for skin care. As with skin traction, the nurse assesses color, sensation, and motion at least every 4 hours. More frequent assessment is necessary immediately after traction is applied or reapplied. If the child is in traction for a spinal condition, assessment of neurologic signs and symptoms is an important indicator of the correct pull and body position.

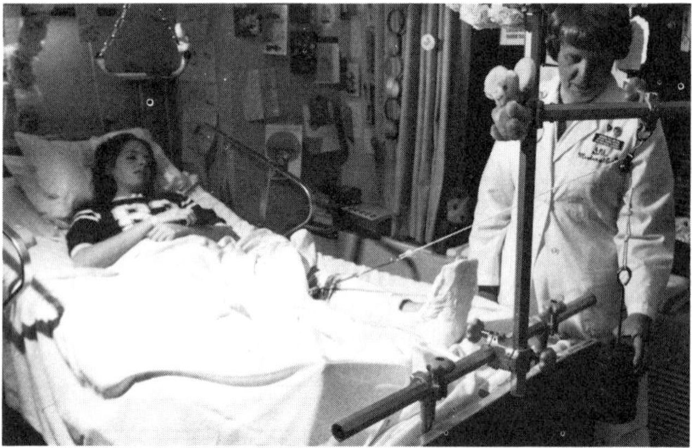

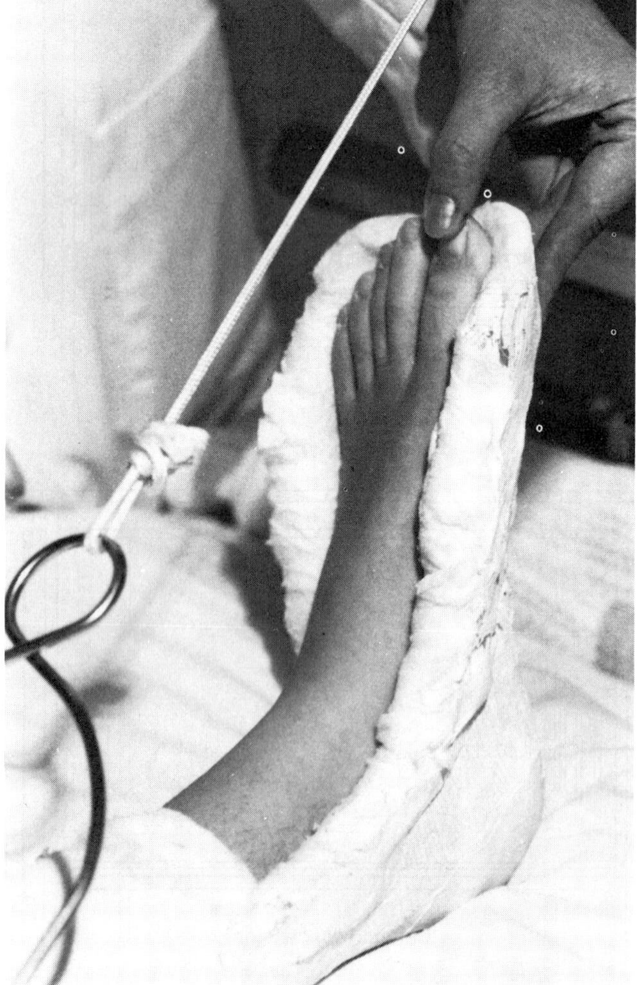

Assessing a child in skeletal traction. (From Swearingen PL: *The Addison-Wesley Photo-Atlas of Nursing Procedures.* Addison-Wesley, 1984, p. 563.)

If possible, the nurse prepares the child and family before traction is applied. Often, however, the child requires traction following an injury, and teaching and demonstrations must be done after traction is applied. Besides pain, which may be present initially, immobility is perhaps the most difficult aspect of traction management for the child and the nurse. Since the success of traction depends on its correct maintenance, the nurse makes certain that the child and family understand the exact purpose of traction, how it works, and what they can do to help maintain it. Marking the bed or side rail with tape to indicate the child's correct position (for example, where head, shoulders, or feet should be) enables the child and family to participate in the child's proper positioning and traction maintenance. The child may also enjoy helping to see that ropes are centered in the pulleys and that weights hang freely. The child can use a trapeze hung from an over-bed frame to pull the body up in bed and help maintain proper body alignment. If countertraction provided by the child's body weight is insufficient, traction can pull the child down in bed or to the side. A jacket restraint or folded sheet used as a sling can help to maintain the correct position. Sometimes, elevating the foot or side of the bed or the Bradford frame on shock blocks suffices to counterbalance traction. See Table 41-2 for nursing considerations appropriate in the management of traction apparatus shown in Figure 41-8.

Braces

Braces are used to immobilize a body part in a position of function, to prevent weight bearing, to stabilize a joint, or to aid in the correction of a deformity, such as clubfoot or scoliosis. Braces allow the child's progress to be monitored and adjustments made on an outpatient basis, a distinct advantage over inpatient casting or traction.

The length of time a brace is worn depends on its purpose. Braces used to correct deformities frequently are worn 23 hours a day, coming off only for skin care and exercises. A brace might also be removed for regular, prescribed periods. For example, if the brace is worn to prevent weight bearing or to stabilize a joint during weight bearing, it may be removed at night.

The brace is fitted to body curves so as not to create friction, skin irritation, or muscle misuse. The nurse needs to assess for circulatory or neurologic compromise. Braces usually exert pressure on the surrounding skin, and regular skin care therefore is required to prevent skin breakdown.

Braces are difficult and expensive to make and require special care if they are to remain functional and not irritate the skin. Leather portions are cleaned periodically with a

(text continued on p. 1484)

TABLE 41-2 Traction Devices Used to Treat Musculoskeletal Conditions in Children

Name and type of traction	Nursing considerations	Indications
Dunlop traction Skin or skeletal (skin traction for lower arm)	Correct alignment is critical because of risk of arm contractures Pain that persists after immobilization might be a sign of circulatory or neurologic compromise	Supracondylar fracture of humerus (fractured elbow), postoperative immobilization, reduction of elbow contractures
Buck's extension Skin	Pull of traction may cause child to slide toward foot of bed; traction is rendered ineffective if weights or ropes do not hang freely	Postoperative immobilization, reduction of hip or knee contractures
Bryant's traction Skin	Frequent assessment of circulation to legs, feet, and toes required because of risk of circulatory impairment due to low blood pressure in ankles, tight leg bandages, vasospasm from traction on blood vessels, or hyperextension of the knee Pain, particularly in the calf, is a sign of impending Volkman's ischemia Child's sacrum must be elevated enough so that nurse can slip hand between child's buttocks and bed or frame	Reduction of fractured femur or congenitally dislocated hip in child less than 2 years of age and weighing less than 25 lb
Russell traction Skin, skeletal, or both	Sling position under knee is checked frequently Hip flexion must remain at correct angle Assess for compromised peroneal nerve Child may need restraint to prevent slipping toward foot of bed	Postoperative immobilization of hip and knee, reduction of fractures of the femur
Split Russell traction Skin or skeletal and skin	Considerations same as for Russell traction	Postoperative immobilization, reduction of hip or knee contractures, dislocated hips
Balance suspension Provides support, sometimes in conjunction with skeletal traction	Involves care of Thomas splint with Pearson attachment Splint and attachment may have separate ropes and weights, allowing greater movement of the knee Child is relatively mobile Slight malalignment can be corrected by repositioning of the ring	Postoperative immobilization of hip or knee, musculoskeletal disease, fractured femur (with skeletal traction)
Ninety-ninety traction Skeletal	Alignment is monitored to ensure that child positioned correctly for pull at a 90° angle Child is quite comfortable Care is simplified by height of traction apparatus above bed	Reduction of fractured femur
Crutchfield tongs Skeletal	Pin sites are monitored for looseness of pins and signs of infection Child may be on a turning frame	Immobilization following spinal fusion, severe injury to cervical spine
Cervical traction Skin	Head of bed is elevated 15–20° Head must be kept straight	Injury or disease of the cervical spine
Halo apparatus Skeletal	Halo apparatus is attached with adjustable bars to a body jacket or cast Pin sites are monitored for looseness of pins and signs of infection	Spinal injury or disease requiring long periods in traction

NURSING CARE GUIDE Child in Traction

Nursing diagnosis	Interventions	Evaluation
1. Potential for alteration in tissue perfusion	Check capillary refill in nail beds of affected extremity every 30 minutes on day of application and every 4 hours thereafter Monitor peripheral pulses when checking capillary refill Notify physician immediately if perfusion status or pulses indicate circulatory compromise	Circulation to the affected extremity is adequate as evidenced by pink nailbeds, rapid capillary refill, and strong peripheral pulses
2. Potential for alteration of sensation and motion	Ask child to identify site of light touch on affected extremity Ask child to move distal parts of affected extremity (for example, wiggle and extend fingers or toes) Ask child to report any unusual sensations in distal parts of affected extremity such as numbness or tingling	There are no signs of sensory or motor deficits in the affected extremity
3. Potential for ineffective traction	Check traction apparatus to be sure that knots are secure and free from pulleys, weights are hanging freely (that is, not touching bed, floors, walls, etc.), and ropes are centered in pulleys Check child's position in bed and correct as necessary Mark head or foot of bed and side rails or sheets with tape to denote correct position of child in relation to traction apparatus Use restraints or elevate bed as necessary to supplement countertraction of child's body weight Monitor pin site for infection or loosening Check elastic bandages to be sure they are smoothly and securely wrapped	Correct traction is maintained by a properly functioning traction apparatus and appropriate positioning of the child
4. Potential for physical alterations related to immobility	Provide nutritious, appetizing, and well-balanced meals and snacks Offer small, frequent meals that include roughage and child's favorite foods; set up tray so that child can feed self Offer fluids frequently to ensure intake beyond daily maintenance requirements Measure fluid intake and output; monitor urine pH and specific gravity daily; record frequency and consistency of stools Have child fully expand lungs by taking several deep breaths at least 4 times per day Encourage deep inspirations by teaching child blowing games, providing harmonica or blow toys, having child use incentive spirometer Monitor breath sounds every shift and report respiratory alterations, such as congestion or cough Change child's position every 2–4 hours, as traction allows	The child demonstrates adequate nutrition, hydration status, respiratory status, skin integrity, elimination patterns, and muscle tone

Nursing diagnosis	Interventions	Evaluation
	Monitor skin condition (including skin under bandages if bandages can be removed); rub skin over bony prominences every 4 hours; note broken skin or redness that does not disappear after skin care or position change Have child do muscle-setting, range-of-motion exercises as prescribed Encourage exercise through use of play (for example, throwing foam balls, bean bags, or Velcro darts; kicking balls with unaffected leg; performing pull-ups on overhead trapeze)	
5. Potential for developmental alteration related to immobility	Have child help to plan a daily routine that alternates rest periods and active periods, time with others and time alone Allow child to choose age-appropriate games and activities, particularly those involving physical activity Encourage child to maintain contacts with peers and facilitate the child's making new friends in the hospital Encourage child to keep up with schoolwork; provide opportunities for child to do so Promote self-care, independence, and self-esteem Assist child in decorating bed space	Child's developmental level is maintained; child demonstrates interest in self-care activities
6. Potential fear related to knowledge deficit	Explain the purpose and function of traction to the child and family Demonstrate approximation and immobilization of bone using models or suitable objects Provide child with doll that is in traction; allow child to manipulate toy traction apparatus Involve child and family in maintaining traction and child's correct position in bed	Child and family understand purpose of traction and can explain how it works. They demonstrate confidence and lack of fear related to traction apparatus
7. Potential for inadequate family coping related to child's condition and treatment	Encourage child and family to express fears, anger, and other negative feelings Offer toys appropriate to expressing aggression Monitor child's response to aggressive activities, setting limits when necessary Provide information and reassurance as appropriate Involve family members in child's care in the hospital and in discharge preparation Encourage family members to visit and support child Advise the family to disrupt home routines and family rituals as little as possible Prepare the family for subsequent phases of treatment by explaining treatments and describing child's expected reactions Explain child's behavior to family members and prepare them to accept some developmental regression during the course of treatment	Family life and relationships are not damaged as a result of the child's condition and treatment

leather cleaner or saddle soap. Plastic portions are wiped off with a mild soap-and-water solution daily. Many children who wear a brace are active, and as a result of this activity, the screws of the brace may become loose. The screws are checked daily and tightened whenever necessary. Metal portions of the brace may be sharp or rough. These may require a protective covering of tape, plastic, or foam rubber to prevent damage to clothing.

The *Denis-Browne splint* is one of many treatment devices used in the correction of in-toeing and clubfoot. The feet fit into special shoes or padded forms into which the feet are taped. The shoes or forms are fastened to an adjustable bar providing the appropriate degree of eversion, rotation, and dorsiflexion needed to achieve a mild degree of overcorrection.

The *abduction brace* is used to keep the hip in abduction. Long-leg casts or leather braces with an abduction bar both accomplish abduction. For an infant with a dislocatable or dislocated hip, devices such as the Paulik harness or Frejka pillow are less rigid and allow some mobility. The Frejka pillow splint fits around the diaper area and between the thighs, so that it is removed and reapplied with each diaper change. The Paulik harness consists of straps passing from the shoulders and chest to the feet and lower legs. The harness is often readjusted to maintain the proper position of the head of the femur in the acetabulum by means of Ortolani and Barlow maneuvers. It is usually not removed by the parent.

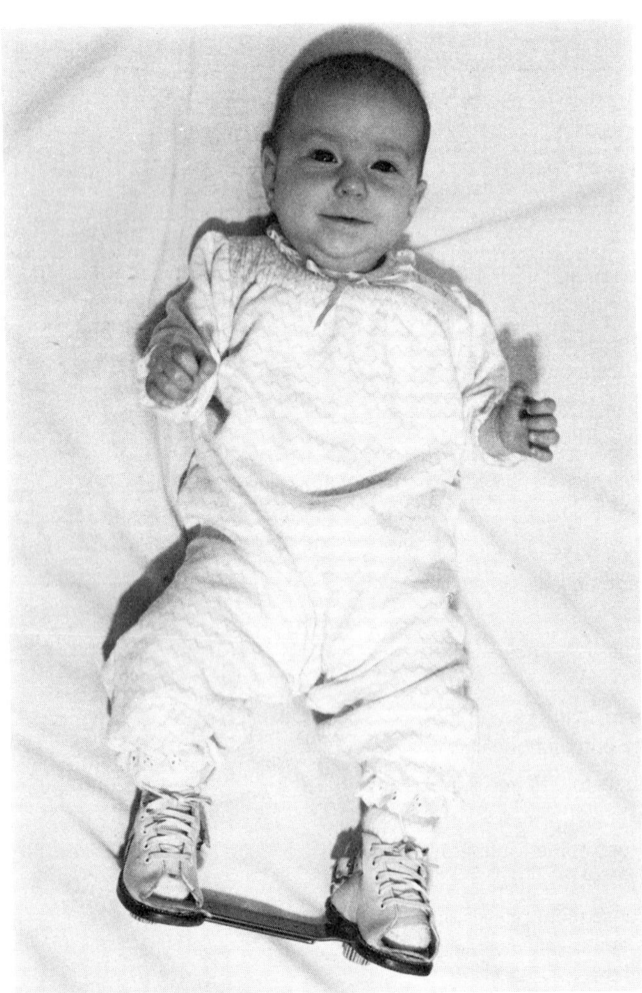

Denis-Browne splint. (From Swearingen PL: *The Addison-Wesley Photo-Atlas of Nursing Procedures.* Addison-Wesley, 1984, p. 528.)

The *Milwaukee brace* is used to treat scoliosis and kyphosis (Fig. 41-9). It is used for some correction of the curve and to prevent further deformity during the pubescent growth period. The brace stretches the spine (that is, provides distraction) between the portion of the brace resting on the occiput and the molded portion at the hips and waist. A holding pad can be used to correct lateral curvature by partially encircling the trunk and attaching to the vertical bars, thus providing pressure on a convex area.

The brace fits the body closely, and so proper skin care is very important. It is generally recommended that the child wear a close-fitting undershirt or stockinet under the brace or at least under the pelvic portion. Although the mandible is completely free from the chin pad, irritation can occur. It may be helpful to cover the chin pad with a smooth cloth.

Continuous Passive Motion

Following certain surgical procedures, proper healing is best promoted by continuous movement of a joint through its range of motion. Continuous passive motion is achieved by securing the child's limb to a device that is set to move

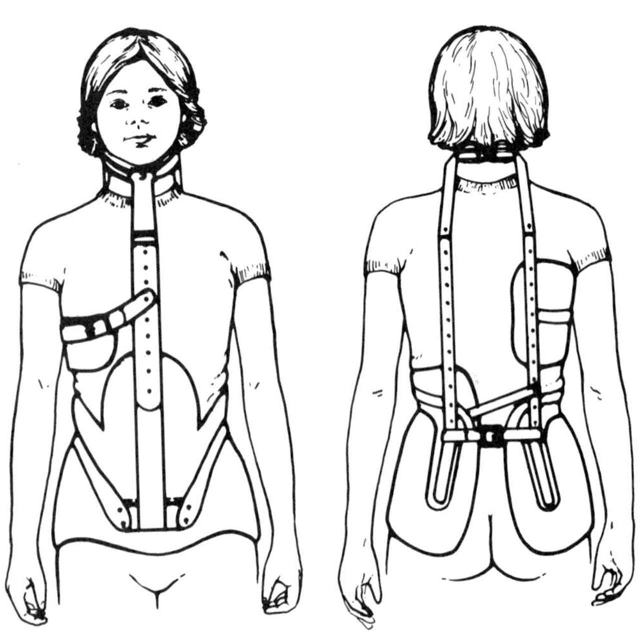

Figure 41-9 Milwaukee brace.

the limb through a specific arc and range of motion at a set rate. The device can be set to increase speed or range of motion as healing progresses. Continuous passive motion promotes healing of tendons, ligaments, and the cartilage of articular joints. It has been used successfully following intraarticular fracture, synovectomy for rheumatoid arthritis or hemophilic arthropathy, arthrotomy for septic arthritis, and other conditions (Salter, 1983).

Continuous passive range of motion is not uncomfortable for the child (Salter, 1983), although some children report mild discomfort when the degree or rate of motion is increased. The nurse ensures that the child's limb remains securely positioned on the device and that the child complies with the treatment. The child who is on bed rest with continuous passive motion requires nursing care appropriate for the child who feels well but has limited mobility and, usually, is recovering from a surgical procedure.

Frames and Beds

Bradford Frame Many different beds and frames facilitate care of the immobilized child. The Bradford frame is a rectangular wooden or metal frame covered with one long or two shorter pieces of canvas separated near the center by 6–8 inches (Fig. 41-10A). The canvas may be covered with water-repellent material and then by blankets or other padding. Sheets or pillow cases are put over the canvas or covering for comfort and cleanliness. The frame may be purchased, rented, or made by the family or facility needing it. The frame should be slightly larger than the child. The frame is usually placed so that its head and foot rest on two large wooden blocks that extend across the width of the bed.

The blocks must rest on a firm surface for stability. If the mattress is not sufficiently firm, a board of approximately the same size may be placed on top of the mattress or the mattress removed and the board placed directly on the bed springs. For safety and stability, the frame is secured at the corners to the bed frame or springs by four long, buckled straps. The child is secured to the frame by some form of restraint. Elevation of the frame facilitates nursing care and allows for overhang of traction or a cast. The frame's elevation at one or both ends depends on the reason for its use. If the child's weight does not provide adequate countertraction, the foot block chosen may be taller than the head block. In this case, the frame with a single long piece

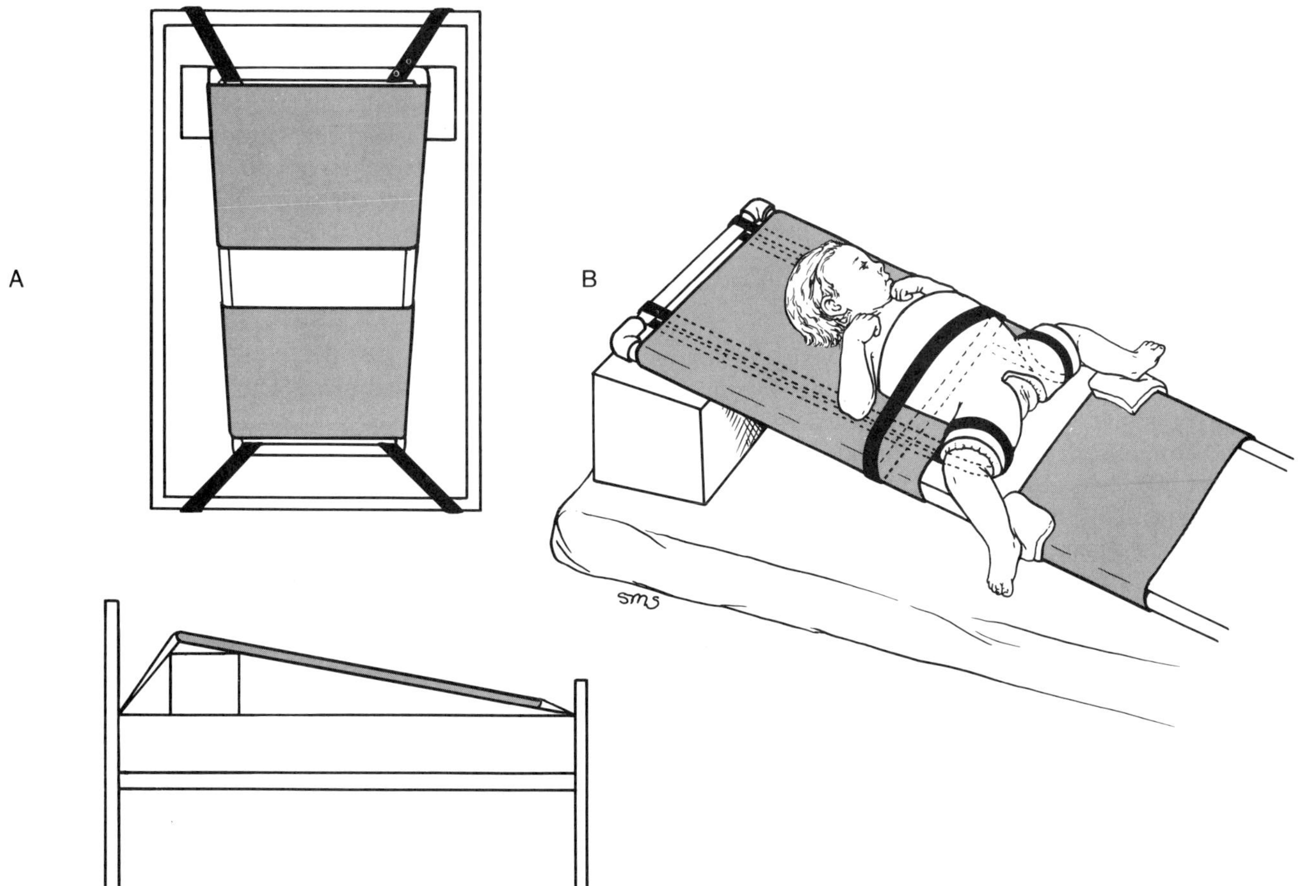

Figure 41-10 *A.* Split Bradford frame. *B.* Child with hip spica cast on Bradford frame.

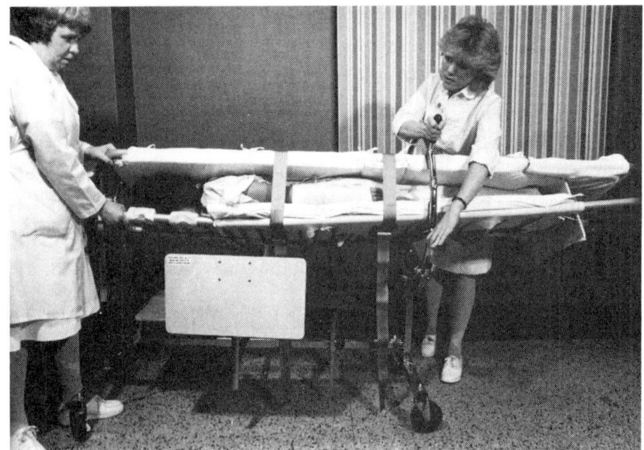

Stryker wedge turning frame. (From Swearingen PL: *The Addison-Wesley Photo-Atlas of Nursing Procedures.* Addison-Wesley, 1984, p. 619.)

of canvas is used. Skin care is extremely important, as this position can cause urine to flow up the child's back.

If the Bradford frame is used for a child in a hip spica cast, the head of the frame is elevated 30–45° above the feet (Fig. 41-10B). This angle is helpful in directing urine and feces away from the body of the cast. The angle is decreased if perineal edema develops or is likely to develop, such as following hip surgery. Sometimes the frame is used for immobilization, as it positions and restrains and helps maintain alignment in the child.

Horizontal Turning Frames Turning frames are special beds that enable the nurse to turn the child horizontally while the child remains immobilized. No weight bearing is experienced by the child during turning, and the risk of injury or pain is greatly reduced.

The Stryker frame consists of a stand into which one or, while turning, two canvas-covered metal frames lock into position. The frame is longer and slightly wider than the child, and arm rests may clamp onto the side of the frame for comfort and change of position. A foot board can be positioned against the feet to maintain functional alignment when the child is supine. Sheepskins, blankets, or egg-carton foam may be placed on top of the canvas to protect skin from pressure. The frame used for the supine position may consist of either one long piece of canvas or two pieces of canvas separated by a space to allow for positioning and use of the bedpan. The frame used for the prone position has one piece of canvas extending from the child's shoulders to the ankles and a small second piece of canvas to support the forehead. This allows the child to look down for reading or eating. A tablelike shelf is positioned under the upper portion of the frame to hold books, food, and supplies. Since the canvas ends at the child's ankle, it allows for functional positioning and full range of motion of the foot and ankle. The Stryker frame is narrow, and so it is important that the child be restrained with a sheet or waist restraint and, if restless, restraints around the chest and thighs.

If possible, the child has seen demonstrated and has experienced being turned on the Stryker frame prior to treatment or surgery. The nurse explains why the frame will be used, describes how it works, and assures the child that turning is not dangerous. Once the child is immobilized on the frame, the nurse ensures that the stabilizer pin is secure and that restraints are kept fastened except during skin care. The nurse enlists the help of trained personnel to turn the child. The child may feel more secure hugging the frame, or may wish to have rolled bath blankets or pillows placed along either side of the body. Before the child is turned, the top half of the frame is applied and fastened securely with safety belts. The nurse then loosens the stabilizer pin, turns the frame smoothly and swiftly, replaces the stabilizer pin immediately, removes the top half (formerly the bottom half) of the frame, and makes the child comfortable.

Vertical Turning Frames The CircOlectric bed enables the nurse to turn the child vertically. It is used for the child in cervical traction and sometimes postoperatively for the child who has undergone spinal fusion with instrumentation. It also helps a child who has been horizontal for an extended period of time to adjust to an upright or vertical position.

The CircOlectric bed consists of two canvas-covered frames that are connected and secured by two large metal circles. The canvas on the posterior frame, on which the child lies supine, is not adjustable, but the canvas on the anterior frame can be adjusted to the child's size. Preparation of the child for turning is similar to that for the horizontal turning frame.

Principles of Nursing Care

Acute-Care Needs

The acute-care needs of the child with a musculoskeletal problem may be related to appliances used to immobilize or exert traction on a body part, to pain, or to surgical procedures.

Casts, Traction, and Braces The acute care needs of a child who is immobilized to some degree by a cast, traction device, or brace are centered around preventing physiologic complications and psychosocial problems related to the immobilization.

Prevention of Skin Breakdown Casts, some traction apparatus, and braces can cause localized skin breakdown as they press or rub the skin. The nurse examines the edges of casts, traction equipment, splints, and braces for any rough areas. Although some problems need to be reported to the physician, brace shop, or cast technician, the nurse can often help smooth cast edges by padding or petalling the edges. The nurse can apply extra padding over bony prominences if skin traction, braces, or splints rub and cause skin irritation. The skin under the extra padding is carefully assessed for signs of undue pressure. The nurse notes and reports any dents in the cast, as these can lead to skin breakdown.

Pressure also results from small objects placed under appliances, most often casts. The nurse instructs the older child to put nothing inside a cast. The younger child is not given any small objects to play with and wears clothing that covers the cast edge. Material, such as loose, soft fluff, can be placed just inside the cast edge to discourage the child from slipping objects inside. The child may scratch dry, itchy skin under a cast with fingernails, pencils, or sharp toys. Scratching can break skin and lead to infection.

Skin care provided to prevent irritation and breakdown varies according to protocols but follows the general principles described in Chapter 29. The nurse keeps the skin clean and dry. Lotions and powders are generally not used on skin that comes in contact with casts, braces, or splints. Lotion softens the skin and thus may hasten breakdown, and powders can lump and cake under appliances, creating irritation and pressure. Alcohol is sometimes used to toughen the skin at cast edges, under removable traction appliances, and over bony prominences that come in contact with removable appliances and apparatus. Toughening with alcohol is particularly useful for children who pull against a cast, brace, splint or traction because of high activity levels or neurologic impairment. The nurse uses alcohol with caution so that the child does not inhale the irritating fumes.

The nurse examines the skin for any signs of actual or potential breakdown, such as redness that does not disappear after skin care. If apparatus can be removed, the nurse examines all skin that comes into contact with the equipment. If the traction apparatus or cast cannot be removed, the nurse inspects the skin around all edges and uses a flashlight to inspect the skin under cast edges or traction apparatus. To assess skin that is not visible, the nurse relies on other data. A child's irritability or complaints of discomfort, especially localized pain not related to the injury or operative site; foul odor; staining on a cast or traction straps; or an elevated temperature can all signal skin breakdown and infection. Sometimes pain decreases as skin breakdown increases and innervated tissue sloughs off. All signs of skin breakdown are reported to the physician, as they may necessitate removal of the appliance or cast.

Control of Infections and Complications Infectious microorganisms can enter the body at sites of skin breakdown or surgical incision and can cause skin infection, bone and tissue infection, or systemic infection. The keys to prevention of infection are correct skin care, preoperative skin preparation, and preoperative administration of antibiotics as ordered by the physician.

With skeletal traction, the site of pin or wire insertion is a potential focus of infection. There is controversy over whether the site should be cleansed daily or left alone following initial placement, and there is great variety among methods of pin care.

Celeste, Folick, and Dumas (1984), in surveying surgical equipment supply companies about recommended methods of pin care, obtained a different protocol from each company. The solutions used and frequency of application generally differed. Povidone-iodine is preferred by a number of orthopedic surgeons for pin care (Celeste, Folick, and Dumas, 1984), although iodine slowly corrodes stainless steel pins. Povidone-iodine, however, contains a surface-active agent and is less corrosive and irritating to the skin than iodine.

Whether or not the nurse cleanses the pin site, several principles are involved in pin care. The nurse assesses the site frequently for signs of infection, such as serosanguineous drainage, crusting, swelling and erythema that persist longer than 72 hours (Celeste, Folick, and Dumas, 1984). Any cleansing technique performed in the hospital should be sterile and performed gently so as not to introduce pathogens or traumatize the skin. A sterile gauze is often cut to fit around the pin. The nurse also assesses the site for any loosening or slipping of the pin.

Control of Circulatory and Neurologic Compromise Pressure exerted on deep arteries by a cast, fracture, or malalignment following fracture reduction or skeletal surgery can cause irreversible neurologic and muscular damage resulting from Volkmann's ischemia. Pain is usually the earliest sign of Volkmann's ischemia. The pain is persistent and severe but will eventually decrease if ischemia goes unchecked. The nurse always assesses for adequate circulation and innervation before medicating or explaining away pain related to a skeletal condition. Other signs of ischemia include puffiness, pallor, and coolness of the extremity, paresthesias, paralysis, and absent pulse.

To detect circulatory or neurologic compromise, the nurse assesses color, sensation, and motion in the body part distal to the cast or traction, and reports any abnormality immediately. (Assessment of color, sensation, and motion is discussed in Chapter 29.) Immediately following application of the cast, traction, brace, or splint, assessment is done every 15–30 minutes. Later, it may only need to be done every 4 hours. The nurse also attempts to decrease edema and increase circulation by elevating the edematous body part or loosening traction if neither intervention is contraindicated by the child's skeletal condition.

Assessment of color, sensation, and motion is continued

as long as the apparatus is in place. A device that fits initially may become too tight as the child grows, exerting pressure that interferes with blood vessels and nerves.

Maintenance of Appliances or Apparatus With active children, casts, splints, and braces can break, loosen, or bend, and traction can become malaligned. Any of these changes can render treatment ineffective or even harmful. The nurse examines casts for breaks or softened areas, splints and braces for breaks, and braces for loose parts. The nurse checks traction against a written description and diagram. If the child's appropriate body position is marked on the bed with tape, the nurse, child, and family can more easily maintain proper body alignment.

Immobility Immobility imposed by casts, traction, or a frame affects every system of the body (see Chapter 29). The nurse counteracts these effects by encouraging the child to move as much as possible, breathe deeply, participate in self-care, and perform prescribed exercises. The child benefits from activities and exercises that maintain muscle strength in noninvolved extremities. Turning, pulling up on an overhead trapeze, and lifting small weights strengthen muscles. The child can usually strengthen muscles of immobilized body parts by doing muscle setting exercises, that is, by contracting and relaxing muscles without moving any joints.

Footdrop, with shortening of the Achilles tendon, can develop if the child must remain in traction and thus be deprived of walking. To prevent footdrop, the nurse helps the child perform passive or active range-of-motion exercises for the ankles and feet, places traction footplates correctly against the feet to maintain them in functional positions, and may use footboards to support the feet.

Control of Pain Often, the pain accompanying skeletal conditions is both intense and severe. Skeletal surgery involves much manipulation, pounding, and application of pressure. The child may experience painful spasms in muscles that have been stretched, pulled, and stabilized in new positions. With any sign or report of pain, the nurse first rules out ischemia as the cause. At first, traction may cause painful muscle spasms that require administration of analgesics. Constant pain, even if it is not severe, creates fatigue and restlessness, and reduces energy needed for coping. See Chapter 29 for a discussion of children's responses to pain and general nursing interventions to control it.

Skeletal Surgery in Children In addition to the preoperative and postoperative nursing interventions discussed in Chapter 29, the nurse considers two major factors for the child undergoing skeletal surgery. First, bone is highly vascular and tends to ooze both intraoperatively and postoperatively. The nurse therefore reviews intraoperative blood loss estimations and blood and fluid replacement. When significant blood loss is anticipated, some facilities use a machine for intraoperative autotransfusion to suction, filter, and reinfuse the child's blood lost during surgery. Blood loss may not end with surgery, however, and the nurse is especially careful to monitor signs of bleeding at the operative site, vital signs, and laboratory values.

The second major factor is that children who undergo musculoskeletal surgery often require care relative to continued treatment with some immobilizing device. If the operative site is casted postoperatively, the nurse assesses the cast for serosanguineous staining and fresh bleeding. The nurse draws a circle around the initial serosanguineous stain and records the date and time. Additional circles are drawn to outline successive increases in staining. Although this practice of circling drainage varies, McFarland's survey (1984) found that most nurses who circled cast drainage found it helpful in assessment. Because bone surgery results in postoperative blood loss and bone oozes for a time following incision, some blood staining on the cast is normal, and for some operations such staining can be considerable. Bleeding may only be apparent on the cast several days after actual blood loss and tends to become brown and spread as plaster casting material dries (Hankin, Gragg, and Kaufer, 1983). Careful monitoring of fresh bleeding, vital signs, and hematocrit enable the nurse to detect signs of excessive blood loss.

Frequent assessment of color, sensation, and motion is important, since edema increases during the first several hours postoperatively, possibly making casts, bandages, or skin traction too tight. The affected body part is often elevated postoperatively on several pillows. This is done to reduce edema and facilitate circulation.

Nutritional Needs

Eating independently is difficult for children who are partially immobilized by casts, traction, or frames. The nurse prepares and positions food on the tray so that it is easy to reach. Use of finger foods and fruit helps maintain the child's independence and control over what is eaten, as do straws inserted into covered cups of liquids. The nurse may find it necessary to cut meat or other large pieces of food for the child or open dishes and packets of salad dressing, jelly, or seasonings. Children who must remain flat in bed, especially in the supine position, require nursing ingenuity during mealtime. Those who may be turned have an easier time eating while lying on their side, with the tray placed on the bed beside them. For children who may be turned prone, such as those on a Stryker frame, the tray can be placed on a shelf underneath. Eating in these positions is fatiguing and often interferes with appetite. Intake is likely to improve if small meals and nutritious in-between-meal snacks are offered. Independence and appropriate control over meals are crucial to the immobilized child, since the need for nutrients is great and the child's opportunities to control the environment are few. The nurse monitors the child's intake to help ensure a diet high in fluids, protein, vitamins, minerals, and fiber to assist healing and combat the effects of immobility.

Developmental Needs

Treatment of skeletal conditions often requires long hospital stays and periods of home care during which the child is deprived of interactions and developmental opportunities normally supplied by school, family life, and association with peers. Chapters 27 and 28 describe nursing interventions for meeting the age-appropriate developmental needs of the hospitalized and immobilized child. Play, participation in self-care and hospital activities, opportunities to socialize, and encouragement with school work all stimulate the child and promote normal growth and development.

Emotional Needs

The emotional needs of children with skeletal conditions have to do with reactions to immobilization, casts and other appliances, and alterations in body image. Nursing interventions relative to body image are described in Chapter 27.

Reactions to Immobilization Some children find immobilization and restrictions difficult to accept, particularly since they feel well. Besides teaching and reteaching about restrictions, the nurse may have to curb inappropriate behavior and set limits firmly. Most children accept immobilization and restrictions quite contentedly, perhaps because equipment, casts, or traction apparatus are concrete and constant reminders of the skeletal condition. The child's apparent acceptance is sometimes superficial, however. Bergmann (1965) has documented dramatic reversals in attitude resulting from seemingly minor changes in the hospital routine or treatment regimen. Some children are unusually quiet while they are immobilized for treatment, thus demonstrating their tenuous adjustment. At the other extreme is the child who becomes so comfortable with the cast or traction apparatus that the eventual return to mobility is resisted.

Once recovery is nearly complete and rehabilitation is about to begin, the previously contented child may become impatient and frustrated. These feelings diminsh as the child begins to regain mobility. At this stage of treatment, many children make up for any setbacks they may have suffered in emotional development.

The child's emotional status throughout treatment depends on the suddenness of the condition's onset, severity of the condition, and length of treatment. The child who has survived an accident in which others have been injured or killed requires special nursing interventions and emotional support.

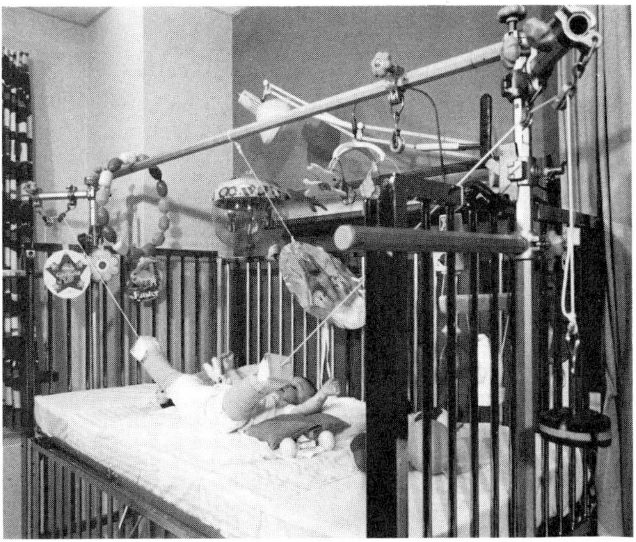

Meeting developmental needs of a child in Bryant's traction by providing visual stimuli, such as toys and mobiles. (From Swearingen PL: *The Addison Wesley Photo-Atlas of Nursing Procedures.* Addison-Wesley, 1984, p. 559.)

Reactions to Casts, Braces, and Traction Apparatus Casts, braces, splints, and traction devices often seem strange and frightening to the child. The nurse carefully explains and, if possible, demonstrates equipment before it is applied or used in the child's treatment (see Chapter 29). The nurse also helps the child to understand the treatment and condition. For example, the child with skeletal traction might wish to believe that a pin or wire does not pass through the bone. Though facts may frighten or alienate the child at first, it is more helpful in the long run to tell the child the truth than to collaborate in deception. While explaining that the pin or wire does pass through the bone, the nurse reassures the child that the bone is not harmed.

The child may refuse to look at the traction apparatus, injury, or stained cast. These sights seem unattractive, and the child may fear that the traction pin will leave holes in the extremity, that the traction weight will make the extremity longer, or that a deformity is permanent. The child needs to express these feelings to someone who can sympathize with these concerns, take them seriously, and answer questions honestly. Some children cannot talk about their fears. For these children, another form of expression, such as doll play, the opportunity to handle equipment, and painting or drawing, are appropriate. (Therapeutic play for the hospitalized child is discussed in Chapter 28.)

Children who are discharged with casts or braces are conscious of their appearance and may fear being teased, stared at, or questioned. Children with these fears need to practice responding to questions about their appearance so that they feel ready to relate to people outside the hospital. The nurse can suggest adaptations for clothing that are attractive and stylish while fitting over or around apparatus.

Health Maintenance Needs

Discharge preparation for the child who is hospitalized for a musculoskeletal condition includes the general principles discussed in Chapter 29 as well as teaching about home care relative to the child's specific problem. Physical aspects of home care might include skin care, assessment, and protection; cast or brace care; turning; and use of crutches, wheelchair, stretcher, scooter, or wagon. The nurse gives the parent instructions in writing. If the parent needs to purchase or construct equipment, such as a Bradford frame, the nurse furnishes written instructions well before the child's discharge.

The nurse helps the family to plan alterations needed in the home to enable the immobilized child to participate in family life, or get around using mobility aids. Environmental hazards, such as throw rugs, stairs, cords, and other obstacles, are safety hazards that are identified and minimized before the child returns home.

The nurse makes arrangements to ensure continuity of care. This may include scheduling follow-up appointments or referring the family to a community health nurse. In many states, the community health nurse, or public health nurse, assists families who need the help provided by Crippled Children's Services.

The Child With a Structural Abnormality

Craniofacial Defects

A variety of craniofacial abnormalities can occur during fetal development. Some of these are severe enough to necessitate later surgery. For such defects as hypertelorism, in which the space between the eyes is abnormally wide or the bony orbits cannot adequately hold the eyes, correction involves delicate resection or grafting of bone.

Not surprisingly, the body image adjustment necessitated by plastic surgery is a major hurdle for the child and family, even when surgery improves the child's appearance. Some undergo supportive therapy before and after making the final decision about surgery.

The incisional areas are chosen so as to minimize or disguise scarring. Often, an incision is made in the scalp. The surrounding hair is shaved and the incision allows, when the skin has been separated, access to many areas of the skull and face. Following surgery, the child's head is bandaged and swollen. Nursing care is meticulous and centers around monitoring and maintaining basic airway function, monitoring for infection, and caring for the incision. Infection can cause sloughing and necessitate removal of grafted bone. The nurse monitors the child's vital signs, the appearance of the face, and any drainage from incisional areas. Careful suture line care according to institution protocol can help prevent scarring. This might include cleaning the sutures with diluted hydrogen peroxide and applying antibacterial ointment to prevent infection and soften crusts. As swelling gradually subsides, the child and family need acceptance, reassurance, and support as well as meticulous physical care.

Clubfoot

Clubfoot is a deformity in which the distal portion of the foot, the forefoot, the proximal portion, the hindfoot, and the ankle are in various nonfunctional positions. The foot and ankle are in either equinus (foot extended, toes lower than heel) or calcaneus (foot flexed and heel lower than toes) positions. The forefoot and hindfoot can be in varus (heel inverted, forefoot adducted and inverted) or valgus (heel everted, forefoot abducted and everted) positions. The most common deformity, and the one that is usually called clubfoot, is talipes equinovarus. In *talipes equinovarus,* the foot twists inward, the forefoot is adducted, and the foot is in plantar flexion. In severe forms, the foot has a clublike appearance. Clubfoot can be unilateral or bilateral, flexible or rigid, mild or severe.

The deformity is almost always congenital. Its exact cause is unknown, though it does seem to have environmental and some inherited components. Incidence is highest in families who already have one child with a clubfoot. Incidence in the general population is 2 in 1000 (Salter, 1983). Clubfoot occurs more frequently in males than in females.

In mild talipes equinovarus, the foot toes inward when the child lies, stands, or walks. The foot is flexible in that it can be passively put through complete range of motion and readily corrects to a neutral position. Heel and leg size are normal. Mild, flexible clubfoot is possibly the result of intrauterine position, especially during the last month or so of gestation.

Severe talipes equinovarus is a rigid deformity. It can be so pronounced that the toes touch the medial side of the lower leg. The foot cannot be passively manipulated to a neutral position. The heel is small, and the leg becomes atrophied to some degree. Soft-tissue changes of the foot include stretched, thin skin on the dorsal lateral aspect of the foot and deeply creased skin on the inner aspect of the ankle and instep. Ligaments on the medial side of the foot and posterior aspect of the ankle are thickened and shortened. Muscles may be contracted.

Medical and Surgical Treatment Treatment for talipes equinovarus is initiated immediately after diagnosis, as the earlier the treatment, the more favorable the results. If deformity is severe, treatment is often begun before the neonate is discharged.

Conservative treatment consists of manipulation of the foot away from the abnormal position and maintenance of the corrected position with adhesive strapping or a plaster cast. Serial restrapping or recasting follows at 1- to 2- week intervals. This routine accommodates the infant's growth, and allows both repositioning and continual, gradual manipulation of the foot to an overcorrected position. An adhesive, nonirritating liquid, such as benzoin, may be applied to the skin before adhesive strapping or casting to prevent slippage and loss of correction. The cast might extend from toes to groin, with the knees flexed so as to control heel position and leg rotation.

Passive stretching exercises may be prescribed alone or in combination with corrective shoes or splints. The parent is taught which exercises to do and how frequently to do them. Many choose to do these exercises during the infant's feedings. Feedings are quite equally spaced, and the parent is less likely to forget the exercises if they are part of another routine aspect of care. Some physicians correct all deformities at once, and others correct them in a distal-to-proximal sequence. Therefore, the choice of exercises and their sequence depends on the treatment sequence chosen. Exercises are frequently prescribed following the completion of serial casting or strapping.

When fully corrected, the foot is held in an overcorrected position by a cast, strap, or splint, such as a Denis-Browne splint, for several weeks. Then a bivalved cast or Denis-Browne splint is commonly worn at night to hold the foot in a slightly overcorrected position. During the day, the child wears special shoes constructed to maintain the desired corrected or overcorrected position.

Treatment continues until walking and shoe wear show no residual or recurring deformity. Surgery and subsequent casting can continue well into adolescence.

A rigid deformity may require surgical intervention. This often includes correcting soft-tissue deformities, for example, lengthening of the heel cord and other tendons, dividing tight ligaments, and restoring bones to normal positions. In older children, bone wedges may be used to realign the bones of the foot. In infants and younger children, surgery is usually confined to the soft tissues so as not to interfere with bone growth. Following surgery, the foot is casted for several months.

Nursing Management Following each application of straps or cast, the nurse assesses the infant's toes for color, sensation, and motion to ensure that the cast or strapping is not too tight. The nurse explains to the parent the rationale for petalling the cast, the importance of frequent diaper changes with a long-leg cast, and the use of plastic pants and plastic wrap to protect the upper edges of the cast from soiling, and instructs the parent about skin care and general care for an infant in a cast.

The infant who is learning to walk must be prevented from attempting to stand, which might damage the foot or cast. The nurse and parent provide stimulating activities to distract the infant. A restraint may also be necessary.

If passive stretching exercises are part of the treatment, the nurse might be the person who teaches the parent how to do them. The nurse then assesses the parent's performance, explains the purpose and desired result of the exercises, and recommends appropriate times to do them.

If surgery is required, the parent might feel guilty and inadequate because nonsurgical intervention was not effective. The nurse who is sensitive to this possibility can help the parent to verbalize such feelings. The parent may need support during frequent visits to the doctor, clinic, or hospital, which can become time-consuming and difficult, depending on the family situation.

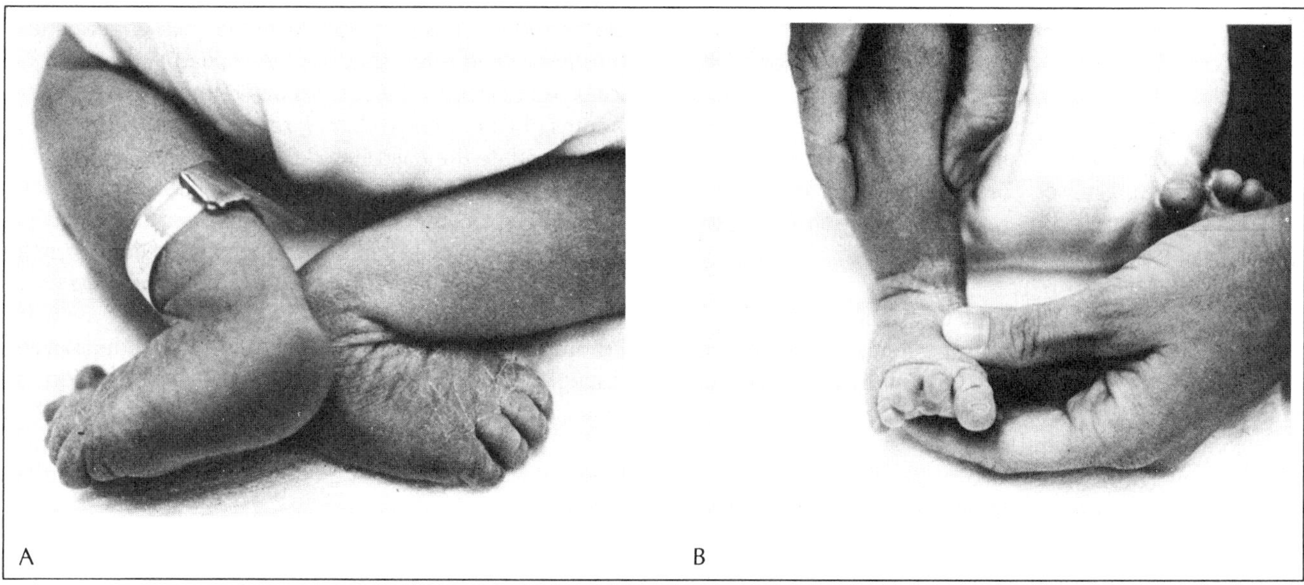

Clubfoot (talipes equinovarus). *A.* With infant in a supine position. *B.* To identify clubfoot, the nurse moves the foot to the midline; resistance indicates clubfoot. (From Olds B, London ML. Ladewig PA: *Maternal-Newborn Nursing.* 2nd ed. Addison-Wesley, 1984, p. 875.

The cast makes the infant somewhat difficult to hold and care for. This influences and occasionally interferes with the parent-child relationship. Assessment and interventions to prevent interference with the parent–child relationship are important nursing functions.

To increase success, treatment must be initiated soon after diagnosis, at a time when the parent is adjusting to the distressing fact that the infant has a deformity. The nurse plays an important role in supporting the parent during initial decision making about treatment choices. By helping the parent to express concerns, providing answers to questions, and maintaining a positive and supportive attitude, the nurse helps the parent to establish coping behaviors necessary during the initial treatment and long follow-up required for the infant with clubfoot.

Congenital Dislocated Hip

Congenital hip dysplasia or the potential for its occurrence is present, although not always diagnosed, at birth. In congenital hip dysplasia, one or both of the femoral heads is displaced from the acetabulum or acetabula. The cause is unknown, but the following factors seem to be relevant:

Familial tendency.

Laxity of the hip joint capsule and associated ligaments.

Breech presentation at birth.

Postnatal positioning. There is low incidence in societies where neonates' legs are maintained in a position of flexion and abduction (for example, in Central Africa, China, and India) and high incidence where neonates' legs are held in a position of extension and adduction (for example, in northern Italy and in Germany and among the Navajo Indians and Canadian Eskimos).

Dislocated hip is one of the most common congenital deformities in the western world. It occurs in approximately 1.5 in 1000 live births (Salter, 1983), and it occurs in girls eight times more often than in boys. Both hips are affected in one-half of the cases (Salter, 1983). Deformity that develops in utero instead of after birth is more severe. Often, the hip is not dislocated at birth but merely shows a tendency to dislocate.

Congenital dislocated hip may be manifested as (a) preluxation, or instability, in which the femoral head can be dislocated by manipulation; (b) subluxation, in which the femoral head has some contact with the acetabulum but has migrated laterally and upward; or (c) dislocation, in which the femoral head has no contact with the acetabulum but lies laterally and superior to it. With dislocation, the femoral head fails to exert appropriate pressure against the acetabulum. This results in both delayed development of the bony nucleus of the femoral head and failure of the acetabulum to form correctly (causing dysplasia). As a result, the femoral head becomes small and flattened and the acetabulum becomes shallow and oblique, eventually becoming small and flat. A secondary false acetabulum may eventually develop above and behind the original acetabulum. The adductor muscles of the hip shorten and contract.

Early detection and treatment can prevent these sequelae. Detection is often the result of nursing assessment of the infant (see Fig. 41-2). If dislocated hip is not diagnosed and treated in infancy, mastery of walking is frequently delayed and the child shows the clinical signs illustrated in Figure 41-3. Radiographic examination confirms the diagnosis.

Treatment initiated in early infancy is more effective and less complicated than later treatment. One-third to one-half of the children whose treatment is initiated after their first birthday experience various complications during life (Adams, 1976). When both hips are affected, the left hip is more resistant to treatment than the right hip (Tachjdian, 1972).

Medical and Surgical Treatment Treatment varies with the severity of clinical manifestations and the age of the child. During the neonatal period, when the adductor muscles have not yet shortened or contracted, treatment consists of carefully positioning and maintaining the hip in abduction with the head of the femur in the acetabulum for several months. This position is maintained by use of a splint such as the Frejka pillow or Paulik harness, or cast. The head of the femur presses against and thus encourages deepening of the acetabulum.

If the dislocation is not treated until 2–3 months but before 12–18 months of age, traction for a number of weeks prior to casting generally facilitates proper positioning. Traction stretches the tightened muscles, allowing better placement of the head of the femur in the acetabulum. Closed reduction is then done with the child under general anesthesia, and a hip spica cast is applied to maintain the abducted position. The cast usually remains on for several months, being removed and reapplied as necessary to accommodate the child's growth.

Once contracture of the adductor muscles and accompanying displacement of the femoral head has occurred, usually after the child's first birthday, more extensive treatment is necessary. If soft tissue and muscle contractures are not severe, bilateral traction may serve to reposition the femoral head and achieve abduction. Closed reduction and casting follow. If the contractures are severe, traction followed by closed or open reduction may yield satisfactory results. While in traction and immediately after cast application, the young child is often positioned on a Bradford frame.

During the course of treatment, periodic radiographs are taken to assess positioning of the head of the femur and depth of the acetabulum. Open reduction is necessary if closed reduction has been ineffective in reducing the dislocation. After reduction, a hip spica cast is worn until healing is complete. If treatment is not begun until after the age of 18 months, increasing rigidity of soft-tissue contractures, changes in the femur, and acetabular abnormality have progressed to a stage that is difficult to correct completely. Open reduction and such bone procedures as osteotomy and arthroplasty may be necessary. If congenital dislocated hip is untreated after the age of 7, treatment is very unsatisfactory and may be limited to preventing or treating degenerative changes and pain (Salter, 1983).

Complications are possible following treatment. Evidence of circulatory impairment or nerve paralysis may develop and must be relieved immediately. Fractures may occur during manipulation in closed or open reduction. If this happens, the fracture may have to be treated and allowed to heal before the dislocation can be corrected. Recurrence of dislocation increases with the age of the child at the time of initial treatment. Avascular necrosis of the head of the femur is another possible complication. It is treated by rest, either in a cast or with treatment similar to that used for Legg–Calvé–Perthes disease.

Nursing Management Nursing management for the child undergoing treatment for congenital hip dysplasia involves direct care and teaching related to splints, spica casts, and Bradford frames. The infant or child is growing and developing quickly, and so nursing and home care are likely to require many adjustments during the months of treatment.

A young infant in a hip spica cast may not be sent home with a Bradford frame. Since the child is not very mobile, the parent is able to keep the child properly positioned and the cast dry by propping the child on pillows. As the child grows, however, care may need to change. One family with a child sent home without a Bradford frame was not successful in keeping the infant and cast dry once the child reached 5 months of age. The cast became very soiled, and the child developed a skin rash. Upon readmission for cast removal, skin healing, and cast reapplication, the family and staff decided that the child should have a Bradford frame. The child's mother roomed in, learned about the frame, and relearned cast care. This was one situation in which the treatment plan needed to be revised to achieve treatment goals and prevent setbacks and complications.

Legg–Calvé–Perthes Disease

Legg–Calvé–Perthes disease, a form of osteochondrosis also known as coxa plana, is a condition produced by avascularity (insufficient supply of blood vessels) in the femoral head. This self-limiting disease, which has the potential for resulting in structural abnormality of the hip, lasts from 2 to 8 years. The cause is unknown. Legg–Calvé–Perthes disease occurs in boys four times more often than in girls. Onset usually occurs when the child is between 4 and 8 years of age, but children as young as 3 and as old as 11 have presented with the disease (Behrman and Vaughan, 1983; Salter, 1983). The disease may affect the entire capital (upper) epiphysis or only the anterior half or two-thirds.

Legg–Calvé–Perthes disease has four stages. A first stage has been described as the incipient, or synovitis, stage, which lasts from 1 to 3 weeks (Tachdjian, 1972). During this stage, there are soft tissue changes, with swelling and edema of the synovial membrane and joint capsule. Hyperemia (vascular engorgement) occurs and may cause some decalcification of the metaphysis adjacent to the epiphyseal plate. The first stage of Legg–Calvé–Perthes disease may or may not be distinguishable from transient synovitis.

The second, or avascular, stage is often the first stage noted and is characterized by interference with the blood supply to the head of the femur and death of osteocytes and bone marrow cells. The second stage is confirmed by radiographs. The ossification center of the head of the femur becomes soft and appears opaque on radiographs. With edema of surrounding joint tissues, the femoral head may be displaced laterally from the acetabulum. This stage lasts from several months to a year.

In the third stage, the regenerative or fragmentation stage, vascular and connective tissue invade the dead bone. The necrotic bone is absorbed and replaced by live though not yet calcified bone.

In the fourth and final stage, ossification (formation of bone substance) occurs. When this happens, the femoral head assumes the shape of the softened tissue. If it has become misshapened, then the newly ossified femoral head is also misshapened. The femoral head may be flattened, the acetabulum enlarged, and the femoral neck widened. If there is incongruity between the femoral head and the acetabular rim, degenerative changes will occur in adult life.

Early manifestations of Legg–Calvé–Perthes disease are a limp and pain, which occur during revascularization (Salter, 1983) and may be present for several months. The pain is usually referred to the knee, thigh, or groin. The child's complaints concerning the severity of pain vary, but severity usually increases with activity and decreases with rest. Symptoms might begin following an injury, but this is not generally the case. The child's antalgic limp is characterized by limited abduction and internal rotation of the hip. The combination of a history of pain, limp, and radiographic evidence of decreased bone cells in the affected femoral head lead to the diagnosis.

Prognosis varies and is related to several factors. First, the earlier the onset, the more favorable the prognosis, since younger children have more cartilage and less osseous bone and thus less risk of deformity. Second, prognosis is better if less than half of the femoral head is involved. Third, the earlier and more effectively the child is treated, the better the outcome.

Medical and Surgical Treatment The goal of medical treatment is to minimize or prevent damage and deformity to the femoral head and keep it congruous with the acetabulum until healing occurs naturally. Some children are merely monitored for proper healing. For others the femoral head is maintained in the acetabulum in a position of moderate abduction. Definitive treatment may or may not involve surgery.

An initial period of bed rest may be followed by application of a cast or brace with the resulting avoidance of weight bearing. If contractures are present as a result of the child's favoring the leg during the initial phases of disease, bilateral traction may be necessary to decrease muscle spasm and return full range of motion to the hip. Sometimes, the child wears a brace during the day, but traction or a bivalved cast might be used to maintain the proper position of the hip during the night.

Children under the age of 4 years, who are more likely to heal without deformity, may be treated with traction until full range of motion is attained in the hip. After that, they might be ambulatory, without cast or brace, but are restricted from strenuous physical activity.

If a cast or brace is selected for treatment, the child's affected leg is maintained so that the femoral head is seated correctly in the acetabulum. A full leg hip spica cast may be used to maintain the legs in abduction. A brace that elevates the affected limb and causes weight bearing on the ischial tuberosities is another means of preventing weight bearing by the head of the femur. An alternative is a sling or stirrup that fits and holds the affected leg up in a flexed position. The child with a brace or sling can ambulate, often with the aid of crutches. This method demands a high degree of cooperation from the child.

The child wears the brace or casts until the bone has reossified, which usually takes about 2 years. If only part of the femoral head is affected, the brace may be worn for less than a year.

Surgical intervention is needed if conservative methods of treatment do not keep the femoral head abducted adequately, if there is incongruity between the reossified head of the femur and the acetabulum, or if conservative treatment is likely to be exceptionally protracted. Whatever surgical procedure is chosen, its goal is to ensure that the acetabulum covers the femoral head and keeps it abducted.

Nursing Management Once the femoral head has been positioned correctly, pain ceases and the child, being comfortable, may also be unconvinced that treatment is necessary. Because the child at the time of diagnosis is likely to associate disease and its accompanying restrictions with punishment, a major nursing goal is to ensure cooperation and understanding of treatment. The nurse may serve as a resource or refer the family to community agencies for additional teaching, answers to questions, reassurance, and support.

Children quickly adapt to wearing treatment devices and may achieve a surprising degree of activity. One 3-year-old was so mobile that his mother refused to have the squeak of his brace repaired. The brace's noise, she said, enabled her to keep track of the child. An active child who wears braces that distribute weight to the ischial tuberosities has the skin in these areas subjected to unusual pressure and stress. The nurse instructs the parent to pay particular attention to skin care in this area.

Some children undergo surgery to shorten the period of immobilization. Others do not choose surgery but need it even though their compliance with treatment was excellent. These children might have to work through feelings of discouragement and sometimes anger or guilt. The parents of one 8-year-old hospitalized for repeated traction and bed rest tried to impress upon the boy that his noncompliance had caused the setback. Adequate teaching and follow-up should prevent such outcomes.

If the femoral head has residual damage (after healing), the hip does not function optimally. The nurse then tailors care to a child who will undergo repeated operations to fashion a congruous femoral head and acetabulum. These children sometimes experience degenerative changes or pain, necessitating corrective surgery for symptomatic relief at a later time.

Slipped Capital Femoral Epiphysis

Slipped capital femoral epiphysis is displacement of the head from the neck of the femur. Usually, the femoral neck moves upward and anteriorly while the capital epiphysis (head) becomes displaced posteriorly and downward. In the preslip phase, the epiphyseal plate widens, but the epiphysis is not displaced. Slippage is classified, according to the amount of displacement, as minimal (less than 1 cm), moderate (less than two-thirds the diameter of the femoral neck but greater than 1 cm), or severe (greater than two-thirds the diameter of the femoral neck). The slip may be acute or chronic.

The exact cause of slipped capital femoral epiphysis is unknown, but endocrine disturbance has been implicated. Slippage tends to occur in children who are either large and obese or tall and thin. It might be related to excess growth hormone or decreased sex hormone. Occasionally acute onset of symptoms follows trauma, but usually symptoms develop gradually.

Slipped capital femoral epiphysis usually occurs during periods of rapid growth in early adolescence (ages 13–16 in boys and 11–14 in girls). Boys are affected more frequently than girls, and a significant number of children, around 30%, suffer slippage on both sides, one side after the other (Salter, 1983).

The child with slipped capital femoral epiphysis complains of intermittent or constant pain and walks with a limp. The pain is described as being in the hip or groin area, the anteromedial aspect of the thigh, or the knee. Thigh or knee pain is generally referred from the hip. The child tends to hold the leg in external rotation, and the range of motion of the hip is restricted. Internal rotation, abduction, and flexion are limited and painful, and, when the hip is flexed, the thighs tend to go into external rotation. Lateral radiographs of the femoral neck confirm the diagnosis.

If the condition is untreated, further slippage can occur. The epiphysis eventually heals to the femoral neck, whether or not it is in an abnormal position. Hip abnormality and sometimes later degenerative changes result.

Medical Treatment Slipped capital femoral epiphysis is treated as an emergency to prevent further slippage. From the time of diagnosis until after treatment, the child does not bear weight on the affected side. Treatment varies according to the acuteness and extent of the condition. If slippage is minimal, the position may be acceptable. Threaded wires are passed into the femoral neck and the epiphysis to promote epiphyseal closure and prevent further slippage. This usually stabilizes the capital femoral epiphysis and prevents further deformity. If slippage is more extensive, the positions of the femoral head and neck must be improved prior to internal fixation with pin or wires.

A child who has experienced symptoms for less than 3 weeks is considered to have acute slippage. A gentle attempt might be made to return the epiphysis to a more normal position. This may be accomplished solely by placing the child in traction or by following traction with gentle manual manipulation. The epiphysis is then fixed into position with pins. A possible complication of this treatment is damage to the epiphyseal blood supply and subsequent avascular necrosis of the femoral head. The child ambulates with crutches until healing is complete.

With chronic slipped capital femoral epiphysis or with moderate to severe acute slippage, open correction (osteotomy) may be done. A wedge of bone is removed, either from the femoral neck or from a site distal to the lesser trochanter. Like the more conservative treatment, this procedure carries the risk of compromising blood supply to the femoral head. The epiphysis may or may not be pinned, depending on the surgical procedure. Some procedures seem to stimulate closure of the epiphyseal plate as the osteotomy heals. Casting or bracing may be all that is needed if epiphyseal closure is about to occur naturally.

Prognosis depends on the degree of slippage and response to treatment: the earlier the diagnosis, the better the prognosis. Complications, such as avascular necrosis of the femoral head, increase the risk of deformity. If healing results in some deformity and incongruity of the joint surfaces, degenerative arthritis or osteoarthritis may develop in adulthood.

Nursing Management Physical care for the child being treated for slipped capital femoral epiphysis might include traction care, cast care, and preoperative and postoperative care. Assessment related to involvement of the opposite hip is important because there is an increased risk that the second hip may become affected. Pain and inadequate range of motion are reported immediately, since rapid initiation of therapy improves the prognosis.

Typically, the child is a large boy in early adolescence who needs reassurance concerning body attractiveness and function and the long-range implications of the condition and its treatment (see Chapter 27).

Scoliosis

Scoliosis is lateral curvature of the spine (see Fig. 41-4). It involves both a lateral deviation from the midline and rotation of a series of vertebrae. Scoliosis may be functional, in which temporary curvature is caused by posture or position changes, or structural, in which curvature results in changes in the bony structure or the soft tissues of the spine or both.

In *functional scoliosis,* which is a postural habit, one long curve involves the thoracolumbar region of the spine. The child can voluntarily correct the curve, and the curve disappears when the child is recumbent. The child with a pelvic tilt due to leg length discrepancy, hip contracture, or other causes frequently has functional scoliosis. Functional scoliosis may also be seen in a child with poor posture. Functional scoliosis may have a neurotic cause, occurring as a conversion reaction. Functional curves do not become structural.

Structural scoliosis may begin at any point in childhood or adolescence. If untreated, tissue changes and deformity may last throughout life. Although the cause is usually unknown, structural scoliosis is sometimes caused by such conditions as vertebral abnormalities, paralysis, or muscle disorders.

Congenital structural scoliosis is caused by abnormal vertebrae. One or more vertebrae may be undeveloped on one side, forming a wedge between other vertebrae. Bars of bone also may keep one or more vertebrae from growing on one side. In infancy, rapid uneven growth of affected vertebrae can cause a severe curve to develop.

In paralytic scoliosis, paralysis causes an imbalance in the way muscles pull on the spine, resulting in curvature. Idiopathic scoliosis, or scoliosis with no recognizable cause, is the most common form of structural scoliosis, occurring in 5 of 1000 persons in the population (Salter, 1983). It has different manifestations in children of different ages. Infantile idiopathic scoliosis usually occurs in boys and frequently resolves by age 3 or 4. Severe curves are braced. Juvenile idiopathic scoliosis occurs in girls and boys and is usually treated with nonsurgical methods. Adolescent idiopathic scoliosis occurs in girls much more frequently than in boys. The curves of adolescent idiopathic scoliosis do not resolve without treatment.

By far the greatest number of children with idiopathic scoliosis have late-onset, adolescent, idiopathic scoliosis, usually occurring after age 10 and as right thoracic scoliosis. Girls are affected five to seven times more frequently than boys. Scoliosis tends to be familial, with incidence being much higher in families where another family member is affected than in the general population. Whites and blacks appear to be equally affected (Tachdjian, 1972). The deformity progresses during periods of growth and stabilizes when vertebral growth ceases. Slight increases (5°) in curvature may occur after childbirth and with aging.

The spine grows so as to maintain the body's balance. When a lateral curve develops, the spine and ribs rotate toward the convex part with the spinous processes rotating toward the concavity of the curve. A compensatory curve develops to maintain erect posture (see Fig. 41-4A). The abnormal forces pressing on the growing spine cause vertebrae to become wedge shaped. They become narrower toward the inside, or concave, side of the curve and wider and thinner on the outside, or convex, side of the curve. Disks undergo degenerative changes. Muscles and ligaments are contracted and thickened on the concave side and thin and atrophied on the convex side of the curve.

Ribs rotate backward on the convex side of the curve, forming a hump. This hump may be mild or so severe that it appears to come to a point in the back and thus is called "razor back." Ribs rotate forward on the concave side, leading to a prominence of the anterior chest wall and the breast. The sternum also rotates and may be displaced laterally from the midline. The thoracic cavity becomes asymmetric. This in severe cases may affect lung ventilation on the convex side, and may disturb cardiac function. With a curve of 50% or more, vital capacity can be affected, and a curve of 100% or more can cause rapid breathing or hypoxia. Pulmonary hypertension and cor pulmonale can result. Very severe scoliosis can be painful, but pain is not common in children, although back pain might occur subsequent to degenerative changes.

After clinical and radiographic examination, curvature is classified according to location, direction, angle, and the degree and direction of vertebral rotation. The age of the child at onset and the type and degree of curvature are major factors affecting the prognosis. The younger the child is at the onset of scoliosis, the more severe the deformity is likely to be. Generally, lumbar scoliosis has a much more favorable prognosis than thoracic scoliosis, which may progress to a sharp, unsightly curve.

Initially, the child almost always has complaints related to asymetric appearance, not to symptoms. Many cases are found during chest radiographs, intravenous pyelograms, well-child screening in schools, and routine physical examinations. Although early diagnosis and treatment do improve the prognosis, prognosis cannot be determined with accuracy for a given child. Some curves cease to progress, whereas others progress rapidly and become severe.

Medical and Surgical Treatment For functional scoliosis, no treatment is necessary unless the curve is marked, in which case postural exercises or correction of hip deformity or leg length discrepancy may be done. Structural scoliosis is treated as early as possible to prevent or lessen progression of the curve. This discussion will focus on treatment of structural adolescent idiopathic scoliosis.

Structural scoliosis may be treated conservatively with exercises and frequent follow-up; with a brace or cast to stretch the spine, relax pressure on the vertebrae, and allow more normal growth; or with spinal fusion to stabilize the spine. Exercises improve posture and help to maintain flexibility of the spine. They may consist of general exercises, bending toward the outside of the curve, and stretching the inside of the curve. Passive stretching exercises are sometimes used, and the child is taught to breathe deeply to improve chest expansion.

For moderate or mild scoliosis, a brace or cast may be worn to provide distraction forces between the head and pelvis and lateral pressure on the convex side of the curve or curves. A Milwaukee brace is frequently used (see Fig. 41-9) and is worn until growth is complete or until another form of treatment is started. The brace is used extensively if the child can be counted on to wear it full-time for as long as it is needed. To be as effective as possible, the brace must be worn for 23 hours a day. It is removed for hygiene and skin care only. A brace can be used to treat curves of less than 40° and is usually worn for several years.

Gradual weaning from the brace begins after growth is complete. The adolescent first removes the brace for a few hours a day, then may go to school without it, and eventually stops wearing it altogether. Periodic follow-up and radiographs enable the physician to determine whether correction is being maintained without the brace.

Spinal fusion stabilizes the spine and arrests progression of the curve. Indications for spinal fusion are cosmetically severe curvature in an adolescent, progressive curvature in a younger child after failure of conservative measures or with potential for complications, and backache that cannot be relieved. Before spinal fusion is done, a cast, brace, or traction may be used to achieve as much correction as possible.

The child with severe scoliosis may have an anterior fusion several weeks before posterior fusion and instrumentation. Through a thoracotomy incision, the anterior portions of compressed, misshapen disks are removed. After disk removal, the spinous processes are stripped to cancellous bone and grafts from a sacrificed rib or donor may be positioned. A chest tube is placed postoperatively, as surgery involves the thoracic cavity when a thoracic curve is fused.

During posterior spinal fusion, the major curve is fused. Fusion encompasses the vertebrae at each end of the curve, to prevent progression. Cancellous bone is exposed, and grafts from the iliac crest, spine, or a donor are added. After healing, mobility is lost in the fused portion of the spine, but the progression of deformity is arrested. Spinal fusion may be done with instrumentation, such as Harrington rods, Dwyer instrumentation, or Luque wires, any of which adds stability and is more effective in correcting curvature than preoperative traction, bracing, or casting.

Harrington rods are telescoping metal rods that, when positioned and anchored on the concave side of the curve, are expanded to provide maximal, safe straightening of the curve. Luque wires are relatively thin and flexible and are threaded through the spinal processes and wrapped around the fusion site and a vertical stable rod. Dwyer instrumentation is applied through an anterior approach; a series of screws are attached to the vertebrae, and a cable is passed through and attached to the screws to maintain proper straightening.

Postoperatively, the spine is immobilized until the fusion is stable. The child is on bed rest until initial healing has begun. Any twisting or bending of the back is scrupulously avoided. The child is often on a turning frame, such as a Stryker frame. Because of the greater stability of instrumentation, the child with fixation devices such as Luque wires or Dwyer instrumentation often is not on a frame but is log-rolled in bed. A child with Luque wires is usually out of bed early in the postoperative period. After about 10 days to 2 weeks, most treatment plans involve removal of stitches and the application of a cast or brace. A localizer cast or silastic-jacket-type brace may be worn to stabilize the fused area and maintain some distraction between the occiput and iliac crests. Radiographs are taken to see if the desired correction has been maintained. If healing and position under the cast are satisfactory, the child can be made ready for discharge and home care. Some children can be ambulatory after discharge, while others require bed rest at home. The child receives periodic medical evaluation and recasting as necessary, usually 3 months after surgery. The child usually is immobilized in the cast or brace for at least 3 months or until healing is complete, at around 6 months.

Nursing Management Teaching is an ongoing nursing responsibility, especially for the child who is undergoing conservative treatment on an outpatient basis. The nurse teaches prescribed treatment routines, determines the child's and parent's understanding of these, and then tries to obtain, on return visits, an honest record of the child's compliance (see Chapter 29). Since it is the child who must do the exercises or wear the brace, and since the child is usually at an age of growing independence, compliance with treatment is primarily determined by the child's motivation and understanding. The nurse gives the parent information needed to reinforce teaching and assist the child with a realistic assessment of compliance.

The child may be expected to do breathing and stretching exercises for the back. Although many children and adolescents believe in the importance of exercises and work them into their daily routine, others confess, usually years later, that they rarely performed their exercises. The child who does not wear an external appliance, such as a brace or cast, may have difficulty believing that a problem exists. Therefore, the nurse needs to reinforce teaching on each return visit.

If the child is to wear a brace, the nurse assesses the child's acceptance of the brace and reinforces teaching about the need for cooperation. If lack of cooperation is identified early, the health care team can consider other approaches to treatment before the deformity has much time to worsen. For example, treatment might begin with a cast that cannot be removed, and the brace might be introduced when the child has accepted the need for treatment. Another alternative is to allow the child to go to school without the brace at first so that the child can become accustomed to the brace gradually.

Compliance is especially difficult for the child who views appearance or athletic participation as more important than a straight back. In teaching the child about activity restrictions, the nurse emphasizes that exercise and activity are very beneficial to the child wearing a Milwaukee brace. Strenuous gymnastics and contact sports are not appropriate, however, as they may endanger the safety of the child and others.

When the child is ready to listen to specific teaching about the brace, the nurse instructs the child about wearing it 23 hours a day and removing it only for hygiene and skin care. The nurse teaches the child how to assess and care for the skin. The child also learns how to check the brace, tighten any loose screws, and determine whether the brace is being outgrown, necessitating adjustment. Without pulling down the top of the brace, the child should be able to lift the chin to one to three finger breadths above the throat mold. When the treatment period is over, and during weaning from the brace, the child may need to learn exercises for little-used muscles.

A child wearing a body cast has many needs similar to those of the child in a Milwaukee brace. Acceptance of altered appearance and care of the skin and cast are areas of concern. Clothing needs to be large and loose fitting. After cast application, the nurse assesses neurologic function, particularly in the hands, and reports any altered sensations or signs of impairment immediately.

If the child is to undergo spinal fusion, extensive preoperative preparation is necessary. (General preoperative preparation is discussed in Chapter 29; a nursing care plan for a child undergoing spinal fusion is included at the end of this chapter.) The nurse ensures that the child is prepared for such experiences as being cared for in an intensive care unit, bivalving a body cast with a cast saw, and immobilization on a turning frame or bed. The child and nurse practice the turning routine to be used postoperatively. If log rolling is to be used, the child practices lying in a bed, being turned like a log, and being placed on a fracture bedpan. The child who will be on a Stryker frame or CircOlectric bed postoperatively needs to be reassured about the safety of the frame and must experience being turned on it before the operation.

Postoperatively, the child is dependent, immobilized, and has experienced a large blood loss. The nurse therefore seeks to reduce the ill effects of these stressors.

Serious postoperative complications are possible. Nursing care includes a careful assessment of cardiopulmonary function, particularly blood pressure, pulse, and respiration. The nurse also monitors hemoglobin and hematocrit values and administers transfusions, as ordered. Elastic stockings help ensure adequate venous return. Auscultation of breath sounds is part of any nursing assessment. The nurse keeps in mind that the child is immobilized, has undergone a lengthy operation, and has an altered thoracic cavity due to correction of the deformity. Coughing and deep breathing, in addition to turning every 2 hours, are crucial. If the child has a chest tube, the nurse monitors the apparatus and assesses the lungs for atelectasis. The nurse inspects the incision frequently, and reports any bleeding beyond a slight oozing of blood in the initial postoperative period.

After manipulation of the vertebral column during surgery, altered neurologic function and paralysis are serious possible complications. Paralysis of the legs can occur following inadvertent injury or overstretching of nerves. The nurse carefully observes and documents color, sensation, and motion in all extremities and reports changes immediately. Prompt relief of stress on the nerves can reverse neurologic compromise and prevent lifelong sequelae.

Immobility may cause gastrointestinal, urinary, and integumentary complications (see Chapter 29). Gastrointestinal function often returns sluggishly after spinal fusion. The child usually has a nasogastric tube at first, and fluids are started very slowly after the return of bowel function. Rectal suppositories may be needed to prevent constipation. Urinary function is monitored, and the child often has an indwelling catheter in the initial postoperative period. Careful positioning and care of the skin over bony prominences, and especially the back, buttocks, heels and elbows, should prevent skin discomfort and breakdown.

Postoperative back pain is at first severe, but after the first few days, is often less severe than pain at the donor site or pain from flatulence. Pain is significant for the child who must be out of bed in the early postoperative period.

To combat weakness for the child who remains in bed, the nurse teaches the child to perform muscle-setting exercises and as much self-care as possible. The nurse involves the child in unit activities when the child feels well enough.

Getting up, when allowed, must be gradual to avoid dizziness and collapse. A tilt table or CircOlectric bed is sometimes used to accustom the child slowly to being upright. A child progressing directly from bed rest to sitting in a chair requires special attention from the nurse, as blood loss, bed rest, and pain all contribute to the potential for dizziness or fainting. The child may be discharged after becoming ambulatory in the hospital, provided that radiographic examination shows that correction is being maintained and the fused area is not compromised. Before discharge, the nurse instructs the child to avoid strenuous activity until healing is complete.

Kyphosis

Kyphosis (hunchback) is an exaggerated posterior curvature of the spine. The deformity may be functional or structural, and may occur at any level of the spine. Functional, or postural, kyphosis is caused by habitual slouching. Structural kyphosis, in which vertebrae become wedge shaped, may be congenital or acquired. Causes of structural kyphosis include myelomeningocele, tuberculosis of the spine, spinal tumors, and osteochondrosis of the vertebrae (Scheuermann's disease, or juvenile kyphosis).

Children with myelodysplasia or a residual neurologic deficit following myelomeningocele repair may have kyphosis severe enough to interfere with brace wearing and trunk support. The defect caused by Scheuermann's kyphosis, which usually begins at puberty, progresses, and eventually heals in a fixed position, remains throughout life. The child with a fixed deformity may experience back pain during growth. With cessation of growth, back pain is less common. Low lumbar disk degeneration may occur in adulthood, particularly if the site of the kyphosis is low or long, affecting the lumbar region of the spine.

Medical and Surgical Treatment Some children with severe fixed deformities require surgery for correction. A child with myelodysplasia may undergo spinal fusion and sometimes fixation of the spine with screws. The usual medical treatment for kyphosis, however, is application of a brace. A Milwaukee brace may be worn 23 hours a day until straightening of the spine occurs (for example, healing of Scheuermann's kyphosis). The brace then may be used only at night. Sometimes, exercises and sleeping on a firm surface without a pillow are all that is needed to minimize deformity. For the many children for whom kyphosis is a postural habit, treatment consists of exploring the reasons for bad posture and teaching the child how to maintain good posture.

Nursing Management Nursing management for the child requiring a brace or spinal fusion is discussed in earlier sections about braces and scoliosis. The child who has undergone myelomeningocele repair can have difficulty with proper skin coverage after spinal fusion. Postoperative assessment of the skin and prevention of pressure on this skin are essential.

The child with functional kyphosis needs help in exploring reasons for poor posture. For example, many girls who are experiencing the body changes of puberty might slouch to disguise such changes as breast development. Others seem to feel that encouraging an exaggerated curve of the spine makes breasts appear larger or shoulders more pronounced. The nurse allows the child to express feelings, honestly discusses how the child can become more attractive with correct posture, and helps the child to feel more comfortable about body changes. The nurse can also teach the child how good posture benefits body mechanics and function.

Leg Length Discrepancy

Leg length discrepancy may be so mild that it is noticed only when fitting and hemming clothing or so severe that it causes a limp or functional scoliosis if the child walks or stands without a corrective wedge under the foot of the shorter leg. Unequal leg length is a common skeletal problem that has many causes. Among them are

1. Congenital anomalies, such as a shortened, absent, or hypoplastic limb; dislocated hip; hemihypertrophy; or localized giantism
2. Skeletal tumors that result in shortening of the affected leg
3. Infection, which can retard or cause excessive growth
4. Legg–Calvé–Perthes disease, in which damage to the femoral head or corrective osteotomy may retard growth
5. Slipped capital femoral epiphysis, in which premature fusion or pinning may result in shortening
6. Trauma, which can cause growth to slow, cease, or speed up
7. Neuromuscular disease, paralysis, or nerve damage in one leg
8. Abnormal decrease or increase in circulation that affects bone growth

Any abnormality or defect that affects only one leg can cause leg length discrepancy.

Medical and Surgical Treatment Treatment varies with the nature and severity of the deformity. No treatment is needed for a minor leg length discrepancy. A lift placed in the shoe can often prevent a limp and strain on the hip. More severe discrepancy may require stopping or retarding growth in one leg, shortening the longer leg, or lengthening the shorter leg. The discrepancy may be so severe that a prosthesis is necessary for the shorter leg. Partial amputation may be needed to fit a prosthesis properly. One goal of treatment is equality of the level of the knees. This goal may influence the choice or site of any surgical procedure.

If the child is not yet skeletally mature, carefully timed interference with the epiphyseal plate of the femur in the longer leg can slow growth in the longer leg, enabling the shorter leg to "catch up." Growth in the longer leg can be stopped by fusing the epiphysis with a bone wedge or screws. Stapling may also retard or stop growth.

After skeletal maturity, the longer leg can be shortened. Although this can be done at any time, there is the risk that surgery will stimulate further growth in the longer limb of the child who is not fully grown.

Leg lengthening is done by separating the diaphysis and applying distraction. An intermedullary rod is often inserted to maintain alignment and stability of the bone fragments. A bone plate may be in place, and grafts may be used to bridge the gap created, especially if the gap is as large as 5 cm. Soft-tissue release is included with some leg lengthening procedures to reduce pressure on bone fragments, knee, nerves, and vessels.

Distraction can be applied with skeletal traction or an apparatus such as the Wagner apparatus. The Wagner apparatus consists of outrigger rods attached to pins inserted into bones of the leg. It can be adjusted postoperatively to increase or decrease distraction. Traction or distraction apparatus remains in place until healing permits its removal and application of a cast. The cast may be applied around the intact pins. The time involved in healing depends on the extent of lengthening and the presence or absence of complications.

Leg lengthening procedures have many potential complications. Infection at pin sites may heal after pin removal and is usually not as grave a complication as infection at the surgical site. Muscle weakening, vascular insufficiency, skin breakdown, and sciatic or peroneal nerve palsy can accompany the stretching of soft tissues. Stretching can also interfere with function of the knee after femoral lengthening or function of the foot after tibial lengthening. The lengthened bone can be bowed, malaligned, weak, or in need of additional grafting.

Nursing Management Nursing management for the child who is undergoing surgical correction of leg length discrepancy involves standard preoperative and postoperative care. The nurse observes strict aseptic technique in wound care, monitors the wound for drainage and odor, assesses circulatory status of the foot, and provides care related to immobilization.

Infection can threaten the skin over the graft and the bone itself. The nurse observes for interference with circulation and innervation by checking color, sensation, motion, and pulses in the foot. The nurse records and reports pain, administers analgesics, and uses other noninvasive measures to relieve pain. Postoperative care also includes observing the appearance of the leg and the equipment.

The child who undergoes surgical treatment for leg length discrepancy has had a chronic functional and cosmetic deformity (see Chapter 30). Although a limp or shoe lift seems like a minor inconvenience, it may be very significant for the growing, often style-conscious child. Some leg length deformities are severe enough to prevent ambulation independent of aids such as crutches. During preoperative teaching, the nurse notes any alterations in body image and offers appropriate reassurance (see Chapter 27). Since surgical correction is planned and scheduled in advance, the child has the opportunity to learn about, see, and touch any apparatus that will be in use during the postoperative recovery period (see Chapter 29). The recovery period can be lengthy, particularly if such complications as infection require repeated hospitalizations. The child needs consistent, well-organized care that integrates opportunities for diversion, learning, creativity, and growth.

Torsional Deformities

Torsional deformities of the femur or tibia are related to embryonic development and intrauterine positioning, and are common in neonates. Often, there is a family history of torsional deformities. After the neonatal period, the child's position, activity, and growth usually cause the bones to assume adult configurations spontaneously.

Femoral anterior torsion is relatively common and leads to in-toeing. Bowing of the legs is noted, and the hindfoot may compensate with a valgus deformity. Spontaneous improvement does not seem to occur after the child is 8 years of age.

Medial tibial torsion usually occurs in conjunction with genu varum (bowlegs). The child toes in and may have some femoral antetorsion. Medial tibial torsion usually is not an isolated condition.

Medical Treatment Since torsional deformities in most children resolve spontaneously, infants usually receive no treatment. If the parent is concerned about the deformity, passive exercises can be taught that decrease soft-tissue contractures that may be maintaining the deformity. With femoral antetorsion, the parent stretches the infant's hip in the direction of external rotation. With medial tibial torsion, the foot is moved to an abducted and everted position.

After age 2, pronounced deformities that are not resolving may be braced. Because early bracing could encourage excessive overcorrection for femoral antetorsion, the brace is worn only at night. A bivalved hip spica cast may be worn to hold the hips in external rotation, flexion, and abduction. The child with tibial torsion may wear a Denis-Browne splint at night. Bracing at night is continued for a long time, as bone changes slowly in response to the stress of positioning. Rotation osteotomies may be done in children over age 8 to prevent further compensatory deformities or degenerative changes in adult life.

Nursing Management The nurse reassures the parent of an infant that the torsional deformity is expected to improve with growth and weight bearing. If stretching exercises are indicated, the nurse may teach the parent the normal range of motion of the hip or foot and how to carry out the exercises gently. The exercise routine, which is carried out several times daily, consists of repeated stretching in which the hip is put into external rotation or the foot abducted and everted. The nurse also teaches the parent about night splints and, if indicated, surgery.

The Child With a Musculoskeletal Injury

Fractures

The factors affecting bone growth in children help explain differences between fractures in children and adults. Bones undergo much remolding as children grow, and there is some natural realignment of poorly united bone fragments as the growing bone responds to the pulls of muscles and stresses for bearing weight. Fractures in young children and fractures that occur relatively close to the epiphyseal plate have more potential for this spontaneous correction. Spinal fractures and fractures in a plane other than the direction of joint movement do not realign spontaneously.

Fractures in children tend to heal more rapidly than those in adults. The blood supply to the bone is rich; the periosteum is thick; and the osteogenic activity is high. As age increases, the time involved in healing also increases. For example, a femoral shaft fracture in a neonate that would heal in 3 weeks heals in an 8-year-old in 8 weeks and in a 12-year-old in 12 weeks (Salter, 1983).

Children's bones, because of their greater flexibility, react to stress in different ways from those of the adult. They deform more before breaking, and so they may simply bend, buckle, or break incompletely. Forces not intense enough to cause a fracture can lead to a bent bone. The bones most commonly bent are the fibula and ulna.

A *buckle fracture,* also called a torus fracture, occurs most frequently in young children. The bone fails with compression forces, usually near the metaphysis. The fracture is seen as a raised or bulging area. In a *greenstick fracture,* forces cause a break through the periosteum and compact bone on one side, while merely bending the other side. Greenstick fractures are commonly seen in the forearm. Despite the flexibility of their bones, children are subject to other types of fractures in which the bone is broken completely.

Fractures that affect the epiphyseal plate can interrupt and alter growth. The implications of these fractures vary depending on the area of the epiphyseal plate affected. The Salter-Harris classification of epiphyseal plate injuries, pictured in Figure 41-11, is commonly used to describe these injuries. One third of skeletal trauma in children involves injury to the epiphyseal plate (Ibiahim, 1984). The degree to which these injuries affect future bone growth is related to (a) the degree of injury to the germinal layer of the

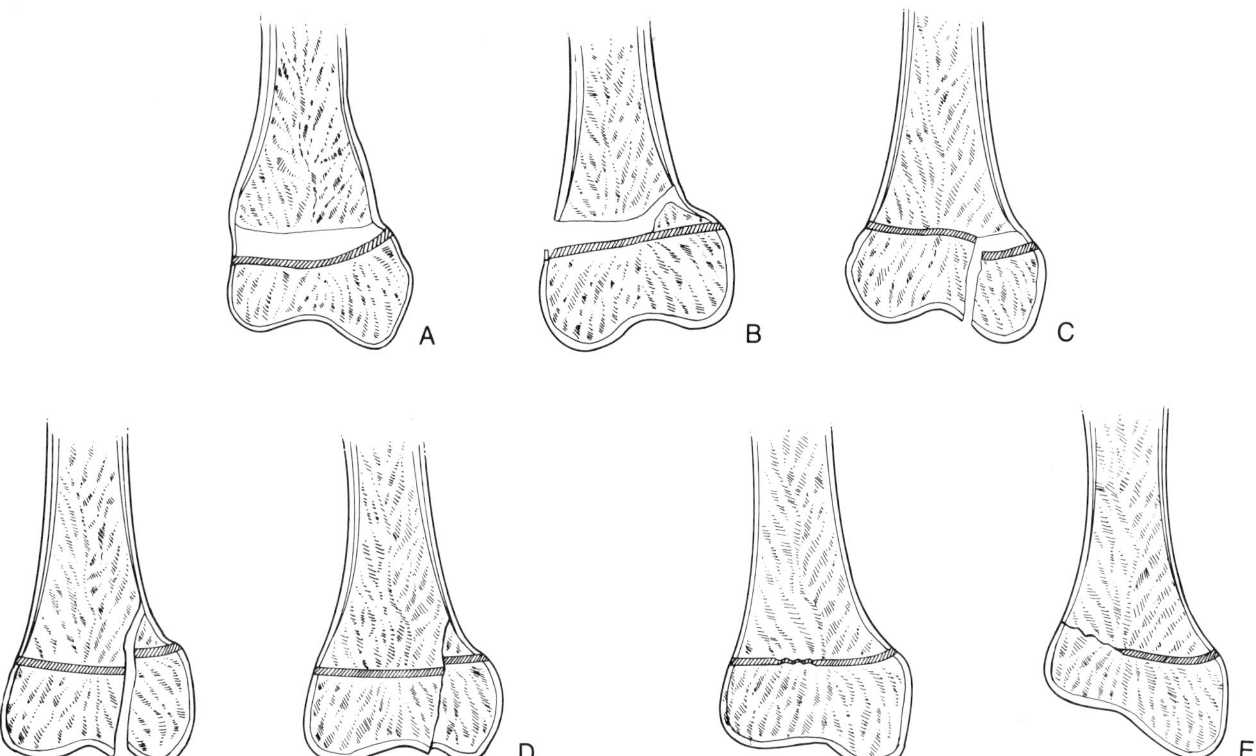

Figure 41-11 Salter-Harris classification of injuries involving the epiphyseal plate (growth plate). *A.* Type I injury: separation of the epiphysis. *B.* Type II injury: fracture separation of epiphysis. *C.* Type III injury: fracture of part of the epiphysis. *D.* Type IV injury: fracture of epiphysis and epiphyseal plate (left) and bony union causing premature closure of the plate (right). *E.* Type V injury: crushing of epiphyseal plate (left) that results in premature closure of the plate on one side (right).

epiphyseal plate and (b) the degree of bony bridge formation between the epiphysis and the metaphyseal area of the diaphysis during fracture healing.

In a Type I injury, the fracture passes through the hypertrophic layer of the epiphyseal plate, leaving the germinal layer intact but with tenderness at the epiphyseal plate. This type of fracture may be mistaken for a sprain. A stress film or comparison roentgenogram can show a gap at the fracture site on the affected side.

A Type II fracture occurs with a shearing or tearing force and is a common epiphyseal plate injury. The germinal layer of the epiphyseal plate and the circulation to the epiphysis remain intact, and so this fracture heals well after it is reduced and immobilized.

An intra-articular shearing force usually causes a Type III fracture. Because this fracture extends into the joint, reduction must establish a regular and congruous joint surface to prevent later joint degeneration. An open reduction with internal fixation may be necessary.

Because a Type IV fracture line passes through the metaphysis, epiphyseal plate, and epiphysis, a bony bridge may form prematurely, fusing the metaphysis and epiphysis. To prevent angular deformity and limb length discrepancy, no displacement or angulation are accepted during reduction and internal fixation of fracture fragments.

A Type V fracture, caused by severe compression force to the epiphyseal plate, crushes the germinal layer. This is a rare fracture and one that causes growth disturbance (Ibrahim, 1984).

Injury that stimulates blood supply to the epiphysis and thus to the epiphyseal plate, or to the metaphyseal area of the diaphysis, may lead to overgrowth of the affected bone. For this reason some fractures, particularly in the long bones, are set with some overriding of fracture fragments so that the healed bone will not be longer than the corresponding bone on the other side of the child's body.

Signs and symptoms of fracture depend on the type of fracture present and whether it affects the diaphysis, epiphyseal plate, or epiphysis. Generally, a fracture causes sudden sharp pain at the time of injury and tenderness at the site thereafter. Pain increases with movement and decreases somewhat with rest. The child usually cannot use the affected body part. Numbness and tingling in the extremity distal to the fracture site is a common occurrence.

There may be obvious deformity at the fracture site and abnormal positioning of the body part. Swelling varies, depending on the degree of soft-tissue damage and the displacement of bone fragments. There may be discoloration around the fracture site or frank bleeding from a wound communicating with a fracture. Bone fragments may be visible in *compound fracture,* which breaks the skin. A possible sign, not generally elicited because of the danger of further injury, is crepitus, grating felt or heard as bone fragments rub together.

Medical and Surgical Treatment Emergency treatment of fractures involves performing an initial assessment of bone injury and soft-tissue damage, preventing further injury, promoting comfort, and keeping the child NPO in case anesthesia or surgery is required. Any deformity is observed and, if only swelling is present, the area is gently palpated for the site of greatest tenderness. Color, sensation, and motion and pulses distal to the injury are monitored to detect neurologic or circulatory compromise. Splinting decreases both discomfort and the chance of further injury. A splint should immobilize the fracture site, including the joints above and below the injury. Outside the hospital or clinic, ingenuity may be needed to devise a splint using materials at hand (see Chapter 19). In the hospital, plaster may be molded to the area or an aluminum splint applied. A lower extremity fracture can be immobilized with a Thomas splint.

The fracture is immobilized after it has been properly reduced or realigned. The fracture may be realigned by (a) closed reduction, or external manipulation of the body part; (b) open reduction, or surgery and internal fixation; or (c) traction. After alignment, the body part is placed in a splint or cast. For proper immobilization, the joint above and the joint below a fracture are included in the cast. Internal fixation devices (rods, pins, or wires) might remain in the child unless they eventually irritate the skin, cause pain, or become superficial. Intermedullary rods frequently remain in. Screws and plates used as internal fixation devices are removed after initial healing if they are thought to weaken the bone.

Radiographs are used to monitor alignment and healing. They may be taken as often as weekly while the child is in traction preceding casting, and during the first few weeks following casting of fractures that are likely to lose alignment, such as displaced or greenstick fractures. Greenstick fractures may spring back to the position of injury, and other fractures may become displaced as swelling decreases and the cast becomes loose.

Follow-up assessment may be done every 3 months for the year following injury, particularly if leg length discrepancy is a risk. This allows early identification of complications of injury and fracture healing.

Nursing Management Fracture usually occurs while the child is engaged in active play or sports or as a result of an accident. In either case, the child is usually frightened by what has happened. The child who is injured in athletic activity often worries about the return of full function. The accident victim may feel in some way responsible for the injury and possibly the injury or even death of another person. The teaching done during emergency treatment may be hurried. All these circumstances may cause the child to understand and remember little of what is said. The nurse therefore repeats teaching and gives reassurances frequently to ensure the child's understanding of the injury and its treatment.

Nursing management may involve splint, cast, or traction care. Whatever treatment is used, the nurse continually monitors color, sensation, and motion in body parts distal to the fracture. Severe pain requires immediate assessment, as pain may indicate neurologic or circulatory compromise. Neurologic or vascular compromise necessitates immediate reporting to the physician and release from cast or traction. Preventing the complications of immobility and watching for signs and symptoms of infection are also essential.

Sprains, Strains, and Contusions

A *sprain* is a joint injury caused by pulling or tearing of a ligament. A *strain* is a muscle or tendon injury caused by stretching or overuse. A *contusion,* or bruise, is a skin and soft-tissue injury caused by a blow that does not break the skin. Although sprains, strains, and contusions make up most of the acute athletic injuries, epiphyseal injuries sometimes occur rather than sprains or strains in children.

Minor sprains cause tenderness at the point of injury and minimal swelling and loss of joint function, but no abnormal movement of the joint. Moderate sprains cause swelling, local hemorrhage, moderate loss of function, and joint pain, particularly with activity or weight bearing. A severe sprain, in which the ligament is completely torn, usually causes less pain than a moderate sprain, but there is severe swelling, hemorrhage, and abnormal joint movement.

The signs of a strain's severity differ, depending on whether the injury affects the point of muscle origin or tendon insertion. Bleeding occurs with an injured muscle belly. Pain and soft-tissue swelling, rather than bleeding, characterize tendon injury. Relatively little pain occurs at the time of tendon or ligament injury, and so complete tears of tendons or ligaments may at first be less obvious than muscle tears. For these reasons, strains or sprains involving the knee, Achilles tendon, finger, or shoulder may be difficult to diagnose unless the child reports that the disturbance in joint stability or function was preceded by a snapping, popping, or tearing noise (Garrick, 1981).

Medical and Surgical Treatment Early treatment reduces recovery time. Ice, compression, elevation, and rest are the emergency treatments for sprains, strains, and contusions. Twenty to thirty minutes of ice and compression applied immediately after the injury may reduce by half the time needed for recovery (Garrick, 1981). Except when surgical intervention is needed, ice, compression, elevation, and rest (ICER) are continued for 24–36 hours. A complete tear is surgically repaired.

During healing, muscle tone is maintained with muscle-setting exercises. After the injury heals and pain is gone, the child works up slowly to preinjury activity levels.

Nursing Management A nurse who witnesses an injury initiates first-aid treatment immediately. If ice is available, it is placed over the injury for at least 20 minutes. The area is wrapped so as to exert compression without interfering with circulation or innervation. While giving first aid, the nurse teaches the child and others who may be at the scene, including parents and coaches, the importance of applying ice and compression immediately to sprains, strains, or contusions.

During recovery, the nurse teaches the child muscle-setting exercises to maintain muscle tone and hasten the return to previous activity levels. The nurse cautions against returning to activities and sports too soon. Only when symptoms and signs have totally disappeared should the child resume strenuous activity. Children and even coaches sometimes try to rush the recovery period, thinking that activity can be resumed if it is not too painful. This could result in reinjury and an even longer recovery period.

Dislocations

Dislocation, or luxation, is displacement of the articular surfaces of a joint. Partial displacement is called subluxation. Dislocation of the femoral head occurs with severe trauma. Dislocation of the elbow and wrist are common in children. Posterior dislocation of the elbow usually results from a fall on the outstretched hand in which the radius and ulna are displaced posteriorly and upward. Dislocation of the wrist occurs commonly in young children who attempt to twist out of a parent's handclasp. Dislocation of the normal knee is not common.

Dislocation is very painful. Deformity at the joint may be obvious. There is often swelling, and joint motion is very painful and restricted. The child with a dislocated knee rarely needs treatment, as the knee usually reduces spontaneously when the leg is extended.

Medical treatment for dislocation is closed, manual reduction or open, surgical reduction. Nursing management depends on medical treatment and the clinical situation. The child and parent need reassurance and support until the joint is reduced. Some children need preparation for general anesthesia and surgery. After reduction of a dislocated elbow, the child rests the elbow, sometimes with a sling. A reduced dislocated hip may require casting or traction. A dislocated knee may be immobilized in a walking cylinder cast until tissues heal. After reduction, the nurse assesses the extremity for color, sensation, and motion to detect any neurologic or vascular compromise.

The Child With Skeletal Inflammation

Infection of the Bone

Infection of the bone, or osteomyelitis, occurs 3–4 times more often in boys than in girls. It usually originates with seeding of bacteria from the blood, but it may be an extension of a local infectious process or, as in a compound fracture, the invasion of microorganisms through an open wound.

The metaphysis of the distal portion of the femur and proximal portion of the tibia are the most frequent sites of osteomyelitis. The next most frequent sites are the proximal metaphysis of the femur and the distal metaphysis of the radius and humerus. Flat bones may also be involved. There is usually pus and necrosis in the metaphyseal area. Abundant vascularity and lowered rate of blood flow in the venous system of the metaphysis provide bacteria with a means of entry and a medium for growth. Purulent material elevates and eventually ruptures the periosteum, and pus surrounds the bone. The joint may become infected. If the infection progresses, pus causes thrombosis of blood vessels in the bone. This and the lifting of the periosteum disrupts blood supply, and the bone dies in affected portions. New bone is then formed around the dead bone by the periosteum. Pus escapes through sinuses, which form in the surrounding live bone. Cavities harboring bacteria, granulation tissue, and dead bone result, and the infection can become chronic.

Signs and symptoms vary considerably with the severity, duration, and location of an infection, and with the age of the child. Severe and constant pain is usual at the site of bone infection. The child may limp or fail to use an extremity. The area over the infection is tender to the touch. Once the periosteum ruptures and pressure exerted on the bone by pus is released, pain lessens. Pain is usually located over the metaphysis, as are local heat and swelling, which is a late sign.

Systemic signs of sepsis, including fever, vomiting, and even dehydration, may occur. The neonate may be irritable and fail to gain weight but may not be febrile. The white count is usually elevated, though it may be normal, even in a severely ill child. Characteristically, the white blood cell differential reveals a high percentage of neutrophils and a shift to the left in the leukocyte count. The sedimentation rate is elevated. As the infection progresses, radiographs reveal local tissue density and then new bone formation and radiolucency in areas of abscess. Dead bone appears dense and sharply outlined.

In a longitudinal study of children having osteomyelitis, Kylberg (1983) reported varying long-term effects on growth. Although many of the 22 children studied showed complete recovery, those who were younger at the time of infection tended to have the most serious sequelae.

Medical and Surgical Treatment Medical treatment for osteomyelitis is rigorous treatment with intravenous antibiotics. Antibiotics are frequently started as soon as blood specimens are withdrawn. Culture and sensitivity tests are done on local aspirates to identify the infectious microorganisms. Once identification is made, an appropriate antibiotic is given. Surgical treatment may be required to release the pressure of pus on the periosteum and to excise dead bone. If a correct diagnosis is not made promptly, the infection worsens and the child is likely to undergo surgical drainage, to experience fever and pain, and to need long-term antibiotic therapy.

Nursing Management Nursing care for the child with osteomyelitis centers around careful assessment of local and systemic signs and symptoms and provision of supportive care. Some children become very ill. The nurse ensures that blood for culture is obtained during temperature elevations. Treatment with intravenous antibiotics is prolonged, and lengthy hospitalization stresses both the child and family (see Chapters 27 and 29). Nursing care may involve bed rest together with a splint or traction to reduce pain.

Infection of the Joint

Infection of the joint, or septic arthritis, may originate from bacteria in the blood; direct extension of an infection, such as osteomyelitis; or direct inoculation from a wound. Infection causes the synovial membrane to produce increased amounts of synovial fluid, and the joint becomes distended. As infection progresses, pus may accumulate in the joint. Destructive and degenerative changes occur, and the joint may eventually dislocate if the joint capsule becomes very distended.

The infected joint is painful, warm, and swollen and has extremely limited range of motion. The symptoms are usually acute. Extremities are moderately flexed due to muscle spasms. If the lower extremities are affected, the child limps or may refuse to walk. Ineffective or late treatment, especially when a major joint is affected, might cause a serious, lifelong disability.

Medical and Surgical Treatment The joint is immobilized. Traction may be applied to relieve muscle spasm, decrease pain, and separate joint surfaces. A splint may be used to immobilize the wrist or ankle. The joint might be aspirated to identify the microorganism and determine which antibiotic will be effective. Systemic administration of antibiotics may control the infection. If it does not, the joint is surgically drained and irrigated with antibiotics. Eventually, range-of-motion exercises are started, but weight-bearing joints are protected from pressure until they again function normally. The child may need crutches temporarily. With early diagnosis and treatment, the prognosis for a return to normal joint function is good.

Nursing Management Nursing management involves caring for a child whose joint may be exquisitely painful, a child who is in traction and needing careful attention to the needs of any immobilized child. As pain and swelling decrease, the nurse teaches the child and family about the importance of continuing to follow the prescribed treatment regimen. Compliance is necessary for a full recovery.

The Child With a Disease of the Bone

Osgood–Schlatter Disease

Osgood–Schlatter disease is tendonitis of the distal portion of the patellar tendon with secondary hypertrophic new bone formation (osteochondrosis) on the proximal tibial tubercle. There is tenderness of the patellar tendon and excessive enlargement of the proximal tibial tubercle. Osgood–Schlatter disease occurs primarily in adolescent males who participate in sports. Symptoms usually follow a rapid growth spurt. The disorder is caused by trauma or repeated stress in the area of the patellar tendon. Soft-tissue swelling and small, free bone particles anterior and superior to the tuberosity are visible on radiographs. The patella may be displaced anteriorly. If the condition has not already resolved, it will do so when the epiphysis closes and the tubercle fuses to the diaphysis. The bony prominence of the tibial tuberosity may be somewhat deformed, which can make kneeling uncomfortable. Rarely, the tubercle fuses early, eventually causing genu recurvatum (hyperextension of the knee). The patella may remain higher on the affected side, causing it to dislocate laterally or contribute to degenerative arthritis.

The child experiences local pain in the anterior aspect of the knee, especially with running, jumping, squatting, use of stairs, and kneeling. Pain diminishes and may disappear with rest. There is excessive enlargement of the tibial tuberosity and thickening of the patellar tendon. No fluid is felt in the knee.

Medical and Surgical Treatment Treatment consists of restricting strenuous physical activities, such as sports, running, jumping, and long walks, for several months. This treatment is adequate in mild cases. In more severe cases, the knee is immobilized in a cylinder cast for several weeks. Strenuous exercise and sports are restricted for several months after cast removal. Anti-inflammatory agents injected into the affected tendon may provide symptomatic relief. Sometimes the tubercle is removed surgically.

Nursing Management The nurse usually sees children with Osgood–Schlatter disease in an outpatient setting. One of the nurse's major goals is to convince the active child of the need for activity restrictions. The child needs to understand the importance of curtailing physical activity for what may seem like a very long time. The nurse can emphasize that time out will prevent complications and help the child or adolescent reach maximum athletic potential in the future.

Osteogenesis Imperfecta

Osteogenesis imperfecta is one condition that results in pathologic bone fractures. Other such conditions include rickets, in which insufficient calcium salts are laid down in developing bone and newly formed cartilage, and malignant tumors affecting the bone (see Chapter 45).

Osteogenesis imperfecta is a connective tissue disorder. It primarily affects the bone, causing fractures to occur with minor stressors. It is usually inherited as an autosomal dominant trait, although it may be inherited as an autosomal recessive trait.

Osteogenesis imperfecta congenita is a severe form of osteogenesis imperfecta that is evident at birth because of multiple fractures that have occurred in utero or during delivery. Children with this form are often stillborn or die soon after birth. They occasionally live through childhood, but they are bedridden. *Osteogenesis imperfecta tarda* is a less severe form of the disease. With this type, some children experience fractures in infancy (gravis form). The fractures heal at the usual rate, but bones are likely to refracture because of disuse atrophy following immobilization.

Some children have a very mild form of the condition, and medical attention is sought because of delayed walking or a fracture. Other children have multiple fractures and may be mistaken for battered children. The extremities may have angular deformities due to fractures. Children experiencing fractures early in life often have shortened stature due to deformities of the legs, overriding of fractures, compression fractures of the spine, and kyphoscoliosis. There is usually little pain with the fractures of osteogenesis imperfecta because there is little soft-tissue trauma.

Other signs of osteogenesis imperfecta include blue sclera. This sign, which is present in almost all children with the disease, is caused by thinness and translucency of the whites of the eyes (sclerae). The color varies from blue-white to deep sky blue. The sclera immediately around the cornea may be white. This ring of white is called "saturn's ring." The outer edge of the cornea may be opaque.

The child's skin is thin, and the muscles have decreased tone. There may be subcutaneous hemorrhages, and any surgical scars are often wide. Ligaments are lax, and joints may have increased mobility. The patella may dislocate.

The forehead is broad, and the shape of the head may be similar to a helmet. There is a deficiency of dentin, and teeth break easily, have poor resistance to caries, and hold fillings poorly. Deafness may result because of otosclerosis or pressure on the auditory nerve.

Medical treatment for osteogenesis imperfecta mainly consists of treating fractures. Proper alignment of fractures may decrease deformity, and intermedullary rods help correct angulation in some children. Immobility is discouraged to lessen disuse atrophy and thus the likelihood of refracture.

Nursing management involves care of a chronically ill child with a deforming, debilitating, inherited condition (see Chapter 30). Nursing considerations vary from family to family because, among other reasons, the condition varies markedly in severity. Parents may be dealing with anger toward health professionals if the parents have been unjustly suspected of child abuse. The nurse allows for expression of feelings of anger or guilt.

Fragility of bones makes cautious handling of the child essential. Encouraging as much activity as possible during periods of immobilization can partially combat disuse atrophy.

Benign Tumors of the Bone

Many tumors and tumor-like conditions affect bone. Pain is a characteristic symptom of malignant tumors. It occurs occasionally with benign tumors, such as osteoid osteoma, and occurs when pathologic fractures result from tumor growth. Osteochondroma is a relatively common benign bone tumor in children. Tumors of the bone are treated to improve appearance or function or to lessen pain. Lesions may be excised if they cause compression on nerves, interfere with joint motion, cause pain, or are cosmetically unacceptable. After excision, any depression in the bone is filled in with chips of bone. Lesions that are potentially cancerous may be excised and the child followed closely.

Nursing care involves reassurance to the child and family concerned about malignancy and preoperative and postoperative care for the child undergoing surgery for excision of the tumor.

NURSING CARE PLAN Child Recovering From Spinal Fusion

Assessment Data

Carrie, a 13-year-old girl with a 70° curvature of the thoracolumbar spine, has undergone a posterior spinal fusion with insertion of Harrington rods. Donor bone was taken from the iliac crest. During surgery she received one unit of packed cells. Postoperatively, she spent the first 2 days in intensive care, but was then transferred to the nursing unit to which she was admitted preoperatively. She is on a Stryker frame. Her indwelling urinary catheter was removed and she has voided independently. Bowel sounds have returned.

Nursing Diagnoses and Goals

1. **Nursing diagnosis:** Potential for ineffective gas exchange.

   Long-term goal: Carrie will not have any respiratory distress or related problems.

   Short-term goals: (a) Carrie will take ten deep breaths and cough effectively every 2 hours. (b) Carrie's lungs will remain clear. (c) Carrie will be afebrile.

2. **Nursing diagnosis:** Potential alteration in tissue perfusion related to blood and fluid loss.

   Long-term goal: Carrie will be free of complications from cardiovascular compromise.

   Short-term goals: (a) Carrie's vital signs will be monitored for stability. (b) Drainage on dressings will be closely observed. (c) Alterations in hemoglobin and hematocrit values will be reported immediately.

3. **Nursing diagnosis:** Potential for decreased sensory perception related to extensive surgery.

   Long-term goal: Carrie will be free of neurologic difficulties.

   Short-term goals: (a) Carrie will wiggle toes and fingers when asked. (b) Carrie will correctly identify area of lower limb touched. (c) Carrie will have full range of motion in distal lower extremities.

4. **Nursing diagnosis:** Potential for alterations in comfort; postoperative pain.

   Long-term goal: Carrie will be relatively free of pain.

   Short-term goals: (a) Carrie will request relief before complaints or signs of pain are severe. (b) Carrie will say that she is less anxious and will trust that medication and comfort measures will alleviate pain.

5. **Nursing diagnosis:** Potential for alteration in patterns of elimination.

   Long-term goal: Carrie will resume normal elimination pattern.

   Short-term goals: (a) Carrie will void in adequate amounts. (b) Carrie will have regular, moderately soft bowel movements.

6. **Nursing diagnosis:** Potential for impairment of skin integrity.

   Long-term goal: Carrie will have smooth, intact skin.

   Short-term goals: (a) Carrie will have no broken areas of skin or areas remaining reddened after turning and skin care. (b) Carrie will cooperate with the turning routine.

7. **Nursing diagnosis:** Fear related to turning sensations and narrowness of Stryker frame.

   Long-term goal: Carrie will feel comfortable and secure while on the Stryker frame.

   Short-term goals: (a) Carrie will show signs of relaxation while on the frame and will say that she feels safe. (b) Carrie will say she is not anxious prior to being turned. (c) Carrie will maintain correct position on the frame.

8. **Nursing diagnosis:** Potential for nutritional deficits related to increased body requirements due to surgery and to impaired mobility.

   Long-term goal: Carrie will have an adequate diet.

   Short-term goals: (a) Carrie will drink more than the maintenance fluid requirement per day. (b) Carrie will identify five good sources of protein. (c) Carrie will choose to eat a well-balanced diet free from most "junk" foods.

9. **Nursing diagnosis:** Deficits related to impaired physical mobility.

   Long-term goal: Carrie will not suffer developmental or physical deficits related to immobility.

   Short-term goals: (a) Carrie will participate in planning each day's routine. (b) Carrie will participate in diversional activities. (c) Carrie will do active range-of-motion exercises of shoulders, arms, hands, fingers, and neck. (d) Carrie will cooperate with passive and active exercises for lower extremities as prescribed.

10. **Nursing diagnosis:** Self-care deficit related to basic hygiene and elimination.

    Long-term goal: Carrie will participate in self-care as she is able and will accept or request needed assistance.

    Short-term goals: (a) Carrie will feed herself. (b) Carrie will wash face and arms, brush teeth, and brush and comb hair. (c) Carrie will state her interest in self-care and appearance. (d) Carrie will talk about feelings and frustrations related to self-care. (e) Carrie will accept assistance with toileting and eating.

11. **Nursing diagnosis:** Potential for disturbance of self-concept because of altered body image.

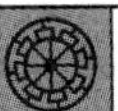

NURSING CARE PLAN Child Recovering From Spinal Fusion (continued)

Long-term goal: Carrie will state positive attributes about self and will talk about treatment realistically.

Short-term goals: (a) Carrie will express feelings verbally and by appropriate activities. (b) Carrie will do 3 hours of schoolwork a day. (c) Carrie will call at least one friend daily. (d) Carrie will talk about feelings of separation and frustration. (e) Carrie will describe treatment and state its purpose accurately. (f) Carrie will talk about her back and her recovery period realistically.

Interventions	Rationale	Evaluation criteria
1. Monitor breath sounds, respiratory rate, depth of respirations, use of accessory muscles, color, and temperature	Early recognition of inadequate air exchange enables health team to prevent severe respiratory distress	Did Carrie remain free of respiratory distress and related problems as evidenced by adequate air exchange and no signs of infection?
Have Carrie breathe deeply and cough at least every 2 hours. Use incentive spirometer or blow bottles	Coughing and deep breathing facilitate lung expansion and prevent pooling of secretions	
Be sure that Carrie is comfortable prior to breathing exercises	Pain can markedly decrease respiratory effort	
Report any respiratory pain or related distress, decreased or absent breath sounds	These could be signs of atelectasis or tension pneumothorax	
2. Observe dressing sites for serosanguineous staining and excessive blood.	Excessive bleeding could lead to hypovolemia and shock	Did Carrie remain free of cardiovascular compromise related to excessive blood loss as demonstrated by adequate hydration, stable vital signs, and no sign of hemmorhage?
Monitor fluid intake and output. Test urine specific gravity	Urine output and specific gravity are excellent indicators of hydration	
Monitor pulse and blood pressure and report changes to the physician	Pulse and blood pressure changes occur relatively late in acute blood loss	
Observe skin color, quality of tissue perfusion (capillary refill), hematocrit, hemoglobin, warmth of extremities and monitor peripheral pulses	Changes may indicate circulatory compromise	
3. Ask Carrie to identify area of limb touched and to move extremities every 2 hours	Inability to perform these tasks may indicate neurologic compromise, which is an extremely serious complication of spinal fusion	Does Carrie remain free of neurologic compromise?
Inquire about tingling or feelings of excessive heaviness in limbs. Observe for bowel or bladder incontinence or dribbling	Altered innervation and resulting feeling and function can occur in extremities or perineal area. Movement of lower legs should be possible, although moving the thigh is probably too painful	
4. Determine Carrie's usual pain tolerance	This provides baseline data for pain assessment	Did Carrie experience relief from postoperative pain?
Identify nonverbal behavior indicative of pain, such as restlessness, withdrawal, anxiety	Child, particularly an adolescent, might not admit to pain. Subtle behavioral changes can indicate increasing pain. Turning redistributes pressure and often lessens pain	

continued on next page

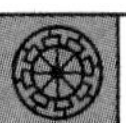

NURSING CARE PLAN Child Recovering From Spinal Fusion (continued)

Interventions	Rationale	Evaluation criteria
Turn Carrie on frame. Teach diversionary measures, such as therapeutic breathing and relaxation techniques. Administer analgesics for severe pain	Diversion helps relieve mild pain. Severe pain is relieved only by analgesics	
Administer muscle relaxants for muscle spasms	Pain from muscle spasms can be relieved by muscle relaxants	
Observe response to pain relief medication	Physician may need to adjust dosage or prescribe another medication	
Remain with child until pain subsides, assist with diversionary tactics, and provide comfort measures	Fear increases the perception of pain. Noninvasive pain relief measures can be very effective when combined with analgesics. Comfort measures improve feelings of well-being	
5. Monitor Carrie's ability to void; particularly note any bladder distention or incomplete bladder emptying as evidenced by small, frequent voids	Bladder distention may occur after catheter removal	Have Carrie's elimination patterns returned to normal?
Measure and note time of voiding; measure intake and output; palpate for bladder distention	Bladder distention with or without overflow can occur after catheter removal	
Encourage Carrie to void by providing privacy, use of running water, spirits of peppermint in bedpan; recatheterize as ordered if measures are ineffective	These measures facilitate bladder emptying by promoting relaxation	
Encourage fluid consumption, particularly fruit juices, and monitor for signs of urinary tract infection (see Chapter 39)	Adequate fluid intake encourages a regular urinary routine and decreases likelihood of urinary tract infection or constipation; juices promote urine acidity, thus decreasing risk of urinary tract infection	
Provide a diet high in roughage; administer stool softeners if ordered; note frequency and consistency of stools	These are measures to prevent constipation; constipation and straining are uncomfortable and potentially harmful in the postoperative period	
6. Provide skin care every 2 hours.	Skin care increases comfort and decreases likelihood of skin breakdown	Is Carrie's skin smooth and intact without evidence of tissue breakdown or infection?
Rub bony prominences. Ensure that child doesn't inhale fumes if alcohol is used for skin care	Alcohol is used in many facilities for skin care but fumes can be irritating	
Use sheepskin if sheets are irritating to skin. Change position on frame (prone or supine) every 2 hours during the day	Sheepskin and turning alleviate prolonged pressure on bony prominences	
When child is prone, check position of feet and forehead. Feet should hang freely over mattress and forehead should rest comfortably on head rest	Correct positioning helps to maintain function and decrease pressure on bony prominences	
7. Explain the frame, how it works, and how its use helps promote healing and stabilization of the Harrington rods	Understanding the purpose and mechanics of the frame increases child's feelings of comfort and control	Is Carrie more relaxed and confident while being turned on the frame?
Keep restraints on except while providing skin care. Have frame stabilizers securely in position	Restraints increase child's safety and feelings of security	

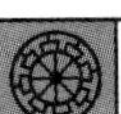

NURSING CARE PLAN Child Recovering From Spinal Fusion (continued)

Interventions	Rationale	Evaluation criteria
Enlist the aid of another knowledgeable person for turning procedures on Stryker frame	Confidence in knowledgeable caregivers and extra assistance helps child relax	
Have Carrie either hug the frame or place arms alongside. Place rolled bath blankets or pillows along the sides	These measures decrease movement and increase child's feelings of control during turning	
Check Carrie more frequently during the night than during the day	Child is likely to forget where she is at night and may even attempt to change position	
8. Maintain intravenous therapy until oral fluid intake is adequate	Total fluid intake must be in excess of maintenance requirements	Does Carrie remain free of nutritional deficits?
Begin oral intake with clear fluids and advance gradually to solid foods	Child has had nothing by mouth for many hours	
Offer small, frequent servings of well-liked foods, frequent snacks. (Carrie likes grilled cheese sandwiches)	Small, frequent servings and favorite foods are most likely to be eaten. Child has poor appetite due to pain, dependence, and immobilization	
Discuss the importance of adequate fluid intake and balanced, high-protein diet	Child should understand that adequate fluid intake is needed to prevent dehydration and hypovolemia; protein is necessary for healing	
Ask Carrie's help in planning menus	Feelings of control over treatment enhance cooperation	
Arrange to have family, friends, or other patients join Carrie for meals	Child is likely to eat better if mealtime is a pleasant and sociable event	
Arrange for family or friends to bring Carrie's favorite foods from home	Food from home can greatly stimulate appetite	
9. Organize Carrie's day and care according to her preferences and maintain routine	The child's maintaining some control over activities and routine is crucial to self-concept and cooperation	Does Carrie remain free of physical, emotional, and developmental deficits related to immobility?
Place personal things, telephone, and call button nearby so Carrie can be as independent as possible	The arrangement of the environment can greatly increase independence, self-control and thus stimulate personal growth	
Plan activities according to position on the turning frame (prone or supine). Provide prism glasses so Carrie can watch television, eat, read, play games, or participate in other diversionary activities while lying flat	Diversions stimulate the child to maintain developmental level	
Encourage family and peers to visit and to discuss daily events of home and school	As the child maintains ties with the outside world, growth increases and jealousy and self-pity decrease	
Do passive and active range-of-motion exercises of the upper extremities at least four times a day	Exercise maintains range of motion and some muscle strength and also reminds the child of eventual recovery and mobility	
Plan with the surgeon and physiotherapist appropriate lower extremity activity, such as quadriceps-setting and knee and hip range-of-motion exercises		

continued on next page

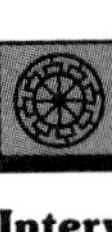

NURSING CARE PLAN Child Recovering From Spinal Fusion (continued)

Interventions	Rationale	Evaluation criteria
Help Carrie to perform the planned exercises at least four times a day		
Place footboard at end of frame	This prevents foot drop	
10. Arrange hygienic and grooming routines for times when pain is minimal (for example, following analgesic administration)	Child is more likely to participate if she is comfortable	Does Carrie participate in self-care to the extent that she is able, and is she able to express a positive outlook about her care after discharge?
Arrange food and utensils for ease in self-feeding	Self-feeding fosters feelings of control and independence	
Anticipate Carrie's needs for help during bathing, grooming, and elimination	Having assistance readily available decreases child's frustration, increases trust, and preserves dignity, while ensuring appropriate care	
Encourage Carrie to verbalize feelings of embarrassment, frustration, or helplessness	Expressing feelings helps child to cope with them	
Assure Carrie that her helpless state is temporary and that results of treatment will be positive	Reassurances remind child that dependence is temporary and help child to keep treatments in perspective	
11. Encourage Carrie to discuss feelings of resentment and anger	Verbal and physical outlets help decrease the effects of dependence, immobility, and surgery that affect body image	Does Carrie remain free of self-concept and body image disturbances?
Provide diversionary activity for tension release, such as latch-hook rug kits, painting, games		
Accept Carrie's need for periods of withdrawal and moodiness as she adjusts to change in body image and separation from peers and normal activities. Explain to parent that these reactions are normal	Child needs understanding and time alone to cope with physical and emotional aspects of treatment	
Help Carrie to keep up with schoolwork. Have parent bring schoolwork to the hospital, arrange for quiet study times, and determine whether a tutor is needed. Praise Carrie for tasks completed and help her to set attainable goals	Keeping up with schoolwork is difficult but important to maintenance or increase in child's feelings of self-worth	
Encourage Carrie to maintain contact with peers via the telephone and visits	Maintaining contact with peers keeps child interested in life outside the hospital, fosters self-esteem, and eases future reentry into normal life	
Arrange to have former patients who have undergone the same procedure come to visit Carrie	Talking to peers who have undergone spinal fusion helps child cope with treatments, provides support and even new friendships, and reassures child that treatment will be "worth it"	
Prepare Carrie for cast application and its significance. Plan with Carrie how to answer peers' questions about cast. Discuss appropriate clothing	The better child is prepared for cast wearing, the less difficult child's adjustment will be	

Key Concepts

- The skeletal system, which is made up of bones, their joints, and attached muscles, ligaments, and tendons, supports and protects the body, enables movement, and contains marrow, which produces blood cells.
- Growth that causes bone to lengthen takes place in a region of the epiphysis called the epiphyseal plate; when bone lengthening ceases in early adulthood, the cartilaginous epiphyseal plate ossifies, thins, and becomes the epiphyseal line.
- Mechanical stress, trauma, circulation, nutrition, metabolism, and infection can affect bone growth and development both before and after birth.
- Bone becomes less flexible, and fractures heal more slowly, as the child grows and ossification takes place.
- Diagnostic tests used in assessing skeletal conditions include radiographs, in which deformities or injuries can be seen; hematologic studies, which are used to assess and monitor infections related to surgery or injury; and serologic studies, which are used to detect congenital deficiencies of hormone secretion.
- Nursing management for the child undergoing internal fixation and fusion involves standard preoperative and postoperative interventions and care appropriate for the child immobilized in a cast, traction, or brace, or on a frame.
- Nursing care related to cast application and removal includes preparing the child by explaining the purpose of casting and describing the sensations caused by wet and drying casting materials and, before removal, demonstrating use of the cast saw to lessen fears.
- Cast maintenance involves assessing the extremity distal to the cast for color, sensation, and motion; observing for edema and cast tightness; preserving skin integrity; and instructing the parent and child in cast care.
- In skin traction, pull is exerted on skin surrounding the body part; in skeletal traction, pull is exerted by means of wires or pins inserted in bone.
- Nursing care for the child in skin traction includes monitoring extremities for color, sensation, and motion; releasing traction, if permitted, to care for skin under bandages; helping the child to adapt to immobilization; and teaching the child and family about the purpose of traction and ways in which they can help to maintain it.
- Skeletal traction requires the same measures as skin traction, except that the nurse does not release traction to provide skin care, but rather observes pin sites for signs of slippage or infection.
- If the child's weight is not sufficient to counterbalance traction, the nurse applies restraints to the child's body or elevates one end of the bed.
- Nursing care for the child with a brace includes maintaining skin integrity, ensuring that the brace fits correctly and comfortably, and teaching the child and parent about compliance with brace wearing and skin and brace maintenance at home.
- For the child who is being treated with a continuous-motion device, nursing care includes ensuring that the extremity is comfortably and securely seated in the device, ensuring that the prescribed rate and range of motion are set, and teaching the child about cooperation.
- Nursing care for the child who is immobilized on a frame includes interventions to prevent physical and developmental complications of immobilization, to ensure that excreta do not remain in contact with the child's skin or soil the cast, to restrain the child to prevent falls or inappropriate movement, and to provide reassurance that being turned on a frame is not dangerous.
- The acute-care needs of the child who is partially immobilized by a cast, traction, or brace include prevention of skin breakdown; control of infections and complications; safety; control of neurologic and circulatory compromise; prevention or detection of appliance or apparatus failure; and prevention of physical, emotional, and developmental complications of immobility.
- Pain due to skeletal conditions or surgery is controlled by analgesics, as prescribed; comfort measures, such as repositioning; and diversion, such as relaxation techniques.
- Nursing care for the child who has undergone skeletal surgery includes frequent postoperative assessment of cast staining; monitoring of vital signs for indications of respiratory complications or excessive blood loss; frequent assessment of color,

sensation, and motion distal to the operative site; control of pain; and prevention of edema.

- The nutritional needs of the child who has a skeletal condition or has undergone bone surgery include high protein intake to promote healing, fluid intake above daily maintenance requirements, and a well-balanced diet containing adequate roughage to prevent constipation.
- The emotional needs of the child with a skeletal condition have to do with reactions to immobilization, casts and other appliances, and altered body image.
- The health maintenance needs of a child with a skeletal condition frequently involve teaching about cooperation with the home treatment plan, ensuring that the home environment is safe for the partially immobilized child, arranging follow-up care, and referring the family to resources in the community.
- Nursing care for the child with a craniofacial defect may involve support during decision making about surgical correction, preoperative and postoperative nursing care, and assistance with adaptations to altered body image.
- For the child with clubfoot, nursing care involves teaching cast or brace care, management and teaching of passive exercises, and, if conservative treatment is not effective, preoperative and postoperative care.
- Nursing management for the child with congenital dislocated hip involves direct care and teaching related to Bradford frames and spica casts.
- Nursing care for the child with Legg–Calvé–Perthes disease may require care related to casting, bracing, traction, or surgery, depending on medical treatment.
- In addition to traction, cast care, and preoperative and postoperative care, the child with slipped capital femoral epiphysis requires careful assessment to detect slippage in the opposite femur.
- For the child undergoing spinal fusion for treatment of severe scoliosis, nursing care involves extensive preoperative teaching, postoperative care of the immobilized child, and careful attention to prevention of developmental setbacks related to immobility and length of treatment.
- Nursing management for the child with postural, or functional, kyphosis is focused on exploring reasons for poor posture, explaining the benefits of good posture, and reinforcing a positive self-image.
- The child undergoing treatment for severe, fixed kyphosis requires brace care and teaching and, occasionally, care related to spinal fusion and postoperative immobilization.
- Besides standard preoperative and postoperative care, nursing care for the child undergoing surgery for leg length discrepancy involves special attention to preventing or detecting infection of skin and bone at the graft site.
- Care of the child with a torsional deformity includes explaining the likelihood of spontaneous resolution to the parent, teaching the parent how to perform passive exercises, and, if spontaneous resolution does not occur, brace care, spica cast care, and care related to surgery.
- The flexibility of children's bones makes them more susceptible than adults to bending, buckle fractures, and greenstick fractures.
- Nursing care for the child with a fracture includes reassuring the injured and often frightened child, repeating teaching and explanations as often as necessary, and interventions related to casts, traction, and, if open reduction is performed, surgery.
- The child who has suffered a sprain, strain, or contusion requires emergency application of ice and compression, elevation of the affected body part, and during recovery muscle-setting exercises to prevent loss of tone.
- Nursing care for the child with a dislocation due to trauma is to offer reassurance and support until the dislocation is reduced and, if open reduction is necessary, provide care related to surgery and cast maintenance.
- The child undergoing treatment for bone infection requires nursing care related to antibiotic administration, assessment of local and systemic signs and symptoms of infection, supportive measures, and, occasionally, surgical intervention.
- Infection of a joint requires nursing care related to traction, immobilization, antibiotic administration, possible surgery, and compliance with range-of-motion exercises.

- For the child with Osgood–Schlatter disease, nursing care focuses on convincing the child to refrain from strenuous physical activities and may involve cast care or care related to surgery.
- Nursing care for the child with osteogenesis imperfecta involves cast care, prevention of muscle atrophy, careful handling of the child, and support of the family (see Chapter 30).
- For the child undergoing surgical excision of a benign bone tumor, nursing care consists of preoperative and postoperative nursing management.

References

Adams J: *Outline of orthopaedics*. 8th ed. Churchill Livingstone, 1976.

Behrman RE, Vaughan V: Nelson Textbook of Pediatrics. Saunders, 1983.

Bergmann T: *Children in the Hospital*. International Universities Press, 1965.

Byrne J et al: *Laboratory Tests*. Addison-Wesley, 1981.

Celeste SM, Folick MA, Dumas KM: Identifying a standard for pin site care using the quality assurance approach. *Orthop Nurs*(July/Aug)1984; 3:17–24.

Garrick J: The sports medicine patient. *Nurs Clin North Am* (Dec)1981; 16:759–767.

Hankin FM, Gragg AJ, Kaufer H: Bleeding beneath postoperative plaster casts. *Orthop Nurs* (Jan/Feb)1983; 2:27–31.

Ibrahim K: An overview of childhood fractures. *Pediatr Nurs* (Jan/Feb)1984; 10:57–65.

Kylberg HK: Descriptions of growth disturbances in children with osteomyelitis at different ages. *Orthop Nurs* (Nov/Dec)1983; 2:28–32.

McFarland MB: Encircling cast drainage: Is it valuable? *Orthop Nurs* (March/April)1984; 3:41–43.

Salter RB: *Textbook of Disorders and Injuries of the Musculoskeletal System*. 2nd ed. Williams & Wilkins, 1983.

Tachdjian M: *Pediatric Orthopedics*. Vol. I and II. Saunders, 1972.

Vick RL: *Contemporary Medical Physiology*. Addison-Wesley, 1984.

Additional Readings

Agee BL, Herman C: Cervical logrolling on a standard hospital bed. *Am J Nurs* (March)1984; 84:315–318.

Allard JL, Dibble, SL: Scoliosis surgery: A look at Luque rods. *Am J Nurs* (May)1984; 84:609–611.

Anderson B: The patient with scoliosis: Carole, a girl treated with bracing. *Am J Nurs* (Sept)1979; 79:1592–1597.

Asher M: Orthopedic screenings especially congenital dislocation of the hip and spinal deformity. *Pediatr Clin North Am* (Nov)1977; 24:713–721.

Beall M: Evaluation of the musculoskeletal system in the pediatric patient. *Iss Compr Pediatr Nurs* (Nov/Dec)1977; 2:1–13.

Bernardo ML: Craniosynostosis: The child's care from detection through correction. *Am J Matern Child Nurs* (July/Aug)1979; 4:234–237.

Brantley P, Cenella M: *The Nurse and Orthopedic Surgery*. The Orthopedic Nurses' Association, Inc., in Cooperation with Howmedica, Inc., 1980.

Bunch W: Common deformities of the lower limbs. *Pediatr Nurs* (July/Aug)1979; 5:18–22.

Chung S: Diseases of the developing hip joint. *Pediatr Clin North Am* (Nov)1977; 24:857–870.

Cohen J: Skeletal problems of children. *Hosp Pract* (July)1977; 12:77–89.

Crossland S, Deyerle W: Broken legs are to be walked on. *Am J Nurs* (Dec)1977; 77:1922–1930.

Davis SE, Lewis SA: Managing scoliosis: Fashions for the body and mind. *Am J Matern Child Nurs* (May/June) 1984; 9:186–187.

Derscheid G: Rehabilitation of common orthopedic problems. *Nurs Clin North Am* (Dec)1981; 16:709–719.

de Toledo C Holt. The patient with scoliosis: The defect, classification and detection. *Am J Nurs* (Sept)1979; 79:1588–1591.

Farrell J: Casts, your patients and you. *Nursing 78* (Oct)1978; 8:65–69.

Farrell J: *Illustrated Guide to Orthopedic Nursing*. 2nd ed. Lippincott, 1982.

Farrell J: Orthopedic pain: What does it mean? *Am J Nurs* (April)1984; 84:466–469.

Gates SJ: Helping your patient on bedrest cope with perceptual/sensory deprivation. *Orthop Nurs* (March/April)1984; 3:35–38.

Goldman L: The injured ankle. *Nurse Pract* (Oct) 1981:51–56.

Guerrein AT: Osteogenesis imperfecta: A disorder that breaks more than our hearts. *Am J Matern Child Nurs* (Sept/Oct)1982; 7:315–318.

Halladay J: Update on scoliosis. *Can Nurse* (Sept) 1984:44–45.

Hensinger R: Congenital dislocation of the hip. *Clin Symp* (Nov)1978; 31:3–31.

Hensinger R: Limp. *Pediatr Clin North Am* (Nov)1977; 24:723–730.

Hill P, Romm L: Screening for scoliosis in adolescents. *Am J Matern Child Nurs* (May/June)1977; 2:156–159.

Hilt N: Care of the child in a hip spica cast. *RN* (April)1976; 39:27–31.

Holland SH: Up-to-date home care of a baby in a hip spica cast. *Ped Nurs* (March/April)1983; 9:114–115.

Hoppenfeld S: Back pain. *Pediatr Clin North Am* (Nov)1977; 24:881–887.

Horoshak I: Auto transfusion: Promising alternative to donor blood. *RN* (May) 1975; 5:33–40.

Jacox A: *Pain: A Source Book for Nurses and Other Health Professionals*. Little, Brown, 1977.

Johnson J, Kirchhoff K, Endress M: Altering children's behavior during orthopedic cast removal. *RN* (Nov/Dec)1975; 24:404–410.

Jones S: Orthopedic injuries: Illness as deviance. *Am J Nurs* (Nov)1975; 75:2030–2033.

Karn MA, Crawford AH: Postoperative nursing management of the patient following posterior spinal fusion. *Orthop Nurs* (March/April)1984; 3:21–25.

Keim H: Back deformities. *Pediatr Clin North Am* (Nov)1977; 24:871–880.

Keim H: Scoliosis. *Clin Symp CIBA* 1978; 30:2–30.

Kelly DJ: The use of fiberglass as reinforcement with plaster casts. *Orthop Nurs* (Nov/Dec)1983; 2:33–36.

King JP: Bones: How to grow new ones. *AORN J* (April)1982; 35:968–975.

Kryschyshen PL, Fischer DA: External fixation for complicated fractures. *Am J Nurs* (Feb)1980; 80:256–260.

Lee BC, Hansen EF, Poppell MR: Facial fractures take a special kind of nursing care. *Nursing 80* (Aug)1980; 10:43–46.

Lentz M: Skeletal aspects of deconditioning secondary to immobilization. *Nurs Clin North Am* (Dec)1981); 16:729–737.

Love-Mignogna S: Scoliosis. *Nursing 77* (May)1977; 7:50–55.

Merservey P: Congenital musculoskeletal abnormalities. *Iss Compr Pediatr Nurs* (Nov/Dec)1977; 2:14–22.

Micheli LJ, Magin MA, Rouvales R: The patient with scoliosis: Surgical management and nursing care. *Am J Nurs* (Sept)1979; 79:1599–1607.

Milazzo V: An exercise class for patients in traction. *Am J Nurs* (Oct)1981; 81:1842–1944.

Miller L: Orthopedic patients in an ambulatory surgery facility. *Nurs Clin North Am* (Dec)1981; 16:749–758.

Mulley D: Harnessing babies. *Am J Nurs* (Aug)1984; 84:1006–1008.

Pashley J, Wahlstrom M: Polytrauma: The patient, the family, the nurse and the health team. *Nurs Clin North Am* (Dec)1981; 16:721–727.

Peterson H: Leg aches. *Pediatr Clin North Am* (Nov)1977; 24:731–736.

Richie JA: Nursing the child undergoing limb amputation. *Am J Matern Child Nurs* (March/April)1980; 5:114–120.

Ross DG: The knee. *Orthop Nurs* (Sept/Oct)1983; 2:23–28.

Salmond SW: Trauma and fractures: Meeting your patient's nutritional needs. *Orthop Nurs* (July/Aug)1984; 3:27–33.

Sawyer J: Fracture dislocations of the elbow. *Am J Nurs* (Aug)1976; 76:1266–1268.

Schatzinger LH, Brower EM, Nash CL: The patient with scoliosis spinal fusion: Emotional stress and adjustment. *Am J Nurs* (Sept)1979; 79:1608–1612.

Segil C: Current concepts in the management of scoliosis. *Nurs Clin North Am* (Dec)1976; 11:691–709.

Smith D, Clarren S: Congenital deformities. *Pediatr Clin North Am* (Nov)1977; 24:664–677.

Smith J: Knee problems in children. *Pediatr Clin North Am* (Nov)1977; 24:841–855.

Spickler LL: Knee injuries of the athlete. *Orthop Nurs* (Sept/Oct)1983; 2:11–19.

Staheli L: Torsional deformity. *Pediatr Clin North Am* (Nov)1977; 24:799–811.

Stepdesign, Inc.: Nursing care of a patient in traction. *Am J Nurs* (Oct)1979; 79:1171–1798.

Stout J, Gibbs K: The child undergoing a leg lengthening procedure. *Am J Nurs* (June)1981; 81:1152–1155.

Strong C, Gavaghan M: Scoliosis and its implications. *Iss Compr Pediatr Nurs* (Nov/Dec)1977; 2:33–45.

Thomas PC: Nursing care of patients undergoing posterior fusion with segmental (Luque) spinal instrumentation. *Orthop Nurs* (May/June)1983; 2:13–20.

Thomassen PF: Helping your scoliosis patient walk tall. *RN* (Feb)1984; 47:34–37.

Thorne BP: A nurse helps prevent sports injuries. *Am J Matern Child Nurs* (July/Aug)1982; 7:236–240.

Tibbits CW: Adolescent idiopathic scoliosis. *Nurse Pract* (March/April)1980:11–20.

Trigueiro M: Pin site care protocol. *Can Nurse* (Sept)1983:24–25.

Varni NA: Osteogenesis imperfecta: The basics. *Pediatr Nurs* (Jan/Feb)1984; 10:29–33.

Villalon D, Smith MN: At home with traction. *Pediatr Nurs* (Jan/Feb)1982; 8:15–16.

Wassell AC: Sports medicine: Acute and overuse injuries. *Orthop Nurs* (March/April)1984; 3:29–33.

Wassel A: Nursing assessment of injuries to the lower extremity. *Nurs Clin North Am* (Dec)1981; 16:739–748.

Webb K: Early assessment of orthopedic injuries. *Am J Nurs* (June)1974; 74:1048–1052.

Wilkins K: The uniqueness of the young athlete: Musculoskeletal injuries. *Am J Sports Med* 1980; 8:377–381.

Williams PF: *Orthopaedic Management in Childhood.* Mosby, 1983.

Innervation and Mobility
Implications of Altered Neurologic and Neuromuscular Function

42

Peggy Smith

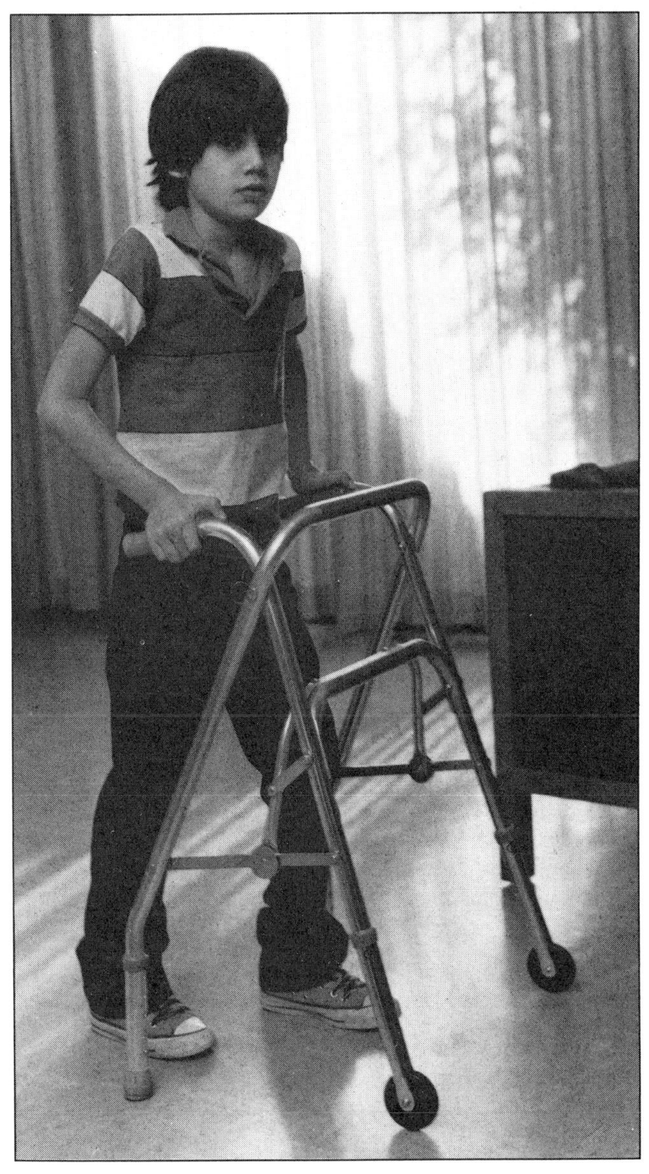

Chapter Outline

continued on next page

Objectives

- Describe the anatomy and physiology of the nervous system.
- Describe the assessment techniques specific to assessment of the nervous system.
- Explain the principles of nursing care common to procedures and treatments for neurologic dysfunction.
- Describe the acute-care needs specific to the child with increased intracranial pressure, the comatose child, and the child requiring neurosurgery.

- Relate the developmental needs of children with neurologic impairments to the effects of long-term neurologic dysfunction.
- Describe the clinical manifestations, treatment, and principles of nursing management for each congenital malformation of the central nervous system.
- Explain the clinical manifestations, methods of diagnostic evaluation, treatment, and principles of nursing management for each infection of the central nervous system.
- Describe the clinical manifestations, diagnostic methods, treatment, and principles of nursing management for the child with a seizure disorder.
- Explain the clinical manifestations, treatment, and principles of nursing management for the child with a head or spinal cord injury and for the child with cerebral palsy.
- Describe the nursing care associated with neurocutaneous syndromes and degenerative neurologic disorders.
- Describe the behavior patterns and clinical manifestations associated with alterations in learning, attention, and activity level.
- Explain the nurse's role in multidisciplinary management for learning, attention, and activity disorders.

The nervous system is the human being's most complex organization of structure and function, influencing virtually all life processes and providing the individual with the primary means of perceiving and interacting with the environment. The child's sensory, motor, and cognitive functions develop through continual neuroregulation and the higher integration of stimuli and responses.

Alterations of neurologic function in children can have significant effects on the child's growth and development, ranging from subtle interferences associated with isolated perceptual weaknesses to the devastating multiple handicaps imposed by severe cerebral insult. In this chapter we review the structure and function of the nervous system, describe the principles of nursing assessment and management common to various neurologic alterations, and introduce the major pathologic conditions encountered in children with nervous system dysfunction.

Anatomy and Physiology of the Nervous System

Central Nervous System

The central nervous system consists of the brain and spinal cord and contains neuronal tissue, which is classified as *gray* (cortical) and *white* (subcortical) *matter.* Contained within the bony structure of the cranium and vertebral column, the brain and spinal cord are covered by the meninges, a three-layer protective membrane. The *dura mater,* or outermost layer of the meninges, is composed of tough, fibrous connective tissue just under the bony skull. Next to the dura is the *arachnoid,* a weblike, thin membrane. The innermost layer is the *pia mater,* a delicate membrane closely surrounding the surface of the brain and spinal cord. Between these layers are the subdural space and subarachnoid space (Fig. 42-1). The subarachnoid space surrounds the surface of the brain and the spinal cord and connects with the ventricles of the brain through the fourth ventricle. It contains the cerebral spinal fluid, which bathes the brain and cord.

The Brain The brain is divided into three main areas: the cerebrum, cerebellum, and brain stem (Fig. 42-2). Their major divisions and functions are listed in Table 42-1.

The *cerebrum* is the largest and most important part of the nervous system and consists of two cerebral hemispheres that are separated incompletely by a deep *medial longitudinal fissure.* They are connected centrally in the brain by a broad band of commissural fibers called the *corpus callosum.* The outer layer of the cerebrum is the cerebral cortex, which is covered by surfaces called *gyri* separated by multiple furrows, or *sulci.* Each hemisphere is divided into four lobes, each of which controls specific integrative functions.

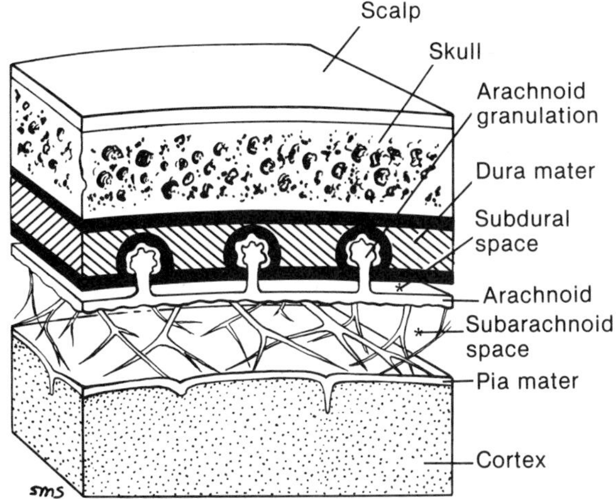

Figure 42-1 Meningeal layers covering the brain surface.

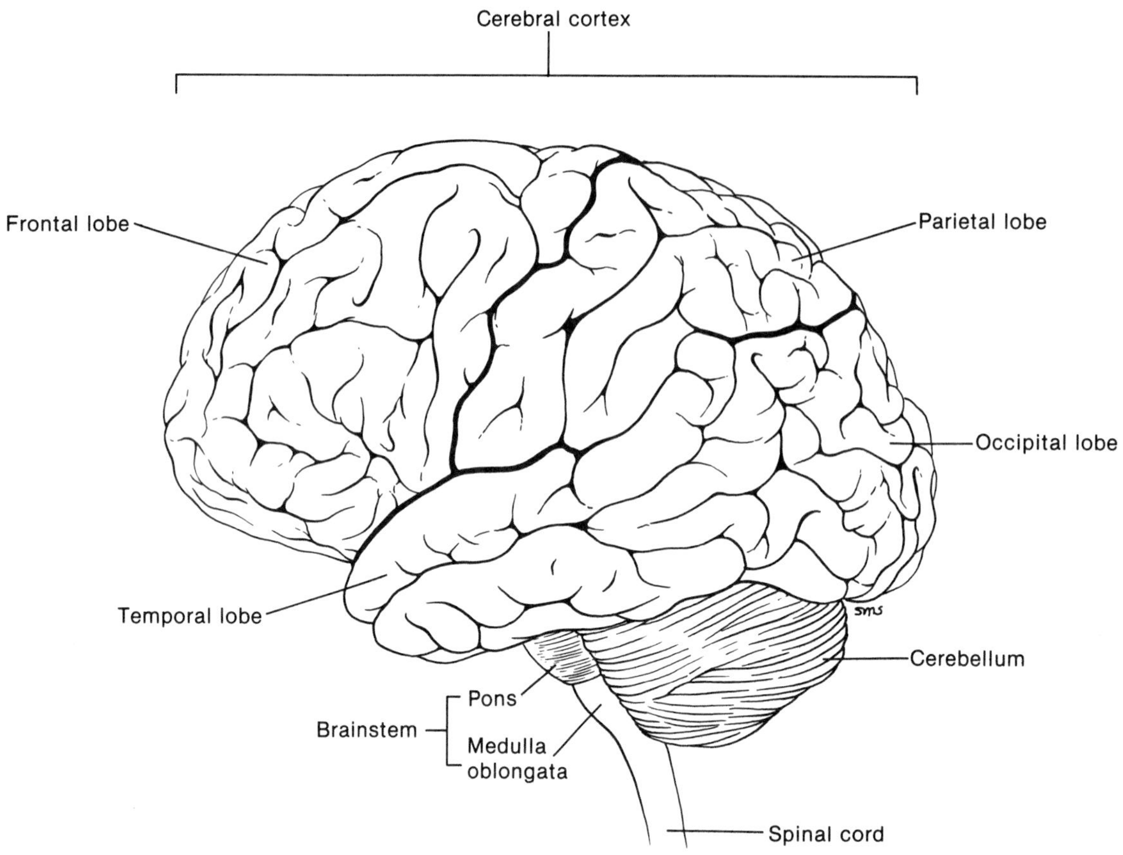

Figure 42-2 Lateral view of the major areas of the brain.

Located at the posterior base of the brain, the *cerebellum* performs integrative functions for refining and coordinating all muscle movements. It receives impulses from all sensory modalities (tactile, auditory, and visual) and modifies body position and movements to allow balanced, smooth performance.

Below the cerebellum is the *brain stem,* which extends from the base of the cerebrum to the spinal cord. The brain stem is the origin of most of the cranial nerves, controls vital life functions, and serves as a receptor and relay center for impulses entering the cerebrum.

The Spinal Cord The spinal cord extends from the medulla oblongata to the lumbar vertebrae, where it ends in the *conus medullaris.* Nerve fibers of the lumbar and sacral spinal nerve roots extend downward from the conus in a formation resembling a horse's tail, which is referred to as the *cauda equina.* The diameter of the spinal cord varies at different points and is larger in the cervical and lumbar areas. Gray and white matter arranged in longitudinal fibers make up the cord, which functions as the conducting pathway for nerve impulses between the brain and periphery. Transverse section of the cord reveals an H shape of gray matter surrounded by white matter divided into sections identified as columns, or *funiculi* (Fig. 42-3). The gray matter of the cord is divided into *posterior* and *anterior horns.*

The segments of the spinal cord are divided into cervical (8), thoracic (12), lumbar (5), sacral (5), and coccygeal (1), numbers of which correspond with the attachment of pairs of spinal nerves at each segment. Because the spinal cord is shorter than the vertebral column in the mature individual, the cord segments do not correspond directly to the adjacent vertebrae.

Spinal nerve pathways are ascending (afferent) or descending (efferent). Afferent tracts carry conscious and unconscious sensory information to receptor sites in the brain. Efferent tracks carry impulses from the brain for the control of motor (somatic) and visceral (autonomic) functions.

Cerebrospinal Fluid System Cerebrospinal fluid (CSF) is a clear, colorless fluid that surrounds the brain and spinal cord and fills the four ventricles of the brain (Fig. 42-4). Small amounts of protein, glucose, trace minerals, and

TABLE 42-1 Areas of the Brain

Area	Anatomic location	Function
Cerebrum		
Frontal lobes	Anterior third of cerebral hemispheres	Anterior part functions in behavior, personality, and cognitive abilities. Posterior part controls initiation of motor activity and speech production
Parietal lobes	Posterior to frontal lobes, above temporal lobes	Function in recognition of sensations and perceptual abilities
Temporal lobes	Inferior to parietal lobes, lower lateral sections of cerebral hemispheres	Center for language processing, auditory association, and interpretation of stimuli. Perceptual area for hearing, taste, and smell
Occipital lobe	Posterior section of cerebrum	Primary visual perception area
Rhinencephalon	Inferior to cerebral cortex	Functions in sense of smell
Basal ganglia	Deep within cerebrum	Exert important influences on refinement and coordination of movement
Cerebellum	Posterior of brain, inferior to occipital lobe	Controls balance, posture, coordination, and refinement of movement
Brain stem	Extends from base of cerebrum to spinal cord	Contains centers for vital life functions; origin of cranial nerves II–XII
Thalamus	Lies on either side of third ventricle	Receives and transmits sensory stimuli to cortex; functions in emotional and instinctual responses
Hypothalamus	Inferior to thalamus	Regulates autonomic system (heart rate, blood pressure, peristalsis); controls appetite, thirst, body temperature, and physical expression of emotion; influences pituitary secretion
Midbrain (Mesencephalon)	Connects hypothalamus and pons	Functions in ocular and postural reflex activity
Pons	Inferior to midbrain, above medulla oblongata	Contains nuclei for cranial nerves: abducens, facial, trigeminal, and acoustic
Medulla oblongata	Forms a pyramid-shaped structure extending from pons downward to spinal cord	Major neural transmission center to and from brain; controls vital life functions of circulation, respiration, and visceral response; regulates attention, arousal, and consciousness through its reticular system

rare lymphocytes ($1-3/mm^3$) are present in CSF, which is formed continuously in the choroid plexuses of the ventricles, enters the CSF circulation, and is absorbed (Table 42-2).

Cerebrospinal fluid flows from two lateral ventricles in the cerebral hemispheres through the *interventricular foramina* (foramina of Monro) to the medial third ventricle. From the third ventricle the CSF enters the smaller fourth ventricle below through the *cerebral aqueduct* (aqueduct of Sylvius). Fluid enters the subarachnoid space through three openings in the fourth ventricle and covers the length of the spinal cord and brain surface. Cerebrospinal fluid is reabsorbed primarily by the *arachnoid villi* over the superior sagittal sinus. The CSF functions as a protective buffer for the central nervous system structures. Any obstruction to its flow or abnormal fluid production increases the intracranial pressure.

Peripheral Nervous System

The peripheral nervous system consists of the cranial and spinal nerves, which connect with the brain and spinal cord to carry neuronal impulses to and from all areas of the body. A functional division of the peripheral system is the autonomic nervous system, which controls subconscious visceral functions. General divisions of peripheral nerve function are as follows:

Somatic afferent—fibers that carry sensory impulses from the body wall, skeletal muscles, tendons, and joints

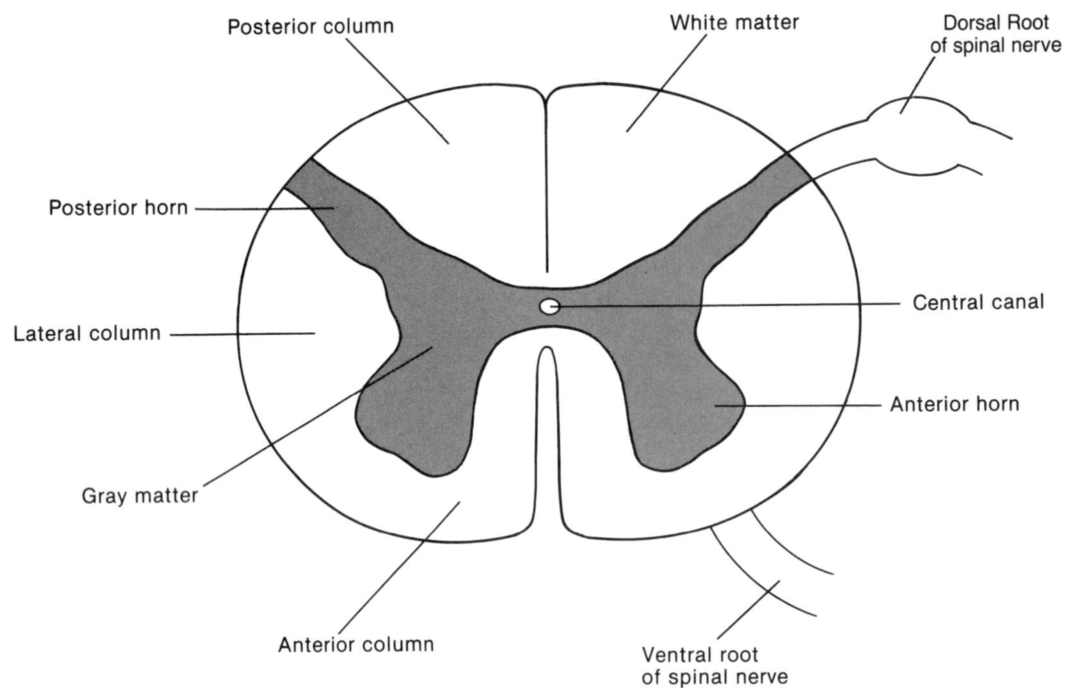

Figure 42-3 Cross section of the spinal cord.

Visceral afferent—fibers that carry sensory impulses from visceral (organs, vasculature) structures

Somatic efferent—motor fibers that innervate skeletal muscle

Visceral efferent—autonomic fibers that innervate smooth and cardiac muscles and control glandular secretion

Each peripheral nerve tract consists of several of these types of nerve fibers bound together by connective tissue, which travel to a common end site in the body.

Cranial and Spinal Nerves Twelve pairs of cranial nerves arise from the brain stem and base of the brain. (Their functions are outlined in Table 14-15).

There are 31 pairs of spinal nerves, each pair corresponding with a spinal cord segment. Each spinal nerve has an efferent (motor) root originating in the anterior (ventral) horn of the spinal cord and an afferent (sensory) root originating in the posterior (dorsal) horn of the spinal cord (Fig. 42-5). The motor and sensory spinal nerve fibers leave the cord separately and join in a single nerve tract immediately outside the vertebral column. Autonomic fibers also connect with spinal nerve tracts to form peripheral nerves.

After leaving the cord, some spinal nerves travel directly to their peripheral sites. Most spinal nerves form an aggregation, or plexus, from which they branch to supply motor and sensory innervation to body parts.

Autonomic Nervous System The autonomic nervous system controls involuntary, unconscious neural functions through innervation of smooth and cardiac muscle and glands of the body. The hypothalamus is the main regulator and integrator of autonomic activity, together with cortical, thalamic, medullary, and local reflex influences.

Sympathetic and parasympathetic divisions of the autonomic nervous system produce opposing physiologic effects in the body and show anatomic and neurotransmission differences as well.

The sympathetic system arises from the thoracic and upper lumbar segments of the spinal cord (thoracolumbar). Its primary neurotransmitter at its effector sites is norepinephrine, and the system is classified as adrenergic. Responses of "fight or flight" characterize the sympathetic system, which mobilizes the body resources in response to pain, cold, strong emotions, or other stresses. Increased heart rate, vasoconstriction, dilatation of coronary arteries and bronchioles, decreased gastrointestinal peristalsis, and sweating are sympathetic responses.

The parasympathetic system arises from cranial and sacral segments of the spinal cord (craniosacral). Its neurotransmitter is acetylcholine, and the system is classified as cholinergic. Parasympathetic effects stabilize and balance the effects of the sympathetic system to achieve homeostasis. Reduced heart rate, bronchial constriction, stimulation of gastrointestinal activity, and bladder emptying are among the parasympathetic functions.

TABLE 42-2 Cerebrospinal Fluid Values

Characteristic	Normal value	Abnormal alterations
Color	Clear	Xanthochromic (yellowish) color is abnormal beyond the neonatal period; indicates hyperbilirubinemia or recent subarachnoid hemorrhage. Cloudy fluid indicates inflammatory purulence
Cell count	Neonate: < 15 leukocytes/mm^3 Child: 0–5 cells/mm^3 (all lymphocytes)	Elevated white blood cell count Bacterial meningitis: often > 1000/mm^3 (predominantly polymorphonuclear leukocytes) Viral meningitis: < 500/mm^3 (predominantly lymphocytes) Red blood cells indicate intracranial hemorrhage; may result from a bloody lumbar puncture
Protein	Neonates: 60–120 mg/dL Child: 15–45 mg/dL	Elevated in inflammatory diseases (meningitis, encephalitis), tumors, or degenerative conditions causing increased permeability of the blood–meningeal barrier
Glucose	One-half to two-thirds serum glucose level	Decreased in bacterial, tubercular, or fungal meningitis or meningeal tumor
Gram's stain	No organisms	Gram-positive or gram-negative organisms in bacterial meningitis

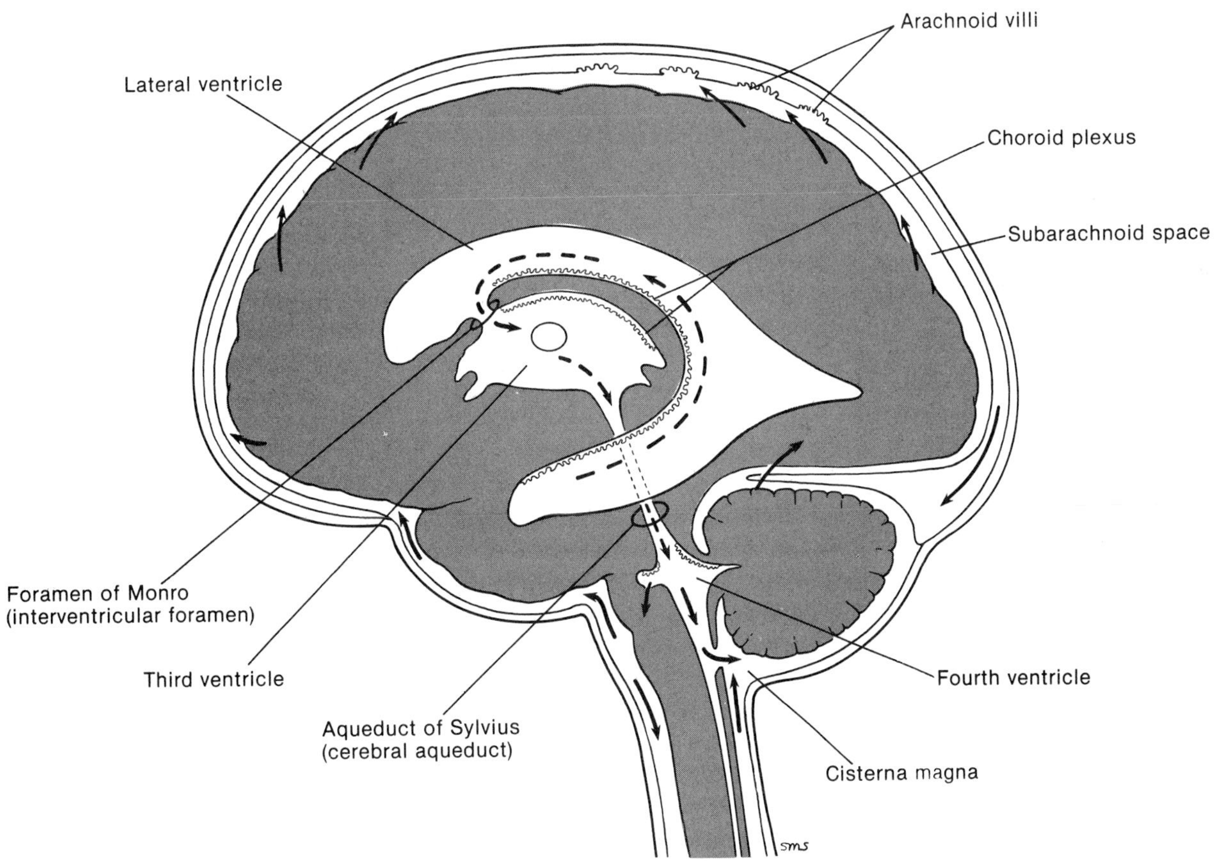

Figure 42-4 Cerebrospinal fluid circulation.

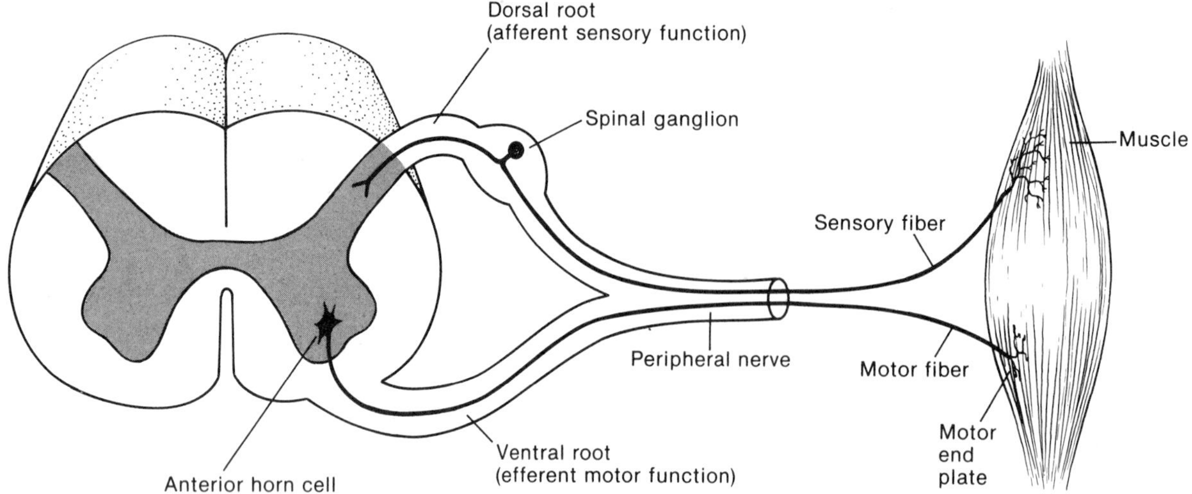

Figure 42-5 Spinal nerve motor and sensory function.

Muscular Function

Muscular function depends on the integrity of the *motor unit,* which is defined as a single motor nerve and the skeletal muscle fibers it innervates. Functional components of the motor unit are the anterior horn cell body of the spinal cord (lower motoneuron), its axon (peripheral nerve), the neuromuscular junction, and the muscle fiber. Cerebral cortical motor cells (upper motoneurons) and subcortical centers control the motor unit by both conscious volition and reflex activity.

The motor unit sends impulses traveling along the peripheral nerve to its termination, the *motor end-plate,* at the junction with muscle fibers. Activation of the peripheral nerve causes the release of acetylcholine at the motor end-plate. Acetylcholine in turn crosses the neuromuscular junction to depolarize the muscle fiber membrane, generating an action potential. Muscle fibers respond to depolarization in a series of structural and chemical changes that cause shortening or contraction.

Two systems of descending pathways govern motor activity. Conscious muscle contraction is controlled primarily by the *pyramidal system.* Impulses originating in the motor areas of the cortex travel along corticospinal tracts to the medulla where the nerve tracts cross (decussate) to the opposite side and descend through the spinal cord. The motor impulses arising from one hemisphere therefore result in muscular activity in the opposite side of the body.

The *extrapyramidal system* refers to those motor pathways that do not pass through the pyramids of the medulla. The basal ganglia, cerebellum, areas of the midbrain, and brain stem regulate the extrapyramidal system, which maintains muscle tone, posture, refinement, and coordination of movements.

The two systems operate in synchrony, using direct or indirect cerebral influence and reflex activity to produce continuous, mild muscle contractions for tone, unconscious muscular activity, and volitional motion.

Assessment of the Child With Neurologic Dysfunction

History

Alterations in neurologic and neuromuscular function might produce a wide variety of subtle or readily apparent difficulties. Other systemic alterations (metabolic, cardiovascular, and others) can accompany neurologic dysfunction, and a thorough history is necessary to determine the possible factors associated with the presenting disorder (see Chapter 14).

The maternal history of previous and subsequent pregnancies includes miscarriage, stillbirth, prematurity, congenital anomalies, or other conditions. The nurse then reviews the prenatal history for factors that might be associated with disorders of neurologic development such as the use of medications, exposure to radiation, nutritional deficiency, alcohol or drug abuse, and maternal endocrine or metabolic disorders (such as hypothyroidism or diabetes). The nurse also reviews the pregnancy for the length of gestation and any abnormalities such as vaginal bleeding, anemia, infection, or toxemia.

The history of labor and delivery includes the length of labor, presence of fetal distress, presentation, type of delivery (vaginal or cesarean section), and umbilical cord prolapse or compression, all of which can be related to perinatal trauma. Birthweight is noted and considered in relation to gestational age. The nurse also notes the Apgar scores, presence of respiratory problems, and congenital anomalies apparent at birth. The neonatal history covers any difficulties such as seizures, jaundice, poor muscle tone, irritability, or feeding problems.

Physical Examination

The nursing evaluation of the child with a neurologic problem includes a wide variety of assessments because virtually all life functions are regulated by the nervous system. The following sections will describe specific neurologic assessments of cerebral function, cranial nerves, cerebellar functions, motor and sensory systems, and reflexes. The nurse does not necessarily need to include all of these aspects in each evaluation but needs to be familiar with the complete neurologic assessment of children to provide knowledgeable management. A variety of diagnostic tests also are used for neurologic assessment (Table 42-3).

Cerebral Function The child's overall cerebral function is assessed by the history, observation, and specific tests. The child's general behavior, level of consciousness, orientation, memory, intellectual performance, and integrative functions of language, sensory, and motor skills are evaluated. The most important aid in assessing cerebral function is a systematic developmental assessment using reliable tests and established norms (see Chapter 16).

The child's level of activity (for example, overactivity, lethargy), mood (irritability, apathy, lability), and social responses are important clues to neurologic function. Behavioral characteristics are assessed according to age. Some behaviors, such as tantrums and a limited attention span, are typical in younger children. Other deviations, including hyperirritability, indifference to environment, or delirium, are abnormal at any age.

Level of consciousness is evaluated by the child's alertness, orientation, and ability to respond to verbal and physical stimuli. Lethargy, drowsiness, lack of orientation to familiar people or places, and decreased responsiveness indicate alterations in consciousness. The levels of altered consciousness can be defined as follows:

Stupor. The child is arousable for brief periods and can make simple verbal and motor responses. Stupor might alternate with periods of delirium, which is characterized by confusion and agitation.

Light coma. The child cannot be aroused and makes primitive and disorganized avoidance movements to painful stimuli.

Deep coma. The child does not respond to painful stimuli or responds with decerebrate posturing (rigid extension and pronation of the arms and extension of the legs).

Flaccid and apneic coma. The child's brain stem functions fail and respiratory effort stops. Artificial ventilation is necessary to support circulation, and electroencephalographic tracings reveal the absence of brain waves (Huttenlocher, 1979).

Although these levels often are used to describe a child's alteration in consciousness, there is considerable observer variability in the use of the terms, and it is important to describe the child's activity and responses accurately and in detail to avoid confusion of terms.

A standardized assessment tool to measure and serially record the level of consciousness has been developed and is now in widespread use. This tool, called the Glasgow Coma Scale (GCS), measures eye opening and best verbal response and best motor response, assigning numeric values to specific observations. The total number of points can range from 3 to 14, with 7 or less considered coma. The tool allows for a rapid, objective evaluation that is easily recorded and is helpful in monitoring for any changes in status (Teasdale and Jennett, 1974; Jones, 1979). These measurements are illustrated in Table 42-4.

In infants and young children, assessment of changes in consciousness must be made on less definitive data, depending on the child's developmental level. Activity level, motor responses, and recognition of familiar faces are helpful assessment criteria in younger children.

Accurate assessment of intellect requires formal psychometric testing procedures that are beyond the scope of the nurse's assessment, but the child's fund of general knowledge, performance of expected age-level tasks, and reasoning abilities can reflect the child's cognitive abilities. Memory problems can be indicated by the child's difficulty in rote repetition (immediate recall), short-term memory (remembering directions or recently presented information), or long-term memory (recall of previously learned material). These functions can be screened by developmental testing and comparison with norms for age. For example, a 3-year-old might be expected to repeat three digits in a test of immediate recall. Memory deficits can reflect language processing disorders, visual memory problems, or more global cerebral dysfunction.

Integrative functions also can be assessed by developmental screening. Language is evaluated both receptively (what the child understands) and expressively (how the child speaks). Following commands, pointing to pictures or objects, and nonverbal responses (gestures and symbols) demonstrate receptive language. The child's speech, vocabulary, naming, and grammar are indicators of expressive language. Deficits of cerebral language function (*aphasia*) are determined by specialized testing. Reading and writing abilities reflect the child's cognitive, language, and visual motor functions.

Functions associated with visual motor and spatial relations can be assessed by such tasks as copying geometric forms, doing puzzles, tying shoes, or catching a ball (see Chapter 16). These tests also assess the child's fine and gross motor skills. The child might have normal cognitive

TABLE 42-3 Radiographic and Other Neurodiagnostic Studies

Study	Organs	Procedure	Nursing management	Implications
Skull radiographs	Cranium	Single radiograph and various views of skull	Preparation for radiographic studies	Detects traumatic fractures and bony changes associated with congenital malformations, space-occupying lesions, and increased intracranial pressure
Computed tomographic (CT) scan	Internal structures of head	Intravenous injection of radiopaque dye (can be done with and without contrast). CT scanner takes multiple cross-sectional views of tissue density with data organized into composite pictures	Explain the procedure and scanning equipment. Administer sedation	Determines the size and position of ventricles, presence of masses, edema, and vascular changes
Cerebral angiography	Cerebral arteries and brain circulation	Sedation or general anesthesia. Injection of dye through femoral or carotid arteries. Radiographs	Explain procedure. Nothing by mouth according to protocol. Administer sedation. Post-test monitoring of vital signs and neurologic signs. Maintain immobility of injection site to reduce potential bleeding and edema—apply sandbag pressure as ordered. Check circulatory status in extremity distal to injection site for signs of obstruction	Detects blood vessel abnormalities, alterations of cerebral blood flow, and vascular tumors
Brain scan	Brain	Intravenous injection of isotope. Radioscanner detects presence of isotope and records the pattern on a chart	Explain procedure and equipment. Administer sedation if needed	Helps to detect intracranial lesions such as tumors and abscesses
Myelography	Spinal cord	Lumbar puncture. Injection of dye into subarachnoid space. Radiographs of spine	Explain procedure and equipment. Administer sedation. Post-test monitoring of vital signs, neurologic signs for indications of adverse reaction	Determines trauma, mass lesion, or other abnormality of the cord
Electroencephalogram (EEG)	Brain	Electrodes applied to head with conductive gel. Recordings taken during sleep, waking, hyperventilation, and stimulation with strobe light	Explain that electrodes do not hurt. Deprive the child of sleep prior to test if ordered. Administer sedation if ordered. Allow trusted adult to remain with child during test	Records electrical activity of the cerebral cortex. Identifies alterations in patterns due to seizures, trauma, or inflammation
Subdural tap	Subdural space of cranium	Performed on infants and young children up to 2 years of age. Needle with stylet is inserted into the subdural space through the anterior fontanel or coronal suture. The stylet is withdrawn and fluid is allowed to flow out.	Explain the procedure to parents. The child is in the supine position with the head held firmly. Monitor the child during the procedure for signs of shock or alteration in consciousness. After the test, maintain pressure dressing to the site, observe for fluid oozing from the site	Detects and removes abnormal fluid collections in subdural space (effusion, hematoma). Collects fluid samples for laboratory analysis

TABLE 42-3 Radiographic and Other Neurodiagnostic Studies

Study	Organs	Procedure	Nursing management	Implications
		The amount of fluid withdrawn is limited to 15–30 mL from each side of the head. The stylet is replaced and the needle is withdrawn		
Lumbar puncture	Cerebrospinal fluid system; lumbar spine	Needle with stylet is inserted into interspace between third and fourth lumbar vertebrae until the dural space is entered. The stylet is removed, and a three-way stopcock with a manometer is attached to measure CSF pressure. Cerebrospinal fluid samples are collected in numbered tubes. The stylet is replaced and the needle is removed	Explain the procedure. Position the child on the side with spine curved. Hold the child firmly with head flexed on chest and knees flexed on abdomen. Give the child constant verbal support and reassurance throughout the procedure. Monitor the child's respiratory status during the procedure. After the test monitor for headache, fever, or fluid leakage from the puncture site. Assist with obtaining a blood sample to measure serum glucose	Determines elevated CSF pressure. Collects CSF samples for culture, cell count, and protein and glucose measurements. Aids in diagnosis of meningitis, encephalitis, central nervous system hemorrhage, and increased intracranial pressure (ICP) (Contraindicated in the presence of acutely increased ICP)
Electromyography (EMG)	Muscle	Needle electrodes are inserted into the muscle to be tested. Electrical activity is recorded at rest and during muscle contraction	Explain the procedure, discomfort, and need to hold still. Administer sedation if ordered. Ensure that the child has an adult support figure during test	Measures electrical activity of muscle—differentiates nerve and muscle disorders
Nerve conduction studies	Peripheral nerves	Electrodes taped to skin at points to be tested. Mild electric shock applied as nerve stimulation. Velocity of transmission of nerve impulses is recorded	Same as for EMG	Measures velocity of nerve impulses along peripheral pathways. Detects nerve damage and demyelination

and visual abilities but lack the motor control necessary to perform the expected tasks.

Cranial Nerve Function Evaluation of the 12 pairs of cranial nerves yields important information about underlying brain function (see Table 14-15) and can help to localize specific deficits. Cranial nerve assessment is outlined in Table 42-5. Examination is difficult in infants and young children, and information is gleaned more readily from careful observation of the child's activity and responses than from formal testing.

Cerebellar Function The cerebellum coordinates and refines motor movements and maintains postural balance. Assessment is directed toward comparing the child's balance and coordination with expectations for age. A variety of tests can be used to determine cerebellar function, and the child's motor movements in play, dressing, and feeding also can be observed. (Tests for cerebellar function are described in Chapter 14.)

The nurse assesses balance by asking the child to stand with the feet together, arms outstretched, and eyes closed. A positive Romberg's sign is demonstrated when the child starts to fall during this test. The arms also are observed for excessive drift or abnormal hand movements.

Motor Function The nurse assesses muscle tone by determining the resistance to passive range of motion of

TABLE 42-4 Glasgow Coma Scale

Numeric value	Eyes open	Best verbal response	Best motor response
5	Yes	Oriented to familiar persons, place, and time	Obeys command to move body part
4	Spontaneously	Able to respond verbally but is disoriented and confused	Purposefully tries to remove painful stimulus
3	To sounds and speech	Inappropriate verbal responses; uses words or phrases that make little or no sense	Arm flexion in response to pain (decorticate)
2	To pain	No intelligible verbalizations; responds with incomprehensible sounds	Arm extension and internal rotation in response to pain (decerebrate)
1	None	None	None

the trunk and extremities. Reduced tone (*hypotonia*) can be seen in the "floppy" infant who lies in a frog-leg position with the hips abducted and legs in external rotation rather than the normal flexed posture. The nurse also can detect hypotonia by suspending the infant in a prone position, supporting the infant under the chest. The infant with decreased muscle tone will hang in a dangling posture without attempting to right the head. Flaccid paralysis is indicated by the child's inability to move or lack of normal resistance to passive movement of a body part.

Increased muscle tone (*hypertonia*) is evidenced by abnormal muscle rigidity when the infant or child is at rest. *Spasticity* refers to prolonged muscular contraction and increased resistance of muscles to passive stretching. Spastic hypertonicity can be noted in a rebound effect when the child's arms or legs are moved through normal range of motion and then released. The child with increased tone of the hip adductors will demonstrate a scissoring motion when attempts are made to separate the legs. When the child is held upright or stands, this scissoring also can be seen with the legs and feet held in extension.

Hypertonia associated with spastic cerebral palsy often results in rigid extensor thrust of the neck, trunk, and legs when the child is lifted or pulled to a sitting position suddenly. Milder degrees of spasticity can be detected in the distal joints (equinus extension of the foot) or consistent fisting of the hand after 5 or 6 months of age. As spastic muscle groups are moved gently through their range of motion, the spastic contraction will suddenly give way, reducing the resistance to the movement (clasp-knife effect). In contrast, persistent rigidity of a joint without relaxation reflects basal ganglia involvement, contracture formation, or inflammation (such as is seen in the neck and spinal rigidity associated with meningitis or poliomyelitis).

Muscle strength is determined by observing the child's spontaneous activity in getting up from lying down or sitting, standing, and walking. The nurse notes symmetry, any weakness, and the degree of ease in movement. Strength also is assessed against resistance. Individual muscle groups are tested by having the child resist the nurse's movements. The child's cooperation can be elicited by making a game of flexing or extending the head, trunk, and extremities against resistance. For example, the nurse might ask the child to keep the arm flexed while the nurse tries to extend it or keep the arms together while the nurse attempts to separate them. Active strength also is assessed by having the child grasp the nurse's fingers and squeeze them. The nurse notes the presence and degree of weakness, paying particular attention to the equality of strength of the muscle groups of the two sides of the body.

Motor control and coordination can be assessed by developmental screening of age-appropriate motor tasks. The nurse assesses head control, sitting balance, standing, walking, and other age-expected motor milestones. The nurse observes the child manipulate toys, reach for objects, and perform bilateral hand activities to evaluate both fine motor control and hand preference. Dominance of one hand or the other normally does not develop before 18 months to 2 years of age. Preferential use of one hand before this age can indicate a weakness of the other hand.

The nurse observes the child's gait for abnormalities of toe-walking, scissoring, unsteadiness, or asymmetric weakness or limp. Other tests of balance and coordination are discussed earlier in the chapter in the section on cerebellar function.

The nurse notes abnormal movements and postures with the child at rest and performing activities. Tremors on

TABLE 42-5 Assessment of Cranial Nerves

Nerve	Assessment	Nursing implications
Olfactory (I)	Test child's ability to smell familiar odors (peppermint, peanut butter) with eyes closed	Impairment usually is related to upper respiratory illness or allergic condition rather than neurologic dysfunction
Optic (II)	Measure visual acuity, visual fields, Fundoscopic exam (see Chapters 14 and 43)	Fundus of eye: optic disk edema (papilledema), retinal hemorrhage, and decreased venous pulsations indicate increased intracranial pressure. Environmental safety precautions and rehabilitation are required for the child with a visual field deficit (blindspot)
Oculomotor (III), trochlear (IV), and abducens (VI) (tested together)	Evaluate size, symmetry, and reaction to light. Test child's ability to move eyes to follow object in all directions (extraocular movements). Note nystagmus (rhythmic jerking of eyes)	Unequal pupils, decreased reaction to light, double vision, or paralysis of eye movement might indicate brain tumor, hemorrhage, inflammation, and increased intracranial pressure. Nystagmus can be associated with toxic reactions to drugs (especially phenytoin and phenobarbital)
Trigeminal (V)	Test facial sensation by child's ability to feel light touch. Assess motor function by strength and symmetry of jaw closure. Test corneal reflex—eyeblink to touching cornea with wisp of cotton	Assess the child's ability to chew and adapt feeding as necessary to avoid possible choking or aspiration. The absence of a corneal reflex requires the instillation of artificial tears (lubricant eye drops) to protect the cornea from abrasion
Facial (VII)	Note symmetry of facial expression and movement. Test facial muscle strength by having the child close eyes tightly and press lips closed. Test the child's ability to taste salt and sugar	Paralysis of the facial nerve (Bell's palsy) might be associated with otitis media and meningitis. Incomplete eye closure might require that a patch be worn to protect the cornea
Acoustic (VIII)	Assess hearing (see Chapter 43)	
Glossopharyngeal (IX), vagus (X)	Test the child's ability to swallow. Assess the gag reflex by stimulating the pharynx with a tongue depressor or cotton-tipped applicator. Note a hoarse or stridorous vocal quality	Impairment can interfere with feeding so the nurse should adapt feeding techniques to reduce the risk of aspiration. Inability to swallow oral secretions requires positioning to facilitate drainage and oropharyngeal suctioning as needed
Accessory (XI)	Test the movement and strength of the trapezius and sternocleidomastoid muscles by having the child turn the head to each side against resistance and elevate the shoulders against resistance	Impairment interferes with head control. Measures are needed to provide head and neck support
Hypoglossal (XII)	Assess tongue movement by having the child protrude the tongue. Note symmetry, tremors, and ability to move tongue	Abnormal tongue movements are common in children with cerebral palsy. Impairment interferes with feeding and speech (Refer to Rehabilitation management, child with cerebral palsy)

reaching, involuntary writhing movements of the extremities (*athetosis*), or irregular jerking movements (*chorea*) might be seen with motor dysfunction. These movements may become more pronounced as the child attempts motor control and diminish or disappear when the child is at rest and during sleep. Other abnormal movements might include tongue thrust, facial twitching or grimacing, and behaviors associated with various seizure activities.

Posturing can reflect alterations in muscle tone. Rigid arching of the back with neck extension is called *opisthotonos* and reflects hypertonic spinal extensors. This posture

(text continued on p. 1530)

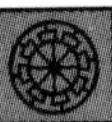

ASSESSMENT GUIDE Child With a Neurologic Impairment

System	Subjective data	Objective data	Validating data: *Diagnostic tests*	Validating data: *Radiographs*	Nursing management
Head and neck	Headache. Stiff neck	Head circumference may be increased if cranial sutures not closed. Fontanelles bulging and tense. Positive Kernig's and Brudzinski's signs. Inabiity to flex neck. Bruising. Soft tissue edema of scalp. Abnormal shape and asymmetry of cranium	Lumbar puncture. Cerebrospinal fluid analysis and culture. Subdural tap	CT scan Skull radiographs	Observe for signs and symptoms of increased ICP. Care of child with meningitis, encephalitis. Care of child with craniocerebral trauma
Eyes and ears	Blurred, double vision. Decreased hearing. Tinnitus	Decreased visual acuity. Abnormal pupil reaction. Unequal or paralysis of extraocular movements. Scleras visible above iris ("setting sun" sign)		CT scan	Observe for signs of intracranial pressure. Monitor level of consciousness Serially measure head and chest circumference. Observe for other signs of hydrocephalus
Nose and throat	Feeding difficulties	Poor or absent suck. Absent gag reflex. Gingival hypertrophy	Serum diphenylhydantoin level		Prevent aspiration by positioning, adapted feeding techniques. Teach oral hygiene measures for child with side effects of anticonvulsant medication
Respiratory	Cough. Dyspnea	Irregular respirations. Gasping respirations. Deep or shallow respirations. Increased or decreased respiratory rate. Cyanosis. Rales. Rhonchi. Absent breath sounds	Arterial blood gases	Chest radiographs	Position for optimal ventilation. Suction airway as needed. Prepare for emergency intubation. Monitor for increased ICP Manually hyperventilate for hypoxia Chest clapping and percussion, postural drainage, frequent position changes

ASSESSMENT GUIDE Child With a Neurologic Impairment (continued)

System	Subjective data	Objective data	Validating data: *Diagnostic tests*	Validating data: *Radiographs*	Nursing management
Cardiovascular		Hypertension. Hypotension. Increased or decreased pulse. Arrhythmias. Widening pulse pressure	Complete blood count Hemoglobin Hematocrit		Monitor vital signs. Monitor for increased ICP
Gastrointestinal	Nausea. Vomiting. Abdominal pain	Projectile vomiting often not preceded by nausea. Abdominal rigidity. Decreased or absent bowel sounds	Complete blood count Electrolyte levels		Nothing by mouth or clear liquids as ordered. Monitor parenteral infusion for fluid maintenance. Measure fluid output
Genitourinary	Urinary incontinence, history of repeated urinary tract infections	Lack of sphincter control. Incomplete bladder emptying. Bladder distention	Blood urea nitrogen level	Urodynamic studies Kidney, ureter, and bladder (KUB) radiographs	Observe for bladder distention. Hygienic care to prevent skin breakdown from incontinence. For the child with a spinal cord lesion, teach urinary tract management
Musculoskeletal	Muscle pain. Weakness. Paralysis	Increased or decreased muscle size or strength. Asymmetry. Paralysis. Hypotonia, hypertonia, spasticity. Abnormal movements. Abnormal postures	Electromyogram Nerve conduction studies	Skeletal radiographs Myelography	Position child to prevent contractures. Perform range-of-motion exercises as ordered. Assist with rehabilitative program
	Reported convulsions. Facial or body twitching	Observed seizure activity, generalized or focal	Electroencephalogram (EEG) Serum anticonvulsant levels Complete blood count Blood chemistries Cerebrospinal fluid culture	CT scan Skull radiographs	Seizure precautions. Teaching and management of the child with a seizure disorder (see Nursing Care Guide)
Integumentary		Petechial rash	Lumbar puncture Cerebospinal fluid culture Nasopharyngeal culture		Strict isolation until meningococcemia is ruled out

continued on next page

ASSESSMENT GUIDE Child With a Neurologic Impairment (continued)

System	Subjective data	Objective data	Validating data: *Diagnostic tests*	Validating data: *Radiographs*	Nursing management
Neuroendocrine	Numbness. Tingling	Decreased superficial sensation. Skin lesions. Café-au-lait spots. Adenoma sebaceum. Spinal dimple or hair tuft	Skin culture		Protect child from trauma caused by insensitivity to pain. Skin care to stimulate circulation and prevent skin breakdown. Management of the child with a neurocutaneous syndrome

can reflect meningeal irritation or cerebral motor insult. Persistent tonic neck reflex posture at any age or elicited tonic neck posture after 6 months of age is atypical. The nurse notes any abnormal posturing of the extremities such as the persistent arm flexion and fisting seen in hemiplegia.

Characteristic postures are associated with severe brain insult and alterations of consciousness. In *decorticate* posturing the arms are held adducted with the elbows flexed and hands fisted over the chest, and the legs are extended. This posture usually reflects diffuse cerebral involvement. *Decerebrate* posturing consists of rigid extension, adduction, and internal rotation of the arms with the legs extended. This posturing indicates brain stem dysfunction.

Nursing Management for Procedures and Treatments

Preparation for Diagnostic Tests

The child with neurologic dysfunction might be functioning at a cognitive level below the chronologic age, and it is important that the nurse perceive the child's level of understanding and any observable behavioral disorder to prepare the child accurately for diagnostic tests.

The *electroencephalogram* (EEG) is a frequently used noninvasive diagnostic test which requires that the child remain still and have electrodes applied to the scalp with a paste. The quality of the recording depends on the child remaining quiet and relaxed, which is more successful when the child is well prepared. Explanation of the procedure should include pictures and description of the "wires," how they are attached to the head, and the assurance that the child will not be hurt. Older children might understand an analogy to a television or radio picking up a "picture" of the brain's activity. Children often fear being shocked electrically by the wires, and they need an opportunity to see the technician or nurse handle the electrodes to see that they are not harmful. The gel or paste used can be likened to a material that the child is familiar with such as toothpaste or petroleum jelly. Sedation might be necessary with infants and very young children. It is extremely helpful to have a trusted adult remain with the child during the EEG for reassurance and to remind the child to stay still.

Radiographic studies include both single radiographs and more specialized procedures such as computerized tomographic (CT) scans and angiography. The CT scanner usually has a device, such as a fluid-filled cap or sandbag and forehead strap, to immobilize the child's head. The nurse tells the child that a special type of hat or headband will help to hold the child still. The scanner can be frightening to the child, and the nurse shows the child pictures of the equipment and explains that the child will lie with the head inside the donut-shaped opening. The machine emits a clicking noise, which also should be explained to the child.

A lumbar puncture is performed to examine the cerebrospinal fluid (CSF) and measure its pressure. The nurse explains the procedure to the child in terms appropriate to the child's level of understanding, telling the child that this special test requires lying in a flexed position curled up like a ball. It is extremely important that the child know that a support figure will be present constantly to help hold the child still. Sedation is occasionally necessary.

The child assumes a side-lying position, and the spine is kept curved by holding the child under the thighs and knees and bringing the child's head forward into flexion (Fig. 42-6). The nurse monitors the child's respiratory status to avoid compromise in the acutely ill child. Once the needle is inserted, the child's flexion is relaxed (still with restraint to

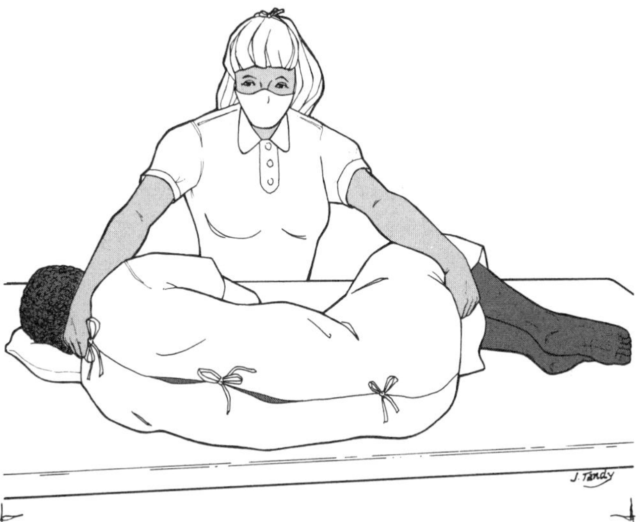

Figure 42-6 Positioning of the child for lumbar puncture.

prevent movement, which could cause trauma) close to a neutral position to reduce postural influences on the CSF pressure measurement. The child is allowed a breather, encouraged to relax, and told that the painful part of the procedure is over. Infants may be given a pacifier to calm them. When the child is quiet, the CSF pressure is measured.

Following the procedure, the child might be required to remain in a flat position for 4–6 hours to reduce headache and discomfort. The nurse monitors the child for headache, fever, pupil changes, or fluid leakage from the puncture site.

A subdural tap might be performed on infants or young children to remove fluid accumulations from the subdural space. The child is restrained securely in the supine position with the head held firmly to prevent movement. Meningeal laceration or cerebral injury can result if the needle moves when in place. The nurse observes the child closely during the procedure for changes indicative of shock or alterations in consciousness caused by removing the fluid too rapidly.

Following the procedure, a pressure dressing is applied to the puncture site, and the child is maintained in a semi-upright position in an infant seat or with pillows to minimize fluid leakage from the site of the tap. The puncture site and surrounding skin are observed for oozing of fluid.

Electromyography and nerve conduction studies require that the child remain still during the placement of electrodes and the recording of electrical activity. The nurse tells the older child that the test will feel like "mosquito bites" and tingling as if the child had hit the funny bone. The procedure can be explained as a picture of the work that muscles do. The nurse tells the child that the needle electrodes cause some discomfort, which prepares and helps the child not to fight the procedure. Younger children might need to be sedated before accurate testing can be performed.

Lumbar Puncture Procedure

- Prepare the child and parent for the procedure
- Child assumes side-lying position with knees tucked and chin flexed to chest. The back is bowed out and resembles the position of the back in a fetal position. Nurse or parent "hugs" child to maintain position.
- Using sterile technique a 6-in circular area of the lumbar region is prepped using a povidone-iodine solution. This feels cold to the child.
- Local anesthetic is injected by needle-syringe or pressurized air gun into the subcutaneous tissue. The child feels a burning, stinging sensation. Occasionally a child will request no anesthetic.
- An 18- to 22-gauge needle with stylet is then inserted between two lumbar vertebrae until the spinal compartment is reached. The child feels pressure and occasionally a shooting pain down a leg.
- The stylet is removed and the child is encouraged to relax. CSF pressure may be measured. A few milliliters of CS fluid are removed for laboratory examination by allowing the fluid to drip into several plastic test tubes.
- The needle is removed and light pressure and a Band-aid are applied to the entry site. The child is comforted and may return to normal activity. Occasionally a headache results. Should this occur, the child should remain in a flat position for 4–6 hours after subsequent LP procedures.

SOURCE: Courtesy of Kathleen Hardin Mooney

Habilitation and Rehabilitation Management

Care of the child with a neurologic disorder often involves special management to improve deficit areas of function, help the child to develop compensatory skills, and maximize the child's overall development. Habilitation and rehabilitation programs for the child must be planned carefully by the child's therapeutic team and based on a thorough assessment of the child's physical and cognitive capabilities, as well as social, family, and environmental strengths and weaknesses. The plan must be realistic but allow for the uncertain prognosis of many childhood neurologic conditions. The child with neuromuscular impairment might develop age-appropriate intellectual abilities, but this can be difficult to determine in infancy or early childhood. Similarly, the child who has suffered head trauma might regain the previous level of function or have permanent residual deficits; the outcome is difficult to predict immediately following the injury.

(text continued on p. 1534)

NURSING CARE GUIDE Rehabilitation for the Child With Neurologic Impairment

Nursing diagnosis	Interventions	Evaluation
1. Potential for multiple alterations in cognitive, motor, sensory, and physiologic functions	Collaborate with multidisciplinary team to assess, plan, implement, and evaluate the child's rehabilitation program Provide for ongoing family participation in child's rehabilitation program	Child's multiple needs are met through coordinated team interventions.
2. Potential for alterations in mobility	Perform exercises as ordered to maintain the child's joint mobility and strengthen muscle function Apply orthoses to stabilize and support the child's trunk and extremities for ambulation Supervise and reinforce the child's ambulation program Provide safety measures as needed (such as helmet and contact guarding) Provide the nonambulatory child with a wheelchair, cart, or stroller Ensure that the child in a wheelchair is adequately supported and is in good sitting alignment Teach the child independent mobility, transfers, and wheelchair safety	Child achieves maximum independent mobility without injury
3. Potential for joint contractures secondary to paralysis, spasticity, and immobility	Perform range-of-motion exercises as indicated Alternate the child's position frequently (positions such as prone on wedge and elevate legs) to prevent prolonged joint flexion and extension Position the child with supports to maintain correct alignment (abduction wedge between legs, footrests, and tray for elbow support, for example) Apply splints, braces, and bivalved casts as ordered	No evidence of joint contractures
4. Potential for alteration in skin integrity secondary to sensory impairment, paralysis, and spasticity	Provide frequent skin care Inspect the skin for pressure areas Check for friction rubs in orthoses, bivalved casts, and shoes Provide measures to protect the skin (such as sheepskin, alternating pressure mattress, flotation seat cushion, shoes without rough seams, protective clothing)	Child shows no evidence of pressure areas, decubitus ulcers, burns, or abrasions
5. Potential alterations in feeding secondary to oromotor impairment or swallowing dysfunction	Position the child in optimal sitting alignment Adapt the consistency of the child's food Provide special assistance as indicated (for example manual jaw closure or placing food between side teeth or at center of tongue) Obtain adapted equipment to facilitate feeding and the child's independence	Child's health status reflects adequate nutritional status; child shows no evidence of feeding complications (airway obstruction or aspiration pneumonia)

NURSING CARE GUIDE Rehabilitation for the Child With Neurologic Impairment (continued)

Nursing diagnosis	Interventions	Evaluation
6. Potential alteration in elimination patterns	Monitor adequacy of bowel and bladder elimination Ensure adequate fluid intake Perform alternate means of bladder emptying as ordered (Credé method and intermittent catheterization) Provide ostomy care for the child with ileal loop diversion (see Chapters 38 and 39) Develop bowel program with regular toileting schedule, dietary adjustment, and use of suppositories Adapt toilet seat to provide support for trunk and extremities	Child is able to feed independently; child shows no evidence of urinary tract infection, bladder distention, or constipation; child achieves maximum possible bladder and bowel continence
7. Potential alterations in communication secondary to oromotor impairment or aphasia	Assist in developing alternative communication systems (gestures, sign language, communication board, typewriter, voice synthesizer, and so on) Exercise patience as the child attempts to communicate Facilitate the use of the communication system by all who interact with the child	Child is able to communicate successfully
8. Potential alteration in developmental progression	Encourage mobility as a means of exploration Adapt play materials to enable the child to manipulate them Provide stimulation appropriate to the child's developmental level Adapt self-care activities to facilitate independence (clothes with Velcro closures, elastic waist, shoes without laces, adapted feeding equipment, support bars in bathroom, and so on) Praise and reinforce the child's attempts at mastery and independence	Child achieves age-appropriate developmental tasks
9. Potential alteration in self-image	Help the child and family to recognize the child's strengths and abilities Set realistic rehabilitation goals to avoid a sense of failure Allow for the expression of frustrations, anger, sadness, and other emotional reactions Encourage opportunities for positive experiences with peers Recognize serious emotional complications and refer the child and family for appropriate intervention	Child demonstrates a positive self-image with no evidence of emotional complications

continued on next page

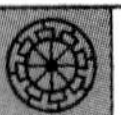

NURSING CARE GUIDE Rehabilitation for the Child With Neurologic Impairment (continued)

Nursing diagnosis	Interventions	Evaluation
10. Potential knowledge deficit related to home rehabilitation management	Teach the child and family specific aspects of the child's rehabilitation (including all of the preceding interventions) Teach the elements of comprehensive child health and not just for the deficit areas Assist the family to prioritize the child's multiple needs; discuss ways that exercises and other therapeutic regimens can be incorporated into daily activities Provide anticipatory guidance and support in helping the family to cope with the impact of the child's disability on siblings, family relationships, and lifestyle Refer the family to community agencies and organizations for children with special needs to provide: Counseling and support Health, educational, and therapy services Recreational opportunities Adapted equipment Advocacy Provide consultation and liaison for school placement	Child and family demonstrate a knowledge of specific rehabilitation measures and health care maintenance. Family copes optimally with the impact of a disabled child. Child and family use resources as needed. Child successfully attends appropriate educational program

The nurse is involved in the therapeutic management of neurologically handicapped children in acute-care settings, rehabilitation centers, and ambulatory and home-based programs. The nurse often coordinates multidisciplinary team efforts and acts as the family's liaison with various specialty services. Depending on the type of disorder, rehabilitative nursing measures include physical care, providing adaptive equipment, developmental stimulation, and behavioral management.

Exercises The child with motor limitations often requires specific exercise programs to maintain joint mobility and strengthen muscle function. Range-of-motion exercises are important for the child with paralysis, muscle weakness, or spasticity. Moving the child's extremities through their full flexion, extension, and rotation both helps to prevent joint contracture from disuse and improves circulation to the affected area. These exercises usually are carried out several times daily and can be incorporated into other care routines (bathing, dressing) and play activities.

Specific therapeutic exercises are determined by the child's orthopedist and physical therapist and usually are directed toward improving strength, endurance, and functional use of particular muscle groups. The paraplegic child might have an exercise program to strengthen the upper body and arms in preparation for walking with crutches and wheelchair mobility, which require considerable shoulder and arm strength. Push-ups and lifting weights in bed using a trapeze are additional muscle strengthening modalities that can be employed.

The exercise program of the child with poor muscular control and alterations in muscle reflex or tone is geared toward improving postural patterns and movement. Mat activities, balancing, and positioning encourage the normal developmental progression of head and trunk control, sitting, crawling, and so on. Young children can be moved through exercises passively, and the nurse obtains cooperation with active exercises by play, positioning, and stimulation. Placing a toy just out of reach and assisting the child to focus on the toy and to move toward it can promote the desired motor movement. Providing visual and auditory stimulation that is pleasing to the child with the child prone or sitting will encourage attempts at head and neck control. Older children are able to follow directions for active and active-assisted exercises and can pay attention to tasks for longer periods. The nurse encourages play and a sense of mastery to increase cooperation with and motivation for exercise programs. Gait training, for instance, can be enhanced by emphasizing the child's independence, using colored tape markers on the floor for goals, and praising the child's accomplishments.

The nurse monitors and reinforces exercise programs, working with the child and family to carry out the specific regimen. The child's attitude toward the exercises often will reflect the attitudes of those around the child, and a positive approach to exercises and incorporating them into meaningful activities will foster cooperation and persistence. Using positive reinforcements, such as achievement charts or goals of walking to the playroom, can help the child to remain engaged in what can otherwise become tiresome exercises.

Casts, Splints, and Braces Assistive devices are used to correct, maintain, and support body parts in a functional position when weakness, paralysis, or spasticity is present. Casts are used following orthopedic corrective surgery (see Chapter 41) and as removable (bivalved) supports for intermittent use. Patients often wear bivalved leg, arm, or body casts at night to maintain joint alignment and prevent contracture formation. The cast is applied in two halves, posterior and anterior, and closed securely with straps and buckles. The child's skin is rubbed with alcohol and inspected for pressure areas before putting the cast on and after removing it. Rubbing inside the cast can result in friction over bony prominences, particularly when the child has spastic muscle movements. It might be necessary to alter the cast or have the child wear it for shorter periods. The child's affected body part is eased into the correct position in the cast following range-of-motion exercises and relaxation and is never forced. The nurse checks circulation, sensation, and movement frequently when the child is adjusting to the cast (see Chapter 41). The casted area is supported with pillows, sandbags, or blanket rolls. A removable bar often is used between long leg casts to maintain hip abduction.

Like casts, splints maintain functional alignment of an affected body part. Handsplints are used frequently when a child's hand is weakened by hemiparesis, paralysis, or spasticity. The splint has a lightweight plastic posterior shell, and Velcro straps are used to hold the hand and wrist in place. As with casts, the nurse moves the extremity gently to the desired position before applying the splint and checks for irritation and pressure sores. Resting splints are removed when the child is actively using the affected part. Assistive splints help to stabilize a joint or joints for functional use. Handsplints provide wrist and hand stability and can be fitted with attachments for eating utensils, pencils, typing pointer, and the like.

Braces of various types are used to stabilize a body part for functional use as well as to maintain alignment. Lower extremity and trunk orthoses (bracing devices) are used to control and support areas of neuromuscular weakness or imbalance for weight bearing, sitting, and ambulation. Below the knee, braces may be molded polypropylene shells that are worn inside the shoes to stabilize the foot and ankle. Other braces might assist motion with adjustable spring joints on vertical supports to aid plantar and dorsiflexion. The supports are attached directly to the shoe or to a molded insert by a band at the upper end around the calf.

More extensive lower extremity orthoses are used for hip and knee control and may be attached to body jackets for maximum support such as for children with spinal cord lesions. Hip and knee joints on the braces have locking pins or slide bars to provide stability for standing but allow sitting with the joints unlocked. The inner surfaces of the brace that come in contact with the skin usually are padded with foam or soft leather to prevent pressure areas. Children should wear absorbent cotton undergarments and socks under braces to prevent skin irritation. The underwear worn beneath the braces must be close fitting and adjusted so that wrinkles do not create friction points.

Skin care is essential when orthoses are worn. Skin breakdowns are prevented by alcohol rubs, inspecting the skin for pressure areas, and applying the braces properly. The braces are adjusted periodically to ensure proper fit, replace worn parts, and change the type of support as the child's needs change. The nurse checks the child who is wearing a new orthosis frequently for areas of redness, friction, and adequacy of circulation. The amount of time that the child wears the brace is increased gradually as the child's ability to tolerate it increases, and the brace is altered as needed.

Other equipment for the child with neuromuscular weakness or imbalance include prone standers, standing tables, chairs with added support and leg abduction wedges, overbed trapezes, and many other devices that are constructed to improve alignment and functional motor skills. The nurse ensures that the child's position is changed at regular intervals to prevent joint contractures and skin breakdown.

Mobilizing Aids In addition to orthoses for stability, children with neuromuscular impairments often need assistive devices for mobility, either ambulatory instruments or wheeled apparatuses. Walkers, crutches, and canes provide added support for standing and walking, and the child's therapist teaches the proper use of these aids and gait technique. The nurse supervises and reinforces the child's ambulation, ensuring that safety measures (helmet, contact guarding) are used as needed to prevent injury from falls. As the child becomes more ambulatory, an important aspect of the teaching program is learning how to fall without injury. Many children with neurologic impairments do not develop normal protective reflexes and need to be taught how to balance, right, and break their fall should they trip or lose their balance. Different types of walkers and crutches give varying degrees of support and are chosen according to the child's strength and motor control. The child might begin ambulation with a rolling walker and progress to crutches as skill and strength develop.

Functional ambulation is possible for many neurologically handicapped children, but for many of these children, ambulation may be slow-paced and require a tremendous energy expenditure. These children and others for whom weight-bearing ambulation is not possible benefit from mobility via wheelchairs, carts, and strollers adapted to their individual needs. Adequate support is needed to maintain these children in correct alignment and provide stability for pushing themselves or engaging in activities with their upper extremities. Adaptations include footrests with straps, pelvic and trunk supports or safety belts, leg abduction wedges, headrests, and one-wheel driven or motorized chairs. The type of chair is selected to allow maximum mobility and independence while providing the necessary stabilization. When positioning the child in a wheelchair, the nurse checks the fit and ensures that the child is adequately supported and in proper sitting alignment. Examples of improper fit include footrests that are too low or high, a seat that is too long and presses on the popliteal space, and a chair size that is too large, preventing the child from reaching the wheels and pushing independently.

The child with upper extremity strength is taught to propel, manipulate doors and ramps, and transfer to and from the chair independently. In all rehabilitative efforts, the goals are to increase the child's freedom and independence while providing adequate safeguards from accidents. The child's age and judgment ability are considered in allowing wheelchair access near such potentially dangerous areas as stoves, stairs, ramps, and so forth. The young child who is mobile on wheels is as capable as the nonimpaired youngster of exploring and being injured accidentally. The nurse teaches safety measures to parents of handicapped children, particularly as previously immobile children learn new means of moving about.

Principles of Nursing Care

Acute-Care Needs

The Child With Increased Intracranial Pressure Increased intracranial pressure (ICP) may accompany a number of neurologic conditions such as craniocerebral trauma, hydrocephalus, brain tumor, meningitis, encephalitis, or intracerebral hemorrhage. Although the primary cause might differ, the physiologic principles of increased ICP in the various conditions are similar.

Normal ICP is a function of balance between the fixed volume of the rigid cranium and the volume of its contents—brain tissue, meninges, CSF, and blood. For the pressure to remain constant once the cranial sutures are closed, an increase in the volume of any one of these intracranial contents must be accompanied by a relative reduction in the volume of one or more of the other contents. The ability of the cerebral structures to compensate for increasing volume is limited to buffer mechanisms of CSF displacement to the spinal subarachnoid space and increased CSF absorption. These compensatory mechanisms allow the brain to tolerate transient elevations in ICP. When the maximal degree of compensation is exceeded by increasing intracranial volume, symptoms of increased ICP are seen.

Cerebral blood flow can be altered by several mechanisms that are important factors in increased ICP. Autoregulation of cerebral blood flow causes vasoconstriction when the arterial carbon dioxide content is low and, conversely, vasodilatation when the carbon dioxide level is elevated (*hypercapnia*). If respiratory insufficiency results in hypoxia and hypercapnia, cerebral blood flow is increased, which further elevates the ICP. Other systemic effects that increase cerebral blood flow include fever and hypertension.

As ICP rises, venous drainage is impeded, which both elevates the pressure further and slows capillary circulation. A progressive loss of vascular autoregulation and reduced cerebral blood flow result in cerebral edema from tissue ischemia, which further raises the ICP. An unchecked cycle decreasing perfusion, increasing edema, and increasing ICP results in complete loss of brain arterial perfusion and death.

The manifestations of increased ICP vary depending on the age of the child, cause of the disorder, and rate (acute or chronic) at which the pressure develops. In infants the skull is able to expand as the volume of its contents expands. A tense, bulging fontanelle, separation of cranial sutures, and head enlargement are signs of increased ICP in infants and young children under 2 years of age. Because of the adaptive ability of the cranial vault, symptoms of disturbed brain function at this age might be minimal. Irritability, poor feeding, and delayed development might occur, but the more classic indicators of increased ICP often are not present.

Older children, whose cranial volume compliance is limited, might develop headache, nausea, vomiting, alterations in behavior and consciousness, *diplopia* (double vision), and *papilledema* (optic disk swelling). As ICP increases, focal neurologic deficits of cranial nerve dysfunction (pupil reactivity changes, loss of oculomotor control), unilateral motor or sensory changes (hemiparesis), and seizures might develop. Advanced increased ICP causes the Cushing triad of slowed pulse, altered respiratory rate, and elevated systemic blood pressure. Progressive lethargy, stupor, and coma accompany untreated increased ICP.

A severe complication of increased ICP is the displacement of brain tissue (*herniation*) into an adjacent space. Herniation of cerebral tissue inferiorly across the *tentorium* (the barrier between the cerebrum and brain stem) can result in the compression of blood vessels, obstruction to the CSF flow, and injury to cerebral and brain stem structures. Cerebellar herniation also can occur, with displacement downward through the foramen magnum. Life-threatening deterioration of vital functions can result from brain stem compression secondary to herniation. Sudden increases in an already elevated ICP from fluid overload or hypercapnia may precipitate herniation as may a sudden reduction of CSF pressure from below (via a lumbar puncture).

The management of increased ICP is directed toward reducing intracranial volume and treating the underlying disorder. Osmotic diuretics (mannitol, glycerol) may be used initially to reduce acute brain edema. These hypertonic agents remove tissue fluid rapidly when renal function is adequate. These agents usually are not continued on a long-term basis because a rebound elevation of ICP results from prolonged use. The child's serum osmolarity, electrolyte levels, and urine output are monitored carefully.

Corticosteroids such as dexamethasone also are given to reduce brain swelling. Slower acting than the osmotic agents, steroids often are started concurrently with diuretics and become effective as the osmotic dehydrating action wears off. Corticosteroids are continued for longer periods than osmotic diuretics, depending on the child's condition. Antacid preparations are given orally or by nasogastric tube to prevent gastric irritation secondary to steroid administration. The nurse also observes the child for signs of gastric bleeding (hematemesis, positive stool guaiac).

Fluid restriction can help to reduce increased ICP by decreasing the circulating blood volume. Fluid amounts below the usual maintenance requirements are ordered, and the child is monitored carefully to prevent fluid overload. The composition of the parenteral fluids administered is determined by the child's electrolyte and serum chemistries, but hypotonic solutions (such as .45% saline) are not used because they increase the blood volume osmotically. The child's state of hydration is monitored continuously by measuring the urine volume and specific gravity, and determining serum osmolarity, electrolyte levels, and blood urea nitrogen and creatinine levels. Strict fluid restriction can potentially result in hypovolemic shock. The nurse therefore is alert for signs of this complication (increased pulse, decreased blood pressure, pallor, thirst, and alterations in levels of consciousness).

Increased ICP also can be treated by hyperventilation by Ambu bag or via tracheal intubation, which decreases arterial carbon dioxide content and results in cerebral vasoconstriction. The nurse monitors the child's respiratory status, including blood gases, during the acute-care period when the early detection of hypoxia and hypercapnia is essential.

Temperature regulation is an important aspect of management. Elevated body temperature increases cerebral blood flow and tissue oxygen requirements. It might be necessary to reduce the child's temperature by administering antipyretics, giving a sponge bath, or using a hypothermia pad. The child's fluid intake is not increased to reduce fever because of the risk of overhydration. In some children with severely increased ICP, hypothermia to subnormal body temperatures can be induced by the use of a cooling mattress or other devices. Intracranial pressure also can be relieved by barbiturate-induced coma (to reduce metabolic demands), removal of ventricular fluid, or decompressive craniectomy in selected cases, but these measures are reserved for the most severe forms of cerebral edema that do not respond to the traditional approaches.

Treatment of the underlying cause of the ICP includes antibiotic therapy for central nervous system infections, neurosurgical excision of accessible masses or lesions, or medical treatment of toxic or metabolic disorders. Conditions that obstruct the flow of CSF and result in hydrocephalus often are treated surgically with shunt procedures to divert the CSF and reduce the ICP.

Nursing care of the child with increased ICP also includes continuous assessment of the child's state of consciousness, monitoring vital and neurologic signs, and employing measures to avoid increasing ICP. The child's level of consciousness is the most sensitive indicator of changes in ICP; altered consciousness precedes other signs and symptoms of more advanced ICP elevations. The nurse is alert to subtle behavioral and mental changes in the child such as decreased responsiveness, confusion, or irritability. The child's condition may deteriorate rapidly, making serial assessments and early detection of changes vital to effective treatment.

Unless contraindicated, (as in a question of spinal injury) the head of the child's bed is elevated 30–45° to improve fluid drainage from the brain. The child's head must be kept in neutral alignment; neck flexion is avoided to prevent airway obstruction or impairment of venous return from the head. Stimulation and emotional agitation increase ICP, and nursing care is organized carefully and carried out gently to avoid unnecessary pressure increases from procedures and manipulations (such as, tracheal suctioning or obtaining rectal temperatures). The nurse evaluates the need for restraints carefully because the child's combativeness will increase ICP. It is best to use the least amount of restraint possible and to apply protective coverings to infusion sites. The child's environment is kept as quiet as possible, and any avoidable stresses are removed.

In the intensive-care setting, more specialized procedures might be performed such as continuous ICP monitoring with intraventricular, subarachnoid, or epidural devices. These devices offer direct or indirect, continuous measurement of ICP to detect fluctuations and sustained elevations. Nursing interventions for children with ICP monitoring devices or other complex therapeutic regimens such as barbiturate coma require specialized critical care skills (Hausman, 1981).

The Comatose Child Alterations in consciousness can accompany a wide range of neurologic and systemic disorders in children, including cerebral trauma, hemorrhage, infection, space-occupying lesions, or seizures. The most important aspect of nursing management of the comatose child involves serial monitoring of neurologic status, including assessing vital signs, level of consciousness, and neurologic signs. The nurse particularly observes the child for changes indicative of improvement or deterioration in condition so that therapeutic interventions can be initiated if needed.

The nurse monitors the child's respiratory status and adequacy of ventilation continuously by assessing respiratory effort, auscultating breath sounds, and observing for fluctuations in arterial blood gases. Changing the child's position and performing chest percussion and postural drainage (unless contraindicated by increased ICP) help to mobilize secretions. The nurse suctions the child's secretions frequently to maintain clear respiratory passages. The child might have an endotracheal or tracheostomy tube in place to ensure a patent airway and may require ventilator assistance. Respiratory care focuses on maintaining adequate arterial oxygenation and preventing complications from hypoxia, pneumonia, and atelectasis (see Chapter 34).

The nurse monitors the child's state of hydration by observing the serum electrolyte levels, urine volume, and measuring specific gravity of the urine. The comatose child might develop water intoxication from inappropriate secretion of antidiuretic hormone (ADH) from the anterior pituitary gland. In this situation the child's urine output drops, the urine is concentrated, serum osmolarity decreases, and hyponatremia develops. This condition can cause elevations in ICP from overhydration and can result in death. Inappropriate ADH secretion is treated by fluid restriction until the child's state of hydration becomes stable. Evaluation of urine output is accompanied by serum chemistries and osmolarity measurements to avoid incorrect fluid therapy.

The management of the comatose child with signs and symptoms of increased ICP is the same as nursing care required for any child with increased ICP. The nurse observes the child carefully for neurologic changes indicative of increasing pressure and brain herniation.

In cases of prolonged coma, the child's nutritional needs are met by nasogastric or gastrostomy tube feedings. The type, amount, and method of feeding might vary, but the nurse assesses the child's ability to tolerate feedings and prevents possible aspiration by positioning the child on the side with the head elevated. As the child's condition improves, oral feeding is begun with soft foods if adequate gag and swallow reflexes are present.

In the acute-care period, an indwelling catheter is used to measure urine output accurately. When the comatose child's condition stabilizes, the catheter is removed to reduce the incidence of bladder infection. Diapers or external collecting devices are used, and the nurse observes the child for bladder distention, changes in output, and frequency of voiding. Stool softeners, bulk agents, or cathartics might be needed to prevent constipation. Loose stools often can be treated by dietary management. The perineum and buttocks of the comatose child who is incontinent must be cleaned thoroughly to prevent excoriation from soiling.

Nursing measures also are directed toward preventing secondary effects of immobility involving the skin and circulatory and musculoskeletal systems. The use of a sheepskin, alternating pressure air mattress, position changes, and skin care to stimulate circulation will prevent the formation of decubitus ulcers. The nurse positions the child with the trunk and extremities in correct postural alignment and changes the child's positions from side to side and to semiprone at 2- to 4-hour intervals. The uppermost extremities are supported by pillows to prevent stress on the major joints (shoulder, elbow, hip, and knee). Antiembolism stockings can be used to improve venous return from the lower extremities. Passive range-of-motion exercises and intermittent splinting or casting to maintain functional position of the extremities can be used to help prevent contractures.

The comatose child's corneal reflexes might be impaired, resulting in incomplete eye closure and subsequent drying and ulceration of the cornea. The nurse instills eye drops frequently because artificial tears might be needed to provide lubrication.

The comatose child's sensory perception is altered, and it might be difficult to determine how aware the child is of environmental stimuli. The nurse prevents sensory deprivation by providing meaningful stimulation for the child through touch, voice, and movement. The child's hearing might be intact, even though the child appears not to respond to auditory stimuli. Radio or television programs or tapes of familiar songs or stories that are selected carefully and geared to the child's developmental level can be played. The parent and those caring for the child are encouraged to talk to and avoid discussing the child or engaging in inappropriate conversation in the child's presence.

The Child Requiring Neurosurgery Children require neurosurgery for a number of pathologic conditions, most notably for the myelodysplasias and hydrocephalus. In addition to routine preoperative and postoperative care, careful monitoring of neurologic status is essential. Complications from neurosurgery, such as increased ICP or infection in the form of meningitis, can have far-reaching consequences for the child's optimal development.

Nutritional Needs

The child with a neurologic disorder may have feeding difficulties associated with impairment of the mechanisms necessary for normal eating and drinking. Feeding techniques are adapted for the child with cerebral palsy or any insult to the nervous system that interferes with motor control, coordination, and reflexes.

Impaired oromotor control can result in problems with sucking, lip closure, ability to move food in the mouth, and

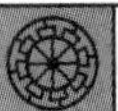

NURSING CARE GUIDE Postoperative Care of the Child Following Neurosurgery

Nursing diagnosis	Interventions	Evaluation
1. Potential for postoperative complications: hemorrhage, respiratory distress/pneumonia, neurologic dysfunction	Provide routine postoperative care (see Chapter 29) Observe for signs of neurologic impairment—abnormal cranial nerve function, motor function, seizures	Neurologic complications are prevented or detected in the early stages
2. Potential for alteration in intracranial pressure (ICP)	Position child with the head of bed flat or slightly elevated as ordered Observe for signs of increased ICP Prevent factors that increase ICP by Maintaining optimal ventilation Monitoring intravenous fluid administration carefully to prevent overhydration Providing comfort and reassurance to decrease agitation Avoiding the use of restraints, which increase combativeness Reporting vomiting immediately and keeping the child on NPO status Using slow, gentle movements when positioning the child	Child shows no evidence of alteration in ICP. Vital signs and neurologic signs are within normal limits
3. Alteration in fluid and electrolyte balance	Maintain ordered intravenous rate Maintain child's NPO status if surgery was done to place a ventriculoperitoneal shunt until bowel sounds return and as ordered Measure and record nasogastric tube output Measure and record urinary output Offer small amounts of oral fluids when allowed	Child shows no evidence of dehydration or fluid overload and has effective resumption of oral intake
4. Potential for postoperative pain	Observe for signs of pain at incision sites, headache, and neck pain Differentiate postoperative pain from signs of meningeal irritation Provide physical measures for pain relief—position changes; cool compresses to the eyes and forehead; and darkening the room Administer analgesics if not contraindicated by the child's neurologic status. If analgesics are permitted, select a medication with the least potential for central nervous system depression	Evaluate the child's pain status (see Chapter 29)
5. Potential infection of incision sites, shunt, and central nervous system	Use aseptic technique for dressing changes Observe for erythema and drainage from incision sites; note the type of drainage; report immediately the drainage of clear fluid (cerebrospinal fluid) Observe for signs of meningitis Provide infection control (see Chapter 29)	Child shows no evidence of infection

continued on next page

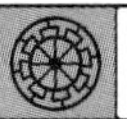

NURSING CARE GUIDE Postoperative Care of the Child Following Neurosurgery (continued)

Nursing diagnosis	Interventions	Evaluation
6. Potential shunt malfunction	Observe for signs of increased ICP Do not position the child with the head lower than the body Do not allow the child to sit upright until ordered Pump the shunt valve as ordered	Child shows no evidence of shunt malfunction. Observations do not indicate any increase in ICP
7. Potential injury from trauma to operative areas	Position the child's head to lie on nonoperative side unless ordered otherwise If operative site is occipital or cervical, do not rotate head when turning; use log roll and move child's head and neck as one unit Use Stryker frame as ordered to immobilize spine	Child shows no evidence of trauma to operative areas such as pain, hemorrhage, or neurologic complications
8. Potential complications secondary to immobility	Provide respiratory, musculoskeletal, and skin care to prevent complications of immobility (see Chapter 29) Use lambswool to pad behind and over the ears under head dressings Avoid overly vigorous chest physiotherapy, postural drainage, suctioning, and range-of-motion exercises if the potential for increased ICP contraindicates these measures	Child shows no evidence of skin breakdown, contracture formation, pneumonia, or other complications secondary to immobility
9. Potential alteration in body image	Prepare the child and family preoperatively for the child's postoperative appearance (shaved head, eye edema, bulky head dressing) Provide a hat or scarf for the child Suggest that the family obtain a wig until the child's hair grows in, if appropriate Support the child and family in coping with the emotional impact of altered body image	Child and family demonstrate the ability to cope optimally with body image alterations
10. Potential knowledge deficit related to postoperative (neurosurgery) management	Teach the child and family the signs of increased ICP, shunt malfunction, central nervous system infection, and wound infection Teach the family to pump the shunt, if indicated Advise the child and family about any activity restrictions and the need for safety precautions such as a helmet Instruct the family about the medications to be given at home (such as anticonvulsants and antibiotics) If indicated, teach the family how to care for the child with seizures Refer the family to community agencies for teaching and support as needed Facilitate the child's reentry to school by continuing schooling during hospitalization; con-	The child and family demonstrate knowledge of home care and importance of follow-up evaluations, and child continues schooling successfully

NURSING CARE GUIDE Postoperative Care of the Child Following Neurosurgery (continued)

Nursing diagnosis	Interventions	Evaluation
	tact the school nurse regarding the operative plan of care for the child Give the family specific information regarding postoperative follow-up plans, particularly neurosurgical appointment	

chewing. The child might exhibit abnormal reflex patterns such as tongue thrust or jaw clamping. Impaired swallow or gag reflexes can increase the risk of aspiration or airway obstruction.

Nursing management includes determining the child's feeding abilities carefully by obtaining a thorough history from the parent and observing the child while eating. Poor suck or food dribbling out of the mouth or being pushed out by tongue thrust are indicative of neuromuscular problems. The nurse gives the child a small amount of water and watches for any swallowing difficulties or choking. The nurse also observes the child's ability to use a bottle and nipple or cup and other eating utensils. Finally, the nurse evaluates the child's ability to self-feed.

Food, equipment, and techniques are adapted to compensate for a variety of feeding problems. Infants who suck and swallow poorly might need gavage feedings (see Chapter 38). Soft nipples or syringe-type feeders are helpful for some infants, as is thickening the formula slightly with a thickener such as baby cereal to aid swallowing.

Manual lip closure and jaw control are feeding techniques used with children with cerebral palsy. The nurse's hand is placed along the side of the child's jaw, and the index and middle fingers gently close the child's lips after food is put in the child's mouth. This is best accomplished by sitting beside or behind the child and using the other hand to feed the child. The child can either sit in the nurse's lap or upright alone with adequate support.

Actual feeding techniques can be adapted to the child's needs. A small Teflon-coated spoon is useful because it is easier for the child to get the food off the spoon, and it avoids trauma from biting down on a hard spoon. The nurse might have to place food part way back on the child's tongue or between the side teeth so that the child can manage it. Feeding programs to facilitate eating and improve the child's oromotor control are developed by a multidisciplinary team that includes the nurse, dietitian, and speech and occupational therapists.

Utensils may be adjusted to help the child with poor motor control to get the food to the mouth (see Fig. 30-2). Cups with double handles, covers with spouts, or a stationary straw aid in handling liquids. Spoons or forks may be attached to a handsplint apparatus or have builtup handles or a swivel mechanism to give the child more control. Devices such as plate guards, scoop dishes, and pads to hold plates or bowls stationary also help to increase the child's independence and control in self-feeding.

The consistency and type of food might have to be adjusted for the child with neuromuscular impairment. Children with difficulties in chewing or swallowing need soft or semisoft food. The chronic feeding problems some children experience can lead to nutritional inadequacies and debilitation. High-protein, high-calorie dietary supplements can be added in forms that the child will tolerate (such as puddings or frappes).

Nasogastric or gastrostomy routes might be used to feed children with impaired consciousness. This form of feeding also might be necessary for severely handicapped children

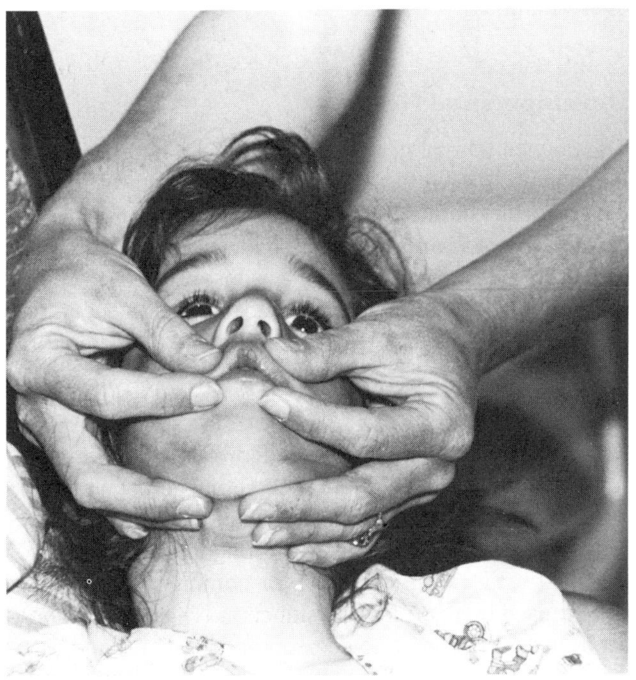

Manual lip closure and jaw control may be used as a feeding technique for children with cerebral palsy.

who cannot handle food orally. The type of formula, procedure, and schedule will vary according to the child's needs and institutional protocols. The general principles for tube feedings include determining the correct placement of the tube, positioning the child to minimize the risks of vomiting and aspiration, and monitoring the child's ability to tolerate both the amount and composition of the feeding. Complications such as high residuals, regurgitation, or diarrhea might require changes in the feeding schedule and type of formula (see Chapter 38).

The dietary needs of some children with neurologic dysfunction are related to obesity caused by excessive food intake and relative physical inactivity. Children with myelodysplasia or spinal cord injury have a particular tendency to gain weight, which complicates their rehabilitative progress by making ambulation and mobility more difficult. In addition, excessive fatty deposits might increase the child's risk for skin breakdown. Because the child with motor impairment expends few calories, dietary management focuses on weight control while ensuring sufficient nutrients for health and growth.

The nurse is sensitive to the child's psychosocial as well as physical needs in developing a dietary plan. Handicapped children and their families might have developed patterns of using food as a form of gratification to replace other pleasures precluded by the children's limitations. The nurse assesses the dynamics contributing to the child's weight problem and develops meaningful incentives to alter dysfunctional behavior patterns associated with food. Dietary planning to prevent obesity in handicapped children is better than treating the handicapped child who is already overweight.

Developmental Needs

The developmental needs of children with neurologic dysfunction are similar to those of all children, but because of their particular deficits, special interventions might be needed to help neurologically impaired children achieve success in developmental tasks. Cognitive, sensory, behavioral, or motor impairments can greatly affect the child's acquisition of skills, adjustment to the environment, and emotional well-being.

Stimulation All infants and children need a variety of sensory and motor experiences to stimulate cognitive and psychosocial growth. The normal exploration of the environment and seeking of stimulation might be impossible for the child with motor, cognitive, or communication limitations caused by neurologic dysfunction. The child can benefit from being exposed to age-appropriate stimuli and given the opportunity to build compensatory strengths such as wheelchair mobility to broaden the possibilities for exploring the environment. Adapting wheelchairs to provide trunk stability and free the child's hands for manipulation and stabilizing toys or books can increase the child's independence and opportunities for stimulation.

Early intervention programs with neurologically impaired children often place a great deal of emphasis on stimulation. When based on a thorough assessment of the child's capabilities and family strengths, individualized programs of sensorimotor stimulation might be recommended by a team with expertise in this field. The nurse is responsible for evaluating the appropriateness of stimulation programs for the child and family. Tudor (1978) cautioned that early intervention programs must be based on realistic evaluations of the child's capabilities and family needs and stresses associated with caring for the neurologically impaired child. In their enthusiasm to stimulate the handicapped child, health care professionals must avoid overwhelming either the child or family with time-consuming and exhausting programs. It is worthwhile working with parents to help them discover opportunities to provide sensorimotor stimulation for the children in their everyday care and recreation activities (such as during bath or mealtimes, while shopping, and so forth).

The child with minimal brain dysfunction (MBD) might need the nurse's help to decrease excessive sensory stimulation. Children with MBD often have difficulty screening out extraneous visual, auditory, or somatic stimuli and respond in a disorganized way to the multiple inputs to which they are exposed. A structured environment that keeps competing stimuli to a minimum helps to keep the child from becoming distracted and overactive. For example, the hospitalized child with MBD cannot be expected to listen adequately to explanations or directions if the television is on or there is an array of play material on hand and commotion in the room.

Learning and Cognitive Needs The educational needs of children with neurologic disorders range from the severely handicapped child's need to learn self-help skills to the learning disabled child's need for compensatory reading instruction.

The neurologically impaired child might continue to require the special treatment of a hospital-based or private school, but these children are being included increasingly in public school programs. School nurses, in particular, face tremendous challenges in educating staff, providing direct health services, and promoting the neurologically impaired child's adjustment in the school setting. The school nurse can act as a liaison between the home, school, and medical care facility regarding the child's health needs. Duties can include monitoring seizures and medication administration, feeding programs, respiratory care, or specialized bowel or bladder programs. The nurse is often a consultant and resource person in coordinating the child's school program, incorporating data from health care assessments and family information to both facilitate the child's adaptation and to ensure communication between home, school, and health care agencies (Igoe, et al., 1980).

Children with neurologic impairments might be hospitalized repeatedly for medical management or surgical procedures. Their school programs can be interrupted frequently, interfering with their academic progress. Whenever possible and as much as possible, educational routines should be part of care for these hospitalized children (see Chapter 29). Collaboration with the family and school is also necessary in discharge planning to prepare for the child's reentry to school.

Socialization The dysfunction in motor control, communication, or cognition that can accompany neurologic disorders might interfere with the child's ability to interact socially and development of social skills. Difficulties can arise not only from the child's limitations but also from the reaction of other people to the child's differences. The child's opportunities for socialization outside the family might be limited by dysfunctional reactions to handicapping conditions. For example, others might be reluctant to socialize with a nonverbal child with cerebral palsy, a child with seizures who wears a helmet, or a child with musculoskeletal or some other deformity who appears "different." Dysfunctional reactions often are based on fear and a lack of understanding about the handicapping condition. Those who do interact with neurologically impaired children tend to relate to them below their level of maturity, treating them as if they were mentally retarded, regardless of their actual cognitive level.

To meet the child's socialization needs, nursing care is based on an assessment of the child's psychosocial developmental level, interactional style, and any physical or emotional barriers to social encounters. During hospitalization, neurologically impaired children might feel even more isolated than they do in their daily lives, surrounded by strangers and in unfamiliar environments. The nurse becomes familiar with any alternate communication system the child uses and ensures that this system is used consistently. The nonverbal child who cannot communicate is particularly vulnerable to social isolation. Devices such as a communication board, mechanical communicator, or description of the child's gesture or signing system should be readily accessible and not put away in a drawer.

The nurse enhances the child's socialization by encouraging interaction with peers, role modeling, providing simple explanations and assistive cues such as "Jenny is a whiz at that game and would like to play it with you. She might have trouble moving the pieces, but I'll bet that you could help her with that." Children can accept individual differences more readily than some adults when adequately guided and can contribute significantly to the overall social adjustment of neurologically impaired children in the hospital, at school, or in the community.

The child whose neurologic dysfunction is manifested behaviorally might exhibit inappropriate social skills such as impulsivity, disinhibited responses, or negativism. Peer interaction is hampered by the child's behavior, and the child often is rejected by other children. Specific behavior management programs developed using a team approach that includes parents and others involved with the child can be helpful. Teaching children how to share, take turns, and recognize other people's needs is undertaken in structured situations, and the goal is for the children to learn a particular social skill, generalize it to other situations, and derive satisfaction from the resulting appropriate interpersonal relationships.

Dependence and Independence The neurologically impaired child often is more dependent because of motor or developmental limitations. Physical dependency might stem from neuromuscular weakness and lack of motor control, with the child requiring assistance with such activities as eating or dressing. The neurologically impaired child might have the same needs for independence as nonimpaired children but has fewer opportunities to achieve independence. Neurologically impaired children often become frustrated by their limitations and necessary reliance on others. Parents might have ambivalent feelings about encouraging independence. They fear for their children's safety, and at times, they are gratified by their children's dependence. The nurse assesses the parent–child relationship and the child's abilities and counsels the family to help them to maximize the child's independence. The child's independence can be enhanced by providing equipment that can be manipulated independently and by giving the child enough time to persevere in attempts to become more independent. Clothes with Velcro closures, builtup spoons or other adapted eating utensils, and stabilizing play materials such as books or games will enable the neurologically impaired child to perform aspects of self-care and learn and play without constant adult attendance. Parents often find it easier to assume the care themselves than to let their children do as much as they can by themselves. The nurse helps the parents to see the value of fostering their children's independence to increase their self-image and future self-sufficiency. (The care of the child with a chronic condition is discussed in Chapter 30.)

In caring for the neurologically impaired child, the nurse provides a balance between allowing the child to perform as many tasks and make as many decisions as possible while preventing frustration and unnecessary failures. Letting children choose when treatments or exercises will be done and select their own menus and giving them the freedom to move in their wheelchairs are some ways to give children the control they might lack in other areas.

The Child With Congenital Malformations of the Central Nervous System

Myelodysplasia

The term *myelodysplasia* encompasses a group of related central nervous system disorders characterized by malformations of the neural tube that occur during embryonic development, including syndromes involving abnormalities in the vertebral column, spinal meninges, and spinal cord (that is, spina bifida occulta, meningocele, and myelomeningocele).

Failure of the midline of the neural plate to close as it forms the neural tube during the third and fourth weeks of gestation is believed to be responsible for these overt and occult spinal defects. The severity of these defects ranges from asymptomatic to severely disabling. Other CNS anomalies might be associated with these defects.

The specific cause of myelodysplasia is not known. Combined hereditary and environmental factors are believed to contribute, and the familial incidence is known to be higher than that for the general population. For families with one affected child, the risk of recurrence increases to 1 in 20–50. With two affected children, the risk of recurrence is 1 in 10 (Carmel, 1982). Siblings and other family members also are at greater risk than the general population of having a child with a neural tube defect.

The incidence estimates vary, but spina bifida occulta is known to occur widely in the general population without evidence of neural dysfunction. A small percentage of affected individuals develop some lower extremity involvement, usually with increasing age (Passo, 1980). Meningocele without neural involvement occurs less often than myelomeningocele. The incidence of these defects, referred to collectively as *spina bifida cystica,* varies worldwide, with the highest number of cases found in Great Britain. In the United States the overall incidence of spina bifida cystica is estimated at 1 per 1000 live births (Shurtleff, 1980).

Clinical Manifestations *Spina bifida occulta* is a defect in closure of the vertebral laminae in which the meninges or neural tissue are not exposed at the skin surface (Fig. 42-7). The usual site of this condition is the lumbosacral area. Underlying malformation of the spinal cord and nerve roots might or might not be present.

Although most cases of spina bifida occulta go undetected throughout life, external cutaneous abnormalities such as a small nevus or hemangioma, dimple, or hair tuft might be present. A dermal sinus often is associated with the vertebral abnormality, forming a blind tract that does not extend to the duramater or spinal cord. This tract, referred to as a pilonidal sinus, might become a focus of infection and require surgical closure.

Meningocele is a defect in which the meninges and CSF protrude through the unfused vertebral arches, appearing as a saclike cyst at the defective area (Fig. 42-7). The spinal cord is not involved. A soft, cystic mass containing meninges and CSF is apparent at birth, usually in the lumbosacral or sacral area. The cyst might be covered with a thick membrane or epithelial tissue and can be completely transilluminated. The spinal nerve roots might be displaced, but their function remains intact. The absence of neurologic involvement is evidenced by normal motor, sensory, reflex, and sphincter function. Hydrocephalus might be present at birth or develop in association with meningocele (Passo, 1980).

Myelomeningocele is a cystlike protrusion at the area of vertebral defect that resembles a meningocele but includes the distended abnormal portion of the spinal cord as well as the meninges and CSF (Fig. 42-7).

When spinal cord segments are involved in the cystic malformation, the most prominent clinical manifestation is flaccid paralysis of the lower extremities. Varying degrees of motor, sensory, reflex, and sphincter dysfunction are present, depending on the location and severity of the spinal abnormality. Eighty percent of myelomeningoceles occur in the lumbar or lumbosacral area (Gabriel, 1980). Less commonly, thoracic or cervical lesions occur. In general, lesions at L3 or above result in total paraplegia, sensory loss, and bowel and bladder incontinence. Involvement at lower spinal cord levels is accompanied by partial preservation of muscular, sensory, or sphincter function; the lower the lesion, the less the neurologic deficit.

Almost all children with lumbar or lumbosacral myelomeningocele develop hydrocephalus of varying severity. This abnormality usually is due to associated embryonic malformations of the CSF circulation in the brain, most often Arnold–Chiari-type malformations (Molnar and Taft, 1977b). Progressive hydrocephalus is manifested by increasing head circumference, separation of sutures, and CT scan evidence of dilated ventricles. (See the section on the child with hydrocephalus.)

Functional motor disability is greatest in children with spinal cord lesions at L3 and above. The motor function disabilities that occur at various levels of spinal cord involvement in myelomeningocele are outlined in Table 42-6. Motor paralysis often results in musculoskeletal deformities, which can compromise the child's mobility further. Partial innervation of muscle groups (flexor and extensor muscles) causes unequal pull at various joints, resulting in dislocation and contractures. Hip dislocation occurs frequently, which in turn contributes to the development of scoliosis. Contractures of the hips, knees, and ankles result from muscle imbalance and are progressive if not prevented through positioning and surgical correction. Various foot deformities, commonly the equinovarus type, occur with myelomeningocele. (Carmel, 1982).

Small muscle bulk and osteoporosis result from the lack

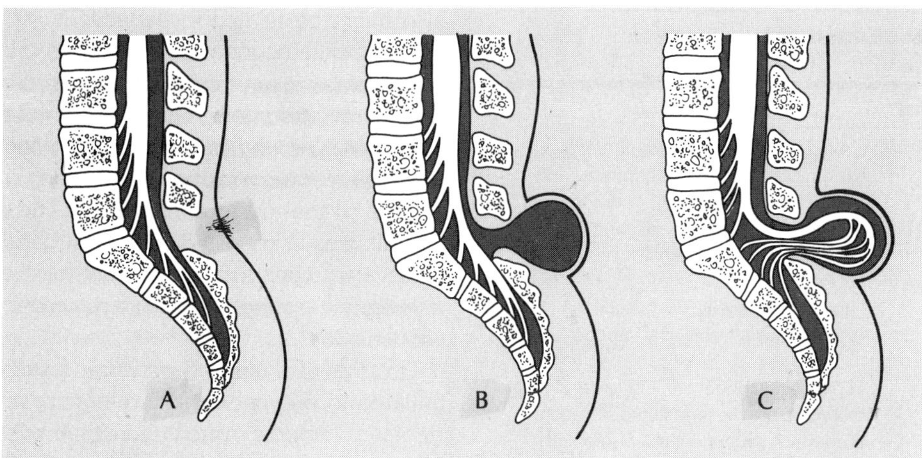

Figure 42-7 Midsagittal view of the spinal column showing various degrees of neural defect. *A.* Spina bifida occulta. Note that the posterior vertebral arches have not fused. There is no herniation of the spinal cord. *B.* Meningocele. The meninges protrude through the spina bifida, forming a saclike cyst that is visible on the infant's back. *C.* Myelomeningocele. Meninges, elements of the spinal cord and its nerves, and cerebrospinal fluid protrude through the spina bifida. Externally, this defect resembles a meningocele.

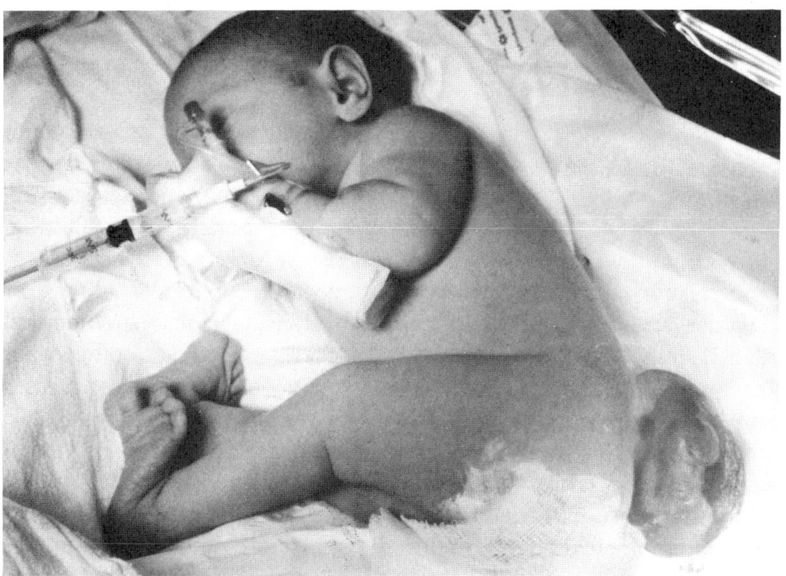

Infant with lumbar myelomeningocele. (Courtesy Dr. Paul Winchester.)

of normal innervation and use. Fractures of the lower extremities are a common complication of bony atrophy in these children. Sensory deficits and circulatory alterations predispose the child to pressure decubiti and unnoticed heat or traumatic injuries of the affected areas of the body.

Bowel and bladder dysfunction usually results in incontinence, with sphincter paralysis, chronic retention of urine, and constipation. The child dribbles urine intermittently or continuously without effective bladder evacuation. Incomplete bladder emptying can lead to the serious urologic complications of recurrent infection, ureteral reflux, and renal impairment. Lack of bowel tone often results in the retention of feces. Rectal prolapse might accompany rectal sphincter paralysis and poor bowel tone.

Other neurologic sequelae might accompany myelomeningocele, caused by structural deformities and neuronal damage. Cognitive, perceptual, and learning disabilities of varying severity can be present, most often associated

TABLE 42-6 Motor Function Disability in Myelomeningocele

Spinal cord lesion	Dysfunction
T6–12	Complete flaccid paralysis of the lower extremities. Weakened abdominal and trunk musculature in higher lesions. Kyphosis and scoliosis are common. Ambulation with maximal support
L1–2	Hip flexion present. Paraplegia. Ambulation with maximal support
L3–4	Hip flexion, adduction, and knee extension are present. Hip dislocation is common. Some control of hip and knee movement is possible. Ambulation with moderate support
L5	Hip flexion, adduction, and varying degrees of abduction. Knee extension and weak knee flexion. Paralysis of the lower legs and feet. Ambulation with moderate support
S1–2	As above, with preservation of some foot and ankle movement. Ambulation with minimal support
S3	Mild loss of intrinsic foot muscular function is possible. Ambulation without support

SOURCE: Data from Kupka J, Geddes N, Carrou NC: Comprehensive management in the child with spina bifida. *Orthop Clin North Am* 1978; 9(1): 97–113.

with hydrocephalus. Some children with myelomeningocele develop a seizure disorder, which tends to disappear in later childhood (Shurtleff, 1980).

Medical and Surgical Treatment Meningocele is treated by surgical closure of the defect at birth. The child is observed carefully for complications of meningitis, hydrocephalus, and spinal cord dysfunction. Close neurologic follow-up is important to monitor the child's head circumference and sensorimotor development.

Management of the child with myelomeningocele is complex, beginning at birth and continuing throughout the child's lifetime. Most neonates with this condition are transferred immediately to tertiary care centers, where surgery is performed to close the myelomeningocele (duramater, connective tissue, and skin) within 24 hours of birth. This reduces the risk of infection and might prevent further neurologic impairment, which occurs as the cyst expands (Gabriel, 1980). Skin grafting often is necessary to repair the defect. The presence of hemorrhage, infection, or rapidly expanding hydrocephalus contraindicate surgery on the myelomeningocele until these conditions are controlled. The decision not to perform surgery in the early neonatal period also might be related to the severity of the malformation and associated congenital anomalies (Shurtleff, 1980).

Prophylactic antibiotics are administered before, during, and following surgery. The operative site is protected from contamination and pressure by positioning. The infant is observed for signs of hydrocephalus, which might follow closure of the myelomeningocele. The obstruction to the CSF flow usually existed prior to surgery, but CSF pressure is elevated when the cystic outlet for the fluid is removed. If indicated, a ventricular shunt is created to divert CSF and reduce ICP.

Urologic evaluation is performed early, and treatment is initiated to prevent urinary retention, infection, and renal damage. Periodic urine cultures, intravenous pyelograms, cystometrograms, and measurement of residual urine are done to monitor the child's urologic status. In infants the bladder often is emptied by Credé's method at regular (2- to 4-hour) intervals. This method is not employed when outlet obstruction or ureteral reflux is present, however, because it might increase retrograde urinary problems (Carmel, 1982). As the child matures, timed voiding with Credé's method and exerting intra-abdominal pressure (using the Valsalva maneuver) might be effective in a bladder-emptying program. Intermittent clean catheterization is used with good results in a large percentage of children. With increasing maturity, the child can be taught to perform this procedure. Medications can be used to alter abnormal bladder tone and promote complete bladder emptying. A hypotonic bladder might respond to cholinergic agents to increase tone, and a hypertonic bladder can benefit from antispasmodic agents. Acute or chronic urinary tract infections are treated with appropriate antibiotics. The child might receive prophylactic urinary antiseptic medication for its bacteriostatic action. When these measures fail to prevent secondary urologic complications, surgical diversion of the urinary tract might be necessary. In an ileal loop bladder procedure, the ureters are diverted to an artificial bladder that is formed from a resected ileal segment, which drains urine through an abdominal stoma to an external collecting bag. Other surgical procedures may be performed, such as sphincterotomy, to improve bladder emptying in the presence of outlet obstruction (Carmel, 1982). Artificial sphincter devices might be implanted in some children (Shurtleff, 1980).

Bowel dysfunction is managed with dietary measures to alter stool consistency and adjunctive methods to help the child achieve continence. Bisacodyl or glycerin suppositories, regular, timed toileting, and abdominal straining are often effective in a bowel program. Enemas and disimpaction might be necessary should constipation become severe.

Promoting the child's mobility and preventing musculoskeletal deformity are early and continuing goals of treatment. Orthopedic care involves exercise, braces, casts, and surgical correction to achieve these goals. Equipment such as body jackets and long or short leg braces maintain good anatomic alignment and give the child more functional posture and support. Ambulation is often possible for young children with myelomeningocele with bracing of the lower extremities and use of a walker or crutches. Older children with higher-level lesions might become more dependent on wheelchairs as functional ambulation becomes more difficult (Carmel, 1982). The child is still encouraged, however, to bear as much weight as possible using assistive devices to prevent osteoporosis and contractures.

Nursing Management Nursing care for the child with myelodysplasia might involve acute care during infancy, care during subsequent hospitalizations, and outpatient or community follow-up in the long-term management of complex needs. The lifelong care of children with these conditions and their families is best achieved with coordinated treatment by a multidisciplinary team to promote optimal development and prevent secondary complications.

Immediate Care at Birth During infancy, the child with myelodysplasia requires intensive care both pre- and postoperatively.

Preoperatively, the meningeal sac is inspected for signs of abrasion, infection, or leakage of CSF. Topical antibiotics and a moist saline dressing to the cele might be prescribed. The infant is positioned on the abdomen with the head turned to the side to protect the sac from irritation, contamination, or rupture. The infant's hips are abducted with a pad to reduce hip dislocation, and the infant's feet are kept in a neutral position with a small blanket roll under the ankles. Sandbags might be used on either side of the infant to prevent rolling. Diapers and clothing are not used, and the infant is kept in an isolette to maintain warmth. The nurse changes the diaper pads beneath the infant frequently to prevent skin excoriation and protect the cele from contamination.

The nurse assesses the infant's sensorimotor function, noting spontaneous movement, response to stimulation, and any changes indicative of neurologic deterioration. The nurse also observes the infant closely for early signs of meningeal infection (elevated or subnormal temperature, irritability, pallor, vomiting, or nuchal rigidity).

Following surgery, the nurse observes the infant's vital signs, head circumference, wound (for leakage of CSF or hemorrhage), and elimination. The infant is kept prone, and the operative site is protected from pressure or contamination until the wound is well healed. Behavioral changes such as restlessness, irritability, lethargy, or fever, vomiting, and pallor could indicate complications of meningitis or hydrocephalus and must be detected early.

Family support and teaching begin with the birth of the infant and continue as the infant matures. Within a short period of time, the family must adjust to the birth of an infant with a serious defect, consent to surgical treatment, and learn how to provide the infant's specialized physical care. Parent–infant bonding is encouraged by allowing the parent to participate in as much of the infant's care as possible. The nurse provides careful, repetitive explanations of the multisystem observations and care required as the family prepares to take the infant home. The nurse establishes liaisons and referrals for long-term care. Ongoing guidance, support, and treatment are best provided by the coordinated efforts of a multidisciplinary team that can communicate effectively with the family.

Chronic Care The nurse teaches the family how to avoid skin breakdown and injury resulting from the child's lack of sensory awareness. The nurse emphasizes the importance of avoiding pressure and temperature extremes and proper positioning and skin care measures. The nurse demonstrates how to perform range-of-motion exercises and apply braces, splints, or casts. The child's ability to explore the environment and development are enhanced by devices to aid sitting and mobility, which are adapted to the individual child's needs. Low-sitting caster carts and prone scooter boards can be employed at early ages to allow children to move about with upper-extremity control. As the child begins ambulation using assistive devices, specialized programs are undertaken to teach the child transfers, gait, self-help skills, and safety measures.

If the child is at risk for hydrocephalus or has a shunt in place, the symptoms of increased ICP are explained to the family, and they are instructed to contact their neurologist or primary care provider should any concerns arise. As is the case with any child with hydrocephalus, shunt malfunctions can occur, requiring revision or removal of the shunt. Other neurologic sequelae, such as seizures, might require specialized therapy and teaching.

Management of elimination is a major focus of care to prevent serious complications. The nurse teaches the family how to carry out the chosen elimination program, explains the rationale for the treatment, and describes the symptoms of urinary tract infection the family should watch for. With increasing maturity, the child can be involved increasingly in the bowel and bladder program. Learning to perform the Credé method, exert intra-abdominal pressure, and insert a urinary catheter independently are realistic goals for many children with myelomeningocele. The nurse stresses the prevention of urinary tract infection by ensuring adequate fluid intake, urine acidification, and frequent bladder emptying. The child with an external urinary diversion (such as an ileal loop) will need to be taught about stoma and skin care and the use of external collecting devices (different types of bags, adhesives, and drainage methods) (see Chapters 38 and 39).

A bowel program is begun when the child is around 2 years of age. The parent is encouraged to develop a regular daily routine of placing the child on the toilet and to use suppositories if needed. Problems with stool consistency are managed by dietary adjustments when possible, and the use of laxatives is avoided.

Incontinence remains a major problem for children with myelomeningocele, and the psychosocial implications become increasingly negative as these children get older. Bowel continence usually can be achieved with some success if regularity is maintained, but bladder continence can be more difficult. The nurse works with the child and family to adapt the frequency and timing of the child's bladder emptying program and provide measures to prevent wetness such as protective incontinence pads for girls or external catheter devices for boys.

Dietary guidance is important in ensuring adequate nutrition and managing elimination problems and also in preventing obesity, a common problem associated with myelomeningocele.

The child with myelomeningocele might be hospitalized repeatedly for orthopedic, urologic, or neurologic treatment. As much as possible, the child's mobility and elimination routines are maintained. When orthopedic surgery is performed, resulting in immobility and casting, the nurse pays special attention to skin care and observes the child carefully for circulatory or pressure complications that the child does not notice immediately because of sensory deficits. Urinary stasis and infection might occur more rapidly in these children, and the nurse observes the children for bladder distention and signs of urinary tract infection. Constipation is avoided with suppositories and enemas, and usual regimens are maintained when possible. Getting these children mobile as soon as possible aids not only elimination but also helps to prevent further osteoporosis and contracture deformities.

Adolescence is a particularly difficult time for children with myelomeningocele. The combination of altered body image, concerns about sexuality, and independence issues accentuates the typical adolescent turbulence. The child's cognitive and social maturity might lag behind physical development, delaying some of the peer-related adolescent issues. Appropriate sex education and sensitive counseling are begun at an earlier age for teenagers with myelodysplasia to help their adjustment during this period.

The lifelong care of children with myelomeningocele requires an interdisciplinary team approach. The nurse plays a major role in both acute care and long-term management through the coordination of specialized programs, child and family teaching, and psychosocial counseling.

The Spina Bifida Association of America (343 South Dearborn Street, Chicago, IL 60604) provides resource and educational materials and can refer families to local support groups.

Hydrocephalus

Hydrocephalus is a condition with multiple causes that results in an increased amount of CSF within the ventricles of the brain. Increased CSF can be caused by obstructions to normal flow of the CSF system, overproduction of CSF, or inadequate reabsorption of CSF in the subarachnoid villa. Hydrocephalus might be present at birth as a result of embryonic malformation or may occur secondary to injury, infection, or space-occupying lesions.

Hydrocephalus can be classified as *noncommunicating* or *communicating* depending on the mechanism of alteration in CSF. Noncommunicating hydrocephalus results from obstruction of CSF flow from the ventricles of the brain to the subarachnoid space. This obstruction can occur at any point in the ventricular system. Communicating hydrocephalus results when CSF flow is not obstructed through the ventricles but is inadequately circulated or reabsorbed in the subarachnoid space.

Aqueductal stenosis is the narrowing or obstruction of the aqueduct of Sylvius between the third and fourth ventricle and is the most common type of hydrocephalus (Conway-Rutkowski, 1982). Congenital stenosis often accompanies other neural tube malformations such as spina bifida. Aqueductal stenosis also can occur as a postinflammatory process (gliosis) following infection or hemorrhage.

Dandy–Walker syndrome is atresia of the foramina of the fourth ventricle (foramina of Magendie and Luschka), which results in a large, dilated fourth ventricle that resembles a cyst. The Dandy–Walker syndrome is believed to result from congenital defects of neural tube closure. This condition often does not become apparent until after infancy; signs include a bulging occipital area and neurologic deficits (Gabriel, 1980).

Arnold–Chiari malformation (ACM) includes four known types, all of which involve malformations of the lower brain stem and cerebellum. These structures are displaced downward into the cervical canal. Hydrocephalus might result from obstruction of the subarachnoid space (communicating), as in ACM Type II. Noncommunicating hydrocephalus also might be present when obstruction to the foramina of the fourth ventricle occurs (Icenogle and Kaplan, 1981). Arnold–Chiari malformations often accompany other anomalies of the nervous system.

Postinfectious, posthemorrhagic hydrocephalus involves meningeal inflammation or subarachnoid hemorrhage and can result in fibrous tissue formation in the subarachnoid space or ventricular obstruction. Bacterial meningitis, toxoplasmosis, and cytomegalic inclusion disease can result in this type of hydrocephalus (Gabriel, 1980). In addition to infection, acquired hydrocephalus of both types can result from cerebral trauma or tumors interfering with CSF circulation at any point in the system.

Clinical Manifestations The signs and symptoms of hydrocephalus depend on the age at onset and the degree of increased CSF volume within the brain. From infancy through 2 years of age, enlarging head size, bulging, nonpulsatile fontanelles, and downward rotation of the eyes with scleras visible above the iris ("setting sun sign") are characteristic signs of hydrocephalus. Scalp veins might be distended and cranial sutures separated. Poor feeding, vomiting, lethargy, irritability, and developmental delays accompany progressive hydrocephalus. A characteristic high-pitched cry and abnormal muscle tone might be present (Gabriel, 1980).

In older children the cranial sutures are closed and head circumference changes are less common. Signs of increased ICP such as vomiting, ataxia, and headache are common. Late signs include alterations in consciousness and papilledema. Intellectual development might be impaired and accompanied by behavioral (hyperactive) and learning disabilities in chronic forms of hydrocephalus.

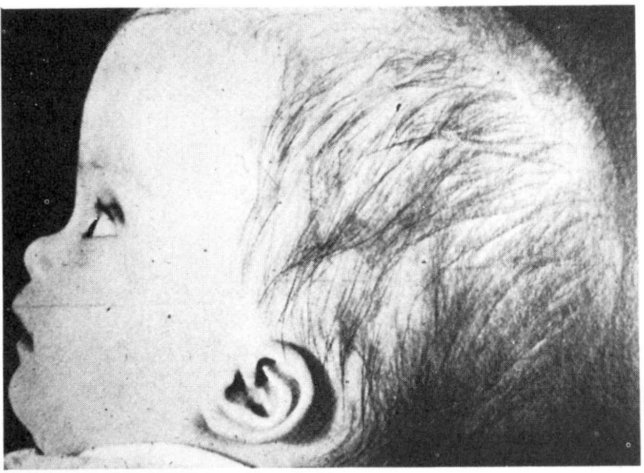

Infant with hydrocephalus. Note enlarged occipital area and lateral view of the sunset eyes.

Diagnostic Evaluation Head circumference changes in infancy that surpass normal parameters indicate the need for further diagnostic assessment of enlarged head size. Transillumination of the skull with a flashlight and special rubber adapter is performed in a darkened room to determine the presence of asymmetric areas of increased light. Transillumination usually does not reveal asymmetric light areas in hydrocephalus but does with subdural hematomas. Serial transilluminations are performed to detect increases in light areas.

Percussion of the skull produces a high-pitched sound (Macewen's sign) in the presence of hydrocephalus.

Computerized tomographic (CT) scanning is performed to determine the size and position of the ventricles and subarachnoid spaces. Dilatation of the ventricles can be determined readily, as well as the presence of tumors or other space-occupying lesions. Cerebrospinal fluid circulation and obstructions to CSF flow or reabsorption can be evaluated by injecting dye into the lumbar subarachnoid space and obtaining CT scans several times to measure the course of the CSF. In most instances the CT scan has replaced pneumoencephalography in the diagnosis of hydrocephalus (Gabriel, 1980). Other studies, such as angiography or radioisotope scanning, might be needed in the diagnosis of hydrocephalus.

Medical and Surgical Treatment Hydrocephalus is treated by surgery to either correct an obstruction to CSF circulation or implant a shunting device to divert the CSF. When a mass, lesion, or adhesions within the CSF system are identified and surgically accessible, they are treated directly. More commonly, progressive hydrocephalus is managed by ventricular shunting procedures.

Both types of hydrocephalus can be treated with bypass shunts, which carry the CSF from the ventricle, divert it extracranially, and drain it into another body compartment. The shunt is made up of a ventricular catheter, one-way valve, and distal catheter. A reservoir might be placed in the ventricular catheter near the valve to give access to the shunt to measure pressure, culture CSF, or instill antibiotics. Various types of valves are used that permit one-way flow of CSF away from the ventricles. The valves are set to open at different intraventricular pressures depending on the degree of increased CSF pressure. The distal catheter attaches to the valve and is directed to the designated body cavity for drainage.

Although other sites occasionally might be used, the majority of ventricular shunts in children drain either into the peritoneum or the superior vena cava. Ventriculoperitoneal (VP) shunts are threaded subcutaneously against the cranium and down the chest to the abdominal wall, where the catheter is inserted to drain the CSF into the peritoneal cavity. The end of the catheter might be coiled to allow the shunt to "grow" with the child without displacing the distal tip (Fig. 42-8). Ventriculovascular shunts are threaded similarly extracranially but then routed into the venous system to the superior vena cava at the T6 level (Gabriel, 1980). The drained CSF enters the vascular flow to the right atrium.

Both types of shunts might require periodic revision as the child grows or if a shunt obstruction occurs. Obstruction might be due to tissue particles, venous clotting, or bacterial colonization. Common shunt complications are obstruction, infection, and disconnection of the tubing. With obstruction, sudden or gradual symptoms of increased ICP develop. Infection might be acute in onset or develop gradually over time. An infected shunt is removed, and the child is treated with appropriate antibiotics. Alternative shunting devices are placed if the child continues to need CSF diversion. One complication of ventriculovascular shunts is bacterial endocarditis and bacteremia, which requires antibiotic treatment and shunt revision. If the shunt becomes disconnected, surgery is performed to reconnect the tubing.

Medical treatment with acetazolamide to decrease CSF production by the choroid plexus has been used in some cases with limited success. Acetazolamide may be used alone

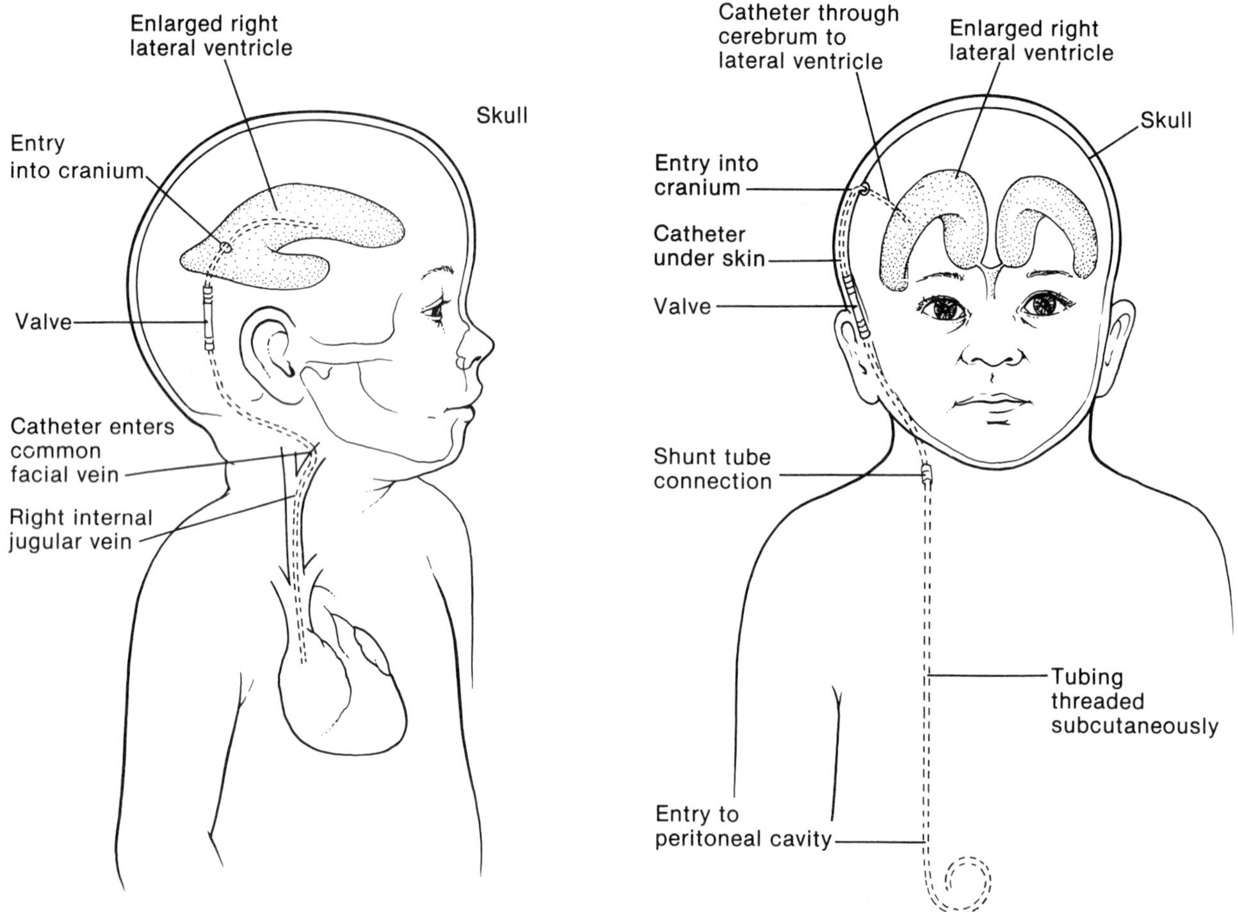

Figure 42-8 Ventriculoperitoneal shunt with the distal end of the tubing located in the superior vena cava and coiled to allow lengthening as the child grows.

or in combination with hyperosmolar agents (urea, mannitol) to reduce increased ICP in hydrocephalus prior to surgical intervention (Gabriel, 1980).

Nursing Management Preoperative nursing care for the child with hydrocephalus is similar to that for any child preoperatively, with several special considerations. The nurse monitors the child's neurologic status periodically. The nurse pays particular attention to the child with acute-onset hydrocephalus, watching for changes indicative of increasing ICP.

The child might have a markedly enlarged head, the weight of which prevents the child from moving or being held easily. The nurse positions the child carefully and uses sheepskin or cushions to prevent skin breakdown. The child can be held with the child's head on a pillow and support from an armchair (McElroy, 1980).

Postoperatively, the nurse assesses the child frequently for changes in vital signs or neurologic status. Operative sites are observed for bleeding or infection, and the nurse positions the child to avoid pressure to these sites. The child usually is kept flat or with the head only slightly elevated to prevent a too rapid reduction in CSF pressure following shunting.

The nurse observes the child carefully for symptoms of increasing ICP. Respiratory complications are avoided by turning and positioning, chest clapping, and suction, if necessary.

The child might complain of headache or postoperative pain, which is treated with analgesics that are less likely to depress consciousness (such as acetaminophen or codeine). Hydration and nutrition initially are provided parenterally. As bowel sounds and consciousness return, the child might be given clear liquids and later progressed in diet depending on individual tolerability. Any preoperative medications, such as anticonvulsants, are continued postoperatively. A follow-up CT scan is done to determine ventricular size.

The child who has had surgery to revise the distal portion of a shunt will have a briefer recovery period than the child who has had an initial shunt placed. In children who demonstrated preoperative lethargy and decreased awareness, it is not uncommon to see marked improvements in the level of consciousness postoperatively.

The family needs a clear explanation of the shunting

procedure, support through the operative period, and education in preparation for discharge. The family might be afraid of displacing the shunt by handling the child or might restrict the child's activity level unnecessarily. The nurse helps the family members to palpate the shunt and valve and reassures them that normal activity will not interfere with shunt function. The physician might recommend that activities that place the child at higher risk for head injury (such as contact sports) be avoided. Guidance is geared to the specific child's age and developmental level.

The nurse describes the signs of shunt obstruction and infection to the family. The family members are taught to observe the child for lethargy, headache, vomiting, eye turning, visual disturbances, or pupil changes. A child with a shunt infection might exhibit the preceding symptoms of increased ICP and fever, stiff neck, nausea, vomiting, and seizures. The family is encouraged to contact the child's primary health care provider if shunt problems are suspected (McElroy, 1980).

The family members might or might not be instructed to "pump" the reservoir of the shunt to check for patency. Some physicians demonstrate this maneuver to parents but advise them not to pump the shunt reservoir routinely. It is important for parents to understand the basic mechanics of the shunt, but it generally is unnecessary or contraindicated for them to compress the reservoir or valves.

Children with hydrocephalus might have developmental or focal neurologic deficits that persist after shunting because of cerebral damage or nervous system malformation. The types and severity of impairment depend on the original disorder (such as, congenital, tumor, trauma, or infection) and the degree of hydrocephalus present before shunting. Frequent follow-up evaluations are essential to monitor the child's development and plan rehabilitative interventions early.

Congenital Vascular Malformations

Malformations of the cerebral vasculature result when abnormal vessel development occurs during gestation. These malformations can take several forms but most often involve arteriovenous malformation (AVM). Abnormal development of capillaries between arteries and veins produces a dilated mass of blood vessels with venous shunting of arterial blood. An AVM can occur anywhere in the brain and range in size from 1 mm to over 10 cm. One-half of AVMs never become symptomatic (Gabriel, 1980). Those AVMs that do become symptomatic usually produce clinical signs in late childhood or adulthood. A smaller percentage become evident in early childhood.

Clinical Manifestations The clinical manifestations of congenital vascular malformations depend on their location and whether they produce symptoms as a result of bleeding or the effects of a space-occupying lesion (Gabriel, 1980). The most common initial presentation is hemorrhage. Characteristically, the sudden onset of severe headache, vomiting, irritability, deterioration of consciousness, focal neurologic deficits, and seizures occur with intracranial hemorrhage. If bleeding extends to the subarachnoid space, signs of meningeal irritation might be present, including nuchal rigidity (Challenor and Gold, 1982). Increasing ICP occurs with progressive bleeding and the formation of hematomas. The onset of childhood stroke from rupture of a vascular malformation is sudden and acute in the majority of cases. Small, recurrent episodes of bleeding that produce focal seizures and neurologic signs occur infrequently (Gabriel, 1980).

Hemiparesis is a common manifestation of congenital vascular malformation and might resolve or persist as a residual deficit. Motor dysfunction is greater in the upper extremities than in the lower extremities, and varying degrees of loss of function and spasticity occur. Sensory deficits might accompany hemiparesis, causing the child to lose awareness of position in space and touch discrimination. The child might actually lose awareness of the affected limbs as a part of the body, a condition called *sensory neglect.*

Speech and language disorders can result from childhood stroke depending on the cerebral area involved. Generally, the younger the child, the better the prognosis for normal language development with lesions involving the dominant cerebral hemisphere. Aphasia might occur initially, but recovery is rapid in children under 5 years of age. The length of the recovery time and degree of residual dysfunction increase with increasing age (Golden, 1978).

Learning and behavior disorders following stroke resemble those of other learning and attention deficits. Hyperactivity, impulsivity, distractibility, and specific learning disabilities might result and require medical and educational intervention.

Seizures often occur at the time of the stroke, with about 50% of affected children developing subsequent seizure disorders (Challenor and Gold, 1982). Focal or generalized seizures might occur and can be difficult to control with anticonvulsant therapy (Menkes, 1980).

Diagnostic Evaluation Diagnosis of the child with sudden stroke involves attempts to determine both the degree of hemorrhage and the underlying vascular disorder. A lumbar puncture is performed unless contraindicated by acutely increased ICP. When a lumbar puncture can be done safely, the CSF pressure is measured, and the CSF is examined for the presence of blood, xanthochromia, and increased protein (Gabriel, 1980).

Intracranial *bruits* (blood flow sounds) can be heard by auscultating the skull. These bruits can be benign but often are heard as harsher and louder when associated with intracranial hemorrhage.

The CT scan is the most important diagnostic tool in defining the extent and localization of the cerebral area involved. Cerebral angiography provides further definitive information about the vascular disorder and usually is performed prior to surgical intervention.

Medical and Surgical Treatment The initial treatment of intracranial hemorrhage is supportive to control cerebral edema, manage increased ICP, and maintain life functions (Conway-Rutkowski, 1982). The child is monitored intensively, and measures such as fluid restriction, hyperventilation and hypothermia therapy, and the administration of steroids or hyperosmolar agents are undertaken to reduce cerebral edema. Anticonvulsant medications are administered to control seizures. If necessary, blood pressure elevations are avoided with antihypertensive medications.

If surgical treatment is indicated to excise a hematoma or ligate vasculature, the procedure usually is deferred until the child's condition has stabilized (Gabriel, 1980). Vasospasm and cerebral edema increase the risk of surgical mortality in the acute phase. Later, when these conditions have subsided, neurosurgical procedures to prevent the recurrence of bleeding might be undertaken in selected cases.

As the child recovers, treatment goals become rehabilitative for persistent sensorimotor, language, cognitive, or other impairments. The child might require orthopedic management for hemiparesis, continued seizure control, and multidisciplinary therapeutic treatment depending on individual needs (Challenor and Gold, 1982).

Nursing Management During the acute phase of rupture of a cerebrovascular malformation, nursing care is the same as that for the child with alterations in consciousness and increased ICP.

The child is confined completely to bed, and the head of the bed is elevated 15–20° to control hemorrhage (Conway-Rutkowski, 1982). If the child is agitated or restless, mild sedation might be given to reduce the risks of an elevated blood pressure and increased bleeding. A quiet atmosphere is essential, and manipulations and irritating stimuli are kept to a minimum.

The nurse takes seizure precautions and describes and reports any seizure activity carefully. Prompt anticonvulsant treatment is undertaken because prolonged seizures can aggravate cerebral edema through hypoxia (Golden, 1978).

Following the acute stage, transient or persistent neurologic deficits require particular attention. The child might experience aphasia, making communication frustrating and a source of anxiety. The nurse anticipates the child's needs, uses a calm approach, and allows the child time to attempt to communicate to help to reduce anxiety. The child might have a receptive language impairment as well. If the child does not seem to understand what has been said, the nurse uses short, simple directions, gestures, and substitutes other words that might be understood more easily. Speech and language therapy is indicated for the child with a communication disorder following a stroke.

Hemiparesis can result in spasticity and contractures of the affected side, requiring exercises, adaptive equipment, and mobilizing aids.

The child with an acquired seizure disorder will continue to require anticonvulsant medication and safety precautions such as a helmet. The child and family are taught about seizures and how to manage them. (See the section on the child with a seizure disorder.)

The nurse provides supportive crisis intervention to the child and family during the acute period. As the child stabilizes, the focus shifts to rehabilitative teaching, utilizing a therapeutic team approach. The deficits that are present can be expected to improve most rapidly in the first 6 months, with some improvement continuing for 3–5 years (Challenor and Gold, 1982).

The Child With an Infection of the Central Nervous System

Acute Bacterial Meningitis

Bacterial meningitis is a significant pediatric health problem, and immediate diagnosis and treatment are necessary to prevent morbidity and mortality. Central nervous system invasion by the causative organism produces inflammation of the meninges, resulting in acute illness. Different organisms are responsible for meningitis, and the prevalence of each organism varies depending on the age of the child. *Hemophilus influenzae* Type B is the primary causative organism of meningitis in children between 3 months and 5 years of age (Weil, 1980). *Streptococcus pneumoniae* (a pneumococcus), *Neisseria meningitidis* (a meningococcus), and staphylococci cause the remainder of the cases of bacterial meningitis in children beyond the neonatal period. Neonatal meningitis differs both in the causative organism and clinical course from that of older infants and children. Gram-negative enteric bacilli (*E-scherichia coli*), other gram-negative rods, and Group B streptococci cause the majority of cases of meningitis in neonates (Gaddy, 1980).

Bacteria most often are carried to the meningeal area in the blood from another site in the body. Direct invasion can occur in traumatic injury, neurosurgical procedures, or from adjacent infections such as sinusitis or otitis (Weil, 1980). Predisposing factors that increase the incidence of meningitis include central nervous system anomalies (myelomeningocele), immune deficiencies, immunosuppression therapy, and sickle cell disease (Gaddy, 1980).

The invading organism most often causes an upper respiratory infection, otitis media, or some other infection. Secondary spread to the meninges occurs when bacteria in the venous drainage from the nasopharynx, ear, or sinus pass into the meningeal vasculature. Meningeal inflammation evolves rapidly, and purulent exudate is released into the CSF system. The infection spreads via vascular and CSF circulation to adjacent brain tissue and nerve roots. Cerebral edema results from vascular congestion and cortical inflammation, and neuronal damage results if the infection is not treated (Weil, 1980).

Clinical Manifestations Acute bacterial meningitis often is preceded by an upper respiratory or gastrointestinal infection. Fever, headache, vomiting, irritability, photophobia, and nuchal and spinal rigidity develop and can progress rapidly to decreased level of consciousness and seizures (Weil, 1980). Irritation of the meninges and spinal roots causes pain and resistance to neck flexion (nuchal rigidity), a positive Kernig's sign (resistance to knee extension in the supine position with the hips and knees flexed against the body), and a positive Brudzinski's sign (flexion of the knees and hips when the neck is flexed forward rapidly). With severe meningeal irritation, the child might demonstrate opisthotonic posturing (rigid arching of the back with the head extended).

Infants and young children often have less specific signs; irritability, crying, poor feeding, and vomiting are the initial manifestations. The fontanelle becomes full and tense and ICP is increased in a later stage of meningitis. Resistance to being held and increased crying when the legs are raised during diapering can indicate meningitis in infancy (Gaddy, 1980).

Neonates (up to 1 month old) exhibit almost no specific clinical signs of meningitis initially, making diagnosis difficult. Fever or subnormal temperature, poor feeding, pallor, lethargy, irritability, and seizures are the possible nonspecific findings. Opisthotonus and a bulging fontanelle occur late in the disease process and indicate a poorer prognosis (Langer and Schott, 1977).

Meningococcal meningitis, which is more common in older children and adults, can produce a characteristic petechial rash. Occasionally, petechiae also are seen with *H influenzae* and pneumococcal meningitis. The course of meningococcal meningitis is more rapidly fulminant and progressive than other forms, with a higher mortality rate when accompanied by septicemia, shock, and disseminated intravascular coagulation (DIC) (Weil, 1980).

Increased ICP results from cerebral edema and might be increased further by obstruction to CSF circulation. Thickened meninges and fibrous exudate in the subarachnoid space at the base of the brain obstruct the CSF, resulting in communicating hydrocephalus. Less commonly, obstruction of a ventricular foramina occurs, producing a noncommunicating hydrocephalus (Sagar, 1978b).

Subdural effusion, a collection of fluid in the subdural space, is a complication of meningitis that occurs primarily in infants under 2 years of age and following *H influenzae* infections. Nonspecific signs of vomiting, irritability, and increasing head circumference together with failure of clinical improvement after 72 hours of antibiotic treatment might indicate subdural effusion.

Inflammation and impaired circulation might cause cranial nerve involvement, resulting in visual, auditory, or other disturbances of head and neck function. Other abnormal neurologic findings include changes in reflexes, muscle tone, sensorimotor alterations, and focal or generalized seizures (Conway-Rutkowski, 1982).

Metabolic alterations in fluid and electrolyte balance might occur as a result of dehydration from vomiting, septic shock, cerebral edema, or inappropriate secretion of ADH. Occurring in about one-third of cases, inappropriate ADH released by the pituitary gland causes hypervolemia, oliguria, high urine osmolality, and dilutional hyponatremia. The child becomes water intoxicated, restless, and irritable and has seizures, all symptoms that might be confused with meningitic symptoms. Cerebral edema is increased further by the inappropriate ADH syndrome (Weil, 1980).

Seizures occur in up to 30% of children with bacterial meningitis, more commonly with *H influenzae* infections than with other types of infection (Gaddy, 1980; Weil, 1980). The seizure activity might be associated with fever, cerebral edema, localized cortical involvement, or metabolic derangements. Seizures might occur only during the period of acute illness or remain as a persistent sequelae.

The incidence of serious residual neurologic deficits has been decreased with early diagnosis and aggressive treatment, but bacterial meningitis continues to result in neurologic sequelae in a significant number of cases. Seizures, vision or hearing loss, cognitive, language, or perceptual deficits, motor dysfunction, and behavioral alterations are possible residual impairments. Neonatal meningitis carries a much poorer prognosis than other forms of meningitis, with a high mortality rate and greater incidence of severe neurologic deficits among survivors (Weil, 1980).

Diagnostic Evaluation When the signs and symptoms suggest meningitis, the diagnosis must be confirmed by examination and culture of the CSF. A lumbar puncture is performed prior to initiating antibiotic therapy to accurately identify the causative organism. If acute increased ICP is suspected, the lumbar puncture is performed cautiously, with a parenteral line in place and emergency equipment available to anticipate brainstem herniation from the sudden reduction of high ICP. This complication occurs rarely but is considered in the acute management process.

Initial CSF pressure is characteristically elevated, and the CSF is cloudy. The white cell count is increased to between 1000 and 10,000 cells/mm^3, predominately polymorphonuclear leukocytes. Protein and lactic acid levels are increased. The CSF glucose level, normally one-half to two-thirds the serum glucose level, is decreased in bacterial meningitis (see Table 42-2). A blood sample is obtained prior to the lumbar puncture to compare the glucose levels.

Gram's stain and culture are performed to determine the causative organism. Specific bacterial antigens may be identified by countercurrent immunoelectrophoresis, a rapid test that is helpful in the initial diagnosis (Rytel, 1975). Nasopharyngeal, blood, and urine cultures are obtained to help identify the causative agent. Positive blood cultures occur in about 40% of cases and are more helpful in diagnosis than nose and throat cultures (Weil, 1980).

Other laboratory tests that are useful include a complete blood count, serum electrolyte levels, blood urea nitrogen, and urinalysis. If other predisposing factors are suspected, additional tests might be performed such as serologic, immunoglobulin, or radiographic studies. CT scan can be used to determine hydrocephalus, subdural effusion, or abscess formation (Sagar, 1978a).

Medical Treatment Acute bacterial meningitis is a pediatric emergency that requires swift diagnosis, antibiotic treatment, and supportive care to reduce the risks of death or permanent disability. The initial antibiotic is broad spectrum, the choice of which is determined by the most likely infecting organism depending on the patient's age, results of CSF Gram's stain, and any known predisposing factors. A combination of ampicillin or penicillin G and chloramphenicol is used in older infants and children. Neonates are treated with ampicillin and gentamycin or kanamycin. Once the specific pathogen has been identified and its sensitivities determined, antibiotic therapy is chosen appropriately.

Antibiotics are administered intravenously in sufficiently high dosages to cross the blood–brain barrier. The dosage is calculated by body surface area or weight, and the drugs are administered by bolus or continual drip. Parenteral antibiotics are continued until the child has been afebrile for 5 days but at least for a total of 7–10 days. The average length of treatment for children is 10–14 days, depending on the clinical response and repeat culture results. The lumbar puncture often is repeated 48 hours after the end of treatment to demonstrate that the CSF is sterile. If clinical improvement is not as good as expected, the CSF is reexamined at any point in the treatment course (Gellis and Kagan, 1982).

Infants with meningitis caused by gram-negative organisms are treated longer, for 2 weeks after repeat CSF cultures are sterile or for a minimum of 3 weeks (Weil, 1980).

The patient's fluid and electrolyte balance is managed with parenteral replacement. Initially, fluid intake usually is kept low (two-thirds of maintenance) to decrease cerebral edema. If the child demonstrates signs of inappropriate secretion of ADH, fluid restrictions are critical to prevent overhydration and a resulting increase in cerebral edema. Hyperosmolar agents (mannitol), steroids, or hyperventilation therapy are used to decrease cerebral edema (Weil, 1980).

Fever is controlled by antipyretics, tepid sponge baths, or a hypothermia mattress, if necessary. If the child becomes febrile after the first 3 or 4 days of treatment, sources of secondary infection must be sought. Seizures are treated promptly with anticonvulsant medication.

The child is monitored continually for the development of complications associated with both the disease process and therapeutic measures. Hypovolemia from septic shock or aggressive fluid restriction, respiratory insufficiency, and renal and metabolic alterations are detected early and treated appropriately. If the bacterial meningitis is associated with other disorders, such as trauma, shunt infection, or other systemic foci of infection, additional treatment is undertaken accordingly (Sagar, 1978a).

Nursing Management Nursing care of the child with acute bacterial meningitis involves continual assessment of status, maintenance of prescribed medical therapies, and supportive measures. An intensive care setting is indicated for neonates, infants, and severely ill older children. The child is isolated and respiratory precautions are taken for 24 hours after specific antimicrobial therapy is initiated to prevent spread of the meningitic infection.

In the diagnostic and initial treatment period, the nurse assists in accomplishing procedures (lumbar puncture, obtaining blood samples, starting intravenous infusions). Required specimens are obtained and other diagnostic tests performed if indicated (such as CT scan, radiographs). A baseline assessment of the child's neurologic and vital signs is made, and the nurse reassesses these parameters frequently to detect changes and the response to treatment. The lumbar puncture can be extremely stressful to the acutely ill, frightened child. During the procedure, the nurse comforts the child as much as possible and observes the child's respirations carefully for signs of distress.

Bedrest is required, with the head of the bed elevated slightly and the child in a position of comfort. This helps to decrease cerebral edema and allows the child to rest. Safety measures are taken to prevent injury should seizures occur and to maintain the patency of the intravenous infusion. Most children with meningitis are irritable, photophobic, and respond with pain to external stimuli. The nurse ensures that excessive manipulations, noise, bright lights, and stressful stimuli are reduced or eliminated during the acute period.

The child's level of consciousness is the most sensitive indicator of neurologic status. The nurse remains alert to subtle changes in responsiveness, behavior, and activity that indicate alterations in consciousness. The nurse assesses the child's vital signs, including temperature, frequently during the initial period.

Temperature elevation increases cerebral metabolic activity and oxygen demands, increases fluid requirements, and places the child at higher risk for febrile seizures. Fever is reduced by external measures (light coverings, tepid sponge baths, and a hypothermia mattress) and by administering antipyretics. Extra fluids usually are not given in the early acute period because they might contribute to increasing cerebral edema.

The nurse monitors the child's blood pressure and pulse for changes indicative of increased ICP or signs of shock. The nurse assesses the child's respiratory effort, rhythm, and rate frequently. Impaired oxygenation can result in cerebral hypoxia, which increases cerebral edema further.

The child's hydration and electrolyte balance are managed by carefully maintaining the fluid intake at the prescribed amount and composition and accurately measuring output. The nurse measures the specific gravity of urine initially and with each void or once each shift. The child is weighed each day to assist in determining hydration. If the child is alert without vomiting, small amounts of clear liquids by mouth might be allowed. After the acute period, the diet might be advanced as the child's condition improves.

The nurse describes and reports any seizures carefully and administers anticonvulsant medications as prescribed. The nurse observes the child for other complicating conditions such as increasing head circumference, motor or sensory deficits, or other infectious sites. Pneumonia, joint effusions, otitis, or abscess formation can develop secondary to meningitis. The prolonged intravenous therapy that is a necessary part of treatment might result in phlebitis. The nurse monitors infusion sites closely and changes them if appropriate.

Within several days, the child usually begins to improve clinically and gradually tolerates increased activity. The nurse offers quiet games, books, and music to provide entertainment while preventing fatigue. Developmentally appropriate stimuli are provided as the child recovers and to the degree warranted by the child's condition. The child works through the traumatic experiences brought about by the meningitis, particularly repeated intravenous insertions and having blood drawn, by hospital play. A follow-up lumbar puncture most likely will be performed to determine the adequacy of treatment. The nurse helps to prepare the child through age-appropriate explanations, play, and rehearsal.

A continuing nursing concern is maintaining the child's intravenous infusion, which is needed for the administration of antibiotics for 10–14 days or longer. Treatment is continued at least 5 days after signs and symptoms subside, when the child has become increasingly active, and even longer for infants. In younger children the intravenous site must be protected, including the use of restraints when the child is unattended. The nurse makes every effort to see that the parent and staff members spend as much time as possible with the child so that restraints can be removed. A heparin lock device is placed to free older children from the constant infusion between medication doses.

The nurse provides emotional support to the child and parent during the initial stages of the child's disease. Parents might feel guilty that they did not recognize the child's illness earlier. The nurse explains the disease process and reassures them that the child's preceding mild illness would not have alerted them to central nervous system infection (Gaddy, 1980). The nurse describes all procedures (such as lumbar puncture, isolation, or treatments) and explains their rationale. First and foremost the parent might be concerned about the child's prognosis and possible neurologic damage. The nurse avoids false reassurances but corrects misconceptions and helps the family to talk about their fears. If neurologic sequelae result, they might not be apparent initially, and the nurse stresses the importance of follow-up appointments to the family.

If residual deficits persist from the recovery period, a specialized rehabilitative treatment might be developed. The nurse evaluates visual, hearing, speech, motor, or other impairments early and makes therapeutic recommendations. (See the section on habilitation and rehabilitation management.) If seizures have occurred and the child is to continue receiving anticonvulsant medication, the nurse teaches the parent and child about seizures and how to manage them.

Aseptic Meningitis

Aseptic meningitis is a usually benign illness that is most often caused by a virus. Coxsackie viruses, echoviruses, and other enteroviruses or mumps viruses are commonly responsible, although arboviruses, herpes viruses, and nonviral (toxic, postinfectious) agents can cause aseptic meningitis (Sagar, 1978a). Seasonal variations in incidence correlate with viral epidemiology, with enteroviruses the most common causative agents during warm weather. The virus is transmitted by enteric means, droplets, or an arthropod vector. Viremia might result, and the organism in turn then invades the meninges. Young adult populations get aseptic meningitis more often than children.

Clinical Manifestations Nonspecific prodromal signs of malaise, gastrointestinal disturbance, and flu symptoms might precede the acute onset of fever, headache, and stiffness and pain in the neck and back. Such mild neurologic signs as lethargy, irritability, and transient reflex changes might occur (Sagar, 1978a). In rare cases motor impairment or cranial nerve involvement occurs (Weil, 1980). A reddened, maculopapular rash can appear with echovirus infections (Conway-Rutkowski, 1982). The disease is self-limited, with complete recovery usually occurring within 7–10 days. Older children and adults might experience transient weakness and fatigue that can last for a few weeks to months, but permanent residual deficits are extremely rare (Weil, 1980).

Because of the similarity in initial manifestations of aseptic meningitis to bacterial meningitis, diagnostic procedures must be performed to rule out other infectious etiologies. A lumbar puncture is done to examine and culture the CSF.

Most often, the CSF is clear, with normal to elevated pressure. Cell counts might range from 100 to several thousand cells per cubic millimeter but is generally less than 500 cells/mm^3 (predominantly lymphocytes). The glucose level is normal, and the protein level can be normal or slightly elevated (Conway-Rutkowski, 1982). Bacterial cultures of CSF are negative. Viral cultures might be performed to identify the specific causative agent, but the results do not affect treatment.

A blood count usually reveals a viral profile, with a normal or decreased white blood cell count and lymphocyte predominance. Other cultures (blood, nasopharyngeal secretions, urine, stool) are obtained to detect a concurrent bacterial infection.

Medical Treatment The child with aseptic meningitis is treated symptomatically with antipyretics, analgesics, and bedrest. Until bacterial meningitis is definitely ruled out, the child might be placed in isolation and treated with intravenous antibiotics. Hospitalization is usually brief, and the child is allowed to recover at home.

Nursing Management Nursing care includes monitoring the child's neurologic status, vital signs, and hydration. The nurse focuses care on regulating the child's temperature, assuring adequate hydration and nutrition, and providing comfort measures. The nurse instructs the parent about how to care for the child at home and advises the family to schedule a follow-up appointment with their primary health care provider.

Encephalitis

Encephalitis is an inflammation of the brain that is caused by an infectious process. Viral agents are most commonly responsible, although encephalitis can be associated with bacterial, fungal, and other infectious agents.

The causative viruses include the arboviruses (those spread to humans by insects), mumps virus, measles virus, varicella-zoster virus, herpesviruses, and enteroviruses. Encephalitis also can occur as a postinfectious complication of a systemic viral illness such as mumps, measles, varicella, or rubella. In rare cases encephalitis occurs following vaccination for measles, pertussis, influenza, or typhoid (Conway-Rutkowski, 1982). In many cases the viral agent responsible for the disease is not known because the organism cannot be isolated from blood or CSF.

Clinical Manifestations The clinical picture of encephalitis can vary from gradual to acute in onset. Often, symptoms of a nonspecific viral illness such as headache, vomiting, and fever appear. Following the nonspecific illness, neurologic signs develop, including behavior changes, lethargy, stiff neck, seizures, or focal neurologic signs. In severe cases alterations in consciousness might progress to coma and death.

Depending on the type and severity of the illness, the clinical course might last days to weeks; the patient might recover completely or suffer permanent neurologic deficits. The permanent sequelae of encephalitis include mental retardation, behavior and personality changes, motor dysfunction, and seizures (Weil, 1980).

Diagnostic Evaluation The diagnosis of encephalitis is based on the patient's neurologic signs and history (especially any known viral exposures) and isolation of the causative organism when possible. Cultures of CSF, blood, feces, and nasopharyngeal secretions are obtained to help identify the etiologic agent.

Medical Treatment Immediate care in the acute stage of the illness is symptomatic, directed toward life support. The child's vital and neurologic signs are monitored continuously to detect changes indicative of increased ICP and cardiac, respiratory, or metabolic derangements.

Cerebral edema may be treated with dehydration therapy, osmotic diuretics, or steroids. Parenteral antibiotics often are administered until a bacterial etiology is ruled out by cultures. Seizures are managed with anticonvulsant medications. Respiratory insufficiency might require ventilatory assistance. Antipyretics and hypothermia therapy are used if necessary to control fever. The child's fluid and electrolyte balance is monitored closely and managed with parenteral therapy.

As the child's condition stabilizes, supportive management continues throughout the recovery period, and rehabilitative care is designed for the child's individual needs. Residual disabilities are treated as appropriate, including orthopedic and physical therapy, neurologic treatment of seizures, and remedial therapy for other deficits.

Nursing Management Nursing care of the child with encephalitis involves intensive monitoring of vital and neurologic signs, including observing the child for signs of increased ICP, meningeal irritation, and cranial nerve involvement. The child's level of consciousness and respiratory and cardiovascular status might change rapidly, and prompt treatment depends on careful and continuous assessment.

If the child's condition progresses to unconsciousness, nursing care of the comatose child is implemented. Preventing the secondary effects of immobility during the acute and recovery stages are continuing goals of nursing intervention (see Chapter 29).

As the child recovers from the acute illness, either transient or permanent neurologic sequelae (such as cognitive impairment, motor dysfunction, or seizures) might become apparent. Both the child and family will need the supportive intervention of rehabilitative management.

Rabies

Rabies is an acute viral infection of the nervous system that is transmitted by the saliva of infected animals. Humans most often are infected by bites from rabid dogs, cats, bats, and wild animals. The virus enters the nervous system at the site of the wound and travels along peripheral nerves to the central nervous system. The disease process is characterized by progressive degeneration of neurons, with phases of encephalopathy and paralysis. The disease usually is fatal. Rabies is relatively uncommon in humans, but the risk of contracting the disease exists when potentially rabid animals are present. The incidence of rabies in animals varies from region to region, and wild animals, particularly skunks, foxes, raccoons, and bats, are common reservoirs of the infection (Plotkin, 1979).

Clinical Manifestations The incubation period is variable, ranging from 1 to 3 months. The severity of the disease and length of incubation are influenced by the amount of exposure and the proximity of the wound to the head. More severe forms of rabies and shorter incubation periods occur with extensive bites of the face and neck.

The symptoms occur in three characteristic phases. In the first, or premonitory, phase numbness or tingling is felt at the site of the wound. Fever, malaise, restlessness, headache, and anorexia might occur. This stage lasts from 2 to 10 days.

In the second, or excitement, phase irritability, apprehension, insomnia, and photophobia gradually develop. Muscle tone and deep tendon reflexes are increased. During the excitement phase, laryngeal spasm characteristically develops. Such manifestations as difficulty swallowing, choking, and inability to handle secretions become severe; in the classic form even the sight or sound of liquids produces violent spasms of the larynx and pharynx (hydrophobia). Periods of delirium and irrational hyperactivity alternate with quiet, lucid periods. Seizures often occur. Death might occur in the acute excitement stage from cardiorespiratory arrest during a seizure or an anoxic episode caused by laryngeal spasm.

The third, or paralytic, phase develops within 1–3 days of the excitement phase. Paralysis, stupor, and coma progress to death within several days (Weil, 1980).

Medical Treatment Treatment for rabies is begun at the time of known or presumed exposure because the disease is almost always fatal once symptoms appear. The wound is cleansed thoroughly and flushed immediately, and an iodine solution or alcohol is applied. Local attempts to remove the virus from the areas of contact must be prompt and thorough.

The long incubation period allows postexposure immunization, both active and passive. Several vaccines are available for active immunization, including human diploid cell vaccine (HDCV), duck embryo vaccine (DEV), and Pasteur brain-fixed virus. The preferred treatment is HDCV because of its greater effectiveness and fewer severe side effects. The vaccine is given intramuscularly in five or six doses over 28–90 days (Ferguson and Roll, 1981). The patient is tested for serum antibody formation, and booster doses are given, if necessary.

Passive immunization with rabies immune globulin (RIG) or hyperimmune rabies serum is given to provide rapid, temporary protection from the virus. Part of the dose is administered directly to infiltrate the wound, and the rest of the dose is given intramuscularly. Passive immunization is indicated for all severe exposures and can be used regardless of the time interval between exposure and treatment (Weil, 1980).

Rabies prophylaxis is administered when exposure is known or cannot reasonably be ruled out. The treatment is painful, and certain vaccines can cause severe adverse reactions, although the newer HDCV appears to be a safer form of effective prophylaxis. Practitioners must base their treatment decisions on local public health epidemiologic data and the US Centers for Disease Control (CDC) recommendations. Guidelines for postexposure antirabies prophylaxis are available from the CDC (1980), and all suspected cases of rabies must be reported to the CDC.

Nursing Management The nurse prepares the child and family for antirabies prophylactic treatment. They need to understand the treatment process, receive ongoing support, and be given opportunities to share their anxieties and fears about both the treatment and the disease.

Rabies infection is prevented by the immunization of domestic animals and avoidance of contact with wild animals. Health teaching of children should include those behaviors that would minimize the risk of animal bites, both domestic and wild. Rabies is a preventable disease, and nurses as well as other health professionals have a responsibility to promote rabies control programs through community education.

Reye's Syndrome

Reye's syndrome is an acute neurologic disorder that causes encephalopathy and fatty degeneration of the viscera. It occurs primarily in children, with a peak incidence between 5 and 15 years of age (Martelli, 1982).

First described in 1963 (Reye, Morgan, and Baral, 1963), the disease is characterized by vomiting, changes in consciousness, hypoglycemia, altered liver function, and seizures. The specific cause is unclear, but Reye's syndrome most often appears following a viral illness such as influenza or chickenpox. Recent research has suggested that the administration of salicylates contributes to Reye's syndrome, and the American Academy of Pediatrics now recommends that aspirin not be given to children with symptoms of influenza or chickenpox (Committee on Infectious Diseases, 1982). Pathologic changes associated with Reye's syndrome include severe cerebral edema, neuronal necrosis, and enlargement and fatty infiltration of the liver (and to a lesser degree of the kidneys, myocardium, and other viscera) (Weil, 1980).

Clinical Manifestations Symptoms usually develop within a few days to several weeks following a viral illness. The child might appear to have a recurrence of the original illness, with lethargy and vomiting. Behavior changes such as irritability, confusion, hostility, and apathy might be noted. Rapid deterioration in neurologic status ensues in 24–48 hours, with decreasing consciousness, hyperventilation, and seizures. The clinical stages of Reye's syndrome are outlined in Table 42-7.

Hepatic dysfunction is determined by laboratory analysis with elevated serum glutamic-oxalacetic transaminase (SGOT) and serum glutamic-pyruvic transaminase (SGPT) levels, prolonged prothrombin time, and high blood ammonia levels. Hypoglycemia is a frequent finding, especially in children under 5 years of age. The acid–base balance is disturbed, and respiratory alkalosis often occurs. Metabolic acidosis develops in severe cases (Trauner, 1981). The diagnosis of Reye's syndrome is made on the basis of the combined history, presenting neurologic signs, and characteristic laboratory findings.

The prognosis depends on the severity of the illness and success of supportive measures in management. The disease has a high mortality rate for those children who develop coma or further progression. The length of the illness is variable, ranging from several days to weeks if the child remains comatose. The majority of children who survive the acute stage of illness will recover completely. Some children who develop deep coma, decerebrate posturing, or seizures and subsequently recover might have neurologic sequelae such as seizures, cognitive impairment, motor dysfunction, or behavioral alterations (VanCaillie, et al., 1977).

Medical Treatment The treatment of Reye's syndrome is supportive and requires an intensive care setting. Therapy is directed toward maintaining life functions, reversing metabolic alterations, and controlling cerebral edema. Hypoglycemia is treated with a 10% or higher intravenous glucose solution. Insulin is given adjunctively, and the child's serum glucose level is monitored frequently. Vitamin K is administered to help correct clotting difficulties caused by hypothrombinemia. In addition, fresh-frozen plasma is given or an exchange transfusion performed if significant bleeding problems occur. Prophylactic anticonvulsant medications might be given to prevent seizures.

Intracranial pressure monitoring devices often are used to directly and continuously measure ICP and detect cerebral edema immediately. Fluids generally are restricted to prevent overhydration and increased edema. Treatment with osmotic diuretics, steroids, and hyperventilation often is undertaken to control cerebral edema.

TABLE 42-7 Clinical Stages of Reye's Syndrome

Stage	Symptoms
Stage I	Vomiting; sleepiness, lethargy
Stage II	Disorientation; delerium; combativeness; hyperventilation; hyperactive reflexes; appropriate response to noxious stimuli; no abnormal posturing
Stage III	Coma; decorticate rigidity; preservation of pupillary light and ocular reflexes
Stage IV	Deepened coma; decerebrate rigidity; loss of oculocephalic reflexes; large, fixed pupils
Stage V	Flaccid paralysis; loss of deep tendon reflexes; seizures; respiratory arrest

SOURCE: Data from Lovejoy FN, et al: Clinical staging in Reye's syndrome. *Am J Dis Child* 1974; 128:36–41.

Various institutions have developed protocols for the treatment of Reye's syndrome, including decreasing high blood ammonia levels through dialysis and reducing ICP by CSF withdrawal, high-dose barbiturates, or decompressive craniotomy (Trauner, 1980; Hilty, 1981).

Nursing Management Children with Reye's syndrome require intensive and highly skilled nursing care. Emergency treatment in a critical-care setting is vital to manage the child's complex and life-threatening problems.

The nurse monitors the child's neurologic status, vital signs, arterial and central venous pressure, blood gases, and ICP continuously. Temperature control is necessary to prevent elevations, which increase cerebral oxygen demand, and the nurse might need to use a hypothermia pad.

Measures are employed to prevent increasing ICP, including elevating the child's head and monitoring fluid intake and output meticulously to prevent overhydration. Hyperventilation therapy by means of intubation frequently is necessary to reduce ICP by raising arterial oxygenation and lowering carbon dioxide levels. The nurse keeps stimulation to an absolute minimum and organizes care to avoid unnecessary manipulations, which could elevate ICP.

Children in the earlier stages of Reye's syndrome are often anxious and disoriented and might demonstrate inappropriate behavior. The nurse talks softly to the child and offers simple, short explanations and calm reassurance to decrease the child's agitation.

If the child's condition progresses to stage III or further (see Table 42-7), the principles of care are like those for the comatose child. The nurse is particularly careful to handle the child gently during respiratory care, positioning, and the like while the child is in the acute stage of cerebral edema. The nurse anticipates the possibility of seizures, and the staff is prepared to manage the child if seizure activity occurs.

The family needs to be updated continuously about the child's condition, and the nurse explains procedures and guides the family to help in keeping the child calm. The nurse also reassures the family that the child's illness was not caused by neglect because the early symptoms often do not indicate such a severe disease (Clark, et al., 1980).

The child recovering from Reye's syndrome needs both physical and emotional support to regain mobility and reduce anxiety. Although the majority of children do not suffer permanent residual disabilities, those who do have permanent deficits will need rehabilitative care.

Efforts to increase public awareness about Reye's syndrome are being undertaken by the National Reye's Syndrome Foundation in cooperation with community health education programs (Belkengren and Sapala, 1981). In addition, increasing media attention and warnings printed on aspirin packages are helping to alert the public about the risk of the disease.

Nurses help parents to recognize the early signs of Reye's syndrome and caution them about giving aspirin to children. These efforts, as well as continued research, are vital to reduce the morbidity and mortality associated with this severe illness.

Postinfectious Polyneuritis (Guillain-Barré Syndrome)

Postinfectious polyneuritis, or *Guillain-Barré syndrome* (GBS), is an acute neuromuscular disease that causes progressive muscular weakness and paralysis. The specific cause is not known, but the disease most often appears following a viral illness such as influenza, gastroenteritis, measles, mumps, or infectious mononucleosis. Guillian-Barré syndrome also has occurred following immunization, particularly with influenza vaccines. The cause of GBS is suspected to be related to a toxic autoimmune reaction to the viral agent (Menkes, 1980). The diesase may occur at any age but is more prevalent in children between 4 and 9 years of age.

The pathologic changes that occur are a diffuse inflammation of the peripheral nerves with progressive myelin breakdown (Menkes, 1980). The disease is self-limiting, and a slow return of neurologic function occurs in most cases. The mortality rate is estimated to be as high as 20%, with deaths most often due to respiratory and cardiac complications (Gellis and Kagan, 1982).

Clinical Manifestations The onset of GBS occurs within 2 weeks following a viral illness in about two-thirds of cases. Sudden pain and weakness of the feet and legs are early symptoms, which progress upward in an ascending motor paralysis to involve the trunk and all four extremities. The muscles of respiration often are affected, resulting in respiratory insufficiency. Cranial nerve paralysis may appear at any point in the disease process, commonly manifested by facial weakness and impaired swallowing.

Muscle weakness and paralysis might progress rapidly over a few hours or days but most often increases for several weeks before reaching a plateau. The paralysis is usually symmetric and is accompanied by the loss of deep tendon reflexes and reduced muscle tone. Sensory function is less affected, but the child might have paresthesias (numbness, tingling, pain) and loss of position sense.

Respiratory failure, secondary to intercostal and phrenic paralysis, is the most serious complication of the acute stage of GBS. Autonomic function might be impaired, resulting in hypertension, postural hypotension, cardiac arrhythmias, and urinary retention. These disturbances can lead to cardiovascular collapse (shock), with a potentially fatal outcome (Gellis and Kagan, 1982).

Cerebrospinal fluid analysis characteristically shows an increased protein level, with a normal cell count and negative culture. The acute stage of progressive paralysis may continue for 2–4 weeks, then plateaus and is followed by a gradual return of function. Recovery is slow and might take up to 2 years. Most children who receive optimal supportive care do, however, recover completely.

Medical Treatment Treatment of GBS is primarily supportive, with the goals of maintaining vital functions and preventing complications. During the acute stage, treatment is best managed in an intensive-care setting.

Respiratory insufficiency frequently requires tracheal intubation and mechanical ventilation. These procedures should be performed when there are early indications of impaired vital capacity to avoid the risk of hypoxia from advanced respiratory failure.

Vasodilators might be required for hypertension, and digoxin occasionally is indicated for the treatment of cardiac arrhythmias. Corticosteroid therapy sometimes is used in the treatment of GBS, but its benefit in altering the outcome of the disease is questionable (Menkes, 1980). In the rehabilitative phase orthopedic care is required to prescribe physiotherapy programs and provide braces, splints, or other assistive devices as needed.

Nursing Management During the acute stage, nursing care of the child with GBS requires intensive support. Management is similar to that for the child with paralysis caused by a spinal cord injury. The nurse pays particular attention to detecting any progression of motor paralysis, respiratory insufficiency, and cranial nerve impairment.

The nurse monitors the child's respiratory status closely for alterations in rate, depth, or pattern and obtains serial measurements of the child's vital capacity. If the child requires a tracheotomy and assisted ventilation, intensive respiratory care is needed (see Chapter 34). Even in the absence of signs of respiratory involvement, the child with GBS needs frequent turning, chest physiotherapy, and inspiratory exercises to prevent pulmonary complications secondary to immobility.

The nurse monitors the child's vital signs frequently to detect cardiovascular complications, particularly alterations in blood pressure and cardiac arrhythmias. The use of a cardiac monitor is indicated in the acute stage. The nurse observes the child closely for signs of impending cardiovascular collapse (restlessness, sweating, cyanosis, hypotension, peripheral coolness, and mottled skin). The nurse avoids postural hypotension in the child by making position changes gradually and using elastic stockings to improve venous return from the legs.

The nurse prevents joint contractures by positioning the child in correct alignment, using resting splints, trochanteric rolls, pillows, and other supports. Active physiotherapy is contraindicated during the period of acute inflammation, but gentle range-of-motion exercises might be permitted depending on the child's condition.

The child often experiences cramping muscular pain and is hypersensitive to touch. The nurse handles the child with extreme gentleness and plans carefully to avoid moving the child unnecessarily and promote the child's rest.

The nurse prevents other complications secondary to immobility through attention to the child's skin care, diet, and elimination. Impaired swallowing might necessitate nasogastric tube feedings to provide adequate nutrition.

As the child recovers, an increasingly active rehabilitation program is developed. Muscle strengthening and stretching exercises are undertaken, and mobilizing aids are provided to help the child get up and about. The child often has a lengthy convalescence, and provisions must be made for developmentally appropriate stimulation and continuation of schooling.

Intrauterine Central Nervous System Infection

Maternal infections can result in abnormalities of the developing fetus's nervous system, depending on the gestational age at the time of fetal exposure and the causative agent. Central nervous system manifestations vary in type and severity, and affected children might require treatment for a number of neurologic deficits. The clinical features and management of intrauterine rubella, cytomegalic inclusion disease, and toxoplasmosis are listed in Table 42-8.

The Child With a Seizure Disorder

Seizures are among the more common manifestations of neurologic dysfunction in childhood and are associated with a variety of acute and chronic conditions. A *seizure* is a sudden, transient alteration in brain function that is caused by the excessive, disorderly discharge of electrical impulses by neuronal tissue. Alterations of consciousness and motor, sensory, or autonomic function are clinical manifestations of seizure activity, which can occur as a single episode or recur intermittently. Different characteristic seizure patterns, such as convulsions, lapses of consciousness, and behavioral disturbances, reflect the type of abnormal electrical activity and area of brain involvement.

Incidence estimates of seizures among children vary depending on age and seizure type. Up to 6% of all children experience one or more seizures by adolescence, but the majority of seizures are single, nonrecurrent episodes associated with acute illness and fever (Conway-Rutkowski, 1982). Chronically recurrent seizures, called a *seizure disorder,* or *epilepsy,* affect approximately 0.5% of children (Muehl, 1979). Seizures are more common in the first 2 years of life than at any other age because of the immaturity of the central nervous system in regulating the brain's electrical activity (Baird, 1979).

Seizures are categorized according to etiology, clinical manifestations, and electroencephalographic pattern. Because seizures are not a specific disease entity but a symptom of an abnormality of brain function, a variety of factors might be responsible. The causes of seizures are summarized in Table 42-9. At different ages, certain causes are more common. In the newborn period, the effects of perinatal insult by anoxia or hemorrhage, and congenital brain defects are frequent causes of seizures. In later infancy and early childhood, febrile convulsions, seizures associated with central nervous system infections, and congenital malformations are common causes. Beginning at about 3 years of age and continuing throughout adolescence, the cause of recurrent seizures cannot be determined in most children, and the disorder is referred to as *idiopathic epilepsy* (Baird, 1979).

Seizures

Clinical Manifestations Seizures are classified as *generalized* (involving both brain hemispheres) or *partial* (involving a localized area of the cerebral cortex). The types and descriptions of seizures observed in children are summarized in Table 42-10.

Depending on the type of seizure, the child might experience an aura or warning sensation just before the onset of the attack. Abdominal pain, nausea, feeling "shaky," dizziness, sudden fear, and visual or auditory sensations are among the auras described by children and adolescents. Grand mal and psychomotor seizures frequently are preceded by an aura.

A seizure episode is usually self-limiting and by itself causes no acute injury. The sudden loss of consciousness and forceful muscle contractions that often accompany seizures, however, can result in injury from falls or striking objects. Children with atonic or myoclonic seizures can suffer severe

TABLE 42-8 Intrauterine Central Nervous System Infections

Infectious agent	Clinical manifestations	Management
Rubella virus	Low birthweight, cataracts, deafness, cardiac defects, encephalitis, retinopathy, hepatitis, thrombocytopenia, psychomotor retardation	Primary prevention through immunization; supportive care for systemic alterations
Cytomegalovirus (CMV)—cytomegalic inclusion disease	Low birthweight, jaundice, hepatosplenomegaly, bone lesions, anemia, cataracts, chorioretinitis, microcephaly, intracranial calcifications, obstructive hydrocephalus, psychomotor retardation, seizures	Antimetabolites and antiviral agents (drug therapy is experimental); supportive care for systemic alterations, including surgical treatment of hydrocephalus and seizure control
Toxoplasma gondii (intracellular protozoan parasite)—toxoplasmosis	Low birthweight, hydrocephalus, chorioretinitis, intracranial calcifications, seizures, hepatosplenomegaly, anemia, psychomotor retardation	Antiprotozoal medication (pyrimethamine, spiramycin, sulfadiazine); supportive care for systemic alterations, including treatment for hydrocephalus and seizures

SOURCE: Data from Devore NE, Jackson VM, Piening SL: TORCH infections. *Am J Nurs* (Dec) 1983; 83(12): 1660–1665 and Weil ML: Infections of the nervous system. In: *Textbook of Child Neurology*. Lea & Febiger, 1980.

TABLE 42-9 Causes of Seizures and Seizure Disorders

Cause	Disorders	Cause	Disorders
Genetic and intrauterine influences	Chromosomal abnormalities Neurocutaneous syndromes (tuberous sclerosis, neurofibromatosis) Cerebral malformations (hydrocephalus, microcephaly) Intrauterine infection, drugs, radiation, hypoxia Familial degenerative disorders		Amino acid and fat metabolism disorders (phenylketonuria, lipid storage disease) Vitamin deficiency
Perinatal influences	Hypoxia Intracerebral hemorrhage Subdural hematoma	Toxic influences	Poisoning (lead, mercury, alcohol, strychnine, hydrocarbons, phosphates, camphor) Drug ingestion (aminophylline, antihistamines, hexachlorophene) Drug withdrawal (barbiturates, benzodiazepines, alcohol) Bacterial toxins Allergic disorders
Trauma	Acute cerebral injuries (contusion, laceration, hemorrhage, fracture) Post-traumatic encephalopathy	Anoxia	Acute asphyxia Postanoxic encephalopathy
Infection	Meningitis Encephalitis Reye's syndrome Intracerebral abscess Postinfectious encephalopathy	Vascular disorders	Arteriovenous malformation Thrombosis Cerebrovascular accident
		Space-occupying lesion	Brain tumor, abscess, cyst
Metabolic disorders	Fluid and electrolyte derangements (overhydration, hyponatremia, hypernatremia, hypocalcemia, alkalosis) Glucose metabolism disorders (hypoglycemia, hepatic dysfunction)	Acute cerebral edema	
		Febrile seizures	
		Unknown	Idiopathic, primary lesions

SOURCES: Data from Baird HW: Convulsive disorders. In: *Nelson's Textbook of Pediatrics*. Behrman RE and Vaughn VC (editors). Saunders, 1983; Jabbour JT, et al: *Pediatric Neurology Handbook*. Medical Examination, 1976; Low NL: Seizure disorders in children. In: *The Child With Disability Illness*. 2nd ed. Downey JA, Low NL (editors). Raven Press, 1982.

TABLE 42-10 Types of Seizures

Type	Description
Generalized seizures Major Motor (grand mal)	May be preceded by an aura. Initial loss of consciousness. Tonic phase involves rigid extension of the body; eye deviation; apnea; cyanosis; increased salivation; and loss of bladder and bowel control. Clonic phase involves rhythmic jerking movements. Postictal phase involves confusion and sleep. Seizure lasts 2–5 minutes or longer. Variable frequency
Absence (petit mal)	Onset between 3 and 8 years of age. Brief (few seconds) staring spell. Loss of awareness, with or without minor muscle twitching (face and hands). No loss of postural tone. Several to hundreds of episodes every day.
Minor motor—atonic	Onset between 3 and 8 years of age. Brief (few seconds) loss of muscle tone. Head drop; upper body drop; or full body drop. Frequency is variable—often daily or weekly episodes.
Minor motor—myoclonic	Onset between 3 and 7 years of age. Brief (few seconds) muscle flexor spasm. Forceful head drop; arm extension; trunk flexion. Variable frequency—daily to weekly episodes.
Infantile spasms	Onset between 3 and 9 months of age. Brief (momentary) flexion of neck, trunk, and legs ("jack-knife" seizures). Recurs in clusters of episodes—up to hundreds of times daily. Disappears after infancy; often replaced by other types of seizures in later childhood; usually accompanied by psychomotor impairment. Characteristic electroencephalographic pattern (hypsarrhythmia).
Partial seizures Focal seizures	Localized motor or sensory disturbance, generally without impairment of consciousness. Often unilateral. Motor—twitching of face, hand, foot may progress to entire side of body (Jacksonian seizure). Sensory—tingling, numbness, or other altered sensation of affected body part. Child might have weakness of the affected muscle group (Todd's paralysis) lasting hours to days following the seizure. The duration usually is several minutes. The frequency is variable.
Psychomotor	May be preceded by an aura. Widely varying manifestations. Behavioral and sensory alterations—most commonly staring; repetitive motor activity (automatisms) such as lip smacking, chewing, eye blinking, and fumbling with hands; confused state, mumbled speech; bizarre behavior (such as purposeless walking or running, undressing, aggression if restrained). Postictal fatigue and sleep. Duration is 5–10 minutes. Frequency is variable—daily to weekly.
Status epilepticus	Prolonged seizure or repeated seizures without regaining consciousness. Usually refers to generalized grand mal seizures. Can result in hypoxia; hypotension; cardiac arrhythmias; respiratory depression. Constitutes a medical emergency that requires immediate treatment.

trauma to the face and teeth from head drop attacks. Another secondary complication from seizures occurs during mealtime aspiration of food. The child also might aspirate excessive oral secretions produced during a generalized seizure.

After a grand mal or psychomotor seizure (the postictal phase), the child is often confused, drowsy, and might sleep for variable periods of time. Some children complain of headache and experience fatigue for a day or two after a grand mal seizure. In contrast, there is usually no postictal drowsiness following absence or minor motor attacks, and the child immediately resumes previous activities.

Diagnostic Evaluation One of the most important aspects in the diagnostic evaluation of seizures is a detailed history, which is obtained from both the parents and, if possible, the child. The purpose of the history is to determine whether the episodes represent seizure activity, the type of seizure, focus (if any), and possible causes for the disorder. The practitioner evaluating the child is seldom present during a seizure and must obtain a detailed clinical description of the episode, including preceding events (illness, fever, injury, and so forth), any aura or warning, and an exact description of the seizure and the child's behavior during the postictal period. The sequence of events, responsiveness of the child, parts of the body involved, and duration of the seizure are helpful in defining the type of seizure. It is important to determine any localizing signs that might indicate a focal origin. The child's age at onset, frequency of seizures, and any factors that precipitate the attacks also are determined. Grand mal seizures usually are not difficult to identify, but petit mal or psychomotor seizures can be difficult to diagnose.

Complete general physical and neurologic examinations are performed. Particular attention is given to determining any localized neurologic signs, head circumference, neurocutaneous lesions, or other findings that might help to diagnose the underlying brain dysfunction.

Various laboratory tests may be performed depending on the indications. These tests include a complete blood count and fasting glucose, serum calcium, phosphorus, and lead levels. Other tests are indicated if an underlying metabolic disturbance is suspected.

An electroencephalogram (EEG) is done to detect any abnormality in electrical activity and determine the type of seizure and focus, if any. The EEG might or might not show alterations between seizures; therefore, a normal EEG does not rule out a seizure disorder. Conversely, an abnormal EEG is not necessarily diagnostic. The EEG is most helpful in differentiating the characteristic patterns of different seizure types such as petit mal or psychomotor seizures.

Radiographic examinations of the skull frequently are performed to rule out intracranial calcifications and asymmetric skull development or when trauma is suspected. A CT scan can help to determine the presence of increased ICP, atrophy, tumors, or other anatomic abnormalities associated with seizures. More definitive studies, such as arteriography or radioisotope brain scans, are used when vascular or focal lesions are indicated that cannot be differentiated by CT scan.

A lumbar puncture is not done routinely, but is indicated for seizures occurring in infants under 6 months of age, children with fever and seizures, and children suspected of having meningitis (Low, 1982).

Medical and Surgical Treatment Children with recurrent seizures are treated with appropriate anticonvulsant medications. Depending on the type of seizure, one drug is chosen to begin treatment, and the dosage is adjusted until the seizures are controlled or the maximum tolerated dose is reached. If the drug is inadequate in controlling seizures, a second drug might be added slowly. For some children, a combination of medications is more effective, and a third or even fourth drug might be added. The goals of treatment are to eliminate seizures or reduce their frequency, without any side effects of drug therapy seriously affecting the child. Many children respond well to medication, with seizures occurring rarely or not at all. Other children's conditions are more difficult to manage, with seizures persisting and varying in frequency or type. Children with mixed seizure disorders, especially minor motor seizures, tend to be more refractive to treatment. Table 42-11 lists the commonly used anticonvulsant medications. All anticonvulsants must be given daily, usually in divided doses, to maintain therapeutic serum levels. Abrupt cessation of medication can lower the seizure threshold and precipitate status epilepticus (see the section on status epilepticus later in the chapter).

Another form of treatment for recurrent seizures is dietary therapy. The ketogenic diet is based on inducing ketosis by high fat and low protein and carbohydrate intake. Its use is reserved for young children (2–5 years of age) with minor motor or petit mal seizures refractive to anticonvulsant medication. This special diet is designed to induce a state simulating the ketosis and acidosis of starvation, which reduces seizure activity by an unknown mechanism. Adequate protein (1–1.5/g/kg of body weight), high fat, and low carbohydrate are calculated in a rigidly controlled diet, and vitamin supplements are given. The fat intake may be partially supplied by medium-chain triglyceride (MCT) oil. The child's urinary excretion of acetone is monitored to ensure that ketosis exists. The amount of fat in the child's diet is adjusted according to the degree of ketosis and clinical response. This diet is difficult to adhere to, with its unpalatable high-fat content, strict regimen of weighing food, and the cooperation necessary. It is useful for some children, but a considerable family commitment is needed to maintain the diet (Baird, 1979; Low, 1982).

Surgical intervention might be indicated if anticonvulsant treatment has been unsuccessful and a seizure focus amenable to surgery is demonstrated by specialized studies. The surgery might involve the removal of an isolated area of tissue or may be as extensive as hemispherectomy in children with hemiplegia and atrophy of one cerebral hemisphere. Neurosurgery is reserved for relatively rare cases with poor seizure control and surgically accessible lesions (Menkes, 1980).

Nursing Management Nurses play an important role in both the acute management of seizures and the ongoing care of the child and family. Seizures can elicit fear, misunderstanding, and feelings of helplessness in the child and those around the child, including nurses and other health care professionals who are unfamiliar with seizures. Nursing responsibilities include not only health supervision and teaching with the child and family but also community education to help reduce the stigmas and negative attitudes associated with seizures.

Acute Care Nursing management begins with being prepared for the occurrence of seizures in any child who is at risk from alteration in cerebral function (such as head trauma, meningitis, Reye's syndrome, brain tumor, or drug ingestion). Seizure precautions include padding side rails to prevent injury and keeping oropharyngeal suctioning equipment, oxygen, and a soft rubber airway at the child's bedside. Additional safety measures involve close supervision during ambulation or mealtimes to protect the child from injury caused by falls or the aspiration of food during a seizure.

During the acute stage of a seizure, nursing care focuses on protecting the child from injury, maintaining an airway, and observing the seizure activity. At the onset of a grand mal seizure, the child becomes rigid and falls. If the child is not in bed, the nurse attempts to break the child's fall and ease the child to the floor. The nurse loosens any tight clothing around the neck and holds the child's head gently to the side with the neck extended to maintain the airway and facilitate the drainage of secretions. Nothing should ever be forced into the child's mouth to prevent tongue biting. Any injury caused by the teeth clenching shut usually occurs at the onset of the seizure, and trying to insert tongue

TABLE 42-11 Commonly Used Anticonvulsant Medications

Medication	Type of seizure	Side effects	Nursing implications
Phenobarbital	Major motor (grand mal) and focal	Drowsiness; irritability; hyperactivity in younger children; skin rashes	Therapeutic serum levels take 2 weeks to develop Effects are potentiated by alcohol, central nervous system sedatives, and depressants; drug should be used with caution When given parenterally in emergencies, patient should be monitored closely for respiratory depression
Diphenylhydantoin (Dilantin)	Major motor and psychomotor	Gingival hypertrophy; hirsutism; megaloblastic anemia; hypocalcemia; allergic morbilliform rash; toxic effects—nystagmus, ataxia, drowsiness, introventricular fibrillation	Good oral hygiene, gum massage with an electric toothbrush, and regular dental examinations will help to decrease gingival hypertrophy. Tablet or capsule form is preferable because the suspension settles, making the dosage unreliable Should not be mixed with 5% dextrose in water for intravenous administration because it will precipitate. May be given in 50–100 ml normal saline given over 30 minutes or by an intravenous push with cardiac monitoring The patient's complete blood count and serum calcium level should be monitored. Folic acid may be supplemented if necessary
Valproic acid (Depakene)	Petit mal, minor motor, major motor, and local	Nausea; transient alopecia; liver toxicity; thrombocytopenia	Causes less sedation than other anticonvulsant medications Should be given with meals to decrease gastric irritation Might increase serum levels of phenobarbital, primidone, or carbamazepine; might increase or decrease serum diphenylhydantoin level Patient's hepatic function, platelet counts, and prothrombin time should be monitored
Carbamazepine (Tegretol)	Psychomotor and major motor	Nausea; vomiting; vertigo; diplopia; liver toxicity; blood dyscrasias	Contraindicated in bone marrow depression; should be used with caution in patients with cardiac, renal, or hepatic dysfunction Frequent monitoring of complete blood counts and platelet counts (every week initially) to detect bone marrow suppression
Ethosuximide (Zarontin)	Petit mal	Nausea; vertigo; skin rash; blood dyscrasias (rare)	Should be used with caution in patients with hepatic or renal dysfunction Might increase major motor seizures Should be given with meals to decrease gastric irritation Complete blood counts and hepatic function tests should be performed periodically to detect bone marrow suppression and hepatic damage, toxic effects of this drug

TABLE 42-11 (continued)

Medication	Type of seizure	Side effects	Nursing implications
Trimethadione (Tridione)	Petit mal	Nausea; photophobia; skin rash; leukopenia; nephrosis	Contraindicated in patients with blood dyscrasias or hepatic dysfunction; should be used with caution in patients with retinal or optic nerve diseases Patients should be advised to use sunglasses for photophobia Complete blood counts and hepatic function tests should be performed to detect bone marrow suppression or hepatic damage
Clonazepam (Clonopin)	Minor motor	Drowsiness; ataxia; irritability; behavioral disturbances; increased salivation; blood dyscrasias	Contraindicated in patients with hepatic dysfunction; should be used with caution in patients with chronic respiratory disease Patient should be monitored for behavioral side effects (belligerence, agitation) or oversedation Periodic complete blood counts and hepatic function tests should be performed to detect bone marrow suppression or hepatic damage
Primidone (Mysoline)	Major motor and focal	Drowsiness; ataxia; irritability	Part of drug metabolized to phenobarbital; should be used cautiously with phenobarbital Patient should be monitored for oversedation Dosage should be increased slowly to decrease side effects
Adrenocorticotropic hormone (ACTH)	Infantile spasms	Gastrointestinal bleeding; immunosuppression; fluid retention; hypertension; muscle weakness	Used for the treatment of infantile spasms Given intramuscularly daily; later given several times per week for periods of 1–6 months Patients should take gastric antacids, have stool guaic level monitored and avoid gastrointestinal irritants High-protein, high-potassium, low-sodium diet should be prescribed to control edema and negative nitrogen balance Patient should be monitored for infections caused by decreased resistance

blades, spoons, or other objects after a seizure has begun can cause more severe damage to the teeth and mouth. If the child's mouth is open, the nurse may place the edge of a soft piece of gauze between the child's side teeth to avoid repetitive biting. If the child can forecast an imminent seizure (from experiencing an aura) the nurse can insert the rubber airway or a padded tongue blade prior to the beginning of seizure activity.

The nurse does not attempt to restrain the child's movements; any attempt to do so can result in musculoskeletal injury. Objects that the child might strike should be moved away, and the nurse places a small pillow or other soft object under the child's head to prevent it from banging against the floor. Unless the child is in a dangerous position (such as near a radiator, stove, or stairs), the nurse does not move the child until the seizure subsides.

The nurse allows the seizure to run its course, attending the child constantly to maintain the airway and prevent injury. The nurse also observes the seizure manifestations, times the duration, and monitors for complications of aspiration or status epilepticus. During a prolonged grand mal seizure, the nurse might need to suction excessive secretions from the child. Oxygen administration and airway placement is indicated when respiratory effort is impaired

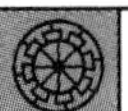

NURSING CARE GUIDE Child With a Seizure Disorder

Nursing diagnosis	Interventions	Evaluation
1. Potential knowledge deficit related to seizures	Teach the child and family about what happens during a seizure; alterations in electrical activity in the brain; and types of seizures Correct misperceptions about etiology, trigger factors, and mental disturbance Teach the family how to care for the child during a seizure: Break child's fall when possible Turn child's head to side Extend child's neck to open airway Remove tight neck clothing Place soft pad under child's head Move surrounding objects *Do not* place anything in the child's mouth Do not restrict the child's movements Institute cardiopulmonary resuscitation and move child when seizure is over Instruct the family to keep a record of seizures and to describe and report them to the child's physician Instruct the family about status epilepticus and when to call for emergency help Teach the child and family about medications. Help them to develop a method and routine of daily medication administration Promote epilepsy education in the schools and community	The child and family demonstrate an accurate awareness about seizures. The family appropriately cares for the child during a seizure. Family members accurately report seizure activity and recognize need for emergency care if status epilepticus occurs. The child receives anticonvulsant medication regularly
2. Potential for injury during a seizure	In hospital maintain seizure precautions—padded side rails, oxygen, suction and airway equipment at bedside; supervise ambulation and mealtimes Teach the family about the potential risks of injury from a seizure while climbing or swimming Help the family to obtain a protective helmet/faceguard for the child who falls frequently Advise the family about safety measures in the home as appropriate: Padded table edge Use of stairs Use of stove Use of sharp utensils Prepare adolescents for possible restrictions in obtaining a driver's license	Child remains free from injury during a seizure
3. Potential for increased seizure activity	Teach the child and family the importance of giving anticonvulsant medication consistently Instruct the family to notify the physician if the child is unable to take medication by mouth Teach the family the methods of fever control	Child has adequate serum levels of anticonvulsant medication. Child's seizure activity is not increased as a result of high fever or drug inducement

NURSING CARE GUIDE Child With a Seizure Disorder (continued)

Nursing diagnosis	Interventions	Evaluation
	Advise the family to check with the child's physician before giving the child any other medication (especially antihistamines)	
	Inform the physician of any increase in seizure frequency or change in the type of seizure	
4. Potential for adverse effects of medication	Teach the family about the possible adverse effects to watch for (see Table 42-11), particularly nausea, vomiting, drowsiness, ataxia, skin rash, bruising, and gum hypertrophy	Adverse effects are recognized early. Child remains free from serious adverse effects of medication
	Teach the family the importance of periodic blood tests to monitor for adverse effects	
	Teach the family oral hygiene measures to help control gingival hypertrophy from diphenylhydantoin	
	Advise the family to administer medication with meals to reduce gastric distress	
5. Potential for emotional response to seizure disorder	Allow the child to express fears, anger, sense of loss of control, and rejection	Child and family demonstrate adequate coping strategies and optimal emotional adjustment to the disorder
	Allow the child to make choices about care and activities whenever possible	
	Encourage the child's independence as much as possible, taking safety precautions as appropriate	
	Provide anticipatory guidance and problem solving to help the child handle seizures at school and reactions from peers	
	Refer the child for individual or peer group counseling	

in status epilepticus. Parenteral anticonvulsant medication might be necessary to halt prolonged or repetitive seizures.

Following the seizure, the nurse helps the child (carries, if necessary) to a private area to rest. The nurse explains simply and calmly that the child has had a seizure, that the child is all right, and that someone will stay with the child. The child often will sleep deeply after a major motor seizure and should not be roused or disturbed unnecessarily. The nurse takes the child's vital signs, which often are altered transiently during and after a seizure. It is important for the nurse to determine whether the child is febrile because an elevated body temperature can trigger seizures. The nurse takes measures to reduce the child's temperature if indicated to prevent repetitive seizures. The nurse identifies other precipitants of seizures, such as an inadequate serum anticonvulsant level, metabolic derangement, or illness, by the history and clinical examination. The child with recurrent seizures does not require medical attention every time a seizure occurs. Most major motor seizures stop spontaneously, without any need for intervention other than protection and observation.

Accurate observation and description of seizure activity are extremely valuable in diagnosis and management. The observations the nurse makes before, during, and following a seizure are outlined in Table 42-12. These observations also can be useful in eliciting a history of the child's seizures and should include the time of day, frequency, and whether the child sustained any injury from the seizure.

Chronic Care The child with a seizure disorder needs long-term monitoring and care directed toward achieving the best possible control of the seizures and promoting optimal adjustment. The nurse's role in both acute and outpatient settings includes teaching the child and family about seizures and anticonvulsant medication, monitoring the child for medication effects and seizure activity, and providing support and counseling to the family.

TABLE 42-12 Nursing Observations During a Seizure

Time	Criteria for observation

Preseizure	Activity or status of the child
	  Awake or asleep
	  Febrile
	  Excited
	Aura
	  Behavior changes
	  Complaints of abdominal pain, fear, or unusual sensations
	Antecedent events
	  Flickering or bright lights
	  Loud or buzzing noises
	  Emotional stress

Seizure activity	Time of onset
	Cry
	Fall—forceful or slow drop
	Description of body movements
	  Localized or full-body involvement
	  Position of head and body
	  Tone—rigid or limp
	  Clonic jerking or twitching
	  Sequence and type of movements
	Facial characteristics
	  Color—cyanotic, or flushed
	  Twitching—parts of face involved
	  Eye position and movements
	  Pupil changes
	  Jaw clencing
	  Frothing of secretions
	Respirations
	  Absence of respiratory effort—length, depth, and quality of respirations
	  Adequacy of airway
	Bladder or bowel incontinence
	Length of seizure

Postseizure (postictal phase)	Activity or status of the child
	  Awake or sleeping
	  Oriented
	  Drowsy
	  Confused
	  Changes in motor function—weakness, movement
	  Complaints of headache or pain
	  Assessment of any injuries sustained at the onset of the seizure

The nurse manages the child with a newly diagnosed seizure disorder and family carefully, helping them to cope with the initial crisis period. The child and family often are frightened by the term epilepsy and are affected by their concept of the stigmas associated with this condition. They will have many questions about the diagnosis, treatment, prognosis, and handling of the child. The nurse offers information, being careful not to overwhelm the child and parents with lengthy, extensive explanations that they might not be ready to hear. The nurse is alert to cues from the family about what they are able to absorb in the early stages. Often, the nurse needs to repeat material over a period of time as the family goes through the process of adjustment.

Instructing the family about the seizures and how to manage the child during a seizure are initial teaching goals. The specific aspects of management will vary depending on the type of seizure disorder. For major motor seizures the parent is instructed to protect the child from injury, maintain the child's airway, and seek emergency medical care if the seizure is prolonged or recurs immediately. A common misconception is that the tongue will be swallowed if something is not placed in the child's mouth, and it is important that the nurse instruct the family not to force anything into the child's mouth during a seizure. The nurse explains that the child usually will sleep or be lethargic following the seizure and encourages the family to allow the child to rest during recovery.

The nurse describes other types of seizures as indicated and teaches the family the appropriate safety precautions. Depending on the seizure manifestations and the degree of

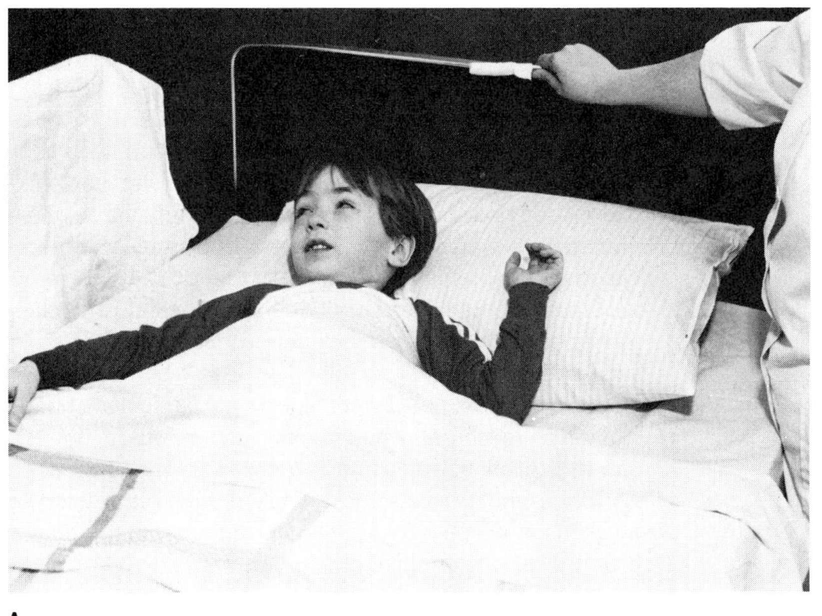

A

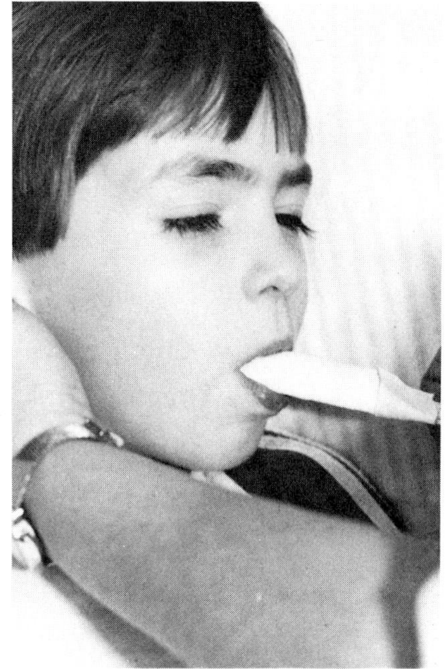

B

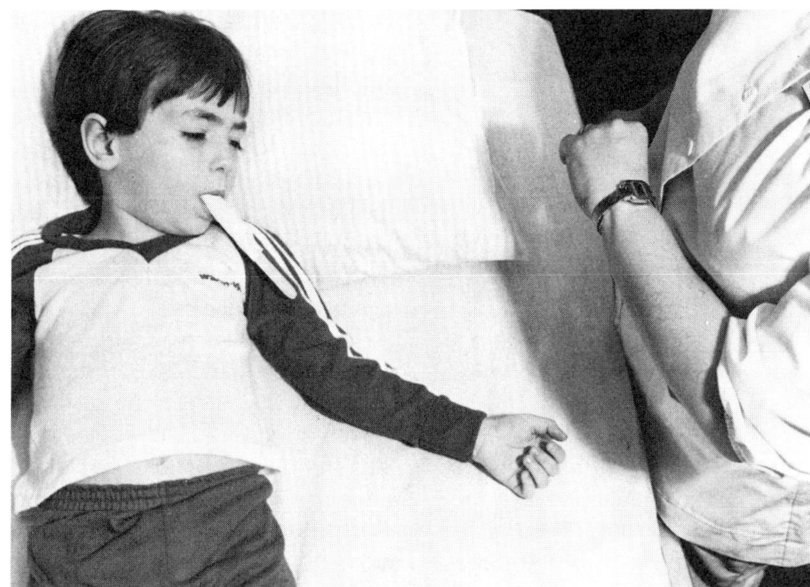

C

Nursing care during a seizure. *A.* The child indicates an impending seizure. *B.* The nurse gently inserts a padded tongue blade between the teeth. *C.* The nurse notes the course and duration of the seizure activity. (From Swearingen PL: *The Addison-Wesley Photo-Atlas of Nursing Procedures.* Addison-Wesley, 1984, p. 612).

control achieved with medication, these precautions might include close supervision in situations where a sudden loss of consciousness could produce injury (such as swimming or climbing to heights). Children who fall frequently because of seizures must wear a protective helmet or faceguard to prevent head and facial injuries.

Teaching about anticonvulsant medication, the effects, side effects, and importance of cooperation is an essential nursing responsibility. The child and family are taught how to take the medication, what side effects to watch for, and why periodic laboratory monitoring is necessary. If the child's seizures are well controlled, the need for continuing to take the anticonvulsant medication might not be apparent to the child and family. The nurse stresses the important fact that the medication be administered regularly to prevent the seizures from recurring. The sudden withdrawal of medication can result in increased seizure activity or status epilepticus. The nurse works out a convenient schedule of

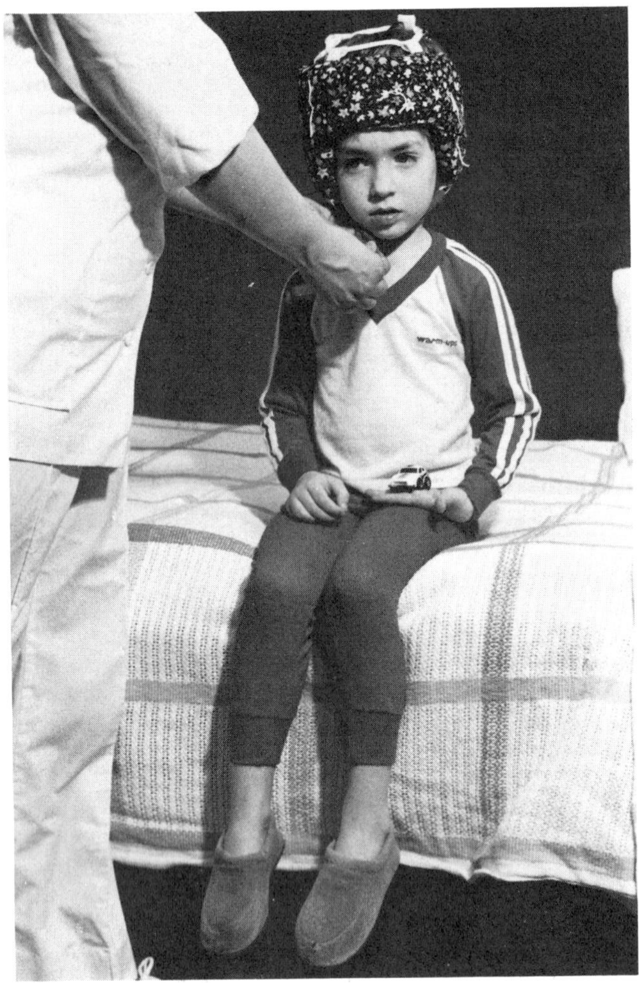

The child who experiences frequent seizures may require a soft, protective helmet to prevent head injury. (From Swearingen PL: *The Addison-Wesley Photo-Atlas of Nursing Procedures.* Addison-Wesley, 1984, p. 611).

medication administration that best fits in with the child's daily routine. Older children can be taught to assume responsibility for taking their own medication.

Families often are concerned about the risks of toxicity, undesirable side effects, and dosage adjustments. The nurse instructs the family to keep a record of the child's seizures and responses to medication because this information is vital to ongoing management. Repeated medication changes are needed to try to control seizures in some children with seizure disorders. At times, the degree of impairment caused by the seizures must be weighed against the impairments caused by the side effects of anticonvulsant medications, such as drowsiness. Achieving a balance of the best control possible with the fewest side effects can be a lengthy, frustrating process, during which the family requires consistent, responsive support and guidance.

The nurse advises the child and family what factors can precipitate seizure activity. A lowered seizure threshold often occurs with fever, and the nurse teaches the family fever control measures, which are important for preventing seizures. The child who has an illness that results in vomiting might be unable to tolerate anticonvulsant medication, which can result in seizures. The nurse advises the family to consult their physician for procedures to follow when the child has missed doses of medication. The child might be given antiemetic medications or parenteral anticonvulsant medications temporarily. Increased seizure activity also can accompany other illnesses, alterations in the fluid and electrolyte balance, excessive fatigue, or severe stress. Certain stimuli, such as flickering lights (such as from televisions, strobe lights, or fluorescent lights) or particular sounds (rhythmic mechanical buzzing or sudden, sharp noises), can precipitate seizures in a few children. The child often is more likely to have seizures while drifting off to sleep or awakening, which is associated with changes in the brain's electrical activity during the transition from sleeping to waking states and vice versa.

Seizure activity might increase during puberty, although many children have fewer seizures as they mature. Premenstrual fluid retention can precipitate seizures, and diuretics might be prescribed for girls who encounter this problem. In addition, some medications can lower the seizure threshold such as antihistamines, central nervous system stimulants, and alcohol. The nurse urges both the child and family to follow prescribed guidelines in taking other medications and encourages them to always ask if they are unsure about a particular drug's effects. Adolescents must be informed adequately about the potential hazards of drug or alcohol use precipitating seizures or interacting with anticonvulsant medications.

The nurse pays particular attention to the psychosocial adaptation of the child and family to the seizure disorder. The family might feel a natural tendency to overprotect and expect less of the child. They might feel guilty about the child's condition or fear that disciplining the child might provoke a seizure. The nurse corrects their misconceptions and stresses the importance that the child's developing independence be fostered. Safety and supervision requirements for each child are determined on an individual basis and depend on the severity and type of seizures and any other disabilities present (such as physical handicaps or cognitive or sensory limitations).

The activities of most children with good seizure control do not need to be limited or restricted beyond the minimal precautions for swimming or climbing previously mentioned. The family often is faced with the dilemma of protecting the child adequately while simultaneously fostering growth. The family often can benefit from the sharing offered by support groups composed of other parents of children with epilepsy. As the family becomes more confident about their ability to care for the child, they often are more receptive to interventions geared toward promoting the child's independence, which might involve some risks. For exam ple, allowing the child to travel on the school bus, stay at a friend's house, or ride a bicycle might provoke intense anxiety and fear that the child might have a seizure. The family needs ongoing support and encouragement in their continual struggle to accept and manage appropriately the child with a seizure disorder.

Public attitudes and acceptance regarding seizures are continuing problems for the child and family. Social stigmas associated with seizures are common and reflect a general misunderstanding of epilepsy. As a liaison and advocate, the nurse promotes the child's acceptance in school and the community by correcting misinformation, dispelling myths, and increasing public awareness of the facts about epilepsy. The Epilepsy Foundation of America (4351 Garden City Drive, Landover, MD 20785) is an excellent resource for educational materials, support groups, and special services. Nurses in community health and school settings can contribute greatly to educating the public about seizures and helping to demystify the disorder. The school nurse is in an ideal position to both monitor the child with a seizure disorder and promote understanding of seizures by teachers and other children. The child who has seizures in school might need a rest period after a major seizure but most often is able to resume class activities and should not be sent home or isolated unnecessarily. Teachers and others dealing with the child must be prepared for the possible occurrence of seizures and instructed in how to manage them. The reactions of other children to a seizure tend to reflect the responsible adult's response. If adults react in a calm and reassuring manner and provide simple explanations about what has occurred, the child's classmates will not be fearful or overreact. If, on the other hand, those in charge respond with panic and revulsion to the child's seizure, the other children will react accordingly, perpetuating the negative attitude toward the disorder. The school staff should be instructed to protect the child from embarrassment by asking curious onlookers not to stand and stare. Following the seizure, the child should be allowed privacy to rest and change clothes if incontinence occurred.

Many children with seizure disorders attend a regular school program and can participate in a range of normal activities with few restrictions. The needs of some children with poorly controlled seizures or other disabilities (physical, cognitive, or sensory deficits) are best met in a specialized educational program that offers individual therapeutic services.

The child with a seizure disorder, like any child with a disability, will experience additional stresses related to poor self-image, dependency needs, and feeling different. The child's sense of self-control and mastery are particularly vulnerable because the loss of control during seizures can leave the child feeling inferior and insecure. The child often is acutely embarrassed after having a seizure, particularly when it occurs in the presence of peers. Being labeled "weird" or different because of seizures is a social catastrophe for the child. Friends might reject the child at a time during childhood or adolescence when peer group acceptance is vitally important. Both the child and family might try to hide the condition in an attempt to avoid others' reactions.

The adolescent with a seizure disorder faces special stresses from restrictions on obtaining a driver's license, worries about getting and keeping a job, peer pressures to try alcohol and drugs, and anxieties about dating. The adolescent's struggle for independence is a difficult task, and the adolescent might react by denying the condition, stopping the medication, and rebelling against parental restrictions.

The nurse caring for the child with a seizure disorder encourages the child and family to share their fears and express their frustrations. The nurse explores coping strategies the family might use. The nurse helps the family to develop a plan for action if a seizure occurs in different situations, allowing them to solve problems ahead of time. Assessing the child's and family's adaptation, and recognizing problems that require referral for more intensive counseling are important nursing functions.

Status Epilepticus

Status epilepticus is a condition in which seizures are prolonged or repeated without the child's regaining consciousness. This condition presents a medical emergency because hypoxia, hypotension, cardiac arrhythmias, and respiratory depression or arrest are potential complications. Failure to adhere to anticonvulsant medication regimens is a frequent cause of status epilepticus in children with a previously diagnosed seizure disorder. Other precipitants include metabolic disturbances (hypoglycemia, hypocalcemia), central nervous system infection, and intracranial trauma or hemorrhage.

Medical Treatment Status epilepticus must be treated promptly to prevent life-threatening complications. Respiratory and cardiovascular functions are rapidly evaluated, any airway obstruction is removed, and an oral airway is inserted. Intubation might be necessary, and resuscitation equipment must be on hand to treat potential cardiorespiratory arrest. Oxygen is administered, with suctioning as needed to maintain a clear airway. An intravenous line is established quickly, and blood samples are drawn to determine serum chemistries, blood counts, and serum anticonvulsant levels.

An anticonvulsant medication (diazepam, phenobarbital, or diphenylhydantoin) is given intravenously, and the patient is monitored closely for adverse effects of respiratory depression and cardiac arrhythmias. Any metabolic alterations are treated such as hypoglycemia, hypocalcemia, and metabolic acidosis. Following the cessation of seizure activity, the child is monitored closely, and anticonvulsant medication is administered parenterally until the child is able to resume oral intake. When the underlying cause of the episode is determined, it is treated appropriately.

Nursing Management When major motor seizure activity persists or recurs without the child regaining consciousness, emergency care for status epilepticus is urgently needed. Nursing responsibilities include establishing an airway, administering oxygen as ordered, and oropharyngeal suctioning of excessive secretions. Recognizing the potential for cardiorespiratory arrest, the nurse ensures that emergency equipment for resuscitation is readily available. The nurse establishes an intravenous route, collects blood specimens, and prepares medications to be given.

Throughout treatment and recovery, the nurse monitors the child's cardiac and respiratory status closely to detect complications from the seizure activity or the anticonvulsant medication administered. Ventricular fibrillation, hypotension, and respiratory depression are possible complications. Prolonged seizure activity often produces hypoglycemia, in which case dextrose is administered. Electrolyte supplement solutions might be ordered, depending on the child's needs. If the child is febrile, tepid sponge baths, rectal antipyretic administration, and hypothermia mattresses may be used to reduce the child's temperature. Causes for the prolonged seizure activity are sought and treated. An insufficient serum anticonvulsant level is a frequent precipitant and might be caused by failure to cooperate with the medication regimen, vomiting, or a recent medication adjustment. The anticonvulsant level is raised to a therapeutic level by parenteral administration of medication and is followed by oral anticonvulsants when the child is able to take them. The nurse must be aware of toxic effects, drug interactions, and correct administration of the anticonvulsants ordered. Diphenylhydantoin (Dilantin) must not be mixed with dextrose and water for intravenous administration because it precipitates. It may be mixed with small amounts of normal saline solution and given intravenously within 30 minutes. Diphenylhydantoin is absorbed poorly from tissue deposits and is not recommended for intramuscular injection. Diazepam is given only by a direct intravenous push or orally; it is never mixed with solutions for intravenous administration. Paraldehyde may be administered intravenously in a 4% solution or rectally. When given rectally, paraldehyde is mixed with mineral oil and administered via a rectal tube.

Following the cessation of status epilepticus, the nurse monitors the child closely, assessing vital signs and level of consciousness and watching for abnormal neurologic signs such as a recurrence of seizure activity or focal neurologic deficits. The child often will be unconscious for prolonged periods following the seizure activity both because of the postictal exhaustion and sedation from medications given.

The Child With a Traumatic Lesion of the Central Nervous System

Cerebral Palsy

Cerebral palsy is a nonspecific term that refers to impairment of motor function resulting from an insult to the brain (motor cortex, basal ganglia, or cerebellum). The disorder is nonprogressive and can have a variety of causes. Prenatal and perinatal factors account for the largest percentage of cases, including maternal infection, toxemia, irradiation, placental insufficiency, and anemia. Prematurity, low birthweight, anoxia, and perinatal trauma are considered high risk factors in the etiology of cerebral motor impairment. Postnatal infection, trauma, or cerebral anoxia can result in damage to upper motor control areas.

Regardless of the specific cause, cerebral palsy carries the essential clinical finding of neuromotor impairment as a result of insult to the immature central nervous system. Sensory, language, perceptual, and cognitive impairments occur frequently. The exact incidence of cerebral palsy is difficult to determine, but estimates vary from 1.5 to 5 cases per 1000 live births. It is considered the most frequent permanent physical disability of childhood (Molnar and Taft, 1977).

Clinical Manifestations Although certain prenatal and perinatal conditions are known to place the infant at higher risk for neuromotor deficits, the diagnosis of cerebral palsy at birth is difficult. Cerebral control of movement develops as the infant matures, and it is during this maturational process that developmental abnormalities and delays are detected (Taft and Barabas, 1982).

The earliest manifestations of cerebral palsy in the neonate who has suffered serious brain injury include poor feeding with weak sucking and swallowing; hypotonia ("floppy infant"); absent or abnormal grasp; Moro, or stepping reflexes; and seizures. As the infant develops, muscle tone might change from hypotonic to hypertonic, which is manifested as spasticity and abnormal rigidity of the extremities (Menkes and Barzdorf, 1980).

More often, the lack of specific neuromotor data in early infancy delays diagnosis until deviations from normal development can be discerned. Delays in gross motor performance are characteristic, with poor head control and failure to sit, crawl, and attain other motor milestones. The delays might range from subtle weaknesses to more obvious impairments accompanied by abnormal posturing and muscle tone.

The infant with cerebral palsy might show signs of increased muscle tone and spasticity, manifested by spinal and leg extensor thrust when the infant is supine or suddenly lifted under the arms. Arching of the back and head, scissoring of the legs, and stiffness or rigidity when held are early manifestations of spasticity. Hands held in a fisted position after 4–5 months of age also indicates spasticity of the upper extremities.

Early hand preference (before 18 months to 2 years of age), asymmetric crawling, using one arm and leg more, and abnormal posturing or weakness of one side of the body might indicate hemiplegia.

Feeding difficulties include poor suck, regurgitation, frequent thrusting of the tongue outward, and swallowing and oromotor incoordination. The infant might exhibit poor lip closure and impaired swallow and gag reflexes, resulting in both trouble with food intake and aspiration of fluids.

As the child develops, other indications of motor dysfunction might become noticeable. Standing on the toes can reflect spasticity of the legs, as can persistent hip adduction and hyperextension of the knees. Crawling using only the upper extremities and dragging the lower extremities might indicate diplegia. Uncoordinated, uncontrolled muscle movements occurring spontaneously or as the child attempts to move to reach for an object reflect underlying motor deficits.

Infantile reflexes persisting beyond the expected ages are a cause to suspect cerebral palsy. A tonic neck reflex or Moro or palmar grasp reflex that remains after 6 months of age indicates neurologic dysfunction. Sustained tonic neck posturing (obligatory) at any age is abnormal. The absence of later developing postural reflexes (neck righting, equilibrium) also suggests impairment of motor mechanisms.

Types of Cerebral Palsy The primary neuromotor dysfunctions seen in cerebral palsy are divided into three types: spastic, athetoid, and ataxic. The differing degrees of involvement of each of these types as well as the combinations of types result in great variation of clinical manifestations.

Spastic Cerebral Palsy Up to 65% of all cases of cerebral palsy are manifested by increased muscle tone, increased stretch reflexes, and muscle weakness (Low and Downey, 1982). Spasticity may be mild or severe, resulting in contractures of affected joints. One side of the body might be affected (hemiparesis), or all four extremities may be involved (quadriparesis).

Hemiparetic cerebral palsy is the most frequent of all the clinical types. The child's extremities are smaller on the affected side, and the arm is usually weaker and more spastic than the leg. The characteristic posturing is flexion at the elbow, wrist, and knee, with equinus extension of the foot. The most severe impairment is fine motor function of the hand. Sensory deficits might accompany the motor dysfunction, as may cortical neglect or unawareness of the paretic side. Affected children almost always become ambulatory and are able to perform most activities with one hand, assisting with the paretic hand and arm (Molnar and Taft, 1977).

In children with quadriparetic cerebral palsy, spasticity and weakness might be present to the same degree in all extremities, but greater involvement of the lower extremities is more common. In rare cases the child's arms might be more affected than the legs. The child's overall motor function often is more severely impaired with spastic cerebral palsy than with other types, with oromotor involvement causing tongue protrusion, impaired swallowing, and dysarthric speech (Low and Downey, 1982). Oculomotor deficits frequently result in strabismus. The usual motor pattern seen is hip adduction spasticity with scissoring of the legs, plantar flexion of the feet, poor trunk control, and fisted hands. Mass flexion–extension spastic movements of the arms, legs, trunk, or head might be the only voluntary motor control present.

Spastic diplegia is a common term that actually refers to a variation of spastic quadriparesis. All four extremities are involved, but the upper extremities are only mildly affected. The child often appears to have normal arm and head function, with subtle alterations in muscle tone, reflex, or fine motor coordination. The lower extremities usually show increased muscle tone of varying severity. Trunk and head control are less affected in spastic diplegia than in spastic quadriparesis (Menkes and Batzdorf, 1980).

Athetoid Cerebral Palsy The second most frequent type of neuromotor abnormality is *athetosis*, or abnormal, involuntary movements. These movements are writhing, uncontrolled muscular activity that first appears when the child is 18 months of age or older. Facial grimacing, tongue and mouth dystonic movements, and rotary or twisting movements of the hands and feet are seen first. Later, the trunk and all extremities show the characteristic involuntary movements of purposeless, "wormlike" writhing, flailing, and distorted positioning. In purely athetotic forms of cerebral palsy, increased muscle tone and spasticity are not present consistently. Muscle tone fluctuates, as does the intensity of abnormal movements. The movements disappear during sleep and become more intense when the child is anxious or physically stimulated. The movements interfere significantly with voluntary control of motor function. Often, elements of spasticity and athetosis are found together in a mixed pattern of cerebral motor deficit (Menkes and Batzdorf, 1980).

Ataxic Cerebral Palsy Ataxic cerebral palsy, which is characterized by cerebellar impairment of balance and coordination, is the least frequent clinical type seen. Children show hypotonia and delay in achieving motor milestones. They have a wide-based, unsteady gait and clumsy, uncoordinated upper extremity function. Most ataxic forms of cerebral palsy improve somewhat as the child matures (Low and Downey, 1982).

Associated Conditions Children with cerebral motor deficits often have other central nervous system impairments. Cognitive impairment occurs in about one-half to three-quarters of children with cerebral palsy; the highest incidence is associated with more severe forms of spastic quadriparesis (Molnar and Taft, 1977). (Nursing care of the child with a mental deficiency is discussed in Chapter 23.) True assessment of learning and reasoning abilities is difficult when the child's motor and speech impairments make standardized testing inappropriate.

Poor attention span, distractibility, hyperactivity, learning disabilities, or any manifestations of the minimal brain dysfunction syndrome can be seen in the child with cerebral palsy. (See the section on the child with alterations in learning, attention, and activity level later in this chapter.) Visual handicaps, hearing impairments, and language or perceptual deficits are other possible associated conditions (Davis and Hill, 1980).

Seizures occur in about one-half of children with cerebral palsy. Grand mal seizures are the most frequent type of seizure, with partial (psychomotor or focal) seizures second in prevalence. Seizures can occur at any time, but the incidence generally peaks between 2 and 6 years of age (Low, 1982). Seizure disorders more often are associated with spastic forms of cerebral palsy and cognitive impairments (Menkes and Batzdorf, 1980).

Children with athetosis and quadriparesis might have respiratory disturbances due to poor function of the respiratory musculature and chronic aspiration (from impaired swallow and gag reflexes). These children have difficulty clearing secretions both because of their inability to cough effectively and their relative inactivity. Scoliosis, a common musculoskeletal complication of cerebral palsy, might further compromise respiratory function (Molnar and Taft, 1977).

Medical and Surgical Treatment Because cerebral palsy is caused by permanent damage to the central nervous system, treatment efforts are directed toward improving motor function and preventing further handicap rather than toward curing the disability. Intervention begins early, is longterm, and is best managed by interdisciplinary methods that are integrated to meet the child's particular needs. Specialists from neurology, orthopedics, pediatrics, nursing, physical therapy, speech and language pathology, occupational therapy, psychology, education, and other disciplines collaborate as a therapeutic team to foster the child's optimal development and functional potential.

Early intervention is desirable and depends on the early detection of initial signs of cerebral motor dysfunction. Most treatment in the early period involves teaching the family and guiding them in the care of the child. The family is taught specialized techniques for handling the child and methods of stimulation to encourage sensorimotor development. Adapted feeding, positioning, musculoskeletal exercises, and appropriate play activities are among the early intervention strategies employed. The importance of sensorimotor experience in developing cognitive and motor skills is emphasized as parents are guided in providing early therapeutic measures (Low and Downey, 1982).

Orthopedic management includes the use of braces, casts, and corrective appliances, which help the child to maintain functional position and prevent contracture formation when supplemented by therapeutic stretching exercises and, when possible, functional use.

Orthopedic surgery may be undertaken to improve the child's functional ability and correct deformities that affect movement or self-care. The child with plantar flexion of the feet might be helped by heel cord lengthening. Other common surgical procedures include hamstring release for knee flexion contractures, obturator neurectomy and adductor myotomy for hip flexion or dislocation, and various wrist and foot procedures to release contractures and provide stabilization. The relative benefits and goals of surgical intervention must be evaluated carefully and communicated clearly to the family to avoid unrealistic expectations of postoperative outcome. Gait, stability, or progressive deformity might be ameliorated, but the underlying motor dysfunction will remain (Low and Downey, 1982).

The use of cerebellar implants with pacemakers providing electrical stimulation to relax spastic muscles is a newer surgical intervention that has been suggested for some children. The long-term effects of such treatment have not yet been evaluated (Conway-Rutkowski, 1982). Other neurosurgical procedures for specific lesions or deformities are indicated in a limited number of cases.

Medications to reduce spasticity or athetotic movements generally have not proven to have sufficient benefit to outweigh their side effects (Menkes and Batzdorf, 1980). Selected children might be helped by diazepam or dantrolene sodium, with careful monitoring for adverse side effects. The child with seizures is treated with appropriate anticonvulsant therapy. Other associated conditions, such as attention deficits, might respond to adjunctive medication therapy. (See the section on the child with alterations in learning, attention, and activity level.)

Physical therapy is an important part of the child's longterm management. The therapist works with the child, family, and other team members to maximize the child's functional motor skills, facilitate mobility, and prevent fixed deformities. The program approaches vary, and the conceptual bases for treatment differ. Active and passive exercise of muscle groups, practice of gross motor activities, and strengthening of equilibrium responses are some of the methods employed.

Adaptive equipment such as seats, prone standers, wedges, and various mobilizing aids are recommended by the therapist to allow the child maximum independent function and provide proper postural and skeletal alignment. The use of equipment, positioning, and activity–exercise programs are taught by the physical therapist to other staff members involved with the child as well as to the child and family.

Occupational therapy offers training in the activities of daily living using adapted techniques and equipment such as modified eating utensils, dressing methods, and self-care skills. The use of a scoop plate and builtup spoon, for example, might help a child achieve independent feeding. Clothing with Velcro closures, handsplints with toothbrush holders, and electric typewriters are some of the many compensatory mechanisms that might be recommended according to the child's developmental level and functional ability. The occupational therapist assesses the child's perceptual skills and visual motor integration and recommends remedial training and compensatory strategies. The therapist collaborates with other team members in developing individual programs such as the use of nonverbal communication systems or environmental control systems. As the child matures, the occupational therapist is a valuable resource in the prevocational assessment of strengths and program planning.

Speech and language pathologists provide evaluation and specific therapy for both speech production and the understanding and use of language. Children with cerebral palsy often have mild to severe problems with oromotor control, breath control, and sound production. Techniques to better articulation and phonation improve the child's speech intelligibility. The child's motor involvement might be so severe that oral communication is impossible. Nonverbal communication methods are used and can range from simple yes or no indicators to multi-item communication boards to electronic devices. The child's cognitive, language, and physical capabilities are considered carefully in planning appropriate nonverbal communication programs. Language disorders are identified early, and interventions are recommended to foster language comprehension, integration, and use.

Vision and hearing assessments must be done early to detect impairments. Strabismus or hemianopia (blindness in one-half the visual field) often are associated with cerebral palsy and can interfere with the child's functioning. Ophthamologic treatment or compensatory training for visual field defects might be indicated. Hearing losses are evaluated and appropriate interventions provided (see Chapter 43).

Educational programming is an integral part of the child's management. The educational plan is individualized for each child depending on the child's motor, cognitive, language, perceptual, and associated abilities. Special settings or partial integration or full participation in a regular school program are appropriate for different children with cerebral palsy. Regardless of the type of program, integration of the various therapeutic goals into the child's educational program is essential to optimal learning.

Nursing Management The nurse's role with children with cerebral palsy and their families involves long-term management in community, home, school, and hospital settings. The nurse's observations of the child's early development might provide the first clues that motor dysfunction exists. Newborn care and contacts in outpatient and hospital visits offer opportunities for developmental screening and the detection of abnormal signs.

The early recognition of potential neuromotor difficulties depends on a sound knowledge of normal development, application of appropriate screening measures, and follow-up with serial assessments. Indicators such as asymmetric strength and movement of the infant's limbs, legs held in extension, rigidity when held, and difficulty sucking and swallowing alert the nurse to the need for more specialized evaluation. Delayed achievement of motor milestones might be the first indication of the disability; often, this does not become apparent until the infant is 6 months of age or older. The family might be the first to suspect that the child is not progressing normally and want rapid diagnosis of the condition and prognosis of the child's function. Caution must be used in interpreting isolated areas of deficit and predicting outcomes because the extent of disability in cerebral palsy cannot be determined early in life.

Parental anxiety and feelings of helplessness can be reduced by offering the concrete services of an early intervention team to develop a home program and provide family support. The family becomes more confident about caring for their child when they are guided carefully by the therapeutic team. Nurses frequently are involved as home visitors in early intervention efforts (Godfrey, 1975). Nurses teach parents stimulation activities, motor exercises, and specialized feeding and handling techniques. At the same time, they encourage these activities as adaptations of normal parent–child interaction and play and not as exhausting "treatments." The nurse role models, demonstrates, and suggests ways to incorporate recommendations into everyday life. As they gain mastery in the care of their children, families feel that they are doing something actively to improve their children's disabilities. This might reduce feelings of guilt and frustration but also carries the danger of raising unrealistic expectations for the child's progress. An unfortunate outgrowth of various therapeutic programs is that parents sometimes believe erroneously that if a little therapy is good, a lot of therapy must be better. Nurses can be extremely helpful in assisting parents to view the child's developmental level realistically, recognize their own and the child's fatigue, and achieve a balance between the demands of the child's particular disability and other aspects of life.

Specific tips and training for handling the child with spasticity focus on promoting relaxation and reducing reflexive postures. The child should not be picked up from a flat position, but rather brought to a flexed sitting position first and then lifted by the underarms with support under the thighs to maintain the flexed position. This technique avoids the reflexive hyperextension thrust. Positioning the child in a sitting position with the head and neck flexed slightly forward, trunk supported, and hips abducted both decreases extensor tone and provides a functional position for activities.

Parents are taught how to apply braces, casts, or splints and the care associated with their use. These and other mobilizing aids such as crutches, walkers, carts, and wheelchairs are adapted to each child's individual needs. Environmental exploration is critical for the development of all children, and early mobilization with adaptive equipment facilitates this exploration for children with cerebral palsy.

The nurse helps the family implement the recommended modifications in feeding techniques. Holding the child in an upright position, preventing hyperextension of the head backward, and facilitating lip and jaw closure by holding them gently are some of the feeding methods that can be used. When the child progresses to self-feeding, the family is encouraged to have the child eat independently, with adapted utensils if necessary. In the area of self-feeding, as in the development of other independent skills, parents often tend to do it for their children rather than watch them struggle. The nurse encourages the family to allow the child's independence as much as possible.

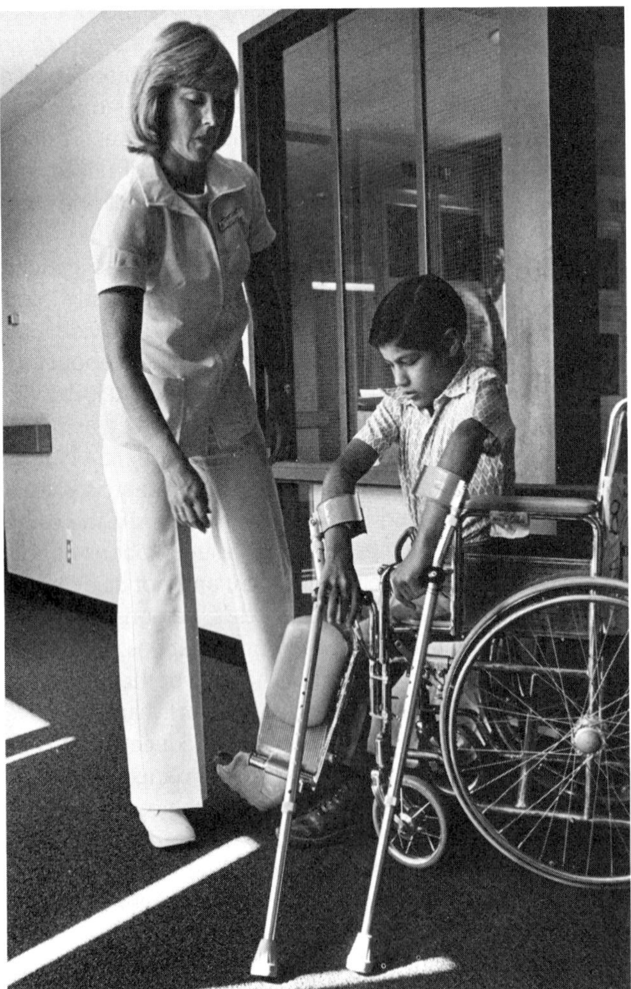
Nursing care for long-term management involves teaching the child to use assistive devices.

Children with more involved forms of spastic quadriparesis are often more susceptible to respiratory congestion and pneumonia. The family can be taught to perform postural drainage and chest percussion prophylactically when the child gets up in the morning and before meals to help the child handle excessive secretions.

Helping the family to adapt to the special demands of caring for a child with cerebral palsy involves emotional support as well as teaching specialized techniques. Many parents describe their child's early years as a nightmare, with conflicting opinions about the child's disability, improper advice, and exhaustive days of appointments, therapy, and basic care. Parents must attempt to cope with the new and changing family organization and with their grief about having a child with defects. The nurse helps the family to mobilize supports within the family and refers them to community agencies for counseling, parent groups, and concrete services such as respite child care. Sharing their concerns with other parents of children with similar problems can reduce the isolation and insecurities many parents feel. The nurse helps the family to find more inventive means of play, interaction, and gratification.

Children with cerebral palsy also face adjustment problems in learning to live with their disabilities. This becomes particularly acute as these children approach adolescence. Difficulty with speech and motor movements set these children apart, often causing peers to misunderstand and shun them. Their understanding and reasoning might be at or above their age level, yet they might be treated like younger children because of their appearance and dependency needs. Especially in unfamiliar situations such as hospitalization, it is important for the nurse to know the child's developmental level, system of communication, and usual routines of activity and care to provide continuity and interact appropriately with the child.

Head Injury

Head injury is one of the leading causes of death and disability in children. Craniocerebral trauma from accidents is the most frequent neurologic condition for which individuals under 19 years of age are hospitalized, with more than 200,000 children hospitalized annually (Walleck, 1980). Many children with minor head trauma are not hospitalized, so the overall incidence of the problem is even higher.

The causes of head injury vary with age. In the perinatal period, birth trauma due to cephalopelvic disproportion and injury from forceps are the primary causes. During infancy and early childhood, falls from heights, (arms, beds, stairs, and so forth) and child abuse account for many of these injuries. Athletic injuries, skateboard and bicycle accidents, and falls are frequent causes of head trauma in older children and adolescents. In all age groups of childen, motor vehicle accidents are a leading cause of serious head trauma (Jabbour, et al., 1976).

Craniocerebral trauma might range from mild head injury to severe, life-threatening nervous system insults. Children have more flexible skulls and tissues, which might enable them to withstand head trauma better than adults, but their greater tissue fragility and proportionally higher cerebral blood volume place them at higher risk for brain damage and complicating hemorrhage (Walleck, 1980).

Trauma results from several types of physical forces acting on the skull and its contents. The mechanism may be direct (coup) when the injury is at the site of impact or indirect (contrecoup) when the injury occurs on the side of the brain contralateral to the blow. The contrecoup phenomenon results when the impact drives the brain contents against the opposite side of the skull. Acceleration and deceleration forces acting on the brain cause pressure changes and shearing forces as different parts of the brain are shifted at different rates. Strain or actual damage to neuronal tissue, dura, bone, and blood vessels occurs, producing various types of injuries (Menkes and Batzdorf, 1980).

Clinical Manifestations Clinical manifestations of head injury depend on the type of injury.

Skull Fractures Skull fractures are less common with head trauma in children than in adults because of the greater elasticity of the child's skull in withstanding impact. Skull fractures alone do not signify underlying cerebral injury and can occur with or without accompanying neurologic manifestations.

Depressed skull fractures occur with direct blunt trauma, directing fragmented bone inward against the brain. In infants and young children, the pliable skull might be depressed on impact, without an actual fracture occurring (Aquino, 1978). The symptoms of depressed fractures depend on the area of the brain compressed and whether blood vessels, dura, or cerebral tissue is lacerated. Cerebral scarring can result from depressed skull fractures.

Basilar skull fractures, which occur infrequently in children, involve anterior fossa or temporobasal fracture. The symptoms might include vertigo, orbital ecchymoses (Raccoon's sign), CSF or blood drainage from the ears or nose, postauricular ecchymoses (Battle's sign), and crainal nerve deficits. Cerebrospinal fluid leakage can predispose the child to meningitis, which is a complication of basilar skull fracture. Diagnosis is confirmed by associated signs because the fracture seldom is visible by radiography. Resolution of symptoms might take days to weeks, (Jabbour, et al., 1976).

Concussion Concussion is the most common type of closed-head injury other than minor head trauma. *Concussion* is defined as an immediate, transient impairment of neural functions due to trauma. The victim characteristically loses consciousness briefly and has no recall of the events surrounding the injury. The loss of memory for events immediately prior to the injury is termed *retrograde amnesia,* and the loss of memory for events following the injury is called *anterograde amnesia.* After consciousness is regained (several minutes), confusion, lethargy, irritability, pallor, headache, and vomiting might be seen. Symptoms usually resolve within 24–48 hours. Subtle behavior changes (attentional problems, personality changes) and dull headaches constitute a postconcussion syndrome, which can occur and might persist for up to 6 months following the injury (Menkes and Batzdorf, 1980).

Contusion and Laceration More severe head injuries can bruise or lacerate brain tissue, causing petechial hemorrhages, edema, and actual tearing of cerebral matter. The clinical manifestations may be the same as those for concussion but are more severe, and focal neurologic deficits are present. Alteration of consciousness is more profound, lasts longer, and may progress rapidly to coma. The focal neurologic deficits seen reflect the contused area of the brain and might be manifested as focal seizures, aphasia, hemiplegia, eye deviations, or other localizing signs. The frontal and temporal lobes are the most frequent sites of contusions. Recovery from cerebral contusion and laceration is variable, depending on the location and severity of the injury, development of complications, and treatment received.

Subdural Hematoma A *subdural hematoma* is a collection of blood between the dura and the brain, which results from the rupture of subdural veins or, less commonly, arteries. It may occur acutely within 24 hours of the initial injury, manifesting symptoms of severe head injury. More often, subdural hematoma develops gradually, taking weeks or months to become symptomatic. The clot tends to encapsulate, and as the protein of the fluid breaks down, the contents become hypertonic and tend to draw more fluid into the formed subdural sac (Aquino, 1978). This transudation and slow bleeding combine to enlarge the hematoma, causing a gradual, insidious onset of symptoms related to compression of an area of the brain and increased ICP.

Subdural hematoma is quite common in infancy, occurring most often in infants between 2 and 6 months of age. Birth trauma and inflicted injury account for most of the cases. The infant often appears chronically ill, with anemia, vomiting, and developmental delays. Seizures, either focal or generalized, and a bulging fontanelle are indicators of cerebral pathology. In older children headache, increasing lethargy, unsteady gait, and seizures occur. A CT scan and subdural tap can be used, if necessary, to diagnose a subdural hematoma (Menkes and Batzdorf, 1980; Walleck, 1980).

Extradural (Epidural) Hematoma *Extradural hematoma* is an acute condition that results from bleeding between the skull and dura, most often due to disruption of the middle meningeal artery. The hemorrhage is usually arterial, with rapid progression compressing the brain and causing the brain to herniate inferiorly through the tentorium. Death results if surgical treatment is not undertaken immediately. A CT scan generally is diagnostic.

The characteristic course is of an initial injury with a temporary recovery (lucid interval) of minutes to several hours, which is followed by progressive deterioration, with headache, seizures, stupor, coma, and focal signs of unequal pupils and contralateral hemiparesis (Jabbour, et al., 1976). In children the initial injury might not be apparent, and the symptoms may take longer (up to several days) to appear (Menkes and Batzdorf, 1980). The manifestations of extradural hematoma are associated with increased ICP and brain stem involvement as the brain is displaced downward.

Intracranial Hematoma Bleeding may occur anywhere within the brain as a result of trauma. Intracerebral hematomas are relatively uncommon in children but are possible; the symptoms are related to the site of involvement. Alterations in consciousness and focal neurologic signs might be seen, depending on the areas of the brain affected and the size of the hematoma (Walleck, 1980).

Complications of Head Injury

Cerebral Edema Contusions, lacerations, and hematomas of the brain are accompanied by cerebral edema, which further jeopardizes the functional integrity of brain tissue by increasing ICP and hypoxia. Focal swelling and vasodilatation with venous stasis decrease cerebral blood flow, resulting in cerebral hypoxia. The hypoxia in turn causes the fluid balance mechanisms to fail, and the resulting accumulation of sodium and water in the cerebral tissues leads to further edema and hence hypoxia. If not treated, the cycle repeats until death occurs (Aquino, 1978).

Increased Intracranial Pressure Both cerebral edema and the mass effect of accumulations of blood can increase ICP. (See the section on the child with increased ICP earlier in the chapter.) Interruption of CSF circulation by trauma also can contribute to increasing ICP.

Posttraumatic Sequelae Posttraumatic seizures may occur early (within 24–48 hours of injury) or late (up to 2 years after the injury). Major cerebral contusions or depressed or compound fractures are more likely to result in post-traumatic seizures, whereas more minor trauma less often leads to a seizure disorder (Low, 1982).

Seizures may be either generalized or focal. Petit mal seizures are not caused by trauma. The seizure manifestations reflect the cerebral area damaged, with cerebral scarring forming a focus for abnormal electrical discharges (Menkes and Batzdorf, 1980).

Anticonvulsant therapy is used to treat posttraumatic seizures and might be employed prophylactically to prevent seizures following severe head trauma. Seizure occurrence tends to regress and cease over time in 50%–75% of cases (Aquino, 1978; Menkes and Batzdorf, 1980).

Focal neurologic deficits following head trauma can include impaired cognitive, language, motor, or sensory function, depending on the area and degree of cerebral injury. Forms of hemiplegia, aphasia, cranial nerve dysfunction, and alterations in memory and cognitive skill can occur. Behavioral changes and emotional disturbances can appear during recovery, which can be either transient or persistent. Anxiety, depression, and phobic reactions have been described following head injury in children, and some authorities have suggested that the symptoms reflect an exacerbation of milder preinjury problems (Schaffer, Chadwick, and Rutter, 1975).

Medical and Surgical Treatment The goal of immediate treatment of head injury is life support, controlling cerebral edema and increased ICP. The child's vital signs are obtained, a thorough neurologic examination is performed, a history of the trauma is elicited, and the indicated diagnostic tests are performed (skull and spine radiographs, CT scan, cerebral angiography, and blood analysis—hematocrit, electrolyte levels, and blood gases).

The child with a concussion is observed for changes in neurologic status for 24–48 hours. The child who has experienced a loss of consciousness or demonstrates abnormal neurologic signs usually is admitted to the hospital for close observation. If the child is allowed to go home, the family is instructed to observe for changes in consciousness, persistent vomiting, motor function changes, or severe headache. The child is seen for periodic neurologic evaluations following a concussion to detect any subsequent changes.

For the child who has suffered more severe head trauma, establishing an airway and providing life-support measures might be the first treatment steps. Emergency measures to decrease cerebral edema through glucocorticoids, hyperosmolar agents, and hyperventilation might be required. Fluid administration is restricted to 75% of the maintenance level to prevent fluid overload and resulting increased edema (Menkes and Batzdorf, 1980).

Efforts to treat increased ICP include the administration of glucocorticoids, primarily dexamethasone, which has an effect in 12–24 hours, and osmotic diuretics, which provide dehydrating effects beginning within 30 minutes and lasting 4–6 hours. Manual hyperventilation reduces hypoxia and cerebral blood volume; parenteral replacement therapy corrects electrolyte and acid–base imbalances; antipyretic measures reduce fever. Anticonvulsant medication might be administered for postinjury seizures. Intravenous diphenylhydantoin is a preferred treatment because it is less likely to cause drowsiness than barbiturates (Menkes and Batzdorf, 1980).

Surgical treatment is undertaken to reduce depressed skull fractures that compress brain tissue. Removal of hematomas and the control of cerebral bleeding also are managed surgically. Subdural hematomas might need to be evacuated repeatedly because they tend to reaccumulate in infants.

Nursing Management The child with head trauma can develop complications related to hemorrhage or cerebral edema rapidly, and continuous neurologic assessments are needed to detect any changes in condition early. The nurses' observations are critical in the management of cerebral trauma to determine interventions and prevent complications.

In the immediate postinjury period, the nurse might be involved with emergency care in placing an airway, establishing parenteral lines, obtaining baseline diagnostic assessments (vital signs, neurologic signs, and radiographic and laboratory tests). Because head trauma often is accompanied by other injuries, the nurse examines the child for other signs of injury. The nurse handles the cervical and spinal areas with particular care until injury to these areas is ruled out.

Following initial assessment and treatment, the nurse monitors the child's vital signs and neurologic status frequently. The child is kept at rest, and stimulation is reduced to a minimum. The head of the child's bed is elevated 30° to increase venous return from the brain. The child's head and neck are maintained in correct alignment. If the child is excessively restless, the nurse applies the fewest restraints necessary to prevent self-injury. Fighting restraints can increase ICP, and the nurse avoids using them whenever possible (Kunkel and Wiley, 1979).

Changes in the child's level of consciousness are the most sensitive indicators of changes in ICP. Subtle alterations in responsiveness might reflect increasing ICP some time before vital sign changes occur (Walleck, 1980). Serial observations describing specific stimuli and responses are the most accurate in noting changes. (See the section on assessment of the child with neurologic dysfunction earlier in the chapter.) The nurse obtains information from the family about the child's normal behavior and responses, which is essential in detecting any changes. The parents are encouraged to remain with the child, and the nurse also observes the child's response to them.

The nurse checks the child's vital signs, symmetry and strength of motor function, and pupil size and reactivity frequently. The nurse monitors the child's respiratory status, including both respiratory rhythm and rate. Brain stem dysfunction can alter the pattern of respirations. The nurse is particularly careful to prevent hypoventilation because it can increase cerebral edema. Respiratory care includes turning and positioning and suctioning for the unconscious child. (See the section on the comatose child earlier in the chapter.)

Motor function assessment depends on the child's age and developmental level. The nurse observes all of the child's extremities for position, movement, increased or decreased muscle tone, sensation, and strength. Any changes in symmetry of the two sides, weakness, or abnormal positioning can indicate focal neurologic deficits.

Seizures might occur, and the nurse takes appropriate seizure precautions. The nurse describes the type and duration of any seizures fully and reports them immediately. (See the section on the child with a seizure disorder.)

The nurse reports the amount and nature of any drainage from the ear or nose (that is, clear, bloody) because it might represent an undetected skull fracture. The nurse monitors the child's fluid intake and output because the child is at risk for cerebral edema. Parenteral fluids are regulated strictly at the prescribed flow. The nurse measures the child's urinary output every hour during acute care. Hyperosmolar agents will produce diuresis but also might lead to severe dehydration and hypovolemic shock unless the fluid level is observed carefully and replacement adjusted accordingly. The nurse weighs the child every day to help determine fluid balance.

The conscious child who is vomiting receives nothing by mouth and then is given clear liquids in small amounts when they are tolerated, depending on fluid allowance or other conditions present (gastrointestinal or renal impairment). As the child improves, the diet is advanced.

The complications of immobility are prevented by position changes, hygienic care, range-of-motion exercises, and respiratory care as described earlier in the chapter. Although excessive stimulation should be avoided in the acute phase of injury, the nurse reassures the child repeatedly in a calm manner and explains briefly everything that is being done. This is important even if the child does not appear to hear because the child might still be perceiving auditory input.

Environmental stimulation in the form of familiar objects, quiet music, positional changes, and interaction is provided as the child recovers. The assessment of possible developmental changes continues past the acute period. Regression or behavioral changes might occur as transient phenomena or as longer term post-traumatic sequelae.

Family support in both the acute and recovery phases is an important aspect of nursing management. During the acute period, the family needs to be informed at all times about the child's condition and have all treatment measures explained to them. They should be allowed to spend as much time as possible with the child, with the staff readily available to answer questions and help them cope with the trauma. Feelings of guilt and anger about the circumstances of the accident and fears that the child will not recover fully can overwhelm the parent. The nurse uses crisis intervention methods, listening supportively, correcting misconceptions, and exploring other supports available to the family.

As the child recovers and the nurse undertakes discharge preparation, the family is informed about the posttraumatic syndrome effects they might encounter. The family should be aware that behavioral changes, mood alterations, and poor concentration are possible transient sequelae following head injury. More significant posttraumatic sequelae such as seizures or sensorimotor or other impairments require specific parent education regarding medication, management, and rehabilitative care. Follow-up evaluations are mandatory for all children who have had cerebral trauma to determine any new or persisting neurologic signs.

Spinal Cord Injury

Traumatic injury to the spinal cord resulting in paraplegia or quadriplegia is relatively uncommon in children, occurring more often in older children and adolescents than in young children. The causes of spinal cord injury vary with age. Although rare, birth injuries can produce traumatic cord damage, usually related to traction of the head and shoulders during a breech delivery (Myers, 1982). Falls from high places or diving or athletic injuries can produce indirect trauma by sudden hyperflexion, hyperextension, or compression of the spinal cord. The most frequent cause of spinal cord trauma at all ages is motor vehicle accidents.

The mechanism of injury is most often indirect trauma. Fracture or dislocation of vertebrae might accompany the injury but are not always present. Common sites of injury in children are the twelfth thoracic and first lumbar segments and the fifth and sixth cervical segments (Menkes and Batzdorf, 1980). Cord injury often is caused by spinal concussion or contusion. Less often, the spinal cord is actually severed. Early changes indicative of cord contusion include edema, petechial hemorrhage, neuronal changes, and an inflammatory reaction. The damaging effects of compression or overstretching on tissue from the initial insult are compounded by the resulting edema and circulatory impairment. Neuronal tissue disruption and ischemia cause necrotic changes in the spinal cord, partially or completely disrupting function (Aquino, 1978).

Clinical Manifestations In spinal concussion a transient loss of cord function follows a traumatic incident. Immediate flaccid paralysis below the injured site occurs, which lasts for minutes to hours. Recovery of function is complete, and pathologic abnormalities of the cord are not seen. The temporary alteration in neuronal tracts is believed to result from violent pressure waves in deep tissues acting on cord elements (Aquino, 1978).

More severe injuries produce permanent neurologic dysfunction of the spinal cord; the manifestations vary depending on the level and degree of damaged neuronal tissue. Complete lesions refer to total loss of functional motor activity and sensation below the level of insult. Incomplete lesions result in varying degrees of functional loss in which partial motor and sensory activities are intact. Types of incomplete lesions include the following:

1. *Anterior cord syndrome*—damage to the anterior section of the spinal cord resulting in complete motor paralysis below the level of the lesion, with scattered preservation of the sensations of touch, motion, and position
2. *Central cord syndrome*—damage to the central gray area of the cord resulting in greater motor impairment of the upper extremities than the lower extremities, with varying degrees of sensory loss
3. *Brown–Séquard syndrome*—damage to one-half of the cord resulting in ipsilateral motor paralysis and loss of pain and temperature sensation on the contralateral side (Menkes and Batzdorf, 1980; Myers, 1982)

Partial lesions might appear as one of these syndromes or as a combination of incomplete forms of injury with a scattered return of function. The spinal cord responds to traumatic insult in characteristic stages. Initially, spinal shock is evidenced by immediate flaccid paralysis and sensory and reflex loss below the level of the lesion. The loss may be either complete or incomplete. Prognosis at this stage is difficult to assess but generally is more favorable if some return of function occurs within 48 hours. The period of spinal shock is highly variable, but often lasts 2–6 weeks. Shorter durations of this stage also are associated with better neurologic outcomes (Molnar and Taft, 1977).

The acute period of spinal shock produces musculoskeletal, autonomic, and metabolic disturbances related both to the neuronal insult and immobility. In high thoracic and lower cervical lesions, respiratory effort can be impaired by loss of accessory muscle function. At level C4 or above, phrenic nerve function is lost, resulting in diaphragmatic paralysis and respiratory failure.

Reflex bladder function is lost, and the bladder becomes atonic and overdistends because of urinary retention. Overflow voiding occurs without bladder emptying. The residual urine stagnation increases the chances of infection and urinary calculi developing. A transient paralytic ileus can occur, resulting in abdominal distention and absent bowel sounds. The bowel becomes atonic and distended, and constipation and impaction result during the period when reflex activity is lost (Aquino, 1978).

Temperature regulation by sweating or shivering is lost below the level of the lesion. The involved areas of the body respond to the environmental temperature without thermoregulation. Excessive sweating above the level of the lesion frequently is seen as a reflex response to bowel or bladder distention or as a compensatory thermoregulatory mechanism.

Cardiovascular changes result both from the loss of vascular reflexes in peripheral venous return and immobilization. Cardiac output and plasma volume are decreased by inactivity. Orothostatic hypotension occurs when postural changes cause blood to pool in the lower extremities due to failure of vasoconstrictive reflexes. Further decrease in cardiac output progressively reduces cerebral blood flow, resulting in syncope (Myers, 1982). Increased autonomic reflexes (hyperreflexia) might cause hypertensive episodes, which often are related to bladder or bowel distention (Aquino, 1978).

Flaccid quadriplegia or paraplegia and immobility cause muscle atrophy and resulting nitrogen loss. This negative nitrogen balance is increased further by poor nutritional intake, which is typical in the acute period (Molnar and Taft, 1977). The loss of calcium from bones, which leads to osteoporosis, also increases the risks of urinary calculi formation and calcium deposition at paralyzed joints. Contractures result from inactivity, paralysis, and joint ossification. Sensory loss, poor protein state, circulatory impairments, and loss of movement combine to promote the rapid development of decubiti from even minimal pressure areas.

The second stage of spinal injury follows spinal shock, with a gradual and increasing return of reflex activity. Exceptions to this reflexive return occur with lesions of the cauda equina or destruction of the distal spinal cord from vascular interference. In these instances flaccid paralysis persists (Menkes and Batzdorf, 1980). Spinal reflex return might be accompanied by varying degrees of functional recovery of movement and sensation. Initially, flexion responses of muscle groups follows external stimulation. Increasing reflexive activity with flexion–extension patterns develops with progressive spasticity of the affected parts (Molnar and Taft, 1977).

Reflex bladder function returns, usually producing hypertonicity of the bladder and partial involuntary emptying. Excessive sphincter resistance can produce outlet obstruction, resulting in bladder distention and retrograde urinary complications. Bowel function returns as reflex or automatic evacuation of the full rectum (Aquino, 1978).

Many of the clinical manifestations of the initial period of spinal shock continue during the second stage as disturbances of motor, sensory, metabolic, and cardiovascular function. The appearance of spastic paralysis increases contracture and decubiti formation by involuntary joint posturing and pressure or shearing forces on bony prominences. Resuming voluntary movement of unaffected parts of the body and the frequent contraction of spastic muscles tend to reduce nitrogen and calcium imbalances and improve cardiovascular status (Molnar and Taft, 1977).

The period of neurologic recovery and reflexive return can continue for months to a year and occasionally longer. The outcomes can range from purely reflexive activity to return of partial motor or sensory function.

Medical Treatment Emergency care of the child with a spinal cord injury involves maintaining cardiovascular and respiratory function and preventing further damage to the neuronal tissue. Initial care and transport is of utmost importance because moving the injured site increases the risk of permanent damage. If resuscitation is necessary in the child with suspected cervical injury, it is accomplished with the head in a neutral position rather than hyperextended. Hasty actions such as the removal of a young athlete's football helmet can seriously aggravate spinal cord injury, as can any flexion, extension, or rotation of the spine. The child is transported on a firm, flat surface, and stabilizing aids such as a cervical collar, straps, and sandbags are used. Airway maintenance, ventilation, and the treatment of associated injuries are carried out with the child's spine immobilized.

A history of the trauma is helpful in determining the site and mechanism of the injury. Neurologic evaluation of motor, sensory, and reflexive functions gives an initial indication of the impairment and serves as a baseline for later comparisons. Only essential diagnostic measures are performed to avoid manipulating the child unnecessarily. The spine is examined radiographically to identify any fractures and dislocations of the spine, and contrast studies are performed to detect compression of the subarachnoid space (Menkes and Batzdorf, 1980).

Glucocorticoids are administered to reduce inflammation and edema, which can compromise neuronal function further. Local hypothermia therapy, hyperbaric oxygen therapy, and drug therapy to block the synthesis of harmful neurohormones are among the experimental treatments under investigation to reduce spinal cord damage (Myers, 1982).

The spine is stabilized by skeletal traction (cervical tongs, halo apparatus), body jackets, or positioning on a horizontal turning frame with sandbags and pads to maintain alignment. Surgical intervention in the acute period usually is avoided except in cases in which debridement of compound injuries is necessary or in which ascending loss of function develops. Fracture reduction and decompressive laminectomy are performed selectively, depending on the type of injury (Menkes and Batzdorf, 1980).

Children with high cervical injuries require respirator-assisted ventilation for an indefinite period of time, depending on the degree of diaphragmatic impairment. Decreased or absent respiratory effort combined with atelectasis and pooling of secretions from inactivity necessitate early and thorough respiratory therapy.

The child's fluid and electrolyte balance is monitored closely, and replacement and correction initially are provided parenterally. Initial paralytic ileus is managed with gastric decompression. Following the return of peristalsis, nutrition is provided by oral or nasogastric feeding (Aquino, 1978). Indwelling or intermittent catheterization is employed for bladder drainage. Bowel atony is managed by rectal tubes or enemas.

Throughout the acute and recovery periods, the child is given frequent neurologic assessments to determine the extent of injury and return of reflex and functional neuronal activity.

Nursing Management Nursing care of children with spinal cord injury in both the acute and rehabilitative phases is an integral part of a multidisciplinary team effort, the goals of which are to maximize postinjury function and prevent secondary complications. If at all possible, care is provided in a regional spinal injury center where specialized management is available.

Acute care is directed first toward maintaining vital functions and immobilizing the injured area. The nurse assesses the child's neurologic and vital signs, frequently with particular attention to motor and sensory functions. Cardiovascular shock is detected early by falling blood pressure, rapid pulse, and associated signs. The child is usually conscious and might be severely agitated and anxious. The nurse needs to comfort and reassure the child calmly, and mild sedation might be employed to help quiet the child.

The nurse monitors the child's respiratory function for adequacy of ventilation and the presence of accumulated secretions. If necessary, the nurse initiates chest physiotherapy, drainage, coughing, and suctioning to maintain pulmonary hygiene. Respiratory therapy may include ventilation assistance, oxygen, nebulizer, intermittent positive pressure breathing, and blow bottles.

The nurse avoids bladder distention in the child, and the Credé method and indwelling and intermittent catheterization are employed to empty the bladder. The specific gravity of the urine is measured to assess hydration, periodic cultures are performed, and the urine is observed closely for sediment, blood, or changes in color or order. The nurse monitors the child's bowel sounds and manages elimination with enemas or suppositories.

If the child undergoes surgery, the same nursing observations are made as those during acute care. In addition, the nurse watches the operative site for drainage, bleeding, or inflammation. Traction or other immobilizing measures are maintained to stabilize the spine during the acute phase (see Chapter 41).

The nurse pays meticulous attention to skin care, turning the child at least every 2 hours and avoiding pressure sites to prevent decubiti formation. Alternating pressure mattresses, sheepskin, and joint protectors (ankle, heel, or elbow) are helpful in reducing pressure over bony prominences. A high-calorie, high-protein diet is important both in reducing nitrogen imbalance and preventing debilitation, tissue breakdown, and urinary complications. Adequate fluid intake and acidification will help to prevent urinary tract infections and calculi formation. The child might refuse food, and the nurse uses ingenuity in providing small, frequent, high-calorie and protein feedings and fluids.

Temperature regulation is lost distal to the level of injury, which makes the child susceptible to effects from changes in the environmental temperature. The nurse adjusts the room temperature, adds or subtracts coverings, and uses external warming or cooling devices to maintain body temperature. The nurse monitors the child's rectal temperature and skin color and temperature to prevent hyperthermia or hypothermia.

Autonomic hyperreflexia episodes occur more often in children with spinal cord lesions above T6. This generalized sympathetic response is characterized by hypertension, flushing, profuse sweating, bradycardia, and headache. It occurs in response to visceral stimuli of bladder or bowel distention or other stimuli such as decubiti, urinary tract infection, or urologic manipulation. The nurse reacts immediately to this paroxysmal response, using interventions to reduce the stimulus and prevent cerebrovascular involvement (King and Dudas, 1980). Urinary drainage is checked, rectal distention is reduced, and other possible stimuli are treated. If these measures do not control the autonomic hyperreflexia, intravenous antihypertensive agents might be administered with close monitoring to reduce dangerously elevated blood pressures (Myers, 1982).

Muscle atrophy, osteoporosis, and contracture formation are treated early with passive range-of-motion exercises of affected and unaffected areas of the body. Active exercises against resistance for functional muscle groups are helpful in reducing the metabolic and cardiovascular effects of immobility and to strengthen the upper body musculature for later mobility strength in children with paraplegia (Molnar and Taft, 1977). As movement restrictions are removed, an overbed trapeze, manipulative and stretching games, and gradual "push-ups" increase shoulder and arm strength and endurance.

When permitted, the child may begin to be placed in upright positions. Assuming an upright posture suddenly can cause a drop in blood pressure and fainting. This is more common with higher thoracic and cervical lesions but can occur with lower lesions. Elastic stockings to help prevent venous pooling of blood and slow, gradual progression to upright positioning increase tolerance. A tilt table or reclining wheelchair with elevating legs are used in a program to progress the child from a horizontal to vertical posture. The tilt table is particularly useful because gravitational weightbearing by the long bones helps to reduce osteoporosis (Myers, 1982). Children might be afraid of falling and not having control as they begin to resume mobility. The tilt table is especially ominous to them, and the nurse supervises them constantly and reassures them to help them gain confidence. The child's tolerance, which is measured by pulse, blood pressure, and subjective discomfort, must be evaluated in the positioning program.

As the child's medical condition stabilizes and the second stage of spinal cord injury evolves, rehabilitation efforts begun during the spinal shock phase are developed into a comprehensive management program. The child's neurologic function is monitored carefully, and the child is observed for secondary complications. Increasing spasticity is treated with slow stretching exercises, braces, splints, and bivalved casts to prevent contractures and allow the child to stand.

Bladder and bowel programs are established, and the importance of preventing bladder distention, urinary stasis, and bowel constipation is emphasized. The child and family are taught techniques of intermittent catheterization or other methods to be used. A regular bowel pattern is developed with toiletsitting and the use of abdominal pressure and suppositories. Problems with stool consistency can be treated by dietary manipulation and adjunctive bulk or stool softening agents.

The nurse stresses repeatedly the importance of a regular program of bladder emptying, adequate fluid intake, and urine acidification because urinary complications remain the most common and serious impairment following spinal cord injury (Myers, 1982). Infections must be recognized and treated promptly and retrograde (reflux) involvement avoided to prevent pyelonephritis and renal failure.

Mobility training is essential to ensure the child's continuing exploration of the environment and optimal development. Depending on the degree of residual paralysis, the child is taught ambulation with braces and walker or crutches or wheelchair mobility using adapted devices such as mouth control. The motivation for mobility is high in children, and they often achieve rehabilitative goals rapidly.

The long-term nursing management of the child with spinal cord injury involves teaching all of the necessary aspects of ongoing care. Musculoskeletal, bladder, bowel, skin, temperature, and respiratory regimens are lifelong concerns, and tremendous energy is needed to maintain these functions. Family adaptations to accommodate the child's physical state are accompanied by major psychosocial changes as the child and family adjust to the new situations they face. The child's self-image changes significantly, as does the family's perception of the child. Support systems provided by the rehabilitation team, referrals, friends, and extended family are vital in promoting optimal postinjury coping mechanisms and maximizing the child's potential.

The Child With a Neurocutaneous Syndrome

Several childhood neurologic disorders, referred to as *phakomatoses,* or neurocutaneous syndromes, commonly have associated skin and nervous system lesions. These syndromes are hereditary diseases, often not apparent at birth, in which the severity of neurologic impairment varies widely. The major features and management of the neurocutaneous syndromes are outlined in Table 42-13.

The Child With a Degenerative Neurologic Disorder

A number of degenerative disorders of the central nervous system occur in childhood. Most of these conditions are hereditary and involve one or more areas of the brain and spinal cord. A specific enzymatic defect can be demonstrated for some children, but in many cases the mechanism of degeneration is obscure. Neurologic manifestations depend on the metabolic or structural changes and the anatomic site affected. Several of the more prevalent types of childhood degenerative disorders are listed in Table 42-14.

TABLE 42-13 Neurocutaneous Syndromes

Diagnosis	Clinical manifestations	Management
Tuberous sclerosis	Characteristic skin lesions (adenoma sebaceum) appearing as a red, papular rash over the nose, cheeks, and chin; areas of depigmented skin; intracranial calcifications; renal, retinal, or other systemic tumors; seizures; mental retardation (mild to severe)	Symptomatic care of involved organ systems Management of seizures Care of the child with mental retardation (see Chapter 23)
Neurofibromatosis	Multiple areas of light brown skin pigmentation (café-au-lait spots); fibrous tumors (neurofibromas) of the peripheral and central nervous system; skeletal abnormalities (scoliosis, overgrowth of bone tissue); seizures (less common than in tuberous sclerosis)	Early detection of tumor formation Surgical excision of tumors causing pain or impairment (see Chapter 45) Orthopedic treatment of skeltal abnormalities (see Chapter 41)

SOURCES: Data from Crawford AH: Neurofibromatosis in the pediatric patients. *Orthop Clin North AM* 1978; 9(1):11–23; Huttenlocker PR: The Nervous System. In: *Nelson's Textbook of Pediatrics.* Vaughn VC, McKay RJ, Behrman RE (editors). Saunders, 1979; Menkes JH (editor): *Textbook of Child Neurology.* 2nd ed. Lea & Febiger, 1980.

TABLE 42-14 Selected Degenerative Neurologic Disorders

Disease	Pathophysiology	Clinical manifestations	Management
Infantile cerebromacular degeneration (Tay-Sachs disease)	Abnormal accumulation of lipid material in the cells of central nervous system due to an enzymatic defect (gangliosidosis)	Onset between 3 and 10 months of age; hypotonia; loss of vision; irritability; cherry-red spot on the macula; exaggerated startle response to noise (hyperacusis); seizures; muscle spasticity, macrocephaly, and deterioration of psychomotor functions in later stages; progresses to death by 2 or 3 years of age	Symptomatic and supportive care Care of the child with vision impairment (see Chapter 43) Gentle handling to decrease reflex spastic responses Care of the child with seizures Care of the terminally ill child (see Chapter 32) Referral for genetic counseling
Familial dysautonomia (Riley-Day syndrome)	Autonomic nervous system dysfunction suggestive of neurohormone metabolism defect	Onset within 0–3 months of age; swallowing difficulties; vomiting; lack of adequate tear formation; excessive perspiration; erratic temperature regulation; skin blotching; labile blood pressure; hypotonia; psychomotor retardation; impaired sensation; chronic respiratory failure due to aspiration and pneumonia; variable course; death usually occurs during childhood from pulmonary complications or unknown causes	Symptomatic and supportive care Adapted feeding techniques Respiratory care to reduce pulmonary complications Eyedrops to protect cornea from ulceration Acute care for persistent vomiting Protection from injury secondary to impaired pain sensation Care of the chronically ill child (see Chapter 30)
Infantile muscular atrophy (Werdnig-Hoffmann disease)	Progressive degeneration of anterior horn cells of the spinal cord and motor nuclei of the brain stem	Present at birth or within the first months of life; Muscle weakness, hypotonia, and atrophy; typical frog-leg position; progressive loss of motor and cranial nerve function; respiratory and feeding difficulties; variable course; most cases are fatal in early childhood	Symptomatic and supportive care Adapted feeding techniques Respiratory care to improve ventilation and decrease congestion Cognitive and sensory stimulation for the child with severe motor deficits Parent–child support for a potentially fatal illness (see Chapter 32)
Spinocerebellar ataxia (Friedreich's ataxia)	Progressive degeneration of spinal cord tracts ("demyelinization" and proliferation of interstitial tissue); degenerative changes in the cerebellum, brain stem, and cortex	Onset in late childhood or early adolescence; ataxia, clumsy gait, easy fatigability; skeletal deformities of the feet and spine; slowly progressive loss of balance and motor control, first of the lower and then of the upper extremities; nystagmus, myocarditis, diabetes; variable course and severity	Orthopedic care for skeletal deformities (see Chapter 41) Rehabilitation management Supportive care for progressive loss of motor function

The Child With Alterations in Learning, Attention, and Activity Level

Often called the *minimal brain dysfunction* (MBD) syndrome, patterns of atypical learning and behavior have received considerable attention in recent years. The diagnostic label MBD includes a group of disorders that are variously referred to as learning disabilities, dyslexia, language disability, cerebral dysfunction, attention deficit disorders, hyperactivity syndrome, perceptual deficit syndrome, and many other terms. The multiplicity of labels and confusion in their application reflect the diversity of diagnostic criteria, presumed causes, and methods of interventions that abound.

Despite the uncertainty of nomenclature, working descriptions of children with such learning and behavior difficulties are helpful in understanding the nature of the disorders and their impact on the child's life. The child has normal intelligence but has one or more areas of specific learning deficit (often reading) and shows poor impulse control, distractibility, and overactivity. The specific types and degrees of dysfunction vary greatly, but these children often share the common characteristics of frustration at their lack of successes, low self-image, and reactive behavior. Interference with academic learning and successful interpersonal relations affect the child's critical years of growth and development, which, if not managed appropriately, can result in maladaptive future adjustment (Hart and Carter, 1982).

Estimates of the incidence of affected children vary widely, again reflecting the heterogeneity and lack of universally accepted diagnostic criteria. Prevalence is reported to be from 5% to 20% of the population, with the number of boys affected far outnumbering the number of girls affected (Huber and Dalldorf, 1980).

The etiology and pathophysiology of most cases of MBD are not clearly known. The central nervous system processing and modulation difficulties seen are felt to reflect neurologic dysfunction. This dysfunction is hypothesized to be caused by brain damage, neuromaturational delays, genetic inheritance, neurochemical alterations, metabolic derangements, and allergic reactions. A combination of factors, including environmental influences on behavior and development, might produce the clinical manifestations of MBD.

Children with a history of prenatal or perinatal insult might exhibit signs of learning and behavior disorders, as may children with cerebral palsy, posthead trauma, and lead poisoning. These findings suggest that in at least some cases, brain damage is the presumed cause (Hart and Carter, 1982). Neuromaturational delays have been proposed as responsible for MBD, with deficit areas resulting from immaturities of one or more central processes (Kinsbourne, 1980). Genetic factors might be responsible because families with affected children have a higher incidence of members with characterisitcs of MBD than nonaffected families (Huber and Dalldorf, 1980). Alterations in neurotransmitters have been studied in an attempt to determine the possible biochemical mechanisms that contribute to MBD (Shaywitz, Cohen, and Shaywitz, 1978). The role of food additives and artificial dyes in the diet has received much attention as a possible cause of hyperactivity (Feingold, 1975). The highly publicized benefits of an additive-free diet remain controversial, but a review of controlled studies suggests that a small percentage of young, hyperactive children might respond somewhat to such a diet (Stare, Whelan, and Sheridan, 1980).

Behavior Patterns in Minimal Brain Dysfunction

The characteristic behavioral manifestations associated with MBD are attention deficits, impulsivity, and hyperactivity. A wide spectrum of behaviors are seen, with children showing severe, subtle, or no atypical behavior patterns, absent or present specific learning disorders, or any combination of these traits. Certain common behavioral features, however, occur with regularity.

Impaired Selective Attention The child has difficulty maintaining attention on one activity or stimulus. The child is readily distracted by visual, auditory, or internal stimuli, shifting rapidly from one focus to another. Poor concentration, inability to screen out extraneous stimuli, and difficulty following directions are seen often.

Impulsivity Impulsive behavior may be noted by the child's inability to take turns, saying or doing whatever comes to mind, and reacting rapidly to emotional stimuli. The child cannot control, modify, or inhibit behavioral responses and has difficulty planning actions. The child is unable to consider the consequences of actions before responding. Disinhibited, disorganized behavior results in inappropriate social responses at home and school and with peers.

Hyperactivity The hyperactive child is in constant motion. Excessive motor activity without purposeful focus characterizes this overactivity. The child has difficulty sitting still, fidgets, and might show a "driven" quality of frenzied behavior. The child often cannot control the restless, perpetual motor output and shifts activities constantly without completing tasks.

These behavioral characteristics are combined in the child's activity and response patterns. The child has difficulty focusing attention and responds impulsively to a bombardment of stimuli, often darting from place to place without apparent motivation. The parent has trouble dealing with the child's behavior, complaining that the child "doesn't listen," cannot be disciplined, and is "always getting into things." The negative consequences of the child's poorly modulated behavior extend to school and social situations. In the classroom the child might be unable to remain seated, concentrate on tasks, or resist talking or acting inappropriately. The child might be rejected because of an inability to share or take turns in play, impulsive aggression, and impatience with others.

Typically, the child's difficulties are more noticeable in situations that require sustained attention and the ability to follow directions and filter environmental stimuli selectively. For this reason, these difficulties often become acute when the child enters school. Toddlers and preschoolers might show the same characteristics, manifested particularly in overactivity and tantrums, but because relatively fewer demands are placed on them to regulate their behavior, the problems might not be as apparent.

Learning Disabilities

Specific learning deficits often are associated with the clinical picture of MBD. Problems in one or more areas of cognitive functioning reflect central processing difficulties in the complex mechanisms of perception, association, integration, and response. The definition of learning disorders excludes those cognitive weaknesses associated with primary visual, hearing, or motor impairments, emotional disturbances, mental retardation, or sociocultural deprivation (Culbertson and Ferry, 1982). The conditions might overlap, however. For example, children with cerebral palsy might exhibit specific language processing difficulties not directly related to their motor dysfunction.

Language Processing The child might have such receptive language deficits as poor verbal memory and auditory comprehension and an inability to understand rapid or complex verbal input. The child might misunderstand or be unable to remember what is said, have a limited vocabulary, and experience difficulties with reading and spelling. Expressive language disorders include word finding problems, syntactical errors, difficulty organizing verbal output, and dysfluency. The child might have great difficulty with self-expression, be unable to name objects, and resort to gestures or pantomime. Other children attempt to compensate by circular descriptions of what they are trying to say (for example, saying, "the white stuff you drink" instead of "milk").

Children with language problems have difficulty making the necessary associations for reading, writing, and spelling.

Visual-Perceptual–Motor Function The child with MBD has difficulty in perceptual tasks that involve discriminating visual information, spatial relationships, and visual–sequential memory. Confusion of directionality, trouble matching similar pictures or symbols, and an inability to recognize part–whole relationships are noted. The child might have trouble with visual motor integration, manifested by such inabilities as tying shoelaces, catching a ball, or copying designs. The child encounters problems when learning to recognize and reproduce letters and numbers.

Visual-spatial processing deficits are not necessarily associated with visual motor problems. The child might perceive information adequately but, for example, lack the fine motor ability to write or do puzzles. Conversely, the child might be able to perform motor tasks well but perceive visual–spatial orientation incorrectly (Levine, Brooks, and Shonkoff, 1980).

Memory and Temporal-Sequential Organization The child might have a short-term memory deficit, which is demonstrated by the inability to repeat what has been said, recall a series of digits, or follow multistep directions. The child might have difficulty recalling previously learned material or may remember things in the wrong order. Sequencing problems also might be evident an in inability to learn number concepts, perform tasks in the right order, or master letter and word formation. Time concepts such as the hours of the day or days of the week and relationships of before, after, next, and so on are difficult to master (Levine, Brooks, and Shonkoff, 1980).

Dyslexia Reading disability, or *dyslexia,* is one of the most commonly encountered isolated learning disorders. Children with reading disorders show different profiles according to their individual deficit areas. According to Mattis (1978), a large percentage of these children have language disorders in naming, comprehension, imitative speech, and speech sound discrimination. A second group of children have deficits in sound blending and coordination skills, although their receptive language is within normal limits. A third group of children have deficit areas in visual perception. Disruption of any of the multiple factors associated with the complex processes required to integrate the auditory and visual information essential to reading, writing, and spelling might interfere with learning to read (Myklebust, 1978).

Secondary Reactive Problems The child with MBD is often poorly understood, frequently in trouble, and generally fails in school and social situations. The child's behavioral characteristics often provoke negative responses from others, which can then perpetuate the child's disinhibited, impulsive reactions. The child often faces embarrassment and isolation, which, combined with the lack of success, can contribute to poor self-image, a sense of inadequacy, and true depression. Sorting out emotional reactivity from "innate" behavioral characteristics is difficult if not impossible (Hart and Carter, 1982). (Nursing care of the child with dysfunctional behavior is discussed in Chapter 24.)

Multidisciplinary Management for Learning, Attention, and Activity Disorders

A comprehensive evaluation of the child's cognitive, language, perceptual, motor, and social and emotional strengths and weaknesses is undertaken by various specialists, depending on the child's needs and areas of dysfunction. Members of the evaluation team might include the psychologist, speech and language pathologist, occupational therapist, special educator, nurse, social worker, and physical therapist.

Evaluative data help to determine both the child's areas of deficit and skills in learning, behavior, and emotional adaptation. Important management data are obtained by history, interview, and observation, as well as by numerous standardized tests.

Diagnostic Evaluation The child with problems of attention, learning, or activity level travel varying routes of referral for diagnostic evaluation. Pediatricians, teachers, psychologists, nurses, or friends are among those that parents might ask for help. Educators often are the first to detect areas of deficit as the child experiences difficulty in school. Regardless of the initial means of referral, the preferred approach to intervention begins with a thorough multidisciplinary assessment of the child's strengths and weaknesses.

History A complete medical, behavioral, and school history is obtained. Prenatal and perinatal influences and a family history of similar problems might provide clues to possible etiologic factors, but specific correlations seldom are found. Any chronic or serious illnesses, head trauma, or toxic episodes that might have caused insult to the central nervous system are determined, as are other health concerns such as allergies and recurrent otitis.

The attainment of developmental milestones is reviewed carefully, as are the child's behavioral characteristics from infancy onward (see Chapter 16). The child's school history is elicited, including academic performance, areas of difficulty, and behavioral adjustment. Exploring the child's presenting concern in detail is one of the most important aspects of the history. How the child functions at home, at school, and in the community are important in determining the child's problem areas and in what context they are present.

Physical and Neurologic Examinations Complete general health examinations are usually normal, but careful physical examination is important to detect underlying medical problems that might explain the child's problem or be an aggravating physical stressor. The child's overall physical maturity for age is assessed, as are the presence or absence of an enlarged thyroid gland, skin lesions, or physical stigmas suggestive of endocrine or neurologic abnormalities.

The child's ears, nose, and throat are examined thoroughly for serous otitis, tympanic membrane scarring, palatal abnormalities, or lesions. Fundoscopic and oculomotor assessments are done to detect eyeground abnormalities, strabismus, or amblyopia (Levine, Brooks, and Shonkoff, 1980). Visual and auditory acuity assessments are essential components of the physical examination.

A neurologic examination is performed to rule out serious neurologic disorders and to document the presence of so-called neurologic "soft signs." The significance of these minor indicators of dysfunction are controversial (Huber and Dalldorf, 1980; Culbertson and Ferry, 1982), but they might be helpful in establishing the diagnosis (Hart and Carter, 1982). The indicators are of two types; those that reflect developmental immaturity at a given chronologic age and those that are borderline signs of neurologic abnormalities at any age. Signs of neurologic immaturity at various ages include difficulty with rapid alternating movements, "mirror" movements of the opposite extremity, fine motor incoordination, and left–right confusion. Borderline neurologic signs are choreiform movements, mild asymmetry of reflexes or muscle tone, or mild tremors (Hart and Carter, 1982).

Ancillary Diagnostic Tests Depending on the findings of the history and physical examinations, other diagnostic tests might be appropriate. Special blood analyses beyond routine pediatric screening tests are seldom needed. Thyroid function tests, chromosome studies, or metabolic tests are indicated in selected cases.

An EEG might be performed but most often yields little diagnostic information. Abnormalities of the tracings tend to appear in a greater percentage of cases than in "normal" controls, but these findings usually do not have therapeutic implications (Levine, Brooks, and Shonkoff, 1980). Children suspected of having seizures or those with focal neurologic signs should have EEGs performed.

Newer electrophysiologic tests currently are being investigated to aid in the diagnostic assessment of MBD. Computerized tomographic mapping of EEG and evoked potential activity has shown physiologic differences between dyslexic and normal subjects (Duffy, et al., 1980). Called Brain Electrical Activity Mapping (BEAM), this new technique might prove helpful in diagnosis in the future.

When a neurologic disorder is suspected, CT scans or other radiographic studies and neurodiagnostic tests might be indicated. Possible diagnoses of hydrocephalus or neurofibromatosis or localizing neurologic signs are indications for further neurologic evaluation.

Medical Treatment Treatment for children with MBD can take many forms but is most successful when it encompasses the various aspects of the child's life at home and school. An interdisciplinary management model addresses the child's educational, behavioral, and emotional needs in a coordinated approach.

Behavioral Counseling Behavior management programs are developed both for parents and for school situations and "target" specific areas of difficulty and suggest modifying techniques. Children with attention deficits and impulsivity have difficulty in highly stimulating situations. Reducing stimuli, offering short, simple directions, and using "time-out" methods can help keep the child from becoming overwhelmed. Most children who have difficulty organizing and controlling their behavior respond better in the presence of consistent routines, structured activities, and clearly defined limits. Counseling is directed toward helping the family understand the child's weaknesses and make adaptations in family interactions to improve the child's behavior and self-esteem.

Educational Programs Adjustments in the child's educational program can range from remedial help in a specific area to placement in a self-contained setting with multitherapeutic support. After evaluation, an individualized educational plan is developed for each child. Special education might be supplemented by speech and language therapy, perceptual–motor training, or psychotherapy. The child is helped to improve deficient skills and develop ways to compensate for areas of weakness. Successful interventions result in both relative academic or functional achievements and improvements in self-concept and social interactions.

Medication Psychoactive medications can be a useful adjunct in the treatment of some children with attention deficit disorders. Central nervous system stimulants (dextroamphetamine, methylphenidate, pemoline) have been demonstrated to improve attention span and reduce hyperactivity, often dramatically, in a number of children (Hart and Carter, 1982). Although the drug treatment of children with MBD has been much debated, when selectively employed and closely monitored, medication therapy is helpful for some children. The specific mechanism of action by which these drugs reduce restless motor activity and improve concentration is not known but is believed to be related to neurotransmitter alterations affecting the reticular activating system of the brain stem (Conway-Rutkowski, 1982). Stimulant medication is not appropriate for all children with attention deficits, but precise criteria to guide practitioners in the decision to try medication are lacking. In general, the child with significant impairment of attention span or impulsivity is a candidate for medication trial, in conjunction with other therapeutic interventions.

The child's response is monitored both for beneficial effects and adverse reactions. Transient appetite suppression or insomnia are frequent occurrences, which often disappear after several weeks or with dosage adjustment. Frequent follow-up evaluations are important to assess dosage and effectiveness. The medication trial is continued for at least 1 month. If minimal or no improvement is observed, the medication is stopped.

Nursing Management Multidisciplinary management of the child with MBD and the family involves nursing interventions in a variety of settings. The nurse initially might detect problem areas and refer the family for further evaluation. As the treatment plan is developed, the nurse participates in health care management, family guidance, and behavioral therapy. The nurse plays a vital role in coordinating medical and educational programs to provide an integrated approach. The nurse often acts as the liaison between the family, school, and specialized treatment settings. In the community the nurse helps families to cope with their children's needs through long-term involvement in home management. Parents are guided in making environmental adjustments to provide structure and safety for their children, as well as to help them experience success. They are taught about their children's disabilities and helped to understand the factors that aggravate or ameliorate their behavior. The principles of behavior modification may be employed in a specific program of reinforcements. Parents are encouraged to use praise as well as criticism and to set realistic goals.

For optimal results, medication treatment must be monitored closely. Communication with school staff and parents is essential to determine the child's response and recognize adverse effects. Often, a behavior checklist is a helpful way for staff and family to note changes in the child's attention span, activity level, impulsivity, and reactivity. This format provides documentation for assessing medication treatment and aids in communication. If side effects develop, the dosage or time of administration may be adjusted. Usually, stimulant medication is given once a day (in the morning) or in the morning and again at noon. If the stimulant is given later in the day, the child frequently experiences insomnia.

The child with learning and behavior dysfunction requires long-term, sensitive care to foster strengths and a positive self-image. Both the child and family will encounter frustrations and setbacks along the way, which can be discouraging. Helping parents to feel competent in their parenting skills, providing anticipatory guidance, and being a supportive listener are valuable nursing interventions.

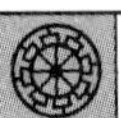

NURSING CARE PLAN The Comatose Child

Assessment Data

Lucy, a 13-year-old girl, suffered severe closed head injury (cerebral contusion) when she was struck by a car while riding her bicycle. Emergency management included tracheal intubation, assisted ventilation, treatment of cerebral edema, and anticonvulsant prophylaxis. Initial loss of consciousness was characterized by flexion response to pain (decorticate posturing) and no eye opening or verbal responses (Glasgow Coma Score 5). Ten days post injury, she no longer requires intubation, her vital signs have stabilized, and she has been transferred from the intensive care unit to the pediatric unit. Although still unconscious, she now opens her eyes in response to verbal stimuli and no longer demonstrates decorticate posturing. Lucy is the youngest of four children; her parents feel guilty about the accident because it followed an argument with Lucy about her curfew.

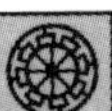

NURSING CARE PLAN The Comatose Child (continued)

Nursing Diagnoses and Goals

1. **Nursing diagnosis:** Alteration in consciousness subsequent to cerebral contusion.

   Long-term goal: Lucy will achieve an optimal level of consciousness.

   Short-term goals: (a) Lucy will be protected from injury while comatose. (b) Any changes in Lucy's neurologic status will be detected promptly. (c) Lucy will receive sensory stimulation.

2. **Nursing diagnosis:** Potential joint contractures as a result of immobility.

   Long-term goal: Lucy will experience no deformity as a result of joint contractures.

   Short-term goals: (a) Lucy's joints will remain flexible. (b) The potential for deformity secondary to spasticity and weakness will be reduced.

3. **Nursing diagnosis:** Potential parental distress related to family crisis.

   Long-term goal: Lucy's parents will be able to cope with the crisis of her accident and comatose condition.

   Short-term goals: (a) Lucy's parents will be able to communicate their feelings about Lucy's accident. (b) Lucy's parents will be supported. (c) The relationship between Lucy and her parents will be maintained.

Intervention	Rationale	Evaluation criteria
1. Position Lucy with her head elevated 15–30°. Support her lying on her side or semiprone	Keeping the head elevated and lying on the side or semiprone reduces intracranial pressure, improves ventilation, and prevents aspiration	Does Lucy remain free of physical injury? Is there any evidence of deterioration in Lucy's neurologic status? Has Lucy achieved an optimal level of consciousness?
Take seizure precautions. Pad the side rails of Lucy's bed	Preventive measures are required for unconscious children at risk for seizures	
Monitor Lucy's neurologic signs and vital signs every 2–4 hours. Include a Glasgow Coma Scale assessment Observe Lucy for associated neurologic signs such as vomiting and seizures	The early detection of changes in neurologic status allows for prompt diagnosis and treatment, which improves the prognosis	
Talk to Lucy while caring for her. Touch her soothingly Have the parents bring tapes to play for Lucy	Sensory stimulation promotes the child's (potential for) increasing orientation and provides comfort	
Refrain from inappropriate discussions within Lucy's hearing	The comatose child might perceive auditory stimuli despite a lack of response	
2. Maintain Lucy's body alignment with pillows and sandbags to support her position	Functional body alignment helps to prevent stress on the joints and contractures	Does Lucy have any evidence of joint contractures?
Change Lucy's position (from side to side and semiprone) every 2 hours	Position changes promote circulation, joint flexibility, and help to prevent respiratory congestion and skin pressure sites	
Perform range-of-motion exercises every 4 hours	Range-of-motion exercises increase circulation and maintain joint mobility	
Apply ankle and foot orthoses and hand splints. Remove every 4 hours for range of motion and skin care	The proper application of orthoses prevents foot drop and wrist drop	

continued on next page

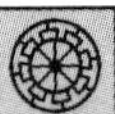

NURSING CARE PLAN The Comatose Child (continued)

Intervention	Rationale	Evaluation criteria
3. Encourage Lucy's parents to express their feelings. Allow them to express their sense of guilt, but reinforce that they did not cause Lucy's accident	The verbalization of feelings helps parents to begin to adapt to a crisis situation and resolve any grief	Are Lucy's parents able to communicate effectively with the health care staff? Do the parents demonstrate adaptive coping behaviors? Has the parent–child relationship been reestablished?
Empathize with the parents' sense of loss and anxiety about Lucy's potential for recovery	Empathic listening will comfort parents in their grief and uncertainty	
Answer the parents' questions sensitively but realistically. Repeat information as needed, and explain all treatments and care	Accurate information will help to prevent parental misperceptions and unrealistic hopes	
Encourage the parents to talk to Lucy and touch and comfort her When the parents indicate their readiness, encourage them to participate in Lucy's care	Interacting with their child and assisting in care reduces the parents' feeling of helplessness and reaffirms the parent–child relationship	
Offer referral to support and counseling (pastoral care, social services)		

Key Concepts

- The nervous system consists of the brain, which is composed of the cerebrum, cerebellum, and brain stem; the spinal cord; the cerebrospinal fluid system; and the peripheral nervous system, which includes the cranial and spinal nerves and the autonomic nervous system.
- Assessment of the child's cerebral function includes observation of the child's behavior, level of consciousness, orientation, memory, and integrative function.
- Assessment of the child's motor function includes examination of muscle tone, muscle strength, motor control and coordination, and movement and posture.
- For the child with neurologic dysfunction, preparation for diagnostic tests involves helping the child become familiar with the equipment, describing the sensations the child will feel, and explaining the position that the child will need to assume for the test.
- Diagnostic tests and procedures common to neurologic function include electroencephalogram, radiographic studies, lumbar puncture, subdural tap, electromyography, and nerve conduction studies.
- Rehabilitation for children with neurologic disorders involves special exercises; assistive devices such as casts, splints, and braces; and mobilizing aids.
- Nursing management for the child requiring rehabilitation to improve neurologic deficits involves physical care, teaching the use of adaptive equipment, developmental stimulation, and behavior management.
- Nursing goals for the child with increased intracranial pressure are to reduce intracranial volume and treat the underlying disorder.
- Nursing management for the child with increased intracranial pressure involves administering diuretics, reducing fluid intake, maintaining an unelevated body temperature, monitoring the child's level of consciousness, and elevating the child's head to promote drainage from the brain.
- Nursing management for the comatose child involves serial monitoring of neurologic status,

which includes assessment of vital signs, neurologic signs, and level of consciousness.

- Nursing measures for the comatose child are directed toward preventing the secondary effects of immobility and altered sensory perception.
- Nutritional needs for children with neurologic dysfunction may be met through adaptive equipment to compensate for impaired motor control and tube feedings for children whose handicaps prevent their handling food orally.
- Children with neurologic dysfunction often require special interventions to provide stimulation within a structured environment, facilitate learning adaptive skills, enhance socialization with peers, and achieve as much independence as possible.
- Myelodysplasia encompasses a group of related central nervous system disorders involving malformations of the neural tube; they include spina bifida occulta, meningocele, and myelomeningocele.
- For the infant with myelodysplasia, nursing care requires intensive preoperative and postoperative observation of vital signs, head circumference, wound, and elimination, together with parent teaching to establish a liaison for long-term care.
- Chronic care for the child with myelodysplasia involves teaching parents to avoid skin breakdown and injury, to avoid extreme temperatures, to enhance mobility through exercise, and to manage elimination to prevent complications.
- Clinical manifestations of hydrocephalus include enlarging head size, downward rotation of the eyes, and signs of increased intracranial pressure.
- Nursing management for the child with hydrocephalus involves close observation of vital signs and neurologic status, prevention of skin breakdown, and parent teaching about shunting procedures and the prevention of obstruction and infection.
- Congenital vascular malformations cause symptoms as a result of bleeding or the effects of space-occupying lesions; common symptoms are hemorrhage, headache, vomiting, irritability, deterioration in consciousness, and focal neurologic deficits.
- Nursing management for the child with intracranial hemorrhage involves observing for alterations in consciousness and increased intracranial pressure, elevating the head to promote drainage, minimizing stimuli to avoid elevating blood pressure, instituting seizure precautions, and reducing anxiety through careful communication.
- Nursing management for the child with acute bacterial meningitis involves observing vital signs, bedrest with head elevated, safety measures, minimizing external stimuli, avoiding temperature elevation, and preventing such complications as infection and motor or sensory deficits.
- Unlike bacterial meningitis, aseptic meningitis is usually a benign illness that is most often caused by a virus; nursing management includes monitoring neurologic status, vital signs, hydration, nutrition, and comfort.
- Nursing management of the child with encephalitis involves monitoring level of consciousness and vital signs and observing for signs of increased intracranial pressure, meningeal irritation, and cranial nerve involvement.
- Because rabies prophylaxis is painful and can cause adverse reactions, the nurse prepares both child and family for treatment and provides ongoing support to minimize anxiety and promote cooperation.
- Nursing management for the child with Reye's syndrome involves monitoring neurologic status, vital signs, and arterial and central venous pressure; preventing overhydration and unnecessary manipulation; instituting hyperventilation therapy as needed; and diminishing anxiety and disorientation with calm, reassuring communication.
- Nursing management for the child with Guillain-Barré syndrome involves monitoring respiratory status, observing for signs of impending cardiovascular collapse, positioning in correct alignment, and preventing muscle pain and complications of immobility.
- Seizures are classified as generalized or partial, are usually self-limiting, are sometimes directly preceded by an aura, and may be followed by varying degrees of headache or fatigue.
- Acute care for the child experiencing a seizure is directed toward protecting the child from injury and maintaining an airway; following the seizure, nursing interventions include calm explanations to the child,

monitoring vital signs and temperature, and documenting seizure activity.

- Chronic care for the child with a seizure disorder is directed toward teaching the child and family to control seizures through anticonvulsant medications and to prevent complications of seizure activity through attention to safety needs and to conditions that lead to the child's seizures.
- Nursing management for the child experiencing status epilepticus involves emergency care directed toward establishing an airway, administering oxygen, providing oropharyngeal suctioning, and preparing for possible cardiorespiratory arrest.
- Cerebral palsy includes a variety of motor impairments caused by insult to the brain.
- Types of cerebral palsy include spastic cerebral palsy—manifested by increased muscle tone and stretch reflexes and muscle weakness—athetoid cerebral palsy—manifested by abnormal, involuntary movements—and ataxic cerebral palsy—characterized by impaired balance and coordination.
- Associated with cerebral palsy are cognitive impairment, hyperactivity, minimal brain dysfunction, seizures, and respiratory disturbances.
- Nursing care for the child with cerebral palsy involves early detection through neurologic and developmental assessment; teaching the child and family about adapting to the condition; ongoing support of parent and child; and referral for physical, occupational or speech therapy.
- Head injuries in children include skull fractures, concussions, contusions and lacerations, subdural hematoma, extradural hematoma, and intracranial hematoma.
- Complications of head injury include cerebral edema, increased intracranial pressure, and posttraumatic sequelae.
- Nursing management for the child with a head injury includes monitoring vital signs and observing for neurologic impairments such as changes in level of consciousness, reducing stimulation, assessing motor function, monitoring fluid status, observing for drainage, and preventing complications of immobility.
- Acute care for the child with a spinal cord injury involves monitoring vital signs, providing skin care, monitoring fluid intake to prevent urinary tract infections and calculi, temperature regulation, and preventing the effects of immobility through range-of-motion exercises and careful positioning.
- Chronic care for the child with spinal cord injury involves rehabilitation to restore as much neuromuscular function as possible, bladder and bowel training as needed, and referral for appropriate long-term support.
- Behavior patterns associated with minimal brain dysfunction include attention deficits, impulsivity, and hyperactivity.
- Learning disabilities include problems in language processing, visual-perceptual–motor function, memory and temporal-sequential organization, reading (a disability known as dyslexia), and secondary problems in socialization.
- Nursing management for the child with learning, attention, and activity disorders is part of a multidisciplinary effort that may involve diagnostic evaluation, behavioral counseling, educational programs, medication, and support for the child and family.

References

Aquino TM: Trauma. In: *Manual of Neurologic Therapeutics*. Samuels MA (editor). Little, Brown, 1978.

Baird HW: Convulsive disorders. In: *Nelson's Textbook of Pediatrics*. Behrman RE, Vaughan VC (editors). Saunders, 1979.

Belkengren RP, Sapala S: Reye's syndrome, clinical guidelines for practitioners in ambulatory care. *Pediatr Nurs* (March/April) 1981; 7(2):26–28.

Carmel PW: Spinal dysraphism. In: *The Child With Disabling Illness*. 2nd ed. Downey JA, Low NL (editors). Raven Press, 1982.

Challenor YB, Gold AP: Cerebrovascular disease in children and remediation of neuromuscular residua. In: *The Child With Disabling Illness*. 2nd ed. Downey JA, Low NL (editor). Raven Press, 1982.

Chee CM: Seizure disorders. *Nurs Clin North Am* (March) 1980; 15(1):71–82.

Clark K, et al: Reye's syndrome nursing protocol. *J Natl Reye's Syndrome Foundation* 1980; 1(2):82–84.

Colon AR: Reye's syndrome: 1980. *J Natl Reye's Syndrome Foundation* 1980; 1(2):54–55.

Committee on Infectious Diseases of the American Academy of Pediatrics: Aspirin and Reye's syndrome. *Pediatrics* (June) 1982; 69(6):810–812.

Conway-Rutkowski BL: *Carini and Owen's Neurological and Neurosurgical Nursing*. 8th ed. Mosby, 1982.

Crawford AH: Neurofibromatosis in the pediatric patient. *Orthop Clin North Am* 1978; 9(1):11–23.

Culbertson JL, Ferry P: Learning disabilities. *Nurs Clin North Am* (Feb) 1982; 29(1):121–136.

Davis GT, Hill PM: Cerebral palsy. *Nurs Clin North Am* (March) 1980; 15(1):35–50.

Devore NE, Jackson VM, Piening SL: TORCH infections. *Am J Nurs* (Dec) 1983; 83(12):1660–1665.

Duffy F, et al: Dyslexia: Regional diffeences in brain electrical activity by topographic mapping. *Ann Neurol* 1980: 7:412–421.

Field G: Social implications of long-term illness in children. In: *The Child With Disabling Illness*. 2nd ed. Downey JA, Low NL (editors). Raven Press, 1982.

Feingold B: *Why Your Child's Hyperactive*. Random House, 1975.

Ferguson CK, Roll LJ: Human rabies. *Am J Nurs* (June) 1981; 81(6):1174–1179.

Gabriel RS: Malformations of the central nervous system. In: *Textbook of Child Neurology*. Menkes JH (editors). Lea & Febiger, 1980.

Gaddy DS: Meningitis in the pediatric population. *Nurs Clin North Am* (March) 1980; 15(1):83–97.

Gellis SS, Kagan BM: *Current Pediatric Therapy*. Vol 10. Saunders, 1982.

Godfrey AB: Sensory–motor stimulation for slow-to-develop children. A specialized program for public health nurses. *Am J Nurs* (Jan) 1975; 75(1):56–59.

Golden GS: Vascular diseases of the brain. *Curr Probl Pediatr* 1978; 8(6):3–28.

Hart EJ, Carter S: Attention deficit disorder, hyperactivity, and learning disabilities: The minimal brain dysfunction syndrome. In: *The Child With Disabling Illness*. 2nd ed. Downey JA, Low NL (editors). Raven Press, 1982.

Hausman KA: Critical care of the child with increased intracranial pressure. *Nurs Clin North Am* (Dec) 1981; 16(4):647–656.

Hilty MD: Treatment and management of Reye's syndrome. *J Natl Reye's Syndrome Foundation* 1981; 2(1):27–32.

Huber CJ, Dalldorf JS: Minimal brain dysfunction syndrome. *Nurs Clin North Am* (March) 1980; 15(1):51–69.

Huttenlocher PR: The nervous system. In: *Nelson's Textbook of Pediatrics*. Behrman RE, Vaughan VC (editors). Saunders, 1979.

Icenogle DA, Kaplan AM: A review of congenital neurologic malformations. *Clin Pediatr* 1981; 20(9):565–576.

Igoe JB, et al: *School Nurses Working With Handicapped Children*. American Nurses' Association Publication No NP-60, 2M. May, 1980.

Jabbour JT, et al: *Pediatric Neurology Handbook*. Medical Examination, 1976.

Jones C: Glasgow coma scale. *Am J Nurs* (Sept) 1979; 79(9):1551–1553.

King RB, Dudas S: Rehabilitation of the patient with a spinal cord injury. *Nurs Clin North Am* (June) 1980; 15(2):225–243.

Kinsborne M: Disorders of mental development. In: *Textbook of Child Neurology*. Menkes JH (editor). Lea & Febiger, 1980.

Kunkel J, Wiley JK: Acute head injury: What to do when . . . and why. *Nursing 79* (March) 1979; 9(3):22–33.

Kupka J, Geddes N, Carrou NC: Comprehensive management in the child with spina bifida. *Orthop Clin North Am* 1978: 9(1):97–113.

Langner BE, Schott JR: Nursing implications of central nervous system infections in children. *Issues Compr Pediatr Nurs* (July/Aug) 1977; 2(2):38–53.

Levine MD, Brooks R, Shonkoff JP: *A Pediatric Approach to Learning Disorders*. Wiley, 1980.

Lovejoy FH, et al: Clinical staging in Reye's syndrome. *Am J Dis Child* 1974; 128:36–41.

Low NL, Downey JA: Cerebral palsy. In: *The Child With Disabling Illness*. 2nd ed. Downey JA, Low NL (editors). Raven Press, 1982.

Low NL, Downey JA: Lower motor neuron diseases. In: *The Child With Disabling Illness*. 2nd ed. Downey JA, Low, NL (editors). Raven Press, 1982.

Low NL: Seizure disorders in children. In: *The Child With Disabling Illness*. 2nd ed. Downey JA, Low NL (editors). Raven Press, 1982.

Martelli ME: Teaching parents about Reye's syndrome. *Am J Nurs* (Feb) 1982; 82(2):260–263.

Mattis S: Dyslexia syndromes: A working hypothesis that works. In: *Dyslexia: An Approach of Current Knowledge*. Benton A, Peral D (editors). Oxford University Press, 1978.

McElroy DB: Hydrocephalus in children. *Nurs Clin North Am* (March) 1980; 15(1):23–34.

Menkes JH (editor): *Textbook of Child Neurology*. 2nd ed. Lea & Febiger, 1980.

Menkes JH, Batzdorf U: Postnatal trauma and injuries by physical agents. In: *Textbook of Child Neurology*. 2nd ed. Menkes JH (editor). Lea & Febiger, 1980.

Molnar GE, Taft LT: Pediatric rehabilitation. Part I: Cerebral palsy and spinal cord injuries. *Curr Prob Pediatr* 1977a; 7(3):6–46.

Molnar GE, Taft LT: Pediatric rehabilitation. Part II: Spina bifida and limb deficiencies. *Curr Probl Pediatr* 1977b; 7(4):3–35.

Muehl JN: Seizure disorders in children: Prevention and care. *Am J Matern Child Nurs* (May/June) 1979; 4(3):154–160.

Myers SJ: The spinal injury patient. In: *The Child With Disabling Illness*. 2nd ed. Downey JA, Low NL (editors). Raven Press, 1982.

Mykelbust HR: Toward a science of dyslexiology. In: *Progress in Learning Disabilities*. Mykelbust HR (editor). Grune & Stratton, 1978.

Passo SD: Malformations of the neural tube. *Nurs Clin North Am* (March) 1980; 15:5–21.

Plotkin SA: Rabies. In: *Nelson's Textbook of Pediatrics*. Behrman RE, Vaughan VC (editors). Saunders, 1979.

Reye, RD, Morgan G, Baral J: Encephalopathy and fatty degeneration of the viscera. *Lancet* 1963; 2:749–752.

Rodgers B, et al: Depression in the chronically ill or handicapped school-aged child. *Am J Matern Child Nurs* (Jul/Aug) 1981; 3(1):34–37.

Rubenstein B: Psychiatric aspects of chronic handicaps. In: *The Child With Disabling Illness*. 2nd ed. Downey JA, Low NL (editors). Raven Press, 1982.

Rytel MW: Counterimmunoelectrophoresis in the diagnosis of infectious disease. *Hosp Pract* 1975; 10:75–82.

Sagar SM: Infectious diseases. In: *Manual of Neurologic Therapeutics*. Samuels MA (editor). Little, Brown, 1978a.

Sagar SM: Toxic and metabolic disorders. In: *Manual of Neurologic Therapeutics*. Samuels MA (editor). Little, Brown, 1978b.

Schaffer D, Chadwick O, Rutter M: Psychiatric outcome of localized head injury in children. In: *Outcome of Severe Damage to the Central Nervous System*. CIBA Foundation Symposium 34. Elsevier, 1975.

Shaywitz S, Cohen DJ, Shaywitz BA: The biochemical basis of minimal brain dysfunction. *J Pediatr* 1978; 92:179–187.

Shurtleff DB: Myelodysplasia: Management and treatment. *Curr Probl Pediatr* 1980: 10(3):1–98.

Stare FJ, Whelan EM, Sheridan M: Diet and hyperactivity: Is there a relationship? *Pediatrics* 1980; 66:521–525.

Taft LT, Barabas G: Infants with delayed motor performance. *Nurs Clin North Am* (Feb) 1982; 29(1):137–149.

Teasdale G, Jennett B: Assessment of coma and impaired consciousness. A practical scale. *Lancet* 1974; 2:81–84.

Trauner DA: Diagnosis of Reye's syndrome. *J Natl Reye's Syndrome Foundation* 1981; 2(1):20–21.

Trauner DA: Treatment of Reye's syndrome. *J Natl Reye's Syndrome Foundation* 1980; 1(2):85–89.

US Centers for Disease Control: Rabies prevention. *MMWR* 1980; 29:279.

VanCaillie M, et al: Reye's syndrome: Relapses and neurological sequelae. *Pediatrics* (Feb) 1977; 59:244–249.

Walleck C: Head trauma in children. *Nurs Clin North Am* (March) 1980; 15(1):115–127.

Weil ML: Infections of the nervous system. In: *Textbook of Child Neurology*. Lea & Febiger, 1980.

Additional Readings

Aadelen SP, Stroebel-Kahn F: Coping with quadriplegia. *Am J Nurs* (Aug) 1981; 81(8):1471–1478.

Ahn H, et al: Developmental equations reflect brain dysfunctions. *Science* 1980; 210:1259–1262.

Algozzine B, Algozzine KM: Some practical considerations of hyperactivity and drugs. *J School Health* 1978; 48(8):479–483.

Apley J (editor): *Care of the Handicapped Child.* Vol 67. *Clinics in Developmental Medicine.* Heinemann, 1978.

Austin JK, McBride AB, Davis HW: Parental attitude and adjustment to childhood epilepsy. *Nurs Res* (March-April) 1984; 33(2):92–96.

Babcock JL: Spinal injuries in children from birth to 18 years. *Pediatr Clin North Am* 1975; 22:487.

Barnard KE, Erikson ML: *Teaching Children With Developmental Problems: A Family Care Approach.* 2nd ed. Mosby, 1976.

Bell WE: Increased intracranial pressure—diagnosis and management. *Curr Probl Pediatr* 1978; 8(4):3–62.

Bell WE, McCormick F: *Increased Intracranial Pressure in Children.* Saunders, 1978.

Benton AL, Pearl D (editors). *Dyslexia. An Appraisal of Current Knowledge.* Oxford University Press, 1978.

Bindler RM, Howry LB: Nursing care of children with febrile seizures. *Am J Matern Child Nurs* (Sept/Oct) 1979; 3(5):270–273.

Black P, Shepard RH, Walker AE: Outcome of head trauma: Age and post-traumatic seizures. In: *Outcome of Severe Damage to the Central Nervous System.* CIBA Foundation Symposium 34. Elsevier, 1975.

Bleck EE, Nagel DA (editors): *Physically Handicapped Children, A Medical Atlas for Teachers.* Grune & Stratton, 1982.

Bobath K: *A Neurophysiological Basis for the Treatment of Cerebral Palsy.* Vol 74. *Clinics in Developmental Medicine.* Spastics International, 1980.

Brown MS: How to tell if a baby has cerebral palsy . . . and what to tell his parents when he does. *Nursing 79* (May) 1979; 9(5):88—93.

Carlson CE: Psychosocial aspects of neurological disability. *Nurs Clin North Am* (June) 1980; 15(2):309–320.

Challenor YB: Orthoses for children. In: *The Child With Disabling Illness.* 2nd ed. Downey JA, Low NL (editors). Raven Press, 1982.

Choi MW: Birth crisis: Parental and professional responses to the birth of a child with a defect. *Issues Compr Pediatr Nurs* (Jan/Feb) 1978; 2(5):1–10.

Chusid JG: *Correlative Neuroanatomy and Functional Neurology.* 17th ed. Lange, 1979.

Clark RG: *Manter and Gatz's Essentials of Clinical Neuroanatomy and Neurophysiology.* 5th ed. Davis, 1975.

Colgan MT: The child with spina bifida, role of the pediatrician. *Am J Dis Child* 1981; 135:854–858.

Connolly R, Zewe GE: Update: Head injuries. *J Neurosurg Nurs* (Aug) 1981; 13(4):195–201.

Conway BL: Neurological assessment during the first year of life. *Curr Pract Pediatr Nurs* 1980; 3:98–113.

Conway BL: *Pediatric Neurological Nursing.* Mosby, 1977.

Coughlin MK: The child with epilepsy: Teaching children about their seizures and medication. *Am J Matern Child Nurs* (May/June) 1979; 4(3):161–162.

Coulter DL, Wu H, Allen RJ: Valproic acid therapy in childhood epilepsy. *JAMA* 1980; 244:785–788.

delCampo EJ: Accommodating the severely retarded child in our schools. *Am J Matern Child Nurs* (Jan/Feb) 1978; 3(1):34–37.

DeLong R, Glick TH: Encephalopathy of Reye's syndrome: A review of pathogenetic hypotheses. *Pediatrics* (Jan) 1982; 69(1):53–65.

Downey JA, Low NL (editors): *The Child With Disabling Illness.* 2nd ed. Raven Press, 1982.

Dubey DR, Kaufman KF: Home management of hyperkinetic children. *J Pediatr* 1978; 93:141.

Eddington C, Lee T: Sensory motor stimulation for slow-to-develop children. A home-centered program for parents. *Am J Nurs* (Jan) 1975; 75(1):59–62.

Farley JN: Valproic acid for children with uncontrolled epilepsy. *Am J Matern Child Nurs* (May/June) 1979; 4(3):163–164.

Finnie N: *Handling the Young Cerebral Palsied Child at Home.* E.P. Dutton, 1975.

Flammang M, Hohm J: The child with Reye's syndrome. *Nursing 76* (March) 1976; 6:80c–80e.

Frye BA: Brain injury and family education needs. *Rehabil Nurs* (July-Aug) 1982:27–28.

Gerson LP, Singleton EB: Computerized tomography in the pediatric patient. *Curr Probl Pediatr Pract* 1979; 9(6):1–32.

Gliebe WA: Involuntary deviance: School and epileptic children. *J School Health* 1979; 5(5):325–329.

Grow DH: Reye's syndrome. *Nursing 81* (Nov) 1981; 11:156–158.

Golden SS: Nonstandard therapies of the developmental disabilities. *Am J Dis Child* 1980; 134(5):487–491.

Haughey CW: What to say . . . and do . . . when your patient asks about CT scans. *Nursing 81* (Dec) 1981; 11(12):72–77.

Hawken M: Epilepsy nurse specialist. *Nursing 78* (Sept) 1978; 8(9):114–119.

Hawken M, Ozuna J: Practical aspects of anticonvulsant therapy. *Am J Nurs* (June) 1979; 79(6):1062–1068.

Hill ML: Meningomyelocele: The child and the family. *Issues Compr Pediatr Nurs* (Jan/Feb) 1978; 2(5):51–63.

Hussey CG: Surviving a handicap in everyday life: How to help. *Am J Matern Child Nurs* (Jan/Feb) 1979; 4(1):46–50.

Jennett B, Teasdale G, Knill-Jones R: Prognosis after severe head injury. In: *Outcome of Severe Damage to the Central Nervous System.* CIBA Foundation Symposium 34. Elsevier, 1975.

Leonidas JC, et al: Mild head trauma in children: When is a roentgenogram necessary? *Pediatrics* (Feb) 1982; 69(2):139–143.

Lepler M: Having a handicapped child. *Am J Matern Child Nurs* (Jan/Feb) 1978; 3(1):32–33.

Levine MB, Melmed RD: The unhappy wanderers: Children with attention deficits. *Pediatr Clin North Am* 1982; 29(1):105–120.

Lynch WJ, Mauss NK: Brain injury rehabilitation: Standard problem lists. *Arch Phys Med Rehabil* (May) 1981; 62:223–227.

MacKeith R: The feelings and behavior of parents of handicapped children. *Dev Med Child Neurol* 1973; 15:524–527.

Manz HJ, Colon AR, McCullogh DC: Neuropathology of Reye's syndrome—acute and chronic changes. *J Natl Reye's Syndrome Foundation* 1980; 1(2):80–82.

Mills G: Preparing children and parents for cerebral computerized tomography . . . in pediatric ambulatory settings and in hospital units. *Am J Matern Child Nurs* (Nov/Dec) 1980; 5:403.

Mitchell PH, Mauss NK: Relationship of patient–nurse activity to intracranial pressure variations: A pilot study. *Nurs Res* (Jan/Feb) 1978; 27(1):4–10.

National Institute of Health (NIH) Consensus Development Conference Summary: *The Diagnosis and Treatment of Reye's Syndrome.* Government Printing Office, 1981.

Nezamis FK: The child with a head, nurse. *Issues Compr Pediatr Nurs* (Jul/Aug) 1977; 2(2):29–37.

Norman SE: Surgical treatment of epilepsy. *Am J Nurs* (May) 1981; 81(5):994–996.

Norman SE, Browne TR: Seizure disorders. *Am J Nurs* (May) 1981; 81(5):984–994.

Parrish MA: A comparison of behavioral side effects related to commonly used anticonvulsants. *Pediatr Nurs* 1984; 10(2):149–152.

Perude P: Urgent priorities in severe trauma: Life-threatening head and spinal injuries. *RN* (June) 1981; 44(6):36–41, 102.

Rimel RW: Emergency management of the patient with central nervous system trauma. *J Neurosurg Nurs* (Dec) 1978; 10(4):185–188.

Ross AJ, et al: Neuromuscular diagnostic procedures. *Nurs Clin North Am* (March) 1979; 14(1):107–121.

Samuels MA (editor): *Manual of Neurologic Therapeutics*. Little, Brown, 1978.

Sands H, Minters FC: *The Epilepsy Fact Book*. Scribners, 1977.

Santilli N, et al: Screening for seizures. *Pediatr Nurs* (March/April) 1981; 7(2):11–15.

Shearer D, Collins B, Creel D: Preparing a patient for EEG. *Am J Nurs* (Jan) 1975; 75(1):63–64.

Sherman FS: Pediatric management problems: Cerebral palsy. *Pediatr Nurs* (March/April) 1981; 7(2):31.

Shonkoff J, et al: Primary care approaches to developmental disabilities. *Pediatrics* (Oct) 1979; 64:506.

Slimmer LW: Helping parents cope with their child's seizure disorder. *J Psychiatr Nurs* (Feb) 1979; 17(2):30–33.

Stone BH: Computerized transaxial brain scan. *Am J Nurs* (Oct) 1977; 77:1601–1604.

Strub RL, Black FW: *Organic Brain Syndromes*. Davis, 1981.

Surveyer JA: Coma in children: How it affects parents. *Am J Matern Child Nurs* (Jan/Feb) 1976; 1(1):17–21.

Surveyer JA: The emotional toll on nurses who care for comatose children. *Am J Matern Child Nurs* (July/Aug) 1976; 1(4):243–248.

Swift N: Helping patients live with seizures. *Nursing 78* (June) 1978; 8(6):24–31.

Swisher JD: Developmental restaging: Meeting the mental health needs of handicapped students in the schools. *J School Health* 1978; 48(9):548–550.

Tucker CA: Complex partial seizures. *Am J Nurs* (May) 1981; 81(5):996–1000.

Tudor M: Nursing intervention with developmentally disabled children. *Am J Matern Child Nurs* (Jan/Feb) 1978; 3(1):25–31.

Volk DM: Reye's syndrome: An update for the practicing physician. *Clin Pediatr* 1978; 20(8):505–511.

Willis JK, Oppenheimer EY: Children's seizures and their management. *Issues Compr Pediatr Nurs* (Jul/Aug) 1977; 2(2):54–67.

Wink D: Bacterial meningitis in children. *Am J Nurs* (April) 1984; 84:456–460.

Wolf S: Controversies in the treatment of febrile convulsions. *Neurology* 1979; 29:287–290.

Perception and Communication

Implications of Impaired Sensory Function

43

Charlotte M. Spicher

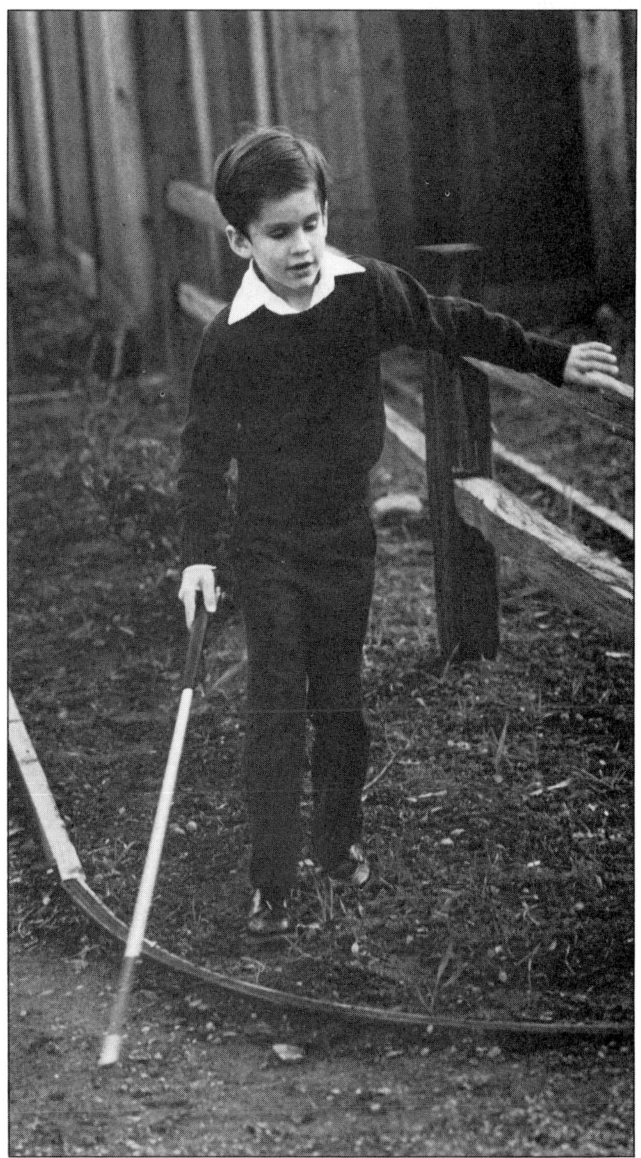

Chapter Outline

continued on next page

Objectives

- Describe how perception and communication are affected by alterations in sensory organs.
- Describe the anatomy and physiology of the eye, ear, and oral cavity.
- Delineate the information obtained from the nursing assessment of a child with a sensory dysfunction, including data from the history, physical assessment, and diagnostic studies.
- List the principles of nursing care related to nursing a child with alterations in sensory function, including acute-care, nutritional, developmental, emotional, and health maintenance needs.
- Describe the nursing approach in the care of a child with a specific problem affecting the eye, the ear, and nasal and oral cavities.
- Identify the interruptions in development of the child who is blind, deaf, or speech impaired.

It is through the perception of events and communication of ideas and feelings that infants and children come to understand the world around them. Any alteration in either perceptive or communicative abilities impinges on successful development and particularly can affect the attachment process between the parent and child.

The senses of vision, hearing, taste, smell, and touch are the vehicles through which children gain perception, whereas language is the major tool of communication. The sensory systems of infants and children are especially sensitive to malfunction, and when malfunction occurs, the potential impact on overall development is great. For this reason, prompt recognition of inadequate or abnormal sensory function is essential.

Nurses are often in a position to first recognize deviations from normal sensory function as they care for newborn infants and practice in primary care settings such as well-child clinics and schools. Nurses also play an important role in minimizing the long-term effects and maximizing rehabilitative efforts after acute, chronic, or permanent changes in sensory function. In this way the impact of sensory malfunctions on the child's development can be reduced.

In this chapter we examine the functions of the sensory system as they relate to perception and communication. This includes a brief review of the anatomy and physiology of the eye, ear, and oral cavity, the nursing assessment of a child with sensory dysfunction, including a description of the common diagnostic and screening tests, and nursing management for selected specific conditions affecting the sensory organs.

Anatomy and Physiology of the Sensory Organs

The Eye

The developing eye is first evident in the twenty-second day of embryonic development. A pair of shallow grooves appears on either side of the forebrain. By the eighth gestational week, the ectoderm, mesoderrn, and neuroderm have differentiated into the tissues of the eye and take the forms described in the following discussion of the normal anatomy of the eye. The retina continues to develop, and myelinization of the optic nerve fibers is complete at the time of birth. During the first 4 months of life, the foveal retinal receptors differentiate, completing eye development. In caucasians the iris usually is blue or dark gray at birth; pigmentation occurs in the early months of life.

The eye is a marvelously compact and complex organ that consists of three layers, each with specific and cooperative functions. The outer layer consists of the *opaque sclera,* or white of the eye, and the transparent *cornea.*

Through the cornea can be seen the *iris,* the round, shutterlike, colored portion of the eye, with its open center, the *pupil.* The iris is a muscular organ that contracts or expands to regulate the passage of light into the eye. The *lens* lies posterior to the iris, positioned behind the pupil. The lens is suspended by the ciliary muscles. The iris, lens, and ciliary body, together with the choroid or vascular lining, constitute the middle layer. The inner layer, the *retina,* can be seen only with the aid of an ophthalmoscope. The retina contains the end-organs of sight, the *rods* and *cones,* which receive the light stimulus and send messages via the optic nerve to the brain, where light stimulus is interpreted into vision. When viewed through an ophthalmoscope, certain important structures can be assessed: the *macula,* in which the greatest concentration of nerve endings is found and the area on which incoming light is focused by the lens, and the *optic disk,* through which the optic nerve enters the orb. In addition, large blood vessels, both arteries and veins, can be seen. These blood vessels branch into smaller vessels in the choroid layer and nourish the eye tissues (see Fig. 14-5).

The ovoid shape and tension of the eye surface is maintained by two separate chambers: the anterior chamber, between the lens and cornea, which is filled with a clear serous fluid *(aqueous humor),* and the posterior chamber, between the lens and the retina, which is filled with the jellylike *vitreous humor.* The integrity of the eye and its functions depend on the maintenance of normal pressure in each chamber.

The eye is attached to the bony structures of the skull with six muscles. These muscles not only hold the orbs in the proper position but also move the two orbs in their sockets in coordination with each other so that binocular vision is achieved. The orb is protected by the upper and lower *eyelids,* muscular sheaths lined with conjunctiva. The *conjunctiva* is the vascular lining, which secretes mucus to lubricate the surface of the eye. The conjunctiva also extends over the surface of the sclera. Additional lubrication is provided by the secretion of tears from the *lacrimal gland,* which is located in the upper outer portion of the orbit. Excess tears are drained through the inner canthus of the eye to the nasal cavity via the lacrimal duct.

The image of an object is focused on the retina when light passes through the lens of the eye and stimulates the nerve endings in the retina. The impulses are transmitted via the optic nerve to the brain, where the sensory data are processed.

The process of focusing light on the retina is called *refraction* and involves the corneal curvature, the shape of the lens, and the length of the eye. *Accommodation,* the ability of the eye to focus on objects at varying distances, is achieved through changes in the lens structure. The shape of the lens curvature changes through tension and relaxation of the ciliary muscles to permit proper focusing of the light from objects at various distances from the eye.

Infants once were believed to have very little visual acuity, but more recent studies reveal the ability of infants to show preferences for patterns and colors (see Chapter 7). Depth perception even has been demonstrated in 2-month-old infants (Franz and Nevis, 1968; Campos, Langer, and Krowitz, 1970).

The Ear

Embryonic development of the ear begins with the internal ear. Early in the fourth week of gestation, a thickened plate of ectoderm appears on each side of the hindbrain. Middle ear development begins as a recess of the first pharyngeal pouch around the sixth week of gestation. The external ear develops from the first branchial groove after the fifth week of gestation. The three divisions of the ear continue to develop and gradually join together. As the mandible forms, the ears move to the sides of the head at the level of the eyes. This process is not completed until about the thirty-second week of gestation. The sensitive period for disruption in ear development extends through the middle of the ninth week of gestation.

The ear is another complex structure, consisting of three parts: the external ear, middle ear, and inner ear. The *outer ear* includes the *cartilaginous shell,* the *auricle,* and the *external ear canal,* which extends from the auricle through the bony skull to the middle ear. The auricle and canal are covered with skin; however, the lining of the canal also contains cells that secrete *cerumen* (earwax). Cerumen prevents the lining tissues of the canal from drying out and forms a barrier against insects and dirt (see Figure 14-9).

The *middle ear* is separated from the ear canal by a membranous structure, the *tympanum,* or eardrum. The middle ear contains three bones or ossicles: the *malleus,* the *incus,* and the *stapes.* The ossicles are connected to one another and suspended in the middle ear, touching the tympanum on one side and the membrane that covers the opening to the inner ear on the other side. The middle ear has a secretory lining. There is also an opening to the *eustachian tube,* a passage from the middle ear to the nasopharynx. This passageway permits excess secretions to drain from the middle ear and allows for air to enter from the throat so that the pressure in the middle ear is identical to that of the external ear canal. This equalized pressure facilitates maximum function of the tympanic membrane. The *inner ear* contains the nerve endings for hearing, which are embedded in the walls of a fluid-filled chamber. There are three additional fluid-filled chambers, called *semicircular canals.* Each semicircular canal is oriented to a different plane (horizontal, vertical, or oblique) and has a secretory lining in which nerve endings are embedded. These nerve endings are receptors for balance.

The function of hearing is accomplished by the conduction of sound through air and fluid. Vibrations are initiated in the source of sound (such as a musical instrument or a voice). Sound waves travel through air to the external ear and impinge on the tympanum. The tympanum vibrates, causing the ossicles to move. The movements of the ossicles are transmitted into the fluid in the inner ear chamber and from there to the auditory nerve endings. It is possible to bypass the external and middle ear air transmission by applying sound wave vibration directly to the bony skull and from there to the inner ear, which is embedded in the cranium (see Chapter 14).

It was once believed that neonates were unable to hear because of amniotic fluid-filled eustachian tubes. It is now known that infants are able to discern sounds and discriminate between sounds, recognizing familiar voices even in utero. Infants respond more readily to high-pitched sounds, which is probably why they respond more readily to a female voice (see Chapter 7). The assessment of auditory acuity of infants is limited to eliciting startle responses or noting alerting responses in infants when a sound is made.

The Oral Cavity

The oral cavity is a rich source of sensations for the infant and child. Taste buds are very sensitive to stimuli and are much more numerous in infants' mouths than in adults' mouths. Taste buds contain the end-organs for the perceptions of salt, sweet, sour, and bitter (Fig. 43-1).

The infant's mouth is shaped to facilitate sucking: thick fat pads in the cheeks, tongue movements, the suck reflex, and the gag reflex are all operational at birth. As infants mature, by about 6 months of age, they are able to control tongue movements to move solid food into their mouths and are able to approximate the edge of a spoon or the rim of a cup with their lips. These new skills signal a readiness to assume more mature eating styles. The infant's production of sound depends on the proper formation of the oral cavity. Immediately after birth, infants can vary the volume and quality of their cry. They soon begin to make sounds that resemble human speech in the range of tone, variation in volume, and cadence. By the end of the first year, many children use words successfully to communicate with adults.

Continued development of the oral cavity during late infancy and early childhood involves the eruption of teeth and the further refinement of the muscular movement of the tongue, cheeks, throat, and diaphragm in the production of sounds and speech. The precise articulation of sounds requires the use of all of the oral structures and control of air past the vocal cords.

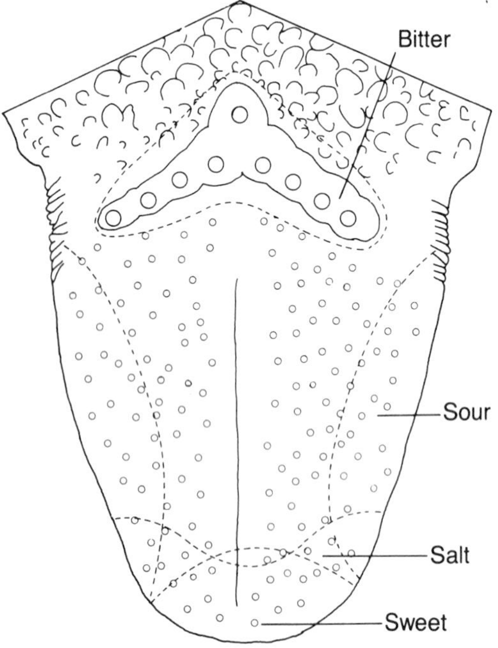

Figure 43-1 Areas of the tongue that are most sensitive to particular taste sensations. (From Vick R: *Contemporary Medical Physiology*. Addison-Wesley, 1984.)

Assessment of a Child With Sensory Dysfunction

History

The nursing history related to a child with sensory dysfunction includes all the elements recommended for the initial interview for any child entering a health care facility (see Chapter 29). For the child with a sensory problem, however, certain aspects of the history deserve special emphasis.

Prenatal history is important because the crucial time of embryonic development of the sensory organs is early in the gestational period, during the first trimester of pregnancy. By the fourth week of gestation, the eyes, ears, nose, and jaws are beginning to form. By the eighth week of gestation, the eyes, ears, jaws, and nose are essentially complete. The palate closes by the twelfth gestational week, thus completing the formation of the oral cavity. Although fully formed, these structures continue to grow larger during fetal life. Interruptions in development during the later weeks of fetal life or alterations in sensory function as a result of premature birth also pose threats to the infant. For example, retrolental fibroplasia and resultant blindness are still potential sequelae of premature birth. Retrolental fibroplasia causes damage to the retina from the high concentrations of oxygen given to a premature infant after delivery.

Information should be obtained about several maternal factors when compiling the history. Maternal infections and the use of drugs or alcohol might either lead to maternal malnutrition or affect fetal development directly. Rubella and other viral infections have the potential to cause hearing, visual, and neurologic deficits in the developing fetus.

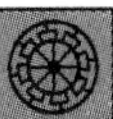

ASSESSMENT GUIDE Child With Impaired Sensory Function

System	Subjective data	Objective data	Validating data	Nursing management
Head	Headache. Tenderness over facial sinuses. Recent upper respiratory infection or allergy	Thick nasal discharge. Elevated temperature. Edema over sinuses	Transillumination of sinus Radiographic studies of sinus	Teach antibiotic compliance and the proper use of decongestants. Encourage the prompt treatment of upper respiratory infections or allergy
Eye, ear, nose, and throat				
Eye	Family history of eye disorders. Decreased visual acuity. Alteration in depth perception. Double vision. Presence of a neuromuscular deficit such as cerebral palsy	Decreased eye contact or exploratory behavior. Squinting for close or distant vision. Observable deviation of one or both eyes (strabismus). Abnormal corneal light reflex. Clumsiness or stumbling behaviors	Tests for visual acuity: Snellen charts Allen cards STYCAR (Screening Test for Young Children and Retardates) test Optokinetic drum DEST (Denver Eye Screening Test) Corneal light reflex Cover test	Prepare the child for the eye examination as appropriate for developmental level. Obtain information from the parent about exploratory behavior and school performance. Describe any routine eye exercises or patching patterns on the nursing care plan and encourage parents to follow through with exercise or patching routines. Review the proper care of eyeglasses or contact lenses. Explore the child's body image concerns
	History of prenatal maternal infection or premature birth. Rapid loss of vision. Sudden, moderate headache. Photophobia. Documented chromosome aberrations. Poor night vision. Blindness	Corneal haze and enlarged corneal diameter in infants. Tonometry readings of over 22 mm Hg (Saxton, et al., 1983). Opacity of the lens. Absence of the red reflex on fundoscopic examination. Inability of the infant to fixate	Ophthalmoscopic examination Tonometry Tests for visual acuity	Prepare the child and family for glaucoma or cataract surgery and postoperative management. Encourage the parent to provide early visual stimulation to maximize visual function in the unaffected eye
	Pain. Photophobia. Itching. Feeling of foreign body in the eye. Fever	Moderate to heavy purulent discharge. Erythematous conjunctiva. Periorbital edema. Corneal ulceration apparent after fluorescein staining	Culture and sensitivity of discharge Fluorescein stain	Teach the family proper medication administration and compliance. Apply warm compresses or irrigations to the affected eye. Teach measures to prevent the spread of infection. Encourage the use of sunglasses for photophobia
	Recent blunt or penetrating trauma to the eye. Pain—often not in proportion to the injury. Feeling of a foreign body in the eye. Headache. History of exposure to chemicals, heat, or ultraviolet light	Visible evidence of eye injury. Presence of blood in anterior chamber (hyphema). Red reflex not visible on fundoscopic examination	Radiographic studies might reveal presence of foreign body or bony damage	See Chapter 19 for first aid and prevention of injury. Refer immediately for ophthalmologic evaluation. Explore feelings of guilt with the child and family. Maintain quiet environment for the child with hyphema. Institute measures to prevent sensory deprivation. Observe closely for signs of retinal detachment

continued on next page

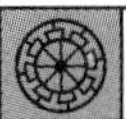

ASSESSMENT GUIDE Child With Impaired Sensory Function (continued)

System	Subjective data	Objective data	Validating data	Nursing management
Eye (cont.)		Failure to discriminate color	Ishihara test (see Chapter 18)	Safety education about alternative methods of recognizing traffic signs and signals
	Pain. Fatigue. Anorexia. Weight loss	Unilateral nystagmus. Strabismus. Change in the color of the iris. Loss of visual acuity. Unequal pupils.		See Chapter 45 for care of the child with aberrant cellular growth
Ear	Familial hearing disorders. Maternal infection during pregnancy. History of neonatal kernicterus or hypoxia. History of mumps, meningitis, or other viral infections. Extensive use of medications known to be toxic to the ear	Abnormalities of the external ear. Delayed or distorted speech. Decrease in babbling after 6 months of age. Abnormal results of routine hearing test. Consistently loud speech. Seeming inattention to environment	Evoked brain stem potential test Crib-o-gram Pure tone audiometry Weber or Rinne tuning fork test Speech reception and discrimination tests	Note the infant's reflex response to sound. Elicit information about early speech development, environmental stimuli, poor school performance, and seeming disregard of parental requests. Attract a deaf child's attention through touch prior to talking. When talking, face the child and speak slowly. Use a sign interpreter if the child has learned signing. Review the principles for proper care and maintenance of a hearing aid
	Fever. Pain in the ear. Repeated ear infections, respiratory allergies, or chronic nasal obstruction. Complaints of poor school performance. History of ear trauma	Bulging, red, or gray tempanic membrane. Decreased auditory acuity. Drainage from the ear. Infant tugging at ear. Feeling of fullness in ear	Otoscopic examination Tympanometry	Teach the importance of following the medication regimen for otitis media. Encourage the prompt treatment of respiratory allergies. Prepare the child for surgery and postoperative management
Nose	Alteration in the sense of smell and taste	Malodorous or blood-tinged discharge. Rhinorrhea		See Chapter 26 for the management of rhinitis. Refer to physician if foreign object is suspected
Throat and mouth	Cleft palate. History of feeding difficulties. History of trauma to the central nervous system. Sore throat	Aphasia. Delayed development of speech. Decreased vocalization. Articulatory or fluency dysfunction. Vocal changes. Tongue thrust not corrected by 7 or 8 years of age	Auditory screening Denver articulation screening examination (DAST)	Examine the child for defects in the palate. Observe for a lack of environmental stimulation or overly high parental expectations. Give slow, careful explanations to children with receptive language disorders

ASSESSMENT GUIDE Child With Impaired Sensory Function (continued)

System	Subjective data	Objective data	Validating data	Nursing management
Gastrointestinal	Anorexia. Alterations in taste. Abdominal pain	Vomiting		Observe for signs of otitis media
Neurologic	Lack of sensation in hands or feet. Decreased sensation of touch. History of spina bifida or other central nervous system disorder			Teach the child and family the principles of safety when in contact with heat or cold. See Chapter 42

The maternal use of alcohol might result in the fetal alcohol syndrome (see Chapter 23), which is a syndrome characterized by irreversibly deficient growth, motor deficiencies, mental retardation, and craniofacial anomalies. Even prescription drugs can cause fetal damage, especially if taken during the first trimester of pregnancy. Increasing concern has focused on the possible adverse influences that environmental pollutants or other environmental factors might have on fetal development.

Sensory dysfunctions might be genetically transmitted, for example, those associated with facial clefts, cataracts, strabismus, glaucoma, and nerve deafness. For this reason, information about family members should be elicited. A pedigree (see Fig. 5-10) should be constructed to include both paternal and maternal families through the two preceding generations and the present generation at least to the identification of first cousins, if possible (see Chapter 5). The nurse elicits information about the presence or history of any congenital anomaly in the family, including those other than the one affecting the patient. Some congenital anomalies are related to one another such as cleft lip, cleft palate, and widely spaced eyes *(hypertelorism)*.

A careful description of the child's development is essential, beginning with very early infancy. Useful information includes when the child first began to attend to the parent's voice or sought eye contact and when the child first began to explore the environment through visual scanning, reaching, and creeping. The Denver Developmental Screening Test (Appendix C) can be used to remind the nurse what questions should be asked to obtain a complete developmental history (see Chapter 16).

The nurse also questions the parent about the specific sensory deficit. For example, if impaired vision is suspected, the nurse asks such questions as whether the child squints while watching television and how far away from the television set the child prefers to sit. The answers to specific questions such as these can yield important information related to the sensory systems of an infant or child. These specific items include reflexive and deliberate responses of the infant or child to stimuli, coordination skills, feeding difficulties, and speech and language patterns. Documentation of these data can be helpful in the diagnosis of neurologic disease, in the assessment of any developmental delay related to the sensory dysfunction, and in the identification of areas of development in which remedial or educational efforts should be applied.

The history includes data about past infections: the site of the infection, course of the illness, treatment and medications used, and age of the child at the time of the illness. These data are useful in understanding the cause of sensory loss or dysfunction. Hearing loss may be caused by recurrent ear infections in which the eardrum was ruptured. The rupture may heal with a scar that reduces the sensitivity of the eardrum to sound waves, resulting in a loss of hearing acuity. Some antibiotics, such as streptomycin, can cause permanent damage to the auditory nerve. The long-term or repeated use of such drugs might be related to nerve deafness. In addition, a history of infections can suggest areas for health teaching to help the parent recognize infections earlier or prevent their occurrence.

A history of trauma can be equally useful as a diagnostic aid or an impetus for anticipatory guidance (see Chapter 21). Data about each trauma should include the child's age at the time of the injury; circumstances surrounding the trauma, such as the time of day, setting, and degree of supervision; site of the injury; treatment and medications used; and the healing process. Head trauma might result in speech, hearing, or vision difficulties. Direct trauma to the eye or ear may cause permanent sequelae. A history of frequent accidents and trauma might be related to an undetected loss of visual or auditory acuity or motor dysfunction in the child. The history and a thorough physical examination of the child are essential to detect sensory deficits and to rule out parental neglect or abuse.

Although health histories generally include queries about the home environment, some home environmental factors are especially important in assessing problems of hearing, vision, or speech. The amount of environmental stimulation can influence the child's attentiveness to stimuli. Some busy, disorganized households include adults who continually shout at the children, and the children soon learn what sounds or messages are safely disregarded. This lack of attention might be puzzling to adults, who become concerned about the children's hearing acuity. On the other hand, if too little stimulation is present, the child might become apathetic and fail to attend or might become fearful and vigilant when in a noisy environment. Children who are not spoken to develop speech more slowly than children whose caregivers talk to them. Children who are spoken to mimic adult speech and receive positive reinforcement from adult responses to their early efforts at language. Children who live in crowded, economically deprived homes might be more vulnerable to ear and eye infections because of close contact with many other people, poor hygiene, or inadequate nutrition. If these environmental factors are identified and changed early, sensory development may be corrected and parental concerns removed. (Assessment of family communication is discussed in Chapter 17. The risk factors associated with dysfunctional family systems are discussed in Chapter 22.)

In addition to general questions, the nurse probes or encourages the parent to provide specific information about the child's behavior that could be related to sensory deficits. Changes in motor skills, decreased attention span, an increase in disruptive behavior, or changes in voice tones or volume might indicate decreased visual or auditory acuity. If changes are noted early and treatment is begun, permanent damage can be avoided or reduced.

A history of specific physical complaints of dizziness, headache, nausea, or vomiting also might serve as a diagnostic aid. It is important to record the onset of the symptom, whether it is continuous or intermittent, concurrent with events or situations, and the frequency and duration of its occurrence. In addition, any other condition or syndrome should be noted, regardless of whether it is associated with the sensory problem. The plan of care must take into account the child's overall physical condition.

Diagnostic Tests

Table 43-1 summarizes the diagnostic tests used to assess sensory function. Two additional objective tests may be included in the assessment of the function of the middle ear. These are static compliance, or balance between mobility and stiffness of the ossicles and the membranes, and acoustic reflex thresholds, or the objective loudness requirement.

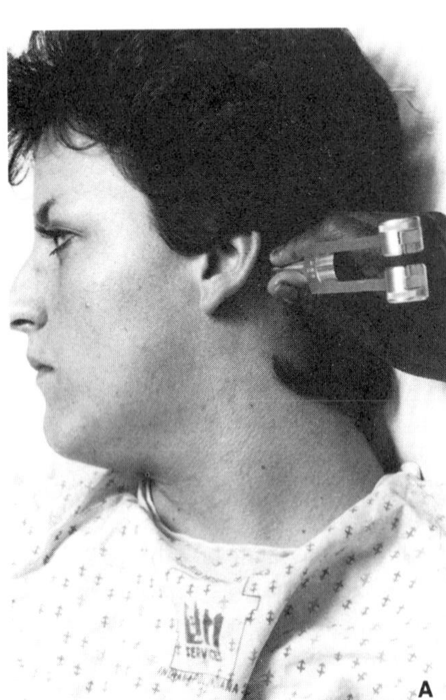

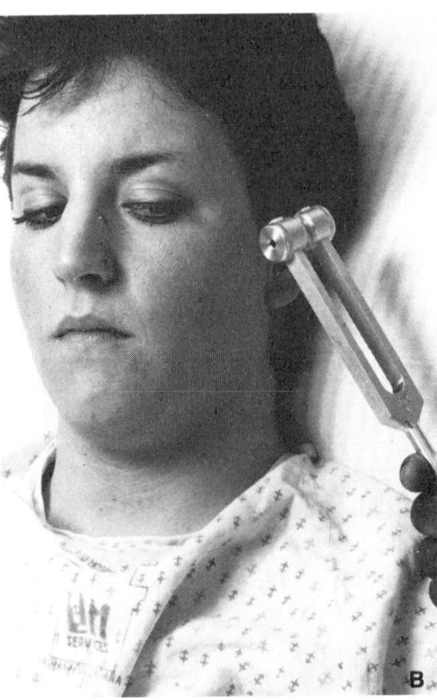

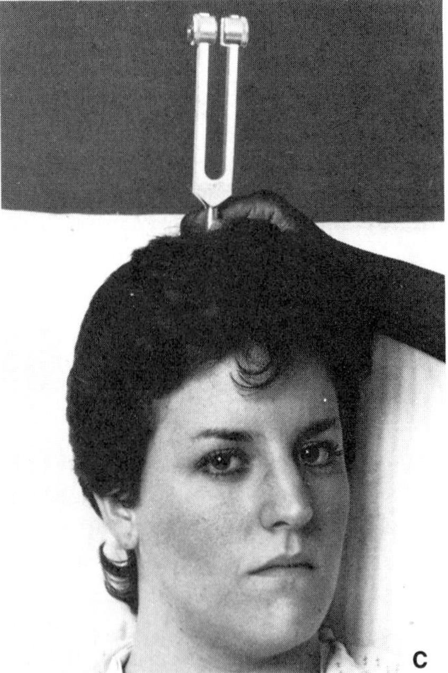

Rinne and Weber tests. *A.* For the Rinne test, the child covers one ear, and the activated tuning fork is placed on the mastoid process of the uncovered ear. The nurse notes the amount of time during which the child heard the sound. *B.* Prongs of the tuning fork are moved in front of the uncovered ear. Unless the child has conductive hearing loss, the child should be able to hear the sound twice as long in this position. *C.* In the Weber test, the activated tuning fork is placed on top of the child's head; normally, the child hears the sound equally in both ears. (From Swearingen PL: *The Addison-Wesley Photo-Atlas of Nursing Procedures.* Addison-Wesley, 1984. p. 627.)

TABLE 43-1 Diagnostic Tests Related to Altered Sensory Function

Test	Description	Preparation
Visual acuity measurement Snellen charts	Alphabet chart; E chart (see Chapter 14)	See Chapter 14; can be used only with children old enough to follow directions
Allen cards	Schematic picture cards (see Chapter 14)	See Chapter 14
STYCAR test (Screening Test for Young Children and Retardates)	Consists of a chart with the letters T, H, V, and O set up in rows of decreasing size letters; also, a set of four cards, each of which is inscribed with one of the four letters; children are asked to match the designated letter with one of the cards in their hands	Children should be encouraged to stand at the prescribed distance from the chart
Optokinetic drum (for infants)	A drum with alternating black and white stripes is rotated before the infant's eyes to elicit nystagmus (involuntary eye movements); stripes of decreasing width are presented and visual acuity is the point at which the nystagmus disappears	The infant should be well rested and fed prior to the test to maintain attention and visual fixation on the drum.
Other tests for infant visual acuity	Involve presenting disks of varied width, alternating black and white stripes against a gray background to the right or left of the infant's visual field; an independent observer judges whether the infant's eyes move in the direction of the disk; facial outlines in black and white stripes have been used instead of striped disks; visual acuity is determined by the infant's ability to discriminate the stripes from the gray background.	The parents need to be informed that the infant's eyes will be patched one at a time; the infant should be well rested and fed prior to the test; the infant may sit on the parent's lap during the test
DEST (Denver Eye Screening Test)	Combination of Snellen E, Allen cards, and tests used to assess eye and extraocular muscle function (see Chapter 14); test distance is 15 ft; the 2- to 3-year-old child's acuity is normal if three of seven Allen cards are identified; older children demonstrate 20/30 vision if the E is correctly positioned in one of three trials; infants are checked for visual fixation by presentation of a moving toy, checking the pupil light reflex, and the cover test (See Fig. 43-2)	
Tonometry	Screens for glaucoma; the child's eyes are anesthetized and the child is placed in a recumbent position; after asking the child to fixate, intraocular pressure is measured with the tonometer	Can only be done with an older, cooperative child. A thorough explanation of the procedure is necessary to ensure cooperation
Auditory acuity measurement Crib-o-gram	Measures the infant's arousal response to sound; the infant is placed on a motion-sensitive recording device; motor activity is recorded before, during, and after the presentation of sounds; infant response includes the presence of a Moro reflex or turning in the direction of the sound	None
Evoked brain stem potential test	Electrodes which record changes in brain stem potential when sounds are introduced are placed on the infant's head	The parent should be aware that the infant might have to be restrained while the electrodes are in place
Audiometry	Headphones or earphones are placed on the child, and tones of varying frequencies are presented one ear at a time; the child indicates by raising a hand when the tone is heard (see Chapter 18 for frequencies measured)	The child must be able to follow directions. The tester needs to check the child's understanding of the directions given
Tuning fork test (Weber)	The tester activates the tuning fork and holds the handle against the midline of the child's head; sound should be equal in both ears; tests for bone and air conduction	The child needs to know what to listen for and that vibrations might be felt on the head
Tuning fork test (Rinne)	Fork tines are placed near the child's ear canal; tests air conduction of sound	
Tympanometry	An airtight probe is fitted into the external ear canal, and pressure and movement of the tympanum are recorded electronically; a flat tracing on the graph (Fig. 43-3b) indicates excessive middle ear pressure	The child should be told that the probe will not hurt. An explanation of the procedure ensures cooperation
Articulation screening DASE (Denver Articulation Screening Examination)	Children age $2\frac{1}{2}$ to 6 years are asked to repeat 22 one- and two-syllable words spoken by the tester; the score is derived from the number of correctly articulated sounds and compared with percentile-ranked scores by age to assess normal language development; the tester makes a judgment regarding overall intelligibility of the child's speech, which also is ranked by age	None. If performance is abnormal, the child should be screened for auditory acuity

DENVER EYE SCREENING TEST

Name
Hospital No.
Ward
Address

Vision Tests	1ST SCREENING:DATE						RESCREENING:DATE					
	Right Eye			Left Eye			Right Eye			Left Eye		
	Normal	Abnormal	Untestable	Normal	Abnormal	Untestable	Normal	Abnormal	Untestable	Normal	Abnormal	Untestable
1. "E" (3 years and above-3 to 5 trials)	3P	3F	U	3P	3F	U	3P	3F	U	3P	3F	U
2. Picture Card (2 1/2 - 2 11/12 yrs.-3 to 5 trials)	3P	3F	U	3P	3F	U	3P	3F	U	3P	3F	U
3. Fixation (6 months - 2 5/12 years)	P	F	U	P	F	U	P	F	U	P	F	U
4. Squinting		yes			yes			yes			yes	

Tests for Non-Straight Eyes	1ST SCREENING: Normal	Abnormal	Untestable	RESCREENING: Normal	Abnormal	Untestable
1. Do your child's eyes turn in or out, or are they ever not straight?	NO	YES	U	NO	YES	U
2. Cover Test	P	F	U	P	F	U
3. Pupillary Light Reflex	P	F	U	P	F	U

Total Test Rating (Both Eyes)	1ST SCREENING	RESCREENING
Normal (passed vision test plus no squint, plus passed 2/3 tests for non-straight eyes)	Normal	Normal
Abnormal (abnormal on any vision test, squinting or 2 of 3 procedures for non-straight eyes)	Abnormal	Abnormal
Untestable (untestable on any vision test or untestable on 2/3 tests for non-straight eyes)	Untestable	Untestable
Future Rescreening Appointment for Total Test Rating (Abnormal or Untestable)	Date:	Date:

Figure 43-2 Denver Eye Screening Test. Reprinted with permission of William K. Frankenburg, MD. University of Colorado Medical Center.

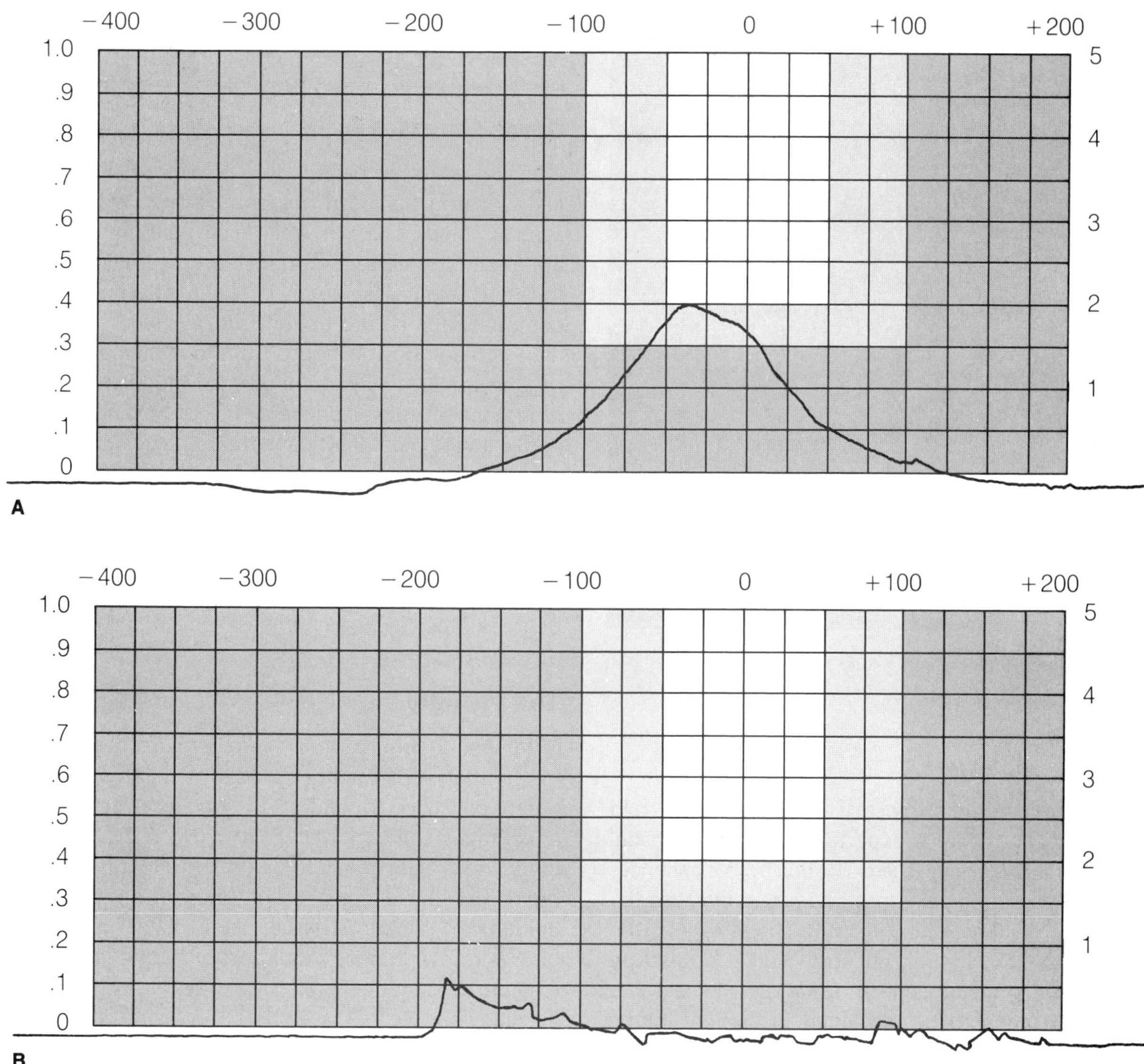

Figure 43-3 *A.* Normal tympanograph. *B.* Abnormal tympanograph.

These are not screening tests but may be used in conjunction with audiometry to supply diagnostic data about the ear and hearing functions. Assessment of speech adequacy depends on listening to a child's verbalizations. When the nurse listens to spontaneous speech, the general intelligibility of the child's speech and the correctness of the articulation of specific vowels and consonants can be identified. These data should be noted in detail in the health record so that any changes can be discerned. The nurse also documents any speech dysfunction such as lisp, stuttering, and consistent substitution of one letter sound for another.

Assessment of taste can be accomplished by giving the child a variety of substances that will elicit a response from the taste buds in the appropriate section of the tongue. Sugar affects taste at the tip; salt is perceived in the forward portion; lemon elicits a sour taste in the middle of the tongue; and quinine's bitterness demonstrates taste bud activity in the back. The child should rinse the mouth with water between each taste for a more accurate response (Systems of Life #88, 1982).

Nursing Management for Procedures and Treatments

The nurse prepares each child for diagnostic tests on an individual basis that is suited to each child's abilities and developmental level (see Chapter 29).

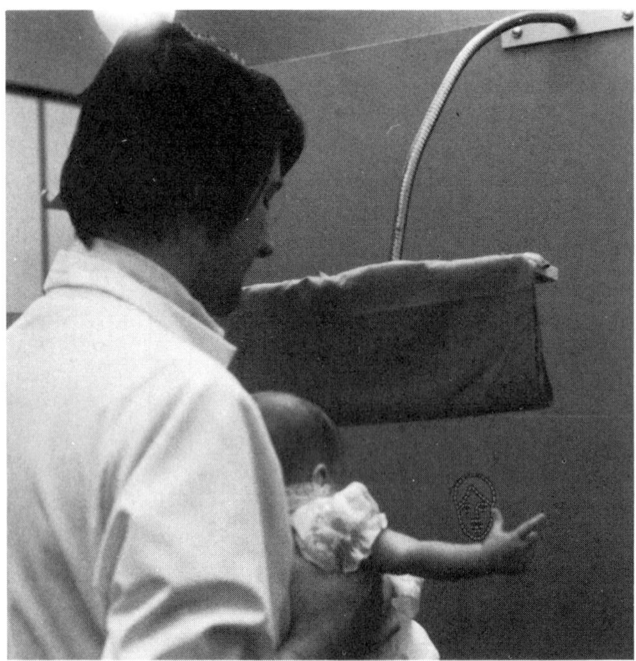

Infant eye examination for visual acuity.

The nurse explains the purpose of the test, what the child will experience, and what is expected of the child. Visual and hearing acuity tests have a gamelike quality that enhances the child's willingness to participate; however, because the results depend on the accuracy of the child's report, the atmosphere should be friendly but businesslike. If otoscopy or ophthalmoscopy or any other intrusive test is to be done, the child might need to be restrained to prevent injury, especially for the child in infancy or early childhood. The restraint should be only as much as is needed for safety, and the child should be reassured that the holding is for only a short time.

Eyedrops and eardrops may be required in the testing and treatment of conditions of the eye or ear. (The procedures and precautions for instilling eyedrops and eardrops are described in Chapter 29.)

Eardrops might be needed to soften impacted cerumen before an ear examination or to treat an external otitis. To soften impacted cerumen, drops might be needed only once or for several days. The cerumen may then be removed by a blunt ear curette or by irrigation with warm water via an ear syringe or Water Pik. Irrigations should be done only when the examiner is sure that the eardrum is intact; if done with a perforated eardrum, infection can be introduced into the middle ear. The removal of cerumen by either method should not be attempted unless the child is able to cooperate or is effectively restrained to prevent injury to the external canal or tympanum.

Principles of Nursing Care

Acute-Care Needs

Nursing care may begin with case finding in a well-child clinic or in a newborn nursery. Deviations from normal, such as blurred vision, deficits in hearing, or abnormal appearance, require medical intervention and are referred to a physician. The urgency of this referral depends, of course, on the nature of the abnormality.

In general, dysfunction or abnormalities of the sensory organs and systems require prompt attention to prevent or reduce the severity of long-term effects. Nursing care includes explaining to parents why the medical referral will be made and stressing the importance of immediate follow-up.

Special nursing measures are required when a child with a chronic or acute sensory deficit is admitted to an ambulatory or inpatient facility for acute health care problems. These special needs and nursing measures depend on the degree of the visual, hearing, or speech impairment.

The Visually Impaired Child

Mild Visual Impairment Nursing care of children with mild visual impairments consists of visual screening and parent education for early detection and referral. The nurse encourages children who have corrective lenses to wear them, not because failure to do so will worsen the vision but because corrected vision promotes safety and the enjoyment of optimal visual acuity. The wearing of eyeglasses or eyepatches should never be a negotiable issue. Children should be taught the proper care and cleaning of eyeglasses.

Parents might have difficulty encouraging children to wear corrective lenses or eyepatches. It is important to discover how the parent feels about the use of these devices; if the parent feels that eyeglasses or eyepatches are stigmatizing or uncomfortable, the child will perceive that attitude and protest or refuse to wear the devices. The parents will be better able to ensure that the devices are used by demonstrating positive attitudes and an expectation that the child will cooperate. Glasses will be more acceptable to the child if the frames are attractive, straight, and fit properly and if the lenses are kept clean and free from scratches. Head straps are useful for small children to keep the glasses from annoying slipping and to prevent breakage. Straps are useful also for older children who participate in athletics. Older children might find glasses more acceptable if they are permitted to chose the style of the frames.

An increasing number of children are wearing contact lenses instead of eyeglasses for the correction of visual impairment. As with eyeglasses, proper care and maintenance of contact lenses is crucial for optimal visual acuity.

Cleaning and storage instructions differ depending on the type of lens used. Because contact lenses are so easily lost, children should be discouraged from wearing them in the hospital if they have eyeglasses available. If lenses are brought to the hospital, the nurse makes certain that the case is well labeled and that the contacts are stored in an easily accessible location. Nurses also should be aware that without the lenses, children, especially those who use contact lenses as cataract replacements, cannot see appropriately and might become disoriented. Families should be encouraged to provide regular eye checkups for all children wearing contact lenses. The risk of corneal abrasions is increased in contact lens wearers; also, children who wear contact lenses for long periods of time can have a decreased supply of oxygen to their corneas. The newer gas-permeable contact lenses seem to alleviate this problem.

Severe Visual Impairment Sudden, traumatic dysfunction of the eyes is a terrifying experience for children and their parents. Blunt trauma or a laceration of the orb may be accompanied by swelling, tearing, and temporary loss of vision. Frequently, both eyes are patched to reduce the movement of the affected eye. This loss of vision adds to the child's confusion, fear, and discomfort.

Nursing care of the child who is temporarily blind includes providing as quiet an environment as possible. The level of distress can be reduced if the child is not bombarded with the sounds of the emergency room or hospital unit when unable to see what is happening. The parent's distress is telegraphed to the child. Prompt attention to the parent's needs and questions can reduce parental anxiety and benefit the child as well. The timely administration of pain medication and treatments such as compresses, ointments, or irrigations reduce the child's pain and discomfort and alleviate anxiety for both the child and parent.

Double patching a child whose sight previously was normal can result in the classic symptoms of sensory deprivation—confusion, withdrawal, nightmares, impaired thought processes and perceptions, and in severe cases hallucination and psychosis (Ashworth, 1979). In a study by Jackson, which was reported by Ashworth (1979) 30%–90% of patients who had both eyes patched experienced some behavioral changes related to the resulting sensory deprivation. Nursing interventions directed toward preventing sensory deprivation include the following:

1. Creating an environment that precludes sensory overload but does not allow for isolation and sensory deprivation
2. Orienting the child to the environment, being as descriptive as possible to help the child create an internal visual image
3. Helping the child to correctly perceive the events that are occurring

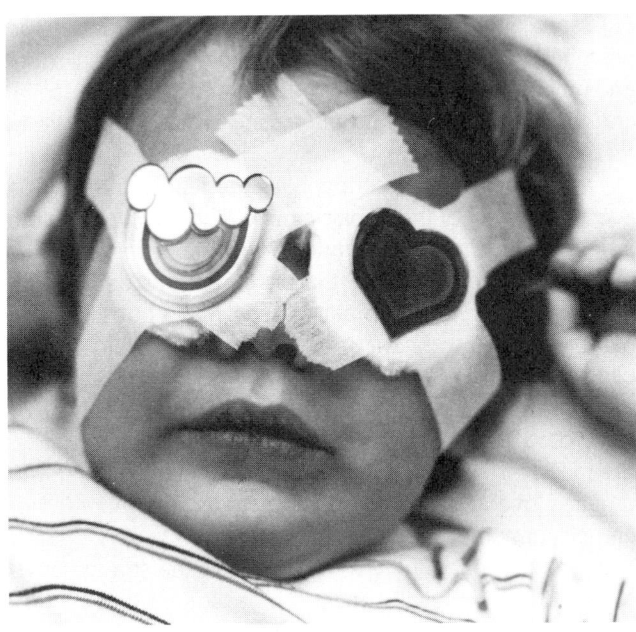

A child with bilateral eyepatches requires careful orientation to the environment.

4. Providing reality orientation, particularly to time, by relating time to events with which the child can identify (such as mealtime, *Sesame Street* time, and so on)
5. Encouraging self-care
6. Facilitating the use of cognitive thought processes by reading stories, playing music, or playing a tape of family members' voices
7. Providing enough sleep and time free from interruptions
8. Varying the external stimuli to maintain the child's attention such as by wheeling the child to a a playroom

When a child with existing severe visual impairment is hospitalized, special attention is needed to orient the child to the new setting. The child's degree of difficulty with orientation will depend on the degree of impairment and how recent its onset. Infants rely on their parents for orientation and a sense of safety; it is especially important that the parent remain with and participate in the care of a blind infant if possible. The older child might be able to accept care by a stranger if the nurse has obtained information from the parent about the child's daily routine and usual manner of communication, as well as the child's preferred arrangement of items in the hospital setting.

The nurse needs to know the degree of visual impairment. If the child cannot see at all, more supervision and assistance will be required in the strange environment than would be required for a child who is able to see shapes and forms and light and dark. On the other hand, the child with a partial loss of vision might be more frightened because of misperception of visual images. In either case the nurse describes the setting in detail to the child—the hospital room and unit for the child who has been admitted to the hospital and the examining room and waiting area for the child in an outpatient setting.

The nature of the description will depend on the child's age at the onset of the impairment. Children who are blind from birth will not understand visual references to colors and abstract measurements that are comprehended by children who are recently impaired. The nurse questions the parent about the means used to orient the child who is blind from birth. Methods include describing distances by referring to familiar settings, the number of steps away, or some other personal referent. The task of describing objects, distances, or persons even to recently impaired children requires inventiveness and patience to be sure that the references or comparisons are understood.

In general, orienting the blind child to the strange environment of a hospital ward can be accomplished best by guiding the child around the rooms and corridors of the patient division and encouraging the child to note sounds, odors, and surface textures to aid in establishing a mental picture of the spatial relationships. Bedside equipment such as the call bell, water glass, and bedside stand should be kept in their usual locations so that the child can learn where to reach for them as needed. The blind child, just like any other new patient, needs to learn how to operate the call bell and the television controls, where the bathroom is, and when and where meals are served.

The need to announce to a blind child any changes in the environment seems self-evident, but it is easy to forget to supply a running commentary on the activities that a sighted child would be able to discern without assistance. It is important to speak to visually impaired children and identify oneself and one's purpose before touching them. Noises in the environment should be identified immediately to prevent worry over their possible meanings, even when the activity is not related to the child's care. For example, the sound of a wheelchair or stretcher being brought into a room for another child might be interpreted by blind children as an indication that they are about to be taken somewhere without warning. The feeling of vulnerability in the strange environment might make blind children even more vigilant and aware of sounds, odors, and skin sensations.

Hospitalized blind children should be encouraged to maintain the same level of independence and self-care that they have achieved at home, within the limitations of the illness and the strange environment. Autonomy and independence are important for any child but will be more difficult to maintain for a blind child. Home routines of hygiene and other self-care activities should be preserved as much as possible, even if the nurse could do things for the child more quickly and effectively. When a child is forced back into dependency because of illness, help should be offered with tact and assurances that the need for assistance is temporary.

Children who have correctable visual impairments might need encouragement or assistance in the use of eyeglasses or contact lenses. It is important to help hospitalized children to keep their lenses clean and in a safe place when not in use.

Documentation of assessment and nursing care is always important, but record keeping is especially important in the care of the visually handicapped child. The nurse notes mobility limitations and aids, the degree of independence in the activities of daily living, and the child's preferences for care to ensure safe and consistent care and to encourage maximum independence.

Preoperative and Postoperative Care The nurse in an acute-care setting offers preoperative preparation to children and families when surgical correction is planned. In addition to the routine preoperative teaching, preparation includes describing the administration of eyedrops to prepare the eyes for surgery and explaining about the possible use of eyepatches immediately after surgery. Parents and older children should be prepared for the typical bloodshot appearance of the eye after surgery. The nurse also determines whether the parent or child holds the common misconception that the eye is removed from the socket during surgery. The physician should describe the incision and sutures accurately, and the nurse can review and clarify the procedures, as needed.

Preoperative preparation should emphasize descriptions of the sounds, odors, and sensations of touch that the child will experience. It might be useful for the nurse to spend some time in the patient unit, operating room, and recovery room with the eyes closed and attending to sounds and sensations to become better able to prepare blind children for these experiences. Blind children benefit from actually handling new equipment or materials that will be used preoperatively and postoperatively such as syringes, cast materials, or arm splints. The nurse tailors the amount of detail used in preoperative preparation to the individual needs and cognitive ability of each child, blind or sighted (see Chapter 29).

Parents need to learn postoperative care. An eyepatch may be recommended for several weeks at naptime and during the night to protect the eye from accidental rubbing and to maintain lubrication during sleep. Antibiotic ointments or eyedrops may be instilled into the eye to prevent infection. Infants and young children will need to be restrained whenever they are not directly supervised by a responsible adult. Elbow restraints are particularly effective (see Chapter 29).

When eyepatches, eyedrops, ointment, or eyeglasses are prescribed postoperatively, parents might need help in enforcing their use. It is important that parents avoid allowing cooperation to become a power issue; they should make

NURSING CARE GUIDE Child Undergoing Eye Surgery

Nursing diagnosis	Interventions	Evaluation
1. Potential for sensory deprivation related to postoperative visual impairment	Preoperatively, familiarize the child with the environment (call light, bed controls, hospital staff) and implement age-appropriate preparation such as puppet play, "dress up" using eyepatches, and audiovisual instruction Postoperatively, minimize unfamiliar environmental stimuli that can increase anxiety and encourage auditory and tactile activities such as story tapes, music, and water play Encourage autonomy through self-care activities and facilitate the verbal and nonverbal expression of frustration through play activities and therapeutic communication	Effects of visual deprivation are minimized by effective intervention Child uses adaptive coping strategies
2. Potential for injury to the affected eye	Maintain eyepatches or shield placement as ordered Restrain as necessary. (Remove the restraints every 1–2 hours to evaluate skin and provide range of motion) Remove blunt objects from the child's reach Pad the side rails of the child's crib or bed If appropriate, minimize intraocular pressure by administering analgesics to decrease agitation and limiting valsalva maneuvers such as straining and coughing	The child avoids additional injury to the affected eye during the postoperative period
3. Potential for infection related to the surgical procedure	Observe, record, and report eye redness, itching, discharge, pain, edema, and change in appearance If appropriate, cleanse the external orbit using aseptic technique, washing from the inner to outer canthus If intraocular pressure is to be minimized, evaluate for hazards of immobility such as pulmonary congestion, urinary stasis, and constipation	The child exhibits no focal and/or systemic signs of infection

SOURCE: Arlene Portale, RN, MS, Pediatric Clinical Specialist, Children's Hospital of San Francisco.

it clear that wearing the patch, receiving the eye medication, or wearing the corrective lens is expected rather than negotiable behavior. It is easy for the parent to slip into the use of bribery and rewards if the nurse does not caution against this practice.

The Hearing-Impaired Child Emergency or acute situations related to the ear may be encountered in the emergency room, outpatient setting, or inpatient facility. Acute conditions include the presence of foreign bodies and acute external and middle ear infections. Each of these conditions is accompanied by pain of varying degrees and, frequently, nausea, vomiting, and vertigo. Nursing management includes the prompt administration of analgesia, medications for vertigo, antibiotics, and other medically prescribed treatments. A quiet and calm environment is also effective in reducing fear and anxiety, which contributes to the vertigo and nausea. Like the child who is visually impaired, however, the child who is hearing impaired is at greater risk for developing the adverse effects of sensory deprivation. The nurse intervenes to prevent this occurrence.

The Child With a Partial Hearing Loss Problems arise for children with partial hearing losses. Strangers might be unaware of the impairment or of the specific loudness or pitch of sounds that can or cannot be perceived. Children who experience temporary losses of hearing from otitis media might have been scolded for a lack of attention or disobedience before the impairment was discovered. These children might be reluctant to say that they did not hear clearly. The speaker must watch closely for facial expressions of confusion, doubt, or strain.

Other signs of hearing loss are disruptive behavior because the child is frustrated and feels unsure about what is expected or passivity and social withdrawal because the child lacks normal auditory stimulation and the usual social engagement. On the other hand, children who wear hearing aids may suffer from persons shouting at them, even though their ability to hear normal tones has been restored.

Careful history taking and recording of the character of the hearing disability can prevent some of these difficulties. In addition, careful, unobtrusive assessment of the child's ability to hear should be part of the admission process. The interviewer may speak the child's name when the child is not watching and note the response or lack of response. The interviewer might ask the child to review what has been said to be sure that the child was able to hear and comprehend.

The Child With Total Hearing Loss When children with total hearing losses are admitted to the hospital, problems similar to those encountered by blind children may arise in dealing with the strange environment. Although deaf children can see, they might have difficulty understanding new activities and in being prepared for surgery or treatments.

The child with a total hearing loss might understand sign language or be able to read lips. If signing is the usual mode of communication, it is important to obtain help from a person skilled in sign language, just as one would enlist the help of a translator to communicate with a client who does not understand English. Pantomime might serve to communicate simple requests, but more complex communications are needed to fully prepare deaf children for surgery or treatments. To assist with simple sign communication, a chart of common positions for finger spelling is helpful. If a deaf child is able to read lips, it is essential that the nurse makes sure before speaking that the child is attending by making eye contact. The nurse stands facing the child at the child's eye level and with the face well lighted. Important communications should be made in a setting with minimal visual distractions.

Additional problems for the hearing impaired child might involve speech development and the ability to communicate with others, especially strangers who are not familiar with the signals and sounds with which the child communicates in the home. Children who are deaf from birth have particular trouble with learning speech because they are unable to hear others talk or their own sound productions. Infants who are deaf from birth do vocalize with the same range and frequency as hearing infants at first, but by 6–9 months of age, their vocalizations decrease markedly.

Early vocalizations occur spontaneously and, in a hearing infant, are reproduced and practiced in a playful manner, each sound serving as a stimulus for the subsequent sound. Deaf children do not perceive this interesting result of their vocalizations and thus have no motivation to continue to make sounds. If the parent responds with smiles and caresses each time the infant vocalizes, the infant may be able to vocalize but will still not be able to use the sounds to communicate.

It is important therefore to remember that deaf children might not only have difficulty perceiving events and interpreting communications but may also experience difficulty communicating their needs to others. If a sign translator is not available, the nurse might supply deaf children with paper and pencil so that they can write down what they want to communicate. Even children who do not read can communicate by drawing or pointing out pictures in a book, so these materials should be readily available.

Another notable point is that deaf children attend more carefully to visual cues. Nurses need to be aware that facial and body language might unintentionally communicate information that may be misinterpreted by the deaf child.

The Child With a Hearing Aid Some children who are hospitalized require hearing aids for auditory assistance. There are four types of hearing aids in general use:

- Behind the ear—the most common type
- In the ear—most compact
- Eyeglass
- Body—for severe hearing loss (Holder, 1982)

All hearing aids have batteries, on–off switches, volume controls, and molds that fit into the outer ear. Hearing aids function by converting sound waves into electrical impulses through the amplification of the sound signals. In children the volume may be set to maximize effectiveness and the volume control taped to prevent the child from turning the volume off and "tuning out" (Kamenir, et al., 1982).

The information the nurse needs to know to care properly for the hearing aid includes the type, make, and serial number (to be recorded on the child's chart); how to insert the hearing aid; how to change the battery; how often the hearing aid is cleaned; and whether the child can clean it (Kamenir, et al., 1982). The ear mold and tube are the only portions of the hearing aid that should be cleaned; cleaning in warm water and mild soap is all that is required. It is important to be certain that the mold and tube are completely dry before they are reinserted into the ear.

If the hearing aid does not appear to be working properly, the nurse checks that the switch is on (and not on the T[telephone] setting), that the battery is not dead, and that it is correctly placed in the ear. If the battery is working, a whistling sound can be heard by covering the mold with a hand prior to insertion. If the hearing aid is inserted incorrectly, a whistling sound can be heard when it is in the ear. The nurse remembers to remove the child's hearing aid prior to any radiographic studies because radiation can adversely affect its function.

Preoperative and Postoperative Care of the Hearing-Impaired Child Orientation to the hospital and preoperative and postoperative preparations are necessary also for the deaf child. Just as for the blind child, the nurse provides concrete descriptions of settings and anticipated events such as preoperative injections, transport by stretcher, and so on. Demonstration and role-play are especially useful for children with minimal verbal ability.

When surgery is contemplated, preoperative preparation includes the expected postoperative conditions of discomfort, drainage, or temporarily reduced hearing acuity. A frequent minor surgical procedure is insertion of plastic tubes in the tympanum *(myringotomy),* which is performed under anesthesia. Children are admitted to the hospital for day surgery or a brief overnight stay. Drainage in the external canal in the immediate postoperative period is common.

Nursing management includes parent education for home care. The ear must be kept dry. Swimming is contraindi-

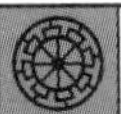

NURSING CARE GUIDE Postoperative Management of the Child With Myringotomy

Nursing diagnosis	Interventions	Evaluation
1. Potential for patient and parent anxiety related to knowledge deficit about surgical procedure, fear of pain and discomfort, and hospitalization	Review with the parents what the physician has told them and what their understanding of the problem is Discuss with the child and family what the procedure involves according to their level of understanding Discuss fears about pain, individual coping mechanisms, and methods of pain management Refer the child for puppet therapy for preparation according to growth and developmental level	The child and parent understand the procedure and possible expected outcomes The child and parent ask questions regarding the procedure and/or hospitalization
2. Potential for drainage from ears related to the surgical procedure	Reinforce to the parents that this drainage is normal—the myringotomy has provided an opening for drainage Note the type of drainage (ie, serous, purulent, or bloody) Remove clots from the ears using sterile cotton swabs soaked in normal saline solution If a large amount of drainage is present, place cotton fluffs over the ear orifice and change as needed Notify the physician if frank bleeding occurs	Any bleeding is recognized early Patient comfort is maintained
3. Potential parental knowledge deficit regarding home care	Instruct the parents and child as appropriate about home care: the child's head should not be immersed in water; cotton fluffs dipped in petroleum jelly should be placed in the ear orifice during bathing; drainage from the ear can be normal for several days; notify the physician if the child develops symptoms of meningitis such as nausea, vomiting, headache, and nuchal rigidity; arrange a follow-up appointment with the physician	The parents and child will understand the principles of home care

SOURCE: Lori J. Howell, RN, MS, Clinical Nurse Specialist, Pediatric Surgery, Assistant Clinical Professor, University of California, San Francisco

cated; even hairwashing and bathing must be done with caution to avoid introducing water into the ear canal and bacteria into the middle ear through the opening in the tympanum. The parent should inspect the external canal regularly for signs of drainage or the presence of the plastic tube. If either are discovered, the physician should be notified.

Occasionally, when damage to the tympanic membrane has been severe, a tympanoplasty might be considered to restore hearing loss. This involves the insertion of a Silastic film to replace the defective tympanic membrane (Bridges, 1982). Postoperatively, the child might have a bulky dressing over the ear and an ear packing. The child should lie on the affected side to facilitate drainage, avoid sudden movement, and be medicated for pain if needed. Sudden nausea, dizziness, or vomiting might indicate disturbance of the cochlea (Bridges, 1982). Home care of the child following tympanoplasty is similar to that of the child following a myringotomy.

Less common ear surgery involves repair of the ossicles. Regardless of the type of ear surgery, nursing interventions are directed toward the prevention of infection, most specifically mastoiditis, which can lead to meningitis.

The Speech-Impaired Child Children develop speech impairments from a variety of causes. The impairment may be a temporary failure to pronounce specific words clearly (articulation defect) or a permanent impairment caused by malformations of the palate or difficulty controlling the passage of air over the vocal cords. Whatever the cause or duration of the problem, it is important for the nurse to assess the amount and type of speech the child understands and the extent of the child's ability to use speech to communicate with others. The nurse cannot assume that a child has equal receptive and expressive speech abilities.

Children with speech impairments might experience much frustration and embarrassment when they enter a new environment and others have difficulty understanding what they say. Nurses can decrease the child's frustration by attending very carefully to the child's speech, asking the child to communicate using other words if the initial words cannot be understood, and remaining calm, pleasant, and accepting of the communication difficulties. Children with speech impairments communicate most clearly when they are unrushed and feel accepted by the listener. Children with sensory deficits who are hospitalized are cared for best by assigning a primary nurse or, at the least, a limited number of persons responsible for care. The nurse who works most closely with the child continually assesses and records the most effective means of communication. Parents can provide additional help and validate the nurse's observations.

Many speech problems can be corrected. Children with cerebral palsy or other neuromuscular problems can be helped to control the expiratory phase of respiration to better increase the quality of speech. Children with malformations of the mouth, palate, posterior pharynx, or vocal cords can be helped by corrective surgery and speech therapy. Some children with chronic hoarseness might be helped by voice training in which they are taught to project the voice without strain and to avoid voice abuse such as shouting.

The effects of any one of these sensory deficits can be devastating to the child and family. Unfortunately, some children have multisensory impairments. Children with congenital rubella syndrome might be deaf, develop glaucoma or cataracts, and be delayed in speech development because of sensory deficits or because of concomitant mental retardation.

These deaf–blind children communicate almost entirely through touch, and the use of touch needs to be heavily incorporated in their nursing care. These children require persistent and vigorous habilitation programs if they are to function with any degree of independence. Children who become impaired in several senses through trauma, brain tumor, or some other cause have the advantage of the learning, orientation, and skills gained before the catastrophe. These achievements can be built on in devising alternative modes of communication with objects, the environment, and other people.

Nutritional Needs

Children with acute infections might have loss of appetite and require frequent, small meals that include the important nutrients of protein, vitamins, and minerals, and increased fluid intake, all of which are essential to restore health and promote healing. Children who have undergone surgery should be in the best possible nutritional condition preoperatively. As soon as the postoperative condition permits, a well-balanced diet should be offered to enhance healing and prevent developmental delays.

Children who are blind have different nutritional needs during hospitalization. These needs are not related to specific nutritional requirements but rather to their eating habits and preferences and the adaptations or modifications that are required because of hospitalization. Children who are blind might have difficulty eating without assistance when hospitalized. Even if the family has developed ways to assist the child, these adaptations might not be communicated to the hospital staff. A careful history obtained and recorded at admission is essential so that successful methods used in home management can be followed in the hospital.

At the very least, a visually impaired child should be assisted to wash before meals, oriented to the type of food and the location of the food on the plate or tray, and provided with pleasant mealtime companions. To orient the young child to the type and location of the food, the nurse secures the plate with a suction cup or places it on a towel if the table is slippery. The nurse guides the child's hand to touch each food as the food is named. The nurse tells older children the location of the food on the plate by referring to the position of the numbers on a clock dial. If the child does not comprehend the clock dial, the nurse shows the location of the food by guiding the child's hand over the plate or tray. Cups and glasses should be placed in the same position at each meal and should be wide based to reduce accidental spilling. It might be necessary to cut, butter, or season food for the young child, but the child's preferences should be learned so that independence can be maintained at the highest possible level.

A child with a hearing impairment caused by chronic ear infections may have a decreased sensitivity to the taste of food because if the chronic infection is related to upper respiratory infections or allergies, the sense of smell is diminished. Smell is an important component of the sensation of taste. Children with chronic ear infections frequently have unpleasant tastes in the mouth caused by drainage from the upper air passages. This unpleasant taste also diminishes pleasure in the taste of food. Because appetite might lag when food is tasteless, color and attractiveness of the food should be enhanced as much as possible. Seasonings such as catsup and spices may be added to the food if not contraindicated by dietary restrictions.

Developmental Needs

Developmental needs are affected whenever a child has a health problem, however brief, but children who experience even temporary disruptions in sight or hearing are vulnerable to developmental delays, especially when these disruptions occur during infancy or early childhood because optimal development is so dependent on sensory input. Early case finding and prompt treatment are the most effective ways of minimizing the impact of temporary sensory dysfunction. However, even when the dysfunction is temporary and brief, nursing management follows the plan of care for children with more prolonged or permanent dysfunction.

Children who are blind or deaf from birth should participate in sensory stimulation programs from the time of diagnosis. Parents of blind infants can help their children to gain mobility and pass other developmental milestones in a timely fashion by focusing on skin stimulation and the use of sound to encourage their infants' hand-to-mouth manipulation of objects and environmental exploration. Parents are encouraged to speak frequently to their infants so that they will begin to recognize their parents by voice and know where their parents are.

Because the blind infant's motor activities cannot be stimulated by visual images, special games and routines are used to encourage the child to use sound and touch to locate objects in space and to manipulate objects and explore the environment. In one study parents participated in teaching sessions every 2 weeks and received much support and counseling as they performed the difficult tasks of caring for their blind infants (Fraiberg, Siegel, and Gibson, 1966; Sharpe, 1973).

Congenitally deaf children require early language training. There is still much controversy over whether deaf children should be taught to communicate by signs or taught to speak. Teachers of deaf children receive special training to learn techniques to communicate with the children and to assist them in making the necessary cognitive connections between the symbols of sign language, the vibrations or amplified sounds of spoken words, or the lip movements of the speaker. Children learn to match the feel of vibrations on their own throats and the shapes of their mouths with those of a speaker to learn to make language sounds. Even when accurate sounds are produced, it is difficult for a deaf child to achieve the variety in tone and inflections of ordinary speech, resulting in monotone speech. Totally deaf children find it very difficult to achieve understandable speech because they are unable to hear their own speech productions and must rely on the reactions of others to determine whether what they have said is comprehensible. On the other hand, the child who has learned to communicate by sign language can communicate only with others who know the hand signals.

Other controversies continue over the comparative value of residential schools, special day schools, or public school education for blind or deaf children. In 1975 Congress passed the Education for All Handicapped Children Act (PL 94-142), which mandates free, appropriate, quality education in the least restrictive environment for all handicapped children between 3 and 21 years of age. Quality education and the least restrictive environment must be defined for each handicapped child individually and a plan devised that is mutually acceptable to the school and the child's parents. For some children, residential school might be necessary, whereas supplemental day school programs may be needed in addition to public school programs for other children. Still other children might be able to be placed exclusively in public schools with the aid of braille books, sign language readers, or other devices. The value of placing handicapped children in regular public schools ("mainstreaming") and the availability of local services so that children can remain at home has been well documented (Lowenfeld, 1975; Koestler, 1976; Heinich, 1979). Children benefit from close family ties and other personal attachments for social development and to obtain a realistic view of the world and the adjustments required for self-care. On the other hand, few families are prepared to offer the intensive training required to enable deaf and blind children to attain that degree of independence. The optimal situation might be local day-care facilities and the supplementation of public school programs so that children can receive both normal socialization experiences and specialized assistance.

Whatever program is carried out and in whatever setting, the aim is to assist children to develop physically, emotionally, cognitively, and socially toward independence and full realization of their potential. To meet these aims, family involvement and support are essential so that the child receives consistent discipline and encouragement in self-care as appropriate to age and physical limitations. (Chapter 30 discusses the effect of chronic conditions on families.)

Emotional Needs

Children whose hearing or sight problems are acute in onset are vulnerable to severe and long-lasting emotional upset. It is difficult for children to believe or comprehend that the loss of sight or hearing is temporary. Even after function has been restored through treatment or surgery, the child might fear recurrence of the loss.

Young children are unable to understand that illness or disability can happen without being caused by someone. A child who is suddenly deprived of sight or hearing might believe that the disability is a punishment for some real or imagined wrongdoing. The child whose sensory disability occurred as a result of an accident such as a firecracker explosion is even more likely to consider the disability as a punishment.

Nurses can explain to children that accidents are not punishments, but the most useful approach to guilt in a child is to continuously demonstrate a nonjudgmental, accepting manner. The nurse can encourage the family to talk to their child about guilty feelings, reassuring the child of continued love and esteem from family members. Because of the nature of their disabilities, children with sensory deficits such as blindness or deafness (with or without communications problems) are vulnerable to delays in emotional development.

Attachment and separation–individuation are developmental concepts that describe the close ties between a child and parent and the loosening of the ties as the child gains skills and abilities in self-care (see Chapter 6). When the child cannot see and obviously needs protection from unseen hazards, it is difficult for both the child and parent to initiate the separation–individuation process. One mechanism used by sighted infants is visual checking back to the parent as the infant gathers the courage to wander farther away. Such checking back is denied the blind child. Parents of blind children can offer the security of the sound of their voices, which the children can use as a form of checking back and reassurance that the parents are still available. Blind children do not initiate this form of checking back at first but might learn to call out to their parents when they feel the need to confirm their presence.

Deaf children can manage the separation–individuation only to the degree that they can see their parents. These children are unable to recapture a sense of their parents' presence by hearing their voices or the sounds of their activity. Both blind and deaf children have difficulty learning how to predict the behaviors of other people, which would help them gain confidence in their parents or other caregivers.

Infants begin to develop notions of body image by gaining mental pictures of their bodies through cutaneous and internal sensations and the perceptions of the love expressed by their parents. The continuous discovery of the potential for action and pride in accomplishment and growth, which are validated by significant people in the child's life, continues throughout childhood. During adolescence, the rapid physical changes and associated temporary clumsiness and uncertainty give way to a relatively stable body image, which persists throughout young adulthood.

Blind children must learn to know their bodies by feel and cutaneous stimulation. They are unable to see admiration or love in the gaze of others; consequently, they need much physical demonstration of the regard their parents have for them. Because blind children frequently are delayed in achieving mobility and autonomy, body image development also might be delayed. It is important for parents or other caregivers to be aware of the need to help blind children establish body boundaries and gain a sense of the potential of their bodies and pride in their accomplishments. Parents can assist their children in these tasks by touching them frequently, naming body parts as they are touched, and deliberately making approving and admiring comments to their children.

Deaf children are able to see their own bodies and can enjoy the tactile stimulation. Deaf children can discern love, caring, and admiration in their parents' expressions. Although deaf children have these advantages as compared with blind children, deafness will always be a part of their body images. The degree of handicap that deaf children perceive will depend on their parents' acceptance and their ability to develop articulate communication with others.

Children with sensory deficits are imperiled by the negative reactions of strangers and others to their handicaps. These responses, either directly or indirectly expressed, become part of the child's self-image. Family members and health care providers can prepare the blind or deaf child for these reactions. Adults can explain that some persons do not know about blindness or deafness and how well children with these conditions can manage, and as a result, they become uncomfortable, feel sorry for the children, and make silly, insensitive remarks.

Children need admiration and respect from their families to foster healthy self-images to counterbalance the negative reactions they receive from others. Families and health care providers can focus on the children's skills and accomplishments and establish plans for continued independence and full realization of the children's potentials. Older children should be encouraged to talk about other people's reactions and their responses to these reactions. Role-play might be helpful in assisting children to develop effective defenses and responses.

Health Maintenance Needs

Health maintenance includes health teaching to prevent illnesses related to the sensory systems and the special primary health needs of children with sensory deficits.

Prevention of Eye Problems Health teaching associated with vision includes accident prevention (see Chapter 19). Eye infections also pose a threat to vision. As part of anticipatory guidance, nurses discuss eye hygiene with parents, explaining that the eye is self-cleansing and that eye washes are not needed. The eyelids should be cleansed with clear water on a clean washcloth, lightly stroking from the inner corner of the eye to the outer corner. A clean portion of the cloth should be used for each eye. If any signs of redness, swelling, or discharge appear, the parent should consult with the nurse or a physician.

The nurse also advises the parents to have their children's visual acuity evaluated before entering school. The child who squints, tilts the head persistently, moves close to objects to see them, has excessive tearing or blinking of the eye, or eyes that do not move together while watching a moving object should be examined sooner. This information is conveyed best while the nurse examines the infant's or child's eyes during a well-child examination. In particular, the nurse demonstrates the child's coordinated eye movements and the proper method of cleansing the eyelids.

The family of a child who has been discharged from the hospital with an artificial eye needs to be taught how to care for the prosthesis. The prosthesis can be removed from the eye socket by depressing the lower lid and allowing the eye to slide out. After washing the artificial eye in soapy water and cleaning the socket, the prosthesis is replaced by lifting the upper lid, depressing the lower lid, and sliding the eye into place (Zucnick, 1975). The eye is held in place by the restraint of both lids. The prosthesis can be cleaned as often as necessary or at the physician's direction. Children can assume care of their own prostheses but must be cautioned against dropping them because this might cause scratches or breakage.

Prevention of Ear Problems New parents need information about ear hygiene. Many parents believe that wax in the external canal should be removed with cotton-tipped applicators, so nurses might need to explain that the wax in the canal is normal and healthy. Only the shell of the ear should be cleansed; nothing should be introduced into the canal. If the external canal should become irritated, inflamed, or swollen, or if the child does not respond to sounds, the parent should consult the nurse or a physician. Parents should not give eardrops or probe the child's ear without medical advice.

Nurses in primary care settings include information about the prevention of ear infections as part of anticipatory guidance for the parents of infants. The nurse describes the relationship between the nasopharynx and the eustachian tube and middle ear and the ease with which infectious material can move from the throat to the ear of an infant or young child (see Chapter 26).

Nurses also can teach parents to prevent ear problems in infants and young children when traveling by air. During takeoff and landing, the parent should offer a bottle to an infant or food to a young child because the sucking or chewing and swallowing will help to keep the eustachian tube open and allow pressure in the middle ear to remain equal with that in the external auditory canal.

Parents should know how to recognize an upper respiratory infection or an allergic response and be alert to possible signs of *otitis media* (middle ear infection), a frequent complication of upper respiratory illnesses (see Chapter 26). Some physicians recommend the use of a decongestant with any upper respiratory infection or allergy to prevent eustachian tube blockage and otitis media. When otitis media is diagnosed, the nurse informs the parent about the treatment prescribed, the expected outcome of the treatment, and the importance of completing the prescribed treatment regimen, even after the child's symptoms have improved. This information will help parents to prevent complications or permanent damage to the eardrum or the middle ear structures and the resultant loss of hearing acuity.

Prevention of Speech Problems During each well-child visit, the nurse assesses the adequacy of the child's speech production and vocabulary. Parental concerns are elicited as part of the interval history.

The Child With a Visual Deficit

Strabismus

A number of visual acuity problems can arise because of structural anomalies of the eye and accessory muscles. *Strabismus* is a neuromuscular incoordination that affects the relative alignment of the two eyes and results in double vision *(diplopia)* or the suppression of vision from one eye to prevent double vision *(amblyopia)*. Strabismus can be normal in very young infants and will disappear as the infant matures and eye muscles become better developed.

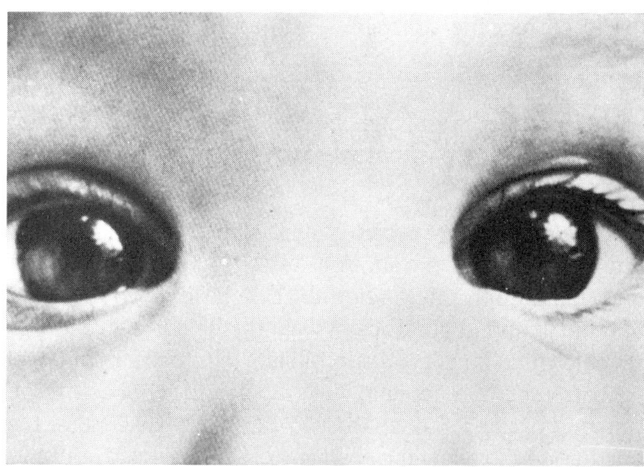

Transient strabismus may be present in the neonate and is caused by poor neuromuscular control. (Courtesy Mead Johnson Laboratories, Evansville, Ind.)

An infant over 4 months of age with strabismus might be referred to an ophthalmologist for evaluation, particularly if there is a family history of strabismus in close relatives. Strabismus must be recognized and treated early in life because the resulting amblyopia and consequent visual deficit can be irreversible.

The type of strabismus is classified according to the position of the affected eyes. In *esotropia* the eyes turn in toward the nose ("cross-eyes"); in *exotropia* the eyes deviate outward ("wall-eyes"); and in *hypertropia* the eyes are at different levels. Estropia is the most common type of strabismus.

Strabismus is diagnosed through observation and the use of the corneal light reflex (see Chapter 14). The cover test will reveal movement of the affected eye when the unaffected eye is covered, indicating abnormal fixation of the affected eye. Visual acuity tests might reveal a vision deficit.

Treatment Neuromuscular coordination may be improved through eye muscle exercises or corrective lenses.

Eye muscle exercises, known as *orthoptics*, requires cooperation from the child and dedication from the parent. The exercises, which are done at least several times each week, consist of the use of a binocular projector or handheld cards. The child consciously contracts the eye muscles to merge the images projected to each eye.

Corrective lenses are ground so that the "lazy eye" receives an image that is compatible with that received by the unaffected eye, thus preventing double vision or amblyopia. Muscle coordination might not be corrected, but vision is restored.

Patching the unaffected eye to force the eye muscles and vision to be used in the affected eye is another method of treatment. Parents might be puzzled at the decision to cover the eye that functions best and will need to have the rationale for the treatment explained to them. If these methods fail to correct the strabismus, surgery might be required. Binocular vision must be restored as soon as possible after the strabismus is recognized. If correction has not been achieved by 6 years of age, the likelihood of restoring vision in the affected eye is remote.

Nursing Management Nurses in outpatient settings are alert for the occurrence of strabismus in young children and make appropriate referrals. Emphasizing to the child and family the importance of wearing the corrective lenses or patch is a nursing responsibility. The child might feel embarrassed by having to wear a patch to school, and the nurse is particularly sensitive to this issue. The parent is encouraged to allow the child to express feelings about this issue at home. The parent needs to emphasize the child's positive qualities because excessive teasing from peers can severely undermine the child's confidence.

If surgery is required, nursing management is comparable to care for any child undergoing eye surgery.

Refractive Errors

Several refractive errors in vision are caused by anomalies in the shape of the orb. Elongation or flattening of the orb may result in hyperopia, myopia, or anisometropia. *Hyperopia* means far-sighted, or the inability to focus on near objects; *myopia* means near-sighted, or the inability to focus on distant objects; and *anisometropia* means inequality of the refractive power of the eyes. Children are mildly hyperopic until 9 years of age and become mildly myopic between 9 and 11 years of age (Chow, et al., 1979). Children with mild hyperopia or myopia might be able to accommodate sufficiently to see clearly until the normal maturational changes increase visual acuity for both near and distant objects. More severe hyperopia or myopia is treated with corrective lenses.

Another common visual deficit is *astigmatism,* asymmetric curvature of the cornea. Astigmatism can occur in one or both eyes; the condition usually is bilateral. Astigmatism must be corrected with glasses or contact lenses to restore visual acuity.

The clinical manifestations of refractive errors are usually complaints by children that they are unable to see clearly, or children are observed squinting, frowning, or holding objects close to their faces or far away. The lenses do not cure or change the condition but do improve visual acuity, and the nurse encourages the proper wear and care of lenses.

Color Blindness

Color blindness occurs almost entirely in boys and is a sex-linked genetic defect (see Chapter 5). Color blindness affects the discrimination of colors within certain groups: red, blue, and green; green and purple; or, more rarely, yellow and blue.

There is no treatment for color blindness. Screening and diagnosis should be done so that parents and teachers understand the limits of a child's ability to discriminate and label colors. Parents and other caregivers need to know whether the child can distinguish the red color on the many warning devices such as car brake lights and traffic signals and the green color on traffic signals. The child who is color blind for these important colors needs to learn other cues for dangers such as the "do not walk" signs and the shapes of traffic signals and other emergency objects.

Cataract

A *cataract* is an opacity of the lens of the eye. It can be detected by shining a light into the eye at an angle or by using an ophthalmoscope. If a cataract is present, the light reflex will be white instead of the usual red color. The cataract may be seen without the use of a light as an "oil droplet" appearance or a dense white opacity that occupies all or part of the lens, visible in the pupillary area. Cataracts are associated with certain syndromes such as muscular dystrophy; metabolic diseases such as galactosemia; congenital infections such as rubella; eye trauma; or the long-term use of cortisone therapy. Cataracts may be present at birth or develop during childhood. Visual impairment also varies widely from no reduction in sight to complete interference with the passage of light to the retina.

Medical and Surgical Treatment When sight is impaired, treatment is surgical removal of the lens. Modern surgical procedures have greatly reduced the risk of infection or other postoperative complications. If the remaining eye structures are normal, sight can be restored after surgery through the use of corrective eyeglasses or contact lenses. Within the past 5 years, artificial lens implants have been used successfully in adults. This surgery holds great promise for children because it not only improves visual acuity but also improves cosmetic appearance since thick glasses are no longer required to substitute for the removed lens.

If a cataract is left in place, untreated for a period of time, irreversible occlusional amblyopia might occur. *Occlusional amblyopia* is the term given to the functional blindness that occurs when the brain "blots out" the confusing double or blurred vision from the affected eye. If a cataract is in one eye only, postoperative treatment is difficult. The corrective lens does not provide the same clarity of vision as the unaffected eye. The child tends not to attend to the faulty image from the affected eye, resulting in permanent suppression of vision from that eye. The part-time use of an eyepatch on the unaffected eye might force sufficient use to preserve vision in the affected eye.

Nursing Management After surgery and discharge, infants and young children are encouraged to return to their usual daily activities, which helps them to recover more quickly. The distraction these activities provide decrease problems with scratching the eye. The parent is instructed to inspect the eye each time the eye ointment or drops are administered to observe for any signs of infection such as thickened discharge, increased inflammation, and increased complaints of itching or soreness and for any signs of opacities in the eye. Any changes in the eye should be reported to the surgeon immediately.

Glaucoma

Glaucoma is a condition caused by elevated intraocular pressure in the anterior chamber. In infancy glaucoma is characterized by enlarged, hazy corneas. Photophobia, tearing, and poor vision are late signs. Glaucoma can occur in association with systemic disease, trauma, infection, or as an isolated disorder. Tonometry reveals an elevated intraocular pressure.

Medical and Surgical Treatment The treatment for children is surgery to remove the obstruction to the aqueous humor flow from the anterior chamber. Careful and frequent medical follow-up is important to detect any recurrence of increased pressure due to inflammation or scarring.

Nursing Management Preoperative and postoperative care of a child who has had surgery for glaucoma might include the administration of miotic eyedrops to enhance the flow of the aqueous humor and antibiotic ointments. Miotic eyedrops cause the pupils to constrict. The parent should know the signs of acute increased intraocular pressure (pain, inflammation of the eye, and nausea and vomiting) and understand that any inflammation, temperature elevation, or signs of increased intraocular pressure should be reported to the surgeon immediately.

Inflammations of the Eye

Three major inflammatory eye diseases are conjunctivitis, orbital cellulitis, and corneal ulcer. Each of these problems has the potential to cause permanent damage to the eye; therefore, prompt detection, referral, and treatment are essential.

Conjunctivitis is an inflammation of the conjunctiva, or lining of the eyelids and covering of the sclera. The inflammation may be caused by mechanical irritation, viral or bacterial organisms, or allergens. The clinical manifestations of conjunctivitis vary depending on the cause but always include erythema, edema of the lids, itching and tearing, and mucoid or purulent discharge. The medical treatment consists of antibiotics, such as erythromycin (Ilotycin), in topical ointments or eyedrops.

Children with conjunctivitis usually are cared for at home, so nursing management includes referral for medical care and parent teaching. The nurse informs the parent about the spread of eye disease and the importance of preventing other children from coming in contact with the discharge from the eye of the affected child. No one else should use the affected child's washcloth or towel. The affected child should not share a pillow or bed if at all possible while the infection is present.

The parent also needs to be instructed about home treatment of the conjunctivitis. The nurse stresses the importance of thorough handwashing before and after cleansing the eyelids and administering the topical medication. The parent cleanses the child's eyelids with plain, warm, tapwater on a clean cloth or cotton balls, being certain to wipe from the inner canthus outward. After treatment, the cloth should be washed thoroughly or the cotton balls discarded. The nurse describes ways to restrain infants and toddlers gently such as safety pin chains from the shirt sleeve wristlet to the diaper or wrapping cardboard around the arms to prevent the child's elbow from bending. If such restraint is needed, the nurse emphasizes the importance of removing the restraints frequently and putting the child's arms through full range of motion before replacing the restraints.

Orbital cellulitis is a more serious inflammation of the tissues behind the orb, usually caused by ethmoid sinusitis or infected skin disruptions or injuries near the eye. The eyelids are swollen, and the orb is displaced anteriorly. Intravenous antibiotics and sinus decongestants are the usual medical treatments to prevent further spread of infection into the cranium.

Nursing management of orbital cellulitis includes monitoring the intravenous infusion, administering the medications, observing for side effects, and noting and recording the sinus drainage and appearance of the eye.

Children and parents might be surprised or frightened at the vigorous treatment of what may appear to be a minor problem. The nurse explains that the infected area is very close to the brain and that the vigorous treatment is necessary to prevent brain abscess. The nurse also keeps the family informed of signs of recovery—normal temperature, reduced inflammation, and changes in the white blood cell count. The parents might be concerned that they did not recognize that the child was ill sooner. The nurse reviews the signs of sinusitis and inflammation in the facial area and encourages parents to seek medical consultation if these signs are noted again.

Children often become restless and bored during the long intravenous therapy regimen, especially after the first day or so when they begin to feel well again. Very young children or infants might require restraints to safeguard the intravenous insertion or to prevent them from rubbing the affected eye. These children need the companionship of their parents and other children. Play and other diversional activities will foster cooperation with the therapy and reduce the boredom of prolonged hospitalization.

Corneal ulcers may develop as a result of infection. The clinical signs of corneal ulceration are moderate to severe pain, blurred vision, and watery or purulent discharge from the eye. Prompt and vigorous medical treatment is essential to prevent permanent scarring and subsequent opacity or loss of visual acuity caused by changes in the refractive surface of the eye. Nursing management includes the administration of topical medications and analgesics and teaching the parent how to administer eyedrops and ointments and prevent infections or irritation caused by the child's rubbing the eye.

Clinical Injury

Trauma to the eye is considered to be an ocular emergency and requires prompt and effective nursing action to prevent severe complications, which might result in the loss of vision. *Chemical burns* of the eye are caused by accidental contact with corrosive agents, usually household cleaning products. These products may be acidic, such as bleach, or alkalis, such as lye and commercial drain cleaners. Regardless of the acidity of the substance, the eye should be flushed as described in Chapter 19. Injuries from alkalis should be flushed for a longer period of time (over 30 minutes) than acids because they penetrate more rapidly and thus are more difficult to remove (Cavalier, 1981). The child should be transported to the hospital immediately for ophthalmologic evaluation.

Treatment After irrigation, the eye is examined for injury. A mydriatic or cycloplegic drug such as atropine sulfate may be administered to relieve pain by resting the ciliary musculature (Tumulty and Resler, 1984). Severely burned corneas no longer have sensation. An antibiotic ointment is instilled to prevent infection, and the affected eye is patched. The eye should be reexamined within 24 hours for injuries that were not apparent at the first examination.

Nursing Management Nursing management includes emergency irrigation or, if the initial inquiry was by telephone, instructing the parent to irrigate the child's eye. Prompt referral to an ophthalmologist is essential. Equally important is prevention of injury. Parent teaching should include the safe storage and use of corrosive liquids or powders (see Chapter 19).

Hyphema

Trauma also can be caused by blunt or penetrating injuries to the eye. Blunt trauma to the eye can result from the child's being hit by a ball or from any other injury likely to result in ecchymosis of the eye. Blunt trauma can cause dislocation of the lens, injury to the retina (detachment or retinal tears), and intraocular bleeding *(hyphema)*. Any of these complications might lead to blindness if not treated quickly.

Hyphema, the presence of blood in the anterior chamber of the eye, is caused by a blunt injury. Such an injury occurs with or without orbital fracture and other injuries to the structures of the eye such as corneal abrasions or a detached retina. Hyphema can result from any head injury, such as from a car accident, or from a direct blow to the eye with an object such as a baseball or bat. These injuries are most common in the active and accident-prone years of early and middle childhood. Hyphema can be observed as a light red color in front of the lower portion of the iris. The presence of blood can be seen by shining a light laterally into the orb. The blood usually is absorbed without further damage, but the bleeding can recur or can cause increased intraocular pressure. For these reasons, it is important to observe a child with hyphema closely for several days.

Treatment Treatment of hyphema includes patching the eye, placing the child on strict bedrest, and instilling ophthalmalogic preparations. Medications might be prescribed for pain, and attention is given to associated injuries.

Nursing Management Nursing care of the child with hyphema includes careful observation, and administration of medications if the child is hospitalized, or teaching parents what to watch for and how to administer medications if the child is cared for at home. Any complaints of diminished vision or sudden flashes of light might indicate retinal detachment and require prompt notification of an ophthalmologist. Severe, sudden headache associated with nausea and/or vomiting might be a sign of glaucoma, another complication of blunt trauma. Acute glaucoma is an ocular emergency and requires immediate attention (Welch, Tyler, and Quinn, 1984). The nurse stresses the importance of observing the child but does so without frightening the parent. If the injury is severe, eyepatches and strict bedrest might be required. The degree to which the child's activity is restricted depends on the severity of the bleeding and other suspected or diagnosed injuries such as a skull fracture. The temporary loss of sight and the restricted activity will be difficult for the child, and the nurse's and family's ingenuity will be taxed to find ways to help the child cope with the restrictions. Storytelling, records, word games, and other activities that can be enjoyed in bed and without sight are helpful. The most important nursing measure is to reduce the child's anxiety by frequent assurances that the restriction and loss of sight are temporary.

The child with hyphema might become withdrawn or be drowsy. For this reason, frequent neurologic checks are essential in trying to discriminate the effects of hyphema from neurologic problems such as concussion. Hyphema usually resolves in less than 1 week, but complications such as retinal detachment, glaucoma, or displaced lens might develop at a later time.

Penetrating Eye Injuries

Injuries to the eye from darts, arrows, or other thin objects can cause severe ocular damage and possible loss of vision, depending on the severity and extent of the injury. As with blunt trauma, the sequlae of penetrating injuries include detachment of the retina and glaucoma. In addition, cataracts can develop from even minor penetrating injuries (Tumulty and Resler, 1984). Infection is an ever-present danger.

Medical and Surgical Treatment Treatment of penetrating injuries includes vigorous antibiotic therapy, tetanus prophylaxis, pain relief, sedation, and the administration of antiemetics because vomiting raises intraocular pressure (Tumulty and Resler, 1984). The penetrating object should be removed surgically and not at the scene of the accident (see Chapter 19). In severe cases of ocular damage, enucleation might be necessary.

Nursing Management First aid for penetrating eye injuries is discussed in Chapter 19. Nursing care of the child with a penetrating eye injury is similar to that of a child with hyphema. The nurse observes for any change in eye drainage, level of pain, or presence of extraordinary ocular edema, all signs of an infection. The child and family might experience psychologic problems related to the injury. Anxiety and guilt are common reactions that might be part of the child's and family's coping repertoire. If loss of vision is documented, the nurse needs to help the child to adjust to the resulting alteration in body image. If the child is to be fitted for a prosthesis, the nurse needs to ensure that both the child and family understand how to take care of it. The prevention of eye injuries is infinitely preferable to treating them (see Chapter 19).

Minor Eye Injuries

Corneal abrasion is a direct injury to the cornea caused when an object such as sand is blown into the eye or a projectile such as a tree limb brushes against the cornea. The protective mechanisms of blinking and tearing are usually but not always adequate to prevent an abrasion. The child will complain of pain and will squeeze the eye tightly shut. Immediate assessment is important. The nurse first examines the conjunctiva and cornea for foreign bodies. Fluorescein stain is used to visualize any abrasions. If an abrasion is found or a foreign body is not removed by the natural action of tears, the nurse refers the child immediately to an ophthalmologist.

Subconjunctival hemorrhage appears as a small red area on the sclera and may be due to increased ocular pressure from something as minor as a cough. Although subconjunctival hemorrhages resolve on their own, they might be associated with other ocular problems and should be evaluated.

The Child With an Auditory Problem

Structural Anomalies of the Ear

Structural anomalies of the external ear might not cause hearing problems but can be a source of embarrassment and unhappiness for the child and family. *Lop ear* is the term used to describe large external ears that protrude from the head in a very noticeable fashion. Other malformations include extra skin tabs in the tragus of the ear, absent skin folds on the helix, and a low-set position on the head. Some of these malformations are associated with syndromes of varying seriousness; therefore, the nurse notes any abnormality of the ear and refers the child for medical diagnosis. Hearing is not affected by these external ear abnormalities, except for those children who have syndromes that include nerve deafness. Arrested development of the external ear sometimes includes failure of the external ear canal to develop, resulting in air conduction deafness.

Structural anomalies of the internal ear include stenosis or atresia of the middle ear and absence or fusion of the ossicles. Some of these anomalies are related to other craniofacial problems.

The treatment for malformed external ears is plastic surgery to achieve as normal an appearance as possible. The surgery should be completed by 6 years of age and prior to the child's entering school, if possible, to reduce the potential for embarrassment by questions from new acquaintances and the sense of being different while making the adjustment to school. Specific postoperative care includes special attention to protecting the operative site by maintaining the integrity of the dressing, observing for circulatory compromise, and discouraging the child from activities that involve roughhousing or have the potential for falls. Parents and children should be prepared for the appearance of the operative site before the dressing is removed. The sight of swollen, ecchymotic structures will be very disappointing if parents do not understand the normal process of healing. Parents and children often have unrealistic expectations of the final results of plastic surgery. Much can be done to construct the external ear, but exact replication is not possible.

Surgery to correct internal structural anomalies should be done as soon as possible to preserve hearing acuity. Microsurgery can be done to replace or realign the ossicles, open an atretic external canal, and replace tympanic membranes. The postoperative course may include vertigo and pain. Nursing care includes the administration of drugs for analgesia and the relief of vertigo and providing safety measures for the ambulatory child. Vertigo is a distressing symptom for children. Vertigo can be reduced by encouraging the child to move slowly as the head is moved or the body is raised or turned. The nurse reassures the child that the symptom is temporary.

Hearing Deficits

Hearing loss in children can be divided into two major categories. *Conductive hearing loss* occurs when the transmission of sound waves between the external ear and the inner ear is interrupted but the inner ear is not affected. For example, conductive hearing loss can be caused by a cerumen-occluded auditory canal, interference with tympanic membrane motility, or ossicle fixation. Many problems that cause conductive hearing loss can be treated successfully medically or surgically (Saxton, et al., 1983).

Sensorineural deafness involves alteration of inner ear function in which sound waves are carried successfully to the inner ear but are improperly analyzed there (Saxton, et al., 1983). Factors contributing to sensorineural deafness include damage from certain medications, head trauma, infections, or noise pollution (Saxton, et al., 1983). Some nerve deafness might be hereditary. Unfortunately, little can be done to treat sensorineural deafness, which forces the child to learn alternate methods of communication.

Ear Infections or Inflammations

Ear infections are common in young children and can cause permanent hearing loss through scarring of the membranes that conduct sound. Temporary hearing loss may occur during the acute phase of the infection or inflammation. The temporary loss of hearing results from the accumulation of fluid in the middle ear, which does not conduct sound waves or allow the same free movement of the ossicles as the normal air media in the middle ear. The permanent loss of hearing results from scarring of the tympanic membrane, which reduces the mobility of the membrane and its sensitivity to sound waves.

Otitis media is the inflammation of the middle ear, which is caused by microorganisms, allergies, or blockage of the drainage from the middle ear through the eustachian tube. Otitis may be either chronic or acute. (Acute otitis media is discussed in Chapter 26.)

Chronic otitis media may result from inadequate treatment of an acute otitis episode or from repeated episodes of acute otitis media. For this reason, the nurse stresses to the parent the importance that the course of antibiotic treatment for acute otitis media be completed, even after the child seems well and the temperature returns to normal. Chronic otitis media can cause *cholesteatoma* (pus and debris in the middle ear), mastoiditis, brain abscess, and permanent hearing loss. Surgery might be needed to remove debris and promote drainage.

Liston and Harbison (1984), in a controlled study of children with recurrent otitis media, demonstrated a significant reduction in the rate of recurrence with the prophylactic administration of sulfisoxasole. Children with severely damaged tympanic membranes from chronic otitis media might recover some hearing with a tympanoplasty.

Serous otitis media occurs as a result of allergic reactions and blockage of the eustachian tube. The treatment for acute serous otitis media includes decongestants to shrink the swollen membranes of the eustachian tube and to allow free drainage of the middle ear and equalization of air pressure on both sides of the tympanum. Children with chronic serous otitis media might benefit from the surgical insertion of small-caliber plastic tubes into the tympanum to reduce the pressure in the middle ear. The insertion of plastic tubes also can be used to treat chronic infection of the middle ear.

Mastoiditis is an infection of the mastoid air cells, which are located in the bony cranium, just behind the ear. The clinical signs are fever, earache, pain, and tenderness over the mastoid area. Facial paralysis is a serious sign which indicates that the infection has spread to the facial nerve sheath. Radiographs of the area might reveal destruction of the bone. Children usually are hospitalized and treated with intravenous antibiotics. If bone destruction has occurred, surgical incision and drainage are done.

Nursing management of a child with mastoiditis might include detection in an outpatient facility and referral to medical care. Nursing care in the hospital includes the maintenance of intravenous infusions, administration of medications, pain management, and preoperative and postoperative management if surgery is required. The nurse explains the condition to the parent, emphasizing the need for vigorous treatment to prevent complications and the spread of infection. Any signs of meningeal irritation should be reported immediately (see Chapter 42). If surgery is done, the nurse observes the dressing for drainage. During convalescence, the nurse assesses the child's hearing acuity to discover if any permanent damage has occurred to the auditory nerve or internal structures of the ear.

A less serious but common and painful condition is infection of the external ear canal *(otitis externa)*. (Otitis externa is discussed in Chapter 26.)

Ear Trauma

The ear may be injured by a sharp blow to the head, laceration of the external ear, and introduction of foreign objects into the external canal. Laceration of the external ear is treated as any other skin injury, with pressure applied to the bleeding site and suturing if needed to achieve clean and undistorted healing.

Sharp blows to the ear or foreign bodies might rupture the eardrum. The child will complain of severe pain and loss of hearing in the affected ear. Prompt medical attention is needed to prevent infection and promote healing of the eardrum without scarring.

Foreign bodies might be introduced into the external canal and be undetected for a time. The object might not be noticed until a discharge appears, the external canal becomes irritated, and hearing acuity is decreased. Removal of the foreign body in the external canal requires professional skill and should not be attempted by the parent. Nursing management includes anticipatory guidance about the potential dangers of allowing toddlers to play with small objects without supervision. Parents might need to be taught the function of earwax; they may not understand that cerumen in the external canal is normal and healthy.

Exposure to loud noises can rupture the eardrum or damage the auditory nerve (Saunders, et al., 1979). Although most of the evidence for damage from loud noises has come from studies of industrial hazards, many researchers believe that similar injuries can occur from stereophonic music turned up to the highest volume. Some loss of hearing acuity might be caused by nerve damage, but the practice also may result in decreased attention to low-volume sounds. Children and parents should know about the potential dangers of exposure to loud noises.

The Child With a Disorder of the Nasal Cavity

Young children, particularly those in early childhood, are prone to putting small objects in their nares, often without subsequent discovery by the parent. The parent should suspect a foreign body when the child exhibits a malodorous or blood-stained nasal discharge. Medical consultation is advised because the object will need to be removed after diagnosis via a nasal speculum.

Anything that causes nasal obstruction, whether it be a foreign object or swollen nasal membranes from the common cold, will not only interfere with the sense of smell but also with the sense of taste. Nurses need to make parents aware of this to decrease parental concern abut anorexia during bouts of upper respiratory infections or during allergy season.

Trauma to the nose is more frequent in children in late childhood or adolescence who participate in athletics. Force from a bat, ball, or other athletic equipment can fracture the nose. If the fracture is not displaced, no treatment is required except to control the resulting epistaxis. Ice packs can be applied for comfort and to reduce edema. Unfortunately, repeated nasal fractures can lead to cosmetic alteration. The child with a deviated septum might require surgery to restore appearance and function.

Postoperative nursing care involves observing for hemorrhage, applying ice packs, and monitoring the fluid and electrolyte balance. The child might have nasal packing and may be discharged shortly after surgery. The nurse instructs the parent regarding the packing and follow-up care.

The Child With a Language Disorder

Language disorders are complex dysfunctions that can adversely affect the child's communicative abilities. Difficulties can be concentrated in any of the following areas of language development:

1. Difficulty formulating ideas or conceptualizing
2. Difficulty learning the symbols that represent ideas
3. Learning symbols that are not congruent with accepted symbols
4. Inability to use symbols for verbal communication
5. Developmental delay in comparison with peers' language development (Bloom and Lahey, 1978)

Normal language development can be interrupted by any number of physical and emotional factors. Language development depends on intact cognitive skills and the ability to process input; therefore, children who have impaired cognitive skills might experience a delay in language development. Emotional stability affects verbal expression, and children with severe psychoses might have unusual speech alterations (see Chapter 25). A stimulating home environment promotes language development, whereas a deprived environment leads to decreased language skills. Articulate, pleasant speech depends on physical health, including auditory acuity, and the absence of any structural or neurologic abnormalities of the mouth or accessory organs of speech.

When managing a child with dysfunctional language development, the nurse needs to be aware of the difference between receptive and expressive language. Children with receptive language problems find it difficult to decode information; that is, they might not understand the verbal symbols of language and/or might have limited ability to comprehend and organize ideas (Goldberg, 1984). Children with expressive disabilities manifest difficulties of speech—poor grammar, alterations in the sound or pattern of speech, or delays caused by environmental deprivation (Goldberg, 1984).

Childhood Aphasia

Childhood aphasia is a disorder of the central nervous system that results in an inability to process symbols and abstract ideas (Emerick and Hatten, 1979). Childhood aphasia also might include an expressive dysfunction in which the child has difficulty translating ideas into speech in a logical manner. Childhood aphasia can be caused by inadequate development in the language realm or by some trauma. Occasionally, the trauma has been minor and the parent is unaware of it until the aphasia is diagnosed (Emerick and Hatten, 1979).

Nurses working with hospitalized aphasic children should be very aware that these children do not process information normally and that they have difficulty relating their past experiences to the present (Emerick and Hatten, 1979). Any explanations of procedures need to be given one piece at a time. A description of even a simple procedure might need to be broken down into component parts and repeated frequently.

Because aphasic children do not express themselves well, it is necessary for the nurse to find out from the parent the child's usual mode of communication. If the child has been in speech therapy, patterns of communication might be established. If at all possible, the parent should remain with the child during hospitalization to reassure and support the child as well as to act as interpreter. The nurse is understanding of the child's difficulties and patient with this often frustrating condition.

Expressive Language Disorders

Speech dysfunctions can be grouped into three distinct categories—articulation disorders, dysfluency, and voice disorders. Voice disorders are variations in pitch that are not considered normal for the child's age and sex. Signs include excessively loud or soft speech, nasal speech, hoarseness, and pitch that is too high or too low. Some voice disorders can be caused by underlying medical problems such as cleft palate or laryngeal nodules. Nurses in outpatient settings can identify voice disorders in children, but more often than not, children with voice disorders are referred for speech therapy by their parents.

Articulation Defects Problems with the articulation of sounds not only makes communication difficult but may be related to other health problems. Proper articulation requires coordination of breathing, sucking, or swallowing; respiratory muscle strength; the ability to control the muscles of the face and lips; the movement of the tongue; and the ability to control the flow of air to the nasal cavity. A number of neuromuscular diseases can contribute to dysfunctional articulation of sounds, as well as structural deformities of the nose, throat, palate, teeth, and tongue. Some children have problems with articulation because of hearing deficits or because they are imitating another person's improper articulation of sounds. Articulation defects also might be idiopathic.

Articulation defects are the most common of the speech disorders. They can take the form of omissions of word syllables, substitutions of incorrect letters for the appropriate ones, distortions such as lisping, or additions of syllables. Consonant sounds are affected most frequently. Some children are born with an abnormally attached lingual frenulum ("tongue tied"). Although this condition can interfere with articulatory speech, it has been found that the frenulum stretches with age. If the child experiences difficulty with developing speech because of severe tongue tie, the frenulum might be clipped after 10 months of age.

Nurses in well-child clinics are in an excellent position to assess children's developing speech patterns early. It is important to discover if the misarticulation is related to other health problems that should be identified and treated. If articulation problems persist, the child's speech should be assessed by a speech specialist and treatment prescribed as appropriate. It is important to treat speech articulation problems as early as possible, certainly before entry into school.

Dysfluency Stuttering is the major problem disrupting the fluency of speech. Stuttering is a speech problem that is particularly troublesome to parents. It is annoying and often appears to be deliberate. A young child under 3 years of age might stutter but be unaware that this form of speech is a problem. After children are 3 or 4 years old they begin to realize that their speech is different, and this self-consciousness might make fluency even more problematic. The major characteristics of stuttering are that the onset is usually prior to 6 years of age; it is more common in boys; it might be familial and related to high parental expectations; it occurs primarily at the beginning of words; and it can cause adverse psychologic effects such as a decrease in self-esteem.

Treatment includes parental guidance. The parent watches for events or situations in which stuttering occurs. When these situations are known, the parent tries to modify or change them to reduce the child's stress. The nurse suggests ways in which the parent can reduce stress. The child should not be scolded for stuttering. The parent should try to be patient and allow the child to complete sentences without interference. The nurse also encourages the parent to identify the child's accomplishments and praise the child as much as possible to build up the child's self-esteem.

Stuttering in the young child can and should be ignored because it is most often a developmental phase of language acquisition. If stuttering continues past the age of 5 years, the child should have professional assistance to help control the stuttering before entering school. The nurse can refer the child and family to a speech specialist.

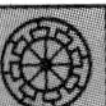

NURSING CARE PLAN Child With Hyphema

Assessment Data

Robert, a 17-year-old high school junior, was admitted to the hospital with a diagnosis of hyphema of the right eye. He suffered a blunt trauma to the eye during football practice and was brought immediately to the hospital when it became apparent that he had sustained an injury. Ophthalmoscopic examination revealed a small area of hemorrhage into the anterior chamber. No other complications were evident at the time other than a right periorbital hematoma. Both eyes were patched, and strict bedrest was ordered. Admission vital signs and laboratory studies were within normal limits, and there was no fracture of the orbital bone. Robert appeared listless and withdrawn.

Nursing Diagnoses and Goals

1. **Nursing diagnosis:** Pain in the right eye and headache subsequent to eye injury.

   Long-term goal: Robert's pain will be relieved through appropriate nursing action.

   Short-term goals: (a) Robert will express the need for pain relief. (b) Robert will understand the reasons for the measures taken to relieve pain.

2. **Nursing diagnosis:** Potential alteration in perception, sensory deprivation, as a result of bilateral eye patching.

   Long-term goal: Robert will not experience any long-term effects from sensory deprivation.

   Short-term goals: (a) Robert will be allowed periods of uninterrupted sleep. (b) Adequate orientation will facilitate Robert's adjustment to the strange environment. (c) Robert will participate in self-care as much as his limitations will allow.

3. **Nursing diagnosis:** Potential for complications secondary to trauma.

   Long-term goal: Long-term sequelae related to eye trauma will be prevented through the prompt recognition of complications.

   Short-term goals: (a) Robert will report any unusual symptoms immediately. (b) Robert will be observed closely for any signs of increased intracranial pressure, glaucoma, or retinal detachment.

4. **Nursing diagnosis:** Potential for psychologic reactions subsequent to injury and hospitalization.

   Long-term goal: Robert will be free from adverse psychologic effects.

   Short-term goals: (a) Robert and his family will experience decreased anxiety as a result of perceiving the event realistically. (b) Robert will experience little interruption in his educational or social life as a result of his injury.

Intervention	Rationale	Evaluation criteria
1. Administer sedatives or analgesics as ordered	Analgesics will provide pain relief. Sedatives promote relaxation and a subsequent decrease in pain. The administration of cycloplegic eyedrops, if ordered, will promote paralysis of the ciliary muscle and provide rest for the eye	Is Robert able to express his need for pain relief? Does the pain appear to be diminishing, as evidenced by increased relaxation, stable vital signs, and decreased anxiety? Are the medications providing the appropriate relief?
Keep both eyes patched	Patching prevents movement of the affected eye by reducing movement of the unaffected eye, thus relieving pain by reducing strain. Patching also prevents the child from rubbing the eye	
Apply ice to the hematoma	The application of cold reduces the injury-induced edema	
Provide quiet diversion such as soft music	See Chapter 29 for an explanation of the use of diversionary strategies to reduce pain	

continued on next page

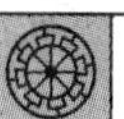

NURSING CARE PLAN Child With Hyphema (continued)

Intervention	Rationale	Evaluation criteria
Explain to Robert the reasons for his pain and encourage him to request pain relief when needed	Realistic explanations decrease anxiety and correspondingly relieve pain	
2. Organize nursing care to allow Robert periods of uninterrupted rest	Lack of sleep contributes to confusion, increased anxiety, and altered perception of events	Is Robert sleeping well? Does he exhibit any signs of sensory deprivation such as nightmares, confusion, withdrawal, or perceptual distortion? Does he express interest in his surroundings and willingness to participate in his care?
Orient Robert to his environment by describing his surroundings as clearly and descriptively as possible; orient Robert frequently to time	Verbal description provides visual images and allows the child to interact with the surroundings; it also identifies spatial limits that enhance safety	
Provide stimulation by changing Robert's environment, allowing family and friends to visit, or providing distraction	Changes in the environment maintain attention and enhance the perception of reality	
Encourage self-care activities such as feeding, bathing, and dressing	Regular participation in care increases the perception of reality and attention to the environment	
3. Take Robert's vital signs frequently and perform regular neurologic checks	Increased blood pressure, severe headache, lethargy, pupil alterations, confusion, and vomiting are signs of increased intracranial pressure caused by head injury	Are there any signs of complications? Do Robert and his family know what to do should symptoms of increased intracranial pressure appear after discharge?
Encourage Robert to report immediately any signs of decreased vision, particles moving across the visual field, or flashes of light	These symptoms might indicate retinal detachment, a complication of blunt trauma to the eye. They will be evident when the patches are removed	
Observe Robert for any signs of severe, sudden headache associated with nausea and vomiting and signs of decreased visual acuity	Glaucoma can occur secondary to trauma	
Alert Robert and his family to the possibility of these complications occurring after discharge	Preparing the family with appropriate information will facilitate the prompt recognition and treatment of complications	
4. Explain to Robert and his family that hyphema usually resolves within several days and that complications are not common	Giving a realistic time frame relieves the anxiety and concern associated with permanent blindness	Do Robert and family appear to be less anxious? Does he interact well with his friends when they come to visit? Is he able to explore an interest in any activity other than football?
Allow Robert to express any feelings he may have relative to missing the rest of the football season	He may have fears that he might lose popularity or social standing by not participating in the sport; verbalizing fears allows the child to deal with them	
Suggest alternative activities which will allow him to continue his social contacts and satisfy his need to participate		

Key Concepts

- It is through the perception of events and communication of ideas and feelings that infants and children gain an understanding of the world, and any alteration in perception or communication impinges on successful development.
- Nurses play an important role in the recognition and referral of children with sensory deficits as well as in minimizing the long-term effects of such deficits.
- The eye, ear, and oral cavity develop early in gestation, and any interference in development results in interference in perception or communication.
- The eye is a complex organ that consists of three layers, each with specific and cooperative functions—the outer layer, consisting of the sclera and cornea; the middle layer, consisting of the iris, lens, ciliary body, and vascular lining; and the inner layer, consisting of the retina.
- The shape and tension of the eye surface are maintained by the anterior and posterior fluid-filled chambers, which facilitate visual function by maintaining normal ocular pressure.
- Visual acuity depends on the proper function of eye structures as well as on the coordination of ocular musculature and proper lubrication.
- The ear consists of three major compartments—the external auricle and auditory canal; the middle ear structures of the tympanum, eustachian tube, and bony ossicles; and the inner fluid-filled semicircular canals, which contain nerve endings.
- Auditory acuity is accomplished through the conduction of sound through air and fluid.
- The oral cavity facilitates taste and supports speech.
- Accessory muscles of the mouth and lips assist in the formation of words.
- The history of a child with a sensory dysfunction includes data regarding the prenatal environment, familial incidence of sensory deficits, child's developmental status, incidences of infections or trauma, and home environmental factors.
- Many diagnostic studies are available to screen children of all ages for sensory deficits, and most of these studies are noninvasive.
- Acute-care needs of the visually impaired child include care of eyeglasses or contact lenses, prevention of sensory deprivation, and meticulous communication via the care plan of the normal routine and self-care skills of the totally blind child.
- Effective preoperative preparation is a nursing challenge with the child who has a sensory deficit.
- Acute-care needs of the hearing-impaired child include relief of pain or vertigo, need for adequate communication via signing or lip reading, prevention of sensory deprivation, and proper care and maintenance of a hearing aid.
- Children with speech deficits experience much frustration and embarrassment when confronted with new situations, and nursing care should be planned accordingly.
- Attention is given to the self-care needs of the blind child regarding feeding to ensure adequate nutrition.
- Children with sensory deficits from birth might experience developmental delays and may have had problems with the attachment process and the development of a healthy self-image.
- Health maintenance needs are directed toward prevention because adequate preventive efforts can reduce the incidence of disease and injury.
- Specific structural conditions that can cause visual deficits in a child include strabismus, refractive errors, cataract, and glaucoma.
- Common eye infections include conjunctivitis, orbital cellulitis, and corneal ulceration.
- Eye injury can be the result of penetrating or blunt eye trauma and chemical burns.
- Complications of eye trauma include hyphema, detached retina, infection, glaucoma, and cataract, any of which could lead to blindness in the affected eye.
- Structural anomalies of the ear may be external, such as abnormal ear placement, or internal, such as the absence or fusion of the ossicles.
- Hearing loss in children can be divided into two major categories—conductive hearing loss and sensorineural hearing loss (nerve deafness).

- Repeated middle ear infections can contribute to conductive hearing loss by damaging the tympanic membrane.
- Foreign bodies in the ear and noise pollution also can contribute to hearing loss.
- Other than inflammation from allergy or virus, difficulties with the nose most often arise from trauma.
- The child with a language disorder may exhibit dysfunction in receptive language, expressive language, or both.
- Speech dysfunction can be identified by nurses in outpatient settings and include disorders of articulation, fluency, or voice.

References

Ashworth P: Sensory deprivation #2—the acutely ill. *Nurs Times* (Feb 15) 1979; 75:290–294.

Bloom L, Lahey M: *Language Development and Language Disorders.* Wiley, 1978.

Bridges M: Extended cortical mastoidectomy and tympanoplasty for chronic otitis media. *Nurs Times* (Jan 20) 1982; Vol 78:101–107.

Campos J, Langer A, Krowitz A: Cardiac responses in the visual cliff in prelocomotor human infants. *Science* 1970; 170:196–197.

Cavalier JP: When moments count . . . the two eye emergencies that demand instant intervention. *RN* (Nov) 1981; 44:41–43.

Chow M, et al: *Handbook of Pediatric Primary Care.* Wiley, 1979.

Emerick L, Hatten J: *Diagnosis and Evaluation in Speech Pathology.* 2nd ed. Prentice-Hall, 1979.

Fanz R, Nevis S: Pattern preferences and perceptual–cognitive development in early infancy. In: *Annual Progress in Child Psychiatry and Child Development.* Chess S, Thomas A (editors). Brunner/Mazel, 1968.

Fraiberg S, Siegel B, Gibson R: The role of sound in search behavior of a blind infant. *Psychoanal Study Child* 1966; 21:327–357.

Goldberg R: Identifying speech and language delays in children. *Pediatr Nurs* (July/Aug) 1984; 10:252–259.

Heinich R: *Educating All Handicapped Children.* Educational Technology Publications, 1979.

Holder L: Hearing aids: Handle with care. *Nursing 82* (April) 1982; 12:64–67.

Kamenir S, et al: Hands-on skills for dealing with hearing aids. *Can Nurse* (Dec) 1982; 78:44–45.

Koestler F: *The Unseen Minority.* David McKay Company, Inc, 1976.

Liston T, Harbison R: Sulfisoxazole chemoprophylaxis and recurrent otitis media. *West J Med* 1984; 140:47–49.

Lowenfeld B: *The Changing Status of the Blind.* Charles C. Thomas, 1975.

Saunders W, et al: *Nursing Care in Eye, Ear, Nose and Throat Disorders.* Mosby, 1979.

Saxton D, et al: *Manual of Nursing Practice.* Addison-Wesley, 1983.

Sharpe A: Helping parents in the developmental rearing of a blind child. *Matern Child Nurs* 1973; 2:23–28.

Systems of Life #88: Examining the cranial nerves completed. *Nurs Times* (Apr 7–13) 1982; center pages.

Tumulty G, Resler M: Eye trauma. *Am J Nurs* (June) 1984; 84:740–743.

Welch J, Tyler J, Quinn B: Dealing with eye injuries. *RN* (March) 1984; 47:53–54.

Zucnick M: Care of an artificial eye. *Am J Nurs* (May) 1975; 75:835–836.

Additional Readings

Adams J, Evans G, Roberts J: Diagnosing and treating otitis media with effusion. *Am J Matern Child Nurs* (May) 1984; 9:22–28.

Bess F, McConnell F: *Audiology, Education, and the Hearing-Impaired Child.* Mosby, 1981.

Brown M, Collar M: Effects of prior preparation on preschoolers' vision and hearing screening. *Am J Matern Child Nurs* (Sept/Oct), 1982; 7:323–328.

Caldarelli D: *Pediatric Otolaryngology.* Medical Examination, 1983.

Clarke M: Psychology: A sense of perception. *Nurs Mirror* (June 12) 1980; 150:41–43.

Crawford J, Morin JD: *The Eye in Childhood.* Grune & Stratton, 1983.

DiChiara E: A sound method for testing children's hearing. *Am J Nurs* (Sept) 1984; 84:1104–1106.

Gerber S: *Audiometry in Infancy.* Grune & Stratton, 1977.

Helveston E: *Pediatric Ophthalmology Practice.* 2nd ed. Mosby, 1984.

Harley R: *Pediatric Ophthalmology.* Vols I and II. 2nd ed. Saunders, 1983.

Harley R, Lawrence G: *Visual Impairment in the Schools.* Thomas, 1977.

Kass J, Beebe M: Serous otitis media. *Nurse Pract* 1979; 25–28.

Lin-Fu J: *Visual Screening of Children.* US Department of Health, Education, and Welfare. DHEW Publication. Government Printing Office, 1971.

Ludington-Hoe S: What can newborns really see? *Am J Nurs* (Sept) 1983; 83:1286–1289.

Maloney: A health care protocol for otitis media. In: *Current Practice in Pediatric Nursing II.* Brandt P, et al (editors). Mosby, 1978.

McDermott J: Immittance screening for aural problems in school children. *J School Health* 1982; 52:462–468.

Meadow K: *Deafness and Child Development.* University of California Press, 1980.

Morgan RH: Breaking through the sound barrier . . . your deaf patient. *Nursing 83* (Feb) 1983; 13:112, 114.

Riddle I: Communicative behaviors of hospitalized school-age children with binocular bandages. *Matern Child Nurs J* 1972; 1:291–354.

Shanks S: *Nursing and the Management of Pediatric Communication Disorders.* College-Hill Press, 1983.

Thompson L: Understanding tympanometry. *Pediatr Nurse* (May/June) 1982; 8:193–197.

Tyers A, Westaby S (editors): Wound care #17–wounds of the eye. *Nurs Times* (March 30) 1983; 79:65–68.

Wassenberg C: Common visual disorders in children. *Nurs Clin North Am* (Sept) 1981; 16:469–485.

Wright K: An update on amblyopia and strabismus. *Consultant* 1982; 22:97–99, 103, 106–107.

Protection
Implications of Inflammation and Altered Skin Integrity

44

Judith A. Surveyer Juanita Fleming Susan Rowen James

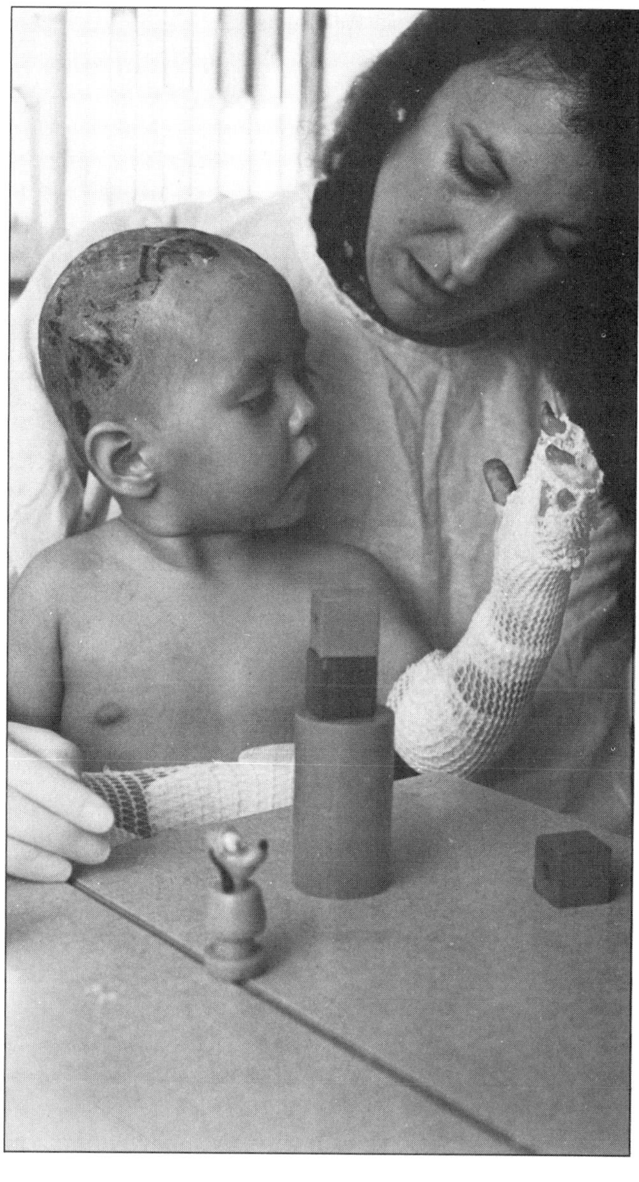

continued on next page

Objectives

- Describe the anatomy and physiology of the skin.
- Describe the history and assessment of lesions required to evaluate the child with altered integument.
- Define the procedures and treatments involved in wound care and skin grafts.
- Explain acute care, nutritional support, and developmental needs of children with skin injuries.
- Outline the standard classification of burns according to the severity of injury and complicating factors.
- Describe the ways in which the medical and nursing management of the child with a burn respond to alterations in the body's systems.
- Outline the basic elements of wound management for the child with a burn.
- State the nurse's responsibilities in the care of specific areas after a burn.
- Describe the chronic-care measures for the child with a burn.
- Explain the physiological processes, medical treatments, and principles of nursing management for the child with frostbite.
- Describe the nursing management for the child with severe surface injuries.
- Explain the physiologic processes, medical treatments, and principles of nursing management for skin infection or infestation.
- Describe the most common types of congenital birthmarks.
- Explain the physiologic processes, medical treatments, and principles of nursing management for skin inflammation.

To find these topics, see the following chapters:

Cradle Cap (Seborrheic Dermatitis)	Chapter 7
Diaper Dermatitis (Diaper Rash)	Chapter 7
Milia	Chapter 7
Miliaria (Prickly Heat)	Chapter 7
Pediculosis	Chapter 26
Scabies	Chapter 26
Moniliasis (Thrush)	Chapter 26

The skin is a complex, essential organ. It is both a physiologic and psychologic protector of the body. As a psychologic protector, the skin is one means of communication, and the appearance of the skin might affect self-image. The integrity of the skin is, therefore, important in ensuring that the individual is protected physiologically and psychologically. Nurses working with children, whether as inpatients or outpatients, are likely to encounter skin alterations because they are one of the most common health problems. Although all skin has similarities, there is considerable variability from individual to individual in terms of color, texture, pH, moisture, and temperature. These variations depend on the care of the skin, age, sex, and racial origin of the individual, and degree of exposure to the elements. The nature of skin also varies in different parts of the body of the same individual and at different times during the life span. The dermis is thinner in newborn infants than it is in adults. Several premises about skin alterations have implications for nursing care. Skin alterations in children and youth may:

- Be major or minor
- Be congenital (such as mongolian spot, birthmark) or acquired
- Be associated with development and, consequently, evident in some age groups and not in others (for example, milia in infants, acne in adolescents)
- Require no specific medical treatment because they are self-limiting (such as erythema infectiosum)
- Be a manifestation of a systemic disease (such as meningococcic meningitis rash, vitamin A deficiency)
- Have prodromal symptoms before skin alteration is noticed (such as measles)
- Affect other organs of the body if not properly treated (such as systemic lupus erythematosus)
- Be caused by any number of agents (viral or bacterial) or autoimmune in origin
- Have psychologic effects on the child (such as psoriasis)
- Be acute or chronic (such as atopic eczema)
- Have a different appearance in children than in adults (such as atopic dermatitis)
- Have a variety of causes (such as unknown systemic disease; foreign substances that are ingested, inhaled, injected, or absorbed; traumas such as burns, falls, or pressure)
- Be affected by many factors that can be interrelated. Some of these factors are age, pH, nutritional status, adequate blood supply, and psychosocial factors

In this chapter we describe nursing care appropriate for children with skin injuries. We first look at the anatomy of the skin to see how its parts function together to provide a protective layer. We discuss how the nurse assesses lesions and the nurse's role in the basic care of wounds and skin grafts. Because care for the child with a burn is such a demanding, specialized area, we explain in depth the nurse's duties in burn treatment. Other areas of skin damage discussed are frostbite, severe surface injuries, infection or infestation, inflammation, and congenital birthmarks.

Anatomy and Physiology of the Skin

The skin is an organ of human attraction and emotional expression. The external appearance of the skin is a part of the child's self-image. It contributes to the physical health and well-being of the child and plays a role in ego development through sensory perception, emotional expression, and outward appearance. Behaviors that might reveal that the child is having difficulty are expressions of low self-esteem, self-blame, and excessive fears. Withdrawal from social contacts and hypochondriacal behavior also might be indicators of difficulty. Consequently, the developing child's self-esteem is a significant concern for the nurse caring for a child with a skin alteration.

The sympathetic nervous system innervates the skin. Some of the physiologic concomitants of emotions that relate to the skin are changes in the skin's temperature, psychogalvanic skin responses, secretion of sebum and fatty acids, thermal sweat production, cutaneous vascular responses, patterns of wheal formation, and changes in the skin's vulnerability to inflammation (Prugh, 1983). Prugh noted that some skin changes are external manifestations of internal psychologic conflicts and represent intermediate phenomena between vegetative disorders (Prugh, 1983). Vegetative disorders are conditions such as eczema, urticaria, and so-called neurodermatitis. Children with eczema and urticaria have the predisposing physiologic factors associated with allergies. The conversion disorders are those skin conditions that occur in response to psychologic or social stimuli.

The skin is an organ of perception. To some extent, strongly felt perceptions are exhibited by the skin. Involuntary mechanisms use the skin to express emotions such as anger (flushing); fear (blanching); anxiety (sweating); and shame or embarrassment (blushing). Montagu's focus on the skin's psychologic aspects is primarily from the perspective of touching. He felt that cutaneous stimulation is important in infancy (Montagu, 1971).

Understanding the structure and function of the skin is necessary to properly assess the changes it undergoes. The skin begins to develop at about the eleventh week of gestation and undergoes developmental changes throughout the life span. A vital and important organ, the skin serves as a physiologic protector, sensor, and thermoregulator. It also aids in secretion, excretion, and absorption. Small amounts of sodium and urea are excreted through the skin. The major function of the skin is to protect the tissues it envelopes against external environmental factors. It forms a barrier to protect the body from various organisms, foreign objects, trauma, radiation, moisture, and humidity. It protects humans by inhibiting excess loss of water, providing an acid covering to protect the surface of the body from irritants and bacteria, acting as a water repellent, and generally protecting the body from the external environment by forming an elastic and resistant covering. The skin is structured so that few substances can pass through it with ease. The internal fluid mechanism of the body is partially maintained by the skin, and it prevents the excess loss of body fluid as long as the surface membrane is intact. When the surface membrane is lost, as in extensive or severe skin conditions, large amounts of fluid, electrolytes, and protein might be lost from the body. Sebum, a protective coating, is secreted by the skin. It has antifungal and antibacterial properties and aids in maintaining skin texture. As a thermoregulator, the skin prevents heat loss from the body by the processes of radiation, conduction, convection, and evaporation. The sensations of pain, temperature, touch, and pressure are discriminated by the skin in conjunction with the cerebral cortex.

The integumentary system is composed of two major tissue layers, hair, nails, sebaceous glands, eccrine glands, sweat glands, and associated structures such as nerves, blood vessels, connective tissue, and muscles.

Epidermis

The outer layer of the skin is a thin, stratified epithelium called the *epidermis*. One of the primary functions of the epidermis is serving as a barrier. The epidermis covers the entire body and gives rise to hair, nails, sebaceous glands, and sweat glands. Its thickness varies little over most of the body, except for the palms and soles, where the skin is thicker. The epidermis is made up of five layers, which are, from outward to inward, the *stratum comeum* (horny layer), *stratum lucidum* (clear layer), *stratum granulosum* (granular layer), *stratum spinosum* (prickly layer), and *stratum germinativum* or *stratum basale* (regenerative layer). Although all of the layers have specific functions, the horny and regenerative layers are the most important. The horny layer consists of keratinized cells, which shed continuously. These cells help to maintain the skin's integrity. Lying between the dead and living cells is a transitional zone that contributes to the impermeability of the skin. This transitional zone prevents the body contents from leaking out and noxious environmental agents from entering the interior of the body. The regenerative layer produces cells that move toward the most superficial layer to replace cells that have been shed from the surface. Regeneration will not occur without an intact stratum germinativum.

The principal pigment of the skin, melanin, also is formed in the stratum germinativum. Skin color varies depending on the melanin content. It has been suggested that darkly pigmented skin does not necessarily mean that there are more *melanocytes* (cells that produce melanin) but rather that the melanocytes that are present are more active (Pillsbury, 1980). The density of melanocytes in the epidermis does not mean that the cells are active to the same degree. The skin of members of darkly pigmented races does not contain more melanocytes; rather, the melanocytes are larger and work harder. In albinism, for example, melanocytes are present but are nonfunctional; consequently, there is a lack of pigmentation. Melanin may be transferred from melanocytes to keratinocytes. Inflammatory reactions may prevent melanin transfer and account in parts for hypopigmentation in certain cutaneous lesions (Laude and Russo, 1983). Other pigments known to influence skin color are carotene, oxyhemoglobin, and reduced hemoglobin (Roach, 1977). To some extent, skin color is associated with the amount of blood in the cutaneous capillaries. Pallor, bluish cast, and redness or flushed appearance of the skin might be caused by the quantity of blood moving through the capillaries, as well as the quality (degree of oxygenation) of the blood. When circulation of the blood is rapid, the skin might appear flushed. When blood circulation is slow, the skin might have a bluish cast, and when blood circulation is impaired or vasoconstriction occurs, pallor results.

Dermis and Subcutaneous Tissue

The *dermis* lies directly beneath the epidermis. Blood vessels, nerves, lymphatic vessels, hair follicles, and sweat glands are found in the dermis. Connective tissue, containing elastic fibers, also is part of the dermis. Two layers divide the dermis, the *papillary layer,* which interdigitates with the epidermis, and the *reticular layer,* which lies between the papillary layer and subcutaneous tissue.

Subcutaneous tissue lies beneath the dermis. This thick, fatty layer attaches the dermis to the underlying structures. Sweat glands also are found in subcutaneous tissue. There are two types of sweat glands. Small sweat glands are called *eccrine glands*. Two to four million eccrine glands are found over almost the entire body (Goldsmith, 1983) and help to control temperature. Eccrine sweat is used when diagnosing cystic fibrosis in children. Large sweat glands are called *apocrine glands*. Apocrine glands are found mainly in the axillas, anal and genitocrural skin, mammary areolas and inframammary regions, and in such areas as the mons pubis, face, scalp, and abdomen. Apocrine glands are found also in the auditory meatus and eyelids (Goldsmith, 1983). The ducts of the apocrine glands parallel the hair follicles. Sebaceous glands, which also are located in the dermis, secrete sebum. The sebum provides a protective coating and is thought to have some bacteriocidal effect; consequently, sebum helps to prevent infection. Many small blood vessels that nourish the skin and carry sensation through the nerves are located in the dermis as well.

Defense System

The stratum corneum serves as the first line of defense against agents from the outside penetrating the skin. The transitional zone is the first line of defense against substances leaving the body. In young children the transitional zone is not as effective a barrier as in the adult. Consequently, more water might seep into the horny layers, making more water available for evaporation in children.

The outer surface of normal skin is acidic, with a pH between 4.5 and 6.5. The acid pH is believed to protect the skin from many pathogenic bacteria because most bacteria require a more alkaline environment to grow. The evaporation of sebum and eccrine sweat, both of which are in contact with keratin, help to lower the skin pH. The pH of the skin decreases with increasing age because there seems to be more sebum and eccrine sweat to evaporate. Consequently, young children, who secrete little sebum and eccrine sweat, are more susceptible to skin infections.

The stratum corneum of infants is thin, the amount of sebum and eccrine sweat secreted is relatively small, and the skin pH is relatively high. As a result, infants are more vulnerable to skin conditions than individuals with more mature skin.

Assessment of the Child With Altered Integument

History

Careful observation and obtaining an accurate history are essential for the nurse before planning care. The history should include changes in life-style, skin alterations in family members, and, particularly, any known allergies of the patient or family. The nurse's initial interview elicits information regarding prodromal symptoms, exposure to substances and persons, length of time lesions have been present, and when the lesions appeared. The nurse also describes the configuration, distribution, type, and color of any lesions. Both the parent and child should provide historical information.

The nurse includes the following critical points in obtaining a history regarding skin alterations:

1. Both the parent and child (if the child is old enough) inform the nurse when the skin alteration first appeared and describe the lesions and any alterations in their appearance. The nurse establishes the size, shape, color, changes, and configuration of the lesions. Perceptions of changes in the appearance of lesions are important. If the lesions are larger, redder, blistered, or have undergone some other changes, this is useful information. Whether the lesions have spread over the body and the direction of the spread are also important. This information is compared with examination of the lesions.

2. The nurse also obtains a description of the sensation experienced from the lesions and the condition of the lesions at various points in time. Are the lesions itchy or painful, or has there been no change in skin sensitivity? Are the lesions dry, scaly, oily, smooth, or rough? Are there secretions from the lesions? If so, the type and amount of secretions should be estimated. This information is compared with examination of the lesions.

3. The nurse asks both the parent and child to describe any symptoms that appeared prior to the skin condition. Specific questions may be posed to help the child and/or parent to remember symptoms because they might not be associated in their minds with the skin alteration. Fever, stomachache, headache, dizziness, nausea, vomiting, runny nose, watery eyes, or cough might be prodromal symptoms.

4. The nurse obtains information regarding contacts with other persons or exposure to substances. The nurse asks for specifics that might give clues to possible allergic reactions. The types of foods, beverages, and medications taken are significant. Recent illnesses and treatments also are noted. Changes in the environment, such as a new pet, and changes in habits, such as the use of a different type of soap or

Obtaining Information in the Assessment of the Integumentary System

1. When did the trouble start? Describe the condition.
2. Where did the condition start? How long has it existed?
3. What other symptoms, if any, did the child have other than the rash when the condition started?
4. Has it spread? If so, how did it spread?
5. Does it come and go? If so, do the lesions come in crops?
6. Does it itch?
7. Does it ever blister? If so, were the blisters filled with clear liquid?
8. What ointments, creams, or lotions have been used on the rash?
9. What makes it worse?
10. What makes it better?
11. Does the child have any contacts with a similar rash?
12. Is there any history of skin conditions? Does anyone in the family have asthma or hay fever or has anyone had either of these conditions in the past?
13. Has the child traveled recently?
14. Have there been any previous illnesses? Describe them.
15. What tablets, medicine, or injections has the child received in the last 6 months?
16. Where does the child play? What does the child play with?

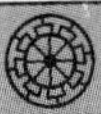

ASSESSMENT GUIDE Child With a Problem of the Integumentary System

System	Subjective data	Objective data	Validating data	Nursing management
Head	Pruritus in head	Small lesions in back of ears and neck		Check head for pediculosis (see Chapter 26)
		Scaly areas on head, ears, eyebrows	Wood's light examination; skin scraping	Watch for alopecia and other signs differentiating tinea, psoriasis, and seborrheic dermatitis
Eyes, ears, nose, and throat	Sore throat, headache, fever	Throat red, inflamed, exudative	Throat culture for β-hemolytic streptococci	Check exposure to scarlet fever or streptococcal pharyngitis; observe for desquamation on hands and feet; watch for skin lesions indicating other communicable diseases
		Adherent white placques on the tongue and mucous membranes		See Chapter 26 for the management of *Candida* infections
Integumentary	Pain	Contusions, lacerations, burns		Observe for associated signs of child abuse if circumstances of injury are questionable
	Fever, pain, heat	Redness, edema, red streaks, enlarged regional lymph nodes	Wound culture; complete blood count	Warm compresses to site of inflammation; observe for more severe cellulitis
	Severe, generalized pruritus	Urticaria	Skin tests, Radioallergosorbant Test	Careful history of allergies, including recent course of antibiotics; watch for signs of anaphylaxis (see Chapter 37)
		Purpura, particularly on the legs, thighs, and buttocks	Complete blood count; erythrocyte sedimentation rate (see Chapter 37)	Observe for gastrointestinal signs as seen in Henoch-Shöenlein purpura (see Chapter 37); check for recent exposure to medications
	Thirsty, restless	Skin and mucous membranes dry, poor turgor, decreased urine output, sunken fontanelles in infant	Serum electrolytes Check for recent exposure to medications	Management for dehydration (see Chapter 33)
		Cyanosis, jaundice, other skin color changes		Observe for signs of underlying disease
Cardiovascular	Numbness and tingling in fingers, toes, and elsewhere	Skin white, cold		Check for exposure to cold; check for butterfly rash on face and other signs of systemic lupus erythematosus (see Chapter 37)
		Generalized edema, decreased blood pressure, increased pulse, pallor, signs of circulatory collapse	Serum electrolytes; central venous pressure monitoring	Vigorous care of child with severe burns to prevent hypovolemic shock

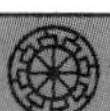

ASSESSMENT GUIDE Child With a Problem of the Integumentary System (continued)

System	Subjective data	Objective data	Validating data	Nursing management
Gastrointestinal	Nausea	Vomiting, gastrointestinal distention, decreased gastrointestinal motility		Nasogastric tube for severe burns; watch for signs of paralytic ileus (see Chapter 38)
Respiratory	Restlessness	Signs of respiratory distress and/or airway obstruction	Blood gases	Ventilation if increased respiratory distress and poor blood gases (severe burn management); chest physical therapy
Genitourinary	Pain in lower abdomen		Urine culture	Foley catheter care (see Chapter 39) for severely burned child; watch for signs of renal failure (see Chapter 39)
Neuroendocrine	Agitation, restlessness	Alteration in consciousness following severe burn; increased blood pressure from release of catecholamines after a burn		Reassure parent if growth or maturation slows during burn healing phase
Musculoskeletal	Pain in joints	Edema of joints with decreased mobility; rash on face or over joints	Blood for Antinuclear Antibody, Rheumatoid Factor (see Chapter 37)	(See Chapter 37 for systemic lupus erythematosus and juvenile rheumatoid arthritis)

shampoo, are worth exploring. Changes in laundry products, use of blankets, or foods ingested also are important to determine. Information about recent travel and where the child plays also are noteworthy.

5. The nurse obtains information about any treatments tried and their results.

6. The nurse also gets a description of the emotional response to skin problems. In this regard the nurse keeps in mind that a variety of adaptive and maladaptive responses might be evident.

Assessment of Lesions

The nurse's eyes and hands are the most effective tools for examining the patient's skin. Using the conceptual base illustrated in Figure 44-1 to observe the skin or any lesions that appear on the skin, the nurse gets an accurate description of skin alterations (Fleming, 1981). The description derived from inspection and palpation of lesions will be essential in helping to obtain solid baseline information about the child's dermatologic condition.

Type and Size Lesions generally are classified as either primary or secondary. *Primary lesions* are those that arise in previously normal skin. *Secondary lesions* result from changes in the primary eruptions. Although useful, the terms primary and secondary lesion are not absolute because the differences between these two types of lesions are not as definitive as the terms suggest. A third type of lesion, *vascular lesions,* contains blood vessels.

It also is important to determine the size of the lesions. Some lesions are smaller than 1 cm, whereas others are larger than 1 cm. Primary skin lesions 1 cm or less in size can be broken down into the following categories and examples:

Macule—circumscribed, flat, discoloration (for example, freckle)

Papule—circumscribed, elevated, solid but superficial, discoloration (for example, individual lesions of lichen planus)

Petechia—circumscribed, sometimes elevated, from minute hemorrhages in the skin (for example, lesions associated with a platelet deficiency)

Vesicle—circumscribed, elevated, filled with serous fluid (for example, lesions of chickenpox)

Lesions 1 cm or greater in size are categorized as follows:

Purpura—circumscribed, elevated, from hemorrhage in skin, similar to petechiae but greater in size (for example, Henoch-Shöenlein purpura)

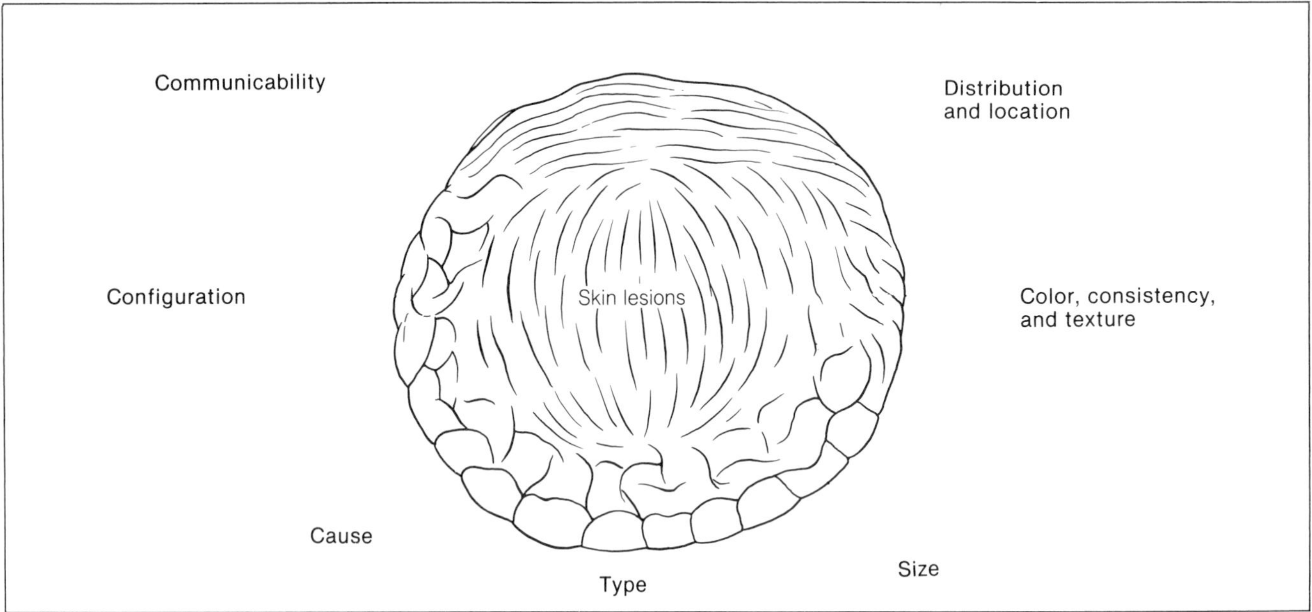

Figure 44-1 Factors used for assessing skin lesions. Reproduced with permission from Fleming, JW, Assessing skin lesions. *AM J Matern Child Nurs* (Sept/Oct); 1981: 6(5). Art by Sutphin E. Copyright © 1981, American Journal of Nursing Company.

Patch—circumscribed, flat, discoloration (for example, salmon patch)

Placque—circumscribed, elevated, solid but superficial, discoloration, similar to papules but larger in size, often results from coalescing of papules (for example, psoriasis)

Tumor—solid with depth, beneath or level with the skin surface, similar to nodules but larger in size (for example, lipoma)

Bulla—circumscribed, elevated, filled with serous fluid, similar to vesicles but larger (for example, contact dermatitis)

Some lesions, however, vary in size and shape, as follows:

Nodule—solid with depth, beneath or level with the skin surface (for example, lymph node)

Wheal—localized, edematous, transitory superficial area (for example, mosquito bite)

Pustule—circumscribed, elevated, filled with purulent fluid (for example, impetigo)

Secondary skin lesions can be classified as follows:

Crust—dried, colored deposits of skin exudates (for example, impetigo)

Excoriation—superficial, traumatic abrasion (for example, scratched insect bites)

Scale—shed, thin, dead epidermal cells, either dry or greasy (for example, psoriasis)

Fissure—linear, sharply defined cracks with abrupt walls

Erosion—loss of epidermis that does not extend into dermis

Ulcer—destruction of epidermis; irregular size and shape

Atrophy—loss of some portion and function of skin

Scar—connective tissue replacing tissue lost through disease or injury

Keloid—nonencapsulated, generally linear mass of hyperplastic fibrous connective tissue that results from a traumatic injury; seen more frequently among blacks

Special lesions are classified as follows because they are for the most part associated with particular conditions:

Comedo (blackhead)—collection of sebum and keratin lodged in the pilosebaceous follicle (for example, acne vulgaris)

Milium (whitehead)—type of papule containing sebaceous or cornfield material (for example, acne vulgaris)

Burrow—tract in the epidermis that appears like a long or short piece of wheat (for example, scabies)

Hemorrhages—extravasations of blood (for example, trauma)

Configuration The configuration, or pattern a group of lesions assumes, can be important in assessing the dermatologic condition. The four common patterns are as follows:

Annular—lesions that have a ringlike pattern

Iris—lesions resembling a bull's eye. The center of the lesion appears cyanotic or hemorrhagic and is surrounded by an area of erythema with a pale, vasoconstricted inner circle

Linear—lesions that assume a straight line, often resembling a streak

Marbling—lesions that resemble swirls; sweeping brush-like patterns

The nurse also determines whether the skin lesions are symmetric or asymmetric in shape.

Distribution and Location The nurse records the areas of the body in which the lesions are found, whether the lesions are generalized or localized, (for example, on the face, trunk, or extremities), and their configuration (clustered, coalesced, or discrete). Some areas of the body have a predilection for particular dermatologic conditions. A localized, discrete rash is seldom caused by a systemic disease or reaction to a food or drug; however, a generalized rash, which often occurs abruptly in hospitalized patients, is frequently a reaction to a drug or some other allergen. The most common appearance of lesions caused by a drug reaction is *urticaria* (hives). These lesions can persist for as long as 1 week or more after the drug that caused the reaction has been discontinued or contact with the allergen has ceased.

Occasionally, skin lesions will seem to disappear, only to reappear elsewhere, especially with bathing or exposure to cold or heat. As one school-aged child with erythema infectiosum (fifth disease) said, "You think it's all gone and the rash comes back somewhere else on your body."

Texture and Color of Skin and Lesions The nurse notes the consistency, texture, and color of the child's skin and any lesions. Moistness, smoothness, and dryness of the skin are considered in determining its texture and consistency. The nurse also considers the skin's color and degree of cleanliness. The skin's turgor can be checked easily by pinching it slightly. Well-hydrated skin will resume its original configuration when released. Dehydrated skin will react like bread dough, retaining the pinched appearance.

The color of the lesions can range from yellow, pink, red, and bluish to gray, brown, and amber. The lesions also can be black or white. The color of the lesions is an important diagnostic guide. To assess color, the nurse considers not only the color of the lesions but also skin color in general. Nonglare daylight is considered the best for examining skin color and will help the nurse to make an objective assessment. The nurse must be astute in making observations on darker-skinned persons because skin coloring can vary the appearance of lesions. The skin color of members of darker-skinned races often varies from black, yellow-brown, and reddish-brown to tones similar to those of whites. Comparing the unaffected skin with the affected skin is one way of observing color alterations.

Yellowish discoloration is seen in individuals with jaundice. During the neonatal period, many infants develop this skin alteration. *Cyanosis,* a bluish discoloration of the skin, is likely to be seen in persons with cardiac and/or pulmonary conditions. It also is noted in some low-birthweight infants. Gunmetal gray purpura is characteristic of meningococcic meningitis rash. When assessing the color of the lesions, the nurse considers not only the present color but also color changes, the length of time the color has been present, and the sequence of the color change. According to Smith and Cairns (1981) the color sequence of reddish-purple to green and yellow commonly is seen in erythema nodosum. A history of prolonged jaundice might be present in individuals with galactosemia. The nurse notes the evenness of the skin pigmentation. Is the skin hyperpigmented or hypopigmented? In phenylketonuria, for example, pigment is underdeveloped (Frankenburg, William, Thornton, and Chors, 1982). The nurse also considers the effect of skin alterations on other body systems.

Nursing Management for Procedures and Treatments

Not all skin conditions are transmissible. Some conditions arise from within the individual, and there is no mode of transmission. A number of skin conditions, however, are transmissible, and the modes of transmission vary. Contaminated, airborne dust particles and direct contact with secretions from an infected person are two ways different types of measles are communicated. The chickenpox virus is spread by airborne droplets and by direct or indirect contact, meningococcic meningitis is spread by direct contact, and the organisms that cause Rocky Mountain spotted fever are carried by ticks.

Inspection of the skin and description of the lesions, as indicated in the assessment guide presented earlier in the chapter, are essential steps in diagnosing a skin condition. Using side lighting or transillumination enables the nurse to visualize the configuration of some lesions. A magnifying lens is useful in helping to determine the topography of a lesion, as well as in locating parasites on the skin. Microscopic examination of a sample of infected skin is another direct means of diagnosing a skin condition.

To obtain a sample for direct microscopic examination, a scraping of the skin is necessary. A smear, culture, or biopsy might be obtained from skin lesions for further examination. Skin scrapings and wound cultures assist in determining causative organisms so that appropriate therapy can be instituted. Before specimens are taken, the skin lesion should be cleansed with a 70% alcohol solution so that topical medication, if present, can be removed.

Complete blood counts and serum electrolyte levels are helpful in diagnosing skin conditions as well as to monitor progress (such as in burn patients). Skin tests are useful in diagnosing allergic reactions (see Chapter 37). Other types of skin tests, such as the tine test for tuberculosis, test for exposure to an infectious organism. When preparing the child for any type of skin test, the nurse explains the purpose of the skin test and the procedure that will be used. The nurse notes on the record if the child is taking steroids or immunosuppressive drugs. The child and family must be told that a positive skin test for an infectious disease does not always indicate an active infectious condition because the organism might be in an inactive, or dormant, state. Skin tests should never be done on inflamed skin. In such a case it is likely that the test would aggravate the skin disorder and also make it difficult to interpret the results accurately.

The diascope, a piece of glass that can be pressed firmly against a skin lesion, is useful in examining erythematous lesions. It helps the examiner to determine if the lesion is caused by vascular dilatation or bleeding into the skin. Lesions that are caused by bleeding in the skin will not blanch under pressure.

The Wood's light is a useful instrument in helping to diagnose certain skin conditions. The fluorescent light reflects a particular color depending on the organism present. For example, the fungi that cause common forms of tinea capitis will reflect a bright blue-green color, enabling the examiner to locate infected hairs. The nurse needs to be careful to remove any topical agents before examination because they might fluoresce as well. Other substances, such as horny material, also might fluoresce. The light may be brighter, weaker, or different from the light produced by the fungi that cause tinea capitis.

Preparation for Diagnostic Tests

Tests used to diagnose skin conditions are relatively benign and noninvasive. A simple explanation to the child that is appropriate for the child's developmental level will ensure cooperation and facilitate the procedure (see Chapter 29). Children like to be included as much as possible in their care. For this reason, allowing them to see their own skin lesions through the magnifying glass or a Wood's light can be a vehicle for describing and explaining the importance of the treatment.

Skin scraping for miscroscopic examination is done with a razor blade but is essentially painless. The child is encouraged to remain still and is told that the procedure feels like being scratched lightly. (The procedure for allergy skin testing is discussed in Chapter 37.)

Wound Care

Cleansing A variety of topical preparations are used to clean minor and severe wounds. The purpose of thoroughly cleansing is to reduce the development of inflammation and infection. Each preparation has its advantages and disadvantages and may be used according to institutional protocol. PHisoDerm and povidone–iodine solutions (Betadine) are commonly used wound-cleansing agents and are readily available for home use. Zephiran Chloride (benzalkonium), although less commonly used, is a nonirritating, painless topical antiseptic. Because Zephiran Chloride is sensitive to light, it must be stored in a dark container. Other solutions used for wound cleansing include Merthiolate (thimerosal) and hydrogen peroxide (Table 44-1).

It is important to remember that children are very concerned about the pain associated with wounds and might resist effective cleansing if they anticipate that the solution will cause additional pain. None of the previously mentioned solutions is painful when applied to wounds, although the effervescence of hydrogen peroxide can be irritating to some children.

Keeping the skin clean and moist and free of irritants promotes healing, helps to prevent infections, and restores skin integrity. Skin irritants include urine, feces, and excessive perspiration, particularly in intertriginous areas. In infants friction from improperly placed diapers might irritate the skin. Diapers washed in certain types of soap and not rinsed sufficiently also might cause irritation. If cloth diapers are worn, a nonirritating soap should be used. The nurse might teach the parent how to diaper the infant so that rubbing does not occur. If too much moisture is a problem after cleaning the skin, exposing the area directly to sunlight or artificial light may help to keep the area dry.

The nurse is careful when cleaning the infant's or child's skin. Bland soap and water and a soft washcloth should be used, and vigorous rubbing should be avoided. Because the intertriginous areas are potential sources of irritation, care should be taken to cleanse them. The folds of the skin should be separated and cleansed. After each diaper change, the nurse does a thorough cleansing. Vigorous rubbing should be avoided and the skin patted dry.

Baths often are helpful in minimizing the inflammatory process of skin lesions. When dryness and chapping are evident, the use of soap should be minimized. The use of bath oils is a simple way to manage dry, scaly skin. Bathing adds moisture to the skin, and the oil helps to retain the moisture. Mineral oil is an inexpensive substitute for bath oil. The disadvantage of mineral oil is that it lacks a surfactant to make it mix with water.

Oil baths such as Alpha Keri or Domol (1–2 tsp per tub of water) might alleviate drying as well as soothe the skin. Other cooling, antipruritic baths such as Aveeno (1 c per tub of water) or tar baths might help to minimize pruritus. Adding baking soda to the bath water is an inexpensive method of relieving pruritus.

Certain shampoos are used to treat skin conditions affecting the head. Available pediculocides can be found in shampoo form, allowing for more effective treatment (see Chapter 26). The many varieties of dandruff shampoo presently on the market also can be used to treat and control seborrheic dermatitis in infants (cradlecap). The major

TABLE 44-1 Some Common Antiseptic and Cleansing Agents

Solution	Actions	Nursing considerations
PHisoDerm	Mild topical antiseptic	Nonirritating; readily available for home use
Povidone–iodine (Betadine)	Antimicrobial; effective against gram-positive and gram-negative organisms, fungi, yeast, and viruses	Available for home use; nonirritating; not to be used on extensive wounds because of the possibility of systemic absorption
Benzalkonium (Zephiran Chloride)	Effective against gram-positive and gram-negative organisms, fungi, and some protozoa	Solution is light sensitive and must be kept in a dark container; incompatible with PHisoDerm and other soaps, so wounds must be thoroughly rinsed of these agents before application; nonirritating to the skin
Thimerosal (Merthiolate)	Bacteriostatic; fungistatic; not as effective an antibacterial agent as others	Nonirritating; needs light-resistant container; used more as an antiseptic than cleansing agent; compatible with soaps
Hydrogen peroxide	Somewhat antibacterial; cleans wounds by release of oxygen (effervescent effect)	Nontoxic; can be used for oral wounds or lesions; must be stored in light-resistant container

Information from: Govoni L., Hayes J.: *Drugs and Nursing Implications*. Appleton-Century-Crofts, 1982 *and* Asperheim M., Eisenhauer L.: *The Pharmacologic Basis of Patient Care*. Saunders, 1981.

difficulty with the use of medicinal shampoos is that they must remain on the scalp for a certain amount of time (usually several minutes) to be effective. This might be difficult to achieve with young children. Shampooing the child's hair during the bath and allowing the child to play with bath toys while the shampoo remains on the child's head usually is successful. However, nurses must caution parents that medicinal shampoos can irritate the eyes and urge them to take care that this does not happen.

Topical Anti-Infectives After thorough wound cleansing, application of a dressing and topical anti-infective agent inhibits bacterial growth in most wounds. The more common anti-infective ointments are presented in Table 44-2.

Dressings Dressings serve a number of purposes. They keep the topical agent in contact with the wound and enable the patient to be ambulatory. They protect the wound from contamination, scratching fingers, bumps, and passing air currents, which might cause pain over exposed nerve endings.

Several different sizes and types of pads can be used to cover wounds. Plain sterile gauze pads come in sizes ranging from 2″ × 2″ to 4″ × 4″. Oversized thick gauze pads may be used on buttocks, back, chest, and abdominal wounds. Oval pads are made specifically for eye wounds. Nonstick Telfa pads are useful for abrasions, although they have limited absorbency. Band-aids come in various shapes and sizes. Many are colorfully decorated to appeal to children.

TABLE 44-2 Topical Anti-Infective Agents

Preparation	Effect	Nursing considerations
Povidone–iodine (Betadine)	Antibacterial for gram-positive and gram-negative organisms; also effective against fungi, viruses, and protozoa	Nonirritating
Bacitracin	Antibiotic; effective against gram-positive and gram-negative bacteria, including streptococci and staphylococci	Should not be used on large surface wounds because of systemic absorption; particularly effective in treating impetigo of staphylococcal or streptococcal origin; nonirritating
Neosporin (polymyxin B–bacitracin–neomycin)	The combination of antibiotics is more effective than any individual one against a broad spectrum of organisms	Nonirritating; also available in generic form—triple antibiotic ointment
Polymyxin B	Effective against gram-negative organisms; not effective against gram-positive organisms or fungi	Sensitivity might cause irritation and burning; usually found in combination with bacitracin
Neomycin	Broad-spectrum antibiotic	Can be irritating to abrasions

SOURCE: Govoni L., Hayes J.: *Drugs and Nursing Implications*. Appleton-Century-Crofts, 1982 *and* Asperheim M., Eisenhauer L.: *The Pharmacologic Basis of Patient Care*. Saunders, 1981.

Depending on the extent of the wounds, dressings may be secured with tape. Adhesive tape is used frequently; however, it can cause a contact dermatitis in susceptible children. Various forms of hypoallergenic tape are available. Tape will adhere to the skin better if tincture of benzoin is applied first. Benzoin serves a secondary purpose of protecting the skin from the irritation of the tape.

Dressing materials also include many kinds of gauze. Fine-mesh or wide-mesh gauze over wounds helps in debridement when the dressings are removed. Kerlix wrap works well on extremities, whereas Kling gauze wrap is needed for small fingers and toes. Stockingette, or tube gauze, also is useful for securing dressings to fingers and is particularly helpful for head dressings.

Removal of even minor dressings can be traumatic to a child. Some children like the tape removed quickly, whereas others prefer the slower method. The nurse inquires about children's preferences and also allows them to remove their own dressings if they so desire. If dressing changes are extensive and frequent, the use of gauze wrap to secure pads is preferable to tape. For major lacerations, particularly lacerations of the abdomen, the use of Montgomery straps reduces irritation from constant tape removal. See the section entitled "Burn Wound Dressings" later in this chapter for specific approaches to burn dressings.

Wound Closure When skin integrity is altered and a wound occurs, healing occurs by primary, secondary, or tertiary intention, depending on the size of the wound, presence or absence of bacteria, adequacy of the individual's diet, and adequacy of blood supply to the area. *Primary intention* healing occurs when there is a good blood supply to the wound, no infection is evident, and the edges of the wound are approximated well. Little granulation tissue forms in the area, and scarring is minimal. *Secondary intention* occurs when the blood supply is not good, infection occurs, and a large amount of granulation tissue forms, resulting in a larger scar. *Tertiary intention* occurs when primary and secondary healing is interrupted.

The healing of an injury to the skin involves the entire body. Temperature and pulse rate become elevated temporarily. Nitrogen and potassium are first lost and then retained. Phagocytes remove debris in the wound. Vasodilatation helps to bring oxygen and nutrients to the injured area. Clot formation results from bleeding into the wound. Fibrin in the clot provides the needed base for cell migration. The epidermis regenerates rapidly to facilitate wound healing. To foster healing, good nutrition, assurance of adequate blood supply to the injured part, and minimizing bacterial contamination are essential.

The wound will not heal until closure occurs, even though some granulation tissue does form. The nurse assesses the healing process by noting the degree of intention and factors that promote or interfere with healing.

The nurse assesses the type and depth of any laceration to determine whether suturing is required (see Chapter 26). In the event that the wound is not severe enough to need sutures, the nurse can use alternate methods to maintain proper closure. Butterfly-shaped bandages can either be bought or made out of adhesive tape. The advantage of this type of closure is that it provides proper tension on the edges of the laceration while leaving enough of the laceration exposed for more rapid healing. Steri-strip closures completely cover the laceration while providing tension for wound closure. They are particularly effective with jagged, uneven lacerations and may be used in place of sutures for this type of wound. When applying either butterfly or steri-strip closures, the nurse might first apply tincture of benzoin to skin areas that will come in contact with the tape but not over the wound itself. The major disadvantage with using both of these types of closures is that children tend to pick at the tape, thus destroying the tension and resulting in a larger scar.

Skin Grafts

The functions of skin grafts include the following:

1. To cover a wound to prevent infection or to decrease fluid loss from the wound
2. To improve cosmetic appearance
3. To improve joint mobility

Skin grafts may be permanent or temporary and are used most often in the approach to a child who has suffered a thermal injury.

Autografts Permanent skin grafts must be *autografts* (those taken from the patient's own skin). The child with extensive burns, however, has little skin that has not been injured and grafting in this child is extremely complex. Once a donor site is used for a split-thickness skin graft, there is a 10- to 14-day waiting period while the site heals and thickens before a graft can be taken again.

In wound grafting survival is the first consideration, function is second, and appearance is third. For example, the child with a 60%–70% full-thickness burn will have large areas such as the chest, back, and extremities grafted before precious donor-site skin is used for the face and hands.

The recipient site is prepared for grafting by hydrotherapy and debridement (described in the section on "Wound Management" later in this chapter) or tangential or primary excision. The bed must be as free from debris and bacteria as possible and must have a good blood supply to ensure that a graft will take.

Most skin grafts are split-thickness in depth, including the epidermis and part of the dermis. They vary in thickness from 0.012 in. to 0.24 in. The surgeon uses a dermatome, a plane-like instrument, to obtain skin from the donor site. This skin is then placed on the recipient bed and often is anchored in place with small, sterile adhesive strips, hemoclips, or sutures. It is essential that the grafted site remain immobile while a vascular network forms between the underlying bed and the graft. Some surgeons prefer to leave the graft site open, whereas others suture thick dressings over the graft site and leave it undisturbed for several days. The aim of any method of treatment is to keep the recipient bed and the skin graft surfaces in touch with each other at all times, thus preventing the graft from sliding and tearing newly formed blood vessels.

When the grafted site is left open, depending on hospital policy, the nurse might "roll" the graft because pockets of serosanguineous or serous drainage collect underneath. Putting gentle pressure on these pockets with cotton-tipped applicators, the nurse rolls the collected exudate out at the graft's edges. The graft might need rolling as often as every 30–60 minutes during the first 24 hours after surgery.

After a day or so, when the skin graft begins to adhere to the underlying bed, rolling can do more harm than good. However, fluid still collects in small pockets under the graft. The skilled nurse again depending on hospital policy may use a small-gauge needle and syringe and aspirate the pocket or make tiny cuts into the top of each bubble and express fluid. This is called "pie-crusting."

When dressings are placed over grafts, they may be left in place for several days or removed down to the last layer of gauze after 1 or 2 days. Procedures vary, but the goals are the same: to prevent infection, disturb the graft as little as possible, support the healing process, and decrease scarring.

Allografts *Allografts* (homografts) are skin grafts from an individual of the same species, which can be used to cover the excised or debrided wound temporarily. The allograft provides some of the functions of an autograft, covering the wound while donor sites heal. It prevents fluid and heat loss from the open wound and serves as a natural barrier against infection.

Skin is one of the body organs that can be donated at the time of death. Using aseptic technique, trained personnel crop skin from carefully screened cadavers. Bacterial cultures are obtained, and the skin is treated, packaged, and frozen for future use.

Some burn centers use allografts or chemically treated amniotic membranes as a biologic dressing over clean partial-thickness burns such as scalds. Experience has shown that these dressings promote reepithelialization of the wound.

The body will begin to reject allografts after approximately 10 days, about the same time the donor sites are ready for recropping.

Heterografts *Heterografts* are skin grafts taken from a species other than humans, often from pigs. With the increased availability of skin banks and allografts, pig skin is being used less often. The heterograft also will protect the patient from infection and fluid and heat loss. Once any biologic graft is applied, nerve endings are no longer exposed, and pain disappears or becomes minimal. These grafts also are removed within 10 days to avoid local and systemic rejection responses.

Donor Sites Donor sites are selected from unaffected areas, excluding joints, the face, and the dorsa of the hands but often including the scalp. Whenever possible, surgeons choose sites that usually can be covered by clothing such as the buttocks and thighs. Some skin discoloration can remain long after donor sites heal.

When donor sites are limited, a mesh graft rather than a sheet graft is used. The surgeon uses an instrument that cuts equidistant slits in the sheet of donor skin. The graft can then be expanded because of the elastic quality of human skin. The graft often is stretched to three times its original size to cover the chest or back. Fluid drains freely through the interstices. Healing occurs as epithelial cells advance across the spaces in this latticework. One disadvantage is that the wound is less smooth in appearance after mesh grafts heal.

From the time the patient is admitted, potential donor sites must be protected from invasive infection and irritating topical agents. For example, often, unburned skin is adjacent to wounds treated with silver nitrate solution. Covering the unburned skin with gauze impregnated with petroleum jelly protects it from the discoloration, silver chloride buildup, and dryness associated with silver nitrate use. There are several ways of managing the donor site once it is cropped, that is, once the graft is taken. The goals are to prevent infection, promote healing, and, often, to ready it rapidly for recropping. Some burn centers cover the wound with a Scarlet Red fine-mesh gauze dressing. This gauze is impregnated with a red dye in an oil base, which has no antiseptic qualities but is thought to promote healing. After 8–12 days, the dressing can be peeled back, revealing a healed wound. Young children often are frightened by this gauze because of its red color and need careful preoperative preparation. As the wound heals, they can help to trim back the gauze using forceps and scissors. When the scalp must be used for a donor site, parents and children need much reassurance that the hair will grow back. The hair follicles are not part of a split-thickness graft from any part of the body.

All donor sites are painful initially but will feel much more comfortable within a few days. As healing progresses, they begin to itch and must be protected from children's scratching and rubbing.

Principles of Nursing Care

Acute-Care Needs

Preventing Itching Pruritus (itching) is the most common reaction in skin conditions. Pruritus is either localized or generalized, depending on the skin condition and other factors. One feature of pruritus is its intermittent character, being more severe in the evening and during the night. This usually is attributed to a higher body temperature and capillary dilatation in the evening, the absence of daily activities to distract the individual, and increased skin temperature in bed (Rajka, 1975). Managing pruritus probably is one of the nurse's key responsibilities in caring for children with dermatologic alterations.

The prevention of secondary infection is important. The child's nails should be cut short and the hands kept meticulously clean. Children who are old enough should cut their own nails. It is essential to explain to the older child the importance of avoiding scratching and the precautions needed to prevent skin breakage. The wearing of mittens to avoid scratching might be useful with both older children and younger children. The use of arm splints and a T-shirt over the hands are ways to help prevent younger children from scratching. The nurse checks the child periodically to ensure that freedom is not completely restricted if these means are used to prevent scratching. Warm, irritating, and tight clothing should be avoided to prevent itching.

Depending on the severity of the condition, the physician might prescribe topical steroids, oral steroids, or antihistamines.

Minimizing or Alleviating Pain Pain is associated with some skin conditions. The nurse assesses the child's perception of pain, its location, and its intensity (see Chapter 29). Pain is a means of protecting the body whenever physiologic or psychosocial disorders occur. Pain warns the individual that some type of trauma is occurring.

When the child is in pain, the nurse's primary responsibility is to reduce or eliminate it. The nurse minimizes or eliminates other discomforts because they might aggravate pain. Noxious stimuli that might intensify the child's reaction to pain should be removed if possible. It is essential to make every effort to ensure that the child is comfortable and safe. If medications for pain are ordered, the nurse and patient decide together when it is needed. Compresses soaked in Burows solution might be helpful in relieving acute inflammation. The nurse needs to recognize factors that enhance comfort and relaxation without medication. The nurse makes every effort to reduce and alleviate pain—reassuring, providing helpful diversions, eliminating stress and distractions that stimulate pain, and providing a climate that is conducive to rest and relaxation. The nurse needs to remember that individuals respond differently to pain because of their pain tolerance and cultural orientation to pain.

Maintaining Fluid Balance Fever might occur with some skin conditions. The relationship between intake and output and fluid and electrolyte balance is complex (see Chapter 33). Alterations in body temperature and maintenance of homeostasis depend to a large extent on the regulation of the fluid balance. The nurse checks the child's temperature periodically to determine whether it is elevated. Antipyretic drugs can be used to lower the temperature, as well as mechanical means to cool the body such as tap water and sponge baths.

The nurse pays particular attention to weeping lesions because fluid loss through the lesions can cause dehydration. Cell production is impaired by dehydration; consequently, healing is slowed. Maintenance of the fluid and electrolyte balance is critical to the nurse caring for the child with a skin condition.

Preventing Tetanus *Clostridium tetani,* an anaerobic organism, is found in dirt and can multiply readily in cuts or wounds. Puncture wounds, which close over quickly, are prime sites for rapid multiplication of the organism. Most commonly, children receive puncture wounds from nails, pins, and wood splinters. Penetration is superficial, and the object can be removed easily. The small puncture wound does not bleed readily, so it should be squeezed gently to promote bleeding and flush out the bacteria. This is especially important if the penetrating object is a dirty, rusty nail. Up-to-date tetanus prophylaxis is essential for preventing tetanus in a dirty, contaminated wound. Table 44-3 outlines the recommended schedule for tetanus prophylaxis. Chemoprophylaxis against tetanus is not practical or useful in wound management. The need for active immunization, with or without passive immunization, depends on the condition of the wound and the patient's immunization history. Rarely have cases of tetanus occurred in persons with a documented primary series of toxoid injections. Evidence indicates that complete primary immunization with tetanus toxoid provides long-lasting protection (10 years or more in most recipients).

Wounds can be contaminated with *C. tetani* depending upon their type. For purposes of decisions regarding tetanus prophylaxis, wounds are classified as non-tetanus prone, moderate tetanus prone, and high tetanus prone. Non-tetanus-prone wounds include wounds that are not yet 24 hours old, are at little risk for bacterial contamination, are not puncture or crushing wounds, do not affect muscle tissue, and do not result in dead tissue (Nurses' Drug Alert, 1984, pp. 493–494). Moderate tetanus-prone wounds are wounds that may be contaminated through wood, cement or asphalt, bites (animal and human), or bullets; crushing or puncture injuries; or wounds involving muscle tissue

TABLE 44-3 Guide to Tetanus Prophylaxis

Immunization status		Type of wound	Prophylaxis
Uncertain immunization status Not previously immunized One known dose of tetanus toxoid		Clean, minor wounds	Give one dose of tetanus toxoid and diphtheria vaccine (Td). If patient is six years old or younger use diphtheria, pertussis, tetanus vaccine (DPT). Complete the series of basic immunizations as appropriate.
		All other wounds	Give one dose of Td (DPT if six years old or younger) and for a wound of average severity, 250 units of human tetanus immune globulin (TIG). Separate sites and syringes should be used for the Td and TIG. Complete the series of basic immunizations as appropriate.
Previously immunized with only two doses of tetanus toxoid		Clean, minor wounds	Give one dose of Td (DPT if patient is six years old or younger).
		All other wounds	Give one dose of Td or DPT. If the wound has been neglected for more than 24 hours, also give one dose of TIG
Previously actively immunized with tetanus toxoid	More than 10 years past	Clean, minor wounds	Give one dose of Td.
		All other wounds	Give one dose of Td.
	Within the past 10 years	Clean, minor wounds	No booster necessary.
		All other wounds	If more than five years since the last dose, give a single dose of Td.

SOURCE: Sebilla A.: When was your last tetanus shot. *RN* (Aug) 1984; 47:23. Reprinted by permission of Medical Economics Co.

(Nurses' Drug Alert, 1984, pp. 493–494). Tetanus-prone wounds have been highly contaminated from contact with animal excrement such as barnyard or stable soil, or sewerage; wounds of the colon; wounds over 24 hours old; or wounds containing dead tissue (Nurses' Drug Alert, 1984, pp. 493–494).

Even minor lacerations or splinters can be contaminated with *C. tetani,* and nurses must consider the recommended prophylaxis when dealing with any wound.

Nutritional Needs

Wound healing is delayed by inadequate nutrition. Cell production is impaired by nutritional deficiencies, particularly vitamin C and protein deficiencies. For wound healing, the following nutritional needs must be met:

1. Sufficient protein and carbohydrate intake to prevent a negative nitrogen balance, hypoalbuminemia, and weight loss.

2. Increased daily intake of vitamins and minerals:
   a. Vitamin A—10,000–50,000 IU
   b. Vitamin B—0.5–1.0 mg/1000 dietary calories
   c. Vitamin B_2—0.25 mg/1000 dietary calories
   d. Vitamin B_6—2 mg
   e. Niacin—15–20 mg
   f. Vitamin B_{12}—400 mg
   g. Vitamin C—75–300 mg
   h. Vitamin D—400 mg
   i. Vitamin E—10–15 IU
   j. Traces of zinc, magnesium, calcium, and copper (Carpenito, 1983).

The nurse encourages the child with a skin condition to eat well-balanced meals. Adequate nutrition is essential to the healing process.

Developmental Needs

Nurses need to continue to foster development leading to independence in self-care tasks for children with skin conditions, just as they would with any other child. The child's energy level, however, is a consideration when planning activities.

Bathing and care of the nails are two important self-care activities related to the skin. Before 4 years of age, the parent or nurse needs to be involved in the bathing process. By the time children are 4 years of age, they can wash and dry themselves with supervision. By the time they are 8 years old, they can bathe themselves independently when reminded to do so and can maintain clean nails and clip the nails on both hands.

Infants with skin conditions need to be talked to, held, and cuddled. They need freedom to move around and mobiles to watch. For the most part, skin lesions should not inhibit the infant's developmental needs. Appropriate nonallergenic toys should be offered to the infant. The nurse provides auditory, visual, tactile, and kinesthetic stimulation for the infant.

For children in early childhood, the nurse might need to ensure that the environment will promote healing rather than exacerbate the skin condition. Preschool children might be more sensitive to their lesions because other people notice them. Dramatic play might help these children decrease the frustrations or negative feelings associated with their skin conditions. Children of early childhood age should be encouraged to engage in age-appropriate activities.

By middle and late childhood, children can understand their skin conditions and follow through with self-care management when it is appropriately demonstrated to them. They might need help in accepting themselves if their peers, family, and other significant others have difficulty accepting them. The child's reaction to skin lesions cannot be predicted. Some children cope well, whereas others respond emotionally and behaviorally. Self-care and other activities appropriate to their age and skin condition should be promoted in these children. Because these children are generally energetic and cooperative, the nurse might find it easy to help them understand the nature and care of their skin conditions.

The stresses on the adolescent's psychic energy are many and varied. A skin condition compounds the complexity of the adolescent's life. Helping adolescents feel good about themselves is crucial. Many adolescents with skin conditions have a significant degree of anxiety. The emotional reactions are manifested in a variety of ways which include self-consciousness, withdrawal, and excessive attention to cleanliness.

Determining the child's and parent's level of knowledge and beliefs and fears about skin alterations helps the nurse in planning care.

The Child With a Burn

Burns are a leading cause of accidental injury in children. Those who survive burn injuries endure pain, lengthy hospitalization, and disfiguring scars (Artzetal, 1979). The patterns of injuries are predictable by age group, coinciding with physical, cognitive, and emotional growth and development. At least 75% of childhood burns are preventable (see Chapter 19). A nursing care plan for a child with a burn is included at the end of this chapter.

Children receive thermal burns from hot liquids, such as soup, coffee, tea, and boiling water; hot surfaces, such as radiators and irons; and contact with flames, as in match play, gasoline play, and house fires. Electrical burns occur when children bite into cords or extension plugs, or when they climb trees or telephone poles and play near high-tension wires. Electrical burns often are deep and disfiguring, damaging muscle and bone and often leading to limb amputation. Chemical burns occur most frequently among toddlers and are caused by handling and ingesting corrosive household cleaners. Overexposure to sunlight and high-dosage radiation also cause burns.

Burns are classified according to the depth of damage to the skin and underlying structures and to the percentage of total body surface area (TBSA) affected (Fig. 44-2).

Classification of Burns

The American Burn Association has classified burns according to the severity of the injury and complicating factors (Arzetal, 1979). The small child with a burn of 10% or more, however, will require as much attention as the older child with a larger burn.

Minor burns include partial-thickness burns involving less than 15% of the TBSA and full-thickness burns involving less than 2% of the TBSA.

Moderate burns include partial-thickness burns involving 15%–30% of the TBSA and full-thickness burns involving less than 10% of the TBSA, except in small children and when the burns involve critical areas.

Major or critical burns include burns complicated by respiratory tract injury, partial-thickness burns involving 30% or more of the TBSA, and full-thickness burns involving 10% or more of the TBSA.

Burns of the face, hands, or feet are considered major because these are critical areas of function and appearance. Burns of the genitals are also in this category because this area harbors many bacteria.

Hospitalization is indicated for any children with moderate or major burns and sometimes children with minor burns involving 10% of the TBSA. Children under 2 years of age, unless the burn is very small and superficial, also should be hospitalized. Other burn categories in which children should be hospitalized include electrical burns; deep chemical burns; burns complicated by fractures or soft tissue injury; burns complicated by concurrent health problems such as obesity, diabetes mellitus, epilepsy, or renal disease; and burns in which child abuse or neglect is suspected (see Chapter 22).

Depth of Injury

Partial-Thickness Burns In partial-thickness (first- and second-degree) burns, the epidermis and part of the dermis are destroyed, leaving hair follicles and sweat glands intact (see Fig. 44-2). Some scalds and flash burns are superficial partial-thickness injuries, which heal in 1–10 days. Deep partial-thickness burns can take up to 6 weeks to heal and might eventually require skin grafting. If protected from injury and infections, partial-thickness burns heal by reepithelialization.

Typically, partial-thickness burns include sunburns, flash burns, and scalds. The shallower partial-thickness burn is

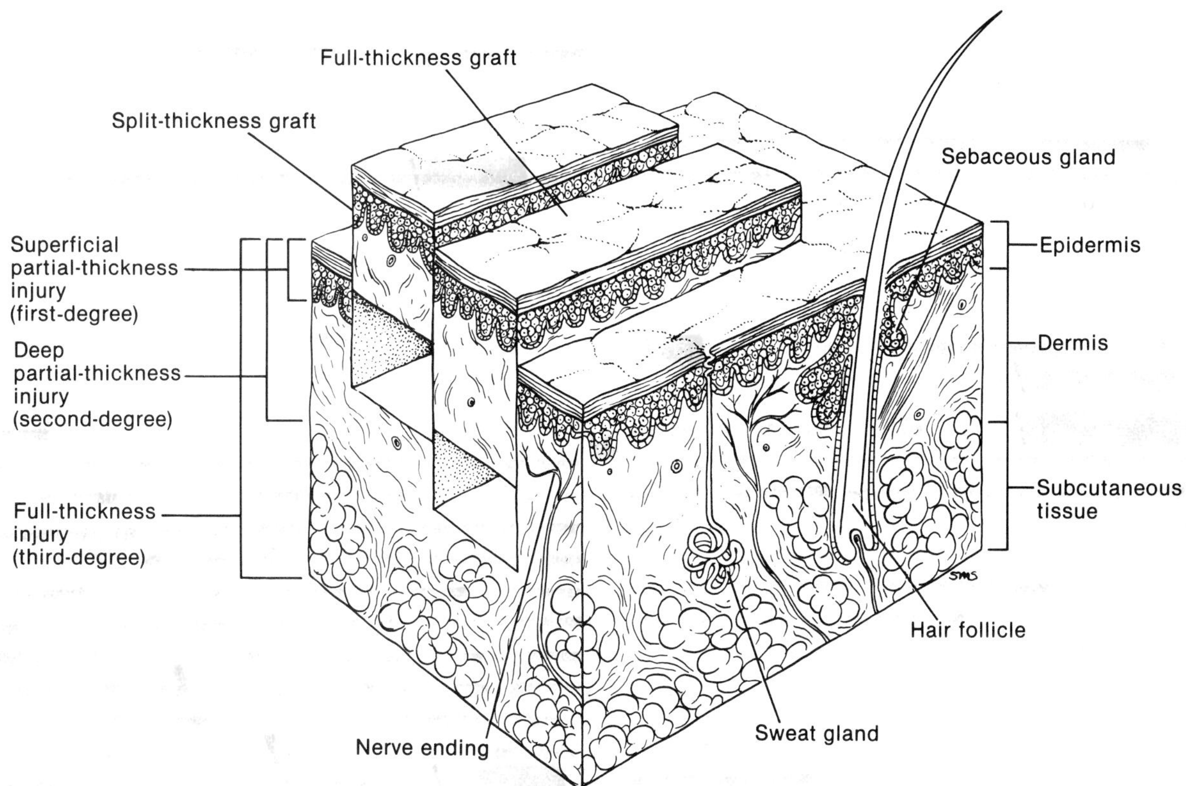

Figure 44-2 Microscopic view of the skin. Superficial partial-thickness (first-degree) burns damage only the epidermis. A deep, partial-thickness injury (second-degree burn) involves the epidermis and part of the dermis. The most serious injury, a full-thickness (third-degree) burn, exposes subcutaneous tissue. Two types of grafts are illustrated—the split-thickness graft, which includes all of the epidermis and part of the dermis, and the full-thickness graft, which includes all of the epidermis and dermis.

reddened, dry, painful, and edematous. The deeper partial-thickness burn is reddened, painful, and edematous and is also moist and often blistered. Tissue blanches and refills with pressure, indicating intact capillaries. (See Color Plate.)

Full-Thickness Burns Full-thickness, or third-degree, burns destroy the dermal layer down to and often including subcutaneous fat. Hair follicles, sweat glands, sebaceous glands, and nerves are destroyed (see Fig. 44-2). Some clinicians classify burn injuries that damage underlying fat, muscle, and bone as fourth degree in depth. The full-thickness burn is pearly white, tan, brown, mahogany, or black in appearance. The tissue feels dry and leathery, does not blanch and refill, and is not painful. The burned tissue of a full-thickness injury is called *eschar.* Once dermis and dermal structures are destroyed, skin regeneration cannot take place. (See Color Plate.) Skin grafting is necessary to close the full-thickness wound.

Percentage of Injury Burns also are classified according to the percentage of total body surface area injured. The rule of nines (Fig. 44-3), useful in estimating burn size

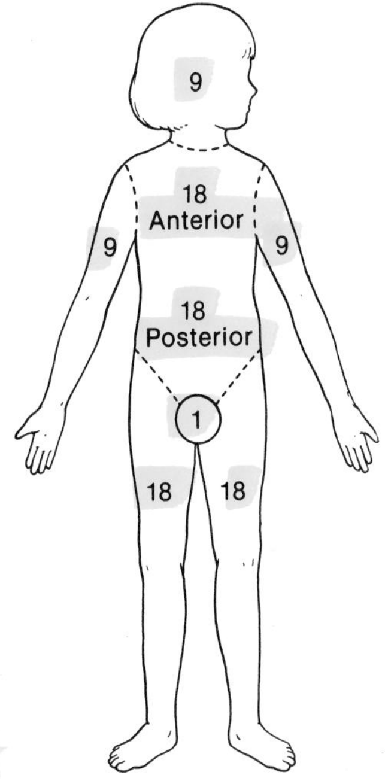

Figure 44-3 Rule of nines.

in children 10 years of age and older, is inaccurate for the younger child. The Lund and Browder chart (Fig. 44-4) takes into account changing body proportions in the growing child. Fluid needs are calculated according to the percentage of injury and the child's body weight, so estimates must be accurate. Diagrams of the body are included in the burn chart. They can be color coded to denote areas of burn and varying depths.

Medical and Nursing Management During the Emergent Phase

The *emergent phase* of care is the time needed to resolve immediate problems resulting from the burn injury. This phase usually lasts from 1 to 5 days depending on the severity of the burn.

The earliest part of the emergent phase is care at the scene of the injury. Stopping the burning process is the first step at the scene of injury. The longer the burning agent is in touch with the skin, the deeper the wound. Children can learn to stop, drop, and roll to extinguish flaming clothing, or a bystander can shout commands or tackle a running, panic-stricken child with a jacket or blanket to smother the flames. Once the flames are extinguished, the clothing must be doused with cool water or any other available nonflammable liquid. Otherwise, clothing continues to smoulder and the burn deepens. Burns caused by contact with a hot surface or hot liquids also should be cooled immediately. Nonadherent clothing should then be removed and the injury assessed. All jewelry, buttons, or buckles, which retain heat and continue to damage the skin, must be removed.

In electrical injury the source of current must be shut off. When high-tension wires are involved, the rescuer must be specially trained and equipped (such as members of the fire and police departments). Once the electrical current is stopped, the victim should be assessed quickly for cardiac arrest and cardiopulmonary resuscitation begun as indicated because electrical current is known to cause ventricular fibrillation and cardiac arrest. Because electrical current can take a variable course throughout the body, the nurse looks for current entrance and exit burns and suspects deep injury when electricity is the causative agent of a burn. On the surface where the electrical current entered and exited, there might only be a small-diameter burn that appears whitened, reddened, or charred. However, massive soft tissue, muscle, and bone damage might be present under the skin, and the area must be assessed carefully for circulation, sensation, and motion. Also, the myoglobin released in the bloodstream from destroyed muscle cells can cause acute renal tubular necrosis (see Chapter 39).

Chemical burns must be flushed with large amounts of water and the victim's clothing removed. Eyes should be flushed for at least 20 minutes while the patient is being transported to an emergency room. Time should not be wasted searching for the causative agent and an antidote. The use of a neutralizing agent might set up another chemical reaction that could deepen the injury.

Once the wound is cooled and clothing removed, the patient is at risk for rapid heat loss. Protective skin that helped to maintain body temperature has been lost or damaged. It is important to keep the child warm during transport to the hospital. Clean sheets and blankets are adequate, although many transporters still use sterile linen with burn victims. Rapid transport to an emergency room is crucial for the burned child because the hypovolemic shock that develops after burns can be life threatening. This is a time of crisis for the family as well as the child, and they too need careful attention (see Chapter 27).

Inhaling smoke in an enclosed space can lead to respiratory failure. Where there is smoke, there is carbon monoxide, which is the end product of the incomplete combustion of organic material. Carbon monoxide is readily absorbed from the lungs into the bloodstream and causes loss of consciousness at certain blood levels. Many burn victims are awake and alert at the scene, but those who have inhaled smoke containing carbon monoxide and other toxins often need cardiopulmonary resuscitation.

The second phase of emergent care involves treatment in the emergency room. Immediate nursing and medical management in the emergency room must focus on providing a secure airway and adequate ventilation and beginning fluid resuscitation. Wound care is not the first priority.

AREA	1 yr.	1–4 yrs.	5–9 yrs.	10–14 yrs.	15 yrs.	Adult	2°	3°
Head	19	17	13	11	9	7		
Neck	2	2	2	2	2	2		
Ant. Trunk	13	13	13	13	13	13		
Post. Trunk	13	13	13	13	13	13		
R. Buttock	2½	2½	2½	2½	2½	2½		
L. Buttock	2½	2½	2½	2½	2½	2½		
Genitalia	1	1	1	1	1	1		
R.U. Arm	4	4	4	4	4	4		
L.U. Arm	4	4	4	4	4	4		
R.L. Arm	3	3	3	3	3	3		
L.L. Arm	3	3	3	3	3	3		
R. Hand	2½	2½	2½	2½	2½	2½		
L. Hand	2½	2½	2½	2½	2½	2½		
R. Thigh	5½	6½	8	8½	9	9½		
L. Thigh	5½	6½	8	8½	9	9½		
R. Leg	5	5	5½	6	6½	7		
L. Leg	5	5	5½	6	6½	7		
R. Foot	3½	3½	3½	3½	3½	3½		
L. Foot	3½	3½	3½	3½	3½	3½		
TOTAL								

Figure 44-4 Lund and Browder method of calculating burn size. (From C.P. Artz and J.A. Moncrief, *The Treatment of Burns,* 2nd ed., Saunders, 1969.) Reprinted with permission.

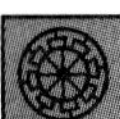

NURSING CARE GUIDE The Burned Child During the Emergent Phase

Nursing diagnosis	Intervention	Evaluation
1. Potential for obstructed upper airway due to edema from burn wounds of face and neck	Observe child for signs of respiratory distress (see Chapter 34) Obtain blood gases Position patient with head elevated Administer humidified oxygen by mask Assist with endotracheal intubation and ventilation as needed (see Chapter 34)	Quiet, comfortable respirations Normal breath sounds Adequate blood gas values
2. Potential for upper and lower airway damage due to smoke and heat inhalation	Determine child's respiratory status Obtain history of injury Observe nose, mouth, and secretions for flecks of soot Observe patient for hoarseness or a dry cough Watch for singed eyebrows, eyelashes, and nasal hairs Assist in obtaining baseline chest radiograph Determine child's level of consciousness Obtain carboxyhemoglobin level Administer 100% humidified oxygen Assist with endotracheal intubation and ventilation as needed	Quiet, comfortable respirations Normal breath sounds Adequate blood gas values
3. Potential for decreased chest excursion due to buildup of wound edema with a full-thickness circumferential injury	Observe child for change in respiratory status, especially note shallow respirations and decreased breath sounds Consult with physician and assist with escharotomy as needed (this is an incision into full-thickness burn eschar that forms a tight, unyielding band around the circumference of the chest or extremities)	Quiet, comfortable respirations Normal breath sounds Adequate blood gas values
4. Alteration in fluid balance from hypovolemia with potential for shock	Monitor child's vital signs and central venous pressure if possible Assist in establishing secure, large-needle bore intravenous lines Administer intravenous fluids to obtain urine output Place Foley catheter and monitor patient's urine output Determine child's weight as soon as possible Estimate the size of burn and time of injury and calculate fluid requirements Monitor any changes in level of consciousness Obtain laboratory studies, usually hematocrit, sodium, potassium, chloride, carbon dioxide, blood urea nitrogen, creatinine, albumin, and globulin levels	Stable vital signs Urine output at least 1 mL/kg of body weight/hr Alert and responsive patient Central venous pressure: 6–12 cm of water Laboratory values within normal limits

continued on next page

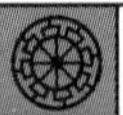

NURSING CARE GUIDE The Burned Child During the Emergent Phase (continued)

Nursing diagnosis	Intervention	Evaluation
5. Potential for nausea, vomiting, and abdominal distention due to decreased gastrointestinal mobility	Listen for bowel sounds Maintain patient on nothing-by-mouth (NPO) status Insert nasogastric tube and attach to low suction, observe amount and characteristics of drainage Administer antacid as ordered	Absence of nausea, vomiting, and abdominal distention Patent nasogastric tube
6. Heat loss due to impairment in skin integrity	Monitor patient's body temperature Maintain room draft-free with temperature and humidity at increased levels Use warming lamps as needed to maintain child's body temperature	Normal body temperature
7. Pain and anxiety	Observe child for verbal and nonverbal signs of pain and anxiety (see Chapter 29) Use comfort measures as possible Administer intravenous medications as ordered (morphine sulfate works well to relieve pain in this phase of care) Encourage parent's participation in giving comfort	Child able to tolerate wound care and other treatments
8. Potential for infection and constricting edema from burn wound	Use careful aseptic technique throughout all wound care Carefully note depth and percentage of injury Obtain baseline wound cultures Obtain baseline wound photographs Cleanse wound with antiseptic (some burn centers use diluted PHisoDerm, which is rinsed off after cleaning) Debride away dead skin Check circulation, sensations, and motion below areas of burns of extremities Assist with escharotomies as needed. Pack incisions with gauze to control bleeding Provide tetanus prophylaxis as ordered (Table 44-3) Apply topical agents and dressings as ordered Administer penicillin prophylaxis if ordered Shave hair from areas close to wound (except for eyebrows) Cleanse around eyes with saline and irrigate as indicated Obtain ophthalmology consult for patients with facial burns and apply ophthalmic ointments as ordered	Wound cleaned Depth and extent of injury noted Dressings securely in place but not constricting to allow for edema increase Bleeding from escharotomies controlled Adequate circulation, sensation, and motion below areas of extremity burns

NURSING CARE GUIDE The Burned Child During the Emergent Phase (continued)

Nursing diagnosis	Intervention	Evaluation
9. Crises of injury, loss, and hospitalization for child and family. Possibility of preexisting family dysfunction	Assess for possibility of abuse when burns appear suspicious (eg, with bathtub immersion burns, the child's feet, ankles, and buttocks may be the only areas damaged) (see Chapter 22) Obtain history of injury and past crises and coping patterns	See Chapter 22

Alterations in Fluid Volume

Burn Shock: Fluid Volume Deficit Capillary permeability alters rapidly after a burn. Plasma proteins, water, and electrolytes leak into interstitial spaces in injured and noninjured tissue and out through the burn wound. In major burns, fluid from the vascular compartment shifts suddenly to interstitial tissue, dangerously reducing the circulating fluid volume. Rapid volume replacement is necessary to restore the patient's pulse and blood pressure and combat life-threatening hypovolemic shock.

The body attempts to compensate for the fluid shift by constricting the blood vessels, increasing the heart rate, and conserving fluid and electrolytes through maximum reabsorption in the kidneys. In the older child with a 10%–20% burn, compensation will prevent a dangerous blood pressure drop and hypoperfusion. With a major burn, however, hypovolemia, if left untreated, quickly leads to shock, organ failure, circulatory collapse, and death. A substance called the myocardial depressant factor is released at the time of injury, further decreasing the patient's cardiac output.

During the first 24–72 hours after injury, fluid continues to leak from vascular to interstitial spaces, with the most dramatic shift occurring in the first 6–12 hours. Edema fluid collects throughout the body. The acute period begins as fluid gradually shifts back into the circulating volume from the interstitial spaces and diuresis begins. This edema fluid drastically alters the child's appearance. Children with facial burns have eyes that are swollen shut and heads that seem to be at least twice their usual size. The nurse reassures the family that the edema will begin to diminish within 72 hours. Nurses can explain that they expect to see swelling in unburned as well as burned areas because of the general increase in capillary permeability that occurs with any major trauma.

Fluid Volume Replacement The fluid that moves from the circulating volume to the interstitial spaces in burn shock consists of water, electrolytes, and albumin. Lactated Ringer's solution, which is similar to plasma in electrolyte composition, is a common replacement crystalloid. Albumin and fresh-frozen plasma are part of fluid therapy in many burn units. Many burn authorities, however, believe that colloid is contraindicated in the first 24 hours. They contend that because protein leaks into the interstitial spaces, colloid will intensify the quantity and duration of peripheral and pulmonary edema.

Fluid resuscitation formulas are used as guidelines for treating burn shock. A formula specifying the amounts of replacement intravenous fluids is used in conjunction with close monitoring of vital signs, urine output, level of consciousness, hematocrit, serum electrolytes, and central venous pressure.

An adequate urine output that reflects proper fluid therapy and hydration is at least 1 mL/kg of body weight/hr. Urine output of more than 1.5–2.0 mL of urine/kg of body weight/hr indicates fluid overload. Too much fluid can lead to pulmonary edema if intravenous infusions are not cut back.

Burns do not bleed, and red blood cells are too large to leak into the interstitial spaces along with plasma proteins. Thus, the hematocrit is elevated initially because of fluid loss and hemoconcentration. With adequate fluid replacement, the hematocrit drops to normal or below normal. Blood loss can occur during escharotomies (see section titled Escharotomies) and might be extensive enough to require transfusions. In deep burns, such as those caused by prolonged flame contact or electrical current, red blood cells hemolyze. Renal tubules can become obstructed with the free hemoglobin that is released. An osmotic diuretic, such as mannitol, is given together with increased intravenous fluids to flush the renal tubules. With this treatment, urine clears from black to reddish-brown to straw-colored, and acute tubular necrosis can be averted.

Because potassium is released from injured cells, serum potassium rises in the first 24–48 hours after burn injury. Once diuresis begins, potassium is excreted and serum levels will drop, necessitating potassium replacement (see Chapter 33).

As capillary permeability returns to normal, reabsorption of edema fluid begins and diuresis follows. Intravenous fluid requirements drop significantly. Daily fluid and electrolyte needs, however, remain increased. Evaporative water loss through the burn wound is far in excess of that lost through

Brooke Formula for Fluid Resuscitation

The Brooke formula, first published in 1953, is a modification of the Evans formula. This formula estimates the following requirements for the first 24 hours after burn injury:

Colloids: 0.5 mL/kg of body weight per percent of body surface burned

Crystalloids: (lactated Ringer's solution) 1.5 mL/kg of body weight per percent of burn

Water: (5% glucose in water) depends on the age and size of the patient, to replace insensible fluid loss

One-half of the estimated fluid requirements for the first 24 hours is given in the first 8 hours, one-quarter of the total in the second 8 hours and one-quarter of the total in the third 8-hour period. The second 24-hour period requirement for colloids and lactated Ringer's solution is about one-half that for the first 24 hours. In applying this formula to burns larger than 50% of total body surface area, requirements must be calculated as though only 50% of the body had been burned.

SOURCE: Feller I, Jones CA: *Nursing the Burned Patient.* Institute for Burn Medicine, 1973. Reprinted with permission.

normal skin, and large amounts of sodium and plasma protein continue to leak through the open wound.

Throughout the entire recovery process, fluid and electrolyte balance fluctuates with surgical procedures, sepsis, and evaporative losses. Careful monitoring is needed until the wound is closed.

Alterations in Respiratory Function

Upper Airway Obstruction Within a few hours after injury, edema from burns of the face and neck might impinge on the upper airway, obstructing respiration. This can occur with or without actual airway burns. Inhalation of superheated air causes upper airway burns. This happens in house fires or accidents in which clothing ignites in enclosed spaces. Heat damage below midtrachea is rare.

Stridor results when the child's airway becomes obstructed. Respiratory rate increases, and other signs of distress, such as restlessness, nasal flaring, and retractions, develop. The physician might examine the airway burns by direct laryngoscopy. In upper airway burns the larynx will be swollen, red, and covered with soot.

The patient needs nasotracheal intubation before edema narrows the airway and makes this procedure difficult. It is important to provide an adequate airway before transporting the patient to a burn center. Edema and obstruction develop rapidly, and an airplane or ambulance is not the best place for emergency intubation.

A tracheostomy is avoided unless oral or nasal tracheal intubation is impossible. Usually, patients with respiratory compromise have neck burns. An incision into burn tissue puts the patient at risk for pulmonary infection due to draining wound exudate and subsequent erosion around the tracheal stoma.

Injury to Bronchi and Lungs Inhalation of smoke containing noxious gases, carbon monoxide, and sooty particles damages the lower airway. Children who sustain flame burns in an enclosed space inevitably inhale smoke. Burns of the face and neck, soot-covered mucous membranes, soot-flecked secretions, singed eyelashes, eyebrows, and nasal hairs, hoarseness, a dry cough, and difficulty swallowing all point to a diagnosis of smoke inhalation injury.

Carbon monoxide is an end product of the incomplete combustion of organic material and is present at virtually every fire. Symptoms of carbon monoxide inhalation depend on the duration of exposure and are systemic rather than local. Carbon monoxide combines much more readily with hemoglobin than does oxygen. Thus, inhalation of smoke from a fire in an enclosed space can result in severe hypoxia. Symptoms range from headache and stupor to collapse, coma, and death depending on carboxyhemoglobin levels. Administration of 100% oxygen greatly reduces the half-life of carboxyhemoglobin and should be started as soon as possible after injury.

Damage to the bronchi and lungs from the noxious gases of smoke is chemical rather than thermal in nature. Smoke is cooled as it passes from the trachea to the bronchi. The irritating gases cause mucosal edema and tissue sloughing in the bronchi. They damage alveolar sacs, altering capillary permeability. This leads to interstitial edema and poor oxygen exchange. Atelectasis and respiratory failure follow if the damage is severe. The injured bronchial walls and boggy atelectatic lungs allow for bacterial invasion and pneumonia. Symptoms of smoke inhalation injury often are not evident immediately but develop 6–24 hours after the fire. Increasing respiratory distress and deteriorating blood gas values indicate the child's need for ventilatory support. Endotracheal intubation and mechanical ventilation are often part of management. Chest radiographs, which are normal at first, will show interstitial edema and decreased aeration within the first day after injury.

Short-term steroid therapy to decrease the inflammatory response after smoke inhalation remains controversial. In a study of 33 burned patients with inhalation injuries, Moylan found that the patients he treated with steroids had a mortality rate four times greater than the patients treated with a saline placebo (Moylan, 1979).

Treatment often includes bronchodilators to reduce bronchospasm. Pulmonary toilet using suctioning, percussion, clapping, postural drainage, and frequent position changes helps to prevent the atelectasis and pooling that leads to infection (see Chapter 34). Athough pressure cannot be applied over a new chest skin graft, modified chest physical therapy and position changes are possible.

Children who survive severe smoke inhalation injuries and their complications might have permanent scarring of lung tissue, but the long-term effect on pulmonary function has not been documented.

Other Pulmonary Problems Infants and small children are susceptible to pulmonary edema if fluid resuscitation is too vigorous. They seem less and less able to tolerate the fluid loads required for the frequent skin grafting procedures. Careful monitoring of urine output and central venous pressure is essential in these patients.

When full-thickness burns encompass the circumference of the chest, constricting eschar might limit chest wall excursions. The child's lungs become more and more difficult to ventilate. Escharotomies, similar to those performed for circumferential digit and limb burns, relieve the pressure.

Alterations in Renal Function The rapid reduction in circulating fluid volume that occurs after a burn reduces blood flow to the kidneys. Adequate fluid resuscitation usually prevents acute tubular necrosis (see Chapter 39). However, the child with underlying kidney disease, a deep extensive thermal burn, or an electrical injury is at risk for acute kidney failure. The lysis of red blood cells and muscle cells that occurs with any deep burn produces free hemoglobin and myoglobin. These substances obstruct renal tubules. Large amounts of resuscitative fluid, along with the osmotic diuretic mannitol, are given to flush clogged renal tubules. Some physicians administer sodium bicarbonate to render the urine alkaline. Hemoglobin is less likely to precipitate in urine with an alkaline pH.

The kidneys also might be damaged later in the course of the burn illness by nephrotoxic antibiotics given in high doses to treat sepsis (see Chapter 39).

Urinary tract infections from ascending bacteria are common in the burn patient. The indwelling Foley catheter often sits in close proximity to the burn wound. Frequent cleansing around the meatus and maintenance of a closed drainage system are preventive nursing measures.

Alterations in the Gastrointestinal System In response to hypovolemia the newly burned child complains of thirst and repeatedly asks for something to drink. Unfortunately, the nurse can give nothing by mouth. Gastric dilatation and paralytic ileus often occur following a major burn, and digestion virtually ceases.

A nasogastric tube is placed and attached to suction in the emergency room to prevent vomiting and aspiration. Antacids are begun soon after admission to avert a Curling's or stress ulcer, a complication of burns in the past. This therapy must continue while a nasogastric tube is in place and while the stress of acute illness persists. Paralytic ileus will resolve and allow for oral intake 2–3 days after injury. The resumption of bowel sounds is one indicator that gastrointestinal function has returned.

Alterations in the Neuroendocrine System Prolonged anoxia caused by smoke inhalation might leave the child in an unresponsive state for days after the burn injury. Most burned children, however, are awake and lucid on admission to the hospital and for a number of days afterward. For the child with a major burn, alterations in consciousness and activity ranging from unresponsiveness to agitation and hallucinations are common phenomena after the first week.

Burn encephalopathy is the term used to classify the symptoms of delirium, coma, and seizures seen in these children. Possible causes include septicemia and fluid and electrolyte imbalances, particularly hyponatremia (Antoon et al., 1972). Less well-defined causes probably account for much of burn encephalopathy. There is a combination of sensory deprivation caused by bulky dressings, eyes swollen shut, immobility, isolation, and sensory overload due to the noisy acute-care setting, sleep deprivation, and frequent, painful treatments. This might account partially for the profound withdrawal or the combativeness seen in many children during the second or third week of hospitalization. Some patients might need psychotropic drugs as part of a behavior management plan.

The adrenal glands respond to the stress of a burn by secreting large amounts of catecholamines. This might account for the hypertension seen in children with major burns. The adrenocortical hormones are also elevated and remain so for most of the hospitalization. Growth might stop or slow down because wound healing demands much of the body's energy. Menses might stop and puberty be delayed until the wound heals. Often, a spurt of growth will occur once the child is in the rehabilitative phase of care.

Alterations in the Hematologic System Platelets decrease markedly in the first few days after injury. This decrease is attributed to the use of platelets at the burn wound site, where they are deposited along arteriole and venule walls. The continued thrombocytopenia seen with burn patients might be caused by depression of blood-forming organs as a result of tissue destruction and infection (Feller and Jones, 1973). The nurse is alert for signs of bleeding at intravenous sites, donor sites, from wounds, or from the urinary or gastrointestinal tract. Disturbances in coagulation are not uncommon in children with major burns during the acute phase of care.

The hematocrit is elevated following a burn because of the decreased circulating fluid volume and hemoconcentration. Once fluid resuscitation begins, the hematocrit will fall and become abnormally low during the diuretic phase, reflecting hemodilution.

Red blood cells are thought to have a shortened half-life in the burn patient. This, combined with blood loss from escharotomies, wound debridement, and surgery, results in anemia. Frequent transfusions are necessary to maintain even low-normal hematocrits and hemoglobin levels throughout the acute-care phase.

Alterations in Metabolism The body responds to the insult of a large, open burn wound by increasing the metabolic rate. Oxygen consumption increases as temperature, respiratory rate, and heart rate rise. At Shriners Burn Institute in Boston, children are placed in bacteria-controlled nursing units. These are plastic tentlike structures with laminar airflow. They protect the child from cross-infection and provide a warm, moist environment. The temperature inside the tent is kept at approximately 86° F with humidity at 85%. Those who recommend this type of environment believe that it reduces evaporative water and heat losses from the wound and unburned skin and in turn reduces the expenditure of calories (Burke et al., 1977).

Medical and Nursing Management During the Acute Phase

Wound Management Once the patients are stabilized in the emergent phase of care, they are said to begin the *acute phase* of burn care. During this phase, the burn team concentrates on preventing wound infection, closing the wound as quickly as possible, and managing the numerous complications that can occur as part of the burn illness.

Any break in the skin weakens one of the body's main defenses against the invasion of microorganisms. Closing the burn wound quickly and thus preventing infection is a high priority.

Wound care can begin as soon as an airway is established, vital signs are stable, and fluid resuscitation is well under way. Personnel performing wound care wear sterile gowns, sterile gloves, caps, and masks to prevent contamination. Initial cultures give baseline data about wound flora. This information might be helpful later on in establishing a time and possible source of contamination. Nurses and physicians collaborate to estimate and record the size and depth of the injury. Many burn centers keep photographic records of the patient's wounds from the time of admission.

Surgical soap solutions are used to clean the wound. Many burn specialists recommend leaving blisters intact as a natural sterile dressing. Dead skin from broken blisters can be debrided with sterile forceps and scissors.

Escharotomy Full-thickness burns that encompass the whole circumference of the extremities, fingers, toes, and chest need careful attention in the first hours after injury. Edema fluid accumulates rapidly under unyielding eschar and puts pressure on underlying blood vessels and nerves. Careful checks of circulation, sensation, and motion are necessary whenever there is a circumferential burn. Children's fingers and toes are very small and thin, and circulation is cut off quite easily. As circulation becomes impaired, hands and feet become cool, pale, or mottled; the child might complain of tingling or numbness. Capillary refill in nail beds is slow or absent, and pulses are difficult to palpate distal to the injury. Pulses might be picked up only by using a Doppler ultrasonic flow detector. When constricting eschar interferes with circulation, the physician performs an *escharotomy* (incision into eschar) to relieve the pressure. Escharotomy is done along the medial and lateral aspects of the extremities, fingers, or toes (see Color Plate). Burns are often of uneven depth, so some bleeding will occur at the site of the escharotomy in the superficial areas. Applying pressure and packing the wound with 4″ × 4″ gauze pads promotes clotting. Similarly, the child with circumferential chest burns will need an escharotomy to relieve pressure and allow full lung expansion. After the escharotomy, it is important to continue checking circulation, sensation, and motion. Even with the extremities elevated, edema fluid continues to accumulate. It is helpful to leave a small window in the dressing where a pulse can be checked and to leave unburned fingers and toes exposed to check temperature and color. Often, the escharotomy incision must be deepened and extended in the first 24 hours to relieve increasing pressure.

Topical Agents Several topical agents are used to treat burns. Each agent has its advantages and disadvantages. All work to protect wounds from the invasion and multiplication of microorganisms. They cannot be totally effective because bacteria become resistant to antimicrobial therapy with repeated exposure, and new agents are always being developed to counteract virulent strains of microorganisms. Table 44-4 describes three topical agents.

Other agents used include povidone-iodine (Betadine), cerium nitrate cream or solution, and nitrofurazone (Furacin).

Burn Wound Dressings Gaining proficiency in changing burn dressings requires time, practice, and attention to detail. During the first hours after a burn, while edema is increasing, the nurse wraps dressings loosely to prevent circulation from being impeded. To avoid interference with respiration, the nurse does not wrap the chest circumferentially in the emergent phase of care. Once the child feels better and is ambulatory, dressings must be secure but allow for maximum mobility. Fingers and toes should be wrapped separately so that surfaces do not adhere, forming weblike scar bands as they heal.

Adhesive tape cannot be used on facial burns. Endotracheal tubes can be secured with cloth tape tied around the tube and then around the head. When the ears are burned, gauze pads placed under each pinna prevent adherence to the scalp during healing. To prevent contamination of the wound, the nurse shaves surrounding hair, except for eye-

TABLE 44-4 Topical Agents Used to Treat Burns

Agent	Information and use	Advantages	Disadvantages
Silver nitrate, 0.5% ($AgNO_3$)	1. Works well with a primary or tangential excision program of care 2. Effective against gram-negative organisms 3. Requires large, bulky dressings, which are kept well moistened. At least six layers of dressing material are required, with rewetting needed approximately every 2 hours 4. Black silver chloride crust builds up on unburned skin, which must be softened with an emollient cream and peeled off with forceps 5. To assess wound: Normal skin becomes black Eschar is stained light brown Partial-thickness wound remains unstained	1. Readily available and inexpensive 2. Painless once the dressing is in place over the wound 3. Can be used over new grafts without disturbing healing	1. Does not penetrate eschar well 2. Requires continuously wet, bulky dressings, which impede mobility 3. Low tonicity causes sodium and chloride electrolytes to be lost at the wound surface, requiring careful monitoring and replacement 4. Stains unburned skin, linen, and most surfaces dark brown or black 5. Color changes of adjacent healthy skin are upsetting to parents and children 6. Wounds are difficult to assess
Silver sulfadiazine cream, 1% (Silvadene)	1. Effective against gram-negative and gram-positive bacteria and *Candida albicans* 2. Apply directly on the wound or impregnate gauze for wound application. Apply about ⅛ in thick 3. May dress wound or leave open 4. Do not use with children who are allergic to sulfa drugs or those with a glucose-6-phosphate dehydrogenase deficiency 5. Remove all old cream before reapplying	1. Little delay in eschar separations 2. Little or no pain from application (ie, the cream does not sting, although touching the wound will hurt) 3. Minimal or no side effects	1. Combines with wound exudate to form a cream-colored buildup on the wound, making assessment difficult 2. Leukopenia is one possible side effect 3. Manipulation of the wound to remove old cream is painful
Mafenide acetate, 10% (Sulfamylon)	1. Effective against gram-positive and gram-negative organisms 2. Apply 3 to 5 mm thick to wound, which usually is left exposed. Occlusive dressings might result in maceration. Reapply twice daily 3. Cleanse wound before reapplying 4. Best used with a hydrotherapy regime	1. Penetrates eschar well; useful in deep full-thickness burns such as electrical injuries 2. Powerful antimicrobial agent	1. Very painful; wound stings for about 30 minutes after application 2. Delays eschar separation 3. Strong carbonic anhydrase inhibitor. Might cause metabolic acidosis

brows. Liquid barrier drapes secured over thigh dressings help to prevent contamination with urine or feces. Splints that maintain joints in a position of function can be made on admission and remodeled to fit over dressings. Kerlix secures splints well.

Elasticized netting material can be used over dressings to keep them in place. This netting can be very useful for the toddler with a scald burn to the chest who is going back and forth to the playroom. Occasionally, infants and toddlers with silver nitrate dressings on their arms and hands will chew or suck on them. A protective drape over the area helps to prevent silver nitrate ingestion.

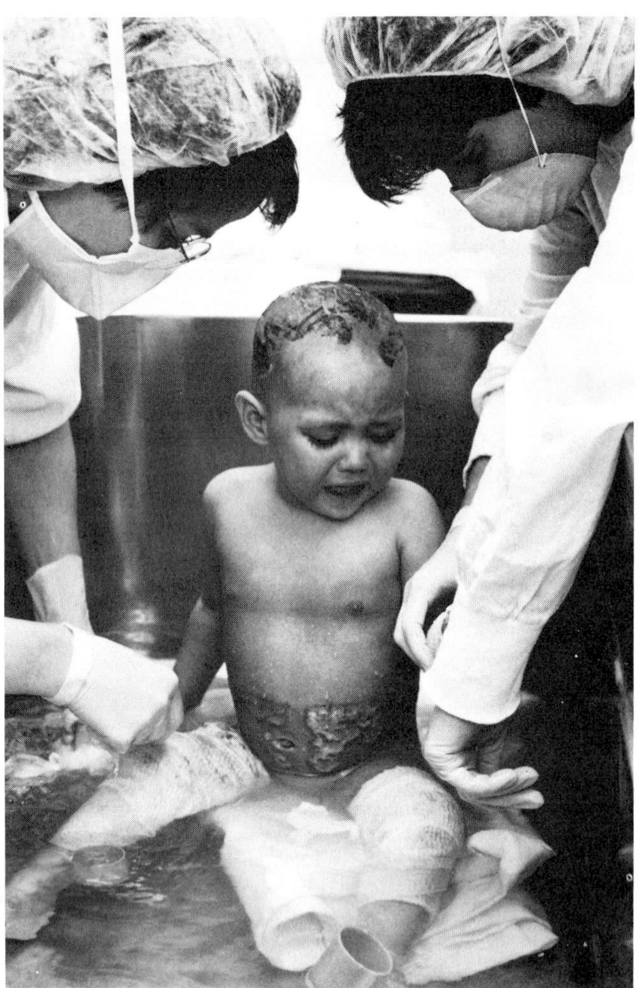

Hydrotherapy to remove dressings and eschar is extremely painful for the child and can be interrupted periodically to allow the child a respite from the procedure. Proper aseptic technique would have all the nurses' hair covered.

Hydrotherapy and Debridement The eschar of full-thickness burns is necrotic tissue, a perfect breeding ground for bacteria. Prompt removal of this eschar and preparation of a healthy bed to receive skin grafts are central to good wound care. Hydrotherapy involves soaking or showering the wound with water once or twice a day for 20–30 minutes. This helps to soften and loosen eschar. Patients who are critically ill, whose body temperatures are abnormally low or high, and those with electrolyte imbalances cannot tolerate hydrotherapy. However, this form of wound care works well for less critically ill patients. Hydrotherapy helps to clean not only the wound but the entire body. It also helps to maintain range of motion. With the open wound, isotonic saline works best to prevent the loss of electrolytes and protect granulation tissue. A detergent is used to promote mild cleansing. The temperature of the solution should be 94–97° F. Patients who undergo hydrotherapy find it painful and frightening, especially at first. As eschar softens, skilled nurses debride the wound with forceps and scissors. Although the task has to be completed, children need breaks to regroup their defenses. The experienced nurse learns how much is "enough" each day for each child, balancing the child's need for control and respite with the need to debride the wound and prepare recipient skin graft sites. Carefully planned teaching and behavior modification programs can help to provide the consistency and predictability needed by children who are enduring this daily suffering (see Chapter 29). Wounds often bleed during debridement. Pressure, sometimes cautery, and occasionally sutures are used to check this bleeding.

As the eschar separates and is debrided away, a bed of granulation tissue forms at the juncture of healthy and necrotic tissue. A healthy, uninfected granulation bed that is ready for grafting is red, flat, vascular, and low in bacteria count. Preparing the deep, full-thickness burn wound for grafting with hydrotherapy and debridement takes a number of weeks. Prompt surgical excision of eschar followed by placement of skin grafts is one treatment method preferred by some burn centers.

Primary and Tangential Excision When the wound is of varying depths, surgeons do a tangential excision. Using a slicing technique, they remove the lifeless, burned tissue layer by layer until they reach a healthy, bleeding bed (Burke et al., 1976).

When primary excision is the surgical technique, the full-thickness wound must be fairly uniform in depth throughout. Using an electrically powered dermatome, the surgeon cuts away as much as 20% of burn eschar per TBSA for each visit to the operating room. Skin grafts obtained from an unburned part of the body are placed over the excised site once the bleeding is controlled. Tangential or primary excision of full-thickness burn wounds is repeated as needed, depending on the patient's condition and availability of donor sites (Burke et al., 1976).

Wound and Systemic Infections In spite of topical agents, early excision and grafting, careful handwashing, and aseptic technique for wound care, burn wounds become infected. Contamination from the body's own flora and cross-contamination between patients are difficult to prevent.

The usual nursing measures to prevent the spread of infection between patients, such as handwashing, are even more important when caring for children with burns. Other measures might include environmental control with laminar airflow rooms and reverse isolation (see Chapter 37). Nurses often wear special clothing while performing wound care. Along with sterile gloves, this attire might include a cap, mask, and plastic, disposable apron, which is removed upon leaving the patient's bedside.

Signs and symptoms of infection are the same for all kinds of skin wounds and include increased pain, swelling, redness in surrounding tissue, heat, and increased exudate that might be purulent or foul smelling. Skin grafts will literally disintegrate if placed on an infected recipient bed.

Wound surface or biopsy cultures give data on predominant flora as well as an estimate of the amount of growth. Topical agents might be changed, grafting delayed or advanced, and frequency of dressing changes increased on the basis of the amount of exudate and type of organism growing on a particular wound.

Systemic sepsis can begin from a number of sites. The burn wound is an obvious site. Other sites include intravenous lines and their insertion sites, Foley catheters, and boggy, atelectatic lungs, where pneumonia organisms breed. Septicemia is a catastrophic illness for any patient. It often begins with subtle changes in the sensorium and decreased gastrointestinal motility but can quickly progress to circulatory collapse, coagulopathies, and even death. Intravenous antibiotic therapy often is begun with the first symptoms, and life supports are initiated to treat shock and respiratory failure. Children do survive sepsis with expert medical and nursing care, but treatment can be difficult because the causative organisms become resistant to antibiotics. There is a race against the clock to cover the burn wound and thus restore an important defense against infection before virulent organisms do irreparable damage.

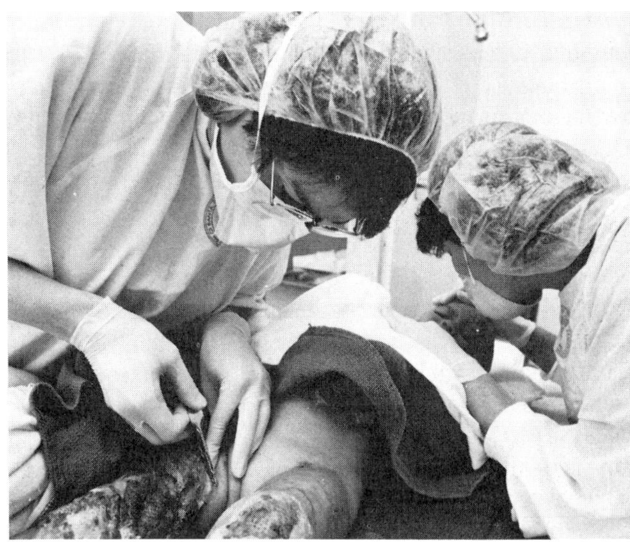

In removing the dressings, the nursing team may find it useful to have one nurse comfort and distract the child while the other concentrates on performing the procedure.

Care of Specific Areas

Eyes The blinking reflex is most efficient in preventing corneal burns even in individuals with facial burns. However, the ophthalmologist examines the patient who suffers facial injury or becomes unconscious at the scene before edema makes lid retraction impossible. Although corneal injury might not be evident, the ophthalmologist often prescribes prophylactic antibiotic ointment.

It is important to keep the eyes clean because burn wound exudate from the facial wounds drains into the eyes. Later, as wounds heal, scar bands and contractures will form and interfere with adequate eyelid closure. Lubricating fluids and antibiotic ointment might be needed to protect exposed corneas. In severe cases surgery will be needed to release these lid contractures within a few weeks of healing.

Ears Cartilage of the external ear becomes infected easily. To avoid this chondritis of the ear and possible tissue loss and infection, the nurse carefully cleans and meticulously debrides the ears. A penetrating topical agent such as mafenide acetate (Sulfamylon) helps to arrest bacterial invasion. Gauze placed behind the ears prevents them from adhering to the scalp as they heal.

Face Many burn centers treat facial burns with topical agents, frequent cleansing, and open technique (no dressings). Some burn centers have used early excision and grafting. The best cosmetic results are achieved with early grafting, using as few pieces of skin as possible and joining seams along normal facial lines or creases.

Nasal cartilage is susceptible to infection and pressure necrosis. A nasogastric tube or endotracheal tube that rubs or pushes against the septum or on the alae nasi can cause disfiguring tissue loss. Changing the tubes regularly from side to side and careful attention to the tightness and placement of tape and ties help to prevent this problem.

Perineum The perineum is a highly contaminated area, and frequent, thorough cleansing and the reapplication of ointment or cream are needed. Children often are incontinent, and it can be a major battle to keep this area free of infection. Keeping the patient in the prone position helps to prevent further tissue damage when there are burns to the buttocks and is the position of choice whenever possible. A Bradford frame might help (see Chapter 41). The child who is placed prone in bed or in a go-cart can be turned to face the activity on the unit and to avoid just looking at the walls and bed frames.

Exposed Tendon, Muscle, and Bone A burn sometimes exposes underlying tendon, muscle, or bone. These structures must be carefully protected and kept moist. A full-thickness skin graft or flap (skin, subcutaneous fat, and blood supply) might be used to cover a large defect.

Ongoing Care of the Child With Burns

Nutritional Management The most expert and vigilant wound care will be fruitless if the patient's nutritional needs are neglected. Caloric requirements increase significantly after burn injury in response to the accelerated metabolic state. Energy stores dwindle rapidly, and catabolism persists if body stores are not replenished and maintained. Protein is lost through the burn wound, along with heat, water, and electrolytes.

As discussed earlier, immediately after a significant injury, the child receives no food or fluid by mouth for 24–48 hours because of decreased gastrointestinal motility. Once peristalsis returns, the nurse can begin feeding the child by mouth or nasogastric tube.

Whether to eat or not can become a control issue with incapacitated children, but even the cooperative child with an adequate appetite has difficulty taking in the amount of calories needed for wound healing. When there is a major burn, tube feedings and hyperalimentation will be needed to provide the necessary nutrients (see Chapter 38).

Often, the hyperalimentation line must pass through burn eschar, providing an easy means of access for bacteria. Because occlusive dressings secured with adhesive tape cannot be used over the burn wound, the site of the hyperalimentation line must be monitored carefully. The nurse cleans it frequently with an antimicrobial solution such as povidone iodine (Betadine) and keeps it covered with gauze impregnated with an antimicrobial ointment. The line site is changed frequently to prevent septicemia.

From the first day of injury onward, nurses need to pay careful attention to the nutritional needs of the burn child. Consultation with a nutritionist and the parent can help the nurse to design a meal plan that will provide the child with maximum calories. The occupational therapist can be called on to fashion adaptive devices to make self-feeding possible. The child should be given as many choices as possible, have food from home brought in if appropriate, and have mealtimes scheduled far apart from dressing changes.

Body weight measured twice a week helps the nurse to evaluate the effectiveness of the nutritional plan. The daily calorie count is an assessment procedure the child can participate in.

The proper mix of fats, proteins, and carbohydrates will vary for each child depending on the size and depth of the injury. The nurse might consult with hospital nutritionists to plan the pattern of meals and snacks that will meet the calculated daily requirements for the child.

Pain Management Pain is one of the first words that comes to mind when burns are mentioned, but little has been written on pain management specific to burns. Having a burn means having pain that recurs and often intensifies. Repeated, painful treatments are also a necessary part of the recovery process.

Nurses speak of how difficult it is to carry out procedures such as hydrotherapy, debridement, and dressing changes day after day. It can be especially difficult to care for children who are too young to understand the reasons for all the pain. Balancing pain control with a number of other nursing goals is challenging. In the emergent phase of care, intravenous narcotics are effective in relieving pain. Morphine sulfate is used commonly. A small amount of morphine can be given intravenously and repeated as needed if the patient's vital signs remain stable. Tranquillizers given along with the narcotics help to decrease the patient's anxiety.

Intramuscular injections are avoided. Because of rapidly accumulating edema throughout the body, medications pool and are absorbed erratically from the intramuscular site. Unburned skin sites must be preserved for donor grafts, and any unnecessary breaks in the skin are portals of entry for infectious organisms.

A variety of different types of oral or intravenous analgesics will be needed throughout the course of hospitalization for hydrotherapy, debridement, and dressing changes. Children might become dependent on narcotics, requiring a gradual tapering of the drugs later on. They also might become tolerant of the drugs, needing larger doses for a period of time to provide adequate pain relief.

As regards pain control and burns, the nurse maintains a difficult balance. The child's pain must be reduced for procedures, but the child must remain alert enough for mealtimes to ensure proper caloric intake.

Touching and stroking, typically used by parents and nurses to express caring and give comfort, might be painful to the burned child. Parents need help to find ways to express their caring, learn to hold their children in a nonpainful position, and find unburned areas and areas not used for donor sites that they can touch and rub.

Even the most gentle and careful wound care can seem like an attack or assault to the child. A young child might interpret dressing changes as punishment in spite of reassurances and explanations. The response to injury from burns and hospitalization parallels the response of different age groups to illness and hospitalization (see Chapter 27). Regression might be more severe, withdrawal more prolonged, and aggressive behavior more pronounced when the injury is severe and wound healing seems to stretch on endlessly. For burn patients, anxiety and the intensity of the pain experience are closely linked. Whatever reduces the child's anxiety level will be helpful in the midst of painful procedures (see Chapter 29).

Kavanagh's (1983) findings in a study with burned children suggest that providing maximum predictability and control will lessen anxiety. Kavanagh applied these concepts to age groups that ranged from toddlers to adolescents. Predictability included doing procedures at the same time and place each day, keeping certain areas and times free and "safe," and wearing a specific object that signaled a dressing change or procedure time.

To give the child maximum control, Kavanagh built in as many choices as possible such as which dressing to do first and how fast to remove the gauze. Children helped remove dressings and even did some of the less painful debriding. Kavanagh asked nurses to explain procedures in a step-by-step manner and to ask the children in the experimental group to watch each part of the care.

Paying attention to each child's level of pain tolerance during a procedure is important in helping the child to stay in control. Pausing to allow the child to take a deep breath, regroup, and get ready for the next few minutes of debridement helps the child to master the situation because it is broken up into manageable parts.

Nurses experienced in burn care wonder about the long-term effects of so much pain and suffering on children. They comment, however, on the resilience and adaptability of children. Hospitalization and illness can be a difficult time for families but a time of growth and positive change as well. Providing opportunities for the child to express anger and hurt during painful procedures and during play, as well as helping the child to maintain control of and master the situations encountered are part of nursing care (Bernstein and Robson, 1983) (see Chapter 29).

Function and Appearance With all major illnesses and injuries, plans for rehabilitation and discharge must begin at the time of admission. Rehabilitation as a third phase of care, however, begins for children when the open wound areas are reduced to less than 10%–15% of the TBSA.

Contractures Burn wounds tend to heal in positions of flexion and nonfunction. Joints must be maintained in neutral positions and in extension (Fig. 44-5). Joints also need range-of-motion exercises at least twice each day from the time of admission onward. After grafts are placed, joints are immobilized for 5–10 days before exercises can resume. The physical therapist, nurse, and recreation therapist collaborate to plan schedules and activities that encourage motion of involved joints as healing progresses.

Flexion contractures are a common problem. To prevent them, joints must be maintained in a position of function and exercised regularly. Physical therapists should be called when a burn patient is admitted to assess the need for splints and plan an exercise schedule. Whenever a burn is present over the surface of a joint, the patient will need some sort of splinting. Splints can be made that will fit over dressings and be secured with Kerlix gauze. New splints are made as burn wound edema subsides, when wounds are grafted, and again after the grafts heal. For example, the child with full-thickness hand burns will need range-of-motion exercises at each dressing change and a splint over the dressings to maintain position of the hands. When skin grafting is done, the hand will be immobilized with a splint until the grafts are well adhered, approximately 7–10 days. After this time, exercises will begin again, and another kind of splint will be used that enables and encourages finger motion and use of the hand for activities such as eating and play.

Once the wound over a joint has healed, the child will continue to need splints to prevent contracture formation. The depth of the burn and severity of scarring will determine how much of the time a splint must be worn. For example, some patients might only need splinting during sleep, whereas others must wear the splint around the clock. With scarring in the axillas, splints are needed that keep the arms at 90° angles, a very awkward position for the child trying to do schoolwork. In this and similar situations, teachers, physicians, physical therapists, and nurses can collaborate with the child and family to plan a splint-wearing and activity schedule that fits in with their daily routine. (See Color Plate).

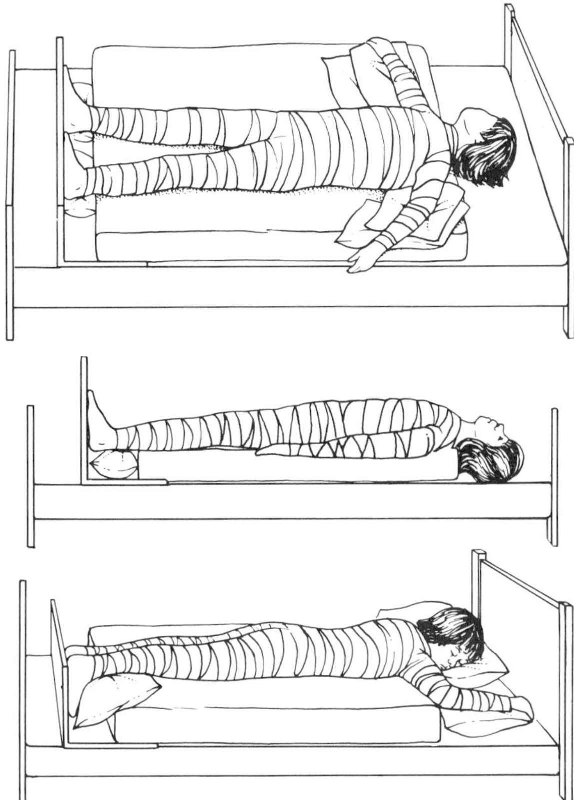

Figure 44-5 For extensive burns, the total body position must be considered. Ideally, the patient is kept on a half mattress so that, in the supine position, the neck is hyperextended; in the prone position, the ankles remain at a 90° angle; and in both positions, the legs and arms are kept abducted.

Scars Scar formation is a major problem as burn wounds heal and for many months following healing. Scar tissue can impinge on joint function and distort the child's appearance. When the inflammatory process is intense and prolonged, as it is with deep partial-thickness and full-thickness burns, hypertrophic scars form. These scars are reddened, raised, firm, and almost woody in appearance. Microscopic examination of hypertrophic scars reveals collagen fibers in a whorl-like pattern rather than the parallel alignment seen in normal tissue. This scar tissue is very active, growing and reshaping itself over several months as it "matures." Eventually, the scar will lose its red color, flatten out, and

Discharge Instructions for Burn Patients

For Healed Superficial Burns and Donor Sites

1. Cleanse daily with mild soap and water. If possible, take a bath or shower and wash the entire skin with a washcloth
2. Use a nonperfumed lubricating cream or ointment, such as petroleum jelly, on the wound after the bath
3. Protect the wound from the sun. Cover healed areas with light, loose clothing. Wear a hat with a brim and apply a sunscreen to areas that are difficult to cover in warm weather such as the face, hands, and feet
4. Feel free to swim in any water—salt, fresh, or pool. Water is a great place for exercise, too. Remember to reapply sunscreen each time you get out of the water

For Healed Deep Burns

1. Follow the instructions for healed superficial burns
2. Liberally apply lubricating cream. Because the burn has destroyed oil-producing glands, cream needs to be applied at least two or three times a day. Check the skin for dryness and flaking, a sign that more lubricating cream is required
3. Once a day, clean the pockets and crevices of scars with cotton-tipped applicators
4. Use medication as prescribed to reduce itching, which is one of the biggest complaints with burn scars
5. Use pain medication as prescribed. Sometimes, scars are painful, possibly as a result of nerve regeneration. In most cases no medication will be needed after discharge
6. Often, blisters on scar tissue break, leaving abrasion-like wounds. Apply Mercurochrome or recommended cream or ointment to those superficial areas of breakdown
7. Clean any open areas, including areas where a blister breaks, with soap and water. Then apply Mercurochrome and cover the area with a gauze bandage before applying the pressure garments. If necessary, use nonirritating paper tape to secure gauze pads
8. If an infection appears to be developing, or if you have any questions about the condition of your skin, wearing and fit of pressure garments, or any other problems, call ____________________

SOURCE: Surveyer JA, Clougherty DM: Burn scars: Fighting the effects. Copyright © 1983, Amerian Journal of Nursing Company. Reproduced with permission from *Am J Nurs*, 1983; 5:746–751.

become more pliable. However, the nurse can do a great deal to prevent or decrease contractures and disfigurement.

Experience in burn centers shows that pressure evenly distributed over the healed wound helps to lessen hypertrophic scar formation. Pressure garments are commercially available that fit any part of the body. When the wound is almost healed, the patient can be measured for pressure garments. The nurse can use ace bandages over healed wounds while waiting for the pressure garments to be made and delivered. Continuous wearing of pressure garments seems to work best for reducing scars. The nurse instructs the family on the care of the elasticized pressure garments and skin care for healed wounds.

Skin Care After Healing Families and patients might be reluctant to touch, wash, and care for healed wounds. The goal of any discharge teaching is to ensure that patients are comfortable caring for themselves or that their families are comfortable with the care before discharge. The nurse can give them written guidelines and the name of someone they can call with questions.

Emotional Needs The first hours and days after a child has been burned are times of repeated crises. For weeks after a major burn injury, the main issue is survival while the wound remains open and the threat of sepsis persists. Children with less serious burns are still caught up with the crises of sudden hospitalization, painful treatments, and surgery. Questions and worries about loss of function, scarring, and disfigurement usually do not appear until the wounds begin to heal.

The nurse draws on knowledge of crisis intervention and grief theory while supporting, guiding, and instructing families through these times of uncertainty and pain (see Chapter 32).

With an accident and something as painful and visible as a burn, the guilt that parents often feel when their children are hospitalized seems doubly intense. Often, the injury occurs because of carelessness or a momentary lapse in parental attention. The guilt is something parents, caregivers, siblings, and victims themselves carry for years to come.

Often, significant losses have occurred in a house fire. Other family members, an entire home, personal possessions, or a pet might have been lost. Parents and other family members of a child with major burns face weeks and months of crises and adjustments.

The nurse learns to listen and offer opportunities for parents and children to express their feelings of guilt, anger, fear, and frustration. Each trip to the operating room might provoke a recurrence of the feelings they experienced when the accident first happened. Parents' groups, siblings' groups, and individual counseling are ways families and burn victims can obtain support and learn to cope.

Children with burns react much as any other child who is hospitalized for an illness (see Chapter 27). Infancy and early childhood are particularly vulnerable times for children with burns, who are unable to understand the need for painful treatments. Infants who see only the masked faces of parents and staff for days on end are missing an important part of the usual stimulation and cues about the world around them. Young children should be allowed to see full faces, especially those of their parents and significant caregivers. Because small children cannot voice their needs and hurts, nurses need to remember that they still require analgesics before painful dressing changes and other procedures.

The nurse is careful to protect the burned child from contact with contaminated objects. Familiar blankets, cuddly toys, and plastic toys can be sterilized and provide comfort and entertainment.

In middle and late childhood children also need the comfort of the familiar. Playtime is doubly important when so much of the child's day is unpleasant and full of pain. Even when extremities, hands, and feet are burned and bandaged, children can play with their eyes and imaginations. For example, one 10-year-old-boy in a major burn center was entirely bandaged except for his face. All other surfaces were burned or used for donor sites. Each day he would ask his nurse to set up his toy people, cars, and trucks on his bedside table in front of him so that he could "play" with them.

Sleep disturbances and nightmares about the accident are common after burn injuries and usually decrease with time and healing. The nurse helps children cope with disturbing dreams by listening, reinforcing reality, and acknowledging the connection between the dreams and the frightening experience they have been through. It is also important to adhere to bedtime routines and provide for periods of undistrubed sleep. For some children, nighttime sedation is necessary.

Living With Disfigurement For all crises, adjustments are made from one phase of recovery to the next. Once the burn wound is covered and scar tissue begins to form, children and their families are faced with the visible and long-lasting effects of burns. Children whose scars are limited and covered easily by clothing usually can resume their normal activities. However, children who have suffered major burns, loss of body parts, or deep burns of the face must cope with problems similar to chronically ill and disabled children (see Chapter 30). Joint contractures that result from scarring cause decreased mobility of fingers, elbows, shoulders, and knees, interfering with simple activities of daily life and self-care.

The visibly scarred burn victim and loved ones will always be in a state of grieving or chronic sorrow. Anniversary of injury dates, birthdays, and developmental milestones will heighten the feelings of sadness and loss. Children whose families were cohesive and well integrated before the injury seem to adjust best to disfigurement and functional losses. Also, clinical experience indicates that children who are expressive and struggle with parents and staff and later with peers and teachers rather than withdrawing are most likely to adapt well in society (Bernstein and Robson, 1983).

It is difficult to predict or measure the adjustment of children and families after a burn injury. Extensive longitudinal studies carried on for years after injuries with large groups of children do not exist. However, caregivers have made observations that help them to understand the process of rehabilitation and adjustment.

Infants and children under 5 years of age are often quite resilient. In the presence of a loving family, they can develop a sense of self-esteem and well-being in spite of severe disfigurement. Their concepts of themselves, their body images, and their ideas about the functioning of their bodies can develop well if parents are encouraging and concentrate on gains and potential rather than on sickness and limitations.

Children in middle childhood focus on the functional aspects of injury, wondering whether they will be able to resume important activities such as playing soccer or ice hockey. Each child develops an individual style of dealing with deformity. Bernstein and Robson described three major areas of concern of children in middle childhood: (1) interacting with peers; (2) dealing with curiosity and staring; and (3) dealing with feelings of guilt and blame (Bernstein and Robson, 1983). In a society that places so much emphasis on appearance, children with visible burn scars, especially facial scars, are often teased or avoided.

Some interventions started soon after hospitalization and continued throughout recovery can help children to make the difficult transition back to school. When a child is first hospitalized, the family and hospital staff can contact the child's teachers and encourage a continued relationship. Classmates can send cards, pictures, letters, and tape recordings to the injured child. This usually happens in the first week or two after hospitalization, but the hospital and school staff need to continue to encourage the activity or it will gradually decline. Once children are well enough, tutoring can begin. In this way children often are able to keep up with their schoolwork and thus return to the class where they are known and accepted.

Consultation and collaboration between the family, burn team, and school will help to prepare the school for the child with disfiguring scars who must wear splints and pressure garments. Shriners Burn Institute in Boston has prepared a booklet on the burned child's return to school (Dumond, et al., n.d.). Along with preparation and contact with teachers and classmates from the time of admission onward, the authors of this booklet advocate that the child return to school as soon as possible after discharge, with careful planning of daily schedules to accommodate the child's therapy and splint-wearing needs.

Often, a classroom of children can be introduced to the subject of burns by an age-appropriate prevention program. The discussion of their own classmate follows naturally, and the classmate's changed appearance and any limitations can be introduced along with a photograph for all to see.

The return home can be both happy and difficult for families. The initial sense of elation may be followed by a let-down, lonely feeling once the realities of daily life become obvious. The nurse can help patients through this transition by careful planning for continued support and service from community agencies, follow-up phone calls, and, sometimes, home visits.

Children preparing to leave the hospital for the first time can benefit from group sessions with other children who already have faced discharge and those first weeks and months afterward. Adolescents, in particular, respond well to this type of peer support. Part of group sessions can be spent rehearsing how to respond to curious stares, jeers, and questions.

Adolescents with new facial injuries or functional losses need much support if they are to readjust their goals and get on with their lives. Injury comes at a time when body image and self-concept are undergoing major changes and growth, when peer regard is so important (see Chapter 11). Some adolescents react by becoming depressed and reclusive, whereas others become hostile and antisocial. Preexisting personality characteristics and coping styles greatly influence adjustment, but skilled psychologic counseling and early vocational counseling are essential for most patients in this age group. Children burned at a younger age might experience a whole new set of adjustment problems when they reach adolescence that will require intervention by school or community mental health staff. Adolescents with facial scars sometimes only feel comfortable in heterosexual relationships with others who have similar scars or disabilities.

Nurses and physicians alike find that parents and children frequently misinterpret the information they receive about the goals and possible outcomes of reconstructive surgery. What the surgeon will describe as possible improvement in appearance or function the parents or children will interpret as a promise of total return to normality. Apparently, they can better maintain hope and courage in the face of repeated surgery and suffering if they deny or distort the limitations of reality.

Disfigured persons will always have parts they wish looked better. Those who are old enough will remember how they looked before they were injured. They will have wishes about how they'd like to look and will daydream about becoming whole and attractive once again (Bernstein and Robson, 1983).

Resources for caring for patients in the acute phase of burn care are available throughout the country, but ongoing, often lifelong services are needed for children who have suffered major burn injuries if they are to develop optimally and lead fulfilling lives.

Alterations in concepts of self-image need careful study to help medical and nursing personnel understand adjustment differences for children at different developmental levels. There might always be a certain amount of denial children with marked facial disfigurement use to cope with life. For example, one adolescent girl who had been burned several years earlier talked of her plans for a modeling career despite obvious facial scars. Reconstructive surgery could never return her face to its former smoothness, and this had been explained to her repeatedly.

Research continues in burn wound care and the prevention of scarring. Synthetic coverings and epithelial cultures of the patient's own cells are now being used at Shriners Burn Institute in Boston as a way to obtain early wound coverage. It is hoped that some of this work will aid in decreasing the inflammatory process and subsequent scarring associated with burns.

Caring for children with burns is a major nursing challenge. Nurses planning to specialize in child health nursing need to examine the stresses and rewards carefully. They need the maturity to face uncertain outcomes, and they must plan supports for themselves that will keep them performing effectively and enjoying their work.

The Child With Frostbite

Children are subject to a second type of thermal injury, *frostbite,* which results from exposure to cold rather than heat. Like burns, frostbite can be mild, moderate, or severe depending on the extent of tissue injury. It is classified as frostnip, superficial frostbite, deep frostbite, or fourth-degree frostbite (Rolnick, Stair, and Silfen, 1980).

Frostnip is mild freezing of the epidermis. The condition appears as a small, pale area and can be rewarmed readily by contact with a warm article of clothing or portion of the body.

Superficial frostbite may be either a partial-thickness or full-thickness injury. A partial-thickness injury is a white, cold area on the skin surface. It feels pliable to the touch, and the involved area is numb. The child might experience severe pain, erythema, burning, and pruritus when the skin is rewarmed. The skin may be edematous and sensitive to cold for several weeks. A full-thickness injury presents symptoms similar to partial-thickness frostbite, although skin involvement is more extensive. Erythema and blistering occur 24–48 hours after rewarming, and the difference between necrotic and healthy tissue is apparent at that time. Within several weeks, the blisters are replaced by dry eschar, which eventually sloughs off (after approximately 1 month), leaving exposed healing tissue. The affected areas are extremely tender.

Deep frostbite affects underlying tissue such as tendons, muscle, and bone. The skin appears white or cyanotic and is cold and hard to the touch. Sensation is absent in the affected area. Rewarming causes severe pain, edema, and extensive blistering. Eschar formation and subsequent sloughing might take up to 3 months. Pain during the healing process indicates a more hopeful prognosis.

Fourth-degree frostbite presents the same symptoms as deep frostbite but without pain on rewarming. It takes approximately 1 month to identify living and dead tissue accurately. After several months, the gangrenous areas of an affected extremity might separate spontaneously. Even in the most severe cases of frostbite, however, more healthy tissues may be present than the appearance of the affected area would suggest. Therefore, many months (may be up to 4 months) usually elapse before any decision to amputate surgically is made.

Several factors contribute to the occurrence of frostbite, the most major of which is hypothermia. *Hypothermia* occurs when body temperatures drop below 95° F. At that point the individual begins shivering. Shivering produces heat and is the body's attempt to compensate for the cold. When core body temperatures drop to below 90° F, the child is considered to be experiencing severe hypothermia. Severe hypothermia is detrimental to all body systems and, if untreated, can cause death. Peripheral vasoconstriction in response to the cold increases the blood flow to the heart. This increased central blood volume causes hormonal changes that result in diuresis. Diuresis and an associated plasma shift increase the viscosity of the blood, resulting in diminished circulation to peripheral tissues. Alterations in hemoglobin also contribute to this general decrease in tissue oxygenation (Bangs, 1982).

As hypothermia progresses, the heart rate decreases, the lungs are unable to rid the body of carbon dioxide, and the liver is unable to process the increased lactic acid produced by the lack of oxygen to the tissues. Increased lactic acid can cause cardiac irregularities and death (Bangs, 1982).

Reduced tissue oxygenation combined with restricted blood flow from tight clothing (for example, boots and gloves) can result in tissue freezing and frostbite. Rewarming the frostbitten area without damaging the tissue further is a nursing and medical challenge. When a child is experiencing frostbite, initial assessment should focus on determining the presence and extent of hypothermia. Mild hypothermia can be treated by moving the child to a warm environment, removing wet clothing, and wrapping the child loosely in blankets. Shivering and environmental warmth might correct the problem. Children with severe hypothermia should be hospitalized and may be treated with fluid volume replacement and warming blankets or other warming techniques (Rolnick, Stair, and Silfen, 1980; Bangs, 1982). Severe hypothermia must be corrected before attention can be given to frostbitten areas.

The frostbitten tissue should be rewarmed by immersion in warm, agitating water (temperature of 110° F). The child can receive medication for pain. All frostbitten areas should be handled gently to minimize additional trauma.

The care of the hospitalized child after rewarming is similar to the care of the child with burns. Protective isolation (see Chapter 37) is required for children with severe blistering and tissue injury. Whirlpool treatments two or three times a day will gently debride injured tissue, and additional debridement is usually unnecessary. Early physical therapy prevents joint contractures. If eschar formation inhibits exercise, escharotomies may be performed. Unlike nursing care for burns, dressings are seldom used. The nurse elevates the child's extremities and uses a bed cradle to reduce pain from the pressure of bed clothing. The child's diet should be high in protein and calories to promote healing. Antibiotic administration or tetanus prophylaxis might be indicated.

Unless the frostbite is fourth degree, the child can be expected to experience pain and can be medicated accordingly. Psychologic alterations caused by severe pain, isolation, and the shock of tissue necrosis are common (Boswick et al., 1983). Signs of depression require understanding and encouragement from the nurse.

Amputation and/or skin grafting might be required after months of healing. Concurrent alterations in body image demand sympathetic and therapeutic nursing care. The long-term effects of frostbite might include scarring, infection, graft rejection, skin sensitivity to cold, and growth retardation in children whose epiphyses are involved.

Teaching the principles of frostbite prevention is a nursing responsibility. Children should be advised to wear appropriate clothing when going out in the cold. Wearing many layers of clothing is preferable to wearing one layer of heavy clothing because air is trapped between layers and acts as an insulator. Hats should always be worn because a large amount of body heat may be lost through the head. Mittens are preferable to gloves because the finger contact allows for more warmth. Tight-fitting boots should be avoided. Children should be advised to come in when their clothing is wet.

Frostbite damage can be more severe if the affected area is rewarmed and then refrozen. If it appears that a continuous source of warmth will soon be available, it is better to wait before attempting a rewarming procedure (Bangs, 1982).

The Child With Severe Surface Injuries

Child victims of automobile or motorcycle accidents are subject to severe contusions, abrasions, and lacerations, along with associated injuries such as fractures, head trauma, and internal organ injury. After initial assessment and management of life-threatening problems, the nurse gives attention to surface injuries. The child's appearance, particularly if injuries are extensive, might daunt even the strongest of nurses.

First priority after stabilization is cleansing of the wounds to prevent infection and the administration of tetanus prophylaxis, if indicated. This becomes a difficult task because in all probability the wounds will be heavily contaminated with dirt and other matter. Miller (1980) recommended the following steps for effective cleansing of contaminated wounds:

1. Soak or scrub abraded and lacerated areas with povidone–iodine for 10 minutes.
2. Follow with sterile water or saline irrigation.
3. Remove contaminated particles with sterile applicator sticks or a small sterile hemostat after anesthetizing the area.
4. Cover with a dry sterile dressing over a topical anti-infective agent.
5. Recommend suturing if necessary.
6. Observe and assess for signs of infection.

Depending on the associated injuries, the child might or might not be able to be sedated for wound cleansing. In all likelihood sedation will be contraindicated because of potential head injury. The nurse explains the procedure to the child and reassures the child that the local anesthetic will limit the pain.

The child with severely denuded skin from extensive abrasions requires careful nursing management. Because fluid seeps through the wounds, nursing care is similar to that for burns, with particular attention to maintaining the fluid and electrolyte balance. Rehabilitative problems of preventing contractures, reducing scar formation, and preventing emotional and social problems are important nursing considerations.

The Child With Infection or Infestation

The common dermatologic alterations discussed in this section will likely be seen primarily in children of early, middle, and late childhood age with the exception of *Candida albicans* infections, which are seen most often in neonates. In early childhood the child's epidermis and dermis are somewhat more cohesive than those of the infant. Consequently, the skin is able to retain body fluids and resist infection better than the infant's skin. The eccrine glands and sebaceous glands are thought to be not totally functional in these children because they have not fully matured.

Wounds become infected when treatment is inadequate or delayed, or when they become contaminated in spite of precautions. Signs and symptoms of infection develop in the first 24–48 hours. Local manifestations of infection are pain, redness, warmth, swelling, drainage, and sometimes enlarged adjacent lymph nodes. General malaise and fever develop later if the infection progresses. When a sutured wound becomes infected, the physician may remove every other stitch to allow for drainage.

Warm saline soaks, frequent dressing changes, and topical antibiotics might be sufficient to treat the infection. However, in case of an abscess, needle aspiration of purulent material or incision and drainage of the wound under local anesthesia might be needed. Oral antibiotics and intramuscular long-acting penicillin help to combat these infections.

An untreated wound infection can lead to invasive local infections and even to septicemia and death.

Cellulitis is an invasive infection that occurs when organisms such as *Staphylococcus aureus*, *β-hemolytic streptococci*, and *Hemophilus influenzae* destroy hyaluronic acid, thus allowing the breakdown of tissue defenses. These microorganisms produce hyaluronidase, which destroys tissue barriers against the invasion and spread of bacteria.

Bacteria can enter through an open wound or at an intravenous site. Often, however, there is just a vague history of recent trauma with no break in the skin or history of injury.

The infected part of the body is red, swollen, warm, and painful. Red streaks from the wound may be present, and adjacent lymph nodes are enlarged and painful.

Treatment includes immobilization and elevation of the infected part, warm, moist packs, fever control, and systemic antibiotics. Intravenous antibiotics such as oxacillin and dicloxacillin are given if the infection is serious. Treatment with oral antibiotics might be adequate to combat less severe cellulitis.

Bacterial and Viral Infections

Impetigo Contagiosa Impetigo is one of the most contagious skin conditions of childhood. It is the most common *pyoderma* (pus in the skin) infection in children. Predisposing factors are crowded living conditions, poor personal hygiene, and a hot, humid environment. Impetigo probably is spread by direct contact with an infected person. The lesions are discrete and coalesced. They begin as papules and progress to pustules, vesicles, and bullae surrounded by narrow areolas of erythema. Lesions tend to be seen primarily on the forearms and lower parts of the leg. Lesions also group around the mouth and nose. The vesicles and bullae rupture easily and release a thin, yellowish fluid. This serous discharge dries and forms a thick, soft, honey-colored crust. The bullous type of impetigo seems to be associated with group II staphylococci, whereas the vesicopustular form seems to be caused by β-hemolytic streptococci. It is sometimes hard to distinguish between impetigo and chickenpox.

Topical treatment might be indicated. Treatment is based on the age of the child and severity of the condition. Cleansing the lesion daily with soap and water or alcohol aids in removing the crusts. Lubricants are helpful in removing crusty scabs. Cleansing of the lesions is sometimes painful but is essential to prevent secondary infection. If the child has a severe case of impetigo, systemic antibiotics might be required since staphylococci or streptococci are the causative organisms. The application of topical antibiotics (such as Neosporin ointment or Mycitracin ointment) might be helpful if the infection is extensive. In extensive conditions the treatment depends on the causative organism. If extensive disease is caused by group A β-hemolytic streptococci, penicillin, 25–40 mg/kg/day, usually divided into several doses for 7–10 days, or erythromycin, 40–50 mg/kg/day in divided doses, is given for 10 days. If the extensive infection is caused by staphylococci, cloxacillin, 50–100 mg/kg/day in divided doses for 7–10 days, or dicloxacillin, 25–50 mg/kg/day in divided doses for 7–10 days, is given. Intravenous antibiotic therapy might be essential for children with disseminated impetigo (involving internal organs). The nurse explains to the child and parent the importance of taking the medication as prescribed. They need to know that the prescribed antibiotic reduces the risk of metastatic complications and decreases the ability of the organism to spread to intimate contacts. Signs of side effects from the drug should be noted. The nurse observes children taking penicillin for allergic reactions, which might include rashes. Children taking erythromycin should be observed for stomatitis and gastrointestinal disturbances. The nurse also notes resistance of the organism, particularly in cases where the antibiotic has been used for an extended period. Fever might be an early indicator of resistance.

If the impetigo is caused by β-hemolytic streptococci, the nurse follows the family to ensure that there are no symptoms that suggest the development of acute glomerulonephritis several weeks after the lesions have healed (see Chapters 37 and 39). Children under 6 years of age seem particularly susceptible to this complication. The problem is presumed to be caused by circulating antigen–antibody complexes that activate complement (Coleman and McBurney, 1981). The nurse avoids alarming the parents by telling them about the possibility of kidney complications; however, parents should be cautioned to be alert for signs of kidney involvement.

Handwashing after caring for a child with impetigo is important to prevent spread. The nurse also teaches the child good hygiene to prevent spread of the infection. The child with impetigo should have daily soap baths, and the child's washcloths and towels should not be interchanged with those of other individuals. The nurse encourages a balanced diet because proper nutrition aids in wound healing. Finally, the nurse helps the child to cope with the condition.

The child's involvement in self-care might be helpful in coping with the condition. Having the child apply topical ointment to lesions when indicated is one way of involving the child. Allowing the child to cleanse the lesions encourages responsibility for self-care. The nurse demonstrates how to perform aspects of care, observes as the child performs the various aspects of care, and reinforces the procedure. Teaching the child that other people might get the condition if good hygiene is not practiced might help the child to begin to learn about the modes of transmission and also encourage the child to assume responsibility for the prevention of health problems in other people.

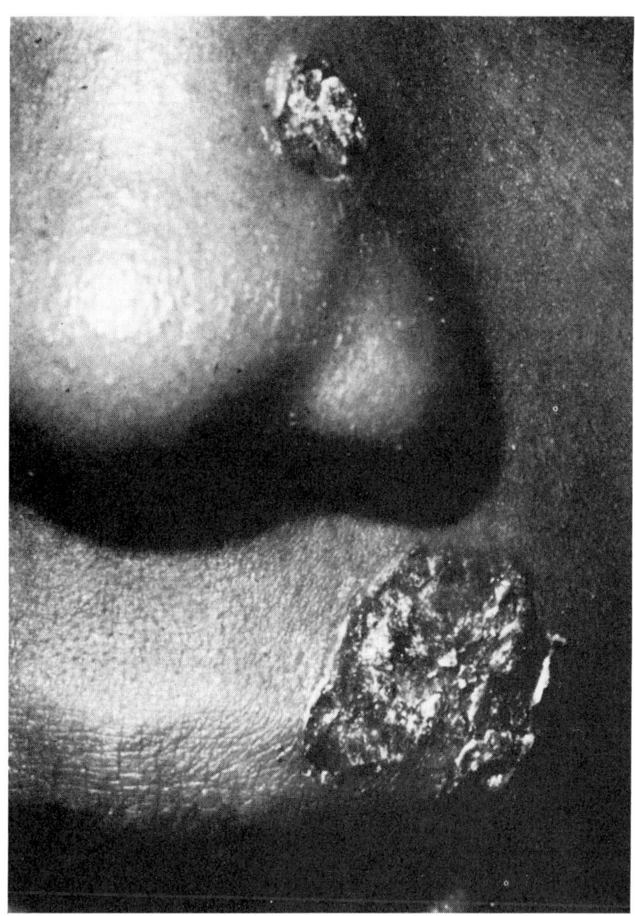

Impetigo. (From Binnick SA: *Skin Diseases: Diagnosis and Management in Clinical Practice.* Addison-Wesley, 1982.)

Viral Warts Plantar warts appear like small, shiny grains of sand imbedded under the skin of the foot. The condition is caused by viral penetration. It is believed that a break in the skin allows the virus to enter. The nurse encourages children to wear shoes or other coverings for their feet and not to go barefoot. Plantar warts may be painful. The use of adhesive foam for padding in the shoes might help to alleviate the pain.

Common warts most frequently are seen on the hands, fingers, and knees. They may be single or multiple. The biggest danger of these warts is that children pick them off.

The nurse informs children that picking warts off is not good because of the risk of viral infiltration into other tissue. Often, a wart will disappear spontaneously if left alone. If the infiltration occurs, medical treatment is necessary.

There is no known treatment for common warts. However, removing warts often is accomplished through surgery, topical administration of liquid nitrogen or a blistering agent such as cantharidin, or chemical destruction. Chemical destruction is used most often in children with multiple warts because it is painless.

Home treatment might include the use of Duofilm, a chemical that can be placed on the wart at bedtime with a toothpick or an applicator. Salicylic acid (40%) ointment is another chemical means of removing a wart at home. Formalin, 10%, increases the potency of the salicylic acid ointment. Extreme caution must be used to avoid getting these preparations on healthy skin.

Mechanical removal of dead wart tissue requires a pumice stone, the tip of a metal nail file, and curved scissors. Following a bath to soften the tissue, the pumice stone is used, after which the tip of the nail file is used to loosen the skin and dislodge the dead wart tissue. The scissors are then used to cut away the dead wart tissue.

Juvenile warts are flat, slightly raised, smooth, brown lesions that appear mainly on the face and hands. They tend to be asymptomatic.

Genital warts are classified as a venereal infection. They might coalesce into a cauliflower-like growth on the genitals. Treatment of all of the types of warts mentioned vary from nothing to curettage to keratolytics to surgical removal. The treatment of choice depends on the dermatologist.

Warts often disappear spontaneously. Occasionally, this phenomenon can be related to an emotional event in the child's life. This might account for the effectiveness of superstitious remedies for curing warts such as scaring the affected child.

Children can be very embarrassed by warts, particularly those that occur on the hands. Many children's games involve holding hands, which leaves an affected child open to teasing. The nurse can assure the child that the warts will disappear eventually. If the child is particularly upset by the warts, removal might be indicated.

Fungal Infections

Tinea Capitis, Corporis, Pedis, and Cruris Tinea infections are caused by fungi. *Tinea capitis* (ringworm of the scalp) is seen frequently in school-age children. It is characterized by patches of alopecia that begin as small papules at the base of the hair follicle. The hair loses its pigmentation, and the scalp becomes scaly and erythematous. A definite diagnosis of tinea capitis can be made using a Wood's light. Ringworm of the body and feet is not as common in children as ringworm of the scalp. In *tinea corporis* (ringworm of the body), multiple lesions are evident, which are ringed with scaly edges. The lesions spread circumferentially and are usually pruritic. In *tinea pedis* (ringworm of the feet), three forms have been noted: (1) intertriginous webspace maceration; (2) vesicular and bullous lesions, usually in the instep; and (3) noninflammatory, diffuse, scaly pedis (Vasarinsh, 1982). Scaly rashes appear on the toes or soles of the feet. Lesions found on the soles of the feet generally are asymmetric and located more anteriorly. When vesicles or bullae are evident, they usually are confined to one foot. *Tinea cruris* (ringworm of the groin) is generally a hyperpigmented eruption of papules and scales. Tight-fitting clothes and obesity are possible contributing factors. The nurse investigates the possibility of diabetes mellitus if the child is not obese or wearing tight-fitting clothes.

The nurse can scrub lesions with tincture of green soap to remove scales and crust. A topical fungicidal agent, which is ordered by the physician, is then applied, usually twice a day for about 2 weeks. Parents and children should be alerted to continue the treatment for at least 2 weeks after healing. An oral fungicide preparation may be given such as griseofulvin, 5–11 mg/kg/day for 2 weeks to 1 month, to eliminate the fungus and promote the growth of healthy tissue. An oral fungicide will likely be given if the condition responds poorly to topical therapy. The nurse informs the child and parent that the drug should be taken with meals containing milk or other fats or shortly after meals because fat enhances its absorption. In addition, the child should avoid prolonged exposure to sunlight and should be monitored for hematologic alterations.

Side effects of topical and systemic drugs are important to note. Maceration at the site is a common side effect with topical agents. Nausea, dizziness, vomiting, allergic reactions, headache, and fatigue are some of the common side effects of griseofulvin. The drug should be discontinued if these side effects occur.

Fungal infections are enhanced by moisture and heat. Therefore, it is important that the infected intertriginous areas be kept dry. A talcum powder applied twice daily helps to keep the area dry. If the lesions are inflamed, with blisters and exudates, warm water compresses might help, applied about four times a day until the lesions are dry.

The nurse informs the child that wearing other children's hats and using other children's combs might help to spread the condition. Good hygiene is the best prevention.

Candida albicans *Candida albicans* infections are caused by a yeast. Forms of intertrigo might be associated with this organism. In child health care this condition is seen most often in neonates. Diaper dermatitis is caused by *C albicans* in a significant percentage of cases (see Chapter 7). A stomatitis referred to as thrush also might be caused by *C albicans* (see Chapter 26). *Candida* infections in older children might be associated with other systemic conditions or with the administration of certain medications. Usually, the physician prescribes systemic drugs such as nystatin along with a topical preparation, depending on the severity of the condition.

Good hygiene is important when caring for a child with a candidal infection (see Chapter 39 for a discussion of vaginal candidiasis).

Parasitic Infestations

Parasitic infestations affecting the skin occur commonly in children. They include flea infestation, scabies, pediculosis, and, less commonly, bedbugs. The nursing care principles for scabies and pediculosis are discussed in Chapter 26. Flea infestations occur in households that have either dogs or cats and are prevalent during the spring, summer, and fall months. Lesions caused by fleabites commonly occur around the foot and ankle area and are subject to secondary infection from scratching.

Because flea infestations are a household rather than a personal condition, such as pediculosis, and transmission is from animals to humans, interventions are directed toward prevention. Pets should be examined regularly for the presence of fleas. The use of flea baths or collars might be helpful. Parents should caution children, particularly young children, not to touch the collar because the insecticide used is poisonous. Frequent vacuuming of carpets and furniture will help to eliminate or prevent infestation. In circumstances where the infestation is severe, the entire house might need to be exposed to a flea-killing preparation.

The Child With Inflammation

Atopic Dermatitis (Eczema)

Atopic dermatitis is a genetically determined condition often associated with allergy (see Chapter 37). It can occur any time from birth to adulthood. This skin condition is characterized by very dry skin, severe pruritus, and erythematous papular and vesicular lesions. There is edema and serous drainage from the lesions and crusting occurs. The primary lesion is difficult to define. It is most common in infancy and can start as early as 2 months of age and might last up to 2 years. This is referred to as the infantile phase. Lesions appear first on the cheeks, forehead, and scalp. The lesions may spread to other parts of the body, including the trunk and extremities. Oozing and crusted eczematous lesions predominate during the infantile phase.

Atopic dermatitis also can occur in late childhood and adolescence. The symptoms differ from those of the infantile phase in that the flexor surfaces of the extremities are involved, particularly the antecubital and popliteal regions. The condition may be mild or severe, acute or chronic.

The management of dry and itchy skin is a critical aspect of the nursing care of children with atopic dermatitis. In severe and intractable cases, hospitalization might be indicated.

The nurse encourages the child to limit the number of baths and to use lubricants that help moisten and rehydrate the skin. Hurwitz (1981) advocated the use of a mild soap such as Dove or Neutrogena for bathing and suggested that lubricants be applied over slightly moist skin. This seals in moisture and rehydrates, lubricates, and moisturizes the skin.

The type of clothing worn is important. Wool near the skin is uncomfortable. Wool garments are undesirable because they irritate the skin. Soft cotton clothing is recommended. Sweaters of acrylic yarn provide warmth without the irritating qualities of wool. Clothes or toys that have potential allergenic properties should be avoided because children with atopic dermatitis are predisposed to other allergic conditions such as asthma.

During the acute phase of atopic dermatitis, warm, wet compresses using Burows solution might have a soothing, antipruritic action on the inflamed skin because they help to rehydrate the skin. It is important to keep the child warm and wet the compresses moderately. A topical steroid ointment, cream, or lotion may be used after the compresses. Caution should be exercised when using topical steroids since systemic effects can result from absorption of steroids through open, draining skin lesions. The child's fingernails should be cut to avoid developing a secondary infection from scratching. Mitts and/or elbow restraints to prevent scratching also have been suggested.

Epstein (1983) described two widely held misconceptions about treating atopic eczema. The first misconception is that atopic eczema is an allergic diathesis that requires extensive diagnostic skin tests and therapy with dietary restrictions and desensitization injections. Neither treatment appears to be of value. Allergies to foods such as eggs, milk, and wheat might, however, complicate the management of infantile atopic eczema. The second misconception is that atopic eczema is a nervous disorder. Epstein (1983) believed that the individual with this condition needs appropriate dermatologic treatment rather than psychotherapy.

Psoriasis

Psoriasis often is confused with seborrheic dermatitis. Psoriasis has an insidious onset and initially resembles seborrhea and atopic dermatitis. The plaques, however, are erythematous, and the scales are not greasy. Psoriasis is an inherited disorder with a complex genetic mechanism. The lesions begin as small, reddish, pinpoint papules surrounded by fine scales. The papules coalesce and form plaques. Sharply demarcated scales that are grayish or silvery white characterize the lesions. The lesions are located on the scalp, ears, forehead, and around the eyebrows, trunk, genitals, elbows, and knees. A sore throat usually precedes the eruption by 2 or 3 weeks. The condition is rare in infants and preschool-age children but may be seen in children 5 years of age and older through adolescence. It is associated with decreased sweating. In individuals with erythroderma from any cause, sweating is reduced and the mechanism of temperature regulation is defective (Burton, 1979).

The treatment of psoriasis is varied and depends on the stage of the condition. Treatment for 90% of the children with this condition requires topical therapy—corticosteroids, tar, or anthralin. Treatment must be vigorous and performed daily and is long term. In severe cases steroid cream and occlusive plastic wraps also might be necessary. When the soles of the feet are involved, the application of corticosteroid cream followed by the use of plastic wrap is an effective treatment.

Topical steroids are the mainstay of treatment for ordinary plaque psoriasis. According to Zackheim (1984), vasoconstrictor assays indicate that ointment bases provide greater activity than cream bases. The use of plastic occlusion enhances the effectiveness of either form. The most common complication of topical steroids is cutaneous atrophy. Intertriginous areas and regions occluded for prolonged periods are particularly susceptible to cutaneous atrophy.

Systemic therapy will depend on the severity of the condition. Systemic treatment might include the use of antimetabolites such as methotrexate. Methotrexate helps to control or minimize psoriasis and psoriatic arthritis. Hepatotoxicity is a side effect of this drug. Exposure to psoralens and ultraviolet light (PUVA) might be effective in some cases of severe and extensive psoriasis. This treatment, however, might be carcinogenic and consequently is used cautiously. Etretinate, a new vitamin A derivative, is also effective in suppressing some severe forms of psoriasis.

The nurse helps the family to adhere to the medical regimen and encourages patience because psoriasis is a difficult condition with which to cope. Progress is often slow. Helping children or adolescents cope with this condition is a challenge. Children of late childhood age and adolescents are particularly vulnerable in terms of having their psychosocial and developmental needs met. During the late childhood period, children are involved in many peer activities. Being selected for teams and participating in structured group activities are important aspects of the child's life. During the late childhood period, children also are learning to be thoughtful and considerate of others. Name calling might occur. Children with psoriasis are not very attractive because of the skin lesions. They might be viewed as being undesirable because of their appearance. Adolescents who are working on self-identity need support in coping because improvement is generally slow.

Erythema Neonatorum Toxicum

Erythema neonatorum toxicum is a self-limiting cutaneous eruption that is characterized by erythematous macules, papules, pustules, or a combination of these lesions. It occurs all over the body, except for the palms and soles of the feet. The rash might first appear as a macular, blotchy erythema. Parents should be reassured that no therapy is necessary and encouraged simply to use good hygiene in handling the infant.

Acne Vulgaris

Acne is the most common skin condition of adolescence. It affects 80%–90% of children in this age group. Acne is particularly distressing to teenagers because it undermines their self-confidence at an age when they already are struggling with their identity and feeling most insecure. As the androgen level rises in the adolescent, the sebaceous glands, which have not been as active before the adolescent years, become more active and produce more sebum. The sebum, along with oxidized fatty acids and accumulated dirt on the skin, form comedones (blackheads). The bacteria on the skin (*Corynebacterium acnes*) thrive in the retained secretions and form pustules. Papule formation also occurs. Acne is thought to be a condition of the sebaceous gland in which changes in keratinization in the wall of the follicle lead to a sequence of pathologic changes that result in the formation of comedones and inflammation.

In addition to comedones, papules, and pustules, cysts and nodules also might occur. The lesions are located primarily on the face, back, and chest. Lesions also might be seen on the neck, back, and arms.

The role of diet in the mangement of acne is highly controversial. Acne is influenced by many factors. Life-style, which includes diet and other factors such as physical and chemical exposures, might influence acne. According to Epstein (1983), the evidence that exposure to halogens such as bromides, iodine, and chlorine can exacerbate an acnelike condition is more compelling than any evidence incriminating particular foods. Epstein noted that in the face of total calorie deprivation, sebum production is maintained at 40%–50% of normal levels. Hitch and Greenburg (1981) found that dietary iodine had no effect on acne. Chocolates also were found to have no effect (Fulton, Pelwig, and Kligman, 1969). A wholesome life-style should be encouraged that includes minimizing stress, getting adequate rest, and eating nourishing foods for a balanced diet.

The nurse encourages the adolescent to keep the skin clean. Alcohol might be useful in helping to cleanse and dry the skin, thus preventing the formation of comedones. Anti-acne soaps and lotions will aid in drying the skin. When the skin dries, the sebum is released more freely. Topical preparations such as benzoyl peroxide and retinoic acid also might be useful in treating acne. The nurse discourages the use of greasy ointments and creams and cautions the adolescent not to pick at or squeeze the lesions. Squeezing might injure underlying tissue and cause scarring. Rubbing the skin too hard also should be avoided to prevent damage.

Estrogens might be prescribed to aid in suppressing sebaceous gland activity. Oral tetracycline has been found effective in treating acne when a large number of pustules and cysts are present (Czernielewski and Skwarczynska-Banys, 1982). The side effects of tetracycline include phototoxicity and an inability to concentrate urine. Therefore, adolescents with renal problems should not be given the drug. The nurse ensures that tetracycline, when ordered for adolescents, is taken with water and on an empty stomach. Tetracycline should be used with caution in adolescent girls who might become pregnant because the drug could damage the fetus. A corticosteroid such as predinisone may be used to reduce inflammation. Ultraviolet light also may be used to treat the condition.

The psychologic aspects of the acne are important to the adolescent's developmental tasks and body image (see Chapter 11). Some authorities believe that stress exacerbates the condition. The rapidity of both physiologic and psychologic changes makes the adolescent extremely vulnerable to identity problems. A number of adolescents with cutaneous alterations are likely to experience anxiety and depression related to feelings about self and self-worth. Successful nursing management depends not only on treating the cutaneous alterations but also on helping adolescents cope with their feelings of frustration and self-consciousness and problems with self-esteem.

Nevus flammeus. (From Binnick SA: *Skin Diseases: Diagnosis and Management in Clinical Practice.* Addison-Wesley, 1982).

The Child With Congenital Birthmarks

Common congenital dermatologic conditions include pigmented nevi, which are caused by pigmentation or hyperplasia.

Vascular nevi, or hemangiomas, include port-wine stain, strawberry nevus, and salmon patch. The port-wine stain (nevus flammeus) appears as flat, red patches that increase in size as the child grows. As the child matures, the port-wine stain might assume a cobblestone appearance. Treatment is not indicated, and cosmetics are useful in covering the lesion. The strawberry nevus resembles a strawberry and generally appears on the head and neck of the infant. It will disappear by the time the child reaches school age with no treatment. Salmon patch is characterized by a macular, pink patch. It appears on the nape of the neck and eyelids of the infant and disappears by the end of the first year without treatment.

Mongolian spots, which appear mainly on the coccygeal area, are seen often in darker-skinned infants. They are dark blue and discolored and often disappear spontaneously.

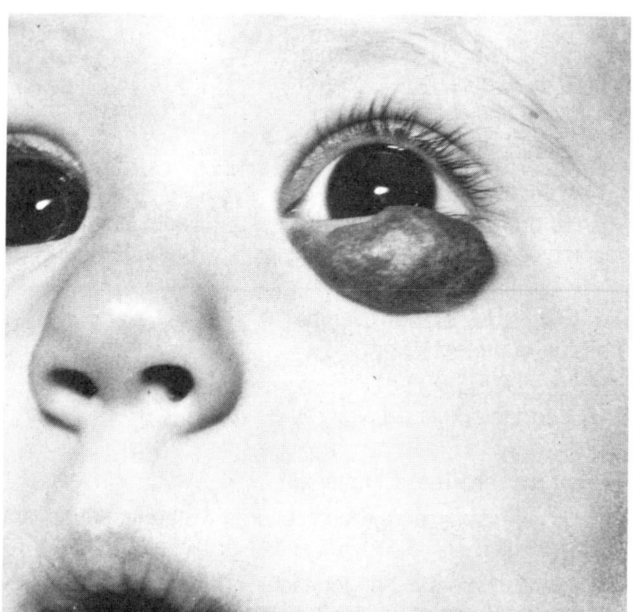

Capillary hemangioma. (From Binnick SA: *Skin Diseases: Diagonosis and Management in Clinical Practice.* Addison-Wesley, 1982.)

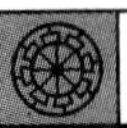

NURSING CARE PLAN Child With a Burn

Assessment Data

Paul is a 10-year-old boy who suffered partial- and full-thickness burns covering 50% of his body surface while reportedly playing with matches and gasoline in his backyard.

Nursing Diagnoses and Goals

1. **Nursing diagnosis:** Abnormal loss of body heat from impairment in skin integrity.

   Long-term goal: Paul's core body temperature will be maintained within the normal range.

   Short-term goal: The loss of heat through Paul's burn wounds will be reduced.

2. **Nursing diagnosis:** Potential infection at site of partial-thickness burns to the right and left anterior thighs.

   Long-term goal: Autocontamination and cross-contamination of burn wounds will be prevented.

   Short-term goals: (a) The burn wounds will be protected from stool and urine contamination. (b) The burn wounds will be protected from cross-contamination from other patients. (c) Infection of the burn wounds will be prevented.

3. **Nursing diagnosis:** Impairment of skin integrity: split-thickness skin graft to the anterior chest and abdomen treated by the open method.

   Long-term goal: Skin graft will adhere and heal.

   Short-term goals: (a) Infection will be prevented. (b) The skin graft will be maintained in contact with underlying tissue.

Interventions	Rationale	Evaluation criteria
1. Increase Paul's room temperature to approximately 80–90° F	Increasing the ambient temperature and humidity will prevent some heat loss from open wounds. Calories needed for healing will be expended on temperature maintenance if loss of heat is not decreased	Is Paul's body temperature maintained at a normal level or slightly elevated?
If possible, increase room humidity to 80%–90%		Are there any complaints of feeling cold from Paul?
Avoid drafts		
Undress and redress one wound at a time to avoid unnecessary exposure		
Use bed cradle when treating wounds by the open method		
Monitor Paul's body temperature every hour. Use a continuous probe if temperature is unstable		
Use warming lights as needed		
2. Use topical agent as ordered		Are signs and symptoms of infection present?
Change dressing immediately if it becomes contaminated with urine or stool	Feces contain many flora that can infect open burn wounds and deepen injury	If present, are they reported immediately to the physician?
Use fluid barrier drapes over the dressing to protect it from contamination.		Is wound clear and healing with signs of epithelialization within 2 weeks of injury?
Offer bedpan and urinal every 2–3 hours		Is pain in the thigh wound decreasing? Is thigh wound drainage decreasing?
Prevent diarrhea (see Chapter 26)		Is Paul's rectal temperature less than 101°F?
Obtain urine, stool, and wound cultures twice a week	Stagnant urine is a good medium for bacterial growth	
Wash hands before caring for each patient and frequently during individual care	The open burn wound is an excellent site for infection and eventual septicemia if not controlled	
Use protective techniques as indicated by hospital policy		

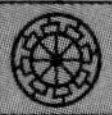

NURSING CARE PLAN Child With a Burn (continued)

Interventions	Rationale	Evaluation criteria
Use aseptic technique for wound care. Dress wounds on each body part separately using new equipment and gloves for each dressing Observe Paul at each dressing change for wound redness, swelling, and increasing pain Note any changes in color, amount, and odor of wound drainage Consult with Paul's physician and increase the number of times the dressings are changed each day if signs and symptoms of infection develop Monitor Paul's vital signs and report a rectal temperature of 101°F or more to the physician Monitor Paul's family and visitors for signs of infection and restrict contact as necessary Instruct Paul's family and visitors in handwashing and protective hand techniques	Early detection of wound infection can lead to prevention of further tissue damage and spread of organisms	
3. Observe the graft frequently for a healthy pink color. Monitor the graft site for the collection of serosanguineous fluid under the graft and at the edges Roll the graft every 30 minutes to 1 hour or as needed during the first 24 hours Once the graft is adherent, do not roll; aspirate any fluid under the graft using tuberculin syringe Restrain the extremities as needed when Paul is awake. Restrain the extremities at all times when Paul is asleep Administer pain medication as indicated Use a sterile gauze pad under the stethoscope bell each time Paul's heart and breath sounds are assessed. Use minimal pressure Maintain Paul's position flat in bed or slightly elevated. No bending at the waist for 10 days	Capillary buds from the recipient bed form a delicate network to help secure the new graft during the first days after placement. Blood flow is established by the third to fourth day The graft must not be manipulated unnecessarily or moved in any way to prevent it from tearing away from the recipient bed	Has the graft taken completely by the tenth day? Are Paul and his family able to tolerate prolonged immobility?

continued on next page

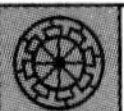

NURSING CARE PLAN Child With a Burn (continued)

Interventions	Rationale	Evaluation criteria
Teach Paul and his family the importance of immobility and other aspects of graft care		
Consult a child-life therapist and provide diversional activities		
Consult mental health nurse clinician to plan behavior management programs as needed		
Monitor Paul for problems associated with prolonged immobility (see Chapter 29)		
For emotional needs see Nursing Care Guide		

Key Concepts

- The major function of the skin, a complex essential organ, is to protect the tissues it encloses against external environmental factors.
- In addition to being a protector, the skin acts as a sensor and thermoregulator and aids in secretion, excretion, and absorption.
- The skin begins to develop around the eleventh gestational week and undergoes developmental changes throughout the individual's life span.
- The major tissue layers of the skin are the epidermis, or outer layer; the dermis, which is the site of the blood vessels, nerves, and sweat glands; and the subcutaneous tissue, which attaches the dermis to the underlying structures.
- The history, which is essential for any treatment of a skin injury, includes changes in life-style, family members' skin alterations, known allergies, exposure to substances or ill persons, length of time lesions have been present, and a thorough description of any lesions.
- The nurse assesses lesions for type and size, configuration, distribution, location, texture, and color.
- The four basic elements of skin wound care are cleansing, administering topical anti-infective agents, applying dressings, and providing for wound closure.
- The three types of skin grafts are autografts, grafts taken from the patient's own skin; allografts, grafts from an individual of the same species; and heterografts, grafts from a species other than humans.
- Acute care for children with skin alterations includes preventing pruritus, minimizing or alleviating pain, maintaining fluid balance, and preventing tetanus.
- Because nutrition is essential to the healing process, the nurse encourages the child with a skin condition to eat well-balanced meals.
- When caring for children with skin conditions, nurses foster development leading to independence in such self-care tasks as bathing and nail care.
- Burns, one of the leading causes of accidental injury in childhood, may be caused by hot liquids, hot surfaces, flames, electrical accidents, or chemical contact.
- Burns are classified according to the severity of injury and complicating factors; general categories include minor burns, moderate burns, and major or critical burns.
- In partial-thickness burns (first- and second-degree burns), the epidermis and part of the dermis are destroyed; in full-thickness burns (third-degree burns), the epidermis, dermis, and frequently even

subcutaneous tissue are destroyed, damaging hair follicles, sweat glands, sebaceous glands, and nerves.

- In burn care management, the emergent phase of care, usually 1–5 days after the injury, is the time needed to resolve immediate problems resulting from the burn injury.
- Immediate nursing and medical management in the emergency room focuses on providing a secure airway, ensuring adequate ventilation, and beginning fluid resuscitation; wound care is not the first priority.
- Because children with burns experience a sudden shift of fluid from the vascular spaces to interstitial tissue, the nurse follows a fluid resuscitation formula for replacing fluids intravenously.
- Upper airway obstruction, caused by edema from burns of the face and neck, may be relieved by nasotracheal intubation; lower airway damage, caused by the inhalation of smoke, is treated with bronchodilators and pulmonary toilet.
- After a burn, alterations can occur in renal function, metabolism, and the gastrointestinal, neuroendocrine, and hematologic systems.
- Wound care can begin once the victim's airway is established, vital signs are stable, and fluid resuscitation is established.
- When constricting eschar inferferes with circulation, the physician performs an escharotomy to relieve the pressure; the nurse subsequently monitors circulation, sensation, and motion.
- The nurse might use topical agents to protect burn wounds from the invasion and multiplication of microorganisms.
- As a part of burn wound care, the nurse learns to apply dressings securely but loose enough to avoid impeding circulation, interfering with respiration, or prohibiting mobility.
- Nursing measures during burn care are designed to prevent infection, most critically, septicemia.
- The nurse follows different cleansing and debridement procedures for specific areas of the body, including the eyes; ears; face; perineum; and exposed tendon, muscle, and bone.
- In the ongoing care of children with burns, the nurse monitors nutritional intake, develops an individualized plan of pain management for each child, and helps to prevent the formation of contractures and scars as the skin heals.
- As the burn wound heals, the nurse offers opportunities for children and parents to express their feelings of guilt, anger, fear, and frustration and assists children in learning to accept their disfigurement.
- Nursing care for the child with frostbite includes determining the extent of hypothermia, rewarming by immersion, and medicating for pain.
- Nursing care for the child with severe surface injuries includes cleansing the contaminated wound, administering tetanus prophylaxis if indicated, and maintaining the fluid and electrolyte balance.
- Nursing care for the child with a bacterial infection includes cleansing the lesion daily, applying topical antibiotics, and administering penicillin if necessary.
- Nursing care for the child with viral warts includes recommending the removal of warts by surgery or the administration of liquid nitrogen or a blistering agent or demonstrating a home treatment for removal.
- Nursing care for the child with fungal infections includes scrubbing with green soap to remove scales and crust and applying a topical fungicidal agent.
- Nursing care for the child with eczema includes recommending a mild, lubricating soap when bathing and cautioning against clothing and toys that might irritate the child's skin.
- Nursing care for the child with psoriasis includes topical therapy with corticosteroids, tar, or anthralin.
- Nursing care for the child with acne includes teaching the proper use of estrogens and recommending a life-style that minimizes stress, offers adequate rest, and provides a balanced diet.
- Congenital birthmarks disappear with time or might be covered effectively with cosmetics.

References

Antoon AY, Volpe JJ, Crawford JD: Burn Encephalopathy in children. *Pediatrics* (Oct) 1972; 50:609–616.

Artz CP, Moncrief JA, Pruitt BA: *Burns: A Team Approach.* Saunders, 1979.

Bangs C: Caught in the cold. *Emerg Med* 1982; 14:29–39.

Bernstein NR, Robson MC (editors): *Comprehensive Approaches to the Burned Person.* Medical Examination, 1983.

Boswick JA, et al: Helping the frostbitten patient. *Patient Care* 1983; 17:90–115.

Burke JF, Quinby WC, Bondoc CC: Primary excision and prompt grafting as routine therapy for the treatment of thermal burns in children. *Surg Clin North Am* 1976; 56:477–494.

Burke, JF, et al: The contribution of a bacterially isolated environment to the prevention of infection in seriously burned patients. *Ann Surg* 1977; 186:377–387.

Burton JL: *Essentials of Dermatology.* Churchill Livingstone, 1979.

Carpenito LJ: *Nursing Diagnosis: Application to Clinical Practice.* Lippincott, 1983.

Coleman WP, McBirney E: *Pediatric Dermatology.* Medical Examination, 1981.

Czernielewski A, Skwarczynska-Banys E: Oral treatment of acne vulgaris and oil acne with tetracycline. *Dermatologist* 1982; 165:62–65.

Dumond JM, et al: *The Burned Child's Return to School.* Unpublished booklet available from Shriners Burn Institute, Boston, MA.

Epstein E: *Common Skin Disorders: A Physician's Illustrated Manual With Patient Instruction Sheets.* Med Economics, 1983.

Feller I, Jones CA: *Nursing the Burned Patient.* Institute for Burn Medicine, 1973.

Fleming J: Common dermatologic conditions in children. *MCN* (Sept/Oct) 1981; 6(5):347.

Frankenburg W, Thornton S, Chors, M: *Pediatric Development Diagnosis.* Thieme-Stratton, 1982.

Fulton JE, Pelwig G, Kigman AM: The effect of chocolate on acne vulgaris. *JAMA* 1969; 210:2071–2074.

Goldsmith LA (editor): *Biochemistry and Physiology of the Skin.* Oxford University Press, 1983.

Hitch JM, Greenburg BG: Adolescent acne and dietary iodine. *Arch Dermatol* 1961; 89:898–911.

Hurwitz S: *Clinical Pediatric Dermatology.* Saunders, 1981.

Kavanagh C: Psychological intervention with the severely burned child: Report of an experimental comparison of two approaches and their effects on psychological sequelae. *Am Acad Psychiatry* 1983; 22:145–156.

Laude TA, Russo R: *Dermatologic Disorders in Black Children and Adolescents.* Medical Examination, 1983.

Miller M: Cycle trauma. *Nursing '80* (July) 1980; 10(7):26–31.

Montagu A: *Touching: The Human Significance of Skin.* Harper & Row, 1971.

Moylan JA: Diagnostic techniques and steroids. *J Trauma* 1979; 19: 917–919.

Nurses' Drug Alert: Tetanus prophylaxis. *Am J Nurs* (April) 1984; 84: 493–494.

Odland G: Structure of skin. In *Biochemistry and Physiology of the Skin.* Goldsmith LA (editor). Oxford University Press, 1983.

Pillsbury DM, Heaton CL: *A Manual of Dermatology.* Saunders, 1980.

Prugh DG: *The Psychosocial Aspects of Pediatrics.* Lea & Febiger, 1983.

Rajka G: *Atopic Dermatitis.* Saunders, 1975.

Roach L: Color changes in dark skin. *Nursing '77* (Jan) 1977; 7:48–51.

Rolnick M, Stair T, Silfen E: Frostbite—easily prevented, responsive to treatment. *Consultant* (Dec) 1980; 20:133–141.

Smith PH, Cairns RJ: *Dermatology: Current Concepts and Practice.* Butterworths, 1981.

Solomon LM, Esterly NB, Loeffel ED: *Adolescent Dermatology.* Saunders, 1978.

Vasarinsh P: *Clinical Dermatology.* Butterworths, 1982.

Zackheim H: Treatment of psoriasis: Use of corticosteroids. In *Controversies in Dermatology.* Epstein E (editor). Saunders, 1984.

Additional Readings

Bernstein N: *Emotional Care of the Facially Burned and Disfigured.* Little, Brown, 1976.

Busby HC: Nursing management of the acute burn patient and nursing management of optimal burn recovery. *J Continuing Educ Nurs* (Jul/Aug) 1979; 10:16–30.

Cahners SS: Group work with parents of burned children. *Health Soc Work* (Aug) 1978; 3:165–172.

Campbell L: Special behavioral problems of the burned child. *Am J Nurs* (Jan) 1976; 76:220–224.

Fagerhaugh SY: Pain expression and control on a burn care unit. *Nurs Outlook.* 1974; 22:645–650.

Frye S, Lander J: The initial management of the acutely burned child. *Issues Compr Pediatr Nurs* (Jul/Aug) 1976; 39–59.

Fujita MT: The impact of illness or surgery on the body image of the child. *Nurs Clin North Am* 1972; 7:641–649.

Jacoby FG: *Nursing Care of the Patient with Burns.* 2nd ed. Mosby, 1976.

Jones CA, Feller I: Burns: Avoiding and coping with complications before and after grafting. *Nursing '77* (Nov) 1977; 7:72–81.

Jones CA, Feller I: Burns: What to do during the first crucial hours. *Nursing '77* (March) 1977; 7:23–30.

Kavanagh C: A new approach to dressing change in the severely burned child and its effect on burn-related psychopathology. *Heart Lung* 1983; 12(6):612–619.

Kavanagh C, Freeman R: Should children participate in burn care. *Am J Nurs* (May) 1984; 84:601.

Parks DH, Carvajal HF, Larson DL: Management of burns. *Surg Clin North Am* 1977; 57:875–894.

Quinby S, Bernstein NR: Identity problems and the adaptation of nurses to severely burned children. *Am J Psychiatry* 1971; 128:90–95.

Sebilia A: When was your last tetanus shot. *RN* (Aug) 1984; 47:18–24.

Surveyer J: Smoke inhalation injuries. *Heart Lung* 1980; 9:825–832.

Aberrant Cellular Growth

Implications for the Child and Family

Kathleen Hardin Mooney

45

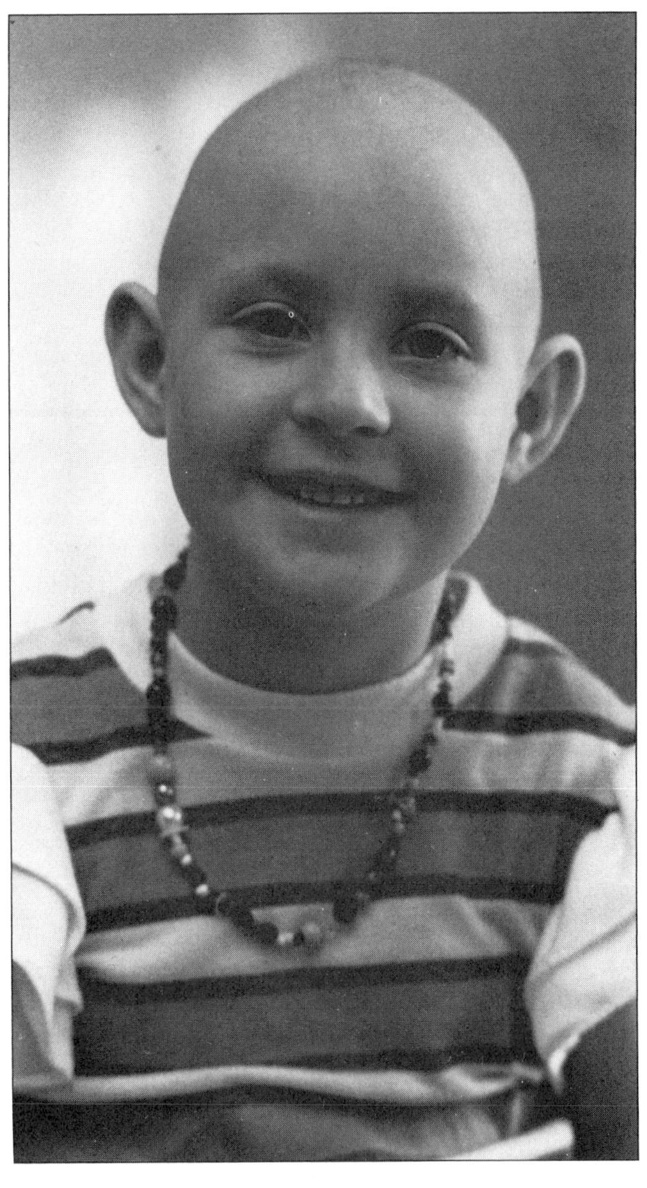

Chapter Outline

continued on next page

Objectives

- Describe tumor characteristics and the types of childhood cancer.
- Describe the assessment criteria related to a child with a neoplasm.
- List the diagnostic tests related to a diagnosis of childhood cancer.
- Describe the main features of medical management of a child with a neoplasm.
- Relate the acute-care needs of the child receiving surgery to preoperative preparation and postoperative nursing care.
- Discuss nursing management related to the side effects of chemotherapy.
- Discuss nursing management related to the side effects of radiation therapy.
- Relate nursing management to the acute-care needs stemming from bone marrow suppression.
- Describe the nursing management of cancer-related pain.
- Discuss the need for optimal nutrition and the nursing strategies to maintain nutritional status.
- Explain the developmental, emotional, and health maintenance needs of the child with a neoplasm.
- Explain the medical treatment and nursing management appropriate for the child with various specific neoplasms.

Aberrant cellular growth refers to pathologic cell proliferation resulting in the development of a neoplasm. A neoplasm may be benign, that is, non-life-threatening, or it may be malignant, that is, life threatening or cancerous. In this chapter we focus on cancer as a malignant disease.

Childhood cancer should be viewed as a chronic disease rather than an inevitably fatal illness. During the past 20 years, tremendous advances have been made in both the diagnosis and successful treatment of childhood cancers (Draper, 1980). Treatment goals are no longer palliation and preparation for death. Instead the emphasis is on total eradication of the disease or significant long-term survival. The overall task for the child and family is nursing care for the child to adapt successfully to the chronic disease and live fully in spite of it. The diagnosis of cancer brings an uncertain prognosis requiring the child and family to continually live from day to day with this unknown while maintaining the family's stability and growth (Spinetta and Deasy-Spinetta, 1981).

The nurse who cares for the child with cancer encounters one of the most challenging situations in nursing. Optimal skill and talent are required to assess and provide effective care for the unique physiologic and psychologic needs that cancer causes. The quality of the nursing care will directly affect the quality of life for the child and family. The nurse who is sensitive to each family's special needs and experiences and who demonstrates skill in physiologic care and supportive counseling will be able to assist the family to adapt successfully to the diagnosis of childhood cancer. If the nurse understands about the diagnosis, medical treatment, and nursing management of childhood cancers, the nurse can offer the family the kind of interaction that will be growth-producing for both family and nurse.

Cancer and Children

Incidence

Cancer in children is relatively rare. There is some discrepancy in reporting statistics about the incidence and mortality rates of childhood cancer. However, according to a British study, 1.36 per 1000 children will develop cancer before they reach 15 years of age (Leck, 1977). This figure is in striking contrast to the rate of cancer in adults. The American Cancer Society (1984) estimated there would be 6000 new cases of childhood cancer annually, yet in adults there would be 870,000 new cases. Children also demonstrate better survival statistics than adults. The American Cancer Society (1984) reported the cancer mortality rate for children declined from 8.3 per 100,000 in 1950 to 4.4 in 1979. Draper (1980) has projected that an excess of 50% of all children diagnosed with cancer will now be cured of the disease.

In spite of the rarity of childhood cancer, it is the leading cause of death from disease in children between 1 and 14 years of age (Vital Statistics of the United States, 1984). Death from childhood cancer is surpassed only by accidents as the major cause of death in children of this age group. Medical advances have virtually eradicated diseases such as scarlet fever and poliomyelitis, which formerly claimed the lives of many children. Even though rare, cancer has replaced the infectious diseases of childhood as a major cause of death.

Tumor Characteristics of Childhood Cancer

Histology Although cancer is often referred to as one disease, it is actually many diseases that share the same pathologic feature of uncontrolled cell growth. The type and location of the abnormal cell accounts for the many different diseases that cancer represents. Depending on the factors of location and cell type, individual cancers demonstrate different characteristics related to growth rate, spread, response to treatment, and prognosis.

The histologic types of cancer differ markedly between childhood and adult tumors. Adult cancers generally involve epithelial tissue and are called *carcinomas*. The etiology of carcinomas is largely environmental. A second type of cancer seen in adults is *sarcoma,* which histologically involves connective tissue. Children also develop sarcomas but rarely develop carcinomas. The absence of carcinomas in childhood is thought to be due to children's limited exposure to environmental carcinogens. Years of exposure to environmental carcinogens are necessary to produce tumor growth; children simply have not lived long enough for carcinomas to appear.

In contrast, a second type of childhood cancer is the embryonal tumors. These tumors probably originate during intrauterine life. The abnormal cells of embryonal tumors appear as immature fetal tissue that is unable to mature or differentiate into fully developed functional cells. Because of their relationships with fetal life, they rarely occur in adults, but usually manifest themselves clinically in early childhood.

Thus childhood and adult cancers have different histologic characteristics and frequencies. The most common adult cancers are carcinomas, which are almost nonexistent in children. Adults also experience some sarcomas and lymphoreticular cancers such as leukemia and lymphoma. Children also develop sarcomas and lymphoreticular cancers, but embryonal tumors are unique to childhood.

Classification Tumors are classified by histology and anatomic site (Table 45-1). A biopsy of the abnormal cells is required to make an accurate diagnosis. The pathologist microscopically examines the tissue to determine whether a malignancy exists and, if so, its histologic type. If a nonmalignant, benign tumor is present, it will generally be named by prefixing of the tissue involved to the term *oma,* which simply means "tumor" or "swelling." For example, a benign tumor of connective fibrous tissue is known as a fibroma. When cancer is found, however, the tumor is called according to its histologic classification and anatomic site of origin. For example, a malignant tumor of the bone that is composed of large spindle cells is known as an *osteosarcoma,* meaning a "malignant connective tissue tumor of the bone." When the tumor is embryonal in origin, the term *blast,* which refers to the immature nature of its cells, is often added to the name of the tissue involved. Thus a malignant embryonal tumor involving neural ganglion tissue is called neuroblastoma, meaning "tumor of immature neural tissue." Occasionally, instead of being named based on its histology and anatomic site, a tumor is named for the medical person who originally described it in the literature. This is the case for three tumors that will be discussed later: Hodgkin's disease, Ewing's sarcoma, and Wilms' tumor.

Properties of Malignant Tumors Malignant cells have escaped the control of orderly cell growth. The exact mechanism by which this happens is not understood. However, it is believed that the DNA contained in the chromosomes of the cell nucleus has somehow been altered, resulting in a mutation. Uncontrolled and inappropriate cell growth occurs from the distorted biologic information. Abnormal cells continue to divide and perpetuate the mutation. Besides inappropriate growth, malignant cells can no longer perform their normal function. Lack of normal function, meaning the cell is not properly differentiated, is called *anaplasia.* Rapidly reproducing, nonfunctional cells result

TABLE 45-1 Classification of Selected Neoplasms

Tissue of origin	Benign tumor	Malignant tumor
Blood cells and related cells		
Hematopoietic cells		Leukemia—all types
Lymphoid tissue		Lymphosarcoma Hodgkin's disease
Connective tissue		
Fibrous tissue	Fibroma	Fibrosarcoma
Cartilage	Chondroma	Chondrosarcoma
Bone	Osteoma	Osteosarcoma
Renal tissue	Nephroma	Nephroblastoma (Wilms' tumor)
Muscle tissue		
Striated muscle	Rhabdomyoma	Rhabdomyosarcoma
Nerve tissue		
Ganglion cells	Ganglioneuroma	Neuroblastoma
Glial cells	Glioma	Glioblastoma

when cells are anaplastic. Thus in leukemia there is not only an overproliferation of white cells but these cells also are unable to fight infection effectively.

Microscopically malignant cells vary in size from normal cells. Their nuclei are larger and irregular; multinucleated cells may be apparent. Generally there is an increase in mitotic activity. The cytoplasm is comparatively scanty and stains more deeply than normal cytoplasm.

Malignant tumors differ in their rate of growth. Generally childhood cancers grow much more rapidly than adult tumors. This rapid growth is thought to occur because childhood cancers involve cells that normally reproduce at a rapid rate, whereas adult cancers occur in tissue that is slower to reproduce and thus has had prolonged contact with carcinogens. The growth rate of a tumor depends on the doubling time (the time it takes for its cells to reproduce themselves) and rate of cell death. These factors in turn depend on the characteristics of the particular cancer and host factors. Nutritional status is particularly important. For a tumor to proliferate rapidly it must have a constant source of nutrition and blood supply. The larger the tumor grows, the more difficult it is to maintain its nutrition and blood supply. Consequently, large tumors grow more slowly than smaller tumors.

Because cancer begins as a single or small group of abnormal cells, a number of doubling times must result before the tumor becomes clinically evident. It is thought that a 1 cm mass is necessary for a tumor to be diagnosed clinically. A 1 cm mass has approximately 1×10^9 tumor cells present (Altman and Schwartz, 1983). Obviously at this point the host has millions of cancer cells, so that early detection is a relative term.

Benign and malignant tumors differ on a number of structural and biologic properties (Table 45-2). *Benign tumors* are composed of mature, functional cells that generally grow within a capsule and a slower rate than cancer cells. Because they are encapsulated, benign tumors do not invade nearby tissue but instead push normal tissue out of the way as they grow. An important difference between benign and malignant tumors is that benign tumors remain localized and do not spread to other areas of the body. In contrast, malignant cells are not encapsulated and cause harm by invading nearby tissue. When benign tumors are surgically removed, they rarely recur; malignant tumors, on the other hand, tend to recur after simple removal. Cancer has the unique property of permitting cells or small groups of cells to break away from the original tumor site and travel to other parts of the body. For these reasons benign tumors generally do not threaten life and are easily treated while malignant tumors are life threatening and difficult to treat. The exceptions to this are some brain tumors that exhibit all the properties of benign tumors but may be lethal because of the pressure they exert on vital brain tissue in the enclosed space of the skull.

Metastasis Normal cells grow in an orderly fashion when in direct contact with other cells. It is thought that cell contact provides a form of communication between cells that limits uncontrolled growth. The mechanism of this communication is probably through electrically charged atoms. This growth-limiting communication between cells is called *inhibition*. When a cell becomes cancerous, it loses contact inhibition. Operating independently of other cells, the cancer cell proliferates at its own rate, growing in irregular groupings of multiple layers. The malignant cells no longer adhere to adjacent cells and have the capacity to break away from the parent tissue and spread to other parts of the body, developing a new site of disease. This property is referred to as *metastasis*.

Cancer may spread in several ways (Fig. 45-1). There may be local extension or invasion of normal tissue directly in the path of tumor growth. Distant metastasis generally

TABLE 45-2 Contrast Between Benign and Malignant Tumors

Property	Benign	Malignant
Microscopic features	Cells usually closely resemble tissue of origin	Cells usually do not closely resemble tissue of origin; poorly differentiated
Rate of growth	Grow slowly	Grow according to individual tumor doubling time, which is dependent on tumor and host factors
Mode of growth	Grow by expansion, compressing adjacent tissue, usually encapsulated	Rarely encapsulated, grow by infiltrating adjacent tissue
Tissue destruction	Minimal tissue destruction	May produce necrosis and extensive tissue damage
Surgical resection	Generally do not recur after surgical removal	Often recur after surgical removal because of infiltration into adjacent tissue
Metastasis	Remain localized, do not spread	Frequently spread from site of origin and establish secondary site of growth in distant organs

occurs through the vascular and lymphatic systems. It may also occur by mechanical spread within a cavity—a process known as *implantation*. This serous spread is seen most commonly in the peritoneal cavity and may occur also in the pleural cavity. Implantation may take place by free malignant cells in the serous fluid transplanting to other organs by gravity. They also may be transplanted during manipulation of the tumor at the time of surgery.

Venous and lymphatic spread are by far the most common routes of distant metastasis. Lymphatic spread occurs when small groups of cancer cells separate from the primary tumor and penetrate the adjacent lymph node chain. Once in a lymphatic vessel, they become emboli and circulate to the peripheral sinus of the adjacent lymph node. As the cells multiply, they penetrate the tissue of the entire node, causing node enlargement. Lymphatic spread is a common route of metastasis in embryonal tumors. Knowing the location and proximity of that part of the lymphatic system near the original tumor site allows determination of the most likely location of lymphatic spread. Eventually tumor cells from the lymphatic system enter the venous system, which provides additional routes for dissemination to distant organ sites.

Venous spread occurs most commonly in sarcomas. Cancer cells may penetrate a vein by forming a thrombus and then developing into emboli. The pathway of tumor

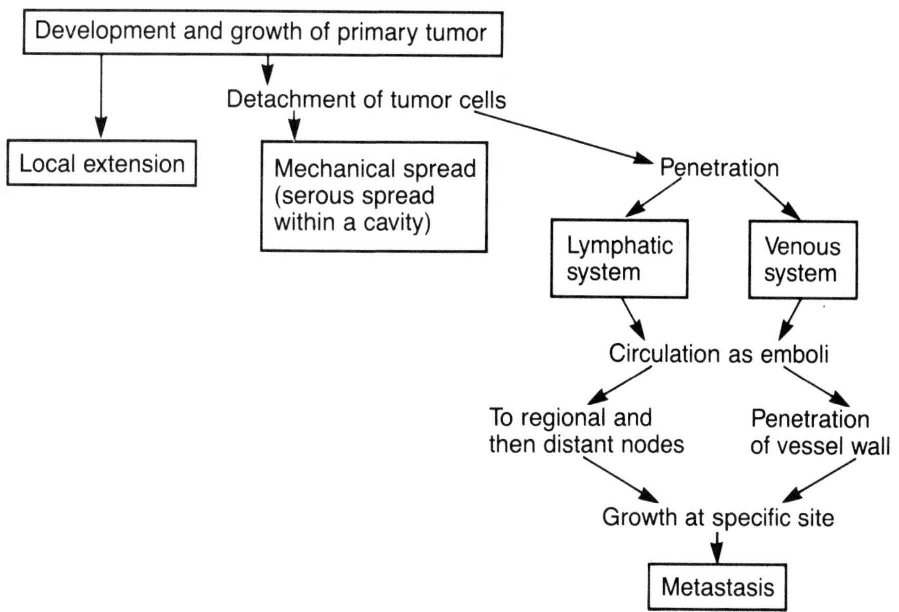

Figure 45-1 Mechanisms of tumor spread.

emboli through the bloodstream depends on the path of the specific veins that are in contact with the tumor. It is unusual for tumor emboli to invade arteries. Tumors involving organs that drain into the portal vein system most frequently metastasize to the liver. Tumors involving organs that drain into systemic veins most frequently metastasize to the lungs.

Many cancer cells may break away from the original tumor and enter the lymphatic or venous system. This does not mean, however, that metastasis has occurred. In fact, experimentally it is estimated that less than 1% of free cancer cells survive to establish an actual site of metastasis (Day et al., 1977). A pathologist generally can determine whether a tumor specimen is a primary tumor of the organ from which the specimen was taken or a metastatic site because a primary tumor will have cells that, although altered, will resemble tissue normally found in that organ. Metastatic lesions do not resemble the tissue of the site from which they were taken but look like tissue of the primary site. Thus when a bone tumor metastasizes to the lung, the biopsy of the tumor from the lung resembles the bone tissue rather than tissue normally found in the lung. When the tumor cells are so radically different from any normal tissue that the pathologist may not be able to identify the parent tissue, they are referred to as poorly differentiated or undifferentiated cells, and the tumor is therefore called "cancer of unknown primary." Metastatic lesions do not necessarily grow at the same rate as the primary tumor, nor are they always proportional in size to that of the primary cancer.

Types of Childhood Cancer

Most childhood cancers occur in every race, but the actual frequency and survival rates vary somewhat. In general cancer incidence is lower in black children, 9.33 per 100,000, than whites, 12.12 per 100,000 (Young et al, 1978). Childhood cancer occurs slightly more often in males than females.

Table 45-3 shows the distribution of cancer during childhood. Leukemia accounts for nearly one-third of all childhood cancers. Tumors of the central nervous system, primarily of the brain, account for the second largest group. The remaining childhood cancers are much less common. Neuroblastoma is an embryonal tumor of the sympathetic nervous system. Wilms' tumor is an embryonal tumor of the kidney. Its histologic name is nephroblastoma. Rhabdomyosarcoma is a tumor of soft tissue, specifically, striated muscle.

Table 45-4 shows the percentage of each tumor occurring during each of three age groupings of childhood. About 45% of all childhood cancers are diagnosed from birth through 4 years of age. This is particularly true of embryonal tumors, because of their relationship with fetal development and therefore their appearance very early in childhood. The remaining incidences of childhood cancers are almost evenly divided between the two remaining age groups. Approximately 27% of childhood malignancies occur between the ages of 5 and 10, and 28% occur between the ages of 10 and 14.

TABLE 45-3 Sites of Cancer in Children Under 15 Years of Age

	Incidence for all tumors in childhood	
Site	*White children*	*Black children*
Leukemia	30.9%	24.3%
Central nervous system	18.3%	21.6%
Lymphoma	13.8%	11.3%
Neuroblastoma	7.8%	7.2%
Rhabdomyosarcoma	6.2%	8.6%
Wilms' tumor	5.8%	9.0%
Bone tumors	4.7%	3.6%
Retinoblastoma	2.5%	4.1%
Others	10.0%	10.3%
	100.0%	100.0%

SOURCE: Based on data in Young et al., 1978.

Genetic and Familial Influence A number of genetic abnormalities are associated with childhood cancer. A tumor of the eye, retinoblastoma, is associated with the deletion of chromosome 13. As an inherited defect, 50% of an affected individual's offspring would be expected to develop the tumor. There is also a high rate of spontaneous mutation of this chromosome abnormality; many children with retinoblastoma do not demonstrate a family history of the disease.

Other congenital factors have been linked with cancer in children. Incidence of leukemia is 15 times higher in children with Down's, or trisomy 21, syndrome than in children who are otherwise healthy. Leukemia is also associated with the hereditary chromosomal abnormalities of Fanconi's anemia and Bloom's syndrome. The kidney tumor, Wilms' tumor, is associated with hemihyptertrophy (muscular overgrowth of half of the body), genitourinary defects, and aniridia (absence of the iris). About 15% of children with Wilms' tumor have a congenital abnormality. Neurofibromatosis, or von Recklinghausen's disease, has been linked to a number of malignancies including some brain tumors.

A familial predisposition may be linked with the development of some cases of childhood leukemia. Children who have a sibling with leukemia have a significantly higher incidence of leukemia. A strikingly higher incidence of leukemia exists for twins when one of the twins has been diagnosed with leukemia (Feinbach, 1984). The risk is highest for identical twins, with a ratio of 1:5, while fraternal twins

TABLE 45-4 Approximate Percentage of Each Tumor Occurring in Three Age Groups

Age	Leukemia	Central nervous system and eye	Lymphoma	Neuroblastoma	Wilms' tumor	Rhabdomyo-sarcoma	Bone tumors	Others
0–4	49%	44%	20%	84%	81%	40%	5%	31%
5–9	30%	30%	38%	11%	18%	34%	27%	32%
10–14	21%	26%	42%	5%	1%	26%	68%	37%
Total	100%	100%	100%	100%	100%	100%	100%	100%

SOURCE: Based on data in Jones and Campbell, 1976.

have a ratio of 1:80. The increased risk period for the unaffected twin generally spans the first few weeks or months after the other twin has been diagnosed with leukemia.

Immune Influence A correlation between the functional status of the immune system and the development of certain malignancies has been postulated (Mulvihill, 1982). Normally the immune system is able to recognize and destroy foreign or abnormal substances in the body by a process known as immune surveillance (see Chapter 37). The individual who develops a malignancy is thought to have a malfunction in this protective function of the immune system so that mutated cells are not recognized and destroyed. It has been suggested that this may be a factor in childhood embryonal tumors. During intrauterine life, the fetus is thought to lack an effective, mature immune surveillance system. With the normal rapid proliferation and differentiation of cells in the developing fetus, a number of cell mutations are likely to occur that result in potential malignancies. Although immature, the fetal immune system may successfully arrest some tumor development. However, in a number of cases it is not effective and an embryonal tumor appears after birth, generally during the first 5 years of life.

Other factors also tend to implicate the status of the immune system with the development of some tumors. The incidence of cancer is higher in children who have immunologic deficiencies, whether inherited or acquired. Ten percent of individuals with congenital or acquired agammaglobulinemia develop leukemia or lymphoma. Children with Wiskott–Aldrich syndrome, a cell-mediated immunologic deficiency, demonstrate a higher incidence of lymphoma. People who have been artificially immunosuppressed so as not to reject an organ transplant have a higher-than-normal incidence of cancer. It is also known that some individuals with cancer are not able to respond when immunologically challenged by antigen skin testing. Those who demonstrate this immunosuppression at the time of diagnosis generally have a less favorable prognosis. (See Chapter 37 for further discussion of the relationship between the immune system and cancer.)

Viruses An understanding of the role of viruses in causing cancer is an intense area of study. There may be an actual oncogenic virus, which does not directly cause cancer but facilitates its development. Studies with mice have linked viruses with the development of leukemia, sarcomas, and a few other tumors, but the link between viruses and human cancer has not as yet been demonstrated and rests only on circumstantial evidence.

The strongest suggestion of a viral role in human cancer is based on evidence of the activity of the Epstein-Barr (EB) virus in Burkitt's lymphoma. Burkitt's lymphoma was first identified in African children who also had antibodies against EB virus. When Burkitt's lymphoma occurs in children in the United States, however, 15%–50% of these children do not have the EB virus titers, and often when levels are present they are within the normal range of healthy individuals. Investigators are presently examining the role of viruses in the development of neuroblastoma, Wilms' tumor, and osteosarcoma. A direct link between viruses and human cancer awaits further research (Mulvihill, 1982).

If there is a viral influence in the development of some cancers, it would be natural to wonder about a communicable factor. At this time there is no cause for concern that cancer is in any way contagious. Although there is some epidemiologic evidence that cancer clusters (a larger-than-expected incidence of cancer in a small geographic area) exist in some communities, further reexamination has shown that these are only coincidental and do not represent a communicable nature. Therefore, there is no evidence that cancer can be transmitted between humans. Those who work with individuals with cancer and the public in general often need to be reassured about this.

Environmental Influence Environmental substances are strongly implicated in the causation of adult cancers. The relationship of such substances to childhood cancer is thought to be minimal. Environmental influence in childhood malignancy is probably a factor only in that environmental carcinogens may affect the fetus through maternal transmission. Diagnostic radiation during pregnancy appears to contribute to leukemia and a few other childhood cancers. Some drugs taken during pregnancy also have been implicated in later development of cancer in the offspring. The most well-documented relationship exists between the use of diethylstilbestrol (DES) to prevent miscarriages and the development of adenocarcinoma of the vagina in female offspring 20 years later (Strong, 1984).

Prognosis

The outlook for survival for the child with cancer is much more positive today than 10–20 years ago. Childhood cancer is more responsive to treatment than most adult tumors, and long-term survival is greater for children than adults. It is estimated that a minimum of 50% of children will be cured of their disease (Draper, 1980). Progress in increasing these survival rates continues. In adults the figure is about 40% (American Cancer Society, 1984). The child is not only more responsive to treatment but also better able to tolerate the therapies.

Determining that a cancer is cured is difficult. Once treatment has been completed, a period of risk remains. In adults the risk period is generally established as 5 years of disease-free survival after therapy has been stopped. A few adult tumors, such as breast cancer, are known to recur or develop secondary sites after this 5-year period and are therefore not considered cured until 10–15 years of disease-free survival. For the child, cure may be calculated by a different method. Childhood malignancy could have been present no longer than the age of the child at diagnosis plus 9 months of uterine life. It could be postulated therefore that cancer cells would multiply to the size where they could be clinically detected in the same amount of time (Jones and Campbell, 1976). Thus a child diagnosed with cancer at the age of 4 years would be considered cured at 4 years and 9 months of disease-free survival after treatment was completed. This theory probably applies best to those childhood cancers of embryonal origin and is based on the assumption that the cancer cells will continue to grow at a constant rate throughout the development, treatment, and posttreatment periods.

With the favorable treatment of many childhood cancers the focus of therapy is on quality of life. Methods for determining the long-term effects of treatment on quality of survival are being investigated. Less toxic treatment regimens are being attempted and their effect on the course of illness assessed. In the past these studies were never attempted because survival statistics were so poor that studies to reduce toxicity seemed inappropriate.

Many people, both in the general public and in the health professions, still assume that childhood cancer is a fatal disease. Education about the advances in treatment therefore is necessary to change this inaccurate perception. The informed nurse should take an active role in reeducating the public and other health professionals about the outlook for childhood malignancy.

The nurse who cares for a child with cancer should provide appropriate care and support consistent with the child's disease status. Preparation for death is only appropriate when it is clear that the child will survive only a limited period of time. Any child should be treated first as a child and second as a child with cancer. The child will continue to grow and strive for developmentally age-appropriate tasks throughout the course of the illness. Many children who face a shortened life expectancy conduct a full and active life in spite of treatment for cancer during childhood, and nursing interventions must therefore be tailored to meet each child's unique needs.

Assessment of a Child With a Neoplasm

Cancer in children is often misdiagnosed. Signs and symptoms of malignancy are, for the most part, identical to many acute, easily treatable childhood illnesses. For this reason and because cancer is so rare in children, the true diagnosis may be missed while other, less serious interpretations are applied to the presenting signs and symptoms.

The delay that results is unfortunate. The earlier a tumor can be identified and appropriate treatment begun, the greater the chance of long-term remission or cure. Childhood cancers generally are rapidly growing malignancies. By the time the abnormal cells have multiplied to cause significant signs and symptoms, several additional weeks of delay have occurred, and many tumors have already metastasized. The earlier the clinician's index of suspicion can be raised and appropriate assessment completed, the greater likelihood of successful treatment.

The signs and symptoms of childhood cancer vary with the type and particularly the location of the presenting malignancy. The nurse who cares for children with cancer must be knowledgeable about pathologic change and the implications of signs and symptoms that encompass the entire body. Skill in total physiologic assessment and a complete understanding of a wide range of diagnostic tools are required when dealing with childhood cancer.

History

Childhood cancer may be identified when the parent brings the child to the physician for examination for a specific complaint, or it may be discovered during a routine physical exam without specific symptoms. The latter has most notably occurred with leukemia or Wilms' tumor. Rarely does the parent or child initially suspect the illness might be cancer.

Once cancer is considered, a systematic history centers around eliciting data regarding the appropriate etiologic factors. A prenatal history of maternal exposure to radiation or specific drugs that have been linked to childhood cancer is carefully noted. A family history is taken to identify hereditary syndromes known to predispose a child to cancer. The child who has a sibling with malignant disease is at higher risk and should raise the clinician's suspicion.

The child who from the history has been determined to have a hereditary or acquired condition linked with sub-

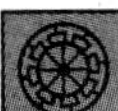

ASSESSMENT GUIDE Child With Cancer

System	Subjective data	Objective data	Validating data	Nursing management
Head, eyes, ears, nose, mouth	Headache; cerebellar signs—ataxia, head tilt, loss of balance; personality changes; learning disabilities; irritability	Signs of increased intracranial pressure; widening cranial sutures; bulging fontanelles; vomiting, often without nausea; nuchal rigidity	Tumor biopsy; CT scan	Elicit information about child's development. Prepare child for diagnostic evaluation (see Chapter 29). Monitor signs associated with tumor site: occular—pupil size, reaction, and equality; headache—pattern, character, severity; monitor other signs of central nervous system involvement (see Chapter 42); institute safety precautions if gait or equilibrium are affected or seizures anticipated
	Visual disturbances	Strabismus, nystagmus, diplopia; whitish glow about the pupil (cat's eye reflex); downward displacement of eyeball (proptosis)	Bilateral indirect ophthalmoscopy (under general anesthesia); bone marrow aspiration and biopsy; lumbar puncture; CT scan; bone scan	Institute safety precautions if vision is limited. Prevent sensory deprivation (see Chapter 43)
	Hypernasal speech; rhinorrhea	Polypoid mass in nasopharyngeal cavity	Complete blood count and blood chemistries; biopsies for primary tumors; radiographic assessment of the primary site, chest radiograph, bone liver and brain scan	Monitor the child for changes in respiratory status if tumor affects head or neck. Provide respiratory support if needed
	Dysphagia; painful mastication	Serous otitis media		
Integumentary	Lethargy; weight loss; fever; pruritis; repeated infections	Pallor; signs of bleeding or bruising; anemia; decreased red blood cells and platelets; increased white blood cells with abnormal differential blood count	Complete blood count with differential; bone marrow aspiration; lumbar puncture; blood chemistries; ESR; CT scan	Monitor degree of anemia (see Chapter 36). Institute infection precautions. Institute bleeding precautions (see Chapter 36). Provide frequent pain medica-

continued on next page

ASSESSMENT GUIDE Child With Cancer (continued)

System	Subjective data	Objective data	Validating data	Nursing management
				tion for bone involvement in acute leukemia. Monitor for respiratory and abdominal symptoms associated with acute leukemia and lymphoma
Cardiovascular	Fatigue; night sweats	Lymphadenopathy—nodes greater than 2.5 cm in size, firm, nontender; alterations in pulse and blood pressure indicating increased intracranial pressure	Lymph node biopsy; lymphangiogram (difficult with children); chest radiograph for mediastinal shift	Observe for signs of intracranial pressure indicating central nervous system involvement
Gastrointestinal	Vomiting; diarrhea; abdominal pain; weight loss	Signs of intestinal obstruction (see Chapter 38); mediastinal or abdominal mass—may be on one side of the midline, movable, smooth (Wilms' tumor), or irregular, nodular, crossing the midline (neuroblastoma); splenomegaly; hepatomegaly; increasing abdominal girth	Blood values; renal and liver function studies; urinalysis; tumor biopsy; 24-hour urine collection for VMA; CEA level; abdominal ultrasound; chest tomography and radiography; skeletal survey; stool for occult blood	Avoid unnecessary abdominal palpation. Monitor temperture elevations. Measure abdominal girth and monitor weight daily. Provide symptomatic management of fever. Provide symptomatic support for nausea, vomiting, and diarrhea. Teach child and family about 24-hour urine collection
Respiratory	Cough; dyspnea	Alterations in respiratory status (see Chapter 34)	Arterial blood gases	Facilitate respiratory efforts
Genitourinary	Straining to void; unusual vaginal bleeding	Hematuria; urinary retention; signs of urinary obstruction (see Chapter 39); polypoid mass from vagina	Urinalysis; urine test for occult blood; IVP; intravenous urography	Test urine for occult blood if Wilms' tumor is suspected; monitor for signs of urinary retention if rhabdomyosarcoma is suspected
Musculoskeletal	Dull pain in bones or joints; limp	Bone mass; edema of joints	White blood cell count; erythrocyte sedimentation rate	Tumor may be masked as athletic injury. Encourage medical evaluation if symptoms persist

sequent malignancy requires a detailed evaluation. These conditions include neurofibromatosis and hereditary or acquired immunodeficiency syndromes such as Wiskott–Aldrich syndrome, agammaglobulinemia, or all types of aplastic anemia. Hereditary chromosomal abnormalities and congenital abnormalities that have been linked with Wilms' tumor should raise concern that a malignancy may be present. When any of these conditions are revealed in the history and the child has presenting symptoms compatible with a malignancy, thorough investigation to establish the diagnosis is warranted.

Presenting Concern

The presenting concern that brings the child in for evaluation varies depending on the location of the malignancy. The child with leukemia or lymphoma generally has fever, lethargy, and pallor, all of which are often initially regarded and treated as the result of a benign childhood infection. Children having bone pain due to leukemia infiltrates might be evaluated for rheumatoid arthritis before leukemia is suspected. If the central nervous system is involved, headache, nausea, and vomiting might also be present. Presenting symptoms of lymphoma include a painless enlarged lymph node, dyspnea, and cough. For those lymphomas that involve the gastrointestinal tract abdominal pain, vomiting and diarrhea are often present.

Tumors of the abdominal cavity, particularly Wilms' tumor and neuroblastoma, generally cause abdominal pain or an abdominal mass. Depending on the rate of tumor growth, there may or may not be pain. The child with Wilms' tumor often appears healthy and asymptomatic except for the abdominal mass. In contrast, the child with neuroblastoma often has diffuse consitutional symptoms, pallor, and lethargy and appears sickly. Rhabdomyosarcoma, a tumor involving soft tissue, varies in presenting symptoms depending on the disease location. Generally symptoms are the result of the compression of adjacent structures or of an actual mass. Bone tumors cause pain at the affected site. The pain is most often described as dull rather than intense. The child may limp or curtail physical activity. These presenting symptoms are often initially treated as muscle pain due to growth or related to recent trauma.

Presenting symptoms of brain tumors also vary with the location and size of the tumor. Symptoms may relate to increased intracranial pressure such as vomiting without preceding nausea. Generalized symptoms include headache, visual disturbance, ataxia, personality change, seizures, and, in infants, enlarging head size with widening of the sutures. Such symptoms as visual change often are not reported by children, and other symptoms may be overlooked by parents. Retinoblastoma, a tumor involving the eye, causes few observable symptoms. A parent may notice a whitish glow about the pupil or may note strabismus. The lack of obvious symptoms increases the likelihood of delay before the diagnosis is made.

The parent and child are carefully questioned about the presenting concern. The onset and duration of the symptoms are noted. A detailed description of the nature of the problem is most helpful. Are there patterns to the symptoms? Does anything aggravate or alleviate the symptoms? The nurse determines whether any treatments, either home remedies or physician-prescribed, have been tried, and the nurse asks about the child's response to those treatments. A thorough description of the problem by the family can provide areas of focus for the physical examination.

Physical Examination

When the history or the presenting concern gives any indication of childhood malignancy, a thorough physical examination is indicated. The evaluation includes both a general health assessment and a detailed examination of the area of concern. (See Chapter 14 for a description of the physical assessment process.) When a brain tumor or central nervous system involvement is suspected, a developmental assessment of the child may also prove useful (see Chapter 16).

Since leukemia involves blood-forming tissue, signs of bone marrow suppression are examined. This includes documenting fever, infection (particularly if it recurs after antibiotic treatment), pallor, spontaneous or prolonged bleeding, petechiae, and bruising. Lymphoma also may be associated with infection.

Lymphadenopathy and splenomegaly can accompany malignant disease. Other less serious conditions than cancer, such as an infection, also involve enlarged spleen and lymph nodes, and so cautious investigation is necessary. Systematic evaluation of lymph nodes should include assessment of all nodes accessible to palpation. Size, location, and character of any enlarged lymph node should be noted. Suspicious nodes are often larger than 2.5 cm. They are firm and nontender, unlike those enlarged because of inflammatory disease, which are movable, tender, and hot. Enlarged nodes located in the supraclavicular or axillary chains are more likely to be involved in malignant disease than tonsillar or inguinal nodes. Benign, palpable lymph nodes are much more common in children than in adults, making assessment by palpation alone inconclusive and further diagnostic evaluation necessary.

Splenomegaly should also be carefully documented. Again, an enlarged spleen may be present in conditions other than cancer. In the child or infant under 4 years of age a palpable spleen may be a normal finding. When the spleen is palpable in the child over 4 years of age, it is usually 2 or 3 times its normal size. Once splenomegaly is documented by palpation, further diagnostic study is warranted.

Abdominal masses are carefully evaluated. A malignant tumor usually feels hard. If it is intraperitoneal, it may move with external pressure or change when the position of the child is altered; if it is retroperitoneal, the mass is nonmovable and requires deep palpation. Abdominal tumors often can be differentiated by palpation. Wilms' tumor tends to be located on one side of the midline and is movable and smooth. Neuroblastoma tends to be attached to adjacent tissue, is irregular in shape and nodular, and often crosses the midline. Palpation of abdominal masses should be gently undertaken and kept to a minimum because abdominal pressure caused by palpation may allow seeding of the tumor resulting in intraperitoneal spread.

Central nervous system signs are evaluated during the neurologic examination and the developmental assessment. Head circumference should be charted and suture closure evaluated. Visual field examination; ophthalmic examination with particular attention for any papilledema; mental status examination evaluating altered sensorium; and examination of cerebellar signs of ataxia, head tilting, and loss of balance are included in the neurologic examination. The child is also evaluated for nystagmus, diplopia, and strabismus.

Validating Diagnostic Tests

To gather further information, a number of diagnostic studies are carried out to delineate the significance of the problem. Together with the results of the history and physical examination, the diagnostic studies provide the basis for determining whether or not to perform a biopsy to establish the diagnosis. Diagnostic studies also provide information about the extent of disease present. Such information is important in determining the type of biopsy and surgical procedure required should a malignancy be confirmed. For example, if during the diagnostic work-up for a bone tumor, lung metastases are suspected based on a radiographic study, a biopsy would be performed on the bone site. Should it prove to be an osteosarcoma, the usual surgical procedure of amputation is often abandoned. The purpose of the amputation is to prevent metastasis from occurring; since metastasis is already present, there is no reason to subject the child to amputation. Diagnostic studies also provide information about the general health status of the child. Because treatment can affect many organ systems, a baseline measure of all organ systems is needed prior to beginning treatment.

Laboratory Tests Suspected malignancies of the hemopoietic system (leukemias and lymphomas) require evaluation by performing a complete and differential blood count. An erythrocyte sedimentation rate (ESR) is useful in evaluating certain lymphomas. These lymphomas produce high sedimentation rates because of the presence of increased amounts of fibrinogen or abnormal globulins.

Blood chemistries provide important baseline information. Of particular importance are chemistries that evaluate renal and liver function. These include measurement of uric acid, blood urea nitrogen (BUN), creatinine, bilirubin, serum glutamic-oxaloacetic transaminase (SGOT), serum glutamic pyruvic transaminase (SGPT), lactate dehydrogenase (LDH), total protein, albumin, and alkaline phosphatase. Tumors with extensive bone involvement are often reflected by increased levels of serum calcium, serum phosphorus, and alkaline phosphatase. There has been increasing interest in identifying tumor-produced substances in the blood that could serve as blood test diagnostic indicators. No universal tumor marker has been identified as of yet, but a few tumors have been found to produce a specific antigen measurable in the blood. This antigen is called carcinoembryonic antigen (CEA), which is present in some cases of neuroblastoma. Although it is not accurate as a diagnostic indicator, it is useful in following children who showed an initial CEA level as they progress through treatment.

A few specialized diagnostic tests using urine collection are helpful in the diagnosis of neuroblastoma. Because this is a tumor of the sympathetic ganglion, increased levels of catecholamines are produced. These catecholamines (epinephrine and norepinephrine) are metabolized to vanillylmandelic acid (VMA) and homovanillic acid (HVA) plus some other by-products excreted in the urine. Most children with neuroblastoma will have abnormally high VMA and HVA levels; thus it is a very useful test during the diagnostic period prior to surgical intervention. A 24-hour urine collection is required to determine accurate levels.

Radiographic Studies Radiologic evaluation assists in determining the exact location and characteristics of a suspected tumor. Simple radiographs of the suspected tumor site usually contribute helpful information. Additionally, a number of more sophisticated techniques are employed during the diagnostic period. Advances in radiologic equipment and techniques have improved accurate noninvasive diagnostic and ongoing evaluation of pediatric malignancies.

Intravenous pyelogram (IVP) is extremely useful in evaluating pediatric abdominal masses because most of these tumors involve the kidney or adjacent tissue. The two most common abdominal tumors of childhood are Wilms' tumor and neuroblastomas. They are often difficult to differentiate by history and physical examination, and use of the IVP can assist in identifying which tumor is most likely present. Two modifications of the IVP, nephrotomography and inferior cavography, may be used to provide further information about the tumor. Nephrotomography combines the IVP with body section tomography. The functional kidney appears well defined while the nonfunctional tumor appears less dense. The inferior cavography allows the kidney and inferior vena cava to appear opaque. This procedure provides additional information about the location and size of the tumor and about whether the vena cava is involved.

Angiography has general application to many childhood tumors. This technique of radiographic visualization of blood vessels after introduction of a contrast material is useful in delineating the blood supply to the tumor and displacement of normal vessels due to tumor growth. Since surgical resection is often attempted, knowledge of blood supply prior to surgery assists in planning the best surgical approach. The pattern and extent of normal blood vessel displacement provides information useful in differentiating benign and malignant disease.

Nuclear medicine techniques have become important methods for diagnosing metastasis and for periodic reevaluations during and after treatment of the primary tumor or metastatic sites. Scanning techniques using radionuclides are available for skeletal survey, brain scan (although this has been largely replaced in favor of computed tomography, or CT), and liver and spleen scan. There are two types of radionuclides used for scanning: (a) indirect agents, which localize in normal tissue and depend on displacement of normal tissue or functions to signal tumor presence, and (b) direct agents, which concentrate in the actual tumor itself. The skeletal survey and brain, liver, and spleen scans are all examples of techniques using indirect agents. The most common direct agent is an isotope of gallium, ^{67}Ga. Lymphomas, especially Hodgkin's disease, Ewing's sarcoma, brain tumors, Wilms' tumor, and neuroblastoma, show increased ^{67}Ga uptake. Although the direct agent scanning technique has implications for diagnosis of childhood malignancy, both false positives and false negatives have been reported.

The CT scan is the newest important diagnostic technique. It is a noninvasive method for determining the geography and characteristics, such as whether a mass is cystic, solid, or lipid, of a suspected tumor. Contrast material may be administered to provide better definition. The CT scan originally was used in evaluating the brain. It has drastically reduced the need for ventriculography and pneumoencephalography in evaluating suspected brain tumors. The CT scan now has the capability of evaluating other body structures and therefore will have a wide range of diagnostic uses. This technique offers a systematic way to visualize and record narrow planes, or "slices," of the structure under study. Thus it is very accurate at locating even small, deep-seated lesions.

Lymphangiography is particularly useful in Hodgkin's disease. Radiopaque material is injected into two lymphatics that have been dissected and cannulated from the top of the feet. The contrast material has an affinity for the lymphatic system and follow-up roentgenograms reveal enlarged nodes suspected of disease involvement. The lymphangiogram is more difficult to perform on the child than adult because the lymphatic vessels of the child are extremely small, making successful location and cannulation difficult.

Ultrasonography Ultrasonography is a technique that allows the visualization of suspected tumor masses by recording the reflection of ultrasonic waves directed into the tissues. It is particularly useful in evaluating masses involving the pelvis, retroperitoneum, and abdominal cavity. The procedure is entirely safe, employing no radiation, and has the added advantage of being painless and noninvasive. Ultrasound can be used when an IVP has not differentiated a Wilms' tumor from multicystic kidneys or hydronephrosis. Characteristic echo patterns can assist in the identification of malignant abdominal lymph nodes and sites of liver metastases. Ultrasound can precisely establish the size, shape, and location of the kidneys, liver, spleen, and major blood vessels. The relationship of normal structures to tumor site can be identified.

Lumbar Puncture Because there can be central nervous system involvement in both childhood leukemia and lymphoma, initial and continued evaluation of cerebrospinal fluid (CSF) is closely followed. A lumbar puncture is performed to obtain the spinal fluid for cytologic examination. When treatment is in progress, the lumbar puncture also serves to instill cytoxic drugs (intrathecal instillation). (See Chapter 42 for discussion of lumbar puncture.)

Biopsy The diagnosis of a malignancy can be confirmed only by a biopsy. This generally surgical procedure allows the removal of all or a portion of the abnormal tissue for pathologic examination and the determination of a precise histologic diagnosis.

Biopsy Procedures

Aspiration The tissue for pathologic examination is obtained by using a needle and syringe and applying suction to collect the specimen

Excisional The entire lesion including a margin of normal tissue is removed for pathologic examination

Exploratory The survey and biopsy of a suspected lesion to determine the exact location and extent of disease

Incisional The biopsy of only a selected portion of the lesion and perhaps some adjacent normal tissue

Needle A biopsy obtained through insertion of a needle into the lesion and withdrawal of a specimen through its adherence to the lumen of the needle

Most biopsies are performed under general anesthetic. The pathologic confirmation of the diagnosis may be determined while the child is still under the anesthesia so that the appropriate surgical intervention may be performed along with the biopsy. Sometimes it is desirable to perform the biopsy only, without planning for subsequent surgery. This provides the pathologist with more time to evaluate the tissue samples before determining the diagnosis. The appropriate surgical procedure can then be selected by the surgical team. Thus the biopsy and surgical intervention are separate procedures.

Needle biopsies and biopsies done under local anesthetic are not commonly used in childhood cancer. Biopsy by aspiration of the bone marrow, however, is used to establish the diagnosis or follow the course of leukemia, lymphoma, and those solid tumors known to metatasize to the bone. This examination of developing blood cells is performed under local anesthetic and is the definitive means to establish histologically the diagnosis of a hematologic malignancy or bone marrow involvement as a metastatic site.

A variety of bone sites are used to obtain the bone marrow sample. In adults the sternum is often used because functioning marrow is usually present. There are, however, risks of penetrating major vessels if the needle slipped off the sternum. In growing children, functioning marrow is present in many other sites. The iliac crest of the pelvis is the most common site for aspiration in the child. The bones of the leg may be used in infants.

Medical Management of the Child With a Neoplasm

The advances made in the treatment of childhood cancer are related to the optimal combination of available treatment modes. Surgery was the sole treatment for cancer in the late 1800s. During the early 1900s radiation was developed as a primary treatment method, and the individual with cancer was treated and followed by the radiation oncologist. Use of chemotherapy was unheard of or considered highly experimental. Chemotherapy as a treatment for cancer emerged in the 1950s and 1960s. Initially, one

Bone Marrow Aspiration Procedure

- Child and parent are prepared for the procedure
- Child is positioned on the stomach. A folded blanket or pillow under the hips may help elevate the hips and expose posterior iliac crest
- Using sterile technique, a circular area approximately 6 in in diameter over the posterior iliac crest is prepped with a povidone-iodine solution. This will feel cold to the child
- Local anesthetic is injected subcutaneously and deep intramuscularly by needle and syringe or pressurized air gun. The child feels a burning, stinging sensation
- The aspiration needle is inserted with a slight twisting motion until it is through the cortex of the bone and into the semisolid marrow. The child feels pressure and perhaps a pop as it enters marrow
- The stylet is removed and a syringe is attached. Suction is applied to withdraw 1 cc of marrow. The child feels sharp pain as the marrow is withdrawn
- The syringe is detached, and the marrow is transferred to a glass slide, where white bone marrow spicules are seen, indicating an adequate specimen. If spicules are not seen, the procedure must be repeated
- The needle is withdrawn, and a pressure dressing is placed on the site. The child is comforted and is encouraged to return to a normal activity level

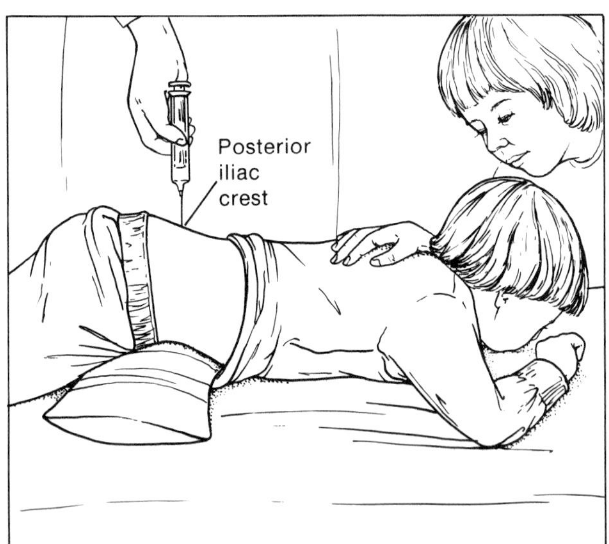

Figure 45-2 Positioning for bone marrow aspiration. A folded blanket, sandbag, or pillow under the hips provides elevation for the hips and exposes the posterior iliac crest.

drug at a time was administered. Gradually, the medical oncologist who managed the chemotherapy became the individual's primary physician with referral when appropriate to the surgeon or radiation oncologist.

The modern era of multimodality therapy, combining surgery, radiation, and chemotherapy, emerged during the 1970s. Procedures and doses are optimally timed and planned to augment each other. No longer is chemotherapy given as a single drug; multiple combinations are administered for the greatest tumor kill. Although a particular drug or procedure may be considered experimental, the concept of treating cancer with surgery, radiation, and chemotherapy is considered conventional therapy. The purpose of these therapies is to either kill malignant cells, as in the case of radiation or chemotherapy, or to remove malignant cells, as in the case of surgery. Surgery and radiation offer treatment for localized disease. This simply means if tumor cells are present in the leg and lung, radiation or surgery to the leg will not alter the growth of the lung disease. Chemotherapy, however, is systemic treatment, having a potential effect on both lung and leg tumors.

There are three approaches to the treatment plan. They are therapy for (a) curative, (b) adjuvant, or (c) palliative purposes. Curative therapy attempts to completely eradicate the disease and is usually the goal for all newly diagnosed childhood cancers. Adjuvant therapy also attempts to eradicate the disease by recognizing that although the child may appear free of disease after an initial surgical procedure, it is highly likely that subclinical micrometastases still exist, requiring additional systemic therapy. This secondary therapy directed at micrometastasis is called adjuvant therapy. The third approach is palliative therapy. This means that the treatments are not able to cure the child but instead provide the child with a long-term quality survival with a significant degree of symptom control.

Two treatment modes are still considered experimental. They are immunotherapy and bone marrow transplantation. The purpose of immunotherapy is to boost the child's own body defenses through stimulation of the immune system. Theoretically, the body's natural defense system then would have a greater capability of recognizing abnormal cancer cells and destroying them. Early laboratory study encouraged cancer specialists to pursue immunotherapy as an important technique in cancer treatment. Most clinical studies that used immunotherapy, however, did not result in significant favorable outcomes. Because of the complexity of the immune system, initial application of immunology to cancer was based on insufficient knowledge. Very few clinical studies of immunotherapy are currently in progress. Additional laboratory study is required before further human trials are conducted.

Although immunotherapy has not played a major role in clinical cancer treatment to date, further study and new laboratory findings may produce significant results in the future. The theoretical role of cancer immunotherapy as a treatment mode is well-documented in the laboratory. Further study is needed to understand and develop practical application of immunotherapy in the clinical treatment of childhood cancer.

Bone marrow transplantation is an investigational technique that allows curative but lethal doses of chemotherapy and total body radiation to be given to persons with cancer. Without transplantation the individual would die of profound bone marrow failure as a result of the treatment, so the individual's bone marrow is reseeded with bone marrow from a donor. The actual transplantation is therefore a rescue procedure after the curative chemotherapy and radiation treatment have been administered. Initial treatment of childhood cancers with bone marrow transplantation has been directed at those diseases involving the bone marrow and lymphatic system, namely leukemia and lymphoma. It has also been used in the nonmalignant hematologic disorder of aplastic anemia.In this disorder, chemotherapy and radiation to destroy abnormal cells is not necessary. This is because aplastic anemia involves life-threatening bone marrow failure without the production of abnormal cells (see Chapter 36).

Bone marrow transplantation may eventually prove useful with other cancers that do not involve the hematologic or lymphatic system. Theoretically, a portion of the individual's own bone marrow could be collected and stored. If potentially lethal doses of chemotherapy and radiation were required to cure the individual of the disease, they could be administered with the subsequent reinfusion of the previously collected bone marrow. (See Chapter 36 for a discussion of bone marrow transplantation.)

In addition to rejection of the transplanted bone marrow a serious hazard of bone marrow transplantation is graft-versus-host disease (GVHD). Because the donor's bone marrow contains immunocompetent lymphocytes that have the capacity to attack and reject foreign tissue, the donor's bone marrow can actually reject the child's body. The donated lymphocytes have the capacity to destroy cells of the skin, liver, and gastrointestinal tract. Severe involvement can cause skin sloughing, serious liver dysfunction, and copious diarrhea and sloughing of the intestinal mucosa. New immunosuppressive drugs are being successfully used to combat this heretofore debilitating and life-threatening complication.

Bone marrow transplantation is considered highly investigational. Progress has been made in recent years to decrease the many life-threatening complications that occur with this procedure. Yet the technology and intensive care that is required makes the procedure available at only selected cancer specialty centers. Currently, bone marrow transplantation is considered only for those children who have a dismal prognosis because conventional treatment does not offer them long-term survival or who have received conventional therapy and it has failed. For these children with refractory disease, bone marrow transplantation offers them hope where no other hope exists.

Communicating the Diagnosis

When the diagnostic tests, investigation of potential metastatic sites, and biopsy have confirmed the presence of a malignancy, the diagnosis and treatment plan are explained to the family. This is the primary responsibility of the physician, but the nurse has an important role at this critical time for the child and family. From the beginning of diagnostic suspicion, the family should know that a serious illness is being investigated. When the diagnosis has been confirmed, a conference should be called with the family when both sufficient time and a private conference room are available. It is important for the nurse to participate in the conference. The physician should gently yet honestly impart the diagnosis to the family. Realism with hope is the basis of the message. Even if the family was anticipating the diagnosis, it will come with profound shock, sadness, and fear. The family's initial shock and numbness often interferes with its ability to listen and understand the discussion of prognosis and treatment plan presented by the physician. The nurse can play a key role in later assessing the family members' understanding of the illness and reinforcing the information and treatment plan outlined by the physician. The nurse assists family members by clarifying understanding and promptly answering innumerable questions they will have in the days ahead.

During the initial conference, plans should be made to tell the child and also the siblings about the diagnosis and the need for long-term treatment. A parent may wish to tell the child or may wish for assistance from the physician. Whatever the parent's decision, the child and other family members need an honest yet hopeful explanation. The information should be age appropriate, and words used should be chosen so that the child can understand. (Parent and child teaching is discussed in Chapter 29.) Withholding the diagnosis or minimizing the actual illness serves only to isolate and frighten the child. Concern should not focus on whether or not to tell the child but on how to tell the child appropriately. (Chapter 30 reviews the psychosocial implications of a chronic illness for both the child and the family.)

Determining Appropriate Treatment

Staging The determination of the extent of disease is called *staging*. The results of the physical examination, diagnostic studies including those documenting metastatic sites, and the biopsy are used to evaluate the stage of the disease. Staging is useful to determine the kind of therapy that would be most effective, and to some extent staging indicates prognosis. Although the stage of disease may be changed throughout the course of the illness, the initial staging at diagnosis is most critical.

There are a wide range of staging criteria and terminology. They vary depending on the specific tumor and the particular treatment facility. Two major classifying systems exist. The first identifies the extent of disease with a Roman numeral system of I through IV. Stage I indicates localized disease without evidence of metastatic spread. Each stage thereafter identifies more extensive disease according to size, structural involvement, and evidence of metastatic disease. Stage IV represents extensive disease with widespread metastatic sites. The child with stage I or II disease generally has a much more favorable prognosis and requires less aggressive therapy than a child with stage III or IV disease.

The second staging system was developed to provide a more precise and universally consistent terminology in cancer treatment. There is often confusion when treatment results are compared among institutions that classify the same tumor and disease status differently. This second staging system, called the TNM system, endeavors to provide a basic language that can be understood by all who treat cancer. The system was initially developed by the International Union Against Cancer and is monitored by the American Joint Committee for Cancer Staging and End Results Reporting (American Joint Committee, 1977). In the TNM system, the *T* identifies primary tumor size, the *N* identifies the presence or absence of regional lymph node involvement, and the *M* identifies the presence or absence of metatastic disease (Table 45-5). After the letters *T* and *N* a rating of 0–4 is indicated. The rating of 0 for the tumor classification conveys that the original tumor site could not be found. The rating of 0 for the lymph node classification means no lymph nodes are involved. Numbers 1–4, like the Roman numeral system, indicate increasing disease involvement of tumor and nodes. Rating for the metastatic classification is either 0, meaning no known metastatic sites, or 1, meaning metastasis is present.

TABLE 45-5 TNM Staging Classification

Area of involvement	Staging criteria
Tumor	
T_0	No evidence of primary tumor
T_1, T_2, T_3, T_4	Progressive increase in tumor size and involvement
T_x	Tumor cannot be assessed
Lymph nodes	
N_0	Regional lymph nodes not demonstrably abnormal
N_1, N_2, N_3, N_4	Increasing degrees of demonstrable abnormality of regional lymph nodes
N_x	Regional lymph nodes cannot be assessed clinically
Metastasis	
M_0	No known distant metastasis
M_1	Distant metastasis present, indicate site

SOURCE: Data from American Joint Committee for Cancer Staging and End Results Reporting, 1977.

Choosing the Treatment Plan The determination of appropriate treatment is based on the results of all initial diagnostic examinations and tests. The specific treatment plan for the child is ideally chosen by an interdisciplinary health team called a tumor board. At the meeting of the board the diagnostic physicians present the pertinent histologic, laboratory, and roentgenographic data. Appropriate developmental and psychosocial assessment of the child and family is presented. It is important for nursing personnel to be represented and their input to be presented. The surgeon, radiation oncologist, and medical oncologist discuss treatment possibilities, and the optimal treatment plan is chosen. The systematic treatment plan, which may include a number of experimental therapies, is referred to as a *protocol*. The protocol outlines the specific treatment, including the surgery, radiation, and chemotherapy, the child will receive. It includes the sequence of treatment and the specific doses that will be administered (Table 45-6). Should initial treatment prove ineffective during the course of the disease, the tumor board may meet again to review the status of the child and recommend further treatment.

Nursing Management for Procedures and Treatments

General principles for preparing the child for invasive and noninvasive procedures are discussed in Chapter 29. Several points, however, are particularly applicable to the child undergoing tests related to aberrant cellular growth.

For the child with cancer, the nurse develops a specific plan for preparation based on the assessment, an understanding of the developmental norms, and the particular procedure the child is to undergo. Generally it is better to explain the sensations and feelings and their duration rather than give a detailed account of the actual procedure. For example, in preparing a child for a bone marrow aspiration, rather than explaining that a 6-in diameter of skin will be cleansed, it is more useful for the child to know that when the area is cleansed, it will feel cold. For the younger child rehearsal may also be useful. If the child will be required to lie still for a long period of time, making a game out of practicing lying still in the appropriate position may aid compliance during the actual procedure. For older children or adolescents, a trip to the laboratory to see their blood cells under a microscope or their actual radiographs often intrigues their developing scientific minds and gains their cooperation.

Because invasive diagnostic tests and treatments are common to the experience of childhood cancer, researchers are investigating additional techniques to reduce the child's distress. Most promising is the use of relaxation technique with visual imagery while the child is undergoing invasive procedures (LaBaw et al. 1975; Dash, 1980). Prior to beginning the procedure, the child participates in a relaxation technique. Visual imagery of a pleasant childhood experience is reinforced while the relaxing child undergoes the invasive procedure.

Principles of Nursing Care

The nursing care of the child with cancer is based on the philosophy that the child should live life fully in spite of life-threatening disease. Every attempt should be made to assist the child to continue developmentally appropriate growth and activities. For this reason, whenever possible, treatment for childhood cancer is delivered on an outpatient basis with hospitalization kept to an absolute minimum. Continued socialization and participation in family activities, school, and peer relationships are encouraged and only restricted if absolutely necessary. The nurse plays a

TABLE 45-6 Example of a Treatment Protocol

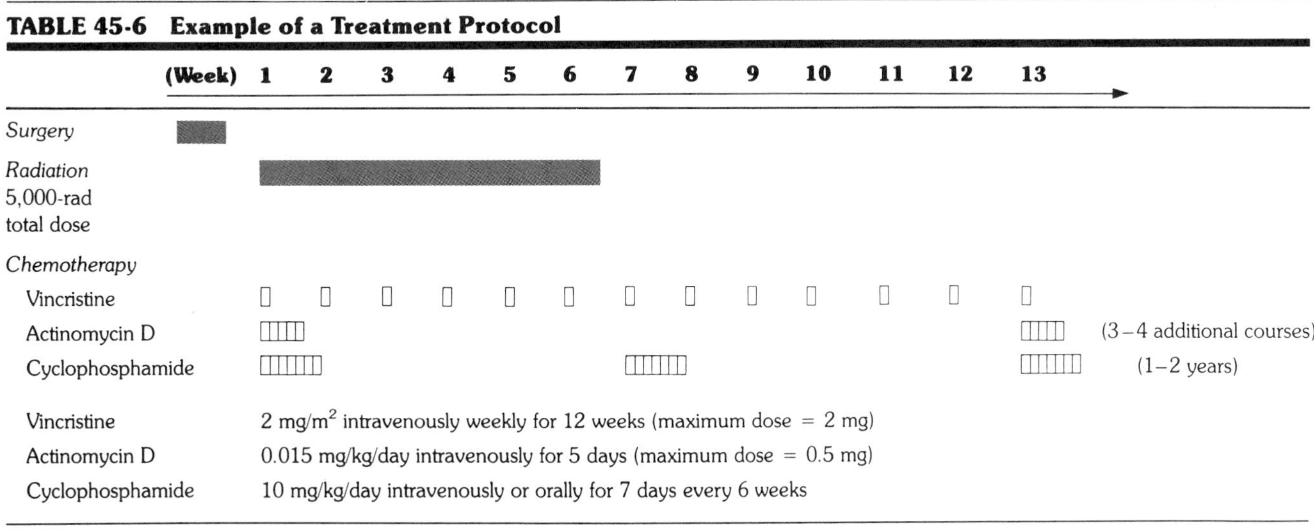

	(Week)	1	2	3	4	5	6	7	8	9	10	11	12	13 →	
Surgery	■														
Radiation 5,000-rad total dose		■	■	■	■	■	■								
Chemotherapy															
Vincristine		□	□	□	□	□	□	□	□	□	□	□	□	□	
Actinomycin D		□□□□□												□□□□□	(3–4 additional courses)
Cyclophosphamide		□□□□□□□						□□□□□□□						□□□□□□□	(1–2 years)

Vincristine	2 mg/m^2 intravenously weekly for 12 weeks (maximum dose = 2 mg)
Actinomycin D	0.015 mg/kg/day intravenously for 5 days (maximum dose = 0.5 mg)
Cyclophosphamide	10 mg/kg/day intravenously or orally for 7 days every 6 weeks

NOTE: □ = number of doses.

major role in assisting the child and family to adapt to the disease and continue normal development. This includes comprehensive education of the child and family so that they may anticipate and effectively deal with complications of the disease and treatment that may occur while the child is at home. Often health professionals concentrate on only the child's immediate treatment needs and fail to assess fully and provide guidance to families in their day-to-day adjustment at home. To provide effective and total nursing care to the child, the nurse integrates a philosophy of quality living in spite of serious illness; the focus is not on the patient as a sick child.

Acute-Care Needs

The Child Receiving Surgery Surgical resection serves as a primary treatment for solid tumors. It is often the initial treatment the child receives, although radiation or chemotherapy or both may precede surgery. Pretreatment with radiation or chemotherapy can decrease the size of the tumor and facilitates the ease of resection.

There are four categories of surgical intervention. The first is a diagnostic and staging procedure for which the primary purpose is to determine the extent of disease and obtain the biopsy. The second category is a definitive or curative procedure. This surgical treatment requires that the tumor mass is completely removable with a margin of normal tissue around it.

The third category is a palliative procedure. The procedure does not involve removal of the entire malignancy but provides a clinical advantage by subtotal resection. Initially it was believed that surgery should be attempted only when total resection is possible, but it is now thought that removing as much tumor as possible, known as a debulking or cytoreductive procedure, allows radiation and chemotherapy to be more effective. This occurs because radiation and chemotherapy destroy cancer cells more effectively when there is a reduced tumor burden present.

Palliative surgery is also used to remove solitary metastatic lesions. This most commonly occurs with lung metastasis from childhood tumors such as osteosarcoma or Wilms' tumors. Over the course of time several such surgeries may be performed to remove new lesions and increase the child's comfort and quality of life. Another use of palliative surgery is removal of obstructions. Obstructions due to tumor growth that are most amenable to this procedure are intestinal, kidney and bladder, and compressions of the spinal cord.

The fourth surgical category is a "second-look" procedure. This is the least common surgical procedure. It is performed after the initial courses of therapy are completed, and the disease status cannot be determined with less invasive tests.

Preoperative Preparation Preoperative care of the child undergoing a surgical procedure is similar to any major surgical procedure during childhood. The child and family need an honest explanation of the expectations of surgery and the anticipated course of recovery. Preoperative rehearsal, orientation to the intensive care unit if the child will be placed there, and the opportunity to see and manipulate appropriate postoperative equipment are beneficial to the child. (Age-appropriate preoperative preparation is discussed in Chapter 29.)

The parent must clearly understand the purpose of the surgery, and complete informed consent should be obtained. The parent should be encouraged to ask questions and should receive honest, complete answers. Parents need to be kept informed during surgical procedures and need to know the anticipated length and where and when children may be seen after surgery is completed. The surgeon should speak to the parent about the outcome of the surgery and the condition of the child as soon as the procedure is finished. The more completely the parent is prepared for the child's surgical procedure and postoperative care, the easier it will be for the child and family to cope with the surgery.

Preoperative physiologic preparation of the child is similar to other pediatric surgical procedures. Depending on the surgeon's routine and the location of the tumor, the actual preparation will vary. Respiratory, cardiovascular, and renal function should be evaluated; drug allergies should be carefully noted. The hematologic status of the child is carefully monitored. Because of the disease process, anemia and bleeding tendencies may be present and must be corrected prior to surgery. Any electrolyte imbalance should be corrected during the preoperative period. Occasionally children with neuroblastoma have severe diarrhea that often ceases after surgery. Preoperative correction of imbalances must therefore be weighed with the surgical outcome.

Postoperative Care Specific areas of postoperative concern and need for monitoring depend on the location and extent of the surgical procedure. (Physiologic needs of hospitalized children are discussed in Chapter 29.) The nurse carefully evaluates respiratory and cardiovascular functioning along with the fluid and electrolyte balance. Dressings are checked frequently for evidence of bleeding. Oral feedings are resumed as tolerated, beginning with clear liquids. If the surgery has involved the intestines or if an ileus is suspected, oral feedings are withheld until bowel sounds are present and the child is passing flatus. The nurse observes the child for evidence of infection.

Pain medication is administered frequently. It is often better to give pain medications on a routine, round-the-clock basis for the first few days rather than when needed. The child is frequently reluctant to ask for injectable pain medication, and so the nurse observes the child and administers medication frequently. As soon as the child can tolerate oral medication, any order for injectable medication should be recalculated for oral usage. The child is generally encouraged to resume former activity level as soon as possible.

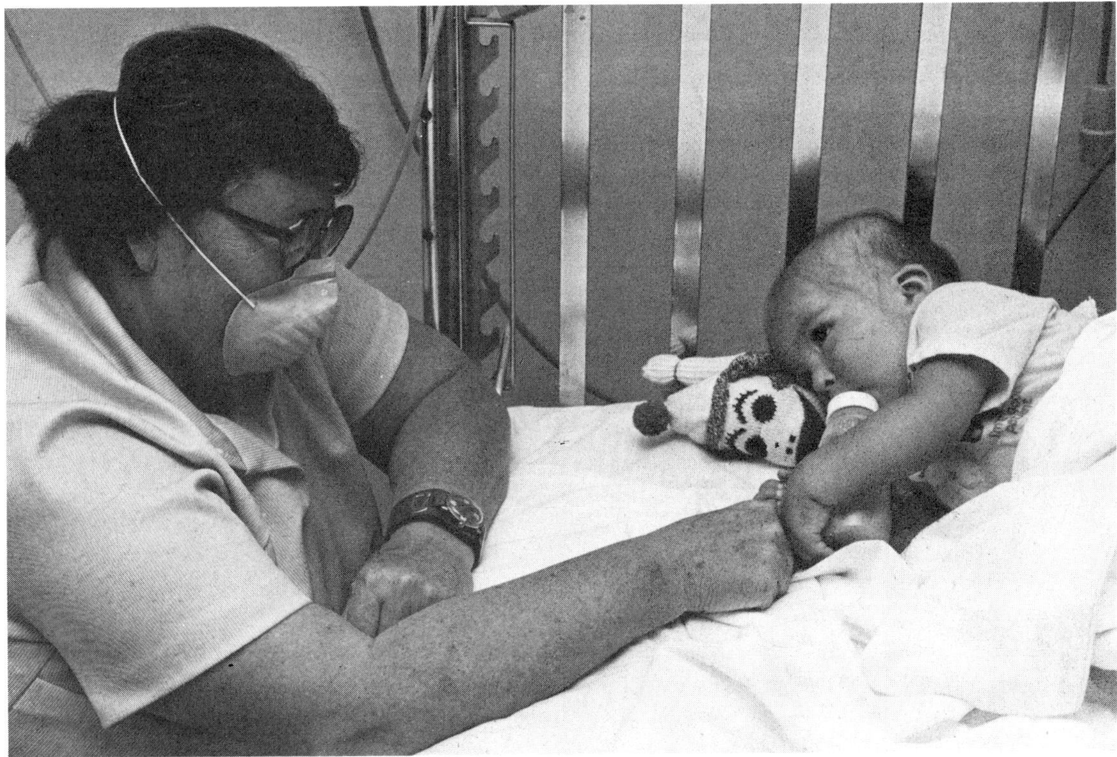

Parents need to maintain physical closeness to their children even when equipment makes this difficult.

By the second postoperative day the child should be allowed to sit upright if this has not already been done. The parents should be encouraged to participate in the child's care. Questions that the parent has about postoperative procedures or treatments should be promptly answered. The nurse also encourages close contact between parent and child. The parent needs to know that the child can still be touched or cuddled in spite of tubings and dressings. The nurse should assist the parent to maneuver the tubing and equipment so that the parent is able to hold or be close to the child.

The Child Receiving Chemotherapy Cancer chemotherapy is the use of cytotoxic drugs to treat malignant disease. The first attempt to administer chemotherapy came in the 1940s after study of the nitrogen mustard gas used in World War I demonstrated its ability to destroy rapidly reproducing cells. Today a form of nitrogen mustard gas, nitrogen mustard, is a major agent in the treatment of Hodgkin's disease. In the late 1940s, further investigation of drugs that might be useful in cancer treatment led to the development of methotrexate. Interest in nutrition established the role of folic acid in normal cell replication. Methotrexate, which is a folic acid antagonist, limits the ability of a cell to replicate. This drug was first used with children who had leukemia. Until its development there was essentially no treatment for these children. Chemotherapeutic drugs currently used in the treatment of childhood cancer are presented in Table 45-7.

Principles of Chemotherapy Chemotherapeutic agents act to kill cancer cells by destroying the cell or preventing the cell from dividing. Unfortunately, these drugs are not tumor-specific, and so they destroy normal cells as well as cancer cells. In giving chemotherapy, the goal is to kill as many cancer cells as possible without sustaining severe damage to normal cells.

The drugs used in chemotherapy act on cells by several different mechanisms that can be categorized into two major methods. Drugs can be identified as either cell cycle–specific, killing cells during a specific phase of cell cycle, or cell cycle–nonspecific, killing cells no matter what phase of the cycle the cells are in. By combining drugs with different actions rather than administering a single drug, greater tumor kill is accomplished. Because of the different activity potentials of cancer cells, however, no tumor can be completely eradicated with one cycle of drugs. Thus groups of drugs are administered over a protracted time and in a specific sequential fashion to coincide with tumor growth and activity. It is hoped that each cycle of drug therapy will continue to reduce the tumor burden, eventually stimulating nondividing cells into the cell cycle. Many cancer cells may be present but clinically undetectable. When the initial disease has been controlled so that no cancer cells can be clinically detected, the child with cancer is said to be in *remission*. Remission does not mean that the child is cured, as many undetectable cells are still present. Thus chemotherapy continues even after remission has been achieved. Because

(text continued on p. 1697)

TABLE 45-7 Chemotherapeutic Drugs Used in the Treatment of Childhood Cancer

Drug classification	Chemotherapeutic agent	Mode of action	Route of administration	Dosage form and preparation	Stability and storage of reconstituted agent	Comments
Antimetabolites		Acts as a fraudulent structure analogue of normal metabolites, mistakenly incorporated into the cell and interferes with DNA and RNA synthesis. Antimetabolites are cell-cycle specific for S phase				
	β = Cytosine arabinoside (Cytosar, Ara-C)		IV, IM, SC, IT	100 and 500 mg powder in vials, reconstituted with 5 mL (100-mg vials) or 10 mL (500-mL vial) of supplied diluent. IT solution should be prepared without preservative in diluent	Refrigerate; however, storage at room temperature acceptable for 48 hours	Hazy solution should be discarded
	Methotrexate (MTX, amethopterin)		PO, IV, IM, IT	2.5-mg tablets; 5-mg and 50-mg/2-mL vials with preservative in solution. Also 20-mg and 100-mg powder vials. Reconstitute with 2–10 mL sterile preservative-free diluent	Diluted with preservative: stable at room temperature 1 week. Diluted without preservative: discard 8 hours after preparation	Very large doses of methotrexate must be followed by "leucovorin rescue," which uses folinic acid in the form of calcium leucovorin as an antidote to the methotrexate
	6-Mercaptopurine (6-MP, Purinethol)		PO	50-mg tablet	Room temperature	
	6-Thioguanine (Thioguan, 6-TG)		PO	10-mg and 40-mg tablet	Room temperature	

TABLE 45-7 continued

Drug classification	Chemotherapeutic agent	Mode of action	Route of administration	Dosage form and preparation	Stability and storage of reconstituted agent	Comments
	5-Azacitidine (5-AZC)		IV	100-mg powder in vials. Add 19.9 mL of sterile water resulting in a 5 mg/mL concentration. May be further diluted	Stable at room temperature only 30 min. Use immediately for maximum potency	
Alkylating agents		Acts by replacing a hydrogen atom in the DNA chain with an alkyl group, resulting in the interference of DNA synthesis and RNA transcription				
	Cyclophosphamide (Cytoxan, CTX)		PO, IV	25-mg and 50-mg tablets. 100 mg, 200 mg, and 500 mg powder in vials for injection. Dilute injectable drug with sterile water as follows: 5 mL to the 100-mg vial, 10 mL to the 200-mg vial, and 25 mL to the 500 mg vial	Stable at room temperature for 24 hours or 6 days under refrigeration	Activated by the liver potentially teratogenic. Administer only a clear solution.
	Nitrogen mustard (Mustargen, HN_2, mechlorethamine		IV	10 mg powder in vial. Reconstitute with 10 mL of sterile water or normal saline	Use immediately; discard any unused solution	Do not use discolored solution

continued on next page

TABLE 45-7 continued

Drug classification	Chemotherapeutic agent	Mode of action	Route of administration	Dosage form and preparation	Stability and storage of reconsti-tuted agent	Comments
Alkylating agents (cont.)	Nitrosureas 3 separate agents:					
	BCNU (carmustine)		IV	100-mL vial for injection with separate 3 mL diluent of absolute alcohol. To mix add diluent and 27 mL of sterile water or normal saline	Relatively unstable. Use immediately and discard unused solution	Protect from light. Dilute solution further to at least 100–200 mL for infusion. Brown staining results if spilled on skin
	CCNU (lomustine)		PO	Available in package of 6 capsules: 2–10 mg capsules, 2–40 mg capsules, and 2–100 mg capsules.	Each package contains sufficient one-time dose. Discard any unused capsules	Protect from heat and moisture
	Methyl-CCNU (semustine, MeCCNU)		PO	10-mg, 50-mg, and 100-mg capsules		Protect from heat and moisture. Administer when client's stomach is empty
	Dacarbazine (imidazole carboxamide, DTIC, DTIC-Dome)		IV	100-mg and 200-mg powder in vials add 9.9 mL sterile water for 100-mg vial and 19.7 mL for 200-mg vial	Stable at room temperature for 8 hours and 72 hours refrigerated	Protect from light. Discard if solution changes color from pale yellow to pink
Antitumor antibiotics		Intercalating with components of the DNA helix				
	Doxorubicin (adriamycin)		IV	10 mg and 50 mg powder in vials. Add 5 mL to 10-mg vial and 25 mL to the 50-mg vial of normal saline or sterile water	Stable for 24 hours at room temperature and 40 hours under refrigeration	Shake vial vigorously for drug to completely dissolve

TABLE 45-7 continued

Drug classification	Chemotherapeutic agent	Mode of action	Route of administration	Dosage form and preparation	Stability and storage of reconstituted agent	Comments
	Daunorubicin (daunomycin, rubidomycin)		IV	20 mg powder in vials add 10 mL of sterile water or normal saline	Stable for 7 days at room temperature; however, since no preservative is used, discard unused portion after 8 hours	Client's urine will turn red for 1–2 days
	Dactinomycin (actinomycin D, Cosmegan)		IV	0.5 mg powder in vials. Reconstitute with 1.1 mL of sterile water without preservatives	Stable for 1 year at room temperature. Because preservative should not be used in preparation, discard unused portion within 8 hours	Protect from light
	Bleomycin (Bleo, Blenoxane)		IV, IM, SC	15 units (15 mg) powder per ampule. For IM, SC preparations dilute with 1–5 mL normal saline or sterile water. For IV use dilute with at least 5 mL normal saline	Because this drug is packaged in ampules, unused portion should be discarded	
Plant alkaloids		Stops the formation of the spindle during the metaphase stage of mitosis				
	Vincristine (Oncovin, VCR)		IV	1 mg and 5 mg powder in vials with a 10-mL diluent vial	Stable for 14 days under refrigeration	
	Vinblastine (Velban, VLB)		IV	10 mg powder in vials. Reconstitute with 10 mL of sodium chloride 0.9% preserved with phenol or benzyl alcohol	Stable for 30 days under refrigeration	

continued on next page

TABLE 45-7 continued

Drug classification	Chemotherapeutic agent	Mode of action	Route of administration	Dosage form and preparation	Stability and storage of reconsti-tuted agent	Comments
Plant alkaloids (cont.)	VM-26 (Teniposide)		IV	50-mg ampules. Dilute ampule solution with 5–20 times the volume of sodium chloride	Stable after dilution for 4 hours at room temperature	Discard if precipitate appears. A slight opalescence of the solution is normal
Hormones		Unclear				
	Corticosteriods Prednisone		PO	2.5-mg and 5-mg tablets	Room temperature	
Miscellaneous agents		Varies with specific drug or action unknown				
	L-Asparginase (L-ASP, Elspar)		IV, IM	10,000 IU powder in vials. Reconstitute with 5 mL preservative-free normal saline or sterile water for IV adminis-tration. For IM use reconstitute with 2 mL of sodium chloride 0.9%.	Use within 8 hours of preparation or discard unused portion. However, the solution is stable for 20 days at room temperature or under refrigeration	Do *not* shake vial vigorously. Discard cloudy solutions
	Procarbazine (Matulane)		PO	50-mg capsules	Room temperature	Protect from moisture
	Hydroxyurea (Hydrea)		PO	500-mg capsules	Room temperature	
	Cisplatin (platinol, platinum, *cis*-platinum)		IV	10 mg and 25 mg powder in vials. Reconstitute with 10 mL to 10-mg vial and 24.5 mL to the 25-mg vial of sterile water. For IV infusion dilute further with 50–250 mL of 5% dextrose in sodium chloride 0.9% or 0.45%	Stable for 20 hours at room temperature	Protect from direct sunlight. This drug must be administered with all infusion equipment, including needles free of aluminum metal, or a black percipitate may form. Stainless steel and plated brass are appropriate substitutes

it is difficult to determine the number of remaining cells, for most childhood cancers chemotherapy is generally administered 1–2 years before therapy is terminated. It is important for parents to understand this accurate definition of remission so they understand the importance of continuing drug treatment even when the child seems well and clinically disease-free.

Once the child is in remission, continual evaluation and diagnostic studies are undertaken to identify recurring disease. Although the cancer may be extremely sensitive to the initial drugs, resistance often develops, and relapse occurs. The reasons that cells become resistant to the cytotoxic effects of chemotherapy are not well-understood. The group of cells currently nondividing but with potential for cell division probably represent the most resistant cells. It is also possible that some cells may be damaged by the chemotherapy but able to repair themselves and continue replication. Large tumors with poor vascularization may have a number of cells escape damage from chemotherapy because sufficient doses of the drug do not reach the poorly vascularized but still active site of cancer growth.By administering a variety of chemotherapeutic agents, resistance should be minimized. Some chemotherapy protocols therefore involve switching to a new combination of drugs once remission has been obtained.

Drug Preparation and Administration Chemotherapeutic agents should be handled with care. Cytotoxic drugs affect both normal and cancer cells; local irritation and allergic reactions can occur with some drugs if they are mishandled or spilled during preparation. Nursing personnel often assume major responsibility for the preparation and administration of many chemotherapeutic drugs. Very little research has focused on the risk to health professionals who handle cytotoxic drugs. The degree of irritation to skin through direct contact or to eyes, mucous membranes, and respiratory system through droplet air transport is not known. Current indications concerning potential for increased mutagenetic or carcinogenic risk for health professionals are not clear (National Study Commission on Cytotoxic Exposure, 1983).

Until further study can clarify risk factors, precautions should be exercised when preparing or administering chemotherapeutic agents (U.S. Department of Health and Human Services, 1983). Ideally drugs should be prepared under a vertical laminar airflow hood. Preparation of cytotoxic drugs under a laminar airflow hood might be assumed by pharmacy staff. If such a system is unavailable, however, several suggestions have been offered (Stolar et al., 1983). First, whenever possible, the nurse should wear protective gloves made of polyvinylchloride. Eye protection is also suggested. When reconstituting drugs in powder form, a mask should be worn to prevent inhalation. Care should be taken to prevent spillage, and particular care should be exercised when removing a needle from a vial so fluid is not ejected. If spillage occurs, the fluid and powder should be cleaned immediately with disposable cloths. Contaminated surface areas should be washed with water, and skin should be cleaned with soap and water.

Appropriate disposal of both unused cytotoxic drugs and the preparation and administration equipment also has not been determined. Until further information is available, waste should be bagged and disposed of separately. The original vial should be used to contain unused drugs, and all materials should be placed in leak-proof and puncture-proof containers and labeled as *hazardous waste*. Disposal should follow guidelines established for hazardous waste by the individual hospital (Oncology Nursing Society, 1984). Additional study of risk factors, if any, for nursing personnel who prepare or administer chemotherapeutic agents should be forthcoming. Until that time, precautions to decrease direct contact with these drugs is advisable.

In addition to personal safety precautions while handling drugs, the nurse's accurate and meticulous caution in preparing and administering chemotherapeutic is imperative for the child's safety. There is no margin for error. Drug doses are calculated for the child's height and weight. Accurate measurement of height and weight must be checked prior to calculation of the dosage. The amount of drug the child will receive is generally close to the known toxicity level. This allows the greatest tumor kill possible without life-threatening side effects. If, however, there is any carelessness in preparing the drug and a higher dose is administered, serious toxicity could result.

The area where drugs are prepared should be well lighted and quiet. Medication orders and dosage should be double-checked. Time and care should be taken when preparing the drug, making sure the proper diluent, proper amount of diluent, and accurate amount of the final drug solution have been prepared for the right child. Another nurse should double-check this for accuracy.

Nursing Management of Chemotherapy Side Effects The side effects of chemotherapy are due to the damage done to normal cells. Because chemotherapy is not selective to only cancer cells, normal cells are vulnerable. Chemotherapy is most destructive to rapidly reproducing cells—both normal and malignant. Therefore normal tissue that is rapidly reproducing is at risk for the toxic effects of chemotherapeutic agents. Rapidly reproducing normal tissues in the body include gastrointestinal epithelial cells, developing blood cells in the bone marrow, and mature reproductive cells (in pubescent children). Thus the side effects of chemotherapy often involve these vulnerable tissues. The degree of toxicity and specific normal tissues affected vary with each drug and with the dose of drug administered. This is another reason that chemotherapeutic drugs are given in combination. Different drugs have toxic effects on different normal tissues. A child therefore may receive a drug that causes moderate bone marrow suppression but limited gastrointestinal toxicity combined with a drug that has the opposite toxicities, limited bone marrow but moderate gastrointestinal effects.

The nurse assumes an important role in assessing the effects of chemotherapy, monitoring side effects, and providing skillful nursing interventions to control the side effects the child is experiencing. The nurse assesses the child daily for new and ongoing problems. Creative intervention strategies are necessary to control side effects effectively.

Nursing Management of Acute Side Effects Hypersensitivity reactions are associated with the administration of some chemotherapeutic agents (see Table 45-8). An immediate anaphylactic reaction can occur. Epinephrine, diphenhydramine (Benadryl), and hydrocortisone should be readily available when these drugs are administered. The child is observed for evidence of urticaria, restlessness, or difficulty in breathing. Urticaria also is occasionally associated with daunorubicin, 6-mercaptopurine, and methotrexate. Photosensitivity occurs with actinomycin D, bleomycin, and methotrexate. The child should avoid prolonged sun exposure for 1–2 days after receiving these drugs.

TABLE 45-8 Acute Side Effects of Specific Chemotherapeutic Agents

Side effect	Chemotherapeutic agents
Hypersensitivity	L-asparginase Bleomycin Cisplatin
Photosensitivity	Actinomycin D Bleomycin Daunorubicin Methotrexate
Urticaria	Daunorubicin 6-Mercaptopurine Methotrexate
Vesicants	Actinomycin D Dacarbazine Daunorubicin Doxorubicin Nitrogen mustard Vinblastine Vincristine
Moderate-to-severe nausea and vomiting	Actinomycin D 5-Azacitidine Carmustine Cisplatin Cyclophosamide Cytosine arbinoside Dacarbazine Daunorubicin Doxorubicin Lomustine Nitrogen mustard Procarbazine Semustine Vinblastine
Fever	Bleomycin Cyclophosphamide Cytosine arbinoside Dacarbazine Daunorubicin Doxorubicin 6-Mercaptopurine Methotrexate Procarbazine Vinblastine Vincristine

Several drugs are extremely toxic if during intravenous administration the solution infiltrates surrounding tissue. Serious vein phlebitis and tissue necrosis may result. When drugs that are vesicants are administered, observation for extravasation is closely monitored. Should infiltration of the solution be suspected, the injection is immediately stopped. A few milliliters of blood and solution are withdrawn. Depending on physician preference, further treatment of the infiltrated site varies. Treatment may include infiltration of the subcutaneous tissue with hydrocortisone and administration of a drug-specific antidote—if one exists for that agent. Cold compresses may be applied. The site is closely observed during the next few days for signs of inflammation and necrosis (Oncology Nursing Society, 1984). Surgical excision, debridement, and skin grafting may be necessary if serious necrosis results (see Chapter 44). Because of the tissue damage risk, vesicant agents should not be injected near a joint such as the wrist or antecubital fossa. Should extravasation occur at these sites, mobility may be impaired as well as tissue damaged. It is also more difficult to determine whether infiltration is occurring when a large deep vein is used in injection.

Many cytotoxic drugs cause nausea and vomiting that generally begin 2–6 hours after they have been administered. This probably does not represent a direct affect on the gastrointestinal lining but rather stimulation of the vomiting center in the brain medulla by the chemoreceptor trigger zone. Vomiting due to chemotherapy generally does not last longer than 48 hours.

Effective treatment to prevent nausea and vomiting has not yet been developed. Currently the most effective drugs come from the phenothiazines. Chlorpromazine (Thorazine) or promethazine (Phenergan) are commonly used with the child. Prochlorperazine (Compazine), which is frequently used with adults, has a high risk of extrapyramidal symptoms in children and should therefore be avoided if possible. Investigational studies are exploring the effectiveness of Δ-9-tetrahydrocannabinol (THC), the active ingredient in marijuana. For research purposes, THC is available in synthetic form, but to date, its usefulness has not been determined. Antihistimines such as Benadryl and hydroxyzine pamoate (Vistaril) have also been used. It is best to begin antiemetic drugs prior to the onset of nausea and vomiting. Children's tolerance to chemotherapy varies. The nurse tries to determine a pattern of nausea and vomiting

TABLE 45-9 Some Chemotherapy Drug Interactions

Drug	Precautions
Cisplatin	Avoid use of aminoglycosides (such as gentamicin), which may increase nephrotoxicity and ototoxicity
6-Mercaptopurine (6-MP)	Avoid the use of allopurinol or reduce the does of 6-MP to one-quarter of the calculated amount. Allopurinol significantly enhances the potency of 6-MP
Methotrexate (MTX)	Avoid ethanol ingestion, which may increase hepatotoxicity. Avoid salicylates, which may increase MTX toxicity. Avoid the use of products containing folate, which may impede the effectiveness of MTX
Actinomycin D Doxorubicin Nitrogen mustard	Radiation "recall" (dermatologic effect) when administered after radiation has been given, mimicking the dermatologic skin manifestations of radiation in areas that have previously been radiated

for each child so that the particular antiemetic drugs and schedule of administration optimal for the individual child can be identified. Antiemetic drugs should be administered on a regular schedule rather than when needed.

The nurse closely monitors intake and output. Fluid and electrolytes are administered to maintain balance. Adequate nutritional intake may be jeopardized during periods of therapy. If possible, small meals are offered rather than large meals consisting of heavy foods. Fluid in the form of Popsicles may be one of the few fluids tolerated. Should the child receive chemotherapy treatment as an outpatient, family members must be instructed on recording intake and output, how to rehydrate the child orally, and how much fluid loss necessitates bringing the child back to the hospital for intravenous hydration.

Fever is associated with the administration of several drugs. The presence of a fever in the child can be confusing because it may result from a number of causes. Infection should always be investigated since immediate treatment is required, particularly in the immunosuppressed and bone marrow–suppressed child. The fever, however, may actually be caused by the chemotherapy, radiation, immunotherapy, or tumor activity; if the fever is related to one of these causes, comfort measures rather than antibiotics are required. Administration of acetaminophen and sponging or other cooling measures may be useful in reducing fever discomfort.

A few chemotherapeutic drugs are known to have either decreased effectiveness or increased toxicity when administered concurrently with some noncytotoxic drugs (see Table 45-9).

Nursing Management of Intermediate Side Effects

Intermediate side effects occur one to several weeks after drug administration. Whether the drugs were administered to the child on an inpatient or outpatient basis, the child is usually at home when symptoms of these side effects develop. Therefore, besides being knowledgeable about potential problems and their management, the nurse teaches the child and family about early recognition of symptoms and appropriate action should side effects occur. Table 45-10 lists intermediate side effects.

Developing blood cells in the bone marrow are rapidly reproducing and are particularly vulnerable to chemotherapy. Most cytotoxic drugs cause some degree of bone marrow suppression. The degree of suppression and specific blood components (erythrocytes, leukocytes, and platelets) affected vary among the different agents and dosage schedules. Generally, peripheral blood counts show signs of suppression 7–10 days after drug administration. The nadir, or lowest, blood count level is reached 14 days after the

TABLE 45-10 Intermediate Side Effects of Specific Chemotherapeutic Agents

Side effects	Chemotherapeutic agents
Moderate-to-severe bone marrow suppression	Actinomycin D 5-Azacitidine Carmustine Cyclophosphamide Cytosine arabinoside Daunorubicin Doxorubicin Hydroxyurea Lomustine Nitrogen mustard Methotrexate Procarbazine Semustine Vinblastine
Stomatitis	Bleomycin Cytosine arabinoside Daunorubicin Doxorubicin 6-Mercaptopurine Methotrexate 6-Thioguanine
Alopecia	Actinomycin-D Bleomycin Cyclophosphamide Daunorubicin Doxorubicin Nitrogen mustard Vincristine

therapy. Recovery and return of blood components to normal levels occur 3–4 weeks after drug administration.

Leukopenia (decreased white blood cells), which predisposes the child to infection, and thrombocytopenia (decreased platelets), which predisposes the child to bruising and bleeding, are the most serious side effects. Anemia due to decreased erythrocyte count is easier to treat.

The rapidly reproducing tissue of the gastrointestinal tract can be destroyed by certain cytotoxic agents. As these cells slough off, inflammation and ulceration occur. Ulcers can develop throughout the entire gastrointestinal tract but are most commonly manifested in the mouth and throat as oral stomatitis. Inflammation and ulcers usually begin 7–10 days after drug administration or about the same time as the peripheral blood counts decrease.

Prevention of stomatitis may be impossible because of the severe damage to the mucosa that results from the use of these cytotoxic drugs. Nursing goals should focus on symptomatic care and prevention of secondary infection of the oral mucosa. The most common infection involves the fungal organism *Candida albicans,* which appears initially as an inflamed patch in the mouth and progresses to white plaques. The organism is treated with the drug nystatin. Lozenges and liquid suspension of the drug are available and should be held in contact with the oral mucosa for as long as possible.

The nurse institutes a systematic schedule of oral hygiene. Researchers have not been able to demonstrate a superior mouth care agent. It is more important to keep the mouth clean and free of debris and mucus than to use a particular agent. Commercial mouth care preparations containing alcohol should be avoided because they tend to dry the mouth. Creativity is often necessary to convince a reluctant child with painful stomatitis to perform mouth care. Soft-sponge applicators rather than stiff toothbrushes may be more comfortable for the child. Use of a tube-feeding bag suspended from a comfortable height and filled with an irrigating solution of a small amount of table salt and baking soda dissolved in water is often a tolerable way for the child to keep the mouth rinsed. Using the bag filled with solution, the child can lean over a sink or bed basin and rinse the mouth while controlling the flow of the solution.

Local pain control may be necessary, and a variety of solutions and sprays may be ordered by the physician. A combination of diphenhydramine (Benadryl Elixir), Maalox antacid, and lidocaine (viscous xylocaine), or Orabase ointment or Vince's mouthwash solution are examples. Each will have varying degrees of acceptability to the individual child. Often, simply having the child suck on Popsicles or ice chips provides a sufficient numbing effect.

The nurse assesses the child's mouth daily. Tenderness or changes in color or texture in any area of the mouth should be recorded. Family members must be instructed about the signs and symptoms of stomatitis and appropriate treatment measures so they may encourage mouth care during hospitalization and maintain treatment at home.

Hair follicles contain rapidly growing cells and are therefore vulnerable to damage from some chemotherapeutic agents. Significant hair loss, or alopecia, can be a devastating side effect even though it is not life-threatening. A child who is to receive a drug that causes alopecia should be prepared for the eventual hair loss. Once the drugs are started, hair begins to thin or come out in large patches within weeks to several months.

The nurse needs to be sensitive to the impact of hair loss on the child and family. Anger and sadness over hair loss also may be compounded because this may be the first visible sign to the family that the child is seriously ill and needs intensive treatment. This is particularly true if the child appeared healthy at diagnosis. Wigs or scarves can be used during periods of alopecia. The child should select a wig before significant hair loss has resulted. The nurse can direct the family to stores that stock child-size wigs. As the hair begins to fall out, the nurse diligently removes the hair that accumulates on the bedding or clothing of the hospitalized child. Cutting the child's hair shorter also makes hair loss less distracting to the child. Parents should be instructed in managing hair loss for the child at home. Some children adjust rather quickly to the hair loss, but their families may need a longer period of adjustment. These children might prefer not to wear a head covering, and this might in turn become a source of conflict to the parent who wants the child to appear "normal" by wearing a wig or scarf.

The child and family should know that hair loss is not permanent and that regrowth will occur once the drugs producing alopecia are discontinued. The new hair may look quite different from the original hair. The texture may be finer, and the color may be a lighter or darker shade. Hair loss can also extend to the entire body. Occasionally the child may lose eyebrows, eye lashes, or even pubic hair. Once the hair has regrown, later disease relapse may necessitate administration of other agents causing alopecia. Hair loss for the second time is usually much more traumatic to the child and family.

Using scalp tourniquets and cooling the scalp with special ice caps have been used to decrease blood flow thereby decreasing drug transport to the scalp to prevent or retard hair loss. The treatment is begun just prior to the child's receiving the drug. The ice cap requires that the scalp be cooled 20 min before the agent is administered. These techniques can be used only when the drug is administered intravenously and clears quickly from the blood plasma. The tourniquet or ice cap remain on the child's head 10–30 minutes after the drug has been injected. A number of researchers have investigated these hair-sparing techniques and found varying degrees of effectiveness. Because the scalp vasoconstriction prevents the cytotoxic drugs from reaching scalp veins, some physicians discourage the use of these techniques because theoretically they allow cancer cells, particularly leukemia and lymphoma cells, to be sequestered in the scalp veins and therefore escape the lethal effects of chemotherapy.

Nursing Management of Cumulative Side Effects Cumulative side effects manifest themselves after several cycles of the chemotherapy program. With time and repeated doses of the drug these toxic effects are more likely to occur. Table 45-11 identifies the most frequent cumulative side effects of chemotherapy.

A few drugs cause some degree of hepatic dysfunction. Clinical signs and symptoms may include elevation of liver function tests, abnormalities in clotting factors, and jaundice. When hepatic dysfunction is identified during its onset, it is reversible within 14–28 days after the drug is withheld. L-Asparginase causes the greatest amount of hepatic toxicity, but this occurs more commonly in adults than in children.

Pulmonary toxicity is associated with a few chemotherapeutic drugs, most notably bleomycin, but toxic effects are more frequent in adults than children and appear to be dose related. Radiologic changes show a diffuse interstitial infiltrate that appears like a pneumonitis or fibrosis. Symptoms include bibasilar rales, cough, and dyspnea. Chest radiograph should be followed closely as the toxicity is usually reversible if identified at onset. The drug should be discontinued and recovery expected in 1–2 months. The use of corticosteroids to aid recovery is controversial.

Cardiac toxicity is a serious side effect of two of the antibiotics and cyclophosphamide. It is related to the cumulative dose of the drugs and concurrent radiation of the chest. Signs and symptoms of cardiotoxicity include abnormalities in the electrocardiogram (ECG) consisting of tachycardia, arrhythmias, and ST-T wave changes and congestive heart failure consisting of tachypnea, cardiomegaly, and hepatomegaly.

Congestive heart failure can be a life-threatening complication and is not always reversible, especially if the diagnosis is not made during the onset. Periodic ECG and echocardiogram may indicate impending toxicity. Because cardiac toxicity is strongly related to cumulative dose, it is recommended that the child not receive more than a lifetime dose of 450 mg/m_2 to 550 mg/m^2 of either daunorubicin or doxorubicin. The nurse carefully assesses the child who is receiving these drugs for signs of impending cardiovascular failure. In many treatment settings, the physician administers daunorubicin or doxorubicin, but the nurse makes sure that each dose has been clearly recorded so that accurate tabulation of the cumulative dose is readily available. The nurse always exercises care in preparing accurate doses of chemotherapeutic drugs, but with cardiotoxic drugs there is even less room for error.

Cytotoxic drugs can produce neurologic toxicity by disrupting peripheral, autonomic, or central nervous system function. Vincristine and vinblastine produce peripheral nerve damage and paralyze autonomic nerves that control the bladder and intestinal motility. Neurologic toxicities occur more frequently with vincristine than with vinblastine. Peripheral nerve damage is manifested by numbness and tingling in the fingers and toes and loss of deep tendon reflexes. At the first sign of numbness, tingling, or weakness, the drug should be discontinued or the dosage reduced. The nurse assesses the child receiving vincristine or vinblastine for signs and symptoms of these peripheral neuropathies. The child who has mastered dressing may demonstrate difficulty in buttoning or snapping clothing. Loss of deep tendon reflexes are noted by observing for foot drop, difficulty in climbing stairs, or inability to walk on the heels.

Paralysis of the autonomic nerves, which control the bladder and intestinal motility, results in urinary retention and constipation. Urinary retention is not common in the child, but constipation can be problematic. Once again, constipation occurs more frequently with vincristine than with vinblastine. Prophylactic stool softeners should be administered to the child receiving vincristine. The nurse assesses bowel function daily. Additional laxatives or enemas may be necessary. The child and caregiver should be aware of this toxicity so that they can report symptoms as soon as they occur. Bowel care will need to be continued at home.

TABLE 45-11 Cumulative Side Effects of Specific Chemotherapeutic Agents

Side effects	Chemotherapeutic agents
Hepatic toxicity	Carmustine 6-Mercaptopurine Methotrexate L-Asparginase
Cardiac toxicity	Cyclophosphamide Daunorubicin Doxorubicin
Renal toxicity	Cisplatin Methotrexate
Pancreatic toxicity	L-Asparginase
Pulmonary Toxicity	Bleomycin Carmustine Cyclophosphamide (uncommon)
Ototoxicity	Cisplatin
Neurologic toxicity	Vincristine Vinblastine Intrathecal methotrexate
Bladder toxicity	Cyclophosphamide

Central nervous system toxicity has been associated with the administration of intrathecal methotrexate, particularly when it is given with concurrent cranial irradiation. Toxicity is manifested by headache, vomiting, irritability, fever, or back pain. This neurotoxic syndrome is generally reversible if recognized early.

Methotrexate in high doses causes renal tubular obstruction from drug precipitation. It is important to prevent obstruction from occurring. Prehydration and fluid administration during and after treatment promotes renal filtration. Alkalinization of the urine, usually by intravenous sodium bicarbonate, will also help prevent tubular obstruction. The nurse is responsible for administering the fluid and sodium bicarbonate therapy. Intake and output are carefully monitored especially since vomiting is associated with high-dose methotrexate infusion. Urine pH is periodically checked to determine whether the urine is sufficiently alkalinized. Serum creatinine, uric acid, and BUN are assessed prior to each methotrexate infusion. A 24-hour urine test for creatinine clearance prior to treatment is the most useful assessment of renal function. If renal function deteriorates, the drug is either discontinued or the dosage is reduced, depending on the severity of the toxicity.

Cisplatin causes tubular necrosis, and assessment of renal functioning prior to drug administration is therefore necessary. Prehydrating the child, attending to fluid and electrolyte balance, and monitoring intake and output are nursing responsibilities. Some physicians administer mannitol and furosemide during therapy as an added precaution against tubular damage. Mannitol may prevent cisplatin from binding with and therefore damaging the renal tubule. Cisplatin also causes significant high-frequency hearing loss in 30% of individuals who receive the drug. This toxicity is irreverisble. Subjective report and audiometric testing document the degree of ototoxicity.

Cyclophosphamide can be toxic to the bladder. Drug metabolites serve as a direct chemical irritant to the bladder epithelium, causing a sterile hemorrhagic cystitis. Hydration and frequent voiding to keep drug metabolites flushed from the bladder are the keys to prevention. Should severe bleeding develop, treatment consists of bladder instillation with formalin or fulguration and appropriate blood replacement. The drug should be discontinued or the dosage reduced if cystitis develops.

L-Asparginase can cause pancreatitis and associated hyperglycemia. The condition is reversible, although the drug should be discontinued or the dosage lowered. Significant hyperglycemia requires insulin therapy. The nurse frequently checks urine sugar and acetone; blood glucose should also be monitored to detect glucose metabolism abnormalities.

Late-appearing, long-term side effects occasionally occur as a result of earlier chemotherapy treatment, although these problems may not be evident for some years after therapy has been discontinued.

The Child Receiving Radiation Therapy Radiation as a potential tool of cancer therapy had its beginning with the discovery of x-rays by Wilhelm Röentgen in 1895. Marie Curie added to this discovery by identifying the radioactive nature of x-rays. Today, radiation therapy is an important mainstay of cancer treatment. The purpose of radiation therapy is to destroy cancer cells in the localized area receiving treatment. Similar to chemotherapy, radiation causes damage to both normal and cancer cells. Rapidly reproducing cells are most vulnerable, resulting in many of the same side effects that are produced by chemotherapy.

External radiation is the most common type of therapy for children. External radiation means the electromagnetic energy sources come from a machine outside the child's body. These machines produce either x-rays, which are generated by electrical machines, or gamma rays, which are emitted from radioisotopes. Of the two classes of available machines—orthovoltage and megavoltage (also called supervoltage)—megavoltage machines are more commonly used in the treatment of childhood cancer. They produce their greatest effect several centimeters into the body, thus having an important skin-sparing function. This allows for higher doses of radiation to be delivered without serious skin damage. Childhood cancers are at some distance from the skin, making this feature of the megavoltage machines most appropriate for therapy with children.

Once the radiation has affected a cell, actual cell death may not occur for a period of time. *Lethal damage* is a term that refers to cells that can no longer divide subsequent to radiation. This may occur immediately, or the cell may still divide a few more times before death takes place. *Sublethally damaged* cells are those disrupted by the radiation but able to repair the damage. Ideally, the goal of radiation therapy is to cause as much lethal damage to cancer cells while producing sublethal damage to normal cells. In fact, normal cells may be better able than cancer cells to repair sublethal damage. Additionally, tumor cells located deep in a mass are often poorly oxygenated. Adequate oxygenation tends to aid sublethal repair. To encourage normal cell recovery, radiation treatment is divided into small exposures over a period of weeks until the total dose to be administered, measured in rad, is reached. For example, a child may receive 3000 rad over 6 weeks of 5-day-a-week treatments or 100 rad per treatment. By delivering radiation therapy over time, normal cells can recover from damaging effects which will reduce toxicity, yet a higher degree of tumor cell death is achieved.

Radiation therapy is not used with all tumors. Although radiation can kill any type of cancer cell, the dose required might be too toxic to surrounding vital tissue. The relationship between tumorcidal doses of radiation and surrounding normal tissue tolerance is referred to as radiosensitivity. In childhood cancer leukemia, lymphoma, Wilms' tumor, and neuroblastoma are most radiosensitive. Osteosarcoma and some brain tumors are least radiosensitive.

Pretherapy Preparation The exact dosage, site, and delivery mechanisms are tailored to the individual child. Calculation is based on a sophisticated knowledge of radiation physics and use of computers. The child is seen in the radiation therapy department for evaluation and a "setup" procedure. When surgery has been performed prior to radiation, radiologic markers may have been attached to the site of residual tumor or around the margins of normal tissue. By viewing diagnostic radiographs, the radiation oncologists can determine the specific area requiring radiation. A simulator machine can also be used to determine the site of radiation. The simulator uses diagnostic x-rays to locate and measure the actual dimensions of the tumor or area to be irradiated. The radiographic film is marked to delineate the margins of radiation therapy. This process is referred to as determining the "ports" or area to be radiated. Then the number and specific sites to receive the radiation beam are determined. Multiple angles spare skin and other tissue not intended for radiation by using a number of lower-dose entry sites while the tumor receives the full dose. Once the final ports are identified, the child's skin is marked with indelible ink to provide an accurate, consistent lineup of the radiation beam for each treatment the child receives. The child and family should be told not to remove or alter the skin markings in any way, as these will serve as a guide for direction of the energy beam.

Shielding to protect vulnerable organs that lie in the path of the radiation is made of lead and prevents the penetration of ionizing radiation. For example, the child receiving chest radiation often has a lead shield designed to protect the heart from the damaging rays. These lead shields must be individually cut to conform to the actual shape of the child's organ.

The child who receives radiation must remain absolutely still during the few minutes of each radiation treatment. This is often difficult for the young or frightened child. The child is left alone during treatment, and although the child feels nothing when the radiation is administered, some children feel frightened by the machine and the isolation. Contact can be continued by voice from the control room, where personnel and the parent can also observe the treatment.

The child and family need an explanation of and orientation to the equipment and purpose of treatment. Rehearsal by lying still on a table for a few minutes and slowly building to the actual period required for immobility during treatment may be useful. Shells, casts, or sandbags may be used to assist the child to remain still. In the very young child, sedation approaching anesthesia may be necessary to ensure cooperation and total immobility.

There are many myths associated with the therapeutic use of radiation. Historically, treatment with low-dose orthovoltage machines did cause severe skin and bone damage. With modern treatment, however, these side effects should be significantly reduced. In spite of advances, therapeutic radiation is still feared. This is probably perpetuated by the association of therapeutic radiation with the destructive use of radiation during nuclear war. Allowing the family to identify their fears and clarify misconceptions is essential. To assist the child and family during radiation therapy, the nurse needs to be knowledgeable about treatment, even though this special therapy is not located on a nursing unit and the nurse may have little knowledge about the process of therapy. Therefore, the nurse who cares for the child receiving radiation also needs to take responsibility for learning about radiation treatment. This is often best accomplished by accompanying a child or several children through the setup and initial treatment procedures.

Radiation Side Effects and Nursing Management Side effects of radiation therapy occur as normal tissue in the radiated field is damaged. The severity of side effects is also dose-related. To anticipate potential side effects, the nurse needs to know the site and dose of radiation administered. Table 45-12 lists potential side effects of radiation therapy in relation to the site receiving radiation; many of the side effects are similar to those associated with chemotherapy.

The child is closely observed for signs and symptoms of developing toxicities. Nausea and vomiting, if the gastrointestinal tract is included in the field of radiation, are the most immediate side effects. Other toxicities develop after one to several weeks of therapy. A few toxicities, such as cataracts, do not occur until months to a year after therapy has been completed. Depending on the severity of toxicity, radiation treatments may be stopped for a few days to allow further recovery of normal tissue.

Nursing management of radiation-induced side effects focuses on symptom control and comfort measures. Radiation effects on epithelial tissue of the skin and mucous membranes result in gastrointestinal side effects and radiation dermatitis. The onset of these symptoms generally begins during the second or third week of therapy. Management of stomatitis from radiation of the head and neck area is like stomatitis caused by chemotherapy.

Radiation to the mouth can cause salivary gland dysfunction. Saliva becomes scanty. Thick, ropy mucus may develop. Frequent mouth care and removal of mucus is imperative. Oral-pharyngeal suctioning may be necessary and should be undertaken carefully as the mucosa is extremely fragile. Because radiation of the mouth causes decreased salivation, dental caries are more likely to develop. The child should have a complete dental evaluation prior to treatment. Fluoride treatments may reduce the incidence of dental caries.

Gastrointestinal effects from radiation of the gut are managed symptomatically. Intake and output are measured carefully. Fluid and electrolytes are replaced as needed. Antiemetics are administered on a routine basis during periods of constant nausea and vomiting. Antidiarrhea drugs such as diphenoxylate hydrochloride (Lomotil) and atro-

TABLE 45-12 Side Effects of Radiation Therapy

Site radiated	Side effects	Nursing management
Brain	*Intermediate:* edema; nausea and vomiting (stimulation of vomiting center in brain stem medulla)	Give steriods as ordered; monitor for headache. Give antiemetic on a round-the-clock schedule; monitor hydration status
	Late: learning disabilities	Follow-up assessment of school achievement; refer for psychologic testing
Scalp, ear, mouth	*Intermediate:* alopecia, otitis media, loss of taste, decreased salivation	Assist with wigs, scarfs, and support; observe for signs and symptoms of otitis media; encourage adequate nutrition and dietary changes to increase taste; consider artificial saliva; offer hard candies to stimulate salivation; offer Popsicles
Throat	Stomatitis, dysphagia, parotitis	Provide frequent oral hygiene; observe for secondary fungal infection; medicate as needed for pain
Eyes, teeth	*Late:* cataracts, dental caries	Encourage follow-up eye examination; promote regular dental examination and treatment with fluoride
Pulmonary area	*Intermediate:* inflammatory pneumonitis *Late:* fibrosis	Observe for signs and symptoms of nonproductive cough, low-grade fever, mild chest pain
Cardiac area	*Intermediate:* pericarditis	Observe for signs and symptoms of chest pain, friction rub; note ECG changes
Gastrointestinal area	Anorexia, nausea and vomiting	Give small frequent feedings; give antiemetic on a round-the-clock schedule
	Intermediate: diarrhea/cramping, dehydration, weight loss	Give antispasmodics and kaolin pectin as needed; monitor intake and output and replace fluids; monitor weight, encourage high calorie feedings and vitamin supplements
	Rectal irritation, tenesmus (spasm of the anal sphincter)	Provide comfort measures (sitz baths, soothing preparations, heat)
	Late (but uncommon): radiation hepatitis, esophageal stricture, pancreatitis	Observe for signs and symptoms
Kidney	*Intermediate (but uncommon):* acute nephritis	Observe for signs and symptoms: malaise, nocturia, leg edema, proteinuria, microhematuria, weight gain
Bladder	*Intermediate:* dysurea, cystitis	Observe for signs and symptoms: malaise, microhematuria, fever, painful urination; encourage hydration, monitor intake and output
Bone	*Possible late (but uncommon):* secondary cancers (sarcomas), pathologic fractures, growth alterations, (growth retardation, asymmetrical growth)	Encourage follow-up medical evaluations after therapy is discontinued
Bone-forming tissue (bone marrow)	*Intermediate:* bone marrow suppression (decreased erythrocytes, decreased leukocytes, decreased platelets)	Observe for signs and symptoms of anemia, infection, bleeding
Skin	*Intermediate:* radiodermatitis (dry desquamation, wet desquamation) *Late:* hyperpigmentation	Keep skin clean, dry, and open to the air; avoid creams (unless prescribed); avoid sun exposure and tight clothing
Testes or ovaries	*Late:* sterility, testicular hypertrophy *Intermediate:* delay in secondary sexual characteristics *Late:* sterility, early menopause	Encourage adequate counseling so family understands potential effects of treatment; assist with referral for fertility evaluations as needed; explain potential sperm banking for adolescent male
Nonspecific	*Intermediate:* radiation fatigue (malaise, weakness, headache, nausea, anorexia)	Encourage rest and good nutrition; provide symptom management as needed; reassure family that this is a treatment effect *not* a disease effect

pine sulfate are sometimes useful in the control of radiation-induced diarrhea.

Toxic skin effects occur because of the destruction of basal cells in the epidermis. This causes an inflammatory reaction that is first apparent over the radiated site approximately 2 weeks after therapy has been initiated. Radiation dermatitis is classified by its severity into one of four groups: first-, second-, third-, and fourth-degree epidermatitis.

A first-degree reaction results in damage to hair roots and causes hair loss. If the skull has received radiation, alopecia will result. Nursing management is the same as outlined for chemotherapy-induced alopecia. If low to moderate doses of radiation are delivered, hair will begin to regrow 2–3 months after therapy. Occasionally, when high-dose radiation is indicated for some brain tumors, hair will not regrow.

Second-degree reactions are characterized by dry desquamation. The radiated skin develops erythema, and the child may complain of itching. The skin may peel in a similar manner to a mild sunburn. Once the skin reaction has healed, a permanent increased pigmentation may result.

Third-degree reactions are characterized by wet desquamation. A deep-purple erythema and blisters form. The blisters eventually erupt, and the moist serum exudate that results is the basis for the reaction to be termed *wet* desquamation. With symptomatic management, healing occurs in about 3 weeks. Again a permanent hyperpigmentation may remain.

The nurse rarely sees a fourth-degree reaction, which is characterized by tissue necrosis and general deep-tissue sloughing. When orthovoltage radiation was the primary method of radiation, these severe reactions occurred more frequently. With the skin-sparing effects of supervoltage machines, however, this type of reaction should not develop.

Symptomatic treatment of skin reactions varies among radiation oncologists. Generally, keeping the skin dry and exposed to air is recommended. Sometimes the physician will prescribe a lotion or spray containing corticosteriods. The child and parent should be instructed not to apply any additional lotions. Tight or restrictive clothing and coverings over the radiation field should be avoided. Because the skin tissue is very fragile, the area should not be scrubbed, rubbed, or scratched. Lukewarm water and gently patting the skin dry should be employed in cleansing the area, taking care not to remove radiation ink markers. Sun exposure or application of hot or cold compresses should be avoided because they may increase the skin reaction.

Similar to the effects of chemotherapy on rapidly dividing blood-forming tissue, bone marrow suppression may result from radiation treatment. The extent of bone marrow suppression is directly related to the dose and extent of bone marrow and lymphoid tissue in the field of irradiation. Reduction of circulating platelets and leukocytes is initially seen in the blood count with a later reduction in circulating erythrocytes. When significant reduction of these blood components results, the child is at risk for developing bruising, bleeding, infection, and anemia.

A nonspecific side effect of radiation is fatigue. The cause of radiation-induced fatigue is not well understood or studied. Cell destruction due to therapy may stimulate the release of toxic by-products that accumulate in the blood and are slow to be excreted. These toxic by-products could serve as an explanation of radiation fatigue. Natural body conservation of energy to direct remaining energy resources to healing normal tissue may be a second explanation. When radiation fatigue is observed in the child undergoing therapy, additional periods of rest must be planned. The child should not be pushed to keep up a busy activity schedule. Parents need to understand that fatigue is a natural reaction to radiation therapy. It does not mean that the disease is getting worse; nor does it mean the child is not responding to treatment.

Acute-Care Needs Related to Bone Marrow Suppression Bone marrow suppression, as a side effect of chemotherapy, or radiation that includes large areas of bone marrow, predisposes the child to anemia, infection, and bleeding. The child with leukemia or lymphoma is at even greater risk because the disease itself can cause bone marrow dysfunction. The child's hematologic status is carefully monitored. Periods of vulnerability can be predicted through evaluation of laboratory findings and knowledge of the time of greatest risk during the treatment cycle. Typically, after chemotherapy and radiation, a decrease in the blood components of the peripheral blood can be detected in 7–10 days. The nadir occurs 14 days after the treatment cycle, and recovery is seen in 21–28 days.

The nurse should be knowledgeable about normal blood values (see Table 36-1) and alterations in those values that indicate the child is at risk. Careful systematic assessment of the child on a daily basis during the periods of vulnerability to determine the presence of these complications is a nursing responsibility. Effective nursing management of the child who is experiencing bone marrow suppression requires judicious attention to both preventive and supportive measures.

Anemia Anemia results from decreased production of red blood cells. This may occur from the effects of treatment, although it is less common than infection and bleeding tendencies. Anemia occurs also from periods of poor nutrition. Additionally, tumor by-products may actually interfere with red blood cell production. At diagnosis and during periods of relapse, the child with leukemia may have significant anemia. This is the result of leukemic cell replacement of normal blood components.

When the hemoglobin value drops below 9 g, the child may begin to show such symptoms of hemoglobin defi-

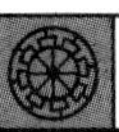

NURSING CARE GUIDE — Child With Bone Marrow Suppression

Nursing diagnosis	Interventions	Evaluation
1. Potential for infection from decreased blood components	Place child with roommate(s) with no infections, and make sure staff and visitors with infections do not enter room Observe child closely for signs of infection, especially temperature variation Follow strict aseptic technique, using reverse isolation or laminar air flow if child is neutropenic Keep hospitalization to minimum to prevent nosocomial infections Examine child regularly for signs of inflammation at all potential sites of infection such as skin breaks (biopsy site, wounds, pierced ears, etc.), oral and rectal mucosa, perineum, groin Monitor vital signs every 4 hours, including respiratory status. Report any signs of upper respiratory infection immediately. Monitor signs of impending sepsis. Do not give live virus vaccines to the immunosuppressed child; and caution parents to avoid exposing the child to chickenpox or measles	Infection does not develop or is detected immediately. Temperature is lower than 101 F and granulocyte count is above 1000 mm
2. Potential for hemorrhage due to thrombocytopenia	Monitor the child for the appearance of petechiae, ecchymoses, or hematomas. Give meticulous skin care; monitor thrombocyte levels.(See Chapter 36 for additional nursing interventions for the child who is bleeding)	Platelet count is above 20,000/ mm^3. Observable areas of bleeding resolve. Child is protected from trauma
3. Fatigue and activity intolerance related to anemia	Arrange furniture and objects in home or hospital room to be within easy reach of child Determine with child which self-care activities will require nursing assistance and offer help in those areas Plan care so that child can rest undisturbed for extended periods Arrange pillows around child's head or elevate the head of the bed to allow optimal breathing Note pallor in skin, oral mucosa, conjunctiva, and nail beds See Chapter 36 for additional nursing care of the child with anemia)	Child does not become excessively tired or short of breath. Activity tolerance is increased. Hemoglobin levels are maintained at greater than 10g during periods of treatment
4. Potential alteration in nutrition related to traumatized oral mucosa	Continue regular and thorough mouth care Apply dry tea bag to gingival bleeding points to control local bleeding Assess child's mouth and gums regularly for changes in mucous membrane Avoid irritating foods, such as extremely dry, hot, or acidic solids and liquids (citrus juices, carbonated sodas, bread, or hot beverages) if the child does not tolerate them. Offer chilled yogurt, gelatin, and nonirritating liquids such as chocolate milk Give small, frequent feedings with high-protein liquids	Child maintains nutrition adequate in proteins and calories. Child is adequately hydrated. Oral mucosa remains intact or suffers only minor breakdown

ciency as fatigue, shortness of breath, and dizziness. Children are able to tolerate low hemoglobin levels quite well, however, and symptoms may not be evident until the child becomes profoundly anemic. The decision to administer packed red blood cells varies among physicians. If the child is asymptomatic and the nadir has passed with recovery expected within a short time, transfusion may not be given. If, however, anemia is profound and complicated by nutritional factors, recovery is not expected to occur for a number of weeks, or the child is symptomatic, transfusions will be administered. There is some theoretical evidence that treatment, in particular radiation therapy, is more effective in the presence of well-oxygenated tissue. Thus there may be some effort to keep the child's hemoglobin above 10 g during periods of treatment. (See Chapter 36 for additional discussion of nursing management of the anemic child and administration of blood components.)

Bleeding and Bruising Platelets, also known as thrombocytes, play a major role in blood coagulation. When the number of available platelets is reduced, the child is at risk for bruising and bleeding tendencies. Circulating platelets may be decreased because of the effects of treatment on bone marrow production, and they may also be consumed during periods of fever and infection. These complications are much more common with leukemia, as platelet production is suppressed because of disease activity as well as treatment.

Bruising may be characterized by petechiae or by ecchymoses. Petechiae occur most frequently over pressure points. If the child has been lying in bed, petechiae may be found on the back and sacrum; if the child has been standing, petechiae may appear on feet and legs; if the child has been crying or coughing, the nurse checks the eyes, head, and chest. Bleeding may vary in amount from mild blood loss to life-threatening hemorrhage. In addition to platelet suppression, bleeding may be caused by liver involvement, which can decrease circulating coagulants; by an enlarged spleen, where platelets are sequestered and therefore not available for circulation; or by a primary bleed due to tumor erosion of vessels.

If bleeding is caused by decreased platelets and cannot be stopped by local pressure, platelet-concentrate transfusion is required. Before platelets could be separated from other blood components and administered separately as a concentrate, bleeding was the primary cause of death in leukemia. The child becomes vulnerable to bleeding episodes when the platelet count drops below 50,000/mm^3, and special caution is warranted when the count is below 20,000/mm^3.

There is disagreement among physicians about the use of "prophylactic" platelet transfusions when the count drops below 20,000/mm^3. Some physicians believe the child is so likely to bleed that platelets should be administered to prevent the possibility of serious hemorrhage. Other physicians believe platelets should be administered only when there is actual bleeding. Because the platelet concentrate contains some leukocytes and antibodies, immune response reactions can develop after a number of transfusions, destroying many of the newly infused platelets. Physicians who discourage prophylactic administration of platelets wish to keep potentially sensitizing transfusions to an absolute minimum. Once the child has become sensitized, even larger volumes of platelet concentrate do not raise the circulating platelet count significantly and still leave the child vulnerable to hemorrhage. Infused platelets are viable for 1–3 days with the peak effect occurring 2 hours after transfusion. For this reason a 2-hour postplatelet infusion blood count may be used to document the platelet rise.

Hemorrhage can be spontaneous or a result of trauma. Any number of sites are prone to bleeding. If sufficient blood has been lost, packed red blood cells or whole blood will be administered. Circulatory volume should be quickly restored. Platelets will be given if the child is thrombocytopenic. Fresh-frozen plasma, which contains clotting factors, may reduce bleeding, especially if there is liver dysfunction. The nurse observes the child with a decreased platelet count for warning signs of impending internal hemorrhage. Sudden restlessness and confusion, often called *air hunger*, loss of consciousness, or drop in blood pressure should alert the nurse to possible hemorrhage. Stool, urine, and emesis are guaiac-tested for the presence of blood. Epistaxis is a common occurrence. (See Chapter 36 for discussion of nursing care during bleeding episodes.)

Infection Many factors contribute to the risk of infection in the child with cancer. These factors are primarily related to four host defense vulnerables: (a) phagocytic, (b) humoral, (c) cell-mediated, and (d) mechanical barrier. Disturbances of phagocytic defenses are associated with marrow suppression caused by chemotherapy and radiation. In addition to treatment effects, children with leukemia are particularly vulnerable because their bone marrow also is dysfunctional as a result of their disease.

The child's immune system also may be dysfunctional (see Chapter 37). Humoral immunity, mediated by cells originating in the bone marrow, is suppressed by treatment and also may be affected by the disease itself. Cell-mediated immunity is altered by treatment, especially by the use of steroids. Similarly, the malignant process plays a role in the disturbance of cell-mediated immunity. This is particularly true with both Hodgkin's disease and non-Hodgkin's lymphoma. Malnutrition, which may be present during times of active treatment or when disseminated disease is present, is another factor in susceptibility to infection. Malnutrition contributes to immune defense dysfunction by affecting both humoral and cell-mediated immunity.

Disturbance of mechanical barrier defense can occur when tissue becomes fragile as a result of chemotherapy and radiation. Stomatitis and fragile erythematous skin, for example, provide easy access to infective agents. Intrusive diagnostic procedures, and supportive care such as hyperalimentation catheters, lumbar punctures, and venipunctures also encourage opportunistic infection.

Children are most vulnerable to infection when their absolute granulocyte count falls below 1000 mm. This is referred to as *neutropenia*. Since the absolute granulocyte count generally is not listed on the laboratory report, it may be calculated by multiplying the percentage of granulocytes by the total white blood count. For example, if a child has 20% granulocytes and 3000 total white blood count, then 0.20 times 3000 equals a 600 absolute granulocyte count, and the child is considered neutropenic.

The nurse observes the neutropenic child closely for signs of infection. Prompt action is required whenever an infection is suspected. If left untreated, a neutropenic child can die of sepsis within 8 hours. Unfortunately, it is often difficult to document the classic signs and symptoms of infection. Because the child has inadequate numbers of functional white blood cells, pus, inflammation, and therefore pain may not be present. A wound that looks clean and healing may actually be a focal point of infection. Careful daily assessment of the neutropenic child to document infectious sites is a nursing responsibility.

Temperature is monitored every 4 hours as an indicator of infection. Occasionally, it is possible to have an infectious process without a significant temperature elevation. For example, the child on long-term steroids may run a subnormal temperature. The septic child also may exhibit a subnormal temperature. In spite of these exceptions, temperature is one of the better indicators and should be followed routinely. Often it is difficult during the night shift to conceive of waking the sleeping child to record the vital signs, but this should not be skipped for the neutropenic child, as treatment for infection must begin immediately, and if no action is taken until morning, the infection may be refractory to treatment.

Whenever infection is suspected and routinely if the temperature is above 39 C (101 F) and the absolute granulocyte count is below 1000 mm (indicating neutropenia), the child should be evaluated for infection. Cultures of blood, throat, sputum, urine, stool, and any specific lesion or suspicious area are collected for examination. Ideally, all cultures should be obtained before antibiotic therapy is begun. A chest radiograph may be ordered to evaluate subclinical pneumonia.

Because the infection may be life threatening and the specific causative agent not known or only suspected, broad-spectrum bacteriocidal coverage with intravenous antibiotics is begun. Although specific drugs may vary among institutions and physician preference, broad coverage is most commonly instituted by triple antibiotic therapy of carbenicillin, gentamicin, and a cephalosporin. Gentamicin and a cephalosporin are useful against gram-negative bacteria, which are common sources of infection. Carbenicillin is recommended because of its activity against *Pseudomonas* infection. Because of heightened susceptibility, the child may have multiple pathogens responsible for the infection and may have multiple repeated infections of the same organism.

At some cancer centers, when treatment of the disease is expected to cause prolonged periods of neutropenia, the child may be placed in a germ-free environment such as a laminar airflow room (see Chapter 37). Nonabsorbable oral antibiotics are administered to sterilize the gut. The child receives only sterilized food. The benefit of the germ-free environment must be weighed against the isolation and psychologic trauma to the child.

Unfortunately, antibiotics are less effective in the neutropenic child. If the child does not respond to systemic antibiotics within 48–72 hours, granulocyte transfusions may be done. These transfusions must be given on a daily basis until the child shows improvement. Infusion of granulocytes can be associated with hypersensitivity blood reactions. The nurse needs to be alert for signs and symptoms of these reactions, such as chills, rash, hives, blood pressure change, and tachycardia.

What initially appears to be a localized infection may quickly become a septicemia. The nurse monitors the child for signs of septic shock. Hypotension, confusion and apprehension, shortness of breath, chills, and a subnormal temperature are classic warning signs. Aggressive treatment is required whenever septic shock is suspected. Treatment includes vasopressors, corticosteroids, antibiotics, and granulocyte transfusion. Oxygen administration and even mechanical ventilatory assistance may be necessary to maintain tissue oxygenation. Renal perfusion must be closely evaluated as hypotension may create renal failure. If renal failure is suspected, the rate of fluid administration is altered and drug doses, particularly potassium and antibiotics, must be lowered to prevent serious toxicity.

Viral, fungal, or protozoal pathogens, rather than bacteria, may be responsible for the infection. Fungal pathogens include *Candida albicans, Aspergillus, cryptococcus,* and, in endemic areas, *Histoplasma*. Amphotericin B is the drug of choice for serious fungal infection. This drug causes both nephrotoxicity and hypokalemia, particularly when prolonged administration is required. The drug is infused daily over a period of hours. The solution is light sensitive so it is covered with a paper bag or aluminum foil during administration. A most unpleasant side effect for the child is severe chills and fever during drug infusion. Premedication with antihistamines, hydrocortisone, and/or meperidine may reduce these symptoms.

The most common protozoal infection is *Pneumoncystis carinii,* which presents as a diffuse pneumonia. It occurs most commonly in individuals who are immunosuppressed and malnourished. It is also likely to occur during periods of remission. The disease is difficult to diagnose and treat. Previously, deep intramuscular injection of pentamidine isethionate was the drug of choice, but use of oral sulfamethoxazole-trimethoprim (Bactrim or Septra) has proved more effective.

Viral infections are also more common in the immunosuppressed child, particularly the child in remission. Serious viral infections in the child with cancer include chickenpox (varicella), measles, herpes zoster, and herpes simplex. Although chickenpox and measles are benign illnesses in normal children, they may be life threatening in the immunosuppressed child with cancer. The child with cancer must carefully avoid exposure to other children with these viruses. When children with measles and chickenpox are present in the child's school or neighborhood, appropriate steps must be taken to isolate the child with cancer. If the child has been exposed to chickenpox, zoster immunoglobulin (ZIG) or zoster immune plasma (ZIP) may be given within the first 72 hours after exposure. Gamma globulin may be given for measles exposure. Measles vaccination or any other childhood immunization with live virus vaccine should not be given to the immunosuppressed child, as this may cause the disease rather than prevent it. Interferon may be useful in the treatment of some viral infections associated with childhood cancer.

Ideally, nursing management of the neutropenic child should focus on prevention of infection. Strict handwashing technique and care in handling intravenous lines and catheters or other tubings is extremely important and must be consistently practiced. Because the child is more vulnerable to nosocomial infections, hospitalization should be kept to a minimum. Parents must be taught preventive care, how to recognize an infection, and when to seek additional care so they can provide proper supervision of the neutropenic child at home.

Reverse isolation may be ordered for the hospitalized child (see Chapter 37). This is particularly important if the child is admitted to a general pediatric unit where children who commonly have chronic infections such as cystic fibrosis may also be hospitalized. Reverse isolation will not, however, prevent many infections. Neutropenic children are infected most often by endogenous organisms found in their natural microbial flora. During periods of neutropenia these organisms become pathogenic so that children actually become infected by their own gut flora.

Meticulous rectal care is performed so that the natural microbial flora, particularly *Escherichia coli,* is not introduced into a break in the mucosa. For this reason, rectal temperature, suppositories, and enemas should be avoided. The child is assessed for the presence of skin lesions or entry sites from diagnostic or treatment procedures. Band-aids and old blood should be promptly removed since they provide excellent media to promote infection.

Should lesions, abscesses, or other sources of infection develop, early treatment and continued close observation are required. The nurse also provides comfort measures to decrease pain from the inflammatory process and discomfort from fever should they be present.

Pain Management During all phases of treatment, comfort measures should be a high nursing priority (see Chapter 29). Discomfort can be caused by many factors, including the disease process, fever, nausea, stomatitis, and diagnostic procedures. The child's perception of the meaning of discomfort is developmentally based. The young child may perceive pain and discomfort as punishment. Play intervention programs should be an integral part of any childhood cancer program. The child strives to deal with the overwhelming demands of the disease and treatment. A structured play program assists the child to gain psychologic mastery over the perceived threats to stability and sense of self. (Therapeutic play is discussed in Chapter 28.)

Cancer-Related Pain There are a number of physiologic and psychologic variables in cancer pain. Pain perception is an individual matter. Perception, meaning, and response to pain vary from child to child. Disease-related causes include tumor infiltration, compression, obstruction, and partial or complete occlusion of pain-sensitive structures. Necrosis, inflammation, and infection as a result of the disease process or side effects of treatment also cause pain. Psychologic aspects related to fear, apprehension, and anxiety may enhance the pain experience.

The initial goal of pain control is to identify the factors causing the pain. Ideally the source of the pain, whether physiologic or psychologic, should be removed. For example, if pain is related to infection, antibiotic therapy may remove the source of pain. Bone pain caused by disease infiltration and stretching of the pain-sensitive periosteum often results in excruciating pain. Several low-dose treatments of radiation therapy reduce the pressure on the periosteum and offer dramatic pain relief. Until therapeutic intervention can remove the source of pain, narcotic treatment and comfort measures should be instituted. When pain is caused by disease-related processes, particularly when advanced disease is present, treatment that removes the source of pain may not be possible. If this occurs, pain control by narcotic treatment and comfort measures is the focus of therapy.

Pain is not synonymous with cancer, although this is a frequent misconception of the public. Since the child and family may fear that severe pain is a part of cancer, reeducation is necessary. The child and family must be assured that should pain develop, effective pain control techniques are available.

Narcotic Management When pain is due to a chronic condition, narcotic treatment should not follow the same guidelines as for acute pain management. Because the cause of the pain is not amenable to treatment and will not go away over time, administering drugs on an as-needed basis is inappropriate. Drugs offered on an as-needed basis require the pain to recur before further drugs are given. This simply increases apprehension and anxiety because the child continues to experience pain periodically throughout the day. Thus drugs should be administered on a routine (not an as-needed) basis so the pain cycle is halted.

There is no one ideal pain control drug. A narcotic should be chosen because of the degree of pain and its effectiveness with the particular child. An appropriate dosage level and schedule must be tailored to the individual child. Sometimes very high doses of drugs must be given and will not cause the drowsiness or significant respiratory suppression that would be expected in an otherwise normal child. The exact reason for this is not known but is thought to relate to an alteration in the pain receptors in the brain.

The route of drug administration should also receive consideration. As long as a drug can be absorbed through the gastrointestinal tract, the oral route should be used. Because the child is receiving the drug on a routine basis, there is no advantage to intramuscular or intravenous injection. The latter routes offer more rapid absorption than oral administration, but since a constant blood level is maintained when the drug is given routinely, absorption speed is not a factor. Several narcotics such as morphine and methadone are available in liquid form. This allows easier individual titration of a therapeutic dose for each child. It may also be easier to swallow than pills or capsules. If nausea, vomiting, or swallowing prevent oral administration, rectal suppositories may be considered if the leukocyte count is adequate. When less invasive methods of drug administration are not effective, then intramuscular injection, if the platelet count is adequate, or intravenous injection may be necessary.

It is important to remember that dosage levels change with the route of administration. An adequate dose must be given if pain control is to be achieved, and the nurse assumes a major role in documenting the effectiveness of pain medication. Data are gathered from the child, the parent, and through observation. The nurse carefully records the child's response to medication and any continuing pain patterns. When pain control is inadequate, the nurse provides additional information to the physician so that the drug or dosage can be adjusted.

Nausea and constipation can be problematic side effects of narcotic administration. An antiemetic may be administered to control nausea. Bowel function should be carefully monitored. The nursing focus should be on preventing constipation rather than treating constipation. Stool softeners or stimulants may be required.

Nonnarcotic Interventions In addition to administration and evaluation of pain medication, the nurse uses other intervention strategies to provide comfort and decrease pain perception. Basic comfort measures should always be a part of nursing care. Bathing and positioning and providing oral hygiene and a clean, noncluttered environment are standard requirements of good nursing care. Encouraging the parent to hold and rock the young child is also therapeutic.

Distraction is another useful intervention (see Chapter 29). The nurse keeps in mind, however, that distraction is not a substitute for adequate pain medication but instead provides an additional resource.

Interventions that promote relaxation are excellent comfort techniques. A warm bath may effectively reduce muscle tension and encourage relaxation. Children are very suggestible and therefore are good candidates for progressive relaxation techniques combined with guided imagery. Relaxation techniques are easy-to-learn, beneficial resources for every nurse to use.

The child is also an excellent candidate for hypnosis. Recent studies have found hypnosis to be a positive adjuvant to other cancer pain-control measures (Barbora and Gitelson, 1980). Before a nurse uses hypnosis as a method of pain control, however, specific training in hypnotic technique is required.

The nurse also needs to remember that psychologic variables play a significant role in pain perception. If the child feels isolated or anxious and fearful about the disease status or family relationships, administration of narcotics will not totally ease the pain. The nurse carefully assesses the child's emotional response to the illness and family interactions. Supportive counseling or referral to child psychologic services are necessary to deal effectively with the psychologic variables of pain control.

Nutritional Needs

The disease process and the effects of treatment contribute to malnutrition in the child with cancer. Because treatment is more effective and potential side effects, such as infection, are less common in the well-nourished child, maintaining optimal nutrition should be a high nursing priority.

Cancer Cachexia Severe weight loss and wasting of body tissue characterize *cancer cachexia*, the general state of ill health and malnutrition associated with a neoplastic illness. Many factors contribute to cancer cachexia, including an increased metabolic rate due to tumor activity. Side effects of treatment, which cause nausea, vomiting, and stomatitis, reduce the child's desire and ability to eat and drink. Additionally, tumor metabolites in the circulation may directly cause anorexia and alteration in taste perceptions. Once cachexia is evident, it is difficult to halt. Intravenous administration of hyperalimentation (total parenteral nutrition) may be necessary (see Chapter 38).

Psychologic factors also contribute to cancer cachexia. When the child does not feel well, is frightened by unfamiliar surroundings, or is receiving foods not usually served at home, food and fluid intake may decrease. The parent may become alarmed when the child continues to eat poorly and lose weight. It is important that eating not become a battle between parent and child. The parent must understand the importance of good nutrition but at the same time must be taught how and when to approach the child about eating so that conflict does not develop.

Nutritional Assessment A complete nutritional assessment includes a dietary history (see Chapter 15), anthropomorphic measurements (muscle circumference and skin-fold thickness), laboratory measurement of serum proteins and total lymphocyte count, skin testing for immune-response capacity, and weight change over time. Any combination of these tests may actually be used in the clinical setting. Lymphocyte count and skin testing may not accurately reflect nutritional status because chemotherapy and radiation may alter the results. If the child is receiving steroids, weight gain or even weight maintenance may only reflect fluid retention. Thus some assessment techniques must be evaluated carefully before they are applied to the child with cancer.

In addition, the nurse observes the child's current eating pattern. Can decreased eating habits be related to fear of impending treatments, pain, or nausea? Would better timing of pain medication or antiemetics increase eating? What is the social setting during meals? Is the child isolated? Is the general setting conducive to eating or are there unpleasant noises or odors? The nurse also observes the child-parent interaction during meals (Principles of care for meeting nutritional needs of hospitalized children are discussed in Chapter 29.)

Dietary Modifications Taste alterations that may occur include intolerance to some meats and an increased threshold for sweets. If a protein aversion develops, the child will refuse meats such as beef and pork. Other sources of protein should be offered, including poultry, fish, cheese, nuts, and protein-rich beans. Children should not be forced to continue eating foods which they cannot tolerate. Besides finding these foods distasteful, forcing the child to eat intolerable foods can create a generalized aversion to all foods. The child may dislike sweet-tasting foods because these foods no longer taste sweet; additional sweetening may make the food more palatable. Some children simply will not eat any sweet foods because of their altered taste.

Meals should be based on the child's individual preference and emphasize maximum calories and nutrients. Calories can be increased by adding butter, cream, mayonnaise, honey, or granola to appropriate foods during cooking. Cheese also can be added to many foods, thus increasing both calories and protein. Milkshakes, puddings, and other nutritional snacks can be offered between meals. Although "junk foods" should not become the mainstay of the child's diet, many of these foods can be made more nutritious. For example, additional cheese and meats (if tolerated) can be added to pizza.

Small, frequent feedings rather than large meals are most acceptable. It may be better to avoid serving liquids with meals since they can quickly make the child feel full. Determining which time of the day is most agreeable to the child helps the child to eat a larger meal. Many children feel better in the morning, and breakfast may be the best time of the day to maximize calories and protein.

Developmental Needs

The child's life should be kept as normal as possible in spite of the illness. Routines should be patterned after the child's preillness activities. Return to school is encouraged. The child's reentry to school is facilitated by the hospital-based or outpatient nurse directly contacting the school or by referral to the school or community health nurse. Teachers need to understand accurately the child's condition and any limitations. They also need reassurance and encouragement to treat the child normally and not single the child out as "special."

The child's body image may be altered by the disease and treatment, and this may result in feelings of self-consciousness and withdrawal from peers and activities. Nurses need to offer sensitive support and encouragement to deal with problems of self-concept and to maintain social contacts. The nursing staff also needs to guard against sheltering the child in the hospital setting, making it so emotionally comfortable for the child that the child resists return to home and community.

In keeping the child's life as normal as possible, discipline should be maintained. This may be very difficult for parents who feel guilty in placing limits on a sick child. Children need the continued security of appropriate discipline and limits. The nurse thus provides anticipatory guidance, allowing parents to express their reluctance to discipline their children but reinforcing the children's need for continued discipline. (See Chapter 30 for further discussion of the implications of chronic illness for the child.)

One way to help meet the child's developmental needs, and especially the need to lead as normal a life as possible, is to continue care of the child at home, particularly when hospitalization and active treatment measures are no longer beneficial. A family who chooses this alternative needs support and education so that the members are comfortable with the child's physiologic care and the family's emotional well-being at home. Hospice programs also provide comprehensive psychosocial and physiologic care in the home setting. (Further discussion of the needs of the dying child and of the role that hospices can play can be found in Chapter 32.)

Emotional Needs

The general emotional needs of the child and family related to aberrant cellular growth vary depending on whether the child is hospitalized (see Chapter 29), is in a state of remission or chronic illness (see Chapter 30), or is in the terminal stages of the disease (see Chapter 32). The following stressors, however, may be particularly significant in cases of childhood cancer:

- The publicity and fear surrounding cancer in today's society may intensify the anxiety felt by parents and children when the diagnosis is communicated.
- The severity of the side effects of many cancer treatments may exacerbate the child's emotional response to the disease.
- The uncertainty over whether a given treatment will be effective will prolong the fear and anxiety of all concerned.
- The treatment for childhood cancer may severely tax the financial resources of the family, creating emotional stress over normal family function.
- The stress of the child's illness may place a strain on the marital relationship of the parents, driving them apart rather than bringing them closer together.
- A sibling may experience not only the normal emotions of fear, guilt, or resentment, but also the fear of contracting the same disease, especially if the sibling and the ill child are twins.

The nurse can play a major role in helping the family meet its own emotional needs by

1. Promoting open and honest communication among all family members, and especially between the parents, to offset any tendency toward individual isolation
2. Referring the family to community resources and parental support groups, such as Candlelighters, to provide financial assistance, needed information, and emotional and social support
3. Providing opportunities for the siblings to express their feelings and to give them as much contact with the ill child as appropriate, while making sure they understand that they cannot "catch" their sibling's disease
4. Being aware of the family's anxieties and thus possibly preventing the members from not hearing or understanding important information (thus the nurse needs to be ready to take more time to prepare the child and family for treatments and procedures, to repeat explanations more frequently, and to answer more questions than usual.)
5. Encouraging parents and siblings to participate as much as possible in the care of the ill child

The family who must face advanced disease and the impending death of the child requires tremendous nursing support and assistance. The nurse encourages open expression of feelings and anticipatory mourning. The death of a child is one of the most profound crises a parent can face. Unfortunately, traditional health care services are often terminated at the death of the child. The family must then deal with their bereavement alone. A parental support group, Compassionate Friends, is available for parents who have experienced the death of a child. Follow-up with bereaved families should be encouraged and integrated into health care services. (See Chapter 32 for further discussion of the family who must face the death of a child.)

Health Maintenance Needs

The Child During Remission The nurse assumes a major role assisting the family to understand the child, the disease, the treatment, and the side effects that may occur. Because the child spends most time at home, parents must be knowledgeable about and comfortable with the care of their child at home. When the child is hospitalized, the parent should also be encouraged to participate in the child's care, continuing the important nurturing and caregiving role. The nursing staff should develop a systematic educational program for parents that can be adapted to each family's unique situation. Written materials and care directions should be given to the family so that the members may refer to them should problems develop at home.

Throughout the course of the illness, parents are confronted with well-meaning friends and relatives and media sources who advocate the use of unproven cancer treatments. Wanting to do everything possible to assure the children's cure, parents may seriously consider alternatives to conventional therapy. Generally, parents choose to investigate unproven treatments (a) during the initial diagnostic period—hoping to find someone who will offer a more favorable diagnosis and treatment or (b) when metastatic disease has been identified—hoping to find someone who can guarantee a cure. Parents need to know that interest in investigating other treatments is normal and that even if they do not actively look for alternatives, friends and relatives or sometimes even unsolicited strangers may contact them. The attitude and sensitivity of the health-care professionals is critical in helping parents to feel comfortable in discussing their concerns about current treatments and alternative methods. The nurse encourages parents to bring in information and assists the parents in finding out what is scientifically known about the treatment. Parents should see the health professional as a supportive ally who may personally discourage the use of unproven treatments but will not condemn and reject the family for investigating other treatments.

The Cured Child Discharging a child cured of cancer is a very satisfying experience, although those cured of childhood cancer still must face residual and late effects of the treatment. The child's growth into adulthood and adjustment in society should be a matter of keen interest to health professionals. The goal in treating the child with cancer is not only to cure the child but also to make the treatment and long-term consequences of the treatment compatible with a normal life-style. Now that many children with cancer can be cured, clinicians are dealing with the new challenges of the cured child.

Physiologic Considerations Permanent physical impairments can result from treatment. If side effects of chemotherapy and radiation have damaged any organ system, normal function may be impaired. Visual and functional defects occur from necessary amputation.

A small percentage of children cured of cancer may be sterile. Chemotherapy and radiation to reproductive organs can result in gonadal failure, causing amenorrhea and testicular failure, but many children mature, marry, and conceive normal offspring. There does not appear to be a significant risk of producing defective children in parents who have been cured of childhood cancer.

Radiation therapy to soft tissue or the bony skeleton can cause atrophy. Radiation to only one side of the vertebral column results in asymmetrical growth, evidenced by scoliosis or kyphosis. Learning disabilities affecting attention span and short-term memory do occur in the child treated for acute leukemia with prophylactic cranial radiation and intrathecal methotrexate (Meadows and Evans, 1976).

An ironic contradiction of many chemotherapy agents and radiation is that they can cause mutations resulting in new cancer formation. This was particularly evident in the early application of radiation therapy with less sophisticated techniques. Secondary malignancies did occur in former sites of radiation. Further study is required to understand the risk and cause of secondary malignancies in individuals cured of childhood cancer. Clinicians are now focusing their attention on developing techniques to not only cure childhood cancer but also prevent late complications of the disease and treatment.

Psychosocial Considerations A number of restrospective studies have been used to document the long-term adjustment of individuals treated for childhood cancer (Holmes and Holmes, 1975; Koocher and O'Malley, 1981; O'Malley, et al., 1979). Most of these researchers have reported that successful adjustment is made by most survivors of childhood cancer. Many social challenges, however, confront the cured individual. Concern over sexuality, ability to bear children, and body image may delay entry into marriage. Discrimination in employment also may occur, particularly if employers are concerned that their insurance premiums may be raised. Employers are also concerned by the amount of sick time or absenteeism the individual may require. A review of the employment records of those cured of childhood cancer, however, showed no increase in leave time from jobs over other workers (Koocher, 1981). Survivors of childhood cancer are able to obtain health insurance and life insurance if they participate in a group plan. Those individuals who seek individual policies are frequently denied coverage. If coverage is offered, the individual must pay much higher premiums or take out policies that exclude any payment for cancer.

To receive satisfaction from curing the child with cancer, consequences after treatment must not be so great as to impair successful social adjustment. Appropriate guidance and advocacy for these individuals should be available so that they may successfully enter into productive adulthood.

The Child With a Neoplasm

Acute Leukemias

Leukemia is a primary malignancy of the bone marrow. It is the most common malignancy of childhood, accounting for 34% of all childhood cancers. There are several types of leukemia, which are divided into two major classifications: (a) acute leukemia and (b) chronic leukemia. Originally, as their names imply, acute leukemia had a sudden onset with a rapid downhill course resulting in death, and chronic leukemia had a more insidious onset and protracted course. Because of the progress in successfully treating acute leukemia, the terms *acute* and *chronic* no longer reflect their original meaning. The acute leukemias constitute 98% of childhood leukemia. The remaining 2% are chronic myelogenous (granulocytic) leukemias. Acute and chronic leukemia are differentiated by the maturity of the involved cell. Acute leukemia involves immature blast cells, whereas chronic leukemia primarily involves mature cells. Table 45-13 identifies the different types of acute leukemia.

Of the acute childhood leukemias, the vast majority (about 80%) are acute lymphocytic (lymphoblastic) leukemia (Fochtman and Foley, 1982). This type of leukemia is characterized by overproliferation of immature lymphocytes known as lymphoblasts. The disease is commonly referred to by its abbreviated letters ALL. The disease can be further subdivided by the predominant immunologic marker of the abnormal lymphocyte involved. Such subdivision also reflects prognosis and intensity of treatment required to control the disease. The subclasses for ALL include T lymphocyte, B lymphocyte, pre–B lymphocyte, and null cell (meaning no definite immunologic marker is present). Pre–B-cell and null cell leukemia have the best prognosis. Fortunately over 75% of children with ALL have null cell disease. Other prognostic factors have been identified. The child with the most favorable diagnosis is, at diagnosis, between the age of 2 and 6; with a peripheral white blood count below 10,000; no lymphadenopathy, hepatosplenomegaly, or central nervous system involvement; and null cell disease. The overall survival rate is 50%; with good prognostic factors the survival rate is closer to 60%–70% (Simone and Rivers, 1984).

There are two other general types of acute leukemia in childhood besides ALL: (a) acute undifferentiated leukemia

TABLE 45-13 Types of Acute Leukemia in Childhood

Type	Abbreviation	Primary involved cell line
Acute lymphocytic leukemia	ALL	Lymphoblast
Subclass by immunologic marker		
T cell		
B cell		
pre–B cell		
null cell		
Acute undifferentiated leukemia	AUL	Unable to determine
Acute nonlymphocytic leukemia	ANLL	
Subclass by involved cell line		
Acute myelocytic leukemia	AML	Myeloblast
Acute myelomonocytic leukemia	AMML	Combination myeloblast and monoblast
Acute monocytic leukemia	AMoL	Monoblast
Erythyrocytic leukemia		Combination erythroblast and myeloblast

(AUL), which is the least common type of acute leukemia, and (b) acute nonlymphocytic leukemia (ANLL), which constitutes approximately 15% of childhood leukemia and includes a number of subclasses. Acute nonlymphocytic leukemia is characterized by the rapid overproliferation of immature cells that come from one of several cell lines, either myeloblasts, monoblasts, a combination of myeloblasts and monoblasts, and (rarely) a combination of erythroblasts and myeloblasts. The subclasses of ANLL are acute myelocytic (myeloblastic) leukemia (AML), acute myelomonocytic leukemia (AMML), acute monocytic leukemia (AMoL), and a very rare form of leukemia involving both erythroblasts and myeloblasts called erythrocytic leukemia. Although ANLL involves a heterogenous group of leukemias, the treatment strategy and prognosis are similar. Generally ANLL carries a much worse prognosis than ALL, although progress is being made. In the past remission duration was usually only 9–16 months with few children alive at 5 years. Recently Weinstein et al. (1983) statistically predicted that 56% of their patients less than 18 years of age would be alive and well 3 years after diagnosis.

The presenting symptoms of leukemia result from the overproliferation of leukemic cells in the bone marrow, which crowd out other normal cell lines. This causes bone marrow failure from decreased production of red blood cells, platelets, and neutrophils, resulting in anemia, bleeding tendencies, and infection. As a direct result of bone marrow failure over 50% of children have fever, pallor, and bruising/bleeding at diagnosis. Leukemia cells can migrate from the bone marrow and inlfiltrate extramedullary sites such as lymph nodes, liver, and spleen. Depending on the location and degree of these infiltrations, lymphadenopathy, mediastinal mass, hepatomegaly, and splenomegaly may be present at diagnosis. Leukemia cells also invade bones and the central nervous system, presenting as bone and joint pain, and meningeal symptoms manifested by vomiting, headache, and papilledema. Extramedullary involvement also can occur in reproductive organs, particularly the testes.

History, physical examination, and peripheral blood count showing the presence of blast cells raises the clinical suspicion of leukemia. The definitive diagnosis and identification of the actual type of leukemia is, however, determined by bone marrow aspiration. Examination of the bone marrow will generally reveal hypercellularity with 80%–90% of the bone marrow replaced with immature blast cells. Normally there are fewer than 5% immature white blood cells in the bone marrow. Because the blast cells have replaced normal cell lines, there is also a decrease in developing red blood cells, platelets, and granulocytes. A lumbar puncture is also performed to determine whether central nervous system disease is present.

Treatment

Acute Lymphocytic Leukemia There are several phases of treatment for ALL. The initial treatment called remission induction is intended to reduce the number of leukemic cells so there is no evidence of leukemia. Currently used are a combination of vincristine and prednisone, with or without a third drug such as L-asparginase. The child with poor prognostic factors may receive an alternative "high-risk" treatment protocol. Approximately 95% of children with ALL obtain a remission in 2–4 weeks after treatment is instituted (Simone and Rivers, 1984).

Once the child is in remission, prophylactic treatment for central nervous system disease is begun. The central nervous system prophylaxis is necessary because systemic treatment does not penetrate the blood–brain barrier. In the past, standard treatment has included both cranial radiation and intrathecal methotrexate. Intrathecal medication administration involves injecting the medication directly into the cerebrospinal fluid through a lumbar puncture. Because of the incidence of learning disabilities in the child who has received this treatment, some clinicians are omitting radiation and administering intrathecal methotrexate over an extended period of time (Klopovich and Cohen, 1984).

The third phase of treatment, maintenance therapy, is intended to reduce leukemic cells further so that a cure is obtained. A common maintenance protocol includes daily doses of 6-mercaptopurine and weekly doses of methotrexate. Periodic pulses (short-term, intermittent drug doses) of additional drugs such as vincristine and prednisone also may be included. Treatment is continued for 30–36 months.

If bone marrow relapse occurs, a second reinduction protocol will be initiated. The likelihood of cure after bone marrow relapse is poor, but second remissions can be achieved in most children. Bone marrow transplantation may be considered after the child has obtained a second remission since further relapse, eventually leading to death, is common.

If relapse occurs in extramedullary sites, bone marrow relapse generally follows. Testicular leukemia infiltrates occur in approximately 10% of males with ALL. Prophylactic therapy is not given because of the relatively low incidence, because presymptomatic treatment does not prevent disease development, and because treatment can result in sterility. When testicular leukemia occurs, radiation to the testes is given (Askin et al., 1981). Aggressive systemic therapy is also begun because of the likelihood of subsequent bone marrow relapse.

Acute Nonlymphocytic Leukemia Because the prognosis for ANLL is worse than ALL, treatment is more intensive. Remission induction includes protocols such as cytosine arabinoside, vincristine, and daunorubicin. In contrast to the 95% remission response in ALL only 60%—70% of children with ANLL ever achieve a first remission (Simone and Rivers, 1984). Because long-term survival was not common with ANLL, prophylactic central nervous system treatment was not routinely given. As the length of survival increases, prophylatic central nervous system treatment has become standard practice.

Bone marrow transplantation can be considered for the child with ANLL when the first remission is achieved. If bone marrow transplant is not an option, additional combinations of chemotherapy are administered. The drugs are given in two phases called early intensification and late intensification. Early intensification is used to provide reduction of leukemia cells. Drugs include doxorubicin and cytosine arabinoside. To prevent drug resistance, late intensification rotates several protocols. The following protocols may be included: 5-azacytidine, doxorubicin, POMP therapy (prednisone, vincristine, methotrexate, and 6-mercaptopurine), and further infusion of cytosine arabinoside.

Nursing Management Nursing management of the child with bone marrow suppression is essential to caring for the child with leukemia. Furthermore, hyperuricemia results from breakdown products during cell death. The leukemic process causes turnover of a large number of cells. Additionally, treatment destroys many cells. The combination of these two processes can cause very high uric acid levels. Urinary excretion of uric acid causes the uric acid to precipitate, leading to obstruction and renal failure. To prevent hyperuricemia, allopurinol, which blocks the formation of uric acid may be ordered. Liberal hydration and alkalinization of the urine by administration of sodium bicarbonate also reduce the renal toxicity of hyperuricemia.

The nurse assists the child and family to adapt to the disease and treatment requirements. Once initial hospitalization to diagnose leukemia has been completed, the child receives most of the ongoing therapy on an outpatient basis. The family and child must quickly learn care requirements at home. Comprehensive care is based on the individual needs of each child during every phase of the disease process.

Lymphomas

The lymphomas are broadly separated into two categories: Hodgkin's disease and non-Hodgkin's lymphoma (also called lymphosarcoma). Hodgkin's disease is characterized by abnormal cellular proliferation in lymph nodes. The predominant cell in Hodgkin's disease is the Reed-Sternberg cell. There also may be proliferation of lymphocytes, eosinophils, histiocytes, and collagen and fibrous tissue. The disease is considered to have one focus of origin with spread to nearby lymph nodes. There are four histologic types described as lymphocytic predominance, nodular sclerosis, mixed cellularity, or lymphocyte depletion.

Hodgkin's disease is more common in males than females. It is rare before the age of 5. There is a gradual increased incidence throughout childhood with a marked increase during adolescence. It accounts for 6.5% of childhood cancers.

Non-Hodgkin's lymphoma represent a group of diseases involving malignant cells of lymphoid tissue. Unlike Hodgkin's disease, they are considered to have no single focal origin and therefore are rarely localized. There is no histologic classification that is generally agreed upon. Subtypes may be identified as lymphocytic, undifferentiated, which includes Burkitt's tumor, convoluted lymphocytic, histiocytic, mixed lymphocytic–histiocytic, and immunoblastic (Lanzkowsky, 1980).

Non-Hodgkin's disease represents 6% of childhood cancers. It also is more common in males than females. The disease occurs equally in children of all ages.

The most common presenting sign of Hodgkin's disease

is painless swelling of a lymph node or several nodes generally in the cervical chain. Axillary, inguinal, mediastinal, and retroperitoneal nodes are less commonly the presenting site. General presenting symptoms include anorexia, lassitude, and malaise.

Staging of the disease is determined by the extent of lymph node and extranodal (disease of lymph nodes) involvement. A more favorable prognosis is associated with disease that is located on just one side of the diaphragm and without extranodal involvement. The presence of a group of systemic symptoms—fever, significant weight loss, and night sweats lends a less favorable prognosis. The presence or absence of systemic symptoms are denoted by adding to the traditional stage I to IV notation the letter *A* when symptoms are not present or adding the letter *B* when symptoms are present.

Extranodal involvement can occur in the spleen, liver, mediastinum, lung, central nervous system, and bones. Laboratory studies of serum copper level and ESR are performed at diagnosis and throughout the course of the illness. Levels are commonly elevated when Hodgkin's disease is present and therefore serum copper and ESR are good indicators of disease activity. Diagnostic studies will also include lymphangiogram or abdominal CT scan, inferior cavogram, liver function tests, bone marrow aspiration, chest radiograph, skeletal survey, and liver and spleen scan. Definitive diagnosis is made by biopsy of the enlarged lymph node with documented evidence of the Reed-Sternberg cell. An abdominal laparotomy is performed to evaluate intraabdominal lymph nodes. A liver biopsy and the bone marrow aspiration also are performed at that time. Traditionally a splenectomy also was performed since abnormal cells are often sequestered in the spleen. This measure is controversial, however, because of the increased risk of life-threatening pneumococcal infection in children who do not have spleens (Sullivan et al., 1984).

The presenting symptoms of non-Hodgkin's lymphoma depend on the specific location of the disease. The most common presentations include lymphadenopathy, abdominal involvement, and mediastinal mass. Symptoms associated with abdominal involvement are abdominal pain, vomiting, and diarrhea. Occasionally a palpable mass can be felt. Abdominal non-Hodgkin's lymphoma is also associated with gastrointestinal bleeding and intussusception. Immediate surgical intervention is required for intussusception. If a mediastinal mass is present, the child may complain of dyspnea and cough. Superior vena cava syndrome and pleural effusions may be present at diagnosis. Superior vena cava syndrome warrants immediate attention. Non-Hodgkin's lymphoma that occurs in the mediastinum often infiltrates the bone marrow, transforming the disease into an acute lymphocytic leukemia.

Burkitt's tumor exhibits a different presentation. The tumor generally involves the jaw and can grow to enormous size around the maxilla or eye. It may also present in the abdomen with disease located in the gastrointestinal tract and often the ovaries in the female. Bone marrow involvement does occur. Burkitt's tumor was originally identified in children living in Africa, where it has a high incidence. The tumor is much less common in the United States. On histologic examination, the American Burkitt's tumor and African Burkitt's tumor appear to be identical but vary in their presentation and disease progression.

Diagnostic studies for non-Hodgkin's lymphoma are similar to those performed for Hodgkin's disease with several exceptions. Serum copper and ESR are not useful disease activity indicators; the staging laparotomy is generally not performed because it offers no therapeutic or prognostic value. A lumbar puncture, however, is performed to identify any central nervous system involvement.

Treatment

Hodgkin's Disease Well-established treatment protocols have been developed for Hodgkin's disease. They are based on the clinical stage of disease. For early-stage disease (stages I, II, and IIIA) radiation therapy may be sufficient to cure the disease. If extensive disease is present (stages IIIB and IV) chemotherapy or a combination of chemotherapy and radiation are given. The most common chemotherapeutic protocol for Hodgkin's disease is MOPP therapy, which uses nitrogen mustard, vincristine, procarbazine, and prednisone. Other drug protocols have been used for the child who has relapsed or not responded to MOPP therapy. The overall prognosis is quite good. The child with early-stage disease has the most favorable prognosis. This is a very treatable tumor with the overall 5-year survival rate range from 75%—90% (Lanzkowsky, 1980).

Non-Hodgkin's Lymphoma Definitive therapy for non-Hodgkin's lymphoma has not been developed. Generally, treatment includes radiation of bulk disease and intensive chemotherapy. Chemotherapy protocols are often similar to those used in the treatment of high-risk leukemia. Remission should occur in 4–6 weeks after therapy has begun. Prophylactic central nervous system treatment identical to acute lymphocytic leukemia protocols may be used for those at risk for central nervous system involvement. As with other cancers, the child with limited disease has a more favorable prognosis. Once relapse occurs, treatment is only palliative. Three year survival rates range from 50%–80% depending on the extent of disease (Weinstein and Link, 1979).

Nursing Management Nursing care of the child with lymphoma will be based on the specific treatment and course of disease for that child. When the spleen has been removed, the child has a long-term risk of infection. These infections are most commonly caused by bacteria. The risk of infection seems to be particularly high in the younger child and less common in the adolescent. Some physicians may prescribe prophylactic penicillin. The nurse observes the child for signs of infection. Since the child is at home during much of the treatment period, the parent must understand the risk of serious infection in the child after the splenectomy.

From the initial contact with the child and family, the nurse prepares them for multiple impending intrusive procedures. Emotional outlets that include therapeutic play allow the child to master the stress of unpleasant diagnostic and treatment measures. If a laparotomy is planned, nursing management also includes preoperative preparation.

Side effects of chemotherapy are related to the specific drugs and doses that the child receives. Because the child with non-Hodgkin's lymphoma receives intensive therapy, side effects are common. Drugs such as cystosine arabinoside may be infused over time, requiring periodic hospitalization. The nurse assists the child to remain active during periods of hospitalization. School tutoring may be necessary so that the child does not get behind in school.

Brain Tumors

Central nervous system tumors constitute the second most common childhood cancer, accounting for approximately 19% of all childhood malignancies. Brain tumors are by far the most common central nervous system tumor. Two-thirds of brain tumors are located below the roof of the cerebellum, usually in the cerebellum or brainstem. They also are referred to as infratentorial, meaning they are below the tentorium in the posterior third of the brain. The remaining third of brain tumors are located above the cerebellum in the anterior two-thirds of the brain. These tumors are referred to as supratentorial (above the tentorium) and generally occupy the cerebrum. In contrast to those in children, most brain tumors in adults are supratentorial. The actual location of the tumor determines the type and extent of presenting signs and symptoms. It also determines how amenable the tumor is to the surgery and therefore ultimately the prognosis. (See Fig. 45-3 for the location of brain tumors in children.)

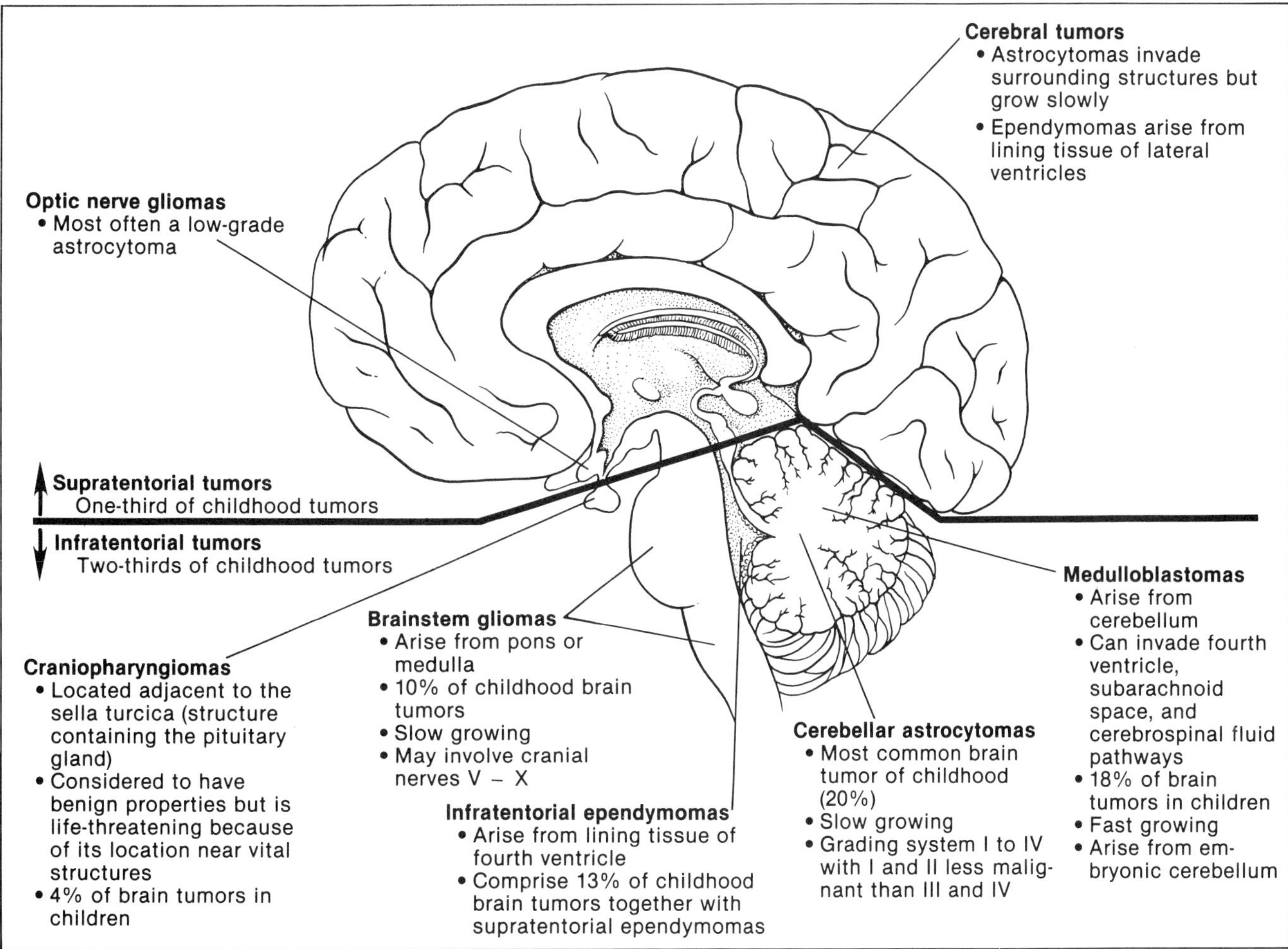

Figure 45-3 Locations of brain tumors in children.

Most childhood brain tumors arise from glial tissue, which is the structural tissue of the brain. Less commonly, tumors may arise from other tissue such as nerve cells, cranial nerves, the pineal gland, blood vessels, or neuroepithelium. Brain tumors are classified by the tissue involved. The specific location should also be noted. Infratentorial tumors of childhood include astrocytomas and medulloblastomas, most commonly found in the cerebellum; gliomas of the brainstem; and ependymomas, located in the lining of the fourth ventricle. The less common, supratentorial tumors of childhood are astrocytomas and ependymomas of the cerebrum, and craniopharyngiomas, located adjacent to the pituitary gland.

It is difficult to determine early signs and symptoms of brain tumors. This is particularly true in the young child, whose skull sutures have not yet closed and thus in whom tumors may be very large before detection. Children are also less likely to report symptoms of visual change or headache, adding to the delay in making a diagnosis.

The most common initial symptoms are often caused by increased intracranial pressure and include headache and vomiting. Headache is most notable in the morning, gradually improving during the day but returning the next morning. Vomiting is often not preceded by nausea. The child may be ready to eat immediately after vomiting. Vomiting also occurs more frequently in the morning and may become projectile. With increased cranial pressure, papilledema may be present.

Because most childhood brain tumors involve the cerebellum, coordination and balance are affected. Cerebellar signs include loss of balance, ataxia, wide-based gait, and head tilting. Widening sutures in the infant will be reflected in enlarging head circumference. Visual defects, altered reflexes, motor deficits due to cranial nerve involvement or paralysis, and altered consciousness and personality are additional signs and symptoms. Seizures are only associated with supratentorial tumors. Brain stem tumors may cause disturbance of the vital sign regulatory mechanisms, resulting in decreased pulse and respirations, increased blood pressure, and difficulty in maintaining normal body temperature.

When signs and symptoms of a brain tumor are present, a complete neurologic, developmental, and ophthalmic examination are indicated. Radiologic studies may include skull radiograph, radioisotope brain scanning, and CT scan. With the development of the CT scan, invasive procedures such as pneumoencephalogram and cerebral angiography are rarely necessary.

Treatment The initial and most useful treatment is surgical resection. Astrocytomas and medulloblastomas may be entirely resectable. If complete resection is not possible, then partial resection is attempted. Because of their location some brainstem tumors are not amenable to resection. Biopsy may even carry too much risk.

Postoperative radiation therapy is employed with many of the brain tumors and serves as either a primary or palliative treatment. Medulloblastomas, brainstem gliomas, and ependymomas are most commonly treated by radiation therapy. Since medulloblastomas and ependymomas tend to spread to the spinal cord, radiation therapy may include the spine.

Chemotherapy has been used for recurrent brain tumors. Some cancer treatment centers also are studying the effectiveness of chemotherapy as a primary treatment. Drugs include vincristine, lomustine (CCNU), procarbazine, and intrathecal methotrexate. Both single-agent and multiple-drugs protocols have been studied. Chemotherapy has not been as effective with brain tumors as with other childhood malignancies. This occurs because many chemotherapy agents do not adequately cross the blood–brain barrier and tumor cell growth may not be sufficient to be affected by the drugs. Until further studies can establish a beneficial role for chemotherapy in childhood brain tumors, surgery and radiation will remain the primary forms of treatment.

The overall 5-year survival rate for the child with a brain tumor is only about 20% (Gumbina, 1983). The most favorable prognosis is the child with a low-grade astrocytoma. The 5-year survival rate for these children is 65%.

Nursing Management The child undergoing brain surgery requires extensive nursing care. On admission, the child and parent may be very apprehensive about the impending diagnostic studies and surgery. Both parents and child should be prepared for each procedure. The nurse assesses the child for developmental and behavioral alterations. Neurologic assessment including vital signs; pupil size, equality, and response to light; level of consciousness; and strength and equality of grip are closely monitored for any changes. Head circumference is measured and followed in the infant. Seizure precautions are followed for the child suspected of a supratentorial tumor (see Chapter 42).

The nurses assist in preparing the child for surgery. The child should be told if hair is to be cut or shaved. Hair may be cut either prior to surgery or after the child has been anesthetized. The child needs to know that the head will be bandaged when the child wakes up after the surgery. There also may be considerable facial edema. Both parent and child should be prepared for the postoperative appearance of the child. The family should know also that the child may experience postoperative headache after awakening. The child who will be transferred to the intensive-care unit should be oriented to the unit and equipment preoperatively.

Postoperative neurologic signs are checked at frequent intervals. Proper positioning and maintenance of a patent airway are important immediate postoperative considerations. Positioning should avoid pressure on the operative site. The head may be elevated without pillows to facilitate cerebrospinal fluid flow and facial edema drainage. If the child's head is kept in the midline position, venous drainage will also be facilitated. Eye care to prevent corneal ulceration and drying should be instituted. Methylcellulose eye drops are administered frequently. Drainage on the surgical dressing is closely monitored. Profuse drainage, frank bleeding, or clear fluid indicating leaking cerebrospinal fluid require immediate physician attention.

Cerebral edema and increased intracranial pressure are postoperative concerns. The nurse monitors fluid balance carefully. Osmotic diuretics and steroids are administered. Headache may be the result of cerebral edema. Occasionally, anticonvulsants may also be necessary. The nurse monitors the child for postoperative seizures, which may develop from infection or intracranial bleeding. Once the child has regained consciousness, orientation and grip strength are frequently assessed and any residual surgical motor deficits are determined. When the child has improved and returned to the original admitting nursing unit, safety precautions should be observed if ataxia, skeletal weakness, or paresthesia are present.

Retinoblastoma

Retinoblastoma is a rare malignant tumor of the eye. The majority of these tumors are diagnosed before the child is 2 years of age. The tumor may result from genetic transmission of a defective gene or spontaneous cell mutation. Most tumors are thought to represent cell mutation rather than hereditary transmission. The disease may be unilateral or, in 29% of cases, bilateral. The child with bilateral disease is considered to have hereditary retinoblastoma.

The tumor may originate in the external retinal layers and extend into the subretinal space causing retinal detachment, or in the internal nuclear retinal layers and extend to the vitreous cavity. Tumors of the internal retinal layers occupying the vitreous cavity are diagnosed more easily because they are readily visible on ophthalmic examination. The tumor may metastasize through blood vessels serving the tumor or extend to the vascular choroid, resulting in bone marrow, liver, lymph node, or bone involvement. Occasionally, the tumor can involve the optic nerve, gain access to the subarachnoid space, and thereby produce brain and spinal metastases.

The most noticeable sign of retinoblastoma is a cat's eye reflex also called leukokoria. This reflex, which makes the child's pupil have a whitish glow, occurs when light is reflected off the tumor. Depending on the location of the tumor, the cat's eye reflex may be seen when the tumor is quite small or not until it is quite large. Strabismus or exophthalmous also are presenting signs. Occasionally, a variety of alterations in the iris may be seen at diagnosis.

Those families who have histories of retinoblastoma should have their young children frequently evaluated. Diagnostic evaluation includes intraocular echography, CT scan, and ophthalmic examination. Diagnosis is made by a special ophthalmic examination under general anesthesia. Liver and bone scans, lumbar puncture, and bone marrow aspiration are used to determine the presence of metastases.

Staging of the tumor indicates the likelihood of retaining useful vision rather than indicating survival or prognosis. The staging system places the child in one of five groups ranging from favorable vision preservation (group I) to unfavorable vision preservation (group V). The overall cure rate of retinoblastoma is 85%–90% (Foley, 1982).

Treatment Radiation is the treatment of choice if curative doses can be delivered while preserving vision. Therefore, unilateral tumors of groups I through III may be treated initially with radiation therapy. Because the child must be absolutely still during treatment to avoid damage to the eye lens, short-acting general anesthesia or heavy sedation and positioning the child's head in a half-cast may be necessary.

In more advanced disease surgical enucleation of the affected eye is the primary treatment. When both eyes are involved, as in bilateral disease, the less affected eye is radiated, and the severely affected eye is enucleated. In bilateral disease, if both eyes are affected equally, treatment depends on the extent of disease. In early disease both eyes will be radiated, and in advanced disease enucleation may be considered as a life-saving procedure. If brain or spinal metastases are present, craniospinal radiation may be given. Potential complications of radiation include retinal detachment, vitreous hemorrhage, glaucoma, cataracts, and secondary malignancies.

Chemotherapy is used for recurrent disease or when the tumor has extended into the choroid. Drugs that may be administered include cyclophosphamide, vincristine, doxorubicin, and intrathecal methotrexate. Additional therapies for localized disease such as laser surgery and cryotherapy are being investigated.

Nursing Management The enucleation of a child's eye is traumatic for parents. Introducing the parent to a family and child who has experienced the surgery and is doing well with an artificial eye eases fears that the procedure leaves a gross deformity. There is usually some postoperative swelling and bruising of the face. After enucleation no deep crater is left in the socket because a sphere is implanted during surgery so that the eye prosthesis may be easily applied. The child returns to the unit with a small bandage covering the eye. The eye socket requires little care. The parent should view the site and learn appropriate care soon after the surgical procedure. Saline irrigation and application of antibiotic cream may be ordered postoperatively. An eye patch is placed over the socket for a number of days primarily to keep the child from touching the site and contaminating the area.

The eye prosthesis is designed to match the color and size of the child's other eye. It may be fitted approximately

3 weeks after surgery. The artificial eye need not be removed except for periodic cleaning if a mucus film develops over the prosthesis (see Chapter 43).

Parents may desire genetic counseling if they are considering additional children (see Chapter 5). The disease cannot be detected by amniocentesis. Risk percentages are available. For unaffected parents there is a 1%–10% risk that additional children may also develop retinoblastoma. For children who survive retinoblastoma, risk for children they might have varies from 7%–15% for previous unilateral disease in the parent and 50% for previous bilateral disease in the parent (Wong and Dornan, 1982).

Neuroblastoma

Neuroblastoma is an embryonal tumor of tissue arising from the neural crest. Normally, in the developing fetus, embryonal neuroblast cells become mature ganglion tissue of the adrenal medulla and sympathetic ganglia. Why the tissue does not differentiate and instead becomes malignant is not known. In contrast to a few other childhood malignancies this tumor is not associated with chromosomal abnormalities or any congenital defects.

Neuroblastoma is the second most frequent solid tumor of childhood, yet it only accounts for between 7% and 8% of all childhood malignancies. Because of its embryonal origin and rapid growth, the tumor is almost always diagnosed before the child is 4 years old. Half of the children with neuroblastoma are diagnosed by 2 years of age. The disease can be present at birth.

Unlike the child with Wilms' tumor, the child with neuroblastoma generally appears quite ill at diagnosis. Because the sympathetic ganglia runs along each side of the spinal cord, the tumor may arise in a variety of locations, including the cervical-mediastinal, intraabdominal, presacral, and pelvic areas. Tumor involvement of the cervical sympathetic ganglia will present as a mass in the neck. Horner's syndrome (exophthalmos, miosis, ptosis, and anhydrosis) may be evident. If the ophthalmic sympathetic nerves are involved, the child's irises may be different colors. Dual eye color is known as heterochromia. Tumors may develop as a posterior mediastinal mass.

Because of the proximity of the spinal column, the tumor may extend into the vertebrae and cause spinal compression and paralysis. Neuroblastoma involving the mediastinum frequently causes airway obstruction, resulting in breathing difficulties. Tumors in the abdomen can originate from the sympathetic ganglia or the adrenal medulla. These retroperitoneal tumors account for approximately 65% of initial sites for neuroblastoma. Unfortunately, this location has the least favorable prognosis. Tumors may also originate in the pelvis. The most common presenting sign is a palpable mass. Many times, however, abnormalities due to a metastatic site may be the first indication of neuroblastoma.

More than 60% of children with neuroblastoma have metastatic disease at diagnosis, possibly involving multiple organs. The liver is a common site of metastasis. Metastases to the long bones and skull are a frequent occurrence. Bone pain or a pathologic fracture may be the presenting symptom. Bone marrow infiltration occurs in over 50% of children and is not necessarily associated with bone involvement. Bone marrow metastasis can result in anemia, bleeding, and infection. Neuroblastoma can also produce profuse diarrhea, which may be caused by tumor metabolites. Skin and soft tissue lesions containing neuroblastoma cells infrequently occur in the infant. General systemic signs and symptoms include weight loss, fatigue, and irritability.

Because neuroblastoma cells can synthesize and metabolize catecholamines, increased levels of metabolites of catecholamines are found in the urine. HVA and VMA are the metabolites most frequently monitored in the urine; HVA and VMA levels are useful both as diagnostic and clinical course indicators.

Diagnostic studies are used to evaluate the tumor site and extent of metastatic disease. Initial studies will include complete blood count, serum chemistries, 24-hour urine for catecholamine metabolites, chest radiographs, skeletal survey, IVP, liver and bone scan, and bone marrow aspiration. Definitive diagnosis is made by pathologic confirmation of neuroblastoma by tissue biopsy.

Unique to neuroblastoma is a relatively high rate of spontaneous regression of the disease. It is thought that spontaneous regression actually represents the disappearance of cancer cells rather than the transformation of cells from malignant to normal. The mechanism of this process is unknown. It occurs more frequently in the child who is under 2 years of age who has either limited- or advanced-stage disease.

Staging of neuroblastoma is based on a I-to-IV scale. There is also a special IV-S classification for tumors that would otherwise be classified as stages I or II (limited disease) but have additional involvement of liver, skin, or bone marrow without direct bone metastases. Interesting is that stage IV-S disease has an excellent prognosis in spite of significant advanced disease. This is attributed to the frequency of spontaneous regression for the child with this particular stage. Overall, the survival rate for neuroblastoma is poor, but infants below 1 year of age, regardless of the disease stage, have a good prognosis.

Treatment Surgery is the initial treatment to obtain a biopsy and remove as much of the tumor as possible. Stage I and II disease are often completely resectable. During surgery metallic clips may be placed around the margins of the tumor site to aid in the delineation of radiation therapy ports and to follow treatment response by radiograph. The child with stage IV disease at diagnosis may not be treated surgically since it has not been determined if debulking the primary tumor will extend survival time.

Radiation therapy is often administered after surgery when residual disease remains. Neuroblastoma is considered to be a radiosensitive tumor. Radiation also may be used initially to shrink large tumors near vital structures so that an inoperable tumor becomes amenable to surgery. Additionally, radiation therapy is the primary treatment for spinal cord compression or respiratory distress due to large mediastinal masses.

Chemotherapy is also used in the treatment of advanced stage IV disease. Drugs that have shown some effectiveness include cyclophosphamide, vincristine, DTIC, VM-26, cisplatin, and doxorubicin. The use of chemotherapy in stages I through III and stage IV-S is controversial and may not contribute to survival. Since spontaneous remission is likely, infants with stage IV-S disease may receive no disease treatment and simply be followed and provided symptomatic support. After an initial waiting period, very small doses of radiation or a short course of small-dose chemotherapy may be given if the disease does not regress in the infant with stage IV-S disease.

Nursing Management It is often difficult for the nurse and parent to care for the very ill young child with neuroblastoma, particularly if a poor prognosis is anticipated. The parent should be encouraged to participate in the day-to-day care and remain close to the child. The nurse facilitates parent–child contact including holding and rocking the child. The parent may be particularly uneasy if the infant has stage IV-S disease, especially if the child looks quite ill and yet no therapy is prescribed. The parent needs reassurance about the favorable outcome for the child.

The nurse is also challenged to carry out 24-hour urine collections on the young child. This often necessitates a bit of creativity to collect the entire urine specimen successfully, particularly with the child who is not toilet-trained (see Chapter 29). Parents also should be taught to collect 24-hour urine samples since once the child is discharged, the parent will be responsible for obtaining these specimens.

Wilms' Tumor

Wilms' tumor, or nephroblastoma according to its historic name, is an embryonal tumor of the kidney. Because it is embryonal, most children are between 1 and 5 years of age at diagnosis. The peak incidence is between 3 and 4 years of age. Approximately 15% of children with Wilms' tumor also have congenital abnormalities such as aniridia, hemihypertrophy, and genitourinary anomalies. The tumor originates from immature renoblast cells located in the kidney parencyma and extends into the renal cavity and often distorts the caliceal system.

The most frequent sign of Wilms' tumor is an increase in abdominal girth or a palpable abdominal mass. The tumor may be discovered in the course of a routine physical examination, or the parent may be the first to note the abdominal enlargement. Often the child appears otherwise healthy and active. The mass is usually smooth, firm, and painless. If pain is evident, it is due to the rapid growth of the tumor. Wilms' tumor is generally unilateral, but bilateral involvement of the kidneys has been reported in up to 10% of children diagnosed with the disease. Gross hematuria is uncommon, but microscopic hematuria may be present, which in either case represents invasion of the renal collecting system. Hypertension due to pressure on the renal artery is evident in 25% of children with Wilms' tumor.

Essential diagnostic evaluation includes IVP and inferior cavogram. Additional studies such as angiography and ultrasonography may be useful. Metastasis most commonly occurs to the lung and secondarily to the liver. Therefore, diagnostic radiographs or scans of the lung and liver are appropriate initial studies. Uncommon but possible sites of metastases include the brain, bone, and bone marrow. Tissue biopsy provides the histologic diagnosis.

The most common staging system is based on the recommendation of National Wilms' Tumor Study classifying the tumor on a group I through group V scale. Groups I and II represent completely resectable disease; Group III represents partial resection but no evidence of metastatic spread; Group IV represents metastatic spread; and Group V represents bilateral kidney disease. Wilms' tumor is one of the most curable solid tumors of childhood. With the latest treatment, the overall survival approaches 90% for localized disease and 50% for advanced disease (Belasco et al., 1984). The specific histology, extent of the disease, and age of the child at diagnosis influence the prognosis for any specific child.

Treatment Initial therapy is begun by laparotomy, definitive biopsy, and total nephrectomy with excision of all tumor. Care is taken not to rupture the tumor or seed the abdominal cavity with tumor cells. If the tumor has spread to regional lymph nodes or involvement of the vena cava is found, a less favorable prognosis is suspected. Metallic clips are placed around any residual tumor that is unresectable so radiation therapy guidelines are evident. The liver is grossly examined for evidence of spread, and lesions are excised if possible. If bilateral kidney involvement is present, the most severely affected kidney will be removed with possible heminephrectomy of the remaining kidney.

Radiation therapy is of value in the treatment of Wilms' tumor since the tumor is considered radiosensitive. Treatments may begin a few days after surgery particularly to destroy any cells that may have seeded the abdominal cavity during surgery. Radiation therapy is generally not necessary in the young child with stage I disease. The radiation field size and appropriate dose is determined by the stage at diagnosis. Radiation therapy is also beneficial to the lungs if pulmonary metastases are evident.

Chemotherapy is useful postsurgically. Successful drug combinations include vincristine and daunorubicin. Doxorubicin has also been used.

Nursing Management Initial nursing goals focus on orienting the child and family to the nursing unit and preparing them for the necessary radiologic studies and surgery. Because diagnosis, surgery, and radiation therapy may occur in rapid succession, the family has little time to adjust to the diagnosis. This may be particularly stressful since the child appears well at diagnosis and may have been quite active before hospitalization.

Preoperatively, the nurse handles the child's abdomen carefully as palpation or manipulation may seed tumor cells through rupture of the renal capsule. All medical personnel should refrain from undue abdominal examination, and a sign may be placed on the child's bed indicating this.

Postoperative care follows normal guidelines after general abdominal surgery. Fluid, electrolytes, and vital signs are monitored. Nasogastric suction is used to preserve gastric decompression. The dressing is checked for drainage, and abdominal girth should be monitored for evidence of distention or internal hemorrhage.

Rhabdomyosarcoma

Rhabdomyosarcoma is a malignant tumor of striated muscle (*rhabdo* = "striated" and *myo* = "muscle"). It accounts for most soft-tissue tumors in childhood. The peak incidence of rhabdomyosarcoma is 2–6 years of age with a second incidence peak during the adolescent years of 15–19.

Because it originates in striated muscle, there are a number of primary sites for tumor growth. The disease also has several histologic categories, including embryonal, alveolar, pleomorphic, and mixed. Embryonal tumors have histologic characteristics similar to those of the muscle tissue of the 2- to 2.5-month old fetus. It often grows into hollow organs of the bladder, vagina, uterus, or nasopharynx. Because it forms as polypoid grapelike clusters, it is often called sarcoma botryoides (*botrys* = "bunch of grapes").

Alveolar rhabdomyosarcoma has histologic characteristics similar to those of the muscle tissue of the 2.5- to 5-month-old fetus. The tumor is more commonly seen in adolescents than younger children. It occurs most readily in the trunk and extremities. Pleomorphic rhabdomyosarcoma is uncommon in childhood and occurs most often in adults who are 30–50 years of age. Mixed rhabdomyosarcoma indicates that the tumor has more than one of the three histologic types.

The most common sites for rhabdomyosarcoma are the head, orbit, and neck, and these account for approximately 40% of tumors. Genitourinary and abdominal sites account for 35%, and trunk or extremity tumors account for 25%. The child under 10 years of age is more likely to have localized disease at diagnosis with tumor location in the head and neck or genitourinary sites. In contrast, adolescents are more likely to have advanced disease and tumors of the trunk, extremity, or paratesticular sites.

The most common presenting sign is a painless mass or functional impairment of the site. Tumors that involve the orbit present with proptosis (downward displacement of the eyeball). Nasopharyngeal tumors are manifested by nasal discharge, serous otitis media, and nasal-sounding speech. The tumor may actually protrude from the nostrils. Urinary tract obstruction or palpable mass occur with urinary rhabdomyosarcoma. Vaginal tumors present with grapelike polypoids extending out of the vaginal canal. Paratesticular tumors are manifested by a firm, painless mass that is often translucent. Rhabdomyosarcoma of the extremity most commonly involves the lower extremities and presents as a painless mass.

Diagnostic studies are determined by the site of the tumor and potential metastatic sites. Head and neck tumors require ENT evaluation, skull radiographs or tomograms, arteriography, and CT scan. Genitourinary and abdominal tumors require cystoscopy, IVP, upper- and lower-GI series, and abdominal CT scan. The evaluation of extremity tumors includes bone radiograph and other radiographic scans.

Rhabdomyosarcoma is a highly malignant disease that demonstrates both blood and lymph node spread. Metastatic sites include lungs, bone marrow, bone, liver, brain, and lymph nodes. Up to 40% of children have metastatic disease at diagnosis. Staging of the disease is based on a standard I-to-IV grading system. Prognosis is based on the primary site, histologic type, stage of the disease at diagnosis, and age of the child. The child with the most favorable diagnosis is between 1 and 7 years of age with sarcoma botryoides of the orbit in its earliest stages. Alveolar rhabdomyosarcoma has the poorest prognosis. The overall survival rate for stage I or II disease is approximately 70%. Two-year survival rates for more advanced stages are poor (about 25%) (Altman and Schwartz, 1983).

Treatment Rhabdomyosarcoma is treated aggressively with combination surgery, radiation, and chemotherapy. Surgery can be curative for localized disease that is amenable to surgical excision. Because radiation therapy and chemotherapy can be effective in controlling disease, mutilating surgeries to the head and neck or pelvic area are not necessary. Amputation for extremity disease may be contraindicated also. Sometimes surgical resection is postponed until radiation therapy and chemotherapy are initially used to shrink or control disease.

Radiation therapy is administered to the tumor site in doses of 5000–6000 rad over a 6-week period. Chemotherapy may be begun concurrently with radiation. The drugs most commonly used are vincristine, cyclophosphamide, and daunorubicin with the occasional addition of doxorubicin.

Nursing Management The care of a child or adolescent with rhabdomyosarcoma requires the utmost nursing skill. Since several treatment modes may be used at one time, side effects are potentiated. This is particularly true in the management of head and neck cancers when combined radiation and chemotherapy in addition to the presence of tumor can obstruct a patent airway. The child is also likely to be quite anxious when these combined effects make breathing difficult and affect appearance. The nurse continually monitors the child's progress and symptoms. Supportive nursing care and comfort measures provide the basis of the care plan.

Osteosarcoma

Primary bone tumors account for about 4.5% of childhood cancer. The peak incidence rate occurs during adolescence. The two most common bone tumors are osteosarcoma and Ewing's sarcoma.

Osteosarcoma, which arises from bone-producing mesenchymal cells, is histologically classified by the appearance of large spindle cells in biopsied tissue. The disease occurs most commonly in the end of long bones with almost 50% located near the knee. The two most frequent sites are the distal ends of the femur and the proximal end of the tibia. The tumor is more common in boys than girls and may be related to the adolescent growth spurt. Some adolescents have reported a recent injury or trauma to the area prior to the tumor appearance, but trauma does not appear to be significantly related to tumor development. Approximately 4% of osteosarcomas can be directly related to previous irradiation of the tumor site. The tumor is uncommon before the age of 10 and is most frequently diagnosed between the ages of 10 and 25.

The most common presenting symptom is pain and possible swelling of the affected area. Delay in diagnosis is a frequent problem since symptoms often are attributed to athletic activity or injury. Other symptoms can include functional limitation, erythema, and warmth in the affected area.

Diagnostic evaluation by radiograph can confirm the suspicion of a malignant tumor. Osteosarcoma normally grows from the center of inside the bone, damaging the cortex and extending into the soft tissue. The lung is the most frequent site of disease spread. Bones may also be secondary sites. Investigation of metastatic sites includes chest radiograph or lung tomograms, bone scan, and skeletal survey. Tissue biopsy confirms the presence of osteosarcoma. Historically the overall survival rate for this tumor has been poor (approximately 20%). With recent therapy advances and better management techniques for lung metastases, the long-term survival rate is about 50% (Gaddy-Cohen, 1982).

Treatment The initial treatment is amputation of the limb above the site of the tumor. Since most lesions appear in the leg, above-the-knee amputation is required for tumors of the tibia, and hip disarticulation is required for tumors of the femur. Some surgeons may avoid total hip disarticulation and instead perform cross-bone amputation around the upper thigh so that the limb prosthesis is easier to fit.

In the adolescent who has passed the growth spurt and nearly attained adult height, limb-sparing bone replacement technique may be indicated rather than amputation. The tumor and often the adjacent joint is removed followed by artificial implant or bone graft. For disease in the distal femur the total femur and knee joint are removed and replaced with a femur implant and total knee prosthesis. This technique is used at only a few cancer treatment centers and is probably appropriate only for a limited number of children who have attained adult height and have small osteosarcoma lesions around the knee. Although limb-sparing techniques show promise, up to a third of adolescents eventually require traditional amputation because of complications of the procedure, such as breakage of the prosthesis, infection, or recurrent disease.

Osteosarcoma is a radioresistant tumor. Very high doses of radiation (6–1200 rad) may not sufficiently control tumor growth and instead cause considerable damage to normal tissue and functional loss. For this reason, radiation therapy is primarily used for nonresectable tumors of the rib, skull, or pelvis.

Micrometastasis of osteosarcoma frequently occurs, resulting in metastasis generally to the lung within a year after amputation. Because of the likelihood of micrometastasis, adjuvant chemotherapy has become an important component of treatment. The agents used for micrometastasis or known residual disease include doxorubicin, cisplatin, and high-dose methotrexate followed by leucovorin rescue. Cyclophosphamide, vincristine, bleomycin, doxorubicin, and daunorubicin have also been utilized in combination.

Prophylactic lung radiation with or without additional chemotherapy also has been attempted because of the likelihood of lung metastases. Whether this substantially contributes to disease-free survival is unclear. For known lung metastases resection of specific lesions by thoracotomy may contribute to longer survival.

Nursing Management The rigorous treatment of osteosarcoma requires skillful psychologic and physiologic nursing intervention. Limb amputation is traumatic and can be particularly damaging to the emerging self-identity of the adolescent. The child must be carefully prepared for the impending amputation with full disclosure of the necessary procedure. Immediate reaction to the news of amputation can range from denial to overt refusal and hostility. The parent and child require time and sensitive support to deal with their feelings. A normal grief reaction generally occurs after surgery as the adolescent adjusts to the loss of the limb. Preoperative or postoperative introduction to another child who has successfully adapted to amputation and has mastered the use of a prosthesis can be very helpful to the child and parent.

Postoperative care of the stump or surgical site depends on the location and extent of surgery. The nurse monitors the stump for evidence of bleeding or drainage. A Hemovac suction may be used to drain the stump postoperatively for a few days. The child is mobilized with physical therapy and rehabilitation as soon as possible after surgery. Crutch walking is taught within the first few postoperative days. The nurse encourges proper crutch-walking techniques. The prosthesis can be fitted within 4–6 weeks after surgery. The child requires instruction on the proper care of the stump and application and maintenance of the prosthesis. Nursing goals focus on successful rehabilitation and ambulation with the prosthetic device.

Aggresive chemotherapy requires judicious skill and monitoring of drug infusions. Treatment with high-dose methotrexate necessitates precise infusion of the drug with accurate follow-up administration of the leucovorin rescue so that life-threatening toxicities do not develop.

Ewing's Sarcoma

In contrast to osteosarcoma, Ewing's sarcoma occurs in the midshaft of long bones and in flat bones such as the pelvis, scapulae, and ribs. The disease was first described by Dr. James Ewing in 1921; hence the name Ewing's sarcoma. Histologically, this tumor has small, round cells rather than the characteristic large spindle cells of osteosarcoma. The peak incidence is in the second decade of life and it is rare after age 30.

Symptoms of Ewing's sarcoma are similar to osteosarcoma, with pain and swelling over the affected site. Metastasis is usually not evident at diagnosis but occurs later in the disease, with spread to the lung and other bones. Diagnostic work-up includes plain radiograph of the bone, bone scan or skeletal survey, and chest radiograph or lung tomograms. Definitive diagnosis is confirmed by tissue biopsy. The best prognosis is associated with localized disease at diagnosis without subsequent relapse. The 3-year disease-free survival rate for children who present without metastatic disease is 50% (Nesbit et al., 1981). Those with metastatic disease at diagnosis or who develop metastatic disease have a poor prognosis.

Treatment Initial surgery is generally not performed except to obtain a tissue biopsy. Surgical resection or amputation has not significantly contributed to long-term survival, but surgical resection after other primary treatment may be indicated. High-dose radiation therapy and chemotherapy offer the best chance of disease control. Adjuvant chemotherapy has been effective with the use of cyclophosphamide, doxorubicin, and daunorubicin in combination. Other chemotherapy protocols have used carmustine (BCNU), mithramycin, and 5-fluorouracil.

Nursing Management The nursing management of the child with Ewing's sarcoma follows the basic guidelines of assisting child and family to adjust to the disease and treatment program. Because the disease rarely necessitates amputation or disfiguring surgery, function and self-image are not altered by a traumatic surgery.

Future Directions

Nurses who care for children with cancer have an exciting opportunity to develop and conduct nursing research. Supportive care or prevention of many of the side effects of treatment come under nursing responsibility. Nurses are only beginning to realize their potential for systematically testing nursing interventions that contribute to the child's quality survival. Studies that explore nursing techniques for the management of stomatitis, alopecia, infection, nondrug pain control, and psychosocial issues, to name a few, are all important areas for investigation. Nurses who specialize in the field of childhood cancer have formed a supportive network known as the Association of Pediatric Oncology Nurses (APON). This organization offers both a supportive contact with other nurse specialists and a mechanism for exchange of the most current ideas and research pertinent to childhood cancer nursing.

Medical research has contributed to the dramatic increase in survival rates over the last several decades. While one simple drug or treatment technique to prevent or cure childhood cancer will not likely be discovered, a number of promising advances are nevertheless taking place. Studies currently being conducted in the laboratory are contributing to an understanding of childhood cancer development, providing new techniques to detect tumors earlier, and with less invasive measure, and developing teatments that are specific for cancer cells.

Basic cancer research is using recombinant DNA (artificially cloned and grown DNA in the laboratory) to study the actual process of normal cell transformation to cancer cell. Unlocking this key should lead to the development of new treatment techniques. Researchers are also developing a technique to grow a child's tumor cells in the laboratory and then subject them to a battery of chemotherapeutic agents. By this method the most effective agents can be tailored to the specific child much like the standard antibiotic sensitivity testing. Another new direction in cancer treatment involves the use of monoclonal antibodies. These antibodies can now be developed to target tumor-specific antigens. The use of monoclonal antibodies should aid both diagnosis and accurate staging of tumors. It offers even more exciting possibilities for treatment because it may exert a direct cytotoxic effect. Additionally, drugs or radiation-sensitized substances may be tagged to the monoclonal antibody, thus providing tumor-specific therapy.

The care of a child with cancer can be taxing and requires the highest level of nursing competence. Yet childhood cancer nursing is an exciting field where new treatments and progress can be seen within short periods of time. It can also be tremendously challenging and rewarding to have a significant impact on the lives of a child and family during this time of crisis, to assist them to adapt to the demands, and to know that they can continue to grow and develop in spite of life-threatening illness.

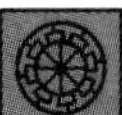

NURSING CARE PLAN Child With Leukemia

Assessment Data

Billy is a 9-year-old boy admitted to the hospital to confirm the diagnosis of acute leukemia. For the past 3 weeks Billy has had an upper respiratory tract infection with fevers that recurred after oral antibiotic treatment. A complete blood count done in the physician's office showed a white blood count of 15,000/mm^3, hemoglobin of 11/g/dL, and platelet count of 30,000/mm^3. Billy appears pale and lethargic and has both bruises and petechiae on his extremities. Physical assessment reveals a fever of 39 C, absence of lymph node adenopathy or bone pain, and moderate hepatosplenomegaly. Chest radiograph reveals no mediastinal mass, and blood chemistries are within acceptable limits with the exception of the uric acid level, which is moderately elevated. Nose, throat, urine, and blood cultures are obtained, and Billy is started on a combination of three broad-spectrum antibiotics. A bone marrow biopsy and lumbar puncture are performed. Results confirm the diagnosis of acute lymphoblastic leukemia with null cell immunologic markers. The bone marrow was hypercellular with 86% blasts. The lumbar puncture showed no evidence of central nervous system disease. Billy is placed in protective isolation because the pediatric unit has a number of children who harbor chronic infections. Billy is considered to be in the most favorable diagnostic category. He begins his remission induction therapy with vincristine, prednisone, and L-asparginase.

An interview with Billy's parents reveals the following information. Billy is the middle child. He has an older brother, Brian, who is 10 and a younger sister, Kerry, who is 6. Up until the present illness Billy has been a healthy, active child who has developed normally in all areas. The other children also are chracterized as completely normal by their parents.

Billy's mother is 33 years old and has been a homemaker since she was married 12 years ago Recently she has been working part-time as salesperson in an antique shop. Billy's father is 35 years old and operates a gas station. Neither parent has had much experience with health professionals and only see a doctor when an illness "doesn't clear up in a few days." Although they have several good friends, neither has relatives close by. They say that Billy's diagnosis of leukemia confirmed their worst fears and is the most devastating thing that has happened to them.

Nursing Diagnosis and Goals

1. **Nursing diagnosis:** Alteration in protective mechanisms—infection related to disease process.

   Long-term goal: Billy will not experience life-threatening infections; infections that do occur will be identified early and receive prompt treatment.

   Short-term goal: Billy's infection will resolve without further complications.

2. **Nursing diagnosis:** Potential alteration in protective mechanisms—potential for bleeding related to disease process.

   Long-term goal: Billy will not experience serious bleeding episodes; minor bleeding will be managed promptly and appropriately.

   Short-term goal: Billy will not experience further bleeding episodes during this admission.

3. **Nursing diagnosis:** Alteration in urinary function related to hyperuricemia secondary to cell lysis as a result of the disease process and chemotherapy.

   Long-term goal: Billy will not experience elevated uric acid levels during chemotherapy treatment.

   Short-term goal: Billy will not experience a further elevation of his uric acid level or renal dysfunction as a result of hyperuricemia.

4. **Nursing diagnosis:** Potential alteration in bowel elimination related to constipation secondary to vincristine administration.

   Long-term goal: Billy will not experience constipation during vincristine treatment.

   Short-term goal. Billy will not experience constipation from induction therapy with vincristine.

5. **Nursing diagnosis:** Potential alteration in peripheral nervous system function related to neurotoxicity from vincristine administration.

   Long-term goal: Billy will not experience serious neuropathy during vincristine treatment.

   Short-term goal: Billy will not experience neuropathies from induction therapy with vincristine.

6. **Nursing diagnosis:** Diversionary activity deficit related to monotony of confinement (hospitalization and protective isolation).

continued on next page

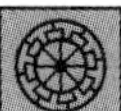

NURSING CARE PLAN Child With Leukemia (continued)

Long-term goal: Billy will return to his normal activity level and maintain normal developmental growth.

Short-term goal: Billy will maintain appropriate activity level, stimulation, and developmental tasks in spite of his hospitalization and protective isolation.

7. **Nursing diagnosis:** Knowledge deficit (parents and child) related to the new diagnosis of leukemia.

   Long-term goal: Billy and his family will possess the knowledge and skill to understand the disease process, treatment, and side effects and their appropriate management so that Billy and his family will participate fully in his care.

   Short-term goal: Billy and his family will understand the purpose and receive support while undergoing diagnostic tests and initial treatment.

8. **Nursing diagnosis:** Fear (parents and child) related to cancer diagnosis.

   Long-term goal: Billy and his family, individually and collectively, will deal appropriately with their fears and develop coping mechanisms that allow them to live fully and grow as individuals and a family in spite of the diagnosis of a life-threatening disease.

   Short-term goal: Billy and his family will express their fears and begin to use helpful coping strategies in dealing with the impact of the diagnosis of a life-threatening illness.

Intervention	Rationale	Evaluation criteria
1. Obtain cultures as ordered	Cultures identify current organisms	Does Billy's temperature return to 37 C within 48 hours of admission? Does the assessment reveal no new evidence of local or systemic infection?
Administer antibiotics as ordered	Antibiotics control current organisms.	
Monitor temperature every 4 hours and as warranted	Early identification prevents serious infection	
Reduce fever if greater than 39 C by promoting cooling of skin and mucous membranes, preventing chilling and administering acetaminophen as ordered	Interventions provide comfort and reduce accelerated metabolic need	
Institute protective isolation as ordered	Preventive measures keep immunosuppressed child from being exposed to others with chronic infection	
Observe potential sites for further infection development	Early identification prevents seriously infected sites	
Achieve and maintain optimal nutrition (Billy likes milkshakes, apple juice, toasted cheese sandwiches, and pizza)	Malnutrition negatively affects immune function. (Children are most likely to eat the foods they like.)	
Maintain the integrity of the skin and mucous membranes. Teach Billy and his family the importance of good personal hygiene. Use aseptic technique when performing intrusive procedures. Avoid rectal temperatures, suppositories, or enemas. Teach Billy and his family about infection risk and preventive treatment	Skin is the first line of defense against microorganisms	
2. Monitor susceptibility to bleeding. Monitor platelet count, presence of additional bruising and petechiae, guiac urine, stool, emesis	Signs indicate potential for bleeding	Is there further evidence of bruising or petechiae? Is there any evidence of bleeding? Is the hospital environment safe and conducive to avoiding trauma?

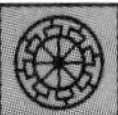

NURSING CARE PLAN Child With Leukemia (continued)

Intervention	Rationale	Evaluation criteria
Maintain skin integrity. Institute safety precautions to decrease likelihood of falls. Hold puncture sites for 5 minutes. Avoid intramuscular injections. Do not take rectal temperatures	Maintaining skin decreases likelihood of capillary damage, skin breakdown, and entry of pathogens	
Protect mucous membranes. Use soft bristle or sponge toothbrush to avoid trauma. Lubricate tips. Avoid forceful nose blowing	Protecting membranes decreases likelihood of capillary damage and mucous membrane breakdown	
Do not give products that contain aspirin. Teach Billy and his parents about bleeding potential and preventive treatment	Aspirin destroys platelets	
3. Monitor serum uric acid level. Encourage fluids (Billy likes apple juice and Popsicles)	Serum uric acid level identifies hyperuricemia. Fluids keep urine dilute	Has the serum uric acid level returned to normal?
Administer allopurinol, bicarbonate, and intravenous fluids as ordered	Allopurinol prevents the formation of uric acid in the kidney	
Check urine pH and specific gravity. Observe for clinical manifestations of hyperuricemia (pain and inflammation in joints, fever, and chills)	Alkalination of urine and fluid discourages formation of uric acid crystals	
4. Begin administration of stool softener before chemotherapy is started. Force fluids and encourage high-fiber diet	Preventive measures combat vincristine-induced constipation	Is Billy constipated?
Monitor frequency and consistency of bowel movements. Teach Billy and his parents about constipation as a side effect of vincristine and as a preventive treatment	Early assessment of constipation allows additional intervention	
5. Observe Billy for signs and symptoms of neurotoxicity (weakness, numbness of extremities, jaw pain, foot drop, decreased deep tendon reflexes). Teach Billy and his parents about signs and symptoms of peripheral neuropathy and importance of prompt reporting of symptoms should they appear	If signs and symptoms of neurotoxicity are identified early, the vincristine dosage may be decreased and toxicity reversed	Is there any sign of peripheral neuropathy?
6. Elicit information about Billy's normal activity pattern. Determine what activities can be continued while in isolation	Identifying normal activity level, interests, and developmental tasks for Billy allow plan to be personalized	Does Billy remain active? Does he keep in contact with outside environment and cope positively with hospitalization and isolation?
Encourage family to bring in special toys such as his puzzles, space creatures, and tape player and headset with his favorite tapes	Billy needs familiar objects and toys	
Refer Billy to child life worker for additional activities	Billy, although confined, needs a therapeutic and recreational outlet	

continued on next page

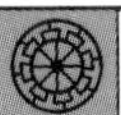

NURSING CARE PLAN Child With Leukemia (continued)

Intervention	Rationale	Evaluation criteria
Explain to Billy the reason for protective isolation. Allow him to express his frustration over his confinement	If medical reason for isolation is clarified, Billy feels less rejected, alienated, or lonely	
Encourage Billy to keep in touch by phone with his friends	Billy needs to maintain contact with normal environment and needs to continue his social development	
Arrange for school tutorial service so that Billy may keep on with his school work	Billy needs to keep up with cognitive development	
Provide for adequate periods of rest	With illness Billy requires additional rest	
Develop a daily routine with Billy	Billy needs structure and consistency in a strange environment	
Encourage family visitation and interaction. Assist siblings to deal with feelings of abandonment and rivalry	Continued contact with family is necessary during period of crisis.	
7. Prepare Billy and his family for each diagnostic procedure (lab work, radiographs, bone marrow, etc.)	Preparation decreases stress and provides positive coping	Does Billy tolerate procedures and demonstrate effective coping? Can family members individually explain basic information about leukemia? Do family members freely ask questions as needed? Can family members correctly decribe treatment plan, side effects which might occur and appropriate management of side effects?
Determine Billy's and his family's understanding of the diagnosis of leukemia by providing them written materials, encouraging Billy (when out of isolation) and his siblings to visit the lab and see blood and bone marrow slides, encourage the family to keep a list of questions that come to mind	The emotional response to the diagnosis of a life-threatening illness often clouds understanding of information. Explanations need to be repeated and additional information given gradually	
Begin teaching program regarding leukemia, its treatment, side effects, and their control. Topics to be covered are leukemia; chemotherapy and how it works; side effects and what to do about infection, bleeding, anemia, constipation, peripheral neuropathies, moon face, mood changes; and follow-up care. Plan follow-up visits for further education after discharge or refer to a visiting nurse for follow-up	A systematic teaching program provides the foundation for parent and child participation in the treatment of childhood cancer	
8. Encourage the family to express fears and feelings. Accept feelings expressed; provide hopeful, realistic support	Expression of feelings is the basis for identifying effective coping mechanism	Are family members able to identify fears, frustrations, guilt and resentments over impact of diagnosis? Do parents spend time together? Are lines of communication kept open? Have parents joined a support group, and do they find it helpful?

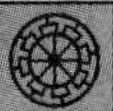

NURSING CARE PLAN Child With Leukemia (continued)

Intervention	Rationale	Evaluation criteria
Encourage the parents to support each other and keep lines of communication open	Parents dealing with the crisis of a child's life-threatening illness can discharge feelings of stress and frustration onto each other unless they are sensitive to each other's needs and share feelings	
Encourage the family to participate in a support group	Group support with people also experiencing a child's life-threatening disease provides a supportive network and a forum for expressing feelings.	

Key Concepts

- Despite the rarity of childhood cancer, it is the leading cause of death from disease in children between 1 and 14 years of age, although half of all children with cancer are cured and the remainder experience significant long-term survival.
- Cancer is a cluster of many diseases that share the same pathologic feature of uncontrolled cell growth.
- Compared to benign tumors, malignant tumors have a faster rate of growth, can invade nearby tissue, and can metastasize to other parts of the body.
- Leukemia and cancers of the central nervous system, particularly the brain, account for the largest proportion of childhood cancers.
- Genetic, immunologic, viral, and environmental factors are all being studied for their relationship to the causes of cancer.
- With the steady improvement in the treatment of childhood cancer over the past 10–20 years, the focus of therapy is on the quality of life.
- The presenting symptoms of a child with a neoplasm will vary, depending on the location and size of the tumor.
- A thorough physical examination of a child suspected of having a malignancy includes a general health assessment, a detailed examination of the area of concern, and careful palpation of the suspected tumor location.
- The diagnostic tests for childhood cancer, especially lumbar puncture and biopsy, can be particularly stressful for the child and require a specific nursing plan for preparation.
- The three approaches to the medical treatment plan are curative therapy, adjuvant therapy, and palliative therapy.
- The medical treatment of the child with cancer is directed toward communicating the diagnosis to the child and family and initiating the treatment plan, which includes determining the stage of the disease and prescribing the appropriate therapeutic regimen.
- The major focus of nursing care is to assist the child and family to adapt to the life-threatening nature of cancer while facilitating normal development.
- Nursing management is directed toward minimizing complications of surgical procedures and alleviating the physical and emotional stresses of chemotherapy and radiation.
- The side effects of chemotherapy are due to the damage of normal cells and will vary depending on the dose, combination of drugs used, and the amount of time after drug administration.
- Acute, intermediate, and cumulative side effects of chemotherapy require a daily assessment for new and ongoing problems leading to creative interventions, strategies, and frequently updated nursing care plans.

- Nursing management during radiation therapy focuses on preparation for the treatment, comfort measures, and the control of side effects affecting the mouth, gastrointestinal tract, skin, and blood.
- Bone marrow suppression, a general side effect of chemotherapy and radiation, predisposes the child to anemia, infection, and bleeding and bruising and requires both preventive and supportive nursing measures.
- In providing narcotic management of the child's pain, the choice of drug, dose, and schedule must be tailored to the individual needs of the child, and the effectiveness of pain medication must be thoroughly documented.
- Nonnarcotic pain management strategies, such as distraction, relaxation techniques, and hypnosis, can be effective nursing measures.
- Cancer cachexia and taste alterations that result in aversions to some meats affect the child's nutritional status and necessitate a thorough and ongoing nutritional assessment.
- The nurse helps the family meet its own emotional needs by promoting communication, referring the family to other resources, and encouraging interaction between other family members, especially siblings, and the ill child.
- During remission the nursing staff should provide a systematic educational program for the parents and children concerning the illness and help them deal with information concerning alternatives to conventional therapy.
- For the child cured of cancer, the nurse can provide assistance in dealing with the physiologic concerns of possible sterility, atrophy or uneven physical growth, learning disabilities, and new cancer formation, and also with the psychosocial concerns of body image, sexuality, and social adjustment.
- The most common childhood neoplasms, which require comprehensive medical and nursing management, are acute leukemias, lymphomas, brain tumors, Wilms' tumor, rhabdomyosarcoma, and osteosarcoma.

References

Altman A, Schwartz A: *Malignant Diseases of Infancy, Childhood and Adolescence.* Saunders, 1983.

Altman A, Schwartz A: The Soft Tissue Sarcomas. In: *Malignant Diseases of Infancy, Childhood and Adolescence.* Altman A and Schwartz A (editors). Saunders, 1983.

American Cancer Society: *Cancer Facts and Figures 1984.* American Cancer Society, 1984.

American Joint Committee for Cancer Staging and End Results Reporting: *Manual for Staging of Cancer.* American Joint Committee, 1977.

Askin F, et al: Occult testicular leukemia: Testicular biopsy at three years of continuous remission of childhood leukemia. *Cancer,* 1981; 47:470.

Barbora J, Gitelson J: Cancer pain: Psychological management using hypnosis. *Cancer J Clin* 1980, 30:130.

Belasco J, et al: Wilms' Tumor. In: *Clinical Pediatric Oncology.* Sutow W, et al. (editors). Mosby, 1984.

Dash J: Hypnosis for Symptom Amelioration. In: *Psychological Aspects of Childhood Cancer.* Kellerman J (editor). Thomas, 1980.

Day S, et al: Cancer Invasion and Metastasis: Biologic Mechanisms and Therapy. *Progress in Cancer Research and Therapy.* Vol. 5. Raven, 1977.

Draper GJ: Population Studies of Incidence, Survival and Followup. In: *Status of the Curability of Childhood Cancers.* Raven, 1980.

Feinbach D: Natural History of Acute Leukemia. In: *Clinical Pediatric Oncology.* Sutow W, Feinbach D, and Vietti T, (editors). Mosby, 1984.

Fochtman D, Foley G: *Nursing Care of the Child with Cancer.* Little, Brown, 1982.

Foley G: Retinoblastoma. In: *Nursing Care of the Child with Cancer.* Fochtman D, Foley G, Little, Brown, 1982.

Gaddy-Cohen D: Nursing care in childhood cancer update. *Am J Nurs* 1982, 82:416.

Gumbina M: Tumors of the Central and Peripheral Nervous System. In: *Malignant Diseases of Infancy, Childhood and Adolescence.* Altman A, Schwartz A, (editors). Saunders, 1983.

Holmes H, Holmes F: After ten years, what are the handicaps and life styles of children treated for cancer? *Clin Pediatr* 1975; 14:819.

Jones P, Campbell P: *Tumours of Infancy and Childhood.* Blackwell, 1982.

Klopovich P, Cohen D: An overview of pediatric oncology for the adult oncology nurse. *Oncology Nurs Forum* 1984; 11:56.

Koocher G, O'Malley J: *The Damocles Syndrome: Psychosocial Consequence of Surviving Childhood Cancer.* McGraw-Hill, 1981.

Koocher G: Surviving Childhood Cancer—Issues in Living. In: *Living with Childhood Cancer.* Spinetta J, Deasy-Spinetta L, (editors). Mosby, 1981.

LaBaw W, et al: The use of self-hypnosis by children with cancer. *Am J Clin Hypn* 1975; 17:233.

Lanzkowsky P: *Pediatric Hematology Oncology.* McGraw-Hill, 1980.

Leck I: Congenital Malformations and childhood neoplasms. *J Med Genet* 1977; 14:321–326.

Meadows A, Evans A: Effects of chemotherapy on the central nervous system, a study of parenteral methotrexate in long-term survivors of leukemia and lymphoma in childhood. *Cancer* 1976; 37:853.

Mulvihill, J: Ecogenetic Origins of Cancer in the Young: Environmental and Genetic Determinants. In: *Cancer in the Young.* Levine A, (editor). Masson USA, 1982.

National Study Commission on Cytotoxic Exposure: *Recommendations for Handling Cytotoxic Agents.* August, 1983.

Nesbit M, et al: Multimodal therapy for the management of primary nonmetastatic Ewing's sarcoma of bone: An intergroup study. *Nat Cancer Inst Monogr* 1981; 56:279.

O'Malley J, et al: Psychiatric sequelae of surviving childhood cancer. *Am J Orthopsychiatry* 1979; 49:608.

Oncology Nursing Society: *Cancer Chemotherapy Guidelines and Recommendations for Nursing Education and Practice,* 1984.

See-Lasley K, Ignoffo R: *Manual of Oncology Therapeutics.* Mosby, 1981.

Simone J, Rivers G: Management of Acute Leukemia. In: *Clinical Pediatric*

Oncology. 3rd ed. Sutow W, Feinbach D and Vietti T (editors). Mosby, 1984.

Spinetta J, Deasy-Spinetta P: *Living with Childhood Cancer.* Mosby, 1981.

Stolar M, Power L, Viele C: Recommendations for handling cytotoxic drugs in hospitals. *Am J Hosp Pharm* (July) 1983; 40: 1163–1171.

Strong L: Genetics, Etiology, and Epidemiology of Childhood Cancer. In: *Clinical Pediatric Oncology*. 3rd ed. Sutow W, Feinbach D, Vietti, T (editors). Mosby, 1984.

Sullivan M, Fuller L, Butler J: Hodgkin's Disease. In: *Clinical Pediatric Oncology*. 3rd ed. Sutow et al. (editors). Mosby, 1984.

U.S. Department of Health and Human Services. Public Health Service. National Institutes of Health: *Recommendations for the Safe Handling of Parenteral Antineoplastic Drugs.* Publication no. 83-2621, 1983.

Vital Statistics of the United States, 1980, Mortality volume. U.S. Department of Health and Human Services, 1984.

Weinstein, H., et al: Chemotherapy for acute myelogenous leukemia in children and adults. VAPA update. *Blood*, 1983; 62:315.

Weinstein H, Link M: Non-Hodgkins lymphoma in children. *Clin Haematol*, 1979; 8:699.

Wong D, Dornan L: Nursing care in childhood cancer—retinoblastoma. *Am J Nurs* (March) 1982; 82:425–431.

Young J, et al: *Cancer Incidence, Survival and Mortality for Children Under 15 years of Age.* American Cancer Society, 1978.

Additional Readings

Association of Pediatric Oncology Nurses: *Standards of Pediatric Oncology Nursing.* American Nurses Association, 1979.

Becker T M: *Cancer chemotherapy: A manual for nurses.* Little, Brown, 1981.

Cleaveland MJ: Nursing care in childhood cancer: Brain tumors. *Am J Nurs*, 1982; 82:422.

Collins M: The leukemia child. *Iss Compr Pediatr Nurs*, 1980; 4:49.

Damon J, Taylor L: Brain Tumors in Children. *Nurs Clin North Am*, 1980; 15:99.

Fochtman D: *Nursing Care of the Child with Cancer.* Little, Brown, 1983.

Griffiths S: Changes in body image caused by antineoplastic drugs. *Iss Compr Pediatr Nurs*, 1980; 4:17.

Hardin K: Solid tumors in children. *Iss Compr Pediatr Nurs*, 1980: 4:29.

Hayes V, Knox JE: Hospital-related stress in parents of children with cancer. *Can Nurs* (Nov), 1983:225–28.

Jenkins D, Sonley M: Soft tissue sarcoma in the young. *Cancer*, 1980; 46:621.

Klopovich P, Suenram D, Cairns N: A common sense approach to caring for children with cancer. *Cancer Nurs*, 1980; 3:201.

Lipman A, Mooney K: Management of Pain. In: *Clinical Pharmacology and Therapeutics in Nursing.* 2nd ed. Weiner M, Pepper G (editors). McGraw-Hill, 1984.

Manchester B: The adolescent with cancer: Concerns for care. *Clin Nurs*, 1981; 2:31

Mills G: Preparing children and parents for cerebral computerized tomography. *Am J Matern Child Nurs*, 1980; 5:403.

Moore I, Triplett J: Students with cancer: A school nurse perspective. *Cancer Nurs*, 1980; 3:265.

Peck B: Effects of childhood cancer on long-term survivors and their families. *Brit Med J*, 1979; 1:1327.

Schorlemer V: Reflections: A mother's and son's struggle with acute lymphocytic leukemia. *Child Health Care* (Spring) 1984; 12(4):163–168.

Sealey A: Getting children to keep still during radiotherapy. *Am J Matern Child Nurs*, 1977; 2:178.

Spinetta J: Behavioral and psychological research in childhood cancer: An overview. *Cancer*, 1982:50:1921.

Stream P et al: Bone marrow transplantation: An option for children with acute leukemia. *Cancer Nurs*, 1980; 3:95.

Van Eys J, Sullivan M: *Status of the Curability of Childhood Cancer.* Raven, 1980.

Walters J: Coping with a leg amputation. *Am J Nurs*, 1981; 81:1349.

Wataru W et al: *Clinical Pediatric Oncology*. 3rd ed. Mosby, 1984.

Wolf W, Bancroft B: Early detection of childhood malignancies. *Pediatr Nurs*, 1980; 5:43.

Appendixes

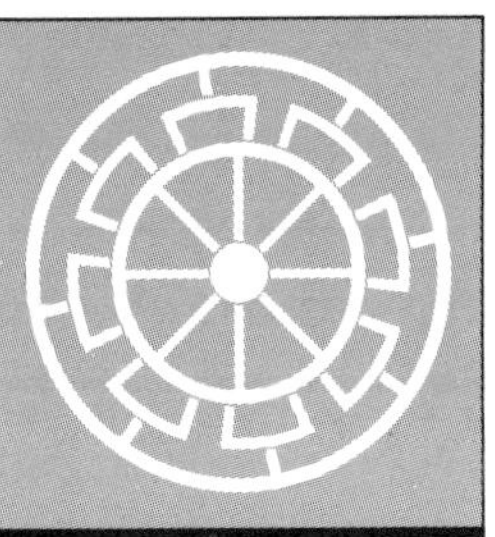

Appendix A

GIRLS FROM BIRTH TO 36 MONTHS

LENGTH FOR AGE

Age (months)

95th
90th
75th
50th
25th
10th
5th

Length (in.) / Length (cm.)

Age (months)

Appendix A continued

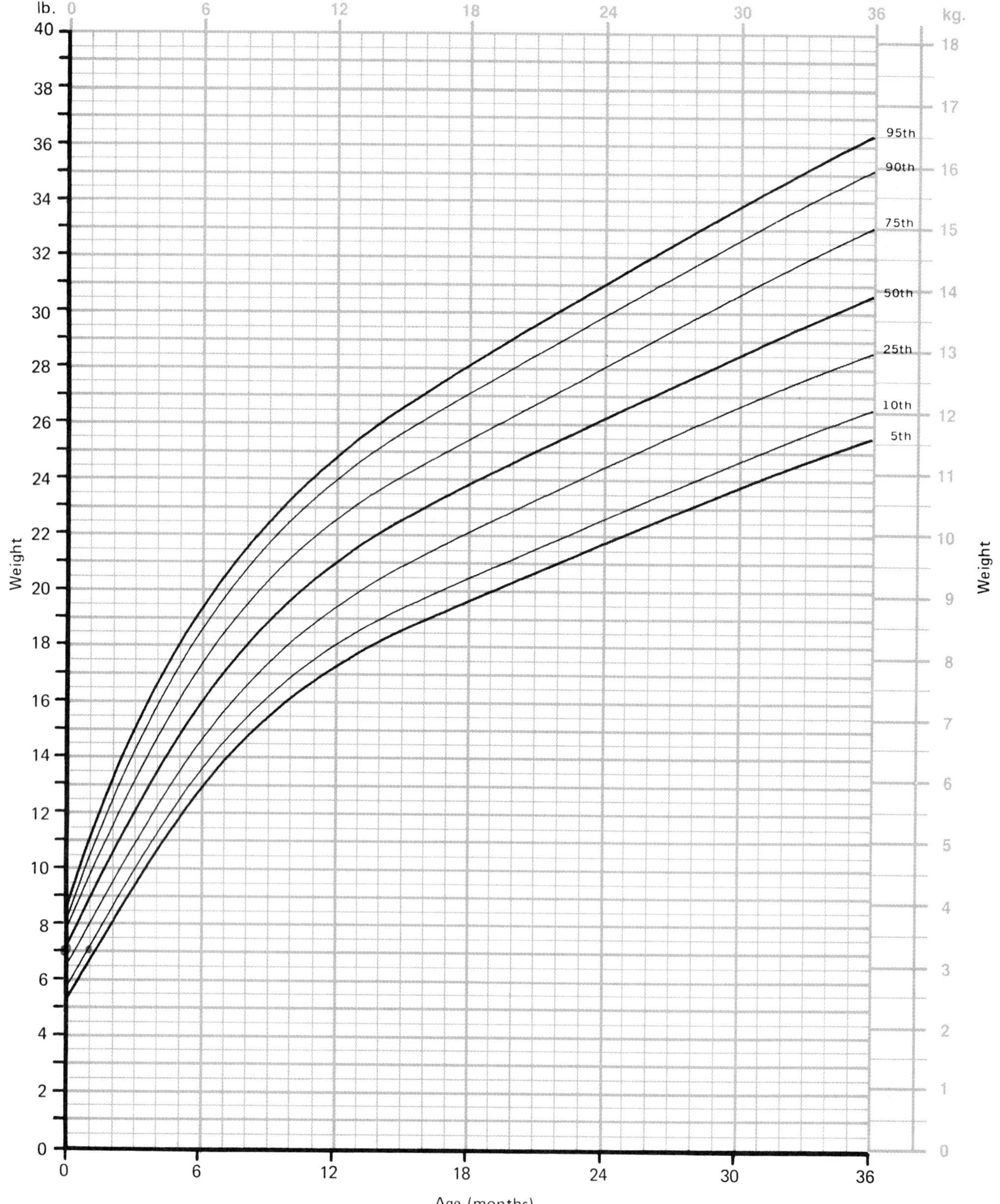

Appendix A continued

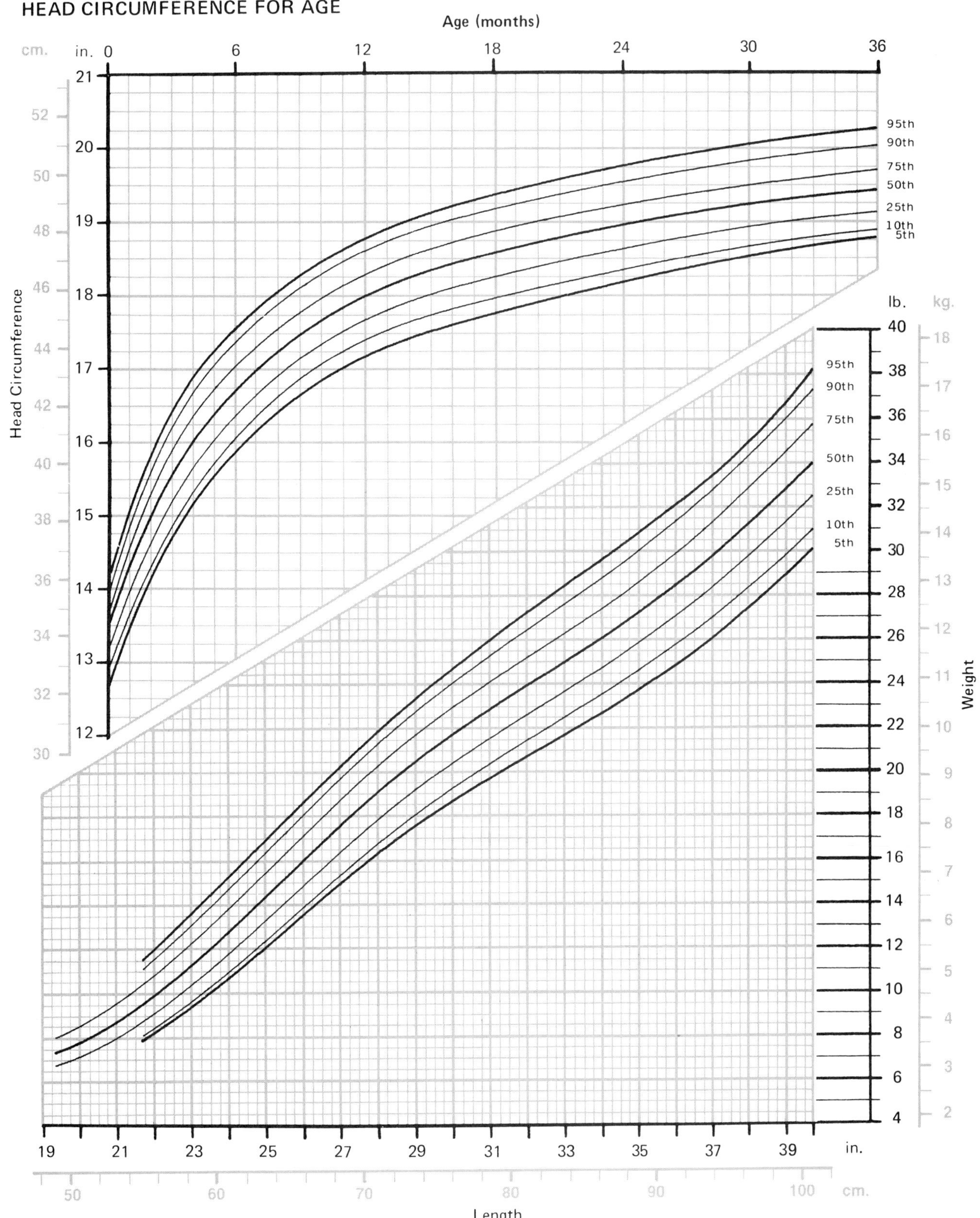

Appendix A continued

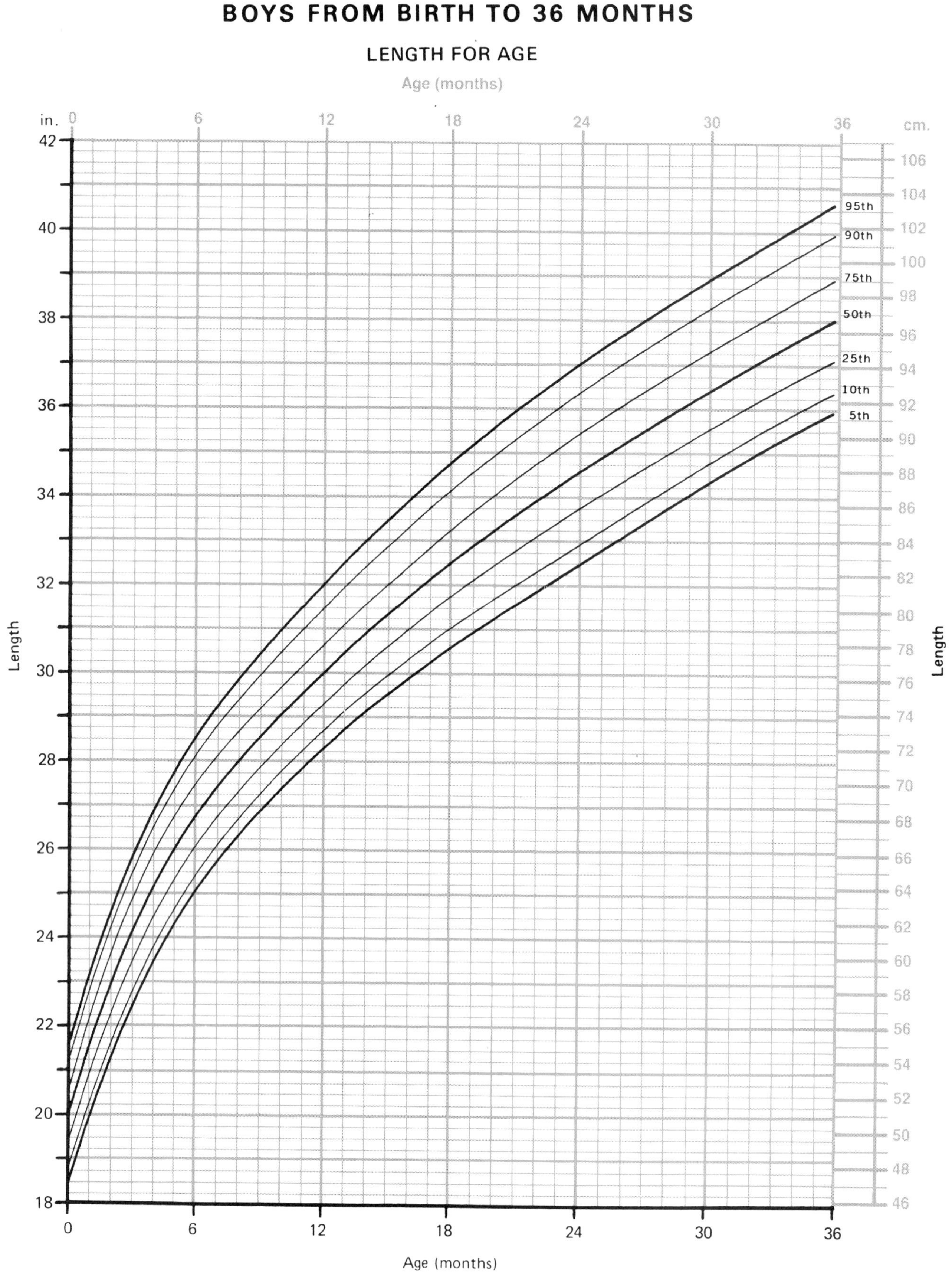

BOYS FROM BIRTH TO 36 MONTHS

LENGTH FOR AGE

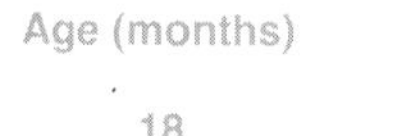

Age (months): 0 6 12 18 24 30 36

in. 42 40 38 36 34 32 30 28 26 24 22 20 18

cm. 106 104 102 100 98 96 94 92 90 88 86 84 82 80 78 76 74 72 70 68 66 64 62 60 58 56 54 52 50 48 46

95th
90th
75th
50th
25th
10th
5th

Length

Length

Age (months)

Appendix A continued

BOYS FROM BIRTH TO 36 MONTHS

WEIGHT FOR AGE

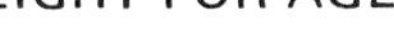

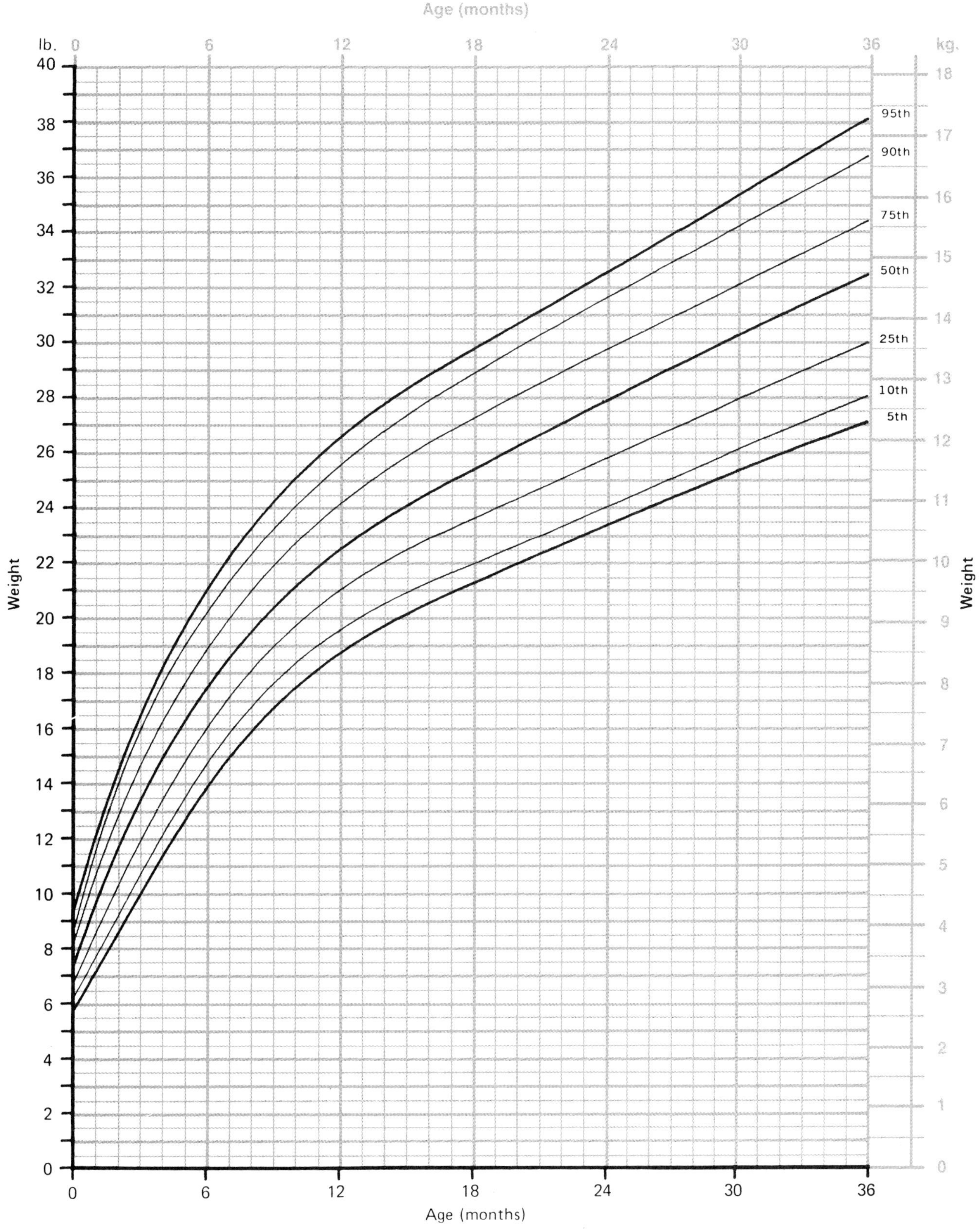

Appendix A continued

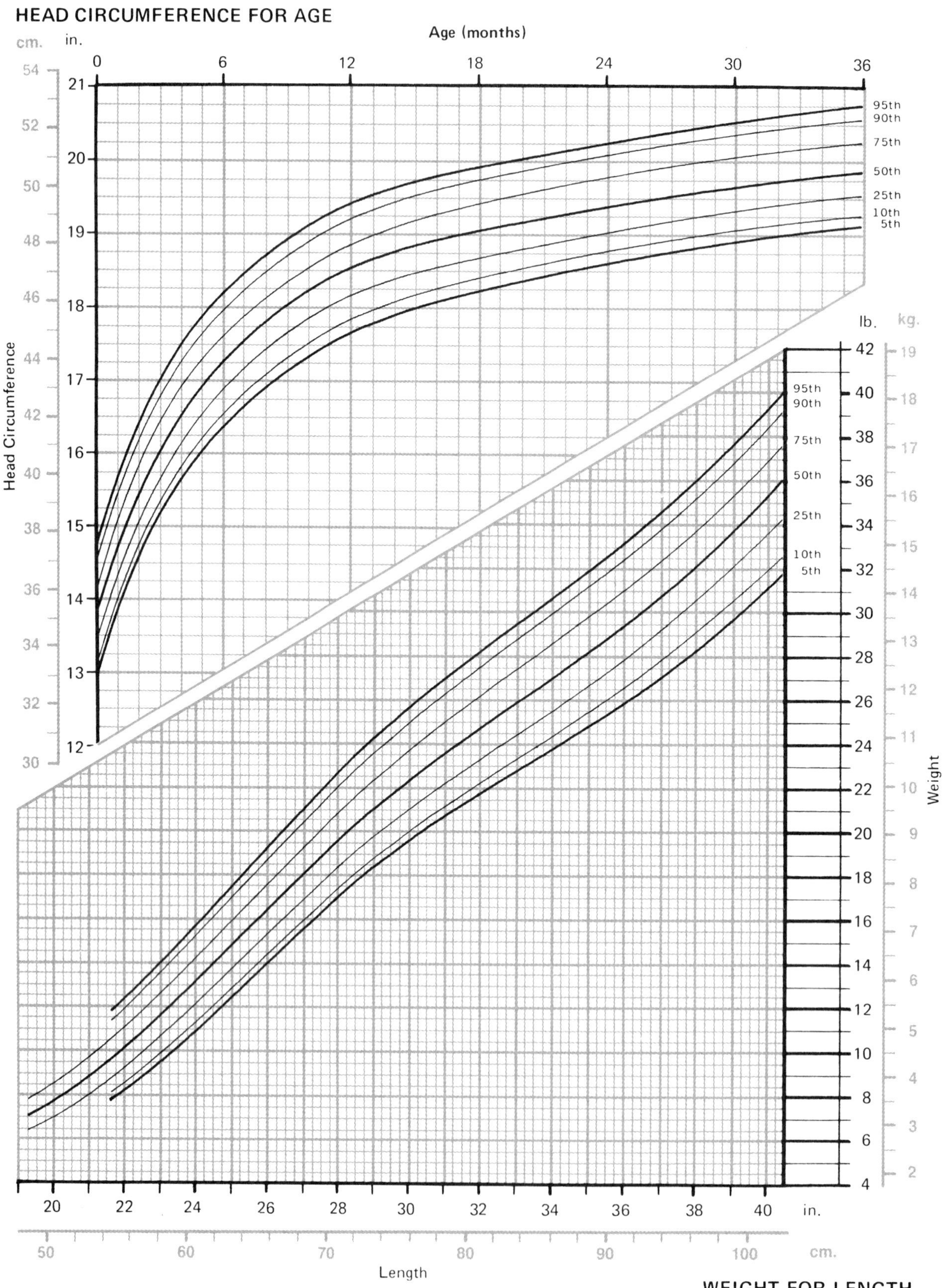

Appendix A continued

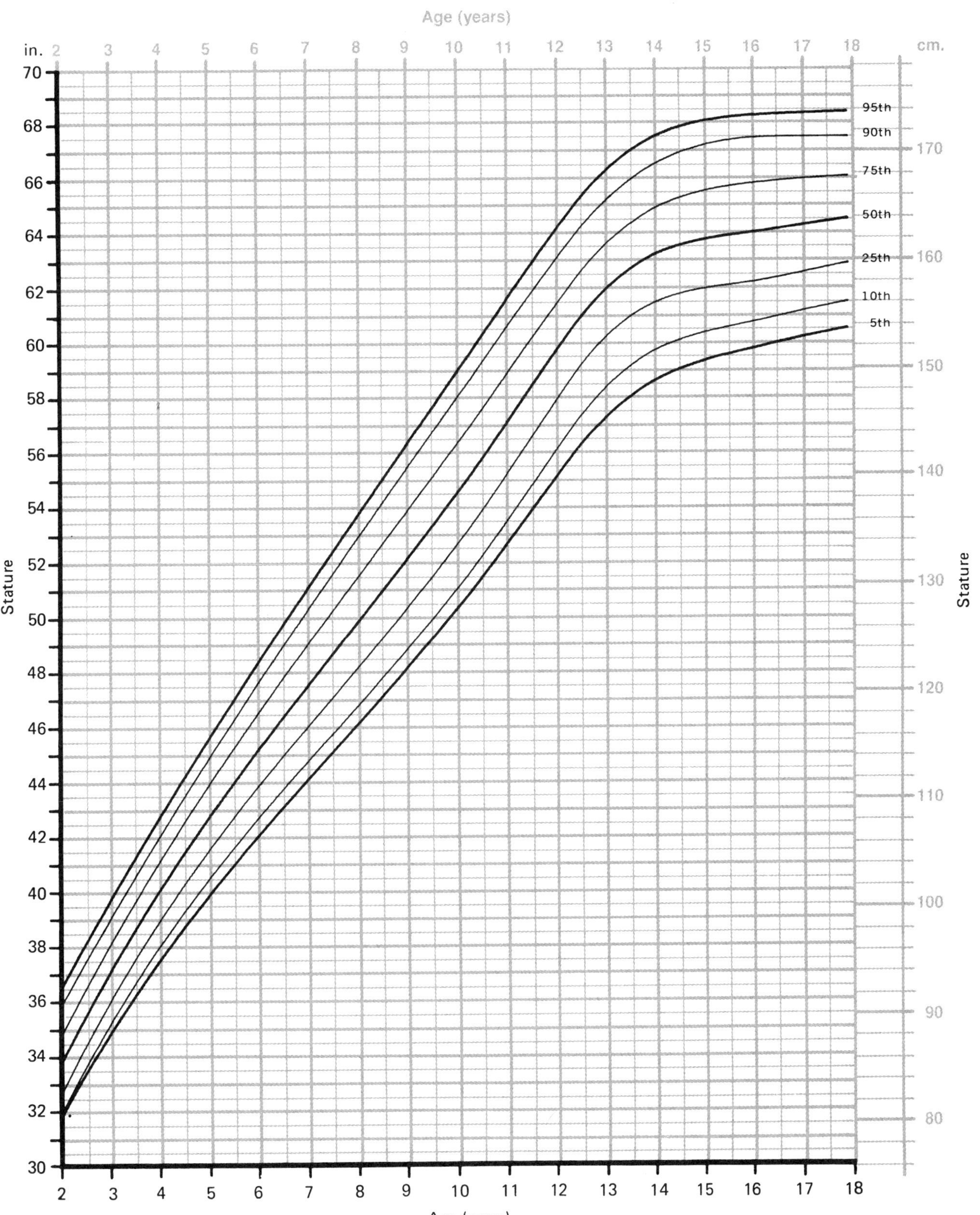

Appendix A continued

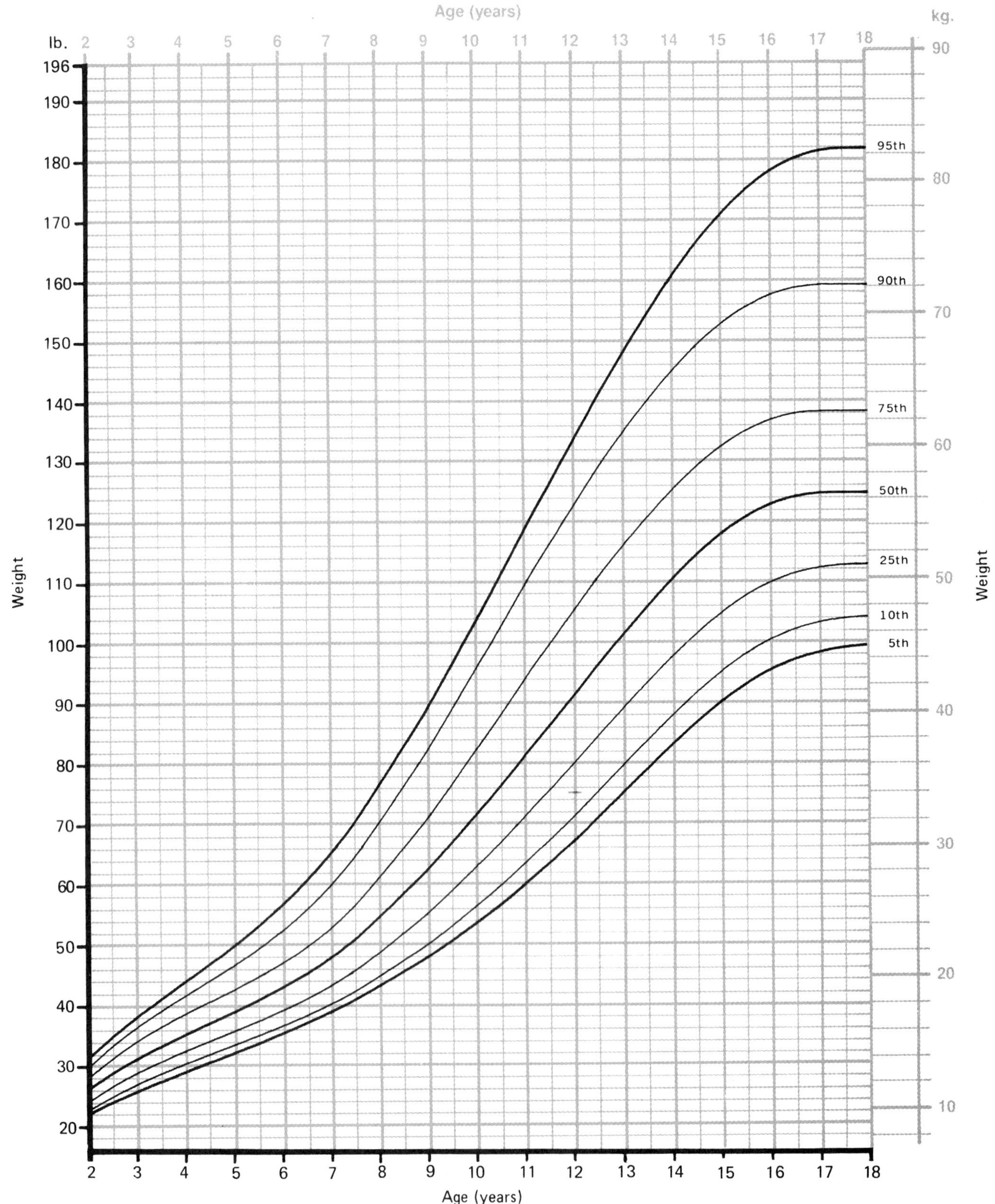

Appendix A continued

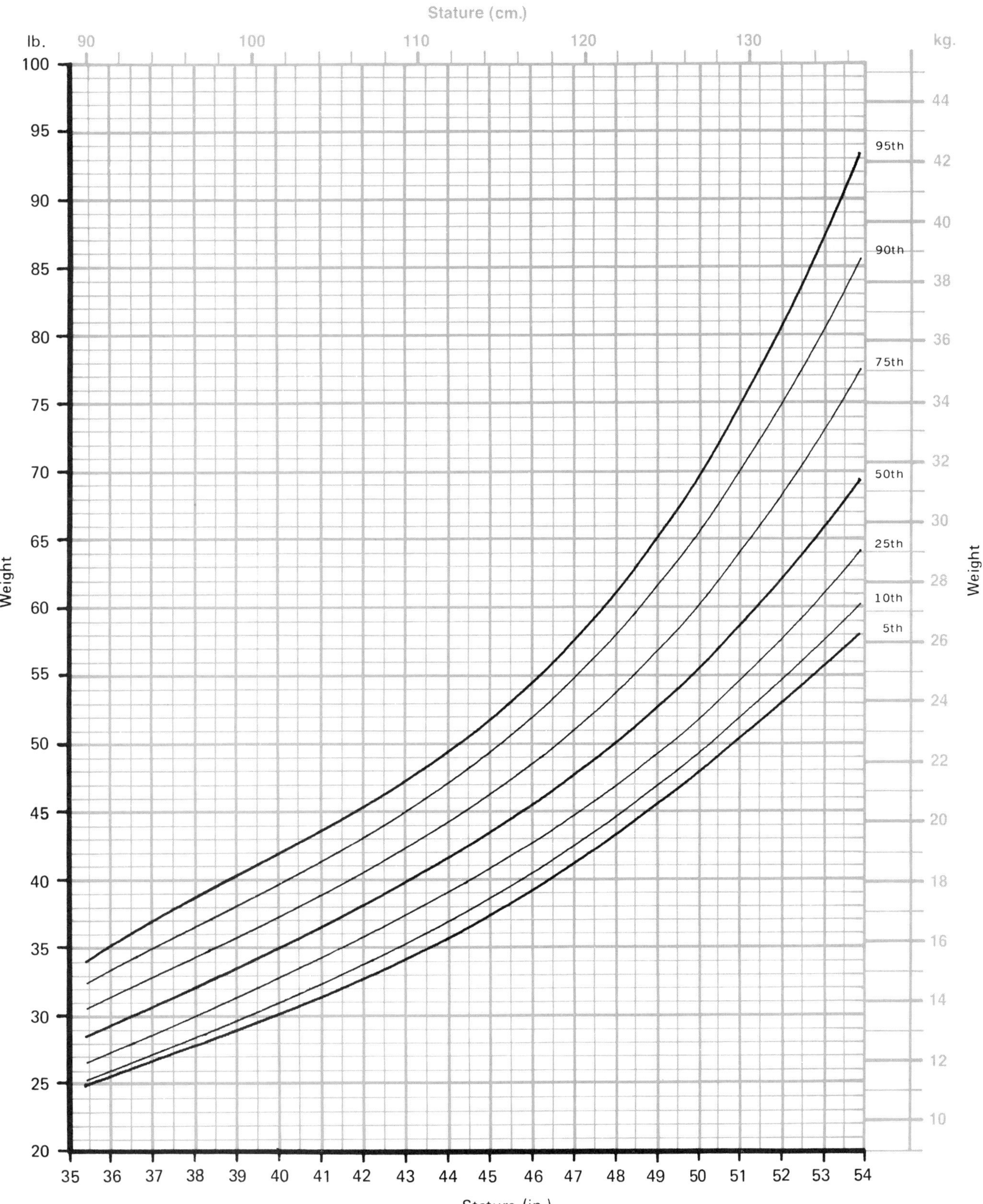

Lit. 504, 1-77

Appendix A continued

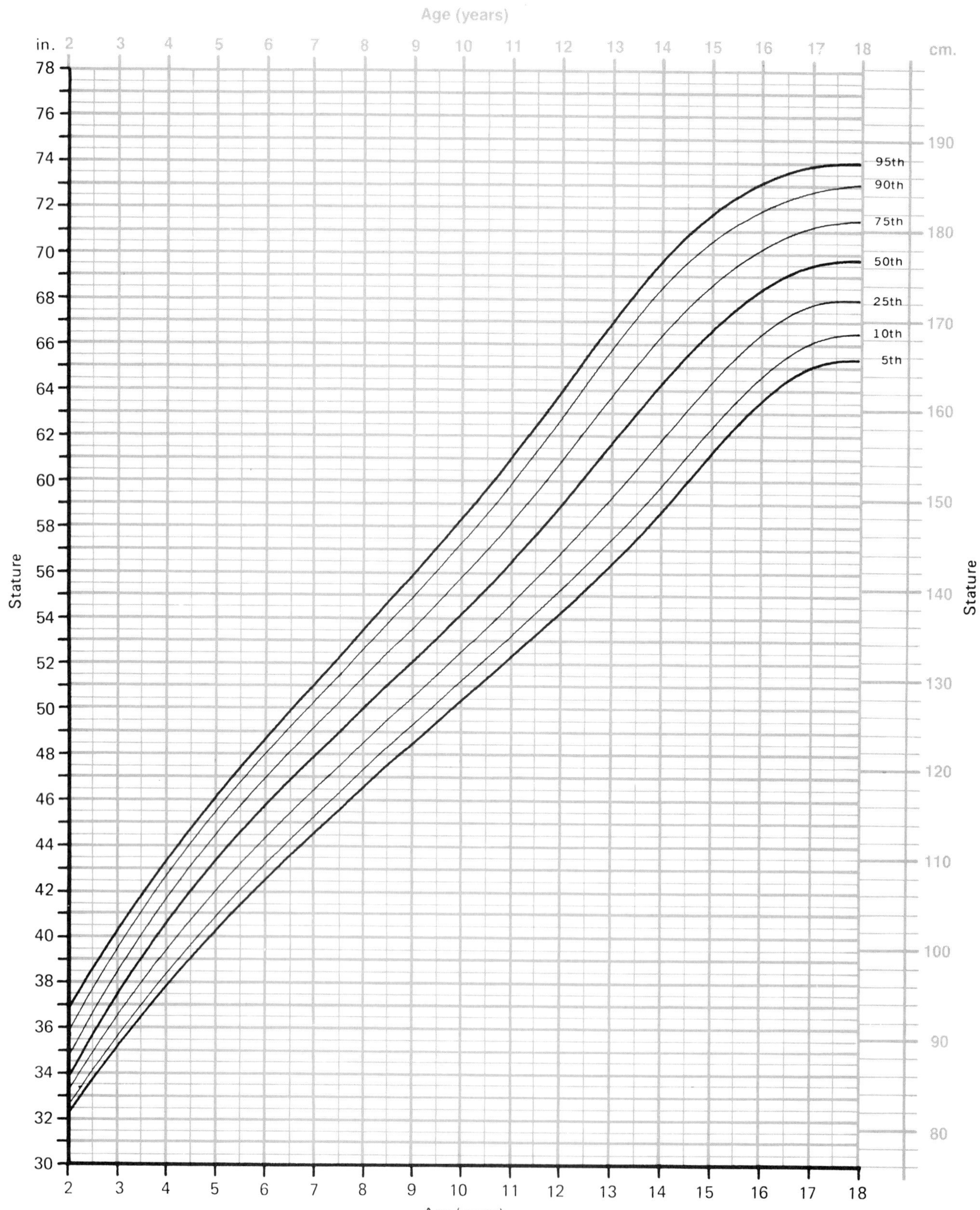

Appendix A continued

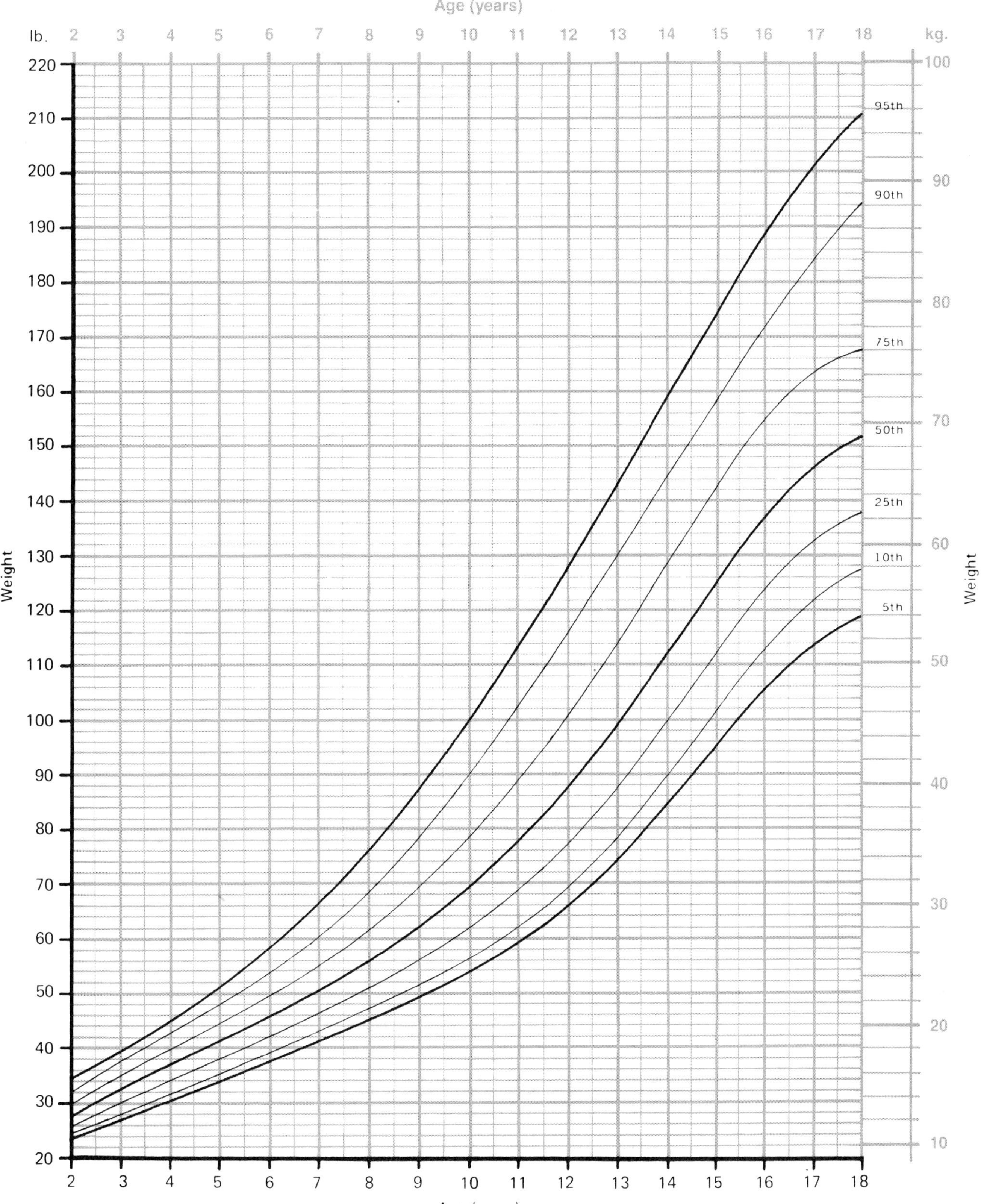

Appendix A continued

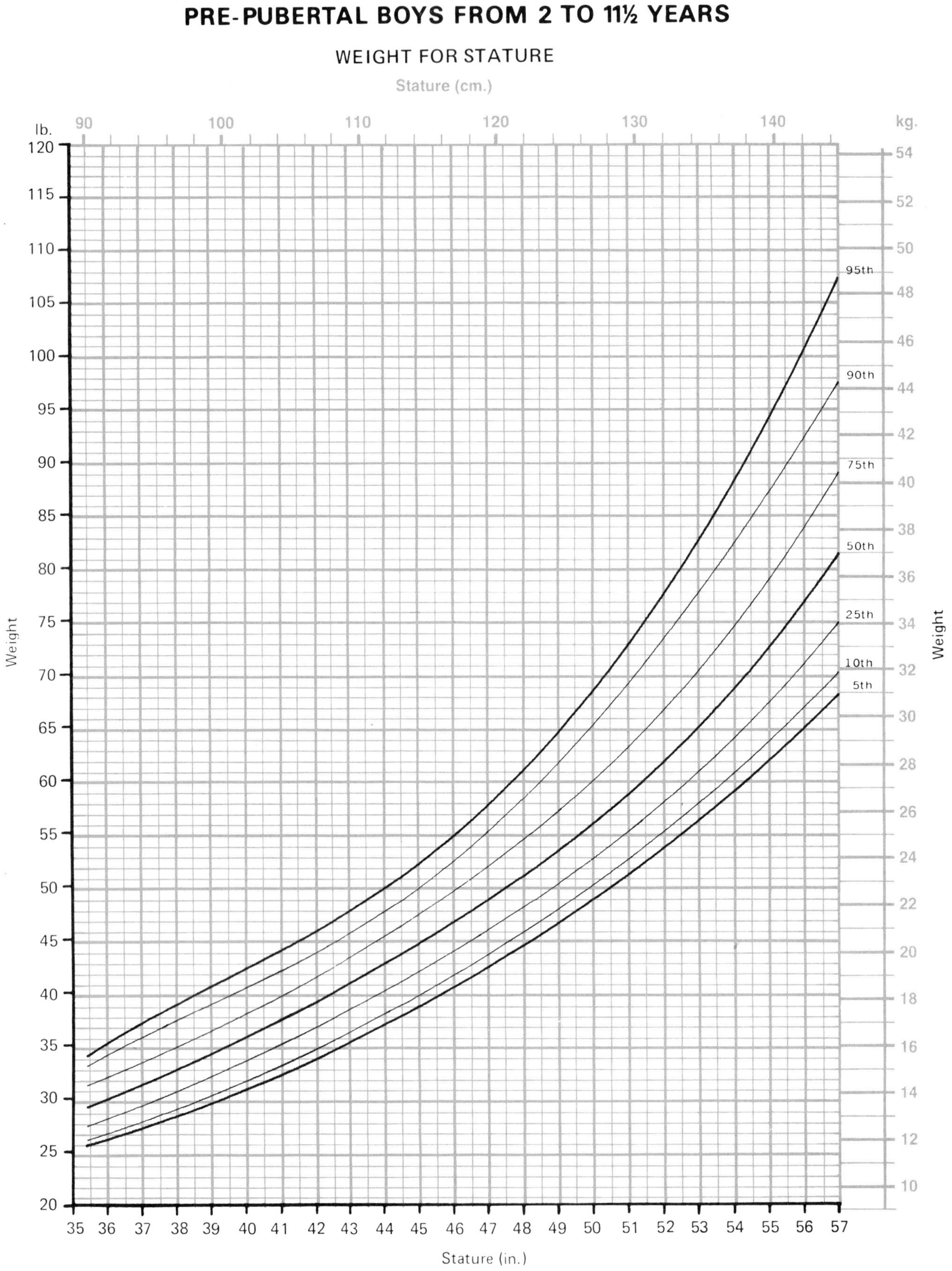

PRE-PUBERTAL BOYS FROM 2 TO 11½ YEARS

WEIGHT FOR STATURE

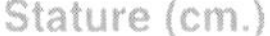

Lit. 502, 1-77

Appendix B Vital Signs—Variations With Age

Average Heart Rate for Children at Rest

Age	Average rate	2 SD
Birth	140	50
1st mo	130	45
1–6 mo	130	45
6–12 mo	115	40
1–2 yr	110	40
2–4 yr	105	35
6–10 yr	95	30
10–14 yr	85	30
14–18 yr	82	25

SOURCE: Reproduced with permission from Lowrey GH: *Growth and Development of Children*. 7th ed. Copyright © 1978 by Year Book Medical Publishers, Inc., Chicago.

Variations in Respiration With Age

Age	Rate/min	Tidal air, cc	Vital capacity, L*
Premature	40–90	12	—
Neonate	30–80	19	—
1 yr	20–40	48	—
2 yr	20–30	90	—
3 yr	20–30	125	—
5 yr	20–25	175	1.0
10 yr	17–22	320	2.0
15 yr	15–20	400	3.7
20 yr	15–20	500	3.8

*These represent mean figures from several sources for both sexes. Vital capacity for boys averages about 6% greater than for girls.

SOURCE: Reproduced with permission from Lowrey GH: *Growth and Development of Children*. 7th ed. Copyright © 1978 by Year Book Medical Publishers, Inc., Chicago.

Normal Blood Pressure for Various Ages (mm Hg)

Infants*		Age	Systolic	2 SD	Diastolic	2 SD
1st day	52	1 day	78	14	42	14
4th day	70	1 mo	86	20	54	18
10th day	80	6 mo	90	26	60	20
2d mo	95	1 yr	96	30	65	25
8th mo	95	2 yr	99	25	65	25
		4 yr	99	20	65	20
		6 yr	100	15	60	10
		8 yr	105	15	60	10
		10 yr	110	17	60	10
		12 yr	115	19	60	10
		14 yr	118	20	60	10
		16 yr	120	16	65	10

*The figures for infants represent averages by the flush method.

SOURCE: Reproduced with permission from Lowrey GH: *Growth and Development of Children*. 7th ed. Copyright © 1978 by Year Book Medical Publishers, Inc., Chicago.

Note: The figures under 1 year were obtained by the Doppler method. From 1 year on, the figures were obtained by auscultation, using the first change in sound to indicate diastolic pressure.

APPENDIX A SOURCE: Department of Health, Education, and Welfare, Public Health Service, Health Resources Administration, National Center for Health Satistics, and Center for Disease Control. Distributed by Mead Johnson Laboratories.

Appendix C Denver Developmental Screening Test

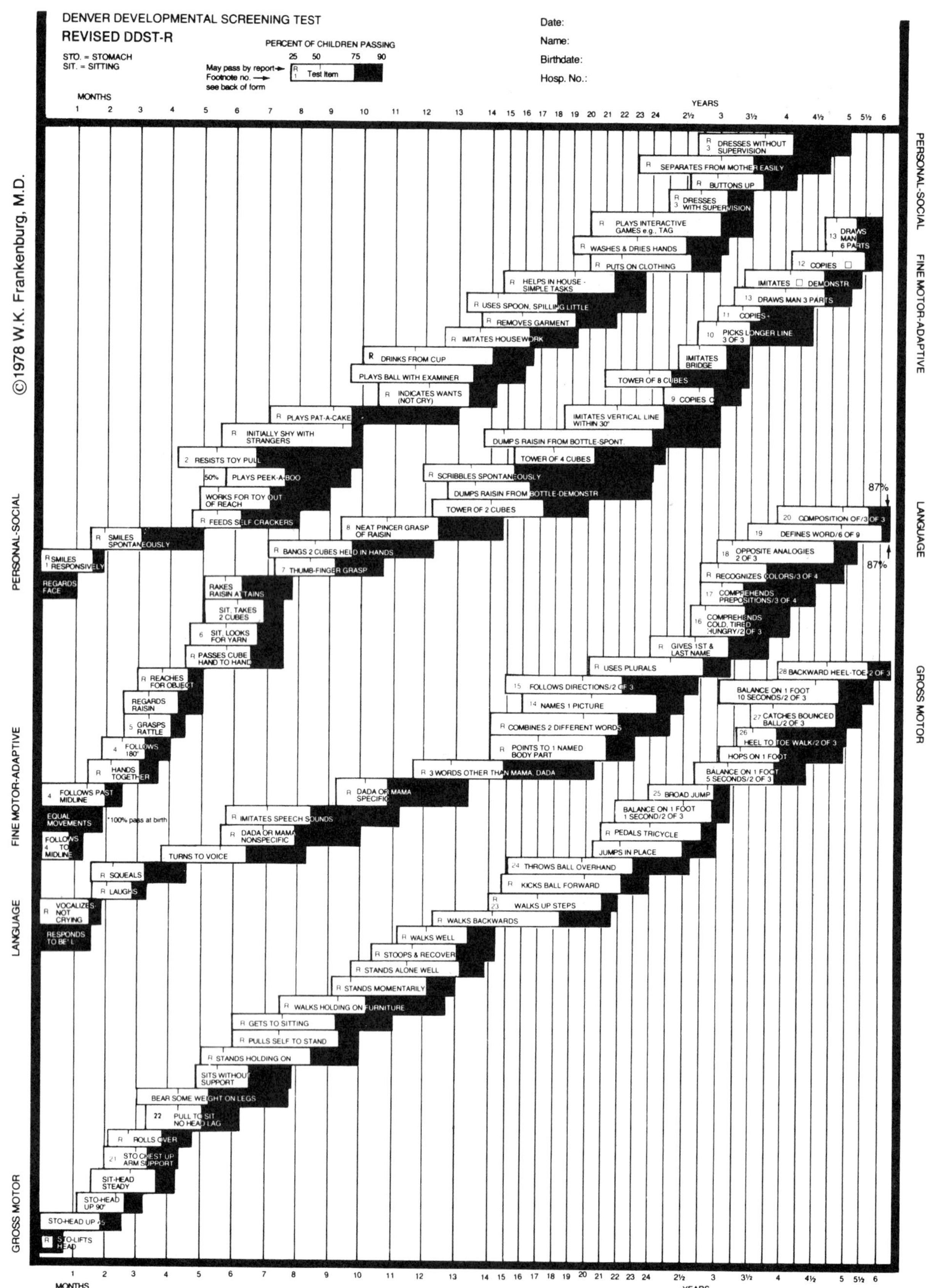

Appendix C continued

DIRECTIONS	DATE NAME BIRTHDATE HOSP. NO.

1. Try to get child to smile by smiling, talking or waving to him. Do not touch him.
2. When child is playing with toy, pull it away from him. Pass if he resists.
3. Child does not have to be able to tie shoes or button in the back.
4. Move yarn slowly in an arc from one side to the other, about 6" above child's face. Pass if eyes follow 90° to midline. (Past midline; 180°)
5. Pass if child grasps rattle when it is touched to the backs or tips of fingers.
6. Pass if child continues to look where yarn disappeared or tries to see where it went. Yarn should be dropped quickly from sight from tester's hand without arm movement.
7. Pass if child picks up raisin with any part of thumb and a finger.
8. Pass if child picks up raisin with the ends of thumb and index finger using an over hand approach.

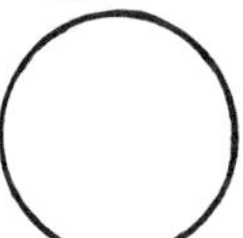

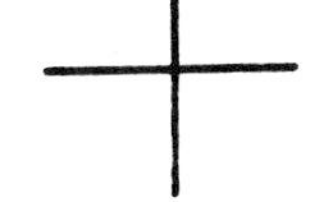
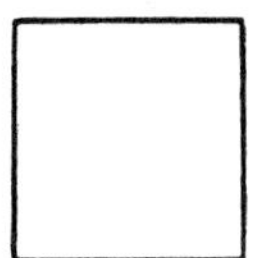

9. Pass any enclosed form. Fail continuous round motions.
10. Which line is longer? (Not bigger.) Turn paper upside down and repeat. (3/3 or 5/6)
11. Pass any crossing lines.
12. Have child copy first. If failed, demonstrate

When giving items 9, 11 and 12, do not name the forms. Do not demonstrate 9 and 11.

13. When scoring, each pair (2 arms, 2 legs, etc.) counts as one part.
14. Point to picture and have child name it. (No credit is given for sounds only.)

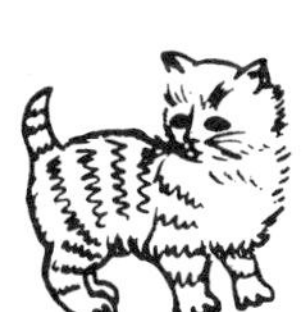
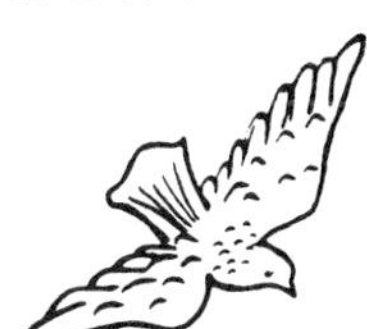
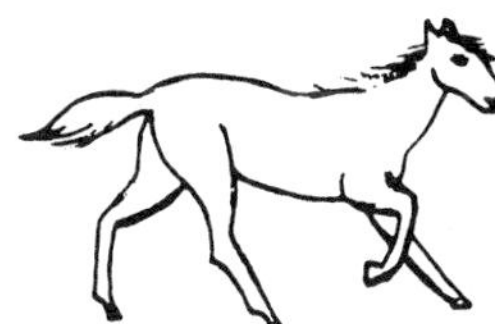
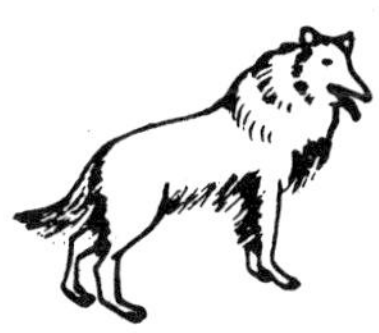
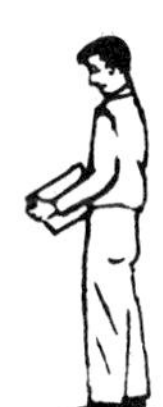

15. Tell child to: Give block to Mommie; put block on table; put block on floor. Pass 2 of 3. (Do not help child by pointing, moving head or eyes.)
16. Ask child: What do you do when you are cold? ..hungry? ..tired? Pass 2 of 3.
17. Tell child to: Put block <u>on</u> table; <u>under</u> table; <u>in front</u> of chair, <u>behind</u> chair. Pass 3 of 4. (Do not help child by pointing, moving head or eyes.)
18. Ask child: If fire is hot, ice is ?; Mother is a woman, Dad is a ?; a horse is big, a mouse is ?. Pass 2 of 3.
19. Ask child: What is a ball? ..lake? ..desk? ..house? ..banana? ..curtain? ..ceiling? ..hedge? ..pavement? Pass if defined in terms of use, shape, what it is made of or general category (such as banana is fruit, not just yellow). Pass 6 of 9.
20. Ask child: What is a spoon made of? ..a shoe made of? ..a door made of? (No other objects may be substituted.) Pass 3 of 3.
21. When placed on stomach, child lifts chest off table with support of forearms and/or hands.
22. When child is on back, grasp his hands and pull him to sitting. Pass if head does not hang back.
23. Child may use wall or rail only, not person. May not crawl.
24. Child must throw ball overhand 3 feet to within arm's reach of tester.
25. Child must perform standing broad jump over width of test sheet. (8-1/2 inches)
26. Tell child to walk forward, ⊂⊃⊂⊃⊂⊃⊂⊃→ heel within 1 inch of toe. Tester may demonstrate. Child must walk 4 consecutive steps, 2 out of 3 trials.
27. Bounce ball to child who should stand 3 feet away from tester. Child must catch ball with hands, not arms, 2 out of 3 trials.
28. Tell child to walk backward, ←⊂⊃⊂⊃⊂⊃⊂⊃ toe within 1 inch of heel. Tester may demonstrate. Child must walk 4 consecutive steps, 2 out of 3 trials.

<u>DATE AND BEHAVIORAL OBSERVATIONS</u> (how child feels at time of test, relation to tester, attention span, verbal behavior, self-confidence, etc,):

Appendix C continued

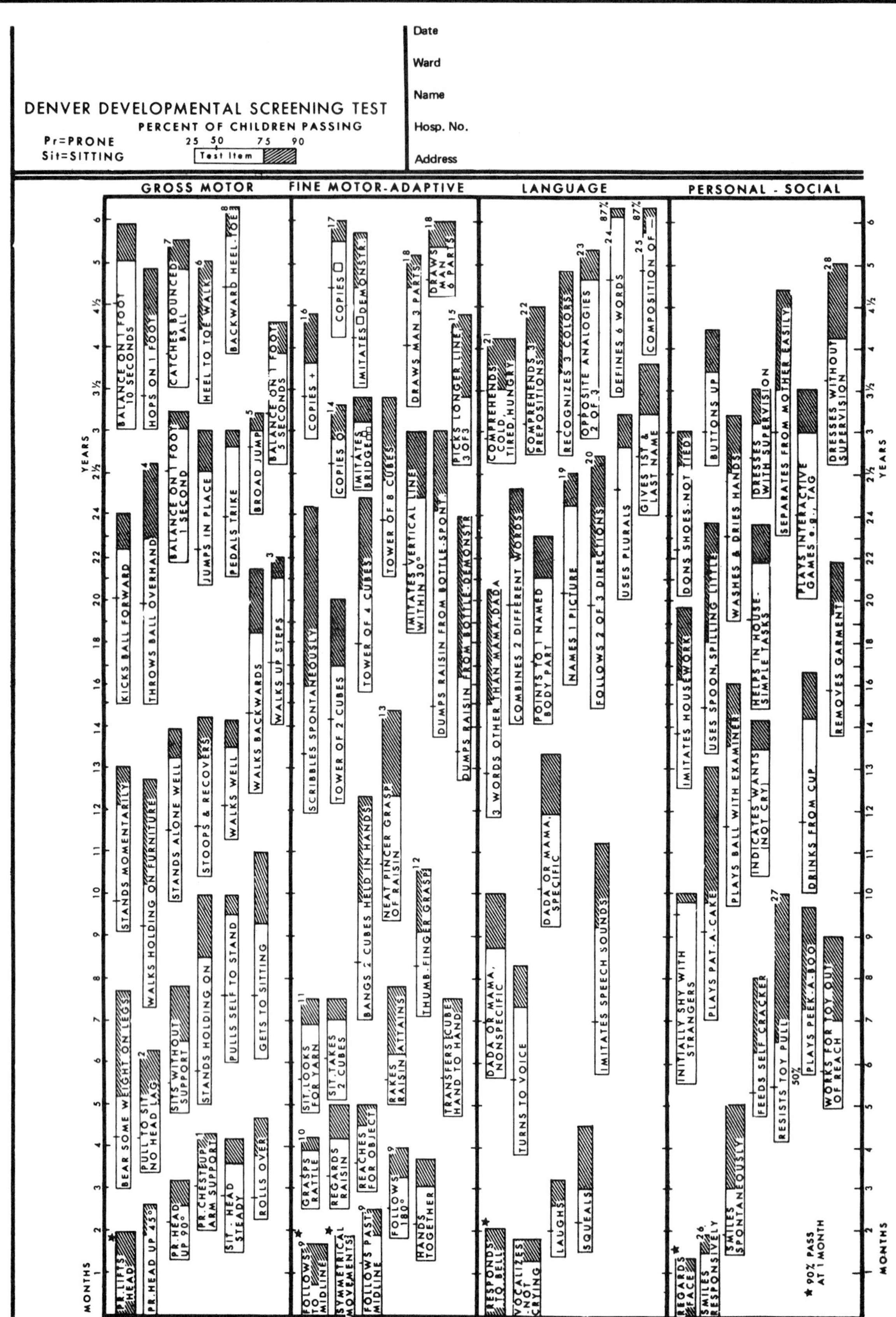

SOURCE: Reprinted with permission of William K. Frankerburg, MD, University of Colorado Medical Center.

Appendix D Home Observations for Measurement of the Environment

Birth to three years

Date of interview ______

Child designee ______
NAME AGE SEX ETHNICITY

Child's birthday ______ Birth order ______
Mother's name ______ Father's name ______
Address ______

Categories	**Raw scores**	**Percentile scores**
I. Emotional and verbal responsivity of mother	______	______
II. Avoidance of restriction and punishment	______	______
III. Organization of physical and temporal environment	______	______
IV. Provision of appropriate play materials	______	______
V. Maternal involvement with child	______	______
VI. Opportunities for variety in daily stimulation	______	______
TOTALS	______	______

I. Emotional and verbal responsivity of mother	**Yes**	**No**
1. Mother spontaneously vocalizes to child at least twice during visit (excluding scolding).	______	______
2. Mother responds to child's vocalizations with verbal response.	______	______
3. Mother tells child the name of some object during visit or says name of person or object in a "teaching style."	______	______
4. Mother's speech is distinct, clear and audible.	______	______
5. Mother initiates verbal interchanges with observer—asks questions, makes spontaneous comments.	______	______
6. Mother expresses ideas freely and easily and uses statements of appropriate length for conversation (eg, gives more than brief answers).	______	______
*7. Mother permits child occasionally to engage in "messy" types of play.	______	______

Example: "Does he sometimes want to play in his food or in his bath?" or "Do you sometimes let him play and be messy?"

8. Mother spontaneously praises the child's qualities or behavior twice during visit.	______	______
9. When speaking of or to child, mother's voice conveys positive feeling.	______	______
10. Mother caresses or kisses child at least once during visit.	______	______
11. Mother shows some positive emotional responses to praise of child offered by visitor.	______	______

II. Avoidance of restriction and punishment	**Yes**	**No**
12. Mother does not shout at child during visit.	______	______
13. Mother does not express overt annoyance with or hostility toward child.	______	______
14. Mother neither slaps nor spanks child during visit.	______	______
*15. Mother reports that no more than one instance of physical punishment occurred during the past week.	______	______

Example: "How do you manage his discipline at this age—what works the best? In general, does he mind pretty well, or do you have to occasionally slap his hands or physically punish him in some way?" If yes, probe for number of times in the past week.

16. Mother does not scold or derogate child during visit.	______	______
17. Mother does not interfere with child's actions or restrict child's movements more than 3 times during visit.	______	______
18. At least ten books are present and visible.	______	______
*19. Family has a pet.	______	______

III. Organization of environment	**Yes**	**No**
20. When mother is away, care is provided by one of three regular substitutes.	______	______

Example: "How about your time outside the home and away from your child; do you have a regular sitter that you can count on or do you have to get someone different each time?" Probe for grocery store (once a week), relatives (monthly).

21. Someone takes child into grocery store at least once a week.	______	______

*Items that may require direct questions

SOURCE: Adapted from Caldwell, BM: Home Observation for Measurement of the Environment (birth to three), Little Rock, Ark., 1970.

Appendix D continued

	Yes	No
22. Child gets out of house at least four times a week.		
23. Child is taken regularly to doctor's office or clinic.		
*24. Child has a special place in which to keep his toys and "treasures."		

Example: Special place for toys; usually ask this at the end of the interview saying, "I'm interested in seeing some of your child's toys, where he keeps them and some of his favorite things to play with."

25. Child's play environment appears safe and free of hazards.		

IV. Provision of appropriate play material	**Yes**	**No**
26. Child has some muscle activity toys or equipment.		
27. Child has push or pull toy.		
28. Child has stroller or walker, kiddie car, scooter or tricycle.		
29. Mother provides toys or interesting activities for child during interview.		
30. Provides learning equipment appropriate to age—cuddly toy or toys for role play.		
31. Provides learning equipment appropriate to age—mobile, table and chairs, high chair, playpen.		
32. Provides eye-hand coordination toys—items to go in and out of receptacle, fit together toys, beads.		
33. Provides eye-hand coordination toys that permit combinations—stacking or nesting toys, blocks or building toys.		
34. Provides toys for literature and music.		

V. Maternal involvement with child	**Yes**	**No**
35. Mother tends to keep child within visual range and to look at him often.		
36. Mother "talks" to child while doing her work.		

Example: "Do you sometimes find yourself making conversation with him while you're working around the house, or is he usually asleep while you're doing your housework?"

37. Mother consciously encourages developmental advance.		
38. Mother invests "maturing toys" with value via her attention.		

Example: "How does he usually get started playing with a new toy—do you show him how to work it and try to get him involved with it or does he usually figure it out for himself?"

39. Mother structures child's play periods.		
40. Mother provides toys that challenge child to develop new skills.		

Example: "How do you usually decide what kinds of toys to select and offer your child to play with at this age? What are some of your guidelines?" (Listen for toys that will challenge child to develop new skills.)

VI. Opportunities for variety in daily stimulation	**Yes**	**No**
41. Father provides some caretaking every day.		
42. Mother reads stories at least three times weekly.		
43. Child eats at least one meal per day with mother and father.		

Example: "What does he do while you and your husband eat your meals? Does he usually eat with you or does he eat at another time?"

44. Family visits or receives visits from relatives (approximately once a month).		
45. Child has three or more books of his own.		

Totals for each category:

Emotional and verbal responsibility of mother	
Avoidance of restriction and punishment	
Organization of environment	
Provision of appropriate play material	
Maternal involvement with child	
Opportunities for variety in daily stimulation	

Three to six years

Date of interview ____________

Child designee ____
NAME AGE SEX ETHNICITY

Child's birthday ____________________ Birth order ____________________

Appendix D continued

Mother's name ____________ Father's name ____________
Address ____________

Categories	Raw scores	Percentile scores
I. Provisions of stimulation through equipment, toys, and experiences		
II. Stimulation of mature behavior		
III. Provision of stimulating physical and language environment		
IV. Avoidance of restriction and punishment		
V. Pride, affection, and thoughtfulness		
VI. Masculine stimulation		
VII. Independence from parental control		
TOTALS		

I. Provision of stimulation through equipment, toys, and experiences	**Yes**	**No**
1–12 The following are present in home and either belong to child subject or he is allowed to play with them:		
1. Toys to learn colors, sizes, shapes—typewriter, pressouts, play school, peg boards, and so on		
2. Toy or game facilitating learning letters (blocks with letters, toy typewriter, letter sticks, books about letters)		
3. Three or more puzzles		
4. Two toys necessitating some finger and whole hand movements (crayons and coloring books, paper dolls)		
5. Record player and at least five children's records		
6. Real or toy musical instrument (piano, drum, toy xylophone or guitar)		
7. Toy or game permitting free expression (finger paints, play dough, crayons or paint and paper)		
8. Toys or game necessitating refined movements (paint by number, dot book, paper dolls, crayons and coloring books)		
9. Toys to learn animals—books about animals, circus games, animal puzzles and so on		
10. Toy or game facilitating learning numbers (blocks with numbers, books about numbers, games with numbers)		
11. Building toys (blocks, tinker toys, Lincoln logs)		
12. Ten children's books		
13. At least 10 books are present and visible in the apartment.		
14. Family buys a newspaper daily and reads it.		
15. Family subscribes to at least one magazine.		
16. Family member has taken child on one outing (picnic, shopping excursion) at least every other week.		
17. Child has been taken out to eat in some kind of restaurant three or four times in the past year.		
18–20 Child has been taken by a family member to the following within the past year:		
18. Airport		
19. A trip more than 50 miles from his home (50 miles radial distance, not total distance)		
20. A scientific, historical, or art museum		
21. Child is taken to grocery store at least once a week.		
SUBSCORE		

II. Simulation of mature behavior	**Yes**	**No**
22–29 Child is encouraged to learn the following:		
22. Colors		
23. Shapes		
24. Patterned speech (nursery rhymes, prayers, songs, TV commercials, and so on)		
25. The alphabet		
26. To tell time		
27. Spatial relationships (up, down, under, big, little, and so on)		
28. Numbers		
29. To read a few words		
30. Tries to get child to pick up and put away toys after play session—without help.		
31. Child is taught rules of social behavior which involve recognition of rights of others.		
32. Parent teaches child some simple manners—to say, "Please," "Thank you," "I'm sorry."		
33. Some delay of food gratification is demanded of the child, e.g., not to whine or demand food unless within ½ hour of meal time.		
SUBSCORE		

Appendix D continued

III. Provision of a stimulating physical and language environment (observation items, except **)	**Yes**	**No**
34. Building has no potentially dangerous structural or health defect (plaster coming down from ceiling, stairway with boards missing, rodents, and so on).	______	______
35. Child's outside play environment appears safe and free of hazards (no outside play area requires an automatic "No").	______	______
36. The interior of the apartment is not dark or perceptibly monotonous.	______	______
37. House is not overly noisy—television, shouts of children, radio, and so on.	______	______
38. Neighborhood has trees, grass, birds—is esthetically pleasing.	______	______
39. There is at least 100 square feet of living space per person in the house.	______	______
40. In terms of available floor space, the rooms are not overcrowded with furniture.	______	______
41. All visible rooms of the house are reasonably clean and minimally cluttered.	______	______
*42. Mother uses complex sentence structure and some long words in conversing.	______	______
43. Mother uses correct grammar and pronunciation.	______	______
44. Mother's speech is distinct, clear, and audible.	______	______
**45. Family has TV and it is used judiciously, not left on continuously (no TV requires an automatic "No"—any scheduling scores "Yes").	______	______
SUBSCORE	______	______

IV. Avoidance of restriction and punishment (observation items, except **)	**Yes**	**No**
46. Mother does not scold or derogate child more than once during visit.	______	______
47. Mother does not use physical restraint, shake, grab, pinch child during visit.	______	______
48. Mother neither slaps nor spanks child during visit.	______	______
49. Mother does not express over-annoyance with or hostility toward child—complain, say child is "bad" or won't mind.	______	______
50. Child is not punished or ridiculed for speech.	______	______
**51. No more than one instance of physical punishment occurred during the past week (accept parental report).	______	______
**52. Child does not get slapped or spanked for spilling food or drink.	______	______
SUBSCORE	______	______

V. Pride, affection, and thoughtfulness (observation items, except**)	**Yes**	**No**
**53. Parent turns on special TV program regarded as "good" for children.	______	______
**54. Someone reads stories to child or shows and comments on pictures in magazines five times weekly.	______	______
**55. Parent encourages child to relate experiences or takes time to listen to him relate experiences.	______	______
**56. Parent holds child close ten to fifteen minutes per day, such as during TV, story time, visiting.	______	______
**57. Parent occasionally sings to child, or sings in presence of child.	______	______
**58. Child has a special place in which to keep his toys and "treasures."	______	______
**59. Child's art work is displayed some place in house (anything that child makes).	______	______
60. Mother introduces interviewer to child.	______	______
61. Mother converses with child at least twice during visit (scolding and suspicious comments not counted).	______	______
62. Mother answers child's questions or requests verbally.	______	______
63. Mother usually responds verbally to child's talking.	______	______
64. Mother provides toys or interesting activities or in other ways structures situation for child during visit when her attention will be elsewhere. (To score "Yes" mother must make an active guiding gesture or suggestion to structure child's play.)	______	______
65. Mother spontaneously praises child's qualities or behavior twice during visit.	______	______
66. When speaking of or to child, mother's voice conveys positive feeling.	______	______
67. Mother caresses, kisses, or cuddles child at least once during visit.	______	______
68. Mother sets up situation that allows child to show off during visit.	______	______
SUBSCORE	______	______

VI. Masculine stimulation	**Yes**	**No**
69. Child sees and spends some time with father or father figure four days a week.	______	______
70. Child eats at least one meal per day, on most days, with mother (or mother figure) and father (or father figure). (One-parent families get an automatic "No".)	______	______
71–73 The following are present in home and either belong to child subject or he is allowed to play with them:		
71. Ride toy (tricycle, scooter, wagon, bike with or without training wheels)	______	______

Appendix D continued

	Yes	No
72. Medium wheel toys—trucks, trains, doll carriage, and so on	______	______
73. Large muscle toy (jump rope, swing, ball, climbing object)	______	______
SUBSCORE	______	______
VII. Independence from parental control	**Yes**	**No**
74. Child is encouraged to try to dress himself.	______	______
75. Child is permitted to choose some of his clothing to be worn except on very special occasions.	______	______
76. Child is permitted some choice in lunch or breakfast menu.	______	______
77. Parent lets child choose certain favorite food products or brands at grocery store.	______	______
78. Child is permitted to go to another house to play without having the caregiver accompany him.	______	______
79. Child can express negative feelings without harsh reprisal.	______	______
80. Child is permitted to hit parent without harsh reprisal.	______	______
SUBSCORE	______	______
TOTAL SCORE	______	______

SOURCE: Adapted from Caldwell BM: Home Observation for Measurement of the Environment (birth to three). College of Education, University of Arkansas at Little Rock.

Appendix E Fluid Intake, Output, and Distribution

Basic Requirements in Relation to Age, Weight, and Surface Area

Age	Weight		Surface area	Basal metabolism		Minimal basal water requirement		
	lb	kg	m^2	Cal/kg	Cal/24 hr	mL/24 hr	mL/m^3	mL/kg
Newborn	7.5	3.3	0.2	45	150	150	750	45
1 wk	7.5	3.3	0.2	60	200	200	1,000	60
2 mo	11	5	0.25	54	270	270	1,080	54
6 mo	17.5	8	0.35	50	400	400	1,140	50
12 mo	22	10	0.45	50	500	500	1,110	50
3 yr	33	15	0.60	47	700	700	1,170	47
5 yr	44	20	0.80	45	900	900	1,120	45
8 yr	66	30	1.05	37	1,100	1,100	1,050	37
13 yr		60	1.70	27	1,600	1,600	840	27

SOURCE: From Rudolph: *Pediatrics,* 16th ed. Appleton-Century-Crofts, New York, 1977, p. 198.

Average Daily Secretion of Urine

Age	mL/24 hr
1 and 2 days	15–50
3–10 days	50–300
10 days to 2 mo	250–400
2 mo to 1 yr	400–500
1–3 yr	500–600
3–5 yr	600–750
5–8 yr	700–1,000
8–14 yr	700–1,500

SOURCE: Lowrey GH: *Growth and Development of Children.* 7th ed. Copyright © 1978 by Year Book Medical Publishers, Inc., Chicago.

Appendix F Admission Assessment—Nursing

A

ADMISSION ASSESSMENT — NURSING

DATE ____ AGE ____ SEX ____

MARITAL STATUS ____ LANGUAGE SPOKEN AT HOME ____

FROM WHOM WAS THIS HISTORY OBTAINED

☐ Patient ☐ Parent(s) ☐ Spouse ☐ Other ____

☐ Legal Guardian/Custody (Name) ____

PREFERRED NAME ____

ATTENDED CHMC PRE-ADMISSION PROGRAM ☐ Yes ☐ No

REASON FOR ADMISSION ____

WHERE DO YOU RECEIVE MEDICAL CARE ____

AGENCIES INVOLVED IN CARE	CONTACT PERSON	TELEPHONE NO.

HT. ____ WT. ____ TEMP. ____ PULSE ____ RESP. ____ B/P ____

RECENT/CURRENT MEDICATIONS ☐ Yes ☐ No (If Yes, give name of medication, frequency taken, who administers medication)

ALLERGIES ☐ Yes ☐ No (Drugs, Food, Environment)

HELPING PATIENT/FAMILY COPE WITH HOSPITALIZATION

PATTERNS OF COPING (Ability to verbalize, comfort measures, identified fears, special needs, words, security objects)

RELIGIOUS OR CULTURAL NEEDS THAT WILL REQUIRE SPECIAL ATTENTION DURING HOSPITALIZATION

EXPRESSED NEED FOR FINANCIAL OR OTHER RESOURCES DURING HOSPITALIZATION

PLANS FOR FAMILY PARTICIPATION IN CARE

03581 5M (Rev. 10/80)

HEALTH CONCERNS/PROBLEMS

REVIEW OF SYSTEMS (Information obtained through interview with patient and/or family)

ASSESSMENT OF PHYSICAL STATUS

Skin ____ Cardiovascular Status ____

Head/Neck ____ Back/Extremities ____

Eyes/Ears/Nose ____ Abdomen ____

Mouth/Teeth ____ Neurological Status ____

Chest/Respiratory Status ____ Genitals/Perineum ____

Psychiatric/Emotional Status ____

Other information important in planning nursing care ____

SIGNATURES OF NURSES COMPLETING FORM

1. ____ Date ____ 2. ____ Date ____

Appendix F continued

FAMILY STAYING ON DIVISION ☐ Yes ☐ No

FAMILY MEMBERS

	NAME	AGE	GENERAL HEALTH
FATHER (or Spouse)			
MOTHER			
SIBLINGS (or Patient's Children)			

SIGNIFICANT OTHERS

PRIMARY CARETAKER

ISSUES RELEVANT TO CARE IN HOSPITAL

ACTIVITIES OF DAILY LIVING (Performed with or without assistance of another person or device – bathing, brushing teeth, feeding, walking, attending school/work, etc.) Explain:

SCHOOL/WORK

Name of School ______ Grade ______

Special Classes/Learning Needs ______

Type of Work ______

HOBBIES/EXERCISE/SPORTS/PLAY

HEALTH MAINTENANCE

DIET ______

☐ Table Food ☐ Baby Food

Favorite Foods ______

Foods Disliked ______

Special Diet – Cultural/Medical ______

Special Feeding Techniques/Problems ______

Drinks from: ☐ Bottle ☐ Special Nurser ☐ Breast Fed ☐ Cup ☐ Tippy Cup

☐ Special Devices ______

SLEEP

Type of Bed ______ Usual Bedtime ______ Usual Rising Time ______ Nap(s) Time ______ How Long ______

Bedwetter ☐ Yes ☐ No Climber ☐ Yes ☐ No

Special Rituals and Sleeping Habits ______

Problems ______

ELIMINATION (Child's usual toileting routines and patterns – techniques or aids used)

☐ Cloth Diapers ☐ Disposable Diapers ☐ Potty Chair ☐ Toilet Trained (☐ Day ☐ Night)

What terminology is used by child to communicate his/her needs ______

Problems ______

OTHER FACTORS THAT MAY AFFECT HEALTH (Tobacco, Alcohol, Drugs, Sexuality – complete this section only if relevant to care)

GROWTH AND DEVELOPMENT (Note milestones and concerns related to gross motor, fine motor, speech/language development and socialization – record when patient sat, walked, spoke first words)

ROUTINE HEALTH SCREENING (Special needs for infection control)

Recent exposure to communicable diseases ☐ Yes ☐ No

Date ______ Describe ______

Congenital Rubella ☐ Yes ☐ No Hepatitis ☐ Yes ☐ No

Cytomegalic Inclusion Virus ☐ Yes ☐ No Other (e.g., parasites) ☐ Yes (describe) ______ ☐ No

Known Antibiotic Resistance ______

Has had Chicken Pox ☐ Yes ☐ No

IMMUNIZATIONS							TUBERCULIN TESTS	
	INITIAL DATE			BOOSTER DATE				
TYPE	1st	2nd	3rd	1st	2nd	3rd	DATE	RESULTS
DPT								
POLIO								
MMR								

SOURCE: The Children's Hospital Medical Center, Boston, Massachusetts 02115 © 1980.

Index

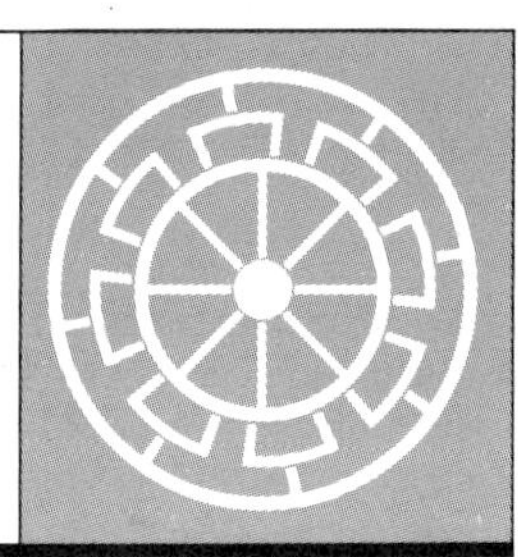

NOTE: A small "f" following a page number refers to a figure; a "t" refers to a table.

Average Heart Rate for Children at Rest

Age	Average rate	2 SD
Birth	140	50
1st mo	130	45
1–6 mo	130	45
6–12 mo	115	40
1–2 yr	110	40
2–4 yr	105	35
6–10 yr	95	30
10–14 yr	85	30
14–18 yr	82	25

SOURCE: Lowrey GH: *Growth and Development of Children.* 7th ed. Year Book, 1978, p. 228.

Variations in Respiration With Age

Age	Rate/min	Tidal air, cc	Vital capacity, L*
Premature	40–90	12	—
Neonate	30–80	19	—
1 yr	20–40	48	—
2 yr	20–30	90	—
3 yr	20–30	125	—
5 yr	20–25	175	1.0
10 yr	17–22	320	2.0
15 yr	15–20	400	3.7
20 yr	15–20	500	3.8

*These represent mean figures from several sources for both sexes. Vital capacity for boys averages about 6% greater than for girls.

SOURCE: Lowrey GH: *Growth and Development of Children.* 7th ed. Year Book, 1978, p. 450.

Normal Blood Pressure for Various Ages (mm Hg)

Infants*		Age	Systolic	2 SD	Diastolic	2 SD
1st day	52	1 day	78	14	42	14
4th day	70	1 mo	86	20	54	18
10th day	80	6 mo	90	26	60	20
2d mo	95	1 yr	96	30	65	25
8th mo	95	2 yr	99	25	65	25
		4 yr	99	20	65	20
		6 yr	100	15	60	10
		8 yr	105	15	60	10
		10 yr	110	17	60	10
		12 yr	115	19	60	10
		14 yr	118	20	60	10
		16 yr	120	16	65	10

*The figures for infants represent averages by the flush method.

SOURCE: Lowrey GH: *Growth and Development of Children.* 7th ed. Year Book, 1978, p. 450.

Note: The figures under 1 year were obtained by the Doppler method. From 1 year on, the figures were obtained by auscultation, using the first change in sound to indicate diastolic pressure.